A PUBLICATION OF THE AMERICAN COLLEGE OF PHYSICIANS

ACP MEDICINE

3RD EDITION

ACP MEDICINE

3RD EDITION

Volume 1

David C. Dale, M.D., F.A.C.P.

Professor of Medicine
University of Washington Medical Center

EDITOR-IN-CHIEF

Daniel D. Federman, M.D., M.A.C.P.

The Carl W. Walter Distinguished Professor of Medicine and Medical Education
and Senior Dean for Alumni Relations and Clinical Teaching
Harvard Medical School

FOUNDING EDITOR

www.acpmedicine.com

WebMD

ISBN 10: 0-9772226-1-6
ISBN 13: 978-0-9772226-1-2
ISSN: 1547-1632

Director of Publishing	Cynthia M. Chevins
Director, Electronic Publishing	Liz Pope
Managing Editor	Maureen O'Sullivan
Development Editors	Nancy Terry, John Heinegg
Art and Design Editor	Elizabeth Klarfeld
Copy Editor	David Terry
Editorial Coordinator	Tiberah Berhanu
Marketing Specialist	Wendy Wels
Electronic Composition	Diane Joiner, Jennifer Smith
Manufacturing Producer	Derek Nash
Indexer	Julia Brooks Figures

Printed in the United States of America

Published by WebMD Inc.

ACP Medicine
WebMD Professional Publishing
111 Eighth Avenue
Suite 700
New York, NY 10011

The authors, editors, and publisher have conscientiously and carefully tried to ensure that recommended measures and drug dosages in these pages are accurate and conform to the standards that prevailed at the time of publication. The reader is advised, however, to check the product information sheet accompanying each drug to be familiar with any changes in the dosage schedule or in the contraindications. This advice should be taken with particular seriousness if the agent to be administered is a new one or one that is infrequently used. *ACP Medicine* describes basic principles of diagnosis and therapy. Because of the uniqueness of each patient and the need to take into account a number of concurrent considerations, however, this information should be used by physicians only as a general guide to clinical decision making.

Editorial Board

Contents

Volume 1

Editorial Board   v

Contributors   xvii

Peer Review Board   xxv

Foreword   xxix
John Tooker, M.D., M.B.A., F.A.C.P., and Steven Weinberger, M.D., F.A.C.P.

Preface   xxxi

On Being a Physician   xxxiii
David C. Dale, M.D., F.A.C.P., and Daniel D. Federman, M.D., M.A.C.P.

Performance Measurement in Clinical Practice   xxxv
*Stephen D. Persell, M.D., M.P.H., David W. Baker, M.D., M.P.H., F.A.C.P.,
and Kevin B. Weiss, M.D., M.P.H., F.A.C.P.*

CLINICAL ESSENTIALS

1   **Contemporary Ethical and Social Issues in Medicine**   1
      Christine K. Cassel, M.D., M.A.C.P., and Ruth B. Purtilo, Ph.D.

2   **Quantitative Aspects of Clinical Decision Making**   7
      Brian Haynes, M.D., Ph.D., F.A.C.P., and Harold C. Sox, Jr., M.D., M.A.C.P.

3   **Reducing Risk of Injury and Disease**   17
      Harold C. Sox, Jr., M.D., M.A.C.P.

4   **Diet and Exercise**   25
      Harvey B. Simon, M.D., F.A.C.P.

5   **Adult Preventive Health Care**   41
      Mark Helfand, M.D., F.A.C.P.

6   **Preoperative Assessment and Care of the Surgical Patient**   50
      Michael F. Lubin, M.D., F.A.C.P.

7   **Occupational Medicine**   58
      Linda Rosenstock, M.D., M.P.H., F.A.C.P., and Mark R. Cullen, M.D.

8   **Health Advice for International Travelers**   69
      Peter F. Weller, M.D., F.A.C.P.

9   **Complementary and Alternative Medicine**   82
      Bimal H. Ashar, M.D., F.A.C.P., and Adrian S. Dobs, M.D., M.H.S.

10   **Palliative Medicine**   92
      Cynthia X. Pan, M.D.

11   **Symptom Management in Palliative Medicine**   100
      Maria Torroella Carney, M.D., and Jennifer Rhodes-Kropf, M.D.

12   **Management of Psychosocial Issues in Terminal Illness**   112
      Jennifer Rhodes-Kropf, M.D., and Ned H. Cassem, M.D., F.A.C.P.

BIOTERRORISM AND MEDICAL EMERGENCIES

13 **Bioterrorism** 121
Jeffrey Duchin, M.D.

14 **Cardiac Resuscitation** 141
Terry J. Mengert, M.D.

15 **Management of Poisoning and Drug Overdose** 155
Kent R. Olson, M.D., and Manish M. Patel, M.D.

16 **Bites and Stings** 180
Lawrence M. Lewis, M.D., William H. Dribben, M.D., and Mark D. Levine, M.D.

CARDIOVASCULAR MEDICINE

17 **Approach to the Cardiovascular Patient** 197
Catherine M. Otto, M.D., and David M. Shavelle, M.D.

18 **Hypertension** 214
Gary L. Schwartz, M.D., F.A.C.P., and Sheldon G. Sheps, M.D., F.A.C.P.

19 **Atrial Fibrillation** 238
Anthony Aizer, M.D., and Valentin Fuster, M.D., Ph.D.

20 **Supraventricular Tachycardia** 250
Melvin M. Scheinman, M.D., F.A.C.P.

21 **Ventricular Arrhythmias** 260
Jonathan J. Langberg, M.D., and David B. DeLurgio, M.D.

22 **Pacemaker Therapy** 273
Jonathan Lowy, M.D., and Roger A. Freedman, M.D.

23 **Chronic Stable Angina** 284
Paul R. Sutton, M.D., Ph.D., F.A.C.P., and Stephan D. Fihn, M.D., M.P.H., F.A.C.P.

24 **Unstable Angina and Non–ST Segment Elevation Myocardial Infarction** 304
Joel Kupersmith, M.D., F.A.C.P., and Amish Raval, M.D.

25 **Acute Myocardial Infarction** 317
Peter B. Berger, M.D., and James L. Orford, M.B., Ch.B., M.P.H.

26 **Heart Failure** 337
Mariell Jessup, M.D.

27 **Valvular Heart Disease** 348
Ronan J. Curtin, M.D., and Brian P. Griffin, M.D.

28 **Diseases of the Aorta** 365
Kim A. Eagle, M.D., F.A.C.P., and William F. Armstrong, M.D.

29 **Diseases of the Pericardium, Cardiac Tumors, and Cardiac Trauma** 377
E. William Hancock, M.D., F.A.C.P.

30 **Congenital Heart Disease** 388
Larry T. Mahoney, M.D., and David J. Skorton, M.D.

31 **Peripheral Arterial Disease** 400
Mark A. Creager, M.D.

32 **Venous Thromboembolism** 410
Clive Kearon, M.B., Ph.D., and Jack Hirsh, M.D., F.A.C.P.

DERMATOLOGY

33 **Approach to the Diagnosis of Skin Disease** 425
Robert T. Brodell, M.D., and Stephen E. Helms, M.D.

34 **Cutaneous Manifestations of Systemic Diseases** 432
Mark Lebwohl, M.D.

35 **Acne Vulgaris and Related Disorders** 446
Mark Lebwohl, M.D.

36 **Papulosquamous Disorders** 452
Elizabeth A. Abel, M.D.

37 **Psoriasis** 461
Elizabeth A. Abel, M.D., and Mark Lebwohl, M.D.

38 **Eczematous Disorders, Atopic Dermatitis, and Ichthyoses** 474
Seth R. Stevens, M.D.

39 **Contact Dermatitis and Related Disorders** 481
James S. Taylor, M.D.

40 **Cutaneous Adverse Drug Reactions** 495
Neil H. Shear, M.D., F.A.C.P., Sandra Knowles, B.Sc. Phm., and Lori Shapiro, M.D.

41	**Fungal, Bacterial, and Viral Infections of the Skin**	504
	Jan V. Hirschmann, M.D.	
42	**Parasitic Infestations**	516
	Elizabeth A. Abel, M.D.	
43	**Vesiculobullous Diseases**	525
	Elizabeth A. Abel, M.D., and Jean-Claude Bystryn, M.D.	
44	**Benign Cutaneous Tumors**	535
	Elizabeth A. Abel, M.D.	
45	**Malignant Cutaneous Tumors**	549
	Allan C. Halpern, M.D., and Patricia L. Myskowski, M.D.	
46	**Disorders of Hair**	563
	David A. Whiting, M.D., F.A.C.P.	
47	**Disorders of the Nail**	571
	James Q. Del Rosso, D.O., and C. Ralph Daniel III, M.D	
48	**Disorders of Pigmentation**	578
	Pearl E. Grimes, M.D.	

ENDOCRINOLOGY AND METABOLISM

49	**Pituitary**	589
	Shlomo Melmed, M.D., F.A.C.P.	
50	**Thyroid**	605
	Paul W. Ladenson, M.D., F.A.C.P.	
51	**Hypoglycemia**	626
	F. John Service, M.D., Ph.D., F.A.C.P.	
52	**Type 1 Diabetes Mellitus**	633
	Saul Genuth, M.D., F.A.C.P.	
53	**Type 2 Diabetes Mellitus**	651
	Matthew C. Riddle, M.D., and Saul Genuth, M.D., F.A.C.P.	
54	**Complications of Diabetes Mellitus**	666
	Mark E. Molitch, M.D., F.A.C.P., and Saul Genuth, M.D., F.A.C.P.	
55	**The Adrenal**	679
	D. Lynn Loriaux, M.D., Ph.D., M.A.C.P.	
56	**Testes and Testicular Disorders**	689
	Peter J. Snyder, M.D.	
57	**Diseases of Calcium Metabolism and Metabolic Bone Disease**	698
	Elizabeth H. Holt, M.D., Ph.D., and Silvio E. Inzucchi, M.D.	
58	**Obesity**	714
	Jonathan Q. Purnell, M.D.	
59	**Diagnosis and Treatment of Dyslipidemia**	729
	John D. Brunzell, M.D., F.A.C.P., and R. Alan Failor, M.D.	
60	**The Porphyrias**	748
	Shigeru Sassa, M.D., Ph.D., and Attallah Kappas, M.D., F.A.C.P.	

GASTROENTEROLOGY

61	**Esophageal Disorders**	757
	Stuart Jon Spechler, M.D.	
62	**Peptic Ulcer Diseases**	776
	Mark Feldman, M.D., F.A.C.P.	
63	**Inflammatory Bowel Diseases**	790
	Stephen B. Hanauer, M.D., F.A.C.P.	
64	**Diverticulosis, Diverticulitis, and Appendicitis**	813
	Willliam V. Harford, M.D., F.A.C.P.	
65	**Diseases Producing Malabsorption and Maldigestion**	824
	Charles M. Mansbach II, M.D.	
66	**Diarrheal Diseases**	837
	Lawrence R. Schiller, M.D., F.A.C.P.	
67	**Gastrointestinal Motility and Functional Disorders**	851
	Henry P. Parkman, M.D.	
68	**Gastrointestinal Bleeding**	863
	Elizabeth Rajan, M.D., and David A. Ahlquist, M.D.	
69	**Acute Viral Hepatitis**	872
	Emmet B. Keeffe, M.D., F.A.C.P.	

70   **Chronic Hepatitis**   882
Peter F. Malet, M.D., F.A.C.P.

71   **Cirrhosis of the Liver**   891
Ramón Bataller, M.D., and Pere Ginès, M.D.

72   **Gallstones and Biliary Tract Disease**   901
Kimberly M. Persley, M.D., and Rajeev Jain, M.D., F.A.C.P.

73   **Diseases of the Pancreas**   913
Peter Draganov, M.D., and Chris E. Forsmark, M.D., F.A.C.P.

74   **Liver and Pancreas Transplantation**   932
Robert L. Carithers, Jr., M.D., F.A.C.P., and James D. Perkins, M.D.

75   **Enteral and Parenteral Nutrition**   940
Khursheed N. Jeejeebhoy, M.B.B.S., Ph.D.

GYNECOLOGY AND WOMEN'S HEALTH

76   **Normal and Abnormal Menstruation**   950
Janet E. Hall, M.D.

77   **Premenstrual Syndrome**   962
Sarah L. Berga, M.D.

78   **Endometriosis**   966
Robert L. Barbieri, M.D., F.A.C.P.

79   **Polycystic Ovary Syndrome**   974
Robert L. Barbieri, M.D., F.A.C.P.

80   **Hirsutism**   987
Robert L. Barbieri, M.D., F.A.C.P.

81   **Contraception**   994
Sarah L. Berga, M.D.

82   **Infertility**   1002
Eric D. Levens, M.D., and Alan H. DeCherney, M.D.

83   **Ectopic Pregnancy and Spontaneous Abortion**   1010
Alan H. DeCherney, M.D.

84   **Medical Complications in Pregnancy**   1016
Ellen W. Seely, M.D., and Jeffrey Ecker, M.D.

85   **Menopause**   1027
Susan D. Reed, M.D., M.P.H., and Eliza Sutton, M.D., F.A.C.P.

86   **Urinary Incontinence and Overactive Bladder Syndrome**   1041
Lennox P. Hoyte, M.D., and Robert L. Barbieri, M.D., F.A.C.P.

87   **Approach to the Patient with a Breast Mass**   1048
Valerie L. Staradub, M.D., and Monica Morrow, M.D.

88   **Approach to the Patient with a Pelvic Mass**   1055
Joseph T. Chambers, M.D., Ph.D., and Carolyn D. Runowicz, M.D.

89   **Approach to the Patient with an Abnormal Pap Smear**   1063
Carolyn D. Runowicz, M.D.

HEMATOLOGY

90   **Approach to Hematologic Disorders**   1070
David C. Dale, M.D., F.A.C.P.

91   **Red Blood Cell Function and Disorders of Iron Metabolism**   1078
Gary M. Brittenham, M.D.

92   **Anemia: Production Defects**   1092
Stanley L. Schrier, M.D., F.A.C.P.

93   **Hemoglobinopathies and Hemolytic Anemias**   1107
Stanley L. Schrier, M.D., F.A.C.P.

94   **The Polycythemias**   1132
Virginia C. Broudy, M.D.

95   **Nonmalignant Disorders of Leukocytes**   1137
David C. Dale, M.D., F.A.C.P.

96   **Hemostasis and Its Regulation**   1153
Lawrence L. K. Leung, M.D.

97   **Platelet and Vascular Disorders**   1163
Lawrence L. K. Leung, M.D.

98	**Coagulation Disorders**	1180
	Lawrence L. K. Leung, M.D.	
99	**Thrombotic Disorders**	1190
	Lawrence L. K. Leung, M.D.	
100	**Transfusion Therapy**	1206
	W. Hallowell Churchill, M.D.	
101	**Hematopoietic Cell Transplantation**	1222
	Frederick R. Appelbaum, M.D.	

IMMUNOLOGY, ALLERGY, AND RHEUMATOLOGY

102	**Deficiencies in Immunoglobulins and Cell-Mediated Immunity**	1226
	Fred S. Rosen, M.D.	
103	**Immunologic Tolerance and Autoimmunity**	1234
	Paul Anderson, M.D., Ph.D.	
104	**Allergic Response**	1240
	Pamela J. Daffern, M.D., and Lawrence B. Schwartz, M.D., Ph.D.	
105	**Diagnostic and Therapeutic Principles in Allergy**	1247
	Mitchell H. Grayson, M.D., and Phillip E. Korenblat, M.D., F.A.C.P.	
106	**Allergic Rhinitis, Conjunctivitis, and Sinusitis**	1253
	Raymond G. Slavin, M.D., F.A.C.P.	
107	**Urticaria, Angioedema, and Anaphylaxis**	1259
	Vincent S. Beltrani, M.D.	
108	**Drug Allergies**	1271
	Mark S. Dykewicz, M.D., F.A.C.P., and Heather C. Gray, M.D.	
109	**Food Allergies**	1278
	A. Wesley Burks, M.D.	
110	**Allergic Reactions to Hymenoptera**	1285
	David B. K. Golden, M.D., F.A.C.P.	
111	**Introduction to the Rheumatic Diseases**	1290
	Shaun Ruddy, M.D., F.A.C.P.	
112	**Rheumatoid Arthritis**	1297
	Gary S. Firestein, M.D.	
113	**Seronegative Spondyloarthritis**	1315
	Frank C. Arnett, M.D., F.A.C.P.	
114	**Systemic Lupus Erythematosus**	1327
	Michael D. Lockshin, M.D., F.A.C.P.	
115	**Scleroderma and Related Diseases**	1342
	George Moxley, M.D.	
116	**Idiopathic Inflammatory Myopathies**	1351
	Nancy J. Olsen, M.D., and Beth L. Brogan, M.D.	
117	**Systemic Vasculitis Syndromes**	1359
	Brian F. Mandell, M.D., Ph.D., F.A.C.P.	
118	**Crystal-Induced Joint Disease**	1371
	Christopher Wise, M.D., F.A.C.P.	
119	**Osteoarthritis**	1382
	Christopher Wise, M.D., F.A.C.P.	
120	**Back Pain and Common Musculoskeletal Problems**	1391
	Christopher Wise, M.D., F.A.C.P.	
121	**Fibromyalgia**	1399
	John Buckner Winfield, M.D.	

INDEX

Volume 2

Editorial Board   v

Contents   vii

INFECTIOUS DISEASE

122   **Hyperthermia, Fever, and Fever of Undetermined Origin**   1407
Harvey B. Simon, M.D., F.A.C.P.

123   **Antimicrobial Therapy**   1420
Timothy H. Dellit, M.D., and Thomas M. Hooton, M.D., F.A.C.P.

124   **Sepsis**   1443
Steven M. Opal, M.D., and Christian E. Huber, M.D.

125   **Bacterial Infections of the Upper Respiratory Tract**   1456
Harvey B. Simon, M.D., F.A.C.P.

126   **Pneumonia and Other Pulmonary Infections**   1468
Harvey B. Simon, M.D., F.A.C.P.

127   **Infective Endocarditis**   1482
David T. Durack, M.B., D.Phil., F.A.C.P., and Adolf W. Karchmer, M.D., F.A.C.P.

128   **Peritonitis and Intra-abdominal Abscesses**   1500
W. Conrad Liles, M.D., Ph.D., F.A.C.P., and E. Patchen Dellinger, M.D.

129   **Urinary Tract Infections**   1508
Kalpana Gupta, M.D., M.P.H., and Walter E. Stamm, M.D., F.A.C.P.

130   **Vaginitis and Sexually Transmitted Diseases**   1520
Matthew R. Golden, M.D., M.P.H.

131   **Septic Arthritis**   1533
Brian F. Mandell, M.D., Ph.D., F.A.C.P.

132   **Osteomyelitis**   1542
Layne O. Gentry, M.D., F.A.C.P.

133   **Bacterial Infections of the Central Nervous System**   1550
Jan V. Hirschmann, M.D.

134   **Infections Due to Gram-Positive Cocci**   1563
Dennis L. Stevens, M.D., Ph.D., F.A.C.P.

135   **Infections Due to Gram-Positive Bacilli**   1584
Frederick S. Southwick, M.D., F.A.C.P.

136   **Anaerobic Infections**   1600
Anthony W. Chow, M.D., F.A.C.P., F.R.C.P.C.

137   **Infections Due to Neisseria**   1617
Jeanne M. Marrazzo, M.D., M.P.H., F.A.C.P.

138   **Infections Due to Escherichia coli and Other Enteric Gram-Negative Bacilli**   1626
Michael S. Donnenberg, M.D.

139   **Enteric Infections Due to Campylobacter, Salmonella, Shigella, Yersinia, Vibrio, and Helicobacter**   1634
Marcia B. Goldberg, M.D.

140   **Infections Due to Haemophilus, Moraxella, Legionella, Bordetella, and Pseudomonas**   1648
Shawn J. Skerrett, M.D.

141   **Infections Due to Brucella, Francisella, Yersinia pestis, and Bartonella**   1664
W. Conrad Liles, M.D., Ph.D., F.A.C.P.

142   **Tuberculosis**   1675
Henry M. Blumberg, M.D., F.A.C.P., and Michael K. Leonard, Jr., M.D.

143   **Syphilis and the Nonvenereal Treponematoses**   1697
Michael Augenbraun, M.D., Ph.D., F.A.C.P.

144   **Lyme Disease and Other Spirochetal Zoonoses**   1712
David C. Tompkins, M.D., and Benjamin J. Luft, M.D., F.A.C.P.

145   **Infections Due to Rickettsia, Ehrlichia, and Coxiella**   1724
Daniel J. Sexton, M.D., F.A.C.P.

146   **Mycoplasma Infections**   1737
R. Doug Hardy, M.D., F.A.C.P.

147   **Diseases Due to Chlamydia**   1745
Walter E. Stamm, M.D., F.A.C.P.

148	**Herpesvirus Infections** *Martin S. Hirsch, M.D.*	1755
149	**Measles, Mumps, Rubella, Parvovirus, and Poxvirus** *Martin S. Hirsch, M.D.*	1768
150	**Respiratory Viral Infections** *Frederick G. Hayden, M.D., F.A.C.P., and Michael G. Ison, M.D., M.Sc.*	1776
151	**Enteric Viral Infections** *Nino Khetsuriani, M.D., Ph.D., and Umesh D. Parashar, M.D., M.P.H.*	1793
152	**Human Retroviral Infections** *Robert W. Coombs, M.D., Ph.D.*	1802
153	**HIV and AIDS** *Robert D. Harrington, M.D., and David H. Spach, M.D.*	1819
154	**Viral Zoonoses** *Lyle R. Petersen, M.D., M.P.H., and Duane J. Gubler, Sc.D.*	1847
155	**Mycotic Infections** *Carol A. Kauffman, M.D., F.A.C.P.*	1861
156	**Mycotic Infections in the Compromised Host** *Jo-Anne van Burik, M.D., F.A.C.P.*	1875
157	**Protozoan Infections** *Wesley C. Van Voorhis, M.D., Ph.D., F.A.C.P., and Peter F. Weller, M.D., F.A.C.P.*	1892
158	**Helminthic Infections** *Wesley C. Van Voorhis, M.D., Ph.D., F.A.C.P., and Peter F. Weller, M.D., F.A.C.P.*	1918

MEDICAL GENETICS

159	**Genetics for the Clinician** *Robb Moses, M.D., and Jone E. Sampson, M.D.*	1944
160	**Genetic Diagnosis and Counseling** *Roberta A. Pagon, M.D.*	1958

NEPHROLOGY

161	**Approach to the Patient with Renal Disease** *Biff F. Palmer, M.D., F.A.C.P.*	1967
162	**Renal Function and Disorders of Water and Sodium Balance** *Richard H. Sterns, M.D., F.A.C.P.*	1975
163	**Disorders of Acid-Base and Potassium Balance** *Robert M. Black, M.D.*	1994
164	**Management of Chronic Kidney Disease** *Biff F. Palmer, M.D., F.A.C.P., and Michael K. Hise, M.D.*	2014
165	**Acute Renal Failure** *Mary Jo Shaver, M.D., and Sudhir V. Shah, M.D., F.A.C.P.*	2026
166	**Chronic Renal Failure and Dialysis** *Eric P. Cohen, M.D.*	2040
167	**Glomerular Diseases** *Raimund H. Pichler, M.D., and Stuart J. Shankland, M.D.*	2051
168	**Vascular Diseases of the Kidney** *Abhijit V. Kshirsagar, M.D., M.P.H., and Ronald J. Falk, M.D., F.A.C.P.*	2071
169	**Tubulointerstitial Diseases** *Gerald B. Appel, M.D., F.A.C.P., and Premila Bhat, M.D.*	2086
170	**Nephrolithiasis** *Fuad N. Ziyadeh, M.D., and Stanley Goldfarb, M.D., F.A.C.P.*	2104
171	**Renal Transplantation** *David K. Klassen, M.D., and Matthew R. Weir, M.D., F.A.C.P.*	2114
172	**Benign Prostatic Hyperplasia** *Michael J. Barry, M.D., F.A.C.P.*	2126

NEUROLOGY

173	**The Dizzy Patient** *David Solomon, M.D., Ph.D., and Elliot M. Frohman, M.D., Ph.D.*	2135
174	**Headache** *Randolph W. Evans, M.D.*	2150

175 **Pain** 2169
Alan Carver, M.D.

176 **Epilepsy** 2187
Jeremy D. Slater, M.D., and Giridhar P. Kalamangalam, M.D.

177 **Cerebrovascular Disorders** 2201
Scott E. Kasner, M.D., and Lewis B. Morgenstern, M.D.

178 **Alzheimer Disease and Other Major Dementing Illnesses** 2217
David S. Knopman, M.D.

179 **Traumatic Brain Injury** 2228
Andres M. Salazar, M.D.

180 **Parkinson Disease and Other Movement Disorders** 2239
Jorge L. Juncos, M.D., and Mahlon R. DeLong, M.D.

181 **Inherited Ataxias** 2263
S. H. Subramony, M.D.

182 **Diseases of Muscle and the Neuromuscular Junction** 2270
Marinos C. Dalakas, M.D.

183 **Diseases of the Peripheral Nervous System** 2291
Colin H. Chalk, M.D., C.M.

184 **Neoplastic Disorders** 2307
Jerome B. Posner, M.D.

185 **Demyelinating Diseases** 2323
J. William Lindsey, M.D., and Jerry S. Wolinsky, M.D.

186 **Anoxic, Metabolic, and Toxic Encephalopathies** 2335
Michael J. Aminoff, M.D., D.Sc.

187 **Acute Viral Central Nervous System Diseases** 2344
Donald H. Gilden, M.D.

188 **Central Nervous System Diseases Due to Slow Viruses and Prions** 2355
Francisco González-Scarano, M.D., F.A.C.P.

189 **Disorders of Sleep** 2362
Sudhansu Chokroverty, M.D., F.R.C.P., F.A.C.P.

ONCOLOGY

190 **Cancer Epidemiology and Prevention** 2373
Alfred I. Neugut, M.D., Ph.D., F.A.C.P., and Frederick P. Li, M.D.

191 **Molecular Genetics of Cancer** 2383
Daniel A. Haber, M.D., Ph.D.

192 **Tumor Immunology** 2400
Bruce G. Redman, D.O., and Alfred E. Chang, M.D., F.A.C.S.

193 **Principles of Cancer Treatment** 2408
Eric H. Rubin, M.D., and William N. Hait, M.D., Ph.D.

194 **Oncologic Emergencies** 2425
Robert W. Carlson, M.D., F.A.C.P.

195 **Head and Neck Cancer** 2437
Everett E. Vokes, M.D., F.A.C.P.

196 **Lung Cancer** 2443
Jeffrey Crawford, M.D.

197 **Breast Cancer** 2459
Nancy E. Davidson, M.D.

198 **Colorectal Cancer** 2474
Bernard Levin, M.D., F.A.C.P.

199 **Pancreatic, Gastric, and Other Gastrointestinal Cancers** 2490
Weijing Sun, M.D., and Daniel Haller, M.D., F.A.C.P.

200 **Bladder, Renal, and Testicular Cancer** 2512
Derek Raghavan, M.D., Ph.D., F.A.C.P.

201 **Prostate Cancer** 2528
Philip W. Kantoff, M.D.

202 **Gynecologic Cancer** 2537
Stephen A. Cannistra, M.D.

203 **Sarcomas of Soft Tissue and Bone** 2549
Haralambos Raftopoulos, M.D., and Karen H. Antman, M.D.

204 **Acute Leukemia** 2561
Richard A. Larson, M.D.

205 **Chronic Myelogenous Leukemia and Other Myeloproliferative Disorders** 2575
Stefan Faderl, M.D., and Hagop M. Kantarjian, M.D.

206 **Chronic Lymphoid Leukemias and Plasma Cell Disorders** 2585
Bruce D. Cheson, M.D., F.A.C.P.

207 **Lymphomas** 2596
Kieron Dunleavy, M.D., and Wyndham H. Wilson, M.D., Ph.D.

PSYCHIATRY

208 **Depression and Bipolar Disorder** 2613
Michael T. Compton, M.D., M.P.H., and Charles B. Nemeroff, M.D., Ph.D.

209 **Alcohol Abuse and Dependency** 2625
Patrick G. O'Connor, M.D., M.P.H.

210 **Drug Abuse and Dependence** 2635
Mark A. Schuckit, M.D.

211 **Schizophrenia** 2647
William T. Carpenter, Jr., M.D., and Gunvant K. Thaker, M.D.

212 **Anxiety Disorders** 2657
M. Katherine Shear, M.D.

213 **The Eating Disorders** 2666
W. Stewart Agras, M.D.

PULMONARY MEDICINE

214 **Pulmonary Function Testing** 2674
E. R. McFadden, Jr., M.D., F.A.C.P.

215 **Invasive Diagnostic and Therapeutic Techniques in Lung Disease** 2687
Martin L. Mayse, M.D., and Kevin L. Kovitz, M.D., M.B.A., F.A.C.P.

216 **Asthma** 2701
Mitchell H. Grayson, M.D., and Michael J. Holtzman, M.D.

217 **Chronic Obstructive Diseases of the Lung** 2720
Gerald W. Staton, Jr., M.D., F.A.C.P.

218 **Focal and Multifocal Lung Disease** 2744
Gerald W. Staton, Jr., M.D., F.A.C.P.

219 **Chronic Diffuse Infiltrative Lung Disease** 2758
Gerald W. Staton, Jr., M.D., F.A.C.P., and Roland H. Ingram, Jr., M.D., F.A.C.P.

220 **Ventilatory Control During Wakefulness and Sleep** 2786
Kingman P. Strohl, M.D.

221 **Disorders of the Chest Wall** 2800
Gerald W. Staton, Jr., M.D., F.A.C.P., and Roland H. Ingram, Jr., M.D., F.A.C.P.

222 **Respiratory Failure** 2809
Marin Kollef, M.D., F.A.C.P

223 **Disorders of the Pleura, Hila, and Mediastinum** 2823
Gerald W. Staton, Jr., M.D., F.A.C.P., and Roland H. Ingram, Jr., M.D., F.A.C.P.

224 **Pulmonary Edema** 2842
Gerald W. Staton, Jr., M.D., F.A.C.P.

225 **Pulmonary Hypertension, Cor Pulmonale, and Miscellaneous Vascular Conditions** 2852
Lewis J. Rubin, M.D., F.A.C.P.

INDEX

Contributors

Elizabeth A. Abel, M.D.   Clinical Professor of Dermatology, Stanford University School of Medicine

W. Stewart Agras, M.D.   Professor of Psychiatry (Emeritus), Department of Psychiatry and Behavioral Sciences, Stanford University School of Medicine

David A. Ahlquist, M.D.   Professor of Medicine, Mayo Medical School

Anthony Aizer, M.D.   Instructor, New York University School of Medicine

Michael J. Aminoff, M.D., D.Sc.   Professor of Neurology, University of California, San Francisco, School of Medicine

Paul Anderson, M.D., Ph.D.   Associate Professor of Medicine, Harvard Medical School, and Rheumatologist, Division of Rheumatology and Immunology, Brigham and Women's Hospital

Karen H. Antman, M.D.   Dean, Boston University School of Medicine

Gerald B. Appel, M.D., F.A.C.P.   Professor of Clinical Medicine, Columbia University College of Physicians and Surgeons, and Director of Clinical Nephrology, New York Presbyterian Hospital

Frederick R. Appelbaum, M.D.   Professor and Head, Division of Medical Oncology, University of Washington School of Medicine, and Member and Director, Clinical Research Division, Fred Hutchinson Cancer Research Center

William F. Armstrong, M.D.   Professor of Internal Medicine, Associate Clinical Chief of Cardiology, and Director of the Echocardiography Laboratory, University of Michigan Health System

Frank C. Arnett, M.D., F.A.C.P.   Chairman, Department of Internal Medicine, and Professor of Internal Medicine and of Pathology and Laboratory Medicine and Elizabeth Bidgood Chair in Rheumatology, University of Texas Health Science Center at Houston

Bimal H. Ashar, M.D., F.A.C.P.   Assistant Professor of Medicine, Johns Hopkins University School of Medicine

Michael Augenbraun, M.D., Ph.D., F.A.C.P.   Associate Professor of Medicine, State University of New York Downstate Medical Center

David W. Baker, M.D., M.P.H., F.A.C.P.   Associate Professor of Medicine; Chief, Division of General Internal Medicine; and Co-Director, Institute for Healthcare Studies, Northwestern University Feinberg School of Medicine

Robert L. Barbieri, M.D., F.A.C.P.   Kate Macy Ladd Professor of Obstetrics, Gynecology, and Reproductive Biology, Harvard Medical School, and Head, Department of Obstetrics, Gynecology, and Reproductive Biology, Brigham and Women's Hospital

Michael J. Barry, M.D., F.A.C.P.   Associate Professor of Medicine, Harvard Medical School, and Chief, General Medical Unit, Massachusetts General Hospital

Ramón Bataller, M.D.   Liver Unit, Institut de Malalties Digestives i Metabòliques, Hospital Clinic, Barcelona, Catlonia, Spain

Vincent S. Beltrani, M.D.   Visiting Professor of Medicine, University of Medicine and Dentistry of New Jersey/Robert Wood Johnson Medical School

Sarah L. Berga, M.D.   Professor of Obstetrics, Gynecology, and Reproductive Sciences and Professor of Psychiatry, University of Pittsburgh School of Medicine, and Director, Division of Reproductive Endocrinology and Infertility, Magee-Women's Hospital

Peter B. Berger, M.D.   Professor of Medicine, Duke University School of Medicine, and Director of Interventional Cardiology, Duke University Medical Center

Premila Bhat, M.D.   Clinical Fellow, Columbia University College of Physicians and Surgeons

Robert M. Black, M.D.   Professor of Clinical Medicine, University of Massachusetts Medical School, and Director, Division of Renal Medicine, Worcester Medical Center

Henry M. Blumberg, M.D., F.A.C.P.   Professor of Medicine, Emory University School of Medicine

Gary M. Brittenham, M.D.   Professor of Pediatrics and Medicine, Columbia University College of Physicians and Surgeons

Robert T. Brodell, M.D.   Professor of Internal Medicine and Dermatopathology, Northeastern Ohio Universities College of Medicine and Case Western Reserve University School of Medicine

Beth L. Brogan, M.D.   Department of Medicine, Vanderbilt University School of Medicine

Virginia C. Broudy, M.D.   Professor of Medicine, Division of Hematology, University of Washington School of Medicine, and Chief, Section of Hematology, Harborview Medical Center

John D. Brunzell, M.D., F.A.C.P.   Professor, Division of Metabolism, Endocrinology, and Nutrition, University of Washington, and Director, Clinical Research Center, University of Washington Medical Center

A. Wesley Burks, M.D.   Professor of Medicine, Duke University School of Medicine, and Chief, Division of Pediatric Allergy and Immunology, Duke University Medical Center

Jean-Claude Bystryn, M.D.   Professor of Dermatology,

New York University School of Medicine, and Director, Melanoma Immunotherapy Clinic, NYU Kaplan Comprehensive Cancer Center

Stephen A. Cannistra, M.D.   Associate Professor of Medicine, Harvard Medical School, and Director, Gynecologic Medical Oncology, Beth Israel Deaconess Medical Center

Robert L. Carithers, Jr., M.D., F.A.C.P.   Professor of Medicine and Director, Hepatology Section, Division of Gastroenterology, Department of Medicine, and Medical Director, Liver Transplantation Program, University of Washington School of Medicine

Robert W. Carlson, M.D., F.A.C.P.   Professor of Medicine, Division of Oncology, Stanford University School of Medicine

Maria Torroella Carney, M.D.   Geriatrics and Adult Development, Mount Sinai School of Medicine

William T. Carpenter, Jr., M.D.   Professor of Psychiatry and Pharmacology, University of Maryland School of Medicine, and Director, Maryland Psychiatric Research Center

Alan Carver, M.D.   Assistant Professor of Neurology, Mount Sinai School of Medicine

Christine K. Cassel, M.D., M.A.C.P.   President, American Board of Internal Medicine

Ned H. Cassem, M.D., F.A.C.P.   Professor of Psychiatry, Harvard Medical School, and Psychiatrist, Massachusetts General Hospital

Colin H. Chalk, M.D., C.M.   Associate Professor, Department of Neurology and Neurosurgery, McGill University Faculty of Medicine, and Associate Physician, Division of Neurology, Montreal General Hospital

Joseph T. Chambers, M.D., Ph.D.   Professor of Clinical Obstetrics and Gynecology, Columbia University, and Director, Gynecologic Oncology, Roosevelt Hospital

Alfred E. Chang, M.D., F.A.C.S.   Hugh Cabot Professor of Surgery and Chief, Division of Surgical Oncology, University of Michigan Medical School

Bruce D. Cheson, M.D., F.A.C.P.   Head, Medicine Section, Clinical Investigations Branch, Cancer Therapy Evaluation Program, National Cancer Institute

Sudhansu Chokroverty, M.D., F.R.C.P., F.A.C.P.   Professor of Neurology, New York Medical College; Clinical Professor of Neurology, University of Medicine and Dentistry of New Jersey/Robert Wood Johnson Medical School; and Associate Chairman and Program Director, Department of Neurology, Chairman, Division of Clinical Neurophysiology, and Director, Center of Sleep Medicine, St. Vincent's Hospital and Medical Center

Anthony W. Chow, M.D., F.A.C.P., F.R.C.P.C.   Professor, Department of Medicine, and Director, MD/PhD Program, University of British Columbia Faculty of Medicine

W. Hallowell Churchill, M.D.   Associate Professor of Medicine, Harvard Medical School, and Medical Director, Therapeutic Services, Brigham and Women's Hospital

Eric P. Cohen, M.D.   Professor of Medicine, Division of Nephrology, Department of Medicine, Medical College of Wisconsin, and Staff Physician, Division of Nephrology, Department of Medicine, Froedtert Memorial Lutheran Hospital

Michael T. Compton, M.D., M.P.H.   Assistant Professor, Department of Psychiatry and Behavioral Sciences, Emory University School of Medicine

Robert W. Coombs, M.D., Ph.D.   Associate Professor, Department of Laboratory Medicine, University of Washington School of Medicine

Jeffrey Crawford, M.D.   Professor of Medicine, Duke University School of Medicine, and Chief, Division of Medical Oncology, Duke University Medical Center

Mark A. Creager, M.D.   Professor of Medicine, Harvard Medical School; and Director, Vascular Center, and Member, Vascular Medicine Section, Cardiovascular Division, Brigham and Women's Hospital

Mark R. Cullen, M.D.   Professor of Medicine and Public Health and Director, Occupational and Environmental Medicine Program, Yale University School of Medicine

Ronan J. Curtin, M.D.   Fellow in Advance Cardiac Imaging, Department of Cardiac Medicine, Cleveland Clinic Foundation

Pamela J. Daffern, M.D.   Assistant Professor of Internal Medicine, Division of Rheumatology, Allergy, and Immunology, Medical College of Virginia at Virginia Commonwealth University

Marinos C. Dalakas, M.D.   Chief, Neuromuscular Diseases Section, National Institute of Neurological Disorders and Stroke, National Institutes of Health

David C. Dale, M.D., F.A.C.P.   Professor of Medicine, University of Washington School of Medicine

C. Ralph Daniel III, M.D.   Clinical Professor of Medicine (Dermatology), University of Mississippi Medical Center

Nancy E. Davidson, M.D.   Professor of Oncology and Breast Cancer Research Chair in Oncology, Johns Hopkins University School of Medicine, and Staff Physician, Breast Cancer Program, Johns Hopkins Hospital

Alan H. DeCherney, M.D.   Professor of Obstetrics and Gynecology, University of California, Los Angeles, School of Medicine

James Q. Del Rosso, D.O.   Clinical Assistant Professor, Department of Dermatology, University of Nevada School of Medicine

E. Patchen Dellinger, M.D.   Vice Chairman, Department of Surgery, and Chief, Division of General Surgery, University of Washington Medical Center

Timothy H. Dellit, M.D.   Assistant Professor of Medicine, Division of Allergy and Infectious Diseases, University of Washington School of Medicine

Mahlon R. DeLong, M.D.   Professor and Director of Neuroscience, Department of Neurology, Emory University School of Medicine

David B. DeLurgio, M.D.   Assistant Professor of Cardiac Electrophysiology, Emory University School of Medicine, and Electrophysiologist, Emory Crawford Long Hospital

Adrian S. Dobs, M.D., M.H.S.   Professor of Medicine and Oncology and Director, Clinical Trials Unit, Johns Hopkins University School of Medicine

Michael S. Donnenberg, M.D.   Professor of Medicine, Professor of Microbiology and Immunology, and Head, Division of Infectious Diseases, University of Maryland School of Medicine

Peter Draganov, M.D.   Associate Professor, Department of Medicine, University of Florida College of Medicine, and Director of Endoscopy, University of Florida Shands Hospital

William H. Dribben, M.D.   Assistant Professor of Medicine, Washington University School of Medicine, St. Louis

Jeffrey Duchin, M.D.   Assistant Professor of Medicine, Division of Allergy and Infectious Disease, University of Washington School of Medicine, and Chief, Communicable Disease Control, Department of Public Health, Seattle and King County, Washington

Kieron Dunleavy, M.D.   Experimental Transplantation and Immunology Branch, National Cancer Institute, National Institutes of Health

David T. Durack, M.D., D. Phil., F.A.C.P.   Consulting Professor, Duke University School of Medicine, and Vice President, Corporate Medical Affairs, Becton Dickinson, Franklin Lakes, New Jersey

Mark S. Dykewicz, M.D., F.A.C.P.   Professor of Internal Medicine, St. Louis University School of Medicine, Director, Allergy and Immunology Fellowship Program, and Medical Staff Physician, St. Louis University Hospital

Kim A. Eagle, M.D., F.A.C.P.   Albion Walter Hewlett Professor of Internal Medicine, Clinical Director, University of Michigan Cardiovascular Center

Jeffrey Ecker, M.D. Associate Professor of Obstetrics and Gynecology, Harvard Medical School, and Director, Clinical Obstetric Research, Massachusetts General Hospital

Randolph W. Evans, M.D. Clinical Professor of Neurology, Joan and Sanford I. Weill Medical College of Cornell University and Methodist Hospital, and Clinical Associate Professor of Neurology, Baylor College of Medicine

Stefan Faderl, M.D. Assistant Professor, Department of Leukemia, University of Texas M. D. Anderson Cancer Center

R. Alan Failor, M.D. Clinical Associate Professor of Medicine, University of Washington School of Medicine

Ronald J. Falk, M.D., F.A.C.P. Professor of Medicine and Chief, Division of Nephrology and Hypertension, University of North Carolina at Chapel Hill School of Medicine

Daniel D. Federman, M.D., M.A.C.P. The Carl W. Walter Distinguished Professor of Medicine and Medical Education and Senior Dean for Alumni Relations and Clinical Teaching, Harvard Medical School

Mark Feldman, M.D., F.A.C.P. William O. Tschumy, Jr., M.D., Chair of Internal Medicine and Clinical Professor of Internal Medicine, University of Texas Southwestern Medical School at Dallas; and Director, Internal Medicine Residency Program, Presbyterian Hospital of Dallas

Stephan D. Fihn, M.D., M.P.H., F.A.C.P. Professor of Medicine and Health Services, University of Washington School of Medicine, and Director, Health Services Research and Development, VA Puget Sound Health Care System

Gary S. Firestein, M.D. Professor of Medicine and Chief, Division of Rheumatology, Allergy and Immunology, University of California, San Diego, School of Medicine

Chris E. Forsmark, M.D., F.A.C.P. Professor and Chief, Division of Gastroenterology and Hepatology, University of Florida College of Medicine

Roger A. Freedman, M.D. Professor of Medicine, University of Utah School of Medicine, and Acting Chief, Division of Cardiology, University Medical Center, Salt Lake City

Elliot M. Frohman, M.D., Ph.D. Director of the Multiple Sclerosis Program and Associate Professor of Neurology, University of Texas Southwestern Medical School at Dallas

Valentin Fuster, M.D., Ph.D. Professor of Medicine and Director, Zena and Michael A. Weiner Cardiovascular Institute, Mount Sinai School of Medicine

Layne O. Gentry, M.D., F.A.C.P. Clinical Professor of Medicine, Baylor College of Medicine; and Chief, Infectious Disease Section, and Medical Director, Infection Control, St. Luke's Episcopal Hospital

Saul Genuth, M.D., F.A.C.P. Professor of Medicine, Division of Clinical and Molecular Endocrinology, Case Western Reserve University School of Medicine

Donald H. Gilden, M.D. Professor and Chairman, Department of Neurology, University of Colorado School of Medicine, and Chairman, Department of Neurology, University of Colorado Hospital

Pere Ginès, M.D. Liver Unit, Institut de Malalties Digestives i Metabòliques, Hospital Clinic, Barcelona, Catlonia, Spain

Marcia B. Goldberg, M.D. Director of Research, Division of Infectious Diseases, Massachusetts General Hospital, and Associate Professor of Medicine, Harvard Medical School

David B. K. Golden, M.D., F.A.C.P. Associate Professor of Medicine, Johns Hopkins University School of Medicine

Matthew R. Golden, M.D., M.P.H. Assistant Professor of Medicine, University of Washington Medical Directory, Public Health, Seattle-King County STD Clinic

Stanley Goldfarb, M.D., F.A.C.P. Professor of Medicine and Interim Chair, Department of Medicine, University of Pennsylvania School of Medicine

Francisco González-Scarano, M.D., F.A.C.P. Professor of Neurology and Microbiology, Department of Neurology, University of Pennsylvania School of Medicine

Heather C. Gray, M.D. Fellow, Allergy and Immunology, St. Louis University College of Medicine, and Fellow, Immunology, St. Louis University Hospital

Mitchell H. Grayson, M.D. Assistant Professor of Medicine, Division of Allergy/Immunology, Washington University School of Medicine, St. Louis

Brian P. Griffin, M.D. Staff Cardiologist, Section of Imaging, and Director, Cardiovascular Training Program, Department of Cardiology, Cleveland Clinic Foundation

Pearl E. Grimes, M.D. Clinical Associate Professor of Dermatology, Division of Dermatology, University of California, Los Angeles, School of Medicine, and Director, Vitiligo and Pigmentation Institute of Southern California

Duane J. Gubler, Sc.D. Adjunct Professor, Department of Microbiology, Colorado State University; Adjunct Professor, Department of International Health, Johns Hopkins University School of Public Health; and Director, Division of Vector-Borne Infectious Diseases, National Center for Infectious Diseases, Centers for Disease Control and Prevention

Kalpana Gupta, M.D., M.P.H. Assistant Professor of Medicine, Yale University School of Medicine

Daniel A. Haber, M.D., Ph.D. Professor of Medicine, Harvard Medical School, and Director, Center for Cancer Risk Analysis, Massachusetts General Hospital Cancer Center

William N. Hait, M.D., Ph.D. Professor of Medicine and Pharmacology and Associate Dean, Oncology Program, University of Medicine and Dentistry of New Jersey/Robert Wood Johnson Medical School, and Director, Cancer Institute of New Jersey

Janet E. Hall, M.D. Associate Professor of Medicine, Harvard Medical School, and Associate Unit Chief, Reproductive Endocrine Unit, Massachusetts General Hospital

Daniel Haller, M.D., F.A.C.P. Professor of Medicine, University of Pennsylvania School of Medicine

Allan C. Halpern, M.D. Associate Professor of Dermatology, Joan and Sanford I. Weill Medical College of Cornell University, and Chief, Dermatology Service, Memorial Sloan-Kettering Cancer Center

Stephen B. Hanauer, M.D., F.A.C.P. Professor of Medicine and Clinical Pharmacology, University of Chicago Pritzker School of Medicine, and Director, Section of Gastroenterology/Nutrition, University of Chicago Hospital

E. William Hancock, M.D., F.A.C.P. Professor of Medicine (Emeritus) (Cardiovascular Medicine), Stanford University School of Medicine

R. Doug Hardy, M.D. Assistant Professor of Internal Medicine and Pediatrics, University of Texas Southwestern Medical School at Dallas

William V. Harford, M.D., F.A.C.P. Professor of Medicine, Department of Medicine, University of Texas Southwestern Medical School at Dallas, and Director, Clinical Gastroenterology Laboratory, Dallas Veterans Affairs Medical Center

Robert D. Harrington, M.D. Associate Professor of Medicine, University of Washington School of Medicine

Frederick G. Hayden, M.D., F.A.C.P. Professor of Internal Medicine and Pathology, University of Virginia School of Medicine

Brian Haynes, M.D., Ph.D., F.A.C.P. Professor of Clinical Epidemiology and Medicine and Chair, Department of Clinical Epidemiology and Biostatistics, McMaster University Health Sciences Centre

Mark Helfand, M.D. Associate Professor, Department of Medicine, Oregon Health and Science University

Stephen E. Helms, M.D. Associate Clinical Professor of Clinical Internal Medicine, Northeastern Ohio Universities College of Medicine

Martin S. Hirsch, M.D. Professor of Medicine, Harvard Medical School, and Director of Clinical AIDS Research and Physician, Massachusetts General Hospital

Jan V. Hirschmann, M.D. Professor of Medicine, University of Washington School of Medicine, and Assistant Chief, Medical Service, Puget Sound Veterans Affairs Medical Center

Jack Hirsh, M.D., F.A.C.P. Professor (Emeritus), McMaster University, and Director, Hamilton Civic Hospitals Research Centre

Michael K. Hise, M.D. Associate Professor of Medicine, University of Maryland School of Medicine

Elizabeth H. Holt, M.D., Ph.D. Assistant Professor of Internal Medicine/Endocrinology and Metabolism, Yale University School of Medicine

Michael J. Holtzman, M.D. Director, Division of Pulmonary and Critical Care Medicine, Washington University School of Medicine, St. Louis

Thomas M. Hooton, M.D., F.A.C.P. Professor, University of Washington Medical Center, and Medical Director, Harborview HIV/AIDS Clinic, Harborview Medical Center

Lennox P. Hoyte, M.D. Assistant Professor of Obstetrics and Gynecology and Reproductive Surgery, Harvard Medical School, and Director, Department of Obstetrics and Gynecology, Brigham and Women's Hospital

Christian E. Huber, M.D. Postdoctoral Research Fellow, Division of Infectious Diseases, Brown Medical School

Roland H. Ingram, Jr., M.D., F.A.C.P. Martha West Looney Professor of Medicine (Emeritus), Emory University School of Medicine

Silvio E. Inzucchi, M.D. Associate Professor of Medicine, Section of Endocrinology, Yale University School of Medicine

Michael G. Ison, M.D., M.Sc. Director, Transplant Infectious Diseases Section, Division of Infectious Diseases, Department of Medicine, Northwestern University Feinberg School of Medicine

Rajeev Jain, M.D., F.A.C.P. Assistant Clinical Professor of Medicine, University of Texas Southwestern Medical School at Dallas, and Chief of Gastroenterology, Presbyterian Hospital of Dallas

Khursheed N. Jeejeebhoy, M.B.B.S., Ph.D. Professor of Medicine, Nutrition and Physiology, University of Toronto

Mariell Jessup, M.D. Professor of Medicine, University of Pennsylvania Medical School, and Medical Director, Heart Failure/Transplant Program, Hospital of the University of Pennsylvania

Jorge L. Juncos, M.D. Associate Professor, Department of Neurology, Emory University School of Medicine, and Wesley Woods Geriatric Center

Giridhar P. Kalamangalam, M.D. Assistant Professor of Neurology, University of Texas Health Science Center at Houston, and Attending Neurologist, Memorial Hermann Hospital

Hagop M. Kantarjian, M.D. Professor of Medicine and Chairman, Department of Leukemia, University of Texas M. D. Anderson Cancer Center

Philip W. Kantoff, M.D. Associate Professor of Medicine, Harvard Medical School, and Director, Lank Center for Genitourinary Oncology, Dana-Farber Cancer Institute

Attallah Kappas, M.D., F.A.C.P. Sherman Fairchild Professor and Physician-in-Chief Emeritus, Rockefeller University

Adolf W. Karchmer, M.D., F.A.C.P. Professor of Medicine, Harvard Medical School, and Chief, Division of Infectious Diseases, Beth Israel Deaconess Medical Center

Scott E. Kasner, M.D. Assistant Professor, Department of Neurology, University of Pennsylvania School of Medicine, and Director, Comprehensive Stroke Center, University of Pennsylvania

Carol A. Kauffman, M.D., F.A.C.P. Professor, Department of Internal Medicine, University of Michigan Medical School

Clive Kearon, M.B., F.R.C.P.C., M.R.C.P.I., Ph.D. Professor of Medicine, McMaster University Faculty of Health Sciences, and Head of the Thromboembolism Service, Henderson General Hospital, McMaster University Clinic

Emmet B. Keeffe, M.D., F.A.C.P. Professor of Medicine, Stanford University School of Medicine; and Co-Director, Liver Transplant Program, and Chief of Hepatology, Stanford University Medical Center

Nino Khetsuriani, M.D., Ph.D. Medical Epidemiologist, Respiratory and Enteric Viruses Branch, Centers for Disease Control and Prevention

David K. Klassen, M.D. Professor of Medicine, University of Maryland School of Medicine

David S. Knopman, M.D. Professor of Medicine, Mayo Clinic College of Medicine

Sandra Knowles, B.Sc. Phm. Pharmacist, Drug Safety Clinic, Sunnybrook and Women's College Health Science Centre

Marin Kollef, M.D., F.A.C.P. Associate Professor, Washington University School of Medicine

Phillip E. Korenblat, M.D., F.A.C.P. Professor of Clinical Medicine, Washington University School of Medicine

Kevin L. Kovitz, M.D., M.B.A., F.A.C.P. Professor of Medicine and Pediatrics, Tulane University School of Medicine

Abhijit V. Kshirsagar, M.D., M.P.H. Assistant Professor, Division of Nephrology and Hypertension, Department of Medicine, University of North Carolina at Chapel Hill School of Medicine

Joel Kupersmith, M.D., F.A.C.P. Chief Research and Development Officer, Department of Veteran Affairs, Washington, D.C.

Paul W. Ladenson, M.D., F.A.C.P. Professor and Director, Division of Endocrinology and Metabolism, Johns Hopkins University School of Medicine

Jonathan J. Langberg, M.D. Professor of Medicine, Cardiology Division, Emory University School of Medicine, and Director, Cardiac Electrophysiology Laboratory, Emory University Hospital

Richard A. Larson, M.D. Professor of Medicine, University of Chicago Pritzker School of Medicine

Mark Lebwohl, M.D. Sol and Clara Kest Professor and Chairman, Department of Dermatology, Mount Sinai Medical Center

Michael K. Leonard, Jr., M.D. Assistant Professor of Medicine, Division of Infectious Diseases, Emory University School of Medicine

Lawrence L. K. Leung, M.D. Maureen Lyles D'Ambrogio Professor of Medicine, Associate Chair, Department of Medicine, Stanford University School of Medicine, and Chief, Medical Service, VA Palo Alto Health Care Systems

Eric D. Levens, M.D. Unit on Reproductive Endocrinology and Infertility, National Institutes of Health

Bernard Levin, M.D., F.A.C.P. Vice President and Division Head, Division of Cancer Prevention, University of Texas M. D. Anderson Cancer Center

Mark D. Levine, M.D. Clinical Instructor in Emergency Medicine, Washington University School of Medicine, St. Louis

Lawrence M. Lewis, M.D. Associate Professor of Medicine, Washington University School of Medicine, St. Louis

Frederick P. Li, M.D. Professor of Clinical Cancer Epidemiology, Harvard School of Public Health, and Professor of Medicine, Harvard Medical School

W. Conrad Liles, M.D., Ph.D., F.A.C.P. Associate Professor of Medicine, University of Washington School of Medicine, and Codirector, Infectious Diseases and Tropical Medicine Clinic, University of Washington Medical Center

J. William Lindsey, M.D.   Assistant Professor of Neurology, University of Texas Health Science Center at Houston

Michael D. Lockshin, M.D., F.A.C.P.   Professor of Medicine and Obstetrics-Gynecology, Joan and Sanford I. Weill Medical College of Cornell University, and Director, Barbara Volcker Center for Women and Rheumatic Disease, and Codirector, Mary Kirkland Center for Lupus Research, Hospital for Special Surgery

D. Lynn Loriaux, M.D., Ph.D., M.A.C.P.   Professor and Chair, Oregon Health and Science University School of Medicine

Jonathan Lowy, M.D.   Director of Electrophysiology, St. John's Hospital/North Cascade Cardiology, Bellingham, Washington

Michael F. Lubin, M.D., F.A.C.P.   Professor of Medicine, Emory University School of Medicine

Benjamin J. Luft, M.D., F.A.C.P.   Professor and Chairman, Department of Medicine, State University of New York at Stony Brook

Larry T. Mahoney, M.D.   Professor of Pediatrics and Director of Pediatric Cardiology, University of Iowa College of Medicine

Peter F. Malet, M.D., F.A.C.P.   Associate Professor of Internal Medicine, Division of Digestive and Liver Diseases, University of Texas Southwestern Medical Center at Dallas

Brian F. Mandell, M.D., Ph.D., F.A.C.P.   Professor and Vice Chairman, Department of Medicine, Cleveland Clinic Lerner College of Medicine of Case Western Reserve University

Charles M. Mansbach II, M.D.   Professor of Medicine and Physiology and Chief, Division of Gastroenterology, Department of Medicine, University of Tennessee, Memphis, College of Medicine

Jeanne M. Marrazzo, M.D., M.P.H., F.A.C.P.   Associate Professor of Medicine, University of Washington School of Medicine

Martin L. Mayse, M.D.   Assistant Professor of Pulmonary and Critical Care Medicine, Washington University School of Medicine

E. R. McFadden, Jr., M.D., F.A.C.P.   Argyl J. Beams Professor of Medicine, Case Western Reserve University School of Medicine, and Director, Pulmonary Research, MetroHealth Medical Center, Cleveland

Shlomo Melmed, M.D.   Professor and Associate Dean, University of California, Los Angeles, School of Medicine, and Senior Vice President of Academic Affairs, Cedars-Sinai Medical Center

Terry J. Mengert, M.D.   Professor of Medicine, University of Washington School of Medicine

Mark E. Molitch, M.D., F.A.C.P.   Professor of Medicine, Northwestern University Feinberg School of Medicine, and Associate Chief, Division of Endocrinology for Clinical Affairs, Northwestern Memorial Hospital

Lewis B. Morgenstern, M.D.   Associate Professor of Neurology and Epidemiology and Co-Director, Stroke Program, University of Texas–Houston Medical School

Monica Morrow, M.D.   Professor of Surgery, Temple University School of Medicine, and Chair, Division of Surgical Oncology, Fox Chase Cancer Center

Robb Moses, M.D.   Professor and Chair, Department of Molecular and Medical Genetics, Oregon Health and Science University School of Medicine

George Moxley, M.D.   Associate Professor, Division of Rheumatology, Allergy and Immunology, Medical College of Virginia at Virginia Commonwealth University, and Chief, Rheumatology Section, McGuire Veterans Affairs Medical Center

Patricia L. Myskowski, M.D.   Associate Professor of Dermatology, Joan and Sanford I. Weill Medical College of Cornell University, and Associate Attending Physician, Dermatology Service, Memorial Sloan-Kettering Cancer Center

Charles B. Nemeroff, M.D., Ph.D.   Chair, Department of Psychiatry, and Reunette W. Harris Professor, Emory University School of Medicine

Alfred I. Neugut, M.D., Ph.D., F.A.C.P.   Myron M. Studner Professor of Cancer Research and Professor of Medicine and Epidemiology, Columbia University College of Physicians and Surgeons; Acting Head, Division of Medical Oncology, and Codirector, Cancer Prevention Program, New York Presbyterian Hospital

Patrick G. O'Connor, M.D., M.P.H.   Professor of Medicine and Chief, Program in Primary Care Medicine, Yale University School of Medicine, and Director, Primary Care, Yale–New Haven Hospital

Nancy J. Olsen, M.D.   Professor of Medicine, Vanderbilt University School of Medicine

Kent R. Olson, M.D.   Clinical Professor of Medicine, Pediatrics and Pharmacy, University of California, San Francisco, Schools of Medicine and Pharmacy, and Medical Director, San Francisco Division, California Poison Control System

Steven M. Opal, M.D.   Professor of Medicine, Department of Medicine, Brown University School of Medicine

James L. Orford, M.B., Ch.B., M.P.H.   Consulting Cardiologist, Mayday University Hospital, London

Catherine M. Otto, M.D.   Professor of Medicine and Acting Director, Division of Cardiology, and Director, Cardiology Fellowship Program, University of Washington School of Medicine

Roberta A. Pagon, M.D.   Professor of Pediatrics, University of Washington School of Medicine; Medical Director, GeneTests Genetic Testing Resource, Children's Hospital and Regional Medical Center; and Editor-in-Chief, GeneClinics: Medical Genetics Knowledge Base, University of Washington

Biff F. Palmer, M.D., F.A.C.P.   Professor of Internal Medicine and Director, Renal Fellowship Program, University of Texas Southwestern Medical Center at Dallas

Cynthia X. Pan, M.D.   Assistant Professor of Palliative Care Education, Mount Sinai School of Medicine, and Staff Attending Physician, Hertzberg Institute of Palliative Care, Mount Sinai Hospital

Umesh D. Parashar M.D., M.P.H.   Medical Epidemiologist, Centers for Disease Control and Prevention

Henry P. Parkman, M.D.   Professor of Medicine, Temple University School of Medicine, and Director, GI Motility Laboratory, Temple University Hospital

Manish M. Patel, M.D.   Assistant Professor, Department of Emergency Medicine, Emory University School of Medicine

James D. Perkins, M.D.   Professor, Department of Surgery, and Chief, Division of Transplantation, University of Washington School of Medicine

Stephen D. Persell, M.D., M.P.H.   Assistant Professor of Medicine, Northwestern University Feinberg School of Medicine

Kimberly M. Persley, M.D.   Assistant Clinical Professor of Medicine, University of Texas Southwestern Medical Center at Dallas, and Staff Physician, Presbyterian Hospital of Dallas

Lyle R. Petersen, M.D., M.P.H.   Deputy Director for Science, Division of Vector-Borne Infectious Diseases, Centers for Disease Control and Prevention

Raimund H. Pichler, M.D.   Assistant Professor of Nephrology, University of Washington School of Medicine

Jerome B. Posner, M.D.   George C. Cotzias Chair in Neuro-Oncology and Member, Memorial Sloan-Kettering Cancer Center

Jonathan Q. Purnell, M.D.   Codirector, Metabolic Clinic, and Assistant Professor, Department of Medicine, Oregon Health and Science University School of Medicine

David Solomon, M.D., Ph.D.   Assistant Professor of Neurology and Otolaryngology, Johns Hopkins University School of Medicine

Frederick S. Southwick, M.D., F.A.C.P.   Professor and Chief, Division of Infectious Diseases, and Associate Chairman, Department of Medicine, University of Florida College of Medicine

Harold C. Sox, Jr., M.D., M.A.C.P.   Editor, *Annals of Internal Medicine*

David H. Spach, M.D.   Associate Professor of Medicine, Division of Allergy and Infectious Diseases, University of Washington School of Medicine

Stuart Jon Spechler, M.D.   Chief, Division of Gastroenterology, Dallas VA Medical Center

Walter E. Stamm, M.D., F.A.C.P.   Professor of Medicine and Head, Division of Allergy and Infectious Disease, University of Washington School of Medicine

Valerie L. Staradub, M.D.   Assistant Professor of Surgery, Northwestern University Feinberg School of Medicine

Gerald W. Staton, Jr., M.D., F.A.C.P.   Professor of Medicine, Emory University School of Medicine, and Medical Director, Long Term Hospital and Respiratory Services, Wesley Woods Geriatric Hospital, Emory Healthcare

Richard H. Sterns, M.D., F.A.C.P.   Professor of Medicine, University of Rochester School of Medicine and Dentistry, and Chief of Medicine, Rochester General Hospital and the Genesee Hospital

Dennis L. Stevens, M.D., Ph.D., F.A.C.P.   Professor of Medicine, University of Washington School of Medicine, and Chief, Infectious Disease Section, Veterans Affairs Medical Center, Boise, Idaho

Seth R. Stevens, M.D.   Director, Global Medical Affairs, Amgen, Inc.

Kingman P. Strohl, M.D.   Professor of Medicine and Anatomy, Case Western Reserve University, and Director, Center for Sleep Disorders Research, Louis Stokes VA Medical Center

S. H. Subramony, M.D.   Professor of Neurology and Vice Chairman, Department of Neurology, University of Mississippi Medical Center

Weijing Sun, M.D.   Assistant Professor, University of Pennsylvania School of Medicine, and Attending Physician, Hospital of the University of Pennsylvania

Eliza Sutton, M.D., F.A.C.P.   Assistant Professor, Department of Medicine, University of Washington School of Medicine, and Staff Physician, Department of Medicine, Women's Health Care Center

Paul R. Sutton, M.D., Ph.D., F.A.C.P.   Associate Professor of Medicine, University of Washington School of Medicine

James S. Taylor, M.D.   Head, Section of Industrial Dermatology, Department of Dermatology, Cleveland Clinic Foundation

Gunvant K. Thaker, M.D.   Professor of Psychiatry, University of Maryland School of Medicine, and Chief, Schizophrenia Related Disorders Program, Maryland Psychiatric Research Center

David C. Tompkins, M.D.   Associate Professor of Clinical Medicine, Stony Brook University Health Sciences Center School of Medicine

Jo-Anne van Burik, M.D., F.A.C.P.   Assistant Professor of Medicine, University of Minnesota Medical School

Wesley C. Van Voorhis, M.D., Ph.D., F.A.C.P.   Professor of Medicine and Adjunct Professor of Pathobiology, University of Washington School of Medicine

Everett E. Vokes, M.D., F.A.C.P.   John E. Ultmann Professor of Medicine and Radiation Oncology and Director, Section of Hematology/Oncology, University of Chicago Pritzker School of Medicine

Matthew R. Weir, M.D., F.A.C.P.   Professor of Medicine, and Director, Division of Nephrology, University of Maryland School of Medicine

Kevin B. Weiss, M.D., M.P.H., F.A.C.P.   Professor of Medicine and Director, Institute for Healthcare Studies, Northwestern University Feinberg School of Medicine

Peter F. Weller, M.D., F.A.C.P.   Professor of Medicine, Harvard Medical School; and Co-Chief, Infectious Diseases Division, and Chief, Allergy and Inflammation Division, Beth Israel Deaconess Medical Center

David A. Whiting, M.D., F.A.C.P.   Associate Professor of Dermatology, University of Texas Southwestern Medical School, and Medical Director, Baylor Hair Research and Treatment Center

Wyndham H. Wilson, M.D., Ph.D.   Senior Investigator and Chief, Lymphoma Section, National Cancer Institute, National Institutes of Health

John Buckner Winfield, M.D.   Smith Professor of Medicine, University of North Carolina at Chapel Hill School of Medicine

Christopher Wise, M.D., F.A.C.P   W. Robert Irby Associate Professor of Internal Medicine, Division of Rheumatology, Allergy and Immunology, Medical College of Virginia at Virginia Commonwealth University School of Medicine

Jerry S. Wolinsky, M.D.   The Bartels Family Professor of Neurology, University of Texas Health Science Center at Houston, and Director, Multiple Sclerosis Research Center, Memorial Hermann Hospital

Fuad N. Ziyadeh, M.D.   Professor of Medicine, Division of Renal-Electrolyte and Hypertension, University of Pennsylvania School of Medicine

Peer Review Board

James E. Gern, M.D.
Professor of Pediatrics, University of Wisconsin School of Medicine and Public Health

Anthony J. Giampolo, M.D., M.B.A.
Clinical Assistant Professor of Neurology, University of Pittsburgh School of Medicine

Aaron E. Glatt, M.D.
Professor of Clinical Medicine, New York Medical College

Dennis Goldfinger, M.D.
Director Emeritus, Division of Transfusion Medicine, Cedars-Sinai Medical Center

Katherine A. Halmi, M.D.
Professor of Medicine, Joan and Sanford I. Weill Medical College of Cornell University

Julie C. Harper, M.D.
Assistant Professor of Dermatology, University of Alabama School of Medicine at Birmingham

R. Brian Haynes, M.D., Ph.D., F.A.C.P.
Professor of Clinical Epidemiology and Medicine and Chair, Department of Clinical Epidemiology and Biostatistics, McMaster University Health Sciences Centre

Alfonso Iorio, M.D.
Assistant Professor of Internal and Cardiovascular Medicine, University of Perugia, Italy

Dennis M. Jensen, M.D.
Professor of Medicine, University of California Los Angeles David Geffen School of Medicine

Stacie M. Jones, M.D.
Associate Professor of Pediatrics and Physiology/Biophysics, University of Arkansas for Medical Sciences College of Medicine

Philip O. Katz, M.D., F.A.C.P.
Clinical Professor of Medicine, Jefferson Medical College of Thomas Jefferson University

Eric B. Larson, M.D., M.P.H., M.A.C.P.
Professor/Adjunct Professor, Medicine Health Services, University of Washington School of Medicine, and Director, Center for Health Studies, Group Health Cooperative, Seattle

Terri M. Laufer, M.D.
Assistant Professor of Medicine, University of Pennsylvania School of Medicine

Karin S. Leder, M.D., M.P.H.
Head, Infectious Disease Epidemiology Unit, Monash University Faculty of Medicine, Melbourne, Australia

Wendy Levinson, M.D., F.A.C.P.
Chair, Department of Medicine, University of Toronto Faculty of Medicine, and Associate Director, Research Administration, Saint Michael's Hospital, Toronto

Beth G. Lewis, M.D.
Instructor of General Medicine, Mount Sinai School of Medicine of New York University

M. Peter Marinkovich, M.D.
Associate Professor of Dermatology, Stanford University School of Medicine

Bruce A. Molitoris, M.D.
Professor of Medicine, Indiana University School of Medicine

Andrew L. Morris, M.D.
Associate Professor of Medicine, Department of Cardiology, University of Manitoba Faculty of Medicine

James L. Mulshine, M.D.
Professor of Internal Medicine, Rush Medical College of Rush University Medical Center

Patrick T. Murray, M.D.
Associate Professor of Medicine, University of Chicago Pritzker School of Medicine

Rick A. Nishimura, M.D., FA.C.P.
Professor of Medicine, Cardiovascular Diseases and Internal Medicine, Mayo Clinic College of Medicine

Brian D. O'Brien, M.D., M.Sc.
Professor of Medicine, University of Alberta Faculty of Medicine

Jeffrey Olin, D.O., F.A.C.P.
Professor of Medicine, Mount Sinai School of Medicine

John E. Pandolfino, M.D.
Assistant Professor of Medicine, Northwestern University Feinberg School of Medicine

Peter G. Pappas, M.D., F.A.C.P.
Professor of Medicine, Division of Infectious Diseases, University of Alabama at Birmingham School of Medicine

Paul Plotz, M.D., M.A.C.P.
Chief, Arthritis and Rheumatism Branch, National Institute of Arthritis and Musculoskeletal and Skin Diseases, National Institutes of Health

Don W. Powell, M.D., M.A.C.P.
Professor, Departments of Internal Medicine and Neuroscience and Cell Biology, and Associate Dean for Research, School of Medicine, University of Texas Medical Branch at Galveston

Jai Radhakrishnan, M.D., M.S.
Assistant Professor of Clinical Medicine, Columbia University College of Physicians and Surgeons

Scott D. Ramsey, M.D., Ph.D.
Professor of Medicine, University of Washington School of Medicine, and Director, Translational and Outcomes Research, Fred Hutchinson Cancer Research Center, Seattle

Susan M. Richman, M.D.
Assistant Professor of Obstetrics, Gynecology and Reproductive Sciences, Yale University School of Medicine

José R. Romero, M.D.
Professor of Pediatrics, Pathology and Microbiology, University of Nebraska College of Medicine, and Director, Section of Pediatric Infectious Diseases and Fellowship Program, University of Nebraska Medical Center

Richard S. Root, M.D., F.A.C.P.
Emeritus Professor of Medicine, University of Washington School of Medicine, and Assistant Director, Graduate Medical Education, Department of Medicine, Swedish Medical Center/Providence

Coleman Rotstein, M.D.
Professor of Medicine, McMaster University Faculty of Medicine

Christopher P. Schaeffer, M.D.
Assistant Professor of Clinical Medicine, State University of New York School of Medicine and Biomedical Sciences at Buffalo

Robert A. Schwartz, D.O.
Professor of Dermatology and Chief of Dermatology, Department of Medicine, Division of Dermatology, University of Medicine and Dentistry of New Jersey/Robert Wood Johnson Medical School

Peter H. Schur, M.D., F.A.C.P.
Professor of Medicine, Harvard Medical School

Marc A. Silver, M.D., F.A.C.P.
Professor of Medicine, University of Illinois College of Medicine

Roland Solensky, M.D.
Staff Physician, Corvallis Clinic, Corvallis, Oregon

Ted S. Steiner, M.D.
Assistant Professor of Medicine, Division of Infectious Diseases, University of British Columbia Faculty of Medicine

William E. Stevens, M.D.
Staff Physician, Department of Internal Medicine, Division of Gastroenterology, Presbyterian Hospital of Dallas

Richard M. Stone, M.D.
Associate Professor of Medicine, Harvard Medical School

Lewis Sudarsky, M.D.
Associate Professor of Neurology, Harvard Medical School

Thoralf Sundt III, M.D.
Professor of Surgery, Mayo Clinic College of Medicine

Jerry W. Swanson, M.D.
Professor of Neurology, Mayo Clinic College of Medicine

Amit Tailor, M.D., M.B.A.
Staff Physician, Hackensack University Medical Center

James Tracy, D.O.
Assistant Clinical Professor, University of Nebraska School of Medicine

James A. Tumlin, M.D.
Assistant Professor of Medicine, Renal Division, Department of Internal Medicine, Emory University School of Medicine

P. J. Utz, M.D.
Assistant Professor and Director, Research Laboratory, Division of Rheumatology and Immunology, Center for Clinical Immunology, Stanford University School of Medicine

Désirée M. van der Heijde, M.D., Ph.D.
Professor of Rheumatology, Universiteit Maastricht, Maastricht, the Netherlands

Kimberly J. Van Zee, M.D., F.A.C.S.
Attending Surgeon, Breast Service, Memorial Sloan-Kettering Cancer Center

Harrison Weed, M.D., M.S., F.A.C.P.
Professor of Clinical Internal Medicine, Ohio State University College of Medicine

Philip Wells, M.D.,
Professor and Chief, Division of Hematology, University of Ottawa Faculty of Medicine, and Director of Clinical Research, Ottawa Hospital

Corrine K. Welt, M.D.
Assistant Professor of Medicine, Harvard Medical School

Arthur P. Wheeler, M.D.
Associate Professor of Medicine, Vanderbilt University School of Medicine

Laura M. Whitman, M.D.
Assistant Professor, Associate Program Director of Internal Medicine, Yale University School of Medicine

L. James Willmore, M.D.
Professor, Departments of Neurology and Pharmacology and Physiology, St. Louis University School of Medicine

John R. Wingard, M.D.
Professor of Medicine, University of Florida College of Medicine

Robert L. Wortmann, M.D., F.A.C.P.
Professor and Chairman, Department of Internal Medicine, University of Oklahoma College of Medicine

Sai-Ching J. Yeung, M.D., Ph.D.
Assistant Professor, Departments of General Internal Medicine, Ambulatory Treatment, and Emergency Care, University of Texas Medical School at Houston and the M. D. Anderson Cancer Center

Foreword

Keeping up with medical knowledge is increasingly challenging. Just pause a minute and think about a few recent changes: the important new roles for biologic therapies in managing cancer, rheumatoid arthritis, and psoriasis; new diagnostic tests for tuberculosis and numerous other diseases; and new vaccines to prevent cervical cancer and herpes zoster. Add to these advancements evidence-based prevention and treatment guidelines; performance measures; quantitative assessments of risk factors for coronary artery disease, stroke, cancer, and complications of surgery; myriads of new drugs and new uses for older agents; and the specific requirement for maintenance of certification. You must wonder, "How can I possibly keep up?"

The American College of Physicians (ACP, www.acponline.org) takes special pride in its role as an advocate for practicing physicians and as a sponsor of continuing medical education courses and materials of the highest quality. One of the College's educational efforts is its sponsorship of the medical reference *ACP Medicine*, which has been published in partnership with the College since 2004. *ACP Medicine* is continually updated and refined by a dedicated team of authors, editors, and staff. Changes in practice recommendations are incorporated as rapidly as possible. David C. Dale, M.D., F.A.C.P., the Editor-in-Chief, reports to the Publication Committee and the Chief Executive Office of ACP regarding content, new developments, and editorial standards for *ACP Medicine*. Most of *ACP Medicine's* editors and authors are actively engaged in the College's educational programs and other activities.

One of the many benefits of the College's sponsorship of *ACP Medicine* is its capacity to serve as a home for new materials and policies from the College, such as ACP guidelines and clinical recommendations. As new requirements for the practice of medicine appear, such as disease-specific performance measures and other quality-improvement initiatives, they are readily incorporated into *ACP Medicine*. Because of the timeliness of performance measures, this important topic is now discussed in the front matter of *ACP Medicine*, and specific content on quality measures appears in chapters throughout this edition. You can receive monthly updated information on this topic and numerous others at the *ACP Medicine* Web site (www.acpmedicine.com). In addition, in support of the College's commitment to continual learning, *ACP Medicine* offers a monthly continuing medical education program as a companion to these monthly updates.

We hope you find *ACP Medicine* to be an authoritative resource that will help you enjoy the practice of medicine and make it easier for you to convert medical information into excellent patient care.

John Tooker, M.D., M.B.A., F.A.C.P.
Executive Vice President and Chief Executive Officer
American College of Physicians

Steven Weinberger, M.D., F.A.C.P.
Senior Vice President, Medical Education and Publishing
American College of Physicians

Preface

Welcome to the 2007 bound edition of *ACP Medicine*, a medical textbook designed for the practicing physician.

The chapters in *ACP Medicine* are written with the goal of supporting the diagnostic and therapeutic decisions that you make daily in clinical practice. Our authors, who are among today's leaders in medicine, base their recommendations on the best current evidence, as well as on their substantial clinical experience. Because our authors realize that medicine is more than just searching for the latest study results, they put recent medical advances into context within existing knowledge and also explain the underlying pathophysiology that is essential for making informed decisions.

The 2007 bound edition of *ACP Medicine* is extremely comprehensive, with more than 3,000 pages, over 1,200 figures and algorithms, nearly 1,000 tables, and over 16,500 references. Performance measurement, a key issue facing physicians in practice today, is addressed in the Front Matter of Volume 1 on page xxxv; the considerations found there inform the discussions of specific topics throughout the book. In addition, all new or revised chapters are now subject to the peer review process that we launched in 2004. Our peer review board is listed in the front matter of Volume 1, starting on page xxv.

The 2007 edition introduces a major reorganization and expansion of our coverage of diabetes mellitus. Instead of a single chapter, we now devote three new chapters to this critically important topic: Type 1 Diabetes Mellitus, written by Saul Genuth, M.D., F.A.C.P., on page 633, Type 2 Diabetes Mellitus, co-authored by Matthew Riddle, M.D., and Saul Genuth, on page 651, and Complications of Diabetes Mellitus, by Mark E. Molitch, M.D., F.A.C.P., and Saul Genuth, on page 666. Together, these chapters provide a comprehensive discussion of the pathophysiology, diagnosis, and treatment of both type 1 and type 2 diabetes and of the measures that can help prevent or minimize such devastating complications as impaired vision, renal insufficiency, neuropathy, and a markedly increased risk of heart disease and stroke.

In addition, for the 2007 edition we have updated our cardiac resuscitation and adult preventive care chapters to include the latest guidelines. Overall, more than 50% of the material in the book either has been updated or is new, and in some sections, an even higher percentage of the chapters—as many as two-thirds in some cases—have been revised since our last edition.

ACP Medicine is available in five formats. In addition to this text, we also publish a quarterly CD-ROM edition, an annual CD-ROM, our original loose-leaf edition, and an online edition, available at www.acpmedicine.com. Both the loose-leaf and the online editions are updated monthly. We recently added two new online features—Special Alerts and Clinical Practice Guidelines—that we believe will significantly enhance the usefulness of *ACP Medicine* for our readers. Special Alerts are reports on recent key studies that are thought to have an important impact on clinical practice. Clinical Practice Guidelines are evidence-based guidelines designed to reduce variation in clinical practice and improve patient care. The Special Alerts and Guidelines appear in the monthly newsletter and can also be accessed online by clicking on a tab in the appropriate chapters.

Included free with the purchase of this bound edition is three months of access to *ACP Medicine Online*. Look for the card inserted at the front of this book to learn more about how to sign up for your free access. (After the trial period, an additional 12-month subscription is available for only $99.) We invite you also to sign up for our free monthly email, What's New in *ACP Medicine*, to receive highlights of new and revised chapters, as well as monthly columns from our editorial board members.

ACP Medicine provides an economical online CME program, through which you can earn up to 120 AMA PRA Category 1 credits. The program is conveniently linked to the related chapters and has an easy-to-use logbook, which bookmarks your tests so that you can return to them later. It also tracks your credits, and you can print out an award certificate as needed.

We want our readers to play a role in the continuing evolution of *ACP Medicine*. We welcome your ongoing comments and questions.

I hope you find *ACP Medicine* to be a convenient and helpful tool for your daily practice of medicine.

David C. Dale, M.D., F.A.C.P.
Editor-in-Chief
ACP Medicine
daviddalemd@webmd.net

On Being a Physician

David C. Dale, M.D., F.A.C.P., and Daniel D. Federman, M.D., M.A.C.P.

Almost all human societies have persons who act in the role of healer. In early societies, the function had only a minimal basis in science, and the practice of the healing arts was highly dependent on a confident, personal relationship between patient and healer. In today's society, medicine combines a progressively enriched science base with an unequaled social connectedness between physician and patient.

In the community and in the patient-doctor relationship, physicians are seen as persons skilled in the art of healing and in teaching others about health and disease. Physicians are the ones who receive the extensive training, the licensure by the state, and the approval of society to provide all levels of care: to give advice for a healthy life, examine and diagnose illness, prescribe drugs to relieve suffering, and care for those who are seriously ill and dying. Although physicians now share the many responsibilities involved in patient care with nurses, physician assistants, pharmacists, technicians, therapists, and family members of patients, it is still the physician who bears most of the responsibility for the care of the patient.

Being a patient's physician carries many responsibilities and requires at least three attributes. First, knowledge of the applicable biomedical science and clinical medicine is necessary to understand a patient's problem. There is no limit to the knowledge that may be needed, but it is important to be able to answer correctly the patient's questions, such as "How did this happen to me?" and "Will I be better soon?" The physician needs to understand disease processes well enough to identify and categorize a patient's problem quickly. It is always important, and sometimes critical, to know whether the problem will resolve spontaneously or whether detailed investigation, consultation, or hospitalization is needed. A thorough and up-to-date understanding of diagnosis and treatment is essential for the day-to-day exchange of information that occurs between physicians as they solve the problems of individual patients and work together to organize systems to improve patient care.

Second, some specific skills are necessary to diagnose and treat a patient. The ability to communicate—both to speak and to listen—is essential, especially for physicians providing primary care. Effective and sensitive communication can be challenging in communities characterized by diverse cultures and languages. This is particularly challenging in the United States, where recent waves of immigration have created a patient community that is extraordinarily diverse, both linguistically and culturally. At times, the physician must be, in part, an anthropologist to grasp the patient's understanding of illness and of the roles of patient and doctor. Knowing how to communicate empathetically is also invaluable: it is important to welcome each patient at every visit, to reach out and hold the hand of a troubled person, and to express understanding and concern. The ability to balance the time spent with the patient and the time required for organizing services for the patient in a busy practice is an increasingly important skill.

The physical examination remains a fundamental skill; the ability to recognize the difference between normal and abnormal findings, adjusting for age, sex, ethnicity, and other factors, is crucial. Good record keeping is essential—with regard to both a written record and a mental record—so that the circumstances of visits are remembered and changes in a patient's appearance or other characteristics that may not have been written down can be recognized. With practice and attention, these skills—history taking, physical examination, and record keeping—can grow throughout a professional lifetime. Other aspects of care, such as selecting and performing diagnostic tests, procedures, and treatments, require evolving expertise. For all physicians, it is necessary both to practice medicine and to study regularly to maintain all of these essential skills.

The third, but by no means least important, attribute is the physician's responsibility to the patient and the medical community to conform to appropriate professional and ethical conduct. The first principle of the doctor-patient relationship is that the patient's welfare is paramount. Putting the patient first necessitates understanding the patient and the patient's values. It often means spending precious personal time explaining illness, determining the best method of treatment, or dealing with emergencies. It places the physician in service to the patient. Ethical conduct includes seeing clearly and acknowledging situations in which the physician's interest may conflict with the interest of the patient. Ethical conduct also requires recognizing and acknowledging conflicts of interest in profiting from the prescribing of services and treatments, in ownership of equities and properties, and in personal and business relationships. Finally, personal exploitation of the intimacy and privacy of the doctor-patient relationship is never allowed. The reassertion of professionalism and of medicine's core ideals has never been more important than in the context of today's constantly changing medical practice.

Almost daily there is new information regarding basic disease mechanisms and new therapies; these advances require us to reconsider how we diagnose and treat both common and rare diseases. The Internet has made available to any computer-savvy patient all the medical information formerly held by doctors; the abundance of information—and, in some cases, misinformation—challenges physicians to be more knowledgeable than any previous generation of medical practitioners.

Population growth, poverty, and emerging infectious diseases, as well as physical inactivity, dietary changes, and obesity, are problems that increase the worldwide burden of illness; these factors have immense implications for the medical profession—both the overall practice of medicine and the work of individual physicians. The aging of the United States' population and the corresponding increase in the prevalence of chronic disease have created new demands that health care be delivered by teams of physicians and other health providers.

The way that hospitals and clinics are organized, how we pay for health care, and how our services are evaluated are also changing. The aggregation of physicians and patients into large organizations places a premium on new systems of behavior, consultation, and communication. The limited supply of resources such as transplantable organs and ICU beds requires new training in distributive ethics. The emphasis on the control of risk factors for disease has allied physicians and their patients in initiatives to prevent or minimize morbidity and mortality.

If some changes in health care are challenging, others promise to benefit physicians by allowing the work of healing to be done with greater ease and precision. New information technologies aid the physician in accessing new findings and updating medical records. Application of discoveries from basic sciences and the human genome project permit a diagnosis to be more precise and treatment more specific. Increased understanding of normal physiology and disease processes has prompted development of new drugs and vaccines. Such benefits have added to the costs and the potential costs of almost every aspect of health care.

Efficiency and cost containment are now watchwords of the payers for health services. Practice guidelines, hospital care pathways, and other efforts to codify the practice of medicine are receiving much attention. When based on good evidence, these efforts are beneficial; they save precious resources—time and money—for both patients and physicians. The development of managed care in the United States has created a new challenge for physicians: to serve as advocates for their patients. In this role, physicians are responsible for overcoming organizational, geographic, and financial barriers to the provision of services that are important for their patients. In organizations in which guidelines for care have been established, it may be necessary for a physician to explain to administrators the specific needs and problems of individual patients—sometimes over and over again, because laypersons may be less apt to recognize that guidelines for clinical practice must remain simply guidelines. Because more and more physicians are salaried and thus bound to the needs of populations of patients, physicians face the problem of balancing the needs of individual patients with the expectations of the employer. This is a delicate and, in some places, even fragile balance. To serve both patients and the employer well, a physician must develop good judgment in managing patient care under conditions in which the allocation of resources is conservative.

The increasing organization of health care on a for-profit basis has raised new issues. The physician's obligation to put the patient first and the increasing costs of diagnostic tests and therapies can collide head-on with health care management's attempts to protect earnings for investors. Professional responsibility to patients and the public good is clear and at times poses difficult challenges for the physician.

A profession is defined by a specialized body of knowledge requiring advanced training and the dedication of its practitioners to the public good over their own enrichment. In exchange, professionals are granted considerable autonomy in setting standards and in the conduct of their work. Circumstances within the medical profession have changed. The public in general and patients in particular have much more knowledge of medicine than at any time in the past, and the modern organization of medicine has severely restricted the autonomy of physicians. But delivery of expert medical care and the welfare of the patient remain central to the physician's professional responsibility. The weight of all these responsibilities may suggest that it is impossible, or nearly impossible, to be a good physician. Quite the contrary; persons with vastly different personalities, interests, and intellects have become and are becoming good physicians and are deeply satisfied in this role. The information necessary for practicing medicine is now more accessible than ever before. The skills the physician needs can be learned through experience, sharpened through practice, and focused through specialization. The ethical requirements of physicians are not onerous. They are, in fact, expectations of all good citizens, regardless of their careers. Being a physician is both exciting and satisfying; it provides a unique opportunity to combine modern scientific knowledge with the traditions of an ancient and honored profession in serving and helping one's fellow man.

ACP Medicine is written and edited by physicians to help other physicians meet the ideals enunciated in this introduction. A principal goal of *ACP Medicine* is to be the most up-to-date textbook of medicine available. The Clinical Essentials section presents the contemporary skills and knowledge needed by all physicians to encourage and maintain good health, analyze medical information, deal compassionately with the end of life, and understand issues of medical ethics. The other sections organize and summarize the most important information on pathophysiology, diagnosis, and treatment for most problems encountered in practicing medicine for adults from general and specialty journals, as interpreted by experienced clinicians. The material is evidence-based, with extensive bibliographic citations that are updated regularly. Authors are selected who understand both the constraints of managed care and the quality of care that is possible with scientific advances. In short, *ACP Medicine* is committed to conveying the information necessary for physicians to provide excellent care to their patients.

Performance Measurement in Clinical Practice

Stephen D. Persell, M.D., M.P.H., *David W. Baker*, M.D., M.P.H., F.A.C.P., *and Kevin B. Weiss*, M.D., M.P.H., F.A.C.P.

Performance in health care is the degree to which desirable objectives are accomplished. Performance measurement can inform quality-improvement activities and allow health care consumers and commercial health care purchasers to hold physicians and health care organizations accountable for the services they provide. Over the past decade, the methodology supporting performance measurement has matured. With this maturity has come an increasing array of performance measures covering a range of care settings and specialties; the increasing information has given rise to an expanded interest in the application of performance measurement. The Centers for Medicare and Medicaid Services (CMS) and large commercial health care purchasers now pay close attention to publicly released performance data. At present, the vast majority of patients in the United States who are enrolled in managed care organizations or Medicare receive health care from health plans, hospitals, nursing homes, or ambulatory care centers for which publicly reported performance data are available; the trend toward the public release of performance information is likely to accelerate in coming years. Physicians may increasingly find themselves the targets of efforts to profile the care provided by group practices or individual physicians. It is likely that the trend toward performance measurement will have increasingly noticeable effects on the ways in which health care is delivered and physicians are compensated.[1]

Why Measure Performance?

Ideally, individual health care professionals would be able to deliver high-quality care as a matter of course, and performance measurement would be unnecessary. Unfortunately, the best practices often are not followed, and patients frequently do not receive indicated services for acute problems, chronic illnesses, and preventive health care.[2] Measurement of clinical performance is needed to assess the quality of care and to compare what is achieved with what is desired. This information can then serve the related but distinct purposes of internal and external quality review. First, measurement can enable internal quality improvement—in other words, deficiencies in health care can be identified and physicians and health care organizations can implement changes to improve quality and track their progress.[3] Second, the public release of performance information can increase accountability of health care providers by (1) allowing health care purchasers and consumers to make informed health care choices and (2) permitting regulators responsible for licensure or accreditation to evaluate the quality of care offered by specific health care organizations. Both purposes figure prominently in the Institute of Medicine's Strategic Framework for a national quality measurement and reporting system.[4]

Performance Measures

In the past, performance measurement was often conducted through the use of implicit review to assess the quality of care provided. In this method, a physician reviewed patient records and judged whether appropriate care had been provided. This approach to performance measurement is poorly reproducible because implicit review involves a level of subjectivity, and physician reviewers frequently do not agree.[5] Currently, the most widely used quality measures define explicit criteria against which performance is judged. Although no performance measure is ideal, well-developed measures share three characteristics[6]: (1) they are based on strong clinical evidence; (2) they depict uncontroversial clinical practices that have broad consensus among physicians; and (3) they incorporate agreed-upon standards for determining satisfactory performance.

For performance measurement to be undertaken, it must be feasible to collect the necessary data. Methods of data collection that are too burdensome limit a measure's utility. When used for comparisons of health care providers, performance measures should be attributable to the physician or organization being assessed. Furthermore, sufficient numbers of patients should be assessed to allow for meaningful statistical comparisons; if required, statistical adjustments should be made to account for confounding variables in the collected data.[6] Several measures are used to assess the quality of health care; these include measures of clinical performance, measures of patient experience, and measures of efficiency.

MEASURES OF CLINICAL PERFORMANCE

Measures of clinical performance can assess health care structures, processes, and outcomes.[7] Structural measures are not measures of clinical performance per se; rather, they describe characteristics of physicians, hospitals, or other health care organizations. Structural characteristics are selected for assessment because they are perceived to be associated with favorable clinical outcomes. Examples of structural measures include the ratio of nurses to patients in the hospital,[8] whether a board-certified critical care physician is available in the intensive care unit of a hospital 24 hours a day,[9] whether a hemodialysis center is operated as a not-for-profit facility,[10] and whether a hospital has a computerized drug-order entry system.[11,12]

Process measures assess specific components of the encounters between physicians and patients: Was a screening test for colon cancer obtained? Was a beta blocker prescribed to a patient with a myocardial infarction? Did a patient who was hospitalized for a mental illness receive an outpatient appointment promptly after discharge?[13]

Outcome measures are direct assessments of patients' health status. Examples include whether a nursing-home patient has a pressure ulcer and whether death occurs within 30 days after coronary artery bypass graft surgery.[14,15]

Structure and process measures have some advantages over outcome measures. Because they are to a greater degree under the control of a single health care organization or individual physician, structure and process measures are less likely than outcome measures to require adjustment for confounding differences between patient groups—a statistical correction referred to as case-mix adjustment, or risk adjustment [*see* Case-Mix Adjustment, *below*]. In addition, structural measures often require very little data collection, as compared with other measures.

Conversely, a limitation of both structure and process measures is that they need to be causally related to desirable health outcomes to be valid measures of health care quality. If structure or process measures are not directly related to desirable health outcomes, efforts made to improve these measures may merely increase the costs of care without improving patients' health status. An advantage of outcome measures is that they directly measure the ultimate objectives of health care—clinical outcomes; however, they are often dependent on the characteristics and actions of individual patients. Observed differences in outcomes may be largely driven by factors that are not under the control of physicians or health care organizations. Patients who receive excellent care may still have bad outcomes, and physicians caring for patients of lower socioeconomic status or educational attainment, who are known to be at higher risk for disease severity and who lack access to care because of mechanisms such as cost sharing of copayments and high deductibles, may falsely appear to be providing inferior care.[16-19]

PATIENT EXPERIENCE AND SATISFACTION MEASURES

Although expert-derived clinical measures may best assess the technical aspects of care, consumers of health care are in the best position to evaluate their own experience and level of satisfaction with the services they receive. Furthermore, care that is timely and well received by patients may lead to better health outcomes. Examples of patient experience measures include the ease with which medical advice can be obtained by phone, the number of times a patient must wait more than 30 minutes past an appointment time to see a physician, and the rating of a personal physician on a scale of 0 to 10.[20] The Consumer Assessment of Health Plans Survey (CAHPS) is a widely used series of surveys to assess patients' experience of health care.[21] CAHPS captures patient satisfaction with the delivery of care occurring during office visits, the level of assistance obtained from health-plan customer service, the perceived accessibility and timeliness of medical and reimbursement services, and the clarity and timeliness of health advice provided by the physician. CAHPS is one form of evaluation used by the National Committee for Quality Assurance (NCQA) to evaluate health plans.[14]

EFFICIENCY MEASURES

Efficiency measures focus on the costs of delivering health care. When combined with measures of clinical performance, efficiency measures assess the value of health care (i.e., the quality of care delivered per unit cost). The methodology for assessing efficiency is less well developed than that of quality measurement.[22] Common units of efficiency measurement (e.g., cost of health plan per member per month and cost per episode of care) do not capture the quality of the care received for that cost.

From Quality Improvement to Accountability

Performance measurement can support quality improvement in several ways. Measuring performance and relaying this information to the physicians who were assessed can produce beneficial, albeit modest, improvements in quality.[23] With-

in health care organizations, reliable measurements of quality are necessary to assess the impact of quality improvement initiatives such as clinical-reminder systems, disease-management programs, clinical-decision support systems, patient-directed programs, and multimodality interventions. Because they are in a position to implement system-level changes, health care organizations may be in a better position than individual physicians to act on performance data and institute quality improvement.[24,25]

Using performance measurement to hold physicians and organizations accountable for the care they provide is a very different undertaking from that of quality improvement. Although publicly released reports on quality performance may prompt physicians to improve performance, they are intended for an audience external to the health care team.[26] The goal of measurement for accountability is to enable comparisons of different health care organizations. For this reason, the measures used in assessing accountability must be standardized across sites. In the United States, private organizations such as the NCQA, the Quality Consortium of the American Medical Association, the Joint Commission on Accreditation of Healthcare Organizations, and the National Quality Forum (NQF) have taken leading roles in the development of standardized performance measures and the dissemination of performance results. Government agencies, such as CMS, are also a major source of performance data. Consumers and commercial health care purchasers can find comparative information on health plans, hospitals, nursing homes, and hemodialysis centers on the Internet or through health insurers.[13-15]

The use of publicly released performance data is not limited to consumers or purchasers of health care. Increasingly, physicians may find their remuneration influenced by their measured performance. The Institute of Medicine has issued a call for government health care payers to reward high-quality care with increased payments.[1] Nongovernmental organizations also are adopting pay-for-performance (PFP or P4P) plans. For example, the Integrated Healthcare Association, a California consortium of medical groups and health plans, distributed $50 million in bonuses to health care providers on the basis of performance in the first year of the consortium's pay-for-performance initiative.[1,27] In the United Kingdom, the government has instituted an ambitious pay-for-performance initiative in which family practitioners will receive from the government an additional £1 billion ($1.8 billion) more than they ordinarily would have received; this represents a 20% increase over the previous year's family-practice budget. The additional funding will be distributed to family practitioners on the basis of a combination of three factors: their performance on a variety of clinical measures, organizational indicators, and patient surveys.[28] Both positive and negative consequences of pay-for-performance have been predicted,[28] but the full impact of the program remains to be seen.

Aside from influencing payments, performance measurement can also be incorporated into the accreditation process. For example, the American Board of Internal Medicine has incorporated a module on self-assessment of the quality of care provided by the physician as an option by which to meet the 2006 practice assessment requirement for recertification in internal medicine.[29]

Methodological Issues

As the use of performance measurement increases, continued awareness of its limitations is vital. There remain both methodological and practical limitations to successful performance measurement.

FACTORS AFFECTING DATA UTILITY

Data Collection

Collecting the data required for performance measurement can be labor-intensive and expensive. Measures that rely on data collected for other purposes (e.g., administrative data) are not burdensome to implement but may not be as reliable as data collected explicitly for quality measurement. Expanded use of clinical computer systems and electronic health records is one way to facilitate the collection of clinical data of high quality,[28] but the implementation of new clinical computer systems is costly.

Use of publicly released data to inform consumer choice or to increase provider accountability also has its drawbacks. One significant problem is that publicly available data may include falsified results. To help maintain the accuracy of data reported to such organizations as the NCQA, auditing is required. Some falsification, however, may be undetectable by audits (e.g., a physician's falsely recording a blood pressure measurement that is below a quality goal). The potential exists for physicians to adjust their performance measures by the selection or dismissal of patients. For example, physicians may dismiss nonadherent or outlier patients (i.e., patients whose data lie far outside the central statistical mass) to improve their measured performance.[30] Physicians who will be judged by clinical outcomes such as mortality following coronary artery bypass graft surgery may avoid taking on patients at high risk for bad outcomes. In one instance, following the release of publicly reported cardiac surgery mortality, cardiologists reported that it became harder to find surgeons willing to operate on high-risk patients who needed surgery.[31]

Sample Size

Another potential problem in performance measurement is insufficient sample size. For any single measure, there may be too few patients for statistically meaningful comparisons, either between providers or between the performances of a single provider over time. An insufficient sample size is frequently a factor when individual physicians are profiled. When statistically meaningful differences cannot be detected because of limited sample size, those who report data should not suggest that providers with statistically insignificant differences in quality scores differ from one another. Combining several years of data is one way to compensate for insufficient sample size; however, this reporting method makes the reported results less timely and may obscure improvements in quality that occur in the short term.

Case-Mix Adjustment

The differences in patient characteristics (referred to as case mix) can introduce systematic biases into quality measurements; case-mix adjustment to correct these biases is an important methodological consideration in the utilization of performance data. Apparent differences in the quality of care received by patients cared for by different physicians may disappear when differences in patients' socioeconomic status or education are taken into account.[16-19] Case-mix adjustment is especially important for measures of clinical outcome or cost

---

Internet Resources for Performance Measures

General Information

Agency for Healthcare Research and Quality (AHRQ)
http://www.ahrq.gov/clinic/epcix.htm

A governmental agency and information clearinghouse on issues of quality, safety, efficiency, and effectiveness of health care

Ambulatory Care Quality Alliance (AQA)
http://www.ahrq.gov/qual/aqaback.htm

Initially convened by the American Academy of Family Physicians, the American College of Physicians, America's Health Insurance Plans, and AHRQ, the Alliance consists of a large body of stakeholders, including physicians, consumers, health care purchasers, and health plans

Centers for Medicare and Medicaid Services (CMS)
http://www.cms.hhs.gov/quality/hospital

Provides hospital quality information to consumers and others in initiatives designed to improve hospital care in the United States

National Committee for Quality Assurance (NCQA)
http://www.ncqa.org

An independent nonprofit organization that provides information on the quality of managed care plans in the United States

National Quality Forum (NQF)
http://www.qualityforum.org

A private, not-for-profit membership organization created to develop and implement a national strategy for measuring and reporting health care quality

Measures and Tools

National Quality Measures Clearinghouse
http://www.qualitymeasures.ahrq.gov

Public repository for evidence-based quality measures and measure sets

Measuring Healthcare Quality
http://www.ahrq.gov/qual/measurix.htm

Includes National Health Care Quality reports, AHRQ quality indicators, and ambulatory care clinical-performance measures

National Voluntary Consensus Standards for Ambulatory Care
http://www.qualityforum.org/pdf/reports/amulatory_care.pdf

Appendix A contains physician standards for ambulatory care pertaining to asthma and respiratory conditions, heart disease, hypertension, prenatal care, and prevention

Quality Profiles
http://www.qualityprofiles.org/quality_profiles/index.asp

Case studies that examine performance measures in such topics as chronic illness, women's health, preventive care, and behavioral health

Quality Improvement Initiative Tools
http://www.qualityprofiles.org/qia_Tools/index.asp

Templates of the tools used by health plans to help implement their health care improvement initiatives

Physician Quality Reports
http://www.ncqa.org/PhysicianQualityReports.htm

Includes measures used to qualify physicians for the Diabetes Physician Recognition Program, the Heart/Stroke Physician Recognition Program, and Physician Practice Connections

Hospital Quality Measures
http://www.qualityindicators.ahrq.gov

Presents hospital quality measures, inpatient quality indicators, and prevention quality indicators

---

efficiency, but it may alter the interpretation of data pertaining to process measures.

Statistical methods can be used to improve the validity of statistical inference when sample sizes are small or when the case mix differs across providers; however, it is not clear whether the methodology to correct for these variables will be generally adopted or, if adopted, applied in uniform ways.[32]

Optional Reporting

Public reporting of performance data may be of limited use to health care purchasers and consumers if poor performers can choose not to report their data. It has been noted that some health plans that participated in the NCQA's Health Plan Employer Data and Information Set (HEDIS) withdrew from HEDIS when they performed poorly.[33]

Inadequate Use of Data

Even when public reports of health care quality are available, purchasers and consumers may not put them to good use.[34] Consumers often do not access the performance data that are available and may have difficulty making sense of the information when they find it.[25,35,36]

METHODS TO IMPROVE PERFORMANCE MEASURES

Although all these methodological issues and limitations are formidable, the organizations developing and promoting such measurement seek to identify and promote only those measures meeting clear criteria. An example of this move toward standardization is the recent development by the NQF of a set of voluntary consensus criteria by which to endorse physician-focused ambulatory care performance measures. The NQF's consensus standards include criteria to judge the importance, scientific acceptability, usability, and feasibility of proposed performance measures.[37]

Issues for the Physician

Although encumbered by methodological and practical issues, performance measurement is a reality of modern medical care. Experts caution physicians that they must be leaders in quality measurement and performance improvement or be vulnerable to challenge by economic or political stakeholders and to the potential loss of patient confidence.[38] Because it is likely that we physicians will increasingly be held accountable for the quality of care we provide, it is to our advantage to have a working knowledge of current performance measurement activities in our specialty [see Sidebar Internet Resources for Performance Measures]. By understanding the types of measures by which we will be judged and knowing how the data are collected, we may be able to improve our performance—as well as the documentation of the data needed for proper measurement of that performance—without greatly increasing our work.

When possible, individual physicians should assess the quality of the care they provide and correct their own deficiencies. They should consider making systematic changes that facilitate quality measurement and internal quality improvement, such as making use of disease registries, flow sheets, or computer systems, to track the quality of chronic disease management and preventive care. It is unlikely that the costs of implementing these changes will be recovered in the short term; however, if pay-for-performance becomes widespread, physicians and health care organizations that have not prepared for it by routinely measuring their own quality of care will find themselves at a distinct disadvantage in comparison with their competitors who have.

References

1. Epstein AM, Lee TH, Hamel MB: Paying physicians for high-quality care. N Engl J Med 350:406, 2004

2. McGlynn EA, Asch SM, Adams J, et al: The quality of health care delivered to adults in the United States. N Engl J Med 348:2635, 2003

3. Kiefe CI, Allison JJ, Williams OD, et al: Improving quality improvement using achievable benchmarks for physician feedback: a randomized controlled trial. JAMA 285:2871, 2001

4. Crossing the Quality Chasm: A New Health System for the 21st Century. Committee on Quality Health Care in America, Institute of Medicine. National Academy Press, Washington, D.C., 2001

5. Hayward RA, McMahon LF Jr, Bernard AM: Evaluating the care of general medicine inpatients: how good is implicit review? Ann Intern Med 118:550, 1993

6. Landon BE, Normand SL, Blumenthal D, et al: Physician clinical performance assessment: prospects and barriers. JAMA 290:1183, 2003

7. Brook RH, McGlynn EA, Cleary PD: Quality of health care. Part 2: Measuring quality of care. N Engl J Med 335:966, 1996

8. Needleman J, Buerhaus P, Mattke S, et al: Nurse-staffing levels and the quality of care in hospitals. N Engl J Med 346:1715, 2002

9. Pronovost PJ, Angus DC, Dorman T, et al: Physician staffing patterns and clinical outcomes in critically ill patients: a systematic review. JAMA 288:2151, 2002

10. Garg PP, Frick KD, Diener-West M, et al: Effect of the ownership of dialysis facilities on patients' survival and referral for transplantation. N Engl J Med 341:1653, 1999

11. Bates DW, Leape LL, Cullen DJ, et al: Effect of computerized physician order entry and a team intervention on prevention of serious medication errors. JAMA 280:1311, 1998

12. Computer Physician Order Entry Fact Sheet: The Leapfrog Group for Patient Safety, Washington, D.C., 2004
http://www.leapfroggroup.org/media/file/Leapfrog-Computer_Physician_Order_Entry_Fact_Sheet.pdf

13. Follow-up after hospitalization for mental illness. State of Health Care Quality Report, 2003. National Committee for Quality Assurance, Washington, D.C., 2003
http://www.ncqa.org/sohc2003/follow_up_after_hospitalization.htm

14. Medicare: The Official U.S. Government Site for People with Medicare: nursing home compare. Department of Health and Human Services, 2005
http://www.medicare.gov/NHCompare

15. Hospital report cards: mortality and complication based outcomes, 2005. Hospital methodologies. Healthgrades, Golden, Colorado
http://www.healthgrades.com

16. Zaslavsky AM, Hochheimer JN, Schneider EC, et al: Impact of sociodemographic case mix on the HEDIS measures of health plan quality. Med Care 38:981, 2000

17. Greenfield S, Kaplan SH, Kahn R, et al: Profiling care provided by different groups of physicians: effects of patient case-mix (bias) and physician-level clustering on quality assessment results. Ann Intern Med 136:111, 2002

18. Fiscella K, Franks P: Influence of patient education on profiles of physician practices. Ann Intern Med 131:745, 1999

19. Franks P, Fiscella K: Effect of patient socioeconomic status on physician profiles for prevention, disease management, and diagnostic testing costs. Med Care 40:717, 2002

20. Zaslavsky AM, Beaulieu ND, Landon BE, et al: Dimensions of consumer-assessed quality of Medicare managed-care health plans. Med Care 38:162, 2000

21. Crofton C, Lubalin JS, Darby C: Consumer Assessment of Health Plans Study (CAHPS). Foreword. Med Care 37(3 suppl):MS1-9, 1999

22. Provider Efficiency White Paper: Measuring Provider Efficiency. Version 1.0. Bridges to Excellence and the Leapfrog Group for Patient Safety, Washington, D.C., 2004
http://www.bridgestoexcellence.org/bte/white_paper_release.htm

23. Thomson O'Brien MA, Oxman AD, Davis DA, et al: Audit and feedback: effects on professional practice and health care outcomes. Cochrane Database Syst Rev (2):CD000259, 2000

24. Berwick DM, James B, Coye MJ: Connections between quality measurement and improvement. Med Care 41(1 suppl):I30, 2003

25. Marshall MN, Shekelle PG, Leatherman S, et al: The public release of performance data: what do we expect to gain? A review of the evidence. JAMA 283:1866, 2000

26. Solberg LI, Mosser G, McDonald S: The three faces of performance measurement: improvement, accountability, and research. Jt Comm J Qual Improv 23:135, 1997

27. Pay-for-performance takes off in California. ACP Observer Online. January-February 2005
http://www.acponline.org/journals/news/jan05/pfp.htm

28. Roland M: Linking physicians' pay to the quality of care: a major experiment in the United Kingdom. N Engl J Med 351:1448, 2004

29. Self-evaluation of practice performance. Maintenance of Certification. American Board of Internal Medicine, Philadelphia, 2005
http://www.abim.org/moc/sempbpi.shtm

30. Hofer TP, Hayward RA, Greenfield S, et al: The unreliability of individual physician "report cards" for assessing the costs and quality of care of a chronic disease. JAMA 281:2098, 1999

31. Schneider EC, Epstein AM: Influence of cardiac-surgery performance reports on referral practices and access to care: a survey of cardiovascular specialists. N Engl J Med 335:251, 1996

32. Zaslavsky AM: Statistical issues in reporting quality data: small samples and casemix variation. Int J Qual Health Care 13:481, 2001

33. McCormick D, Himmelstein DU, Woolhandler S, et al: Relationship between low quality-of-care scores and HMOs' subsequent public disclosure of quality-of-care scores. JAMA 288:1484, 2002

34. Hibbard JH, Jewett JJ, Legnini MW, et al: Choosing a health plan: do large employers use the data? Health Aff (Millwood) 16:172, 1997

35. Schneider EC, Epstein AM: Use of public performance reports: a survey of patients undergoing cardiac surgery. JAMA 279:1638, 1998

36. Hibbard JH, Jewett JJ: Will quality report cards help consumers? Health Aff (Millwood) 16:218, 1997

37. Pre-voting review for "National Voluntary Consensus Standards for Ambulatory Care: An Initial Physician-Focused Measure Set." The National Quality Forum. Washington, D.C., 2005
http://www.qualityforum.org/txWEBambreport04-29-05.pdf

38. Blumenthal D: Quality of care: what is it? Part 1. N Engl J Med 335:891, 1996

1 Contemporary Ethical and Social Issues in Medicine

Christine K. Cassel, M.D., M.A.C.P., *Ruth B. Purtilo*, PH.D

In the past, medical ethics was thought to refer solely to pro-scriptions against physicians advertising their services and fees or engaging in questionable economic arrangements such as fee-splitting. Within the past 20 years, however, medical ethics has evolved into a discipline in which clinicians (physicians, nurses, and other health professionals), philosophers, theologians, and social scientists speak knowledgeably about value conflicts that arise in the practice of medicine.[1,2] Physicians have come to recognize the need to be knowledgeable about complex and wide-ranging moral issues as the result of advances in biomedical science and technology; changes in the delivery of health care; changing worldwide demographic trends; epidemics (e.g., the AIDS and severe acute respiratory syndrome epidemics) and new or reemerging infectious illnesses (e.g., avian influenza and Marburg viruses); and a growing understanding of the interconnectedness of individual and public health concerns. The AIDS pandemic has brought awareness that global health threats and cross-cultural contacts can present clinical, epidemiologic, and ethical challenges. For example, what responsibility does the international community have to provide assistance to severely underprivileged, impoverished countries experiencing an AIDS epidemic when treatment of the disease is readily available but out of reach of millions of people who suffer from its ravages?

Ethical issues in the clinical setting persist, and physicians need to be aware of legal decisions and new technologies that affect clinical practice. The rapid, continuing advances of medical technology have raised a host of moral issues around such fundamental questions as when does life begin, when and how does life end, which services can patients require of physicians, and which requests can physicians legitimately refuse. These questions become even more complex in a society as diverse and multicultural as our own, where moral norms may conflict. Respect for the personal values of our patients requires physicians to examine ethical dilemmas carefully and analytically. Consider the following ethical dilemmas and the questions that each one raises for physicians today:

- A 90-year-old woman, totally disabled from several strokes, lives at home, where she receives 24-hour care. Her strokes have left her cognitively impaired and unable to communicate. She signed a living will 15 years ago, and her husband is her designated health care proxy. She was hospitalized because she had stopped eating, and while in the hospital, she developed aspiration pneumonia. Four days into her hospitalization, she developed a bleeding ulcer and hemorrhaged several units of blood. She had a cardiac arrest, was resuscitated after 45 minutes of asystole, and is now unresponsive and ventilator dependent. Her husband insists that she be kept alive by whatever means possible. The hospital team is strongly divided about the morally appropriate course of action. Some agree with the patient's husband and argue that the patient should receive life-sustaining treatment, even though she has virtually no chance of recovery. Others argue that it would be more respectful to discontinue intrusive medical care—an action consistent with her advance directive—and allow her to die. What clinical and moral value considerations should govern their final decision?

- A 58-year-old man living in Oregon is suffering from end-stage AIDS with lymphopenia, multiple refractory fungal infections, and Kaposi sarcoma. He has significant pain from mucosal lesions and skin breakdown and has sustained fractures, including one from a spinal metastasis that has led to paraplegia and urinary and fecal incontinence. He is cognitively intact and has given oral and written directives indicating that he does not want to be kept alive any longer. He has repeatedly asked his physician to give him an overdose of sedative so that he will die and be released from his intractable suffering. The physician is convinced that this patient is competent, that he is well-informed about his condition, and that his wish to die is made in good faith. The patient's companion of 15 years agrees with the patient's decision. Both have known the physician for a long time and trust her judgment. Physician-assisted suicide is currently legal in Oregon. Should the physician comply with this patient's wishes? If she cannot do so in good conscience, must she refer her patient to a physician who can? Why or why not?

- Science allows physicians to transplant hearts, livers, kidneys, and other living organs, tissues, and cells. Overall, there are drastic shortages of donors. Hundreds, sometimes thousands, of people die each year before an organ match becomes available. Currently in the United States, people who wish to donate organs are encouraged to indicate that wish on their driver's licenses. In the absence of such clear evidence of consent, physicians and other hospital staff are often reluctant to ask bereaved family members for donations because many people, understandably, cannot deal with such a request in a time of crisis. Should the United States adopt a policy—already practiced in other countries—of allowing hospitals to harvest organs upon the death of a patient unless that person has specified otherwise? Could one policy ever work to everyone's benefit in a diverse society in which there may be differing attitudes about treatment of the dead, the moral use of animals, and other culturally derived considerations? Would therapeutic cloning or xenotransplantation provide ethically preferable alternatives?

- A woman whose family has a strong history of breast and ovarian cancer wants to be tested to determine whether she is a carrier of the *BRCA* family of genes, which confer high risk for these malignancies. She is between jobs and is about to apply for a position with a small, innovative firm that has a self-insured health care plan. She knows that the disclosure of this information would dramatically skew the insurance risk and insurance costs for this company, which is largely composed of young people who have relatively low health care costs. She might be denied the job for these reasons. The patient wants to undergo *BRCA* screening but asks you not to note the results in her medical record. You know that her fears are well founded. What should you do?

These examples highlight the complexity of ethical dilemmas and the need for a common language by which clinicians and society can openly deliberate about ethical issues. Often, there is not a single right answer to an ethical dilemma; in almost all cases, there are competing values that need to be weighed against each other before a decision is made that most fully upholds the moral values by which physicians must guide their practice. As in many other areas of medicine, there may be a high degree of uncertainty. For that reason alone, it is useful to have a framework for ethical decision making.

A Context and Process for Ethical Decision Making

A conflict of values lies at the center of each ethical dilemma. Most medical ethicists agree that several fundamental ethical norms can be drawn from the overarching principle that patients should be treated with respect. These ethical norms include the responsibility to act in a way that benefits the patient (beneficence); the responsibility, whenever possible, to do no harm (nonmaleficence); the responsibility to acknowledge the autonomy of the patient and his or her right to self-determination; and the responsibility to treat people fairly and equitably. Although it would be hard to argue against any of these values taken individually, they come into conflict with one another every day in medical practice. Three steps are useful for making decisions when ethical conflicts arise.

First, the clinician needs to gather all available relevant information regarding the patient. Inadequate information can result in decisions that do not reflect the interests and desires of the patient. However, the clinician must be aware that cultural differences and language barriers may limit a patient's understanding of the choices that need to be addressed.[3] Key information includes not only information about the medical condition of the patient but also information about the patient's values and preferences, the family and social situation, and the realities of the options open to the patient.

Second, ethical dilemmas must be clarified and presented clearly to all those involved in the decision-making process. For example, a spouse of an incompetent patient who argues for aggressive, clinically futile treatment in the face of an imminently terminal and untreatable illness can present the physician with a conflict between respecting the considered wishes of family members and doing what the physician judges is best for the patient.[4] Sometimes, enhanced communication between physician, patient, and family helps bring the matter to resolution.[5,6] For example, having a discussion with the family that is focused on the likelihood that aggressive measures would only prolong the suffering of the patient may convince them to end life-prolonging interventions. In other circumstances, however, the patient's and family's beliefs may necessitate that the physician take aggressive measures to preserve life at all costs.[7,8] It may be important to discuss the spiritual and moral dimensions of the impending decision explicitly. It is often helpful to involve other physicians or nonphysician mediators, such as the hospital ethicists, patient advocates, social workers, and clergy members, in the decision-making process.[9] Once values are explicitly discussed and differences clarified, a plan may be agreed upon by which all parties can abide.

Third, once a decision has been made, it is essential that the decision be carried out effectively, compassionately, and with continuing respect for the patient's needs and wishes. For example, if genetic testing is indicated and there are potential consequences regarding the patient's future eligibility for health insurance, the physician must ensure the confidentiality of information about the tests.[10,11] If complete confidentiality is not possible, the physician should be sure that the patient understands and accepts the risks.[12,13] Whatever the topic at hand, the physician must employ the clinical and interpersonal skills necessary to carry out the patient's wishes respectfully and compassionately.

Areas of Current Ethical Debate

Three broad societal concerns that have important implications for clinical practice lie at the center of many current ethical dilemmas.

DIFFERENCES OF OPINION ABOUT THE MORAL LIMITS OF MEDICAL INTERVENTION IN AN ERA OF TECHNOLOGICAL IMPERATIVES

Modern medicine has been criticized for generating an ethos in which clinicians assume that if an intervention is available, it should always be used. A physician might offer a new intervention as a way of either sustaining hope for the patient and family or avoiding the reality of a poor prognostic situation. In these circumstances, the chances of success can sometimes be overestimated. There are times when the better course is to help patients and families deal realistically with their losses. Physicians' ethics should allow them to consider each medical intervention in the light of their patient's values and wishes and with due regard for the appropriateness of the treatment in that particular setting.[14,15] Several questions frame the current debate about the appropriate use of medical technology—among them, questions as to when life begins and ends, what constitutes quality of life, and is it appropriate to withhold interventions in the face of medical futility.

THE ENIGMA OF WHAT CONSTITUTES A PERSON AND WHEN LIFE BEGINS AND ENDS

Physicians sometimes face extreme and unfamiliar situations in discharging their duty to respect a patient's autonomy. Current research in genetics, for example, challenges traditional assumptions of the uniqueness of individual identity and the acceptability of genetic interventions.[16] Germline interventions were considered completely ethically unacceptable just a few years ago because of the reluctance on the part of geneticists to create changes that would persist through subsequent generations. However, research has now progressed to the point of growing human stem cells under laboratory conditions, and stem cell research is thought to be one of the most promising new areas for clinical interventions.[17] Although the debate has become intensely political and national funding of stem cell research by the National Institutes of Health is strictly proscribed, many in the scientific community are actively supporting stem cell research and are taking steps to address some of the ethical concerns raised by the use of these cells. This shift has occurred in part because stem cell techniques do not create permanent germline changes. Scientific research is ongoing, especially in other countries[18]; in the United States, interest in the clinical promise of stem cell technology continues to grow. Legislators in California and Massachusetts have created and funded state-level research centers, and other states are considering whether to undertake similar initiatives.

Attempts to promulgate practice guidelines for governing the conduct of stem cell research engender extensive debate; such debate generates rich ethical discourse that addresses the very essence of personhood. Reproductive technologies, including the potential for cloning, have an impact on this issue and have spurred new questions about the ethics of medical intervention in human reproduction. The debate about abortion in the United States continues to encompass many points of controversy that directly affect the practice of medicine, sometimes violently.

At the other end of the continuum of care is the question of when life ends. This question is brought into sharp focus by dramatic life-extending technologies. For example, although rational criteria for brain death have served to guide organ transplantation, the extreme shortage of donor organs and evolving technological capabilities have prompted new ethical considerations regarding organ recovery. As utilization of organ donations from non–brain-dead but irreversibly comatose persons has become an increasingly common practice, commitment to clarifying and addressing the ethical dilemmas associated with the use of such donors remains warranted.[19,20] Finally, the debate about assisted suicide raises profound questions of quality of life and the limits of personal choice [see Chapter 186].[21-24]

APPROPRIATE APPROACHES TO ASSESSING QUALITY OF LIFE

Discussions of quality of life gain broader clinical relevance as technical advances make it easier to extend life beyond a point where many people would consider it meaningful. When a patient or family member raises the issue, it is important for the physician to learn more about what that person means by "quality of life." Physicians, family members, and patients may disagree about what constitutes an acceptable quality of life. Often, the phrase is used in the context of how long clinicians should continue attempts to extend life. The ideal setting for gathering this key information is in an ongoing caregiving relationship that allows the patient time to think about the issues, discuss them with those close to him or her, and come back to the physician for a fuller discussion.[25] Unfortunately, this ideal relationship is becoming increasingly rare. Crucial decisions must often be made among relative strangers in times of great stress (for example, in an intensive care unit or when the patient is on the brink of having a cardiac arrest precipitated by critical illness).[26]

For that reason, physicians should be amenable to such discussions and should try to open the door to these discussions with patients ahead of time whenever appropriate.[27] Increasingly frequent discussions of death and dying in the popular media have set the stage for patients and families to be receptive to such discussions and to be better informed about the facts and issues involved.

In general, questions related to acceptable quality of life should be answered by the patient.[28] Often, however, the patient is unable to speak for himself or herself when the answer is needed.[29,30] For example, patients with advanced dementia from Alzheimer disease or with irreversible coma cannot make these decisions, and few such patients have written detailed and specific advance directives. A proxy decision maker, usually a family member or a friend, should be asked about the patient's likely wishes in such a situation. It is crucial to emphasize to a proxy that it is the patient's values, not the proxy's, that should be conveyed in these situations. In addition to providing clear information about prognosis and likely outcomes, it is important for the clinician to recognize that a proxy is in a very difficult position—often, the proxy is in the midst of acute grief or anxiety—and should be provided a comforting context in which to make a decision. A proxy should not be made to feel that he or she is alone in making this decision, especially in the common situation in which the patient is likely to die in any case. Written advance directives—so-called living wills—can be helpful in this regard, mostly as adjuncts to discussions between patient and physician. Assigning a trusted proxy is still recommended, however, because situations are often more complex than can be adequately addressed in a written document.

Traditional Medical Ethics and the Changing World of Medicine

Among the various reasons the medical profession has been able to maintain a strong ethical standard for more than 2,000 years is the fact that the standard has been so simple. From the Hippocratic oath to the prayer of Moses Maimonides, statements of medical ethics have required the physician to do what is best for the patient, putting the patient's interest before the physician's own. Admittedly, there have been breaches of the standard. Many physicians became rich selling unproven patent medicines before the advent of scientific medicine. More recently, some have overcharged patients or have ordered unnecessary tests, medications, and procedures to further their own financial interests. Overtreatment can be as unethical as undertreatment, for two reasons: (1) all treatments carry some degree of risk to the patient and (2) rising health care costs contribute to the difficulty our nation faces in extending health care access to the uninsured and underinsured. Generating costs to enhance one's own income, with no benefit to the patient, adds to the barriers facing populations who are underserved by the health care system. Physicians have a responsibility for societal health, as well as the health of their individual patients.[31]

In the past, the accountability structure for health care was clearly delineated between physician and patient. Today, changes in the economics and delivery systems of managed care have so affected this classic ethical construct of undivided loyalty to the patient that even previously inviolable ethical relationships are being challenged.[32,33]

Managed care has been criticized for withholding care from patients, and physicians have been seen as the agents of rich insurance companies rather than as advocates for the best health care for their patients. Good managed care, however, allows physicians to limit risk to patients and reduce waste and cost. Physicians are challenged to examine whether their role in such managed care programs is truly in the patients' best interest; to do so could ameliorate the loss of public trust in the profession.[34] Studies by the Institute of Medicine and the RAND Corporation have spurred new approaches in the provision of quality care.[35,36] Physicians are being asked to measure the quality of their care and make this information available to payers, consumers, certifying/accrediting organizations, and others. Such measures are imperfect but will reveal to patients and others standards for ideal care. How should physicians respond to these new demands for transparency? Understanding the fundamental responsibility of the profession to the welfare of the patient is an important starting point for dealing with any ethical problems arising from social change, technological innovation, and changes in the delivery and financing of health care. The Physician Charter on Medical Professionalism identifies a modern framework that may be used to clarify professional standards in this more complex world.[37,38]

POPULATION-BASED MEDICINE AND THE RIGHTS OF THE INDIVIDUAL

Although simple in the abstract, the physician's responsibility to the patient is not always clear in actual practice. For example, the traditional standard requires a physician to do everything possible for patients directly in his or her care. Arguing that a more utilitarian standard is needed, some theorists have suggested changes to meet the requirements of population-based medicine, in which some treatments that are potentially beneficial to the individual patient are forgone to benefit larger numbers of patients with the available resources.

Utilitarian considerations are sometimes discussed in the context of a communitarian philosophy, which holds that all members of the society are better off if standards are based on the benefit to communities rather than to individuals exclusively.[39] Many European governments base policies on communitarian premises, whereas in the United States, policy makers have traditionally focused more sharply on the rights of the individual. However, it may be that the rights of a far greater number of individuals would be better served with a health care structure that emphasizes more collective responsibility and resolution.

One area where this tension can be seen is in end-of-life care. In recent decades, there has been a presumption and a legal standard in the United States that patients may make their own decisions about the care they receive at the end of life and, in particular, that every person has the right to refuse life-sustaining treatment. This freedom of choice is the thrust of the Patient Self-Determination Act of 1990, which requires hospitals and nursing homes to inform patients of local laws regarding advance directives and to help them prepare advance directives if they choose to do so. In several well-publicized cases (e.g., the Quinlan, Cruzan, and Schiavo cases),[40,41] courts supported families or patients who wished to end life-sustaining treatment. However, attention is now being drawn to instances in which patients or their proxies ask for life-sustaining treatment over objections from health care payers and, sometimes, providers. In the relatively few cases in which such conflicts have been brought to litigation, courts, again, have been generally supportive of patients' and families' desires. Interestingly, these cases conflict with the recent judgments that financial incentives to restrict care are acceptable in the context of insurance law.

In recent years, some ethicists have worked to define a standard of medical futility that would give physicians the right to withhold treatment in specific cases.[42,43] There is profound disagreement, however, about the definition of futility and its statistical basis. For example, the chances of success with cardiopulmonary resuscitation (CPR) are remarkably small in patients of very advanced age who have debilitating illness and poor functional status, particularly in cases of an unwitnessed cardiac arrest; however, many physicians would be uncomfortable making the decision to withhold CPR without consulting the patient's family.[44] From one perspective, this inclination to involve and communicate with patient and family is a sound one, motivated by respect and caring.[45] In other cases, however, an insistence on family permission in the context of medical futility is a misguided gesture, perhaps driven by liability con-

Biomedical Ethics Information on the Internet

Federal Government

Bioethicsline
http://www.nih.gov/sigs/bioethics
The National Library of Medicine's database of peer-reviewed bioethics literature.

National Bioethics Advisory Commission
http://bioethics.gov
Agendas and transcripts of meetings, online publications, and other information primarily regarding genetics research and research involving humans.

Ethical, Legal and Social Implications Program, National Human Genome Research Institute
http://www.genome.gov/page.cfm?pageID=10001618
Information on policy and legislation, research opportunities, grant products and publications, education and training activities.

Professional Societies

American College of Physicians Center for Ethics and Professionalism
http://www.acponline.org/ethics
Position papers, educational programs, and other resources on end-of-life care, managed care, and other issues related to medical ethics.

American Medical Association Institute for Ethics
http://www.ama-assn.org/ama/pub/category/2416.html
Educational and outreach programs for physicians, including the Education for Physicians on End-of-life Care Project.

American Society for Bioethics and Humanities
http://www.asbh.org
Consolidation of the Society for Health and Human Values, the Society for Bioethics Consultation, and the American Association of Bioethics; meeting agendas, position papers.

American Society of Law, Medicine & Ethics
http://www.aslme.org
Conference agendas, publications, online forum.

Bioethics Council
http://www.bioethics.org.nz/about-bioethics/international-links.html
Comprehensive guide to international resources in bioethics.

Institutes and Centers

Case Western Reserve University Center for Biomedical Ethics
http://www.cwru.edu/med/bioethics/bioethics.html
Program news, events, online newsletter.

Georgetown University Kennedy Institute of Ethics
http://kennedyinstitute.georgetown.edu/index.htm
Information on symposia, publications, and services, including the National Reference Center for Bioethics Literature. (http://www.georgetown.edu/nrcbl)

The Hastings Center
http://www.thehastingscenter.org
Research and educational programs on ethical issues in medicine, the life sciences, and the environment.

University of Chicago MacLean Center for Clinical Medical Ethics
http://ethics.bsd.uchicago.edu/resources.html
Comprehensive guide to online resources in biomedical ethics; online newsletter.

University of Pennsylvania Center for Bioethics
http://www.med.upenn.edu/bioethic
Online bioethics tutorial, publications, discussion groups; special sections on genetics, cloning, and physician-assisted suicide.

cerns. Ethicists have asserted the physician's duty to regain the responsibility of prognostication and decision making inherent in the older paternalistic model of medical practice.[46,47] This belief can be supported by two arguments: (1) there is a responsibility to avoid wasteful use of scarce resources and (2) the attitude of caring means to avoid inflicting unrealistic choices on grieving families and to offer reassurances of aggressive palliative care and relief from suffering for patients who are dying.

Outside of the context of life and death, the allocation of medical resources is an area in which the tensions between wasteful expenditure and appropriate care are regularly played out. For example, the high cost of brand-name medications would lead a physician to prescribe equally effective generic agents whenever possible; however, direct-to-consumer advertising and drug detailing to physicians have created a demand for brand-name medications, even when there is no evidence that they are better than older formulations. On the basis of biomedical and clinical evidence, government agencies (e.g., the Centers for Medicare and Medicaid Services, the Veterans Administration, and certain state agencies) and health care plans have created formularies that determine the most cost-effective medications. These formularies are regularly used in the filling of prescriptions covered by health care payers. When these formularies are used, patients may not be given the brand of medication they request; however, they receive a formulation that is equally effective. The savings resulting from the adjustment in prescription allows health care plans to cover the health care costs of larger numbers of people. Patients who prefer the more expensive brand-name medication may have it if they pay for it. In these instances, does the physician's responsibility to avoid waste override the responsibility to respect the patient's values? The Physician Charter calls on physicians to reduce waste and improve quality. The achievement of this dual goal may require concerted effort to educate patients—and possibly policy makers—about the best uses of their health care resources.[31,37,38]

A BROADER CONTEXT FOR CLINICAL DECISION MAKING

The role of the physician and the nature of the doctor-patient relationship may be challenged, not only by changes in the practice of medicine but also by the increasing interconnectedness of communities and societies and the emergence of public health as a global concern. Regional and national health care systems are commonplace; epidemics can occur worldwide because of widespread international travel, immigration, and dislocation caused by war and civil strife.

The global, multicultural aspect of modern medicine will have increasingly significant implications for ethical decision making in clinical practice in coming years. For example, in seeking to honor a patient's right to autonomy, a physician may have to balance the traditional standard of care with a patient's desire to choose an alternative or complementary therapy; or following the traditional Hippocratic model, a physician may feel justified in using the most powerful antibiotic available to treat a patient's infection, despite the fact that the widespread use of powerful antibiotics leads to the emergence of new and more resistant organisms throughout the world.

Caring for patients in this new environment raises challenges for modern physicians that their predecessors never faced. Physicians must now analyze ethical issues systematically, understand the conflicts modern medicine poses for some

traditional Hippocratic precepts, and come to terms with the conflict between their responsibility to their patients and the consequences of individual clinical decisions for the broader population. Even as electronic communication systems evolve to keep physicians abreast of new global realities, the moral and ethical framework of clinical decision making must begin to encompass those realities [see Sidebar Biomedical Ethics Information on the Internet]. It is critical that physicians learn the language of medical ethics and follow its literature closely so that their voices will help shape basic medical values in the future, even as they cope with complex ethical challenges in their daily practice.

The authors have no commercial relationships with manufacturers of products or providers of services discussed in this chapter.

References

1. Pellegrino ED: The metamorphosis of medical ethics: a 30-year retrospective. JAMA 269:1158, 1993

2. Pellegrino ED: Ethics. JAMA 275:1807, 1996

3. Davis TC, Williams MV, Marin E, et al: Health literacy and cancer communication. CA Cancer J Clin 52:134, 2002

4. Hines SC, Glover JJ, Babrow AS, et al: Improving advance care planning by accommodating family preferences. J Palliat Med 4:481, 2001

5. Quill TE, Brody H: Physician recommendations and patient autonomy: finding a balance between physician power and patient choice. Ann Intern Med 125:763, 1996

6. Medical futility in end-of-life care: report of the Council on Ethical and Judicial Affairs. JAMA 281:937, 1999

7. Asch DA, Hansen-Flaschen J, Lanken PN: Decisions to limit or continue life-sustaining treatment by critical care physicians in the United States: conflicts between physicians' practices and patients' wishes. Am J Respir Crit Care Med 151:288, 1995

8. Cantor NL: Can healthcare providers obtain judicial intervention against surrogates who demand "medically inappropriate" life support for incompetent patients? Crit Care Med 24:883, 1996

9. DuVal G, Clarridge B, Gensler G, et al: Experiences with ethical dilemmas and ethics consultation. J Gen Intern Med 19:251, 2004

10. Dressler L: Genetic testing for the *BRCA1* gene and the need for protection from discrimination: an evolving legislative and social issue. Breast Dis 10:127, 1998

11. Gostin LO: National health information privacy: regulations under the Health Insurance Portability and Accountability Act. JAMA 285:3015, 2001

12. Geller G, Botkin JR, Green MJ, et al: Genetic testing for susceptibility to adult-onset cancer: the process and content of informed consent. JAMA 277:1467, 1997

13. Ensenauer RE, Michels VV, Reinke SS: Genetic testing: practical, ethical, and counseling considerations. Mayo Clin Proc 80:63, 2005

14. Sharpe VA, Faden AI: Appropriateness in patient care: a new conceptual framework. Milbank Q 74:115, 1996

15. Brett AS, Jersild P: "Inappropriate" treatment near the end of life: conflict between religious convictions and clinical judgment. Arch Intern Med 163:1645, 2003

16. Kaji E, Leiden J: Gene and stem cell therapies. JAMA 285:545, 2001

17. Daar AS, Bhatt A, Court E, et al: Stem cell research and transplantation: science leading ethics. Transplant Proc 36:2504, 2004

18. Ethics can boost science. Nature 408:275, 2000

19. Herdman R, Beauchamp TL, Potts JT: The Institute of Medicine's report on non–heart-beating organ transplantation. Ken Inst Ethics J 8:83, 1998

20. DeVita MA, Snyder JV, Arnold RM, et al: Observations of withdrawal of life-sustaining treatment from patients who became non–heart-beating organ donors. Crit Care Med 28:1709, 2000

21. Physician-assisted suicide: toward a comprehensive understanding: report of the Task Force on Physician-Assisted Suicide of the Society for Health and Human Values. Acad Med 70:583, 1995

22. Drickamer MA, Lee MA, Ganzini L: Practical issues in physician-assisted suicide. Ann Intern Med 126:146, 1997

23. Muskin PR: The request to die: role for a psychodynamic perspective on physician-assisted suicide. JAMA 279:323, 1998

24. Kohlwes RJ, Koepsell TD, Rhodes LA, et al: Physicians' responses to patients' requests for physician-assisted suicide. Arch Intern Med 161:657, 2001

25. Meier DE, Morrison RS, Cassel CK: Improving palliative care. Ann Intern Med 127:225, 1997

26. Schneiderman LJ, Gilmer T, Teetzel HD, et al: Effect of ethics consultations on non-beneficial life-sustaining treatments in the intensive care setting: a randomized controlled trial. JAMA 290:1166, 2003

27. Searight HR, Gafford J: Cultural diversity at the end of life: issues and guidelines for family physicians. Am Fam Physician 71:515, 2005

28. Garrett JM, Harris RP, Norburn JK, et al: Life-sustaining treatments during terminal

illness: who wants what? J Gen Intern Med 8:361, 1993

29. Cranford RE: The vegetative and minimally conscious states: ethical implications. Geriatrics 53(suppl 1):S70, 1998

30. Rubenfeld GD: Principles and practice of withdrawing life-sustaining treatments. Crit Care Med 20:435, 2004

31. Gruen R, Pearson S, Brennan T: Physician-citizens: public roles and professional obligations. JAMA 291:94, 2004

32. Quill TE, Cassel CK: Nonabandonment: a central obligation for physicians. Ann Intern Med 122:368, 1995

33. Mechanic D, Schlesinger M: The impact of managed care on patients' trust in medical care and their physicians. JAMA 275:1693, 1996

34. Mechanic D: Changing medical organization and the erosion of trust. Milbank Q 74:171, 1996

35. Crossing the quality chasm: a new health system for the 21st century/Committee on Quality Health Care in America. Institute of Medicine. National Academy Press, Washington, DC, 2001

36. McGlynn EA, Asch SM, Adams J, et al: The quality of health care delivered to adults in the United States. N Engl J Med 348:2635, 2003

37. Medical professionalism in the new millennium: a physician's charter. ABIM Foundation, American Board of Internal Medicine; ACP-ASIM Foundation, American College of Physicians-American Society of Internal Medicine; European Federation of Internal Medicine. Ann Intern Med 136:243, 2002

38. Brennan TA: Physicians' professional responsibility to improve the quality of care. Acad Med 77:973, 2002

39. Luce JM: The changing physician-patient relationship in critical care medicine under health care reform. Am J Respir Crit Care Med 150:266, 1994

40. Gostin LO: Deciding life and death in the courtroom: from Quinlan to Cruzan, Glucksberg, and Vacco: a brief history and analysis of constitutional protection of the 'right to die.' JAMA 278:1523, 1997

41. Annas G: "Culture of life" politics at the bedside: the case of Terri Schiavo. N Engl J Med 352:1710, 2005

42. Schneiderman LJ, Jecker NS, Jonsen AR: Medical futility: response to critiques. Ann Intern Med 125:669, 1996

43. Marco CA, Larkin GL, Moskip JC, et al: Determination of "futility" in emergency medicine. Ann Emerg Med 35:604, 2000

44. Hofmann JC, Wenger NS, Davis RB, et al: Patient preferences for communication with physicians about end-of-life decisions. Study to Understand Prognoses and Preferences for Outcomes and Risks of Treatment (SUPPORT) investigators. Ann Intern Med 127:1, 1997

45. Doukas DJ, McCullough LB: A preventive ethics approach to counseling patients about clinical futility in the primary care setting. Arch Fam Med 5:589, 1996

46. Helft PR, Siegler M, Lantos J: The rise and fall of the futility movement. N Engl J Med 343:293, 2000

47. Schneiderman LJ, Capron AM: How can hospital futility policies contribute to establishing standards of practice? Camb Q Healthc Ethics 9:524, 2000

Practice Guidelines and Consensus Statements

American Society of Clinical Oncology policy statement update: genetic testing for cancer susceptibility. J Clin Oncol 21:2397, 2003

Consensus statement of the Society of Critical Care Medicine's Ethics Committee regarding futile and other possibly inadvisable treatments. Crit Care Med 25:887, 1997

Emanuel LL: A professional response to demands for accountability: practical recommendations regarding ethical aspects of patient care. Working Group on Accountability. Ann Intern Med 124:240, 1996

Ethical considerations in the allocation of organs and other scarce medical resources among patients. Council on Ethical and Judicial Affairs, American Medical Association. Arch Intern Med 155:29, 1995

Fletcher JC, Siegler M: What are the goals of ethics consultation? A consensus statement. J Clin Ethics 7:122, 1996

Karlawish JH, Quill T, Meier DE: A consensus-based approach to providing palliative care to patients who lack decision-making capacity. ACP-ASIM End-of-Life Care Consensus Panel. American College of Physicians–American Society of Internal Medicine. Ann Intern Med 130:835, 1999

Lo B, Quill T, Tulsky J: Discussing palliative care with patients: ACP-ASIM End-of-Life Care Consensus Panel. American College of Physicians–American Society of Internal Medicine. Ann Intern Med 130:744, 1999

Position paper of the Ethics Committee of the International Xenotransplantation Association. Sykdes M, d'Apice A, Sandrin M, et al: Transplantation 78:1101, 2004

Practice parameters: assessment and management of patients in the persistent vegetative state (summary statement). The Quality Standards Subcommittee of the American Academy of Neurology. Neurology 45:1015, 1995

Snyder L, Leffler C: Ethics manual: fifth edition. Human Rights Committee of the American College of Physicians. Ann Intern Med 142:560, 2005
http://www.acponline.org/ethics/ethicman5th.htm

2 Quantitative Aspects of Clinical Decision Making

Brian Haynes, M.D., PH.D., F.A.C.P., Harold C. Sox, M.D., M.A.C.P.

BRIAN HAYNES, M.D., PH.D.
HAROLD C. SOX, M.D.

An increasing amount of very useful quantitative evidence from health care research is available to practitioners. New research findings continually expand the knowledge base of what does more good than harm for patients, and institutional forces, both professional and financial, are accelerating the adoption of research findings. More and more information is available on issues related to such important clinical topics as screening and diagnostic tests, preventive and therapeutic interventions, prognosis and clinical prediction, risk of adverse outcomes, improvement in quality of care, and cost-effectiveness of tests and treatments. Clinical application of this evidence has lagged, however, for a number of reasons.[1] First, evidence from research is often not definitive or covers only some aspects of practice. Second, clinicians are often slow to adopt research findings, even those that are well validated. Third, resources may be inadequate or too poorly organized in the local setting to permit implementation. Fourth, clinicians may be unfamiliar with the concepts that lie behind the application of quantitative reasoning to clinical care. This chapter addresses the last of these barriers: principles and methods for quantitative reasoning.

Lack of precision in clinical thinking is beginning to yield to several encouraging developments—in particular, clinicians increasingly applying principles of critical appraisal to evidence in the medical literature; formulation of methods for medical decision analysis; increasing clinical comfort with terms such as sensitivity, specificity, likelihood ratio, number needed to treat, and confidence interval (CI); and creation of print and electronic resources that minimize the effort that clinicians must make to find and interpret valid quantitative evidence when it is needed. These developments notwithstanding, the possibility of miscommunication is still considerable. A 2003 study of primary care physicians reported that just over 50% of respondents were able to answer questions about critical appraisal of methods and interpretation of results of studies focusing on treatments and diagnostic tests.[2] Patients are entitled to expect clearer thinking from their physicians, especially because many patients have difficulty themselves interpreting information about risks, benefits, and prognoses provided by their doctors.[3] Moreover, the current health care environment increasingly demands that physicians be able to justify clinical policies and decisions with an evidence-based, quantitative approach.

We have two principal goals in this chapter. The first is to provide a basic explanation of the measurements used in critical appraisal of the literature and the ways in which physicians interpret these measurements in evidence-based clinical decision making. With the advent of electronic access to MEDLINE and its clinical subsets, specialized compendia of studies (e.g., Clinical Evidence[4] and Physicians' Information and Education Resource [PIER][5]), systematic reviews of studies (e.g., the Cochrane Library[6]), and alerting services for new, clinically relevant evidence (e.g., bmjupdates+[7] and MEDSCAPE Best

Evidence alerts[8]), the current best evidence for clinical practice is becoming more and more accessible to clinicians.

The second goal is to introduce the topic of medical decision analysis. Clinicians use decision analysis in two ways. One way is essentially indirect: reliance on products of decision analyses conducted by others. For example, practice guidelines increasingly influence many of the quick, straightforward decisions that occur in daily practice. Many of these guidelines are based on formal decision analyses. The second way of employing decision analysis is more direct: using the tools of decision analysis to assist in making major decisions about the care of an individual patient. Although few physicians spend the hours required to conduct a formal decision analysis from scratch, some tools of decision analysis (e.g., likelihood ratios of test results) are easy to apply; moreover, some decision analyses are accessible on a desktop or palmtop computer and only require the clinician to enter the clinical findings required by the decision tree.

It is important to understand the intent of this effort to achieve precision and quantitation in measurement and decision making: to enhance the quality of care by making it more tailored to the individual patient. Anything that can be measured, even if only qualitatively, can be counted and turned into a clinically useful quantitative measure. For example, a study might classify clinical outcomes only qualitatively (e.g., as satisfactory or unsatisfactory), but if the numbers of participants in the study who fall into one or the other of the two outcome states are counted, the result then becomes quantitative. If physicians can define individual states and measure them quantitatively (e.g., by using a continuous scale to assess functional status), they can describe individual patient status more precisely and therefore can make finer distinctions between groups of patients. By placing patients in distinctive groups, physicians can achieve one of the great goals of patient care: to inform patients of the choices between alternative treatments by the known predictors of response to those treatments.

What is the role of the individual practitioner in retrieving and evaluating evidence from research and incorporating it into individual clinical decisions? The answer to this innocuous question distills the angst of contemporary health care. In some settings, the practitioner has the freedom to act as circumstances dictate, whereas in others (e.g., certain managed care settings), someone else tries to dictate how to translate research results into patient care. We believe that practitioners cede their responsibility for clinical decision making to others at great risk to their patients and themselves, because any clinical decisions must take into account not only the evidence available and the guidelines in force but also the patient's unique circumstances and individual wishes. In today's world, the freedom to determine the content of one's practice is increasingly precious. To use this freedom responsibly, practitioners must have ready access to information that is based on current best evidence, must understand the basic principles of quantitative decision making and decision analysis, must be able to determine whether others have applied these principles appropriately in published works or in practice,

Table 1   Abbreviated Users' Guides for Appraisal of Medical Journal Articles

Purpose of Study	Source of Data	Method of Arriving at Findings	Method of Reducing Bias of Findings
Diagnosis	Clearly identified comparison groups, all suspected of having the disorder, but one of which is free of the disorder	Objective or reproducible diagnostic standard applied to all participants	Blinded assessment of test and diagnostic standard
Therapy	Random allocation of patients to comparison groups	Outcome measure of known or probable clinical importance	Follow-up of ≥ 80% of subjects
Prognosis	Inception cohort, early in the course of the disorder and initially free of the outcome of interest	Objective or reproducible assessment of clinically important outcomes	Follow-up of ≥ 80% of subjects
Causation	Clearly identified comparison group for those who are at risk for, or for those having, the outcome of interest	Blinding of observers of outcome to exposure; blinding of observers of exposure to outcome	—
Review	Comprehensive search for relevant articles	Explicit criteria for rating relevance and merit of studies	Inclusion of all relevant studies

and must be able to understand how to use evidence from research to make decisions in clinical practice.

How to Critically Evaluate Research Reports

To use numbers wisely in making decisions about patients, the physician must have some way of determining whether the numbers are derived from sound research. Detailed users' guides for interpreting the medical literature are available[9]; in an effort to simplify this issue, we have provided an abbreviated set of such guides [*see Table 1*].[10] Physicians may find these guides especially useful when reading research reports in the primary literature. However, when physicians are not getting and interpreting evidence themselves, they should look to evidence-based publications, such as *Clinical Evidence* and *PIER*; systematic review articles, such as those from the Cochrane Collaboration and clinical journals; and practice guidelines that use explicit criteria for evaluating evidence [*see Table 1*].

How to Apply Research Results to Patient Care

Once a physician is satisfied that the quantitative results from the relevant research were derived through sound methods, he or she can interpret them in light of the patient's circumstances and use them to help determine the best way to proceed with management. The interpretation of research results takes five main forms: (1) measures of disease frequency, (2) measures of diagnostic certainty, (3) measures of diagnostic test performance and interpretation, (4) measures of the effects of treatment, and (5) measures of treatment outcomes adjusted for quality of life.

MEASURES OF DISEASE FREQUENCY

Clinically useful measures of disease frequency include incidence, prevalence, the case-fatality rate, the *P* value, and the CI [*see Table 2*]. The use of such terms is illustrated in more detail elsewhere (see below).

MEASURES OF DIAGNOSTIC CERTAINTY: USE OF PROBABILITIES

When asked how sure they are of their diagnoses, most physicians express their degree of certainty in words rather than numbers. A classic study illustrates the difficulty of this approach.[11] The authors examined pathology and radiology reports and recorded various terms expressive of the probability of a disorder, such as "compatible with," "consistent with," "likely," "probably," and "pathognomonic." They then asked a group of clinicians to assign numerical probabilities to all of these terms. For each term (even "pathognomonic"), the range of probabilities stretched over half the scale. For example, to one physician, "likely" meant there was a 45% chance that the disease in question was present, whereas to another, "likely" meant the probability was higher than 90%. When diagnostic-test specialists were asked on two different occasions what they meant by these terms, the earlier and later answers were highly consistent for each individual specialist but highly inconsistent from one specialist to the next.

An alternative to using words to express the degree of diagnostic certainty is to use a number—namely, the probability that the diagnosis is present. A probability is a number between 0 and 1 that expresses the likelihood that an event will occur; 0 represents certainty that it will not occur, and 1 represents certainty that it will. Using probability to express diagnostic certainty has two key advantages. First, it facilitates precise communication. Comparison of probability estimates is a far more precise method of comparing degrees of diagnostic certainty than ex-

Table 2   Clinically Useful Measures of Disease Frequency

- Incidence: the proportion of new cases of a disorder occurring in a defined population during a specified period of time, typically 1 year.
- Prevalence: the proportion of cases of a disorder at a designated point in time in a specified population.
- Case-fatality rate: the proportion of cases of a specified disorder that are fatal during a specified period of follow-up (typically 1 yr) from the onset of the disorder.
- Quality-adjusted life year (QALY): a measure of survival in which each year of a patient's survival is discounted according to a measure (usually an index) of the patient's quality of life.
- *P* value: the probability of obtaining the observed data, or more unlikely data, when the null hypothesis is true. The *P* value does not indicate the magnitude of the effect of interest, or even its direction, nor does it indicate how much uncertainty is associated with the results.
- Confidence interval (CI): the range of values of a true effect that is consistent with the data observed in a study. A common (although not entirely correct) interpretation of a 95% confidence interval is that 95% of the time, the true value lies within the stated range of values.

changing verbal assessments. Second, there exists an accurate method of calculating changes in the likelihood of disease as new information (e.g., a test result) becomes available. This method, Bayes' theorem, should be one of the central principles that underlie medical practice. This claim may seem audacious to some readers, but we all recognize that the interpretation of new information about the patient moves us either away from or closer to a diagnosis and, therefore, away from or closer to the decision to use a specific treatment.

The probability of an event is not precisely the same thing as the odds of an event occurring, even though the two are mathematically equivalent ways of expressing diagnostic uncertainty. Habitués of the racetrack are reputed to use odds directly, but most clinicians are likely to find probabilities easier to use. Each of these measures can be readily converted to the other, as follows:

$$\text{Odds} = \frac{\text{probability}}{1 - \text{probability}}$$

$$\text{Probability} = \frac{\text{odds}}{1 + \text{odds}}$$

To use a test result quantitatively, a physician must first estimate the pretest probability of the disease. Unaided, physicians are not particularly good at this task. In a 1982 study, when primary care physicians were given clinical scenarios and asked for their estimates of the probabilities of given disorders, they provided estimates—quite confident ones—but their estimates did not agree with those of their fellow clinicians.[12] Indeed, when individual physicians were tested subsequently with the same scenarios, their later estimates did not agree with their initial ones.

How does a physician estimate the probability that a patient's chief complaint is a manifestation of a particular disease? The first step is to take a careful history and do a physical examination. From this point, the physician may take any of three basic approaches to estimating the probability of a disease[13]: (1) subjective estimation, (2) estimation based on the prevalence of disease in other patients with the same syndrome, or (3) application of clinical prediction rules.

Subjective Estimation

In principle, the physician can draw on personal experience with similar patients and use the estimated frequency of the disease in those patients. In practice, this approach is little more than a semiquantitative guess and is prone to error because of defective recall, as well as to bias in the application of the heuristics (i.e., the rules of thumb) for estimating probability. Examples of such heuristics are representativeness, by which one estimates a probability on the basis of the similarity of the patient's signs and symptoms to the features of the classic description of the disease, and availability, by which one estimates a probability partly on the basis of how easy it is to recall similar cases. One very useful heuristic is anchoring and adjustment, by which one establishes an initial estimate (e.g., the prevalence of pulmonary embolism in 100 patients presenting to the emergency department with pleuritic chest pain) and then adjusts the estimate upward or downward by taking into account the patient's findings (e.g., hypoxemia, unilateral leg swelling, or a history of cancer). Physicians can, in principle, calculate the extent of such adjustments by using Bayes' theorem (see below).

Estimation Based on the Prevalence of Disease in Other Patients with the Same Syndrome

One antidote to the failures of subjective probability estimation is to base the estimate on accurate diagnoses established in a series of patients with the same clinical syndrome as the patient under consideration. The best example is the diagnosis of suspected coronary artery disease in patients with chronic chest pain. On the basis of the clinical history, the physician can place the patient in one of three categories: typical angina pectoris, atypical angina, or nonanginal chest pain. Many published studies have reported the frequency of angiographically proven coronary disease in patients with these syndromes. These studies have shown, for example, that in a man with atypical angina, the probability of significant coronary artery disease is approximately 0.70 (see below).

Application of Clinical Prediction Rules

Clinical prediction rules describe the key clinical findings that predict a disease and show how to use these findings to estimate the probability of disease in a patient. Such rules are based on analysis of a standardized set of data, including clinical findings and the final diagnosis, for each of many patients with a diagnostic problem. One type of clinical prediction rule uses regression analysis to identify the best clinical predictors and their diagnostic weights. The sum of the diagnostic weights corresponding to a patient's findings is a score, and the probability of disease for each patient is equivalent to the prevalence of disease among patients with a similar score. A well-known example of this approach is the rule for estimating the probability of cardiac complications from noncardiac surgery.[14] Another interesting example showed that the prevalence of coronary artery disease in patients with similar chest pain scores varied systematically according to the overall prevalence of coronary artery disease in several study populations.[15] This study suggested that the probability of disease corresponding to a patient's clinical history varies depending on whether the setting of care is a primary care practice or a referral practice. *Diagnostic Strategies for Common Medical Problems*[16] is an excellent source of pretest probabilities, as is *Evidence-Based Physical Diagnosis.*[17]

MEASURES OF DIAGNOSTIC TEST PERFORMANCE AND INTERPRETATION

Clinically useful measures of diagnostic test performance include sensitivity, specificity, and the likelihood ratio; clinically useful measures of test interpretation include pretest odds, pretest probability, probability after a positive test result, and probability after a negative test result [*see Table 3*]. Physicians should memorize and internalize the definitions of these terms to avoid becoming muddled when attempting to use information from diagnostic tests in decision making.

In the past, articles usually described the performance of a diagnostic test only in terms of sensitivity and specificity. These familiar terms do not directly describe the effect of a test result on the probability of disease. To correct this shortcoming, many articles now use the likelihood ratio (LR), which is the amount by which the odds of a disease change with new information. This value is calculated as follows:

$$\text{LR} = \frac{P \text{ [test result if disease present]}}{P \text{ [test result if disease absent]}}$$

Because physicians often express test results as either positive or negative, there is a likelihood ratio for a positive test re-

Table 3 Definitions of Clinically Useful Measures of Diagnostic Test Performance and Interpretation

The typical approach to evaluation of most diagnostic tests, particularly those with so-called binary outcomes (e.g., a positive or a negative test result, with no other categories), makes use of a 2 × 2 table, as follows:

Diagnostic Test Result	Presence or Absence of Disease on a Reference Test (Gold Standard)		No. of Patients with Given Test Result
	Present	Absent	
Positive	a	b	a + b
Negative	c	d	c + d
Total	a + c	b + d	

Measures of diagnostic test performance, defined below, are calculated from this table.

- Sensitivity: the proportion of people with a disease of interest who are detected by a diagnostic test; calculated as $a/(a+c)$.
- Specificity: the proportion of people who do not have a disease who are correctly identified by a negative result on a diagnostic test; calculated as $d/(b+d)$.
- Likelihood ratio: the amount by which the odds of having a disease change after a test result; calculated as $[a/(a+c)]/[b/(b+d)]$ for a positive test result and as $[c/(a+c)]/[d/(b+d)]$ for a negative test result.
- Pretest probability: the proportion of people with the disorder of interest in a group suspected of having the disorder; calculated as $(a+c)/(a+b+c+d)$.
- Odds: calculated as probability/(1 – probability).
- Probability: calculated as odds/(1+ odds).
- Posttest odds: calculated as pretest odds × likelihood ratio.
- Probability after a positive test: the proportion of people with a positive test result who have the disease of interest; calculated as $a/(a+b)$.
- Probability after a negative test: the proportion of people with a negative test result who have the disease of interest; calculated as $c/(c+d)$.

sult (LR^+) and a likelihood ratio for a negative test result (LR^-). The formula for the likelihood ratio for a positive test result is as follows:

$$LR^+ = \frac{sensitivity}{1 - specificity}$$

The formula for the LR for a negative test is as follows:

$$LR^- = \frac{1 - sensitivity}{specificity}$$

The likelihood ratio is generally a better descriptor than sensitivity or specificity because it more directly describes the effect of a test result on the odds of disease. The probability after obtaining new information is an application of Bayes' theorem. The most useful form of Bayes' theorem for this purpose is the odds ratio format:

Posttest odds = pretest odds × likelihood ratio

This form of Bayes' theorem illustrates a very powerful concept that clinicians often overlook: new information has meaning only in context. Operationally, the statement means that a physician should never interpret a test result in isolation but should always take into account the individual patient's pretest probabili-

ty. Simply stated, the posttest probability after a positive test result will be greater if the pretest index of suspicion was high than if the pretest index of suspicion was low. The most important practical application of this reasoning is to be suspicious when a test result is negative in a patient whose clinical findings strongly point toward a disease—that is, the probability of the disease may still be high, even after the negative test. One should also be suspicious when a test is positive in a patient for whom the likelihood of disease is very low.

The evaluation of suspected pulmonary embolism (PE) is a good example of the practical use of these statistical terms and methods. A 37-year-old woman presents to the emergency department (ED) with pleuritic chest pain and new dyspnea. She has a low-grade fever and has no cough or hemoptysis, but the ED physician believes it necessary to rule out PE. The patient has none of the other known risk factors for PE (e.g., recent surgery or prolonged bed rest, previous deep vein thrombosis [DVT], coagulopathy, malignancy, pregnancy, and use of oral contraceptives), and physical examination reveals no evidence of DVT. The arterial oxygen tension (P_aO_2) is 92 mm Hg on room air. The patient is quite distressed. The ED physician orders a chest x-ray and a helical CT scan. The CT scan is interpreted as negative for PE. The resident wishes to explain this result to the patient and then to take the appropriate next steps.

A useful flowchart for working up patients with suspected PE is provided elsewhere [*see Chapter 32*]; however, this chart provides no guidance on how to estimate the clinical probability of PE. It is particularly instructive to examine how the results of a quantitative, evidence-based approach to this patient's case relate to the recommendations outlined in the flowchart.

The initial step is to estimate the pretest probability of PE by one of two approaches. The first is to use the anchoring and adjustment heuristic. The anchor, or starting point, is the prevalence of PE in adults who present to the ED with pleuritic chest pain. One very careful study found that 21% of such patients (36/173) had a positive pulmonary angiogram.[18] The physician should use this 21% initial probability as the starting point (the anchor) for the patient under discussion and adjust it on the basis of the history and the physical examination. As noted, this patient has no predisposing factors for PE and no evidence of DVT, and her P_aO_2 is greater than 90 mm Hg. Using this approach, the ED physician concludes that the probability of PE before helical CT is quite low, perhaps 10%.[19]

The second approach is to use a clinical prediction rule.[20] This model places patients into three categories on the basis of clinical findings (typical for PE, atypical for PE, severe PE), the likelihood of alternative diagnoses, and the presence of risk factors for DVT. The prevalence rates of PE in the three categories are 3.4%, 27.8%, and 78.4%, respectively. The algorithm for placing patients into one of the three categories is somewhat complex but is easy to use when represented on the screen of a palmtop computer. Assuming that the ED physician did not identify an alternative diagnosis that seemed more likely than PE, the patient's pretest probability of PE was 28%, considerably higher than the ED physician's subjective probability.

With an estimate for the pretest probability of PE, the next step is to obtain the likelihood ratio for a negative helical CT scan. The sensitivity and specificity of the helical CT scan have varied considerably among studies. A recent meta-analysis of studies of diagnostic tests for pulmonary embolism found the likelihood ratio for a positive chest CT scan to be 24.1 (95% CI,

12.4 to 46.7). The likelihood ratio for a negative scan was 0.04 (95% CI, 0.03 to 0.06).[21]

To calculate the posttest odds of PE, the ED physician must combine the patient's pretest odds with the test's likelihood ratio by means of the odds ratio format of Bayes' theorem mentioned earlier (posttest odds = pretest odds × likelihood ratio). An alternative to converting the pretest probability to odds and doing the calculation of posttest odds is to use a nomogram [*see Figure 1*]. To estimate posttest probability, anchor a straightedge at a pretest probability of 28% (corresponding to the clinical predictive rule's estimate of pretest probability) in the left-hand column; then pass the straightedge through a likelihood ratio for a negative helical CT scan, 0.04, in the middle column. Read the posttest probability from the right-hand column: about 1.5%. The math for this estimate is as follows, with the 0.28 pretest probability of PE first needing to be converted to pretest odds:

$$\text{Pretest odds} = \text{pretest probability}/(1 - \text{pretest probability})$$
$$= 0.28/(1 - 0.28)$$
$$= 0.28/0.72$$
$$= 0.39$$

Now, the post–helical CT scan odds of PE for this patient must be determined by multiplying the pretest odds of PE, 0.39, by the likelihood ratio for a negative helical CT, 0.04:

$$\text{Posttest odds} = \text{pretest odds} \times \text{likelihood ratio}$$
$$= 0.39 \times 0.04$$
$$= 0.0156$$

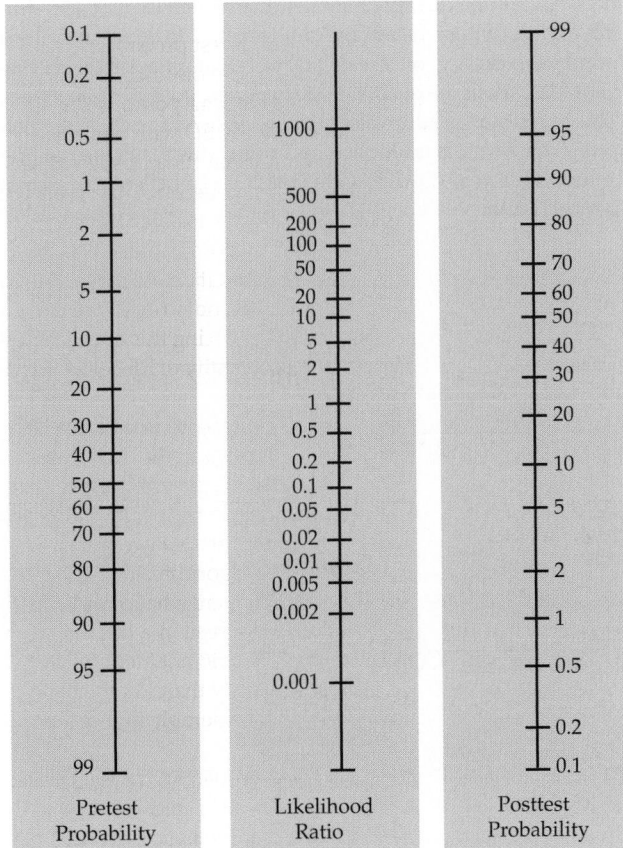

Figure 1 **Nomogram for converting pretest probabilities to posttest probabilities when test results are presented as likelihood ratios.**

Table 4 Definitions of Clinically Useful Measures of Treatment Effects from Clinical Trials

Like evaluation of diagnostic tests, evaluation of treatment effects often makes use of a 2 × 2 table, as follows:

Treatment Group	Treatment Outcome		No. of Patients in Treatment Group
	Bad	Good	
Experimental	a	b	a + b
Control	c	d	c + d
Total	a + c	b + d	

Measures of treatment effects when treatment reduces the risk of bad outcomes are calculated from this table.

- Experimental event rate (EER): the rate of an adverse clinical outcome in the experimental group; calculated as $a/(a+b)$.
- Control event rate (CER): the rate of an adverse clinical outcome in the control group; calculated as $c/(c+d)$.
- Absolute risk reduction (ARR): the absolute arithmetic difference in outcome rates between control and experimental groups in a trial; calculated as CER − EER, or $[c/(c+d)] - [a/(a+b)]$.
- Relative risk reduction (RRR): the proportional reduction in the rate of an adverse clinical outcome in the experimental group in comparison with the control group in a trial; calculated as ARR/CER, or (CER − EER)/CER, or $\{[c/(c+d)] - [a/(a+b)]\}/[c/(c+d)]$.
- Number needed to treat (NNT): the number of patients to whom one would have to give the experimental treatment to prevent one adverse clinical outcome; calculated as 1/ARR, or $1/\{[c/(c+d)] - [a/(a+b)]\}$, and reported as a whole number rounded to the next highest integer.
- Odds ratio: the odds that an experimental patient will experience an adverse event relative to the odds that a control subject will experience such an event; calculated as $(a/b)/(c/d)$.

Convert the posttest odds to the posttest probability, as follows:

$$\text{Posttest probability} = \text{posttest odds}/(1 + \text{posttest odds})$$
$$= 0.0156/(1 + 0.0156)$$
$$= 0.0154$$

At a posttest probability of PE of 1.5%, only 15 patients per 1,000 would have PE. Anticoagulating patients with a 1.54% probability of PE would mean exposing 65 patients (i.e., 1/0.0154) to the harms of anticoagulation to benefit one patient with a PE. Most physicians would follow this patient closely without giving specific treatment for PE. This same logic can be applied to all screening and diagnostic tests for PE, including D-dimer testing (high sensitivity and low specificity), which is therefore more useful for ruling out PE (when it is negative) than ruling it in (when it is positive).[22] D-dimer tests can also be used for calibrating clinical observations to enhance the quantitation of pretest probabilities.[23]

MEASURES OF TREATMENT EFFECTS

One of the most important tasks of clinicians is to advise patients about the current best treatment for their condition. Such advice should be based on the best evidence available. Clinically useful measures of treatment effects reported in clinical trials include the experimental event rate (EER), the control event rate (CER), relative risk reduction (RRR), absolute risk reduction (ARR), the number needed to treat (NNT), and the number needed to harm [*see Table 4*]. These measures can be effective tools for quantifying the magnitude of treatment benefits and risks, provided that there is a statistically significant difference in the clinical event rate between experimental subjects and control subjects (i.e., between the EER and the CER).

Again, we illustrate the practical application of these terms by a specific example. A 69-year-old hypertensive male smoker has experienced a partial left hemispheric stroke, with good recovery of function. He has a 75% ipsilateral internal carotid artery stenosis. One option would be to give this patient aspirin or clopidogrel and manage his risk factors for cerebrovascular disease; another would be to offer him carotid endarterectomy in addition to medical treatment. The question is, how and on what evidentiary basis does the clinician choose one treatment over another? It is tempting to think of treatments in black-and-white terms, as either working or not working, but the reality is rarely so absolute; often, the choice is between two or more treatments, each of which works after a fashion in certain situations. To apply the available evidence to the decision-making process in the most effective manner, the clinician must interpret it quantitatively, offering accurate, relevant figures instead of gut feelings when the patient asks what his chances are with each therapeutic approach.

Three randomized, controlled trials of carotid endarterectomy for symptomatic carotid artery stenosis[24-26] can inform our choice of treatment in this hypothetical patient. Examination of the North American Symptomatic Carotid Endarterectomy Trial (NASCET)[24] in the light of the users' guides discussed earlier [see Table 1] reveals that this study meets the three criteria for a study focusing on therapy. First, patients with symptomatic hemispheric transient ischemic attacks or partial strokes and ipsilateral carotid stenoses of 70% to 99% were randomly assigned to either an experimental group that underwent carotid endarterectomy or a control group that did not. All patients received continuing medical care, with special attention given to risk factors for cerebrovascular disease. Second, the study assessed the effect of carotid endarterectomy on important clinical events—namely, recurrence of stroke or perioperative stroke or death. Third, none of the patients were lost to follow-up. Consequently, the data from the study are likely to be valid guides in determining which treatment is best for this patient.

In the NASCET report, the risk of major or fatal ipsilateral stroke within a 2-year follow-up period was 2.5% in the group that underwent carotid endarterectomy and 13.1% in the control group. The absolute risk reduction, therefore, was 13.1% – 2.5%, or 10.6% ($P < 0.001$; CI, 5.5% to 15.7%), and the relative risk reduction was 10.6%/13.1%, or 81%. The number needed to treat was 10 (1/0.106); that is, 10 patients (CI, 7 to 18) would have to be treated with carotid endarterectomy (rather than medical treatment alone) to ensure that one major or fatal ipsilateral stroke would be prevented. The NASCET report indicates that this benefit is somewhat lower for patients with less severe stenosis (70% to 79%) and somewhat higher for patients with multiple risk factors for cerebrovascular disease—circumstances that offset one another in the case of the patient under consideration here.

Having determined the NNT, the next question is whether an NNT of 10 for major or fatal stroke over a 2-year period is a small benefit or a large one. By contrast, treatment of elevated diastolic blood pressures that do not exceed 115 mm Hg is associated with an NNT of 167 to prevent one stroke over a 5-year period.[25] Thus, for patients who have symptomatic, severe carotid artery stenosis, carotid endarterectomy is highly beneficial.

Given this conclusion, the next question is, do these research results apply to a specific patient, hospital, and surgeon? For example, the NASCET data reflect operative procedures performed by highly competent surgeons in specialized centers. One would have to know the perioperative complication rates for local surgeons to be able to assess a patient's level of risk if referred to any of those surgeons. If the local surgeons' perioperative complication rates for carotid endarterectomy are lower than 7%, the results are comparable to the NASCET results. On the other hand, patients with a stenosis of less than 70% are at substantially less risk for subsequent stroke to begin with. Potential benefit is similar to potential harm for patients with stenoses of 50% to 70%; for patients with stenoses of less than 50%, current evidence indicates that carotid endarterectomy would not yield any net reduction of this risk, even when the procedure is done by a highly skilled surgeon.[26,27]

MEASURES OF TREATMENT OUTCOME, ADJUSTED FOR QUALITY OF LIFE

Measures of treatment outcome, such as reduction in mortality, are important in deciding whether to start a medication or perform an operation, but they do not answer a question that is important to many patients: How much longer can they expect to live if treatment is started? One way of responding is to frame the answer in terms of life expectancy, the average length of life after starting treatment, which has a simple relation to the annual mortality in patients undergoing treatment.[13]

Although life expectancy is a useful measure of treatment outcome, it has one shortcoming: it places the same value on years in perfect health as on years in poor health. Arguably, a year with partially treated chronic disease is not equivalent to a year in perfect health. A solution to this problem is to adjust life expectancy for the quality of life that the patient experiences during a year of poor health by multiplying life expectancy by a number, expressed on a scale of 0 to 1, that reflects how the patient feels about the quality of life experienced during an illness. This number is usually called a utility. When life expectancy, expressed in years, is multiplied by a utility, the result is a quality-adjusted life year (QALY). One QALY is equivalent to a year in perfect health.

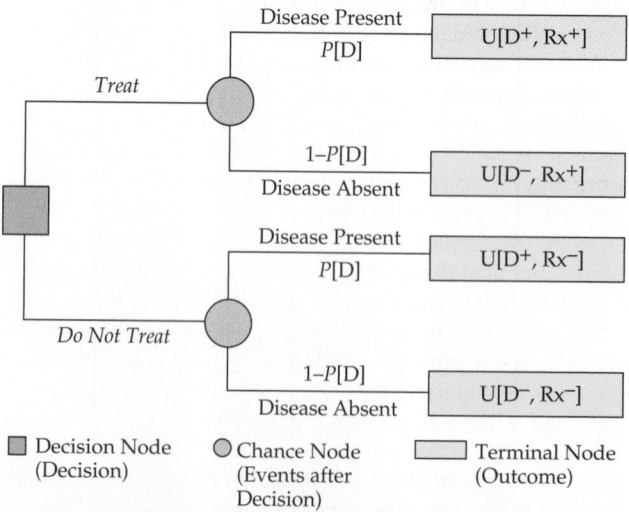

Figure 2 Shown is a decision tree for calculating the treatment threshold probability in a patient who is a possible candidate for carotid endarterectomy. (D—disease; U—utility)

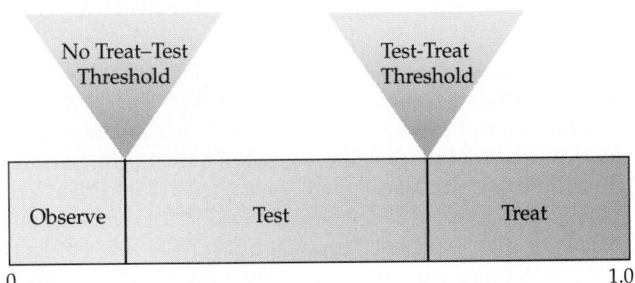

Figure 3   **Probability scale showing the ranges of probability corresponding to different actions following the initial history and physical examination.**

Medical Decision Analysis

Clearly, there is more to clinical decision making than simply collecting numbers that measure treatment effects. Reports of treatment effects in randomized, controlled trials are important starting points that help determine whether a treatment has merit in its own right, but the actual decision whether to offer a given patient a particular treatment is complex and must take into account each patient's specific clinical circumstances and individual wishes. For example, if the patient has significant comorbidity that would result in an especially high risk of perioperative complications, surgical therapy might not be the best choice. Even if the patient is well enough to undergo operation, individual preferences and values must be taken into account: the patient might be strongly averse to the immediate risks posed by surgery or might lack the resources to pay for the procedure.

THE THRESHOLD MODEL OF DECISION MAKING

At the conclusion of every history and physical examination, the clinician must choose one of three options: to treat, to observe, or to obtain more information. The optimal approach to making this choice starts with the assumption that the physician will seek more information (i.e., order diagnostic tests) only if the results may alter the treatment decision. Although occasional exceptions are easily justified, this rule is a good guiding principle for a lean style of practice. It is also the central assumption behind the threshold model of decision making.

When a diagnosis is uncertain, the decision whether to start treatment depends on the probability of the diagnosis. If the probability is 0, no one would start treatment; if the probability is 1, everyone would start treatment. Therefore, there must be a probability between 0 and 1 at which a physician would have no preference between treating and not treating. This probability is called the treatment threshold probability.

The treatment threshold probability is a key to solving the important decision-making problem of whether to treat, to observe, or to obtain more information. The most elegant way of obtaining the treatment threshold probability is to construct a decision tree that represents the choice between starting treatment and withholding treatment [*see Figure 2*]. In a decision tree, decisions are represented by squares (decision nodes), and the chance events that follow a decision are represented by circles (chance nodes). The probabilities of the events after a chance node must total 1.0. A terminal node (represented by a rectangle enclosing the name of the state) represents a state in which there are no subsequent chance events. Each terminal node has a value, which is a measure of the outcome associated with the event.

In a decision tree for starting or withholding treatment, each branch of the two chance nodes ends in a terminal node whose value is the utility (U) for being in the state specified. For example, U[D$^+$, Rx$^+$] is the utility for having the disease (D) and being treated for it, which one could calculate by representing that state as a tree with chance nodes and terminal nodes. To obtain the treatment threshold probability, one sets the expected utility of treatment at a value equal to the value for the expected utility of no treatment and then solves for the probability of disease. The general solution to the equation is as follows:

$$\text{Treatment threshold probability} = \frac{\text{harm}}{\text{harm} + \text{benefit}}$$

where harm is the net utility of being treated when disease is absent (U[D$^-$, Rx$^+$] – U[D$^-$, Rx$^-$]) and benefit is the net utility of being treated when disease is present (U[D$^+$, Rx$^+$] – U[D$^+$, Rx$^-$]). This relationship between harms and benefits of treatment is fundamental to solving the common decision problem of deciding about treatment when the diagnosis is not known with certainty. Because the treatment threshold depends on the benefits and harms of the treatment, it will vary from treatment to treatment. When the benefits of a treatment exceed harms, which is usually the case, the treatment threshold probability must be less than 0.50.

To make the choice between treating, not treating, and ordering tests to obtain additional information, the physician needs to know the range of probabilities of disease within which testing is the preferred action. The probability scale can be divided into three ranges [*see Figure 3*], one of which is the test range. The first step in defining the test range is to establish the treatment threshold probability. For the next step, we must invoke the principle that the physician should seek more information only if the results might alter the treatment decision. Translated to the threshold model, this principle takes the following form: testing is indicated only if the result of the test might move the probability of disease from one side of the treatment threshold (the do-not-treat side) to the other (the treat side). A physician can use this principle to decide whether to obtain a test in an individual patient. If the patient's pretest probability is below the treatment threshold and therefore in the do-not-treat zone, the physician should order the test only if the posttest probability of disease after a positive test result would be higher than the treatment threshold probability.

To obtain the test range, we must extend this example to a more general solution, which is to use the test's likelihood ratio and Bayes' theorem to calculate the pretest probability at which the posttest probability is exactly equal to the treatment threshold probability [*see Figure 3*]. This probability is called the no treat–test threshold probability. Clearly, if the pretest probability is lower than the no treat–test threshold probability, the test should not be done, because the posttest probability will be lower than the treatment threshold probability (i.e., a positive result will not change the management decision); conversely, if the pretest probability is higher than the no treat–test threshold probability, the test should be done, because the posttest probability will be higher than the treatment threshold probability (i.e., a positive test result would change the management decision from do not treat to treat).

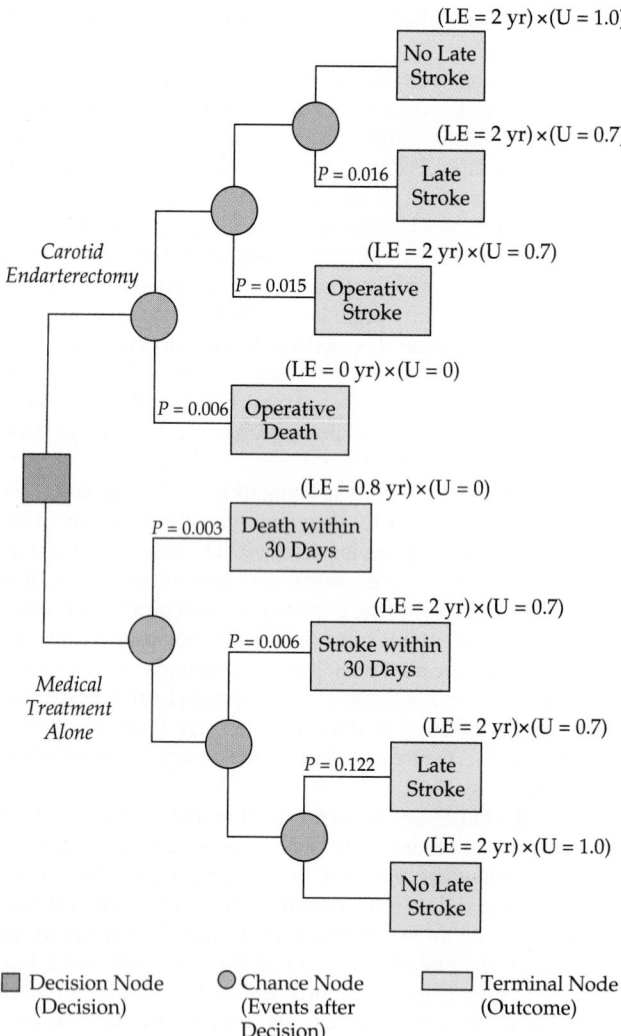

$(LE = 2 \text{ yr}) \times (U = 1.0)$ — No Late Stroke

$(LE = 2 \text{ yr}) \times (U = 0.7)$ — Late Stroke

$P = 0.016$

$(LE = 2 \text{ yr}) \times (U = 0.7)$ — Operative Stroke

$P = 0.015$

$(LE = 0 \text{ yr}) \times (U = 0)$ — Operative Death

$P = 0.006$

Carotid Endarterectomy

$(LE = 0.8 \text{ yr}) \times (U = 0)$ — Death within 30 Days

$P = 0.003$

$(LE = 2 \text{ yr}) \times (U = 0.7)$ — Stroke within 30 Days

$P = 0.006$

$(LE = 2 \text{ yr}) \times (U = 0.7)$ — Late Stroke

$P = 0.122$

$(LE = 2 \text{ yr}) \times (U = 1.0)$ — No Late Stroke

Medical Treatment Alone

■ Decision Node (Decision)   ○ Chance Node (Events after Decision)   ▭ Terminal Node (Outcome)

Figure 4 **Shown is a decision tree depicting the application of expected-outcome decision analysis to the same patient referred to in Figure 2. (LE—life expectancy; U—utility)**

The size of the test range depends on the likelihood ratios reported for the test. If LR⁻ is close to zero and LR⁺ is much greater than 1.0, the test range will be very wide. In general, the better the test, the larger the test range. If the posttest probability falls within the treat zone, the physician must then decide which treatment to offer. The choice among treatments offers a good opportunity to explore the principles of decision making under conditions of uncertainty.

MEASURES OF EXPECTED-OUTCOME DECISION MAKING: THE TREATMENT DECISION

The purpose of decision analysis is to help with those decisions for which the outcome cannot be foretold (e.g., the decision whether to treat carotid artery stenosis surgically). Even when randomized trial results indicate that one treatment generally gives better results than another, some degree of uncertainty remains: individual patients may still exhibit idiosyncratic outcomes or may experience unusual but serious side effects of treatment. Faced with this uncertainty, most physicians choose the treatment that gives the best results averaged over a large number of patients. In so doing, they become, perhaps unwittingly, what are known as "expected-value decision makers." Expected value is the value of an intervention when the outcomes of that intervention are averaged over many patients. A more general term might be "expected-outcome decision maker," which would denote a physician who chooses the treatment that gives the best outcome when averaged over many patients. This concept is the basis of expected-outcome decision analysis, which is a method of framing a decision problem in terms of the expected outcome of each decision alternative. Thus, in a patient with stable angina, the physician would decide between medical management, coronary angioplasty, and coronary artery bypass surgery by first calculating a patient's life expectancy, expressed in years in good health, after undergoing each of these treatment options; then, the physicial would choose the treatment with the highest life expectancy.

We can illustrate the application of expected-outcome decision making by returning to the example of the 69-year-old man who has recovered from a hemispheric stroke and has a 75% carotid stenosis. The question to be answered is the same: Should the patient be offered carotid endarterectomy in addition to best medical treatment? The first step is to represent the problem by a decision tree [*see Figure 4*]. Each of the terminal nodes in this decision tree is associated with a life expectancy, as well as a utility representing the value of life in the outcome state, represented by the terminal node. As noted earlier [*see* How to Apply Research Results to Patient Care, Measures of Treatment Outcome Adjusted for Quality of Life, *above*], life expectancy by itself is not a sufficiently precise measure: clearly, 2 years of life after a major stroke is not equivalent to 2 years in perfect health. The decision maker needs a quantitative measure of the patient's feelings about being in an outcome state. The physician can obtain the patient's utility for that state by asking the patient to indicate the length of time in perfect health that he would consider equivalent to his life expectancy in a disabled state (e.g., after a major stroke). This technique is called time trade-off. Other techniques used to obtain this utility include linear scaling and the standard reference gamble.[13]

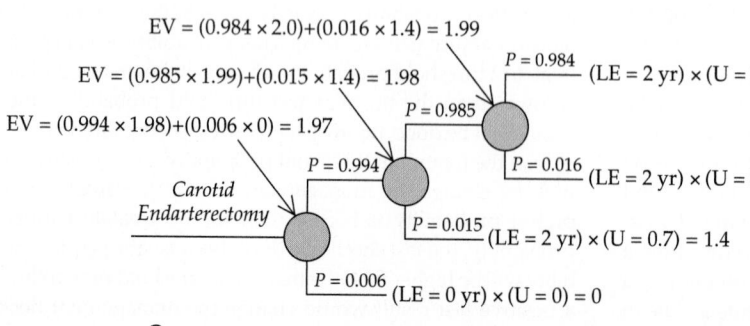

$EV = (0.984 \times 2.0)+(0.016 \times 1.4) = 1.99$

$EV = (0.985 \times 1.99)+(0.015 \times 1.4) = 1.98$

$EV = (0.994 \times 1.98)+(0.006 \times 0) = 1.97$

Carotid Endarterectomy

$P = 0.984$ $(LE = 2 \text{ yr}) \times (U = 1.0) = 2.0$

$P = 0.985$

$P = 0.994$

$P = 0.016$ $(LE = 2 \text{ yr}) \times (U = 0.7) = 1.4$

$P = 0.015$ $(LE = 2 \text{ yr}) \times (U = 0.7) = 1.4$

$P = 0.006$ $(LE = 0 \text{ yr}) \times (U = 0) = 0$

○ Chance Node (Events after Decision)

Figure 5 **Illustrated is the process of averaging out at a chance node, as applied to the upper (carotid endarterectomy) portion of the decision tree depicted in Figure 2. (EV—expected value; LE—life expectancy; U—utility)**

To calculate the expected value of surgical management, the decision maker starts at the chance nodes that are farthest from the decision node (the tips of the branches of the decision tree), multiplies the probability of each event at each chance node by the value of the event, and sums these products over all the events at the chance node. This calculation is known as averaging out at a chance node [see Figure 5]. The value obtained for each chance node by means of this process becomes the outcome measure for the next step, which is to repeat the averaging-out process at the next chance node to the left.

With either therapeutic option—aspirin combined with carotid endarterectomy or continued management with aspirin alone—there is a chance of death within 30 days, stroke within 30 days, or stroke within 2 years [see Figure 4]. As noted [see How to Apply Research Results to Patient Care, Measures of Treatment Effects, above], reliable data on the probabilities of these adverse events are available in the NASCET report.[24] To simplify the presentation of the decision analysis, we measure survival only within the 2-year time frame addressed in the NASCET report, and we assume that all late strokes occur at the start of this 2-year period. Further, we assume that a patient would value 2 years of disability resulting from a stroke as equivalent to 17.5 months of healthy life, which means that the utility representing the state of having experienced a major stroke is 0.70.

The decision analysis indicates that the decision maker should prefer surgical treatment to medical treatment. The expected value of carotid endarterectomy for this patient is 1.96 QALY, whereas the expected value of medical treatment is 1.91 QALY. Admittedly, this difference is not very large, indicating a close call, and it is reasonable to ask how high the operative mortality would have to be to make medical treatment the favored approach. Sensitivity analysis, one of the most powerful features of decision analysis, shows that the operative mortality would have to increase considerably before medical treatment would become preferable. The baseline figure for operative mortality in the NASCET report was 0.6%. The sensitivity analysis indicates that medical treatment would have a higher expected value than surgical treatment only if the operative mortality were 3.2% or higher, which might be the case if considerable comorbidity were present or if the surgeon seldom performed carotid endarterectomy. Although most physicians would not have the time or expertise to carry out this decision analysis, storing the appropriate decision tree in a palmtop computer would make it possible to do the decision analysis easily in the office setting, using values specific to the clinical setting and the patient.

COST-EFFECTIVENESS ANALYSIS

Cost-effectiveness analysis is a method for comparing the impact of expenditures on different health outcomes. Cost-effectiveness analysis assesses the trade-off between added benefit and added cost by examining costs and benefits at the margin (i.e., comparing one intervention with another or with no intervention). The cost-effectiveness of one intervention (A) versus another (B) is calculated as follows:

$$\text{Cost-effectiveness (A vs. B)} = \frac{\text{cost A} - \text{cost B}}{\text{effectiveness A} - \text{effectiveness B}}$$

In the carotid endarterectomy example, the costs would include all costs associated with a subsequent stroke. If we assume that the average lifetime cost associated with carotid endarterectomy is $10,000 and the average lifetime cost associated with medical treatment is $8,000, then the cost-effectiveness of surgical treatment, as compared with medical treatment, would be calculated as follows:

$$\text{Cost-effectiveness (surgery vs. no surgery)}$$
$$= (\$10,000 - \$8,000)/(1.96 - 1.91 \text{ QALY})$$
$$= \$2,000/0.05 \text{ QALY}$$
$$= \$40,000/\text{QALY}$$

One may then ask, is a treatment choice that costs $40,000 for each extra QALY cost-effective? There is no absolute answer to this question. In practice, a physician compares the cost-effectiveness of carotid endarterectomy with that of other interventions. How this information should affect the decision whether to offer surgical treatment to any given patient is an even more difficult question. Indeed, most experts would say that cost-effectiveness is a technique for deciding policies that would apply to many patients. An organization with limited resources would choose policies that prescribe interventions with the lowest cost per added QALY. The organization would not offer interventions that have a high cost relative to the magnitude of the anticipated benefit.

Conclusion

Quantitative approaches to clinical reasoning are still evolving. By combining better evidence from health care research with today's burgeoning information technology, physicians can apply evidence effectively to individual patient care. As requirements for efficiency and accountability continue to increase, physicians are under more and more pressure to adopt a quantitative, evidence-based approach to patient care. Physicians who can back up their decisions with sound research and sound reasoning will be in a better position to provide their patients with optimal care.

The authors have no commercial relationships with manufacturers of products or providers of services discussed in this chapter.

References

1. Antman EM, Lau J, Kupelnick B, et al: A comparison of results of meta-analyses of randomized control trials and recommendations of experts. JAMA 268:240, 1992

2. Godwin M, Seguin R: Critical appraisal skills of family physicians in Ontario, Canada. BMC Med Educ, 2003
http://www.biomedcentral.com/1472-6920/3/10

3. Lobb EA, Butow PN, Kenny DT, et al: Communicating prognosis in early breast cancer: do women understand the language used? Med J Aust 171:290, 1999

4. Clinical Evidence: A Compendium of the Best Available Evidence for Effective Health Care (Online). BMJ Publishing Group, Serial Electronic Publication, London, 1999
http://www.clinicalevidence.org

5. Physicians' Information and Education Resource (Online). American College of Physicians, Philadelphia, 2005
http://pier.acponline.org/info/?hp

6. The Cochrane Library (Online). Serial Electronic Publication, Oxford
http://www.update-software.com/cochrane

7. BMJupdates+(Online). BMJ Publishing Group and McMaster University Health Information Research Center, Hamilton, Ontario, Canada, 2005
http://www.bmjupdates.com

8. MEDSCAPE Best Evidence alerts (Online). WebMD, New York, 2005
https://profreg.medscape.com/px/newsletter.do

9. Sackett DL, Straus S, Richardson SR, et al: Evidence-Based Medicine: How to Practice and Teach EBM, 2nd ed. Churchill Livingstone, London, 2000

10. Haynes RB, Sackett DL, Cook DJ, et al: Transferring evidence from health care research into medical practice: 2. Getting the evidence straight. ACP J Club 126:A14, 1997

11. Bryant G, Norman G: Expression of probability: words and numbers (letter). N Engl J Med 302:411, 1980

12. Feightner JW, Norman GR, Haynes RB: The reliability of likelihood estimates by physicians. Clin Res 30:298A, 1982

13. Sox HC, Blatt M, Marton KI, et al: Medical Decision Making. Butterworths, Stoneham, Massachusetts, 1988

14. Goldman L, Caldera DL, Nussbaum SR, et al: Multifactorial index of cardiac risk in noncardiac surgical procedures. N Engl J Med 297:845, 1977

15. Sox HC, Hickam DH, Marton KI, et al: Using the patient's history to estimate the probability of coronary artery disease: a comparison of referral and primary care practice. Am J Med 89:7, 1990

16. Black E, Bordley DR, Tape TG, et al: Diagnostic Strategies for Common Medical Problems, 2nd ed. ACP Publications, Philadelphia, 1999

17. McGee S: Evidence-Based Physical Diagnosis. WB Saunders Co, Philadelphia, 2001

18. Hull RD, Raskob GE, Carter CJ, et al: Pulmonary embolism in outpatients with pleuritic chest pain. Arch Intern Med 148:838, 1988

19. Mayewski RJ: Respiratory problems: pulmonary embolism. Diagnostic Strategies for Common Medical Problems. Panzer R, Black E, Griner P, Eds. ACP Library on Disk (CD-ROM publication). American College of Physicians, Philadelphia, 1996

20. Wells PS, Ginsberg JS, Anderson DR, et al: Use of a clinical model for safe management of patients with suspected pulmonary embolism. Ann Intern Med 129:997, 1998

21. Roy PM, Colombet I, Durieux P, et al: Systematic review and meta-analysis of strategies for the diagnosis of suspected pulmonary embolism. BMJ 331:259, 2005

22. Stein PD, Hull RD, Patel KC, et al: D-dimer for the exclusion of acute venous thrombosis and pulmonary embolism. Ann Intern Med 140:589, 2004

23. Chunilal SD, Eikelboom JW, Attia J, et al: Does this patient have pulmonary embolism? JAMA 290:2849, 2003

24. Beneficial effect of carotid endarterectomy in symptomatic patients with high-grade carotid stenosis. North American Symptomatic Carotid Endarterectomy Trial collaborators. N Engl J Med 325:445, 1991

25. Cook RJ, Sackett DL: The number needed to treat: a clinically useful measure of treatment effect. BMJ 310:452, 1995

26. Analysis of pooled data from the randomised controlled trials of endarterectomy for symptomatic carotid stenosis. Carotid Endarterectomy Trialists' Collaboration. Lancet 361:107, 2003

27. Cina CS, Clase CM, Haynes RB: Carotid endarterectomy for symptomatic carotid stenosis. Cochrane Database Syst Rev (2):CD001081, 2000

3 Reducing Risk of Injury and Disease

Harold C. Sox, Jr., M.D., M.A.C.P.

Prevention: A Brief Overview

During the past 2 decades, disease and injury prevention has occupied an expanding share of medical practice. Public interest in prevention is very high, driven by a steady accumulation of high-quality evidence that preventive interventions do reduce cause-specific death rates. The purpose of these interventions is to eliminate the root causes of diseases that precede death (e.g., heart disease, cancer, and stroke), which in the United States in 2000 were tobacco use (435,000 deaths), poor diet and inadequate physical activity (400,000 deaths), alcohol consumption (85,000 deaths), microbial agents (75,000 deaths), toxic agents (55,000 deaths), firearms (29,000 deaths), unprotected sexual intercourse (20,000 deaths), motor vehicle accidents (43,000 deaths), and use of illicit drugs (20,000 deaths).[1] These causes of death are the targets of disease and injury prevention. They contribute to 50% of the deaths in the United States. Most are simply bad habits, and changing those habits reduces the risk of dying.

Physicians have two principal roles in prevention: they identify risk factors for disease and injury, and they act as teachers and counselors. Physicians must expand their routine questioning beyond diet, exercise, and substance abuse to include recreational activities that increase the risk of death (e.g., boating, bicycling, and riding motorcycles), gun ownership, use of swimming pools, smoke detectors in the home, and domestic violence. In counseling patients about a healthy diet (including vitamin supplements), exercise, and other elements of a healthy lifestyle, physicians must often help patients adopt healthy living habits. Some patients simply require reinforcement of a chosen lifestyle. Others need help in changing harmful habitual behaviors to healthy behaviors.

The report of the second United States Preventive Services Task Force (USPSTF)[2] contains evidence-based guidelines on 70 prevention topics [see Table 1]. As they become available, the third USPSTF reports will appear on its Web site (http://www.ahcpr.gov/clinic/cps3dix.htm). Other literature is also helpful [see Chapters 4, 5, 153, 209, and 210].

CAVEATS IN DISEASE AND INJURY PREVENTION

Although disease and injury prevention can have a significant effect on the health of the public, physicians should observe several caveats. First, the baseline risk of most diseases is very low in the average person. Each year, colon cancer occurs in 165 per 100,000 men 60 to 64 years of age. The low baseline risk means that the number needed to screen or treat to prevent one death is often very high. Annual fecal occult blood testing must be performed on more than 300 people for 12 years to prevent one death from colon cancer. Whether this inefficiency is important depends partly on the cost of the intervention. Fecal occult blood testing can be costly because it must be performed annually and because abnormal results trigger costly diagnostic tests. Seat belts and smoke alarms are very cost-effective because they incur a onetime cost.

Second, disease prevention does not prevent death. At best, it postpones death by shifting the cause of death from the targeted disease to another disease that strikes later in life. In the Minnesota Colon Cancer Control Study, a randomized trial of fecal occult blood testing, annual testing reduced deaths from colon cancer during 18 years of surveillance. However, the total mortality was the same in the control group and the intervention groups. Our preventive efforts may reduce the likelihood of death from the target disease, whose identity and natural his-

---

Table 1 **Recommendations of the United States Preventive Services Task Force[2]**

Tobacco Use

Provide tobacco cessation counseling to patients who use tobacco products. Counsel pregnant women and parents about the potentially harmful effects of smoking on fetal and child health. Prescribe nicotine patches or gum to selected patients as an adjunct to counseling. Give antitobacco messages to young people as part of health promotion counseling.

Alcohol Abuse

Screen all adults and adolescents for problem drinking, using a careful history or a standardized screening questionnaire. Advise pregnant women to limit or abstain from drinking. Counsel all persons who use alcohol about the dangers of operating a motor vehicle or engaging in other potentially dangerous activities while drinking.

Drug Abuse*

Although the evidence is insufficient for a strong recommendation to be made, it is reasonable to ask adolescents and adults about drug use and drug-related problems. All pregnant women should be advised of the potential adverse effects of drug use on fetal development. Refer drug-abusing patients to specialized treatment facilities where available.

Preventing Motor Vehicle Injuries†

Counsel all patients and the parents of young people to use occupant restraints (lab/shoulder safety belts and child safety seats), to wear helmets when riding motorcycles, and to refrain from driving while under the influence of alcohol or other drugs.

Preventing Falls‡

Counsel elderly patients on specific measures to reduce the risk of falls. Effective measures include exercise, balance training, environmental hazard reduction, and monitoring and adjusting medications. Provide multifactorial individualized interventions to elderly patients at especially high risk for falls.

Fires

Advise homeowners to install smoke detection devices and test them periodically. Infants and children should wear flame-resistant nightclothes. Smokers should cease or reduce smoking.

Drowning

Families with swimming pools should install four-sided 4-ft isolation fences with self-latching gates.

Firearm Injuries

Remove firearms from the home or store them unloaded in a locked compartment.

---

*There is insufficient evidence to recommend routine screening for drug abuse with standardized questionnaires or biologic assays.
†There is insufficient evidence to recommend for or against counseling patients to avoid pedestrian injuries.
‡There is insufficient evidence of effectiveness of external hip protectors.

tory we know. Inevitably, we raise the lifetime probability of dying from another disease.

Third, we know little about the age at which we should stop our efforts to prevent disease. Our studies provide good information on effectiveness in the study population, which is usually in middle age, but we do not know how the results apply to older people, whose care will occupy an increasing amount of the primary care physician's time.[3] Interventions that take years to show their impact may be ill suited to people whose life expectancy is measured in years rather than decades.

The decision to do a screening test on an older person should depend on the person's general health, which may be quantified as the person's physiologic age. The physician can determine a patient's physiologic age by asking the patient to rate his or her health as excellent, good, fair, or poor.[3] The most likely age at death is the sum of the patient's actual age and the life expectancy that corresponds to the patient's physiologic age. For example, a 75-year-old man in excellent health has a physiologic age of 67 years, which corresponds to a 14.7-year life expectancy [see Figure 1]. The most likely age at death is 75 years plus 14.7 years, or 90 years. This information can be very helpful in deciding how hard to press preventive efforts. With a life expectancy of almost 15 years, a 75-year-old man has plenty of time in which to experience gains from preventive efforts.

CHANGING BEHAVIOR

Many interventions of proven efficacy are not completely effective because patients are reluctant to change long-established risky behaviors. The USPSTF recommends the following steps for helping patients use their ability to change (self-efficacy)[4]:

1. Match teaching to the patient. Identify a patient's beliefs about a behavior, and adjust advice to the patient's lifestyle. Building the patient's confidence in his or her ability to change requires recognizable successes; define success in terms of goals the patient can achieve.

2. Tell why, what, and when. Patients need to know the reason for a recommendation and the results of following the recommendation. They must also know the time scale for the results so that they do not become discouraged when results do not occur immediately.

3. Small changes succeed. As the patient achieves small successes, propose larger but achievable goals.

4. Be specific. Couch suggestions in terms of current behavior, and give precise instructions in writing.

5. Add new behaviors. Adopting good habits is often easier than discarding bad ones.

6. Link positive behaviors with the daily routine. For example, patients can be encouraged to exercise before lunch or to take medication immediately after brushing teeth.

7. Do not mince words. Tell the patient directly, simply, and specifically what you want and why.

8. Extract promises. Get explicit commitments from the patient. Have the patient tell you exactly how he or she will achieve a goal. Assess the patient's self-confidence and address concerns about succeeding.

9. Use combination strategies. An approach that combines several strategies is more likely to succeed than a single strategy.

10. Involve others. Members of the physician's office staff can become educators. Anyone can offer encouragement to patients.

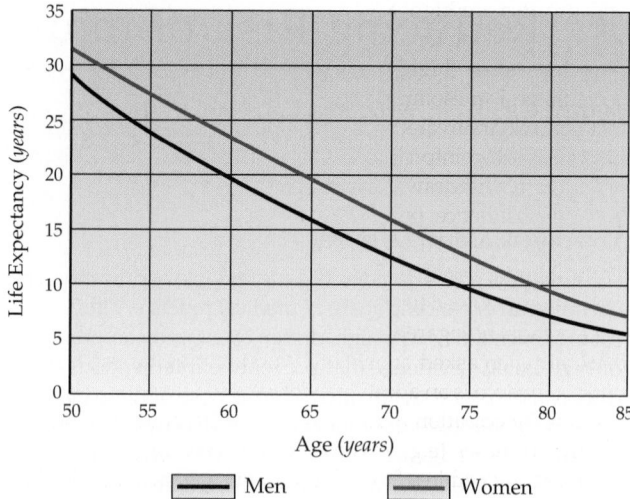

Figure 1   **Life expectancy of men and women in the United States.**

11. Refer. Subspecialists in many chronic diseases have trained teams that can educate patients far more effectively than individual physicians can. Another form of referral is sending novice patients to talk with successful patients.

12. Stay interested. According to research findings, a call from a health professional to inquire about progress is very effective in changing a behavior. A well-organized office will have a protocol for making these calls a matter of routine.

Health Risks from Substance Abuse

Substance abuse exacts a large toll on the health of the American people, accounting for at least 520,000 deaths in 1990, or 24% of all deaths.[1] Unfortunately, many physicians do not place diseases resulting from self-abuse in the same category as diseases that strike seemingly by chance. Two factors make helping patients shed their habitual use of tobacco, alcohol, and illicit drugs a very efficient way for physicians to add healthy years to patients' lives. First, there is a high baseline risk that substance abuse will lead to serious disease. Therefore, the absolute reduction in risk from a successful intervention is high. This principle is especially true of substance abuse during pregnancy. Second, substance abuse is primarily a problem of youth and middle age, so a successful intervention can add many years of healthy life.

TOBACCO USE

Tobacco contains an addictive drug, nicotine, as well as other substances that contribute to death from cardiovascular disease, cancer, and chronic lung disease. Smoking also contributes to 10% of infant deaths and 20% to 30% of low-birth-weight infants.[5] Tobacco use contributed to one in every five deaths in the United States in 1990 (420,000 deaths a year). In one 40-year cohort study of male physicians in the United Kingdom, half of the deaths after age 35 were smoking related, and smoking caused 25% of the residential fires that resulted in death.[5] Tobacco use is less common than it was several decades ago, but 25% of adults smoke, and an increasing number of smokers are women. Women are starting to smoke earlier—many as high-school students—and they are heavier smokers; nearly twice as many women smoked at least 25 cigarettes a day in 1985 as in 1965.[6]

Cigarettes are highly addictive. Fewer than 10% of people who quit smoking for a day are still abstinent 1 year later. Nicotine, like other highly addictive substances, acts on the dopaminergic mesolimbic pathway, the brain reward pathway that controls motivated behaviors [see Chapter 210]. The use of nicotine is self-reinforcing, leading to compulsive use. Nicotine produces a withdrawal syndrome that begins within a few hours of abstinence, peaks within the first week, and continues for several weeks. The withdrawal syndrome includes dysphoria, insomnia, irritability, anxiety, difficulty in concentrating, restlessness, slowed heart rate, and increased appetite.[7]

Detection of cigarette smoking is easy; most smokers are truthful when asked about their habit and its extent, and the odor of tobacco is an additional diagnostic clue.

Smoking cessation reduces mortality dramatically. The risk of some diseases (e.g., myocardial infarction and stroke) declines rapidly within a few years after quitting [see Table 2].[8] This information is important when one is trying to convince long-term smokers to quit.

Research has shown that a strong message from a personal physician is the most important factor in successful quitting. The elements of successful quitting are consistent, repeated, and strong advice to stop smoking; setting a specific quit date; and follow-up visits to reinforce behavior [see Table 3]. However, not all physicians counsel smokers to quit. In one study, only 78% of cigarette smokers reported that their physician had advised them to quit.[9]

A current theory in behavioral psychology suggests that changes in behavior reflect predictable stages in the readiness to change, ranging from no intention to change, to definite plans to change in the near future, to active attempts at change. A stage of readiness to change is predictive of quitting,[10] and this behavioral model may help clinicians shape smoking-cessation efforts to the patient's state of mind.

School-based prevention has received extensive study, and it is effective for at least 2 to 4 years. Clinicians, especially those caring for adolescents, must reinforce the messages of school-based programs.

Nicotine products are an important adjunct to counseling.[11] Drugs are most reinforcing when the level in the brain rises very rapidly, as with inhaled nicotine. Nicotine in medication form, especially transdermal products, appears in the blood much more slowly than inhaled nicotine and produces much less of the reinforcing effect that leads to craving for cigarettes. Plasma nicotine concentrations after transdermal administration reach stable levels in 2 to 3 days. Nicotine medications reduce the symptoms of withdrawal, so that symptoms in the first week are reduced to the level of symptoms at 5 to 10 weeks. Nicotine medications may also provide some nicotine-like effects, such as helping patients to sustain concentration and deal with stress.

Nicotine medications improve abstinence rates, but abstinence at 1 year is still the exception. A meta-analysis summarized the results of 46 trials of nicotine gum and 20 trials of nicotine patches.[12] At 12 months, 19% of patients who received nicotine gum were abstinent, as compared with 11% of patients who did not receive gum. The number needed to treat to achieve one success at 1 year (NNT) was 17 ($P < 0.001$). Transdermal nicotine led to similar rates. At 12 months, 16% of patients who received a transdermal nicotine patch had quit smoking, as compared with 9% who did not receive the patch (NNT, 16). Clonidine also increases the rate of abstinence at 12

Table 2 Years of Smoking Abstinence Needed to Reduce Risk of Disease[2,8]

Disease	Years until Risk Is Half of a Current Smoker's Risk	Years until Risk Is Equal to a Never-smoker's Risk
Recurrent myocardial infarction or death from coronary artery disease	1	15
Stroke	2–4	5–15
Oral and esophageal cancer	5	—
Lung cancer	10	20

months. Weight gain is a common occurrence in patients who have stopped smoking. The average weight gain in a national sample of adults who had stopped smoking was 4.4 kg for men and 5.0 kg for women.[13]

The dose of nicotine medications should depend on the degree of nicotine dependence.[11] The score on the Fagerstrom questionnaire[14] and the number of cigarettes a day are measures of dependence. Follow-up calls at prearranged times will help the patient to maintain abstinence. It is best to designate a specific member of the physician's office staff to be the smoking-cessation coordinator.

The starting dose of nicotine gum (nicotine polacrilex) is 2 mg per two cigarettes; in patients who smoke more than 20 cigarettes a day, the dose should be 4 mg per three or four cigarettes. Patients may take additional unit doses if their withdrawal symptoms are unpleasant. The medication should be taken at regular intervals throughout the waking hours. The patient should compress the gum a few times with the teeth and then hold it in the mouth, repeating the cycle every minute or so for 15 to 30 minutes for each dose. After 1 to 2 months, weaning can begin with a reduction of 1 unit dose a week.

With transdermal nicotine, patients who smoke more than 10 cigarettes a day should use the largest patch (21 mg). After 1 to 2 months, weaning can begin with each of the lower doses (usually 14 mg and 7 mg, respectively), prescribed for 2 to 4 weeks. Patients who smoke fewer than 10 cigarettes a day can start with the 14 mg dose. A hairless site allows the best absorption. The patient should rotate sites to avoid skin irritation.

Nicotine medications are quite safe[11]—certainly safer than cigarette smoking—even for patients with cardiovascular disease. The only contraindication is hypersensitivity to nicotine or to a component of the delivery system. Twenty-four-hour application of transdermal medication can result in sleep distur-

Table 3 Elements of a Successful Smoking Cessation Strategy

Direct, face-to-face advice and suggestions
Reinforcement, especially in first 2 weeks
Office reminders: a sticker on chart of smokers may stimulate physician to deliver antitobacco message at each visit
Self-help materials
Community programs for additional help
Drug therapy

bance, which subsides if the medication is removed before sleep. Nicotine medication during pregnancy is of concern but probably of less concern than heavy smoking during pregnancy. Medication during pregnancy should be reserved for women who have failed to quit without medication and who smoke more than 10 to 15 cigarettes a day. Dependence on nicotine medications is most likely with delivery systems such as a nasal spray, which causes a rapid rise in the plasma nicotine concentration, and a small number of patients will still be using nicotine medication 1 year after starting treatment.

Nicotine therapy is not the only pharmacologic approach to smoking cessation. Another approach focuses on dopamine. Nicotine releases norepinephrine in the brain and increases dopamine in areas of the brain associated with reinforcing the effects of addictive substances, such as opioids. Bupropion potentiates the effect of norepinephrine and dopamine by acting as a weak inhibitor of their neuronal uptake. Thus, bupropion can mimic some of the central nervous system effects of nicotine and act as a substitute for nicotine in people who are trying to quit cigarettes. Randomized clinical trials have shown that abstinence rates are approximately twice as high with bupropion as with placebo.[15] In one trial, for example, the rates of abstinence from tobacco at 1 year were 12% for those taking placebo and 23% for those taking 150 or 300 mg of bupropion.[16] Side effects of bupropion include agitation and insomnia. Seizures are very uncommon when the daily dose of bupropion is 300 mg or less.

The recommended dose of bupropion is 150 mg/day for the first 3 days and then 150 mg twice daily. The patient should wait to stop smoking until he or she has been on bupropion for 1 week. There are no peer-reviewed reports comparing nicotine-replacement products with bupropion or detailing possible synergy between the two drugs.

ALCOHOL ABUSE

Habitual excessive alcohol consumption causes 100,000 deaths annually in the United States.[1] Although more than one million adults are under treatment for alcoholism, a far greater number engage in drinking that injures their health or has social consequences. The Institute of Medicine estimates that 20% of the population of the United States are problem drinkers, but only 5% are alcohol dependent.[17] Therefore, it is important to distinguish alcohol dependence from problem drinking. Alcohol dependence is associated with major withdrawal symptoms, tolerance, complete loss of self-control, and preoccupation with drinking. Problem drinking, on the other hand, is a less severe condition. Problem drinkers are younger, have a shorter drinking history, have fewer alcohol-related job problems, and have better social resources. In community surveys,

the prevalence of problem drinking has been shown to be highest in young men (17% to 24% in 18- to 29-year-olds) and lowest in men and women older than 65 years (1% to 3% and less than 1%, respectively). Women are more frequently problem drinkers than alcohol dependent.

Problem drinking has consequences that affect others, such as motor vehicle accidents, fetal-alcohol syndrome, unsafe sex, domestic violence, and psychological damage to children of problem drinkers. Binge drinking, which is especially prevalent in young adults, leads to violence, unsafe sex, and drunk driving.

Screening for problem drinking and alcohol dependence can be time consuming, and most methods are inaccurate. The gold-standard test for alcoholism is the *Diagnostic and Statistical Manual of Mental Disorders* (DSM-IV) criteria, which require a detailed interview and do not constitute a suitable screening instrument. Results of physical examination and laboratory tests are often normal in problem drinkers. Screening questionnaires such as the modified Michigan Alcoholism Screening Test (MAST), the Alcohol Use Disorders Identification Test (AUDIT), and the CAGE test are the most accurate instruments for detecting problem drinking[2] [see Tables 4 and 5 and Chapter 209]. The questions in the MAST and CAGE instruments focus on alcohol dependence and are much less sensitive or specific for binge drinking. The AUDIT screening instrument[2] may be more generally useful because it also asks about quantity of alcohol imbibed, frequency of drinking, and binge behavior. The CAGE and MAST questionnaires may also fail to detect a level of alcohol use that is dangerous during pregnancy.

The treatment of problem drinking depends on the severity of the problem. Problem drinkers often respond to brief office interventions (as short as 10 or 15 minutes), which use motivational techniques such as goal setting, contracts, and enhancing self-efficacy. In most instances, the goal is usually controlled moderate drinking rather than abstinence. The first step toward successful counseling is to get the patient to recognize that there is a problem. It is important to help the patient see a relationship between drinking and current medical or psychosocial problems. Strong advice to reduce consumption is also important. Regular follow-up visits to monitor progress are just as important for problem drinkers as they are for patients with high blood pressure.[18] One meta-analysis of brief intervention trials for nondependent problem drinkers showed a reduction of 24% in average alcohol consumption.[19] Another meta-analysis of nine studies showed somewhat smaller effects. In five of nine studies in men, the number of drinks a week decreased (range of decrease, five to 20 a week). The effects in women were smaller.[20] A third meta-analysis of nine randomized trials found that brief interventions

Table 4 Test Performance of Screening Questionnaires for Alcohol Abuse[2]

Screening Instrument	Number of Items	Sensitivity (%)	Specificity (%)	Likelihood Ratio Positive	Likelihood Ratio Negative
MAST	25	84–100	87–95	10.2	0.10
CAGE	4	74–89	79–95	6.3	0.21
AUDIT*	10	96	96	24	0.04
AUDIT†	10	61	90	6.1	0.43

*In inner-city clinic population.
†In rural clinic.
AUDIT—Alcoholism Use Disorders Identification Test   CAGE—see Table 5   MAST—Michigan Alcoholism Screening Test

Table 5 The CAGE Questionnaire

C: Have you ever felt you ought to **C**ut down on drinking?

A: Have people **A**nnoyed you by criticizing your drinking?

G: Have you ever felt bad or **G**uilty about your drinking?

E: Have you ever had a drink in the morning to steady your nerves or get rid of a hangover (**E**ye-opener)?

were associated with alcohol moderation 6 to 12 months later (pooled odds ratio, 1.91; 95% confidence interval = 1.61 to 2.27).[21] An excellent guide to managing problem drinking is available from the National Institute on Alcohol Abuse and Alcoholism (http://pubs.niaaa.nih.gov/publications/arh23-2/138-143.pdf).

In contrast to the success of brief office-based interventions for problem drinking, successful treatment of alcohol dependence requires intensive therapy from specialists in substance abuse. A randomized trial of employees with alcohol dependence showed the importance of intervening intensively. Participants were randomly allocated to compulsory 3-week hospitalization followed by 1 year of attendance at Alcoholics Anonymous (AA) meetings, mandatory attendance at AA meetings at least three times a week, or a choice of treatment. Rates of being fired from work were similar in all groups, but rates for hospitalization for additional alcohol treatment were much lower in the mandatory-hospitalization group.[22]

The personal physician does have an important role to play in the management of patients with alcohol dependence. In addition to managing medical complications of alcoholism, physicians should be able to use adjunctive therapy for alcohol dependence, such as naltrexone. Another key role for the personal physician is encouragement. Patients need to know that the abstinence rate can be as high as 60% at 10 years after intensive treatment. Finally, the personal physician can lead efforts to help patients solve life problems that are contributing to alcohol dependence.

DRUG ABUSE

The abuse of illicit and legal drugs is a large problem in the United States. A 2001 household survey showed that use of illicit drugs within the previous month peaked among 18 to 20 year olds, at 22.4%, and declined steadily with increasing age. Casual use of marijuana accounts for most of these reports, but as many as 1.7 million Americans use cocaine weekly and 130,000 use heroin. The drug abuser is at risk for many medical complications, but the social cost of drug abuse far outweighs the personal costs. Illicit drug use plays a major role in spreading HIV infection and in homicide, suicide, and motor vehicle accidents. The health care costs of drug abuse are estimated to be $3.2 billion annually, and the cost of federal and state government efforts to stem the flow of illicit drugs is several times higher [*see Chapter 210*].

Many professional organizations recommend that physicians ask about drug abuse as part of a periodic health examination of a well person. However, learning about drug abuse may be difficult in the office setting. Patients may be unwilling to acknowledge drug abuse until presented with incontrovertible evidence or after persistent questioning by an alerted physician. There is little information about the accuracy of the history or questionnaires in detecting drug abuse.

Toxicologic testing is the best way to detect illicit drug use.

Compared with reference tests, current tests can detect drugs in the urine with 99% sensitivity. However, detection depends on when the patient supplies the specimen relative to the last drug exposure. Marijuana is detectable up to 14 days after use, whereas cocaine, opiates, amphetamines, and barbiturates are present for only 2 to 4 days after use.

Although physicians sometimes test for illicit drugs without obtaining the patient's consent, they do so in the context of trying to determine the cause of a clinical problem that could be caused by an illicit drug. Whether it is ethical to test for illicit drugs in an apparently healthy person who is at high risk for drug abuse is an open question. Regardless of the circumstances leading to testing, abnormal results deserve the physician's best efforts to maintain confidentiality, because they may affect the patient's employability, insurability, and personal relationships. At present, no professional organization recommends drug testing in apparently healthy people.

Physicians must learn to think of drug abuse as a chronic disease. Recidivism after intensive treatment programs is very common, no doubt in part because psychiatric disorders, unemployment, and homelessness often coexist with drug abuse. On the other hand, treating heroin abuse with maintenance methadone, an opioid agonist, can dramatically reduce the social effects of abusing the drug. Heroin addicts in methadone maintenance programs report less use of heroin and reduced rates of HIV infection, criminal behavior, and unemployment. There is no similarly effective treatment for cocaine addiction. Changes in the law now encourage methadone maintenance in office practice. Physicians who wish to treat their regular patients will need to learn about the new regulations.[23]

Health Risks from Accidents and Violence

A person's environment contains many threats to health: motor vehicle accidents, accidents in the home, recreation-related accidents, and domestic violence. Passive strategies, which change the environment in which accidents can occur, are generally more successful at accident prevention than active strategies, which require people to change their behavior. Improving roads saves more lives than exhorting people to drive carefully. For a fuller account, refer to the report of the USPSTF[2] and to a comprehensive review published in 1997.[24]

MOTOR VEHICLE INJURIES

Motor vehicle accidents are the leading cause of loss of potential years of life before age 65. Alcohol-related accidents account for 44% of all motor vehicle deaths. One can experience a motor vehicle accident as an occupant, as a pedestrian, or as a bicycle or motorcycle rider.

Injuries to Motor Vehicle Occupants

In 2000, 37,409 people died of injuries sustained in motor vehicle accidents in the United States.[25] The two greatest risk factors for death while one is driving a motor vehicle are driving while intoxicated and failing to use a seat belt. The physician's role is to identify patients with alcoholism [*see Alcohol Abuse, above*], to inquire about seat-belt use, and to counsel people to use seat belts and child car seats routinely. In one study, 53.5% of patients in a university internal medicine practice did not use seat belts. Problem drinking, physical inactivity, obesity, and low income were indicators of nonuse. The prevalence of nonuse was 91% in people with all four indicators and only

25% in those with no indicators.[26] Seat belts confer considerable protection, yet in one survey, only 3.9% of university clinic patients reported that a physician had counseled them about using seat belts.[27]

Three-point restraints reduce the risk of death or serious injury by 45%.[27] Air bags reduce the risk of death by an additional 6% in drivers using seat belts.[28] Because air bags reduce the risk of death by only 14% in unbelted drivers,[28] physicians must tell their patients not to rely on air bags.

Injuries to Motorcyclists

Motorcycle deaths in the United States have been rising since 1997, reaching 3,181 in 2001.[29] The chance of death per mile when one is riding a motorcycle is 35 times higher than when one is riding in an automobile. Most deaths are caused by head injuries. Helmets reduce the risk of a fatal head injury by 27%, but only 50% of riders use helmets. Laws mandating helmet use are quite effective; the rate of helmet use rose to 95% in California after passage of a law, and the rate of head injuries dropped by 34%. Substance abuse is very common among injured motorcyclists.

Physicians should inquire about motorcycle use. They should redouble their efforts to screen for substance abuse in motorcyclists and should recommend using helmets.

Injuries to Pedestrians

Pedestrian injuries caused by motor vehicles accounted for 4,739 deaths in 2000, a 27% decrease from 1990. Children are at greatest risk for injury. Among adults, the elderly are at greatest risk, principally because of sensory deficits, locomotor disability, and inability to process simultaneous stimuli.

Injuries to Cyclists

Each year, there are approximately 900 deaths from bicycle injuries in the United States.[30] Children are at greatest risk. Head injuries account for two thirds of hospitalizations and three quarters of deaths related to bicycling. A meta-analysis of case-control studies showed that use of safety helmets reduced the risk of head injuries by 63% to 88%.[30] Helmets are effective for all ages and provide protection even in collisions with motor vehicles. Community-based education efforts have raised the rate of helmet use to 50%. Physicians should ask about bicycle use and counsel riders to use safety helmets.

INJURIES FROM FALLING

Falling is a serious health risk for older persons [see Table 6]. The lifetime risk of hip fracture, perhaps the most important consequence of a fall, is 40% for a 50-year-old woman. One approach to reducing the risk of hip fracture is to prevent osteoporosis. Strategies for prevention of osteoporosis include vitamin D and supplementation of dietary calcium intake,[31] drugs that increase bone mass, such as etidronate and alendronate, and estrogen replacement after menopause. In a cohort study, weight-bearing exercise, such as walking, was associated with a 40% lower risk of hip fracture in women and a 50% lower risk in men.[32] Exercise works in part by increasing bone mass and in part by reducing the likelihood of a fall. Combined interventions that included home visits, modifying home hazards, and exercise and gait programs reduced the risk of falls by 31% in a randomized clinical trial.[33] Physicians should identify patients who are at greatest risk for falling [see Table 6], treat osteoporosis, and link the patient to community-based programs for im-

Table 6 Risk Factors for Falls among the Elderly[32]

Prior falls	Low body mass index
Cognitive impairment	Female sex
Chronic illness	General frailty
Balance and gait impairment	Hazards in the home

proving mobility and reducing hazards in the home. Hip pads are also effective; in a randomized trial, a pad worn over each hip reduced the risk of hip fracture from 46 per 1,000 patient-years to 21.3 per 1,000 patient-years ($P = 0.008$).[34]

INJURIES FROM FIRE

Prevention of death from fires is an example of a successful passive strategy. Smoke detectors prevent fire injury. A study in Oklahoma City measured the effects of door-to-door distribution of smoke detectors to residents of an area that had much higher rates of burn injuries than the rest of the city. The fire-injury rate declined 80%, to the same level as that in the rest of the city. The injury rate per fire also declined dramatically.[35] Physicians should inquire about smoke detectors in the home and recommend them to people who don't have them. Persons who are alcohol dependent or who smoke in bed are at high risk and need special effort.

DROWNING

In most instances of witnessed drowning, bystanders report that the victim becomes motionless while swimming or simply fails to surface after a dive. Struggle is unusual. This observation raises the possibility that many cases of drowning occur when something such as a seizure, an arrhythmia, or an injury occurs.[36]

All victims of immersion have hypoxemia. Aspirated freshwater is hypotonic and therefore rapidly absorbed by the pulmonary circulation and distributed throughout the body water compartment. Freshwater alters pulmonary surfactant and causes alveolar collapse and atelectasis. Saltwater is hypertonic and draws water into the alveoli, causing perfused but poorly ventilated alveoli and hypovolemia with concentration of electrolytes. The end result with both types of water is venous admixture and hypoxemia, often resulting in metabolic acidosis. Saltwater drowning often leads to hypovolemia as well.

The main goal of treatment is to prevent brain injury.[36] The first step is to initiate cardiopulmonary resuscitation if the victim is apneic and pulseless. The American Heart Association recommends abdominal thrusts only to clear the airway in case of suspected foreign-body aspiration or failure to respond to artificial ventilation. Supplemental oxygen is indicated as long as the patient is hypoxemic. The most effective single treatment of hypoxemia is continuous positive airway pressure (CPAP), using mechanical ventilation to expand collapsed alveoli caused by freshwater immersion.[36] Hypothermia, which often accompanies near-drowning, can protect the brain from injury by reducing its metabolic requirements when the patient is hypoxemic.

Most efforts to prevent drowning focus on children, for whom the passive strategy of requiring fencing around swimming pools is associated with reduced drowning rates. In adults, alcohol ingestion is a risk factor for drowning. The efficacy of personal flotation devices is not known. Relatively few boaters (14%) wear personal flotation devices, but this rate is

Domestic Violence Information on the Internet

Medical Resources
  Family Peace Project
  http://www.family.mcw.edu/d_FamilyPeace.htm
  Domestic Violence: A Practical Approach for Clinicians
  http://www.sfms.org/domestic.html

Legal Resources
  Women's Law Initiative
  http://www.womenslaw.org
  American Bar Association Commission on Domestic Violence
  http://www.abanet.org/domviol/home.html

similar to that of drowning victims. Physicians should ask patients whether they use boats recreationally and advise avoiding alcohol and using a personal flotation device while boating.

DOMESTIC VIOLENCE

For women especially, the home is the most dangerous place. In one large study of women in a primary care clinic, one in 20 had experienced domestic violence in the previous year, one in four had experienced it as adults, and one in three had experienced it in their lifetime.[37,38] A condition so prevalent in primary care practice demands the attention of the physician.

Among those abused in the previous year, approximately equal numbers had been abused once, two or three times, or four or more times. In this study, the definition of domestic violence was an affirmative answer to the question "Have you been hit, slapped, kicked, or otherwise physically hurt by someone?" or "Has anyone forced you to have sexual activities?" Generally, a husband, ex-husband, boyfriend, or relative is the abuser in domestic violence.

Most of the rapidly developing literature on domestic violence focuses on screening, diagnosis, and management, and there is little on preventing the first episode. Screening for domestic violence typically occurs in the office setting. Many authorities recommend that physicians routinely ask about domestic violence as part of the screening history.[38,39] Domestic violence occurs in homosexual relationships as well, so it is best to ask both men and women. Some physicians introduce the question by saying that they are now asking all their patients about domestic abuse, in view of the growing awareness of the problem. Then they ask, "At any time [or since I last saw you] has your husband [lover, partner, boyfriend] hit, kicked, threatened, or otherwise frightened you?" If the patient replies in the affirmative, the physician should gather more information, including the name of the abuser, and record it. Because many people are ashamed of their situation and their inability to break out of it, the physician should avoid any judgmental statements other than to confirm that what is being done to the patient is wrong.

In many cases, patients will not disclose an abusive relationship but their medical and social history contains clues to the true situation. Somatic symptoms that are particularly indicative (prevalence ratio > 2.5) of an abusive relationship include multiple symptoms (especially with no apparent physical cause), poor appetite, nightmares, eating binges, pain in the pelvic region, vaginal discharge, musculoskeletal injuries, and diarrhea.[36] Even more indicative are emotional symptoms such

as high anxiety, severe depression, a high level of somatization, and low self-esteem; current or past use of street drugs; positive items on the CAGE questionnaire for alcohol abuse; a current or past drinking problem; a husband or partner who abuses alcohol or uses street drugs; a history of suicide attempt; and abuse as a child (prevalence ratio > 10.0 for all of these).[37,40] Pregnancy is often associated with an escalation of violence.

Some abused patients will disclose a history of abuse, but many will not. Therefore, during the physical examination, the physician should be alert to signs of injury. One expert states that a woman who presents with any injury should be considered a victim of domestic abuse until proved otherwise.[39] Trauma to the face, abdomen, breasts, or genitals is especially likely to be from domestic abuse, as are bilateral or multiple injuries, injuries in different stages of healing, and injuries that occurred well before the patient sought help. Injuries to the ulnar aspect of the elbows may occur as a woman raises her hands to protect herself during an assault.

Older persons are subject to several forms of abuse: self-neglect or caregiver neglect, emotional and psychological abuse, fiduciary exploitation, and physical abuse. Signs of elder abuse include bruising and other signs of trauma, malnutrition, volume depletion, and poor hygiene.

The physician should communicate concern and validate the patient's belief that domestic abuse is wrong. The physician should not only provide medical treatment of injuries but also talk with the patient about how to avoid serious injury during an assault, review the patient's options, and facilitate referral to community and other resources for abused partners [*see Sidebar* Domestic Violence Information on the Internet].

INJURIES FROM FIREARMS

The rate of death by firearms in the United States peaked at 39,595 in 1993, and it has since declined, reaching 28,663 in 2000.[41,42] Firearms accounted for 992 accidental deaths, 13,677 homicides, and 17,767 suicides in 1997. In two large communities, 58% of suicide victims used a firearm. Seventy percent of the suicides occurred at home. Firearms kill more teenagers than all natural causes of death combined. The Bureau of Alcohol, Tobacco and Firearms estimates that there are 192 million firearms in private hands. Firearms, often bought for protection in the home, are far more dangerous to the occupants than to an intruder. After controlling for other suicide risk factors, the odds of suicide are 1.9 times greater in homes in which there is at least one gun.[43,44] The odds of homicide are 2.2 times higher in homes in which there is a firearm.[45]

Physicians strongly support regulation of firearms and community efforts to restrict ownership.[46] Physicians also have a role to play in preventing injury from firearms.[47] They should inquire about firearms in the home and counsel owners about storing their firearms in a safe place. With the increased number of teenagers who own guns and commit homicide with guns, the need to educate parents is urgent. The American Academy of Pediatrics has developed an information kit for physicians to use in counseling parents and children. The kits, called Steps To Prevent Firearm Injury In The Home, are available without charge from the Brady Center to Prevent Gun Violence, 1225 Eye Street NW, Suite 1100, Washington, DC 20005, or they can be obtained on the Internet, at http://www.bradycenter.com/stop2/.

The author has no commercial relationships with manufacturers of products or providers of services discussed in this chapter.

References

1. Mokdad AH, Marks JS, Stroup DF, et al: Actual causes of death in the United States, 2000. JAMA 291:1238, 2004

2. United States Preventive Services Task Force: Guide to Clinical Preventive Services. Williams & Wilkins, Baltimore, 1996

3. Welch HG, Albertsen PC, Nease RF, et al: Estimating treatment benefits for the elderly: the effect of competing risks. Ann Intern Med 124:577, 1996

4. Lorig K: Patient Education and Counseling. United States Preventive Services Task Force. Williams & Wilkins, Baltimore, 1996.

5. American Academy of Pediatrics: Tobacco's toll: implications for the pediatrician. Committee on Substance Abuse. Pediatrics 107:794, 2001

6. Bartecchi CE, MacKenzie TD, Schrier RW: The human costs of tobacco use. N Engl J Med 330:907, 1994

7. Diagnostic and Statistical Manual of Mental Disorders, 4th ed.: DSM-IV. American Psychiatric Association, Washington, DC, 1994

8. Kawachi I, Colditz GA, Stampfer MJ, et al: Smoking cessation and decreased risk of stroke in women. JAMA 269:232, 1993

9. Dietrich AJ, O'Connor GT, Keller A, et al: Cancer: improving early detection and prevention: a community practice randomised trial. BMJ 304:687, 1992

10. Djikstra A, Roijackers J, De Vries H: Smokers in four stages of readiness to change. Addict Behav 23:339, 1998

11. Henningfield JE: Nicotine medications for smoking cessation. N Engl J Med 333:1196, 1995

12. Silagy C, Lancaster T, Stead L, et al: Nicotine replacement therapy for smoking cessation. Cochrane Database Syst Rev (4):CD000146, 2002

13. Flegal KM, Troiano RP, Pamuk ER, et al: The influence of smoking cessation on the prevalence of overweight in the United States. N Engl J Med 333:1165, 1995

14. Heatherton TF, Kozlowski LT, Frecker RC, et al: The Fagerstrom test for nicotine dependence: a revision of the Fagerstrom Tolerance Questionnaire. Br J Addict 86:1119, 1991

15. Holm KJ, Spencer CM: Bupropion: a review of its use in the management of smoking cessation. Drugs 59:1007, 2000

16. Hurt RD, Sachs DPL, Glover ED, et al: A comparison of sustained-release bupropion and placebo for smoking cessation. N Engl J Med 337:1195, 1997

17. Institute of Medicine. Broadening the base of treatment for alcohol problems. National Academy Press, Washington, DC, 1990

18. Bien TH, Miller WR, Tonigan JS: Brief interventions for alcohol problems: a review. Addiction 88:315, 1993

19. Brief interventions and alcohol use. Effective Health Care, Bulletin No. 7. Nuffield Institute for Health Care, University of Leeds, Leeds, England, 1993

20. Kahan M, Wilson L, Becker L: Effectiveness of physician-based interventions with problem drinkers: a review. Can Med Assoc J 152:851, 1995

21. Wilk AI, Jensen NM, Havighurst TC: Meta-analysis of randomized control trials addressing brief interventions in heavy alcohol drinkers. J Gen Intern Med 12:274, 1997

22. Walsh DC, Hingson RW, Merrigan DM, et al: A randomized trial of treatment options for alcohol-abusing workers. N Engl J Med 325:775, 1991

23. Fiellin DA, O'Connor PG: Clinical practice: office-based treatment of opioid-dependent patients. N Engl J Med 347:817, 2002

24. Rivara FP, Grossman DC, Cummins P: Medical progress: injury prevention. N Engl J Med 337: 536, 1997

25. Traffic safety facts 2000. A compilation of motor vehicle crash data from the fatality analysis reporting system and the general estimates system (DOT HS 809 337). National Highway Traffic Safety Administration, US Department of Transportation. December, 2001
http://www-fars.nhtsa.dot.gov/pubs/1.pdf

26. Hunt DR, Lowenstein SR, Badgett RG, et al: Safety belt nonuse by internal medicine patients: a missed opportunity in preventive medicine. Am J Med 98:343, 1995

27. Effectiveness of occupant protection systems and their use: third report to Congress. National Highway Traffic Safety Administration, US Department of Transportation. Washington, DC, December 1996
http://www.nhtsa.dot.gov/people/injury/airbags/208con2e.html

28. Kahane CJ: Fatality reduction by airbags: analyses of accident data through early 1996 (DOT HS 808 470). National Highway Traffic Safety Administration, US Department of Transportation. Washington, DC, August 1996
www.nhtsa.dot.gov/cars/rules/regrev/evaluate/808470.html

29. The National Highway Traffic Safety Administration Motorcycle Safety Program. National Highway Traffic Safety Administration, US Department of Transportation, January 2003
http://www.nhtsa.dot.gov/people/injury/pedbimot/motorcycle/motorcycle03

30. Thompson DC, Rivara FP, Thompson R: Helmets for preventing head and facial injuries in bicyclists. Cochrane Database Syst Rev (2):CD001855, 2000

31. Bischoff HA, Stahelin HB, Dick W, et al: Effects of vitamin D and calcium supplementation on falls: a randomized controlled trial. J Bone Miner Res 18:343, 2003

32. Paganini-Hill A, Chao A, Ross RK, et al: Exercise and other risk factors in the prevention of hip fracture: the Leisure World Study. Epidemiology 2:16, 1991

33. Tinetti ME, Baker DI, McAvay G, et al: A multi-factorial intervention to reduce the risk of falling among elderly people living in the community. N Engl J Med 331:821, 1994

34. Kannus P, Parkkari J, Niemi S, et al: Prevention of hip fracture in elderly people with use of a hip protector. N Engl J Med 343:1506, 2000

35. Mallonee S, Istre GR, Rosenberg M, et al: Surveillance and prevention of residential-fire injuries. N Engl J Med 335:27, 1996

36. Bierens JJ, Knape JT, Gelissen HP: Drowning. Curr Opin Crit Care 8:578, 2002

37. McCauley J, Kern DE, Kolodner K, et al: The "battering syndrome": prevalence and clinical characteristics of domestic violence in primary care internal medicine practices. Ann Intern Med 123:737, 1995

38. Barrier PA: Domestic violence. Mayo Clin Proc 73:271, 1998

39. Alpert EJ: Violence in intimate relationships and the practicing internist: new "disease" or new agenda? Ann Intern Med 123:774, 1995

40. Kyriacou DN, McCabe F, Anglin D, et al: Emergency department–based study of risk factors for acute injury from domestic violence against women. Ann Emerg Med 31:502, 1998

41. Nonfatal and fatal firearm-related injuries—United States, 1993–1997. MMWR Morb Mortal Wkly Rep 48:1029, 1999

42. Deaths: Final Data for 2000. National vital statistics reports, vol 50, no 15. National Center for Health Statistics, Hyattsville, Maryland, 2002

43. Miller M, Azrael D, Hemenway D: Household firearm ownership and suicide rates in the United States. Epidemiology 13:517, 2002

44. Cummings P, Koepsell TD: Does owning a firearm increase or decrease risk of death? JAMA 280:471, 1998

45. Kellerman AL, Rivera FP, Rushforth NB, et al: Gun ownership as a risk factor for homicide in the home. N Engl J Med 329:1084, 1993

46. Cassel CK, Nelson EA, Smith TW, et al: Internists' and surgeons' attitudes toward guns and firearm injury prevention. Ann Intern Med 128:224, 1998

47. American College of Physicians: Firearm injury prevention. Ann Intern Med 128:236, 1998

Acknowledgment

Figure 1   Marcia Kammerer. Adapted from life table from the Vital Statistics of the United States, 1999.

4 Diet and Exercise

Harvey B. Simon, M.D., F.A.C.P.

Many chronic diseases result from unhealthful eating and a sedentary lifestyle. Poor nutrition and inadequate exercise substantially increase the risk of such maladies as coronary artery disease, hypertension, stroke, diabetes, obesity, osteoporosis, and certain cancers and account for about 400,000 deaths in the United States each year.[1] Dietary factors also contribute to cholelithiasis, hemorrhoids, hernias, constipation, irritable bowel syndrome, and diverticulosis. A rigorous program that combines a low-fat, high-fiber diet with daily exercise can produce dramatic improvement in cardiovascular risk factors in as little as 3 weeks' time.[2]

Diet

In the 20th century, the average American diet shifted from one based on fresh, minimally processed vegetable foods to one based on animal products and highly refined, processed foods. As a result, Americans now consume far more calories, fat, cholesterol, refined sugar, animal protein, sodium, and alcohol and far less fiber and starch than is healthful.

In the United States, 35% of adults are overweight (body mass index [BMI] of 25 to 29.9), 30% are obese (BMI of 30 to 39.9), and 5% are extremely obese (MBI > 40).[3] The consequences include a substantial decrease in life expectancy and an increase in morbidity similar in magnitude to the burden imposed by smoking.[4]

Obesity is a complex, multifactorial disorder, but an element common to all cases is a positive energy balance in which more calories are consumed than expended. During the obesity epidemic of the past 4 decades, portion size and caloric intake have increased,[5] but exercise has not. Excess calories are stored in body fat; each pound of adipose tissue contains 3,500 calories. Weight loss is accomplished only by achieving a negative energy balance.

ENERGY

Genetic, metabolic, and behavioral variables make it difficult to predict an individual's caloric requirements with precision. However, physicians can provide estimates: sedentary adults require about 30 cal/kg/day to maintain body weight; moderately active adults require 35 cal/kg/day; and very active adults require 40 cal/kg/day. On average, therefore, a 70 kg (154 lb) person can expect to maintain body weight by consuming 2,100 to 2,800 calories daily.

Although any source of dietary energy, including carbohydrate, protein, and alcohol, can be converted in the body to fatty acids and cholesterol, the caloric value of foods varies considerably; for example, fat provides 9 cal/g and alcohol provides 7 cal/g, but protein and carbohydrates each provide only 4 cal/g. Patients with excess body fat should be encour-aged to reduce their caloric intake by reducing portion size and restricting the intake of calorie-dense foods. As an example, to lose 1 lb a week, patients must consume 500 fewer calories than they expend each day; in almost all cases, sustained weight loss requires both an energy-restricted diet and regular vigorous exercise.

FAT AND CHOLESTEROL

Structure

Most dietary lipids are triglycerides, in which three fatty acids are joined to one glycerol molecule. At the core of every fatty acid is a chain of carbon atoms with a methyl group at one end and a carboxyl group at the other [see Figure 1]. The biologic properties of fatty acids are determined by the presence or absence of double bonds between carbon atoms, the number and location of the double bonds, and the configuration of the molecules.

Most of the fatty acids in foods are composed of an even number of carbon atoms, generally in chains of 12 to 22 atoms. The number of double bonds between carbon atoms determines the saturation of fats. Fatty acids with no double bonds are fully saturated; they have no room for additional hydrogen atoms. Fatty acids with one double bond are monounsaturated, and those with two or more double bonds are polyunsaturated.

Fatty acids contain zero to six double bonds, where additional hydrogen atoms can be attached. The location of the double bonds is of great physiologic importance; an unsaturated fatty acid's group (i.e., omega-3, omega-6, or omega-9) is determined by the position of the double bond closest to the methyl group. In omega-3 fatty acids, for example, three carbon atoms lie between the methyl end of the chain and the first double bond.

Most of the fatty acids in natural foods are in the curved, or *cis*, configuration. When hydrogen is added back to unsaturated fats during food manufacturing, however, the molecules assume a straightened, or *trans*, configuration [see Figure 1].

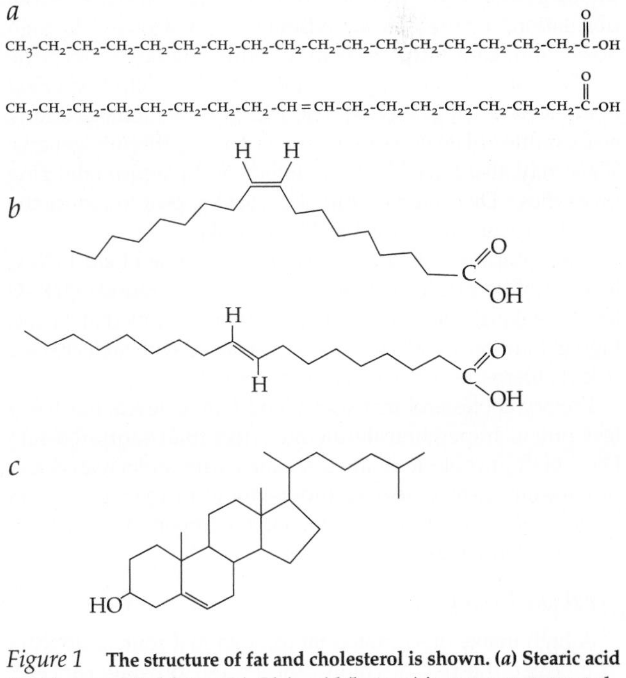

Figure 1 The structure of fat and cholesterol is shown. (*a*) Stearic acid (top) is a saturated fatty acid. Oleic acid (bottom) is a monounsaturated omega-9 fatty acid. (*b*) Oleic acid (top) displays a *cis* double bond. Elaidic acid (bottom) displays a *trans* double bond. (*c*) Cholesterol has a structure similar to that of fatty acids.

Cholesterol is a waxy, fatlike molecule that is present in the membranes of all animal cells but is absent from plant cells. Although cholesterol is a sterol rather than a true fat, its metabolism is intimately linked to the dietary intake of fatty acids.

Effects on Blood Lipid Levels and Cardiovascular Risk

Although all fats have the same caloric value (9 cal/g), their effects on human health vary greatly, largely because of their disparate effects on blood cholesterol levels. Saturated fats stimulate hepatic cholesterol production, thus increasing blood cholesterol levels. Of the four saturated fatty acids that predominate in the American diet, myristic acid (14 carbons) has the most potent hypercholesterolemic effect, followed by palmitic acid (16 carbons) and lauric acid (12 carbons). Stearic acid (18 carbons) has little effect on blood cholesterol levels. Evidence strongly suggests that the degree to which saturated fat and cholesterol intake increase the risk of coronary artery disease depends on their effects on blood cholesterol concentration.[6]

Unsaturated fatty acids are generally derived from vegetable and marine sources; they are often called oils rather than fats because they are liquid at room temperature. When monounsaturated or polyunsaturated fatty acids are substituted for saturated fats, blood cholesterol levels fall. Neither type of unsaturated fat, however, has a direct ability to lower low-density lipoprotein cholesterol (LDL-C) or raise high-density lipoprotein cholesterol (HDL-C) levels. Although monounsaturated and polyunsaturated fats have a similar, generally neutral, effect on blood cholesterol levels, monounsaturated fats are less susceptible to oxidation and may therefore be less atherogenic. Omega-3 polyunsaturated fatty acids in particular have been shown to have a cardioprotective effect.

Consumption of omega-3 fatty acids is inversely related to the incidence of death from coronary artery disease,[7] atrial fibrillation,[8] ventricular arrhythmias,[9] and strokes.[10] In high doses, omega-3 fatty acids may reduce blood triglyceride levels,[11] but in dietary amounts, they have little effect on blood lipid levels. Even in modest amounts, however, omega-3 fatty acids reduce platelet aggregation, impairing thrombogenesis. They may also have antiarrhythmic[8,9] and plaque-stabilizing properties.[12] Diets high in α-linolenic acid appear to reduce the risk of coronary artery disease[13,14] and stroke.

Like saturated fats, trans-fatty acids increase blood LDL-C levels; unlike saturated fats, trans-fatty acids reduce HDL-C levels, making trans-fatty acids even more detrimental.[15] Diets high in trans-fatty acids have been associated with an increased risk of atherosclerosis and coronary events.[6]

Dietary cholesterol increases blood LDL-C levels but has a less potent hypercholesterolemic effect than saturated fat.[6] Diets high in cholesterol are associated with an increased risk of coronary artery disease independent of their effects on blood cholesterol levels,[13] reinforcing the importance of reducing cholesterol intake.

Fat and Health

A high intake of saturated fat from animal sources appears to increase the risk of colon cancer[16] and prostate cancer.[17] However, a modest reduction in total dietary fat does not reduce the risk of colon cancer.[18]

Some dietary fat is essential. For example, omega-3 and omega-6 fatty acids cannot be synthesized endogenously and therefore must be obtained from food. Dietary fat is required for the absorption of fat-soluble vitamins. Lipids are essential components of cell membranes and steroid hormones; adipose tissue is the body's major energy depot, and it provides insulation against heat loss. As little as 15 to 25 g of dietary fat a day can provide essential physiologic functions.

Dietary Recommendations

The American Heart Association (AHA) dietary guidelines[19] for healthy adults suggest that no more than 30% of calories should come from fat, with less than 10% coming from saturated fat and the remainder coming from unsaturated fat in vegetables, fish, legumes, and nuts. The AHA guidelines also specify consumption of less than 300 mg of cholesterol a day. Patients with atherosclerosis or diabetes and persons who are hyperlipidemic or obese should follow more stringent limits, such as a saturated-fat intake of no more than 7% of daily calories, with a corresponding decrease in cholesterol consumption to less than 200 mg a day. In some persons, very low fat diets providing 15% to 22% of calories from fat can reduce blood HDL levels and produce other adverse effects[20,21]; however, in carefully monitored high-risk persons, diets with about 10% fat and virtually no cholesterol have been beneficial.[22] Although reductions in total fat intake can help reduce body fat and serum cholesterol levels, the risk of coronary artery disease may depend more on the type of fat in the diet; saturated fats and trans-fatty acids are the most atherogenic, whereas monounsaturated and omega-3 fatty acids are the most desirable [see Table 1].[6,19]

Food labels list the fat, saturated fat, trans-fatty acid, and cholesterol contents of packaged foods; consumers should be advised to read them carefully and to be sure the portion sizes used for the computations are realistic.

Table 1 Recommended Daily Intake of Fat and Other Nutrients*

Nutrient	Recommended Intake
Total fat	20%–35% of total calories
Saturated fat[†]	< 7% of total calories
Polyunsaturated fat	≤ 10% of total calories
Monounsaturated fat	≤ 20% of total calories
Cholesterol	< 300 mg/day 50%–60% of total calories
Carbohydrate[††]	≥ 25 g/day
Fiber	15% of total calories
Protein	—
Total calories[§]	Balance energy intake and expenditure to maintain desirable body weight and prevent weight gain

*See reference 19.
[†]Trans-fatty acids, which raise low-density lipoprotein (LDL) and lower high-density lipoprotein (HDL) cholesterol, should also be kept at low levels.
[††]Carbohydrates should be derived predominantly from foods rich in complex carbohydrates, including grains, especially whole grains, fruits, and vegetables. Simple sugars should contribute no more than 25% of total calories.
[§]Daily energy expenditure should include at least moderate physical activity (consuming 200 kcal/day).

Table 2 Types of Dietary Fiber
and Representative Food Sources

Fiber Type	Food Sources
Gums*	Oats, beans, legumes, guar
Pectin*	Apples, citrus fruits, soybeans, cauliflower, squash, cabbage, carrots, green beans, potatoes
Mucilage*	Psyllium
Hemicellulose*†	Barley, wheat bran and whole grains, brussels sprouts, beet roots
Lignin†	Green beans, strawberries, peaches, pears, radishes
Cellulose†	Root vegetables, cabbage, wheat and corn, peas, beans, broccoli, peppers, apples

*Soluble fiber.
†Insoluble fiber.

CARBOHYDRATES

Carbohydrates are a vital source of energy for metabolic processes. They are also vital constituents of nucleic acids, glycoproteins, and cell membranes.

Plants are the principal dietary sources of carbohydrates. The only important carbohydrates that originate from animal sources are the lactose in milk and the glycogen in muscle and liver. Carbohydrate-rich foods contain varying amounts of simple and complex carbohydrates. Simple carbohydrates include monosaccharides such as glucose, fructose, and galactose and disaccharides such as sucrose (table sugar), maltose, and lactose. Complex carbohydrates include polysaccharides (e.g., starch and glycogen that can be digested into sugars by intestinal enzymes) and fiber (i.e., high-molecular-weight carbohydrates that cannot be split into sugars by human intestinal enzymes). Sugars, starches, and glycogen provide 4 cal/g; because fiber is indigestible, it has virtually no caloric value.

Carbohydrates contribute about 50% of the calories in the average American diet—half from sugar and half from complex carbohydrates. Because sugars are more rapidly absorbed, they have a higher glycemic index than starches. In addition to provoking higher insulin levels, carbohydrates with a high glycemic index appear to reduce HDL-C levels[23] and may increase the risk of coronary artery disease, diabetes, and obesity.[24,25] Processed foods containing simple sugars are often calorie dense, whereas foods that are rich in complex carbohydrates provide vitamins, trace minerals, and other valuable nutrients. A healthful diet should provide 55% to 65% of calories from complex carbohydrates found in fresh fruits and vegetables, legumes, and whole grains.[19]

DIETARY FIBER

Dietary fiber is a heterogeneous mix of very long chain branched carbohydrates that resist digestion by human intestinal enzymes because of the ways their monosaccharide components are linked to one another. Fiber is found only in plants, particularly in the bran of whole grains, in the stems and leaves of vegetables, and in fruits, seeds, and nuts. The two general categories of dietary fiber are soluble and insoluble.

Soluble fiber delays gastric emptying, which produces a sensation of satiety, and slows the absorption of digestible carbohydrates, which reduces insulin levels. Soluble fiber also lowers blood cholesterol levels, probably by inhibiting bile

acid and nutrient absorption in the small intestine and by promoting bile acid sequestration by colonic bacteria.[26] Because soluble fiber is metabolized by these bacteria, it has little effect on fecal bulk. In contrast, insoluble fiber increases the water content and bulk of feces and shortens intestinal transit time [*see Table 2*].

Diets that are high in fiber also tend to be low in fat. Such diets have been associated with a reduced risk of intestinal disorders, including constipation, irritable bowel syndrome, cholelithiasis, hemorrhoids, and diverticulosis. Although studies have suggested that a very high intake of fiber may substantially reduce the risk of colorectal cancer,[27,28] a pooled analysis of 13 trials reported that the apparent protective effect of fiber was attenuated by corrections for other dietary factors.[29] However, a dietary pattern that includes a high intake of fruits, vegetables, legumes, fish, poultry, and whole grains but little red meat, processed meats, sweets, or refined grains appears protective.[30] A high intake of fiber is associated with a reduced risk of diabetes[31]; in patients with diabetes, it is associated with improved glycemic control and decreased blood lipids.[32] It is also associated with a reduced risk of obesity[33] and coronary artery disease[34,35] and a lower all-cause mortality.[36] The Institute of Medicine recommends 38 g of fiber a day for men younger than 50 years and 30 g a day for older men; for women, the recommended intake of fiber is 30 g a day before age 50 and 21 g a day thereafter.[37]

PROTEINS

Unlike reserves of fat (which is stored in large amounts as triglyceride in adipose tissue) and reserves of carbohydrate (which is stored in small amounts as glycogen in liver and muscle), there are no endogenous reserves of amino acids or protein; all the proteins in the body are serving a structural or metabolic function. As a result, bodily function can be impaired if proteins are catabolized because of energy deficiency, wasting diseases, or dietary protein intake that is not sufficient to replace protein losses.

All proteins in human cells are continuously catabolized and resynthesized. In a healthy 70 kg adult, about 280 g of protein is degraded and replaced daily. In addition, about 30 g of protein is lost externally through the urine (urea), feces, and skin.

In healthy adults, daily protein losses can be fully replaced by as little as 0.4 g/kg. Because not all dietary proteins are fully digestible, the recommended dietary allowance (RDA) of protein for healthy adults is 0.8 g/kg. People who exercise strenuously on a regular basis may benefit from extra protein to maintain muscle mass; a daily intake of about 1 g/kg has been recommended for athletes. Women who are pregnant or lactating require up to 30 g/day in addition to their basal requirements. To support growth, children should consume 2 g/kg/day.

A healthful diet should provide 10% to 15% of its calories from protein.[19] For healthy, nonpregnant women, an intake of 44 to 50 g/day of protein is required; for men, an intake of 45 to 63 g/day of protein is needed. Although excessive protein intake has not been proved to be harmful, there are several potential disadvantages to a very high protein intake. The protein in foods derived from animals is often accompanied by large amounts of fat. In the body, excessive protein can be transaminated to carbohydrate, adding to the energy surplus responsible for obesity. When excess protein is eliminated from the body as urinary nitrogen, it is often accompanied by increased urinary calcium, perhaps increasing the risk of nephrolithiasis and osteoporosis. Because nitrogen is excreted in the urine, high dietary protein intake is associated with an increase in renal plasma flow and glomerular filtration rates and, eventually, with increased renal size. In some animal models, increased dietary protein is associated with accelerated renal aging; and in humans with kidney disease, high dietary protein intake is associated with more rapid disease progression.[38] On the other hand, high dietary protein intake appears linked to somewhat reduced blood pressure readings,[39] possibly because of increased urinary sodium losses; protein supplements may be beneficial for patients with acute or chronic illnesses.[40]

The thousands of proteins in the human body are synthesized from just 21 amino acids. Most amino acids can be synthesized endogenously, but nine cannot. Not all dietary proteins contain all nine essential amino acids; in particular, vegetable proteins may be incomplete. However, by eating a varied diet with foods that contain a mix of proteins, even strict vegetarians can obtain all the amino acids they need. In fact, diets high in vegetable proteins are associated with a lower risk of coronary artery disease than diets high in animal proteins (e.g., red meats).[41]

VITAMIN AND MINERAL CONSUMPTION

Vitamins

Vitamins are either fat soluble or water soluble. Vitamins A, D, E, and K are fat soluble. They are found in fatty foods and are absorbed, transported, and stored with fat. Because excretion is minimal and storage in fat is abundant, deficiencies of fat-soluble vitamins are rare, but toxic amounts can accumulate if intake is excessive. Vitamin C and the B-complex group are water soluble; they are absorbed in the intestine, bound to transport proteins, and excreted in the urine. Because storage is minimal, water-soluble vitamins should be ingested regularly; toxicity is rare except in cases involving the ingestion of large doses of vitamin B_3 and B_6 [see Table 3].

Although there is great disparity between popular beliefs about vitamins and their known physiologic effects, new medical information may narrow the gap. It is clear that many persons in the United States, particularly the elderly and the poor, do not consume adequate amounts of vitamin-rich foods. Laboratory and animal experiments demonstrate that antioxidant vitamins can retard atherogenesis and suggest that antioxidants may lower the risk of carcinogenesis. Epidemiologic and observational studies have indicated an association between a low dietary intake or low plasma levels of antioxidants and an increased risk of atherosclerosis and certain cancers; however, randomized clinical trials have failed to demonstrate benefit from antioxidant supplements.[42,43] Moreover, β-carotene supplements actually appear to increase the risk of lung cancer in smokers,[44] and hypervitaminosis A is linked to an increased risk of fractures.[45] Similarly, studies have linked low levels of folic acid, vitamin B_6, and vitamin B_{12} with elevated blood homocysteine levels and a heightened risk of coronary artery disease,[46] stroke, and dementia,[47] but early trials of folic acid supplements have not demonstrated benefit.[48,49] It is clear that additional studies are required to clarify the impact of vitamins on health.

Women of childbearing age, the elderly, and people with suboptimal nutrition should take a single multivitamin tablet daily; others may benefit as well.[50] Strict vegetarians should take vitamin B_{12} in the recommended daily amount (2–4 μg); because many people older than 60 years have atrophic gastritis and cannot absorb B_{12} bound to food protein, they may also benefit from supplementary B_{12}. Multivitamin supplements may also be necessary to avert vitamin D deficiencies, particularly in the elderly.[51] A supplement that combines antioxidants with zinc can slow the progression of age-related macular degeneration.[52] Use of so-called megadose vitamins should be discouraged. Expensive brand-name and so-called all-natural preparations are no more effective than reputable generic preparations. In any case, vitamin supplements should never be used as a substitute for a balanced, healthful diet that provides abundant amounts of vitamin-rich foods.

Minerals

Although minerals are chemically the simplest of nutrients, their roles in metabolism and health are complex. At least 16 minerals are essential for health [see Table 4]; 10 are classified as trace elements because only small amounts are required. Other minerals, such as boron, nickel, vanadium, and silicon, have been shown to be essential in various animal studies but have not been found to be necessary for humans. Many persons in the United States consume too little of some minerals (e.g., calcium and iron) or too much of others (e.g., sodium).

Sodium The body can conserve sodium so effectively that only small amounts are required in the diet. The Food and Nutrition Board of the National Academy of Science estimates that an intake of no more than 500 mg of sodium a day is needed for health; the average American diet contains more than 4,000 mg a day.

Population studies have demonstrated conclusively that a high sodium intake increases blood pressure, especially in older people.[53] The Dietary Approaches to Stop Hypertension (DASH) trial demonstrated that reduction of sodium intake from high amounts to moderate amounts will result in lower blood pressures and that further reductions in sodium intake will produce additional benefits.[54] When combined with other elements of the DASH diet (i.e., increased consumption of fruits, vegetables, whole grains, and low-fat dairy products, along with decreased consumption of saturated fat and sugar), sodium restriction can lower systolic blood pressure by an average of 7.1 mm Hg in normotensive persons and 11.5 mm Hg in patients with hypertension. Hence, reductions in dietary sodium could substantially reduce the risk of stroke and coronary artery disease. A high sodium intake also increases urinary calcium excretion, which in turn increases the risk of osteoporosis.

There is no RDA for sodium, and additional controlled clinical trials are needed to provide conclusive evidence that sodium restriction is beneficial to normotensive persons. Pending such information, the AHA recommends that daily consumption of sodium not exceed 2,400 mg.[19] Dietary guidelines published by the United States Department of Agriculture (USDA) recommend a 2,300 mg daily maximum intake of sodium[55]; the Institute of Medicine proposes a limit of 1,500 mg of dietary sodium a day.[56] Patients with illnesses such as hypertension, congestive heart failure, cirrhosis, and nephrotic syndrome may benefit from substantially lower sodium intakes.

Table 3 The Vitamins

Vitamin	Functions	Deficiency Effects	Toxic Effects	Sources	RDA for Adults*
A (retinol, retinoic acid)	Vision, epithelial integrity; possible protection against epithelial cancers and atherosclerosis	Night blindness; increased susceptibility to infection	Teratogenicity, hepatotoxicity, cerebral edema, desquamation; yellowish skin discoloration by carotenoids; increased fracture risk	Liver, dairy products, eggs; dark-green and yellow-orange vegetables (carotenoids)	Men, 3,000 IU or 900 µg Women, 2,333 IU or 700 µg
B_1 (thiamine)	Metabolism of carbohydrates, alcohol, and branched-chain amino acids	Beriberi, Wernicke-Korsakoff syndrome	None	Grains, legumes, nuts, poultry, meat	Men, 1.2 mg Women, 1.1 mg
B_2 (riboflavin)	Cellular oxidation-reduction reactions	Stomatitis, dermatitis, anemia	None	Grains, dairy products, meat, eggs, dark-green vegetables	Men, 1.3 mg Women, 1.1 mg
B_3 (niacin, nicotinic acid)	Oxidative metabolism; reduces LDL cholesterol; increases HDL cholesterol	Pellagra	Flushing, headaches, pruritus, hyperglycemia, hyperuricemia, hepatotoxicity	Meat, poultry, fish, grains, peanuts; synthesized from tryptophan in foods	Men, 16 mg Women, 14 mg
B_6 (pyridoxine)	Amino acid metabolism and heme synthesis; neuronal excitability; reduces blood homocysteine levels	Anemia, cheilosis, dermatitis	Neurotoxicity	Meat, poultry, fish, grains, soybeans, bananas, nuts	Men 19–50 yr, 1.3 mg; men ≥ 50 yr, 1.7 mg Women 19–50 yr, 1.3 mg; women ≥ 50 yr, 1.5 mg
B_{12} (cobalamin)	DNA synthesis (with folate); myelin synthesis (without folate); reduces blood homocysteine levels	Megaloblastic anemia, neuropathies	None	Meat (especially liver), poultry, fish, dairy products	2.4 µg
Folic acid	DNA synthesis (with B_{12}); reduces blood homocysteine levels	Megaloblastic anemia, birth defects	None	Vegetables, legumes, grains, fruit, poultry, meat	400 µg
Biotin	Metabolic processes	Rare	None	Many foods	30 µg
Pantothenic acid	Metabolic processes	Rare	None	Many foods	5 mg
C (ascorbic acid)	Collagen synthesis; possible protection against certain neoplasms	Scurvy	Nephrolithiasis, diarrhea	Fruits, green vegetables, potatoes, cereals	Men, 90 mg Women, 75 mg
D (calciferol)	Intestinal calcium absorption	Osteomalacia and rickets	Hypercalcemia	Fortified dairy products, fatty fish, egg yolks, liver	< 50 yr, 200 IU; 50–70 yr, 400 IU; > 70 yr, 600 IU
E (α-tocopherol)	Reduces peroxidation of fatty acids: possible protection against atherosclerosis	Rare	Antagonism of vitamin K, possible headaches	Vegetable oils, wheat germ, nuts, broccoli	15 mg
K	Synthesis of clotting factors VII, IX, X, and possibly V	Hemorrhagic diathesis	None	Leafy green vegetables (K_1), intestinal bacteria (K_2)	Men, 120 µg Women, 90 µg

*RDAs during pregnancy and lactation may differ.
HDL—high-density lipoprotein   IU—international units   LDL—low-density lipoprotein   RDA—recommended dietary allowance

About 80% of dietary sodium comes from processed foods. Physicians should review these hidden sources of salt with patients who would benefit from sodium restriction.

Calcium   A high intake of calcium, either from dairy products or supplements,[57] improves bone density but does not appear to provide protection from bone fracture[58]; high-dose vitamin D may be effective in reducing fracture risk.[59] Dietary calcium intake is inversely related to blood pressure[60] and to the risk of stroke[60,61]; calcium supplements, on the other hand, produce only small reductions in systolic blood pressure.[62] Calcium supplements appear to reduce the risk of colorectal adenomas,[63] but high doses may increase the risk of prostate cancer.[64]

At present, fewer than 50% of persons in the United States consume the RDA of calcium [*see Table 4*]. Persons who do not consume enough calcium from foods should consider a supplement such as calcium carbonate or calcium citrate. High-calcium diets do not increase the risk of nephrolithiasis,[65] but prolonged overdoses of supplements may produce hypercalcemia (milk-alkali syndrome) or nephrolithiasis.

Iron   Iron deficiency is the most common cause of anemia. In the United States, 9% to 11% of women of childbearing age are iron deficient, and 2% to 5% have iron deficiency anemia; only 1% of men are iron deficient. Routine administration of

Table 4 Essential Minerals and Trace Elements

Minerals and Elements	RDA/ESADDI for Healthy Individuals
Macrominerals	
Calcium	1,000 mg before age 50; 1,200 mg after age 50
Phosphorus	700 mg
Magnesium	Men, 350 mg; women, 280 mg
Potassium	1,700–5,100 mg
Trace elements	
Iron	Men and postmenopausal women, 8 mg; premenopausal women, 18 mg; pregnant women, 27 mg
Chromium	Men 19–50 yr, 35 µg; men ≥ 50 yr, 30 µg; women 19–50 yr, 25 µg; women ≥ 50 yr, 20 µg
Cobalt	Required in small amounts as a component of vitamin B_{12}
Copper	900 µg
Fluoride	Men, 4 mg; women, 3 mg
Iodine	150 µg
Manganese	Men, 2.3 mg; women, 1.8 mg
Molybdenum	45 µg
Selenium	55 µg
Zinc	Men, 11 mg; women, 8 mg

ESADDI—estimated safe and adequate daily dietary intake   RDA—recommended dietary allowance

iron supplements is recommended only for infants and pregnant women[66]; dietary sources should provide adequate amounts of iron for other healthy people. However, vegetarians who exclude all animal products from their diet may need almost twice as much dietary iron each day as nonvegetarians because of the lower intestinal absorption of the nonheme form of iron derived from plant foods.[67] Good sources of nonheme iron include chick peas, spinach, molasses, figs, and apricots.

A high intake of iron is harmful for patients with hemochromatosis and for others at risk for iron overload. A Finnish study linked high iron levels to cardiac risk. However, studies in the United States have not confirmed these observations, and one study indicated a possible inverse association between iron stores and mortality from cardiovascular disease and other causes.[68]

Potassium   Dietary potassium is inversely related to blood pressure and to stroke mortality in hypertensive men.[69] Although potassium supplements may assist in the treatment of hypertension,[70] current data do not justify the routine use of potassium supplements. Physicians should encourage a high dietary potassium intake in most individuals,[19,54] but low-potassium diets may be necessary for patients with renal disease or other conditions that cause hyperkalemia. For most people, a diet rich in vegetables and fruits provides all of the potassium needed.

Selenium   Selenium is a cofactor of the free radical scavenger enzyme glutathione peroxidase. A randomized clinical trial reported that selenium supplements of 200 µg/day appear to reduce mortality from various cancers.[71] Selenium levels have been inversely associated with mortality from prostate cancer[72] and gastroesophageal malignancies.[73] These data, however, do not yet support the routine use of selenium supplements, which can be toxic in high doses. Selenium is present in many foods, including tomatoes, poultry, shellfish, garlic, meat, egg yolks, and grains grown in selenium-rich soil.

Chromium   Chromium plays a role in glucose metabolism,[74] and low chromium levels are associated with an increased risk of coronary artery disease.[75] There is no scientific basis for the claims that chromium supplements contribute to weight loss or increased energy. Chromium supplements may be beneficial for persons with low HDL-C levels, but more study is needed. Dietary sources of chromium include brewer's yeast, whole grains, legumes, peanuts, and meats.

Magnesium   Magnesium deficiency is common in diabetic patients, persons with alcoholism, patients who take diuretics, and hospitalized patients. Persons with hypomagnesemia may require magnesium supplements, but others can rely on foods such as green vegetables, whole grains, bananas, apricots, legumes, nuts, soybeans, and seafood to provide magnesium.

WATER AND FOOD CONSUMPTION

Water

On average, adults consume about 2 L/day of water, with two thirds coming from beverages and the remainder coming from food. Healthy people have no need to track their water intake. Patients with conditions such as nephrolithiasis and urinary tract infections may benefit from consciously increasing their fluid intake; patients who are at risk for hyponatremia should restrict their water consumption.

Foods

Fruits and vegetables   Fruits and vegetables provide many desirable nutrients, including complex carbohydrates, fiber, vitamins, and minerals. Deep-green and yellow-orange vegetables may be particularly beneficial because of their carotenoids, and citrus fruits may be valuable because of their vitamin C, soluble fiber, and potassium. Cruciferous vegetables, such as cabbage, may reduce the risk of certain cancers. Vegetables and fruits are low in sodium and calories; none contain cholesterol, and only coconut, palm oil, and cocoa butter contain saturated fat.

Findings of many case-control and cohort studies strongly suggest that the consumption of fruits and vegetables is inversely related to the risk of coronary artery disease,[76] stroke,[77] malignancies of the respiratory and digestive tracts,[29] chronic obstructive pulmonary disease,[78] and all-cause mortality[79]; however, an observational study did not support these findings.[80] A dietary-intervention trial demonstrated that a diet rich in vegetables, fruits, and low-fat dairy products can substantially reduce blood pressure.[54] The USDA dietary guidelines recommend eating two to four servings of fruit and three to five servings of vegetables a day; at present, only 35% of women and 19% of men meet these standards.[81]

Legumes   Often neglected in the Western diet, legumes (beans, peas, and lentils) are rich in complex carbohydrates with low glycemic indices, iron, and B vitamins. Legumes are an excellent source of dietary fiber, including soluble fiber that can reduce blood cholesterol levels. Because of their high protein content, legumes are an excellent meat substitute. Soy protein can reduce blood cholesterol[82] and blood pressure[83] levels, and soy intake is inversely related to the risk of prostate and breast cancers.

Legumes can increase intestinal gas, causing bloating, flatulence, and cramps. Distress can be minimized by use of the nonprescription α-galactosidase preparation Beano.

Grains The seed-bearing fruits of grains, called kernels, consist of three layers: the inner germ, which contains vitamins and polyunsaturated fats; the middle endosperm, which contains complex carbohydrates; and the outer bran, which contains dietary fiber. Because milling removes the bran and endosperm, whole grains are nutritionally superior to refined grain; whole-grain consumption is inversely related to the risk of diabetes,[31] coronary artery disease,[34,35] all-cause mortality,[36] and possibly stroke.[84,85] Whole-grain flour can be used to make cereals, baked goods, and even pasta. Whole grains such as brown rice, couscous, and yellow cornmeal (polenta) are easily prepared and healthful side dishes. Oats and barley contain soluble fiber that can lower blood cholesterol levels.

Meat and poultry Although meat is a source of protein, vitamins, and iron and other minerals, its high content of saturated fat, cholesterol, and calories makes it a potentially unhealthy food. Patients who eat meat should be encouraged to select lean cuts, trim away visible fat, and use cooking methods that remove, rather than add, fat. It is even more beneficial to reduce the amount of meat consumed by reducing portion size and frequency; a reasonable goal is to eat about 4 oz one to three times a week.

Poultry is a more healthful source of protein and other nutrients. Chicken and turkey are best, but the skin should be removed before cooking to reduce the fat content.

Dairy products and eggs To reduce the intake of saturated fat and cholesterol, nonfat or low-fat dairy products can be substituted for whole-milk products. The use of nondairy creamers, imitation cheese, margarine, and other products that contain *trans*-fatty acids in partially hydrogenated vegetable oils should be limited. The consumption of up to one egg a day does not appear to increase the risk of cardiovascular disease in healthy, nondiabetic people,[86] but additional egg-yolk consumption should be limited. One egg yolk contains about two thirds of the total amount of cholesterol that is recommended for an entire day. Egg whites and egg substitutes are good alternatives to egg yolks.

Fish Fish consumption is inversely related to the risk of coronary artery disease[9] and stroke.[10] A 1989 intervention trial that randomized 2,033 myocardial infarction survivors to usual care or usual care plus fish consumption found that eating two or three fish meals a week reduced 7-year mortality by 29%.[87] Fish consumption has also been associated with a reduced risk of primary cardiac arrest,[88] hypertension,[15] and prostate cancer.[89] As little as 4 oz of fish twice a week may provide protection.[90] Fish should be baked, broiled, grilled, steamed, or poached rather than fried, and high-fat sauces should be avoided. Because of their higher content of omega-3 fatty acids, oily deep-water fish may be best. People who are reluctant to eat fish may benefit from fish oil supplements in the modest dose of about 1 g/day.[90]

Cooking oils Canola oil contains an omega-3 fatty acid, α-linolenic acid. High serum levels of α-linolenic acid have been associated with a decreased risk of stroke, and consumption of canola oil is inversely related to the risk of myocardial infarction.[13] Canola oil and olive oil have a high content of oxidation-resistant monounsaturated fatty acids. Olive oil may be a cardioprotective element in the Mediterranean diet. Although more study is needed, canola and olive oils appear to be the most beneficial oils for food preparation.

Nuts Nuts are high in monounsaturated and polyunsaturated fatty acids and fiber. Nut consumption appears to be inversely related to the risk of coronary artery disease[91] and diabetes.[92]

Garlic Medical studies of garlic have shown mixed results. Some meta-analyses suggest that garlic extracts can improve blood cholesterol levels, but others do not.[93] The putative benefits of garlic on blood pressure and coagulation are even less clear.

Flavonoid-rich foods Flavonoids are polyphenolic antioxidants that are found in a variety of foods, including apples, onions, tea, and red wine. Although not all studies agree, consumption of these foods has been inversely related to the risk of coronary artery disease and stroke.[94]

Alcohol Rarely regarded as a nutrient, alcohol should be considered when dietary recommendations are formulated. Containing 7 cal/g, alcohol is a calorie-dense food. Numerous studies demonstrate that low to moderate alcohol consumption substantially reduces the risk of coronary artery disease, peripheral vascular disease, and all-cause mortality.[95] The major mechanism of protection is alcohol's ability to increase HDL-C levels; favorable effects on blood coagulation mechanisms may also contribute. Protective doses of alcohol can be obtained from one to two drinks a day; 5 oz of wine, 12 oz of beer, or 1.5 oz of spirits is counted as one drink. Despite its antioxidant content, red wine is no more protective than other alcoholic beverages.[96]

Caffeine Studies have failed to confirm putative links between caffeine and hypertension,[97] peptic ulcers, coronary artery disease, breast disease, or cancer. Caffeine can trigger migraines in sensitive individuals, and caffeine withdrawal can precipitate headaches or depression in habitual consumers. Caffeine can cause anxiety, insomnia, and gastroesophageal reflux. Brewed coffee can increase blood cholesterol levels, but filtered coffee does not. The effects of caffeine on pregnancy are not fully understood, but it is wise to discourage consumption.[98] Caffeine restriction does not reduce palpitations in patients with idiopathic premature ventricular contractions.[99]

DIET AND HEALTH

Much remains to be learned about the complex relation between nutrition, health, and disease. Dietary preferences are no less complex and individual. Despite these uncertainties, a dietary pattern characterized by a high intake of vegetables, fruits, legumes, whole grains, fish, and poultry is associated with major health benefits for men[100] and women.[101] Physicians have an important role in educating patients about healthful nutrition and in providing dietary guidelines [*see* Table 5].

Table 5 Dietary Guidelines for Healthy People

Eat more vegetable products than animal products
Eat more fresh and homemade foods than processed foods
Less than 30% of calories should come from fat
Limit cholesterol to less than 300 mg a day
Eat at least 30 g of fiber a day
55%–65% of calories should come from complex carbohydrates
10%–15% of calories should come from protein
Limit sodium to less than 2,400 mg a day
Obtain 1,200–1,500 mg of calcium a day from food or supplement
Eat 6 or more servings of grain products a day
Eat 3–5 servings of vegetables and legumes a day
Eat 2–4 servings of fruit a day
Eat two 4 oz servings of fish a week
Eat no more than two 4 oz servings of red meat a week
Chicken and turkey should be eaten in moderation with skin removed
Eat no more than one egg yolk a day, including those used in cooking and baking
Use vegetable oils, preferably olive and canola oils, in moderation
Have no more than two alcoholic drinks a day
Adjust caloric intake and exercise level to maintain a desirable body weight
Avoid fad diets and extreme or unconventional nutrition schemes
Avoid untested nutritional supplements, including megavitamins, herbs, food extracts, and amino acids

Exercise

Numerous observational studies have demonstrated an inverse relation between the amount of habitual physical activity and the risk of many of the chronic illnesses that afflict people in industrialized societies.[102] The protective effect of exercise is strongest against coronary artery disease but is also significant against hypertension, stroke, type 2 (non–insulin-dependent) diabetes mellitus, obesity, anxiety, depression, osteoporosis, and cancers of the colon and breast. Despite these proven benefits, only 25% of adults in the United States exercise at recommended levels. Of all deaths in the United States, as many as 12%, or about 250,000 annually, can be attributed to a sedentary lifestyle.[103]

EXERCISE PHYSIOLOGY

The physiologic effects of exercise depend on the type of exercise, its intensity, its duration, and its frequency. Exercise is either isometric or isotonic. Isometric contraction of muscle is characterized by an increase in muscle tension without a significant change in fiber length. No external work is accomplished, but substantial energy is expended. Examples of isometric work include handgrip exercises, pushing or pulling against a fixed resistance, and holding a heavy weight. In contrast, isotonic work involves a shortening of muscle fibers with little increase in tension; examples include swimming, bicycling, and running. Most exercise includes both isometric elements and isotonic elements.

Isometric and isotonic exercises differ substantially in their physiologic effects. Isometric work increases total peripheral resistance; both systolic blood pressure and diastolic blood pressure rise substantially, with relatively little increase in stroke volume or cardiac output. Isotonic work lowers total peripheral resistance, but heart rate and cardiac output rise. Systolic blood pressure rises substantially, but diastolic pres-

sure changes little, resulting in a small increase in mean arterial pressure. Isometric work places a pressure load on the heart, whereas isotonic work imposes a volume load.

Isometric exercise increases muscle strength and bulk, which is desirable for competitive athletes, for patients recovering from musculoskeletal injuries, and for individuals who wish to attenuate the loss of muscle mass and bone strength that accompanies sedentary aging and certain chronic illnesses.[104] However, static exercises produce minimal cardiovascular conditioning, and the circulatory demands of intense isometric work can be hazardous to patients with heart disease. In contrast, dynamic exercises enhance endurance and can produce adaptive cardiovascular changes in healthy individuals and cardiac patients.

Cardiovascular Response to Dynamic Exercise

The acute circulatory response to maximal dynamic exercise is a dramatic rise in cardiac output, from about 5 L/min to 20 L/min in healthy young men. The increased cardiac output results from a 300% increase in heart rate. This increased transport of oxygen is matched by a threefold increase in peripheral oxygen extraction. Total peripheral resistance falls, and blood is shunted away from nonworking muscles and the viscera toward exercising muscles and the coronary circulation, where blood flow increases fourfold.

The physiologic adaptations produced by repetitive dynamic exercise are known collectively as the training effect. The magnitude of the training effect depends on the intensity, duration, and frequency of exercise. Training requires rhythmic, repetitive use of large muscle groups for prolonged periods. Aerobic fitness can be developed and maintained in healthy adults with three to five exercise sessions a week. Each day's exercise should involve isotonic work at 60% to 90% of maximal heart rate for 20 to 60 minutes, either continuously or in increments of 10 minutes or longer.[105] Obviously, sedentary persons and patients with cardiopulmonary disease must initiate training at lower intensities and shorter durations and build up gradually. In addition, most of the health benefits of regular exercise can be attained by moderate exercise at intensities well below the aerobic intensity level[106]; gardening and walking during golf are examples of activities that have major health benefits without producing major gains in aerobic fitness.

Perhaps the most obvious effect of aerobic training is resting bradycardia; heart rates of 40 to 50 beats/min are common in highly trained endurance athletes. The mechanisms responsible are not fully understood but probably involve increased vagal tone, decreased sympathetic activity, and increased stroke volume. The best overall measurement of the aerobic training effect and of physical fitness is the maximal oxygen uptake ($\dot{V}O_{2MAX}$).

Oxygen consumption relates directly to the amount of muscular work; maximal oxygen uptake therefore reflects maximal work capacity. Many factors determine an individual's $\dot{V}O_{2MAX}$, including age, gender, lean body mass, genetics, and, most important, the level of habitual aerobic exercise. Just 3 weeks of bed rest will cause a 20% to 25% decline in $\dot{V}O_{2MAX}$. It is no wonder that patients are debilitated after being confined to bed by illness or treatment regimens. In contrast, regular aerobic training lasting weeks or months will increase $\dot{V}O_{2MAX}$, typically by 30% to 40%.

Both central (cardiac) and peripheral (muscular) adaptations are involved in the aerobic training effect. In healthy individuals, training produces dramatic changes in cardiac structure. The dimensions of all cardiac chambers increase by up to 20%, and myocardial mass may increase as much as 70%.[107] Although increased coronary blood flow and collateralization have not been demonstrated directly in humans, echocardiographic studies show that elite athletes have increased proximal coronary artery size, which is proportional to their increased left ventricular mass. Cardiac function is also enhanced by training; left ventricular contractility, stroke volume, and compliance[108] increase, and angiographic studies have demonstrated increased dilating capacity in the coronary arteries of endurance athletes. Exercise training also improves endothelial function in patients with coronary artery disease and in elderly persons[109]; this improvement in endothelial function is achieved, in part, by an increase in nitric oxide production.[110] In addition, exercise increases the number of circulating endothelial progenitor cells,[111] which appears to protect against cardiovascular events.[112]

In addition to these cardiac changes that allow enhanced O_2 delivery, exercise training improves peripheral O_2 extraction by enhancing O_2 extraction by the skeletal muscles themselves. This effect on skeletal muscle is specific for the muscles that have been trained; if only leg muscles are trained, the circulatory response to strenuous leg exercise will improve, but the response to vigorous arm exercise will not change.

Exercise training decreases the risk of hypertension. A meta-analysis of 72 controlled intervention studies concluded that isotonic exercise training in normotensive patients lowers systolic blood pressure by about 3 mm Hg and diastolic blood pressure by about 2 mm Hg; in hypertensive patients, isotonic training reduces systolic pressure by about 7 mm Hg and diastolic pressure by about 5 mm Hg.[112] With regular exercise, the benefit can be maintained for 3 years or more.[113] Regular exercise can even reduce left ventricular hypertrophy and blood pressure in patients with severe hypertension. Regular exercise also lowers catecholamine levels, protecting against arrhythmias, and it reduces myocardial oxygen demands.

Isotonic exercise reduces peripheral resistance and lowers blood pressure at rest and during exercise[112]; however, intense isometric exercise increases total peripheral resistance and acutely elevates blood pressure. Sustained hypertension is not a complication of resistance training, and moderate resistance training can even reduce resting blood pressure.[114] Unsupervised isometric exercising should be avoided by patients with cardiovascular disease; with appropriate precautions, however, it can be safe for selected cardiac patients and can produce favorable effects on muscular function.[115]

Pulmonary Response

Except in people with intrinsic lung disease, the pulmonary diffusion capacity does not limit exercise. At heavy workloads, however, skeletal muscle oxygen demands exceed oxygen delivery. As a result, muscle metabolism becomes anaerobic; the lactic acid that accumulates is buffered by bicarbonate, so that the pH remains nearly normal. The CO_2 that is liberated by the buffering reaction produces an increased ventilatory drive and tachypnea. Athletes know when they have crossed the anaerobic threshold by a markedly increased respiratory rate and a sensation of dyspnea. Habitual exercise does not improve pulmonary function in healthy people, but exercise training may be helpful in patients with chronic lung disease as a result of adaptations in muscles rather than in the lungs.

Musculoskeletal Response

Isotonic exercises increase muscle endurance. Training increases capillary density, and it can increase muscle mitochondria and oxidative capacity more than twofold. These changes account for the greater oxygen extraction that is an important element of the training effect. Isometric training builds muscle mass, which improves performance and may decrease the risk of injuries. Isometric exercises involving slow repetitions of work against high resistance produce fiber hypertrophy and strength but do not alter muscle enzyme content.

Exercise training affects tissues in addition to muscles. Of great importance, weight-bearing exercises increase bone mineral density, reducing the risk of osteoporosis. Repetitive performance of athletic tasks improves coordination and efficiency; changes in neuromuscular recruitment may be partially responsible. Tendon strength and bone density increase as a result of repetitive use. Joint wear and tear remains a concern, but as long as there is no trauma, habitual exercise probably does not produce degenerative joint disease.[116] In fact, aerobic and resistance exercise may help reduce disability in patients with osteoarthritis and fibromyalgia.[117,118]

Metabolic Effects

Skeletal muscle contains only very limited energy stores; preformed adenosine triphosphate (ATP) and creatine phosphate (CP) can supply less energy than that which is consumed in a 100-yard dash. Clearly, ATP and CP must be generated during exercise. Only three sources of fuel are available to skeletal muscle for this purpose: endogenous muscle glycogen, blood glucose, and free fatty acids (FFAs) derived either from muscle triglyceride or from adipose tissue. Normally, the body's skeletal muscle contains only 120 g of glycogen, and the liver, only 70 g. The 600 kcal of energy available from these two sources could sustain running for only 6 miles. The blood glucose provides only 40 kcal more. In contrast, the average person's 15,000 g of adipose tissue provides 100,000 kcal of energy— theoretically, enough to fuel a run from Boston to Atlanta.

At rest and during low-intensity exercise, both FFAs and muscle glycogen provide energy. As exercise begins, catecholamines stimulate adipose lipase, which cleaves triglyceride into glycerol and three FFA molecules [see Figure 2]. In muscle cells, FFAs are metabolized to acetyl coenzyme A (acetyl CoA); in the presence of oxygen, acetyl CoA undergoes oxidative metabolism by enzymes of the citric acid (Krebs) cycle in mitochondria.

As the intensity of exercise increases, the relative contribution of FFAs decreases and glycogen becomes more important; at maximum work, muscle depends entirely on glycogen. When oxygen is available, glycogen is metabolized in the cytoplasm to pyruvate, which then undergoes oxidation in the mitochondria via the citric acid cycle to water and CO_2. However, when the demands of muscle outstrip the availability of oxygen, energy can be generated only anaerobically via glycolysis. Anaerobic metabolism is much less efficient: from a gram of glycogen, anaerobic metabolism generates only 5% of the energy that aerobic metabolism generates. In addition, pyruvate cannot be converted to acetyl CoA. Instead, pyruvate

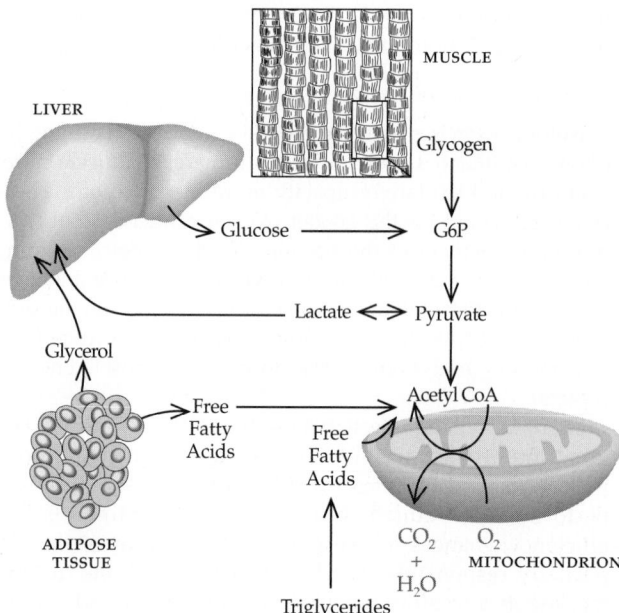

Figure 2 **During exercise, catecholamine stimulation of adipose tissue rapidly mobilizes free fatty acids to achieve blood levels that are six times the normal level, which are far higher than the muscle can use. Glucose derived from the liver and muscle glycogen are initially phosphorylated to yield glucose-6-phosphate (G6P). The G6P, the free fatty acids from adipose tissue, and the muscle's own triglycerides are metabolized to acetyl coenzyme A (acetyl CoA). This compound then undergoes oxidative metabolism in the mitochondrial Krebs cycle (blue), thus providing energy for exercising muscle.**

is reduced to lactate. Acidosis limits muscular performance, and buffering by the bicarbonate system generates CO_2, causing tachypnea.

Although the blood glucose itself constitutes only a modest caloric reserve, glucose turnover is greatly accelerated by exercise. During exercise, the liver releases glucose by both glycogenolysis and gluconeogenesis. Simultaneously, peripheral glucose uptake is enhanced. As a result of these metabolic events, blood glucose can account for 10% to 30% of exercising muscle's metabolic needs. The blood glucose level remains normal and may even rise during modest exertion. However, hypoglycemia can occur if hepatic glycogen stores are depleted and high-intensity exercise continues to consume blood glucose and muscle glycogen.

These changes in glucose metabolism are moderated by a number of hormonal alterations. Circulating catecholamines, growth hormone, cortisol, and glucagon levels rise. Insulin levels fall. All of these factors tend to elevate blood glucose levels. Glucose that is ingested during exercise will also tend to maintain blood glucose levels, but ingestion of glucose before exercise may actually raise insulin levels, thus impeding energy mobilization. Contrary to popular so-called instant-energy theories, preexercise meals should not contain concentrated sweets. Indeed, preexercise meals should be sparse, and people should probably ingest little other than water during the 2 hours before exercise.

Exercise increases the insulin sensitivity of muscle, thereby increasing glucose transport and muscle glycogen synthesis. Even moderate physical activity such as walking can help prevent the development of type 2 diabetes mellitus[119] and the metabolic syndrome.[120] Because exercise improves glucose

tolerance in diabetic patients, patients taking insulin may require special precautions to exercise safely [*see* Medical Complications of Exercise, *below*].

During exercise, the rate of protein synthesis is depressed. As a result, amino acids are available for anabolic processes, including hepatic gluconeogenesis. Amino acids also may directly provide a small fraction of the energy needed for muscle contraction. It is not clear whether athletes have higher nutritional protein requirements than sedentary persons; the ingestion of protein and amino acid supplements does not enhance athletic performance.

Regular exercise also alters body weight and body composition. Even if dietary caloric intake remains constant, regular exercise will produce weight loss and a reduction in central adiposity[121]; moderately intensive activities are beneficial if they are sustained.[122] It takes 35 miles of walking or jogging to consume the calories present in 1 lb of adipose tissue. Intense exercise also stimulates both energy expenditure and lipid oxidation for up to 17 hours after exercise itself, thus further contributing to a reduction in body fat. Even as body fat declines, muscle mass increases; because muscle is denser than fat, net weight loss may be slight. Swimming appears to be less effective than land exercise for reducing body fat and increasing bone mineral content. Although weight loss is an important goal for people who are obese, regular physical activity will reduce mortality independent of weight loss.[123]

Effects on Blood Lipid Levels

Exercise increases serum levels of HDL-C, probably by increasing the formation apo A-I, which is the major structural protein of HDL, and cellular lipids.[124] The amount of exercise appears to be the major determinant of the magnitude of the increase in HDL-C. As little as 5 to 10 miles of jogging a week will elevate HDL-C levels, which rise with increasing exercise in a dose-response fashion. Beyond about 35 miles a week, however, additional training does not produce a further increase in HDL-C levels[125]; the mean increase in HDL-C is about 8%.[6] Similar changes in HDL-C levels have also been demonstrated in walkers, cross-country skiers, tennis players, bicyclists, and other endurance athletes. The effects of exercise are independent of other factors known to alter HDL-C levels, such as diet, body weight, smoking, and alcohol consumption. Exercise must be sustained to maintain high HDL-C levels.

The effects of exercise on HDL-C levels are observed consistently, but changes in the other blood lipid levels have varied. In general, exercise reduces chylomicron levels and produces a fall in triglyceride levels that averages 24%.[6] Total cholesterol and LDL-C levels are less likely to decline in the absence of weight loss. Heritable factors, in part, determine lipid profile responses to exercise.[126]

Hematologic Effects

A mild decrease in hematocrit is commonly observed in endurance athletes. This so-called sports anemia is usually a pseudoanemia, because red blood cell mass is normal but plasma volume is increased; decreased viscosity has also been observed. Exercise-related hemolysis or gastrointestinal blood loss may be an additional factor in some cases of anemia in athletes. No consistent long-term changes in polymorphonuclear leukocytes, lymphocytes, or immunoglobulins have been noted.

Hemostatic mechanisms are influenced by exercise. Endurance exercise acutely increases fibrinolytic activity, and repetitive exercise is associated with reduced fibrinogen levels. In contrast, intense exercise can activate platelets, perhaps contributing to a prothrombotic state that may contribute to exertion-induced cardiac events [*see* Medical Complications of Exercise, *below*]. The effects of exercise on platelet function require further study.

Effects on Vascular Inflammation

It has become clear that atherosclerosis is accompanied by vascular inflammation that contributes importantly to arterial damage and occlusive events. Elevated serum levels of C-reactive protein and other inflammatory markers predict cardiovascular risk in persons without known atherosclerosis and indicate an adverse prognosis in patients with the disease. Both cross-sectional and longitudinal studies show that regular exercise reduces blood levels of C-reactive protein and other inflammatory markers.[127] Similar benefits have been documented in cardiac patients during exercise-based rehabilitation.[128]

Effects on Body Fluids

During exercise, skeletal muscle generates a tremendous amount of heat. Sweating is necessary to dissipate this heat. During strenuous exercise in a warm environment, up to 2 L can be lost each hour. Because sweat is hypotonic, the serum sodium concentration rises. Even in the absence of systemic acidosis, serum potassium levels may rise because of an efflux of potassium from muscle cells, but potassium levels normalize within minutes after exertion ceases.

The decline in blood volume, together with a shift in blood flow from the kidneys to skeletal muscle, produces a sharp decline in urine volume during exercise. The rise in plasma osmolarity increases thirst. However, thirst lags behind volume requirements, and fluid intake is often inadequate during athletic events. Volume depletion impairs athletic performance and can contribute to renal dysfunction or heatstroke. Unfortunately, coaching lore often limits fluid intake for fear of cramps, when, in fact, athletes can tolerate large volumes of fluids during brief pauses in exercise. Although water is an excellent fluid replacement, excessive amounts during prolonged exercise can produce severe, even fatal, hyponatremia.[129] Athletes do not require supplemental potassium or salt, so popular glucose-sodium-potassium solutions make little sense physiologically.

Psychological Effects

Endurance exercise produces improvements in mood, self-esteem, and work behavior both in healthy people and in patients undertaking cardiac rehabilitation; exercise training can help treat depression.[130] Several mechanisms have been suggested to explain the psychological effects of exercise. Purely psychological factors, such as distraction, may be involved. The serum levels of β-endorphin, monoamines, and other neuropeptides are affected by exercise in direct relation to the intensity and duration of exercise. Changes in endogenous opioid peptides may mediate the subjective effects of exercise (so-called runner's high).

EXERCISE AND THE ELDERLY

Many physiologic changes attributed to aging closely resemble those that result from inactivity.[131] In both circumstances, bone calcium wastage occurs, and there are decreases in $\dot{V}O_{2MAX}$, cardiac output, red blood cell mass, glucose tolerance, and muscle mass; total peripheral resistance and systolic blood pressure are increased, as are body fat and serum cholesterol levels. Regular exercise appears to retard these age-related maladies. Exercise training improves left ventricular systolic function and increases stroke volume to maintain exercise cardiac output in healthy older people.[108,132] The age-related decline in $\dot{V}O_{2MAX}$ has been found to be twice as great for sedentary men as for active men, and even low-intensity training can improve $\dot{V}O_{2MAX}$ in the elderly. Exercise training also helps blunt the age-related decline in peripheral vascular function experienced by sedentary people. Endurance training improves glucose tolerance and serum lipid levels in older men and women, and regular exercise appears to blunt the age-related decline in resting metabolic rate. Physical activity in the elderly is associated with increased functional status and decreased mortality. Exercise is safe in the elderly if simple precautions are observed [*see* Prescribing Exercise, *below*]. Walking programs increase aerobic capacity in persons 70 to 79 years of age, with few injuries; healthy elderly persons who are randomly assigned to aerobic exercise acquire fewer new cardiovascular disorders than control subjects. Appropriate resistance weight programs are not hemodynamically stressful in the elderly and produce increases in muscle strength, functional mobility, and walking endurance. Even frail nursing home residents (mean age, 87 years) responded to resistance training with an increase in muscle mass and strength, as well as improved gait velocity, stair-climbing power, and spontaneous activity. Although more studies are needed to clarify correlations between aging, inactivity, and exercise, enough information is available to warrant a recommendation of carefully planned exercise programs for the elderly.[133]

EXERCISE AND LONGEVITY

Primary Prevention of Atherosclerosis

Exercise training can favorably modify many of the conditions associated with an increased risk of coronary artery disease, including hypercholesterolemia, elevated blood pressure, glucose intolerance, obesity, elevated levels of C-reactive protein, and the less firmly incriminated traits of hypertriglyceridemia, hyperinsulinemia, hyperfibrinogenemia, and psychological stress. Studies conducted in men, women, and children demonstrated a consistent inverse relation between physical fitness and body weight, percent body fat, systolic blood pressure, and serum levels of cholesterol, triglycerides, and glucose.[134]

Is a sedentary way of life itself a risk factor independent of these other traits? Investigators at the Centers for Disease Control and Prevention (CDC) reviewed 43 methodologically sound studies of exercise and coronary artery disease.[135] Collectively, these studies showed that sedentary living increases coronary risk by 1.9 times. An independent meta-analysis derived the same relative risk.[136] The magnitude of this excess risk is similar to that conferred by other risk factors: hypertension, 2.1 times; hypercholesterolemia, 2.4 times; and cigarette smoking, 2.5 times.[135] Because sedentary living is at least two to three times more prevalent than any of these other risk factors, it can be argued that physical inactivity makes the most significant contribution to the epidemic of coronary artery disease in the United States. Maintaining a physically active way of life can be expected to reduce the risk of myocardial infarction by 35% to 70%. Even mild to moderate exercise that is started later in life is highly protective.[137]

Although reductions in coronary artery disease account for the great majority of the improvements in survival conferred by exercise, other factors may play a role. Physical activity protects against stroke[138] and hip fracture.[139] Exercise also reduces the risk of colon cancer[140] and breast cancer.[141] It may confer some protection against cancer of the reproductive organs in women and prostate cancer. Large studies have demonstrated that there is a graded, inverse association between activity and mortality.[142]

Secondary Prevention of Ischemic Heart Disease

A growing body of evidence supports the role of exercise in the rehabilitation of patients after myocardial infarction and in the prevention of recurrent cardiac events.[143] Certain benefits of supervised exercise programs have been clearly established, including physiologic and symptomatic improvements and the reduction of risk factors. Patients completing exercise programs demonstrate the training effect, including a lower heart rate at rest and both a lower heart rate and a lower systolic blood pressure at submaximal workloads. These changes reduce myocardial oxygen demands, thereby increasing the angina threshold. Significant improvements in maximal oxygen uptake and work capacity can also be demonstrated. Exercise training can improve walking distances in patients with claudication.[144] Exercise can be useful even for patients with severe ischemic left ventricular dysfunction and chronic congestive heart failure,[145] although extra precautions should be taken in these patients; cardiac exercise programs are safe. Most important, randomized trials have demonstrated that cardiac exercise programs reduce mortality by 20% to 25%.[143,146] Unsupervised moderate exercise, such as walking or gardening, also appears to reduce mortality in older patients with coronary artery disease.[147]

PRESCRIBING EXERCISE

Physicians can provide important incentives for their patients by educating them about the benefits, as well as the risks, of habitual exercise. Healthy, sedentary individuals are the largest group in need of such advice. In addition, physicians may be responsible for the medical screening of competitive athletes or for prescribing exercise for patients with chronic illnesses.

A careful history and physical examination are central to the medical evaluation of all potential exercisers. Particular attention should be given to a family history of coronary disease, hypertension, stroke, or sudden death and to symptoms suggestive of cardiovascular disease. Cigarette smoking, sedentary living, hypertension, diabetes, and obesity all increase the risks of exercise and may indicate the need for further testing. Physical findings suggestive of pulmonary, cardiac, or peripheral vascular disease are obvious causes for concern. A musculoskeletal evaluation is also important.

The choice of screening tests for apparently healthy individuals is controversial. A complete blood count and urinalysis are reasonable in all cases. Determination of blood glucose, serum cholesterol, and creatinine levels may also be useful in screening for risk factors or occult disease. The Valsalva maneuver and the isometric handgrip may be useful additions to the workup.

Young adults who are free of risk factors, symptoms, and abnormal physical findings do not require further evaluation. It is not at all clear that more aggressive medical screening can prevent sudden cardiac death. Although echocardiography and electrocardiography might reveal asymptomatic hypertrophic cardiomyopathy in some patients, the infrequency of this problem makes routine screening impractical.

The role of exercise electrocardiography as a screening test before an individual begins an exercise program is controversial. The AHA no longer recommends routine exercise testing for asymptomatic individuals.[102] In fact, a study of 3,617 asymptomatic men 35 to 59 years of age casts doubt on the value of exercise electrocardiography for routine preexercise screening.[148] None of the men had known coronary artery disease on entry into the study, but all were at increased risk because of hypercholesterolemia. Each individual had an exercise test on entry; the tests were repeated annually over a mean follow-up period of 7.4 years. Exercise proved safe in this group, with approximately 2% experiencing exercise-related cardiac events. Only 11 of the 62 men who experienced such events had abnormal exercise tests on entry—a sensitivity of only 18%. The cumulative sensitivity of annual tests was also low (24%). Even in elderly people, routine exercise testing before starting a moderate exercise program may not be necessary.[149]

Despite its limitations as a screening test for silent coronary artery disease, exercise testing can be useful for detecting exercise-induced arrhythmias, establishing a maximal heart rate for the exercise prescription, and determining work capacity. Serial testing may help motivate a patient by demonstrating increased work capacity. Specialized tests such as pulmonary function tests and exercise ergometry, Holter or telemetric monitoring during exercise, and echocardiography may be very useful in the evaluation of patients who have known or suspected cardiovascular abnormalities.

Screened patients will fall into one of three groups:

1. Healthy persons who can exercise without supervision. (Medical guidelines [see below] may still be helpful.)
2. Patients with ischemic heart disease or other significant

Table 6 Exercise Time Required to Consume 2,000 kcal

Activity	Time (hr)
Strolling	10
Bowling	8.5
Golf	8
Raking leaves	7
Doubles tennis	6
Brisk walking	5.5
Biking (leisurely)	5.5
Ballet	4.5
Singles tennis	4.5
Racquetball, squash	4
Biking (hard)	4
Jogging	4
Downhill skiing	4
Calisthenics, brisk aerobics	3.3
Running	3
Cross-country skiing	3

cardiovascular abnormalities who should have medically supervised, graded exercise programs. (If structured programs are not available, such patients should engage in milder forms of exercise, such as walking or bicycling, with appropriate precautions.)

3. Patients for whom physical exertion is contraindicated because of decompensated congestive heart failure, complex ventricular irritability, unstable angina, significant aortic valve disease, aortic aneurysm, uncontrolled diabetes, or uncontrolled seizure disorders.

People can exercise in the course of daily life or in formal exercise programs. Although most physicians have recommended structured exercise, studies demonstrate that even modest levels of physical activity are beneficial.[106,136,147] Walking and gardening are good examples[150]; such activities are protective even if they are not started until midlife or late in life.[145] In one study, for example, elderly men who walked less than 1 mile a day had nearly twice the mortality of men who walked more than 2 miles a day.[151] Compliance with walking is good,[152] and lifestyle interventions appear to be as effective as formal exercise programs of similar intensity in improving cardiopulmonary fitness, blood pressure, and body composition.[153]

People should be encouraged to exercise nearly every day. Formal, intense exercise is not necessary; even moderate exercise that consumes about 150 kcal/day or 1,000 kcal/wk is very beneficial to health. Warm-ups, stretches, and a graded increase in exercise intensity can help prevent musculoskeletal problems.[106]

Whereas all people can benefit from moderate daily activity, additional benefit can be obtained from more intense exercise; people who consume about 2,000 kcal in exercise a week obtain the greatest reduction of cardiovascular risk and mortality[142] [see Table 6]. On average, people can obtain optimal health benefits from about 30 minutes of aerobic exercise or 45 to 60 minutes of mild to moderate exercise a day.

Physicians who provide specific practical advice are most likely to motivate their patients to adopt better health habits, including diet and exercise [see Table 7].

The success of a structured fitness program depends on the frequency, duration, and intensity of exercise. At least three sessions a week are needed. An alternate-day schedule will help prevent muscle soreness, but as fitness improves, individuals should be encouraged to increase exercise sessions to five or even seven times a week. Each session consists of 15 to 60 minutes of activity. Untrained individuals may not be able to sustain even 15 minutes at first, but they should be encouraged to progress slowly as they improve. Each exercise session should be preceded by a 5- to 10-minute warm-up period and followed by a 5- to 10-minute cool-down period; stretching, gentle calisthenics, and walking are ideally suited for this purpose. These same exercises are excellent for a 5- to 10-minute cool-down period.

The intensity of exercise can best be judged by the target heart rate. A heart rate of 60% to 85% of maximum is considered optimal for aerobic training. If an exercise test has not been performed, a maximal heart rate can be calculated by subtracting the patient's age from 220. Unfit people should start at the lower end of the target heart rate range. Healthy people need not monitor pulse rate. Instead, they can adjust the intensity of effort to a talking pace: they are working hard but still able to talk to a companion without a sensation of dyspnea.

Table 7 Exercise Advice for Patients

Get a medical checkup before beginning a formal exercise program

Warm up before each exercise session, and cool down afterward with 10 min of stretching and light calisthenics

Start slowly and build up to 30 min of moderate to intense exercise or 45–60 min of mild to moderate exercise

Begin with aerobic-type exercise, and later add stretching exercises for flexibility and low-resistance weight training for strength

Exercise daily if possible, and alternate harder workouts with easier ones

Dress comfortably

Use good equipment, especially good shoes

Do not eat during the 2 hr before you exercise, but drink plenty of water before, during, and after exercise, particularly in warmer weather

Do not ignore aches and pains that may signify injury

Do not exercise if you are feverish or ill

Learn warning signals of heart disease, including chest pain or pressure, disproportionate shortness of breath, fatigue, sweating, erratic pulse, light-headedness, or even indigestion

Consider getting instruction or joining a health club

Many kinds of exercise can be used to attain fitness. Dynamic (i.e., isotonic or aerobic) exercises in which large muscle groups are used continuously in a rhythmic, repetitive fashion for prolonged periods are ideal. The energy requirements of various activities have been measured. An energy expenditure of 5 to 6 metabolic equivalents (METs) or more is desirable for aerobic training (1 MET is equal to the energy expenditure at rest or equivalent to approximately 3.5 ml O_2/kg body weight/min). Brisk walking, jogging, swimming, cross-country skiing, skating, bicycling, and vigorous singles racket sports all provide good conditioning. Sports that allow prolonged periods of inactivity, such as doubles tennis, golf, bowling, and baseball, are much less desirable for aerobic fitness but can still make important contributions to health. Activities requiring sudden bursts of intense isometric activity, such as weight lifting, provide little cardiovascular conditioning and are contraindicated for patients with hypertension or heart disease. Contact sports cannot be recommended for health.

Although physicians should encourage patients to choose the sports that appeal most to them, medical considerations may also be important. For example, swimming is particularly desirable for individuals who have various musculoskeletal problems, and it is also ideal for people who experience exercise-induced asthma (EIA). Walking and bicycling are ideal for older individuals or for anyone who is starting from a low level of fitness. Jogging can be recommended because it is convenient and because the participants can easily adjust intensity and duration upward as fitness develops. Most desirable of all is a balanced program containing a variety of activities that exercise different muscle groups. People who have several activities at their command find it easier to remain active despite constraints of climate, schedules, and minor injuries. Although moderate or aerobic exercise is most important for metabolic improvement and cardiovascular health, exercises for flexibility and strength should be part of a balanced fitness program.[106] Stretching exercises promote flexibility and help prevent injuries. A stretching routine should be performed at least two to three times a week, but it is best when incorporated in the warm-up and cool-down periods that should surround aerobic exercise. Low-resistance strength training is important to preserve muscle mass and power in the face of the aging process; two to three sessions a week are ideal.

COMPLICATIONS OF EXERCISE

Reducing Risk of Injury and Complications

Physicians can minimize injuries and medical complications associated with exercise by educating patients about potential health-related problems. Physicians should stress the need for such safety devices as helmets for biking, eye guards when playing squash and racquetball, and elbow and knee pads for roller-skating. Diet, weight control, stress management, smoking cessation, and other preventive health measures should be discussed [*see Chapter 3*], as should the warning signs of cardiac disease and the precautions for exercising in cold or hot climates.

Medical Complications of Exercise

Exercise promotes health, but it can also have adverse consequences. In some cases, the physiologic adaptations to exercise produce changes that may be misinterpreted as pathologic; athlete's heart is one example. In other cases, however, exercise can precipitate clinically important problems.

The cardiac complications of exercise include ischemia, infarction, and sudden death, often caused by rupture of an atherosclerotic plaque. These dire events are infrequent and can be minimized by proper patient screening and instruction [*see Prescribing Exercise, above*]. Exercise-induced cardiac events are less common in people who exercise regularly than in sedentary individuals.[154] On balance, exercise is clearly beneficial for the heart.

The most common pulmonary complication of exercise is EIA, which usually responds well to treatment.[155] A much less common problem that can mimic hypersensitivity disorders is exercise-induced anaphylaxis.

The gastrointestinal response to exercise may produce reflux, diarrhea, or bleeding, which is usually occult and transient. Women who exercise very strenuously may experience oligomenorrhea or amenorrhea; the menstrual dysfunction is reversible but may be accompanied by osteoporosis. With appropriate precautions, exercise is safe during pregnancy. Precautions are also in order for prevention of hypoglycemia in diabetic patients who exercise.

People who exercise regularly can experience increased plasma volume that produces hemodilution or pseudoanemia. True anemia is less common but may result from a shortening of the life span of red cells caused by vascular trauma or iron deficiency. Exercise can produce proteinuria or hematuria; both are benign but are indications for performing studies to rule out renal disease. In warm, humid weather, exercise can produce heat cramps, hyperthermia, or heatstroke, all of which are preventable.

Exercise does not appear to cause or accelerate osteoarthritis.[116] Acute muscle injury, manifested by transient elevations of creatine phosphokinase levels, is common, but exertional rhabdomyolysis is rare. Extremely prolonged exercise can elevate troponin levels without other evidence of injury to cardiac muscle.[156] Musculoskeletal problems, however, are the most frequent side effects of exercise.[157] Overstress, overuse, or trauma is usually responsible. Poor technique, faulty equipment, or fatigue often contributes to injury. Soft tissue injuries such as sprains, strains, and tendinitis usually respond well to simple treatment regimens. The same is true of stress fractures. Primary care physicians can manage many of these problems, but more serious injuries may merit referral to a sports medicine facility.

The author has no commercial relationships with manufacturers of products or providers of services discussed in this chapter.

References

1. Mokdad AH, Marks JS, Stroup DF, et al: Actual causes of death in the United States, 2000. JAMA 291:1238, 2004

2. Roberts CK, Vaziri ND, Barnard RJ: Effect of diet and exercise intervention on blood pressure, insulin, oxidative stress, and nitric oxide availability. Circulation 106:2530, 2002

3. Hedley AA, Ogden CL, Johnson CL, et al: Prevalence of overweight and obesity among U.S. children, adolescents, and adults, 1999–2002. JAMA 291:2847, 2004

4. Peeters A, Barendregt JJ, Willekens F, et al: Obesity in adulthood and its consequences for life expectancy: a life-table analysis. Ann Intern Med 138:24, 2003

5. Nielsen SJ, Popkin BM: Patterns and trends in food portion sizes, 1977–1998. JAMA 289:450, 2003

6. Fletcher B, Berra K, Ades P, et al: Managing abnormal blood lipids: a collaborative approach. Circulation 112:3184, 2005

7. He K, Song Y, Daviglus ML, et al: Accumulated evidence on fish consumption and coronary heart disease mortality: a meta-analysis of cohort studies. Circulation 109:2705, 2004

8. Mozaffarian D, Pstay BM, Rimm EB, et al: Fish intake and risk of incident atrial fibrillation. Circulation 110:368, 2004

9. Kang JX, Leaf A: The cardiac antiarrhythmic effects of polyunsaturated fatty acid. Lipids 31:S41, 1996

10. He K, Song Y, Daviglus, et al: Fish consumption and incidence of stroke: a meta-analysis of cohort studies. Stroke 35:1538, 2004

11. Omega-3 polyunsaturated fatty acids (Omacor) for hypertriglyceridemia. Med Lett Drugs Ther 47:91, 2005

12. Thies F, Garry JM, Yaqood P, et al: Association of n-3 polyunsaturated fatty acids with stability of atherosclerotic plaques: a randomized controlled trial. Lancet 361:477, 2003

13. de Lorgeril M, Salen P, Martin JL, et al: Mediterranean diet, traditional risk factors, and the rate of cardiovascular complications after myocardial infarction: final report of the Lyon Diet Heart Study. Circulation 99:779, 1999

14. Hu FB, Stampfer MJ, Manson JE, et al: Dietary intake of α-linolenic acid and risk of fatal ischemic heart disease among women. Am J Clin Nutr 69:890, 1999

15. Lichtenstein AH, Ausman LM, Jalbert SM, et al: Effects of different forms of dietary hydrogenated fats on serum lipoprotein cholesterol levels. N Engl J Med 340:1933, 1999

16. Cummings JH, Bingham SA: Diet and the prevention of cancer. BMJ 317:1636, 1998

17. Kolonel LN, Nomura AMY, Cooney RV: Dietary fat and prostate cancer: current status. J Natl Cancer Inst 91:414, 1999

18. Beresford SA, Johnson KC, Ritenbaugh C, et al: Low-fat dietary pattern and risk of colorectal cancer. The Women's Initiative Randomized Controlled Dietary Modification Trial. JAMA 295:643, 2006

19. Krauss RM, Eckel RH, Howard B, et al: AHA dietary guidelines: revisions 2000: a statement for healthcare professionals from the nutritional committee of the American Heart Association. Circulation 102:2284, 2000

20. Knopp RH, Walden CE, Retzlaff BM, et al: Long-term cholesterol-lowering effects of 4 fat-restricted diets in hypercholesterolemic and combined hyperlipidemic men. The Dietary Alternatives Study. JAMA 278:1509, 1997

21. Barnard ND, Scialli AR, Berton R, et al: Effectiveness of a low-fat vegetarian diet in altering serum lipids in healthy premenopausal women. Am J Cardiol 85:969, 2000

22. Ornish D, Scherwitz LW, Billings JH, et al: Intensive lifestyle changes for reversal of coronary heart disease. JAMA 280:2001, 1998

23. Frost G, Leeds AA, Dore CJ, et al: Glycaemic index as a determinant of serum HDL-cholesterol concentration. Lancet 353:1045, 1999

24. Pereira MA, Swain J, Goldfine AB, et al: Effects of a low-glycemic load diet on resting energy expenditure and heart disease risk factors during weight loss. JAMA 292:2482, 2004

25. Schulze MB, Manson JE, Ludwig DS, et al: Sugar-sweetened beverages, weight gain, and incidence of type 2 diabetes in young and middle-aged women. JAMA 292:927, 2004

26. Spiller RC: Cholesterol, fibre, and bile acids. Lancet 347:415, 1996

27. Bingham SA, Day NE, Luben R, et al: Dietary fibre in food and protection against colorectal cancer in the European Prospective Investigation into Cancer and Nutrition (EPIC): an observational study. Lancet 361:1496, 2003

28. Peters U, Sinha R, Chatterjee N, et al: Dietary fibre and colorectal adenoma in a colorectal cancer early detection programme. Lancet 361:1491, 2003

29. Park Y, Hunter DJ, Spiegelman D, et al: Dietary fiber intake and risk of colorectal cancer: a pooled analysis of prospective cohort studies. JAMA 294:2849, 2005

30. Slattery ML, Curtin KP, Edwards SL, et al: Plant foods, fiber, and rectal cancer. Am J Clin Nutr 79:274, 2004

31. Montonen J, Knekt P, Jarvinen R, et al: Whole-grain and fiber intake and the incidence of type 2 diabetes. Am J Clin Nutr 77:622, 2003

32. Chandalia M, Garg A, Lutjohann D, et al: Beneficial effects of high dietary fiber intake in patients with type 2 diabetes mellitus. N Engl J Med 342:1391, 2000

33. Ludwig DS, Pereira MA, Kroenke CH, et al: Dietary fiber, weight gain, and cardiovascular disease risk factors in young adults. JAMA 282:1539, 1999

34. Bazzano LA, He J, Ogden LG, et al: Dietary fiber intake and reduced risk of coronary heart disease in U.S. men and women. The National Health and Nutrition Examination Survey 1 Epidemiologic Follow-up Study. Arch Intern Med 163:1897, 2003

35. Pereira MA, O'Reilly E, Augustsson K, et al: Dietary fiber and risk of coronary heart disease: a pooled analysis of cohort studies. Arch Intern Med 164:370, 2004

36. Liu S, Sesso HD, Manson JE, et al: Is intake of breakfast cereals related to total and cause-specific mortality in men? Am J Clin Nutr 77:594, 2003

37. Dietary reference intakes for energy, carbohydrate, fiber, fat, fatty acids, cholesterol, protein, and amino acids (macronutrients). Institute of Medicine, Washington, D.C., 2002
http://www.iom.edu/CMS/3788/4576/4340.aspx

38. Pedrini MT, Levey AS, Lau J, et al: The effect of dietary protein restriction on the progression of diabetic and nondiabetic renal diseases: a meta-analysis. Ann Intern Med 124:627, 1996

39. Stamler J, Elliott P, Kesteloot H, et al: Inverse relation of dietary protein markers with blood pressure: findings for 10,020 men and women in the INTERSALT study. Circulation 94:1629, 1996

40. Potter J, Langhorne P, Roberts M: Routine protein energy supplementation in adults: systematic review. BMJ 317:495, 1998

41. Kelemen LE, Kush LH, Jacobs DR, et al: Associations of dietary protein with disease and mortality in a prospective study of postmenopausal women. Am J Epidemiol 161:239, 2005

42. Lonn E, Bosch J, Yusuf S, et al: Effects of long-term vitamin E supplementation on cardiovascular events and cancer: a randomized controlled trial. The HOPE and HOPE-TOO Trial Investigators. JAMA 293:1338, 2005

43. Lee I-M, Cook NR, Gaziano JM, et al: Vitamin E in the primary prevention of cardiovascular disease and cancer: the Women's Health Study: a randomized controlled trial. JAMA 294:56, 2005

44. Omenn GS, Goodman GE, Thornquist MD, et al: Effects of a combination of beta carotene and vitamin A on lung cancer and cardiovascular disease. N Engl J Med 334:1150, 1996

45. Michaelsson K, Lithell H, Vessby B, et al: Serum retinol levels and the risk of fracture. N Engl J Med 348:287, 2003

46. Wald DS, Law M, Morris JK: Homocysteine and cardiovascular disease: evidence on causality from a meta-analysis. BMJ 325:1202, 2002

47. Ravaglia G, Forti P, Maioli F, et al: Homocysteine and folate as risk factors for dementia and Alzheimer disease. Am J Clin Nutr 82:636, 2005

48. Liem A, Reynierse-Buitenwerf GH, Zwinderman AH, et al: Secondary prevention with folic acid: effects on clinical outcomes. J Am Coll Cardiol 41:2105, 2003

49. Toole JF, Malinow MR, Chambless LE, et al: Lowering homocysteine in patients with ischemic stroke to prevent recurrent stroke, myocardial infarction, and death: the Vitamin Intervention for Stroke Prevention (VISP) randomized controlled trial. JAMA 291:565, 2004

50. Vitamin supplements. Med Lett Drugs Ther 40:75, 1998

51. Utiger RD: The need for more vitamin D. N Engl J Med 338:828, 1998

52. A randomized, placebo-controlled, clinical trial of high-dose supplementation with vitamins C and E, beta carotene, and zinc for age-related macular degeneration and vision loss: AREDS Report No. 8. Arch Ophthalmol 119:1417, 2001

53. Elliott P, Stamler J, Nichols R, et al: INTERSALT revisited: further analyses of 24 hour sodium excretion and blood pressure within and across populations. BMJ 312:1249, 1996

54. Sacks FM, Svetkey LP, Vollmer WM, et al: Effects on blood pressure of reduced dietary sodium and the Dietary Approaches to Stop Hypertension (DASH) diet. N Engl J Med 344:3, 2001

55. Sodium and potassium. Dietary Guidelines for Americans 2005. Department of Health and Human Services and U.S. Department of Agriculture. January 12, 2005
http://www.healthierus.gov/dietaryguidelines/

56. Dietary reference intakes: water, potassium, sodium, chloride, and sulfate. Food and Nutrition Board, Institute of Medicine, Washington, D.C., 2004
http://www.iom.edu/?id=18495&redirect=0

57. Dawson-Hughes B, Harris SS, Krall EA, et al: Effect of calcium and vitamin D supplementation on bone density in men and women 65 years of age or older. N Engl J Med 337:670, 1997

58. Porthouse J, Cockayne S, King C, et al: Randomized controlled trial and supplementation with cholecalciferol (vitamin D3) for prevention of fractures in primary care. BMJ 330:1003, 2005

59. Bischoff-Ferrari HA, Willect WC, Wong JB, et al: Fracture prevention with vitamin D supplementation: a meta-analysis of randomized controlled trials. JAMA 293:2257, 2005

60. Iso H, Stampfer MJ, Manson JE, et al: Prospective study of calcium, potassium, and magnesium intake and risk of stroke in women. Stroke 30:1772, 1999

61. Abbott RD, Curb JD, Rodriguez BL, et al: Effect of dietary calcium and milk consumption on risk of thromboembolic stroke in older middle-aged men: the Honolulu Heart Program. Stroke 27:813, 1996

62. Allender PS, Cutler JA, Follmann D, et al: Dietary calcium and blood pressure: a meta-analysis of randomized clinical trials. Ann Intern Med 124:825, 1996

63. Baron JA, Beach M, Mandel JS, et al: Calcium supplements for the prevention of colorectal adenomas. Calcium Polyp Prevention Study Group. N Engl J Med 340:101, 1999

64. Giovannucci E, Rimm EB, Wolk A, et al: Calcium and fructose intake in relation to risk of prostate cancer. Cancer Res 58:442, 1998

65. Curhan GC, Willett WC, Speizer FE, et al: Comparison of dietary calcium with supplemental calcium and other nutrients as factors affecting the risk for kidney stones in women. Ann Intern Med 126:497, 1997

66. U.S. Department of Health and Human Services: Recommendations to prevent and control iron deficiency in the United States. MMWR Morb Mortal Wkly Rep 47:1, 1998

67. Dietary reference intakes for vitamin A, vitamin K, arsenic, boron, chromium, copper, iodine, iron, manganese, molybdenum, nickel, silicon, vanadium and zinc. Food and Nutrition Board, Institute of Medicine, Washington, D.C., 2001
http://www.iom.edu/Object.File/Master/7/294/0.pdf

68. Danesh J, Appleby P: Coronary heart disease and iron status: meta-analyses of prospective studies. Circulation 99:852, 1999

69. Whelton PK, He J, Cutler JA, et al: Effects of oral potassium on blood pressure: meta-analysis of randomized controlled clinical trials. JAMA 277:1624, 1997

70. Fang J, Madhavan S, Alderman MH: Dietary potassium intake and stroke mortality. Stroke 31:1532, 2000

71. Clark LC, Combs GF Jr, Turnbull BW, et al: Effects of selenium supplementation for cancer prevention in patients with carcinoma of the skin: a randomized controlled trial. Nutritional Prevention of Cancer Study Group. JAMA 276:1957, 1996

72. Yoshizawa K, Willett WC, Morris SJ, et al: Study of prediagnostic selenium level in toenails and the risk of advanced prostate cancer. J Natl Cancer Inst 90:1219, 1998

73. Mark SD, Qiao YL, Dawsey SM, et al: Prospective study of serum selenium levels and incident esophageal and gastric cancers. J Natl Cancer Inst 92:1753, 2000

74. Cefalu WT, Hu FB: Role of chromium in human health and in diabetes. Diabetes Care 27:2741, 2004

75. Guallar E, Jimenez J, van't Veer P, et al: Low toenail chromium concentration and increased risk of nonfatal myocardial infarction. Am J Epidemiol 162:157, 2005

76. Joshipura KJ, Hu FB, Manson JE, et al: The effect of fruit and vegetable intake on risk for coronary heart disease. Ann Intern Med 134:1106, 2001

77. Joshipura KJ, Ascherio A, Manson JE, et al: Fruit and vegetable intake in relation to risk of ischemic stroke. JAMA 282:1233, 1999

78. Romieu I, Trenga C: Diet and obstructive lung disease. Epidemiol Rev 23:268, 2001

79. Gillman MW: Enjoy your fruits and vegetables: eating fruits and vegetables protects against the common chronic diseases of adulthood (editorial). BMJ 313:765, 1996

80. Hung HC, Joshipura KJ, Jiang R, et al: Fruit and vegetable intake and risk of major chronic disease. J Natl Cancer Inst 96:1577, 2004

81. DeBoer SW, Thomas RJ, Brekke MJ, et al: Dietary intake of fruits, vegetables, and fat in Olmstead County, Minnesota. Mayo Clin Proc 78:161, 2003

82. Zhan S, Ho S: Meta-analysis of the effects of soy protein containing isoflavones on the lipid profile. Am J Clin Nutr 81:397, 2005

83. He J, Gu D, Wu X, et al: Effect of soybean protein on blood pressure: a randomized controlled trial. Ann Intern Med 143:1, 2005

84. Liu S, Manson JE, Stampfer MJ, et al: Whole grain consumption and risk of ischemic stroke in women: a prospective study. JAMA 284:1534, 2000

85. Steffen LM, Jacobs DR Jr, Stevens J, et al: Associations of whole-grain, refined grain, and fruit and vegetable consumption with risks of all-cause mortality and incident coronary artery disease and ischemic stroke. The Atherosclerosis Risk in Communities Study. Am J Clin Nutr 78:383, 2003

86. Hu FB, Stampfer MJ, Rimm EB, et al: A prospective study of egg consumption and risk of cardiovascular disease in men and women. JAMA 281:1387, 1999

87. Burr ML, Fehily AM, Gilbert JF, et al: Effects of changes in fat, fish, and fibre intakes on death and myocardial reinfarctions: diet and reinfarction trial (DART). Lancet 2:757, 1989

88. Albert CM, Hennekens CH, O'Donnell CJ, et al: Fish consumption and risk of sudden cardiac death. JAMA 279:23, 1998

89. Augustsson K, Michaud DS, Rimm EB, et al: A prospective study of intake of fish and marine fatty acids on prostate cancer. Cancer Epidemiol Biomarkers Prev 12:64, 2003

90. Kris-Etherton PM, Harris WS, Appel LJ: Fish consumption, fish oil, omega-3 fatty acids, and cardiovascular disease. Circulation 106:2747, 2002

91. Nash SD, Westpfal M: Cardiovascular benefits of nuts. Am J Cardiol 95:963, 2005

92. Jiang R, Manson JE, Stampfer MJ, et al: Nut and peanut butter consumption and risk of type 2 diabetes in women. JAMA 288:2554, 2002

93. Neil HA, Silagy CA, Lancaster T, et al: Garlic powder in the treatment of moderate hyperlipidaemia: a controlled trial and meta-analysis. J R Coll Physicians Lond 30:329, 1996

94. Keli SO, Hertog MGL, Feskens EJ, et al: Dietary flavonoids, antioxidant vitamins, and incidence of stroke: the Zutphen Study. Arch Intern Med 156:637, 1996

95. Mukamal KJ, Conigrave KM, Mittleman MA, et al: Roles of drinking pattern and type of alcohol consumed in coronary heart disease in men. N Engl J Med 348:109, 2003

96. Rimm EB, Stampfer MJ: Wine, beer, and spirits. Are they really horses of a different color? Circulation 105:2806, 2002

97. Winkelmayer WC, Stampfer MJ, Willett WC, et al: Habitual caffeine intake and the risk of hypertension in women. JAMA 294:2330, 2005

98. Bech BH, Nohr EA, Vaeth M, et al: Coffee and fetal death: a cohort study with prospective data. Am J Epidemiol 162:983, 2005

99. Newby DE, Neilson JM, Jarvie DR, et al: Caffeine restriction has no role in the management of patients with symptomatic idiopathic ventricular premature beats. Heart 76:355, 1996

100. Hu FB, Rimm EB, Stampfer MJ, et al: Prospective study of major dietary patterns and risk of coronary heart disease in men. Am J Clin Nutr 72:912, 2000

101. Kant AK, Schatzkin A, Graubard BI, et al: A prospective study of diet quality and mortality in women. JAMA 283:2109, 2000

102. Thompson PD, Buchner D, Pina H, et al: Exercise and physical activity in the prevention and treatment of atherosclerotic cardiovascular disease: a statement from the Council on Clinical Cardiology (Subcommittee on Exercise, Rehabilitation, and Prevention) and the Council on Nutrition, Physical Activity, and Metabolism (Subcommittee on Physical Activity). Circulation 107:978, 2003

103. Myers J: Cardiology patient pages: exercise and cardiovascular health. Circulation 107:e2, 2003

104. Castaneda C, Gordon PL, Uhlin KL, et al: Resistance training to counteract the catabolism of a low-protein diet in patients with chronic renal insufficiency: a randomized, controlled trial. Ann Intern Med 135:965, 2001

105. The recommended quantity and quality of exercise for developing and maintaining cardiorespiratory and muscular fitness, and flexibility in healthy adults. Med Sci Sports Exerc 30:975, 1998

106. Simon HB: The No Sweat Exercise Plan. McGraw-Hill, New York, 2005

107. Huonker M, Halle M, Keul J: Structural and functional adaptations of the cardiovascular system by training. Int J Sports Med 17:S164, 1996

108. Vona M, Rossi A, Capodaglio P, et al: Impact of physical training and detraining on endothelium-dependent vasodilation in patients with recent acute myocardial infarction. Am Heart J 147:1039, 2004

109. Hambrecht R, Adams V, Erbs S, et al: Regular physical activity improves endothelial function in patients with coronary artery disease by increasing phosphorylation of endothelial nitric oxide synthase. Circulation 107:3152, 2003

110. Laufs U, Werner N, Link A, et al: Physical training increases endothelial progenitor cells, inhibits neointima formation, and enhances angiogenesis. Circulation 109:220, 2004

111. Werner N, Kosiol S, Schiegl T, et al: Circulating endothelial progenitor cells and cardiovascular outcomes. N Engl J Med 353:999, 2005

112. Cornelissen VA, Fagard RH: Effects of endurance training on blood pressure, blood pressure-regulating mechanisms, and cardiovascular risk factors. Hypertension 46:667, 2005

113. Ketelhut RG, Franz IW, Scholze J: Regular exercise as an effective approach in antihypertensive therapy. Med Sci Sports Exerc 36:4, 2004

114. Cornelissen VA, Fagard RH: Effect of resistance training on resting blood pressure: a meta-analysis of randomized controlled trials. J Hypertension 23:251, 2005

115. Pollock ML, Franklin BA, Balady GJ, et al: Resistance exercise in individuals with and without cardiovascular disease: an advisory from the committee on exercise, rehabilitation, and prevention, Council on Cardiology, American Heart Association. Circulation 101:828, 2000

116. Sutton AJ, Muir KR, Mockett S, et al: A case-control study to investigate the relation between low and moderate levels of physical activity and osteoarthritis of the knee using data collected as part of the Allied Dunbar National Fitness Survey. Ann Rheum Dis 60:756, 2001

117. Penninx BW, Messier SP, Rejeski WJ, et al: Physical exercise and the prevention of disability in activities of daily living in older persons with osteoarthritis. Arch Intern Med 161:2309, 2001

118. Richards SC, Scott DL: Prescribed exercise in people with fibromyalgia: parallel group randomized controlled trial. BMJ 325:185, 2002

119. Sigal RJ, Wasserman DH, Kenney GP, et al: Physical activity/exercise and type 2 diabetes. Diabetes Care 27:2518, 2004

120. Laaksonen DE, Lakka HM, Salonen JT, et al: Low levels of leisure-time physical activity and cardiorespiratory fitness predict development of the metabolic syndrome. Diabetes Care 25:1612, 2002

121. Slentz CA, Duscha BD, Johnson JL, et al: Effects of the amount of exercise on body weight, body composition, and measures of central obesity. STRRIDE: a randomized controlled study. Arch Intern Med 164:31, 2004

122. Littman AJ, Kristal AR, White E: Effects of physical activity intensity, frequency, and activity type on 10-y weight change in middle-aged men and women. Int J Obes (Lond) 29:524, 2005

123. Hu FB, Willett WC, Li T, et al: Adiposity as compared with physical activity in predicting mortality among women. N Engl J Med 351:2694, 2004

124. Olchawa B, Kingwell BA, Hoang A, et al: Physical fitness and reverse cholesterol transport. Arterioscler Thromb Vasc Biol 24:1087, 2004

125. Williams PT: Relationship of distance run per week to coronary heart disease risk factors in 8,283 male runners. The National Runners' Health Study. Arch Intern Med 157:191, 1997

126. Rice T, Despres JP, Perusse L, et al: Familial aggregation of blood lipid response to exercise training in the health, risk factors, exercise training, and genetics (HERITAGE) Family Study. Circulation 105:1904, 2002

127. Kasapis C, Thompson PD: The effects of physical activity on serum C-reactive protein and inflammatory markers: a systematic review. J Am Coll Cardiol 45:1563, 2005

128. Milani RV, Lavie CJ, Mehra MR: Reduction in C-reactive protein through cardiac rehabilitation and exercise training. J Am Coll Cardiol 43:1056, 2004

129. Noakes TD: Overconsumption of fluids by athletes. BMJ 327:113, 2003

130. Blumenthal JA, Babyak MA, Moore KA, et al: Effects of exercise training on older patients with major depression. Arch Intern Med 159:2349, 1999

131. Cassel CK: Use it or lose it: activity may be the best treatment for aging. JAMA 288:2333, 2002

132. McGuire DK, Levine BD, Williamson JW, et al: A 30-year follow-up of the Dallas bed rest and training study: II. Effect of age on cardiovascular adaptation to exercise training. Circulation 104:1358, 2001

133. Young A, Dinan S: Activity in later life. BMJ 330:189, 2005

134. LaMonte MJ, Eisenman PA, Adams TD, et al: Cardiorespiratory fitness and coronary heart disease risk factors: the LDS Hospital Fitness Institute Cohort. Circulation 102:1623, 2000

135. Protective effect of physical activity on coronary heart disease. MMWR Morb Mortal Wkly Rep 36:426, 1987

136. Berlin JA, Colditz GA: A meta-analysis of physical activity in the prevention of coronary heart disease. Am J Epidemiol 132:612, 1990

137. Gregg EW, Cauley JA, Stone K, et al: Relationship of changes in physical activity and mortality among older women. JAMA 289:2379, 2003

138. Hu G, Sarti C, Jousilahti P, et al: Leisure time, occupational, and commuting physical activity and the risk of stroke. Stroke 36:1994, 2005

139. Feskanich D, Willett W, Colditz G: Walking and leisure-time activity and risk of hip fracture in postmenopausal women. JAMA 288:2300, 2002

140. Batty D, Thune I: Does physical activity prevent cancer? Evidence suggests protection against colon cancer and probably breast cancer. BMJ 321:1424, 2000

141. McTiernan A, Kooperberg C, White E, et al: Recreational physical activity and the risk of breast cancer in postmenopausal women. JAMA 290:1331, 2003

142. Lee IM, Paffenbarger RS Jr: Associations of light, moderate and vigorous intensity physical activity with longevity. The Harvard Alumni Health Study. Am J Epidemiol 151:293, 2000

143. Leon AS, Franklin BA, Costa F, et al: Cardiac rehabilitation and secondary prevention of coronary heart disease: an American Heart Association scientific statement from the Council on Clinical Cardiology (Subcommittee on Exercise, Cardiac Rehabilitation, and Prevention) and the Council on Nutrition, Physical Activity, and Metabolism (Subcommittee on Physical Activity), in collaboration with the American Association of Cardiovascular and Pulmonary Rehabilitation. Circulation 111:369, 2005

144. Stewart KJ, Hiatt WR, Regensteiner J: Exercise training for claudication. N Engl J Med 347:1941, 2002

145. Smart N, Marwick TH: Exercise training for patients with heart failure: a systemic review of factors that improve mortality and morbidity. Am J Med 116:693, 2004

146. Taylor RS, Brown A, Ebrahim S, et al: Exercise-based rehabilitation for patients with coronary heart disease: systemic review and meta-analysis of randomized controlled trials. Am J Med 116:682, 2004

147. Wannamethee SG, Shaper G, Walker M: Physical activity and mortality in older men with diagnosed coronary heart disease. Circulation 102:1358, 2000

148. Siscovick DS, Ekelund LG, Johnson JL, et al: Sensitivity of exercise electrocardiography for acute cardiac events during moderate and strenuous physical activity. Arch Intern Med 151:325, 1991

149. Gill TM, DiPietro L, Krumholz HM: Role of exercise stress testing and safety monitoring for older persons starting an exercise program. JAMA 284:342, 2000

150. Manson JE, Greenland P, LaCroix AZ, et al: Walking compared with vigorous exercise for the prevention of cardiovascular events in women. N Engl J Med 347:716, 2002

151. Hakim AA, Petrovitch H, Burchfiel CM, et al: Effects of walking on mortality among nonsmoking retired men. N Engl J Med 338:94, 1998

152. Pereira MA, Kriska AM, Day RD, et al: A randomized walking trial in postmenopausal women: effects on physical activity and health 10 years later. Arch Intern Med 158:1695, 1998

153. Dunn AL, Marcus BH, Kampert JB, et al: Comparison of lifestyle and structured interventions to increase physical activity and cardiorespiratory fitness: a randomized trial. JAMA 281:327, 1999

154. Albert CM, Mittleman MA, Chae CU, et al: Triggering of sudden death from cardiac causes by vigorous exertion. N Engl J Med 343:1355, 2000

155. Steinshamn S, Sandsund M, Sue-Chu M, et al: Effects of montelukast and salmeterol on physical performance and exercise economy in adult asthmatics with exercise-induced bronchoconstriction. Chest 126:1154, 2004

156. Urhausen A, Scharhag J, Herrmann M, et al: Clinical significance of increased cardiac troponins T and I in participants of ultra-endurance events. Am J Cardiol 94:696, 2004

157. Hootman JM, Macera CA, Ainsworth B, et al: Epidemiology of musculoskeletal injuries among sedentary and physically active adults. Med Sci Sports Exerc 34:838, 2002

Acknowledgments

Figure 1   Marcia Kammerer.

Figure 2   Talar Agasyan.

5 Adult Preventive Health Care

Mark Helfand, M.D., F.A.C.P.

Over the past 20 years, prevention has become a major activity in primary care. During a typical day, primary care clinicians spend much of their time managing asymptomatic conditions in which the main goal is to prevent death or complications (e.g., hypertension, hyperlipidemia, osteoporosis). Many chapters in *ACP Medicine* include information on screening or prevention of specific disorders in asymptomatic patients or those at increased risk [*see Table 1*]. This chapter focuses primarily on preventive screening recommendations from the United States Preventive Services Task Force (USPSTF).

Rationale and Evolution of Preventive Care Guidelines

The rationale for delivering preventive care during an office visit is strong. In 2002, life expectancy in the United States was 77.4 years, an all-time high.[1] Behavioral risk factors, including tobacco use, diet, and alcohol use, as well as factors such as hyperlipidemia and hypertension, contributed to the most frequent causes of death [*see Table 2*]. From the viewpoint of clinical preventive services, modifiable risk factors such as these, rather than the diseases they affect, are the true causes of death.[2]

Primary care visits provide an opportunity to assess risk, discuss options, and recommend behaviors and treatments that have been proved to reduce the risks of diseases and death. During 2002, an estimated 558 million visits were made to primary care physicians in the United States, an overall rate of about two visits per person per year.[3] On average, these physicians spent 20 minutes with the patient at each visit.

In 1975, Frame and Carlson published a series of articles that examined the quality of evidence for periodic screening conducted in the routine physical examination.[4] These authors argued that any preventive strategy should meet certain criteria of accuracy and usefulness [*see Table 3*]. The criteria are helpful in understanding the controversy about screening proposals. Several scholars have pointed out that clinical intuition about screening is often wrong, leading to errors in inference about the effects of screening. Some of these logical fallacies and hidden assumptions are now well recognized and even find their way into board examinations [*see Table 4*].

The work of Frame and Carlson gave rise to evidence-based decision making in prevention. The Canadian Task Force on the Periodic Health Exam used independent reviews of the scientific literature and a set of rules to grade the strength of evidence supporting a clinical service.

The USPSTF, founded in 1984, was modeled on the Canadian Task Force. It published its first set of guidelines for clinical preventive services in 1989.[5] The current USPSTF has experts from the specialties of family medicine, pediatrics, internal medicine, obstetrics and gynecology, geriatrics, preventive medicine, public health, behavioral medicine, and nursing.

Other expert panels also make recommendations about prevention [*see Table 5*]. Despite general agreement that recommendations should be evidence based, opinions about the effectiveness of specific preventive services differ. These differences arise because interpretation of the evidence is ultimately a subjective process, especially regarding the balancing of benefits and risks—an equation that includes such disparate factors as mortality reduction, costs or burden of illness, and patient discomfort.

To avoid errors in judging the evidence and weighing benefits and harms, expert panels, as well as individual clinicians, should do the following: (1) use an independent systematic review to distinguish assertions based on evidence from those based on other grounds, (2) make the rationale for a recommendation explicit, and (3) be free from financial and political conflicts of interest. Although the use of these measures does not guarantee a correct decision, they represent the best safeguards against bias.

USPSTF Evidence Ratings

The USPSTF assigns an overall grade of A, B, C, D, or I to each prevention service. The grades reflect the overall strength of evidence and the magnitude of benefit, defined as benefits minus harms [*see Table 6*].[6]

A grade of A indicates services that have solid supporting evidence and at least a moderate net benefit. A grade of B suggests that there are information gaps (so-called fair evidence) or that the benefits are only moderately greater than the harms for all patients. A grade of C denotes a toss-up, whereas a D grade indicates a service that is either proven ineffective or unlikely to provide benefits that outweigh the harms.

When there is too little evidence to determine whether or not a service works, the USPSTF assigns a grade of I for insufficient evidence. Some of the services with an I grade make good clinical sense and some are very promising, but without better research, it is not possible to say with confidence that they improve outcomes. Other grade I services have uncertain benefits but definite harms.

Noncancer Prevention Imperatives

Several preventive measures have earned an A grade on the strength of their good supportive evidence, substantially greater benefits than harms, and broadest applicability to primary care practice [*see Table 7*]. Implementation of these measures is described in detail in other *ACP Medicine* chapters [*see Table 1*].

IMMUNIZATION

The USPSTF has not issued recommendations about immunization since 1996, and those recommendations are now out of date. The Advisory Committee on Immunization Practices (ACIP), which consists of 15 experts in fields associated with immunization, is currently the only entity in the United States federal government that makes recommendations about immunizations. In contrast to the USPSTF, the ACIP does not use systematic reviews and does not usually describe the quality of evidence supporting a recommendation.

The ACIP publishes schedules for vaccination against certain infectious diseases in adults, depending on age and risk factors; these recommendations are discussed in individual *ACP Medicine* chapters and are available on the Internet (http://www.cdc.gov/nip/recs/adult-schedule.pdf). For example, general recommendations include a tetanus-diphtheria booster every 10

Table 1 Selected Prevention-Related Content in *ACP Medicine*

Chapter	*Relevant Content*
Ch. 3 Reducing Risk of Injury and Disease	Alcohol, tobacco, and other drug abuse; injury; violence; cites USPSTF
Ch. 4 Diet and Exercise	AHA recommendations
Ch. 8 Health Advice for International Travelers	CDC-recommended pretravel immunizations, other prophylactic measures
Ch. 18 Hypertension	Prevention
Ch. 25 Acute Myocardial Infarction	Secondary prevention; drugs and risk-factor modification
Ch. 27 Valvular Heart Disease	Prophylactic drug therapy for endocarditis; drugs and surgery for valvular disease
Ch. 32 Venous Thromboembolism	Primary and secondary prophylaxis
Ch. 39 Contact Dermatitis and Related Disorders	Prevention
Ch. 45 Malignant Cutaneous Tumors	Prevention
Ch. 57 Diseases of Calcium Metabolism and Metabolic Bone Disease	Osteoporosis prevention
Ch. 69 Acute Viral Hepatitis	Immunization
Ch. 106 Urticaria, Angioedema, and Anaphylaxis	Prevention of anaphylaxis
Ch. 109 Allergic Reactions to Hymenoptera	Prevention
Ch. 133 Infections Due to Gram-Positive Cocci	Prevention of spread of staphylococcal infection
Ch. 141 Tuberculosis	Tuberculosis prevention
Ch. 136 Infections Due to Neisseria	Prophylaxis for meningococcal disease
Ch. 134 Infections Due to Gram-Positive Bacilli	Prevention of diphtheria, listeria, anthrax
Ch. 135 Anaerobic Infections	Tetanus prevention
Ch. 143 Lyme Disease and Other Spirochetal Zoonoses	Prevention of Lyme disease
Ch. 139 Infections Due to Haemophilus, Moraxella, Legionella, Bordetella, and Pseudomonas	*H. influenzae* immunization and secondary prevention; pertussis immunization
Ch. 144 Infections Due to Rickettsia, Ehrlichia, and Coxiella	Prevention of Rocky Mountain spotted fever, typhus
Ch. 126 Infective Endocarditis	Prevention for high-risk patients/procedures
Ch. 129 Vaginitis and Sexually Transmitted Diseases	Screening recommendations for sexually transmitted diseases
Ch. 149 Respiratory Viral Infections	Prevention of influenza and other respiratory viral infections
Ch. 147 Herpesvirus Infections	Prevention of herpes simplex, varicella-zoster, and cytomegalovirus infections
Ch. 150 Enteric Viral Infections	Polio prevention
Ch. 148 Measles, Mumps, Rubella, Parvovirus, and Poxvirus	MMR, smallpox vaccination

(continued)

years in all adults, influenza vaccination every year in adults 50 years of age and older, and pneumococcal vaccination once in adults 65 years and older. The ACIP has made specific recommendations for vaccination of health care workers [*see Table 8*].[7]

Cancer Prevention

Only two cancer screening tests meet the USPSTF criteria for a strong recommendation: (1) Papanicolaou (Pap) smears for cervical cancer and (2) fecal occult blood testing or endoscopic procedures for colorectal cancer [*see Table 9*]. With both of these conditions, the aim of screening is to remove precancerous lesions, which prevents invasive cancer, saves the involved organ,

and reduces disease-specific mortality. By contrast, the more controversial cancer screening tests, such as prostate-specific antigen (PSA) and mammography, detect invasive cancers and lead to aggressive treatments (prostatectomy and mastectomy) that often destroy the involved organ and that have more substantial morbidity than cone biopsy for cervical cancer and polypectomy for colorectal cancer.

CERVICAL CANCER

Although no data from randomized, controlled trials support the value of the Pap smear in reducing mortality from cervical cancer, indirect evidence suggests that it is among the most effective cancer screening techniques.[8] By current standards, the sensi-

Table 1   *(continued)*

Chapter	Relevant Content
Ch. 153 Viral Zoonoses	Vaccination for yellow fever, Japanese encephalitis, and rabies
Ch. 152 HIV and AIDS	Prevention of HIV infection
Ch. 156 Protozoan Infections	Prevention of malaria, toxoplasmosis, giardiasis, and amebiasis
Ch.155 Mycotic Infections in the Compromised Host	Prevention of several opportunistic fungal infections
Ch. 16 Bites and Stings	Prophylactic antibiotics for bites
Ch. 6 Preoperative Assessment and Care of the Surgical Patient	Assessing operative risk and preventing complications
Ch. 13 Bioterrorism	Vaccination and postexposure prophylaxis
Ch. 59 Diagnosis and Treatment of Dyslipidemia	Primary and secondary prevention
Chs. 52–54 Diabetes Mellitus	ADA screening recommendations, prevention of type 2 diabetes, prevention of diabetic complications
Ch. 164 Acute Renal Failure	Prevention
Ch. 169 Nephrolithiasis	Prevention of recurrent kidney stones
Ch. 176 Cerebrovascular Disorders	Risk reduction for stroke
Ch. 173 Headache	Migraine prophylaxis
Ch. 189 Cancer Epidemiology and Prevention	Screening of asymptomatic patients for prevention and early detection; ACS recommendations
Ch. 197 Colorectal Cancer	Risk reduction, screening tests; ACS recommendations
Ch. 196 Breast Cancer	Screening and prophylaxis
Ch. 195 Lung Cancer	Prevention
Ch. 200 Prostate Cancer	Risk reduction, screening; ACS recommendations
Ch. 208 Alcohol Abuse and Dependency	Screening for alcoholism and treatment to prevent relapse
Ch. 84 Medical Complications in Pregnancy	Limited discussion of screening
Ch. 85 Menopause	Prevention and screening per USPSTF
Ch. 89 Approach to the Patient with an Abnormal Pap Smear	Prevention and screening per USPSTF

ACS—American Cancer Society   ADA—American Diabetes Association   AHA—American Heart Association   CDC—Centers for Disease Control and Prevention
MMR—measles, mumps, rubella vaccine   USPSTF—United States Preventive Services Task Force

tivity of traditional Pap testing is low (51%).[9,10] Cervical dysplasia is slow to progress to invasive carcinoma, however, so periodic screening can make up for the low sensitivity of a single exam.

The USPSTF recommends screening with Pap smears at least every 3 years, beginning within 3 years after the start of sexual activity or age 21 (whichever comes first). The Task Force recommends against annual screening. In women who have had consistently negative Pap smear results, continuing screening past age 65 is unnecessary because of the declining incidence of high-grade cervical lesions and an increased risk for potential harms, including false positive results and invasive procedures. The USPSTF also recommends against routine Pap smear screening in women who have had a total hysterectomy for benign disease.

The specificity of Pap smears for detection of dysplasia and cancer is 98%. False positive results occur infrequently, but Pap smears may correctly detect a large number of low-grade lesions that, without treatment, would remain stable or regress.[11] As a consequence, many women who would never develop invasive cervical cancer are subjected to anxiety and to colposcopy and biopsy.

In a systematic review, the effectiveness of liquid-based cytology, computerized rescreening, and algorithm-based screening have been compared with that of conventional Pap smear screening in reducing the incidence and mortality of invasive cervical cancer. The review concluded that the liquid-based monolayer preparation (ThinPrep) appears to offer higher sensitivity but lower specificity than conventional Pap smears.[10] However, the USPSTF could not determine whether the potential benefits of the three new screening approaches relative to conventional Pap smears are sufficient to justify a possible increase in potential harm or cost. They also found insufficient evidence to recommend for or against the routine use of human papillomavirus testing as a primary screening test for cervical cancer.

COLORECTAL CANCER

Screening modalities for colorectal cancer include fecal occult blood testing (FOBT), sigmoidoscopy, double-contrast barium enema, colonoscopy, and computed tomographic colonography [*see Chapter 197*]. FOBT is the only screening modality that

Table 2   Major Causes of Death in the
United States[1]*

Cause of Death	Number of Deaths	Age-Adjusted Death Rate (per 100,000 population)
Diseases of the heart	695,754	204.4
Malignant neoplasms	558,847	194
Cerebrovascular diseases	163,010	56.3
Chronic lower respiratory diseases	125,500	43.7
Accidents (unintentional injuries)	102,303	35.3
Diabetes mellitus	73,119	25.4
Influenza and pneumonia	65,984	22.7
Alzheimer disease	58,785	20.2

*Preliminary data for 2002; these causes account for three quarters of all deaths.

has been shown in randomized controlled trials to reduce colorectal cancer mortality. In the Minnesota Colon Cancer Control Study, 33 volunteers 50 to 80 years of age were randomized to annual FOBT, biennial FOBT, or a control group. After 18 years of follow-up, colorectal cancer mortality was 33% lower in the annual FOBT group and 21% lower in the biennial group than in the control group.[12] In this study, the slides were rehydrated, a technique that increases sensitivity but reduces specificity; during the trial, 38% of patients in the annual FOBT group underwent colonoscopy because of a positive test result. Two randomized, controlled trials from Europe have demonstrated 16% and 18% reductions in colorectal cancer mortality using FOBT.[13,14] In the European trials, unlike in the Minnesota study, patients were drawn from the general population, the slides were not rehydrated, and all testing was biennial.

In the screening trials, FOBT reduced mortality from colon cancer but did not reduce all-cause mortality. For example, the Minnesota trial findings indicate that 10 years of screening would result in 12 (95% confidence interval, 1 to 24) fewer colon cancer deaths per 10,000 persons screened. In that trial, however, the 95% confidence interval for all-cause mortality was 334 to 350 with annual screening, 333 to 348 with biennial screening, and 336 to 351 in control subjects.[12]

Evidence for the efficacy of sigmoidoscopy comes from case-control studies, which suggest that the protective effect of a single sigmoidoscopy lasts at least 6 years. The results of a large United Kingdom trial of screening with flexible sigmoidoscopy are not yet complete. Preliminary results suggest that flexible sigmoidoscopy is safe and that about 5% of persons 55 to 64 years of age have high-risk polyps (three or more adenomas; size 1 cm or greater; villous, severely dysplastic, or malignant).[15]

Because of the imperfect sensitivity of FOBT and sigmoidoscopy and because many patients who undergo these procedures end up requiring colonoscopy anyway, many clinicians are advising their average-risk patients to undergo colonoscopy as a screening test, either as a one-time procedure or periodically (e.g., every 10 years) beginning at age 50. Colonoscopy is the most sensitive test for detecting polyps; however, as for

other slow-growing lesions, such as cervical dysplasia, it is not clear whether improved sensitivity for polyps at a single point in time will translate into fewer invasive cancers in the long run.

In 2002, for the first time, the USPSTF included screening colonoscopy as an option, but with the qualification that the potential added benefits of colonoscopy may not always be great enough to justify the increased risks and inconvenience.[16] All colon cancer screening tests have a low yield—over 500 patients must be screened to prevent one invasive cancer[17]—so even a slightly increased rate of serious complications with colonoscopy might negate the benefit. Several gaps in the evidence base for colonoscopy can also be mentioned. First, the frequency of one procedure every 10 years was arrived at by means of mathematical models; in fact, no one knows how many patients will develop invasive cancer less than 10 years after a negative colonoscopy. Second, surveys suggest that gastroenterologists overuse colonoscopy for surveillance in patients who have clinically insignificant hyperplastic polyps or low-risk lesions, such as small adenomas. As a result, colonoscopic screening may lead to the use of a scarce, expensive resource, primarily in patients who have little chance of benefit. Third, the accuracy of colonoscopy when performed by the so-called average colonoscopist is not known. The primary advantage of colonoscopy, visualization of the entire colon, is negated if the operator cannot reach the cecum consistently or does not view the entire circumference of the lumen during the procedure.

No direct evidence supports the use of double-contrast barium enema for screening, and patients find it more uncomfortable than other alternatives. CT colonography may prove to be more sensitive and better tolerated than double-contrast barium enema and safer than colonoscopy; as of yet, however, there are insufficient data to determine whether it would result in better outcomes.[18]

BREAST CANCER

It was predicted that in the United States in 2004, invasive breast cancer would be diagnosed in an estimated 215,990 women; in situ disease would be diagnosed in 55,700 women; and 40,110 women would die of the disease.[19] A 40-year-old woman has a 13.2% (approximately one in eight) chance of developing invasive breast cancer during her life, but her risk of developing breast cancer within 10 years is only 1.47% (approximately one in 68). Modalities for breast cancer screening include mammography, clinical breast examination, and breast self-examination.

Table 3   Criteria for Evaluating a
Screening Program

1. Does the program target a disease that causes serious morbidity and mortality that might be prevented by the service?
2. Can the screening test accurately identify healthy people who are at high risk for developing advanced disease?
3. Is the screening test feasible to use in primary care?
4. Does treatment given before symptoms occur result in better outcomes than treatment given later?
5. Do the overall benefits outweigh the harms of screening and treatment?

Table 4 Sample Board Examination Questions About Screening

Question	Answer and Explanation
A screening test correctly identifies 95% of patients who have prexerostosis and 95% of patients who are well. If 1 of every 500 patients has prexerostosis, what is the likelihood that a patient who has a positive test has the disease?	The correct answer is 3%; the positive predictive value is commonly overestimated because of neglecting Bayes theorem.
The 5-year survival of stage 0 lung cancer is 95%, versus 10% for more advanced stages. In usual care, 70% of patients present in advanced stages. When screening with a CT scan, 90% of patients have stage 0 disease. By how much will screening reduce mortality?	The correct answer is that the effect of screening on survival cannot be determined; increasing detection of disease in a "curable stage" may improve 5-yr survival but does not necessarily reduce mortality because of overdiagnosis bias, length bias, and lead-time bias—for example, screening may detect slower-growing cancers that would never have become lethal.
With improvements in treatment, mortality from advanced HIV infection has dropped by 63%. Because effective treatment is now available, screening and early treatment should result in even greater mortality reductions. True or false?	The conclusion may be, but is not necessarily, true. If treatment of advanced disease is very effective, screening may not confer any additional advantage. Screening is most likely to improve outcomes when advanced disease is untreatable but treatment of earlier, asymptomatic disease can result in cure.

Mammography

In 2000, a Danish meta-analysis of the major randomized trials of mammography concluded that there was no evidence that mammography reduced mortality from breast cancer.[20] However, another analysis of the same trials conducted for the USPSTF concluded that mammography reduced breast cancer mortality in women 40 to 70 years of age.[21] The controversy centered on disagreement about the quality of the randomized trials of mammography: the Danish investigators excluded five of the eight trials that showed mammography to be beneficial, whereas the United States investigators excluded only two of those eight trials on grounds of quality.

The USPSTF demoted mammography from grade A to grade B to reflect their view that the quality of the evidence was fair and that the net benefit (benefits minus harms) was moderate. Coming after the widely publicized Danish study, the USPSTF recommendation of grade B for mammography received a mixed reception. One independent review, published in 2003, confirmed the USPSTF view that although the trials were flawed, the balance of the evidence still favored screening mammography in women 40 years of age and older at least every 2 years.[22] Conversely, the National Cancer Institute's Physician Data Query program largely endorsed the idea that most of the mammography trials were seriously flawed.

The USPSTF's most controversial decision regarding mammography was to promote screening in women 40 to 50 years of age from a grade C to a grade B. This was done because with several additional years of follow-up since the previous recommendations, in 1996, the pooled risk reduction for women who began screening at this age had become statistically significant. Nevertheless, the number needed to screen is higher, and the balance of benefits and harms narrower, in women 40 to 50 years of age than in older women.

For clinicians, the most difficult question is how to present information about the risks and benefits clearly and fairly to patients. At the time of an earlier controversy over the effectiveness of mammography in women 40 to 49 years of age, a survey of 509 women in the United States found that most believed the

Table 5 Government-Sponsored Preventive Guidelines Programs

Organization	Sponsorship	Focus	Web Site
U.S. Preventive Services Task Force	Agency for Healthcare Research and Quality	Clinical preventive services	http://www.ahrq.gov/clinic/uspstfix.htm
Canadian Task Force on Preventive Health Care	Health Canada (Canadian Federal Government)	Clinical prevention, periodic health examination	http://www.ctfphc.org
Physician Data Query Program	National Cancer Institute	Cancer prevention	http://cancernet.nci.nih.gov/cancertopics/pdq/screening
Task Force on Community Preventive Services	CDC	Community, population, and health care system strategies	http://www.thecommunityguide.org
Advisory Committee on Immunization Practices	DHHS and CDC	Immunizations, bioterrorism response	http://www.cdc.gov/nip/recs/adult-schedule.pdf
National Heart, Lung, and Blood Institute	National Institutes of Health	Asthma, cholesterol, hypertension, obesity	http://www.nhlbi.nih.gov/guidelines
Board on Health Promotion and Disease Prevention	Institute of Medicine	Population-based public health measures and the public health infrastructure	http://www.iom.edu/board.asp?id=3793

CDC—Centers for Disease Control and Prevention DHHS—Department of Health and Human Services

Table 6   United States Preventive Services Task
Force Grading System[6]

Grade*	Strength of Evidence	Magnitude of Benefit
A	Good	Large
B	Good Fair	Moderate Moderate to large
C	Fair to good	Small
D	Fair to good	None
I	Poor	None to large

*A—Service strongly recommended   B—Service recommended
C—No recommendation for or against   D—Service not recommended
I—Insufficient evidence

controversy was really about cost.[23] Women may interpret the lifetime risk of one in eight to be their immediate risk of developing breast cancer if they defer or miss their next mammogram.[24] In deciding how to inform patients, clinicians should carefully consider the major criticisms of the USPSTF recommendation. These criticisms represent differences in values rather than disagreements over the facts. There are four principal issues:

1. Is reducing breast cancer mortality important? In the trials, which involved nearly half a million women, mammography clearly had no effect on all-cause mortality. The USPSTF, although fully aware of this fact, chose to base their assessment of the benefits on the narrower grounds of breast cancer mortality. They chose to let women decide for themselves whether reducing the risk of dying of breast cancer was important to them.
2. How large is the reduction in breast cancer mortality? Judging from the trials, about 1,200 women 40 to 70 years of age must be invited to be screened four to five times over 10 years to prevent one death from breast cancer. Of women 40 to 49 years of age, 1,792 (95% CI, 764 to 10,540) must be invited to be screened to prevent one death from breast cancer, a death that would not have occurred until about 20 years after screening began. The specification "invited to" is important: it is likely that the trials underestimated the true benefit because they are diluted by a large number of subjects who were assigned to have mammography but did not.[25] Nevertheless, to benefit even one woman, a large number of women must have a large number of mammograms over many years.
3. Are these estimates from the randomized trials still valid? Evidence from the trials may be out of date. The first trial began in 1963, and the others began between 1976 and 1982. Improvements in mammography since then might translate into better outcomes than were seen in the trials. On the other hand, improved systemic treatment for clinically detected breast cancer may have eliminated the advantage that earlier detection conferred in the era of the trials.
4. How large are the harms? The USPSTF was criticized for ignoring or underestimating harms. In fact, the USPSTF considered the harms, but it was also influenced by evidence that many healthy women stated that they would be willing to take on these risks, as well as the morbidity associated with treatments, to avoid a breast cancer death.[26]

What are the harms? Women who get 10 annual mammograms have about a 50% chance that at least one of them is a false positive result; many of these false positive results necessitate a biopsy. Of women who are found to have invasive cancer, about 30 must undergo major surgery, or surgery plus radiation or tamoxifen, to prevent one death from breast cancer. In addition, screening identifies many women with ductal carcinoma in situ, and many of these women also undergo surgery, with uncertain benefit. In sum, many women experience immediate morbidity from treatment; without screening, most of them would not have had consequences of their breast cancer (and no morbidity from mastectomy) for many years, if ever.

Table 7   Strongly Recommended Noncancer Preventive Services in Adults*

Service	Candidates	Established Benefits
Aspirin for primary prevention of cardiovascular events	Adults at high cardiovascular risk	Reduces the risk of stroke
Blood pressure screening	All adults	Reduces the risk of stroke
Screening for lipid disorders	Men 35 yr of age and older; women 45 yr of age and older; and younger adults at increased risk for coronary artery disease	Reduces overall mortality, as well as mortality from cardiovascular disease
Chlamydial infection screening	Sexually active women 25 yr of age and younger; other asymptomatic women at increased risk for infection	Reduced the risk of pelvic inflammatory disease in one randomized trial[36]
Hepatitis B virus (HBV) infection screening	Pregnant women	Reduces prenatal transmission of HBV
Syphilis screening	Persons at increased risk for infection; all pregnant women	Penicillin treatment during pregnancy reduces the risk to the fetus of acquiring congenital syphilis
HIV screening†	Pregnant women High-risk men and women	Reduces prenatal transmission of HIV Delays mortality from HIV disease and permits counseling to reduce transmission
Screening for asymptomatic bacteriuria	Pregnant women (urine culture at 12–16 weeks' gestation)	Prevents symptomatic urinary tract infections, low birth weight, and preterm delivery

*As per the United States Preventive Services Task Force. †As per the CDC.[37,38]

Table 8   Recommended Vaccination Schedule for Health Care Workers[7]*

Vaccine	Schedule
Tetanus-diphtheria	Every 10 yr after complete primary series or for persons lacking documentation of vaccination
Influenza	Annual
Pneumococcal (polysaccharide)	For persons with medical indications[†] or at risk for exposure
Hepatitis B	For persons lacking documentation of vaccination or evidence of disease
Hepatitis A	No data to support a recommendation
Measles, mumps, rubella (MMR)	For persons lacking documentation of vaccination or history of disease[‡]
Varicella	For persons lacking documentation of vaccination or history of disease

*As per the Advisory Committee on Immunization Practices.

[†]*Medical indications:* Chronic pulmonary disorders, excluding asthma; cardiovascular disease; diabetes mellitus; chronic liver disease, including liver disease as a result of alcohol abuse (i.e., cirrhosis); chronic renal failure; chronic renal failure or nephrotic syndrome; functional or anatomic asplenia (e.g., sickle cell disease or splenectomy); lymphoma, multiple myeloma, generalized malignancy, or organ or bone marrow transplantation; chemotherapy with alkylating agents, antimetabolites, or long-term systemic corticosteroids; or cochlear implants.

[‡]*Measles component:* Adults born before 1957 can be considered immune to measles. Health care workers born during or after 1957 should receive two doses of MMR vaccine unless they have a medical contraindication, documentation of one or more dose, or other acceptable evidence of immunity. *Mumps component:* One dose of MMR vaccine should be adequate for protection. *Rubella component:* Administer one dose of MMR vaccine to women whose rubella vaccination history is unreliable, and counsel women to avoid becoming pregnant for 4 wk after vaccination. For women of childbearing age, routinely determine rubella immunity and counsel regarding congenital rubella syndrome. Do not vaccinate pregnant women or those planning to become pregnant during the next 4 wk. For women who are pregnant and susceptible, vaccinate as early as possible in the postpartum period.

Clinical Breast Examination

The USPSTF could not determine the benefits of clinical breast examination (CBE) alone or the incremental benefit of adding CBE to mammography (grade I recommendation). No screening trial has examined the benefits of CBE alone (without accompanying mammography). Four of the eight trials of screening used mammography alone, and four used mammography plus CBE. In the trials that used both methods, CBE detected 40% to 69% of breast cancers. It is not clear from the trials whether CBE contributed to the reduction in breast cancer mortality observed in some of the trials.

Breast Self-examination

A randomized trial from China failed to show a reduction in breast cancer mortality or an improvement in tumor stage at presentation in women receiving instruction in breast self-examination.[27] Results from a Russian trial were similar.[28] In both trials, women who had been instructed in breast self-examination were more likely to seek medical advice for benign breast lesions.

Genetic Risk Assessment

In women whose family history suggests an increased risk of deleterious *BRCA1* or *BRCA2* mutations, the USPSTF recommends referral for genetic counseling and evaluation for *BRCA* testing (grade B recommendation). However, the USPSTF recommends against routine testing for breast cancer susceptibility genes (i.e., *BRCA1* or *BRCA2*) or routine referral for genetic counseling in women whose family history does not suggest an increased risk of deleterious mutations in these genes (grade D recommendation). Such screening and counseling have few or no benefits and could have important adverse ethical, legal, social, and medical consequences.

Cancer Screening Measures That Are Not Recommended

The USPSTF recommended against screening for bladder, ovarian, pancreatic, and testicular cancers. In each case, the deciding factor was that screening and treatment caused serious, immediate harms, whereas evidence of a benefit was inconclusive. As with mammography for breast cancer, screening for

Table 9   Recommended and Strongly Recommended Measures for Cancer Prevention*

Service	Recommendation Grade	Candidates	Comment
Cervical cancer screening	A	Women who have been sexually active and have a cervix; begin screening within 3 yr of onset of sexual activity or at age 21 (whichever comes first) and screen at least every 3 yr, stopping at age 65	Reduces the risk of invasive cervical cancer and mortality from cervical cancer
Colorectal cancer screening	A	Adults 50 yr and older (earlier in patients with a strong family history)	Reduces the risk of invasive colon cancer and mortality from colon cancer
Breast cancer screening	B	Women 40 yr and older	Reduces mortality from breast cancer
Breast cancer chemoprophylaxis	B	Women at high risk for developing breast cancer	Reduces the incidence of invasive breast cancer

*As per the United States Preventive Services Task Force [*see Table 6*].

Table 10   Recommended Preventive Noncancer Screening*

Condition	Screening Measure	Comments
Abdominal aortic aneurysm	Abdominal palpation, ultrasonography	Men 65 to 70 yr of age who have ever smoked should be screened one time by ultrasonography
Depression	Standardized questionnaire	In most trials, screening alone had nonsignificant effects on treatment rates and on clinical outcome; however, larger benefits were observed in studies in which the communication of screening results was coordinated with effective follow-up and treatment; in such settings, 110 patients would need to be screened to produce one additional remission after 6 mo of treatment
Obesity	Measurement of body mass index (BMI)	Screening can identify obesity (BMI ≥ 30 kg/m²); programs that combined diet and physical activity produced modest weight loss (6.4 lb on average for 1 yr or more); most trials did not report the proportion of subjects who lost weight
Osteoporosis	Dual–energy x-ray absorptiometry	Women older than 65 yr and high-risk women 50 yr of age and older should be screened; alendronate reduces the risk of fracture over 3–5 yr, but the longer-term benefit of treatment is unclear

*"B" recommendations, United States Preventive Services Task Force.

these cancers is aimed at detection of early invasive disease, and treatment has substantial morbidity. This degree of morbidity is in contrast to that associated with screening for colonic polyps or cervical dysplasia, for which treatment is relatively safe and is aimed at preserving, rather than removing, the involved organ.

Prostate Cancer Screening

The USPSTF concluded that evidence was insufficient to recommend for or against prostate cancer screening. This conclusion was based on the following considerations: (1) there are no completed randomized, controlled trials of screening, although studies are ongoing in the United States[29] and in Europe[30]; (2) although prostate cancer is a major cause of cancer death in men, many cases are clinically indolent (in autopsy studies, the prevalence of histologic prostate cancer in men older than 50 years is about 30%, but only 3% of men die of prostate cancer)[31]; (3) the value of treatment for the localized cancers targeted by screening is unknown; the one randomized, controlled trial of radical prostatectomy, which found no improvement in the 15-year survival rates of patients undergoing surgery, has been criticized for methodological problems[32] (another randomized, controlled trial comparing expectant management with radical prostatectomy for the treatment of localized cancer is under way)[33]; (4) aggressive treatments for localized disease are associated with significant morbidity; and (5) mortality from prostate cancer has not declined in the United States despite 15 years of widespread use of PSA testing.

Lung Cancer Screening

The USPSTF concluded that evidence was insufficient to recommend for or against screening asymptomatic patients for lung cancer with low-dose CT, chest x-ray, sputum cytology, or a combination of these tests. Although there is fair evidence that screening with these measures can result in detection of lung cancer at an earlier stage, there is poor evidence that any screening strategy for lung cancer decreases mortality. Moreover, the invasive nature of diagnostic testing and the possibility of a high number of false positive tests in certain populations raises the potential for significant harms from screening.

Noncancer Screening

Selected screening tests for diseases other than cancer are rec-

ommended for all adults, or for groups defined by age and sex. These diseases include abdominal aortic aneurysm in older men, depression, obesity, and osteoporosis [see Table 10].

Behavioral-Counseling Interventions

Unhealthy behaviors have a huge impact on mortality and morbidity. Tobacco use remains the leading preventable cause of death in the United States, contributing to more than 440,000 deaths each year. Misuse of alcohol is responsible for 100,000 more deaths. Although tobacco use has decreased, alcohol abuse, obesity, and diabetes have increased in recent years, bringing new attention to the need to eat, drink, and exercise sensibly.

The evidence base supporting brief counseling by primary care physicians has grown substantially in the past 10 years. To date, however, efficacy has been proved only for counseling on tobacco cessation and alcohol use [see Table 11]. Evidence to support counseling on diet, exercise, and other behaviors (e.g., use of sunscreens, seat-belt use) is limited. In many instances, follow-up in the available studies was too short to confirm that behavior change is sustained long enough to reduce the risk of developing disease or injury.

Table 11   Selected Recommendations for Counseling and Patient Education

Counseling Topic	USPSTF Grade*
Tobacco use	B
Alcohol use/driving after drinking	B
Healthy diet	I
Physical activity	I
Seat-belt use	I
Regular dental care	I
Avoidance of sun exposure/use of protective clothing	I
Adequate calcium intake (women)	I
Use of sunscreens	I

*See Table 6.
USPSTF—United States Preventive Services Task Force

SMOKING CESSATION

There is strong evidence that actions such as the instituting of smoking bans, increasing the price of tobacco products, and conducting public-information campaigns can discourage people from starting to smoke and encourage them to stop. Smoking cessation rapidly decreases the risk of stroke and heart disease and slowly decreases the risk of lung cancer [*see Chapter 3*]. In patients with peripheral vascular disease, smoking cessation reduces the risk of limb amputation and recurrent stroke.

Brief counseling by clinicians can help smokers take action. Counseling by physicians becomes increasingly important as more patients become motivated to quit. Because many patients have tried and failed before, brief messages should emphasize that repeated efforts often bring success.

ALCOHOL USE

Screening and counseling of alcohol use in primary care is aimed at drinkers who are at risk for harm from alcohol consumption that exceeds daily, weekly, or per-occasion norms (i.e., risky or hazardous drinking) [*see Chapter 208*]. Unlike harmful drinking and alcohol abuse or dependence, risky drinking behavior has not yet resulted in physical, social, or psychological harm to the drinker, and such drinkers do not meet diagnostic criteria for alcohol dependence.[34] In contrast to persons who engage in risky drinking, alcohol-abusing and alcohol-dependent drinkers may require intense addiction treatment and are unlikely to respond to brief advice from a physician.

Self-administered questionnaires or brief interviews can be used to assess average quantity or frequency and binge use. In the United States, about 8% to 18% of patients screen positive for binge drinking. CAGE is a four-item screening questionnaire to detect alcohol abuse and dependence. Its name derives from the topics of the four questions: Have you ever felt you ought to **C**ut down on drinking? Have people **A**nnoyed you by criticizing your drinking? Have you ever felt bad or **G**uilty about your drinking? Have you ever had a drink in the morning to steady your nerves or get rid of a hangover (**E**ye-opener)? In contrast, the Alcohol Use Disorders Identification Test (AUDIT), a 10-item instrument, is designed to identify risky and harmful use. In several controlled trials conducted in primary care settings, it was found that brief, multicontact behavioral-counseling interventions reduced risky and harmful alcohol use. About one in 10 risky drinkers reduced their alcohol use to sensible levels for up to 1 year.[35]

Reminder Systems

The USPSTF has created patient pocket guides that are based on its guidelines and that clinicians can use as reminder systems to promote patients' involvement in their own preventive care. These pocket guides are available on the Internet. There is one for all adults (http://www.ahrq.gov/ppip/adguide), one for adults older than 50 years (http://www.ahrq.gov/ppip/50plus/index.html), and one for women (http://www.ahrq.gov/ppip/healthywom.htm).

The author has no commercial relationships with manufacturers of products or providers of services discussed in this chapter.

References

1. Kochanek KD, Smith BD: Deaths: Preliminary Data for 2002. National Center for Health Statistics, Hyattsville, Maryland, 2004
http://www.cdc.gov/nchs/data/nvsr/nvsr52/nvsr52_13.pdf
2. McGinnis M: Actual causes of death in the United States. JAMA 270:2207, 1993
3. Woodwell DA, Cherry DK: National Ambulatory Medical Care Survey: 2002 Summary. Advance data from vital and health statistics; no. 346. National Center for Health Statistics, Hyattsville, Maryland, 2004
http://www.cdc.gov/nchs/data/ad/ad346.pdf
4. Frame PS, Carlson SJ: A critical review of periodic health screening using specific criteria. J Fam Pract 2:29, 1975
5. Guide to Clinical Preventive Services: An Assessment of the Effectiveness of 169 Interventions, 1st ed. US Preventive Services Task Force. Williams & Wilkins, Baltimore, 1989
6. Harris R, Helfand M, Woolf SH, et al: Current methods of the third US Preventive Services Task Force: a review of the process. Am J Prev Med 20:21, 2001
7. Recommended adult immunization schedule—United States, October 2004–September 2005. MMWR Morb Mortal Wkly Rep 53:Q1, 2004
http://www.cdc.gov/nip/recs/adult-schedule.pdf
8. Guzick D: Efficacy of screening for cervical cancer: a review. Am J Public Health 68:125, 1978
9. McCrory DC, Matcher DB, Bastian L: Evaluation of Cervical Cytology: Evidence Report Number 5, Summary Agency for Health Care Policy and Research. Agency for Health Care Policy and Research, Rockville, Maryland, 1999
10. Nanda K, McCrory DC, Myers E, et al: Accuracy of the Papanicolaou test in screening for and follow-up of cervical cytologic abnormalities: a systematic review. Ann Intern Med 132:810, 2000
11. Holowaty P, Miller AB, Rohan T, et al: Natural history of dysplasia of the uterine cervix. J Natl Cancer Inst 91:252, 1999
12. Mandel JS, Church TR, Ederer F, et al: Colorectal cancer mortality: effectiveness of biennial screening for fecal occult blood. J Natl Cancer Inst 91:434, 1999
13. Kronborg O, Fenger C, Olsen J, et al: Randomised study of screening for colorectal cancer with faecal-occult-blood test. Lancet 348:1467, 1996
14. Hardcastle J, Chamberlain J, Robinson M, et al: Randomised controlled trial of faecal-occult-blood screening for colorectal cancer. Lancet 348:1472, 1996
15. Single flexible sigmoidoscopy screening to prevent colorectal cancer: baseline findings of a UK multicentre randomised trial. UK Flexible Sigmoidoscopy Screening Trial Investigators. Lancet 359:1291, 2002
16. Screening for colorectal cancer: recommendation and rationale. US Preventive Services Task Force. Ann Intern Med 137:129, 2002
17. Pignone M, Rich M, Teutsch SM, et al: Screening for colorectal cancer in adults at average risk: a summary of the evidence for the U.S. Preventive Services Task Force. Ann Intern Med 137:132, 2002
18. van Dam J, Cotton P, Johnson CD, et al: AGA future trends report: CT colonography. Gastroenterology 127:970, 2004
19. Cancer Facts and Figures. American Cancer Society. American Cancer Society, Atlanta, 2004
20. Gøtzsche PC, Olsen O: Is screening for breast cancer with mammography justifiable? Lancet 355:129, 2000
21. Humphrey LL, Helfand M, Chan BK, et al: Breast cancer screening: a summary of the evidence for the U.S. Preventive Services Task Force. Ann Intern Med 137:347, 2002
22. Green BB, Taplin SH: Breast cancer screening controversies. J Am Board Fam Pract 16:233, 2003
23. Woloshin S, Schwartz LM, Byram SJ, et al: Women's understanding of the mammography screening debate. Arch Intern Med 160:1434, 2000
24. Baines CJ: Mammography screening: are women really giving informed consent? J Natl Cancer Inst 95:1508, 2003
25. Berry D: Commentary: screening mammography: a decision analysis. Int J Epidemiol 33:68, 2004
26. Schwartz LM, Woloshin S, Sox HC, et al: US women's attitudes to false positive mammography results and detection of ductal carcinoma in situ: cross sectional survey. BMJ 320:1635, 2000
27. Thomas DB, Gao DL, Ray RM, et al: Randomized trial of breast self-examination in Shanghai: final results. J Natl Cancer Inst 94:1445, 2002
28. Semiglazov VF, Manikhas AG, Moiseenko VM, et al: [Results of a prospective randomized investigation [Russia (St. Petersburg)/WHO) to evaluate the significance of self-examination for the early detection of breast cancer]. Voprosy Onkologii 49:434, 2003
29. Gohagan JK, Prorok PC, Kramer BS, et al: Prostate cancer screening in the Prostate, Lung, Colorectal and Ovarian Cancer Screening Trial of the National Cancer Institute. J Urol 151:1283, 1994
30. Schroder FH, Kranse R, Rietbergen J, et al: The European randomized study of screening for prostate cancer (ERSPC): an update. Eur Urol 35:539, 1999
31. Coley CM, Barry MJ, Fleming C, et al: Early detection of prostate cancer: part I: prior probability and effectiveness of tests. Ann Intern Med 126:394, 1997
32. Graversen PH, Corle DK, Nielsen KT, et al: Radical prostatectomy versus expectant primary treatment in stages I and II prostatic cancer: a fifteen-year follow-up. Urology 36:493, 1990
33. Wilt TJ, Brawer MK: The prostate cancer intervention versus observation trial (PIVOT). Oncology 8:1133, 1997
34. Diagnostic and Statistical Manual of Mental Disorders, 4th ed. American Psychiatric Association, Washington, DC, 1994
35. Whitlock EP, Polen MR, Green CA, et al: Behavioral counseling interventions in primary care to reduce risky/harmful alcohol use by adults: a summary of the evidence for the U.S. Preventive Services Task Force. Ann Intern Med 140:557, 2004
36. Scholes D, Stergachis A, Heidrich FE, et al: Prevention of pelvic inflammatory disease by screening for cervical chlamydial infection. N Engl J Med 334:1362, 1996

6 Preoperative Assessment and Care of the Surgical Patient

Michael F. Lubin, M.D., F.A.C.P.

Surgery is changing, and so too is the preoperative evaluation of surgical patients. Newer surgical procedures (e.g., laparoscopic cholecystectomy), along with many common, well-established procedures, are being done in outpatient facilities and on increasingly older and much sicker patients. Increasing numbers of patients are having elective surgical procedures. The evaluation of a patient who is being considered for surgery has changed a great deal in the years since the first papers on cardiac risk assessment were published in the late 1970s.[1] Despite much progress and new data, expert opinion and clinical judgment are still critical in this area of medicine. This chapter reviews risk assessment and provides current recommendations for the evaluation and management of perioperative medical problems [*see Sidebar* Approach to the Preoperative Consultation].

Goldman and coworkers developed the first systematic method to evaluate surgical patients for potential cardiac complications [*see Table 1*].[1] Their cardiac risk index for noncardiac surgery factored in decompensated heart failure, recent myocardial infarction, and arrhythmias, all of which were found to significantly contribute to the risk of cardiac complications and cardiac death. Impairment of pulmonary, renal, or hepatic function added additional risk; other risk factors included age, certain surgical sites (e.g., abdomen, thorax, and aorta), and emergency procedures. A subsequent study confirmed these risk factors and emphasized that severe and unstable angina added significantly to the risk of cardiac complications and cardiac death [*see Table 2*].[2]

Although these methods could identify groups of patients for whom surgery posed higher risk, they were not very helpful in selecting out individual patients who were at increased risk. Except in the highest risk group, the chances of cardiac complications varied from only 1% to 11%, and the risk of death varied from 0 to 2%[2]; these data demonstrate that a large majority of patients can tolerate surgery without problems, even if they have higher risk scores. Since the original indices were published, other methods to assess risk have been developed that employ a variety of information.[3,4] Although the use of any of these indices yields results that are better than the results that come from chance alone, all of them have a high false positive rate that limits their usefulness.[5]

How then should a physician proceed in evaluating a patient for surgery? Initially, two very important questions that have nothing to do with individual risk assessment need to be asked: First, is the surgical procedure being contemplated important to the patient's health and well-being? Second, what are the intrinsic risks of the anesthesia and proposed surgery?

It is quite clear that in a young patient who has a compound fracture, surgical repair is essential to the patient's health, and the risk of the surgery itself is rather low. On the other hand, extensive liposuction in a patient with advanced heart failure who also has renal failure is unlikely to have an acceptable risk-to-benefit ratio no matter how stable the patient appears to be. Many procedures fall between these two extremes, however, and risk assessment in such cases can be much more challenging. For example, bypass surgery for moderately severe angina in an 80-year-old patient with diabetes may or may not be useful, and the risks of the operation are not low.

Therefore, the decision to proceed with surgery requires the input of all the medical personnel involved. The internist or family physician has a critical role in assessing the findings from the history and physical examination; such an assessment will determine the degree of risk in the contemplated operation and the need for further testing to define risk. The surgeon must evaluate the risk-to-benefit ratio for the proposed procedure. The anesthesiologist needs to evaluate the risks of anesthesia and present this assessment to the patient. Finally, of course, the patient will have to understand the risks of the procedure and have confidence that they are outweighed by the potential benefits.

Approach to the Preoperative Consultation*

Assessment

Cardiac risk

Use Goldman or Detsky score [*see Tables 1 and 2*] but provide explanation if the score does not reflect the true assessed risk (e.g., patient does not have angina but has many risk factors, including being wheelchair bound)

Pulmonary risk

Assess as low, medium, or high, using clinical judgment

Other risks

Hypertension (well or poorly controlled)

Diabetes mellitus

Heart failure (uncontrolled)

Bleeding risk
Use of aspirin or other NSAIDs

DVT risk
Assess as low, medium, or high [*see Chapter 32*]

Plan

Cardiac risks

Use routine cardiac monitoring or monitor as if for stable coronary disease; consider perioperative beta blockade

Pulmonary risks

Use routine pulmonary care or preoperative and postoperative incentive spirometry with or without preoperative and postoperative chest physiotherapy

Hypertensive patients

Continue hypertensive medications; hold diuretics on day of surgery

Diabetic patients

Monitor blood glucose and treat with sliding-scale regular insulin, q. 4 hr, or give NPH insulin half dose, then follow with sliding-scale regular insulin

Thrombosis risk

Hold aspirin for 5 days preoperatively; if DVT prophylaxis is necessary, give low-dose heparin, 5,000 U q. 12 hr, or LMWH

---

*This sidebar presents an example of possible assessments and plans.
DVT—deep vein thrombosis   LMWH—low-molecular-weight heparin
NSAIDs—nonsteroidal anti-inflammatory drugs

Table 1   Calculating Operative Morbidity and Mortality[1]

Information Source	Criterion	Points
History	Age > 70 yr	5
	MI < 6 mo ago	10
	Chronic liver disease	3
	Bedridden	3
Physical examination	S$_3$ heart sound or JVD	11
	Significant aortic stenosis	3
Electrocardiogram	Rhythm other than sinus or PACs; > 5 PVCs/min	7
Laboratory tests	Po$_2$ < 60 mm Hg or Pco$_2$ > 50 mm Hg	3
	Serum potassium < 3 mmol/L	3
	Serum bicarbonate < 20 mEq/L	3
	Serum creatinine > 3 mg/dl	3
	BUN > 50 mg/dl	3
	Elevated AST	3
Intended operation	Peritoneal, thoracic, or aortic	3
	Emergency	4

Risk Class (Total Points)	Morbidity	Mortality
1 (0–5)	0.7%	< 0.2%
2 (6–12)	5%	2%
3 (13–25)	11%	2%
4 (> 25)	22%	56%

AST—aspartate aminotransferase BUN—blood urea nitrogen JVD—jugular venous distention MI—myocardial infarction PAC—premature atrial contraction PVC—premature ventricular contraction

Decisions about proceeding to surgery require good clinical judgment. High-risk patients need individual assessment. Despite high risk, those with life-threatening indications, such as an uncontrollable upper gastrointestinal bleed, will usually proceed to surgery. Less important procedures that are not likely to sustain or enhance life will more likely be postponed to permit treatment of alterable conditions, replaced with a lower-risk procedure, or canceled if the risks appear to be too high and the benefits not high enough.

Clinical Evaluation

In determining surgical risk, the history and physical examination are of great importance. The systems most involved in postoperative morbidity and mortality are the cardiovascular and pulmonary systems.[1,2] It is also essential to evaluate renal, hepatic, and endocrine function.

ASSESSING CARDIOVASCULAR RISK

The most critical parts of the cardiac assessment are those that involve heart failure and coronary artery disease (CAD). Assessment of anginal chest pain is particularly important because proper management of CAD can decrease the risks of surgery. On the other hand, extensive cardiac testing in a patient who is unlikely to have significant CAD will delay procedures that may be important and will increase the cost of care.

Heart Failure

Uncontrolled heart failure is the most important risk factor for cardiac death or complications. A history of functional limitation appears to be the most helpful of all the historical points in this assessment. Patients who can perform activities that require four metabolic equivalents (METs) have a good chance of survival for most surgical procedures [*see Table 3*]; such patients require no further testing. Some authors have used stair climbing to assess patients' functional capacity; the ability to walk up approximately two flights of stairs or to walk four level city blocks has proved helpful.[6] The presence of such symptoms as orthopnea and paroxysmal nocturnal dyspnea in a patient with poor functional capacity increases the likelihood of heart failure but does not have predictive value for perioperative outcome.

The physical examination should identify signs of heart failure, such as distended neck veins, an S$_3$ gallop, rales, and edema. Other signs of cardiovascular disease, such as hypertension, decreased pulses, or bruits, should be recorded. These signs will help identify patients with ventricular dysfunction and peripheral vascular disease that may increase overall risk.

The use of echocardiography as a predictive tool is controversial. Although many experts advocate echocardiography as a good tool for assessing heart failure control, the procedure may provide little prognostic information beyond that available from a careful history and physical examination.

The most important preoperative use of echocardiography is in the differentiation of systolic dysfunction from diastolic dysfunction in patients with new-onset heart failure. A careful history and physical examination can suggest which is more likely, but the echocardiographic differentiation is significantly more reliable. The distinction is important, because data clearly show that systolic dysfunction, in a patient with substantial clinical manifestations (i.e., overt congestive failure), adds significantly to the risk of surgery.[1] On the other hand, there are no data showing that echocardiographic evidence of systolic dysfunction in a patient without symptoms or signs of heart failure has any prognostic implications.[7]

There are also no good data indicating that diastolic dysfunction increases risk significantly. Although diastolic dysfunction probably adds some degree of risk, patients with echocardiographic findings of diastolic dysfunction but who have no signs and symptoms are probably not at substantially higher risk. Thus, there is no reason to order preoperative echocardiography when the diagnosis of diastolic dysfunction has already been established.

Patients who are able to perform tasks that require more than four METs can undergo most surgery without a significant increase in risk[8]; therefore, such patients would not benefit from an echocardiogram. Additionally, patients who have no clear-cut symptoms or signs of heart failure are unlikely to benefit from the test. Patients who do have symptoms and signs (e.g., elevated neck veins, S$_3$ gallop, orthopnea, or paroxysmal nocturnal dyspnea) are definitely at increased risk; preoperative echocardiography is unnecessary in such cases because it provides no additional information on risk.[7] Treating the heart failure until the symptoms have stabilized and the signs have improved will lower risk substantially.

Coronary Artery Disease

The preoperative evaluation of the patient with established or probable CAD is of great importance. In general, most patients who will be having cardiac surgery or major vascular

surgery are evaluated by cardiologists. Recent myocardial infarction is second only to decompensated heart failure as a risk
factor for perioperative complications.[1] Decisions regarding the
evaluation of chest pain in patients without a history of CAD
can be difficult under any circumstance. Preoperatively, a decision must be made about the likelihood of CAD; again, if the
chances of having the disease are low, there will be many false
positive tests [see General Laboratory Testing, below], delays in
surgery, and interventions that will not help many patients and
may actually harm some of them. If a patient has known CAD
or if angina is a serious consideration, however, then the severity and stability of the CAD must be ascertained. The clinician
should then proceed with the evaluation process (see below).

The American College of Cardiology and the American Heart
Association (ACC/AHA) have developed guidelines for preoperative cardiovascular evaluation for noncardiac surgery
(http://www.acc.org/qualityandscience/clinical/guidelines/
perio/clean/perio_index.htm).[8] These guidelines are widely
used. The ACC/AHA guidelines include an eight-step algorithm for patient risk stratification and subsequent determination of appropriate cardiac evaluation[9]; this algorithm is available
on the ACC Web site (http://www.acc.org/qualityandscience/
clinical/guidelines/perio/clean/fig1.htm).

The American College of Physicians has also developed
guidelines on the perioperative assessment and management of

Table 2 Calculating the Likelihood of Postoperative Events[2]

Risk Factor	Points
CAD	
MI < 6 mo ago	10
MI > 6 mo ago	5
Canadian CVS angina	
Class III	10
Class IV	20
Unstable angina < 6 mo	10
Alveolar pulmonary edema	
< 1 wk	10
Ever	5
Critical aortic stenosis	20
Arrhythmia	
Other than sinus or PACs	5
> 5 PVCs/min	5
Poor medical status	5
Age > 70 yr	5
Emergency surgery	10

Class (Total Points)	Likelihood Ratio*
1 (0–15)	0.42
2 (16–30)	3.58
3 (> 30)	14.93

*Likelihood ratio for postoperative events, defined as myocardial infarction, pul-
monary edema, ventricular tachycardia or fibrillation, and cardiac death.
CAD—coronary artery disease CVS—Cardiovascular Society MI—myocardial
infarction PAC—premature atrial contraction PVC—premature ventricular
contraction

Table 3 Metabolic Equivalents of Selected Activities*

Activity	METs
Baking	2
Golfing with cart	2.5
Playing a musical instrument (various)	1.8–2.3
Mowing lawn (power mower)	3
Bicycling (leisurely)	3.5
Calisthenics (no weights)	4
Golfing without cart	5
Chopping wood	5

*A metabolic equivalent (MET) is an approximation of the energy expenditure
involved in a particular physical activity, expressed as a unit of oxygen uptake;
1 MET is defined as 3.5 ml O_2/kg/min. Representative levels are as follows:
1 MET, resting; 2 METs, walking on level ground at 2 mph; 4 METs, walking on
level ground at 4 mph.

risk from CAD.[10] Perhaps the most important message in the
ACP's clinical guideline is the following: most patients who do
not have an independent clinical need for coronary revascularization can proceed to surgery without further cardiac investigation.[10] In other words, if there is no prior reason to perform
coronary artery bypass surgery, further cardiac investigation
usually does not need to be carried out for the anticipated
surgery, unless there is some other overriding consideration.
This guideline does not apply to the patient with significant peripheral vascular disease, particularly if the patient is to undergo major vascular surgery.

Unstable angina or severe angina needs evaluation before
surgery if the procedure is not immediately lifesaving. For patients who have stable, less than severe angina and for those
whose symptoms occur only after significant exertion (e.g.,
walking at 4 miles an hour or engaging in moderate lifting), it is
not necessary to proceed with coronary artery evaluation for
most surgical procedures.[8] This is particularly true if the operative procedure is of low risk (see above). It may also be true in
those at moderately higher risk when the following factors are
considered: there may be an unacceptable increase in risk because of the delay induced by the bypass surgery, if such
surgery is done before the anticipated operation (e.g., resection
of potentially curable lung cancer or repair of a hip fracture); the
combined mortality of bypass surgery and of the planned procedure may exceed the risk of simply proceeding with the operation (e.g., hip arthroplasty or herniorrhaphy).

The preoperative use of noninvasive testing for CAD is controversial. Despite the indications given in the ACC/AHA algorithm, it is important to consider the consequences of doing
these tests, along with their rate of false positive and false negative results. Specifically, it is important to determine whether
bypass surgery is truly an option before testing for CAD; if it is
not an option, there is no need to test, because surgery will not
be done no matter what the result. Some patients refuse bypass
surgery even when significant disease is found.

Another consideration is the reliability and accuracy of the
test or tests being considered. Exercise tests can be helpful, but
only for those patients who can exercise enough to have a valid
result. Those whose capacity to exercise is limited by weight,
age, arthritis, or other physical or mental ailments will not
achieve the level of exercise necessary to give valid results.

Thallium testing, particularly in women, can also be quite
difficult. The specificity of these tests may be as low as 50% in

women[11]; that is, half of the patients without disease may test positive. These patients will be subjected to invasive catheterization despite the absence of clinically significant disease.

Dobutamine echocardiography is now being used to identify patients with reversible ischemia. This test appears to have fairly good sensitivity and specificity when an adequate test can be done, but it is not definitive, and no controlled studies have proved its usefulness.[12,13] The results of dobutamine echocardiography may also be less accurate in patients in whom the study is difficult (e.g., obese patients).

ELECTROCARDIOGRAPHY

There is general agreement on indications for electrocardiography, and there is some additional clinical support for its use.[1,2] ECG testing is recommended for men older than 45 years and women older than 55 years, although these age limits are arbitrary. Many elderly patients (arbitrarily defined as those older than 65 years) will have ECG abnormalities even without a history of any cardiovascular disease.[14] The ECG has been shown to have modest predictive value in anticipating morbidity and mortality; it is also useful as a baseline to guide care in patients who develop postoperative symptoms or complications. In addition, any patient with hypertension, cardiovascular disease, or pulmonary disease should have an ECG. For these latter indications, it is probable that an ECG done within the past 3 to 6 months can be used, provided there has been no intervening clinical change.

ASSESSING PULMONARY RISK

The pulmonary evaluation process is unfortunately much more subjective than the cardiac evaluation. Despite many attempts to find methods to identify patients at increased pulmonary risk, no method has been shown to be definitively useful for an individual patient; thus, clinical judgment is critical. The importance of the surgery is often the deciding factor, even in those who are thought to be at high risk.

Significant lung disease, particularly from smoking, is often identified at the time of surgery. For that reason, taking a smoking history is an important part of the preoperative assessment. In the pulmonary assessment, it is important to note any dyspnea on exertion, wheezing, or coughing with sputum production, particularly if acute. Acute reversible disease, such as asthma or a respiratory tract infection, must be identified so that it can be treated and reversed before the procedure, if possible. Patients who can exercise without significant symptoms are at low risk.[3] Shortness of breath on exercise, in the absence of heart disease, identifies patients at higher risk. In general, the ability to climb a flight of stairs or walk several blocks without stopping indicates a lower risk level. Advancing age is a minor risk factor.[1,2] On physical examination, a respiratory rate above normal; poor chest wall movement; use of accessory muscles on inspiration; and poor breath sounds, wheezes, or rales on lung auscultation suggest significant underlying disease.

Clinical detection of obstructive airway disease has not been carefully studied. One study in 309 patients found only four clinical elements that were significantly associated with the diagnosis of obstructive airway disease: smoking for more than 40 pack-years, a self-reported history of chronic obstructive airway disease, a maximum laryngeal height of 4 cm (corrected) or less, and an age of 45 years or older.[15] In this study, the presence of all four findings indicated obstructive airways disease (likelihood ratio, 220); the absence of all four ruled out obstructive airways

disease (likelihood ratio, 0.13). In patients with more severe chest disease, formal testing of respiratory function is indicated.

Pulmonary Function Tests

Preoperative use of pulmonary function tests (PFTs) is controversial.[16,17] PFTs do not readily identify individual patients who are at prohibitive risk for mortality; there is poor correlation between PFT results and mortality, despite some statistical correlation.[18] If the history and physical examination do not suggest significant pulmonary disease, there is no advantage in performing PFTs. If the intended surgery is of major importance, such surgery will have to be done regardless of the PFT results. The most important place for PFTs is in patients whose surgery may be of some benefit but whose risks may be prohibitively high. Many patients with very poor PFT results have been shown to survive surgery despite serious underlying disease.[19]

Exercise tolerance may be a good way to test for risk of death from pulmonary causes. It appears that for patients who can walk up two to four flights of stairs without stopping, the risk associated with major surgery is reasonable.[18]

Patients with chronic obstructive pulmonary disease and asthma should have their condition under the best possible control before surgery is attempted. In those whose symptoms are not controlled, surgery should be delayed until control is maximized; if this is not possible, additional drugs, including steroids, can be given before admission or in hospital to achieve as much control as possible before the procedure. It may be necessary to admit patients to the hospital one day or more before the operation to control their disease if it is particularly resistant to treatment.

Chest X-ray

Most experts believe that any patient older than 60 years should have a baseline chest x-ray. This has been shown to be clinically useful in elderly patients, who often have abnormalities that would not have been expected from history and physical examination.[20] Although the results of the chest x-ray may have little impact on preoperative risk assessment, I have found them to be useful in the care of patients who have postoperative pulmonary complications.

Clearly, any patient with cardiovascular or pulmonary disease needs a chest x-ray. Those with acute pulmonary symptoms and perhaps those with a history of tuberculosis or tuberculosis exposure probably derive some benefit from a chest x-ray. Again, in the absence of a change in symptoms or signs, a recent x-ray is usually adequate; a repeat x-ray is not needed in the immediate preoperative period.

ASSESSING RENAL RISK

Decreased renal function, most commonly defined as a serum creatinine concentration of approximately 2.0 mg/dl or higher, increases the risk of morbidity and mortality.[3] Because most renal disease results from hypertension and diabetes, a history of these diseases should lead to testing of renal function. Polyuria and nocturia may also indicate underlying kidney disease.

ASSESSING FOR LIVER DISEASE

Although significant liver disease is not common, failure to identify underlying liver disease can lead to catastrophic complications, particularly bleeding. The leading cause of significant liver disease is ethanol, so a history of alcohol intake is very important. Hepatitis B and C are also important risk factors for impaired hepatic function; these diseases may be suggested by a history of bleeding episodes, transfusions, drug abuse, or sexual promiscuity.

ASSESSING FOR ENDOCRINE DISEASE

Endocrine abnormalities affect surgical risks. Diabetes is the most common endocrine abnormality; it is especially important because of its association with cardiovascular disease, which may be silent in diabetic patients.[21] Consequently, a history of hyperglycemic symptoms should be sought.

A history of thyroid disease is important, although most patients with hypothyroidism are at low risk unless they are profoundly affected.[22,23] On the other hand, identifying patients with undiagnosed or undertreated hyperthyroidism is very important, because it is well known that surgery can precipitate thyroid storm.[24] Thus, a history of hyperthyroidism or its symptoms (e.g., tremor, palpitations, weight loss, and anxiety) must be sought. Physical findings of tremor, lid lag, hyperreflexia, and tachycardia are useful clues. If there is any indication that the patient may be hyperthyroid, the thyroid-stimulating hormone level should be measured.

Addison disease is uncommon but can be deadly with the stress of surgery.[25] Profound weakness, orthostatic hypotension, and hyperpigmentation suggest adrenal insufficiency. For patients with adrenal insufficiency and those receiving long-term corticosteroid therapy, supplementary doses of corticosteroids must be given during the perioperative period.

ASSESSING FOR NEUROLOGIC DISEASE

Neurologic disease may significantly increase surgical risks. The most common and important neurologic disease is cerebrovascular disease. Hypertension, atherosclerosis, and diabetes are important antecedent processes. A history of episodic or fixed neurologic deficits, as well as a history of stroke, is important to identify. A history of memory loss or other cognitive deficits must also be sought, because strokes and dementia increase the risk of postoperative delirium.[26]

On examination, neurologic deficits must be noted and an etiology sought. I believe a baseline mini–mental status examination should be done on any patient suspected of having a dementing illness. With elderly patients, I recommend a mini–mental status examination even in those with no clear evidence of dementia. Particularly in elderly patients, any signs of dementia on mental status examination should be noted and clearly documented so that any suspected change after surgery can be compared with the presurgical state.

Medication Review and Adjustment

Review of medications, particularly in the elderly, is critical. In some cases, it may be necessary to discontinue a drug or adjust its dosage before surgery. As a side benefit, the medication review may reveal that the patient is taking unnecessary medications; this may be especially likely in elderly patients, many of whom are on multiple medications. Stopping unnecessary drugs simplifies the care of all patients.

The most commonly prescribed medications that require adjustment of dosages with surgery are those for hypertension and diabetes. Diuretics and oral diabetic medications are usually not administered on the day of surgery.[27,28]

Anticoagulant therapy obviously requires thoughtful periop-

erative management [see Thrombosis, below]. There are good reviews of the management of perioperative anticoagulation.[29] Because of their antiplatelet actions, nonsteroidal anti-inflammatory drugs (NSAIDs), including aspirin, should be discontinued 5 days before surgery. NSAIDs also increase the risk of acute renal failure, particularly in patients with renal insufficiency.

Many patients take over-the-counter medications or herbal remedies. It is important to specifically ask about such products when taking a medication history. These products may affect coagulation or interact with medications the patient will receive perioperatively. All such products should be stopped before surgery.

The clinician should review any previous surgery the patient has undergone. This review may reveal problems with anesthetic agents, such as malignant hyperthermia, that might otherwise be missed.

General Laboratory Testing

Laboratory testing before surgery has been studied extensively over the past 2 decades. Unfortunately, there are few data to help clinicians determine which patients truly need specific tests; most published recommendations are based on expert opinion. Many clinicians worry about the medicolegal risks of not performing tests before surgery, but preoperative testing also has drawbacks. Testing subjects the patient to increased risks from more invasive procedures such as catheterization and may even erroneously indicate disease that is not present.

Noninvasive tests are often far from perfect for predicting the presence or absence of disease. Most of these tests have rather good sensitivity but only moderate specificity. The lower the prevalence of a disease in the population being tested for it, the greater the odds of false-positive results, which almost inevitably lead to further costly, invasive, and perhaps risky testing. This limitation of testing underlines the importance of a good history and physical examination for selecting patients for testing. Methods for calculating the likelihood of disease on the basis of a given test result are discussed in detail elsewhere [see Chapter 2].

For many years, most preoperative patients at most institutions underwent a standard panel of tests: a complete blood count (CBC), including platelets; electrolytes and renal panel; extended serum chemistry studies with liver function tests; prothrombin time and partial thromboplastin time; and chest x-ray and electrocardiogram. Kaplan and colleagues showed that many tests were not needed for the care of these patients and that many of the abnormal test results were only slightly out of the normal range.[30] Almost all of those abnormal results were ignored without consequence or were pursued with no benefit to the patients. Pursuing these abnormal results simply added more tests and caused delays in surgery. A number of subsequent studies confirmed these findings.[31,32]

Most experts agree that patients who are older than 60 years and those undergoing procedures that pose a substantial risk of bleeding should have their hematocrit measured. It is not clear, however, that even this limited testing makes a clinical difference. Obviously, patients with a history of anemia should have a CBC; those with any underlying disease associated with anemia should also be tested. Measurement of renal function and electrolyte levels may be indicated for all patients older than 60 years, but there are no data to support this recommendation. Such tests should be performed on the following patients: those with hypertension, diabetes, cardiovascular disease, or renal disease; those who are taking diuretics, angiotensin-converting enzyme (ACE) inhibitors, or angiotensin receptor blockers (ARBs); and those who will undergo bowel preparation for surgery. The Cockcroft-Gault equation should to used to estimate renal function from the serum creatinine; this equation estimates creatinine clearance, corrected for age and weight:

$$\text{Creatinine clearance (ml/min)} = \frac{(140 - \text{age}) \times \text{wt (in kg)}}{(\text{serum creatinine} \times 72)}$$

Routine measurement of the platelet count, prothrombin time, and partial thromboplastin time are not necessary.[30] Indications for testing include a history of prolonged bleeding, easy bruising, postoperative bleeding, or a family history of bleeding.[33] Patients on anticoagulants obviously also need testing.

Other areas of testing are more controversial. Liver enzyme, bilirubin, and albumin measurements are not needed unless there are indications of liver dysfunction on history and physical examination. Other serum chemistry tests, such as calcium and phosphate concentrations, are rarely indicated.

Management of Surgical Risk Factors

CORONARY ARTERY DISEASE

It is now clear that the use of perioperative beta blockers can prevent complications after surgery, both short term and long term.[34-36] Patients with known CAD who can tolerate beta blockers should already be taking these drugs. If they are not, a beta blocker should be started. Many experts recommend starting beta blockade before surgery in patients at high risk for CAD; such patients include those older than 70 years and those who have symptomatic heart failure, a history of stroke, renal insufficiency (i.e., a serum creatinine concentration greater than 2.0), or diabetes.[20] A number of agents have proved useful for perioperative treatment, including labetolol, esmolol, and bisoprolol. Because only a few studies have been done, no specific recommendations can be made; both intravenous and oral regimens have been used with success.[36]

BLOOD PRESSURE

Patients with diastolic blood pressures below 110 mm Hg are not at significant added risk and do not require specific blood pressure management.[1] For elective surgery, however, I believe it is useful that blood pressure be reasonably controlled (i.e., that diastolic blood pressure be lower than 100 mm Hg). It is clear that in patients with poorly controlled blood pressure who undergo surgery, blood pressure may swing widely, both in hypertensive and hypotensive directions. High blood pressure and low blood pressure can each cause problems perioperatively. Unless surgery is urgent or emergent, hurried attempts at blood pressure control are not advised. Excessive diuretic use can lead to volume depletion and hypokalemia; heavy doses of other medications can lead to unanticipated hypotension. Maintaining reasonable control for a period of about a week on an outpatient basis appears to be quite safe. Diuretics are usually withheld on the day of surgery to avoid preoperative volume decrease.[27] Other antihypertensive medications should be taken as usual. Patients with very high blood pressure who need surgery may require treatment with intravenous doses of drugs such as nitroprusside, labetolol, or enalaprilat.

RENAL INSUFFICIENCY

Although patients with significant renal disease are known to be at increased risk for perioperative morbidity and mortality, including increased cardiac complications,[1,2] there is little that can be done to decrease the risks for most of these patients. Foreknowledge aids in watching for complications, however. Perhaps the most common problem seen is volume depletion from high doses of diuretics. A blood urea nitrogen:creatinine ratio of approximately 10 is usually optimal; higher levels should increase suspicion of volume depletion. The presence of such signs as tachycardia, orthostatic changes in blood pressure and pulse, and poor skin turgor help to confirm this suspicion.

Other problems that are seen frequently in patients with renal insufficiency include hyponatremia, hyperkalemia, volume overload, and metabolic acidosis. These abnormalities should be treated to the extent possible before the operation. In patients with acute renal insufficiency, acute complications should be anticipated. Delirium from uremia, serositis (particularly pericarditis), and severe acidosis may be present or may develop quickly. Some of these patients may require dialysis before surgical intervention.

The management of patients on replacement therapy can be quite complicated. In general, to be in optimal condition for the operation, most patients undergo dialysis either on the day before or the day of surgery.

HYPERGLYCEMIA AND DIABETES MELLITUS

Hyperglycemia can lead to poor wound healing and perioperative infections, particularly wound infections.[37] Control of blood sugars to below approximately 200 mg/dl appears to be sufficient. There is now evidence that controlling blood sugars, even in patients without previous diabetes, can improve outcomes in patients in intensive care units.[38]

Oral antidiabetic agents should be discontinued on the day of surgery. In patients whose diabetes is controlled by diet and oral agents, normoglycemia can usually be maintained by giving regular insulin every 4 hours on a sliding scale, until diet and oral medications can be resumed.[39] Patients on insulin generally must be given insulin during and after surgery. It is best to perform surgery in the morning in these patients so that the dose of insulin can be more easily determined.

There are a number of methods of giving insulin.[39] There are no good studies to prove that one method gives better clinical results than another. The most expensive and time consuming but the one that provides the best glucose control is an intravenous drip of regular insulin. This method is probably not necessary in most cases, but in difficult, brittle cases, it will give the best glucose control. In most cases, it is reasonable to give one half to two thirds of the usual dose of neutral protamine Hagedorn (NPH) or other long-acting insulin, monitor regularly, and give regular insulin or glucose as needed.[39] Patients with hyperglycemia or acidosis will require more intensive dosing with regular insulin.

DECREASED HEMATOCRIT

The hematocrit level necessary for minimizing surgical risk has been controversial for many years. There are no good data to support any specific limits for all patients, although young, healthy patients clearly can tolerate much lower hematocrits than older patients with multiple underlying diseases, particularly those of the heart, vascular system, and lungs. Most patients without underlying disease can tolerate surgery if their hematocrit is above 28%; those with underlying heart or lung disease, particularly elderly patients, may need to undergo transfusion to raise the hematocrit above 35%.[40] Transfusion appears to decrease the development of postoperative delirium.

THYROID DISEASE

Patients with hypothyroidism do not have significant problems with surgery and do not require special treatment, provided they are functional.[23] Patients who are clinically hyperthyroid are at risk for thyroid storm perioperatively, so hyperthyroidism should be well controlled before surgery is undertaken. If surgery is necessary, it is best to consult an endocrinologist to manage the hyperthyroidism perioperatively.[41]

LIVER DISEASE

Underlying liver disease does not appear to be a major risk factor for surgery under most circumstances,[1] nor do elevated levels of liver enzymes appear to be associated with increased risk. Active inflammation from alcoholic hepatitis, however, substantially increases the risk of mortality. Patients with fever, elevated white blood cell counts, and jaundice should not have surgery unless their condition is clearly not the result of alcoholic hepatitis and they are facing a surgical emergency.[42] The main risks from underlying liver disease are variceal bleeding in patients with varices and hepatic encephalopathy in those at risk. Ascites also presents difficult management problems, with many complicated issues that are beyond the scope of this chapter [see Chapter 69].

CORTICOSTEROID THERAPY

Patients who are taking corticosteroids (e.g., for rheumatic disease or asthma) usually need replacement therapy perioperatively.[25] In normal persons, the daily output of cortisone is approximately 30 mg; peak stress levels are approximately 300 mg a day. Unfortunately, no good studies have been done to determine which patients definitely need supplementation and how long the increase in dose should be maintained. Current practice is to give additional medication to patients who are taking the equivalent of 30 mg or more of hydrocortisone a day. For patients at lower dose ranges, supplemental doses (e.g., 50 mg) given twice daily are adequate; for those taking more than 150 mg a day, three doses a day of 50 to 100 mg are usually recommended. It is unusual to give more than 100 mg three times a day. For most patients, the dose can be tapered back to baseline in 2 to 3 days.

ALCOHOL ABUSE

Patients who abuse alcohol are at risk for withdrawal syndromes when admitted for surgery. It is best to get patients to stop drinking at least a week before surgery. If efforts to get a patient to stop do not succeed (or if such efforts were not made, because the patient gave a misleading drinking history), then therapy should be begun for withdrawal as soon as the initial signs and symptoms are noted. Most often, these consist of tremor and tachycardia with agitation. Oral benzodiazepines (e.g., chlordiazepoxide, lorazepam, diazepam), are the usual choice for treating withdrawal; they may be given every 4 to 6 hours until symptoms abate.[43] The dose will depend on the patient's alcohol consumption; the dose can be remarkably high, as compared with the dose in patients who do not abuse alcohol. Requiring the equivalent of 400 mg of chlordiazepoxide is not uncommon.

THROMBOSIS

All surgical procedures increase the risk of deep vein thrombosis (DVT), and most major surgery carries a significant risk of both DVT and pulmonary embolism. Patients older than 40 years who will have an operation lasting longer than 30 minutes will require DVT prophylaxis. Most general and gynecologic surgery patients require low-dose heparin at 5,000 U every 12 hours; some experts believe that 5,000 U every 8 hours should be given for patients having long and complicated surgical procedures. In orthopedic surgery, particularly hip and knee operations, low-molecular-weight heparin is the agent of choice. There is increasing and convincing evidence that continuing DVT prophylaxis, particularly after orthopedic hip and knee surgery, for 4 to 6 weeks postoperatively prevents morbidity and mortality from late thromboses and pulmonary emboli. This is particularly true in light of the shorter hospitalizations of patients after surgical procedures.[44,45] Warfarin can be used as well. For surgical procedures in which any increased risk of bleeding is unacceptable (e.g., neurosurgery or open prostatectomy), intermittent compression stockings are most often used to prevent DVT.

ADVANCED AGE

Surgery in elderly patients has become routine over the past decade or so. Improvements in anesthetic techniques, better understanding of the management of medical diseases, and improved and less invasive surgical techniques have allowed older and much sicker patients to undergo surgery. Many studies have shown that an elderly patient can undergo most procedures that are important to survival or quality of life without being exposed to a large increase in perioperative risk.

The author has no commercial relationships with manufacturers of products or providers of services discussed in this chapter.

References

1. Goldman L, Caldera DL, Nussbaum SR et al: Multifactorial index of cardiac risk in noncardiac surgical procedures. N Engl J Med 297:845, 1977

2. Detsky AS, Abrams HB, McLaughlin JR, et al: Predicting cardiac complications in patients undergoing noncardiac surgery. J Gen Intern Med 1:211, 1986

3. Lee TH, Marcantonio ER, Mangione CM, et al: Derivation and prospective validation of a simple index for prediction of cardiac risk of major noncardiac surgery. Circulation 100:1043, 1999

4. Palda VA, Detsky AS: Perioperative assessment and management of risk for CAD. Ann Intern Med 127:313, 1997

5. Gilbert K, Larocque BJ, Patrick LT: Prospective evaluation of cardiac risk indices for patients undergoing noncardiac surgery. Ann Intern Med 133:356, 2000

6. Reilly DF, McNeely MJ, Doerner D, et al: Self reported exercise tolerance and the risk of serious perioperative complications. Arch Intern Med 159:2185, 1999

7. Halm EA, Browner WS, Tubau JF, et al: Echocardiography for assessing cardiac risk in patients having non-cardiac surgery. Ann Intern Med 125:433, 1996

8. Eagle KA, Berger PB, Calkins H, et al: ACC/AHA guideline update for perioperative cardiovascular evaluation of noncardiac surgery—executive summary: a report of the ACC/AHA task force on practice guidelines (Committee to Update the 1996 Guidelines on Perioperative Cardiovascular Evaluation for Noncardiac Surgery). J Am Coll Cardiol 39:542, 2002

9. Mukherjee D, Eagle KA: Perioperative cardiac assessment for noncardiac surgery: eight steps to the best possible outcome. Circulation 107:2771, 2003

10. Guidelines for assessing and managing the perioperative risk from CAD associated with major non-cardiac surgery. American College of Physicians. Ann Intern Med 127:309, 1997

11. Kwok Y, Kim C, Grady D et al: Meta-analysis of exercise testing to detect CAD in women. Am J Cardiol 83:660, 1999

12. Grayburn PA, Hillis LD: Cardiac events in patients undergoing noncardiac surgery: shifting the paradigm from noninvasive risk stratification to therapy. Ann Intern Med 138:506, 2003

13. Geleijnse ML, Elhendy A, Fioretti PM, et al. Dobutamine stress myocardial perfusion imaging. J Am Coll Cardiol 36:2017, 2000

14. Seymour DG, Pringle R, MacLennan WJ: The role of the routine preoperative elec-

trocardiogram in the elderly surgical patient. Age Ageing 12:97, 1983

15. Straus SE, McAlister FA, Sackett DL, et al: The accuracy of patient history, wheezing, and laryngeal measurements in diagnosing obstructive airway disease. CARE-COAD1 Group. Clinical Assessment of the Reliability of the Examination—Chronic Obstructive Airways Disease. JAMA 283:1853, 2000

16. Lawrence V, Page CP, Harris GD: Preoperative spirometry before abdominal operations. Arch Intern Med 149:280, 1989

17. Kocabas A, Kara A, Ozgur G, et al: Value of preoperative spirometry to predict postoperative pulmonary complications. Respir Med 90:25, 1996

18. Smetana GW: Preoperative pulmonary evaluation. N Engl J Med 340:937, 1999

19. Arozullah A, Daley J, Henderson W, et al: Multifactorial risk index for predicting postoperative respiratory failure in men after noncardiac surgery. Ann Surg 232:242, 2000

20. Seymour DG, Pringle R, Shaw JW: The role of the routine chest x-ray in the elderly general surgical patient. Postgrad Med 58:742, 1982

21. Consensus development conference on the diagnosis of coronary heart disease in people with diabetes. American Diabetes Association. Diabetes Care 12:1551, 1998

22. Ladenson PW, Levin AA, Ridgeway EC, et al: Complications of surgery in hypothyroid patients. Am J Med 77:261, 1984

23. Drucker DJ, Burrows GN: Cardiovascular surgery in the hypothyroid patient. Arch Intern Med 145:1585, 1985

24. Lamphier TA, Wickman W: Postoperative thyroid storm. Postgrad Med 15:493, 1954

25. Salassa RM, Bennett WA, Keating FR, et al: Postoperative adrenal cortical insufficiency: occurrence in patients previously treated with cortisone. JAMA 152:1509, 1953

26. Winawer N: Postoperative delirium. Med Clin North Am 85:1229, 2001

27. Kroenke K, Gooby-Toedt D, Jackson JL: Chronic medications in the perioperative period. South Med J 91:358, 1998

28. Lawrence R, Walter RM: Diabetes mellitus. Medical Management of the Surgical Patient. Lubin MF, Walker HK, Smith RB III, Eds. Lippincott Williams & Wilkins, Philadelphia, 1995, p 317

29. Geerts W, Heit J, Claggett G, et al: Prevention of venous thromboembolism. Chest 119:132s, 2001

30. Kaplan EB, Sheiner LB, Boeckmann AJ, et al: The usefulness of preoperative laboratory screening. JAMA 253:3576, 1985

31. Narr BJ, Hansen TR, Warner MA: Preoperative laboratory screening in healthy Mayo patients. Mayo Clinic Proc 66:15, 1991

32. McKee RF, Scott EM: The value of routine preoperative investigation. Ann R Coll Surg Engl 69:160, 1987

33. Rapaport SI: Preoperative hemostatic evaluation: which tests if any? Blood 61:229, 1983

34. Mangano DT, Layug EC, Wallace A, et al: Effect of atenolol on mortality and cardiovascular morbidity after non-cardiac surgery. N Engl J Med 335:1713, 1996

35. Poldermans D, Boersma E, Bax JJ, et al: The effect of bisoprolol on perioperative mortality and myocardial infarction in high risk patients undergoing vascular surgery. N Engl J Med 341:1789, 1999

36. Auerbach AD, Goldman L: Beta blockers and reduction of cardiac events in noncardiac surgery: scientific review. JAMA 287:1435, 2002

37. Golden SH, Peart-Vigilance C, Kao WH, et al: Perioperative glycemic control and the risk of infectious complications in a cohort of adults with diabetes. Diabetes Care 22:1408, 1999

38. Van den Berghe G, Wouter R, Weekers F, et al: Intensive insulin therapy in critically ill patients. N Engl J Med 345:1359, 2001

39. Hoogwerf BJ: Management of the diabetic patient. Med Clin North Am 85:1213, 2001

40. Carson JL, Duff A, Berlin JA, et al: Perioperative blood transfusion and postoperative mortality. JAMA 279:199, 1998

41. Langley RW, Burch HB: Perioperative management of the thyrotoxic patient. Endocrinol Metab Clin North Am 32:519, 2003

42. Powell-Jackson P, Greenway B, Williams R: Adverse effects of exploratory laparotomy in patients with unsuspected liver disease. Br J Surg 69:449, 1982

43. Chang PH, Steinberg MB: Alcohol withdrawal in postoperative patients. Med Clin North Am 85:1191, 2001

44. Hull RD, Pineo GF, Stein PD, et al: Extended out-of-hospital low-molecular-weight heparin prophylaxis against deep vein thrombosis in patients after elective hip arthroplasty: a systematic review. Ann Intern Med 135:858, 2001

45. Eikelboom JW, Quinlan DJ, Couketis JD: Extended-duration prophylaxis against venous thromboembolism after total hip or knee replacement: a meta-analysis of the randomised trials. Lancet 358:9, 2001

7 Occupational Medicine

Linda Rosenstock, M.D., M.P.H., F.A.C.P., and Mark R. Cullen, M.D.

Awareness of the impact of the work environment on health has increased dramatically in the past few decades. Common clinical problems, such as carpal tunnel syndrome and respiratory irritation and allergy, are increasingly being related to physical, chemical, and biologic hazards at work.[1] In this chapter, we cover some of the most common occupational disorders diagnosed in industrialized countries, and we present examples of known or suspected causes [*see Table 1*]. More extensive descriptions of specific disorders are presented in other chapters of *ACP Medicine* and in textbooks of occupational medicine.[2-4] An increasing amount of information about occupational medicine is available on the Internet from the National Institute for Occupational Safety and Health (http://www.cdc.gov) and the Occupational Safety and Health Administration (http://www.osha.gov).

Data on the frequency of occurrence of most occupational disorders are limited; however, data demonstrating the extent of the problem are available. Recent estimates are that each year, approximately 55,000 deaths result from occupational illness, and 3.8 million disabling occupation-related injuries occur.[5] Costs of occupational deaths and related injuries have been estimated to be $125 billion to $155 billion a year.[5,6] Occupational illness is common and has substantial clinical ramifications.

Basic Principles of Occupational Disease

It is important to debunk the widespread and erroneous perception that most occupational disorders are pathologically unique. Although some disorders, such as silicosis, do have distinguishing pathologic characteristics, the majority do not. Most occupational diseases—such as lung cancer induced by ionizing radiation, bladder cancer caused by fumes from coke ovens, asthma triggered by the inhalation of platinum salts, and fatty liver resulting from the absorption of the solvent dimethylformamide through the skin—are pathologically indistinguishable from disorders with more familiar causes. However, it is virtually always possible to differentiate occupational diseases from their nonoccupational counterparts. Laboratory testing and data gathering provide the best clues for the diagnosis of occupational disease, but to recognize these disorders, it is critical to ask appropriate questions when taking the medical history [*see* Clinical Evaluation, *below*].

Workplace toxins and hazards, when adequately studied, have predictable and discrete pathologic consequences. Although other diseases share common final pathways, the initial mechanisms of injury are generally highly specific for each agent. Aside from the possibility of idiosyncratic responses, as occur with pharmacologic agents, the actual potential effects of most toxins are few. For example, beryllium may cause an acute inflammatory pneumonia (acute beryllium disease) within hours after intense exposure, or it may cause a delayed hypersensitivity response with granulomatous lung disease (chronic beryllium disease [CBD]) in persons with recurrent or long-term exposures; no other form of nonmalignant lung disease is known to be caused by this metal or its salts.

Both the likelihood that workplace hazards will produce effects and the severity of those effects are determined by the amount of toxin to which the patient is exposed (hereafter referred to as dose). The nature of the relation between dose and response depends on the mechanism of action of the agent. For direct-acting toxins, which cause effects by directly disrupting cellular function or cell death at the target-organ level, there is usually a dose beneath which no biologic effects are observed—a so-called threshold level. Above this level, there is typically a sigma-shaped dose-response correlation as dose rises, until a lethal dose is reached. Similarly, an increasing percentage of the exposed population is affected as dose rises; eventually, everyone is affected. This is characteristic of heavy metals, organic solvents, and pesticides. For agents that cause allergic-type or idiosyncratic responses, such as latex and epoxy resins, which affect only susceptible people, dose contributes to the likelihood of sensitization, though not necessarily to the severity of the reaction. Further, once a worker has become sensitized, a very low dose may be sufficient to induce a full-blown clinical response. For mutagens and carcinogens, current knowledge presumes a linear dose-response model, with each increment in cumulative dose resulting in a proportional increase in the risk of cancer. The severity of the resultant cancer bears no predictable relation to the induction dose, though the time from exposure to onset generally is shorter when doses are higher.

The temporal relation between exposure and effect is highly predictable for each agent and each effect. For many direct toxins, effects occur within minutes or hours after exposure to an appropriate dose, such as the syndrome of cholinergic storm after organophosphate pesticide poisoning. Similarly, immunologically mediated responses, such as asthma and dermatitis, will occur within minutes or hours after exposure. Conversely, other effects are predictably delayed. Asbestos and silica rarely cause pneumoconiosis in less than 10 years after first exposure, except after very high exposure levels. Solid tumors, such as lung cancer associated with these same dusts, emerge, on average, 20 to 30 years after first exposure. Other effects occur in an intermediate time frame: some organophosphates cause a paralysis whose onset is delayed by weeks to months after an intense overexposure. The presentations of acute lead, mercury, or arsenic poisoning are insidious, coming after the poison accumulates to a dangerous level, usually after weeks or months of exposure.

When the clinician is approaching patients with new medical problems, consideration should be given to occupational causes. If the problem is acute, such as the relatively sudden onset of a rash or of liver function abnormalities or hemolysis, the search for a possible occupational cause should focus on recent events: Has there been a new or increased exposure to an agent that can cause such toxicity in the hours, days, or, at most, weeks before onset? On the other hand, for chronic disorders, such as pulmonary fibrosis and cancer, the search for causes should begin with a work history that goes back years.

With regard to work histories, it is important to note that host factors may modify temporal and dose-response correlations; all workers do not react alike to comparable exposures.

Table 1   Common Occupational Disorders

	Disorders	Examples of Causal Factors
Respiratory tract	Pneumoconiosis Asthma Allergic alveolitis Metal fume fever	Coal, silica, asbestos Latex, polyurethane Vegetable matter, machining fluids Metal fumes
Skin	Contact dermatitis Acne Urticaria	Oils, rubber, metals Herbicides, oils, friction Latex
Urinary tract	Glomerular disease Tubulointerstitial disease	Organic solvents, mercury Cadmium, lead
Liver	Acute or subacute necrosis Cholestatic hepatitis Acute and chronic hepatitis Steatosis Hepatoportal sclerosis Hepatocellular injury	Organic solvents, TNT, 2-nitropropane Methylene dianiline Viruses (hepatitis B, C) Organic solvents Vinyl chloride, arsenical compounds Lead, arsenic, phosphorus, dioxin
Musculoskeletal	Carpal tunnel syndrome Raynaud phenomenon Scleroderma	Repetitive trauma Repetitive vibrations, vinyl chloride Coal mining
Nervous system	Parkinsonism Peripheral neuropathy Acute encephalopathy Acute or subacute cholinergic crisis Subacute encephalopathy Subacute peripheral neuropathy Chronic basal gangliar disorder Chronic encephalopathy	Manganese Solvents, lead, acrylamide, arsenic Organic solvents, asphyxiants Organophosphate and carbamate pesticides Mercury, lead, arsenic, manganese, carbon disulfide Organophosphates Manganese, carbon monoxide (postasphyxiation) Recurrent organic solvent exposures

Hematologic conditions	Hemolysis
	Accelerated red cell destruction
	  Acute hemolysis
	  Subacute hemolysis
	Disorders of oxygen transport
	  Methemoglobinemia
	  Carboxyhemoglobinemia
	Disorders of red cell production
	  Hyperplastic anemia
	  Aplastic anemia, hypoplastic anemia
	  Myelodysplasia
	  Polycythemia
		Lead, organic nitrites
		
		Nitro and amine compounds
		Lead
		
		Nitro and amine compounds
		Carbon monoxide
		
		Lead
		Ethylene glycol ethers, benzene, arsenic, ionizing radiation
		Benzene, ionizing radiation
		Cobalt

Infectious	Hepatitis B, C Influenza A (H5N1) SARS Anthrax	Health care Poultry workers Health care Animal handling
Endocrine and reproductive	Hypogonadism Azoospermia, oligospermia Teratogenesis	Lead DBCP, ionizing radiation Organic mercury, PCBs

DBCP—1,2-dibromo-3-chloropropane (pesticide)   PCBs—polychlorinated biphenyls   SARS—severe acute respiratory syndrome

In every workplace, some people appear to be immune to the effects of even the most toxic agents, and others seem to react to low doses, often lower than the threshold deemed toxic by regulatory authorities. These differences may be caused by genetic, dietary, or constitutional factors or by the preexistence of other illnesses.

In addition, many workplace hazards and toxins interact with one another and with nonoccupational factors to cause disease. Dose-response correlations for industrial hazards may be markedly shifted in the presence of other hazards, habits, or medications. An important example is the likelihood of disease resulting from thermal stress (i.e., heat or cold) in the presence of hemodynamically active agents, such as calcium channel blockers, autonomic agents, and diuretics.[7] Likewise, the effects of vibration trauma on wrists and digits may be amplified by nicotine.[8] The effects of one hazard may be significantly altered in the presence of another; for example, the combined effect of noise and solvents on hearing loss[9] and of asbestos and smoking on lung cancer[10] are greater than the effect of exposure to each hazard alone.

CLINICAL EVALUATION

Defining the Pathophysiologic Basis of the Patient's Complaints

When searching for the pathophysiologic basis of a patient's complaints, it is important to ascertain the following: Is the process an acute or relapsing process, with precipitous changes in physiologic status, reflecting a recent or ongoing exposure? Or is it a chronic process, more likely the result of noxious exposure in the distant past? Dysfunction of what organ or organs best explains symptoms? Is there evidence of physiologic disruption, or is the disorder predominantly one of subjective difficulties?

Taking the Occupational History

Every patient should be questioned regarding the essentials of occupation, including current and past workplaces, job type, and materials used. Open-ended questions are always appropriate (e.g., "Are there dangerous materials or hazards in your workplace?" and "Do you believe that your work is causing you any health problems?").[11] The exploration of work as the basis for a complaint or medical problem entails an incisive approach and depends on the nature of the clinical problem being investigated. Evidence suggests that physicians need to become more adept at assessing a patient's occupational history.[12]

Approach to the Patient with an Acute Disorder

The emphasis should be on new exposures, increased exposures, and accidental exposures. Has the patient recently begun a new job or task involving hazards? Were new materials recently introduced at work? Has there been a change in working conditions, such as a failure of the ventilation system? Has there been a leak, spill, or accident? If the answer to all of these questions is no, the likelihood is low that the acute illness is related to work processes or chemicals.

Other than acute effects that are immunologically mediated, most effects are not idiosyncratic and will follow a sigma-shaped dose-response correlation like that discussed for direct-acting toxins (see above). In such circumstances, it would be expected that a high proportion of exposed persons would be affected, although individual thresholds and dose responses may differ. Questions probing effects in other exposed persons are extremely helpful, as in the investigation of food poisoning or respiratory infections. Although a negative answer does not exclude a work-related effect, the suggestion of an outbreak or a cluster makes the probability of an association high and increases the urgency of a prompt, correct diagnosis.

Approach to the Patient with Recurrent Manifestations

A patient may have repeated or recurring manifestations, such as intermittent cough, rash, or nausea. Although the cause may be difficult to establish in some situations, especially when symptoms have been very persistent or chronic, the time course, particularly at the onset of recurring manifestations, is often extremely revealing. For example, a new asthma patient whose symptoms occur on vacations and weekends is unlikely to have an occupationally related disorder.

Approach to the Patient with Chronic Disease

When patients present with evidence of irreversible organ damage or malignancy, the approach is altogether different. Although the longer latency between initial exposure and disease onset is useful in determining whether occupational exposures have played an important role, questions directed at temporal associations between symptoms and exposures are not helpful. Rather, the first step is to establish a clear pathophysiologic picture of the disease process itself. Sometimes, knowledge of past exposures may assist in directing this evaluation. For example, a worker who has been exposed to asbestos and who presents with a malignant pleural effusion should be carefully evaluated for mesothelioma, which is otherwise an uncommon disorder.

Once the disease process is characterized, a role for occupational factors can be more seriously considered by obtaining a more detailed history of exposures. Because only a handful of agents are suspected of causing or have been proved to cause any single chronic disease, the goal of this history is to determine whether exposure to any of those agents has occurred and whether the exposure occurred at a time and dose that suggest a causal connection to the disease.

Approach to Subacute and Insidious Disease

The greatest diagnostic challenge in clinical occupational medicine is the clinical disorder of gradual onset over days to weeks for which none of the above approaches are effective. Examples include peripheral neuropathies, anemia, and a change in bowel habit in the absence of evidence of malignant or irreversible organ system damage. Often, in such cases, the search for the underlying pathophysiologic process and the search for its cause seem intricately related and must proceed simultaneously. Lessons from these paradigms may be helpful. If indeed the subacute process is toxic, it most likely reflects the effects of a recent exposure, typically of an agent that is accumulating slowly. Heavy metals, pesticides, and various toxic organic chemicals often accumulate in this fashion; under typical conditions of exposure, it may take weeks or months for these agents to accrue to levels of pathogenic significance. Although it is unnecessary to identify an accidental leak or spill to make a diagnosis in such cases, it is essential to note any enhanced opportunity for exposure or any novel exposure that may have occurred relatively recently. The distant exposure history is not likely to be helpful, because the subacute disorders almost always present at the point of maximal accumulation; once the worker is removed from the site of the exposure, latency or delay in onset is unusual.

CONFIRMING AND QUANTIFYING EXPOSURE

There are two basic approaches to obtaining additional exposure information. The first involves the collection of independent information about present or former work (depending on which is relevant). After the physician obtains consent from the patient (to ensure that the patient is protected from unwanted consequences), information about exposures is requested from the employer, a trade union, or a regulatory agency. Such information is usually reported through the use of a material safety data sheet (MSDS). The MSDS provides generic chemical names, compositions, and basic toxicity information of all materials used. In addition, employers may be able to provide evidence of objective sampling that may have been done to test air levels of hazardous substances. Job descriptions, results of medical tests performed at work, information about other workers with health problems, and the use of protective equipment or other methods to limit exposure may all be of value in assessing workplace exposures.

The second potential source of dose information is biologic testing. For a few hazards, testing of urine, blood, or hair may enable the physician to determine the body burden of the agent;

Table 2 Common Occupational Hazards for Which There Are Widely Available Biologic Tests of Exposure

Hazard	Comments
Metals	
Arsenic	Hair sampling can detect historic exposures
Cadmium	Detectable in urine for many years if there is renal injury
Fluorides	Transient in urine
Lead	Half-life 40 days in blood
Mercury	Detectable in urine for days to weeks
Asphyxiants	
Carbon monoxide	Half-life 4 hr in blood
Pesticides	
Organophosphates	Detectable indirectly, by measurement of cholinesterase, which may be depressed for days to months
Organochlorines (e.g., DDT, chlordane, dieldrin)	Persists in blood
Organic solvents	
Benzene and toluene	Metabolites transiently in urine
Antigens	IgE antibodies measurable by RAST
Miscellaneous	
PCBs	Persists in blood

PCBs—polychlorinated biphenyls   RAST—radioallergosorbent test

the results of such testing correlate with current or recent levels and, less commonly, with remote exposures [*see Table 2*]. Most of these tests cannot detect chemicals that have been cleared from the body or deposited in bodily organs; this substantially limits their usefulness for diagnostic decision making. Of course, there are no simple tests for chemicals that cause topical injury to skin or respiratory mucosa but are not absorbed. For agents that act by immune sensitization, radioallergosorbent testing or skin-patch testing may be useful both for documenting exposure and for subsequent elicitation of an immune response.

Most important of all is to remember that a test for exposure can be interpreted only in the context of the history and the clinical problem. It should not be directly interpreted as a test for disease, regardless of how the laboratory reports the data. For example, a whole blood lead level of 25 mg/dl is clear evidence of excess lead exposure. If the history indicated that the patient had recently been exposed for the first time, this level would suggest a modest, generally subtoxic dose of lead. If, however, the patient had worked around lead for many years and quit a year before the test was performed, this same value would suggest a very high previous exposure and might well be associated with health effects caused by high long-term exposure. Similarly, a large proportion of bakers working around flour dust may have IgE antibodies to wheat, rye, or other grain antigens, even though the vast majority of those bakers are symptom free and will most likely remain so. Given all these limitations, biologic testing plays only a limited role in occupational medicine and can never be a substitute for the occupational history.

DIAGNOSTIC DECISION MAKING

The determination that a patient's symptoms are work related often entails extensive ramifications for the patient's employer,

as well as potentially serious public health and medicolegal implications. These may present a significant challenge to the clinician, because for many occupational disorders, there is no gold standard for diagnosis.

The decision-making process should address the following questions:

1. Is the clinical illness—including the history, physical examination, and laboratory findings—consistent with other case descriptions?
2. Is the timing between exposure and clinical onset compatible with the known biologic facts about the hazard?
3. Is the exposure dose within the range of doses believed to cause such effects?
4. Are there special attributes of the particular patient that make it more or less likely that he or she would be so affected?
5. Are there alternative ways of constructing the case that better fit the available facts?
6. Where there remains significant uncertainty about the cause, how important is it to be certain?

Regarding the certainty of identifying the cause, the general legal standard for workers' compensation purposes is "more likely than not," which is a relatively low hurdle of certainty (i.e., at least 50% certain). However, there may be other situations that demand a higher level of confidence, irrespective of the standard for obtaining compensation benefits. In general, problems involving current working conditions demand a far greater level of certainty than historical ones. For example, a diagnosis of occupational asthma in a spray painter would likely dictate removing the patient completely from exposure to the offending paint or constituent; correct identification of that agent might be crucial to saving his or her career. Similarly, if a surgeon presented with recurrent anaphylactic reactions, it would be very important to determine whether the reactions were to latex, an anesthetic agent, or some extrinsic factor.

In situations where a high level of certainty is needed, it is often worth the effort to refine the diagnostic impression by serial observations, usually while the patient remains exposed, or by utilizing diagnostic challenges of removal followed by reexposure. Using serial functional measurements, such as peak expiratory flow records or serial blood tests, a more certain judgment can be made. This may also be an appropriate circumstance for referral to occupational physicians who specialize in evaluating challenging cases.

Major Occupational Disorders in Developed Countries

The spectrum of occupational disorders of clinical importance is rapidly shifting as a result of several factors: these include changes in the economy, which have brought about a decline in traditional manufacturing and a rise in service-sector activities; better control of many hazards, such as mineral dusts (e.g., asbestos, silica, coal), heavy metals (e.g., lead, arsenic, mercury), and the most toxic solvents (e.g., benzene); rapid introduction of many new technologies whose health risks remain inadequately characterized; and changing demographics in the workplace, in which the proportion of women, minority, and older workers is increasing. In the sections that follow, the disorders that are most important in clinical practice in developed countries are briefly discussed by organ system.

OCCUPATIONAL CANCER

Only a small fraction of known chemical agents and a handful of physical and biologic hazards appear capable of inducing neoplastic change in mammalian tissues. In general, the risk of cancer being induced increases in direct proportion to total dose of toxin to which the person is exposed. Typically, the target organ is relatively specific and is determined by metabolism and transport of the agent. However, a few agents, including ionizing radiation and asbestos, appear to have potential to cause malignancy at more than one human site. There is invariably a long lag time between initial exposure and onset of clinical disease. Only a small number of hazards found in the workplace have been clearly established as carrying substantive cancer risk for workers. An additional group of hazards are suspected, but additional studies are needed. The list of potential carcinogens is expanding; for example, evidence suggests that exposure to cadmium may play a role in the development of prostate cancer.[13] Studies provide some indication that workers in print shops, service-station employees, farm-product vendors, horticulturists, farmers, and aircraft mechanics are at increased risk for renal cell carcinoma[14,15] [see Table 3].

Table 3 Established Occupational Carcinogens

Cancer Site	Hazard	Setting
Lung	Asbestos	Insulation, textiles
	Ionizing radiation	Uranium mining
	Arsenic	Refining
	Polyaromatic hydrocarbons	Coke ovens
	Nickel	Nickel refining
	Chromium	Tanning, pigments
	Alkylating agents	Chemical industry
	Silica	Mining, stonecutting
	Ceramic fibers	Insulation
	Formaldehyde	Chemicals, plastics
	Beryllium	Nuclear weapons, aerospace industry
	Cadmium	Batteries
	Acrylonitrile	Plastics
	1,3-Butadiene	Rubber, plastics
Pleura and peritoneum	Asbestos	Construction materials
Upper respiratory tract	Wood dust	Carpentry
	Nickel	Refining
	Chromium	Plating
	Asbestos	Friction products
	Formaldehyde	Chemicals, plastics
Urinary bladder	Benzidine and related amines	Dyes, chemicals
	Polyaromatic hydrocarbons	Aluminum reduction
Liver	Vinyl chloride monomer	Plastics
	Arsenic	Pesticides
Upper GI tract	Asbestos	Shipbuilding
	Coal dust	Mining
	Acrylonitrile	Plastics
Hematologic system	Benzene	Chemicals, rubber
	Ionizing radiation	Defense industry
	Ethylene oxide	Chemicals, sterilizers
Soft tissue	Dioxin	Chemical industry
Brain	Vinyl chloride	Chemical industry
	Formaldehyde	Chemical industry

RESPIRATORY TRACT DISORDERS

The respiratory tract is a frequent target of toxic effects. Complaints referable to the lungs or upper respiratory tract often require a careful evaluation for occupational causes. The presence of other possible causal factors, such as common allergy and smoking, does not exclude the possibility of an occupational cause and may, in fact, increase the likelihood of one.

Acute Disorders and Recurrent Disorders

The most prevalent acute effects—inflammatory reactions of the mucosae of the upper or lower airway system—are caused by environmental irritants.[16] An extraordinary array of agents are irritating, including simple inorganic gases (e.g., ammonia and chlorine), organic solvents, acid and alkaline mists, metal fumes (i.e., tiny particles of metal and metal oxide that occur when vaporized metals hit cool air), mineral dusts (e.g., fibrous glass and coal), and almost all the pyrolytic products of combustion. The anatomic site of irritation for dusts, mists, and fumes depends on the deposition of particles; for gases, it depends on water solubility (i.e., the more water soluble the gas, the more it will dissolve in the upper respiratory tract). Expression of symptoms, from mild burning of the eyes, nose, and throat to small airway and alveolar injury associated with the acute respiratory distress syndrome, depends on dose, duration of exposure, and the potency and composition of the irritant; there is also substantial host variability. The period from the time of exposure to the onset of symptoms is very brief for the upper respiratory structures and can be from minutes to hours for lower structures.

Most of the consequences of acute irritation are self-limited; the upper respiratory tract is particularly resilient, although patients who work in areas of poor air quality will experience frequent recurrences, punctuated by commonplace complications such as sinusitis. Such cases require steps to modify exposure. More severe insults may result in fixed scarring of airways or lung parenchyma; late inflammatory sequelae such as bronchiolitis obliterans are occasionally reported. A newly recognized and probably common outcome of significant lower airway injury is the occurrence of persistent mucosal irritation and bronchospasm, a variant of asthma induced by a single exposure or repeated exposures to irritants. Initially dubbed reactive airways dysfunction syndrome,[17] this disorder is best classified as nonimmune occupational asthma or simply asthma without latency. Unfortunately, the condition tends to be highly resistant to therapy, and patients derive only modest benefit from inhaled steroids or other bronchodilators. Typically, cough with some phlegm, chest discomfort, and occasionally even dyspnea persist despite early and intensive therapy. Reassurance and reduction of further exposures to irritants are the mainstays of treatment.

Occupational asthma, including the nonimmune- and the immune-mediated varieties, is prevalent.[18] There are now over 200 established causes of presumed immune-mediated asthma[19]; these are usually categorized as proteins and other high-molecular-weight antigens (e.g., animal danders, latex antigens, and grains) and small molecules such as the isocyanates—the ubiquitous chemicals used in polyurethane products. Typically, the classic antigens differentially affect those with atopy and are associated with identifiable IgE antibody responses to the sensitizer.[20] In such cases, the greatest diagnostic dilemma is distinguishing occupational sources from other causes of asthma, though the periodicity as documented by history or peak expiratory flow records (PEFR) aid in identifying a relation to work. Latex has become a particularly important cause, especially when rendered airborne in association with the use of powdered gloves.[21,22] More troublesome are the low-molecular-weight agents such as toluene-2,4-diisocyanate (TDI) and other isocyanates, for which atopy is not a risk factor.[19,23] Onset is often insidious, with cough and chest discomfort relatively more common than in asthma of other causes. Far more often than with the IgE-mediated agents, symptoms may be delayed some hours after exposure, so patterns may include nocturnal complaints. Once the physiologic hallmarks of asthma are established, the history and PEFR are the keys to specific diagnosis. Studies have shown that detailed histories can be inconclusive; in some cases, objective measurements can establish the diagnosis of occupational asthma.[24] Specific inhalation tests may be valuable, but they should be performed only under medical supervision.

Current evidence suggests that correct diagnosis of occupational asthma makes a difference. People who are removed early from further contact have a better likelihood of reducing their dependence on medication; many will become nonasthmatic over time.[19,20] Most who remain exposed will develop persistent nonspecific bronchial hyperreactivity, as well as possible fixed obstructive changes. These patients will typically fail to recover after they are removed from contact with the agent, and their conditions may even worsen; this is the basis for an aggressive posture toward early evaluation and management.

Acute infectious diseases occur in an extraordinarily wide variety of workplaces, from health care to industrial and agricultural settings. Anthrax and other agents of bioterrorism, as well as emerging infectious diseases such as severe acute respiratory syndrome and influenza A (H5N1) are of particular concern to workers.[25,26]

Allergic alveolitis, with its more benign variants, such as humidifier fever, continues to occur sporadically in a wide range of settings. This disorder was traditionally associated with agricultural exposures to molds and bacilli. Cases are now reported to occur in manufacturing and other industrial settings because of the appearance of a few chemicals that appear capable of inducing the immune response (e.g., plastic resin constituents) and because of the contamination of many industrial processes with microorganisms.[27] The office environment continues to be an occasional source of this condition as well, though the reservoir of causal microbes may be obscure; such organisms may potentially reside in heating and air-conditioning systems remote from the patient's work area.[28]

Chronic Conditions

The pneumoconioses continue to occur, in part because of their very long latency from first exposure and because pockets of very poor industrial conditions continue to exist even in developed countries. Construction activities have been particularly problematic. In general, asbestosis, silicosis, and coal workers' pneumoconiosis are diseases that occur after extensive work exposures. The diagnosis can usually be made on the basis of clinical findings and the history of exposure, once the patient's lifetime job history is obtained.

The granulomatous diseases, including CBD and so-called hard metal disease, are less common but important and increasingly recognized disorders of sensitization. CBD is clinically almost identical to idiopathic sarcoidosis except that all cases involve the lung and that the prognosis—even after the patient is removed from exposure to beryllium metal, compound, or fumes—is generally unfavorable. All patients with sarcoidosis

should be asked if they work with metals, and the least suspicion should prompt specific testing; there is a highly sensitive test that can distinguish sarcoidosis from CBD on blood or bronchoalveolar lavage (BAL) fluid.[29] Hard metal disease is a giant cell alveolitis induced through an idiosyncratic reaction in workers exposed to the metal cobalt.[30] Most often, it occurs in workers making or using tungsten carbide, the very hard metal used for machine tools. Onset may be insidious and may include asthmatic symptoms, because cobalt is asthmogenic as well. Recognition of the parenchymal process by BAL or biopsy is crucial because hard metal disease is progressive, often refractory to treatment with steroids, and often lethal; there is anecdotal evidence favoring the use of cytotoxic drugs. Once hard metal disease is diagnosed, the patient should be promptly removed from any further exposure.

In 1998, a novel form of interstitial fibrosis related to an industrial exposure was reported: flock worker's lung, named after the nylon flocking used for making feltlike textiles.[31] Cases of flock worker's lung are distinctive, with pathologic evidence of both parenchymal fibrosis and lymphocytic bronchiolitis. The reporting of flock worker's lung underscores a key principle of occupational medicine: that new occupational diseases and other clinical consequences of work continue to be uncovered.[32]

DERMATOLOGIC DISORDERS

Despite increased recognition of the need to reduce contact between the skin and the chemical and physical environment, dermal conditions remain responsible for significant morbidity in the workplace. Most disorders are caused by direct exposure of the skin to workplace irritants, sensitizers, pigments, carcinogens, and materials that interfere with normal dermal function by disrupting sebaceous and follicular secretions (e.g., oils that cause acne) or solvents that erode protective lipids. Trauma, foreign bodies, ionizing and nonionizing radiation, and extremes of temperature may modify or disrupt skin growth, vascular integrity, or both. On occasion, systemic exposure may have a dermal consequence, as in urticarial responses to inhaled antigens, pigmentary alterations from the deposition of metals (e.g., silver), and the much-described though rarely seen chloracne, a variant of acne induced by dioxins and related chemicals. Workers who are at increased risk for allergic contact dermatitis include tanners, cast-concrete product workers, leather-goods workers, footwear workers, machine and metal product assemblers, electrical and telecommunications equipment assemblers, print-shop workers, and machine and engine mechanics.[33] Several excellent texts of occupational skin diseases are available.[34-36]

Overwhelmingly, the major skin problem in the workplace remains dermatitis, either irritant induced or caused by allergy. Many agents may be responsible, including organic and inorganic chemicals, plastics and rubber, oils and lubricants, metals and construction materials, paints, and coatings.[37] Both allergic dermatitis and irritant-induced dermatitis are more likely to affect persons with atopic conditions, dry skin, or other dermal risk factors. Distinguishing between the two is less important than recognizing occupational precipitants in the first place; both are difficult to differentiate from other commonplace skin disorders, such as eczema. The key to correct diagnosis is the history of skin contact and the temporal relation between contact and manifestations. Unfortunately, there is seldom a perfect or obvious correlation between the two, and some sleuthing is necessary, especially to discern the extent to which chemical contact may spread to places like the groin or areas where hand contact occurs. Airborne exposure may cause lesions in apparently untouched areas, such as the face; such occurrences are signs of likely hypersensitivity. Vexingly, symptoms do not always abate dramatically over weekends or during short periods in which exposure is avoided; removing the patient from the toxin for a week or two may be necessary to observe response. This, combined with observation of the patient during reexposure, is often the most valuable diagnostic test. Patch testing, performed by an experienced clinician aware of the exposures of concern, may be useful in difficult cases, though the clinician should keep in mind that irritants may yield false negative results and that even many healthy atopic persons will experience reactions to common contactants, such as nickel.[38] Often, complete isolation from offending agents is economically infeasible, and materials that previously were well tolerated become sources of irritation and exacerbation. Combinations of work modification, aggressive treatment of flares and complications, and careful attention to routine skin care are necessary to control disease.

DISORDERS OF THE URINARY TRACT

Although innumerable toxins are known to cause acute injury to the kidney, exposures to chemical and physical agents at concentrations found in the workplace rarely cause such effects (exceptions include cases involving overwhelming accidental overexposure or ingestion). Of far greater concern are recurring exposures to agents at more typical workplace exposure levels that have subclinical effects but can lead to late nephropathy. Although there remains a vast burden of unexplained nephropathology in the population and despite epidemiologic data suggesting an occupational cause,[39,40] chronic renal injury resulting from workplace exposures remains poorly characterized.

The best-established effects on the urinary tract are those caused by exposure to heavy metals, especially lead, mercury, and cadmium; each of these metals is associated with a unique pattern of effects. Workers whose jobs entail exposure to lead include traffic police, hazardous-waste incineration workers, industrial workers, and furniture strippers; workers at risk for exposure to mercury include gold-mine workers, workers at chloral-kali plants, workers exposed to hazardous waste, and construction workers; workers at risk for exposure to cadmium include those involved in the manufacture of batteries. Long-standing heavy-lead exposure results in a pattern of injury difficult to distinguish pathologically and clinically from the effects of hypertension; signs and symptoms include nephrosclerosis and evidence of both glomerular and tubular defects. The ability to clear urate is impaired early in the course and may be a clue; saturnine gout may occur a decade later. There is debate about the possibility of low-level or brief exposures to lead predisposing to hypertension or enhancing the degree of renal injury associated with essential hypertension or gout.[41,42] Proponents of this view stress the importance of assessment of lead exposure in patients with mild chronic renal insufficiency.[43]

Long-term occupational exposure to inorganic mercury—principally through exposure to mercury vapor—may result in renal alterations involving the tubules and glomeruli. The monitoring of urinary mercury is useful for controlling such risk.[44]

Cadmium exposure in jewelry making, battery production, and other metal-processing operations leads to bioaccumulation of cadmium in the kidney, which results in proximal tubular injury with excessive excretion of β_2-microglobulin and other tubular proteins. Later, a pattern of renal tubular acidosis may

occur, which subsequently may lead to the development of renal insufficiency. Because the tubular dysfunction is only partially reversible,[45] it is important to carefully monitor cadmium exposure, which is best done with regular blood and urine cadmium testing.[46] Renal damage can occur at relatively low levels of cadmium exposure.[47]

Organic solvents have been implicated in renal tubular and renal parenchymal injury[48]; despite uncertainty of their role in renal toxicity, growing evidence suggests the need for evaluation of these substances in all new cases of unexplained nephropathy.

LIVER DISEASE

The liver is highly sensitive to effects of numerous organic and inorganic substances used in the workplace [see Table 1]. Despite the impressive potential for harm, often at exposure levels not uncommon in the workplace, occupational liver diseases are rarely recognized except during outbreaks.[49] This is almost certainly because the clinical presentation is nonspecific, most often consisting of unsuspected elevations of hepatocellular enzymes occasionally associated with mild gastrointestinal symptoms. The single exception to this is the now extremely rare vascular disorder resembling veno-occlusive disease that is caused by vinyl chloride.

The more common hepatic effects of occupational hazards—steatosis and nonspecific hepatocellular injury—have numerous causes and are prevalent in the general population; a given case may be readily attributed to infection, alcohol use, drug toxicity, biliary tract disease, diabetes, obesity, or weight change. When persistent elevations of hepatic enzymes prompt more extensive workup with radiographic studies and biopsy, results rarely provide specific evidence of an occupational cause. Only high suspicion of a workplace culprit, combined with evidence of exposure to a suspect agent, serves to distinguish etiology.

CENTRAL AND PERIPHERAL NERVOUS SYSTEMS

Most pesticides,[50] organic solvents,[51] and many metals[52] are neurotoxic at doses that may be seen in the workplace [see Table 1]. A handful of other chemicals used in plastics, lubricating fluids, and chemical operations are also neurotoxic; most cases occur after accidental or unusual exposures. In addition, persons exposed to asphyxiants, such as carbon monoxide and cyanide, may present with acute or recurring central nervous system symptoms. Both acute and late effects may occur—the former typically occurring immediately after an intense exposure, the latter often after prolonged periods of exposure. Importantly, the late or chronic effects usually result from prolonged periods of bioaccumulation or recurrent mild or subclinical acute exposures or as sequelae of acute intoxication. A direct consequence of this toxicologic fact is that neurotoxicity almost invariably presents during the time of occupational exposure to the offending agent and not long afterward, as may occur with carcinogenic substances or dusts causing pneumoconiosis.

Because of the extraordinarily diverse range of clinical symptoms that may herald CNS toxicity, including subtle changes in cognitive and affective function, the evaluation of suspected cases follows the general principles for all occupational disease, with increased attention given to recent exposures. The acute disorders usually occur as mild alterations of CNS function,[53] often with associated GI or other systemic effects; they are often recurrent, cycling with periods of work exposure, as might be seen in a painter (through exposure to solvents) or a pest-control worker. The key to recognition is the temporal pattern, with remission of symptoms occurring over a course of time consistent with the metabolism of the toxin. There may also be evidence of symptoms associated with withdrawal, similar to the effects associated with ethyl alcohol. For the subacute and chronic effects, the key to diagnosis is identification of evidence of substantial exposure occurring over a course of time consistent with the evolving neurotoxic picture. None of the neurologic disorders appear to involve allergy or idiosyncrasy; thus, the doses of exposure involved must be substantive.

In many cases, the exposure to the agent can be biologically confirmed with measurement of the levels of metal in the urine or blood, measurement of cholinesterase levels, or identification of a metabolite of an organic chemical in urine. There may also be some clinical or pathophysiologic clues. For example, the constellation of cerebellar ataxia, personality change, and salivary gland hypersecretion should prompt consideration of inorganic mercurialism, possibly with associated renal effects. An asymmetrical motor neuropathy should always raise the specter of lead poisoning. Insidious symmetrical distal sensory neuropathies, on the other hand, are far more common with solvents and acrylamide; electrophysiologic or pathologic evaluation reveals almost pure axonal degeneration, with minimal secondary demyelination—an important differential feature. Highly localized neuropathies, either unilateral or bilateral, should raise the possibility of a compressive etiology, not uncommon with repetitive work activities [see Musculoskeletal Disorders, below].[54]

Although diagnosis may be straightforward once the possibility of a workplace agent is considered, management remains challenging. Treatment of acute disorders involves ending the exposure and providing support where clinically necessary. Several hazards, such as certain cholinesterase inhibitors and cyanide, have specific antidotes that should be administered under medical supervision. The subacute and chronic conditions all require removal from further exposure. In addition, patients with heavy-metal exposure may be given chelation therapy when signs and symptoms of severe intoxication are evident; this, too, must be done under very close supervision in view of the risk of enhancing CNS effects early in treatment. Moreover, the possibility of rebound effects from reequilibration of metal into the nervous system must be anticipated when chelation is stopped. Most important, whatever strategy is chosen, physician and patient must be aware that the prognosis for full recovery from all but the most acute effects is somewhat guarded. Axons regrow very slowly, and higher integrative functions, such as affective or cognitive functions of the CNS, resolve even more slowly or not completely. Early efforts at functional rehabilitation, as may be used for trauma or stroke patients, are indicated when impairments limit work or other major life activities.

Possibly the most challenging diagnostic situation in occupational neurology is the worker who presents with CNS-related complaints that exhibit a temporal pattern consistent with a workplace origin but who does not have substantial exposure to neurotoxic agents. Such symptoms are a common part of the so-called sick-building syndrome, now referred to as nonspecific building-related illness, and are universal among persons who have acquired intolerance to low levels of chemicals (multiple chemical sensitivities).[55] It is important to recognize early that these syndromes are different from the neurotoxic disorders discussed here with regard to evaluation, prognosis, and treatment. They are discussed more fully later in this chapter [see Clinical Problems Associated with Low-Level Environmental Exposures, below].

MUSCULOSKELETAL DISORDERS

There has been a marked increase in the awareness of the role that work factors play in musculoskeletal disorders, ranging from such well-defined clinical problems as arthropathies and nerve compression syndromes to the less well characterized ailments causing pain of the trunk and extremities.[54,56] In developed countries, such disorders account for billions of dollars of costs in medical care and lost productivity. The overwhelming bulk of this epidemic relates to suspected consequences of physical stressors and trauma that occur at work. A number of systemic occupational disorders may also have expression in the muscles, bones, joints, and connective tissues; important examples of such disorders are the arthralgias and gouty consequences of lead intoxication, bony pain in association with systemic fluorosis, and the apparent increased risk of scleroderma in miners.[57]

It is clinically useful to divide potential occupational musculoskeletal disorders into those that have a well-defined anatomic structure of involvement, such as carpal tunnel syndrome, and those that lack such a clear-cut pattern, such as low back pain.[58,59] Although extensive data suggest that physical aspects of work, such as overall force, repetition, awkward posture, and vibration, contribute in a cumulative fashion to the development of both localizable and nonspecific symptoms, the approach to diagnosis and treatment is somewhat different for each. There is also evidence that factors other than physical strain, such as work stress, work fatigue, and adverse relationships in the workplace, may be important contributory factors, partially explaining high rates of musculoskeletal disorders among certain white-collar workers.[60,61]

For disorders of new onset involving the trunk or extremities or for clinically mild disorders, the initial approach should be short-term palliation with minimal workup. Rest from physically demanding tasks, use of nonsteroidal anti-inflammatory drugs or other nonnarcotic pain relievers, reassurance, and follow-up after a few days of treatment are suggested; further evaluation is indicated only if suggested by physical findings. If conservative steps fail to alleviate symptoms rapidly, additional examination and laboratory evaluation may be appropriate to rule out an anatomically discrete lesion that could be amenable to treatment. Where specific lesions are identified, such as compression of a nerve or disk or tenosynovial inflammation, longer-term efforts at elimination of strain in the affected region combined with anti-inflammatory drugs or other therapies are appropriate, followed by surgical intervention should these fail. In such cases, it is crucial to remember that the work-related stressors that caused the problem will complicate recovery unless they are modified.[62-64]

The most perplexing problem is the management of patients whose complaints cannot be specifically localized by physical examination or, when necessary, electrophysiologic or radiologic evaluation. Such complaints are no less real than those that are more readily understood and treated. Modification of work activities is often necessary but is rarely sufficient to resolve the problem. Pain may be persistent and refractory to treatment, and the value of physical therapy or pain medications is questionable. Rather, it is important for the treating physician to establish early that the symptoms are troublesome but not the result of a progressive process and that the patient may have to adapt to them despite discomfort. Expectation of cure often leads to unnecessary treatment, prolonged (and clinically unhelpful) loss of work time, and, ultimately, frustration on the part of the employer, the insurance company, the patient, and the physician.

HEMATOLOGIC DISORDERS

A host of disturbances of red cell function, survival, and production have been attributed to workplace exposures, including acute, subacute, and chronic processes [see Table 1]. Effects involving other cell lines have seldom been reported and will not be discussed. In clinical practice, the biggest concerns are the risk of acute hemolysis in workers exposed to nitrogen-containing oxidant chemicals in pharmaceutical, chemical, and explosives manufacturing; the effects of lead, which remains ubiquitous in the work environment; and the potential for solvent-induced marrow injury. The problem of oxidant stressors is somewhat difficult. Although workers with marked deficiency of glucose-6-phosphate dehydrogenase (G6PD) should probably avoid significant contact with such chemicals, there is not a clear relation between any of the measurable enzyme levels and risk. It is prudent to periodically screen all exposed workers for subclinical evidence of hemolysis, as well as for subclinical accumulation of methemoglobin, which is often induced by the same agents; workers who show evidence of early effects should probably be removed from harm's way, irrespective of identifiable factors.[65]

The hematologic effects of lead are widely misunderstood.[66,67] Although there is a dose-related inhibition of heme synthetase by lead that can be readily quantified by determining the accumulation of the precursor protoporphyrin (usually measured as whole blood zinc protoporphyrin), this biochemical effect of lead on blood hemoglobin or hematocrit is minimal until very high levels are reached, and there is almost no impact on red cell volume. In other words, anemia associated with hypoproliferation of red cells is very rare, and the absence of anemia should never be used to exclude a role for lead in causing toxicity to organs and systems that are far more sensitive, such as the nervous system and renal tubules. Furthermore, microcytosis can only occasionally be attributed to lead alone; when it is seen, especially in children, it most often signifies coincident iron deficiency. On the other hand, rapid accumulation of lead in acute lead poisoning, typically heralded clinically by the onset of abdominal pain, is almost always associated with evidence of rapid hemolysis; reticulocyte counts are in the range of 5% to 20%. In this setting, the notorious basophilic stipples are frequently seen as well, though they are by no means pathognomonic for lead toxicity. In general, this syndrome will occur only after lead levels have exceeded 60 mg/dl in whole blood. The hemolysis tends to abruptly stop after effective chelation therapy, which is usually indicated in this acute symptomatic form of lead poisoning.

The bone marrow effects of workplace chemicals are only slowly being unraveled, but certain conclusions seem warranted. Benzene, the aromatic constituent of petroleum products, was once widely prevalent in the work environment as a solvent and a component of gasoline. It can cause hypoplastic injury to the marrow, which may directly progress to a chronic blood dyscrasia (i.e., myelodysplasia or leukemia), or dyscrasia may occur after apparent recovery.[68] In other words, an exposed worker may show depressed cell counts, be removed from the source of toxicity, improve, and years later (possibly long after exposure ceases) develop myelodysplasia or a myeloproliferative syndrome. It is likely that some workers will develop the obviously more serious dyscrasias without direct marrow injury having been recognized while exposure was ongoing. There are no hallmark features of either the hypoplastic state (occurring during ongoing exposure) or the myelodysplastic state (occurring later) that distinguish benzene toxicity from other causes of

such disorders; this differentiation depends on the history of substantial benzene exposure, because the disorders are not believed to be idiosyncratic but dose related. Although there is some evidence that a few other solvents, such as the glycol ethers that are widely used in paints and coatings,[69] may cause such injury, the vast majority of solvents, including many benzene congeners such as toluene and xylene, do not appear to have potential for marrow injury. For this reason, most products that formerly contained benzene that are used in developed countries have been modified, and benzene is not used directly except for specific purposes in the manufacture of chemicals and pharmaceuticals. Obviously, exposed persons should be carefully monitored for hematologic effects, the presence of which would be clear evidence of overexposure.

ENDOCRINE AND REPRODUCTIVE EFFECTS

Despite an exceptional upsurge in interest in the endocrine-disrupting effects of environmental contaminants, there is little evidence that occupational exposures to chemical hazards cause clinically relevant endocrinopathies in adults.[70] Lead has been shown to impair hypothalamic–pituitary axis secretions and probably testosterone regulation in men heavily exposed, but the clinical relevance of these observations is unclear. Several compounds used in the pharmaceutical industry and other industries have been shown to have estrogenic activity, with predictable clinical consequences in both men and women.

The effects of work on male and female reproduction are a more formidable concern.[71] Although data are far from complete because many chemicals have never been studied adequately, several substances at occupational levels of exposure have been proved to cause infertility and decreases in sperm counts; such substances include lead, the pesticides 1,2-dibromo-3-chloropropane (DBCP) and ethylene dibromide (EDB), ethylene glycol ethers, and carbon disulfide. Heat and ionizing radiation have also been associated with infertility and decreased sperm counts. In addition, a host of other metals, anesthetic agents, and plastic reagents have been shown to cause worrisome gonadal effects in toxicologic experiments on male animals. For this reason, infertile men should be carefully questioned about work exposures; they should be observed for signs of improvement for about 9 months (which equals four cycles of spermatogenesis) should suspicion of an occupational cause be entertained.

Female reproduction is harder to study for lack of a single body fluid to analyze and because of the absence of a simple animal model. There is evidence that several common exposures, including waste anesthetic gases, lead, glycol ethers, ethylene oxide, and antineoplastic drugs, have the potential to increase the risk of miscarriage. Lead, organic mercury, polychlorinated biphenyls (PCBs), heat, and ionizing radiation are established teratogens; organic solvents are also suspect on the basis of animal studies and new epidemiologic reports.[72] Most of the agents that cause human cancer [see Table 3] are considered likely fetal hazards as well. In most cases, there is risk of adverse effects at doses considered acceptable in the workplace, because regulations have not traditionally been developed on the basis of reproductive concern. To a disturbing degree, knowledge of the reproductive effects of thousands of additional chemicals is unknown. Even the effects of hard physical work during pregnancy remain unclear, though there is evidence that excessive lifting and standing late in the third trimester may induce prematurity.

With the majority of women of reproductive age now in the workforce, many are questioning the safety of work during pregnancy, and clinicians are being confronted with trade-offs between fetal risks and the worker's economic security. Although each case must be studied individually, a reasonable guideline is to rigorously protect patients from the established teratogens or ensure the levels of exposure below those established for pregnancy. For others, reasonable steps can be taken to minimize exposure, including job transfer if the patient prefers and the employer has alternative work. For the patient for whom any risk represents an unacceptable psychological impediment, transfer or removal is probably in the best interest of all parties.

CLINICAL PROBLEMS ASSOCIATED WITH LOW-LEVEL ENVIRONMENTAL EXPOSURES

One of the most common problems emerging in developed countries is the constellation of respiratory and systemic complaints that are appearing with increasing frequency in office workers and others in what are traditionally considered safe jobs.[73,74] Typical symptoms of sick-building syndrome, or nonspecific building-related illness, include upper and lower respiratory symptoms, often combined with neurologic problems, such as fatigue, headache, and cognitive deficits, as well as rashes and other nonspecific complaints.[74] Usually, the patient will relate that others in the environment are experiencing similar difficulties and that the symptoms improve when the patient is away from work and return upon reexposure. Although in a minority of cases, investigation may reveal a specific allergy (e.g., in patients with asthma, rhinitis, or allergic alveolitis) or a specific hazard (e.g., fibrous glass released during a renovation or from a ventilation duct, causing pruritus), in the majority of cases, the environment is usually best described as poorly ventilated.[74,75] At present, there is no specific treatment of this syndrome other than palliative care and reassurance that it is neither progressive nor life threatening.[76,77] Expensive testing of either the patient or the work environment is rarely necessary or beneficial.[74] Ideally, remediation of both should be undertaken as soon as more dire possibilities are excluded by history and a walk-through of the workplace by an industrial hygienist or comparable environmental professional. In the vast majority of cases, improvement of ventilation will result in symptomatic improvement for most workers.[74]

On occasion, a patient in an affected building will start to experience similar discomfort in other situations, such as driving behind a bus, being in a store, or using a perfume or detergent.[55] The net impression is that the patient has become reactive to everything that has an odor. Many also have fatigue or other asthenic symptoms between exposures. Symptoms reminiscent of those in panic disorder may also occur. Dubbed multiple chemical sensitivities (MCS), this disorder is not associated with measurable abnormalities of organ system function but may be highly disabling.[55] Although there are many physical and psychological theories regarding the origin of MCS, present knowledge is limited. Patients do not easily tolerate pharmacologic agents and usually do not respond to treatment for anxiety or depression. Avoidance is equally fruitless, with shorter and more trivial exposures causing problems in those who quit work and minimize human contact. At present, the recommended treatment is supportive care coupled with moderate life modifications to avoid the most provocative exposures while preserving everyday functioning, including work if possible. Unrealistic expectations of cure or remission are as harmful as unwarranted fears of deterioration; neither outcome appears common among patients followed for many years.

Linda Rosenstock, M.D., M.P.H., F.A.C.P., has no commercial relationships with manufacturers of products or providers of services discussed in this chapter. Mark R. Cullen, M.D., is a consultant for Alcoa, Inc.

References

1. Palmer K, Coggon D: ABC of work related disorders: investigating suspected occupational illness and evaluating the workplace. BMJ 313:809, 1996
2. Encyclopedia of Occupational Health and Safety, 4th ed. Stellman JM, Ed. International Labor Office, Geneva, Switzerland, 1999
3. Maxcy Rosenau Textbook of Public Health and Preventive Medicine, 14th ed. Last WB, Ed. Appleton & Lange, Norwalk, Connecticut, 1998
4. Textbook of Clinical Occupational and Environmental Medicine, 2nd ed. Rosenstock L, Cullen M, Brodkin CA, et al, Eds. Elsevier Saunders, 2005
5. Schulte P: Characterizing the burden of occupational injury and disease. J Occup Environ Med 47:607, 2005
6. Injury Facts, 1998. National Safety Council. Itasca, Illinois, 1999
7. Epstein Y, Albukrek D, Kalmovitc B, et al: Heat intolerance induced by antidepressants. Ann NY Acad Sci 813:553, 1997
8. Tanaka S, Wild DK, Cameron LL, et al: Association of occupational and non-occupational risk factors with the prevalence of self-reported carpal tunnel syndrome in a national survey of the working population. Am J Ind Med 32:550, 1997
9. Lataye R, Campo P: Combined effects of a simultaneous exposure to noise and toluene on hearing function. Neurotoxicol Teratol 19:373, 1997
10. Erren TC, Jacobssen M, Piekarski C: Synergy between asbestos and smoking on lung cancer. Epidemiology 10:405, 1999
11. Lax MB, Grant WD, Manetti FA, et al: Recognizing occupational disease: taking an effective occupational history. Am Fam Physician 58:935, 1998
12. Politi BJ, Arena VC, Schwerha J, et al: Occupational medical history taking: how are today's physicians doing? A cross-sectional investigation of the frequency of occupational history taking by physicians in a major US teaching center. J Occup Environ Med 46:550, 2004
13. Achanzar WE, Diwan BA, Liu J, et al: Cadmium-induced malignant transformation of human prostate epithelial cells. Cancer Res 61:455, 2001
14. Parent ME, Hua Y, Siemiatycki J: Occupational risk factors for renal cell carcinoma in Montreal. Am J Ind Med 38:609, 2000
15. Zhang Y, Cantor KP, Lynch CF, et al: A population-based case-control study of occupation and renal cell carcinoma risk in Iowa. J Occup Environ Med 46:235, 2004
16. Baur X, Chen Z, Liebers V: Exposure-response relationships of occupational inhalative allergens. Clin Exp Allergy 28:537, 1998
17. Brooks SM, Bernstein IL: Reactive airways dysfunction syndrome or irritant induced asthma. Asthma in the Workplace. Bernstein IL, Chan-Yeung M, Malo JL, et al, Eds. Marcel Dekker, New York, 1993, p 533
18. Rabatin JT, Cowl CT: A guide to the diagnosis and treatment of occupational asthma. Mayo Clin Proc 76:633, 2001
19. Chan-Yeung M, Malo JL: Occupational asthma. N Engl J Med 333:107, 1995
20. Wild LG, Lopez M: Occupational asthma caused by high-molecular-weight substances. Immunol Allergy Clin North Am 23:235, 2003
21. Liss GM, Sussman GL: Latex sensitization: occupational versus general population prevalence rates. Am J Ind Med 35:196, 1999
22. Zeiss CR, Gomaa A, Murphy FM, et al: Latex hypersensitivity in Department of Veterans Affairs health care workers: glove use, symptoms, and sensitization. Ann Allergy Asthma Immunol 91:510, 2003
23. Meredith SK, Bugler J, Clark RL: Isocyanate exposure and occupational asthma: a case-referent study. Occup Environ Med 57:830, 2000
24. Malo JL, Chan-Yeung M: Occupational asthma. J Allergy Clin Immunol 108:317, 2001
25. Drazen J: SARS: looking back over the first 100 days. N Engl J Med 349:319, 2003
26. Bridges CB, Lim W, Hu-Primmer J, et al: Risk of influenza A (H5N1) infection among poultry workers. J Infect Dis 185:1005, 2002
27. Hodgson MJ, Bracker A, Yang C, et al: Hypersensitivity pneumonitis in a metalworking environment. Am J Ind Med 39:616, 2001
28. Hoffman RE, Wood RC, Kreiss K: Building-related asthma in Denver office workers. Am J Public Health 83:89, 1993
29. Middleton DC: Chronic beryllium disease: uncommon disease, less common diagnosis. Environ Health Perspect 106:765, 1998
30. Cugell DW: The hard metal diseases. Clin Chest Med 13:269, 1992
31. Kern DG, Crausman RS, Durand KT, et al: Flock worker's lung: chronic interstitial lung disease in the nylon flocking industry. Ann Intern Med 129:261, 1998
32. Kern DG, Kuhn C 3rd, Pransky GS, et al: Flock worker's lung: broadening the spectrum of clinicopathology, narrowing the spectrum of suspected etiologies. Chest 117:251, 2000

33. Kanerva L, Jolanki R, Estlander T, et al: Incidence rates of occupational allergic contact dermatitis caused by metals. Am J Contact Dermat 11:155, 2000

34. Hogan DJ: Occupational Skin Disorders. Igaku-Shoin, New York, 1994

35. Adams R: Occupational Skin Disease, 3rd ed. WB Saunders Co, Philadelphia, 1999

36. Marks JG, DeLeo VA: Contact and Occupational Dermatology, 3rd ed. Mosby, St. Louis, 2001

37. Pratt MD, Belsito DV, DeLeo VA, et al: North American Contact Dermatitis Group patch-test results, 2001–2002 study period. Dermatitis 15:176, 2004

38. Krob HA, Fleischer AB Jr, D'Agostino R Jr, et al: Prevalence and relevance of contact dermatitis allergens: a meta-analysis of 15 years of published T.R.U.E. test data. J Am Acad Dermatol 51:349, 2004

39. de Broe ME, D'Haese PC, Nuyts GD, et al: Occupational renal diseases. Curr Opin Nephrol Hypertens 5:114, 1996

40. Wedeen RP: Occupational and environmental renal disease. Semin Nephrol 17:46, 1997

41. Batuman V, Landy E, Maesaka JK, et al: Contribution of lead to hypertension with renal impairment. N Engl J Med 309:17, 1983

42. Lin JL, Lin-Tan DT, Hsu KH, et al: Environmental lead exposure and progression of chronic renal diseases in patients without diabetes. N Engl J Med 23:277, 2003

43. Erhlich R, Robins T, Jordaan E, et al: Lead absorption and renal dysfunction in a South African battery factory. Occup Environ Med 55:453, 1998

44. Roels HA, Hoet P, Lison D: Usefulness of biomarkers of exposure to inorganic mercury, lead, or cadmium in controlling occupational and environmental risks of nephrotoxicity. Ren Fail 21:251, 1999

45. Roels HA, Van Assche FJ, Overstseyns M, et al: Reversibility of microproteinuria in cadmium workers with incipient tubular dysfunction after reduction of exposure. Am J Ind Med 31:645, 1997

46. Jarup L, Persson B, Elinder CG: Blood cadmium as an indicator of dose in a long-term follow-up of workers previously exposed to cadmium. Scand J Work Environ Health 23:31, 1997

47. Jarup L, Hellstrom L, Alfven T, et al: Low level exposure to cadmium and early kidney damage: the OSCAR study. Occup Environ Med 57:668, 2000

48. Ravnskow U: Hydrocarbons may worsen renal function in glomerulonephritis. Am J Ind Med 37:599, 2000

49. Hoet P, Graf MI, Bourdi M, et al: Epidemic of liver disease caused by hydrochlorofluorocarbons used as ozone-sparing substitutes of chlorofluorocarbons. Lancet 350:556, 1997

50. Keifer MC, Mahurin RK: Chronic neurologic effects of pesticide overexposure. Occup Med 12:291, 1997

51. Rutchik JS, Whittman RI: Neurologic issues with solvents. Clin Occup Environ Med 4:621, 2004

52. Manzo L, Artigas F, Martinez E, et al: Biochemical markers of neurotoxicity: a review of mechanistic studies and applications. Hum Exp Toxicol 15(suppl):S20, 1996

53. Stallones L, Beseler C: Pesticide illness, farm practices, and neurological symptoms among farm residents in Colorado. Environ Res 90:89, 2002

54. Musculoskeletal Disorders and Workplace Factors: A Critical Review of Epidemiologic Evidence for Work-Related Musculoskeletal Disorders of the Neck, Upper Extremity, and Low Back. Publication no. 97-141, U.S. Department of Health and Human Services. National Institute for Occupational Health and Safety, Cincinnati, Ohio, 1997 http://www.cdc.gov/niosh/ergosci1.html

55. Cullen MR: Low-level environmental exposures. Textbook of Clinical Occupational and Environmental Medicine, 2nd ed. Rosenstock L, Cullen MR, Brodkin CA, et al, Eds. Elsevier Saunders 2005, p 1127

56. Tanaka S, Petersen M, Cameron L: Prevalence and risk factors of tendinitis and related disorders of the distal upper extremity among U.S. workers: comparison to carpal tunnel syndrome. Am J Ind Med 39:328, 2001

57. Katz JN, Brissot R, Liang MH: Systemic rheumatologic disorders. Textbook of Clinical Occupational and Environmental Medicine, 2nd ed. Rosenstock L, Cullen MR, Brodkin CA, Eds. WB Saunders Co, Philadelphia, 2005, p 533

58. Pascarelli EF, Hsu YP: Understanding work-related upper extremity disorders: clinical findings in 485 computer users, musicians, and others. J Occup Rehabil 11:1, 2001

59. Hoogendoorn WE, Bongers PM, de Vet HC, et al: Flexion and rotation of the trunk and lifting at work are risk factors for low back pain: results of a prospective cohort study. Spine 25:3087, 2000

60. Macfarlane GJ, Hunt IM, Silman AJ: Role of mechanical and psychosocial factors in the onset of forearm pain: prospective population based study. BMJ 321:676, 2000

61. Haufler AJ, Feuerstein M, Huang GD: Job stress, upper extremity pain and functional limitations in symptomatic computer users. Am J Ind Med 38:507, 2000

62. Jayson MI: ABC of work related disorders: back pain. BMJ 313:355, 1996

63. Hagberg M: ABC of work related disorders: neck and arm disorders. BMJ 313:419, 1996

64. Buckle PW: Work factors and upper limb disorders. BMJ 315:1360, 1997

65. Luster MI, Wierda D, Rosenthal GJ: Environmentally related disorders of the hematologic and immune systems. Med Clin North Am 74:425, 1990

66. Nelson JC, Westwood M, Allen KR, et al: The ratio of erythrocyte zinc-protoporphyrin to protoporphyrin IX in disease and its significance in the mechanism of lead toxicity on haem synthesis (pt 3). Ann Clin Biochem 35:422, 1998

67. Solliway BM, Schaffer A, Pratt H, et al: Effects of exposure to lead on selected biochemical and haematological variables. Pharmacol Toxicol 78:18, 1996

68. Smith MT: Overview of benzene-induced aplastic anaemia. Eur J Haematol 57:107, 1996

69. Cullen MR, Solomon L, Pace PE, et al: Morphologic, biochemical and cytogenetic studies of bone marrow and circulating blood cells in painters exposed to ethylene glycol ethers. Environ Res 59:250, 1992

70. Cullen MR: Endocrine disorders. Textbook of Clinical Occupational and Environmental Medicine, 2nd ed. Rosenstock L, Cullen M, Brodkin CA, et al, Eds. WB Saunders Co, Philadelphia, 2005, p 609

71. Reproductive Hazards. U.S. Department of Labor. Occupational Health and Safety Administraiton, Washington, DC, 2005 http://www.osha.gov/SLTC/reproductivehazards

72. Khattak S, Moghtader GK, McMartin K, et al: Pregnancy outcome following gestational exposure to organic solvents. JAMA 281:12, 1999

73. Seltzer JM: Effects of the Indoor Environment on Health. Occupational Medicine: State of the Art Reviews, Vol 10, No 1. OEM Press, 1995

74. Redlich CA, Sparer JS, Cullen MR: Sick building syndrome. Lancet 349:1013, 1997

75. Mitchell LS, Donnay A, Hoover DA, et al: Immunologic parameters of multiple chemical sensitivity. Occup Med State Art Rev 15:539, 2000

76. Husman T: Health effects of indoor-air microorganisms. Scand J Work Environ Health 22:5, 1996

77. Bascom R, Kesavanathan J, Swift DL: Human susceptibility to indoor contaminants. Occup Med 10:119, 1995

8 Health Advice for International Travelers

Peter F. Weller, M.D., F.A.C.P.

The provision of health advice and the administration of prophylactic measures can help reduce the morbid and, at times, mortal risks of infectious illnesses that may be acquired during international travel. The Centers for Disease Control and Prevention (CDC) publishes *Health Information for International Travel*, which provides information on required and recommended vaccinations and malaria prophylaxis, as well as general advice.[1] *Health Information for International Travel 2003–2004* is available for purchase on the Internet, at http://bookstore.phf.org/cat24.htm, or by phone, at 1-877-252-1200. Other information regarding international travel is readily available on the CDC Web site (http://www.cdc.gov), such as the Green Sheet, which provides reports of cruise-ship sanitation inspections; detailed guidelines on the need for yellow fever immunizations; guidelines on international health issues for travelers by country; recently recognized disease outbreaks; and general guidelines on immunizations and other medical issues for travelers. Information may also be obtained from state public health departments, local physicians or clinics catering to travelers, the embassies of individual countries, and Internet-based advisory services. Even the most up-to-date information sources, however, may not be able to provide precise information on specific diseases prevalent in specific locales, because mechanisms for recognizing and reporting diseases are often lacking in developing areas.

Pretravel Evaluation and Immunizations

Medical consultation should be obtained at least 1 month before international travel to allow time for immunizations [*see Table 1*]. A general patient medical history should be obtained to define pertinent underlying medical conditions. For instance, splenectomy predisposes a person to more severe malaria, babesiosis, and infections with encapsulated bacteria, including meningococcal infections. A history of allergies to antimicrobial agents or to other components of vaccines should be determined. Knowledge of the duration and purpose of a trip, as well as of the countries and locales to be visited, can help in estimating the risks of exposure to endemic diseases. In addition, specific groups of travelers—including pregnant women; persons with HIV; persons with chronic diseases such as chronic obstructive pulmonary disease, diabetes mellitus, hypercoagulable states, and cardiovascular disease; and health care workers—may require more time before travel to address their potentially altered needs for immunization and prophylaxis.

Table 1 Guidelines for Immunizations for Travelers

	Asia	Eastern Mediterranean, North Africa	Middle East	Sub-Saharan Africa	Pacific Islands	Caribbean, Mexico, Central and South America	North America, Europe, Japan, Australia, New Zealand
Yellow fever				X (some countries)		X (some South American countries)	
Cholera*							
Polio	X (some countries			X (some countries			
Tetanus/diphtheria (booster every 10 yr)	X	X	X	X	X	X	X
Measles (if born after 1957 and not recipient of 2 doses of vaccine)	X	X	X	X	X	X	X
Typhoid	X	X	X	X	X	X	
Rabies (for prolonged visits)	X	X	X	X		X	
Hepatitis A	X	X	X	X	X	X	
Hepatitis B (especially for prolonged visits)	X	X	X	X	X	X	
Meningococci	X (during outbreaks)	X (during outbreaks)	X (especially Mecca, during Hajj)	X (especially in meningococcal "belt" countries)		X (during outbreaks)	
Japanese encephalitis	X[†]						

*Only if required by a country.
[†]Prolonged visits to some regions.

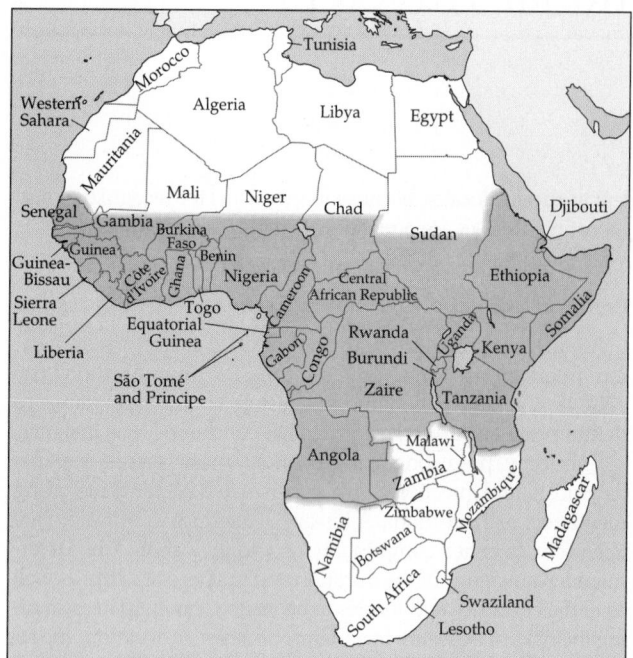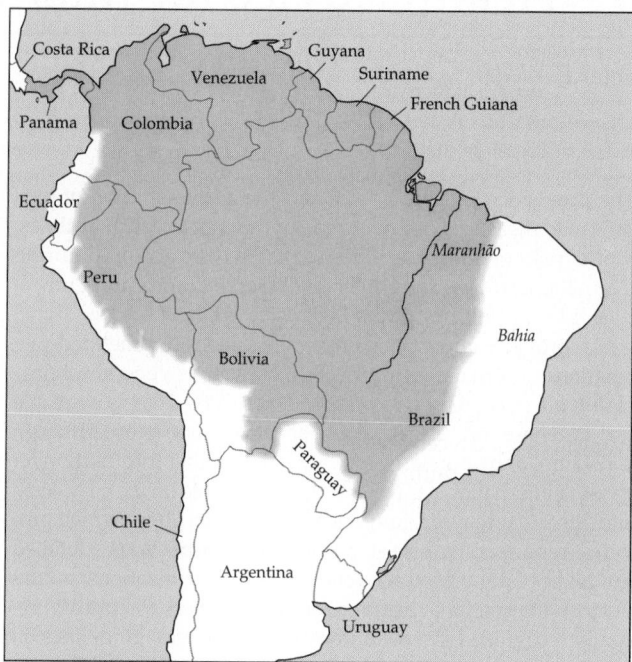

Figure 1 Yellow fever (gray areas) is endemic in parts of Africa (left) and South America (right). Several countries consider these zones infected areas and require an International Certificate of Vaccination against yellow fever from travelers from these zones.

REQUIRED IMMUNIZATION

The only immunization legally required for entrance into specific countries is that for yellow fever.

Yellow Fever

Yellow fever is a mosquito-transmitted viral infection, whose severity may range from an influenzalike illness to potentially fatal hepatitis and hemorrhagic fever. Yellow fever occurs only in equatorial Africa and in areas of tropical South America [*see Figure 1*].[1] Persons older than 6 months visiting countries where yellow fever is known to exist should be immunized. In addition, those traveling outside of urban areas in countries that are in the yellow fever endemic zones but are not officially reporting the infection should be immunized because the disease may be underrecognized. Some countries, especially in Asia, may require yellow fever immunizations for entry, especially for persons who have traveled in potentially endemic countries.[1] Yellow fever vaccine, a live virus vaccine grown in chick embryos, is effective.

Although generally safe, yellow fever vaccines are uncommonly associated with encephalitis (referred to as yellow fever vaccine–associated neurotropic disease [YEL-AND]) and a potentially fatal multiorgan system failure (referred to as yellow fever vaccine–associated viscerotropic disease [YEL-AVD]). In the United States, estimated rates of these two complications are four to six cases per million doses for encephalitis and three to five cases per million doses for multiorgan failure.[1] However, the risks of illness and death due to yellow fever in an unvaccinated traveler are greater, estimated to be one per 1,000 and one per 5,000 a month, respectively.[1] Thus, for those entering yellow fever endemic areas, yellow fever vaccination is indicated; however, vaccine use should be limited to those who are truly at risk. This is especially true for travelers older than 60 years, because they appear to be at greater risk for developing YEL-AVD.[2] For these travelers, vaccine may be indicated only if the risk of potential exposure is high (e.g., when travel in endemic areas outside urban centers is anticipated). A history of thymus disorders appears to be a contraindication for vaccine. In an analysis of 23 vaccinated persons who developed YEL-AVD, four (17%) had a history of thymus disease.[2] Travelers with a history of thymus disorders or dysfunction, including myasthenia gravis, thymoma, thymectomy, or DiGeorge syndrome, should not receive yellow fever vaccine. If travel to yellow fever–endemic regions cannot be deferred, persons with thymus disorders should be advised to use N,N-diethyl-m-toluamide (DEET) and permethrin to reduce mosquito bites [*see* Insect Repellents and Avoidance, *below*].[2]

Initially, a single subcutaneous dose of 0.5 ml is given. A booster dose is required every 10 years. Immunizations, which are recorded on the International Certificate of Vaccination, are available only from designated physicians and centers, an updated listing of which can be found on the Internet at http://www2.ncid.cdc.gov/travel/yellowfever. Yellow fever vaccine, which contains both egg proteins and gelatin, rarely causes anaphylaxis.[3] For those persons allergic to egg proteins or gelatin, skin testing with yellow fever vaccine (per directions included on the package insert) may help determine whether vaccine can be given safely.

Because yellow fever vaccine is a live virus vaccine, cautions and potential contraindications to its use apply to those who are pregnant, lactating, or immunocompromised. In these persons, if the sole indication for administration of yellow fever vaccine is to satisfy legal requirements for entry, a physician's letter documenting the contraindications to vaccination can be provided to the traveler; in addition, advice should be sought from the embassy or consulate of the country or countries to be visited.

Influenza

Travelers are at increased risk for influenza infection.[1] Influenza, like hepatitis A, has become one of the more common infections in travelers that are preventable by vaccine. In temperate countries, influenza is prevalent in the winter months; whereas in the tropics, influenza transmission occurs year-round. For travelers to the Northern Hemisphere, the risk is greatest during December through February; and for travelers to the Southern Hemisphere, the risk is greatest from April through September. Summertime outbreaks of influenza have occurred on cruise ships in the Northern and Southern hemispheres. For travelers to tropical countries, the risk of influenza exists throughout the year.[1]

Persons at high risk for influenza, including those older than 50 years, should receive influenza vaccine (1) if influenza vaccine was not received during the preceding fall or winter, (2) if travel is planned to the tropics, (3) if travel is planned with large groups of tourists (e.g., on cruise ships), or (4) if travel is planned during seasons in which influenza is prevalent.[1,4] In North America, travel-related influenza vaccination should be administered in the spring, if possible, because vaccine may be unavailable in the summer.

Cholera

Cholera is caused by toxigenic *Vibrio cholerae* groups 01 and 0139. Although the number of cases of cholera seen in the United States has increased in recent years, many of the cases have been the result of the illness being imported into the United States by travelers from other countries; tourists from the United States visiting other countries have only rarely been infected. Cholera is acquired by ingestion of contaminated water, ice, or food, including raw or undercooked fish and shellfish. Travelers in endemic regions should be advised of the precautions to be followed to minimize risks of acquiring cholera and other enteric infections [see Travel-Related Illness, *below*] and of the importance of rehydration in the treatment of cholera. Dietary precautions include consuming only boiled or treated water, eating thoroughly cooked food, avoiding all fruit not peeled by onself, and avoiding undercooked or raw fish or shellfish, including seviche.

Routine immunization is not recommended for travelers.[1] In the unlikely event that a locale requires immunization for cholera, immunization would need to be obtained outside the United States in countries in which current cholera vaccine is available. Currently, no country requires proof of cholera immunization as a condition for entry, and the World Health Organization recommends against such a requirement. Some local authorities, however, may require immunization (to determine local requirements, travelers may consult the embassies of the countries to which they will be traveling). The only cholera vaccine licensed for use in the United States is no longer manufactured. In other countries, two cholera vaccines (Dukoral, from Biotec AB, and Mutacol, from Berna) have been licensed for use, but neither of these vaccines is indicated for most travelers.[1] Travelers who are at risk for cholera and who expect to travel to areas remote from medical care should take with them packets of oral rehydration salts. Antimicrobial agents often employed for therapy for traveler's diarrhea, such as ciprofloxacin, are usually very effective in helping terminate cholera infections.[5]

Poliomyelitis

Travelers to countries in which polio is endemic or in which there is a current epidemic are at risk for the disease and should be immunized. Countries considered to be free of wild poliovirus are all countries in the Western Hemisphere, the Western Pacific Region (which includes China), and the European region.[1] Polio transmission continues in some developing countries, including Afghanistan, India, Pakistan, Nigeria, and Niger, although efforts to achieve global eradication of polio are ongoing.

Travelers who were immunized previously should receive one booster dose of polio vaccine. Oral live virus vaccine is no longer recommended for immunizations in the United States.[6] The inactivated vaccine is preferred to avoid the small risk of paralytic disease from the oral vaccine. Patients with an altered immune status should receive inactivated vaccine. Children who have not been immunized should receive a full series of immunizations with inactivated polio vaccine. Adults who have not been immunized should receive a series of three doses of enhanced-potency inactivated vaccine.[1] If there is insufficient time before travel for at least three doses of inactivated vaccine to be given at intervals of 1 to 2 months, the following alternatives are recommended[1]: if less than 1 month is available before travel, a single dose of inactivated vaccine is given; if between 1 and 2 months is available before travel, two doses of inactivated vaccine are administered 4 weeks apart. Travelers who were incompletely immunized previously should receive the remaining required doses of vaccine.

Tetanus and Diphtheria

A tetanus-diphtheria booster should be administered every 10 years [see Chapter 140].[1] Older persons and women are more likely to lack the tetanus and diphtheria antibodies and thus are more likely to require boosters.[7,8]

Pneumococcal Infections

There are no data on the risk to travelers of acquiring pneumococcal infections; however, those at risk, including those older than 65 years [see Chapter 134], are recommended as candidates to receive pneumococcal vaccinations.

Measles

Because of the declining prevalence of measles in the United States, disease imported by immigrants and by returning residents accounts for an increasing proportion of cases in this country. Measles may be acquired during travel in developed countries, including those in Europe and Asia, as well as in less developed countries.[1] Most persons who were born before 1957 are immune because of natural exposure and do not require vaccination. Persons who were born after 1956 who either have not been immunized or were immunized before 1980 and who have neither serologic evidence of infection nor a history of physician-diagnosed measles should be immunized with a single subcutaneous dose of measles vaccine before travel. Measles vaccine is contraindicated for both pregnant and immunodeficient patients. HIV-infected patients, unless they are severely immunocompromised, should be immunized before travel because measles can be severe and even fatal in persons with HIV infection.[1,9]

Typhoid

Salmonella typhi infection is prevalent in many areas of Asia, Africa, and Latin America. Typhoid is acquired from contaminated food or water. Although the overall risk of acquiring typhoid during travel remains low (2.3 million cases per million travelers),[10] foreign travel accounted for 74% of 1,393 cases of typhoid reported to the CDC between 1994 and 1999.[11] The risk was greatest for those traveling to the Indian subcontinent (India, Pakistan, and Bangladesh) and Haiti. Of note, even those traveling for no more than a couple of weeks were at risk of acquiring typhoid. Given the safety of current typhoid vaccines, typhoid vaccination should be considered for short-term travel in high-risk areas, as well as for any travel to areas off the usual tourist itinerary.[11]

Two typhoid vaccines are available for use in the United States. One typhoid vaccine is an oral vaccine (Vivotif Berna, from Berna) that uses the attenuated Ty21a strain of *S. typhi;* this vaccine does not cause the local and systemic side effects frequently produced by the older, parenteral vaccine. The oral vaccine is supplied as a packet of four enteric-coated capsules that must be refrigerated. Patients need explicit guidance on refrigerating the vaccine because failure to do so might compromise its efficacy.[12] At least 2 weeks before departure, the traveler takes one capsule every other day until all four capsules have been taken. Because mefloquine and antibiotics inhibit the growth in vitro of *S. typhi* strains, including Ty21a, it is prudent to separate the oral administrations of mefloquine and antibiotics and of Ty21a vaccine by 24 hours.[1] It is recommended that a booster dose of Ty21a vaccine, consisting of four capsules taken on alternate days, be given every 5 years to persons who continue to be at risk for exposure to typhoid. The safety of the oral vaccine has not been established for patients with deficient humoral or cell-mediated immunity, and thus, patients with congenital or acquired immunodeficiencies should not receive it. It may be given to children 6 years of age or older.

The second typhoid vaccine is a capsular polysaccharide vaccine for parenteral use (Typhim Vi, from Aventis Pasteur). Primary vaccination consists of one I.M. dose of 0.5 ml; the same dose is administered as a booster every 2 years. The vaccine is well tolerated but, like the oral vaccine, protects only 50% to 80% of recipients.[1,13] This vaccine is safe for immunocompromised persons, including HIV-infected patients.[1] The only contraindication to its use is a history of serious reactions to the vaccine. It may be given to children 2 years of age and older.

Rabies

Rabies vaccine—either human diploid cell rabies vaccine (HDCV), purified chick embryo cell vaccine (PCEC), or rabies vaccine adsorbed (RVA)—is an inactivated viral preparation. Immunizations with either of the three vaccine preparations consists of three I.M. doses, 1 ml each, administered on days 0, 7, and 21 or 28.[1] Preexposure immunization with rabies vaccine is not indicated for most travelers but should be strongly considered for persons who anticipate contact with wild animals or who are living for a month or more where rabies is endemic. Dog rabies is present in most countries of Asia, Africa, and Central and South America and is prevalent in parts of Brazil, Bolivia, Mexico, El Salvador, Guatemala, Colombia, Ecuador, Peru, India, Nepal, the Philippines, Sri Lanka, Thailand, and Vietnam.[1] Preexposure immunization does not eliminate the need for postexposure immunization but abbreviates its course and eliminates the need to administer rabies immune globulin. If left untreated, rabies is fatal, and postexposure rabies immune globulin and postexposure vaccine are frequently unavailable in many areas of the world.

Plague

Plague vaccine is no longer commercially available. Vaccina-tion against plague is not indicated for most travelers.[1] However, prophylaxis should be considered for travelers to areas in which plague is epidemic or actively epizootic. For adults, tetracycline or doxycycline is appropriate prophylactic therapy; for children younger than 8 years, trimethoprim-sulfamethoxazole is recommended.[1]

Hepatitis A

Hepatitis A is prevalent in many less-developed countries [*see Figure 2*] and is the most common infection acquired by travelers that is preventable by vaccine. In visitors to developing countries, even those staying in luxury hotels, the incidence of hepatitis A in unprotected travelers is about 3 per 1,000 travelers per month of stay, and this rate rises to 20 per 1,000 travelers per month for those eating or drinking under poor hygienic conditions.[14]

Immunization for hepatitis A is recommended for persons who will be traveling or working in countries with intermediate or high endemicity for hepatitis A infection.[1] Although hepatitis A previously was prevented solely by the administration of immune globulin, two monovalent inactivated hepatitis A vaccines and a combined hepatitis A and hepatitis B vaccine are now available. The monovalent vaccines, HAVRIX (GlaxoSmithKline) and VAQTA (Merck), have proved safe and highly effective.[15] For adults, two I.M. 1.0 ml doses should be administered in the deltoid muscle at 0 and 6 to 12 months. For persons between 2 and 18 years of age, two doses, 0.5 ml each, should be administered at 0 and 6 to 12 months. VAQTA contains no preservative, whereas HAVRIX contains 2-phenoxyethanol. The bivalent hepatitis A and hepatitis B vaccine, TWINRIX (GlaxoSmithKline), is likewise safe and effective and is administered to those 18 years of age or older in three I.M. 1.0 ml doses at 0, 1, and 6 months. TWINRIX contains 2-phenoxyethanol.

With the monovalent vaccines, many persons who have been vaccinated will have detectable antibody responses within 2 weeks after the first dose; 94% to 100% of persons treated will have protective levels of antibody by 1 month after the first dose. The second dose of vaccine provides longer-term protection. If the immunization schedule is unduly interrupted, it is not necessary to restart the full regimen; the second dose may simply be administered. A vaccination series started with one brand of vaccine may be completed with the same or the other brand of hepatitis A vaccine. Travelers who receive vaccine less than 2 weeks before travel are at risk for acquiring hepatitis and should also receive immune globulin, given at an injection site different from the one for vaccine.

For travelers who are allergic to vaccine components or who opt not to receive the vaccine, immune globulin should be administered. Administration of immune globulin should begin shortly before departure in a dose of 2.0 ml I.M. for adults (1.0 ml for patients, including children, weighing 23 to 45 kg; 0.5 ml for those weighing less than 23 kg). If the stay is to be longer than 3 months, the adult dose is 5.0 ml (2.5 ml for patients weighing 23 to 45 kg; 1.0 ml for those weighing less than 23 kg). If the duration of stay is prolonged, the latter dosage schedule should be repeated every 4 to 6 months. Immune globulin should be given at least 2 weeks after measles, mumps, or rubella live virus vaccines. Conversely, these vaccines should be given at least 3 months after immune globulin. Immune globulin does not interfere with the immune response to killed virus vaccines or to yellow fever or polio vaccines.

Because immune globulin has been in limited supply and because the hepatitis A vaccines have proved to be highly effective against hepatitis A infection, which is frequent in travelers, immunization with hepatitis A vaccine has become the principal approach for preventing hepatitis A infection in travelers. The hepatitis A vaccines are safe in pregnancy and immunosuppression.

Hepatitis B

The risk to travelers of acquiring hepatitis B is generally low, compared with the risk of acquiring hepatitis A. The risk increases, however, in regions where hepatitis B is highly prevalent [see Figure 3], if there is contact with blood or bodily secretions, if sexual contact with infected persons occurs, or if travel is prolonged.[1] Immunization for hepatitis B, which is recommended for all persons who work in health care fields with potential exposure to human blood, is especially important for medical workers traveling in countries with high or intermediate hepatitis B endemicity. Hepatitis B immunization should be considered for persons residing for more than 6 months in regions where hepatitis B is endemic and for persons with potential contact with blood (including those receiving tattoos or body piercing), potential sexual contact, or potential need for medical or dental procedures.

Two monovalent hepatitis B vaccines are available, both of which include recombinant HBsAg (hepatitis B surface antigen) protein produced in yeast. Except for rare hypersensitivity reactions to vaccine components, including yeast proteins, the two recombinant vaccines are safe and efficacious; there are no other medical contraindications, including pregnancy and immunosuppression, for administration of these vaccines. The two vaccines, Recombivax HB (Merck) and Engerix-B (GlaxoSmithKline), are administered in three I.M. doses: at 0, 1, and 6 months. Engerix-B may also be given in four doses: at 0, 1, 2, and 12 months. Immunization should start 6 months before travel, but if this schedule is not feasible, some protection is afforded by one or two doses administered before travel. Full protection will be achieved in most cases by completion of the three-dose or four-dose schedule.[1] For travelers who will depart before the recommended series can be completed, an accelerated regimen, involving doses given on days 0, 7, and 14, can be administered; the accelerated regimen is not approved by the Food and Drug Administration. Travelers receiving the accelerated course should receive a booster at least 6 months later to provide long-term immunity.[1]

An additional vaccine for hepatitis B is TWINRIX, a combined hepatitis A and hepatitis B vaccine. Primary immunization with TWINRIX consists of three doses administered at 0, 1, and 6 months. The bivalent vaccine can be used to complete immunization series started with monovalent hepatitis A and B vaccines.

Meningococcal Disease

Although acquisition of meningococcal disease is uncommon in travelers from the United States, immunization should be considered for travelers to areas with recognized epidemics or to regions where such disease is hyperendemic, especially if prolonged contact with the local populace is anticipated. Epidemics of meningococcal disease are frequent in the area of sub-Saharan Africa extending from Guinea in the west to Ethiopia in the east [see Figure 4]. Vaccination against meningococcal disease is legally required only for pilgrims who make the Hajj pilgrimage to Mecca, Saudi Arabia. Routine immunization is also indicated for persons who have either deficiencies of terminal complement components or functional or anatomic asplenia. The currently available quadrivalent vaccine is composed of meningococcal

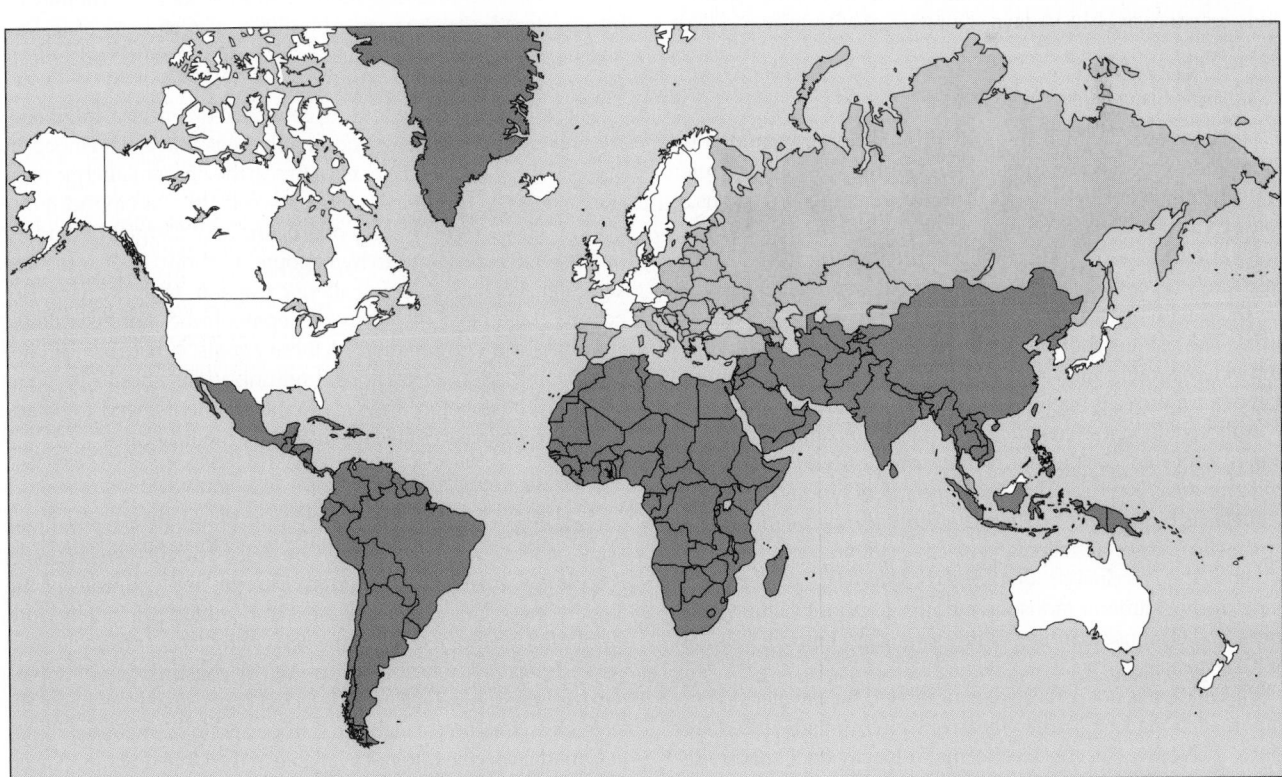

Figure 2   **The prevalence of hepatitis A is high in those countries shaded blue, intermediate in those shaded gray, and low in the white areas of the map.**

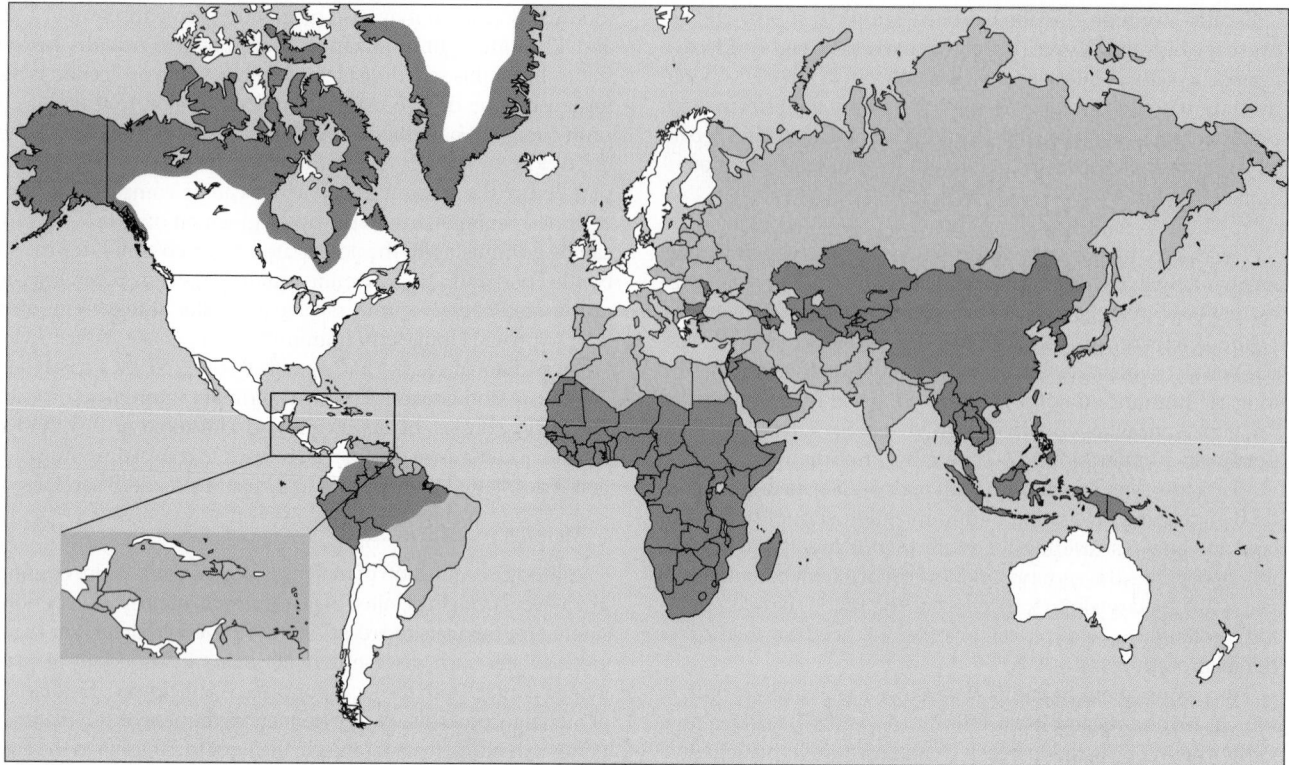

Figure 3 Hepatitis B is highly endemic in those countries shaded blue (prevalence > 8%). Those regions shaded gray, where the prevalence is 2% to 7%, are considered to be of intermediate endemicity. The prevalence of hepatitis is less than 2% in the white areas of the map.

polysaccharides from *Neisseria meningitidis* serogroups A, C, Y, and W-135. A single 0.5 ml subcutaneous dose of vaccine is administered to both adults and children and will induce an antibody response in 10 to 14 days.[1] Duration of immunity is at least 3 years.

Japanese Encephalitis

Japanese encephalitis, an arboviral infection transmitted by mosquitoes, may occur in epidemics during the late summer and autumn in northern tropical areas and temperate regions of some countries. The risk of acquiring Japanese encephalitis infection varies by season and geographic area [*see Table 2*].[1] The disease rarely occurs in Hong Kong or Japan. Persons at highest risk are those who live for extended periods in endemic or epidemic areas. The risk for short-term travelers to urban centers is low, and in temperate countries, the risk for travelers to either an urban or a rural area is negligible during the winter.

Although Japanese encephalitis is highly uncommon, prevention is important for those traveling specifically to epidemic or endemic areas [*see Table 2*], because the risk of serious neurologic sequelae is high. Exposure to mosquitoes should be minimized by the use of insect repellents, protective clothing, and mosquito screens. Also, vaccination should be considered for persons traveling during summer monsoon months, for those visiting rural areas, and for those planning to stay more than 1 month in urban or rural areas.

Vaccination is not usually recommended for travelers to Singapore or Hong Kong, urban Japan or China, or high-altitude regions in Nepal. An effective formalin-inactivated, mouse-derived vaccine (JE-Vax, Aventis Pasteur) has been licensed by the FDA. Primary immunization for persons older than 3 years consists of three doses, 1 ml each, administered subcutaneously on days 0, 7, and 30. An abbreviated schedule of 0, 7, and 14 days can be used if there is insufficient time before travel to administer the standard immunization. A booster dose of 1 ml may be administered after 2 years. About 20% of recipients of JE-Vax vaccine experience local reactions and mild systemic side effects (e.g., fever, headache, myalgias, and malaise).[1]

Allergic reactions, including generalized urticaria, angioedema, respiratory distress, and anaphylaxis, have developed in about six per 1,000 recipients; at times, the onset of allergic reaction is delayed for hours or even a week after vaccine administration. Those with a history of urticaria and allergies (including hay fever and reactions to hymenoptera venom) appear to have a greater risk of developing allergic reactions to the vaccine. Reactions have been responsive to epinephrine, antihistamines, steroids, or a combination of these agents.[1,16] Because of late-developing allergic reactions, immunizations should be completed 10 days before travel; vaccine recipients need to be advised to remain accessible to emergency medical care.

Tick-Borne Encephalitis

Tick-borne encephalitis is a viral infection of the central nervous system that is transmitted by ticks. The disease occurs in Scandinavia, western and central Europe, and countries of the former Soviet Union. The disease is transmitted principally from April through August, when the tick vector, *Ixodes ricinus*, is most active. Infections may also be acquired by consumption of unpasteurized dairy products from infected cows, goats, or sheep. Effective vaccines are available in Europe and in many travel clinics in Canada; vaccines are not available in the United States. Vaccination should be considered for travelers who anticipate extensive outdoor exposure (e.g., camping or related activities) in the endemic regions during the spring and summer months.[1]

VACCINE CONTRAINDICATIONS

Vaccines that contain live attenuated viruses (i.e., oral polio, measles, mumps, rubella, and yellow fever vaccines) should not be given to pregnant women or to persons who have known or potential immunodeficiencies (e.g., leukemia, lymphoma, or a generalized malignant disorder) or who are receiving corticosteroids, alkylating agents, antimetabolites, or irradiation. Oral polio vaccine, which is no longer recommended in the United States, should not be given to a patient if an immunodeficient person resides in the same household. If a pregnant woman cannot defer travel to areas of high risk for yellow fever, yellow fever vaccine may be given.[1] For travelers infected with HIV, immunization with live oral polio and attenuated oral typhoid vaccines should be avoided in favor of killed parenteral vaccines. The risks of live yellow fever vaccine have not been defined for HIV-infected persons, but persons with asymptomatic HIV infection who cannot avoid exposure in areas endemic for yellow fever should be offered the choice of immunization.[1] Because measles can be severe in patients with HIV, measles immunization should be provided, unless the patient is severely immunocompromised (i.e., total CD4+ T cell count < 200/µl).[9]

Contraindications to vaccination also include hypersensitivity to components of the vaccine. Neomycin and gelatin are present in some vaccines. Persons who have immediate hypersensitivity reactions to neomycin, gelatin, or preservative agents should avoid vaccines containing these substances. Yellow fever vaccine, which contains egg proteins and gelatin, may be contraindicated in patients who have allergic reactions to these proteins. In general, there is a poor correlation between a history of egg sensitivity and skin-test reactivity to egg antigen. The most reliable predictor of reactions to egg-containing vaccines is skin testing with the vaccine itself.[1] If travel plans cannot be changed, persons who have positive skin tests or known egg hypersensitivity (i.e., urticaria, oropharyngeal swelling, bronchospasm, or hypotension) should be given a letter documenting the contraindication to immunization and obtain a waiver before travel from the embassy of any country requiring yellow fever immunization.

INSECT REPELLENTS AND AVOIDANCE

To reduce the risk of all mosquito-borne infections (e.g., malaria, yellow fever, and dengue fever), travelers should be instructed about the importance of minimizing the potential for insect bites. The most effective insect repellents contain DEET.[17,18] DEET is available in many products in concentrations ranging from 25% to more than 75% and repels mosquitoes, ticks, fleas, and biting flies. Protection lasts for several hours but is shortened by losses from swimming, washing, rainfall, sweating, and wiping. A long-acting formulation, which contains polymer to limit the losses of DEET that result from dermal absorption and evaporation, has been developed by the military and is available in the United States as Ultrathon (3M).

The absorption of DEET through the skin can cause such adverse reactions as dermatitis, allergic reactions, and neurotoxicity. Potential toxicity can be avoided by using solutions of 30% to 35% DEET and following instructions for its use. The repellent should be applied sparingly to clothing and exposed skin only. The product should be applied carefully to avoid introducing it into the eyes, to avoid contact with wounds and sensitive skin, and to prevent inhalation or ingestion. Clothing and bed netting can also be treated with permethrin for protection against mosquitoes and ticks.[19] Treated clothing will effectively repel mosquitoes for more than 1 week even with washing and field use. Permethrin is available, often in outdoor supply stores, as a nonstaining aerosol clothing spray (e.g., Permanone Tick Repellent).

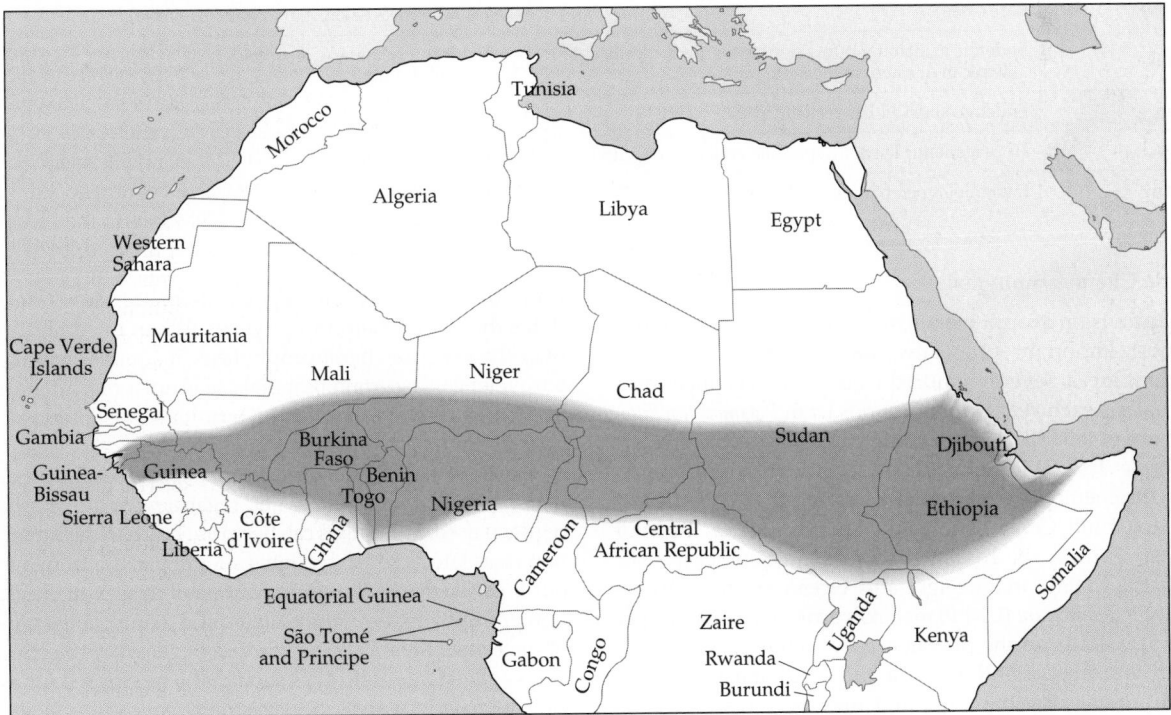

Figure 4 **Epidemics of meningococcal disease are frequent in the area of sub-Saharan Africa that extends from Guinea in the west to Ethiopia in the east.**

Table 2   Risk of Japanese Encephalitis by Country, Region, and Season[1]

Country	Affected Areas	Transmission Season
Australia	Islands of Torres Strait	Probably year-round transmission
Bangladesh	Few data, probably widespread	Possibly July through December
Bhutan	No data	No data
Brunei	Presumed to be sporadic-endemic, as in Malaysia	Presumed year-round transmission
Myanmar (Burma)	Presumed to be endemic-hyperendemic countrywide	Presumed to be May through October
Cambodia	Presumed to be endemic-hyperendemic countrywide	Presumed to be May through October
India	Reported cases from many states	South India: May through October in Goa, October through January in Tamil Nadu, and August through December in Karnataka Andhra Pradesh: September through December North India: July through December
Indonesia	Kalimantan, Bali, Nusa, Tenggara, Sulawesi, Mollucas, Irian, Jaya, and Lombok	Probably year-round risk (varies by island); peak risks associated with rainfall, rice cultivation, and presence of pigs Peak periods of risk are November through March and, in some years, June through July
Japan	Rare, sporadic cases on all islands, except Hokkaido	June through September; Ryukyu Islands (Okinawa), April through October
Korea	Sporadic in South Korea; endemic with occasional outbreaks	July through October
Laos	Presumed to be endemic-hyperendemic countrywide	Presumed to be May through October
Malaysia	Sporadic-endemic in all states of Malay Peninsula, Sarawak, and probably Sabah	No seasonal pattern; year-round transmission
Nepal	Hyperendemic in southern lowlands (Terai)	July through November
People's Republic of China	Hyperendemic in southern China; periodically epidemic in temperate areas	Northern China: May through September Hong Kong and southern China: April through October
Pakistan	May be transmitted in central deltas	Presumed to be June through January
Philippines	Presumed to be endemic on all islands	Uncertain
Russia	Far eastern maritime areas south of Khabarovsk	Peak period July through September
Singapore	Rare cases	Year-round transmission; April peak
Sri Lanka	Endemic in all but mountainous areas; periodically epidemic in northern and central provinces	October through January; secondary peak of enzootic transmission May through June
Taiwan	Endemic-sporadic cases island-wide	April through October; June peak
Thailand	Hyperendemic in north; sporadic-endemic in south	May through October
Vietnam	Endemic-hyperendemic in all provinces	May through October

Malaria Chemoprophylaxis

The provision of appropriate malaria chemoprophylaxis is the most important preventive measure for travelers to malarious areas. Several hundred United States civilians contract malaria each year,[1] and infections from *Plasmodium falciparum* are potentially lethal and do cause deaths in travelers [*see Chapter 157*].[20] Morbidity and mortality are largely avoidable with chemoprophylaxis. Malaria is prevalent in parts of Mexico, Haiti, Central and South America, Africa, the Middle East, Turkey, the Indian subcontinent, Southeast Asia, China, the Malay archipelago, and Oceania. Chloroquine-resistant *P. falciparum* (CRPF) malaria occurs in most areas [*see Figure 5*]. Details on the prevalence by country and regions with-in countries of both malaria and CRPF malaria are reported annually by the CDC and may be accessed online (www.cdc.gov/travel/yb/index.htm).[1] Because even brief exposures to infected mosquitoes can transmit malaria infec-

tions, travel in malarious regions, no matter how brief, mandates the use of chemoprophylaxis. When uncertainty exists over the need for chemoprophylaxis, it should be initiated. If a traveler can ascertain that malaria is not a risk after arriving in an area, prophylaxis can be terminated as long as further travel into malarious areas is not planned.

Travelers should be advised that it is possible to acquire malaria despite prophylaxis and regardless of the prophylactic regimen used. Symptoms can begin as early as 8 days after infection or as late as several months after departure from a malarious area. Travelers should be cautioned to seek medical attention promptly for any febrile illness and to inform the physician of their prior itinerary. The wisdom of general protective measures against mosquito bites should also be stressed for all travelers to malarious areas. Because the vector mosquitoes usually feed at night, it is advisable to diminish exposure between dusk and dawn by remaining in screened areas; using mosquito net-

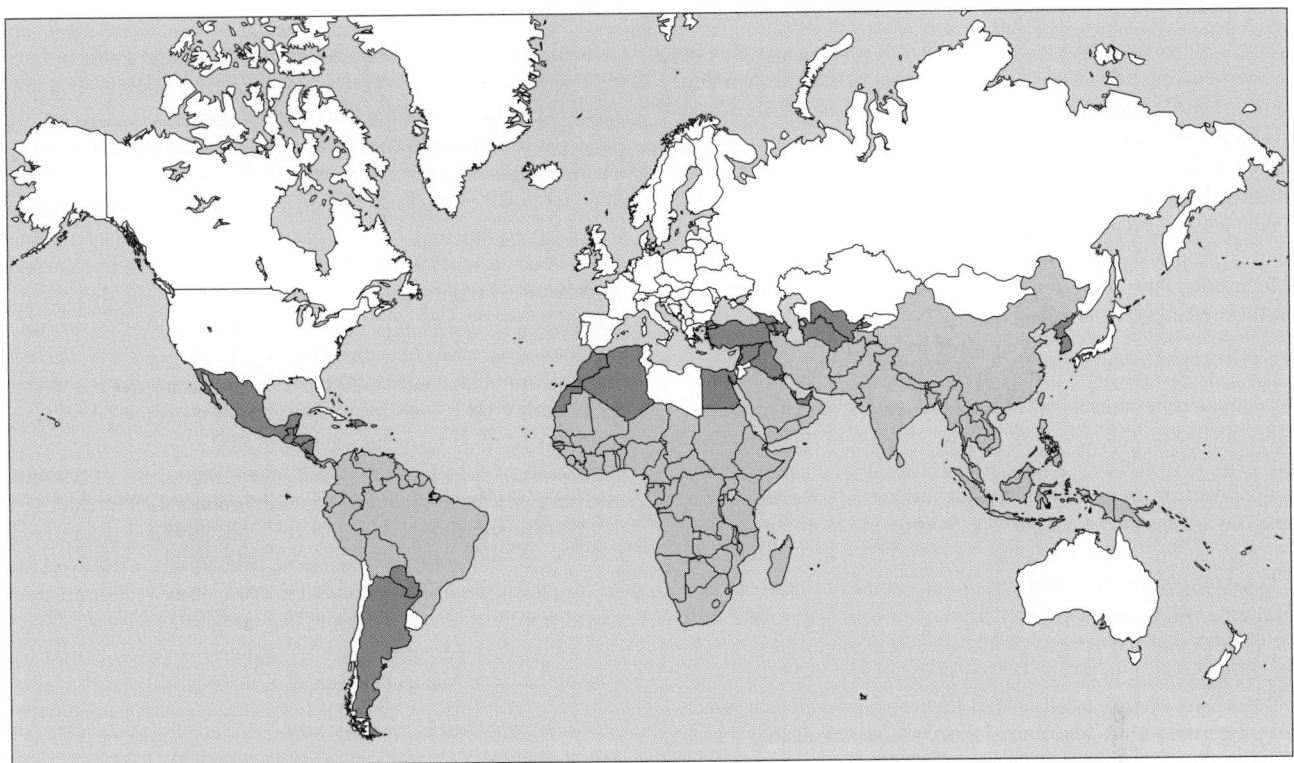

Figure 5 **This map displays the distribution of the chloroquine-resistant malaria (gray areas) and chloroquine-sensitive malaria (blue areas) in the Americas and in Asia, Europe, and Africa.**

ting, ideally treated with permethrin; covering exposed skin with clothing; and using insect repellent.

The choice of appropriate chemoprophylactic agents against malaria depends on the geographic areas to be visited and, importantly, whether these areas are endemic for CRPF [*see Figure 5*]. If travel is not to include areas where CRPF has been reported (e.g., Central America and the Caribbean), chloroquine remains the chemoprophylactic agent of choice. For most of the world, however, alternatives to chloroquine are required. Mainline alternatives to chloroquine include mefloquine and atovaquone-proguanil (Malarone).

Chloroquine

For those limited geographic regions not yet experiencing CRPF [*see Figure 5*], the chemoprophylactic agent of choice is chloroquine, given as either chloroquine phosphate (Aralen) or hydroxychloroquine sulfate (Plaquenil).[1] Chloroquine phosphate, 500 mg (300 mg of chloroquine base), or hydroxychloroquine sulfate, 400 mg (310 mg of hydroxychloroquine base), should be taken once weekly beginning 1 to 2 weeks before travel and continuing during the stay and for 4 weeks after departure from malarious areas. Minor side effects, including gastrointestinal disturbances, dizziness, blurred vision, and headache, may be alleviated by taking the drug after meals. Serious side effects are rare. Specifically, retinal injury, which can occur when high doses of chloroquine are used to treat rheumatoid arthritis, does not occur with the weekly dosages used for malaria prevention, even when such a regimen is continued for 5 years. However, deaths from malaria have occurred among tourists from the United States who avoided chloroquine prophylaxis out of a misguided concern for ocular toxicity.

Mefloquine

Mefloquine (Lariam) is active against CRPF and against *P. falciparum* that is resistant to sulfadoxine with pyrimethamine (Fansidar). With the now-widespread geographic prevalence of CRPF [*see Figure 5*], either mefloquine or atovaquone-proguanil is for many travelers the mainstay of malarial chemoprophylaxis. Strains of *P. falciparum* that are resistant to mefloquine, however, have been recognized in Africa and along the border between Thailand and Cambodia. Mefloquine, 250 mg, is taken once a week, beginning 1 to 2 weeks before travel and continuing during the stay and for 4 weeks after departure from a malarious area.[1] (This schedule is similar to that for chloroquine.) For travelers who will be immediately arriving in malarious areas, a loading dose of mefloquine (250 mg daily for the first 3 days) is advisable.

Despite the benefits of mefloquine to travelers in regions with CRPF malaria, mefloquine has acquired an unsalutary reputation. Mefloquine causes side effects, including nausea, dizziness, vertigo, light-headedness (described as an inability to concentrate), bad dreams, seizures, and psychosis. These reactions occur principally when the drug is given at therapeutic doses, which are higher than those given for prophylaxis. The incidence of psychosis or seizures has been about one per 10,000 travelers treated with chemoprophylactic mefloquine, which is comparable to the incidence associated with chloroquine use.[21] Other controlled trials have demonstrated that mefloquine is reasonably well tolerated in groups receiving this agent.[22-24] Thus, the uncommon and self-limited, but bothersome, side effects of mefloquine are to be weighed against the very real risks of serious and fatal malaria in many nonimmune travelers.

Mefloquine use has also been associated with sinus bradycardia and prolongation of the QT interval. Therefore, mefloquine probably should not be used by persons with cardiac conduction abnormalities but may be used by patients without arrhythmias who are taking beta blockers.[1] Other contraindications to mefloquine include a history of serious neuropsychiatric disorders or seizures. Mefloquine appears to be safe and effective for young children.[25] Studies indicate that use of mefloquine in pregnancy during the second and third trimesters is not associated with adverse fetal or pregnancy outcomes; more limited data suggest that mefloquine is probably safe during the first trimester.[26-28] Mefloquine has no deleterious effects on fine motor skills, such as those required by airplane pilots.[29]

Atovaquone-Proguanil

Atovaquone-proguanil (Malarone) is available in many countries, including the United States, for the chemoprophylaxis of malaria. Atovaquone-proguanil is formulated as a fixed-dose tablet in adult strength (250 mg atovaquone/100 mg proguanil) and in pediatric strength (62.5 mg atovaquone/25 mg proguanil). For prophylaxis, one tablet is taken daily, beginning 1 to 2 days before travel and continuing for the duration of travel and for 1 week after departure from malarious areas. One, two, or three pediatric-strength tablets are taken by children weighing 11 to 20 kg, 21 to 30 kg, or 31 to 40 kg, respectively.

Atovaquone-proguanil is well tolerated; side effects, which are uncommon, are abdominal pain, nausea, vomiting, headache, and rash. Atovaquone-proguanil is safe and efficacious for prophylaxis of *P. vivax* and *P. falciparum* malaria, including CRPF. For *P. vivax* and *P. ovale* malaria, atovaquone-proguanil, like mefloquine and chloroquine, does not prevent development of hepatic hypnozoite stages, so treatment with primaquine (so-called terminal prophylaxis) may be necessary to prevent relapses with these species [see Primaquine, below]. Atovaquone-proguanil, therefore, is an alternative to mefloquine for malaria chemoprophylaxis[1] in regions of Thailand, Myanmar (Burma), and Cambodia where mefloquine-resistant *P. falciparum* malaria is present.

Doxycycline

Doxycycline, taken alone, is an alternative chemoprophylactic agent.[1] It should be taken in a dosage of 100 mg daily, beginning 1 to 2 days before travel and continuing for 4 weeks after departure from malarious areas. The use of doxycycline is appropriate for persons who are intolerant of sulfonamides, pyrimethamine, chloroquine, or mefloquine and for persons who are planning short-term visits in forested areas of Thailand, Myanmar (Burma), or Cambodia, where strains of malaria that are resistant to chloroquine, mefloquine, and sulfadoxine with pyrimethamine (Fansidar) are present.[1] Doxycycline may cause photosensitivity skin reactions and is contraindicated in pregnant women and in children younger than 8 years.

Proguanil

Proguanil (Paludrine) is not available in the United States but is available in Canada, Europe, and much of Africa. This agent, like pyrimethamine, is a dehydrofolate reductase inhibitor, and some strains of malaria are resistant to it. Proguanil (200 mg) is taken daily in combination with a weekly dose of chloroquine. The combination of proguanil and chloroquine, however, is much less effective than mefloquine or atovaquone-proguanil against chloroquine-resistant *P. falciparum* malaria and hence is not recommended.[1,30]

Primaquine

Primaquine may be used either as a single agent taken daily for chemoprophylaxis against all species of malaria or as an agent to eradicate residual intrahepatic stages of *P. vivax* and *P. ovale*. For the latter purpose, primaquine is administered during the last weeks of or just after a course of prophylaxis with either chloroquine or mefloquine. When intended as terminal prophylaxis, primaquine may be administered as 30 mg of the base daily for 14 days. Such terminal prophylaxis is generally reserved for persons who have had more than a casual potential exposure to *P. vivax* or *P. ovale*; other persons may be followed clinically and evaluated if they become symptomatic. For use as a primary chemoprophylactic agent, 30 mg of primaquine base is taken daily starting 1 day before travels and continuing for 2 days after departure from a malarious area.[31]

Because primaquine can cause severe hemolysis in patients who have glucose-6-phosphate dehydrogenase (G6PD) deficiency, this disorder must be excluded before the drug is administered. As a chemoprophylactic agent, primaquine is reserved for the rare individual who is unable to take other recommended chemoprophylactic regimens. CDC suggests primaquine be used only after consultation with malaria experts, including those at the CDC Malaria Hotline (1-770-488-7788).[1]

Sulfadoxine with Pyrimethamine

For chemoprophylaxis in areas where CRPF malaria occurs, it was formerly recommended that a single tablet of Fansidar, which contains 500 mg of long-acting sulfadoxine and 25 mg of pyrimethamine, be taken once a week along with chloroquine beginning 1 to 2 weeks before arrival in an endemic area and continuing for 4 weeks after departure from such an area. However, severe mucocutaneous reactions, including erythema multiforme, Stevens-Johnson syndrome, and toxic epidermal necrolysis, have developed after the use of two or more doses of Fansidar. These reactions produced fatalities with an incidence of about one per 11,000 to 20,000 travelers from the United States. Moreover, *P. falciparum* malaria is increasingly resistant to antifolate agents. Consequently, Fansidar is not recommended for chemoprophylactic use.

PROPHYLAXIS DURING PREGNANCY

Malaria infections represent a major health hazard to the mother and fetus.[32,33] Infections are potentially more serious during pregnancy and increase the risks of stillbirths, abortions, and other adverse pregnancy outcomes. For pregnant women who cannot defer travel or residence in malarious areas, chloroquine, which is without established teratogenicity, may be used.[1] Mefloquine appears to be safe in pregnancy.[26-28] For the pregnant traveler in regions with CRPF malaria, the benefits of effective mefloquine chemoprophylaxis need to be balanced with any potential, but as yet not recognized, adverse effects of mefloquine in pregnancy. Sulfadoxine should be avoided before delivery because of the risk of neonatal jaundice. Pyrimethamine, which is teratogenic in animals because it interferes with folate metabolism, is generally avoided but probably could be used. Doxycycline should not be used during pregnancy because of the effects of tetracyclines on the fetus, which include dental discoloration and dysplasia and inhibition of bone growth. To avoid the risk of inducing hemolytic anemia in utero in a G6PD-deficient fetus, primaquine should not be taken during pregnancy. The safety of malarone in pregnancy has not been established.

Travel-Related Illness

In a study of more than 10,000 Swiss who had traveled in developing countries for less than 3 months, 15% experienced health problems, and 3% were unable to work for an average of 15 days.[34] Infections with the greatest incidence per month abroad included giardiasis (seven cases per 1,000 months abroad), amebiasis (four cases per 1,000), hepatitis (four cases per 1,000), and gonorrhea (three cases per 1,000). Malaria, syphilis, and helminthic infections occurred at a lower incidence (fewer than one case per 1,000). No cases of typhoid fever or cholera were reported. The most common modes of acquisition of infection were enteral and sexual. Travelers should be cautioned about sexual contacts, especially in areas where hepatitis B or HIV is prevalent, and be advised to use condoms and barrier protection during sexual encounters.

Because of the global prevalence of HIV, postexposure antiretroviral prophylaxis may be germane for travelers who may have occupational exposures (e.g., health care workers) and for students and workers who are traveling and may be at risk for HIV exposure. The availability of local postexposure prophylactic medications should be ascertained at overseas work or study sites. Options for two- or three-drug regimens of postexposure antiretroviral therapy are discussed elsewhere [see Chapter 158]. If selected antiretroviral therapy is not assuredly available at work or study sites, sufficient medication should be carried by the traveler to ensure that a 28-day course of antiretroviral therapy is available.

Stays at major resorts and first-class hotels are associated with less risk than stays in less frequented locales or rural dwellings or encampments. In areas where sanitation and personal hygiene may be poor, it is prudent to be careful of food and water, although such care does not necessarily diminish the risk of diarrheal disease. Fruit that is peeled by the traveler is safe, whereas vegetables may be contaminated with fecally passed organisms in the soil and should not be consumed raw. Unpasteurized dairy products should be avoided, as should inadequately cooked fish or meat. If water is of uncertain quality, travelers should avoid drinking it or using ice made from it. Boiling will render water safe. Chlorination will kill most bacterial and viral pathogens, but protozoal cysts of *Giardia lamblia* and *Entamoeba histolytica* may survive. Carbonated beverages, beer, wine, and drinks made from boiled water are safe.

In areas where schistosomiasis is prevalent, swimming in freshwater should be avoided, although swimming in chlorinated or saltwater is safe. Even short exposures to infested water during rafting or swimming have caused the onset of acute schistosomiasis.

Most infections acquired during travels will present within weeks of travel, but some may not manifest themselves until much later; hence, knowledge of a patient's travel history is important.

ALTITUDE ILLNESS

Altitude illnesses may develop in travelers who arrive at heights between 6,000 and 8,000 ft (1,829 and 2,438 m) above sea level.[1] Travelers may arrive at these altitudes rapidly by flying into an airport at these elevations or more slowly by driving or climbing. Altitude illness includes three syndromes: acute mountain sickness (AMS), high-altitude pulmonary edema (HAPE), and high-altitude cerebral edema (HACE). AMS, the most common form of altitude illness, may occur at altitudes between 4,000 and 6,000 ft. Symptoms include headache, fatigue, loss of appetite, nausea, and, sometimes, vomiting. AMS usually develops 6 to 12 hours after arrival at the higher altitude. HACE is a progression of AMS characterized by extreme lethargy, confusion, and an ataxic gait during a tandem gait test.

HAPE may develop alone or in conjunction with HACE. Symptoms include increasing breathlessness. HAPE is more likely than HACE to be fatal. Travelers who develop HACE or HAPE must immediately descend to lower altitudes. Travelers to elevated altitudes need to be cautioned about the symptoms of these syndromes [see Chapter 224], advised about the gravity of HACE and HAPE, and admonished not to delay descent to lower altitudes if these potentially lethal syndromes develop.

Three medications can be used to prevent and treat altitude illnesses. Acetazolamide can prevent AMS if taken before ascent; it also can hasten recovery. Dosing is 125 mg every 12 hours beginning the day of ascent. Dexamethasone (4 mg every 6 hours) can be used to prevent and treat AMS and HACE. Some investigators recommend relying on acetazolamide for prophylaxis and reserving dexamethasone for treatment of symptoms.[1] Persons who have experienced HAPE are at increased risk of its recurrence. If travel to high altitudes is unavoidable, nifedipine (10 to 20 mg every 8 hours) can prevent and ameliorate HAPE in those prone to experience this syndrome.

TRAVELER'S DIARRHEA

Diarrhea is the most common illness of travelers.[35] Infectious agents, primarily bacterial but also viral and parasitic pathogens, are responsible for traveler's diarrhea. Over 75% of cases of traveler's diarrhea are caused by bacteria, with enterotoxigenic *Escherichia coli* being the most frequent cause. Other common bacterial causes of traveler's diarrhea include *Shigella* species, *Campylobacter jejuni*, *Aeromonas* species, *Plesiomonas shigelloides*, *Salmonella* species, and noncholera *Vibrio* species.[35] Rotavirus and Norwalk agent are the most common viral causes; *Giardia, Cryptosporidium, Cyclospora,* and, less commonly, *Dientamoeba fragilis, Isospora belli, Balantidium coli, Strongyloides stercoralis,* and *E. histolytica* are parasitic causes.

In addition to exercising caution about food and water,[36] travelers may take either of two approaches: chemoprophylaxis and postonset treatment.

Chemoprophylaxis

The benefits of chemoprophylaxis may be offset by the risks of taking chemoprophylactic agents. Side effects of short-term prophylactic doses of bismuth subsalicylate may include tinnitus, blackening of the stool and tongue, and impaired absorption of doxycycline, which is important if doxycycline is used as daily antimalarial chemoprophylaxis. Side effects of antibiotics may include skin rashes and vaginal candidiasis, photosensitivity skin eruptions (especially with doxycycline), and, in rare instances, potentially life-threatening bone marrow suppression, mucocutaneous reactions, or anaphylaxis. Although these potential side effects temper the routine use of chemoprophylaxis, specific needs or wishes of travelers may dictate its use. Patients with underlying medical conditions that may be aggravated by a serious diarrheal illness, including active inflammatory bowel disease, type 1 (insulin-dependent) diabetes mellitus, and heart disease in the elderly, as well as patients whose activities during travel cannot tolerate interruption by an episode of diarrheal illness, should consider chemoprophylaxis. Several regimens are available [see Table 3]. Bismuth subsalicylate, which should not

Table 3   Chemoprophylaxis and
Treatment of Traveler's Diarrhea

Drug	Dose
Prophylaxis	
Bismuth subsalicylate	Two 262 mg tablets chewed q.i.d. with meals and at bedtime
Quinolone antibiotics	
Norfloxacin	400 mg/day
Ciprofloxacin	500 mg/day
Ofloxacin	300 mg/day
Levofloxacin	500 mg/day
Doxycycline	100 mg/day
Treatment	
Loperamide	4 mg loading dose, then 2 mg after each loose stool, to a maximum of 16 mg/day
Quinolone antibiotics	
Norfloxacin	400 mg b.i.d. for up to 3 days
Ciprofloxacin	500 mg b.i.d. for up to 3 days
Ofloxacin	300 mg b.i.d. for up to 3 days
Levofloxacin	500 mg/day for up to 3 days
Azithromycin	1,000 mg single dose or 500 mg/day for 3 days
Rifaximin	200 mg t.i.d. for 3 days

be taken by persons with peptic ulcer disease, coagulopathies, or allergies to salicylates, is not as completely effective as quinolone antibiotics but has fewer side effects and enables the use of quinolone antibiotics, if they are needed for therapy. Resistance among bacterial causes of traveler's diarrhea is not common at present for the quinolone antibiotics (except for quinolone-resistant *Campylobacter* infection prevalent in Thailand) but is quite common for trimethoprim-sulfamethoxazole and doxycycline, limiting their efficacy. Chemoprophylactic medications should be started on the first day of arrival and continued for 1 to 2 days after returning home but not for more than 3 weeks.

Postonset Treatment

A generally preferable alternative to chemoprophylaxis is early therapy for traveler's diarrhea [*see Table 3*]. Because of the likelihood of bacterial resistance, trimethoprim-sulfamethoxazole is less effective than regimens employing quinolone antibiotics. Antibiotics will shorten the duration of traveler's diarrhea to a range of 16 to 30 hours, compared with a range of 59 to 93 hours in those not receiving antibiotics. The use of loperamide, which diminishes intestinal motility and fluid and electrolyte losses, together with antibiotics can further abbreviate symptoms. In a study of patients with dysentery caused by *Shigella* or enteroinvasive *E. coli*, the use of loperamide with ciprofloxacin, in comparison with ciprofloxacin alone, led to briefer (median, 19 hours versus 42 hours) and milder (median, two stools versus 6.5 stools) diarrheal illness, without untoward effects.[37] Loperamide has not been studied in children, and adults with prolonged fever or bloody stools should be advised to cease loperamide use and seek medical attention. Azithromycin is an alternative to quinolone antibiotics that can be used by pregnant patients; it is the agent of choice where quinolone-resistant *Campylobacter* infection is prevalent. Rifaximin (Xifaxan, from Salix), a nonabsorbable agent, is approved by the FDA for traveler's diarrhea caused by noninvasive strains of *Escherichia coli*.[38] Rifaximin should not be used if dysentery is suspected (i.e., if symptoms include fever and bloody stools) or if other causes of diarrhea (e.g., *Campylobacter*, *Shigella*, or invasive *E. coli*) are possible or isolated.

For any diarrheal illness, maintenance of hydration is of cardinal importance and can often be achieved by oral replacement of lost fluid and electrolytes. Convenient and inexpensive packets of oral rehydration salts formulated according to World Health Organization recommendations (i.e., 3.5 g of sodium chloride, 1.5 g of potassium chloride, 20 g of glucose, and 2.9 g of trisodium citrate in each packet) are available in both developed and developing countries. Each packet of oral rehydration salts is added to a liter of boiled or treated water and should be consumed or discarded within 12 hours if kept at ambient temperature or within 24 hours if kept refrigerated.

MEDICAL ISSUES DURING TRANSIT

Cruise ships that dock at ports in the United States are inspected for sanitation by officials from the CDC. Inspections are aimed at minimizing the potential for outbreaks of gastrointestinal disease on board. Travelers may obtain information on whether specific cruise ships meet sanitation standards from travel agents, state health departments, or the CDC.[1] Outbreaks of influenza have occurred aboard cruise ships in the past 10 years in various regions, including Alaska and the Yukon Territory. Travelers older than 50 years should consider influenza vaccination.

Because jet aircraft are not pressurized to sea level, passengers will be exposed to high-altitude environments. The atmospheric pressure maintained within the cabin of an airplane flying at 27,000 to 42,000 ft is equivalent to the pressure at an altitude of 3,000 to 8,000 ft, so that at a cruising altitude of 35,000 ft, the cabin pressure is about 600 mm Hg. Because of the decreased pressure, the arterial oxygen tension (P_aO_2) of normal persons will fall to about 68 mm Hg. In patients with chronic obstructive lung disease, the P_aO_2 will fall even lower. However, despite a fall in P_aO_2, patients may not show symptoms of hypoxia. Although hypoxia occurs in pregnant women, jet air travel has no deleterious effects on them or their fetuses. It is difficult to establish precise criteria for the use of supplemental oxygen for air travelers. Caution is indicated, however, for patients with impaired cardiopulmonary function: supplemental oxygen may be administered during flights at altitudes higher than 22,500 ft.

Scuba divers should wait 12 to 48 hours, depending on the length of their diving exposures, before boarding a commercial aircraft. This measure is important for avoiding the occurrence of aeroembolism, commonly known as the bends, which could develop in an underpressurized cabin if nitrogen gas dissolved in the person's fat cells is mobilized.

In patients with upper respiratory tract infections, differential air pressures between blocked eustachian tubes or sinuses and the cabin may develop on ascent or descent and impair hearing or cause pain in the ears or sinuses; symptoms can be relieved by the use of decongestants. Persons prone to motion sickness should take a prophylactic medication. Prolonged immobilization during flight may cause venous thrombosis in persons with preexisting thrombotic or venous disease [*see Chapter 32*]. The exact risks and rates for developing venous thromboembolism during air travel are not yet defined.[39] Leg exercise and walking during the flight and use of below-the-knee stockings have been suggested to be beneficial, but evidence is lacking.

The author has received grant or research support from and is an advisor to GlaxoSmithKline.

References

1. Centers for Disease Control and Prevention: Health information for international travel 2003-2004. US Department of Health and Human Services, Atlanta, 2003 (http://www.cdc.gov)

2. Rachel Barwick: History of thymoma and yellow fever vaccination (correspondence). Eidex for the Yellow Fever Vaccine Safety Working Group. Lancet 364:936, 2004

3. Kelso JM, Mootrey GT, Tsai TF: Anaphylaxis from yellow fever vaccine. J Allergy Clin Immunol 103:698, 1999

4. Prevention and control of influenza. Recommendations of the Advisory Committee on Immunization Practices (ACIP). MMWR Morb Mortal Wkly Rep 53(RR-6):1, 2004 (http://www.cdc.gov/mmwr/preview/mmwrhtml/rr5306a1.htm)

5. Khan WA, Bennish ML, Seas C, et al: Randomised controlled comparison of single-dose ciprofloxacin and doxycycline for cholera caused by Vibrio cholerae 01 or 0139. Lancet 348:296, 1996

6. Poliomyelitis prevention in the United States. Updated recommendation of the Advisory Committee on Immunization Practices (ACIP). MMWR Morb Mortal Wkly Rep 49(RR-5):1, 2000 (http://www.cdc.gov/mmwr/PDF/RR/RR4905.pdf)

7. Maple PA, Jones CS, Wall EC, et al: Immunity to diphtheria and tetanus in England and Wales. Vaccine 19:167, 2000

8. Leder K, Weller PF, Wilson ME: Travel vaccines and elderly persons: review of vaccines available in the United States. Clin Infect Dis 33:1553, 2001

9. Measles immunization in HIV-infected children. American Academy of Pediatrics. Committee on Infectious Diseases and Committee on Pediatric AIDS. Pediatrics 103:1057, 1999

10. Mermin JH, Townes JM, Gerber M, et al: Typhoid fever in the United States, 1985-1995: changing risks of international travel and antimicrobial resistance. Arch Intern Med 158:633, 1998

11. Steinberg EB, Bishop R, Haber P, et al: Typhoid fever in travelers: who should be targeted for prevention? Clin Infect Dis 39:186, 2004

12. Stubi CL, Landry PR, Petignat C, et al: Compliance to live oral Ty21a typhoid vaccine, and its effect on viability. J Travel Med 7:133, 2000

13. Plotkin SA, Bouveret-Le Cam N: A new typhoid vaccine composed of the Vi capsular polysaccharide. Arch Intern Med 155:2293, 1995

14. Steffen R, Kane MA, Shapiro CN, et al: Epidemiology and prevention of hepatitis A in travelers. JAMA 272:885, 1994

15. Prevention of hepatitis A through active or passive immunization: recommendations of the Advisory Committee on Immunization Practices (ACIP). MMWR Morb Mortal Wkly Rep 48(RR-12):1, 1999

16. Plesner A, Ronne T, Wachmann H: Case-control study of allergic reactions to Japanese encephalitis vaccine. Vaccine 18:1830, 2000

17. Fradin MS, Day JF: Comparative efficacy of insect repellents against mosquito bites. N Engl J Med 347:13, 2002

18. Insect repellents. Med Lett Drugs Ther 24:41, 2003

19. D'Allessandro V: Insecticide treated bed nets to prevent malaria. BMJ 322:249, 2001

20. Shah S, Filler S, Causer LM, et al: Malaria surveillance—United States, 2002. MMWR Surveill Summ 53(1):21, 2004

21. Steffen R, Fuchs E, Schildknecht J, et al: Mefloquine compared with other chemoprophylactic regimens in tourists visiting East Africa. Lancet 341:1299, 1993

22. Jaspers CA, Hopperus Buma AP, van Thiel PP, et al: Tolerance of mefloquine chemoprophylaxis in Dutch military personnel. Am J Trop Med Hyg 55:230, 1996

23. Davis TM, Dembo LG, Kaye-Eddie SA, et al: Neurological, cardiovascular and metabolic effects of mefloquine in healthy volunteers: a double-blind, placebo-controlled trial. Br J Clin Pharmacol 42:415, 1996

24. Croft AM, Clayton TC, World MJ: Side effects of mefloquine prophylaxis for malaria: an independent randomized controlled trial. Trans R Soc Trop Med Hyg 91:199, 1997

25. Luxemburger C, Price RN, Nosten F, et al: Mefloquine in infants and young children. Ann Trop Paediatr 16:281, 1996

26. Smoak BL, Writer JV, Keep LW, et al: The effects of inadvertent exposure of mefloquine chemoprophylaxis on pregnancy outcomes and infants of US Army servicewomen. J Infect Dis 176:831, 1997

27. Steketee RW, Wirima JJ, Slutsker L, et al: Malaria treatment and prevention in pregnancy: indications for use and adverse events associated with use of chloroquine or mefloquine. Am J Trop Med Hyg 55(suppl 1):50, 1996

28. Schlagenhauf P: Mefloquine for malaria chemoprophylaxis 1992-1998: a review. J Travel Med 6:122, 1999

29. Schlagenhauf P, Lobel H, Steffen R, et al: Tolerance of mefloquine by SwissAir trainee pilots. Am J Trop Med Hyg 56:235, 1997

30. Bradley DJ, Bannister B: Guidelines for malaria prevention in travelers from the United Kingdom for 2003. Health Protection Agency Advisory Committee on Malaria Prevention for UK Travellers. Commun Dis Public Health 6:180, 2003

31. Schwartz E, Rgev-Yochay G: Primaquine as prophylaxis for malaria for nonimmune travelers: a comparison with mefloquine and doxycycline. Clin Infect Dis 29:1502, 1999

32. Steketee RW, Wirima JJ, Hightower AW, et al: The effect of malaria and malaria prevention in pregnancy on offspring birthweight, prematurity, and intrauterine growth retardation in rural Malawi. Am J Trop Med Hyg 55(suppl):33, 1996

33. Steketee RW, Wirima JJ, Slutsker L, et al: Malaria parasite infection during pregnancy and at delivery in mother, placenta, and newborn: efficacy of chloroquine and mefloquine in rural Malawi. Am J Trop Med Hyg 55(suppl 1):24, 1996

34. Steffen R, Rickenbach M, Wilhelm U, et al: Health problems after travel to developing countries. J Infect Dis 156:84, 1987

35. Ryan ET, Kain KC: Health advice and immunizations for travelers. N Engl J Med 342:1716, 2000

36. Herwaldt BL, de Arroyave KR, Roberts JM, et al: A multiyear prospective study of the risk factors for and incidence of diarrheal illness in a cohort of Peace Corps volunteers in Guatemala. Ann Intern Med 132:982, 2000

37. Murphy GS, Bodhidatta L, Echeverria P, et al: Ciprofloxacin and loperamide in the treatment of bacillary dysentery. Ann Intern Med 118:582, 1993

38. Infante RM, Ericsson CD, Jiang ZD, et al: Enteroaggregative Escherichia coli diarrhea in travelers: response to rifaximin therapy. Clin Gastroenterol Hepatol 2:135, 2004

39. Mendis S, Yach D, Alwan A: Air travel and venous thromboembolism. Bull World Health Organ 80:403, 2002

Acknowledgment

Figures 1 through 5 Tom Moore.

9 Complementary and Alternative Medicine

Bimal H. Ashar, M.D., F.A.C.P., and Adrian S. Dobs, M.D., M.H.S.

Definitions

The term alternative medicine encompasses a spectrum of approaches to medical conditions not routinely used by conventional practitioners. Historically, the term has been associated with negative conceptions about medical practices that did not conform to accepted standards of care. The term complementary medicine has since evolved to describe a more positive, symbiotic relationship between unconventional medicine and conventional medicine. The field of complementary and alternative medicine (CAM) now encompasses a multitude of different approaches and beliefs that are generally linked by their emphasis on so-called natural modalities of healing and wellness. More and more, the term integrative medicine is being used, suggesting that CAM should be integrated into conventional care. This chapter describes modalities that are complementary to conventional medicine in the United States; in other countries, many of these modalities are part of mainstream medical practice.

Classification

Patient demand, media attention, and the growth of an approximately $40 billion industry[1] have stimulated leaders in governmental agencies and academic medicine to recognize and categorize CAM and to direct research initiatives on the subject. Although there is currently no universally accepted classification of CAM modalities, the National Center for Complementary and Alternative Medicine (NCCAM) has grouped CAM practices into five domains [see Table 1]. It should be recognized that these categories are not mutually exclusive. Certain practices will overlap (e.g., qigong is considered an energy therapy but is part of Chinese medicine, which is an alternative medical system). Also, as evidence emerges regarding mechanisms of action, safety, and efficacy, certain modalities will naturally move beyond the CAM label and become part of mainstream medicine.

Use of CAM

PREVALENCE AND DEMOGRAPHICS

The widespread use of CAM by the public has been well documented. In 2002, about 62% of adults in the United States reported using at least one form of alternative medicine within the previous year.[1] It has been estimated that 75% of people in the United States have used at least one CAM therapy over their lifetime.[1] Public-opinion surveys have suggested similar overall patterns of use in European countries, although the popularity of specific CAM modalities varies greatly from country to country.[2] Patients across all demographic groups use alternative medicine. However, some surveys have noted that predictors of CAM use may include female gender, white race (as opposed to African-American or Hispanic), higher socioeconomic status, and higher levels of education.[3,4] Many CAM users have chronic, non–life-threatening medical conditions,[3,5] and they may have an interest in spirituality.[6] A number of diagnosis-based surveys suggested exceptionally high usage of alternative medicine in patients with cancer,[7] HIV infection,[8] fibromyalgia,[9] and inflammatory bowel disease.[10]

PUBLIC PERCEPTION

The alternative-medicine movement has clearly been a public-driven process that has spanned decades. It was initially thought that this movement was primarily the result of dissatisfaction with conventional medicine.[11] Subsequent studies have shown that this is not the case[6,12] and that patients continue to see their conventional health care practitioners while using CAM therapies; however, about 27% of CAM users believe that conventional medicine will not help their health care problem.[1] Two disturbing observations are that most patients do not disclose their use of alternative therapies to their physicians and that such patients are never asked about CAM use by their physicians.[13] Furthermore, many patients feel no need to communicate their CAM use to their physicians because they believe that their physicians would be unable to understand and incorporate that information into their treatment plan.[12,14] On the other hand, current data suggest that about one quarter of patients who use CAM do so on the advice of a conventional medical professional.[1]

A number of other factors have stimulated public use of alternative medical therapies. The fact that many CAM modalities emphasize natural forms of healing seems to form the fundamental basis for its use. Many patients desire a more holistic approach to their medical care.[6] They may feel that conventional medicine focuses excessively on suppression of symptoms (e.g., pharmacologic lowering of elevated blood pressure) rather than addressing the root cause of symptoms. They believe that so-called natural products are better and safer than synthetic medications. In many cases, they may turn to alternative medical practices to get relief from chronic conditions that have not responded to conventional symptomatic therapy. Additionally, media hype, direct-to-consumer advertising, and the wide-

Table 1 NIH/NCCAM Classification of Complementary and Alternative Medicine Practices

Category	Examples
Alternative medical systems	Ayurveda (traditional Indian medicine), traditional Chinese medicine, homeopathy
Mind-body interventions	Biofeedback, hypnosis, meditation, prayer
Biologic-based therapies	Dietary therapy, herbal medicine, megavitamins, shark cartilage
Manipulative and body-based methods	Chiropractic, massage therapy, craniosacral therapy
Energy therapies	Therapeutic touch, qigong, bio-electric field manipulation, reiki

NIH/NCCAM—National Institutes of Health/National Center for Complementary and Alternative Medicine

spread availability of information over the Internet have all played a role in the popularity of CAM and have served to expand the public's health care choices. Of concern to many physicians is that these choices are frequently based on insufficient basic science or clinical evidence.

Research Concerns

SCIENTIFIC ISSUES

One of the defining characteristics of alternative medicine is the paucity of definitive evidence supporting mechanism of action, efficacy, and safety. Although a number of clinical trials on CAM have been published, the overall quality of those trials is quite poor, primarily because of inadequate sample size, randomization, and blinding.[15,16] Additionally, publication bias may be common in the international literature. Critical reviews of published studies on CAM therapies from a number of countries have shown that the studies almost universally report positive findings pertaining to CAM. This suggests that studies reporting negative findings may never make it to press.[17,18]

There are a number of barriers to the proper evaluation of CAM studies. First, the establishment of adequate control groups is frequently very difficult. Studies on acupuncture, for example, have attempted to incorporate a placebo control by stimulating nonacupuncture points, stimulating actual points unrelated to the treated condition, or applying pressure instead of inserting needles. Some critics argue that so-called sham acupuncture is an inadequate placebo that does not preserve subject blinding. Proponents of acupuncture may argue that such control methods are still potentially therapeutic because of their possible positive effect on the flow of subtle energy through the body. Similar pitfalls are inherent in mind-body research. In the study of personal prayer, of prayer groups, or of intercessory prayer that occurs in the presence of the patient, the intervention group can be compared with those who do not partake in organized prayer. Such a design clearly does not lend itself to adequate blinding. Additionally, any positive results could reflect aspects of prayer that are unrelated to its spiritual qualities (e.g., relaxation), making definitive conclusions difficult.

Another major problem with interpreting CAM research stems from inconsistencies in the intervention groups. Drawing meaningful conclusions from herbal-medication studies is difficult because extracts are not standardized. For example, although positive effects have been seen in a number of published clinical trials with the plant genus *Echinacea* for treatment of upper respiratory tract infections, definitive conclusions cannot be drawn because of variation in the species of plant studied, the part of the plant utilized (root, leaf, or flower), and extraction methods.[19] In addition, the manufacturing processes within and between companies vary widely, so that the concentration of active product in an over-the-counter preparation is rarely known.

Lack of standardization is also a flaw in acupuncture research. Many different types of acupuncture are practiced around the world, and each type may utilize a completely different set of points for the same condition. Even among providers who practice the same type of acupuncture, variation in point selection is common because approaches differ on the basis of the patient's history and physical examination and on the acupuncturist's personal style. This individualization of therapy is alluring to patients, but the unwillingness of practitioners to agree on what constitutes acceptable technique challenges conventional study methodology. CAM practitioners often criticize the typical scientific model that employs randomized clinical trials because in clinical practice, there are multiple interventions, such as mind-body and herbal treatments, that occur simultaneously. Thus, any research in the area may have to be multidimensional.

FINANCIAL ISSUES

Unlike conventional pharmaceutical and medical-device research, large-scale studies in CAM derive their funding almost exclusively from government sources. Modalities such as prayer, acupuncture, and massage therapy are not lucrative enough endeavors to support large, privately funded trials. Dietary supplements, such as herbs, may have a significant profit potential, but the incentive for research is weakened by the fact that herbs, like other natural substances, cannot be patented. In addition, the rules and regulations under which foods and natural products are regulated differ from those for pharmaceuticals, which must meet stringent standards of efficacy and safety.

In an effort to boost CAM research, the United States Government set up NCCAM (http://nccam.nih.gov), under the National Institutes of Health (NIH). With an annual working budget of about $120 million, NCCAM has funded a number of individual projects, as well as specialty centers around the country [see Table 2].

Specific CAM Modalities

ALTERNATIVE MEDICAL SYSTEMS

Traditional Chinese Medicine

Acupuncture Acupuncture has been used for centuries as a component of traditional Chinese medicine (TCM). It involves the insertion of thin needles into specific points on the skin to facilitate the movement of energy (qi). Chinese medicine posits that qi (pronounced *chee*) flows along distinct channels (called meridians) in the body and that balanced circulation of qi is a prerequisite for good health. A block in the flow of qi can result in either a deficiency or an excess of qi along a meridian; those imbalances can be corrected by accurate needle placement (or pressure, in the case of acupressure) at specific points on the body. Acupuncture practitioners often enhance the effect of the needles by electrical stimulation; manual manipulation (e.g., twirling); or moxibustion, which involves burning mugwort (*Artemisia vulgaris*) on the acupuncture point or the end of the needle. Practitioners of TCM frequently combine acupuncture with other modalities, including herbal remedies, to achieve the desired physiologic response. Each treatment is individualized on the basis of the patient's history and physical examination, including pulse and tongue examinations. Many types of acupuncture are practiced today; a few examples are traditional Chinese acupuncture, five-elements acupuncture, and auricular acupuncture.

To date, no clear physical mechanism of action has emerged to explain the potential therapeutic response to acupuncture. Changes in blood flow and biologic mediators (e.g., hormones, neurotransmitters, and endorphins) have been shown to occur with needle manipulation.[20-23] There are numerous published clinical studies on acupuncture treatment for a variety of ailments. Most are small in size and have methodologic flaws that make consensus difficult. Nevertheless, in 1997, an NIH consensus panel concluded that there is clear evidence to support the use of acupuncture for postoperative, chemotherapy-induced, and probably pregnancy-associated nausea and vomiting.[23] Although the data are less compelling, evidence also suggests a positive effect of acupuncture on idiopathic headache,[24] fibromyalgia,[25,26] and osteoarthritis of the knee.[27] Current evidence does not support its use for smoking cessation,[28] asthma,[29] or low back pain.[30]

If done correctly, acupuncture is quite safe.[31] Rare case reports of serious adverse events, including skin infections, hepatitis, pneumothorax, and cardiac tamponade, seem to stem from inadequate sterilization of needles and practitioner negligence.[32,33]

Table 2   Government-Funded Specialty Centers for Research into Complementary and Alternative Medicine

Specialty	Center and Location
Acupuncture—addiction	Minneapolis Medical Research Foundation, Minneapolis; New England School of Acupuncture, Watertown, Massachusetts
Acupuncture—neuroimaging	Massachusetts General Hospital, Charlestown
Aging and women's health	Columbia University, New York
Antioxidants	Oregon State University, Corvallis
Arthritis	University of Maryland, Baltimore
Botanical treatment of age-related diseases	Purdue University, West Lafayette, Indiana
Botanical dietary supplements for women's health	University of Illinois, Chicago
Botanical dietary supplements	UCLA, Los Angeles
Cancer	Johns Hopkins University, Baltimore
Cancer and hyperbaric oxygen	University of Pennsylvania, Philadelphia
Cardiovascular diseases	University of Michigan, Ann Arbor
Cardiovascular disease and aging in African Americans	Maharishi University of Management, Fairfield, Iowa
Chiropractic	Palmer Center for Chiropractic Research, Davenport, Iowa
Craniofacial disorders	Kaiser Foundation Hospitals, Portland, Oregon
Frontier medicine (biofield science)	University of Arizona, Tucson
Frontier medicine (therapeutic touch)	University of Connecticut, Farmington
Neurodegenerative diseases	Emory University School of Medicine, Atlanta
Neurologic disorders	Oregon Health Sciences University, Portland
Pediatrics	University of Arizona Health Sciences Center, Tucson
Phytomedicine	University of Arizona, Tucson
Phytonutrient and phytochemical studies	University of Missouri, Columbia

To prevent transmission of infection, most practitioners now use disposable needles. Minor side effects, including insertion-site pain or bleeding, fatigue, and vasovagal syncope, are probably more common.[34]

Homeopathy

Homeopathy is one of the most controversial modalities in CAM, primarily because of its theoretical implausibility. The roots of homeopathy trace back to the 1700s, when it was first described by Samuel Hahnemann. Homeopathic principles revolve around two basic tenets: the law of similars and the principle of serial dilutions. According to the law of similars, substances that cause symptoms in healthy people can cure those same symptoms in people who are sick. A number of examples of this principle exist in conventional medicine. Digoxin is used to treat the same arrhythmias that it is capable of inducing. Similarly, methylphenidate, which is a stimulant, has been used to treat attention-deficit/hyperactivity disorder.[35]

The principle of serial dilutions (or the minute dose) is another controversial aspect of homeopathy. According to this principle, medications can have a biologic effect even if diluted to levels at which the original substance is undetectable (a so-called homeopathic dose).

A homeopath's approach to patients differs from that of the conventional physician. Homeopaths concentrate almost exclusively on subjective symptoms and sensations. They choose medications on the basis of the patient's symptomatology, rather than on the objective medical diagnosis. This results in the use of a wide array of different medications for any one conventionally diagnosed condition. A number of homeopathic encyclopedias (*materia medica*) are available that describe symptoms induced by different remedies when given to healthy individuals (provings). These provings are matched to a patient's symptoms to determine the therapeutic regimen. Patients are typically followed closely so that the homeopath can titrate dosing schedules.

Meta-analyses of a number of trials of homeopathic remedies have suggested an effect superior to placebo.[36,37] However, many studies and reviews on specific medications have shown negative or inconclusive results.[37-39] Given the conflicting clinical data and the lack of evidence regarding mechanism of action, it is difficult to support the general use of homeopathy until more high-quality research is available.

Because homeopathic remedies typically contain little or no detectable active ingredients, serious side effects are rare. Homeopathic preparations are generally marketed as over-the-counter remedies and are usually exempt from government requirements for finished product testing or expiration dating. In the United States, the Food and Drug Administration requires that all homeopathic remedies list the indications for their use, the ingredients, instructions for safe use, and dilutions. Dilutions in a ratio of 1:10 are labeled with an X, and dilutions in a ratio of 1:100 are labeled with a C. For example, a 3X product has been diluted 1:10 three times; a 3C product has been diluted 1:100 three times. It should also be noted that these remedies are not restricted to the 10% alcohol limit of conventional drugs.[40]

MIND-BODY INTERVENTIONS

The relationship between psychological stress and physical health has been studied extensively over the past 30 years. Despite positive results from some trials, interventions designed to alter the stress response have not become part of mainstream medical practice. The reluctance of physicians to incorporate

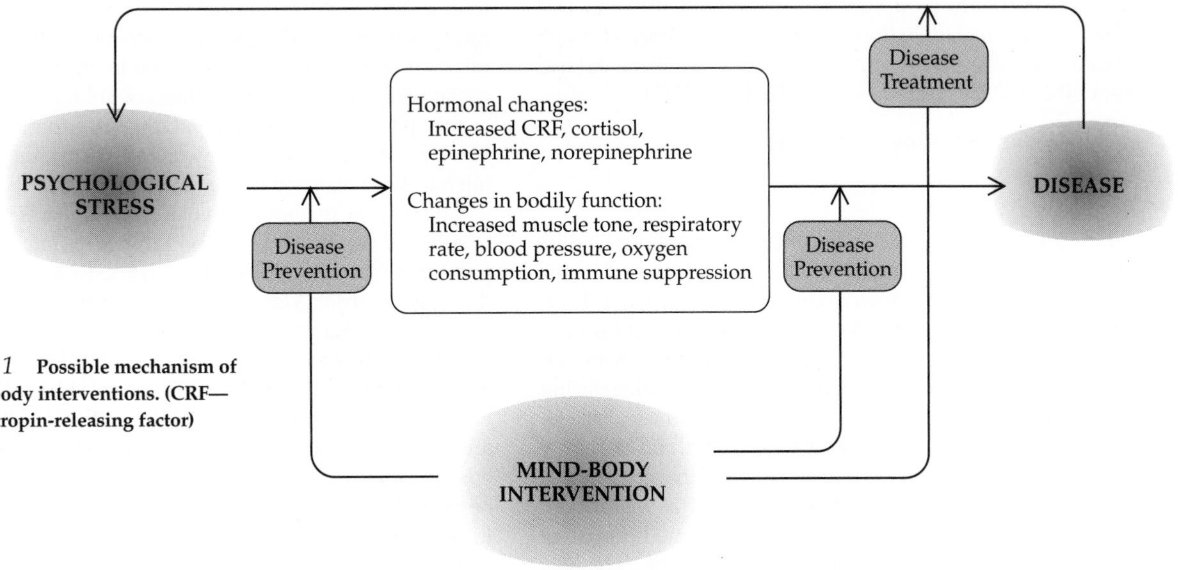

Figure 1 **Possible mechanism of mind-body interventions. (CRF—corticotropin-releasing factor)**

mind-body strategies into their therapeutic armamentarium likely stems from their unfamiliarity with such interventions; time constraints; and the lack of a clear mechanistic pathway to disease. Furthermore, many physicians may feel that these therapies need to be patient driven rather than physician driven, because they require significant changes in self-care.

The proposed theory of mind-body medicine stems from work done in the early 1900s. The fight-or-flight response was described as physiologic preparation for combating or fleeing an external threat.[41] Stimulation of the hypothalamus and increased sympathetic nervous system activity lead to neurohormonal stimulation and increases in blood pressure, heart rate, respiratory rate, and muscle tension. This response has historically been protective, ensuring survival in the face of physical danger. In today's society, however, we are continually faced with innumerable stressors that can elicit the fight-or-flight response, yet fighting or running away is inappropriate or impossible. The body is primed for action but can take none. This chronic physiologic stimulation is thought to increase the likelihood of disease. Furthermore, the development of a chronic disease may stimulate the response through a feedback mechanism, potentially worsening the condition. The effect of the chronic fight-or-flight response on immunosuppression and cytokine and hormone production needs greater elucidation.

Mind-body interventions can elicit a relaxation response that may prevent or aid in the treatment of a number of medical ailments[42] [*see Figure 1*]. A number of modalities can be used for this purpose. Many people have incorporated yoga, meditation, or self-hypnosis into their daily self-care regimen. Several clinical studies have suggested that there are positive results from mind-body modalities for many conditions [*see Table 3*]. As with other CAM interventions, however, limitations in study methodology and sample size, as well as lack of an adequate control, make definitive conclusions difficult.

The mind-body category also encompasses techniques for which a mechanism is not even remotely understood. No physical explanation for distant healing modalities—such as intercessory prayer, spiritual healing, and mental healing—is currently accepted, despite some evidence for positive treatment effects.[43] No harmful effects are seen when most mind-body interventions are used as an adjunct to conventional care. However, there is

concern that patients might choose exclusive use of one or more of these methods in lieu of appropriate diagnosis and therapy.

BIOLOGIC-BASED THERAPIES

Biologic therapy is the most popular of all fields of CAM. Its popularity stems from its similarity to the process of using conventional medications. Some people consider biologics to be a possible quick fix for their ailments, without the need for physician visits or potentially harmful prescription medications. Others turn to biologics in the hope of preventing potentially serious diseases through the use of so-called natural substances.

Dietary supplements, including herbal and nonherbal products, make up the preponderance of medications in this category. The supplement industry has become a billion-dollar business, largely as a result of the loosening of federal regulations. The Dietary Supplement Health and Education Act (DSHEA) of 1994 expanded the definition of dietary supplements to include vitamins, amino acids, herbs, and other botanicals. Furthermore, under DSHEA, supplements no longer require premarket testing for safety and efficacy. Supplements are assumed to be safe unless proved otherwise by the FDA. Given the number and variety of products currently available, the FDA's ability to effectively regulate all products after they have been marketed is limited. An example of the regulatory process was the banning of products containing ephedra. The FDA first expressed concern over the herb in 1997, when it proposed limitations on its use. The General Accounting Office viewed these limitations as inappropriate, because of insufficient evidence proving harm. It took 7 years (and a few high-profile deaths) for the FDA to be able to effect a ban on ephedra.[44] Although most dietary supplements are well tolerated and are associated with few adverse effects, the potential for harm from the lack of regulation can be seen from examples of misidentification of plant species,[45] contamination with heavy metals, and addition of pharmaceutical agents.[46,47]

Overall, there is only limited evidence supporting the use of most dietary supplements. Most clinical trials have been small, nonrandomized, or unblinded. In general, physicians and patients should view herbs as medications. Physicians should advise patients to be wary of products for which grandiose claims are made, because misleading advertising is common.[48] The potential for significant toxicity and drug interactions does exist.

The list of currently used supplements is immense, and this chapter can touch on only the most popular [*see Tables 4 through 6*]. More comprehensive resources for dietary supplements (and other CAM modalities) are now available [*see Table 7*].

MANIPULATIVE AND BODY-BASED THERAPIES

Chiropractic

Many would argue that chiropractic medicine should not be considered alternative therapy. Patients, physicians, and insurance companies have all shown some degree of support for chiropractic care in recent years. Between 10% and 20% of the population have used chiropractors.[6] Health care insurance plans, including Medicare, cover many of the services performed during chiropractic visits. Most chiropractor visits are for musculoskeletal problems, including low back pain, neck pain, and extremity pain. However, a small proportion of patients currently seek out chiropractic care for a variety of other conditions, as well as general health concerns.[49] The tenets of chiropractic medicine place the spinal cord and nervous system at the center of a person's well-being. The nervous system is thought to control and influence all other bodily systems. Malalignments (subluxations) of the vertebrae are thought to cause or perpetuate disease. Once these subluxations are identified and corrected (via manipulation), the body uses its natural healing abilities to restore physiologic balance and health. Chiropractors typically look for spinal pain, asymmetry, impaired range of motion, or abnormalities in tone, texture, and temperature when evaluating patients.[50] Laboratory testing, including x-rays, electromyography (EMG), and ultrasonography, may be used to aid in diagnosis. Actual spinal manipulation is performed by direct or indirect delivery of thrusts to the spine. Frequently, the patient will experience a cracking noise. Some chiropractors may use adjunctive therapies, including massage, heat, and trigger-point injections.[50]

Chiropractic manipulation has been touted as treatment for a number of conditions, including hypertension, asthma, pelvic pain, and fibromyalgia. Very little data exist to support its use for these conditions.[51,52] Use of chiropractic therapy for neck pain and headaches is also weakly supported.[53,54] Much of the current use of chiropractic care stems from its utility in cases of low back pain. A number of controlled trials on chiropractic treatment for low back pain have been done, with conflicting results. A meta-analysis concluded that spinal manipulation appears to be more effective than sham therapy or treatments previously judged to be ineffective, but not to be superior to other standard treatments for acute or chronic low back pain, such as analgesics, physical therapy, or exercises.[55] Patient satisfaction also seems to be high with such therapy.[56]

Serious complications from lumbar spinal manipulation seem to be uncommon, although there are reports of cauda equina syndrome.[57] Many patients, however, experience mild to moderate side effects, including localized discomfort, headache, or tiredness. These reactions usually disappear within 24 hours.[58] Brain stem or cerebellar infarction, vertebral fracture, tracheal

Table 3   Selected Mind-Body Interventions

Modality	Description	Potential Applications	Comments
Aromatherapy	The use of essential oils (e.g., jasmine, chamomile, lavender) to enhance physical or psychological well-being; often combined with massage	Anxiety, agitation	Long-term efficacy data (independent of massage) are lacking[71]
Biofeedback	Voluntary control of physiologic processes—e.g., brainwaves, smooth muscle contraction, vasodilation—learned and reinforced with the aid of instrumentation (EEG, EMG, skin temperature/sweat monitors)	Asthma, ADHD, back pain, fibromyalgia, headache, hypertension, incontinence, neuromuscular disorders, Raynaud disease	Effective for fecal incontinence[72]; techniques utilized may vary between patients and practitioners; learning process can be slow, requiring multiple sessions with therapist and regular practice by patient
Guided imagery	Use of the imagination to positively stimulate the senses to bring about emotional and physiologic change	Chronic pain, perioperative management, headaches, nausea, posttraumatic stress disorder	Small studies suggest a positive impact on surgical and cancer treatment outcomes[73]
Hypnotherapy	The induction of a trancelike state to induce relaxation and susceptibility to positive suggestion; used as a diagnostic and therapeutic tool	Anesthesia, headache, irritable bowel syndrome, smoking cessation	Success of therapy may depend on patient susceptibility and attitude toward hypnosis; no conclusive data on most conditions
Intercessory prayer	Request to God (or other spiritual beings) for the benefit of others; can take place in the presence of the patient or at a distance	Cardiac disease, HIV infection, RA	Studies are conflicting and inconclusive[74]; mechanism is unclear
Meditation	Release of the mind from attachment to discursive thought, typically aided by focusing on the breath or a mantra	Anxiety, chronic pain, hypertension, substance abuse	Many types of meditation exist; large-scale studies are needed to prove the absolute impact of this simple intervention on health
Music therapy	Use of music to improve psychological, physical, cognitive, or social functioning	Anxiety, dementia, chronic pain, Parkinson disease	Treatment is guided by a trained music therapist; may have a short-term effect on anxiety and mood during treatments or procedures[75]
Writing therapy	Creative writing exercise about an emotionally traumatic event	General emotional health, asthma, RA, HIV infection	Short-term studies show positive response in asthma and RA[76,77]

ADHD—attention-deficit/hyperactivity disorder   EEG—electroencephalography   EMG—electromyography   RA—rheumatoid arthritis

Table 4 Commonly Used Herbal Dietary Supplements

Herb	Suggested Uses	Potential Toxicity	Potential Drug Interactions	Comments
Black cohosh (*Cimicifuga racemosa*)	Menopausal symptoms	Gastrointestinal discomfort	None known	Scant efficacy data, long-term safety unknown[78]
Chaste tree berries (*Vitex agnus-castus*)	Premenstrual syndrome, mastodynia	Pruritus	May have dopaminergic activity; therefore, avoid with use of dopamine-receptor antagonists (e.g., neuroleptics)	Small, short-term studies suggest efficacy[79]
Cranberry (*Vaccinium macrocarpon*)	Urinary tract infections	Nephrolithiasis (with cranberry concentrate tablets)[80]	Possible interaction with warfarin[81]	No clear role in treatment of UTIs; may be effective for prophylaxis[82]
Dong quai (*Angelica sinensis*)	Menopausal symptoms	Rash	Increased INR in patients taking warfarin	No clinical evidence of efficacy[78]
Echinacea (*E. purpurea, E. pallida, E. angustifolia*)	Upper respiratory infections	Hypersensitivity reactions	Theoretically, may antagonize the effect of immunosuppressive medications	Variations in plant species studied, part of plant used, and extraction methods make conclusions regarding efficacy difficult[83]
Ephedra (*E. sinica,* mahuang)	Asthma, congestion, weight loss	Hypertension, arrhythmia, myocardial infarction, stroke	Interaction with monoamine oxidase inhibitors and cardiac glycosides; potential for serious toxicity when combined with other stimulants	Banned by the FDA, effective April 2004, but still available internationally over the Internet
Evening primrose (*Oenothera biennis*)	Eczema, irritable bowel syndrome, mastalgia, premenstrual syndrome, rheumatoid arthritis	Nausea, vomiting, diarrhea, flatulence	Possible lowering of seizure threshold in patients taking antiepileptic medications[84]	Conflicting efficacy data for a number of conditions
Feverfew (*Tanacetum parthenium*)	Migraine prophylaxis	Hypersensitivity reactions	Theoretical risk of increased bleeding when combined with anticoagulants	No clear evidence to support efficacy[85]
Garlic (*Allium sativum*)	Cardiovascular protection	Gastrointestinal upset, bleeding	Theoretical risk of increased bleeding when combined with anticoagulants	Possible short-term improvement in cardiovascular risk factors, but impact on disease unknown; active ingredient unclear[86]
Ginger (*Zingiberis rhizoma*)	Nausea, motion sickness, dyspepsia	None known	Theoretical risk of increased bleeding when combined with anticoagulants	May be useful for nausea and vomiting of pregnancy[87]

(continued)

rupture, internal carotid artery dissection, and diaphragmatic paralysis are rare but have all been reported with cervical manipulation.[59] Given the lack of efficacy data and the risk (although small) of catastrophic adverse events, it is difficult to advocate routine use of this technique for treatment of neck or headache disorders. Physicians should also recognize potential contraindications to chiropractic therapy. Patients with coagulopathy, osteoporosis, rheumatoid arthritis, spinal neoplasms, or spinal infections should be advised against such treatments.[59]

Massage Therapy

A number of different types of massage are in practice today. Many therapists combine aspects of Swedish massage (stroking and kneading), shiatsu (pressure-point manipulation), and neuromuscular massage (total body, deeper therapy) to relieve stress, anxiety, and muscle tension, as well as improve circulation. Frequently, aromatic oils are employed to enhance the relaxation response. A number of small studies have suggested a potential beneficial effect of massage on fibromyalgia, headaches, and anxiety,[60] although the paucity of data precludes definitive conclusions. Massage therapy does seem to be effective for subacute and chronic back pain.[30] No significant adverse ef-

fects are seen with properly performed massage, although caution must be advised for patients with coagulation disorders.

Structural integration (rolfing) is a system of deep-tissue manipulation that involves stretching of the fascial planes. In this system, the fascia is thought to be the key supporting structure for bones and muscles. When injury or stress occurs, the fascia tends to become shorter and thicker. Manipulation of the fascia with fingers, thumbs, and elbows is supposed to relieve tension, restore structural integrity, and improve physiologic and psychological function. Limited data exist to support the efficacy of rolfing for any particular condition.

ENERGY THERAPIES

Many traditional cultures describe the physical body as existing within a field of energy. Such energy is called prana by Indians and qi by the Chinese; English terms include subtle energy, vital energy, and life energy. Many ancient and modern CAM techniques involve the manipulation of this energy or the transfer of additional energy into the patient's field in an effort to restore or maintain balance. Because the field extends beyond the body, energy therapies do not always involve physical contact between practitioner and patient. Further, the presumed connec-

Table 4 *(continued)*

Herb	Suggested Uses	Potential Toxicity	Potential Drug Interactions	Comments
Ginkgo biloba	Dementia, claudication, tinnitus	Gastrointestinal upset, headache, dizziness, bleeding, seizure	Theoretical risk of increased bleeding when combined with anticoagulants	May have modest effects on cognitive performance and functioning in patients with Alzheimer disease or multi-infarct dementia[88]; no evidence to support prevention of memory loss or dementia
Ginseng (*Panax* species; Asian ginseng, Korean ginseng, American ginseng)	Fatigue, diabetes	Generally considered safe; rare reports of hypertension, insomnia, headache, and mastalgia	May interact with monoamine oxidase inhibitors and warfarin (decreased prothrombin time)	Currently, little data to support its use[89]
Kava kava (*Piper methysticum*)	Anxiety	Rash, sedation, liver toxicity	May potentiate effects of benzodiazepines; best to avoid with other anxiolytics or alcohol because of risk of excess sedation	Studies suggest efficacy for short-term treatment of anxiety[90]; no data on addiction potential; banned in many European countries because of cases of hepatic failure
Kola nut (*Cola nitida*)	Fatigue	Irritability, insomnia	Caution when used with other stimulants	Contains caffeine
Milk thistle (*Silybum marianum*)	Chronic liver disease	Rare mild laxative effect, gastrointestinal upset	None known	Appears to be safe and well tolerated; efficacy data too limited to exclude a substantial benefit or harm[91]
Saw palmetto (*Serenoa repens*)	BPH	Mild gastrointestinal effects	None known	Short-term studies show improvement in symptoms[89,92]; no evidence for prevention of BPH or its complications, or prevention of prostate cancer
St. John's wort (*Hypericum perforatum*)	Depression, anxiety	Headache, insomnia, dizziness, gastrointestinal irritation	Can decrease levels of cyclosporine, digoxin, oral contraceptives, theophylline, and indinavir; serotonin syndrome can occur when combined with prescription SSRIs	May be effective for mild to moderate depression[89,93]
Valerian (*Valeriana officinalis*)	Insomnia	Headaches	Avoid use with benzodiazepines because of sedation	Efficacy data inconclusive[94]; theoretical risk of addiction with prolonged use

BPH—benign prostatic hyperplasia FDA—Food and Drug Administration INR—international normalized ratio SSRI—selective serotonin reuptake inhibitor UTI—urinary tract infection

tion of these individual fields with a universal field is believed to permit the use of some of these therapies at a distance.

Qigong

Qigong is a branch of traditional Chinese medicine designed to affect the flow of energy (qi) to preserve health. This system combines relaxation techniques with movement to achieve a meditative state designed to ensure mental and physical health. Tai chi (tai chi chuan) is a type of movement-oriented qigong that utilizes a sequence of slow, dancelike maneuvers to enhance the flow of qi through the body. In the course of a tai chi session, the person shifts body weight constantly from one foot to the other. Studies of tai chi in elderly persons have shown that long-term regular practice may improve balance, flexibility, and cardiovascular fitness and, possibly, decrease the risk of falls in older individuals.[61,62] Meditative qigong is accomplished without movement and is intended to establish inner harmony. Breathing exercises can also be part of qigong. They are designed to enhance circulation of qi and expel negative energy. Qigong has been used extensively in China for a number of conditions, including hypertension, anxiety, asthma, and nausea and vomiting.[63] Data to support use for any individual condition are lacking, despite historical successes. Although the principles of qigong seem simple, it involves a complex set of processes that are not clearly understood. Inappropriate training has reportedly been associated with physical and mental disturbances.[64]

Yoga

Yoga is an ancient Indian philosophical practice that uses postures or stretching exercises (asanas), breathing exercises (pranayama), and meditation to help unite the body and the mind. It was developed as a means of enlightenment through self-realization and self-mastery. Only recently, with its migration to the West, has yoga come to be seen as a means to heal illness or reduce anxiety. As with most CAM modalities, there are limited data for or against the use of yoga for particular conditions. Studies on the use of yoga in patients with carpal tunnel syndrome seem promising.[65] Yogic breathing exercises may have

Table 5 Commonly Used Nonherbal Dietary Supplements

Supplement	Common Uses	Potential Toxicity	Potential Drug Interactions	Comments
Coenzyme Q10	Heart failure, hypertension, angina, Parkinson disease	Nausea, heartburn, diarrhea	Decreased INR in patients on warfarin	Data inconclusive for treatment or prevention of cardiovascular disease[95]; early data promising for slowing the progression of Parkinson disease[96]
Glucosamine and chondroitin	OA	Hyperglycemia in diabetic patients	Theoretical risk of increased bleeding in patients taking chondroitin and anticoagulants	Current data suggest symptomatic improvement for OA of the hips and knees,[97] with a slowed progression of joint space narrowing[98]
Melatonin	Jet lag, insomnia	Fatigue, drowsiness, headache	Theoretical risk of bleeding in patients taking anticoagulants	Data suggest efficacy for jet lag[99]; no data on long-term use
SAMe (S-adenosylmethionine)	OA, depression, liver disease	Nausea, abdominal discomfort	Can lead to serotonin syndrome when used with tricyclic antidepressants	Early data promising[100]; poor oral bioavailability; very expensive; marketed doses are much lower than studied doses

INR—international normalized ratio   OA—osteoarthritis

some beneficial effect on the symptoms of asthma and may reduce bronchodilator use, but they do not decrease airway reactivity or improve lung function.[66]

Therapeutic Touch

Therapeutic touch is the use of the hands, without actual physical touching, to influence or direct life energy throughout the body in an effort to promote healing. Therapeutic touch was codeveloped by a nurse, Dolores Krieger,[67] and many of its practitioners are nurses who use the technique for hospital inpatients.

In a therapeutic-touch session, which generally lasts 20 to 30 minutes, the practitioner enters a meditative state (centering) and then assesses the patient's energy field. To do so, the practitioner holds his or her hands a few inches from the patient's body and moves from head to foot. Downward sweeping movements are then used to remove any blockages of energy and correct any energy-field imbalances. The practitioner then transfers energy to the patient's field and finishes the session by smoothing the field.

A number of small trials have suggested a positive effect of therapeutic touch on conditions such as osteoarthritis, tension headache, and anxiety.[43] However, most of these trials are quite small and suffer from methodologic weaknesses that make definitive conclusions difficult.[68] A critical evaluation of relevant trials concluded that the data did not support the hypothesis that therapeutic touch promoted wound healing.[69] More vigorous trials need to be performed to determine the true efficacy of this technique.

CAM and the Practicing Physician

The field of research in CAM is in its infancy. Current levels of evidence are insufficient to support or disprove a majority of CAM modalities. Despite these limitations, the public continues to embrace CAM therapies as alternatives or adjuncts to conventional care. Given that many patients currently do not inform their physician of their use of CAM, it is imperative that physicians take the lead in inquiring about such therapies. Open dialogue needs to be established to uncover the types of modalities being utilized, reasons for pursuing such therapy, and patient experiences. From there, a discussion of the current data on level of efficacy and toxicity can follow. Ultimately, primary care physicians may need to develop referral networks of trusted CAM practitioners who are open to reciprocal communication.

Table 6 Popular Uses for Common Dietary Supplements*

Use	Supplement
Anxiety	Kava kava, St. John's wort, valerian
Benign prostatic hyperplasia	Saw palmetto, *Pygeum africanum*
Claudication	*Ginkgo biloba*
Dementia	*Ginkgo biloba*, pyridoxine
Depression	SAMe, St. John's wort
Diabetes	Aloe vera, chromium picolinate, ginseng, *Gymnema sylvestre*
Fatigue	Ginseng, licorice root
Heart failure	Coenzyme Q10, hawthorn extract
Hypercholesterolemia	Fenugreek, garlic, guggulipid, red yeast rice
Hypertension	Coenzyme Q10, garlic
Insomnia	Melatonin, valerian
Irritable bowel syndrome	Acidophilus, aloe, evening primrose, peppermint oil
Jet lag	Melatonin
Liver disease	Milk thistle, SAMe
Menopausal symptoms	Black cohosh, dong quai, red clover, soy
Migraine prophylaxis	Butterbur root, feverfew, riboflavin
Nausea and vomiting	Ginger, pyridoxine
Osteoarthritis	Ginger, glucosamine and chondroitin, SAMe
Premenstrual syndrome	Calcium, chaste tree berries, evening primrose, pyridoxine
Tinnitus	*Ginkgo biloba*
Upper respiratory infections	Ascorbic acid, *Echinacea*
Urinary tract infections	Ascorbic acid, cranberry
Weight loss	Chitosan, chromium picolinate, *Garcinia cambogia*

*See Tables 4 and 5 for potential toxicity, drug interactions, and comments.

Table 7 Sources of Information on Complementary and Alternative Medicine

Medium	Listing	Description (Price)
Internet	Natural Medicine Comprehensive Database www.naturaldatabase.com	Monographs on a multitude of natural products ($92/year)
	Natural Standard www.naturalstandard.com	Monographs on a multitude of natural products and CAM modalities; grades the level of evidence currently available for each potential application ($99/year)
	Memorial Sloan Kettering Cancer Center Integrative Medicine www.mskcc.org/aboutherbs	Brief descriptions of popular herbs/supplements (free)
	National Center for Complementary and Alternative Medicine http://nccam.nih.gov/index.htm	Describes ongoing CAM research; contains links to governmental resources on popular modalities and supplements (free)
	United States Pharmacopeia (USP) www.usp.org	Dietary supplement verification program identifies ingredients and absence of contaminants of specific brands that undergo testing (free)
	ConsumerLab.com www.consumerlab.com	Tests individual supplements and reports on purity and accuracy of labeling ($24/year)
	National Cancer Institute PDQ Cancer Information Summaries: Complementary and Alternative Medicine www.cancer.gov/cancertopics/pdq/cam	Overviews of selected CAM products used in cancer treatment (free)
Print	Essentials of Complementary and Alternative Medicine. Jonas W, Levin J, Eds. Lippincott Williams & Wilkins, Philadelphia, 1999	Concise overview of popular CAM therapies
	Herbal Medicine: Expanded Commission E Monographs. Blumenthal M, Goldberg A, Brinckmann J, Eds. American Botanical Council, Austin, Texas, 2000	Expanded English translation of the German compendium on herbs
	Evidence-Based Herbal Medicine. Rotblatt R, Ziment I, Eds. Hanley & Belfus, Philadelphia, 2001	Pocket-sized handbook that contains a summary of clinical trials as well as a rating of efficacy, evidence, and safety levels of common herbs

These steps should serve to strengthen the physician-patient relationship while limiting the potential for adverse outcomes.

Specific emphasis should be placed on the role of dietary supplements, which pose a risk of significant toxicity and drug interactions. To ensure patient safety, the medication history should include specific questioning about what vitamins, herbs, or other supplements the person is taking. Unfortunately, supplements are often sold as combination products that are identified only by their catchy trade names. Patients should be encouraged to bring in all new medications and supplements at each visit. Depending on their side-effect profile or potential for drug interactions, certain supplements should be discontinued in the perioperative period.[70] Finally, any suspected adverse reactions or drug-supplement reactions should be reported to the FDA's MedWatch program at their web site (http://www.fda.gov/medwatch) or by calling them at 1-800-FDA-1088.

The authors have no commercial relationships with manufacturers of products or providers of services discussed in this chapter.

References

1. Barnes PM, Powell-Griner E, McFann K, et al: Complementary and alternative medicine use among adults: United States, 2002. Advance data from vital and health statistics; no 343. Hyattsville, Maryland: National Center for Health Statistics, 2004 http://www.cdc.gov/nchs/data/ad/ad343.pdf

2. Fisher P, Ward A: Medicine in Europe: complementary medicine in Europe. BMJ 309:107, 1994

3. Bausell RB, Lee WL, Berman BM: Demographic and health-related correlates of visits to complementary and alternative medical providers. Med Care 39:190, 2001

4. Population-based survey of complementary and alternative medicine usage, patient satisfaction, and physician involvement. South Carolina Complementary Medicine Program Baseline Research Team. South Med J 93:375, 2000

5. Eisenberg DM, Kessler RC, Foster C, et al: Unconventional medicine in the United States. N Engl J Med 328:246, 1993

6. Astin JA: Why patients use alternative medicine. JAMA 279:1548, 1998

7. Bernstein BJ, Grasso J: Prevalence of complementary and alternative medicine use in cancer patients. Oncology 15:1267, 2001

8. Sparber A, Wootton JC, Bauer L, et al: Use of complementary medicine by adult patients participating in HIV/AIDS clinical trials. J Altern Complement Med 6:415, 2000

9. Pioro-Boisset M, Esdaile JM, Fitzcharles MA: Alternative medicine use in fibromyalgia syndrome. Arthritis Care Res 9:13, 1996

10. Rawsthrone P, Shanahan F, Cronin NC, et al: An international survey of the use and attitudes regarding alternative medicine by patients with inflammatory bowel disease. Am J Gastroenterol 94:1298, 1999

11. Campion EW: Why unconventional medicine? N Engl J Med 328:282, 1993

12. Eisenberg DM, Kessler RC, Van Rompay MI, et al: Perceptions about complementary therapies relative to conventional therapies among adults who use both: results from a national survey. Ann Intern Med 135:344, 2001

13. Eisenberg DM, Davis RB, Ettner SL, et al: Trends in alternative medicine use in the United States, 1990–1997. JAMA 280:1569, 1998

14. Blendon RJ, DesRoches CM, Benson JM, et al: Americans' views on the use and regulation of dietary supplements. Arch Intern Med 161:805, 2001

15. Bloom BS, Retbi A, Dahan S, et al: Evaluation of randomized controlled trials on complementary and alternative medicine. Int J Technol Assess Health Care 16:13, 2000

16. Linde K, Jonas WB, Melchart D, et al: The methodological quality of randomized controlled trials of homeopathy, herbal medicines and acupuncture. Int J Epidemiol 30:526, 2001

17. Vickers A, Goyal N, Harland R, et al: Do certain countries produce only positive results? A systematic review of controlled trials. Control Clin Trials 19:159, 1998

18. Tang JL, Zhan SY, Ernst E: Review of randomized controlled trials of traditional Chinese medicine. BMJ 319:160, 1999

19. Melchart D, Linde K, Fischer P, et al: *Echinacea* for preventing and treating the common cold (review). Cochrane Database Syst Rev (2):CD000530, 2000

20. Lee JD, Chon JS, Jeong HK, et al: The cerebrovascular response to traditional acupuncture after stroke. Neuroradiology 45:780, 2003

21. Sandberg M, Lindberg LG, Gerdle B: Peripheral effects of needle stimulation (acupuncture) on skin and muscle blood flow in fibromyalgia. Eur J Pain 8:163, 2004

22. Han JS: Acupuncture and endorphins. Neurosci Lett 361:258, 2004

23. Acupuncture. NIH Consensus Statement 15(5):1, 1997

24. Linde K, Melchart D, Fischer P, et al: Acupuncture for idiopathic headache (review). Cochrane Database Syst Rev (1):CD001218, 2001

25. Berman BM, Ezzo J, Hadhazy V, et al: Is acupuncture effective in the treatment of fibromyalgia? J Fam Pract 48:213, 1999

26. Holdcraft LC, Assefi N, Buchwald D: Complementary and alternative medicine in fibromyalgia and related syndromes. Best Pract Res Clin Rheumatol 17:667, 2003

27. Ezzo J, Hadhazy V, Birch S, et al: Acupuncture for osteoarthritis of the knee: a systematic review. Arthritis Rheum 44:819, 2001

28. White AR, Rampes H, Ernst E: Acupuncture for smoking cessation (review). Cochrane Database Syst Rev (2):CD000009, 2000

29. McCarney RW, Brinkhaus B, Lasserson TJ, et al: Acupuncture for chronic asthma. Cochrane Database Syst Rev (1):CD000008, 2004

30. Cherkin DC, Sherman KJ, Deyo RA, et al: A review of the evidence for the effectiveness, safety, and cost of acupuncture, massage therapy, and spinal manipulation for back pain. Ann Intern Med 138:898, 2003

31. Lao L, Hamilton GR, Fu J, et al: Is acupuncture safe? A systematic review of case reports. Altern Ther Health Med 9:72, 2003

32. Ernst E, White A: Life-threatening adverse reactions after acupuncture? A systematic review. Pain 71:123, 1997

33. Yamashita H, Tsukayama H, Tanno Y, et al: Adverse events related to acupuncture. JAMA 280:1563, 1998

34. Ernst E, White AR: Prospective studies of the safety of acupuncture: a systematic review. Am J Med 110:481, 2001

35. Chapman EH: Homeopathy. Essentials of Complementary and Alternative Medicine. Jonas W, Levin JS, Eds. Lippincott Williams & Wilkins, Philadelphia, 1999, p 472

36. Kleijnen J, Knipschild P, ter Riet G: Clinical trials of homeopathy. BMJ 302:316, 1991

37. Linde K, Clausius N, Ramirez G, et al: Are the clinical effects of homoeopathy placebo effects? A meta-analysis of placebo-controlled trials. Lancet 350:834, 1997

38. Jonas WB, Kaptchuk TJ, Linde K: A critical overview of homeopathy. Ann Intern Med 139:393, 2003

39. Ernst E: A systematic review of systematic reviews of homeopathy. Br J Clin Pharmacol 54:577, 2002

40. Stehlin I: Homeopathy: real medicine or empty promises? FDA Consumer 30, 1996 http://www.fda.gov/fdac/features096_home.html

41. Cannon WB: The emergency function of the adrenal medulla in pain and the major emotions. Am J Physiol 33:356, 1914

42. Benson H: The Relaxation Response. William Morrow, New York, 1975

43. Astin JA, Harkness E, Ernst E: The efficacy of "distant healing": a systematic review of randomized trials. Ann Intern Med 132:903, 2000

44. Rados C: Ephedra ban: no shortage of reasons. FDA Consum 38:6, 2004

45. Nortier JL, Martinez MC, Schmeiser HH, et al: Urothelial carcinoma associated with the use of a Chinese herb (Aristolochia fangchi). N Engl J Med 342:1686, 2000

46. Ko RJ: Adulterants in Asian patent medicines. N Engl J Med 339:847, 1998

47. Fugh-Berman A: Herb-drug interactions. Lancet 355:134, 2000

48. Ashar BH, Miller RG, Getz KJ, et al: A critical evaluation of Internet marketing of products containing ephedra. Mayo Clin Proc 78:944, 2003

49. Meeker WC, Haldeman S: Chiropractic: a profession at the crossroads of mainstream and alternative medicine. Ann Intern Med 136:216, 2002

50. Lawrence DJ: Chiropractic medicine. Essentials of Alternative and Complementary Medicine. Jonas WB, Levin JS, Eds. Lippincott Williams & Wilkins, Philadelphia, 1999, p 275

51. Hondras MA, Linde K, Jones AP: Manual therapy for asthma. Cochrane Database Syst Rev (4):CD001002, 2002

52. Ernst E: Chiropractic manipulation for non-spinal pain: a systematic review. N Z Med J 116:U539, 2003

53. Ernst E: Chiropractic spinal manipulation for neck pain: a systematic review. J Pain 4:417, 2003

54. Astin JA, Ernst E: The effectiveness of spinal manipulation for the treatment of headache disorders: a systematic review of randomized clinical trials. Cephalgia 22:617, 2002

55. Assendelft WJ, Morton SC, Yu EI, et al: Spinal manipulative therapy for low back pain: a meta-analysis of effectiveness relative to other therapies. Ann Intern Med 138:871, 2003

56. Cherkin DC, Deyo RA, Battie M, et al: A comparison of physical therapy, chiropractic manipulation, and provision of an educational booklet for the treatment of patients with low back pain. N Engl J Med 339:1021, 1998

57. Kaptchuk TJ, Eisenberg DM: Chiropractic: origins, controversies, and contributions. Arch Intern Med 158:2215, 1998

58. Senstad O, Leboeuf-Yde C, Borchgrevink C: Frequency and characteristics of side effects of spinal manipulative therapy. Spine 22:435, 1997

59. Ernst E: Adverse effects of spinal manipulation. Essentials of Complementary and Alternative Medicine. Jonas WB, Levin JS, Eds. Lippincott Williams & Wilkins, Philadelphia, 1999, p 176

60. Field T: Massage therapy. Med Clin North Am 86:163, 2002

61. Lee CT, Lei T: Qigong. Essentials of Complementary and Alternative Medicine. Jonas W, Levin JS, Eds. Lippincott Williams & Wilkins, Philadelphia, 1999, p 392

62. Ng BY: Qigong-induced mental disorders. Aust N Z J Psychiatry 33:197, 1999

63. O'Connor D. Marshall S, Massy-Westropp N: Non-surgical treatment (other than steroid injection) for carpal tunnel syndrome. Cochrane Database Syst Rev (1):CD003219, 2003

64. Cooper S, Oborne J, Newton S, et al: Effect of two breathing exercises (Buteyko and pranayama) in asthma: a randomised controlled trial. Thorax 68:674, 2003

65. Wang C, Collet JP, Lau J: The effect of Tai Chi on health outcomes in patients with chronic conditions: a systematic review. Arch Intern Med 164:493, 2004

66. Wolf SL, Sattin RW, Kutner M, et al: Intense Tai Chi training and fall occurrences in older, transitionally frail adults: a randomized, controlled trial. J Am Geriatr Soc 51:1693, 2003

67. Krieger D: Accepting Your Power to Heal: The Personal Practice of Therapeutic Touch. Bear & Company, Rochester, Vermont, 1993

68. O'Mathuna: Evidence-based practice and reviews of therapeutic touch. J Nurs Scholarsh 32:279, 2000

69. O'Mathuna DP, Ashford RL: Therapeutic touch for healing acute wounds. Cochrane Database Syst Rev (4):CD002766, 2003

70. Ang-Lee MK, Moss J, Yuan CS: Herbal medicines and perioperative care. JAMA 286:208, 2001

71. Cooke B, Ernst E: Aromatherapy: a systematic review. Br J Gen Pract 50:493, 2000

72. Hinninghofen H, Enck P: Fecal incontinence: evaluation and treatment. Gastroenterol Clin North Am 32:685, 2003

73. Barrows KA, Jacobs BP: Mind-body medicine: an introduction and review of the literature. Med Clin North Am 86:11, 2002

74. Roberts L, Ahmed I, Hall S: Intercessory prayer for the alleviation of ill health. Cochrane Database Syst Rev (2):CD000368, 2000

75. Cassileth BR, Vickers AJ, Magill LA: Music therapy for mood disturbance during hospitalization for autologous stem cell transplantation: a randomized controlled trial. Cancer 98:2723, 2003

76. Smyth JM, Stone AA, Hurewitz A, et al: Effects of writing about stressful experiences on symptom reduction in patients with asthma or rheumatoid arthritis. JAMA 281:1304, 1999

77. Petrie KJ, Fontanilla I, Thomas MG, et al: Effect of written emotional expression on immune function in patients with human immunodeficiency virus infection: a randomized trial. Psychosom Med 66:272, 2004

78. Kronenberg F, Fugh-Berman A: Complementary and alternative medicine for menopausal symptoms: a review of randomized, controlled trials. Ann Intern Med 137:805, 2002

79. Fugh-Berman A, Kronenberg F: Complementary and alternative medicine in reproductive-age women: a review of randomized controlled trials. Reprod Toxicol 17:137, 2003

80. Terris MK, Issa MM, Tacker JR: Dietary supplementation with cranberry concentrate tablets may increase the risk of nephrolithiasis. Urology 57:26, 2001

81. Suvarna R, Pirmohamed M, Henderson L: Possible interaction between warfarin and cranberry juice. BMJ 327:1454, 2003

82. Jepson RG, Mihaljevic L, Craig J: Cranberries for preventing urinary tract infections (review.) Cochrane Database Syst Rev (4):CD001321, 2004

83. Melchart D, Linde K, Fischer P, et al: Echinacea for preventing and treating the common cold. Cochrane Database Syst Rev (2):CD000530, 2000

84. Miller LG: Herbal medicinals: selected clinical considerations focusing on known or potential drug-herb interactions. Arch Intern Med 158:2200, 1998

85. Pittler MH, Ernst E: Feverfew for preventing migraine. Cochrane Database Syst Rev (1):CD002286, 2004

86. Ackermann RT, Mulrow CD, Ramirez G, et al: Garlic shows promise for improving some cardiovascular risk factors. Arch Intern Med 161:813, 2001

87. Vutyavanich T, Draisarin T, Ruangsri R: Ginger for nausea and vomiting in pregnancy: randomized, double-masked, placebo-controlled trial. Obstet Gynecol 97:577, 2001

88. LeBars PL, Katz MM, Berman N, et al: A placebo-controlled, double-blind, randomized trial of an extract of Ginkgo biloba for dementia. JAMA 278:1327, 1997

89. Ernst E: The risk-benefit profile of commonly used herbal therapies: ginkgo, St. John's wort, ginseng, Echinacea, saw palmetto, and kava. Ann Intern Med 136:42, 2002

90. Pittler MH, Ernst E: Kava extract for treating anxiety. Cochrane Database Syst Rev (1):CD003383, 2003

91. Jacobs BP, Dennehy C, Ramirez G, et al: Milk thistle for the treatment of liver disease: a systematic review and meta-analysis. Am J Med 113:506, 2002

92. Wilt TJ, Ishani A, Stark G, et al: Saw palmetto extracts for the treatment of benign prostatic hyperplasia: a systematic review. JAMA 280:1604, 1999

93. Gaster B, Holroyd J: St John's wort for depression: a systematic review. Arch Intern Med 160:152, 2000

94. Stevinson C, Ernst E: Valerian for insomnia: a systematic review of randomized clinical trials. Sleep Med 1:91, 2000

95. Shekelle P, Morton SC, Hardy M, et al: Effect of supplemental antioxidants vitamin C, vitamin E, and coenzyme Q10 for the prevention and treatment of cardiovascular disease. Evid Rep Technol Assess June (83):1, 2003

96. Shults CW, Oakes D, Kieburtz K, et al: Effects of coenzyme Q10 in early Parkinson disease: evidence of slowing of the functional decline. Arch Neurol 59:1541, 2002

97. McAlindon TE, LaValley MP, Gulin JP, et al: Glucosamine and chondroitin for treatment of osteoarthritis. JAMA 283:1469, 2000

98. Richy F, Bruyere O, Ethgen O, et al: Structural and symptomatic efficacy of glucosamine and chondroitin in knee osteoarthritis: a comprehensive meta-analysis. Arch Intern Med 163:1514, 2003

99. Herxheimer A, Petrie KJ: Melatonin for the prevention and treatment of jet lag. Cochrane Database Syst Rev (2):CD001520, 2002

100. Hardy M, Coulter I, Morton SC, et al: S-adenosyl-L-methionine for treatment of depression, osteoarthritis, and liver disease. Evidence Report/Technology Assessment no. 64. AHRQ publication no. 02-E034, 2002

10 Palliative Medicine

Cynthia X. Pan, M.D.

One unanticipated result of the advances in health care during the past century has been the emergence of chronic illness as the leading cause of death [*see Table 1*]. At the same time, the enhanced ability to significantly extend life for patients with chronic diseases has blurred the boundary between curable illnesses and illnesses that inevitably result in death. As a result, over the course of the 20th century, Western society increasingly attributed near-miraculous powers to medical science—and increasingly avoided the subject of death. Many patients and physicians came to regard the prolongation of life and the cure of disease as the fundamental and exclusive goals of modern medicine. Viewed from this perspective, death is a medical failure.

Recent decades, however, have seen a growing recognition that this view is unrealistic and potentially harmful. This recognition has supported the emergence of the field of palliative care. Unlike curative care, which focuses on the disease process, palliative care focuses on the patient, striving to minimize the patient's burden and maximize the patient's quality of life. A distinguishing feature of palliative care is that it openly acknowledges dying as part of living and does not consider death an enemy.[1]

This chapter describes the general concepts of palliative care, reviews the clinical skills needed to provide competent palliative care to patients who are chronically ill or near the end of life, and discusses some of the challenging legal and ethical issues often encountered in palliative and terminal care.

History and Rationale

Palliative medicine was first recognized as a medical specialty in Great Britain in 1987. This discipline grew out of the hospice care movement, a special interdisciplinary system of comprehensive care for the dying and for their families.[1] Over time, the palliative care model has been extended. It now applies not only to patients who are clearly at the end of life but also to those with chronic illnesses that, although not imminently fatal, cause significant impairment in function, quality of life, and in-

Table 1 Leading Causes of Death in the United States: 2000[46]

Rank	Condition	Percent of Total Deaths
1	Heart disease	29.6
2	Malignant neoplasm	23.0
3	Cerebrovascular diseases	7.0
4	Chronic lower respiratory tract diseases	5.1
5	Accidents	4.1
6	Diabetes mellitus	2.9
7	Influenza and pneumonia	2.7

Note: These conditions account for approximately 75% of all deaths.

dependence. Palliative medicine for patients with serious illness thus should no longer be seen as the alternative to traditional life-prolonging care. Instead, it should be viewed as part of an integrated approach to medical care. Palliative care is not characterized by less care or by withdrawal of care. On the contrary, palliative care may involve intensive and highly sophisticated medical interventions, albeit ones intended to relieve suffering or improve quality of life.

Settings for Delivery of Palliative Care

Palliative care may be delivered in a variety of settings, including a hospital, nursing home, hospice, or private home. In some cases, the level of care required will dictate the choice of setting. For the most part, however, palliative care depends more on the attitude of the clinician than on the setting.

HOSPITALS

Increasing numbers of hospital-based palliative care programs have been developed in recent years to meet the needs of people who are chronically and critically ill and eventually die in hospitals.[2] A national Center to Advance Palliative Care has been created to provide technical support and resources for hospitals that want to establish such programs [*see Sidebar* Palliative Care Information and Resources on the Internet].

HOSPICE

Hospice is one way to deliver palliative care [*see Table 2*]. Hospice care traditionally has been characterized as low tech, high touch. Hospice provides home nursing, support for the family, spiritual counseling, pain treatment, medications for the illness that prompted the referral, medical care, and some inpatient care. The National Hospice and Palliative Care Organization (NHPCO) estimates that in the United States, hospices admitted 775,000 patients in 2001 (compared with approximately 340,000 persons in 1994) and that, in 2000, one in four persons who died of all causes were receiving hospice care at the time of death.[3]

Palliative care and hospice share similar philosophies, and both are delivered by an interdisciplinary team of health care professionals. Palliative care differs from hospice care in that palliative care can be provided at any time during an illness and in a variety of settings, may be combined with curative treatments, and is independent of the third-party payer. In the United States, hospice is paid through the Medicare Hospice Benefit. Medicare requires that recipients spend 80% of hospice care days at home, which means that to qualify for hospice, the patient must have a home and have caregivers (e.g., family members) capable of providing care. In addition, primarily for financial reasons, Medicare requires that recipients have an estimated survival of 6 months or less and that their care be focused on comfort rather than cure.[4] These eligibility rules were created at a time when hospice programs principally served patients with cancer or AIDS, in which the trajectory of dying is relatively predictable; in 1994, for example, 80% of hospice patients had cancer, and the average patient enrolled about 1 month before death.[5] Because hospice increasingly serves pa-

Palliative Care Information and Resources on the Internet

American Academy of Hospice and Palliative Medicine (AAHPM)

http://www.aahpm.org

Organization for physicians dedicated to the advancement of hospice/palliative medicine.

Americans for Better Care of the Dying (ABCD)

http://www.abcd-caring.org

Nonprofit public charity dedicated to social, professional, and policy reform aimed to improve the care system for patients with serious illness and their families.

Center to Advance Palliative Care (CAPC)

http://www.capcmssm.org

For hospitals and health systems interested in developing palliative care programs.

Death and Dying: MEDLINEplus

http://www.nlm.nih.gov/medlineplus/endoflifeissues.html

Links from the U.S. National Library of Medicine and the National Institutes of Health.

Education for Physicians on End-of-life Care (EPEC)

http://www.epec.net

Provides a core curriculum for physicians on the basic knowledge and skills needed to appropriately care for dying patients.

End of Life/Palliative Education Resource Center (EPERC)

http://www.eperc.mcw.edu

Identifies and disseminates information on end-of-life care education and training materials, publications, conferences, and other resources.

End-of-life Nursing Education Consortium (ELNEC) Project

http://www.aacn.nche.edu/elnec

Provides a comprehensive national education program to develop a core of expert nursing educators and to coordinate national nursing efforts in end-of-life care.

Growth House

http://www.growthhouse.org

Gateway to international resources for life-threatening illness and end-of-life care; intended to improve the quality of care for dying people through public education and global professional collaboration; includes links and search engine on reviewed resources for end-of-life care.

National Hospice and Palliative Care Organization (NHPCO)

http://www.nhpco.org

Nonprofit membership organization representing hospice and palliative care programs and professionals in the United States. Offers information in Spanish and English on local hospice and palliative care programs across the country. Toll-free telephone number: 800-658-8898.

Project on Death in America (PDIA)

http://www.soros.org/death

Strives to increase understanding and transform the culture and experience of dying and bereavement through initiatives in research, scholarship, the humanities, and the arts, and to foster innovations in the provision of care, public education, professional education, and public policy.

governing the coordination of palliative care in nursing homes vary according to reimbursement venues and availability of trained staff. Many nursing homes coordinate palliative care through local hospices, taking advantage of the skilled hospice nurses and other health care professionals.

Demographics of Death and Dying in the United States

Most people in the United States can now expect to die in old age. Of the over 2 million deaths per year in the United States, 73% occur in persons 65 years of age or older: 49% in persons 65 to 84 years of age, and 24% in persons 85 years of age or older. In 2001, the estimated life expectancy at birth reached 77.2 years, compared with less than 50 years in 1900.[10]

The median age of death in the United States is 77 years of age; of persons who survive to 65 years of age, median age at death is 84 years for women and 80 years for men.[11] Persons 65 years of age or older constitute an increasingly large number and proportion of the United States population, and those persons 85 years of age or older constitute the most rapidly growing segment. In 1999, persons 65 years of age or older accounted for about 13% of the population; this proportion is projected to rise to 20% by the year 2030.[12]

The elderly population is extremely heterogeneous, varying in socioeconomic status, educational level, and cultural and ethnic background. This diversity is likely to increase in the coming years. For example, African Americans 65 years of age and older numbered 2.5 million in 1990 (constituting 8% of the population of persons older than 65 years), and their number is expected to more than triple, to 8.4 million (or 10.5% of that population) by 2030. Similarly, there were approximately 1.1 million Hispanic elderly persons in 1990 (3.5% of the population of persons older than 65 years), but by 2030 this number will skyrocket to 12.5 million (15.6% of that group).[12]

Compared with the current elderly population, elderly baby boomers will be far more knowledgeable about health care and far more demanding of health care providers. Their expectations are likely to lead them to challenge the health care profession to deliver high quality end-of-life care tailored to patients' individual need and to provide that care in a culturally sensitive manner.

Although most deaths occur in the elderly, people can become critically ill at any point in their lives and can die at any age. In fact, the persons whose cases were the basis for establishing important precedents for ethical and legal decisions related to death and dying were young adults: 26-year-old Nancy Cruzan,[13] whose case involved the issue of artificial feeding of patients in a persistent vegetative state; and 21-year-old Karen Ann Quinlan,[14] whose case involved the withdrawal of artificial ventilation from patients in a persistent vegetative state.

LEADING CAUSES AND SETTINGS OF DEATH

The three leading causes of death in adults in the United States in 2001 were heart disease, malignant neoplasm, and stroke.[10] Chronic obstructive pulmonary disease (COPD), pneumonia, and accidents each accounted for less than 10% of all deaths. Most adult deaths in the United States occur in hospitals (56%), followed sequentially by deaths occurring at home (21%), in nursing homes (19%), and in other settings (4%).[15] These statistics vary substantially according to geographic site, primarily because of regional variations in hospital, hospice, and nursing home bed supply.

tients with chronic conditions in which prognostication remains inaccurate, these eligibility rules now limit access to care.[6,7] Asking patients and families to choose between curative care and palliative care is difficult for all concerned and is inconsistent with the current model of care, which views palliative care on a continuum with life-prolonging therapy [see Figure 1].[8] Also, this either/or situation contributes to late referrals and underutilization of hospice services.[9]

Palliative care can be provided in nursing homes, and increasing numbers of nursing homes strive to do so. Policies

Table 2 Comparison of Hospice and Palliative Care

Feature	Hospice	Palliative Care
Initiation	Prognosis of < 6 mo survival	Any time during illness
Clinical focus	Comfort care; no curative care	May involve both comfort care and curative care
Third-party payment	Medicare hospice benefit	Independent of payer
Personnel	Volunteers integral and required	Health care professionals
Setting	> 90% provided at home; inpatient hospice for acute deterioration, very short life expectancy (e.g., < 2 wk), or high symptom burden	Anywhere (hospital, home, nursing home)
Do not resuscitate (DNR) orders	Not required	Not required

Prognosis and Palliative Care

Traditionally, palliative care has been narrowly conceptualized as an alternative to standard life-prolonging therapy and has been provided to patients whose disease no longer responds to curative treatment. Although this model may be appropriate for patients dying of metastatic cancer, in which prognosis is relatively predictable and response to treatment is typically well defined, fewer than a quarter of persons in the United States die of cancer; the majority die of chronic diseases (e.g., heart disease) in which the prognosis is often uncertain, functional decline is nonlinear, and life-prolonging therapies coexist with or are identical to therapies directed at palliation and comfort (e.g., diuresis for fluid overload in heart failure).

One of the barriers to initiating palliative care is the uncertainty of predicting prognosis in these complex, chronic medical illnesses. For example, timing of death in heart failure is far less predictable than in many other fatal disorders. A patient dying of colon cancer usually has a long period of functional stability, then several months of progressive functional decline and weight loss just before death. In contrast, most heart failure patients experience a lengthy decline in daily function, with periodic bouts of severe symptoms and disability and multiple hospital admissions for exacerbation and for adjustment of therapy. Death may occur during a severe exacerbation but often occurs suddenly and relatively unpredictably from cardiac arrhythmia [*see Figure 2*]. In the SUPPORT project (Study to Un-

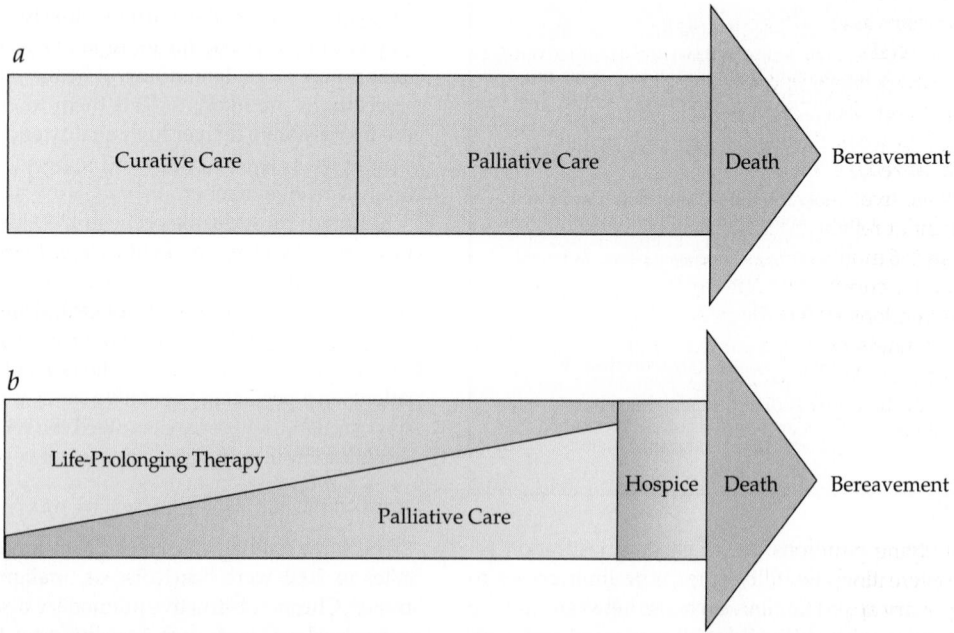

Figure 1 (*a*) Formerly, curative care and palliative care were viewed as mutually exclusive; when death became inevitable, curative care was abandoned and palliative care begun. This model of care is now outdated, because prognosis is so difficult to determine. (*b*) The current model views palliative care on a continuum with life-prolonging therapy, with palliative care assuming increasing importance as the patient's illness progresses and curative options are exhausted. Also, many chronic and life-threatening illnesses have no cures; the goals of treatment are to contain the illness and maintain an acceptable level of function and quality of life.

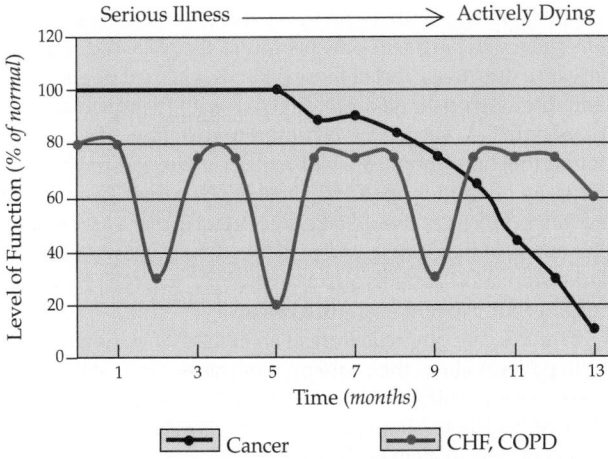

Serious Illness ————————➔ Actively Dying

Figure 2 **Prognosis is relatively predictable in metastatic cancer; these patients typically have a long period of functional stability, then several months of progressive functional decline and weight loss just before death. In contrast, prognosis can be difficult to predict in diseases such as chronic heart failure (CHF), chronic obstructive pulmonary disease (COPD), and Alzheimer disease; these patients typically experience a lengthy decline in daily function, with periodic bouts of severe symptoms and disability and multiple hospital admissions for exacerbation and for adjustment of therapy. Death may occur during a severe exacerbation, but—especially in CHF—often occurs suddenly and relatively unpredictably from cardiac arrhythmia.**

derstand Prognoses and Preferences for Outcomes and Risks of Treatments),[16] heart failure patients were given surprisingly long prognoses even up to the day before death. The median prognosis on the day before death was a 50% chance of living 2 months.[17] Dementia is another condition that often progresses over years rather than months.

To help clinicians assess prognosis in various nonneoplastic conditions, the NHPCO has compiled guidelines describing factors associated with poor prognosis; these guidelines can promote discussion about preferences for care and advance care planning.[18] However, SUPPORT data indicate that for seriously ill, hospitalized patients with advanced COPD, heart failure, or end-stage liver disease, recommended clinical-prediction criteria cannot reliably identify those patients whose survival prognosis is 6 months or less.[19] Because it is not possible to consistently and accurately predict the timing of death, palliative care interventions should be incorporated early in a patient's course of illness, even in the face of substantial uncertainty about prognosis. As disease progresses, the goals of care should change accordingly, with the balance shifting from curative to palliative.

Clinical Skills

Caring for dying patients and for those who suffer from chronic and severe illnesses with uncertain prognoses requires an interdisciplinary approach and specific clinical skills. In particular, the clinician who provides palliative care must be competent in clinical communication, management of symptoms (physical, emotional, and psychological), and planning for continuity of care.

COMMUNICATION

The ability to communicate well with both patient and fami-

ly is paramount in palliative care. In the beginning, it enables the physician to deliver bad news, assess the patient's and the family's knowledge and understanding of the disease process, determine the factors that they consider important to quality of life, and discuss goals and preferences for future care. As the illness progresses, regular communication about the course of illness and the patient's needs and expectations enables the physician to provide the most appropriate care for the patient and support for the family. Communication continues to be important after the patient's death, because the period of bereavement poses major challenges and increased risks of medical illness and psychiatric illness for family members.[1]

Patients whose cultural background and language differ from that of the physician present special challenges and rewards and need to be approached in a culturally sensitive manner [*see* Accounting for Cultural Differences, *below*]. Physicians also need to communicate effectively with colleagues and interdisciplinary team members to achieve optimal care for their patients. Communication in palliative care is discussed in detail elsewhere [*see Chapter 12*].

SYMPTOM MANAGEMENT

Symptom management in palliative care encompasses the assessment and treatment not only of physical symptoms but of emotional and psychological symptoms as well. Physical symptoms that can contribute to discomfort, disability, and dependence include pain, dyspnea, constipation, nausea and vomiting, delirium, fatigue, and anorexia. Emotional and psychological symptoms include depression, anxiety, delirium, cognitive impairment, fear, and agitation or sedation, as well as spiritual and existential angst.

Pain is the most common symptom of terminal illness, reported by 84% of patients with cancer and 67% of patients dying of other causes.[11] Surprisingly, the leading cause of physical distress in patients dying of heart failure is also pain, followed by fatigue and shortness of breath. Other common symptoms reported by dying patients include trouble with breathing (49%), nausea and vomiting (33%), sleeplessness (40%), depression (36%), loss of appetite (47%), and constipation (36%). Apart from illness, symptoms that become more prevalent with increasing age include mental confusion, loss of bladder and bowel control, difficulty seeing and hearing, and dizziness.

At present, the identification and management of many symptoms, including pain, remain suboptimal. Undertreatment of symptoms is common in elderly patients whether they have cancer[20] or other chronic conditions, whether they reside in long-term care settings (45% to 80% prevalence)[21,22] or in the community, and whether they are white or are members of minority groups.[20,23] Undertreatment of pain in the elderly may be more common in patients who are women, are members of minority groups, or have mild to moderate cognitive impairment.[24] Clinicians may contribute to undertreatment of pain through lack of proper pain-assessment procedures, misconceptions regarding both the efficacy of nonpharmacologic pain-management strategies and the attitudes of the elderly toward such treatments,[25] and legitimate concerns about drug interactions and side effects.

Education and involvement of the patient and family as partners in care are key to the successful management of symptoms. Specific strategies for symptom management include both pharmacologic and nonpharmacologic measures. These strategies are discussed in detail elsewhere [*see Chapters 11 and 175*].

ACCOUNTING FOR CULTURAL DIFFERENCES

The United States is a culturally heterogeneous country. Culture can broadly include race and ethnicity, as well as country of origin, religion, spirituality, and profession.[26] Medicine has its culture as well, with its attendant values, beliefs, behaviors, and language. Thus, in some cases, patients may be encountering two unfamiliar cultures: that of the United States mainstream and that of Western medicine.

Cultural traits may have a far-reaching impact on a patient's views on illness, preferences, and ultimate decisions.[27] Compared with patients from mainstream United States culture (most of whom are whites of European descent), people from other cultural backgrounds may be less willing to discuss resuscitation status,[27] less likely to forgo life-sustaining treatment,[27-29] and more reluctant to complete advance directives.[30]

Although many individual variations exist, some frequently encountered examples of cultural differences include the following:

(1) Hindus traditionally respect the doctor's medical opinion and may request the physician, rather than a family member, be appointed as health care proxy. They may prefer to die at home, preferably on the floor near the earth. After death, the relatives may want to wash the body themselves and dress it in new clothes. Autopsy is not forbidden but is considered distasteful, and cremation is usual.

(2) Traditional Chinese (and some other Asian) families usually will ask the clinician not to inform the patient about a terminal diagnosis (especially cancer) for fear that the patient will lose hope and die. In these cultures, the patient ideally will be informed after a period of adjustment. Decision-making is often entrusted to the eldest child, usually a son. Patients may seek traditional therapies, such as acupuncture and herbal medicine, often in conjunction with allopathic care.

(3) African Americans may decline participation in research studies, because of their long history of abuse as experimental subjects in research. Because of their history of receiving inappropriate undertreatment, they may continue to request aggressive care, even in terminal illness.[31]

With patients who do not speak English, it is extremely helpful to have access to a trained interpreter who can provide an objective translation and shift the translation burden from family members. This can prevent awkward and inappropriate situations, such as having to ask a male teenager to interpret for his mother who has cervical cancer. Translators may also be able to provide valuable information about patients' cultural attitudes and expectations.

Although it is important to learn about and respect different cultural practices, it is even more important not to stereotype or assume that membership in a group determines preferences. Instead, the physician should treat each patient as an individual. When in doubt, ask: "I have had patients from your cultural group who told me…. Does this apply to you?" Or, "I don't know much about medical practices or beliefs in your culture; can you tell me more about this?"

Advance Directives

Public opinion polls have revealed that close to 90% of adults in the United States would not want to be maintained on life-support systems without prospect of recovery. Yet a survey of emergency department patients found that 77% did not have advance directives, and of those patients who had one, only 5% had discussed their advance directive with their primary care physician.[32] A survey of community-dwelling older adults found that only about 16% had written advance directives.[33] In a survey of adult outpatients, most felt that discussions about advance directives should take place at an earlier age, earlier in the course of the disease, and earlier in the patient-physician relationship; most subjects also agreed that it was the physician's responsibility to initiate the discussion.[34]

Primary care physicians are in an excellent position to speak with patients about their care preferences because of the therapeutic relationship that already exists between patient and doctor. Conversations about preferences of care should be a routine aspect of care, even in healthy older patients. Determination of the patient's preferences can be made over two or three visits and then updated on a regular basis (e.g., annually). Reevaluation is indicated if the patient's condition changes acutely. In general, it is preferable that a close family member or friend accompany the patient during these discussions, so that these care preferences can be witnessed and any potential surprises or conflicts can be explored with the family.

Such discussions have particular urgency in patients who are showing early signs of cognitive impairment, because advancing impairment may render these discussions impossible. In older persons with existing cognitive impairment, it is important to assess both their current degree of decision-making capacity and any evidence, written or verbal, of previously stated preferences.

Decision-making capacity refers to the capacity to provide informed consent to treatment. This is different from competence, which is a legal term; competence is determined by a court. Any physician who has adequate training can determine capacity. It does not need to be determined by a psychiatrist. Primary care physicians often have more insight and knowledge about their patients than a psychiatrist, who might be seeing the patient for the first time.[35] The more complicated and serious the decision, the more stringent the requirements for understanding. For instance, a demented patient may have the capacity to appoint a trusted family member to serve as health care proxy but may not have the capacity to decide whether to have a permanent feeding tube placed.

A patient must meet three key criteria to demonstrate decision-making capacity: (1) the ability to understand information about diagnosis and treatment; (2) the ability to evaluate, deliberate, weigh alternatives, and compare risks and benefits; and (3) the ability to communicate a choice, whether verbally, in writing, or with a nod or gesture.

In eliciting patient preferences, the clinician should explore the patient's values—what is important to the patient and what makes life worth living or what makes life intolerable. The clinician should help the patient identify and set realistic goals, then direct treatment decisions according to these goals. More specifically, it is important to evaluate whether the patient would prefer to focus on length of life or quality of life if faced with a serious illness. In older persons who have chronic conditions that are not immediately life threatening, there is more time to explore these issues and to modify decisions over time. Outlining the available treatment options (e.g., probability and extent of response to treatment, duration and quality of extended life, anticipated side effects), identifying patients' short- and long-term goals and needs, uncovering their expectations about therapy, evaluating their coping strategies, and identifying their support networks are critical components of this discussion.

Discussions of care preferences should cover specific life-sustaining treatments such as cardiopulmonary resuscitation (CPR), artificial nutrition and hydration, and mechanical intubation and ventilation. Physicians should review with the patient the potential indications for such therapies and, if possible, offer an explicit appraisal of the outcome in their situation. A helpful strategy is to ask patients how long they think they would want a particular treatment to be continued if it did not seem to be helping. For example, the physician might ask, "If you had a brain injury that left you in a coma and the neurologists determined that only a miracle would restore your brain function, how long would you want to stay on treatments that were keeping you alive?" Some patients may specify a week, some a month, and still others, a year. Such discussions help clarify the patient's preferences and tolerance for uncertainty.

In eliciting patient preferences for care, it is critical to consider the person's cultural, ethnic, and religious background.[26] For example, it is fairly well known that Jehovah's Witnesses will not accept blood transfusions, even in the face of life-threatening conditions, but may want all other invasive treatments. Such differences can make a patient unwilling to accept a physician's recommendations and can make a physician angry at the patient's resistance to those recommendations. With patience and training, however, it is usually possible to uncover these beliefs and negotiate treatment plans that are acceptable to all concerned.

TYPES OF ADVANCE DIRECTIVES

There are three types of advance directives: (1) do not resuscitate (DNR) orders, (2) directives involving health care proxies, and (3) living wills. All are legal instruments. The federal Patient Self-Determination Act of 1990 requires hospitals, skilled nursing facilities, home health agencies, hospice programs, and health maintenance organizations to maintain written policies and procedures guaranteeing that every adult receiving medical care be given written information concerning advance directives. Although forms for designating health care proxies and living wills are completed by patients themselves, physicians may wish to secure copies of the forms used in their state and assist their patients in completing these forms.

A health care proxy is a person appointed by the patient to make health care decisions in the patient's stead, in the event that the patient loses the capacity to make those decisions. In general, it is preferable for the physician to speak to the patient first, ask the patient to think about appointing a health care proxy, and then ask the patient to bring the potential proxy to a follow-up meeting. The proxy should be aware of and advised about the patient's goals of care and preferences and should be able and willing to assume the responsibilities of serving as proxy. Typically, an alternative proxy is also appointed.

A living will is a document that directs health care personnel to withhold or withdraw life-sustaining treatment in the event that the patient is in an incurable or irreversible condition with no reasonable expectation of recovery. Not all states have statutes recognizing living wills. However, courts have recognized and upheld the use of living wills as long as these documents provide "clear and convincing evidence" of a competent patient's wishes.

Ethical Issues in Palliative Care

Chronic illness and end-of-life care bring into focus some compelling ethical issues. These include limiting life-sustaining treatments, physician-assisted suicide, and euthanasia. Guidelines and principles on these issues have been established to enable patients, families, and physicians to reach medically sound, ethical treatment decisions in cases of irreversible illness. As a result, and despite widespread physician feeling to the contrary, these treatment decisions are almost devoid of litigation danger. Nevertheless, physicians should work with their hospital attorneys to clarify the status of legislation and case law on these issues in their particular jurisdiction.

LIMITING TREATMENT (REFOCUSING GOALS OF CARE)

In the discussion of treatment goals and plans with patients or family members, the language a physician uses can make a tremendous difference. If the physician says, "It is time to stop [or limit] the treatments," the patient or family will likely feel abandoned and hopeless and therefore ask for more interventions that may not be appropriate or useful. However, if the physician says, "It is time to refocus our efforts; let's strive to maximize comfort and dignity rather than prolong the dying process," the patient and family are more likely to feel validated and reassured. Similarly, if the physician refers to mechanical ventilation, dialysis, or artificial nutrition as "life-sustaining" treatments, it is a rare individual who will elect to forgo them. Rather, the physician should refer to them as medical interventions used to achieve specific goals. For example, one might speak of instituting mechanical ventilation to support breathing, in the hope that the patient will regain spontaneous breathing; if this hope is not realized, it is then time to discuss what the goals of care are and whether they need to be modified.

Ordinarily, discussions of goals of care involving limitation of life-sustaining treatment occur in three categories of patients. The first category includes patients whose illness is judged irreversible and who are moribund; these patients usually do not benefit from aggressive medical interventions, which can become invasive and burdensome. For patients who will die with or without treatment, such as a patient with advanced metastatic cancer or a patient with end-stage cardiomyopathy for whom a transplant is not possible, interventions often pose more burdens and risks than benefit. The second category consists of patients with capacity who are not moribund but have an irreversible illness, such as amyotrophic lateral sclerosis or multiple sclerosis. These patients often wish to discuss their ultimate goals of care and their right to refuse medical treatments so as to retain control over their health care as their disease progresses. The third category includes patients with capacity who have a reversible illness. As with any patient with capacity, the principle of autonomy guarantees these patients the right to refuse any treatment, even a lifesaving one, although physicians obviously will question these refusals much more vigorously than refusals in cases of irreversible and progressive illnesses.

An important caveat here is that although supreme autonomy of the patient is valued by mainstream culture in the United States, it is not the guiding value of many other cultures. In fact, most ethnic groups in the United States (e.g., Hispanic Americans, Asian Americans, Orthodox Jews, African Americans) favor a family-based decision-making process. Furthermore, autonomy does not always mean that the patient must be informed or must participate in decision making. Autonomy means that patients should be asked whether they wish to be informed or participate in decision making; they may refuse to do either.

In some cases, a limited trial of life-prolonging treatment may clarify the patient's chances of recovery. The treatment can be stopped if it becomes clear that health (or the extent of recovery acceptable to the patient) cannot be restored. However, sometimes it is psychologically more difficult to stop such a treatment once it has been started, even if its original justification no longer applies.

When the patient does not have capacity, there are several ways to resolve treatment decisions. Advance directives are the most helpful. Otherwise, common sense should be followed, and the patient's next of kin should be asked to provide a substituted judgment about what the patient would have wanted or what decision would be in the patient's best interest.

Ethically and legally, there is no difference between forgoing or withholding a medical treatment (such as mechanical ventilation) and stopping or withdrawing it. However, family members and health care providers may feel that withholding and withdrawing interventions are emotionally different. It is therefore critical to counsel families and health care professionals that the decisions about any medical treatment should be guided by overall goals of care. Consultation with the hospital's palliative care service or ethics committee may be valuable for resolving conflicts over life-prolonging treatments.

FUTILE TREATMENT

Conflicts that require arbitration often center on treatments that either the family or the treatment team regard as futile or ineffective. Futility is a narrowly applied term that is used in the setting of CPR to describe a resuscitation attempt that would not succeed in resuscitating the patient or that, if successful, would likely be followed shortly afterward by another arrest. In many cases, when a patient is irreversibly ill and dying, CPR would be futile. Application of it is contrary to the standards of medical practice; it is unethical and inhumane. In such a case, the physician does not have a duty to consult anyone before writing a DNR order but should inform the family that a DNR order is being implemented. This is an opportunity for the physician to remind the family just how severe the illness is and to refocus attention to meeting other needs of the patient and the family.

Defining futility is currently a major goal of medical ethics.[36] The negative right of refusal has become transformed by some into a positive right to demand of physicians any life-sustaining treatment. Others argue that physicians have a duty not to offer or provide treatments that are ineffective.[37] Because most risk-versus-benefit considerations of life-sustaining treatment involve value judgments and because the principle of autonomy requires that the patient's values come first, some argue that so-called objective standards for futility are impossible to formulate and that physicians should make no such judgments.[38] However, for patients in an irreversible coma and, increasingly, for those in a persistent vegetative state, life-sustaining treatments are seen to be futile.

Controversial questions about defining treatments as futile will most likely be resolved city by city by a panel of experts set up to judge whether a treatment is futile after hearing all evidence presented by the family, the medical team, and others. This was the approach used by the Houston citywide consortium of hospitals.[39]

THE REQUEST FOR ASSISTED SUICIDE OR EUTHANASIA

In the United States, the public increasingly accepts physician-assisted suicide and euthanasia as moral practices and believes that these practices should be legal.[40] These views can be seen as the public's condemnation of at least two things: the way hospitals and physicians overtreat sick patients in their last days, making death a painful journey; and medicine's inadequate and ineffective treatment of suffering. These views also reflect a demand for more control in decisions about the end of life. Some people equate physician-assisted suicide with euthanasia, but they are different concepts. In physician-assisted suicide, the patient requests the physician's help in dying, usually in the form of a prescription of a lethal dose of medication to be taken at home. Euthanasia occurs when there is no patient request but the physician (or other health care professional) decides to hasten the patient's dying process in order to relieve suffering (the patient's or the physician's).

In June 1997, the United States Supreme Court ruled that there is no constitutional right to physician-assisted suicide.[41] This opinion did not remove the authority of individual states to outlaw or decriminalize physician-assisted suicide, however; and in November 1997, Oregon voters confirmed their acceptance of the Death with Dignity Act, which allows terminally ill Oregon residents to obtain from their physicians and to use prescriptions for self-administered, lethal medications. The act states that ending one's life in accordance with the law does not constitute suicide, and it specifically prohibits euthanasia (i.e., direct administration of a medication to end another person's life).

Many, if not most, of those patients who want physician-assisted suicide want it not to relieve suffering as ordinarily understood but to maintain control over their dying.[42] As of 1999 (2 years after legalization of physician-assisted suicide in Oregon), a survey of Oregon physicians found that they granted about one in six requests for a prescription for a lethal medication and that one in 10 requests actually resulted in suicide. Substantive palliative interventions led some—but not all—patients to change their minds about assisted suicide.[43,44] As of 2002, a total of 129 people had committed physician-assisted suicide in Oregon, corresponding to a rate of 8.8 per 10,000 deaths from any cause in the state.[45] Compared with Oregon residents who died of similar underlying causes, rates of physician-assisted suicide decreased with age and were higher among those who had been divorced and among those with higher levels of education. The rate of physician-assisted suicide was also higher among those afflicted with amyotrophic lateral sclerosis and cancer. The majority of patients using physician-assisted suicide were non-Hispanic whites, but a significant minority were Asian Americans. Overall, the number of Oregon residents using physician-assisted suicide has increased over the years, but it remains a very small minority relative to overall deaths.

Regardless of legal issues, however, when a patient requests a prescription for enough medication to commit suicide or to hasten death, the physician has the ethical responsibility to try to learn why. What is it that now makes death seem a better option than life? What is it that the patient feels must be avoided? From what is the patient trying to escape? Is the patient depressed? Why does the patient feel that that he or she can no longer be someone who matters? Are there financial considerations—that is, does the patient fear becoming a financial burden, a burden to care for, or both? Has any of this been discussed with the family? How would the family understand the patient's requests and be affected by them? If the patient considers life to be devoid of value and meaning, does the patient's life still have meaning for other persons? Does this affect the patient? Has the patient made any effort to achieve consensus so that his or her death can be a meaningful, shared family experience?

FEAR OF LEGAL REPRISAL

When a physician makes a reasonable clinical judgment of irreversible illness and decides to forgo or stop life-sustaining treatment—whether on the wish of the patient or, if the patient is incompetent, with the agreement of the patient's proxy or surrogates—fear of litigation is neither a reasonable nor a legitimate excuse not to proceed. The courts have made it clear that these decisions are valid and that the persons involved in those decisions should not be brought to trial. It is irrational to demand guarantees that no litigation will follow, however. It is hoped that physicians' energies will be spent doing the best they can for the patient, in accord with the patient's wishes. Should litigation follow an action taken in accord with the above guidelines, the physician will be well prepared to defend the decisions in court.

The author has no commercial relationships with manufacturers of products or providers of services discussed in this chapter.

References

1. Billings J: Recent advances: palliative care. BMJ 321:555, 2000

2. Pan CX, Morrison RS, Meier DE, et al: How prevalent are hospital-based palliative care programs? Status report and future directions. J Palliat Med 4:315, 2001

3. NHPCO facts and figures. National Hospice and Palliative Care Organization, 2003 http://www.nhpco.org

4. Health Care Financing Administration: Medicare hospice benefits. U.S. Dept. of Health and Human Services, Baltimore, 1999

5. Lynn J: Caring at the end of our lives. N Engl J Med 335:201, 1996

6. Davis MP, Walsh D, Nelson KA, et al: The business of palliative medicine. Part 2: The economics of acute inpatient palliative medicine. Am J Hosp Palliat Care 19:89, 2002

7. Covinsky KE, Eng C, Lui LY, et al: The last 2 years of life: functional trajectories of frail older people. J Am Geriatr Soc 51:492, 2003

8. Good care of the dying patient. Council on Scientific Affairs, American Medical Association. JAMA 275:474, 1996

9. Christakis NA: Timing of referral of terminally ill patients to an outpatient hospice. J Gen Intern Med 9:314, 1994

10. Deaths: Preliminary Data for 2001. National Vital Statistics Reports 51:1, 2003 http://www.cdc.gov/nchs/data/nvsr/nvsr51/nvsr51_05.pdf

11. Seale C, Cartwright A: The Year Before Death. Ashgale Publishing Co, Brookfield, Vermont, 1994

12. National Population Projections. United States Census Bureau, 2002 http://www.census.gov/population/www/projections/natproj.html

13. Fairman RP: Withdrawing life-sustaining treatment: lessons from Nancy Cruzan. Arch Intern Med 152:25, 1992

14. Healey JM: Decisions at the end of life: the legacy of Karen Ann Quinlan. Conn Med 49:549, 1985

15. National Mortality Followback Survey. National Center for Health Statistics, 1998 http://www.cdc.gov/nchs/about/major/nmfs/nmfs.htm

16. A controlled trial to improve care for seriously ill hospitalized patients: the study to understand prognoses and preferences for outcomes and risks of treatments (SUPPORT). The SUPPORT Principal Investigators. JAMA 274:1591, 1995

17. Lynn J, Harrell F Jr, Cohn F, et al: Prognoses of seriously ill hospitalized patients on the days before death: implications for patient care and public policy. New Horiz 5:56, 1997

18. Koretz B, Whiteman E: Hospice eligibility. University of California Office of the President Academic Geriatric Resource Plan, 2002 http://www.ucop.edu/agrp/docs/la_hospice.pdf

19. Evaluation of prognostic criteria for determining hospice eligibility in patients with advanced lung, heart, or liver disease. SUPPORT Investigators. Study to Understand Prognoses and Preferences for Outcomes and Risks of Treatments. JAMA 282:1638, 1999

20. Management of pain in elderly patients with cancer. SAGE Study Group. Systematic Assessment of Geriatric Drug Use via Epidemiology. JAMA 279:1877, 1998

21. Ferrell BA, Ferrell BR, Rivera L: Pain in cognitively impaired nursing home patients. J Pain Symptom Manage 10:591, 1995

22. Sengstaken EA, King SA: The problems of pain and its detection among geriatric nursing home residents. J Am Geriatr Soc 41:541, 1993

23. Pain and treatment of pain in minority patients with cancer. The Eastern Cooperative Oncology Group Minority Outpatient Pain Study. Ann Intern Med 127:813, 1997

24. Feldt KS, Warne MA, Ryden MB: Examining pain in aggressive cognitively impaired older adults. J Gerontol Nurs 24:14, 1998

25. Gagliese L, Melzack R: Chronic pain in elderly people. Pain 70:3, 1997

26. Culture and Nursing Care: A Pocket Guide. Lipson JDS, Minarik PA, Eds. UCSF Nursing Press, San Francisco, 1996

27. Caralis PV, Davis B, Wright K, et al: The influence of ethnicity and race on attitudes toward advance directives, life-prolonging treatments, and euthanasia. J Clin Ethics 4:155, 1993

28. Leggat JE Jr, Bloembergen WE, Levine G, et al: An analysis of risk factors for withdrawal from dialysis before death. J Am Soc Nephrol 8:1755, 1997

29. Blackhall LJ, Frank G, Murphy ST, et al: Ethnicity and attitudes towards life sustaining technology. Soc Sci Med 48:1779, 1999

30. Garrett JM, Harris RP, Norburn JK, et al: Life-sustaining treatments during terminal illness: who wants what? J Gen Intern Med 8:361, 1993

31. Crawley L, Payne R, Bolden J, et al: Palliative and end-of-life care in the African American community. JAMA 284:2518, 2000

32. Llovera I, Ward MF, Ryan JG, et al: Why don't emergency department patients have advance directives? Acad Emerg Med 6:1054, 1999

33. Kvale JN, Melloh JR, Oprandi A, et al: Use of advance directives by community-dwelling older adults. J Clin Outcomes Meas 6:39, 1999

34. The discussion about advance directives: patient and physician opinions regarding when and how it should be conducted. End of Life Study Group. Arch Intern Med 155:1025, 1995

35. Carney MT, Neugroschl J, Morrison RS, et al: The development and piloting of a capacity assessment tool. J Clin Ethics 12:17, 2001

36. Pellegrino ED: Ethics. JAMA 270:202, 1993

37. Jecker NS, Schneiderman LJ: Medical futility: the duty not to treat. Camb Q Health Ethics 2:151, 1993

38. Truog RD, Brett AS, Frader J: The problem with futility. N Engl J Med 326:1560, 1992

39. Halevy A, Brody BA: Medical futility in end-of-life care. JAMA 282:1331, 1999

40. Paul P: Euthanasia and assisted suicide. Am Demogr 24:20, 2002

41. Vacco v. Quill. 521 US 793, 1997

42. Ganzini L, Harvath TA, Jackson A, et al: Experiences of Oregon nurses and social workers with hospice patients who requested assistance with suicide. N Engl J Med 347:582, 2002

43. Ganzini L, Nelson HD, Schmidt TA, et al: Physicians' experiences with the Oregon Death with Dignity Act. N Engl J Med 342:557, 2000

44. Ganzini L, Nelson HD, Lee MA, et al: Oregon physicians' attitudes about and experiences with end-of-life care since passage of the Oregon Death with Dignity Act. JAMA 285:2363, 2001

45. Hedberg K, Hopkins D, Kohn M: Five years of legal physician-assisted suicide in Oregon. N Engl J Med 348:961, 2003

46. Deaths: Final Data for 2000. National Vital Statistics Reports 50:8, 2002 http://www.cdc.gov/nchs/data/nvsr/nvsr50/nvsr50_15.pdf

11 Symptom Management in Palliative Medicine

Maria Torroella Carney, M.D., and Jennifer Rhodes-Kropf, M.D.

The goal of palliative care is to provide comfort and support for both patient and family through the course of a life-threatening illness. Symptom control is essential to meeting that goal. This chapter discusses symptoms that commonly contribute to patients' suffering in terminal illness. These symptoms include pain; respiratory, gastrointestinal, mouth, and skin problems; and delirium.

Although this chapter focuses on physical and psychological symptoms, achieving symptom control requires the physician to address the patient's suffering in all its aspects: physical, psychological, social, and spiritual. Physical distress cannot be effectively treated in isolation from the emotional and spiritual components that contribute to it, nor can these sources of suffering be addressed adequately when patients are in physical distress. The various components of suffering must be addressed simultaneously [*see Chapter 12*].

Symptom Assessment

A full and formal symptom assessment is necessary before effective treatment can be instituted.[1] Symptoms are inherently subjective[2]; therefore, patient self-reporting must be the primary source of information, and the clinician must believe what the patient says. If the patient is unable to report, a family member or professional can provide a surrogate assessment. However, several studies have demonstrated that observer and patient assessments are not well correlated.[3,4]

To compensate for this inherent subjectivity, researchers have developed symptom measurement systems that are intended to quantify patients' perceptions in a manner that is valid and reliable. These systems have the further benefit of eliciting symptoms that the patient might not have volunteered. In one study of palliative care patients, the median number of symptoms found using systematic assessment was 10-fold higher than that found on open-ended questioning.[5]

Often, symptom measurement systems have taken the form of symptom checklists.[6,7] For example, the Edmonton Symptom Assessment Scale[6] comprises 14 questions that evaluate eight physical and psychological symptoms [*see Table 1*]. This scale has been extensively employed in palliative care research, in part because of its ease of use. Although the scale yields a numerical score (the higher the score, the more severe the patient's condition), the formal scoring mechanism is used only in research. In clinical practice, the scale can be used informally to evaluate a patient's status and follow it over time.

The Memorial Symptom Assessment Scale[8] characterizes 32 physical and psychological symptoms in terms of intensity and frequency, as well as the level of distress from the symptoms [*see Table 2*]; it is valid for palliative care patients with or without cancer.[9] Although the Memorial Symptom Assessment Scale provides a greater range of information than the Edmonton Symptom Assessment Scale, the former is correspondingly more time consuming to use.

Physical Symptoms

PAIN

Diagnosis

Management of pain begins with a careful and detailed assessment [*see Chapter 175*]. The goal of this assessment is to determine the location and character of the pain, define its cause (or causes), and develop a plan of care.

Pain cannot be measured objectively, and several studies have shown that medical care providers' estimates of patients' pain severity are significantly lower than the patients' self-reports.[10,11] Pain is independent of age, gender, marital status, physical function, and cognitive function.[12] Therefore, the central guiding principle of pain assessment is to ask the patient and believe the patient's description of pain.

Pain assessment in the elderly is often complicated by coexistent cognitive impairment. The cognitively impaired patient may be unable to express pain adequately or request analgesics and, therefore, is at increased risk for undertreatment of pain.[13,14] As with cognitively intact patients, the first step in the assessment of pain in demented patients is to ask them about their pain. Although patients with severe dementia may be incapable of communicating, many patients with mild or moderate impairment can accurately localize and grade the severity of their pain,[15] and these self-reports should be regarded as valid.

Untreated pain can result in agitation and disruptive behavior, and it may worsen or precipitate delirium, particularly in cognitively impaired patients.[16,17] When delirium prevents communication with the patient, the physician may have to infer that pain is present and proceed with treatment.

Treatment

Opioids are the standard choice for treating pain in terminally ill patients. The physician who provides palliative care needs to have the confidence and competence to prescribe opioids at whatever dose is needed to control pain, as well as the skill to determine when adjuvant analgesics (e.g., antidepressant or antiseizure medication) are needed to manage certain types of pain.[18,19] Terminally ill patients are a special population, often suffering chronic pain and taking pain medications over longer periods and at higher dosages.[20] Indeed, tolerance to opioids may require that these agents be used in amounts that would be fatal to the opioid-naive patient.

In a multisite study of terminally ill patients in the United States, Weiss and colleagues[21] found that half of terminally ill patients experienced moderate to severe pain but that less than one third wanted additional pain treatment from their primary care physician. Reasons for not wanting additional therapy included dislike of analgesic side effects and not wanting to take more pills or injections. Some patients, however, mentioned fear of addiction. This is a common—and unwarranted—concern not only of patients but of some medical personnel, as well.

Several strategies can be used to improve pain relief when opioids are insufficiently effective or cause significant side effects. Adding the nonsteroidal anti-inflammatory drug ketorolac

---

Table 1   Modified Edmonton Symptom Assessment Scale[6]

1a. Please rate your *pain* now.
  1. ☐ No pain
  2. ☐ Mild pain
  3. ☐ Moderate pain
  4. ☐ Severe pain

1b. Please rate your *pain* over the past 3 days.
  1. ☐ No pain
  2. ☐ Mild pain
  3. ☐ Moderate pain
  4. ☐ Severe pain

1c. Is your *pain control* acceptable to you?
  1. ☐ Very acceptable
  2. ☐ Acceptable
  3. ☐ Not acceptable

2. How would you describe your *activity level* over the past 3 days?
  1. ☐ Very active
  2. ☐ Somewhat active
  3. ☐ Minimally active
  4. ☐ Not active

3. How would you describe your amount of *nausea* over the past 3 days?
  1. ☐ Not nauseated
  2. ☐ Mildly nauseated
  3. ☐ Moderately nauseated
  4. ☐ Very nauseated

4a. How would you describe your level of *constipation* over the past 3 days?
  1. ☐ No constipation
  2. ☐ Mild constipation
  3. ☐ Moderate constipation
  4. ☐ Severe constipation

4b. When was your *last bowel movement*?
  1. ☐ Today
  2. ☐ Yesterday
  3. ☐ 2–3 days ago
  4. ☐ More than 4 days ago

5. How would you describe your feelings of *depression* over the past 3 days?
  1. ☐ Not depressed
  2. ☐ Mildly depressed
  3. ☐ Moderately depressed
  4. ☐ Very depressed

6. How would you describe your feelings of *anxiety* over the past 3 days?
  1. ☐ Not anxious
  2. ☐ Mildly anxious
  3. ☐ Moderately anxious
  4. ☐ Very anxious

7. How would you describe your level of *fatigue* over the past 3 days?
  1. ☐ Not fatigued
  2. ☐ Mildly fatigued
  3. ☐ Moderately fatigued
  4. ☐ Very fatigued

8. How has your *appetite* been over the past 3 days?
  1. ☐ Very good appetite
  2. ☐ Moderate appetite
  3. ☐ Poor appetite
  4. ☐ No appetite

9. How would you describe your sensation of *well-being* over the past 3 days?
  1. ☐ Very good sensation of well-being
  2. ☐ Moderately good sensation of well-being
  3. ☐ Not very good sensation of well-being
  4. ☐ Poor sensation of well-being

10. How *short of breath* have you been over the past 3 days?
  1. ☐ No shortness of breath
  2. ☐ Mild shortness of breath
  3. ☐ Moderate shortness of breath
  4. ☐ Very short of breath

11. How has your *physical discomfort* been over the past 3 days?
  1. ☐ No physical discomfort
  2. ☐ Mild physical discomfort
  3. ☐ Moderate physical discomfort
  4. ☐ Severe physical discomfort

(60 mg orally three times a day) may reduce opioid requirements and opioid-related constipation, although at the price of greater gastric discomfort.[22] Use of implantable systems that deliver drugs intrathecally can provide better pain control (i.e., less escalation of pain medication at week 1), less toxicity (i.e., fatigue and depressed level of consciousness), and even improved survival at 6 months.[23] Nerve blocks (e.g., celiac plexus block for patients with terminal pancreatic cancer[24]) can be effective in selected patients with regional pain. Relaxation techniques may be useful adjuncts to other forms of analgesia.[25]

In patients who are still ambulatory, pain control can be enhanced by having the patient keep a daily pain diary. Nursing interventions (i.e., clinical reassessment and dose adjustment) can be made on the basis of diary entries that indicate fluctuation in pain levels.[26]

As the goals of care change in the course of a life-threatening illness, higher dosages of pain medication may be needed to achieve comfort. In the last days of life, relief of suffering may require sedation to the point of unconsciousness, a technique referred to as palliative sedation (see below).

RESPIRATORY SYMPTOMS

Dyspnea

Shortness of breath has been described in 70% of cancer patients during the last 6 weeks of life and in 50% to 70% of patients dying of other illnesses.[27-29] Like pain, dyspnea is a subjective symptom that may not correlate with any objective signs of respiratory compromise,[30] and hence, its management can be challenging.

It is important to diagnose and treat any underlying reversible causes of dyspnea. For example, dyspnea caused by congestive heart failure will require diuretics and possibly inotropic support [*see Chapter 26*].

When therapy specific to the underlying cause is unavailable or ineffective, several techniques may alleviate breathlessness. Simple measures include pursed-lip breathing and diaphragmatic breathing, leaning forward with arms on a table, cool-air ventilation (from a fan or an open window), and nasal oxygen.

Opioids are highly effective in the amelioration of dyspnea.[31-34] In one study, morphine in doses sufficient to relieve dyspnea had no measurable adverse effect on respiratory rate or effort, oxygen saturation, and carbon dioxide concentration.[31] Therefore, morphine is the drug of choice for treating dyspnea in terminal illness.

Lorazepam and other benzodiazepines are also widely used, especially in terminally ill patients whose dyspnea has an anxiety component, although evidence to support this practice is limited.[35] In addition, steroids and oxygen therapy may be of benefit [see Table 3]. Although oxygen therapy may alleviate dyspnea and improve quality of life, only limited evidence of its efficacy is available; therefore, oxygen therapy should be prescribed on the basis of patient report of benefit.[36]

Cough

Cough can be an annoyance or can develop into a major source of suffering by causing muscle strain and increasing fatigue and by interrupting sleep. In one study of lung cancer patients, cough was the most common symptom, affecting 80% of patients until just before death.[37] Because the causes of cough are varied, the optimal approach is treatment of the underlying problem, if possible. When such treatment is not possible, however, a productive cough may improve with chest physiotherapy, oxygen, humidity, and suctioning [see Figure 1].[38] Antibiotics for infection, N-acetylcysteine, bronchodilators, and guaifenesin are also effective.[39,40] Opioids, antihistamines, and anticholinergics decrease mucus production, which can decrease the stimulus for cough. Cough suppressants can be harmful if used in patients with productive cough by causing mucus retention,[39,40] which may lead to the formation of mucous plugs and airway obstruction. A patient with a nonproductive cough may benefit from a cough-suppressing agent such as a local anesthetic (e.g., nebulized bupivacaine), bronchodilators, opioids, or a soothing agent such as a lozenge. Benzonatate, steroids, and opiates are effective treatments. Opioids act centrally and are one of the most effective agents against cough.[41] Nonopioid antitussives, such as dextromethorphan, may work synergistically with opiates.[40]

GASTROINTESTINAL SYMPTOMS

Anorexia, nausea and vomiting, constipation, bowel obstruction, and diarrhea are common and potentially devastating in terminal illness.

Anorexia

Anorexia is nearly universal in patients with a terminal illness.[42] Evaluation of anorexia should be concentrated on finding a reversible or treatable cause. It is important to note that cognitive impairment, which is also highly prevalent in advanced disease, may cause a person to be misdiagnosed as anorexic, because the person may be unable to obtain, prepare, or eat meals.[43] Often in terminal disease, however, the patient simply loses the desire to eat.

Patients themselves may complain of anorexia because they find the resulting cachexia unacceptable. In such cases, the decision whether to treat is straightforward. Anorexia, however, can often be of more concern to family, friends, and medical staff than to patients themselves. The family may be concerned because loss of appetite is seen as a certain sign of impending death.[44] Concern about anorexia may also be rooted in the emotional and psychological meanings that surround food and its consumption: not feeding the patient may be considered equivalent to not caring about the patient. The family should be reassured that anorexia in terminal disease is usually not associated with suffering[45]; especially at the end of life, patients rarely feel hunger or thirst, and many patients who stop eating experience analgesia and even euphoria. Excessive proteins and lipids can induce nausea and vomiting, and excessive hydration can result in edema and dyspnea.[46] In the early stages of terminal illness, however, studies have shown that the treatment of anorexia with appetite stimulants may improve patients' quality of life.[47,48] Treatment can begin with simple measures. The patient should be encouraged to eat without any restrictions on sugar, salt, or fats, when possible. Alcohol has appetite-stimulating properties, so patients may wish to consider a cocktail or glass of wine before the evening meal.[49]

Appetite stimulants with proven efficacy in palliative care include dexamethasone, in dosages of 2 to 20 mg/day (recommended because its long half-life permits once-daily dosing and because it has minimal mineralocorticoid effects) and megestrol acetate (beginning with 200 mg every 8 hours and titrating to 800

Table 2   Memorial Symptom Assessment Scale[16]

For physical symptoms, patients are instructed to check off all symptoms experienced during the past week and the degree to which the symptom bothered or distressed them. Categories and scores are as follows: Not at all (0), A little bit (1), Somewhat (2), Quite a bit (3), and Very much (4). Patients may also add symptoms not listed and rate them on the same scale. For psychological symptoms, patients are instructed to check off all symptoms experienced during the past week and how often each occurred. Categories and scores are as follows: Rarely (1), Occasionally (2), Frequently (3), and Almost constantly (4). Patients may also add symptoms not listed and rate them on the same scale.

Physical Symptom	Severity				
	0	1	2	3	4
Difficulty concentrating					
Pain					
Lack of energy					
Cough					
Changes in skin					
Dry mouth					
Nausea					
Feeling drowsy					
Numbness or tingling in hands and feet					
Hair loss					
Constipation					
Swelling of arms or legs					

Psychological Symptom	Frequency				
	0	1	2	3	4
Feeling sad					
Worrying					
Feeling irritable					
Feeling nervous					

Table 3 Drug Treatment for Dyspnea[44]

Drug (Trade Name)	Dosage	Comment
Oral morphine	2.5–5 mg p.o., q. 4 hr while awake	Doses for opiate-naive patients
I.V. morphine	0.5 mg/hr; titrate to relief	Once dose requirement established, switch to long-acting oral opiate or fentanyl patch
Nebulized morphine	2.5–10 mg injectable in 2 ml NS	—
Nebulized hydromorphone	0.25–1 mg injectable in 2 ml NS	—
Nebulized albuterol	0.083% (3 ml)	Possible adjunct to opioid
Nebulized methylprednisolone (Solu-Medrol)	10 mg	Possible adjunct to opioid
Dexamethasone	Day 1: 16 mg p.o.; days 2–3: 8 mg b.i.d.; days 3–4: 4 mg b.i.d.; subsequent: 2 mg b.i.d.	Possible adjunct to opioid
Prednisone	40 mg b.i.d. for 5–7 days	Possible adjunct to opioid
Lorazepam (Ativan)	1–10 mg/day in two or three divided doses; usual dose, 2–6 mg/day in divided doses. Elderly: 0.5–4 mg/day	For patients whose dyspnea has an anxiety component
Oxygen	2 L/min by nasal cannula; titrate to relief	—

NS—normal saline

mg/day).[50] In addition, dronabinol is approved for the treatment of anorexia associated with weight loss in patients with AIDS (starting with 2.5 mg twice daily, before lunch and supper, and titrating to effect and tolerability).

Anorexia in patients with dementia Many patients with Alzheimer disease progress to a stage at which they are unable to eat on their own or even chew and swallow reliably. Before agreeing to gastrostomy tube placement for such patients, family members must be made aware of the many complications of tube feeding, such as repeated infections. The needle sticks, transfer to a hospital, and restraints that such infections require are especially burdensome for a confused patient who cannot understand the reason for such interventions.[51] In addition, patients with advanced neurologic impairment are at high risk for pneumonia from a variety of causes, including but not limited to aspiration. There is no evidence that tube feeding reduces the risk of pneumonia in such patients; it may even increase the risk.[52] One study of hospitalized patients with advanced dementia found that insertion of a feeding tube had no measurable influence on survival; regardless of feeding tube placement, median mortality was 50% at 6 months.[53] Nevertheless, placement of a feeding tube was very common in the study, especially in patients who were African American or who had previously lived in a nursing home.

Of note, forgoing artificial nutrition and hydration does not seem to result in high levels of discomfort for patients with severe dementia who have mostly or completely stopped eating or drinking.[54] Because of the terminal and irreversible nature of end-stage dementia and the substantial burden that continued artificial nutrition and hydration may pose for these patients, they are better served by palliative care that focuses predominantly on their comfort. Comfort care is viewed as preferable to life-prolonging measures by a substantial proportion of nursing home patients and family members.[55] Families should be reassured that it is never unethical to forgo artificial nutrition and hydration if these interventions are unlikely to help the patient.

Nausea and Vomiting

Nausea and vomiting occur in up to 62% of patients with terminal cancer[56] and 27% of patients dying of other causes. There are multiple potential causes for both nausea and vomiting [see Table 4].[49] Once the cause has been determined, symptomatic relief is relatively easy to achieve with the appropriate medications [see Table 5].[38] The anatomic sites most involved in the physiology of nausea are the gastric lining, the chemoreceptor trigger zone in the base of the fourth ventricle, the vestibular apparatus, and the cortex. Stimulation of the vomiting center in the brain from one or more of these areas is mediated through the neurotransmitters acetylcholine and histamine. Serotonin and dopamine are important neurotransmitters in the gastric lining and the chemoreceptor trigger zone; acetylcholine acts in the vestibular apparatus. Cortical responses are mediated via both neurotransmitters and learned responses (e.g., nausea related to anxiety or anticipatory nausea with chemotherapy).[57]

The major causes of nausea and vomiting can be classified by the mechanisms' principal site of action. Dopamine-mediated nausea is probably the most common form of nausea and the most frequently targeted one for initial symptom management. Antidopamine medications are phenothiazines and butyrophenone neuroleptics (metoclopramide and prochlorperazine). They may cause drowsiness and extrapyramidal symptoms. Haloperidol is a highly effective antinausea agent and may be less sedating. Antihistamines such as diphenhydramine can be used to control nausea, but they may cause sedation. Antihistamines also have anticholinergic properties. Serotonin has been implicated in chemotherapy-associated nausea. Antiserotonin medications (e.g., ondansetron) can be effective, but they are expensive.

Nausea can also result from slow gastric and intestinal motility; so-called squashed stomach syndrome from mechanical compression of the stomach; and constipation. Hence, prokinetic agents (e.g., metoclopramide) and aggressive fecal disimpaction and institution of a bowel regimen (see below) should be considered as therapeutic modalities. In some patients, hyperacidity and mucosal erosion may also be associated with significant

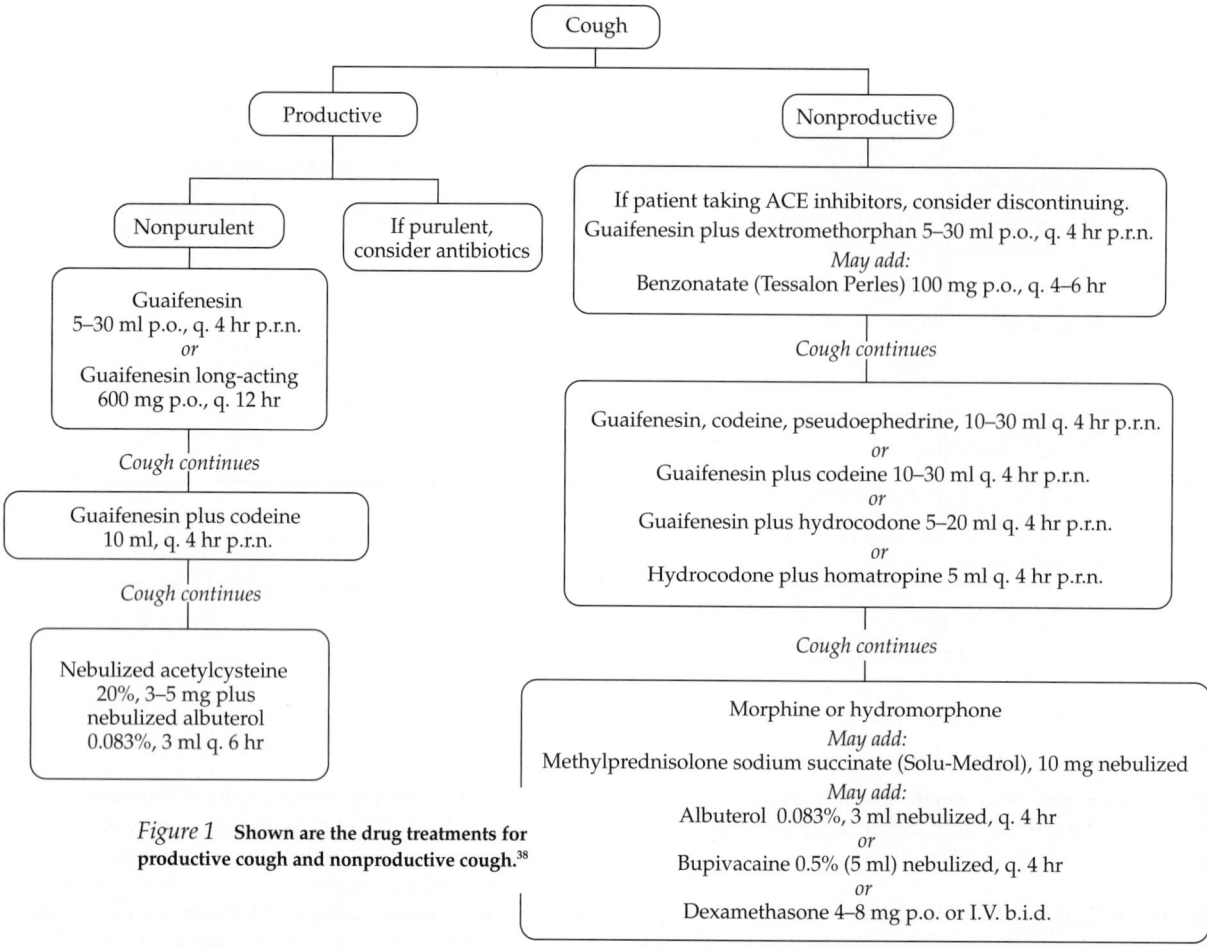

Figure 1   **Shown are the drug treatments for productive cough and nonproductive cough.**[38]

nausea. In these patients, one should consider the use of antacids, histamine$_2$ blockers, proton-pump inhibitors, and misoprostol [*see Chapter 67*].

Constipation

Constipation can lead to serious complications, such as bowel obstruction, ulceration, or perforation, as well as delirium. Because constipation is so common in terminal illness, appropriate management includes the institution of preventive measures in patients at high risk for this complication.

Diagnosis   Assessment of constipation begins with inquiry about the frequency and consistency of stools; possible contributing factors, such as medications, reduced mobility, and a low-fiber diet; and any accompanying symptoms that suggest complications, such as nausea, vomiting, abdominal pain, distention, and discomfort.[58] As with any symptom, the search for a reversible cause is primary. A plain x-ray can be useful to evaluate for ileus or bowel obstruction. Invasive evaluation with colonoscopy should be considered in difficult, refractory, or complicated cases.

Many medications can contribute to constipation. These include beta blockers, calcium channel blockers, anticholinergic agents, and diuretics.[58,59] First and foremost, however, are opioid analgesics: constipation is a universal side effect of opioid therapy, especially in the terminally ill. For that reason, every terminally ill patient who is placed on opioids should also be started

on a preventive regimen for constipation. The bowel regimen in these patients starts with stool softeners and stimulant laxatives and progresses through hyperosmotic agents and enemas, as necessary [*see Table 6*].[60] This regimen can also be utilized for treatment of constipation from other causes, once intestinal obstruction is ruled out.

Treatment   Treatment of constipation is with oral agents or rectal suppositories and can focus on softening the stool, enlarging stool volume, or promoting bowel peristalsis. Laxative categories include detergents, stimulants, osmotic agents, prokinetic agents, lubricant stimulants, and large-volume enemas [*see Table 7*]. Polyethylene glycol solution (GoLYTELY) or powder (MiraLax) is an osmotic agent that is marketed as a bowel cleanser to prepare patients for colonoscopy, but it is often effective in relieving constipation and may cause less cramping than other laxatives. Whichever laxative is chosen, the clinician should prescribe the maximum therapeutic dose of the agent before switching to another one.

Fecal impaction   Although impaction of stool in the rectum is a complication of constipation, the typical clinical manifestation is so-called overflow diarrhea from leakage of unformed stool around the obstruction. A digital rectal examination may confirm fecal impaction in the distal rectum, but abdominal x-rays may be required for the diagnosis of more proximal impaction. Treatment of fecal impaction is from below, utilizing

Table 4 Management of Nausea and Vomiting[49]

Etiology	Pathophysiology	Therapy
Mechanical obstruction—intraluminal	Constipation, obstipation	Laxatives; disimpaction
Mechanical obstruction—extraluminal	Tumor, fibrotic stricture	Surgery, fluid management, steroids, octreotide, scopolamine
Medications—chemotherapy	Chemoreceptor trigger zone, GI tract	Antiserotonin, antidopamine, steroids
Medications—NSAIDs	GI tract irritation	Cytoprotective agents, antacids
Medications—opioids	Chemoreceptor trigger zone, vestibular effect, GI tract	Antidopamine, anticholinergic, prokinetic agents, stimulant cathartics
Medications—other	Chemoreceptors	Antidopamine, antihistamine
Meningeal irritation	Increased intracranial pressure	Steroids
Mentation (e.g., anxiety)	Cortical	Anxiolytics
Metabolic—hypercalcemia	Chemoreceptor trigger zone	Antidopamine, antihistamine
Metabolic—hyponatremia	Chemoreceptor trigger zone	Antidopamine, antihistamine
Metabolic—hepatic/renal failure	Chemoreceptor trigger zone	Rehydration, steroids
Metastases—cerebral	Increased intracranial pressure	Steroids, mannitol
	Chemoreceptor trigger zone	Antidopamine, antihistamine
Metastases—liver	Toxin buildup	Antidopamine, antihistamine
Microbes—gastroenteritis	GI tract	Anti-infectives, antacids
Microbes—sepsis	Chemoreceptor trigger zone	Antidopamine, antihistamine, anti-infectives
Movement	Vestibular stimulation	Anticholinergic
Mucosal irritation	GI hyperacidity, GERD	Cytoprotective agents, antacids
Myocardial—ischemia, CHF	Vagal stimulation, cortical, chemoreceptor trigger zone	Oxygen, opioids, antidopamine, antihistamine, anxiolytics

CHF—congestive heart failure   GERD—gastroesophageal reflux disease   NSAIDs—nonsteroidal anti-inflammatory drugs

digital disimpaction and rectal laxatives (suppositories, enemas, or both); only if those fail should oral treatment be attempted.[58]

Bowel Obstruction

The prevalence of bowel obstruction is as high as 40% in bowel and pelvic cancers.[61] Constipation and fecal impaction are the most common causes of bowel obstruction in terminal illness. Symptoms of bowel obstruction include anorexia, confusion, nausea and vomiting, constipation, and pain. Diagnosis is made on the basis of the clinical presentation and abdominal x-rays.

Consultation with a surgeon is advisable to establish a treatment plan. In addition to aggressive measures to prevent or treat constipation and fecal impaction (see above), treatment of bowel obstruction may involve endoscopic decompression,[62] insertion of a self-expandable metal stent,[63] surgical relief of obstruction, nasogastric suction, and pharmacologic measures. Colicky or cramping pain may respond to dicyclomine, opioids (parenteral or rectal), and warm soaks to the abdomen. The obstruction and associated nausea and vomiting may respond to metoclopramide, haloperidol, or dexamethasone. Parenteral octreotide is also useful in this setting to decrease the volume of bowel secretions.

Diarrhea

Diarrhea, which is often secondary to fecal impaction or an-

tibiotic-associated colitis, is a particularly distressing and exhausting symptom in the terminally ill patient.[58] Once impaction, overgrowth, and other causes (e.g., gastrointestinal bleeding, malabsorption, and medications) have been ruled out, kaolin-pectin, psyllium, loperamide, or tincture of opium may be tried. Octreotide (see above) is an effective means of reducing gastrointestinal secretions.

MOUTH SYMPTOMS

Oral problems can cause altered taste, pain, and difficulty swallowing, which may lead to reduced food and fluid intake. Good hydration, hygiene, and regular observation can keep oral problems to a minimum. The patient's teeth should be brushed twice daily with toothpaste. Daily observation of the oral mucosa is recommended.

Dentures also require regular cleansing. Dentures may cease to fit properly in patients who lose a significant amount of weight. Some of those patients may wish to have their dentures refitted; others (especially those nearing death) will choose to forgo this arduous process.

Key questions to ask regarding the mouth [see Table 8] include the following: Is the mouth dry? Is infection present? Is the mouth dirty? Is the mouth painful? Are oral ulcerations present?[64]

Dry Mouth

The presence of saliva is usually taken for granted, but the lack of it can seriously damage the quality of life. Xerostomia (the subjective sensation of dry mouth) may result from salivary gland disease or systemic conditions such as Sjögren syndrome, Parkinson disease, AIDS, or diabetes[65]; it may also be a side effect of medications, including agents with anticholiner-gic action, benzodiazepines, diuretics, and interleukin-2.[66] Regardless of the cause, xerostomia almost always requires symptomatic treatment. The goal of therapy is to moisten the oral mucosa, and the best, simplest way is for the patient to sip water frequently. However, mouth moisteners and artificial salivas exist and may be preferred by some patients.[64,66] Pilocarpine tablets may be used, at a dosage of 5 to 10 mg every 8 hours, if

Table 5 Medications for Nausea and Vomiting[38]

Administration	Category	Drug (Trade Name)	Dosage
Oral	Corticosteroid	Dexamethasone	2–8 mg q. 6–12 hr
	Antidopamine	Haloperidol (Haldol)	0.5–5 mg q. 6–8 hr
		Prochlorperazine (Compazine)	5–10 mg q. 4–6 hr
		Prochlorperazine SR	10–15 mg b.i.d.
	Antihistamine	Diphenhydramine (Benadryl)	25–50 mg q. 4–6 hr
		Hydroxyzine (Atarax)	25–50 mg t.i.d.–q.i.d.
		Promethazine (Phenergan)	12.5–25 mg t.i.d.–q.i.d.
	Anticholinergic	Hyoscyamine (Levsin)	0.125–0.25 S.L. q. 4 hr
		Meclizine (Antivert)	12.5–25 mg b.i.d.–q.i.d.
	Anxiolytic	Lorazepam (Ativan)	1–2 mg q. 2–4 hr
	Prokinetic	Metoclopramide (Reglan)	10–40 mg q.i.d.
	Antiserotonin	Ondansetron (Zofran)	8 mg p.o., t.i.d.–q.i.d.
	Other	Dronabinol (Marinol)	2.5–10 mg b.i.d., t.i.d.
		Thiethylperazine (Torecan)	10 mg q.d.–t.i.d.
		Trimethobenzamide (Tigan)	250 mg t.i.d.–q.i.d.
Rectal suppositories	Antidopamine	Prochlorperazine (Compazine)	25 mg q. 6 hr
	Antihistamine	Promethazine (Phenergan)	12.5, 25, 50 mg t.i.d.–q.i.d.
	Other	Trimethobenzamide (Tigan)	200 mg t.i.d.–q.i.d.
Continuous intravenous infusion	Corticosteroids	Dexamethasone	8–100 mg/24 hr
	Antidopamine	Haloperidol (Haldol)	2.5–10 mg/24 hr
	Anticholinergic	Hyoscyamine (Levsin)	1–2 mg/24 hr
		Scopolamine	0.8–20 mg/24 hr
	Antiserotonin	Ondansetron (Zofran)	0.45 mg/kg/24 hr
	Prokinetic	Metoclopramide (Reglan)	20–80 mg/24 hr
Intermittent intravenous infusion	Corticosteroids	Dexamethasone	2–8 mg q. 4–6 hr
	Antidopamine	Haloperidol (Haldol)	0.5–2 mg q. 4–6 hr
		Prochlorperazine (Compazine)	5–10 mg q. 4–6 hr
	Antihistamine	Diphenhydramine (Benadryl)	25–50 mg q. 6 hr
	Anxiolytic	Lorazepam (Ativan)	1–2 mg q. 6–8 hr
	Prokinetic	Metoclopramide (Reglan)	10–20 mg q. 6 hr
	Antiserotonin	Ondansetron (Zofran)	4–8 mg q. 8 hr
		Granisetron (Kytril)	10 μg/kg q.d.
	Other	Dronabinol (Marinol)	5 mg/m^2 q. 4 hr (maximum, six doses/day)

the above measures fail. Side effects may include nausea, diarrhea, urinary frequency, and dizziness. Other nonpharmacologic treatments include eating ice chips and sucking on hard candy.

Oral Ulcers/Mucositis

Oral infection can have multiple causes. Aphthous ulcers are common and can be eased by topical corticosteroids, tetracycline mouthwash, or thalidomide. Oral candidiasis usually presents as adherent white plaques but can also present as erythema or angular cheilitis. Nystatin suspension is the usual treatment, but a 5-day course of oral ketoconazole, 200 mg daily, can also be used. Severe viral infection (herpes simplex or zoster) requires treatment with acyclovir, 200 mg every 4 hours for 5 days. Malignant ulcers are often associated with anaerobic bacteria and may respond to metronidazole, 400 to 500 mg orally or rectally every 12 hours or as a topical gel.[64]

SKIN SYMPTOMS

Pressure Ulcers

Pressure ulcers typically result from both intrinsic and extrinsic factors [see Table 9]. Major sites of pressure ulcers in terminally ill patients include the ear and the skin overlying the spine (apex of kyphosis), sacrum, greater femoral trochanter, head of the fibula, and malleolus. Prevention should emphasize these sites and should include daily visual inspection of them in patients at risk for pressure sores.

Prevention and treatment of pressure sores require targeting risk factors and minimizing them.[67] Caregivers need to minimize pressure by turning and repositioning the patient frequently and avoiding shear (sliding movement) and friction. They should be aware that even crumpled bedclothes can impair circulation. How a patient moves or is moved by caregivers needs to be assessed and monitored. Even with regular turning and careful lifting and positioning, special pressure surfaces or mattresses are sometimes needed.[64] Fragile skin that is at risk for breakdown should be covered with clear, occlusive dressings; pressure points should be covered with thin, hydrocolloid dressings.

Caregivers must keep the patient's skin clean and dry. Absorbent surfaces, urinary catheters, and rectal tubes may be helpful, but they must be used carefully because of their attendant complications.[49]

Nutrition is an important factor in both prevention and treatment. Good hydration, a diet that is high in protein and carbohydrates, and vitamin C supplements help maintain skin integrity and encourage healing.

If pressure ulcers develop, they should be covered with gel or colloid dressings, which keep the area moist, reduce pain, and can be left in place for several days. The pain of dressing changes can be eased by extra analgesia before each change.[64] The clinician should instruct caretakers to give oral pain medication one-half hour before the dressing change. The dose is determined by whether or not the patient is on regular opioid medications. If the patient is not on regular pain medications, start with 15 mg of immediate-release morphine. If the patient is on a regular opioid regimen, the predressing dose should be the same as the rescue dose.

Pressure ulcer management needs to be consistent with the overall goals of care. If maintenance or improvement of function is the goal and the patient's life expectancy is weeks to months, the ulcer should be treated according to the usual management guidelines. If the patient's life expectancy is very limited (e.g., days), the intent should be to optimize quality of life and minimize pain and discomfort (such as from excessive dressing changes or debridement).

Malignant Ulcers

For uncomplicated malignant ulcers, pain relief and wound care are managed in the same way as pressure ulcers. Malignant wounds can present special problems, however, which may include bleeding, exudate, infection, odor, and disfigurement. A bleeding malignant ulcer should be treated with radiation therapy, topical sucralfate, or topical tranexamic acid. Dirty ulcers should be debrided, which can be accomplished chemically. Altered body image from disfiguring wounds can be lessened with cavity foam dressings. Furthermore, empathetic listening is often therapeutic in itself. Anxiety, anger, or depression needs specific support, however[64] [see Chapter 12].

Foul-Smelling Wounds

Odors from wounds may be very distressing to patients, families, and caregivers and may lead to poor quality of care, as even professional caregivers tend to avoid sickening smells. Wound odors are usually the result of anaerobic infections or poor hygiene. Treat superficial infections with topical metronidazole or

---

Table 6 A Progressive Bowel Regimen for Patients Receiving Opioid Therapy[60]*

Step 1
Docusate, 100 mg b.i.d.
Senna, 1 tablet q.d. or b.i.d.

Step 2
Docusate, 100 mg b.i.d.
Senna, 2 tablets b.i.d.
Bisacodyl rectal suppositories, 1–2 after breakfast

Step 3
Docusate, 100 mg b.i.d.
Senna, 3 tablets b.i.d.
Bisacodyl rectal suppositories, 3–4 after breakfast

Step 4
Docusate, 100 mg b.i.d.
Senna, 4 tablets b.i.d.
Lactulose or sorbitol, 15 ml b.i.d.
Bisacodyl suppositories, 3–4 after breakfast

Step 5
Sodium phosphate or oil-retention enema; if no results, add a high-colonic tap-water enema

Step 6
Docusate, 100 mg b.i.d.
Senna, 4 tablets b.i.d.
Lactulose or sorbitol, 30 ml b.i.d.
Bisacodyl rectal suppositories, 3–4 after breakfast

Step 7
Docusate, 100 mg b.i.d.
Senna, 4 tablets b.i.d.
Lactulose or sorbitol, 30 ml q.i.d.
Bisacodyl rectal suppositories, 3–4 after breakfast

*The bowel regimen is started at the time of or before the initiation of opioid therapy, and it should be continued for the duration of opioid therapy. The clinician should start with step 1 and progress through higher steps until an effective regimen is found.

Table 7   Treatments for Constipation

Laxative Type	Mechanism	Agent	Dosage	Comment
Stimulant	Irritate the bowel and increase peristaltic activity	Prune juice	120–240 ml q.d. or b.i.d.	
		Senna	1–2 tablets p.o., q.h.s.	Titrate to effect; ≤ 8 tablets b.i.d.
		Bisacodyl	10–15 mg p.o., h.s.; or 10 mg p.r., after breakfast	Titrate to effect
Osmotic	Draw water into the bowel lumen, increase overall stool volume	Lactulose	30 ml p.o., q. 4–6 hr	Titrate to effect
		Sorbitol, 70% solution	2 ml/kg, up to 50 ml p.o., q.d.–t.i.d.	
		Milk of magnesia	1–2 tbsp, q.d.–t.i.d.	
		Magnesium citrate	1–2 bottles p.r.n.	
		Polyethylene glycol solution	1–4 L p.o.	Drink 8 oz q. 10 min until consumed
		Polyethylene glycol powder	17 g (1 tbsp) powder in 8 oz water, q.d.	2–4 days may be required to produce a bowel movement; increase dose as needed
Detergent (stool softeners)	Increase water content in stool by facilitating the dissolution of fat	Docusate sodium	1–2 capsules p.o., q.d.–b.i.d.	Titrate to effect
		Docusate calcium*	1–2 capsules p.o., q.d.–b.i.d.	Titrate to effect
Prokinetic agents	Stimulate the bowel's myenteric plexus, and increase peristaltic activity and stool movement	Metoclopramide	10–20 mg p.o., q. 6 hr	
Lubricant stimulants	Lubricate the stool and irritate the bowel, increasing peristaltic activity and stool movement	Glycerin suppositories	Daily	
		Mineral oil or peanut oil enema	Daily	
Large-volume enemas	Soften stool by increasing its water content; distend the colon and induce peristalsis	Warm-water enema	Daily	Addition of soapsuds irritates bowel wall to induce peristalsis
High-colonic enemas	Utilize gravity to bring fluid to more proximal parts of bowel	2 L of water or saline warmed to body temperature, hung on I.V. pole at ceiling level	Run in over 30 min, repeat q. 1 hr	

*Not available in the United States.

silver sulfadiazine. These agents are expensive, however; if a less costly alternative is required, a diluted hydrogen peroxide solution can be used.[49] For soft tissue infections, systemic metronidazole can be added to topical management.

To control odors, caregivers can place a pan containing kitty litter or activated charcoal under the patient's bed, provide adequate room ventilation, place an open cup of vinegar in the room, or burn a candle. Special charcoal-impregnated dressings placed over the odorous wound may also be helpful.[49]

Psychiatric Symptoms

Adjustment disorders, depression, anxiety, dementia, and delirium are the most common psychiatric problems encountered in dying patients.[68,69] Depending on the severity of the psychiatric problems, their management may be within the capacity of the primary care physician or may require referral [*see Chapter 12*].

DELIRIUM

Delirium occurs in 28% to 83% of terminally ill patients.[70] Symptoms of delirium include inability to maintain attention, waxing and waning of consciousness, psychomotor changes,

disturbance of sleep-wake cycle, disorientation, visual or auditory hallucinations, and problems with memory and language.[71] Other terms often used synonymously with delirium include acute confusional state, metabolic encephalopathy, and sundowning. In contrast to dementia, delirium is more rapid in onset (developing over hours to days), fluctuates in severity, is potentially reversible, and is associated with a lesser degree of memory impairment.

Delirium is a multifactorial syndrome, involving preexisting risk factors and precipitating factors that occur during hospitalization. Factors that predispose a patient to delirium include vision impairment, severe illness, cognitive impairment, and dehydration.[72] In older patients, cognitive impairment that is so mild as to be inapparent when such patients are well may nevertheless increase the risk of delirium. Precipitating factors include the use of physical restraints, malnutrition, taking more than three drugs, bladder catheter use, and any iatrogenic event.[72] Prevention of delirium can be accomplished by targeting risk factors.[72]

Management of delirium in the terminally ill patient includes correction of the cause and provision of symptomatic relief. In patients with morphine-induced delirium, opioid rotation from morphine to fentanyl may be effective in alleviating the delirium; because fentanyl works through different receptors, the

Table 8 Local Measures for Oral Problems[64]

Dry mouth
  Semifrozen fruit juice
  Frequent sips of cold water or water sprays
  Petroleum jelly rubbed on lips
Dirty mouth
  Regular brushing with soft toothbrush and toothpaste
  Pineapple chunks
  Cider and soda mouthwash
Infected mouth
  Tetracycline mouthwash, 250 mg every 8 hr (one capsule
    dissolved in 5 ml water)
Painful mouth
  Topical corticosteroids: betamethasone, 0.5 mg in 5 ml water,
    as mouthwash; or triamcinolone in carmellose paste
  Coating agents: sucralfate suspension as mouthwash,
    carmellose paste, carbenoxolone
  Topical anesthesia: benzocaine or lozenges containing local
    anesthetics

same degree of pain control may be accomplished with lower doses of narcotics.[73] Identification and treatment of underlying diseases or conditions are paramount—for example, give antibiotics for sepsis or oxygen for shortness of breath. In patients with underlying dementia, the possibility of untreated pain deserves special consideration. In the past, physicians were taught that the use of narcotic analgesics is dangerous in patients with dementia because those agents cause delirium. That is not true of a demented patient who becomes agitated or belligerent because of pain, however; in those cases, a dose of a narcotic analgesic may calm the patient within an hour or so. One study demonstrated that in patients 85 years of age or older with advanced dementia, treatment with low-dose, long-acting opioids can lessen agitation that is otherwise difficult to control.[74] The risk of undertreating severe pain should be of greater concern, both medically and ethically, than the risk of worsening delirium with analgesic medications.

Additional means of treating delirium include minimizing any sensory impairments by providing appropriate eyeglasses or hearing aids and maintaining a quiet, familiar, and reassuring setting. It is important to maintain communication with the patient, using frequent reorientation; familiar objects, places, and people; and avoidance of stimulus overload or deprivation.[75]

Pharmacologic symptom relief is best achieved with the use of an antipsychotic agent such as haloperidol or risperidone [*see Table 10*]. Benzodiazepines or sedatives should be used only if antipsychotic agents fail.[76]

Terminal Delirium

Delirium may be an irreversible part of the dying process. Many terminally ill patients have escalating restlessness, agitation, or hallucinations that can be relieved only with sedation.[77] When death is imminent, reversing the underlying causes of delirium is not possible. Instead, the clinician should focus on the management of the symptoms associated with the terminal delirium and bring comfort to the patient and family.

Benzodiazepines are widely used in the management of terminal delirium because they are anxiolytics, amnestics, skeletal muscle relaxants, and antiepileptics. Oral lorazepam (1 to 2 mg as an elixir, or the tablet predissolved in 0.5 to 1.0 ml of water and administered against the buccal mucosa) should be given every hour as needed; it will settle most patients at a daily dose of 2 to 10 mg. The lorazepam can then be given in divided doses, every 3 to 4 hours, to keep the patient settled. For a few extremely agitated patients, high doses of lorazepam—20 to 50 mg or more per 24 hours—may be required. A midazolam infusion (1 to 5 mg S.C. or I.V. every 1 hour, preceded by repeated loading boluses of 0.5 mg every 15 minutes to effect) may be a rapidly effective alternative.[49]

Palliative sedation When terminal delirium cannot be adequately controlled despite aggressive efforts to identify a tolerable therapy that does not compromise consciousness, it may be necessary to resort to palliative sedation. Most physicians define palliative sedation as the act of purposely inducing and maintaining a pharmacologically sedated and unconscious state, without the intent to cause death. A Japanese study of palliative sedation therapy in terminally ill cancer patients found that the technique is usually effective and safe, but that fatal complications related to sedation occur in a small number of patients.[78]

Palliative sedation is usually accomplished with benzodiazepines, neuroleptics, or barbiturates. Propofol may be useful for patients in whom traditional sedating agents have failed, such as patients with intractable nausea and vomiting.[79]

Once palliative sedation is initiated, the dosage of the sedative agent should not be increased unless the patient awakens or becomes restless, tachypneic, or tachycardic. Increasing the level of sedation in the absence of a clinical indication might imply that the physician is intending to hasten death, which if true would cross the line between palliative sedation and physician-assisted suicide or euthanasia [*see Chapter 10*].[80]

Terminal Wean

Mechanical ventilation is often tried in patients with respiratory distress, when there is hope that their condition will improve. This is best referred to as a time-limited trial. If reversal of the acute medical condition proves unsuccessful, the physician needs to discuss discontinuance of ventilation with the family.

Terminal ventilation withdrawal should be approached with attention to ensuring the patient's comfort and to enhancing the

Table 9 Risk Factors for Pressure Ulcers

Intrinsic	Extrinsic
Malnutrition	Pressure
Protein	Shear
Vitamin C	Trauma
Zinc	Friction
Diminished mobility	Crumpled bedclothes
Tissue fragility	Restraints
Anemia	Bed rails
Dehydration	Poor hygiene
Hypotension	Hospital equipment
Poor peripheral perfusion	Oxygen tubing
Incontinence	Heart monitor wires
Neurologic deficit	
Sensory	
Motor	
Older age	
Coma	
Moribund state	

Table 10 Drug Treatment for Agitation or Delirium[33]

Acute	Haloperidol, 0.5–5 mg p.o., p.r., I.M., I.V., or S.C.; titrate until calm
	Chlorpromazine, 1 mg I.V. q. 2 min until calm
Chronic	Haloperidol, 0.5–5 mg p.o. or p.r., b.i.d. (maximum dose, 100 mg/day)
	Thioridazine, 10–25 mg p.o., b.i.d. (maximum dose, 800 mg/day)
	Risperidone, 0.5 mg p.o., b.i.d.; increase by 0.5 mg b.i.d., q. 24 hr (maximum dose, 6 mg/day)
	Chlorpromazine, 10–50 mg p.o. or p.r., b.i.d. (maximum dose, 500 mg/day)
	Olanzepine, 2.5–15 mg p.o., q.d.

family's access to the bedside.[81] Miles[82] recommends a 10-step protocol, which applies to unconscious patients dependent on a ventilator:

1. Shut off and remove all monitors and alarms from the patient's room.
2. Remove equipment that impedes access to the patient's hands (e.g., intravenous lines, pulse oximeter, restraints). Hands are for holding.
3. Remove encumbering or disfiguring devices from the bedside.
4. Invite the family to be with the patient.
5. Quietly and personally request that pressors be turned off and that intravenous infusions be set to keep veins open.
6. Watch for distressing symptoms, such as agitation, tachypnea, or seizures; treat appropriately (e.g., with diazepam) if they appear.
7. Turn the fraction of inspired oxygen (F_IO_2) down to 20% and observe the patient for respiratory distress.
8. If the patient appears comfortable, remove the endotracheal tube with a clean towel in hand.
9. Educate and debrief the house staff and nursing staff about the process.
10. Consider contacting the family during the bereavement period, whether by letter or visit.

The goal is for a peaceful, pain-free death for the patient and a supportive, comfortable environment for the family and friends. It is important to warn family that a patient removed from the ventilator may live for hours to days afterward and to reassure them that all measures necessary to ensure comfort during the dying process will be used.

Symptom Management in the Last Hours of Life

The final hours of living can be some of the most important ones for the patient and for family. Managed well, they can lead to a peaceful death and healthy grief and bereavement.[49]

During the final hours, patients usually need skilled care around the clock. Ideally, the environment will allow family and friends both easy access to their loved one and privacy. All who are present should presume that the unconscious patient hears everything.[49]

It is important to be knowledgeable about the normal physiologic changes that occur in the last hours of life and to educate the patient's family about them. Reassure the family that dehydration in the final hours of living does not cause distress and

may stimulate endorphin release that adds to the patient's sense of well-being. Moaning and groaning, although frequently misinterpreted as pain, is often terminal delirium (see above). Decreased hepatic and renal function lead to the accumulation of metabolites, which may cause terminal delirium. Only essential medications should be used, at appropriate doses as needed.[49]

In the final hours of life, many persons in semiconscious or unconscious states are unable to swallow saliva reflexively or to cough up mucus. This inability to clear secretions from the oropharynx and trachea results in the so-called death rattle—noisy respiration as the secretions move up and down with expiration and inspiration. The cause and meaning of death rattle should be explained to the family, and an anticholinergic drug should be administered to the patient to reduce pharyngeal secretions (e.g., hyoscine as a single parenteral dose or by continuous infusion, or scopolamine by patch).[83] At times, it may be necessary to reposition the patient or to gently administer suction to the airway with the use of a soft catheter. Reassure the family that despite the way the breathing sounds, the patient is not uncomfortable.

The removal of the body too soon after death can be even more upsetting to the family than the moment of death; the family should be allowed time with the body.[49] After the patient has died, follow-up with the family is important to ensure that grief and bereavement are progressing normally [*see Chapter 12*].

The authors have no commercial relationships with manufacturers of products or providers of services discussed in this chapter.

References

1. O'Neill B, Fallon M: Principles of palliative care. BMJ 315:801, 1997
2. Ingham J, Portenoy RK: The measurement of pain and other symptoms. Oxford Textbook of Palliative Medicine. Doyle D, Hanks GW, MacDonald N, Eds. Oxford University Press, Oxford, England, 1993, p 202
3. Grossman SA, Sheidler VR, Swedeen K, et al: Correlation of patient and caregiver ratings of cancer pain. J Pain Symptom Manage 6:53, 1991
4. Clipp EC, George LK: Patients with cancer and their spouse caregivers: perceptions of the illness experience. Cancer 69:1074, 1992
5. Homsi J, Walsh D, Rivera N, et al: Symptom evaluation in palliative medicine: patient report vs systematic assessment. Support Care Cancer 14:1, 2006
6. Bruera E, Kuehn N, Miller M, et al: Symptom Assessment System: a simple method for the assessment of palliative care patients. J Palliative Care 7:6, 1991
7. Donnelly S, Walsh D: The symptoms of advanced cancer. Semin Oncol 22(suppl 3):67, 1995
8. Portenoy RK, Thaler HT, Kornblith AB, et al: The Memorial Symptom Assessment Scale: an instrument for the evaluation of symptom prevalence, characteristics and distress. Eur J Cancer 30A:1326, 1994
9. Tranmer JE, Heyland D, Dudgeon D, et al: Measuring the symptom experience of seriously ill cancer and noncancer hospitalized patients near the end of life with the Memorial Symptom Assessment Scale. J Pain Symptom Manage 25:420, 2003
10. Camp L: A comparison of nurses' record assessment of pain with perceptions of pain as described by cancer patients. Cancer Nurs 11:237, 1988
11. Teske K, Daut R, Cleeland C: Relationships between nurses' observations and patients' self-reports of pain. Pain 16:289, 1983
12. Bernabei R, Gambassi G, Lapane K, et al: Management of pain in elderly patients with cancer. SAGE Study Group. Systematic Assessment of Geriatric Drug Use via Epidemiology. JAMA 279:1877, 1998
13. Feldts KS, Ryder MB, Miles S: Treatment of pain in cognitively impaired compared with cognitively intact older patients with hip fracture. J Am Geriatr Soc 46:1069, 1998
14. Morrison RS, Siu AL: A comparison of pain and its treatment in advanced dementia and cognitively intact patients with hip fracture. J Pain Symptom Manage 19:240, 2000
15. Ferrell B, Ferrell B, Rivera L: Pain in cognitively impaired nursing home patients. J Pain Symptom Manage 10:591, 1995
16. Duggleby W, Lander J: Cognitive status and postoperative pain: older adults. J Pain Symptom Manage 9:19, 1994
17. Lynch EP, Lazor MA, Gellis JE, et al: The impact of postoperative pain on the development of postoperative delirium. Anesth Analg 86:781, 1998
18. Super A: Going one step further: skilled pain assessment and the art of adjuvant analgesia. Am J Hosp Palliat Care 14:279, 1997
19. Ahmedzai S: Current strategies for pain control. Ann Oncol 8(suppl 3):521, 1997

20. Sallerin-Caute B, Lazorthes Y, Deguine O, et al: Does intrathecal morphine in the treatment of cancer pain induce the development of tolerance? Neurosurgery 42:44, 1998

21. Weiss SC, Emanuel LL, Fairclough DL, et al: Understanding the experience of pain in terminally ill patients. Lancet 357:1311, 2001

22. Mercadante S, Fulfaro F, Casuccio A: A randomised controlled study on the use of anti-inflammatory drugs in patients with cancer pain on morphine therapy: effects on dose-escalation and a pharmacoeconomic analysis. Eur J Cancer 38:1358, 2002

23. Smith TJ, Staats PS, Deer T, et al: Randomized clinical trial of an implantable drug delivery system compared with comprehensive medical management for refractory cancer pain: impact on pain, drug-related toxicity, and survival. J Clin Oncol 20:40, 2002

24. Mercadante S, Catala E, Arcuri E, et al: Celiac plexus block for pancreatic cancer pain: factors influencing pain, symptoms and quality of life. J Pain Symptom Manage 26:1140, 2003

25. Plews-Ogan M, Owens JE, Goodman M, et al: A pilot study evaluating mindfulness-based stress reduction and massage for the management of chronic pain. J Gen Intern Med 20:1136, 2005

26. Allard P, Maunsell E, Labbe J, et al: Educational interventions to improve cancer pain control: a systematic review. J Palliat Med 4:191, 2001

27. Reuben DB, Mor V: Dyspnea in terminally ill cancer patients. Chest 89:234, 1986

28. Hockely JM, Dunlop R, Davies RJ: Survey of distressing symptoms in dying patients and their families in hospital and their response to a symptom control team. BMJ 296:1715, 1988

29. Ventafridda V, De Conno F, Ripamonti C, et al: Quality-of-life assessment during a palliative care programme. Ann Oncol 1:415, 1990

30. Carrieri VK, Janson-Bjerklie S: The sensation of dyspnea: a review. Heart Lung 13:436, 1984

31. Bruera E, Macmilan K, Pither J, et al: Effects of morphine on the dyspnea of terminal cancer patients. J Pain Symptom Manage 5:341, 1990

32. Cohen MH, Anderson AJ, Krasnow SH, et al: Continuous intravenous infusion of morphine for severe dyspnea. South Med J 84:229, 1991

33. Jennings AL, Davies AN, Higgins JP, et al: A systematic review of the use of opioids in the management of dyspnoea. Thorax 57:939, 2002

34. Abernethy AP, Currow DC, Frith P, et al: Randomised, double blind, placebo controlled crossover trial of sustained release morphine for the management of refractory dyspnoea. BMJ 327:523, 2003

35. Bruera E, Neumann CM: Management of specific symptom complexes in patients receiving palliative care. CMAJ 159:1242, 1998

36. Booth S, Wade R, Johnson M, et al: The use of oxygen in the palliation of breathlessness: a report of the expert working group of the Scientific Committee of the Association of Palliative Medicine. Respir Med 98:66, 2004

37. Muers MF, Round CE: Palliation of symptoms in non–small cell lung cancer: a study by the Yorkshire Regional Cancer Organization Thoracic Group. Thorax 48:339, 1993

38. Stegman MB: Non-pain symptoms. Pain and Symptom Control in Palliative Medicine. Stegman MB, Ed. Hospice Resources, Fort Myers, Florida, 1997, p 6.1

39. Fuller RW, Jackson DM: Physiology and treatment of cough. Thorax 45:425, 1990

40. Estfan B, LeGrand S: Management of cough in advanced cancer. J Support Oncol 2:523, 2004

41. Homsi J, Walsh D, Nelson KA, et al: A phase II study of hydrocodone for cough in advanced cancer. Am J Hosp Palliat Care 19:49, 2002

42. Bruera E: ABC of palliative care: anorexia, cachexia, and nutrition. BMJ 315:1219, 1997

43. Bruera E, Miller L, MacCallion J, et al: Cognitive failure in patients with terminal cancer: a prospective study. Proc Am Soc Clin Oncol 9:308, 1990

44. Holden CM: Anorexia in the terminally ill cancer patient: the emotional impact on the patient and the family. Hosp J 7:73, 1991

45. Ganzini L, Goy ER, Miller LL, et al: Nurses' experiences with hospice patients who refuse food and fluids to hasten death. N Engl J Med 349:359, 2003

46. Strang P: Quality of life is the most important goal in nutritional support of the dying. Lakartidningen 97:1141, 2000

47. Bruera E, Macmillan K, Hanson J, et al: A controlled trial of megestrol acetate on appetite, caloric intake, nutritional status, and other symptoms in patients with advanced cancer. Cancer 66:1279, 1990

48. Tchekmedyian NS, Hariri L, Siau J, et al: Megestrol acetate in cancer anorexia and weight loss. Proc Am Soc Clin Oncol 9:336, 1990

49. Emanuel LL, von Gunten CF, Ferris FD: The Education for Physicians on End-of-Life Care (EPEC) Curriculum, Institute for Ethics at the American Medical Association, 1999, p 14

50. Yavuzsen T, Davis MP, Walsh D, et al: Systematic review of the treatment of cancer-associated anorexia and weight loss. J Clin Oncol 23:8500, 2005

51. Volicer L: Ethical issues in the treatment of advanced Alzheimers dementia: hospice approach. Clinical Management of Alzheimers Disease. Aspen Publishers, Rockville, Maryland, 1988, p 167

52. Finucane TE, Christmas C, Travis K: Tube feedings in patients with advanced dementia: a review of the evidence. JAMA 284:1365, 1999

53. Meier DE, Ahronheim JC, Morris J, et al: High short-term mortality in hospitalized patients with advanced dementia: lack of benefit of tube feeding. Arch Intern Med 161:594, 2001

54. Pasman HR, Onwuteaka-Philipsen BD, Kriegsman DM, et al: Discomfort in nursing home patients with severe dementia in whom artificial nutrition and hydration is forgone. Arch Intern Med 165:1729, 2005

55. Luchins DJ, Hanrahan P: What is appropriate health care for end-stage dementia? J Am Geriatr Soc 41:25, 1993

56. Reuben DB, Mor V: Nausea and vomiting in terminally ill cancer patients. Arch Intern Med 146:2021, 1986

57. Baines MJ: ABC of palliative care: nausea, vomiting and intestinal obstruction. BMJ 315:1148, 1997

58. Fallon M, O'Neill B: ABC of palliative care: constipation and diarrhea. BMJ 315:1293, 1997

59. Meiring PJ, Joubert G: Constipation in elderly patients attending a polyclinic. S Afr Med J 88:888, 1998

60. Carney MT, Meier DE: Palliative care and end-of-life issues. Anaesthesiol Clin North America 18:183, 2000

61. Ripamonti C: Malignant bowel obstruction in advanced and terminal cancer patients. European Journal of Palliative Care 1:23, 1994

62. Adler DG: Management of malignant colonic obstruction. Curr Treat Options Gastroenterol 8:231, 2005

63. Baron TH: Colonic stenting: technique, technology, and outcomes for malignant and benign disease. Gastrointest Endosc Clin N Am 15:757, 2005

64. Regnard C, Allport S, Stephenson L: ABC of palliative care: mouth care, skin care, and lymphoedema. BMJ 315:1002, 1997

65. Atkinson JC, Grisius M, Massey W: Salivary hypofunction and xerostomia: diagnosis and treatment. Dent Clin North Am 49:309, 2005

66. Narhi TO, Meurman JH, Ainamo A: Xerostomia and hyposalivation: causes, consequences and treatment in the elderly. Drugs and Aging 15:103, 1999

67. Brem H, Lyder C: Protocol for the successful treatment of pressure ulcers. Am J Surg 188(1A suppl):9, 2004

68. Breitbart W, Passik SD: Psychiatric aspects of palliative care. Oxford Textbook of Palliative Medicine. Doyle D, Hanks GW, MacDonald N, Eds. Oxford University Press, Oxford, England, 1993, p 609

69. Barraclough J: ABC of palliative care: depression, anxiety, and confusion. BMJ 315:1365, 1997

70. Casarett DJ, Inouye SK, American College of Physicians-American Society of Internal Medicine End-of-Life Care Consensus Panel: Diagnosis and management of delirium near the end of life. Ann Intern Med 135:32, 2001

71. Lipowski ZJ: Delirium. Acute Confusional States. Oxford University Press, New York, 1990

72. Inouye SK: Prevention of delirium in hospitalized older patients: risk factors and targeted intervention strategies. Ann Med 32:257, 2000

73. Tajima T, Tani K, Matsubara T, et al: Opioid rotation from morphine to fentanyl in delirious cancer patients: an open-label trial. J Pain Symptom Manage 30:96, 2005

74. Manfredi PL, Breuer B, Wallenstein S, et al: Opioid treatment for agitation in patients with advanced dementia. Int J Geriatr Psychiatry 18:700, 2003

75. Rummans TA, Evans JM, Krahn LE, et al: Delirium in elderly patients: evaluation and management. Mayo Clin Proc 70:989, 1995

76. Pan CX, Meier DE: Clinical aspects of end-of-life care. Annual Review of Gerontology and Geriatrics, Year 2000: Focus on the End-of-life: Scientific and Social Issues, Lawton P, Ed. Springer-Verlag, New York, 2000, p 273

77. Fainsinger RL, Waller A, Bercovici M, et al: A multicentre international study of sedation for uncontrolled symptoms in terminally ill patients. Palliat Med 14:257, 2000

78. Morita T, Chinone Y, Ikenaga M, et al: Efficacy and safety of palliative sedation therapy: a multicenter, prospective, observational study conducted on specialized palliative care units in Japan. J Pain Symptom Manage 30:320, 2005

79. Lundstrom S, Zachrisson U, Furst CJ: When nothing helps: propofol as sedative and antiemetic in palliative cancer care. J Pain Symptom Manage 30:570, 2005

80. Rousseau P: Existential suffering and palliative sedation: a brief commentary with a proposal for clinical guidelines. Am J Hospice Palliat Care 18:299, 2001

81. von Gunten C, Weissman DE: Ventilator withdrawal protocol. J Palliat Med 6:773, 2003

82. Miles S: Protocol for rapid withdrawal of ventilator support in anticipation of death. Ethical Currents 45(Spring), 1996

83. Doyle D: Domiciliary Terminal Care. Churchill Livingstone, Edinburgh, Scotland, 1987

12 Management of Psychosocial Issues in Terminal Illness

Jennifer Rhodes-Kropf, M.D., and Ned H. Cassem, M.D., F.A.C.P.

Like all good medical care, palliative care addresses patients' needs at many levels. The physical deterioration as death approaches can challenge the ingenuity and equanimity of health care professionals [*see Chapters 10 and 11*]. Yet symptom management is only one aspect of the care that these patients need; the psychosocial and spiritual problems that arise at the end of life also require attention.

A fatal illness—such as untreatable heart disease, terminal cancer, or AIDS—brings with it not only physical pain but also emotional suffering. Fear is prominent. The body, once regarded as a friend, may seem more like a dormant adversary programmed for betrayal. Even innocuous bodily changes may be interpreted as ominous. Patients who have been diagnosed with a disease become fearful before disease symptoms occur. Cancer patients, for example, fear pain, shortness of breath, nausea and vomiting, anorexia, dyspnea, and isolation.[1] Well before the terminal stages of an illness, patients fear the unknown, losing autonomy, disfigurement, dementia, and, last but not least, becoming a burden to their families.

The stress of terminal illness may manifest itself in many ways. Patients may deny or be unable to accept diagnosis or treatment; they may have unrealistic hopes of being cured, and they may persistently ask why there is no improvement. They may express anxiety, often extreme, with near panic and unspecified fears about dying. They may experience intense feelings of ambivalence and guilt regarding their personal relationships.

Considering the severe distress that is frequently involved, it is remarkable how well most patients do cope with a terminal illness and its treatments. The unique set of coping mechanisms that they have used to maintain self-esteem and stability in the past plays a vital role in this process. Religion and spirituality may be most helpful to patients and families at the end of a patient's life and should therefore be recognized and encouraged.

When a patient is dying, the entire family is the appropriate focus of treatment. A family member may be the first to notice a symptom, such as a personality change, in the patient or in another family member and can thus serve as an indispensable historian. The physician must also contend with the psychosocial forces that can lead to family fragmentation and interfere with care. A family member may have more difficulty than the patient in coping with the illness; this may irritate and distract caregivers and ultimately disrupt the relationship between the physician and the family. For example, the physician may be inclined to schedule visits to the patient so as to avoid encounters with the family. This could seriously jeopardize the patient's treatment and the chance to make the patient's death meaningful and dignified. After the patient's death, the survivors may experience abnormal grieving patterns that deserve medical attention.

Most of the psychosocial aspects of palliative care are within the capability of the primary care physician. In some cases, however, psychiatric consultation may be necessary to help the dying patient cope with major depression, personality disorders, continuous treatment-resistant pain, substance abuse, or grieving.

Preliminary Considerations

BREAKING BAD NEWS

Psychosocial care of the patient with terminal illness begins with delivery of the diagnosis. Because there are so many possible reactions a patient may have when informed of the diagnosis, it is helpful to have some plan of action in mind that will permit the greatest range and freedom of response by the patient. Guidelines have been developed for communicating bad news.[2] When the diagnosis is made and it is time to inform the patient, the physician should meet with the patient in a private place. The spouse (and sometimes the family) should be included in the discussion, unless there is a good reason not to do so. If possible, the patient should be informed ahead of time that after all the tests are completed the physician will review the results and discuss treatment plans in detail. With inpatients, the physician should sit down at the bedside to deliver bad news. Standing while conveying bad news may be regarded by a patient as unkind and expressive of wanting to leave as quickly as possible. If the patient is tested as an outpatient and returns home before the results are known, he or she should be told that the diagnostic information is too important to convey by phone, and a meeting to discuss the results should be arranged. Relaying bad news by phone may be perceived by patients as thoughtless, even though they may have asked for information. A physician must also be prepared to respond to a patient who wishes no or minimal information about the diagnosis.

When the findings are life threatening (e.g., a biopsy positive for malignancy), how can the news best be conveyed? A good opening statement is one that is (1) rehearsed so that it can be delivered calmly, (2) brief (three sentences or less), (3) designed to encourage further dialogue, and (4) reassuring of continued attention and care. A typical delivery might go as follows: "The tests confirmed that your tumor is malignant. I have therefore asked the surgeon (or radiotherapist or oncologist) to speak with you, examine you, and make recommendations for treatment. After this, we can discuss how we should proceed." Silence and quiet observation at this point will yield more valuable information about the patient than any other part of the exchange. What are the emotional reactions? What sort of coping is seen at the very start? While observing, one can decide how best to continue with the discussion. Just sitting with the patient for a period of time, however, is the most important part of this initial encounter with a grim reality that both patient and physician will continue to confront together, possibly for a long time.

TELLING THE TRUTH

Given the difficulties that can follow the disclosure of a life-threatening illness, it may be tempting to avoid telling the patient the diagnosis. This tactic has ancient roots: Hippocrates himself recommended concealing bad news from patients, lest they become discouraged.[3] Nevertheless, most empirical studies in which patients were asked whether they wanted to be told the truth about malignancy have indicated an overwhelming desire in the affirmative. Of 740 patients in a cancer-detection clinic who were asked before diagnosis whether they wanted to be told their diagnosis, 99% said that they did.[4] Another group of patients in this clinic were asked the same question after the diagnosis was established, and 89% of them replied affirmatively, as did 82% of patients in still another group who had been examined and found to be free of malignancy.

Truth telling entails eliciting the patient's concerns. Studies indicate the clinician's use of specific communication skills enhances a patient's disclosure of his or her concerns.[5] Such communications skills include making eye contact with the patient, asking open-ended questions, responding to the patient's affect, and demonstrating empathy. The desire for truth telling may vary among different ethnic groups.[6] In a study of elderly persons in the United States, Korean Americans and Mexican Americans were less likely than African Americans and European Americans to believe that a patient should be told the diagnosis of metastatic cancer.[7] However, a population study in Hong Kong reported that the majority of persons canvassed would want to know if they had terminal cancer; this finding is at odds with the cultural preference of many Chinese, who usually prefer to withhold diagnostic information from terminally ill family members.[8] This study emphasizes that cultural preferences give only general indications of a patient's readiness to hear bad news; truth telling ultimately depends on the physician's assessment of what the patient wants to know and is prepared to know about the diagnosis. Socioeconomic factors may also be involved in a patient's willingness to hear bad news: younger age and higher income and education make patients more likely to want detailed diagnostic information.[9]

Is the truth harmful? Gerle and colleagues[10] studied 101 patients who were divided into two groups, with one group, along with their families, being told the frank truth of their diagnoses and the other group being excluded from discussion of the diagnosis (although the patients' families were informed). Initially, there appeared to be greater emotional upset in the group of patients and families who were informed together. The investigators observed in follow-up, however, that the emotional difficulties of the families of the patients who were shielded from the truth far outweighed those of the patients and families that were told the diagnosis simultaneously. In general, empirical studies support the idea that the truth about the diagnosis is desired by terminally ill patients and does not harm those to whom it is told. Honesty sustains the relationship with a dying person rather than jeopardizing it.[11] Individual variations in willingness to hear the initial diagnosis are extreme, however, and diagnosis is entirely different from prognosis. Many patients have said that they were grateful to their physician for telling them they had a malignancy. Very few, however, reacted positively to being told that they were dying. In our experience, "Do I have cancer?" is a common question, whereas "Am I dying?" is a rare one. The question about dying is more commonly heard from patients who are dying rapidly, such as those in cardiogenic shock.

Honest communication of the diagnosis by no means precludes later avoidance or even denial of the truth of the diagnosis. In two studies, patients who had been explicitly told their diagnosis (using the words cancer or malignancy) were asked 3 weeks later what they had been told: in both studies, about 20% of the patients sampled denied that their condition was cancerous or malignant.[12,13] Croog and colleagues[14] interviewed 345 men 3 weeks after myocardial infarction; 20% of those patients said they had not had a heart attack. All had been explicitly told their diagnosis. For a person to function effectively, truth's piercing voice may be muted or even excluded from awareness. Denial can reduce psychological distress, and preliminary evidence

suggests that in women with nonmetastatic breast cancer, it may be associated with prolonged survival.[15] However, information-seeking behavior and fighting spirit have been more consistently associated with higher rates of recurrence-free survival 5 and 10 years after diagnosis of breast cancer.[16,17] Communicating a diagnosis honestly, though difficult, is easier than the labors that lie ahead. Telling the truth is merely a way to begin, but it provides a firm basis on which to build a relationship of trust.

COMMUNICATING WITH THE PATIENT

The most important component of communication is listening. The real issue is not what you tell your patients but, rather, what you let your patients tell you.[1] Most people are afraid to let dying patients say what is on their minds. If a patient who is presumed to be 3 months from death says, "My plan was to buy a new car in 6 months, but I guess I won't have to worry about that now," a poor listener might say nothing or, "Right. Don't worry about it." A better listener might ask, "What kind of car were you thinking about?" In a study of 126 patients with incurable cancer, 98% wanted their physicians to be realistic about their health status, to provide an opportunity to ask questions, and to acknowledge them as an individual when discussing prognosis.[18]

It is essential to get to know the patient as a person. The best way to recognize and acknowledge the person's worth is to learn those features of his or her history and nature that make him or her unique. Encourage dying persons to tell their stories. Learn about significant areas of the patient's life—such as family, work, or school—and chat about common interests. This is the most natural way to give the patient the sense that she or he is known and appreciated.

Patients occasionally complain about professionals and visitors who regard them as "the dying patient," not as a unique person. The physician can help dissolve communication barriers for staff members by showing them the remarkable qualities of each patient. Comments such as, "She has 34 grandchildren," or, "This woman was an Olympic sprinter," convey information that helps other members of the health care team appreciate their patient and to find something to talk about with them. Listen for the patient's own conversational cues whenever possible. Awkwardness subsides when a patient is appreciated as a real person and not merely "a breast cancer patient." This rescue from anonymity is essential to prevent a sense of isolation. The most important communication is often not verbal. A pat on the arm, a wave, a wink, or a grin communicates important reassurances. Back rubs and physical examinations can also be an opportunity to convey reassurance.

Psychosocial Support during Terminal Illness

The diagnosis of a terminal illness impacts the patient's relationships with family, friends, and coworkers and can thus undermine the patient's sense of self. Although death is a natural part of life, the adjustment to diminished function and role in relationships can be stressful, both for the patient and the patient's family.

FAMILY AND FRIENDS

Family members and friends must be helped to support the patient and one another. To provide this help, the physician must get to know both the patient and the family members. When patients are permitted to give support to their families, they often feel they are less of a burden.

One must appreciate the fact that for family and close friends, a fatal illness of a loved one may be the only event important enough to resolve long-standing conflicts. Peacemaking should be a priority. Specific plans for the family are important. The writing of wills, the clarification of family history, the review of memorable family gatherings and achievements, the carrying out of such family projects as trips or photo-album reviews, and planning a funeral or memorial service are all important activities.

The care of a dying person can be a process of mutual growth for the patient and the family. Just as the deterioration of a person with a fatal disease can be threatening (family members may feel both horrified at the prospect of the same thing happening to them and helpless to assist), the response of the dying person to the challenge may be not only edifying but also an invaluable lesson in coping. Indeed, family members who act as caregivers report strong positive emotions regarding the opportunity to express their love through care. Those caregivers may experience extreme grief after the patient's death, however, and may require special support and attention from health care providers at that time.[19]

Near the end of life, a patient may be too weak to communicate by speech, and sometimes, consciousness itself may be difficult to assess. Most patients who have lost the ability to communicate have a period when they can still hear or perceive those in attendance. Family feelings of helplessness can be minimized by reading especially meaningful passages to the dying person (e.g., the daily headlines, articles by favorite authors or columnists, poetry, passages from the Bible, the Dow-Jones average, sports scores, and letters new and old). Conversations should make natural reference to the person as though hearing and understanding were intact. Singing favorite songs, playing favorite music, or praying aloud may increase the sense of unity and purpose for the family. Although the patient may never be able to tell us how important that time is, an occasional incident will do so dramatically, as when a supposedly unconscious person suddenly smiles appropriately, gestures, or even speaks. Often, this conveys gratitude for the attention given to him or her, which is very rewarding for the loved ones in attendance.

The end of life is an opportunity to educate the younger generation. Whenever possible, children should be included in all the planning, meetings, discussions, activities, and care, as well as the final attendance at death. Children can learn that death need not be violent or terrifying and that we face our losses best when we face them together.

Investigators have consistently learned that the visits of children are as likely as any other intervention to bring consolation and relief to the terminally ill patient. How can one determine whether a particular child should visit a dying patient? No better approach has been found than asking the child directly whether he or she wants to visit.

Ideally, this mutual work at the end of life will confirm the dying person's sense of self. It also can give family, friends, and caregivers the wonderful feeling that they have provided good care and safe passage.

OCCUPATION AND WORK

Work is critical for the self-esteem of many people. Many people begin to feel less valuable when work ceases or they retire, and the approaching end of life may intensify a sense of failure. The continuation of work for as long as feasible, as well as continued contact with work colleagues, can remind the dying of who they are and what they have accomplished. It encourages

the belief that they are remembered and respected, regardless of their illness. Similarly, continued involvement in recreational activities can be very satisfying.

Near the end of life, a person is often too disabled to get around or to contact colleagues and friends. Wherever possible, such contact should be arranged for and encouraged.

RELIGION AND SPIRITUALITY

Studies find that people who have a strong internalized faith possess a resource that helps significantly in coping with a fatal illness.[1,20-23] It is a well-documented finding that religious persons usually belong to a community that can be unusually thoughtful and generous in providing support. However, the community may not know of the patient's plight and may need to be contacted. Thus, the appreciation of a person's religion or spirituality is extremely important.

The Physician's Psychological Role in Patient Care

The first responsibility of the caregiver, as Saunders[24] points out, is "above all to listen." A suffering person often wants to communicate just how awful a fatal illness is. Words from the caregiver may be irrelevant: "When no answers exist," says Saunders, "one can offer silent attention."

It is important to be aware of the impact that patients' feelings can have on one's own mood and the amount of time spent with the patient. The relentless approach of death from cancer or AIDS may leave a patient with feelings of terror, hopelessness, and despair. Those feelings tend to be contagious, intensifying our feelings of impotence. A caregiver's own helplessness and despair may result in neglect or avoidance of the patient or feelings that the patient would be better off dead. Sensing that a patient is burdensome to caregivers can be devastating to the patient who looks to a doctor or nurse for some sense of hope.[25] In one study of terminal cancer patients, the majority of patients (87%) indicated that seeing their physician nervous or uncomfortable in their presence did not promote hope.[16] Thus, it is of the utmost importance that caregivers remain empathetic and reassure patients that they will continue to be there for them at all stages of their illness and that caregivers learn to live with negative feelings and resist the urge to avoid certain patients—attitudes that could convey that care of a patient is difficult for us or that the patient no longer matters to us.

COMPASSION

Of all attributes in physicians and nurses, none is more highly valued by terminally ill patients than compassion. Although they may never convey it precisely by words, some physicians and nurses are able to tell the patient that they are genuinely touched by his or her predicament. Although universally praised as a quality for a health professional, compassion exacts a cost that is usually overlooked in professional training. This cost is conveyed by its two Latin roots: *com*, meaning with, and *passio*, from *pati*, meaning to suffer—that is, to suffer with another person. It is important for caregivers to have a source of support for themselves—such as colleagues, friends, and family—so that they can continue to be there for their patients.[26]

CHEERFULNESS

The possessor of a gentle and appropriate sense of humor can bring relief to all parties involved. Often, patients provide this, and their wit may soften many a difficult incident. Humor needs to be used sensitively, however: forced or inappropriate mirth with a sick person can increase feelings of distance and isolation.

CONSISTENCY AND PERSEVERANCE

Dying patients have a realistic fear of progressive isolation. The physician or nurse who regularly visits the sickroom provides tangible proof of continued support and concern. A brief visit is far better than no visit at all; the patient may not even be able to tolerate a prolonged visit. Do continue to visit: patients are quick to identify those who show interest at first but gradually disappear from the scene. Stay the course even if this means that you must listen to repeated or irrelevant complaints.

The Patient's Psychological Response to Terminal Illness

Any serious illness inflicts some loss on the patient. A diagnosis itself, with no change in subjective symptoms, can cause a feeling of loss, as concepts of self and plans for the future are swept away.

The emotional reactions to a myocardial infarction serve as a model for the reactions of a person who has experienced physical loss. In a series of 149 coronary patients whose emotional difficulties were severe enough to warrant psychiatric consultation, the majority of problems during the first 2 days stemmed from fear and anxiety. These patients generally showed a sequence of emotions beginning with anxiety, followed shortly thereafter by denial (at this stage, a few wanted to sign out of the hospital) and then by despondency, which sometimes persisted. A final group of management problems, related mostly to dependency or personality disorders, rounded out the sequence.[27]

In essence, this reaction pattern suggests that the most common difficulty for a patient immediately after admission is fear. The patient fears imminent death, the presence or return of pain or breathlessness, or some vague but ominous threat to well-being. As symptoms stabilize or subside, the patient is likely to imagine that admission symptoms were false alarms and, in some cases, to insist on signing out of the hospital. When the diagnostic tests confirm the presence of myocardial infarction, however, the patient is confronted with the reality of the illness and feels demoralized. As hospitalization continues, any personality flaws (e.g., passive aggression) further complicate interactions between the patient and the hospital personnel. The sequence of acute onset of illness, fear, stabilization, denial, confirmation of illness, and depression provides a convenient framework for assessing the mental state of an individual hospitalized for any serious illness.

FEAR

Anxiety and despondency are the most common emotional reactions to illness. Panic distorts personality as nothing else does. Yet fear assumes many guises. If a patient seems impossible to deal with on the first day of hospitalization, the reason very likely is underlying fright. However, if difficult behavior continues after 4 or 5 days in the absence of new events that are frightening, it is probably because of the patient's personal style. Excessive talkativeness or mute withdrawal is a typical sign of fear in the acute phase.

Medication, quiet reassurance, or both can relieve a patient's fear and anxiety. Minor tranquilizers are the agents most commonly employed, but explanation and reassurance can be even more effective than medication.

When the physician senses that the patient is afraid, it is safe to assume that the patient regards the illness as an overwhelming threat to well-being. This threat is based on what the patient already knows or presumes about the disease. The physician, therefore, may ask questions designed to uncover erroneous concepts about the patient's condition, such as, "Have you ever known anyone with this disease?" or, "What is your notion of this disease?" If any family member has died of the disease, his or her age at death may also contribute heavily to the patient's fear of the same fate.

After false notions have been corrected, it is important to emphasize the positive aspects of the treatment plan. Even when the prognosis is grave, a calm statement of the treatments planned to counteract and contain the disorder is of value to the anxious patient. The more ominous the prognosis, the more important it is to encourage the patient to specify the fear, so that correspondingly true reassurances (e.g., "the medication can control pain") can be given. False comfort is not recommended. It robs the physician of credibility and, therefore, of the ability to reassure the patient as the illness progresses. An empathetic yet silent presence can sometimes be more helpful than well-meant counsel.[28]

DENIAL AND PANIC

Denial is a common defense mechanism in the initial stage of life-threatening illness. The ability to minimize or to completely deny the threatening implications of the disease ("There's nothing to worry about; I'll be all right.") is essential for controlling panic. When panic sets in, denial fails and people want to flee. Panic is the most common reason why acutely sick patients sign out of a hospital. Although it may simply mean that the patient does not take his or her illness seriously enough, the threat to sign out should be considered a panic reaction. The patient's panic conviction is, "I'll die if I don't get out of here."

Because patients who are experiencing a panic reaction are feeling desperate, they may become antagonistic to efforts to detain them. A gentle approach is essential. For example, the doctor, seated if possible, may begin with "Mr. Jordan, I'm not here to force you to do anything; I just ask that you hear me out." Then the patient needs to hear the truth—that he is seriously ill—expressed in direct but reassuring terms. To quiet the panic, it is most important to explain that the illness is manageable. As the patient calms down, other questions designed to reduce fear can be asked. Even if calmed, however, an anxious patient will not remain calm for long and should be promptly medicated. Family members should also be mobilized and informed.

ANXIETY

Anxiety disorders may or may not intensify during a terminal illness, but they clearly require psychiatric attention when they do. The four most common anxiety-provoking fears associated with death are (1) helplessness or loss of control, (2) being considered bad (guilt and punishment), (3) physical injury or symbolic injury (castration), and (4) abandonment.[29]

In the clinical examination, a severely anxious patient usually does not know what it is about death that is so frightening. Increased anxiety may result from specific memories and associations related to the death of parents or others with whom one identifies; patients may picture the same fate for themselves (e.g., agonizing pain or excessive use of technology). Memories of someone who died of the same illness (e.g., a woman with breast cancer who had relatives who died of breast cancer or a patient with AIDS who tended to a lover dying of AIDS) or particular associations with the illness may produce specific reasons for anxiety (e.g., the disease will be disfiguring). For the sake of the patient's mental health, it is important to explore these issues.

Pharmacologic therapy with an antidepressant such as a selective serotonin reuptake inhibitor (SSRI) or benzodiazepine may be warranted for patients with moderate levels of anxiety. The effect of benzodiazepine is immediate, whereas the therapeutic effect of an SSRI is delayed, occurring 2 weeks after initiation of treatment. Benzodiazepines (e.g., lorazepam and clonazepam) are therefore the preferred class of drug. Lorazepam (0.5 to 2 mg, given orally two to four times a day) peaks in 1 to 6 hours and is available in tablet, elixir, sublingual, rectal, or I.V. formulations. Clonazepam (0.25 to 0.5 mg, given orally two to four times a day) has a slightly longer half-life; it is available in tablet formulation. Patients who have anxiety in the setting of dyspnea respond well to morphine [see Chapter 11].[30] If psychotic symptoms accompany anxiety, a neuroleptic agent such as haloperidol (0.5 to 5 mg, given orally, I.V., or S.C. every 2 to 12 hours) is helpful.[31]

DESPONDENCY

Despondency—a mixture of dread, bitterness, and despair—is the result of an attack on the patient's self-image. The patient feels broken, scarred, and ruined. Work and personal relationships appear jeopardized. It may seem too late to realize cherished goals. The patient is haunted by disappointment with both what has been done and what has been missed. He or she may feel old and that life has been a failure.

Despondency is a contagious feeling, and in most cases, the physician can sense that the patient is depressed. Simply asking about the depression is helpful: "You look a bit blue today. What's on your mind?" The patient is likely to respond with the feelings already described. The patient should be told that such feelings are a normal part of any serious illness. It is important to remind even those who deny despondency that there is nothing unusual about feeling low from time to time in the struggle with any illness and that these feelings are time-limited. When the patient has acknowledged feelings of depression, even in the first few days of illness, it is very helpful if the physician describes future plans for medical treatment.

DEPRESSION

The more seriously ill a patient becomes, the more likely it is that a major depression will develop.[32] In a review of the literature, major depression was reported to affect as many as 29% of palliative care patients[33]; however, this figure may be low. Researchers identified depression in 62% of patients in a palliative care unit in Winnipeg, Canada.[34] Standard depression inventories (e.g., Beck) are not as useful for diagnosing depression in terminal patients, because some of the physical symptoms of depression that these inventories target can occur in terminal illness without depression. At present, there is no validated instrument to assess depression in patients with terminal illness, although research is under way. Emotional symptoms remain helpful, however.[35] These include anhedonia, depressed mood, suicidal thoughts, and guilt.

Patients in pain have a significantly higher rate of depression than comparable patients without pain.[36] Extreme depression and hopelessness are the strongest predictors that patients may develop a desire for hastened death.[29] Ganzini and colleagues[37] documented that severely depressed patients make more re-

stricted advance directives when depressed and change them when the depression is in remission.

Dignity therapy, a novel psychotherapeutic intervention, may hold promise as a treatment for depression in palliative care patients. As part of the intervention, patients are asked to discuss issues that matter most to them or that they most want remembered by their families; these discussions are recorded and transcribed for the patients and their families. In a multicenter study, the majority of patients who received dignity therapy reported a heightened sense of dignity (76%) and an increased sense of purpose (68%) after the intervention.[38] These results suggest dignity therapy may be useful in treating depression and distress common in palliative care patients.

Pharmacologic options for depression in palliative care extend beyond the traditional agents [see Table 1]. Because standard antidepressant medications typically require several weeks to take effect, psychostimulants such as methylphenidate (Ritalin) and pemolin (Cylert) are increasingly being used for short-term treatment of depression for terminally ill patients in pain. They may be used instead of traditional antidepressants, in patients whose life expectancy is less than 3 weeks, or as an interim measure until traditional antidepressants take effect.[39] They

Table 1 Antidepressant Medications Used in Patients with Advanced Disease[37,56]

Class	Agent (Trade Name)	Dosage
Tricyclic antidepressants	Amitriptyline (Elavil)	10–150 mg p.o./I.M./p.r., q.d.
	Clomipramine (Anafranil)	10–150 mg p.o., q.d.
	Desipramine (Norpramin)	12.5–150 mg p.o./I.M. q.d.
	Doxepin (Sinequan)	12.5–150 mg p.o./I.M. q.d.
	Imipramine (Tofranil)	12.5–150 mg p.o./I.M. q.d.
	Nortriptyline (Pamelor)	10–125 mg p.o., q.d.
Second-generation antidepressants	Bupropion (Wellbutrin)	200–450 mg p.o., q.d.
	Citalopram (Celexa)	10–60 mg p.o., q.d.
	Fluoxetine (Prozac)	10–60 mg p.o., q.d.
	Fluvoxamine (Luvox)	50–300 mg p.o., q.d.
	Mirtazepine (Remeron)	15–45 mg p.o., q.d.
	Paroxetine (Paxil)	10–60 mg p.o., q.d.
	Sertraline (Zoloft)	25–200 mg p.o., q.d.
	Trazodone (Desyrel)	25–300 mg p.o., q.d.
	Venlafaxine (Effexor)	37.5–225 mg p.o., q.d.
Psychostimulants	Dextroamphetamine (Dexedrine)	2.5–20 mg p.o. in the morning and at noon*
	Lithium carbonate	600–1,200 mg p.o., q.d.
	Methylphenidate (Ritalin)	2.5–20 mg p.o. in the morning and at noon*
	Pemoline (Cylert)	37.5–75 mg p.o. in the morning and at noon*

*Give last dose at noon to avoid insomnia at night.

are also useful to counteract opiate-induced sedation and may potentiate opiate analgesia.

Of the antidepressant agents, the selective serotonin reuptake inhibitors (SSRIs) are associated with fewer side effects than traditional tricyclic agents, which are associated with a high incidence of anticholinergic toxicity, including constipation, urinary retention, confusion, and altered cardiac conduction. The SSRIs (fluoxetine, sertraline, and paroxetine) are effective antidepressants and are generally well tolerated. Major side effects include anorexia, nausea, restlessness, and insomnia. Antidepressants with demonstrated efficacy as adjuvant therapy for treatment of pain include the tricyclic antidepressants and paroxetine.

PERSONALITY DISORDERS

Seriously ill people share common objectives with their physician: the relief of suffering and, as far as possible, the restoration of health. Dysfunctional personality traits (e.g., passive, hysterical, obsessive, dependent) that are the residue of past problems, such as parental conflicts, can distract both patient and doctor from those shared objectives. The doctor has enough to do to care for the physical illness and its normal emotional consequences to the patient (e.g., fear, anger, or despondency) without trying to alter personality traits. If reasonable efforts do not suffice, further intervention is best left to a consulting psychiatrist.

Preparation for the End of Life

THE CHOICE OF WHERE TO DIE

Where a person wishes to spend the end of his or her life is a very personal decision. The options are to remain at home, to move to an inpatient hospice [see Chapter 10], or to die in the hospital. Factors that influence this decision include the degree of support at home to care for the patient (emotional and physical), how comfortable the caretakers are with the care of a person who is dying, financial resources, and the technical support needed to keep the patient comfortable. In most cases, special equipment and services can be set up in the home, but this can be prohibitively expensive.

If it is anticipated that the patient has less than 6 months before death, this is an appropriate time to discuss hospice, whether inpatient or at home [see Chapter 10].

Health care providers frequently overlook the financial burden for patients and families resulting from terminal illness. Financial costs can be devastating. It is important to address this issue with patients and families and to refer them to appropriate financial counseling. Social workers can provide invaluable assistance in facilitating the provision of the home services to which patients are entitled under Medicare or Medicaid, and they can usually tell the patient and family what services will have to be paid for out of pocket.

Remember that while patients are in the hospital, caregivers surround them. When they return home, they often feel isolated and abandoned. Every effort should be made to maintain channels of communication among patients, family, and home health care workers.

ADVANCE DIRECTIVES

It is a mistake to delay the discussion of advance directives until the patient is in the terminal stages of illness. Rather, this issue should be dealt with soon after the diagnosis of terminal illness [see Chapter 10].

FINAL CLOSURE

The end of life is the opportunity for closure in relationships with loved ones. Relationship completion comprises five types of communications: I forgive you; forgive me; thank you; I love you; and good-bye.[40] These messages are vital to the peace of mind of the patient and the patient's family and should be encouraged by the physician as an aspect of standard palliative care.

Other actions that help with life's closure are a discussion of personal preferences for a memorial service, the settlement of financial affairs, and, if applicable, the completion of a plan for care of the children.

The physician should instruct the family in practical considerations concerning their loved one's death. For instance, the family should be told that there is no need to call 911 when the patient dies; instead, they should contact the funeral director. If a patient is dying at home and the family panics and calls 911, it is important that they have a "Do Not Resuscitate (DNR)" form in the home. Otherwise, the emergency medical services in some states are required to automatically intubate the patient.

Grief and Bereavement

In one respect, life can be described as one loss after another. The degree of recovery from each loss determines whether an individual regains a stable life or remains disabled. When losses occur, the resulting sadness can eventually give way to a process of reorganization that restores the person's ability to function normally. For example, the death of a parent can cause a child to become self-reliant. Some persons maintain a satisfying, productive life despite seemingly overwhelming losses, whereas others never recover from less severe losses. What makes the difference?

NORMAL GRIEVING

Grief is the psychological process by which an individual copes with loss, struggles to understand it, regains perspective, and goes on with life. Causes of grief include not only the loss of a loved one, of valued possessions, or of employment but also the loss of good health that occurs with major illness or injury. Serious illness or injury challenges personal integrity; it could be said, for example, that every myocardial infarction causes an ego infarction. Therefore, recovery from major illness is not complete until the patient has also recovered from the accompanying emotional damage to the self.

Surrounded daily by the sick and injured, physicians see grief-work in process. It is important for the physician to realize that grief is a normal reaction serving an important restitutive function, that it follows a typical pattern, and that marked deviation from this pattern may be a sign that psychological intervention is required.

The normal grieving process follows a similar course in individuals suffering from any serious loss. Several prominent features of normal grieving have been identified.[41,42] Because these features are often mistakenly labeled as pathologic, familiarity with their correlation to grief can prevent well-meaning but misguided efforts to intervene in a necessary process.

Somatic symptoms of grieving may be prominent, including sighing respirations, exhaustion, gastrointestinal symptoms of all kinds, restlessness, yawning, and choking. Feelings of guilt, especially early in the wake of loss, seem to be universal. "What more could I have done?" or other references to unresolved emotional conflicts are common expressions of these feelings.

Preoccupation with the image of the deceased person, often seeming bizarre even to the griever, is a sure sign that normal mourning is under way. The intense focus on the deceased may be manifested in several ways: by continual mental conversations with the dead person; by a sense of the dead person's presence so vivid, especially at night, that the griever hears, sees, or is touched by the person; or by the simultaneous feeling that all other persons are emotionally distant.

Hostile reactions and irritability also seem to be the rule, combined with a disconcerting loss of warm feelings toward others. Some disruption of normal patterns of conduct is present, such as a desire to be alone, uncharacteristic procrastination, and indecisiveness toward others. The style, traits, mannerisms, or even the physical symptoms of the dead person may alarmingly appear in the mourner; such identification phenomena signify only that grief is in process. Finally, it is routine for the griever to feel that part of the self has been destroyed or mutilated.

How long will it take for the acute symptomatology of grieving to subside? Although the usual estimate is 1 to 3 months, many factors affect the actual time required. They include the number of strong remaining relationships, the intensity and duration of the bond with the lost person, the number and severity of any unresolved conflicts, the degree of dependence on the lost person, and how much of the survivor's mental life habitually assumed the dead person's physical or emotional presence. The main signs of resolution of acute grief are the reappearance of normal functioning, the capacity to experience pleasure, and the ability to enter new relationships.

The acute phase is followed by the disorganization phase. In this phase, the pain of the experience becomes foremost in the person's consciousness. Turmoil, emptiness, despair, and thoughts about the pointlessness of life and the reasonableness of suicide are common. Social interaction seems impossible and is avoided, even though solitude itself is dreaded and intolerable.

Finally, there is reorganization, characterized by a return of normal functioning and behavior. Reversals during this time are the rule, and reappearance of the earlier two phases should be expected. The bereaved person is caught off guard by sudden reminders of the lost person (e.g., a special coat discovered in storage) or by new and painful realizations (e.g., no more shared holidays) that reopen the wound of loss.

The grieving process is often delayed when death follows a prolonged and difficult illness. In such circumstances, death is entirely acceptable, even welcomed as the end of suffering. Later, especially when returning to a scene that sharply evokes the memory of the dead person when healthy, death becomes unacceptable, and feelings of protest or resentment spontaneously emerge.

ABNORMAL GRIEVING

Preexisting personality traits in survivors can interfere with the normal grief process. Additionally, survivors are at heightened risk of abnormal or complicated bereavement if the loved one died suddenly or unexpectedly, if the death was violent, or if no bodily remains were found. Because grief serves an important restitutive function, failure to grieve normally may result in serious psychological symptoms.

Some markers of abnormal grief are evident immediately; others do not appear for 3 months or longer after the loss. An inability to grieve immediately after the loss, typically manifested by absence of weeping, is the best predictor of later problems. Prolonged hysterical grieving that is defined as excessive by the individual's own subcultural norms (not those of the physician) is an equally ominous prognostic sign. Overactivity without a sense of loss is an early sign of distorted grieving. Furious hostility against specific persons—for example, the doctor or hospital staff—which may assume true paranoid proportions, can be regarded as a sign of abnormality when the individual dwells on it to the exclusion of the other concerns of normal grief. A suppression of hostility to the degree that the person's affect and conduct appear frozen (masklike appearance, stilted robotlike movements, and no emotional expressiveness) and self-destructive behavior (giving away belongings, foolish business deals, or other self-punitive actions with no attendant guilt feelings) are also early indicators of abnormal grieving.

Ultimately, it may become apparent that social isolation has become progressive, with a lasting loss of interpersonal initiative. When symptoms of the deceased person appear in the survivor as conversion symptoms or have become the focus of hypochondriacal complaints overshadowing all other manifestations of grief, pathologic grief is likely. Unresolved grief can also be suspected when the dead person is portrayed either as a saint who had no shortcomings or as one who never occasioned the least feeling of anger, burden, or disagreement in the survivor. In such cases, the mourner usually harbors intense feelings that are in conflict with those feelings outwardly expressed, and fear that these feelings will be discovered immobilizes the grieving process.

The result of prolonged grieving may be prolonged sadness, social isolation, somatic complaints, or loss of ability to function. A few sessions with a psychiatrist, aimed at helping the patient bring his or her own feelings into the open so that the process of grieving can be completed, often provide great relief.

Helping the Bereaved

Mourners tend to be outcasts from society. Their presence is painful to many around them, and efforts to silence, impede, or stop the manifestations of their grief are common. Allowing the grieving person to express feelings is essential, however. Most important is avoidance of maneuvers that negate grieving, such as clichés ("It's God's will"), efforts to distract ("After all, you've got three other children"), and outright exhortations to stop grieving ("Cheer up, life must go on").

Seeing the body of the deceased facilitates grieving, probably by establishing the irrevocable fact of death.[39] Permitting survivors to express their feelings and reminders that grief is a normal process are helpful. Gentle review of the deceased person's last days of life, last conversations, and final exchange of words, as well as talking about the deceased's general lifestyle, help initiate grieving. The memories most obstructive of grieving are those of hostile interactions with the deceased and any other interactions that leave the survivor feeling guilty. The more negative these interactions were, the longer it takes to begin recalling and discussing them.

In helping the bereaved, presence means more than words. Someone who can remain calm and accepting in the presence of a weeping, angry, or bitter mourner is highly valued. A hand on the shoulder can be just what is needed. Over time, helping the griever complete memories of the deceased also facilitates mourning. Old photograph albums and letters can be helpful in this regard. Anniversaries are key points in the grieving process, and special attention to the bereaved on these days is a basic element in the care of mourners.

A return to a job is an essential feature of the recovery process because it brings the mourner back into contact with concerned fellow workers. In addition, the therapeutic effects of work on self-esteem play an important part in alleviating the narcissistic component of the response to the loss. Most bereaved persons benefit from returning to work within 2 to 4 weeks after the death of a loved one.

Self-help groups can be extremely effective for permitting expression of emotion, showing that grief is universal, and supplying the compassion and respect necessary for rebuilding self-esteem. Books that recount events such as losing a spouse or that give instructions for the surviving spouse and children may be helpful.

SPECIFIC TYPES OF LOSS

Each type of loss carries specific challenges to mourners, and each type has a specific literature that can be helpful.[43] Loss of a parent by an adult, although a nearly universal occurrence, is not trivial, and loss of the second parent may leave the bereaved feeling particularly alone and vulnerable. Loss of a parent by a child invariably worries the adult survivors responsible for the child's care because successful mourning in a child is a more complex process than in an adult.[44,45] For example, the child may face adjustment to parental surrogates, to a parent stressed by the responsibility of raising the child alone, to the loss of a gender role model, or, eventually, to the replacement of the deceased parent by remarriage and competition for the affection of the surviving parent. However, studies of bereaved children from stable families have shown optimistic results: 8 weeks after the death of a parent, children 5 to 12 years of age were similar to nonbereaved children in school behavior, interest in school, peer involvement, peer enjoyment, and self-esteem.[46]

Research on loss of a sibling appears to be lacking, but the available data indicate that death of a sibling forces surviving siblings to reorganize their roles and relationships with their parents and with one another.[43]

Loss of a spouse, ranked on life-event scales as the most stressful of all possible losses,[47] is more detrimental for men than for women and leads to increased morbidity and mortality in elderly men.[48] The bereaved spouse is left with sole responsibility for children, finances, management, and planning; faced with possible loss of income; and forced to cope with a changed social role in the community.

Each year, about 800,000 parents lose a child younger than 25 years. This loss is particularly traumatic because it is so contrary to life-cycle expectancies.[49]

Sudden death, such as death in an emergency ward, stillbirth, sudden infant death, accidental or traumatic death, cardiac arrest, or death during or after surgery, inflicts a uniquely intense trauma on the survivors. Shock is dramatically intensified. Guilt is likely to be a much more serious problem than it is with nonsudden death because of the total absence of preparation. Violence or disfigurement further intensifies the survivor's feelings.

General rules for dealing with the bereaved also apply here, with certain specific emphases. The chance to view the body, even when mutilated, should be offered to the family members. If there is severe mutilation, the family should be warned. The need to view the body, an aid to normal mourning, is greater when death is sudden.

Suicide is an especially difficult way to lose a loved one. Feeling abandoned and rejected, the survivor often experiences unsettling anger or, if the relationship had been hostile and stormy,

equally unsettling relief. The bereaved scours through memories for an action that might have caused or prevented the suicide. Guilt is such an inevitable consequence of suicide that even casual acquaintances wonder what they might have done that contributed to the death. Shame can cause avoidance of others, falsification of the event as an accident, or unwillingness to let others know that a family member has died. A scapegoat may be sought, such as the deceased's therapist, spouse, or boss or the medical examiner who labeled the death a suicide.[50]

Loss by homicide also produces especially intense grief reactions.[51] Flashbacks of the violent death are unavoidable. Survivors tend to avoid locations associated with the death and to stop watching television news because of possible reports of violence. Rage and desire for proportional revenge may cause intense discomfort for the bereaved, if suppressed, or for those around the bereaved, if excessively expressed. Children who witness the murder of one parent by another are afflicted with traumatic intrusive memories of the parents, massive conflicts of loyalty, and the intense need for secrecy because of the stigmatizing nature of their loss. They may inadvertently become so-called neglected victims and are at risk for perpetuating an intergenerational cycle of violence.[52,53]

Patience and gentleness with the family's prolonged numbness and shock are essential features of caring for bereaved family members. Physical acts of kindness may be the only avenue of communication at first. Leading the family to a quiet room, providing comfortable seats, bringing beverages, and making sure that all possible members are included are all helpful and may lay the groundwork for dialogue.

Immediately after imparting the news of death, the physician may be able to bring the family together and start a dialogue by offering to give them as detailed an account as possible. Teamwork is usually required to get everyone present and seated with beverages, ashtrays, and any other comforts that seem appropriate. Survivors may benefit from very gentle questions about the last hours of the deceased: Were there any prodromal syndromes? Any premonitions? Who saw the deceased last? Families who do not wish to explore these crucial questions at this time should not be pushed, however.

A chaplain, nurse, or other team member with counseling skills, present from the time the physician begins communicating the bad news, may be able to address sensitive issues that arise. Family members or other supportive figures (e.g., family doctor or clergyman) who are absent should be notified and asked to come to the hospital when appropriate. When the family members are too shaken to sit down or participate in any dialogue, it is important to leave them a telephone contact at the hospital should any questions arise.

MEDICATIONS AND BEREAVEMENT

Treatment of bereavement-related major depressive episodes has recently been shown to be beneficial. In one trial, persons who had lost their spouses within 6 to 8 weeks and met the *Diagnostic and Statistical Manual of Mental Disorders*, fourth edition (DSM-IV) criteria for a major depressive episode were treated with sustained-release bupropion. Improvement was noted in both depression and grief intensity.[54] In another study, persons with major depressive episodes that began within 6 months before or 12 months after the loss of a spouse were randomly assigned to a 16-week double-blind trial of one of four treatments: nortriptyline plus interpersonal psychotherapy, nortriptyline alone in a medication clinic, placebo plus interpersonal psychotherapy, or placebo alone in a medication clinic. Nortriptyline proved superior to placebo in achieving remission of bereavement-related major depressive episodes, but the combination of medication and psychotherapy was associated with the highest rate of treatment completion. The investigators concluded that the results support the use of pharmacologic treatment of major depressive episodes in the wake of a serious life stressor such as bereavement.[55]

The authors have no commercial relationships with manufacturers of products or providers of services discussed in this chapter.

References

1. Magni KG: The fear of death. Death and Presence: The Psychology of Death and the After-Life. Godin A, Ed. Lumen Vitae, Brussels, Belgium, 1972, p 125

2. The EPEC Project: Education on Palliative Care and End-of-Life Care. Feinberg School of Medicine, Northwestern University, Chicago http://www.epec.net

3. Hippocrates: Decorum, XVI. Hippocrates with an English Translation, Vol 2. Jones WH, Ed. Heinemann, London, England, 1923

4. Kelly WD, Friesen SR: Do cancer patients want to be told? Surgery 27:822, 1950

5. Morrison RS, Meier DE: Palliative Care. N Engl J Med 350:2582, 2004

6. Searight HR, Gafford J: Cultural diversity at the end of life: issues and guidelines for family physicians. Am Fam Physician 71:515, 2005

7. Blackhall LJ, Murphy ST, Frank G, et al: Ethnicity and attitudes toward patient autonomy. JAMA 274:820, 1995

8. Tse CY, Chong A, Fok SY: Breaking bad news: a Chinese perspective. Palliat Med 17:339, 2003

9. Sullivan RJ, Menapace LW, White RM: Truth-telling and patient diagnoses. J Med Ethics 27:192, 2001

10. Gerle B, Lunden G, Sandblom P: The patient with inoperable cancer from the psychiatric and social standpoints. Cancer 13:1206, 1960

11. Emanuel LL, Alpert HR, Baldwin DC, et al: What terminally ill patients care about: toward a validated construct of patients' perspectives. J Palliat Med 3:419, 2000

12. Aitken-Swan J, Easson EC: Reactions of cancer patients on being told their diagnosis. Br Med J 1:779, 1959

13. Gilbertsen VA, Wangensteen OH: Should the doctor tell the patient that the disease is cancer? Surgeon's recommendation. The Physician and the Total Care of the Cancer Patient. American Cancer Society, New York, 1962, p 80

14. Croog SH, Shapiro SD, Levine S: Denial among male heart patients. Psychosom Med 33:385, 1971

15. Greer S: The management of denial in cancer patients. Oncology (Williston Park) 6:33, 1992

16. Watson M, Homewood J, Haviland J, et al: Influence of psychological response on breast cancer survival: 10-year follow-up of a population-based cohort. Eur J Cancer 41:1710, 2005

17. Nelson DV, Friedman LC, Baer PE, et al: Attitudes of cancer: psychometric properties of fighting spirit and denial. J Behav Med 12:341, 1989

18. Hagerty RG, Butow PH, Ellis PM, et al: Communicating with realism and hope: incurable cancer patients' views on the disclosure of prognosis. J Clin Oncol 23:1278, 2005

19. Grbich C, Parker D, Maddocks I: The emotions and coping strategies of caregivers of family members with a terminal cancer. J Palliat Care 17:30, 2001

20. Koenig HG, George LK, Titus P: Religion, spirituality, and health in medically ill hospitalized older patients. J Am Geriatr Soc 52:554, 2004

21. Larson DB, Swyers JP, McCullough ME: Scientific research on spirituality and health: a consensus report. National Institute for Healthcare Research, Rockville, Maryland, 1998

22. Mueller PS, Plevak DJ, Rummans TA: Religious involvement, spirituality and medicine: implications for clinical practice. Mayo Clin Proc 76:1225, 2001

23. McClain CS, Rosenfeld B, Breibart W: Effect of spiritual well-being on end-of-life despair in terminally-ill patients. Lancet 362:1603, 2003

24. Saunders CM: Foreword. Mortally Wounded: Stories of Soul, Pain, Death, and Healing. Kearney M, Ed. Simon & Schuster, New York, 1997, p 11

25. Wilson KG, Curran D, McPherson CJ: A burden to others: a common source of distress for the terminally ill. Cogn Behav Ther 34:115, 2005

26. Kash KM, Holland JC, Breitbart W, et al: Stress and burnout in oncology. Oncology (Williston Park) 14:1621, 2000

27. Cassem NH, Hackett TP: Psychiatric consultation in a coronary care unit. Ann Intern Med 75:9, 1971

28. Penson RT, Partridge RA, Shah MA, et al: Fear of death. Oncologist 10:160, 2005

29. Breitbart W, Rosenfeld B, Pessin H, et al: Depression, hopelessness, and desire for hastened death in terminally ill patients with cancer. JAMA 284:2907, 2000

30. Brurera E, MacEachern T, Ripamonti C, et al: Subcutaneous morphine for dyspnea in cancer patients. Ann Intern Med 119:906, 1993

31. Massie MJ: Anxiety, panic and phobias. Handbook of Psycho-oncology: Psychological Care of the Patient with Cancer. Holland JC, Rowland JH, Eds. Oxford University Press, New York, 1989, p 300

32. Cassem NH: Depression and anxiety secondary to medical illness. Psychiatry Clin North Am 13:597, 1990

33. Hotopf M, Chidgey J, Addington-Hall J, et al: Depression in advanced disease: a systematic review. Part 1. Prevalence and case finding. Palliat Med 16: 81, 2002

34. Chochinov HM: Management of grief in the cancer setting. Psychiatric Aspects of Symptom Management in Cancer Patients. Breitbart W, Holland JC, Eds. American Psychiatric Press, Washington, DC, 1993, p 231

35. Block SD: Assessing and managing depression in the terminally ill patient. ACP-ASIM End of Life Care Consensus Panel. American College of Physicians-American Society of Internal Medicine. Ann Intern Med 132:209, 2000

36. Plumb MM, Holland JC: Comparative studies of psychological function in patients with advanced cancer. Psychosom Med 39:264, 1977

37. Ganzini L, Lee MA, Heintz RT, et al: The effect of depression treatment on elderly patients' preferences for life-sustaining medical therapy. Am J Psychiatry 151:1631, 1994

38. Chochinov HM, Hack T, Hassard T, et al: Dignity therapy: a novel psychotherapeutic intervention for patients near the end of life. J Clin Oncol 23:5520, 2005

39. Clinical practice guidelines for quality palliative care, executive summary. National Consensus Project for Quality Palliative Care. J Palliat Med 7:611, 2004

40. Byock I: Dying Well: Peace and Possibilities at the End of Life. Riverhead Books, Berkley Publishing Group, New York, 1997, p 140

41. Parkes CM, Weiss RS: Recovery from Bereavement. Basic Books Inc, New York, 1983

42. Lindemann E: Symptomatology and management of acute grief. Am J Psychiatry 101:141, 1944

43. Bereavement: Reactions, Consequences, and Care. Osterweis M, Solomon F, Green M, Eds. National Academy Press, Washington, DC, 1984

44. Furman E: Child's Parent Dies: Studies in Childhood Bereavement. Yale University Press, New Haven, Connecticut, 1988

45. Geis HK, Whittlesey SW, McDonald NB, et al: Bereavement and loss in childhood. Child Adolesc Psychiatr Clin N Am 7:73, 1998

46. Fristad MA, Jedel R, Weller RA, et al: Psychosocial functioning in children after the death of a parent. Am J Psychiatry 150:511, 1993

47. Holmes TH, Rahe RH: The social readjustment rating scale. J Psychosom Res 11:213, 1967

48. Schaefer C, Quesenberry CP Jr, Wi S: Mortality following conjugal bereavement and the effects of a shared environment. Am J Epidemiol 141:1142, 1995

49. Cassem NH: The person confronting death. The New Harvard Guide to Psychiatry. Harvard University Press, Cambridge, Massachusetts, 1988, p 728

50. Ness DE, Pfeffer CR: Sequelae of bereavement resulting from suicide. Am J Psychiatry 147:279, 1990

51. Rynearson EK, McCreery JM: Bereavement after homicide: a synergism of trauma and loss. Am J Psychiatry 150:258, 1993

52. Black D, Kaplan T: Father kills mother: issues and problems encountered by a child psychiatric team. Br J Psychiatry 153:624, 1989

53. McCune N, Donnelly P: Child surviving parental murder (letter). Br J Psychiatry 154:889, 1989

54. Zisook S, Shucter SR, Pedrelli P, et al: Bupropion sustained release for bereavement: results of an open trial. J Clin Psychiatry 62:227, 2001

55. Reynolds CF 3rd, Miller MD, Pasternak RE, et al: Treatment of bereavement-related major depressive episodes in later life: a controlled study of acute and continuation treatment with nortriptyline and interpersonal psychotherapy. Am J Psychiatry 156: 202, 1999

56. Massie MJ: Depression: Handbook of Psycho-oncology. Holland JC, Rowland JH, Eds. Oxford University Press, New York, 1989, p 283

13 Bioterrorism

Jeffrey Duchin, M.D.

Well before the 2001 anthrax outbreak, public health and government leaders in the United States recognized the need for increased preparedness to detect and respond to acts of biologic terrorism. Concern about the vulnerability of the United States to a biologic attack grew with revelations about the offensive biologic weapons programs of the former Soviet Union and Iraq, as well as uncertainty about the whereabouts of and accountability for biologic agents produced through those programs; the successful chemical attack on the Tokyo subway system by the Aum Shinrikyo cult, coupled with information that the cult was actively experimenting with biologic agents; and information about the potential for domestic bioterrorism.[1-5]

In April 2000, the Centers for Disease Control and Prevention (CDC) published a strategic plan for preparedness and response to biologic and chemical terrorism.[6] This subsection describes the clinician's role in recognizing and responding to biologic terrorism, as presented in the CDC plan; summarizes current information on the diagnosis and management of the most likely agents of bioterrorism; and describes current resources for authoritative information and guidelines related to bioterrorism.

The Clinician's Role in Bioterrorism Preparedness and Response

For clinicians, the response to a bioterrorism attack is in many ways the same as the response to naturally occurring outbreaks of communicable disease.[7,8] Both situations typically require early identification of ill or exposed persons, rapid implementation of preventive therapy, special infection control considerations, and collaboration or communication with the public health system. Examples of naturally occurring communicable diseases that require such a response include meningococcal disease[9]; enteric infection with *Escherichia coli* 0157:H7, *Salmonella,* or *Shigella*[10]; pertussis, rubella, measles, or chickenpox occurring in health care facilities and clinics[11-14]; unusual or newly emerging infections such as West Nile virus and hantavirus pulmonary syndrome[15-17]; and the inevitable reappearance of pandemic influenza.[18] The 2002 outbreak of severe acute respiratory syndrome (SARS) exemplifies the type of unexpected, naturally occurring disease for which the need for preparedness and the impact on clinicians have much in common with that of biologic terrorism.[19,20]

The first indication of an unannounced biologic attack will likely be an increase in the number of persons seeking care from primary care physicians. In the 2001 anthrax outbreak, as well as in outbreaks of *E. coli* 0157:H7 disease and hantavirus pulmonary syndrome in 1993 and West Nile virus in 1999, alert clinicians initiated the public health response by recognizing an unusual clinical syndrome, ordering appropriate laboratory tests, and notifying public health officials.[10,16,17] Similarly, primary care physicians and subspecialists alike must be familiar with both the specific clinical syndromes associated with agents of bioterrorism and the ways to rapidly notify public health authorities. In addition to identifying cases and treating ill patients, clinicians also play a critical role in managing postexposure prophylaxis and its complications, as well as psychological and mental health problems brought on by the event.

During both bioterrorism attacks and naturally occurring outbreaks, clinicians are faced with the challenge of excluding the outbreak disease in persons who are worried about potential exposure or who are ill with signs and symptoms similar to those of the outbreak disease. The clinician must have knowledge of the signs and symptoms, modes of transmission, incubation periods, and communicable periods of these diseases, as well as skill in both clinical evaluation and eliciting an appropriate and thorough history, including relevant occupational, social, and travel information. In both the 2001 anthrax bioterrorism attack and the 2002 SARS outbreak, the epidemiologic setting of cases played an important role in guiding clinical management, diagnostic tests, and treatment.[21-23] The primary care clinician has the best opportunity to obtain relevant information early in the evaluation; this is important because such information may be more difficult to obtain as time goes on, particularly if the patient's condition deteriorates.

Physicians and other health care providers should have a working knowledge of the basic classes of isolation and infection control measures recommended for patients exposed to agents of potential bioterrorism. Again, these measures are also used in the management of common communicable diseases.[14,24-26]

Recognition of Potential Bioterrorism Agents

The CDC has developed a list of bacteria, viruses, and toxins thought to pose the greatest risk for use in a bioterrorist attack [see Table 1].[27] Agents were included in the list on the basis of their ability to cause disease that (1) is easily disseminated or transmitted from person to person; (2) has high mortality, with potential for major public health impact; (3) may result in panic and social disruption; and (4) requires special action for public health preparedness. Category A agents are thought to pose the highest immediate risk for use as biologic weapons; and category B agents, the next highest risk. Category C agents are thought to pose a potential, but not immediate, risk for use as biologic weapons.

As in naturally occurring outbreaks, early recognition of a bioterrorist attack is critical for rapid implementation of preventive measures and treatment. Early recognition can be challenging, however, because patients presenting for medical care after exposure to a biologic agent may initially exhibit nonspecific symptoms, and pathogens that ordinarily occur in the community, particularly enteric organisms, may be used in a biologic attack.[28,29] A heightened level of suspicion, plus knowledge of the relevant epidemiologic clues, should help physicians recognize changes in illness patterns, including clusters and increases in observed cases over the number expected [see Table 2].[30] Physicians should also be able to recognize diagnostic clues in single cases of a syndrome of concern (e.g., inhalational anthrax, plague and tularemia, botulismlike illness, and possible smallpox).[31] Familiarity with the clinical features of diseases from potential bioterrorist agents and diseases prevalent in the community will allow recognition of potentially significant differences from naturally occurring cases. One of the most important lessons learned from the 2001 anthrax attack was that clinical ill-

Table 1   Critical Biologic Agent Categories for Public Health Preparedness

Category	Biologic Agent	Disease
A (highest immediate risk)	Variola major *Bacillus anthracis* *Yersinia pestis* *Clostridium botulinum* (botulinum toxins) *Francisella tularensis* Filoviruses and arenaviruses (e.g., Ebola virus, Lassa virus)	Smallpox Anthrax Plague Botulism Tularemia Viral hemorrhagic fevers
B (next highest risk)	*Coxiella burnetii* *Brucella* species *Burkholderia mallei* *Burkholderia pseudomallei* Alphaviruses (VEE, EEE, WEE) *Rickettsia prowazekii* Toxins (e.g., ricin, staphylococcal enterotoxin B) *Chlamydia psittaci* Food-safety threats (e.g., *Salmonella* species, *E. coli* 0157:H7) Water-safety threats (e.g., *Vibrio cholerae*, *Cryptosporidium parvum*)	Q fever Brucellosis Glanders Melioidosis Encephalitis Typhus fever Toxic syndromes Psittacosis
C (potential, but not immediate, risk)	Emerging-threat agents (e.g., Nipah virus, hantavirus)	

EEE—eastern equine encephalitis   VEE—Venezuelan equine encephalitis   WEE—western equine encephalitis

ness caused by agents prepared as biologic weapons may differ from typical natural infections.

The identification of a bioterrorist attack requires clinicians to be prepared, alert, and open-minded [*see Sidebar* Internet Resources on Bioterrorism]. Many local and state health departments post current information about communicable diseases on their Web sites and distribute informational newsletters with relevant data. The CDC's weekly bulletin, *Morbidity and Mortality Weekly Report (MMWR),* contains current information on medical conditions of public health importance in the United States. Subscriptions to MMWR are available online at http://www.cdc.gov/mmwr/mmwrsubscribe.html.

Communication with Authorities

Once a potential outbreak or significant cluster or event has been detected, prompt consultation with appropriate medical specialists and public health authorities is indicated. Clinicians must have reliable, around-the-clock contact information for emergency resources in the geographic area where they practice; these resources include specialist consultants (e.g., consultants in infectious disease, dermatology, or pulmonary medicine) and infection control professionals or hospital epidemiologists. All clinicians should know how to contact their local or state public health department 24 hours a day to report suspicious or otherwise immediately notifiable cases or for consultation. Many local and state health departments have such contact numbers on their Web sites. Clinicians should have these numbers readily accessible and keep them current.

Clinicians must also ensure that they have a reliable way to promptly receive urgent communications from public health authorities, both for naturally occurring outbreaks of local significance and for a bioterrorist event or outbreak. Increasingly, public health authorities are disseminating health alerts over the Internet, through Web sites and e-mail listserves.

Smallpox

Smallpox is caused by variola virus, an orthopox virus unique to humans. No known animal or insect reservoirs or vectors exist.[32] Related orthopox viruses infecting humans include vaccinia (smallpox vaccine), monkeypox, and cowpox. Smallpox existed in two forms: variola major, which accounted for most morbidity and mortality, and a milder form, variola minor. Variola major is the type of concern in the context of biologic terrorism.

Smallpox was declared eradicated in 1980, 3 years after the last naturally occurring case was reported from Somalia. Stocks of smallpox virus were retained, however, by World Health Organization (WHO) reference laboratories at the Institute of Virus Preparations in Moscow, Russia, and at the CDC in Atlanta, Georgia. In the late 1990s, allegations were published describing the production of large quantities of smallpox virus by the former Soviet Union. These stores, which may have become dis-

Table 2   Epidemiologic Clues of a Biologic Attack

Presence of a large epidemic
Unusually severe disease or unusual routes of exposure
Unusual geographic area, unusual season, or absence of normal vector
Multiple simultaneous epidemics of different diseases
Outbreak of zoonotic disease
Unusual strains of organisms or antimicrobial-resistance patterns
Higher attack rates in persons with common exposures
Credible threat, as determined by authorities, of biologic attack
Direct evidence of biologic attack

Internet Resources on Bioterrorism

General

CDC portal to bioterrorism information for laboratory and health professionals
http://www.bt.cdc.gov/index.asp

Contact information for U.S. state and local health departments
http://www.cdc.gov/other.htm#states

CDC Emergency Response Hotline (24 hours): 770-488-7100

American College of Physicians–American Society of Internal Medicine (ACP-ASIM) bioterrorism resources
http://www.acponline.org/bioterro/?hp

Association for Professionals in Infection Control and Epidemiology, Inc.
http://www.apic.org/Content/NavigationMenu/PracticeGuidance/Topics/Bioterrorism/Bioterrorism.htm

Center for Biosecurity of the University of Pittsburgh Medical Center
www.upmc-biosecurity.org

Center for Infectious Disease Research & Policy (CIDRAP), University of Minnesota
http://www1.umn.edu/cidrap/content/bt/bioprep

FDA bioterrorism site
http://www.fda.gov/oc/opacom/hottopics/bioterrorism.html

Infectious Diseases Society of America
bioterrorism: **http://www.idsociety.org/BT/ToC.htm**
practice guidelines: **http://www.idsociety.org/PG/toc.htm**

National Academies' Expert-selected Web Resources for "First Responders" on Bioterrorism
http://www.nap.edu/shelves/first

National Institute of Allergy and Infectious Diseases
http://www.niaid.nih.gov/publications/bioterrorism.htm

National Library of Medicine Specialized Information Services
http://www.sis.nlm.nih.gov/enviro/biologicalwarfare.htm

St. Louis University Center for Study of Bioterrorism
http://bioterrorism.slu.edu

Treatment of Biological Warfare Agent Casualties (July 17, 2000), U.S. Army Field Manual on Treatment of Biological Warfare Casualties
http://www.globalsecurity.org/wmd/library/policy/army/fm/8-284/fm8-284.pdf

USAMRIID's Medical Management of Biological Casualties Handbook (Blue Book)
http://www.usamriid.army.mil/education/bluebookpdf/USAMRIID%20Blue%20Book%205th%20Edition.pdf

seminated after the breakup of the Soviet Union, would presumably be the source for a bioterrorist attack involving smallpox.

Smallpox is stable and highly infectious in the aerosol form. The risk for a smallpox attack currently is considered low but not zero.[1,4,33,34]

CLASSIFICATION

On the basis of a study from India, the WHO has classified smallpox into five clinical forms: ordinary, flat-type, hemorrhagic, modified, and sine eruptione.[35] These forms reflect different host reactions to the same strain of virus.

Ordinary Smallpox

Ordinary smallpox is the most common form seen in nonimmune persons; it accounted for 90% of cases in the WHO study and had an average case-fatality rate of 30%. The incubation period is 7 to 17 days (mean, 10 to 12 days). Symptoms of the pro-

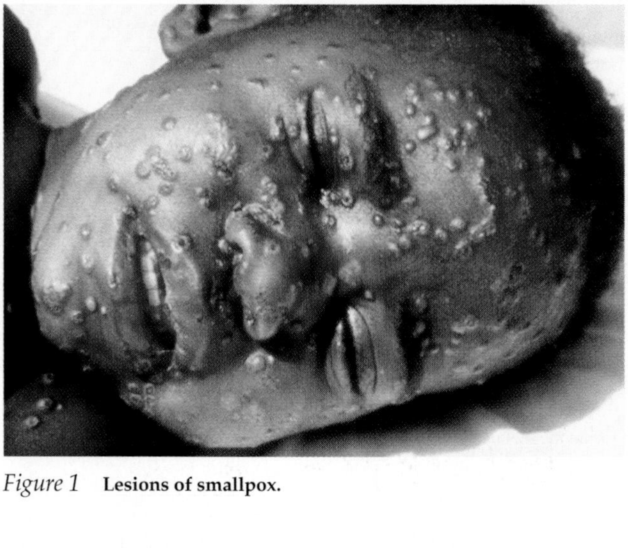

Figure 1   **Lesions of smallpox.**

dromal phase include the acute onset of high fever, malaise, headache, backache, and prostration. Other prominent symptoms include vomiting and abdominal pain.

The characteristic rash occurs 2 to 3 days later, appearing first on the face and forearms. An enanthem involving the oropharyngeal mucosa precedes the rash by a day. The rash progresses slowly, from macules to papules to vesicles and pustules and finally to scabs, with each stage lasting 1 to 2 days. The lesions are firm, discrete vesicles or pustules (4 to 6 mm in diameter) deeply embedded in the dermis; they may become umbilicated or confluent as they evolve [*see Figure 1*]. The patient remains febrile throughout the evolution of the rash, which may become painful as pustules enlarge. A second fever spike 5 to 8 days after onset of the rash may signify a secondary bacterial infection. Pustules remain for 5 to 8 days, after which umbilication and crusting occur. Lesions are in the same stage of development on any given part of the body. They are peripherally distributed, more concentrated on the face and distal extremities than on the trunk, and may involve the palms and soles. Scarring occurs with scab separation from destruction of sebaceous glands.

Experience during the global smallpox eradication program suggests that the onset of communicability coincides with the development of rash, approximately 2 days after the onset of the acute febrile prodrome. However, because the oropharyngeal enanthem and associated release of virus into oral secretions may precede rash onset, it is recommended that for the purposes of postexposure management, anyone who has contact with smallpox patients from the time of onset of fever should be considered potentially exposed [*see* Infection Control, *below*].[36]

Complications of smallpox include fluid and electrolyte disturbances; extensive desquamation that clinically resembles burns; bronchitis and pneumonitis; panophthalmitis and blindness from viral keratitis or secondary infection of the eye; arthritis (developing in up to 2% of children); and encephalitis (less than 1% of cases). Death results from toxemia associated with circulating immune complexes and variola antigens.[37]

Other Forms of Smallpox

Flat-type (or malignant) smallpox occurs in 5% to 10% of cases and is severe, with a 97% case-fatality rate among unvaccinated persons. In this form, lesions are flat and become densely confluent, evolving slowly and coalescing with a soft, velvety texture. Hemorrhagic smallpox was reported in less than 3% of cases, occurring particularly in pregnant women. It is a severe, rapidly progressive, uniformly fatal illness. A dusky erythema develops, followed by hemorrhages into the skin and mucous membranes. Both hemorrhagic and flat-type smallpox have an accelerated and more severe prodromal phase and are thought to be associated with underlying immune dysfunction.

Modified smallpox is a mild form that accounted for 2% of cases in unvaccinated patients and 25% in previously vaccinated patients. This form rarely resulted in death, and these patients had fewer, smaller, more superficial, and more rapidly evolving lesions. Smallpox sine eruptione (without rash) occurs in previously vaccinated persons or children with maternal antibodies to smallpox. It is a mild or asymptomatic illness that has not been documented to be transmissible.[35,37-39]

DIAGNOSIS

A suspected case of smallpox is a public health emergency. Local and state health authorities, the hospital epidemiologist, and other members of a hospital response team for biologic emergencies should be notified immediately (see the CDC Smallpox Response Plan and Guidelines at http://www.bt.cdc.gov/agent/smallpox/response-plan/index.asp).

The differential diagnosis of smallpox includes other illnesses that can cause fever and a rash [see Table 3]. Severe varicella is the disease most likely to be confused with smallpox. However, familiarity with the clinical features of the two diseases, particularly the rash, should help differentiate them [see Table 4]. Additional information that may be useful in differentiating smallpox from chickenpox includes a history of exposure to persons with chickenpox, a personal history of chickenpox, a history of vaccination

against varicella or smallpox, and the clinical course of illness.

If shingles or disseminated herpes infection is a consideration, direct fluorescent antibody testing for varicella-zoster virus can rapidly confirm varicella-zoster virus and herpes simplex virus infection in patients not considered at high risk for smallpox. Such testing should not be done in patients who are considered at high risk, to avoid exposing laboratory workers to smallpox virus. Certain laboratories can also perform polymerase chain reaction (PCR) testing for herpes simplex virus and varicella-zoster virus. Consultation with an infectious disease specialist, a dermatology specialist, or both is recommended.

Flat-type and hemorrhagic smallpox may be difficult to recognize because of the absence of the characteristic rash of ordinary smallpox, yet these cases are highly infectious. Hemorrhagic smallpox cases may be mistaken for meningococcemia or acute leukemia. All patients with potential smallpox should be asked about their travel history, history of varicella and vaccinia vaccination, level of immunocompetence, and current medications.

The local or state health department should be contacted to facilitate specimen collection for smallpox testing (http://www.statepublichealth.org). CDC protocols for specimen collection for smallpox testing are available on the Internet (http://www.bt.cdc.gov/agent/smallpox/response-plan/files/guide-d.pdf).

Diagnostic testing is available at designated biosafety level 4 (BSL-4) laboratories and includes electron microscopy, immunohistochemical tests, and viral culture with PCR and restriction fragment length polymorphism (RFLP) testing. Only personnel who have undergone successful smallpox vaccination recently (within 3 years) and who are wearing appropriate barrier protection (gloves, gown, and shoe covers) should be involved in specimen collection for suspected cases of smallpox. Respiratory protection is not needed for personnel with recent, successful vaccination. Masks and eyewear or face shields should be used if splashing is anticipated. If unvaccinated personnel must collect specimens, only those who are without contraindications to vaccination

Table 3 Diagnosis of Smallpox

Incubation Period	Clinical Presentation	Differential Diagnosis	Diagnostic Testing
7–17 days; mean, 10–12 days	Severe, acute febrile prodrome 1–4 days before rash onset, with temperature ≥ 101° F (38.3° C), headache, backache, chills, vomiting, abdominal pain, prostration Enanthem on oropharyngeal mucosa, followed by rash on face, forearms, distal extremities, then trunk; lesions most concentrated on face and distal extremities Lesions evolve slowly from macules to papules to deep-seated, firm, nodular, round, well-circumscribed vesicles or pustules to scabs over 1–2 days per stage; are in same stage of evolution on a given area of the body; may become umbilicated or confluent Hemorrhagic smallpox: bleeding into skin and mucous membranes Flat-type/malignant smallpox: lesions remain soft and flattened, coalesce Modified smallpox: less severe with fewer, more superficial and rapidly evolving lesions	Varicella (chickenpox); disseminated herpes zoster and simplex; drug eruptions; erythema multiforme; enteroviral infections; secondary syphilis; contact dermatitis; impetigo; scabies; molluscum contagiosum Hemorrhagic smallpox: meningococcemia, Rocky Mountain spotted fever, ehrlichiosis, gram-negative bacterial sepsis, severe acute leukemia Malignant smallpox: hemorrhagic chickenpox	Diagnostic testing at BSL-4 laboratory, including skin biopsy, electron microscopic examination of vesicular and pustular fluid, culture, PCR; serology Appropriate infection control precautions

Note: The clinical manifestations of infections acquired during a biologic attack may differ from those of naturally occurring infections. Clinicians should remain alert for compatible syndromes that vary from the descriptions given.
BSL-4—biosafety level 4   PCR—polymerase chain reaction

Table 4 Differentiating Features of Smallpox and Chickenpox

Clinical Feature	Smallpox	Chickenpox
Prodromal illness	Febrile prodrome lasting 1–4 days; patient appears ill or toxic	No or mild prodrome; patients typically do not appear ill
Appearance of lesions	Firm, round, well-circumscribed, deep-seated lesions; may be umbilicated	Superficial lesions
Stage of lesions on any one part of the body	Lesions are all at the same stage of development on a given area of the body	Lesions occur in crops with various stages of development evident on a given area of the body
Initial lesions	Oral mucosa, face, or forearms	Face, then trunk
Oral lesions	Early; may not be evident	May occur
Severity of illness	Typically severe	Typically not severe
Distribution of rash	Centrifugal: lesions concentrated on the face and extremities, with relative sparing of the trunk	Centripetal: lesions concentrated on the trunk with relative sparing of the face and extremities
Lesions on palms or soles	Lesions on palms and soles in majority of cases	Lesions on palms and soles uncommon
Rate of evolution of rash	Slow evolution of lesions from macules to papules to pustules over days	Rapid evolution from macules to papules to crusted lesions within 24 hours
Presence of pruritus	Lesions may be painful and are not usually pruritic until scabbing occurs	Often pruritic, typically not painful in the absence of secondary infection
Hemorrhagic lesions	Can occur	Can occur

should do so, because they would require immediate vaccination if the diagnosis of smallpox were confirmed. Vesicular or pustular fluid, scabs, punch biopsies of skin lesions, blood, and tissue from autopsy specimens should be obtained, packaged, and transported according to CDC protocol (http://www.bt.cdc.gov/agent/smallpox/lab-testing/#collection, http://www.cdc.gov/agent/smallpox/response-plan/#guided).[36,39]

The CDC has developed a protocol in poster format for evaluating patients with an acute vesicular or pustular rash illness and for determining the risk of smallpox. The protocol, including color pictures of smallpox lesions, is available on the Internet at the CDC smallpox Web site (http://www.bt.cdc.gov/agent/smallpox/index.asp).

INFECTION CONTROL AND POSTEXPOSURE ISOLATION

In the event of a limited outbreak, patients should be admitted to the hospital and confined to rooms that are under negative atmospheric pressure and equipped with high-efficiency particulate air (HEPA) filtration. Standard, contact, and airborne precautions, including use of gloves, gowns, and masks, should be strictly observed. Unvaccinated personnel caring for patients suspected of having smallpox should wear fit-tested N95 or higher-quality respirators. Once successful vaccination is confirmed, care providers are no longer required to wear an N95 mask.[39] Patients should wear a surgical mask and be wrapped in a gown or sheet to cover the rash when they are not in a negative-airflow room. All laundry and waste should be placed in biohazard bags and autoclaved before being laundered or incinerated. Surfaces that may be contaminated with smallpox virus can be decontaminated with disinfectants that are used for standard hospital infection control, such as hypochlorite and quaternary ammonia.

Persons suspected of being infected with smallpox should be immediately isolated, and all their household members and others who have had face-to-face contact with the infected patient after the onset of fever should be vaccinated and placed under surveillance. Because persons who have had contact with an infected patient would not be contagious until the onset of rash, they should take their temperatures at least once daily, preferably in the evening. Any temperature higher than 101° F (38.3° C) during the 17-day period after the last exposure to the infected patient would suggest the possibility of the development of smallpox. This would be cause for immediate isolation until the diagnosis can be determined clinically, by laboratory examination, or both.

In the event of an outbreak, the following high-risk groups should be given priority for vaccination: (1) persons exposed to the initial release of the virus; (2) contacts of suspected or confirmed smallpox patients; (3) personnel who are directly involved in medical or public health evaluation of suspected or confirmed smallpox patients, as well as the care or transportation of such patients; (4) laboratory workers involved in the collection or processing of possible smallpox specimens; (5) other persons who may be in contact with infectious material, such as hospital laundry, medical waste, and mortuary workers; (6) other groups essential to response activities, such as law enforcement, emergency response, or military personnel; and (7) all persons in a hospital where there is a smallpox patient who is not isolated appropriately. Employees for whom vaccination would be contraindicated (see below) should be furloughed.[36,39]

Smallpox Vaccine

Vaccinia vaccine does not contain smallpox (variola) virus. The only currently available vaccine was prepared from calf lymph with a seed virus derived from the New York City Board of Health (NYCBOH) strain of vaccinia virus (Dryvax vaccine, Wyeth Laboratories, Marietta, Pennsylvania). A supply of licensed Dryvax vaccine was used in 2003 to immunize smallpox health care and public health teams as part of the National Smallpox Vaccination Plan. A reformulated vaccine, produced by using cell-culture techniques, is being developed.

The immune status of those vaccinated more than 27 years ago is not clear. Studies have demonstrated persistence of T cell and humoral responses, but absolute levels of neutralizing antibodies decline substantially during the first 5 to 10 years after vaccination. Interpretation of the data is complicated by the fact that the laboratory correlates of immunologic protection against smallpox infection are not currently established. Epidemiologic studies demonstrate that an increased level of protection against smallpox persists for less than 5 years after primary vaccination, and substantial but waning immunity can persist for longer than 10 years. Antibody levels after revaccination can remain high longer, conferring a greater period of immunity than occurs after primary vaccination alone.[32,35]

Complications of smallpox vaccination Current data on complication rates after primary vaccination are derived from observations made when smallpox vaccine was in routine use in the United States, over 30 years ago, and from the initial reports from the 2002 to 2003 United States military and civilian smallpox vaccination programs, involving 450,293 and 38,257 vaccinees, respectively. In these vaccination programs from 2002 to 2003, licensed undiluted Dryvax vaccine was used.[32,40-42] No cases of eczema vaccinatum or progressive vaccinia or vaccine-attributable deaths occurred. These reports suggest that for selected healthy vaccinees who have been carefully screened for vaccine contraindications and educated about adverse effects, adverse-event rates can be comparable to or less than historical rates. Should smallpox vaccine need to be administered to the general public, higher rates of vaccine complications could occur, given the increased number of persons with vaccine contraindications, including atopic dermatitis and other medical conditions, as well as the number of persons receiving medications that compromise the immune system. Contact transmission of vaccinia from immunized persons to close contacts, particularly those at risk for serious adverse events, is of particular concern.[43] Twenty-one cases of contact transmission were reported from the military program (47 per million vaccinees); no cases of transmission from health care providers to patients occurred.

Cell-mediated immunity is important in controlling smallpox and vaccinia infection. However, the level of immunosuppression that correlates with increased risk of adverse events is not known with certainty. In HIV-infected persons, progressive vaccinia infection after smallpox vaccination is the adverse event of greatest concern (see below); the risk presumably correlates with CD4 cell count.[44] During the 2002 to 2003 United States military smallpox vaccination program, 10 service members with HIV infection and CD4 cell counts ranging from 303 to 752 cells/μl were inadvertently vaccinated before recognition of their HIV infection. All 10 responded successfully to vaccination without adverse events.[40]

Moderate and severe complications of vaccinia vaccination include eczema vaccinatum, generalized vaccinia, progressive vaccinia, and postvaccinial encephalitis. These complications are rare but are at least 10 times more common after primary vaccination than after revaccination; they occur more frequently in infants than in older children and adults.

The most common complication of smallpox vaccination, occurring in 529.2 cases per million doses, is localized vaccinia infection resulting from inadvertent transfer (autoinoculation) of vaccinia from the vaccination site to other parts of the body. In addition, transmission of vaccinia virus can occur when a recently vaccinated person has contact with a susceptible person;

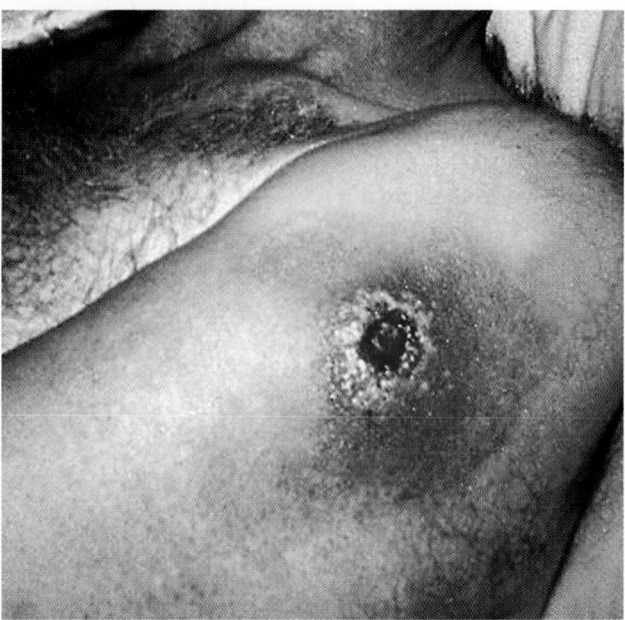

Figure 2   **Progressive vaccinia (vaccinia necrosum) at the site of smallpox vaccination in a 64-year-old man.**

in one study, approximately 30% of eczema vaccinatum cases were persons who had had such contact.[32,45] Inadvertent transfer of vaccinia from the vaccination site to other parts of the body can be prevented by careful hand washing after touching the vaccination site and by keeping the site covered.

Eczema vaccinatum (38.5/million doses) is a localized or systemic dissemination of vaccinia virus that occurs in persons who have eczema or a history of eczema or other chronic or exfoliative skin conditions (e.g., atopic dermatitis). Illness is usually mild and self-limited but can be severe or fatal. Severe cases have also been observed in persons with active eczema or a history of eczema, after contact with recently vaccinated persons.

Generalized vaccinia (241.5/million doses) is characterized by a vesicular rash of varying extent that can occur in persons without underlying illness. The rash is generally self-limited and requires minor or no therapy except in patients whose condition might be toxic or who have serious underlying immunosuppressive illnesses.

Progressive vaccinia (vaccinia necrosum, 1.5/million doses) is a severe, potentially fatal illness characterized by progressive necrosis in the area of vaccination, often with metastatic lesions [*see Figure 2*]. It has occurred almost exclusively in persons with cellular immunodeficiency.

The most common serious complication is postvaccinial encephalitis (12.3/million doses). It occurs mostly in infants younger than 1 year and, less often, in adolescents and adults receiving a primary vaccination. Rates of this complication were influenced by the strain of virus used in the vaccine and were higher in Europe than in the United States. The principal strain of vaccinia virus used in the United States—the NYCBOH strain—was associated with the lowest incidence of postvaccinial encephalitis. Approximately 15% to 25% of affected vaccinees with this complication die, and 25% have permanent neurologic sequelae.

Fatal complications caused by vaccinia vaccination are rare, with approximately one death per million primary vaccinations and 0.25 deaths per million revaccinations. Death is most often the result of postvaccinial encephalitis or progressive vaccinia.

In 2003, cases of myocarditis, pericarditis, or both (myoperi-carditis) occurred at higher than expected rates in both the civilian and the military smallpox vaccination programs. Cases of cardiac ischemic events, including myocardial infarction and angina, were also reported in persons who had received vaccinations; however, the rates of ischemic events were not clearly elevated above expected background rates, and the association between smallpox vaccination and cardiac ischemic events is unclear.[46,47]

Among 450,293 United States military service members vaccinated from December 2002 to May 2003, 37 cases of suspected, probable, or confirmed myopericarditis were observed; the rate was 1:12,195 among male primary vaccinees 21 to 33 years of age. No cases were reported among 132,836 previously vaccinated vaccinees.[40] Through May 9, 2003, 21 cases of myopericarditis (90% of revaccinees) were reported among 36,217 civilian vaccinees, representing a rate of 1:1,700 vaccinees (the rate decreases to 1:36,000 vaccinees when vaccinees without elevations in cardiac enzyme levels are excluded).[46]

Symptoms of myopericarditis after smallpox vaccination began 7 to 19 days after vaccination (range, 1 to 42 days). Symptoms included prodromal myalgias, arthralgias, or both, as well as subsequent pleuritic precordial chest pain with variable shortness of breath, dry cough, or both. Electrocardiogram findings varied; such findings included ST segment and T wave abnormalities and dysrhythmias, including paroxysmal atrial fibrillation, atrial ectopy, supraventricular tachycardia, and ventricular ectopy. ECG findings included pleural effusion and wall motion abnormalities; these findings were not seen in all patients. All patients among the United States military vaccinees, as well as one civilian patient, were reported to have had elevated cardiac enzyme levels. All the patients who were reported to have myopericarditis recovered. In cases where alternative etiologies were sought, none were established, and in no case was a virologic diagnosis made. The biologic mechanism for myopericarditis after smallpox vaccination is not established; it may involve the viral cytopathic effect, an immune-mediated reaction, or both.[47] A surveillance case definition for myopericarditis has been developed to monitor smallpox vaccine adverse events (this definition is not to be used for clinical diagnosis). That surveillance case definition is available on the Internet.[46]

In response to these reports, new cardiovascular screening and exclusion criteria were published for use of smallpox vaccine in persons not exposed to smallpox.[48] Vaccinees experiencing chest pain, shortness of breath, or other symptoms of cardiac disease within 2 weeks of smallpox vaccination are advised to seek medical attention. Although myopericarditis after smallpox vaccination had been previously reported, a causal association with the vaccine had not been recognized.

Focal folliculitis and generalized folliculitis were reported after smallpox vaccination in 7.4% and 2.7%, respectively, of 148 primary vaccinees enrolled in a clinical trial of a smallpox vaccine that is not currently in use but that was derived from the same strain of vaccinia virus as the NYCBOH strain used in Dryvax.[49] Follicular erythematous papules developed from 9 to 11 days after vaccination; these papules progressed to pustules that lasted 3 to 5 days. Lesions appeared primarily in areas where there were larger numbers of hair follicles or sebaceous glands (e.g., the extremities, face, and back); concurrent lesions were in different stages of development. Vaccinia was not isolated from specimens that were available for culture. This new observation is significant because of the potential for this apparently benign condition to be confused with generalized vaccinia.

Contraindications Groups at special risk for complications include persons with eczema or other acute, chronic, or exfoliative skin conditions; patients with immune system suppression, including leukemia, lymphoma, or generalized malignancy who are receiving therapy with alkylating agents, antimetabolites, radiation, or large doses of corticosteroids; patients with HIV infection and persons with hereditary immune disorders; children younger than 1 year; and women who are pregnant or breast-feeding (because of the risk of contact transmission to the child). On the basis of reports of adverse cardiac events in 2003, persons should currently be excluded from preexposure smallpox vaccination if they have known underlying heart disease or three or more known cardiac risk factors (i.e., hypertension, smoking, diabetes, hypercholesterolemia, and heart disease occurring by 50 years of age in a first-degree relative). Deferring vaccination of persons with active inflammatory disease of the eye requiring steroid treatment is advised until the condition resolves and treatment is complete.[48] In persons with contraindications who require vaccination because of exposure to smallpox virus from a bioterrorist attack, the risk of complications can be reduced by giving vaccinia immune globulin (VIG; see below) simultaneously with the vaccine. However, current stores of VIG are insufficient to allow its prophylactic use. Even if VIG is not available, vaccination may still be warranted, given the far higher risk of an adverse outcome from smallpox than from vaccination.

Current information about smallpox vaccine, including recommendations for vaccine use, contraindications, screening of potential vaccinees, prevention of contact transmission, and management of adverse effects, is available on the CDC Web site (http://www.cdc.gov).

Vaccinia immune globulin Complications of vaccinia vaccination can be prevented or treated with VIG, which is an isotonic sterile solution of the immunoglobulin fraction of plasma from persons vaccinated with vaccinia vaccine. For prophylactic use, in persons with contraindications who require vaccination, VIG is given along with vaccinia vaccine.[32] Very large amounts are required: VIG is administered intramuscularly in a dose of 0.3 ml/kg (e.g., 22.5 ml I.M. for a 75 kg patient) At present, however, supplies of VIG are so limited that its use should be reserved for treatment of patients with the most serious vaccine complications.

For treatment of vaccinia vaccination complications, VIG is administered intramuscularly; 0.6 ml/kg is given in divided doses over a 24- to 36-hour period. A repeat dose may be given 2 to 3 days later if improvement does not occur. VIG is effective for treatment of eczema vaccinatum and certain cases of progressive vaccinia; it might be useful also in the treatment of ocular vaccinia resulting from inadvertent implantation. VIG is contraindicated for the treatment of vaccinial keratitis. VIG is recommended for severe generalized vaccinia if the patient is extremely ill or has a serious underlying disease. VIG provides no benefit in the treatment of postvaccinial encephalitis and has no role in the treatment of smallpox.[32,36]

Anthrax

Anthrax is a zoonotic disease caused by the spore-forming bacterium *Bacillus anthracis,* a large, nonmotile, nonhemolytic, gram-positive rod [*see Chapter 135*]. The organism is distributed worldwide in soil. Animals, primarily herbivores, become infected through grazing in contaminated areas. Under natural conditions, humans contract the disease after close contact with infected animals or contaminated animal products such as hides, wool, or meat.[50] Hardy spores resistant to heat and environmental degradation are the usual infective form. The spores develop in response to exposure to ambient air. On exposure to favorable, nutrient-rich environmental conditions such as tissues or blood of an animal or human host, the spores germinate, producing vegetative cells.[51]

CLASSIFICATION AND EPIDEMIOLOGY

Anthrax occurs in three clinical forms in humans: inhalational, cutaneous, and gastrointestinal. In a biologic attack, aerosol exposure to anthrax spores would be most likely.[33] Only 18 cases of inhalational anthrax were reported in the United States in the 20th century, none of them after 1976. Sixteen of these cases were attributable to an industrial source of infection, and two cases were laboratory associated.[52] Before 2001, exposure to powdered anthrax spores in an envelope or package was not thought to be an efficient means of causing inhalational disease. However, exposure to anthrax spores sent through the United States mail in the 2001 anthrax attack resulted in 11 cases of inhalational anthrax and 11 cases of cutaneous disease.[21,53,54] Research has demonstrated the unanticipated potential for significant dispersion of respirable aerosol particles of spores through opening of a contaminated envelope.[55] In addition, expected clinical findings based on previous experience with naturally occurring anthrax infections did not entirely correspond to the clinical presentation in persons exposed to anthrax in the context of a biologic attack, although there was considerable overlap between the two.

Cutaneous anthrax accounts for the majority of naturally occurring anthrax cases worldwide. It results from inoculation of spores subcutaneously through a cut or abrasion.[56] Given that cutaneous anthrax cases occurred during the 2001 anthrax outbreak, it is possible that a bioterrorist attack could be detected through recognition of cutaneous anthrax cases.[21] Gastrointestinal and oropharyngeal anthrax occur in rural parts of the world where anthrax is endemic. They result from ingestion of meat contaminated with spores or large numbers of vegetative cells.[57] No cases of gastrointestinal anthrax occurred during the 1979 accidental release of anthrax from a military facility in Sverdlovsk, Russia, in which 77 inhalational cases occurred, or during the 2001 outbreak in the United States. Because of the logistic difficulty of effectively contaminating food and water supplies, it is thought that this form of anthrax would be less likely to occur as a result of a biologic attack.[33]

PATHOPHYSIOLOGY

Anthrax is a toxin-mediated disease. In inhalational anthrax, 1 to 5 μm particle–bearing spores are deposited in the terminal airways or alveoli, phagocytized by alveolar macrophages, and transported to mediastinal and peribronchial lymph nodes. Spores may stay in the mediastinal lymph nodes for extended periods and can germinate for up to 60 days or longer.[58] Cases of inhalational anthrax occurred up to 43 days after exposure in the Sverdlovsk outbreak.[59] Spores germinate into vegetative cells, which escape from the macrophages, multiply in the lymphatics, and ultimately gain access to the bloodstream, where they can reach high concentrations (107 to 108 organisms per milliliter of blood). Hemorrhagic meningitis is a complication of bacteremic spread; it develops in up to one half of cases.

In anthrax, tissue damage is mediated by two toxins: edema toxin and lethal toxin. These two toxins are composed of various combinations of edema factor, lethal factor, and protective antigen. The three components of edema toxin and lethal toxin are produced by vegetative cells. Vegetative cells also produce an antiphagocytic capsule that is necessary for virulence.[60] Lethal toxin is a combination of lethal factor and protective antigen that interferes with cellular protein synthesis; it causes macrophages to release tumor necrosis factor and interleukin-1. In severe cases, it contributes to sudden death from toxemia. Edema toxin is a combination of edema factor and protective antigen that causes increased cellular levels of cyclic adenosine monophosphate (cAMP) and altered water homeostasis, resulting in massive edema. Together, edema toxin and lethal toxin cause edema, hemorrhage, necrosis, and shock. In cutaneous and gastrointestinal anthrax, toxin production results in a similar pathophysiologic process that causes edema and hemorrhagic necrosis in the skin and gastrointestinal mucosa, respectively. Pathologic studies of eight cases of inhalational anthrax related to the bioterrorism attack of 2001 demonstrated hemorrhagic mediastinitis without pneumonia; pulmonary infiltrates seen on chest radiographs corresponded to pulmonary edema and hyaline membrane formation. Large numbers of anthrax bacilli and cell wall and capsular antigens were observed in pleural tissues—findings that related to persistent pleural effusions seen clinically.[61]

INHALATIONAL ANTHRAX

Clinical Presentation and Diagnosis

Information on the clinical manifestations of inhalational anthrax derived from the 2001 anthrax outbreak both confirms many of the features reported in naturally occurring anthrax cases and reveals unanticipated differences.[52,58,62-64] The infectious dose of anthrax is not known with certainty. Animal data suggest that the median lethal dose (LD_{50}, which is the dose sufficient to kill 50% of exposed subjects) is 2,500 to 55,000 inhaled spores. Data from naturally occurring cases and from two cases in the 2001 outbreak suggest that the infectious dose may be very low in some persons, particularly those with underlying pulmonary disease.[58,63,65]

Clinical symptoms develop rapidly after germination of anthrax spores. The incubation period for inhalational disease is most commonly reported as 1 to 6 days but may be prolonged by antibiotic administration or, presumably, a low infectious dose.[66,67] In the 2001 anthrax outbreak, the median incubation period was 4 days (range, 4 to 6 days) for the six cases in which it could be calculated.

Inhalational anthrax has been described as a two-stage disease. The initial stage is a nonspecific, flulike illness lasting from several hours to a few days. In the 2001 bioterrorism-associated anthrax cases, symptoms at presentation included some combination of fever, chills, weakness, cough, dyspnea, chest discomfort, nausea or vomiting, myalgia, and headache. Profound malaise and drenching sweats were prominent symptoms, and most patients reported nausea or vomiting. Tachycardia was the most consistent clinical sign. Fever was documented in the majority of patients, although it was sometimes low grade. Sore throat, nasal symptoms, and abdominal pain were common. Classically, the initial stage is followed 1 to 3 days later, sometimes after brief improvement, by the rapidly progressive second stage, characterized by fever, dyspnea, diaphoresis,

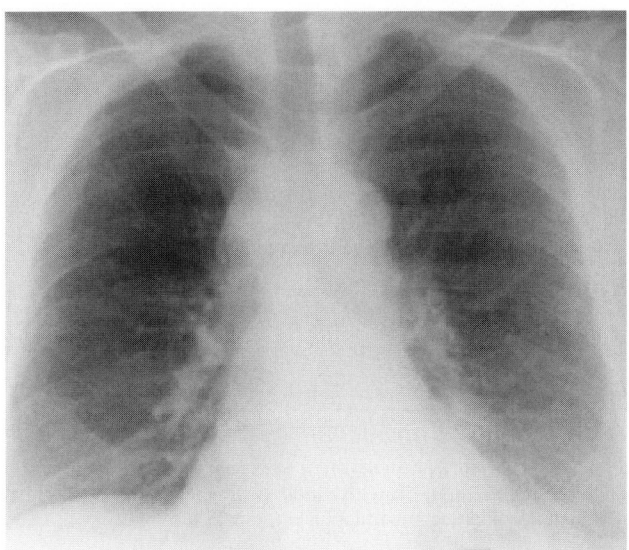

Figure 3   **Chest x-ray of a patient with inhalational anthrax showing mediastinal widening and a small left pleural effusion.**

cyanosis, and shock. In the 2001 cases, no brief improvement between stages was observed.

Laboratory studies are nonspecific or unremarkable during the early stage of disease. The majority of patients experienced elevations in hepatic transaminase levels; neutrophilia without leukocytosis; hyponatremia; hypoalbuminemia; and hypocalcemia.[62,68] Chest x-rays were abnormal on initial presentation in all 11 cases in 2001, although one patient had subtle abnormalities that were initially interpreted as normal. Only seven patients had the classic finding of mediastinal widening [*see Figure 3*]. Pleural effusions were present in all cases. These effusions were often small on presentation and were progressive, requiring drainage in the majority of patients. In contrast to previous descriptions, seven patients had pulmonary infiltrates consistent with pneumonia at presentation, and one patient was thought to have heart failure with pulmonary congestion. Other abnormalities included paratracheal and hilar fullness. The CT scan was valuable in further characterizing abnormalities in the lungs and mediastinum and was more sensitive than the chest x-ray in revealing mediastinal changes. Blood cultures can be diagnostic, although appropriate antibiotic therapy rapidly reduces the likelihood of isolating the organism. In the 2001 cases, *B. anthracis* was isolated from blood cultures obtained before antibiotic therapy was given, but not from those obtained afterward.

The initial manifestations of inhalational anthrax are nonspecific and are consistent with flulike illnesses caused by a variety of respiratory viruses, as well as with community-acquired bacterial infections. Adults can average one to three episodes of flulike illness a year, and millions of cases occur throughout the United States.[69] Because of the high frequency of flulike illnesses and the low likelihood of inhalational anthrax in a given patient, a combination of epidemiologic, clinical, and (if indicated) laboratory testing should be used to evaluate potential cases of inhalational anthrax [*see Figure 4*]. According to CDC guidelines, consideration of inhalational anthrax hinges on a history of exposure or occupational/environmental risk within 2 to 5 days before illness onset.[19] Whenever possible, exposure and risk determinations should be made in consultation with public health authorities before initiating treatment or preventive therapy.

The clinical presentation of inhalational anthrax may be difficult to distinguish from that of community-acquired pneumonia.[68] According to the CDC, diagnostic testing for anthrax should be done in patients whose signs and symptoms are consistent with anthrax and when one or more of the following conditions are present: a history of a recent anthrax case or outbreak in the community; a credible threat of anthrax exposure, as determined by law enforcement and public health authorities; a cluster of anthraxlike cases characterized by rapid deterioration. Anthrax should also be considered in any patient with compatible symptoms and rapid deterioration. Alternatively, a set of five symptoms that are compatible with inhalational anthrax, in combination with fever and tachycardia, have been suggested as criteria for pursuing additional diagnostic evaluation for patients with possible inhalational anthrax who are without epidemiologic risk factors.[70] All cases of *suspected* anthrax should be reported immediately to local or state public health authorities and the hospital epidemiologist (http://www.statepublichealth.org). The clinical laboratory should also be alerted when diagnostic specimens of suspected anthrax are submitted to ensure that appropriate precautions are taken to protect laboratory staff, facilitate proper evaluation of the isolate, and expedite confirmatory testing at the nearest laboratory that belongs to the public health Laboratory Response Network.[6]

There is no rapid screening test to diagnose inhalational anthrax in its early stages. In persons with a compatible clinical illness for whom there is a heightened suspicion of anthrax based on clinical and epidemiologic data, the appropriate initial diagnostic tests are a chest x-ray or chest CT scan, or both, and culture and smear of peripheral blood. On chest x-rays, the posteroanterior and lateral view may be more sensitive than the anteroposterior (portable) view in detecting pulmonary abnormalities. Mediastinal widening or hyperdense mediastinal lymphadenopathy (secondary to hemorrhagic lymph nodes) on a nonenhanced CT scan should raise the suspicion of pulmonary anthrax [*see Figure 5*]. Most persons with flulike illnesses do not have radiologic findings of pneumonia; such findings occur most often in the very young, the elderly, and persons with chronic lung disease.

Pleural fluid and cerebrospinal fluid, as well as biopsy specimens taken from the pleura and lung, are also potentially useful for culture and other testing when disease is present in these sites, whereas sputum culture and Gram stain are unlikely to be useful. In highly suspicious cases, local or state health departments can arrange for additional diagnostic testing, including immunohistochemical staining and PCR at the CDC. Serologic testing is not useful in clinical management but may be used in epidemiologic investigations. Similarly, nasal swabs are of potential value in epidemiologic investigations for determining the route and extent of spread of anthrax in a population, but they have no role in clinical management.

A rapid influenza test can be used when influenza itself is a consideration in a patient with flulike illness, but these kits have limited value because their sensitivity can be relatively low (45% to 90%). However, rapid influenza testing with viral culture can help indicate whether influenza viruses are circulating among certain populations, and this epidemiologic information can be useful in diagnosing flulike illnesses.[69]

Treatment

Early intravenous antibiotic treatment may improve survival in inhalational anthrax.[71] In contrast to the reported case-fatality

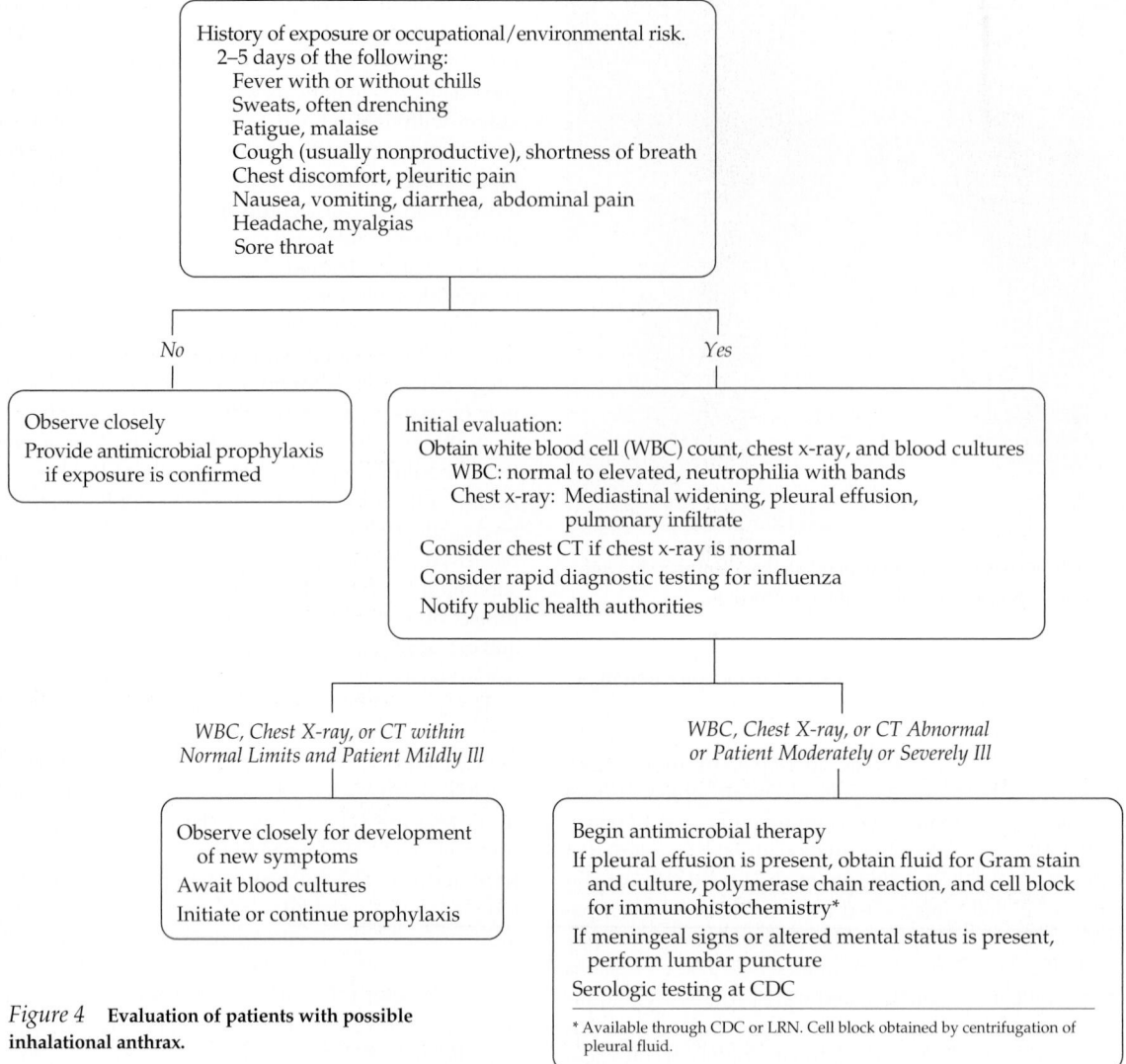

Figure 4 **Evaluation of patients with possible inhalational anthrax.**

rate of 85% for 20th-century inhalational anthrax cases, 6 of 11 patients in the 2001 outbreak survived; all the survivors presented during the initial phase of the illness and received treatment the same day with antibiotics active against *B. anthracis.* Fatal cases occurred in patients who had severe disease by the time they first received antibiotics with activity against *B. anthracis.* Aggressive supportive care—including attention to fluid, electrolyte, and acid-base disturbances and drainage of pleural effusions—also played an important role in treatment.[62]

Current CDC treatment recommendations and related guidelines and information can be obtained at http://www.bt.cdc.gov/agent/anthrax/index.asp. Before initiating treatment, clinicians should review this site to stay informed of revisions and updates. The Working Group on Civilian Biodefense has published similar recommendations with a detailed accompanying text.[58]

At present, intravenous ciprofloxacin or doxycycline plus one or two additional antimicrobials with in vitro activity against *B. anthracis* are recommended for initial empirical treatment [*see Table 5*]. Antibiotic therapy should be modified according to the results of antimicrobial susceptibility testing to ensure that the most effective and least toxic regimen is used. The duration of antimicrobial therapy should be at least 60 days. Once clinical improvement occurs, it may be possible to complete the course of treatment with one or two agents given orally. Corticosteroid therapy has been suggested as adjunct therapy for inhalational anthrax associated with extensive edema, respiratory compromise, and meningitis.[21,56,58]

Prevention

Ciprofloxacin and doxycycline are recommended first-line agents for prophylaxis in persons exposed to inhalational anthrax. In vivo data suggest that other fluoroquinolone antibiotics would have efficacy equivalent to that of ciprofloxacin.[58] High-dose amoxicillin is an option when ciprofloxacin or doxycycline is contraindicated [*see Table 6*]. Postexposure prophylaxis should continue for at least 60 days.[72] Given the uncertainty about the length of time viable spores can persist in the lungs, patients should be instructed to seek prompt medical evaluation if symptoms compatible with anthrax develop after discontinuance of postexposure prophylaxis. Because of uncertainty about the length of time that anthrax spores can remain viable in the lungs, the United States Department of Health and Human Services made two additional options available for preventive treatment for persons exposed to inhalational anthrax in the 2001 outbreak. These options were to follow a 60-day course of antibiotic treatment with either (1) an additional 40 days of an-

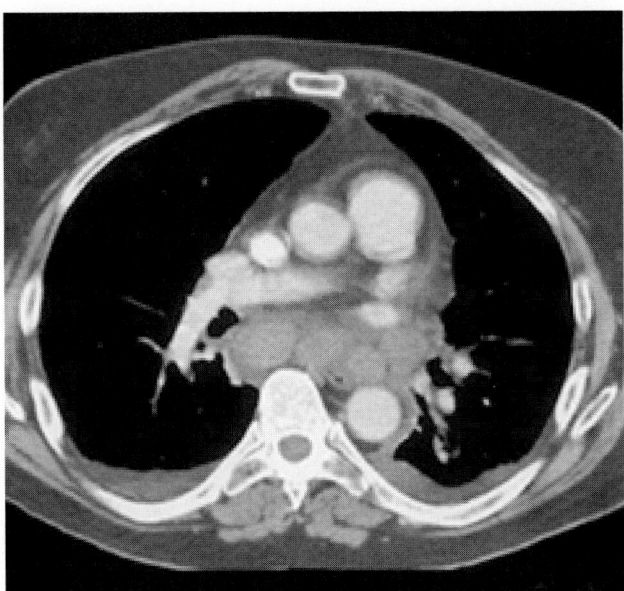

Figure 5   CT scan of the chest of a patient with inhalational anthrax showing mediastinal lymphadenopathy and small bilateral pleural effusions.

tibiotic treatment or (2) an additional 40 days of antibiotic treatment plus three doses of anthrax vaccine over a 4-week period.[73]

Anthrax vaccine   The only licensed human anthrax vaccine available in the United States is anthrax vaccine adsorbed (AVA). This is an inactivated, cell-free filtrate of a nonencapsulated attenuated strain of *B. anthracis* (BioPort Corporation, Lansing, Michigan).[67] Primary vaccination consists of three subcutaneous injections at 0, 2, and 4 weeks and three booster vaccinations at 6, 12, and 18 months. To maintain immunity, the manufacturer recommends an annual booster injection. The basis for this recommended schedule of vaccination is not well defined.

Vaccination of adults with the licensed vaccine induced an immune response, as measured by indirect hemagglutination, in 83% of vaccinees 2 weeks after the first dose and in 91% of vaccinees who received two or more doses. Approximately 95% of vaccinees undergo seroconversion after three doses, with a fourfold rise in titers of IgG against protective antigen (the principal antigen responsible for inducing immunity). However, the precise correlation between antibody titer (or concentration) and protection against infection is not defined. The vaccine has shown efficacy in experiments involving animal models of inhalational anthrax in preexposure settings and, in combination with antibiotics, in postexposure settings.[58,69]

Anthrax vaccine is considered acceptably safe by the Advisory Committee on Immunization Practices and the Institute of Medicine.[67,74] Supplies of anthrax vaccine are limited and are held by the United States Department of Defense. A combination of antibiotics and anthrax vaccine, if available, is recommended for exposed persons after a biologic attack.[58,75,76] At this time, preexposure use of anthrax vaccine is recommended only for certain laboratory workers and others at occupational risk for repeated exposures to *B. anthracis* spores; it is not recommended for the general public.

CUTANEOUS ANTHRAX

After an incubation period of approximately 7 days (range, 1 to 12 days), the primary lesion of cutaneous anthrax appears as a nondescript, painless, pruritic papule, usually on an exposed area such as the face, head, neck, or upper extremity. The papule enlarges and develops a central vesicle or bullae with surrounding brawny, nonpitting edema. The central vesicle enlarges and ulcerates over 1 to 2 days, becoming hemorrhagic, depressed, and necrotic and leading to a central black eschar [*see Figure 6*]. Satellite vesicles may be present. The eschar dries and falls off over the next 1 to 2 weeks. The findings of a painless lesion and edema out of proportion to the size of the lesion and the fact that pustules are rarely present in cutaneous anthrax are clinically useful. Tender regional lymphadenopathy, fever, chills, and fatigue may occur. Systemic disease has been

Table 5   Treatment of Inhalational Anthrax

Patients	*Medication and Dosage*	*Comments*
Adults, including pregnant women and immunocompromised persons	Ciprofloxacin, 400 mg I.V., q. 12 hr *or* Doxycycline, 100 mg I.V., q. 12 hr *and* One or two additional antimicrobials*	If meningitis is suspected, doxycycline may be less optimal because of poor central nervous system penetration Modify regimen on the basis of susceptibility testing of isolate; can switch to p.o. after patient is clinically stable; continue treatment for at least 60 days Consider corticosteroids for meningitis, severe edema, or respiratory compromise
Children, including those who are immunocompromised	Ciprofloxacin, 10–15 mg/kg I.V., q. 12 hr, not to exceed 1 g/day *or* Doxycycline If > 8 yr and > 45 kg, give adult dosage If ≤ 8 yr or if > 8 yr but ≤ 45 kg, give 2.2 mg/kg q. 12 hr (maximum, 200 mg/day) *and* One or two additional antimicrobials*	If meningitis is suspected, doxycycline may be less optimal because of poor central nervous system penetration Modify regimen on the basis of susceptibility testing of isolate; can switch to p.o. after patient is clinically stable; continue treatment for at least 60 days Consider corticosteroids for meningitis, severe edema, or respiratory compromise

Note: Treatment recommendations may change over time and according to antimicrobial susceptibility test results during a biologic attack and to availability of selected antimicrobial agents. Before initiating treatment, clinicians should consult with an infectious disease specialist and public health authorities and should check for revisions and updates at http://www.bt.cdc.gov/index.asp. This information is adapted from CDC and Working Group on Civilian Biodefense recommendations and may not represent FDA-approved uses.
*Other agents with in vitro activity against anthrax include rifampin, vancomycin, penicillin, ampicillin, chloramphenicol, imipenem, clindamycin, and clarithromycin.

Table 6 Postexposure Prophylaxis for Anthrax in the Setting of a Bioterrorist Attack

Patients	Medication	Comments
Adults, including immuno-compromised persons	Ciprofloxacin, 500 mg p.o., q. 12 hr *or* Doxycycline, 100 mg p.o., q. 12 hr *or, if strain proved susceptible,* Amoxicillin, 500 mg p.o., q. 8 hr	Give prophylaxis for at least 60 days
Pregnant women	Ciprofloxacin, 500 mg p.o., q. 12 hr *or, if strain proved susceptible,* Amoxicillin, 500 mg p.o., q. 8 hr	Give prophylaxis for at least 60 days
Children, including those who are immunocom-promised	Ciprofloxacin, 10–15 mg/kg p.o., b.i.d., not to exceed 1g/day *or, if strain proved susceptible,* Amoxicillin If ≥ 20 kg: 500 mg p.o., q. 8 hr If < 20 kg: 80 mg/kg/day p.o., in divided doses q. 8 hr (maximum, 500 mg/dose)	Give prophylaxis for at least 60 days

Note: Prophylaxis recommendations may change over time and according to antimicrobial susceptibility test results during a biologic attack and to availability of selected antimicrobial agents. Before initiating prophylaxis, clinicians should consult with an infectious disease specialist and public health authorities and should check for revisions and updates at http://www.bt.cdc.gov/index.asp. This information is adapted from CDC and Working Group on Civilian Biodefense recommendations and may not represent FDA-approved uses.

reported to have a mortality of 20% if untreated. Cutaneous anthrax of the face or neck may lead to respiratory compromise from massive edema.[56,58,60,77]

The differential diagnosis of cutaneous anthrax includes other causes of eschar and ulceration and the ulceroglandular syndrome.[75] Guidelines for the diagnosis of cutaneous anthrax have been published by the American Academy of Dermatology (http://www.aad.org).

For patients with the typical appearance and progression of cutaneous anthrax, a Gram stain and culture of the skin lesion should be obtained using a dry swab for unroofed vesicle fluid and a moist swab for the base of the ulcer and edges underneath the eschar. Blood cultures are also recommended. If the patient is taking antimicrobial drugs or if the Gram stain and culture are negative for *B. anthracis* or clinical suspicion remains high, two punch biopsies for culture (with the specimen placed in saline) and immunohistochemical staining should be performed; PCR (with the specimen placed in formalin) should be performed, or both should be considered [*see Figure 7*]. Immunohistochemical staining and PCR testing at the CDC should be arranged through local public health authorities.[21,58]

Management

Antibiotic treatment is curative in cutaneous anthrax and can be initiated pending confirmation of anthrax infection. Ciprofloxacin and doxycycline are first-line agents for the empirical treatment of cutaneous anthrax and may be administered orally. Intravenous therapy with multiple drugs, as for inhalational anthrax (see above), is recommended for patients with signs of systemic involvement, extensive edema, or lesions of the face and neck.[71]

GASTROINTESTINAL AND OROPHARYNGEAL ANTHRAX

Symptoms appear 2 to 5 days after ingestion of contaminated food and include nausea, vomiting, fever, malaise, and abdominal pain. Severe bloody diarrhea with rebound abdominal tenderness develops. Ulcerative lesions occur primarily in the terminal ileum and cecum. Gastric ulcers with hematemesis, hemorrhagic mesenteric lymphadenitis, and marked ascites may

occur. Mediastinal widening has also been reported with gastrointestinal anthrax. Morbidity results from blood loss, fluid and electrolyte imbalances, and shock. The case-fatality rate is reportedly greater than 50%; death results from toxemia or intestinal perforation.[33,57,58]

Oropharyngeal anthrax is characterized by sore throat, fever, dysphagia, and marked edema and lymphadenitis. Ulcerative lesions may have an associated pseudomembrane. Specimens for diagnosis of gastrointestinal anthrax may include ascitic fluid for Gram stain and culture, blood cultures, and tissue samples from affected mucosal sites.

Treatment for gastrointestinal anthrax and oropharyngeal anthrax is the same as that for inhalational anthrax (see above).

INFECTION CONTROL

Person-to-person transmission of anthrax is not known to occur. Patients may be hospitalized in a standard hospital room

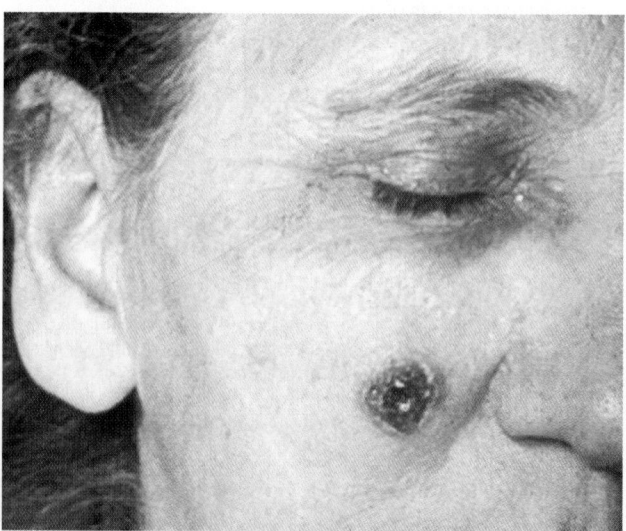

Figure 6   Cutaneous anthrax lesion, 11 days old.

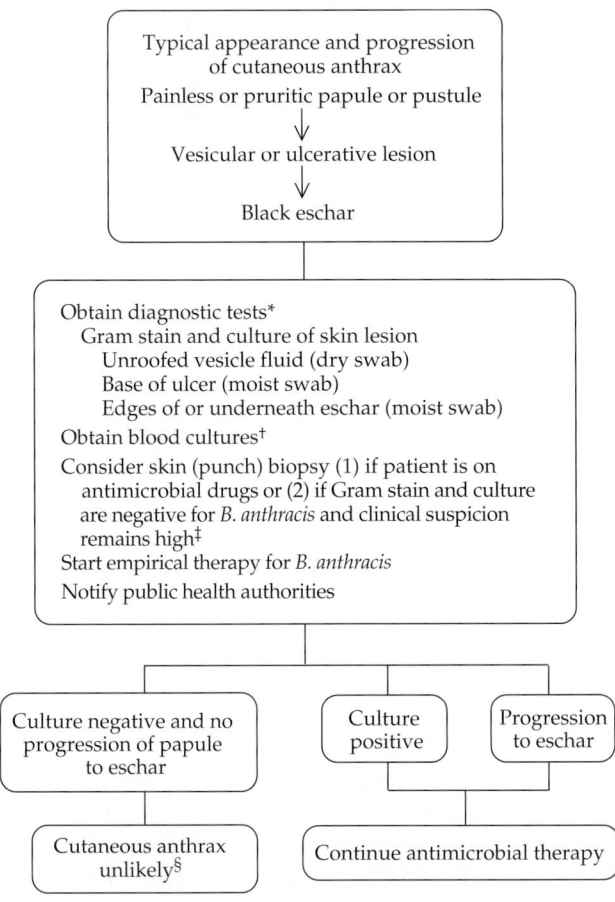

Typical appearance and progression
of cutaneous anthrax
Painless or pruritic papule or pustule
↓
Vesicular or ulcerative lesion
↓
Black eschar

Obtain diagnostic tests*
  Gram stain and culture of skin lesion
    Unroofed vesicle fluid (dry swab)
    Base of ulcer (moist swab)
    Edges of or underneath eschar (moist swab)
Obtain blood cultures†
Consider skin (punch) biopsy (1) if patient is on
  antimicrobial drugs or (2) if Gram stain and culture
  are negative for *B. anthracis* and clinical suspicion
  remains high‡
Start empirical therapy for *B. anthracis*
Notify public health authorities

Culture negative and no
progression of papule
to eschar

Culture
positive

Progression
to eschar

Cutaneous anthrax
unlikely§

Continue antimicrobial therapy

* Serologic testing available at CDC may be an additional diagnostic technique for confirmation of cases of cutaneous anthrax.

† If blood cultures are positive for *B. anthracis*, treat with antimicrobials as for inhalational anthrax.

‡ Punch biopsy should be submitted in formalin to CDC. Polymerase chain reaction can also be done on formalin-fixed specimen. Gram stain and culture are frequently negative for *B. anthracis* after initiation of antimicrobials.

§ Continue antimicrobial prophylaxis for inhalational anthrax for 60 days if aerosol exposure to *B. anthracis* is known or suspected.

Figure 7 **Evaluation of patients with possible cutaneous anthrax.**

with standard barrier isolation precautions. No treatment is necessary for contacts of cases.

The microbiology laboratory should be notified upon suspicion of anthrax to ensure that appropriate precautions are taken under BSL-2 conditions when specimens are processed for culture.[78] Sporicidal solutions approved for use in hospitals and commercially available bleach or a 0.5% hypochlorite solution (1:10 dilution of household bleach) are effective for decontamination of contaminated areas. Precautions should be taken during autopsies, and cremation of human remains should be considered to prevent further transmission of disease.[24]

Plague

Plague is caused by the gram-negative coccobacillus *Yersinia pestis*, of the family Enterobacteriaceae. Wild rodents are the animal reservoir for the disease. Under natural conditions, plague is transmitted to humans by the bite of an infectious flea and, less frequently, by direct contact with infectious body fluids or tissues of an infected animal or by inhaling infectious droplets.[79]

Plague has a long history of use and development as a biologic weapon, including the catapulting of plague victims' corpses over the walls of a besieged city in the 14th century. The most likely presentation after a biologic attack is primary pneumonic plague.[33] Additional information on plague, including the nonpneumonic forms (bubonic and septicemic plague), microbiology, and pathogenesis, is available elsewhere [*see Chapter 141*].

CLINICAL PRESENTATION

Plague is a severe febrile illness. Pneumonic plague, the most fatal form of the infection, can develop from inhalation of plague bacilli (primary pneumonic plague) or from hematogenous spread secondary to septicemic plague. Approximately 12% of cases of bubonic and primary septicemic plague develop into secondary pneumonic plague. Conversely, septicemic plague can be secondary to primary pneumonic plague.

The incubation period for pneumonic plague is typically 2 to 4 days (range, 1 to 6 days). Presenting symptoms typically include the acute onset of malaise, high fever, chills, headache, chest discomfort, dyspnea, and cough concomitant with or followed rapidly by clinical sepsis. Hemoptysis is a classic sign that should suggest plague in the appropriate clinical context, but sputum may be watery or purulent. Gastrointestinal symptoms may be prominent with pneumonic plague; these include nausea, vomiting, diarrhea, and abdominal pain. A cervical bubo is infrequently present.

The disease is rapidly progressive, with increasing dyspnea, stridor, and cyanosis. Rapidly progressive respiratory failure and sepsis within 2 to 4 days of onset of illness is typical of pneumonic plague. Abnormalities on chest x-ray are variable but frequently show bilateral patchy infiltrates or consolidation. The mortality for pneumonic plague is reported to be 57% and is extremely high when initiation of treatment is delayed beyond 24 hours after symptom onset.[80] Complications of septicemic plague include disseminated intravascular coagulation (DIC), purpuric skin lesions and gangrene of extremities (so-called black death), acute respiratory distress syndrome (ARDS), meningitis, and multiorgan failure with shock.[33,81-83]

DIAGNOSIS

During a confirmed outbreak of pneumonic plague after a biologic attack, a presumptive diagnosis can be made on the basis of symptoms, especially if there is a high index of suspicion. However, other causes of severe pneumonia or rapidly progressive respiratory infection with or without sepsis should be considered. Suspected cases of plague should be immediately reported to the local public health department and the hospital epidemiologist.

There are no widely available, rapid confirmatory tests for *Y. pestis*. Specimens for bacteriologic and serologic testing should be collected before initiating therapy. Sputum, blood, and lymph node aspirate should be submitted for Gram stain and culture. Microscopic examination of clinical specimens or buffy coat may show a gram-negative coccobacillus; Wright, Giemsa, or Wayson stains may show bipolar (safety pin) staining. Sera for acute and convalescent antibody detection should be obtained, but findings are primarily of epidemiologic value. Additional diagnostic testing, including antigen detection, IgM immunoassay, immunostaining, PCR testing, and antimicrobial susceptibility testing, is available through the CDC and through designated public health laboratories (http://www.

Table 7   Antimicrobial Treatment of Pneumonic Plague

Patients	Drug	Comments
Adults	Streptomycin, 1 g I.M., b.i.d. *or* Gentamicin, 5 mg/kg I.M. or I.V., q.d., or 2 mg/kg loading dose followed by 1.7 mg/kg I.M. or I.V., t.i.d. *Alternative choices:* Doxycycline, 100 mg I.V., b.i.d., or 200 mg I.V., q.d. Ciprofloxacin, 400 mg I.V., b.i.d. Chloramphenicol, 25 mg/kg I.V., q.i.d.	Treat for 10 days; during a community outbreak of pneumonic plague, all persons developing a temperature ≥ 101.3° F (38.5° C) or a new cough should begin parenteral antibiotic treatment; oral treatment may be given when resources for parenteral treatment are limited; pregnant women should not receive streptomycin or chloramphenicol; tetracycline may be substituted for doxycycline
Children	Streptomycin, 15 mg/kg I.M., b.i.d. (maximum, 2 g/day) *or* Gentamicin, 2.5 mg/kg I.M. or I.V., t.i.d. *Alternative choices:* Doxycycline: if ≥ 45 kg, adult dosage; if < 45 kg, 2.2 mg/kg b.i.d. (maximum, 200 mg/day) Ciprofloxacin, 15 mg/kg I.V., b.i.d. Chloramphenicol, 25 mg/kg I.V., q.i.d.; maintain serum concentration between 5 and 20 µg/ml	Use chloramphenicol in plague meningitis

Note: Treatment recommendations may change over time and according to antimicrobial susceptibility test results during a biologic attack and to availability of selected antimicrobial agents. Before initiating treatment, clinicians should consult with an infectious disease specialist and public health authorities and should check for revisions and updates at http://www.bt.cdc.gov/index.asp. This information is adapted from CDC and Working Group on Civilian Biodefense recommendations and may not represent FDA-approved uses.

statepublichealth.org). Specimen submission should be arranged through local public health authorities. The laboratory should be notified whenever plague is suspected, to help prevent exposures to staff and to facilitate appropriate testing.[33,80,83]

Laboratory findings are consistent with the systemic inflammatory response syndrome. The leukocyte count is elevated and the differential shows a neutrophil predominance, including immature forms. Platelets may be normal or low. Coagulation abnormalities include increased fibrin degradation products, hypofibrinogenemia, and prolongation of the prothrombin time (PT) and partial thromboplastin time (PTT). Elevated liver function tests and abnormal renal function tests are seen with systemic disease.

TREATMENT

When plague is suspected, antibiotic treatment should begin before laboratory confirmation of the diagnosis [*see Table 7*]. Whenever possible, specimens should be collected for bacteriologic and serologic testing before the start of therapy. Antibiotic resistance is rare with naturally occurring *Y. pestis* but may be present in strains used as biologic weapons. Treatment should be continued for 10 days or for 3 days after defervescence and improvement in symptoms. The route of administration can be changed from intravenous to oral after the patient is clinically stable. The choice of antibiotic may be modified after microbial sensitivity testing is completed. The CDC bioterrorism Web site or local public health authorities should be consulted for updated treatment recommendations.[33,80,83]

Postexposure Prophylaxis for Pneumonic Plague

All persons potentially exposed to aerosolized *Y. pestis* and all persons in close contact with pneumonic plague patients (close contact is defined as exposure within 2 m [6.5 ft]) should be treated for 7 days after the last exposure [*see Table 8*]. Persons receiving prophylactic antibiotic treatment should seek medical evaluation immediately if fever or illness with cough develops.

There is no currently available vaccine for pneumonic plague. The previously available licensed plague vaccine in the United States was discontinued in 1999. That vaccine was demonstrated to reduce the severity of illness with bubonic plague but not pneumonic plague.[81]

Communicability and Infection Control Considerations

Pneumonic plague is transmitted person to person through respiratory droplets. Aerosol transmission has not been demonstrated. For patients with pneumonic plague, respiratory droplet precautions as well as standard precautions are recommended, including the use of gowns, gloves, eye protection, and surgical masks for the first 48 hours of antimicrobial therapy and until clinical improvement occurs. Hospitalized patients should remain in isolation for the first 48 hours of antimicrobial therapy and until clinical improvement occurs. Hospitalized patients should wear a mask during transport.

Y. pestis is rapidly destroyed by sunlight and drying. Environmental surfaces can be decontaminated with a standard disinfectant. Persons exposed to aerosolized plague bacilli during a biologic attack should shower with warm water and soap. Clothing of persons exposed to an aerosol of *Y. pestis* and linens of plague patients should be washed in hot water.[24,81,82]

Botulism

Botulism is a paralytic illness caused by a potent neurotoxin produced by *Clostridium botulinum,* an anaerobic, spore-forming bacterium. Natural forms of the disease are foodborne botulism, wound botulism, and infant botulism. Foodborne botulism results from ingestion of improperly processed foodstuffs containing preformed toxin produced by *C. botulinum.* Wound botulism results from production of botulinum toxin by *C. botulinum* organisms that contaminate wounds. Infant botulism results from the colonization of the intestinal tract of infants after ingestion of spores. Botulinum toxin has been developed as a biologic weapon. An aerosol attack is considered the most likely use of botulinum toxin for bioterrorism, although intentional contamination of food supplies is possible.[33,84] Additional information about the pathogenesis and epidemiology of noninhalational forms of botulism is available elsewhere [*see Chapter 136*].

Botulinum toxin is the most potent lethal toxin known. The estimated toxic dose of type A botulinum toxin is 0.001 μg/kg of body weight. There are seven distinct antigenic types of botulinum neurotoxins—types A through G—produced by different strains of *C. botulinum*. Human botulism is caused primarily by toxin types A, B, and E. Botulinum toxin acts to block neurotransmission by binding irreversibly to the presynaptic nerve terminal at the neuromuscular junction and preventing the release of acetylcholine, resulting in bulbar palsies and skeletal muscle weakness. The toxin is colorless, odorless, and presumably tasteless.[33,85,86]

CLINICAL PRESENTATION

The incubation period for foodborne botulism is 2 hours to 8 days; the typical incubation period is 12 to 72 hours. The incubation period for inhalational botulism is not established. Aerosol exposures of monkeys and accidental aerosol exposure of humans have resulted in clinical illness developing 12 to 80 hours after exposure. Type A toxin is associated with more severe disease and a higher fatality rate than type B or E. The neurologic features of all forms of botulism are similar.[33,85,86] Although initial symptoms in foodborne botulism may include nausea, vomiting, abdominal cramps, and diarrhea, these symptoms are thought to result from other bacterial metabolites in contaminated food and may not occur in inhalational botulism.

The so-called classic triad of botulism summarizes the clinical presentation: an afebrile patient, symmetrical descending flaccid paralysis with prominent bulbar palsies, and a clear sensorium.[85-87] Symptoms of cranial nerve abnormalities nearly always begin in the bulbar musculature; patients typically present with difficulty seeing, speaking, or swallowing. Clinical hallmarks include ptosis, blurred vision, and the so-called four Ds: diplopia, dysarthria, dysphonia, and dysphagia. Cranial nerve abnormalities and bulbar weakness are followed by symmetrical descending weakness and paralysis with progression from the head to the arms, thorax, and legs. The extent of paralysis and rapidity of onset of symptoms are proportional to the dose of toxin absorbed into the circulation. Recovery depends on the regeneration of new motor axon twigs to reinnervate paralyzed muscle fibers; recovery may take weeks to months.

Anticholinergic symptoms are common, including dry mouth, ileus, constipation, nausea and vomiting, urinary retention, and mydriasis. Other symptoms include dizziness and sore throat. Sensory findings are not present, with the exception of circumoral and peripheral paresthesias secondary to hyperventilation resulting from anxiety. Botulinum toxin does not cross the blood-brain barrier. Cranial nerve dysfunction and facial nerve weakness may make communication difficult; these symptoms may be mistaken for lethargy and signs of central nervous system involvement.

DIAGNOSIS

Initiation of treatment with botulinum antitoxin should be based on the clinical diagnosis and should not await laboratory confirmation. A clinician who suspects botulism should immediately contact the local or state health department to facilitate procurement of antitoxin for treatment; arrangements should be made for confirmatory diagnostic testing and initiation of an epidemiologic investigation to identify the source of infection. In cases of potential foodborne botulism, any leftover foodstuffs or containers should be held for testing by the public health laboratory.

Demonstration of botulinum toxin in serum samples by mouse bioassay is diagnostic. Samples of serum (in adults, > 30 ml blood in a tiger-top or red-top tube) obtained before administration of botulinum antitoxin should be submitted for testing. For potential foodborne botulism, samples of stool, gastric aspirate, emesis, and suspect foods should also be submitted.[86] The likelihood of finding toxin in the sera of affected patients decreases with time; it is detectable in only 13% to 28% of patients more than 2 days after ingestion.[88]

The possibility of a bioterrorist attack should be considered in any outbreak of botulism. A bioterrorist attack should especially be considered when a cluster of cases occurs; when an outbreak has a common geographic location but there is no common dietary exposure (suggestive of possible aerosol exposure); when there is an outbreak of an unusual botulinum toxin type; or when multiple simultaneous outbreaks occur. A careful dietary and travel history must be taken to help identify the

Table 8 Postexposure Prophylaxis of Pneumonic Plague

Patients	Drug	Comments
Adults, including pregnant women	Doxycycline, 100 mg p.o., b.i.d. Ciprofloxacin, 500 mg p.o., b.i.d. *Alternative:* Chloramphenicol, 25 mg/kg p.o., q.i.d.	Asymptomatic household contacts, hospital contacts, or other close contacts should receive postexposure prophylaxis for 7 days; contacts who develop fever or cough while receiving prophylaxis should begin antibiotic treatment for plague.
Children	Doxycycline: if ≥ 45 kg, adult dosage; if < 45 kg, 2.2 mg/kg p.o., b.i.d. (maximum, 200 mg/day) Ciprofloxacin, 20 mg/kg p.o., b.i.d. *Alternative:* Chloramphenicol, 25 mg/kg p.o., q.i.d.	Asymptomatic household contacts, hospital contacts, or other close contacts should receive postexposure prophylaxis for 7 days; contacts who develop fever or cough while receiving prophylaxis should begin antibiotic treatment for plague.

Note: Prophylaxis recommendations may change over time and according to antimicrobial susceptibility test results during a biologic attack and to availability of selected antimicrobial agents. Before initiating prophylaxis, clinicians should consult with an infectious disease specialist and public health authorities and should check for revisions and updates at http://www.bt.cdc.gov/index.asp. This information is adapted from CDC and Working Group on Civilian Biodefense recommendations and may not represent FDA-approved uses.

source. Patients should be asked if they know of others with similar symptoms.

The differential diagnosis of botulism includes stroke and other neuromuscular disorders.[85,86] A CT scan of the head may be used to exclude cerebrovascular accident, although it is relatively insensitive in early ischemic stroke [see Chapter 177]. Patients with myasthenia gravis will often have characteristic electromyographic findings and serum antibody tests. A test dose of edrophonium (Tensilon) may briefly reverse paralysis in patients with myasthenia gravis but also, reportedly, in some cases of botulism. Guillain-Barré syndrome typically results in ascending paralysis and sensory abnormalities. Cerebrospinal fluid protein is normal in patients with botulism and is normal or elevated in patients with Guillain-Barré syndrome. The rare Miller-Fisher variant of Guillain-Barré syndrome is characterized by descending paralysis and may be confused with botulism. Other conditions that mimic botulism include tick paralysis; poliomyelitis; Eaton-Lambert syndrome; paralytic shellfish poisoning; pufferfish ingestion; and anticholinesterase intoxication with organophosphates, atropine, carbon monoxide, or aminoglycosides.

The electromyogram (EMG) can help distinguish different causes of paralysis. The EMG in botulism demonstrates normal nerve conduction velocity, normal sensory nerve function, and small amplitude motor potentials with facilitation to repetitive stimulation at 50 Hz.[89]

TREATMENT

The mainstay of treatment for botulism is supportive care, including intensive care, mechanical ventilation, and parenteral nutrition. Morbidity and mortality are usually from pulmonary aspiration secondary to loss of the gag reflex and dysphagia leading to inability to control secretions, respiratory failure secondary to inadequate tidal volume from diaphragmatic and accessory respiratory muscle paralysis, and airway obstruction from pharyngeal and upper airway muscle paralysis. Careful and frequent monitoring of the gag and cough reflexes, swallowing, oxygen saturation, vital capacity, and inspiratory force are critical. Airway intubation is indicated for inability to control secretions and impending respiratory failure. Secondary infections are common and should be sought in patients who develop fever.

Trivalent (ABE) equine antitoxin is available from the CDC through state and local health departments and should be administered as soon as possible after clinical diagnosis. Antitoxin can prevent progression of disease caused by subsequent binding of toxin but does not reverse the effects of already bound toxin. For this reason, antitoxin is not useful if the patient is no longer showing progression of disease or is improving from maximum paralysis. The amount of neutralizing antibody present in the standard treatment dose of antitoxin far exceeds maximum serum toxin concentrations in foodborne botulism patients, and repeat doses are usually not required. In a biologic attack, however, patients may be exposed to unusually high concentrations of toxin, so serum toxin levels should be assessed after initiation of treatment in such cases to determine the need for repeat doses. Botulism caused by toxin types other than A, B, or E would not respond to the trivalent antitoxin. Limited quantities of an investigational heptavalent (A-G) antitoxin are held by the United States Army. However, because of the time delay involved in typing the toxin, the utility of this product in a biologic attack is probably minimal.[85,87]

Hypersensitivity reactions, including anaphylaxis, have occurred after administration of botulism antitoxin. For that reason, all patients should undergo a skin test before receiving the antitoxin, and resuscitation equipment should be immediately available. Patients showing a positive hypersensitivity reaction on the skin test can be desensitized over several hours.[90,91]

Before administering antitoxin, physicians should carefully review the package insert for dosage and adverse effects. Standard regimens can be used in children, pregnant women, and immunocompromised persons with botulism. Botulism immune globulin intravenous is an investigational human-derived neutralizing antibody that is available only for treatment of infant botulism from the California Department of Health Services, Berkeley. The CDC bioterrorism Web site or local public health authorities should be consulted for updated treatment recommendations.[33,85,86]

Transmissibility and Infection Control

Botulism is an intoxication, not an infection, and thus is not transmitted from person to person. Botulinum toxin does not penetrate intact skin. Standard infection-control precautions are adequate unless meningitis is suspected, in which case droplet precautions are indicated. Clothes of persons exposed to an aerosol release of botulinum toxin should be removed and washed. Exposed persons should shower with soap and hot water. Exposed environmental surfaces can be decontaminated with 0.1% hypochlorite bleach solution.[86]

Tularemia

Tularemia is a zoonotic infection caused by Francisella tularensis, a small, nonmotile, gram-negative, pleomorphic coccobacillus. The disease is typically acquired through contact with blood or tissue fluids of infected animals or through the bite of an infected deerfly, tick, or mosquito.[92] Inhalation of organisms aerosolized from the environment and the drinking of contaminated water can also result in human infection.[93] F. tularensis was developed for use as a biologic weapon by the United States (before its offensive biologic weapons program was terminated) and other countries.[33] The epidemiology, pathogenesis, and clinical manifestations of the naturally occurring forms of tularemia are discussed in more detail elsewhere [see Chapter 141].

CLINICAL PRESENTATION

Tularemia can take several forms in humans, depending on the route of infection. Ulceroglandular, oculoglandular, glandular, typhoidal, and pharyngeal tularemia are discussed elsewhere [see Chapter 141]. Inhalational tularemia is a term used to describe infection resulting from an aerosol release of F. tularensis.[94] Most patients with inhalational tularemia develop pleuropulmonary tularemia (tularemia pneumonia), but many patients may present with an undifferentiated febrile illness. The infectious dose is as low as one to 50 organisms, and the incubation period is typically 3 to 5 days (range, 1 to 14 days).[33]

The clinical course of inhalational tularemia is less rapidly progressive than that of pulmonary anthrax or plague. Illness onset is acute, with some combination of fever, chills, sweats, myalgias, headache, coryza, and sore throat. Nausea, vomiting, diarrhea, and abdominal pain are common. Anorexia and weight loss may occur as the illness continues. Cough may be dry or mildly productive. Hemoptysis is uncommon. Pleuritic chest pain, substernal chest discomfort, and dyspnea may be present. Chest x-rays may be normal or minimally abnormal or show a variety of abnormalities, including peribronchial patchy infiltrates, effusions, and hilar adenopathy.[95]

F. tularensis infection may be mild and nonspecific or rapidly progressive. Any form of tularemia may result in hematogenous spread with secondary pleuropneumonia, sepsis, and, rarely, meningitis. If left untreated, tularemia can progress to respiratory failure; liver, kidney, and splenic involvement; meningitis; sepsis; shock; and death. There is usually complete recovery with early diagnosis and treatment. Mortality is less than 2% if the patient is treated; it can be as high as 60% for untreated severe disease and pneumonia.[94,96,97]

DIAGNOSIS

A clustering of sudden, severe pneumonias in previously healthy patients should raise the possibility of an intentional aerosolized release of tularemia. Clusters of patients with tularemia and cases in which there is no natural explanation for the disease should be reported immediately to the local or state health department (http://www.statepublichealth.org). There are no rapid confirmatory tests for *F. tularensis*. Gram stain of sputum is not diagnostic but may identify other potential etiologies.[97,98] In the context of a known or suspected outbreak, a presumptive diagnosis can be made on the basis of symptoms. A chest x-ray should be obtained for patients with suspected pleuropulmonary tularemia. The x-ray may show infiltrates, effusion, hilar adenopathy, or subtle abnormalities, or it may be normal. Recent experience with inhalational anthrax suggests that chest CT scans of patients with tularemia may show pulmonary abnormalities, including infiltrates, effusions, and adenopathy, before they are evident on x-ray.[62]

Specimens of respiratory secretions and blood for bacteriologic and serologic testing should be collected before initiating therapy. Pharyngeal washings, sputum specimens, fasting gastric aspirates, and blood can be cultured for *F. tularensis*. Growth may be slow, so cultures should be held for 10 days. Cysteine-enriched culture media should be used to improve yield. Direct examination (by direct fluorescent antibody staining or immunohistochemical testing, antigen detection, microagglutination antibody testing, PCR, and other research tests) is available through designated public health laboratories. Acute and convalescent serologies are valuable for epidemiologic purposes.[94,98]

TREATMENT AND POSTEXPOSURE PROPHYLAXIS

When the index of suspicion is high, antibiotic treatment should be started before diagnosis is confirmed. Streptomycin or gentamicin is the preferred agent. All persons potentially exposed to aerosolized *F. tularensis* should be treated with doxycycline or ciprofloxacin. Close contacts of patients with tularemia pneumonia do not need prophylactic antibiotics. No vaccine for tularemia is currently available. The CDC bioterrorism Web site, local public health authorities, or both should be consulted for updated treatment recommendations.[33,94,99]

Transmissibility and Infection Control

Tularemia is not transmitted from person to person, and isolation of patients with tularemia is not necessary. Standard precautions are recommended for all patients with tularemia. Microbiology staff must be alerted when tularemia is suspected, so they can take precautions to prevent laboratory-acquired infection from culture plates and other infectious materials. Contaminated environmental surfaces can be disinfected with a 10% bleach solution followed by cleansing with 70% alcohol.[94]

Hemorrhagic Fever Viruses

Hemorrhagic fever viruses (HFVs) are RNA viruses classified in several taxonomic families. HFVs cause a variety of disease syndromes with similar clinical characteristics, referred to as acute hemorrhagic fever syndromes [*see Chapter 154*]. The pathophysiologic hallmarks of HFV infection are microvascular damage and increased vascular permeability. HFVs that are of concern as potential biologic weapons include Arenaviridae (Lassa, Junin, Machupo, Guanarito, and Sabia viruses, which are the causative agents of Lassa fever and Argentine, Bolivian, Venezuelan, and Brazilian hemorrhagic fevers, respectively); Filoviridae (Ebola and Marburg viruses); Flaviviridae (yellow fever, Omsk hemorrhagic fever, and Kyasanur Forest disease viruses); and Bunyaviridae (Rift Valley fever [RVF]). Under natural conditions, humans are infected through the bite of an infected arthropod or through contact with infected animal reservoirs. Hemorrhagic fever viruses are highly infectious by aerosol; are associated with high morbidity and, in some cases, high mortality; and are thought to pose a serious risk as biologic weapons.[33] All suspected cases of HFV infection should be reported immediately to the local or state health department and the hospital epidemiologist.

PATHOPHYSIOLOGY

The exact pathogenesis for HFVs varies according to the etiologic agent. The major target organ is the vascular endothelium. Immunologic and inflammatory mediators are thought to play an important role in the pathogenesis of HFVs. All HFVs can produce thrombocytopenia, and some also cause platelet dysfunction. Infection with Ebola and Marburg viruses, Rift Valley fever virus, and yellow fever virus causes destruction of infected cells. DIC is characteristic of infection with Filoviridae. Ebola and Marburg viruses may cause a hemorrhagic diathesis and tissue necrosis through direct damage to vascular endothelial cells and platelets with impairment of the microcirculation, as well as cytopathic effects on parenchymal cells, with release of immunologic and inflammatory mediators. Arenaviridae, on the other hand, appear to mediate hemorrhage via the stimulation of inflammatory mediators by macrophages, thrombocytopenia, and the inhibition of platelet aggregation. DIC is not a major pathophysiologic mechanism in arenavirus infections.[100,101]

CLINICAL PRESENTATION

The incubation period of HFVs ranges from 2 to 21 days. The clinical presentations of these diseases are nonspecific and variable, making diagnosis difficult. It is noteworthy that not all patients will develop hemorrhagic manifestations. Even a significant proportion of patients with Ebola virus infections may not demonstrate clinical signs of hemorrhage.[102]

Initial symptoms of the acute HFV syndrome may include fever, headache, myalgia, rash, nausea, vomiting, diarrhea, abdominal pain, arthralgias, myalgias, and malaise. Illness caused by Ebola, Marburg, Rift Valley fever virus, yellow fever virus, Omsk hemorrhagic fever virus, and Kyasanur Forest disease virus are characterized by an abrupt onset, whereas Lassa fever and the diseases caused by the Machupo, Junin, Guarinito, and Sabia viruses have a more insidious onset. Initial signs may include fever, tachypnea, relative bradycardia, hypotension (which may progress to circulatory shock), conjunctival injection, pharyngitis, and lymphadenopathy. Encephalitis may occur, with delirium, seizures, cerebellar signs, and coma. Most HFVs cause cutaneous flushing or a macular skin rash, although the rash may be difficult to appreciate in dark-skinned persons and varies according to the causative virus. Hemorrhagic symptoms, when they occur, develop later in the course of illness and include petechiae, purpura, bleeding into mucous membranes and conjunctiva, hematuria, hematemesis, and melena. Hepatic involvement is common, and renal involvement is proportional to cardiovascular compromise.[33,100,102,103]

Laboratory abnormalities include leukopenia (except in some cases of Lassa fever), anemia or hemoconcentration, and elevated liver enzymes; DIC with associated coagulation abnormalities and thrombocytopenia are common. Mortality ranges from less than 1% for Rift Valley fever to 70% to 90% for Ebola and Marburg virus infections.[33,100,102-104]

DIAGNOSIS

The nonspecific and variable clinical presentation of the HFVs presents a considerable diagnostic challenge. Clinical diagnostic criteria based on WHO surveillance standards for acute hemorrhagic fever syndrome include temperature greater than 101° F (38.3° C) of less than 3 weeks' duration; severe illness and no predisposing factors for hemorrhagic manifestations; and at least two of the following hemorrhagic symptoms: hemorrhagic or purple rash, epistaxis, hematemesis, hematuria, hemoptysis, blood in stools, or other hemorrhagic symptom with no established alternative diagnosis. Any suspected case of HFV should result in immediate notification of the hospital epidemiologist, local public health department, and clinical laboratory personnel.[101,105] Laboratory testing is currently available only at the CDC and the United States Army Medical Research Institute for Infectious Diseases. Laboratory techniques for the diagnosis of HFVs include antigen detection, IgM antibody detection, isolation in cell culture, visualization by electron microscopy, immunohistochemical techniques, and reverse transcriptase–polymerase chain reaction. Submission of clinical specimens, including processing and transport, should be arranged through consultation with local public health authorities. The CDC's Packaging Protocols for Biologic Agents/Diseases are available at (http://www.bt.cdc.gov/agent/vhf/index.asp).

TREATMENT

Therapy for HFVs is largely supportive. Treatment of other suspected causes of infection should be administered pending confirmation of HFV infection. Hypotension and shock may require early administration of vasopressors and hemodynamic monitoring with attention to fluid and electrolyte balance, circulatory volume, and blood pressure. HFV patients tend to respond poorly to fluid infusions and rapidly develop pulmonary edema.

Secondary infections may occur and should be diagnosed and treated. Intravenous lines, catheters, and other invasive procedures should be avoided unless they are clearly indicated. The management of bleeding is controversial. Recent recommendations include not treating mild bleeding and use of replacement therapy and heparin for severe bleeding with DIC.[33] Intramuscular injections and medications that interfere with platelet function or coagulation should be avoided.

No treatments of HFVs have been approved by the Food and Drug Administration. Ribavirin is a nucleoside analogue with activity against some Arenaviridae and Bunyaviridae (includ-ing the viruses that cause Lassa fever, Argentine hemorrhagic fever, and Crimean-Congo hemorrhagic fever) but not against Filoviridae or Flaviviridae. Ribavirin may be used under an IND protocol for the empirical treatment of HFV patients while awaiting identification of the etiologic agent. Current treatment protocols and dosing recommendations for ribavirin should be obtained through local public health authorities or the CDC's bioterrorism Web site.

Postexposure Prophylaxis

Postexposure prophylaxis is currently recommended only for persons potentially exposed to HFV and for known high-risk contacts or close contacts of HFV patients who develop fever or other clinical criteria of HFV infection with no alternative diagnosis, unless the etiologic agent is known to be a filovirus or a flavivirus.[100]

Infection Control Considerations

Ebola virus, Marburg virus, Lassa fever virus, and the New World arenaviruses are transmissible from person to person through direct contact with blood and body fluids. Airborne transmission of HFVs is unlikely but cannot be completely ruled out. The risk of person-to-person transmission is highest during the latter stages of illness, which are characterized by vomiting, diarrhea, shock, and, often, hemorrhage. The most important step in preventing transmission of HFVs is strict attention to implementation of appropriate barrier infection control measures, including double gloves, impermeable gowns, face shields, eye protection, and leg and shoe coverings.

Airborne precautions are recommended during care of patients with possible HFV infections. Airborne precautions include high-efficiency particulate respirators such as N-95 masks or powered air-purifying respirators (PAPRs) for all persons entering the patient's room. Patients should be placed in a negative-pressure isolation room with 6 to 12 air changes per hour.[101,106]

High-risk contacts of HFV patients include persons having contact with mucous membranes (e.g., through kissing or sexual intercourse) or with secretions, excretions, or blood (through percutaneous injury) of the infected person. Close contacts are persons who have other direct contact with the patient (e.g., shaking hands or hugging), provide medical care to the patient, or process laboratory specimens from a patient with HFV before initiation of infection-control precautions.

Persons potentially exposed to HFVs in a bioterrorist attack and their close and high-risk contacts should be placed under medical surveillance for 21 days from the day of exposure. Temperatures should be recorded twice daily, and any temperature of 101° F (38.3° C) or higher should be reported to the designated clinical or public health authority. Therapy with ribavirin should be initiated promptly unless an alternative diagnosis is established or the etiologic agent is known to be a filovirus or a flavivirus [*see* Treatment, *above*].[100]

HFVs are highly infectious in the laboratory setting through small-particle aerosols generated through procedures such as centrifugation. Laboratory personnel should be alerted when HFV infections are suspected, and appropriate personal-protection precautions and laboratory biosafety procedures should be implemented.

The author has no commercial relationships with manufacturers of products or providers of services discussed in this chapter.

References

1. Davis CJ: Nuclear blindness: an overview of the biological weapons programs of the former Soviet Union and Iraq. Emerg Infect Dis 5:509, 1999

2. Stern J: The prospect of domestic bioterrorism. Emerg Infect Dis 5:517, 1999

3. Kortepeter MG, Parker GW: Potential biological weapons threats. Emerg Infect Dis 5:523, 1999)

4. Alibek K: Biohazard. Random House, Inc. New York, 1999

5. Henderson DA: The looming threat of bioterrorism. Science 283:1279, 1999

6. Biological and chemical terrorism: strategic plan for preparedness and response. Recommendations of the CDC Strategic Planning Workgroup. MMWR Morb Mortal Wkly Rep 49:1, 2000

7. Gerberding JL, Hughes JM, Koplan JP: Bioterrorism preparedness and response: clinicians and public health agencies as essential partners. JAMA 287:898, 2002

8. Lane HC, Fauci AS: Bioterrorism on the home front: a new challenge for American medicine. JAMA 286:2595, 2001

9. Meningococcal disease and college students. Recommendations of the Advisory Committee on Immunization Practices (ACIP). MMWR Morb Mortal Wkly Rep 49:13, 2000

10. Bell BP, Goldoft M, Griffin PM, et al: A multistate outbreak of Escherichia coli 0157:H7-associated bloody diarrhea and hemolytic uremic syndrome from hamburgers: the Washington experience. JAMA 272:1349, 1994

11. Weber DJ, Rutala WA: Pertussis: a continuing hazard for healthcare facilities. Infect Control Hosp Epidemiol 22:736, 2001

12. Measles, mumps, and rubella: vaccine use and strategies for elimination of measles, rubella, and congenital rubella syndrome and control of mumps. Recommendations of the Advisory Committee on Immunization Practices (ACIP). MMWR Morb Mortal Wkly Rep 47:1, 1998

13. Prevention of varicella. Updated Recommendations of the Advisory Committee on Immunization Practices (ACIP). MMWR Morb Mortal Wkly Rep 48:1, 1999

14. Bolyard EA, Tablan OC, Williams WW, et al: Guideline for infection control in healthcare personnel, 1998. Hospital Infection Control Practices Advisory Committee. Infect Control Hosp Epidemiol 19:386, 1998

15. Suspected brucellosis case prompts investigation of possible bioterrorism-related activity–New Hampshire and Massachusetts, 1999. MMWR Morb Mortal Wkly Rep 49:509, 2000

16. Duchin JS, Koster FT, Peters CJ, et al: Hantavirus pulmonary syndrome: a clinical description of 17 patients with a newly recognized disease. The Hantavirus Study Group. N Engl J Med 330:949, 1994

17. Fine A, Layton M: Lessons from the West Nile viral encephalitis outbreak in New York City, 1999: implications for bioterrorism preparedness. Clin Infect Dis 32:277, 2001

18. Pandemic influenza: confronting a re-emergent threat. Proceedings of a meeting. Bethesda, Maryland, 11-13 December 1995. J Infect Dis 176:S1, 1997

19. Rota PA, Oberste MS, Monroe SS, et al: Characterization of a novel coronavirus associated with severe acute respiratory syndrome. Science 300:1394, 2003

20. Wenzel RP, Edmond MB: Managing SARS amidst uncertainty. N Engl J Med 348:1947, 2003

21. Update: investigation of bioterrorism-related anthrax and interim guidelines for clinical evaluation of persons with possible anthrax. MMWR Morb Mortal Wkly Rep 50:941, 2001

22. Updated interim surveillance case definition for severe acute respiratory syndrome (SARS)—United States, April 29, 2003. MMWR Morb Mortal Wkly Rep 52:391, 2003

23. Interim guidance on infection control precautions for patients with suspected severe acute respiratory syndrome (SARS) and close contacts in households. Centers for Disease Control and Prevention, Atlanta, August 18, 2003
http://www.cdc.gov/ncidod/sars/ic-closecontacts.htm.

24. Control of Communicable Diseases Manual, 17th ed. Chin JE, Ed. American Public Health Association, Washington DC, 2000

25. Garner JS: Guideline for isolation precautions in hospitals. Infect Control Hosp Epidemiol 17:53, 1996

26. Immunization of health-care workers. Recommendations of the Advisory Committee on Immunization Practices and the Hospital Infection Control Practices Advisory Committee. MMWR Morb Mortal Wkly Rep 46:1, 1997

27. Rotz LD, Khan AS, Lillibridge SR, et al: Public health assessment of potential bioterrorism agents. Emerg Infect Dis 8:225, 2002

28. Torok TJ, Tauxe RV, Wise RP, et al: A large community outbreak of salmonellosis caused by intentional contamination of restaurant salad bars. JAMA 278:389, 1997

29. Kolavic SA, Kimura A, Simons SL, et al: An outbreak of Shigella dysenteriae type 2 among laboratory workers due to intentional food contamination. JAMA 278:396, 1997

30. Pavlin JA: Epidemiology of bioterrorism. Emerg Infect Dis 5:528, 1999

31. Recognition of illness associated with the intentional release of a biologic agent. MMWR Morb Mortal Wkly Rep 50:893, 2001

32. Vaccinia (smallpox) vaccine. Recommendations of the Advisory Committee on Immunization Practices (ACIP), 2001. MMWR Morb Mortal Wkly Rep 50:1, 2001

33. Franz DR, Jahrling PB, Friedlander AM, et al: Clinical recognition and management of patients exposed to biological warfare agents. JAMA 278:399, 1997

34. Draft Supplemental Recommendation of the ACIP. Use of Smallpox (Vaccinia) Vaccine. Centers for Disease Control and Prevention, Atlanta, June 2002

35. Fenner F, Henderson DA, Arita I, et al: Smallpox and its eradication. World Health Organization, Geneva, 2001
http://www.who.int/csr/en/

36. Smallpox as a biological weapon: medical and public health management. Working Group on Civilian Biodefense. JAMA 281:2127, 1999

37. Breman, JG, Henderson DA: Diagnosis and management of smallpox. N Engl J Med 346:1300, 2002

38. Henderson DA: Smallpox: clinical and epidemiologic features. Emerging Infect Dis 5:537, 1999

39. Smallpox response plan and guidelines. Centers for Disease Control and Prevention, Atlanta, November 26, 2002
http://www.bt.cdc.gov/agent/smallpox/response-plan/index.asp

40. Grabenstein JD, Winkenwerder W: US military smallpox vaccination program experience. JAMA 289:3278, 2003

41. Update: cardiac and other adverse events following civilian smallpox vaccination—United States, 2003. MMWR Morb Mortal Wkly Rep 52:639, 2003

42. Update: adverse events following civilian smallpox vaccination—United States, 2003. MMWR 52:819, 2003

43. Neff JM, Lane JM, Fulginetti VA, et al: Contact vaccinia: transmission of vaccinia from smallpox vaccination. JAMA 288:1901, 2003

44. Bartlett J: Smallpox vaccination and patients with human immunodeficiency virus infection or acquired immunodeficiency syndrome. Clin Infect Dis 36:468, 2003

45. Lane JM, Ruben FL, Neff JM, et al: Complications of smallpox vaccination, 1968: results of ten statewide surveys. J Infect Dis 122:303, 1970

46. Update: cardiac-related events during the civilian smallpox vaccination program—United States, 2003. MMWR Morb Mortal Wkly Rep 52:492, 2003
http://www.cdc.gov/mmwr/preview/mmwrhtml/mm5221a2.htm

47. Halsell JS, Riddle JR, Atwood JE, et al: Myopericarditis following smallpox vaccination among vaccinia naive US military personnel. JAMA 289:3283, 2003

48. Supplemental recommendations on adverse events following smallpox vaccine in the pre-event vaccination program: recommendations of the Advisory Committee on Immunization Practices. MMWR Morb Mortal Wkly Rep 52:282, 2003

49. Talbot TR, Bredenberg HK, Smith M, LaFleur BJ, Boyd A, Edwards KM. Focal and generalized folliculitis following smallpox vaccination among vaccinia-naive recipients. JAMA 289:3290, 2003

50. Acha PN, Szyfres B: Zoonoses and Communicable Disease Common to Man and Animals, 3rd ed. Vol I. Pan American Health Organization, Washington, DC, 2001

51. Swartz MN: Recognition and management of anthrax: an update. N Engl J Med 345:1621, 2001

52. Brachman PS: Bioterrorism: an update with a focus on anthrax. Am J Epidemiol 155:981, 2002

53. Update: investigation of bioterrorism-related anthrax and adverse events from antimicrobial prophylaxis. MMWR Morb Mortal Wkly Rep 50:973, 2001

54. Cieslak TJ, Eitzen HM Jr: Bioterrorism: agents of concern. J Public Health Manag Pract 6:19, 2000

55. Kournikakis B, Armour SJ, Boulet CA, et al: Risk assessment of anthrax threat letters. Technical Report 2001-048. Defense Research Establishment, Suffield, Canada, 2001

56. Dixon TC, Meselson M, Guillemin J, et al: Anthrax. N Engl J Med 341:815, 1999

57. Sirisanthana T, Brown AE: Anthrax of the gastrointestinal tract. Emerg Infect Dis 8:649, 2002

58. Inglesby TV, O'Toole T, Henderson DA, et al: Anthrax as a biological weapon, 2002: updated recommendations for management. JAMA 287:2236, 2002

59. Meselson M, Guillemin J, Hugh-Jones M, et al: The Sverdlovsk anthrax outbreak of 1979. Science 266:1202, 1994

60. LaForce FM. Anthrax. Clin Infect Dis 19:1009, 1994

61. Guarner J, Jernigan JA, Sheih W, et al: Pathology and pathogenesis of bioterrorism-related inhalational anthrax. Am J Pathol 163:701, 2003

62. Jernigan JA, Stephens DS, Ashford DA, et al: Bioterrorism-related inhalational anthrax: the first 10 cases reported in the United States. Emerg Infect Dis 7:933, 2001

63. Barakat LA, Quentzel HL, Jernigan JA, et al: Fatal inhalational anthrax in a 94-year-old Connecticut woman. JAMA 287:863, 2002

64. Mina B, Dym JP, Kuepper F, et al: Fatal inhalational anthrax with unknown source of exposure in a 61-year-old woman in New York City. JAMA 287:858, 2002

65. Brachman PS: Inhalation anthrax. Ann NY Acad Sci 353:83, 1980

66. USAMRIID's Medical Management of Biological Casualties Handbook (USAMRIID Blue Book), 4th ed. United States Army Medical Research Institute of Infectious Diseases, Fort Detrick, Maryland, February, 2001
http://www.usamriid.army.mil/education/bluebookpdf/USAMRIID%20Blue%20Book%205th%20Edition.pdf

67. Use of anthrax vaccine in the United States. Recommendations of the Advisory Committee on Immunization Practices. MMWR Morb Mortal Wkly Rep 49:1, 2000

68. Kuehnert MJ, Doyle TJ, Hill HA, et al: Clinical features that discriminate inhalational anthrax from other acute respiratory diseases. Clin Infect Dis 36:328, 2003

69. Considerations for distinguishing influenza-like illness from inhalational anthrax. MMWR Morb Mortal Wkly Rep 50:984, 2001

70. Mayer TA, Morrison A, Bersoff-Matcha S, et al: Inhalational anthrax due to bioterrorism: would current Centers for Disease Control and Prevention guidelines have identified the 11 patients with inhalational anthrax from October through November 2001? Clin Infect Dis 36:1275, 2003

71. Update: investigation of bioterrorism-related anthrax and interim guidelines for exposure management and antimicrobial therapy, October 2001. MMWR Morb Mortal Wkly Rep 50:909, 2001

72. Update: investigation of anthrax associated with intentional exposure and interim public health guidelines, October 2001. MMWR Morb Mortal Wkly Rep 50:889, 2001

73. Statement by the Department of Health and Human Services: Regarding additional options for preventive treatment for those exposed to inhalational anthrax. US Department of Health and Human Services, December 18, 2001
http://www.bt.cdc.gov/DocumentsApp/Anthrax/12182001/hhs12182001.asp

74. Committee to Assess the Safety and Efficacy of the Anthrax Vaccine. Medical Follow-Up Agency: The Anthrax Vaccine: Is It Safe? Does It Work? Joellenbeck LM, Zwanziger LL, Durch JS, et al, Eds: Institute of Medicine, National Academy Press, Washington, DC, 2002
http://www.iom.edu/CMS/3795/4324.aspx

75. Additional options for preventive treatment for persons exposed to inhalational anthrax. MMWR Morb Mortal Wkly Rep 50:1142, 2001

76. Use of anthrax vaccine in response to terrorism. Supplemental recommendations of the Advisory Committee on Immunization Practices. MMWR Morb Mortal Wkly Rep 51:1024, 2002

77. Cutaneous anthrax management algorithm. AAD Ad Hoc Task Force on Bioterrorism. American Academy of Dermatology, November 21, 2001
http://www.aad.org/professionals/educationcme/bioterrorism/CutaneousAnthrax.htm

78. Biosafety in Microbiological and Biomedical Laboratories (BMBL) 4th Edition. U.S. Department of Health and Human Services Centers for Disease Control and Prevention and National Institutes of Health, May 1999. US Government Printing Office, Washington, DC, 1999
http://www.cdc.gov/od/ohs/biosfty/bmbl/bmbl3toc.htm

79. Perry RD, Fetherston JD: Yersinia pestis—etiologic agent of plague. Clin Microbiol Rev 10:35, 1997

80. Gage KL, Dennis DT, Orloski KA, et al: Cases of cat-associated human plague in the western U.S., 1977–1998. Clin Infect Dis 30:893, 2000

81. Inglesby TV, Dennis DT, Henderson DA, et al: Plague as a biological weapon: medical and public health management. Working Group on Civilian Biodefense. JAMA 283:2281, 2000

82. Prevention of plague. Recommendations of the Advisory Committee on Immunization Practice. MMWR Morb Mortal Wkly Rep 45:1 1996

83. McGovern TW, Friedlander AM: Plague. Medical Aspects of Chemical and Biological Warfare. Textbook of Military Medicine Series. Part I, Warfare, Weaponry and the Casualty. Sidell FR, Takafuji ET, Franz DR, Eds. TMM Publications, Washington, DC, 1997

84. Shapiro RL, Hatheway C, Becher J, et al: Botulism surveillance and emergency response: a public health strategy for a global challenge. JAMA 278:433, 1997

85. Shapiro RL, Hatheway C, Swerdlow DL: Botulism in the United States: a clinical and epidemiologic review. Ann Intern Med 129:221, 1998

86. Arnon SS, Schechter R, Inglesby TV, et al: Botulinum toxin as a biological weapon: medical and public health management. JAMA 285:1059, 2001

87. Cherington M: Clinical spectrum of botulism. Muscle Nerve 21:701, 1998

88. Woodruff BA, Griffin PM, McCroskey LM, et al: Clinical and laboratory comparison of botulism toxin types A, B and E in the United States, 1975–1988. J Infect Dis 166:1281, 1992

89. Angulo FJ, Getz J, Taylor JP, et al: A large outbreak of botulism: the hazardous baked potato. J Infect Dis 178:172, 1998

90. Eitzen E: Medical management of biological casualties, 3rd ed. U.S. Army Medical Research Institute of Infectious Diseases, Fort Detrick, Frederick, Maryland, 1998

91. Black RE, Gunn RA: Hypersensitivity reactions associated with botulinal antitoxin. Am J Med 69:567, 1980

92. Tularemia—United States, 1999–2000. MMWR Morb Mortal Wkly Rep 51:181, 2002

93. Feldman KA, Enscore RE, Lathrop SL, et al: An outbreak of primary pneumonic tularemia on Martha's Vineyard. N Engl J Med 345:1601, 2001

94. Dennis DT, Inglesby TV, Henderson DA, et al: Tularemia as a biological weapon: medical and public health management. JAMA 285:2763, 2001

95. Choi E: Tularemia and Q fever. Med Clinics North Am 86:393, 2002

96. Evans ME, Gregory DW, Schaffner W, et al: Tularemia: a 30-year experience with 88 cases. Medicine (Baltimore) 64:251, 1985

97. Gill V, Cunha BA: Tularemia pneumonia. Semin Respir Infect 12:61, 1997

98. Evans ME, Friedlander AM: Tularemia. Medical Aspects of Chemical and Biological Warfare. Textbook of Military Medicine Series. Part I, Warfare, Weaponry and the Casualty. Sidell FR, Takafuji ET, Franz DR, Eds. TMM Publications, Washington, DC, 1997

99. Limaye AP, Hooper CJ: Treatment of tularemia with fluoroquinolones: two cases and review. Clin Infect Dis 29:922, 1999

100. Borio L, Inglesby T, Peters CJ, et al: Hemorrhagic fever viruses as biological weapons: medical and public health management. JAMA 287:2391, 2002

101. Khan AS, Sanchez A, Pflieger AK: Filoviral hemorrhagic fevers. Br Med Bull 54:675, 1998

102. Bwaka MA, Bonnet MJ, Calain P, et al: Ebola hemorrhagic fever in Kikwit, Democratic Republic of the Congo: clinical observations in 103 patients. J Infect Dis 179:S1, 1999

103. Jahrling PB: Viral hemorrhagic fevers. Textbook of Military Medicine Series. Part I, Warfare, Weaponry and the Casualty. Sidell FR, Takafuji ET, Franz DR, Eds. TMM Publications, Washington, DC, 1997

104. Isaacson M: Viral hemorrhagic fever hazards for travelers in Africa. Clin Infect Dis 33:1707, 2001

105. Acute hemorrhagic fever syndrome. World Health Organization.
http://www.who.int/topics/haemorrhagic_fevers_viral/en/

106. Update: management of patients with suspected viral hemorrhagic fever—United States. MMWR Morb Mortal Wkly Rep 44:475, 1995

Acknowledgments

Figures 1, 3, 4, and 5   Centers for Disease Control and Prevention Public Health Image Library.

Figure 2   Centers for Disease Control and Prevention Public Health Image Library (Dr Duma).

14 Cardiac Resuscitation

Terry J. Mengert, M.D.

Out-of-hospital sudden cardiac arrest claims the lives of more than 300,000 persons in the United States each year, making it the leading cause of death.[1-4] In fact, approximately 50% of all cardiac deaths are sudden deaths.[5] In hospitals, a minimum of 370,000 patients also suffer a cardiac arrest, followed by an attempted, but only sometimes successful, resuscitation.[6] Although most victims of sudden death have underlying coronary artery disease (70% to 80%), sudden death is the first manifestation of the disease in half of these persons.[2] Other causes and contributing factors include abnormalities of the myocardium (e.g., chronic heart failure or hypertrophy from any cause), electrophysiologic abnormalities, valvular heart disease, congenital heart disease, and miscellaneous inflammatory and infiltrative disease processes (e.g., myocarditis, sarcoidosis, and hemochromatosis).[7-9]

The pathophysiology that culminates in a sudden cardiac death is complex and poorly understood. It likely represents a mix of electrical abnormalities combined with acute functional triggers, such as myocardial ischemia, central and autonomic nervous system effects, electrolyte abnormalities, and even pharmacologic influences.[1] Classically, most sudden deaths that occur in adults in the community are thought to be secondary to ventricular tachycardia (VT) that quickly degenerates into ventricular fibrillation (VF). In a 10-year study in the Seattle area, the different arrhythmias found in prehospital cardiac arrest patients presumed to have underlying cardiovascular disease were VF (45%), asystole (31%), pulseless electrical activity (PEA; 10%), VT (1%), and other arrhythmias (14%).[3] Studies indicate that the out-of-hospital incidence of VF has decreased in recent years, probably because of the decrease in mortality from coronary artery disease.[10] In a 4-year study of in-hospital cardiac arrest involving almost 37,000 adults in 253 hospitals in the United States and Canada, initial rhythms identified were asystole (40%), PEA (24%), unknown by documentation (22%), and VF or pulseless VT (14%).[11]

The Chain of Survival

The resuscitation of an adult victim of sudden cardiac arrest should follow an orderly sequence, no matter where the patient's collapse occurs. This sequence is called the chain of survival.[12] It comprises four elements, all of which must be instituted as rapidly as possible: (1) activation of the emergency medical services (EMS) network, (2) prompt and technically competent cardiopulmonary resuscitation (CPR) with as few subsequent interruptions in chest compressions as is possible, (3) early defibrillation, and (4) provision of advanced care.

ACTIVATION OF EMERGENCY MEDICAL SERVICES

A person in cardiac arrest is unresponsive and pulseless, although agonal respirations may last for minutes. Confirm unresponsiveness by speaking loudly and gently shaking the patient. If the patient is truly unresponsive, immediately call for help by activating the EMS system in the community (in most locales, this means calling 911); or if the patient is already in the hospital, call a code (e.g., code blue, code 199). The exception is when a lone rescuer encounters a victim of an unwitnessed and presumed asphyxial arrest; in such cases, the rescuer should perform CPR for about 2 minutes before pausing to activate the EMS system.[13] If an automated external defibrillator (AED) is available, have it brought to the resuscitation scene. AEDs are both easily used and lifesaving.[14-18]

INITIATION OF CPR

While awaiting the arrival of a defibrillator and advanced help, the rescuer assesses the patient's airway, breathing, and circulation [*see* The Primary Survey, *below*] and initiates CPR [*see Table 1*]. When CPR is started within 4 minutes of collapse, the likelihood of patient survival at least doubles.[19,20] Throughout the resuscitation, the provision of quality CPR with as few interruptions to chest compressions as possible is key to optimizing the patient's possibility of survival.

INITIATION OF DEFIBRILLATION

When the AED or monitor-defibrillator arrives, attach it appropriately to the patient and analyze the patient's rhythm; if the patient is in VF or pulseless VT, a defibrillatory shock should be rapidly applied [*see Tables 2 and 3*], followed by immediate resumption of CPR. The importance of rapid access to defibrillation cannot be overemphasized. In a patient who is dying from a shockable rhythm, the chance of survival declines by 7% to 10% for every minute that defibrillation is delayed.[21]

INITIATION OF ADVANCED CARE

If the patient remains pulseless despite the steps described above, continue quality CPR; establish a definitive airway, confirm its correct placement, and then secure it. Simultaneously, establish intravenous access, and then administer vasopressor medications (either epinephrine or vasopressin) followed by oth-

---

Table 1 Initial Resuscitation Steps in the Unresponsive Patient 8 Years of Age or Older

Confirm unresponsiveness
Activate the emergency medical system
   In most community locales, call 911
   In the hospital, activate a "code" response
Call for an automatic external defibrillator (AED)
Begin basic life support (CPR)
   Open airway (maintain spinal stability and alignment in suspected victims of trauma)
   Check breathing; if not breathing, deliver two initial breaths (each over 1 sec, allowing exhalation between each)
   Check for a carotid pulse (allow < 10 sec to assess); if pulseless, do the following:
      Begin chest compressions ("push hard and fast") at the rate of 100 compressions/min, depressing the sternum 1.5–2 in. per compression and allowing full chest recoil between each compression
      Intersperse ventilations with chest compressions: in nonintubated patients, deliver 30 compressions, pause for two breaths (i.e., one cycle of CPR), then repeat; in intubated patients, deliver one breath every 5 sec with no pause in the compression rate, which is ongoing at 100/min
When defibrillator arrives, immediately analyze and treat arrhythmia; minimize any interruptions to chest compressions
   Attach patient to AED [*see Table 2*] or the monitor-defibrillator [*see Table 3*]
   Analyze arrhythmia and treat as appropriate [*see Figure 2*]

Table 2   Using an Automatic External Defibrillator in Patients 8 Years of Age or Older

Automatic external defibrillator (AED) arrives (CPR is in progress)
  Place AED beside patient.
  Turn on the AED.
  Attach the electrodes to the AED (they may already be attached).
  Attach the electrode pads to the patient (as diagrammed on the pads).
AED analyzes patient's rhythm
  Pause CPR (and ensure no one is touching the patient). Press the Analyze button on the AED (some devices analyze the rhythm automatically as soon as the pads are placed on the patient).
AED instructs rescuers (via an audible voice prompt and/or on-screen instructions)
  Shock is indicated: clear the patient (ensure no one is touching the patient) and push the Shock button.
  After delivering the shock, immediately resume CPR and perform five cycles (30 compressions to two ventilations per cycle in nonintubated patients) or about 2 min of CPR in intubated patients; then pause CPR to reanalyze rhythm. If the AED instructs rescuers to shock again, do so. If shock is not indicated, assess the patient for evidence of return of spontaneous circulation; if none, resume CPR.
  Key concept: the pattern of shock delivery and CPR interspersion is as follows: shock, CPR for 2 min, then reanalyze rhythm; this pattern is repeated as indicated.
or
  Shock not indicated: reassess the patient for signs of circulation; if present, assess the adequacy of breathing; if there are no signs of circulation, resume CPR for five cycles (nonintubated patients) or 2 min (intubated patients). After 2 min of CPR, reanalyze the rhythm, followed (if indicated) by shock, followed immediately by CPR steps as outlined above. If shock is not indicated, assess the patient for signs of spontaneous circulation; if present, assess for adequacy of breathing. If the patient is still pulseless, repeat rhythm analysis, followed (if indicated) by shock steps.

er appropriate interventions, as determined by the rhythm and the arrest circumstances [*see* Cardiac Resuscitation Based on Rhythm Findings, *below*]. If the patient is in VF or pulseless VT, repeated attempts at defibrillation are made approximately every 2 minutes, combined with delivery of vasoactive and antiarrhythmic drugs [*see* Table 4].

RESUSCITATION OUTCOME

When every link in the chain of survival is quickly and sequentially available, the patient is provided an optimal opportunity for return of spontaneous circulation.[21-24] In the United States, individual communities report survival rates of 4% to 40% or more in cases of sudden cardiac death.[25-29] Prehospital victims of VF have had survival rates to hospital discharge of greater than 50% when an AED was expeditiously used.[30] Many other factors also influence patient survival, however; these include whether the patient's collapse was witnessed, the rapidity and effectiveness of bystander CPR, the number and length of interruptions to CPR, the rhythm associated with the cardiac arrest, and underlying comorbidities.[31,32] With inpatient cardiac arrest, for example, overall survival rates vary from 9% to 32%[32-39]; in one study, survival to hospital discharge was 30% for patients with primary heart disease, 15% for patients with infectious diseases, and only 8% for patients with other end-stage diseases (e.g., cancer, lung disease, liver failure, or renal failure).[40]

Such statistics underline the importance of using cardiac resuscitation appropriately and with discrimination. Cardiac resuscita-

tion provides rescuers with powerful tools that save the lives of thousands of people every year. These techniques are capable of returning patients who would otherwise die to productive and meaningful lives. However, cardiac resuscitation should not be employed to reverse timely and natural death. Under those circumstances, it has the potential to lengthen the dying process and to increase human suffering. All practitioners are well advised to

Table 3   Using a Manual Defibrillator[54,92]

Defibrillator arrives (CPR is in progress)
  Place defibrillator beside patient.
  Turn defibrillator on (initial energy level setting for defibrillators is typically 200 J).*
  Set Lead Select switch to Paddles. Alternatively, if patient is already attached to monitor leads, set Lead Select switch to lead I, II, or III; ensure all three leads are correctly attached to the patient and the defibrillator: white to right shoulder, black to left shoulder, red to ribs on left side.
  Apply gel to paddles or place conductor pads on patient's chest. Some devices use disposable electrode patches that are prepasted with a conducting gel. In either case, the appropriate positions of the paddles with applied gel, conductor pads, or disposable paddles are as follows: sternal paddle is placed to the right of the sternum, just below the right clavicle; apex paddle is placed to the left of the left breast, centered in the left midaxillary line at roughly the fifth intercostal space.
Briefly pause CPR and analyze rhythm
  If using paddles to assess rhythm, apply paddles as described with firm pressure (25 lb of pressure to each paddle) and visually assess rhythm on monitor (if using leads, assess rhythm in leads I, II, or III). If rhythm is either pulseless VT or VF, proceed as follows:
    Defibrillate, then immediately resume CPR.
    Announce to resuscitation team, "Charging defibrillator!" and press Charge button on either paddles or defibrillator (360 J, not synchronized, recommended for monophasic defibrillators).*
    Warn resuscitation team that a defibrillatory shock is coming:
    "I am going to shock on three! ONE, I'm clear; TWO, you're clear, THREE, everybody's CLEAR!" Simultaneously with these statements, visually ensure that no resuscitation team member is in contact with patient.
    Press the Discharge buttons on both paddles simultaneously to deliver a defibrillatory shock. Immediately resume CPR after shock delivery (do not attempt to analyze for rhythm change after the shock); perform five cycles of CPR in nonintubated patients (about 2 min of CPR in intubated patients). Recharge defibrillator (360 J)* in preparation for next step.
    Pause CPR and reassess rhythm on monitor; if patient is still in VT or VF, recharge defibrillator (now 300 J)* and repeat process of loudly informing team members by giving the warning statements as above, and then apply defibrillatory shock.
    Reassess rhythm on monitor; if patient is still in VT or VF, recharge defibrillator (now 360 J)* and repeat process of loudly informing team members by giving the warning statements as above, and then apply defibrillatory shock.
    Reassess rhythm on monitor; if patient is still in VT or VF, resume CPR and continue with resuscitation sequence [*see* Figure 2].

*Note: if using a biphasic defibrillator, a lower initial defibrillatory energy level (< 200 J) without energy escalation on subsequent shocks is acceptable.
VF—ventricular fibrillation   VT—ventricular tachycardia

remember that "death is not the opposite of life, death is the opposite of birth. Both are aspects of life."[41] It is untimely death that requires immediate intervention with cardiac resuscitation.

The Primary and Secondary Surveys of Cardiac Resuscitation

A cardiac resuscitation is a stressful event for everyone involved. Too often, clinic and inpatient cardiac arrests and their management are episodes of chaos in the busy lives of resident and attending physicians. Yet, it has been eloquently stated that a good resuscitation team should function like a fine symphony orchestra.[42] Such skill levels require dedicated individual and team practice and careful code-team organization. Mastery in cardiac resuscitation is in fact a lifelong pursuit that requires training and retraining in advanced cardiac life support (ACLS); regular practice and review; and leadership and team skill development. Its key elements include not only the resuscitation itself but also the response to the announcement of a code, postresuscitation stabilization of the patient, notification of the family and primary care provider, and code critique and debriefing. To help practitioners learn and apply some of the most essential techniques used in cardiac resuscitation more easily and effectively, the American Heart Association (AHA) has developed the concepts of primary and secondary surveys of a patient in atraumatic cardiac arrest.[43]

THE PRIMARY SURVEY

The primary survey for the victim of sudden cardiac arrest consists of the appropriate assessment of the patient's airway (A), breathing (B), and circulation (C) and the simultaneous application of expert CPR until defibrillation (D) becomes possible (assuming the patient is in VF or pulseless VT). Thus, the primary survey includes the second and third links in the chain of survival (see above).

In 1958, Kouwenhoven noted that when his research fellow forcefully applied external defibrillating electrodes on a dog's chest in the laboratory, an arterial pressure wave occurred.[44] Further study and refinements led to the technique of closed-chest CPR, the careful description of which was published in 1960.[45] The first report of the use of this technique in patients was in 1961.[46] Since those early days, the fundamentals of closed-chest CPR have remained relatively unchanged. Mouth-to-mouth, mouth-to-mask, or bag-valve-mask ventilation oxygenates the blood. Chest compressions produce forward blood flow. This flow appears to result from a combination of direct compression of the heart and intrathoracic pressure changes with both chest compression and subsequent chest recoil.[47,48]

CPR in isolation does not defibrillate the heart. Its main benefit is to extend patient viability until a defibrillator and advanced interventions become available and, one hopes, succeed in restoring spontaneous circulation in the patient. CPR is not nearly as effective as a contracting heart; systolic arterial pressure peaks of 60 to 80 mm Hg may be generated, but diastolic blood pressure remains low, and a cardiac output of only 25% to 30% of normal can be achieved even under optimal conditions.[49] Still, effective CPR is critical to keeping the patient alive. It is worth remembering that the most important rescuers at a cardiac resuscitation are those who are performing expert CPR, because it is only through their efforts that the patient's heart and brain are kept viable until defibrillation and other advanced interventions can restore spontaneous circulation. Quality CPR, including expertly delivered chest compressions, should take place with as few interruptions as is possible throughout the resuscitation effort.

After unresponsiveness is confirmed, the EMS is activated and an AED is called for; the primary survey (A, B, C, and D) proceeds as described (see below) until the AED arrives.

Airway Optimization

Open the patient's mouth and optimize the airway in the nontrauma patient by use of the head-tilt and chin-lift maneuver. A jaw-thrust maneuver should be used instead of the head-tilt technique if cervical spine injury is suspected. In patients with suspected spine injury, proper spine alignment must be maintained throughout all phases of the resuscitation. In such circumstances, as equipment becomes available, the patient's spine requires immobilization with a padded backboard, hard cervical collar, appropriate bolstering around the patient's head to prevent movement, and strapping of the patient to the backboard.[50]

Breathing Assessment

To assess breathing, the rescuer places his or her cheek close to the patient's mouth and looks, listens, and feels for patient respirations. If the respirations are agonal or the patient is apneic, the rescuer then delivers two initial breaths. Each breath is delivered over 1 second. The patient's chest should rise with each delivered breath, and exhalation is allowed for between breaths. Breaths may be delivered using the mouth-to-mouth technique with appropriate barrier precautions (the patient's nose should be pinched if the mouth-to-mouth technique is used) or mouth-to-mask technique. The ideal device, if available, is a bag-valve-mask device attached to high-flow oxygen; this allows the delivery of a substantially higher oxygen concentration to the patient. If the patient cannot be ventilated, the rescuer repositions the airway and attempts the technique again. If the airway is still obstructed, up to five abdominal thrusts are then applied, followed by a look in the mouth for a foreign body (with a finger sweep of the oropharynx if a foreign body is seen), and then repeat ventilation attempts. Definitive intervention for an obstructed airway in the hospital setting may involve laryngoscopic visualization of the cause of obstruction and foreign-body removal. If an adequate airway cannot be established by less invasive means, cricothyrotomy may be required.

CPR Initiation

The health care rescuer next checks for a carotid pulse in the unresponsive patient but should allow no more than 10 seconds to do so. (The AHA no longer recommends pulse checks for rescuers who are not health care providers[51]; instead, lay rescuers should initiate chest compressions if the patient is not breathing, coughing, or moving after the initial two breaths.) If the patient has no carotid pulse, begin chest compressions. The patient should be on a firm surface, and the heel of the rescuer's hand should be in the center of the inferior half of the patient's sternum (but cephalad to the xiphoid process) at approximately the nipple level. The rescuer's other hand is placed on top of the lower hand, with the fingers interlocked.

The rescuer's arms are held straight, with the force of each compression coming from the rescuer's trunk. In patients 8 years of age and older, the sternum is firmly compressed by 1.5 to 2.0 inches, then released. The rate of recommended chest compression is 100 per minute in patients 8 years of age or older. The chest should be allowed to rebound to its precompression dimensions between compressions, but the heel of the resuscitator's hand that is closest to the patient should remain in contact with the sternum.

Table 4   Drugs Useful in Cardiac Arrest[3,93]

Category	Drug and Doses Supplied	Indications in Cardiac Arrest	Adult Dosage	Comments
Vasopressors	Epinephrine, 1 mg in 10 ml emergency syringe; 1 mg/ml (1 ml and 30 ml vials)	Pulseless VT or VF unresponsive to initial defibrillatory shocks; PEA; asystole	1 mg I.V. push; may repeat every 3–5 min for as long as patient is pulseless; can also be given via the endotracheal route: 2–2.5 mg diluted with NS to 10 ml total volume	I.V. boluses of epinephrine (1 mg) are appropriate only in pulseless cardiac arrest patients; if continued epinephrine is required postresuscitation, a continuous infusion should be started (1–10 µg/min). High-dose epinephrine (up to 0.2 mg/kg I.V. per dose) does not improve survival to hospital discharge in cardiac arrest patients and is no longer recommended in adults (except in certain rare settings, such as beta blocker overdose).
	Vasopressin, 20 IU/ml (1 ml vial)	May use in place of the first and/or second doses of epinephrine in cardiac arrest	40 IU I.V. push, single dose only; can also be given via endotracheal tube: same dose, diluted with NS to 10 ml total volume	If no response after 10 min of continued resuscitation, administer epinephrine subsequently, as above.
Antiarrhythmics	Amiodarone, 50 mg/ml (3 ml vial)	Pulseless VT or VF unresponsive to initial defibrillatory shocks and epinephrine (or vasopressin) plus shock(s)	VT/VF: 300 mg diluted in 20–30 ml; NS or D5W rapid I.V. push; a repeat dose of 150 mg may be given if required; maximum dose in 24 hr should not exceed 2,200 mg	Side effects may include hypotension and bradycardia in the postresuscitation phase.
	Lidocaine, 50 or 100 mg in 5 ml emergency syringes; premixed bag, 1 g/250 ml or 2 g/250 ml	Pulseless VT or VF unresponsive to initial defibrillatory shocks and epinephrine (or vasopressin) plus shock(s)	Initial dose: 1–1.5 mg/kg I.V.; for refractory VF or unstable VT, additional doses of 0.5–0.75 mg/kg I.V. may be given at 5–10 min intervals; maximum dose, 3 mg/kg. May also be given endotracheally: 2–4 mg/kg diluted with normal saline to 10 ml total volume	If lidocaine is effective, initiate continuous I.V. infusion at 2–4 mg/min when patient has return of a perfusing rhythm (but do not use if this rhythm is an idioventricular rhythm or third-degree heart block with an idioventricular escape rhythm). Continuous infusion should begin at 1 mg/min in congestive heart failure or chronic liver disease or in elderly patients.
	Magnesium sulfate, 500 mg/ml (2 ml and 10 ml vials), or 10 ml emergency syringe	Pulseless VT or VF associated with torsade de pointes, suspected QT prolongation problem, or other suspected hypomagnesemic condition	Administer 1–2 g diluted in 100 ml D5W I.V. over 1–2 min. Total body magnesium deficits should be replaced gradually after initial therapy has stabilized the emergency: administer 0.5–1 g/hr for 3–6 hr, then reassess continued need	Measured magnesium levels correlate only approximately with the actual level of deficiency. Patients with renal insufficiency are at risk for dangerous hypermagnesemia; use appropriate caution. Side effects may include bradycardia, hypotension, generalized weakness, and temporary loss of reflexes.
Anticholinergic	Atropine, 1 mg in 10 ml emergency syringe	Asystole or PEA (if rate of rhythm is slow)	For asystole or PEA: 1 mg I.V. every 3–5 min up to 3 mg. May be given via ET tube: 2–3 mg diluted with normal saline to 10 ml	Minimal adult dose is 0.5 mg. Avoid use in type II second-degree heart block or third-degree heart block.
Miscellaneous	Bicarbonate, 50 mEq in 50 ml emergency syringe	Significant hyperkalemia. Significant metabolic acidosis unresponsive to optimal CPR, oxygenation, and ventilation. Certain drug overdoses, including tricyclic antidepressants and aspirin	Hyperkalemia therapy: 50 mEq I.V. Metabolic acidosis: 1 mEq/kg slow I.V. push; may repeat half initial dose in 10 min; ideally, ABGs should help guide further therapy. Use in overdose: discuss with toxicologist	In non–dialysis-dependent hyperkalemic patients, bicarbonate is most useful if metabolic acidosis is also present; bicarbonate is less effective in dialysis-dependent renal failure patients. The use of bicarbonate in metabolic acidosis management in cardiac arrest patients is controversial. Side effects may include sodium overload, hypokalemia, and metabolic alkalosis.
	Calcium chloride, 100 mg/ml in 10 ml prefilled syringe	Significant hyperkalemia. Calcium channel blocker drug overdose. Profound hypocalcemia of other causes	In hyperkalemia: 5–10 ml slow I.V. push; may repeat if required. In calcium channel blocker overdose: discuss with toxicologist	Do not use if hyperkalemia is suspected to be caused by acute digoxin poisoning. Do not combine in same I.V. with sodium bicarbonate. Calcium chloride is not a routine medication in cardiac arrest.

Note: All medications used during cardiac arrest, when given via a peripheral venous site in an extremity, should be followed by a 20 ml I.V. saline bolus and elevation of the extremity for 10 to 20 sec.

ABG—arterial blood gases   D5W—5% dextrose in water   ET—endotracheal   NS—normal saline   PEA—pulseless electrical activity   VF—ventricular fibrillation   VT—ventricular tachycardia

In nonintubated patients, chest compressions are briefly paused for the delivery of ventilations. The sequence is the same, regardless of whether one-rescuer or two-rescuer CPR is being performed: the rescuer delivers 30 compressions, pauses for two breaths (each given over 1 second), then resumes compressions. A sequence of 30 compressions and two breaths is called one CPR cycle. In endotracheally intubated patients, no pause for ventilation is necessary; instead, every 5 seconds, one ventilation is delivered over a period of 1 second, while compressions continue at the rate of 100 per minute.[20]

The optimal timing and ratio of ventilations to compressions in CPR is an ongoing area of research and has led to changes from the older ratio of 15 compressions for every two ventilations to the 2005 recommendation of 30 compressions for every two ventilations.[52] In the porcine model, for example, optimal neurologic outcome was achieved with the use of chest compressions alone for the first 4 minutes, followed by the use of both compressions and ventilations at a compression-to-ventilation ratio of 100:2.[53] In the prehospital setting, when rapid advanced care is available within minutes, bystander-initiated mouth-to-mouth ventilation combined with chest compressions offers no advantage over chest compressions alone.[54]

Good technique is critical throughout CPR delivery. The patient should have carotid pulses with chest compressions and should have appropriate breath sounds and chest movement with ventilations. Interestingly, femoral pulsations with CPR do not necessarily indicate effective CPR; these pulsations often are venous rather than arterial. Quantitative end-tidal carbon dioxide levels can be monitored, if practical. Higher levels correlate with more effective CPR and increased survival[55] [see Table 1].

Defibrillation

When the monitor-defibrillator or AED arrives, it is attached to the patient; the rhythm is analyzed, and if the patient is in VF or pulseless VT, defibrillation is provided [see Tables 2 and 3]. CPR should be immediately resumed; rescuers should not stop to determine the effect of defibrillation until five cycles of CPR have been completed. Again, the goal is to maximize chest compressions and minimize interruptions to CPR. After five cycles, reassess the rhythm and, if a potentially perfusing rhythm appears to be present, assess for a carotid pulse.

Defibrillation is thought to work by simultaneously depolarizing a sufficient mass of cardiac myocytes to make the cardiac tissue ahead of the VT or VF wavefronts refractory to electrical conduction. Subsequently, the sinus node or another appropriate pacemaker region of the heart with inherent automaticity can resume orderly depolarization-repolarization, with return of a perfusing rhythm.[17,56] The sooner defibrillation occurs, the higher the likelihood of resuscitation. When defibrillation is provided immediately after the onset of VF, its success rate is extremely high.[57] In a study of patients who experienced sudden cardiac arrest in Nevada gambling casinos, the survival rate to hospital discharge was 74% for patients who received their first defibrillation no later than 3 minutes after a witnessed collapse.[30] In this study, defibrillation was delivered via an AED operated by casino security officers.

Early defibrillation is so critical that if a defibrillator is immediately available, its use traditionally takes precedence over CPR for patients in VF or pulseless VT of witnessed onset. If CPR is already in progress, it should of course be briefly halted while defibrillation takes place.

Newer defibrillators can compensate for thoracic impedance, ensuring that the selected energy level is in fact the energy that is delivered to the myocardial tissue. In addition, defibrillators that deliver biphasic defibrillation waveforms instead of the standard monophasic damped sinusoidal waveforms allow effective defibrillation at lower energy levels (< 200 joules) without the need for energy-level escalation during subsequent shocks.[17,58-61] In the Optimized Response to Cardiac Arrest (ORCA) study, which involved 115 patients with prehospital VF, the 150-joule biphasic-shock AED was more effective than the traditional high-energy

monophasic-shock AED in four respects: it was more successful in producing defibrillation with the first shock (96% versus 59%); it led to a higher rate of ultimate success with defibrillation (100% versus 84%); it had a better rate of return of spontaneous circulation (76% versus 54%); and its use was associated with a higher rate of good cerebral performance in the survivors (87% versus 53%).[62] There were no differences, however, in terms of survival to hospital admission or discharge, and replication of the ORCA findings is lacking at this time. Current AHA guidelines state that lower-energy biphasic waveform defibrillators are safe and have equivalent or higher efficacy for termination of VF, as compared with the standard monophasic waveform defibrillator.[17,52]

Ongoing research suggests that the duration of VF is a consideration in deciding whether to defibrillate immediately and as soon as a defibrillator is available or to perform CPR for a brief period first to "prime the pump" before proceeding to defibrillation. In the porcine model in the setting of prolonged VF (> 10 minutes), CPR before countershock provided several physiologic benefits.[63] Studies have found that patients with VF of longer than 5 minutes' duration had better return of spontaneous circulation, survival to hospital discharge, and 1-year survival if ambulance personnel provided 3 minutes of CPR before performing defibrillation than if ambulance personnel performed defibrillation immediately after arriving at the scene; however, some experts question the validity of these results, on the basis of study design.[64,65] In the 2005 guidelines, CPR for approximately five cycles before calling for help is recommended for the lone rescuer of a victim of an unwitnessed and presumed asphyxial cardiac arrest (e.g., from near-drowning).[64,65]

THE SECONDARY SURVEY

The secondary survey for a victim of persistent cardiac arrest takes place after completion of the primary survey. Again, ongoing CPR with as few interruptions to chest compressions as possible is key throughout. Like the primary survey, the secondary survey follows an ABCD format, which in this case consists of advanced airway interventions (A); optimized oxygenation and ventilation by confirmation of endotracheal (ET) tube placement and repeated reassessment of the adequacy of delivered breaths (B); intravenous access and appropriate medication delivery to the patient's circulation (C); and definitive therapy (D), determined on the basis of a differential diagnosis that considers the specific disease processes thought to be responsible for, or contributing to, the cardiac arrest. The secondary survey includes the fourth link in the chain of survival, rapid advanced care (see above).

Placement of an Advanced Airway

Patients who remain in cardiac arrest after completion of the primary survey require placement of an advanced airway. Depending on the setting and the experience of the rescuers, this advanced airway may be a laryngeal mask airway, an esophageal-tracheal Combitube (a tracheal tube bonded side by side with an esophageal obturator), or an ET tube.[38,66,67] The laryngeal mask airway and the Combitube can be placed by personnel with less training than that required for ET intubation, and they do not require additional special equipment or visualization of the vocal cords. Nevertheless, oral ET intubation is generally the preferred advanced airway technique for an ongoing cardiac resuscitation, especially in the hospital setting, where experienced intubators are generally present; in the prehospital setting, the evidence supporting ET intubation remains inconsistent. ET intubation isolates the airway, maintains airway patency, helps protect the trachea from the ever-present risk of aspiration, helps permit optimal oxygenation and ventilation of the patient, allows for tracheal suctioning, and even provides a route for delivery of some medications to the systemic circulation (via the pulmonary circulation) if intravenous access is unobtainable or lost.[66]

Optimization of Breathing and Ventilation

When a patient in cardiac arrest undergoes ET intubation, correct positioning of the ET tube must be immediately confirmed and regularly reconfirmed during and after the resuscitation [see Table 5]. Routine use of an esophageal detector device or end-tidal CO_2 detector is recommended, along with careful patient examination. Caution is necessary with qualitative colorimetric end-tidal CO_2 detectors because both false positive and false negative results have been documented during cardiac arrests.[68] Breath sounds should be present during auscultation over the anterior and lateral chest walls, and the patient's chest should rise and fall with delivered ventilations. No gurgling should be heard when the epigastrium is auscultated. The ET tube should be inserted to the appropriate depth marking: for average-size adults, this is 21 cm at the corner of the mouth in a woman and 23 cm in a man. The patient's skin color should be reasonable (i.e., not dusky or cyanotic), provided that the patient's pigmentation allows such assessment.

Once correct positioning is confirmed, the ET tube is then appropriately secured to prevent its dislodgment. When feasible, an arterial blood gas (ABG) measurement will help further confirm the adequacy of oxygenation and ventilation as the resuscitation proceeds.

Establishment of Circulation Access

Access to the patient's venous circulation is mandatory. Such access may be achieved by a code-team member or members simultaneously while other resuscitators pursue steps A and B of the secondary survey. Ideally, a large intravenous cannula is placed in a prominent upper-extremity vein or the external jugular vein to optimize delivery of needed medications. If a peripheral line is not achievable, additional access possibilities include central line placement via the internal jugular, the subclavian (via the supraclavicular approach), or, less ideally, the femoral vein; even intraosseous access is possible (the intraosseous route is commonly used for vascular access in pediatric emergencies, but it is an unusual route of access in adults). It is useful to remember, as already noted, that some important resuscitation medications can be delivered via the ET tube in cases of failed intravenous access; such medications include naloxone, atropine, vasopressin, epinephrine, and lidocaine (mnemonic: NAVEL).

The commonly used medications in cardiac resuscitation may be grouped into the following general categories: vasopressors (epinephrine or vasopressin), antiarrhythmics (amiodarone, lidocaine, and magnesium), anticholinergic agents (atropine, if the arrest arrhythmia is asystole or PEA is slow), and miscellaneous drugs used to treat specific problems contributing to the arrest state, such as sodium bicarbonate (for severe metabolic acidosis, hyperkalemia, and certain drug overdoses) and calcium chloride (for hyperkalemia, calcium channel blocker drug overdose, or severe hypocalcemia) [see Table 4]. The antiarrhythmic agent procainamide is no longer recommended for use in cardiac arrest.

Persons in cardiac arrest (which can result from pulseless VT, VF, PEA, or asystole) require a vasopressor for as long as they remain pulseless. Typically, this consists of 1 mg of epinephrine

---

Table 5   Confirmation of Oral Endotracheal Tube Placement

Intubation process
  Vocal cords are visualized by intubator
  Tip of ET tube is seen passing between the cords
  Cuff of ET tube also passes cords by 1 cm
Postintubation checks
  Esophageal detector device or end-tidal CO_2 detector confirms ET tube placement in trachea
  Breath sounds are symmetrical (auscultate over lateral anterior chest and in midaxillary line bilaterally)
  No gurgling heard with auscultation over epigastrium
  Patient's chest rises and falls appropriately with ventilation
  ET tube depth is appropriate: 21 cm at the corner of the mouth in women, 23 cm in men
Secure the ET tube to prevent dislodgment
Reassess the adequacy of oxygenation and ventilation throughout the resuscitation (bedside patient assessment; also obtain ABGs when feasible)
Postresuscitation, obtain a portable chest radiograph

ABG—arterial blood gas   ET—endotracheal

---

intravenously every 3 to 5 minutes. Epinephrine stimulates adrenergic receptors, which leads to vasoconstriction and optimization of CPR-generated blood flow to the heart and brain. Vasopressin (40 IU I.V. once only) is a reasonable alternative to epinephrine, at least initially. Vasopressin in the recommended dose is a potent vasoconstrictor. It also has the theoretical advantage over epinephrine of not increasing myocardial oxygen consumption or lactate production in the arrested heart.[69] Despite its potential advantages, however, in a study of 200 inpatient cardiac arrest patients, vasopressin did not result in a better survival rate than epinephrine.[70] Vasopressin was found to be comparable to epinephrine in out-of-hospital cardiac arrests when the rhythm was VF or PEA but superior to epinephrine for patients in asystole.[71,72]

During resuscitation with ongoing CPR, medication delivery through an intravenous cannula needs to be followed by a 20 ml saline bolus; if the cannula is in a peripheral vein, the extremity containing the cannula should then be elevated for 10 to 15 seconds to augment delivery of the medication to the central circulation. This is especially important because of the low-flow circulatory state with closed-chest CPR.

Differential Diagnosis and Definitive Care

The most challenging part of the secondary survey, as well as cardiac resuscitation management in general, is the problem-solving required when spontaneous circulation does not return despite appropriate initial interventions. This situation poses a critical question to the resuscitators: Why is this patient dying right now? The intellectual challenge of that question, which the resuscitators must try to answer expeditiously and at the bedside, is compounded by the emotional intensity that pervades most cardiac resuscitations.

The solvable problems that may interfere with resuscitation can be grouped into three broad categories: technical [see Table 6], physiologic, and anatomic [see Table 7]. Technical problems consist of difficulties with the resuscitators' equipment or skills; such difficulties include ineffective CPR, allowing too many interruptions to CPR, inadequate oxygenation and ventilation, ET tube complications, intravenous access difficulties, and monitor-de-

Table 6 Technical Problems That May Prevent a Successful Resuscitation

Problem	*Patients at Risk*	*Recommendations*
Ineffective CPR	All cardiac arrest patients	Minimize any interruptions to chest compressions. Ensure technically perfect CPR. Confirm carotid pulses with CPR ("push hard, push fast"). If arterial line was in place before cardiac arrest, confirm adequate arterial waveform with CPR on arterial line monitor. Monitor end-tidal CO_2 if available (higher levels correlate with better CPR and improved patient survival). Confirm adequate oxygenation with an ABG when feasible.
Inadequate oxygenation and ventilation	All cardiac arrest patients	Ensure optimal airway positioning and control. Have suction immediately available to manage pharyngeal and airway secretions. Ensure use of properly fitting, tightly sealed face mask for bag-valve mask (BVM) ventilation until a definitive airway is established. In nonintubated patients, the sequence is 30 chest compressions:two ventilations, then repeat. Apply cricoid pressure to prevent gastric distention during BVM ventilation until a definitive airway is established. Ensure that supplemental oxygen is flowing to BVM at 15 L/min. Deliver an appropriate tidal volume per breath (6–7 ml/kg if oxygen is available) at the rate of 12–15 breaths/min. Confirm bilateral and equal breath sounds with ventilation. Confirm that patient's chest rises with each ventilation. Allow adequate time for exhalation between breaths. Confirm optimal oxygenation and ventilation with an ABG when feasible.
ET tube difficulties	All patients intubated with ET tube	Allow ≤ 20–30 sec/intubation attempt. Intubator should see tip of ET tube and cuff pass between vocal cords at time of intubation. After intubation, immediately confirm correct ET tube placement [*see Table 5*]; regularly reconfirm ET tube placement throughout resuscitation. Confirm adequacy of oxygenation and ventilation with an ABG. After intubation, consider nasogastric tube placement to decompress stomach and optimize diaphragmatic excursions with ventilation.
Intravenous line difficulties	All cardiac arrest patients	Place one or more 18-gauge or larger I.V. cannulas in an antecubital or external jugular vein site. Check for I.V. infiltration regularly throughout the resuscitation. Follow all medications administered through a peripheral I.V. site with a 20 ml saline bolus and elevation of the extremity containing the I.V. for 10–15 sec (if possible). Consider central line placement if the resuscitation is prolonged. Be aware of every I.V. infusion the patient is receiving. Stop all nonessential medications that had been started before the cardiac arrest (e.g., nitroglycerin). During the resuscitation, the only infusions the patient should receive are normal saline, blood products (if clinically indicated), and pertinent medications necessary to assist with return of spontaneous circulation. Pulmonary artery catheters and central lines occasionally act as an arrhythmogenic focus within the right ventricle. If applicable, deflate all relevant balloons on the catheter and withdraw the catheter to a superior vena cava position.
Monitor-defibrillator difficulties	All cardiac arrest patients	Make sure Synchronization Mode button is in the off position when defibrillating patients in pulseless VT or VF. Make sure electricity is not arcing over the patient's chest because of perspiration or smeared conducting gel; dry patient's chest with a towel except for areas directly beneath pads or paddles. Do not administer shock through nitroglycerin paste or patches. If the patient has an internal cardioverter-defibrillator (ICD) or a pacemaker, the patient may still be manually defibrillated, but do not shock directly over the internal device. Under these circumstances, place the pads or paddles at least 1 in. away from the patient's internal device. If the ICD is intermittently firing but not defibrillating the patient and if the ICD is thought to be compromising the resuscitation, turn the device off with a magnet so that manual defibrillation may take place without interference. Maximize the gain or electrocardiography "size" and check the rhythm in several leads (or change the axes of the paddles if reading the rhythm in Paddles mode) to confirm asystole when the initial rhythm appears to be asystole.

ABG—arterial blood gas   ET—endotracheal   VF—ventricular fibrillation   VT—ventricular tachycardia

fibrillator malfunction or misuse. The physiologic and anatomic problems consist of life-threatening but potentially treatable conditions that may have led to the cardiac arrest in the first place. This differentiation between physiology and anatomy is admittedly artificial, given that physiology is always involved in a cardiac arrest, but it has some usefulness as a teaching and problem-solving tool. Physiologic problems classically include hypoxia, acidosis, hyperkalemia, severe hypokalemia, hypothermia, hypoglycemia, and drug overdose. Anatomic problems are hypovolemia/hemorrhage, tension pneumothorax, cardiac tamponade, myocardial infarction, and pulmonary embolism.[43]

Whenever possible, the patient's medical and surgical history

Table 7   Potentially Treatable Conditions That May Cause or Contribute to Cardiac Arrest[3]

Condition	Clinical Setting	Diagnostic and Corrective Actions
Acidosis	Preexisting acidosis, diabetes, diarrhea, drugs, toxins, prolonged resuscitation, renal disease, shock	Obtain stat ABG. Reassess technical quality of CPR, oxygenation, and ventilation. Confirm correct endotracheal tube placement. Hyperventilate patient (P_aCO_2 of 30–35 mm Hg) to partially compensate for metabolic acidosis. If pH < 7.20 despite above interventions, consider I.V. sodium bicarbonate, 1 mEq/kg I.V. slow push.
Cardiac tamponade	Hemorrhagic diathesis, malignancy, pericarditis, postcardiac surgery, postmyocardial infarction, trauma	Initiate large-volume I.V. crystalloid resuscitation. Confirm diagnosis with emergent bedside echocardiogram, if available. Perform pericardiocentesis. Immediate surgical intervention is appropriate if pericardiocentesis is unhelpful but cardiac tamponade is known or highly suspected clinically.
Hypoglycemia	Adrenal insufficiency, alcohol abuse, aspirin overdose, diabetes, drugs, toxins, liver disease, renal disease, sepsis, certain tumors	Consider clinical setting and obtain finger-stick glucose or stat blood glucose measurements (may be obtained on ABG specimen). If glucose < 60 mg/dl, treat: 50 ml = 25 g of D50W I.V. Follow glucose levels closely posttreatment.*
Hypomagnesemia	Alcohol abuse, burns, diabetic ketoacidosis, severe diarrhea, diuretics, drugs (e.g., cisplatin, cyclosporine, pentamidine), malabsorption, poor intake, thyrotoxicosis	Obtain stat serum magnesium level. Treat: 1–2 g magnesium sulfate I.V. over about 5 min in patients with pulseless VT or VF in the setting of suspected prolonged QT interval problems, torsade de pointes, or hypomagnesemia. Follow magnesium levels over time, because blood levels correlate poorly with total body deficit.
Hypothermia	Alcohol abuse, burns, central nervous system disease, debilitated and elderly patients, drowning, drugs, toxins, endocrine disease, exposure history, homelessness, poverty, extensive skin disease, spinal cord disease, trauma	Obtain core body temperature. If severe hypothermia (< 30° C), limit initial shocks for pulseless VT/VF to one, initiate active internal rewarming and cardiopulmonary support, and hold further resuscitation medications or shocks until core temperature > 30° C.† If moderate hypothermia (30°–34° C), proceed with resuscitation (space medications at intervals greater than usual), provide active external rewarming (e.g., forced air, warmed infusions).
Hypovolemia, hemorrhage, anemia	Major burns, diabetes, gastrointestinal losses, hemorrhage, hemorrhagic diathesis, malignancy, pregnancy, shock, trauma	Initiate large-volume I.V. crystalloid resuscitation. Obtain stat hemoglobin level on ABG specimen. Emergently transfuse packed red blood cells (O negative if type-specific blood not available) if hemorrhage or profound anemia is contributing to arrest. Emergently consult necessary specialty for definitive care. Emergent thoracotomy with open cardiac massage is a consideration if experienced providers are available for the patient with penetrating truncal trauma and cardiac arrest.
Hypoxia	All cardiac arrest patients are at risk	Reassess technical quality of CPR, oxygenation, and ventilation. Confirm correct ET tube placement. Obtain stat ABG to confirm adequate oxygenation and ventilation.
Myocardial infarction	Consider in all cardiac arrest patients, especially those with risk factors for coronary artery disease, a history of ischemic heart disease, or prearrest picture consistent with an acute coronary syndrome	Review prearrest clinical presentation and ECG. Continue resuscitation algorithm; proceed with definitive care as appropriate for the immediate circumstances (e.g., thrombolytic therapy, cardiac catheterization/coronary artery reperfusion, circulatory assist device, emergent cardiopulmonary bypass).

(continued)

and the circumstances and symptoms immediately before the cardiac arrest should be sought from family members, bystanders, or hospital staff as the resuscitation proceeds. This information may contain important clues to the principal arrest problem and how it may be expeditiously treated. For example, a patient who presents to an emergency department with chest pain and then suffers a VF cardiac arrest is in all likelihood experiencing of a massive myocardial infarction, pulmonary embolism, or aortic dissection, with tension pneumothorax or cardiac tamponade also being possibilities.

Specific questions to consider include the following: Does the patient have risk factors for heart disease, pulmonary embolism, or aortic disease? What was the quality of the patient's pain and its radiation before the cardiac arrest? What were the prearrest vital signs and physical examination findings? What did the prearrest electrocardiogram show (if available)? Can any of this information be used now, at the bedside, to dictate the needed resuscitation interventions during the D phase of the secondary survey? For example, if the prearrest ECG showed prominent ST segment elevation in leads V1 through V4 consistent with a large anterior myocardial infarction, if the patient's resuscitation is failing despite appropriate interventions, and if there appear to be no technical problems hampering the resuscitation, a working diagnosis of massive myocardial infarction can be made; intravenous thrombolytic therapy may then be a reasonable and needed step in such a resuscitation.[73]

Thoughtful consideration of the possible reasons why a resuscitation is failing will regularly push the code-team captain's and resuscitation team's expertise and clinical skills to the limits. Nevertheless, the failure to consider these formidable issues will deprive the patient of an optimal opportunity to survive the cardiac arrest.

Table 7 (*continued*)

Condition	Clinical Setting	Diagnostic and Corrective Actions
Poisoning	Alcohol abuse, bizarre or puzzling behavioral or metabolic presentation, classic toxic syndrome, occupational or industrial exposures, history of ingestion, polysubstance abuse, psychiatric disease	Consider clinical setting and presentation; provide meticulous supportive care. Emergently consult toxicologist (through regional poison center) for resuscitative and definitive care advice, including appropriate antidote use. Prolonged resuscitation efforts are appropriate. If available, immediate cardiopulmonary bypass should be considered.
Hyperkalemia	Metabolic acidosis, excessive administration, drugs and toxins, vigorous exercise, hemolysis, renal disease, rhabdomyolysis, tumor lysis syndrome, significant tissue injury	Obtain stat serum potassium level on ABG specimen. Treatment: calcium chloride 10% (5–10 ml I.V. slow push [do not use if hyperkalemia is secondary to digitalis poisoning]), followed by glucose and insulin (50 ml of D50W and 10 U regular insulin I.V.); sodium bicarbonate (50 mEq I.V.); albuterol (15–20 mg nebulized or 0.5 mg I.V. infusion).‡
Hypokalemia	Alcohol abuse, diabetes, diuretic use, drugs and toxins, profound gastrointestinal losses, hypomagnesemia, excess mineralocorticoid states, metabolic alkalosis	Obtain stat serum potassium level on ABG specimen. If profound hypokalemia (K^+ < 2–2.5 mEq/L) is contributing to cardiac arrest, initiate urgent I.V. replacement (2 mEq/min I.V. for 10–15 mEq), then reassess.§
Pulmonary embolism	Hospitalized patients, recent surgical procedure, peripartum, known risk factors for venous thromboembolism (VTE), history of VTE, prearrest presentation consistent with acute pulmonary embolism	Review prearrest clinical presentation; initiate appropriate volume resuscitation with I.V. crystalloid and augment with vasopressors as necessary. Attempt emergent confirmation of diagnosis, depending on availability and clinical circumstances; consider emergent cardiopulmonary bypass to maintain patient viability. Continue resuscitation algorithm; proceed with definitive care (thrombolytic therapy, embolectomy via interventional radiology, or surgical thrombectomy) as appropriate for immediate circumstances and availability.
Tension pneumothorax	Post–central line placement, mechanical ventilation, pulmonary disease (including asthma, COPD, necrotizing pneumonia), postthoracentesis, trauma	Consider risks and clinical presentation (prearrest history, breath sounds, neck veins, tracheal deviation). Proceed with emergent needle decompression, followed by chest tube insertion.

*Unrecognized hypoglycemia can cause significant neurologic injury and can be life threatening, but caution with I.V. glucose is appropriate in the setting of cardiac arrest. Available evidence indicates that hyperglycemia may contribute to impaired neurologic recovery in cardiac arrest survivors.

†Active internal or core rewarming includes warm (42°–46° C) humidified oxygen delivered through the endotracheal tube; warm I.V. fluids; peritoneal lavage; esophageal rewarming tubes; bladder lavage; and extracorporeal rewarming if immediately available. Active external rewarming includes warming beds, forced hot air, hot-water bottles, heating pads to groin/neck/axilla, and radiant heat sources applied externally to the patient.

‡Glucose is not necessary initially if patient is already hyperglycemic, but glucose levels should be followed closely after administration of I.V. insulin because of the risk of hypoglycemia (especially in patients with renal failure, because of the long duration of action of I.V. insulin in such patients). Sodium bicarbonate is most helpful in patients with concomitant metabolic acidosis; it is less effective in lowering serum potassium in dialysis-dependent renal failure patients. High-dose nebulized albuterol should lower serum potassium by 0.5 to 1.5 mEq/L within 30 to 60 min, but administration during cardiac arrest may be difficult.

§In a non–cardiac arrest situation, usual I.V. potassium replacement guidelines for patients requiring parenteral therapy are generally 10 to 20 mEq/hr with continuous electrocardiographic monitoring. If profound hypokalemia is contributing to cardiac arrest, however, these usual replacement rates are impractical, given the critical nature of the situation. Under these circumstances, potassium chloride, 2 mEq/min I.V. for 10 to 15 mEq, is reasonable, but reassessment and careful attention to changing levels, redistribution, and ongoing clinical circumstances are essential to prevent life-threatening hyperkalemia from developing.

ABG—arterial blood gas   COPD—chronic obstructive pulmonary disease   D50W—50% dextrose in water   ET—endotracheal   VF—ventricular fibrillation VT—ventricular tachycardia

Cardiac Resuscitation Based on Rhythm Findings

When a monitor-defibrillator arrives at the scene of a cardiac arrest, the patient's rhythm is immediately analyzed. This step constitutes the beginning part of the defibrillation stage, or step D, of the AHA's primary survey. There are four rhythm possibilities [*see Figure 1*]: (1) pulseless VT; (2) VF; (3) organized or semi-organized electrical activity despite the absence of a palpable carotid pulse, which defines PEA; and (4) asystole. The detailed management of these different cardiac resuscitation scenarios is based on the recommendations of the AHA[52] and the International Liaison Committee on Resuscitation.[74] Those recommendations were revised in the 2005 guidelines.[75] In following these guidelines, the clinician should remember that, with the exception of early CPR and early defibrillation for VF and pulseless VT, many of the recommendations that form the foundation of modern resuscitation are evidence supported or consensus based (rather than evidence based, as would be ideal). Because of the nature of cardiac arrest and the multiple variables involved, it is exceptionally difficult to perform high-quality, prospectively designed research in cardiac resuscitation.

PULSELESS VENTRICULAR TACHYCARDIA OR VENTRICULAR FIBRILLATION

The appearance of either VF or pulseless VT on the rhythm monitor in a patient with ongoing CPR is a relatively favorable finding, because there is reasonable hope for a successful outcome with these rhythms. In addition, the interventions and medications sequentially used in the resuscitation are plainly delineated, and the initial course of action is clear. VF and pulseless VT are managed identically.

Initiation of Defibrillation

Defibrillation with 120 to 200 joules (biphasic) or 360 joules (monophasic) should be attempted immediately. However, if the time from onset of arrest to CPR to the availability of defibrillation is estimated to be longer than 5 minutes, it is reasonable to continue CPR for another 2 to 3 minutes before initiating defibrillation [*see* Defibrillation, *above*]. Unlike earlier guidelines, however, current guidelines recommend that after an attempt at defibrillation, CPR should immediately be restarted. No attempt is made to assess the rhythm response to defibrillation or return of

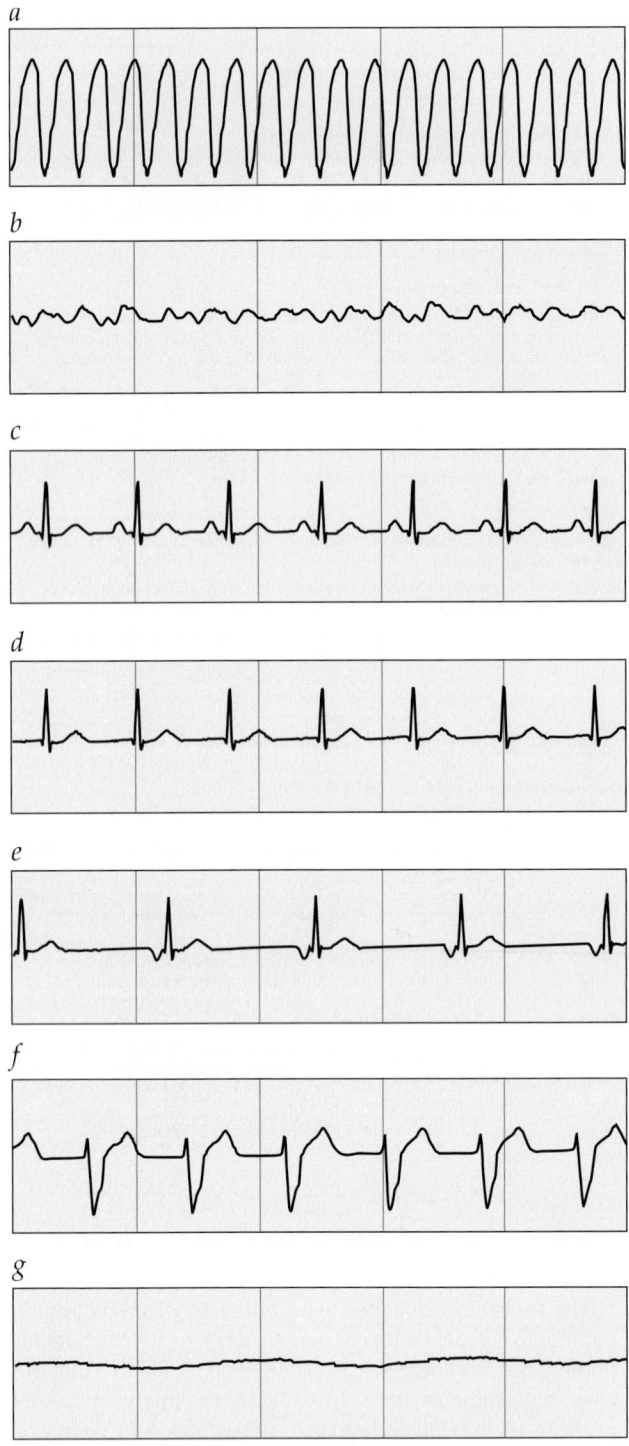

Figure 1 The sudden cardiac arrest arrhythmias. (*a*) Ventricular tachycardia. (*b*) Ventricular fibrillation. Pulseless electrical activity encompasses any of several forms of organized electrical activity in the pulseless patient; these include (*c*) normal sinus rhythm, (*d*) junctional rhythm, (*e*) bradycardic junctional rhythm, and (*f*) idioventricular rhythm. (*g*) Asystole.

spontaneous circulation until five cycles of CPR have been completed (or after about 2 minutes of CPR in intubated patients). This recommendation is intended to minimize the unnecessary pauses to chest compression that characterized resuscitations in the past. If the VF or VT persists after the initial shock (followed by five cycles of CPR), another defibrillation attempt should be

made with 120 to 200 joules (biphasic) or 360 joules (monophasic), again followed immediately by five cycles of CPR and then assessment of rhythm response to the shock [*see Figure 2*].

A lower, nonescalating equivalent biphasic energy level is acceptable, if the defibrillator offers this option. After shock delivery followed by five cycles of CPR, the displayed rhythm on the monitor must be carefully assessed; if it appears to be a potentially perfusing rhythm, the patient's carotid pulse should be checked to confirm return of spontaneous circulation. If VF or pulseless VT persists, CPR is immediately resumed, the patient is endotracheally intubated, correct ET tube placement is confirmed, and the tube is secured. Simultaneously, intravenous access should be established. After intubation, subsequent shocks for VF or pulseless VT should be delivered roughly every 2 minutes. Again, after each shock is delivered, resume CPR and do not assess for rhythm change or the presence of a pulse until CPR has been employed for approximately 2 minutes.

Initiation of Drug Therapy

In patients with ongoing VF, drug therapy starts with a vasoconstrictor (either epinephrine or vasopressin) [*see Table 4*]. The drug is given as soon as intravenous access is established; in the absence of intravenous access, the drug can be given endotracheally. After each intravenous dose, drug delivery is followed by a 20 ml saline bolus and the extremity containing the intravenous line is elevated. Drug delivery may precede or follow shock delivery. As long as the patient remains pulseless, epinephrine is administered every 3 to 5 minutes. When vasopressin is the chosen initial drug, only a single dose is given; if the resuscitation continues 10 minutes or longer after vasopressin is administered, epinephrine (1 mg I.V. push every 3 to 5 minutes) should be substituted for vasopressin for the remainder of the code. If VF or pulseless VT persists despite the initial administration of a vasoconstrictor and a repeated defibrillation attempt, parenteral antiarrhythmic drug therapy is added; amiodarone or lidocaine is an appropriate agent [*see* Choice of Antiarrhythmic Drugs, *below*]. Antiarrhythmic drug delivery may precede or follow an attempt at defibrillation. Throughout all of these steps, the code-team leader is also actively looking for and correcting any technical and physiologic or anatomic problems that may be preventing a successful resuscitation [*see Tables 6 and 7*].

Emergency Laboratory Tests

If spontaneous circulation does not return after the first round of antiarrhythmic drug therapy, the resuscitation team must endeavor to identify and treat the clinically relevant conditions causing or contributing to the cardiac arrest [*see Table 7*]. In theory, the interventions conducted to this point should have resulted in a perfusing rhythm. The code team must ask why this has not occurred and then attempt to answer this question as the resuscitation continues. Emergency laboratory studies that may prove helpful include a stat ABG measurement and measurements of hemoglobin, potassium, magnesium, and blood glucose levels (most of which can be obtained from the ABG specimen).

Choice of Antiarrhythmic Drugs

Three antiarrhythmic drugs are used in cardiac resuscitation in the setting of VF or pulseless VT: amiodarone, lidocaine, and magnesium (this last is used if the patient is thought or proved to have hypomagnesemia, torsade de pointes, or a prearrest prolonged QT interval).[76] It is not known which one of these drugs or which combination of them will optimize the chances of pa-

Rapid access
    Confirm unresponsiveness
    If out of hospital, call EMS (911)
    If in hospital, activate a "code" response
    Call for a defibrillator
If lone rescuer and unwitnessed and presumed asphyxial
    arrest, perform five cycles of CPR before EMS activation
    (one cycle = 30 compressions followed by two ventilations)

Primary survey
    Begin CPR; when defibrillator arrives, attach
    to patient and briefly pause to assess rhythm

Pulseless VT or VF
Administer shock (biphasic, 120–200 J; monophasic, 360 J)
Immediately resume CPR for five cycles before assessing rhythm
    response (simultaneously recharge defibrillator in preparation for
    next shock)
Pause CPR and reassess rhythm: if still pulseless
    VT or VF, shock again (biphasic: 120–200 J; monophasic, 360 J),
    then resume CPR for five cycles before assessing rhythm response
    (simultaneously recharge defibrillator in preparation for next shock)

PEA
Resume CPR

Asystole
Resume CPR
Confirm asystole by ensuring that all
    leads are in place on the patient and are
    appropriately attached to monitor-
    defibrillator, that ECG gain control on
    the monitor is at maximum, and that
    the rhythm is assessed in several leads

Secondary survey
    Establish I.V. access and administer either epinephrine (1 mg I.V. push) or vasopressin (40 U I.V. push, one time)
    Endotracheally intubate, confirm tube placement, and secure tube
    With subsequent steps, concomitantly identify and correct technical difficulties hampering resuscitation
    [*see Table 6*] and initiate emergency therapy for conditions contributing to cardiac arrest [*see Table 7*]

Pulseless VT or VF
Subsequent steps assume continuing pulseless
    VT or VF; do not interrupt CPR except as
    absolutely necessary for rapid performance of
    lifesaving procedures
While continuing CPR, administer epinephrine
    (1 mg I.V. push every 3–5 min, or 10 min after
    initial dose of vasopressin); medication may be
    given before or after shocks
Deliver an appropriate shock approximately every
    2 min; then immediately perform CPR for 2 min
    before assessing for rhythm change and return
    of spontaneous circulation

If no response to CPR, shock(s), and vasopressor
    plus shock, consider antiarrhythmic drug therapy
Antiarrhythmic drugs may be given before or after
    shocks; after any shock, perform 2 min of CPR
    before assessing for rhythm change and return of
    spontaneous circulation
Amiodarone 300 mg I.V. push; if a second dose is
    needed, 150 mg after 5 min
        or
Lidocaine, 1–1.5 mg/kg I.V. push; subsequent
    doses are 0.5–0.75 mg/kg I.V. push at 5–10 min
    intervals, to a maximum of 3 mg/kg
        or
If torsade de pointes, long QT process, or
    hypomagnesemia is suspected:
        Magnesium sulfate, 1–2 g I.V. over 5–20 min
        Follow drug delivery with a 20 ml saline bolus;
        elevate extremity with I.V. line; CPR is ongoing

PEA
Subsequent steps assume continuing
    PEA despite interventions; do
    not interrupt CPR except as
    required for rapid performance
    of lifesaving procedures
Administer epinephrine, 1 mg I.V.
    push, with ongoing CPR; repeat
    every 3–5 min as long as CPR is
    required (or 10 min after initial
    dose of vasopressin)
If heart rate as shown on monitor
    is slow, administer atropine,
    1 mg I.V. push, with ongoing
    CPR; may repeat every 3–5 min
    to a total dose of 3 mg
Follow medication delivery with
    a 20 ml saline bolus and
    elevation of the extremity
    containing the I.V. line

Asystole
Subsequent steps assume
    continuing asystole despite
    interventions; do not interrupt CPR
    except as required for the rapid
    performance of lifesaving procedures
Consider attempting transcutaneous
    pacing early (reasonable intervention,
    but no clear evidence of efficacy)
Administer medications with ongoing
    CPR:
        Epinephrine 1 mg I.V. push;
        repeat every 3–5 min for as long
        as patient requires CPR (or 10 min
        after initial dose of vasopressin)
            and
        Atropine, 1 mg I.V. push, with
        ongoing CPR; may repeat every
        3–5 min to a total dose of 3 mg
Follow medication delivery with a
    20 ml saline bolus and elevation of
    the extremity containing the I.V. line
End resuscitation attempt if patient
    remains in confirmed asystole for
    > 10 min and there is no technical
    problem preventing resuscitation,
    no imminently treatable cause,
    and no extenuating circumstance

Figure 2   **Treatment algorithm for patients with VT, VF, PEA, or asystole. (PEA—pulseless electrical activity; VF—ventricular fibrillation; VT—ventricular tachycardia)**

tient survival to hospital discharge. Despite many years of routine use, there are no controlled studies demonstrating a survival benefit with lidocaine, versus placebo, in the management of VF or pulseless VT. Two studies in patients with shock-refractory prehospital VF showed that survival to hospital admission was better with amiodarone than with placebo (44% versus 34%; P = 0.03)[7] or with lidocaine (22.8% versus 12.0%; P = 0.009).[78] Neither of these studies demonstrated an improved survival to hospital discharge in the amiodarone groups, but neither study had the statistical power to demonstrate such a difference. Amiodarone is considerably more expensive than lidocaine.

The optimal role and the exact benefit of antiarrhythmic medications in cardiac resuscitation are yet to be fully elucidated. According to AHA guidelines, either amiodarone or lidocaine is an acceptable initial antiarrhythmic drug for the treatment of patients with VF or pulseless VT that is unresponsive to initial shock, CPR, airway management, and administration of epinephrine or vasopressin plus shocks. On the basis of available evidence, however, amiodarone may be the antiarrhythmic agent of first choice in the setting of prehospital refractory VF, allowing for optimal survival to hospital arrival.[76-78]

PULSELESS ELECTRICAL ACTIVITY

Community ACLS providers are encountering nonventricular arrhythmias (i.e., PEA and asystole) with increasing frequency. Classically, the prognosis for PEA has been poor, with outpatient survival rates generally reported as 0% to 7%.[79,80] In the hospital setting, only 11% of adult PEA arrest victims survive to hospital discharge.[11] The sequence of resuscitation steps in the management of PEA is as follows: activation of the emergency medical or code response, primary survey (CPR and rhythm evaluation), and secondary survey (intubation and confirmation of correct ET tube placement, optimal oxygenation and ventilation, establishment of I.V. access, epinephrine or vasopressin administration, and, finally, problem solving for technical difficulties and establishment of the cause of the cardiac arrest) [see Figure 2]. The core drugs for PEA management are epinephrine (repeated every 3 to 5 minutes for as long as the patient is pulseless) or vasopressin (40 IU I.V. push, one dose only) and atropine (up to 3 mg over time if the PEA rhythm on the monitor is inappropriately slow). The best hope for a successful resuscitation is to find and treat the cause of PEA; therein lies the exceptionally challenging aspect of PEA resuscitation management [see Tables 6 and 7]. Because coronary artery thrombosis and pulmonary thromboembolism are common causes of cardiac arrest, a trial evaluated the efficacy of tissue plasminogen activator (t-PA) in the setting of PEA of unknown or presumed cardiovascular cause in 233 patients in prehospital and emergency department settings.[81] No benefit was found with thrombolytic therapy for PEA in this study; the proportion of patients with return of spontaneous circulation was 21.4% in the t-PA group and 23.3% in the placebo group.

ASYSTOLE

The prognosis for asystole is generally regarded as dismal unless the patient is hypothermic or there are other extenuating but treatable circumstances. For in-hospital cardiac arrest victims of asystole, the rate of hospital survival to discharge is about 10%.[11] The sequence of resuscitation steps in the management of asystole is as follows: activation of the emergency medical or code response (a lone rescuer facing a presumed asphyxial arrest should perform five cycles of CPR before EMS activation), primary survey (CPR, rhythm evaluation, and asystole confirmation), and

secondary survey (intubation and confirmation of correct ET tube placement, optimal oxygenation and ventilation, establishment of I.V. access, administration of epinephrine or vasopressin and atropine, immediate transcutaneous pacing if available, and problem solving for technical difficulties and establishment of the cause of cardiac arrest) [see Figure 2]. The core drugs for asystole management are epinephrine (repeated every 3 to 5 minutes for as long as the patient is pulseless) or vasopressin (40 IU I.V. push), along with atropine (up to 3 mg over time). As with PEA, vasopressin appears to be a reasonable and possibly beneficial substitute for epinephrine in asystole. A single dose of aminophylline (250 mg I.V.) may also be beneficial in atropine-resistant asystole.[82] Potentially treatable causes of asystole include hypoxia, acidosis, hypothermia, hypokalemia, hyperkalemia, and drug overdose. Resuscitation efforts should stop if asystole persists for longer than 10 minutes despite optimal CPR, oxygenation and ventilation, and epinephrine or vasopressin and atropine administration; if there are no extenuating circumstances (e.g., hypothermia, cold-water submersion, or drug overdose); and if no other readily treatable condition is identified.

Immediate Postresuscitation Care

Even when the resuscitation is successful, the patient's situation remains tenuous, and continued meticulous patient care is essential. When the cardiac monitor indicates what should be a perfusing rhythm, the rescuer should immediately confirm that the patient has a palpable pulse. If there is a pulse, the patient's blood pressure is then obtained. Simultaneously, resuscitation team members need to quickly reassess the adequacy of the patient's airway, the ET tube position, oxygenation and ventilation, and the patient's level of consciousness and comfort.

If the patient is hypotensive, appropriate blood pressure management depends on the presence or absence of fluid overload, as judged at the bedside. If the patient is clinically volume overloaded or in frank pulmonary edema and is hypotensive, dopamine is started at inotropic doses (5 µg/kg/min I.V.) and titrated to a target systolic blood pressure of 90 to 100 mm Hg. If the patient's clinical status suggests normovolemia or hypovolemia, intravenous crystalloid boluses (in 250 to 500 ml increments) can be administered instead of dopamine to optimize intravascular volume and support adequate tissue perfusion. In patients who are regaining consciousness, their level of comfort mandates careful assessment and administration of analgesia and sedation, as appropriate.

If the arrest rhythm was either VT or VF, the parenteral antiarrhythmic drug used immediately before the return of spontaneous circulation is continued as a maintenance infusion (amiodarone, 1 mg/min for 6 hours, then 0.5 mg/min for 18 hours as blood pressure allows; or lidocaine, 2 to 4 mg/min). If an antiarrhythmic drug has not yet been administered, it is usually started at this point to prevent the recurrence of VF or pulseless VT. There are important exceptions to this guideline, however. If the perfusing postarrest arrhythmia is an idioventricular rhythm or third-degree heart block accompanied by an idioventricular escape rhythm, an antiarrhythmic medication should not be started at this time, because the antiarrhythmic agent could eliminate the ventricular perfusing focus and return the patient to a pulseless state.

Initial postresuscitation studies usually include an ECG; portable chest radiography; and measurement of ABGs, a serum electrolyte panel, fingerstick or blood glucose, serum magnesium and cardiac enzyme levels, and hemoglobin and hematocrit. The resuscitated patient requires urgent transfer to the optimal site for continued definitive care. Depending on the circumstances, this may be either the cardiac catheterization laboratory or the intensive care unit.

Ongoing research continues to look at optimal postresuscitation management strategies to improve neurologic outcome and survival to hospital discharge.[83] Hyperthermia and hyperglycemia compromise postresuscitation neurologic outcome, whereas mild to moderate induced hypothermia appears to improve neurologic outcome and decrease mortality.[84-87]

Ending a Resuscitation Attempt

Throughout the resuscitation, the team leader must speak with calmness and authority, and all resuscitations should be orchestrated with clarity and finesse. If possible, the code captain should make clinical decisions without directly performing specific procedures. When a procedure is performed or a drug is delivered, the team member should immediately inform the team captain of the completed order (e.g., "1 mg of epinephrine has just been given as an I.V. push"). Cardiac arrests are emotionally charged, but the leader must insist on a composed, orderly, and technically sound resuscitation. It is appropriate to invite suggestions from team members and to ensure that all members are comfortable with the decision to stop the resuscitation, should that time arrive.

The decision whether to stop a cardiac resuscitation is burdensome. Clearly, the circumstances of the event, patient comorbidities, the nature of the lethal arrhythmia, and the resuscitation team's ability to correctly identify and treat potential contributing causes of the arrest circumstance are all important considerations. Resuscitation efforts beyond 30 minutes without a return of spontaneous circulation are usually futile unless the cardiac arrest is confounded by intermittent or recurrent VF or pulseless VT, hypothermia, cold-water submersion, drug overdose, or other identified and readily treated contributing conditions.[88,89]

With nontraumatic cardiac arrest in the prehospital setting (assuming proper equipment and medications are available and no extenuating circumstances suggest otherwise), full resuscitation efforts take place at the scene of the arrest in preference to rapid transport to an emergency department. A prehospital resuscitation that has been appropriately conducted but has not resulted in at least temporary return of spontaneous circulation to the patient may be discontinued in the field. It is important that certain criteria be adhered to, however, including the following: high-quality CPR with as few interruptions as possible, successful placement of an adequate airway, delivery of appropriate oxygenation and ventilation, establishing of intravenous access, administration of appropriate medications specific to the arrest scenario, and resuscitation attempted for at least 10 minutes; in addition, the patient must not be in persistent VF, and there can be no extenuating circumstances that mandate in-hospital continuation of the resuscitation (e.g., hypothermia, drug overdose). The decision whether to cease resuscitation efforts in the field is bolstered by direct discussion with EMS physicians. It is also essential that social services be available to provide immediate assistance and support to the family and loved ones of the patient who has now died.

Discontinuing in-hospital resuscitations is advisable when three criteria are met: (1) the arrest was unwitnessed, (2) the initial rhythm was other than VF or VT, and (3) spontaneous circulation does not return after 10 minutes of ongoing resuscitation.[38] In a study of this three-component decision rule, only 1.1% of patients (three out of 269) who met these criteria survived to hospital dis-

charge, and none of the three survivors were capable of independent living.[90] In a study of 445 prospectively recorded resuscitation attempts in hospitalized patients, no patient survived who suffered a cardiac arrest between 12 A.M. and 6 A.M. if the arrest was unwitnessed and if it occurred in an unmonitored bed.[40]

A resuscitation attempt in a persistently asystolic patient should not last longer than 10 minutes, assuming all of the following conditions apply: asystole is confirmed through proper rhythm monitoring and assessment; high-quality CPR is taking place with as few interruptions as possible; ET intubation is correctly performed and confirmed; adequate oxygenation and ventilation are provided; intravenous access is secured; appropriate medications (atropine and either epinephrine or vasopressin) have been administered; and the patient is not the victim of hypothermia, cold-water submersion, drug overdose, or other readily identified and reversible cause.

After all resuscitation attempts, the code-team captain should debrief the team so that all may learn from the experience. Finally, marked empathy and skill are needed to carefully and compassionately inform family members about the outcome of the resuscitation.[91]

The author has no commercial relationships with manufacturers of products or providers of services discussed in this chapter.

References

1. Callans DJ: Management of the patient who has been resuscitated from sudden cardiac death. Circulation 105:2704, 2002
2. Zipes DP, Wellens HJ: Sudden cardiac death. Circulation 98:2334, 1998
3. Eisenberg MS, Mengert TJ: Cardiac resuscitation. N Engl J Med 344:1304, 2001
4. 1999 Heart and Stroke Statistical Update. American Heart Association, Dallas, 1998
5. Huikuri HV, Castellanos A, Myerburg R: Sudden death due to cardiac arrhythmias. N Engl J Med 345:1473, 2001
6. Ballew KA, Philbrick JT: Causes of variation in reported in-hospital CPR survival: a critical review. Resuscitation 30:203, 1995
7. Myerburg RJ, Castellanos A: Cardiac arrest and sudden cardiac death. Heart Disease: A Textbook of Cardiovascular Medicine. Braunwald E, Ed. WB Saunders Co, Philadelphia, 1997, p 742
8. Osborn LA: Etiology of sudden death. Cardiac Arrest: The Science and Practice of Resuscitation Medicine. Paradis NA, Halperin HR, Nowak RM, Eds. Williams & Wilkins, Philadelphia, 1996, p 243
9. Maron BJ: Sudden death in young athletes. N Engl J Med 349:1064, 2003
10. Cobb LA, Fahrenruch CD, Olsufka M, et al: Changing incidence of out-of-hospital ventricular fibrillation, 1980–2000. JAMA 288:3008, 2002
11. Nadkarni VM, Larkin GL, Peberdy MA, et al: First documented rhythm and clinical outcome from in-hospital cardiac arrest among children and adults. JAMA 295:50, 2006
12. Cummins RO, Ornato JP, Thies W, et al: Improving survival from cardiac arrest: the chain of survival concept: a statement for health professionals from the Advanced Cardiac Life Support Subcommittee and the Emergency Cardiac Care Committee, American Heart Association. Circulation 83:1832, 1991
13. 2005 American Heart Association guidelines for cardiopulmonary resuscitation and emergency cardiovascular care. Part 4: adult basic life support. ECC Committee, Subcommittees and Task Forces of the American Heart Association. Circulation 112(24 suppl):IV19, 2005
14. Capussi A, Aschieri D, Piepoli MF, et al: Tripling survival from sudden cardiac arrest via early defibrillation without traditional education in cardiopulmonary resuscitation. Circulation 106:1065, 2002
15. Callaham M, Madsen CD: Relationship of timeliness of paramedic advanced life support interventions to outcome in out-of-hospital cardiac arrest treated by first responders with defibrillators. Ann Emerg Med 27:638, 1996
16. Marenco JP, Wang PJ, Link MS, et al: Improving survival from sudden cardiac arrest: the role of the automated external defibrillator. JAMA 285:1193, 2001
17. Peberdy MA: Defibrillation. Cardiol Clin 20:13, 2002
18. Public-access defibrillation and survival after out-of-hospital cardiac arrest. The Public Access Defibrillation Trial Investigators. N Engl J Med 351:637, 2004
19. Cummins RO, Eisenberg MS: Prehospital cardiopulmonary resuscitation: is it effective? JAMA 253:2408, 1985
20. Stapleton ER: Basic life support cardiopulmonary resuscitation. Cardiol Clin 20:12, 2002
21. Valenzuela TD, Roe DJ, Cretin S, et al: Estimating effectiveness of cardiac arrest interventions: a logistic regression survival model. Circulation 96:3308, 1997
22. Eisenberg MS, Bergner L, Hallstrom A: Cardiac resuscitation in the community: the

importance of rapid delivery of care and implications for program planning. JAMA 241:1905, 1979

23. Weaver WD, Cobb LA, Hallstrom AP, et al: Considerations for improving survival from out-of-hospital cardiac arrest. Ann Emerg Med 15:1181, 1986

24. Larsen MP, Eisenberg MS, Cummins RO, et al: Predicting survival from out-of-hospital cardiac arrest: a graphic model. Ann Emerg Med 270:1211, 1993

25. Eisenberg MS, Horwood BT, Cummins RO, et al: Cardiac arrest and resuscitation: a tale of 29 cities. Ann Emerg Med 19:179, 1990

26. Lombardi G, Gallagher J, Gennis P: Outcome of out-of-hospital cardiac arrest in New York City: the Pre-Hospital Arrest Survival Evaluation (PHASE) study. JAMA 271:678, 1994

27. Becker LB, Ostrander MP, Barrett J, et al: Outcome of CPR in a large metropolitan area: where are the survivors? Ann Emerg Med 20:355, 1991

28. Killien SY, Geyman JP, Gossom JB, et al: Out-of-hospital cardiac arrest in a rural area: a 16-year experience with lessons learned and national comparisons. Ann Emerg Med 28:294, 1996

29. Bunch TJ, White RD, Gersh BJ, et al: Long-term outcomes of out-of-hospital cardiac arrest after successful early defibrillation. N Engl J Med 348:2626, 2003

30. Valenzuela TD, Roe DJ, Nichol G, et al: Outcomes of rapid defibrillation by security officers after cardiac arrest in casinos. N Engl J Med 343:1206, 2000

31. Eisenberg M, Bergner L, Hallstrom A: Sudden Cardiac Death in the Community. Praeger, Philadelphia, 1984

32. Becker L: The epidemiology of sudden death. Cardiac Arrest: The Science and Practice of Resuscitation Medicine. Paradis NA, Halperin HR, Nowak RM, Eds. Williams & Wilkins, Philadelphia, 1996, p 28

33. Jastremski MS: In-hospital cardiac arrest. Ann Emerg Med 22:113, 1993

34. Rosenberg M, Wang C, Hoffman-Wilde S, et al: Results of cardiopulmonary resuscitation: failure to predict survival in two community hospitals. Arch Intern Med 153:1370, 1993

35. Ballew KA, Philbrick JT, Caven DE, et al: Predictors of survival following in-hospital cardiopulmonary resuscitation: a moving target. Arch Intern Med 154:2426, 1994

36. de Vos R, Koster RW, de Haan RJ, et al: In-hospital cardiopulmonary resuscitation: prearrest morbidity and outcome. Arch Intern Med 159:845, 1999

37. Goodlin SJ, Zhong Z, Lynn J, et al: Factors associated with use of cardiopulmonary resuscitation in seriously ill hospitalized adults. JAMA 282:2333, 1999

38. van Walraven C, Forster AJ, Stiell IG: Derivation of a clinical decision rule for the discontinuation of in-hospital cardiac arrest resuscitations. Arch Intern Med 159:129, 1999

39. Zoch TW, Desbiens NA, DeStefano F, et al: Short- and long-term survival after cardiopulmonary resuscitation. Arch Intern Med 160:1969, 2000

40. Dumot JA, Burval DJ, Sprung J, et al: Outcome of adult cardiopulmonary resuscitations at a tertiary referral center, including results of "limited" resuscitations. Arch Intern Med 161:1751, 2001

41. Meade M: Men and the Water of Life. Harper, San Francisco, 1993, p 442

42. Burkle FM Jr, Rice MM: Code organization. Am J Emerg Med 5:235, 1987

43. ACLS Provider Manual. American Heart Association, Dallas, 2001

44. Safar P: On the history of modern resuscitation. Anesthesiol Clin North Am 13:751, 1995

45. Kouwenhoven WB, Jude JR, Knickerbocker GG: Closed-chest cardiac massage. JAMA 173:1064, 1960

46. Jude JR, Kouwenhoven WB, Knickerbocker GG: Cardiac arrest: report of application of external cardiac massage on 118 patients. JAMA 178:1063, 1961

47. Halperin HR: Mechanisms of forward flow during external chest compression. Cardiac Arrest: The Science and Practice of Resuscitation Medicine. Paradis NA, Halperin HR, Nowak RM, Eds. Williams & Wilkins, Philadelphia, 1996, p 252

48. Ornato JP, Peberdy MA: Cardiopulmonary resuscitation. Textbook of Cardiovascular Medicine. Topol EJ, Ed. Lippincott-Raven, Philadelphia, 1998, p 1779

49. Paradis NA, Martin GB, Goetting MG, et al: Simultaneous aortic, jugular bulb, and right atrial pressures during cardiopulmonary resuscitation in humans: insights into mechanisms. Circulation 80:361, 1989

50. Daya MR, Mariani RJ: Out-of-hospital splinting. Clinical Procedures in Emergency Medicine, 3rd ed. Roberts JR, Hedges JR, Eds. WB Saunders Co, Philadelphia, 1998, p 1297

51. Guidelines 2000 for cardiopulmonary resuscitation and emergency cardiovascular care: international consensus on science. Circulation 102(suppl I):1, 2000

52. 2005 American Heart Association guidelines for cardiopulmonary resuscitation and emergency cardiovascular care. Part 3: overview of CPR. ECC Committee, Subcommittees and Task Forces of the American Heart Association. Circulation 112(24 suppl):IV12, 2005

53. Sanders AB, Kern KB, Berg RA, et al: Survival and neurologic outcome after cardiopulmonary resuscitation with four different chest compression–ventilation ratios. Ann Emerg Med 40:553, 2002

54. Hallstrom A, Cobb L, Johnson E, et al: Cardiopulmonary resuscitation by chest compression alone or with mouth-to-mouth ventilation. N Engl J Med 342:1546, 2000

55. Levine RL, Wayne MA, Miller CC: End-tidal carbon dioxide and outcome of out-of-hospital cardiac arrest. N Engl J Med 337:301, 1997

56. Hedges JR, Greenberg MI: Defibrillation. Clinical Procedures in Emergency Medicine, 3rd ed. Roberts JR, Hedges JR, Eds. WB Saunders Co, Philadelphia, 1998, p 1297

57. Hossack KF, Hartwig R: Cardiac arrest associated with supervised cardiac rehabilitation. J Cardiac Rehab 2:402, 1982

58. Bardy GH, Marchlinski FE, Sharma AD, et al: Multicenter comparison of truncated biphasic shocks and standard damped sine wave monophasic shocks for transthoracic ventricular defibrillation. Circulation 94:2507, 1996

59. Gliner BE, White RD: Electrocardiographic evaluation of defibrillation shocks delivered to out-of-hospital sudden cardiac arrest patients. Resuscitation 41:129, 1999

60. Gliner BE, Jorgenson DB, Poole JE, et al: Treatment of out-of-hospital cardiac arrest with a low-energy impedance-compensating biphasic waveform automatic external defibrillator. Biomed Instrum Technol 32:631, 1998

61. Poole JE, White RD, Kanz KG, et al: Low-energy impedance-compensating biphasic waveforms terminate ventricular fibrillation at high rates in victims of out-of-hospital cardiac arrest. J Cardiovasc Electrophysiol 8:1373, 1997

62. Schneider T, Martens PR, Paschen H, et al: Multicenter, randomized, controlled trial of 150-J biphasic shocks compared with 200- to 360-J monophasic shocks in the resuscitation of out-of-hospital cardiac arrest victims. Circulation 102:1780, 2000

63. Berg RA, Hilwig RW, Kern KB, et al: Precountershock cardiopulmonary resuscitation improves ventricular fibrillation median frequency and myocardial readiness for successful defibrillation from prolonged ventricular fibrillation: a randomized, controlled swine study. Ann Emerg Med 40:563, 2002

64. Wik L, Hansen TB, Fylling F, et al: Delaying defibrillation to give basic cardiopulmonary resuscitation to patients with out-of-hospital ventricular fibrillation. JAMA 289:1389, 2003

65. Weisfeldt ML, Becker LB: Resuscitation after cardiac arrest: a 3-phase time sensitive model. JAMA 288:3035, 2002

66. Aehlert B: ACLS: Quick Review Study Guide, 2nd ed. CV Mosby, St Louis, 2001

67. Rumball CJ, MacDonald D: The PTL, Combitube, laryngeal mask, and oral airway: a randomized prehospital comparative study of ventilatory device effectiveness and cost-effectiveness in 470 cases of cardiorespiratory arrest. Prehosp Emerg Care 1:1, 1997

68. Garnett AR, Ornato JP, Gonzales ER, et al: End-tidal carbon dioxide monitoring during cardiopulmonary resuscitation. JAMA 257:512, 1987

69. Paradis NA, Wenzel V, Southall J: Pressor drugs in the treatment of cardiac arrest. Cardiol Clin 20:61, 2002

70. Stiell IG, Hebert PC, Wells GA, et al: Vasopressin versus epinephrine for inhospital cardiac arrest: a randomized controlled trial. Lancet 358:105, 2001

71. Wenzel V, Krismer AC, Arntz HR, et al: A comparison of vasopressin and epinephrine for out-of-hospital cardiopulmonary resuscitation. N Engl J Med 350:105, 2004

72. McIntryre KM: Vasopressin in asystolic cardiac arrest. N Engl J Med 350:179, 2004

73. Tiffany PA, Schultz M, Stueven H: Bolus thrombolytic infusions during CPR for patients with refractory arrest rhythms: outcome of a case series. Ann Emerg Med 31:124, 1998

74. Cummins RO, Chamberlain DA: Advisory statements of the International Liaison Committee on Resuscitation. Circulation 95:2172, 1997

75. 2005 American Heart Association guidelines for cardiopulmonary resuscitation and emergency cardiovascular care, part 7: advanced cardiovascular life support. ECC Committee, Subcommittees and Task Forces of the American Heart Association. Circulation 112(24 suppl):IV51, 2005

76. Kudenchuk PJ: Advanced cardiac life support antiarrhythmic drugs. Cardiol Clin 20:79, 2002

77. Kudenchuk PJ, Cobb LA, Copass MK, et al: Amiodarone for resuscitation after out-of-hospital cardiac arrest due to ventricular fibrillation. N Engl J Med 341:871, 1999

78. Dorian P, Cass D, Schwartz B, et al: Amiodarone as compared with lidocaine for shock-resistant ventricular fibrillation. N Engl J Med 346:884, 2002

79. Myerburg RJ, Conde CA, Sung RJ, et al: Clinical, electrophysiologic, and hemodynamic profile of patients resuscitated from prehospital cardiac arrest. Am J Med 68:568, 1980

80. Stratton SJ, Niemann JT: Outcome from out-of-hospital cardiac arrest caused by nonventricular arrhythmias: contribution of successful resuscitation to overall survivorship supports the current practice of initiating out-of-hospital ACLS. Ann Emerg Med 32:448, 1998

81. Abu-Laban RB, Christenson JM, Innes GD, et al: Tissue plasminogen activator in cardiac arrest with pulseless electrical activity. N Engl J Med 346:1522, 2002

82. Mader TJ, Smithline HA, Durkin L, et al: A randomized controlled trial of intravenous aminophylline for atropine-resistant out-of-hospital asystolic cardiac arrest. Acad Emerg Med 10:192, 2003

83. Angelos MG, Menegazzi JJ, Callaway CW: Bench to bedside: resuscitation from prolonged ventricular fibrillation. Acad Emerg Med 8:909, 2001

84. Zeiner A, Holzer M, Sterz F, et al: Hyperthermia after cardiac arrest is associated with an unfavorable neurological outcome. Arch Intern Med 161:2007, 2001

85. Moghissi E: Hospital management of diabetes: beyond the sliding scale. Cleve Clin J Med 71:801, 2004

86. Bernard SA, Gray TW, Buist MD, et al: Treatment of comatose survivors of out-of-hospital cardiac arrest with induced hypothermia. N Engl J Med 346:557, 2002

87. Mild therapeutic hypothermia to improve the neurologic outcome after cardiac arrest. The Hypothermia after Cardiac Arrest Study Group. N Engl J Med 346:549, 2002

88. Bonnin MJ, Pepe PE, Kimball KT, et al: Distinct criteria for termination of resuscitation in the out-of-hospital setting. JAMA 270:1457, 1993

89. Kellermann AL, Hackman BB, Somes G: Predicting the outcome of unsuccessful prehospital advanced cardiac life support. JAMA 270:1433, 1993

90. van Walraven C, Forster AJ, Parish DC, et al: Validation of a clinical decision aid to discontinue in-hospital cardiac arrest resuscitations. JAMA 285:1602, 2001

91. Iserson K: Grave Words: Notifying Survivors about Sudden, Unexpected Deaths. Galen Press, Tucson, Arizona, 1999

92. Cummins RO, Field JM, Hazinski MF, et al: ACLS Provider Manual. American Heart Association, Dallas, 2001, p 36

93. Part 1: introduction to the International Guidelines 2000 for CPR and ECC: a consensus on science. Circulation 102(8 suppl):I1, 2000

15   Management of Poisoning and Drug Overdose

Kent R. Olson, M.D., and Manish M. Patel, M.D.

Drug overdose and poisoning are leading causes of emergency department visits and hospital admissions in the United States, accounting for more than 500,000 emergency department visits[1] and 11,000 deaths[2] each year. Exposure to poison can occur in several ways. The patient may have ingested it accidentally or for the purpose of committing suicide, may be a victim of accidental intoxication from acute or long-term exposure in the workplace, may be suffering from unexpected complications or overdose after intentional drug abuse, or may be a victim of an assault or terrorist attack. Poisons can include drugs, chemicals, biotoxins in plants or foods, and toxic gases. In all cases of poisoning, the clinician has several priorities: (1) immediately stabilize the patient and manage life-threatening complications; (2) perform a careful diagnostic evaluation, which includes obtaining a directed history, performing a physical examination, and ordering appropriate laboratory tests; (3) prevent further absorption of the drug or poison by decontaminating the skin or gastrointestinal tract; and (4) consider administering antidotes and performing other measures that enhance the elimination of the drug from the body. For expert assistance with identification of poisons, diagnosis and treatment, and referral to a medical toxicologist, the clinician should consider consulting with a regional poison-control center.

Initial Stabilization

In many cases of poisoning, the patient is awake and has stable vital signs, which allows the clinician to proceed in a stepwise fashion to obtain a history and to perform a physical examination. In other cases, however, the patient is unconscious, is experiencing convulsions, or has unstable blood pressure or cardiac rhythm, thus requiring immediate stabilization [*see Table 1*].

The first priority is airway patency. The airway's reflex protective mechanisms may be impaired because of drug-induced central nervous system depression (e.g., from opioids or sedative-hypnotic agents), excessive bronchial and oral secretions (e.g., from organophosphate insecticides), or swelling or burns (e.g., from corrosive agents or irritant gases). The airway should be cleared by the use of suction and by repositioning the patient; if the patient has an impaired gag reflex or other evidence of airway compromise, a cuffed endotracheal tube should be inserted. The adequacy of ventilation and oxygenation should be determined by clinical assessment, pulse oximetry, measurement of arterial blood gases, or a combination of these techniques. Supplemental oxygen should be administered, and if necessary, ventilation should be assisted with a bag/valve/mask device or a ventilator.[3] Even if the patient is not unconscious or hemodynamically compromised on arrival in the emergency department, continued absorption of the ingested drug or poison may lead to more serious intoxication during the next several hours. Therefore, it is prudent to keep the patient under close observation, with continuous or frequent monitoring of alertness, vital signs, the electrocardiogram, and pulse oximetry.

Management of Common Complications

COMA

Poisoning or drug overdose depresses the sensorium, the symptoms of which may range from stupor or obtundation to unresponsive coma. Deeply unconscious patients may appear to be dead because they may have nonreactive pupils, absent reflexes, and flat electroencephalographic tracings; however, such patients may have a complete recovery without neurologic sequelae as long as they receive adequate supportive care, including airway protection, oxygenation, and assisted ventilation.[4]

All patients with a depressed sensorium should be evaluated for hypoglycemia because many drugs and poisons can directly reduce or contribute to the reduction of blood glucose levels. A finger-stick blood glucose test and bedside assessment should be performed immediately; if such testing and assessment are impractical, an intravenous bolus of 25 g of 50% dextrose in water should be administered empirically before the laboratory report arrives.[5] For alcoholic or malnourished patients, who may have vitamin deficiencies, 50 to 100 mg of vitamin B_1 (thiamine) should be administered I.V. or I.M. to prevent the development of Wernicke syndrome.[5] If signs of recent opioid use (e.g., suspicious-looking pill bottles or I.V. drug paraphernalia) are in evidence or if the patient has clinical manifestations of excessive opioid effect (e.g., miosis or respiratory depression), the administration of naloxone may have both therapeutic and diagnostic value. Naloxone is a specific opioid antagonist with no intrinsic opioid-agonist effects.[6,7] Initially, a dose of 0.2 to 0.4 mg I.V. should be administered; if there is no response, repeated doses of up to 4 to 5 mg should be given. Doses as high as 15 to 20 mg may be administered if overdose with a resistant opioid (e.g., propoxyphene, codeine, or some fentanyl derivatives) is suspect-

---

Table 1   The ABCDs of Initial
Stabilization of the Poisoned Patient

Airway
  Position the patient to open the airway; suction any secretions or vomitus; evaluate airway-protective reflexes; consider endotracheal intubation

Breathing
  Determine adequacy of ventilation; assist ventilation, if necessary; administer supplemental oxygen

Circulation
  Evaluate perfusion, blood pressure, and cardiac rhythm; determine QRS complex; attach continuous cardiac monitor

Dextrose
  Quickly determine blood glucose by finger-stick test; give dextrose if patient is suspected of having hypoglycemia

Decontamination
  Perform surface and gastric decontamination to limit absorption of poisons

Table 2 Mechanisms of Drug-Induced Hypotension

Mechanism	Selected Causes
Hypovolemia	
Vomiting and diarrhea	Iron; arsenic; food poisoning; organophosphates and carbamates; mushroom poisoning; thallium
Sweating	Organophosphates and carbamates
Venodilatations	Barbiturates; other sedative-hypnotic agents
Depressed cardiac contractility	Tricyclic antidepressants; beta blockers; calcium antagonists; class IA and class IC antiarrhythmic agents; sedative-hypnotic agents
Reduced peripheral vascular resistance	Theophylline; beta$_2$-adrenergic stimulants; phenothiazines; tricyclic antidepressants; hydralazine

ed.[6,7] Patients with opioid intoxication usually become fully awake within 2 to 3 minutes after administration of naloxone. Failure to respond to naloxone suggests that (1) the diagnosis is incorrect [*see* Differential Diagnosis, *below*]; (2) other, nonopioid drugs may have been ingested; (3) a hypoxic insult may have occurred before the victim was found and resuscitated; or (4) an inadequate dose of naloxone was given.

Flumazenil, a short-acting, specific benzodiazepine antagonist with no intrinsic agonist effects, can rapidly reverse coma caused by diazepam and other benzodiazepines.[5,7] However, it has not found a place in the routine management of unconscious patients with drug overdose, because it has the potential to cause seizures in patients who have been consuming large quantities of benzodiazepines on a long-term basis or who have ingested an acute overdose of benzodiazepines and a tricyclic antidepressant or other potentially convulsant drug [*see* Sedative-Hypnotic Agents, *below*].[5,7,8]

HYPOTENSION AND CARDIAC DYSRHYTHMIAS

The hypotension that commonly complicates drug intoxication has many possible causes [*see* Table 2].[9,10] Hypotension may result from volume depletion caused by severe drug-induced vomiting or diarrhea. In addition, relative hypovolemia may be caused by the venodilating effects of many drugs. Certain drugs or poisons can have direct negative inotropic or chronotropic effects on the heart, reducing cardiac output. Others can cause a severe reduction in peripheral vascular resistance. Some drugs or poisons can cause shock by a combination of these mechanisms.

Treatment of drug-induced shock includes rapid assessment of the likely cause, which is suggested by the history of exposure and the clinical findings. Hypotension with tachycardia suggests that the cause is volume depletion or reduced peripheral vascular resistance, whereas hypotension with bradycardia suggests that the cause is a disturbance of cardiac rhythm or that shock is a result of the generalized cardiodepressant effects of the drug. Regardless of the etiology, most patients benefit from an I.V. bolus of fluid (e.g., 0.5 to 1 L of normal saline) and empirical pressor therapy with dopamine or norepinephrine.[11] However, if hypoperfusion persists, it may be necessary to insert a pulmonary arterial catheter to obtain more specific information about volume and hemodynamic status.

A variety of cardiac dysrhythmias may occur as a result of drug intoxication or poisoning [*see* Table 3]. In addition to the direct pharmacologic actions of the drug or poison, impaired ventilation and oxygenation may trigger disturbances of cardiac rhythm.[11] Treatment of a cardiac dysrhythmia depends on its etiology.

Because conventional advanced cardiac life support (ACLS) protocols were not designed with poisoning in mind, use of these guidelines may have inappropriate or dangerous effects.[12] For example, a patient with tricyclic antidepressant intoxication (see below) may have wide-complex tachycardia resulting from severe depression of sodium-dependent channels in the myocardial cell membrane. However, use of the ACLS protocols for wide-complex tachycardia or possible ventricular tachycardia may lead the treating physician to administer procainamide, a class IA antiarrhythmic agent with cardiodepressant effects that are additive to those of the tricyclic antidepressants.[11] A patient with multiple premature ventricular contractions or who experiences episodes of ventricular tachycardia after intoxication with chloral hydrate or inhalation of a chlorinated solvent would respond more readily to a beta blocker than to lidocaine, the drug recommended by the ACLS protocols.[13] Finally, cardiac dysrhythmias from digitalis intoxication are most appropriately treated with digoxin-specific antibodies (see below).

HYPERTENSION

Although hypertension is not commonly recognized as a serious pharmacologic effect of drug intoxication, it may have life-threatening consequences and requires aggressive treatment. Hypertension may result from generalized CNS and sympathetic stimulation (e.g., by amphetamines or cocaine) or from the peripheral actions of drugs such as phenylpropanolamine, a potent alpha-adrenergic agonist.[14] (Although the Food and Drug Administration removed phenylpropanolamine from the market in the United States in November 2000, phenylpropanolamine is still available in other countries.) In addition, hypertension may result from the pharmacologic interaction of two agents, such as in the use of a stimulant or the ingestion of an inappropriate food by a person taking monoamine oxidase (MAO) inhibitors.[15] Severe hypertension can lead to intracranial hemorrhage, aortic dissection, or other catastrophic complications.[16,17]

Hypertension may be accompanied by tachycardia, as commonly occurs in cases of intoxication with generalized stimu-

Table 3 Causes of Cardiac Disturbances

Type of Disturbance	Selected Causes
Sinus tachycardia	Anticholinergic agents (e.g., diphenhydramine, atropine, tricyclic antidepressants); theophylline and caffeine; cocaine and amphetamines; volume depletion
Bradycardia or atrioventricular block	Beta blockers; calcium antagonists; tricyclic antidepressants; class IA and class IC antiarrhythmic agents; organophosphate and carbamate insecticides; digitalis glycosides; phenylpropanolamine (hypertension with reflex bradycardia)
Widening of the QRS complex	Tricyclic antidepressants; class IA and class IC antiarrhythmic agents; diphenhydramine; thioridazine; propoxyphene; hyperkalemia; hypothermia
Ventricular tachycardia or ventricular fibrillation	Tricyclic antidepressants; cocaine and amphetamines; theophylline; digitalis glycosides; fluoride or hydrofluoric acid burns (hypocalcemia); trichloroethane and numerous other chlorinated, fluorinated, and aromatic solvents; chloral hydrate; agents that cause prolongation of the QT interval (e.g., quinidine, sotalol)

lants such as cocaine and amphetamine derivatives. Hypertension may also be accompanied by bradycardia or even atrioventricular (AV) block, which may occur after phenylpropanolamine overdose because of the reflex baroreceptor response.

Treatment is directed at the cause of the hypertension. In patients who have taken cocaine, amphetamines, or other generalized stimulants, mild or moderate increases in blood pressure may be reduced simply by providing a quiet environment and administering a sedative agent such as diazepam. In persons who have taken an overdose of phenylpropanolamine or other alpha-adrenergic stimulant, administration of a specific alpha-adrenergic antagonist, such as phentolamine (2 to 5 mg I.V.), is extremely effective and usually leads to normalization of the slow heart rate or reversal of the AV block.[14] In general, beta blockers should not be used as single agents in the treatment of drug-induced hypertension, because their use may lead to unopposed alpha-adrenergic activity with paradoxically worsened hypertension.[18]

SEIZURES

Seizures may result from a number of factors, including a variety of drugs and poisons. The drugs that most commonly induce seizures are tricyclic antidepressants, bupropion, cocaine and related stimulants, antihistamines, and isoniazid [see Table 4].[19,20] Prolonged or repeated convulsions can lead to serious complications, including hyperthermia, rhabdomyolysis, brain damage, and death. In addition, seizure activity causes metabolic acidosis, which may worsen cardiotoxicity in patients who have taken an overdose of a tricyclic antidepressant.[11,19] Seizures can also result from hypoxia, hypoglycemia, head trauma, stroke, or serious CNS infections [see Differential Diagnosis, below].

Treatment of seizures includes taking immediate steps to protect the airway and provide oxygen while administering anticonvulsant drugs. The blood glucose level should be determined and dextrose administered if needed [see Coma, above]. Initial anticonvulsant therapy consists of diazepam (5 to 10 mg I.V.), lorazepam (1 to 2 mg I.V.), or midazolam (3 to 5 mg I.V. or, if I.V. access is not immediately available, 5 to 10 mg I.M.). Repeated doses are given if the initial therapy is ineffective. Because it is often ineffective, phenytoin is not a first-line anticonvulsant agent for drug- or toxin-induced seizures.[19] If convulsions persist, phenobarbital should be administered at a dosage of 15 to 20 mg/kg (1 to 1.5 g) I.V. over 20 to 30 minutes.[21] If seizure activity continues, the physician should consult with a neurologist and consider administering pentobarbital, another short-acting barbiturate, or propofol.[21] In addition, inducing neuromuscular paralysis (e.g., with pancuronium) should be considered to control the muscle hyperactivity, which may be necessary for controlling hyperthermia, rhabdomyolysis, or metabolic acidosis. If neuromuscular paralysis is induced, however, the physician should be aware that seizure activity in the brain may persist but may not be apparent.[21] If isoniazid poisoning is suspected, 5 g of pyridoxine (vitamin B$_6$) should be administered intravenously; or if more than 5 g of isoniazid was ingested, pyridoxine should be administered in an amount (in grams) equal to that of the isoniazid overdose.

HYPERTHERMIA

Hyperthermia is an underrecognized complication of poisoning and drug overdose that is associated with high morbidity and mortality.[22] It may result from the pharmacologic effects of

Table 4 Drug-Induced Seizures

Common Causes	Comments
Tricyclic antidepressants	Seizure activity and resulting metabolic acidosis often aggravate cardiotoxicity; protracted seizures with absent sweating may lead to hyperthermia; phenytoin worsens cardiotoxicity in animal models; treat with benzodiazepines or phenobarbital
Cocaine and amphetamines	Seizures are usually brief and self-limited and are often preceded by tremors, agitation, hallucinations, or tachycardia; bupropion most commonly implicated in seizures, sometimes even with therapeutic use
Theophylline	Seizures are often prolonged, recurrent, and refractory to anticonvulsant therapy; phenytoin is ineffective in animal models; administer high-dose phenobarbital (at least 15–20 mg/kg I.V.); for patients with serum theophylline levels > 100 mg/L or status epilepticus, consider hemoperfusion or hemodialysis
Diphenhydramine	Seizures are usually brief and self-limited; in patients with massive intoxication (e.g., > 4–5 g), tricycliclike cardiotoxicity may also occur
Isoniazid	Seizures are often accompanied by severe lactic acidosis; the specific antidote for seizures and coma is vitamin B$_6$ (pyridoxine), 5–10 g I.V.; or, if the amount of ingested isoniazid is known, the equivalent gram-for-gram amount of vitamin B$_6$

the agent or as a consequence of prolonged muscle hyperactivity or seizures [see Table 5]. Severe hyperthermia (rectal temperature > 104° F [40° C]) that goes untreated may lead to brain damage, coagulopathy, rhabdomyolysis, hypotension, and, ultimately, death.[22]

Because it is immediately life threatening, hyperthermia warrants immediate and aggressive treatment.[22] Therapy is directed at the underlying cause, which is usually excessive muscle activity or rigidity. For mild or moderate cases, the physician should use appropriate pharmacologic agents (e.g., sedatives for cases of stimulant-induced psychosis and hyperactivity and anticonvulsants for cases of seizure), remove the patient's clothing, and maximize evaporative cooling by spraying the exposed skin with tepid water and fanning the patient. For severe cases, the most rapidly effective treatment is neuromuscular paralysis accompanied by maximal evaporative cooling.[22] In some cases, a specific antidote or therapeutic agent may be available [see Table 5].

HYPOTHERMIA

Hypothermia may accompany drug overdose and is usually caused by environmental exposure combined with inadequacy of the patient's response mechanisms. These inadequate mechanisms may include impaired judgment (in patients who have taken opioids, sedative-hypnotic agents, or phenothiazines or who have underlying mental disorders), a reduced shivering response (in those who have taken phenothiazines or sedative-hypnotic agents), and peripheral vasodilatation (in those who have taken phenothiazines or vasodilators).[23] Severe hypothermia (core temperature < 82° F [28° C]) may cause the patient to appear to be dead and may be associated with barely perceptible blood pressure, heart rate, or neurologic reflexes. Hypotension, bradycardia, and ventricular arrhythmias may fail to respond to pharmacologic treatment until the patient is warmed.[23,24] Because no controlled trials comparing rewarming methods exist, man-

Table 5 Drug-Induced Hyperthermia

Mechanisms	Selected Causes and Comments
Increased metabolic activity	Causes include salicylates, dinitrophenol, and cocaine and amphetamines
Reduced sweating	Causes include anticholinergic agents (e.g., tricyclic antidepressants, antihistamines, many plants, and some mushrooms)
Increased muscle activity or exertion	Causes include cocaine and amphetamines, phencyclidine, and exertional heatstroke
Neuroleptic malignant syndrome	Causes include haloperidol, related antipsychotic agents, and lithium; patients have lead-pipe rigidity, acidosis, and an elevated creatine kinase level that are caused by CNS dopamine blockade; specific treatment is bromocriptine (2.5–10.0 mg by nasogastric tube two to six times daily)[157]; treat severe hyperthermia with neuromuscular paralysis
Malignant hyperthermia	An inherited disorder of muscle cell function, commonly triggered by certain anesthetic agents (e.g., succinylcholine or halothane); causes severe muscle rigidity and acidosis not responsive to neuromuscular paralysis; treatment is dantrolene (2–5 mg/kg I.V.)[158]
Serotonin syndrome	Associated with the use of serotonin-enhancing agents (e.g., meperidine, dextromethorphan, fluoxetine, paroxetine, sertraline, L-tryptophan, or trazodone), especially in patients taking monoamine oxidase inhibitors; causes muscle rigidity, acidosis, and hyperthermia; treatment is neuromuscular paralysis; for mild cases, consider cyproheptadine (4 mg p.o. every hour for three or four doses)[159] or methysergide (2 mg p.o. every 6 hr for three or four doses)[160]

agement protocols vary institutionally and are often controversial.[23] Treatment of hypothermia is generally administered gradually because more aggressive management may precipitate cardiac dysrhythmias. Passive external rewarming is an acceptable treatment if the patient's condition is stable. Administration of a warmed mist inhalation or warmed I.V. fluids may be helpful, as may gastric or peritoneal lavage with warmed fluids, although the heat transfer involved in these measures is variable. For profound hypothermia accompanied by evidence of severe hypoperfusion (e.g., cardiac arrest or ventricular fibrillation), more aggressive measures, such as partial cardiopulmonary or femorofemoral bypass, may be required.[23,24] Of note is that patients with severe hypothermia can withstand cardiorespiratory arrest longer than normothermic patients—hence the old adage, "No one is dead until warm and dead."

RHABDOMYOLYSIS

Rhabdomyolysis, a common complication of severe poisoning or drug overdose, may result from direct myotoxic effects of the agent, from prolonged or recurrent muscle hyperactivity or rigidity, or from prolonged immobility with mechanical compression of muscle groups.[25] Severe rhabdomyolysis (usually associated with markedly elevated serum creatine kinase levels) may cause massive myoglobinuria that results in acute tubular necrosis and renal failure. Myoglobinuria is usually recognized by the pink or reddish hue of spun serum or by a positive dipstick test for hemoglobin in the urine, with few or no red blood cells seen on microscopic examination. Severe rhabdomyolysis may also cause hyperkalemia, which results from loss of potassium from dead or injured cells.

Treatment of rhabdomyolysis includes measures to prevent further muscle breakdown (e.g., control of muscle hyperactivity and treatment of hyperthermia) and to prevent deposition of toxic myoglobin in the renal tubules. Unequivocally, the mainstay of treatment in rhabdomyolysis is aggressive volume expansion with normal saline early in the disease to maintain urine output of 200 ml/hr in those who can tolerate the fluid load.[25] Nonrandomized trials have also shown alkalinization of urine to be beneficial, but the role of mannitol and furosemide in rhabdomyolysis is less clear.[25]

Clinical Evaluation

Although the history recounted by patients who have intentionally taken a drug overdose may be unreliable, it should not be overlooked as a valuable source of information. If the patient is unwilling or unable to specify which drugs were taken and when they were ingested or to provide a pertinent medical history, family and friends may be able to do so. Family members should be asked about other medications available in the household and about exposure in the workplace and through hobbies. In addition, paramedics should be asked for any pill bottles or drug paraphernalia that they may have obtained at the scene.

A directed toxicologic physical examination may yield important clues about the drugs or poisons that have been taken. Pertinent variables include the patient's vital signs, pupil size, lung sounds, peristaltic activity, skin moisture and color, and muscle activity; the presence or absence of unusual odors; and the presence or absence of track marks associated with I.V. drug

Table 6 Autonomic Syndromes Induced by Drugs or Poisons

Autonomic Syndrome	Selected Causes	Empirical Interventions
Sympathomimetic (agitation; dilated pupils; elevated BP and HR; sweaty skin; hyperthermia)	Cocaine; amphetamines; pseudoephedrine	Induce sedation; initiate aggressive cooling; treat hypertension with phentolamine; treat tachycardia with beta blockers
Sympatholytic (lethargy or coma; small pupils; normal or low BP and HR; low temperature)	Barbiturates; opioids; clonidine; benzodiazepines	Give naloxone for suspected opioid overdose; consider flumazenil for benzodiazepine overdose
Cholinergic (pinpoint pupils; variable HR; sweaty skin; abdominal cramps and diarrhea)	Organophosphate and carbamate insecticides; chemical warfare nerve agents	Give atropine and pralidoxime; obtain measurements of serum and RBC cholinesterase activity
Anticholinergic (agitation; delirium; dilated pupils; tachycardia; decreased peristalsis; dry, flushed skin)	Atropine and related drugs; antihistamines; phenothiazines; tricyclic antidepressants	Obtain immediate ECG tracing to evaluate for poisoning with tricyclic antidepressants; consider physostigmine only if tricyclics are not involved

Table 7 Use of the Clinical Laboratory in the Initial Diagnosis of Poisoning

Test	Finding	Selected Causes
Arterial blood gases	Hypoventilation (elevated Pco_2) Hyperventilation	CNS depressants (e.g., opioids, sedative-hypnotic agents, phenothiazines, and ethanol) Salicylates; carbon monoxide; other asphyxiants
Electrolytes	Anion-gap metabolic acidosis Hyperkalemia Hypokalemia	Salicylates; methanol; ethylene glycol; carbon monoxide; cyanide; iron; isoniazid; theophylline Digitalis glycosides; fluoride; potassium Theophylline; caffeine; beta-adrenergic agents (e.g., albuterol); soluble barium salts
Glucose	Hypoglycemia	Oral hypoglycemic agents; insulin; ethanol
Osmolality and osmolar gap	Elevated osmolar gap*	Ethanol; methanol; ethylene glycol; isopropyl alcohol; acetone
ECG	Wide QRS complex Prolongation of the QT interval Atrioventricular block	Tricyclic antidepressants; quinidine and other class IA and class IC antiarrhythmic agents Quinidine and related antiarrhythmic agents Calcium antagonists; digitalis glycosides
Plain abdominal x-ray	Radiopaque pills or objects	Iron; lead; potassium; calcium; chloral hydrate; some foreign bodies
Serum acetaminophen	Elevated level (> 140 mg/L 4 hr after ingestion)	Acetaminophen (may be the only clue to a recent ingestion)

*Osmolar gap = measured osmolality – calculated osmolality. Measured osmolality is performed in the laboratory using a freezing-point-depression device (do not use the vaporization method). Calculated osmolality = 2(Na) + [BUN/2.8] + [glucose/18]. The normal osmolar gap is 0 ± 5 mOsm/L.
BUN—blood urea nitrogen Pco_2—carbon dioxide tension

abuse. Signs of one of the so-called autonomic syndromes [*see Table 6*] may suggest diagnostic possibilities and potential empirical interventions.[10]

The clinical laboratory may provide useful information that obviates an expensive and time-consuming toxicology screen. Recommended laboratory tests in the patient with an overdose of unknown cause include a complete blood count; measurements of glucose, electrolytes, blood urea nitrogen, creatinine, aspartate aminotransferase (AST), and serum osmolality (both measured and calculated); ECG; and plain abdominal x-ray (KUB [kidneys, ureters, and bladder] view) [*see Table 7*]. A quantitative serum acetaminophen level should be obtained immediately because acetaminophen overdose may be difficult to diagnose in the absence of a complete and reliable history, does not produce suggestive clinical or laboratory findings, and requires prompt administration of an antidote in patients with a serious acute ingestion if hepatic injury is to be prevented.[10,26,27]

Obtaining a thorough history, performing a careful physical examination, and using the clinical laboratory in a logical manner can often enable the physician to make a tentative diagnosis and to order specific quantitative measurements of certain drugs (e.g., salicylates, valproic acid, or digoxin) when the results of such tests may alter therapy. It is rarely useful, especially in the emergency management of a poisoning victim, to order a comprehensive toxicology screen. Generally, this test is performed at an outside reference laboratory at considerable expense, and patients often awaken and confirm the tentative diagnosis before results are available (usually 1 to 2 days after testing). In addition, many common dangerous drugs and poisons (e.g., isoniazid, digitalis glycosides, calcium antagonists, beta blockers, metals, and pesticides) are not included in the screening procedure; thus, a negative toxicology screen does not rule out the possibility of poisoning.[28] So-called drugs-of-abuse screens for opioids, amphetamines, and cocaine are commonly performed by hospital laboratories and are useful in identifying intoxication by these substances, but they should not be mistaken for a comprehensive toxicologic screening test.

Differential Diagnosis

Whenever a patient with suspected poisoning or drug overdose is evaluated, the possibility that other illnesses are mimicking or complicating the presentation should always be considered. These illnesses include head trauma (e.g., in the ethanol-intoxicated patient, who often falls); cerebrovascular accident; meningitis; metabolic abnormalities, such as hypoglycemia, hyponatremia, and hypoxemia; underlying liver disease; and the postictal state. In any patient with altered mental status, computed tomography of the head and lumbar puncture should be considered.

Management Issues

DECONTAMINATION AFTER ACUTE INGESTION

Nowhere in the field of toxicology is there more controversy than in the debate about gastrointestinal decontamination.[29-31] Techniques for gut decontamination include emesis, gastric lavage, administration of activated charcoal, and whole bowel irrigation [*see Table 8*].

Ipecac-induced emesis has been almost completely abandoned in the clinical setting.[32] In 2003, the American Academy of Pediatrics advised against routine home use of ipecac and recommended disposing of all ipecac found in the home.[33] One reason it has fallen out of favor is that treated patients run the risks of sudden, unexpected deterioration from the effects of the overdose and subsequent pulmonary aspiration; more important, however, is the lack of evidence of the efficacy of ipecac-induced emesis, especially when emesis is induced more than 1 hour after the ingestion.[29,30]

Gastric lavage is still an accepted method for gut decontamination in hospitalized patients who are obtunded or comatose, but several prospective, randomized, controlled trials failed to show that lavage in conjunction with the administration of activated charcoal provides better clinical results than administration of activated charcoal alone. In one study, patients given a

Table 8   Methods of Gastrointestinal Decontamination

Method and Technique	Useful Situations	Comments
Emesis: give syrup of ipecac, 30 ml p.o. in adults (15 ml in children), along with one to two glasses of water; may repeat after 30 min if no emesis occurs; alternatively, give 1–2 tbsp of liquid handwashing or dishwashing soap	Possible benefit in rare circumstances after a potentially lethal ingestion when medical care is more than 60 min away, but only under the guidance of a poison control center	No longer used in emergency departments; American Academy of Pediatrics recommends against routine home use of ipecac[32]; contraindicated in ingestions of corrosive agents and most hydrocarbons, when the patient is lethargic, or when the ingested substance is likely to cause abrupt onset of coma or seizures
Gastric lavage: insert large-bore nasogastric or orogastric tube, empty stomach contents, and lavage with 100–200 ml aliquots of water or saline until clear	Useful in obtunded or comatose patients, in recent ingestions (< 1 hr), or in ingestion of anticholinergic agents or salicylates (delayed gut emptying)	Obtunded patient should have prior endotracheal intubation to protect airway; best position is left lateral decubitus to reduce movement of poison into small intestine
Activated charcoal: give 50–60 g of charcoal slurry p.o. or by gastric tube; goal is approximately 10:1 ratio of charcoal to ingested poison; usually given with one dose of a cathartic agent	Often useful because it adsorbs most drugs and poisons; may be equally effective when given alone as when given after emesis or lavage	Not effective for ingestions of iron, lithium, potassium, sodium, or alcohols; may need to repeat two or three times or more for large ingestions; repeated dosing may also enhance elimination of some drugs
Whole bowel irrigation: give Colyte or GoLYTELY, 1–2 L/hr p.o. or by gastric tube, until rectal effluent is clear or x-ray is negative for radiopaque materials	Useful in ingestions of iron, lithium, sustained-release or enteric-coated pills, and drug packets or other foreign bodies	Generally well tolerated; no significant fluid or electrolyte gain or loss occurs; most useful in awake, ambulatory patients; may reduce effectiveness of activated charcoal

regimen of activated charcoal and patients given a combination regimen of gastric lavage and charcoal showed no significant differences in all outcome parameters, including clinical deterioration, length of hospital stay, complications, and mortality.[34] Studies of volunteers have shown that only about 30% of ingested material is returned with gastric lavage.[29,31] However, many authors agree that it may still be useful if the ingested material has caused slowing of peristalsis (e.g., in the case of anticholinergic agents or opioids) or pyloric spasm (e.g., in the case of salicylates) or if a potentially life-threatening amount of poison (e.g., 5 g of a tricyclic antidepressant) was ingested.[29] Some investigators have suggested that gastric lavage is associated with an increased rate of complications, although adverse events are rare in clinical practice.[31,35]

Activated charcoal—a fine powder produced from the distillation of various organic materials—has a large surface area that is capable of adsorbing many drugs and poisons.[31] Studies of volunteers and clinical trials have suggested that administration of activated charcoal without gastric lavage may be as effective as, or superior to, its administration after gut emptying.[29,31,34] Although it seems logical that gastric lavage in combination with the use of activated charcoal would be more effective than the use of activated charcoal alone, this hypothesis has not been proved. Most clinicians now employ oral activated charcoal without prior gut emptying in the awake patient who has taken a moderate overdose of a drug or poison; some clinicians still recommend lavage after a massive ingestion of a highly toxic drug.

There is no consensus about the use of cathartic agents with activated charcoal, although it seems logical to hasten passage of the charcoal-drug material from the intestinal tract. If a cathartic agent is used, it should be limited to a single dose, and the potential adverse effects should be taken into account.[36] Adverse effects may more likely occur in the very young or old (who may not be able to tolerate fluid shifts associated with osmotic cathartics such as sorbitol) or in patients with renal insufficiency (who may not be able to tolerate large doses of magnesium or sodium).

Whole bowel irrigation is a technique that was introduced for

gut cleansing before surgical or endoscopic procedures and that has recently been adopted for gut decontamination after certain ingestions.[31,37] It involves the use of a large volume of an osmotically balanced electrolyte solution, such as Colyte or GoLYTELY, that contains nonabsorbable polyethylene glycol and that cleans the gut by mechanical action without net gain or loss of fluids or electrolytes. Whole bowel irrigation is well tolerated by most awake patients. Although no controlled clinical trials to date have demonstrated improved outcome, it is recommended for those who have ingested large doses of poisons that are not well adsorbed to charcoal (e.g., iron or lithium), for those who have ingested sustained-release or enteric-coated products, and for those who have ingested drug packets or other potentially toxic foreign bodies.[31,38]

ENHANCED ELIMINATION

Measures to enhance the elimination of drugs and poisons are less popular than they were 20 years ago, primarily because it has since been recognized that the available techniques do not have a significant effect on total drug elimination of many of the most commonly ingested products and that they have little effect on the clinical course of intoxication.[9] In addition, hemodialysis is an invasive procedure that requires systemic anticoagulation and that is associated with potential morbidity. For a drug or poison to be considered for removal by hemodialysis, it should have a relatively small volume of distribution, have a slow intrinsic rate of removal (clearance), and cause life-threatening intoxication that is poorly responsive to supportive measures.[9] Only a few drugs and poisons meet these criteria [*see Table 9*]. Continuous renal replacement therapy has been utilized for enhanced removal of a few poisons (e.g., lithium), but data on its efficacy are limited.[39]

Repeated oral doses of activated charcoal can reduce the elimination half-life of some drugs and poisons by interrupting enterohepatic or enteroenteric recirculation.[29,40] This technique was introduced in the late 1970s, after studies reported its efficacy in volunteers, and it was considered a benign, noninvasive treatment. However, reports of fluid depletion and shock caused by excessive coadministration of sorbitol, as well as the paucity of evidence of clinical benefit, have reduced the initial optimism about this treatment.[29,40]

Specific Drugs and Poisons

ACETAMINOPHEN

Acetaminophen is a widely used analgesic and antipyretic drug that is found in a number of over-the-counter and prescription products. When it is taken in combination with another drug that has acute toxic effects (e.g., an opioid), the more obvious and more rapidly apparent manifestations of the second drug may cause the clinician to overlook the subtle and nonspecific symptoms of acetaminophen poisoning. As a result, the opportunity to administer the highly effective prophylactic antidote acetylcysteine may be missed.

Acetaminophen is metabolized by various processes in the liver and, to a lesser extent, in the kidneys. One of the minor pathways of acetaminophen metabolism in the liver involves the cytochrome P-450 system (CYP 2E1), which generates a highly reactive intermediate metabolite. Normally, this toxic intermediate metabolite is readily scavenged by the intracellular antioxidant glutathione. In overdose, however, exhaustion of glutathione stores by production of the toxic intermediate metabolite allows the metabolite to react with cellular macromolecules, leading to cell injury and death. A similar process occurs in kidney cells.

The minimum acutely toxic single dose of acetaminophen is

approximately 150 to 200 mg/kg, or about 7 to 10 g in adults.[41] Alcoholics are at risk for toxicity at lower doses, particularly when the drug is taken for several days, presumably because they have increased cytochrome P-450 metabolic activity and reduced glutathione stores.[42] Enhanced susceptibility to toxic effects has also been reported in persons who are fasting and in patients receiving long-term anticonvulsant therapy[43] or taking isoniazid.[42] Severe toxicity may result in fulminant hepatic and renal failure.[41]

Diagnosis

Early after acute ingestion of acetaminophen, the patient may have few or no symptoms.[44] Vomiting is not uncommon in those who have taken large doses. Other than what can be found in the patient's history, the only reliable early diagnostic clue is provided by a quantitative measurement of the serum acetaminophen level, which can be provided immediately by most hospital laboratories. Clinical evidence of liver and kidney damage is usually delayed for 24 hours or more after ingestion. An acute massive overdose of acetaminophen (i.e., levels greater than 500 to 600 mg/L) can cause transient metabolic acidosis.[45]

The earliest evidence of toxicity in most patients is elevated levels of hepatic aminotransferases (i.e., AST and alanine aminotransferase [ALT]), followed by a rising prothrombin time (PT) and bilirubin levels. Hypoglycemia, metabolic acidosis, and encephalopathy are signs of a poor prognosis.[41]

Treatment

Oral activated charcoal should be administered. Ipecac-induced emesis is not recommended, because it often leads to protracted vomiting, which makes administration of the oral antidote difficult. A serum acetaminophen level should be obtained approximately 4 hours after ingestion, and the result should be plotted on the Rumack-Matthew nomogram [see Figure 1]. Ingestion of massive quantities of acetaminophen or a modified-release preparation or the coingestion of a drug that slows gastric emptying may result in delayed peak serum acetaminophen levels; in such cases, repeated measurements of serum concentrations should be obtained. If the acetaminophen level is above the "probable toxicity" line (many clinicians use the "possible toxicity" line instead), treatment should be initiated with acetylcysteine. If the patient has additional risk factors for hepatotoxicity (e.g., long-term alcohol abuse, long-term use of anticonvulsants or isoniazid, or an unreliable history of time of ingestion), it is prudent to treat for toxicity even with levels below the lower possible toxicity line. Acetylcysteine, an antioxidant that substitutes for glutathione as a scavenger, is highly effective in preventing liver damage from acetaminophen toxicity, especially if therapy is initiated within 8 to 10 hours after the ingestion of acetaminophen.[44] It is less effective when initiated 12 to 16 hours after acetaminophen ingestion; but it should be given in such cases anyway because it still has beneficial effects, presumably owing to its antioxidant and anti-inflammatory properties and because it increases survival in patients with hepatic failure.[44] The dose of oral acetylcysteine is 140 mg/kg initially (diluted in soda or juice) followed by 70 mg/kg every 4 hours. The treatment protocol approved by the FDA for the oral administration of acetylcysteine stipulates that 17 doses (approximately 3 days of therapy) be administered; however, shorter courses have been shown to be equally effective in patients who were treated within 8 to 10 hours after ingestion of acetaminophen.[44,46] At our institution, we usually administer oral acetylcysteine until 36 hours after the in-

Table 9 Methods of and Indications for Enhanced Drug Removal

Drug or Poison	Preferred Elimination Method and Indications
Carbamazepine	Hemoperfusion is indicated for severe poisoning with status epilepticus or cardiotoxicity; repeated doses of charcoal are of possible benefit for mild to moderate poisoning and for gut decontamination
Ethanol, isopropyl alcohol	Hemodialysis is rarely indicated because supportive care is generally successful; consider hemodialysis for deep coma with refractory hypotension
Lithium	Hemodialysis is indicated for severe neurologic manifestations (deep coma or seizures); I.V. saline is fairly effective for mild to moderate intoxication
Methanol, ethylene glycol	Hemodialysis is indicated for severe acidosis or for estimated or measured drug levels > 20–50 mg/dl
Phenobarbital	Hemoperfusion is indicated for refractory shock and drug levels > 200 mg/dl; repeated doses of charcoal are of questionable clinical benefit
Salicylates	Hemodialysis is indicated for severe acidosis and drug levels > 100 mg/dl; consider hemodialysis at lower salicylate levels (> 60 mg/dl) in elderly patients with chronic, accidental intoxication
Theophylline	Hemoperfusion or hemodialysis is indicated for drug levels > 100 mg/L or status epilepticus; repeated doses of charcoal are indicated for less severe cases
Valproic acid	Hemodialysis or hemoperfusion is indicated for severe cases (coma, acidosis, and drug levels > 1,000 mg/L); repeated doses of charcoal are of theoretical benefit

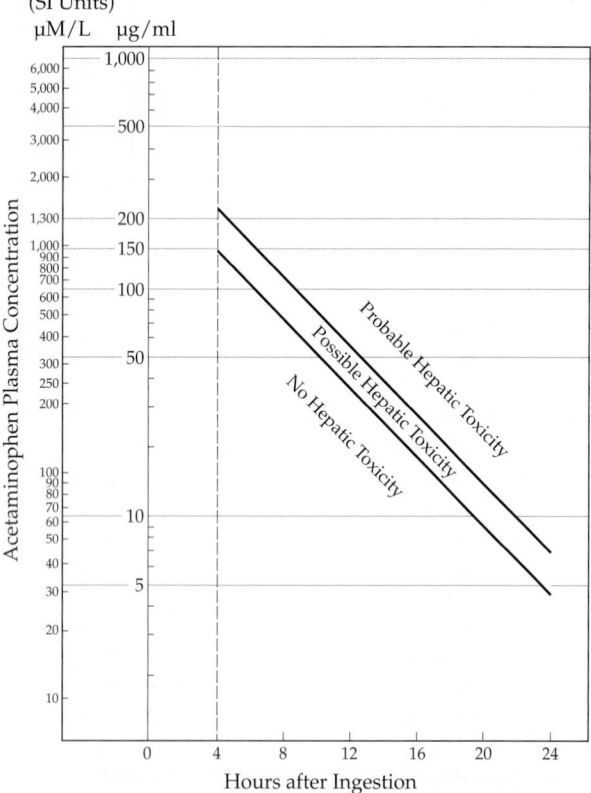

Figure 1   **The Rumack-Matthew nomogram for acetaminophen poisoning.**

gestion and then stop its administration if the liver enzymes (e.g., AST and ALT) reach normal levels. A retrospective study showed that the 36-hour regimen has a safety and efficacy profile similar to that of the traditional 72-hour protocol.[47] A longer course may be given to high-risk patients (e.g., patients who arrive in the emergency department late in the course of overdose or who have evidence of liver injury).[44]

Aggressive intervention is recommended to ensure that the loading dose is given within the first 8 hours of overdose. Occasionally, however, patients cannot tolerate oral acetylcysteine because the drug has a disagreeable odor and they are already vomiting. In such cases, it is advisable to administer the drug by the I.V. route. In 2004, the FDA approved a 20-hour acetylcysteine protocol for the treatment of acetaminophen overdose.[48] The initial loading dose is 150 mg/kg in 200 ml of 5% dextrose in water (D5W) over 15 minutes. This is followed by 50 mg/kg in 500 ml D5W over 4 hours, then 100 mg/kg in 1 L D5W over the next 16 hours. Intravenous administration can cause an anaphylactoid reaction (i.e., skin flushing and hypotension), and we usually slow the rate of the initial loading dose, administering it over 45 to 60 minutes.[49]

ANTICHOLINERGIC AGENTS AND ANTIHISTAMINES

Intoxication with anticholinergic agents can involve a variety of over-the-counter and prescription products, including antihistamines, antispasmodic agents, antipsychotic drugs, and antidepressants. In addition, several plants and mushrooms (e.g., *Datura stramonium* [angel's trumpet],[50] *Atropa belladonna,* and *Amanita phalloides*) contain potent anticholinergic alkaloids [*see Amanita phalloides* Mushrooms, *below*]. Anticholinergic agents competi-

tively inhibit the action of acetylcholine at muscarinic receptors. Antihistamines are commonly found in a variety of over-the-counter and prescription medications for the treatment of cough and cold symptoms, itching, dizziness, nausea, and insomnia. The most commonly used nonprescription antihistamine is diphenhydramine.

Diagnosis

Clinical manifestations of intoxication with anticholinergic agents include delirium, flushed skin, dilated pupils, tachycardia, ileus, urinary retention, jerky muscle movements, and, occasionally, hyperthermia. Coma and respiratory arrest may occur. Tricyclic antidepressants (see below) and phenothiazines may also cause seizures and quinidinelike cardiac conduction abnormalities. Therefore, an ECG should be obtained and the QRS complex and cardiac rhythm monitored in any patient who displays anticholinergic manifestations of intoxication.

Antihistamine intoxication is similar to anticholinergic poisoning and may also be associated with seizures[19] and tricyclic-like cardiac conduction abnormalities.[51] The older nonsedating antihistamines terfenadine and astemizole were associated with prolongation of the QT interval and the occurrence of atypical (torsade de pointes) ventricular tachycardia both after overdose and after coadministration of macrolide antibiotics or other drugs that interfere with their elimination.[52] Because safer agents are available, both of these drugs were removed from the United States market by the manufacturers in 1999.[53]

Treatment

Activated charcoal and a cathartic agent should be administered to patients with anticholinergic or antihistamine intoxication. Gastric lavage should be considered in cases of a large ingestion; this measure may be appropriate even if some time has passed since ingestion, because ileus may delay gastric emptying. Coma and respiratory depression should be treated with the usual supportive measures. The physician should consider administering physostigmine, 0.5 to 2.0 mg in a slow I.V. infusion, in patients with pure anticholinergic intoxication (i.e., intoxication with agents other than tricyclic antidepressants or antihistamines) and severe delirium.[54] Drowsiness, confusion, and sinus tachycardia usually resolve without aggressive intervention. Prolongation of the QT interval and atypical ventricular tachycardia can be treated with magnesium, 1 to 2 g I.V., or overdrive pacing.

ANTICOAGULANTS

The anticoagulants include warfarin and the so-called superwarfarin rodenticides. Accidental intoxication with warfarin may result from long-term therapeutic overmedication or from the addition of a drug that interacts with it (e.g., allopurinol, cimetidine, nonsteroidal anti-inflammatory drugs, quinidine, salicylates, or sulfonamides). Acute ingestion of a single dose of warfarin rarely causes significant anticoagulation. However, a single dose of brodifacoum or one of the other superwarfarins can cause severe and prolonged anticoagulation that lasts for weeks to months.[55]

Diagnosis

All anticoagulants inhibit the hepatic production of clotting factors II, VII, IX, and X and prolong the PT. Circulating factors are not affected; the peak effect of anticoagulants on the PT is not seen until 36 to 48 hours after administration, when circulating factors are degraded. Severe anticoagulation can result in hemorrhage, which may be fatal.[55]

Treatment

Acute superwarfarin overdose should be treated with oral activated charcoal and a cathartic agent. A baseline PT should be obtained on presentation and 24 and 48 hours later. If prolongation of the PT occurs, the physician should administer oral vitamin K$_1$ (phytonadione), 25 to 50 mg/day, and monitor the PT; in rare instances, as much as 150 to 200 mg/day may be necessary to correct the PT. It may also be necessary to continue treatment for several weeks or even months.[56] Patients should not be treated prophylactically with vitamin K$_1$ after an acute ingestion, because such treatment would mask the rise in PT for about 3 to 5 days or more, preventing early diagnosis. As a result, the patient would require prolonged follow-up even in the case of a subtoxic ingestion.

Vitamin K$_1$ may be given subcutaneously or, cautiously, by the I.V. route to patients with severe prolongation of the PT. However, because vitamin K$_1$ does not restore clotting factors immediately, patients who have active bleeding may require fresh frozen plasma or whole blood. Because coagulopathy after a superwarfarin overdose may last for weeks to months, high-dose oral vitamin K$_1$ therapy (5 mg/kg over 24 hours) may be necessary for outpatient therapy.[57]

Beta Blockers

Beta blockers are used for the treatment of hypertension, angina pectoris, migraine, and cardiac arrhythmias. Propranolol is the prototypical beta blocker but is also the most toxic [see Table 10].[58] All of these agents act competitively at beta-adrenergic receptors; at therapeutic doses, some have a degree of selectivity for beta$_1$- or beta$_2$-adrenergic receptors that is not apparent at high doses. Propranolol and a few of the other agents also have depressant effects on the myocardial cell membrane that are similar to those of quinidine and the tricyclic antidepressants.[59]

Beta blockade typically causes hypotension and bradycardia. Severe overdose may cause cardiogenic shock and asystole. Bronchospasm and hypoglycemia may also occur. In addition, propranolol overdose may cause widening of the QRS complex and CNS intoxication, including seizures and coma.[59] Most patients with beta-blocker poisoning manifest symptoms within 6 hours after an acute ingestion.[60]

Treatment

Treatment of overdose with a beta blocker includes aggressive gut decontamination. In cases of a large or recent ingestion, gastric lavage and the administration of activated charcoal and a cathartic agent should be initiated.

Hypotension and bradycardia are unlikely to respond to beta-adrenergic–mediated agents such as dopamine and isoproterenol; instead, the patient should receive high dosages of glucagon (5 to 10 mg I.V. followed by 5 to 10 mg/hr). Glucagon is a potent inotropic agent that does not require beta-adrenergic receptors to activate cells.[59,61] When glucagon fails, an epinephrine drip may be more beneficial in increasing heart rate and contractility than isoproterenol or dopamine. If pharmacologic therapy is unsuccessful, transvenous or external pacing should be used to maintain heart rate.[59,61] Use of hemodialysis in atenolol poisoning has been reported.[59]

CALCIUM ANTAGONISTS

Calcium channel blockers are used for the treatment of angina pectoris, hypertension, hypertrophic cardiomyopathy, migraine, and supraventricular tachycardia. These agents have a relatively low toxic-to-therapeutic ratio, and life-threatening toxicity can occur after accidental or intentional overdose. Calcium antagonists block the influx of calcium through calcium channels and act mainly on vascular smooth muscle, resulting in vasodilatation, reduced cardiac contractility, and slowed AV nodal conduction and sinus node activity. The most commonly used calcium antagonists in the United States are nifedipine, verapamil, diltiazem, and amlodipine. Although each of these agents has a different spectrum of activity, this selectivity is usually lost in overdose.[59]

Diagnosis

Manifestations of intoxication with a calcium antagonist include hypotension and bradycardia. Bradycardia may result from AV block or sinus arrest with a junctional escape rhythm. The QRS complex is usually normal. Severe poisoning may cause profound shock followed by asystole. Overdose with sustained-release products, which are very popular, may be associated with delayed onset of toxicity.[62]

Treatment

Treatment of overdose of an orally administered calcium antagonist includes aggressive gut decontamination. Gastric lavage and administration of activated charcoal are recommended. For patients who have ingested a large dose of a sustained-release preparation, the physician should consider whole bowel irrigation[62] in combination with administration of repeated doses of activated charcoal; in such cases, the patient should be observed closely for possible delayed-onset effects.

Hypotension should be initially treated with boluses of fluid, vasopressors, and I.V. calcium chloride (10 ml of a 10% solution) or calcium gluconate (20 ml of a 10% solution).[12] Doses of calcium should be repeated as needed; in some case reports, as much as 10 g of calcium has been given.[63] Calcium administration may improve cardiac contractility but has less effect on AV nodal conduction or peripheral vasodilatation. Infusion of glucagon (5 to 10 mg I.V.) or epinephrine has been recommended for patients with unresponsive hypotension; in one reported case, cardiopulmonary bypass was also shown to be effective. In a verapamil-toxic canine model, the survival rate was higher with high-dose insulin therapy (i.e., insulin-dextrose infusion) than with high doses of epinephrine, calcium chloride, or glucagon. A small, uncontrolled case series of patients with calcium channel blocker poisoning showed improvement with high-dose insulin therapy,

Table 10   Toxicity of Common Beta Blockers[161]

Drug	Usual Daily Dose (mg)	Cardioselective	Myocardial Cell Membrane Depression
Acebutolol	400–800	+	+
Atenolol	50–100	+	–
Labetalol	200–800	–	+
Metoprolol	100–450	+	Variable
Nadolol	40–240	+	–
Propranolol	40–360	–	++

but a prospective, controlled trial is still pending.[64] Hemodialysis is not effective.[59]

CARBON MONOXIDE

Carbon monoxide is a colorless, odorless, nonirritating gas that is produced by the combustion of organic material. It is responsible for more than 5,000 deaths in the United States each year, most occurring from suicidal inhalation. Sources of carbon monoxide include motor vehicle exhaust, improperly vented gas or wood stoves and ovens, and smoke generated by fire. Children riding under closed canopies in the backs of pickup trucks have been poisoned from the exhaust, and campers have been poisoned by using propane stoves or charcoal grills inside their tents.[65] The blizzards that hit the eastern United States in the winter of 1996 produced reports of carbon monoxide poisoning associated with snow-obstructed vehicle exhaust systems.[66] In 2005, use of portable generators in hurricane-damaged areas of Florida led to increased cases of carbon monoxide poisoning.[67]

Tissue hypoxia, which occurs as a consequence of the high affinity of carbon monoxide for hemoglobin, is the major pathophysiologic disturbance in carbon monoxide poisoning: at a carbon monoxide concentration of only 0.1%, as many as 50% of hemoglobin binding sites may be occupied by carbon monoxide. In addition to reducing the oxygen-carrying capacity of the blood, carbon monoxide interferes with the release of oxygen to the tissues. Carbon monoxide may also inhibit intracellular oxygen utilization by binding to myoglobin and cytochromes.[68]

Diagnosis

Carbon monoxide poisoning produces the symptoms and signs commonly associated with hypoxia, such as headache, confusion, tachycardia, tachypnea, syncope, hypotension, seizures, and coma. Clinical manifestations depend on the duration and intensity of exposure: an acute, sizable exposure may produce rapid unconsciousness, seizures, and death, whereas prolonged, low-level exposure may cause vague and nonspecific symptoms such as headache, dizziness, nausea, and weakness. Mild cases may be mistakenly diagnosed as influenza or migraine headache. So-called classic features of carbon monoxide poisoning, such as cherry-red skin coloring and bullous skin lesions, are not always present. Survivors of severe carbon monoxide poisoning may be left with permanent neurologic sequelae. These sequelae can include gross deficits, such as a permanent vegetative state or parkinsonism, or more subtle deficits, such as memory loss, depression, and irritability. In some cases, delayed neurologic deterioration may occur after 1 to 2 weeks.[68,69]

Laboratory findings may include metabolic acidosis and cardiac ischemia on ECG. The oxygen tension is usually normal because carbon monoxide binds to hemoglobin but does not disturb levels of dissolved oxygen; therefore, the calculated oxygen saturation is falsely normal. Furthermore, indirect measurement of oxygen saturation by pulse oximetry is inaccurate because of the similar absorption characteristics of oxyhemoglobin and carboxyhemoglobin.[70] Thus, correct diagnosis depends on direct spectrophotometric measurement of oxyhemoglobin and carboxyhemoglobin in a blood sample or direct measurement of exhaled carbon monoxide. Carboxyhemoglobin levels greater than 20% to 30% are usually associated with moderate symptoms of intoxication, and levels greater than 50% to 60% are associated with a serious or fatal outcome. There is considerable variability, however, and levels do not always correlate with symptoms.[68]

Treatment

The victim of carbon monoxide poisoning should immediately be removed from the site of exposure and given supplemental oxygen in the highest available concentration. Oxygen competes with carbon monoxide for hemoglobin binding sites, and administration of 100% oxygen can reduce the half-life of carboxyhemoglobin to approximately 40 to 60 minutes, thereby restoring normal oxygen saturation within about 2 to 3 hours. It should be noted that it is difficult to deliver 100% oxygen unless the patient is endotracheally intubated. Hyperbaric oxygen (HBO) administered in a sealed chamber can deliver oxygen at a pressure of 2.5 to 3.0 atm and has been reported to speed recovery and reduce neurologic sequelae.[68,71] Proponents of HBO therapy assert that this treatment can reduce cerebral edema and quell lipid peroxidation and other postinjury mechanisms of cellular destruction.[68,72] However, hyperbaric chambers are not readily available, and until recently, the few clinical studies to have compared HBO therapy with 100% oxygen at ambient pressure produced conflicting or inconclusive results or were otherwise unsatisfactory.[73]

In Australia in 1999, a randomized, double-blind, placebo-controlled trial (using sham HBO treatments) compared HBO with normobaric oxygen in a large number of patients with significant carbon monoxide poisoning; the authors found that HBO provided no greater benefit than normobaric oxygen.[74] A more recent study of similar design from the United States found a small but statistically significant reduction in cognitive sequelae 6 weeks after treatment.[71] Proponents of HBO generally advise its use for patients who have a history of unconsciousness, a detectable neuropsychiatric abnormality on bedside testing, or a carboxyhemoglobin level greater than 25%.[68] Because of concerns about the higher affinity of carbon monoxide for fetal hemoglobin, the recommended threshold for treatment of young infants and pregnant women is usually lower.[75] However, there are no controlled studies evaluating HBO therapy in pregnancy. It also remains unclear whether HBO may be useful in patients presenting many hours after exposure or with milder degrees of poisoning.

In patients with carbon monoxide poisoning associated with smoke inhalation, consideration should be given to the potential role of other toxic gases produced during combustion, such as cyanide, phosgene, nitrogen oxides, and hydrogen chloride, as well as the possibility that inhaled soot or steam has caused direct thermal injury to the airway and respiratory tract.

COCAINE, AMPHETAMINES, AND OTHER STIMULANTS

The 2004 National Survey on Drug Use and Health reports that 5.7 million Americans used cocaine in the past year.[76] This figure is down from 5.9 million in 2003. In 2002, there were an es-

Table 11 Common Stimulant Drugs

Drug	Street Names
Cocaine	Coke, crack (free-base cocaine)
Methamphetamine	Speed, crystal, ice
3,4-Methylenedioxymethamphetamine (MDMA)	Ecstasy
Methylphenidate	Ritalin*
Methcathinone†	Cat

*Ritalin is the trade name, not the street name.
†An illegally synthesized ephedrine derivative.

Table 12 Corrosive Agents

Corrosive or Caustic Agent	Comments
Mineral acids (e.g., hydrochloric, sulfuric, nitric, and phosphoric acids)	Produce rapidly painful coagulation necrosis of skin and eyes; inhalation of mists or vapors can cause irritation, bronchospasm, and chemical pneumonitis
Hydrofluoric acid	Highly electronegative fluoride ion causes deep tissue injury, which may have a delayed onset; systemic absorption from the skin or after ingestion may cause fatal hypocalcemia or hyperkalemia[162,163]
Caustic alkalis (e.g., sodium, potassium, calcium, and ammonium hydroxides)	Injury is often progressive and deep because of tissue saponification and resulting liquefaction necrosis
Phenol (carbolic acid)	Liquid and vapor are rapidly absorbed across the skin, causing severe systemic toxicity (shock, convulsions, and coma)[164]; isopropyl alcohol may speed its removal from skin[165]
Paraquat	Ingestion causes severe corrosive injury; systemic absorption leads to progressive and ultimately fatal pulmonary fibrosis[166]

timated 199,198 cocaine-related emergency department visits.[1]

Cocaine and the amphetamines [*see* Table 11] stimulate the CNS and the sympathetic nervous system and may act directly on peripheral adrenergic receptors.[76,77] Although cocaine also has local anesthetic properties and may cause sodium channel blockade in high doses, the clinical manifestations and treatment of cocaine overdose are essentially the same as those of amphetamine overdose. These drugs can be taken orally or can be snorted, smoked, or injected. So-called crack cocaine is a crudely prepared nonpolar derivative of the hydrochloride salt that is more easily volatilized and is thus the preferred form for smoking. The combined use of ethanol and cocaine may create the highly potent metabolite cocaethylene, which has a longer half-life than does cocaine and may contribute to the development of delayed toxic effects.[77,78]

Another common drug of abuse, particularly among teenagers and young adults, is methylenedioxymethamphetamine (MDMA), or ecstasy. National surveys suggest a marked increase in the prevalence of MDMA use in the United States. In 1993, there were 168,000 new users of MDMA; in 2001, the number of new users had soared to 1.8 million.[79] The 2001 National Survey on Drug Use and Health reports that 3.2% of teenagers (aged 12 to 17) and 13.1% of young adults (aged 18 to 25) have used MDMA.[79] Additionally, MDMA-related emergency department visits increased significantly from 253 visits in 1999 to 5,542 visits in 2001 and then declined to 4,026 in 2002.[80] Although MDMA is an amphetamine derivative with psychoactive properties similar to those of the hallucinogen mescaline, MDMA toxicity appears to be related to its stimulant properties. The subjective effects of MDMA include euphoria, sexual arousal, enhanced sensory perception, increased endurance, and greater sociability.[81] Adverse reactions from MDMA abuse reported in the literature include hyperthermia, hyponatremia, seizures, hepatitis, cerebrovascular accidents, and cardiac arrhythmias.[81] As MDMA use rises, health care providers are likely to see more patients with adverse reactions from this drug.[82]

Very limited national data regarding abuse of prescription stimulants, particularly methylphenidate (Ritalin), indicate that rates of abuse in children and teenagers are declining. Past-year rates of abuse have been tracked only since 2001; the data indicate an overall decrease from 2001 to 2004 among eighth graders (2.9% to 2.5%) and 10th graders (4.8% to 3.4%). Among 12th graders, past-year rates of abuse fluctuated between 5.1% and 4.0%. Data show that the past-year rate of abuse of methylphenidate among young adults was 2.9% in both 2002 and 2003.[83] Methylphenidate toxicity is most commonly the result of therapeutic error in children treated with the drug.[84] Abuse of methylphenidate has been reported; a national survey indicated the prevalence among college students in the United States varies by region, ranging from zero to 25%.[85]

Diagnosis

Clinical manifestations of mild stimulation include euphoria, alertness, and anorexia. More severe intoxication causes agitation, psychosis, tachycardia, hypertension, and diaphoresis. The pupils are usually dilated. Severe poisoning may result in convulsions, hypertensive crisis (e.g., intracerebral hemorrhage or aortic dissection), and hyperthermia.[17,18] Consequences of severe hyperthermia include shock, brain damage, coagulopathy, and hepatic and renal failure.[22]

The differential diagnosis includes acute functional psychosis, acute exertional heatstroke, and intoxication with other drugs. Phencyclidine, a ketaminelike dissociative anesthetic, may produce stimulant effects, but victims of overdose often have a waxing-and-waning encephalopathy with periods of flaccid stupor or coma.[17] Anticholinergic agents (see above) may also cause dilated pupils, tachycardia, and agitation, but these toxins usually cause the skin to be dry and flushed; stimulants generally cause the skin to be pale, clammy, and diaphoretic.

Treatment

Mild or moderate intoxication with a stimulant can often be successfully managed by administering a sedative agent, such as diazepam or lorazepam, and by providing the patient with a quiet room. If hypertension is severe and does not improve after sedation, phentolamine (2 to 5 mg I.V. at 5- to 10-minute intervals) or nitroprusside (0.5 to 10 μg/kg/min) should be administered. For patients with tachycardia or ventricular arrhythmias, a short-acting beta blocker such as esmolol (50 to 100 μg/kg/min) is recommended, although it should be cautioned that beta blockers may worsen hypertension because of unopposed alpha-adrenergic effects of the stimulant drug.[18] Wide-complex dysrhythmias in cases of cocaine overdose should be treated with sodium bicarbonate.[76] Severe hyperthermia should be treated aggressively to prevent brain damage and multiorgan complications [*see* Hyperthermia, *above*].

Because acute myocardial infarction may occur even in young persons with normal coronary arteries, all patients with chest pain should be evaluated carefully for evidence of ischemia.[18] Other causes of chest pain in these patients may include mechanical trauma to the chest wall, pneumomediastinum from hard coughing or the Valsalva maneuver, or pectoral muscle ischemia.[18]

CORROSIVE AGENTS

A number of agents with caustic or corrosive properties [*see* Table 12] are used for a variety of purposes in industry, as cleaning agents in the home, and in hobbies. Exposure to these agents may occur accidentally or as a result of suicidal ingestion. In some cases, the corrosive effect of these agents is a direct result of the high concentration of hydrogen (H^+) or hydroxyl (OH^-) ions and can be predicted from the very low or very high pH of the product. In other cases, toxicity may result from the product's oxidizing or alkylating or from other cytotoxic effects. Systemic toxicity can occur as a result of absorption across burned skin or after ingestion (e.g., in the case of hydrofluoric acid, phenol, or paraquat) [see Table 12].[86]

Diagnosis

Manifestations of toxicity usually occur immediately after exposure to the corrosive or caustic agent and include burning pain and erythema at the site of exposure. Immediate effects occur most commonly with acids. Injury caused by alkali burns can evolve over several hours and takes the form of a penetrating liquefaction necrosis. Burns may also be delayed in cases of exposure to hydrofluoric acid (hydrogen fluoride in aqueous solution); the toxicity of this agent is mediated through its fluoride component, which combines with calcium and magnesium ions. With hydrofluoric acid burns, pain and swelling may not be apparent until several hours after exposure, especially after exposure to relatively dilute solutions.

Treatment

Treatment of toxicity from corrosive or caustic agents must be initiated rapidly to reduce injury. Exposed areas should be flushed with copious amounts of plain water and any contaminated clothing removed (health providers must be careful not to become exposed while assisting victims). For patients whose eyes have been exposed to the agent, the physician should use an eyewash fountain or should splash water into the face, then pour water directly over the eyes from a pitcher or glass. Patients who have ingested a corrosive agent should drink one to two glasses of water. Although use of gastric lavage is controversial because of concerns about possible mechanical damage to the esophagus, our gastrointestinal consultants recommend gastric intubation with a small flexible tube as soon as possible after corrosive-liquid ingestion, to remove as much of the injurious material as possible. Neutralizing agents should not be administered in an attempt to normalize the pH; they may modify the pH too far in the opposite direction, and the heat of neutralization may cause thermal injury. There are a few exceptions to this rule; for example, after exposure to hydrofluoric acid, soaking the skin in a solution or gel that contains calcium (e.g., 2.5% calcium gluconate gel) or magnesium or in benzalkonium chloride may bind the toxic fluoride ion before it can be absorbed[87]; calcium is sometimes injected subcutaneously or by the intra-arterial route for deeper burns. For management of exposure to hydrofluoric acid, the physician should consult a regional poison-control center, a medical toxicologist, or a plastic or hand surgeon.

CYANIDE

Cyanide (the CN⁻ anion or a salt that contains this ion) is a highly toxic chemical that is used in a variety of industries, including electroplating, chemical synthesis, and laboratory analysis.[88] Cyanide is also released in the I.V. administration of nitroprusside. Acetonitrile, which is found in some glue removers for artificial fingernails, is metabolized to cyanide and has caused death in children.[88] Natural sources of cyanide (cyanogenic glycosides) include cassava, apricot pits, and several other plants and seeds. Hydrogen cyanide gas is generated from the combustion of many natural and synthetic materials that contain nitrogen and is a common component of the smoke generated by fire [see Smoke Inhalation, below].[89]

Cyanide is a highly reactive chemical that binds to intracellular cytochrome, blocking the utilization of oxygen. The resulting cellular asphyxia leads to headache, confusion, dyspnea, syncope, collapse, and death.[88,90] Although these effects occur rapidly after inhalation of hydrogen cyanide gas, symptoms of intoxication may be delayed for minutes after the ingestion of cyanide salts or even for hours after the ingestion of cyanogenic glycosides or acetonitrile.[88]

Diagnosis

A diagnosis of cyanide poisoning is based on a history of possible exposure (e.g., in a laboratory worker who attempts to commit suicide; in a person who has ingested laetrile, a cyanogenic glycoside; in a victim of smoke inhalation; or in a patient who has received a rapid high-dose infusion of nitroprusside) and the presence of characteristic symptoms. Any victim of smoke inhalation who has altered mental status should be suspected of having been poisoned with cyanide as well as with carbon monoxide. After cyanide ingestion, the victim may detect a smell of bitter almonds, but only about 50% of the general population has the ability to perceive this odor. Severe lactic acidosis is usually present. Because cyanide blocks the cellular utilization of oxygen, the oxygen content of venous blood may be elevated; a venous oxygen saturation of greater than 90% suggests the diagnosis.

Treatment

Once cyanide poisoning is suspected, immediate measures must be taken to prevent further exposure and to provide an antidote. For an ingestion, oral activated charcoal should be immediately administered; although the adsorption of cyanide to charcoal is relatively low, a standard dose of charcoal (e.g., 50 to 60 g) is sufficient to adsorb several hundred milligrams of cyanide salts. If charcoal is not available and there will be a delay before the patient reaches the hospital, emesis should be induced with ipecac. If ipecac is not available, emesis should be induced by mechanical gagging.

The antidotes for cyanide poisoning consist of nitrites, which oxidize hemoglobin to methemoglobin; in turn, methemoglobin binds free cyanide ions. If I.V. access is not immediately available, a pearl of amyl nitrite should be broken and the victim should inhale the contents. As soon as possible, sodium nitrite, 300 mg I.V., should be administered. The other antidote is sodium thiosulfate (12.5 g I.V.), which enhances the conversion of cyanide to the less toxic thiocyanate by the endogenous enzyme rhodanese. Although nitrites produce serious side effects (e.g., methemoglobinemia reduces the oxygen-carrying capacity, and vasodilatation may cause hypotension), sodium thiosulfate is relatively benign and can be used empirically as a single agent when the diagnosis is uncertain. Other potential antidotes include cobalt ethylenediaminetetraacetic acid (cobalt EDTA) and vitamin B_{12a} (hydroxocobalamin), but these agents have not been approved for use in the United States, and hydroxocobalamin, although used in the United States for the treatment of pernicious anemia, is not available in a concentrated high-strength form needed for antidotal treatment of cyanide poisoning.[88,91]

DIGITALIS GLYCOSIDES

Digitalis glycosides are found in a variety of plants, including foxglove, oleander, and rhododendron,[92] and have been used for centuries to treat heart failure. Digoxin is the most commonly prescribed digitalis glycoside. Digitalis poisoning may occur af-

Table 13   Dosing of Digoxin-Specific Antibodies

Type of Intoxication	Dose Needed to Provide Complete Binding of Digoxin
Acute ingestion*	Administer one vial (40 mg) for each 0.5 mg of digoxin expected to be absorbed (because bioavailability is 80%, multiply ingested dose by 0.8 to estimate absorbed dose)
Chronic intoxication†	Use the following formula to calculate the number of vials needed: $$\frac{\text{Serum digoxin level (ng/ml)} \times \text{body weight (kg)}}{100}$$

*Dose of digoxin-specific antibodies is based on the estimated amount of digoxin ingested.
†Dose of digoxin-specific antibodies is based on the steady-state serum digoxin level.

ter accidental or suicidal acute overdose, as a result of long-term accumulation (usually because of renal insufficiency or overmedication), or as a drug interaction. There have been many reports of elevated digoxin levels resulting from the interaction of digoxin with commonly used drugs, such as quinidine, amiodarone, and macrolide antibiotics.[93] Digitalis glycosides inhibit the sodium pump (Na^+,K^+-ATPase), which returns potassium to cells and increases the intracellular calcium concentration.[94]

Diagnosis

After an acute overdose, serum potassium levels are often elevated and AV nodal conduction is impaired, leading to varying degrees of AV block. Additionally, gastrointestinal symptoms of nausea, vomiting, and anorexia are often described after acute digitalis poisoning. With chronic poisoning, in contrast, ventricular dysrhythmias (e.g., ventricular ectopic beats or bidirectional ventricular tachycardia) predominate, and the potassium level is often normal or low, perhaps in part because of long-term coadministration of diuretic agents. The digitalis level is usually markedly elevated; however, if the sample is drawn within a few hours of overdose or within a few hours after receiving the last therapeutic dose, the result may be misleading because the drug would not have been fully distributed to tissues.[95]

Treatment

Management of acute digitalis poisoning includes gut decontamination with the oral administration of activated charcoal and, if the ingestion was large and occurred shortly before presentation, gastric lavage. Activated charcoal administered in multiple doses is effective in reducing deaths and life-threatening cardiac arrhythmias after yellow oleander poisoning.[96] This treatment has important implications for areas of the world where antidotal therapy with digoxin-specific antibodies is not available. Initially, sinus bradycardia or uncomplicated AV block should be treated with atropine (0.5 to 2 mg I.V.). A temporary pacemaker may be needed in patients with persistent symptomatic bradycardia; however, such patients should also receive digoxin-specific antibodies.

Digoxin-specific antibodies (e.g., Digibind, DigiFab) are indicated for patients with manifestations of severe intoxication (i.e., marked hyperkalemia and symptomatic dysrhythmias). These antibodies are derived from sheep and then cleaved so as to leave only the Fab fragment, which is small enough to be filtered and eliminated by the kidney after binding to digoxin. Extensive clinical experience with dixogin-specific antibodies has shown

that they are safe and highly effective, with peak activity occurring within 20 to 30 minutes after administration.[7] The dose of digoxin-specific antibodies depends on the type of intoxication [*see Table 13*]. After acute ingestion, the serum level of drug does not predict the body burden because of ongoing tissue distribution[95]; therefore, the dose of digoxin-specific antibodies is calculated by estimating the amount of drug ingested. In patients with chronic poisoning in whom a steady-state digoxin level can be obtained, the body burden can be estimated on the basis of the serum level and the average apparent volume of distribution. When the ingested dose is not known or a steady-state level cannot be obtained, patients should be treated empirically: initially, one to five vials should be administered, depending on the severity of toxicity. It may also be appropriate to start with small doses and to titrate them to clinical effect in patients who have preexisting disease that requires residual digitalis effect (e.g., those with congestive heart failure or atrial fibrillation).

ETHANOL, METHANOL, AND ETHYLENE GLYCOL

Ethanol (grain alcohol) is probably the most widely used drug in the United States, and complications related to acute intoxication, as well as related medical illness and trauma, are commonly encountered. Ethanol-related illnesses account for nearly 20% of the national expenditure for hospital care, and ethanol is involved in about 50% of all fatal motor vehicle accidents.[97] Ethanol is frequently ingested with other drugs, both in suicide attempts and in recreational drug abuse. Ethylene glycol (antifreeze) and methanol (wood alcohol) are other alcohols that cause profound and often fatal poisoning when mistakenly ingested as substitutes for ethanol.

Ethanol

Diagnosis Acute ethanol intoxication produces an easily recognized state of inebriation that includes disinhibition, slurred speech, ataxia, stupor, and coma.[17] Loss of protective reflexes in the airway may permit pulmonary aspiration of gastric contents, possibly causing respiratory arrest in those who are in a deep coma. In most states, a blood ethanol level above 80 to 100 mg/dl is considered sufficient evidence to charge a driver of a car with the crime of driving while intoxicated. A level above 300 mg/dl is generally considered sufficient to cause deep coma and respiratory arrest; however, because tolerance to ethanol develops, persons with a long history of ethanol abuse who have ethanol blood levels above 300 mg/dl are often awake and even able to ambulate.[17] Acute ethanol ingestion can also cause hypoglycemia because of the inhibitory effect of ethanol on gluconeogenesis.

Treatment Treatment of ethanol intoxication usually consists of supportive care. The blood ethanol level decreases at an average (but variable) rate of about 20 mg/dl/hr,[17] and most patients are awake and ambulatory within 6 to 12 hours or less. The physician should protect the airway and, if necessary, intubate the trachea and assist ventilation. The patient should be evaluated for hypoglycemia, and glucose-containing fluids should be given as necessary; vitamin B_1, 100 mg I.V. or I.M., should be administered to malnourished patients or patients with chronic alcoholism. Hypotension, although uncommon, may result from vasodilatation and dehydration and usually responds to an I.V. bolus of fluid. Although such patients often come to medical attention because of falls, even those without a history of trauma should be examined for occult injuries (especially to the head, neck, and abdomen) because inebriated patients often have such injuries. In addition, serious infections, vitamin deficiencies (especially of vitamin B_1 and folic acid), and metabolic abnormalities also occur frequently in patients with chronic alcoholism[18]; if any of these are present, they should be treated.

Methanol and Ethylene Glycol

Diagnosis Methanol or ethylene glycol poisoning produces an initial clinical picture that is similar to that of ethanol intoxication. However, these alcohols are gradually metabolized to highly toxic organic acids that can have disastrous effects [see Table 14]. After a delay of up to several hours, the patient develops severe metabolic acidosis and evidence of end-organ injury from the accumulation of the toxic acid metabolites. A diagnosis of methanol or ethylene glycol poisoning is based on the patient's history of exposure and the presence of severe metabolic acidosis. The osmolar gap is usually elevated, especially early after ingestion when the parent compounds are present, but toxic products can be present with a seemingly normal osmolar gap.[98] The serum lactate level is relatively low despite a large anion gap.[99]

Treatment If methanol or ethylene glycol poisoning is suspected, immediate measures should be instituted to reduce absorption, prevent metabolism, and remove the toxic acid metabolites.[99] If the ingestion occurred shortly before presentation (i.e., < 1 hour), gastric aspiration should be performed to remove as much of the ingested liquid as possible; activated charcoal does not efficiently adsorb the alcohols. Metabolism of the alcohols can be prevented by giving ethanol or fomepizole (4-methylpyrazole), which competitively inhibits the enzyme alcohol dehydrogenase. If ethanol is used, a loading dose of approximately 750 mg/kg orally or I.V. usually produces an ethanol level of about 100 mg/dl[99]; an infusion of 100 to 150 mg/kg/hr is given to maintain this level. An ethanol drip is difficult to manage, and the ethanol may contribute to obtundation. Fomepizole is easier to administer, has few side effects, and, if initiated early after ethylene glycol ingestion, may eliminate the need for dialysis (this is not the case for methanol). Although costly, fomepizole therapy may be less expensive than the combined costs of hemodialysis, intensive care, and serial blood work during an ethanol drip.[99] Administration of folic acid (50 mg I.V. every 4 hours), vitamin B_1 (100 mg I.M. or I.V. every 6 hours), and pyridoxine (50 mg I.V. every 6 hours) is also recommended to enhance the metabolism of the toxic organic acids. In addition, sodium bicarbonate should be given as needed to restore normal serum pH and enhance renal elimination of the toxic acid metabolites.

If the measured or estimated serum level of the toxic alcohol is greater than 50 mg/dl or if severe metabolic acidosis is present, hemodialysis is indicated to remove the parent compounds and their metabolites. During hemodialysis, the ethanol infusion is usually increased twofold, and fomepizole is administered every 4 hours to replace the respective drugs that are lost during the procedure.[99]

γ-HYDROXYBUTYRIC ACID

γ-Hydroxybutyric acid (GHB) is a naturally occurring four-carbon compound that was first synthesized in 1960. Since then, the drug has been used for various clinical purposes, including induction of general anesthesia, treatment of alcohol withdrawal and narcolepsy, and even as a protective agent during tissue ischemia.[100] In the United States, it has been available only under an FDA investigational new drug exemption for the treatment of narcolepsy. However, in the late 1980s, GHB gained popularity among some bodybuilders who believed it could enhance muscle mass through stimulation of growth hormone release. It is now promoted popularly as a sleep aid, a diet agent, and a euphorigenic drug. Its increasing use has been accompanied by a number of reports of severe and fatal effects. Its illegal recreational abuse has become a part of the underground drug culture (e.g., at rave parties and dance clubs). It has also been used to facilitate rape and assault because it produces rapid loss of consciousness. Innovative ways to continue GHB use despite FDA and Drug Enforcement Administration restrictions have included the sale of precursors of the drug such as γ-butyrolactone (GBL) and 1,4-butanediol, marketed as dietary supplements at health food stores and on the Internet under several trade names (e.g., Renewtrient and Revivarant). These precursors are metabolized to GHB in the body, and toxic effects are similar or identical to those of GHB.[101] After numerous reports of adverse reactions to these agents, including one death, the FDA asked manufacturers on January 21, 1999, to recall their GBL-containing products and warned consumers to avoid taking these products.[101]

Diagnosis

Clinically, patients poisoned by GHB or its analogues usually present with profound CNS and respiratory depression, with possible loss of laryngeal reflexes and apnea. Symptoms usually last less than 4 to 6 hours, and patients often have sudden awakening and agitation, particularly in response to painful stimuli (e.g., intubation).[102] Concurrent sinus bradycardia, myoclonic movements, and vomiting are common. Delirium and tonic-clonic seizures have been reported. There is an additive effect of GHB when it is taken in conjunction with sedative agents or al-

Table 14 Poisoning with Ethylene Glycol, Isopropyl Alcohol, or Methanol

Alcohol	Metabolic Products	Treatment
Ethylene glycol	Oxalic, hippuric, and glycolic acids cause severe anion-gap metabolic acidosis; calcium oxalate crystals precipitate in tissues and kidneys[167]	Fomepizole or ethanol infusion; perform hemodialysis if there is severe acidosis, if serum level > 20–50 mg/dl, or if osmolar gap > 10 mOsm/L
Isopropyl alcohol	Acetone causes characteristic odor; toxicity includes CNS depression, but there are no toxic acid by-products[168]	Isopropyl alcohol is a potent CNS depressant and gastric irritant, but its toxicity is usually managed supportively
Methanol	Formic acid causes severe anion-gap metabolic acidosis and visual disturbances that can lead to blindness and death[169]	Fomepizole or ethanol infusion; perform hemodialysis if there is severe acidosis, if serum level > 20–50 mg/dl, or if osmolar gap > 10 mOsm/L

cohol. GHB is absorbed within 10 to 15 minutes, and because of its short half-life of 27 minutes, plasma blood levels are undetectable within 4 to 6 hours of therapeutic ingestion.[100] Evidence suggests that GHB dependence may lead to severe withdrawal after sudden discontinuance.[100] Symptoms are similar to those of alcohol withdrawal but may last 7 to 14 days; these patients often require very large doses of benzodiazepines and barbiturates to control agitation.[103]

Treatment

There is no specific antidote for GHB. Therapy consists of airway protection, with rapid-sequence intubation if needed [*see* Initial Stabilization, *above*]. Because of the short half-life of GHB, patients without complications from GHB (e.g., prolonged hypoxia, aspiration, or untoward effects of mechanical ventilation) are often extubated and discharged from the emergency department within 3 to 7 hours.[102] Symptomatic bradycardia can be successfully treated with atropine.[102] Decontamination measures, such as gastric lavage and activated charcoal, are of little benefit because of GHB's rapid absorption, although it should be considered for large overdoses or if a coingestion is suspected. GHB withdrawal can be treated in the same manner as alcohol withdrawal, although physicians should recognize the potential need for higher doses of benzodiazepines and a longer treatment period.[104]

IRON

Iron poisoning is typically seen in children who accidentally ingest their parents' iron supplements, but intentional overdose occasionally occurs in adults.[105] Iron in large quantities is corrosive to the gastrointestinal tract, causes nausea and vomiting, and sometimes causes bloody emesis and diarrhea. Intestinal perforation occasionally occurs. Shock may result from volume loss and fluid shifts, as well as from iron-induced peripheral vasodilatation. In addition, free iron is cytotoxic, and coma, metabolic acidosis, and liver failure may develop from excessive, acute systemic absorption.[105]

Diagnosis

The diagnosis of acute iron poisoning may be based on a history of exposure or may be suspected in a patient with severe gastroenteritis and hypotension, especially if such a patient also has metabolic acidosis, hyperglycemia, and leukocytosis.[105] A plain x-ray of the abdomen (KUB view) may reveal radiopaque iron tablets. Serum iron levels in patients with severe poisoning are usually higher than 600 to 1,000 μg/dl, although lower levels may be seen if the sample is drawn late in the course of intoxication. In the past, it was common to estimate the quantity of free iron by subtracting the total iron-binding capacity (TIBC) from the serum iron level. However, it has since been shown that the TIBC is falsely elevated during iron poisoning, and this value is no longer considered useful for the purpose.[106]

Treatment

Treatment of acute iron overdose includes gut decontamination, I.V. administration of fluids, and, possibly, chelation with deferoxamine. Patients who are in shock should receive vigorous I.V. fluid replacement. Because activated charcoal does not bind iron, it should not be given unless an overdose of other drugs is also suspected. Gastric lavage may be useful in patients who have taken liquid iron preparations or chewable products; however, if intact tablets are seen on x-ray, it is unlikely that they

can be removed through even the largest-bore gastric hose. Attempts to render the iron insoluble by gastric lavage with bicarbonate- or phosphate-containing solutions have proved ineffective or dangerous. Currently, the recommended method of gut decontamination in patients with large ingestions is whole bowel irrigation,[26,31] which is achieved by administering polyethylene glycol-electrolyte solution (e.g., GoLYTELY or Colyte), 1 to 2 L/hr by nasogastric tube for several hours, until the rectal effluent is clear and the x-ray shows no radiopacities.

Therapy with deferoxamine, a specific chelator of iron, is indicated in patients who have evidence of severe poisoning, but such therapy should not replace thorough gut decontamination and aggressive volume replacement.[105] The I.V. route is preferred, and an initial dosage of 10 to 15 mg/kg/hr should be given. Dosages as high as 40 to 50 mg/kg/hr may be given in particularly severe cases of poisoning. The iron-deferoxamine complex imparts an orange or vin rosé color to the urine; this discoloration is sometimes used as evidence of the continued presence of chelatable (free) iron. Inasmuch as serum iron levels are readily available in most hospitals, the so-called vin rosé test is seldom used as an indication to continue therapy. Many clinicians stop administering deferoxamine as soon as the serum iron level is lower than 350 μg/dl, because prolonged infusions have been associated with acute respiratory distress syndrome (ARDS).[7]

ISONIAZID

Isoniazid is widely used in the treatment of tuberculosis. Long-term use of isoniazid has been associated with hepatitis and peripheral neuropathy [*see Chapters 70 and 123*]. Acute overdose of isoniazid is a well-known cause of seizures and metabolic acidosis.[107] Isoniazid causes acute toxicity by competing with pyridoxal 5′-phosphate (the active form of vitamin B_6), resulting in lowered γ-aminobutyric acid (GABA) levels in the brain. It also inhibits the hepatic metabolism of lactate to pyruvate. As little as 1.5 g of isoniazid may cause toxicity, with severe toxicity likely to occur after administration of 5 to 10 g.

Diagnosis

Acute overdose of isoniazid causes confusion, seizures, and coma; the onset is abrupt, often occurring within 30 to 60 minutes of ingestion. Lactic acidosis is often severe, and its severity is disproportional to the duration or intensity of seizure activity. Diagnosis is based on a history of isoniazid ingestion and should be suspected in any person who experiences the acute onset of seizures and who may be taking the drug (e.g., persons who have tuberculosis or AIDS and recent immigrants who test positive on the purified protein derivative [PPD] skin test). Results of testing for serum isoniazid levels are not generally available immediately, and routine toxicology screens do not ordinarily test for the drug.

Treatment

Activated charcoal should be administered to any person who is suspected of having isoniazid intoxication. Emesis should not be induced because of the risk of the abrupt onset of seizures and coma. Gastric lavage is appropriate in cases of large, recent ingestion. Seizures should be treated initially with diazepam, 5 to 10 mg I.V., or with lorazepam, 1 to 2 mg I.V. Vitamin B_6 is a specific antidote and should be given to all patients who have taken more than 3 to 5 g of isoniazid. In cases in which the amount of isoniazid ingested is unknown, the dose is 5 to 10 g I.V.; if the amount is known, an equivalent gram-for-gram amount of vitamin B_6 should be given.[107] Administration of vitamin B_6 effectively stops resistant seizures and improves metabolic acidosis. It has also reportedly reversed isoniazid-induced coma.[108]

LEAD

Lead poisoning primarily occurs in the occupational setting, with exposure occurring over a period of months or years. However, lead is a ubiquitous metal found in the paint of older houses, car batteries and radiators, some pottery glazes and solders, and some folk medicines[109]; thus, it may be encountered by hobbyists, home-repair buffs, and those who use ceramic cookware.

Diagnosis

The clinical manifestations of lead poisoning are sufficiently variable and nonspecific that lead poisoning should be suspected in any patient who has multisystem illness, especially if the illness involves the neurologic, hematopoietic, and gastrointestinal systems.[109] Lead poisoning rarely results from a single ingestion, although such occurrences have been reported.[38] More commonly, exposure occurs repeatedly and gradually. Patients typically have cramplike abdominal pain or nausea and may have chronic systemic symptoms such as irritability, malaise, and weight loss. Other manifestations of lead poisoning include peripheral motor neuropathy (wristdrop) and anemia, which is often microcytic and accompanied by basophilic stippling. Lead encephalopathy, manifested by coma and seizures, is rare.

Chronic lead poisoning has been misdiagnosed as porphyria, in part because they both involve alteration of heme metabolism.[110] Diagnosis of lead poisoning is usually based on the lead level in whole blood. Symptoms generally occur in patients with lead levels above 25 to 40 µg/dl, but lower levels have been associated with impaired neurobehavioral development in children.[111] Lead levels above 80 µg/dl are often associated with severe overt toxicity. The free erythrocyte protoporphyrin (FEP) concentration, which is elevated (> 35 µg/dl) in persons with chronic intoxication, has been used to screen large populations for lead poisoning but is not sufficiently sensitive for the identification of low blood lead levels (< 30 µg/dl) in children.

Treatment

For patients with an acute ingestion of lead (e.g., a fishing weight, bullet, or curtain weight), a plain x-ray of the abdomen should be obtained. If the object is in the stomach, there is a risk that the action of stomach acid may create enough absorbable lead to cause systemic toxicity; therefore, the object should be removed by the use of cathartic agents, whole bowel irrigation, or endoscopy. Objects that clearly lie beyond the pylorus are likely to pass uneventfully into the stool, but confirmation of this supposition should be obtained by close follow-up with repeated x-rays and measurement of blood lead levels.[38]

Several chelating agents are available for the treatment of patients with acute or chronic intoxication who are symptomatic and have elevated blood lead levels.[111] The oldest chelating agent, dimercaprol, is reserved for patients with lead encephalopathy (but even this use is controversial). For less severe intoxication, the physician should administer I.V. calcium EDTA or oral succimer (meso-2,3-dimercaptosuccinic acid [DMSA]). Triple-chelation therapy with dimercaprol, EDTA, and oral succimer has been used in conjunction with whole bowel irrigation following an extremely high lead level in a 3-year-old child with encephalopathy.[111] A recent trial suggests that succimer does not provide any benefit in children with chronically elevated blood lead levels between 20 and 44 µg/dl.[112] However, the findings of this study, the indications for treatment, and the recommended agents and doses are controversial; the physician should consult with a specialist in occupational medicine or toxicology or contact a regional poison-control center for specific advice about the doses and side effects of these drugs.

Health care providers should be aware that the Occupational Safety and Health Administration (OSHA) has provided specific guidelines for monitoring and managing workers who have been exposed to lead [see Chapter 7]; these guidelines stipulate that such workers be removed from exposure if a single blood lead level exceeds 60 µg/dl or if the average of a series of three successive periodic screening levels exceeds 50 µg/dl.[113] For further information, a regional OSHA office or an occupational medicine specialist should be consulted. (A directory of regional offices is available at the OSHA Web site, at http://www.osha.gov.) Finally, because household members of persons who have been occupationally exposed to lead may be contaminated by the poisoned individual, household members should also be evaluated for lead poisoning even if they are apparently asymptomatic, and measures should be taken to reduce or prevent further exposure.

LITHIUM

Lithium is a simple cation that is widely used for the treatment of manic-depressive illness and other psychiatric disorders. It is also used to elevate the white blood cell count in patients with severe leukopenia. Lithium is excreted renally, and severe intoxication usually results from drug accumulation caused by renal impairment or excessive overmedication. An acute single overdose, however, is less likely to result in severe poisoning.

Diagnosis

The usual therapeutic level of lithium is 0.6 to 1.2 mEq/L. Chronic intoxication can occur with levels only slightly above 1.2 mEq/L, but patients with acute overdose may remain asymptomatic despite having much higher levels early after ingestion of the drug.[114] Manifestations of lithium intoxication include confusion, lethargy, tremors, and muscle twitching. The ECG may show flattening of T waves, the presence of U waves, and prolongation of the QT interval. In severe cases, coma and convulsions may occur.[114] Symptoms may take several days to weeks to resolve, and some patients are left with permanent neurologic impairment.[115] Other toxic effects of lithium intoxication are nephrogenic diabetes insipidus and neuroleptic malignant syndrome [see Table 5]. These effects can also occur at therapeutic levels of the drug.

Treatment

Treatment of acute lithium overdose consists mainly of gut decontamination and fluid therapy. Because lithium is poorly adsorbed to activated charcoal, administration of this agent is not necessary unless the physician suspects that another drug has also been ingested. Gastric lavage may reduce the gastric burden of lithium. Whole bowel irrigation should be considered, especially if the patient has ingested a sustained-release form of the drug.[114] Limited experimental and anecdotal evidence suggests that administration of sodium polystyrene sulfonate reduces absorption and enhances elimination of lithium, although its role in acute lithium overdose remains to be established.[116]

Fluid therapy is an essential part of treatment of lithium intoxication. Volume should be restored with 1 to 2 L of normal saline; the I.V. administration of fluids should be continued at a rate sufficient to produce urine at a rate of about 100 ml/hr. The indications for hemodialysis in the setting of lithium toxicity are controversial. A recent review article recommends the following guidelines for hemodialysis: a lithium level greater than 6 mEq/L in any patient; a lithium level greater than 4 mEq/L in any patient on long-term lithium therapy (in contrast to an acute overdose); or a lithium level of 2.5 to 4.0 mEq/L in any patient with severe neurologic symptoms, renal insufficiency, hemodynamic instability, or neurologic instability.[114] However, a poison-control center–based study did not report any significant difference in patients with lithium toxicity in whom hemodialysis was recommended by the poison-control center but not performed and in those for whom hemodialysis was performed.[117] These authors recommended reserving hemodialysis for severe cases of lithium toxicity. Blood should be drawn at least 8 to 12 hours after the last dose of lithium is given to prevent misinterpretation, which can occur as a result of the serum level being falsely elevated before the drug is distributed in tissues. Serial lithium measurements should be obtained until the level clearly drops, to exclude ongoing absorption or rebound after hemodialysis. Consultation with a regional poison-control center, medical toxicologist, and nephrologist should be obtained early to help manage a lithium-toxic patient.

METHEMOGLOBINEMIA-INDUCING AGENTS

Methemoglobin is an oxidized form of hemoglobin that is incapable of carrying and delivering oxygen normally. A number of oxidant drugs and chemicals can convert hemoglobin to its oxidized form, causing methemoglobinemia.[118] These agents include local anesthetics (e.g., benzocaine and lidocaine), antimicrobial agents (e.g., chloroquine, dapsone, primaquine, and sulfonamides), analgesics (e.g., phenazopyridine and phenacetin), nitrites and nitrates (e.g., amyl nitrite, butyl nitrite, isobutyl nitrite, and sodium nitrite), and several miscellaneous drugs and chemicals (e.g., aminophenol, aniline dyes, bromates, chlorates, metoclopramide, nitrobenzene, nitrogen oxides, and nitroglycerin). Benzocaine-containing sprays used for topical anesthesia before certain procedures (e.g., endoscopy, intubation, and nasogastric lavage) are a common cause of methemoglobinemia.[119] Persons with glucose-6-phosphate dehydrogenase (G6PD) deficiency and congenital methemoglobin reductase deficiency are more likely than persons without these conditions to accumulate methemoglobin after exposure to an oxidant.

Diagnosis

Methemoglobinemia causes cellular asphyxia. Symptoms of mild to moderate methemoglobinemia include headache, nausea, dizziness, and dyspnea. Methemoglobin levels as low as 15% can cause the patient to appear cyanotic despite having a normal oxygen tension. The blood usually has a dark or chocolate-brown appearance. Although pulse oximetry is abnormal, the reported drop in oxygen saturation does not correlate with the actual reduction in oxyhemoglobin saturation, and specific testing for methemoglobinemia should be performed.[120]

Treatment

Mild methemoglobinemia (methemoglobin levels < 15% to 20%) usually resolves spontaneously and requires no treatment. Patients who have more severe intoxication should be given the antidote methylene blue (1 to 2 mg/kg I.V. [0.1 to 0.2 ml/kg of a 1% solution] over several minutes).[118] The dosage may be repeated once. Although symptoms and signs usually resolve quickly, methemoglobinemia may recur with the administration of long-acting oxidants such as dapsone [*see Chapter 93*].[118]

OPIOIDS

The opioids and opiates include several synthetic and naturally occurring compounds that are widely used for their analgesic properties. Common opium derivatives include morphine, heroin, hydrocodone, and codeine. Synthetic opioids include fentanyl, methadone, and butorphanol. Preparations of hydrocodone or codeine for oral use commonly contain aspirin or acetaminophen, which may themselves be responsible for serious toxicity in an overdose. Opioids stimulate several receptors in the CNS, resulting in sedation and reduced sympathetic outflow.[6,7] Excessive opioid effect may cause coma and blunting of the respiratory response to hypercapnia. Buprenorphine is a mixed opioid agonist-antagonist that has been introduced as an alternative to methadone in outpatient drug-treatment programs. The use of buprenorphine in a patient addicted to opioids may precipitate acute withdrawal symptoms.[121] The opioids meperidine and dextromethorphan may cause serious rigidity and hyperthermia in persons who are taking MAO inhibitors or other serotoninergic drugs (e.g., selective serotonin reuptake inhibitors [SSRIs]).[122]

Diagnosis

Patients may have opioid intoxication as a result of unintentional overdose or attempted suicide. Signs of intoxication include lethargy or coma, pinpoint pupils, and respiratory depression. Acute noncardiogenic pulmonary edema may occur.[6] Seizures are not typical but may occur with acute propoxyphene overdose; repeated therapeutic doses of meperidine can also cause seizures, especially in persons with renal failure because of the accumulation of the metabolite normeperidine.

Diagnosis of opioid intoxication is usually not difficult in a person who is in a coma and has pinpoint pupils and apnea.[5,6] Paramedics may discover I.V. drug paraphernalia or empty prescription bottles at the scene. Exposure to other drugs, however, may complicate the clinical picture.

Treatment

The physician should immediately establish that the airway is not obstructed and that ventilation is adequate. Supplemental oxygen should then be administered as necessary. After these initial measures, the specific opioid antagonist naloxone should be given (0.2 to 2 mg I.V. or S.C.). A recent trial has shown similar results with subcutaneous and intravenous naloxone.[123] Persons who are suspected of long-term narcotic abuse should be started with smaller doses of naloxone to minimize the severity of an acute withdrawal reaction. Patients usually become fully awake within a few minutes after administration. If the initial dose is not effective, additional doses (up to 15 to 20 mg if opioid intoxication is strongly suspected) should be given until a satisfactory response is achieved. The plasma half-life of naloxone is about 60 minutes, which is shorter than that of most of the opioids whose actions it reverses; therefore, patients who respond to the antidote should be observed for at least 3 hours after the last dose for the recurrence of sedation. Traditionally thought to be an innocuous drug, naloxone has been associated with an approximately 1.6% complication rate. Complications include asystole, seizures, pulmonary edema, and severe agitation.[6]

Oral ingestion of an opioid should be treated with activated charcoal. Gastric lavage should be considered in cases of large or recent overdose. There is no role for hemodialysis or other enhanced removal procedures in the treatment of opioid overdose.

ORGANOPHOSPHATES AND RELATED AGENTS

Organophosphates and carbamates are widely used as pesticides,[124] and several of the nerve agents (e.g., VX, soman, sarin) developed for chemical warfare[125] are potent organophosphates. All of these poisons inhibit the enzyme acetylcholinesterase, preventing the breakdown of acetylcholine at cholinergic synapses. Whereas the organophosphates may cause permanent damage to the enzyme, carbamates have a transient and reversible effect. Many of these agents are well absorbed through intact skin. Persons may be exposed accidentally while working with or transporting the chemicals or as a result of accidental or suicidal ingestion.

Diagnosis

Excessive activity of acetylcholine may occur at nicotinic, muscarinic, and CNS cholinergic receptors. The most common presenting symptoms of poisoning are abdominal cramps and vomiting accompanied by sweating and hypersalivation [see Table 15]. The patient usually has small or pinpoint pupils. Because of the mixed effects of poisoning on sympathetic ganglia and parasympathetic synapses, the heart rate may be either slow or fast. Life-threatening manifestations of acetylcholinesterase inhibition include muscle weakness with respiratory arrest, as well as severe bronchospasm. Significant volume loss may result from excessive sweating, salivation, vomiting, and diarrhea.[124]

Treatment

Contaminated clothing should be removed immediately and all exposed areas washed thoroughly with soap and water. Rescue personnel should take precautions to avoid secondary contamination from direct contact with the victim's skin, clothing, or vomitus. Xylene or other solvent vapors emanating from the victim are not life threatening to medical personnel but may cause dizziness, nausea, and headache. In patients who have ingested an organophosphate or a carbamate, gastric lavage should be performed with the use of a closed-container unit, and activated charcoal should be administered.

Specific therapy includes administration of atropine and pralidoxime (2-PAM). Atropine is not a physiologic antidote but can reverse excessive muscarinic stimulation, thereby alleviating abdominal cramps, bronchospasm, and hypersalivation. It does not reverse muscle weakness. All patients with organophosphate poisoning should also be given 2-PAM because it can chemically restore the enzyme acetylcholinesterase; in persons who go untreated, the organophosphate's binding to acetylcholinesterase may become permanent (the so-called aging effect). Because carbamates have a transient effect, 2-PAM therapy is not needed in patients who have been poisoned with these agents. However, because the exact product causing cholinergic excess is often not known initially or because the cholinergic excess may be the the result of a mix of organophosphate and carbamate, 2-PAM may be initiated empirically. Additionally, several case reports suggest that 2-PAM may be useful in carbamate poisoning.[126]

Table 15 Manifestations of Excessive Activity of Acetylcholine

Site of Activity	Clinical Manifestations
Postganglionic muscarinic receptors	Bradycardia; miosis; salivation; lacrimation; bronchorrhea; increased peristalsis; sweating
Autonomic ganglia	Tachycardia; hypertension
Skeletal muscle nicotinic receptors	Muscle fasciculations followed by weakness; neuromuscular paralysis
CNS cholinergic receptors	Agitation; seizures

The dosage of 2-PAM is 1 to 2 g I.V. initially, followed by a continuous infusion of 200 to 500 mg/hr, depending on the patient's response. The infusion should be continued until the patient can be weaned from the drug without experiencing recurrence of weakness or muscarinic manifestations. This process may take several days in persons who have been exposed to highly lipid-soluble agents such as fenthion or dichlorvos.[7] A so-called intermediate syndrome has been described in which some patients experience recurrent muscle weakness several days after initially successful treatment[127]; this syndrome may be caused by neurotoxic components of the agent, continued toxicity from a lipid-soluble product, or inadequate 2-PAM therapy.

SALICYLATES

Aspirin (acetylsalicylic acid) and other salicylates are widely used for their antipyretic, anti-inflammatory, and analgesic effects and can be found alone or in combination in a number of prescription and over-the-counter products (e.g., oil of wintergreen, Pepto-Bismol). Salicylates interfere with the metabolism of glucose and fatty acids; they also uncouple oxidative phosphorylation, leading to inefficient production of adenosine triphosphate, accumulation of lactic acid, and production of heat. Poisoning may result from an acute single ingestion (usually in a dose > 200 mg/kg) or from long-term overmedication.[128] Long-term poisoning occurs most commonly in elderly persons who regularly take large doses of aspirin (e.g., for osteoarthritis) and who gradually begin to take larger doses or in whom renal insufficiency develops. In such cases, the diagnosis of salicylism is often overlooked, and patients may be assumed to have sepsis, gastroenteritis, or pneumonia on admission to the hospital.[128]

Diagnosis

The most common initial manifestation of salicylate poisoning is hyperventilation, which occurs largely as a result of central stimulation of the respiratory drive and partly in response to metabolic acidosis. Measurement of arterial blood gases usually reveals respiratory alkalosis with predominant alkalemia and underlying metabolic acidosis. Other findings include tinnitus, confusion, and lethargy. Patients with severe intoxication may experience coma, seizures, hyperthermia, noncardiogenic pulmonary edema, and circulatory collapse. The serum salicylate level in such cases usually exceeds 100 mg/dl (1,000 mg/L), although patients with chronic intoxication may experience severe effects with much lower serum levels.[129]

Treatment

For patients with an acute ingestion, activated charcoal

should be administered and gastric lavage considered if the ingestion was large (e.g., > 10 to 15 g). Because salicylates cause pylorospasm and delay gastric emptying, lavage may be successful even after a delay of several hours. For a patient who has taken a massive ingestion, extra dosages of activated charcoal (50 to 60 g every 4 to 6 hours for the first 1 to 2 days) may be needed to achieve the desired 10-to-1 ratio of charcoal to drug. Massive ingestions, as well as those involving enteric-coated aspirin, may lead to prolonged or delayed absorption and the potential for catastrophic worsening after 1 to 2 days.[128] In such cases, close observation of the patient should be maintained, and measurement of the serum salicylate level should frequently be performed until the level clearly drops into the therapeutic range (10 to 20 mg/dl).

Enhanced elimination procedures can effectively reduce elevated salicylate levels. Alkalinization of the urine traps the ionized form of salicylate in the kidney tubules, increasing renal elimination.[120] To initiate alkalinization, the physician should add 100 mEq of sodium bicarbonate to 1 L of 5% dextrose in quarter-normal (0.225%) saline, then infuse the solution at 200 ml/hr while monitoring the pH of the urine (the goal is to achieve a pH of 7 to 8). It may be difficult to perform alkalinization in patients with volume and potassium deficits without first replacing these losses. Hemodialysis rapidly lowers serum salicylate levels and can restore fluid and electrolyte balances. Hemodialysis is recommended for patients who are unable to tolerate fluid challenges (e.g., as in cerebral edema or pulmonary edema) and those who have worsening renal insufficiency, severe metabolic acidosis, or a serum salicylate level greater than 100 mg/dl (1,000 mg/L).

SEDATIVE-HYPNOTIC AGENTS

The sedative-hypnotic agents include the barbiturates (e.g., phenobarbital, pentobarbital, butalbital, and amobarbital) and the benzodiazepines (e.g., alprazolam, diazepam, lorazepam, and triazolam), as well as several other drugs, such as meprobamate, glutethimide, ethchlorvynol, chloral hydrate, zolpidem, zaleplon, and buspirone. These drugs cause generalized depression of CNS activity and are commonly used to alleviate anxiety or to induce sleep. The mechanisms of action and pharmacokinetics are different for each drug group.[13,130,131]

Diagnosis

Overdose of a sedative-hypnotic drug causes lethargy, ataxia, and slurred speech. In patients with severe poisoning, coma and respiratory arrest may occur, especially when sedative-hypnotic drugs are combined with other depressants, such as ethanol. The blood pressure and pulse rate are usually decreased, the temperature may be low because of exposure and venodilatation, and the pupils are usually small (although they may be dilated in patients with glutethimide overdose). Patients who are in a deep coma may appear to be dead because they may have absent reflexes, fixed pupils, and even flat EEG tracings.[132] In patients with chloral hydrate overdose, ventricular ectopy and ventricular tachycardia may develop; these effects are caused by generation of the metabolite trichloroethanol, which, like other chlorinated hydrocarbons, can sensitize the myocardium to the effects of epinephrine.[133] In cases of phenobarbital overdose, blood levels of the drug can be obtained in most hospital laboratories, but in cases of overdose of most of the other sedative-hypnotic agents, blood levels are neither clinically useful nor readily available.

Treatment

An unobstructed airway should be maintained and supplemental oxygen should be administered. The trachea should then be intubated and assisted ventilation initiated, if necessary. Uncomplicated hypothermia should be treated with gradual passive external rewarming. I.V. crystalloids should be administered to patients with low blood pressure; if necessary, dopamine and other pressor agents should be given. For patients with ventricular arrhythmias caused by chloral hydrate overdose, propranolol (1 to 5 mg I.V.) or esmolol (25 to 100 µg/kg/min) should be given.[134] Activated charcoal should be administered. For cases of massive ingestion, gastric lavage should be considered.

Flumazenil is a specific benzodiazepine antagonist that has been proved effective in reversing the coma caused by benzodiazepine overdose. It has a rapid onset of action after I.V. administration (0.5 to 3.0 mg); because its effects last for only about 2 to 3 hours, resedation may occur. Flumazenil is contraindicated in patients with a known or suspected overdose of a tricyclic antidepressant and in patients who have been given a benzodiazepine for the control of status epilepticus, because flumazenil may induce seizures in these patients. It should also not be used in patients who have increased intracranial pressure and who are receiving benzodiazepines for sedation. The use of flumazenil in persons who have been taking large quantities of benzodiazepines for long periods may provoke an acute withdrawal syndrome.[5,7,8]

Enhanced removal procedures are rarely needed in patients with sedative-hypnotic overdose because most will recover with airway management, assisted ventilation, and other supportive measures. When supportive measures fail, hemodialysis can effectively reduce blood concentrations of phenobarbital.[134]

THEOPHYLLINE

Although no longer a first-line drug, theophylline is still occasionally used for the treatment of asthma and other bronchospastic disorders, congestive heart failure, and neonatal apnea. It is available in regular and sustained-release formulations for oral use. Aminophylline, the ethylenediamine salt of theophylline, is used for I.V. infusions. Theophylline intoxication may occur after an acute single overdose or as a result of long-term overmedication.[135] Chronic intoxication may also be caused by reduced theophylline metabolism resulting from the addition of an interfering drug (e.g., cimetidine or erythromycin) or from an intercurrent illness (e.g., congestive heart failure or liver failure). The normal elimination half-life, 4 to 6 hours, may be prolonged to more than 20 hours in theophylline overdose.

Diagnosis

Acute theophylline overdose causes vomiting, tremors, and tachycardia. Laboratory findings include hypokalemia, hypophosphatemia, and hyperglycemia. These metabolic effects, as well as tachycardia and vasodilatation, are thought to be mediated through excessive beta$_2$-adrenergic stimulation. If serum theophylline levels exceed 100 mg/L, seizures, hypotension, and ventricular arrhythmias are likely to develop.[135] The seizures are often refractory to anticonvulsant therapy. Serum drug levels may not peak for 16 to 24 hours after theophylline ingestion, especially if the drug was in a sustained-release formulation.

Chronic intoxication may develop gradually, with toxicity possibly occurring at serum drug levels that are much lower than those associated with acute overdose: seizures have been reported to occur at levels as low as 14 to 35 mg/L.[135] Unlike the findings in acute overdose, hypokalemia and hypotension are not common.

Treatment

In cases of acute ingestion of theophylline, activated charcoal should be given. Gastric lavage should be considered for large ingestions (i.e., more than 15 to 20 tablets). However, it is unlikely that lavage will remove intact sustained-release tablets, and severe or fatal intoxication may ensue despite aggressive attempts at decontamination.[136] Although some toxicologists have suggested administering repeated doses of activated charcoal in combination with whole bowel irrigation for massive ingestions of sustained-release medications, this approach remains controversial.[136]

Hypotension should be treated with esmolol (25 to 100 μg/kg/min) rather than a beta-adrenergic agonist because the hypotension is probably caused by beta$_2$-adrenergic–mediated vasodilatation.[137] Seizures should be treated with phenobarbital (15 to 20 mg/kg I.V.) rather than with phenytoin, which is ineffective.[136] For patients with recurrent seizures and for those with serum theophylline levels of around 100 mg/L or greater, excess theophylline should be removed as quickly as possible by hemodialysis or hemoperfusion.[138] Administration of multiple repeated doses of activated charcoal [see Enhanced Elimination, above] can effectively shorten the elimination half-life of theophylline, but such administration is often not practical in the critically ill patient.

TRICYCLIC ANTIDEPRESSANTS AND RELATED COMPOUNDS

Tricyclic antidepressants, also known as cyclic antidepressants, were once a leading cause of seizures and death from acute drug overdose.[134] Although most of the newer SSRI antidepressants are much less toxic [see Table 16], tricyclic antidepressants are still commonly used for the treatment of depression, enuresis, and other disorders.

The toxicity of the tricyclic antidepressants is caused by various pharmacologic properties of this class of agents, including anticholinergic activity, inhibition of norepinephrine reuptake, alpha-adrenergic blockade, and, most important, depression of the fast sodium channel in cardiac cells (the so-called quinidine-like or membrane-depressant effect). This last property is responsible for prolongation of conduction and depressed cardiac contractility.[139] Ingestion of approximately 1 g of a tricyclic antidepressant is likely to produce severe toxicity.

Diagnosis

Initially, persons with tricyclic antidepressant overdose have anticholinergic signs, including tachycardia; dilated pupils; reduced peristalsis; muscle twitching; and dry, flushed skin. Lethargy and slurred speech are common. The abrupt onset of seizures, coma, and hypotension signals severe toxicity, which may occur within 30 to 60 minutes of ingestion or may be delayed because of slowed gut absorption. In patients with severe intoxication, the ECG shows a QRS complex that is usually wider than 0.12 second[139,140]; however, this finding may initially be absent if the drug has not been absorbed or in cases of overdose with amoxapine or another noncardiotoxic drug. In some patients, right-axis deviation of the terminal 40 msec of the QRS complex may represent early evidence of a conduction disturbance.[140] Death may result from profound depression of cardiac conduction and contractility; respiratory arrest; or complications

---

> *Table 16*   Common Tricyclic and Other Antidepressants
>
> *Tricyclic antidepressants and related agents (may induce cardiotoxicity, including widening of the QRS complex)*
> Amitriptyline
> Desipramine
> Doxepin
> Imipramine
> Maprotiline
> Nortriptyline
>
> *Newer-generation antidepressants (cardiotoxicity is unlikely but seizures may occur)*
> Amoxapine
> Bupropion
> Fluoxetine
> Paroxetine
> Sertraline
> Trazodone
> Venlafaxine

of pulmonary aspiration, aspiration pneumonia, or hyperthermia (caused by muscle twitching and seizures coupled with the absence of sweating).

Treatment

The physician should administer activated charcoal. Gastric lavage should be considered for patients with massive ingestions (e.g., > 4 to 5 g), especially if less than 1 hour has elapsed since the overdose. All patients should be monitored closely for at least 6 hours; any person with altered mental status, evidence of anticholinergic toxicity, or cardiac conduction abnormalities should be admitted to the hospital and monitored closely. The physician should maintain an unobstructed airway, intubate the trachea, and assist ventilation if needed.

Seizures should be treated with benzodiazepines and phenobarbital (see above). Physostigmine should not be administered, because it may cause seizures and can worsen cardiac conduction disturbances. Initially, hypotension should be treated with I.V. boluses of normal saline. If there is evidence of depression of the sodium channel (i.e., a wide QRS complex), sodium bicarbonate should be administered at a dosage of 50 to 100 mEq I.V.[11,139] Repeated doses may be given as needed, although the serum pH should be monitored for excessive alkalemia. If hypotension does not respond to administration of fluids and sodium bicarbonate, dopamine or norepinephrine should be given. Norepinephrine may be more effective than dopamine in some patients, possibly because of tricyclic antidepressant–induced depletion of norepinephrine, but in one study, no difference between these agents was found.[139] Partial cardiopulmonary bypass has been suggested for patients with refractory hypotension and agonal cardiac rhythm, although there is little likelihood of survival.[12] There is no known role for hemodialysis in this setting.

Food Poisoning

A variety of toxins may produce illness after consumption of fish, shellfish, or mushrooms. Illness caused by bacterial or viral contamination of food, including botulism, is discussed elsewhere [see Chapter 136].

SEAFOOD

The mechanism of toxicity varies with each toxin [*see Table 17*]. In general, the seafood-associated toxins are heat stable; therefore, cooking does not render the food safe to eat. In some cases (e.g., ciguatera and paralytic shellfish poisoning [PSP]), the poisons are highly potent neurotoxins elaborated by dinoflagellates, which are then consumed by fish or concentrated by filter-feeding clams and mussels. Scombroid poisoning results from bacterial overgrowth in inadequately refrigerated fish (although the fish may look and smell fresh); scombrotoxin is a mixture of histamine and histaminelike compounds produced by the breakdown of histidine in the fish flesh. Tetrodotoxin is produced by microorganisms associated with the puffer fish (as well as the California newt and some species of South American frogs) and concentrated in various internal organs. Although the fish is deadly and ranks as the leading cause of fatal food poisoning in Japan, it is also considered a delicacy; extreme care is required in preparation of this fish by specially trained chefs to separate the edible muscle from the toxin-containing organs. Poisoning from saxitoxin (the culprit in PSP) has recently been reported in persons who ate puffer fish caught in waters near Titusville, Florida.[141]

Diagnosis

Signs and symptoms of seafood poisoning vary with the toxin [*see Table 17*]. Diagnosis is based on the clinical presentation and history of ingested seafood. In some cases, laboratory confirmation can be carried out with the assistance of the regional or state health department.

Treatment

In general, treatment is supportive. For neurotoxic poisonings such as PSP and tetrodotoxin, prompt medical attention may be required to prevent death from sudden respiratory arrest. Scombroid poisoning is often treated with H_1 and H_2 histamine blockers (e.g., diphenhydramine and cimetidine). For ciguatera poisoning, previous anecdotal reports have suggested benefit from mannitol, but a recent randomized, controlled blinded trial showed that mannitol did not relieve symptoms of ciguatera poisoning and resulted in more side effects than normal saline.[142] Ciguatera poisoning can produce chronic symptoms, which may resemble multiple sclerosis or chronic fatigue syndrome.[143] Improvement in chronic symptoms has been reported in patients treated with amitriptyline or fluoxetine[144,145]; polyneuropathy has responded to gabapentin.[146] Recurrence of symptoms, which may be worse than the initial attack, can be triggered by ingestion of fish or alcohol.

AMANITA PHALLOIDES MUSHROOMS

The *A. phalloides* mushroom ("death cap") has been known and feared for at least two millennia and continues to cause serious illness and death, although in recent years, mortality has declined because of the availability of orthotopic liver transplantation for patients with fulminant liver failure. This mushroom, as well as several others that contain the cellular toxin amanitin (also known as amatoxin), are found throughout Europe and the United States. Most victims are amateur or novice mushroom hunters who mistake this mushroom for another, edible species. The toxin is heat stable and is not destroyed by cooking. Once absorbed, it binds to RNA polymerase and inhibits cellular protein synthesis. Hepatocytes and rapidly dividing cells are most sensitive.

Diagnosis

Severe abdominal cramps, vomiting, and diarrhea begin about 8 to 12 hours or longer after a meal. Diarrhea can be so severe that it results in severe volume depletion and cardiovascular collapse. After apparent recovery from the gastrointestinal syndrome, patients can develop rapidly progressive hepatic failure.

Treatment

Treatment of suspected amatoxin poisoning includes aggressive fluid replacement and administration of activated charcoal by mouth to bind any unabsorbed toxin in the gut and to prevent enterohepatic reabsorption, which can be significant.[147] Patients who develop severe liver injury with encephalopathy are candidates for emergency liver transplantation. Various antidotes have been described over the years, including high-dose intravenous penicillin G, corticosteroids, thioctic acid, and silibinin (an extract of the milk thistle plant), but none have proved to be effective in controlled studies, and neither thioctic acid nor silibinin is available as a pharmaceutical in the United States.[147] (Milk thistle extract can be found in some stores selling dietary and nutritional supplements, however.)

MONOSODIUM GLUTAMATE

Monosodium glutamate (MSG) is a food additive used to enhance flavor and add body to prepared foods. It is also found as a component of hydrolyzed vegetable protein. Consumption of MSG can invoke, in susceptible persons, a syndrome originally

Table 17   Seafood Poisonings[170]

Type	Onset	Common Sources	Syndrome	Treatment
Ciguatera	1–6 hr	Barracuda, red snapper, grouper	Gastrointestinal upset, paresthesias, sensation of hot and cold reversal, itching, weakness, myalgias, orthostatic hypotension	Supportive; ?mannitol
Paralytic shellfish poisoning	30 min	Bivalve mollusks (mussels, clams), associated with algae bloom (red tide)	Gastrointestinal upset, paresthesias, ataxia, weakness, respiratory muscle paralysis, respiratory arrest	Supportive
Scombroid	Minutes to hours	Tuna, mahi-mahi, bonito, mackerel	Gastrointestinal upset, flushed skin, urticaria, wheezing	Antihistamines
Tetrodotoxin	30 min	Puffer fish (fugu), sunfish, porcupine fish	Vomiting, paresthesias, perioral tingling, muscle weakness, respiratory paralysis, respiratory arrest	Supportive

coined the Chinese-restaurant syndrome and now known as the MSG symptom complex. The syndrome, which begins about 15 to 30 minutes after ingestion, includes a burning sensation or pressure in the face, behind the eyes, and in the chest, neck, shoulders, forearms, and abdomen. Headache, syncope, and, rarely, cardiac arrhythmias have been described. Not everyone who ingests MSG experiences the reaction. The etiology of the syndrome is not clearly understood. Symptoms usually last no more than 2 to 3 hours, and there is no specific treatment.[148,149]

HERBAL REMEDIES AND DIETARY SUPPLEMENTS

In 2002, about 62% of adults in the United States reported using at least one form of alternative medicine within the previous year[150] [see Chapter 9]. Herbal products are not subject to FDA approval, because they do not undergo the scientific testing required of conventional therapies. They cannot be promoted specifically for treatment, prevention, or cure of a disease. However, the Dietary Supplement Health and Education Act of 1994 allows these products to be sold and labeled with statements describing their professed effects. With the increasing use and availability of herbal medications, poison-control centers and health care providers are commonly encountering patients who have experienced adverse effects from impure products, drug interactions, and intentional ingestions. Ginkgo biloba has been suggested to have antiplatelet effects, and cases of spontaneous hyphema and bilateral subdural hematomas have been reported.[151] The additional risk of warfarin must be considered in patients taking Ginkgo biloba. Ephedra (ma huang) is a common ingredient in herbal weight-loss products (herbal fen-phen), stimulants (herbal ecstasy), decongestants, and bronchodilators. The active moiety in ephedra is ephedrine and related alkaloids. Serious adverse reactions, including hypertension, seizures, arrhythmias, heart attack, stroke, and death, have been reported.[152] In 2004, the FDA declared dietary supplements containing ephedra to be unsafe and banned ephedra-containing supplements.[153] However, a federal judge reversed the ban in early 2005; the future of this substance remains uncertain. St. John's wort (Hypericum perforatum), touted as a natural antidepressant, has been shown to inhibit serotonin, dopamine, and norepinephrine reuptake and thus presents the possibility of interaction with MAO inhibitors and other serotoninergic drugs.[152]

Adverse events associated with most herbal products are largely undescribed, and there are few specific antidotes. Emergency and supportive measures should therefore be instituted as necessary [see Management of Common Complications, above]. To enhance research and knowledge in this area, all such events should be reported to poison-control centers and to the FDA's MedWatch Program (800-FDA-1088; http://www.fda.gov/medwatch).

Smoke Inhalation

Smoke inhalation injury is the most common cause of mortality among fire victims, accounting for up to 75% of deaths.[90] Fires produce heat and smoke, although the latter is the chief culprit in inhalation injuries.[154] Smoke comprises a varying mixture of particles and gaseous chemicals that are pyrolysis products of substances that become toxic only when burned.[155] Smoke components can be broken down into simple asphyxiants, chemical asphyxiants, and irritants. Simple asphyxiants (e.g., methane and carbon dioxide) displace oxygen, thus decreasing fraction of inspired oxygen (F_IO_2) and resulting in hypoxemia. Chemical as-

phyxiants (e.g., carbon monoxide, cyanide, and hydrogen sulfide) cause systemic toxicity and cellular hypoxia by interrupting transport or utilization of oxygen [see Specific Drugs and Poisons, above].

Irritant gases have a direct cytotoxic effect on the oropharynx and the respiratory tract. Toxicity depends on the physical and chemical properties of the gas, which are often divided into two major groups on the basis of their water solubility. Highly water-soluble gases (e.g., ammonia, acrolein, hydrogen chloride, and sulfur dioxide) are readily absorbed in the mucous membranes along the upper respiratory tract, causing local irritation of the eyes, nose, and throat. Compounds with intermediate solubility (e.g., chlorine and isocyanates) cause upper and lower respiratory tract injury. Substances that are less water soluble (e.g., phosgene and nitrogen dioxide) do not dissolve readily in the mucous membranes of the upper respiratory tract and can reach the distal airway, producing delayed-onset pulmonary toxicity.[90,155]

Diagnosis

Clinical symptoms vary with the location of tissue injury, which in turn depends on the solubility and the concentration of exposure. Manifestations of toxicity may include conjunctival irritation, rhinitis, oropharyngeal erythema and burns, coryza, hoarseness, stridor, wheezing, coughing, and noncardiogenic pulmonary edema. Onset of pulmonary edema may be delayed from 12 to 24 hours or longer when the patient has been exposed to low-solubility gases such as phosgene and nitrogen dioxide.[90]

Treatment

Management at the scene of the exposure should include evacuation of all persons from further exposure to the smoke. Rescuers should take precautions to avoid personal exposure and should use a self-contained breathing apparatus. Although the clinician rarely has access to information regarding the constituents of the smoke, initial treatment of all victims should focus on the airway [see Initial Stabilization, above]. All patients should receive supplemental oxygen in the highest concentration while arterial blood gas and carboxyhemoglobin levels are pending [see Carbon Monoxide, above]. For patients who do not require immediate airway protection (e.g., those who are without respiratory distress, coma, or stridor), a careful plan should be sought for identifying those at high risk for potential deterioration. Many authors recommend fiberoptic bronchoscopy to help identify supraglottic and subglottic airway injury.[90] An important caveat is that lack of upper airway injury (e.g., oropharyngeal burns or singed nasal hairs) neither precludes nor predicts future airway demise. Patients should be risk-stratified on the basis of history (e.g., closed-space fire, particular materials in the fire, loss of consciousness, or history of reactive airway disease) before final disposition. Patients with any sign of airway injury or clinically significant smoke inhalation should be observed overnight. A normal initial chest radiograph is not a reliable indicator of pulmonary injury.[156] If exposure to a low-solubility toxin is likely (e.g., phosgene or nitrogen dioxide), manifestation of pulmonary injury may be delayed for 12 to 24 hours. Bronchodilators should be used for bronchospasm, but unlike treatment of patients with asthma and chronic obstructive pulmonary disease, use of steroids has not been shown to be beneficial in patients with smoke inhalation.[90] Patients with suspected cyanide poisoning should receive sodium thiosulfate [see Cyanide, above].

Kent R. Olson, M.D., has served as a paid expert consultant to McNeil Con-

sumer Products, the makers of Tylenol-brand acetaminophen.

Manish M. Patel, M.D., has no commercial relationships with manufacturers of products or providers of services discussed in this chapter.

References

1. Emergency department trends, final estimates 1995–2002: data from the Drug Abuse Warning Network (DAWN). US Department of Health and Human Services, Public Health Service, Alcohol, Drug Abuse, and Mental Health Administration (DHS Publication No [SMA] 03-3780), Rockville, Maryland, 2003
http://dawninfo.samhsa.gov/old_dawn

2. Mortality data: Data from the Drug Abuse Warning Network (DAWN). US Department of Health and Human Services, Public Health Service, Alcohol, Drug Abuse, and Mental Health Administration (DHS Publication No [SMA] 02-3633), Rockville, Maryland, 2002
http://dawninfo.samhsa.gov/old_dawn

3. Kharasch M, Graff J: Emergency management of the airway. Crit Care Clin 11:53, 1995

4. Powner DJ: Drug-associated isoelectric EEGs: a hazard in brain-death certification. JAMA 236:1123, 1976

5. Hoffman RS, Goldfrank LR: The poisoned patient with altered consciousness: controversies in the use of a 'coma cocktail.' JAMA 274:562, 1995

6. Sporer KA: Acute heroin overdose. Ann Intern Med 130:584, 1999

7. Bowden CA, Krenzelok EP: Clinical applications of commonly used contemporary antidotes: a US perspective. Drug Saf 16:9, 1997

8. Seger DL: Flumazenil: treatment or toxin. J Toxicol Clin Toxicol 42:209, 2004

9. Vernon DD, Gleich MC: Poisoning and drug overdose. Crit Care Clin 13:647, 1997

10. Krenzelok EP, Leikin JB: Approach to the poisoned patient. Dis Mon 42:509, 1996

11. Kolecki PF, Curry SC: Poisoning by sodium channel blocking agents. Crit Care Clin 13:829, 1997

12. Albertson TE, Dawson A, de Latorre F, et al: TOX-ACLS: toxicologic-oriented advanced cardiac life support. Ann Emerg Med 37:S78, 2001

13. Sing K, Erickson T, Amitai Y, et al: Chloral hydrate toxicity from oral and intravenous administration. J Toxicol Clin Toxicol 34:101, 1996

14. Leo PJ, Hollander JE, Shih RD, et al: Phenylpropanolamine and associated myocardial injury. Ann Emerg Med 28:359, 1996

15. Volz HP, Gleiter CH: Monoamine oxidase inhibitors: a perspective on their use in the elderly. Drugs Aging 13:341, 1998

16. Hsue PY, Salinas CL, Bolger AF, et al: Acute aortic dissection related to crack cocaine. Circulation 105:1592, 2002

17. Brust JC: Acute neurologic complications of drug and alcohol abuse. Neurol Clin 16:503, 1998

18. Hoffman RS, Hollander JE: Evaluation of patients with chest pain after cocaine use. Crit Care Clin 13:809, 1997

19. Olson KR, Kearney TE, Dyer JE, et al: Seizures associated with poisoning and drug overdose. Am J Emerg Med 12:392, 1994

20. Shepherd G, Velez LI, Keyes DC: Intentional bupropion overdoses. J Emerg Med 27:147, 2004

21. Bleck TP: Management approaches to prolonged seizures and status epilepticus. Epilepsia 40(suppl 1):S59, 1999

22. Halloran LL, Bernard DW: Management of drug-induced hyperthermia. Curr Opin Pediatr 16:211, 2004

23. Kempainen RR, Brunette DD: The evaluation and management of accidental hypothermia. Respir Care 49:192, 2004

24. Antretter H, Dapunt OE, Bonatti J: Management of profound hypothermia. Br J Hosp Med 54:215, 1995

25. Huerta-Alardin AL, Varon J, Marik PE: Bench-to-bedside review: rhabdomyolysis: an overview for clinicians. Crit Care 9:158, 2005

26. Salgia AD, Kosnik SD: When acetaminophen use becomes toxic: treating acute accidental and intentional overdose. Postgrad Med 105:81, 1999

27. Kirk M, Pace S: Pearls, pitfalls, and updates in toxicology. Emerg Med Clin North Am 15:427, 1997

28. Belson MG, Simon HK: Utility of comprehensive toxicologic screens in children. Am J Emerg Med 17:221, 1999

29. Manoguerra AS: Gastrointestinal decontamination after poisoning. Where is the science? Crit Care Clin 13:709, 1997

30. Bond GR: The role of activated charcoal and gastric emptying in gastrointestinal decontamination: a state-of-the-art review. Ann Emerg Med 39:273, 2002

31. Krenzelok E, Vale A: Position statements: gut contamination. American Academy of Clinical Toxicology: European Association of Poisons Centres and Clinical Toxicologists. J Toxicol Clin Toxicol 35:695, 1997

32. Position paper: ipecac syrup. J Toxicol Clin Toxicol 42:133, 2004

33. Poison treatment in the home. American Academy of Pediatrics Committee on Injury, Violence, and Poison Prevention. Pediatrics 112:1182, 2003

34. Pond SM, Lewis-Driver DJ, Williams GM, et al: Gastric emptying in acute overdose: a prospective randomised controlled trial. Med J Aust 163:345, 1995

35. Vale JA, Kulig K: Position paper: gastric lavage. J Toxicol Clin Toxicol 42:933, 2004

36. Position paper: cathartics. J Toxicol Clin Toxicol 42:243, 2004

37. Position paper: whole bowel irrigation. J Toxicol Clin Toxicol 42:843, 2004

38. Mowad E, Haddad I, Gemmel DJ: Management of lead poisoning from ingested fishing sinkers. Arch Pediatr Adolesc Med 152:485, 1998

39. van Bommel EF, Kalmeijer MD, Ponssen HH: Treatment of life-threatening lithium toxicity with high-volume continuous venovenous hemofiltration. Am J Nephrol 20:408, 2000

40. Bradberry SM, Vale JA: Multiple-dose activated charcoal: a review of relevant clinical studies. J Toxicol Clin Toxicol 33:407, 1995

41. Makin AJ, Wendon J, Williams R: A 7-year experience of severe acetaminophen-induced hepatotoxicity (1987–1993). Gastroenterology 109:1907, 1995

42. Whitcomb DC, Block GD: Association of acetaminophen hepatotoxicity with fasting and ethanol use. JAMA 272:1845, 1994

43. Bray GP, Harrison PM, O'Grady JG, et al: Long-term anticonvulsant therapy worsens outcome in paracetamol-induced fulminant hepatic failure. Hum Exp Toxicol 11:265, 1992

44. Jones AL: Mechanism of action and value of N-acetylcysteine in the treatment of early and late acetaminophen poisoning: a critical review. J Toxicol Clin Toxicol 36:277, 1998

45. Roth B, Woo O, Blanc P: Early metabolic acidosis and coma after acetaminophen ingestion. Ann Emerg Med 33:452, 1999

46. Brok J, Buckley N, Gluud C: Interventions for paracetamol (acetaminophen) overdoses (Cochrane Review). Cochrane Database Syst Rev (3):CD003328, 2002

47. Woo OF, Mueller PD, Olson KR, et al: Shorter duration of oral N-acetylcysteine therapy for acute acetaminophen overdose. Ann Emerg Med 35:363, 2000

48. Safety labeling changes approved by FDA Center for Drug Evaluation and Research (CDER)—April 2004. Acetadote (acetylcysteine) injection, accessed 2005
http://www.fda.gov/medwatch/SAFETY/2004/apr_PI/Acetadote_PI.pdf

49. Bailey B, McGuigan MA: Management of anaphylactoid reactions to intravenous N-acetylcysteine. Ann Emerg Med 31:710, 1998

50. Greene GS, Patterson SG, Warner E: Ingestion of angel's trumpet: an increasingly common source of toxicity. South Med J 89:365, 1996

51. Doig JC: Drug-induced cardiac arrhythmias: incidence, prevention and management. Drug Saf 17:265, 1997

52. de Abajo FJ, Rodriguez LA: Risk of ventricular arrhythmias associated with nonsedating antihistamine drugs. Br J Clin Pharmacol 47:307, 1999

53. Gottlieb S: Antihistamine drug withdrawn by manufacturer. BMJ 319:7, 1999

54. Burns MJ, Linden CH, Graudins A, et al: A comparison of physostigmine and benzodiazepines for the treatment of anticholinergic poisoning. Ann Emerg Med 35:374, 2000

55. Chua JD, Friedenberg W: Superwarfarin poisoning. Arch Intern Med 158:1929, 1998

56. Sheen SR, Spiller HA, Grossman D: Symptomatic brodifacoum ingestion requiring high-dose phytonadione therapy. Vet Hum Toxicol 36:216, 1994

57. Bruno GR, Howland MA, McMeeking A, et al: Long-acting anticoagulant overdose: brodifacoum kinetics and optimal vitamin K dosing. Ann Emerg Med 36:262, 2000

58. Love JN, Litovitz TL, Howell JM, et al: Characterization of fatal beta blocker ingestion: a review of the American Association of Poison Control Centers data from 1985 to 1995. J Toxicol Clin Toxicol 35:353, 1997

59. DeWitt CR, Waksman JC: Pharmacology, pathophysiology, and management of calcium channel blocker and beta-blocker toxicity. Toxicol Rev 23:223, 2004

60. Love JN, Handler JA: Toxic psychosis: an unusual presentation of propranolol intoxication. Am J Emerg Med 13:536, 1995

61. Miller MB: Arrhythmias associated with drug toxicity. Emerg Med Clin North Am 16:405, 1998

62. Ashraf M, Chaudhary K, Nelson J, et al: Massive overdose of sustained-release verapamil: a case report and review of literature. Am J Med Sci 310:258, 1995

63. Buckley N, Dawson AH, Howarth D, et al: Slow-release verapamil poisoning: use of polyethylene glycol whole-bowel lavage and high-dose calcium. Med J Aust 158:202, 1993

64. Yuan TH, Kerns WP, Tomaszewski CA, et al: Insulin-glucose as adjunctive therapy for severe calcium channel antagonist poisoning. J Toxicol Clin Toxicol 37:463, 1999

65. Carbon monoxide poisoning deaths associated with camping—Georgia, March 1999. MMWR Morb Mortal Wkly Rep 48:705, 1999

66. Carbon monoxide poisonings associated with snow-obstructed vehicle exhaust systems in Philadelphia and New York City, January 1996. MMWR Morb Mortal Wkly Rep 45:1, 1996

67. Carbon monoxide poisoning from hurricane-associated use of portable generators—Florida, 2004. MMWR Morb Mortal Wkly Rep 54:697, 2005

68. Hardy KR, Thom SR: Pathophysiology and treatment of carbon monoxide poisoning. J Toxicol Clin Toxicol 32:613, 1994

69. Weaver LK: Carbon monoxide poisoning. Crit Care Clin 15:297, 1999

70. Hampson NB: Pulse oximetry in severe carbon monoxide poisoning. Chest 114:1036, 1998

71. Weaver LK, Hopkins RO, Chan KJ, et al: Hyperbaric oxygen for acute carbon monoxide poisoning. N Engl J Med 347:1057, 2002

72. Van Meter KW, Weiss L, Harch PG, et al: Should the pressure be off or on in the use of oxygen in the treatment of carbon monoxide-poisoned patients? (editorial). Ann Emerg Med 24:283, 1994

73. Buckley NA, Isbister GK, Stokes B, et al: Hyperbaric oxygen for carbon monoxide poisoning: a systematic review and critical analysis of the evidence. Toxicol Rev 24:75, 2005

74. Scheinkestel CD, Bailey M, Myles PS, et al: Hyperbaric or normobaric oxygen for acute carbon monoxide poisoning: a randomised controlled clinical trial. Med J Aust 170:203, 1999

75. Elkharrat D, Raphael JC, Korach JM, et al: Acute carbon monoxide intoxication and hyperbaric oxygen in pregnancy. Intensive Care Med 17:289, 1991

76. Results from the 2004 National Survey on Drug Use and Health: national findings. Substance Abuse and Mental Health Services Administration, US Department of Health and Human Services, Public Health Service, Alcohol, Drug Abuse, and Mental Health Administration, 2005
http://oas.samhsa.gov/nsduh/2k4nsduh/2k4Results/apph.htm

77. Benowitz NL: Clinical pharmacology and toxicology of cocaine. Pharmacol Toxicol 72:3, 1993

78. Henning RJ, Wilson LD, Glauser JM: Cocaine plus ethanol is more cardiotoxic than cocaine or ethanol alone. Crit Care Med 22:1896, 1994

79. Ecstasy, LSD, PCP, and other hallucinogens: data from 2001 National Household Survey on Drug Abuse. Substance Abuse and Mental Health Services Administration, US Department of Health and Human Services, Public Health Service, Alcohol, Drug Abuse, and Mental Health Administration.
http://oas.samhsa.gov/ecstasy.htm#Trends

80. Club Drugs, 2002 Update. Drug Abuse Warning Network [DAWN]. The DAWN Report, 2002
http://oas.samhsa.gov/2k4/clubdrugs/clubdrugs.cfm

81. Kalant H: The pharmacology and toxicology of "ecstasy" (MDMA) and related drugs. CMAJ 165:917, 2001

82. Patel MM, Wright DW, Ratcliff JJ, et al: Shedding new light on the "safe" club drug: methylenedioxymethamphetamine (ecstasy)-related fatalities. Acad Emerg Med 11:208, 2004

83. Pharmaceuticals: national drug threat assessment 2005. National Drug Intelligence Center, February 2005
http://www.usdoj.gov/ndic/pubs11/12620/pharma.htm

84. White SR, Yadao CM: Characterization of methylphenidate exposures reported to a regional poison control center. Arch Pediatr Adolesc Med 154:1199, 2000

85. McCabe SE, Knight JR, Teter CJ, et al: Non-medical use of prescription stimulants among US college students: prevalence and correlates from a national survey. Addiction 100:96, 2005

86. Kao WF, Dart RC, Kuffner E, et al: Ingestion of low-concentration hydrofluoric acid: an insidious and potentially fatal poisoning. Ann Emerg Med 34:35, 1999

87. Matsuno K: The treatment of hydrofluoric acid burns. Occup Med (Lond) 46:313, 1996

88. Beasley DM, Glass WI: Cyanide poisoning: pathophysiology and treatment recommendations. Occup Med (Lond) 48:427, 1998

89. Shusterman D, Alexeeff G, Hargis C, et al: Predictors of carbon monoxide and hydrogen cyanide exposure in smoke inhalation patients. J Toxicol Clin Toxicol 34:61, 1996

90. Bizovi KE, Leikin JD: Smoke inhalation among firefighters. Occup Med 10:721, 1995

91. Sauer SW, Keim ME: Hydroxocobalamin: improved public health readiness for cyanide disasters. Ann Emerg Med 37:635, 2001

92. Dasgupta A, Emerson L: Neutralization of cardiac toxins oleandrin, oleandrigenin, bufalin, and cinobufotalin by digibind: monitoring the effect by measuring free digitoxin concentrations. Life Sci 63:781, 1998

93. Marik PE, Fromm L: A case series of hospitalized patients with elevated digoxin levels. Am J Med 105:110, 1998

94. Derlet RW, Horowitz BZ: Cardiotoxic drugs. Emerg Med Clin North Am 13:771, 1995

95. Williamson KM, Thrasher KA, Fulton KB, et al: Digoxin toxicity: an evaluation in current clinical practice. Arch Intern Med 158:2444, 1999

96. de Silva HA, Fonseka MM, Pathmeswaran A, et al: Multiple-dose activated charcoal for treatment of yellow oleander poisoning: a single-blind, randomised, placebo-controlled trial. Lancet 361:1935, 2003

97. Freedland ES, McMicken DB, D'Onofrio G: Alcohol and trauma. Emerg Med Clin North Am 11:225, 1993

98. Glaser DS: Utility of the serum osmol gap in the diagnosis of methanol or ethylene glycol ingestion. Ann Emerg Med 27:343, 1996

99. Jacobsen D, McMartin KE: Antidotes for methanol and ethylene glycol poisoning. J Toxicol Clin Toxicol 35:127, 1997

100. Galloway GP, Frederick SL, Staggers FE Jr, et al: Gamma-hydroxybutyrate: an emerging drug of abuse that causes physical dependence. Addiction 92:89, 1997

101. Adverse events associated with ingestion of gamma-butyrolactone—Minnesota, New Mexico, and Texas, 1998–1999. MMWR Morb Mortal Wkly Rep 48:137, 1999

102. Chin RL, Sporer KA, Cullison B, et al: Clinical course of gamma-hydroxybutyrate overdose. Ann Emerg Med 31:716, 1998

103. Dyer JE, Roth B, Hyma BA: Gamma-hydroxybutyrate withdrawal syndrome. Ann Emerg Med 37:147, 2001

104. Addolorato G, Caputo F, Capristo E, et al: A case of gamma-hydroxybutyric acid withdrawal syndrome during alcohol addiction treatment: utility of diazepam administration. Clin Neuropharmacol 22:60, 1999

105. McGuigan MA: Acute iron poisoning. Pediatr Ann 25:33, 1996

106. Siff JE, Meldon SW, Tomassoni AJ: Usefulness of the total iron binding capacity in the evaluation and treatment of acute iron overdose. Ann Emerg Med 33:73, 1999

107. Romero JA, Kuczler FJ Jr: Isoniazid overdose: recognition and management. Am Fam Physician 57:749, 1998

108. Temmerman W, Dhondt A, Vandewoude K: Acute isoniazid intoxication: seizures, acidosis and coma. Acta Clin Belg 54:211, 1999

109. Graeme KA, Pollack CV Jr: Heavy metal toxicity, part II: lead and metal fume fever. J Emerg Med 16:171, 1998

110. Markowitz SB, Nunez CM, Klitzman S, et al: Lead poisoning due to hai ge fen: the porphyrin content of individual erythrocytes. JAMA 271:932, 1994

111. Gordon RA, Roberts G, Amin Z, et al: Aggressive approach in the treatment of acute lead encephalopathy with an extraordinarily high concentration of lead. Arch Pediatr Adolesc Med 152:1100, 1998

112. Rogan WJ, Dietrich KN, Ware JH, et al: The effect of chelation therapy with succimer on neuropsychological development in children exposed to lead. N Engl J Med 344:1421, 2001

113. Staudinger KC, Roth VS: Occupational lead poisoning. Am Fam Physician 57:719, 1998

114. Timmer RT, Sands JM: Lithium intoxication. J Am Soc Nephrol 10:666, 1999

115. Kores B, Lader MH: Irreversible lithium neurotoxicity: an overview. Clin Neuropharmacol 20:283, 1997

116. Gehrke JC, Watling SM, Gehrke CW, et al: In-vivo binding of lithium using the cation exchange resin sodium polystyrene sulfonate. Am J Emerg Med 14:37, 1996

117. Bailey B, McGuigan M: Comparison of patients hemodialyzed for lithium poisoning and those for whom dialysis was recommended by PCC but not done: what lesson can we learn? Clin Nephrol 54:388, 2000

118. Coleman MD, Coleman NA: Drug-induced methaemoglobinaemia: treatment issues. Drug Saf 14:394, 1996

119. Moore TJ, Walsh CS, Cohen MR: Reported adverse event cases of methemoglobinemia associated with benzocaine products. Arch Intern Med 164:1192, 2004

120. Sinex JE: Pulse oximetry: principles and limitations. Am J Emerg Med 17:59, 1999

121. Gowing L, Ali R, White J: Buprenorphine for the management of opioid withdrawal. Cochrane Database Syst Rev 18:CD002025, 2004

122. Mills KC: Serotonin syndrome: a clinical update. Crit Care Clin 13:763, 1997

123. Wanger K, Brough L, Macmillan I, et al: Intravenous vs subcutaneous naloxone for out-of-hospital management of presumed opioid overdose. Acad Emerg Med 5:293, 1998

124. Bardin PG, van Eeden SF, Moolman JA, et al: Organophosphate and carbamate poisoning. Arch Intern Med 154:1433, 1994

125. Holstege CP, Kirk M, Sidell FR: Chemical warfare: nerve agent poisoning. Crit Care Clin 13:923, 1997

126. Lifshitz M, Rotenberg M, Sofer S, et al: Carbamate poisoning and oxime treatment in children: a clinical and laboratory study. Pediatrics 93:652, 1994

127. De Bleecker J, Van den Neucker K, Colardyn F: Intermediate syndrome in organophosphorus poisoning: a prospective study. Crit Care Med 21:1706, 1993

128. Yip L, Dart RC, Gabow PA: Concepts and controversies in salicylate toxicity. Emerg Med Clin North Am 12:351, 1994

129. Chui PT: Anesthesia in a patient with undiagnosed salicylate poisoning presenting as intraabdominal sepsis. J Clin Anesth 11:251, 1999

130. Fraser AD: Use and abuse of the benzodiazepines. Ther Drug Monit 20:481, 1998

131. Coupey SM: Barbiturates. Pediatr Rev 18:260, 1997

132. Hojer J, Baehrendtz S, Gustafsson L: Benzodiazepine poisoning: experience of 702 admissions to an intensive care unit during a 14-year period. J Intern Med 226:117, 1989

133. Zahedi A, Grant MH, Wong DT: Successful treatment of chloral hydrate cardiac toxicity with propranolol. Am J Emerg Med 17:490, 1999

134. Herrington AM, Clifton GD: Toxicology and management of acute drug ingestions in adults. Pharmacotherapy 15:182, 1995

135. Shannon M: Hypokalemia, hyperglycemia and plasma catecholamine activity after severe theophylline intoxication. J Toxicol Clin Toxicol 32:41, 1994

136. Shannon M: Life-threatening events after theophylline overdose: a 10-year prospective analysis. Arch Intern Med 159:989, 1999

137. Kempf J, Rusterholtz T, Ber C, et al: Haemodynamic study as guideline for the use of beta blockers in acute theophylline poisoning. Intensive Care Med 22:585, 1996

138. Shannon MW: Comparative efficacy of hemodialysis and hemoperfusion in severe theophylline intoxication. Acad Emerg Med 4:674, 1997

139. Shanon M, Liebelt E: Targeted management strategies for cardiovascular toxicity from tricyclic antidepressant overdose: the pivotal role for alkalinization and sodium loading. Pediatr Emerg Care 14:293, 1998

140. Harrigan RA, Brady WJ: ECG abnormalities in tricyclic antidepressant ingestion. Am J Emerg Med 17:387, 1999

141. Update: Neurologic illness associated with eating Florida pufferfish, 2002. MMWR Morb Mortal Wkly Rep 51:414, 2002

142. Schnorf H, Taurarii M, Cundy T: Ciguatera fish poisoning: a double-blind randomized trial of mannitol therapy. Neurology 58:873, 2002

143. Ting JY, Brown AF: Ciguatera poisoning: a global issue with common management problems. Eur J Emerg Med 8:295, 2001

144. Davis RT, Villar LA: Symptomatic improvement with amitriptyline in ciguatera fish poisoning. N Engl J Med 315:65, 1986

145. Berlin RM, King SL, Blythe DG: Symptomatic improvement of chronic fatigue with fluoxetine in ciguatera fish poisoning. Med J Aust 157:567, 1992

146. Perez CM, Vasquez PA, Perret CF: Treatment of ciguatera poisoning with gabapentin. N Engl J Med 344:692, 2001

147. Yamada EG, Mohle-Boetani J, Olson KR, et al: Mushroom poisoning due to amatoxin. Northern California, Winter 1996–1997. West J Med 169:380, 1998

148. Yang WH, Drouin MA, Herbert M, et al: The monosodium glutamate symptom

complex: assessment in a double-blind, placebo-controlled, randomized study. J Allergy Clin Immunol 99:757, 1997

149. Tarasoff L, Kelly MF: Monosodium L-glutamate: a double blind study and review. Food Chem Toxicol 31:1019, 1993

150. Barnes PM, Powell-Griner E, McFann K, et al: Complementary and alternative medicine use among adults: United States, 2002. Advance Data from Vital and Health Statistics, no 343. National Center for Health Statistics, Hyattsville, Maryland, 2004 http://www.cdc.gov/nchs/data/ad/ad343.pdf

151. Matthews MK Jr: Association of Ginkgo biloba with intracerebral hemorrhage (letter). Neurology 50:1933, 1998

152. Haller CA, Benowitz NL: Adverse cardiovascular and central nervous system events associated with dietary supplements containing ephedra alkaloids. N Engl J Med 343:1833, 2000

153. Final rule declaring dietary supplements containing ephedrine alkaloids adulterated because they present an unreasonable risk: final rule. Fed Regist 69:6787, 2004

154. Hill IR: Reactions to particles in smoke. Toxicology 115:119, 1996

155. Weiss SM, Lakshminarayan S: Acute inhalation injury. Clin Chest Med 15:103, 1994

156. Wittram C, Kenny JB: The admission chest radiograph after acute inhalation injury and burns. Br J Radiol 67:751, 1994

157. Harpe C, Stoudemire A: Aetiology and treatment of neuroleptic malignant syndrome. Medical Toxicology 2:166, 1987

158. Sessler DI: Malignant hyperthermia. J Pediatr 109:9, 1986

159. Goldberg RJ, Huk M: Serotonin syndrome from trazodone and buspirone (letter). Psychosomatics 33:235, 1992

160. Sternbach H: The serotonin syndrome. Am J Psychiatry 148:705, 1991

161. Benowitz NL: Beta-adrenergic blockers. Poisoning & Drug Overdose, 4th ed. Olson KR, Ed. Appleton & Lange, Norwalk, Connecticut, 2004

162. Stremski ES, Grande GA, Ling LJ: Survival following hydrofluoric acid ingestion. Ann Emerg Med 21:1396, 1992

163. Bertolini JC: Hydrofluoric acid: a review of toxicity. J Emerg Med 10:163, 1992

164. Spiller HA, Quadrani-Kushner DA, Cleveland P: A five year evaluation of acute exposures to phenol disinfectant (26%). J Toxicol Clin Toxicol 31:307, 1993

165. Hunter DM, Timerding BL, Leonard RB, et al: Effects of isopropyl alcohol, ethanol, and polyethylene glycol/industrial methylated spirits in the treatment of acute phenol burns. Ann Emerg Med 21:1303, 1992

166. Suzuki K, Takasu N, Arita S, et al: Evaluation of severity indexes of patients with paraquat poisoning. Hum Exp Toxicol 10:21, 1991

167. Karlson-Stiber C, Persson H: Ethylene glycol poisoning: experiences from an epidemic in Sweden. J Toxicol Clin Toxicol 30:565, 1992

168. Gaudet MP, Fraser GL: Isopropanol ingestion: case report with pharmacokinetic analysis. Am J Emerg Med 7:297, 1989

169. Becker CE: Methanol poisoning. J Emerg Med 1:51, 1983

170. Kim S: Food poisoning: fish and shellfish. Poisoning & Drug Overdose, 4th ed. Olson KR, Ed. Appleton & Lange, Stamford, Connecticut, 2004

Acknowledgment

Figure 1   Tom Moore. Data from "Acetaminophen poisoning and toxicity," by B. H. Rumack and H. Matthew, in *Pediatrics* 55:871, 1975.

16 Bites and Stings

Lawrence M. Lewis, M.D., William H. Dribben, M.D., and Mark D. Levine, M.D.

Mammalian Bites

EPIDEMIOLOGY

There were an estimated four and a half million cases of dog bites in the United States in 1994, the most recent year for which published statistics are available.[1] Over a lifetime, over half of all Americans are bitten by a dog or cat.[2] Although the majority of victims with bite wounds treat themselves, nearly 370,000 dog-bite victims required medical attention in an emergency department in 2001.[3] This is an increase of 10% to 15% over that reported for 1992 to 1994.[4] The highest incidence of dog-bite injuries is in boys 5 to 9 years of age (60.7 per 10,000 person-years).[4] Children are also more likely to be bitten on the face, head, and neck than are adults.[4] Infection, the most common complication of bite wounds, arises from microbes either on the victim's skin or in the mouth of the human or animal inflicting the bite wound. The relative risk of infection is determined by a number of factors, including the species of animal inflicting the wound, the location of the bite, the size and depth of the wound, host factors, and the type of wound care given.[5-7] Most infections that result from mammalian bites are polymicrobial, with mixed aerobic and anaerobic species.[8] Nonetheless, certain species tend to cause infections with characteristic bacteriologic pathogens. In addition, transmission of the rabies virus may occur through bites from mammals of certain species.

DOMESTIC ANIMALS

Dog Bites

Dogs are responsible for more bite wounds in patients who seek medical attention than all other animals combined.[9] Most bites are inflicted by animals known to the victim, with strays accounting for less than 10% of reported bite-wound injuries.[9] Wounds occur most frequently on the extremities, except in young children, in whom bite wounds to the face, head, and neck are most common.[4,10] Specifically, bite wounds to the hand occur in anywhere from one fifth to one half of reported cases; such wounds are associated with an increased risk of infection, particularly tenosynovitis, closed-space compartment infection, and septic arthritis.[11] Although deaths from dog attacks are rare, this tragic scenario occurs about 12 to 15 times a year in the United States (238 dog-bite–related deaths from 1979 through 1998). Pit-bull–type dogs and Rottweilers are responsible for over half of the reported deaths.[12]

The oral bacterial flora of dogs includes *Pasteurella multocida*, *Staphylococcus aureus*, *Capnocytophaga canimorsus*, *S. epidermidis*, *Streptococcus* species, and a number of anaerobes. Mixed aerobic and anaerobic infection is present in about half of infected dog bites.[8] The aerobic organisms most commonly isolated from infected dog bites include *Pasteurella*, *Staphylococcus*, and *Streptococcus* species.[8,13] The anaerobic organisms most commonly isolated from dog bites include *Fusobacterium*, *Bacteroides*, *Porphyromonas*, and *Prevotella* species.[8,13] Anaerobic organisms are significantly more common in cultures from abscesses than from other types of infection.[6]

Dog bites are unlikely to become infected, with infection rates usually reported to be on the order of 5% to 10%.[14,15] However, the risk of infection is higher in older persons and in persons with diabetes, vascular disease, chronic alcoholism, or immunosuppression. Infection risk is also higher in puncture wounds, in wounds on the hand or foot or over a joint, and in wounds associated with crush injuries.[11]

Dog bites infected with *Capnocytophaga canimorsus* may cause an overwhelming sepsislike picture associated with high fever, leukocytosis, disseminated intravascular coagulation (DIC), and multiorgan failure. This complication of dog-bite injuries is seen most commonly in immunocompromised patients (e.g., those with asplenia, alcoholism, or hematologic malignancy) and carries a 25% mortality.[11]

Globally, dogs are the major reservoirs for rabies.[16] In developed countries, however, vaccination programs have reduced the prevalence of canine rabies; for example, only 117 rabid dogs were reported in the United States in 2003.[17] Rabies is discussed in detail elsewhere [*see Chapter 154*].

Cat Bites

Cat bites are the second most common mammalian bites in the United States, accounting for 5% to 15% of all reported bites. About two thirds of all cat bites occur on the upper extremity. Cat bites are more often puncture wounds than tearing lacerations and often appear innocuous initially. However, the infection rate for cat bites is reported to be 15% to 30%, or almost triple that for dog bites.[18,19] *P. multocida* is the major pathogen associated with cat bites, being found in about three fourths of infected cat-bite wounds.[8] *P. multocida* infection progresses rapidly, with pain, swelling, and erythema usually occurring within 24 hours.[9] The types of anaerobic organisms found in cat bites are similar to those found in dog bites (see above), although anaerobic isolates are somewhat more common in cat bites. Penetration into deep tissues with resultant osteomyelitis or septic arthritis is more common with cat bites than dog bites.[13] Cat-scratch disease (CSD) is an infection arising from a rickettsia-like organism, *Bartonella henselae*; CSD is discussed in detail elsewhere [*see Chapter 141*].

Cats continue to outnumber dogs by more than 2 to 1 as the most common domestic rabid animal.[15,20] Overall, however, domestic animals account for only a small minority of animal rabies cases in the United States; about 90% occur in wildlife [*see Chapter 154*].

Ferret Bites

Ferrets have become increasingly popular as pets; a 1996 survey suggested that there are almost 800,000 ferrets in the United States.[21] Ferret attacks are uncommon but can result in severe injury, especially to infants and small children.[22,23] These attacks (in contrast to dog or cat bites) are usually unprovoked.[22,23]

The bacteriologic flora in ferrets has not been well studied. One study showed that facultative anaerobic gram-positive cocci were the predominant organisms, followed by *Pasteurella* and *Corynebacterium* species; few strict anaerobes were detected.[24]

Ferrets are clearly capable of contracting and carrying the rabies virus.[25] However, it is not known how long infected ferrets can shed virus before showing clinical signs of disease, thus making quarantine recommendations problematic. Although there is an approved rabies vaccine for use in ferrets, its efficacy in preventing rabies is currently not known.[26] For ferret bites involving animals suspected of being rabid, current recommendations are to give the patient rabies postexposure prophylaxis immediately. For cases involving ferrets that are not suspected of being rabid, the recommendation is to withhold vaccination and to observe the animal for 10 days; the patient should be vaccinated only if the animal shows signs of rabies during that period.[27]

HUMAN BITES

Human bites are the third most common mammalian bite in the United States, accounting for approximately 5% to more than 20% of bite wounds seen in urban emergency departments.[11,18,28] Most human-bite wounds occur on the extremities, with an unusually high percentage being over the metacarpal-phalangeal joint secondary to a clenched fist contacting a tooth. Traditionally, human-bite wounds have had a reputation for frequent and severe complications. Current data, however, suggest an infection rate from human-bite wounds on the order of 10% to 50%, depending on the wound type and location.[11,16,28] Occlusional/simple bite wounds to areas other than the hand probably are no more at risk for infection than any other type of bite wound and minimally more than for nonbite lacerations.[11,16,17,29,30] However, human-bite wounds to the hand are associated with infection rates of almost 50%.[18] A clenched-fist injury is considered the most serious of all human-bite wounds.[1] These injuries may appear innocent at first but progress to serious infections that may include the joint, tendons, or various compartments of the hand. These injuries require meticulous wound care, appropriate antibiotic therapy, and consultation with a hand surgeon. Bacterial pathogens associated with human-bite wounds include a number of anaerobes similar to those recovered from dog and cat bites, but with a much higher percentage of β-lactamase producers.[19,31,32] The predominant aerobes are *Staphylococcus* and *Streptococcus* species. About 10% to 30% of human-bite wounds have been shown to contain *Eikenella corrodens*, a facultative anaerobe.[18,28,33,34] *E. corrodens* is present in 25% of clenched-fist injuries and often causes serious, chronic infections.[34] Besides bacterial infection, human bites can transmit the hepatitis B virus, HIV, herpes simplex virus, tuberculosis, and even syphilis.[11,13,28,35] Prophylactic therapy against hepatitis B or HIV should be considered for patients bitten by persons considered at high risk for these diseases.

NONDOMESTIC ANIMALS

Rats

Rat bites are uncommon, representing less than 2% of the bite wounds seen in one urban emergency department.[36] Although the list of potential pathogens that could be transmitted from rat bites is daunting, infections from rat bites, including rabies, are, in fact, very infrequent.[37] Rat-bite fever is a disease caused by *Streptobacillus moniliformis*, a gram-negative rod. It is associated with fever, chills, headache, myalgia, and rash and usually begins abruptly about 3 to 10 days after inoculation [*see Chapter 144*].

Bats

Although bat bites typically produce only trivial trauma, bat bites were responsible for almost 75% of all human rabies cases

Table 1 Bite Wounds Requiring Prophylactic Antibiotics

Wound characteristics	Puncture wounds Full-thickness wounds Hand or foot wounds Wounds requiring surgical repair Treatment delay (> 24 hr) Human bites* Cat bites*
Patient characteristics	Age > 50 yr Immunosuppression (e.g., asplenia, alcoholism, corticosteroid use) Diabetes mellitus Peripheral vascular disease

*There is debate, but many authors recommend prophylactic antibiotic treatment for virtually all human and cat bites because of the high rate of infection.

reported in the United States since 1990 and for 90% of all cases acquired in the United States from 1981 through 1998.[37,38] Studies suggest that cleaning a bite wound with soap and a virucidal agent is effective in lowering the risk of rabies transmission.[39] Rabies prophylaxis is recommended for any bat exposures unless immediate brain testing of the animal can be performed.

Other Mammals

Skunks, raccoons, and foxes are also important animal reservoirs of rabies in the United States.[38] Bites from raccoons, skunks, and foxes should be regarded as likely to be rabid until proved otherwise, and the use of rabies immune globulin and rabies vaccine is warranted, particularly if rabies is endemic to the area or the animal's behavior is deemed abnormal.[39]

Bite wounds from wild animals are rare; most occur from exposure at zoos or from owning or harboring exotic animals.[40] The incidence of serious injury from wild-animal attacks among the three million visitors to Yellowstone National Park is reported to be lower than the chance of being struck by lightning.[40]

Bite wounds from nonhuman primates are rare. In addition to transmitting bacterial infection, these bites may transmit *Herpesvirus simiae* or monkey B virus [*see Chapter 154*]. If left untreated, monkey B virus infection often causes encephalitis, resulting in death or permanent neurologic impairment.[41] Monkey B virus is enzootic in North African and Asian monkeys, including the macaque and rhesus. Thorough scrubbing of bites or scratches with soap or detergent and irrigation for 15 minutes have been shown to reduce the viral inoculum.[42]

TREATMENT

The goals of bite-wound care are to recognize and treat serious injury (e.g., nerve or tendon laceration), avoid infection (both local and systemic), and achieve a good cosmetic result. The treatment of mammalian-bite wounds begins with a history and physical examination. The history should include when and where the bite occurred, the events leading to the bite, what type of animal was responsible for the bite, and any background information on the animal. Any treatment rendered before arrival at the facility, as well as the patient's tetanus immunization history, should be documented.

A careful physical examination to assess for arterial or major venous injury and nerve, joint, bone, or tendon involvement should be performed and documented. The wound should be explored for foreign bodies, including teeth or tooth fragments.

Table 2   Common and Important Pathogens and Antibiotic Selection for Various Mammalian Bite Wounds

Animal	Pathogen	Antibiotics
Dog	*Staphylococcus, Streptococcus, Capnocytophaga canimorsus, Pasteurella multocida,* anaerobes	Amoxicillin–clavulanic acid, third-generation fluoroquinolones, doxycycline*
Cat	*P. multocida, Staphylococcus, Streptococcus,* anaerobes	Amoxicillin–clavulanic acid, third-generation fluoroquinolones, doxycycline*
Human	*Staphylococcus, Streptococcus,* anaerobes, *Eikenella corrodens*	Amoxicillin–clavulanic acid, third-generation fluoroquinolones
Rodents	*Staphylococcus, Streptococcus, S. moniliformis*	Penicillin G (for *S. moniliformis*), amoxicillin–clavulanic acid, doxycycline*
Nonhuman primates	*Staphylococcus, Streptococcus,* monkey B virus	Amoxicillin–clavulanic acid; third-generation fluoroquinolones; acyclovir, valacyclovir, or famciclovir (for monkey B virus)

*Consider doxycycline in penicillin-allergic patients but do not use in pregnant patients or young children.

After the examination and provision of adequate anesthesia, the wound should be meticulously cleaned and irrigated. Wound soaking or scrubbing is to be avoided. Irrigation with 200 to 250 ml of normal saline or dilute povidone-iodine solution using moderate pressure (20 psi, the pressure generated using a syringe and a 19-gauge needle) has been shown to decrease wound infection fivefold.[16,43] Careful debridement of nonviable or grossly contaminated tissue may be necessary. If the risk of rabies is high, a benzalkonium chloride scrub should be used, because povidone-iodine irrigation has not been shown to be effective in reducing viral load.[16] Benzalkonium chloride should be rinsed out to avoid tissue irritation.

Whether lacerations associated with bite wounds should be treated with primary closure is an area of debate. A number of studies suggest that it is safe to suture bite-wound lacerations that are greater than 1 to 2 cm in length and less than 12 hours old—especially those about the head and face, where there is good circulation and greater concern for a good cosmetic result.[44,45] Bite wounds to the hand and to the lower extremities often result in complications and probably have increased rates of infection with primary closure.[44,46]

The use of prophylactic antibiotics for any bite wound is debatable,[47] but there is general consensus that certain wounds in all patients and most wounds in certain patients deserve prophylactic antibiotics [*see Table 1*]. The antibiotic of choice for prophylaxis of most mammalian-bite wounds is amoxicillin–clavulanic acid. For the penicillin-allergic patient, a third-generation fluoroquinolone (e.g., moxifloxacin)[48] or a cephalosporin (e.g., ce-

fotaxime)[49] serves as a good alternative [*see Table 2*]. The timing of prophylactic antibiotics is important. Prophylactic antibiotics should be given as soon after the bite injury as possible. A systematic review suggests that prophylactic antibiotics may reduce the incidence of infection in all hand-bite wounds and human bites, regardless of location.[49]

Tetanus prophylaxis should be given to those patients who have not been immunized in the previous 10 years [*see Table 3*]. The standard adult dose is 0.5 ml of tetanus and diphtheria toxoids adsorbed, given intramuscularly. If tetanus immune globulin is required, it is usually given in a single dose of 250 units intramuscularly, but not in the same arm as the tetanus toxoid.

Postexposure rabies prophylaxis consists first and foremost of appropriate wound care. The use of rabies immune globulin and vaccine administration depend on local epidemiology, the animal involved (species and behavior), and the type of exposure[16] [*see Chapter 154*]. Postexposure rabies prophylaxis for domestic animal bites is warranted in any of the following circumstances: (1) the animal is observed to be abnormal, (2) the animal is not available for observation and the rate of endemic rabies in domestic animals for the region is not exceedingly low, or (3) the animal exhibited abnormal behavior, including an unprovoked attack [*see Table 4*].[26]

Snakebites

EPIDEMIOLOGY

Over 3,000 species of snakes exist worldwide. Snakes are found everywhere on Earth except for the Arctic and Antarctic, New Zealand, Madagascar, and a few small islands. Snakes live in almost all land environments and in both saltwater and freshwater.

Approximately 10% of snakes are venomous. Of the 14 families of snakes, only five include venomous species: the Colubridae, Hydrophidae (sea snakes), Elapidae (cobras, kraits, mambas, and coral snakes), Viperidae (Russell viper, puff adder, Gaboon viper, saw-scaled viper, and European viper), and Crotalidae (rattlesnake, water moccasin, copperhead, bushmaster, and fer-de-lance). Snakes are carnivores; venomous snakes use their venom to immobilize prey for digestive purposes.

The number of snakebites in the United States is estimated to be approximately 8,000 a year. Many bites occur when patients are hiking, walking, or handling a snake. Frequently, the patient is intoxicated at the time of the bite.[50] Most snakebites do not result in envenomation, but nine to 15 deaths occur annually from

Table 3   Recommendations for Tetanus Prophylaxis after Animal Bites

Primary Tetanus Immunization Series Received?	Wound	Time since Last Tetanus Toxoid Dose	Recommended Prophylaxis
Yes	Clean, minor	> 10 yr	Td*
	All other	> 5 yr	Td*
Uncertain	Clean, minor	—	Td*
	All other	—	Td*, TIG†

*Adult (> 7 yr) Td dose is 0.5 ml I.M.; DTaP (diphtheria, tetanus, acellular pertussis) vaccine may be used in patients younger than 7 yr.
†Dose of TIG is 250 units I.M.; give in opposite arm from Td.

Td—diphtheria and tetanus toxoids adsorbed   TIG—tetanus immune globulin

Table 4   Recommendations for Rabies Postexposure Prophylaxis[27]

Animal Type	Evaluation and Disposition of Animal	Postexposure Prophylaxis Recommendations
Dogs, cats, ferrets	Healthy and available for 10 days of observation Rabid or suspected rabid Unknown (e.g., escaped)	Do not begin prophylaxis unless animal develops clinical signs of rabies* Immediately vaccinate Consult public health officials
Skunks, raccoons, foxes, most other carnivores; bats	Regarded as rabid unless animal proved negative by laboratory tests†	Consider immediate vaccination
Livestock, small rodents, lagomorphs (rabbits and hares), large rodents (woodchucks and beavers), other mammals	Consider individually	Consult public health officials; bites of squirrels, hamsters, guinea pigs, gerbils, chipmunks, rats, mice, other small rodents, rabbits, and hares almost never require antirabies postexposure prophylaxis

*During the 10-day observation period, begin postexposure prophylaxis at first sign of rabies in a dog, cat, or ferret that has bitten someone. If the animal exhibits clinical signs of rabies, it should be euthanized immediately and tested.

†The animal should be euthanized and tested as soon as possible. Holding for observation is not recommended. Discontinue vaccine if immunofluorescence test results of the animal are negative.

bites that do result in envenomation.[51] In the United States, rattlesnake bites most frequently result in significant envenomation and death.

Snakes are most active in the spring, when they begin to mate and are no longer hibernating[52]; however, the incidence of snakebite is highest in the summer months. Snakes remain active throughout the day and night, but because they are poikilothermic, they must contain their activity within a narrow temperature range of approximately 25° to 35° C.

CORAL SNAKES

The range of the eastern coral snake extends from North Carolina south and west to Texas. The western coral snake is found mainly in Arizona and New Mexico. Coral snakes are nocturnal and shy away from human contact.

Coral snakes are identified by their color, pattern, and permanently erect fangs. The nose of the coral snake is black, and the body has black, red, and yellow bands. The black bands do not separate the red and yellow bands, as they do on the nonvenomous but similarly banded kingsnake. This pattern is commonly remembered through the rhyme "red on black, venom lack; red on yellow, kills a fellow" [see Figure 1]. Coral snakes release their venom slowly, so they attach themselves to their prey and envenomate through a chewing motion. Instead of the puncture wounds typical of most snakebites, the chewing leaves what appear to be scratches on the skin.[52,53]

The bite of the eastern coral snake can be fatal. There are no confirmed fatalities from western coral snake envenomations.

PIT VIPERS

In the United States, pit vipers (Crotalidae) are found in all states except Maine, Alaska, and Hawaii. South America has nine subspecies of rattlesnakes; Mexico and Central America have four subspecies of rattlesnakes. These snakes can be found in a variety of habitats and at elevations up to 14,000 ft. The eastern and western diamondback rattlesnakes (*Crotalus adamanteus* and *C. strox*) [see Figure 2] are the largest and most dangerous in the United States and are found in the southwestern states and in Nevada, California, and Oklahoma.[54,55] The timber rattlesnake (*C. horridus*) is the second most dangerous rattlesnake common to the eastern United States, but it is rarely found in Delaware, Maine, Michigan, or Washington, D.C. Pigmy rattlesnakes (*Sistrurus catenatus* and *S. miliarius*) are found in areas ranging from New York to Michigan and from Texas to Arizona; they

have the least toxic venom of all the rattlesnakes.[51] Overall, rattlesnakes are responsible for 65% of envenomations in the United States. Their venom is 2.5 to 5 times more toxic than other North American species of venomous snakes.[50] Cottonmouths (*Agkistrodon piscivorus*), also known as water moccasins, live in the southern and southeastern states along streams and in low-lying trees. Copperheads (*A. contortix*) [see Figure 3] are found in mountains, rock piles, and sawdust piles. Their range extends from Massachusetts southwest to Texas. Cottonmouths and copperheads have only moderately toxic venom; their bite is painful but rarely fatal. In a study of 400 copperhead bites, 32 of which were treated with antivenin, 88% of bites responded to the antivenin, as evidenced by a cessation of local tissue injury progression.[56]

Pit vipers are identified by a small depression (pit) between the eyes and the nostrils bilaterally. They have a triangular-shaped head, an elliptical pupil, and fangs that fold back when the mouth is closed and unfold via a hingelike mechanism when the mouth is opened. The pit is a heat-sensitive organ that enables the snake to locate live, warm-blooded prey. Snakes can detect movement at a distance of about 40 ft. They can strike at a distance of approximately half their body length. Rattlesnakes use their rattle when threatened or endangered, not necessarily just when they are about to attack. The pit viper is aggressive and will stand its ground when provoked or cornered.[54,55] The venom is stored in glands that are located on each side of the head above the maxillae and behind the eyes. The glands are similar in function to the human submaxillary glands. The snake may discharge anywhere from 25% to 75% of its venom when biting a human. The fangs are either hollow or grooved. Even young snakes are venomous, and the venom of young snakes may be 12 times as strong as the venom of adult snakes.

ENVENOMATION

Toxicology

Snake venom has both neurotoxic and hematotoxic properties. The venom is a complex mixture of hydrolases, polypeptides, glycoproteins, and low-molecular-weight compounds. Snake venom, especially that of the Elapidae and Hydrophidae families, contains polypeptides that produce neuromuscular blockade at the presynaptic or postsynaptic terminals, or both, causing a flaccid paralysis. Composition of the venom varies greatly between species and between individual snakes. Viper venom is mainly cytotoxic, Elapidae (cobra, coral) venom is usu-

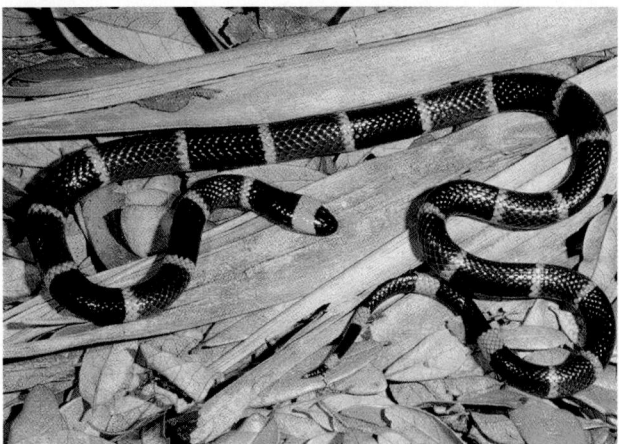

Figure 1 **The nose of the coral snake is black, and the body has black, red, and yellow bands. The black bands do not separate the red and yellow bands, as they do on the nonvenomous but similarly banded kingsnake. Snake shown is an eastern coral snake,** *Micrurus fulvius.*

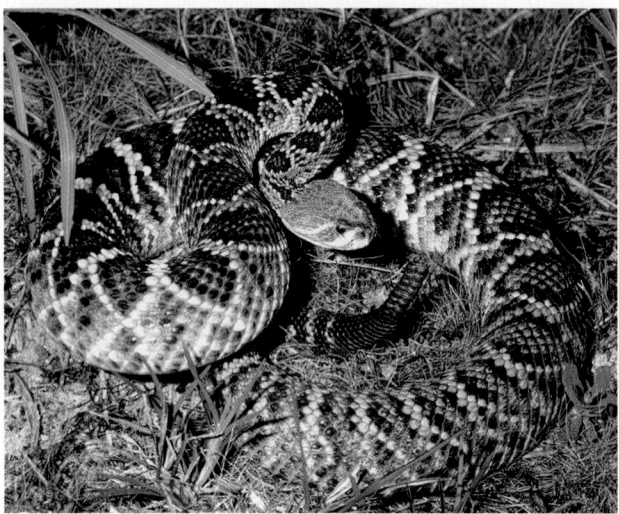

Figure 2 **Diamondback rattlesnakes are the largest and most dangerous rattlesnakes in the United States. Shown is an eastern diamondback rattlesnake,** *Crotalus adamanteus.*

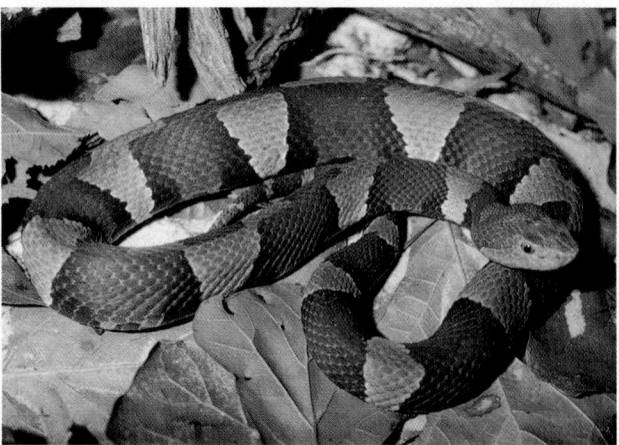

Figure 3 **The copperhead (***Agkistrodon contortix***) has a geographic range that extends from Massachusetts southwest to Texas. Bites from these snakes are painful but rarely fatal.**

ally neurotoxic, and Hydrophidae (sea snake) venom is mainly myotoxic.[57]

Snake venom has profound effects on coagulation pathways, causing a hypercoagulable state. Over the first few hours after a person is bitten, thrombocytopenia occurs, with a platelet count of less than $10,000/mm^3$, a decrease in fibrinogen, and an increase in fibrin degradation products. The venom proteins may induce distention of the vascular basement membrane and capillary matrix.[58] Prothrombin time and partial thromboplastin time increase with severe envenomation. Usually, these increases occur because consumption of coagulation factors results in clinical anticoagulation. In dog experiments, activation of fibrinolysis may be preceded by thrombus formation, with clotting of critical vessels in the coronary vasculature, which can lead to cardiac arrest and death. This may also explain pulmonary emboli, as the thrombus formation may occur in the legs and cause deep vein thrombosis.[59] Drops in hematocrit may also occur, along with so-called burring of erythrocytes.[54] Approximately 53% of patients experience coagulopathy 2 to 14 days after envenomation. In one study, 76% of patients with pit viper envenomations developed coagulopathy during their hospital course.[60] The coagulopathy may last up to 26 days.[59]

Clinical Features

From 30% to 50% of snakebites do not result in envenomation. The snake can control the amount of venom injected and may inject up to 90% of its venom to immobilize its prey. Other factors involved in the injection of venom include the health of the snake; its satiety; the condition of the fangs; the toxicity of the venom; whether the snake is injured; and the size, age, and health of the victim.

Minor pit viper envenomation causes local pain and swelling (edema with a diameter of approximately 1 to 5 in.), without systemic symptoms or signs. Moderate envenomation is characterized by greater edema (diameter of 6 to 12 in.), weakness, sweating, nausea, fainting, dizziness, ecchymoses, and tender adenopathy.[51] As the envenomation becomes more severe, the symptoms increase to include tachycardia, tachypnea, hypothermia, hypotension, ecchymoses, paresthesias, fasciculations, gingival bleeding, hematemesis, hematuria, melena, oliguria, epistaxis, intracerebral hemorrhage, or coma.[58] Fasciculations are a characteristic manifestation of bites from the eastern diamondback rattlesnake.[61] The skin around and over the snakebite will develop a tense, discolored bulla with serous or hemorrhagic fluid. Death usually results from hemorrhage, increased vascular permeability, and thromboembolic events secondary to disruption of the coagulation pathways.

Coral snake envenomation is painful and has the appearance of scratch marks with no surrounding edema. Systemic symptoms are delayed by about 1 to 6 hours. They begin with paresthesias around the wound margins, followed by weakness, apprehension, giddiness, nausea, vomiting, and a sense of euphoria. Excess salivation is nearly always present.[61] Bulbar and cranial nerve paralysis and ptosis may develop. Ptosis is very common and is often the first sign of coral snake envenomation. Diplopia, papillary dilatation, salivation, dysphagia, and respiratory failure may occur. The paralysis may last up to 14 hours, and full strength may not return for 6 to 8 weeks. In fatal cases, the usual cause of death is respiratory failure.

Viperid venom may increase vascular permeability, leading to bleeding into the gastrointestinal or genitourinary tract. In addition to the obvious signs and symptoms, renal failure may occur secondary to hemorrhage, coagulopathy, or secondary shock. Intracranial hemorrhage, especially into the anterior pituitary gland (leading to Sheehan syndrome) has been seen in envenomation by the Russell viper. Nephrotic syndrome, glomerulonephritis, hemolytic-uremic syndrome, and DIC have an incidence of 1.4% to 28%, especially in envenomations by the Russell viper, puff adder, and sea snake.[59,62]

TREATMENT

First Aid

Treatment in the field should focus on preventing systemic absorption of the toxin. This may be done with compressive dressings and immobilization of the bitten extremity. Stabilization may be accomplished via an inflatable splint. Nothing should be given by mouth.

If signs of envenomation begin to occur, a constriction band to impede lymphatic flow should be placed on the extremity, proximal to the bite.[63] The Commonwealth Serum Laboratory technique (Australia) uses an elastic band or air splint for wrapping the extremity. The Monash method uses a thick pad and tight bandage over the wound site to impede flow of the venom. Both of these methods have proven efficacy only with Elapidae bites. Transport to a hospital should take place immediately, because the absorption of neurotoxic venoms may result in respiratory compromise or arrest. In patients with a facial envenomation, edema may cause airway obstruction, so emergency response personnel may have to establish immediate airway control.[64]

The site should be wiped off and cleaned. However, the old practice of incising the bite site and applying suction to remove the snake venom should not be used. This practice, which dates from the 1920s, was tested in animal models and found not to increase survival. In fact, incision and suction at the wound site poses more hazard than benefit. The incision may aggravate bleeding, damage nerves and tendons, introduce infection, and delay healing. Cryotherapy (e.g., placing ice on the bite site), which was once thought to lower venom enzyme activity and absorption into the systemic circulation, has also been shown to provide no significant benefit; rather, it causes tissue loss, cold injury, and possible permanent disability.

Extraction therapy has also fallen out of favor. In this procedure, a suction device is placed over the fang wounds, and suction is applied to remove the venom from the bite site and the surrounding tissue without an incision. Prehospital personnel who find a suction device already in place when they arrive at the scene should remove the device, provided there is no fluid accumulating in the cup.[64] The use of field first-aid methods such as incision and suction, tourniquets, and cryotherapy has been associated with a threefold increase in the likelihood of the need for surgical intervention.[50]

Although popular belief has it that snakebites kill within minutes, in fact, the toxicity from snake venom usually does not even begin to affect the body for several hours. In one review, 64% of deaths from snakebite occurred between 6 and 48 hours after the patient was bitten.[65]

Emergency Department Management

History When a snakebite victim arrives at the hospital, the history of the bite should be obtained. This should include (1) a description of the snake, (2) the time elapsed since the bite, (3) the circumstances surrounding the bite, (4) the number of bites, (5) the location of the bite, (6) the type of first aid administered,

and (7) any symptoms that have occurred since the bite. The patient's past medical history and allergy history should be reviewed briefly. In particular, the clinician should ask whether the patient has ever experienced allergic symptoms around horses or on exposure to horse serum and whether the patient has asthma, hay fever, or urticaria.

Physical examination Special attention should be paid to the area around the snakebite. The wound should be examined for fang marks, edema, petechiae, ecchymoses, and bullae. Thorough neurologic and cardiovascular examinations are indicated. If the patient was bitten on an extremity, circumferential measurements of the extremity should be taken at the site of injury and 5 in. proximal to the site. Distal pulses and neurologic status should be assessed and recorded, because edema from snakebites may result in elevated compartment pressures, leading to compartment syndrome.[50,64] The patient should be monitored in an intensive care setting.

Laboratory tests All patients should have baseline laboratory studies performed, including a complete blood count, urinalysis, electrocardiogram, prothrombin time, partial thromboplastin time, fibrinogen levels, fibrin split products, serum electrolytes, blood urea nitrogen, and serum creatinine. Blood should be typed and screened. In severe envenomations, arterial blood gas determinations also are indicated. In patients with extremity edema, arterial Doppler evaluation and, in some cases, compartmental pressure determinations may be necessary.

Antivenin Therapy

Antivenins are available for bites of North American pit vipers and eastern coral snakes. Water moccasin and copperhead bites are typically managed without the use of antivenin. The choice whether to use antivenin is based on many factors, including clinical signs and symptoms of envenomation and the physiologic status of the victim. Antivenin is indicated only for severe envenomations.[66]

Antivenin can be obtained through hospital pharmacies, veterinarians, local zoos, and poison control centers. Antivenin is most therapeutic when given within 4 hours after the bite. It is of limited value when given after 12 hours.[52]

Classification of envenomation Envenomations are classified according to a five-level system. The amount of antivenin given correlates with the grade of envenomation.

In grade 0 envenomations, the patient may have fang marks or superficial abrasions of the skin at the bite site but has minimal local edema or pain and no associated systemic manifestations.

Grade 1 envenomations involve some pain or throbbing at the bite site, with 1 to 5 in. of edema and erythema surrounding it. There are no systemic manifestations.

Grade 2 envenomations produce more severe pain over a larger area. The edema spreads toward the trunk, and petechiae and ecchymosis are present in the edematous area. There may be systemic involvement consisting of nausea, vomiting, and temperature elevation.

Grade 3 envenomation is considered severe. Edema spreads up the extremity and may move to the trunk. There may be generalized ecchymosis and petechiae. The patient may have a rapid pulse, hypotension, and hypothermia and may go into shock.

Grade 4 envenomation is very severe and usually results from the bite of a large snake or from a very large venom load. Edema, petechiae, ecchymosis, and necrosis rapidly overtake the extremity and a large portion of the trunk. Muscle fasciculations, sweating, nausea, vomiting, cramping, pallor, weak pulse, incontinence, convulsions, and coma may all occur.

Antivenins Multiple types of antivenin are on the market. The first marketed antivenin (Antivenin [Crotalidae] polyvalent [ACP]) was a horse-serum–based, whole antibody preparation. The dosage for that preparation was three to five ampules of antivenin diluted in 500 ml of intravenous fluid. Up to 54% of patients treated in studies were allergic to the ACP antivenin. Rash, hypotension, wheezing, and phlebitis occurred in 20% of patients.[67] Nevertheless, clinicians would frequently forgo skin testing for allergy to ACP because it delayed administration of the antivenin.

Although the ACP antivenin is still produced and is used in some areas, a polyvalent crotalid (ovine) Fab antivenin (CroFab) has been introduced. This antivenin minimizes the risk of immediate hypersensitivity and prevents delayed serum sickness. It is based on sheep serum and is four to five times more potent than ACP.[60] CroFab is made by immunizing sheep with crotaline snake venom and digesting the immune serum with papain to produce antibody fragments (Fab and Fc); the antigenic Fc segment is removed during purification.[66] In a study of 1,000 treated patients, none showed evidence of true anaphylaxis.[68] Each vial of CroFab contains 750 mg of Fab and is reconstituted in 10 ml of normal saline; four vials are diluted in 250 ml of normal saline. Studies have shown improvement at the 4-hour mark in all patients given this regimen, although some patients subsequently worsened.[68] The half-life of Fab antivenin is less than 12 hours, compared with 61 to 194 hours for ACP,[69,70] so repeat dosing of Fab may be needed to maintain therapeutic serum levels.[71] In studies, only 16% of patients experienced serum sickness after administration of Fab antivenin, and the severity of the serum sickness was classified as only mild to moderate; in one study, the only reaction in 64 of 65 patients receiving antivenin was simple urticaria.[72] The Fab antivenin is given in interval doses, with the first dose given to achieve initial control (defined as cessation of all symptoms—local, systemic, and coagulopathy) and subsequent doses given 6, 12, and 18 hours after the first dose. It is presumed that in some cases, coagulopathy may recur after initial neutralization of the venom. Recurrence may result from a depot of unneutralized venom at the bite site that is released into the circulation after the venom-antivenin complexes are cleared. A combination of edema, circulatory injury, and a lesser amount of subcutaneous tissue at the site of the bite may inhibit the antivenin from reaching the venom depot.[60,73] Alternatively, uncleared complexes may dissociate, leaving free venom to recirculate.[60,68]

Adjunctive Therapy

A number of adjunctive therapies have been proposed for snakebite envenomations. Excision of tissue around the snakebite to remove the depot of venom was proposed at one time, but this approach is no longer used. The strategy of excising only necrotic-appearing tissue has likewise proved inadvisable, because histologic examination of the excised tissue revealed live muscle fibers interwoven with the macroscopically necrotic tissue. Aggressive debridement and antibiotic therapy may be indicated in the event of complications from infection. This may be seen with necrotizing fasciitis from either *Vibrio vulnificans* or *Aeromonas hydrophila*.[74]

Extremity edema from a snakebite may mimic compartment syndrome, but true compartment syndrome is rare in such cases.

Most often, the subcutaneous tissue rather than the deep compartmental space is involved. When a deep envenomation occurs and a true compartment syndrome does develop, first-line treatment is antivenin administration, which diminishes the compartmental pressure and swelling. Compartmental pressures greater than 30 mm Hg may indicate a need for fasciotomy, but fasciotomy and debridement should be avoided if possible because this procedure is associated with worse functional results. Fasciotomy is recommended only if a patient's fingertip was bitten and has swelled, with loss of neurovascular or functional activity. Such patients are candidates for so-called digit dermotomy. The incision should be made on the lateral or medial aspect of the finger, through the skin only, and should extend from the web to the middle of the distal phalanx.[61,75]

General Management

A regional poison control center or the local zoo should be used as a resource when dealing with a venomous snakebite. This is especially true if the snake is not believed to be native to the area, as might occur with hobbyists who keep exotic snakes as pets. For cases in which an expert is not available, the Department of Surgery at the University of California, San Diego, School of Medicine has established a Web site that lists protocols (including antivenin availability) for management of snakebites from venomous species around the world. This information is available online at http://www.surgery.ucsd.edu/ENT/DAVIDSON/snake/index.htm.

Other therapeutic measures are keyed to specific symptoms. Isotonic fluid replacement should be given if the patient is hypotensive. Abnormalities of the clotting mechanism should be corrected with blood product replacement as necessary, but this should be done only after antivenin therapy has been started. In fact, common treatments for standard coagulopathies are ineffective or dangerous for snakebite-induced coagulopathies. Instead, the effects of the venom should be treated (with antivenin) before usual coagulopathy treatment is initiated.[59] Corticosteroids are contraindicated during the acute stages of envenomation, but they may be used if the patient experiences serum sickness from antivenin use. Studies in Costa Rica have shown that in viper bites, the release of inflammatory cytokines leads to clinical and pathologic alterations similar to those found in trauma patients.[76] Further research on this reaction and on the potential use of steroids is indicated. Patients should be placed on oxygen and should be given mechanical support if necessary for signs of trismus, laryngeal spasm, or excessive salivation. Tetanus therapy should be given if indicated [*see Table 3*]. Antibiotics are recommended only if signs of infection are present. In one study, there were no wound infections in patients with nonenvenomated snakebite.[77]

The wounds should be examined daily. Superficial necrosis and hemorrhagic blebs should be debrided at days 3 through 10. Debridement may need to be done in stages.

SPECIAL CONSIDERATIONS

Snakebite in Pregnancy

In pregnant women who have been bitten by snakes, what is best for the mother will usually be best for the fetus. Fetal outcome may depend on the gestational age of the fetus, with younger age associated with a negative outcome. The miscarriage rate after snake envenomation may be as high as 43%.[78] Miscarriage may result from shock, uterine contractions, pyrexia, or placental or uterine bleeding. Venom may cross the placental barrier and cause some systemic poisoning of the fetus, even if the mother remains symptom free.[78]

In pregnant snakebite victims, airway compromise and shock states should be corrected to ensure perfusion of the placenta and uterus and thereby prevent fetal hypoxia. Circulatory support with vasopressors should be avoided because they reduce uterine blood flow and are detrimental to the fetus. Pregnant women are already in a hypercoagulable state and therefore are even more susceptible to DIC.[78] Abruptio placentae from hypercoagulability has occurred after snakebites.

Antivenin is the therapy of choice in pregnant patients, but there is no reliable information regarding the risks of administration of antivenin during pregnancy. Serum sickness and anaphylactic reactions remain the highest risks associated with antivenin administration.[79]

Snakebite in Children

Snakebites in children are often on the lower extremities or—if the child was handling the snake—on the hands. Signs and symptoms are typically similar to those in adults.[80] Because of their smaller blood volume, however, children may experience a more severe envenomation syndrome.[81] In a study of 67 children with severe envenomation, 72% had systemic involvement and 50% developed coagulopathy; 61% received antivenin, and 36% of those treated experienced adverse reactions.[82] In another case study of 12 children with rattlesnake envenomation who were treated with with CroFab, no evidence of acute or delayed hypersensitivity was noted.[83] Recurrence of local swelling was seen in one patient despite repeated treatment with antivenin. In children, dosing of antivenin should be based on venom load and severity of signs and symptoms rather than on patient age or weight.[82] Although envenomation can lead to multiorgan failure in children, most of the symptoms are localized and limited to erythema, edema, and blisters at the snakebite site.[83] Although most patients are admitted to an intensive care unit, only hemodynamically unstable patients must be admitted to such a setting. Mild and moderate symptoms can be treated in the emergency department or the floor setting.[83]

Disposition

All victims of suspected snakebites should be observed for a minimum of 4 to 6 hours. If there is no sign of envenomation after 6 hours and it is believed that the snake was either nonvenomous or a pit viper, the patient can be discharged. The patient should be given instructions to return to the emergency department immediately if any symptoms of envenomation occur. A patient who has minimal edema and pain should be observed for at least 12 hours. If the swelling has begun to diminish and the pain has resolved, the patient may be discharged with the same discharge instructions.

Pit viper envenomation may result in significant hypofibrinogenemia and thrombocytopenia lasting up to 2 weeks, which may lead to complications from surgery or trauma.[84] If coagulation abnormalities have resolved, however, no further workup of the coagulation system is needed. The best predictor of late hypofibrinogenemia is early hypofibrinogenemia.[60]

Any patient who has been bitten by a Mojave rattlesnake, coral snake, or other exotic snake should be admitted to the intensive care unit, with cardiorespiratory and dialysis equipment readily available. Antivenin should be administered to such patients.[52]

Snakes should not be handled except by a professional herpetologist. Even a dead snake can envenomate its handler. Persons spending time outdoors in areas known to be heavily populated with snakes should wear long pants and closed shoes. Because of the varying size of snake fangs, loose pants are preferred to tight-fitting trousers. Heavy leather boots are recommended rather than sandals, open-toed shoes, or sneakers. Persons who are going to handle snakes, even dead ones, should also wear protective gloves.

Spider Bites

The class Arachnida contains the largest number of known venomous species, including 20,000 venomous spiders. In the United States, only 50 species can envenomate humans, partly because most spiders' fangs are not long enough to penetrate human skin. All spiders are carnivorous; they capture their prey either by hunting or trapping it. Trappers spin webs and wait for prey to become ensnared. They have limited vision and sense prey on their web with their jaw, which can detect movement. Hunters have better eyesight than trappers, and most hunters eat their prey on the spot. For a true diagnosis of a spider bite with possible envenomation, there should be evidence of a bite with pain or discomfort (except with bites from *Loxosceles* species, which are considered painless), collection of the spider at the time of the bite, and identification of the spider by an expert arachnologist. Other signs should be the appearance of fang marks, redness at the site of injury, immediate or delayed itching, and the presence of spines and swelling (which may not be seen in all cases).[85]

BLACK WIDOW SPIDERS

The black widow spider, *Latrodectus mactans* [*see Figure 4*], is found throughout the United States and southern Canada, with other closely related species found mainly in the western United States. There have been no recorded findings of the spider in Alaska. The female is twice the size of the male and is the only sex that is able to envenomate. The male does have venom, but because of its smaller size and less powerful fangs, it is unable to bite and envenomate a human. The female is glossy black, with a bright-red marking on the abdomen that may appear to be two spots or have an hourglass shape. Occasionally, it has red stripes. Immature females are red, brown, and cream colored. The spider's body is about $1/2$ in. long; with the legs, it measures approximately $1^1/_2$ in. in length. It is usually found under rocks and in woodpiles, outhouses, and stables, and it is not aggressive unless guarding its eggs. The black widow is a trapper. The webs are close to the ground to have access to crawling insects and are usually in secluded, dim areas.

Envenomation

Toxicology Black widow venom contains various proteinaceous compounds. The venom paralyzes the prey and begins the digestive process by liquefying the victim's tissues. The toxin depletes acetylcholine from the presynaptic nerve terminals, thereby destabilizing nerve cell membranes and opening ionic channels. The toxin of the black widow is thought to cause a massive release of acetylcholine and then block its reuptake, which leads to both sympathetic and parasympathetic stimulation.[86] There is a patchy paralysis of skeletal muscles with various changes in the autonomic nervous system. This paralytic syndrome has been likened to polio.[87]

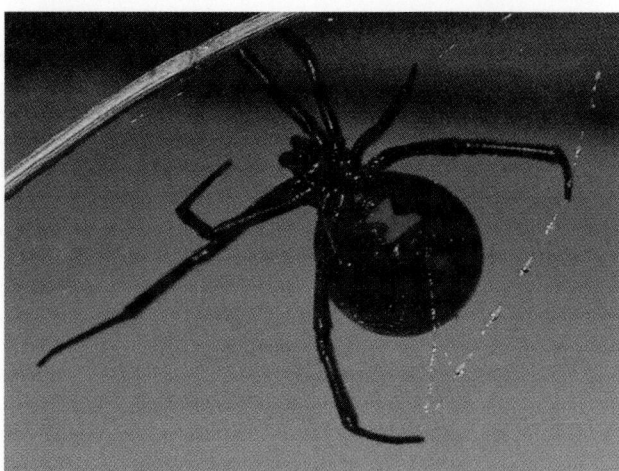

Figure 4 **The mature female black widow spider is glossy black, with a bright-red marking on the abdomen that may appear to be two spots or have an hourglass shape.**

Clinical features On being bitten by a black widow spider, a person may feel a pinprick sensation, with minimal local swelling and erythema. Two small fang marks may be visible. The middle of the bite site may be white, with surrounding erythema and a reddish-blue border. Within an hour, the patient may feel a dull ache or crampy pain in the area of envenomation. This feeling may spread throughout the body shortly thereafter. The pain will increase over the first hour in approximately one half of the cases.[85] The pain spreads to the chest from upper extremity bites and to the abdomen from lower extremity bites. This pain may mimic pancreatitis, appendicitis, or a peptic ulcer. The abdomen may have boardlike rigidity but will not necessarily be painful to palpation. In addition, there may be other myopathic signs such as facial trismus, muscle fibrillation, tonic contractions, or so-called facies latrodectismica, a constellation of symptoms that includes blepharoconjunctivitis, flushing, and contortions.[88] Other systemic symptoms may include dizziness, nausea, vomiting, headache, itching, conjunctivitis, diaphoresis, piloerection, priapism, anxiety, and dyspnea. There is wide variability in the percentage of each symptom experienced by people bitten by the spider.[85] The symptoms may last for 2 to 3 days, abating slightly after a few hours. Patients with preexisting hypertension, cerebrovascular disease, or cardiovascular disease are at risk for a worsening of those conditions. Rare complications of the bites also include compartment syndrome, rhabdomyolysis, and obstruction of the venous outflow in the affected extremity.[89]

Treatment

First aid Patients bitten by a black widow spider should have cool compresses applied to the bite and be transported to a hospital. Laboratory experiments have shown that a Sawyer extraction device may be helpful in removing venom if applied to the skin within 3 minutes after the bite.[88] Basic or advanced life support should be given on the way to the hospital. If possible, the spider should be brought along with the patient, because many nonvenomous species may resemble the black widow.

Emergency department management A complete history and physical examination should be done, with attention paid to the circumstances surrounding the bite, a description of the spider, and allergies to other bites or to horse serum. The site should be inspected and cleansed. Tetanus immunization should be updated, if necessary. Laboratory studies should be obtained, including a complete blood count, serum electrolytes, clotting studies, urinalysis, electrocardiogram, blood urea nitrogen, and serum creatinine.

Patients with envenomations should be treated symptomatically. Nitroprusside may be used for hypertensive episodes related to the envenomation. Abdominal cramps may be alleviated with calcium gluconate (10 ml of a 10% solution given intravenously over 20 minutes). Serum calcium levels should be followed. Diazepam may be given to alleviate muscle spasms.[90] Dantrolene has also been shown to provide muscle relaxation in these patients.[91]

Antivenin therapy *Latrodectus* antivenin exists and is indicated for patients who have hypertensive heart disease, underlying respiratory disease, or severe envenomation. Patients between 16 and 65 years of age may receive the antivenin. The antivenin is derived from horse serum and may cause allergic reactions. The intravenous route is preferred. The contents of the vial are diluted in 50 ml of normal saline and given over 15 minutes. The typical dose is one to two vials. Widow antivenin is available in Australia, South Africa, and the United States, which are the primary locations of the widow spiders. Intramuscular administration in Australian studies has shown few adverse reactions. However, American black widow antivenin has a higher incidence of early allergic reactions.[92]

Special Considerations

Spider bites in children Children who are bitten by a black widow spider may have severe symptoms that may lead to death. Possibly because of the smaller volume in which the venom is circulated, a dose that would be tolerable in an adult may cause fatal cardiovascular or respiratory decompensation in a child. A retrospective Australian study of red-back spider bites showed systemic symptoms of diaphoresis, irritability, and hypertension in 85% of pediatric patients admitted to the hospital.[93]

Spider bites in pregnancy A pregnant woman who is bitten by a black widow spider will have signs and symptoms that are otherwise typical, but she may not have a rigid abdomen because of the stretching and laxity of the gravid abdominal wall. However, the cramping may be severe enough to induce miscarriage. The toxin does not seem to have a direct effect on the fetus, possibly because it is not able to cross the placental barrier, nor is it able to cross the blood-brain barrier. Antivenin is indicated for the symptomatic pregnant patient.[78]

Disposition

Patients with signs or symptoms of black widow spider envenomation should be admitted to the hospital. The patient should be observed for a minimum of 2 hours and, if totally asymptomatic, may be discharged with instructions to return if any symptoms develop.

BROWN RECLUSE SPIDERS

The brown recluse spider, *Loxosceles reclusa* [*see Figure 5*], is approximately 1 in. long and ranges in color from tan to dark brown. The female has a violin-shaped dark-brown spot on its abdomen. Males and young spiders may also have a darkened violin pattern on the thorax.[94] The brown recluse has three sets of eyes arranged in pairs called dyads.

The brown recluse is frequently found in clothing, bedsheets, and blankets in a closet; in woodpiles in a shed; or under rocks. The brown recluse hunts for its food but can live for 6 months without food or water.[95] It forages at night but is not aggressive unless threatened, hence the "recluse" name.[95]

The brown recluse is found in the south central United States, especially in Missouri, Kansas, Arkansas, Louisiana, east Texas, and Oklahoma. It is occasionally found in other states, but these cases likely represent spiders uprooted and transported from the endemic areas.[94] The diagnosis of true *Loxosceles* spider bites in the United States is considered to be far less than the number of patients who are treated for recluse spider envenomations.[95] Strict inclusion criteria for recluse envenomation include sighting of the biting spider and identification of that specific spider. In studies from areas endemic for *Loxosceles*, patients present with almost no true *Loxosceles* bites or envenomations despite exposure to dozens to hundreds of spiders; these results suggest that nonendemic areas should have minimal to no true *Loxosceles* bites.[85,96]

Loxosceles spiders are also found outside of North America, most notably in Brazil and elsewhere in South America. *L. laeta* is the most toxic of these species.[97]

Envenomation

Toxicology Brown recluse venom is protein based, and it has antigenic and locally destructive properties. Esterases, hyaluronidases, and proteases have been isolated from recluse spider venom.[95] The components of the venom are cytotoxic to endothelial cells and red blood cells. Sphingomyelinase-D acts directly on red blood cells to cause lysis.[98] Unlike black widow venom, brown recluse venom has no known neurotoxic effects.

Clinical features Brown recluse spider venom produces both localized and systemic symptoms. These are referred to as cutaneous and viscerocutaneous symptoms.[85] Cutaneous loxoscelism presents initially as pain in the area of the bite, or pain may be absent at first and then develop over the next 3 to 4 hours. Soon thereafter, a ring of pallor from vasoconstriction appears around the bite, with a surrounding area of erythema. A bleb develops in the center and, after a few days, becomes necrotic. The bleb may spread with gravity-dependent flow. This necrotic area spreads over the next few days, involving both superficial and deep tissues. An eschar usually forms days later, and the wound may not heal for months after the eschar separates.[99,100] Subcutaneous fat may liquefy below the eschar, leaving a depressed scar. This occurs in areas with more subcutaneous tissue, such as the thigh. Healing of the eschar takes from 5 days to 17 weeks.[101] Viscerocutaneous loxoscelism may present as systemic effects that include fever, chills, rash, nausea, vomiting, shock, renal failure, hemorrhage, DIC, or pulmonary edema. There have been case reports of transverse myelitis and paralysis from the brown recluse spider bite; these are believed to result from microthrombosis at the anterior vertebral artery.[102] Also, loss of cutaneous sensation may be caused by damage to or destruction of a nerve or its branch by the venom itself or ischemia from the edema.[98]

The differential diagnosis of the skin changes caused by brown recluse spider envenomation includes Stevens-Johnson syndrome, toxic epidermal necrolysis, erythema nodosum, purpura fulminans, diabetic ulcer, allergic dermatitis, Lyme disease, and pyoderma gangrenosum.[88] Patients who have had numerous brown recluse spider bites have demonstrated an antibody

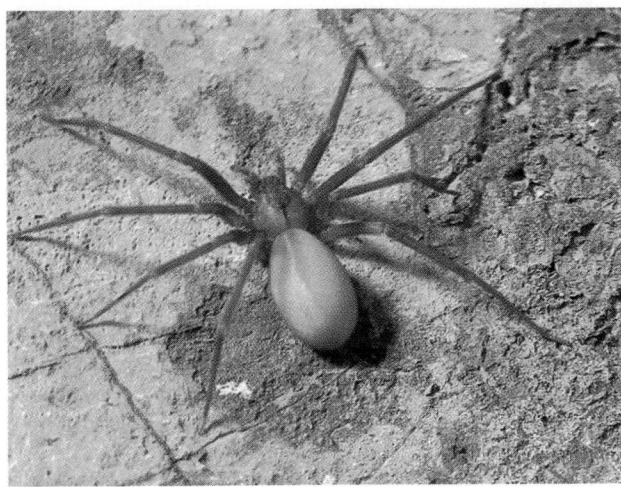

Figure 5 **The brown recluse spider (7 to 12 mm body length) is a timid arachnid that may be encountered in basements, closets, and woodpiles.**

response and may have a decreased response to subsequent bites.[95]

In the few cases of fatal bites, death usually results from DIC and renal failure. In the United States, however, brown recluse spider envenomations frequently result in little more than an inflammatory reaction.[94]

Spider bites in children Brown recluse spider bites in children may result in severe systemic reactions, among which are hemolytic anemia, hypotension, and anemia.[103] It is thought that sphingomyelinase-D in the venom leads to hemolysis, platelet aggregation, thrombosis, and vasoconstriction in children. The severity of any reaction is a function of the amount of venom injected and the location of the bite. Swelling of the neck and subsequent airway obstruction has been reported in a child.[104] Death is a rare but known complication.

Treatment

Prehospital care should include basic or advanced life support, cool compresses, and immobilization of the extremity. On the patient's arrival at the emergency department, a complete history and physical examination should be done, with attention paid to the circumstances surrounding the bite, the description of the spider, and allergies to other bites or to horse serum. Early diagnosis is most easily accomplished if the patient brings the spider to the emergency department. The site should be inspected and cleansed. Tetanus toxoid should be administered, if appropriate.

Brown recluse antivenin is available and has been shown in some studies to be successful in limiting necrosis, but it must be given within the first 24 hours of the bite. During this time, however, it is difficult to assess the future severity of the cutaneous lesion.[105] A 1983 study found some evidence that systemic steroids should be used with brown recluse bites if the patient is seen within 24 hours.[106] Other studies have shown that the intralesional injection of steroids may help control inflammation or thrombosis but does not alter eschar size or outcome[107,108] Dapsone has also been shown to be helpful in treating the local effects of the venom. However, it should be used only in adults who have been screened for glucose-6-phosphate dehydrogenase (G6PD) deficiency. Dapsone is most effective in the first few hours after a bite, but its side effects usually outweigh its benefits for prophylactic use.[105] The complications of dapsone use include hemolysis, agranulocytosis, aplastic anemia, methemoglobinemia, rashes, toxic epidermal necrolysis, and fatal reactions.[106] Phentolamine has not been shown to have any appreciable effect on the necrotic activity.[95] In animal models, hyperbaric oxygen therapy has not been conclusively proved to be effective, but studies have shown some positive outcomes.[109] In one study, electric-shock treatment of the envenomation site in a human showed a potentially positive outcome to the lesion; however, no benefit was shown in animal models, and delayed healing was actually found to occur in some cases. Therefore, electric-shock therapy has not been supported by the literature.[94,110] Excision has not been shown to improve outcome and, in fact, may be detrimental. Antibiotics may be prescribed if signs of infection are present. Analgesia should also be offered to the patient.[98] Patients who have signs or symptoms of envenomation should be admitted to the hospital. If acute renal failure develops, dialysis may be necessary. Tissue necrosis at the wound site may necessitate surgical intervention, but only if the lesion is large, has persisted for 6 to 8 weeks, and has stopped progressing in size.

Disposition

A patient who has been bitten by a brown recluse spider should be observed in the emergency department for a minimum of 6 hours. If no local or systemic symptoms develop, the patient may be discharged with instructions to return if any symptoms appear.

TARANTULAS

At least 30 species of tarantula (*Theraphosidae*) live in the deserts of the western United States. Tarantulas are hunters that eat nocturnal insects. Because of the location of its fangs, a tarantula must raise itself on its hind legs to inflict a bite. In addition, when it is handled, a tarantula releases the hairs of its abdomen, which cause a local urticarial reaction in humans.

Bites from the tarantula are relatively innocuous and result in a low-grade histamine reaction. However, they should be cleansed, and tetanus immunization should be updated if necessary.

Bites from tarantulas from the Panama Canal Zone may cause paresthesias and local discomfort. The South American tarantula has a more toxic bite, for which antivenin is available.

Treatment of all tarantula bites should be supportive, with the administration of antihistamines and oral analgesics. The tarantula hairs, which may be barbed, can be removed with adhesive tape.

Scorpion Stings

EPIDEMIOLOGY

Scorpion stings are common in tropical and subtropical regions of the world. For example, Tunisia reports almost 40,000 stings a year, which result in approximately 1,000 hospitalizations and 100 deaths.[111] Deaths from severe envenomation are the result of cardiogenic shock and pulmonary edema.[112]

Scorpion envenomation is not rare in the United States, with 14,569 consultations for scorpion stings reported in 2001 by the American Association of Poison Control Centers.[113] Most scorpion stings occur in the southwestern states. The scorpion responsible for severe envenomations in the United States is *Centruroides exilicauda*.[114]

Table 5 Grading System for Severity of *Centruroides exilicauda* Envenomation[117]

Grade	Features
I	Pain or paresthesia at the site of envenomation
II	Local findings plus pain or paresthesia remote from the sting site
III	Cranial nerve dysfunction* or somatic-skeletal neuromuscular dysfunction†
IV	Cranial nerve dysfunction* and somatic-skeletal neuromuscular dysfunction†

*Blurred vision, wandering eye movements, hypersalivation, trouble swallowing, tongue fasciculation, problems with upper airway, slurred speech.
†Restlessness, severe involuntary shaking, and jerking of extremities (may be mistaken for seizures).

ENVENOMATION

Toxicology

The toxin of *C. exilicauda* is a heat-stable neurotoxin that increases permeability of neuronal sodium channels, causing depolarization of the nerve and myocyte.[115] Severe envenomation results in stimulation of both cholinergic and adrenergic neurons by its action on presynaptic cell membranes.[116] Increased permeability of neuronal sodium channels in the autonomic nervous system results in tachycardia, agitation, hypertension, hypersalivation, dysphagia, and gastrointestinal symptoms.[117,118]

Clinical Features

Scorpion envenomation can produce effects ranging from local to life threatening. Envenomations are categorized by severity from grade I (pain or paresthesia at the sting site) to grade IV (combined cranial nerve and somatic-skeletal neuromuscular dysfunction) [*see Table 5*].[116]

Treatment

Most adults stung by *C. exilicauda* experience only local pain and paresthesia and can be managed as outpatients.[119] Young children, however, often present with severe involuntary motor activity, agitation, and respiratory symptoms requiring intensive supportive care.[119,120]

Initial hypertension and tachycardia may occur in close to half the patients with milder envenomation.[121] These patients normally respond well to treatment with an antihypertensive agent such as prazosin[121] or captopril.[122]

Patients with severe envenomation may have hypotension, left ventricular failure, and pulmonary edema.[122] Supportive care and afterload reduction with vasodilators appear to reduce mortality.[121,122]

The use of specific antivenin in scorpion stings is controversial.[123-127] Antivenin specific to *C. exilicauda* is not available except in Arizona,[115] where it is commonly used for severe grade III and almost all grade IV envenomations.[128] It is rarely associated with anaphylaxis but commonly results in mild serum sickness.[115,128] A majority of opinions recommend the treatment of scorpion stings with antivenin, but this recommendation depends on the dose of the antivenin and its route of administration. Intravenous administration is recommended because of the slow absorption of the intramuscular route compared with the rapid distribution and absorption of scorpion venom. In studies using the intravenous administration of antivenin, overall mortality was reduced to less than 0.05%.[129] However, some of the symptoms, such as pulmonary edema, labile vital signs, and dysrhythmias, were still seen in envenomated patients.

The use of sedative-hypnotics has been advocated for the severe agitation and motor restlessness associated with *C. exilicauda* envenomation. Careful assessment (to ensure adequate airway, breathing, and circulation) and monitoring of patients treated with sedative-hypnotics is essential because respiratory depression and even respiratory arrest have been reported with this therapy.[115,120]

Insect Bites and Stings

Insect bites are medically important primarily because insects can act as vectors for pathogenic microorganisms by directly inoculating their human hosts while feeding on blood or tissue fluids. In addition, stinging insects have venom, and the exoskeleton, hair, and secretions may act as irritants or allergens. Allergic reactions to Hymenoptera venom are discussed elsewhere [*see Chapter 110*].

Although insect bites and stings are an essentially universal human experience, the exact incidence of serious morbidity and mortality is difficult to determine because of different reporting practices, regional differences of endemic species, and the wide spectrum of clinical effects, particularly severity. In 2003, the American Association of Poison Centers reported 94,247 bites and envenomations (representing 3.5% of all toxic exposures), with six deaths (0.25% fatal exposure cases).[130] These statistics include bites and stings not only from insects but also from marine species and mammals.

FIRE ANTS

Two species of fire ants were imported into Alabama in the early part of the 1900s. Since that time, they have spread throughout the southeastern United States and Texas.[131] Fire ants both bite and sting, anchoring themselves with their mandibles to leverage the thrust of their stinger. Their venom is primarily composed of an insoluble alkaloid that has local hemolytic and necrotic effects.[132] Fire ants have a propensity to swarm, resulting in multiple bites. Initially, stings cause an erythematous papule or wheal that develops into a pruritic sterile pustule over the course of 6 to 24 hours and may persist for weeks [*see Chapter 110*]. Because of the alkaloid nature of the venom, reactions typically remain local; systemic or anaphylactic reactions are rare. Occasionally, secondary infection occurs.[133]

Treatment consists of local wound care, cold packs, antihistamines, and topical steroids. Extensive involvement may necessitate oral steroids. Anaphylactic reactions are managed in the same manner as those from other causes. Secondary infection requires treatment with antibiotics. Desensitization therapy should be considered for patients who experience life-threatening reactions.[134]

KISSING BUGS AND BEDBUGS

The kissing bug (*Triatoma* species), also known as the assassin, cone-nosed, or reduviid bug, is found mostly in the southern and western regions of the United States. It feeds on the blood of vertebrates, including humans, mostly at night. Kissing bugs possess a long proboscis from which they suck blood from the victims without pain. Bites commonly occur on the face because that area is usually exposed during the night.[132] In Central and South America, kissing bugs are the vector for *Trypanosoma cruzi*, the causative agent of Chagas disease.[135]

Bedbugs (*Cimex* species) are also nocturnal bloodsucking insects that have adapted to human environments. They are found throughout the United States and live in baseboards, furniture, clothing, and bedding. Bedbugs are not known to be vectors for human disease, but allergic reactions to their bites can present as multiple clustered, erythematous, pruritic papules that can last over a week.[136] Systemic effects are rarely encountered. Treatment consists of symptomatic care with antihistamines and topical steroids.

CATERPILLARS AND MOTHS

The order *Lepidoptera* includes venomous caterpillars and moths. Some of these caterpillars have hollow spines among their body hairs; injection of venom through these spines can cause symptoms ranging from local dermatitis to generalized systemic reactions.[137] The puss caterpillar, or woolly slug, is found in the southeastern United Sates and Texas and accounts for most of the envenomations from this insect family for which patients seek medical care. Stings produce small, erythematous, painful papules at the site of contact. Fever and muscle cramps may occur, but serious systemic effects are rare.[137]

Gypsy moths infest much of the eastern United States but also are present elsewhere in the country. Skin contact with gypsy moth caterpillars can cause dermatitis from delayed hypersensitivity. Treatment is symptomatic, with topical steroids and oral antihistamines. Analgesics occasionally are needed for pain control.[135]

BLISTER BEETLES

The blister beetle is found throughout the United States.[132] Blister beetles do not have a toxic bite or sting, but they secrete cantharidin, which acts as a vesicating agent, causing skin irritation and blisters several hours after contact.[132] The blisters can range from a few millimeters to several centimeters in diameter. Pulverized blister beetles were used as an aphrodisiac known as Spanish fly, which causes urethral irritation when ingested orally. Local blisters from blister beetle contact are treated as a chemical burn, with diligent wound care and prevention of secondary infection.[135]

TICKS

Ticks are found throughout the world and are members of the class Arachnida. They painlessly attach to their host (mostly mammals) to feed on blood. The primary medical importance of ticks is as vectors for infection. Infectious diseases carried by ticks include Lyme disease, Rocky Mountain spotted fever, babesiosis, ehrlichiosis, tularemia, Colorado tick fever, and relapsing fever.[138]

Some *Ixodid* species of ticks produce a neurotoxin in their salivary gland that can induce a syndrome known as tick paralysis.[139] The toxin is usually transmitted by an engorged, gravid female and causes an ascending flaccid paralysis approximately 2 to 7 days after the tick begins feeding. Children are the ones who are most often affected. Respiratory failure may occur, and ventilatory support is required in some cases. The diagnosis is confirmed by finding an embedded tick on the victim. Removal of the tick is essential to recovery. Symptoms improve several hours to days after the tick is removed.[140]

Ticks generally attach themselves to their hosts after approximately 1 to 2 hours, so persons in tick-infested areas should perform frequent checks of their clothing and body. If a tick does attach, it should be removed promptly to minimize the risk of disease transmission. The tick should be grasped as close to the skin as possible, using blunt forceps, tweezers, or protected fingers. Steady pressure should be applied while pulling out the tick. After removal, standard wound care should be employed. If the mouth parts are only partially removed, foreign-body reactions, secondary infections, and granuloma formation can occur.

Marine Envenomations

Almost 75% of the earth's surface is covered with water, and approximately 80% of our planet's organisms live in this environment. Only a few of these marine creatures pose a threat to humans, but the dangers have been recognized since ancient times. Significant human morbidity and mortality, ranging from minor dermatitis to life-threatening infections, envenomations, and trauma, may result from exposure to marine life.

Over recent decades, human exposure to the aquatic environment has greatly increased, thanks to scientific and technological advancement and exploration, increased sport diving and recreational activities, increased harvesting of marine resources for food, private and commercial saltwater aquariums, and more travel to and greater accessibility of exotic locations. These factors have increased the risk of exposure to marine organisms. Consequently, it is imperative for clinicians, not only in coastal areas but also inland, to be familiar with the hazards.

Marine organisms that are harmful to humans range from one-celled diatoms and dinoflagellates that cause poisoning by being bioamplified up the food chain (e.g., ciguatera and amnestic shellfish poisoning) to invertebrates with lethal toxins (e.g., jellyfish poisoning) to large vertebrates, such as sharks, that can inflict massive trauma. This discussion reviews some of the more common and clinically relevant envenomations (and their associated injuries and infections) that humans may incur in freshwater and saltwater around the United States.

TOXIC INVERTEBRATES

Coelenterates

The phylum Cnidaria (which includes the former phylum Coelenterata) is divided into three classes: (1) *Hydrozoa* (which includes Portuguese man-of-war, feather hydroids, and fire coral); (2) *Schyphozoa* (true jellyfish, sea nettles, and box jellyfish); and (3) *Anthozoa* (sea anemones, stony corals, and soft corals).[141]

Coelenterates are characterized by venomous stinging organoids called nematocysts. The nematocyst is a fluid-filled capsular structure that encloses a tightly coiled, hollow, sharply pointed tubule that bursts forth into the victim when it is discharged after contact. The venom is a complex mixture of proteins, carbohydrates, and other nonproteinaceous substances.[142]

Clinical effects The clinical features of coelenterate envenomation are fairly constant but have a range of severity from mild dermatitis to rapid cardiovascular collapse resulting in death. Factors that determine severity include the following: species (the Australian box jellyfish is the most deadly of all stinging marine life[143]); season; number of nematocysts triggered; size and age of the victim; location and surface area of the sting; and the sensitivity of the victim to the venom.[141,144] Knowledge of the species of coelenterates indigenous to the geographic location is important in predicting the potential severity of the envenomation. Most hydroids and hydroid corals (which inhabit both temperate and tropical waters off the Atlantic and Pacific coasts of the

United States) initially produce a stinging sensation, paresthesias, and pruritus, with local edema, blistering, and wheal formation. Occasionally, the injury can progress over several days to local necrosis, ulceration, and secondary infection.

Physalia physalis (Portuguese man-of-war) consists of a violet-blue floating sail with several nematocyst-bearing tentacles that can be up to 30 m in length.[145] They are widely distributed but are prevalent in the tropical and semitropical waters off the southeastern coast of the United States and in the Gulf of Mexico.

The man-of-war's sting produces an intense pain radiating up the involved extremity, with the development of linear, edematous, erythematous, cutaneous eruptions. Systemic involvement can occur, involving multiple organ systems, with nausea, vomiting, headache, myalgias, respiratory distress, hypotension, anaphylaxis, and cardiovascular collapse.[145,146]

Jellyfish from the class Scyphozoa display a wide variety of colors, shapes, and sizes and vary in toxic potential. They are the most common coelenterates that produce clinical injuries and that cause people to seek medical attention. They have a worldwide distribution and can range in size from a few millimeters to greater than 2 m at the bell with tentacles up to 36 m in length.[147] Because the tentacles are so long in some species, it is possible to undergo a significant envenomation without ever seeing the bell. Organisms that have washed ashore also pose a risk, because undischarged nematocysts can fire if an unwary person steps on or picks up a tentacle or part of it. Envenomations from most jellyfish are of mild to moderate severity, with clinical symptoms similar to those of the hydroids and *Physalia* species.[148]

Treatment Treatment of coelenterate stings includes advanced-life-support measures, symptomatic care, pain control, and prevention of further envenomation by nematocyst inactivation. In the case of box jellyfish envenomations, an antivenin is available (Commonwealth Serum Laboratories, Melbourne, Australia) and should be administered as soon as possible.[149] Anaphylaxis and bronchospasm should be treated with epinephrine, oxygen, intravenous fluids, glucocorticoids, antihistamines, bronchodilators, and vasopressors if needed. The area of the sting should immediately be rinsed with saltwater (not freshwater) or 5% acetic acid (vinegar) for nematocyst inhibition. In the case of a Portuguese man-of-war sting, vinegar should be avoided and only saltwater used. Tentacles should then be removed with a gloved hand, hemostats, or a towel to prevent envenomation of the treating individual.[141] Alternatively, isopropyl alcohol (40% to 70%) may be effective. For *Chrysaora* (sea nettle) or *Cyanea* (lion's mane) stings, a baking-powder slurry applied to the affected area is an effective treatment.[144] In patients with seabather's eruption, a vesicular or morbilliform, pruritic dermatitis caused by larval forms of certain coelenterates [see Chapter 42], a papain (meat tenderizer) solution is effective.[150] Topical anesthetics, antihistamines, and corticosteroids may be of benefit. Prophylactic antibiotics are generally not indicated, but appropriate tetanus prophylaxis and proper wound care should be provided.

Echinodermata

The phylum Echinodermata consists of poisonous species of starfish, sea urchins, and sea cucumbers. Toxic sea urchins (mostly found in the Pacific and Indian oceans and the Red Sea) have sharp, brittle, venom-filled spines and may also possess pincerlike seizing organs termed pedicellariae.[147] Spines can easily penetrate wet suits and skin to lodge in the victim.[151] The immediate reaction consists of intense local pain, erythema, edema, and bleeding. Subcutaneous staining from pigments in the spine can also occur. If multiple spines have penetrated the skin, the patient may develop systemic envenomation symptoms, such as nausea, vomiting, paresthesias, muscular paralysis, hypotension, and respiratory distress. Nontoxic sea urchins can also cause significant morbidity by foreign-body reactions and soft tissue infections or septic arthritis if a spine enters a joint.[145]

Most starfish are nontoxic, but the crown-of-thorns sea star (*Ancanthaster planci*) is covered with thorny spines that deliver a secreted venom produced in specialized glandular tissue.[152] Sea cucumbers are free-living bottom dwellers that produce a mild toxin that is concentrated in the tentacular organs. Direct contact can cause dermatitis. The venom is usually diluted in the seawater, and the greatest risk is exposure of the corneas and conjunctiva, resulting in an intense inflammation.[148] Treatment consists of immersion in hot water (110° to 115° F) for 30 to 90 minutes or until the patient has significant relief of pain. Spines should be localized under direct visualization or by appropriate radiographic technique and carefully removed; retained spines may produce a granulomatous reaction requiring surgical excision. Routine antibiotics are not necessary, but diligent wound care and tetanus prophylaxis should be employed.[147]

Mollusca

Two classes in the phylum Mollusca that have potential toxicities include gastropods (coneshells) and cephalopods (octopuses). Coneshells are univalve animals found in shallow Indo-Pacific waters.[147] They inject potent neurotoxins (conotoxins) into their victims via a detachable, dartlike, radular tooth.[153] Local symptoms resemble a bee or wasp sting, followed by ischemia, cyanosis, and numbness in the area surrounding the wound. In severe envenomations, local paralysis can progress to generalized weakness, paralysis, and respiratory failure.[145] Octopus bites are rare, but deaths have been reported from the Australian blue-ringed octopus. This creature possesses a potent neurotoxin with at least one fraction identical to tetrodotoxin (also found in tissues from the pufferfish), which blocks neuronal sodium conduction.[153] Local symptoms are usually minimal, but significant envenomations can lead to generalized paresthesias, followed by paralysis and respiratory failure.[145] Treatment of octopus envenomation is mostly supportive, with close attention to the need for respiratory support.

Porifera

The phylum Porifera consists of over 5,000 species of sponges. Sponges are stationary acellular animals that attach to the ocean floor or coral beds and may be colonized by other animals.[147] Sponges inhabit waters off both the Atlantic and Pacific coasts of the United States, as well as Hawaii. Sponge diver's disease is usually caused by colonization of the sponges by coelenterates and manifests as a dermatitis or a local necrotic skin reaction.[152] Two primary syndromes can also occur from contact with sponges.[145] The first is a contact dermatitis similar to that caused by plants. The second is an irritant dermatitis caused by the penetration of small spicules of silica or calcium carbonate into the skin. Because it is difficult to distinguish between the two different reactions, treatment of both should be initiated. The skin should be dried, and the spicules should be removed with adhesive tape or a facial peel. Acetic acid 5% soaks should be applied for 10 to 30 minutes three or four times a day (isopropyl alcohol,

40% to 70%, may be substituted). Topical steroids may help with secondary inflammation but should not be used initially.[145]

Annelida

The phylum Annelida includes bristleworms, or fireworms, which are covered by cactuslike bristles and spines. On contact, these bristles easily enter the skin and break off, causing an intense inflammation with a burning sensation and erythema. Bristles should be removed with adhesive tape or a facial peel, with subsequent treatment similar to that used for sponge envenomations (see above).[145,147]

TOXIC VERTEBRATES

Stingrays

Stingrays are found in temperate to tropical waters worldwide and represent the most common source of human envenomations from vertebrates.[145] The stingray is armed with one to four venomous spines on a whiplike tail. Envenomations usually occur when an unwary swimmer steps on a buried stingray. The fish reflexively whips its tail upward, thrusting its spine into the victim. The venomous spine has a sharp tip with serrated edges that often cause a jagged laceration in addition to a puncture wound. Occasionally, a spine breaks off and remains in the wound.[154] Most envenomations occur on the ankle or foot. Initial symptoms include an intense, localized pain that may radiate centrally. Local edema and variable bleeding may occur. The pain intensifies, peaking after approximately 30 to 60 minutes.[155] The wound often appears dusky or cyanotic and progresses to an erythematous, hemorrhagic stage, occasionally with deep tissue involvement and frank necrosis.[154] Systemic effects can occur and include muscle cramps, nausea, vomiting, weakness, headache, diaphoresis, dizziness, and, in rare cases, seizures, paralysis, cardiovascular collapse, and death.[145] Initial treatment consists of hot-water immersion for 60 minutes to deactivate the venom, which is heat labile, and to provide pain relief. The wound should then be thoroughly irrigated and debrided, if needed. Hot-water immersion often provides adequate pain relief, but if pain continues, analgesics should be given, as well as tetanus prophylaxis. These wounds are at risk for infection, and antibiotics are often necessary, along with diligent wound care and close follow-up.[155]

Scorpionfish and Lionfish

The Scorpaenidae family consists of over 80 species and includes stonefish, lionfish, and zebrafish. Most Scorpaenidae species are reef-dwelling fish found in tropical waters of the Pacific and Indian oceans and the Red Sea.[156] They are exquisitely camouflaged, and envenomations occur when a victim inadvertently grasps or steps on one of these fish. Lionfish are often kept in home saltwater aquariums because of their beauty and, therefore, may be involved in accidental envenomations. These fish possess venomous spines covered by an integumentary sheath. The venom consists of a complex mixture of inflammatory mediators and heat-labile proteins and is injected after the spine punctures the skin.[154] The spine may also fracture and remain in the puncture site, causing a foreign-body reaction or acting as a nidus for secondary infection.

Clinical manifestations of envenomation vary from mild toxicity with the lionfish to severe life-threatening toxicity with the stonefish.[156] Initial symptoms include an intense pain at the sting site, with central radiation, that can continue to intensify for several hours. The wound appears ecchymotic and cyanotic initially; subsequently, it often becomes erythematous and swollen. Localized tissue necrosis and skin sloughing can occur after several days.[155] Systemic symptoms can include nausea, vomiting, abdominal pain, headache, myalgias, weakness, tremor, syncope, hypotension, paralysis, seizures, cardiac arrhythmias, hypotension, cardiopulmonary arrest, and death.[154] Initial treatment is immediate immersion of the affected area in hot water (110° to 115° F) for 60 to 90 minutes in an attempt to denature the venom proteins and provide pain relief.[155] Supportive care for systemic symptoms, diligent local wound care (including evaluation for retained spines), tetanus prophylaxis, and analgesics are also the mainstay of treatment. An antivenin is available but is usually reserved for the more serious stonefish envenomations.[156]

Catfish

There are over 1,000 species of catfish worldwide that inhabit both freshwater and saltwater environments.[156] Freshwater catfish are typically sedentary bottom dwellers of slow-moving and often dirty waters. Saltwater catfish, on the other hand, travel in schools and typically stay on the move. Catfish have a smooth, scaleless skin and derive their name from the perioral barbels (which, contrary to popular belief, are incapable of inflicting any stings or envenomation). However, catfish do possess serrated dorsal and pectoral spines that have venom glands enclosed in an integumentary sheath. The spines can produce a deep puncture wound, and the glands release their venom after being traumatized.[157] Most stings occur when the fish is handled after capture, although occasionally, a wader will be stung on the foot. The initial symptom is intense pain, which radiates up the affected limb and is out of proportion to the mechanical trauma. The pain is followed by an intense inflammatory reaction that can include erythema, swelling, local hemorrhage, and tissue necrosis.[158] Systemic reactions are rare but can include nausea, vomiting, weakness, hypotension, syncope, and respiratory distress.[155]

The main concern with catfish stings, as with all aquatic trauma, is the risk of secondary infection. Catfish spines can be retained in the puncture site. Because spines are often radiopaque, x-rays should be obtained to locate them.[157] If there is evidence of a retained spine, the wound should be surgically explored and the foreign matter removed. Initial treatment includes immersion of the affected site in hot water (100° to 115° F) for 60 to 90 minutes, meticulous wound care and debridement, tetanus prophylaxis, and analgesics.[155]

Weeverfish

The weeverfish is the most venomous fish of the temperate zone and is found in the Mediterranean Sea, the Black Sea, and the eastern Atlantic coastal waters from North Africa to the North Sea.[156] It has four to eight sharp dorsal spines and two opercular spines, with which it can cause one of the most painful envenomations known. Weeverfish inhabit flat sandy or muddy bays and hide on the bottom with only their head exposed. Injuries usually occur to the hands or feet of fishermen or unwary swimmers. Weeverfish are typically sedentary but can be aggressive when provoked and can remain alive for many hours after removal from the water.[155]

Initially, weeverfish envenomations cause an intense pain that spreads to involve the entire limb; the pain is often so severe that the victim acts irrationally or loses consciousness. The wound becomes swollen, ecchymotic, and warm and may take months to heal. Systemic symptoms may occur, and secondary infection

Table 6 Pathogens Associated with Aquatic Sources of Infections

Freshwater Organisms	Saltwater Organisms
Aeromonas hydrophila	Aeromonas hydrophila
Agrobacterium sanguineum	Bacteroides fragilis
Chromobacterium violaceum	Clostridium perfringens
Escherichia coli	Erysipelothrix rhusiopathiae
Pseudomonas aeruginosa	Mycobacterium marinum
Staphylococcus aureus	Salmonella enteritidis
Streptococcus species	Staphylococcus aureus
Vibrio parahaemolyticus	Streptococcus species
	Vibrio species

is common.[145] The affected area should be immediately placed in hot water, as for other marine invertebrate envenomations (see above), although this may not be as effective for weeverfish envenomations. The wound should be cleaned and gently explored, although retention of spines is uncommon. Tetanus prophylaxis should be administered. Systemic analgesics and possibly infiltration of local anesthetics or regional nerve blocks may be needed for pain relief.[155]

WATER-BORNE INFECTIONS

Freshwater and saltwater environments provide a medium for a host of microbes not typically encountered in traumatic wounds of nonaquatic origin. The concentration and diversity of these organisms vary, depending on temperature, sunlight, depth, salinity, nutrients, coexisting lifeforms, and pollutants. However, most aquatic microbes are heterotrophic, motile, gram-negative rods that are facultative anaerobes [see Table 6].[159,160] Antibiotic coverage should include gram-negative organisms, as well as S. aureus and Streptococcus species, which are the pathogens in most secondary aquatic wound infections.

The authors have no commercial relationships with manufacturers of products or providers of services discussed in this chapter.

References

1. Sacks JJ, Kresnow M, Houston B: Dog bites: how big a problem? Inj Prev 2:52, 1996
2. Statistical Abstracts of the United States, 112th ed. United States Department of Commerce, 1992
3. Nonfatal dog bite–related injuries treated in hospital emergency departments—United States, 2001. MMWR Morb Mortal Wkly Rep 52:605, 2003
4. Weiss HB, Friedman DI, Coben JH: Incidence of dog bite injuries treated in emergency departments. JAMA 279:51, 1998
5. Boenning DA, Fleisher GR, Campos JM: Dog bites in children: epidemiology, microbiology, and penicillin prophylactic therapy. Am J Emerg Med 1:17, 1983
6. Rest JG, Goldstein EJ: Management of human and animal bite wounds. Emerg Med Clin North Am 3:117, 1985
7. Goldstein EJ: Bite wounds and infection. Clin Infect Dis 14:633, 1992
8. Talan DA, Citron DM, Abrahamian FM, et al: Bacteriologic analysis of infected dog and cat bites. Emergency Medicine Animal Bite Infection Study Group. N Engl J Med 340:85, 1999
9. Garcia VF: Animal bites and *Pasteurella* infections. Pediatr Rev 18:127, 1997
10. Dire DJ: Emergency management of dog and cat bite wounds. Emerg Med Clin North Am 10:719, 1992
11. Griego RD, Rosen T, Orengo IF, et al: Dog, cat, and human bites: a review. J Am Acad Dermatol 33:1019, 1995
12. Sacks JJ, Sinclair L, Gilchrist J, et al: Breeds of dogs involved in fatal human attacks in

the United States between 1979 and 1998. J Am Vet Med Assoc 217:836, 2000

13. Goldstein EJ, Richwald GA: Human and animal bite wounds. Am Fam Physician 36:101, 1987

14. Dire DJ, Hogan DE, Riggs MW: A prospective evaluation of risk factors for infections from dog-bite wounds. Acad Emerg Med 1:258, 1994

15. Medeiros I, Saconato H: Antibiotic prophylaxis for mammalian bites. Cochrane Database Syst Rev (2):CD001738, 2001

16. Rupprecht CE, Gibbons RV: Prophylaxis against rabies. N Engl J Med 351:2626, 2004

17. Krebs JW, Mandel EJ, Swerdlow DL, et al: Rabies surveillance in the United States during 2003. J Am Vet Med Assoc 225:1837, 2004

18. Callaham M: Human and animal bites. Top Emerg Med 4:1, 1982

19. Glaser C, Lewis P, Wong S: Pet-, animal-, and vector-borne infections. Pediatr Rev 21:219, 2000

20. Compendium of animal rabies prevention and control, 2000. National Association of State Public Health Veterinarians, Inc. MMWR Recomm Rep 49(RR-8):21, 2000

21. Gehrke C: Results of the AVMA survey of US pet-owning households on companion animal ownership. J Am Vet Med Assoc 211:169, 1997

22. Paisley JW, Lauer BA: Severe facial injuries to infants due to unprovoked attacks by pet ferrets. JAMA 259:2005, 1988

23. Applegate JA, Walhout MF: Childhood risks from the ferret. J Emerg Med 16:425, 1998

24. Fischer RG, Edwardsson S, Klinge B, et al: The effect of cyclosporin-A on the oral microflora at gingival sulcus of the ferret. J Clin Periodontol 23:853, 1996

25. Krebs JW, Strine TW, Smith JS, et al: Rabies surveillance in the United States during 1994. J Am Vet Med Assoc 207:1562, 1995

26. Compendium of animal rabies control, 1996. National Association of State Public Health Veterinarians, Inc. J Am Vet Med Assoc 208:214, 1996

27. Human rabies prevention—United States, 1999. Recommendations of the Advisory Committee on Immunization Practices (ACIP). MMWR Recomm Rep 48(RR-1):1, 1999

28. Callaham M: Controversies in antibiotic choices for bite wounds. Ann Emerg Med 17:1321, 1988

29. Lindsey D, Christopher M, Hollenbach J, et al: Natural course of the human bite wound: incidence of infection and complications in 434 bites and 803 lacerations in the same group of patients. J Trauma 27:45, 1987

30. Broder J, Jerrard D, Olshaker J, et al: Low risk of infection in selected human bites treated without antibiotics. Am J Emerg Med 22:10, 2004

31. Goldstein EJ, Citron DM, Vagvolgyi AE, et al: Susceptibility of bite wound bacteria to seven oral antimicrobial agents, including RU-985, a new erythromycin: considerations in choosing empiric therapy. Antimicrob Agents Chemother 29:556, 1986

32. Brook I: Microbiology of human and animal bite wounds in children. Pediatr Infect Dis J 6:29, 1987

33. Goldstein EJ: Infectious complications and therapy of bite wounds. J Am Podiatr Med Assoc 79:486, 1989

34. Glass KD: Factors related to the resolution of treated hand infections. J Hand Surg [Am] 7:388, 1982

35. Wiley JF, 2nd: Mammalian bites: review of evaluation and management. Clin Pediatr (Phila) 29:283, 1990

36. Ordog GJ, Balasubramanium S, Wasserberger J: Rat bites: fifty cases. Ann Emerg Med 14:126, 1985

37. Smith JS, Fishbein DB, Rupprecht CE, et al: Unexplained rabies in three immigrants in the United States: a virologic investigation. N Engl J Med 324:205, 1991

38. Krebs JW, Smith JS, Rupprecht CE, et al: Mammalian reservoirs and epidemiology of rabies diagnosed in human beings in the United States, 1981–1998. Ann N Y Acad Sci 916:345, 2000

39. Moran GJ, Talan DA, Mower W, et al: Appropriateness of rabies postexposure prophylaxis treatment for animal exposures. Emergency ID Net Study Group. JAMA 284:1001, 2000

40. Freer L: North American wild mammalian injuries. Emerg Med Clin North Am 22:445, 2004

41. Ostrowski SR, Leslie MJ, Parrott T, et al: B-virus from pet macaque monkeys: an emerging threat in the United States? Emerg Infect Dis 4:117, 1998

42. Holmes GP, Chapman LE, Stewart JA, et al: Guidelines for the prevention and treatment of B-virus infections in exposed persons. B-Virus Working Group. Clin Infect Dis 20:421, 1995

43. Callaham ML: Treatment of common dog bites: infection risk factors. JACEP 7:83, 1978

44. Maimaris C, Quinton DN: Dog-bite lacerations: a controlled trial of primary wound closure. Arch Emerg Med 5:156, 1988

45. Chen E, Hornig S, Shepherd SM, et al: Primary closure of mammalian bites. Acad Emerg Med 7:157, 2000

46. Garbutt F, Jenner R: Best evidence topic report: wound closure in animal bites. Emerg Med J 21:589, 2004

47. Cummings P: Antibiotics to prevent infection in patients with dog bite wounds: a meta-analysis of randomized trials. Ann Emerg Med 23:535, 1994

48. Talan DA, Abrahamian FM, Moran GJ, et al: Clinical presentation and bacteriologic analysis of infected human bites in patients presenting to emergency departments. Clin Infect Dis 37:1481, 2003

49. Turner TW: Evidence-based emergency medicine/systematic review abstract. Do mammalian bites require antibiotic prophylaxis? Ann Emerg Med 44:274, 2004

50. Offerman SR, Smith TS, Derlet RW: Does the aggressive use of polyvalent antivenin

for rattlesnake bites result in serious acute side effects? West J Med 175:88, 2001

51. Gold BS, Barish RA: Venomous snakebites: current concepts in diagnosis, treatment and management. Emerg Med Clin North Am 10:249, 1992

52. Smith TA, Figge HL: Treatment of snakebite poisoning. Am J Hospital Pharm 48:2190, 1991

53. Norris R: Snake envenomations: coral. eMedicine Jan 19, 2005 http://www.emedicine.com/emerg/topic542.htm

54. Sanford JP: Snakebites. Cecil Textbook of Medicine. Wyngaarden JB, Smith LH, Bennett JC, Eds. WB Saunders Co, Philadelphia, 1992

55. Bush SP: Snake envenomations: rattle. eMedicine Nov 2, 2004 http://www.emedicine.com/emerg/topic540.htm

56. White J: Snake venoms and coagulopathy. Toxicon 45:951, 2005

57. Nasu K, Ueda T, Miyakawa M: Intrauterine fetal death caused by pit viper poisoning in early pregnancy. Gynecol Obstet Invest 57:114, 2004

58. Bartholdi D, Selic C, Meier J, et al: Viper snakebite causing symptomatic intracerebral haemorrhage. J Neurol 251:889, 2004

59. Lavonas EJ, Gerardo CJ, O'Malley G: Initial experience with Crotalidae polyvalent immune Fab (ovine) antivenom in the treatment of copperhead snakebite. Ann Emerg Med 43:200, 2004

60. Boyer LV, Seifert SA, Clark RF, et al: Recurrent and persistent coagulopathy following pit viper envenomation. Arch Intern Med 159:706, 1999

61. Watt CH: Treatment of poisonous snakebite with emphasis on digit dermotomy. South Med J 78:694, 1985

62. Karthik S, Phadke KD: Snakebite-induced acute renal failure: a case report and review of the literature. Pediatr Nephrol 19:1053, 2004

63. McKinney PE: Out-of-hospital and interhospital management of crotaline snakebite. Ann Emerg Med 72:168, 2001

64. Lewis JV, Portera CA: Rattlesnake bite of the face: case report and review of the literature. Am Surgeon 60:681, 1994

65. Parrish HM: Analysis of 460 fatalities from venomous animals in the United States. Am J Med Sci 245:129, 1963

66. Dart RC, McNally J: Efficacy, safety, and use of snake antivenoms in the United States. Ann Emerg Med 37:181, 2001

67. Jurkovich GJ, Luterman A, McCullar K, et al: Complications of Crotalidae antivenin treatment. J Trauma 28:1032, 1988

68. Dart RC, Seifert SA, Carroll L, et al: Affinity-purified, mixed monospecific crotalid antivenom ovine Fab for the treatment of crotalid venom poisoning. Ann Emerg Med 30:33, 1997

69. Gillissen A, Theakston RD, Barth J, et al: Neurotoxicity, haemostatic disturbances and haemolytic anaemia after a bite by a Tunisian saw-scaled or carpet viper (Echis 'pyramidium'-complex): failure of antivenom treatment. Toxicon 32:937, 1994

70. Hardy DL, Jeter M, Corrigan JJ: Envenomation by the Northern blacktail rattlesnake (Crotalus molossus molossus): report of two cases and the in vitro effects of the venom on fibrinolysis and platelet aggregation. Toxicon 20:487, 1982

71. Seifert SA, Boyer LV, Dart RC, et al: Relationship of venom effects to venom antigen and antivenom serum concentrations in a patient with Crotalus atrox envenomation treated with a Fab antivenom. Ann Emerg Med 30:49, 1997

72. LoVecchio F, DeBus DM: Snakebite envenomation in children: a 10-year retrospective review. Wilderness Environ Med 12:184, 2001

73. Berlinger FG, Flowers HH: Some observations of the treatment of snakebites in Vietnam. Military Med 138:139, 1973

74. Wu CH, Hu WH, Peng YC, et al: Snakebite complicated with Vibrio vulnificus infection. Vet Hum Toxicol 34:283, 2001

75. Hall EL: Role of surgical intervention in the management of crotaline snake envenomation. Ann Emerg Med 37:175, 2001

76. Avila-Aquero ML, Paris MM, Hu S, et al: Systemic cytokine response in children bitten by snakes in Costa Rica. Snakebite Study Group. Pediatr Emerg Care 17:425, 2001

77. Weed HG: Nonvenomous snakebite in Massachusetts: prophylactic antibiotics are unnecessary. Ann Emerg Med 22:220, 1993

78. Pantanowitz L, Guidozzi F: Management of snake and spider bite in pregnancy. Obstet Gynecol Survey 51:615, 1996

79. Parrish HM, Kahn MS: Snakebite during pregnancy. Obstet Gynecol 27:468, 1966

80. Cruz NS, Alvarez RG: Rattlesnake bite complications in 19 children. Pediatr Emerg Care 10:30, 1994

81. Weber RA, White RR: Crotalidae envenomation in children. Ann Plast Surg 31:141, 1993

82. Schmidt JM: Antivenom therapy for snakebites in children: is there evidence? Curr Opin Pediatr 17:234, 2005

83. Offerman SR, Bush SP, Moynihan JA, et al: Crotaline Fab antivenom for the treatment of children with rattlesnake envenomation. Pediatrics 110:968, 2002

84. Mammen EF: Fibrinogen abnormalities. Semin Thromb Hemost 9:1, 1983

85. Isbister GK, White J: Clinical consequences of spider bites: recent advances in our understanding. Toxicon 43:477, 2004

86. Zukowski CW: Black widow spider bite. J Am Board Fam Pract 6:279, 1993

87. Sternlicht H, Fosson A: Partial paralysis following a black widow spider bite. J Kentucky Med Assoc 9:531, 1987

88. Allen C: Arachnid envenomations. Emerg Med Clin North Am 19:269, 1992

89. Isbister GK, White J, Currie BJ: Letter to the editor: spider bites: addressing mythology and poor evidence. Am J Trop Med Hyg 72:361, 2005

90. Otten EJ: Venomous animal injuries. Emergency Medicine—Concepts and Clinical Practice. Rosen P, Barkin RM, Braen GR, et al, Eds. Mosby Year Book, St. Louis, 1992

91. Ryan PG: Preliminary report: experience with the use of dantrolene sodium in the treatment of bites by the black widow spider *Latrodectus hesperus*. J Toxicol Clin Toxicol 21:487, 1984

92. Jelinek GA: Widow spider envenomation (latrodectism): a worldwide problem. Wilderness Environ Med 8:226, 1997

93. Trethewy CE, Bolisetty S, Wheaton G: Red-back spider envenomation in children in Central Australia. Emerg Med (Fremantle) 15:170, 2003

94. Swanson DL, Vetter RS: Bites of brown recluse spiders and suspected necrotic arachnidism. N Engl J Med 352:700, 2005

95. Young VL, Pin P: The brown recluse spider bite. Ann Plast Surg 20:447, 1988

96. Vetter RS, Cushing PE, Crawford RL, et al: Diagnoses of brown recluse spider bites (loxoscelism) greatly outnumber actual verifications of the spider in four western American states. Toxicon 42:413, 2003

97. de Oliveira KC, Goncalves de Andrade RM, Piazza RM, et al: Variations in *Loxosceles* spider venom composition and toxicity contribute to the severity of envenomation. Toxicon 45:421, 2005

98. Gross AS, Wilson DC, King LE: Persistent segmental cutaneous anesthesia after a brown recluse spider bite. South Med J 83:1321, 1990

99. Wasserman G: Wound care of spider and snake envenomations. Ann Emerg Med 17:1331, 1988

100. Wong R, Hughes S, Voorhees J: Spider bites. Arch Dermatol 123:99, 1987

101. Sams HH, Hearth SB, Long LL, et al: Nineteen documented cases of *Loxosceles reclusa* envenomation. J Am Acad Dermatol 44:603, 2001

102. Sauer GC: Transverse myelitis and paralysis from a brown recluse spider bite. Missouri Med 72:603, 1975

103. Elbahlawan LM, Stidham GL, Bugnitz MC: Severe systemic reaction to *Loxosceles reclusa* spider bites in a pediatric population. Pediatr Emerg Care 21:177, 2005

104. Goto CS, Abramo TJ, Ginsburg CM: Upper airway obstruction caused by brown recluse spider envenomization of the neck. Am J Emerg Med 14:660, 1996

105. Glenn JB, Lane JE, Clark EK: Arachnid envenomation from the brown recluse spider. Clin Pediatr (Phila) 42:567, 2003

106. King LE, Rees RS: Dapsone treatment of brown recluse bite. JAMA 250:648, 1983

107. Gutowicz M, Fritz RA, Sonoga AL: Brown recluse spider bite: a literature review and case report. J Am Podiatric Med Assoc 79:142, 1979

108. Elston DM, Miller SD, Young RJ, et al: Comparison of colchicine, dapsone, triamcinolone, and diphenhydramine therapy for the treatment of brown recluse spider envenomation: a double-blind, controlled study in a rabbit model. Arch Dermatol 141:595, 2005

109. Wright SW, Wrenn KD, Murray L: Clinical presentation and outcome of brown recluse spider bites. Ann Emerg Med 30:28, 1997

110. Ben Welch E, Gales BJ: Use of stun guns for venomous bites and stings: a review. Wilderness Environ Med 12:111, 2001

111. Abroug F, Nouira S, Haguiga H, et al: High-dose hydrocortisone hemisuccinate in scorpion envenomation. Ann Emerg Med 30:23, 1997

112. Abroug F, Boujdaria R, Belghith M, et al: Cardiac dysfunction and pulmonary edema following scorpion envenomation. Chest 100:1057, 1991

113. Litovitz TL, Klein-Schwartz W, Rodgers GC Jr, et al: 2001 annual report of the American Association of Poison Control Centers Toxic Exposure Surveillance System. Am J Emerg Med 20:391, 2002

114. Bush SP, Gerardo C: Scorpion envenomations. eMedicine July 30, 2003 http://www.emedicine.com/emerg/topic524.htm

115. Gibly R, Williams M, Walter FG, et al: Continuous intravenous midazolam infusion for *Centruroides exilicauda* scorpion envenomation. Ann Emerg Med 34:620, 1999

116. Sofer S: Scorpion envenomation. Intensive Care Med 21:626, 1995

117. Curry SC, Vance MV, Ryan PJ, et al: Envenomation by the scorpion *Centruroides sculpturatus*. J Toxicol Clin Toxicol 21:417, 1983

118. Likes K, Banner W, Chavez M: *Centruroides exilicauda* envenomation in Arizona. West J Med 141:634, 1984

119. Rachesky IJ, Banner W, Dansky J, et al: Treatments for *Centruroides exilicauda* envenomation. Am J Dis Child 138:1136, 1984

120. Berg RA, Tarantino MD: Envenomation by the scorpion *Centruroides exilicauda* (*C. sculpturatus*): severe and unusual manifestations. Pediatrics 87:930, 1991

121. Bawaskar HS, Bawaskar PH: Prazosin for vasodilator treatment of acute pulmonary oedema due to scorpion sting. Ann Tropic Med Parasitol 81:719, 1987

122. Karnad DR: Haemodynamic patterns in patients with scorpion envenomation. Heart 79:485, 1998

123. Abroug F, ElAtrous S, Nouira S, et al: Serotherapy in scorpion envenomation: a randomised controlled trial. Lancet 354:906, 1999

124. Belghith M, Boussarsar M, Haguiga H, et al: Efficacy of serotherapy in scorpion sting: a matched-pair study. J Toxicol Clin Toxicol 37:51, 1999

125. Amaral CF, Rezende NA: Treatment of scorpion envenoming should include both a potent specific antivenom and support of vital functions. Toxicon 38:1005, 2000

126. Bond GR: Antivenin administration for *Centruroides* scorpion sting: risks and benefits. Ann Emerg Med 21:788, 1992

127. de Rezende NA, Chavez-Olortegui C, Amaral CF: Is the severity of *Tityus serrulatus* scorpion envenoming related to plasma venom concentrations? Toxicon 34:820, 1996

128. LoVecchio F, Welch S, Klemens J, et al: Incidence of immediate and delayed hypersensitivity to *Centruroides* antivenom. Ann Emerg Med 34:615, 1999

129. Hamed MI: Treatment of the scorpion envenoming syndrome: 12 years experience with serotherapy. Int J Antimicrob Agents 21:170, 2003

130. Watson WA, Litovitz TL, Klein-Schwartz W, et al: 2003 annual report of the American Association of Poison Control Centers Toxic Exposure Surveillance System. Am J Emerg Med 22:335, 2004

131. Kemp SF, DeShazo RD, Moffitt JE, et al: Expanding habitat of the imported fire ant (*Solenopis invicta*): a public health concern. J Allergy Clin Immunol 105:683, 2000

132. Handbook of Clinical Toxicology and Animal Venoms and Poisons. Meier J, White J, Eds. CRC Press, New York, 1995, p 331

133. deShazo RD, Williams DF, Moak ES: Fire ant attacks on residents in health care facilities: a report of two cases. Ann Intern Med 131:424, 1999

134. Elgart GW: Ant, bee, and wasp stings. Dermatol Clin 8:229, 1990

135. Sherman AM, Bechtel HB, EricksonTB: North American arthropod envenomation and parasitism. Wilderness Medicine, 4th ed. Mosby, St. Louis, 2001, p 863

136. Elston DM, Stockwell S: What's eating you? Bedbugs. Cutis 65:262, 2000

137. Rosen T: Caterpillar dermatitis. Dermatol Clin 8:245, 1990

138. Spach DH, Liles WC, Campbell GL, et al: Tick-borne diseases in the United States. N Engl J Med 329:936, 1993

139. Grattan-Smith PJ, Morris JG, Johnston HM, et al: Clinical and neurophysiological features of tick paralysis. Brain 120:1975, 1997

140. Dworkin MS, Shoemaker PC, Anderson DE: Tick paralysis: 33 human cases inWashington State. Clin Infect Dis 29:1435, 1999

141. Fenner PJ: Dangers in the ocean: the traveler and marine envenomation. I. Jellyfish. J Travel Med 5:135, 1998

142. Burnett JW, Calton GJ: Venomous pelagic coelenterates: chemistry, toxicology, immunology and treatment of their stings. Toxicon 25:581, 1987

143. Bonnet MS: The toxicology of the *Chironex fleckeri* jellyfish. Br Homeopath J 88:62, 1999

144. Burnett JW: Human injuries following jellyfish stings. Maryland Med J 41:509, 1992

145. Auerbach PS: Envenomation by aquatic invertebrates, envenomation by aquatic vertebrates.Wilderness Medicine, 4th ed. Auerbach PS, Ed. Mosby, St. Louis, 2001, p 1450

146. Kaufman MB: Portuguese man-of-war envenomation. Pediatr Emerg Care 8:27, 1992

147. Handbook of Clinical Toxicology and Animal Venoms and Poisons. Meier J, White J, Eds. CRC Press, New York, 1995, p 27

148. Brown CK, Shepherd SM: Marine trauma, envenomations, and intoxications. Emerg Med Clin North Am 10:385, 1992

149. Fenner PJ, Williamson JA, Burnett JW, et al: First aid treatment of jellyfish stings in Australia: response to a newly differentiated species. Med J Aust 158:498, 1993

150. Kumar S, Hlady WG, Malecki JM: Risk factors for seabather's eruption: a prospective cohort study. Public Health Rep 112:59, 1997

151. Baden HP, Burnell JW: Injuries from sea urchins. South Med J 70:459, 1997

152. Auerbach PS: Marine envenomations. N Engl J Med 325:486, 1991

153. Wu CH, Narahashi T: Mechanism of action of novel marine neurotoxins on ion channels. Annu Rev Pharmacol Toxicol 28:141, 1998

154. Cooper NK: Stone fish and stingrays: some notes on the injuries that they cause to man. J R Army Med Corps 137:136, 1991

155. McGoldrick J, Marx JA: Marine envenomations. J Emerg Med 9:497, 1991

156. Gwee MC, Gopalakrishnakone P, Yuen R., et al: A review of stonefish venoms and toxins. Pharmacol Ther 64:509, 1994

157. Shepherd S, Thomas SH, Stone K: Catfish envenomation. J Wilderness Med 5:67, 1994

158. Bolmkalns AL, Otten EJ: Catfish spine envenomation: a case report and literature review. Wilderness Environ Med 10:242, 1999

159. Auerbach PS, Yajko DM, Nassos PS, et al: Bacteriology of the freshwater environment: implications for clinical therapy. Ann Emerg Med 16:1016, 1987

160. Auerbach PS, Yajko DM, Nassos PS, et al: Bacteriology of the marine environment: implications for clinical therapy. Ann Emerg Med 16:643, 1987

Acknowledgments

Figures 1, 2, and 3   Photography by Bill Love/Blue Chameleon Ventures.

Figure 4   Photography from Animals Animals/Jim Bockowski. Used by permission.

Figure 5   Photography by B. J. Kaston (Trans. no K13623). Courtesy of the Department of Library Services, the American Museum of Natural History, New York.

17 Approach to the Cardiovascular Patient

Catherine M. Otto, M.D., and David M. Shavelle, M.D.

The complete evaluation of the cardiovascular patient begins with a thorough history and a detailed physical examination. These two initial steps will often lead to the correct diagnosis and assist in excluding life-threatening conditions. The history and physical examination findings should be assessed in the context of the overall clinical status of the patient, including lifestyle, comorbidities, and expectations. Cardiovascular conditions that frequently require evaluation include chest pain, dyspnea, palpitations, syncope, claudication, and cardiac murmurs. Each of these conditions will be discussed separately, with an emphasis on a diagnostic algorithm and the appropriate use of invasive and noninvasive cardiac testing.

Chest Pain

BACKGROUND

Chest pain is perhaps the most common cardiovascular symptom encountered in clinical practice. Establishing a cardiac origin of chest pain in a patient with multiple cardiovascular risk factors is essential because it allows initiation of appropriate therapy, thereby reducing the risk of myocardial infarction and death. Similarly, excluding a cardiac origin of chest pain in a low-risk patient is no less essential to avoid costly and potentially risky diagnostic testing that will neither add to the care of the patient nor relieve the patient's discomfort.[1] Cardiac disorders that result in chest pain include myocardial ischemia, myocardial infarction, acute pericarditis, aortic stenosis, hypertrophic cardiomyopathy, and aortic dissection. Noncardiac disorders that may result in chest pain include pulmonary embolism, pneumonia, pleural effusion, reactive airway disease, gastrointestinal and biliary disease, anxiety, and musculoskeletal disorders.

Angina most frequently is caused by atherosclerosis of the coronary arteries. Less common causes of angina include coronary artery spasm (e.g., Prinzmetal angina or spasm secondary to drug use, as with cocaine), coronary artery embolism (from aortic valve endocarditis), congenital coronary anomalies, spontaneous coronary artery dissection, coronary arteritis, and aortic dissection when the right coronary artery is involved. Angina may also occur in the presence of angiographically normal coronary arteries and is referred to as syndrome X. The underlying pathophysiology is thought to be related to microvascular dysfunction; the prognosis is generally good despite frequent episodes of chest pain.[2]

HISTORY AND PHYSICAL EXAMINATION

Essential features of the history include an accurate description of the chest pain, including the severity, frequency, location, radiation, quality, alleviating and aggravating factors, and duration of symptoms [*see Table 1*]. Anginal chest pain is often described as pressure or a heavy sensation. Symptoms may be difficult for the patient to describe and may be better characterized as discomfort, not pain. Angina typically is described as substernal with radiation to the left neck, jaw, or arm; is mild to moder-

ate in severity; and lasts for 5 to 15 minutes. Classically, angina occurs with exercise, stress, or exposure to cold weather and is relieved with rest or use of nitroglycerin. Some of the most useful features of the patient history that help establish that chest pain is angina are (1) reproducibility of the pain with a given degree of activity, (2) brief duration, and (3) alleviation of the pain with rest or use of nitroglycerin. In patients with a history of coronary artery disease (CAD), an accurate characterization of the quality and frequency of the pain is essential to determine whether a change in the anginal pattern has occurred (i.e., a patient with chronic stable angina now has unstable angina) or if a noncardiac origin of pain is now present (e.g., a patient with chronic stable angina now has musculoskeletal pain). Elderly patients, diabetic patients, and women experiencing angina often present with atypical symptoms that may appear to be noncardiac in nature.

Anginal chest pain may also be seen in patients with aortic stenosis or hypertrophic cardiomyopathy secondary to the supply-demand imbalance caused by excessive myocardial hypertrophy. Pericarditis commonly results in a sharp type of chest pain that occurs in the substernal region and worsens on inspiration (pleuritic) when the patient is in a supine position and improves when the patient is in an upright position. The pain of aortic dissection is also substernal, but typically, it is described as a tearing or ripping sensation, radiates to the back or interscapular area, begins abruptly, and fails to improve with rest or use of nitroglycerin. Musculoskeletal pain may be located anywhere on the chest wall, is often reproducible with palpation, and frequently worsens with rotation of the thorax. If the pain is musculoskeletal in origin, recent episodes of excessive lifting or activity may be elicited in the history. Esophageal spasm and gastroesophageal reflux disease are frequent causes of noncardiac chest pain.[3]

Cardiovascular risk factors should be reviewed in all patients presenting with chest pain. These risk factors include (1) a history of hypertension, hyperlipidemia, diabetes mellitus, or cigarette smoking,[4] and (2) a family history of CAD (i.e., a first-degree male relative with myocardial infarction or sudden death occurring before 55 years of age or a first-degree female relative with these events occurring before 65 years of age). Relatively uncommon factors that may also result in angina include prior radiation therapy, drug use (e.g., cocaine and amphetamines), and the presence of a systemic disease (e.g., lupus erythematosus, polyarteritis nodosum, or rheumatoid arthritis) that is associated with coronary arteritis.

The physical examination is usually unremarkable in patients presenting with anginal chest pain. However, certain physical findings can be very helpful in supporting the diagnosis of CAD. Elevated blood pressure by cuff sphygmomanometry and retinal abnormalities on fundoscopic examination (e.g., arteriovenous nicking, microaneurysms, arteriolar narrowing, or hemorrhages) may indicate previously undiagnosed hypertension. Xanthomas (cholesterol-filled nodules that occur subcutaneously or over tendons) indicate severe elevations in serum cholesterol levels. Femoral, carotid, or renal artery bruits and diminished peripheral pulses signify peripheral vascular disease and markedly increase the probability of CAD.[5] Tenderness to palpation of the chest wall, especially at the costochondral and chondrosternal articulations, suggests a musculoskeletal etiology of chest pain. Occasionally, patients with anginal chest pain also have a component of reproducible pain with palpation. A third heart sound and a holosystolic murmur of mitral regurgitation (secondary to ischemia of a papillary muscle) may be present if a patient with CAD is examined during an episode of anginal pain.

Physical examination also is directed toward findings that suggest an alternative cause of chest pain. Asymmetrical peripheral pulses, an early diastolic murmur, and the appropriate clinical history (tearing chest pain with radiation to the back) indicate an aortic dissection. A systolic murmur that radiates to the base of the neck (aortic stenosis) or a systolic murmur that increases in intensity with the strain phase of the Valsalva maneuver (hypertrophic cardiomyopathy) are uncommon but useful findings. A so-called leatherlike or scratchy series of sounds indicates a pericardial rub and supports a diagnosis of pericarditis. The intensity of the rub may increase with inspiration, indicating associated inflammation of the pleura, or pleuritis. Examination of the lung fields may disclose diminished breath sounds associated with dullness to percussion (pleural effusion), rhonchi, and egophony (pneumonia) or expiratory wheezes (asthma).

DIAGNOSTIC TESTS

On the basis of the history, chest pain is characterized as anginal, atypical anginal (some features of angina combined with some noncharacteristic features), or nonanginal. Estimates of the pretest probability of CAD can be accurately derived from a description of the chest pain syndrome and the presence or absence of cardiovascular risk factors.[6,7] The most widely used method for determining pretest likelihood of CAD is the Duke University Database formula, which considers the patient's age, sex, cardiovascular risk factor profile, description of chest pain, and information from the resting electrocardiogram.[8]

Although the diagnostic yield from the baseline ECG is low, it provides useful information on the advisability of pursuing additional diagnostic testing [see Figure 1]. Notable findings include Q waves consistent with a prior myocardial infarction and left ventricular hypertrophy that may be secondary to aortic stenosis, hypertrophic cardiomyopathy, or long-standing hypertension. ST segment depression, T wave abnormalities, and arrhythmias may be present if the ECG is obtained during an episode of anginal chest pain. A normal resting ECG predicts normal left ventricular function with a high degree of certainty (i.e., > 95%).

As with the ECG, a routine chest roentgenogram is usually normal. However, the presence of cardiomegaly, a left ventricular aneurysm, significant coronary or aortic calcification, or pulmonary venous congestion would be useful information and may warrant additional diagnostic testing.

Some physicians have started to use portable or handheld echocardiographic devices to evaluate patients with chest pain. Pertinent findings by echocardiography that would assist in establishing the etiology of chest pain include a pericardial effusion (pericarditis), hypokinesis or akinesis of a left ventricular wall segment (acute coronary ischemia), a dilated right ventricle (pulmonary embolism), and calcification and impaired excursion of the aortic valve leaflets (aortic stenosis).

Noninvasive stress testing is most likely to influence clinical decision making when the pretest probability of CAD is in the intermediate range. Patients with a low risk of CAD should not undergo noninvasive cardiac stress testing, because an abnormal test result would likely be a false positive one, and a negative test result would simply confirm the low probability of CAD. However, if patient reassurance is a consideration, a normal test result may be very useful. In addition, exercise stress testing provides information regarding symptom status, exercise capacity, and the hemodynamic response to exercise if the history is unclear (e.g., the patient denies symptoms but has decreased exercise capacity for "other reasons"). Absolute and relative contraindications to exercise testing should be reviewed in all patients before testing is begun [see Table 2].[8]

Similarly, patients with a high risk of CAD in general should not undergo noninvasive cardiac stress testing for the purpose of diagnosing CAD, because a negative test result would likely be a false negative one, and a positive result would simply confirm the high probability of CAD. In such patients, coronary angiography should be used to establish a diagnosis of CAD. However, noninvasive cardiac stress testing in certain patients at high risk for CAD may be useful. Indications for noninvasive stress testing in these patients include (1) assessment of the ef-

Table 1 Differentiating Features in the Patient's History of Chest Pain

Condition	Location	Radiation	Quality	Alleviating Factors	Aggravating Factors	Duration
Angina pectoris	Substernal	Jaw, arm	Pressure	Rest, nitroglycerin	Exercise, cold weather	5–15 minutes
Pericarditis	Left-sided, substernal	Neck, trapezius ridge	Sharp	Sitting up and leaning forward	Inspiration, supine position	Hours
Musculoskeletal	Variable over entire chest wall	None	Sharp or aching	Rest, anti-inflammatory or analgesic medications	Movement, palpation	Variable, but usually constant
Aortic stenosis	Substernal	Occasionally to jaw, arm	Pressure	Rest, nitroglycerin	Exercise, cold weather	Minutes
Hypertrophic cardiomyopathy	Substernal	Occasionally to jaw, arm	Pressure	Rest, nitroglycerin	Exercise, cold weather	Minutes
Aortic dissection	Substernal	Back	Tearing	None	None	Minutes to hours

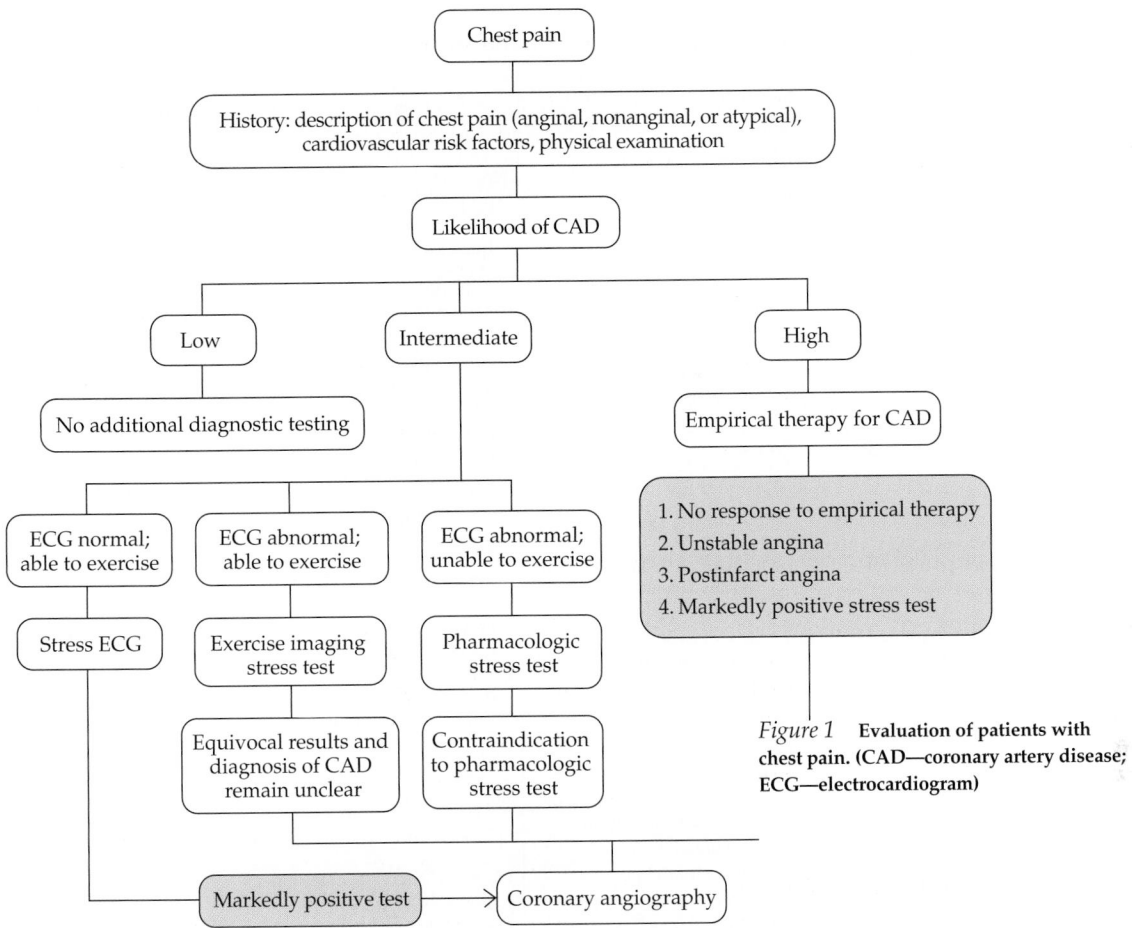

Figure 1 **Evaluation of patients with chest pain. (CAD—coronary artery disease; ECG—electrocardiogram)**

fectiveness of current medical therapy, (2) objective measurement of exercise capacity, (3) evaluation of the extent and location of ischemia or infarction with nuclear or echocardiographic imaging, (4) preoperative risk assessment in patients with known CAD who are undergoing noncardiac surgery, and (5) assessment of prognosis in patients with symptoms consistent with CAD or in patients with known CAD.

To establish the diagnosis of CAD in intermediate-risk patients, a number of noninvasive testing methods are available.[9] The decision whether to perform a specific test is based on various patient characteristics (e.g., body size, associated medical conditions, and ability to exercise), findings on the baseline ECG, and institutional experience with specific testing methods [see Table 3].[10-16] The most appropriate noninvasive stress test is chosen on the basis of each of these factors, as indicated in the chest pain algorithm [see Figure 1]. For most patients who are able to exercise with a normal baseline ECG, treadmill-ECG stress testing is indicated [see Table 2].[14,15,17] Women have a higher incidence of false positive results; therefore, many physicians recommend that, for all women, exercise be combined with an imaging method (e.g., echocardiography or nuclear imaging).[11] In general, to establish the diagnosis of CAD, exercise is preferred over pharmacologic stress agents. For patients who are unable to exercise because of physical limitations (e.g., arthritis or orthopedic problems), severe coexisting pulmonary disease, or general disability, pharmacologic stress agents such as dobutamine, adenosine, or dipyridamole can be employed. Each of these agents has specific contraindications [see Table 4].

Coronary angiography is considered the gold standard for the diagnosis of CAD. Although the incidence of major compli-

cations is low (< 2%), coronary angiography is costly and has some risk; thus, it is reserved for (1) patients with markedly positive noninvasive tests (i.e., hypotension and significant ST segment depression on ECG stress testing on a treadmill), (2) patients at high risk for CAD in whom a course of empirical antianginal therapy has failed, (3) patients with unstable or postinfarction angina, (4) patients with a contraindication to ex-

Table 2 **Absolute and Relative Contraindications to Exercise Testing**[8]

Absolute	*Relative*
Recent myocardial infarction (within 48 hr)	Left main coronary stenosis
Unstable angina not previously stabilized with medical therapy	Moderate stenotic valvular heart disease
Uncontrolled cardiac arrhythmias causing symptoms or hemodynamic compromise	Electrolyte abnormalities
Symptomatic severe aortic stenosis	Severe arterial hypertension
Uncontrolled symptomatic heart failure	Tachycardia or bradyarrhythmias
Acute pulmonary embolism or pulmonary infarction	Hypertrophic cardiomyopathy and other forms of outflow tract obstruction
Acute myocarditis or pericarditis	Mental or physical impairment leading to inability to exercise adequately
Acute aortic dissection	High degree of atrioventricular block

Table 3   Diagnostic Testing Methods Available for Evaluating Chest Pain[10-17]

Diagnostic Test	Indications	Information Obtained	Limitations	Sensitivity	Specificity
Exercise electrocardiographic stress test (stress ECG)	Initial test for most males with chest pain to establish diagnosis of CAD; females have higher rate of false positive test results Assess prognosis and functional capacity in patients with prior MI or known CAD Assess efficacy of current medical therapy in patients with known CAD	Exercise duration and functional aerobic capacity Amount of ST segment depression as indication of extent of ischemia Hemodynamic response to exercise	Normal baseline ECG Ability to exercise (patients who cannot attain adequate cardiopulmonary stress because of respiratory or musculoskeletal problems should receive a pharmacologic stress agent) Contraindications [see Table 2] False positives occur with left ventricular hypertrophy, bundle branch block, preexcitation syndromes, electrolyte abnormalities, and digoxin use	68%[1] (females, 61%[2])	77%[1] (females, 70%[2])
Thallium-201 perfusion scintigraphy	Often used when increased diagnostic accuracy for CAD required Can be combined with pharmacologic stress agents such as dobutamine, adenosine, or dipyridamole	Diagnosis of CAD with higher sensitivity and specificity than stress ECG Extent of ischemia Extent of infarction Left ventricular cavity size	Higher cost and longer testing time than stress ECG Imaging artifacts (attenuation) from diaphragm, breast, and intestine Contraindications [see Table 2 if exercise; see Table 4 if pharmacologic stress agent]	Ex thall 89%[5] Ph thall 90%[5] Dob thall 88%[4]	Ex thall 76%[5] Ph thall 70%[5] Dob thall 74%[4]
Technetium-99m perfusion scintigraphy	Often used when increased diagnostic accuracy for CAD required Can be combined with pharmacologic stress agents such as dobutamine, adenosine, or dipyridamole	Higher sensitivity and specificity for diagnosis of CAD than stress-ECG Extent of ischemia Extent of infarction Left ventricular cavity size ECG-gated SPECT allows calculation of left ventricular ejection fraction and evaluation of wall motion; evaluation of wall motion reduces false positive scans caused by imaging artifacts (attenuation) Used when excessive body weight precludes thallium imaging	Higher cost and longer testing time than stress ECG Imaging artifacts (attenuation) from diaphragm, breast, and intestine Contraindications [see Table 2 if exercise; see Table 4 if pharmacologic stress agent]	Ex tech 89%[5] Ph tech 90%[5] Dob tech 88%[4]	Ex tech 76%[5] Ph tech 70%[5] Dob tech 74%[4]
Exercise or dobutamine echocardiography	Exercise echocardiography often used when patient can exercise and has good-quality echocardiographic images Dobutamine used when exercise not possible	Higher sensitivity and specificity for diagnosis of CAD than stress ECG Left and right ventricular chamber size and function, presence of valve disease and pulmonary arterial pressures	Inadequate image quality may occur in patients with obesity, chronic obstructive pulmonary disease, and chest wall deformities Contraindications [see Table 2 if exercise; see Table 4 if pharmacologic stress agent]	Ex echo 85%[6] Dob echo 82%[6]	Ex echo 86%[6] Dob echo 82%[6]
Holter monitoring	Prinzmetal angina	Transient ST segment elevation in presence or absence of chest pain	Difficult to interpret because of baseline abnormalities		
Coronary angiography	Chest pain of unclear etiology despite noninvasive testing Angina not responsive to medical therapy Unstable and postinfarction angina Unclear diagnosis of CAD despite noninvasive stress testing	Anatomic severity of CAD Completely exclude cardiac origin of chest pain—gold standard of diagnostic tests Left ventricular function if left ventricular angiography also performed	Invasive procedure with low (< 2%) but inherent risk of MI, stroke, and death Represents a luminogram; does not evaluate functional significance of arterial narrowing	100%	100%

CAD—coronary artery disease Dob tech—dobutamine technetium Dob thall—dobutamine thallium ECG—electrocardiogram Ex echo—exercise echocardiography Ex tech—exercise technetium Ex thall—exercise thallium MI—myocardial infarction Ph stress—pharmacologic stress Ph tech—pharmacologic (adenosine or dipyridamole) stress combined with technetium Ph thall—pharmacologic (adenosine or dipyridamole) stress combined with thallium SPECT—single-photon emission computed tomography

Table 4   Mechanism of Action, Side Effects, and Contraindications of Pharmacologic Stress Agents

Pharmacologic Stress Agent	Mechanism of Action	Side Effects	Contraindications
Dobutamine	Increase myocardial oxygen demand by increasing heart rate, blood pressure, and myocardial contractility	78% of patients experience side effects: chest pain, palpitations, headache, flushing, malaise, and dyspnea; ventricular and atrial arrhythmias may occur	Severe hypertension at baseline, recent history of ventricular and/or atrial arrhythmias, and current beta-blocker use
Dipyridamole	Coronary artery vasodilatation—indirect response by blocking adenosine uptake and degradation	Increase in heart rate (average, 5–10 beats a minute), decrease in systolic blood pressure (average, 10–15 mm Hg); approximately 50% of patients experience side effects: chest pain, flushing, dizziness, headaches, or nausea; may provoke bronchospasm	Severe reactive airway disease (not contraindicated with chronic obstructive pulmonary disease unless a significant component of reactive airway disease is present), current theophylline use; avoid caffeine use 1 day before testing
Adenosine	Coronary artery vasodilatation—direct response	79% of patients experience side effects (more than with dipyridamole); side effects are chest, throat or jaw pain, headache, flushing, malaise, nausea, and bradyarrhythmias	Similar to dipyridamole; avoid caffeine use 1 day before testing; may cause bradyarrhythmias and is therefore contraindicated with baseline second- or third-degree heart block

ercise or pharmacologic stress testing, and (5) patients with equivocal results on noninvasive stress testing when the diagnosis of CAD remains unclear. Coronary angiography has certain limitations, including the inability to determine (1) the functional significance of a coronary artery stenosis and (2) which coronary plaque is likely to rupture (i.e., the so-called vulnerable plaque) and result in an acute coronary syndrome. Intravascular ultrasound studies have shown that coronary angiography may occasionally underestimate the severity of an area of narrowing, because it represents a so-called luminogram (shadow image) and not the size of the atherosclerotic plaque.[18] Despite these shortcomings, the extent and severity of CAD and measurement of left ventricular function by left heart catheterization are powerful predictors of clinical outcome.[14]

Dyspnea

BACKGROUND

Dyspnea refers to difficulty with breathing and can occur with a wide variety of cardiac, pulmonary, and systemic conditions [*see Table 5*]. Dyspnea can be classified as occurring (1) at rest, (2) with exertion, (3) during the night, awakening a patient from sleep (paroxysmal nocturnal dyspnea), or (4) during episodes of recumbency (orthopnea). Paroxysmal nocturnal dyspnea and orthopnea result from similar mechanisms. Specifically, the recumbent position augments venous return to the right heart. This increase in cardiac filling further increases the pulmonary capillary pressure and results in interstitial (and possibly intra-alveolar) pulmonary edema. Patients find relief by sitting upright, which reduces venous filling and transiently decreases the pulmonary interstitial pressure.

Dyspnea may be acute or chronic. An acute presentation suggests a pulmonary embolism, acute asthma exacerbation, pneumothorax, or rapidly developing pulmonary edema, as occurs with ischemic mitral regurgitation. Chronic dyspnea suggests heart failure resulting from systolic or diastolic dysfunction.

HISTORY AND PHYSICAL EXAMINATION

The history will often exclude less likely conditions and establish the etiology of dyspnea. A history of reactive airway disease, bronchodilator use, or corticosteroid use suggests asthma. Reactive airway disease tends to occur in children and young

adults; therefore, in older patients given this diagnosis, a cardiac cause for dyspnea (e.g., new onset of congestive heart failure) should be considered. A significant history of tobacco use, wheezing, chronic cough, and sputum production suggests obstructive airway disease.[19] A recent history of fever, chills, and

Table 5   Causes of Dyspnea

Cardiac
  Valve disease
    Aortic stenosis
    Aortic regurgitaion
    Mitral stenosis
    Mitral regurgitation
  Myocardial disease
    Hypertensive heart disease
    Dilated cardiomyopathy
    Restrictive cardiomyopathy
    Hypertrophic cardiomyopathy
  Pericardial disease
    Constrictive pericarditis
    Pericardial tamponade
    Pericardial effusion
  Coronary disease
    Myocardial infarction and ischemia
  Arrhythmia
    Ventricular and supraventricular arrhythmias
  Congenital heart disease
Pulmonary
  Reactive airway disease
  Chronic obstructive lung disease (chronic bronchitis and emphysema)
  Interstitial lung disease
  Infection (acute bronchitis and pneumonia)
  Pulmonary embolism
  Chest wall disease
  Pleural effusion
Deconditioning
Obesity
Malingering
Psychogenic
  Anxiety and panic disorders
Anemia

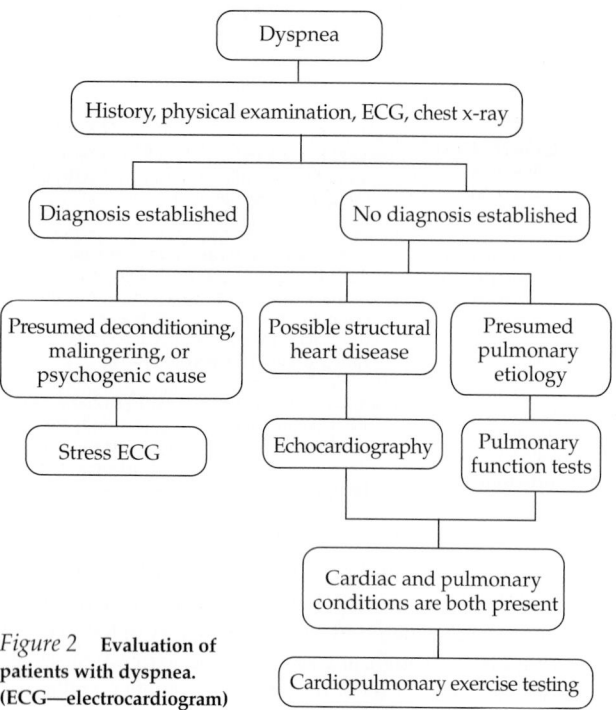

Figure 2 **Evaluation of patients with dyspnea. (ECG—electrocardiogram)**

productive cough may indicate bronchitis or pneumonia. The acute onset of dyspnea associated with pleuritic chest pain after a period of immobilization suggests pulmonary embolism. Paroxysmal nocturnal dyspnea, orthopnea, nocturia, recent weight gain, and lower extremity edema suggest a cardiac cause for dyspnea. Patients with chronic obstructive pulmonary disease may also awaken at night with dyspnea, but they usually have a history of sputum production and expectoration that improves with the patient in the upright position. Occasionally, on the basis of the history alone, it may not be possible to determine whether a cardiac or pulmonary cause of dyspnea is present.[20] In up to one third of patients being evaluated, dyspnea may have more than one cause.[21] In elderly patients, dyspnea may be the only symptom of a myocardial infarction. Hemoptysis may indicate the presence of severe underlying pulmonary disease (e.g., pulmonary embolism or lung cancer) but must be differentiated from hematemesis and nasopharyngeal bleeding.

Several findings on physical examination can assist in excluding a cardiac cause for dyspnea. These findings include a normal level of the jugular venous pressure, a normal point of maximal cardiac impulse, the lack of a third heart sound or cardiac murmurs, the absence of rales on lung examination, and the absence of peripheral edema. Alternatively, elevated jugular venous pressure, a displaced point of maximal cardiac impulse, a third heart sound, a holosystolic murmur of mitral regurgitation, basilar rales, and peripheral edema suggest congestive heart failure. A positive abdominojugular reflux maneuver may also identify dyspnea of cardiac origin.[22]

Obese patients and those with chest wall deformities may experience dyspnea secondary to the increased workload of breathing from the mechanical limitation imposed on the chest wall. Patients with emphysema frequently have an increased anteroposterior chest diameter, prolonged expiratory phase, expiratory wheezes, and diminished breath sounds. Central cyanosis, a normal anteroposterior chest diameter, and expiratory

wheezes or rhonchi on lung examination suggest chronic bronchitis. Expiratory wheezing can occur in both cardiac and pulmonary conditions and is therefore not helpful in establishing an etiology. Stridor may result from an upper airway obstruction or vocal cord paralysis and at times may resemble wheezing. Tachypnea, a loud pulmonic component of the second heart sound, and calf tenderness suggest a pulmonary embolism.

DIAGNOSTIC TESTS

An ECG and a chest roentgenogram should be the initial tests in the evaluation of dyspnea. Pertinent ECG findings include Q waves (prior myocardial infarction), a bundle branch block (structural heart disease), left ventricular hypertrophy (aortic stenosis, hypertension), and evidence of atrial chamber enlargement (valvular heart disease). Notable chest roentgenogram findings include an enlarged cardiac silhouette; interstitial or alveolar edema (congestive heart failure); aortic valve calcification (valvular heart disease); lung mass (lung cancer); focal infiltrate (pneumonia); pleural effusion (congestive heart failure, infectious process); and hyperinflation, bullae, and flattened hemidiaphragms (emphysema). Screening laboratory tests may be useful to exclude anemia as a potential cause of dyspnea.

If the diagnosis of dyspnea remains unclear, additional testing can be pursued [*see Figure 2*]. For patients with cardiovascular risk factors, with findings on physical examination that suggest structural heart disease, or with abnormal ECGs, echocardiography is indicated to exclude valvular heart disease and assess systolic and diastolic ventricular function. Patients with a presumed pulmonary etiology for dyspnea that remains undiagnosed should undergo pulmonary function testing to exclude reactive airway and restrictive and chronic obstructive pulmonary disease. Stress-ECG may be useful to objectively evaluate the degree of limitation and may be particularly helpful for patients with presumed deconditioning, malingering, or a psychogenic cause for dyspnea. For patients who may have a component of dyspnea from both a cardiac and a pulmonary source, cardiopulmonary exercise testing can be considered. Serum brain natriuretic peptide (BNP) levels are useful in distinguishing cardiac from noncardiac causes of dyspnea; a BNP greater than 100 pg/ml has a sensitivity of 90% but a specificity of only 73% for establishing the diagnosis of heart failure.[23] Other factors that affect BNP levels include renal failure, acute coronary syndrome, and female gender.

Palpitations

BACKGROUND

Palpitations are a nonspecific symptom associated with severity ranging from an increased awareness of the normal heartbeat to life-threatening ventricular arrhythmias [*see Table 6*]. Although palpitations represent one of the most common complaints requiring evaluation in the outpatient setting,[24] consensus guidelines describing the appropriate evaluation have not yet been established.

For patients with an underlying cardiac disease associated with palpitations, long-term outcome is poor. In contrast, clinical outcome is excellent for those with a noncardiac origin for palpitations, despite a high rate of recurrent episodes.[25] The key, then, in the evaluation of palpitations is to establish or exclude the presence of underlying structural heart disease. This determination can often be made by use of information from the history, physical examination, and ECG, but it may require additional evaluation with ambulatory ECG monitoring and possibly electrophysiologic testing. Psychiatric illnesses (anxiety, panic, and somatization disorders) account for a certain number of patients who seek medical attention for palpitations[25]; these disorders can initially be screened by use of simple and rapid patient-administered questionnaires. Although an underlying psychiatric illness should be considered in appropriate patients, it does not obviate the need for a complete evaluation to exclude a cardiac origin.[26] A diagnostic algorithm is presented that utilizes a rational approach to diagnostic testing [see Figure 3].

HISTORY AND PHYSICAL EXAMINATION

Palpitations are often described as a fluttering, a pounding, or an uncomfortable sensation in the chest. Occasionally, patients may complain only of a sensation of awareness of the heart rhythm. Patients may be able to discern whether the episodes are rapid and regular or rapid and irregular. Tapping a finger on the patient's chest in either a regular or an irregular manner may occasionally lead to an accurate description of the events.

A history of palpitations since childhood suggests a supraventricular arrhythmia and possibly an atrioventricular bypass tract, such as in the Wolff-Parkinson-White syndrome. Patients with congenital long QT syndrome typically begin to manifest symptoms in adolescence. A family history of sudden cardiac death, congestive heart failure, or syncope may suggest an inherited dilated or hypertrophic cardiomyopathy.

Knowing the circumstances in which palpitations occur may be useful in determining their origin. Palpitations associated only with strenuous physical activity are normal, whereas episodes occurring at rest or with minimal activity suggest un-

Table 6 Causes of Palpitations

General Category	Prognosis
Hyperdynamic state	Anemia, thyrotoxicosis, and exercise—all leading to sinus tachycardia
Increase in cardiac stroke volume	Aortic regurgitation, patent ductus arteriosus
Arrhythmia Ventricular	Frequent ventricular premature beats, ventricular tachycardia
Supraventricular	Frequent atrial premature beats, atrial fibrillation, atrial flutter, multifocal atrial tachycardia, atrial tachycardia, atrioventricular nodal reentry tachycardia, atrioventricular reentry tachycardia
Psychiatric	Anxiety, panic, or somatization disorder

derlying pathology. Episodes associated with a lack of food intake suggest hypoglycemia, and episodes after excessive alcohol intake suggest the toxic effects of alcohol. The resolution of symptoms with vagal maneuvers (breath-holding or the Valsalva maneuver) suggests paroxysmal supraventricular tachycardia. The onset of an episode of palpitations on assuming an upright position after bending over suggests atrioventricular nodal tachycardia.[27] Emotional stress and strenuous exercise may precipitate episodes in patients with long QT syndrome. Palpitations associated with anxiety or a sense of doom or panic suggest, but do not confirm, an underlying psychiatric disorder. An odds-ratio analysis found that regular palpitations, palpitations

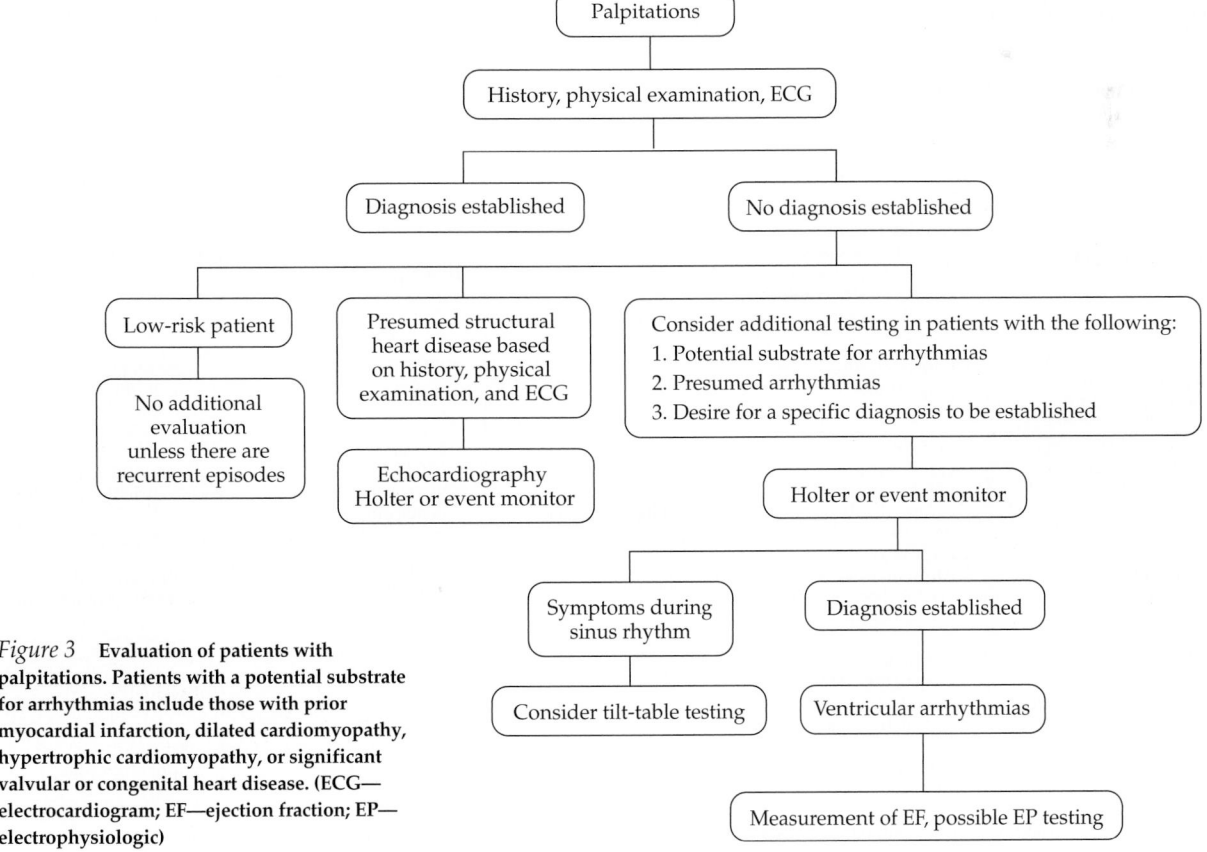

Figure 3 Evaluation of patients with palpitations. Patients with a potential substrate for arrhythmias include those with prior myocardial infarction, dilated cardiomyopathy, hypertrophic cardiomyopathy, or significant valvular or congenital heart disease. (ECG—electrocardiogram; EF—ejection fraction; EP—electrophysiologic)

Table 7 Medications Associated with Prolongation of the QT Interval

Antibiotics
  Tetracycline
  Erythromycin
  Trimethoprim and
    sulfamethoxazole
  Pentamidine
Antihistamines
  Terfenadine
  Astemizole
  Diphenhydramine
Antiarrhythmic agents
  Quinidine
  Procainamide
  Disopyramide
  Sotalol
  Amiodarone
  Dofetilide

Other cardiac drugs
  Bepridil
Gastrointestinal
  Cisapride
Antifungal drugs
  Ketoconazole
  Fluconazole
  Itraconazole
Psychotropic drugs
  Tricyclic antidepressants
  Phenothiazines
  Haloperidol
  Resperidone
Diuretics
  Indapamide

experienced at work, and those affected by sleeping were more likely to indicate cardiac origin.[28]

Symptoms associated with an episode of palpitations should also be explored. Syncope or presyncope after an episode suggests ventricular arrhythmias. However, patients with structural heart disease (e.g., severe left ventricular systolic dysfunction) may also experience these symptoms after supraventricular arrhythmias because of dependence on atrial filling. Additional mechanisms of syncope in patients with supraventricular arrhythmias have also been reported.[29] Regardless of the mechanism, syncope and presyncope are worrisome symptoms and merit a complete cardiovascular evaluation. Occasionally, patients may experience an episode of polyuria that follows the

palpitations. This condition may suggest supraventricular arrhythmias as the cause of palpitations, although studies have found this to be uncommon.[30]

The physical examination should focus on establishing whether underlying structural heart disease is present. Evidence of cardiac enlargement, third heart sound, and holosystolic murmur of mitral regurgitation suggest an underlying dilated cardiomyopathy. A midsystolic click, often followed by a systolic murmur, indicates mitral valve prolapse, which may be associated with both ventricular and supraventricular arrhythmias. A midsystolic murmur along the left sternal border that varies in intensity with alterations in left ventricular filling (e.g., Valsalva maneuver or changes in body position) is consistent with hypertrophic cardiomyopathy. Although atrial fibrillation is common in hypertrophic cardiomyopathy, ventricular arrhythmias may also occur.

DIAGNOSTIC TESTS

The ECG is the first step in the diagnostic evaluation of a patient with palpitations [see Figure 3]. A short PR interval and delta wave (Wolff-Parkinson-White syndrome), prolonged QT interval (long QT syndrome), and left bundle branch block (structural heart disease) are notable findings. Certain medications [see Table 7] may result in prolongation of the QT interval (i.e., acquired prolonged QT) and increase the risk of arrhythmias. Extreme voltage amplitudes and Q waves in leads I, aVL, and V4 through V6 are seen with hypertrophic cardiomyopathy. Pathologic Q waves indicate prior myocardial infarction and therefore a substrate for ventricular arrhythmias. Left ventricular hypertrophy or atrial abnormalities are nonspecific findings but suggest underlying structural heart disease. Many pertinent findings for various causes of palpitations can be obtained from the history, physical examination, and ECG [see Table 8].

If the cause of palpitations is not apparent after the initial evaluation (history, physical examination, and ECG), additional

Table 8 Diagnosis of the Underlying Etiology of Palpitations

Condition	History	Physical Examination	ECG	Underlying Etiology of Palpitations
Congenital long QT syndrome	Symptom onset in adolescence; episodes may be triggered by emotional stress and strenuous exercise	Normal	Prolonged QT interval	Ventricular arrhythmias
Atrioventricular bypass tract (e.g., Wolf-Parkinson-White syndrome)	Childhood episodes of palpitations	Normal	Short PR interval, delta wave	Supraventricular arrhythmias
Inherited dilated cardiomyopathy	Family history of cardiomyopathy, syncope, or sudden cardiac death	Abnormal cardiac impulse, systolic murmur (MR), third heart sound	Atrial enlargement, IVCD, LBBB, ventricular ectopic beats, or Q waves	Supraventricular or ventricular arrhythmias
Hypertrophic cardiomyopathy	Family history of cardiomyopathy, syncope, or sudden cardiac death	Systolic murmur	Increased voltage amplitude (LVH), Q waves in V4-V6, I, aVL	Supraventricular or ventricular arrhythmias
Anxiety, panic, or somatization disorder	Sense of doom, panic, or anxiety associated with episodes; coexisting psychiatric illness	Normal	Normal	Psychiatric
Mitral valve prolapse	Associated fatigue, dyspnea	Midsystolic click, systolic murmur (MR)	Normal or left atrial enlargement	Supraventricular arrhythmias

IVCD—interventricular conduction defect   LBBB—left bundle branch block   LVH—left ventricular hypertrophy   MR—mitral regurgitation

diagnostic testing is indicated for certain patients [*see Figure 3*].[27] Such patients include those with presumed arrhythmias that remain undiagnosed and those with prior myocardial infarction, dilated cardiomyopathy, hypertrophic cardiomyopathy, or significant valvular or congenital heart disease. In addition, patients who desire a specific diagnosis should be considered for additional testing.

Ambulatory ECG devices include Holter monitoring and continuous-loop event recorders. Holter monitors continuously record the heart rhythm for 24 or 48 hours. Patients are asked to maintain a diary documenting the time and describing the symptoms during the monitoring period. The key is to correlate patient symptoms with documented rhythm abnormalities. Patients with significant complaints of palpitations that correlate with periods of normal sinus rhythm should be further evaluated for underlying psychiatric disorders. Event monitors also continuously record the heart rhythm but require the patient to trigger the device to save the information. These devices can be kept by patients for several weeks and are especially useful when symptoms are infrequent. Event monitors are more cost-effective than Holter monitors for evaluating palpitations.[31,32] For patients with underlying structural heart disease and documented ventricular arrhythmias on ambulatory ECG monitoring, additional evaluation is warranted, including determination of left ventricular function and, occasionally, electrophysiologic testing.

Syncope

BACKGROUND

Syncope refers to a transient loss of consciousness accompanied by loss of postural tone. Roughly one third of all persons have an episode of syncope during their lifetime. It is a particularly common problem encountered in emergency departments and accounts for approximately 6% of all hospital admissions.[33] Determining which patients require hospital admission is difficult, given the large number of potential causes of syncope. Although many conditions that result in syncope are life threatening, other common etiologies, such as medication side effects, orthostatic hypotension, and psychiatric disorders, are benign.

Syncope is classified on the basis of the underlying etiology [*see Table 9*]. In elderly patients, the etiology may be multifactorial and related to medication side effects (particularly antihypertensives and antidepressants),[34] orthostatic hypotension, and bradyarrhythmias. Various medications are associated with prolongation of the QT interval and the development of ventricular arrhythmias and resulting syncope [*see Table 7*]. Vasovagal syncope is particularly common in otherwise healthy patients and has a benign prognosis. Episodes often occur in response to injury and are characterized by a sudden decline in blood pressure with or without associated bradycardia.

Establishing the presence of structural heart disease in the evaluation of patients with syncope is essential because such patients may have a 1-year mortality as high as 30%.[35,36] Structural heart disease is usually apparent on the basis of history, physical examination, and information from the baseline ECG. Occasionally, additional diagnostic testing with echocardiography, tilt-table testing, or electrophysiologic testing may be required.

HISTORY AND PHYSICAL EXAMINATION

The first step in establishing the presence of structural heart disease is to obtain an accurate description of the episode of syn-

Table 9 Classification of Syncope Based on Etiology

Cardiac
  Blood flow obstruction
    Aortic stenosis
    Pulmonic stenosis
    Left atrial myxoma
    Hypertrophic cardiomyopathy
    Massive pulmonary embolism
  Reduction in forward cardiac output
    Pericardial tamponade
    Severe pump failure
  Arrhythmia
    Tachyarrhythmias
      Ventricular tachycardia
      Supraventricular tachycardia
    Bradyarrhythmias
      Sinus bradycardia
      Sick sinus syndrome
      Atrioventricular block
      Carotid sinus hypersensitivity (can also be considered neurologic cause)
Neurologic
  Vasovagal
  Situational (micturition)
  Seizures
  Cerebrovascular accident
  Cerebrovascular insufficiency
  Orthostatic hypotension—autonomic dysfunction
Other
  Volume depletion
  Drugs
  Hypoglycemia
  Anxiety attack
  Psychogenic

cope. Key elements of the history include the presence of postural or exertional symptoms; associated chest pain, shortness of breath, or palpitations; and the situation in which the episode occurred (e.g., during micturition). Neurologic symptoms such as focal motor weakness, arm or leg movement, tongue biting, or a postictal state suggest a neurologic rather than cardiac event. However, seizures can occur from cardiac causes if a patient is kept upright during an episode (usually the result of a well-meaning bystander) because of cerebral hypoperfusion. A witness to the episode of syncope may provide a clear description of the event and should be questioned if possible. Medications associated with QT prolongation [*see Table 7*], blood pressure lowering (antihypertensives), and volume depletion (diuretics) should be reviewed. A family history of sudden cardiac death, syncope, or heart failure suggests hypertrophic cardiomyopathy, an inherited dilated cardiomyopathy, or long QT syndrome. A history of myocardial infarction or congestive heart failure raises the possibility of ventricular arrhythmias.

The physical examination focuses on determining whether structural heart disease is present and excluding common causes of syncope. Orthostatic vital signs should be obtained in all patients. Focal neurologic findings such as a motor deficit or a visual-field defect may indicate a neurologic cause for syncope. Pertinent findings on cardiovascular examination include a delayed carotid upstroke (aortic stenosis), an abnormal point of maximal cardiac impulse (cardiomyopathy), an irregular or

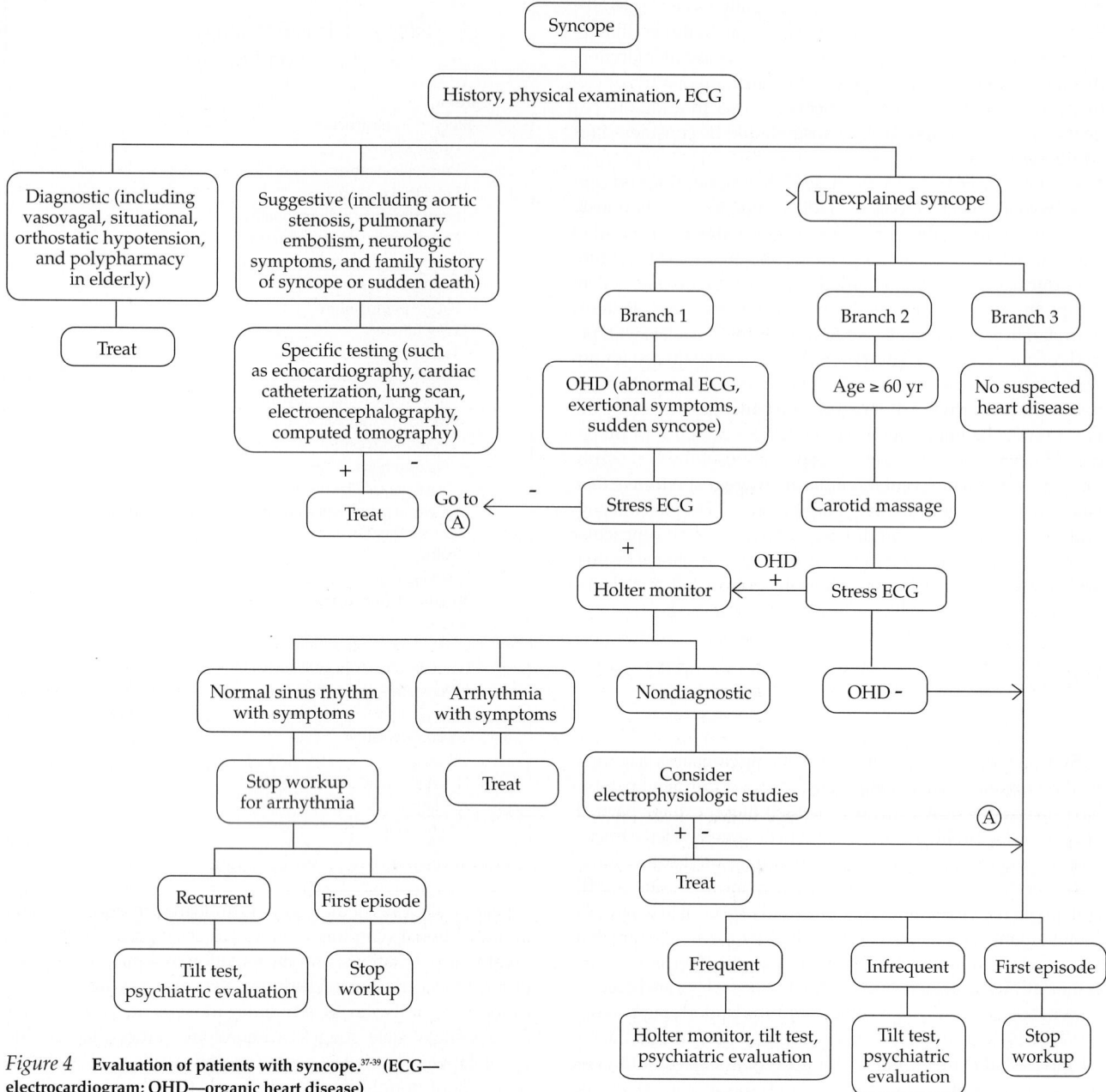

Figure 4 **Evaluation of patients with syncope.**[37-39] **(ECG—electrocardiogram; OHD—organic heart disease)**

bradycardiac rhythm (arrhythmias), a third heart sound (cardiomyopathy), a midsystolic murmur (aortic stenosis, hypertrophic cardiomyopathy), and a holosystolic murmur (mitral regurgitation secondary to left ventricular dilatation). Less common findings include an early diastolic sound (so-called tumor plop, indicating a left atrial myxoma), asymmetrical peripheral pulses (aortic dissection), and a loud second heart sound (pulmonary hypertension secondary to pulmonary embolism). Information from the history and physical examination yields a cause for syncope in approximately 45% of patients.[37]

DIAGNOSTIC TESTS

An ECG is the initial diagnostic test for all patients with syncope. Although the yield of the baseline ECG is low (approximately 5%), a number of potential findings are useful,[37] including bundle branch block, Q waves indicating prior myocardial infarction, left ventricular hypertrophy, prolonged QT interval, or evidence of atrioventricular block. The presence of sinus bradycardia, first-degree atrioventricular block, and bundle branch block suggests bradyarrhythmias as the cause of syncope. Extreme voltage amplitudes and Q waves in leads I, aVL, and V4 through V6 suggest hypertrophic cardiomyopathy and therefore the possibility of ventricular arrhythmias. An uncommon but unique ECG abnormality is the combination of a right bundle branch block, T wave inversions in leads V1 through V3, and an epsilon wave (a positive wave on the terminal portion of the QRS complex)—findings that indicate right ventricular dysplasia, which is associated with ventricular arrhythmias. Ventricular arrhythmias are also seen in the Brugada syndrome, which can be identified on the ECG by an incomplete right bundle branch block and ST segment elevation in leads V1 through V3.[38] A short PR interval and slurring of the initial portion of the

Table 10   Differential Diagnosis of Claudication

Condition	History	Physical Examination	Diagnostic Tests	Comments
Peripheral vascular disease	Symptoms occur with exercise and are relieved by rest	Diminished or absent peripheral pulses	ABI, arterial duplex ultrasound	Angiography reserved for those with severe disease who are considering surgical or percutaneous revascularization
Lumbar spinal stenosis	Paresthesias occur with standing and walking Symptoms are relieved by sitting and/or leaning forward History may include chronic low back pain and prior lumbar surgery	Normal peripheral pulses	Computed tomography or magnetic resonance imaging of the lumbar spine	Referred to as pseudoclaudication
Arthritis	Pain localized to the joint area as opposed to adjacent muscles	Normal peripheral pulses	Radiograph of affected joint	
Myalgia	Pain within a muscle group at rest and with exertion No relief with rest	Tenderness to palpation of the affected muscle group; reduced muscle strength	Laboratory evaluation of muscle inflammation with CPK, aldolase	Associated with hypothyroidism and end-stage renal disease; may be related to drug side effect (e.g., HMG-CoA reductase inhibitors)

ABI—ankle-brachial index   CPK—creatinine phosphokinase

QRS complex (the delta wave) suggests preexcitation (i.e., Wolff-Parkinson-White syndrome), with the possibility of rapid antegrade conduction via the accessory pathway.

If the etiology of syncope remains unclear after reviewing the history, physical examination, and ECG, additional diagnostic testing should be pursued. For patients with findings suggestive of an underlying cardiac cause, echocardiography and coronary angiography can be performed; for those with a possible neurologic cause, brain imaging (computed tomography or magnetic resonance imaging), neurovascular studies (carotid and transcranial Doppler ultrasound studies), and electroencephalography can be performed; and for those with a presumed pulmonary cause, lung scanning can be considered [see Figure 4]. If the diagnosis remains uncertain despite these tests, one of three pathways can be followed.[39]

The first pathway is for patients with structural heart disease or an abnormal ECG, who therefore have an increased likelihood for underlying arrhythmias or valve disease as a cause for syncope. Echocardiography, noninvasive stress testing, and ambulatory ECG monitoring using either a Holter monitor or continuous-loop event recorder should be considered for these patients. Event recorders have been found to be more accurate than Holter monitors in the diagnosis of syncope and presyncope; however, some patients find event recorders difficult to operate correctly.[40] If ambulatory ECG monitoring documents normal sinus rhythm in the setting of reported syncope, psychiatric evaluation and possibly tilt-table testing are warranted.

The second pathway is for patients older than 60 years, who are more likely to have valve disease (aortic stenosis), ischemic heart disease, carotid sinus syncope, cerebrovascular disease (transient ischemic attacks), and situational events (micturition, defecation, postural) as a basis for syncope. Carotid sinus massage (in the absence of carotid bruits, recent myocardial infarction, or stroke) should be the initial diagnostic test for these patients.[41,42] A positive test is defined as asystolic arrest lasting 3 seconds or longer and may identify those with cardioinhibitory hypersensitivity of the carotid sinus who will benefit from pacemaker placement. For

those with a negative test result, echocardiography, noninvasive stress testing, and ambulatory ECG monitoring can be performed.

The third pathway is for patients with unexplained syncope and no suspected structural heart disease. For those who have had a single episode, additional evaluation can be deferred until a second episode occurs. In patients with more than one episode, ambulatory ECG monitoring or tilt-table testing and, possibly, psychiatric evaluation should be considered.

Tilt-table testing was initially developed in the 1980s to evaluate patients with presumed vasovagal syncope. The passive portion of the test involves quickly raising a patient from the supine position to an angle of 60° (the tilt angle) for approximately 45 minutes, which causes pooling of venous blood in the lower extremities, a decrease in venous return, compensatory tachycardia, and enhanced ventricular contraction. For individuals with vasovagal syncope, augmented ventricular contraction causes activation of vasodepressor reflexes that result in hypotension, bradycardia, or both. Approximately 49% of patients referred for evaluation of

Table 11   Ankle-Brachial Index (ABI) Values and Accompanying Findings in Peripheral Vascular Disease (PVD)

Condition	Symptoms	Physical Findings	ABI
Normal	None	None	> 1.0
Mild PVD	Mild claudication on exertion	Diminished pulses	0.8–0.9
Moderate PVD	Moderate or severe claudication on exertion	Diminished or absent pulses; nonhealing ulcers or skin wounds	0.5–0.8
Severe PVD	Severe claudication; symptoms may occur at rest	Absent pulses; nonhealing ulcers or skin wounds	< 0.5

vasovagal syncope have positive responses, compared with 9% of control patients.[43] The active portion of tilt-table testing uses an isoproterenol infusion to enhance the vasodepressor reflex.

Claudication

BACKGROUND

Claudication is a condition of muscle pain or weakness associated with compromised blood flow to the extremities. It is a common complaint of patients who have peripheral vascular disease (PVD). Claudication is also a common symptom of CAD, a disease that shares risk factors with PVD. PVD is associated with an increased risk of stroke, cardiovascular death, and all-cause mortality[44]; it is most frequently caused by atherosclerosis. Studies suggest that PVD is infrequently diagnosed and often undertreated in the primary care setting.[45]

Intermittent claudication associated with PVD is a reproducible discomfort of a muscle group that is induced by exercise and relieved by rest. It is frequently manifested during ambulation as pain in the buttocks, upper thighs, and calves. The differential diagnosis of claudication [see Table 10] can be challenging and requires a detailed history and physical examination supplemented with diagnostic testing.

HISTORY AND PHYSICAL EXAMINATION

Claudication is described by patients as pain or cramping in the buttocks, thighs, and calf muscles. Symptoms typically occur during ambulation and are relieved by rest. Patients may also describe generalized weakness or a tired sensation within the legs. Depending on the extent of disease, men may experience impotence. Patients with severe disease may experience pain at rest. Patients with pain originating from compression of a nerve root describe an electric shock–like discomfort that frequently involves both legs and may be relieved by sitting down and leaning forward. More than one cause for leg symptoms may exist in a given patient, necessitating careful and clear delineation of each individual patient. Lumbar stenosis is another common cause of these symptoms (i.e., pseudoclaudication). The pain of pseudoclaudication is often poorly localized and may affect the leg from thigh to calf. Additional information that should be elicited from the history include the presence of a nonhealing ulcer or wound and previous manifestations of PVD, such as prior carotid endarterectomy. Risk factors associated with PVD are similar to those associated with CAD and include older age, cigarette smoking, diabetes mellitus, hypertension, and hyperlipidemia.

Physical examination should focus on assessment of all peripheral pulses, including the carotid, femoral, popliteal, dorsal pedis, and posterior tibial. Peripheral pulses should be described as normal, diminished, or absent, and the presence or absence of a bruit should be noted. For patients with severe PVD, the skin distal to the area of occlusion may be cold, and elevation of the legs may result in pallor of the soles of the feet. The presence and location of ulcers, skin wounds, and gangrene should be noted. Auscultation over the neck and abdomen may reveal bruits suggesting carotid artery stenosis and renal artery stenosis, repectively.

DIAGNOSTIC TESTS

The key diagnostic test in the evaluation of claudication is the ankle-to-brachial systolic pressure index (ABI). This involves measuring the systolic blood pressure in the ankle and the upper arm (brachial artery) in the supine position. The ankle systolic pressure is measured with a standard blood pressure cuff placed around the ankle, with the lower edge of the cuff situated above the malleoli. The blood pressure cuff is inflated to approximately 30 mm Hg above the systolic pressure to temporarily occlude flow. As the cuff is slowly deflated, a Doppler probe is used to monitor the signal; the pressure at which the Doppler flow signal is heard is recorded as the systolic pressure. A normal ABI is greater than 1.0; a value of less than 1.0 indicates the presence of PVD [see Table 11]. In addition to establishing the diagnosis of PVD, the ABI gives an assessment of disease severity and has prognostic implications for future cardiovascular and cerebrovascular events.[46,47] Additional noninvasive imaging to evaluate the extent and severity of PVD may include an arterial duplex ultrasound. The vasculature from the abdominal aorta to the distal tibial arteries can be imaged to localize the area of stenosis and assess hemodynamic significance using the Doppler flow signals or Doppler velocity spectra.

Diagnostic angiography involves the use of cineangiographic imaging and radiographic contrast to image the peripheral vessels. Because angiography is an invasive procedure that carries a 1% risk of vascular complications, it is usually reserved for patients being considered for surgical or percutaneous (angioplasty and stenting) revascularization procedures; such procedures are undertaken to relieve limiting claudication, nonhealing ulcers, and severe ischemia [see Figure 5]. Magnetic resonance angiography is potentially useful in the initial evaluation of patients with renal insufficiency.

A normal ABI excludes PVD as the cause of claudication and prompts investigation of alternative conditions as the underlying disorder [see Figure 6].

For patients with an abnormal ABI and mild symptoms, medical therapy can be initiated and risk factors modified.[48] Patients with moderate to severe symptoms should undergo additional noninvasive testing using arterial Duplex ultrasound. Patients with limiting symptoms or threatened limb loss should undergo angiography in anticipation of surgical or percutaneous revascularization.

Cardiac Murmurs

BACKGROUND

The increased access to health care and the widespread use and availability of echocardiography have resulted in a large number of patients being diagnosed and evaluated for various cardiac murmurs. A cardiac murmur may indicate underlying valvular, congenital, or myocardial disease, but it may also be caused by systemic illnesses and occur in the setting of a structurally normal heart.

Cardiac murmurs result from disturbed or turbulent blood flow, often through diseased cardiac valves or intracardiac structures. The presence of a cardiac murmur, however, does not always indicate underlying cardiac pathology. Hyperthyroidism, anemia, and a febrile illness may all result in increased blood flow through the aortic valve and produce a soft, crescendo-decrescendo, systolic murmur over the aortic area. In this setting, the aortic valve is structurally normal, and the murmur is the result of augmented blood flow (i.e., a flow murmur) caused by the systemic illness. Another common cause of a systolic murmur is calcification of the aortic valve, which is referred

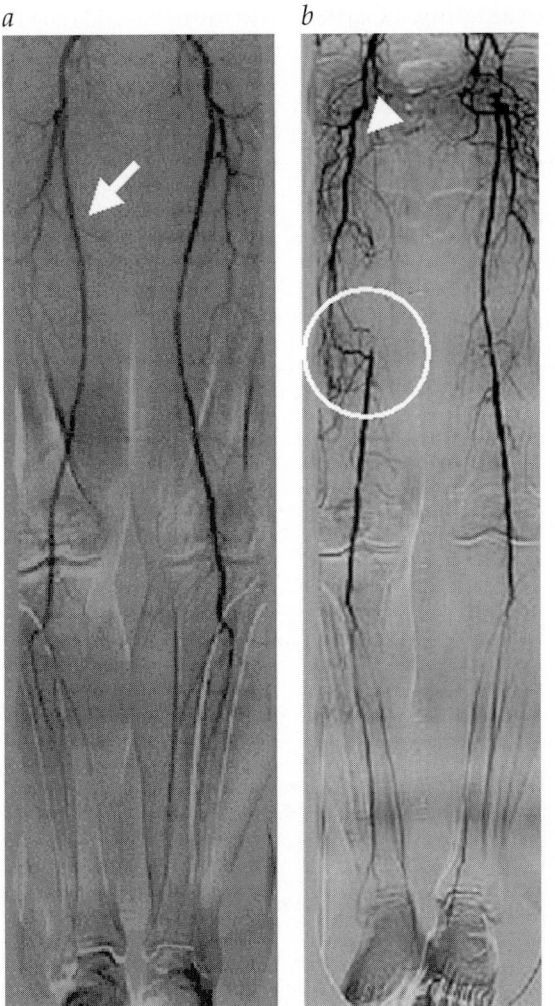

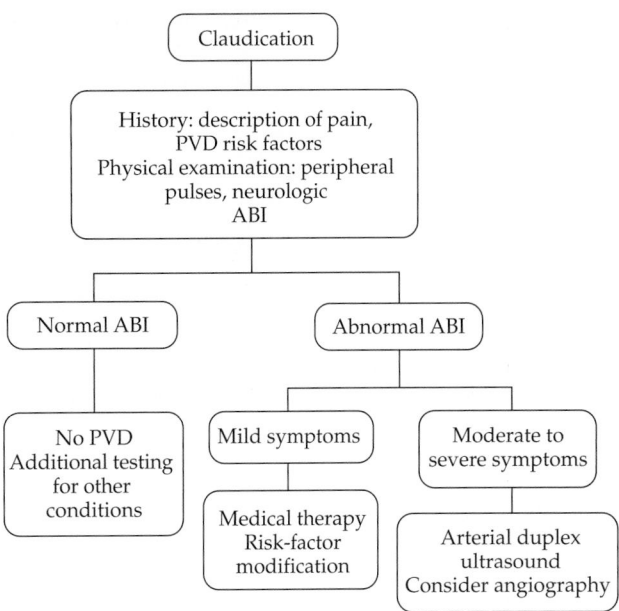

Figure 6   Evaluation of patients with claudication.

Figure 5   **Abdominal aortogram showing peripheral runoff. (*a*) Mild irregularities of the peripheral vessels are present, but there is no evidence of severe disease. The arrow indicates mild irregularities of the right superficial femoral artery. (*b*) Severe peripheral vascular disease with occlusion of proximal right superficial femoral artery (arrowhead) is evident. The midportion of the right superficial femoral artery is reconstituted from collateral vessels supplied by the right profunda femoralis artery (circle).**

aortic valve. A febrile illness occurring in childhood should raise the suspicion of rheumatic fever, possibly resulting in rheumatic mitral stenosis. Although rheumatic fever is uncommon in the United States, it may still be seen in immigrants from Asia, Latin America, and the Caribbean.

Establishing the presence or absence of cardiovascular symptoms is essential in the evaluation of a cardiac murmur. Otherwise healthy young adults without cardiac symptoms, with a systolic flow murmur and no other cardiac findings on examina-

to as aortic sclerosis when there is no obstruction to left ventricular outflow. Aortic sclerosis is a common finding in elderly patients; 25% of those older than 65 years are affected.[49] This condition is often diagnosed when a systolic murmur is detected in an otherwise asymptomatic patient during a routine physical examination. In addition to being caused by diseases of the cardiac valves, murmurs may result from intracardiac communications (atrial and ventricular septal defects), congenital abnormalities (patent ductus arteriosus), and disease of the myocardium (hypertrophic cardiomyopathy).

A thorough history and physical examination can often provide the etiology of a murmur. Additional diagnostic tests, such as the ECG, chest roentgenogram, and echocardiogram, are used to confirm the diagnosis and establish the severity of the abnormality.

HISTORY AND PHYSICAL EXAMINATION

A history of a childhood murmur may indicate a congenital abnormality of a cardiac valve, such as a bicuspid or unicuspid

Table 12   Differential Diagnosis of a Cardiac Murmur Based on Timing of Cardiac Cycle

Systolic
   Midsystolic
      Innocent flow murmur
      Aortic stenosis
      Pulmonic stenosis
      Atrial septal defect
   Holosystolic
      Ventricular septal defect
      Tricuspid regurgitation
      Hypertrophic cardiomyopathy
      Mitral regurgitation
Diastolic
   Early diastolic
      Aortic regurgitation
      Pulmonic regurgitation
   Middiastolic
      Mitral stenosis
      Tricuspid stenosis
      Austin Flint murmur associated with chronic
         aortic regurgitation
      Severe mitral regurgitation (augmented
         antegrade mitral valve flow)
Continuous
   Patent ductus arteriosus

Table 13 Physical Findings Useful for Evaluating a Cardiac Murmur

Condition	Timing	Location	Radiation	Characteristics	Effects of Maneuvers	Associated Findings
Innocent flow murmur	Midsystolic	Base	Variable or none	Soft, ejection	No change	None
Aortic stenosis	Systolic	Base (right second ICS)	Carotid arteries	Crescendo-decrescendo	Decrease with hand-grip or standing	Single S_2, delayed and decreased carotid upstroke, ES if mobile valve leaflets
Mitral regurgitation	Systolic	Apex	Axilla (sometimes back)	Holosystolic	Increase with hand-grip	Hyperdynamic apical impulse
Ventricular septal defect	Systolic	Left sternal border	None	Holosystolic	No change	Palpable thrill
Atrial septal defect	Systolic	Left second ICS	None	Crescendo-decrescendo	Possible increase with inspiration	Fixed split S_2
Hypertrophic cardiomyopathy	Systolic	Base	Carotid arteries	Late-peaking crescendo	Increase with standing and strain phase of Valsalva maneuver	Brisk carotid upstroke
Tricuspid regurgitation	Systolic	Left lower sternal border	Right lower sternal border	Holosystolic	Increase with inspiration	Prominent v waves in JVP, pulsatile liver
Pulmonic stenosis	Systolic	Left second ICS	None	Crescendo-decrescendo	No change	ES if mobile valve leaflets
Aortic regurgitation	Diastolic	Left sternal border	None	Decrescendo, high-pitched	Increase with handgrip	Wide pulse pressure, displaced and enlarged apical impulse
Mitral stenosis	Diastolic	Apex	None	Low-pitched rumble, presystolic accentuation	Best heard in left lateral decubitus position	Loud S_1, opening snap
Pulmonic regurgitation	Diastolic	Left second ICS	Left sternal border	Decrescendo	May increase with inspiration	—
Tricuspid stenosis	Diastolic	Right lower sternal border	Right upper abdomen	Low-pitched rumble	Increase with inspiration	Right ventricular heave
Patent ductus arteriosus	Continuous	Left second ICS	Back	Machinery-like	None	Wide pulse pressure, bounding pulses

ES—ejection sound   ICS—intercostal space   JVP—jugular venous pulse S_1, S_2—first, second heart sounds

tion, often require no additional evaluation.[50] In contrast, the finding of a cardiac murmur in patients with cardiovascular symptoms must be further explored and a diagnosis established.

Aortic stenosis may result in the triad of angina, syncope, and impaired exercise tolerance or dyspnea on exertion. Patients with hypertrophic cardiomyopathy experience similar symptoms but may also complain of palpitations from associated atrial or ventricular arrhythmias. Hypertrophic cardiomyopathy is most commonly familial, with an autosomal dominant inheritance pattern; therefore, the patient should be questioned about a family history of sudden cardiac death, heart failure, and syncope. Symptoms of mitral stenosis include shortness of breath, impaired exercise tolerance, palpitations (from associated atrial fibrillation), and hemoptysis. These symptoms may occur during episodes of tachycardia, volume overload, or both as mitral valve flow is increased and the stenotic mitral valve impairs filling of the left ventricle. Asymptomatic women with mitral stenosis may develop symptoms during pregnancy. Mitral and aortic regurgitation cause a volume overload to the left atrium and left ventricle, respectively, and may result in shortness of

breath, orthopnea, paroxysmal nocturnal dyspnea, lower extremity edema, and impaired exercise capacity. A ventricular septal defect is either congenital or ischemic (e.g., occurring after a myocardial infarction). The congenital form often becomes apparent during adolescence; the ischemic form presents several days after a myocardial infarction as a new holosystolic murmur associated with significant respiratory distress.

The physical examination begins with determining the timing of the murmur in the cardiac cycle—systolic, diastolic, or continuous [*see Table 12*]. The grade, quality, location, area of radiation, and change in intensity with maneuvers should then be described. Murmurs are graded on a scale of 1 to 6. Grade 1 is a soft intermittent murmur, grade 4 is a palpable murmur, and grade 6 is a murmur that can be appreciated without a stethoscope. Thus, most murmurs are classified as grade 2 or 3. Midsystolic murmurs are derived from the aortic or pulmonic valves or occur in association with hypertrophic cardiomyopathy. In contrast, holosystolic murmurs are the result of regurgitant blood flow through either the mitral or the tricuspid valves or a ventricular septal defect. The murmur of a ventricular septal

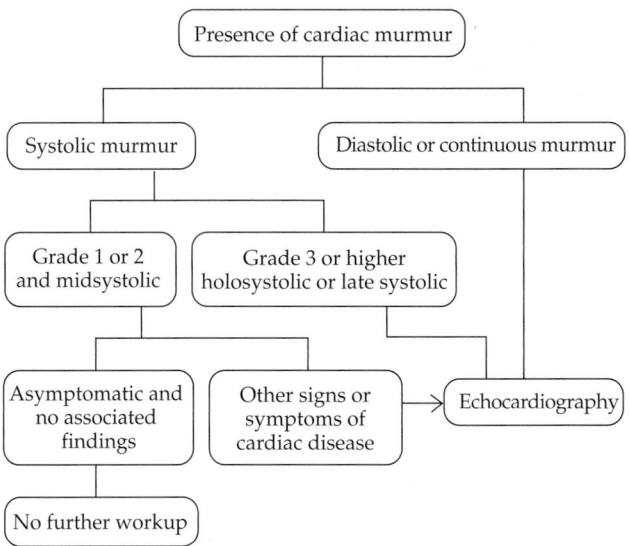

Figure 7 **Evaluation of patients with cardiac murmurs.**[45]

defect is usually well localized to the fourth left intercostal space, does not radiate significantly, and is often associated with a thrill (i.e., grade 4 or higher). Late systolic murmurs occur from mitral regurgitation that is secondary to (1) ischemia or infarction to the papillary muscles (ischemic mitral regurgitation), (2) left ventricular dilatation with functional mitral regurgitation, or (3) mitral valve prolapse. Additional findings on cardiac auscultation, such as a fixed, split second heart sound or an ejection sound, may be helpful in determining the etiology of a systolic murmur [*see Table 13*]. Electronic stethoscopes and handheld ultrasound devices have begun to supplement the bedside evaluation of cardiac murmurs.

Diastolic murmurs always indicate underlying cardiac pathology and commonly occur in either early diastole or middiastole. Early diastolic murmurs begin at the onset of diastole (i.e., with the second heart sound) and originate from regurgitant flow across the pulmonic and aortic valves. Aortic regurgitation occurs because of failure of the aortic valve leaflets to adequately coadapt during diastole and may be the result of disease processes affecting the aortic valve (e.g., endocarditis) or the aortic root (e.g., aortic dissection). Pulmonary regurgitation is most commonly seen in patients with pulmonary hypertension and is therefore associated with a loud second heart sound. Middiastolic murmurs occur from either mitral or tricuspid stenosis; the Austin Flint murmur associated with chronic aortic regurgitation or occurring in the setting of severe mitral regurgitation arises from augmented antegrade flow across the mitral valve in diastole.

In adults, continuous murmurs are usually from a previously undiagnosed patent ductus arteriosus. Occasionally, a patient with chronic aortic regurgitation may have a prominent systolic murmur in addition to the early diastolic murmur, thus simulating a continuous murmur. The systolic murmur in this case is the result of enhanced stroke volume from increased diastolic filling of the left ventricle. Whereas both conditions are associated with a widened pulse pressure and murmurs that occur during both systole and diastole, the murmur of a patent ductus arteriosus is continuous and peaks on the second heart sound; with chronic aortic regurgitation, there is a so-called silent period at the end of systole as the systolic murmur fades, before the beginning of the diastolic murmur.

Additional findings on physical examination can assist in determining the severity of the valve lesion and in excluding other conditions that result in similar murmurs. For patients with a midsystolic murmur presumed to be aortic stenosis, the carotid upstroke and splitting of the second heart sound should be carefully evaluated. A delayed carotid upstroke and single splitting of the second heart sound indicate hemodynamically severe aortic stenosis. However, physical examination has a low sensitivity for diagnosis of severe aortic stenosis, and overreliance on examination findings can lead to serious errors. The threshold for diagnostic imaging should be low in a patient with possible aortic valve stenosis. In contrast, hypertrophic cardiomyopathy results in a brisk carotid upstroke (the so-called spike-and-dome configuration) and normal splitting of the second heart sound. Severe mitral regurgitation can be identified by a holosystolic murmur associated with a third heart sound and a middiastolic murmur that results from the increased blood flow crossing antegrade across the mitral valve in diastole.

Several bedside maneuvers may also be useful in the evaluation of cardiac murmurs.[51] Right-sided murmurs (e.g., tricuspid regurgitation) increase in intensity during inspiration because of augmented right heart filling. The murmur of hypertrophic cardiomyopathy is extremely dependent on left ventricular filling, such that both the strain phase of the Valsalva maneuver and moving from squatting to the standing position augment the intensity of the murmur.

DIAGNOSTIC EVALUATION

An ECG should be obtained to evaluate for the presence of cardiac chamber enlargement and hypertrophy. Aortic stenosis imposes a pressure overload to the left ventricle, resulting in left ventricular hypertrophy by ECG in approximately 50% of patients. Hypertrophic cardiomyopathy is characterized by increased ventricular muscle mass, which is usually apparent on the ECG with extreme voltage amplitudes and small Q waves in leads I, aVL, and V4 through V6, referred to as septal Q waves. Mitral stenosis results in left atrial enlargement and occasionally right axis deviation and right ventricular hypertrophy.

Pertinent Web Sites

http://www.aha.org
The American Heart Association maintains this site with information on recent cardiovascular trials, local and national meetings, information for patients, and clinical guidelines.

http://www.acc.org
The American College of Cardiology maintains this site with information on recent cardiovascular trials, local and national meetings, and clinical guidelines.

http://www.theheart.org
This excellent site has current information on clinical trials, pertinent articles, clinical cases, discussion forums, cybersessions, and links to other cardiovascular sites. It frequently has summaries of clinical trials recently reported at the major cardiology meetings.

http://www.vasgbi.com
The Vascular Surgical Society of Great Britain and Ireland maintains this site, which provides patient information.

http://www.tasc-pad.org
The Trans-Atlantic Inter-Society Consensus on the Management of Peripheral Arterial Disease offers management recommendations for intermittent claudication, acute limb ischemia, and critical limb ischemia.

A chest roentgenogram should be reviewed for chamber enlargement and the presence of calcification. Chronic aortic and mitral insufficiency cause a volume overload to the left ventricle and left atrium, respectively. Left atrial enlargement, without enlargement of the left ventricle, and mitral valve calcification suggest mitral stenosis. Calcification of the aortic valve frequently occurs with valvular aortic stenosis but is rarely apparent on the chest roentgenogram.

In the absence of cardiovascular symptoms and other physical findings, a grade 1 or grade 2 midsystolic murmur does not require additional evaluation [see Figure 7].[50] Midsystolic murmurs of grade 3 and higher, holosystolic murmurs, or late systolic murmurs should be further evaluated by echocardiography. All patients with a diastolic or continuous murmur should be referred for echocardiography because these murmurs always indicate underlying cardiac pathology. In addition to confirming the etiology of a cardiac murmur, echocardiography provides evaluation of left ventricular systolic and diastolic function, wall motion abnormalities (that may indicate associated CAD), and estimation of pulmonary arterial pressures. For patients with valvular, congenital, or myocardial diseases, echocardiography provides a baseline from which additional studies can be obtained and used to follow disease progression over time.

Cardiovascular Information on the Internet

There are numerous sources of cardiovascular information on the Internet. The most useful general information sites are listed [see Sidebar Pertinent Web Sites].

The authors have no commercial relationships with manufacturers of products or providers of services discussed in this chapter.

References

1. Lee TH, Goldman L: Evaluation of the patient with acute chest pain. N Engl J Med 341:1187, 2000
2. Ammann P, Sabine M, Kraus M, et al: Characteristics and prognosis of myocardial infarction in patients with normal coronary arteries. Chest 117:333, 2000
3. Goyal RK: Changing focus on unexplained esophageal chest pain. Ann Intern Med 124:1008, 1996
4. Khot UN, Khot MB, Bajzer CT, et al: Prevalence of conventional risk factors in patients with coronary heart disease. JAMA 290:898, 2003
5. Hertzer NR, Beven EG, Young JR, et al: Coronary artery disease in peripheral vascular patients: a classification of 1,000 coronary angiograms and results of surgical management. Ann Surg 199:223, 1984
6. Diamond GA, Forrester JS: Analysis of probability as an aid in the clinical diagnosis of coronary artery disease. N Engl J Med 300:1350, 1979
7. Pryor DB, Shaw L, McCants CB, et al: Value of the history and physical in identifying patients at increased risk for coronary artery disease. Ann Intern Med 118:81, 1993
8. Gibbons RJ, Balady GJ, Bricker JT, et al: ACC/AHA 2002 guideline update for exercise testing: summary article. A report of the American College of Cardiology/American Heart Association Task Force on Practice Guidelines (Committee to Update the 1997 Exercise Testing Guidelines). J Am Coll Cardiol 40:1531, 2002
9. Chou TM, Amidon TM: Evaluating coronary artery disease noninvasively: which test for whom? West J Med 161:173, 1994
10. Gianrossi R, Detrano R, Mulvihil D, et al: Exercise-induced ST depression in the diagnosis of coronary artery disease: a meta-analysis. Circulation 80:87, 1989
11. Kwok Y, Kim C, Grady D, et al: Meta-analysis of exercise testing to detect coronary artery disease in women. Am J Cardiol 83:660, 1999
12. Garber AM, Solomon NA: Cost effectiveness of alternative test strategies for the diagnosis of coronary artery disease. Ann Intern Med 130:719, 1999
13. Kim C, Kwok YS, Heagerty P, et al: Pharmacologic stress testing for coronary disease diagnosis: a meta-analysis. Am Heart J 142:934, 2001
14. Gibbons RJ, Chatterjee K, Daley J, et al: ACC/AHA/ACP-ASIM guidelines for the management of patients with chronic stable angina: a report of the American College of Cardiology/American Heart Association Task Force on Practice Guidelines (Committee on the Management of Patients with Chronic Stable Angina). J Am Coll Cardiol 33:2092, 1999

15. Gibbons RJ, Abrams J, Chatterjee K, et al: ACC/AHA 2002 guideline update for the management of patients with chronic stable angina: summary article: a report of the American College of Cardiology/American Heart Association Task Force on practice guidelines (Committee on the Management of Patients With Chronic Stable Angina). J Am Coll Cardiol 41:159, 2003
16. Cheitlin MD, Alpert JS, Armstrong WF, et al: ACC/AHA Guidelines for the clinical application of echocardiography. A report of the American College of Cardiology/American Heart Association Task Force on Practice Guidelines (Committee on Clinical Application of Echocardiography). Developed in collaboration with the American Society of Echocardiography. Circulation 95:1686, 1997
17. Morise AP, Olson MB, Merz CN, et al: Validation of the accuracy of pretest and exercise test scores in women with a low prevalence of coronary disease: the NHLBI-sponsored Women's Ischemia Syndrome Evaluation (WISE) study. Am Heart J 147:1085, 2004
18. Nissen SE, Grines CL, Gurley JC, et al: Application of a new phased-array ultrasound catheter in the assessment of vascular dimensions: in-vivo comparison to cineangiography. Circulation 82:660, 1990
19. Holleman DR Jr, Simel DL, Goldberg JS: Diagnosis of obstructive airways disease from the clinical examination. J Gen Intern Med 8:63, 1993
20. Manning HL, Schwartzstein RM: Mechanism of disease: pathophysiology of dyspnea. N Engl J Med 333:1547, 1995
21. Schmitt BP, Kushner MS, Wiener SL: The diagnostic usefulness of the history of the patient with dyspnea. J Gen Intern Med 1:386, 1986
22. Mulrow CD, Lucey CR, Farnett LE: Discriminating causes of dyspnea through clinical examination. J Gen Intern Med 8:383, 1993
23. Mueller C, Scholer A, Laule-Kilian K, et al: Use of B-type natriuretic peptide in the evaluation and management of acute dyspnea. N Engl J Med 350:647, 2004
24. Kroenke K, Arrington ME, Mangelsdorff AD: The prevalence of symptoms in medical outpatients and the adequacy of therapy. Arch Intern Med 150:1685, 1990
25. Weber BE, Kapoor WN: Evaluation and outcomes of patients with palpitations. Am J Med 100:138, 1996
26. Lessmeier TJ, Gamperling D, Johnson-Liddon V, et al: Unrecognized paroxysmal supraventricular tachycardia: potential for misdiagnosis as panic disorder. Arch Intern Med 157:537, 1997
27. Zimetbaum P, Josephson ME: Current concepts: evaluation of patients with palpitations. N Engl J Med 338:1369, 1998
28. Summerton N, Mann S, Rigby A, et al: New-onset palpitations in general practice: assessing the discriminant value of items within the clinical history. Fam Pract 18:383, 2001
29. Leitch JW, Klein GJ, Yee R, et al: Syncope associated with supraventricular tachycardia: an expression of tachycardia rate or vasomotor response? Circulation 85:1064, 1992
30. Brugada P, Gursoy S, Brugada J, et al: Investigation of palpitations. Lancet 341:1254, 1993
31. Kinlay S, Leitch JW, Neil A, et al: Cardiac event recorders yield more diagnoses and are more cost-effective than 48-hour Holter monitoring in patients with palpitations: a controlled clinical trial. Ann Intern Med 124:16, 1996
32. Fogel RI, Evans JJ, Prystowsky EN: Utility and cost of event recorders in the diagnosis of palpitations, presyncope and syncope. Am J Cardiol 79:207, 1997
33. Hayes OW: Evaluation of syncope in the emergency department. Emerg Med Clin North Am 16:601, 1998
34. Hanlon JT, Linzer M, MacMillan JP, et al: Syncope and presyncope associated with probable adverse drug reactions. Arch Intern Med 150:230, 1990
35. Kapoor WN: Evaluation and outcome of patients with syncope. Medicine (Baltimore) 69:160, 1990
36. Brieger D, Eagle KA, Goodman SG, et al: Acute coronary syndromes without chest pain, an underdiagnosed and undertreated high-risk group: insights from the Global Registry of Acute Coronary Events. Chest 126:461, 2004
37. Linzer M, Yang EH, Estes M III, et al: Diagnosing syncope: value of history, physical examination and electrocardiography (pt 1). Ann Intern Med 126:989, 1997
38. Littmann L, Monroe MH, Kerns WP 2nd, et al: Brugada syndrome and "Brugada sign": clinical spectrum with a guide for the clinician. Am Heart J 145:768, 2003
39. Linzer M, Yang EH, Estes M III, et al: Diagnosing syncope: unexplained syncope (pt 2). Ann Intern Med 127:76, 1997
40. Sivakumaran S, Krahn AD, Klein GJ, et al: A prospective randomized comparison of loop recorders versus Holter monitors in patients with syncope or presyncope. Am J Med 115:1, 2003
41. Brignole M, Menozzi C, Gianfranchi L, et al: Neurally mediated syncope detected by carotid sinus massage and head-up tilt table test in sick sinus syndrome. Am J Cardiol 68:1032, 1991
42. McIntosh SJ, Lawson J, Kenny RA: Clinical characteristics of vasodepressor, cardioinhibitory, and mixed carotid sinus syndrome in the elderly. Am J Med 95:203, 1993
43. Kapoor WN, Smith MA, Miller NL: Upright tilt testing in evaluating syncope: a comprehensive literature review. Am J Med 97:78, 1994
44. Newman A, Shemanski L, Manolio T, et al: Ankle-arm index as a predictor of cardiovascular disease and mortality in the Cardiovascular Health Study. Arterioscler Thromb Vasc Biol 19:538, 1999
45. Hirsch AT, Criqui M, Treat-Jacobson D, et al: Peripheral arterial disease detection, awareness, and treatment in primary care. JAMA 286:1317, 2001
46. Leng GC, Fowkes FGR, Lee AJ, et al: Use of the ankle brachial pressure index to predict cardiovascular events and death: a cohort study. BMJ 313:1440, 1996
47. Lee AJ, Price JF, Russell MJ, et al: Improved prediction of fatal myocardial infarction using the ankle brachial index in addition to conventional risk factors: the Edinburgh

Artery Study. Circulation 110:3075, 2004

48. Hiatt WR: Medical treatment of peripheral arterial disease and claudication. N Engl J Med 344:1608, 2001

49. Stewart BF, Siscovick D, Lind BK, et al: Clinical factors associated with calcific aortic valve disease. J Am Coll Cardiol 29:630, 1997

50. Bonow RO, Carabello B, de Leon AC Jr, et al: ACC/AHA guidelines for the man-

agement of patients with valvular heart disease: a report of the American College of Cardiology/American Heart Association Task Force on Practice Guidelines (Committee on Management of Patients with Valvular Heart Disease). J Am Coll Cardiol 32:1486, 1998

51. Lembo NJ, Dell'Italia LJ, Crawford MH, et al: Bedside diagnosis of systolic murmurs. N Engl J Med 318:1572, 1988

18 Hypertension

Gary L. Schwartz, M.D., F.A.C.P., and Sheldon G. Sheps, M.D., F.A.C.P.

Hypertension is the most common chronic disorder in the United States, affecting over 31% of the adult population.[1] It is the most common reason adults visit the doctor's office. In the year 2000, hypertension accounted for more than 1 million office visits to health care providers. The prevalence increases with age: for a normotensive middle-aged person in the United States, the lifetime risk of developing hypertension approaches 90%.[2] With the increasing age of the population in most developed and developing societies, it seems safe to assume that hypertension will become steadily more widespread in the coming years.

Hypertension is a major risk factor for stroke, myocardial infarction, heart failure, chronic kidney disease, progressive atherosclerosis, and dementia.[3-5] The treatment of hypertension is highly effective in reducing cardiovascular (CV) morbidity and mortality.[6,7] However, despite widespread public and professional education regarding the risks of hypertension and the benefits of treatment, and despite the ready availability of effective therapies, only 58% of adults with hypertension are receiving treatment, and in only 31% is hypertension controlled.[8,9] A number of factors have been identified that contribute to poor control rates for hypertension.[10] Improving these rates depends on setting appropriate, patient-specific, evidence-based therapeutic goals, understanding and using available treatment options in an efficient and cost-effective manner, involving the patient in goal setting and the care process in an empathetic manner, and employing timely follow-up to monitor and adjust therapy as necessary. It is important to recognize that multiple classes of drugs are often needed for control; that patient education, communication, and involvement in the process are vital to long-term compliance; and that systematic approaches to therapy are required to achieve and maintain control over time.

Definition

Blood pressure (BP) is a quantitative trait that is continuously distributed in the population. Essential hypertension represents the upper end of the distribution of this trait and is defined by the BP level associated with a threshold value of increased CV risk. Any definition of hypertension is arbitrary because the risk of CV disease related to BP level increases steadily across the spectrum of BP values. On the basis of a meta-analysis of studies relating BP level to vascular mortality, optimum BP is defined as less than 115/75 mm Hg.[11] According to the Seventh Report of the Joint National Committee on Prevention, Detection, Evaluation, and Treatment of High Blood Pressure (JNC 7), normal BP (the level associated with minimal risk) for adults 18 years of age or older is a systolic BP of less than 120 mm Hg and a diastolic BP of less than 80 mm Hg [see Table 1].[8] Blood pressures ranging from 120 to 139 mm Hg systolic or 80 to 89 mm Hg diastolic are considered prehypertensive. Patients with BP in this range are at increased risk for the development of target organ injury and for progression to definite hypertension over time.[11,12] Therefore, these patients should have annual BP checks and be educated in strategies to lower BP and CV risk and to prevent the development of hypertension [see Prevention of Hypertension, below]. For patients with diabetes or renal disease, BP in the prehypertensive range poses a significantly higher risk than for healthy persons, and a lower threshold for intervention is indicated for these patients: above 130 mm Hg systolic or 80 mm Hg diastolic.

For the general population, hypertension is defined as a systolic BP of 140 mm Hg or higher or a diastolic BP of 90 mm Hg or higher. Hypertension is further divided into two stages, defined on the basis of the highest level of either the systolic or diastolic BP. Prospective drug intervention trials have demonstrated the benefit of treatment for patients with a diastolic BP of 90 mm Hg or higher. Isolated systolic hypertension (ISH), which occurs mainly in persons older than 55 years, is defined as a systolic BP of 140 mm Hg or higher and a diastolic BP of less than 90 mm Hg. ISH is the most common hypertension subtype in older adults, who are the most rapidly growing segment of the population.[13] Epidemiologic data clearly demonstrate elevated and graded risk associated with systolic BP higher than 115 mm Hg.[11] However, those drug intervention trials that showed a benefit enrolled only subjects whose systolic BP was 160 mm Hg or higher[7]; the benefits of drug intervention for patients with ISH whose pretreatment systolic BP is below 160 mm Hg is inferred.

Epidemiology

Currently, it is estimated that at least 65 million adults in the United States have hypertension or are taking antihypertensive medications.[1] In addition to definitive hypertension, an additional 45 million adults in the United States have prehypertension.

In developed societies, BP increases with age. Diastolic BP plateaus in the fifth decade and may decline thereafter, but systolic BP continues to rise through the seventh decade. In persons younger than 50 years, diastolic BP level is the major predictor of CV risk, whereas in persons older than 60 years, systolic BP is the major predictor.[14] Individual risk is related to the level and duration of BP, as well as to the presence of other CV risk factors and of injury to so-called target organs—brain, heart, kidneys, peripheral arteries, and retina.[3]

The relationship between BP and CV morbidity and mortality begins in patients whose BP is higher than optimal levels (115/75 mm Hg) and is strong, continuous, graded, consistent, and independent. The relationship between BP and CV risk has largely been determined in middle-aged and older people, but

Table 1 Classification of Blood Pressure for Adults 18 Years of Age and Older[8]

Category	Blood Pressure Level (mm Hg)
Normal	Systolic < 120 and diastolic < 80
Prehypertension	Systolic 120–139 or diastolic 80–89

Hypertension
  Stage 1
  Stage 2
	
	Systolic 140–159 or diastolic 90–99
	Systolic ≥ 160 or diastolic ≥ 100

Note: These categories apply to patients who are not taking antihypertensive drugs and are not acutely ill. When systolic and diastolic blood pressures fall into different categories, the higher category should be selected to classify the person's blood pressure status.

above-normal BP in young adulthood is also related to increased long-term CV and all-cause mortality.[15] In young adulthood and early middle age, hypertension is more common in men than in women, but the opposite is the case in persons 60 years of age and older.[9] At all ages, hypertension is more common in African Americans than in whites; in all ethnic and racial groups, it is more common in the economically disadvantaged. At any given level of BP, CV risk is greater in men than women, in blacks than whites or members of other racial or ethnic groups, in older persons than younger ones, and in patients with target organ disease and longer duration of hypertension.[3]

Etiology and Genetics

Essential hypertension develops as the consequence of a complex interplay over time between susceptibility genes and environmental factors. Numerous family and population studies suggest a significant role for genetic factors. Hypertension in persons younger than 55 years is four times more common in individuals with a family history of hypertension than in those with no family history of it. Estimates of the genetic contribution to BP variation range from 30% to 50%. However, the genetic contribution to essential hypertension is complex. Multiple genes are likely involved, and although the effects of some genes may affect BP independently, most genetic effects involve both gene-gene interaction (epistasis) and gene-environment interaction. Important interactions between the effects of specific genes and environments may occur at a particular time (perinatal life) or over the lifetime of an individual. Thus, sorting out the genetic contribution to essential hypertension is complex and challenging.

Some insight into the genetic contribution to essential hypertension has been gained from the identification of rare monogenic forms of hypertension.[16] Interestingly, most of these forms of hypertension arise from gene mutations that result in impairment of renal sodium excretion; impairment occurs either through the disruption of the renal sodium transport systems or through interference with mineralocorticoid receptor activity. Additional insight has come from studies that employ a candidate gene approach, in which genes are chosen on the basis of animal studies or previous knowledge of genes that encode proteins involved in BP regulatory pathways. Polymorphisms of candidate genes have been studied in association and linkage studies to assess their potential role in essential hypertension in humans. Most extensively studied have been genes encoding components of the renin-angiotensin-aldosterone system. Results of this line of investigation have implicated polymorphisms of the angiotensinogen (AGT) gene *(AGT)* and the angiotensin-converting enzyme (ACE) gene *(ACE)* in human essential hypertension.[17,18] The M235T variant of *AGT* has been associated with higher circulating levels of AGT and is found more often in hypertensive than in normotensive persons.[18] An insertion/deletion polymorphism of *ACE* has been associated with differences in ACE activity, with higher levels associated with the deletion allele.[19] The deletion allele has also been associated with several cardiovascular phenotypes, including higher BP levels and greater risk of target organ complications in hypertensive individuals.[17,20] In large samples, the observed associations have frequently been gender specific, suggesting interaction between the effects of the insertion/deletion polymorphism and gender.[17,21]

Variants of other genes have been implicated in essential hypertension. Adducin is a membrane skeleton protein consisting of α and β subunits that may influence ion transport across membranes. A variant of the α-adducin gene (Gly 460 Trp) has been associated with essential hypertension in case-control studies and may play a role in salt-sensitive hypertension.[22] Linkage studies have also found evidence indicating a role for variants of adrenergic and dopamine receptor genes.[23] Some evidence supports a possible role for variants in genes encoding the epithelial sodium channel, atrial naturetic peptide, G-proteins, the glucagon receptor, insulinlike growth factor 1, the endothelin system, endothelial nitric oxidase synthase, apolipoproteins and cytokines.[24] Experts expect that the number of gene polymorphisms associated with essential hypertension will continue to grow. However, because of the limitations of candidate gene studies and of linkage and association studies, there is a need for new approaches that can assess the effects of multiple genes and environments. These types of studies will be difficult to perform but will be necessary if we are to someday be able to determine the specific genotypes and environments present in the majority of persons destined to develop hypertension.[25]

Regarding the role of genetics in hypertension, it is important to note that hypertension is virtually nonexistent in primitive peoples who follow a preagricultural hunter-gatherer lifestyle. This lifestyle involves significant daily physical activity and a diet rich in potassium and low in fat and sodium. Obesity is uncommon. Dietary patterns involve periods of feasting interspersed with long periods with minimal food. Given that the human gene pool has changed little over the past 30,000 years, some suggest that hypertension is the consequence of a human genome selected for a hunter-gatherer lifestyle but now interacting with a modern one. In contrast to primitive societies, modern societies are characterized by a low level of physical activity and constant availability of abundant food that is rich in sodium and fat and low in potassium; the result is an increase in body weight with aging and a high incidence of obesity. Genetic adaptation to the hunter-gatherer lifestyle provided survival advantages in that environment but may now be contributing to many modern diseases such as obesity and hypertension.

Pathophysiology and Pathogenesis

Simplistically, BP is the product of cardiac output and peripheral vascular resistance (BP = cardiac output × peripheral vascular resistance). Thus, variations in extracellular fluid volume, the contractile state of the heart, and vascular tone determine variation in BP level. The hemodynamic hallmark of established essential hypertension is elevated peripheral vascular resistance. An increase in cardiac output is occasionally noted early but is not a persistent finding. Hypertension can be viewed as the final outcome of a complex interaction between genetic and environmental factors that act on intermediate physiologic systems involved in BP regulation (i.e., those that influence fluid volume, heart contractility, and vascular tone).

A central hypothesis for the pathogenesis of essential hypertension involves an interaction between the high dietary sodium intake typical of industrial society and defects in renal sodium excretion. Evidence of a role for dietary sodium comes from animal studies and from epidemiologic and experimental studies in humans.[26,27] Guyton hypothesized that hypertension develops when the kidneys require a higher BP to maintain extracellular volume within normal limits.[28] This would occur in persons with impaired renal sodium excretion. Studies support the possibility of an inherited defect in renal sodium excretion as the basis of human essential hypertension. Most monogenic forms of hypertension discovered so far involve mutations that impair renal sodium excretion by increasing mineralocorticoid activity or by influencing tubular sodium transport systems.[16] Moreover, renal sodium excretion can be influenced by variations in activity of both the renin-angiotensin-aldosterone system and the sympathetic nervous system. Angiotensin II enhances renal tubular sodium reabsorption directly and indirectly through stimulation of aldosterone release and the sympathetic nervous system. Additional mechanisms that may explain defective renal sodium excretion include an inherited reduction in the number of nephrons, as well as the presence of a subpopulation of so-called ischemic nephrons, which occur as a result of increased afferent renal artery tone and lead to increased renin activity.[29,30] Extracellular volume expansion could lead to chronic increases in vascular resistance through mechanisms of organ autoregulation of blood flow (i.e., variation in the tone of vessels that occurs so as to regulate organ blood flow to meet metabolic needs). Some studies have suggested that volume expansion stimulates the release of a sodium-potassium-adenosine triphosphatase (Na^+,K^+-ATPase) inhibitor (i.e., an ouabainlike substance) that facilitates renal sodium excretion but increases vascular tone by interfering with sodium-calcium exchange in vascular smooth muscle cells.[31]

Other evidence suggests that increased sympathetic nervous system activity has a role in causing hypertension in some persons.[32] These cases could be the result of a genetic tendency toward increased sympathetic activity interacting with repetitive psychogenic stress, obesity, or high sodium intake. Hypertension could also arise or be sustained by defects in baroreceptor function.[33]

Weight gain and obesity (especially abdominal fat accumulation) are associated with an increased risk of hypertension. A number of humoral factors may be responsible, including increased activity of the sympathetic nervous system and the renin-angiotensin system.[34] In addition, obesity is associated with insulin resistance and hyperinsulinemia. Hyperinsulinemia may directly stimulate sympathetic activity, in addition to promoting vascular hypertrophy (increased vascular tone) and re-

nal sodium retention.[35] In addition, leptin levels are increased in obese individuals. Leptin may also increase BP by stimulation of the sympathetic nervous system.[36]

More general abnormalities of cell membranes or multiple ion transport systems acting across cell membranes could contribute to the development of hypertension. In addition to impairing sodium excretion in the kidneys, these defects could act in a variety of ways to influence vascular structure and tone.[37] Vascular tone could also be influenced by variation in vascular endothelial function through an imbalance in the production of substances that cause vasodilation (e.g., nitric oxide) and those that cause vasoconstriction (e.g., endothelin).[38]

The role of progressive stiffness in the aorta and its major branches as a cause of the progressive rise in systolic BP with age has received increasing attention in recent years.[39,40] In younger persons, the aorta is elastic, and expands as blood is ejected into it during systole. This retained blood is then transmitted to the periphery during diastole, supporting diastolic BP. As the aorta and its main branches stiffen, in association with aging and other factors, the aorta dilates less during systole. This leads to a higher systolic pressure. In addition, because more blood is forced into the periphery during systole, less is available during diastole, and diastolic pressure decreases. This causes the familiar widening of pulse pressure (i.e., the difference between systolic and diastolic BP) with age. Moreover, as blood is ejected into the aorta, a forward pressure wave is generated that travels along the vessel and into the periphery. The forward wave is partially reflected at points of vessel branching and by smaller vessels in the periphery. These reflections summate to form a composite reflected pressure wave that returns to the central aorta in late systole or early diastole and is referred to as the augmentation pressure. Forward pulse-wave velocity increases with progressive aortic stiffness. Consequently, the reflected wave (i.e., the augmentation pressure) arrives earlier at the central aorta, which further increases the peak central aortic pressure.[41]

Diagnosis

The diagnosis of hypertension relies on multiple office measurements of BP performed in a rigorous manner with a validated and well-maintained mercury or aneroid sphygmomanometer and a cuff of appropriate size. Several expert groups have published guidelines for proper BP measurement; unfortunately, these guidelines are rarely complied with in most clinics [see Table 2].[42,43] The diagnosis of hypertension requires findings of an elevated average BP on at least two office visits, with at least two standardized measures of BP made at each visit. For most patients, confirmation can occur over a 1- to 2-month period. If an initial BP is severely elevated, confirmation should occur over a shorter period. Self-measurements of BP outside the office setting can be used to distinguish sustained hypertension from isolated clinic hypertension; self-measurement has the further advantages of involving patients in the process of care (which often improves compliance) and aiding in the assessment of response to therapy. On average, home readings are lower than office readings; therefore, values above 135 mm Hg systolic or 85 mm Hg diastolic are considered elevated.[8] BP devices for home use (aneroid or oscillometric) need to be validated twice yearly by the health care provider, and patients need to be educated in the technique of proper BP measurement [see Table 2].

Table 2   Proper Blood Pressure Measurement Technique

Patient should refrain from smoking or caffeine ingestion for 30 min before measurement

Patient should be at rest, seated in a chair with back and feet supported, for at least 5 min before measurement is taken

Patient should not speak while blood pressure is being measured

Patient's arm should be bare, with no tight clothing constricting the upper arm

Select a proper cuff size for the arm: bladder should encircle at least 80% of arm (many adults will require a large cuff)

Position patient's arm so cuff is at the level of the heart

Place stethoscope bell over brachial artery

Inflate cuff to occlude the pulse

Deflate at rate of 2–3 mm/sec

Measure systolic (first sound) and diastolic (last sound) to nearest 2 mm Hg

Repeat measurement after 2 min

Under special circumstances, measure blood pressure with patient in standing position

Table 3 Classic Features of Essential Hypertension

Onset of hypertension in the fourth or fifth decade of life
Family history of hypertension
BP < 180/< 110 mm Hg at diagnosis
Asymptomatic
History, physical examination, and routine laboratory studies are normal (no target organ damage at time of diagnosis)
BP control achieved with lifestyle changes and one or two drugs
BP control is maintained once achieved

AMBULATORY BLOOD PRESSURE MONITORING

Cross-sectional studies show that BP averages from ambulatory BP monitoring (ABPM) correlate better with the presence of target organ injury (especially left ventricular hypertrophy [LVH]) than office BP measurements.[44] Also, prospective studies and population-based observational studies have shown that average BP derived from ABPM predicts additional risk for CV events after adjustment for clinic or office BP.[45] This is true for both untreated as well as treated patients.[46,47] ABPM is the best method of establishing the presence of isolated clinic hypertension (so-called white-coat hypertension), which is defined as an elevation in BP that occurs only in the clinic setting, with normal BP in all other settings, in the absence of evidence of target organ injury.[8] Screening for white-coat hypertension is currently a reimbursable indication for ABPM by Medicare.[48] The possibility of a white-coat effect should be considered in selected patients with resistant hypertension, in elderly patients with significant office systolic hypertension, and in some pregnant women. Although white-coat hypertension is associated with lower risk than sustained hypertension, it is a predictor of future sustained hypertension in some persons.[49] Other uses for ABPM include assessment of hypotensive symptoms, episodic hypertension, and suspected autonomic dysfunction in patients with postural hypotension.[8] ABPM is also useful in the evaluation of the occasional patient with hypertensive target organ injury (e.g., LVH, stroke) whose office BP is normal. Some of these patients have so-called white-coat normotension, or masked hypertension; for these patients, BP is normal in the office but is elevated outside the office setting.[50] This important group is often missed in routine practice unless target organ injury is manifested.

INITIAL EVALUATION

The initial evaluation of patients with elevated BP has four major objectives: (1) to identify lifestyle factors contributing to elevated BP and higher CV disease risk, (2) to identify associated modifiable CV risk factors, (3) to assess for target organ injury or clinical CV disease, and (4) to identify any secondary causes of hypertension.[8] The second and third objectives are important for risk stratification, which defines the BP threshold for initiation of drug therapy and establishes the BP goal to achieve with therapy.[51,52]

The overall frequency of secondary hypertension is 5% to 10% in primary care practices. The classic picture of essential hypertension should be compared with the individual patient's presentation [see Table 3]. Secondary hypertension should be suspected on finding features that are not consistent with essential hypertension. Such features include age at onset younger than 30 or older than 50 years; BP higher than 180/110 mm Hg at di-

agnosis; significant target organ injury at diagnosis; hemorrhages and exudates on retinal examination; renal insufficiency; LVH; poor response to appropriate three-drug therapy; and the presentation of accelerated or malignant hypertension. Specific features that suggest secondary causes of hypertension vary with the individual condition [see Table 4].

HISTORY

The clinician should inquire about a family history of hypertension, premature CV disease, and disorders that would increase the possibility of secondary hypertension (e.g., polycystic kidney disease or other renal disease, medullary cancer of the thyroid, hyperparathyroidism, or pheochromocytoma). The patient should be questioned about lifestyle habits that influence BP (e.g., level of physical activity, sodium intake, use of caffeine and alcohol, history of weight gain), and CV risk (e.g., tobacco use); in addition, the patient should be asked about symptoms suggesting target organ disease (e.g., angina, symptoms of heart failure, transient cerebral ischemia, or renal disease) or secondary hypertension (e.g., spells suggesting pheochromocy-

Table 4 Features Suggesting Specific Causes of Secondary Hypertension

Condition	Features
Primary aldosteronism	Unprovoked hypokalemia
Pheochromocytoma	Labile BP with episodic headache, sweats, tachycardia, pallor, abdominal pain, weight loss, diabetes Neurofibromas, café-au-lait spots Orofacial neuromas (multiple endocrine neoplasia type II) Retinal angiomas (von Hippel–Lindau syndrome)
Renovascular hypertension	Abdominal or flank bruits Peripheral bruits/diminished pulses from atherosclerosis Elevated serum creatinine level, hypokalemia Flash pulmonary edema Hypertension in a patient younger than 30 yr (fibromuscular dysplasia) Sudden onset or worsening of systolic-diastolic hypertension after age 50 yr (atheromatous disease) Accelerated malignant hypertension Treatment-resistant hypertension Unexplained subacute decline in renal function
Cushing syndrome	Truncal obesity, proximal muscle weakness and atrophy Stria, acne, thin skin, bruises, hyperpigmentation Elevated plasma glucose, hypokalemia
Coarctation of the aorta	Headaches Cold feet, claudication Delay of femoral pulse compared to radial pulse Weak or absent femoral pulses High BP in arms/low BP in legs Murmurs in front/back chest
Polycystic renal disease	Abdominal/flank masses, family history of renal disease

toma). A known history of dyslipidemia, diabetes, or cerebrovascular, heart, or renal disease also should be documented. In addition, a thorough medication review (including prescription and over-the-counter drugs, herbs and herbal compounds, and street drugs) is important to identify drugs that can raise BP or interfere with the antihypertensive effect of planned drug therapy [see Table 5].[53] In patients with a history of hypertension, the physician should ascertain the duration of hypertension, the previous BP levels, and the specific drugs used for treatment, together with the efficacy of those drugs and the reasons for discontinuing them. Other comorbid conditions and their treatments need to be documented, because they may influence antihypertensive drug selection.

PHYSICAL EXAMINATION

The examination should include at least two standardized measurements of BP with the subject in the seated position. Initially, BP should also be measured in the opposite arm (to identify arterial narrowing, which can cause an inaccurately low reading in one arm) and in the standing position, especially in diabetic patients and older patients (to identify orthostatic declines). Height and weight should be determined to permit calculation of body mass index, and waist circumference (a potential CV risk factor) should be recorded.

The physical examination is directed toward identifying target organ injury or features suggesting secondary hypertension [see Table 4]. Retinal examination should be performed, primarily to identify changes resultling from diabetes or severe hypertension (i.e., hemorrhages, exudates, papilledema). Arteriolar narrowing, focal constrictions, and arteriovenous nicking on retinal examination are more closely associated with atherosclerosis and are of limited value for predicting the severity of hypertension or assessing overall CV risk.[52,54]

LABORATORY TESTS

Laboratory studies are performed to support the general goals of the initial evaluation [see Table 6]. In addition, they provide baseline information for monitoring in patients who are subsequently treated with antihypertensive drugs that can influence laboratory values (i.e., diuretics, beta blockers, ACE inhibitors, and angiotensin receptor blockers [ARBs]). Additional studies are not advised unless the history, physical examination, or initial laboratory studies are inconsistent with essential hypertension or suggest a specific secondary etiology.

If the initial assessment suggests renal dysfunction, the patient should be evaluated for chronic kidney disease by measuring 24-hour urinary protein excretion and estimating glomerular filtration rate (GFR). Equations are available to estimate GFR [see Table 6].[55,56] The Modification of Diet in Renal Disease (MDRD) equation requires measurement of blood urea nitrogen and serum albumin concentrations in addition to serum creatinine concentration. The estimate of GFR can also be calculated with an online tool (available at www.hdcn.com/calcf/gfr.htm).

RISK STRATIFICATION

At any given level of BP, specific factors in an individual patient may result in deviations above or below the average CV risk observed in population studies. These factors are used to determine the BP threshold and timing of drug therapy and the BP goal for the individual patient. Individual specific factors that determine risk include the presence of other CV risk factors and the presence of injury to the target organs of hypertension or clinical CV disease.[3] A simple and clinically useful scheme modified from the JNC 6 report separates patients into three levels of risk [see Table 7].[51] This scheme suggests aggressive treatment and lower

Table 5   Drugs That Can Increase Blood Pressure or Interfere with Antihypertensive Drug Efficacy

Drug	Mechanism
Oral contraceptives	Sodium retention, increase level of angiotensinogen, facilitate action of catecholamines
Alcohol (moderate or heavy intake)	Activate sympathetic nervous system, increase cortisol secretion and intracellular calcium levels
Sympathomimetics and amphetamine-like substances (over-the-counter cold or allergy formulas, diet pills)	Increase peripheral vascular resistance
Nonsteroidal anti-inflammatory drugs	Sodium retention, renal vasoconstriction; interfere with efficacy of all antihypertensive drugs, especially diuretics, beta blockers, angiotensin-converting enzyme inhibitors, angiotensin receptor blockers
Corticosteroids	Iatrogenic Cushing disease
Tricyclic antidepressants	Inhibit action of centrally acting sympatholytics (clonidine, guanfacine)
Serotoninergics (antidepressants)	Systemic vasoconstriction (increased peripheral vascular resistance)
Cyclosporine	Renal and systemic vasoconstriction (sodium retention, increased peripheral vascular resistance)
Erythropoietin	Systemic vasoconstriction (increased peripheral vascular resistance)
Monoamine oxidase inhibitors + tyramine-containing foods (aged cheeses, red wine)	Prevents degradation of norepinephrine released by tyramine-containing foods; increase in BP with reserpine
Cocaine	Systemic vasoconstriction (increased peripheral vascular resistance)
Marijuana	Increases systolic blood pressure
Glycyrrhizinic acid (chewing tobacco, imported licorice, health food products)	Inhibits renal metabolism of cortisol to cortisone (increased mineralocorticoid activity causing sodium retention, loss of potassium)
Grapefruit products	Inhibit cytochrome P-450 metabolism of some drugs
Herbs	
Bloodroot	CNS stimulant
Blue cohosh	Action of methylcytisine
Broad bean	Unknown
Scotch broom	Sympathomimetic
Kola nut	Sympathomimetic
Ephedra	Sympathomimetic, CNS stimulant
Foxglove	Cardiac inotrope
Gentian	Unknown
Ginseng	CNS stimulant, glucocorticoid effect
Goldenseal	Systemic vasoconstriction
Grindelia	CNS stimulant
Jimson weed	Anticholinergic effect
Juniper	Aquaretic
Kava	Unknown
Yohimbe	Central alpha blocker

Table 6 Laboratory Evaluation of Newly Diagnosed Hypertensive Patients

Purpose	Tests
Identify cardiovascular risk factors	Cholesterol (total, HDL), triglycerides, fasting blood glucose
Identify target-organ injury	Chest x-ray, ECG, urinalysis, serum creatinine or BUN, uric acid, urine microalbumin
Screen for secondary hypertension	Serum creatinine, potassium, calcium; urinalysis
Calculate kidney function	Cockcroft and Gault equation: $$GFR = (140 - \text{age in yr}) \times (\text{weight in kg}) \times 0.85 \ (\text{if patient is female}) / 72 \times S_{Cr}$$ Modification of Diet in Renal Disease (MDRD) equation: $$GFR = 170 \times (S_{Cr})^{-0.999} \times (\text{age in yr})^{-0.176} \times 0.762 \ (\text{if patient is female}) \times 1.18 \ (\text{if patient is black}) \times (BUN)^{-0.17} \times (alb)^{0.318}$$

alb—serum albumin concentration (g/dl)   BUN—blood urea nitrogen (mg/dl) ECG—electrocardiogram   GFR—glomerular filtration rate (ml/min) HDL—high-density lipoprotein S_{Cr}—serum creatinine (mg/dl)

BP goals for patients at the highest level of risk and more conservative treatment and BP goals for patients at the lowest level of risk. For example, in a patient with diabetes, drug therapy is indicated initially (along with lifestyle changes) when BP exceeds 130/80 mm Hg. In contrast, in a young patient who has no other CV risk factors or evidence of target organ injury or CV disease, a 6- to 12-month trial of lifestyle changes rather than drugs is indicated as initial therapy unless BP is stage 2 (≥ 160 mm Hg systolic or ≥ 100 mm Hg diastolic). In these low-risk cases, the goal BP is less than 140/90 mm Hg. Guidelines from Europe provide an even more detailed approach to risk stratification.[52]

Prevention of Hypertension

In many cases, the assessment will show BP in the prehypertensive range (i.e., 120 to 139/80 to 89 mm Hg); in the United States, 22% of adults, or approximately 45 million persons, fit this category. Preventive care is indicated in these patients.[57]

Multiple studies support the effectiveness of environmental manipulation in preventing or delaying the onset of hypertension.[58-63] Prevention of hypertension is important, given that treatment of established hypertension is only partly effective in reducing the associated morbidity and mortality.[64] Furthermore, the relationship between BP level and CV morbidity and mortality is continuous and extends into nonhypertensive levels; approximately one third of the coronary artery disease deaths attributable to BP occur in persons whose BP is in the prehypertensive range. Prevention strategies that lower BP in prehypertensive patients extend the benefits of BP reduction to this large group.

Currently, the use of pharmacologic interventions for the treatment of prehypertension is limited to high-risk patients with diabetes or chronic kidney disease when BP exceeds 130/80 mm Hg. Pharmacologic treatment of prehypertension can delay the development of high blood pressure.[65] However, use of drug therapy for all patients with prehypertension cannot be justified at this time.

The risk of developing hypertension is increased in African Americans and in all persons with prehypertension or a family history of hypertension. Reversible patient characteristics associated with an increased risk of developing hypertension include being overweight or obese; having a sedentary lifestyle; ingesting a high-sodium, low-potassium diet; using excessive amounts of alcohol; and manifesting the so-called metabolic syndrome. The metabolic syndrome is defined as three or more of the following conditions: abdominal obesity (waist circumference > 40 inches in men or > 35 inches in women), glucose intolerance (fasting blood glucose ≥ 110 mg/dl [or 100 mg/dl, depending on the organization]), BP of 130/85 mm Hg or higher, elevated triglycerides (≥ 150 mg/dl), or low high-density lipoprotein (HDL) cholesterol (< 40 mg/dl in men or < 50 mg/dl in women).[66] Clinical trials support the efficacy of seven interventions in such people for the primary prevention of hypertension [*see Table 8*].[57-59,61] Combining interventions is beneficial.[67,68] For patients with the metabolic syndrome, in addition to intensive lifestyle modifications, drug therapy is recommended for management of each of its components when appropriate.

Treatment

The overall goal of treatment in hypertensive patients is to reduce the risk of CV morbidity and mortality by lowering BP and treating other modifiable risk factors. In general, the goal is to lower BP to below 140/90 mm Hg. In patients with heart failure,

Table 7 Risk Stratification and Treatment in Hypertensive Patients[8,51,52]

Blood Pressure Stage (mm Hg)	Risk Group A (no risk factors, no TOD/CCD*)	Risk Group B (≥ 1 risk factor, not including diabetes; no TOD/CCD)	Risk Group C (TOD/CCD and/or diabetes ± other risk factors)
Prehypertension (120–139/80–89)	Lifestyle modification	Lifestyle modification	Lifestyle modification, drug therapy‡
Stage 1 (140–159/90–99)	Lifestyle modification (up to 12 mo)	Lifestyle modification (up to 6 mo)†	Lifestyle modification, drug therapy
Stage 2 (≥ 160/≥ 100)	Lifestyle modification, drug therapy	Lifestyle modification, drug therapy	Lifestyle modification, drug therapy

*Risk factors are cigarette smoking, dyslipidemia, diabetes, age > 55 yr in men and > 65 yr in women, male sex, postmenopausal status in women, family history of premature cardiovascular disease (women < 65 yr, men < 55 yr), nephropathy (microalbuminuria or glomerular filtration rate < 60 ml/min), obesity (body mass index ≥ 30 kg/m²; waist circumference ≥ 102 cm in men and ≥ 88 cm in women), C-reactive protein level ≥ 1 mg/dl, physical inactivity. TOD/CCD includes left ventricular hypertrophy, angina, prior myocardial infarction, heart failure, previous coronary revascularization procedure, stroke, transient ischemic attack, nephropathy, peripheral arterial disease, retinopathy.
†For patients with multiple risk factors, consider drugs initially in addition to lifestyle modifications.
‡Use drugs if BP > 130 mm Hg systolic or > 80 mm Hg diastolic and patient has heart failure, chronic kidney disease, or diabetes.
TOD/CCD—target-organ disease/clinical cardiovascular disease

Table 8 Lifestyle Modifications for Hypertension
Prevention and Management

Lose weight if overweight

Reduce sodium intake to ≤ 100 mmol/day (2.4 g sodium,
  6 g salt)

Increase aerobic exercise (30–45 min/day)

Limit daily alcohol intake to no more than 1 oz (30 ml; e.g., 24 oz
  of beer, 10 oz of wine, 2 oz of 100-proof whiskey) or to 0.5 oz for
  women and lighter-weight people

Maintain adequate intake of potassium (90 mmol/day)

Ingest a diet rich in fruits and vegetables and low-fat dairy products but reduced in saturated and total fat (e.g., Dietary
  Approaches to Stop Hypertension [DASH] diet)

Discontinue tobacco use

diabetes, or renal disease, the goal is to lower BP to below 130/80 mm Hg. In older patients with ISH, the goal is to lower systolic BP to below 140 mm Hg.

These goals are achieved through lifestyle modification and, in most cases, drug therapy [*see Table 9*]. In addition, comorbid conditions such as dyslipidemia or diabetes should be addressed.[66] Low-dose aspirin should be considered once BP is controlled.[69] Self-measurement of BP should be encouraged.[43]

LIFESTYLE FACTORS

Observational studies have identified several environmental factors associated with hypertension, and prospective studies have demonstrated BP lowering with manipulation of these factors [*see Table 8*].[58,59,61,67,68,70-74] In addition to lowering BP, lifestyle recommendations are designed to reduce overall CV risk. These measures should be advised for all patients with BP above the normal level. Tobacco use should be discouraged because, in addition to being a powerful CV risk factor, each cigarette smoked elevates BP for 15 to 30 minutes, and multiple cigarettes can raise BP for most of the day. A device that facilitates deep-breathing exercises (RESPeRATE) has been shown to lower BP and can be considered as an adjunct to lifestyle and drug treatments.[75]

PHARMACOLOGIC TREATMENT

The JNC 7 report recommends thiazide diuretics as initial drugs of choice for most patients; this recommendation is based on the totality of data from randomized trials, including the Antihypertensive and Lipid Lowering Treatment to Prevent Heart Attack Trial (ALLHAT).[8,76-78] Critics of diuretics have cited evidence suggesting that diuretic-based treatment does not provide protection from coronary artery disease events to the degree predicted from epidemiologic studies. The ALLHAT was designed to determine whether treatment with a diuretic would be inferior to treatment with an alpha blocker, a calcium antagonist, or an ACE inhibitor in preventing fatal and nonfatal coronary artery disease events in a high-risk group of adults with essential hypertension. The study showed no difference among the drugs for the outcome of fatal and nonfatal coronary artery disease or total mortality, regardless of the patient's race.[79] Moreover, diuretic treatment was superior to alpha blocker, calcium antagonist, or ACE inhibitor treatment with some CV disease outcomes. The alpha-blocker arm of the trial was terminated early because of an almost twofold increase in the risk of heart failure compared with the diuretic group. On the basis of these results, alpha blockers are no longer considered an appropriate initial

therapy for hypertension. Compared with the diuretic group, the calcium antagonist group also had a higher risk of heart failure. Compared with the diuretic group, the ACE inhibitor group had an increased risk of stroke and combined CV disease, but much of the increased risk occurred in blacks, in whom BP control with the ACE inhibitor was inferior to the control achieved with the diuretic. In addition, there was no evidence that calcium channel blockers or ACE inhibitors are superior to a thiazide diuretic as initial therapy in patients with diabetes mellitus or chronic kidney disease.[80,81]

Alternative medications should be considered if diuretics are contraindicated or are poorly tolerated or there is a compelling indication for a drug from a different class. Alternative drug choices are beta blockers, ACE inhibitors, ARBs, and calcium antagonists.

A subsequent study contradicted the results of ALLHAT and suggested that ACE inhibitors are superior to diuretics in older men.[82] In truth, differences in outcomes by drug choice likely reflect differences in achieved BP rather than unique effects of specific agents.[83] Therefore, achieving the BP goal is more important than the specific agents used to achieve it.

The role of beta blockers as an alternative initial treatment of uncomplicated primary hypertension is controversial. One meta-analysis found that the effect of beta blockers is less than optimum compared with that of other antihypertensive drugs, with an increased risk of stroke; these reviewers concluded that beta blockers should not remain a first-choice option in the treatment of primary hypertension.[84] Another meta-analysis also found relatively increased risk, particularly of stroke, in patients 60 years of age and older, but concluded that in younger patients, beta blockers are associated with a significant reduction in cardiovascular morbidity and mortality.[85]

Randomized clinical trials suggest that the presence of certain comorbid conditions constitutes a so-called compelling indication for selection of specific drugs [*see Table 10*]. Other considerations that should influence drug selection include concomitant conditions for which some agents may be beneficial and others contraindicated [*see Tables 10 and 11*], potential drug-drug interactions, concerns about quality of life, and cost (generic formulations are available for diuretics, beta blockers, calcium antagonists, and ACE inhibitors). Finally, demographics should be considered: in general, older patients and blacks respond better to diuretics and calcium antagonists, whereas younger patients and whites respond better to beta blockers, ACE inhibitors, and ARBs. Blacks are more likely to sustain oxidative stress from endothelial dysfunction. Nebivolol, a new beta blocker that also has vasodilating and antioxidant properties, has proved especially effective in blacks; however, this agent is not yet available in the United States.[86]

In general, the drug chosen should have a long half-life (once-daily dosing is preferable). It should be continued only if the patient tolerates it and is comfortable with its cost, because these are important factors in long-term compliance. To achieve currently recommended goal BP levels, many patients will require more than one drug; this possibility should be discussed at the outset with the patient. Regardless of the agent chosen, BP should be reassessed after 2 to 4 weeks of treatment [*see Figure 1*].

Combination Therapy

The JNC 7 report suggests initiation of therapy with two drugs (combination therapy) rather than a single agent if BP is

Table 9   Antihypertensive Drugs

Attributes	Agent	Dosage	Costs/mo ($)	Comment
Diuretics — General side effects: hyponatremia, hypokalemia, hypomagnesemia, hyperglycemia, hypercalcemia (decrease in urinary calcium excretion), hyperuricemia, increased triglycerides and cholesterol, decreased lithium secretion Contraindications: avoid in pregnancy and in patients with gout Long-term use associated with increased risk of type II diabetes	HCTZ	Initial dose: 12.5 mg/day; range: 12.5–50 mg/day	9	First choice in uncomplicated hypertension and isolated systolic hypertension
	Chlorthalidone	Initial dose: 12.5 mg/day; range: 12.5–25 mg/day	9	First choice in uncomplicated hypertension and isolated systolic hypertension
	Indapamide	Initial dose: 1.25 mg/day; range: 1.25–5.0 mg/day	16	Use in presence of renal insufficiency
	Metolazone	Initial dose: 1.25 mg/day; range: 1.25–5.0 mg/day	66	Use in presence of renal insufficiency
	Furosemide	Initial dose: 20 mg/day; range: 20–320 mg/day	11	Alternate diuretic in renal insufficiency; increases urinary calcium excretion
	Bumetanide	Initial dose: 0.5 mg/day; range: 0.5–5.0 mg/day	37	Alternate diuretic in renal insufficiency; increases urinary calcium excretion
	Ethacrynic acid	Initial dose: 25 mg/day; range: 25–100 mg/day	32	Alternate diuretic in renal insufficiency or sulfa-based diuretic allergy; only non–sulfa-based diuretic; increases urinary calcium excretion
	Torsemide	Initial dose: 5 mg/day; range: 5–20 mg/day	23	Alternate diuretic in renal insufficiency; long-acting loop diuretic; increases urinary calcium excretion
	Spironolactone	Initial dose: 25 mg/day; range 25–100 mg/day	40	Potassium sparing; aldosterone antagonist (mineralocorticoid receptor blocker); avoid in renal insufficiency; specific side effects: hyperkalemia, hyponatremia, painful gynecomastia, menstrual irregularities; available combined with HCTZ
	Eplerenone	Initial dose: 50 mg/day; range: 50–100 mg/day	472	Potassium sparing; aldosterone antagonist (mineralocorticoid receptor blocker); fewer antiandrogen side effects than spironolactone; avoid in renal insufficiency; specific side effects: hyperkalemia, hyponatremia; reduce dose by half if patient is on verapamil
	Triamterene	Initial dose: 50 mg/day; range: 50–150 mg/day	18	Potassium sparing; usually used for prevention of diuretic-induced hypokalemia; specific side effects: hyperkalemia, nephrolithiasis; available combined with HCTZ
	Amiloride	Initial dose: 5 mg/day; range: 5–10 mg/day	36	Potassium sparing; usually used for prevention of diuretic-induced hypokalemia; specific side effect: hyperkalemia; available combined with HCTZ
Calcium antagonists — Alternative first-line drugs; general side effects: headache, edema, gingival hyperplasia	Diltiazem extended release	Initial dose: 120 mg/day; range: 120–480 mg/day	34	Additional side effects: constipation, AV block, bradycardia, heart failure
	Verapamil extended release	Initial dose: 120 mg/day; range: 120–480 mg/day	26	Additional side effects: constipation, AV block, bradycardia, heart failure
	Nifedipine extended release	Initial dose: 30 mg/day; range: 30–120 mg/day	66	Additional side effects: flushing, tachycardia
	Amlodipine	Initial dose: 2.5 mg/day; range: 2.5–10 mg/day	61	Additional side effects: flushing, tachycardia
	Nicardipine extended release	Initial dose: 60 mg/day; range: 60–120 mg/day	98	Additional side effects: flushing, tachycardia
	Felodipine	Initial dose: 2.5 mg/day; range: 2.5–10 mg/day	60	Additional side effects: flushing, tachycardia
	Isradipine extended release	Initial dose: 5 mg/day; range: 5–10 mg/day	67	Additional side effects: flushing, tachycardia
	Nisoldipine	Initial dose: 10 mg/day; range: 10–60 mg/day	96	Additional side effects: flushing, tachycardia

(continued)

Table 9 *(continued)*

Attributes	Agent	Dosage	Costs/mo ($)	Comment
Beta blockers — Alternative first-line drugs in younger patients; general side effects: fatigue, bradycardia, reduced exercise tolerance, bronchospasm, vivid dreams, reduction in HDL cholesterol, increase in triglycerides, insomnia, masked symptoms and delayed recovery from hypoglycemia in diabetics. Long-term use associated with increased risk of type II diabetes	Propranolol	Initial dose: 40 mg/day; range: 40–240 mg/day	19	
	Propranolol extended release	Initial dose: 60 mg/day; range: 60–240 mg/day	112	
	Metoprolol fumarate	Initial dose: 50 mg/day; range: 50–200 mg/day	14	
	Metoprolol succinate	Initial dose: 50 mg/day; range: 50–400 mg/day	118	
	Atenolol	Initial dose: 25 mg/day; range: 25–100 mg/day	11	
	Bisoprolol	Initial dose: 5 mg/day; range: 5–20 mg/day	68	
	Nadolol	Initial dose: 20 mg/day; range: 20–320 mg/day	55	
	Timolol	Initial dose: 10 mg/day; range: 10–40 mg/day	32	
	Acebutolol	Initial dose: 200 mg/day; range: 200–1,200 mg/day	58	Additional side effects: intrinsic sympathomimetic activity, resulting in less bradycardia and lipid changes. Associated with positive ANA and drug-induced lupus
	Pindolol	Initial dose: 10 mg/day; range: 10–60 mg/day	38	Additional side effects: intrinsic sympathomimetic activity, resulting in less bradycardia and lipid changes
	Labetalol	Initial dose: 200 mg/day; range: 200–1,200 mg/day	78	Alpha$_1$-blocking activity; additional side effects: orthostatic hypotension, hepatotoxicity
	Carvedilol	Initial dose: 12.5 mg/day; range: 12.5–50 mg/day	95	Alpha$_1$-blocking activity; additional side effects: orthostatic hypotension, hepatotoxicity
ACE inhibitors — Alternative first-line drugs; general side effects: cough, angioedema, hyperkalemia, acute renal failure if there is bilateral renal artery stenosis; contraindicated in pregnancy	Captopril	Initial dose: 12.5 mg/day; range: 12.5–100 mg/day	9	Additional side effects: taste disturbance, leukopenia, proteinuria with membranous glomerular lesion secondary to sulfhydryl group; only sulfa-based ACE inhibitor
	Enalapril	Initial dose: 2.5 mg/day; range: 2.5–40 mg/day	22	
	Lisinopril	Initial dose: 5 mg/day; range: 5–40 mg/day	25	
	Benazepril	Initial dose: 10 mg/day; range: 10–80 mg/day	24	
	Fosinopril	Initial dose: 10 mg/day; range: 10–40 mg/day	30	
	Moexipril	Initial dose: 7.5 mg/day; range: 7.5–30 mg/day	46	
	Perindopril	Initial dose: 4 mg/day; range: 4–8 mg/day	49	
	Quinapril	Initial dose: 5 mg/day; range: 5–80 mg/day	72	
	Ramipril	Initial dose: 1.25 mg/day; range: 1.25–20 mg/day;	93	
	Trandolapril	Initial dose: 1 mg/day; range: 1–4 mg/day	30	

(continued)

Table 9 (*continued*)

	Attributes	Agent	Dosage	Costs/mo ($)	Comment
Angiotensin II receptor antagonists	Alternative first-line drug; alternatives to ACE inhibitors; general side effects: angioedema (rare); do not cause cough	Losartan	Initial dose: 25 mg/day; range: 25–100 mg/day	58	
		Valsartan	Initial dose: 80 mg/day; range: 80–320 mg/day	63	
		Irbesartan	Initial dose: 150 mg/day; range: 150–300 mg/day	53	
		Candesartan	Initial dose: 8 mg/day; range: 8–32 mg/day	56	
		Eprosartan	Initial dose: 400 mg/day; range: 400–800 mg/day	61	
		Telmisartan	Initial dose: 40 mg/day; range: 40–80 mg/day	46	
		Olmesartan	Initial dose: 20 mg/day; range: 20–40 mg/day	43	
Alpha₁ blockers	Add-on therapy; not first-line drugs as monotherapy; general side effects: orthostatic hypotension; edema; syncope with first dose (take at bedtime)	Prazosin	Initial dose: 1 mg/day; range: 1–20 mg/day	52	
		Doxazosin	Initial dose: 1 mg/day; range: 1–16 mg/day	48	
		Terazosin	Initial dose: 1 mg/day; range: 1–20 mg/day	28	
Central alpha-adrenergic agonists	Add-on therapy; use as second drug with diuretic; general side effects: sedation, fatigue, dry mouth, bradycardia, heart block, fluid retention, rebound hypertension with sudden discontinuance	Clonidine	Initial dose: 0.1 mg/day; range: 0.1–0.6 mg/day	12	
		Clonidine transdermal patch	Initial dose: 0.1 mg/day; range, 0.1–0.3 mg/day	121	Rebound hypertension less likely than with oral form; additional side effect: contact dermatitis from patch
		Methyldopa	Initial dose: 250 mg/day; range: 250–2,000 mg/day	25	Additional side effects: can cause hepatitis, Coombs-positive hemolytic anemia, lupuslike syndrome, blood dyscrasias
		Guanfacine	Initial dose: 1 mg/day; range: 1–2 mg/day	61	Take at bedtime to lessen sedation
		Guanabenz	Initial dose: 4 mg/day; range: 4–64 mg/day	362	
Direct vasodilators	Use as third drug in combination with diuretic and adrenergic inhibitor; general side effects: headache, fluid retention	Hydralazine	Initial dose: 40 mg/day; range: 40–200 mg/day	11	Additional side effects: flushing, tachycardia, nasal congestion, hepatitis, lupuslike syndrome
		Minoxidil	Initial dose: 2.5 mg/day; range: 2.5–40 mg/day	72	Use for resistant hypertension; additional side effects: tachycardia; significant fluid retention requiring loop diuretic for control; pericardial effusion; hair growth

ACE—angiotensin-converting enzyme   ANA—antinuclear antibody   HCTZ—hydrochlorothiazide   HDL—high-density lipoprotein

more than 20 mm Hg systolic or 10 mm Hg diastolic above the treatment goal.[8] Generally, a two-drug regimen should include a diuretic appropriate for the level of renal function. However, a 2005 study in high-risk hypertensive patients 40 to 79 years of age demonstrated that combination therapy with a calcium channel blocker and an ACE inhibitor prevented more major cardiovascular events and induced less diabetes than therapy with a beta blocker and a diuretic.[87]

An increasing number of antihypertensive combination products are available in a number of dosing options.[8] Although combination products may be more convenient, it is often less expensive to use individual agents, because generic forms of the component drugs are frequently available. In addition, titration of doses of the two agents may be easier when the two drugs are prescribed separately. Once BP control is

achieved with given doses of two agents, switching to the same therapy in combination form can be considered to enhance compliance, if cost is not prohibitive.

The advantages and disadvantages of using combination products have been reviewed.[88] Caution is advised when using combination drugs as initial therapy in older persons and diabetic patients, because of the increased risk of precipitous declines in BP or aggravation of orthostatic hypotension.

Improving Control Rates

In general, significant progress has been made in lowering BP in patients with hypertension. Although the proportion of patients with BP lower than 160/95 mm Hg has increased significantly since the 1970s, the percentage of patients with controlled hypertension (defined as systolic BP maintained below 140 mm

Hg and diastolic BP below 90 mm Hg) remains low. It is estimated that control of hypertension was accomplished in 31% of patients for the period from 1999 to 2000.[9] This is well below the Healthy People 2010 goal of at least 50% of patients achieving control. It is commonly believed that the major factors responsible for lower control rates are lack of access to health care and patient noncompliance. It is also believed that the population of patients with uncontrolled hypertension comprises disproportionately large numbers of ethnic and racial minorities. However, studies suggest that other factors are also important. Analyses of the Third National Health and Nutrition Examination Survey (NHANES III) identified factors associated with the likelihood both of attaining control of hypertension and of failing to attain control.[89] Factors associated with an increased likelihood of controlling hypertension included being married (greater social support), having private health insurance, visiting the same health care facility or having the same provider over time, having had BP measured within the previous 6 to 11 months, and using lifestyle modifications in the treatment program. On the other hand, factors associated with an increased likelihood of uncontrolled hypertension included being 65 years of age or older, being male, being black, and failing to see a physician in the preceding year. Interestingly, not having health insurance or not having a source of health care was not predictive of uncontrolled hypertension.

Table 10 Patient Condition and Choice of Antihypertensive Drugs

Conditions	Drug Choice
No comorbid conditions	Diuretics
Isolated systolic hypertension (elderly patients)	Diuretics (preferred), calcium antagonists (DHP)*
Angina	Beta blockers,* calcium antagonists (non–short-acting DHP)
Angina (with diabetes or LV dysfunction)	ACE inhibitors† (in addition to beta blockers and calcium antagonists)
Atrial fibrillation	Beta blockers,* calcium antagonists (rate limiting)*†
Cough with ACE inhibitors	ARBs*
Diabetes mellitus type 1 with proteinuria	ACE inhibitors*; calcium antagonists (non-DHP); diuretics, beta blockers†
Diabetes mellitus type 2 with proteinuria	ARBs*†; calcium antagonists (non-DHP)†; diuretics, beta blockers†
High risk of type 2 diabetes	ACE inhibitors†
Essential tremor	Beta blockers (noncardioselective)†
Heart failure, LV dysfunction	ACE inhibitors, beta blockers, diuretics, aldosterone antagonists*; ARBs†; hydralazine (in combination with long acting nitrates); generally, an ACE inhibitor with an approved beta blocker in asymptomatic patients with decreased LVEF (stage B); diuretic used to treat congestion; aldosterone antagonist used only in advanced disease in combination with other agents (combined use of ACE inhibitor, ARB, and aldosterone antagonist not recommended); hydralazine with a long-acting nitrate alternative in stage C patients with decreased LVEF who are intolerant of ACE inhibitors and ARB [*see 1:II Heart Failure*]
High risk of cardiovascular disease or type 2 diabetes	ACE inhibitor†
Hyperlipidemia	Alpha blockers (not considered first-line therapy)†
Intolerance to other antihypertensive drugs	ARBs†
Left ventricular hypertrophy (by ECG)	ARBs†
Migraine	Beta blockers (noncardioselective), calcium antagonists (non-DHP)†
Myocardial infarction	Beta blocker (non-ISA) most often drug of choice, with ACE inhibitor added if LV function impaired*; aldosterone antagonist can be added to standard therapy in patients with LV dysfunction*; diltiazem (non–Q wave infarction)†; verapamil†
Osteoporosis	Thiazide diuretics†
Peripheral vascular disease	Calcium antagonists†
Preoperative hypertension if at increased cardiovascular risk	Beta blockers†
Previous stroke	Diuretic + ACE inhibitor*; ACE inhibitor as monotherapy had no effect on BP or outcome; benefit noted only with combination that lowered BP
Prostatism	Alpha blockers (not considered first-line therapy)†
Renal insufficiency with proteinuria from any cause	ACE inhibitors, ARBs, calcium antagonists (non-DHP)†

*Compelling indication.
†Specific indication.
ACE—angiotensin-converting enzyme   ARB—angiotension II receptor blocker   DHP—dihydropyridine   ISA—intrinsic sympathomimetic activity   LV—left ventricle
LVEF—left ventricular ejection fraction

Table 11   Contraindications to Antihypertensive Drugs

Class of Drug	Possible Contraindications	Compelling Contraindications
Diuretics	Dyslipidemia (high doses), allergy to sulfa-based antibiotics, patient is sexually active man, diabetes mellitus (high doses)	Gout, allergy to sulfa-based diuretics
Beta blockers	Bronchospastic disease (asthma, COPD, noncardioselective agents), dyslipidemia (non-ISA agents), severe peripheral vascular disease, athletes	Bronchospastic disease (noncardioselective agents) second- or third-degree heart block
ACE inhibitors, ARBs	Renovascular disease (bilateral renal artery stenosis), renal insufficiency	Pregnancy, hyperkalemia
Calcium antagonists	—	Second- or third-degree heart block (non-DHP agents); heart failure (except amlodipine, felodipine)
Alpha blockers	Postural hypotension	Urinary incontinence
Reserpine	Peptic ulcer, nasal allergy	Depression
Methyldopa	Liver disease	—
Labetalol	Liver disease	—
Central alpha agonists	Depression, sleep disorders	—

ACE—angiotensin-converting enzyme   ARBs—angiotensin receptor blockers   COPD—chronic obstructive pulmonary disease   DHP—dihydropyridine
ISA—intrinsic sympathomimetic activity

Most cases of uncontrolled hypertension occur in older persons and represent mild ISH (systolic BP, 140 to 160 mm Hg).[90] In a study of self-reported treatment practices among primary care physicians, 43% of physicians would neither start drug therapy for a patient whose systolic BP is between 140 and 160 mm Hg nor intensify treatment for a patient whose systolic BP is 158 mm Hg.[91] In this study, 41% of the caregivers were unfamiliar with national hypertension guidelines. Further analysis showed that providers who were familiar with the guidelines had a lower BP treatment threshold. Other studies of physician practices have shown similar results. Emerging from these studies is the realization that a major factor in continued poor control rates for hypertension is a tolerance by the health care provider of elevated systolic BP, especially in older patients. On the basis of these study results, health care providers should consider steps to improve control rates in their practice [*see Table 12*]. Familiarity with the epidemiology of uncontrolled hypertension may be useful in this regard.[10]

REFRACTORY/RESISTANT HYPERTENSION

Studies conducted to determine what causes resistant hypertension have used different definitions of the term. In most studies, hypertension was considered resistant or refractory if control was not achieved with a combination of lifestyle modifications and the rational use of full therapeutic doses of two or three antihypertensive medications, one of which was a diuretic appropriate for the level of renal function. Studies suggest five issues to consider when evaluating patients with resistant hypertension[51]: noncompliance with therapy, interfering substances, an inappropriate drug regimen, office hypertension or pseudohypertension, and secondary hypertension. In most cases, causative factors will be identified if these five issues are given careful attention.

Noncompliance

Lack of BP control often results from noncompliance with the drug regimen or diet. Common reasons for noncompliance with drug therapy include drug costs, side effects, complex dosing schedules, and inadequate follow-up. Patients are reluctant to admit noncompliance with drug treatment, so a high degree of vigilance is required. Asking an open-ended question such as, "Many people have problems remembering their drug schedule; do you?" is occasionally effective. Clues to noncompliance include failure to keep follow-up appointments or renew prescriptions, or complaints about the cost of drugs or side effects. Certain drugs are expected to cause effects observable on physical examination or laboratory evaluation. An absence of these findings may indicate noncompliance. Examples are slowing of the heart rate with beta blockers, electrolyte changes with diuretics, or dry mouth with clonidine. Noncompliance with a low-salt diet can also be important. A high-salt diet can interfere with the effectiveness of almost all of the currently used antihypertensive drugs.

Interfering Substances

Certain prescription drugs, over-the-counter medications, herbals, and street drugs can raise BP or interfere with the BP-lowering effect of antihypertensive drugs [*see Table 5*]. Taking a complete medication history and asking patients to bring in all their medication bottles is essential for identifying interfering substances. Alcohol abuse should also be considered, because in addition to its physiologic effects, alcohol abuse is often associated with poor compliance and lack of BP control.

Inappropriate Drug Regimens

The drug regimen should be carefully reviewed. Full therapeutic doses of drugs should be employed. In general, it is preferable to use drugs that have complementary actions and that work by interfering with different BP regulatory pathways. In compliant patients, inadequate control of extracellular volume is the most common cause of resistant hypertension.[92] Extracellular volume expansion tends to occur as BP is lowered and is a secondary effect of some drugs (e.g., centrally acting sympatholytics in modest doses and some direct vasodilators). In patients with renal dysfunction, impaired renal excretion of sodium often is an important factor in raising BP. The filtered load of sodium declines in parallel with declining renal function. Because the thiazide diuretics impair reabsorption of sodium in the distal nephron, where only 7% of the filtered load of sodium is reabsorbed, they are often ineffective when serum creatinine is higher than 2.0 mg/dl or creatinine clearance is less than 30 ml/min. In such patients, loop diuretics are required; loop diuretics interfere with sodium reabsorption in the loop of Henle, where 30% of the filtered load of sodium is reabsorbed. For patients on multidrug regimens, the lack of a diuretic or the use of low doses of short-acting loop diuretics given only once daily may explain the resistant state. It should be noted that thiazide and loop diuretics are organic acids that gain access to their site of action in the kidney by active secretion into the proximal renal tubule. As renal function declines, less of an oral dose reaches the site of action, as a result of reduced renal blood flow and competition for secretory sites by accumulating endogenous organic acids. Thus, higher doses of diuretics are needed as renal function declines. In some patients with renal disease, combinations of loop agents and thiazide diuretics in adequate doses are required to control fluid volume.

Office Hypertension/Pseudohypertension

Office measures of BP may overestimate the usual or average level [*see* Ambulatory BP Monitoring, *above*]. Before embarking on further evaluation, the clinician should consider using out-of-office BP readings or ABPM to exclude a white-coat effect. Pa-

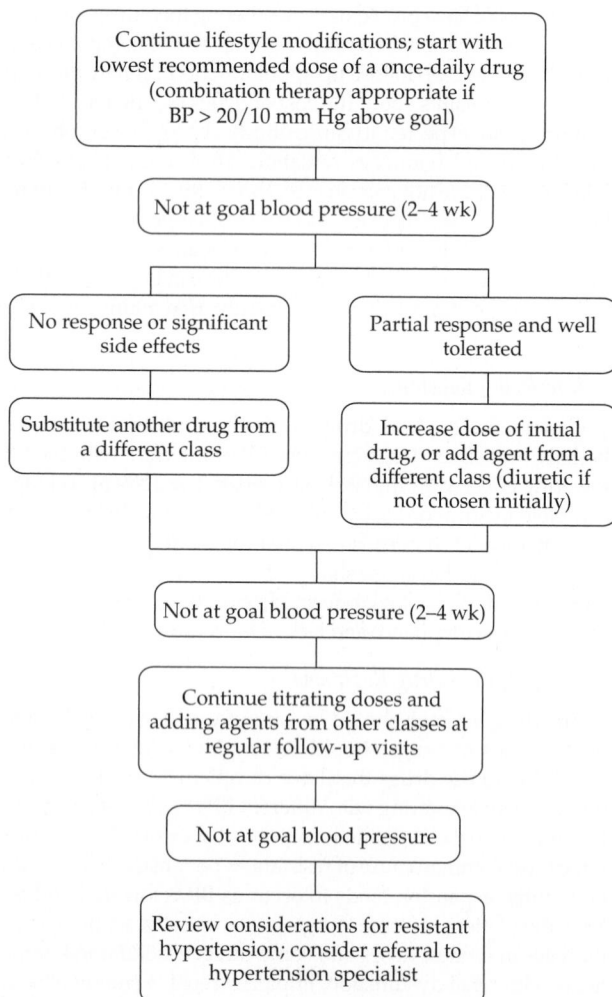

Figure 1   **Overview of drug treatment for hypertension.**

Table 12   Considerations for Improving Blood Pressure Control Rates

Become familiar with national guidelines (set a BP goal with the patient)
Schedule regular follow-up visits
Recommend self-monitoring of BP (involve patients in the treatment process)
Measure BP at every follow-up office visit and articulate a treatment recommendation if BP is above goal (be more aggressive, especially with systolic hypertension in older patients)
Emphasize lifestyle factors as part of the treatment program (involve patients in the treatment process); review progress and barriers at each visit
Use adequate doses of antihypertensive drugs; be willing to use multiple drugs
Encourage communication regarding medication costs and side effects
Be aware of poor control rates in men and African Americans

tients with white-coat hypertension are more likely to be younger (although cases of white-coat ISH do occur in elderly patients), female, and of normal weight. They often have no target organ injury and complain of fatigue and weakness (which are symptoms of hypotension) when drug doses are increased. One study suggested that up to 50% of hypertensive patients deemed resistant by office determinations of BP in fact had controlled hypertension.[93]

Some elderly patients may have pseudohypertension—falsely elevated systolic and diastolic BP as determined by cuff measurement. Pseudohypertension results from atherosclerosis of the brachial artery. Because of the excessive stiffness of the vessel wall, higher cuff pressure must be applied to produce vascular occlusion. In addition, the accuracy of oscillometric devices is impaired under these circumstances. Such patients often have evidence of severe generalized atherosclerosis and remarkable elevations of systolic BP without concomitant symptoms. They may complain of weakness and fatigue with increases in drug doses. The ability to palpate the pulseless radial artery after cuff inflation (i.e., a positive Osler sign) increases the likelihood of pseudohypertension, but this is not a sensitive test.[94] Confirmation of pseudohypertension requires intra-arterial measures of BP.

Secondary Hypertension

Secondary forms of hypertension are relatively uncommon in the general hypertensive population but may account for a significant proportion of cases of resistant hypertension. Once the other considerations have been eliminated, patients with resistant hypertension should be considered for further evaluation of secondary causes [*see* Secondary Hypertension, *below*].

HYPERTENSIVE CRISIS

An acute and severe rise in BP is a serious medical concern. Prompt therapy may be lifesaving. Clinically, acute and severe increases in BP can be classified as either hypertensive urgencies or emergencies (crises).[51]

The term hypertensive emergency or hypertensive crisis is defined as severely elevated BP associated with acute injury to target organs (i.e., brain, heart, kidneys, vasculature, and retina). Prompt hospitalization and reduction of BP with parenteral therapy is required. Examples of hypertensive emergencies include malignant hypertension, hypertensive encephalopathy, aortic dissection, eclampsia, unstable angina or acute myocardial infarction, pulmonary edema, and acute renal failure.

Malignant hypertension is an old term that describes a clinical syndrome associated with acute severe elevation of BP that may be fatal if not promptly treated. It is associated with a marked increase in peripheral vascular resistance caused by systemic vasoconstrictors (e.g., angiotensin II) or locally generated vasoconstrictors (e.g., endothelin). Any form of hypertension can progress to the malignant phase. Clinical characteristics include severe hypertension (diastolic BP $\geq$ 130 mm Hg); hemorrhages, exudates, and papilledema on retinal examination; encephalopathy (i.e., headache, confusion, somnolence, stupor, visual loss, focal neurologic deficits, seizure, or coma); oliguria and azotemia; nausea, vomiting, and dyspnea; and physical findings of heart failure (e.g., rales, an S_3 heart sound). Encephalopathy arises from the failure of cerebral autoregulation of blood flow at critically high pressures, which results in cerebral vasodilation, hyperperfusion, vascular leakage, and cerebral edema. The hallmark vascular lesion of malignant hypertension is fibrinoid necrosis of arterioles that, in turn, increases both ischemic injury and further vasoactive substance release, setting up a vicious cycle. Microangiopathic hemolytic anemia with fragmentation of red cells and intravascular coagulation may occur in the setting of fibrinoid necrosis.

Hypertensive urgency is defined as severe hypertension without evidence of acute target organ injury that requires BP reduction over 24 to 48 hours. Oral therapy in the outpatient setting is often adequate. Examples include severe hypertension in a patient with known coronary artery disease, an aortic aneurysm (or aneurysm at another site), or a history of heart failure. The term accelerated hypertension is often used to describe a state of acute, severe hypertension with hemorrhages and exudates on retinal examination (but not papilledema) but without other findings of acute organ injury. This condition can be managed with oral therapy but may progress to malignant hypertension if left untreated.

The causes of hypertensive urgencies and emergencies include neglected essential hypertension (approximately 7% of untreated hypertension can progress to the malignant phase), sudden discontinuance of drug therapy (especially multiple drug regimens or regimens containing clonidine or beta blockers), renovascular disease, collagen vascular disease (especially scleroderma), eclampsia, acute glomerulonephritis, and pheochromocytoma. Approximately 50% of hypertensive crises occur in patients with preexisting hypertension.

The goals of the initial evaluation are to assess for target organ injury and to define potential causes. The evaluation begins with a focused medical history and physical examination. In taking the history, the clinician must ask about compliance with prescribed antihypertensive medications and the use of drugs that can raise BP [see Table 5]. Retinal examination is a mandatory aspect of the physical examination. Immediate laboratory studies include a complete blood count (to check for anemia); blood smear (to look for fragmented red blood cells); serum creatinine and blood urea nitrogen assays; urinalysis; serum sodium, potassium, and glucose assays; a chest x-ray; and an electrocardiogram. In hypertensive crisis, evaluation for secondary hypertension should be deferred until the patient is stable. If a cause of the crisis is not apparent, such patients should eventually have an evaluation to exclude renal vascular disease, pheochromocytoma, scleroderma, and primary aldosteronism.

Patients with hypertensive crisis should be hospitalized in an intensive care unit. The challenge of treatment is to lower BP without aggravating ischemia to vital organs. Parenteral therapy should be used [see Table 13]. Sodium nitroprusside is generally the drug of choice. Diazoxide is considered obsolete, because of the availability of newer and safer drugs. Mean BP should be lowered by 20% in the first hour (diastolic BP should be reduced to 100 to 110 mm Hg). As BP is lowered, the patient should be monitored for evidence of worsening cerebral, renal, or cardiac function. If the patient is stable, BP should be further lowered over the next 24 hours. Oral therapy can be started, and parenteral therapy gradually discontinued.

TREATMENT FOR SPECIFIC PATIENT GROUPS

The Elderly

Approximately 60% to 70% of persons 60 years of age or older have hypertension.[1] In this age group, systolic BP is the dominant predictor of adverse events, and ISH is the most common type of blood pressure disturbance.[13,14] Treatment of hypertension in the elderly reduces CV disease event rates and lessens the risk of development and progression of cognitive dysfunction and dementia.[7,95] The benefits of treatment have been shown for persons with either systolic-diastolic hypertension or ISH and for those older than 80 years. Although most elderly persons have primary hypertension, secondary forms of hypertension should be considered if the onset is recent or the hypertension is resistant.

There are special concerns regarding BP measurement in the elderly. Systolic BP is often quite variable, and the phenomenon of white-coat hypertension may be common in the elderly, especially in older women. Thus, readings of BP outside the office should be encouraged, as should selective use of ambulatory monitoring, especially if the patient has no target organ changes related to hypertension or complains of side effects that suggest hypotension with treatment. As noted, white-coat hypertension is an indication for ambulatory monitoring that is covered under Medicare.[49] Orthostatic hypotension and postprandial hypotension are more common in the elderly, in most cases because of dysautonomia of aging. Systolic hypertension is a predictor of orthostatic hypotension, and diabetic patients are at greater risk because of autonomic neuropathy. Thus, BP measurement in the standing position is required in all elderly patients at all office visits. Pseudohypertension should be considered in elderly patients who have palpably stiff vessels, who lack significant target organ changes despite very high BP readings, and who complain of hypotensive symptoms with treatment. Such patients may require a direct intra-arterial measure of BP for clarification.

In general, treatment of hypertension in the elderly follows the same principles as treatment in younger patients. The BP goals are the same as for the general hypertensive population. However, because the benefit of treatment on longevity is less in most elderly patients, the costs of drugs, side effects, and quality of life are important considerations. Goal BP may be difficult to achieve in some patients with systolic hypertension, but any reduction is beneficial. Thus, in some patients, a higher systolic goal may be reasonable.

Modification of adverse lifestyle factors is beneficial in the elderly and should be encouraged.[96] Salt sensitivity increases with age and with the reduction in renal function that is common in the elderly.[97] In patients who require drugs, lower initial doses should be considered, especially in the presence of orthostatism or comorbid vascular diseases. However, many elderly patients ultimately require multiple drugs for BP control.

Table 13   Parenteral Therapy for Hypertensive Crisis

Drug	Dosage	Comments
Sodium nitroprusside	0.25–10.0 µg/kg/min I.V. infusion	General drug of choice; produces direct arteriolar and venous dilation; immediate onset and offset; side effects include metabolic acidosis, nausea, vomiting, agitation, psychosis, tremor (monitor thiocyanate levels)
Labetalol	Repetitive I.V. boluses of 20–80 mg q. 10 min or constant infusion of 0.5–2.0 mg/min	Combination alpha/beta blocker; onset 5–10 min, offset 3–6 hr; useful in most settings, especially postoperative state, hypertensive crisis of pregnancy; avoid in acute heart failure; take beta-blocker precautions; side effects include scalp tingling, vomiting, heart block, orthostatic hypotension
Glyceryl trinitrate	5–100 µg/min I.V. infusion	Produces direct arteriolar and venous dilation; onset 5–10 min, offset 3–5 min; especially useful in acute coronary ischemia, CHF; tolerance with prolonged infusion; side effects include headache, flushing, nausea, methemoglobinemia
Esmolol	50–300 µg/kg/min I.V.	Cardioselective beta blocker, onset 1–2 min, offset 10–20 min; especially useful in postoperative state, aortic dissection, ischemic heart disease; take beta-blocker precautions; side effects include bradycardia, nausea
Hydralazine	10–20 mg I.V. bolus	Causes direct arteriolar vasodilation; onset 10–20 min, offset 3–8 hr; used primarily for hypertensive crisis of pregnancy; avoid in acute MI, angina, aortic dissection; side effects include headache, flushing, nausea, vomiting, tachycardia, angina
Enalapril	1.25–5 mg I.V. bolus, q. 6 hr	ACE inhibitor; onset 15 min, offset 6 hr; especially useful in acute heart failure in postoperative state; lower doses in renal disease; side effects include precipitous decline in BP (high-renin states), acute renal failure (presence of renal vascular disease)
Nicardipine	5–15 mg/hr I.V. infusion	Dihydropyridine calcium antagonist; onset 5–10 min, offset 1–4 hr; especially useful in postoperative state; avoid in acute heart failure; side effects include headache, nausea, flushing, phlebitis
Fenoldopam	0.1–1.6 µg/kg/min I.V. infusion	Dopamine (DA1) agonist; onset 5 min, offset 30–60 min; especially useful in patients with impaired renal function because it increases renal blood flow and sodium excretion; side effects include nausea, vomiting, headache, flushing
Phentolamine	5–15 mg I.V. bolus	Alpha blocker; onset instantaneous, offset 3–10 min; drug of choice for pheochromocytoma crisis; side effects include flushing, tachycardia
Trimethaphan	0.5–15 mg/min I.V. infusion	Ganglionic blocker; onset 1–5 min, offset 10 min; tachyphylaxis common with prolonged infusion; side effects include urinary retention, paralytic ileus, dry mouth, blurred vision, orthostatic hypotension
Diazoxide	1–150 mg/kg I.V. bolus over 10 min; repeat at 10–15 min intervals if needed	Considered obsolete; direct arteriolar dilator; onset 1 min, offset 3–18 hr; avoid in acute MI, aortic dissection; side effects include hyperglycemia, hyperuricemia, fluid retention

ACE—angiotensin-converting enzyme   CHF—chronic heart failure   MI—myocardial infarction

In the elderly with systolic-diastolic hypertension, placebo-controlled studies have shown that initial therapy with a diuretic or a beta blocker is beneficial. In one trial, treatment using newer drugs (calcium antagonists or ACE inhibitors) was not superior to treatment using diuretics and beta blockers.[98] In another study, however, starting treatment with an ACE inhibitor rather than a diuretic was associated with better outcomes, particularly in men.[82] Studies in patients with ISH have shown efficacy of thiazide diuretics and long-acting dihydropyridine calcium antagonists.[7] In elderly patients with LVH, the LIFE (Losartan Intervention For Endpoint reduction in hypertension) trial demonstrated that, compared with therapy using a beta blocker (atenolol), use of an ARB (losartan) was associated with fewer CV events, including strokes.[99] This observation was noted overall and in the subset of elderly patients with ISH. In elderly patients with a history of stroke or transient ischemic attack, the combination of indapamide and perindopril reduced the risk for subsequent stroke and progression to dementia.[100] In many elderly patients, comorbid conditions will determine the use of specific drugs. Because of the problem of polypharmacy in the elderly, a goal should always be to keep the program as simple as possible.

Diabetic Patients

Patients who have both hypertension and diabetes have twice the risk of CV disease as nondiabetic hypertensive patients. In addition, hypertension increases the risk of diabetic retinopathy and nephropathy.[101] Epidemiologic and observational studies have shown that the risk of BP-related CV disease and mortality in diabetic patients begins to rise when BP exceeds 120/70 mm Hg.[101,102] There does not appear to be a threshold value for risk associated with systolic BP in diabetic patients. In the Hypertension Optimal Treatment Trial (HOT), diabetic patients randomized to the lowest diastolic BP goal (≤ 80 mm Hg; the achieved diastolic BP was 82.6 mm Hg) had the best outcomes.[69] In the United Kingdom Prospective Diabetes Study (UKPDS), a mean achieved diastolic BP of 82 mm Hg was beneficial, as compared with less aggressive BP reduction.[103] On the basis of these data, the American Diabetes Association, the National Kidney Foundation, and the JNC 7 report recommend a goal BP of less than 130/80 mm Hg in hypertensive diabetic patients.[8,102,104]

All patients with diabetes should be encouraged to adopt lifestyle modifications [*see Table 8*]. Weight loss (if the patient is overweight or obese) and moderate exercise are especially beneficial in diabetic patients because in addition to lowering BP, these interventions improve insulin sensitivity and blood lipid levels. Many patients will require lifestyle modifications and three or more drugs to achieve the BP goals. Meeting these goals may be difficult in some patients. The clinician must balance benefit from lower BP with cost of medication, side effects, and risks associated with the lower goals in some patients. The American Diabetes Association recommends a trial of lifestyle modifications alone for up to 3 months if the initial systolic BP is 130 to 139 mm Hg or the diastolic BP is 80 to 89 mm Hg. Drug monotherapy should be considered initially along with lifestyle modifications if the initial systolic BP is 140 mm Hg or higher or if the diastolic BP is 90 mm Hg or higher.[102] The JNC 7 report suggests that if the initial systolic BP is 150 mm Hg or higher or the initial diastolic BP is 90 mm Hg or higher, consideration should be given to starting therapy with a combination of two drugs, one of them a thiazide diuretic.[8] Before initiating drug therapy, it is important to measure BP in the standing position to detect orthostatism, the presence of which may be a clue to autonomic neuropathy and would necessitate a modification to the treatment approach.

Placebo-controlled trials in diabetic patients have shown the efficacy of ACE inhibitors, ARBs, diuretics, and beta blockers as initial therapy. Although thiazides, ACE inhibitors, and calcium channel blockers provide equivalent cardiovascular benefit in this setting,[80] numerous studies have shown the effectiveness of ACE inhibitors and ARBs in retarding progression of diabetic nephropathy.[105,106] For diabetic patients with nephropathy, the American Diabetes Association guidelines recommend ACE inhibitors as initial drugs of choice in type 1 diabetes but ARBs in type 2 diabetes.[102] It is unclear whether ARBs are as cardioprotective in diabetic patients as ACE inhibitors have been shown to be. In some studies, the incidence of cardiac events has been higher in diabetic patients treated with dihydropyridine calcium antagonists, as compared with ACE inhibitors.[107] Beta blockers should be considered in the setting of coronary artery disease, a common comorbidity in patients with diabetes. On balance, treatment data suggest that reaching the goal BP in diabetic patients is probably more important than the choice of drugs used to achieve it.

Patients with Heart Disease

Ischemic heart disease is the most common cause of death in patients with hypertension. Poorly controlled hypertension also results in the development of LVH. Both LVH and ischemic injury lead to the development of heart failure from either systolic or diastolic dysfunction.[108] Hypertension is the most common antecedent of heart failure.[109] Hypertensive effects on the heart also increase the risk for atrial fibrillation.

For asymptomatic patients with known coronary artery disease, an ACE inhibitor should be considered initially because some studies (but not all) suggest that their use may be associated with a reduced risk of cardiovascular events.[110] An ACE inhibitor would also be the initial drug of choice for patients with concomitant reduced systolic function or concomitant diabetes with renal involvement.[102,105,111] If there is a history of myocardial infarction, the first drug should be a beta blocker.[112] For hypertensive patients with previous myocardial infarction and reduced left ventricular function, combination therapy with a beta blocker and an ACE inhibitor should be considered.[113] In addition, the aldosterone antagonist eplerenone has been shown to be effective.[114] If eplerenone is used, serum potassium levels should be monitored carefully, especially in patients with renal dysfunction or if ACE inhibitors or ARBs are used.

The drug of choice in hypertensive patients with stable angina, both to lower BP and to relieve symptoms and ischemia, is a beta blocker. Long-acting dihydropyridine or nondihydropyridine calcium antagonists have been shown to relieve symptoms and are alternative agents if beta blockers are contraindicated; these alternative agents are also suitable as additional therapy for BP or symptom control. Newer vasoselective, long-acting dihydropyridine calcium antagonists such as amlodipine or felodipine can be used safely to lower BP in patients with impaired left ventricular function. Nitrates can be used in combination with either beta blockers or calcium antagonists for symptomatic relief and may lower systolic BP. Beta blockers should be avoided in pure vasospastic angina, a disorder best managed with long-acting calcium antagonists or nitrates. Diuretics are safe antihypertensives for patients with coronary artery disease; they work well with other agents to lower BP. Hypokalemia should be avoided.

LVH is associated with a doubling of the risk of myocardial infarction and death in hypertensive patients.[115] Effective BP control causes regression of LVH and improves prognosis. Weight loss and the use of antihypertensive drugs of all major classes have been shown to induce regression of LVH; however, increasing evidence suggests that ACE inhibitors and ARBs may be more effective than other agents.[116]

The goal of treating hypertension in patients with heart failure is a BP of less than 130/80 mm Hg. The American College of Cardiology and the American Heart Association have developed guidelines for the evaluation and management of heart failure in adults that encompass a staging system and evidence-based treatment recommendations for patients with heart failure [*see Chapter 26*].

The goal of hypertension treatment in patients with coronary artery disease is also a BP of less than 130/80 mm Hg; however, concern has been raised that excessive decreases of diastolic BP may be associated with a paradoxical increase in morbidity and mortality (referred to as the J-curve hypothesis). A secondary analysis of a study of hypertensive patients with coronary artery disease demonstrated a progressively increased risk of all-cause death and myocardial infarction with low diastolic BP (< 84 mm Hg).[117]

Patients with Chronic Kidney Disease

Kidney disease is both a cause and a consequence of hypertension. Hypertension is the second most common cause of the development of end-stage kidney disease, and most people with kidney disease have hypertension. Aggressive control of elevated BP can slow the progression of renal damage and delay or prevent the development of end-stage disease.[104-106,118,119] The currently recommended BP goal for patients with kidney disease is a level below 130/80 mm Hg. In addition to elevated BP, other modifiable CV risk factors require management, because patients with chronic kidney disease are also at high risk for CV morbidity and mortality. A study of hypertensive patients who were 55 years of age or older found that a low GFR was independently predictive of an increased risk of coronary artery disease; those patients with a reduced GFR proved more likely to develop coronary artery disease than to develop end-stage renal disease.[120] In this study, neither a calcium channel blocker nor an ACE inhibitor proved superior to a thiazide diuretic in preventing coronary artery disease, stroke, or combined CV disease, and chlorthalidone was superior to both for preventing heart failure, independent of the level of renal function.

Chronic kidney disease is defined as either a GFR of less than 60 ml/min/1.73 m² or the presence of albuminuria (> 300 mg/day or > 200 mg albumin per gram of creatinine).[104] The GFR can be estimated using the Cockcroft-Gault or MDRD equation [see Table 6]. Determination of creatinine clearance using timed urine collections generally does not improve upon the estimates of GFR obtained using these equations.

ACE inhibitors and ARBs may be more effective than other drugs in slowing progression of proteinuric kidney disease. Whether these agents provide a specific advantage in the absence of proteinuria is less certain.[104] Serum creatinine concentrations often increase acutely when these drugs are used, so serum creatinine and potassium should be measured within several days of initiating treatment. An increase in creatinine is not a reason to stop the drug unless it is excessive (> 30% from baseline) or associated with severe hyperkalemia (> 5.5 mEq/dl). Concomitant use of potassium-sparing diuretics, potassium supplements, or nonsteroidal anti-inflammatory drugs should be avoided. A persistent increase in creatinine with treatment raises the possibility of renal artery stenosis. Most patients with kidney disease will require a diuretic as part of the treatment regimen. If GFR is estimated to be less than 30 ml/min, thiazide diuretics are usually ineffective, and loop diuretics are required. Often, three or more drugs are required to control BP.

Patients with Acute Stroke

The majority of patients presenting with either acute ischemic or hemorrhagic stroke have hypertension.[121] The temporal profile is that of an initial acute rise in BP in the first 24 hours, followed by a slow decline over the next several days. On the whole, observational studies show that high BP at stroke onset is associated with an increased risk of death or dependency.[122] However, this association is not evident in some studies, especially studies in patients with ischemic stroke.[123]

Unfortunately, at present there is little evidence from clinical trials to provide clear recommendations for the appropriate management of BP during acute stroke. Currently, there is consensus that in patients with acute intracranial hemorrhage, BP should be lowered if it exceeds 200/120 mm Hg, to prevent growth of the hematoma or rebleeding. Lowering of BP by less than 20% is suggested in this setting.[124] Guidelines for BP management in acute ischemic stroke from the Stroke Council of the American Heart Association suggest that in patients who are not candidates for thrombolytic therapy, hypertension should be managed with observation alone if BP is less than 220 mm Hg systolic and 120 mm Hg diastolic, unless there is evidence of other acute target-organ injury (e.g., aortic dissection, acute myocardial infarction, pulmonary edema, hypertensive encephalopathy).[125] For patients with systolic BP higher than 220 mm Hg or diastolic BP of 121 to 140 mm Hg, treatment with intravenous labetalol or nicardipine is recommended. Labetalol is given in a dosage of 10 to 20 mg over 1 to 2 minutes; the dose is repeated or doubled as needed every 10 minutes to a maximum dose of 300 mg. Nicardipine is given in an initial 5 mg/hr infusion and titrated to desired effect by increasing the dosage by 2.5 mg/hr every 5 minutes, to a maximum rate of 15 mg/hr. It is suggested that BP be lowered by 10% to 15%.

Nitroprusside is recommended if diastolic BP is higher than 140 mm Hg; the dose should be titrated to lower BP by 10% to 15%.

In patients who are eligible for thrombolytic therapy, the Stroke Council suggests lowering BP before initiating thrombolysis if the BP is higher than 185 mm Hg systolic or 110 mm Hg diastolic. Treatment with labetalol, 10 to 20 mg intravenously over 1 to 2 minutes, is advised. If needed, this dose can be repeated once; or nitroglycerin paste, 1 to 3 inches, can be applied. If antihypertensive treatment does not reduce BP to below 185/110 mm Hg, thrombolytic therapy is not advised. During and after thrombolytic treatment, BP should be monitored frequently (every 15 minutes for 2 hours, then every 30 minutes for 6 hours, and then every hour for 16 hours). During this period, treatment with nitroprusside is advised for diastolic BP higher than 140 mm Hg. For systolic BP higher than 180 mm Hg or diastolic BP of 105 to 140 mm Hg, intravenous labetalol in a dosage of 10 mg administered over 1 to 2 minutes is recommended; the dosage should be repeated or doubled every 10 minutes to a maximum of 300 mg, or a drip at a rate of 2 to 8 mg/min should be started.

Women

Prospective cohort studies have shown that lower dietary intake of folate or increased intake of sugared or diet cola beverages is associated with an increased risk of hypertension in women; however, there was no association between caffeine consumption overall and risk of hypertension.[126,127]

It has long been recognized that the use of ACE inhibitors during the second and third trimesters of pregnancy increases the risk of fetal malformations. However, a 2006 case-control study found that the risk of fetal malformations—specifically, cardiovascular and central nervous system malformations—is also increased with ACE inhibitor use during the first trimester.[128] For that reason, it would be prudent to avoid this class of drugs in women who may become pregnant. A larger body of evidence suggests, however, that the risk of inducing fetal anomalies is greatest when exposure is during the second or third trimesters. For this reason, exposure during the first trimester is not in itself an indication for elective termination of pregnancy.

In postmenopausal women who have hypertension, hormone therapy with a combination of drospirenone—a progestin with antialdosterone activity—and 17-β-estradiol (Angeliq) has been found to reduce BP without inducing significant increases in serum potassium. This product is approved for the treatment of moderate to severe vasomotor symptoms associated with menopause.[129]

Secondary Hypertension

Detection of secondary hypertension is important because, depending on the cause, it may be possible to cure the underlying condition or tailor therapy to achieve optimal BP control. Certain features suggest the presence of specific secondary forms of hypertension [see Table 4], which should then direct further testing [see Table 14].

Common reversible causes of hypertension include obesity, the use of drugs that raise BP [see Table 5], obstructive sleep apnea, and renal disease. Obstructive sleep apnea is prevalent in the population and is often associated with hypertension; treatment with continuous positive airway pressure can significantly lower both daytime and nighttime BP in these patients.[130] Renal insufficiency from any etiology causes BP to rise. Elevated BP in turn accelerates loss of renal function, and a vicious cycle ensues. Traditional secondary causes of hypertension include renal vascular disease, coarctation of the aorta, the adrenal causes of primary aldosteronism, pheochromocytoma, and Cushing syndrome.

Table 14   Screening and Diagnostic Options for Secondary Hypertension

Disorder	*Screening Tests (Sensitivity/Specificity)*	*Comments*
Renovascular hypertension[146-148]	Captopril radionuclide renal scan (75%/85%)	Advantage: no contrast allergy Disadvantages: renal dysfunction impairs interpretation, may miss accessory- or branch-vessel disease
	Duplex ultrasound (80%–90%/90%)	Advantages: no contrast allergy, can be used in patients with renal dysfunction; calculation of resistive index identifies patients with renal dysfunction likely to benefit from intervention Disadvantages: failure to visualize both renal arteries; may miss accessory- or branch-vessel disease
	Spiral CT angiography	Advantages: excellent images of renal arteries; can identify dissection, accessory vessels, and fibromuscular disease Disadvantage: considerable contrast load precludes use in presence of renal dysfunction
	Magnetic resonance angiography (85%–100%/79%–98%)	Advantages: no contrast allergy, can be used in patients with renal dysfunction; no radiation exposure Disadvantages: cost, may overstate degree of stenosis, claustrophobic patients may not tolerate test
	Renal angiography	Gold standard Advantages: identifies accessory- and branch-vessel disease; percutaneous interventions can be performed as part of study Disadvantages: cost, contrast exposure, invasive (atheroemboli)
Primary aldosteronism[139,149]	Measurement of serum sodium, potassium, PRA, and PAC; 24-hr urinary aldosterone, sodium, and PRA after 3 days of 200 mEq sodium diet	Diagnosis confirmed if $U_{Na} > 200$ mEq, $U_{aldo} > 12$, and PRA < 1.0; 30% of patients with primary aldosteronism will be normokalemic at presentation Ratio of PAC/PRA > 20 (PAC >15 ng/dl and PRA < 2.0 ng/ml) Advantage: simple Disadvantages: many antihypertensive drugs can influence values of PRA and PAC; sensitive screen but not specific
Pheochromocytoma[141]	Plasma free metanephrine (highly sensitive); 24-hr fractionated urinary metanephrines	—
Cushing syndrome	24-hr urinary free cortisol (95%–100%/97%–100%)	Diagnosis certain if 24-hr urinary free cortisol level > 3× normal; diagnosis excluded if level normal; use low-dose dexamethasone suppression test if elevation < 3× normal
Coarctation of the aorta	Chest x-ray; transesophageal echocardiogram; CT or MRI of the aorta	Diagnostic findings on chest x-ray: "3" sign from dilation of aorta above and below the coarctation, rib notching from collateral vessels

RENOVASCULAR HYPERTENSION

Renovascular hypertension is the most common form of potentially curable secondary hypertension. It probably occurs in 1% to 2% of the overall hypertensive population. The prevalence may be as high as 10% in patients with resistant hypertension, and 30% in patients with accelerated or malignant hypertension.

Stenosing lesions of the renal circulation cause hypertension through ischemia-mediated stimulation of the renin-angiotensin-aldosterone axis. Correcting renal ischemia eliminates excess renin production and improves or cures the hypertension. In unilateral disease, prolonged hypertension can cause nephrosclerosis in the nonischemic kidney; nephrosclerosis lessens the likelihood of benefit from correction of the renal vascular lesion.

Fibromuscular disease is the most common cause of renovascular hypertension in younger patients, especially women between 15 and 50 years of age[131]; it accounts for approximately 10% of cases of renovascular hypertension.[132] Vascular lesions typically affect the middle and distal portions of the renal artery and often extend into branches. Three subtypes are defined on the basis of the layer of the vascular wall affected: (1) intimal hyperplasia (1% to 2% of cases), (2) medial fibromuscular dysplasia (95% of cases), and (3) periadventitial fibrosis (1% to 2% of cases). The most common subtype, medial fibromuscular dysplasia, presents as a classic string-of-beads (i.e., aneurysmal dilatations) on angiography; it progresses in 30% of cases. It is rarely associated with dissection or thrombosis. In contrast, the rarer forms can progress rapidly, and dissection and thrombosis are common. Fibromuscular dysplasia is a rare cause of renal artery occlusion.

Atheromatous disease is the most common cause of renovascular hypertension in middle-aged and older patients and accounts for approximately 90% of renovascular hypertension.[132,133] Vascular lesions are usually in the proximal third of the renal arteries, often near or at the orifice. The prevalence of atheromatous renal artery disease increases with age and is common in older hypertensive patients, especially in those with diabetes or with atherosclerosis in other vascular beds. Most patients with atheromatous renal vascular disease and hypertension have essential hypertension and may not benefit from correction of the disorder. Sorting out the subset of patients with renovascular disease who have renovascular hypertension is a challenge. The disease is frequently bilateral (30%) and is often progressive. The likelihood of progression can be decreased by aggressive control of risk factors (e.g., dyslipidemia, cigarette smoking, and hypertension). Patients with atheromatous renal artery disease are at increased risk for cardiovascular morbidity and mortality, including stroke, congestive heart failure, and myocardial infarction.[134] This increased risk can be explained in part by the observation that atheromatous renal artery disease is often a marker of more generalized atherosclerotic vascular disease. In addition, increased angiotensin II levels from a critical renal artery lesion may act in a variety of ways to accelerate the atherosclerotic process. Whether interventional therapy and correction of the underlying renal artery stenosis improves prognosis over optimum medical management in the majority of these patients is uncertain and is currently the subject of a major clinical trial.[135]

The presentations of hemodynamically significant bilateral renal artery disease (i.e., ischemic nephropathy) include the following: an acute decline in renal function with use of an ACE inhibitor or ARB or with a sudden decrease in blood pressure; acute hypertension and pulmonary edema (i.e., flash pulmonary edema); recurrent or resistant heart failure; or an unexplained subacute decline in renal function with or without worsening of hypertension.[136] Bilateral atherosclerotic renal artery disease accounts for a small but increasing number of cases of end-stage renal disease in older persons.[137]

A variety of screening tests for renal artery disease are available [see Table 13]; however, duplex renal ultrasonography, magnetic resonance angiography (MRA), and spiral computed tomographic angiography are considered the initial screening tests of choice [see Chapter 168]. In general, spiral CT and MRA have superior diagnostic accuracy compared with duplex ultrasonography. Duplex ultrasonography and MRA do not involve the use of iodinated contrast and therefore are safe in patients with chronic kidney disease. MRA is not highly sensitive for the identification of fibromuscular disease. The gold standard for the diagnosis of renal artery disease remains contrast angiography. In settings of renal disease, alternative contrast agents (e.g., CO_2 or gadolinium) can be used.

For lesions from fibromuscular dysplasia, percutaneous intervention with balloon angioplasty is the treatment of choice. For lesions from atheromatous disease, stent-supported angioplasty is the treatment of choice. Surgery is employed for both types if the lesions are not amenable to angioplasty; for the rare subtypes of fibromuscular dysplasia that usually are unresponsive to angioplasty; and for atheromatous disease in settings where aortic replacement is required.

Atheroembolic renal disease can mimic renovascular hypertension and ischemic nephropathy, in that it may present as hypertension of acute onset or as a worsening of hypertension in conjunction with a subacute decline in renal function. Atheroembolic renal disease often occurs after angiography or vascular surgery. Physical findings include the presence of distal livido reticularis and peripheral emboli. Laboratory findings include an elevated erythrocyte sedimentation rate, anemia, hematuria, eosinophilia, and eosinophiluria.

PRIMARY ALDOSTERONISM

The classic syndrome of primary aldosteronism consists of hypertension, hypokalemia from excessive renal excretion, alkalosis, suppressed plasma renin activity, and increased aldosterone secretion.[138] Hypokalemia is the abnormality that most often raises suspicion of this disorder, but approximately 30% of patients with primary aldosteronism present with normal serum potassium levels.

Although several subtypes of primary aldosteronism have been identified, the most common are unilateral aldosterone-producing adenoma, which comprises 30% to 40% of cases; and bilateral adrenal zona glomerulosa hyperplasia (also known as idiopathic hyperaldosteronism [IHA]), which comprises 60% to

70% of cases. Rare subtypes include glucocorticoid-suppressible hyperplasia, unilateral hyperplasia, and aldosterone-producing cortical carcinoma. The prevalence of primary aldosteronism is probably around 2%, but studies have suggested the prevalence to be as high as 13% of the hypertensive population, which would make it the most common secondary form of hypertension.[139] The higher prevalence estimates reflect an increase in the number of patients being diagnosed with IHA, a condition that may be part of the spectrum of essential hypertension.

Patients for whom the diagnosis of primary aldosteronism should be considered include the following: all hypertensive patients with spontaneous hypokalemia of renal origin (for a hypokalemic patient, a 24-hour urinary potassium level higher than 30 mEq/L is consistent with renal potassium wasting); most patients with excessive hypokalemia who are receiving usual doses of diuretics (serum potassium < 3.0 mEq/L); most patients with resistant hypertension, even if normokalemic; all patients with hypertension and an adrenal mass; and patients receiving treatment with ACE inhibitors or ARBs, with or without concomitant diuretic therapy, who have hypokalemia or who require potassium supplements.

Screening is usually carried out by simultaneous measurement of plasma aldosterone concentration and plasma renin activity with calculation of the aldosterone-to-renin ratio [see Table 13]. Values that exceed 15 are suggestive of this disorder. This screening test has only fair diagnostic accuracy, with a sensitivity of 75% to 85% and a specificity of 75%.[138] Because of the low specificity of the ratio test, confirmation testing is required for the diagnosis to be established. Confirmation is made by demonstrating an inability to suppress aldosterone production by extracellular volume expansion [see Table 13]. After the diagnosis is confirmed, the subtype is determined with CT imaging of the adrenal glands. Occasionally, adrenal vein sampling is required to confirm the presence of an aldosterone-producing adenoma. Treatment for an adenoma is usually with a laparoscopic adrenalectomy. Treatment of idiopathic hyperaldosteronism is pharmacologic and employs aldosterone antagonists, usually with additional drugs as needed for adequate BP control.

PHEOCHROMOCYTOMA

Pheochromocytomas are rare tumors of chromaffin cell origin that produce excess amounts of catecholamines, which leads to paroxysmal or sustained hypertension [see Chapter 55]. The incidence in the general population is 2 to 8 cases per million persons per year. The prevalence is about 0.5% in patients with hypertension who have suggestive symptoms, and approximately 4% in hypertensive patients with an adrenal mass. Most tumors are benign, but approximately 10% are malignant. Symptomatic paroxysms occur in less than 50% of patients. Episodes are characterized by symptoms of headache, diaphoresis, palpitations, and pallor associated with increases in blood pressure.[140] Such paroxysms are usually rapid in onset and offset and can be precipitated by a variety of activities (e.g., exercise, bending over, urination, defecation, induction of anesthesia, infusion of intravenous contrast media, smoking). A history of unintended weight loss is not uncommon, as is the presence of glucose intolerance. The hypertension may be associated with marked BP lability and orthostatic hypotension. Rarely, patients may present with catecholamine-induced cardiomyopathy, fever, or peripheral vasospasm. The hypertension can be severe and resistant to control.

Table 15   Causes for False Positive Screening Results for Plasma Free Metanephrines
and 24-Hour Urinary Metanephrines

Category	Sources	Tests Affected
Diet	Coffee (including decaffeinated)	Plasma metanephrines/urinary HPLC electrophoresis
	Acetaminophen (direct effect)	Plasma metanephrines/urinary HPLC electrophoresis
	Caffeine (increases plasma catecholamines)	All
	Unknown diet sources	Plasma metanephrines/urinary HPLC electrophoresis
Drugs	Nicotine (increases plasma catecholamines)	All
	Tricyclic antidepressants (norepinephrine and its metabolites)	All
	Dibenzyline (norepinephrine and its metabolites)	All
	Drugs containing catecholamines (decongestants)	All
	Labetalol	Urinary HPLC electrophoresis
	Withdrawal from clonidine	All
	Withdrawal from alcohol	All
	Withdrawal from benzodiazepines	All
	Levodopa	All
	Cyclobenzaprine	All
	Amphetamines	All
	Phenothiazines	Unknown
	Benzodiazepines	Unknown
Physiologic stress	Obstructive sleep apnea, heart failure	All

HPLC—high-pressure liquid chromatography

Most pheochromocytomas are sporadic, but 10% are familial. The inheritance pattern for all familial cases is autosomal dominant, with variable penetrance. Familial syndromes include a simple form not associated with other abnormalities; the multiple endocrine neoplasias, in which the risk of pheochromocytoma is 50% (type IIA [medullary thyroid carcinoma, hyperparathyroidism] and type IIB [medullary thyroid carcinoma, mucosal neuromas, marfanoid habitus, thickened corneal nerves, intestinal gangliomatosis]); neurofibromatosis (risk of pheochromocytoma is 0.1% to 5.7%); the von Hippel-Lindau syndrome (retinal hemangiomatosis, cerebellar hemangioblastomas, renal cell carcinoma; risk of pheochromocytoma is 10% to 20%); and the familial paraganglioma syndrome (tumors of the head or neck [glomus tumors] or carotid body; risk of pheochromocytoma is 20%). Familial pheochromocytomas can be bilateral. Persons with suspected familial pheochromocytoma should undergo genetic testing.

Most pheochromocytomas (90%) are located in one or both adrenal glands. Extra-adrenal pheochromocytomas can occur anywhere along the sympathetic chain and, rarely, in other sites (i.e., the superior para-aortic region, the glomus jugulare, the inferior para-aortic region, the bladder, or the thorax). About 98% of pheochromocytomas are located in the abdomen.

Screening for pheochromocytoma should be selective and based on suggestive clinical features. Screening tests include measurement of catecholamines (i.e., epinephrine, norepinephrine, dopamine) and their metabolites (i.e., metanephrine, normetanephrine, and vanillylmandelic acid [VMA]) in the plasma and urine. Traditionally, most experts have considered measurement of 24-hour urinary catecholamines or catecholamine metabolites to be the screening tests of choice.[140] However, studies now suggest that measurement of plasma free metanephrines is a much more sensitive screening test (for hereditary tumors, sensitivity is 97%, versus 60% for urinary metanephrines; for sporadic tumors, sensitivity is 99%, versus 88% for urinary metanephrines).[141] Also, this screening test ob-

viates the concerns associated with obtaining an adequate 24-hour urine collection. Although the sensitivity of the plasma screen is higher than that of urinary tests, its specificity is lower with regard to screening for sporadic tumors (for sporadic tumors, specificity is 82% with the plasma test versus 89% with the urinary test; in hereditary tumors, specificity is 96% with the plasma test versus 97% with the urinary test). Plasma metanephrine assay should be strongly considered as the screening test of choice if a hereditary form of pheochromocytoma is suspected; it should also be considered the test of choice for patients with a history of pheochromocytoma and for patients in whom the clinical suspicion is high. A negative result on either a plasma or urinary metanephrine test excludes the diagnosis in most cases. Measurement of catecholamines in the plasma or urine is quite insensitive and should not be used alone as a screening test.

Because of the low prevalence of pheochromocytomas in patients screened for this disorder, false positive results outnumber true positive results. This is of major concern because positive results from screening tests often lead to additional tests and anxiety on the part of the both the physician and the patient. There are three main factors associated with false positive results: diet, drugs, and physiologic stressors [see Table 15]. Specific dietary factors and drugs affect plasma screens and urinary metanephrine screens differently. Moreover, for urinary metanephrine screens, different drugs affect the results differently depending on the method of analysis used (i.e., high-pressure liquid chromatography [HPLC] versus mass spectrophotometry). Anticipation of these potential problems and proper preparation of the patient can prevent many false positive results.

A positive screening test should prompt a search for the tumor if sources of a false positive result have been excluded. Abdominal imaging with CT or magnetic resonance imaging is the initial test of choice, given that 90% of pheochromocytomas are on the adrenal glands and 98% are in the abdomen. Additional studies may be required if a tumor is not found with initial imaging.[142] Medical treatment is required before surgical intervention. The mainstay of treatment is alpha blockade with phenoxybenzamine. Beta blockers can be used to control the tachycardia that occasionally follows adequate alpha blockade. Because pheochromocytomas can recur in 10% of patients, long-term biochemical follow-up is required.

CUSHING SYNDROME

Cushing syndrome arises from excess production of glucocorticoids. It is rare: the incidence of the ectopic adrenocorticotropic hormone (ACTH) syndrome is about 660 cases per million population; in 50% of these cases, the underlying cause is small cell lung cancer. The incidence of adrenal tumors is one to five cases per million population per year. The incidence of pituitary ACTH-dependent disease is estimated to be five to 25 cases per million population per year. The signs and symptoms of Cushing syndrome arise from long-term exposure to excess glucocorticoids. They include central obesity, skin atrophy, striae, acne, slow wound healing, proximal muscle wasting and weakness, osteoporosis, menstrual irregularity, hyperpigmentation (ACTH dependent), glucose intolerance, hypokalemia, and hypertension. Clinical manifestations vary on the basis of the degree and duration of glucocorticoid excess, the presence or absence of androgen excess (in women, androgen excess produces hirsutism, decreased libido, virilization, and oily skin), and the cause of hypercortisolism (hyperpigmentation results from excessive ACTH; androgen excess is more common in adrenal carcinomas). States of pseudo–Cushing syndrome can result from significant stress, severe obesity, depression, and chronic alcoholism.[143]

Patients suspected of having Cushing syndrome should undergo measurement of 24-hour urinary free cortisol. Normal levels exclude the diagnosis, and levels higher than threefold normal confirm it. In patients with equivocal results, a low-dose dexamethasone suppression test can be used. For this test, the patient is given a 1 mg tablet at 11 P.M. Serum cortisol is measured on a specimen drawn the next morning at 8 A.M. A normal response is a serum cortisol level of less than 5 μg/dl. An alternative method is to give a 0.5 mg tablet every 6 hours for eight doses and to measure 24-hour urinary cortisol excretion on the second day. A normal response is a urinary cortisol excretion of less than 10 μg/24 hr and a serum cortisol level of less than 5 μg/dl.

COARCTATION OF THE AORTA

Congenital constriction of the aorta accounts for approximately 7% of congenital cardiovascular diseases. Coarctation can occur anywhere along the aorta but most often occurs just distal to the takeoff of the left subclavian artery. The disorder is usually detected in childhood, but occasionally it escapes detection until adulthood. Symptoms include headache, cold feet, and claudication. The classic feature of coarctation is elevated blood pressure in the arms and low or unobtainable blood pressure in the legs. This finding can be identified by direct measurement. The presence of weak femoral pulses or a delay in sensing the femoral pulse when simultaneously palpating the radial pulse is cause to suspect coarctation. Other findings include visible pulsations in the neck or chest wall and murmurs in the front and back of the chest from collateral vessels. Physical findings may be subtle. If the diagnosis is suspected, screening tests include transesophageal echocardiography or MRI or CT imaging of the aorta. Treatment is surgical in most cases [see Chapter 28].

Complications

Left untreated, hypertension leads to premature death or disability from complications of CV diseases, especially atherosclerosis.[3-5] Hypertension affects blood vessels directly, inducing endothelial dysfunction, and acts in concert with other factors (e.g., smoking, hyperlipidemia, and diabetes) to promote the atherosclerotic process. Although the effect of hypertension on blood vessels is systemic, it expresses itself by characteristic effects on target organs—the heart, brain, kidneys, and eyes.

Hypertension increases the risk of myocardial infarction and sudden cardiac death twofold.[3] It contributes to the risk of atrial fibrillation and is the single most important antecedent to the development of heart failure.[108,109] These adverse effects of hypertension reflect both acceleration of atherosclerosis and the development of structural adaptation of the heart (LVH and left atrial enlargement) to increased afterload. The structural changes limit coronary reserve.

Heart failure can be the result of either systolic or diastolic dysfunction. Hypertension is commonly associated with abnormal diastolic relaxation, which can be demonstrated by echocardiography. Progression of these effects on the heart can lead to symptoms of heart failure with preserved systolic function, a condition known as diastolic heart failure [see Chapter 26]. In addition, long-standing hypertension leads to LVH and ventricular remodeling, which progresses to systolic dysfunction. This process is aggravated by myocardial infarction.

Hypertension is the single most important cause of stroke, which itself is the third leading cause of death in the United States.[144] Hypertension increases the risk of stroke by aggravating atherosclerosis in the aortic arch and carotid and cerebral arteries (causing thrombotic or embolic ischemic strokes) and by inducing arteriosclerosis in small, penetrating subcortical cerebral vessels, leading to leukoaraiosis (periventricular leukoenceophalopathy) and lacunar strokes. Severe hypertension is also associated with intraparenchymal and subarachnoid hemorrhage.

Hypertension in midlife is associated with an increased risk of cognitive dysfunction and dementia in later life.[5] This may be a complication of multiple cerebral infarctions (multi-infarct dementia), but it also occurs in the absence of previous strokes. In some persons, cognitive dysfunction may arise from the effects of elevated BP on the small penetrating subcortical arterioles, leading to ischemic injury to white matter (visible as leukoaraiosis on brain imaging studies). Although vascular dementia in the elderly is strongly related to hypertension, the relationship between BP and cognition is less clear in persons older than 75 years. In some cases, an inverse relationship has been noted. This may reflect a shift in cerebral autoregulation to a higher range in patients with hypertension-induced small vessel disease, making these patients more vulnerable to further ischemic brain injury when BP is lowered.

Hypertension is a risk factor for abdominal aortic aneurysm. In addition, the majority of patients with aortic dissection have hypertension. Aortic dissection arises from the combined effects of accelerated aortic atherosclerosis and increased pulsatile stress on the aortic wall. Hypertension increases the risk of peripheral vascular disease, especially in cigarette smokers and diabetic patients.

Hypertension is the second leading cause of end-stage renal disease.[137] Arteriosclerotic changes lead to ischemic injury and loss of glomeruli and tubular elements, ultimately leading to the shrunken kidney of nephrosclerosis. End-stage kidney disease from hypertension is much more common in blacks. Malignant hypertension induces fibrinoid necrosis of renal arterioles and can lead to acute renal failure.

Hypertension-related vascular disease causes loss of vision through a variety of mechanisms.[145] Chronic hypertension causes arteriosclerosis of retinal vessels. These changes at the site of arterial-venous crossings can lead to branch retinal vein occlusion. Central retinal vein occlusion can also occur. Ischemic optic neuropathy can be a complication of chronic hypertension or acute severe hypertension. Acute, severe elevations in BP can also cause retinal hemorrhages, exudates, and papilledema. Hypertension accelerates atherosclerosis. Atherosclerotic emboli can occlude central or branch retinal arteries, with sudden and irreversible visual loss. Severe atherosclerosis can lead to venous stasis retinopathy as a result of a reduction in blood flow in the carotid or ophthalmic artery. Occlusive disease of retinal vessels can lead to cystoid macular edema, epiretinal membrane formation, and collateral vessel formation.

Prognosis

Effective treatment has a dramatic effect on the prognosis of patients with hypertension. Prospective treatment trials have established that BP reduction with drug therapy markedly reduces CV morbidity and mortality. Active treatment of hypertension lessens the tendency for BP to increase over time. For patients whose diastolic BP is 90 mm Hg or more or whose systolic BP is 160 mm Hg or more, drug intervention has been shown to reduce the risk of stroke by 35% to 40%; the risk of myocardial infarction is reduced by 20% to 25%; and the risk of heart failure is reduced by over 50%. In hypertensive patients with chronic kidney disease, drug intervention reduces the risk of progression to dialysis, transplantation, and death. However, even when BP is brought down to current recommended levels, hypertensive individuals remain at higher risk for CV disease events compared with normotensive individuals. Patients with target-organ disease remain at even higher risk, despite good BP control. These observations argue for application of public health and individual patient strategies to prevent the development of hypertension and for early detection and effective treatment of high BP.

The authors have no commercial relationships with manufacturers of products or providers of services discussed in this chapter.

References

1. Fields LE, Burt VL, Cutler JA, et al: The burden of adult hypertension in the United States, 1999 to 2000: a rising tide. Hypertension 44:398, 2004

2. Vasan RS, Beiser A, Seshadri S, et al: Residual lifetime risk for developing hypertension in middle-aged women and men: the Framingham Heart Study. JAMA 287:1003, 2002

3. Kannel WB: Blood pressure as a cardiovascular risk factor: prevention and treatment. JAMA 275:1571, 1996

4. Whelton PK, He J, Perneger TV, et al: Kidney damage in "benign" essential hypertension. Curr Opin Nephrol Hypertens 6:177, 1997

5. Launer LJ, Masaki K, Petrovitch H, et al: The association between midlife blood pressure levels and late-life cognitive function: the Honolulu-Asia Aging Study. JAMA 274:1846, 1995

6. Staessen JA, Wang JG, Thijs L: Cardiovascular protection and blood pressure reduction: a meta-analysis. Lancet 358:1305, 2001

7. Staessen JA, Gasowski J, Wang JG, et al: Risks of untreated and treated isolated systolic hypertension in the elderly: meta-analysis of outcome trials. Lancet 355:865, 2000

8. Chobanian AV, Bakris GL, Black HR, et al: The seventh report of the Joint National Committee on Prevention, Detection, Evaluation, and Treatment of High Blood Pressure: the JNC 7 report. JAMA 289:2560, 2003

9. Hajjar I, Kotchen TA: Trends in prevalence, awareness, treatment, and control of hypertension in the United States, 1988–2000. JAMA 290:199, 2003

10. Wang TJ, Vasan RS: Epidemiology of uncontrolled hypertension in the United States. Circulation 112:1651, 2005

11. Lewington S, Clarke R, Qizilbash N, et al: Age-specific relevance of usual blood pressure to vascular mortality: a meta-analysis of individual data from one million adults in 61 prospective studies. Lancet 360:1903, 2002

12. Vasan RS, Larson MG, Leip EP, et al: Assessment of frequency of progression to hypertension in non-hypertensive participants in the Framingham Heart Study: a cohort study. Lancet 358:1682, 2001

13. Franklin SS, Jacobs MJ, Wong ND, et al: Predominance of isolated systolic hypertension among middle-aged and elderly US hypertensives: analysis based on National Health and Nutrition Examination Survey (NHANES) III. Hypertension 37:869, 2001

14. Franklin SS, Larson MG, Khan SA, et al: Does the relation of blood pressure to coronary heart disease risk change with aging? The Framingham Heart Study. Circulation 103:1245, 2001

15. Miura K, Daviglus ML, Dyer AR, et al: Relationship of blood pressure to 25-year mortality due to coronary heart disease, cardiovascular diseases, and all causes in young adult men: the Chicago Heart Association Detection Project in Industry. Arch Intern Med 161:1501, 2001

16. Lifton RP, Gharavi AG, Geller DS: Molecular mechanisms of human hypertension. Cell 104:545, 2001

17. O'Donnell CJ, Lindpainter K, Larson MG, et al: Evidence for association and genetic linkage of the angiotensin-converting enzyme locus with hypertension and blood pressure in men but not in women in the Framingham Heart Study. Circulation 97:1766, 1998

18. Caulfield M, Lavender P, Farrall M, et al: Linkage of the angiotensinogen gene to essential hypertension. N Engl J Med 330:1629, 1994

19. Rigat B, Hubert C, Alhenc-Gelas F, et al: An insertion/deletion polymorphism in the angiotensin I–converting enzyme gene accounting for half the variance of serum enzyme levels. J Clin Invest 86:1343, 1990

20. Cambien F, Poirier O, Lecerf L, et al: Deletion polymorphism in the gene for angiotensin-converting-enzyme is a potent risk factor for myocardial infarction. Nature 359:641, 1992

21. Turner ST, Boerwinkle E, Sing CF: Context-dependent associations of the ACE I/D polymorphism with blood pressure. Hypertension 34(4 pt 2):773, 1999

22. Cusi D, Barlassina C, Azzani T, et al: Polymorphisms of alpha-adducin and salt sensitivity in patients with essential hypertension. Lancet 349:1353, 1997

23. Krushkal J, Xiong M, Ferrell R, et al: Linkage and association of adrenergic and dopamine receptor genes in the distal portion of the long arm of chromosome 5 with systolic blood pressure variation. Hum Mol Genet 7:1379, 1998

24. Marteau JB, Zaiou M, Siest G, et al: Genetic determinants of blood pressure regulation. J Hypertens 23:2127, 2005

25. Sing CF, Stengard JH, Kardia SL: Genes, environment, and cardiovascular disease. Arterioscler Thromb Vasc Biol 23:1190, 2003

26. Intersalt: an international study of electrolyte excretion and blood pressure: results for 24 hour urinary sodium and potassium excretion. Intersalt Cooperative Research Group. BMJ 297:319, 1988

27. Cutler JA, Follmann D, Allender PS: Randomized trials of sodium reduction: an overview. Am J Clin Nutr 65(2 suppl):643S, 1997

28. Guyton AC: Kidneys and fluids in pressure regulation: small volume but large pressure changes. Hypertension 19(suppl):I2, 1992

29. Brenner BM, Chertow GM: Congenital oligonephropathy and the etiology of adult hypertension and progressive renal injury. Am J Kidney Dis 23:171, 1994

30. Sealey JE, Blumenfeld JD, Bell GM, et al: On the renal basis for essential hypertension: nephron heterogeneity with discordant renin secretion and sodium excretion causing a hypertensive vasoconstriction-volume relationship. J Hypertens 6:763, 1988

31. Blaustein MP: Endogenous ouabain: role in the pathogenesis of hypertension. Kidney Int 49:1748, 1996

32. Esler M, Rumantir M, Kaye D, et al: The sympathetic neurobiology of essential hypertension: disparate influences of obesity, stress, and noradrenaline transporter dysfunction? Am J Hypertens 14(6 pt 2):139S, 2001+

33. Izzo JL, Taylor AA: The sympathetic nervous system and baroreflexes in hypertension and hypotension. Curr Hypertens Rep 1:254, 1999

34. Grassi G, Seravalle G, Dell'Oro R, et al: Adrenergic and reflex abnormalities in obesity-related hypertension. Hypertension 36:538, 2000

35. Landsberg L: Insulin-mediated sympathetic stimulation: role in the pathogenesis of obesity-related hypertension (or, how insulin affects blood pressure, and why). J Hypertens 19(3 pt 2):523, 2001

36. Haynes WG, Morgan DA, Walsh SA, et al: Cardiovascular consequences of obesity: role of leptin. Clin Exp Pharmacol Physiol 25:65, 1998

37. Jackson WF: Ion channels and vascular tone. Hypertension 35(1 pt 2):173, 2000

38. Cosentino F, Lüscher TF: Effects of blood pressure and glucose on endothelial function. Curr Hypertens Rep 3:79, 2001

39. Tomiyama H, Arai T, Koji Y, et al: The age-related increase in arterial stiffness is augmented in phases according to the severity of hypertension. Hypertension Res 27:465, 2004

40. Franklin SS, Pio JR, Wong ND, et al: Predictors of new-onset diastolic and systolic hypertension: the Framingham Heart Study. Circulation 111:1121, 2005

41. Mitchell GF: Arterial stiffness and wave-reflection in hypertension: pathophysiological and therapeutic implications. Curr Hypertens Rep 6:436, 2004

42. Recommendations for routine blood pressure measurement by indirect cuff sphygmomanometry. American Society of Hypertension. Am J Hypertens 5(4 pt 1):207, 1992

43. Pickering TG, Hall JE, Appel LJ, et al: Recommendations for blood pressure mea-

surement in humans and experimental animals. Part 1: Blood pressure measurement in humans: a statement for professionals from the subcommittee on professional and public education of the American Heart Association Council on High Blood Pressure Research. Circulation 111:697, 2005

44. Gosse P, Ansoborlo P, Jullien V, et al: Ambulatory blood pressure and left ventricular hypertrophy. Blood Press Monit 2:70, 1997

45. Verdecchia P, Porcellati C, Schillaci G, et al: Ambulatory blood pressure: an independent predictor of prognosis in essential hypertension. Hypertension 24:793, 1994

46. Clement DL, De Buyzere ML, De Bacquer DA, et al: Prognostic value of ambulatory blood pressure recordings in patients with treated hypertension. N Engl J Med 348:2407, 2003

47. Dolan E, Stanton A, Thijs L, et al: Superiority of ambulatory over clinic blood pressure measurement in predicting mortality: the Dublin Outcome Study. Hypertension 46:156, 2005

48. Updated policy and claims processing instructions for ambulatory blood pressure monitoring (ABPM). Centers for Medicare & Medicaid Services, 2004 http://www.cms.hhs.gov/MLNMattersArticles/downloads/MM2726.pdf

49. Ugajin T, Hozawa A, Ohkubo T et al: White-coat hypertension as a risk factor for the development of home hypertension: the Ohasama Study. Arch Intern Med 165:1541, 2005

50. Pickering T, Davidson K, Gerin W, et al: Masked hypertension. Hypertension 40:795, 2002

51. The sixth report of the Joint National Committee on prevention, detection, evaluation, and treatment of high blood pressure. Arch Intern Med 157:2413, 1997

52. 2003 European Society of Hypertension–European Society of Cardiology guidelines for the management of arterial hypertension. J Hypertens 21:1011, 2003

53. Kaplan NM: Other secondary forms of hypertension. Kaplan's Clinical Hypertension, 8th ed. Kaplan NM, Ed. Lippincott Williams & Wilkins, Philadelphia, 2002, p 495

54. Fuchs FD, Maestri MK, Bredemeier M, et al: Study of the usefulness of optic fundi examination of patients with hypertension in a clinical setting. J Hum Hypertens 9:547, 1995

55. Cockcroft DW, Gault MH: Prediction of creatinine clearance from serum creatinine. Nephron 16:31, 1976

56. Levey AS, Bosch JP, Lewis JB, et al: A more accurate method to estimate glomerular filtration rate from serum creatinine: a new prediction equation. Modification of Diet in Renal Disease Study Group. Ann Intern Med 130:461, 1999

57. Svetkey LP: Management of prehypertension. Hypertension 45:1056, 2005

58. The effects of nonpharmacologic interventions on blood pressure of persons with high normal levels: results of the Trials of Hypertension Prevention, phase I. Trials of Hypertension Prevention Collaborative Research Group. JAMA 267:1213, 1992

59. Effects of weight loss and sodium reduction intervention on blood pressure and hypertension incidence in overweight people with high-normal blood pressure: the Trials of Hypertension Prevention, phase II. Trials of Hypertension Prevention Collaborative Research Group. Arch Intern Med 157:657, 1997

60. Xin X, He J, Frontini MG, et al: Effects of alcohol reduction on blood pressure: a meta-analysis of randomized controlled trials. Hypertension 38:1112, 2001

61. Appel LJ, Moore TJ, Obarzanek E, et al: A clinical trial of the effects of dietary patterns on blood pressure. DASH Collaborative Research Group. N Engl J Med 336:1117, 1997

62. Moore LL, Visioni J, Mustafa M, et al: Weight loss in overweight adults and the long-term risk of hypertension. Arch Intern Med 165:1298, 2005

63. Elmer PJ, Obarzanek E, Vollmer WM, et al: Effects of comprehensive lifestyle modification on diet, weight, physical fitness, and blood pressure control: 18-month results of a randomized trial. Ann Intern Med 144:485, 2006

64. Andersson OK, Almgren T, Persson B, et al: Survival in treated hypertension: follow-up study after two decades. BMJ 317:167, 1998

65. Julius S, Nesbitt SD, Egan BM, et al: Feasibility of treating prehypertension with an angiotensin-receptor blocker. Trial of Preventing Hypertension (TROPHY) Study Investigators. N Engl J Med 354:1685, 2006

66. Executive summary of the third report of the National Cholesterol Education Program (NCEP) Expert Panel on Detection, Evaluation, and Treatment of High Blood Cholesterol in Adults (Adult Treatment Panel III). JAMA 285:2486, 2001

67. Effects on blood pressure of reduced dietary sodium and the Dietary Approaches to Stop Hypertension (DASH) diet. DASH-Sodium Collaborative Research Group. N Engl J Med 344:3, 2001

68. Appel LJ, Champagne CM, Harsha DW, et al: Effects of comprehensive lifestyle modification on blood pressure control: main results of the PREMIER clinical trial. Writing Group of the PREMIER Collaborative Research Group. JAMA 289:2083, 2003

69. Hansson L, Zanchetti A, Carruthers SG, et al: Effects of intensive blood-pressure lowering and low-dose aspirin in patients with hypertension: principal results of the Hypertension Optimal Treatment (HOT) randomized trial. Lancet 351:1755, 1998

70. He J, Whelton PK, Appel LJ, et al: Long-term effects of weight loss and dietary sodium reduction on incidence of hypertension. Hypertension 35:544, 2000

71. Chobanian AV, Hill M: National Heart, Lung, and Blood Institute Workshop on Sodium and Blood Pressure: a critical review of current scientific evidence. Hypertension 35:858, 2000

72. Kelley GA, Kelley KS: Progressive resistance exercise and resting blood pressure: a meta-analysis of randomized controlled trials. Hypertension 35:838, 2000

73. Whelton SP, Chin A, Xin X, He J: Effect of aerobic exercise on blood pressure: a meta-analysis of randomized, controlled trials. Ann Intern Med 136:493, 2002

74. Dickinson HO, Mason JM, Nicolson DJ, et al: Lifestyle interventions to reduce raised blood pressure: a systematic review of randomized controlled trials. J Hypertens 24:215, 2006

75. Schein MH, Gavish B, Herz M, et al: Treating hypertension with a device that slows and regularises breathing: a randomized double-blind controlled study. J Hum Hypertens 15:271, 2001

76. Major cardiovascular events in hypertensive patients randomized to doxazosin vs chlorthalidone: the Antihypertensive and Lipid-Lowering Treatment to Prevent Heart Attack Trial (ALLHAT). ALLHAT Officers and Coordinators for the ALLHAT Collaborative Research Group. JAMA 283:1967, 2000

77. Major outcomes in high-risk hypertensive patients randomized to angiotensin-converting enzyme inhibitor or calcium channel blocker vs diuretic: the Antihypertensive and Lipid-Lowering Treatment to Prevent Heart Attack Trial (ALLHAT). ALLHAT Officers and Coordinators for the ALLHAT Collaborative Research Group. JAMA 288:2981, 2002

78. Psaty BM, Lumley T, Furberg CD, et al: Health outcomes associated with various antihypertensive therapies used as first-line agents: a network meta-analysis. JAMA 289:2534, 2003

79. Wright JT Jr, Dunn JK, Cutler JA, et al: Outcomes in hypertensive black and nonblack patients treated with chlorthalidone, amlodipine, and lisinopril. JAMA 293:1595, 2005

80. Whelton PK, Barzilay J, Cushman WC, et al: Clinical outcomes in antihypertensive treatment of type 2 diabetes, impaired fasting glucose concentration, and normoglycemia: Antihypertensive and Lipid-Lowering Treatment to Prevent Heart Attack Trial (ALLHAT). Arch Intern Med 165:1401, 2005

81. Mahboob R, Pressel S, Davis BR, et al: Renal outcomes in high-risk hypertensive patients treated with an angiotensin-converting enzyme inhibitor or a calcium channel blocker versus a diuretic: a report from the Antihypertensive and Lipid-Lowering Treatment to Prevent Heart Attack Trial (ALLHAT). Arch Intern Med 165:936, 2005

82. Wing LM, Reid CM, Ryan P, et al: A comparison of outcomes with angiotensin-converting-enzyme inhibitors and diuretics for hypertension in the elderly. N Engl J Med 348:583, 2003

83. Wang J, Staessen JA: Benefits of antihypertensive pharmacologic therapy and blood pressure reduction in outcome trials. J Clin Hypertens 5:66, 2003

84. Lindholm LH, Carlberg B, Samuelsson O: Should beta blockers remain first choice in the treatment of primary hypertension? A meta-analysis. Lancet 366:1545, 2005

85. Khan N, McAlister FA: Re-examining the efficacy of beta-blockers for the treatment of hypertension: a meta-analysis. CMAJ 174:1737, 2006

86. Mason RP, Kalinowski L, Jacob RF, et al: Nebivolol reduces nitroxidative stress and restores nitric oxide bioavailability in endothelium of black Americans. Circulation 112:3795, 2005

87. Dahlof B, Sever PS, Poulter NR, et al: Prevention of cardiovascular events with an antihypertensive regimen of amlodipine adding perinopril as required versus atenolol adding bendroflumethazide as required, in the Anglo-Scandinavian Cardiac Outcomes Trial-Blood Pressure Lowering Arm (ASCOT-BPLA): a multicentre randomised controlled trial. Lancet 366:895, 2005

88. Moser M, Pickering T, Sowers JR: Combination drug therapy in the management of hypertension: when, with what, and how? J Clin Hypertens 2:94, 2000

89. He J, Muntner P, Chen J, et al: Factors associated with hypertension control in the general population of the United States. Arch Intern Med 162:1051, 2002

90. Hyman DJ, Pavlik VN: Characteristics of patients with uncontrolled hypertension in the United States. N Engl J Med 345:479, 2001

91. Hyman DJ, Pavlik VN: Self-reported hypertension treatment practices among primary care physicians: blood pressure thresholds, drug choices, and the role of guidelines and evidence-based medicine. Arch Intern Med 160:2281, 2000

92. Taler SJ, Textor SC, Augustine JE: Resistant hypertension: comparing hemodynamic management to specialist care. Hypertension 39:982, 2002

93. Redon J, Campos C, Narciso ML, et al: Prognostic value of ambulatory blood pressure monitoring in refractory hypertension: a prospective study. Hypertension 31:712, 1998

94. Messerli FH: Osler's maneuver, pseudohypertension, and true hypertension in the elderly. Am J Med 80:906, 1986

95. Di Bari M, Pahor M, Franse LV, et al: Dementia and disability outcomes in large hypertension trials: lessons learned from the Systolic Hypertension in the Elderly Program (SHEP) trial. Am J Epidemiol 153:72, 2001

96. Whelton PK, Appel LJ, Espeland MA, et al: Sodium reduction and weight loss in the treatment of hypertension in older persons: a randomized controlled trial of nonpharmacologic interventions in the elderly (TONE). TONE Collaborative Research Group. JAMA 279:839, 1998

97. Midgley JP, Matthew AG, Greenwood CM, et al: Effect of reduced dietary sodium on blood pressure: a meta-analysis of randomized controlled trials. JAMA 275:1590, 1996

98. Hansson L, Lindholm LH, Ekbom T, et al: Randomised trial of old and new antihypertensive drugs in elderly patients: cardiovascular mortality and morbidity in the Swedish Trial in Old Patients with Hypertension–2 study. Lancet 354:1751, 1999

99. Dahlof B, Devereux RB, Kjeldsen SE, et al: Cardiovascular morbidity and mortality in the Losartan Intervention For Endpoint reduction in hypertension study (LIFE): a randomised trial against atenolol. Lancet 359:995, 2002

100. Randomized trial of a perindopril-based blood-pressure-lowering regimen among 6,105 individuals with previous stroke or transient ischemic attack. PROGRESS Collaborative Group. Lancet 358:1033, 2001

101. Adler AI, Stratton IM, Neil HA, et al: Association of systolic blood pressure with macrovascular and microvascular complications of type 2 diabetes (UKPDS 36): prospective observational study. BMJ 321:412, 2000

102. Treatment of hypertension in adults with diabetes. American Diabetes Association.

Diabetes Care 26(suppl 1):S80, 2003

103. Efficacy of atenolol and captopril in reducing risk of macrovascular and microvascular complications in type 2 diabetes: UKPDS 39. UK Prospective Diabetes Study Group. BMJ 317:713, 1998

104. K/DOQI clinical practice guidelines for chronic kidney disease: evaluation, classification, and stratification. Kidney Disease Outcome Quality Initiative. National Kidney Foundation (NKF) Disease Outcome Quality Initiative (K/DOQI) Advisory Board. Am J Kid Dis 39(2 suppl 2):S1, 2002

105. Lewis EJ, Hunsicker LG, Bain RP, et al: The effect of angiotensin-converting-enzyme inhibition on diabetic nephropathy. N Engl J Med 329:1456, 1993

106. Brenner BM, Cooper ME, de Zeeuw D, et al: Effects of losartan on renal and cardiovascular outcomes in patients with type 2 diabetes and nephropathy. N Engl J Med 345:861, 2001

107. Estacio RO, Jeffers BW, Hiatt WR, et al: The effect of nisoldipine as compared with enalapril on cardiovascular outcomes in patients with non–insulin-dependent diabetes and hypertension. N Engl J Med 338:645, 1998

108. Vasan RS, Levy D: The role of hypertension in the pathogenesis of heart failure: a clinical mechanistic overview. Arch Intern Med 156:1789, 1996

109. Levy D, Larson MG, Vasan RS, et al: The progression from hypertension to heart failure. JAMA 275:1557, 1996

110. Effects of an angiotensin-converting-enzyme inhibitor, ramipril, on cardiovascular events in high-risk patients. The Heart Outcomes Prevention Evaluation Study Investigators. N Engl J Med 342:145, 2000

111. Effect of enalapril on survival in patients with reduced left ventricular ejection fractions and congestive heart failure. The SOLVD investigators. N Engl J Med 325:293, 1991

112. Freemantle N, Cleland J, Young P, et al: Beta blockade after myocardial infarction: systematic review and meta regression analysis. BMJ 318:1730, 1999

113. Tepper D: Frontiers in congestive heart failure: effect of metoprolol CR/XL in chronic heart failure: Metoprolol CR/XL Randomized Intervention Trial in Congestive Heart Failure (MERIT-HF). Congest Heart Fail 5:184, 1999

114. Pitt B, Remme W, Zannad F, et al: Eplerenone, a selective aldosterone blocker, in patients with left ventricular dysfunction after myocardial infarction. Eplerenone Post-Acute Myocardial Infarction Heart Failure Efficacy and Survival Study Investigators. N Engl J Med 348:1309, 2003

115. Vakili BA, Okin PM, Devereaux RB: Prognostic implications of left ventricular hypertrophy. Am Heart J 141:334, 2001

116. van Zwieten PA: The influence of antihypertensive drug treatment on the prevention and regression of left ventricular hypertrophy. Cardiovasc Res 45:82, 2000

117. Messerli FH, Mancia G, Conti CR, et al: Dogma disputed: can aggressively lowering blood pressure in hypertensive patients with coronary artery disease be dangerous? Ann Intern Med 144:884, 2006

118. Effect of ramipril vs amlodipine on renal outcomes in hypertensive nephrosclerosis: a randomized controlled trial. African American Study of Kidney Disease and Hypertension (AASK) Study Group. JAMA 285:2719, 2001

119. Sarnak MJ, Greene T, Wang X, et al: The effect of a lower target blood pressure on the progression of kidney disease: long term follow-up of the modification of diet in renal disease study. Ann Intern Med 142:342, 2005

120. Rahman M, Pressel S, Davis BR, et al: Cardiovascular outcomes in high-risk hypertensive patients stratified by baseline glomerular filtration rate. Ann Intern Med 144:172, 2006

121. Morfis L, Schwartz RS, Poulos R, et al: Blood pressure changes in acute cerebral infarction and hemorrhage. Stroke 28:1401, 1997

122. Wilmot M, Leonardi-Bee J, Bath PMW: High blood pressure in acute stroke and subsequent outcome: a systematic review [abstract]. Cerebrovasc Dis 13(suppl 3):95, 2002

123. Semplicini A, Maresca A, Boscolo G, et al: Hypertension in acute ischemic stroke: a compensatory mechanism or an additional damaging factor? Arch Intern Med 163:211, 2003

124. Bath P, Chalmers J, Powers W, et al: International Society of Hypertension (ISH): statement on the management of blood pressure in acute stroke. International Society of Hypertension Writing Group. J Hypertens 21:665, 2003

125. Adams HP Jr, Adams RJ, Brott T, et al: Guidelines for the early management of patients with ischemic stroke: a scientific statement from the Stroke Council of the American Heart Association. Stroke 4:1056, 2003

126. Winkelmayer WC, Stampfer MJ, Willet WC, et al: Habitual caffeine intake and the risk of hypertension in women. JAMA 294:2330, 2005

127. Forman JP, Rimm EB, Stampfer MJ, et al: Folate intake and the risk of incident hypertension among US women. JAMA 293:320, 2005

128. Cooper WO, Hernandez-Diaz S, Arbogast PG, et al: Major congenital malformations after first-trimester exposure to ACE inhibitors. N Engl J Med 354:2443, 2006

129. White WB, Hanes V, Chauhan V, Pitt B: Effects of a new hormone therapy, drospirenone and 17-β-estradiol, in postmenopausal women with hypertension. Hypertension June 26, 2006 [Epub ahead of print]

130. Norman D, Loredo JS, Nelesen RA, et al: Effects of continuous positive airway pressure versus supplemental oxygen on 24-hour ambulatory blood pressure. Hypertension 47:840, 2006

131. Slovut DP, Olin JW: Current concepts: Fibromuscular dysplasia. N Engl J Med 350:1862, 2004

132. Safian RD, Textor SC: Renal-artery stenosis. N Engl J Med 344:431, 2001

133. Garovic VD, Textor SC: Renovascular hypertension and ischemic nephropathy. Circulation 112:1362, 2005

134. Conlon PJ, Little MA, Pieper K, et al : Severity of renal vascular disease predicts mortality in patients undergoing coronary angiography. Kidney Int 60:1490, 2001

135. Cooper CJ, Murphy TP, Matsumoto A, et al: Stent revascularization for the prevention of cardiovascular and renal events among patients with renal artery stenosis and systolic hypertension: rationale and design of the CORAL trial. Am Heart J 152:59, 2006

136. Alcazar JM, Rodicio JL: Ischemic nephropathy: clinical characteristics and treatment. Am J Kid Dis 36:883, 2000

137. Fatica RA, Port FK, Young EW: Incidence trends and mortality in end-stage renal disease attributed to renovascular disease in the United States. Am J Kid Dis 37:1184, 2001

138. Schwartz GL, Turner ST: Screening for primary aldosteronism in essential hypertension: diagnostic accuracy of the ratio of plasma aldosterone concentration to plasma renin activity. Clin Chem 51:386, 2005

139. Young WF Jr: Primary aldosteronism: a common and curable form of hypertension. Cardiol Rev 7:207, 1999

140. Young WF Jr: Pheochromocytoma: issues in diagnosis & treatment. Compr Ther 23:319, 1997

141. Lenders JW, Pacak K, Walther MM, et al: Biochemical diagnosis of pheochromocytoma: which test is best? JAMA 287:1427, 2002

142. Pacak K, Linehan WM, Eisenhofer G, et al: Recent advances in genetics, diagnosis, localization, and treatment of pheochromocytoma. Ann Intern Med 134:315, 2001

143. Newell-Price J, Trainer P, Besser M, et al: The diagnosis and differential diagnosis of Cushing's syndrome and pseudo-Cushing's states. Endocr Rev 19:647, 1998

144. Deaths: Preliminary Data for 2004. National Vital Statistics Reports 54:1, 2006 http://www.cdc.gov/nchs/data/nvsr/nvsr54/nvsr54_19.pdf

145. Lock LC: Ocular manifestations of hypertension. Optometry Clin 2:47, 1992

146. Radermacher J, Chavan A, Bleck J, et al: Use of doppler ultrasonography to predict the outcome of therapy for renal-artery stenosis. N Engl J Med 344:410, 2001

147. Vasbinder GB, Nelemans PJ, Kessels AG, et al: Diagnostic tests for renal artery stenosis in patients suspected of having renovascular hypertension: a meta-analysis. Ann Intern Med 135:401, 2001

148. Carman TL, Olin JW, Czum J: Noninvasive imaging of the renal arteries. Urologic Clin North Am 28:815, 2001

149. Mulatero P, Rabbia F, Milan A, et al: Drug effects on aldosterone/plasma renin activity ratio in primary aldosteronism. Hypertension 40:897, 2002

19 Atrial Fibrillation

Anthony Aizer, M.D., and Valentin Fuster, M.D., PH.D.

Atrial fibrillation (AF) is a supraventricular tachyarrhythmia defined by rapid, irregular atrial activation. This disordered atrial activation results in loss of coordinated atrial contraction; irregular electrical input to the atrioventricular (AV) node typically leads to sporadic ventricular contractions. On an electrocardiogram, AF is characterized by the absence of visible discrete P waves, the presence of irregular fibrillatory waves, or both, and an irregularly irregular ventricular response [*see Figure 1*].

AF may occur by itself or with other arrhythmias, notably, atrial flutter. Atrial flutter is more organized than AF, involving regular atrial activation that often produces a characteristic sawtooth pattern on ECG. Cardiac rhythm may alternate between AF and atrial flutter, AF may trigger atrial flutter, or atrial flutter may degenerate into AF.

Classification

Numerous classification schemes have been used to characterize AF patients, and the lack of a consistent classification scheme across studies has led to difficulties in comparison of analyses and an inability to extrapolate results to all patients. Consequently, the American College of Cardiology (ACC), the American Heart Association (AHA), and the European Society of Cardiology (ESC), in collaboration with the North American Society of Pacing and Electrophysiology, have established guidelines for the classification of AF.[1] The ACC/AHA/ESC guidelines include the following categories:

- Recurrent—AF occurring in a patient who has experienced an episode of AF in the past.
- Lone—AF occurring in a patient younger than 60 years who has no clinical or echocardiographic evidence of cardiopulmonary disease.
- Valvular or nonvalvular—Valvular AF is AF that occurs in a patient who has evidence or history of rheumatic mitral valve disease or who has a prosthetic heart valve; all other forms of AF are classified as nonvalvular.
- Paroxysmal—AF that typically lasts 7 days or less and that converts spontaneously to sinus rhythm.
- Persistent—AF that typically lasts longer than 7 days or requires pharmacologic or direct current (DC) cardioversion.
- Permanent—AF that is refractory to cardioversion or that has persisted for longer than 1 year.

Paroxysmal, persistent, and permanent AF categories do not apply to episodes of AF lasting 30 seconds or less or to episodes precipitated by a reversible medical condition. Reversible conditions include acute myocardial infarction, cardiac surgery, pericarditis, myocarditis, hyperthyroidism, pulmonary embolism, and acute pulmonary disease.

Epidemiology

AF is the most common sustained arrhythmia, currently affecting more than 2.2 million persons in the United States.[2] The incidence is approximately 0.1% per year for the entire population; however, the incidence of AF increases steadily with age. As a result, one out of 11 Americans older than 80 years has AF.[3-5]

AF is associated with significant morbidity and mortality. The annual incidence of ischemic stroke in patients with AF is 5%, which is two to seven times higher than the incidence in the general population. In addition, the mortality in patients with AF is approximately twice that of patients without AF.[3,6,7] AF frequently leads to reduced functional capacity, dyspnea, palpitations, fatigue, tachycardia-induced cardiomyopathy, heart failure, and angina, significantly impairing quality of life.[8]

Finally, AF results in tremendous health care expenditures. There are more than 370,000 hospital admissions for AF annually.[9] After the first diagnosis of AF, hospitalization costs are typically 35% higher for patients with AF than for age-matched control subjects.[10]

Pathophysiology

Central to the pathophysiology of AF are two factors: the electrical trigger that initiates the arrhythmia and the abnormal myocardial substrate that allows AF to be maintained. A spectrum of triggers is thought to initiate AF, ranging from premature atrial contractions to atrial tachycardias; ultimately, AF may be self triggering.[11-13] Ectopic atrial foci, frequently located in the pulmonary veins, have been shown to trigger AF.

For AF to persist, the atrial tissue must be primed to allow the propagation of multiple wavelets of electrical depolarization throughout the atria.[14] If a wavelet encounters refractory tissue, the wavelet can extinguish, divide into additional wavelets, or change direction. If the underlying atrial substrate leads to the extinction of the wavelets, then AF will not persist. In contrast, if the underlying atrial substrate promotes the generation of additional wavelets or the maintenance of the existing wavelets, then AF will continue. Fibrosis, hypertrophy, and fatty infiltration of atrial tissue likely allow for abnormal atrial electrical conduction and the maintenance of AF wavelets.

Diagnosis

CLINICAL MANIFESTATIONS

AF can result in a wide variety of signs and symptoms. Some patients are asymptomatic, although they may have an irregularly irregular pulse. Other patients experience strokes, palpitations, fatigue, dyspnea, reduced exercise capacity, heart failure, angina, presyncope, or syncope. Additional complications include

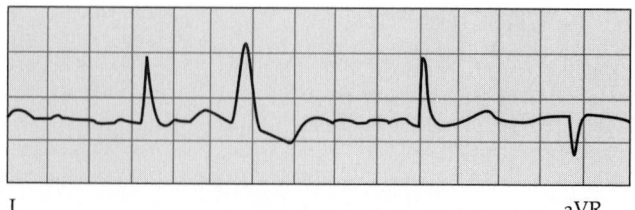

I   aVR

Figure 1   **An electrocardiographic tracing shows characteristic features of atrial fibrillation, with absent P waves, irregular fibrillatory waves, and an irregularly irregular ventricular response.**

Table 1 Initial Clinical Evaluation of Atrial Fibrillation[10]

Evaluation	Features to Assess
History and physical examination	Presence, frequency, onset, duration, termination, exacerbating and alleviating factors of AF; date of AF onset; AF classification; associated symptoms; reversible and irreversible contributing conditions; thromboembolic and hemorrhagic risk factors; response to pharmacologic or mechanical interventions
Laboratory studies	Thyroid function,* serum electrolytes, hemoglobin or hematocrit
Chest radiography	Lung parenchyma for intrinsic lung disease; abnormal pulmonary vasculature for pulmonary hypertension; cardiac size and shape for heart failure and pericardial disease
ECG	AF verification; P wave morphology for atrial flutter; preexcitation; atrial arrhythmias besides AF, as possible AF triggers; LVH, for hypertension and hypertrophic cardiomyopathy; bundle branch block and previous MI as markers for CAD, left ventricular dysfunction, and conduction system disease; RR, QRS, and QT intervals to guide antiarrhythmic drug therapy
Transthoracic echocardiography	Left and right atrial size and function; left ventricular size, function, and hypertrophy; valvular heart disease, including rheumatic heart disease; right ventricular systolic pressure for pulmonary hypertension; left atrial thrombus; spontaneous echocardiographic contrast (low sensitivity); pericardial disease; aortic plaque (low sensitivity)

*Reassessment of thyroid function should be considered if ventricular rate becomes difficult to control or atrial fibrillation recurs unexpectedly after conversion to sinus rhythm.
AF—atrial fibrillation CAD—coronary artery disease ECG—electrocardiogram
LVH—left ventricular hypertrophy MI—myocardial infarction

thromboembolism and tachycardia-induced cardiomyopathy.[15] The effect of AF on the patient's quality of life is often a critical component that guides decisions regarding AF management.

CLINICAL EVALUATION

The initial evaluation of a patient with AF focuses on the following tasks: (1) confirming the diagnosis of AF, (2) classifying the type of AF, (3) identifying factors (both reversible and irreversible) that contribute to or cause AF, (4) establishing the risk of thromboembolism and additional adverse outcomes, and (5) defining the most effective treatment strategy. In taking the history, the clinician should try to determine whether this is the first episode of AF. If more than one episode of AF has occurred, the AF is defined as recurrent. If no reversible condition is detected in recurrent AF, the clinician may be able to classify the AF as paroxysmal, persistent, or permanent [see Classification, *above*].

LABORATORY STUDIES

The standard blood tests that are recommended by the ACC/AHA/ESC are thyroid function tests and measurement of serum electrolytes and hemoglobin or hematocrit. Other recommended laboratory studies include chest radiography, ECG, and transthoracic echocardiography [see Table 1]. Additional tests that may be indicated in specific situations are event and Holter monitoring, exercise testing, transesophageal echocardiography (TEE), and electrophysiologic study (EPS).

Event and Holter Monitors

Event monitors are of particular use for documenting infrequent symptomatic episodes in patients in whom AF has not been confirmed previously. In addition to their diagnostic utility for documenting AF, Holter monitors may be used for therapeutic follow-up to evaluate rate control.[16]

Exercise Testing

Exercise testing can confirm the presence of ischemic heart disease and may unmask exercise-mediated AF. In addition, exercise testing can be used to explore the safety of using specific antiarrhythmic medications and to assess rate control.

Transesophageal Echocardiography

TEE is of greatest use in establishing the risk for embolic stroke, most notably in association with cardioversion to sinus rhythm. Risk factors for cardiogenic embolism that are best identified with TEE include the following: left atrial and left atrial appendage thrombus, left atrial and left atrial appendage spontaneous echo contrast (smoke), left atrial appendage flow velocity, and aortic plaque.[17]

Electrophysiologic Study

EPS can define specific forms of AF that are amenable to catheter-based intervention (i.e., radiofrequency ablation). In addition, EPS allows for assessment of the underlying conduction system to determine the etiology of wide-complex tachycardias, whether supraventricular or ventricular in origin.

Management

Treatment of AF includes either restoration and maintenance of sinus rhythm or control of ventricular rate if AF is persistent or if future paroxysmal events are likely to occur. In ad-

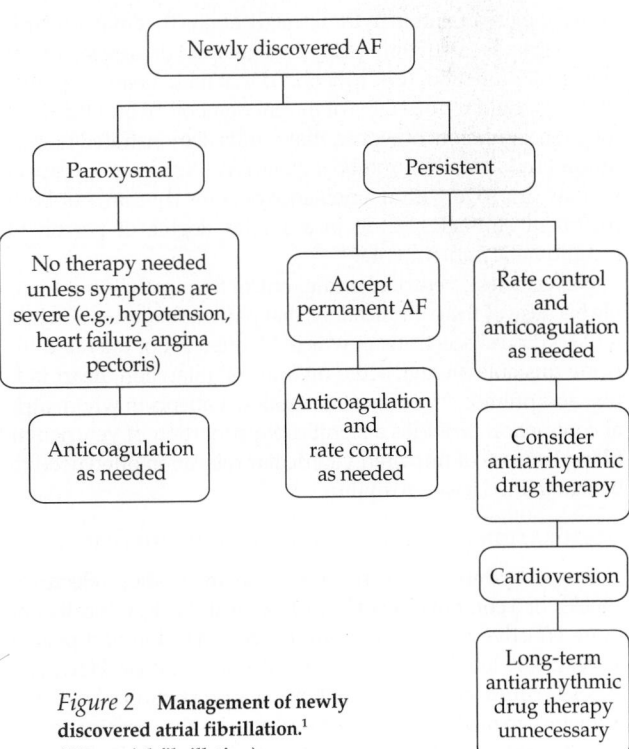

Figure 2 **Management of newly discovered atrial fibrillation.[1] (AF—atrial fibrillation)**

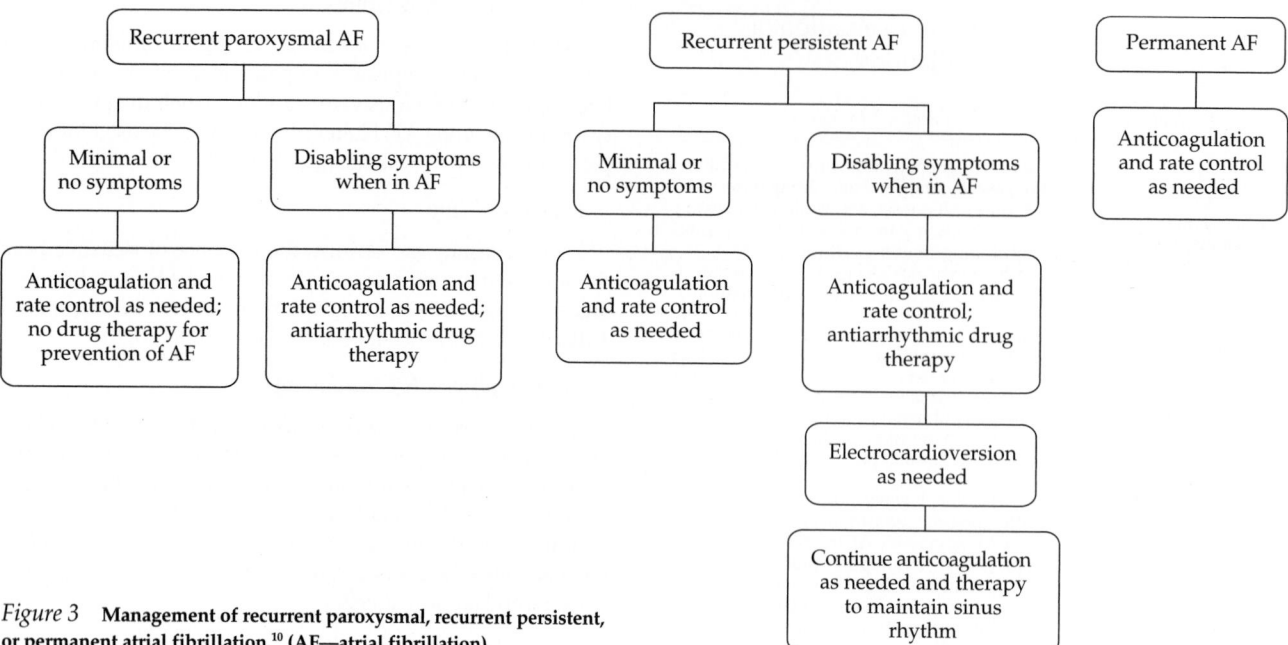

Figure 3   **Management of recurrent paroxysmal, recurrent persistent, or permanent atrial fibrillation.[10] (AF—atrial fibrillation)**

dition, antithrombotics are used to reduce embolic risk [*see Figures 2 through 4*].[10] Treatment decisions involve a synthesis of research results with the characteristics of the individual patient.

Several trials have compared restoration of sinus rhythm with control of ventricular rate in patients with AF. Outcomes evaluated have included overall mortality, stroke, symptoms, and quality of life. Contrary to the expectations of many experts, maintenance of sinus rhythm provided no survival advantage and possibly a higher mortality when compared with ventricular rate control.[18,19] Maintenance of sinus rhythm frequently requires the use of antiarrhythmic medications that may precipitate ventricular arrhythmias, bradycardia, and depression of left ventricular function. It was theorized that maintenance of sinus rhythm would reduce rates of thromboembolism and the need for anticoagulation; however, trial results demonstrated no significant reduction in thromboembolic risk. Peak exercise capacity may improve with maintenance of sinus rhythm, but both treatment strategies result in a similar degree of perceived symptomatic impairment.[8,20,21]

Nevertheless, ventricular rate control frequently is not feasible because of the complications that patients experience while in AF. Clinical scenarios in which AF often is not tolerated include unstable angina, acute myocardial infarction, heart failure, and pulmonary edema. In addition, patients in whom atrial contraction provides a significant proportion of ventricular filling because of impaired ventricular relaxation often need to be maintained in sinus rhythm.

RESTORATION AND MAINTENANCE OF SINUS RHYTHM

Sinus rhythm can be restored with medication, electrical shocks, or a combination of both. Electrical shocks typically are more effective than medication for cardioversion and pose a lower risk of life-threatening ventricular arrhythmias. However, shocks require conscious sedation. In a proportion of patients refractory to medication or electrical shocks, the combination of both therapies results in return of sinus rhythm.

Pharmacologic Cardioversion

Antiarrhythmic medications typically alter the conduction properties of both diseased and normal atrial tissue, suppressing AF triggers or inhibiting the propagation of AF electrical wavelets. Although pharmacologic cardioversion might seem simpler than electrical cardioversion, it has a lower success rate and it poses a risk of life-threatening arrhythmias; the latter risk often precludes use of this strategy. The efficacy of medications for cardioversion of AF typically declines as the duration of AF increases.[22]

A number of medications can be used for cardioversion or for maintenance of sinus rhythm [*see Tables 2 and 3*]. Some medications can be used for both purposes, but others should be used for cardioversion only or for maintenance of sinus rhythm only.

Medication selection for pharmacologic cardioversion must be based on individual patient characteristics. Amiodarone, dofetilide, and ibutilide (agents with potassium channel blocking effects) can be given safely to patients with heart failure or reduced left ventricular systolic function. In contrast, flecainide and propafenone may exacerbate heart failure and should be avoided in such patients. Dofetilide and ibutilide have higher success rates for conversion of atrial flutter than of AF, whereas flecainide and propafenone have higher success rates with conversion of AF than of atrial flutter. Flecainide, propafenone, disopyramide, procainamide, and quinidine also may increase ventricular rate response, especially if patients convert from AF to atrial flutter. Before receiving one of these medications, the patient should be pretreated with an AV nodal blocking agent (typically, diltiazem or verapamil, or possibly digoxin).

Disopyramide, procainamide, and quinidine have either limited efficacy for cardioversion of AF or are associated with significant adverse effects that preclude their use except in rare circumstances. Sotalol effectively maintains sinus rhythm and controls ventricular rate in patients who have undergone cardioconversion from AF, but it has not been shown to effectively convert AF to sinus rhythm. Similarly, beta blockers, verapamil, diltiazem, and digoxin are effective for control of ven-

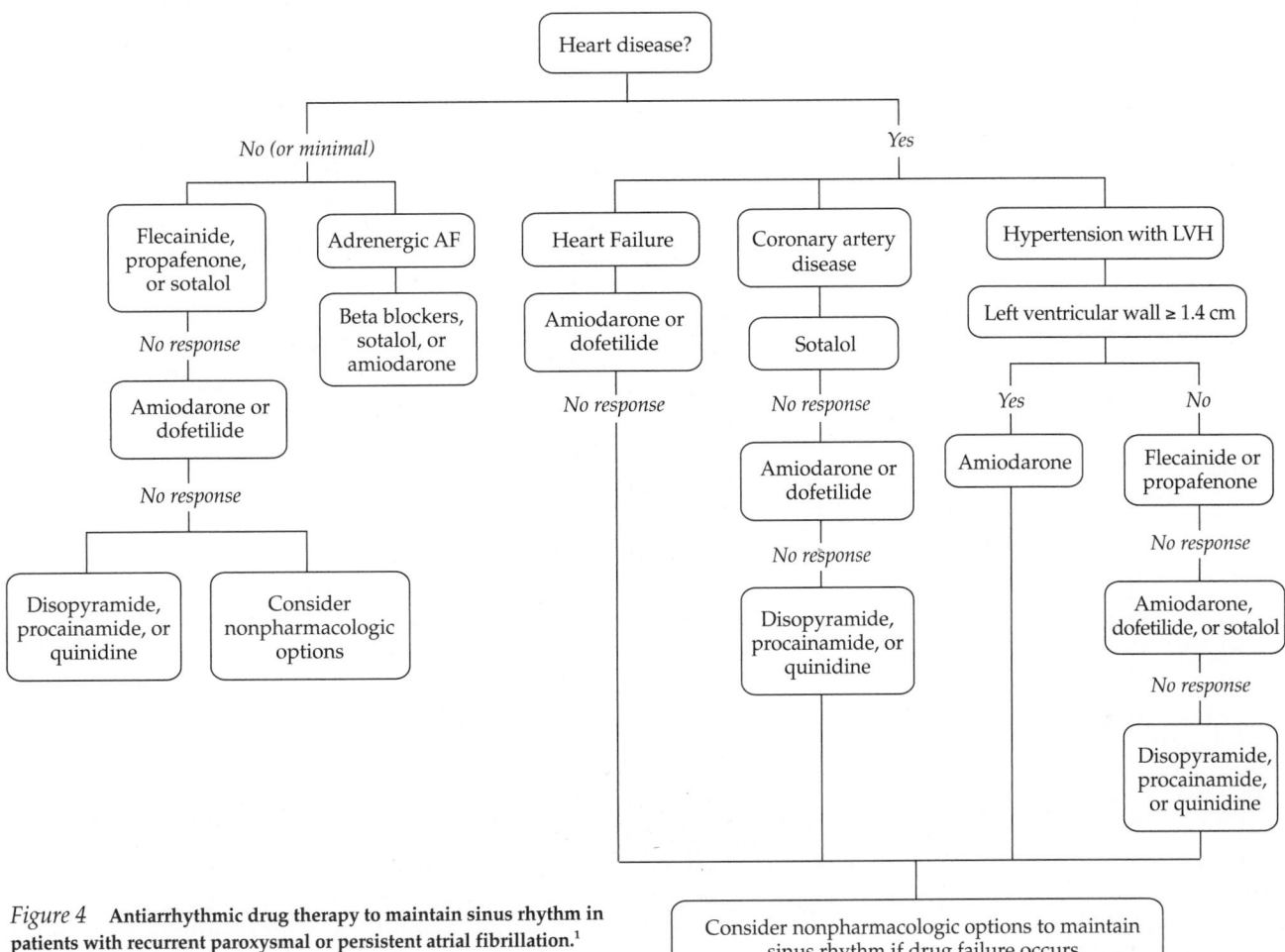

Figure 4 **Antiarrhythmic drug therapy to maintain sinus rhythm in patients with recurrent paroxysmal or persistent atrial fibrillation.[1] (AF—atrial fibrillation; LVH—left ventricular hypertrophy)**

tricular rate in patients with AF, but these medications have little role in AF cardioversion.

Electrical Cardioversion

DC cardioversion is the most effective mechanism for achieving sinus rhythm, with success rates of approximately 70% to 90%.[23,24] DC cardioversion has an even greater rate of success with atrial flutter, approximating 95%.[25] The efficacy of DC cardioversion can be optimized by enhancing delivery of energy to the atrial myocardium. This is achieved through a number of maneuvers:

- Electrode paddle positioning. Anteroposterior positioning is more effective than anterolateral positioning.[26] In addition, applying pressure to the paddles during conversion reduces transthoracic impedance, improving energy conduction.
- Timing of cardioversion. Application of the energy when the patient has fully exhaled reduces pulmonary resistance to the current.[27]
- Use of rectilinear biphasic energy. Traditional energy sources supply monophasic energy. Biphasic energy transfers more efficiently to atrial tissue, leading to higher cardioversion success rates and lower cumulative energy discharge.[28]

Although numerous protocols have been validated, a reasonable protocol that uses monophasic energy to convert AF is to start at 200 joules (J), followed by 300 J, then by 360 J or 400 J.[29]

For patients with atrial flutter, cardioversion is frequently achieved with 50 J of monophasic energy; therefore, the monophasic AF protocol can be modified for AF by starting with 50 J, followed by 100 J. If biphasic energy is utilized for AF, a protocol of 70 J or 100 J followed by 150 J and then by 200 J may be utilized.[28,30]

Although success rates are high with DC cardioversion, a number of risk factors for cardioversion failure have been identified. These include longer duration of AF (notably, greater than 1 year), older age, left atrial enlargement, cardiomegaly, rheumatic heart disease, and transthoracic impedance.[25,28] Pretreatment with amiodarone, ibutilide, sotalol, flecainide, propafenone, disopyramide, and quinidine have been shown to increase DC cardioversion success rates.[1] Transvenous cardioversion also may be successfully used for cardioversion for patients in whom transthoracic cardioversion fails.[31,32]

DC cardioversion of AF is extremely safe, typically resulting in no significant myocardial damage if cardioversion attempts are separated by at least 1 minute. Nevertheless, clinicians must give consideration to two types of adverse events[33,34]:

- Reprogramming or malfunction of permanent pacemakers or implantable cardioverter-defibrillators (ICDs). Electricity transmitted from endocardial wires to myocardium can lead to tissue scarring and an increased threshold for tissue capture.[35] In addition, cardioversion energy can erase or alter the programming of permanent pacemakers or ICDs. For that

Table 2 Drugs for Cardioversion of Atrial Fibrillation and Maintenance of Sinus Rhythm[10]

Medication	Route	Time to Conversion	Precautions	Drug Interactions	Side Effects	Comments
Amiodarone	Oral/ I.V.	Hours to weeks	—	Increases digoxin, procainamide, quinidine, and warfarin levels	Bradycardia, visual disturbances, nausea, constipation, phlebitis (I.V. form); hepatic, ocular, pulmonary, thyroid, neurologic toxicity	Safe for use in patients with left ventricular dysfunction; TdP/VT less common than with dofetilide, ibutilide, or sotalol
Dofetilide	Oral	Days to weeks	—	Levels increased by cimetidine and verapamil	—	Safe for use in patients with left ventricular dysfunction; associated with TdP
Ibutilide	I.V.	< 1 hr	Check serum potassium, magnesium levels; requires 4 hr of monitoring for TdP	—	—	Safe for use in patients with left ventricular dysfunction; associated with TdP; not used for maintenance of sinus rhythm
Sotalol	Oral	Incompletely studied; reduced efficacy or no proven efficacy for cardioversion of AF	May exacerbate CHF and/or COPD	—	Bradycardia	Use with caution in patients with reduced left ventricular function; associated with TdP
Flecainide	Oral	3 hr	Pretreat with AV nodal blocking agents* to avoid accelerated ventricular response; avoid in patients with heart failure, left ventricular dysfunction, or CAD	Levels increased by amiodarone	—	
Propafenone	Oral/I.V.	< 6 hr	Pretreat with AV nodal blocking agents* to avoid accelerated ventricular response; avoid in patients with heart failure, left ventricular dysfunction, or CAD; may exacerbate COPD	Increases digoxin and warfarin levels	Blurred vision, hypotension	Efficacy reduced in patients with structural heart disease
Quinidine	Oral/I.V.	2–6 hr	Pretreat with AV nodal blocking agents* to avoid accelerated ventricular response; avoid in patients with heart failure or left ventricular dysfunction	Increases digoxin levels; levels increased by verapamil	Hypotension, nausea, diarrhea, fever, hepatic dysfunction, thrombocytopenia, hemolytic anemia	Safety limits use in cardioversion; side effects limit use; associated with TdP
Disopyramide	Oral/I.V.	< 12 hr	Incompletely studied, reduced efficacy or no proven efficacy for cardioversion of AF; pretreat with AV nodal blocking agents* to avoid accelerated ventricular response; avoid in patients with heart failure or left ventricular dysfunction	—	Dry mucous membranes, constipation, urinary retention; significant reduction of left ventricular function	Side effects limit use; associated with TdP
Procainamide	I.V.	< 24 hr	Incompletely studied, reduced efficacy or no proven efficacy for cardioversion of AF; pretreat with AV nodal blocking agents* to avoid accelerated ventricular response; avoid in patients with heart failure or left ventricular dysfunction	—	Drug-induced lupus, vasculitides, blood dyscrasias, central nervous system disturbances	Reduced efficacy, side effects limit use; associated with TdP

*AV nodal blocking agents typically used are verapamil or diltiazem, and possibly digoxin.
AF—atrial fibrillation   CAD—coronary artery disease   CHF—chronic heart failure   COPD—chronic obstructive pulmonary disease   TdP—torsade de pointes
VT—ventricular tachycardia

Table 3 Dosages of Drugs for Pharmacologic Cardioversion of Atrial Fibrillation and Maintenance of Sinus Rhythm[10,80]

Drug	Dosage for Cardioversion	Daily Dosage for Maintenance of Sinus Rhythm

Amiodarone	Oral, inpatient
	    1.2–1.8 g/day in divided doses until 10 g total, then 200–400 mg/day maintenance; or 30 mg/kg as single dose
	Oral, outpatient
	    600–800 mg/day in divided doses until 10 g total
	Intravenous/oral
	    5–7 mg/kg over 30–60 min, then 1.2–1.8 g/day continuous I.V. or in divided oral doses until 10 g total
		100–400 mg

Dofetilide	Oral dosages for specified C_{Cr} values
	    500 µg b.i.d. for C_{Cr} > 60 ml/min
	    250 µg b.i.d. for C_{Cr} 40 to 60 ml/min
	    125 µg b.i.d. for C_{Cr} 20 to 40 ml/min
	    Contraindicated for C_{Cr} < 20 ml/min
		500–1,000 µg; dosage adjustment based on QTc

Ibutilide	I.V.: 1 mg over 10 min; repeat once, if necessary	Not available
Sotalol	Not effective for cardioversion	240–320 mg; dosage adjustment based on QTc; reduced dosing with renal insufficiency
Flecainide	Oral: 200–300 mg	200–300 mg; reduced dosing with renal insufficiency
Propafenone	Oral: 450–600 mg I.V.: 1.5–2.0 mg/kg over 10–20 min; reduced dosing with renal insufficiency	450–900 mg; reduced dosing with hepatic dysfunction
Quinidine	Oral: 0.75–1.5 g in divided doses over 6–12 hr I.V.: 1.5–2.0 mg/kg over 10–20 min	600–1,500 mg
Disopyramide	Oral: 200 mg q. 4 hr, up to 800 mg	400–750 mg; reduced dosing with renal insufficiency
Procainamide	I.V.: 100 mg q. 5 min, up to 1,000 mg	1,000–4,000 mg; reduced dosing with renal insufficiency or hepatic dysfunction

Note: Dosages given may differ from those recommended by the manufacturer; see Table 2 for guidance regarding medication selection and dosing adjustments.
C_{Cr}—creatinine clearance QTc—corrected QT interval

reason, all such devices should be interrogated before and after DC cardioversion. Distancing of paddles from implanted devices may limit these adverse events.

• Arrhythmias. Life-threatening arrhythmias are more common with pharmacologic conversion but can occur with DC cardioversion. Ventricular tachycardia and ventricular fibrillation can result from cardioversion in patients with hypokalemia or digoxin toxicity. Failure to synchronize DC energy with ventricular rhythm can lead to ventricular fibrillation if energy is applied during ventricular repolarization.

Finally, many patients with AF have underlying sinus node dysfunction that may require permanent pacing once cardioversion is completed.[36]

Pharmacologic Approaches to Maintaining Sinus Rhythm

Except for patients in whom the cause of AF is reversible, pharmacologic therapy likely will be required to maintain sinus rhythm after cardioversion. In approximately 50% of AF patients who undergo cardioversion to sinus rhythm, AF will return within 1 year if prophylactic drug therapy is not employed; AF will recur in approximately 75% of patients within 4 years.[24] Before prescribing medication to maintain sinus rhythm, the clinician must assess the patient for underlying cardiovascular disease [see Table 1]. The presence of heart failure, coronary artery disease (CAD), or hypertension with left ventricular hy-

pertrophy has a critical impact on the selection of antiarrhythmic medications [see Figure 4].

Class I antiarrhythmics frequently suppress left ventricular function. Randomized clinical trials have demonstrated that amiodarone and dofetilide maintain sinus rhythm without reducing survival in AF patients with heart failure.[37-39] As a result, these two drugs have become first-line therapy in this patient subgroup. In patients with ICDs, sotalol may be used safely.[40,41]

Agents with beta-blocking properties are preferred for patients with CAD. Sotalol has the advantage of blocking both beta-adrenergic receptors and potassium channels. In addition, sotalol has been shown to reduce reinfarction rates after a myocardial infarction, and its use has been associated with a trend toward reduced mortality.[42] However, in patients with concomitant heart failure or reduced ventricular function, amiodarone or dofetilide is preferable.

Hypertension and left ventricular hypertrophy may affect drug selection. If the left ventricular wall thickness is 14 mm or greater, amiodarone is recommended.

Although these recommendations can be applied to the majority of patients with AF, a number of distinct clinical scenarios require a tailored approach. In patients who do not have structural heart disease but who experience AF during exercise or under adrenergic stimulation, beta blockers are the treatment of choice, followed by sotalol or amiodarone. Vagally mediated AF that is not associated with structural heart disease often responds to disopyramide, a vagolytic medication. Second-line therapy includes flecainide and amiodarone.

Combination therapy may be used when a single medication fails to maintain sinus rhythm. With the combination of medications comes the increased risk of drug-induced side effects, notably, torsade de pointes and heart failure. Monitoring of symptoms and the width of the QTc and QRS intervals is critical.

Monitoring of antiarrhythmic therapy ECG monitoring is necessary in all patients receiving antiarrhythmic medications for maintenance of sinus rhythm. If flecainide or propafenone is used, QRS widening should not exceed 150% of pretreatment QRS width. QRS width should be assessed during exercise ECG testing, typically within 3 days after starting the medication. With all antiarrhythmics except amiodarone, QTc width should not exceed 520 msec. In addition, renal function and levels of serum potassium and serum magnesium should be monitored periodically, because abnormalities in these levels may predispose to arrhythmias.

Outpatient Initiation of Antiarrhythmic Drugs

In a subset of patients with AF, drugs for restoration and maintenance of sinus rhythm can be started safely in the outpatient setting. Advantages of this approach are elimination of the need for DC cardioversion, reduction of hospitalization time, and a decrease in early recurrences of AF after conversion to sinus rhythm. Although outpatient pharmacologic therapy to restore sinus rhythm is appealing, the concern for induction of life-threatening arrhythmias often precludes use of this approach.

Flecainide and propafenone may be initiated on an outpatient basis if the patient has no history of heart failure; if there is no left ventricular dysfunction; if the QRS width is normal; and if the QTc interval is not prolonged. Patients should have both a normal ECG (without any evidence of bradycardia, sinus node disease, or AV nodal disease) and a documented history of at least one episode of inpatient cardioversion with these medications during which no conduction abnormality was unmasked. Amiodarone and sotalol may be started in the ambulatory setting, provided there is no history of structural heart disease, left ventricular hypertrophy, reduced left ventricular function, bradycardia, sinus node or AV nodal conduction disease, hypokalemia, hypomagnesemia, or previous arrhythmias other than AF or atrial flutter. Flecainide, propafenone, amiodarone, or sotalol should not be started if the patient is also taking other medications that may prolong the QTc interval or predispose to electrolyte abnormalities. Dofetilide, disopyramide, procainamide, and quinidine typically should not be started in the ambulatory setting.[1]

Nonpharmacologic Approaches to Maintaining Sinus Rhythm

Several mechanical techniques offer the benefit of reducing the use of antiarrhythmics. The need for anticoagulation with these techniques remains uncertain, however.

Catheter-based ablation Radiofrequency energy emitted from intravascular catheters promotes the generation of endocardial scars to eliminate AF. These procedures focus primarily on elimination or isolation of ectopic foci, many of which are located in the pulmonary veins. Although these procedures have the potential to cure AF, many patients experience recurrence of AF. The risks of catheter-based ablation include thromboembolism, pulmonary vein stenosis, and cardiac perforation.[43]

Endovascular radiofrequency ablation is less suited to AF than to atrial flutter, which it can cure with minimal risks and a high rate of success. Ablation of atrial flutter typically involves creating a scar within the right atrium and therefore has a lower risk of complications than AF ablation of the pulmonary veins. Radiofrequency ablation for atrial flutter is curative in more than 90% of cases and should be considered primary therapy for these patients.[44]

Surgical ablation Surgical ablation of AF is similar in concept to catheter-based ablation. During open thoracotomy, linear lesions are created across atrial tissue to generate scars that will act as electromechanical obstacles, extinguishing the reentrant circuits needed for the maintenance of AF. There is a greater than 90% rate of success in eliminating AF with this procedure; however, approximately 25% of patients require a permanent pacemaker for sinus node dysfunction postoperatively.[45-47] This approach has an operative mortality of less than 1% but involves the morbidity of an invasive surgical procedure. The procedure is most often utilized when patients are undergoing cardiac surgery for other indications. The techniques utilized to generate the scars, as well as the location and number of scars created, continue to be modified to reduce surgical time while maintaining efficacy.

Atrial pacing In patients requiring ventricular pacing, the addition of atrial pacing reduces the risk of AF. However, the use of atrial pacing as the primary treatment to prevent AF has not been validated.[48-50]

Atrial defibrillators Implantable devices to detect and provide DC cardioversion for AF have been shown to successfully terminate AF in more than 95% of episodes.[51] Although promising, the use of atrial defibrillators is limited by the generation of pain associated with the release of the electrical shock, as well as the risks associated with device implantation (typically, bleeding and infection). As a result, atrial defibrillators have been used in patients who are unable to tolerate a strategy of ventricular rate control and whose condition is refractory to pharmacologic and ablative therapies.

CONTROL OF VENTRICULAR RATE

Ventricular rate control must be addressed both in the acute and the chronic setting. Medication selection in these scenarios is influenced by the rate of onset of the medication, its potential side effects, and its convenience of use.

Hemodynamically unstable patients with angina, myocardial infarction, heart failure, or symptomatic hypotension should be considered for acute conversion to sinus rhythm rather than rate control. In contrast, acute rate control can often be achieved rapidly in hemodynamically stable patients through the use of intravenous beta blockers, diltiazem, verapamil, or digoxin. Oral formulations of these medications are utilized for transition to long-term rate control [*see Table 4*]. More than one medication is often required to achieve ventricular rate control. Although digoxin is available orally and intravenously, its onset of action is at least 1 hour after infusion, so it is rarely sufficient for stand-alone therapy in the acute clinical setting.

Depending on the clinical scenario, specific agents may be more or less preferable for rate control. This is true of patients with reduced ventricular function, CAD, high sympathetic tone, pulmonary disease, and atrial flutter.

Table 4   Drugs for Ventricular Rate Control in Atrial Fibrillation[10]

Drug	I.V. Loading Dose	I.V. Onset	I.V. Maintenance Dose	Oral Loading Dose	Oral Onset	Oral Maintenance Dose	Drug Interactions and Precautions
Esmolol*	0.5 mg/kg over 1 min	5 min	5–20 µg/kg/min	Available in I.V. form only	—	—	—
Metoprolol*	2.5–5 mg over 2 min, up to 15 mg	5 min	Bolus every 4–6 hr	Not applicable	4–6 hr	50–200 mg daily in divided doses	—
Propranolol*	0.15 mg/kg over 1 min, repeat once	5 min	Bolus every 4 hr	Not applicable	1–1.5 hr	80–240 mg daily in divided doses	—
Diltiazem	0.25 mg/kg over 2 min	2–7 min	5–15 mg/hr	Not applicable	2–4 hr	120–360 mg daily in divided doses	Increases levels of digoxin, quinidine, simvastatin
Verapamil	75–150 µg/kg over 2 min	3–5 min	Bolus q. 3–6 hr	Not applicable	1–2 hr	120–360 mg daily in divided doses	Increases levels of digoxin, dofetilide, quinidine, simvastatin
Digoxin	0.25 mg q. 2 hr, up to 1.5 mg	2 hr	0.125–0.25 mg daily	0.25 mg q. 2 hr, up to 1.5 mg	2 hr	0.125–0.250 mg/day	Reduce dosing with renal insufficiency; levels increased by amiodarone, propafenone, quinidine, diltiazem, verapamil, spironolactone
Amiodarone	1.2–1.8 g/day until 10 g total	1–3 wk	720 mg/day up to 3 wk; limited data on continuous infusion beyond 3 wk	800 mg/day × 1 wk, 600 mg/day × 1 wk, 400 mg/day × 4–6 wk	1–3 wk	200 mg/day	Increases levels of digoxin, procainamide, quinidine, and warfarin

Note: Typical dosing regimens are provided; however, adjustments are necessary based on individual patient characteristics.
*Other beta-blocking medications may also be used.

Reduced Ventricular Function

Diltiazem and verapamil can significantly exacerbate left ventricular dysfunction and associated heart failure and so should be avoided in the acute setting. Beta blockers can also have this effect but are preferable for acute rate control. Intravenous esmolol has the advantage of rapid onset and clearance and so may be used to determine whether a patient with left ventricular dysfunction tolerates intravenous beta blockade. However, the large infusion of saline given with esmolol makes long-term intravenous use unattractive for patients with heart failure. If the patient tolerates intravenous esmolol, the clinician should consider changing to another intravenous beta blocker or to oral beta blockade. In addition, digoxin can be utilized in patients with left ventricular dysfunction without concern for exacerbating heart failure. Intravenous amiodarone may also be used in the subacute setting for rate control of patients with AF and reduced ventricular function.

Chronic rate control can be achieved through the oral administration of beta blockers. Bisoprolol, extended-release metoprolol, and carvedilol improve symptoms and survival in patients with systolic dysfunction and heart failure independent of atrial rhythm.[52-54] These medications should be first-line therapy for long-term rate control in these patients. If these medications are not tolerated, oral amiodarone should be considered. In addition, digoxin is effective and well tolerated in heart failure patients with AF.

Coronary Artery Disease

Beta blockers have been shown to reduce mortality in patients with CAD. Because of this additive benefit, beta blockers typically should be selected for CAD patients.

High Sympathetic Tone

The effects of digoxin are attenuated in patients with high sympathetic tone, so this agent rarely provides significant control of heart rate in acute, high sympathetic tone states.

Pulmonary Disease

Patients with asthma can experience significant exacerbation of their lung disease with the use of beta blockers. In these patients, diltiazem and verapamil should be used. Patients with chronic obstructive pulmonary disease without reactive airway disease may or may not tolerate beta blockers. Use of beta blockers in this population should be carefully monitored.

Atrial Flutter

It is often more difficult to achieve ventricular rate control in patients with atrial flutter than in those with AF. If rate control cannot be achieved easily in patients with atrial flutter, radiofrequency ablation should be reconsidered.

Monitoring Rate Control

Adequacy of rate control should be assessed both with the patient at rest and under stress. The history, physical examination, and ECG provide significant data for this assessment, but Holter monitoring and exercise stress testing also can be used. The ventricular rate should be maintained between 60 and 80 beats/min during rest and 90 to 115 beats/min during moderate exercise.[55,56] If rate control cannot be achieved with pharmacologic therapy, AV nodal ablation, combined with permanent pacemaker insertion, should be considered. In addition, permanent pacemaker insertion may be necessary for patients with AF who have labile responses to pharmacologic therapy to avoid episodes of symptomatic bradycardia.

Table 5 Data Collection for Assessment of Thromboembolic Risks and Need for Antithrombotic Therapy in Atrial Fibrillation

Characteristic	Comments
Age	
Sex	
History of hypertension	Patients with medically treated hypertension are considered hypertensive for risk-stratification guidelines
Diabetes mellitus	Irrespective of control with insulin or oral medications
Coronary artery disease	
Heart failure	Past or current
Hyperthyroidism	Treatment varies depending on whether currently euthyroid
Rheumatic heart disease	Defined as involving the mitral valve
Previous thromboembolism	Includes strokes, transient ischemic attacks, and other emboli
Prosthetic heart valves	
LVEF less than 35%	

LVEF–left ventricular ejection fraction

ANTITHROMBOTIC THERAPY

AF (including paroxysmal, permanent, and chronic forms) is associated with an increased risk of stroke and other embolic phenomena. The risk of stroke for an individual AF patient varies according to the presence or absence of a number of thromboembolic risk factors. These factors can be garnered from the baseline history, physical examination, laboratory evaluation, ECG, and transthoracic echocardiogram; assessment of these thromboembolic risk factors can serve to guide antithrombotic therapy [see Table 5].

Current ACC/AHA/ESC guidelines for anticoagulation recommend the use of aspirin or warfarin [see Table 6]. Clinical trials have shown that both aspirin and warfarin significantly reduce AF-related strokes in high-risk patients.[57-59] Warfarin reduces the risk of stroke by greater than 60%, whereas aspirin reduces stroke risk by 19%. However, the increased benefits of warfarin must be counterbalanced by the increased risk of hemorrhage.[60] Use of lower-intensity warfarin in combination with aspirin provides no additional stroke prevention over aspirin alone, and the combination of full-dose warfarin with aspirin further increases the risk of intracranial hemorrhage.[61,62] After warfarin therapy is started, the international normalized ratio (INR) of prothrombin time should be measured at least weekly until stable dosing is reached, and monthly thereafter [see Chapter 32].

Atrial Flutter

Although clinical trial data are limited, epidemiologic studies demonstrate that the risk of stroke with atrial flutter, although less than that with AF, remains elevated.[63] As a result, use of warfarin and aspirin in atrial flutter should be based on the current AF guidelines.

Elderly Patients

Patients who are 75 years of age or older are at increased risk for both stroke with AF and bleeding with AF anticoagulation.[64] As a result of these increased risks, anticoagulation must be tightly monitored in elderly patients, with a goal of maintaining the INR at 2.

Surgical Procedures

Anticoagulation may need to be discontinued in patients scheduled for elective surgical procedures. AF anticoagulation can be discontinued for up to 1 week for surgical procedures in patients without mechanical heart valves. In patients with mechanical valves, the practice has been to discontinue warfarin 1 week before surgery but to maintain anticoagulation with either unfractionated or low-molecular-weight heparin (LMWH). However, current case reports suggest that LMWH may not provide sufficient anticoagulation for patients with mechanical valves, irrespective of concomitant AF.[65] Until further data become available, intravenous unfractionated heparin should be utilized.[66]

Anticoagulation and Cardioversion

Cardioversion from AF or atrial flutter to sinus rhythm—whether it occurs spontaneously or is accomplished with drugs or electricity—is associated with a 1% to 5% risk of thromboembolism. Therefore, strategies for cardioversion of AF should include consideration of anticoagulation; the anticoagulation may start before cardioversion, extend after it, or both [see Figure 5].

If warfarin anticoagulation (to an INR of 2 to 3) is used for 3 to 4 weeks before and after cardioversion, the risk of stroke is reduced to 0.5% in the immediate follow-up period.[36,67,68] For that reason, anticoagulation before cardioversion has been strongly advocated.

TEE has been validated as an alternative mechanism to gauge the risk of thromboembolism at the time of cardioversion and immediately afterward. If TEE reveals no evidence of thrombus in the left atrium or left atrial appendage, cardioversion can be performed immediately, with a risk of thromboembolism comparable to that in patients pretreated with 3 to 4

Table 6 ACC/AHA/ESC Recommendations for Antithrombotic Therapy in Atrial Fibrillation Based on Underlying Risk Factors[1]

Patient Characteristics	Antithrombotic Therapy
Age < 60 yr, no heart disease (lone atrial fibrillation)	Aspirin, 325 mg daily, or no therapy
Age < 60 yr, heart disease but no risk factors	Aspirin, 325 mg daily
Age ≥ 60 yr but no risk factors	Aspirin, 325 mg daily
Age ≥ 60 yr with DM or CAD	Warfarin (INR, 2.0–3.0); consider addition of aspirin, 81–162 mg daily
Age ≥ 75 yr, especially in women	Warfarin (INR, 2.0)
Heart failure	Warfarin (INR, 2.0)
LVEF ≤ 0.35	Warfarin (INR, 2.0–3.0)
Thyrotoxicosis	Warfarin (INR, 2.0–3.0)
Hypertension	Warfarin (INR, 2.0–3.0)
Rheumatic heart disease (mitral stenosis)	Warfarin (INR, 2.5–3.5 or possibly higher)
Prosthetic heart valves	Warfarin (INR, 2.5–3.5 or possibly higher)
Prior thromboembolism	Warfarin (INR, 2.5–3.5 or possibly higher)
Persistent atrial thrombus on TEE	Warfarin (INR, 2.5–3.5 or possibly higher)

ACC/AHA/ESC—American College of Cardiology/American Heart Association/European Society of Cardiology   CAD–coronary artery disease   DM—diabetes mellitus   INR—international normalized ratio   LVEF–left ventricular ejection fraction   TEE–transesophageal echocardiography

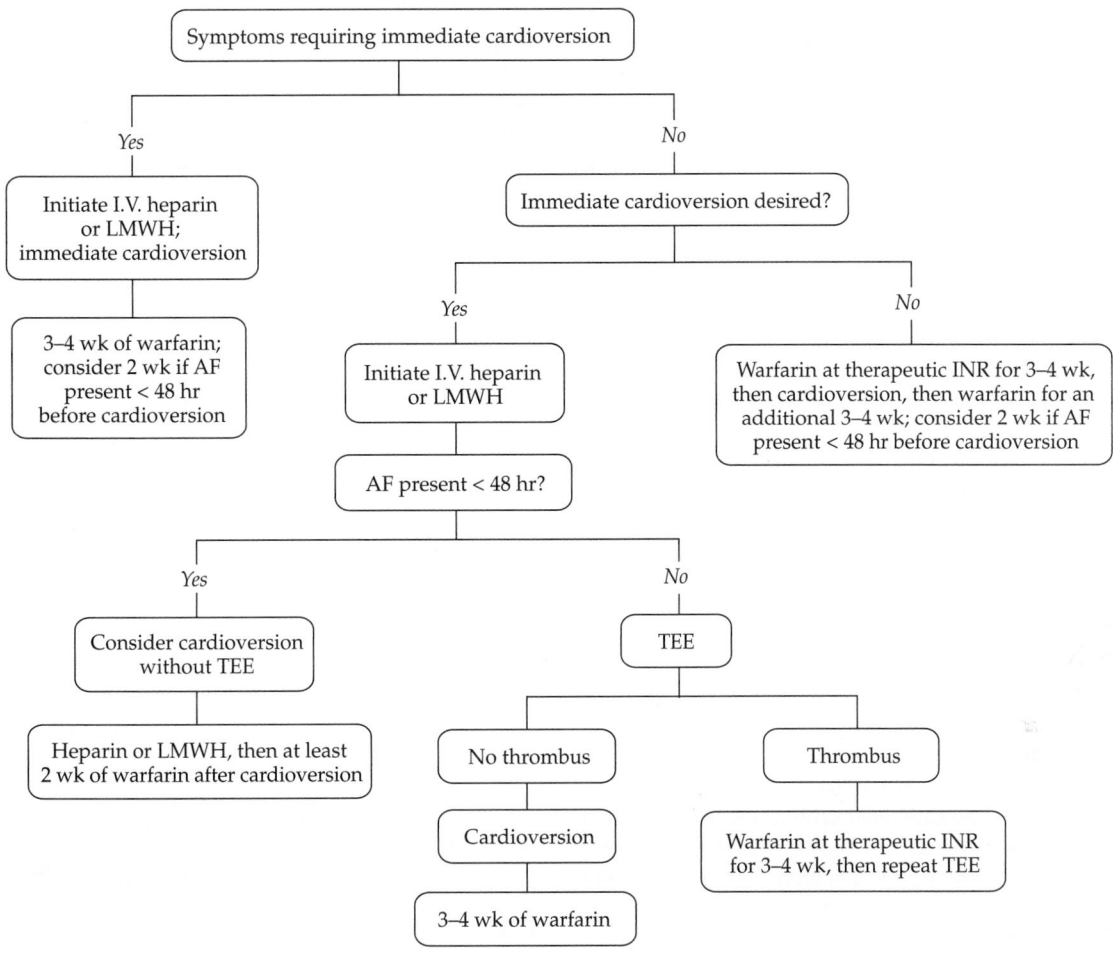

Figure 5 **Cardioversion and anticoagulation strategy for atrial fibrillation. Symptoms that frequently require cardioversion include hypotension, altered mental status, heart failure, pulmonary edema, angina, and myocardial infarction. Adjustment of warfarin intensity and therapy duration is based on individual patient characteristics; the anticoagulation goal is typically an INR of 2–3. (AF—atrial fibrillation; INR—international normalized ratio; LMWH—low-molecular-weight heparin; TEE— transesophageal echocardiography)**

weeks of warfarin therapy.[69] This approach allows for immediate cardioversion; however, because cardioversion frequently results in so-called stunning of left atrial and left atrial appendage tissue (a condition that may predispose to thrombus formation), warfarin anticoagulation is required for 3 to 4 weeks after cardioversion, even when TEE performed before cardioversion showed no thrombus. If TEE does identify thrombus, cardioversion should be postponed for 3 to 4 weeks of anticoagulation therapy with warfarin, after which TEE should be repeated.

Cardioversion without 3 to 4 weeks of warfarin pretreatment and without TEE assessment can be considered if the cardioversion can be done within 48 hours of the onset of AF or if the patient is started on heparin within 48 hours of AF initiation. Limited data suggest that LMWH may be used instead of intravenous unfractionated heparin, allowing both simplified dosing and transition to warfarin therapy on an outpatient basis.[70,71] This strategy should be most strongly considered in AF patients with significant symptoms of cardiac compromise, including hemodynamic instability, angina, myocardial infarction, heart failure, and shock. The need for anticoagulation after cardioversion in this scenario is unclear, but considering that more than 95% of postcardioversion thromboemboli occur

within 10 days after cardioversion, at least 2 weeks of warfarin therapy should be strongly considered if the patient has no contraindications.[72]

Even if heparin was not started until more than 48 hours after the onset of AF, immediate cardioversion also may be necessary if the patient has symptoms of cardiac compromise. Unlike patients who present less than 48 hours after onset of AF, patients with AF of longer duration should receive 3 to 4 weeks of warfarin therapy after cardioversion.

Prolonged anticoagulation after cardioversion should be considered in patients at high risk for both AF recurrence and thromboembolic complications. Atrial flutter is associated with a risk of thromboembolism in the setting of elective cardioversion and should be treated in the same manner as AF.[67]

TREATMENT IN SPECIFIC CLINICAL SCENARIOS

Cardiac Surgery

AF occurs after 25% of all coronary artery bypass surgeries and after more than 60% of combined coronary artery bypass and mitral valve surgeries.[73] Additional risk factors in these cases included advanced age, male sex, preoperative atrial arrhythmias, left atrial enlargement, chronic lung disease, and previous cardiac surgery.[74] AF after cardiac surgery leads to a significant increase in length of hospital stay and cost.[75] A number of prophylactic therapies to prevent postoperative AF have been examined and validated, including use of beta blockers, sotalol, amiodarone, and postoperative temporary atrial pacing.[76] The incremental cost of prophylactic therapy must be balanced against the potential savings achieved by reducing length of stay if AF is prevented. Unless contraindicated, beta blockers should be given to all patients scheduled for cardiac surgery. Sotalol, amiodarone, and biatrial pacing should be considered if patients are at high risk for postoperative AF because of additional risk factors.

Anticoagulation should be given if AF occurs after cardiac surgery and lasts longer than 48 hours. Although sinus rhythm returns spontaneously within 6 weeks in 95% of patients with postoperative AF, pharmacologic or DC cardioversion is often performed, particularly in patients who are symptomatic or hemodynamically unstable.[77] Medications to maintain sinus rhythm or to achieve ventricular rate control can be selected on the basis of patient characteristics.

Acute Myocardial Infarction

In patients with acute myocardial infarction, AF is an independent predictor of mortality and stroke. Immediate DC cardioversion should be performed in patients with severe hemodynamic compromise or persistent ischemia. If rate control is possible, digoxin can be combined with a beta blocker if left ventricular function is preserved. Because of the thromboembolic risk, heparin should be given acutely and followed with warfarin if AF persists or significant left ventricular dysfunction develops.

Wolff-Parkinson-White Syndrome

Wolff-Parkinson-White syndrome (WPW) in association with AF can be a life-threatening condition. The bypass tract of WPW may allow rapid conduction of atrial activity to the ventricles, precipitating hemodynamic compromise or ventricular fibrillation. In the acute setting, DC cardioversion should be pursued if hemodynamic compromise is present. If the patient is hemodynamically stable, the clinician may consider pharmacologic cardioversion to sinus rhythm with intravenous procainamide or ibutilide.[78] Agents that slow AV conduction are contraindicated, including digoxin, diltiazem, and verapamil. Beta blockers should be used rarely and with extreme caution. Once stabilization is achieved, catheter ablation of the WPW bypass tract should be pursued in all symptomatic WPW patients with AF.

Hyperthyroidism

Hyperthyroidism may cause AF and is associated with an increased risk of stroke. Hence, these patients require anticoagulation. Rate control should be attempted with beta blockers, supplemented with diltiazem, verapamil, or digoxin as needed. Warfarin should be given while the patient is thyrotoxic. Once the euthyroid state has returned, use of aspirin or warfarin should be based on underlying risk factors.

Hypertrophic Cardiomyopathy

AF in patients with hypertrophic cardiomyopathy is associated with a high risk of death and stroke.[79] Warfarin therapy is recommended (INR, 2 to 3).

Pulmonary Disease

In patients with pulmonary disease, hypoxia and other metabolic disturbances frequently initiate AF. Initial therapy focuses on treating the underlying lung disease. Beta blockers, propafenone, sotalol, and adenosine are contraindicated in patients with reactive airway disease. Diltiazem or verapamil, with or without digoxin, should be utilized for rate control in these patients.

The authors have no commercial relationships with manufacturers of products or providers of services discussed in this chapter.

References

1. Fuster V, Ryden LE, Asinger RW, et al: ACC/AHA/ESC guidelines for the management of patients with atrial fibrillation: executive summary. A report of the American College of Cardiology/American Heart Association Task Force on Practice Guidelines and the European Society of Cardiology Committee for Practice Guidelines and Policy Conferences (Committee to Develop Guidelines for the Management of Patients With Atrial Fibrillation): developed in collaboration with the North American Society of Pacing and Electrophysiology. J Am Coll Cardiol 38:1231, 2001

2. Atrial fibrillation as a contributing cause of death and Medicare hositalization—United States, 1999. MMWR Morb Mortal Wkly Rep 52:128, 2003

3. Krahn AD, Manfreda J, Tate RB, et al: The natural history of atrial fibrillation: incidence, risk factors, and prognosis in the Manitoba Follow-up Study. Am J Med 98:476, 1995

4. Psaty BM, Manolio TA, Kuller LH, et al: Incidence of and risk factors for atrial fibrillation in older adults. Circulation 96:2455, 1997

5. Wolf PA, Abbott RD, Kannel WB: Atrial fibrillation as an independent risk factor for stroke: the Framingham Study. Stroke 22:983, 1991

6. Kannel WB, Abbott RD, Savage DD, et al: Coronary heart disease and atrial fibrillation: the Framingham Study. Am Heart J 106:389, 1983

7. Flegel KM, Shipley MJ, Rose G: Risk of stroke in non-rheumatic atrial fibrillation. Lancet 1:526, 1987

8. Gosselink AT, Crijns HJ, van den Berg MP, et al: Functional capacity before and after cardioversion of atrial fibrillation: a controlled study. Br Heart J 72:161, 1994

9. Wattigney WA, Mensah GA, Croft JB: Increasing trends in hospitalization for atrial fibrillation in the United States, 1985 through 1999: implications for primary prevention. Circulation 108:711, 2003

10. Wolf PA, Mitchell JB, Baker CS, et al: Impact of atrial fibrillation on mortality, stroke, and medical costs. Arch Intern Med 158:229, 1998

11. Haissaguerre M, Jais P, Shah DC, et al: Spontaneous initiation of atrial fibrillation by ectopic beats originating in the pulmonary veins. N Engl J Med 339:659, 1998

12. Franz MR, Karasik PL, Li C, et al: Electrical remodeling of the human atrium: similar effects in patients with chronic atrial fibrillation and atrial flutter. J Am Coll Cardiol 30:1785, 1997

13. Bennett MA, Pentecost BL: The pattern of onset and spontaneous cessation of atrial fibrillation in man. Circulation 41:981, 1970

14. Moe G: On the multiple wavelet hypothesis of atrial fibrillation. Arch Int Pharmacodyn Ther 140:183, 1962

15. Grogan M, Smith HC, Gersh BJ, et al: Left ventricular dysfunction due to atrial fibrillation in patients initially believed to have idiopathic dilated cardiomyopathy. Am J Cardiol 69:1570, 1992

16. Gillis AM, Klein GJ, MacDonald RG: Investigation of the patient with atrial fibrillation. Can J Cardiol 12(suppl A):12A, 1996

17. Zabalgoitia M, Halperin JL, Pearce LA, et al: Transesophageal echocardiographic correlates of clinical risk of thromboembolism in nonvalvular atrial fibrillation. Stroke Prevention in Atrial Fibrillation III Investigators. J Am Coll Cardiol 31:1622, 1998

18. Wyse DG, Waldo AL, DiMarco JP, et al: A comparison of rate control and rhythm control in patients with atrial fibrillation. N Engl J Med 347:1825, 2002

19. Van Gelder IC, Hagens VE, Bosker HA, et al: A comparison of rate control and rhythm control in patients with recurrent persistent atrial fibrillation. N Engl J Med 347:1834, 2002

20. Atwood JE, Myers J, Sullivan M, et al: The effect of cardioversion on maximal exercise capacity in patients with chronic atrial fibrillation. Am Heart J 118:913, 1989

21. Gosselink AT, Bijlsma EB, Landsman ML, et al: Long-term effect of cardioversion on peak oxygen consumption in chronic atrial fibrillation: a 2-year follow-up. Eur Heart J 15:1368, 1994

22. Suttorp MJ, Kingma JH, Lie AHL, et al: Intravenous flecainide versus verapamil for acute conversion of paroxysmal atrial fibrillation or flutter to sinus rhythm. Am J Cardiol 63:693, 1989

23. Lundstrom T, Ryden L: Chronic atrial fibrillation: long-term results of direct current conversion. Acta Med Scand 223:53, 1988

24. Van Gelder IC, Crijns HJ, Tieleman RG, et al: Chronic atrial fibrillation: success of serial cardioversion therapy and safety of oral anticoagulation. Arch Intern Med 156:2585, 1996

25. Van Gelder IC, Crijns HJ, Van Gilst WH, et al: Prediction of uneventful cardioversion and maintenance of sinus rhythm from direct-current electrical cardioversion of chronic atrial fibrillation and flutter. Am J Cardiol 68:41, 1991

26. Botto GL, Politi A, Bonini W, et al: External cardioversion of atrial fibrillation: role of paddle position on technical efficacy and energy requirements. Heart 82:726, 1999

27. Ewy GA, Hellman DA, McClung S, et al: Influence of ventilation phase on transthoracic impedance and defibrillation effectiveness. Crit Care Med 8:164, 1980

28. Mittal S, Ayati S, Stein KM, et al: Transthoracic cardioversion of atrial fibrillation: comparison of rectilinear biphasic versus damped sine wave monophasic shocks. Circulation 101:1282, 2000

29. Joglar JA, Hamdan MH, Ramaswamy K, et al: Initial energy for elective external cardioversion of persistent atrial fibrillation. Am J Cardiol 86:348, 2000

30. Page RL, Kerber RE, Russell JK, et al: Biphasic versus monophasic shock waveform for conversion of atrial fibrillation: the results of an international randomized, double-blind multicenter trial. J Am Coll Cardiol 39:1956, 2002

31. Schmitt C, Alt E, Plewan A, et al: Low energy intracardiac cardioversion after failed conventional external cardioversion of atrial fibrillation. J Am Coll Cardiol 28:994, 1996

32. Levy S, Lauribe P, Dolla E, et al: A randomized comparison of external and internal cardioversion of chronic atrial fibrillation. Circulation 86:1415, 1992

33. Lund M, French JK, Johnson RN, et al: Serum troponins T and I after elective cardioversion. Eur Heart J 21:245, 2000

34. Jakobsson J, Odmansson I, Nordlander R: Enzyme release after elective cardioversion. Eur Heart J 11:749, 1990

35. Levine PA, Barold SS, Fletcher RD, et al: Adverse acute and chronic effects of electrical defibrillation and cardioversion on implanted unipolar cardiac pacing systems. J Am Coll Cardiol 1:1413, 1983

36. Mancini GB, Goldberger AL: Cardioversion of atrial fibrillation: consideration of embolization, anticoagulation, prophylactic pacemaker, and long-term success. Am Heart J 104:617, 1982

37. Roy D, Talajic M, Dorian P, et al: Amiodarone to prevent recurrence of atrial fibrillation. Canadian Trial of Atrial Fibrillation Investigators. N Engl J Med 342:913, 2000

38. Singh S, Zoble RG, Yellen L, et al: Efficacy and safety of oral dofetilide in converting to and maintaining sinus rhythm in patients with chronic atrial fibrillation or atrial flutter: the symptomatic atrial fibrillation investigative research on dofetilide (SAFIRE-D) study. Circulation 102:2385, 2000

39. Torp-Pedersen C, Moller M, Bloch-Thomsen PE, et al: Dofetilide in patients with congestive heart failure and left ventricular dysfunction. Danish Investigations of Arrhythmia and Mortality on Dofetilide Study Group. N Engl J Med 341:857, 1999

40. Pinto JV Jr, Ramani K, Neelagaru S, et al: Amiodarone therapy in chronic heart failure and myocardial infarction: a review of the mortality trials with special attention to STAT-CHF and the GESICA trials. Grupo de Estudio de la Sobrevida en la Insuficiencia Cardiaca en Argentina. Prog Cardiovasc Dis 40:85, 1997

41. Pacifico A, Hohnloser SH, Williams JH, et al: Prevention of implantable-defibrillator shocks by treatment with sotalol. D,L-Sotalol Implantable Cardioverter-Defibrillator Study Group. N Engl J Med 340:1855, 1999

42. Julian DG, Prescott RJ, Jackson FS, et al: Controlled trial of sotalol for one year after myocardial infarction. Lancet 1:1142, 1982

43. Wellens HJ: Pulmonary vein ablation in atrial fibrillation: hype or hope? Circulation 102:2562, 2000

44. Natale A, Newby KH, Pisano E, et al: Prospective randomized comparison of antiarrhythmic therapy versus first-line radiofrequency ablation in patients with atrial flutter. J Am Coll Cardiol 35:1898, 2000

45. Cox JL, Jaquiss RD, Schuessler RB, et al: Modification of the maze procedure for atrial flutter and atrial fibrillation. II. Surgical technique of the maze III procedure. J Thorac Cardiovasc Surg 110:485, 1995

46. Cox JL, Boineau JP, Schuessler RB, et al: Modification of the maze procedure for atrial flutter and atrial fibrillation. I. Rationale and surgical results. J Thorac Cardiovasc Surg 110:473, 1995

47. Cox JL, Schuessler RB, D'Agostino HJ Jr, et al: The surgical treatment of atrial fibrillation. III. Development of a definitive surgical procedure. J Thorac Cardiovasc Surg 101:569, 1991

48. Gillis AM, Wyse DG, Connolly SJ, et al: Atrial pacing periablation for prevention of paroxysmal atrial fibrillation. Circulation 99:2553, 1999

49. Andersen HR, Nielsen JC, Thomsen PE, et al: Long-term follow-up of patients from a randomised trial of atrial versus ventricular pacing for sick-sinus syndrome. Lancet 350:1210, 1997

50. Delfaut P, Saksena S, Prakash A, et al: Long-term outcome of patients with drug-refractory atrial flutter and fibrillation after single- and dual-site right atrial pacing for arrhythmia prevention. J Am Coll Cardiol 32:1900, 1998

51. Wellens HJ, Lau CP, Luderitz B, et al: Atrioverter: an implantable device for the treatment of atrial fibrillation. Circulation 98:1651, 1998

52. The Cardiac Insufficiency Bisoprolol Study II (CIBIS-II): a randomised trial. Lancet

353:9, 1999

53. Packer M, Bristow MR, Cohn JN, et al: The effect of carvedilol on morbidity and mortality in patients with chronic heart failure. U.S. Carvedilol Heart Failure Study Group. N Engl J Med 334:1349, 1996

54. Hjalmarson A, Goldstein S, Fagerberg B, et al: Effects of controlled-release metoprolol on total mortality, hospitalizations, and well-being in patients with heart failure: the Metoprolol CR/XL Randomized Intervention Trial in congestive heart failure (MERIT-HF). MERIT-HF Study Group. JAMA 283:1295, 2000

55. Rawles JM: What is meant by a "controlled" ventricular rate in atrial fibrillation? Br Heart J 63:157, 1990

56. Resnekov L, McDonald L: Electroversion of lone atrial fibrillation and flutter including haemodynamic studies at rest and on exercise. Br Heart J 33:339, 1971

57. Hart RG, Benavente O, McBride R, et al: Antithrombotic therapy to prevent stroke in patients with atrial fibrillation: a meta-analysis. Ann Intern Med 131:492, 1999

58. Hart RG, Halperin JL: Atrial fibrillation and thromboembolism: a decade of progress in stroke prevention. Ann Intern Med 131:688, 1999

59. Hylek EM, Skates SJ, Sheehan MA, et al: An analysis of the lowest effective intensity of prophylactic anticoagulation for patients with nonrheumatic atrial fibrillation. N Engl J Med 335:540, 1996

60. Hylek EM, Singer DE: Risk factors for intracranial hemorrhage in outpatients taking warfarin. Ann Intern Med 120:897, 1994

61. Adjusted-dose warfarin versus low-intensity, fixed-dose warfarin plus aspirin for high-risk patients with atrial fibrillation. Stroke Prevention in Atrial Fibrillation III randomised clinical trial. Lancet 348:633, 1996

62. Hart RG, Benavente O, Pearce LA: Increased risk of intracranial hemorrhage when aspirin is combined with warfarin: a meta-analysis and hypothesis. Cerebrovasc Dis 9:215, 1999

63. Biblo LA, Yuan Z, Quan KJ, et al: Risk of stroke in patients with atrial flutter. Am J Cardiol 87:346, 2001

64. Bleeding during antithrombotic therapy in patients with atrial fibrillation. The Stroke Prevention in Atrial Fibrillation Investigators. Arch Intern Med 156:409, 1996

65. Ginsberg JS, Chan WS, Bates SM, et al: Anticoagulation of pregnant women with mechanical heart valves. Arch Intern Med 163:694, 2003

66. Hirsh J, Fuster V, Ansell J, et al: American Heart Association/American College of Cardiology Foundation guide to warfarin therapy. J Am Coll Cardiol 41:1633, 2003

67. Gallagher MM, Hennessy BJ, Edvardsson N, et al: Embolic complications of direct current cardioversion of atrial arrhythmias: association with low intensity of anticoagulation at the time of cardioversion. J Am Coll Cardiol 40:926, 2002

68. Prystowsky EN, Benson DW Jr, Fuster V, et al: Management of patients with atrial fibrillation: a statement for healthcare professionals. Subcommittee on Electrocardiography and Electrophysiology, American Heart Association. Circulation 93:1262, 1996

69. Klein AL, Grimm RA, Murray RD, et al: Use of transesophageal echocardiography to guide cardioversion in patients with atrial fibrillation. N Engl J Med 344:1411, 2001

70. Wodlinger AM, Pieper JA: Low-molecular-weight heparin in transesophageal echocardiography–guided cardioversion of atrial fibrillation. Pharmacotherapy 23:57, 2003

71. Wu LA, Chandrasekran K, Friedman PA, et al: Safety of expedited anticoagulation in patients undergoing transesophageal echocardiographic-guided cardioversion. Am J Med 119:142, 2006

72. Berger M, Schweitzer P: Timing of thromboembolic events after electrical cardioversion of atrial fibrillation or flutter: a retrospective analysis. Am J Cardiol 82:1545, 1998

73. Creswell LL, Schuessler RB, Rosenbloom M, et al: Hazards of postoperative atrial arrhythmias. Ann Thorac Surg 56:539, 1993

74. Zimmer J, Pezzullo J, Choucair W, et al: Meta-analysis of antiarrhythmic therapy in the prevention of postoperative atrial fibrillation and the effect on hospital length of stay, costs, cerebrovascular accidents, and mortality in patients undergoing cardiac surgery. Am J Cardiol 91:1137, 2003

75. Crystal E, Connolly SJ, Sleik K, et al: Interventions on prevention of postoperative atrial fibrillation in patients undergoing heart surgery: a meta-analysis. Circulation 106:75, 2002

76. Kowey PR, Stebbins D, Igidbashian L, et al: Clinical outcome of patients who develop PAF after CABG surgery. Pacing Clin Electrophysiol 24:191, 2001

77. Glatter KA, Dorostkar PC, Yang Y, et al: Electrophysiological effects of ibutilide in patients with accessory pathways. Circulation 104:1933, 2001

78. Maron BJ, Olivotto I, Bellone P, et al: Clinical profile of stroke in 900 patients with hypertrophic cardiomyopathy. J Am Coll Cardiol 39:301, 2002

79. Halperin JL: SPORTIF III: a long-term randomized trial comparing ximelagatran with warfarin for prevention of stroke and systemic embolism in patients with nonvalvular atrial fibrillation. American College of Cardiology Annual Scientific Session, Chicago, 2003

80. Falk RH: Atrial fibrillation. N Engl J Med 344:1067, 2001

20 Supraventricular Tachycardia

Melvin M. Scheinman, M.D., F.A.C.P.

Over the past decade, enormous strides have been made in the treatment of patients with supraventricular tachycardia (SVT). Although acute therapy for SVT continues to require drugs or cardioversion, advances in the understanding of the mechanisms of SVT have led to the development of catheter ablation procedures for most forms of SVT.[1] These procedures often cure the condition, freeing the patient from the need for lifelong drug therapy. This chapter focuses on the most common forms of SVT—excluding atrial fibrillation, which is discussed in detail elsewhere [*see Chapter 19*].

Classification

SVT is often paroxysmal (PSVT). Clinically, PSVT is marked by palpitations, occurring in episodes that start and end abruptly. During these episodes, the 12-lead ECG shows a heart rate greater than 100 beats/min and, typically, narrow QRS complexes. For almost all patients with PSVT, the underlying mechanism of the tachycardia is atrioventricular node reentry (AVNRT), reentry involving an accessory pathway (AVRT), or atrial tachycardia. AVNRT and AVRT are the most common and the second most common causes of PSVT, respectively. Atrial flutter

also presents as a rapid regular tachycardia, but this arrhythmia usually does not begin and end abruptly.

The clinician has a variety of tools to distinguish the various mechanisms of SVT [*see Figure 1*]. The use of carotid massage[2] or intravenous adenosine[3] [*see Figure 2*] may be diagnostic, therapeutic, or both. If vagal maneuvers terminate the arrhythmia acutely or produce no effect, the patient probably has AVNRT or AVRT. In patients with atrial tachycardia, these maneuvers will frequently result in transient AV block. Perpetuation of the arrhythmia in the face of AV block strongly suggests atrial tachycardia or atrial flutter.[3] Intravenous adenosine will almost always terminate tachycardia from AVNRT or AVRT, but focal atrial tachycardia may also terminate abruptly after adenosine. Hence, the use of adenosine does not reliably distinguish those disorders from atrial tachycardia unless it produces AV block.[3]

Paying careful attention to the relationship between the P wave and the QRS complex during tachycardia is also very helpful in distinguishing tachycardia mechanisms[4] [*see Figure 1*]. If the retrograde P wave falls within or just after the QRS, the most likely diagnosis is AVNRT [*see Figure 3*]. If the tachycardia shows a retrograde P wave in the ST segment [*see Figure 4*], AVRT is

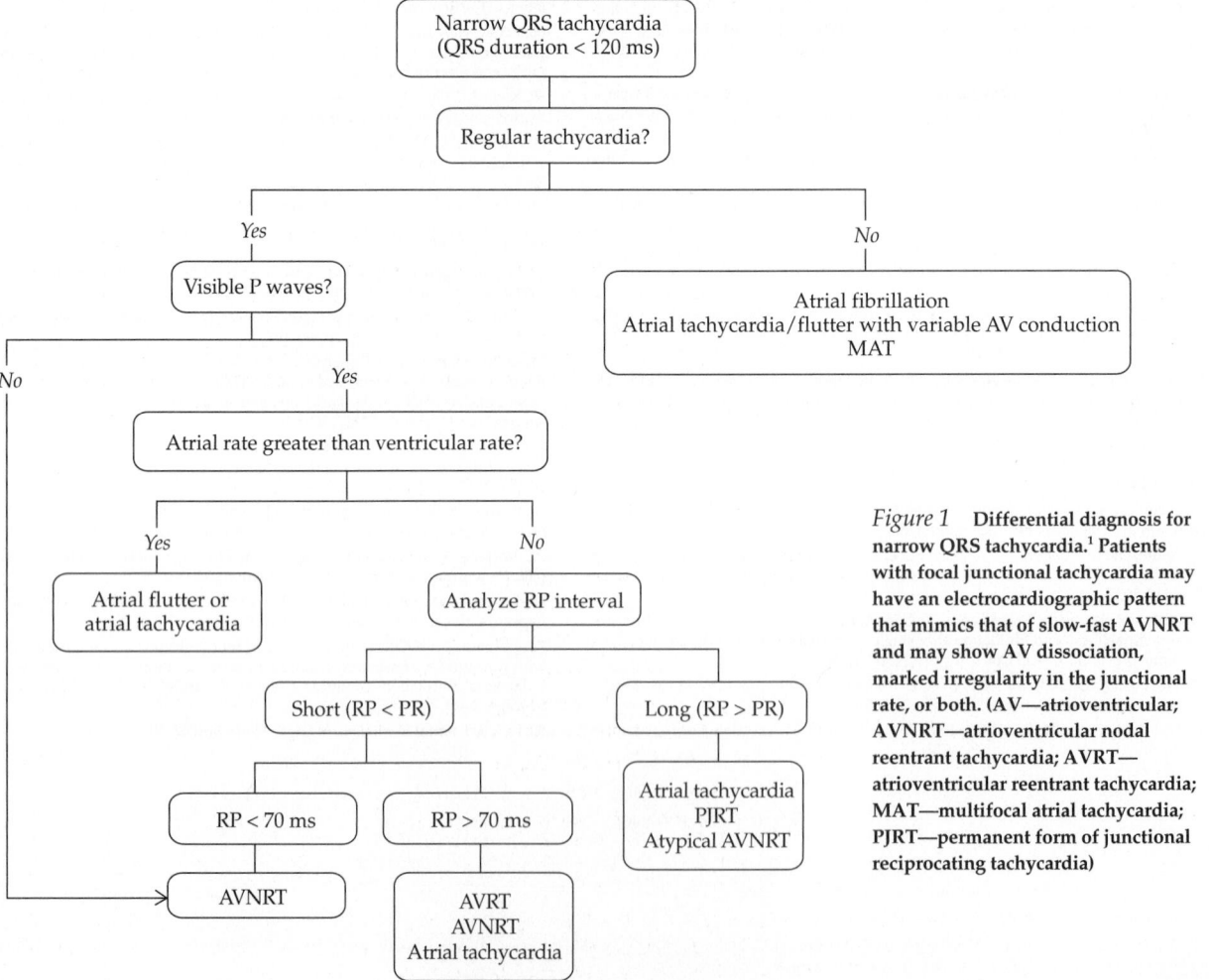

Figure 1 **Differential diagnosis for narrow QRS tachycardia.[1] Patients with focal junctional tachycardia may have an electrocardiographic pattern that mimics that of slow-fast AVNRT and may show AV dissociation, marked irregularity in the junctional rate, or both. (AV—atrioventricular; AVNRT—atrioventricular nodal reentrant tachycardia; AVRT—atrioventricular reentrant tachycardia; MAT—multifocal atrial tachycardia; PJRT—permanent form of junctional reciprocating tachycardia)**

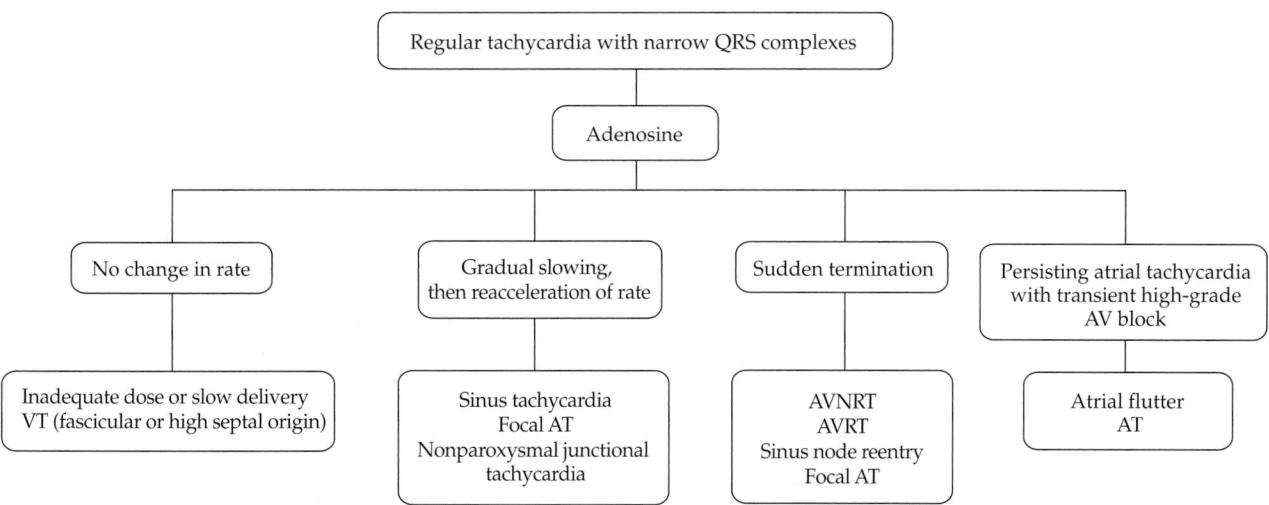

Figure 2 The response to intravenous adenosine can be useful in determining the cause of tachycardia.[1] (AT—atrial tachycardia; AV—atrioventricular; AVNRT—atrioventricular nodal reentrant tachycardia; AVRT—atrioventricular reentrant tachycardia; VT—ventricular tachycardia)

most likely. Finally, atrial tachycardia is characterized by the presence of P waves immediately in front of the QRS (long RP tachycardia) [*see Figure 5*].

Although the QRS complex is usually narrow in SVT, it may be broad (> 120 ms) in patients who have either bundle branch block or aberrant conduction. A number of ECG findings have been found very helpful in distinguishing SVT with a broad QRS complex from ventricular tachycardia (VT).[5,6] For example, AV dissociation (i.e., independent atrial activity during tachycardia), fusion beats, or capture beats prove the presence of VT. Unfortunately, AV dissociation is not apparent in 80% to 85% of patients with rapid VT, because the P wave is obscured by the QRS complex and T waves.[6] In this setting, morphologic criteria may be very helpful in distinguishing SVT from VT.

Use of morphologic criteria begins with careful attention to the precordial leads [*see Figure 6*]. Any of the following features in the precordial tracings will favor the diagnosis of VT: (1) Concordance of all the precordial leads (i.e., all are positive or all are negative); (2) absence of an initial positive deflection (r wave) followed by a negative deflection (s wave; recall that in ECG nomenclature, upper-case letters denote dominance; small waves are designated by lowercase letters); (3) an r/s pattern is present but the time from the initial r to the nadir of the s wave is greater than 60 ms; (4) presence of a right bundle branch pattern in lead V1, with an r greater than s or a qr pattern, where q indicates the initial negative deflection; (5) presence of a left bundle branch pattern in V1, with a broad r wave (> 30 ms) or an interval of greater than 60 ms from the onset of the r wave to the nadir of the s wave; (6) extreme left axis deviation; or (7) very broad QRS complexes (> 160 ms).

Atrioventricular Nodal Reentry Tachycardia

PATHOGENESIS

Normally, sinus impulses are discharged into the surrounding atria and directed to the region of the node that resides in the atrial septum. The AV nodal impulses then propagate through the ventricles over the His-Purkinje system. The normal AV node has a single transmission pathway. In two to three persons

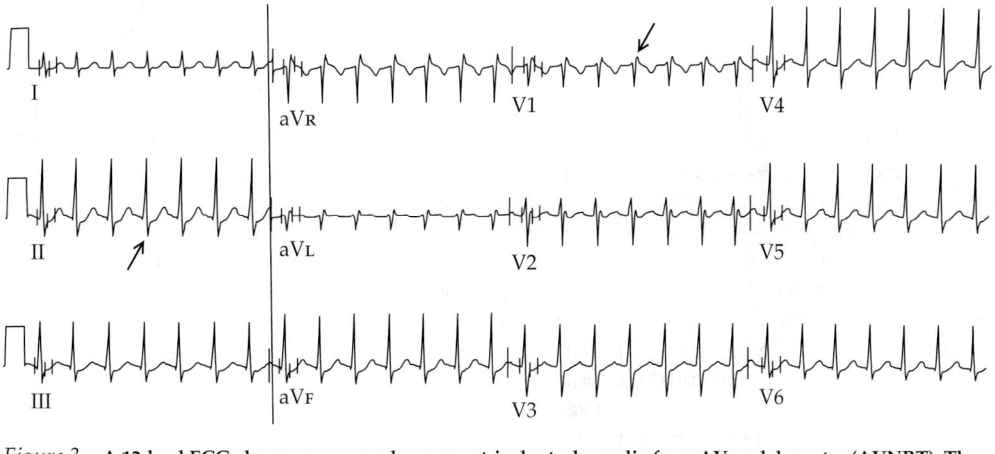

Figure 3 A 12-lead ECG shows paroxysmal supraventricular tachycardia from AV nodal reentry (AVNRT). The arrows point to a pseudo r[1] in lead V1 and S waves in the inferior leads (II, III, and aVF), which disappeared with conversion to sinus rhythm.

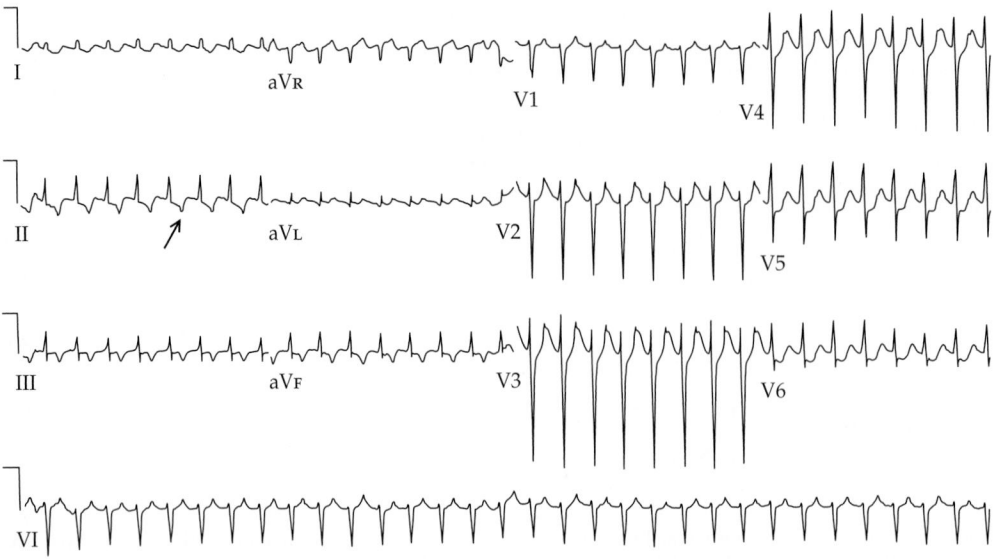

Figure 4   A 12-lead ECG showing narrow complex tachycardia with P waves (arrow) inscribed well after the QRS, taken from a patient who had paroxysmal supraventricular tachycardia supported by an accessory pathway.

per 1,000 population, however, the AV node has both a normal (fast) pathway and a second, slow pathway.[7,8] In such persons, the sinus impulse is ordinarily transmitted over the fast pathway to the ventricle, and slow pathway conduction is preempted. However, if an atrial premature complex (APC) occurs at a critical point in the conduction cycle, the impulse can block in the fast pathway, thus allowing for anterograde (forward) conduction over the slow pathway and retrograde (backward) conduction over the fast pathway [*see Figure 7*]. The latter situation may produce a single echo beat (a beat that returns to the chamber of origin) or stabilize into a circus-movement tachycardia.

DIAGNOSIS

The diagnosis of AVNRT can usually be made by careful analysis of the 12-lead ECG.[4] Because retrograde conduction over the AV node is occurring more or less simultaneously with anterograde conduction to the ventricles, the P wave is either buried within the QRS complex or inscribed just after the QRS. The P wave inscribed by retroconduction over the AV node will be negative in the inferior leads and positive in lead V1; therefore, PSVT from AVNRT may manifest as small negative deflections in the inferior leads and a small positive deflection in V1—the so-called pseudo r' pattern[5] [*see Figure 3*].

MANAGEMENT

Acute Therapy

AVNRT may respond to carotid sinus massage[2] but is highly responsive to intravenous adenosine,[3] beta blockers,[9] or calcium channel blockers[10] [*see Table 1*].

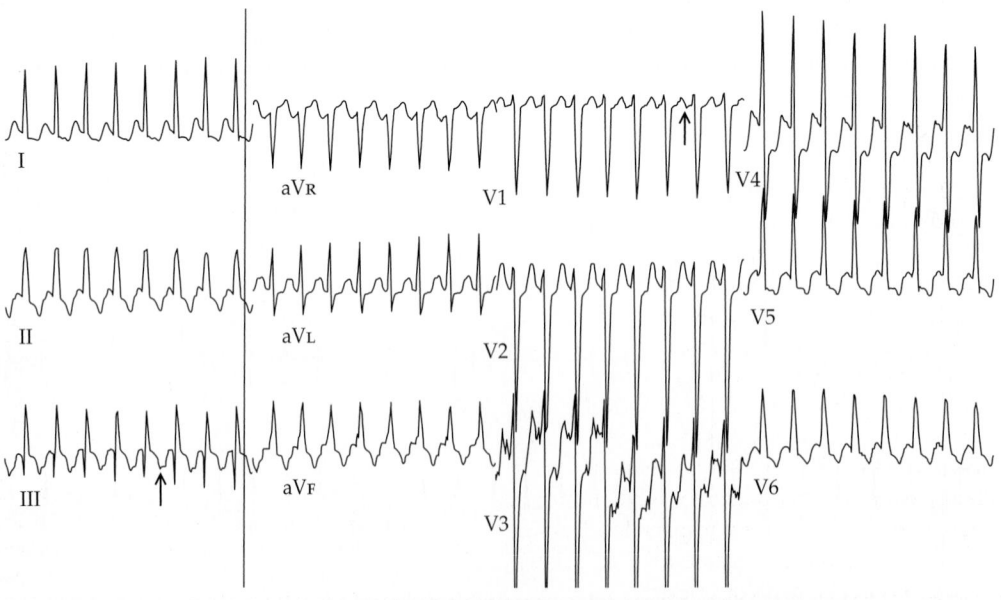

Figure 5   A 12-lead ECG shows tachycardia with P waves (arrows) just preceding the QRS complex. The patient in this case had a focal atrial tachycardia emanating from the lateral tricuspid annulus.

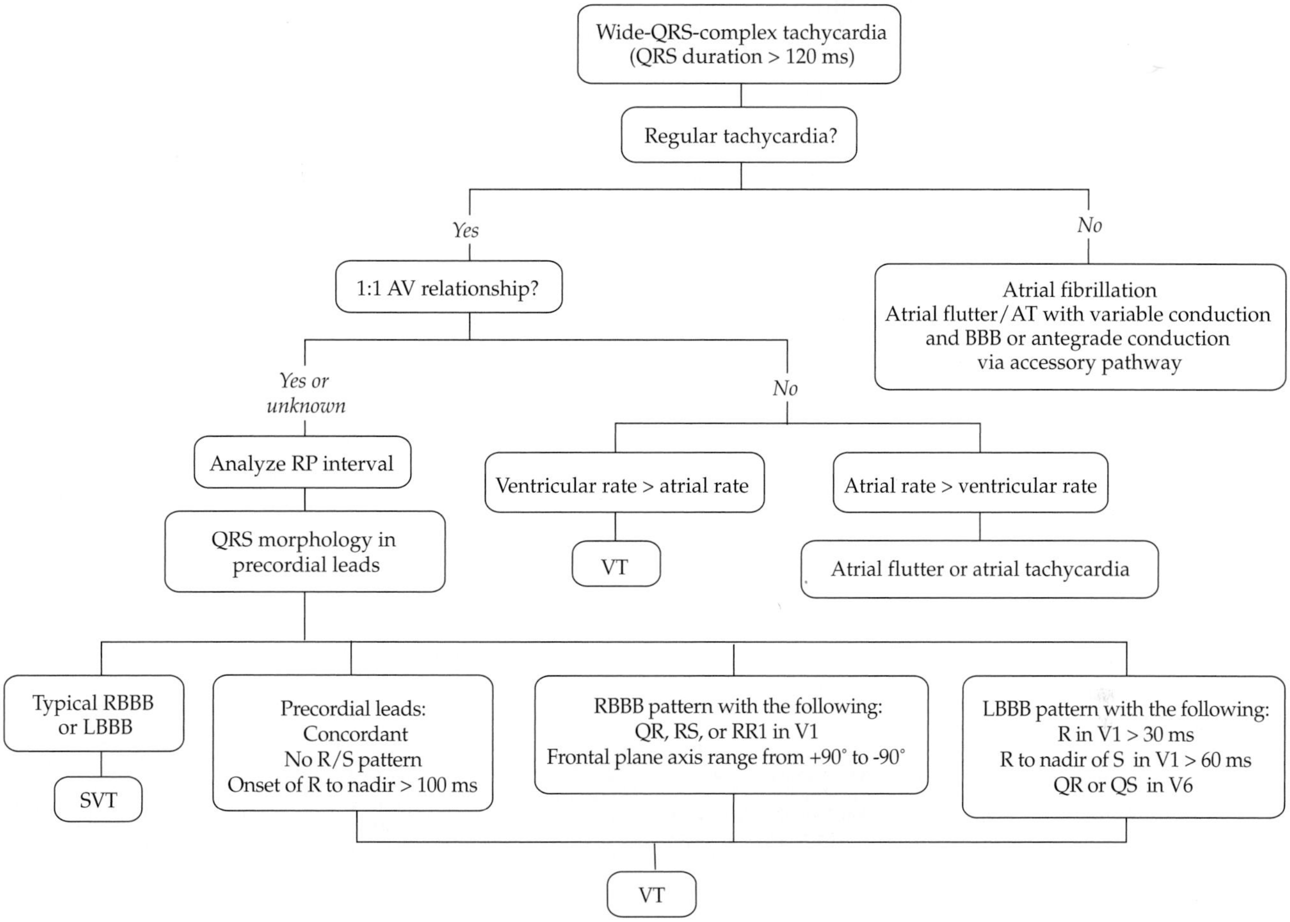

Wide-QRS-complex tachycardia
(QRS duration > 120 ms)

Regular tachycardia?

Yes

No

1:1 AV relationship?

Atrial fibrillation
Atrial flutter/AT with variable conduction
and BBB or antegrade conduction
via accessory pathway

*Yes or
unknown*

No

Analyze RP interval

Ventricular rate > atrial rate

Atrial rate > ventricular rate

QRS morphology in
precordial leads

VT

Atrial flutter or atrial tachycardia

Typical RBBB
or LBBB

Precordial leads:
Concordant
No R/S pattern
Onset of R to nadir > 100 ms

RBBB pattern with the following:
QR, RS, or RR1 in V1
Frontal plane axis range from +90° to -90°

LBBB pattern with the following:
R in V1 > 30 ms
R to nadir of S in V1 > 60 ms
QR or QS in V6

SVT

VT

Figure 6 **Differential diagnosis for wide (> 120 ms) QRS complex tachycardia.[1] If the tachycardia is regular and comparison with a baseline electrocardiogram shows that the QRS complex is identical to that during sinus rhythm, the patient may have supraventricular tachycardia (SVT) with bundle branch block (BBB) or antidromic atrioventricular reentrant tachycardia (AVRT). If the patient has a history of myocardial infarction or has structural heart disease, ventricular tachycardia (VT) is likely. Vagal maneuvers or adenosine may convert regular tachycardia, although adenosine should be used with caution when the diagnosis is unclear, because this drug may produce ventricular fibrillation (VF) in patients with coronary artery disease and patients with alternative pathways who have atrial fibrillation with a rapid ventricular rate. Precordial leads are concordant when all show either positive or negative deflections. Fusion complexes are diagnostic of VT. In preexcited tachycardias, the QRS is generally wider (i.e., more preexcited) than during sinus rhythm. (AT—atrial tachycardia; AV—atrioventricular; LBBB—left bundle branch block; RBBB—right bundle branch block)**

Adenosine If carotid massage fails to convert SVT, the drug of choice is intravenous adenosine, which is effective in 95% of cases.[10,11] The initial dose is given as a rapid bolus infusion of 6 mg, followed by 12 mg and finally 18 mg if necessary. The bolus must be given rapidly and then followed by a saline flush. If administration is too slow, the adenosine may be metabolized before it reaches the AV node. Possible adverse effects include headache, wheezing, and flushing. These effects disappear within 45 to 60 seconds. It is important to note that atrial, ventricular, and junctional premature beats are commonly observed after adenosine. In 3% to 5% of cases, the APCs trigger atrial fibrillation,[3] which may result in serious problems for patients with accessory pathways (see below). If possible, an external defibrillator should be readily available when adenosine is administered.

The most common reason for failure to respond to adenosine is that multiple premature beats are retriggering the tachycardia. In this setting, a longer-acting intravenous preparation (i.e., 5 mg of metoprolol or 0.1 mg/kg of verapamil) is indicated. Agents that more selectively block purogenic receptors have been

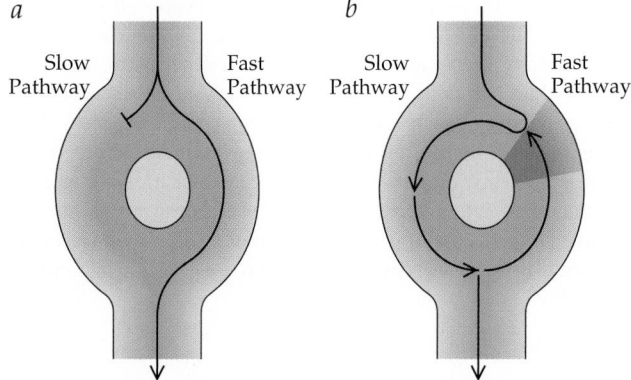

Figure 7 **In persons with dual pathways in the AV node, the sinus impulse is normally transmitted over the fast pathway to the ventricle and slow pathway conduction is preempted (*a*). However, if an atrial premature complex occurs during the fast pathway's refractory period, the impulse can block in the fast pathway. This may allow for anterograde (forward) conduction over the slow pathway and retrograde (backward) conduction over the fast pathway (*b*).**

Table 1 Drugs Used to Maintain Sinus Rhythm in Patients with Supraventricular Tachycardia[55]

Drug	Typical Daily Dose	Potential Adverse Effects
Amiodarone	100–400 mg*	Photosensitivity, pulmonary toxicity, polyneuropathy, GI upset, bradycardia, torsade de pointes (rare), hepatic toxicity, thyroid dysfunction
Disopyramide	400–750 mg	Torsade de pointes, heart failure, glaucoma, urinary retention, dry mouth
Dofetilide	500–1,000 µg	Torsade de pointes
Flecainide	200–300 mg	Ventricular tachycardia, heart failure, enhanced AV nodal conduction (conversion to atrial flutter)
Procainamide	1,000–4,000 mg	Torsade de pointes, lupuslike syndrome, GI symptoms
Propafenone	450–900 mg	Ventricular tachycardia, heart failure, enhanced AV nodal conduction (conversion to atrial flutter)
Quinidine	600–1,500 mg	Torsade de pointes, GI upset, enhanced AV nodal conduction
Sotalol	240–320 mg†	Torsade de pointes, heart failure, bradycardia, exacerbation of chronic obstructive or bronchospastic lung disease

*A loading dose of 600 mg/day is usually given for 1 month, or a dose of 1,000 mg/day is given for 1 week.
†Adjust dose for renal function and QT-interval response during in-hospital initiation phase
AV—atrioventricular   GI—gastrointestinal

shown to be very effective and associated with fewer side effects than older agents. Selective purogenic blockers are currently under investigation.

Long-term Therapy

A wide variety of drugs have proved effective for controlling episodes of AVNRT, including beta blockers,[9] calcium channel blockers,[12] and digoxin[13] [*see Table 1*]. Long-term drug therapy is associated with frequent recurrences and adverse effects, however. In patients without structural cardiac disease, class IC antiarrhythmic agents (e.g., flecainide, propafenone) are more effective than drugs that act by blocking AV nodal conduction, but recurrence rates nevertheless range from 25% to 35%.[14-16] For patients who have episodes infrequently and tolerate them well, some cardiologists will prescribe medication for use as needed—the "pill in the pocket" approach. For example, single-dose diltiazem (120 mg) and propranolol (80 mg) have been shown to be more effective than placebo or flecainide in patients with PSVT.[17]

Catheter Ablation

Current catheter ablative techniques involve placement of an electrode catheter between the tricuspid annulus and coronary sinus in the so-called slow pathway region.[18] One or more applications of radiofrequency energy are delivered through the catheter to destroy or attenuate the slow pathway. The success rate of ablation is over 96%, and the only significant complication is AV block, which occurs in approximately 1% of patients.[19]

Catheter ablation for AVNRT has proved so safe and effective that it is clearly the procedure of choice for patients in whom drug therapy fails. Moreover, it can be offered to those with milder symptoms who prefer to avoid long-term drug therapy. Precise recommendations for drug therapy versus ablative therapy are provided in the American College of Cardiology/American Heart Association/European Society of Cardiology guidelines.[1]

Atrioventricular Reentry Tachycardia

PATHOGENESIS

The normal conduction system of the heart limits the propagation of electrical impulses from the atria to a single pathway through the AV node and the His-Purkinje system. This limitation delays ventricular activation and thus optimizes mechanical function. The presence of an alternative pathway of atrioventricular conduction creates the potential for reentrant tachycardia.

The most prominent manifestation of accessory atrioventricular pathways is the Wolff-Parkinson-White (WPW) syndrome. In this syndrome, the accessory pathway can be located at various regions around the tricuspid and the mitral atrioventricular rings, but it is most commonly sited at the left free wall of the mitral annulus. The next most common pathway sites are the posteroseptal and right free wall areas. Pathways in the anteroseptal and the midseptal regions are relatively rare. Occasionally, posteroseptal pathways can be associated with a branching vein from the coronary sinus. On occasion, a patient will have more than one accessory pathway.

The basic mechanism of tachycardia in AVRT is similar to that of AVNRT. Electrical impulses can travel down both the AV node and the accessory pathway to activate the ventricles, with ventricular activation occurring earlier at sites near the accessory pathway than at sites activated normally (i.e., ventricular preexcitation). An APC may block in the accessory pathway but conduct over the normal pathway to activate the ventricle. After ventricular depolarization, the impulse may return to the atrium via retrograde conduction over the accessory pathway, leading to a sustained tachycardia.[20]

The most feared arrhythmia in the WPW syndrome involves atrial fibrillation with dominant conduction over an accessory pathway that has rapid conduction properties[21,22] [*see Figure 8*]. These patients may experience extraordinarily rapid ventricular rates and are at risk for sudden cardiac death from ventricular fibrillation.[23] In one large series, atrial fibrillation developed in 30% of patients with the WPW syndrome.[24]

DIAGNOSIS

Clinical Presentation

Symptomatic tachyarrhythmias associated with the WPW syndrome generally begin in the teenage years or during early adulthood. Pregnancy may produce an initial attack in some women. Pregnancy can also be associated with an increasing frequency of attacks and more symptomatic episodes. Symptoms are generally paroxysmal palpitations with or without dizziness, syncope, shortness of breath, weakness, or chest pain. Diuresis is another frequently described symptom; it occurs 30 minutes to an hour after onset of tachycardia and may be related to production of atrial natriuretic factor during the arrhythmia.

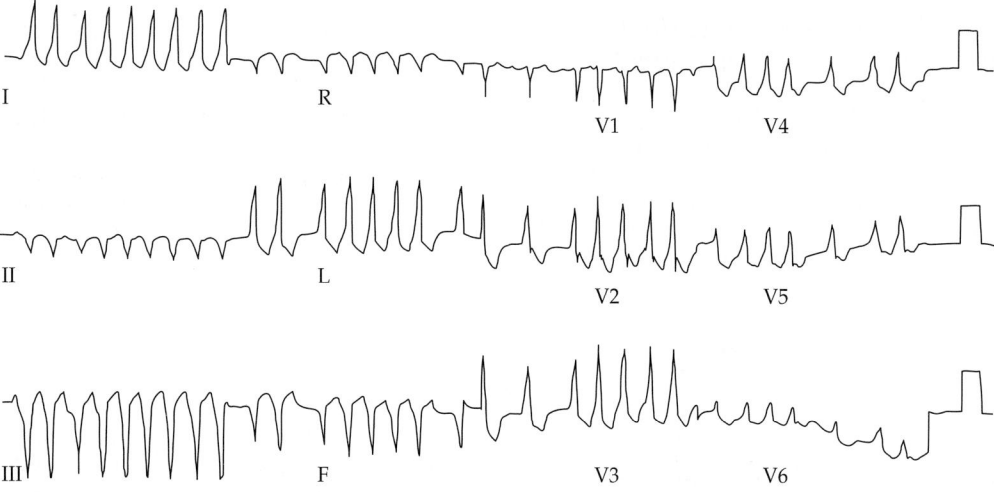

Figure 8 **A 12-lead ECG in a patient with Wolff-Parkinson-White syndrome shows the rapid, irregularly irregular ventricular rate and wide QRS complexes of atrial fibrillation with a very short refractory period. This is an especially dangerous arrhythmia.**

Electrocardiographic Findings

Ventricular preexcitation may be evident on a baseline ECG as fusion complexes (WPW pattern). The WPW pattern comprises a short PR interval and an earlier than normal deflection on the QRS complex (delta wave).[25] The ECG during AVRT will usually show a narrow complex with the retrograde P wave falling in the ST segment because atrial activation occurs well after ventricular depolarization[4] [*see Figure 4*]. Of interest is that a subset of patients with AVRT never show manifest anterograde conduction over the accessory pathway yet still have this form of tachycardia.[20] The only evidence that the tachycardia is supported by an accessory pathway is that the retrograde P wave clearly occurs after the QRS during tachycardia. On rare occasions, patients may have slowly conducting retrograde pathways[26]; their ECG will show a long RP–short PR relationship. These patients tend to have persistent tachycardias that have been referred to as the permanent form of junctional tachycardia (PJRT). In addition, approximately 5% of patients with the WPW syndrome (WPW pattern and arrhythmias) will show anterograde conduction over the accessory pathway with retrograde conduction through the AV node or over a separate accessory pathway. The ECG in these patients will show a wide-complex tachycardia with retrograde P waves preceding the QRS complex.

MANAGEMENT

Acute Therapy

Acute management of AVRT is similar to that for AVNRT: adenosine is the drug of choice,[11] but calcium channel blockers[13] or beta blockers[9] are also effective. Again, because adenosine usually provokes APCs and thus may in rare instances precipitate atrial fibrillation,[3] it is advisable to have ready access to an external defibrillator when using this agent.

Long-term Therapy

Long-term therapy for AVRT may be directed at interfering with conduction either through the AV node (i.e., with beta blockers or calcium channel blockers[27]) or through the accessory pathway (i.e., with class IC or class III antiarrhythmic agents[28-32]). Oral digitalis therapy is contraindicated because very rapid ven-

tricular rates may occur if atrial fibrillation develops. Class IC agents appear to be more effective than AV nodal blockers, but their use is restricted to patients who do not have significant cardiac disease. Class III agents (particularly amiodarone) are limited by long-term systemic toxicity and modest efficacy for patients with WPW and atrial fibrillation.[30] In general, drug therapy is attended by a significant risk of arrhythmic recurrence and adverse drug effects.

Treatment of WPW and Atrial Fibrillation

The treatment of WPW and atrial fibrillation is different from the treatment of AVRT. Because atrial fibrillation may precipitate a life-threatening arrhythmia, urgent therapy is required. If the patient presents with hemodynamic collapse, emergency direct current (DC) cardioversion is the first step. If the patient is less ill, trials of intravenous drug therapy are in order.[33] The drug of choice is procainamide, 50 mg/min to a total of 1 g, or ibutilide, 2 mg infused over 15 minutes. Ibutilide is very effective but should be used only in patients without significant structural cardiac disease. Intravenous digoxin or calcium channel blockers may result in an inordinate increase in heart rate and so should be avoided. Beta blockers, lidocaine, and adenosine are not likely to be effective, and their use will tend only to delay effective therapy.

Catheter Ablation

Reports from both single centers[34,35] and multicenter prospective registries[36,37] have documented the efficacy and possible adverse effects of ablative therapy in AVRT. Current techniques allow for successful ablation of accessory pathways that traverse the AV annulus or the anterior or posteroseptal spaces. For pathways over the left AV groove, current ablation techniques involve use of either transseptal or retrograde aortic approaches.[38] The overall success rate for ablation is approximately 95%.

Complications of ablation are primarily related to the site of the accessory pathway. For example, patients with an anteroseptal accessory pathway are at risk for injury to the AV node (5%), whereas ablations of left-sided accessory pathways carry a risk of cerebrovascular accident, myocardial perforation, or coronary artery occlusion.[36,37] The overall incidence of significant adverse effects varies from 2% to 4%. Death associated with ablative procedures is quite rare, occurring in 0.13% to 0.2% of cases.[36,37,39]

Treatment Selection

The remarkable efficacy and safety of ablation make this mode of therapy more attractive than long-term drug therapy for symptomatic patients. Drug therapy carries the possibility of recurrent arrhythmias, including atrial fibrillation. Hence, ablation is currently recommended for all patients with symptomatic WPW. Patients with mild symptoms and without manifest pre-excitation can be managed with drug therapy, but even in these cases ablation would appear to be a favored approach. Some of these patients decline long-term drug therapy, leaving ablation as the only alternative.

Asymptomatic preexcitation The management of asymptomatic preexcitation remains controversial. The vast majority of these patients have an overall good prognosis; sudden cardiac death is a rare initial manifestation. Leitch and colleagues followed asymptomatic WPW subjects in whom atrial fibrillation was induced during invasive electrophysiologic study; although approximately 20% demonstrated the capacity for rapid ventricular conduction, on follow-up few became symptomatic and none died suddenly.[39] A later study, however, emphasized findings on electrophysiologic testing (e.g., inducible AVRT, atrial fibrillation, and multiple pathways) that indicated increased risk for subsequent spontaneous development of atrial fibrillation or even sudden death.[40] Whether to treat an asymptomatic patient can also be decided on an individual basis[1]; for example, patients judged to be in high-risk occupations (e.g., airplane pilots, bus drivers) might well be considered for ablative therapy.

Focal Atrial Tachycardia

Regular tachycardias emanating in an atrial area and showing a centripetal pattern of spread are designated as focal atrial tachycardias (FATs). These arrhythmias are the least common cause of PSVT but nevertheless can cause significant morbidity. This is particularly true if the arrhythmia is incessant, which can result in the development of so-called tachycardia myopathy.

Atrial tachycardia may arise from sites in either the right or left atrium. The most common site of FAT is in the right atrium, with predilection for sites over the crista terminalis, tricuspid annulus, or coronary sinus.[41,42] In the left atrium, FAT is more apt to develop at the ostium of the pulmonary veins or over the mitral annulus.[42]

ELECTROCARDIOGRAPHIC DIAGNOSIS

In patients with FAT, the P wave may appear anywhere in the diastolic cycle but most often appears in front of the QRS (long RP tachycardia) [see Figure 5]. The ectopic P wave has a different shape than the sinus P wave unless the tachycardia originates from the high cristal or right pulmonary vein area. The P wave morphology gives excellent clues to tachycardia localization.[43,44] For example, P waves from left atrial foci will show negative deflection in leads I or aVL and positive deflections in the precordial leads. Right atrial foci tend to show negative P waves in lead V1 but positive or biphasic deflection in aVL. As a rule, foci from superior atrial sites generally produce strongly positive P waves in the inferior leads, whereas those arising from the inferior atrium produce negative P waves.

MANAGEMENT

Acute Therapy

Acute treatment of FAT attempts either to convert the arrhythmia or to slow the heart rate. Drugs used to slow the rate are the AV nodal blockers (i.e., digoxin, beta blockers, or calcium channel blockers). In contrast, class IC antiarrhythmic agents (e.g., flecainide, propafenone) or class III agents (e.g., amiodarone or sotalol) may terminate the tachycardia. Intravenous adenosine may be effective in terminating FAT and should be tried early. DC cardioversion may not be effective, particularly if the tachycardia results from an automatic mechanism.

Long-term Therapy

Long-term oral therapy for FAT is not well defined.[1] The general approach is empirical, with initial use of AV nodal blockers followed by class IC or III antiarrhythmic agents if the AV nodal blockers are ineffective.

Catheter Ablation

Catheter ablative procedures have been successfully applied to patients with FAT. Ablation has proved more effective for patients with right atrial foci (in whom the success rate is approximately 90%) than for those with left atrial foci (in whom the success rate is approximately 70%). A study of pooled data that included 514 patients showed an overall success rate of 86%, with an incidence of significant complications from 1% to 2%.[45]

Multifocal Atrial Tachycardia

Multifocal atrial tachycardia, generally regarded as automatic in origin, is characterized by atrial rates of 100 to 130 beats/min, three or more morphologically distinct (nonsinus) P waves, and variable AV conduction. It is commonly associated with respiratory disease and heart failure. Hypoxemia is a frequent finding. The arrhythmia may be exacerbated by digitalis excess, theophylline toxicity, or hypokalemia.

Treatment of multifocal atrial tachycardia is usually directed at the underlying precipitants. Metoprolol (used cautiously in patients with bronchospasm) or verapamil may slow atrial and ventricular rates and, occasionally, may restore sinus rhythm. Potassium and magnesium supplements may help suppress the arrhythmia. Amiodarone has also been useful in restoring sinus rhythm.

Atrial Flutter

Rapid reentrant atrial arrhythmias are referred to as atrial flutter. The most common circuit involves reentry around the tricuspid annulus. The reentrant circuit is usually counterclockwise (in the left anterior oblique projection) but may be clockwise.[46] Other circuits may involve the upper portion of the right atrium.[47] Less commonly, left atrial (LA) circuits are operative. LA circuits may involve the mitral annulus or scars around the posterior LA wall, pulmonary veins, or the foramen ovale.[47]

DIAGNOSIS

Clinical Presentation

Atrial flutter generally occurs in older patients who have associated cardiopulmonary disease. Atrial flutter may appear acutely during acute myocardial infarction, after cardiac surgery, or

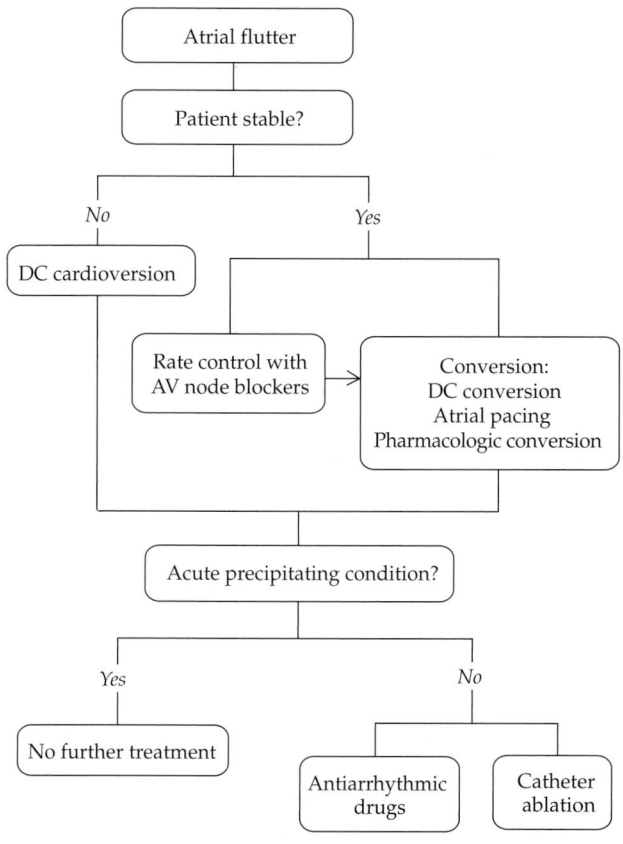

Figure 9 **Management of atrial flutter. With patients whose condition is unstable (e.g., because of heart failure, shock, or acute myocardial infarction), atrial flutter typically does not recur once the underlying disorder is resolved. Anticoagulant precautions, as per atrial fibrillation, should be taken in patients undergoing elective attempts to convert atrial flutter to sinus rhythm. (AV—atrioventricular; DC—direct current)**

with acute pulmonary insufficiency; in such cases, the arrhythmia usually does not recur once the inciting event has resolved. In contrast, atrial flutter in patients without concomitant acute illness tends to recur; like atrial fibrillation, it is usually a relapsing and remitting disease.

Electrocardiographic Findings

The ECG in patients with atrial flutter usually shows a flutter rate of 300 beats/min with 2:1 AV block. The most common atrial flutter pattern—a counterclockwise loop around the annulus—manifests as negative flutter waves in the inferior leads and positive waves in V1.[48] The ECG shows a continuous or so-called picket-fence appearance. In contrast, patients with a clockwise pattern will have positive flutter waves in the inferior leads and negative waves in V1. The ECG is much more variable for nonannular types of flutter circuits.[47]

MANAGEMENT

Acute Therapy

Treatment of atrial flutter is directed at attempts to convert the arrhythmia or use of AV nodal blockers to slow the ventricular response [*see Figure 9*]. Acute conversion of atrial flutter can be accomplished electrically by use of external DC shocks[49] or by

pacing.[50,51] Atrial flutter is usually exquisitely responsive to a small "dose" of DC shock (i.e., 25 to 50 joules).[49] Atrial overdrive pacing is also quite effective for terminating flutter, especially when the patient has been pretreated with drugs (i.e., ibutilide or procainamide).[51] Overdrive pacing is particularly appropriate for atrial flutter that occurs after cardiac surgery, because atrial wires are routinely left in place postoperatively in such patients. Transesophageal pacing has also been used to terminate flutter,[52] but its popularity has been limited by the need for analgesics to alleviate the associated chest pain.

Ibutilide (a class III antiarrhythmic agent) may be used to convert atrial flutter to sinus rhythm. Randomized prospective studies have shown that ibutilide is approximately 70% effective for this purpose.[53] In addition, ibutilide has been shown to be far more effective than intravenous procainamide.[54] Ibutilide is given in 1 mg aliquots over 10 minutes separated by a 10-minute rest period. A total of 2 mg of the drug is used, and the patient must remain under telemetry monitoring for approximately 4 hours after drug delivery. Ibutilide should not be given to patients with severe structural cardiac disease (i.e., those with a left ventricular ejection fraction less than 30%) because the risk of torsade de pointes becomes significant in this setting.

Patients with atrial flutter are at risk for thromboembolism. The current recommendations for anticoagulant therapy are the same as those for patients with atrial fibrillation.[55] For example, if the flutter duration is less than 48 hours, the risk of left atrial clot is small, and one may proceed with chemical or electrical cardioversion without full anticoagulation. Anticoagulant therapy is still required for 4 to 6 weeks after conversion because of the increased risk of thromboembolism secondary to decreased left atrial flow velocity after conversion. If the flutter duration is greater than 48 hours, a transesophageal echocardiogram to exclude clot is recommended before cardioversion. Complete guidelines for antithrombotic therapy in patients with atrial flutter are described elsewhere [*see Chapter 19*].

As an alternative to cardioversion, AV nodal blocking agents can be used to decrease the ventricular response in patients with flutter. Controlled trials have demonstrated the efficacy of intravenous calcium channel blockers (verapamil or diltiazem) in producing prompt decreases in heart rate.[56] Calcium channel blockers have been shown to reduce the heart rate below 100 beats/min more promptly than digoxin or amiodarone.

Long-term Therapy

Drug therapy for chronic atrial flutter is notoriously unreliable, and long-term rate control alone usually requires large doses of AV nodal blocking agents. A more effective intervention involves an ablative procedure in which radiofrequency lesions are applied in a line from the tricuspid annulus to the inferior vena cava.[57] This area is the critical isthmus for the usual type of atrial flutter circuit. Ablation of this area resulting in total conduction block of the isthmus is associated with a 90% to 100% cure rate in flutter.[58] Non–isthmus-dependent flutter circuits may involve either the right or the left atrium and usually require sophisticated mapping tools to determine the tachycardia circuit and the critical isthmus needed for curative ablation. These patients should be referred to experienced centers for evaluation.

Many patients have both atrial flutter and atrial fibrillation. For example, atrial flutter may deteriorate into atrial fibrillation, or bursts of atrial fibrillation may trigger atrial flutter. In addition, approximately 15% to 30% of patients treated with class IC antiarrhythmics or amiodarone for atrial fibrillation will develop stable atrial flutter.[59] In these patients, radiofrequency ablation of the flutter circuit together with continuance of drug therapy is usually quite effective in controlling both atrial fibrillation and flutter. Ablation of the flutter usually does not cure the atrial fibrillation.[60]

Sinus Tachycardia

Sinus tachycardia is usually a normal reflex response to changes in physiologic, pharmacologic, or pathophysiologic stimuli, such as exercise, emotion (e.g., anxiety, anger), fever, hemodynamic or respiratory compromise, anemia, thyrotoxicosis, poor physical condition, sympathomimetic or vagolytic agents, and abnormal hemoglobins. Heart rate during sinus tachycardia generally does not exceed 180 beats/min, except perhaps in young persons, who may achieve sinus rates greater than 200 beats/min during vigorous exercise.

When sinus tachycardia is a reflex response to altered physiology, the resulting increase in cardiac output is usually beneficial. Tachycardia resolves when conditions return to normal.

Inappropriate Sinus Tachycardia

An infrequent but troublesome problem, inappropriate sinus tachycardia (IST) appears to be a true syndrome with cardiac, neurologic, and psychiatric components. It affects women more often than men. Structural heart disease is generally absent. In one series of 475 patients, IST was the indication for catheter ablation in 2.3%.[61]

DIAGNOSIS

Clinical Presentation

IST may be persistent or episodic. It is often precipitated by arising from a reclining or sitting position (postural orthostatic tachycardia).[62] Very rapid rates (> 170 beats/min) may be triggered by minimal exertion.

The tachycardia is frequently accompanied by symptoms of dizziness, near-syncope, or syncope. Fatigue and atypical chest pain may also accompany IST. Peculiar but inconsistent autonomic and hemodynamic findings may be seen in these patients. This suggests that the syndrome is not uniform in etiology.

Electrocardiographic Findings

Because tachycardia rates may arise from higher foci, the P waves seen during IST may differ slightly from those seen at rest.

MANAGEMENT

Drug Therapy

Beta blockers and calcium channel blockers (i.e., verapamil or diltiazem) may be used to alleviate tachycardia in IST. Unfortunately, these drugs are often not effective and tend to exacerbate the nonspecific symptoms that accompany this syndrome. Agents that alter sinus node automaticity, autonomic tone, or both, such as flecainide, propafenone, and amiodarone, may be tried in selected patients.[63]

Catheter Ablation

Radiofrequency ablation has been employed to ablate or modify the sinus node in IST. Large-tipped (8 to 10 mm) catheters are often required to create more sizable lesions. Successful modification or ablation has been achieved in 70% to 100% of patients.[64] Sinus nodal modification is associated with a 10% to 27% risk of sinus node damage necessitating permanent pacing.

Both intracardiac electrograms and intracardiac ultrasonography have been used to target lesion delivery. Intracardiac ultrasonography targets the fastest portions of the sinus node by ablating the uppermost portion of the crista terminalis. This approach seems to require fewer radiofrequency applications than do electrogram-guided approaches. It may also reduce the need for permanent pacing.

Long-term follow-up after radiofrequency modification has been less encouraging. Recurrence rates are high. Ablation to the extent that permanent pacing is required may be necessary for sustained success. Thus, patients require careful follow-up for recurrent tachycardia or progressive sinus node dysfunction. Surgical isolation of the sinus node for IST has also been followed by recurrent tachycardia at new foci.

The author has received a grant for educational activities from the National Association for Sport and Physical Education and has during the past 12 months owned stock in or served as a consultant or member of the speakers' bureaus for AstraZeneca Pharmaceuticals LP; Bristol-Myers Squibb Company; Guidant Corporation; Medtronic, Inc.; The Procter & Gamble Company; Solvay Pharmaceuticals, Inc.; 3M; and Wyeth-Ayerst Laboratories, Inc.

References

1. Blomstöm-Lundqvist C, Scheinman MM, Aliot EM, et al: ACC/AHA/ESC Guidelines for the management of patients with supraventricular arrhythmias—executive summary: a report of the American College of Cardiology/American Heart Association Task Force on Practice Guidelines and the European Society of Cardiology Committee for Practice Guidelines (Writing Committee to Develop Guidelines for the Management of Patients with Supraventricular Arrhythmias). Circulation 108:1871, 2003

2. Mehta D, Wafa S, Ward DE, et al: Relative efficacy of various physical manoeuvres in the termination of junctional tachycardia. Lancet 1:1181, 1988

3. Glatter KA, Cheng J, Dorostkar P, et al: Electrophysiologic effects of adenosine in patients with supraventricular tachycardia. Circulation 99:1034, 1999

4. Kay GN, Pressley JC, Packer DL, et al: Value of the 12-lead electrocardiogram in discriminating atrioventricular nodal reciprocating tachycardia from circus movement atrioventricular tachycardia utilizing a retrograde accessory pathway. Am J Cardiol 59:296, 1987

5. Brugada P, Brugada J, Mont L, et al: A new approach to the differential diagnosis of a regular tachycardia with a wide QRS complex. Circulation 83:1649, 1991

6. Wellens HJ, Bar FW, Lie KI: The value of the electrocardiogram in the differential diagnosis of a tachycardia with a widened QRS complex. Am J Med 64:27, 1978

7. Akhtar M, Jazayeri MR, Sra J, et al: Atrioventricular nodal reentry: clinical, electrophysiological, and therapeutic considerations. Circulation 88:282, 1993

8. Sung RJ, Waxman HL, Saksena S, et al: Sequence of retrograde atrial activation in patients with dual atrioventricular nodal pathways. Circulation 64:1059, 1981

9. Amsterdam EA, Kulcyski J, Ridgeway MG: Efficacy of cardioselective beta-adrenergic blockade with intravenously administered metoprolol in the treatment of supraventricular tachyarrhythmias. J Clin Pharmacol 31:714, 1991

10. Lee KL, Chun HM, Liem LB, et al: Effect of adenosine and verapamil in catecholamine-induced accelerated atrioventricular junctional rhythm: insights into the underlying mechanism. Pacing Clin Electrophysiol 22:866, 1999

11. Overholt ED, Rheuban KS, Gutgesell HP, et al: Usefulness of adenosine for arrhythmias in infants and children. Am J Cardiol 61:336, 1988

12. Mauritson DR, Winniford MD, Walker WS, et al: Oral verapamil for paroxysmal supraventricular tachycardia: a long-term, double-blind randomized trial. Ann Intern Med 96:409, 1982

13. Winniford MD, Fulton KL, Hillis LD: Long-term therapy of paroxysmal supraventricular tachycardia: a randomized, double-blind comparison of digoxin, propranolol and verapamil. Am J Cardiol 54:1138, 1984

14. Flecainide acetate prevents recurrence of symptomatic paroxysmal supraventricular tachycardia. The Flecainide Supraventricular Tachycardia Study Group. Circulation 83:119, 1991

15. Long-term safety and efficacy of flecainide in the treatment of supraventricular tachyarrhythmias: the United States experience. The Flecainide Supraventricular Tachyarrhythmia Investigators. Am J Cardiol 70:11A, 1992

16. A randomized, placebo-controlled trial of propafenone in the prophylaxis of paroxysmal supraventricular tachycardia and paroxysmal atrial fibrillation. UK Propafenone PSVT Study Group. Circulation 92:2550, 1995

17. Yeh SJ, Lin FC, Chou YY, et al: Termination of paroxysmal supraventricular tachycardia with a single oral dose of diltiazem and propranolol. Circulation 71:104, 1985

18. Clague JR, Dagres N, Kottkamp H, et al: Targeting the slow pathway for atrioventricular nodal reentrant tachycardia: initial results and long-term follow-up in 379 consecutive patients. Eur Heart J 22:82, 2001

19. Scheinman MM, Huang S: The 1998 NASPE prospective catheter ablation registry. Pacing Clin Electrophysiol 23:1020, 2000

20. Ross DL, Uther JB: Diagnosis of concealed accessory pathways in supraventricular tachycardia. Pacing Clin Electrophysiol 7:1069, 1984

21. Dreifus LS, Haiat R, Watanabe Y, et al: Ventricular fibrillation: a possible mechanism of sudden death in patients and Wolff-Parkinson-White syndrome. Circulation 43:520, 1971

22. Klein GJ, Bashore TM, Sellers TD, et al: Ventricular fibrillation in the Wolff-Parkinson-White syndrome. N Engl J Med 301:1080, 1979

23. Timmermans C, Smeets JL, Rodriguez LM, et al: Aborted sudden death in the Wolff-Parkinson-White syndrome. Am J Cardiol 76:492,1995

24. Campbell RW, Smith RA, Gallagher JJ, et al: Atrial fibrillation in the preexcitation syndrome. Am J Cardiol 40:514, 1977

25. Krahn AD, Manfreda J, Tate RB, et al: The natural history of electrocardiographic preexcitation in men. The Manitoba Follow-up Study. Ann Intern Med 116:456, 1992

26. Murdock CJ, Leitch JW, Teo WS, et al: Characteristics of accessory pathways exhibiting decremental conduction. Am J Cardiol 67:506, 1991

27. Lai WT, Voon WC, Yen HW, et al: Comparison of the electrophysiologic effects of oral sustained-release and intravenous verapamil in patients with paroxysmal supraventricular tachycardia. Am J Cardiol 71:405, 1993

28. Flecainide acetate treatment of paroxysmal supraventricular tachycardia and paroxysmal atrial fibrillation: dose-response studies. The Flecainide Supraventricular Tachycardia Study Group. J Am Coll Cardiol 17:297, 1991

29. Cockrell JL, Scheinman MM, Titus C, et al: Safety and efficacy of oral flecainide therapy in patients with atrioventricular re-entrant tachycardia. Ann Intern Med 114:189, 1991

30. Kappenberger LJ, Fromer MA, Steinbrunn W, et al: Efficacy of amiodarone in the Wolff-Parkinson-White syndrome with rapid ventricular response via accessory pathway during atrial fibrillation. Am J Cardiol 54:330, 1984

31. Kunze KP, Schluter M, Kuck KH: Sotalol in patients with Wolff-Parkinson-White syndrome. Circulation 75:1050, 1987

32. Rosenbaum MB, Chiale PA, Ryba D, et al: Control of tachyarrhythmias associated with Wolff-Parkinson-White syndrome by amiodarone hydrochloride. Am J Cardiol 34:215, 1974

33. Glatter KA, Dorostkar PC, Yang Y, et al: Electrophysiological effects of ibutilide in patients with accessory pathways. Circulation 104:1933, 2001

34. Jackman WM, Wang XZ, Friday KJ, et al: Catheter ablation of accessory atrioventricular pathways (Wolff-Parkinson-White syndrome) by radiofrequency current. N Engl J Med 324:1605, 1991

35. Kuck KH, Schluter M, Geiger M, et al: Radiofrequency current catheter ablation of accessory atrioventricular pathways. Lancet 337:1557, 1991

36. Scheinman MM: NASPE Survey on Catheter Ablation. Pacing Clin Electrophysiol 18:1474, 1995

37. The Multicentre European Radiofrequency Survey (MERFS): complications of radiofrequency catheter ablation of arrhythmias. Multicentre European Radiofrequency Survey (MERFS) investigators of the Working Group on Arrhythmias of the European Society of Cardiology. Eur Heart J 14:1644, 1993

38. Lesh MD, Van Hare GF, Scheinman MM, et al: Comparison of the retrograde and transseptal methods for ablation of left free wall accessory pathways. J Am Coll Cardiol 22:542, 1993

39. Leitch JW, Klein GJ, Yee R, et al: Prognostic value of electrophysiology testing in asymptomatic patients with Wolff-Parkinson-White pattern. Circulation 82:1718, 1990

40. Pappone C, Santinelli V, Rosanio S, et al: Usefulness of invasive electrophysiologic testing to stratify the risk of arrhythmic events in asymptomatic patients with Wolff-Parkinson-White pattern: results from a large prospective long-term follow-up study. J Am Coll Cardiol 41:239, 2003

41. Kalman JM, Olgin JE, Karch MR, et al: "Cristal tachycardias": origin of right atrial tachycardias from the crista terminalis identified by intracardiac echocardiography. J Am Coll Cardiol 31:451, 1998

42. Natale A, Breeding L, Tomassoni G, et al: Ablation of right and left ectopic atrial tachycardias using a three-dimensional nonfluoroscopic mapping system. Am J Cardiol 82:989, 1998

43. Tang CW, Scheinman MM, Van Hare GF, et al: Use of P wave configuration during atrial tachycardia to predict site of origin. J Am Coll Cardiol 26:1315, 1995

44. Tada H, Nogami A, Naito S, et al: Simple electrocardiographic criteria for identifying the site of origin of focal right atrial tachycardia. Pacing Clin Electrophysiol 21:2431, 1998

45. Hsieh MH, Chen SA: Catheter ablation of focal AT. Catheter Ablation of Arrhythmias. Zipes DP, Haissaguerre M, Eds. Futura Publishing Co, Armonk, New York, 2002

46. Waldo AL: Pathogenesis of atrial flutter. J Cardiovasc Electrophysiol 9:S18, 1998

47. Yang Y, Cheng J, Bochoeyer A, et al: Atypical right atrial flutter patterns. Circulation 103:3092, 2001

48. Kalman JM, Olgin JE, Saxon LA, et al: Electrocardiographic and electrophysiologic characterization of atypical atrial flutter in man: use of activation and entrainment mapping and implications for catheter ablation. J Cardiovasc Electrophysiol 8:121, 1997

49. Lown B: Electrical reversion of cardiac arrhythmias. Br Heart J 29:469, 1967

50. Zeft HJ, Cobb FR, Waxman MB, et al: Right atrial stimulation in the treatment of atrial flutter. Ann Intern Med 70:447, 1969

51. Stambler BS, Wood MA, Ellenbogen KA: Comparative efficacy of intravenous ibutilide versus procainamide for enhancing termination of atrial flutter by atrial overdrive pacing. Am J Cardiol 77:960, 1996

52. Doni F, Manfredi M, Piemonti C, et al: New onset atrial flutter termination by overdrive transoesophageal pacing: effects of different protocols of stimulation. Europace 2:292, 2000

53. Ellenbogen KA, Stambler BS, Wood MA, et al: Efficacy of intravenous ibutilide for rapid termination of atrial fibrillation and atrial flutter: a dose-response study. J Am Coll Cardiol 28:130, 1996

54. Volgman AS, Carberry PA, Stambler B, et al: Conversion efficacy and safety of intravenous ibutilide compared with intravenous procainamide in patients with atrial flutter or fibrillation. J Am Coll Cardiol 31:1414, 1998

55. Fuster V, Ryden LE, Asinger RW, et al: ACC/AHA/ESC guidelines for the management of patients with atrial fibrillation: executive summary. A report of the American College of Cardiology/American Heart Association Task Force on Practice Guidelines and the European Society of Cardiology Committee for Practice Guidelines and Policy Conferences (Committee to Develop Guidelines for the Management of Patients with Atrial Fibrillation) developed in collaboration with the North American Society of Pacing and Electrophysiology. Circulation 104:2118, 2001

56. Ellenbogen KA, Dias VC, Plumb VJ, et al: A placebo-controlled trial of continuous intravenous diltiazem infusion for 24-hour heart rate control during atrial fibrillation and atrial flutter: a multicenter study. J Am Coll Cardiol 18:891, 1991

57. Cosio FG, Goicolea A, Lopez-Gil M, et al: Catheter ablation of atrial flutter circuits. Pacing Clin Electrophysiol 16:637, 1993

58. Chen SA, Chiang CE, Wu TJ, et al: Radiofrequency catheter ablation of common atrial flutter: comparison of electrophysiologically guided focal ablation technique and linear ablation technique. J Am Coll Cardiol 27:860, 1996

59. Nabar A, Rodriguez LM, Timmermans C, et al: Radiofrequency ablation of "class IC atrial flutter" in patients with resistant atrial fibrillation. Am J Cardiol 83:785, 1999

60. Natale A, Newby KH, Pisano E, et al: Prospective randomized comparison of antiarrhythmic therapy versus first-line radiofrequency ablation in patients with atrial flutter. J Am Coll Cardiol 35:1898, 2000

61. McKenzie JP, Frazier DW, Smith JM, et al: Successful radio frequency ablation of inappropriate sinus tachycardia (abstr). Circulation 92:I, 1995

62. Low PA, Opfer-Gehrking TL, Textor SC, et al: Postural tachycardia syndrome (POTS). Neurology 45(4 suppl 5):S19, 1995

63. Kanjwal MY, Kosinski DJ, Grubb BP: Treatment of postural orthostatic tachycardia syndrome and inappropriate sinus tachycardia. Curr Cardiol Rep 5:402, 2003

64. Shen WK: Modification and ablation for inappropriate sinus tachycardia: current status. Card Electrophysiol Rev 6:349, 2002

21 Ventricular Arrhythmias

Jonathan J. Langberg, M.D., and David B. DeLurgio, M.D.

Ventricular tachyarrhythmias characteristically are sudden in onset, unpredictable, and transitory. Consequently, their assessment and treatment present extraordinary challenges to the clinician. Moreover, the prognosis for patients with these arrhythmias is quite variable. In some patients, ventricular ectopic activity may be benign and without sequelae, but in other patients, comparable ectopy is a harbinger of ventricular fibrillation and sudden cardiac death.[1] This chapter summarizes the practical aspects of evaluation and treatment of patients with ventricular arrhythmias.

Pathophysiology

Ventricular tachyarrhythmias are mediated by one of three basic mechanisms: reentry, abnormal automaticity, and triggering. Although causation cannot be directly determined in individual patients, experimental and clinical observations make it possible to infer the mechanism underlying many of the ventricular arrhythmia syndromes encountered in practice.

VENTRICULAR TACHYCARDIA CAUSED BY REENTRY

Reentrant arrhythmias (also called circus-movement tachycardias) are produced by a continuous circular or looping pattern of myocardial activation. Reentry can occur around lines of anatomic or functional block or occur as spinning wavefronts or

rotors that lack a fixed anatomic path. When reentry occurs around lines of block, two features must be present for reentry to occur: (1) a barrier around which the wavefront circulates, either a fixed region of inexcitability caused by scarring or a dysfunctional region resulting from local refractoriness, and (2) unidirectional block at the entrance of the circuit. If activation spreads down both sides of the barrier, the impulses will collide distally and reentry will not occur; however, if propagation is blocked in one limb and proceeds in an anterograde direction over the other, the activation wavefront may be capable of retrograde invasion of the initially blocked pathway, thereby initiating sustained reentry.

In patients with structural heart disease, most symptomatic ventricular arrhythmias are mediated by reentry.[2,3] Sustained monomorphic ventricular tachycardia often occurs after transmural myocardial infarction (MI). The arrhythmia usually arises in the border zone of the scar [*see Figure 1*]. The larger the extent of this heterogeneous border zone, the greater the probability of a circuit capable of mediating reentrant ventricular tachycardia. This is consistent with the observation that the risk of malignant ventricular arrhythmias is proportional to the volume of the scar and the severity of left ventricular dysfunction after MI.[4]

Ventricular fibrillation is also a reentrant phenomenon.[5] Unlike ventricular tachycardia, during which a single activation wavefront circulates around a fixed barrier, ventricular fibrilla-

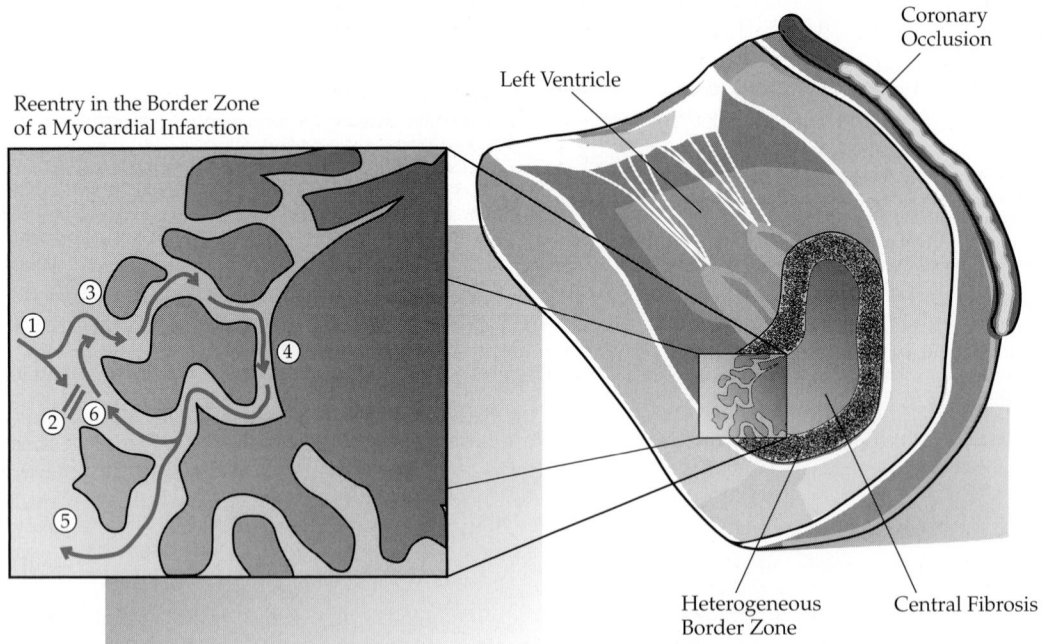

Figure 1 **Reentrant ventricular tachycardia usually arises as the result of reentry within the border zone of a myocardial infarction. This region consists of strands of viable myocytes interspersed with inexcitable fibrous tissue. Reentry begins when a wavefront of activation (1) encounters a bifurcation and blocks in one of the two pathways around an obstacle (2). The activation wavefront then conducts exclusively through the orthodromic pathway (3) and encounters a region of relatively slow conduction within the tachycardia circuit (4). The activation wavefront may exit from the tachycardia circuit at a site quite different from the entrance point (5). Although the anterograde limb of the circuit is initially refractory, it recovers excitability by the time it is depolarized by the reentrant wavefront (6). The activation wavefront reenters the orthodromic limb of the circuit, and the circus movement is established.**

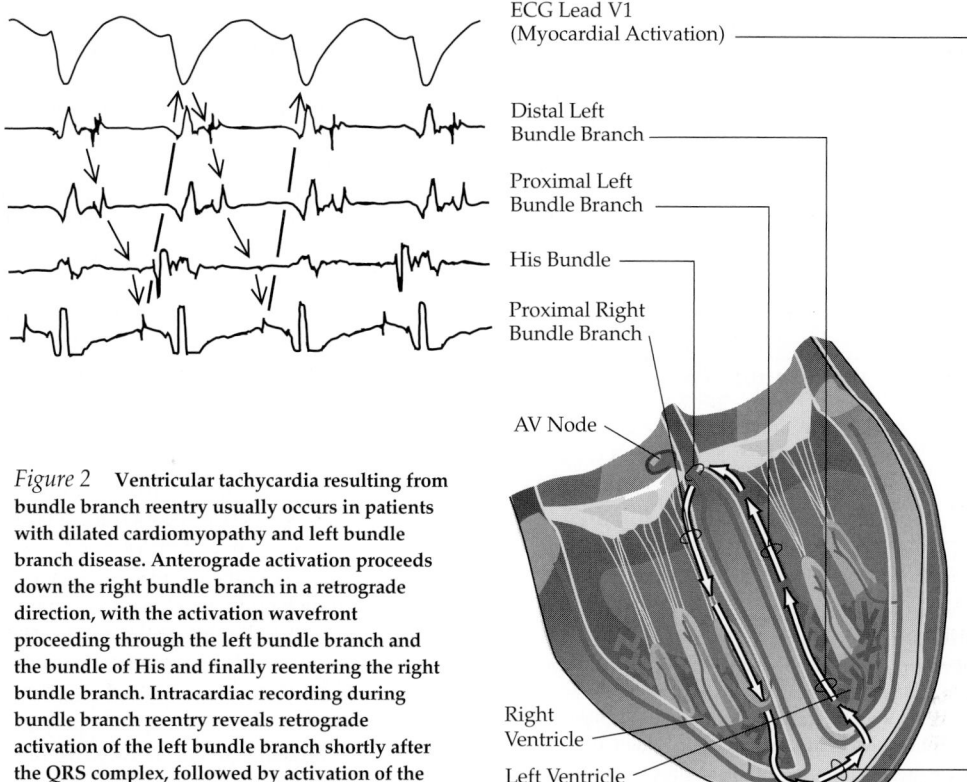

ECG Lead V1
(Myocardial Activation)

Distal Left
Bundle Branch

Proximal Left
Bundle Branch

His Bundle

Proximal Right
Bundle Branch

AV Node

Right
Ventricle

Left Ventricle

Figure 2 Ventricular tachycardia resulting from bundle branch reentry usually occurs in patients with dilated cardiomyopathy and left bundle branch disease. Anterograde activation proceeds down the right bundle branch in a retrograde direction, with the activation wavefront proceeding through the left bundle branch and the bundle of His and finally reentering the right bundle branch. Intracardiac recording during bundle branch reentry reveals retrograde activation of the left bundle branch shortly after the QRS complex, followed by activation of the His bundle and right bundle branch.

tion is caused by multiple simultaneous impulses that travel around functional barriers of refractory tissue, moving continuously throughout the myocardium to create very rapid, irregular, and ineffective activation. Alternatively, in some patients, ventricular fibrillation may be initiated by very early ectopic beats in the specialized conduction system.[6]

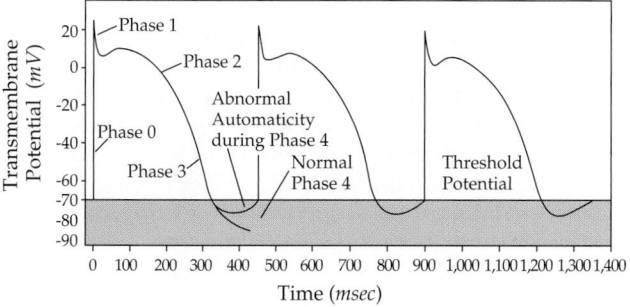

Figure 3 The resting transmembrane potential of the myocardial cell is created by active maintenance of sodium and potassium gradients. The cell is depolarized (phase 0) by an electrical stimulus that allows a sudden influx of sodium (Na^+). Repolarization, phases 1 through 3, requires an early rapid chloride influx, a plateau phase mediated by calcium currents, and reestablishment of the resting transmembrane potential via potassium (K^+) efflux. Between action potentials, the resting potential is designated as phase 4. In cells with automaticity, depolarization mediated by calcium (Ca^{2+}) and Na^+ currents may occur during phase 4, resulting in spontaneous generation of the next action potential. In normal ventricular myocytes, the resting potential during electrical diastole (phase 4) remains in the region of −80 to −90 mV. The rate of automatic firing is determined by the resting potential, the slope of phase 4, and the threshold potential.

Like postinfarction arrhythmias, the ventricular tachycardia in patients with nonischemic cardiomyopathy is often the result of reentry in a zone of patchy fibrosis. However, in patients with left ventricular dilatation and slowed conduction in the specialized conduction system, the tachycardia may be mediated by bundle branch reentry, characterized by anterograde conduction over the right bundle branch, activation of the septum, and retrograde conduction over the left bundle branch [*see Figure 2*].[7] Although an infrequent cause of ventricular tachycardia, bundle branch reentry is of interest to cardiac electrophysiologists because it can be cured by selective destruction of either the right or the left bundle branch by use of radiofrequency catheter ablation [*see Chapter 22*].

VENTRICULAR TACHYCARDIA MEDIATED BY ABNORMAL AUTOMATICITY

Normal ventricular myocytes maintain a steady transmembrane resting potential of −80 to −90 mV, depolarizing only when stimulated by an activation wavefront. Extrinsic factors, such as electrolyte imbalance and ischemia, or intrinsic disease may reduce the resting potential and produce simultaneous diastolic (phase 4) depolarization [*see Figure 3*].

Unlike reentry, which can usually be induced and terminated by premature beats, automatic rhythms tend not to be influenced by pacing. Changes in heart rate at the onset of ventricular tachycardia may also provide insight into the arrhythmia mechanism. Reentrant tachycardias are usually stable because of a fixed conduction time around the circuit. In contrast, automaticity often shows warm-up, with progressive acceleration during the first few seconds of the tachycardia.

Abnormal automaticity may play a role in a number of clinical arrhythmia syndromes. An accelerated idioventricular rhythm

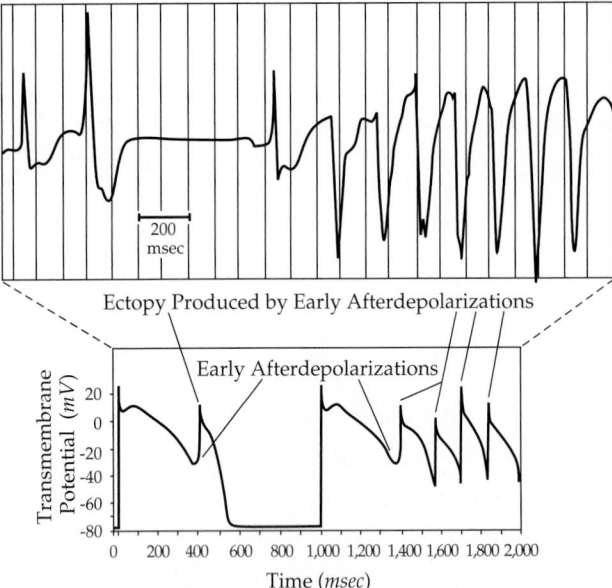

Ectopy Produced by Early Afterdepolarizations

Early Afterdepolarizations

Figure 4 **In ventricular tachycardia caused by triggering, prolongation of the action potential (and the QT interval) results in depolarization during phase 3. Such early afterdepolarizations are manifested as positive deflections at the end of the phase 2 plateau or during the phase 3 rapid repolarization of the action potential. If this deflection exceeds the threshold potential, one or more triggered beats will occur. Bradycardia-dependent torsade de pointes is an example of an arrhythmia caused by early afterdepolarizations. The electrocardiogram of a patient with quinidine intoxication reveals an extrasystole and polymorphic ventricular tachycardia.**

(60 to 100 beats/min) or episodes of slow ventricular tachycardia (100 to 140 beats/min) occur in approximately 20% of patients who are monitored after transmural MI.[8] These slow-fast rhythms are probably the result of abnormal automaticity in ischemic Purkinje fibers.

More rapid ventricular tachycardia is also a frequent complication of acute ischemia, reperfusion, or both. These arrhythmias are often polymorphic, characterized by QRS complexes that change in amplitude and cycle length, with heart rates that may approach 300 beats/min. Abnormal automaticity in ischemic myocardium probably causes many of these episodes.

Ventricular tachycardia occasionally occurs in patients without apparent structural heart disease.[9] This idiopathic arrhythmia generally originates in the right ventricular outflow tract, just beneath the pulmonary valve. A number of observations suggest that it, too, is sometimes mediated by abnormal automaticity. It can develop spontaneously in response to increased adrenergic tone and, as a rule, cannot be induced or terminated by pacing. It may occur as a pattern of recurrent short bursts of tachycardia interspersed with equally short interludes of sinus rhythm, a pattern more consistent with automaticity than reentry.[10]

VENTRICULAR TACHYCARDIA CAUSED BY TRIGGERING

Early Afterdepolarization

Triggered activity, defined as premature activation caused by one or more preceding impulses, is the result of afterdepolarizations that occur either during (early afterdepolarization) or just after (delayed afterdepolarization) completion of the repolarization process [*see Figure 4*]. Factors that slow the heart rate tend to

prolong the duration of depolarization, which is identified by a lengthened QT interval on the electrocardiogram, often sufficiently to bring early afterdepolarizations to threshold. Thus, triggered ventricular tachycardia that results from early afterdepolarizations is characteristically bradycardia dependent or pause dependent.

Early afterdepolarizations have been produced experimentally under a variety of conditions, including ischemia, hypokalemia, and antiarrhythmic drug toxicity. The arrhythmias seen in these studies are bradycardia dependent and, typically, are both rapid and polymorphic. Slowing of the tachycardia rate just before spontaneous termination is another characteristic feature of early afterdepolarization–mediated ventricular tachycardia.

Although it is difficult to prove, it seems likely that early afterdepolarizations mediate a variety of clinical arrhythmias. Prolongation of the QT interval—whether congenital or acquired as a result of drugs (class IA antiarrhythmic agents or, more commonly, other drugs such as haloperidol or erythromycin) or electrolyte depletion—increases the risk of a polymorphic ventricular tachycardia. As in the experimental situation, patients with QT prolongation tend to develop polymorphic ventricular tachycardia as a result of slowing of the heart rate, heart rate pauses, or sudden surges in adrenergic tone. Unlike rhythms mediated by automaticity or reentry, ventricular tachycardia in the setting of QT prolongation is almost always polymorphic, sometimes with the twisting pattern that characterizes torsade de pointes.

Delayed Afterdepolarization

Arrhythmias mediated by delayed afterdepolarization are distinctly different from those associated with early afterdepolarization and appear to be caused by abnormal accumulation and oscillation of cytosolic calcium concentration. The amplitude of these arrhythmias is augmented by acceleration rather than slowing of the heart rate. Delayed afterdepolarizations have been implicated in the genesis of ventricular tachycardia in patients with digitalis toxicity, and in some patients with ventricular tachycardia who have no apparent structural heart disease. Verapamil may be therapeutic in this subset of patients.[11] Although these arrhythmias have been recorded from surviving Purkinje fibers and infarcted canine myocardium, their role in clinical arrhythmias during and after MI is less well established.

Delayed afterdepolarizations are induced at a critical heart rate range, which is patient specific, either spontaneously or during atrial or ventricular pacing. As with reentrant arrhythmias, tachycardia resulting from delayed afterdepolarizations is often terminated by overdrive pacing, although it will frequently persist for several cycles after cessation of pacing.

Asymptomatic Ventricular Ectopy

Ventricular ectopy is recorded in more than half of normal persons undergoing ambulatory electrocardiographic monitoring. Complex ectopy (multifocal premature ventricular complexes and nonsustained ventricular tachycardia) is less frequent but is still observed in 5% to 10% of healthy persons with no apparent heart disease.[12]

The prognostic significance of ventricular ectopy depends on the severity of left ventricular dysfunction. In the absence of structural heart disease, asymptomatic ventricular ectopic activity is benign, with no demonstrable risk of sudden death, even in the presence of ventricular tachycardia. In patients with structural heart disease, however, ventricular ectopic activity is associated with an increased risk of sudden cardiac death. This risk is markedly increased with progressive left ventricular dysfunction.[13] For example, post-MI patients with a left ventricular ejection fraction (LVEF) greater than 40% who experience fewer than 10 ventricular premature complexes (VPCs) an hour after MI have a mortality of 5% to 7% a year. Those patients who experience more than 10 VPCs an hour, however, have a mortality of 12% to 18%. The combination of an LVEF of less than 40% and more than 10 VPCs an hour raises the annual mortality to between 27% and 40%.

The presence of frequent ventricular premature beats 7 to 10 days after MI is associated with a fivefold increase in the risk of symptomatic or fatal arrhythmias during follow-up.[4] Because many patients with frequent ectopy do not develop malignant ventricular arrhythmias, the positive predictive accuracy of this finding is only 16%. Conversely, because the majority of patients without frequent ectopy remain free of fatal arrhythmias, its absence is associated with a negative predictive accuracy of 82%. The occurrence of nonsustained ventricular tachycardia (fewer than three consecutive rapid beats over a period of less than 30 seconds) during monitoring appears to confer an even greater risk than does the presence of frequent isolated ventricular premature beats.[4,12,13]

The association between ambient ventricular ectopy and the risk of arrhythmic death is less well established in patients with nonischemic (i.e., valvular, hypertensive, or idiopathic) cardiomyopathy. However, most reports in the literature do suggest that the presence of high-grade ventricular arrhythmias, defined as multifocal VPCs or nonsustained ventricular tachycardia, confers an increased risk of sudden death that is independent of the severity of left ventricular dysfunction.[14,15]

Because the significance of ventricular ectopy depends on the degree of ventricular function impairment, cardiac imaging should be part of the initial evaluation. Echocardiography is the most versatile test; it provides information regarding regional wall motion abnormalities and valvular lesions as well as the LVEF. Radionuclide ventriculography also gives precise information regarding ejection fraction and may be of value in patients whose heart disease is already well characterized. If ventricular function is normal or close to normal, reassurance or treatment with beta blockers or calcium channel blockers to suppress bothersome symptoms is appropriate. In contrast, if patients have evidence of significant ventricular dysfunction or other significant structural heart disease such as hypertrophic cardiomyopathy, further evaluation and therapy may be appropriate. This evaluation may include additional tests that can help define the risk of a sustained arrhythmic event and the need for a prophylactic implantable cardioverter-defibrillator (ICD).

SIGNAL-AVERAGED ELECTROCARDIOGRAPHY

Signal-averaged electrocardiography may be useful for estimating risk in patients with heart disease and ventricular ectopy. This noninvasive test detects signals from areas of slow conduction in the arrhythmogenic regions on the periphery of an MI. The surface ECG is recorded for approximately 250 beats, and the signal is averaged by a computer and filtered, resulting in dramatic reduction of the signal-to-noise ratio. This allows detection of low-amplitude, high-frequency late potentials that result from the activation of zones of slow conduction just after the offset of the QRS complex.

Low-amplitude, high-frequency late potentials are recorded in about one third of patients after MI. These patients have a 20% incidence of life-threatening ventricular arrhythmias during the first year after infarction, compared with a 3% incidence in patients without late potentials.[16] Signal-averaged ECG findings are independently predictive of adverse events after MI and provide additional information regarding risks in patients with frequent ventricular premature contractions and impaired left ventricular function. A limitation of signal-averaged ECG is that it cannot be used in patients with bundle branch block or atrial fibrillation.

MICROVOLT T WAVE ALTERNANS

Another screening test that may be useful for assessing risk of sudden cardiac death in patients with left ventricular dysfunction is microvolt T wave alternans.[17] In this technique, signal processing is used to detect minute beat-to-beat variation in T wave amplitude that takes place during low-level exercise. Like signal-averaged ECG, microvolt T wave alternans has been approved by the Food and Drug Administration,[18] although currently it has little role in the selection of patients for ICDs. Unlike signal-averaged ECG, microvolt T wave alternans appears to have prognostic value in nonischemic as well as ischemic cardiomyopathy. A limitation of the test is that patients must be able to exercise for 5 minutes to a heart rate of at least 110 beats a minute.

ELECTROPHYSIOLOGIC TESTING

Electrophysiologic study can be used to assess the inducibility of sustained ventricular arrhythmias in patients with structural heart disease.[4] Electrode catheters are introduced percutaneously into the venous system, usually via the femoral vein, and advanced under fluoroscopic guidance into the right ventricle. Programmed electrical stimulation is performed in an attempt to elicit ventricular tachycardia or fibrillation. This usually consists of a drive train at a constant paced cycle length followed by one, two, or three extra stimuli (premature beats). The stimuli are introduced at progressively more premature coupling intervals until tachycardia is induced or the stimuli fail to capture as the result of local refractoriness [see Chapter 22].

Programmed stimulation can induce sustained monomorphic ventricular tachycardia in about 20% of patients with reduced left ventricular function after MI and can induce ventricular fibrillation in an additional 10% to 15% of such patients. During follow-up, arrhythmic events occur in 5% of the noninducible patients, in 10% of patients with inducible ventricular fibrillation, and in 50% of patients with inducible ventricular tachycardia.

Although electrophysiologic study has reasonable sensitivity for prediction of subsequent arrhythmic events, the positive predictive value of the test is probably no better than that of the signal-averaged ECG, T wave alternans testing, or both, especially when such tests are combined with measurements of left ventricular systolic function and quantification of ambient ectopy. Electrophysiologic study is invasive and relatively expensive. Moreover, there is no evidence to suggest that treatment of this group of patients with antiarrhythmic drugs improves survival. Thus, it is difficult to justify routine electrophysiologic testing in asymptomatic patients after MI. The role of invasive electrophysiologic study for risk stratification in asymptomatic patients after MI has diminished with the increasing use of ICDs for primary prevention of sudden cardiac death.

Electrophysiologic testing is of uncertain value for stratification of risk in patients with nonischemic cardiomyopathy and asymptomatic ventricular ectopy. In this population, induction of sustained monomorphic ventricular tachycardia is infrequent and does not appear to be predictive of subsequent sudden cardiac death.

Currently, electrophysiologic studies are perhaps most useful in patients who have an LVEF of 30% to 40% and evidence of nonsustained ventricular tachycardia. In this select group, electrophysiologic testing can help determine whether the risk of sudden cardiac death is sufficiently high to merit prophylactic implantation of an ICD [see The Implantable Cardioverter-Defibrillator, below].

Syncope and Ventricular Arrhythmias

Syncope, defined as transient loss of consciousness, is a common phenomenon, accounting for about 3% of all emergency room visits.[19] Because the spells usually resolve by the time the patient is initially evaluated, determination of the cause of loss of consciousness is difficult but extremely important, because prognosis depends on the nature of the episode. If ventricular arrhythmias are detected during subsequent monitoring, additional evaluation should be undertaken to determine whether the syncope was produced by a paroxysm of ventricular tachycardia.

HISTORY AND PHYSICAL EXAMINATION

A thorough history may provide important clues to the diagnosis of ventricular tachycardia. The onset of syncope mediated by ventricular tachycardia is usually abrupt, with only a brief prodrome of light-headedness or no premonitory symptoms at all. The absence of rapid heartbeat does not exclude the diagnosis, because only about one half of patients with documented sustained ventricular tachycardia experience this symptom. The duration of unconsciousness is brief, rarely lasting longer than several minutes. Because of the abrupt onset, traumatic injury is common.

Spontaneous movements during syncope often cause confusion and misdiagnosis. Cerebral hypoperfusion from any cause, including ventricular tachycardia, may produce one or more clonic jerks of the extremities. However, syncopal episodes differ from seizure activity in three respects: (1) the movements in syncopal episodes are not reciprocating (tonic-clonic), (2) they are much briefer in duration, and (3) bladder or bowel incontinence rarely occurs.

Historical information regarding the patient's condition after awakening is frequently overlooked but may be very helpful. Patients typically recover quickly from ventricular tachycardia–mediated syncope. Postictal confusion lasting longer than 5 minutes suggests a grand mal event rather than an arrhythmic one. Similarly, persistent residual malaise, nausea, and weakness are characteristic of a faint produced by the vasodepressor syndrome rather than arrhythmic syncope.

Ventricular tachycardia of sufficient rate or duration to produce loss of consciousness is rare in patients with normal ventricular function. Thus, patients in whom ventricular arrhythmias are identified after a syncopal episode must be thoroughly evaluated for structural heart disease. The presence of severe left ventricular dysfunction in these patients is associated with an ominous prognosis.

Patients with coronary artery disease, syncope, or ventricular arrhythmias require evaluation of myocardial ischemia with a functional study (e.g., thallium scintigraphy), coronary angiography, or both, in addition to quantification of ventricular function. Acute ischemia may precipitate rapid ventricular tachycardia that is sufficient to cause loss of consciousness. In such cases,

exercise treadmill testing may induce ventricular ectopy, thereby suggesting the diagnosis, especially if premonitory symptoms are reproduced.

ELECTROCARDIOGRAPHY

On occasion, findings on a 12-lead ECG will suggest the cause of the loss of consciousness in a patient with unexplained syncope. A prolonged QT interval can indicate congenital long QT syndrome; ST segment elevation in lead V1 can indicate the Brugada syndrome; and a short QT interval may indicate short QT syndrome [see Heritable Ventricular Arrhythmias, below].

Signal-averaged electrocardiography plays a limited but important role in the evaluation of patients with syncope and ventricular arrhythmias. The positive predictive accuracy of this test is inadequate to confirm the diagnosis of an arrhythmic event. However, a negative result makes the possibility of sustained ventricular tachycardia unlikely enough that additional, more invasive studies are probably not justified.

Ambulatory electrocardiography is useful in selected patients with a history of syncope and ventricular arrhythmias. The yield of 24-hour or 48-hour Holter monitoring is low in patients with infrequent arrhythmic episodes, however. In such patients, a transtelephonic loop recorder is more likely to provide diagnostic information. This device is worn by the patient for 4 to 6 weeks, continuously recording and storing several minutes of the ECG in an endless loop. Immediately after presyncope or a syncopal spell, the patient presses the event button on the device to stop the recording and store the preceding ECG in memory. The output of the device is then transmitted over the telephone to a receiving station. This system has been shown to be more cost-effective than Holter monitoring and is preferable unless symptoms are present on a daily basis.

ELECTROPHYSIOLOGIC TESTS

Electrophysiologic testing can be useful in determining whether an episode of loss of consciousness was produced by ventricular tachycardia.[20] Assessment of sinus node function and atrioventricular conduction should be performed during electrophysiologic testing even when ventricular tachycardia is suspected, because episodic bradyarrhythmias may produce spells with very similar symptoms.

The induction of sustained monomorphic ventricular tachycardia during programmed stimulation increases the probability that the patient's spontaneous episode was mediated by ventricular tachycardia and increases the likelihood that therapy will be effective. Several studies have shown a lower rate of recurrent syncope in patients whose therapy is based on results of electrophysiologic testing, compared with those in whom the study was unrevealing or for whom no effective treatment could be found.[20,21]

Evaluation of the Patient Rescued from Cardiac Arrest

In 80% to 90% of patients who develop out-of-hospital cardiac arrest, the precipitating event is either primary ventricular fibrillation or a rapid ventricular tachycardia that degenerates into ventricular fibrillation. Bradyarrhythmic events occur occasionally, but when asystole is recorded as the initial rhythm, it is usually indicative of a prolonged downtime interval and is associated with a very poor prognosis.

The majority of patients who sustain cardiac arrest have structural heart disease. In industrialized societies, this is most often the result of coronary atherosclerosis. Studies of both victims and survivors of cardiac arrest show significant coronary obstruction in 75% to 80% of patients. Unfortunately, sudden cardiac death is the initial manifestation of coronary artery disease in 10% to 20% of patients, making it the most common cause of mortality in adults younger than 65 years.[22]

Despite the close association between coronary artery disease and sudden cardiac death, acute MI is an infrequent cause of cardiac arrest. Only about 20% of patients rescued from an episode of ventricular fibrillation have evidence of an evolving MI during their subsequent hospitalization.[23] The prognosis is favorable for cardiac arrest survivors in whom the event can be clearly linked to acute myocardial ischemia, with a recurrence rate of only 2% during the subsequent year. In contrast, patients with ventricular fibrillation not related to an ischemic event have an annual recurrence rate of greater than 20%, presumably because they have a chronic substrate capable of mediating malignant ventricular arrhythmias.[22,23]

All patients rescued from cardiac arrest require serial ECGs and enzyme measurements to determine whether the event was a consequence of acute MI. Coronary angiography should be performed in all patients as well, except those in whom the precipitating factor has already been unequivocally identified.

ELECTROCARDIOGRAPHY

Laboratory evaluation of patients rescued from cardiac arrest should be directed at the identification of specific reversible causative factors. As in patients who have experienced syncope, the postresuscitation ECG may provide important information. A prolonged QT interval suggests the possibility of drug-induced torsade de pointes or the congenital long QT syndrome. A short PR interval and slurring of the QRS onset (a delta wave) are manifestations of the Wolff-Parkinson-White (WPW) syndrome [see Chapter 20]. Patients with WPW syndrome have an accessory connection linking the atrium and ventricle across either the mitral or the tricuspid annulus. A subset of patients with the WPW syndrome are capable of very rapid anterograde conduction over the accessory connection. If these patients develop atrial fibrillation, the ventricular response may be in excess of 300 beats/min and can degenerate into ventricular fibrillation.

LABORATORY TESTS

The initial evaluation of serum electrolytes is sometimes revealing, because severe depletion of serum potassium, serum magnesium, or both may precipitate ventricular arrhythmias. Such depletions are characteristic of patients with chronic heart failure who are maintained on long-term diuretic therapy with inadequate electrolyte supplementation.

ELECTROPHYSIOLOGIC TESTS

Electrophysiologic study was once an important part of the evaluation of cardiac arrest survivors in whom a reversible cause cannot be identified. With ICD therapy becoming commonplace for such patients, however, the usefulness of electrophysiologic testing has become limited to patients in whom the exact nature of the arrhythmia that precipitated the arrest remains uncertain. In a study of electrophysiology testing in 572 patients with ventricular fibrillation, ventricular tachycardia with syncope, or sustained ventricular tachycardia in the setting of left ventricular dysfunction, 67% of patients had inducible sustained ventricular tachycardia or ventricular fibrillation, but inducibility of these arrhythmias did not predict death or arrhythmia recurrence. These investigators concluded that electrophysiologic testing may not

be worth the risks and costs of the procedure in this patient population, particularly in those patients likely to receive an ICD.[24]

Heritable Ventricular Arrhythmias

Alterations in the duration of the QT interval are most often acquired, typically from drugs.[25] In rare cases, however, ventricular arrhythmias result from genetic disorders that alter ventricular repolarization. These disorders include long QT syndrome, Brugada syndrome, and short QT syndrome.

LONG QT SYNDROME

A familial disorder with distinct clinical features, the congenital long QT syndrome usually presents as syncope (or, in rare instances, as cardiac arrest) during childhood or the teenage years, mediated by recurrent bouts of rapid, polymorphic ventricular tachycardia. Many patients are incorrectly diagnosed with a grand mal seizure disorder. Loss of consciousness characteristically occurs with a sudden surge in adrenergic tone caused by abrupt physical, emotional, or auditory stimulation. There is often a family history of unexplained syncope or premature sudden cardiac death.

The hallmark of this disorder is abnormal prolongation of the QT interval on the ECG. Prolongation is present if the heart rate–corrected QT interval (QT/RR interval) exceeds 0.47 in children, 0.46 in men, or 0.48 in women. Other depolarization abnormalities are often present in the long QT syndrome. The T wave is flattened and may have a bifid, or double-hump, appearance. In addition, a prominent U wave may be seen. About one third of patients will have a resting heart rate of less than 60 beats/min.

Congenital long QT syndrome has two principal phenotypes. The originally described Jervell and Lange-Nielsen syndrome, an autosomal recessive disorder with associated deafness, has proved to be quite rare.[26] The more common Romano-Ward syndrome is an autosomal dominant disorder and is not associated with hearing loss. Genomic studies in families with congenital long QT syndrome have shown that the disorder is produced by mutations of membrane ion channel proteins. To date, more than 300 of these mutations have been identified in seven genes, accounting for approximately 70% of affected patients.[27] Interestingly, the different mutations seem to produce slightly different ECG appearances.

Evaluation of a patient for the long QT syndrome should include screening of all first-degree relatives. A careful history regarding unexplained syncope and a 12-lead ECG should be obtained. A point system has been developed that combines ECG findings, clinical history, and family history (e.g., unexplained sudden death at a young age in an immediate family member) into a score that indicates the likelihood of disease.[28] Genetic testing for long QT syndrome is now commercially available and includes analysis of five major cardiac ion channel genes. The sensitivity of this test is approximately 70%, and its role in the management of affected patients and their families has not been established. Treatment of long QT syndrome is with beta blockers, ICD placement in high-risk patients, and left thoracic sympathectomy in selected cases.[29] Treatment of asymptomatic family members should be considered if screening uncovers a prolonged QT interval.

BRUGADA SYNDROME

Brugada syndrome is an inherited disorder that is manifested by syncope or sudden cardiac death. It is characterized by an

ECG that shows an incomplete right bundle branch block and ST segment elevation in leads V1 through V3.[30] However, these ECG findings also occur in many patients who do not have Brugada syndrome. Because of the low specificity of the ECG characteristics, the diagnosis should not be made on the basis of the ECG alone.[31] A set of diagnostic criteria that includes history, ECG and electrophysiologic test results, and family history has been proposed.[32] As with the long QT syndrome, genetic testing for Brugada syndrome is commercially available, but it is of uncertain utility. ICD placement is recommended for patients with Brugada syndrome who have experienced symptoms; recommendations for ICD placement are less well established for patients with Brugada syndrome who are asymptomatic or have inducible arrhythmias.

SHORT QT SYNDROME

Short QT syndrome is an inherited disorder characterized by a family history of sudden death (perhaps including sudden infant death syndrome), an abnormally short QT (QTc < 300 msec), and inducible ventricular fibrillation.[33,34] The syndrome has been traced to mutations in the cardiac ion channel genes.[35] Because short QT syndrome has only recently been recognized, its incidence remains uncertain. It is important to remember that electrolyte and drug effects that cause QT shortening (e.g., hypercalcemia and digitalis) need to be excluded before this diagnosis is entertained.

Pharmacologic Therapy

As a result of changes in the medical care system, more primary care practitioners bear direct responsibility for treatment decisions in patients with cardiac arrhythmias. The use of antiarrhythmic drugs in patients with ventricular arrhythmias presents a growing challenge, especially given that the medical literature contains reports of real and potential harm associated with the use of antiarrhythmic drugs.

CLASSIFICATION AND MECHANISMS OF
ANTIARRHYTHMIC DRUGS

Antiarrhythmic drugs directly alter the electrophysiologic properties of myocardial cells. Therefore, an understanding of basic cellular electrophysiology is critical for an informed use of these compounds [see Figure 5].[36]

The most widely accepted classification of antiarrhythmic drugs, originally proposed by Vaughan Williams in 1970, involves four main classes of drugs, with the first class further divided into three subgroups [see Table 1].[37] This classification is based primarily on the ability of the drug to control arrhythmias by blocking ionic channels and currents. Few drugs demonstrate pure class effects, however, and other characteristics, such as influence of the drug on autonomic tone, contractility, and adverse effects, may be more important clinically and will be discussed as they pertain to individual drugs.

Class I agents inhibit the fast Na^+ channel during depolarization (phase 0) of the action potential, with resultant decreases in depolarization rate and conduction velocity [see Figure 5]. Agents in class IA (quinidine, procainamide, disopyramide, and moricizine) significantly lengthen both the action potential duration and the effective refractory period (and therefore the QT interval) through a combination of the class I effect of Na^+ channel inhibition and the lengthening of repolarization by K^+ channel blockade, a class III effect.

Class IB drugs (lidocaine, mexiletine, and phenytoin) are less powerful Na^+ channel blockers and, unlike class IA agents, shorten the action potential duration and refractory period in normal ventricular tissue, probably by inhibition of a background Na^+ current during phase 3 of the action potential.[38,39] In ischemic tissue, lidocaine may also block an adenosine triphosphate (ATP)–dependent K^+ channel, thus preventing ischemically mediated shortening of depolarization.[40]

Class IC drugs (flecainide and propafenone), the most potent Na^+ channel blockers, markedly decrease phase 0 depolarization rate and conduction velocity. Unlike other class I agents, they have little effect on the action potential duration and the effective refractory period in ventricular myocardial cells, but they do shorten the action potential of the Purkinje fibers.[41,42] This inhomogeneity of depolarization combined with marked slowing of conduction may contribute to the proarrhythmic effects of this class of drugs.

Class II agents are the beta-adrenergic antagonists. The efficacy of these drugs in the reduction of arrhythmia-related morbidity and mortality has become more evident in recent years, but the precise ionic bases for their salutary effects have not been fully elucidated. Beta-adrenergic antagonism has been shown to decrease spontaneous phase 4 depolarization and, therefore, to decrease adrenergically mediated automaticity, an effect that may be of particular importance in the prevention of ventricular arrhythmias during ischemia and reperfusion. Beta blockade also results in the slowing of heart rate and decreased oxygen consumption, effects long recognized as desirable in MI patients.[43] Effects on the cardiac action potential differ in atrial, ventricular, and specialized conduction tissues. For example, conduction velocity is slowed most profoundly in specialized conduction tissue, resulting in prolongation of the PR interval, whereas action potential duration in ventricular myocardium is generally not affected.

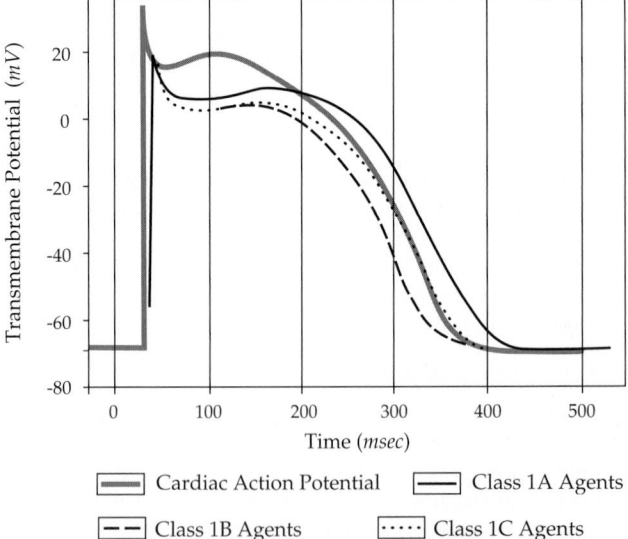

Figure 5 The electrophysiologic hallmark of class I antiarrhythmic drugs is inhibition of the fast Na^+ channel, which results in a decrease in the slope and amplitude of phase 0 of the cardiac action potential. Class IA agents (quinidine, procainamide, and disopyramide) also prolong the action potential duration, whereas class IB agents (lidocaine and mexiletine) may shorten the action potential duration, particularly in ischemic tissue. Class IC agents (flecainide and propafenone) have little effect on action potential duration.

Table 1 Classification of Antiarrhythmic Drugs

Class (Agents)	Action	I.V. Dosage	Oral Dosage	Route of Elimination	Side Effects
I	Inhibit membrane sodium channels; affect Purkinje fiber action potential during depolarization (phase 0)				
IA Quinidine	Slow the rate of rise of the action potential and prolong its duration; slow conduction; increase refractoriness	6–10 mg/kg (I.M. or I.V.) over 20 min	200–400 mg every 4–6 hr or every 8 hr (long-acting)	Hepatic	GI, ↓LVF, ↑Dig, torsade de pointes
Procainamide		100 mg every 1–3 min to 500–1,000 mg; maintain at 2–6 mg/min	50 mg/kg/day in divided doses every 3–4 hr or every 6 hr (long-acting)	Renal	SLE, hypersensitivity, ↓LVF, torsade de pointes
Disopyramide			100–200 mg every 6–8 hr	Renal	Urinary retention, dry mouth, markedly ↓LVF
Moricizine			200–300 mg every 8 hr	Hepatic	Dizziness, nausea, headache, ↓theophylline level, ↓LVF
IB Lidocaine	Shorten action potential duration; do not affect conduction or refractoriness	1–2 mg/kg at 50 mg/min; maintain at 1–4 mg/min		Hepatic	CNS, GI
Mexiletine			100–300 mg every 6–12 hr; maximum, 1,200 mg/day	Hepatic	CNS, GI, leukopenia
IC Flecainide	Slow the rate of rise of the action potential and slow repolarization (phase 4); slow conduction; increase refractoriness		100–200 mg twice daily	Hepatic	CNS, GI, ↓↓LVF, incessant VT, sudden death
Propafenone			150–300 mg every 8–12 hr	Hepatic	CNS, GI, ↓↓LVF, ↑Dig
II Beta blockers Esmolol	Inhibit sympathetic activity; decrease automaticity; prolong atrioventricular conduction and refractoriness	500 µg/kg over 1–2 min; maintain at 25–200 µg/kg/min	Other beta blockers may be used	Hepatic	↓LVF, bronchospasm
Propranolol		1–5 mg at 1 mg/min	40–320 mg in 1–4 doses (depending on preparation)	Hepatic	↓LVF, bradycardia, AV block, bronchospasm
Acebutolol			200–600 mg twice daily	Hepatic	↓LVF, bradycardia, positive ANA, lupuslike syndrome
III Amiodarone	Block potassium channels; predominantly prolong action potential duration, prolong repolarization, widen QRS complex, prolong QT interval, decrease automaticity and conduction, and prolong refractoriness	150 mg I.V. over 10 min, then 1 mg/min for 6 hr; maintain at 0.5 mg/min; overlap with initiation of oral treatment	800–1,600 mg/day for 7–21 days; maintain at 100–400 mg/day (higher doses may be needed)	Hepatic	Pulmonary fibrosis, hypothyroidism, hyperthyroidism, corneal and skin deposits, hepatitis, ↑Dig, neurotoxicity, GI
Sotalol			80–160 mg every 12 hr (higher doses may be used for life-threatening arrhythmias)	Renal (dosing interval should be extended if creatinine clearance < 60 ml/min)	↓LVF, bradycardia, fatigue and other side effects associated with beta blockers
Dofetilide			125–500 µg b.i.d.	Renal (dosing based on creatinine clearance)	Infrequent (rare CNS)
IV Verapamil	Slow calcium channel blockers; block the slow inward current; decrease automaticity and atrioventricular conduction	10–20 mg over 2–20 min; maintain at 5 µg/kg/min	80–120 mg every 6–8 hr; 240–360 mg once daily with sustained-release preparation (not approved for arrhythmia)	Hepatic	↓LVF, constipation, ↑Dig
Diltiazem		0.25 mg/kg over 2 min; second 0.35 mg/kg bolus after 15 min if response is inadequate; infusion rate, 5–15 mg/hr	180–360 mg daily in 1–3 doses, depending on preparation (oral forms not approved for arrhythmias)	Hepatic metabolism, renal excretion	Hypotension, ↓LVF

ANA—antinuclear antibodies AV—atrioventricular CNS—central nervous system ↑Dig—elevation of serum digoxin level GI—gastrointestinal (nausea, vomiting, diarrhea) ↓LVF—reduced left ventricular function SLE—systemic lupus erythematosus VT—ventricular tachycardia

The primary actions of class III agents (amiodarone, sotalol, and dofetilide) are prolongation of depolarization, the action potential duration, and the effective refractory period by K^+ channel blockade. These effects may prevent arrhythmias by decreasing the relative proportion of the cardiac cycle during which the myocardial cell is excitable and therefore susceptible to a triggering event. Reentrant tachycardias may be suppressed if the action potential duration becomes longer than the cycle length of the tachycardia circuit and if the leading edge of the wavefront suddenly impinges on inexcitable tissue. Class III agents have proven efficacy and an incidence of proarrhythmia lower than that seen with class IA agents.

Class IV agents act by inhibiting the inward slow Ca^{2+} current, which may contribute to late afterdepolarizations and therefore to ventricular tachycardia. These Ca^{2+} channel blockers reduce afterdepolarizations and are useful in the treatment of idiopathic ventricular tachycardia.[11,44,45] They have no appreciable effect on conduction velocity or repolarization and tend to evoke sympathetic activation. Thus, their role in the treatment of ventricular tachycardia in the setting of structural heart disease is limited.

Antiarrhythmic drugs in clinical use today have activity in multiple classes. For example, in addition to its class III effects, amiodarone also exhibits prominent Na^+ channel blockade (class I), beta blockade (class II), and Ca^{2+} channel blockade (class IV). Sotalol is a racemic mixture of d and l isomers, which have similar class III effects, whereas the l-isomer is essentially a beta blocker. d-Sotalol has been shown to increase mortality in patients with left ventricular dysfunction and recent MI.[46] The lower incidence of proarrhythmia seen with amiodarone or racemic sotalol therapy may be related to beneficial class II effects.

PROARRHYTHMIA

Proarrhythmia refers to the worsening of an existing arrhythmia or the induction of a new one by an antiarrhythmic drug. Three types of proarrhythmia have been described: torsade de pointes (the most common), incessant ventricular tachycardia, and extremely wide complex ventricular rhythm.

Torsade de Pointes

Torsade de pointes is triggered by early afterdepolarizations in a setting of delayed repolarization and increased dispersion of refractoriness. Class IA and class III drugs, which prolong refractoriness (and thus the QT interval) by K^+ channel blockade, provide the milieu for torsade de pointes. Drug-induced torsade de pointes is often pause dependent or bradycardia dependent, because the QT interval is longer at slower heart rates and after pauses. Exacerbating factors, such as hypokalemia, hypomagnesemia, and the concomitant use of other QT-prolonging drugs, are particularly important in this type of proarrhythmia.

Incessant Ventricular Tachycardia

Incessant ventricular tachycardia may be induced by drugs that markedly slow conduction (class IA and class IC) sufficiently to make the patient's own ventricular tachycardia continuous.[47,48] The arrhythmia is generally slower because of the drug effect, but it may become resistant to drugs or cardioversion, with potentially disastrous consequences in the presence of hemodynamic instability. This proarrhythmia is rarely associated with class IB drugs, which affect weaker Na^+ channel blockades.

Extremely Wide Complex Ventricular Rhythm

Extremely wide complex ventricular rhythm is usually associated with class IC agents, also in the setting of structural heart disease, and has been linked to excessive plasma drug levels or a sudden change in dose. The arrhythmia is not thought to represent a preexisting reentrant tachycardia and easily degenerates to ventricular fibrillation.

EFFICACY AND OUTCOMES OF ANTIARRHYTHMIC DRUG USE

Suppression of ambient ventricular ectopy by an antiarrhythmic agent does not prevent future life-threatening arrhythmias. In fact, patients effectively treated with class IC agents in the Cardiac Arrhythmia Suppression Trial (CAST) had a greater risk of sudden cardiac death than those who received placebo, a finding that underlines the proarrhythmic potential of these agents.[49] Conversely, beta blockers, which typically do not suppress ambient ectopy, appear to reduce the risk of malignant ventricular arrhythmias. A retrospective analysis of the CAST data showed that mortality related to arrhythmias, as well as from all causes, was reduced in patients who received beta blockers. The Electrophysiologic Study versus Electrocardiographic Monitoring (ESVEM) trial compared seven antiarrhythmic drugs and found that the risk of arrhythmia recurrence and cardiac mortality was greater with the class I agents than with sotalol.

As mentioned, patients with a history of MI and ventricular arrhythmias have an increased risk of fatal arrhythmias during follow-up. Meta-analysis of 138 trials involving 98,000 patients showed increased mortality with class I drugs.[50] Beta blockers have been conclusively associated with short-term and long-term survival in this population.[51] Therefore, all such patients should receive a beta blocker unless it is specifically contraindicated. In contrast, evidence that class IA and class IC agents increase mortality suggests that these drugs should be avoided in MI patients. Class IV agents have shown neither benefit nor harm.

Amiodarone is not associated with a significant survival benefit in MI patients, nor does it seem to be associated with an increased risk of sudden death. For example, the randomized, double-blind, placebo-controlled Canadian Amiodarone Myocardial Infarction Arrhythmia Trial (CAMIAT) was conducted in 1,202 MI patients with frequent or repetitive ventricular premature depolarizations. Resuscitated ventricular fibrillation or arrhythmic death occurred in 6.9% of patients in the placebo group and in 4.5% of those in the amiodarone group.[52]

Treatment of ventricular arrhythmias in patients with chronic heart failure is particularly challenging. The presence of a reduced ejection fraction and ventricular ectopy significantly increases the risk of sudden death. No antiarrhythmic drug has been shown to produce a significant survival benefit in this population. The proarrhythmic and negative inotropic effects of class IA and class IC drugs preclude their use in these patients. Amiodarone, overall, appears to be neutral in its effects. The Survival Trial of Antiarrhythmic Therapy in Congestive Heart Failure did not show significantly greater improvement in survival in patients treated with amiodarone than in those who received placebo, despite an antiarrhythmic effect.[15] Similarly, in the European Myocardial Infarct Amiodarone Trial (EMIAT), a randomized, double-blind, placebo-controlled trial conducted in 1,486 MI survivors with an LVEF of 40% or less, neither all-cause mortality nor cardiac mortality differed between the amiodarone and the placebo groups. The investigators noted, however, that the 35% risk reduction in arrhythmic deaths in the amiodarone group support the use of amiodarone in patients for whom antiarrhythmic therapy is indicated.[53] Therefore, the only indication for the use of amiodarone in patients with chronic heart failure appears to be to suppress symptoms from frequent ectopy and nonsustained ventricular tachycardia. Improvement in survival requires ICD therapy.

Nonpharmacologic Therapy

SURGERY AND CATHETER ABLATION OF VENTRICULAR TACHYCARDIA

Surgical techniques for the treatment of ventricular tachycardia after MI were introduced in the late 1970s. However, these procedures are associated with relatively high perioperative mortality and require ventriculotomy, which can further compromise an already damaged ventricle. For these reasons, along with the increased simplicity of ICD implantation, surgical treatment is now rarely performed.

Radiofrequency catheter ablation has a role in selected patients with idiopathic ventricular tachycardia. Ablation is also useful for palliation in patients who have had an ICD implanted and are experiencing frequent shocks.

THE IMPLANTABLE CARDIOVERTER-DEFIBRILLATOR

The ICD automatically detects ventricular tachycardia or fibrillation and terminates the arrhythmia by overdrive pacing, high-energy shocks, or both. Since the first implantation of an ICD in a human, in 1980, the device has been utilized in hundreds of thousands of patients worldwide, and its use is growing exponentially.

All ICD systems contain three elements: the generator, rate-sensing leads, and electrodes to deliver high-energy shocks. In the early ICDs, defibrillating shocks were delivered via wire-mesh patch electrodes applied directly to the epicardial surface, and the generator was implanted subcutaneously in the abdomen. The implantation procedure required a thoracotomy and was associated with considerable morbidity and a perioperative mortality of 3% to 5%.[54] Current ICD models use transvenous leads, and the generator is implanted in a subcutaneous pocket in the anterior chest wall [see Figure 6].[55] ICD implantation is simple and safe, with a median duration of less than an hour and a median postoperative stay of 24 hours or less. The incidence of surgical complications is less than 2%—similar to that with routine pacemaker implantation.[55] As with modern pacemakers, the current generation of ICDs are multiprogrammable, microprocessor-based devices capable of automatically detecting ventricular tachycardia or fibrillation on the basis of timing information. The heart rate and duration of a tachycardia episode that will trigger overdrive pacing or shock therapy can be programmed. Additional detection enhancements can be used to reduce the probability that inappropriate pacing or shock will be delivered during episodes of sinus tachycardia or atrial fibrillation that exceed the programmed rate cutoff. The device can also be programmed to initiate therapy only if the heart rate increases abruptly during one cycle and only if the rate variability during the episode is less than a specified amount.

The ICD's output can also be tailored to suit patients' individual needs. For patients with a history of primary ventricular fibrillation, the ICD is programmed to deliver high-energy shocks when it detects tachycardia. Patients with a history of stable monomorphic ventricular tachycardia may benefit from overdrive pace termination. Cardioverting shocks will be delivered only if the specified number of pacing trains fails to terminate or if pacing accelerates the arrhythmia. Because overdrive pacing is associated

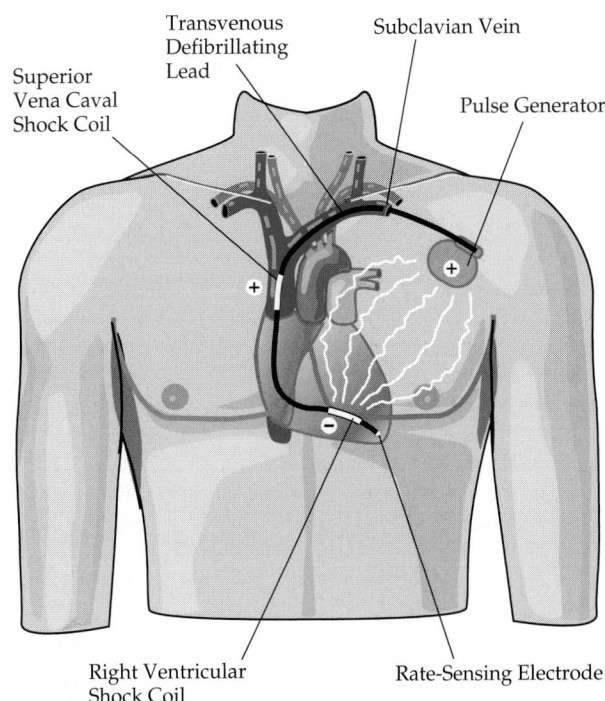

Figure 6 An implantable cardioverter-defibrillator (ICD) consists of a pulse generator and one or more leads for cardioversion and defibrillation. The pulse generator is usually installed in a subcutaneous pocket in the pectoral region. It comprises a battery, capacitors, memory chips, integrated circuits and microprocessors, and a telemetry module, which are sealed within a titanium casing. A transvenous defibrillating lead from the pulse generator is inserted into the subclavian vein and advanced into the apex of the right ventricle. When a persistent ventricular tachyarrhythmia with a rate faster than the programmed rate cutoff is detected by the rate-sensing electrode in the lead's tip, the device charges and delivers a high-voltage defibrillating shock. For this purpose, the shock coil in the right ventricle serves as the cathode, whereas the proximal shock coil in the superior vena cava portion of the lead, plus the metal casing of the generator, serve as the anode. In older ICD models, the metal casing alone serves as the anode.

with little or no discomfort, the device may be considered in patients with recurrent episodes of tolerated ventricular tachycardia.

The ICD also functions as a ventricular demand pacemaker, obviating a second device in patients with symptomatic bradyarrhythmias. This feature is also useful for prevention of the transitory bradycardia that sometimes occurs after delivery of a defibrillating shock.

The ICD has the capability of recording individual arrhythmia episodes. When tachycardia is detected, the device stores the electrograms in memory that can then be played back through the programmer at the time of a follow-up visit. This Holter function provides valuable diagnostic information regarding arrhythmia frequency, duration, rate, and response to therapy.

ICD Trials

ICDs were initially used for secondary prevention in survivors of cardiac arrest and in patients with documented life-threatening ventricular arrhythmias. Three large randomized trials have compared ICD therapy with pharmacologic treatment for the prevention of death in survivors of ventricular fibrillation or sustained ventricular tachycardia: the Antiarrhythmics vs Implantable Defibrillator (AVID) study,[56] the Cardiac Arrest Study

Table 2   Recommendations for Implantable Cardioverter-Defibrillator Therapy[66]

Recommendation Class	Indication	Level of Evidence
I	Cardiac arrest due to VF or VT not due to a transient or reversible cause	A
	Spontaneous sustained VT in association with structural heart disease	B
	Syncope of undetermined origin with clinically relevant, hemodynamically significant sustained VT or VF induced at electrophysiologic study when drug therapy is ineffective, not tolerated, or not preferred	B
	Nonsustained VT in patients with coronary disease, prior MI, LV dysfunction, and inducible VF or sustained VT at electrophysiologic study that is not suppressible by a class I antiarrhythmic drug	BA
	Spontaneous sustained VT in patients without structural heart disease not amenable to other treatments	C
IIa	LVEF ≤ 30% at least 1 mo after MI and 3 mo after coronary artery revascularization surgery	B
IIb	Cardiac arrest presumed to be due to VF when electrophysiologic testing is precluded by other medical conditions	C
	Severe symptoms (e.g., syncope) attributable to ventricular tachyarrhythmias in patients awaiting cardiac transplantation	C
	Familial or inherited conditions with a high risk for life-threatening ventricular tachyarrhythmias such as long QT syndrome or hypertrophic cardiomyopathy	B
	Nonsustained VT with coronary artery disease, prior MI, LV dysfunction, and inducible sustained VT or VF at electrophysiologic study	B
	Recurrent syncope of undetermined origin in the presence of ventricular dysfunction and inducible ventricular arrhythmias at electrophysiologic study when other causes of syncope have been excluded	C
	Syncope of unexplained origin or family history of unexplained sudden cardiac death in association with typical or atypical right bundle branch block and ST segment elevations (Brugada syndrome)	C
	Syncope in patients with advanced structural heart disease in whom thorough invasive and noninvasive investigations have failed to define a cause	C
III	Syncope of undetermined cause in a patient without inducible ventricular tachyarrhythmias and without structural heart disease	C
	Incessant VT or VF	C
	VF or VT resulting from arrhythmias amenable to surgical or catheter ablation (e.g., atrial arrhythmias associated with the Wolff-Parkinson-White syndrome, right ventricular outflow tract VT, idiopathic left ventricular tachycardia, or fascicular VT)	C
	Ventricular tachyarrhythmias due to a transient or reversible disorder (e.g., acute MI, electrolyte imbalance, drugs, or trauma) when correction of the disorder is considered feasible and likely to substantially reduce the risk of recurrent arrhythmia	CB
	Significant psychiatric illnesses that may be aggravated by device implantation or may preclude systematic follow-up	C
	Terminal illness with projected life expectancy less than 6 mo	C
	Patients with coronary artery disease with LV dysfunction and prolonged QRS duration in the absence of spontaneous or inducible sustained or nonsustained VT who are undergoing coronary bypass surgery	B
	NYHA class IV drug-refractory congestive heart failure in patients who are not candidates for cardiac transplantation	C

LV—left ventricular   LVEF—left ventricular ejection fraction   MI—myocardial infarction   NYHA—New York Heart Association   VF—ventricular fibrillation   VT—ventricular tachycardia

Hamburg (CASH),[57] and the Canadian Implantable Defibrillator Study (CIDS).[58] A meta-analysis of the three trials showed consistent benefit from ICDs: patients who received ICDs had a significant reduction in death from any cause, with a summary hazard ratio (ICD:amiodarone) of 0.72; for arrhythmic death, the hazard ratio was 0.50.[59] Furthermore, 11-year follow-up of a subset of CIDS patients found that the benefit of the ICD over amiodarone increases with time; eventually, most amiodarone-treated patients develop side effects, experience recurrences of arrhythmia, or die.[60]

More recently, ICDs have been used for the primary prevention of sudden death. The first Multicenter Automatic Defibrillator Implantation Trial (MADIT I) compared ICD therapy with conventional medical therapy in MI patients with reduced ejection fraction, nonsustained ventricular tachycardia, and inducible nonsuppressible ventricular tachycardia on electrophysiologic testing. MADIT I showed that compared with conventional therapy, ICD therapy saved lives, with an ICD to non-ICD hazard ratio of 0.46.[61] The magnitude of the survival benefit increased with the severity of cardiac dysfunction.[62]

To study the role of ICDs in primary prevention, MADIT II enrolled MI patients with advanced left ventricular dysfunction (LVEF, 30% or less) who did not necessarily have manifest or inducible ventricular tachycardia. ICD implantation also increased survival in this population: over 20 months of follow-up, the ICD to non-ICD hazard ratio for death from any cause was 0.69.[63]

Additional trials have been performed to determine whether prophylactic ICD implantation is beneficial in all patients with chronic heart failure of any cause, ischemic or nonischemic. In the Sudden Cardiac Death in Heart Failure Trial (SCD-HeFT), patients were evenly divided between those with ischemic and those with nonischemic cardiomyopathy. Patients who were receiving conventional treatment for heart failure were randomly assigned to supplemental therapy with amiodarone, placebo, or an ICD. Amiodarone did not increase survival, but simple, shock-only ICDs decreased mortality by 23%. The protective effect of the device was independent of the cause of the heart failure.[64] The Comparison of Medical Therapy, Pacing and Defibrillation in Heart Failure (COMPANION) trial was designed to compare medical therapy with a biventricular pacemaker and with a ventricular ICD in patients with advanced chronic heart failure and a wide QRS. Cardiac resynchronization with a biventricular pacemaker improved outcome, compared with medical therapy. Compared with biventricular pacing, biventricular ICD had an additional 21% survival benefit.[65]

Indications for ICD Implantation

Guidelines for the selection of patients for ICD implantation have been developed by the American College of Cardiology, the American Heart Association, and the National Association for Sport & Physical Education [see Table 2].[66] Since the 2002 revision of these guidelines, the indications for ICD implantation have expanded to include patients with nonischemic cardiomyopathy and an LVEF of less than 30%, even in the absence of symptomatic arrhythmias.[64]

AUTOMATED EXTERNAL DEFIBRILLATORS

An automated external defibrillator (AED) is a compact, easily portable device that can automatically analyze a patient's cardiac rhythm and, if it detects ventricular fibrillation, direct the rescuer to apply a shock. AEDs require minimal training to operate and are achieving widespread distribution.

Public-Access AEDs

AEDs can now be found in many public places, such as airports, stadiums, casinos, and large office buildings. Preliminary data suggest that these devices may confer a survival benefit,[67] although cost-effectiveness is difficult to calculate. It seems safe to say that the availability of public-access AEDs will result in increased numbers of patients successfully resuscitated from cardiac arrest, who will then require follow-up treatment.

Home AEDs

The FDA has approved several AED models for consumer use in the home, without a prescription, and these devices are now being marketed directly to the public for this purpose. The utility of home AEDs is uncertain, but the patients for whom these devices should be considered are those who meet the criteria for prophylactic ICD therapy but either have declined the implantation procedure or have comorbidities that make the implantation procedure inadvisable. The cost-effectiveness of these devices will be difficult to measure, and the potential medicolegal liability issues involved may be complex.

Wearable Automatic Defibrillators

An automatic defibrillator that is worn as a vest has been approved by the FDA.[68] This device is typically worn by patients who are awaiting heart transplants or who recently experienced an MI or underwent coronary revascularization. At our institution, we have used the device to provide temporary prophylaxis for a patient who required removal of an ICD because of site infection.

The authors serve as clinical investigators for Medtronic, Inc, Guidant Corporation, and St. Jude Medical, Inc.

References

1. Zipes DP: An overview of arrhythmias and antiarrhythmic approaches. J Cardiovasc Electrophysiol 10:267, 1999

2. de Bakker JM, van Capelle FLJ, Janse MJ, et al: Reentry as a cause of ventricular tachycardia in patients with chronic ischemic heart disease: electrophysiological and anatomic correlation. Circulation 77:589, 1988

3. de Bakker JM, Coronel R, Tasseron S, et al: Ventricular tachycardia in the infarcted, Langendorff-perfused human heart: role of the arrangement of surviving cardiac fibers. J Am Coll Cardiol 15:1594, 1990

4. Callans DJ, Josephson ME: Ventricular tachycardias in the setting of coronary artery disease. Cardiac Electrophysiology: From Cell to Bedside. Zipes DP, Jalife J, Eds. WB Saunders Co, Philadelphia, 1995, p 732

5. Kenknight BH, Bayly PV, Gerstle RJ, et al: Regional capture of fibrillating ventricular myocardium: evidence of an excitable gap. Circ Res 77:849, 1995

6. Haissaguerre M, Shoda M, Jais P, et al: Mapping and ablation of idiopathic ventricular fibrillation. Circulation 106:962, 2002

7. Caceres J, Jazayeri M, McKinnie J, et al: Sustained bundle branch reentry as a mechanism of clinical tachycardia. Circulation 79:256, 1989

8. Kaplinsky E, Ogawa S, Michelson EL, et al: Instantaneous and delayed ventricular arrhythmias after reperfusion of acutely ischemic myocardium: evidence for multiple mechanisms. Circulation 63:333, 1981

9. Wall TS, Freedman RA: Ventricular tachycardia in structurally normal hearts. Curr Cardiol Rep 4:388, 2002

10. Nibley C, Wharton JM: Ventricular tachycardias with left bundle branch block morphology. Pacing Clin Electrophysiol 18:334, 1995

11. Ohe T, Shimomura K, Aihara N, et al: Idiopathic left ventricular tachycardia: clinical and electrophysiological characteristics. Circulation 77:560, 1988

12. Gordon T, Kannel WB: Premature mortality from coronary heart disease: the Framingham Study. JAMA 215:1617, 1971

13. Myerburg RJ, Kessler KM, Castellanos A: Sudden cardiac death: epidemiology, transient risk and intervention assessment. Ann Intern Med 119:1187, 1993

14. Doval HC, Nul DR, Grancelli HO, et al: Randomized trial of low-dose amiodarone in severe congestive heart failure. Lancet 344:493, 1994

15. Singh SN, Fletcher RD, Fisher SG, et al: Amiodarone in patients with congestive heart failure and asymptomatic ventricular arrhythmia. Survival Trial of Antiarrhythmic Therapy in Congestive Heart Failure. N Engl J Med 333:77, 1995

16. Breithardt G, Schwarzmaier J, Borggrefe M, et al: Prognostic significance of late ventricular potentials after acute myocardial infarction. Eur Heart J 4:487, 1983

17. Hohnloser SH, Klingenheben T, Li YG, et al: T wave alternans as a predictor of recurrent ventricular tachyarrhythmias in ICD recipients: prospective comparison with conventional risk markers. J Cardiovasc Electrophysiol 9:1258, 1998

18. Kunavarapu C, Bloomfield DM: Role of noninvasive studies in risk stratification for sudden cardiac death. Clin Cardiol 27:192, 2004

19. Schnipper JL, Kapoor WK: Diagnostic evaluation and management of patients with syncope. Med Clin North Am 85:423, 2001

20. Krol RB, Morady FF, Flaker GC, et al: Electrophysiological testing in patients with unexplained syncope: clinical and noninvasive predictors of outcome. J Am Coll Cardiol 10:358, 1987

21. Denes P, Ezri MD: The role of electrophysiological studies in the management of patients with unexplained syncope. Pacing Clin Electrophysiol 8:424, 1985

22. Zheng ZJ, Croft JB, Giles WH, et al: Sudden cardiac death in the United States, 1989 to 1998. Circulation 104:2158, 2001

23. Bardy GH, Olsen WH: Clinical characteristics of spontaneous-onset sustained VT and VF in survivors of cardiac arrest. Cardiac Electrophysiology: From Cell to Bedside. Zipes DP, Jalife J, Eds. WB Saunders Co, Philadelphia, 1995, p 778

24. Brodsky MA, Mitchell LB, Halperin BD, et al: Prognostic value of baseline electrophysiology studies in patients with sustained ventricular tachyarrhythmia: the Antiarrhythmics Versus Implantable Defibrillators (AVID) trial. Am Heart J 144:478, 2002

25. Roden DM: Drug-induced prolongation of the QT interval. N Engl J Med 350:1013, 2004

26. Wehrens XH, Vos MA, Doevendans PA, et al: Novel insights in the congenital long QT syndrome. Ann Intern Med 137:981, 2002

27. Chiang CE: Congenital and acquired long QT syndrome: current concepts and management. Cardiol Rev 12:222, 2004

28. Schwartz PJ: The long QT syndrome. Curr Probl Cardiol 22:297, 1997

29. Khan IA: Long QT syndrome: diagnosis and management. Am Heart J 143:7, 2002

30. Brugada P, Brugada J: Right bundle branch block, persistent ST segment elevation and sudden cardiac death: a distinct clinical and electrocardiographic syndrome: a multicenter report. J Am Coll Cardiol 20:1391, 1992

31. Hermida JS, Lemoine JL, Aoun FB, et al: Prevalence of the Brugada syndrome in an apparently healthy population. Am J Cardiol 86:91, 2000

32. Wilde AA, Antzelevitch C, Borggrefe M, et al: Proposed diagnostic criteria for the Brugada syndrome. Eur Heart J 23:1648, 2000

33. Brugada R, Hong K, Dumaine R, et al: Idiopathic short QT interval: a new clinical syndrome? Cardiology 94:99, 2000

34. Faita F, Giustetto C, Bianchi F, et al: Short QT syndrome: a familial cause of sudden death. Circulation 108:965, 2003

35. Brugada R, Hong K, Dumaine R, et al: Sudden death associated with short-QT syndrome linked to mutations in HERG. Circulation 109:30, 2004

36. Singh SN, Patrick J, Patrick J: Antiarrhythmic drugs. Curr Treat Options Cardiovasc Med 6:357, 2004

37. Vaughan Williams EM: Cardiac Arrhythmias. Sandoe E, Fiensted-Jensen E, Olson KH, Eds. Astra, Sodertalje, Sweden, 1970, p 449

38. Singh BN, Opie LH, Marcus FI: Antiarrhythmic agents. Drugs for the Heart, Third Edition. Opie LH, Ed. WB Saunders Co, Philadelphia, 1991, p 180

39. Opie LH: The Heart: Physiology, Metabolism, Pharmacology and Therapy. Grune & Stratton, Orlando, 1984

40. Olschewski A, Brau ME, Olschewski H, et al: ATP-dependent potassium channel in rat cardiomyocytes is blocked by lidocaine. Circulation 93:656, 1996

41. Cowan JC, Vaughan Williams EM: Characterization of a new oral antiarrhythmic drug, flecainide (R818). Eur J Pharmacol 73:333, 1981

42. Ikeda N, Singh BN, Davis LD, et al: Effects of flecainide on the electrophysiological properties of isolated canine and rabbit myocardial fibers. J Am Coll Cardiol 5:303, 1985

43. Expert consensus document of beta-adrenergic receptor blockers. Task Force on Beta-Blockers of the European Society of Cardiology. Eur Heart J 25:1341, 2004

44. Takanaka C, Singh BN: Barium induced nondriver action potential as a model of triggered potentials from early afterdepolarizations: significance of slow channel activity and differing effects of quinidine and amiodarone. J Am Coll Cardiol 15:213, 1990

45. Gaita F, Giustetto C, Leclercq JF, et al: Idiopathic verapamil-responsive left ventricular tachycardia: clinical characteristics and long-term follow-up of 33 patients. Eur Heart J 15:1252, 1994

46. Waldo AL, Camm AJ, deRuyter H, et al: Survival with oral d-sotalol in patients with left ventricular dysfunction after myocardial infarction: rationale, design, and methods (the SWORD trial). Am J Cardiol 75:1023, 1995

47. Levine JH, Morganroth J, Kadish AH: Mechanisms and risk factors for proarrhythmia with type Ia compared with Ic antiarrhythmic drug therapy. Circulation 80:1063, 1989

48. Chaudhry GM, Haffajee CI : Antiarrhythmic agents and proarrhythmia. Crit Care Med 28(10 suppl):N158, 2000

49. Preliminary report: effect of encainide and flecainide on mortality in a randomized trial of arrhythmia suppression after myocardial infarction. The Cardiac Arrhythmia Suppression Trial (CAST) investigators. N Engl J Med 321:406, 1989

50. Teo KK, Yusuf S, Furburg CD: Effects of prophylactic antiarrhythmic drug therapy in acute myocardial infarction. JAMA 270:1589, 1993

51. Kennedy HL, Brooks MM, Barker AH, et al: Beta blocker therapy in the Cardiac Arrhythmia Suppression Trial. CAST Investigators. Am J Cardiol 74:674, 1994

52. Cairns JA, Connolly SJ, Roberts R, et al: Randomised trial of outcome after myocardial infarction in patients with frequent or repetitive ventricular premature depolarisations: CAMIAT. Canadian Amiodarone Myocardial Infarction Arrhythmia Trial Investigators. Lancet 349:675, 1997

53. Julian DG, Camm AJ, Frangin G, et al: Randomised trial of effect of amiodarone on mortality in patients with left-ventricular dysfunction after recent myocardial infarc-tion: EMIAT. European Myocardial Infarct Amiodarone Trial Investigators. Lancet 349:667, 1997

54. Bardy GH, Hofer B, Johnson G, et al: Implantable transvenous cardioverter-defibrillators. Circulation 87:1152, 1993

55. DiMarco JP: Implantable cardioverter-defibrillators. N Engl J Med 349:1836, 2003

56. A comparison of antiarrhythmic-drug therapy with implantable defibrillators in patients resuscitated from near-fatal ventricular arrhythmias. The Antiarrhythmics versus Implantable Defibrillators (AVID) Investigators. N Engl J Med 337:1576, 1997

57. Kuck KH, Cappato R, Siebels J, et al: Randomized comparison of antiarrhythmic drug therapy with implantable defibrillators in patients resuscitated from cardiac arrest: the Cardiac Arrest Study Hamburg (CASH). Circulation 102:748, 2000

58. Connolly SJ, Gent M, Roberts RS, et al: Canadian implantable defibrillator study (CIDS): a randomized trial of the implantable cardioverter defibrillator against amiodarone. Circulation 101:1297, 2000

59. Connolly SJ, Hallstrom AP, Cappato R, et al: Meta-analysis of the implantable cardioverter defibrillator secondary prevention trials: AVID, CASH and CIDS studies. Eur Heart J 21:2071, 2000

60. Bokhari F, Newman D, Greene M, et al: Long-term comparison of the implantable cardioverter defibrillator versus amiodarone: eleven-year follow-up of a subset of patients in the Canadian Implantable Defibrillator Study (CIDS). Circulation 110:112, 2004

61. Moss AJ, Hall WJ, Cannom DS, et al: Improved survival with an implanted defibrillator in patients with coronary disease at high risk for ventricular arrhythmia. Multicenter Automatic Defibrillator Implantation Trial Investigators. N Engl J Med 335:1933, 1996

62. Moss AJ, Fadl Y, Zareba W, et al: Survival benefit with an implanted defibrillator in relation to mortality risk in chronic coronary heart disease. Am J Cardiol 88:516, 2001

63. Moss AJ, Zareba W, Hall WJ, et al: Prophylactic implantation of a defibrillator in patients with myocardial infarction and reduced ejection fraction. Multicenter Automatic Defibrillator Implantation Trial II Investigators. N Engl J Med 346:877, 2002

64. Bardy GH, Lee KL, Mark DB, et al: Amiodarone or an implantable cardioverter-defibrillator for congestive heart failure. N Engl J Med 352:225, 2005

65. Bristow MR, Saxon LA, Boehmer J, et al: Cardiac-resynchronization therapy with or without an implantable defibrillator in advanced chronic heart failure. Comparison of Medical Therapy, Pacing, and Defibrillation in Heart Failure (COMPANION) Investigators. N Engl J Med 350:2140, 2004

66. ACC/AHA/NSAPE 2002 Guideline Update for Implantation of Cardiac Pacemakers and Antiarrhythmia Devices: a report of the American College of Cardiology/American Heart Association Task Force on Practice Guidelines (ACC/AHA/NASPE Committee on Implantation). American College of Cardiology, 2002 http://www.acc.org/clinical/guidelines/pacemaker/II_implantable.htm

67. Caffrey SL, Willoughby PJ, Pepe PE, et al: Public use of automated external defibrillators. N Engl J Med 347:1242, 2002

68. Auricchio A, Klein H, Geller CJ, et al: Clinical efficacy of the wearable cardioverter-defibrillator in acutely terminating episodes of ventricular fibrillation. Am J Cardiol 81:1253, 1998

Acknowledgments

Figures 1, 2, and 7   Joseph Bloch, CMI.

Figures 3 through 6   Marcia Kammerer.

22　Pacemaker Therapy

Jonathan Lowy, M.D., and Roger A. Freedman, M.D.

Worldwide, more than 250,000 permanent cardiac pacemakers are implanted each year. As the population ages and as indications for pacemakers expand, the number of implants continues to increase. Advances in technology have played an important role in the evolution of pacemaker therapy: currently available pacemakers are smaller and more reliable than older models and contain a multitude of sophisticated programmable features.

Normal Cardiac Electrical System

The primary role of cardiac pacing is to augment or replace the heart's intrinsic electrical system. This specialized system consists of structures capable of automaticity and conduction and provides the timing and synchrony needed to maintain appropriate cardiac output.

SINOATRIAL NODE

In normal circumstances, the sinoatrial (SA) node (also referred to as the sinus node) is the origin of impulse generation and dictates the intrinsic heart rate. The SA node is located in the superior aspect of the right atrium. It is composed of specialized tissue that demonstrates the fastest rate of spontaneous depolarization (automaticity) of any of the cardiac tissues.

ATRIOVENTRICULAR NODE

The atrioventricular (AV) node is the junction between the atria and the ventricular conduction system. This node is a dense and complex structure that plays three important roles. First, it demonstrates spontaneous depolarization and is capable of acting as an auxiliary pacemaker. Second, it delays propagation of the impulse between the atria and the ventricles, thereby allowing normal atrioventricular synchrony. Third, it acts as a filter, limiting the number of impulses that can be propagated from the atria to the ventricles and protecting the heart from rapid ventricular rates.

HIS-PURKINJE SYSTEM

The His-Purkinje system originates at the inferior border of the AV node. From this point, the bundle of His courses down the interventricular septum, where it diverges into the left and right bundle branches and terminates in the Purkinje fiber network. The bundle of His and the bundle branches provide rapid and synchronous depolarization of the ventricles. The Purkinje fibers serve as the interface between the specialized conduction system and the local ventricular myocardium.

MODULATION OF HEART RATE

The basal heart rate is maintained by the balance between sympathetic and parasympathetic tone. Changes in the heart rate are mediated by the autonomic nervous system and circulating catecholamines. There is a normal physiologic acceleration of the heart rate that results from increased demand for cardiac output. This acceleration is mediated by both increased sympathetic tone and reduced parasympathetic tone. Inability to increase the heart rate in response to increased demand for cardiac output can result in a number of symptoms, including fatigue, poor exercise tolerance, and exertional dyspnea.

Disruption or imbalance of sympathetic and parasympathetic inputs to the SA node or the AV node can cause profound abnormalities in the heart rate, resulting in inappropriate increases or decreases that give rise to significant symptoms. SA node dysfunction may be caused by intrinsic abnormalities of the conduction system or by imbalances in autonomic tone.

Indications for Permanent Pacing

GENERAL CONSIDERATIONS

The cardiac conduction system can be affected by any of a wide variety of pathologic states, ranging from benign abnormalities to conditions that can lead to severe symptoms and substantial morbidity and mortality.

Guidelines for permanent pacemaker implantation were established by a joint task force of the American College of Cardiology and the American Heart Association and were first published in 1984.[1] These guidelines were subsequently revised in 1991,[2] 1998,[3] and 2002.[4] The North American Society of Pacing and Electrophysiology (NASPE) was also involved in the 2002 revision [see Table 1]. Current recommendations are divided into the following three broad categories on the basis of (1) the strength of the available data and (2) the consensus of experts in the field:

- Class I: conditions for which there is evidence or general agreement that a given procedure or treatment is beneficial, useful, and effective.
- Class II: conditions for which there is conflicting evidence or a divergence of opinion about the usefulness or efficacy of a procedure or treatment.
  IIa: conditions for which the weight of the evidence or expert opinion is in favor of usefulness/efficacy.
  IIb: conditions for which usefulness or efficacy is less well established by evidence or opinion.
- Class III: conditions for which there is evidence or general agreement that a procedure or treatment is not useful or effective and, in some cases, may be harmful.

GUIDELINES FOR SPECIFIC PACEMAKER INDICATIONS

Acquired Atrioventricular Block

AV block is defined as delayed or failed conduction from the atria to the ventricles.[5-9] It is usually categorized as occurring either at or below the level of the AV node. First-degree AV block describes conduction delay from the sinus impulse to the ventricles and is defined as prolongation of the PR interval without a dropped QRS complex. Usually, first-degree AV block occurs at the level of the AV node, though it may also occur in the His-Purkinje system.

Second-degree AV block is present when some, but not all, P waves are conducted to the ventricles. It can be further subdivided into Mobitz type I (Wenckebach) and Mobitz type II. In type I second-degree AV block, there is a progressive prolongation of the PR interval preceding a nonconducted P wave. The anatom-

Table 1   Guidelines for Permanent Pacemaker Implantation

Condition	Indications for Pacing			
	Class I	Class IIa	Class IIb	Class III
Acquired AV block	Third-degree AV block or advanced second-degree AV block associated with any of the following: Symptomatic bradycardia Medical conditions requiring medications that result in symptomatic bradycardia (e.g., beta blockers, calcium channel blockers, antiarrhythmic agents) Asymptomatic asystole ≥ 3 sec or escape rate < 40 beats/min in awake patient Ablation of AV junction Postoperative AV block not expected to resolve after cardiac surgery Neuromuscular disease, including myotonic muscular dystrophy, Kearns-Sayre syndrome, Erb dystrophy, and peroneal muscular atrophy, with or without symptoms of bradycardia Second-degree AV block, regardless of type, with documented associated bradycardia	Asymptomatic third-degree AV block with average ventricular rate ≥ 40 beats/min when awake Asymptomatic type II second-degree AV block with narrow QRS complex Asymptomatic type I second-degree AV block found during electrophysiologic study performed for another reason First- or second-degree AV block with symptoms similar to those of pacemaker syndrome	Marked first-degree AV delay > 30 msec in patients with left ventricular dysfunction and congestive symptoms of heart failure Neuromuscular disease, including myotonic muscular dystrophy, Kearns-Sayre syndrome, Erb dystrophy, and peroneal muscular atrophy, with any degree of AV block, with or without symptoms	Asymptomatic first-degree AV block Asymptomatic type I (Wenckebach) second-degree AV block Any AV block that is expected to resolve and does not
Chronic bifascicular and trifascicular block	Intermittent third-degree AV block Type II second-degree AV block Alternating bundle-branch block	Syncope in which other causes (specifically, ventricular tachycardia) have been excluded but that has not been demonstrated to be due to AV block Asymptomatic patients in whom electrophysiologic study reveals prolonged HV interval Electrophysiologic study finding of nonphysiologic block below His bundle	Neuromuscular diseases with any degree of fascicular block, with or without symptoms, in which there is unpredictable progression	Fascicular block without AV block or symptoms Fascicular block with first-degree AV block without symptoms
Myocardial infarction	Persistent second-degree AV block in His-Purkinje system with bifascicular block or third-degree AV block within or below His-Purkinje system after acute MI Persistent and symptomatic second- or third-degree AV block Transient advanced second- or third-degree infranodal AV block and associated bundle-branch block; electrophysiologic study may be indicated to identify level of block	None	Persistent second- or third-degree block at level of AV node	Transient AV block in absence of intraventricular conduction delay Transient AV block in presence of isolated left anterior fascicular block Acquired left anterior hemiblock in absence of AV block Persistent first-degree AV block in presence of old bundle-branch block
SA node dysfunction	SA node dysfunction with documented symptomatic bradycardia Symptomatic SA node dysfunction resulting in bradycardia that occurs as consequence of essential drug therapy to which there is no acceptable alternative Symptomatic chronotropic incompetence	SA node dysfunction occurring either spontaneously or as a result of drug therapy with heart rates < 40 beats/min where there is clear association between symptoms but where actual presence of bradycardia during symptoms has not been documented Syncope of unexplained origin in which major abnormalities of SA node are elicited during electrophysiologic studies	Patients with minimal symptoms with resting heart rates < 40 beats/min while awake	Asymptomatic patients, including those on drug therapy with resting heart rates < 40 beats/min Patients with symptoms of bradycardia in which SA node dysfunction is clearly not associated with symptoms SA node dysfunction with symptomatic bradycardia caused by unnecessary drug therapy
Neurocardiogenic syncope and hypersensitive carotid sinus syndrome	Recurrent syncope caused by carotid sinus massage that results in ventricular asystole ≥ 3 sec (must occur in absence of any medication that depresses SA node or AV conduction)	Recurrent syncope without another cause and cardioinhibitory response to carotid sinus massage Symptomatic and recurrent neurocardiogenic syncope associated with documented bradycardia	None	Hyperactive cardioinhibitory response to carotid sinus massage in absence of symptoms or in presence of vague symptoms Recurrent symptoms in absence of documented cardioinhibitory response Situational vasovagal syncope in which avoiding behavior or environmental factors is effective

ic site of the block is usually the AV node, and the QRS complex is usually narrow. In type II second-degree AV block, there is a fixed PR interval preceding the dropped QRS complex. Type II block is often accompanied by bundle branch block, and its anatomic location is usually below the AV node in the His-Purkinje system.

When every other P wave is conducted, 2:1 AV block is present; 2:1 block cannot be classified as either type I or type II block, because there are not consecutive PR intervals preceding the nonconducted P wave. When 2:1 block is accompanied by bundle branch block, the site of the block is likely to be below the AV node in the His-Purkinje system. High-degree (or advanced) type II AV block is defined as blockage of two or more consecutive P waves. Complete heart block, or third-degree block, denotes a complete absence of conduction from the atria to the ventricles.

The anatomic location of AV block has important prognostic implications. Typically, a block occurring at the level of the AV node—such as first-degree block, type I second-degree block, and 2:1 block at the level of the AV node—does not typically lead to abrupt complete heart block, though gradual progression is common. A block occurring below the level of the AV node, on the other hand, can often progress quickly to complete heart block. In addition, high-degree or complete heart block at the level of the AV node is often ameliorated by junctional escape rhythms, whereas escape rhythms are much less reliable when the block is at the level of the His-Purkinje system.

Chronic Bifascicular and Trifascicular Block

The conduction system below the AV node is composed of three fascicles: the right bundle branch, the left anterior fascicle, and the left posterior fascicle. The left anterior and left posterior fascicles are divisions of the left bundle branch. Bifascicular block denotes blockage of the right bundle and either the left anterior or the left posterior fascicle; trifascicular block is present when alternating bundle branch block is seen or when right bundle branch block occurs in conjunction with alternating left anterior and left posterior hemiblock.[10] Trifascicular block may also be present when bifascicular block is accompanied by first-degree AV block. More commonly, however, this electrocardiogram pattern is the result of bifascicular block combined with conduction delay at the AV node.

Acute Myocardial Infarction

Conduction abnormalities are common in the setting of acute myocardial infarction.[11-15] Pathophysiologic mechanisms include ischemia, necrosis, autonomic influences, and the neurohumoral response to injury. Temporary transvenous pacing is often required during the acute phase of an infarction. The need for temporary pacing does not, however, predict the need for permanent pacing, given that many of the conduction abnormalities are transient and resolve after revascularization or upon recovery from the acute phase of the infarction.

Patients with acute inferior infarction can manifest a variety of abnormalities, including SA node dysfunction, first-degree AV block, type I second-degree block, and third-degree block at the level of the AV node. It is uncommon for any of these conduction disturbances to persist after the acute phase of the infarction. These patients often require temporary pacing if they manifest hemodynamic instability, but they rarely require permanent pacing.

Patients with anterior infarction can manifest bundle branch block, bifascicular block, trifascicular block, type II second-de-

gree block, or complete heart block. These patients are much more likely to require permanent pacing than those with inferior infarction are. Although conduction abnormalities are associated with higher mortality in the setting of anterior infarction, the increased mortality is a consequence of the larger infarct size and is not directly related to the conduction abnormality.

SA Node Dysfunction

SA node dysfunction is a loose term that includes a number of different arrhythmias, including sinus bradycardia, sinus arrest, sinoatrial block, and the bradycardia-tachycardia syndrome.[16-20] The bradycardia-tachycardia syndrome is characterized by atrial tachyarrhythmias (usually atrial fibrillation) alternating with periods of bradycardia or sinus pauses. SA node dysfunction must be differentiated from the physiologic sinus bradycardia seen in trained athletes. During sleep, sinus rates as low as 30 beats/min and type I second-degree AV block are commonly seen in normal persons.

Pacing for Neurocardiogenic Syncope and Hypersensitive Carotid Syndrome

Neurocardiogenic syncope is syncope secondary to vasodilatation or bradyarrhythmias resulting from abrupt imbalance of autonomic input to the heart and the vascular system.[21-25] Classic neurocardiogenic syncope involves sinus tachycardia followed by bradycardia, vasodilatation, and syncope. Some patients have primarily a vasodepressive (vasodilatation) syndrome, whereas others have a syndrome with a significant cardioinhibitory component (bradycardia). Thus, bradycardia is not always a contributing component in neurocardiogenic syncope. Head-up tilt testing is often useful for diagnosing the presence and type of neurocardiogenic syncope.

The hypersensitive carotid syndrome is characterized by a similar abnormal response of the autonomic nervous system, in which baroreceptors in the carotid sinus trigger a vasodepressive or cardioinhibitory response. A hyperactive carotid sinus response is defined as a sinus pause longer than 3 seconds or a substantial symptomatic decrease in systolic blood pressure.

Other Pacemaker Indications

Besides those already mentioned, there are several indications for which pacemakers are implanted that warrant mention, including treatment of hypertrophic cardiomyopathy, prevention or suppression of tachyarrhythmias, and resynchronization therapy for congestive heart failure. Cardiac resynchronization therapy is an exciting new development in the treatment of heart failure but lies outside the scope of this chapter.

Pacemaker Systems

A basic pacemaker system is made up of three main components: the pulse generator, the pacemaker lead(s), and the programmer.

PULSE GENERATOR

Over the past 30 years, pulse generators have evolved from large, bulky devices into small, sophisticated systems [*see Figure 1*]. All pulse generators contain hardware, software, and a battery; however, the systems currently available can differ from one another with respect to a number of factors, including number of chambers, biventricular pacing capability, presence and type of activity sensor, size, battery life, and cost. All of these fac-

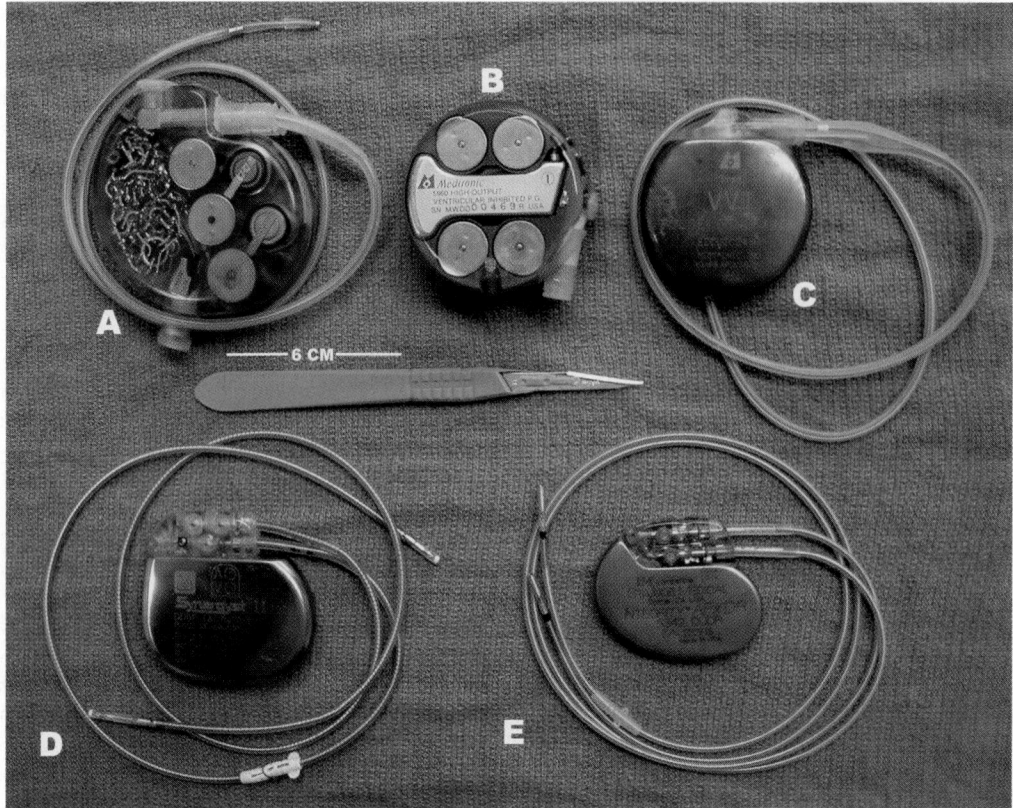

Figure 1 Shown are five different pacemaker generators. The first three are older single-chamber devices from (*a*) 1972, (*b*) 1977, and (*c*) 1983. The last two are modern dual-chamber devices from (*d*) 1994 and (*e*) 2000.

tors are taken into account in selecting a specific generator for a specific patient.

Generators are usually described as being either single-chamber or dual-chamber. Single-chamber systems have one lead, which is usually placed in the right ventricle (though it may, on occasion, be placed in the atrium). Dual-chamber systems have two leads, one of which is implanted in the right atrium and the other in the right ventricle. The biventricular pacemaker devices currently used in patients with heart failure have a third lead that is usually placed in a branch of the coronary sinus to provide left ventricular pacing. Dual-chamber systems can be programmed to single-chamber modes of operation.

At present, most generators currently use lithium iodine batteries that have a typical life span of 5 to 10 years. These batteries are not rechargeable or replaceable; accordingly, when the battery reaches the end of its life, a new generator must be implanted.

PACEMAKER LEADS

Pacemaker leads are the conduits from the generator to the myocardium. Most leads are implanted transvenously. There are still occasional applications for epicardial leads, but these are generally limited to patients with mechanical tricuspid valves, certain congenital heart abnormalities, or other conditions that preclude transvenous leads. Like pulse generators, leads have gone through a complex evolution since they were first developed. Various types are currently used [*see Figure 2*]; the major differences among them have to do with type of insulation, fixation mechanism, and polarity.

Most pacemaker leads are insulated with either silicone or polyurethane. In the past, there were significant differences between the two materials with respect to durability and handling. Today, however, the differences are minimal, and the choice of material is usually operator dependent.

Leads can be attached to the myocardium via either passive or active fixation. Passive-fixation leads usually have tines at the distal tip to help maintain stability. Active-fixation leads have a corkscrew helix mechanism at the distal end, which inserts into the myocardium. Both fixation mechanisms are reliable, and lead dislodgment is uncommon with either one.

Finally, leads can be either unipolar or bipolar. Unipolar leads have a single conductor and a single electrode; the unipolar pacing circuit involves the single electrode and the metal housing of the generator. Bipolar leads have two conductors and two electrodes; the pacing circuit is between the two electrodes. Advantages of unipolar leads include decreased diameter and reduced susceptibility to lead fracture. Advantages of bipolar leads include reduced risk of inappropriate sensing of myopotentials, greater resistance to electromagnetic interference (EMI), less likelihood of pectoral muscle stimulation, and better compatibility with implanted defibrillators. At present, bipolar leads are more commonly used, but unipolar leads are still employed on occasion.

Currently available lead systems are very reliable: failure rates at 5 years are typically 5% or lower.

PACEMAKER PROGRAMMER

The programming computer allows telemetric communication with the implanted pulse generator and serves as the interface between the health care provider and the pacemaker. Because there is no standardization among pacemaker manufacturers, each company's device requires its own programmer.

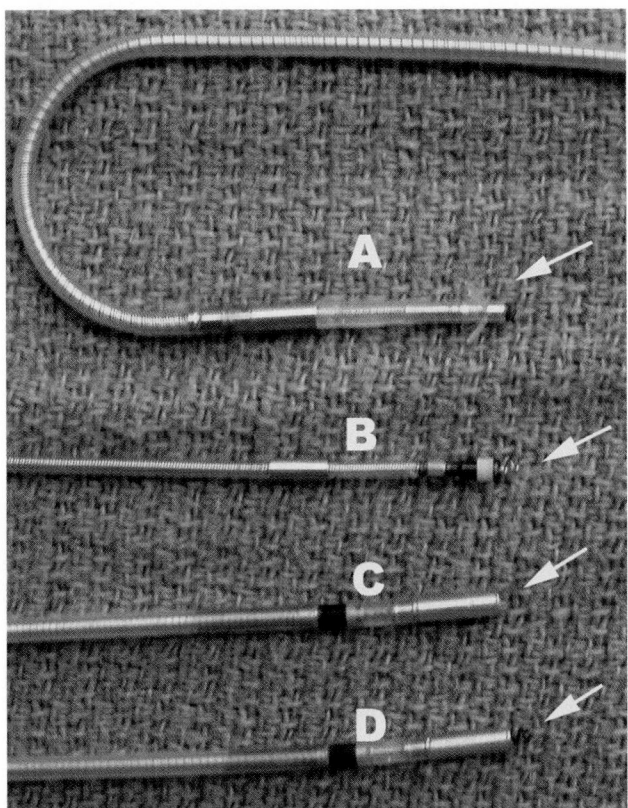

Figure 2 **Shown are four different pacemaker leads. The first (*a*) is a passive-fixation lead with soft tines at the tip (arrow); it is also a preformed J lead used for atrial pacing. The second (*b*) is an active-fixation lead with a fixed helix. The third (*c*) and fourth (*d*) are active-fixation leads with a retractable helix; the fourth has the helix mechanism exposed.**

Programmers are equipped with a wand that provides external telemetry through the skin, thus allowing direct communication with the pacemaker generator and access to the software contained within it. The pacemaker programmer is used to perform a multitude of functions, including assessing battery status, modifying pacemaker settings, and providing access to diagnostic information the pacemaker has stored (e.g., heart rate trends and tachyarrhythmia documentation).

PACEMAKER MAGNETS

Pacemaker generators are designed to respond to the placement of a strong magnet over the device. The response of most pacemakers is to pace at a set "magnet rate" in an asynchronous

mode. Magnets also can be used to perform any of a number of functions designated by the manufacturer, including checking battery life, threshold testing, and obtaining event snapshots (in much the same way as an event monitor). Magnets should be available in the hospital and clinic, as well as on code carts for immediate access.

Although such use is beyond the scope of this chapter, it is worth mentioning that magnets can also temporarily turn off defibrillation therapy in implantable cardioverter-defibrillators.

Pacemaker Programming

Detailed description of specific programming techniques and indications is beyond the scope of this chapter; however, familiarity with the basic functions and nomenclature is critical for understanding how pacemakers function.

BASIC FUNCTIONS

A pacemaker has three basic functions: pacing, sensing, and action. Its other, more complicated functions are based on these three. Pacing is the delivery of an electrical impulse to the myocardium to elicit depolarization. Sensing is the ability to "see" intrinsic depolarization (i.e., the local intrinsic electrical signal that passes by the tip of the lead). Action is the response of the pacemaker to a sensed event—namely, either inhibition or triggering of a paced event.

CODES

The basic functions—pacing, sensing, and action—are determined by basic pacemaker programming. In 1974, the American Heart Association and the American College of Cardiology proposed a three-letter code for describing the basic functions of pacemakers. Under the guidance of NASPE and the British Pacing and Electrophysiology Group (BPEG), this code evolved into the five-position code currently in use [*see Table 2*].[26] The first position denotes the chamber or chambers paced; the second denotes the chamber or chambers sensed; the third denotes the action or actions performed; the fourth denotes rate response; and the fifth denotes multiple-site pacing. The simplest mode of pacing is VVI, otherwise known as ventricular demand pacing or ventricular inhibited pacing. The most commonly used mode in dual-chamber pacing is DDD.

TIMING CYCLES

A pacemaker is governed by timing cycles, which are a hierarchy of clocks that regulate how the pacemaker functions. The most basic timing cycle is the lower rate, which reflects how long the pacemaker will wait after a paced or sensed beat before initi-

Table 2 NASPE-BPEG Generic Five-Position Code for Antibradycardia Pacing

	Position				
	I	*II*	*III*	*IV*	*V*
Parameter measured	Chamber(s) paced	Chamber(s) sensed	Response or action	Rate modulation	Multisite pacing
Possible values	O = None A = Atrium V = Ventricle D = Dual (A + V)	O = None A = Atrium V = Ventricle D = Dual (A + V)	O = None I = Inhibited T = Triggered D = Dual (I + T)	O = None R = Rate response on	O = None A = Atrium V = Ventricle D = Dual (A + V)

NASPE—North American Society of Pacing and Electrophysiology   BPEG—British Pacing and Electrophysiology Group

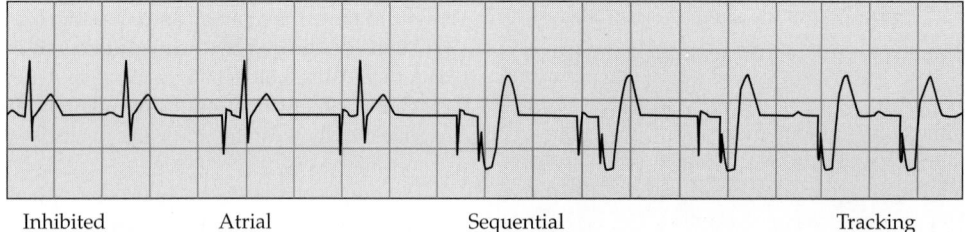

Inhibited   Atrial   Sequential   Tracking

Figure 3 Illustrated are different forms of DDD pacing. In the first two beats (labeled "Inhibited"), the pacemaker senses both the intrinsic P wave and the QRS complex; the result is inhibition of pacing. In the next two beats (labeled "Atrial"), there is a pacing spike preceding each P wave; the result is atrial pacing. The intrinsic QRS complex is then sensed, and ventricular pacing is inhibited. In the third set of beats (labeled "Sequential"), there are pacing spikes preceding both the P wave and the QRS complex. Both chambers are paced. The paced QRS morphology is noticeably different from the intrinsic complexes seen in the previous examples. In the final set of beats (labeled "Tracking"), an intrinsic P wave is followed by a paced QRS. The intrinsic atrial beat is sensed and triggers ventricular pacing.

ating pacing. If the pacemaker is set to VVI mode at a lower rate of 60 beats/min, then as long as the interval between intrinsic beats is less then 1,000 msec, the pacemaker will reset the lower rate clock with each sensed QRS complex, and pacing will not occur. If, however, the intrinsic heart rate falls below 60 beats/min, the pacemaker's lower-rate clock will time out before an intrinsic beat is sensed, and pacing will occur. After a paced beat, the lower-rate clock is reset and the cycle repeats. In a modern dual-chamber pacemaker, there are a number of additional timing cycles that regulate how the pacemaker responds to these paced and sensed events [*see Figure 3*].

Patients with chronic atrial fibrillation and slow ventricular response are generally treated with single-chamber ventricular pacemakers. Such devices are also occasionally used in patients with isolated SA node dysfunction.

Pacemaker Implantation

Most pacemakers are implanted by cardiologists, and most implantation procedures are performed in the cardiac catheterization laboratory.[27]

PREPROCEDURAL CONSIDERATIONS

There are several issues that should be considered after the need to implant a pacemaker has been established. In particular, the patient's underlying health must be assessed and any comorbid conditions evaluated.

In select patients, the issue of reversal and reinitiation of oral anticoagulation must be addressed before implantation. In the past, all patients receiving warfarin had their international normalized ratios (INRs) normalized before the procedure. Furthermore, patients with a strong indication for anticoagulation (e.g., a mechanical heart valve) required prolonged hospitalization for reinitiation of oral anticoagulation after the procedure. In the past few years, however, favorable results have been reported with routine pacemaker implantation in patients undergoing therapeutic anticoagulation with warfarin. These results suggest that preprocedural reversal of anticoagulation may not be necessary.[28-29]

Pacemakers can interfere with or preclude certain imaging procedures, such as mammography and magnetic resonance imaging. In the case of elective pacemaker implants, a baseline mammogram should be performed beforehand.[30] Any MRI pro-

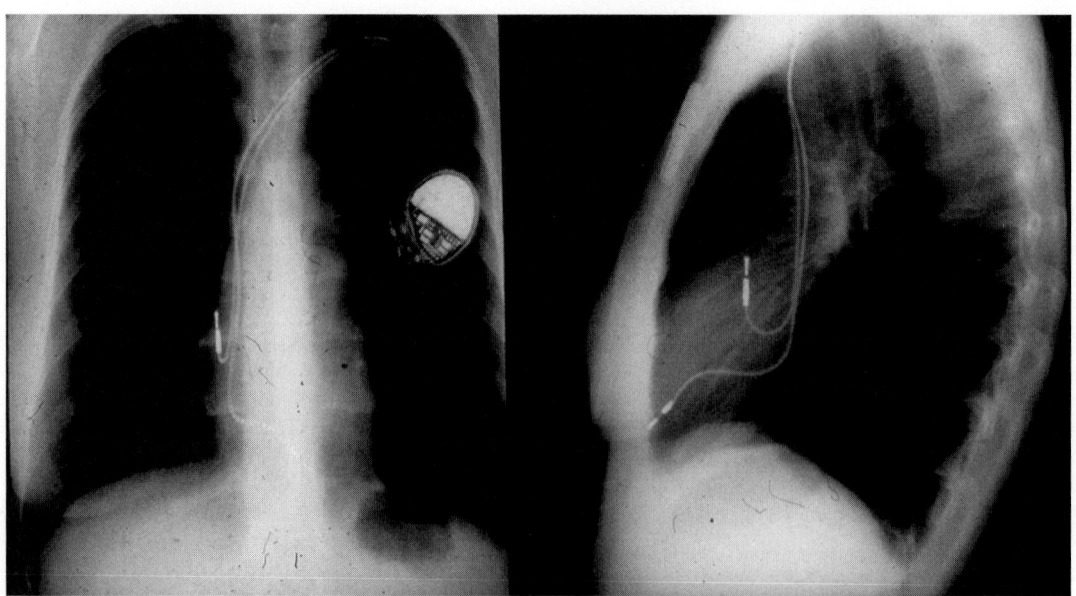

Figure 4 Shown is the typical appearance of a dual-chamber pacemaker on posteroanterior (left) and lateral (right) chest x-rays. The RV lead is at the apex, and the RA lead is in the right atrial appendage.

cedures that may be indicated should also be performed before implantation.

Local anesthesia is typically employed in conjunction with parenteral sedation. In certain circumstances (e.g., in pediatric patients or other patients who would tolerate the procedure poorly under local anesthesia), an anesthetist should be involved, but such circumstances are relatively uncommon. Antibiotic prophylaxis is commonly employed, but not in a uniform manner. There are no strict guidelines, and antibiotic regimens vary greatly.[31]

PACEMAKER POCKET PLACEMENT

The pulse generator pocket is usually placed on the upper left aspect of the chest, just medial to the angle of the deltopectoral grove and 2 to 3 cm below the clavicle. In the case of left-handed patients or in certain other specific situations (e.g., when left subclavian vein acclusion is present or the patient has undergone a left mastectomy), the pacemaker may be located on the right side. It is important to locate the generator medially enough that it does not interfere with normal shoulder function. The pocket is formed deep to the subcutaneous tissue and above the plane of the pectoral fascia. Occasionally, if the patient is extremely thin or if cosmetic considerations are a priority, the generator may be placed either below the pectoral muscle or via a retromammary approach.

VASCULAR ACCESS

Vascular access is most frequently gained by means of the Seldinger technique. The subclavian vein remains the most common venous access site; however, the axillary vein is becoming an increasingly popular site. Venous access may also be obtained via the cephalic vein or the internal jugular vein. In addition, leads may be tunneled subcutaneously from a remote entry site (e.g., the internal jugular vein) to the site of the generator pocket. Occasionally, thoracotomy and the use of epicardial lead systems are still necessary.

RISKS

Overall, transvenous pacemaker implantation is both safe and well tolerated. The risk of major adverse events (e.g., death, myocardial infarction, stroke, and the need for emergency thoracotomy) is approximately 0.1%. Other complications sometimes encountered include pneuomothorax, vascular injury, cardiac perforation, tamponade, local bleeding, pocket hematoma, infection, and venous thrombosis. There is also a small risk that one or more leads may become dislodged and have to be repositioned in a second procedure.

POSTPROCEDURAL CARE

At most institutions, it is standard practice to admit patients for overnight observation after routine pacemaker implantation. Routine exchange of the pacemaker generator because of battery depletion is often performed as a same-day outpatient procedure. Longer hospitalizations may be required in certain specific situations, as when anticoagulation must be reversed and reinitiated or when a major comorbid condition must be treated.

After implantation of new devices or leads, the ipsilateral arm is placed in a sling or a soft restraint for 12 to 24 hours. Nonnarcotic analgesics are usually sufficient for pain control, but occasionally, oral narcotics are indicated. Patients are monitored via continuous telemetry. We routinely obtain a portable chest x-ray and a 12-lead ECG immediately after implantation.

The day after the procedure, the pacemaker is interrogated and the final settings confirmed. Posteroanterior and lateral chest x-rays are obtained both to verify the positioning of the leads and to rule out the possibility of a slowly accumulating pneumothorax [see Figure 4].

Before discharge, the patient receives instruction about the pacemaker teaching and is given a temporary pacemaker card that lists the manufacturer, the specific generator and lead(s) used, and complete serial-number information. Later, the manufacturer mails the patient a permanent identification card, which the patient is asked to keep on hand at all times.

POSTDISCHARGE INSTRUCTIONS AND RESTRICTIONS

Postoperative care focuses on averting hematoma and preventing lead dislodgment. Patients are prohibited from showering for the first 48 to 72 hours. After this period, they may shower, but for the first week, they are advised to cover the implantation site with plastic wrap to protect it from contamination. When 24 hours have passed after implantation, minimal range-of-motion restrictions are placed on the ipsilateral arm and shoulder. Patients are asked to refrain from raising the arm above shoulder level and to perform only limited heavy lifting for the first few weeks. After this period, patients may return to normal activity levels without having to be concerned about displacing the leads or the generator system.

Usually, a follow-up visit is scheduled 7 to 10 days after implantation. During this visit, a wound check is performed to ensure proper healing and to remove the skin suture if it is nonresorbable. As a rule, the pacemaker pocket heals completely within 2 to 4 weeks.

LONG-TERM FOLLOW-UP

Pacemaker patients need routine follow-up care, including interrogation of the pacemaker. Follow-up care can be provided during office visits, via transtelephonic monitoring (TTM), or both. Guidelines for follow-up have been published by NASPE,[32] as well as by the Canadian Working Group in Cardiac Pacing.[33] We recommend that patients either be seen in the office or undergo TTM every 3 months. As the battery approaches the end of its life, more frequent visits may be required.

Complications

Pacemaker complications are infrequent but can lead to serious situations. To minimize adverse consequences, it is important to identify problems early in their course, initiate appropriate workup and treatment, and refer when necessary [see Table 3]. Generally, pacemaker complications can be classified according to whether they primarily affect the pocket, the generator, or the leads.

GENERATOR POCKET COMPLICATIONS

Pocket hematomas can occur in any patient but are especially likely to occur in those receiving anticoagulants. These hematomas are usually self-limited, and intervention is rarely necessary. Acute management includes direct manual compression, sandbag compression, pressure dressings, or a combination thereof. Needle aspiration and opening the pocket to drain the hematoma are discouraged because of the risk of introducing infection. Reoperation is generally limited to situations in which there is impending compromise of the incision, uncontrollable bleeding, uncontrollable pain, or suspected infection. Other possible pocket problems include erosion of the underlying hardware, infection, pocket pain, migration of the pulse generator,

Table 3   Common Findings Related to Pacemaker Problems

Findings	*Potential Causes*	*Treatment/Workup*	*When to Refer*
Ecchymoses Hematoma Oozing at incision site	Local bleeding Anticoagulation	External compression; avoid needle aspiration or surgical drainage if possible Withhold anticoagulation	Impending wound dehiscence, uncontrolled pain Signs of infection
Palpable hardware, including header or leads	Benign unless findings consistent with impending erosion	No treatment Cushion with gauze or dressing to avoid irritation from clothing Pocket revision	Signs of impending erosion Pain requiring consideration of pocket revision
Adhesion of skin Thinning or atrophy of skin Scaling of skin Erythema	Impending generator or lead erosion	Pocket revision	Early If hardware becomes exposed, extraction may be required
Exposed hardware	Erosion with infection	Blood cultures Blood count Antibiotics Hardware extraction	Immediately
Pocket erythema Pocket swelling Purulent discharge	Infection Local inflammatory reaction Local trauma	Blood cultures Chest x-ray Blood counts	Early
Pocket pain	Superficial implant Infection Generator migration Pacemaker allergy Superficial irritation from bra strap or clothing	Chest x-ray Examination of generator pocket for signs of migration or infection	Signs of infection Continued pain despite mild analgesics
Fever, chills, or other signs of systemic infection or bacteremia, even without signs of pocket infection	Systemic infection, including bacteremia, bloodstream infection, or endocarditis	Blood cultures Chest x-ray Blood counts Echocardiography	Immediately
Ipsilateral arm swelling Arm heaviness Superior vena cava syndrome	Venous thrombosis	Doppler ultrasonography Arm elevation Anticoagulation	Early
Pectoral muscle twitching Diaphragmatic stimulation	Lead fracture Unipolar pacing Autocapture feature Phrenic nerve stimulation	Chest x-ray Pacemaker interrogation	Early

and misplacement of the generator (so that it interferes with shoulder movement).

Erosion of the underlying hardware can be quite serious, in that it usually leads to infection of the system. In normal circumstances, the underlying hardware, including the leads, can be felt during palpation of the pacemaker pocket, especially if the patient is thin. In extreme cases, the outlines of the generator and the leads can be clearly seen through the skin. It is important to be able to distinguish between normal palpability or visibility and impending pacemaker pocket erosion. Normally, the skin overlying the pacemaker is freely mobile, without discoloration or tenderness to palpation. Fixation, erythema, thinning, atrophy, and scaling of the skin over the underlying hardware are signs of impending erosion. It is crucial to identify early signs of erosion before the hardware breaks the skin. If the skin is intact, surgical revision of the pocket is often all that is needed to protect the hardware from contamination and infection. Once the hardware has been exposed, however, the device must be assumed to be infect-

ed, and treatment usually involves a much more complex procedure that includes removal of all the hardware.[34]

Device migration is unusual but can cause significant discomfort. In some cases, surgical revision of the pocket is required to restore an appropriate position.

Chronic pacemaker pocket pain is also infrequent. There is normally some postoperative discomfort while the site heals and the capsule of scar tissue develops. Chronic pain may indicate that the device is not properly located in relation to the shoulder joint and the clavicle or may be an early sign of subacute infection.

GENERATOR COMPLICATIONS

On the whole, pacemaker generators are highly reliable: normal battery depletion aside, failure is unusual. True allergy to pacemaker materials does occur but is rare.

LEAD COMPLICATIONS

Pacemaker lead complications include dislodgment, fracture,

and infection. Fractures can occur throughout the body of the lead, but the most common location is the area where the lead passes between the first rib and the clavicle; fracture at this site leads to the so-called subclavian crush syndrome. Lead fractures may be asymptomatic or may give rise to symptoms related to failure to pace or sense appropriately. Extracardiac stimulation and changes in measured parameters of lead function may be noted. Some lead fractures may be evident on chest x-ray; however, only the conductors are radiopaque, and thus, simple disruption of the outer insulation will not be visible.

A common lead complication is the so-called twiddler's syndrome, which refers to patients who, whether intentionally or subconsciously, continually manipulate the generator within the pocket, eventually causing lead damage or dislodgment.

PACEMAKER INFECTIONS

Bacterial infections can affect any part of the pacemaker system, and the consequences can be devastating. The most com-

Table 4 Sources of Electromagnetic Interference That Can Affect Pacemakers

	Source	Safe with Pacemaker	Specific Recommendations
Medical sources	MRI	No	Rarely done; restricted to life-threatening situations with close monitoring
	CT scanning	Yes	Pacemaker may interfere with images of thorax
	Lithotripsy	Yes	Activity sensors should be disabled Pacemaker-dependent patients should be programmed to asynchronous mode Shocks should be synchronized to R wave Contraindicated in patients with abdominal implants
	External direct current cardioversion	Yes	Avoid placing patches or paddles directly over pacemaker Have transcutaneous pacing available Use lowest possible energy and biphasic waveform when possible Interrogate pacemaker after procedure
	Neurostimulation	Yes	Test at highest output for pacemaker inhibition before discharge
	Peripheral nerve stimulation	Yes	Nerve conduction studies below the elbow or knee are safe
	Transcutaneous electric nerve stimulation (TENS)	Yes	May require increasing sensing threshold Avoid placing TENS electrodes parallel to pacing vector
	Radiation therapy	Yes	Avoid direct irradiation; maximize shielding If total dose is expected to exceed 10 Gy, device may have to be relocated out of field Reprogram to asynchronous mode if patient is pacemaker dependent Initiate continuous monitoring if patient is pacemaker dependent Check device function after each session and for first few weeks after therapy
	Diagnostic ultrasonography, including echocardiography	Yes	No precautions needed
	Surgical electrocautery	Yes	[*See Figure 5*]
Household and industrial sources	Microwave ovens, TV remote-control devices, cordless telephones, other household appliances	Yes	All devices considered safe; controlled studies lacking
	Slot machines	Yes	May cause interaction and spurious shocks with ICDs
	Walk-through metal detectors	Yes	Do not dwell in scanner; device will probably set off alarm Patients should be advised to carry pacemaker ID card as proof
	Handheld security wand	Yes	Patient should instruct person conducting search not to put wand directly over pacemaker generator
	Cellular telephones	Yes	Keep phone at least 10 cm from pacemaker; do not keep phone in shirt pocket above pacemaker; try to use contralateral ear when using phone
	Electronic article surveillance devices	Yes	Do not dwell in scanner
	Industrial sources, including large electric motors, magnets, and high-voltage power	Yes/No	Depends on source and proximity of pacemaker; site visit may be needed to determine safety
	Arc-welding equipment	No	Cannot be used because of magnetic field of cable

ICD—implantable cardioverter-defibrillator

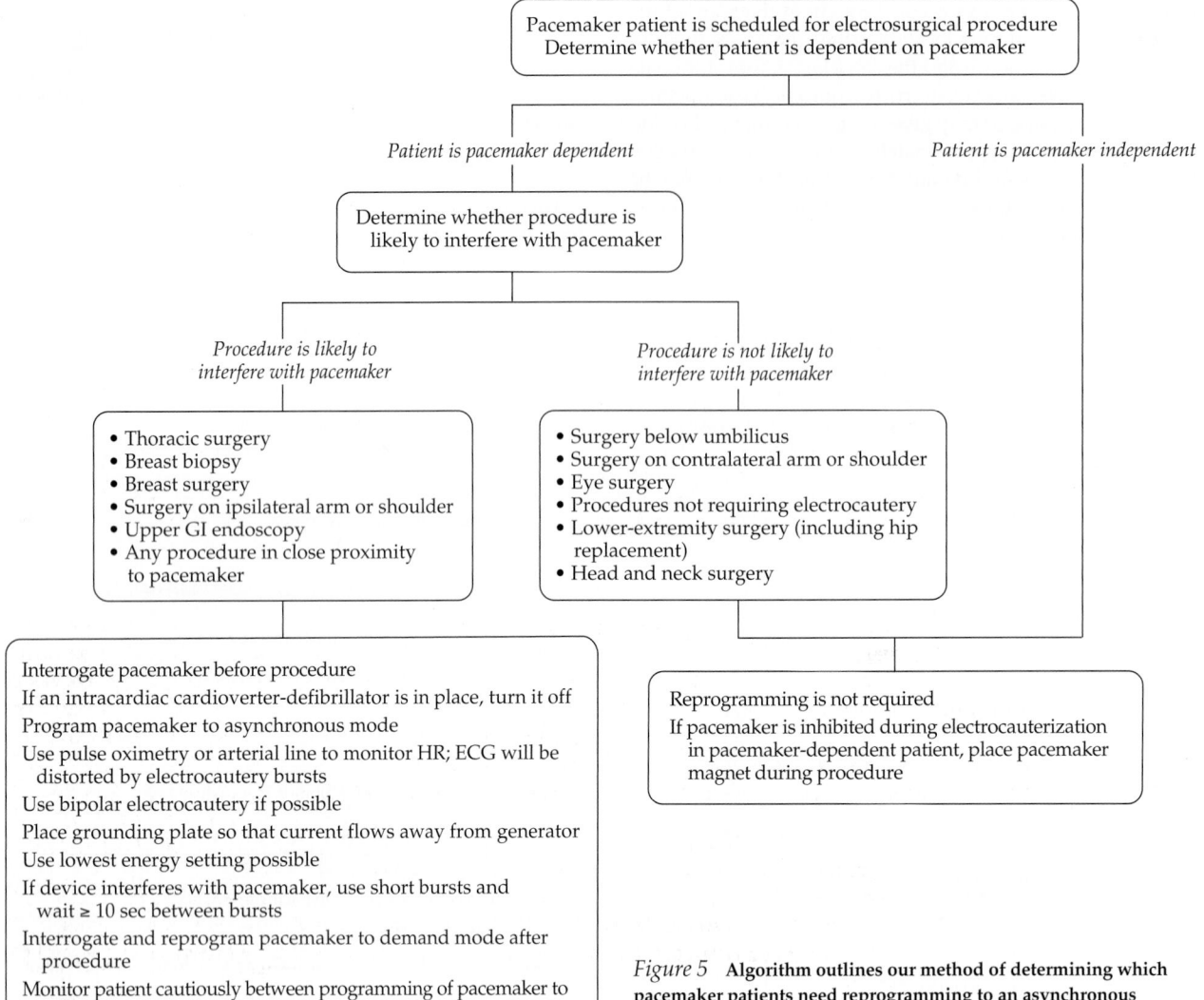

Figure 5 Algorithm outlines our method of determining which pacemaker patients need reprogramming to an asynchronous mode before procedures involving electrosurgery.

mon pathogens are staphylococci, especially *Staphylococcus epidermidis.* Once a pacemaker infection is established, it is difficult to eradicate with antibiotics; thus, infected pacemaker systems usually must be removed in their entirety. Patients with pacemakers in place who acquire *S. aureus* bacteremia are at significant risk for a secondary device infection.[35] If infection of an implanted cardiac device is suspected, prompt referral to an experienced center is critical.

External Interference with Pacemaker Function

To function appropriately, pacemakers must be able to sense a clean signal from the myocardium. A number of potential sources can interfere with such signals and thereby affect pacemaker function.[36,37] The most significant of these is EMI, which can have several detrimental effects on pacing systems. The most common detrimental effect of EMI is inhibition of pacing: the pacemaker senses the EMI and interprets it as cardiac activity. In a pacemaker-dependent patient, this misinterpretation can have catastrophic consequences. Other detrimental effects include reversion to an asynchronous pacing mode, reversion to a backup pacing mode, inappropriate activation of other features, and damage to the pacemaker circuitry. Modern pacemakers with

bipolar leads are less susceptible to EMI; in addition, they often contain filters and other features designed to protect the patient from device malfunction.

SOURCES OF EMI

Sources of EMI can be divided into household sources, industrial sources, and medical sources [*see Table 4*]. In general, household appliances such as microwave ovens, hairdryers, and television remote controls are safe for pacemaker recipients to use.[38-40] Medical sources of EMI are common in both noninvasive and invasive procedures. MRI scans are generally contraindicated in pacemaker patients; they should be performed only in life-threatening situations and with close monitoring.[41,42] Surgical procedures involving electocauterization are important sources of EMI and often necessitate pacemaker reprogramming before and after the procedure.[43] As a rule, only patients who are pacemaker dependent require reprogramming. The location of the procedure in relation to the pacemaker generator is also an important consideration in deciding whether reprogramming is indicated. On the basis of case reports and our own clinical experience, we have developed an approach we use to determine who needs pacemaker reprogramming before surgery [*see Figure 5*].

The Future

Pacemaker technology is advancing on many fronts.[44,45] Devices are becoming smaller and more sophisticated. Improvements in pacemaker software are allowing closer imitation of normal physiologic cardiac function. New automatic features (e.g., automatic mode switching in response to atrial fibrillation, automatic capture verification, and automatic sensing) are leading to greater reliability and simplified follow-up. New indications for pacing (including cardiac resynchronization therapy for heart failure and treatment of sleep apnea) are evolving. Pacemaker and implantable cardioverter-defibrillator technologies are converging. New information technology is allowing improved collection, storage, and analysis of pacemaker patient data. Internet-based patient management systems are being developed that will include automatic wireless interrogation performed at the patient's home.

Roger A. Freedman, M.D., has received grants for clinical research from Guidant Corporation, Medtronic Inc., and St. Jude Medical, Inc., has served as a consultant to Guidant Corporation and St. Jude Medical, Inc., has received program support from Guidant Corporation and Medtronic Inc., and has served as a speaker for Guidant Corporation.

Jonathan Lowy, M.D., has received grants for clinical research from Guidant Corporation.

References

1. Frye RL, Collins JJ, DeSanctis RW, et al: Guidelines for permanent cardiac pacemaker implantation, May 1984: a report of the Joint American College of Cardiology/American Heart Association Task Force on assessment of cardiovascular procedures (Subcommittee on Pacemaker Implantation). Circulation 70:331A, 1984

2. Dreifus LS, Fisch C, Griffin JC, et al: Guidelines for implantation of cardiac pacemakers and antiarrhythmia devices: a report of the American College of Cardiology/American Heart Association Task Force on assessment of diagnostic and therapeutic cardiovascular procedures. Circulation 84:455, 1991

3. Gregoratos G, Cheitlin MD, Conill A, et al: ACC/AHA Guidelines for implantation of cardiac pacemakers and antiarrhythmia devices: a report of the American College of Cardiology/American Heart Association Task Force on practice guidelines (Committee on Pacemaker Implantation). JACC 31:1175, 1998

4. Gregoratos G, Abrams J, Epstein AE, et al: ACC/AHA/NASPE 2002 guideline update for implantation of cardiac pacemakers and antiarrhythmia devices. Circulation 106:2145, 2002

5. Mymin D, Mathewson FA, Tate RB, et al: The natural history of primary first-degree atrioventricular block. N Engl J Med 315:1183, 1986

6. Shaw DB, Kekwick CA, Veale D, et al: Survival in second degree atrioventricular block. Br Heart J 53:587, 1985

7. Strasberg B, Amat-Y-Leon F, Dhingra RC, et al: Natural history of chronic second-degree atrioventricular nodal block. Circulation 63:1043, 1981

8. Connelly DT, Steinhaus DM: Mobitz type I atrioventricular block: an indication for permanent pacing? Pacing Clin Electrophysiol 19:261, 1996

9. Barold SS: Indications for permanent cardiac pacing in first degree AV block: class I, II, or III? Pacing Clin Electrophysiol 19:747, 1996

10. McAnulty JH, Rahimtoola SH, Murphy E, et al: Natural history of "high risk" bundle-branch block: final report of a prospective study. N Engl J Med 307:137, 1982

11. Ryan TJ, Antman EM, Brooks NH, et al: 1999 update: ACC/AHA guidelines for the management of patients with acute myocardial infarction: executive summary and recommendations: a report of the American College of Cardiology/American Heart Association Task Force on practice guidelines (Committee on Management of Acute Myocardial Infarction). Circulation 100:1016, 1999

12. Nicod P, Gilpin E, Dittrich H, et al: Long-term outcome in patients with inferior myocardial infarction and complete atrioventricular block. J Am Coll Cardiol 12:589, 1988

13. Dubois C, Pierard LA, Smeets JP, et al: Long-term prognostic significance of atrioventricular block in inferior acute myocardial infarction. Eur Heart J 10:816, 1989

14. Goldberg RJ, Zevallos JC, Yarzebski J, et al: Prognosis of acute myocardial infarction complicated by complete heart block (the Worcester Heart Attack Study). Am J Cardiol 69:1135, 1992

15. Spencer FA, Jabbour S, Lessard D, et al: Two-decade-long trends (1975–1997) in the incidence, hospitalization, and long-term death rates associated with complete heart block complicating acute myocardial infarction: a community-wide perspective. Am Heart J 145:500, 2003

16. Kusumoto FM, Goldschlager N: Cardiac pacing. N Engl J Med 334:89 1996

17. Anderson HR, Nielson JC, Thomsen PEB, et al: Long-term follow-up of patients from a randomized trial of atrial versus ventricular pacing for sick sinus syndrome. Lancet 350:1210, 1997

18. De Marneffe M, Gregoire JM, Waterschoot P, et al: The sinus node function: normal and pathological. Eur Heart J 14:649, 1993

19. Santini M, Alexidou G, Ansalone G, et al: Relation of prognosis in sick sinus syndrome to age, conduction defects and modes of permanent cardiac pacing. Am J Cardiol 65:729, 1990

20. Lamas GA, Lee KL, Sweeney MO, et al: Ventricular pacing or dual chamber pacing for sinus node dysfunction. N Engl J Med 346:1854, 2002

21. Grubb BP, Kosinski DJ: Syncope resulting from autonomic insufficiency syndromes associated with orthostatic intolerance. Med Clin North Am 85:457, 2001

22. Connolly SJ, Sheldon R, Roberts RS, et al: The North American vasovagal pacemaker study (VPS): a randomized trial of permanent cardiac pacing for the prevention of vasovagal syncope. J Am Coll Cardiol 33:16, 1999

23. Ammirati F, Colivicchi F, Santini M: Permanent cardiac pacing versus medical treatment for the prevention of recurrent vasovagal syncope: a multicenter, randomized, controlled trial. Circulation 104:52, 2001

24. Connolly SJ, Sheldon R, Thorpe KE, et al: Pacemaker therapy for the prevention of syncope in patients with recurrent severe vasovagal syncope: Second Vasovagal Pacemaker Study (VPS II). JAMA 289:2224, 2003

25. Morillo CA, Camacho ME, Wood MA, et al: Diagnostic utility of mechanical, pharmacological and orthostatic stimulation of the carotid sinus in patients with unexplained syncope. J Am Coll Cardiol 34:1587, 1999

26. Bernstein AD, Daubert JC, Fletcher RD, et al: The Revised NASPE/BPEG generic code for antibradycardia, adaptive-rate, and multisite pacing. Pacing Clin Electrophysiol 25:260, 2002

27. Hayes DL, Naccarelli GV, Furman S, et al: Report of the NASPE Policy Conference training requirements for permanent pacemaker selection, implantation, and follow-up. North American Society of Pacing and Electrophysiology. Pacing Clin Electrophysiol 17:6, 1994

28. al-Khadra AS: Implantation of pacemakers and implantable cardioverter defibrillators in orally anticoagulated patients. Pacing Clin Electrophysiol 26:511, 2003

29. Michaud GF, Pelosi F Jr, Noble MD, et al: A randomized trial comparing heparin initiation 6 h or 24 h after pacemaker or defibrillator implantation. J Am Coll Cardiol 35:1915, 2000

30. Roelke M, Rubinstein VJ, Kamath S, et al: Pacemaker interference with screening mammography. Pacing Clin Electrophysiol 22:1106, 1999

31. Da Costa A, Kirkorian G, Cucherat M, et al: Antibiotic prophylaxis for permanent pacemaker implantation: a meta-analysis. Circulation 97:1796, 1998

32. Bernstein AD, Irwin ME, Parsonnet V, et al: Report of the NASPE policy conference on antibradycardia pacemaker follow-up: effectiveness, needs, and resources. North American Society of Pacing and Electrophysiology. Pacing Clin Electrophysiol 17:1714, 1994

33. Fraser JD, Gillis AM, Irwin ME, et al: Guidelines for pacemaker follow-up in Canada: a consensus statement of the Canadian Working Group on Cardiac Pacing. Can J Cardiol 16:355, 2000

34. Chua JD, Wilkoff BL, Lee I, et al: Diagnosis and management of infections involving implantable electrophysiologic cardiac devices. Ann Intern Med 133:604, 2000

35. Chamis AL, Peterson GE, Cabell CH, et al: *Staphylococcus aureus* bacteremia in patients with permanent pacemakers or implantable cardioverter-defibrillators. Circulation 104:1029, 2001

36. Pinski SL, Trohman RG: Interference in implanted cardiac devices, part I. Pacing Clin Electrophysiol 25:1367, 2002

37. Pinski SL, Trohman RG: Interference in implanted cardiac devices, part II. Pacing Clin Electrophysiol 25:1496, 2002

38. Niehaus M, Tebbenjohanns J: Electromagnetic interference in patients with implanted pacemakers or cardioverter-defibrillators. Heart 86:246, 2001

39. Hayes DL, Wang PJ, Reynolds DW, et al: Interference with cardiac pacemakers by cellular telephones. N Engl J Med 336:1473, 1997

40. McIvor ME, Reddinger J, Floden E, et al: Study of pacemaker and implantable cardioverter defibrillator triggering by electronic article surveillance devices (SPICED TEAS). Pacing Clin Electrophysiol 21:1847, 1998

41. Hayes DL, Holmes DR Jr, Gray JE: Effect of 1.5 Tesla nuclear magnetic resonance imaging scanner on implanted permanent pacemakers. J Am Coll Cardiol 10:782, 1987

42. Lauck G, von Smekal A, Wolke S, et al: Effects of nuclear magnetic resonance imaging on cardiac pacemakers. Pacing Clin Electrophysiol 18:1549, 1995

43. Madigan JD, Choudhri AF, Chen J, et al: Surgical management of the patient with an implanted cardiac device. Ann Surg 230:639, 1999

44. Bryce M, Spielman SR, Greenspan AM, et al: Evolving indications for permanent pacemakers. Ann Intern Med 134:1130, 2001

45. Gold MR: Permanent pacing: new indications. Heart 86:355, 2001

23 Chronic Stable Angina

Paul R. Sutton, M.D., PH.D., F.A.C.P., and Stephan D. Fihn, M.D., M.P.H., F.A.C.P.

Definitions

Angina pectoris is the cardinal symptom of myocardial ischemia. Ischemia occurs when the coronary blood supply is inadequate to meet the metabolic demands of the myocardium. This mismatch of coronary blood supply and myocardial metabolic demand usually results from narrowing or occlusion of one or more coronary arteries, but in rare cases, it may be caused by coronary vasospasm or solely by excessive myocardial oxygen demand in the absence of significant coronary atherosclerosis.

Angina is typically a substernal, pressurelike discomfort or pain, but it may also take the form of discomfort in the jaw, shoulder, back, or arm. Usually, it is precipitated by physical exertion or emotional stress, and it is promptly relieved by rest or by taking nitroglycerin. Chronic stable angina refers to a pattern of chest pain or discomfort that does not change appreciably in frequency or severity over 2 months or longer and in which the episodes of pain are provoked by exertions or stresses of similar intensity.[1] Unstable angina, by contrast, is defined as rest angina, severe angina of new onset, or an increase in the severity or frequency of previously stable angina. Certain patients with symptoms of unstable angina are at an increased risk for myocardial infarction (MI) or death [see Epidemiology, below]. Chronic stable angina precedes MI in about half of cases and is common afterward. Although angina is a cardinal symptom of ischemic heart disease (IHD), MI or sudden death is the initial presentation of IHD in as many as half of patients.

Epidemiology

IHD is the leading cause of mortality in the United States and the rest of the developed world; it is responsible for more than 20% of deaths.[2] In the United States, approximately one million persons suffer an MI, and 500,000 coronary deaths occur each year. IHD is the leading cause of death in the United States for both sexes in both white and black populations.

The prevalence of IHD increases with age and is higher in men than in women in every age group. The American Heart Association (AHA) conservatively estimates that more than six million persons in the United States experience angina.[3]

In addition to posing an increased risk of MI and premature death, chronic stable angina often limits affected persons' capacity for work and other activities, which, in turn, negatively affects their quality of life. The direct and indirect costs of hospitalization, diagnostic procedures, and revascularization related to angina are substantial. Estimates of direct hospital costs for Medicare patients with a history of chronic stable angina exceed $7 billion annually.[1] Of patients with angina who undergo a coronary revascularization procedure, 30% or more never return to work.[4]

The major modifiable risk factors for IHD are dyslipidemias—in particular, elevated levels of low-density lipoprotein (LDL) cholesterol and low levels of high-density lipoprotein (HDL) cholesterol—as well as hypertension, diabetes mellitus, and cigarette smoking.[5,6] Other important, but immutable, risk factors are increasing age, a family history of premature coronary disease, and male sex. Obesity, physical inactivity, and atherogenic dietary habits also contribute to cardiovascular risk, although it is difficult to distinguish the risks conferred by these risk factors independently of the risks conferred by the major cardiovascular risk factors because of the potential interaction of these factors. Patients with combinations of risk factors may be at particular risk for developing IHD. Patients with the metabolic syndrome, which consists of obesity (particularly abdominal adiposity), hypertension, dyslipidemia (i.e., elevated triglyceride levels and low HDL levels), and insulin resistance, are at particularly high risk for IHD.[7] It is estimated that in the United States, the metabolic syndrome affects nearly 25% of all persons and 43.5% of adults 60 years of age or older.[8]

Numerous clinical trials have identified important risk factors and effective therapies for coronary artery disease; however, few of these studies have included sufficient numbers of women to draw meaningful conclusions about coronary disease in women.[9] Thus, much of the evidence that supports contemporary recommendations for testing, prevention, and treatment of coronary disease in women is extrapolated from studies conducted predominantly in middle-aged men.

Although it has been proposed that 50% or more of patients with IHD lack any of the traditional major risk factors, two studies have challenged this notion; these studies indicate that the vast majority of patients who experience cardiac events (either fatal or nonfatal) have one or more major risk factors.[10,11] Nevertheless, interest remains in identifying additional laboratory markers of risk of IHD and, in particular, risk of acute coronary syndromes. In observational studies, several measures of inflammation, including C-reactive protein (CRP) levels, interleukin-6 (IL-6) levels, and levels of soluble cellular adhesion molecules, have been associated with risk of IHD and cardiovascular events.[12,13] Measures of fibrinogen, platelet activator inhibitor, and components of the coagulation/fibrinolysis cascade may ultimately be of use in predicting risk of cardiovascular events.[12] A number of genetic polymorphisms and candidate genes that may increase the risk of MI have been identified in specific populations. Currently, however, it is uncertain whether these or other laboratory measurements represent truly independent risk factors or whether they will prove useful in clinical practice.[14]

Pathophysiology and Pathogenesis

Angina occurs as a result of myocardial ischemia, which occurs when cardiac blood supply is insufficient to meet myocardial oxygen demand. Stable angina commonly occurs in the setting of narrowing or partial occlusion of segments of coronary arteries by atherosclerotic plaque. Significant occlusion is defined as a reduction of the diameter of a major coronary artery by 70%, which corresponds to a 50% reduction in vessel lumen surface area; such occlusion is often sufficient to cause angina. Coronary atherosclerosis and angina often progress over time, reflecting both gradual and more abrupt changes in luminal diameter of coronary vessels. Incremental changes in coronary atherosclerosis reflect the progression of existing lesions and the appearance of new stenoses. Abrupt changes in vessel diameter may be associated with sudden changes in anginal symptoms, termed unstable angina. Unstable angina is commonly caused by rupture of vulnerable atherosclerotic plaque with associated platelet thrombosis. Unstable angina may also be caused by endothelial injury, thrombosis of severely stenotic coronary arteries, or coronary artery spasm. Although angina is usually associated with coronary artery disease (CAD), it may also occur in persons with normal or near-normal coronary arteries; in these settings, angina may occur as a result of increased myocardial oxygen demand associated with aortic stenosis, hyperthyroidism, or anemia.

Myocardial ischemia, regardless of cause, is associated with intracardiac release of adenosine. Adenosine release slows atrioventricular conduction and reduces contractility, which are adaptive changes in the setting of myocardial ischemia. Stimulation of adenosine receptors in the chest is believed to be responsible for the sensation of angina.

Angina occurs most often in the setting of coronary atherosclerosis. Atherosclerosis occurs as a result of vascular injury and subsequent responses to injury. Vascular injury may result from the mechanical stress of blood flow or from direct endothelial injury from toxins, such as those in cigarette smoke. Traditional cardiovascular risk factors, such as smoking, hypertension, hyperlipidemia, and diabetes, increase coronary risk, at least in part by potentiating vascular injury or altering the subsequent response to injury. Direct endothelial injury produces a sequence of events similar to chronic inflammation: the endothelium elaborates procoagulants, vasoactive molecules, growth factors, and cytokines. Platelets, inflammatory cells (e.g., monocytes and T cells), and smooth muscle cells are attracted to the site of injury.[15] This cascade of events is initially adaptive, resulting in repair of endothelial injury; however, repeated cycles of injury and repair can result in progressive atherosclerosis and luminal narrowing.

Support for the inflammatory hypothesis of atherosclerosis comes from clinical studies that suggest a correlation between the risk of future cardiovascular events and the presence of markers of inflammation, including CRP.[12,13] Inflammation may also play a role in acute coronary syndromes (i.e., unstable angina and acute MI). In some studies, levels of CRP during episodes of unstable angina are associated with a greater risk of MI or death,[16] although it is not clear whether inflammation (and corresponding elevations of CRP) contributes to the etiology of unstable coronary syndromes or is simply a consequence of myocardial ischemia and injury.[17]

Histologically, atherosclerotic plaques are composed of a fibrous cap derived from smooth muscle cells; the cap covers a core of oxidized lipids, inflammatory cells, and cellular debris. Immature plaques consist of a necrotic, lipid-rich core surrounded by a thin, fibrous capsule. These so-called vulnerable plaques may not be visible angiographically, but they are prone to disruption and thrombus formation and, thus, are associated with unstable coronary syndromes. In fact, many of the plaques responsible for myocardial infarction may not be associated with significant coronary stenosis.[18] Mature atherosclerotic plaques, by contrast, have less necrotic cores and thicker, more stable fibrous caps. These plaques tend to cause greater degrees of coronary stenosis and are the lesions typically identified by coronary angiography; they are generally less susceptible to fracture and are associated less with acute coronary syndromes than are immature plaques. Atherosclerotic lesions may be associated with chronic stable angina, either because of luminal narrowing or because of dysfunctional vascular reactivity.

Table 1 Grading of Angina Pectoris by the Canadian Cardiovascular Society Classification System[18]

Class I

Ordinary physical activity, such as walking and climbing stairs, does not cause angina. Angina occurs with strenuous, rapid, or prolonged exertion at work or recreation.

Class II

Slight limitation of ordinary activity. Angina occurs while walking or climbing stairs rapidly; while walking uphill; while walking or climbing stairs after meals in cold or in wind; while under emotional stress; or only during the first several hours after waking. Angina occurs while walking more than two blocks on level grade and climbing more than one flight of ordinary stairs at a normal pace and in normal condition.

Class III

Marked limitations of ordinary physical activity. Angina occurs while walking one or two blocks on level grade and climbing one flight of stairs in normal conditions and at a normal pace.

Class IV

Inability to engage in any physical activity without discomfort. Anginal symptoms may be present at rest

---

Clinical Manifestations

A cardinal manifestation of IHD, angina is characterized by substernal pain or discomfort that may radiate to the neck, jaw, epigastrium, back, or arms. Words characteristically used to describe the sensation of angina include "squeezing," "vicelike," "heavy," "griplike," and "suffocating." Angina ordinarily lasts only a few minutes. Typical angina has three key characteristics: (1) substernal chest discomfort of characteristic quality and duration that is (2) provoked by exertion or emotional stress and is (3) relieved by rest or nitroglycerin. Atypical angina has two of the three characteristics of typical angina; noncardiac chest pain has one or none of the characteristics of typical angina.

The severity of angina is graded according to the Canadian Cardiovascular Society (CCS) classification [*see Table 1*].[19] Angina grade provides a useful way to evaluate functional limitation, treatment efficacy, and stability of symptoms over time.

Anginal chest pain is further characterized as stable or unstable. Unstable angina presents as prolonged angina at rest; new-onset angina that is severe, prolonged, or frequent; and established angina that has become distinctly more frequent, longer in duration, or more easily provoked. Some patients with unstable angina are at increased risk for acute MI and death [*see Table 2*]; the pathophysiology of unstable angina in these patients is often the result of plaque rupture and thrombosis. Patients with unstable angina and intermediate-risk or high-risk clinical features are best evaluated in the hospital.[20]

Differential Diagnosis

Given the potentially life-threatening sequelae of angina and the availability of effective therapies, it is important to consider angina in all patients presenting with chest pain. One approach to chest pain is to consider the differential diagnosis anatomically [*see Table 3*]. Various diseases of the heart and pericardium cause chest pain. Arrhythmias and valvular heart disease cause typical angina; pericarditis often causes pleuritic pain (i.e., pain that worsens on inspiration), but it may produce angina that is relieved by sitting up and leaning forward. Dissection of the great vessels can cause a characteristic, sudden, excruciating "tearing" pain in the chest or back. Diseases of the esophagus, such as esophageal spasm and acid reflux, may cause chest pain that is often postprandial or that occurs with recumbence. Esophageal spasm, in particular, can mimic angina and may respond to nitrates or calcium channel blockers. Diseases of lungs and pleura, including pulmonary embolism, pneumonia, pleuritis, and empyema, can cause chest pain that is often pleuritic. Chest wall syndromes, such as costochondritis, can cause substernal chest pain, typically reproduced with palpation. Herpes zoster may cause neuralgia that is localized to the chest; the pain may precede the appearance of the characteristic rash. Patients with panic disorder may describe chest pain or tightness accompanied by shortness of breath, diaphoresis, and other symptoms suggesting cardiac disease.

Diagnosis and Risk Stratification

PRELIMINARY EVALUATION

The evaluation of patients with chest pain should take into account symptom characteristics and cardiovascular risk factors, because these indicate the probability of angina and IHD [see Patient History and Its Use in Determining Risk for IHD, below]. If the history and physical examination suggest the presence of angina and IHD, patients are further evaluated by noninvasive tests, such as exercise treadmill testing or coronary angiography. Noninvasive testing serves to refine the probability of the diagnosis of IHD and stratify patients according to their risk for near-term cardiovascular events [see Noninvasive Testing, below].[21]

Patient History and Its Use in Determining Risk for IHD

Determining the pretest probability of significant IHD, which is defined as greater than 70% stenosis of one or more of the major epicardial coronary arteries, is an essential step in the evaluation of patients with suspected IHD. Decisions regarding testing and management are strongly influenced by estimates of the probability of significant IHD [see Figure 1].[21]

Estimates of the pretest probability of significant IHD can be accurately derived from a description of the chest pain syndrome and the presence or absence of cardiovascular risk fac-

tors.[22] It is important to characterize suspected angina by location, quality, duration, associated symptoms, and factors that exacerbate or relieve the pain [see Table 4]. Typical angina is substernal, lasts less than 5 minutes, is dull and aching, and is worse with exertion or emotional stress. Atypical angina has some but not all features of anginal chest pain. For example, a patient with aching substernal chest pain that lasts minutes but is unrelated to exertion is considered to have atypical angina. Similarly, a patient with sharp, exertional chest pain may also have atypical angina. Nonanginal pain is chest pain that does not have any features of angina: it is pleuritic or positional, unrelated to exertion, and is fleeting or lasts for many minutes. A detailed chest pain history allows the clinician to classify a patient's chest pain syndrome as typical angina, atypical angina, stable angina, unstable angina, or nonanginal chest pain. Among patients presenting to a clinician with chest pain, the presence of typical angina substantially increases the probability of significant IHD (likelihood ratio, 5.6), whereas the presence of atypical angina does not substantially alter the probability of significant IHD (likelihood ratio, 1.3).[23]

Once a detailed history of chest pain is obtained, cardiovascular risk factors are assessed; risk factors include increased age, male sex, menopausal status, cigarette smoking, hyperlipidemia, diabetes, hypertension, cerebrovascular disease, peripheral vascular disease, and a family history of premature coronary disease.[24] Cardiovascular risk factors greatly affect the pretest probability of significant IHD, particularly for women, younger patients, and patients with atypical chest pain syndromes [see Table 5]. For example, a 55-year-old man with atypical angina and no risk factors has a pretest probability of clinically significant IHD of 45%, whereas a 55-year-old man with typical angina and multiple cardiovascular risk factors has a 95% pretest probability of significant IHD.

Estimating the pretest probability of significant IHD is essential to determine whether further testing is warranted. For example, further diagnostic testing of the patient with a 45% probability of IHD would likely clarify the presence or absence of IHD. On the other hand, further testing of the patient with a 95% probability of IHD would be unlikely to alter the diagnosis of IHD, although further testing might help assess risk of cardiovascular events [see Risk Stratification in Patients with Chronic Stable Angina, below]. In general, further testing is not recommended for patients with a

Table 2 Short-Term Risk of Death or Nonfatal Myocardial Infarction in Patients with Unstable Angina[19]

High Risk	Intermediate Risk	Low Risk
At least one of the following features must be present: Prolonged ongoing (> 20 min) rest pain Pulmonary edema, most likely related to ischemia Angina with new or worsening MR murmur Angina with S$_3$ or new/worsening rales Angina with hypotension	No high-risk features but must have any of the following: Prolonged (> 20 min) rest angina, now resolved, with moderate or high likelihood of CAD Rest angina (> 20 min or relieved with sublingual nitroglycerin) Nocturnal angina New-onset CCSC III or IV angina in the past 3 wk with moderate or high likelihood of CAD Pathologic Q waves or resting ST depression ≤ 1 mm in multiple lead groups (anterior, inferior, lateral) Age > 65 yr	No high- or intermediate-risk feature but may have any of the following: Increased angina frequency, severity, or duration Angina provoked at a lower threshold New-onset angina with onset 2 wk to 2 mo before presentation Normal or unchanged ECG

Note: Estimation of the short-term risks of death and nonfatal myocardial infarction in unstable angina is a complex multivariable problem that cannot be fully specified in a table such as this. Therefore, the table is meant to offer general guidance and illustration rather than rigid algorithms.
CAD—coronary artery disease   CCSC—Canadian Cardiovascular Society Classification   MR—mitral regurgitation

very low pretest probability of significant IHD, as determined by a clinical assessment of patient history and risk factors.

Estimates of the risk of cardiovascular events can also be determined from clinical variables; the Framingham risk equations are commonly used for this purpose [see Figure 2].[25] This multivariate model estimates the 10-year risk of developing IHD on the basis of a patient's age; gender; total cholesterol level; and history of diabetes, hypertension, and smoking. This model is widely used, is readily available, and has been validated across a variety of populations.

The decision to pursue further testing in patients with possible angina appropriately incorporates patient preferences regarding diagnosis or intervention and an assessment of comorbidities [see Patients Warranting Noninvasive Testing, below].

Physical Examination

The physical examination of patients with chronic stable angina is often normal but may indicate the presence of hypertension (e.g., elevated blood pressure, enlarged or laterally displaced point of maximum impulse, S_4 gallop, or retinal vascular chang-es) or coexisting peripheral vascular disease (e.g., diminished pulses or bruits). In younger patients with premature coronary disease, there may be stigmata of genetic dyslipidemia syndromes (e.g., xanthelasma associated with familial hypercholesterolemia). For patients with chest pain, the presence of any of these findings increases the likelihood of significant IHD.

It is particularly helpful to examine a patient during an episode of angina. The presence of an S_4 or S_3 gallop, a mitral regurgitation murmur, a paradoxically split S_2 heart sound, bibasilar crackles, or a chest wall heave makes IHD more likely, particularly if the finding disappears when the pain goes away.[26] Physical examination findings that wax and wane with anginal symptoms are of particular significance, because they may indicate significant myocardial dysfunction at low work loads.

Laboratory Tests

A resting 12-lead electrocardiogram should be performed in all patients with suspected angina, although the results are normal in 50% of patients with chronic stable angina.[27] The presence of pathologic Q waves is virtually pathognomonic of

Table 3 Differential Diagnosis of Chest Pain

Diagnosis	Characteristics	Comments
Ischemic heart disease	Typical or atypical angina	Caused by diminished coronary blood flow and/or increased myocardial oxygen demand
Nonischemic heart disease		
Arrhythmias	Palpitations or typical angina	Tachycardia
Valvular heart disease	Typical angina, often exertional	Heart murmur present
Aortic dissection	"Tearing" pain, often abrupt onset	Widened mediastinum, often with hypertension
Pericarditis	Often pleuritic pain, but may be anginal; relieved by sitting up and leaning forward	Friction rub may be present; diffuse ST segment elevation (PR segment depression) on ECG
Pulmonary disease		
Pulmonary embolus	Pleuritic pain, associated dyspnea	Hypoxia/hypoxemia, pulsus paradoxus, and risk factors for thromboembolic disease
Pneumothorax	Acute onset, pleuritic pain, associated dyspnea	Hyperresonance on examination; tension pneumothorax is associated with distended neck veins, hypotension, and tachycardia
Pneumonia	Pleuritic pain	Associated with fever and productive cough
Gastrointestinal disease		
Esophageal disease	May be indistinguishable from angina	Often diagnosed following a negative evaluation for ischemic heart disease
Acid peptic disease	May be indistinguishable from angina	Pain often related to meals
Biliary disease	Right upper quadrant pain that radiates to the back or scapula	Typically worse following meals; right upper quadrant tenderness may be present
Pancreatitis	"Boring" epigastric pain, may radiate to the back	Chronic pancreatitis pain may occur without signs of systemic illness
Chest wall or dermatologic pain	Characteristically reproduced with palpation or movement	Reproduction of pain does not exclude angina
Costochrondritis		
Rib fracture		
Sternoclavicular arthritis		
Herpes zoster		Pain may precede rash
Fibrositis		Characteristic point tenderness
Psychiatric disorders	May be indistinguishable from angina	Often diagnosed following a negative evaluation for angina
Anxiety disorders		Often associated with palpitations, sweating, and anxiety
Affective disorders (e.g., depression)		
Somatoform disorders		
Thought disorders (e.g., fixed delusions)		
Factitious disorders (e.g., Munchausen syndrome)		

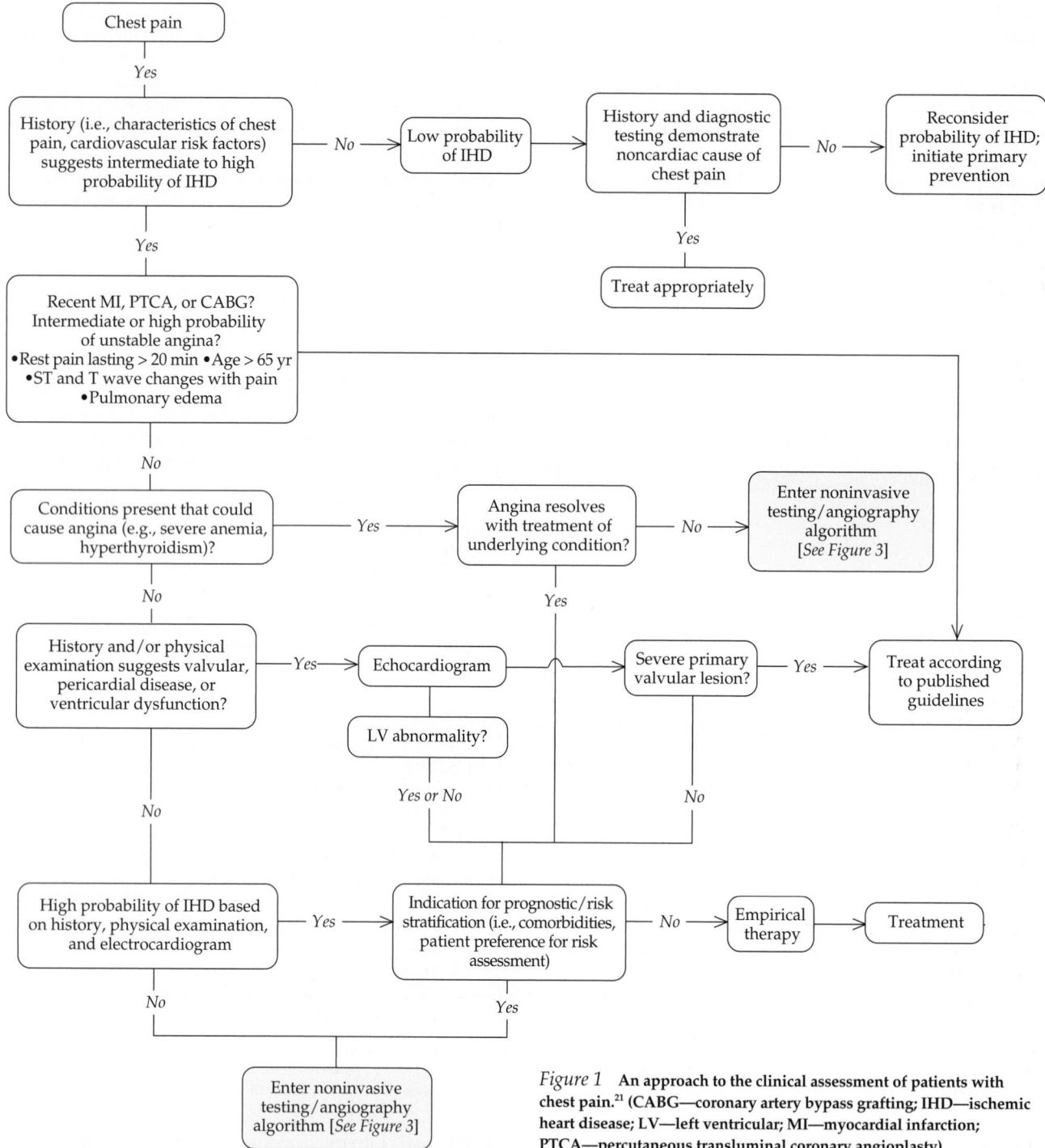

Figure 1 **An approach to the clinical assessment of patients with chest pain.**[21] **(CABG—coronary artery bypass grafting; IHD—ischemic heart disease; LV—left ventricular; MI—myocardial infarction; PTCA—percutaneous transluminal coronary angioplasty)**

clinically significant IHD, although isolated Q waves in lead III or a QS pattern in leads V1 and V2 is nonspecific. Several other ECG findings increase the clinical probability of IHD; ST segment depression, T wave inversions, and left ventricular hypertrophy (LVH) favor the diagnosis of angina.[28] Arrhythmias, including atrial fibrillation, ventricular tachyarrhythmias, bundle branch blocks, and atrioventricular block, increase the likelihood of IHD somewhat but are nonspecific.

As with the physical examination, an ECG obtained during an episode of pain may be particularly informative. About half of patients with a normal resting ECG will have an abnormality suggestive of ischemia during an episode of chest pain. Sugges-

tive abnormalities include ST segment depression, T wave inversion, or "pseudonormalization" of these abnormalities during pain.[29] Abnormalities on a resting ECG that disappear with resolution of pain may indicate severe IHD, because they suggest ischemia at low work loads or unstable coronary syndromes.

Recommended laboratory tests include measurement of hemoglobin and fasting glucose levels and a fasting lipid panel (including measurement of levels of total cholesterol, HDL cholesterol, triglycerides, and calculated LDL cholesterol).[1] Hyperlipidemia is an important risk factor for IHD; the risk for IHD increases 1% for each 1 mg/dl increase in serum LDL cholesterol.[30] Similarly, patients with impaired glucose tolerance or

Table 4 Features of Typical Angina

Feature	Typical Angina	Comments
Location	Substernal but may radiate to neck, jaw, shoulder, or arms	The symptom of angina is typically felt below the ears and above the umbilicus
Duration	Typically less than 5 min	Longer-lasting chest pain raises concern for MI but may also be nonanginal
Quality	Dull, aching, pressurelike pain that is difficult to localize precisely	Levine sign, a clenched fist held over the chest well, represents the location and quality of typical angina
Exacerbating or relieving factors	Worsens with exertion or emotional stress and is relieved by rest or nitroglycerin; pain is often precipitated by a reproducible amount of exertion	Typical angina that occurs at lower than the usual amounts of exertion raises concern for unstable angina
Associated symptoms	Diaphoresis, nausea, palpitations, light-headedness, and dyspnea	Palpitations and light-headedness raise concern for arrhythmia; dyspnea suggests left ventricular or valvular dysfunction

frank diabetes are at increased risk for IHD. Normal hemoglobin excludes anemia. Thyroid function tests are indicated in patients who have signs or symptoms compatible with hyperthyroidism.

Imaging Studies

Chest radiography is of limited value in most patients with suspected angina[31]; however, a chest radiograph or other imaging study, such as computed tomography, is indicated in patients with signs or symptoms of congestive heart failure (CHF), valvular heart disease, or pericardial disease or in patients with possible aortic dissection or aneurysm. Echocardiography or multigated equilibrium radionuclide angiography should be obtained in any patient with suspected left ventricular impairment.

Patients Warranting Noninvasive Testing

Noninvasive testing usually has two objectives: to ascertain the probability of clinically important IHD and to estimate the risk of a serious cardiovascular event (e.g., MI or death) in the near future. These two objectives are often pursued concurrently, but it is useful to distinguish between diagnostic testing and testing for purposes of risk stratification.

Noninvasive testing is most likely to influence clinical decision making when the pretest probability of IHD is in the intermediate range. For example, a positive exercise treadmill test in a 55-year-old man with atypical chest pain and no other risk fac-

tors (pretest probability of clinically significant IHD, approximately 50%) would significantly increase the suspicion of clinically important IHD (posttest probability, 85%), whereas a negative exercise treadmill test would significantly reduce the suspicion of clinically significant IHD (posttest probability, 15%).

On the other hand, an abnormal exercise treadmill test in a 35-year-old woman with atypical chest pain and no other risk factors (pretest probability of clinically significant IHD, < 5%) would likely be falsely positive and could prompt use of unnecessary medications or potentially invasive diagnostic testing; a negative test would simply support a low clinical suspicion of disease. Therefore, further testing in such a low-risk patient would not be indicated. Similarly, further testing of high-risk patients is not likely to provide information that would alter the diagnosis of IHD. For example, because of the likelihood of significant coronary disease in a 65-year-old man with typical angina (pretest probability, 94%), a positive exercise test would only confirm the high clinical suspicion of IHD; a negative result would only lower the estimate into the moderate range and would not exclude the diagnosis of significant IHD.

Noninvasive testing is commonly obtained in persons with a high clinical probability of having significant IHD. In this setting, however, noninvasive testing is useful to assess risk and establish prognosis but not to establish or refute the diagnosis of coronary disease, as is the case for patients with an intermediate clinical probability of significant IHD.

Table 5 Comparison of Pretest Likelihood of IHD in Low-Risk Symptomatic Patients and High-Risk Symptomatic Patients[49]

Age (yr)	Nonanginal Chest Pain (%)*		Atypical Angina (%)*		Typical Angina (%)*	
	Men	Women	Men	Women	Men	Women
35	3–35	1–19	8–59	2–39	30–88	10–78
45	9–47	2–22	21–70	5–43	51–92	20–79
55	23–59	23–59	45–79	10–47	80–95	38–82
65	49–69	49–69	71–86	20–51	93–97	56–84

*Each value represents the percentage with significant IHD. The first number given in each range (e.g., 3–35) is the percentage for a low-risk, mid-decade patient who does not have diabetes, does not smoke, and does not have hyperlipidemia. The second number in each range is the percentage for a same-age patient who does have diabetes, does smoke, or does have hyperlipidemia. Both high- and low-risk patients have normal resting ECGs. If ST-T wave changes or Q waves are present, the likelihood of IHD is higher in each entry of the table.

IHD—ischemic heart disease

Estimate of 10-Year Risk for Men

Age (yr)	Points
20–34	−9
35–39	−4
40–44	0
45–49	3
50–54	6
55–59	8
60–64	10
65–69	11
70–74	12
75–79	13

Total Cholesterol (mg/dl)	Points				
	Age 20–39 yr	Age 40–49 yr	Age 50–59 yr	Age 60–69 yr	Age 70–79 yr
< 160	0	0	0	0	0
160–199	4	3	2	1	0
200–239	7	5	3	1	0
240–279	9	6	4	2	1
≥ 280	11	8	5	3	1

	Points				
	Age 20–39 yr	Age 40–49 yr	Age 50–59 yr	Age 60–69 yr	Age 70–79 yr
Nonsmoker	0	0	0	0	0
Smoker	8	5	3	1	1

HDL (mg/dl)	Points
≥ 60	−1
50–59	0
40–49	1
< 40	2

Systolic Blood Pressure (mm Hg)	Untreated	Treated
< 120	0	0
120–129	0	1
130–139	1	2
140–159	1	2
≥ 160	2	3

Total Points	10-Year Risk (%)
< 0	< 1
0–4	1
5–6	2
7	3
8	4
9	5
10	6
11	8
12	10
13	12
14	16
15	20
16	25
≥ 17	≥ 30

Estimate of 10-Year Risk for Women

Age (yr)	Points
20–34	−7
35–39	−3
40–44	0
45–49	3
50–54	6
55–59	8
60–64	10
65–69	12
70–74	14
75–79	16

Total Cholesterol (mg/dl)	Points				
	Age 20–39 yr	Age 40–49 yr	Age 50–59 yr	Age 60–69 yr	Age 70–79 yr
< 160	0	0	0	0	0
160–199	4	3	2	1	1
200–239	8	6	4	2	1
240–279	11	8	5	3	2
≥ 280	13	10	7	4	2

	Points				
	Age 20–39 yr	Age 40–49 yr	Age 50–59 yr	Age 60–69 yr	Age 70–79 yr
Nonsmoker	0	0	0	0	0
Smoker	9	7	4	2	1

HDL (mg/dl)	Points
≥ 60	−1
50–59	0
40–49	1
< 40	2

Systolic Blood Pressure (mm Hg)	Untreated	Treated
< 120	0	0
120–129	1	3
130–139	2	4
140–159	3	5
≥ 160	4	6

Total Points	10-Year Risk (%)
< 9	< 1
9–12	1
13–14	2
15	3
16	4
17	5
18	6
19	8
20	11
21	14
22	17
23	22
24	27
≥ 25	≥ 30

Figure 2 **Estimates of major cardiovascular risk for men and women, based on the Framingham risk equations.**[25]

For purposes of deciding on a course of noninvasive testing, there is no precise definition of the upper and lower boundaries of intermediate probability of IHD; rather, this is a matter of clinical judgment in individual situations. Relevant issues include the degree of uncertainty acceptable to the physician and patient, the probability of an alternative diagnosis, the costs and risks of additional testing, and the benefits and risks of treatment in the absence of additional testing.[32] It is reasonable to consider a risk of clinically significant IHD of 10% to 20% or lower as low probability and of 80% to 90% risk or greater as high probability.[32]

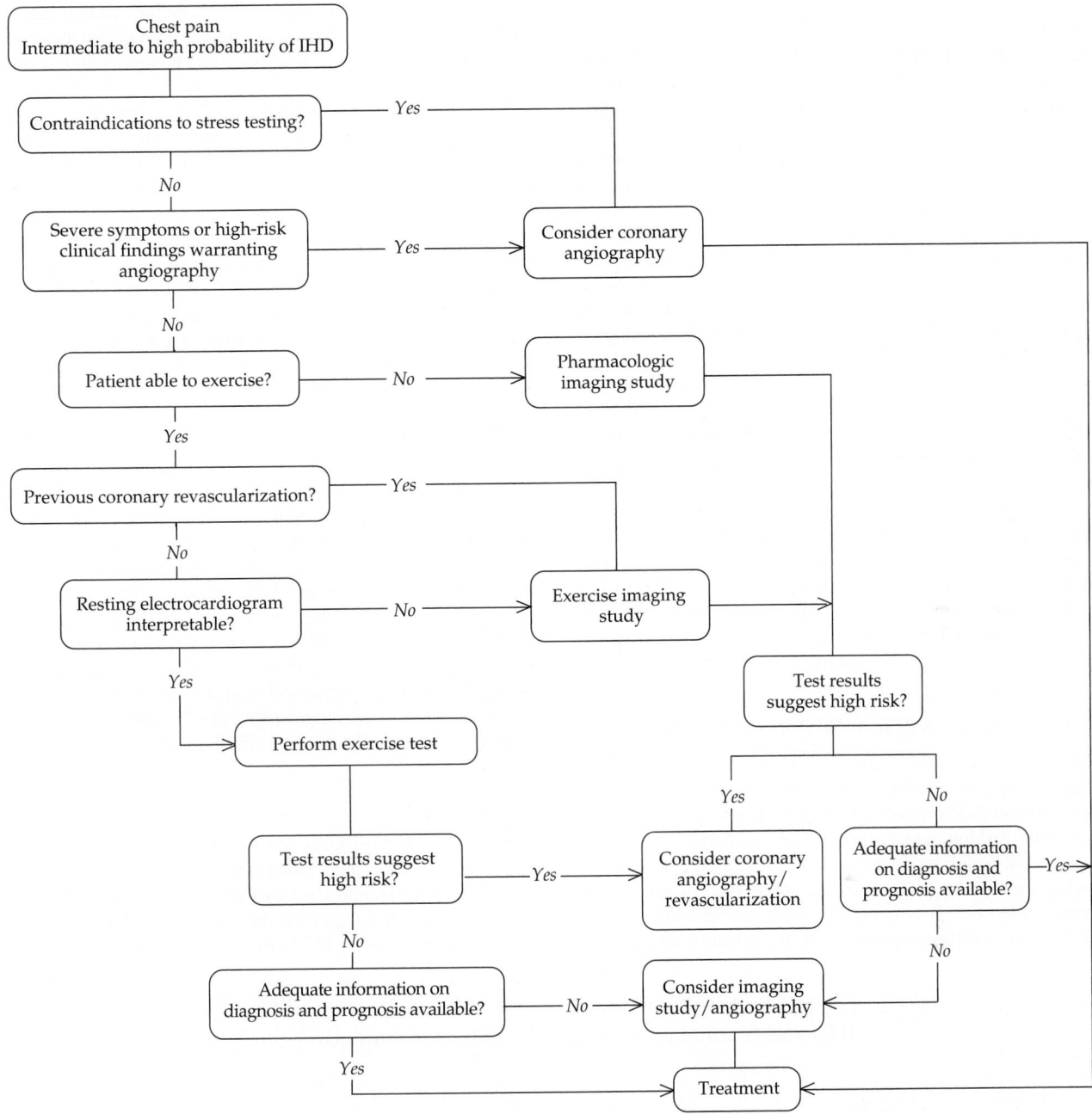

Figure 3 **Noninvasive testing and angiography in the evaluation of patients suspected of having ischemic heart disease.**[21]

NONINVASIVE TESTING

Patients whose history, physical examination, and ECG results indicate an intermediate or high probability of IHD usually should undergo further diagnostic evaluation [*see Figure 3*]. Noninvasive testing in patients with an intermediate probability of IHD provides important information about diagnosis (i.e., the presence or absence of coronary disease). In patients with an intermediate or high probability of IHD, noninvasive testing helps to stratify risk for major cardiovascular events. This stratification helps determine treatment strategies.

Commonly performed noninvasive studies include exercise ECG testing, stress radionuclide myocardial perfusion imaging, and stress echocardiography. The performance characteristics of various noninvasive tests and posttest probabilities of IHD for a range of pretest probabilities are listed [*see Table 6*].

ECG Exercise Testing

Guidelines from the American College of Cardiology/American Heart Association/American College of Physicians (ACC/AHA/ACP) recommend exercise ECG as the first-choice diagnostic test for the average patient with an intermediate pretest probability of IHD and a normal resting ECG.[32,33] Exercise testing has imperfect sensitivity and specificity (68% and 77%, respectively), but it is widely available and inexpensive. In addition, it readily identifies patients at high risk for IHD and provides important prognostic information [*see* Risk Stratification in Patients with Chronic Stable Angina, *below*]. Exercise testing is generally safe; MI or death occurs with a frequency of less than 1 in 2,500 tests.[34] Symptom-limited exercise testing is safe in patients with unstable angina who lack evidence of MI and CHF and who are free of chest pain at the time of testing.[32] Specific absolute and relative contraindications for exercise testing can be found in guidelines from the ACC/AHA.[1] Other noninvasive tests are preferred in patients who are unable to exercise, in those who previously underwent coronary revascularization, and in those with specific resting ECG abnormalities that would interfere with the interpretation of an exercise ECG (such abnormalities include ST segment depression of greater than 1 mm at rest, preexcitation syndrome, electronically paced rhythm, left bundle branch block, and left ventricular hypertrophy with repolarization abnormalities).[32]

Interpretation of the exercise test depends on the patient's exercise capacity, symptoms, the reasons for stopping the test, the hemodynamic response, any pertinent findings on physical examination (e.g., exercise-induced S_3 heart sound or mitral regurgitation), and any changes in the ECG. Patients who stop the test because of the onset of angina are very likely to have significant IHD. Exercise-induced falls in blood pressure or the development of an exercise-induced S_3 heart sound are strongly suggestive of ischemic left ventricular dysfunction. Specific exercise-induced ECG changes suggestive of IHD include a horizontal or downward-sloping ST segment depression or elevation of greater than 1 mm during or after exercise.[1] Exercise-induced changes in lead V5 are most reliable for the diagnosis of IHD.[1]

Stress Radionuclide Myocardial Perfusion Imaging

Although exercise ECG continues to be recommended as the diagnostic test of choice for most patients with suspected angina, stress myocardial perfusion imaging using single-photon emission computed tomography (SPECT) is the most common noninvasive test performed in the United States. SPECT imaging following exercise or pharmacologic stress (e.g., using dipyridamole, adenosine, or dobutamine) has greater sensitivity for IHD than exercise testing, particularly in patients with an abnormal resting ECG; in addition, SPECT can define vascular regions in which stress-induced coronary flow is limited. Furthermore, SPECT imaging allows an estimation of left ventricular (LV) systolic size and function.

Exercise myocardial perfusion SPECT is preferred for patients who have baseline ECG abnormalities that interfere with the interpretation of an exercise ECG. Such abnormalities include a resting ST segment depression greater than 1 mm and LVH; digoxin therapy and ventricular preexcitation can also cause ECG abnormalities.[35] Myocardial perfusion SPECT with pharmacologic stress is preferred in the setting of left bundle branch block or ventricular pacing.[35] Because of its greater sensitivity, stress myocardial perfusion imaging is an option after a nondiagnostic exercise ECG. Stress myocardial perfusion imaging can also further stratify the risk of IHD in patients with an abnormal exercise ECG.[36]

Stress Echocardiography

Stress echocardiography (i.e., echocardiography performed after exercise or dobutamine administration) is another option for noninvasive testing to establish the diagnosis of IHD. Stress induces regional wall motion abnormalities in the myocardial regions supplied by stenotic coronary vessels; stress echocardiography defines such regions of the left ventricular wall. Stress echocardiography, like myocardial perfusion imaging, is a good choice for patients with ECG abnormalities that might interfere with the interpretation of an exercise ECG.[37] The sensitivity of stress echocardiography, as with that of stress myocardial perfusion imaging, is in the range of 80% to 85%. Exercise echocardiography is marginally more specific than other noninvasive diagnostic tests.[38]

Test Selection

Although exercise ECG remains the recommended initial noninvasive test for most patients with suspected IHD, clinical decision making should also take into account individual patient characteristics, local expertise, and availability. Stress echocardiography and exercise ECG can be performed in a physician's

Table 6 Posttest Probability of Significant IHD Based on Pretest Probabilities of IHD and Normal or Abnormal Results of Noninvasive Studies

Test Result	20% Pretest Probability		50% Pretest Probability		80% Pretest Probability	
	Men	Women	Men	Women	Men	Women
Exercise ECG						
Abnormal	71	43	91	75	98	92
Normal	13	16	38	43	71	75
ECG with SPECT						
Abnormal	85	71	96	91	99	98
Normal	3	4	11	13	33	36
Exercise echocardiography						
Abnormal	38	37	71	70	91	82
Normal	15	17	41	44	74	76
Dobutamine echocardiography*						
Abnormal	46	—	77	—	93	—
Normal	3	—	11	—	32	—

Note: calculations are based on point estimates of the sensitivities and specificities of noninvasive studies abstracted from Gibbons.[21]

*Available studies did not include women in sufficient numbers to accurately estimate sensitivity and specificity for these tests.

IHD—ischemic heart disease   SPECT—single-photon emission computed tomography

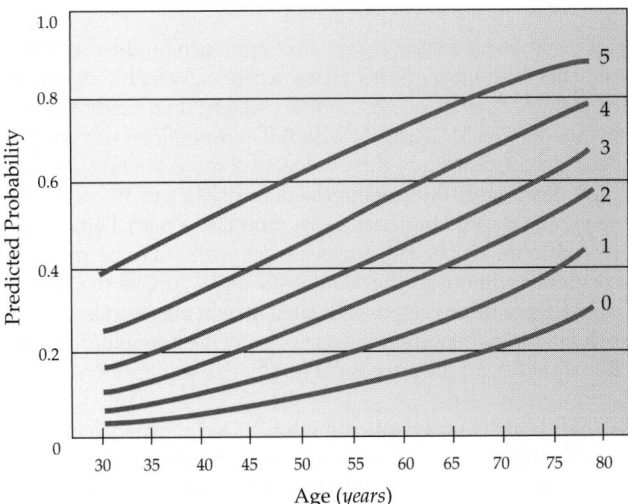

Figure 4 Nomogram showing the probability of severe coronary disease (i.e., three-vessel disease or left main coronary artery disease) on a five-point score. One point is awarded for each of the following variables: male gender; typical angina; history or electrocardiographic evidence of myocardial infarction; diabetes; and use of insulin. Each curve shows the probability of severe coronary disease as a function of age.[50]

office, whereas radionuclide myocardial perfusion imaging requires a specialized setting. In addition, myocardial perfusion imaging is considerably more expensive than exercise ECG.

Specific noninvasive tests are preferred in certain patient subsets. Patients unable to exercise should undergo some form of pharmacologic noninvasive test. Pharmacologic stress echocardiography using dipyridamole, adenosine, or, less commonly, dobutamine is an option for patients who are unable to exercise. Nonspecific perfusion image defects may be more common with exercise myocardial perfusion imaging in patients with left bundle branch block; pharmacologic stress imaging or echocardiography is preferred in these patients.[32] Exercise ECG is less accurate in establishing the diagnosis of IHD in women, and some authors have suggested that SPECT imaging and stress echocardiography are more accurate diagnostic tests for women with an intermediate probability of having IHD.[39,40] The ACC/AHA/ACP expert panel concluded, however, that insufficient data are available to recommend stress imaging or echocardiography over standard exercise ECG in women with suspected angina.[32]

Echocardiography is less sensitive in very obese patients, and examination tables used for SPECT imaging often have weight limitations. Planar scintigraphy, positron-emission tomography, and coronary angiography are testing options for obese patients. Planar scintigraphy is less sensitive than SPECT, and positron emission tomography is less well characterized than other modalities. There is some rationale for performing stress imaging or echocardiography in patients with angina whose histories suggest they are at high risk for major cardiovascular events (e.g., patients who experience angina at low work loads or whose angina is progressive); in such patients, determination of LV systolic function and anatomic distribution of IHD are important considerations in anticipation of a possible need for revascularization. For these patients, it may be appropriate to proceed directly to coronary angiography [*see* Invasive Testing, *below*].

Beta blockade reduces the sensitivity of all noninvasive tests, particularly exercise ECG[41]; it is recommended that, whenever possible, beta blockers be withheld for four half-lives (approximately 48 hours) before noninvasive testing is undertaken. Digoxin causes resting ST segment depression and reduces the specificity of exercise ECG.

In general, it is cost-effective to perform exercise ECG as the initial test in most patients, followed by additional imaging for patients in whom further diagnostic or prognostic testing is warranted.[42] Noninvasive testing is not generally recommended as a screening test in asymptomatic persons. Specific exceptions include patients whose occupation requires periodic stress testing (e.g., pilots, firefighters, competitive athletes, and police).

Imaging Studies under Investigation

Several CT and magnetic resonance imaging techniques are currently under study for use in diagnosing patients with suspected angina or in stratifying such patients for risk of cardiac events. Of these techniques, the most widely used is electron-beam computed tomography (EBCT), which detects coronary artery calcification. Although the sensitivity of EBCT for the diagnosis of significant coronary artery stenosis is high, the specificity of EBCT for significant coronary artery stenoses ranges from only 41% to 76%, yielding many false positive results. Some studies suggest that the "calcium score" derived from EBCT predicts the extent of angiographically detected CAD.[43] Studies that correlate calcium scores with risk of future cardiac events have been fraught with methodologic problems[44,45]; it is not clear whether EBCT adds significantly to clinical risk assessment using validated tools such as the Framingham risk score.[46] To date, no prospective, population-based studies have investigated a potential association between calcium score derived from EBCT and risk of future coronary events; likewise, no studies have shown that screening for IHD with EBCT reduces mortality.

Asymptomatic patients identified as being at potentially high risk for cardiac events on the basis of EBCT may suffer anxiety and undergo unnecessary procedures as a result of the study. Estimates of the cost efficacy of EBCT relative to current strategies for diagnosis and risk stratification are varied and are sensitive to the prevalence of disease in a screened population; currently, the clinical benefits of screening asymptomatic patients are uncertain.[47] The ACC/AHA guidelines do not recommend EBCT and other imaging procedures, such as MRI angiography, in asymptomatic patients.[48] Although EBCT testing is currently not recommended as a screening test, it is reasonable to evaluate patients who have undergone EBCT and who have been found to have severe coronary calcification with some form of noninvasive testing.

INVASIVE TESTING

Coronary angiography provides unequaled detail of coronary anatomy, including detail sufficient to enable evaluation for possible revascularization; however, angiography is invasive and expensive compared with noninvasive testing. In addition, although angiography identifies the degree and distribution of coronary stenoses, it provides inconsistent assessment of the functional significance and stability of a particular coronary lesion[32]; for example, plaques that can possibly rupture and thereby cause acute coronary syndromes are commonly angiographically insignificant.[18] Moreover, studies have called into question the reliability of angiographic measurements of coronary stenosis in some settings.[49]

The decision to pursue angiography should be based on preferences of the patient and provider, coexisting illnesses, estimates of the probability of high-risk IHD, and the urgency to confirm or refute a possible diagnosis of IHD.

Direct referral for coronary angiography is recommended for patients who have survived sudden death, because of the high probability of multivessel IHD in these patients.[32] Other patients for whom angiography is recommended as a diagnostic test include those for whom the diagnosis of IHD remains uncertain despite noninvasive testing, provided the benefit of a more certain diagnosis outweighs the risk and cost of angiography; patients who cannot undergo noninvasive testing because of disability, illness, or morbid obesity; patients with suspected nonatherosclerotic angina (e.g., coronary dissection, coronary anomaly, Kawasaki disease, and coronary artery spasm); and patients with a high pretest probability of disease of the left main coronary artery or three-vessel IHD [see Prognostic Value of Coronary Angiography, below].[32]

DIAGNOSIS OF CHRONIC STABLE ANGINA

The presence of clinically stable, typical angina for a period of 2 or more months is adequate to establish the diagnosis of chronic stable angina. As mentioned [see Preliminary Evaluation, above], an accurate estimate of the likelihood of significant IHD can be established from simple clinical criteria (i.e., characteristics of chest pain and cardiovascular risk factors). For patients with an uncertain diagnosis after undergoing clinical assessment, particularly patients with some cardiovascular risk factors and an atypical angina syndrome, noninvasive testing is valuable for establishing the diagnosis of IHD. IHD can be confirmed by coronary angiography, which is also helpful in defining the severity of coronary atherosclerosis [see Risk Stratification in Patients with Chronic Stable Angina, below].

RISK STRATIFICATION IN PATIENTS WITH CHRONIC STABLE ANGINA

Risk stratification that determines the prognosis for MI or death is essential in determining treatment recommendations for patients with chronic stable angina. In general, a patient's coronary risk is determined by the interplay of four factors[32]: (1) left ventricular systolic function; (2) the extent and severity of atherosclerotic occlusion of the coronary tree (i.e., ischemic burden); (3) plaque stability (i.e., risk of plaque rupture); and (4) coexisting medical conditions. Clinical parameters, results of noninvasive testing, and coronary angiography provide important prognostic and diagnostic information.

Clinical Parameters Indicating High Risk

Although noninvasive testing and coronary angiography are the mainstays of risk stratification, clinical parameters alone are sufficient to identify some patients as having a high probability of severe IHD (i.e., three-vessel disease or left main CAD). Hubbard and colleagues developed a simplified algorithm for predicting the probability of severe IHD on the basis of six clinical parameters: age, gender, presence of typical angina, presence of diabetes, insulin use, and prior MI (as indicated by history or ECG) [see Figure 4].[50] Older patients with multiple risk factors have a greater than 50% chance of having severe IHD and should be considered for direct referral for coronary angiography. In one study, a previous history of MI and the presence of a carotid bruit (a marker for peripheral vascular disease) more than doubled the probability of severe IHD.[51] Direct referral for coronary angiography is estimated to be cost-effective when the pretest probability of severe IHD is high.[52]

Follow-up Noninvasive Testing

Noninvasive testing is a sensible approach for the majority of patients without high-risk characteristics. Available diagnostic modalities predict death more accurately than cardiovascular events such as MI. Patients with IHD are stratified according to their risk of death into three categories: those at low risk (< 1% mortality a year); those at intermediate risk (1% to 3% mortality a year); and those at high risk (> 3% mortality a year). Persons estimated to be at low risk for death generally may be managed medically without further diagnostic testing unless their condition deteriorates.[32] Persons estimated to be at intermediate or high risk after initial noninvasive testing may need to undergo additional studies for the purpose of further risk stratification.

Left ventricular systolic function Declining left ventricular systolic function is the strongest single predictor of long-term mortality in patients with IHD.[53] Patients with an ejection fraction of less than 35% have a mortality in excess of 3% a year. Left ventricular function can be assessed by echocardiography, stress myocardial perfusion imaging with SPECT, angiographic ventriculography, or gated nuclear medicine studies. As noted, not all patients with angina require evaluation of left ventricular function. Patients with a normal resting ECG and no history of MI or CHF are very likely to have normal left ventricular systolic function (92% to 95% probability).[54] Patients with a history of CHF, MI, or ECG evidence of prior MI should undergo evaluation of left ventricular function.

Exercise treadmill ECG In addition to the diagnostic information it provides, exercise treadmill ECG testing supplies useful prognostic information. Exercise capacity during a treadmill test is one of the strongest predictors of cardiovascular risk. Exercise capacity is influenced, in part, by LV function, both at rest and with exercise. Several measures of exercise capacity are used: exercise duration, maximum heart rate, exercise duration × heart rate, and estimates of work measured in metabolic equivalents (METs). Other important variables include ECG measures of exercise-induced ischemia, as reflected in ST segment depression or elevation, and the duration of ST segment deviation during the recovery phase of the exercise protocol.

The Duke treadmill score (DTS) combines these exercise test variables and is the most widely used prognostic treadmill score.[55] The DTS is calculated as follows:

Exercise time (in min) – (5 × the ST segment deviation [in mm]) – (4 × the angina index)

The angina index equals 2 when angina is the reason for stopping the exercise test; it equals 1 when angina occurs during the test or the recovery period; and it equals 0 if no angina occurs. In patients with a low-risk DTS (i.e., ≥ +5), the 4-year survival is 99% (average annual mortality, 0.25%) [see Table 7]. Patients with a high-risk DTS (< –10) have a 4-year survival rate of 79% (average annual mortality, 5%). In one study, more than two thirds of outpatients with suspected IHD had low-risk scores, and only 4% of patients had high-risk scores.[55] Available data suggest that patients with frequent ventricular ectopy or a slow heart rate recovery time following exercise testing are also at increased risk for death during subsequent follow-up,[56] although it remains uncertain how best to incorporate this information into the stratification of risk.

Stress testing Stress myocardial perfusion imaging and stress echocardiography are commonly used in risk stratification

Table 7 Survival According to Risk Groups
Based on Duke Treadmill Score (DTS)

Risk Group (DTS)	Overall Survival (%)	4-Year Survival (%)	Annual Mortality (%)
Low risk (≥ +5)	62	0.99	0.25
Moderate risk (−10 to +4)	34	0.95	1.25
High risk (< −10)	4	0.79	5.0

of patients with IHD, although their prognostic value is less known than that of exercise ECG.[57] In patients with an intermediate-risk exercise ECG (DTS < + 5 and ≥ −10), annual mortality is between 1% and 3%; these patients are usually referred for additional diagnostic testing, either stress imaging or coronary angiography. In patients with a high-risk exercise ECG result (DTS < −10), annual cardiac mortality is estimated to exceed 3%; these patients are generally referred for coronary angiography. Patients with a low-risk exercise ECG (DTS ≥ +5) require no further testing and may be medically managed. It is also appropriate to obtain a stress imaging study for purposes of risk stratification for patients who are unable to exercise and for patients with uninterpretable rest ECGs. Stress imaging studies are preferred over exercise ECG for evaluating ischemia in symptomatic patients who have previously undergone revascularization.

A normal poststress myocardial perfusion imaging study, as with a low-risk exercise ECG, indicates an excellent prognosis, even among patients with chronic stable angina.[58] The number, size, and location of abnormalities on stress myocardial perfusion studies indicate the distribution and severity of coronary artery stenoses; larger and more numerous perfusion defects are associated with more severe CAD. Stress-induced LV dysfunction—a marker of severe multivessel IHD—is indicated by LV dilatation or lung uptake of radionuclide tracer.[59,60] Patients with two or more moderate to large stress-induced perfusion defects or evidence of stress-induced LV dysfunction are considered to have a high probability of severe IHD; these patients are candidates for referral for coronary angiography.

A negative stress echocardiogram also indicates a good prognosis.[61] In the presence of significant IHD, stress induces regional wall motion abnormalities in the myocardial regions supplied by the stenotic coronary vessel. Stress-induced wall motion abnormalities involving two or more segments at lower levels of stress predict high-risk IHD. As with stress myocardial perfusion imaging, stress-induced LV dilatation suggests multivessel IHD. Abnormal stress echocardiography provides diagnostic and prognostic information that is incremental to that obtained by exercise ECG,[62] although there are relatively fewer follow-up data for this test than for myocardial perfusion studies.

Prognostic Value of Coronary Angiography

The anatomic extent of IHD is a powerful indicator of prognosis. Referral for coronary angiography should be considered for patients with a high-risk exercise ECG (DTS < −10), a high-risk stress myocardial perfusion imaging study, or a high-risk stress echocardiogram, provided the patient is a candidate for revascularization.

In the Coronary Artery Surgery Study database of patients with suspected IHD who were referred for coronary angiography, the 12-year survival rate for patients with normal coronary arteries was 91%, compared with 74% for patients with one-vessel disease, 59% for patients with two-vessel disease, and 40% for patients with three-vessel disease.[63] Proximal lesions are associated with greater risk than more distal lesions.[64] LV function remains crucially important. For example, the 5-year survival of a 65-year-old man with stable angina, three-vessel coronary stenoses, and normal LV function is 93%, compared with 5-year survival of only 58% in a similar patient with an LV ejection fraction of 30%.[64] Although angiography provides detailed information about the extent and severity of stenoses, it does not define which ones are actually responsible for anginal symptoms. Furthermore, the atherosclerotic plaques most likely to rupture and to thereby cause acute coronary syndromes, including MI and death, are often missed by coronary angiography.[18]

In summary, for patients with IHD, the strongest predictor of long-term survival is LV systolic function. A second determinant of survival is the severity and distribution of coronary lesions. A third determinant is the stability of coronary plaques; plaque instability and rupture increase the short-term risk of unstable coronary syndromes and death. Currently, there is no satisfactory means to measure this third determinant.

Treatment

The two overarching goals of the treatment of patients with chronic stable angina are to reduce the likelihood of untoward clinical events (i.e., acute coronary syndromes and sudden death) and to improve quality of life by reducing anginal symptoms and enhancing function. Treatment options include lifestyle modifications, medications, and revascularization. Evidence-based guidelines have been published, and a general approach to the treatment of patients with chronic stable angina is outlined below. However, management should be individualized in accordance with a patient's risk of adverse outcomes, coexisting conditions, and preferences, as well as in consideration of the cost and effectiveness of therapeutic alternatives. An ACC/AHA/ACP expert panel developed an mnemonic for the treatment of patients with chronic stable angina [*see Table 8*].[21]

LIFESTYLE MODIFICATION

Smoking Cessation

Among nonpharmacologic interventions, smoking cessation has the greatest impact on total mortality and cardiovascular risk. A systematic review of prospective cohort studies of smokers with IHD found a striking 29% to 36% relative risk reduction in all-cause mortality for patients who were able to quit smoking.[65] Most patients in these cohort studies had previous MI, angioplasty, or coronary artery bypass grafting (CABG) at the time

---

Table 8 The "ABCDEs" of Treatment
for Patients with Chronic Stable Angina[20]

A = Aspirin and antianginal therapy; ACE inhibitors should be considered for most patients

B = Beta blocker and blood pressure

C = Cigarette smoking and cholesterol

D = Diet and diabetes

E = Education and exercise

ACE—angiotensin–converting enzyme

of entry into the study. The magnitude of the risk reduction for smoking cessation was as great as or greater than that expected to result from use of aspirin, statins, beta blockers, or angiotensin-converting enzyme (ACE) inhibitors. Smoking cessation should be strongly and repeatedly recommended to all patients with known or suspected IHD who smoke. Physicians should become accustomed to applying effective techniques for counseling patients and using effective medications such as nicotine replacement and bupropion. Patients' efforts to quit are often more effective in the setting of a formal smoking-cessation program; therefore, internists should be familiar with local smoking-cessation resources and programs.

Physical Activity and Dietary Modifications

Physical activity Regular physical activity and dietary modifications also reduce cardiovascular risk. Physical fitness during middle age is associated with lower long-term cardiovascular mortality[66]; in addition, self-reported increases in physical activity is associated with reduced all-cause and cardiovascular mortality in elderly men.[67] In the Health Professionals Follow-up Study, half an hour or more of brisk walking each day was associated with an 18% relative risk reduction in cardiovascular events; in addition, greater duration and intensity of exercise were associated with greater reductions in risk.[68] This study also suggested that weight training was associated with a decreased cardiovascular risk. Although these observational studies are potentially subject to bias, the preponderance of evidence strongly supports recommending regular physical activity to patients.

Patients with chronic stable angina should be encouraged to include moderate aerobic activity in their daily lives.[21] Moderate physical activity consists of walking briskly for 30 minutes or more five to seven times a week or the equivalent. Unresolved questions include whether more vigorous physical activity provides greater risk reduction than moderate exercise; whether sustained aerobic exercise of 30 or more minutes is necessary for cardiovascular benefit or whether an accumulation of 30 or more minutes of physical activity during the day is sufficient; and to what extent physical activity provides reductions in risk above and beyond those achieved simply through modification of specific risk factors, such as dyslipidemia, hypertension, and diabetes.

Dietary modification Diet also has the potential to modify multiple coronary risk factors—namely, lipid levels, obesity, insulin resistance, and hypertension. Although trials assessing the effects of dietary modification on stable IHD have not uniformly demonstrated benefit, several trials have shown reductions in cardiac mortality. In the Lyon Diet Heart Study, patients who had had an MI were randomized either to adopt a Mediterranean diet rich in fresh fruits and vegetables, whole grains, olive oil, fish, and relatively little meat or to adopt a prudent Western diet low in saturated fats. At 4 years' follow-up, patients randomized to the Mediterranean diet enjoyed a 2.5% to 3% per year reduction in cardiac death and nonfatal MI.[69] Another trial randomized patients with IHD (about half of whom had a history of MI) either to adopt an Indo-Mediterranean diet rich in fresh fruits, vegetables, legumes, nuts, and whole grains and supplemented with omega-3 fatty acids or to adopt a prudent Indian diet low in saturated fats. Moderate exercise was recommended for all patients. Patients randomized to the Indo-Mediterranean diet had a 7.4% absolute reduction in the risk of MI or cardiac death at 2 years' follow-up.[70] Patients randomized to the inter-

vention diet had significant reductions in daily intake of calories, protein, fat (mostly saturated), cholesterol, and salt; they ingested significantly more complex carbohydrates, fiber, monounsaturated and polyunsaturated fats, fruits, vegetables, legumes, nuts, and omega-3 polyunsaturated oils.

Other studies demonstrate evidence of the protective benefit of fresh fruits and vegetables. The Nurses' Health Study and Health Professionals Follow-up Study found that persons in the highest quintile of fruit and vegetable intake had a 20% relative risk reduction for nonfatal MI or cardiac death compared with the lowest quintile.[71] A review of diet and IHD concluded that three dietary strategies are effective at reducing the risk of IHD: (1) substituting unsaturated fats (particularly polyunsaturated fats) for saturated fats (e.g., animal fats) and *trans*-fatty acids (e.g., stick margarine, vegetable shortenings, many commercially prepared baked goods, and deep-fried foods); (2) increasing consumption of omega-3 fatty acids (e.g., oily fish, canola oil, soybean oil, and flaxseed oils); and (3) consuming a diet high in fruits, vegetables, nuts, and whole grains and low in refined grains.[72]

MEDICAL THERAPY TO REDUCE CARDIOVASCULAR RISK

Antiplatelet Agents

Aspirin Acute coronary events commonly result from rupture of an atherosclerotic plaque and subsequent platelet aggregation and thrombosis. Aspirin inhibits cyclooxygenase and the synthesis of prothrombotic platelet thromboxane A_2. In studies of more than 3,000 patients with chronic stable angina that compared treatment with aspirin to placebo, the use of aspirin reduced the risk of adverse cardiovascular events by 33% over 6 months.[73,74] This reduction in relative risk corresponds to a reduction in absolute risk of approximately 5%. In other words, five cardiovascular events would be prevented for every 100 persons with known cardiovascular disease treated with aspirin for 6 months.[73] In the Swedish Angina Pectoris Aspirin Trial, which involved patients with stable angina, the addition of aspirin (75 mg daily) to a regimen of sotalol resulted in a 34% decrease in MI and sudden death[75]; most of this decrease involved reductions in the incidence of first MI. In the Physician's Health Study, which involved asymptomatic middle-aged men, the use of aspirin (325 mg every other day) was associated with a decrease in the incidence of MI.[76] Doses ranging from 75 to 325 mg daily were found to offer equivalent benefit,[77] although the incidence of gastrointestinal toxicity was dose-dependent. All patients with chronic stable angina should be treated with aspirin unless there is a history of documented aspirin allergy or life-threatening gastrointestinal hemorrhage.

Aspirin alternatives Two thienopyridine derivatives, clopidogrel and ticlopidine, inhibit adenosine diphosphate–mediated activation of platelet glycoprotein IIb/IIIa. These agents, particularly clopidogrel, are reasonable alternatives for aspirin-intolerant patients with chronic stable angina. In a randomized, controlled trial of patients with symptomatic vascular disease (including patients with chronic stable angina), clopidogrel was slightly more effective than aspirin in reducing the risk of MI, vascular death, and ischemic stroke.[78] Clopidogrel is much more expensive than aspirin; in addition, approximately 200 more patients would need to be treated with clopidogrel than with aspirin for 2 years to prevent one major vascular event.[79] There are no studies demonstrating that ticlopidine reduces cardiovascular events in outpatients with chronic stable angina. Ticlopidine can cause cytopenia, and there is a reported rare association with thrombotic thrombocytopenic purpura.

Lipid-Lowering Agents

There are abundant data showing the beneficial effects of lipid-lowering therapy in patients with chronic stable angina. Each 1% reduction in total cholesterol is associated with an approximately 2% reduction in coronary events.[80] In the Scandinavian Simvastatin Survival Study, patients with documented ischemic heart disease (including chronic stable angina) and elevated total cholesterol levels (i.e., levels of 212 to 308 mg/dl) were randomized to receive either a statin or placebo.[81] A 30% to 35% reduction in mortality and major coronary events was observed in patients receiving a statin. In the Cholesterol and Recurrent Events Trial, patients with prior MI and somewhat lower cholesterol levels (i.e., mean total cholesterol and LDL cholesterol of 209 mg/dl and 139 mg/dl, respectively) had a 25% relative risk reduction in the composite outcome of fatal or nonfatal MI when treated with a statin.[82] In the Heart Protection Study, patients with IHD or conditions that confer a similarly high risk of MI or coronary death (e.g., peripheral vascular disease, cerebrovascular disease, or diabetes) were randomized to receive either simvastatin (40 mg) or placebo, irrespective of baseline LDL level.[83] Statin therapy reduced total mortality; the incidence of first MI, coronary death, and stroke; and the use of revascularization procedures among all groups of patients, including those with LDL cholesterol levels of less than 116 mg/dl at entry (3.0 mmol/L). From this study, it may be concluded that all patients with chronic stable angina should be treated with a statin, barring specific allergy. Detailed recommendations for lipid-lowering therapy are provided by the National Cholesterol Education Program Adult Treatment Program III (NCEP ATP III).[30]

The target for therapy for patients with known IHD, including patients with chronic stable angina, is a serum LDL cholesterol level of less than 100 mg/dl. Patients with diabetes, peripheral vascular disease, and cerebrovascular disease are regarded as having a risk of cardiovascular events equivalent to patients with established IHD; the target for therapy in these patients is an LDL cholesterol level of less than 100 mg/dl, which is the same as in patients with known IHD. For other patients, including patients with possible IHD (e.g., a patient with atypical angina and a nondiagnostic exercise treadmill test) or two or more cardiovascular risk factors, the aggressiveness of lipid-lowering therapy is determined by calculating cardiovascular risk from the Framingham risk calculator[30] and the Third Report of the Expert Panel on Detection, Evaluation, and Treatment of High Blood Cholesterol in Adults (http://www.nhlbi.nih.gov/guidelines/cholesterol/index.htm) [see Figure 2].

Available data suggest a potential benefit for more aggressive lowering of LDL cholesterol. In one study, low-risk patients with stable, mild to moderate angina were randomized to receive either atorvastatin, 80 mg daily, or percutaneous coronary intervention (PCI) followed by usual care (including lipid-lowering treatment). Patients receiving atorvastatin required fewer revascularization procedures or admissions for worsening angina with objective evidence of ischemia (13.4% versus 20.9%).[84] Patients in the atorvastatin-treated group reached an average LDL cholesterol level of 77 mg/dl, as compared with 119 mg/dl in the PCI group. A second study compared the effects of intensive lipid-lowering therapy using atorvastatin (80 mg/day) with

moderate lipid-lowering therapy using pravastatin (40 mg/day).[85] Patients treated with atorvastatin (80 mg/day) achieved an average LDL cholesterol level of 79 mg/dl (2.05 mmol/L) and showed less progression of coronary atherosclerosis than patients treated with pravastatin (40 mg/day), who achieved an average LDL cholesterol level of 110 mg/dl (2.85 mmol/L).

Statin therapy is associated with several important potential adverse reactions. Elevations of liver transaminase levels have been described in patients taking statin drugs, although elevations to levels greater than three times the upper limit of normal (necessitating discontinuance) occur in fewer than 0.3% to 0.5% of patients.[86]

Rhabdomyolysis from statins is an uncommon dose-related phenomenon that usually occurs within the first few weeks of therapy, but it may occur at any time; rhabdomyolysis resolves after withdrawal of the offending drug. Clinically significant myopathy with 10-fold elevations of creatine kinase (CK) occurs in about 0.5% of patients treated with statins.[86] Massive rhabdomyolysis usually occurs only with concomitant use of clofibrate, niacin, or gemfibrozil. The incidence appears to be higher with drugs that interfere with the cytochrome P-450 system (e.g., simvastatin, lovastatin, and atorvastatin) and lower with less potent agents (e.g., pravastatin and fluvastatin). Predispositions to this adverse effect include certain P-450 polymorphisms (CYP3A4), renal failure, liver disease, hypothryoidism, concomitant medications (e.g, macrolides, azole antifungals, cyclosporine, protease inhibitors, selective serotonin reuptake inhibitors, nefazodone, verapamil, diltiazem, and amiodarone), and ingestion of grapefruit juice in quantity.[87] Myopathy can also occur without elevation of CK.[88]

Niacin, fibric acid derivatives (e.g., gemfibrozil and clofibrate), and bile acid sequestrants (e.g., cholestyramine and colestipol) reduce cholesterol an average of 6% to 15%. Niacin raises the HDL cholesterol, lowers the LDL cholesterol, and reduces the level of triglycerides. A meta-analysis of 37 studies suggests that the lipid-lowering effect of these agents is associated with reduced coronary mortality and total mortality.[89] In high-risk patients with a low HDL cholesterol level or hypertriglyceridemia, it is reasonable to consider the use of niacin or a fibric acid derivative, alone or in combination with a statin.[90-92] In the Veterans Affairs HDL Intervention Trial (VA-HIT), patients with established IHD and low HDL cholesterol levels who were randomized to receive gemfibrozil experienced a significant reduction in major cardiovascular events and cardiovascular mortality, as compared with patients who received placebo.[90] In another study, patients with established IHD and low levels of HDL cholesterol who were randomized to receive simvastatin plus niacin had fewer first cardiovascular events, as compared with patients who received placebo or simvastatin alone.[91]

Ezetimibe represents a new class of agent that inhibits intestinal absorption of cholesterol and produces moderate reductions in LDL cholesterol. Its principal indication at this time, as with the bile-acid sequestrants, is to augment the lipid-lowering efficacy of a statin.[93] Ezetimibe is associated with fewer gastrointestinal side effects than bile-acid sequestrants. Niacin commonly causes flushing, a side effect that can be mitigated by gradual titration toward a target dose and by pretreatment with aspirin. Extended-release preparations of niacin are associated with less flushing. Niacin modestly increases glucose intolerance and can cause hyperuricemia. As with statins, niacin and fibric acid derivatives are associated with a risk of elevations in transaminase levels, as well as with infrequent hepatitis and rare myositis. Although the manufacturers of these drugs recommend routine laboratory evaluation of liver function, routine monitoring was shown to have a low yield in a primary care practice.[94]

Reduction of non-LDL cholesterol lipid fractions may also reduce cardiovascular risk, particularly in patients who have the metabolic syndrome. Although definitions vary, the metabolic syndrome is a constellation of cardiovascular risk factors, including insulin resistance, obesity, hypertension, and dyslipidemia.[95] The dyslipidemia characteristic of the metabolic syndrome consists of elevated triglycerides, a low HDL cholesterol level, and a normal (or near-normal) LDL cholesterol level. Retrospective analysis of the VA-HIT, which studied patients with established coronary disease and low HDL cholesterol levels, suggested that the benefits of treatment with gemfibrozil are most pronounced in patients with insulin resistance (whose fasting plasma insulin levels were comparable to those found in patients with the metabolic syndrome).[96] Because patients with the metabolic syndrome have elevated cardiovascular risk despite often having unremarkable LDL cholesterol levels, NCEP ATP III recommends measuring non-HDL cholesterol in patients with elevated triglyceride levels (i.e., triglyceride levels ≥ 200 mg/dl or 2.25 mmol/L) through use of the following formula:

$$\text{Non-HDL cholesterol} = \text{measured total cholesterol} - \text{HDL cholesterol}$$

The level of non-HDL cholesterol determined by this formula corresponds to the sum of LDL cholesterol and atherogenic remnant lipoproteins containing apolipoprotein B (very low density lipoprotein cholesterol). Among patients with hypertriglyceridemia, the target level for non-HDL cholesterol is less than 130 mg/dl for patients with IHD or IHD equivalent conditions, as well as for patients with two or more cardiovascular risk factors and a 10-year risk of cardiovascular events greater than 20%, as determined by the Framingham risk estimates [see Figure 2].[30]

In summary, numerous studies demonstrate that patients with IHD benefit from treatment with statins; this includes IHD patients with relatively normal LDL cholesterol levels. The vast majority of patients with chronic stable angina should be treated with a statin. Treatment with niacin or fibric acid derivatives should be considered in patients with a low HDL cholesterol level or an elevated triglyceride level. In view of the consistent benefits of statins across many patient subsets, it would be most reasonable to consider adding niacin or fibric acid derivatives to statin therapy.

Antihypertensive Therapy

Hypertension contributes to cardiovascular risk by increasing myocardial wall stress, oxygen demand, and endothelial injury. Treatment of hypertension in patients with IHD reduces the risk of future cardiovascular events.[97] A reduction in systolic blood pressure of 2 mm Hg is associated with a 7% reduction in mortality from IHD.[98] By lowering myocardial oxygen demand, treatment of hypertension may also improve anginal symptoms. The therapeutic target for patients with IHD is to maintain blood pressure at levels below 140/90 mm Hg.[99]

Two groups of patients with hypertension and chronic stable angina warrant particular consideration: patients with specific coexisting chronic conditions (e.g., diabetes, heart failure, or renal insufficiency) and patients with LVH. Guidelines from the Joint National Committee for the Diagnosis, Evaluation, and Treatment of Hypertension (JNC) recommend a lower therapeutic target blood pressure for hypertensive patients who have diabetes, heart failure, or renal insufficiency—namely, a level below 130/85 mm Hg.[99] Although no specific target has been promulgated for therapy for hypertension and LVH, the latter is a marker for the severity and chronicity of hypertension and is a risk factor for MI, CHF, and cardiac sudden death.[100] Treatment of hypertension results in the regression of LVH; ECG evidence of LVH regression is associated with a significantly reduced risk of cardiovascular events.[101] Patients with LVH should therefore be targeted for aggressive antihypertensive therapy.

Two classes of antihypertensives—beta-adrenergic receptor antagonists (i.e., beta blockers) and calcium channel blockers—are also effective antianginal medications. Beta blockers confer mortality benefit in patients after MI[102] and are recommended as first-line therapy for most patients with chronic stable angina.[32] Calcium channel blockers (e.g., diltiazem, verapamil, and long-acting dihydropyridines) are also effective antihypertensive and antianginal medications. Current ACC/AHA/ACP guidelines recommend beta blockers as first-line antihypertensive therapy in patients with chronic stable angina. Long-acting calcium channel blockers are an acceptable alternative, particularly in patients without a history of MI.[102]

ACE Inhibitors

Results of the Heart Outcomes Prevention Evaluation (HOPE) trial demonstrated that ACE inhibitors reduced MI, stroke, and cardiovascular death in patients at high cardiovascular risk. In this study, patients with a history of IHD, diabetes, stroke, or peripheral vascular disease and at least one additional cardiovascular risk factor (e.g., hypertension, dyslipidemia, cigarette smoking, or microalbuminuria) were randomized to receive either ramipril (10 mg daily) or placebo; patients were followed for an average of 4 years. Total mortality was reduced 1.8% in the ramipril-treated group; in terms of numbers needed to treat (NNT), this means that 56 patients would need to be treated for 4 years to prevent one death. The primary outcome of MI, stroke, or cardiovascular death was reduced by 3.8% (NNT of 26). This study indicated that a broad range of patients at high risk for IHD who had normal left ventricular function obtained an impressive survival benefit from the use of ACE inhibitors. The magnitude of benefit was greater than might have been expected for the small decrement in average blood pressure observed in the study, suggesting a mechanism at work other than reduction in blood pressure.[103] In the European Trial on Reduction of Cardiac Events with Perindopril in Stable Coronary Artery Disease (EUROPA), patients with stable coronary disease and no known congestive heart failure or uncontrolled hypertension were randomized to receive either the ACE inhibitor perindopril or placebo.[104] Combined cardiovascular end points were significantly reduced in the perindopril group; in addition, there was a nonsignificant reduction in total mortality. On the basis of the HOPE and EUROPA trials, it can be concluded that most patients with chronic stable angina should be treated with an ACE inhibitor, barring renal insufficiency, hyperkalemia, or an allergy to ACE inhibitors. Angiotensin receptor blockers may offer a similar benefit, but these agents have not been extensively studied in this regard.

MEDICAL THERAPY FOR ANGINAL SYMPTOMS

The major classes of medications for the treatment of angina include beta blockers, calcium channel blockers, and nitroglycerin/nitrates. Randomized trials demonstrate that beta blockers and calcium channel blockers are equally effective in relieving angina and improving exercise tolerance.[105,106] Current guidelines, however, recommend beta blockers as first-line therapy[32,33] because they improve survival and reduce cardiac events in patients who have had a previous acute MI[107] and in elderly patients with systolic hypertension[108]; no similar benefits have been demonstrated for calcium channel blockers or nitrates. In addition, beta blockers improve survival and reduce the risk of stroke and congestive heart failure in patients with hypertension.[109] Beta blockers should be considered as initial antianginal therapy in patients with chronic stable angina.

Beta Blockers

Beta blockers decrease heart rate, myocardial contractility, blood pressure, and myocardial oxygen demand by inhibiting cardiac and peripheral beta-adrenergic receptors. Beta blockers delay the onset of angina and increase exercise capacity in patients with exertional angina.[110,111] They are titrated to a dose adequate to reduce the resting heart rate to 55 to 60 beats/min. Titration to lower heart rates may be necessary in patients with more severe angina, provided patients do not develop heart block or symptoms of severe bradycardia.

Beta blockers are generally well tolerated by patients with chronic obstructive pulmonary disease; however, they may exacerbate bronchospasm in patients with severe asthma. Beta blockers are well tolerated in patients with diabetes, and in these patients, they can reduce macrovascular events[112]; theoretically, however, beta blockers can mask the adrenergically mediated symptoms of hypoglycemia insulin (e.g., tachycardia).

Beta blockers are contraindicated in the presence of severe bradycardia, high-degree atrioventricular block, sinus node dysfunction, and uncompensated congestive heart failure. Patients with extensive peripheral vascular disease and claudication may experience worsening of their symptoms. Beta blockers are also contraindicated in the small subset of patients with pure variant or vasospastic angina (i.e., angina occurring in the absence of fixed obstruction of the coronary arteries), in whom beta blockade is unlikely to alleviate symptoms. In these patients, beta blockers may actually worsen angina as a result of unopposed alpha-adrenergic effects. Calcium channel blockers are the preferred first-line agent in this patient group [see Calcium Channel Blockers, below].

Calcium Channel Blockers

Calcium channel blockers reduce smooth muscle tone and cause coronary and peripheral vasodilatation, improving coronary blood flow and reducing peripheral vascular resistance. Calcium channel blockers can be used as monotherapy in the treatment of chronic stable angina, although combinations of beta blockers and calcium channel blockers relieve angina more effectively than either agent alone. Combination therapy with a beta blocker may blunt the reflex tachycardia that can occur with dihydropyridine calcium channel antagonists. All calcium channel blockers exert some negative inotropic effect, although this effect is typically most significant clinically with the nondihydropyridine agents verapamil and diltiazem. Calcium channel blockers are contraindicated in the presence of decompensated congestive heart failure, although the vasoselective dihydropyridine agents amlodipine and felodipine are tolerated in patients with clinically stable LV dysfunction.[113] Verapamil and diltiazem have a pronounced effect on heart rate and conduction; they should be used with caution in combination with beta blockers

because of the increased risk of heart block associated with the combined use of these agents. Constipation and peripheral edema are common side effects of calcium channel blockers.

Nitrates and Nitroglycerin

Nitrates and nitroglycerin dilate coronary arteries and their collateral vessels, directly improve myocardial perfusion, diminish afterload, and increase venous capacitance. These agents exert antianginal effects by improving coronary blood flow and by reducing myocardial oxygen demand. Long-acting nitrate preparations, in tablet or patch form, reduce the severity and frequency of angina and improve exercise tolerance; however, they often induce a reflexive increase in sympathetic tone and increase heart rate. Therefore, long-acting nitrates are often used in combination with beta blockers or calcium channel blockers. Short-acting nitroglycerin tablets or spray is appropriate for the immediate relief of exercise-induced or rest angina. They may also prevent angina when taken several minutes before exertion sufficient to cause angina.

Nitroglycerin and nitrates should not be used within 24 hours of taking sildenafil (Viagra) or other phosphodiesterase inhibitors used in the treatment of erectile dysfunction, because of the potential for life-threatening hypotension.[114] It is important to discuss this interaction with patients taking nitrates or sildenafil. Nitroglycerin and nitrates are relatively contraindicated in patients with severe aortic stenosis or hypertrophic obstructive cardiomyopathy because of an increased risk of syncope resulting from diminished cardiac output. Continued use of long-acting nitrates results in tachyphylaxis; the mechanism of this is unclear. An adequate nitrate-free period (8 to 12 hours each day) is necessary to minimize this effect. Headaches are common and often limit nitroglycerin and nitrate therapy; with continued use, headaches will diminish in up to 80% of patients. Hypotension may occur, particularly in hypovolemic patients.

In general, patients who are found to be at low or moderate risk for cardiovascular complications during risk stratification should be treated aggressively with medical therapy. Medical therapy should not be considered to have failed until the patient has been treated with full therapeutic doses of a beta blocker, a calcium channel blocker, and a long-acting nitrate and continues to experience angina or develops unacceptable adverse effects.

PATIENTS WITH DIABETES MELLITUS

IHD therapy for patients with diabetes merits special consideration. Cardiovascular events are the leading cause of death in patients with diabetes, and this patient group is at particularly high risk for MI. Middle-aged persons with diabetes and no history of MI have a risk of MI and cardiac death equivalent to that of nondiabetic patients with a history of MI.[115] A substudy of the Heart Protection Study demonstrated that treatment with statins reduced major coronary and major vascular events, even among diabetic patients without a prior diagnosis of ischemic heart disease and among diabetic patients with LDL cholesterol levels lower than 116 mg/dl (3 mmol/L).[116] Treatment with statins resulted in a relative risk reduction for major coronary events (nonfatal MI and coronary death [27%]), stroke (25%), and first revascularization procedures (17%). A HOPE substudy demonstrated the benefits of ACE inhibitors in patients with diabetes and one or more cardiovascular risk factors.[117] Treatment with an ACE inhibitor resulted in a 25% reduction in MI, stroke, or cardiovascular death. Total mortality was reduced 24%; progression to overt nephropathy was reduced by 24%. In the United Kingdom

Prospective Diabetes Study, beta blockers were found to be equivalent to ACE inhibitors in reducing the risk of macrovascular complications.[112] Another study found that cardiovascular events were more common in patients with type 2 diabetes mellitus and hypertension who were randomized to receive a dihydropyridine calcium channel blocker, as compared with patients who received an ACE inhibitor.[118] It remains uncertain whether to attribute this result to a higher risk of cardiovascular events among the group taking the calcium channel blocker amlodipine or to a reduced risk of cardiovascular events among the group taking the ACE inhibitor fosinopril. Nevertheless, most experts consider calcium channel blockers to be third-line agents for patients with diabetes and hypertension. Results of the Hypertension Optimal Treatment (HOT) study support aggressive blood pressure reduction in patients with diabetes; the target blood pressure for these patients is 135/80 mm Hg or lower.[119]

Although it remains uncertain when to initiate antiplatelet therapy in diabetic patients, it is reasonable to treat diabetic patients who have any additional cardiovascular risk factor with aspirin or an equivalent antiplatelet therapy.[120] The American Diabetes Association and the NCEP recommend a target LDL cholesterol level of 100 mg/dl (2.59 mmol/L) or lower.[31,121]

REVASCULARIZATION

Techniques for revascularization include PCI, using catheter-based methods with or without placement of intracoronary stents, and CABG. For most patients with angina, survival with optimal medical therapy is equivalent to that resulting from revascularization; in addition, CABG results in excellent symptom relief. For a select few patients with chronic stable angina, revascularization is associated with improved survival, as compared with that achieved with medical therapy.[122] Among 2,649 patients with left main coronary stenoses or multivessel coronary artery disease and reduced LV systolic function, those who were treated with CABG in randomized trials had an absolute mortality at 5 years that was more than 5% lower than that of patients assigned to medical management (10.2% versus 15.8%).[123] This benefit persisted at 10 years' follow-up. There is much weaker evidence to suggest that patients with proximal stenoses of the left anterior descending coronary artery and normal LV function also experience lower mortality with CABG. One randomized trial showed no difference in mortality among patients assigned to CABG, PCI, or medical management.[124] In two trials comparing CABG with PCI, survival was equivalent; however, the patients who underwent surgery had fewer symptoms and required fewer antianginal medications and subsequent revascularization procedures.[125,126] Initial costs and short-term (procedure-related) mortality were higher in patients who underwent CABG. Most of the patients enrolled had two-vessel CAD and normal LV systolic function. In one study, survival was improved in patients with diabetes who underwent CABG, as compared with patients who underwent PCI.[125]

Randomized trials comparing PCI with medical management in patients with one- or two-vessel CAD and normal LV systolic function have demonstrated equivalent survival.[127,128] Relief of symptoms was generally greater with PCI than that seen with medical therapy, although PCI was associated with an increased risk of procedure-related MI and death[127,128] and substantially greater cost.[129]

On the basis of a limited number of randomized trials, it appears that only the subgroup of patients with severe coronary disease (defined as two- or three-vessel disease) and impaired LV function can confidently expect improved average survival after revascularization and that improvement is seen only with CABG. Thus, evaluation for revascularization is generally recommended for patients who are at moderate or high risk of death and who are willing to undergo a revascularization procedure.[32] Patients meeting these criteria who are found to have either extensive areas of ischemia on noninvasive testing or reduced LV systolic function should then be considered candidates for angiography. It should be recognized, however, that the results of currently available studies comparing PCI, CABG, and medical therapy do not reflect recent advancements in all three forms of treatment. For example, restenosis rates with PCI using stents, drug-eluting stents, and platelet inhibitors are lower than previously reported rates with angioplasty techniques.

In general, medical therapy is preferred in patients who are determined through risk stratification by noninvasive testing to be at low risk for death. There is no evidence that revascularization improves survival in such patients. For this reason, currently available evidence suggests that many revascularization procedures conducted in the United States may not be warranted.

NEW THERAPIES

Newer procedures, such as transmyocardial revascularization, enhanced external counterpulsation, and gene therapy, are all under investigation. These procedures are reserved for patients who are refractory to drug therapy and unsuitable for traditional revascularization procedures. Another approach for the treatment of angina has been the use of drugs that modify myocardial metabolism. The heart employs free fatty acids, glucose, and lactate as sources of energy. Inhibition of fatty acid oxidation results in an increase in glucose oxidation and an increase in the efficiency of oxygen use by the myocardium. This alteration in myocardial metabolism may improve anginal status. Ranolazine, a fatty acid oxidation inhibitor, has been approved for clinical use. This drug has shown efficacy as monotherapy or in combination with other antianginal agents in improving exercise tolerance, decreasing electrocardiographic evidence of ischemia, and reducing the frequency of angina and the need for sublingual nitroglycerin.[130] Because of possible QT interval prolongation, its use is limited to patients who have failed all other antianginal therapies.[130]

FOLLOW-UP

Patients with chronic stable angina should be regularly followed in a primary care setting. There is little evidence to recommend a particular frequency of follow-up visits, although ACC/AHA/ACP guidelines suggest regular visits at 4- to 12-month intervals for patients with chronic stable angina.[21] The expert panel recommends addressing the following questions at each visit[21]:

• Has there been a change in the level of activity since the last visit?
• Have anginal symptoms increased in severity or frequency?
• Is current therapy well tolerated?
• Has the patient been successful at modifying cardiac risk factors?
• Has the patient developed new or worsening comorbid illnesses that may have an impact on the patient's angina?

It is important to inquire about changes in anginal symptoms or activity levels to identify patients who require increased intensity of antianginal therapy or further risk stratification. For example, it would be reasonable to repeat noninvasive testing in a patient with stable class II angina who developed new class III anginal symptoms since the last clinic visit. Similarly, in a patient with new symptoms of CHF, it would be appropriate to perform echocardiography and consider referral for coronary angiography; multiple-vessel CAD with reduced left ventricular function would be an indication for CABG.

Medical therapy should be reviewed at each visit to assess adherence to recommended therapy, knowledge about doses and indications, and potential side effects. In addition, it is worth considering whether recent evidence for benefit from new therapies or new indications for existing therapies support a modification of IHD management. Patients with chronic stable angina should be encouraged to quit smoking, to eat a prudent diet, and to regularly engage in moderate exercise. Successful adoption of these interventions is challenging, but repeated encouragement from a personal physician enhances success.[131]

Vital signs (i.e., heart rate, blood pressure, and weight) should be regularly followed. The physical examination is focused on the heart, lungs, and vasculature. Findings of particular note include signs of CHF, new or changing heart murmurs, arrhythmias, or evidence of carotid or peripheral vascular disease.

Laboratory assessment should include periodic measurements of fasting lipid levels. Regular measurements of liver transaminase and CK levels are not recommended in the absence of symptoms. Other laboratory testing is indicated by comorbid conditions or changes in the patient's history and physical examination.

There is no evidence showing that regular ECG studies are helpful in the management of patients with chronic stable angina in the absence of changes in history or physical examination. ECGs are indicated when new medications are introduced that may affect cardiac conduction. Changes in anginal or syncopal symptoms and findings suggestive of dysrhythmia or conduction abnormalities should also prompt a repeat ECG.

There is little evidence to guide the use of repeat stress testing in patients with chronic stable angina. Recommendations for follow-up stress testing vary according to initial assessments of a patient's cardiovascular risk.[21] For example, patients with class II angina whose exercise treadmill test places them at low risk have an annual risk of mortality of less than 1%; these patients do not require follow-up stress testing for a period of 3 to 4 years in the absence of new and concerning symptoms or signs. Similarly, patients who underwent PCI more than 6 months earlier and who have minimal residual stenosis are unlikely to benefit from regular stress testing. It is not known whether patients at intermediate or high cardiovascular risk benefit from periodic stress testing.

Follow-up noninvasive tests are selected according to the approach outlined (see above). When possible, the same form of stress (exercise or pharmacologic) and testing (ECG or imaging) should be repeated, because this permits the most valid comparison with the original study.[21]

Patients should be referred to a cardiologist when appropriate for consideration of revascularization. Candidates for referral include patients with valvular disorders that require repair, patients with angina that is refractory to maximal medical therapy, and patients with comorbidities that complicate therapy.

The authors have no commercial relationships with manufacturers of products or providers of services discussed in this chapter.

References

1. Gibbons RJ, Balady GJ, Beasley JW, et al: ACC/AHA Guidelines for Exercise Testing. A report of the American College of Cardiology/American Heart Association Task Force on Practice Guidelines (Committee on Exercise Testing). J Am Coll Cardiol 30:260, 1997
2. 1997 Biostatistical Fact Sheets. American Heart Association, Dallas, 1997, p 1
3. 1999 Heart and Stroke Statistical Update. American Heart Association, Dallas, 1999, p 1
4. Five-year clinical and functional outcome comparing bypass surgery and angioplasty in patients with multivessel coronary disease: a multicenter randomized trial. Writing Group for the Bypass Angioplasty Revascularization Investigation (BARI) Investigators. JAMA 277:715, 1997
5. Grundy SM, Pasternak R, Greenland P, et al: Assessment of cardiovascular risk by use of multiple-risk-factor assessment equations: a statement for healthcare professionals from the American Heart Association and the American College of Cardiology. Circulation 100:1481, 1999
6. Pasternak RC, Grundy SM, Levy D, et al: 27th Bethesda Conference: matching the intensity of risk factor management with the hazard for coronary disease events. Task Force 3. Spectrum of risk factors for coronary heart disease. J Am Coll Cardiol 27:978, 1996
7. Isomaa B, Almgren P, Tuomi T, et al: Cardiovascular morbidity and mortality associated with the metabolic syndrome. Diabetes Care 24:683, 2001
8. Scott CL: Diagnosis, prevention, and intervention for the metabolic syndrome. Am J Cardiol 92:35i, 2003
9. Lee PY, Alexander KP, Hammill BG, et al: Representation of elderly persons and women in published randomized trials of acute coronary syndromes. JAMA 286:708, 2001
10. Greenland P, Knoll MD, Stamler J, et al: Major risk factors as antecedents of fatal and nonfatal coronary heart disease events. JAMA 290:891, 2003
11. Khot UN, Khot MB, Bajzer CT, et al: Prevalence of conventional risk factors in patients with coronary heart disease. JAMA 290:898, 2003
12. Naghavi M, Libby P, Falk E, et al: From vulnerable plaque to vulnerable patient: a call for new definitions and risk assessment strategies: Part II. Circulation 108:1772, 2003
13. Koenig W, Sund M, Frohlich M, et al: C-reactive protein, a sensitive marker of inflammation, predicts future risk of coronary heart disease in initially healthy middle-aged men: results from the MONICA (Monitoring Trends and Determinants in Cardiovascular Disease) Augsburg Cohort Study, 1984 to 1992. Circulation 99:237, 1999
14. Danesh J, Wheeler JG, Hirschfield GM, et al: C-reactive protein and other circulating markers of inflammation in the prediction of coronary heart disease. N Engl J Med 350:1387, 2004
15. Ross R: Atherosclerosis: an inflammatory disease. N Engl J Med 340:115, 1999
16. Morrow DA, Rifai N, Antman EM, et al: C-reactive protein is a potent predictor of mortality independently of and in combination with troponin T in acute coronary syndromes: a TIMI 11A substudy. Thrombolysis in Myocardial Infarction. J Am Coll Cardiol 31:1460, 1998
17. Kennon S, Price CP, Mills PG, et al: Cumulative risk assessment in unstable angina: clinical, electrocardiographic, autonomic, and biochemical markers. Heart 89:36, 2003
18. Ambrose JA, Tannenbaum MA, Alexopoulos D, et al: Angiographic progression of coronary artery disease and the development of myocardial infarction. J Am Coll Cardiol 12:56, 1988
19. Campeau L: Letter: grading of angina pectoris. Circulation 54:522, 1976S
20. Braunwald E, Antman EM, Beasley JW, et al: ACC/AHA 2002 guideline update for the management of patients with unstable angina and non-ST-segment elevation myocardial infarction: summary article: a report of the American College of Cardiology/American Heart Association task force on practice guidelines (Committee on the Management of Patients with Unstable Angina). J Am Coll Cardiol 40:1366, 2002
21. Gibbons RJ, Chatterjee K, Daley J, et al: ACC/AHA/ACP-ASIM guidelines for the management of patients with chronic stable angina: executive summary and recommendations. A Report of the American College of Cardiology/American Heart Association Task Force on Practice Guidelines (Committee on Management of Patients with Chronic Stable Angina). Circulation 99:2829, 1999
22. Pryor DB, Shaw L, McCants CB, et al: Value of the history and physical in identifying patients at increased risk for coronary artery disease. Ann Intern Med 118:81, 1993
23. Chun AA, McGee SR: Bedside diagnosis of coronary artery disease: a systematic review. Am J Med 117:334, 2004
24. Swan HJ, Gersh BJ, Graboys TB, et al: 27th Bethesda Conference: matching the intensity of risk factor management with the hazard for coronary disease events. Task Force 7. Evaluation and management of risk factors for the individual patient (case management). J Am Coll Cardiol 27:1030, 1996
25. Wilson PW, D'Agostino RB, Levy D, et al: Prediction of coronary heart disease using risk factor categories. Circulation 97:1837, 1998
26. Levine HJ: Difficult problems in the diagnosis of chest pain. Am Heart J 100:108, 1980
27. Connolly DC, Elveback LR, Oxman HA: Coronary heart disease in residents of Rochester, Minnesota: IV. Prognostic value of the resting electrocardiogram at the time of initial diagnosis of angina pectoris. Mayo Clin Proc 59:247, 1984
28. Levy D, Garrison RJ, Savage DD, et al: Prognostic implications of echocardiographically determined left ventricular mass in the Framingham Heart Study. N Engl J Med 322:1561, 1990
29. Fisch C: Electrocardiography and vectorcardiography. Heart Disease. Braunwald E, Ed. WB Saunders Co, Philadelphia, 1992, p 145
30. Executive Summary of The Third Report of The National Cholesterol Education Program (NCEP) Expert Panel on Detection, Evaluation, and Treatment of High Blood

Cholesterol in Adults (Adult Treatment Panel III). Expert Panel on Detection, Evaluation, and Treatment of High Blood Cholesterol in Adults. JAMA 285:2486, 2001

31. Tape TG, Mushlin AI: The utility of routine chest radiographs. Ann Intern Med 104:663, 1986

32. Gibbons RJ, Chatterjee K, Daley J, et al: ACC/AHA/ACP-ASIM guidelines for the management of patients with chronic stable angina: a report of the American College of Cardiology/American Heart Association Task Force on Practice Guidelines (Committee on Management of Patients With Chronic Stable Angina). J Am Coll Cardiol 33:2092, 1999 [erratum, J Am Coll Cardiol 34:314, 1999]

33. Gibbons RJ, Abrams J, Chatterjee K, et al: ACC/AHA 2002 guideline update for the management of patients with chronic stable angina: summary article: a report of the American College of Cardiology/American Heart Association Task Force on practice guidelines (Committee on the Management of Patients with Chronic Stable Angina). J Am Coll Cardiol 41:159, 2003

34. Stuart RJ Jr, Ellestad MH: National survey of exercise stress testing facilities. Chest 77:94, 1980

35. Klocke FJ, Baird MG, Lorell BH, et al: ACC/AHA/ASNC guidelines for the clinical use of cardiac radionuclide imaging: executive summary: a report of the American College of Cardiology/American Heart Association Task Force on Practice Guidelines (ACC/AHA/ASNC Committee to Revise the 1995 Guidelines for the Clinical Use of Cardiac Radionuclide Imaging). J Am Coll Cardiol 42:1318, 2003

36. Shaw LJ, Hachamovitch R, Peterson ED, et al: Using an outcomes-based approach to identify candidates for risk stratification after exercise treadmill testing. J Gen Intern Med 14:1, 1999

37. Cheitlin MD, Alpert JS, Armstrong WF, et al: ACC/AHA guidelines for the clinical application of echocardiography: executive summary. A report of the American College of Cardiology/American Heart Association Task Force on practice guidelines (Committee on Clinical Application of Echocardiography). Developed in collaboration with the American Society of Echocardiography. J Am Coll Cardiol 29:862, 1997

38. Fleischmann KE, Hunink MG, Kuntz KM, et al: Exercise echocardiography or exercise SPECT imaging? A meta-analysis of diagnostic test performance. JAMA 280:913, 1998

39. Amanullah AM, Kiat H, Friedman JD, et al: Adenosine technetium-99m sestamibi myocardial perfusion SPECT in women: diagnostic efficacy in detection of coronary artery disease. J Am Coll Cardiol 27:803, 1996

40. Kim C, Kwok YS, Saha S, et al: Diagnosis of suspected coronary artery disease in women: a cost-effectiveness analysis. Am Heart J 137:1019, 1999

41. Gauri AJ, Raxwal VK, Roux L, et al: Effects of chronotropic incompetence and beta-blocker use on the exercise treadmill test in men. Am Heart J 142:136, 2001

42. Ladenheim ML, Kotler TS, Pollock BH, et al: Incremental prognostic power of clinical history, exercise electrocardiography and myocardial perfusion scintigraphy in suspected coronary artery disease. Am J Cardiol 59:270, 1987

43. Bielak LF, Rumberger JA, Sheedy PF 2nd, et al: Probabilistic model for prediction of angiographically defined obstructive coronary artery disease using electron beam computed tomography calcium score strata. Circulation 102:380, 2000

44. Redberg RF: Coronary artery calcium and cardiac events. Circulation 108:E167, 2003

45. O'Malley PG, Taylor AJ: Prognostic value of coronary artery calcification. Circulation 108:E169, 2003

46. Detrano RC, Wong ND, Doherty TM, et al: Coronary calcium does not accurately predict near-term future coronary events in high-risk adults. Circulation 99:2633, 1999

47. Mark DB, Shaw LJ, Lauer MS, et al: 34th Bethesda Conference: task force #5: is atherosclerosis imaging cost effective? J Am Coll Cardiol 41:1906, 2003

48. O'Rourke RA, Brundage BH, Froelicher VF, et al: American College of Cardiology/American Heart Association Expert Consensus Document on electron-beam computed tomography for the diagnosis and prognosis of coronary artery disease. J Am Coll Cardiol 36:326, 2000

49. Kussmaul WG 3rd, Popp RL, Norcini J: Accuracy and reproducibility of visual coronary stenosis estimates using information from multiple observers. Clin Cardiol 15:154, 1992

50. Hubbard BL, Gibbons RJ, Lapeyre AC 3rd, et al: Identification of severe coronary artery disease using simple clinical parameters. Arch Intern Med 152:309, 1992

51. Pryor DB, Shaw L, Harrell FE Jr, et al: Estimating the likelihood of severe coronary artery disease. Am J Med 90:553, 1991

52. Patterson RE, Eisner RL, Horowitz SF: Comparison of cost-effectiveness and utility of exercise ECG, single photon emission computed tomography, positron emission tomography, and coronary angiography for diagnosis of coronary artery disease. Circulation 91:54, 1995

53. Mock MB, Ringqvist I, Fisher LD, et al: Survival of medically treated patients in the coronary artery surgery study (CASS) registry. Circulation 66:562, 1982

54. O'Keefe JH Jr, Zinsmeister AR, Gibbons RJ: Value of normal electrocardiographic findings in predicting resting left ventricular function in patients with chest pain and suspected coronary artery disease. Am J Med 86:658, 1989

55. Mark DB, Shaw L, Harrell FE Jr, et al: Prognostic value of a treadmill exercise score in outpatients with suspected coronary artery disease. N Engl J Med 325:849, 1991

56. Cole CR, Blackstone EH, Pashkow FJ, et al: Heart-rate recovery immediately after exercise as a predictor of mortality. N Engl J Med 341:1351, 1999

57. Gibbons RJ, Balady GJ, Bricker JT, et al: ACC/AHA 2002 guideline update for exercise testing: summary article. A report of the American College of Cardiology/American Heart Association Task Force on Practice Guidelines (Committee to Update the 1997 Exercise Testing Guidelines). J Am Coll Cardiol 40:1531, 2002

58. Brown KA: Prognostic value of thallium-201 myocardial perfusion imaging; a diagnostic tool comes of age. Circulation 83:363, 1991

59. Boucher CA, Zir LM, Beller GA, et al: Increased lung uptake of thallium-201 during exercise myocardial imaging: clinical, hemodynamic and angiographic implications in patients with coronary artery disease. Am J Cardiol 46:189, 1980

60. Cox JL, Wright LM, Burns RJ: Prognostic significance of increased thallium-201 lung uptake during dipyridamole myocardial scintigraphy: comparison with exercise scintigraphy. Can J Cardiol 11:689, 1995

61. McCully RB, Roger VL, Mahoney DW, et al: Outcome after normal exercise echocardiography and predictors of subsequent cardiac events: follow-up of 1,325 patients. J Am Coll Cardiol 31:144, 1998

62. Marwick TH: Use of stress echocardiography for the prognostic assessment of patients with stable chronic coronary artery disease. Eur Heart J 18(suppl D):D97, 1997

63. Emond M, Mock MB, Davis KB, et al: Long-term survival of medically treated patients in the Coronary Artery Surgery Study (CASS) Registry. Circulation 90:2645, 1994

64. Mark DB, Nelson CL, Califf RM, et al: Continuing evolution of therapy for coronary artery disease: initial results from the era of coronary angioplasty. Circulation 89:2015, 1994

65. Critchley J, Capewell S: Smoking cessation for the secondary prevention of coronary heart disease. Cochrane Database Syst Rev (4):CD003041, 2003

66. Sandvik L, Erikssen J, Thaulow E, et al: Physical fitness as a predictor of mortality among healthy, middle-aged Norwegian men. N Engl J Med 328:533, 1993

67. Bijnen FC, Caspersen CJ, Feskens EJ, et al: Physical activity and 10-year mortality from cardiovascular diseases and all causes: the Zutphen Elderly Study. Arch Intern Med 158:1499, 1998

68. Tanasescu M, Leitzmann MF, Rimm EB, et al: Exercise type and intensity in relation to coronary heart disease in men. JAMA 288:1994, 2000

69. de Lorgeril M, Salen P, Martin JL, et al: Mediterranean diet, traditional risk factors, and the rate of cardiovascular complications after myocardial infarction: final report of the Lyon Diet Heart Study. Circulation 99:779, 1999

70. Singh RB, Dubnov G, Niaz MA, et al: Effect of an Indo-Mediterranean diet on progression of coronary artery disease in high risk patients (Indo-Mediterranean Diet Heart Study): a randomised single-blind trial. Lancet 360:1455, 2002

71. Joshipura KJ, Hu FB, Manson JE, et al: The effect of fruit and vegetable intake on risk for coronary heart disease. Ann Intern Med 134:1106, 2001

72. Hu FB, Willett WC: Optimal diets for prevention of coronary heart disease. JAMA 288:2569, 2002

73. Collaborative overview of randomised trials of antiplatelet therapy: I. Prevention of death, myocardial infarction, and stroke by prolonged antiplatelet therapy in various categories of patients. Antiplatelet Trialists' Collaboration. BMJ 308:81, 1994 [erratum BMJ 308:1540, 1994]

74. Ridker PM, Manson JE, Gaziano JM, et al: Low-dose aspirin therapy for chronic stable angina: a randomized, placebo-controlled clinical trial. Ann Intern Med 114:835, 1991

75. Double-blind trial of aspirin in primary prevention of myocardial infarction in patients with stable chronic angina pectoris. The Swedish Angina Pectoris Aspirin Trial (SAPAT) Group. Lancet 340:1421, 1992

76. Final report on the aspirin component of the ongoing Physicians' Health Study. Steering Committee of the Physicians' Health Study Research Group. N Engl J Med 321:129, 1989

77. Collaborative meta-analysis of randomised trials of antiplatelet therapy for prevention of death, myocardial infarction, and stroke in high risk patients. Antithrombotic Trialists' Collaboration. BMJ 324:71, 2002

78. A randomised, blinded trial of clopidogrel versus aspirin in patients at risk of ischaemic events (CAPRIE). CAPRIE Steering Committee. Lancet 348:1329, 1996

79. Gaspoz JM, Coxson PG, Goldman PA, et al: Cost effectiveness of aspirin, clopidogrel, or both for secondary prevention of coronary heart disease. N Engl J Med 346:1800, 2002

80. The cholesterol facts. A summary of the evidence relating dietary fats, serum cholesterol, and coronary heart disease. A joint statement by the American Heart Association and the National Heart, Lung, and Blood Institute. The Task Force on Cholesterol Issues, American Heart Association. Circulation 81:1721, 1990

81. Randomised trial of cholesterol lowering in 4444 patients with coronary heart disease: the Scandinavian Simvastatin Survival Study (4S). Lancet 344:1383, 1994

82. The effect of pravastatin on coronary events after myocardial infarction in patients with average cholesterol levels. Cholesterol and Recurrent Events Trial investigators. N Engl J Med 335:1001, 1996

83. MRC/BHF Heart Protection Study of cholesterol lowering with simvastatin in 20,536 high-risk individuals: a randomised placebo-controlled trial. Heart Protection Study. Lancet 360:7, 2002

84. Aggressive lipid-lowering therapy compared with angioplasty in stable coronary artery disease. Atorvastatin versus Revascularization Treatment Investigators. N Engl J Med 341:70, 1999

85. Nissen SE, Tuzcu M, Schoenhagen P, et al: Effect of intensive compared with moderate lipid-lowering therapy on progression of coronary atherosclerosis: a randomized controlled trial. JAMA 291:1071, 2004

86. Rosenson RS: Lipid lowering with HMG CoA reductase inhibitors (statins). UpToDate Online, 2004
http://www.uptodate.com

87. Thompson PD, Clarkson P, Karas RH: Statin-associated myopathy. JAMA 289:1681, 2003

88. Phillips PS, Haas RH, Bannykh S, et al: Statin-associated myopathy with normal creatine kinase levels. Ann Intern Med 137:581, 2002

89. Gould AL, Rossouw JE, Santanello NC, et al: Cholesterol reduction yields clinical benefit: impact of statin trials. Circulation 97:946, 1998

90. Gemfibrozil for the secondary prevention of coronary heart disease in men with low levels of high-density lipoprotein cholesterol. Veterans Affairs High-Density Lipoprotein Cholesterol Intervention Trial Study Group. N Engl J Med 341:410, 1999

91. Brown BG, Zhao XQ, Chait A, et al: Simvastatin and niacin, antioxidant vitamins, or the combination for the prevention of coronary disease. N Engl J Med 345:1583, 2001

92. Bays HE, McGovern ME: Once-daily niacin extended release/lovastatin combination tablet has more favorable effects on lipoprotein particle size and subclass distribution than atorvastatin and simvastatin. Prev Cardiol 6:179, 2003

93. Ballantyne CM, Houri J, Notarbolo A, et al: Effect of ezetimibe coadministered with atorvastatin in 628 patients with primary hypercholesterolemia: a prospective, randomized, double-blind trial. Circulation 107:2409, 2003

94. Smith CC, Bernstein LI, Davis RB, et al: Screening for statin-related toxicity: the yield of transaminase and creatine kinase measurements in a primary care setting. Arch Intern Med 163:688, 2003

95. Wilson PW, Grundy SM: The metabolic syndrome: a practical guide to origins and treatment: Part II. Circulation 108:1537, 2003

96. Rubins HB, Robins SJ, Collins D, et al: Diabetes, plasma insulin, and cardiovascular disease: subgroup analysis from the Department of Veterans Affairs High-Density Lipoprotein Intervention Trial (VA-HIT). Arch Intern Med 162:2597, 2002

97. Smith SC Jr, Blair SN, Criqui MH, et al: AHA consensus panel statement: preventing heart attack and death in patients with coronary disease. The Secondary Prevention Panel. J Am Coll Cardiol 26:292, 1995

98. Lewington S, Clarke R, Qizilbash N, et al: Age-specific relevance of usual blood pressure to vascular mortality: a meta-analysis of individual data for one million adults in 61 prospective studies. Lancet 360:1903, 2002

99. Chobanian AV, Bakris GL, Black HR, et al: The Seventh Report of the Joint National Committee on Prevention, Detection, Evaluation, and Treatment of High Blood Pressure: the JNC 7 report. JAMA 289:2560, 2003

100. Kannel WB, Gordon T, Offutt D: Left ventricular hypertrophy by electrocardiogram: prevalence, incidence, and mortality in the Framingham study. Ann Intern Med 71:89, 1969

101. Levy D, Salomon M, D'Agostino RB, et al: Prognostic implications of baseline electrocardiographic features and their serial changes in subjects with left ventricular hypertrophy. Circulation 90:1786, 1994

102. Heidenreich PA, McDonald KM, Hastie T, et al: Meta-analysis of trials comparing beta-blockers, calcium antagonists, and nitrates for stable angina. JAMA 281:1927, 1999

103. Effects of an angiotensin-converting-enzyme inhibitor, ramipril, on cardiovascular events in high-risk patients. The Heart Outcomes Prevention Evaluation Study Investigators. N Engl J Med 342:145, 2000 [errata, N Engl J Med 342:748, 2000, and N Engl J Med 342:1376, 2000]

104. Fox KM: Efficacy of perindopril in reduction of cardiovascular events among patients with stable coronary artery disease: randomised, double-blind, placebo-controlled, multicentre trial (the EUROPA study). Lancet 362:782, 2003

105. Dargie HJ, Ford I, Fox KM: Total Ischaemic Burden European Trial (TIBET). Effects of ischaemia and treatment with atenolol, nifedipine SR and their combination on outcome in patients with chronic stable angina. The TIBET Study Group. Eur Heart J 17:104, 1996

106. Rehnqvist N, Hjemdahl P, Billing E, et al: Effects of metoprolol vs verapamil in patients with stable angina pectoris. The Angina Prognosis Study in Stockholm (APSIS). Eur Heart J 17:76, 1996

107. The beta-blocker heart attack trial. Beta-Blocker Heart Attack Study Group. JAMA 246:2073, 1981

108. Prevention of stroke by antihypertensive drug treatment in older persons with isolated systolic hypertension: final results of the Systolic Hypertension in the Elderly Program (SHEP). SHEP Cooperative Research Group. JAMA 265:3255, 1991

109. MacMahon S, Peto R, Cutler J, et al: Blood pressure, stroke, and coronary heart disease: Part 1. Prolonged differences in blood pressure: prospective observational studies corrected for the regression dilution bias. Lancet 335:765, 1990

110. Double-blind comparison of once daily betaxolol versus propranolol four times daily in stable angina pectoris. Betaxolol Investigators Group. Am J Cardiol 65:577, 1990

111. Comparison of celiprolol and propranolol in stable angina pectoris. Celiprolol International Angina Study Group. Am J Cardiol 67:665, 1991

112. Efficacy of atenolol and captopril in reducing risk of macrovascular and microvascular complications in type 2 diabetes: UKPDS 39. UK Prospective Diabetes Study Group. BMJ 317:713, 1998

113. Effect of amlodipine on morbidity and mortality in severe chronic heart failure. Prospective Randomized Amlodipine Survival Evaluation Study Group. N Engl J Med 335:1107, 1996

114. Cheitlin MD, Hutter AM Jr, Brindis RG, et al: ACC/AHA expert consensus document: use of sildenafil (Viagra) in patients with cardiovascular disease. American College of Cardiology/American Heart Association. J Am Coll Cardiol 33:273, 1999

115. Haffner SM, Lehto S, Ronnemaa T, et al: Mortality from coronary heart disease in subjects with type 2 diabetes and in nondiabetic subjects with and without prior myocardial infarction. N Engl J Med 339:229, 1998

116. Collins R, Armitage J, Parish S, et al: MRC/BHF Heart Protection Study of cholesterol-lowering with simvastatin in 5963 people with diabetes: a randomised placebo-controlled trial. Lancet 361:2005, 2003

117. Effects of ramipril on cardiovascular and microvascular outcomes in people with diabetes mellitus: results of the HOPE study and MICRO-HOPE substudy. Heart Outcomes Prevention Evaluation (HOPE) Study Investigators. Lancet 355:253, 2003

118. Tatti P, Pahor M, Byington RP, et al: Outcome results of the Fosinopril versus Amlodipine Cardiovascular Events Randomized Trial (FACET) in patients with hypertension and NIDDM. Diabetes Care 21:597, 1998

119. Effects of intensive blood-pressure lowering and low-dose aspirin in patients with hypertension: principal results of the Hypertension Optimal Treatment (HOT) randomised trial. HOT Study Group. Lancet 351:1755, 1998

120. Colwell JA: Aspirin therapy in diabetes. Diabetes Care 26(suppl 1):S87, 2003

121. Haffner SM: Management of dyslipidemia in adults with diabetes. Diabetes Care (26 suppl 1):S83, 2003

122. Coronary artery surgery study (CASS): a randomized trial of coronary artery bypass: survival data. Circulation 68:939, 1983

123. Yusuf S, Zucker D, Peduzzi P, et al: Effect of coronary artery bypass graft surgery on survival: overview of 10-year results from randomised trials by the Coronary Artery Bypass Graft Surgery Trialists Collaboration. Lancet 344:563, 1994 [erratum, Lancet 344:1446, 1994]

124. Hueb WA, Soares PR, Almeida De Oliviera S, et al: Five-year follow-up of the medicine, angioplasty, or surgery study (MASS): a prospective, randomized trial of medical therapy, balloon angioplasty, or bypass surgery for single proximal left anterior descending coronary artery stenosis. Circulation 100(19 suppl):II107, 1999

125. Comparison of coronary bypass surgery with angioplasty in patients with multivessel disease. The Bypass Angioplasty Revascularization Investigation (BARI) Investigators. N Engl J Med 335:217, 1996 [erratum, N Engl J Med 336:147, 1997]

126. King SB 3rd, Kosinski AS, Guyton RA, et al: Eight-year mortality in the Emory Angioplasty versus Surgery Trial (EAST). J Am Coll Cardiol 35:1116, 2000

127. Coronary angioplasty versus medical therapy for angina: the second Randomised Intervention Treatment of Angina (RITA-2) trial. RITA-2 trial participants. Lancet 350:461, 1997

128. Parisi AF, Folland ED, Hartigan P: A comparison of angioplasty with medical therapy in the treatment of single-vessel coronary artery disease. Veterans Affairs ACME Investigators. N Engl J Med 326:10, 1992

129. Sculpher M, Smith D, Clayton T, et al: Coronary angioplasty versus medical therapy for angina: health service costs based on the second Randomized Intervention Treatment of Angina (RITA-2) trial. Eur Heart J 23:1291, 2002

130. Chaitman BR: Ranolazine for the treatment of chronic angina and potential use in other cardiovascular conditions. Circulation 113:2462, 2006

131. Duncan CL, Cummings SR, Hudes ES, et al: Quitting smoking: reasons for quitting and predictors of cessation among medical patients. J Gen Intern Med 7:398, 1992

24 Unstable Angina and Non–ST Segment Elevation Myocardial Infarction

Joel Kupersmith, M.D., F.A.C.P., and Amish Raval, M.D.

Definition

Acute coronary syndromes are the constellation of symptoms, signs, and electrocardiographic and laboratory findings associated with new-onset or worsening myocardial ischemia. They include the spectrum of acute ST segment elevation myocardial infarction (MI) with or without Q waves, non–ST segment elevation MI (NSTEMI), and unstable angina. The main difference between NSTEMI and unstable angina is that in the latter, the ischemia is not severe enough to cause cardiac enzyme elevation and tissue injury; however, this difference may not be apparent on initial presentation.[1,2]

Pathophysiology

Unstable angina/NSTEMI results from an acute reduction in myocardial oxygen supply caused by rupture or erosion of an atherosclerotic coronary plaque; this plaque disruption is associated with inflammation, thrombosis, vasoconstriction, and microvascular embolization. The plaques implicated in these syndromes usually had previously produced only minor obstruction to blood flow (on angiography, up to 70% of affected vessels have less than 50% stenosis of the lumen); in addition, these plaques are characterized by a large lipid pool, reduced collagen content, a thin fibrous cap, and inflammatory cells.[3-9] Embolization of platelets and clot fragments into the microvasculature results in microcirculatory ischemia, which may account for the slight elevation of cardiac biomarkers. The events leading to unstable angina/NSTEMI also affect atherosclerotic plaques in the rest of the coronary vascular tree and other vascular territories.[10-12]

Less common causes of unstable angina/NSTEMI include intense focal epicardial spasm, cardiac emboli, and severe progressive atherosclerotic narrowing without superimposed thrombus.[1] Rarely, secondary unstable angina can be precipitated by conditions that increase myocardial demand, such as thyrotoxicosis, sepsis, fever, tachycardia, and anemia. Secondary unstable angina usually occurs in patients who also have underlying stable coronary atherosclerosis. Cocaine and amphetamines can also induce the syndrome.

Diagnosis

CLINICAL PRESENTATION

Unstable angina/NSTEMI has three principal presentations: (1) prolonged angina at rest, usually lasting less than 20 minutes; (2) new-onset angina that is severe, disabling, and prolonged or frequent; and (3) established angina that has become distinctly more frequent, longer in duration, or more easily provoked.[13]

HISTORY AND PHYSICAL EXAMINATION

Five clinical factors are key to establishing the diagnosis and the prognosis in patients with suspected unstable angina/ NSTEMI: the anginal symptoms; any history of coronary artery disease (CAD); patient sex; patient age; and traditional risk factors for CAD [see Table 1].[1]

In the initial evaluation of a patient with suspected unstable angina/NSTEMI, the clinician should elicit a full description of the chest pain, including its character, onset, severity, and duration. Jaw pain, neck pain, epigastric pain, and arm pain may be experienced in isolation or in concert with the chest discomfort. In the National Registry of Myocardial Infarction, which included 440,000 patients, one third had atypical symptoms.[14] In the Alabama Unstable Angina Study of Medicare beneficiaries, which included over 4,000 patients, 51.7% of patients with unstable angina had the following atypical symptoms: dyspnea (69.4%), nausea (37.7%), diaphoresis (25.2%), syncope (10.6%), arm pain (11.5%), epigastric pain (8.1%), shoulder pain (7.4%), and neck pain (5.9%).[15] Atypical symptoms were more common in young patients (i.e., those 25 to 40 years of age), the elderly (i.e., those older than 75 years), diabetic patients, and women.[14]

Although it is important to inquire about the traditional risk factors for CAD, both to assess current risk and to guide future risk reduction, these factors are only weakly predictive of unstable angina/NSTEMI.[1] Important secondary or precipitating causes of unstable angina/NSTEMI should be ruled out, including a history of cocaine or amphetamine abuse, severe hypertension, and hyperthyroidism. Myopericarditis, hypothyroidism, and renal failure are among the conditions that may mimic acute coronary syndrome and can be associated with elevated cardiac enzyme levels.

In many cases, the physical examination will be normal. The examination is nevertheless useful to establish the presence of certain prognostic factors for the purpose of risk stratification and also to rule out such potentially devastating conditions as aortic dissection, pulmonary embolus, pneumothorax, and pericarditis.

The pulse is carefully evaluated to assess for significant bradycardia, tachycardia, or irregularity. Blood pressure is measured, to look for uncontrolled hypertension or significant hypotension (suggesting cardiogenic shock); pressure should be

---

Table 1 Clinical Factors for Determining Diagnosis and Prognosis in Patients with Suspected Unstable Angina or Non–ST Segment Myocardial Infarction

Nature of the anginal symptoms
History of coronary artery disease
Sex
Age ≥ 65 years
Number of traditional risk factors (smoking, diabetes, hypertension, hyperlipidemia, family history)

measured in both arms, to assess for aortic dissection [*see Chapter 28*]. Examination of the thyroid may suggest hypothyroidism or hyperthyroidism. Heart failure should be suspected if there is evidence of pulmonary rales, an elevated jugular venous impulse, an S_3 gallop, or a displaced and diffuse apical impulse. A murmur of acute mitral regurgitation may be a consequence of ischemia. Thrills, bruits, or pulse deficits may indicate coexisting peripheral vascular disease.

LABORATORY TESTS

Biochemical Cardiac Markers

Cardiac biomarkers—specifically, troponins, cardiac creatine kinase, and myoglobin—have important diagnostic, prognostic, and therapeutic implications in unstable angina/NSTEMI and for detection of MI generally. After ischemia-induced myocardial injury, loss of myocyte membrane integrity results in the release of various intracellular molecules into the interstitial space, lymphatics, and, eventually, into the peripheral circulation. Critical to the interpretation of these tests is the precise time of onset of ischemic symptoms.

Troponin Troponin I and T (TnI and TnT) are cardiac-specific subunits of the thin filament-associated troponin-tropomyosin complex, which regulates striated muscle contraction. Troponins have become the primary biomarkers in the evaluation of patients with acute coronary syndromes. These markers are detected in about one third of patients without elevation in the level of creatine kinase–myocardial band (CK-MB). Troponins may be detectable 3 to 4 hours after the onset of ischemic symptoms; they peak at 12 to 48 hours and persist for 4 to 10 days.[16,17] Generally, they are not detectable in the blood of healthy persons. However, both TnI and TnT are exceptionally sensitive to the presence of even minor myocardial necrosis, such as in supraventricular tachycardia, heart failure, and myocarditis, and they may also be elevated in severe renal impairment. Therefore, they should be evaluated in the context of the patient's clinical presentation.

Creatine kinase Before the advent of troponin assays, CK-MB was the primary cardiac biomarker. The CK-MB assay has considerable sensitivity and specificity for detecting myocardial necrosis at 6 to 48 hours after symptom onset or earlier. Abnormal CK-MB levels can be occasionally found in patients with high total CK levels; on clinical grounds, the CK-MB in such cases is thought to originate from skeletal muscle. Elevations in levels of the CK-MB isoforms CK-MB2 and CK-MB1 are very early markers of myocardial necrosis, but these assays are generally not part of the clinical routine.[18]

Myoglobin Myoglobin is a nonspecific biomarker found both in cardiac and skeletal muscle. It is released rapidly in response to muscle injury and is detectable 2 hours after the onset of ischemia.[17] Serial determination of myoglobin is not useful, but because of its high sensitivity in early ischemia, a negative myoglobin assay could potentially rule out myocardial necrosis.

Twelve-lead electrocardiogram ECG results may be important for determining treatment; patients with acute ST segment elevation should be considered for immediate reperfusion therapy.[19] In patients with suspected unstable angina/NSTEMI, ST segment depression of 0.05 mV or more in two or more contigu-

ous leads is highly consistent with myocardial ischemia (this is especially the case if the ST segment depression is present during chest pain and resolves with the easing of pain). Deep, symmetrical T wave inversion is also highly consistent with myocardial ischemia. Other nonspecific abnormalities, such as transient bundle branch block, atrial or ventricular arrhythmias, and QT prolongation, can also occur with unstable angina/NSTEMI but are not useful for diagnosis. Interestingly, a quarter of patients diagnosed with unstable angina/NSTEMI will go on to develop Q waves,[2] and up to 60% may have a normal 12-lead ECG.[20]

RISK STRATIFICATION

Determining whether a patient is at low, medium, or high risk for ischemic complications (e.g., full-blown MI) is important for deciding treatment of unstable angina/NSTEMI. Depending on whether the therapeutic strategy will be invasive or conservative (see below), the degree of risk can be used to determine the level of therapy. Older age, positive cardiac biomarkers, rales, ST segment depression, hypotension and tachycardia,[21] and reduced left ventricular ejection fraction (< 40%) have been associated with increased mortality. Clinical diabetes mellitus is also associated with higher risk. One specific and widely used method of risk stratification, the Antman/Thrombolysis in Myocardial Infarction (TIMI) risk score, is a seven-point scoring system that helps to predict death, reinfarction, or recurrent ischemia requiring revascularization [*see Table 2*].[22] This risk score was developed from the TIMI 11B[23] and Efficacy and Safety of Subcutaneous Enoxaparin in Non–Q-wave Coronary Events (ESSENCE)[24] trial and has been validated in two other large trials: Therapy with an Invasive or Conservative Strategy—Thrombolysis (TACTICS)–TIMI 18 and Platelet Receptor Inhibition in Ischemic Syndrome Management in Patients Limited by Unstable Signs and Symptoms (PRISM-PLUS).[25,26] The risk of adverse outcomes ranges from 5% to 41%, according to the simple sum of the individual variables.

Table 2 Thrombolysis in Myocardial Infarction (TIMI) Risk Score for Unstable Angina or Non–ST Segment Myocardial Infarction*

Variable	Points
Age ≥ 65 years	1
More than three coronary risk factors	1
History of coronary artery disease	1
ST segment deviation	1
More than two anginal events within 24 hr	1
Use of aspirin within past 7 days	1
Elevated cardiac markers	1

Total Score	Risk of a Cardiac Event (%) Within 14 Days†
0/1	5
2	8
3	13
4	20
5	26
6/7	41

*To determine a patient's level of risk, the clinician determines the total score, based on the presence of specific risk markers.
†Death, recurrent myocardial infarction, or recurrent ischemia requiring urgent revascularization.

Electrocardiographic Changes

Patients with unstable angina/NSTEMI and ECG findings of bundle branch block, ventricular hypertrophy, paced rhythm, or severe ST segment depression (> 0.2 mV) in multiple leads are independently at high risk for subsequent adverse events.[1,20] Considered at low risk are those with isolated T wave abnormalities or a normal ECG pattern. Continuous ECG monitoring may detect transient ischemic episodes, which have been shown in small studies to have prognostic value, but the use of this technique as a risk marker is not widely recommended.[1,27,28]

Blood Tests

Both TnI and TnT are markers of increased risk in that they reflect the presence and level of myocardial necrosis.[1,16] High-sensitivity C-reactive protein (hsCRP), which is produced by the liver in response to inflammation,[29,30] and other acute-phase reactants such as plasma fibrinopeptide, fibrinogen, serum amyloid A, and interleukin-6, have demonstrated similar predictive value for adverse outcomes.[31-33] B-type natriuretic peptide (BNP), released in response to ventricular wall stress, may also independently predict mortality.[34] Measurement of hsCRP and BNP may be of use at times, but more studies are needed to clarify the roles of these markers in routine care.

Stress Testing

Stress testing for assessment of risk may be performed in patients who have been stable and asymptomatic for 24 to 48 hours and in all patients before discharge. Stress testing is a necessary component of an early conservative strategy (see below). Briefly, stress test results that show the patient to be at high risk for significant ischemia are as follows:

1. Treadmill ECG: inability to achieve a workload of greater than two metabolic equivalents (mets); early and persistent ST segment depression of greater than 2 mm; symptom onset at less than 6.5 mets; or hypotension or ST segment elevation during exercise in the absence of Q waves
2. Stress nuclear scintigraphy: evidence of left ventricular dilation or thallium lung uptake during stress, or moderate to large reversible perfusion defects
3. Stress echocardiography: more than two myocardial wall segments demonstrating reversible impairment of thickening with stress or evidence of left ventricular dilation with stress[35]

Treatment

WHERE TO HOSPITALIZE

In most medical centers in the United States, patients with definite features of unstable angina/NSTEMI are admitted to a cardiac care unit that provides continuous ECG monitoring and specialized nursing. Patients with less than definite features of unstable angina or those in whom the chest pain has ceased by the time of arrival may be admitted to a chest pain unit with telemetry (sometimes called a step-down cardiac unit).

Ideally, patients with unstable angina/NSTEMI should be hospitalized in an institution that offers mechanical revascularization, because these procedures are frequently needed in such patients, especially those who have high-risk features. If this is not possible, high-risk patients should receive interim treatment with an intensive pharmacologic regimen until arrangements can be made for transfer to a facility with interventional capability.

INITIAL THERAPY

The initial management of unstable angina/NSTEMI includes resuscitation and supportive measures for patients who present with hemodynamic instability, as well as prompt administration of medication of proven, evidence-based value [see Pharmacologic Therapy, below, and Figure 1]. Bed rest with continuous ECG monitoring for ischemia and arrhythmia detection is a class I rec-

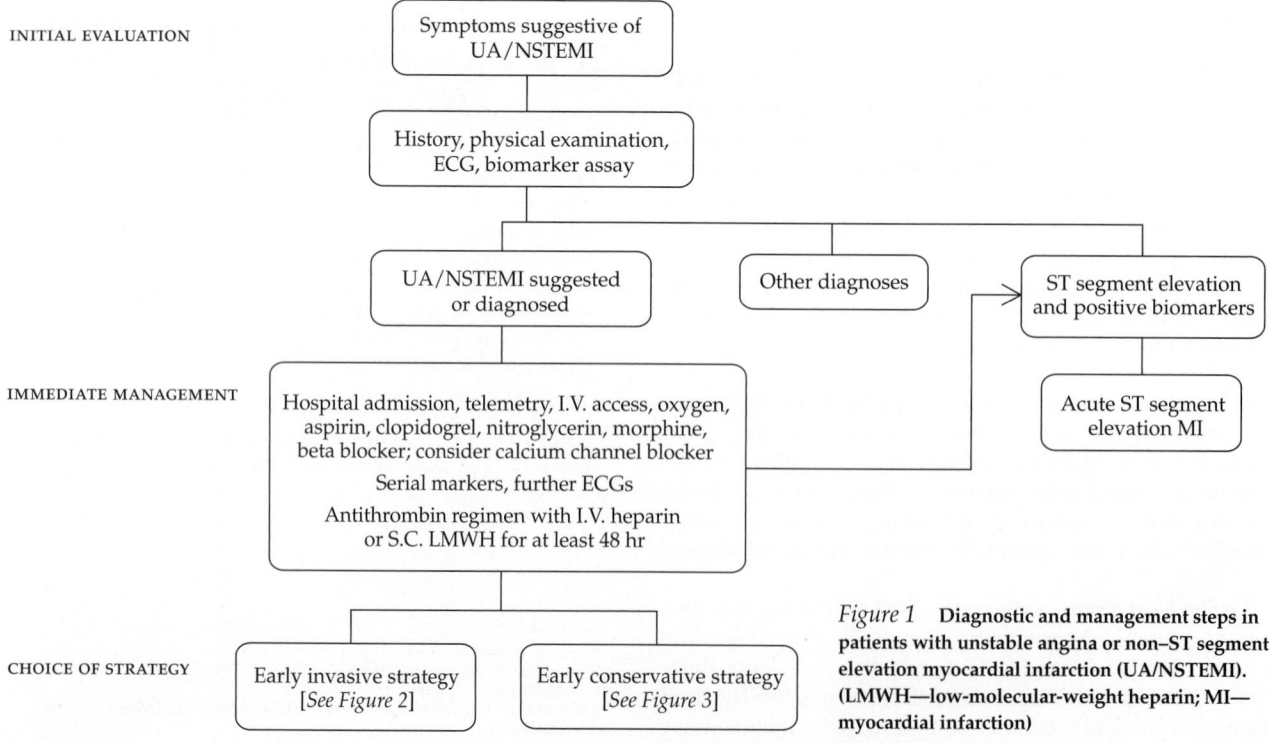

INITIAL EVALUATION

Symptoms suggestive of UA/NSTEMI

History, physical examination, ECG, biomarker assay

UA/NSTEMI suggested or diagnosed

Other diagnoses

ST segment elevation and positive biomarkers

Acute ST segment elevation MI

IMMEDIATE MANAGEMENT

Hospital admission, telemetry, I.V. access, oxygen, aspirin, clopidogrel, nitroglycerin, morphine, beta blocker; consider calcium channel blocker

Serial markers, further ECGs

Antithrombin regimen with I.V. heparin or S.C. LMWH for at least 48 hr

CHOICE OF STRATEGY

Early invasive strategy [See Figure 2]

Early conservative strategy [See Figure 3]

Figure 1 **Diagnostic and management steps in patients with unstable angina or non–ST segment elevation myocardial infarction (UA/NSTEMI). (LMWH—low-molecular-weight heparin; MI—myocardial infarction)**

ommendation for patients who have ongoing anginal pain at rest, on the basis of level C evidence [*see Table 3*]. The strictness of the bed rest requirement can be tailored to the severity of symptoms. For instance, patients can be mobilized to a chair or bedside commode when symptom free.

Oxygen Inhaled oxygen therapy should be reserved for those patients with clear respiratory distress, cyanosis, or arterial hypoxemia. In the absence of these high-risk features, time and resources need not be spent for the sole purpose of oxygen administration. Supplemental oxygen is recommended for patients with cyanosis or respiratory distress. Finger pulse oximetry or arterial

blood gas measurements should be done to determine whether the patient has adequate arterial oxygen saturation ($S_aO_2 > 90\%$) or has hypoxemia and requires supplemental oxygen. These class I recommendations are supported by level C evidence.

EARLY INVASIVE VERSUS EARLY CONSERVATIVE STRATEGY

The first decision in management (and one that is often a matter of dispute) is to choose between the two reigning strategies for unstable angina/NSTEMI: early invasive management and early conservative management [*see Figures 2 and 3*]. In the early invasive strategy, early coronary angiography is performed unless contraindicated. In the early conservative strategy, angiography is reserved for those patients who have indications of being at high risk for cardiac events; such indications include evidence of significant ischemia on a noninvasive stress test and recurrent ischemia despite adequate medical therapy. It should be noted that although many patients assigned to the conservative strategy undergo angiography and receive interventions (e.g., in one study, 51% of patients underwent angiography and 36% received subsequent revascularization[25]), in these patients there was an additional indication for the angiography, based on risk, besides the diagnosis of unstable angina/NSTEMI.

Advocates of an early conservative strategy suggest that angiography—and its associated risks—can be avoided in low-risk patients and that costs and resources can be conserved by not performing these procedures in all patients. Advocates of an early invasive strategy suggest that this approach can result in superior clinical outcomes through early identification of patients with high-risk lesions, including those with critical left main coronary artery stenosis or triple-vessel coronary disease. In addition, advocates of an early invasive strategy argue that such intervention results in shorter hospital stays for patients found to have low-risk anatomy; these proponents also note that cardiac

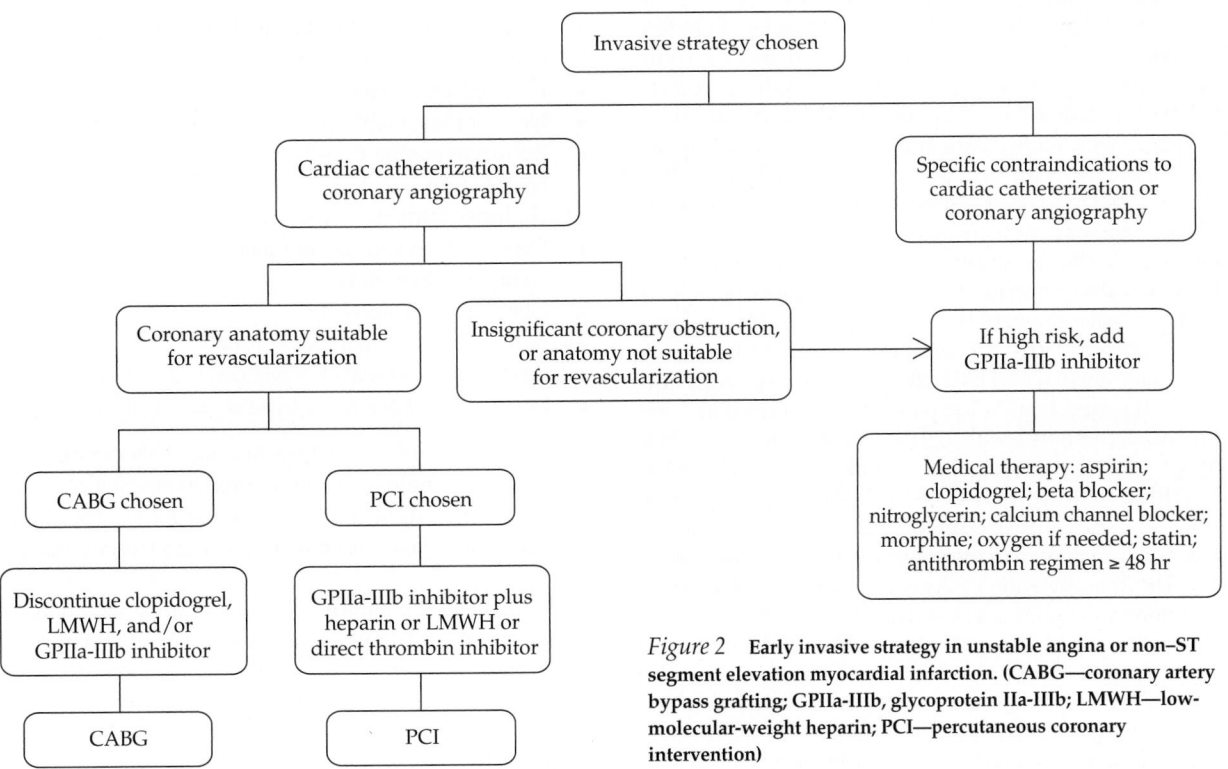

Figure 2 **Early invasive strategy in unstable angina or non–ST segment elevation myocardial infarction. (CABG—coronary artery bypass grafting; GPIIa-IIIb, glycoprotein IIa-IIIb; LMWH—low-molecular-weight heparin; PCI—percutaneous coronary intervention)**

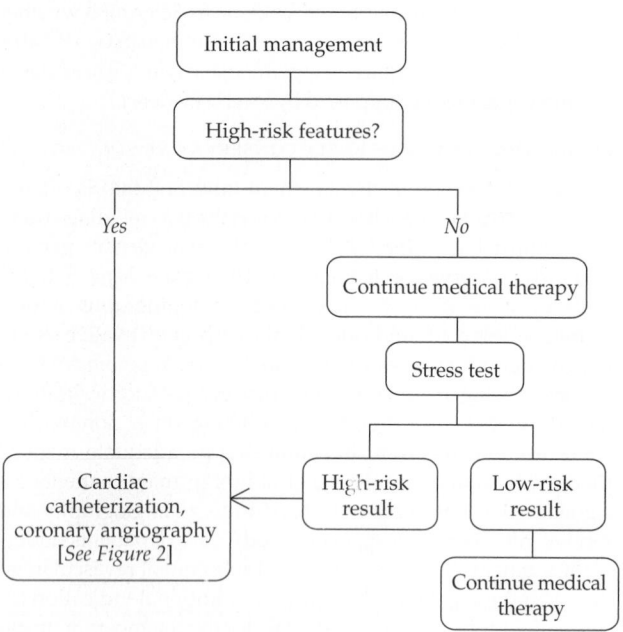

Figure 3 **Early conservative strategy in unstable angina/non–ST segment elevation myocardial infarction.**

catheterization is now available to almost all patients and that catheterization has a very low procedural risk.

Trial Results

Three initial multicenter, randomized trials found that there was no difference in outcome between an early invasive strategy and an early conservative strategy, whereas three subsequent trials showed benefit in favor of the invasive strategy. TIMI IIIB showed no difference in death or MI at 42 days with either strategy in patients with unstable angina/NSTEMI[36]; the Veterans Affairs Non–Q-Wave Myocardial Infarction Strategies In-Hospital (VANQWISH) trial showed no difference in death or recurrent MI in the early invasive versus the conservative group at 2 years' average follow-up (32.9% versus 30.3%; P = 0.35), although there were more deaths in the early invasive group at 1 year[37]; and the Medicine versus Angiography in Thrombolytic Exclusion (MATE) trial, conducted in patients with acute coronary syndrome who were ineligible for thrombolysis, showed no difference in clinical outcome between either strategy.[38]

The three subsequent studies have begun to move opinion toward the invasive strategy. The Fragmin in Unstable Coronary Artery Disease II (FRISC II) study was conducted in patients with unstable angina/NSTEMI who were receiving dalteparin; death or MI occurred in 9.4% of patients who received invasive treatment, as compared with 12.1% of those treated conservatively (P < 0.031; risk ratio, 0.78; confidence interval, 0.62 to 0.98).[39] However, a substudy of FRISC II showed that the most benefit of the early invasive strategy accrued to those patients with an ST segment shift of more than 2.5 mm or in five or more leads.[40] The Therapy with an Invasive or Conservative Strategy–Thrombolysis—TIMI 18 (TACTICS-TIMI 18) trial involved patients with unstable angina/NSTEMI who had ST or T wave changes, increased cardiac markers, and a history of coronary artery disease and who were taking aspirin, heparin, and tirofiban. This trial showed a combined end point (death, MI, or rehospitalization at 6 months) of 15.9% in the early invasive

group, as compared with 19.4% in the early conservative group (P = 0.025; relative risk, 0.78; confidence interval, 0.62 to 0.97). Major bleeding was similar in both groups (1.9% versus 1.3%; P = 0.24). Subgroup analysis of the trial suggested that early invasive treatment benefited only patients whose TnI or TnT level was initially elevated.[41] Of note, median length of stay was somewhat shorter with the invasive strategy (3.9 days versus 4.3 days; P < 0.001). The cost of care in the invasive group was somewhat higher for the initial hospitalization ($15,714 versus $14,047 in year 2000 dollars), though the 6-month average total costs did not differ between the two groups ($21,813 for the invasive group versus $21,227 for the conservative group; P = nonsignificant).[42] In the Randomized Intervention Trial of unstable Angina–3 (RITA-3) in unstable angina/NSTEMI patients treated with enoxaparin, rates of death or MI at 4 months were lower in the early invasive group (9.6% versus 14.5%; P = 0.001; relative risk, 0.66; confidence interval, 0.51 to 0.85).[43]

Although the results of these three trials differed, patients who were considered to be at high risk for death or MI consistently seemed to benefit the most from a strategy of early angiography and revascularization. Because of the low event rate in patients considered to be at low risk, it is not clear that the early invasive approach offers a clear advantage over an early conservative strategy for this population. Therefore, until further evidence becomes available, an early conservative strategy may be a reasonable initial approach for the management of low-risk patients with unstable angina/NSTEMI.

Treatment Recommendations

High-risk patients A class I recommendation and level A evidence support the use of an early invasive strategy in patients with unstable angina/NSTEMI who have no serious comorbidity and have any of the following high-risk indicators:

- Recurrent angina at rest or with low-level activity despite intensive medical therapy.
- Elevated TnI or TnT levels.
- New, or presumably new, ST segment depression.
- Recurrent angina or ischemia with symptoms or signs of heart failure.
- High-risk findings on noninvasive stress testing.
- Depressed left ventricular function (ejection fraction < 40%) on noninvasive study.
- Hemodynamic instability.
- Sustained ventricular tachycardia.
- Percutaneous coronary intervention within the past 6 months.
- Previous coronary artery bypass grafting (CABG).

In the absence of any of these findings, either a conservative or an invasive strategy may be offered to hospitalized patients without contraindications for revascularization. This option is supported by a class 1 recommendation and level B evidence.

Women and the elderly There should be no difference in the management of men and women. The elderly should be treated no differently than younger patients, although management should take into consideration general health, comorbid conditions, cognitive status, life expectancy, and altered pharmacokinetics of and sensitivity to hypotensive drugs.

Table 4   Antiplatelet Therapy in Unstable Angina or Non–ST Segment Elevation Myocardial Infarction

Drug (Trade Name)	Initial Dose	Route	Duration	Adverse Effects	Adverse Drug Reactions	Contraindications
Aspirin	81–325 mg q.d.	Oral (first dose chewed)	Indefinite	Bleeding, tinnitus, rash, GI intolerance	None	Active, severe bleeding
Clopidogrel (Plavix)	300 mg loading dose, then 75 mg q.d.	Oral	1 yr	Bleeding, rare TTP	Partial inhibition of effect with statin drugs	Active, severe bleeding; major surgery within < 5 days
Ticlopidine (Ticlid)	250 mg b.i.d.	Oral	1 yr	Bleeding, TTP, rash, neutropenia, diarrhea	None	Active, severe bleeding; major surgery planned
Abciximab (ReoPro)	0.25 mg/kg bolus, then 0.125 µg/kg/min; max 10 µg/min	I.V.	12 hr	Bleeding, thrombocytopenia	None	Active, severe bleeding; major surgery planned
Eptifibatide (Integrilin)	180 µg/kg bolus, then 2 µg/kg/min	I.V.	72–96 hr or 18 hr if PCI performed	Bleeding	None	Active, severe bleeding; major surgery planned
Tirofiban (Aggrastat)	0.4 µg/kg/min bolus (× 30 min), then 0.1 µg/kg/min	I.V.	48 hr	Bleeding	None	Active, severe bleeding; major surgery planned

PCI—percutaneous coronary intervention   TTP—thrombotic thrombocytopenic purpura

PHARMACOLOGIC THERAPY

Antiplatelet Drugs

Antiplatelet medications used in unstable angina/NSTEMI include aspirin, thienopyridines (clopidogrel and ticlopidine), abciximab, eptifibatide, and tirofiban [*see Table 4*].

Aspirin   Aspirin is considered the benchmark antiplatelet agent for the treatment of unstable angina/NSTEMI. A class I recommendation and level A evidence suggest that aspirin be started immediately in these patients and continued indefinitely.[1,2]

Aspirin's mechanism of action is to decrease the formation of the potent platelet aggregator thromboxane A_2 by irreversibly binding cyclooxygenase-1 in platelets. The effect on platelets is rapid (occurring within 15 to 30 minutes), and it is achieved with an oral dose as low as 81 mg.

Four pivotal randomized trials that evaluated the effectiveness of aspirin in the treatment of acute coronary syndrome showed consistent and durable long-term benefit at doses ranging from 75 to 325 mg daily.[44-47] The Antiplatelet Trialists' Collaboration meta-analysis of more than 100,000 patients in 145 trials showed such benefits in several cardiovascular disorders. For example, in 4,000 patients with unstable angina, rates of so-called vascular events (nonfatal MI, nonfatal stroke, or vascular death) were reduced from 14% to 9% ($P < 0.00001$) after 6 months.[48] Furthermore, the benefit of aspirin in these high-risk patients was sustained for at least 2 years.

Aspirin dosages have varied among several trials; no dosage has been definitively shown to be preferable. For patients with suspected MI in the International Studies of Infarct Survival–2 (ISIS-2) trial, the effective dosage was 160 mg daily.[49] A dose of aspirin between 160 and 325 mg should be administered immediately; the first dose should be chewed, for rapid absorption, and subsequent doses swallowed.

Adverse effects of aspirin include allergy, which may manifest as rash, angioedema, or asthma; a tendency to bleed; gastrointestinal effects, including gastric ulcer; and, rarely, precipitation of acute gout. Contraindications include allergy (especially if the allergic reaction is in the form of asthma), active bleeding, a serious bleeding disorder, severe untreated hypertension, and an active peptic ulcer.

Thienopyridines   Thienopyridines irreversibly bind the adenosine diphosphate receptor on platelets, preventing fibrinogen binding and platelet aggregation. The two thienopyridines that have been used clinically are ticlopidine (Ticlid) and clopidogrel (Plavix).

In a single open-label trial in patients with unstable angina, ticlopidine (250 mg twice daily) significantly reduced vascular death and nonfatal MI at 6 months (13.6% versus 7.3%; $P = 0.009$), compared with standard aspirin therapy.[50] Several trials have shown the value of clopidogrel. In 12,562 patients with unstable angina, all of whom were also treated with aspirin, clopidogrel (300 mg followed by 75 mg daily), administered for 3 to 12 months, reduced a combined end point of cardiovascular death, nonfatal MI, and stroke from 11.4% to 9.3% ($P < 0.001$) and also decreased the incidence of ischemia, heart failure, and revascularization procedures. Benefit occurred as early as 24 hours after initiating treatment and persisted for up to 1 year. Clopidogrel increased major bleeding from 2.7% to 3.7% ($P = 0.003$), but there was no difference in life-threatening bleeding or hemorrhagic shock. Importantly, bleeding was increased in patients who underwent CABG within 5 days after stopping clopidogrel.[51] Two other studies found that clopidogrel benefited patients treated with percutaneous coronary intervention.[52,53] The Clopidogrel for the Reduction of Events During Observation (CREDO) study examined the timing of therapy with a combination of clopidogrel and aspirin. In one arm of the study, patients received a bolus load of aspirin and clopidogrel 6 to 24 hours before undergoing percutaneous coronary intervention. In the other arm of the study, patients received a bolus load less than 6 hours before the procedure. Benefit was observed in those patients who received the bolus 6 to 24 hours before the procedure.

The dosage of ticlopidine is 250 mg orally, twice daily; the dosage of clopidogrel is 300 mg orally. Both agents should be started immediately on presentation. The duration of therapy, which has been better defined for clopidogrel, is up to 1 year at a dose of 75 mg daily.

The principal adverse reaction that has limited the clinical use of ticlopidine is severe neutropenia; rarely, thrombotic thrombocytopenic purpura develops within the first 3 months of therapy. Both conditions are life threatening unless the drug is discontinued promptly. Clopidogrel has been associated with increased bleeding complications when administered with other antithrombotic agents, particularly when arterial puncture is performed for intervention. Bleeding during surgery is an important complication of clopidogrel use; for this reason, surgery should be avoided for 5 and preferably 7 days after the last dose, because of the prolonged duration of action.

Recommendations for the use of clopidogrel are as follows:

1. Patients with unstable angina/NSTEMI in whom a noninterventional approach is planned should receive clopidogrel for at least 1 month (this class I recommendation is supported by level A evidence) and for up to 9 months (class I recommendation, level B evidence).
2. Patients with unstable angina/NSTEMI for whom a percutaneous coronary intervention is planned and who are not at high risk for bleeding should receive clopidogrel for at least 1 month (class I recommendation, level A evidence) and for up to 9 months (class I recommendation, level B evidence).
3. Clopidogrel should be stopped for 5 to 7 days before elective surgical revascularization (class I recommendation, level B evidence).
4. When used to pretreat patients undergoing percutaneous coronary intervention, clopidogrel should be given more than 6 hours before the procedure (level B evidence).[53]

Glycoprotein IIb-IIIa receptor antagonists Abciximab, eptifibatide, and tirofiban act by specifically binding the glycoprotein (GP) IIb-IIIa receptor on platelet surfaces, thereby preventing fibrinogen binding and ultimately preventing platelet aggregation. Abciximab is the Fab fragment of a monoclonal antibody that has a short plasma half-life but irreversibly binds the GPIIb-IIIa receptor for 24 to 48 hours. The half-lives of eptifibatide and tirofiban are 2 to 3 hours, with platelet aggregation returning to normal 4 to 8 hours after drug discontinuance.

In three large clinical trials of patients with unstable angina/NSTEMI who underwent percutaneous coronary intervention, all of these GPIIb-IIIa inhibitors provided significant benefit in the composite outcome of death, MI, or urgent repeat revascularization, with the major benefit seen in recurrent MI and urgent repeat revascularization.[26,54,55] The Do Tirofiban and Reopro Give Similar Efficacy Trial (TARGET), which was conducted in patients with unstable angina/NSTEMI who underwent percutaneous coronary intervention with stenting, found that abciximab conferred greater benefit than tirofiban (although tirofiban was administered at a suboptimal dosage).[56]

For patients not undergoing planned percutaneous intervention, the results with GPIIb-IIIa inhibitors have been less impressive. Abciximab, given for 24 or 48 hours, was found to be no better than placebo in the Global Use of Strategies to Open Occluded Coronary Arteries IV (GUSTO IV) trial in patients with acute coronary syndrome.[57] On the other hand, two trials with tirofiban and eptifibatide demonstrated modest benefit in patients who did not undergo an interventional procedure[26,54]; the benefit was greatest in high-risk patients.

Abciximab, which is recommended for use during percutaneous coronary intervention, is administered as a 0.25 mg/kg in-

travenous bolus, followed by an infusion at 0.125 µg/kg/min for 12 hours. Eptifibatide is administered as a 180 µg/kg intravenous bolus, followed by a second bolus after 10 minutes. Thereafter, it is infused at a rate of 2 µg/kg/min for 72 to 96 hours if no percutaneous intervention is performed or for 18 hours if such a procedure is performed. Tirofiban is given in an intravenous 0.4 µg/kg/min bolus over 30 minutes, then infused at a rate of 0.1 µg/kg/min for 48 hours.

Bleeding is the most common complication of GPIIb-IIIa inhibitors. Special care should be taken to prevent bleeding in high-risk patients such as the elderly, women, those with low body weight, and those who require arterial puncture for an intervention. Because of their short half-lives, eptifibatide or tirofiban may be better suited for patients who may require surgical revascularization. Abciximab results in serious thrombocytopenia in about 0.3% of patients,[56] so serial platelet measurements are recommended in patients receiving this agent. In a meta-analysis, GPIIb-IIIa inhibitors were found to increase major bleeding from 1.4% to 2.4 % ($P < 0.0001$). There was no increase in the rate of intracranial hemorrhage.[58]

Three evidence-based recommendations can be made for the use of GPIIb-IIIa inhibitors:

1. In patients with unstable angina/NSTEMI who are to undergo a planned percutaneous coronary intervention, a GPIIb-IIIa inhibitor should be given either before or during the procedure. This class I recommendation is supported by level A evidence.
2. Patients with unstable angina/NSTEMI who have high-risk features and who are not to undergo a planned percutaneous intervention should receive eptifibatide or tirofiban (class IIa recommendation, level A evidence).
3. Patients with unstable angina/NSTEMI in whom percutaneous intervention is not planned should not receive abciximab (class III recommendation, level A evidence).

Fibrinolytic Drugs

Fibrinolytic therapy is not indicated for patients with unstable angina/NSTEMI. Level A evidence indicates that intravenous fibrinolytic therapy should not be administered to patients who do not have acute ST segment elevation, unless they have a true posterior MI or a presumed new left bundle branch block (class III recommendation).[59]

Anticoagulants

Heparin, low-molecular-weight heparin (LMWH), bivalirudin, or warfarin can be used for anticoagulant therapy in patients with unstable angina/NSTEMI [see Table 5].

Heparin Unfractionated heparin is composed of a number of chains of varying molecular weights that differ with regard to anticoagulant activity. Heparin generally increases the action of circulating antithrombin, which inactivates factor IIa, factor IXa, and factor Xa and prevents thrombus formation.[60]

Three randomized, placebo-controlled trials suggested that early intravenous administration of heparin leads to a modest reduction in the incidence of MI or recurrent ischemia.[61-63] A meta-analysis of six trials showed a relative risk of 0.67 (95% confidence interval, 0.44 to 1.02) in favor of the combination of heparin and aspirin.[64]

Heparin should be given in an initial intravenous bolus of 60 to 70 U/kg (maximum, 5,000 U), followed by an infusion of 12 to

Table 5 Anticoagulant Therapy in Unstable Angina/ Non–ST Segment Elevation Myocardial Infarction

Drug	Dose	Route	Duration	Adverse Effects	Adverse Drug Reactions	Contraindications
Unfractionated heparin	60–70 U/kg bolus (max 5,000 U); 12–15 U/kg/hr (max 1,000 U/hr)	I.V.	48–72 hr	Bleeding, HIT, mild thrombocytopenia	None	Active, severe bleeding; HIT
Enoxaparin	1 mg/kg b.i.d.	S.C.	48–72 hr	Bleeding, HIT	None	Active bleeding; major surgery planned
Bivalirudin	0.75 mg/kg bolus; 1.75 mg/kg/hr	I.V.	Duration of PCI	Bleeding	None	Active, severe bleeding
Warfarin	5–10 mg; dose adjusted to maintain desired INR, typically 2–3	Oral	Varies with indication	Bleeding, warfarin skin necrosis	Dose adjustment with macrolides, cimetidine, digoxin, amiodarone, other drugs	Active, severe bleeding; major surgery planned

HIT—heparin-induced thrombocytopenia   INR—international normalized ratio   PCI—percutaneous coronary intervention

15 U/kg/hr (maximum, 1,000 U/hr). Doses should be adjusted to maintain an activated partial thromboplastin time (aPTT) of 1.5 to 2.5 times control values.[1]

As with any anticoagulant, heparin is contraindicated in patients with active severe bleeding or who are to undergo imminent surgery. Heparin-induced thrombocytopenia (HIT) is a serious but rare (< 0.2% incidence) antibody-mediated reaction leading to reduced platelet counts and thrombosis [*see Chapter 98*]. HIT mandates immediate cessation of heparin, including heparinized solutions used for the flushing of intravenous ports. From 10% to 20% of patients receiving heparin may experience mild thrombocytopenia that is not associated with severe thrombosis or excessive bleeding.[1] For serious bleeding, heparin anticoagulation can be immediately reversed with intravenous protamine sulfate.

Low-molecular-weight heparin LMWHs are produced by enzymatic depolymerization of unfractionated heparin, resulting in smaller chain units. Advantages include less protein binding; longer half-life; more stable, dose-dependent clearance; and a greater anti–factor Xa effect that is associated with more thrombin inhibition. The standard aPTT assay cannot be used for LMWH, because this assay is not sensitive to the anti-Xa effects of LMWHs. Rapid factor Xa assays are not widely available, but the stable kinetics of LMWH tends to reduce the need for monitoring.

A number of trials have compared individual LMWHs with unfractionated heparin. Meta-analysis of two trials revealed a modest benefit of enoxaparin over heparin in terms of death and MI at 45 days (7.1% versus 8.6%; $P = 0.02$).[65] In trials with dalteparin and nadroparin, neither showed benefit.[66,67] FRISC showed a significant improvement in death, MI, or urgent revascularization with dalteparin (1.8% versus 4.8%; $P = 0.001$) for up to 43 days.[68] In the Integrilin and Enoxaparin Randomized Assessment of Acute Coronary Syndrome Treatment (INTERACT) trial, enoxaparin was found to be associated with less ischemia, as evidenced on ECG (14.3% versus 25.4%; $P = 0.002$), and to lead to an improvement in the composite end point of death or MI at 30 days (5% versus 9%; $P = 0.031$).[69] Several trials showed evidence of a small increase in minor bleeding with LMWH, as compared with heparin, but no difference in major bleeding was seen.[66-69] One small trial demonstrated that enoxaparin was safe with regard to serious bleeding in unstable angina/NSTEMI patients undergoing percutaneous

coronary intervention.[70] Another trial showed significantly lower rates of major CABG–related bleeding with LMWH, as compared with enoxaparin, by 96 hours after percutaneous coronary intervention (1.8% versus 4.6%; $P = 0.03$).[23] When enoxaparin was added to abciximab, no difference in the rate of bleeding events and adverse ischemic outcomes was seen, as compared with historical controls.[71]

In summary, evidence to date suggests that LMWH is at least as effective as unfractionated heparin and is generally safe in patients with unstable angina/NSTEMI in whom surgery or percutaneous coronary intervention is not planned. The dosing of LMWH is simpler than that of unfractionated heparin, and LMWH therapy does not require monitoring with coagulation studies. Abundant data (e.g., from the TIMI 11B, ESSENCE, and INTERACT studies) suggest that enoxaparin is the preferred agent.[23,24,69] In patients for whom percutaneous coronary intervention is planned, LMWH may be started or continued, provided that meticulous attention is given to dosing and the timing of its administration. Enoxaparin has not found wide use in contemporary interventional practice, however, because of practitioners' uneasiness over the inability to monitor the level of anticoagulation. In patients in whom surgery is planned, LMWH should be avoided; if an LMWH has already been started, the patient should be switched to unfractionated heparin, whose effects can be monitored closely.

Enoxaparin is given subcutaneously at a dosage of 1 mg/kg every 12 hours for at least 48 hours. Percutaneous coronary intervention may be performed within 8 hours of starting the drug, without additional anticoagulation therapy. If the percutaneous procedure is performed 8 to 12 hours after starting the drug, an additional intravenous bolus of 0.3 mg/kg may be given. Dose adjustment must be made in patients with moderate to severe renal impairment.

Compared with unfractionated heparin, LMWH has a slightly higher rate of minor bleeding complications and the same rate of major bleeding complications. Although the risk of HIT seems to be lower with LMWH than with unfractionated heparin, LMWH is absolutely contraindicated in patients with a history of HIT because of the danger posed by this reaction.

A class I recommendation and level A evidence support the use of anticoagulation with intravenous heparin or subcutaneous LMWH in patients with unstable angina/NSTEMI; the anticoagulant is given in addition to aspirin, clopidogrel, or both.

Level A evidence indicates that enoxaparin is preferable to unfractionated heparin in patients without renal failure, unless CABG is planned within 24 hours (class IIa recommendation).

Direct thrombin inhibitors These agents directly bind to the fibrinogen-recognition and catalytic sites of thrombin, neutralize clot-bound thrombin, and inhibit thrombin-mediated platelet aggregation; the result is sustained anticoagulation. Hirudin and bivalirudin are the two principal agents that have undergone clinical testing, but hirudin is not used.

In the Randomized Evaluation in Percutaneous Coronary Intervention Linking Angiomax to Reduced Clinical Events–2 (REPLACE-2) trial, which involved patients undergoing percutaneous coronary intervention, bivalirudin in combination with provisional GPIIb-IIIa inhibition was found to be equivalent to unfractionated heparin plus GPIIb-IIIa inhibition in terms of death, MI, urgent repeat revascularization, and in-hospital major bleeding after 30 days of therapy.[72] Rates of in-hospital major bleeding were significantly lower with bivalirudin (2.4% versus 4.1%; $P < 0.001$), although it has been noted that activated clotting time (ACT) values in the patients who received unfractionated heparin and a GpIIb-IIIa inhibitor were higher than was seen in other trials.

Bivalirudin is given as an intravenous bolus of 0.75 mg/kg at the start of percutaneous coronary intervention; for the duration of the procedure, an infusion of 1.75 mg/kg/hr is given. Because of the predictable profile of bivalirudin, measurement of ACT levels is usually not necessary. If the ACT is measured, typical values are 300 to 400 seconds.

Although bleeding seems to occur less commonly with bivalirudin than with unfractionated heparin or GPIIb-IIIa inhibitors, any serious bleeding that does occur could be disastrous because there is no effective way to immediately reverse the anticoagulation (as can be done with protamine sulfate for heparin). However, thrombocytopenia is not a problem, and the offset of bivalirudin's effect is relatively more rapid than that of heparin (1 hour), permitting sheaths to be pulled sooner after the procedure. Mainly because of its better safety profile, some interventional cardiologists have embraced the use of bivalirudin in the catheterization laboratory, but its general use awaits further trials.

If percutaneous coronary intervention is planned, level B evidence indicates that bivalirudin may be used as an alternative to unfractionated heparin and a GPIIb-IIIa inhibitor.

Warfarin Warfarin works by inhibiting the vitamin K–dependent clotting factors II, VII, IX, and X. Achievement of the desired antithrombotic effect takes 4 to 7 days.

In a few small pilot studies, starting warfarin therapy shortly after presentation in patients with unstable angina/NSTEMI showed benefit.[1] In a large trial of patients with unstable angina/NSTEMI who had previously undergone CABG, warfarin provided no advantage over aspirin alone and was associated with excess minor and major bleeding complications.[73]

Warfarin is taken orally once daily. The dose is titrated to maintain the desired international normalized ratio (INR), which is from 2 to 3 for most indications.

Bleeding is the main complication associated with warfarin therapy. Several drugs (e.g., cimetidine, amiodarone) can markedly increase warfarin's effect. Warfarin anticoagulation is reversed by stopping the drug; reversal by administration of vitamin K or of fresh frozen plasma is usually reserved for emergent and life-threatening bleeding.

The available evidence does not support the routine use of warfarin in patients with unstable angina/NSTEMI unless there are other indications for warfarin (e.g., atrial fibrillation, mechanical prosthetic heart valve).

Anti-ischemia Therapy

The agents used for treating ischemia in patients with unstable angina/NSTEMI include nitrates, morphine sulfate, and beta blockers (e.g., metoprolol) [see Table 6].

Nitrates Nitroglycerin is an endothelium-independent general arterial and venous dilator. It decreases myocardial oxygen demand through increased venous capacitance and peripheral artery dilation—factors that reduce preload and afterload, respectively, and thereby reduce myocardial wall stress. Epicardial coronary vasodilation and increased collateral flow act to enhance myocardial oxygen delivery.

No large, placebo-controlled clinical trials addressing reductions in major cardiac events or symptoms in unstable angina/NSTEMI have been performed. Multiple small, uncontrolled trials, a well-characterized biologic effect, and decades of experience have made nitrates a standard of care in the early treatment of these patients.[1]

Table 6 Anti-ischemia Therapy

Drug	Dosage	Route	Duration	Adverse Effects	Adverse Drug Reactions	Contraindications
Nitrates	S.L.: 0.4 mg q. 5 min × 3; I.V.: 10 mg/min, titrate up q. 5 min; paste: 2–6 cm; patch: 0.4 mg/hr	S.L., I.V., paste, patch	15–20 min until side effects occur or symptoms resolve	Hypotension, headache, nausea, tolerance	None	Hypotension; sildenafil or vardenafil within 24 hr of nitrate use
Morphine sulfate	1–5 mg every 10–15 min	I.V.	Until side effects or symptoms resolve	Hypotension, respiratory depression, rash, pruritus, nausea	None	Severe ventilatory failure, hypotension
Metoprolol*	5 mg q. 5 min to max 3 doses, then 25–100 mg b.i.d. with titration	I.V., then oral	Symptom resolution (if MI, then indefinite)	Hypotension, bradycardia, bronchospasm, worsened claudication	None	Hypotension, bradycardia, asthma, decompensated heart failure

*Other beta blockers are equally effective, although agents with intrinsic sympathomimetic activity should be avoided. Calcium channel blockers may be used for patients in whom beta blockers are contraindicated.
MI—myocardial infarction

In the emergency department, the initial nitrate dosage in a nonhypotensive patient is typically 0.4 mg of sublingual nitroglycerin (tablet or spray) repeated approximately every 5 minutes if ischemic symptoms do not subside. If this fails to terminate the ischemia, intravenous nitroglycerin at an infusion rate of 10 µg/min is recommended. The dose is titrated upward in increments of 10 to 20 µg/min until symptoms or signs of ischemia subside, hypotension develops, or the recommended maximal dose of 200 µg/min is achieved. After the acute period, topical nitrates, such as a 0.4 mg/hr nitrate patch, can be used for long-term therapy if necessary.

Nitroglycerin can result in significant hypotension, necessitating withdrawal of the agent. It should be avoided in patients who have taken sildenafil (Viagra) or vardenafil (Levitra) in the past 24 hours, because very severe hypotension can occur. Nitrate tolerance develops with prolonged nitrate administration, so patients should have nitrate-free intervals. Other adverse reactions, including intermittent headaches and nausea, are common.

A class I recommendation and level C evidence support the use of nitroglycerin to terminate or prevent ischemic episodes. Nitroglycerin therapy should serve as a bridge to the use of other evidence-based therapies, such as revascularization.

Morphine sulfate Almost a century of experience in acute coronary syndrome (albeit in the absence of clinical trial data) has established morphine sulfate as a useful adjunct to the early management of unstable angina/NSTEMI. Besides its potent analgesic and anxiolytic effect, morphine sulfate causes venodilation and mild arterial dilation, leading to reduced preload and afterload, and it may increase vagal tone to modestly reduce heart rate. These effects make it useful for treating patients with severe pulmonary congestion.

Morphine sulfate is given in a dose of 1 to 5 mg intravenously every 10 to 15 minutes until ischemic symptoms dissipate. At the same time, consideration for intravenous nitroglycerin treatment should be made. Morphine sulfate often causes hypotension, nausea, vomiting, and respiratory depression. Effects are quickly reversible with naloxone. A class I recommendation and level C evidence support the use of morphine sulfate to relieve chest pain that is refractory to sublingual nitroglycerin, to reverse acute pulmonary edema, and to ease severe agitation.

Beta blockers Beta blockers reduce myocardial oxygen demand by reducing heart rate and contractility. Slowing of the heart rate may also permit increased coronary filling during a prolonged diastole.

Much of the evidence in favor of beta-blocker therapy for unstable angina/NSTEMI is extrapolated from the large benefit shown in major clinical trials of acute MI. A meta-analysis of trials of threatened or evolving MI revealed a 13% reduction in progression to acute MI,[74] but there was insufficient power for mortality analysis.

There is no evidence of any difference in efficacy between the various beta blockers available, although agents with intrinsic sympathomimetic activity should be avoided. The dose will vary with the agent selected. In unstable angina/NSTEMI, intravenous loading doses titrated to a target resting heart rate of 50 to 60 beats/min may be used, with rapid conversion to an oral regimen. In patients who may have difficulty tolerating the adverse effects of beta blockers, the initiating dose should be small and titration should proceed more slowly.

Bronchospasm and severe asthma are contraindications to the use of beta blockers. Significant sinus bradycardia, AV nodal block, and hypotension can also occur, typically in patients with preexisting disease of cardiac conductive tissue.

A class I recommendation and level B evidence support the use of beta blockers in patients with ongoing chest pain; in such patients, an initial intravenous dose is followed by oral therapy.

Calcium channel blockers These agents are primarily vasodilators, but they also have effects on atrioventricular nodal conduction and left ventricular contractility. The dihydropyridine calcium channel blockers (e.g., nifedipine and amlodipine) have the most peripheral vasodilatory capability and the least negative inotropic effect.

To date, the trial data generally suggest that calcium channel blockers offer symptom relief in patients with unstable angina, but a meta-analysis found no improvements with regard to death or the occurrence of MI.[75] Nifedipine, compared with a beta blocker (metoprolol), demonstrated a trend toward increased MI.[76] In unstable angina/NSTEMI, the nondihydropyridine agents are used for coronary artery spasm and may be chosen for patients who cannot tolerate beta blockade.

Doses of calcium channel blockers vary with the agent chosen. For diltiazem, the usual immediate dose is a 20 mg/kg intravenous bolus, followed 15 minutes later by a 20 to 25 mg/kg bolus. Thereafter, the drug is administered orally, in a dosage of 30 mg three to four times a day, titrated to a total daily dose of 360 mg if necessary. Long-acting formulations exist as well.

Hypotension occurs with all calcium channel blockers. Bradycardia and negative inotropic effects accompany the nondihydropyridine agents; these agents should be avoided in patients with heart failure. The dihydropyridine agents may cause reflex tachycardia and other sympathomimetic effects.

Recommendations for the use of calcium channel blockers are as follows:

1. Nondihydropyridine calcium channel blockers (i.e., verapamil, diltiazem) may be initiated in patients with continuing or frequently recurring ischemia for whom beta blockers are contraindicated, in the absence of severe left ventricular dysfunction or other contraindications of calcium channel blockade. This class I recommendation is supported by level B evidence.

2. Extended-release forms of nondihydropyridine calcium channel blockers may be used instead of a beta blocker (class IIa recommendation, level B evidence).

3. Immediate-release dihydropyridine calcium channel blockers (i.e., nifedipine) should not be used in the absence of beta-blocker treatment (class III recommendation, level B evidence).

4. Immediate-release dihydropyridine calcium channel blockers may be used, if specifically indicated, in patients who are receiving a beta blocker (class II recommendation, level B evidence).

Lipid-Lowering Agents

There is evidence indicating that the use of lipid-lowering agents in hospital confers a benefit for patients with unstable angina/NSTEMI, and intensive lipid-lowering therapy appears to confer greater protection against death and major cardiovascular events than standard regimens.[77] In addition, patients given such therapy in the hospital are much more likely to continue it out of hospital, and in-hospital use has therefore been recommended.[78,79] The use of a fibrate or niacin in patients with a high-density lipoprotein cholesterol level of less than 40 mg/dl is supported by a class I recommendation and level B evidence. A class IIa recommendation and level B evidence support treatment with statins and diet for patients whose low-density lipoprotein cholesterol is greater than 100 mg/dl; treatment should begin 24 to 96 hours after admission and continue after hospital discharge.

Angiotensin-Converting Enzyme Inhibitors

Angiotensin-converting enzyme (ACE) inhibitors may block inflammatory processes and encourage plaque stability. In the Heart Outcomes Prevention Evaluation (HOPE) trial, use of the ACE inhibitor ramipril was associated with significant reductions in death, MI, or stroke in moderate- to high-risk patients, most of whom had normal left ventricular function.[80] The American College of Cardiology/American Heart Association (ACC/AHA) recommends ACE inhibitors for patients with unstable angina/NSTEMI and heart failure; left ventricular systolic dysfunction (ejection fraction less than 40%); hypertension; or diabetes. This class I recommendation is supported by level B evidence.

MECHANICAL REVASCULARIZATION

Coronary revascularization with percutaneous procedures or CABG is performed to relieve symptoms and improve prognosis [see Early Invasive versus Conservative Strategy, above]. Several factors influence the decision to proceed with coronary revascularization, including risk, absence of relevant comorbid conditions, disabling symptoms, viable myocardium at risk, and whether the patient's coronary anatomy is suitable for the procedure.

Percutaneous Coronary Intervention

Advances in percutaneous coronary intervention techniques and devices have improved safety and long-term vessel patency rates. Several changes in the evolution of coronary stent design, including smaller profile, increased flexibility, small strut diameter, and, the newest development, drug-eluting technology, have improved deliverability and reduced the rate of in-stent restenosis. Furthermore, the use of adjunctive antiplatelet and antithrombotic therapies, particularly in the setting of acute coronary syndrome, has improved outcomes.

The ACC/AHA guidelines for the use or avoidance of percutaneous coronary intervention in unstable angina/NSTEMI are as follows[1]:

1. Percutaneous coronary intervention (or CABG) is recommended for patients with single-vessel or two-vessel CAD without significant involvement of the proximal left anterior descending coronary artery (LAD) who have large areas of viable myocardium and high-risk features on noninvasive testing. This class I recommendation is supported by level B evidence.
2. Percutaneous coronary intervention is recommended for patients who have single-vessel or multivessel CAD, have suitable coronary anatomy, have normal left ventricular function, and do not have diabetes (class 1 recommendation, level A evidence).
3. Percutaneous coronary intervention (or CABG) is recommended for patients who have single-vessel or two-vessel CAD without significant proximal LAD involvement but who have a moderate area of viable myocardium and ischemia on noninvasive testing (class IIa recommendation, level B evidence).
4. Percutaneous coronary intervention (or CABG) is recommended for patients who have single-vessel disease with significant proximal LAD involvement (class IIa recommendation, level B evidence).
5. Percutaneous coronary intervention (or CABG) is not indicated for patients who have atypical symptoms or have no evidence of ischemia on noninvasive testing or have not received an adequate trial of medical therapy (class III recommendation, level C evidence).
6. Percutaneous coronary intervention (or CABG) is not indicated for patients with significant left main CAD who are suitable candidates for CABG (class III recommendation, level B evidence).

Surgical Revascularization

Surgical revascularization techniques and perioperative outcomes have improved over the years. Particular advances include use of internal mammary artery conduits, off-pump procedures, minithoracotomy, and, the newest development, robot-assisted procedures.

The ACC/AHA guidelines for CABG in patients with unstable angina/NSTEMI are as follows[1]:

1. CABG is indicated for patients with significant left main CAD. This class I recommendation is supported by level A evidence.
2. CABG is indicated for patients with triple-vessel CAD and abnormal left ventricular function (class 1 recommendation, level A evidence).
3. CABG is indicated for patients who have two-vessel disease with significant proximal LAD disease and abnormal left ventricular function (class 1 recommendation, level A evidence).
4. CABG or percutaneous intervention is indicated for patients who have single-vessel or two-vessel CAD without significant proximal LAD involvement but with large areas of viable myocardium and high-risk features on noninvasive testing (class 1 recommendation, level B evidence).

Diabetes and Revascularization

Overall, patients with diabetes are more likely to require repeat revascularization after percutaneous intervention, because of increased rates of restenosis; in addition, there is a trend toward higher mortality 1 year after both CABG and percutaneous intervention with stents in diabetic patients.[81] In the Bypass Angioplasty Revascularization Investigation (BARI) trial, diabetic patients with multivessel CAD were found to have better survival rates with CABG than with percutaneous intervention.[82] However, analysis of the diabetic subgroup of a randomized trial and registry of percutaneous intervention with bare metal stents versus CABG in unstable angina patients revealed no difference in 3-year survival between the groups.[83] Drug-eluting stents display markedly reduced rates of in-stent restenosis, as compared with traditional bare-metal stents, particularly in diabetic patients.[84,85]

Currently, the available evidence suggests that surgical revascularization should be offered to diabetic patients with CAD in three or more vessels, particularly if they have left ventricular dysfunction. However, it is common practice to offer percutaneous intervention as the revascularization strategy for diabetic patients with CAD involving one or two vessels. Trials are needed to compare the most advanced drug-eluting stent technology with the most advanced surgical management to define their roles in diabetic patients with CAD.

POSTHOSPITAL CARE

Preparation for the posthospital care of a patient with unstable angina/NSTEMI should begin during the hospitalization, with appropriate education, dietary advice, psychosocial counseling, weight loss advice, exercise prescription, cardiac rehabilitation referral (if appropriate), smoking cessation counseling, and the initiation of drug therapy. Given the importance of aggressive risk modification, the entire medical staff has a responsibility to ensure that all of these therapies and advice are offered, encouraged, and established for the future.[78]

Aspirin therapy should be maintained indefinitely, and clopidogrel should be taken for 9 months. For patients who have had an MI or who have left ventricular dysfunction, beta-blocker therapy is recommended indefinitely, in the absence of contraindications. ACE inhibitor treatment is recommended indefinitely for secondary prevention in moderate- to high-risk patients with atherosclerotic disease, diabetes, a low ejection fraction, or other specific indications. Lipid-lowering therapy (e.g., with a statin drug) should be administered if the patient has a low-density lipoprotein level higher than 100 mg/dl post diet (class I, level B), or a high-density lipoprotein level lower than 40 mg/dl (class IIa, level B).[79] Blood pressure should be kept below 140/90 mm Hg unless the patient has renal disease or diabetes, in which case the target is a pressure lower than 130/80 mm Hg.[86] All patients should be prescribed sublingual nitroglycerin and instructed in its use; in particular, they should understand the importance of returning to the hospital immediately if symptoms persist despite three doses of nitroglycerin. Finally, follow-up should take place 2 to 6 weeks after discharge in low-risk and revascularized patients, or 1 to 2 weeks after discharge in higher-risk patients.[1]

The authors have no commercial relationships with manufacturers of products or providers of services discussed in this chapter.

References

1. Braunwald E, Antman E, Beasley J, et al: ACC/AHA 2002 guidelines update for the management of patients with unstable angina and non–ST-segment elevation myocardial infarction. J Am Coll Cardiol 40:1366, 2002

2. Braunwald E, Antman EM, Beasley JW, et al: ACC/AHA guidelines for the management of patients with unstable angina and non–ST segment elevation myocardial infarction: a report from the American College of Cardiology/American Heart Association Task Force guidelines. J Am Coll Cardiol 36:970, 2000

3. Stary HC, Chandler AB, Dinsmore RB, et al: A definition of advanced types of atherosclerotic lesions and a histological classification of atherosclerosis: a report from the Committee on Vascular Lesions of the Council on Arteriosclerosis, American Heart Association. Circulation 92:1355, 1995

4. Fuster V, Badimon JJ, Chesebro JH, et al: The pathogenesis of coronary artery disease and the acute coronary syndromes. N Engl J Med 326:242, 1992

5. Falk E, Shah PK, Fuster V: Coronary plaque disruption. Circulation 92:657, 1995

6. Gutstein DE, Fuster V: Pathophysiology and clinical significance of atherosclerotic plaque rupture. Cardiovasc Res 41:323, 1999

7. Moons AH, Levi M, Peters RJ: Tissue factor and coronary artery disease. Cardiovasc Res 53:2:313, 2002

8. Little WC, Constantinescu M, Applegate RJ, et al: Can coronary angiography predict the site of a subsequent myocardial infarction in patients with mild to moderate coronary artery disease? Circulation 78:1157, 1988

9. Levin DC, Fallon JT: Significance of angiographic morphology of localized coronary stenoses: histopathologic correlations. Circulation 66:312, 1982

10. Buffon A, Biasucci LM, Liuzzo G, et al: Widespread coronary inflammation in unstable angina. N Engl J Med 347:1:5, 2002

11. Goldstein A, Demetrou D, Grines CL, et al: Multiple complex coronary plaques in patients with acute myocardial infarction. N Engl J Med 343:915, 2000

12. Rioufol G, Finet G, Ginon I, et al: Multiple atherosclerotic plaque rupture in acute coronary syndrome: a three-vessel intravascular ultrasound study. Circulation 106:804, 2002

13. Braunwald E: Unstable angina classification. Circulation 80:410, 1989

14. Canto JG, Shilpak MG, Rogers WJ, et al: Prevalence, clinical characteristics and mortality among patients with myocardial infarction presenting without chest pain. JAMA 283:3223, 2000

15. Canto JG, Fincher C, Kiefe CI, et al: Atypical presentations among Medicare beneficiaries with unstable angina pectoris. Am J Cardiol 90:248, 2002

16. Bertrand M, Simoons M, Fox K, et al: Management of acute coronary syndromes in patients without persistent ST-segment elevation: Task Force Report. Eur Heart J 23:1809, 2002

17. Panteghini M: Acute coronary syndrome: biochemical strategies in the troponin era. Chest 122:1428, 2002

18. Puleo P, Meyer D, Wathen C, et al: Use of a rapid assay of subforms of creatine kinase MB to diagnose or rule out acute myocardial infarction. N Engl J Med 331:561, 1994

19. ACC/AHA guidelines for the management of patients with acute myocardial infarction: 1999 update. American College of Cardiology/American Heart Association Task Force on Practice Guidelines. J Am Coll Cardiol 34:3:890, 1999

20. Cannon CP, McCabe CH, Stone PH, et al: The electrocardiogram predicts one-year outcome of patients with unstable angina and non-Q myocardial infarction: results of the TIMI III Registry ECG Ancillary Study. Thrombolysis in Myocardial Ischemia. J Am Coll Cardiol 30:133, 1997

21. Predictors of outcome in patients with acute coronary syndromes without persistent ST segment elevation: results from an international trial of 9146 patients. The PURSUIT Investigators. Circulation 101:2557, 2000

22. Antman E, Cohen M, Bernink P, et al: The TIMI risk score for unstable angina/non–ST elevation MI: a method of prognostication and therapeutic decision making. JAMA 284:835, 2000

23. Antman EM, McCabe CH, Gurfinkel EP, et al: Enoxaparin prevents death and cardiac ischemic events in unstable angina/non–Q wave myocardial infarction: results of the thrombolysis in myocardial infarction (TIMI) 11B trial. Circulation 100:1593, 1999

24. A comparison of low molecular weight heparin with unfractionated heparin for unstable coronary artery disease. Efficacy and Safety of Subcutaneous Enoxaparin in Non-Q Wave Coronary Events Study Group. N Engl J Med 337:447, 1997

25. Cannon CP, Weintraub WS, Demopoulos LA, et al: Comparison of early invasive and conservative strategies in patients with unstable coronary syndromes treated with the glycoprotein IIb/IIIa inhibitor tirofiban. N Engl J Med 344:1879, 2001

26. Inhibition of the platelet glycoprotein IIb/IIIa receptor with tirofiban in unstable angina and non–Q wave myocardial infarction. PRISM-PLUS investigators. N Engl J Med 338:1488,1998

27. Patel DJ, Holdright DR, Knight CJ, et al: Early continuous ST segment monitoring in unstable angina: prognostic value additional to the clinical characteristics and the admission electrocardiogram. Heart 75:222, 1996

28. Patel DJ, Knight CJ, Holdright DR, et al: Long-term prognosis in unstable angina: the importance of early risk stratification using continuous ECG monitoring. Eur Heart J 19:240, 1998

29. Haverkate F, Thompson SG, Pyke SD, et al: Production of C-reactive protein and risk of coronary events in stable and unstable angina. Lancet 349:462, 1997

30. Morrow DA, Rifai N, Antman EM, et al: C-reactive protein is a potent predictor of mortality independently of and in combination with troponin T in acute coronary syndromes: a TIMI 11A substudy. J Am Coll Cardiol 31:1460, 1998

31. Becker RC, Cannon CP, Bovill EG, et al: Prognostic value of plasma fibrinogen concentration in patients with unstable angina and non–Q wave myocardial infarction (TIMI IIIB trial). Am J Cardiol 78:142, 1996

32. Morrow DA, Rifai N, Antman EM, et al: Serum amyloid A predicts early mortality in acute coronary syndromes: a TIMI 11A substudy. J Am Coll Cardiol 35:358, 2000

33. Biasucci LM, Vitelli A, Liuzzo G, et al: Elevated levels of interleukin-6 in unstable angina. Circulation 94:874, 1996

34. Morrow DA, de Lemos JA, Sabatine MS, et al: Evaluation of B-type natriuretic peptide for risk assessment in unstable angina/non–ST elevation myocardial infarction. J Am Coll Cardiol 41:1264, 2003

35. Cannon CP, Braunwald E: Unstable angina. Heart Disease: A Textbook of Cardiovascular Medicine, 6th ed. Braunwald E, Zipes DP, Libby P, Eds. WB Saunders Co, Philadelphia, 2001, p 890

36. Effects of tissue plasminogen activator and a comparison of early invasive and conservative strategies in unstable angina and non-Q myocardial infarction: results of the TIMI IIIb trial. TIMI IIIB Trial Investigators. Circulation 89:1545, 1994

37. Boden WE, O'Rourke RA, Crawford MH, et al: Outcomes in patients assigned with acute non–Q-wave myocardial infarction randomly assigned to an invasive as compared with a conservative management strategy. Veterans Affairs Non–Q Wave Infarction Strategies. N Engl J Med 338:1785, 1998

38. McCullough PA, O'Neill WW, Graham M, et al: A prospective randomized trial of triage angiography in acute coronary syndromes ineligible for thrombolytic therapy: results of Medicine versus Angiography in Thrombolytic Exclusion (MATE). J Am Coll Card 32:596, 1998

39. Invasive compared with non-invasive treatment in unstable coronary artery disease: FRISC II prospective randomized multicenter study. Fragmin and Fast Revascularisation during Instability in Coronary Artery Disease Investigators. Lancet 354:708, 1999

40. Holmvang L, Clemmensen P, Lindahl B, et al: Quantitative analysis of the admission electrocardiogram identifies patients with unstable coronary artery disease who benefit the most from early invasive treatment. J Am Coll Card 41:905, 2003

41. Morrow DA, Cannon CP, Rifai N, et al: Ability of minor elevations of troponins I and T to predict benefit from an early invasive strategy in patients with unstable angina and non–ST elevation myocardial infarction: results from a randomized trial. JAMA 286:2405, 2001

42. Mahoney EM, Jurkovitz CT, Chu H, et al: Cost and cost-effectiveness of an early invasive vs conservative strategy for the treatment of unstable angina and non–ST-segment elevation myocardial infarction. JAMA 288:1851, 2002

43. Fox KA, Poole-Wilson PA, Henderson RA, et al: Interventional versus conservative treatment for patients with unstable angina or non–ST segment elevation myocardial infarction: the British Heart Foundation RITA 3 randomised trial. Lancet 360:743, 2002

44. Lewis HD, Davis JW, Archibald DG, et al: Protective effects of aspirin against acute myocardial infarction and death in men with unstable angina: results of a Veterans Administration Cooperative Study. N Engl J Med 309:396, 1983

45. Theroux P, Ouimet H, McCans J, et al: Aspirin, heparin, or both to treat acute unstable angina. N Engl J Med 319:1105, 1988

46. Cairns JA, Gent M, Singer J, et al: Aspirin, sulfinpyrazone, or both in unstable angina. N Engl J Med 313:1369, 1985

47. Risk of myocardial infarction and death during treatment with low dose aspirin and intravenous heparin in men with unstable coronary artery disease. The RISC Group. Lancet 336:827, 1990

48. Collaborative overview of randomized trials of antiplatelet therapy—1: Prevention of death, myocardial infarction, and stroke by prolonged antiplatelet therapy in various categories of patients. Antiplatelet Trialists' Collaboration. BMJ 308:81, 1994

49. Randomised trial of intravenous streptokinase, oral aspirin, both or neither among 17,187 cases of suspected acute myocardial infarction. ISIS-2 Investigators. Lancet 2:349, 1988

50. Balsano F, Rizzon P, Violi F, et al: Antiplatelet treatment with ticlopidine in unstable angina: a controlled multicenter trial. Circulation 82:17, 1990

51. Effects of clopidogrel in addition to aspirin in patients with acute coronary syndromes without ST-segment elevation. The Clopidogrel in Unstable Angina to Prevent Recurrent Events (CURE) Trial Investigators. N Engl J Med 345:494, 2001

52. Mehta SR, Yusuf S, Peters RJG, et al: Effects of pretreatment with clopidogrel and aspirin followed by long-term therapy in patients undergoing percutaneous coronary intervention: the PCI-CURE study. Lancet 358:527, 2001

53. Steinhubl SR, Berger PB, Mann T, et al: Early and sustained dual oral antiplatelet therapy following percutaneous coronary intervention. JAMA 288:2411, 2002

54. Inhibition of platelet glycoprotein IIb/IIIa in unstable angina: receptor suppression using integrilin therapy. PURSUIT trial investigators. N Engl J Med 339:436, 1998

55. Randomised placebo-controlled trial of abciximab before and during coronary intervention in refractory unstable angina. CAPTURE Investigators. Lancet 349:1429, 1997

56. Topol EJ, Moliterno DJ, Hermann HC, et al: Comparison of two platelet glycoprotein IIb/IIIa inhibitors, tirofiban and abciximab, for the prevention of ischemic events with percutaneous coronary revascularization. N Engl J Med 344:1888, 2001

57. Effect of glycoprotein IIb/IIIa receptor blocker abciximab on outcome in patients with acute coronary syndromes without early coronary revascularization. GUSTO-IV ACS investigators. Lancet 357:1915, 2001

58. Boersma E, Harrington RA, Moliterno DJ, et al: Platelet glycoprotein IIb/IIIa inhibitors in acute coronary syndrome: a meta-analysis of all major randomized clinical trials. Lancet 9302:189, 2002

59. Effects of tissue plasminogen activator and a comparison of early invasive and conservative strategies in unstable angina and non–Q wave myocardial infarction. Circulation 97:1195, 1994

60. Hirsh J: Heparin. N Engl J Med 324:1565, 1991

61. Theroux P, Waters D, Qiu S, et al: Aspirin versus heparin to prevent myocardial infarction during the acute phase of unstable angina. Circulation 88:2045, 1993

62. Neri SG, Gensini GF, Poggesi L, et al: Effect of heparin, aspirin or alteplase in reduction of myocardial ischemia in refractory unstable angina. Lancet 335:615, 1990

63. Telford AM, Wilson C: Trial of heparin versus atenolol in prevention of myocardial infarction in intermediate coronary syndrome. Lancet 1:1225, 1981

64. Oler A, Whooley MA, Oler J, et al: Adding heparin to aspirin reduces the incidence of myocardial infarction and death in patients with unstable angina: a meta-analysis. JAMA 276:10:811, 1996

65. Antman EM, Cohen M, Radley D, et al: Assessment of the treatment effect of enoxaparin for unstable angina/non–Q wave myocardial infarction: TIMI 11B – ESSENCE meta-analysis. Circulation 100:1602, 1999

66. Klein W, Buchwald A, Hillis SE, et al: Comparison of low-molecular weight heparin with unfractionated heparin acutely and with placebo for 6 weeks in the management of unstable coronary artery disease: Fragmin in Unstable Coronary Artery Disease Study (FRIC). Circulation 96:61, 1997

67. Comparison of two treatment durations (6 days and 14 days) of a low molecular weight heparin with a 6 day treatment of unfractionated heparin in the initial management of unstable angina or non–Q wave myocardial infarction. The FRAXIS Investigators. Eur Heart J 20:1553, 1999

68. Low molecular weight heparin during instability in coronary artery disease. The FRISC Study Group. Lancet 347:561, 1996

69. Goodman SG, Fitchett D, Armstrong PW, et al: Randomized evaluation of the safety and efficacy of enoxaparin versus unfractionated heparin in high-risk patients with non–ST-segment elevation acute coronary syndromes receiving the glycoprotein IIb/IIIa inhibitor eptifibatide. Circulation 107:238, 2003

70. Collet JP, Montelalescot G, Lison L, et al: Percutaneous coronary intervention after subcutaneous enoxaparin pretreatment in patients with unstable angina pectoris. Circulation 103:658, 2001

71. Kereiakes DJ, Grines C, Fry E, et al: Enoxaparin and abciximab adjunctive pharmacotherapy during percutaneous coronary intervention. J Invasive Cardiol 13:272, 2001

72. Lincoff AM, Bittl JA, Harrington RA, et al: Bivalirudin and provisional glycoprotein IIb/IIIa blockade compared with heparin and planned glycoprotein IIb/IIIa blockade during percutaneous coronary intervention: REPLACE-2 randomized trial. JAMA 289:853, 2003

73. Huynh T, Theroux P, Bogaty P, et al: Aspirin, warfarin or the combination for secondary prevention of coronary events in patients with acute coronary syndromes and prior coronary artery bypass surgery. Circulation 103:3069, 2001

74. Yusuf S, Wittes J, Friedman L: Overview of results of randomized clinical trials in heart disease, II: unstable angina, heart failure, primary prevention with aspirin, and risk factor modification. JAMA 260:2259, 1988

75. Held PYS, Furberg CD: Calcium channel blockers in acute myocardial infarction and unstable angina: an overview. Br Med J 299:1187, 1989

76. Lubson JTJ: Efficacy of nifedipine and metoprolol in the early treatment of unstable angina in the coronary care unit: findings from the Holland Interuniversity Nifedipine/metoprolol Trial (HINT). Am J Cardiol 60:18A, 1988

77. Cannon CP, Braunwald E, McCabe CH, et al: Intensive versus moderate lipid lowering with statins after acute coronary syndromes. N Engl J Med 350:778, 2004

78. Fonarow GC, Gawlinski A, Moughrabi S, et al: Improved treatment of coronary heart disease by implementation of a Cardiac Hospitalization Atherosclerosis Management Program (CHAMP). Am J Cardiol 87:819, 2001

79. Third report of the National Cholesterol Education Program Expert Panel on detection, evaluation and treatment of high blood cholesterol in adults (Adult Treatment Panel III) final report. NCEP Expert Panel. Circulation 106:3143, 2002

80. Effect of an angiotensin-converting enzyme inhibitor, ramipril, on cardiovascular events in high risk patients. The Heart Outcomes Prevention Evaluation Study Investigators. N Engl J Med 342:145, 2000

81. Lincoff AM: Important triad in cardiovascular medicine: diabetes, coronary intervention, and platelet glycoprotein IIb/IIIa receptor blockade. Circulation 107:1556, 2003

82. Comparison of coronary bypass surgery with angioplasty in patients with multivessel disease. Bypass Angioplasty Revascularization Investigation (BARI) Investigators. N Engl J Med 335:217, 1996

83. Sedlis SP, Morrison DA, Lorin JD, et al: Percutaneous coronary intervention versus coronary bypass graft surgery for diabetic patients with unstable angina and risk factors for adverse outcomes with bypass: outcome of diabetic patients in the AWESOME randomized trial and registry. J Am Coll Cardiol 40:1555, 2002

84. Morice MC, Serruys PW, Sousa E, et al: A randomized comparison of a sirolimus-eluting stent with a standard stent for coronary revascularization. N Engl J Med 346:1773, 2002

85. Moses JW, Leon MB, Popma JJ, et al: Sirolimus-eluting stents versus standard stents in patients with stenoses in a native coronary artery. N Engl J Med 349:1315, 2003

86. Chobanian A, Bakris G, Black H, et al: The seventh report of the Joint National Committee on Prevention, Detection, Evaluation and Treatment of High Blood Pressure. JAMA 289:2560, 2003

25 Acute Myocardial Infarction

Peter B. Berger, M.D., and James L. Orford, M.B., ChB., M.P.H.

In the 1970s, coronary angiography demonstrated that almost all cases of acute myocardial infarction were caused by thrombotic occlusion of a coronary artery. This discovery has led to the development of therapies to restore coronary blood flow in the occluded artery, which has dramatically reduced the morbidity and mortality associated with acute myocardial infarction.

Epidemiology

In the past decade, the number of people who die each year of myocardial infarction has decreased significantly. Both in-hospital mortality and out-of-hospital mortality have declined as a result of substantial increases in the use of aspirin, heparin, thrombolytic therapy, and coronary angioplasty, as well as a reduction in the risk factors for coronary artery disease (e.g., hypertension, hyperlipidemia, smoking, and sedentary lifestyle) [*see* Risk-Factor Modification, *below*]; however, it must be emphasized that there is, unfortunately, persistent discordance between existing guidelines for management of acute coronary artery disease syndromes and current clinical practice.[1,2]

Despite these advances, approximately 1.5 million people in the United States suffer acute myocardial infarction each year, and nearly 500,000 of these patients die of coronary artery disease.[3] Nearly half of these deaths occur before the patients receive medical care either from emergency medical technicians or in a hospital.[3,4]

Pathogenesis

The factors responsible for the sudden thrombotic occlusion of a coronary artery have only recently been elucidated.[5-7] Atherosclerotic plaques rich in foam cells (lipid-laden macrophages) are susceptible to sudden plaque rupture and hemorrhage into the vessel wall, which may result in the sudden partial or total occlusion of the coronary artery. Although severe stenosis of a coronary artery (i.e., stenosis ≥ 70% of the diameter of the artery) is generally required to produce anginal symptoms, such stenoses tend to have dense fibrotic caps and are less prone to rupture than mild to moderate stenoses, which are generally more lipid laden. Studies of patients in whom angiography was performed before and after a myocardial infarction revealed that in most cases, acute coronary artery occlusion occurred at sites in the coronary artery circulation with stenoses of less than 70%, as demonstrated on the preinfarction angiogram.[8] Although patients who have unstable anginal syndromes with increasingly frequent and severe angina are clearly at increased risk for myocardial infarction, the ability of physicians to predict which patients with stable anginal syndromes are likely to experience infarction and which coronary artery stenoses are likely to result in acute thrombotic occlusion is poor.

Diagnosis

According to the World Health Organization, the diagnosis of myocardial infarction requires at least two of the following three criteria: (1) a clinical history of ischemic-type chest discom-fort, (2) serial electrocardiographic tracings indicative of myocardial infarction, and (3) a rise and fall in serum cardiac markers.[9] However, the advent and widespread adoption of novel diagnostic tools, including highly sensitive and specific serologic biomarkers and precise imaging techniques, have necessitated reevaluation of this established definition. The Joint European Society of Cardiology/American College of Cardiology Committee for the Redefinition of Myocardial Infarction has integrated these diagnostic modalities and published updated definitions of acute myocardial infarction, evolving or recent myocardial infarction, and established myocardial infarction that more accurately reflect current clinical practice [*see Table 1*].[10]

CLINICAL MANIFESTATIONS

Patients with acute myocardial infarction often describe a heaviness, pressure, squeezing, or tightness in the chest that has persisted for more than 30 minutes. The discomfort may radiate or be located primarily in the arms, neck, or jaw. Chest pain, particularly severe or stabbing chest pain, and pain that causes writhing are unusual for coronary artery ischemia and should lead the clinician to consider causes other than myocardial infarction. Many patients with acute myocardial infarction, particularly those with inferior infarction, are diaphoretic; nausea and emesis are common as well. Dyspnea is also a common associated symptom. Syncope may occur and is more frequent with inferior than anterior infarction, in part because of the more frequent occurrence of bradyarrhythmias, heart block, and tachyarrhythmias with inferior infarction. Elderly patients with

---

Table 1 Clinical Definitions of Myocardial Infarction as Determined by the Joint European Society of Cardiology/American College of Cardiology Committee[10]

Acute, Evolving, or Recent Myocardial Infarction

Biochemical markers of myocardial necrosis (i.e., typical rise and gradual fall of troponin or more rapid rise and fall of CK-MB) with at least one of the following:

   Ischemic symptoms

   Development of pathologic Q waves on the ECG

   ECG changes indicative of ischemia (ST segment elevation or depression)

   Coronary artery intervention (e.g., primary coronary angioplasty)

Pathologic findings of an acute myocardial infarction

Established Myocardial Infarction

Development of new pathologic Q waves on serial ECGs; the patient may or may not remember previous symptoms; biochemical markers of myocardial necrosis may have normalized, depending on the length of time that has passed since the infarct developed

Pathologic findings of a healed or healing myocardial infarction

CK-MB—creatine kinase–myocardial band

---

infarction often present with symptoms that differ from the symptoms of infarction in younger patients; more than half of elderly patients present with shortness of breath as their main complaint, and many others present with dizziness or symptoms of arrhythmia rather than the classic symptoms of acute myocardial infarction.[11]

Approximately two thirds of patients describe the new onset of angina or a change in their anginal pattern in the month preceding infarction.[12] However, in approximately one fourth of patients, myocardial infarction is associated with only mild symptoms or no symptoms at all.[13]

PHYSICAL EXAMINATION

The patient with acute myocardial infarction often appears anxious and in distress. Vital signs are often normal, but sinus tachycardia is not uncommon. The pulse may be rapid or slow if arrhythmias are present. Either hypotension caused by left or right ventricular dysfunction or arrhythmia or hypertension caused by adrenergic discharge may be present. The respiratory rate may be elevated because of anxiety or pain or because of hypoxia in patients with significant congestive heart failure. The jugular venous pressure may be elevated, reflecting right ventricular dysfunction caused by right ventricular involvement (more common with inferior infarction); arrhythmia in which atrioventricular dissociation is present may produce so-called cannon A waves, which are abnormally high jugular venous waves caused by atrial systole occurring when the atrioventricular valves are closed. The lung examination is typically normal, but moist rales indicative of congestive heart failure resulting from left ventricular dysfunction may be present. The cardiac examination may reveal a dyskinetic apical pulsation on palpation; a fourth and, less commonly, a third heart sound may be audible. The murmur of ischemic mitral regurgitation may be present. If a left bundle branch block is present, abnormal splitting of the second heart sound may be heard.

It must be emphasized that the physical examination in acute myocardial infarction is generally most useful in excluding other potentially serious causes of the patient's chest discomfort, including pulmonary embolism, aortic dissection, spontaneous pneumothorax, pericarditis, and cholecystitis, rather than in confirming a diagnosis of acute myocardial infarction.

ELECTROCARDIOGRAPHY

ECG is a valuable tool both in confirming the diagnosis of acute myocardial infarction and in selecting the most appropriate therapy for the patient. Although rhythm and conduction disturbances may be present, the presence and type of repolarization abnormalities are most useful in identifying myocardial infarction. If ST segment elevation is present in a patient with chest pain typical of acute myocardial infarction, the likelihood that the patient has acute myocardial infarction is greater than 90%.[14] Other findings, such as ST segment depression, T wave inversion, and bundle branch block, are less specific but may also support a diagnosis of acute myocardial infarction, particularly when typical symptoms are present [see Figure 1]. Fully 50% of patients with myocardial infarction do not have ST segment elevation on their ECGs, although the ECG is seldom normal even at an early stage.[15] In such patients, the ECG can help predict complications and early mortality.[16] Patients with ST segment depression are at high risk; 30-day mortality in such patients is nearly as high as in patients with anterior ST segment elevation.[17] Patients with other nonspecific ECG abnormalities are at lesser

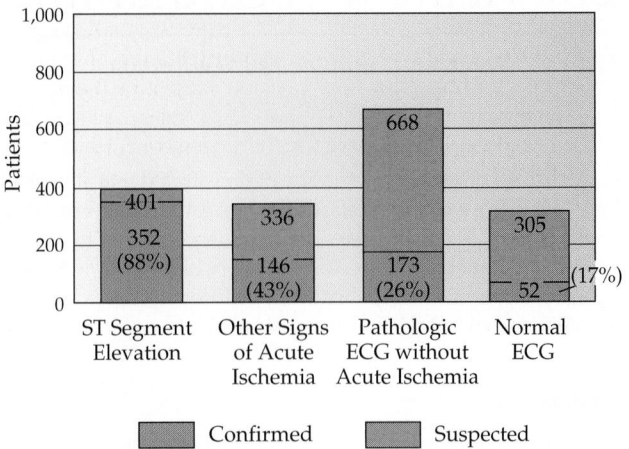

Figure 1   **Relation between the initial electrocardiographic changes and the development of infarction in 1,715 patients strongly suspected of having an acute myocardial infarction. Each column shows the total number of patients and the number of patients later found to have had an infarction. Although infarction is less frequently confirmed in patients without ST segment elevation than in those with ST segment elevation, even patients with normal ECG findings may suffer acute myocardial infarction.[14]**

risk; those with normal ECGs who suffer infarction generally have the best prognosis [see Figure 2]. Regardless of the findings on the initial ECG, the most important element in the evaluation of a patient with suspected acute myocardial infarction is the patient's description of symptoms. All patients suspected of having acute myocardial infarction should be admitted to the hospital and receive rapid and appropriate therapy.

LABORATORY FINDINGS

Injury to myocardial cells results in the release of intracellular enzymes into circulating blood, permitting their detection by blood tests. Traditionally, the serum cardiac marker creatine kinase (CK) and an isoenzyme, creatine kinase–myocardial band (CK-MB), which are found in high concentration in myocardial cells, have been used to diagnose myocardial infarction in its earliest stages.[18] Rapid assays of these enzymes have been developed, permitting the determination of the blood levels of these enzymes within 30 to 60 minutes. Drawbacks to the use of CK-MB include its lack of specificity for cardiac muscle and the time required for CK-MB levels to rise during myocardial infarction. CK and CK-MB usually require at least 3 hours of profound ischemia to rise above normal levels; patients who present early in their infarction would not be expected to have elevated CK levels. Furthermore, patients may have only partial obstruction of the infarct-related artery, or there may be extensive collateralization of the infarct-related artery, which further delays the release of these enzymes. In patients suspected of having acute myocardial infarction, it is not appropriate to delay treatment until an elevation of CK or CK-MB is present, because the goal of treatment is to prevent injury to the myocardium. The challenge facing physicians is to identify patients suffering myocardial infarction even before CK becomes elevated, because these patients require emergency therapy and stand to benefit the most from reperfusion therapy.

To overcome these limitations and more accurately and rapidly identify patients in need of emergency reperfusion therapy, other blood tests have been developed to help identify patients with ischemia. Myoglobin is a low-molecular-weight heme protein found in cardiac muscle. Its advantage for diagnosis is that it is released more rapidly from infarcted myocardium than is CK-MB. However, myoglobin is also found in skeletal muscle, and the lack of specificity is a drawback.[19] Troponin is a cardiac-specific marker for acute myocardial infarction; an increase in serum levels of troponin occurs soon after myocardial cell injury. An elevated cardiac troponin level on admission is a predictor of subsequent cardiac events.[20,21] Changes to the definition of acute myocardial infarction reflect the increased emphasis on these specific biomarkers of myocardial injury [see Table 1].[10]

IMAGING STUDIES

Echocardiography

Echocardiography may be useful in identifying patients with myocardial infarction in the emergency department. Regional wall motion abnormalities occur within seconds of coronary occlusion and well before myocyte necrosis,[22-26] and most patients with acute myocardial infarction have regional wall motion abnormalities readily seen on echocardiography. However, echocardiographic evidence of myocardial infarction is not required in patients with symptoms and electrocardiographic evidence typical of acute myocardial infarction, and treatment should not be delayed, so that an echocardiogram can be performed. Similarly, wall motion abnormalities are not specific for acute myocardial infarction and may be caused by ischemia or prior infarction. Echocardiography may be useful in patients with left bundle branch block or abnormal ECGs without ST segment elevation whose symptoms are atypical and in whom the diagnosis is uncertain.[27]

Radionuclide Imaging

Perfusion imaging with both thallium and sestamibi in the emergency department has been reported to be both sensitive and specific in the evaluation of patients in whom the diagnosis is uncertain.[27-29] A prospective randomized trial of 2,475 patients found that resting technetium-99m sestamibi imaging reduced unnecessary hospitalization in patients with acute ischemia without reducing admission of patients with acute ischemia.[30]

Emergent Therapy

Treatments have been developed that reduce the morbidity and mortality of acute myocardial infarction, particularly when initiated early; it is therefore important to avoid delay in administering therapy.[4,31] Much of the emphasis on reducing delay has focused on the time between a patient's presentation to the emergency department and the administration of reperfusion therapy. The 2004 ACC/AHA guidelines recommended that all initial therapy be carried out in the emergency department based upon a predetermined, institution-specific, written protocol.[31] A patient with symptoms suggestive of myocardial infarction should be evaluated within 10 minutes after arrival in the emergency department. Early steps should include the assessment of hemodynamic stability by measurement of the patient's heart rate and blood pressure; the performance of a 12-lead ECG; and the administration of oxygen by nasal prongs, I.V. analgesia (most commonly morphine sulfate), oral aspirin, and sublingual nitroglycerin if the blood pressure is greater than 90 mm Hg. The challenge facing physicians who work in emergency departments is that more than 90% of patients who present to the emergency department complaining of chest pain are not suffering myocardial infarction; many do not have a cardiac etiology for their chest pain.

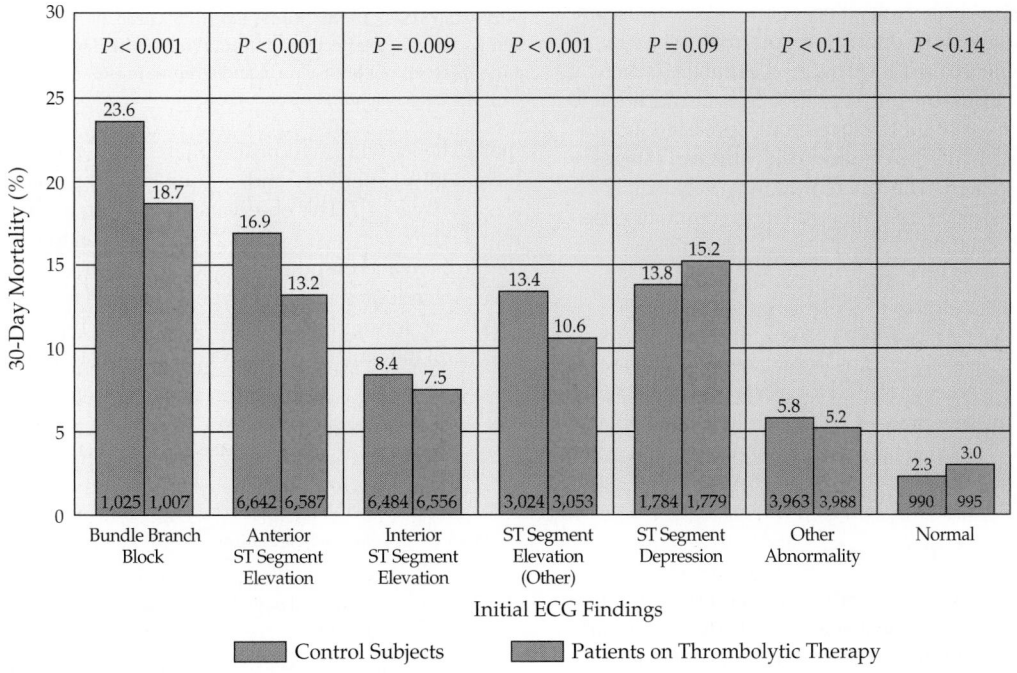

Figure 2 **Thirty-day mortality in patients with suspected acute myocardial infarction from placebo-controlled trials of thrombolytic therapy on the basis of their initial ECGs. Patients with ST segment depression are at high risk, nearly as high as patients with anterior ST segment elevation. The mortality among such patients is not reduced (and may be increased) by thrombolytic therapy. Patients with other nonspecific electrocardiographic abnormalities are at lesser risk, and those with normal ECG findings have the best prognosis.**

All patients with definite or suspected myocardial infarction should be admitted to the hospital, undergo preparation for I.V. access, and be placed on continuous ECG monitoring. High-risk patients should be admitted to a coronary care unit. In many hospitals, patients at low risk for major complications are admitted to a telemetry unit, where emergency medical care can be quickly administered, rather than to a coronary care unit. Tachyarrhythmias and bradyarrhythmias may occur even in low-risk patients, particularly in the first 24 hours. Lidocaine, atropine, an external or internal pacemaker, and a defibrillator should be readily available.

OXYGEN

Oxygen is generally recommended for all patients with acute myocardial infarction for the first several hours after admission and is mandatory for patients with pulmonary congestion or evidence of oxygen desaturation.

ASPIRIN

Aspirin should be given to all patients as soon as a diagnosis of myocardial infarction is made.[17] In the second International Study of Infarct Survival (ISIS-2), aspirin was found to be nearly as effective as streptokinase, reducing 30-day mortality 23% in 17,000 patients with acute myocardial infarction; the benefit was additive in patients receiving both aspirin and streptokinase [*see Figure 3*].[17] Other studies have revealed similar benefit from immediate aspirin therapy.[32]

Patients should be maintained on aspirin indefinitely. Prolonged administration of aspirin in patients with a history of myocardial infarction is associated with a 25% reduction in death, nonfatal reinfarction, and stroke.[32]

ANALGESIA

Pain relief should be among the initial therapies offered to patients with acute myocardial infarction. Persistent chest discomfort is generally caused by ongoing myocardial ischemia; although the ultimate goal of therapy is to eliminate ischemia, analgesia should be administered without delay. In addition to making patients more comfortable, pain relief may reduce the outpouring of catecholamines characteristic of the early stages of acute myocardial infarction and thereby reduce myocardial oxygen demand. Intravenous morphine sulfate is commonly used for pain relief in this setting.

Reperfusion Therapy

Reperfusion may be achieved by percutaneous coronary intervention (PCI) (previously referred to as primary coronary angioplasty, percutaneous transluminal coronary angioplasty [PTCA], or balloon angioplasty) or thrombolytic therapy.

REPERFUSION STRATEGIES AND OUTCOMES

Importance of Time to Reperfusion

Many important predictors of early clinical outcome in myocardial infarction are independent of treatment. Most of the early mortality is explained by factors such as the age of the patient, initial heart rate and blood pressure, initial Killip classification [*see Table 2*], and infarct location. However, the time to administration of reperfusion therapy is a critical determinant of outcome and one of the few determinants of early clinical outcome under the control of the physician. Many studies have revealed

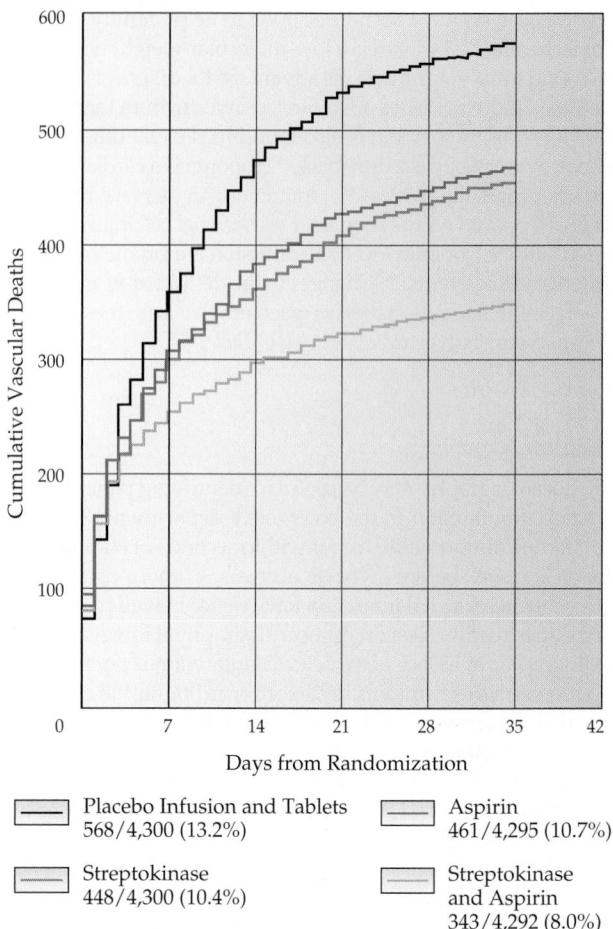

| Placebo Infusion and Tablets 568/4,300 (13.2%) | Aspirin 461/4,295 (10.7%) |
| Streptokinase 448/4,300 (10.4%) | Streptokinase and Aspirin 343/4,292 (8.0%) |

Figure 3 **Mortality at 35 days in 17,187 cases of suspected acute myocardial infarction in the second International Study of Infarct Survival (ISIS-2). In this study, aspirin reduced 30-day mortality by 23% and was nearly as effective as streptokinase; the benefit was additive in patients receiving both aspirin and streptokinase.[17]**

that patients with myocardial infarction treated most rapidly have a lower mortality and, among survivors, reduced infarct size [*see Figure 4*].[33] This observation has led to recommendations that the time between a patient's presentation to the emergency department and the administration of thrombolytic therapy not exceed 60 minutes; ideally, this period should not exceed 30 minutes.[34] The most critical interval is the time between symptom onset and the achievement of reperfusion, not the time to the ini-

Table 2 Killip Classification of Acute Myocardial Infarction

Class I	No clinical heart failure
Class II	Findings consistent with mild or moderate heart failure (e.g., isolated S_3 gallop, bilateral rales in up to 50% of lung fields)
Class III	Pulmonary edema, rales in all lung fields, acute mitral regurgitation
Class IV	Cardiogenic shock (e.g., stuporous state of consciousness, systolic blood pressure < 90 mm Hg, decreased urine output, pulmonary edema, and cold, clammy skin)

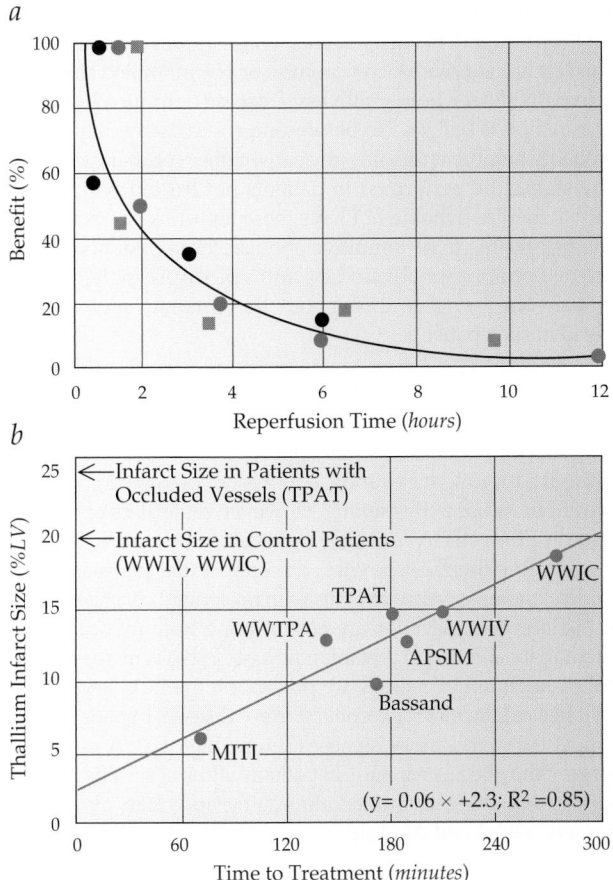

Figure 4 **Many studies have revealed lower mortality (*a*) and reduced infarct size among survivors (*b*) of myocardial infarction treated most rapidly. The equation shows the linear relation between infarct size and time to treatment.[33] (APSIM—APSAC dans l'Infarctus du Myocarde; Bassand—Bassand study; MITI—Myocardial Infarction Triage and Intervention; TPAT—Tissue Plasminogen Activator, Toronto trial; WWIC—Western Washington Intracoronary streptokinase trial; WWIV—Western Washington Intravenous streptokinase trial; WWTPA—Western Washington Tissue Plasminogen Activator trial)**

tiation of therapy. Thus, therapy that takes longer to initiate may actually be superior if it achieves reperfusion more rapidly than another therapy that can be initiated more rapidly (e.g., thrombolytic therapy). The ACC/AHA task force gave a class I recommendation to the use of PCI for any patient with an acute ST-segment elevation myocardial infarction (STEMI) who presents within 12 hours of symptom onset and who can undergo the procedure within 90 minutes of presentation by clinicians skilled in the procedure.[31] When primary PCI is not available or its implementation is delayed, use of thrombolytic therapy is recommended. The ACC/AHA task force gave a class I recommendation to the use of thrombolytic therapy for any patient with an acute STEMI without contraindications for thrombolysis, who presents to a facility without the capability for expert, prompt intervention with primary PCI within 90 minutes of first medical contact.[31] The delay from patient arrival to administration of thrombolytics should be less than 30 minutes.[31] Reperfusion therapy, whether PCI or thrombolytics, should not await the availability of results of cardiac biomarkers. The immediate implementation of reperfusion therapy without awaiting biomarker data was given a class I recommendation.[31]

The importance of avoiding hospital delay in performing pri-

mary coronary angioplasty was evident in the Global Use of Strategies to Open Occluded Arteries (GUSTO-IIb) substudy, which compared primary coronary angioplasty with tissue plasminogen activator (t-PA) therapy.[35] There was a clear relation between the length of time until angioplasty was performed after enrollment in the study and 30-day mortality [*see Figure 5*]. Analysis of 27,080 patients in the second National Registry of Myocardial Infarction also revealed a relation between time to treatment with primary PTCA and survival, even after adjusting for other mortality risk factors.[36] In that study, the volume of patients treated with angioplasty at the hospital was also a predictor of outcome; a lower mortality was seen at hospitals in which a high number of patients with acute myocardial infarction were treated with coronary angioplasty. There have been studies in which unacceptably high mortality was seen at hospitals when primary angioplasty was not performed rapidly; reducing delay led to a reduction in mortality.[37] Therefore, as is the case with thrombolytic therapy, the speed with which reperfusion is achieved appears to be an important determinant of clinical outcome. The best reperfusion therapy (coronary angioplasty or thrombolytic therapy) is not necessarily the one that can be most rapidly initiated but, rather, the one that achieves coronary patency most rapidly. In general, the therapy that restores flow most rapidly should be preferred.[38-40]

Transfer for Primary Angioplasty versus Immediate Thrombolytic Therapy

Time to reperfusion is an important modifiable predictor of clinical outcome for both thrombolysis and primary angioplasty, although it has the greatest impact on patients treated with thrombolytic therapy. An alternative treatment strategy for patients with STEMI initially assessed at a hospital without on-site cardiac surgery facilities is immediate transfer for primary PCI.

The PRAGUE-2 investigators randomized 850 patients with acute STEMI presenting within 12 hours to a hospital without a catheterization laboratory to either immediate thrombolysis or transfer for primary PCI.[41] The investigators determined that in the acute phase of STEMI, long-distance transport from a community hospital to a facility with PCI is safe and is associ-

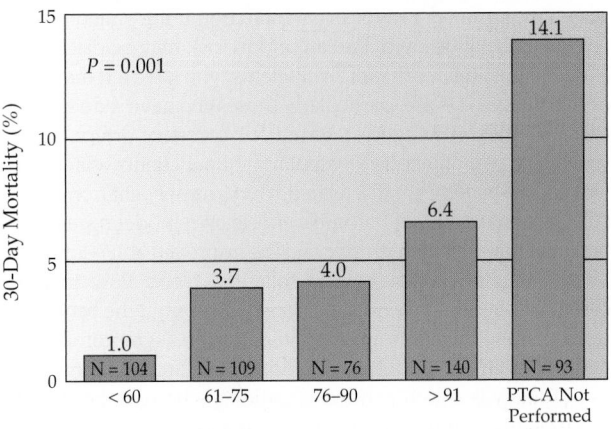

Figure 5 **Relation between the time from study enrollment to the first balloon inflation and 30-day mortality in the GUSTO-IIb substudy. Patients assigned to angioplasty in whom angioplasty was not performed are also shown.[35] (PTCA—percutaneous transluminal coronary angioplasty)**

ated with decreased mortality in patients presenting more than 3 hours after symptom onset. Similarly, the Danish Trial in Acute Myocardial Infarction (DANAMI)–2 trial investigators concluded that immediate transfer for primary PCI, in preference to immediate thrombolysis, was safe and efficacious.[42]

However, data from these trials need to be understood within the context of the individual trial designs and their actual conduct. The maximum transport distance in the PRAGUE-2 trial was 120 kilometers, and the time from transport to balloon inflation was only 97 ± 27 minutes. In the DANAMI-2 trial, the time from arrival to initiation of treatment in the thrombolysis arm of the study was 51 minutes, whereas the time required to transfer patients for primary PCI was 155 minutes ($P < 0.0001$). It is reasonable to assume that the reported benefit associated with this particular treatment strategy in the aforementioned randomized, controlled clinical trials (i.e., PRAGUE-2 and DANAMI-2) can be realized only if similar transfer times and door-to-balloon times are reproduced in clinical practice; the findings of the NRMI 4 investigators are not reassuring in this regard.

Coronary Angiography after Uncomplicated Myocardial Infarction

The role of coronary angiography after uncomplicated myocardial infarction remains controversial for patients who have received thrombolytic therapy. Coronary angiography in patients initially treated with thrombolytic agents has been studied in the second Thrombolysis in Myocardial Infarction (TIMI II) study, the Should We Intervene Following Thrombolysis? (SWIFT) study, the Treatment of Post-thrombolytic Stenoses (TOPS) study, and, most recently, a German study.[43-46] It is clear from these studies that patients treated with thrombolytic therapy in whom complications do not occur are at low risk for reinfarction and death after discharge and that the routine performance of coronary angiography and coronary angioplasty does not reduce the occurrence of these adverse events. Despite the publication of these well-designed studies, there has been considerable reluctance among physicians to accept their results, and there remains considerable variability throughout the United States and the world in the frequency with which coronary angiography is performed in such patients.

Many cardiologists feel more comfortable caring for patients who have suffered a myocardial infarction if the patient's coronary anatomy is known. Patients at low risk may be discharged from the hospital more rapidly. Patients who have left mainstem or multivessel disease, particularly those who have reduced ventricular function, may be referred for coronary artery bypass surgery or percutaneous revascularization. Patients with persistent occlusion of the infarct-related artery may benefit from revascularization because of favorable effects on remodeling, a reduction in ventricular arrhythmia, and the improved ability of the infarct-related artery to provide collateral blood flow to other coronary arteries in the future. Nonetheless, until the benefits of cardiac catheterization are demonstrated in asymptomatic patients after an uncomplicated myocardial infarction, a conservative strategy is recommended in patients who have been given thrombolytic therapy, and coronary angiography is recommended only for patients with hemodynamic instability or for patients in whom spontaneous or exercise-induced ischemia occurs; such a strategy is safe and is associated with a good clinical outcome.

Patients who are not given thrombolytic therapy are at higher risk for reinfarction and death than those receiving thrombolytic therapy. The role of coronary angiography in patients with acute myocardial infarction not receiving thrombolytic therapy has not been studied. In such patients whose infarctions are complicated by hemodynamic compromise or postinfarction chest pain or in patients in whom multivessel disease or reduced ventricular function is believed to be present, coronary angiography is probably helpful. It remains unclear whether coronary angiography should be performed in patients not treated with thrombolytic therapy who do not have these high-risk characteristics. It is impossible to be definitive about recommendations in the absence of appropriate studies, and not surprisingly, practice patterns vary widely throughout the United States and the world in such patients.

Reperfusion Therapy in Patients without ST Segment Elevation

Primary PTCA has not been appropriately studied in patients without ST segment elevation, and it is not possible to be definitive about its use in this setting. However, regardless of the findings on ECG, PTCA is widely believed to be beneficial in patients with ischemic-type chest discomfort that persists despite medical therapy. Many patients with prolonged chest pain without ST segment elevation are not suffering from myocardial infarction; the likelihood that infarction is present is increased if repolarization abnormalities are present on the ECG and the patient has risk factors for coronary artery disease. In patients with critical coronary artery stenoses, immediate PTCA or bypass surgery may be appropriate. In patients without significant coronary artery disease, immediate angiography can also be extremely useful and can lead to the withdrawal of cardiac med-

---

Table 3   Class I Recommendations for the Use of an Invasive Strategy in the Management of Patients with Unstable Angina or Non–ST Segment Elevation Myocardial Infarction

An early invasive strategy is recommended for patients who have unstable angina or non–ST segment elevation myocardial infarction (NSTEMI) without serious comorbidity and who have any of the following high-risk indicators (level of evidence: A):

  Recurrent angina/ischemia at rest or with low-level activities despite intensive anti-ischemic therapy

  Elevated levels of troponin T or troponin I

  New or presumably new ST segment depression

  Recurrent angina/ischemia with symptoms of congestive heart failure, an S_3 gallop, pulmonary edema, worsening rales, or new or worsening mitral regurgitation

  High-risk findings on noninvasive stress testing

  Depressed left ventricular systolic function (e.g., ejection fraction < 0.40 on noninvasive study)

  Hemodynamic instability

  Sustained ventricular tachycardia

  Percutaneous coronary intervention within 6 mo

  Prior coronary artery bypass grafting

In the absence of any of these findings, an early conservative strategy or an early invasive strategy may be offered in hospitalized patients without contraindications for revascularization (level of evidence: B)

Note: Class I recommendations pertain to conditions for which there is evidence or general agreement that a given procedure is useful and effective. Level A evidence (highest)—Derived from multiple randomized clinical trials. Level B evidence (intermediate)—Derived from limited number of randomized clinical trials, nonrandomized studies, or observational registries.

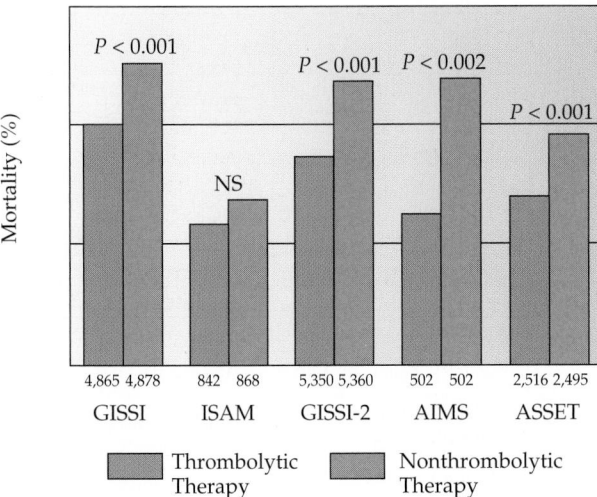

Figure 6 **Data from five controlled megatrials of thrombolytic therapy large enough to detect a mortality difference between the thrombolytic and nonthrombolytic control arms of the trials. Pooled data from these five trials (not shown) reveal a 29% mortality reduction in patients treated within 6 hours of symptom onset.[53] (AIMS—APSAC International Mortality Study; ASSET—Anglo-Scandinavian Study of Early Thrombosis; GISSI—Gruppo Italiano per lo Studio della Streptochinasi nell'Infarto Miocardico; GISSI-2—Gruppo Italiano per lo Studio della Sopravvivenza nell'Infarto Myocardico; ISAM— Intravenous Streptokinase in Acute Myocardial Infarction; NS—not significant)**

ications, discharge from the coronary care unit, and appropriate diagnostic evaluation, in many cases as an outpatient. Immediate angiography is recommended in all patients with hypotension, severe congestive heart failure, or cardiogenic shock regardless of the initial ECG results, because immediate revascularization appears to reduce mortality in this setting.[47] In addition, there is a compelling case to be made for routine invasive evaluation of all patients who are admitted with unstable angina or non–ST segment elevation myocardial infarction (NSTEMI).[48]

In the TIMI-IIIb study, an early intervention strategy was compared with a conservative strategy in 3,000 patients with either unstable angina, recent non–Q wave myocardial infarction, or prolonged chest pain without ST segment elevation on ECG.[49] Patients were randomized to receive either early angiography or medical therapy; only those patients who subsequently experienced recurrent chest pain or had an exercise test underwent angiography. Although death and myocardial infarction occurred with similar frequency in the two groups, the study showed that the initial hospitalization was longer and the need for rehospitalization more frequent in the group receiving conservative therapy. More recently, in the second Fragmin and Fast Revascularization during Instability in Coronary Artery Disease (FRISC-II) trial, an early invasive strategy was shown to reduce both mortality and myocardial infarction at 1 year.[50] In the Treat Angina with Aggrastat [tirofiban] and Determine Cost of Therapy with Invasive or Conservative Strategy—Thrombolysis in Myocardial Infarction–18 (TACTICS-TIMI-18) study, an early invasive strategy was found to reduce the combined end point of death or myocardial infarction.[51] In both the FRISC-II and TACTICS-TIMI-18 studies, patients at greatest risk, such as those with positive troponin values and with ST segment depression at study entry, had the highest event rates and derived the greatest benefit from an invasive strategy.

The 2002 ACC/AHA unstable angina guideline update has summarized the data regarding early invasive versus early conservative strategies in patients with unstable angina or NSTEMI and issued an updated set of recommendations to guide clinical decision making in this setting [*see Table 3*].[52]

THROMBOLYTIC THERAPY

Thrombolytic therapy has been widely studied in prospective, randomized, controlled trials involving more than 50,000 patients and has been proved to reduce mortality 29% in patients with ST segment elevation treated within 6 hours after the onset of chest pain [*see Figure 6*].[53] The survival benefit of thrombolytic therapy is maintained for years.[54] The benefit of thrombolytic therapy is achieved through rapid restoration of blood flow in an occluded coronary artery.[55-57]

Thrombolytic therapy is strongly recommended for patients with ST segment elevation in two or more contiguous leads who have had less than 6 hours of chest pain; for patients with classic symptoms of infarction in whom a bundle branch block precludes detection of ST segment elevation[53]; and for patients presenting with 6 to 12 hours of chest pain, although the expected benefits for this last group of patients are fewer. The potential benefits should be weighed against the potential risks in patients with relative contraindications to thrombolytic therapy (see below).[17,58] It is important to calculate the duration of infarction as the time from the last pain-free interval. The infarct-related artery often opens and closes spontaneously during the early stages of infarction, which the patient may experience as alternating pain-free and painful intervals; the window of benefit from thrombolytic therapy may be greater than 12 hours if antegrade flow was even briefly restored.

Contraindications to Thrombolytic Therapy

Contraindications to thrombolytic therapy include all conditions that predispose a patient to significant bleeding. The most feared bleeding complication is intracerebral hemorrhage, which is fatal in over half of cases. Risk factors for intracerebral bleeding include advanced age, low body weight, hypertension, warfarin use, and previous stroke.[53,59] Patients with gastrointestinal bleeding and those who have recently undergone surgery are also at increased risk for bleeding. Even when risk factors for bleeding are present, however, the potential benefits of thrombolytic therapy may still outweigh the risks. For example, although the elderly have a higher risk of intracerebral bleeding than younger patients, elderly patients should certainly be considered candidates for thrombolytic therapy, because their increasing absolute mortality results in a greater reduction in absolute mortality with thrombolytic therapy than is seen in younger patients.[53]

In patients with ECG findings other than ST segment elevation or bundle branch block, thrombolytic therapy has been found to be either of no use or deleterious; its use is not recommended in such patients.[17,53]

Choice of Thrombolytic Agent

Many different thrombolytic regimens have been proved effective for the treatment of acute myocardial infarction, and many more are being studied. In principle, the preferred thrombolytic regimen would restore normal antegrade blood flow to an occluded coronary artery most rapidly and in the greatest number of patients, would have the lowest reocclusion rate, and would be associated with the lowest risk of severe hemorrhagic complications. The first Global Utilization of Streptokinase and Tissue Plasminogen Activator for Occluded Arteries (GUSTO-I) trial evaluated four thrombolytic regimens to determine which was associated with the greatest overall survival and stroke-free survival at 30 days: (1) a regimen of front-loaded, weight-adjusted t-PA and I.V. heparin, (2) a regimen of streptokinase and I.V. heparin, (3) a regimen of streptokinase and subcutaneous heparin, and (4) a combination of I.V. t-PA and streptokinase given concurrently with I.V. heparin. Front-loaded t-PA was found to be moderately superior to the other thrombolytic regimens [*see Figure 7*].[56] However, because of the approximately 10 times greater cost of t-PA than I.V. streptokinase and the low margin of superiority of t-PA (one life saved per thousand patients treated), some physicians prefer the less expensive streptokinase therapy, particularly for patients at low risk of dying (such as those with uncomplicated inferior infarctions) and the elderly, who are more likely to have hemorrhagic complications with t-PA than with streptokinase; t-PA is associated with a greater frequency of intracerebral hemorrhage than streptokinase.[56] The recommendation of streptokinase in these patient groups is largely driven by its lower cost; if the costs of t-PA and streptokinase were similar, t-PA would most likely be the preferred therapy in all patient subgroups, with the possible exception of those at increased risk for intracerebral hemorrhage, in whom streptokinase might be preferred.

Streptokinase therapy is contraindicated in patients who have recently received a dose of streptokinase because of antibodies that form against the drug; these antibodies limit the efficacy of repeat doses and increase the risk of allergic reactions. It has been suggested that the drug not be readministered for at least 2 years.

New thrombolytic agents are continuously being developed in the hope of finding safer and more effective therapies. One such agent, reteplase, is a recombinant tissue plasminogen activator (rt-PA) that is a mutant of alteplase. Reteplase is easier to administer than alteplase; because of its longer half-life, it can be administered as two 10 mU boluses given 30 minutes apart, with concomitant aspirin and I.V. heparin administration. Several pilot studies suggest that reteplase has an early patency rate that is superior to the patency rates of streptokinase and alteplase. In the International Joint Efficacy Comparison of Throm-

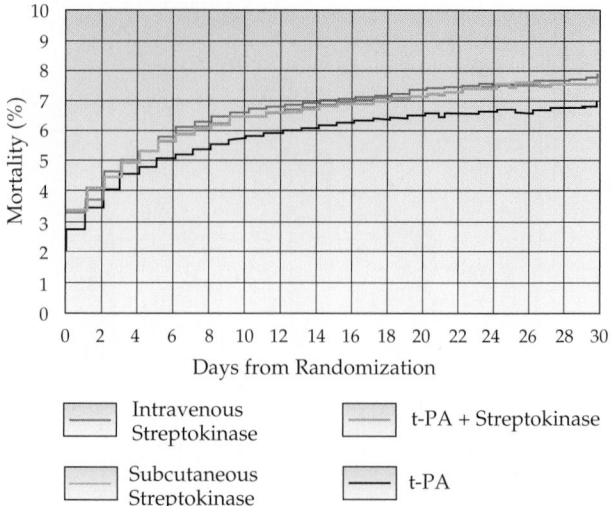

Figure 7   The frequency of death or disabling stroke in the 30 days after enrollment in 41,021 patients in the Global Utilization of Streptokinase and Tissue Plasminogen Activator for Occluded Arteries (GUSTO-I) trial. Front-loaded t-PA was found to be superior to the other thrombolytic regimens.[56]

bolytics (INJECT) trial, 6,010 patients with acute myocardial infarction received either reteplase or streptokinase within 12 hours after the onset of symptoms.[60] Mortality at 35 days, the primary end point of the study, was 9.02% for patients given reteplase, compared with 9.53% for patients given streptokinase, a nonsignificant difference (95% confidence interval, 1.98 to 0.96). This lack of significant difference indicates that reteplase was at least as effective as streptokinase.

In the GUSTO-III trial, reteplase was compared with t-PA in 15,059 patients with acute myocardial infarction who presented within 6 hours of symptom onset.[61] Patients received either reteplase or an accelerated infusion of t-PA. For patients receiving reteplase, the mortality at 30 days was 7.47%, compared with 7.24% for patients receiving t-PA ($P = 0.54$; odds ratio, 1.03; 95%

a

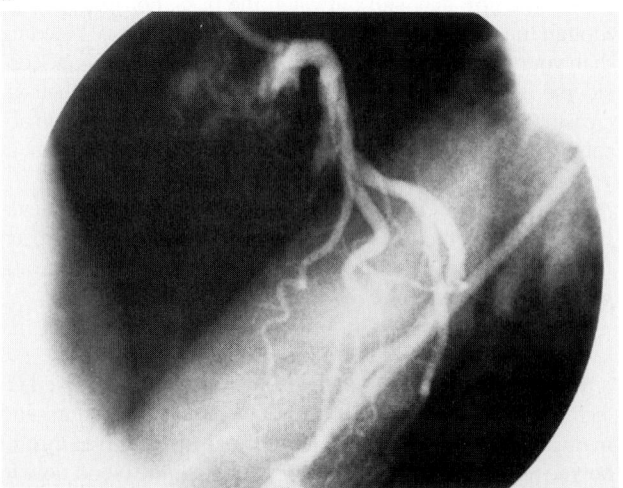

b

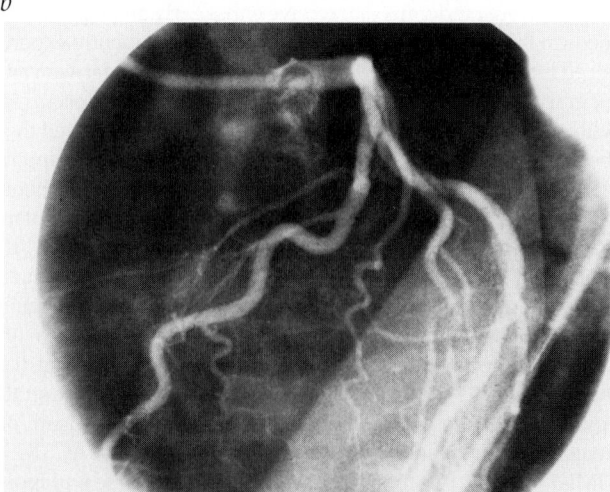

Figure 8   (*a*) Left anterior oblique view of an occluded left anterior descending artery in a patient suffering an acute anterior myocardial infarction. (*b*) Patency was restored with direct coronary angioplasty 17 minutes after the patient had arrived in the catheterization laboratory, and the patient had immediate resolution of his symptoms.

confidence interval, 0.91 to 1.18). The mortality rates with the two agents were therefore similar, and the two agents are probably, although not definitely, equivalent in efficacy.

Combination Therapy

Combination therapy, defined as the use of a thrombolytic agent and a glycoprotein IIb/IIIa inhibitor, has been proposed as an alternative to thrombolytic therapy alone for the primary treatment of STEMI. This strategy is supported by data from a number of trials that demonstrated improved rates of TIMI-3 flow after combination therapy, as compared with thrombolytic therapy alone.[62,63] However, the results of two randomized, controlled trials evaluating clinical outcomes after the respective aforementioned reperfusion strategies have been somewhat disappointing.

The GUSTO-V trial randomized 16,588 patients who presented within 6 hours after symptom onset with STEMI to either standard-dose reteplase or half-dose reteplase and full-dose abciximab.[64] At 30 days, the incidence of death in the reteplase arm was 5.9%, compared with 5.6% in the combination-therapy arm ($P = 0.43$), suggesting no mortality benefit associated with combination therapy. However, five of 16 prespecified secondary end points were reduced to a statistically significant degree ($P < 0.05$), suggesting a beneficial impact of combination therapy on the incidence of recurrent ischemic events and the mechanical and electrical complications of acute myocardial infarction (e.g., nonfatal reinfarction, recurrent ischemia, ventricular fibrillation, sustained ventricular tachycardia, and atrioventricular block). However, these clinical benefits were offset by an increased incidence of bleeding of any kind (13.7% with monotherapy versus 24.6% with combination therapy; $P < 0.0001$); severe or moderate, spontaneous, nonintracranial bleeding (1.9% versus 4.3%, $P < 0.0001$); severe bleeding (0.5% versus 1.1%; $P < 0.0001$), and bleeding sufficient to require blood transfusion (4.0% versus 5.7%; $P < 0.0001$). Furthermore, there were subgroups of patients in whom intracranial bleeding was increased by combination therapy; there was a significant ($P = 0.033$) association between age (< 75 or ≥ 75 years) and intracranial hemorrhage in the combination-therapy arm.

The Assessment of the Safety and Efficacy of a New Thrombolytic (ASSENT)–3 trial randomized 6,095 patients to one of

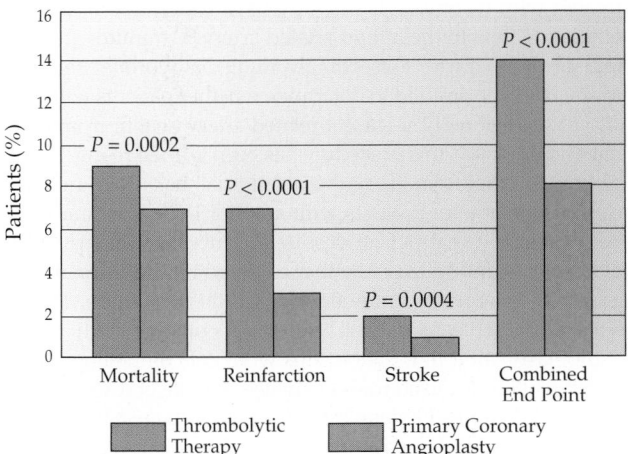

Figure 9   **Results from a quantitative review of 23 randomized trials of primary angioplasty versus intravenous thrombolytic therapy for acute myocardial infarction.[72] Clinical outcome was improved in patients who received angioplasty.**

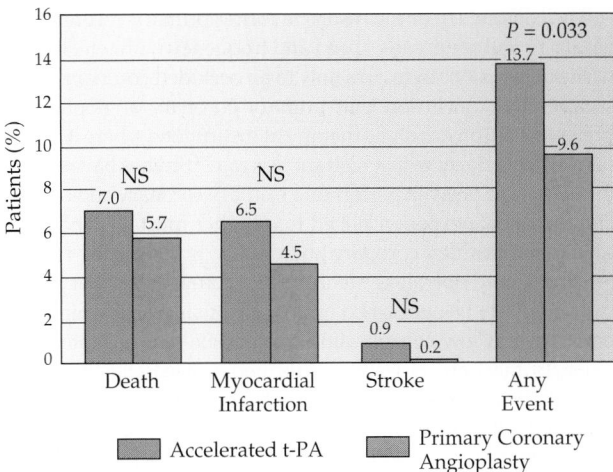

Figure 10   **Results from the GUSTO-IIb substudy trial comparing primary coronary angioplasty and accelerated t-PA indicate that primary angioplasty was associated with a lower mortality, reinfarction rate, and frequency of stroke in the 30 days after enrollment than was accelerated t-PA.[73] (NS—not significant)**

three treatment regimens: full-dose tenecteplase and enoxaparin, half-dose tenecteplase and weight-adjusted low-dose unfractionated heparin infusion plus 12-hour infusion of abciximab, or full-dose tenecteplase and weight-adjusted unfractionated heparin infusion for 48 hours.[65] In-hospital mortality was not significantly different between the three groups. The abciximab treatment regimen reduced in-hospital rates of reinfarction and refractory ischemia. Although rates of intracranial hemorrhage were similar, other types of major bleeding were significantly higher in the abciximab arm of the trial. The enoxaparin arm suggested that there is a higher rate of intracranial bleeding in the elderly; this finding was corroborated by the ASSENT-PLUS study, which necessitated a change in dose of enoxaparin when administered with a thrombolytic agent in elderly patients.[66]

PRIMARY CORONARY ANGIOPLASTY

In prospective, randomized trials comparing primary coronary angioplasty [*see Figure 8*] with different thrombolytic agents, primary coronary angioplasty was associated with a lower morbidity and mortality than thrombolytic therapy.[67-71] Although most of the individual trials were too small to detect statistically significant differences in mortality, pooled data from these trials suggest that primary coronary angioplasty is the preferred therapy for acute myocardial infarction at institutions where it can be performed without delay [*see Figure 9*].[72]

The GUSTO-IIb trial was designed to be large enough to confirm the reduction in mortality found in the smaller randomized trials.[73] The results of the study indicate that compared with thrombolytic therapy, primary coronary angioplasty is associated with a lower mortality, reinfarction rate, and frequency of stroke in the 30 days after enrollment [*see Figure 10*]. However, the degree of benefit associated with primary coronary angioplasty was much smaller than that seen in the earlier randomized studies; this finding was in part related to the lower frequency with which patients assigned to undergo angioplasty in GUSTO-IIb actually underwent the procedure and in part related to the lower frequency with which normal antegrade coronary blood flow was achieved in patients who did undergo coronary angioplasty.

The consistency of the results favoring primary coronary angioplasty and the greater speed and frequency with which coronary angioplasty can restore flow to an occluded coronary artery support the conclusion that primary coronary angioplasty is preferable to thrombolytic therapy at institutions where it can be performed quickly with a high success rate.[74] Studies have shown that excessive delay in performing primary coronary angioplasty and operator inexperience lead to a higher mortality than that seen when primary coronary angioplasty is performed rapidly by experienced operators.[36] It has been recommended that primary angioplasty be performed only in hospitals where a high success rate and low complication rate can be demonstrated and where primary angioplasty is performed in at least 80% to 90% of patients in whom acute myocardial infarction is confirmed.[72,75] The need for surgical backup is controversial, as excellent results have been obtained at centers without surgical backup.[76] However, surgical backup is recommended because approximately 5% of patients with acute myocardial infarction who undergo immediate coronary angiography require emergency surgery either for angioplasty that has failed or, more commonly, because lethal coronary anatomy precludes primary angioplasty.

Immediate transfer for primary angioplasty is an alternative treatment strategy for patients with STEMI initially assessed at a hospital without on-site cardiac surgery facilities.

Antiplatelet Therapy

Aspirin and clopidogrel therapy   Aspirin should be given to patients with suspected STEMI as early as possible and continued indefinitely. True aspirin allergy is the only exception to this recommendation.[31] The 2004 ACC/AHA guidelines gave a class I recommendation to the use of clopidogrel in all patients treated with primary PCI.[31] Clopidogrel may be given in a loading dose of 300 mg or 600 mg; limited trial data suggest that 600 mg works within 2 to 3 hours and that outcomes may be better than with 300 mg. There are no data available regarding the combination of fibrinolytic agents and clopidogrel, but ongoing trials will provide this information. However, clopidogrel is probably indicated in patients receiving fibrinolytic therapy who are unable to take aspirin because of hypersensitivity or major gastrointestinal intolerance.

Glycoprotein IIb/IIIa inhibitor therapy   The 2004 ACC/AHA guidelines gave a class IIa recommendation to treatment with abciximab as early as possible prior to PCI (with or without implantation of stents) in patients with STEMI.[31] This recommendation was based on several studies including the Randomized, Placebo-Controlled Trial of Abciximab with Primary Angioplasty for Acute Myocardial Infarction (RAPPORT), the Intracoronary Stenting and Antithrombotic Regimen–2 (ISAR-2) study, the Abciximab before Direct Angioplasty and Stenting in Myocardial Infarction Regarding Acute and Long-term Follow-up (ADMIRAL) study, and, most recently, the Controlled Abciximab and Device Investigation to Lower Late Angioplasty Complications (CADILLAC) study.[77-80] The results of the four studies differ, in part because the trials used different end points, in part because of the high frequency of noncompliance with the protocol in some trials, and in part because of differences in the treatments utilized (balloon angioplasty alone versus balloon angioplasty followed by stent placement).

The largest of the four studies, the CADILLAC study, found that abciximab is beneficial at reducing major adverse events, but the benefit appeared to be limited to patients undergoing balloon angioplasty without stent placement. The apparent lack of benefit following treatment with abciximab in patients in the CADILLAC trial who received a coronary stent is contrary to the results of the ISAR-2 and ADMIRAL trials, in which abciximab was found to be beneficial in patients receiving stents. There are data suggesting that stent placement in the setting of acute myocardial infarction slightly reduces the frequency with which normal antegrade blood flow in the infarct-related artery is achieved.[81] This would suggest that glycoprotein IIb/IIIa inhibitors should be beneficial in this setting. Taken together, the results of these studies that are currently available suggest that abciximab is beneficial in patients with acute myocardial infarction but that the benefit in patients undergoing balloon angioplasty alone may differ from that in patients who undergo balloon angioplasty with stent placement. Clearly, however, stents markedly reduce the frequency with which a repeat revascularization procedure is needed in the months after the angioplasty procedure.[81] The combined use of stents and platelet glycoprotein inhibitors may maximize the frequency with which normal antegrade blood flow is achieved while reducing the need for repeat procedures in the following year.

One study compared the outcome of thrombolytic therapy using t-PA with that of primary angioplasty utilizing both stents and abciximab.[82] The reduction in infarct size was far greater in the group undergoing primary angioplasty; the clinical outcome was also better in the patients who underwent angioplasty.

CORONARY ARTERY BYPASS SURGERY

Coronary artery bypass surgery can restore blood flow in an occluded infarct-related artery. However, because of the time required to perform coronary angiography and to transport patients to the operating room, reperfusion is achieved more slowly with bypass surgery than with thrombolytic therapy and primary coronary angioplasty.[83] Emergency coronary artery bypass surgery should generally be reserved for patients in whom immediate angiography reveals coronary anatomy that precludes primary coronary angioplasty; for patients in whom angioplasty has failed; and for patients with a ventricular septal defect, severe mitral regurgitation, or myocardial rupture.

RESCUE CORONARY ANGIOPLASTY

Depending on the regimen used, only 33% to 60% of patients treated with thrombolytic therapy have restoration of normal antegrade flow in the infarct-related artery 90 minutes after the initiation of therapy.[55] Accordingly, immediate coronary angiography has been studied to determine whether patients with persistent occlusion of the infarct-related artery benefit from coronary angioplasty; this procedure has been termed rescue angioplasty. A single small, randomized trial has examined the clinical outcome of patients with anterior infarction and coronary occlusion that persist despite thrombolytic therapy.[84] Patients were randomized to either undergo rescue coronary angioplasty or receive continued medical therapy alone. The results of the trial suggested improved outcome with rescue angioplasty, although the benefits were not compelling. Three additional randomized trials evaluated the role of rescue angioplasty.[85-87] Analyzed together, the four trials suggest that rescue angioplasty offers benefit, although the data are not compelling. Although use of coronary stents and platelet glycoprotein inhibitors improves the results of percutaneous revascularization procedures and would be expected to further increase the benefit of angioplasty after failed thrombolytic therapy, this has not yet been proved. There are insufficient data to recommend immediate angiography and angioplasty in all patients early after thrombolytic therapy. Immediate angiography is most likely to be beneficial in patients with large myocardial infarctions in whom persistent pain, ST segment elevation, or hemodynamic compromise is present more than 90 minutes after the administration of a thrombolytic agent.

The routine performance of angioplasty immediately after the administration of thrombolytic therapy in all patients with a significant residual stenosis (not just those patients with occluded coronary arteries) has been well studied in three prospective, randomized trials and has been found to be either of no benefit or deleterious.[43,88] Angioplasty should not be routinely performed in such patients.

Stents appear to improve the ability to achieve arterial patency early after thrombolytic therapy, as compared with balloon angioplasty alone[89]; therapy with a glycoprotein IIb/IIIa inhibitor may also do so, although an increase in bleeding has been seen when glycoprotein IIb/IIIa inhibitors are used early after full-dose thrombolytic therapy.[90] Data from several pilot studies suggest that the combination of a fibrin-specific thrombolytic agent, either t-PA or reteplase, combined with the glycoprotein IIb/IIIa inhibitor abciximab, may actually facilitate the performance of angioplasty rather than reduce its safety and efficacy, as was seen when balloon angioplasty was performed after thrombolytic therapy.[62,63] Hence, the term facilitated angioplasty has been coined for the routine performance of angioplasty after the combination of half-dose thrombolytic therapy with a glycoprotein IIb/IIIa inhibitor.

The Plasminogen-activator Angioplasty Compatibility Trial (PACT) investigators randomized 606 patients to a reduced dose of a short-acting fibrinolytic regimen (50 mg bolus of reteplase) or a placebo followed by immediate angiography with angioplasty, if needed.[91] In the group receiving reduced-dose reteplase, there was no increase in the incidence of stroke or major bleeding, and convalescent left-ventricular ejection fraction was higher, as evidenced by a patent infarct–related artery (TIMI-3 flow) on arrival in the catheterization laboratory (62%) or a TIMI-3 flow that was achieved by angioplasty within 1 hour after administration of the drug bolus (58%). However, only 12% of successful angioplasty procedures resulted in a patent infarct–related artery within 1 hour, because of routine delay in transfer to the catheterization laboratory, and there was no difference between the two treatment groups by a traditional intention-to-treat analysis.

The Southwest German Study in Acute Myocardial Infarction III (SIAM III) investigators randomized 163 patients initially treated with thrombolysis at a community hospital with no on-site PCI facilities either to hospital transfer and immediate stenting within 6 hours of thrombolysis or to delayed, elective stenting approximately 2 weeks after acute myocardial infarction.[92] Transfer and immediate stenting were associated with a statistically significant reduction in the incidence of the composite primary end point (i.e., death, reinfarction, ischemic events, and target-lesion revascularization at 6 months), as compared with delayed stenting (25.6% versus 50.6%; P = 0.001). The difference in outcome was driven by events occurring during the 2 weeks that patients waited for elective stenting in the deferred PCI group. This trial design does not address whether PCI performed 1 to 2 days after thrombolytic therapy, as is usual in the United States, is as effective as PCI performed immediately after thrombolytic therapy. A randomized trial that analyzed the use of combination therapy

(half-dose thrombolytic therapy with full-dose abciximab) before routinely performing primary PCI was reported.[93] In the Bavarian Reperfusion Alternatives Evaluation (BRAVE) Trial, patients with STEMI were randomly assigned to receive either half-dose reteplase and full-dose abciximab or abciximab alone, and all patients underwent PCI as rapidly as possible. No advantage was seen with combination therapy; in fact, more bleeding complications occurred in this group. The results argue against the use of a facilitated PCI approach using the combination regimen of reteplase and abciximab.

Adjunctive Medical Therapy

INTRAVENOUS HEPARIN

The need for I.V. heparin after thrombolytic therapy varies with the thrombolytic agents used. A retrospective analysis of the GUSTO-I trial suggested that I.V. heparin with a partial thromboplastin time of 50 to 70 seconds was associated with the best clinical outcome in patients treated with t-PA.[94] Data from GUSTO-I also suggest that I.V. heparin is not required when I.V. streptokinase is used, although heparin is recommended in patients with large anterior infarctions to prevent the development of apical mural thrombus and embolization.[56] In patients in whom I.V. heparin is not administered, subcutaneous heparin should be administered during the period of bed rest to reduce the risk of deep vein thrombosis.[95]

The optimal duration of I.V. heparin therapy is unclear. Standard practice was to administer I.V. heparin for 3 to 5 days, although patients are now often discharged after only 3 days. It is recommended that heparin be discontinued more than 24 hours before patient discharge from the hospital because of the possibility of a rebound effect and recurrent thrombosis within 24 hours after cessation of heparin therapy.[96]

Randomized studies from the prethrombolytic era suggested that administration of I.V. heparin reduces mortality and reinfarction in patients not treated with thrombolytic agents.[95] Aspirin and beta blockers were not routinely administered in those early trials; consequently, the true benefits of heparin when these drugs are administered are unknown. However, on the basis of the early data, I.V. heparin is generally recommended for patients with suspected myocardial infarction who are not treated with thrombolytic therapy.[75]

LOW-MOLECULAR-WEIGHT HEPARIN

Low-molecular-weight heparins (depolymerized unfractionated heparin with a mean molecular weight of approximately 5,000) have a number of potential pharmacokinetic advantages over the parent molecule, including decreased binding to plasma proteins, decreased sensitivity to platelet factor 4, enhanced factor Xa activity, and improved bioavailability. These factors are associated with a predictable dose-response relationship and, combined with the ease of administration (once or twice daily S.C. dosing regimens) and lower rates of heparin-induced thrombocytopenia, have increased investigators' interest in low-molecular-weight heparins in preference to unfractionated heparin for the treatment of myocardial infarction. The results of four large randomized trials comparing three different low-molecular-weight heparins with unfractionated heparin have suggested that low-molecular-weight heparin is at least as effective in reducing ischemic events in patients with NSTEMI acute coronary syndromes. Following patients with STEMI, the second trial of Heparin and Aspirin Reperfusion Therapy (HART II) and the Acute Myocardial Infarction–Streptokinase (AMI-SK) trial demonstrated evidence of improved rates of reperfusion when the low-molecular-weight heparin enoxaparin was combined with t-PA or streptokinase, respectively.[97,98] The ASSENT-3 trial compared three regimens: full-dose tenecteplase and enoxaparin, full-dose tenecteplase and unfractionated heparin, and half-dose tenecteplase and abciximab for the treatment of thrombolytic-eligible STEMI; the study revealed that enoxaparin fared better than unfractionated heparin in terms of 30-day mortality, in-hospital reinfarction, and in-hospital refractory ischemia ($P = 0.0001$) at 30 days.[99] However, at 1 year, the benefits had diminished, and the mortality with enoxaparin was identical to that with unfractionated heparin. In addition, when the data from ASSENT-3 and ASSENT-3–PLUS (a study examining the administration of tenecteplase with enoxaparin in the prehospital setting) were pooled, a marked and prohibitive increase in the risk of intracerebral hemorrhage was seen in the elderly.[66,99] As a result, ongoing trials utilizing enoxaparin with a fibrinolytic agent have adjusted the dose of enoxaparin downward in elderly patients. At present, the adjunctive anticoagulant that should be administered with fibrinolytic therapy and its optimal dose are not known.

DIRECT THROMBIN INHIBITORS

Direct thrombin inhibitors are an attractive alternative to indirect thrombin inhibitors, such as heparin or low-molecular-weight heparins, particularly because they block both circulating and clot-bound thrombin. A collaborative meta-analysis of phase-3 trials of direct thrombin inhibitors for the treatment of acute coronary artery syndromes demonstrated superiority over unfractionated heparin for the prevention of the composite end point of death or myocardial infarction.[100] The Hirulog and Early Reperfusion or Occlusion (HERO)–2 trial demonstrated a similar benefit in a comparison of bivalirudin with heparin in patients with STEMI.[101] Bivalirudin was associated with a 30% reduction in the incidence of reinfarction, but mortality did not decrease; however, the bivalirudin arm of the study exhibited a trend toward more bleeding events.

BETA BLOCKERS

The 2004 ACC/AHA guidelines recommended that oral beta blockers be administered to all STEMI patients for whom treatment is not contraindicated, irrespective of whether they are undergoing fibrinolytic therapy or primary PCI.[31] Early administration of beta blockers is recommended because it may reduce infarct size by reducing heart rate, blood pressure, and myocardial contractility, all of which diminish myocardial oxygen demand. Meta-analysis of the effects of early administration of I.V. beta blockers in 27,486 patients with acute myocardial infarction enrolled in 28 randomized trials revealed a 14% reduction in mortality during the first week of therapy; reinfarction was reduced by 18%.[102]

The TIMI-II study compared immediate beta-blocker therapy with deferred beta-blocker therapy in acute myocardial infarction; all patients also received I.V. t-PA.[103] Results indicated that immediate beta-blocker therapy reduced the incidence of nonfatal reinfarction and recurrent ischemia, compared with oral metoprolol therapy begun on the sixth hospital day; as in earlier studies, only about 40% of patients with acute myocardial infarction were eligible for acute beta-blocker therapy.[43] There are also data suggesting that immediate beta-blocker

therapy reduces the risk of intracranial hemorrhage after lytic therapy.[104]

In patients in whom contraindications preclude early beta-blocker therapy, reevaluation should take place before discharge. Many patients will no longer have contraindications at the time of discharge. Patients without contraindications should be routinely started on beta-blocker therapy before discharge from the hospital. The optimal duration of benefit remains unclear, but it appears that the benefit of beta-blocker therapy is maintained for years. Patients with the largest infarctions benefit the most from the use of beta blockers. Current recommendations are that beta-blocker therapy be continued indefinitely in the absence of contraindications or side effects.

ANGIOTENSIN-CONVERTING ENZYME INHIBITORS

Several large randomized, controlled clinical trials evaluating the use of angiotensin-converting enzyme (ACE) inhibitors early after acute myocardial infarction have been performed; all but one trial revealed a significant reduction in mortality. Meta-analysis of these large trials and many smaller trials, which together included over 100,000 patients, suggested a 6.5% reduction in deaths, with an absolute reduction in mortality of 4.6 deaths per 1,000 patients among those treated with an ACE inhibitor.[105] All patients with significant ventricular dysfunction (an ejection fraction < 40%) without contraindications should be treated with an ACE inhibitor; treatment should begin within the first 48 hours of infarction and be increased cautiously to avoid hypotension. If hypotension results from the early administration of ACE inhibitors, short-term mortality may be increased.[106]

The benefit of ACE inhibitors is clear in patients with large anterior infarctions and an ejection fraction less than 40%; whether patients with an ejection fraction greater than 40% benefit from ACE inhibitor therapy is less clear. However, the results of two large trials suggest that patients with a normal ejection fraction after myocardial infarction, as well as even patients with coronary artery disease without a previous myocardial infarction, have a reduction in mortality when treated with an ACE inhibitor. In the Heart Outcomes Prevention Evaluation (HOPE) study, 9,297 patients 55 years of age or older with vascular disease (or with diabetes and another cardiovascular risk factor) without a low ejection fraction or congestive heart failure were randomly assigned to receive either the ACE inhibitor ramipril or placebo for a mean of 5 years.[107] The reduction in the combined end point of death from cardiovascular causes, myocardial infarction, or stroke with ramipril was remarkable; it occurred in 17.7% of placebo-treated patients versus 14.1% of patients receiving ramipril (relative risk, 0.78; 95% confidence interval, 0.70 to 0.86; $P < 0.001$). A statistically significant reduction was also present in the individual end points of cardiovascular death, myocardial infarction, and stroke. The study was stopped prematurely by the Data Safety Monitoring Board when clear evidence of a beneficial effect of ramipril was found. These findings are supported by the results of the European Trial on Reduction of Cardiac Events with Perindopril in Patients with Stable Coronary Artery Disease (EUROPA) trial, which randomized 12,218 patients with stable coronary artery disease and no evidence of congestive heart failure to 8 mg of perindopril or conventional therapy.[108] Treatment with perindopril was associated with a highly statistically significant reduction in the incidence of fatal and nonfatal myocardial infarction at 4 years. Whether these favorable results are unique to tissue-specific ACE inhibitors or represent a class effect is unknown.

INTRAVENOUS NITROGLYCERIN

Randomized studies examining the role of I.V. nitroglycerin in acute myocardial infarction revealed beneficial effects on left ventricular function and a reduction in infarct size and mortality.[109] However, these studies were small and were performed before the reperfusion era. To determine whether nitroglycerin therapy is beneficial in patients treated with reperfusion, 58,050 patients with acute myocardial infarction in the fourth International Study of Infarct Survival (ISIS-4) were randomized to receive either oral controlled-release mononitrate therapy or placebo; thrombolytic therapy was administered to patients in both groups.[105] The results of this study revealed no benefit to the routine administration of oral nitrate therapy in this setting. Similar results were seen among 19,000 patients in the third Gruppo Italiano per lo Studio della Sopravvivenza nell'Infarto Miocardico (GISSI-3) study, in whom I.V. nitroglycerin was administered for the first 24 hours, followed by transdermal nitrates.[110] Whether these disappointing results in the ISIS-4 and GISSI-3 trials were caused by the routes of administration of the nitroglycerin preparation or the administration of thrombolytic therapy is unknown. However, on the basis of existing data, it does not appear that the routine administration of nitroglycerin to patients receiving early thrombolytic therapy is beneficial. I.V. nitroglycerin is probably most likely to be beneficial in patients with persistent or recurrent chest pain after reperfusion therapy and in patients in whom reperfusion therapy is not administered.

PROPHYLACTIC ANTIARRHYTHMIC THERAPY

Previously, routine prophylactic antiarrhythmic therapy with I.V. lidocaine was recommended for all patients in the early stages of acute myocardial infarction. However, studies have revealed that prophylactic therapy with lidocaine does not reduce and may actually increase mortality because of an increase in the occurrence of fatal bradyarrhythmia and asystole.[111] Neither I.V. lidocaine nor other antiarrhythmic agents are recommended as prophylactic therapy for patients without malignant ventricular ectopy.[111,112]

STATIN THERAPY

Statin therapy in the early management of acute myocardial infarction is under investigation; current evidence indicates such therapy may be beneficial. A study of more than 300,000 patients in the National Registry of Myocardial Infarction found that statin use within the first 24 hours of admission for acute myocardial infarction was associated with a significantly lower rate of early complications and in-hospital mortality.[113] Statin therapy in the follow-up management of acute myocardial infarction is recommended.[31,114,115] The 2004 ACC/AHA gave a class I recommendation to the initiation of statin therapy prior to hospital discharge in all STEMI patients [see Secondary Prevention, below].[31,114,115]

CALCIUM CHANNEL ANTAGONISTS

Calcium channel antagonists should not be routinely administered for acute myocardial infarction. Calcium channel antagonists have been studied in prospective, double-blind, placebo-controlled trials; and neither verapamil,[116,117] nifedipine,[118,119] nor diltiazem[120] appears to reduce postinfarction mortality. Verapamil and diltiazem may be useful in patients with preserved left ventricular function and no heart failure in whom contraindications to beta blockers exist.[121,122] However, the data are insufficient to recommend the routine administration of these agents. On the basis of existing data, treatment with calcium channel blockers should be reserved for patients with ischemia that persists despite use of aspirin, beta blockers, nitrate therapy, and I.V. heparin and for patients with other indications for their administration.

MAGNESIUM

Magnesium has been studied in many prospective, randomized trials of acute myocardial infarction, and the results have been conflicting. Magnesium is involved in hundreds of enzymatic steps and produces systemic and coronary vasodilatation, inhibits platelet function, and reduces reperfusion injury. Meta-analysis of seven prospective, randomized trials revealed a significant reduction in mortality with the use of magnesium (odds ratio, 0.44; confidence interval, 0.27 to 0.71).[123] In ISIS-4, in which 58,050 patients were randomized to receive either I.V. magnesium or no magnesium, there was no reduction in 30-day mortality.[105] It is possible that the later administration of magnesium in this study, compared with the previous studies, and the concomitant use of thrombolytic therapy in 70% of patients contributed to the lack of efficacy of magnesium in ISIS-4; only one third of patients in the LIMIT-2 study received thrombolytic therapy. Therefore, on the basis of the existing evidence, current recommendations are that magnesium not be routinely given to patients in whom reperfusion therapy is administered. It is possible that magnesium is of benefit, particularly in patients not receiving reperfusion therapy. Magnesium is clearly indicated in patients with myocardial infarction who have torsade de pointes–type ventricular tachycardia and in patients with magnesium deficiency.

Complications of Acute Myocardial Infarction

VENTRICULAR ARRHYTHMIAS

Ventricular arrhythmias are a frequent cause of death in the earliest stages of acute myocardial infarction. The development of coronary care units, continuous ECG surveillance, and defibrillators in the 1960s led to a reduction in mortality from acute myocardial infarction through the prompt identification and treatment of ventricular arrhythmia; and emergency medical technicians have reduced outpatient mortality in the earliest minutes of myocardial infarction. In cities with well-developed emergency response systems, such as Seattle, Washington, and Rochester, Minnesota, where the average response time is less than 5 minutes, survival of patients with myocardial infarction complicated by cardiac arrest has increased.[4] In fact, long-term survival of patients who have undergone rapid defibrillation after out-of-hospital cardiac arrest is similar to that of age-, sex-, and disease-matched patients who did not have out-of-hospital cardiac arrest; the quality of life of the majority of survivors is similar to that of the general population.[124]

Ventricular Fibrillation

In the setting of acute myocardial infarction, ventricular fibrillation is often described as either primary, when it occurs in the absence of hypotension or heart failure, or secondary, when hypotension or heart failure is present. Primary ventricular fibrillation occurs in approximately 3% to 5% of patients with acute myocardial infarction; the peak incidence is in the first 4 hours of infarction. Primary ventricular fibrillation is infrequent more than 24 hours after symptom onset. Mortality is increased in patients who suffer this complication.[125,126] In patients who are successfully resuscitated and survive to hospital discharge, however, the long-term prognosis does not appear to be affected.[125] Although lidocaine was shown to reduce the occurrence of primary ventricular fibrillation, mortality in patients receiving lidocaine increased because of an increase in fatal bradycardia and asystole; therefore, prophylactic lidocaine is no longer recommended if defibrillation can rapidly be performed.[111] Beta blockers may reduce the early occurrence of ventricular fibrillation and should be administered to patients who have no contraindications.

Hypokalemia is a risk factor for primary ventricular fibrillation and should be rapidly corrected if present. When ventricular fibrillation occurs, rapid defibrillation with 200 to 300 joules should be attempted, and repeated shocks of 360 joules should be administered. The Advanced Cardiac Life Support (ACLS) guidelines recommend medical therapy, including epinephrine, lidocaine, and bretylium; in addition, I.V. amiodarone should be considered in patients in whom defibrillation is initially unsuccessful.

Secondary ventricular fibrillation is associated with a high mortality, in part because of the underlying hypotension and heart failure. Treatment must be aimed not only at terminating the arrhythmia but also at treating the hemodynamic abnormalities and their causes.

Ventricular Tachycardia

Ventricular tachycardia (three or more consecutive ventricular ectopic beats) is common in patients with acute myocardial infarction; however, short runs of nonsustained ventricular tachycardia are no longer believed to predispose a patient to sustained ventricular tachycardia or ventricular fibrillation. In patients in whom sustained or hemodynamically significant ventricular tachycardia occurs, prompt electrical cardioversion should be performed. If the ventricular tachycardia is monomorphic, synchronic cardioversion with 100 joules should first be attempted. As with ventricular fibrillation, polymorphic ventricular tachycardia should be treated with unsynchronized discharge. Prolonged runs of asymptomatic ventricular tachycardia can be initially treated with I.V. lidocaine, procainamide, or amiodarone. These medications may also be helpful in reducing recurrent ventricular tachycardia.

ATRIAL ARRHYTHMIA

Atrial Fibrillation

Atrial fibrillation is the most common atrial arrhythmia in acute myocardial infarction, occurring in 10% to 16% of patients. Atrial fibrillation may result either from an acute increase in left atrial pressure caused by left ventricular dysfunction or from atrial ischemia as a result of occlusion of a coronary artery (usually the right coronary artery) proximal to the origin of atrial branches. The incidence of atrial fibrillation is decreased in patients given thrombolytic therapy.[56]

The treatment of atrial fibrillation in acute myocardial infarction should be similar to the treatment of atrial fibrillation in other settings. When there is hemodynamic compromise caused by loss of atrial systole or a rapid ventricular response with a reduction in cardiac output, cardioversion should be performed immediately. In patients with preserved left ventricular function in whom the atrial fibrillation is well tolerated, beta-blocker therapy is indicated. Verapamil and diltiazem may also be effective in such patients. In patients with congestive heart failure, digoxin is a reasonable alternative and may slow the ventricular response. If

atrial fibrillation recurs, antiarrhythmic agents may be used, although their impact on clinical outcomes is unproved. The Atrial Fibrillation Follow-up Investigation of Rhythm Management (AFFIRM) investigators randomized 4,060 patients to either rhythm-control or rate-control treatment strategies.[127] The rhythm-control strategy achieved no survival advantage over the rate-control strategy and there were both fewer hospital admissions and fewer adverse drug reactions in the rate-control group.

BRADYARRHYTHMIAS AND HEART BLOCK

Sinus bradycardia is common in acute myocardial infarction, particularly in patients with inferior myocardial infarction. However, treatment with atropine and a temporary pacemaker is required infrequently and, generally, only in patients with significant hemodynamic compromise manifested by increased angina, hypotension, or congestive heart failure.

High-degree (second- or third-degree) heart block occurs in approximately 20% of patients with inferior infarction; it is uncommon with infarction at other sites.[128] About half of the cases of heart block seen with inferior infarction are Wenckebach-type second-degree heart block; the remainder are cases of third-degree heart block. The heart block is often easily treated with atropine, but a temporary pacemaker is required in as many as 50% of cases. The heart block generally lasts for hours to days; placement of a permanent pacemaker is needed in fewer than 1% of cases. However, the development of heart block with inferior infarction is associated with a threefold to fourfold increase in in-hospital mortality over inferior infarction without heart block.[128,129] The increased mortality appears to result from the association between heart block and more severe left and right ventricular infarction rather than from the heart block itself or treatment of the heart block.

Heart block during anterior infarction is uncommon, occurring in fewer than 1% of cases. It is generally associated with extensive left ventricular myocardial infarction involving the conduction system below the atrioventricular node and carries a very poor prognosis.

MITRAL REGURGITATION

Mitral regurgitation may result from injury to any of the components of the mitral valve apparatus, including the papillary muscles and ventricular walls to which they attach. Mild mitral regurgitation is common in acute myocardial infarction and is present in nearly 50% of patients. Severe mitral regurgitation caused by acute myocardial infarction is rare and generally results from partial or complete rupture of a papillary muscle. The characteristic murmur of severe chronic mitral regurgitation may not be present with acute rupture of a papillary muscle. Instead, a decrescendo systolic murmur is often present, extending less throughout systole as systemic arterial pressure falls and left arterial pressure rises. In many cases, the significance of the murmur is not recognized. The blood supply of the anterior papillary muscle arises from branches of both the left anterior descending and the circumflex arteries; therefore, rupture of the anterior papillary muscle is rare. However, the posterior papillary muscle receives blood only from the dominant coronary artery (the right coronary artery in nearly 90% of patients); thrombotic occlusion of this artery may cause rupture of the posterior papillary muscle, resulting in severe mitral regurgitation. Severe mitral regurgitation is 10 times more likely to occur with inferior infarction than with anterior infarction. Acute severe mitral regurgitation is poorly tolerated and generally results in pulmonary edema, often with cardiogenic shock. Prompt surgical repair is recommended. Although the mortality associated with mitral valve surgery is high in this setting, approaching 50%, survival appears to be greater than with medical therapy alone. Therapy aimed at reducing left ventricular afterload, such as use of I.V. nitroprusside and an intra-aortic balloon pump, reduces the regurgitant volume and increases forward blood flow and cardiac output and may be helpful as a temporizing measure.

VENTRICULAR SEPTAL DEFECTS

Ventricular septal defects are slightly more frequent in patients with anterior infarction than in patients with inferior infarction. The characteristic holosystolic murmur of ventricular septal defects may be difficult to distinguish from that of severe mitral regurgitation; however, ventricular septal defects are generally better tolerated and less frequently result in severe congestive heart failure. Surgical repair is recommended and results in the best outcome when repaired emergently in the hemodynamically compromised patient. As with acute severe mitral regurgitation, therapy aimed at reducing afterload, including I.V. nitroprusside and an intra-aortic balloon pump, may be beneficial. Repair of the septum is generally more difficult when associated with inferior infarction, because there may not be a viable rim of myocardial tissue beneath the defect to facilitate repair. The surgical mortality associated with repair of a postinfarction ventricular septal defect is approximately 20% but is largely related to the age of the patient, whether cardiogenic shock is present, the infarction site, and the severity of the underlying coronary artery disease.

MYOCARDIAL RUPTURE

As more and more patients survive the acute phase of myocardial infarction because reperfusion therapy reduces myocardial infarct size, myocardial rupture has increased in frequency as a cause of early death. Myocardial rupture has been reported to account for more than 20% of in-hospital deaths in some series in the thrombolytic era. Physicians must have a heightened awareness of the diagnosis if a patient is to survive this catastrophic occurrence, because emergency surgery is required. Symptoms suggestive of rupture include repetitive vomiting, pleuritic chest pain, restlessness, and agitation. ECG evidence of rupture includes a deviation from the normal pattern of ST segment and T wave evolution. Resolution of ST segment elevation and T wave inversion, with maximal T wave negativity in the leads with maximal ST segment elevation, should normally occur; however, in patients with rupture, there is progressive or recurrent ST segment elevation and persistently positive T wave deflections or reversal of initially inverted T waves.[130] Echocardiography can quickly confirm the diagnosis. Even when emergency surgery is performed, fewer than 50% of patients survive to discharge.

RIGHT VENTRICULAR INFARCTION

Right ventricular infarction occurs in approximately one third of patients with acute inferior left ventricular infarction and is hemodynamically significant in approximately 50% of affected patients.[131] Hemodynamically significant right ventricular infarction associated with anterior infarction or isolated right ventricular infarction is rare. The classic findings associated with hemodynamically significant right ventricular infarction are hypotension with clear lung fields and an elevated jugular venous pressure, often with the Kussmaul sign. Although nearly all patients with right ventricular infarction suffer both right and left ventricular infarc-

tion, the characteristic hemodynamic findings of right ventricular infarction generally dominate the clinical course and must be the main focus of therapy. Right ventricular involvement during inferior myocardial infarction is associated with a significant increase in mortality, and aggressive attempts at early reperfusion should be pursued.[128,131] Prompt recognition of right ventricular involvement is clinically important because therapy that reduces right ventricular filling, such as use of nitrates or diuretics, should be avoided. Volume therapy should be administered to maintain cardiac output; in patients whose hypotension is refractory to volume therapy, dopamine may be beneficial. Heart block, which occurs in as many as 50% of patients with right ventricular infarction, should be treated rapidly, and maintenance of atrioventricular synchrony with dual atrial and ventricular pacing is often required to maintain filling of the ischemic noncompliant right ventricle and an adequate cardiac output.

Cardiogenic shock resulting from right ventricular infarction is generally reversible with these measures. Improvement in right ventricular function generally occurs over time, particularly in patients in whom reperfusion therapy was successful in achieving vessel patency.[125] In patients who survive the initial hospitalization, left ventricular function is the most potent predictor of long-term outcome.

STROKE

Extensive infarction of the anterior wall and apex of the left ventricle leads to thrombus formation in the apex of the left ventricle in approximately 30% of patients; systemic embolization occurs in about 15% of these patients. Left ventricular thrombus formation is much less common after inferior infarction. The thrombus generally appears within the first several days after infarction; it is more likely to embolize and cause stroke if it is pedunculated, protrudes into the left ventricular cavity, or is mobile. Left ventricular thrombus is an indication for anticoagulation with I.V. heparin, followed by warfarin therapy for 3 to 6 months.

Therapy that reduces infarct size, such as thrombolytic therapy, reduces the frequency of thrombus formation and therefore the risk of systemic embolization and stroke. However, in 0.3% to 1.0% of patients, thrombolytic therapy causes hemorrhagic stroke, most commonly in the 24 hours after its administration, which is fatal in more than 50% of cases. Hemorrhagic stroke is rare in acute myocardial infarction except as a consequence of thrombolytic therapy, although an ischemic stroke may become hemorrhagic because of thrombolytic, antiplatelet, and anticoagulation therapy. Hemorrhagic stroke, the most feared complication of thrombolytic therapy, is more likely in elderly patients; in patients with low body weight, with hypertension, or who have previously had a stroke; and in those on warfarin.[53,59] Although thrombolytic therapy decreases the risk of ischemic stroke, there is a slight net increase in the overall risk of stroke because of the risk of hemorrhagic stroke. Primary coronary angioplasty is believed to reduce the incidence of ischemic stroke without increasing the risk of hemorrhagic stroke.

Predischarge Exercise Testing

In patients with spontaneous postinfarction angina, congestive heart failure, hypotension, or malignant ventricular arrhythmia, exercise testing should generally be deferred and coronary angiography should be performed. However, in patients without these high-risk characteristics, exercise testing is generally recommended before discharge from the hospital to assess a patient's functional capacity and ability to return to activities of daily living and work.[132] Most data indicating that predischarge exercise testing can identify patients at increased risk for cardiac events after discharge are from the prethrombolytic era, when the risk of adverse cardiac events was much higher. In the modern era, in which thrombolytic therapy or primary coronary angioplasty is frequently performed and in which aspirin, beta blockers, ACE inhibitors, and lipid-lowering agents are routinely administered—all of which reduce the frequency of adverse events in the years after discharge—it is difficult to identify patients at risk, because the adverse event rate is so low. Nonetheless, exercise testing is generally recommended to provide a measure of comfort to both the patient and the physician, to help determine the appropriateness of medical therapy, and to facilitate entry of the patient into a cardiac rehabilitation program.

Although predischarge exercise testing has been the standard of care in the United States for some time, only recently has a study examined whether therapy based on the results of a predischarge exercise test improves clinical outcome. The Danish Trial in Acute Myocardial Infarction (DANAMI) was the first study to examine the usefulness of exercise testing in patients treated with thrombolytic agents (a low-risk group) and to provide support for what has been the standard of care in the United States [see Figure 11].[133] The results of this study revealed that clinical outcome was improved in patients who received angiography and coronary angioplasty, compared with those who received medical therapy alone. Use of the results of exercise testing to decide whether or not to employ revascularization in patients without spontaneous angina is less common outside of the United States.

Patients with acute myocardial infarction who do not receive thrombolytic therapy or do not undergo primary angioplasty are at greater risk for adverse events after discharge from the hospital, and predischarge exercise testing is of even greater utility in such patients.

Prognostic variables indicating increased risk during exercise testing are exercise-induced angina or ST segment depression, particularly when it occurs during exercise at a low work load, and an abnormal drop in systolic blood pressure. However, electrocardiographic, symptomatic, and scintigraphic risk markers of ischemia (e.g., ST segment depression, angina, or a reversible perfusion defect) are less sensitive for identifying morbid and fatal outcomes than markers of left ventricular dysfunction or heart failure (e.g., exercise duration, impaired systolic blood pressure response, and peak left ventricular ejection fraction).[134] The patients at greatest risk are those unable to exercise; such patients have the highest mortality after discharge.[135]

The type of exercise test that should be performed has been the subject of controversy. It is generally recommended that only simple treadmill testing be performed before discharge; in patients with abnormalities in the baseline ECG, stress testing with perfusion imaging or stress echocardiography may be helpful. In patients without widespread abnormalities on the ECG, perfusion imaging or stress echocardiography is generally deferred until at least 4 weeks after discharge, when a more vigorous exercise test can be performed. Whether the predischarge treadmill test should be a low-level test or a more vigorous symptom-limited test is unclear. It has been shown that a symptom-limited Bruce protocol exercise test detects ischemia more frequently than a submaximal test; however, it is not known which test has the greater positive and greater negative predictive value for identifying patients at risk. Currently, a lower-level exercise test

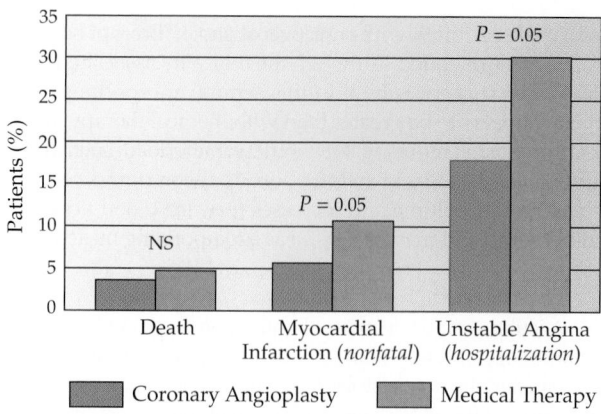

Figure 11   In the Danish Acute Myocardial Infarction (DANAMI) study, 1,008 patients treated with thrombolytic therapy in whom exercise-induced ischemia was present on a predischarge exercise test were randomized to receive either coronary angioplasty or medical therapy alone. Clinical outcome was improved in patients in the invasive arm of the study. (NS—not significant)

is preferred, although a more vigorous test may be appropriate in patients likely to resume a more active and vigorous lifestyle shortly after discharge and in whom a low-level test may not cause the patient to expend the amount of energy he or she will be using during activities of daily living.

There has been concern that the use of beta blockers before the predischarge exercise test may mask the presence of significant coronary artery disease and prevent the identification of high-risk patients. This concern does not appear to be significant enough to outweigh the benefits of early beta-blocker therapy.

Secondary Prevention

PHARMACOTHERAPY

Lipid-Lowering Therapy

Recent studies have demonstrated that in patients with coronary artery disease, lipid-lowering therapy with HMG-CoA (3-hydroxy-3-methylglutaryl coenzyme A) reductase inhibitors reduces not only fatal and nonfatal infarction but also mortality from all causes. The Scandinavian Simvastatin Survival Study revealed a 42% reduction in cardiac mortality and a 30% reduction in all-cause mortality in 4,444 men and women with coronary artery disease over the 5.4 years of the study.[136] The reductions in mortality were similar in patients in the lowest and those in the highest quartiles of serum low-density lipoprotein (LDL) cholesterol. It has been demonstrated that postinfarction patients with an LDL cholesterol level at or above 130 mg/dl benefit from lipid-lowering therapy within as little as 2 years after the initiation of such therapy.[137] Initial measurement of cholesterol should be made within 24 hours after myocardial infarction; measurement of lipids 24 hours or more after myocardial infarction can be misleading in that cholesterol levels may be reduced below baseline levels during this period and remain low for up to 1 month. Early initiation of statins may be more beneficial than later initiation.[138] Exercise, weight reduction in overweight patients, avoidance of dietary saturated fat and cholesterol, and smoking cessation have all been reported to favorably influence blood lipid levels and should be recommended whether or not lipid-lowering medications are prescribed [*see Chapters 3 and 4*].

Anticoagulation Therapy

Several prospective, randomized trials revealed that warfarin therapy reduces mortality after discharge from the hospital in patients with acute myocardial infarction. However, in these studies, in which warfarin therapy was compared with placebo, aspirin was not administered in either arm of the study.[139,140] The Coumadin Aspirin Reinfarction Study (CARS) revealed that the risk of reinfarction in patients treated with aspirin alone was similar to that in patients treated with aspirin and either low-dose (1 mg) or higher-dose (3 mg) warfarin.[141] Warfarin is also ineffective at preventing coronary reocclusion in patients in whom thrombolytic therapy was successful.[142] The routine administration of warfarin is not currently recommended to prevent reinfarction in patients who have survived myocardial infarction.

Antiarrhythmic Therapy

Although Holter monitoring before discharge can help identify patients at increased risk for sudden cardiac death, antiarrhythmic therapy has not been shown to decrease the risk of death in such patients, and in fact, it increased mortality in the Cardiac Arrhythmia Suppression Trial (CAST).[143] Since CAST, several prospective, randomized studies have been performed that have examined the role of amiodarone in patients at increased risk for sudden death. Taken together, the results of those studies do not indicate that amiodarone reduces mortality. Further studies are needed before the routine use of amiodarone can be recommended in high-risk patients, such as those included in these trials.

Automated, Implantable Cardioverter-Defibrillator

Automated implantable cardioverter-defibrillators are of proven benefit in patients with coronary artery disease, reduced left ventricular ejection fraction, nonsustained ventricular tachycardia, and inducible ventricular tachycardia.[144] It has been proposed that patients with a prior myocardial infarction and advanced left ventricular dysfunction may benefit from prophylactic implantation of a defibrillator (in the absence of electrophysiologic testing to induce arrhythmias). The Multicenter Automatic Defibrillator Implantation Trial (MADIT)–II investigators randomized 1,232 patients with a prior myocardial infarction and a left ventricular ejection fraction of 0.30 or less to an implantable defibrillator or conventional medical therapy. During an average follow-up of 20 months, the mortality rates were 19.8% in the conventional-therapy group and 14.2% in the defibrillator group (*P* = 0.016). Prophylactic implantation of a defibrillator is a recommended therapy in this patient population.[145]

RISK-FACTOR MODIFICATION

An important and often neglected aspect of medical care after a myocardial infarction is the identification and modification of risk factors for atherosclerosis. Hypertension and hypercholesterolemia should be treated. Cessation of smoking [*see Chapter 3*] has been shown to prolong life in patients who have survived a myocardial infarction; behavior modification and group therapy can increase the likelihood of kicking the habit. Cardiac rehabilitation and the establishment of a healthier lifestyle with an exercise program[146] [*see Chapter 4*] can further reduce the likelihood of

a return to smoking. Hypercholesterolemia should be aggressively treated as described above.

Although there are few data that conclusively indicate that patients who participate in a cardiac rehabilitation program after discharge have increased survival, an exercise rehabilitation program appears to improve a patient's sense of well-being and hasten return to work and leisure activities. A cardiac rehabilitation program can also help improve diet and aid weight reduction in overweight patients, help smokers refrain from smoking, and help establish an exercise program that the patient can maintain long after the formal rehabilitation program has ended. In summary, participation in a cardiac rehabilitation program often leads to the establishment of a healthier lifestyle.

Long-term Prognosis

Long-term prognosis after myocardial infarction is determined primarily by the severity of left ventricular dysfunction, the presence and degree of residual ischemia, and the potential for malignant ventricular arrhythmia. These adverse prognostic factors are related to each other but are also independently associated with death after discharge. Age is also an important determinant of outcome. Most deaths that occur in the first year after discharge occur in the first 3 months, a fact that stresses the importance of assessing risk and optimizing therapy before discharge from the hospital. However, there can be substantial improvement in ventricular function in the weeks and months after acute myocardial infarction, particularly in patients in whom early reperfusion was achieved. Therefore, measurement of ventricular function 2 to 3 months after myocardial infarction is a more accurate predictor of long-term prognosis than measurement of left ventricular function in the acute stages.

The authors have no commercial relationships with manufacturers of products or providers of services discussed in this chapter.

References

1. Rogers WJ, Canto JG, Lambrew CT, et al: Temporal trends in the treatment of over 1.5 million patients with myocardial infarction in the U.S. from 1990 through 1999: the National Registry of Myocardial Infarction 1, 2 and 3. J Am Coll Cardiol 36:2056, 2000

2. Eagle KA, Goodman SG, Avezum A, et al: Practice variation and missed opportunities for reperfusion in ST-segment-elevation myocardial infarction: Findings from the Global Registry of Acute Coronary Events (GRACE). Lancet 359:373, 2002

3. Mortality from coronary heart disease and acute myocardial infarction—United States, 1998. MMWR Morb Mortal Wkly Rep 50:90, 2001

4. Patient/bystander recognition and action: rapid identification and treatment of acute myocardial infarction (NIH Publication No 93-3303). National Heart Attack Alert Program (NHAAP). National Heart, Lung, and Blood Institute. National Institutes of Health, Bethesda, Maryland, 1993

5. Fuster V: Lewis A. Conner Memorial Lecture. Mechanisms leading to myocardial infarction: insights from studies of vascular biology. Circulation 90:2126, 1994

6. Libby P: Molecular bases of the acute coronary syndromes. Circulation 91:2844, 1995

7. Libby P: Current concepts of the pathogenesis of the acute coronary syndromes. Circulation 104:365, 2001

8. Ambrose JA, Tannenbaum MA, Alexopoulos D, et al: Angiographic progression of coronary artery disease and the development of myocardial infarction. J Am Coll Cardiol 12:56, 1988

9. Tunstall-Pedoe H, Kuulasmaa K, Amouyel P, et al: Myocardial infarction and coronary deaths in the World Health Organization MONICA Project. Circulation 90:583, 1994

10. Myocardial infarction redefined: a consensus document of The Joint European Society of Cardiology/American College of Cardiology Committee for the Redefinition of Myocardial Infarction. J Am Coll Cardiol 36:959, 2000

11. Aronow WS: Prevalence of presenting symptoms of recognized acute myocardial infarction and of unrecognized healed myocardial infarction in elderly patients. Am J Cardiol 60:1182, 1987

12. Kouvaras G, Bacoulas G: Unstable angina as a warning symptom before acute myocardial infarction. Q J Med 64:679, 1987

13. Kannel WB, Abbott RD: Incidence and prognosis of unrecognized myocardial infarction: an update on the Framingham study. N Engl J Med 311:1144, 1984

14. Karlson BW, Herlitz J, Edvardsson N, et al: Eligibility for intravenous thrombolysis in suspected acute myocardial infarction. Circulation 82:1140, 1990

15. Grijseels EW, Deckers JW, Hoes AW, et al: Prehospital triage of patients with suspected acute myocardial infarction. Evaluation of previously developed algorithms and new proposals. Eur Heart J 16:325, 1995

16. Cragg DR, Friedman HZ, Bonema JD, et al: Outcome of patients with acute myocardial infarction who are ineligible for thrombolytic therapy. Ann Intern Med 115:173, 1991

17. Randomised trial of intravenous streptokinase, oral aspirin, both, or neither among 17,187 cases of suspected acute myocardial infarction: ISIS-2. Second International Study of Infarct Survival Collaborative Group. Lancet 2:349, 1988

18. Roberts R, Kleinman N: Earlier diagnosis and treatment of acute myocardial infarction necessitates the need for a "new diagnostic mind-set." Circulation 89:872, 1994

19. Zabel M, Hohnloser SH, Koster W, et al: Analysis of creatine kinase, CK-MB, myoglobin, and troponin T time-activity curves for early assessment of coronary artery reperfusion after intravenous thrombolysis. Circulation 87:1542, 1993

20. Ohman EM, Armstrong P, Califf RM, et al: Risk stratification in acute ischemic syndromes using serum troponin T. The GUSTO Investigators. J Am Coll Cardiol 25(suppl):148A, 1995

21. Ravkilde J, Nissen H, Horder M, et al: Independent prognostic value of serum creatine kinase isoenzyme MB mass, cardiac troponin T and myosin light chain levels in suspected acute myocardial infarction: analysis of 28 months of follow-up in 196 patients. J Am Coll Cardiol 25:574, 1995

22. Hauser AM, Gangadharan V, Ramos RG, et al: Sequence of mechanical, electrocardiographic and clinical effects of repeated coronary arterial occlusion in human beings: echocardiographic observation during coronary angioplasty. J Am Coll Cardiol 5:193, 1985

23. Sabia P, Abbott RD, Afrookteh A, et al: Importance of two-dimensional echocardiographic assessment of left ventricular systolic function in patients presenting to the emergency room with cardiac-related symptoms. Circulation 84:1615, 1991

24. Fleischmann KE, Lee TH, Come PC, et al: Echocardiographic prediction of complications in patients with chest pain. Am J Cardiol 79:292, 1997

25. Talreja D, Gruver C, Sklenar J, et al: Efficient utilization of echocardiography for the assessment of left ventricular systolic function. Am Heart J 139:394, 2000

26. St John Sutton M, Pfeffer MA, Plappert T, et al: Quantitative two-dimensional echocardiographic measurements are major predictors of adverse cardiovascular events after acute myocardial infarction: the protective effects of captopril. Circulation 89:68, 1994

27. Hilton TC, Thompson RC, Williams HJ, et al: Technetium-99m sestamibi myocardial perfusion imaging in the emergency room evaluation of chest pain. J Am Coll Cardiol 23:1016, 1994

28. Duca MD, Giri S, Wu AH, et al: Comparison of acute rest myocardial perfusion imaging and serum markers of myocardial injury in patients with chest pain syndromes. J Nucl Cardiol 6:570, 1999

29. Radensky PW, Hilton TC, Fulmer H, et al: Potential cost effectiveness of initial myocardial perfusion imaging for assessment of emergency department patients with chest pain. Am J Cardiol 79:595, 1997

30. Udelson JE, Beshansky JR, Ballin DS, et al: Myocardial perfusion imaging for evaluation and triage of patients with suspected acute cardiac ischemia. JAMA 288:2693, 2002

31. Antman EM, Anbe DT, Armstrong PW, et al: ACC/AHA guidelines for the management of patients with ST-elevation myocardial infarction: executive summary: a report of the American College of Cardiology/American Heart Association Task Force on Practice Guidelines (Writing Committee to Revise the 1999 Guidelines for the Management of Patients with Acute Myocardial Infarction). Circulation 110:588, 2004

32. Secondary prevention of vascular disease by prolonged antiplatelet treatment. Antiplatelet Trialists Collaboration. Br Med J 296:320, 1988

33. Weaver WD: Time to thrombolytic treatment: factors affecting delay and their influence on outcome. J Am Coll Cardiol 25(suppl 7):3S, 1995

34. Emergency department rapid identification and treatment of patients with acute myocardial infarction. National Heart Attack Alert Program Coordinating Committee 60 minutes to Treatment Working Group. Ann Emerg Med 23:311, 1994

35. Berger PB, Ellis SG, Holmes DR Jr, et al: The relationship between delay in performing direct coronary angioplasty and early clinical outcome in patients with acute myocardial infarction: results from the global use of strategies to open occluded arteries in acute coronary syndromes (GUSTO-IIb) trial. Circulation 100:14, 1999

36. Cannon CP, Gibson CM, Lambrew CT, et al: Relationship of symptom-onset-to-balloon time and door-to-balloon time with mortality in patients undergoing angioplasty for acute myocardial infarction. JAMA 283:2941, 2000

37. Caputo RP, Ho KKL, Stoler RC, et al: Effect of continuous quality improvement on the delivery of primary percutaneous transluminal coronary angioplasty for acute myocardial infarction. Am J Cardiol 79:1159, 1997

38. Jhangiana AH, Jorgenson MB, Kotlewski A, et al: Community practice of primary angioplasty for myocardial infarction. Am J Cardiol 80:209, 1997

39. Patel S, Reese C, O'Connor RE, et al: Adverse outcomes accompanying primary angioplasty (PTCA) for acute myocardial infarction (AMI)—dangers of delay. J Am Coll Cardiol 27(suppl A):62A, 1996

40. Rosman HS, Ciolino D, Nerenz D, et al: Primary PTCA and thrombolysis for acute myocardial infarction: observations from the community. J Am Coll Cardiol 27(suppl A):26A, 1996

41. Widimsky P, Budesinsky T, Vorac D, et al: Long distance transport for primary angioplasty vs immediate thrombolysis in acute myocardial infarction. Final results of the randomized national multicentre trial—PRAGUE-2. Eur Heart J 24:94, 2003

42. Andersen HR, Nielsen TT, Rasmussen K, et al: A comparison of coronary angioplasty with fibrinolytic therapy in acute myocardial infarction. N Engl J Med 349:733, 2003

43. Immediate versus delayed catheterization and angioplasty following thrombolytic therapy for acute myocardial infarction. The TIMI Study Group. JAMA 260:2849, 1988

44. SWIFT trial of delayed elective intervention v conservative treatment after thrombolysis with anistreplase in acute myocardial infarction. SWIFT Study Group. BMJ 302:555, 1991

45. Ellis SG, Mooney MR, George BS, et al: Randomized trial of late elective angioplasty versus conservative management for patients with residual stenoses after thrombolytic treatment of myocardial infarction. Treatment of Post-Thrombolytic Stenoses (TOPS) Study Group. Circulation 86:1400, 1992

46. Zeymer U: The ALKK Trial. Oral presentation at the Late Breaking Clinical Trials Session of the 49th Annual Scientific Sessions of the American College of Cardiology, March 2000

47. Berger PB, Holmes DR Jr, Stebbins AL, et al: Impact of an aggressive invasive catheterization and revascularization strategy on mortality in patients with cardiogenic shock in the Global Utilization of Streptokinase and Tissue Plasminogen Activator for Occluded Coronary Arteries (GUSTO-I) trial: an observational study. Circulation 96:122, 1997

48. Prasad A, Mathew V, Holmes DR, et al: Current management of non-ST-segment-elevation acute coronary syndrome: reconciling the results of randomized controlled trials. Eur Heart J 24:1544, 2003

49. Effects of tissue plasminogen activator and a comparison of early invasive and conservative strategies in unstable angina and non-Q-wave myocardial infarction: results of the TIMI IIIB Trial. The TIMI IIIB Investigators. Circulation 89:1545, 1995

50. Wallentin L, Lagerqvist B, Husted S, et al: Outcome at 1 year after an invasive compared with a non-invasive strategy in unstable coronary-artery disease: the FRISC II invasive randomised trial. Lancet 356:9, 2000

51. Cannon CP, Weintraub WS, Demopolous LA, et al: Comparison of early invasive and conservative strategies in patients with unstable coronary syndromes treated with the glycoprotein IIb/IIIa inhibitor tirofiban. N Engl J Med 344:1879, 2001

52. Braunwald E, Antman EM, Beasley JW, et al: ACC/AHA 2002 guideline update for the management of patients with unstable angina and non-ST-segment elevation myocardial infarction – summary article: A report of the American College of Cardiology/American Heart Association task force on practice guidelines. J Am Coll Cardiol 40:1366, 2002

53. Indications for fibrinolytic therapy in suspected acute myocardial infarction: collaborative overview of early mortality and major morbidity results from all randomised trials of more than 1000 patients. Fibrinolytic Therapy Trialists' (FTT) Collaborative Group. Lancet 343:311, 1994

54. French JK, Hyde TA, Patel H, et al: Survival 12 years after randomization to streptokinase: the influence of thrombolysis in myocardial infarction flow at three to four weeks. J Am Coll Cardiol 34:62, 1999

55. The effects of tissue plasminogen activator, streptokinase, or both on coronary-artery patency, ventricular function, and survival after acute myocardial infarction. The GUSTO Angiographic Investigators. N Engl J Med 329:1615, 1993

56. An international randomized trial comparing four thrombolytic strategies for acute myocardial infarction. The GUSTO Investigators. N Engl J Med 329:673, 1993

57. Simes RJ, Topol EJ, Holmes DR Jr, et al: Link between the angiographic substudy and mortality outcomes in a large randomized trial of myocardial reperfusion: importance of early and complete infarct artery reperfusion. Circulation 91:1923, 1995

58. Late Assessment of Thrombolytic Efficacy (LATE) study with alteplase 6 to 24 hours after onset of acute myocardial infarction. Lancet 342:759, 1993

59. de Jaegere PP, Arnold AA, Balk AH, et al: Intracranial hemorrhage in association with thrombolytic therapy: incidence and clinical predictive factors. J Am Coll Cardiol 19:289, 1992

60. Randomised double-blind comparison of reteplase double-bolus administration with streptokinase in acute myocardial infarction (INJECT): trial to investigate the equivalent. International Joint Efficacy Comparison of Thrombolytics. Lancet 346:329, 1995

61. A comparison of reteplase with alteplase for acute myocardial infarction. The Global Use of Strategies to Open Occluded Coronary Arteries (GUSTO III) Investigators. N Engl J Med 337:1118, 1997

62. Antman EM, Giugliano RD, Gibson CM, et al: Abciximab facilitates the rate and extent of thrombolysis: results of the Thrombolysis in Myocardial Infarction (TIMI 14) Trial. Circulation 99:2720, 1999

63. Ohman EM, Lincoff AM, Bode C, et al: Enhanced early reperfusion at 60 minutes with low-dose reteplase combined with full-dose abciximab in acute myocardial infarction: preliminary results from the GUSTO-IV Pilot (SPEED) Dose-ranging Trial (abstr). Circulation 98(suppl I):I-504, 1998

64. Topol EJ: Reperfusion therapy for acute myocardial infarction with fibrinolytic therapy or combination reduced fibrinolytic therapy and platelet glycoprotein IIb/IIIa inhibition: the GUSTO V randomised trial. Lancet 357:1905, 2001

65. Assessment of the Safety and Efficacy of a New Thrombolytic regimen (ASSENT-3) Investigators. Efficacy and safety of tenecteplase in combination with enoxaparin, abciximab, or unfractionated heparin: the ASSENT-3 randomized trial of acute myocardial infarction. Lancet 358:605, 2001

66. Wallentin L, Goldstein P, Armstrong PW, et al: Efficacy and safety of tenecteplase in combination with the low-molecular-weight heparin enoxaparin or unfractionated heparin in the prehospital setting: the Assessment of the Safety and Efficacy of a New Thrombolytic Regimen (ASSENT)-3 PLUS randomized trial in acute myocardial infarc-

tion. Circulation 108:135, 2003

67. O'Neill W, Timmis G, Bourdillon P, et al: A prospective randomized clinical trial of intracoronary streptokinase versus coronary angioplasty for acute myocardial infarction. N Engl J Med 314:812, 1986

68. de Boer MJ, Hoorntje JCA, Ottervanger JP, et al: Immediate coronary angioplasty versus intravenous streptokinase in acute myocardial infarction: left ventricular ejection fraction, hospital mortality, and reinfarction. J Am Coll Cardiol 23:1004, 1994

69. de Boer MJ, Suryapranata H, Hoorntje JC, et al: Limitation of infarct size and preservation of left ventricular function after primary coronary angioplasty compared with intravenous streptokinase in acute myocardial infarction. Circulation 90:753, 1994

70. Zijlstra F, de Boer MJ, Hoorntje JCA, et al: A comparison of immediate coronary angioplasty with intravenous streptokinase in acute myocardial infarction. N Engl J Med 328:680, 1993

71. Grines CL, Browne KF, Marco J, et al: A comparison of immediate angioplasty with thrombolytic therapy for acute myocardial infarction. N Engl J Med 328:673, 1993

72. Keeley EC, Boura JA, Grines CL: Primary angioplasty versus intravenous thrombolytic therapy for acute myocardial infarction: a quantitative review of 23 randomized trials. Lancet 361:13, 2003

73. A clinical trial comparing primary coronary angioplasty with tissue plasminogen activator for acute myocardial infarction. The Global Use of Strategies to Open Occluded Coronary Arteries in Acute Coronary Syndromes (GUSTO IIb) Angioplasty Substudy Investigators. N Engl J Med 336:1621, 1997

74. Berger PB, Bell MR, Holmes DR Jr, et al: Time to reperfusion with direct coronary angioplasty and thrombolytic therapy in acute myocardial infarction. Am J Cardiol 73:231, 1994

75. Ryan TJ, Anderson JL, Antman EM, et al: ACC/AHA guidelines for the management of patients with acute myocardial infarction: a report of the American College of Cardiology/American Heart Association task force on practice guidelines (Committee of Management of Acute Myocardial Infarction). J Am Coll Cardiol 28:1328, 1996

76. Wharton TP, McNamara SN, Fedele FA, et al: Primary angioplasty for the treatment of acute myocardial infarction: experience at two community hospitals without cardiac surgery. J Am Coll Cardiol 33:1257, 1999

77. Brener SJ, Barr LA, Burchenal JE, et al: Randomized, placebo-controlled trial of platelet glycoprotein IIb/IIIa blockade with primary angioplasty for acute myocardial infarction. ReoPro and Primary PTCA Organization and Randomized Trial (RAPPORT) Investigators. Circulation 98:73, 1998

78. Neumann FJ, Blasini R, Schmitt C, et al: Effect of glycoprotein IIb/IIIa receptor blockade on recovery of coronary flow and left ventricular function after placement of coronary-artery stents in acute myocardial infarction. Circulation 98:2695, 1998

79. Montalescot G, Barragan P, Wittenberg O, et al: Platelet glycoprotein IIb/IIIa inhibition with coronary stenting for acute myocardial infarction. N Engl J Med 344:1895, 2001

80. Stone GW, Grines CL, Cox DA, et al: Comparison of angioplasty with stenting, with or without abciximab, in acute myocardial infarction. N Engl J Med 346:957, 2002

81. Grines CL, Cox DA, Stone GW, et al: Coronary angioplasty with or without stent implantation for acute myocardial infarction. Stent Primary Angioplasty in Myocardial Infarction Study Group. N Engl J Med 341:1949, 1999

82. Schomig A, Kastrati A, Dirschinger J, et al: Coronary stenting plus platelet glycoprotein IIb/IIIa blockade compared with tissue plasminogen activator in acute myocardial infarction. Stent versus Thrombolysis for Occluded Coronary Arteries in Patients with Acute Myocardial Infarction Study Investigators. N Engl J Med 343:385, 2000

83. Berger PB, Stensrud PE, Daly RC, et al: Emergency coronary artery bypass surgery following failed coronary angioplasty: time to reperfusion and other procedural characteristics. Am J Cardiol 76:565, 1995

84. Ellis SG, Ribeiro da Silva E, Heyndrickx G, et al: Randomized comparison of rescue angioplasty with conservative management of patients with early failure of thrombolysis for acute anterior myocardial infarction. Circulation 90:2280, 1994

85. Belenkie I, Traboulsi M, Hall CA, et al: Rescue angioplasty during myocardial infarction has a beneficial effect on mortality: a tenable hypothesis. Can J Cardiol 8:357, 1992

86. Widimsky P, Groh L, Ascherman M, et al: The "PRAGUE" study: a national multicenter randomized study comparing primary angioplasty vs thrombolysis vs both in patients with acute myocardial infarction admitted to the community hospitals: results of the pilot phase (abstr). Eur Heart J 19(suppl):56, 1998

87. Vermeer F, Brunninkhuis L, van de Berg E, et al: Prospective randomized comparison between thrombolysis, rescue PTCA, and primary PTCA in patients with extensive myocardial infarction admitted to a hospital without PTCA facilities: a safety and feasibility study. Heart 82:426, 1999

88. Simoons ML, Arnold AE, Betriu A, et al: Thrombolysis with tissue plasminogen activator in acute myocardial infarction: no additional benefit from immediate percutaneous coronary angioplasty. Lancet 1:197, 1988

89. Dirschinger J, Kastrati A, Neumann FJ, et al: Influence of balloon pressure during stent placement in native coronary arteries on early and late angiographic and clinical outcome: a randomized evaluation of high-pressure inflation. Circulation 100:918, 1999

90. Miller JM, Smalling R, Ohman EM, et al: Effectiveness of early coronary angioplasty and abciximab for failed thrombolysis (reteplase or alteplase) during acute myocardial infarction: results from the GUSTO-III trial. Am J Cardiol 84:779, 1989

91. Ross AM, Coyne KS, Reiner JS, et al: A randomized trial comparing primary angioplasty with a strategy of short-acting thrombolysis and immediate planned rescue angioplasty in acute myocardial infarction: the PACT trial. PACT investigators. Plasminogen-activator Angioplasty Compatibility Trial. J Am Coll Cardiol 34:1954, 1999

92. Scheller B, Hennen B, Hammer B, et al: Beneficial effects of immediate stenting after thrombolysis in acute myocardial infarction. J Am Coll Cardiol 42:634, 2003

93. Kastrati A, Mehilli J, Schlotterbeck K, et al: Early administration of reteplase plus abciximab versus abciximab alone in patients with acute myocardial infarction referred for percutaneous coronary intervention. JAMA 291:947, 2004

94. Granger CB, Hirsh J, Califf RM, et al: Activated partial thromboplastin time and outcome after thrombolytic therapy for acute myocardial infarction: results from the GUSTO-I trial. Circulation 93:870, 1996

95. Chesebro JH, Fuster V: Antithrombotic therapy for acute myocardial infarction: mechanisms and prevention of deep venous, left ventricular, and coronary artery thromboembolism. Circulation 74:1, 1986

96. Granger CB, Miller JM, Bovill EG, et al: Rebound increase in thrombin generation and activity after cessation of intravenous heparin in patients with acute coronary syndromes. Circulation 91:1929, 1995

97. Ross AM, Molhoek P, Lundergan C, et al: Randomized comparison of enoxaparin, a low-molecular-weight heparin, with unfractionated heparin adjunctive to recombinant tissue plasminogen activator thrombolysis and aspirin: second trial of Heparin and Aspirin Reperfusion Therapy (HART II). Circulation 104:648, 2001

98. Simoons M, Krzeminska-Pakula M, Alonso A, et al: Improved reperfusion and clinical outcome with enoxaparin as an adjunct to streptokinase thrombolysis in acute myocardial infarction. The AMI-SK study. Eur Heart J 23:1282, 2002

99. Assessment of the Safety and Efficacy of a New Thrombolytic Regimen (ASSENT)-3 Investigators. Efficacy and safety of tenecteplase in combination with enoxaparin, abciximab, or unfractionated heparin: the ASSENT-3 randomised trial in acute myocardial infarction. Lancet 358:605, 2001

100. Direct thrombin inhibitors in acute coronary syndromes: principal results of a meta-analysis based on individual patients' data. Direct Thrombin Inhibitor Trialists' Collaborative Group. Lancet 359:294, 2002

101. Thrombin-specific anticoagulation with bivalirudin versus heparin in patients receiving fibrinolytic therapy for acute myocardial infarction: the HERO-2 randomised trial. Hirulog and Early Reperfusion or Occlusion (HERO)-2 Trial Investigators. Lancet 358:1855, 2001

102. Gersh BJ, Rahimtoola SH: Acute myocardial infarction. Pharmacological Management of Acute Myocardial Infarction. Warnica JW, Ed. Elsevier, New York, 1991, p 205

103. Comparison of invasive and conservative strategies after treatment with intravenous tissue plasminogen activator in acute myocardial infarction: results of the Thrombolysis in Myocardial Infarction (TIMI) phase II trial. The TIMI Study Group. N Engl J Med 320:618, 1989

104. Barron HV, Rundle AC, Gore JM, et al: Intracranial hemorrhage rates and effect of immediate beta-blocker use in patients with acute myocardial infarction treated with tissue plasminogen activator. Participants in the National Registry of Myocardial Infarction–2. Am J Cardiol 85:294, 2000

105. ISIS-4: a randomised factorial trial assessing early oral captopril, oral mononitrate, and intravenous magnesium sulphate in 58,050 patients with suspected acute myocardial infarction. Fourth International Study of Infarct Survival Collaborative Group. Lancet 345:669, 1995

106. Sigurdsson A, Swedberg K: Left ventricular remodelling, neurohormonal activation and early treatment with enalapril (CONSENSUS II) following myocardial infarction. Eur Heart J 15(suppl B):14, 1994

107. Yusuf S, Sleight P, Pogue J, et al: Effects of an angiotensin-converting-enzyme inhibitor, ramipril, on cardiovascular events in high-risk patients. The Heart Outcomes Prevention Evaluation Study Investigators. N Engl J Med 342:145, 2000

108. Efficacy of perindopril in reduction of cardiovascular events among patients with stable coronary artery disease: randomised, double-blind, placebo-controlled, multicentre trial (the EUROPA study). European Trial on Reduction of Cardiac Events with Perindopril in Stable Coronary Artery Disease Investigators. Lancet 362:782, 2003

109. Judgutt BI, Warnica JW: Intravenous nitroglycerin therapy to limit myocardial infarct size, expansion, and complications: effect of timing, dosage, and infarct location. Circulation 78:906, 1988

110. GISSI-3: effects of lisinopril and transdermal glyceryl trinitrate singly and together on 6-week mortality and ventricular function after acute myocardial infarction. Gruppo Italiano per lo Studio della Sopravvivenza nell'Infarto Miocardico. Lancet 343:1115, 1994

111. MacMahon S, Collins R, Peto R, et al: Effects of prophylactic lidocaine in suspected acute myocardial infarction: an overview of results from the randomized, controlled trials. JAMA 260:1910, 1988

112. Teo KK, Yusuf S, Furberg CD: Effects of prophylactic antiarrhythmic drug therapy in acute myocardial infarction: an overview of results from randomized controlled trials. JAMA 270:1589, 1993

113. Fonarow GD, Wright RS, Spencer FA, et al: Effect of statin use within the first 24 hours of admission for acute myocardial infarction on early morbidity and mortality. Am J Cardiol 96:611, 2005

114. Schwartz GG, Olsson AG, Ezekowitz MD, et al: Effects of atorvastatin on early recurrent ischemic events in acute coronary syndromes the MIRACL study: a randomized controlled trial. JAMA 285:1711, 2001

115. Cannon CP, Braunwald E, McCabe CH, et al: Intensive versus moderate lipid lowering with statins after acute coronary syndromes. N Engl J Med 350:1495, 2004

116. Gheorghiade M: Calcium channel blockers in the management of myocardial infarction patients. Henry Ford Hosp Med J 39:210, 1991

117. Held PH, Yusuf S: Effects of beta-blockers and calcium channel blockers in acute myocardial infarction. Eur Heart J 14(suppl F):18, 1993

118. Secondary Prevention Reinfarction Israeli Nifedipine Trial (SPRINT): A randomized intervention trial of nifedipine in patients with acute myocardial infarction. The Israeli SPRINT Study Group. Eur Heart J 9:354, 1988

119. Goldbourt U, Behar S, Reicher-Reiss H, et al: Early administration of nifedipine in suspected acute myocardial infarction. The Secondary Prevention Reinfarction Israel

Nifedipine Trial 2 Study. Arch Intern Med 153:345, 1993

120. The effect of diltiazem on mortality and reinfarction after myocardial infarction. The Multicenter Diltiazem Postinfarction Trial Research Group. N Engl J Med 319:385, 1988

121. Gibson RS, Hansen JF, Messerli F, et al: Long-term effects of diltiazem and verapamil on mortality and cardiac events in non-Q-wave acute myocardial infarction without pulmonary congestion: post hoc subset analysis of the multicenter diltiazem postinfarction trial and the second Danish verapamil infarction trial studies. Am J Cardiol 86:275, 2000

122. Boden WE, van Gilst WH, Scheldewaert RG, et al: Diltiazem in acute myocardial infarction treated with thrombolytic agents: a randomised placebo-controlled trial. Incomplete Infarction Trial of European Research Collaborators Evaluating Prognosis post-Thrombolysis (INTERCEPT). Lancet 355:1751, 2000

123. Teo KK, Yusuf S, Collins R, et al: Effects of intravenous magnesium in suspected acute myocardial infarction: overview of randomised trials. BMJ 303:1499, 1991

124. Bunch TJ, White RD, Gersh BJ, et al: Long-term outcomes of out-of-hospital cardiac arrest after successful early defibrillation. N Engl J Med 348:2626, 2003

125. Berger PB, Ruocco NA, Ryan TJ, et al: Incidence and prognostic significance of ventricular tachycardia and ventricular fibrillation in the absence of hypotension or heart failure in acute myocardial infarction treated with recombinant tissue-type plasminogen activator: results from the TIMI II trial. J Am Coll Cardiol 22:1773, 1993

126. Behar S, Goldbourt U, Reicher-Reiss H, et al: Prognosis of acute myocardial infarction complicated by primary ventricular fibrillation. Am J Cardiol 66:1208, 1990

127. Wyse DG, Waldo AL, DiMarco JP, et al: A comparison of rate control and rhythm control in patients with atrial fibrillation. N Engl J Med 347:1825, 2002

128. Berger PB, Ryan TJ: Inferior infarction: high risk subgroups. Circulation 81:401, 1990

129. Berger PB, Ruocco NA, Frederick MM, et al: The incidence and significance of heart block during inferior infarction: results from the TIMI II trial. J Am Coll Cardiol 20:533, 1992

130. Oliva PB, Hammill SC, Edwards WD: Cardiac rupture, a clinically predictable complication of acute myocardial infarction: report of 70 cases with clinicopathologic correlations. J Am Coll Cardiol 22:720, 1993

131. Zehender M, Kasper W, Kauder E, et al: Right ventricular infarction as an independent predictor of prognosis after acute inferior myocardial infarction. N Engl J Med 328:981, 1993

132. Flapan AD: Management of patients after their first myocardial infarction. BMJ 309:1129, 1994

133. Madsen JK, Grande P, Saunamaki K, et al: Danish Multicenter Randomized Study of Invasive Versus Conservative Treatment in Patients with Inducible Ischemia after Thrombolysis in Acute Myocardial Infarction (DANAMI). Danish Trial in Acute Myocardial Infarction. Circulation 96:748, 1997

134. Shaw LJ, Peterson ED, Kesler K, et al: A metaanalysis of predischarge risk stratification after acute myocardial infarction with stress electrocardiographic, myocardial perfusion, and ventricular function imaging. Am J Cardiol 78:1327, 1996

135. Chaitman BR, McMahon RP, Terin M, et al: Impact of treatment strategy on predischarge exercise test in the Thrombolysis in Myocardial Infarction (TIMI) II trial. Am J Cardiol 71:131, 1993

136. Randomised trial of cholesterol lowering in 4444 patients with coronary heart disease: the Scandinavian Simvastatin Survival Study (4S). Scandinavian Simvastatin Survival Study Group. Lancet 344:1383, 1994

137. Sacks FM, Pfeffer MA, Moye LA, et al: The effect of pravastatin on coronary events after myocardial infarction in patients with average cholesterol levels. N Engl J Med 335:1001, 1996

138. Stenestrand U, Wallentin L: Early statin treatment following acute myocardial infarction and 1-year survival. JAMA 285:430, 2001

139. Effect of long-term oral anticoagulant treatment on mortality and cardiovascular morbidity after myocardial infarction. Anticoagulants in the Secondary Prevention of Events in Coronary Thrombosis (ASPECT) Research Group. Lancet 343:499, 1994

140. Smith P, Arnesen H, Holme I: The effect of warfarin on mortality and reinfarction after myocardial infarction. N Engl J Med 323:147, 1990

141. Randomised double-blind trial of fixed, low-dose warfarin with aspirin after myocardial infarction. Coumadin Aspirin Reinfarction Study (CARS) Investigators. Lancet 350:389, 1997

142. Meijer A, Verheugt FWA, Wester CPJP, et al: Aspirin versus coumadin in the prevention of reocclusion and recurrent ischemia after successful thrombolysis: a prospective placebo-controlled angiographic study: results of the APRICOT study. Circulation 87:1524, 1993

143. Epstein AE, Hallstrom AP, Rogers WL, et al: Mortality following ventricular arrhythmia suppression by encainide, flecainide, and moricizine after myocardial infarction: the original design concept of the Cardiac Arrhythmia Suppression Trial (CAST). JAMA 270:2451, 1993

144. Moss AJ, Hall WJ, Cannom DS, et al: Improved survival with an implanted defibrillator in patients with coronary disease at high risk for ventricular arrhythmia. Multicenter Automatic Defibrillator Implantation Trial Investigators. N Engl J Med 335:1933, 1996

145. Moss AJ, Zareba W, Jackson Hall W, et al: Prophylactic implantation of a defibrillator in patients with myocardial infarction and reduced ejection fraction. N Engl J Med 346:877, 2002

146. Rana JS, Mukamal KJ, Morgan JP, et al: Obesity and the risk of death after acute myocardial infarction. Am Heart J 147:841, 2004

Acknowledgment

Figures 1 through 7, 8, and 11   Marcia Kammerer.

26 Heart Failure

Mariell Jessup, M.D.

Definition

Heart failure is a clinical syndrome resulting from a structural or functional cardiac disorder that impairs the ability of the ventricle to fill with or eject blood to meet the needs of the body. This syndrome, which is a constellation of signs and symptoms, is primarily manifested by dyspnea, fatigue, fluid retention, and decreased exercise tolerance. Heart failure may result from disorders of the pericardium, myocardium, endocardium, valvular structures, or great vessels of the heart or from rhythm disturbances. It is important to emphasize that not all patients with heart failure symptoms have similar cardiac structural abnormalities. Indeed, the major aim of an initial evaluation of a patient with heart failure is to define the cardiac abnormalities responsible for the symptoms.

Classification

Heart failure has been classified in many ways. One useful framework involves describing the underlying cardiomyopathy, which frequently will suggest the etiology [*see Table 1 and Figure 1*].[1-4] Some examples of the World Health Organization (WHO) classification are ischemic, hypertrophic, restrictive, and idiopathic dilated cardiomyopathy. In the United States, the most common cause of heart failure is ischemic cardiomyopathy resulting from coronary artery disease (CAD).[5,6]

Another practical approach for classification is to divide patients with heart failure into groups of patients with primarily systolic dysfunction and those with diastolic dysfunction. For the clinician, this usually means assessing the patient's left ventricular ejection fraction (LVEF), most commonly with echocardiography.[7-10] Patients with systolic heart failure typically have a low LVEF (usually less than 40% to 45%), a dilated left ventricular cavity, and a reduced cardiac output because of diminished contractility of the myocardium. In contrast, patients with diastolic heart failure have a normal LVEF and normal contractility, but filling of the heart is impaired by a variety of pathophysiologic abnormalities, and salt and water homeostasis is abnormal.[11-14] Despite an increased understanding of the etiologies and pathophysiology of heart failure and significant advances in treatment, morbidity and mortality from this disorder remain unacceptably high.[15-18] Most experts agree that earlier recognition of the syndrome or better identification of patients at risk for heart failure may offer the best hope for the future reduction of heart failure's death toll. This is analogous to the concerted efforts to screen for cancer at its earliest stages, before the disease can defy therapy. Consequently, in 2001, the committee charged with revising the American College of Cardiology/American Heart Association (ACC/AHA) Guidelines for the Evaluation and Management of Heart Failure took the bold step of developing a new classification for patients with heart failure.[19] These guidelines can be obtained from the ACC Web site (http://content.onlinejacc.org/cgi/reprint/46/6/e1.pdf) or the AHA Web site (http://circ.ahajournals.org/cgi/content/full/104/24/2996). The guidelines were updated in 2005, and once again this new approach was used to craft specific recommendations.[20]

The ACC/AHA classification emphasizes the evolution and progression of heart failure; it defines four stages of the disorder [*see Table 2 and Figure 2*]. Stage A identifies patients who are at high risk for developing heart failure but who have no apparent structural abnormality of the heart. This includes patients with hypertension, diabetes, or CAD; patients with a history of rheumatic fever, alcohol abuse, or exposure to cardiotoxic drugs; and patients with a family history of cardiomyopathy. Stage B denotes patients with a structural abnormality of the heart but in whom symptoms of heart failure have not yet developed. This group includes patients who have left ventricular hypertrophy or dilatation, a decreased LVEF, or valvular disease, as well as patients with prior myocardial infarction. Stages A and B can be viewed as preclinical stages. Stage C refers to patients with a structural abnormality of the heart and symptoms of clinical heart failure. This group includes patients with dyspnea, fatigue, or fluid overload, as well as patients with a prior diagnosis of heart failure who are receiving treatment that has relieved their symptoms. Importantly, once patients have had symptoms of heart failure, they remain in stage C even if they subsequently experience clinical improvement. Stage D includes patients with end-stage heart failure that is refractory to standard treatment. Typical stage D patients include those who require frequent hospital admissions for heart failure, are awaiting a heart transplant, are being supported with intravenous agents or mechanical assist devices, or are receiving hospice care for end-stage heart failure.

The ACC/AHA classification is a departure from the traditional New York Heart Association (NYHA) classification, which characterizes patients by symptom severity.[21] Patients with heart failure may progress from stage A to stage D, but never the reverse. In contrast, many patients with NYHA class IV symptoms can be restored to class II with appropriate therapy. The ACC/AHA classification highlights the importance of known risk factors and structural abnormalities in the development of heart failure. Additionally, it reinforces the concept that heart failure is a progressive disease whose onset can be prevented, or its progression halted, by early identification and intervention.

It is important to note that other guidelines have been published that do not use this stage classification, including a revision of the guidelines from the Heart Failure Society of America.[22,23] Irrespective of the guidelines used, all sources agree on the fundamental value of heart failure prevention and the recognition of those risk factors that can be modified. In addition, there is unanimity about the dynamic nature of heart failure symptoms and the poor correlation between functional capacity and structural abnormalities in the syndrome.

Epidemiology

Heart failure is one of the most important cardiac disorders in the United States, both in terms of the number of patients affected and the health care dollars spent. Nearly five million people have heart failure, and almost 500,000 new patients are diagnosed with the disease each year. The estimated direct and indirect costs of heart failure were $21 billion in 2001, more than 5% of the total amount spent on health care[24]; annual spending on drugs for heart failure is about $500 million.[19] Hos-

Table 1   Examples of Descriptive and Etiologic Classifications of Heart Failure

Classification Scheme	Disorder or Disease Process	Comments
By disorder	Dilated cardiomyopathy	Dilatation and impaired function of left ventricle or both ventricles; multiple etiologies: ischemia, valvular disease, infectious process, inflammatory process, toxins, familial/genetic cause, idiopathic
	Hypertrophic cardiomyopathy	Hypertrophy of left ventricle or both ventricles, often asymmetrical and involving the interventricular septum; often associated with mutations in sarcoplasmic proteins; associated with arrhythmias and sudden death
	Restrictive cardiomyopathy	Usually associated with normal systolic function and impaired diastolic function; can be idiopathic or associated with infiltrative diseases, such as amyloidosis, sarcoidosis, and endomyocardial fibrosis
	Arrhythmogenic right ventricular cardiomyopathy	Replacement of myocardium with fatty tissue; can involve left ventricle as well; associated with ventricular arrhythmias; may have a genetic component
By underlying disease process	Ischemic heart disease	Secondary to coronary artery disease
	Valvular disease	Caused by primary valvular disease
	Hypertension	Usually associated with left ventricular hypertrophy; can involve systolic and/or diastolic dysfunction
	Diabetes mellitus	Associated with systolic and/or diastolic dysfunction and left ventricular hypertrophy, even independent of coexisting hypertension or coronary artery disease
	Inflammatory/infectious disease	Systolic dysfunction from myocarditis; multiple infectious etiologies, both viral (e.g., coxsackievirus, echovirus, HIV) and bacterial (rheumatic fever)
	Metabolic disorders	Associated with endocrine abnormalities (e.g., hyperthyroidism, hypothyroidism), electrolyte deficiencies (potassium, magnesium), nutritional deficiencies (e.g., beriberi), and glycogen storage disease (e.g., Pompe disease, Gaucher disease)
	General systemic disease	Associated with connective tissue diseases (e.g., systemic lupus erythematosus, rheumatoid arthritis) and infiltrative diseases (e.g., sarcoidosis, amyloidosis)
	Muscular dystrophies	Includes Duchenne, Becker, and myotonic muscular dystrophies
	Neuromuscular disease	Includes Friedreich ataxia and Noonan syndrome
	Toxins	Associated with alcohol and cocaine abuse, treatment with cardiotoxic chemotherapeutic agents (e.g., anthracyclines), and radiation therapy
	Tachycardia	Associated with uncontrolled tachycardias (e.g., atrial fibrillation and other supraventricular tachycardias)
	Genetic/familial disorders	Associated with a family history of cardiomyopathy and/or sudden death; many cardiomyopathies previously designated as idiopathic may fall into this category
	Pregnancy	Manifests in peripartum period

pitalizations for heart failure increased by 159% from 1979 to 1998,[24] and this trend will likely continue as the United States population ages.

Heart failure is primarily a disease of the elderly.[25] Approximately 6% to 10% of people older than 65 years have heart failure,[26] and roughly 80% of patients hospitalized with heart failure are older than 65 years.[27] More Medicare dollars are spent on heart failure than on any other disease, and heart failure is the most common Medicare diagnosis–related group.[5]

It is important to recognize that heart failure has diverse causes and affects diverse populations. Until recently, this diversity was not reflected in the composition of heart failure trials in the United States, which typically enrolled middle-aged white men with ischemic cardiomyopathy. In fact, the heart failure population in the United States includes significant numbers of women, elderly persons, and members of racial minorities—and these patients tend to have various forms of heart failure. For example, in an estimated 20% to 50% of patients with heart failure, ventricular systolic function is preserved (i.e., the patients have diastolic heart failure), and these patients are more likely to be elderly women.[28-31] Moreover, there are substantial data to suggest that the etiology and natural history of heart failure in African Americans and whites may be different.[32] Heart failure therapy has also been shown to have different efficacies depending on racial, ethnic, and genetic backgrounds. It is clear that the role of pharmacogenomics will continue to expand in the near future.[33]

Etiology

CAD is responsible for roughly two thirds of cases of heart failure in the United States.[34] Coronary ischemia or infarction can lead to heart failure through a variety of mechanisms: acute coronary syndromes or infarction can cause acute heart failure in an otherwise normal heart; likewise, repeated insults of ischemia or infarction can cause a chronic cardiomyopathy. Moreover, many patients with diastolic heart failure, or heart failure with a preserved LVEF, have underlying CAD.

Ventricular dysfunction can result from a multitude of nonischemic causes [*see Table 1*]. These include hypertension, diabetes, valvular disease, arrhythmias, myocardial toxins, myocarditis from a variety of infectious agents (including HIV), and hypothyroidism. Infiltrative causes of ventricular dysfunction, which are usually associated with restrictive cardiomyopathy, include amyloidosis, hemochromatosis, and sarcoidosis. Myocardial systolic dysfunction for which there is no apparent cause is labeled idiopathic cardiomyopathy. Over the past several years, there has been increased recognition that

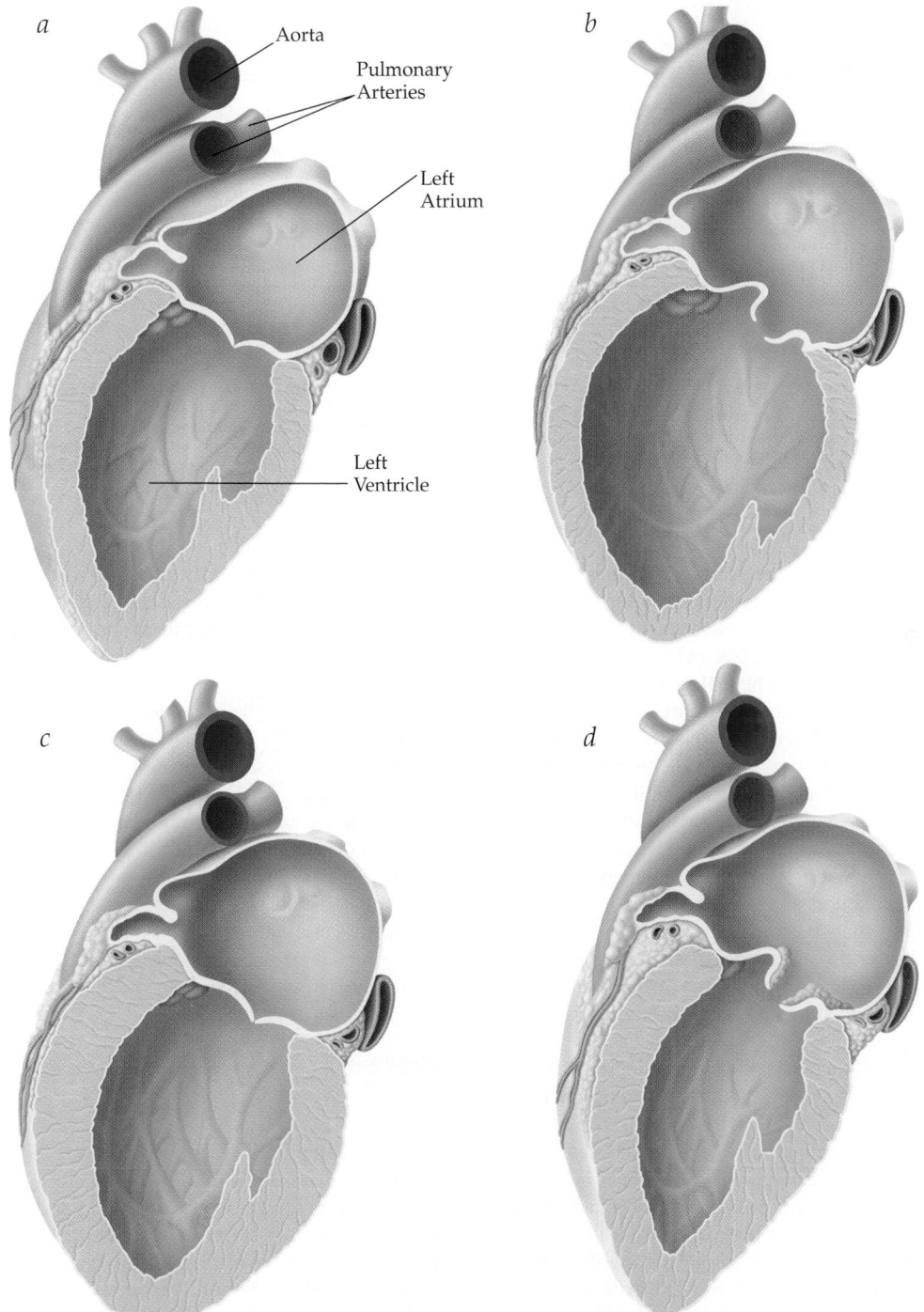

Figure 1 **The different cardiac morphologies in heart failure: (*a*) normal, (*b*) dilated cardiomyopathy, (c) hypertrophic cardiomyopathy, and (d) diastolic dysfunction. The heart is viewed from the left side, with the mitral valve partially cut away; the aortic valve is visible in the upper portion of the left ventricle.**

many of these so-called idiopathic dilated cardiomyopathies are familial; a number of centers are actively focusing on the identification of the genetic irregularities responsible for the abnormal phenotypes.[35]

Pathophysiology

There is no single, simple model that effectively explains the syndrome of heart failure; currently, the consensus view integrates multiple pathophysiologic models to explain the complex cascade of events leading to this clinical syndrome.[36,37] The different structural, functional, and biologic changes that culminate in heart failure have led to a variety of treatment modalities to target this array of causative factors.[38] For example, for many years, beta blockers were contraindicated in patients with heart failure because the disorder was thought to be primarily a result of decreased myocardial contractility that would worsen with negative inotropic therapy. However, that

Table 2   Stages of Heart Failure[19]

Stage	Description	Examples
A	Patients at high risk for heart failure because of the presence of conditions strongly associated with the development of heart failure; no identified structural or functional abnormalities of the pericardium, myocardium, or cardiac valves; no current or previous history of signs or symptoms of heart failure	Patients with systemic hypertension, coronary artery disease, diabetes mellitus, history of cardiotoxic drug therapy or alcohol abuse, history of rheumatic fever, family history of cardiomyopathy
B	Patients with structural heart disease that is strongly associated with the development of heart failure but who have no current or previous history of signs or symptoms of heart failure	Patients with left ventricular hypertrophy or fibrosis, left ventricular dilatation or hypocontractility, asymptomatic valvular heart disease, previous myocardial infarction
C	Patients who currently have or who in the past have had symptoms of heart failure associated with underlying structural heart disease	Patients with dyspnea or fatigue due to left ventricular systolic dysfunction; asymptomatic patients undergoing treatment for prior symptoms of heart failure
D	Patients with advanced structural heart disease and marked symptoms of heart failure at rest despite maximal medical therapy; need for specialized interventions	Patients who are frequently hospitalized for heart failure and cannot be safely discharged from the hospital; patients in hospital awaiting heart transplantation; patients at home receiving continuous intravenous support for symptom relief or support with a mechanical circulatory assist device; patients in a hospice setting for the management of heart failure

older model of heart failure has been replaced by one that gives a central role to pathologic sympathetic activation—the maladaptive mechanisms that lead to vasoconstriction, arrhythmias, and ventricular remodeling (see below). This model explains the therapeutic benefits of beta blockade.

The hemodynamic model of heart failure concentrated on the role of increased load on a failing ventricle; this conceptual approach led to the successful use of vasodilators and inotropes. Later, the neurohormonal model of heart failure identified the critical importance of the renin-angiotensin-aldosterone axis and the sympathetic nervous system in the progression of cardiac dysfunction, leading to widespread use of angiotensin-converting enzyme (ACE) inhibitors and beta blockers.

The recognition that progressive ventricular dilatation serves as a marker for disease progression has focused attention on the myocyte and on the role of the cardiac interstitium. Both medical and surgical therapies have been directed at this mechanism.

Left ventricular dysfunction begins with an injury to the myocardium. The unanswered question is why ventricular systolic dysfunction continues to worsen in the absence of recurrent insults. This pathologic process, which has been termed remodeling, is the structural response to the initial injury. Mechanical, neurohormonal, and possibly genetic factors alter ventricular size, shape, and function to decrease wall stress and compensate for the initial injury. Remodeling involves hypertrophy, loss of myocytes, and increased fibrosis and is secondary to both neurohormonal activation and other mechanical factors.[39-41] Ultimately, the changes in ventricular shape lead to a less efficient cardiac pump. Functional mitral regurgitation often occurs as the left ventricle dilates and becomes more globular, increasing volume overload. Remodeling seems to beget more adverse remodeling.

Arrhythmias often contribute to myocardial dysfunction and are an unwelcome side effect of heart failure. Supraventricular arrhythmias, particularly atrial fibrillation, often unmask systolic or diastolic dysfunction in a previously asymptomatic patient.[42] In addition, intraventricular conduction delays and bundle branch block are often present in patients with heart failure. Abnormal ventricular conduction, particularly left bundle branch block, has significant detrimental hemodynamic ef-

fects.[43-47] In addition to contributing to worsening heart failure, ventricular arrhythmias are likely a direct cause of death in many of these patients; the rate of sudden cardiac death in persons with heart failure is six to nine times that seen in the general population.[48]

These pathophysiologic models do not easily explain diastolic heart failure.[49] In the 20% to 50% of patients who have heart failure with normal systolic function, cardiac output is limited by abnormal filling and disordered relaxation of the ventricles, especially during exercise. Ventricular pressures are elevated for a given ventricular volume, leading to pulmonary congestion, dyspnea, and peripheral edema identical to that seen in patients with a dilated, poorly contracting heart.[11,13,14,50,51] CAD or ischemia frequently compounds the impairment of ventricular performance in patients with diastolic heart failure, who typically are elderly women[28] with hypertension, diabetes, and obesity.

Diagnosis

STAGE A

The first step in the diagnosis of heart failure is to identify patients who are at risk for developing the syndrome; this concept was part of the reasoning behind the ACC/AHA staging system.[19] Patients in stage A are those with CAD, hypertension, diabetes, a history of alcohol abuse or exposure to cardiotoxic drugs (e.g., certain chemotherapeutic agents, cocaine), a history of rheumatic fever, or a family history of cardiomyopathy or sudden death. In these high-risk patients, reversible risk factors should be aggressively treated to prevent heart failure from developing.[52,53]

STAGE B

Stage B patients have asymptomatic, structural heart disease. Echocardiography is easily the best diagnostic tool to uncover left ventricular hypertrophy or dilatation, valvular disease, or wall motion abnormalities indicative of previous myocardial infarction. Patients in stage B represent a significant portion of the heart failure population and constitute a key opportunity for intervention. In a community-based survey, less than half of patients with moderate or severe systolic or diastolic dysfunction, as defined by echocardiographic parameters, had recognized heart failure.[54] Current ACC/AHA guidelines do not recommend routine screening echocardiography for the large number of patients at risk for the development of heart failure. The guidelines do, however, include a class I recommendation that a noninvasive evaluation of left ventricular function be performed in patients who have a strong family history of cardiomyopathy or have been exposed to cardiotoxic therapies.[20]

STAGES C AND D

Stages C and D represent the traditional definition of heart failure. Patients in stage C or D usually present with decreased exercise tolerance, fluid retention, or both. Initial assessment of these patients should focus on the structural abnormality leading to heart failure, as well as evaluation of its etiology. Initial testing should include a 2-D echocardiogram with Doppler flow studies, a chest x-ray, electrocardiography, and laboratory studies, including urinalysis, complete blood count, serum chemistries, liver function studies, and thyroid-stimulating hormone measurement. These tests serve primarily to exclude other potential causes of dyspnea or fatigue.[19] In patients with dyspnea, measurement of serum brain natriuretic peptide (BNP) may aid in the diagnosis; marked elevation of BNP levels suggests that the dyspnea is cardiac rather than pulmonary in origin.[55,56] Strong consideration should be given to excluding significant CAD, because CAD is the leading cause of left ventricular dysfunction.[34] The ACC/AHA guidelines strongly encourage coronary angiography rather than noninvasive testing for the evaluation of patients with heart failure, even if they do not have a known history of CAD; the guidelines cite the fact that noninvasive testing can often lead to inaccurate results in patients with cardiomyopathies (e.g., perfusion defects or wall motion abnormalities in patients with a nonischemic cardiomyopathy).[20] Some clinicians argue that there is little evidence that revascularization changes the outcome or prognosis in patients with left ventricular dysfunction and that it should therefore be used only to relieve angina.[57]

Several clinical parameters are useful for the subsequent evaluation and management of heart failure. A patient's weight

Table 3   Treatment of Heart Failure[20]

Stage A	Treat hypertension Encourage smoking cessation Treat lipid disorders Encourage regular exercise Discourage alcohol intake, illicit drug use Prescribe ACE inhibitors or ARBs in appropriate patients with vascular disease or diabetes
Stage B	All measures used for stage A ACE inhibitors or ARBs if appropriate Beta blockers if appropriate

Stage C	All measures used for stage A
	Dietary salt restriction
	Drugs for routine use:
	    ACE inhibitors or ARBs
	    Beta blockers
	    Diuretics for fluid retention
	Drugs or devices for selected patients:
	    Aldosterone antagonists
	    Digitalis
	    Other vasodilators
	    Biventricular pacing
	    Implantable defibrillators

Stage D	All measures used for stages A, B, and C Mechanical assist devices Heart transplantation Continuous (not intermittent) I.V. inotropic infusions for palliation Hospice care Experimental surgery or drugs

ACE—angiotensin-converting enzyme   ARBs—angiotensin receptor blockers

should be measured in the office, and patients should be taught to follow their weight at home to assess for fluid retention. Office evaluation of jugular venous pressure, hepatojugular reflux, gallop rhythm, and peripheral edema can aid in making the initial diagnosis and guiding the need for diuresis. In addition, these signs of heart failure may be prognostically important.[58]

DIASTOLIC HEART FAILURE

There is no universally accepted definition of diastolic heart failure,[11,13,59,60] although a number of investigators have suggested options. The diagnosis is usually made by a clinician who recognizes the typical signs and symptoms of heart failure despite the finding of normal systolic function (i.e., a normal LVEF) on an echocardiogram. Doppler echocardiographic techniques can also aid in establishing the diagnosis of diastolic dysfunction.[10,61]

Treatment

Treatment for heart failure is keyed to the stage of the syndrome as defined by the ACC/AHA guidelines [*see Table 3*]. Treatment in all stages is aimed at preventing or palliating the remodeling process [*see Pathophysiology, above*]. In addition, therapy for stages C and D heart failure is intended to relieve the disabling symptoms of the disease.

STAGE A

The goal of treatment of stage A heart failure is to prevent structural heart disease. This is achieved by controlling risk fac-

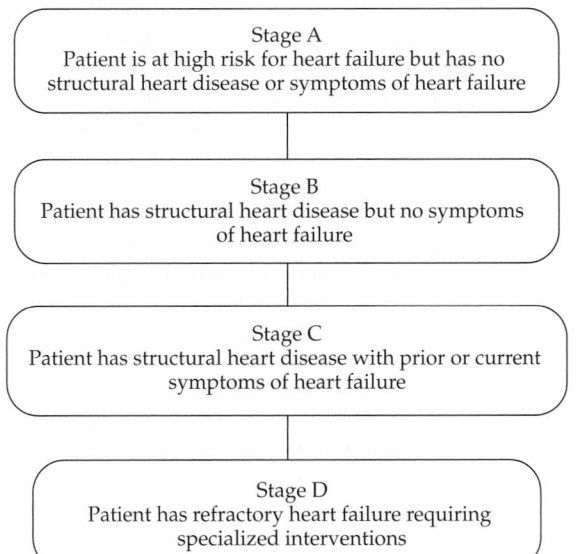

Figure 2   The evolution of heart failure by stage.[19]

tors (e.g., hypertension, CAD, diabetes mellitus, hyperlipidemia, smoking, alcohol ingestion, and use of cardiotoxic drugs), which lowers the incidence of later cardiovascular events. For example, effective treatment of hypertension decreases left ventricular hypertrophy and cardiovascular mortality; it can also reduce the incidence of heart failure by 30% to 50%.[52,53]

Diabetes deserves particular attention because patients with diabetes mellitus have a high incidence of CAD and of heart failure in the absence of CAD; diabetes causes many detrimental biochemical and functional cardiac changes independent of ischemia.[62,63] ACE inhibitors and angiotensin receptor blockers (ARBs) have assumed a major role in risk reduction for diabetes patients (see below). In asymptomatic high-risk patients with diabetes or vascular disease who have no history of heart failure or left ventricular dysfunction, treatment with these agents has been shown to yield significant reductions in death, myocardial infarction, and stroke,[64,65] as well as delays in the first hospitalization for heart failure.[66]

STAGES B, C, AND D

The goals of therapy for patients with heart failure and a low LVEF are to decrease the progression of disease and the number of hospitalizations, improve symptoms and survival, and minimize risk factors. Simple interventions can help patients control their disease. For example, basic habits of moderate sodium restriction, weight monitoring, and adherence to medication schedules serve to prevent hospitalizations for rapid fluid overload. Other frequent causes of decompensation in heart failure include anemia, arrhythmias (especially atrial fibrillation), noncompliance with medications and diet, and the use of nonsteroidal anti-inflammatory drugs (NSAIDs).[67,68]

Medical Therapy

Pharmacologic treatment of heart failure with low LVEF routinely includes diuretics, angiotensin antagonists, and beta blockers. Digoxin and aldosterone antagonists or inotropes may be utilized in some cases [see Table 4].

Diuretics In symptomatic patients in stages C and D, diuretics are often the first drugs prescribed to decrease fluid overload and congestive symptoms. Loop diuretics are most often given to these patients, either as maintenance therapy or on an as-needed basis. Loop diuretics can be combined with thiazides to optimize diuresis.[69,70]

ACE inhibitors ACE inhibitors are recommended for all patients with low LVEF in stages B, C, and D. By decreasing the conversion of angiotensin I to angiotensin II, ACE inhibitors minimize the multiple pathophysiologic effects of angiotensin II, such as vasoconstriction and fibrosis. ACE inhibitors (but not ARBs) also decrease the degradation of bradykinin, a substance that causes vasodilatation and natriuresis. In patients with heart failure, ACE inhibitors have been shown to increase survival, improve cardiac performance, decrease symptoms and hospitalizations, and decrease or slow the remodeling process.[71-73]

It is not clear whether all ACE inhibitors are equally effective in all forms of heart failure. There are few data from controlled trials, for example, regarding the efficacy of ACE inhibitors in diastolic heart failure. Moreover, although several guidelines have emphasized the need to maximize the dose of an ACE in-

hibitor to target levels (rather than using blood pressure alone to guide dose titration), current recommendations underscore the need to add beta blockers to the regimen of patients in stage C early in the course of treatment, even if target ACE inhibitor doses have not been achieved.

Angiotensin receptor blockers What is the role of ARBs in heart failure? These agents block the effects of angiotensin II at the angiotensin II type 1 receptor site. Initially, recommendations for the use of ARBs were limited to patients who cannot tolerate ACE inhibitors because of cough or angioedema[19]; the guidelines stress that ARBs are comparable, but not superior, to ACE inhibitors.[74-76] Several key trials, however, have reported successful intervention with ARBs in stage B and C patients.[77-79] Possible roles for ARBs in patients who are already on beta blockers, with or without an ACE inhibitor, have likewise been explored in trials.[80-82] There is considerable debate about the appropriate sequence of the addition of drugs to the regimens of patients who remain symptomatic after treatment with a diuretic, an ACE inhibitor, and a beta blocker. Some clinicians add an ARB, whereas others add aldosterone antagonists, digoxin, or other vasodilators.[82,83]

Beta blockers Although it was once taught that beta blockers were contraindicated in patients with heart failure secondary to systolic dysfunction, multiple studies have shown remarkable effects of these drugs on many aspects of heart failure at all stages. The primary action of these agents is to counteract the harmful effects of the increased sympathetic nervous system activity in heart failure. Beta blockers increase survival and improve ejection fraction and quality of life; they also decrease morbidity, hospitalizations, sudden death, and the maladaptive effects of remodeling.[84,85] Long-term, placebo-controlled trials have shown improvement in systolic function and reversal of remodeling after 3 to 4 months of treatment with beta blockers.[86-88] A topical analysis showed that even in the sickest of heart failure patients, beta-blocker therapy was well tolerated and led to decreases in mortality and hospitalizations as early as 14 to 21 days after initiation of therapy.[89] Clinicians should be extremely cautious, however, about starting beta blockers in patients with significant reactive airway disease, in diabetic patients with frequent episodes of hypoglycemia, and in patients with bradyarrhythmias or heart block who do not have a pacemaker implanted.

In the United States, two beta blockers are specifically approved for treatment of heart failure: carvedilol and long-acting metoprolol. Beta blockers should be started at the lowest possible dose and titrated up slowly at 2- to 4-week intervals. Patients should be closely monitored for worsening of symptoms or fluid retention, which can sometimes occur early in therapy with these agents. If patients do have exacerbations during initiation of beta blockade, diuretic therapy can be increased, and titration of the beta blocker can proceed more slowly.

Digoxin Digoxin has long been a mainstay of treatment of left ventricular dysfunction in symptomatic patients, despite a lack of data from clinical trials showing survival benefit.[90] A large randomized study demonstrated that digoxin was successful in decreasing hospitalizations for heart failure—an important clinical end point—but did not decrease mortality.[91] Post hoc analysis of data from this trial showed that in the patients randomized to receive digoxin therapy, mortality may

Table 4 Pharmacotherapy of Heart Failure

| Category | Drug (Trade Name) | Dosage | | Comment |
		Initial Daily Dose	Maximum Daily Dose	
Loop diuretics	Bumetanide (Bumex) Furosemide (Lasix) Torsemide (Demadex)	0.5–1 mg q.d. or b.i.d. 20–40 mg q.d. or b.i.d. 10–20 mg q.d. or b.i.d.	Up to 10 mg Up to 400 mg Up to 200 mg	Titrate to achieve dry weight; carefully monitor serum potassium and creatinine levels
ACE inhibitors	Captopril (Capoten) Enalapril (Vasotec) Fosinopril (Monopril) Lisinopril (Prinivil, Zestril) Quinapril (Accupril) Ramipril (Altace)	6.25 mg t.i.d. 2.5 mg b.i.d. 5–10 mg 2.5–5 mg 10 mg b.i.d. 1.25–2.5 mg	50 mg t.i.d. 10–20 mg b.i.d. 40 mg 20–40 mg 40 mg b.i.d. 10 mg	Carefully monitor serum potassium and creatinine levels
Beta blockers	Bisoprolol (Zebeta) Carvedilol (Coreg) Metoprolol tartrate (Lopressor) Metoprolol succinate extended release (Toprol-XL)	1.25 mg 3.125 mg b.i.d. 6.25 mg b.i.d. 12.5–25 mg	10 mg 25 mg b.i.d. (50 mg b.i.d. for patients > 85 kg) 75 mg b.i.d. 200 mg	Titrate dosage up over 2- to 4-week intervals, carefully monitoring for signs and symptoms of fluid overload
Digitalis glycosides	Digoxin (Lanoxin)	0.125–0.25 mg	0.125–0.25 mg	Narrow therapeutic window; monitor levels carefully in older patients and those with renal insufficiency
Aldosterone inhibitors	Spironolactone (Aldactone) Eplerenone (Inspra)	25 mg 25 mg	50 mg 50 mg	50 mg q.d. was maximum spironolactone dosage used in RALES trial[78]; use carefully with concurrent ACE inhibitor or ARB; carefully monitor serum potassium and creatinine levels; use if potassium < 5.0 mmol/L, creatinine < 2.5 mg/dl
Angiotensin receptor blockers	Candesartan (Atacand) Irbesartan (Avapro) Losartan (Cozaar) Valsartan (Diovan)	8 mg 75 mg 25 mg 80 mg	32 mg 300 mg 100 mg 320 mg	Use if patients have cough or angioedema on ACE inhibitor; may be used as first-line therapy

ACE—angiotensin-converting enzyme   ARB—angiotensin receptor blocker   RALES—Randomized Aldosterone Evaluation Study

have been higher in women than in men.[92] It is hypothesized that the therapeutic windows for digoxin may be different in men and women, with women perhaps needing a lower dose of the drug.[93] Indeed, data suggest that digoxin improves morbidity as effectively at low serum concentrations (0.5 to 0.9 ng/ml) as it does at higher levels, with less toxicity at the lower concentrations.[94] Clinicians should carefully monitor all patients for signs and symptoms of digoxin toxicity, especially patients who are elderly or have renal dysfunction. Physicians and patients should also keep in mind that digoxin interacts with numerous other drugs.

Aldosterone antagonists The aldosterone antagonists (i.e., spironolactone and eplerenone) are another relatively old class of drugs with new data to support use in heart failure.[95] Because of the activation of the renin-angiotensin-aldosterone axis, which is incompletely suppressed by ACE inhibitors, patients with heart failure have increased circulating levels of aldosterone, leading to sodium retention and potassium loss. Aldosterone also works locally in the myocardium, contributing to hypertrophy and fibrosis in the failing heart.[96] A large randomized trial showed that the addition of low-dose spironolactone to standard treatment reduces morbidity and mortality in patients with NYHA class III and IV heart failure (stage C and

stage D patients).[97] Subsequently, eplerenone was shown to be efficacious in a slightly different heart failure population.[98] Despite the noteworthy results, these drugs are associated with a smaller safety margin than ACE inhibitors and beta blockers. Clinicians are urged to use caution in the selection of patients for this class of therapy and to follow serum electrolyte levels and renal function carefully after initiation of the drug.[82]

Other vasodilators Symptomatic patients who cannot tolerate ACE inhibitors or ARBs, usually because of renal insufficiency, may benefit from a combination of hydralazine and isosorbide dinitrate for afterload reduction.[99] In a study of advanced heart failure in black patients, the addition of this drug combination to standard heart failure therapy resulted in a lower rate of death and of first hospitalization for heart failure, as well as an improvement in the quality of life; indeed, the trial was terminated early because of significantly higher mortality in the placebo group.[100] It is not clear whether this benefit will be operative in other ethnic or racial groups, however.

Intravenous inotropes Patients with refractory heart failure (stage D patients) often require intermittent intravenous inotropic therapy to aid in diuresis and to improve symptoms.[101] No survival benefit has been demonstrated with inotropic

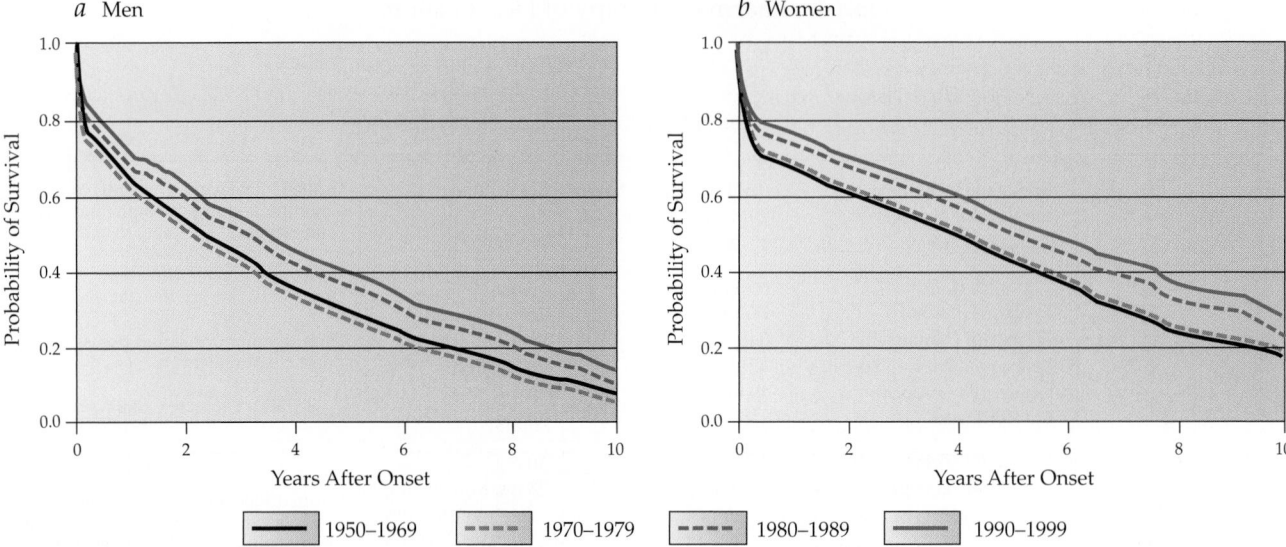

Figure 3 Data from the Framingham Heart Study indicate a steady upward trend since the 1950s in age-adjusted survival after the onset of heart failure.[133] Estimates shown are for patients 65 to 74 years of age.

treatment given in any form. These agents should be regarded as palliative or as maintenance therapy for patients awaiting heart transplantation.[19]

DIASTOLIC HEART FAILURE

Despite the large number of patients with primarily diastolic heart failure, few clinical trials have addressed the management of these cases. Physiologic principles used to guide treatment of these patients include control of blood pressure, heart rate, myocardial ischemia, and blood volume.[19,20,22]

REVASCULARIZATION AND SURGICAL THERAPY

Patients in all stages of heart failure must be evaluated for CAD. Angioplasty and surgical revascularization improve ischemic symptoms and can lead to improved ejection fraction and decreased incidence of sudden death.[102]

Clinical trials to investigate the role of surgical interventions in halting or reversing the remodeling process are now under way. Such interventions include mitral valve repair or replacement, mechanical devices to reduce wall stress, and surgical excision of infarcted tissue.[103-106]

Cardiac transplantation remains the only definitive treatment for stage D patients, but it is available only to roughly 2,500 patients a year in the United States.[107] Left ventricular assist devices are available to support patients waiting for a heart transplant. There is growing evidence supporting the use of these devices as destination therapy for stage D patients, many of whom are not eligible for cardiac transplantation.[108-110] One such left ventricular assist device has been approved for use as permanent replacement therapy for stage D heart failure.

IMPLANTED ELECTRICAL DEVICES

Biventricular Pacing Systems

Many heart failure patients have intraventricular conduction delays that may contribute to altered myocardial contractility or dyssynchrony. Biventricular pacing is a novel therapy for patients with left ventricular systolic dysfunction, particularly those with left bundle branch block. In this procedure, pacing leads are placed in the right atrium and the right ventricle and into a cardiac vein in the lateral wall of the left ventricle via the coronary sinus. The goal of this therapy is to restore the usual pattern of electrical activation of the left ventricle and thereby restore ventricular synchrony.[111,112] There is evidence that with restored ventricular synchrony from a biventricular pacing system, the remodeling process is halted and reversed. Trials have shown that implantation of a biventricular pacer results in decreased ventricular size and volumes, improved ventricular function, and less mitral regurgitation. This has led to improved exercise tolerance, decreased hospitalizations, and improved quality of life.[113-115] A meta-analysis of the largest trials showed a 51% decrease in death from progressive heart failure.[116] In addition, a large clinical trial of biventricular pacing in patients with heart failure was stopped early because resynchronization therapy was found to confer a statistically significant benefit regarding the combined end point of mortality and hospitalization.[117] Finally, a large randomized trial examining the role of biventricular pacing showed a significant reduction in mortality with the pacing system alone, in the absence of a concomitant defibrillator.[118]

A number of ongoing trials are exploring alternative methods of identifying appropriate candidates for this therapy (e.g., by identifying dyssynchrony). In addition, there are continued efforts to understand why certain patients fail to respond to pacing.

Cardioverter-Defibrillators

The use of implantable cardioverter-defibrillators (ICDs) for the primary prevention of sudden death in patients with left ventricular dysfunction has grown enormously [*see Chapter 21*]. There is increasing evidence that ICD placement reduces mortality in patients with ischemic cardiomyopathy, irrespective of whether they have nonsustained ventricular arrhythmias.[119] The role of these devices in patients with heart failure of a nonischemic cause has likewise been expanded after several important trials.[117,120] All patients with an LVEF less than 35% and stage B or C heart failure, regardless of etiology, should be considered for ICD therapy. Important exclusions for consideration include shortened life expectancy, end-stage heart failure symptoms, or psychiatric disorders. A current debate centers on the extent and duration of medical therapy that should be given before the ICD is implanted.[20,22]

Prognosis

Despite many advances in the management of heart failure, it remains life threatening. Symptomatic heart failure continues to confer a worse prognosis than the majority of cancers in the United States, with 1-year mortality averaging 45%.[15,16] Nonetheless, it is difficult to discuss the prognosis of heart failure as a whole, because an individual patient's likelihood of survival is related to the cause of the heart failure, as well as multiple other clinical factors.[121-125] For example, given the same severity of heart failure symptoms, an 85-year-old woman with ischemic cardiomyopathy would have a lower likelihood of survival than a 45-year old man with idiopathic cardiomyopathy. One study of 1,230 patients with cardiomyopathy found that survival was significantly worse in patients with cardiomyopathy from ischemia, infiltrative disease, cardiotoxic chemotherapy, HIV infection, or connective tissue disease than in patients with idiopathic cardiomyopathy.[126]

There are conflicting data about the prognosis of patients with diastolic heart failure. Studies have shown, however, that mortality in these patients may be as high as the mortality in patients with systolic heart failure, and hospitalization rates are equal.[54,123,127-130]

It is also important for clinicians to remember that a low LVEF is not universally predictive of poor outcome. In patients referred for cardiac transplantation, survival has correlated more closely with other variables—notably, peak exercise oxygen consumption.[131] One prospectively validated model for predicting survival in patients with severe heart failure incorporates LVEF with six other clinical factors: presence of coronary disease, resting heart rate, mean arterial blood pressure, presence of intraventricular conduction delays, serum sodium concentration, and peak exercise oxygen consumption.[132] These tools can be used to stratify patients according to risk and to make the most appropriate use of modern therapies and treatment modalities.

How can physicians improve the prognosis of patients with heart failure? A 2002 report from the Framingham Heart Study showed promising evidence of increased survival after the diagnosis of heart failure [see Figure 3].[133] To further this trend, physicians must work toward widespread implementation of the therapies known to decrease morbidity and mortality in heart failure. Researchers must also investigate more completely the impact of medical therapy on the survival of patients with diastolic heart failure. There should be continued effort to increase the number of traditionally underrepresented patients (e.g., women and minorities) enrolled in heart failure trials. Finally, in keeping with the emphasis of the ACC/AHA guidelines, clinicians must concentrate on identifying and treating those patients at greatest risk for heart failure to prevent it from occurring.

The author has received grants for clinical research from, and served as an advisor or consultant to, Acorn Cardiovascular, Inc.; Medtronic, Inc.; GlaxoSmithKline; AstraZeneca Pharmaceuticals LP; and Ventracor.

References

1. Boffa GM, Thiene G, Nava A, et al: Cardiomyopathy: a necessary revision of the WHO classification. Int J Cardiol 30:1, 1991

2. Goodwin JF: Overview and classification of the cardiomyopathies. Cardiovasc Clin 19:3, 1988

3. Keren A, Popp RL: Assignment of patients into the classification of cardiomyopathies. Circulation 86:1622, 1992

4. Pisani B, Taylor DO, Mason JW: Inflammatory myocardial diseases and cardiomyopathies. Am J Med 102:459, 1997

5. Massie B, Shah N: Evolving trends in the epidemiologic factors of heart failure: rationale for preventive strategies and comprehensive disease management. Am Heart J 133:701, 1997

6. Wilhelmsen L, Rosengren A, Eriksson H, et al: Heart failure in the general population of men: morbidity, risk factors and prognosis. J Intern Med 249:253, 2001

7. Gadsboll N, Hoilund-Carlsen P, Neilsen G, et al: Interobserver agreement and accuracy of bedside estimation of right and left ventricular ejection fraction in acute myocardial infarction. Am J Cardiol 63:1301, 1989

8. Ghali JK, Kadakia S, Cooper RS, et al: Bedside diagnosis of preserved versus impaired left ventricular systolic function in heart failure. Am J Cardiol 67:1002, 1991

9. Mosterd A, de Bruijne MC, Hoes AW, et al: Usefulness of echocardiography in detecting left ventricular dysfunction in population-based studies (The Rotterdam Study). Am J Cardiol 79:103, 1997

10. Ommen S, Nishimura R, Appleton C, et al: The clinical utility of Doppler echocardiography and tissue Doppler imaging in estimation of left ventricular filling pressures: a comparative simultaneous Doppler-catheterization study. Circulation 102:1788, 2000

11. Aurigemma GP, Gaasch WH: Clinical practice. Diastolic heart failure. N Engl J Med 351:1097, 2004

12. Dahlstrom U: Can natriuretic peptides be used for the diagnosis of diastolic heart failure? Eur J Heart Fail 6:281, 2004

13. Vasan R, Levy D: Defining diastolic heart failure: a call for standardized diagnostic criteria. Circulation 101:2118, 2000

14. Zile MR, Brutsaert DL: New concepts in diastolic dysfunction and diastolic heart failure: part II: causal mechanisms and treatment. Circulation 105:1503, 2002

15. Khand A, Gemmel I, Clark A, et al: Is the prognosis of heart failure improving? J Am Coll Cardiol 36:2284, 2000

16. Konstam MA: Progress in heart failure management? Lessons from the real world. Circulation 102:1076, 2000

17. Bouvy ML, Heerdink ER, Leufkens HG, et al: Predicting mortality in patients with heart failure: a pragmatic approach. Heart 89:605, 2003

18. Baker DW, Einstadter D, Thomas C, et al: Mortality trends for 23,505 Medicare patients hospitalized with heart failure in Northeast Ohio, 1991 to 1997. Am Heart J 146:258, 2003

19. Hunt SA, Baker DW, Chin MH, et al: ACC/AHA guidelines for the evaluation and management of chronic heart failure in the adult: executive summary. A report of the American College of Cardiology/American Heart Association Task Force on Practice Guidelines (Committee to revise the 1995 Guidelines for the Evaluation and Management of Heart Failure). J Am Coll Cardiol 38:2101, 2001

20. Hunt SA, Abraham WT, Chin MH, et al: ACC/AHA 2005 guideline update for the diagnosis and management of chronic heart failure in the adult: a report of the American College of Cardiology/American Heart Association Task Force on Practice Guidelines (Writing Committee to Update the 2001 Guidelines for the Evaluation and Management of Heart Failure): developed in collaboration with the American College of Chest Physicians and the International Society for Heart and Lung Transplantation: endorsed by the Heart Rhythm Society. Circulation 112:e154, 2005
http://content.onlinejacc.org/cgi/reprint/46/6/e1

21. Gibelin P: An evaluation of symptom classification systems used for the assessment of patients with heart failure in France. Eur J Heart Fail 3:739, 2001

22. Adams K, Lindenfeld J, Arnold J, et al: Executive summary: HFSA 2006 comprehensive heart failure practice guidelines. J Cardiac Fail 12:10, 2006

23. Nieminen MS, Bohm M, Cowie MR, et al: Executive summary of the guidelines on the diagnosis and treatment of acute heart failure: the Task Force on Acute Heart Failure of the European Society of Cardiology. Eur Heart J 26:384, 2005

24. American Heart Association: 2001 Heart and Stroke Statistical Update. American Heart Association, Dallas, 2000

25. Kannel WB, Belanger A: Epidemiology of heart failure. Am Heart J 121:951, 1991

26. Kannel WB: Epidemiology and prevention of cardiac failure: Framingham Study insights. Eur Heart J 8(suppl F):23, 1987

27. Haldeman GA, Croft JB, Giles WH, et al: Hospitalization of patients with heart failure: National Hospital Discharge Survey, 1985 to 1995. Am Heart J 137:352, 1999

28. Masoudi FA, Havranek EP, Smith G, et al: Gender, age, and heart failure with preserved left ventricular systolic function. J Am Coll Cardiol 41:217, 2003

29. Senni M, Tribouilloy CM, Rodeheffer RJ, et al: Congestive heart failure in the community: a study of all incident cases in Olmsted County, Minnesota, in 1991. Circulation 98:2282, 1998

30. Vasan RS, Larson MG, Benjamin EJ, et al: Congestive heart failure in subjects with normal versus reduced left ventricular ejection fraction. J Am Coll Cardiol 33:1948, 1999

31. Kitzman DW, Gardin JM, Gottdiener JS, et al: Importance of heart failure with preserved systolic function in patients > or = 65 years of age. CHS Research Group. Cardiovascular Health Study. Am J Cardiol 87:413. 2001

32. Aronow WS, Ahn C, Kronzon I: Comparison of incidence of congestive heart failure in older African-Americans, Hispanics, and whites. Am J Cardiol 84:611, 1999

33. Feldman AM: The emerging role of pharmacogenomics in the treatment of patients with heart failure. Ann Thorac Surg 76:S2246, 2003

34. Gheorghiade M, Bonow RO: Chronic heart failure in the United States: a manifestation of coronary artery disease. Circulation 97:282, 1998

35. Schonberger J, Seidman CE: Many roads lead to a broken heart: the genetics of dilated cardiomyopathy. Am J Hum Genet 69:249, 2001

36. Mann D: Mechanisms and models in heart failure. Circulation 100:999, 1999

37. Mann DL, Bristow MR: Mechanisms and models in heart failure: the biomechanical model and beyond. Circulation 111:2837, 2005

38. McMurray J, Pfeffer MA: New therapeutic options in congestive heart failure: part I. Circulation 105:2099, 2002

39. Eichhorn EJ, Bristow MR: Medical therapy can improve the biological properties of the chronically failing heart: a new era in the treatment of heart failure. Circulation 94:2285, 1996

40. Mann DL: Basic mechanisms of left ventricular remodeling: the contribution of wall stress. J Cardiac Fail 10(6 suppl):S202, 2004

41. Sutton MGSJ, Sharpe N: Left ventricular remodeling after myocardial infarction: pathophysiology and therapy. Circulation 101:2981, 2000

42. Benjamin EJ, Wolf PA, D'Agostino RB, et al: Impact of atrial fibrillation on the risk of death: the Framingham Heart Study. Circulation 98:946, 1998

43. Gerber T, Nishimura R, Holmes D, et al: Left ventricular and biventricular pacing in congestive heart failure. Mayo Clin Proc 76:803, 2001

44. Hultgren H, Craige E, Fujii J, et al: Left bundle branch block and mechanical events of the cardiac cycle. Am J Cardiol 52:755, 1983

45. Sadaniantz A, Saint Laurent L: Left ventricular Doppler diastolic filling patterns in patients with isolated left bundle branch block. Am J Cardiol 81:643, 1998

46. Xiao H, Lee C, Gibson D: Effect of left bundle branch block on diastolic function in dilated cardiomyopathy. Br Heart J 66:443, 1991

47. Ozdemir K, Altunkeser B, Danis G, et al: Effect of the isolated left bundle branch block on systolic and diastolic functions of left ventricle. J Am Soc Echocardiogr 14:1075, 2001

48. Stevenson WG, Stevenson LW: Prevention of sudden death in heart failure. J Cardiovasc Electrophysiol 12:112, 2001

49. Burkhoff D, Maurer M, Packer M: Heart failure with a normal ejection fraction: is it really a disorder of diastolic function? Circulation 107:656, 2003

50. Banerjee P, Banerjee T, Khand A, et al: Diastolic heart failure: neglected or misdiagnosed? J Am Coll Cardiol 39:138, 2002

51. Brutsaert DL, Sys SU: Diastolic dysfunction in heart failure. J Cardiac Fail 3:225, 1997

52. Deedwania PC: Hypertension and diabetes: new therapeutic options. Arch Intern Med 160:1585, 2000

53. Mosterd A, D'Agostino RB, Silbershatz H, et al: Trends in the prevalence of hypertension, antihypertensive therapy, and left ventricular hypertrophy from 1950 to 1989. N Engl J Med 340:1221, 1999

54. Redfield M, Jacobsen SJ, Burnett JC Jr, et al: Burden of systolic and diastolic ventricular dysfunction in the community. JAMA 289:194, 2003

55. Morrison LK, Harrison A, Krishnaswamy P, et al: Utility of a rapid B-natriuretic peptide assay in differentiating congestive heart failure from lung disease in patients presenting with dyspnea. J Am Coll Cardiol 39:202, 2002

56. Silver MA, Maisel A, Yancy CW, et al: BNP Consensus Panel 2004: A clinical approach for the diagnostic, prognostic, screening, treatment monitoring, and therapeutic roles of natriuretic peptides in cardiovascular diseases. Congest Heart Fail 10(5 suppl 3):1, 2004 (erratum, Congest Heart Fail 11:102, 2005)

57. Cleland JG, Alamgir F, Nikitin NP, et al: What is the optimal medical management of ischemic heart failure? Prog Cardiovasc Dis 43:433, 2001

58. Drazner M, Rame E, Stevenson L, et al: Prognostic importance of elevated jugular venous pressure and a third heart sound in patients with heart failure. N Engl J Med 345:574, 2001

59. Cohen-Solal A: Diastolic heart failure: myth or reality? Eur J Heart Fail 4:395, 2002

60. How to diagnose diastolic heart failure. European Study Group on Diastolic Heart Failure. Eur Heart J 19:990, 1998

61. Nishimura RA, Tajik J: Evaluation of diastolic filling of left ventricle in health and disease: Doppler echocardiography is the clinician's Rosetta Stone. J Am Coll Cardiol 30:8, 1997

62. Taegtmeyer H, McNulty P, Young ME: Adaptation and maladaptation of the heart in diabetes: part I. Circulation 105:1727, 2002

63. Dries DL, Sweitzer NK, Drazner MH, et al: Prognostic impact of diabetes mellitus in patients with heart failure according to the etiology of left ventricular systolic dysfunction. J Am Coll Cardiol 38:421, 2001

64. Effects of ramipril on cardiovascular and microvascular outcomes in people with diabetes mellitus: results of the HOPE study and MICRO-HOPE substudy. Heart Outcomes Prevention Evaluation Study Investigators. Lancet 355:253, 2000

65. Tight blood pressure control and risk of macrovascular and microvascular complications in type 2 diabetes. UKPDS 38. UK Prospective Diabetes Study Group. BMJ 317:703, 1998

66. Dargie HJ: Effect of carvedilol on outcome after myocardial infarction in patients with left ventricular dysfunction: the CAPRICORN randomised trial. Lancet 357:1385, 2001

67. Feenstra J, Heerdink ER, Grobbee DE, et al: Association of nonsteroidal anti-inflammatory drugs with first occurrence of heart failure and with relapsing heart failure: the Rotterdam Study. Arch Intern Med 162:265, 2002

68. Merlo J, Broms K, Lindblad U, et al: Association of outpatient utilisation of non-steroidal anti-inflammatory drugs and hospitalised heart failure in the entire Swedish population. Eur J Clin Pharmacol 57:71, 2001

69. Brater DC: Drug therapy: diuretic therapy. N Engl J Med 339:387, 1998

70. Ellison D: Diuretic drugs and the treatment of edema: from clinic to bench and back again. Am J Kidney Dis 23:623, 1994

71. Garg R, Yusuf S: Overview of randomized trials of angiotensin-converting enzyme inhibitors on mortality and morbidity in patients with heart failure. Collaborative Group on ACE inhibitor Trials. JAMA 273:1450, 1995

72. Khalil M, Basher A, Brown EJ Jr, et al: A remarkable medical story: benefits of angiotensin-converting enzyme inhibitors in cardiac patients. J Am Coll Cardiol 37:1757, 2001

73. Munzel T, Keaney JF Jr: Are ACE inhibitors a "magic bullet" against oxidative stress? Circulation (Online) 104:1571, 2001

74. Havranek E, Thomas I, Smith W, et al: Dose-related beneficial long-term hemodynamic and clinical efficacy of irbesartan in heart failure. J Am Coll Cardiol 33:1174, 1999

75. Pitt B, Poole-Wilson PA, Segal R, et al: Effect of losartan compared with captopril on mortality in patients with symptomatic heart failure: randomised trial—the Losartan Heart Failure Survival Study ELITE II. Lancet 355:1582, 2000

76. Pitt B, Segal R, Martinez FA, et al: Randomised trial of losartan versus captopril in patients over 65 with heart failure (Evaluation of Losartan in the Elderly Study, ELITE). Lancet 349:747, 1997

77. Cohn JN, Tognoni G, Valsartan Heart Failure Trial Investigators: A randomized trial of the angiotensin-receptor blocker valsartan in chronic heart failure. N Engl J Med 345:1667, 2001

78. McMurray JJ, Pfeffer MA, Swedberg K, et al: Which inhibitor of the renin-angiotensin system should be used in chronic heart failure and acute myocardial infarction? Circulation 110:3281, 2004

79. Young JB, Dunlap ME, Pfeffer MA, et al: Mortality and morbidity reduction with Candesartan in patients with chronic heart failure and left ventricular systolic dysfunction: results of the CHARM low-left ventricular ejection fraction trials. Circulation 110:2618, 2004

80. Jong P, Demers C, McKelvie RS, et al: Angiotensin receptor blockers in heart failure: meta-analysis of randomized controlled trials. J Am Coll Cardiol 39:463, 2002

81. Martin J, Krum H: Role of valsartan and other angiotensin receptor blocking agents in the management of cardiovascular disease. Pharmacol Res 46:203, 2002

82. McMurray J, Cohen-Solal A, Dietz R, et al: Practical recommendations for the use of ACE inhibitors, beta-blockers, aldosterone antagonists and angiotensin receptor blockers in heart failure: putting guidelines into practice. Eur J Heart Fail 7:710, 2005

83. Gring CN, Francis GS: A hard look at angiotensin receptor blockers in heart failure. J Am Coll Cardiol 44:1841, 2004

84. Farrell M, Foody J, Krumholz H: Beta-blockers in heart failure: clinical applications. JAMA 287:890, 2002

85. Foody J, Farrell M, Krumholz H: Beta-blocker therapy in heart failure: scientific review. JAMA 287:883, 2002

86. Bristow M: Beta-adrenergic receptor blockade in chronic heart failure. Circulation 101:558, 2000

87. Groenning B, Nilsson J, Sondergaard L, et al: Antiremodeling effects on the left ventricle during beta-blockade with metoprolol in the treatment of chronic heart failure. J Am Coll Cardiol 36:2072, 2000

88. Hall S, Cigarroa C, Marcoux L, et al: Time course of improvement in left ventricular function, mass and geometry in patients with congestive heart failure treated with beta-adrenergic blockade. J Am Coll Cardiol 25:1154, 1995

89. Krum H, Roecker EB, Mohacsi P, et al: Effects of initiating carvedilol in patients with severe chronic heart failure: results from the COPERNICUS study. JAMA 289:712, 2003

90. Rahimtoola SH: Digitalis therapy for patients in clinical heart failure. Circulation 109:2942, 2004

91. The effect of digoxin on mortality and morbidity in patients with heart failure. Digitalis Investigators Group. N Engl J Med 336:525, 1997

92. Rathore S, Wang Y, Krumholz HM: Sex-based differences in the effect of digoxin for the treatment of heart failure. N Engl J Med 347:1403, 2002

93. Eichhorn EJ, Gheorghiade M: Digoxin—new perspective on an old drug. N Engl J Med 347:1394, 2002

94. Adams KF, Gheorghiade M, Uretsky BF, et al: Clinical benefits of low serum digoxin concentrations in heart failure. J Am Coll Cardiol 39:946, 2002

95. McMurray JJ, O'Meara E: Treatment of heart failure with spironolactone—trial and tribulations. N Engl J Med 351:526, 2004

96. Weber KT: Aldosterone in congestive heart failure. N Engl J Med 345:1689, 2001

97. Pitt B, Zannad F, Remme W, et al: The effect of spironolactone on morbidity and mortality in patients with severe heart failure. N Engl J Med 341:709, 1999

98. Pitt B, Remme W, Zannad F, et al: Eplerenone, an aldosterone-receptor blocker, in patients with left ventricular dysfunction after myocardial infarction. N Engl J Med 348:1309, 2003

99. Gomberg-Maitland M, Baran DA, Fuster V: Treatment of congestive heart failure: guidelines for the primary care physician and the heart failure specialist. Arch Intern Med 161:342, 2001

100. Taylor AL, Ziesche S, Yancy C, et al: Combination of isosorbide dinitrate and hydralazine in blacks with heart failure. N Engl J Med 351:2049, 2004 (erratum, N Engl J Med 352:1276, 2005)

101. Stevenson LW: Clinical use of inotropic therapy for heart failure: looking back-

ward or forward? Part II: chronic inotropic therapy. Circulation 108:492, 2003

102. Baumgartner WA: What's new in cardiac surgery. J Am Coll Surg 192:345, 2001

103. Bishay ES, McCarthy PM, Cosgrove DM, et al: Mitral valve surgery in patients with severe left ventricular dysfunction. Eur J Cardiothoracic Surg 17:213, 2000

104. Bitran D, Merin O, Klutstein MW, et al: Mitral valve repair in severe ischemic cardiomyopathy. J Cardiac Surg 16:79, 2001

105. Raman JS, Hata M, Storer M, et al: The mid-term results of ventricular containment (ACORN WRAP) for end-stage ischemic cardiomyopathy. Ann Thorac Cardiovasc Surg 7:278, 2001

106. Starling RC, McCarthy PM, Buda T, et al: Results of partial left ventriculectomy for dilated cardiomyopathy: hemodynamic, clinical and echocardiographic observations. J Am Coll Cardiol 36:2098, 2000

107. Hosenpud JD, Bennett LE, Keck BM, et al: The Registry of the International Society for Heart and Lung Transplantation: eighteenth official report–2001. J Heart Lung Transplant 20:805, 2001

108. Jessup M: Mechanical cardiac-support devices—dreams and devilish details. N Engl J Med 345:1490, 2001

109. Frazier OH: Mechanical circulatory support: new advances, new pumps, new ideas. Semin Thorac Cardiovasc Surg 14:178, 2002

110. Stevenson LW, Rose EA: Left ventricular assist devices: bridges to transplantation, recovery, and destination for whom? Circulation 108:3059, 2003

111. Abraham WT: Cardiac resynchronization therapy: a review of clinical trials and criteria for identifying the appropriate patient. Rev Cardiovasc Med 4(suppl 2):S30, 2003

112. Boehmer JP: Device therapy for heart failure. Am J Cardiol 91:53D, 2003

113. Abraham WT, Fisher WG, Smith AL, et al: Cardiac resynchronization in chronic heart failure. N Engl J Med 346:1845, 2002

114. Cazeau S, Leclercq C, Lavergne T, et al: Effects of multisite biventricular pacing in patients with heart failure and intraventricular conduction delay. N Engl J Med 344:873, 2001

115. Touiza A, Etienne Y, Gilard M, et al: Long-term left ventricular pacing: assessment and comparison with biventricular pacing in patients with severe congestive heart failure. J Am Coll Cardiol 38:1971, 2001

116. Bradley D, Bradley E, Baughman KL, et al: Cardiac resynchronization and death from progressive heart failure: a meta-analysis of randomized controlled trials. JAMA 289:730, 2003

117. Bristow MR, Saxon LA, Boehmer J, et al: Cardiac-resynchronization therapy with or without an implantable defibrillator in advanced chronic heart failure. N Engl J Med 350:2140, 2004

118. Cleland JG, Daubert JC, Erdmann E, et al: The effect of cardiac resynchronization on morbidity and mortality in heart failure. N Engl J Med 352:1539, 2005

119. Moss AJ, Zareba W, Hall WJ, et al: Prophylactic implantation of a defibrillator in patients with myocardial infarction and reduced ejection fraction. N Engl J Med 346:877, 2002

120. Bardy GH, Lee KL, Mark DB, et al: Amiodarone or an implantable cardioverter-defibrillator for congestive heart failure. N Engl J Med 352:225, 2005

121. Gustafsson I, Brendorp B, Seibaek M, et al: Influence of diabetes and diabetes-gender interaction on the risk of death in patients hospitalized with congestive heart failure. J Am Coll Cardiol 43:771, 2004

122. Hillege HL, Girbes AR, de Kam PJ, et al: Renal function, neurohormonal activation, and survival in patients with chronic heart failure. Circulation 102:203, 2000

123. Jones RC, Francis GS, Lauer MS: Predictors of mortality in patients with heart failure and preserved systolic function in the Digitalis Investigation Group trial. J Am Coll Cardiol 44:1025, 2004

124. McAlister FA, Ezekowitz J, Tonelli M, et al: Renal insufficiency and heart failure: prognostic and therapeutic implications from a prospective cohort study. Circulation 109:1004, 2004

125. Rudiger A, Harjola VP, Muller A, et al: Acute heart failure: clinical presentation, one-year mortality and prognostic factors. Eur J Heart Fail 7:662, 2005

126. Felker GM, Thompson RE, Hare JM, et al: Underlying causes and long-term survival in patients with initially unexplained cardiomyopathy. N Engl J Med 342:1077, 2000

127. Senni M, Redfield M: Heart failure with preserved systolic function: a different natural history? J Am Coll Cardiol 38:1277, 2001

128. Burkhoff D, Maurer MS, Packer M: Heart failure with a normal ejection fraction: is it really a disorder of diastolic function? Circulation 107:656, 2003

129. Chen HH, Lainchbury JG, Senni M, et al: Diastolic heart failure in the community: clinical profile, natural history, therapy, and impact of proposed diagnostic criteria. J Cardiac Fail 8:279, 2002

130. Gaasch WH, Zile MR: Left ventricular diastolic dysfunction and diastolic heart failure. Annu Rev Med 55:373, 2004

131. Mancini DM, Eisen H, Kussmaul W, et al: Value of peak exercise oxygen consumption for optimal timing of cardiac transplantation in ambulatory patients with heart failure. Circulation 83:778, 1991

132. Aaronson K, Schwartz S, Chen T, et al: Development and prospective validation of a clinical index to predict survival in ambulatory patients referred for cardiac transplant evaluation. Circulation 95:2660, 1997

133. Levy D, Kenchaiah S, Larson M, et al: Long-term trends in the incidence of and survival with heart failure. N Engl J Med 347:1397, 2002

Acknowledgment

Figure 1   Alice Y. Chen

27 Valvular Heart Disease

Ronan J. Curtin, M.D., and Brian P. Griffin, M.D.

Valvular heart disease is an important cause of cardiac morbidity in developed countries despite a decline in the prevalence of rheumatic disease in those countries. Valvular heart disease can give rise to stenosis, regurgitation, or a combination of lesions at one or more valves. The more common significant anomalies that are currently encountered are mitral regurgitation, caused by mitral valve prolapse (MVP); aortic stenosis, caused by a congenital bicuspid valve or by senile valvular calcification; and aortic regurgitation, caused by a bicuspid aortic valve or dilatation of the aorta. Valvular lesions can occur as a result of pathologic changes in the valvular leaflets or supporting structures (i.e., the chordae or papillary muscles). Ventricular or aortic enlargement can also produce valvular regurgitation as a result of annular dilatation and inadequate leaflet coaptation in the absence of any specific valve pathology. Valvular heart disease tends to progress over time as degenerative changes are superimposed on the primary pathology. Iatrogenic causes of valvular disease are increasingly recognized. Common causes of major valvular lesions are listed [see Table 1].[1]

Etiology

CONGENITAL DISORDERS

Bicuspid aortic valve, a condition in which the aortic valve has two leaflets instead of three, is the most common congenital cardiac disorder, affecting 1% to 2% of the population [see Figure 1].[2] Patients with bicuspid aortic valve tend to present with significant aortic stenosis or regurgitation in their fifth or sixth decade of life. The exact cause of bicuspid aortic valve is unknown, but there is a large heritable component and a significant association with other cardiovascular developmental disorders, including coarctation of the aorta, ventricular and atrial septal defect, mitral valvular abnormalities, and hypoplastic left heart.[3] Many patients with a bicuspid aortic valve have an associated aortopathy with age-dependent aortic dilatation; by 40 years of age, the majority (77%) of patients have significant dilatation of the ascending aorta and aortic arch.[4] A further insight into the complexity of bicuspid aortic valve was provided by the discovery that mutations in the *NOTCH1* gene, a signaling and transcriptional regulator, were found to be associated with bicuspid aortic valve and other congenital cardiac disorders in two families.[5]

Unlike bicuspid aortic valve, unicuspid aortic valve is rare. The latter typically causes significant aortic stenosis by the third

decade of life,[6] and it is associated with dilatation of the ascending aorta in almost 50% of patients. Pulmonary stenosis, a relatively common disorder, usually presents in childhood. Much less common are the congenital abnormalities of the atrioventricular valves, including cleft mitral valve and tricuspid atresia. Valvular abnormalities can be seen in specific developmental syndromes, such as pulmonary stenosis in rubella syndrome and supravalvular aortic stenosis in Williams syndrome.

MYXOMATOUS DEGENERATION

Myxomatous degeneration most often involves the mitral or tricuspid valve. In this condition, leaflet tissue, particularly chordal tissue, is abnormally extensible and weak. The affected valves are therefore more likely to prolapse, leading to significant regurgitation. On echocardiography, features of myxomatous degeneration include elongated and thickened mitral leaflets with interchordal hooding and chordal elongation. Chordal rupture is common and may precipitate a rapid clinical deterioration resulting from sudden, severe regurgitation. The precise abnormality in valvular tissue is unknown, but it is thought to involve dysregulation of the extracellular matrix proteins.[7] A familial tendency is often noted in this disease.[8] Three genetic loci for autosomal dominant inherited myxomatous mitral valve disease have been described, but the precise genes and mutations responsible have not yet been delineated.[9-11] Inherited connective tissue diseases such as Marfan syndrome produce valvular abnormalities similar to those found in myxomatous degeneration.

RHEUMATIC HEART DISEASE

Rheumatic fever is now rare in the United States, with approximately 100 cases reported each year; however, it remains a major health problem in developing countries, particularly sub-Saharan Africa and Southeast Asia.[12] About 60% of people with rheumatic carditis develop chronic rheumatic heart disease. Rheumatic heart disease remains the most common cause of mitral stenosis in the United States; it is also a common cause of aortic regurgitation and multivalvular heart disease.[13]

Rheumatic fever appears to cause valvular heart disease by an autoimmune phenomenon whereby antibodies against streptococcal antigens cross-react with valvular tissue. Valvular involvement can present acutely as a result of edema of valvular tissue. Chronic rheumatic heart disease is caused by progressive fibrosis, superimposed calcification, and scarring with retraction of leaflet tissue—a process leading to valvular

Table 1 Causes of Specific Valvular Lesions

	Mitral	Aortic	Tricuspid	Pulmonary
Stenosis	Rheumatic disease, calcification, SLE	Calcification, congenital disease, rheumatic disease	Rheumatic disease, carcinoid tumor	Congenital disease, carcinoid tumor
Regurgitation	Myxomatous degeneration, ischemia, secondary causes, rheumatic disease, annular calcification, endocarditis, SLE	Congenital disease, secondary causes, rheumatic disease, endocarditis, SLE	Secondary causes, rheumatic disease, endocarditis	Secondary causes

SLE—systemic lupus erythematosus

a

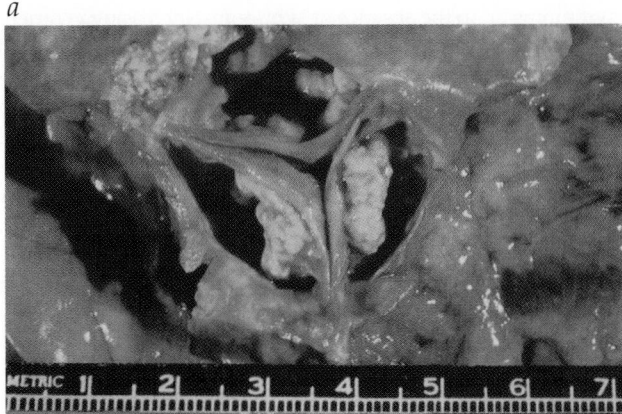

b

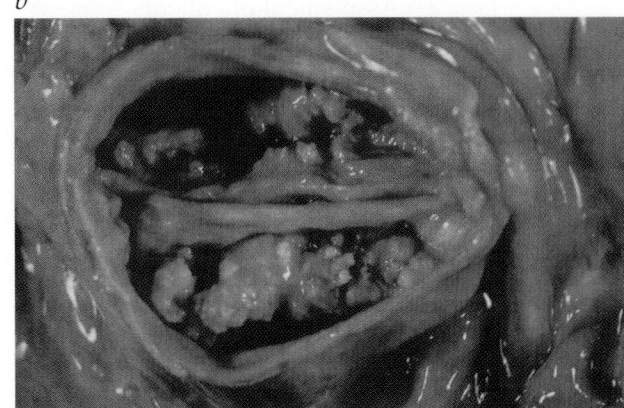

Figure 1   Pathologic specimens showing degenerative calcification of (*a*) a tricuspid aortic valve and (*b*) a congenital bicuspid valve.[62]

stenosis, incompetence, or both. The mitral and aortic valves are usually involved. The interval between the occurrence of rheumatic fever and occurrence of chronic rheumatic heart disease varies, as does the degree of involvement.

DEGENERATIVE HEART DISEASE

Degenerative calcification is a cause of aortic stenosis in the elderly and in patients with renal dysfunction; it results from calcium deposition on the body of the valvular leaflets rather than on the commissures [*see Figure 1*].[2] Factors that have been found to promote degenerative valvular changes are increasing age, a low body mass index, hypertension, and hyperlipidemia. Histologic changes that simulate atheroma and involve lipid deposition and inflammatory cell infiltration of the leaflets have been described in patients with early degenerative changes in the aortic leaflets. Even mild degenerative changes in the aortic valve have been reported to be adverse prognostic factors.[14] Calcification of the mitral annulus is common in the elderly; it is more common in women than in men and can produce mitral regurgitation. Occasionally, mitral annular calcification extends onto the valvular leaflets, causing stenosis.

ENDOCARDITIS

Endocarditis usually occurs on previously abnormal valves, although overwhelming sepsis can infect normal valves. The predominant hemodynamic manifestation of endocarditis is valvular regurgitation. Contributory causes of endocarditis-related valvular regurgitation include leaflet prolapse (resulting from a large vegetation), leaflet perforation, and chronic scarring of infected tissue. In rare cases, large vegetations lead to valvular stenosis.

CORONARY ARTERY DISEASE

Mitral regurgitation is common in coronary artery disease (CAD) and has a number of causal mechanisms. Acute ischemia or infarction of a papillary muscle or of the wall to which the papillary muscle is attached leads to impaired leaflet coaptation and mitral regurgitation. Regurgitation can be severe and can vary with the severity of the ischemia. Papillary head rupture or, more rarely, muscle rupture leads to catastrophic regurgitation that is often fatal.

CONNECTIVE TISSUE DISEASE

Libman-Sacks endocarditis consists of noninfected warty vegetations involving predominantly the mitral valve; it is charac-

teristic of systemic lupus erythematosus.[15] Significant regurgitation and stenosis rarely occur acutely but are seen with scarring from chronic disease. Valvular involvement in rheumatoid arthritis is common and leads to valvular thickening but is usually not of hemodynamic significance. Aortitis in ankylosing spondylitis may produce significant aortic regurgitation.

IATROGENIC CAUSES OF VALVULAR HEART DISEASE

Iatrogenic causes include radiation therapy, drug therapy, and complications of permanent cardiac pacing devices. Radiation leads to scarring and calcification of valvular leaflets many years after the initiating radiation. This usually follows a typical pattern, affecting predominantly the aortic valve and anterior mitral leaflet. Treatment with serotonin agonists such as methysergide or treatment with anorexiants such as fenfluramine and phentermine in combination (fen-phen) can cause valvular injury [*see* Anorexiant-Induced Valvular Disorder, *below*].[16-18] One report has suggested that implantation of right ventricular pacemaker and implantable cardioverter-defibrillator (ICD) leads can cause an injury to the tricuspid valve that results in severe symptomatic tricuspid regurgitation.[19] The incidence of device-induced tricuspid regurgitation is not known and appears to be underestimated by transthoracic echocardiography.

OTHER CAUSES OF VALVULAR HEART DISEASE

Amyloid disease causes valvular thickening but rarely causes significant stenosis. The carcinoid syndrome most often involves the valves on the right side of the heart and leads to stenosis or incompetence of the tricuspid or pulmonary valve.

SECONDARY INVOLVEMENT

Left ventricular dilatation can cause dilatation of the mitral annulus and, thereby, mitral regurgitation. Common secondary causes of mitral regurgitation include CAD, aortic valvular disease, and dilated cardiomyopathy. Similarly, tricuspid regurgitation results from right ventricular enlargement secondary to pulmonary hypertension or an atrial septal defect. Dilatation of the ascending aorta, especially involving the annulus of the aortic valve, can lead to aortic regurgitation. This condition is seen in hypertension and in aneurysms of the ascending aorta.

Assessment and Management

Valvular heart disease often remains asymptomatic for many years, but once symptoms develop, survival is reduced if the le-

Table 2 Assessment of Patients
with Valvular Heart Disease

Parameters	Tools
Symptom severity	History, stress testing
Nature of valve lesion	Auscultation, Doppler echocardiography
Hemodynamic severity of lesion	Physical examination, Doppler echocardiography, cardiac catheterization
Effects of lesion on cardiac chamber size and function	Echocardiography, cardiac catheterization, stress echocardiography
Determination of the optimal time for intervention	Echocardiography, stress echocardiography
Selection of appropriate procedure/prosthesis	Echocardiography

sion is not corrected. The assessment of patients with valvular heart disease can be summarized [*see Table 2*]. Patients should be carefully questioned regarding any limitation of physical activity. The evaluation of exercise capacity may require a stress test in some cases. The physical examination, which includes cardiac auscultation [*see Table 3*], is important in characterizing the lesion and its hemodynamic severity; however, all significant murmurs should be further assessed by echocardiography.[20] Valvular stenosis is readily quantified by continuous wave Doppler echocardiography using the modified Bernoulli equation (P = $4v^2$, where P is the pressure gradient measured in mm Hg and v is the flow velocity measured in m/sec). For example, if the peak velocity recorded across the aortic valve by Doppler echocardiography is 4 m/sec, then the peak pressure gradient will be estimated as $4(4^2)$, or 64 mm Hg. Valvular regurgitation can be more difficult to assess and requires an integrated approach that includes color flow Doppler, continuous wave Doppler, pulsed wave Doppler, and two-dimensional echocardiographic measurements.[21] The effects of valvular heart disease on chamber size and function are best assessed serially by echocardiography or, at the time of cardiac catheterization, by ventriculography. In cases of stenotic lesions, intervention is rarely required until symptoms occur. Indications for intervention in regurgitant lesions are more complex; such indications include significant

symptoms or, in the absence of symptoms, increasing ventricular size, overt ventricular contractile dysfunction, or both.[20] All patients with even mild valvular heart disease require prophylaxis against endocarditis at the time of dental procedures or other procedures that can produce significant bacteremia. The American Heart Association has recommended several prophylactic regimens [*see Table 4*].[22]

Despite the increase in intravascular volume that occurs during pregnancy, pregnancy is usually well tolerated in previously asymptomatic patients with valvular heart disease.[23] During pregnancy, regurgitant lesions are better tolerated than stenosis. Prophylactic intervention to increase the valvular area is recommended in patients with hemodynamically severe stenosis before pregnancy.

Patients with hemodynamically significant valvular heart disease should generally avoid participation in competitive sports. Reference should be made to the recommendations of the American College of Cardiology for more information about specific lesions.[20] Valvular heart disease is a chronic disease requiring periodic examination and follow-up, even in asymptomatic patients and in those who have had corrective surgical or other procedures. Patients with prosthetic valves should be seen at least yearly.

Specific Valvular Lesions

MITRAL STENOSIS

Normally, the cross-sectional area of the mitral valve is at least 4 cm². Mitral stenosis leads to a reduction in valvular area; stenosis is considered severe when the valvular area is less than 1 cm². To maintain flow through the valve, left atrial pressure rises, leading to an increase in the pressure gradient across the valve and increased pulmonary venous and capillary pressures, with resultant dyspnea. Flow through the stenotic valve is dependent on the duration of diastole. Tachycardia shortens diastole disproportionately and causes a further elevation in left atrial pressure and can precipitate symptoms even in patients with relatively mild stenosis. Elevated left atrial pressure contributes to left atrial enlargement, which in turn predisposes the patient to atrial fibrillation, atrial thrombus formation, and thromboembolism, all of which are common complications of mitral stenosis. Severe mitral stenosis is often associated with an increase in pulmonary arterial pressure, leading to right-sided heart failure and secondary tricuspid and pulmonary incompetence. In pa-

Table 3 Auscultatory Findings Associated with Common Valve Problems

Lesion	Cardiac Cycle	Quality	Location	Other Sounds
Aortic stenosis	Systolic, mid-peaking to late peaking	Harsh	Aortic area, left sternal border, apex	Soft S_2, S_4
Aortic regurgitation	Diastolic, early decrescendo	Blowing	Left sternal border, aortic area	—
Mitral stenosis	Diastolic, mid-peaking to late peaking, increases with atrial contraction if rhythm is normal	Rumble	Apex	Opening snap, loud S_1
Mitral regurgitation	Systolic, holosystolic, late systolic with MVP, papillary muscle dysfunction	Blowing	Apex, axilla	Click, soft S_1, S_3
Tricuspid regurgitation	Systolic, increase with inspiration	Blowing	Lower left sternal border, xiphisternum	—
Pulmonary stenosis	Systolic, mid-peaking	Harsh	Pulmonary area, left sternal border	—

MVP—mitral valve prolapse

Table 4 Summary of American Heart Association Recommendations for Endocarditis Prophylaxis[22]

Procedure	Patient Condition	Drug	Regimen*
Dental, oral, respiratory tract, or esophageal†	At risk	Amoxicillin	Adults, 2.0 g; children, 50 mg/kg; orally 1 hr before procedure
	At risk and unable to take oral medications	Ampicillin	Adults, 2.0 g; children, 50 mg/kg. I.M. or I.V. within 30 min before procedure
	At risk and allergic to amoxicillin, ampicillin, and penicillin	Clindamycin *or* Cephalexin‡ or cefadroxil‡ *or* Azithromycin or clarithromycin	Adults, 600 mg; children, 20 mg/kg; orally 1 hr before procedure Adults, 2.0 g; children, 50 mg/kg; orally 1 hr before procedure Adults, 500 mg; children, 15 mg/kg; orally 1 hr before procedure
	At risk and allergic to amoxicillin, ampicillin, and penicillin and unable to take oral medications	Clindamycin *or* Cefazolin	Adults, 600 mg; children, 20 mg/kg. I.V. within 30 min before procedure Adults, 1.0 g; children, 25 mg/kg. I.M. or I.V. within 30 min before procedure
Genitourinary/ gastrointestinal	High risk	Ampicillin plus gentamicin	Ampicillin: adults, 2.0 g; children, 50 mg/kg *plus* Gentamicin: 1.5 mg/kg (for both adults and children, not to exceed 120 mg) I.M. or I.V. within 30 min before starting procedure *Then, 6 hr later,* Ampicillin: adults, 1 g; children, 25 mg/kg. I.M. or I.V. *or* Amoxicillin, orally: adults, 1.0 g; children, 25 mg/kg
	High risk and allergic to ampicillin and amoxicillin	Vancomycin plus gentamicin	Vancomycin: adults, 1.0 g; children, 20 mg/kg I.V.; over 1–2 hr *plus* Gentamicin: 1.5 mg/kg (for both adults and children, not to exceed 120 mg) I.M. or I.V. Complete injection/infusion within 30 min before starting procedure
	Moderate risk	Amoxicillin *or* Ampicillin	Adults, 2.0 g; children, 50 mg/kg; orally 1 hr before procedure Adults, 2.0 g; children, 50 mg/kg. I.M. or I.V. within 30 min before starting procedure
	Moderate risk and allergic to ampicillin and amoxicillin	Vancomycin	Adults, 1.0 g; children, 20 mg/kg; over 1–2 hr; complete infusion within 30 min of starting the procedure

Note: For patients already taking an antibiotic or for other special situations, see reference 22.
*Total children's dose should not exceed adult dose.
†Follow-up dose no longer recommended.
‡Cephalosporins should not be used in patients with immediate-type hypersensitivity reaction to penicillins.

tients with severe pulmonary hypertension, cardiac output at rest is reduced; this output reduction can cause a relatively low pressure gradient across the mitral valve even in patients with severe stenosis.

Diagnosis

Clinical manifestations Mitral stenosis is often asymptomatic at presentation and for many years thereafter. Symptomatic patients often present with dyspnea, but they can also present with angina, right-sided heart failure, atrial arrhythmia, or embolism. The physical findings in mitral stenosis depend on the severity of the stenosis, the mobility of the valve, and the cardiac rhythm. The principal sign is a rumbling diastolic murmur that is best heard at the apex with the stethoscope bell. Such a murmur is accentuated by having the patient lie on the left side and by using provocative maneuvers, such as exercise, to increase the heart rate. In sinus rhythm, the murmur increases in intensi-

ty with atrial contraction (presystolic accentuation). Increased severity of stenosis is associated with a longer murmur and a thrill. With a pliable valve, an opening sound (the opening snap) is heard and the sudden closure of the stenotic valve at end diastole gives rise to a loud first heart sound that lends a tapping quality to the apex beat. When the valve calcifies and becomes less mobile, the opening snap and loud first heart sound disappear. A loud pulmonary component of the second heart sound is heard with pulmonary hypertension. The signs and symptoms of mitral stenosis are simulated by left atrial myxoma. In this condition, functional mitral stenosis results from a mobile tumor arising from the interatrial septum and prolapsing into the mitral valve opening.

Imaging studies Electrocardiography can reveal left atrial enlargement if the patient is in sinus rhythm. Left atrial enlargement, mitral valve calcification, and signs of pulmonary conges-

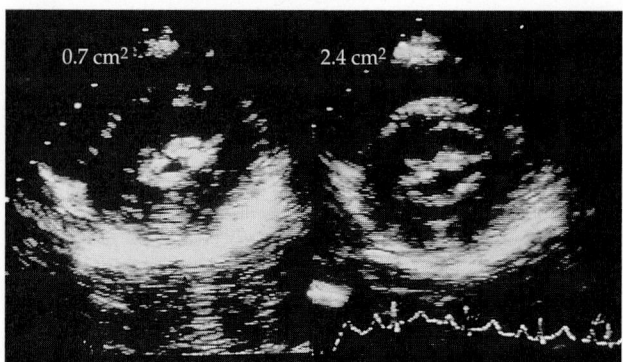

Figure 2 Two-dimensional echocardiographic parasternal short-axis image of a mitral valve before (left) and after (right) percutaneous balloon mitral valvuloplasty. The valve area is estimated by planimetry and increases from 0.7 cm² before valvuloplasty to 2.4 cm² after valvuloplasty.

tion can all be present on chest x-ray. Echocardiography is the test of choice in confirming the diagnosis, establishing the severity of stenosis, detecting complications, and determining the most appropriate treatment. Echocardiography also allows accurate differentiation of mitral stenosis from a left atrial myxoma.

Typically, the stenotic mitral valve leaflets are thicker and less mobile than normal, and they are fused at the commissures. The severity of stenosis is determined by measuring the pressure gradient across the valve with Doppler echocardiography and by calculating the valvular area. Mitral stenosis should be suspected if the mean gradient exceeds 5 mm Hg; the pressure can exceed 20 mm Hg in severe stenosis. Valvular area is measured by tracing the smallest opening of the valve in cross section [*see Figure 2*]. This method is the most accurate way of defining the severity of stenosis, although it is technically demanding and sometimes impossible to perform by two-dimensional echocardiography.[24] Three-dimensional echocardiography is better at identifying the true mitral valve orifice, and it allows very accurate measurement of mitral valve area; however, its availability is limited.[25] Mitral valve area is most readily estimated by Doppler echocardiography. Such evaluation is made on the basis of an empirical formula that calculates the time it takes for the pressure gradient to fall to half its initial value (the pressure half-time). Valvular area is estimated as 220 divided by the pressure half-time. Pulmonary arterial systolic pressure (PAP) can be determined from the tricuspid regurgitant velocity (TRv) and the estimated right atrial pressure (RAP) (usually estimated as 5 mm Hg) by the following equation:

$$PAP = 4(TRv^2) + RAP$$

If the tricuspid regurgitant velocity is 3 m/sec and if RAP is estimated to be 5 mm Hg, then the estimated PAP is $4(3^2) + 5 = 41$ mm Hg. The likelihood that the valve may be successfully dilated, either with percutaneous balloon valvuloplasty or open surgical procedure, is estimated by use of a scoring system based on the echocardiographic appearance of the valvular leaflets and supporting structures.[26]

Transesophageal echocardiography is more useful than transthoracic echocardiography in excluding atrial thrombus and determining the severity of mitral regurgitation and is usually performed if balloon valvuloplasty is being considered. Cardiac catheterization is rarely needed to establish the diagnosis but is used to confirm the severity of stenosis. The valvular gradient is the difference between the left atrial pressure or the pulmonary arterial wedge pressure and the left ventricular diastolic pressure. Valvular area can be calculated from the pressure gradient and the cardiac output.

Stress echocardiography can be very helpful when there is a discrepancy between symptoms and baseline hemodynamic data. It provides an objective assessment of symptoms and functional capacity, as well as transmitral and pulmonary pressures at rest and with exercise. An exercise mean transmitral gradient of 15 mm Hg or higher and a peak right ventricular systolic pressure greater than 60 mm Hg indicate hemodynamically significant mitral stenosis.[20]

Treatment

Once symptoms develop in mitral stenosis, the chance of survival decreases without surgical or balloon dilatation or replacement of the valve. In the absence of symptoms, management is directed at preventing recurrence of rheumatic fever.[27]

Medical therapy Patients in atrial fibrillation require heart-rate control with a beta blocker (e.g., atenolol, 50 mg daily), a calcium channel blocker (e.g., diltiazem CD, 100 mg daily), digoxin (0.125 to 0.25 mg daily), or a combination of these therapies. Systemic anticoagulation with warfarin is indicated to prevent thromboembolism when (1) atrial fibrillation is present, (2) there is a history of embolism, or (3) a thrombus is detected in the atrium. Anticoagulation should be considered for patients with paroxysmal atrial fibrillation, a dilated left atrium (> 50 to 55 mm in diameter on echocardiography), or severe atrial stasis (as evidenced by swirling echoes or smoke in the left atrium on echocardiography).[28,29] In symptomatic patients for whom surgical intervention poses a relatively high risk, the judicious use of diuretics and drugs to control heart rate (i.e., digoxin, calcium channel blockers, or beta blockers) may allow symptomatic relief without the need for surgical intervention.

Surgical intervention Intervention to increase valvular area is indicated before the onset of symptoms of dyspnea in the following patients: (1) women with severe stenosis who wish to become pregnant but are unlikely to tolerate the volume load of pregnancy, (2) patients who experience recurrent thromboembolic events, and (3) patients who have severe pulmonary hypertension. A number of interventions are currently available to increase the valvular area in mitral stenosis. These interventions include percutaneous balloon valvuloplasty, which is performed in the cardiac catheterization laboratory; surgical commissurotomy; and replacement of the mitral valve with a prosthesis.

Balloon valvuloplasty, which is performed by inflating a specially designed balloon catheter in the mitral orifice to split the fused commissures,[30] provides excellent symptomatic relief in suitable patients[31]; it is currently the intervention of choice in mitral stenosis. Balloon valvuloplasty typically doubles the mitral valve area, from 1.0 cm² to 2.0 cm², and provides a concomitant reduction in the pressure gradient [*see Figure 3*]. Complications of mitral balloon valvuloplasty include severe mitral regurgitation (3%), thromboembolism (3%), and residual atrial septal defect with significant shunting (10% to 20%). Mortality associated with the procedure is less than 1%.[32,33] Contraindications to mitral balloon valvuloplasty include significant mitral regurgitation, which is likely to increase after balloon inflation; the presence of a left atrial thrombus, which can be dislodged at the time of the procedure; and significant subvalvular involvement or

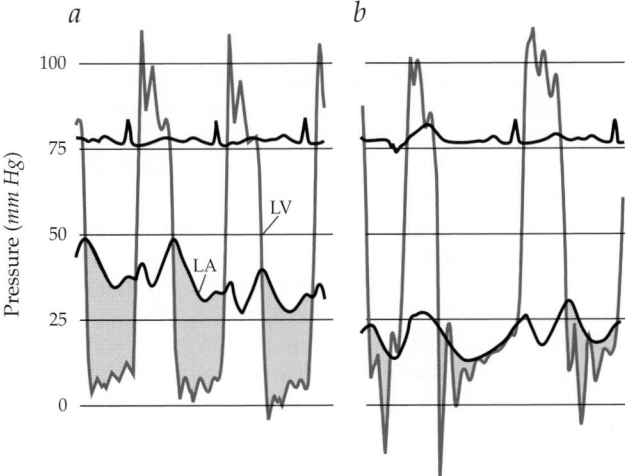

Figure 3 Simultaneous left atrial pressure (LA, black line) and left ventricular pressure (LV, blue line) are shown before (*a*) and after (*b*) percutaneous mitral valvuloplasty. The shaded area shows the pressure gradient across the mitral valve; the pressure falls after valvuloplasty.

leaflet calcification, each of which increases the risk of complications and limits the degree of dilatation produced.[34] In pregnant patients with symptomatically severe mitral stenosis that is not responsive to conservative measures (e.g., bed rest and heart-rate control), balloon valvuloplasty is the intervention of choice.[35]

Surgical commissurotomy is usually performed under direct vision after cardiopulmonary bypass. Surgical commissurotomy may be feasible when balloon valvuloplasty is impossible (e.g., in patients with significant mitral regurgitation, subvalvular stenosis, or atrial thrombus). A number of studies comparing surgical commissurotomy with balloon commissurotomy have shown equivalent immediate, medium-term (3- to 4-year), and long-term (7-year) results with regard to increase in valvular area, improvement in symptoms, and freedom from repeat intervention in appropriately selected patients.[34,36] At 7 years after balloon commissurotomy, 50% to 69% of patients remain free of major cardiovascular events, and up to 90% of patients remain free of reintervention.[36-38] However, commissurotomy, whether effected by a balloon or surgically, is a palliative procedure; in most cases, further intervention is eventually required. Repeat commissurotomy is sometimes feasible; most often, mitral valve replacement is necessary.[39]

A prosthetic replacement is indicated if the valve is heavily scarred or calcified or if severe mitral regurgitation is present. Morbidity and mortality are higher with prosthetic replacement than with either surgical or balloon commissurotomy.

MITRAL REGURGITATION

Mitral regurgitation leads to volume overload of the left ventricle, which must increase in size to achieve a normal stroke output to accommodate the leakage of blood back into the left atrium. Progressive left ventricular dilatation eventually leads to an increase in afterload, contractile impairment, reduction of cardiac output, and heart failure. In acute mitral regurgitation (such as that which can occur with chordal rupture, ischemia, or endocarditis), left atrial and pulmonary venous and arterial pressures increase quickly, giving rise to dyspnea and, often, acute pulmonary edema. In more chronic forms of mitral regurgitation, an increase in left atrial pressure is often offset by a concomitant

increase in atrial compliance; hence, symptoms appear late in the course of the disease. Left atrial enlargement predisposes the patient to atrial fibrillation and atrial thromboembolism. In long-standing mitral regurgitation, pulmonary hypertension can develop, which in turn leads to tricuspid regurgitation and right-sided heart failure.

Diagnosis

Clinical manifestations In most patients, mitral regurgitation remains asymptomatic for many years. Dyspnea, fatigue from low cardiac output, and edema occur late in the course of the disease. Mitral regurgitation is recognized clinically by a systolic murmur at the apex, radiating to the axilla and increasing on expiration. In patients with a posteriorly directed jet of mitral regurgitation, the murmur is heard well at the back. In more severe cases, the murmur lasts throughout systole, the first and second heart sounds are soft or difficult to hear, and a third heart sound is present. A midsystolic click can be present in myxomatous disease; in less severe cases, this click can precede the murmur. The murmur can also be confined to late systole with papillary muscle dysfunction. Mitral regurgitant murmurs caused by ischemia can be variable in duration and intensity, depending on the degree of ischemia and the loading conditions.

Imaging studies Doppler echocardiography is the noninvasive method of choice in confirming the presence of mitral regurgitation. Doppler echocardiography is used both to diagnose the mechanism of the regurgitation (e.g., prolapse or annular dilatation) and to provide a measure of its severity [*see* Assessment of Regurgitation Severity, *below*]. Transesophageal echocardiography is very sensitive in the detection of mitral regurgitation; it is used mainly in patients who are difficult to evaluate by the transthoracic approach or when the valvular morphology and regurgitant severity are still in question after transthoracic echocardiography. Contrast ventriculography is used to determine the severity of mitral regurgitation in patients undergoing cardiac catheterization. This procedure involves injecting radiopaque contrast medium into the left ventricle and assessing the extent and duration of opacification of the left atrium. In patients undergoing hemodynamic monitoring, large systolic V waves on the pulmonary arterial wedge tracing raise the suspicion of acute severe mitral regurgitation, as can occur in acute ischemia; however, such systolic V waves can occur in the absence of severe regurgitation.

Assessment of regurgitation severity Measuring the severity of regurgitation by echocardiography requires an integrated assessment of several parameters. These include color flow Doppler to assess the regurgitant jet; continuous wave Doppler to assess jet density; pulsed wave Doppler to assess transmitral and pulmonary venous flow; and two-dimensional echocardiography to assess structural features (e.g., left atrial size, left ventricle size, and contractile function).[21] Quantitative measurements of regurgitation—such as the regurgitant volume, regurgitant fraction (i.e., regurgitant volume divided by [regurgitant volume plus stroke volume]), and regurgitant orifice area (ROA) (i.e., the area through which the valve leaks)—are now possible with newer Doppler techniques. An accurate measurement of ROA and regurgitant volume can be achieved in most patients by the flow convergence (also called the proximal isovelocity surface area (PISA)) method of calculation. This method is based on the principle that as blood approaches the regurgitant orifice, its velocity increases and its volume remains constant. This can be represented graphically as a series of hemispheres of increasing velocity and decreasing surface area on the ventricular aspect of the mitral regurgitant orifice [see Figure 4]. Knowing the velocity of one of these hemispheres (Nyquist limit) and its radius allows us to calculate the ROA by using the following formula:

$$ROA = 2\pi r^2 \times Va/Pk\ Vreg$$

where r is the radius, Va is the Nyquist limit of blood flow in the direction of the regurgitant jet, and Pk Vreg is the maximal velocity of the regurgitant jet on continuous wave Doppler. This method of calculation, when properly applied, is useful in determining the true severity of the lesion; repeated calculations can be used to evaluate the changes of the lesion over time.[40]

Calculation of ROA may prove useful in determining the appropriate timing of surgery in asymptomatic patients [see Indications for Surgery in Asymptomatic Patients, below]. However, size and volume of the left ventricle and contractile function, as assessed by the ejection fraction, are the standard parameters used to determine the need for surgical intervention.

Treatment

Indications for surgery in asymptomatic patients Asymptomatic mitral regurgitation is more difficult to assess than other valvular lesions because in this condition, the true contractile function of the left ventricle is difficult to determine with conventional measures such as the ejection fraction. Left ventricular dysfunction is often latent, and once present, the dysfunction may not be corrected by operative intervention.[41] Conventional measurements of contractility are confounded by the increase in ventricular preload caused by the extra volume of blood in the left atrium and the variable effect on afterload. Afterload is increased by left ventricular dilatation, but this effect is offset as the ventricle ejects much of its blood into a relatively low pressure

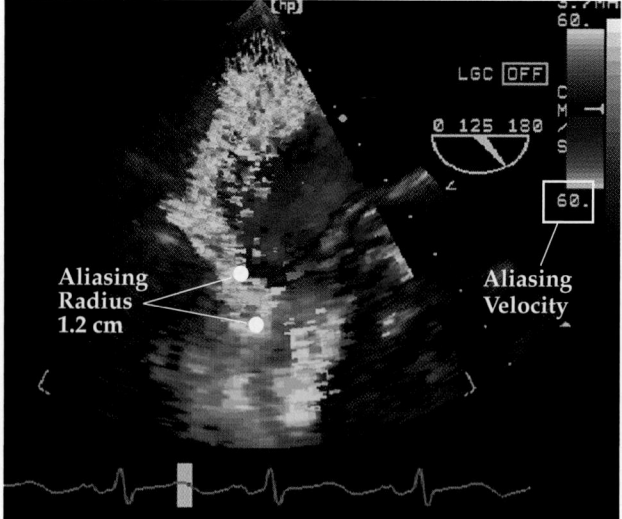

Figure 4 **Transesophageal echocardiogram of a patient with severe, posteriorly directed mitral regurgitation (MR). An aliasing radius of 1.2 cm was measured at a Nyquist limit of 60 cm/sec. Peak MR velocity by color flow Doppler measured 540 cm/sec (not shown). Using the formula ROA = 2πr² × Va/Pk Vreg, the ROA was calculated at 1 cm² (6.28 × (1.2)² × 60/540). (ROA—regurgitant orifice area; r—radius; Va—Nyquist limit; Pk Vreg—maximal velocity of regurgitant jet on continuous wave Doppler)**

system (the left atrium). The left ventricular ejection fraction can appear falsely elevated in mitral regurgitation and usually falls after surgical correction. An ejection fraction of less than 60% should be considered abnormally low in patients with mitral regurgitation. The American Heart Association/American College of Cardiology (AHA/ACC) guidelines recommend referral for mitral valve repair or replacement when the left ventricular end-systolic dimension is greater than 4.5 cm and resting ejection fraction is less than 60%.[20] There is evidence, however, suggesting that a left ventricular end-systolic dimension greater than 4.0 cm is more sensitive to contractile reserve and that its use as an indication for surgery leads to improved postoperative outcomes.[42,43] Stress echocardiography is useful in detecting latent left ventricular dysfunction not evident on a resting study. Failure of the left ventricular ejection fraction to increase or failure of the left ventricular end-systolic volume to decrease on exercise is predictive of incipient left ventricular dysfunction, but this finding is not a well-established indication for early surgery.[44,45] Data indicate that quantitative measurements of mitral regurgitation are also important in making a decision on the appropriate timing of surgery for patients with asymptomatic mitral regurgitation. An ROA greater than 0.4 cm² indicates severe mitral regurgitation and, in asymptomatic patients, is associated with a high risk of cardiovascular events, including death.[46] Serial echocardiographic evaluation should be performed at least yearly and should be performed more frequently as ventricular dilatation progresses in patients with severe asymptomatic mitral regurgitation. Studies indicate a better long-term survival rate in patients with severe mitral regurgitation when surgery is performed early.[47,48]

Indications for surgery in symptomatic patients Symptomatic severe mitral regurgitation is considered an indication for surgical intervention if the valve is primarily involved. Symptomatic patients with ischemic mitral regurgitation often require mitral valve surgery in addition to revascularization [see Surgical Intervention, below]. Mitral regurgitation secondary to left ventricular dilatation often improves with afterload reduction, and surgical intervention is not usually indicated.

Patients with moderately severe or severe left ventricular dysfunction (ejection fraction < 35%) and significant mitral regurgitation were once thought to be poor surgical candidates because of high operative risk; however, studies have shown that there is acceptable risk associated with operations in these patients.[49,50] Surgery usually improves symptoms in these patients, but a survival benefit has not yet been demonstrated.[51,52]

Nonsurgical intervention Patients who are not considered suitable for surgery because of left ventricular dysfunction often benefit from afterload reduction and diuretics.[53] However, in patients who have primary asymptomatic mitral regurgitation with preserved left ventricular function, afterload reduction has not been shown to delay surgery or improve left ventricular function in the few small studies that have addressed this issue; afterload reduction is not currently recommended to treat such patients.[54] Afterload reduction is beneficial for stabilizing patients with hemodynamically significant acute mitral regurgitation in preparation for surgery.

Surgical intervention Mitral valve repair is currently the technique of choice in the surgical management of mitral regurgitation caused by degenerative mitral valve disease, bacterial endocarditis, and, in select patients, ischemic mitral regurgitation [see Figure 5]. Mitral valve repair is less useful for patients with rheumatic mitral disease because of the limited durability of valve repair in this patient group.[55]

Valve repair is accomplished by use of a variety of techniques, depending on the mechanism and etiology of the regurgitation. Such techniques include partial leaflet resection, chordal shortening or transfer, and insertion of an annuloplasty ring to reduce the size of the annulus. In patients with degenerative valve disease, the benefits of valve repair over valve replacement include lower operative and long-term mortality, better preservation of ventricular function, reduced need for warfarin therapy, and a lower risk of serious hemorrhage.[56,57] Reoperation rates for valve repair and valve replacement are similar (1% to 2% a year). Valve repair is most successful in patients who have degenerative mitral valve disease with severe mitral regurgitation caused by segmental posterior leaflet prolapse; in these patients, valve repair is enhanced by intraoperative echocardiography.[58]

Mitral valve repair for anterior leaflet prolapse is more challenging for the surgeon, and the risk of reoperation is higher than that associated with surgery for posterior leaflet prolapse.[57] Nevertheless, the results remain more favorable for anterior leaflet repair than for mitral valve replacement. Long-term success with mitral valve repair for bacterial endocarditis is excellent, and evidence supports early consideration of surgery if indications are present.[59]

Mitral valve repair for ischemic mitral regurgitation remains controversial, but it may be successful in select patients.[60,61] In patients with ischemic mitral regurgitation, valve repair generally consists of insertion of an undersized annuloplasty ring. Survival has increased dramatically for combined coronary artery and mitral valve surgery, and some of this improvement may be attributable to increasing rates of valve repair versus valve replacement.[61,62] Some observational studies have shown that the addition of mitral annuloplasty to coronary artery bypass surgery in patients with ischemic mitral regurgitation results in an improvement in functional class and survival; however, other studies have not supported this finding.[60,63]

The decision whether to proceed with mitral valve repair or with mitral valve replacement should ideally include consultation with a surgeon who is skilled in mitral valve repair. If mitral valve repair is not possible, a mitral prosthesis is implanted.[64] Prosthetic implantation procedures increasingly include preservation of chordal and papillary muscles, because evidence indicates that preservation of these muscles conserves left ventricular function after surgery.[65] Percutaneous catheter repair of degenerative and ischemic mitral regurgitation is currently under investigation; various technologies have been used, including a clip that is deployed to improve coaptation of the valvular leaflets at their midpoint and an annuloplasty ring that is placed around the mitral valve annulus by way of the coronary sinus.[66,67]

MITRAL VALVE PROLAPSE

MVP is a common condition in which the mitral valve leaflets are displaced in systole into the left atrium.[8] MVP has a highly variable natural history and can occur in some form in up to 2.4% of the general population.[68,69] In the majority of cases, MVP represents a benign abnormality; in patients who develop significant mitral regurgitation, the disorder is associated with increased cardiovascular morbidity and mortality and requires surgical intervention.[68] A variety of symptoms (e.g., atypical chest pain, palpitations, anxiety, and syncope) and clinical findings (e.g., low body weight, low blood pressure, pectus excavatum, and electrocardiographic abnormalities)—the so-called MVP syndrome—were attributed to MVP in the past.[70] However, the association between MVP and most of these clinical findings is erroneous; most likely, the presumed association was drawn on the basis of selection bias and overdiagnosis of MVP in older studies. Only the association of MVP with low body weight was reproduced in the Framingham community-based study.[71]

Diagnosis

A midsystolic click at the mitral area during cardiac auscultation is often the finding that first brings MVP to the attention of the examiner. The click has been attributed to tensing of the redundant valvular tissue with cardiac contraction. A late systolic murmur can follow the click. Maneuvers that reduce intracardiac volume, such as having the patient stand or perform the Valsalva maneuver, cause the click to occur earlier in systole and cause an increase in the duration of the murmur. The typical auscultatory findings and their response to these maneuvers are sufficient to make a diagnosis of MVP. Two-dimensional echocardiography is the method of choice to confirm the diagnosis. Overdiagnosis of MVP by M-mode and two-dimensional echocardiography was common before the realization that the mitral valve annulus is nonplanar and saddle shaped. True MVP is diagnosed on two-dimensional echocardiography by leaflet prolapse beyond the annular plane, as seen in a long-axis view.[72] Two-dimensional echocardiography can also be used to determine whether the valvular leaflets are thickened and redundant, which indicates the presence of myxomatous mitral valve disease. Color flow Doppler echocardiography can establish the presence of associated mitral regurgitation.[71] Patients with prolapse but with otherwise anatomically normal leaflets and no mitral regurgitation are at low risk for complications.

Treatment

Asymptomatic mitral valve prolapse requires no specific treatment. Periodic examination is indicated to detect any progression in the severity of mitral regurgitation. Prophylaxis for endocarditis is indicated if both a click and a murmur are present, but it is not indicated in the absence of mitral regurgitation.[22] Treatment of mitral regurgitation is discussed elsewhere [see Mitral Regurgitation, above].

AORTIC STENOSIS

The normal aortic valve area (AVA) is 3 to 4 cm^2 in area when the valve is fully open. Aortic stenosis is considered severe when the AVA is 1 cm^2 or less and is considered critical when the AVA is less than 0.75 cm^2. Aortic stenosis causes concentric left ventricular hypertrophy as a compensatory mechanism that maintains cardiac output at rest despite the increased pressure gradient across the valve. Eventually, this compensatory mechanism is overcome, causing the left ventricle to fail and dilate and the resting cardiac output to decline.

Diagnosis

Clinical manifestations There is a variable relation between the severity of stenosis and symptoms. Many patients with critical aortic stenosis are asymptomatic, whereas patients in states of volume overload, such as pregnancy, may have symptoms with stenosis of lesser severity. Dyspnea is often the presenting feature; it reflects increased left atrial pressure and pulmonary ve-

a

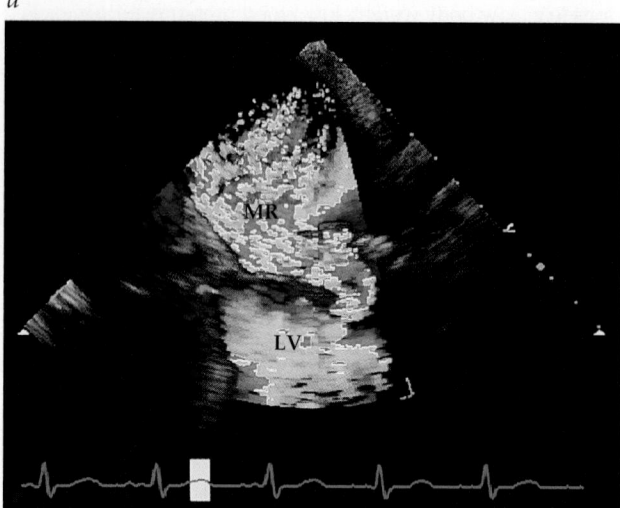

b

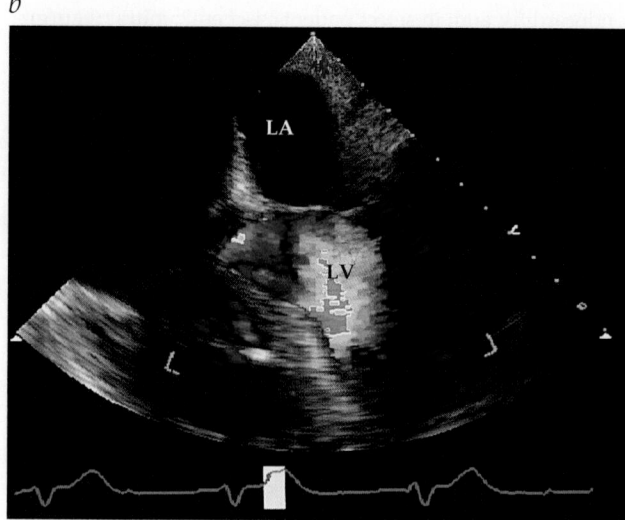

Figure 5   Transesophageal echocardiogram of a patient with severe myxomatous mitral regurgitation (MR) before (*a*) and after (*b*) mitral valve repair.

nous hypertension from the increased left ventricular pressure in systole and the diastolic ventricular dysfunction imposed by left ventricular hypertrophy. Angina is common even in the absence of significant obstruction in the epicardial coronary blood vessels because of impaired supply of blood to the subendocardium in the hypertrophied left ventricle. Exertional syncope also occurs with stenosis and can result from the inability to increase cardiac output sufficiently to supply both skeletal muscle and the cerebral vasculature, resulting in impaired cerebral blood supply, or from abnormal baroreceptor reflexes. Serious arrhythmia can also cause syncope and, in severe aortic stenosis, even sudden death. Fatigue is common because of low cardiac output.

In severe aortic stenosis, the carotid pulse typically is reduced in intensity and has a slow delayed upstroke. Aortic stenosis gives rise to a systolic murmur that is heard over the aortic area and that can radiate to the carotid arteries and to the apex. In severe stenosis, the murmur peaks later in systole and can be associated with a thrill. A fourth heart sound is usually present. In mobile congenitally abnormal valves, an ejection click can precede the murmur. Severe calcific aortic stenosis is often associated with a diminished intensity of the aortic component of the second heart sound. Although the physical findings are important in alerting the clinician to the presence of aortic valve disease, the degree of hemodynamic severity is more reliably determined with Doppler echocardiography.

Imaging studies   The presence of left ventricular hypertrophy on electrocardiography provides useful supporting evidence for significant aortic stenosis. Doppler echocardiography is used to determine the mechanism and the hemodynamic severity of the stenosis and the effects of disease on left ventricular size and function. In aortic stenosis, the opening of the aortic valve is reduced, as seen on the echocardiogram.

Assessment of stenosis severity   Using two-dimensional and Doppler echocardiography, the modified Bernoulli equation can be used to measure the aortic pressure gradient, and the AVA can be calculated by using the continuity equation. In patients with severe aortic stenosis, the mean pressure gradient across the valve is usually more than 50 mm Hg, and the AVA

is less than 1.0 cm^2. The transvalvular gradients are typically overestimated in patients with coexisting aortic regurgitation and underestimated in patients with reduced cardiac output. The measurement of the AVA by use of the continuity equation is relatively unaffected by either of these scenarios; therefore, measurement of AVA by this method is a useful complement to the measurement of peak and mean gradients. However, in two patient groups—namely, patients with very severe left ventricular dysfunction and patients with very low flow rates—the AVA measured by the continuity equation tends to underestimate the true AVA.[73,74] In patients with low cardiac output, dobutamine stress echocardiography can help differentiate true aortic stenosis from pseudoaortic stenosis.[75] Truly severe aortic stenosis is suggested by an AVA that does not increase with dobutamine infusion. In addition, low-dose dobutamine stress echocardiography can detect contractile reserve—a feature that is associated with a lower operative risk and better long-term prognosis after aortic valve replacement in patients with severe left ventricular dysfunction.[76,77]

Invasive evaluation   Because of the accuracy of echocardiography, invasive assessment of aortic stenosis by right and left heart catheterization using the Gorlin equation is necessary only when there is a discrepancy between the clinical and the echocardiographic findings [*see Figure 6*].[78] It should be noted that in patients with low cardiac output, the AVA calculated by echocardiography is more accurate than invasive assessment using the Gorlin equation.[79] Because there is a high incidence of CAD in patients with aortic valve stenosis, cardiac catheterization is frequently performed before aortic valve replacement to assess for CAD.[80]

Treatment

Medical treatment   Currently, there is no specific medical treatment for aortic stenosis. Because degenerative aortic stenosis has many features in common with atherosclerosis, including similar risk factors, statin therapy has been postulated as a possible treatment. Initial retrospective studies suggested a clinical benefit of statin therapy in slowing aortic stenosis progression, but this finding has not been reproduced in one relatively small

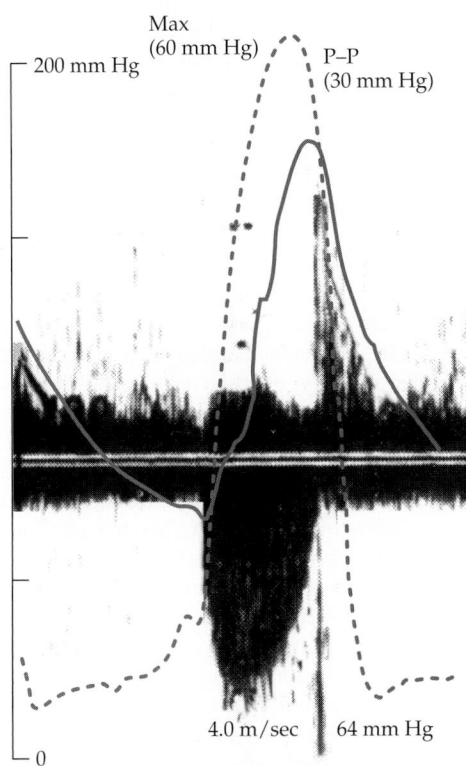

Figure 6 Simultaneous left ventricular (broken blue line) and aortic (solid blue line) pressure tracings and continuous wave Doppler tracing in a patient with severe aortic stenosis. The pressure gradient (P–P; 30 mm Hg) is the area between the aortic and left ventricular (LV) tracings. Maximal pressure gradient (Max) by cardiac catheterization (60 mm Hg) is similar to that measured by Doppler echocardiography (64 mm Hg).[78]

randomized, controlled trial.[81-83] Larger clinical trials are currently under way.

Indications for surgery Aortic stenosis is a progressive disease, and patients with the disease can remain asymptomatic for many years. The rate of progression varies greatly but increases with age, associated CAD, and the severity of the stenosis.[84] Progression to symptoms is more likely when the AVA is relatively small or when left ventricular hypertrophy is present.[85] Once symptoms become manifest, the survival rate without surgical treatment is reduced; mean survival is 5 years in patients with angina, 3 years in patients with syncope, and 2 years or less in patients with heart failure.[84] Operative mortality increases with severe symptoms, advanced age, and the presence of left ventricular dysfunction. The onset of symptoms, therefore, is the major indication for surgical intervention. Left ventricular dysfunction attributable to aortic stenosis is another indication for intervention, because it demonstrates the failure of compensatory mechanisms and the presence of incipient symptoms. Sudden death occurs without symptoms in about 4% of patients who have an initial peak systolic velocity of 4 m/sec or greater, as detected by Doppler echocardiography, and who are followed for 5 years. Patients should be instructed to report the onset of any symptoms and should undergo regular follow-up evaluations with physical examination and Doppler echocardiography. Doppler examination should be performed at least yearly in patients with

moderate or severe aortic stenosis. Asymptomatic patients with severe aortic stenosis who have moderate or severe calcification, left ventricular systolic dysfunction, hypotension on exercise, ventricular tachycardia, excessive left ventricular hypertrophy, or an AVA less than 0.6 cm^2 are at higher risk for adverse outcomes and should either be monitored more closely until symptoms supervene or be considered for elective surgery.[20,86] Brain natriuretic peptide (BNP) measurement appears to be an independent predictor of mortality in patients with severe aortic stenosis; in asymptomatic patients, regular BNP measurement may supplement assessment of symptoms in determining the timing of aortic valve replacement.[87,88] More experience with measurement of BNP in aortic stenosis is required before any firm recommendations can be made.

The decision whether to perform prophylactic aortic valve replacement in a patient with mild to moderate asymptomatic aortic stenosis who is undergoing coronary bypass surgery is a difficult one; it is dependent on the characteristics of the individual patient, including age, the grade of severity of aortic stenosis on echocardiography, and the rate of disease progression. In general, for patients younger than 70 years, concomitant aortic valve replacement should be recommended if the peak aortic gradient is greater than 25 to 30 mm Hg.[89] Aortic valve surgery in the very elderly is associated with increased mortality, but it provides excellent palliation of symptoms; surgery should be considered for such patients provided they are otherwise good candidates.[85] Patients with severe left ventricular dysfunction resulting from aortic stenosis should also be considered for surgery, because significant improvement in ventricular function and symptoms is often achieved by surgery and because the survival rate in these patients is poor without surgery.

Surgical intervention Surgical intervention for patients with aortic stenosis usually involves insertion of a prosthesis or a human valve. In congenital aortic stenosis, valve repair or commissurotomy can be feasible, although significant aortic regurgitation can result. Balloon valvuloplasty has proved to be disappointing in the long-term treatment of adult calcific aortic stenosis. Balloon valvuloplasty typically increases AVA from 0.5 cm^2 to 0.8 cm^2 and is associated with improvement of symptoms in the majority of cases[30]; however, stenosis recurs in as many as 50% of patients within 6 months, and fewer than 25% survive more than 3 years.[90] Balloon valvuloplasty is now indicated in the palliative treatment of adult patients with aortic stenosis who are not surgical candidates because of significant comorbidity; it is also used to stabilize critically ill patients for whom surgery is planned at a later stage. Balloon dilatation is effective in young patients with congenital aortic stenosis and is an alternative to surgery in symptomatic aortic stenosis during pregnancy. Successful percutaneous deployment of an aortic valve prosthesis has been reported in humans and is currently under clinical investigation.[91]

AORTIC REGURGITATION

Aortic regurgitation causes volume overload of the left ventricle. In chronic aortic regurgitation, the volume overload is well tolerated for years. The left ventricle dilates to accommodate the increased volume load and thereby maintains a normal resting cardiac output. In aortic regurgitation, unlike in mitral regurgitation, the left ventricle must expel all of the increased volume of blood into the systemic circulation; severe enlargement of the left ventricle is common. Because of a compensatory increase in ventricular compliance, left ventricular diastolic pressure often remains in the normal range despite the increase in ventricular size. The ventricle hypertrophies to maintain normal wall stress. Eventually, compensatory mechanisms fail, and contractile impairment and increased diastolic pressure result in elevated left atrial and pulmonary venous pressures and symptoms. Acute aortic regurgitation can develop as a result of sudden disruption of the valve apparatus with endocarditis or aortic dissection. This condition is poorly tolerated because the left ventricle is unable to dilate fast enough to compensate for the volume load. Left ventricular diastolic pressure rises rapidly and leads to pulmonary congestion and edema. Cardiac output falls, and shock and even death can follow.

Diagnosis

Clinical manifestations In chronic aortic regurgitation, symptomatic presentation occurs late in the course of disease; dyspnea and fatigue are the usual findings. Angina can occur in the absence of CAD because of the increased demand for oxygen caused by severe left ventricular enlargement and hypertrophy together with the reduced supply of oxygen resulting from the underperfusion of the coronary arteries. Such underperfusion is caused by the low diastolic pressure that is characteristic of this condition.

The cardinal physical sign of aortic regurgitation is a diastolic murmur that is high pitched and best heard with the diaphragm of the stethoscope with respiration suspended in expiration. The murmur is loudest immediately after aortic valve closure; it progressively diminishes in intensity throughout diastole, paralleling the decline in the pressure gradient between the aorta and the left ventricle. The murmur is best heard on the left of the sternal border in disease of the aortic cusps and on the right of the sternal border in disease of the aortic root. Even in the absence of significant stenosis, an aortic systolic murmur is audible, reflecting the increased flow through the valve. Severe chronic aortic regurgitation is characterized by a wide pulse pressure and an elevated systolic pressure caused by the increased stroke output; also characteristic is a reduction in the diastolic pressure, which occurs as blood leaks back into the left ventricle throughout diastole. If the aortic regurgitant jet hits the mitral valve leaflet, it can cause partial closure of the valve, creating an apical diastolic murmur that simulates mitral stenosis (Austin Flint murmur). The ejection of a large volume of blood into the systemic circulation and its rapid leak backward into the heart cause many peripheral circulatory manifestations that confirm rather than establish the diagnosis. Acute aortic regurgitation can be more difficult to recognize because the murmur is often short, and the reduced cardiac output leads to reduced intensity of the murmur.

Imaging studies Marked cardiomegaly and prominence of the ascending aorta are often present on chest x-ray in patients with chronic severe aortic regurgitation. Doppler echocardiography confirms the mechanism and severity of aortic regurgitation and its effect on left ventricular size and function. Regurgitant volume and fraction can be quantified by echocardiographic Doppler techniques. More often, the severity of regurgitation is graded on the basis of several qualitative and semiquantitative measures, including the dimensions of the regurgitant jet in the left ventricular outflow tract, as determined by color flow Doppler mapping, and the presence of diastolic flow reversal in the descending thoracic aorta, as determined by pulsed wave Doppler echocardiography [*see Figure 7*].[21] In severe aortic regurgitation, early closure of the mitral valve and diastolic mitral regurgitation can occur as a result of the increased pressure in the left ventricle in diastole [*see Figure 7*]. Confirmation of the severity of aortic regurgitation is obtained by aortography, a process in which contrast medium is injected into the aortic root and the retrograde filling and clearing of contrast dye from the left ventricle are examined. Aortography should be performed if there is any discrepancy between the clinical findings and the findings on Doppler echocardiography. Stress ventriculography and echocardiography have both been used to determine the response of the left ventricle to the effects of exercise. A significant fall in left ventricular ejection fraction or an increase in end-systolic volume suggests incipient contractile dysfunction; however, this is not a well-established indication for early surgical intervention.

Treatment

Chronic aortic regurgitation is well tolerated for many years.[92] Operative mortality is increased and long-term survival reduced

a

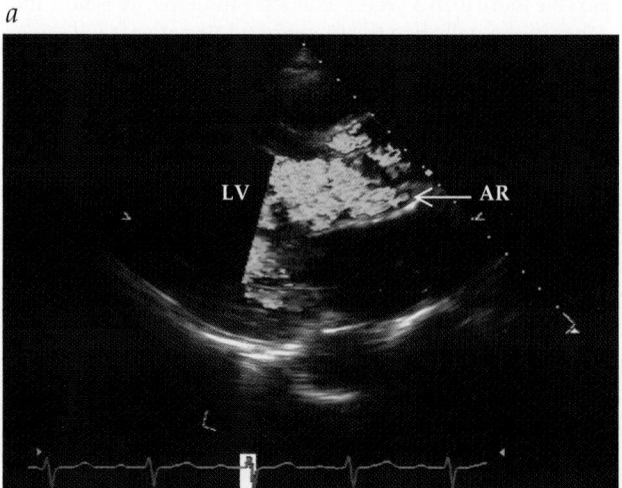

b

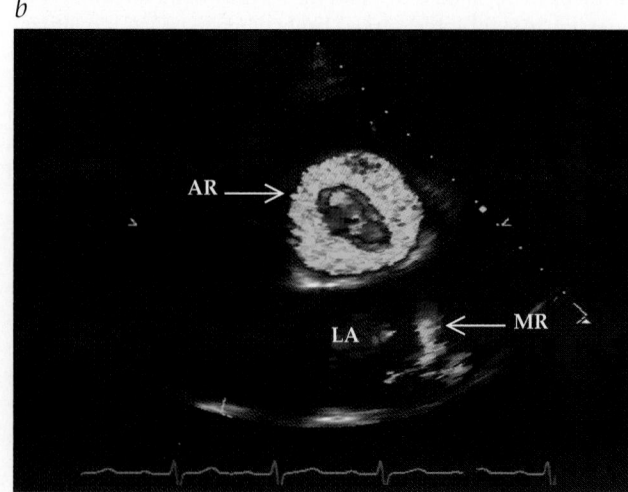

Figure 7 **Parasternal long-axis view (*a*) and short-axis view (*b*) of a severely regurgitant aortic allograft. Aortic regurgitation (AR) is seen circumferentially around the insertion site. Diastolic mitral regurgitation (MR) is also seen.**

if the left ventricle is greatly enlarged or if left ventricular dysfunction has been present for more than 1 year. Left ventricular dysfunction that is present for a shorter period is likely to improve and even resolve after surgery. Several studies have shown that asymptomatic patients with normal left ventricular function can be safely followed for a long period (up to 11 years in one study) when serial physical examination and Doppler echocardiographic examination are performed at least yearly and then performed more frequently as left ventricular dilatation progresses.[93] Surgery is indicated when symptoms develop. In asymptomatic patients, surgery is indicated when resting left ventricular function declines or if severe left ventricular dilatation (end-systolic dimension > 5 cm; end-diastolic dimension > 7 cm) occurs.[20,94] Evidence suggests that these dimensions should be normalized for body size and that surgery should be considered at an earlier stage, especially in women. Afterload reduction with vasodilators such as hydralazine, captopril, and nifedipine has been shown to reduce left ventricular volume and mass and increase ejection fraction in aortic regurgitation.[54] However, vasodilator treatment for aortic regurgitation has yielded variable results in clinical trials.

Whereas one series has suggested that treatment with nifedipine delays the need for surgical intervention and improves recovery of myocardial contractility postoperatively, another showed no benefit with either nifedipine or enalapril in asymptomatic aortic regurgitation.[95-97] Acute severe aortic regurgitation necessitates urgent surgery. Intravenous vasodilatation with sodium nitroprusside or another vasodilator can reduce the regurgitant volume and help stabilize the patient awaiting surgery.

Surgical intervention for aortic regurgitation usually leads to improvement in symptoms and left ventricular size. Although the operative risk is increased when severe left ventricular dilatation or dysfunction is present, significant improvement in symptoms and ventricular function often occurs after surgery; the prognosis without surgery is very poor.[94] Aortic regurgitation usually requires insertion of a prosthesis or a human valve. Occasionally, repair is feasible, especially in cases of a prolapsing bicuspid valve or a dilated aortic ring.

TRICUSPID AND PULMONARY DISEASE

Specific Lesions

Tricuspid regurgitation Tricuspid regurgitation is most often secondary to right ventricular dilatation and is the most common valvular problem of the right heart. Tricuspid regurgitation may be caused by damage to or disruption of the valvular apparatus resulting from transvenous permanent pacing and ICD leads. Tricuspid regurgitation is recognized on physical examination by the characteristic large V waves in the jugular venous pulse and by a systolic murmur heard at the base of the xiphisternum that increases on inspiration. In severe cases, pulsatile hepatomegaly is present. Doppler echocardiography allows rapid detection and assessment of the severity of the regurgitation. Presentation often includes fatigue from reduced forward output and peripheral edema. Severe tricuspid regurgitation is usually treated with surgical repair. If a repair is not possible, a biologic prosthesis is usually implanted because of the increased risk of thrombosis of a mechanical prosthesis at this position. Secondary tricuspid regurgitation can improve if the primary condition causing pulmonary hypertension is treated and leads to a decrease in right heart size.

Tricuspid stenosis Tricuspid stenosis occurs in approximately 5% to 10% of patients with severe mitral stenosis. The characteristic physical findings are a large A wave in the jugular venous pressures and a diastolic murmur over the tricuspid area. Doppler echocardiography and right heart catheterization are both used to assess severity. The mean gradient across the tricuspid valve is typically greater than 5 mm Hg. In patients with significant stenosis, either balloon dilatation, surgical repair, or valve replacement is indicated.

Pulmonary disease Congenital pulmonary stenosis occurs in isolation or as part of various syndromes and is usually detected before adulthood. Significant pulmonary stenosis is treated with balloon dilatation or surgery. Significant pulmonary insufficiency is rare but can occur with a carcinoid tumor or endocarditis or secondary to pulmonary hypertension. Pulmonary allograft implantation is indicated for severe cases.

Valve Replacement

Prosthestic valves can be classified into two groups—mechanical and biologic—each having different properties, problems, and indications.[98]

Mechanical prostheses Mechanical prostheses are of two main types: ball-in-cage and tilting-disk [*see Figure 8*]. The Starr-Edwards valve is the prototypical ball-in-cage valve that has been implanted with various modifications since the 1960s. Tilting-disk valves can consist of one or two leaflets. Single-leaflet models include the Björk-Shiley and Medtronic-Hall valves. The most commonly implanted bileaflet models are the St. Jude valve and the CarboMedics valve. The major advantage of mechanical prostheses is durability. Mechanical prostheses can remain functional for decades and are used especially in young or middle-aged patients to reduce the need for reoperation.[99] Their chief disadvantage is the associated risk of thromboembolism, which necessitates long-term anticoagulation and carries a risk of hemorrhage. An increased incidence of subsequent infection, hemolysis, thrombosis of the valve, and mechanical failure is another problem associated with mechanical prostheses.

Biologic prostheses Three classes of biologic valves are currently available: xenografts, allografts, and autografts. A xenograft is a prosthesis fashioned from animal tissue [*see Figure 9*]. Most xenografts consist of modified porcine valves that are preserved in glutaraldehyde and mounted on a stent.[100] Prostheses have also been constructed of pericardium and other biologic materials.[101] Stentless biologic prostheses are postulated to improve the effective size of the prosthetic valve opening and enhance regression of left ventricular hypertrophy[102]; however, not all studies have confirmed this.[103,104] Allografts (homografts) are human valves that have been harvested post mortem and either cryopreserved or treated with antibiotics.[105] An autograft is a valve from the patient's own body that is removed from its original position and inserted at a different anatomic site.[106,107] The most common autograft is the pulmonary valve inserted at the aortic position. A pulmonary allograft is inserted in its place.

Patients with biologic valves have a lower risk of thromboembolism than those with mechanical prostheses, and they do not usually require long-term anticoagulation. Biologic valves are indicated for patients in whom anticoagulation is inappropriate. Xenografts are less durable than mechanical prostheses. Xenograft durability is greatest in patients older than 60 years and improves

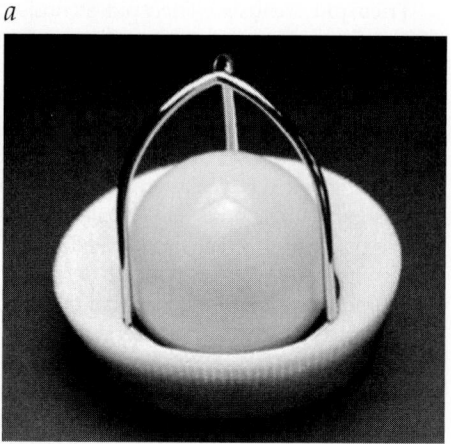 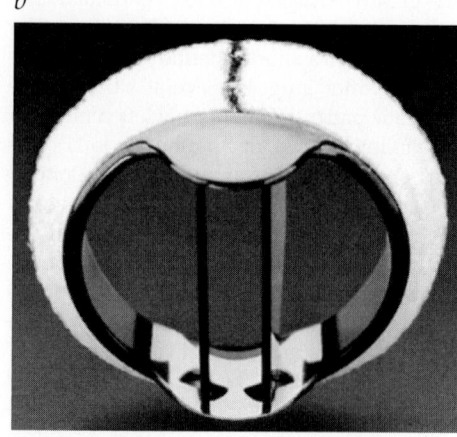

Figure 8   Two aortic mechanical prostheses. (*a*) Starr-Edwards ball-in-cage prosthesis and (*b*) St. Jude bileaflet tilting-disk prosthesis.

with age.[108] Xenografts are not usually inserted in patients younger than 60 years because of the poor survival record of such grafts in this patient group. Allografts and autografts are alternatives to mechanical prosthetic implantation at the aortic or pulmonary positions in younger patients. Insertion of these valves is technically more demanding and is not widely done. No long-term survival benefit has been demonstrated for allografts over xenografts. Autografts have proved to be durable and have the potential to grow in situ.[106,107] They are used in the management of pediatric and adolescent patients with aortic valve disease.[109] Both allografts and autografts result in a low reinfection rate when used in the treatment of prosthetic aortic endocarditis; they are considered the valve replacement of choice for this condition.[105]

Problems and Complications of Valvular Prostheses

Thromboembolism   Systemic anticoagulation with warfarin or dicumarol decreases the incidence of, but does not eliminate the occurrence of, thromboembolism with mechanical valves.[110] The incidence of thromboembolic events is lowest in patients younger than 50 years, lower with aortic prostheses than with mitral or multiple prostheses, and lower with bileaflet disk valves than with single-leaflet valves.[111] Hemorrhagic events

are more common in older patients. Anticoagulation is generally monitored using the international normalized ratio (INR). Studies have indicated that the level of anticoagulation required to prevent thromboembolism is less than was previously thought. A large study of anticoagulation in patients with mechanical prostheses has suggested that an INR of between 2.5 and 4.0 is desirable in most instances and minimizes hemorrhagic and thromboembolic complications.[111] The appropriate INR for an individual patient will vary depending on the history of embolic or bleeding events; age; and type, position, and number of prostheses. Antiplatelet agents such as aspirin (81 mg q.d.) or clopidogrel (75 mg once daily) may be added to the anticoagulation regimen in patients who have sustained recurrent thromboembolic events despite adequate anticoagulation. Thromboembolic risk with xenografts is greatest in the first 3 months after surgery.[112] During this period, oral anticoagulation medications are recommended for high-risk patients (e.g., those with mitral prostheses or paroxysmal atrial fibrillation); for patients who are not at high risk, aspirin, 325 mg/day, is recommended.

Valvular thrombosis   Acute thrombosis of a mechanical valve is more common with a single tilting-disk valve. The inci-

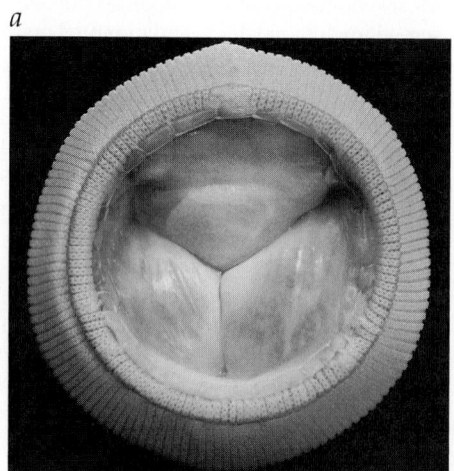 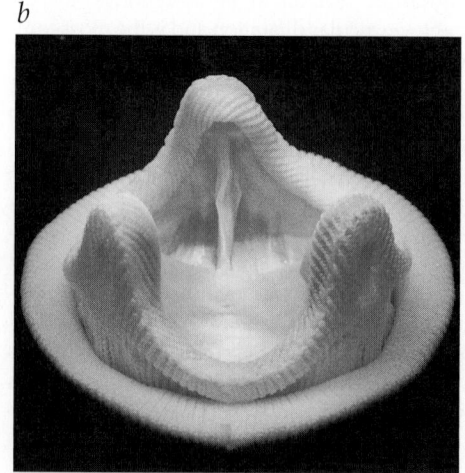

Figure 9   (*a*) Top view of an aortic porcine xenograft that has been preserved in glutaraldehyde and mounted on a flexible plastic stent. (*b*) Bottom view of the same valve.

dence is highest at the tricuspid position, followed by the mitral position and then the aortic position. Thrombosis of left-sided valves can lead to acute pulmonary edema and systemic thromboembolism. Reduced motion of the disk or ball is characteristic of valvular thrombosis and can be demonstrated with transesophageal echocardiography or fluoroscopy.[113,114] There is usually an increased pressure gradient across the valve. Acute thrombosis of a mechanical valve is an indication for emergency surgery to remove the thrombus and to implant another prosthesis. In patients who are not surgical candidates or who are considered at high operative risk, thrombolysis has been used successfully to increase the valvular opening and motion and to reduce the valvular gradient. Success rates greater than 70% have been reported in a number of series.[114] Thromboembolism is the most common complication of thrombolysis in this setting and occurs in 12% to 22% of patients. Further episodes of valvular thrombosis after initial successful thrombolysis have been reported.[114]

Valvular failure In mechanical prostheses, failure of one of the mechanical parts is rare but can have catastrophic consequences. Failure is most common with tilting-disk valves, particularly the Björk-Shiley single-leaflet tilting-disk valve, which is no longer available commercially in the United States.[115] Failure of the outlet strut in several of these models led to embolization of the disk and acute valvular failure, with high morbidity and mortality. Because even advanced imaging techniques have poor sensitivity to detect strut fracture, prophylactic repeat surgery was recommended for certain groups of patients in whom the failure rate was highest.[115,116] These predictive models based on patient and implantation characteristics appear to have been successful.[117] Valvular failure is expected with bioprostheses and allografts. Fortunately, degeneration is a slow process with biologic prostheses; significant hemodynamic consequences do not occur for years after implantation. Leaflet calcification can give rise to stenosis, whereas cusp degeneration can lead to perforation with resultant regurgitation. Degeneration of a biologic prosthesis is managed in the same way as stenosis or regurgitation of a native valve. Repeat surgery is indicated for significant symptoms or progressive ventricular enlargement or dysfunction.

Failure of either a mechanical or a biologic prosthesis can occur because of problems with the sutures holding the valve in place. Suture-related failures can occur spontaneously or because of associated infection. A St. Jude valve in which the sewing ring was impregnated with silver nitrate to reduce the likelihood of infection was recalled because of a high incidence of paravalvular leak. The paravalvular leak resulting from suture failure can begin as a relatively mild lesion, but progression is common. In severe instances, partial or complete dehiscence can result in a characteristic rocking motion of the valve, as revealed by echocardiography. Paravalvular leaks are often accompanied by significant hemolysis as red blood cells are destroyed at the site of increased shear stress.[118] Hemodynamically significant paravalvular leaks are considered an indication for reoperation.

Infection There is a greater risk of endocarditis with mechanical prostheses and xenografts than with native valves or allografts. Prosthetic valve endocarditis is often associated with abscess formation. Prosthetic vegetation and abscess formation are best evaluated by using transesophageal echocardiography, which should be performed if prosthetic valve endocarditis is being considered as a diagnosis. Prosthetic valve endocarditis is

extremely difficult to eradicate with medical treatment alone; operative intervention is usually required.

Inherent or acquired prosthetic stenosis All prosthetic valves are inherently stenotic, but in an appropriately selected prosthesis, the degree of stenosis is mild and not of clinical significance. Occasionally, a smaller-than-desirable prosthesis is implanted because the native valve annulus is small; a so-called patient-prosthesis mismatch has been described for both mitral and aortic valve replacements.[119,120] In such cases, patients can manifest symptoms and signs of valvular stenosis; severely increased pressure gradients across the valve can also be present in these patients, especially during exercise. In severe cases, explantation of the prosthesis and annular reconstruction may be necessary to accommodate a prosthesis of sufficient size. Where possible, care should be taken to insert an appropriately sized prosthesis at the time of initial surgery.[121] In some patients with mechanical prostheses, prosthetic stenosis is acquired because of ingrowth of a fibrous pannus that can impede blood flow and may require reoperation.

Problems associated with pregnancy Pregnancy is contraindicated in women with mechanical prostheses because of considerable risk to mother and fetus. The risk to the mother is associated with difficulty in maintaining effective anticoagulation; the risk to the fetus is associated with potential teratogenic effects of warfarin.[122] If possible, valve repair or insertion of an allograft or autograft should be attempted in a woman of childbearing age who wishes to become pregnant. Xenografts are less durable in young patients, especially during pregnancy, and are best avoided.[123]

The management of patients with mechanical prostheses who become pregnant or desire pregnancy is controversial. None of the three available anticoagulants have been adequately studied in pregnancy. Warfarin is associated with embryopathy and increases the risk of fetal wastage. Optimal anticoagulation is also difficult with unfractionated heparin, especially when given subcutaneously, and is associated with increased maternal risk of thromboembolism and hemorrhage.[23] High rates of thromboembolism have been reported with use of low-molecular-weight heparin in pregnant women, which prompted the Food and Drug Administration to issue a black-box warning—the FDA's most serious warning in the labeling of a prescription medication. However, thromboembolism associated with use of low-molecular-weight heparin in pregnancy seems to be related to inadequate dosing and inadequate monitoring.[124] Self-administration of either unfractionated or low-molecular-weight heparin subcutaneously throughout pregnancy (ideally, from the time of conception) is one approach to the management of pregnant patients with mechanical prostheses.[23] Unfractionated or low-molecular-weight heparin is administered every 8 to 12 hours, and patients are monitored by their physician at least every 2 weeks. For patients treated with unfractionated heparin, the recommended level of the activated partial thromboplastin time is 2.0 to 3.0 times the control value 6 hours after administration. Because of an increased and changing dose requirement in pregnancy, weight-based dose calculation of low-molecular-weight heparin is inadequate. It is recommended that the patient's plasma level of low-molecular-weight heparin be measured before administration of each dose; the anti-Xa assay is used for this purpose. A predose anti-Xa level of 0.6 to 0.7 U/ml is recommended. Peak levels of anti-Xa (4 hours after dosing) should also be measured to detect excessive anticoagulation (> 1.5 U/ml). Subcutaneous heparin should be replaced by intravenous unfractionated heparin 18 to 24 hours before elective delivery. Low-dose aspirin may be considered for additional prophylaxis of thromboembolism in high-risk patients.[125]

ANOREXIANT-INDUCED VALVULAR DISORDER

Drugs that suppress appetite (anorexiants) have been reported to cause a valvular disorder similar to that caused by ergot derivatives and carcinoid syndrome. This finding was first reported in 1997, and a number of large studies since then have confirmed an increased prevalence of valvular disorders in populations treated with fenfluramine, dexfenfluramine, phentermine, or a combination of these drugs.[16-18] Over 18 million prescriptions were filled for these drugs in 1996 alone. The precise pathophysiology of the valvular disorder is still unclear. All of these anorexiants affect central serotoninergic receptors. A causal relation of serotonin in this disorder is also suggested by the disorder's similarity to carcinoid disease, in which serotonin is also implicated as a causative factor. Initial reports suggested a high prevalence of valvular disease in patients treated with these anorexiants, and they were withdrawn from the market in September 1997. The prevalence of clinically symptomatic valve-related disease in patients receiving these drugs has been reported to be 1 in 1,000.[126] Anorexiant-drug valvulopathy affects mainly the aortic and mitral valve. Leaflet thickening, restricted leaflet motion, chordal thickening, and valvular regurgitation without stenosis are the most common abnormalities seen.[127] Although valvular disease severe enough to warrant surgery has been reported, the valvular lesion, in many instances, has appeared to be mild or moderate in severity. Factors thought to increase the likelihood of more severe disease are longer duration of treatment with anorexiant therapy, use of drug combinations, and higher dosages of drugs. Patients receiving less than 3 months of treatment appear to have a relatively low likelihood of significant valvular disease.[126] Studies also suggest that the valvular lesions may not progress and may even regress after discontinuance of the drug.[128] Patients exposed to anorexiants should undergo a thorough cardiovascular examination for signs of mitral or aortic regurgitation. Echocardiography is indicated if the physical findings suggest valvular disease or if the duration of treatment has been more than 3 months. Patients with evidence of valvular disease on echocardiography should be followed serially and receive prophylactic antibiotics for dental and other procedures associated with significant bacteremia.

Ronan J. Curtin, M.D., has no relationships with manufacturers of products or providers of services discussed in this chapter.

Brian P. Griffin, M.D., has received grants for clinical research from Pfizer, Inc.

References

1. Rose AG: Etiology of valvular heart disease. Curr Opin Cardiol 11:98, 1996

2. Weyman AE: The left ventricular outflow tract. Principles and Practices of Echocardiography, 2nd ed., rev. Weyman AE, Ed. Lea & Febiger, Philadelphia, 1994, p 513

3. Cripe L, Andelfinger G, Martin LJ, et al: Bicuspid aortic valve is heritable. J Am Coll Cardiol 44:138, 2004

4. Cecconi M, Manfrin M, Moraca A, et al: Aortic dimensions in patients with bicuspid aortic valve without significant valve dysfunction. Am J Cardiol 95:292, 2005

5. Garg V, Muth AN, Ransom JF, et al: Mutations in NOTCH1 cause aortic valve disease. Nature 437:270, 2005

6. Novaro GM, Mishra M, Griffin BP: Incidence and echocardiographic features of congenital unicuspid aortic valve in an adult population. J Heart Valve Dis 12:674, 2003

7. Rabkin E, Aikawa M, Stone JR, et al: Activated interstitial myofibroblasts express

catabolic enzymes and mediate matrix remodeling in myxomatous heart valves. Circulation 104:2525, 2001

8. Hayek E, Gring CN, Griffin BP: Mitral valve prolapse. Lancet 365:507, 2005

9. Disse S, Abergel E, Berrebi A, et al: Mapping of a first locus for autosomal dominant myxomatous mitral-valve prolapse to chromosome 16p11.2-p12.1. Am J Hum Genet 65:1242, 1999

10. Freed LA, Acierno JS Jr, Dai D, et al: A locus for autosomal dominant mitral valve prolapse on chromosome 11p15.4. Am J Hum Genet 72:1551, 2003

11. Nesta F, Leyne M, Yosefy C, et al: New locus for autosomal dominant mitral valve prolapse on chromosome 13: clinical insights from genetic studies. Circulation 112:2022, 2005

12. Carapetis JR, Steer AC, Mulholland EK, et al: The global burden of group A streptococcal diseases. Lancet Infect Dis 5:685, 2005

13. Feldman T: Rheumatic heart disease. Curr Opin Cardiol 11:126, 1996

14. Otto CM, Lind BK, Kitzman DW, et al: Association of aortic-valve sclerosis with cardiovascular mortality and morbidity in the elderly. N Engl J Med 341:142, 1999

15. Roldan CA, Shively BK, Crawford MH: An echocardiographic study of valvular heart disease associated with systemic lupus erythematosus. N Engl J Med 335:1424, 1996

16. Connolly HM, Crary JL, McGoon MD, et al: Valvular heart disease associated with fenfluramine-phentermine. N Engl J Med 337:581, 1997

17. Gardin JM, Schumacher D, Constantine G, et al: Valvular abnormalities and cardiovascular status following exposure to dexfenfluramine or phentermine/fenfluramine. JAMA 283:1703, 2000

18. Shively BK, Roldan CA, Gill EA, et al: Prevalence and determinants of valvulopathy in patients treated with dexfenfluramine. Circulation 100:2161, 1999

19. Lin G, Nishimura RA, Connolly HM, et al: Severe symptomatic tricuspid valve regurgitation due to permanent pacemaker or implantable cardioverter-defibrillator leads. J Am Coll Cardiol 45:1672, 2005

20. Bonow RO, Carabello B, de Leon AC Jr, et al: Guidelines for the management of patients with valvular heart disease: executive summary: a report of the American College of Cardiology/American Heart Association Task Force on Practice Guidelines (Committee on Management of Patients with Valvular Heart Disease). Circulation 98:1949, 1998
http://circ.ahajournals.org/cgi/content/full/98/18/1949

21. Zoghbi WA, Enriquez-Sarano M, Foster E, et al: Recommendations for evaluation of the severity of native valvular regurgitation with two-dimensional and Doppler echocardiography. J Am Soc Echocardiogr 16:777, 2003

22. Dajani AS, Taubert KA, Wilson W, et al: Prevention of bacterial endocarditis: recommendations by the American Heart Association. Circulation 96:358, 1997

23. Elkayam U, Bitar F: Valvular heart disease and pregnancy part I: native valves. J Am Coll Cardiol 46:223, 2005

24. Faletra F, Pezzano A Jr, Fusco R, et al: Measurement of mitral valve area in mitral stenosis: four echocardiographic methods compared with direct measurement of anatomic orifices. J Am Coll Cardiol 28:1190, 1996

25. Zamorano J, Cordeiro P, Sugeng L, et al: Real-time three-dimensional echocardiography for rheumatic mitral valve stenosis evaluation: an accurate and novel approach. J Am Coll Cardiol 43:2091, 2004

26. Wilkins GT, Weyman AE, Abascal VM, et al: Percutaneous balloon dilatation of the mitral valve: an analysis of echocardiographic variables related to outcome and the mechanism of dilatation. Br Heart J 60:299, 1988

27. Dajani A, Taubert K, Ferrieri P, et al: Treatment of acute streptococcal pharyngitis and prevention of rheumatic fever: a statement for health professionals. Committee on Rheumatic Fever, Endocarditis, and Kawasaki Disease of the Council on Cardiovascular Disease in the Young, the American Heart Association. Pediatrics 96:758, 1995

28. Gohlke-Barwolf C, Acar J, Oakley C, et al: Guidelines for prevention of thromboembolic events in valvular heart disease. Study Group of the Working Group on Valvular Heart Disease of the European Society of Cardiology. Eur Heart J 16:1320, 1995

29. Salem DN, Stein PD, Al-Ahmad A, et al: Antithrombotic therapy in valvular heart disease—native and prosthetic: the Seventh ACCP Conference on Antithrombotic and Thrombolytic Therapy. Chest 126:457S, 2004

30. Vahanian A: Balloon valvuloplasty. Heart 85:223, 2001

31. Palacios IF, Tuzcu ME, Weyman AE, et al: Clinical follow-up of patients undergoing percutaneous mitral balloon valvotomy. Circulation 91:671, 1995

32. Dean LS, Mickel M, Bonan R, et al: Four-year follow-up of patients undergoing percutaneous balloon mitral commissurotomy a report from the National Heart, Lung, and Blood Institute Balloon Valvuloplasty Registry. J Am Coll Cardiol 28:1452, 1996

33. Orrange SE, Kawanishi DT, Lopez BM, et al: Actuarial outcome after catheter balloon commissurotomy in patients with mitral stenosis. Circulation 95:382, 1997

34. Reyes VP, Raju BS, Wynne J, et al: Percutaneous balloon valvuloplasty compared with open surgical commissurotomy for mitral stenosis. N Engl J Med 331:961, 1994

35. Gupta A, Lokhandwala YY, Satoskar PR, et al: Balloon mitral valvotomy in pregnancy: maternal and fetal outcomes. J Am Coll Surg 187:409, 1998

36. Ben Farhat M, Ayari M, Maatouk F, et al: Percutaneous balloon versus surgical closed and open mitral commissurotomy: seven-year follow-up results of a randomized trial. Circulation 97:245, 1998

37. Hernandez R, Banuelos C, Alfonso F, et al: Long-term clinical and echocardiographic follow-up after percutaneous mitral valvuloplasty with the Inoue balloon. Circulation 99:1580, 1999

38. Hildick-Smith DJ, Taylor GJ, Shapiro LM: Inoue balloon mitral valvuloplasty: long-term clinical and echocardiographic follow-up of a predominantly unfavourable population. Eur Heart J 21:1690, 2000

39. Pathan AZ, Mahdi NA, Leon MN, et al: Is redo percutaneous mitral balloon valvuloplasty (PMV) indicated in patients with post-PMV mitral restenosis? J Am Coll Cardiol 34:49, 1999

40. Pu M, Vandervoort PM, Griffin BP, et al: Quantification of mitral regurgitation by the proximal convergence method using transesophageal echocardiography: clinical validation of a geometric correction for proximal flow constraint. Circulation 92:2169, 1995

41. Enriquez-Sarano M, Schaff HV, Orszulak TA, et al: Congestive heart failure after surgical correction of mitral regurgitation: a long-term study. Circulation 92:2496, 1995

42. Flemming MA, Oral H, Rothman ED, et al: Echocardiographic markers for mitral valve surgery to preserve left ventricular performance in mitral regurgitation. Am Heart J 140:476, 2000

43. Matsumura T, Ohtaki E, Tanaka K, et al: Echocardiographic prediction of left ventricular dysfunction after mitral valve repair for mitral regurgitation as an indicator to decide the optimal timing of repair. J Am Coll Cardiol 42:458, 2003

44. Lee R, Haluska B, Leung DY, et al: Functional and prognostic implications of left ventricular contractile reserve in patients with asymptomatic severe mitral regurgitation. Heart 91:1407, 2005

45. Leung DY, Griffin BP, Stewart WJ, et al: Left ventricular function after valve repair for chronic mitral regurgitation: predictive value of preoperative assessment of contractile reserve by exercise echocardiography. J Am Coll Cardiol 28:1198, 1996

46. Enriquez-Sarano M, Avierinos JF, Messika-Zeitoun D, et al: Quantitative determinants of the outcome of asymptomatic mitral regurgitation. N Engl J Med 352:875, 2005

47. Ling LH, Enriquez-Sarano M, Seward JB, et al: Early surgery in patients with mitral regurgitation due to flail leaflets: a long-term outcome study. Circulation 96:1819, 1997

48. Ling LH, Enriquez-Sarano M, Seward JB, et al: Clinical outcome of mitral regurgitation due to flail leaflet. N Engl J Med 335:1417, 1996

49. Bach DS, Bolling SF: Improvement following correction of secondary mitral regurgitation in end-stage cardiomyopathy with mitral annuloplasty. Am J Cardiol 78:966, 1996

50. Bolling SF, Pagani FD, Deeb GM, et al: Intermediate-term outcome of mitral reconstruction in cardiomyopathy. J Thorac Cardiovasc Surg 115:381, 1998

51. Romano MA, Bolling SF: Update on mitral repair in dilated cardiomyopathy. J Card Surg 19:396, 2004

52. Wu AH, Aaronson KD, Bolling SF, et al: Impact of mitral valve annuloplasty on mortality risk in patients with mitral regurgitation and left ventricular systolic dysfunction. J Am Coll Cardiol 45:381, 2005

53. Rosario LB, Stevenson LW, Solomon SD, et al: The mechanism of decrease in dynamic mitral regurgitation during heart failure treatment: importance of reduction in the regurgitant orifice size. J Am Coll Cardiol 32:1819, 1998

54. Levine HJ, Gaasch WH: Vasoactive drugs in chronic regurgitant lesions of the mitral and aortic valves. J Am Coll Cardiol 28:1083, 1996

55. Skoularigis J, Sinovich V, Joubert G, et al: Evaluation of the long-term results of mitral valve repair in 254 young patients with rheumatic mitral regurgitation. Circulation 90:II167, 1994

56. Enriquez-Sarano M, Schaff HV, Orszulak TA, et al: Valve repair improves the outcome of surgery for mitral regurgitation: a multivariate analysis. Circulation 91:1022, 1995

57. Mohty D, Orszulak TA, Schaff HV, et al: Very long-term survival and durability of mitral valve repair for mitral valve prolapse. Circulation 104:I1, 2001

58. Gillinov AM, Cosgrove DM, Blackstone EH, et al: Durability of mitral valve repair for degenerative disease. J Thorac Cardiovasc Surg 116:734, 1998

59. Zegdi R, Debieche M, Latremouille C, et al: Long-term results of mitral valve repair in active endocarditis. Circulation 111:2532, 2005

60. Di Donato M, Frigiola A, Menicanti L, et al: Moderate ischemic mitral regurgitation and coronary artery bypass surgery: effect of mitral repair on clinical outcome. J Heart Valve Dis 12:272, 2003

61. Gillinov AM, Wierup PN, Blackstone EH, et al: Is repair preferable to replacement for ischemic mitral regurgitation? J Thorac Cardiovasc Surg 122:1125, 2001

62. Miller DC: Ischemic mitral regurgitation redux—to repair or to replace? J Thorac Cardiovasc Surg 122:1059, 2001

63. Diodato MD, Moon MR, Pasque MK, et al: Repair of ischemic mitral regurgitation does not increase mortality or improve long-term survival in patients undergoing coronary artery revascularization: a propensity analysis. Ann Thorac Surg 78:794, 2004

64. Gillinov AM, Cosgrove DM, Lytle BW, et al: Reoperation for failure of mitral valve repair. J Thorac Cardiovasc Surg 113:467, 1997

65. Corin WJ, Sutsch G, Murakami T, et al: Left ventricular function in chronic mitral regurgitation: preoperative and postoperative comparison. J Am Coll Cardiol 25:113, 1995

66. Feldman T, Wasserman HS, Herrmann HC, et al: Percutaneous mitral valve repair using the edge-to-edge technique: six-month results of the EVEREST Phase I Clinical Trial. J Am Coll Cardiol 46:2134, 2005

67. Daimon M, Shiota T, Gillinov AM, et al: Percutaneous mitral valve repair for chronic ischemic mitral regurgitation: a real-time three-dimensional echocardiographic study in an ovine model. Circulation 111:2183, 2005

68. Avierinos JF, Gersh BJ, Melton LJ 3rd, et al: Natural history of asymptomatic mitral valve prolapse in the community. Circulation 106:1355, 2002

69. Freed LA, Levy D, Levine RA, et al: Prevalence and clinical outcome of mitral-valve prolapse. N Engl J Med 341:1, 1999

70. Devereux RB, Kramer-Fox R, Brown WT, et al: Relation between clinical features of the mitral prolapse syndrome and echocardiographically documented mitral valve prolapse. J Am Coll Cardiol 8:763, 1986

71. Freed LA, Benjamin EJ, Levy D, et al: Mitral valve prolapse in the general population: the benign nature of echocardiographic features in the Framingham Heart Study. J Am Coll Cardiol 40:1298, 2002

72. Levine RA, Stathogiannis E, Newell JB, et al: Reconsideration of echocardiographic standards for mitral valve prolapse: lack of association between leaflet displacement isolated to the apical four chamber view and independent echocardiographic evidence of abnormality. J Am Coll Cardiol 11:1010, 1988

73. Burwash IG, Thomas DD, Sadahiro M, et al: Dependence of Gorlin formula and continuity equation valve areas on transvalvular volume flow rate in valvular aortic stenosis. Circulation 89:827, 1994

74. Kadem L, Rieu R, Dumesnil JG, et al: Flow-dependent changes in Doppler-derived aortic valve effective orifice area are real and not due to artifact. J Am Coll Cardiol 47:131, 2006

75. deFilippi CR, Willett DL, Brickner ME, et al: Usefulness of dobutamine echocardiography in distinguishing severe from nonsevere valvular aortic stenosis in patients with depressed left ventricular function and low transvalvular gradients. Am J Cardiol 75:191, 1995

76. Monin JL, Monchi M, Gest V, et al: Aortic stenosis with severe left ventricular dysfunction and low transvalvular pressure gradients: risk stratification by low-dose dobutamine echocardiography. J Am Coll Cardiol 37:2101, 2001

77. Zuppiroli A, Mori F, Olivotto I, et al: Therapeutic implications of contractile reserve elicited by dobutamine echocardiography in symptomatic, low-gradient aortic stenosis. Ital Heart J 4:264, 2003

78. Currie PJ, Seward JB, Reeder GS, et al: Continuous-wave Doppler echocardiographic assessment of severity of calcific aortic stenosis: a simultaneous Doppler-catheter correlative study in 100 adult patients. Circulation 71:1162, 1985

79. Burwash IG, Dickinson A, Teskey RJ, et al: Aortic valve area discrepancy by Gorlin equation and Doppler echocardiography continuity equation: relationship to flow in patients with valvular aortic stenosis. Can J Cardiol 16:985, 2000

80. Vandeplas A, Willems JL, Piessens J, et al: Frequency of angina pectoris and coronary artery disease in severe isolated valvular aortic stenosis. Am J Cardiol 62:117, 1988

81. Novaro GM, Tiong IY, Pearce GL, et al: Effect of hydroxymethylglutaryl coenzyme A reductase inhibitors on the progression of calcific aortic stenosis. Circulation 104:2205, 2001

82. Bellamy MF, Pellikka PA, Klarich KW, et al: Association of cholesterol levels, hydroxymethylglutaryl coenzyme-A reductase inhibitor treatment, and progression of aortic stenosis in the community. J Am Coll Cardiol 40:1723, 2002

83. Cowell SJ, Newby DE, Prescott RJ, et al: A randomized trial of intensive lipid-lowering therapy in calcific aortic stenosis. N Engl J Med 352:2389, 2005

84. Otto CM, Burwash IG, Legget ME, et al: Prospective study of asymptomatic valvular aortic stenosis: clinical, echocardiographic, and exercise predictors of outcome. Circulation 95:2262, 1997

85. Pellikka PA, Sarano ME, Nishimura RA, et al: Outcome of 622 adults with asymptomatic, hemodynamically significant aortic stenosis during prolonged follow-up. Circulation 111: 3290, 2005

86. Rosenhek R, Binder T, Porenta G, et al: Predictors of outcome in severe, asymptomatic aortic stenosis. N Engl J Med 343:611, 2000

87. Lim P, Monin JL, Monchi M, et al: Predictors of outcome in patients with severe aortic stenosis and normal left ventricular function: role of B-type natriuretic peptide. Eur Heart J 25:2048, 2004

88. Nessmith MG, Fukuta H, Brucks S, et al: Usefulness of an elevated B-type natriuretic peptide in predicting survival in patients with aortic stenosis treated without surgery. Am J Cardiol 96:1445, 2005

89. Smith WT 4th, Ferguson TB Jr, Ryan T, et al: Should coronary artery bypass graft surgery patients with mild or moderate aortic stenosis undergo concomitant aortic valve replacement? A decision analysis approach to the surgical dilemma. J Am Coll Cardiol 44:1241, 2004

90. Wang A, Harrison JK, Bashore TM: Balloon aortic valvuloplasty. Prog Cardiovasc Dis 40:27, 1997

91. Cribier A, Eltchaninoff H, Tron C, et al: Early experience with percutaneous transcatheter implantation of heart valve prosthesis for the treatment of end-stage inoperable patients with calcific aortic stenosis. J Am Coll Cardiol 43:698, 2004

92. Bonow RO: Chronic aortic regurgitation: role of medical therapy and optimal timing for surgery. Cardiol Clin 16:449, 1998

93. Bonow RO, Lakatos E, Maron BJ, et al: Serial long-term assessment of the natural history of asymptomatic patients with chronic aortic regurgitation and normal left ventricular systolic function. Circulation 84:1625, 1991

94. Klodas E, Enriquez-Sarano M, Tajik AJ, et al: Aortic regurgitation complicated by extreme left ventricular dilation: long-term outcome after surgical correction. J Am Coll Cardiol 27:670, 1996

95. Scognamiglio R, Rahimtoola SH, Fasoli G, et al: Nifedipine in asymptomatic patients with severe aortic regurgitation and normal left ventricular function. N Engl J Med 331:689, 1994

96. Scognamiglio R, Negut C, Palisi M, et al: Long-term survival and functional results after aortic valve replacement in asymptomatic patients with chronic severe aortic regurgitation and left ventricular dysfunction. J Am Coll Cardiol 45:1025, 2005

97. Evangelista A, Tornos P, Sambola A, et al: Long-term vasodilator therapy in patients with severe aortic regurgitation. N Engl J Med 353:1342, 2005

98. Vongpatanasin W, Hillis LD, Lange RA: Prosthetic heart valves. N Engl J Med 335:407, 1996

99. Zellner JL, Kratz JM, Crumbley AJ 3rd, et al: Long-term experience with the St. Jude Medical valve prosthesis. Ann Thorac Surg 68:1210, 1999

100. Cohn LH, Collins JJ Jr, Rizzo RJ, et al: Twenty-year follow-up of the Hancock modified orifice porcine aortic valve. Ann Thorac Surg 66:S30, 1998

101. Banbury MK, Cosgrove DM 3rd, Lytle BW, et al: Long-term results of the Carpentier-Edwards pericardial aortic valve: a 12-year follow-up. Ann Thorac Surg 66:S73, 1998

102. Walther T, Falk V, Langebartels G, et al: Prospectively randomized evaluation of stentless versus conventional biological aortic valves: impact on early regression of left ventricular hypertrophy. Circulation 100:II6, 1999

103. Cohen G, Christakis GT, Joyner CD, et al: Are stentless valves hemodynamically superior to stented valves? A prospective randomized trial. Ann Thorac Surg 73:767, 2002

104. Doss M, Martens S, Wood JP, et al: Performance of stentless versus stented aortic valve bioprostheses in the elderly patient: a prospective randomized trial. Eur J Cardiothorac Surg 23:299, 2003

105. Ross DN: Evolution of the homograft valve. Ann Thorac Surg 59:565, 1995

106. Chambers JC, Somerville J, Stone S, et al: Pulmonary autograft procedure for aortic valve disease: long-term results of the pioneer series. Circulation 96:2206, 1997

107. O'Brien MF, Harrocks S, Stafford EG, et al: The homograft aortic valve: a 29-year, 99.3% follow up of 1,022 valve replacements. J Heart Valve Dis 10:334, 2001

108. Milano A, Guglielmi C, De Carlo M, et al: Valve-related complications in elderly patients with biological and mechanical aortic valves. Ann Thorac Surg 66:S82, 1998

109. Lupinetti FM, Warner J, Jones TK, et al: Comparison of human tissues and mechanical prostheses for aortic valve replacement in children. Circulation 96:321, 1997

110. Vink R, Kraaijenhagen RA, Hutten BA, et al: The optimal intensity of vitamin K antagonists in patients with mechanical heart valves: a meta-analysis. J Am Coll Cardiol 42:2042, 2003

111. Cannegieter SC, Rosendaal FR, Wintzen AR, et al: Optimal oral anticoagulant therapy in patients with mechanical heart valves. N Engl J Med 333:11, 1995

112. Heras M, Chesebro JH, Fuster V, et al: High risk of thromboemboli early after bioprosthetic cardiac valve replacement. J Am Coll Cardiol 25:1111, 1995

113. Barbetseas J, Nagueh SF, Pitsavos C, et al: Differentiating thrombus from pannus formation in obstructed mechanical prosthetic valves: an evaluation of clinical, transthoracic and transesophageal echocardiographic parameters. J Am Coll Cardiol 32:1410, 1998

114. Binder T, Baumgartner H, Maurer G: Diagnosis and management of prosthetic valve dysfunction. Curr Opin Cardiol 11:131, 1996

115. Kallewaard M, Algra A, Defauw J, et al: Prophylactic replacement of Bjork-Shiley convexo-concave valves at risk of strut fracture. Bjork-Shiley Study Group. J Thorac Cardiovasc Surg 115:577, 1998

116. Hopper KD, Gilchrist IC, Landis JR, et al: In vivo accuracy of two radiographic systems in the detection of Bjork-Shiley convexo-concave heart valve outlet strut single leg separations. J Thorac Cardiovasc Surg 115:582, 1998

117. van Gorp MJ, Steyerberg EW, Van der Graaf Y: Decision guidelines for prophylactic replacement of Bjork-Shiley convexo-concave heart valves: impact on clinical practice. Circulation 109:2092, 2004

118. Garcia MJ, Vandervoort P, Stewart WJ, et al: Mechanisms of hemolysis with mitral prosthetic regurgitation: study using transesophageal echocardiography and fluid dynamic simulation. J Am Coll Cardiol 27:399, 1996

119. Blais C, Dumesnil JG, Baillot R, et al: Impact of valve prosthesis–patient mismatch on short-term mortality after aortic valve replacement. Circulation 108:983, 2003

120. Li M, Dumesnil JG, Mathieu P, et al: Impact of valve prosthesis–patient mismatch on pulmonary arterial pressure after mitral valve replacement. J Am Coll Cardiol 45:1034, 2005

121. Pibarot P, Dumesnil JG, Cartier PC, et al: Patient-prosthesis mismatch can be predicted at the time of operation. Ann Thorac Surg 71:S265, 2001

122. Chan WS, Anand S, Ginsberg JS: Anticoagulation of pregnant women with mechanical heart valves: a systematic review of the literature. Arch Intern Med 160:191, 2000

123. Elkayam U, Bitar F: Valvular heart disease and pregnancy: part II: prosthetic valves. J Am Coll Cardiol 46:403, 2005

124. Oran B, Lee-Parritz A, Ansell J: Low molecular weight heparin for the prophylaxis of thromboembolism in women with prosthetic mechanical heart valves during pregnancy. Thromb Haemost 92:747, 2004

125. Cappelleri JC, Fiore LD, Brophy MT, et al: Efficacy and safety of combined anticoagulant and antiplatelet therapy versus anticoagulant monotherapy after mechanical heart-valve replacement: a metaanalysis. Am Heart J 130:547, 1995

126. Jick H: Heart valve disorders and appetite-suppressant drugs. JAMA 283:1738, 2000

127. Weissman NJ, Tighe JF Jr, Gottdiener JS, et al: An assessment of heart-valve abnormalities in obese patients taking dexfenfluramine, sustained-release dexfenfluramine, or placebo. Sustained-Release Dexfenfluramine Study Group. N Engl J Med 339:725, 1998

128. Weissman NJ, Tighe JF Jr, Gottdiener JS, et al: Prevalence of valvular-regurgitation associated with dexfenfluramine three to five months after discontinuation of treatment. J Am Coll Cardiol 34:2088, 1999

28 Diseases of the Aorta

Kim A. Eagle, M.D., F.A.C.P., and William F. Armstrong, M.D.

The Normal Aorta

The normal aorta is composed of three distinct layers: the inner intima, an elastic middle layer called the media, and a thin outer layer called the adventitia. In the media, layers of elastic elements intertwine with collagen and smooth muscle cells, providing the elastic strength that enables the aorta to withstand the pulsatile stress produced by the ejection of blood during ventricular systole. During systole, the aorta is distended by the force of blood ejected into the lumen. The kinetic energy of the ejected blood is transmitted to the wall of the aorta. In diastole, the potential energy stored in the aortic wall is transformed to kinetic energy as it propels the blood forward in the aorta and to its branches. With age, the normal elastic elements of the aorta degenerate, reducing its elasticity and distensibility. The aorta is considered to consist of three anatomic segments: the ascending aorta, the aortic arch, and the descending aorta. The ascending aorta consists of the aortic annulus, the aortic cusps, the sinuses of Valsalva, the sinotubular ridge, and the tubular portion of the ascending aorta. The ascending aorta connects the cardiovascular outflow tract at the aortic valve to the aortic arch, which begins at the brachiocephalic artery. The arch provides branches to the head and neck vessels, coursing just in front of the trachea and then proceeding to the left of the esophagus and the trachea. The descending aorta begins in the posterior mediastinum at the ligamentum arteriosum and courses in front of the vertebral column as it descends to the bifurcation of the leg vessels.

Aortic Aneurysms

Aneurysms may occur at any location in the aorta but are most common in the abdominal segments. Aortic aneurysm is a potentially life threatening entity for which both effective screening and curative therapy are available.

ABDOMINAL AORTIC ANEURYSMS

An aorta is considered aneurysmal when its diameter exceeds 1.5 times the expected normal diameter at any location along its length. Aneurysms are divided into those that affect the abdominal cavity and those that affect the thoracic cavity. More extensive aneurysms (termed thoracoabdominal) involve both aortic areas. In addition, aneurysms are defined as either fusiform or saccular.

Aneurysms of the abdominal aorta are more common than thoracic aortic aneurysms. Among the risk factors for aneurysms, perhaps the most important is age. The incidence of aneurysms increases in men older than 55 years and in women older than 70 years. Overall, men are four to five times more likely to develop aortic aneurysms. Additional risk factors are hypertension, smoking, elevated cholesterol, and a family history suggesting a genetic predisposition to aneurysms.[1] Several reports show that aneurysms develop in as many as 25% of first-degree relatives of patients with abdominal aortic aneurysms.[2] The infrarenal aorta is the most commonly affected region.

SCREENING FOR ABDOMINAL AORTIC ANEURYSMS

Current recommendations are for noninvasive screening of patients of appropriate age, which is typically defined as older than 65 years but younger if there is a significant family history of or risk factors for aneurysms. Screening may be particularly effective for obese patients, in whom abdominal palpation is of limited value. A large-scale (67,900 patients) randomized trial of ultrasound screening in men 65 to 74 years of age demonstrated a substantial reduction (i.e., 43%; 95% CI, 22 to 58; $P = 0.0002$) in aneurysm-related death with a strategy of routine testing.[3] The cost-effectiveness of various screening strategies has yet to be demonstrated.[4] Careful abdominal palpation is probably cost-effective, particularly in men older than 55 years who are at risk for developing vascular disease. A related issue concerns which patients should undergo noninvasive imaging when the abdominal examination is difficult to perform.

Clinical Presentation

Most abdominal aortic aneurysms produce no symptoms and are discovered during a routine physical examination or as a result of noninvasive screening. The most common symptom is pain, often described as a steady, gnawing discomfort in the lower back or hypogastrium. Generally, the pain is not affected by movement.

In some patients, the abdominal aortic aneurysm is first discovered during a period of rapid expansion or an impending rupture, which is often marked by severe discomfort in the lower abdomen or back, radiating to the buttocks, groin, or legs. Rupture is accompanied by the abrupt onset of back and abdominal pain, abdominal tenderness, the presence of a palpable pulsatile mass, hypotension, and shock. However, only one third of aneurysms present in this fashion. Of note, a ruptured aneurysm may mimic other conditions, including abdominal colic, renal colic, diverticulitis, and gastrointestinal hemorrhage. Not surprisingly, more than 25% of patients presenting with rupture or expansion of an aortic aneurysm are initially misdiagnosed.

Patients with impending or actual rupture must be managed as a surgical emergency in a manner similar to that used for patients with major trauma. Such patients rapidly experience hemorrhagic shock, manifested by peripheral vasoconstriction, hypotension, mottled skin, diaphoresis, oliguria, disorientation, and cardiac arrest. Patients with retroperitoneal rupture may show evidence of hematomas on the flank and in the groin. Although rare, rupture into the duodenum may present as massive upper or lower gastrointestinal hemorrhage.

Diagnostic Evaluation

Physical examination The abdominal aorta is usually detectable on deep palpation, particularly in thin persons. In obese patients, the normal aortic impulse may not be palpable. Obese patients may harbor a large aneurysm without any symptoms or findings on physical examination, unless the aneurysm is exerting pressure on an adjacent structure. Thin patients, in contrast, often feel a pulsatile mass in the abdomen when an abdominal aneurysm has developed.

When palpable, an aneurysm will be identified as a pulsatile mass extending from as high as the xiphoid process to the suprapubic area. Because of the layers of tissue between the examiner's fingers and the aneurysm, measurements of the transverse diameter of the aneurysm are typically overestimated. Also, it is difficult to differentiate ectatic aorta from aneurysm. Some aneurysms are sensitive to palpation and may be tender if they have recently expanded or are in impending rupture. Thus, palpation should be done with consideration of patient discomfort. Patients with aneurysms often have evidence of other peripheral vascular disease, such as femoral bruits and poor peripheral pulses.

Imaging studies   Several diagnostic tools can help identify and measure the size of abdominal aortic aneurysms. For years, aortography was considered the gold standard of diagnostic techniques for evaluating aortic aneurysms. One advantage of aortography is that it can be used to evaluate associated iliofemoral disease and involvement of the renal and mesenteric branches of the aorta. However, aortography is invasive and requires intravascular contrast, which carries a risk of nephrotoxicity. Its use has declined with the development of abdominal ultrasonography, computed tomography, and especially magnetic resonance angiography.

Abdominal ultrasonography is the most frequently used method and the most practical.[5] Ultrasonography has a sensitivity of nearly 100% for diagnosing aneurysms of significant size and can discriminate size to within ± 3 mm. Ultrasonography is inexpensive and noninvasive but may be inadequate for evaluating the most superior or inferior extent of an aneurysm and is generally considered inadequate as a sole diagnostic technique for planning surgical resection.

CT can discriminate aneurysm size to within ± 2 mm. Because CT scanning can determine the inferior and superior extent of the aneurysm and its shape, this method is more useful for planning surgical repair. However, the need for radiographic contrast is a relative disadvantage. When a CT image is compared with an image derived from abdominal ultrasonography, the size of the aneurysm determined by CT is larger by approximately 2.7 mm.[6] New diagnostic techniques such as fast spiral CT have improved the resolution of CT scanning. Magnetic resonance angiography can be successfully used for both screening and surgical planning. It identifies the size and extent of an aneurysm with a high degree of accuracy.

Anatomic landmarks are easily distinguished in the three-dimensional images created with MR angiography, which correctly defines the distal and proximal extent of an aneurysm in more than 75% of the cases examined.[7]

Management to Reduce Risk of Aneurysm Rupture

Current management of abdominal aortic aneurysm is directed at reducing the risk of rupture by intervening with timely surgical resection. Natural history studies show that the likelihood of rupture is greatest in patients with symptomatic, large, or rapidly expanding aneurysms. Aneurysms smaller than 4 cm in diameter have a low (< 2%) risk of rupture. Aneurysms exceeding 10 cm in diameter have a 25% risk of rupture over 2 years. Because aneurysms tend to expand with time, current strategies call for identifying and observing aneurysms that are asymptomatic and are small enough to have a low risk of rupture. The median rate of expansion is slightly less than 0.5 cm a year.[8] However, the tendency for expansion is variable and may not be linear. The more rapidly expanding aneurysms are more likely to rupture than are the stable

aneurysms. Aneurysms larger than 6 cm in diameter are generally referred for surgery, whereas aneurysms less than 4 cm in diameter are generally watched.[9-11] Evidence of expansion, particularly if the diameter of the aneurysm has exceeded 5.0 to 5.5 cm, is often taken as an indication to operate.[12] Current data support careful observation and serial noninvasive testing of patients with aneurysms between 4.0 and 5.5 cm in diameter.[13]

Surgical Treatment

Surgical treatment consists of resection of the aneurysm with insertion of a synthetic (Dacron) graft. Additional distal surgery is often necessary, with resection and interposition of grafts into one or both iliac arteries. For most large aneurysms, the aneurysm wall is left intact, and the Dacron graft is placed inside the aneurysm. The surgical treatment of abdominal aneurysms carries an average operative mortality of 4% to 6%. Surgical mortality is 2% in low-risk patients but may be as high as 20% in patients with impending rupture. For patients in shock with aneurysm rupture who require emergency surgery, operative and perioperative mortality may be as high as 50%.

A therapeutic option is percutaneous placement of implantable endovascular stents, which are similar to those used in patients with coronary artery, renal artery, and peripheral artery stenoses. Some centers are using endovascular stents in nearly 50% of patients referred for treatment of abdominal aortic aneurysms.[14] Larger stents have been used successfully to isolate abdominal aortic aneurysms in patients for whom the risk of surgical resection is unacceptable. However, widespread application of stenting awaits further evaluation of long-term outcomes.[15]

Preoperative evaluation and management   Appropriate preoperative evaluation and management of a patient before undergoing elective aortic aneurysm resection are critical. Reports suggest that one third to two thirds of perioperative deaths can be attributed to coronary artery disease. A guideline published by the American College of Cardiology and the American Heart Association reviewed the literature regarding preoperative assessment and presents a simple algorithm to help determine which patients should be considered for preoperative noninvasive testing for coronary disease [see Figure 1].[16]

The first consideration is whether the vascular surgery is urgent or emergent. By definition, emergent surgery cannot be delayed, and risk will be higher. In either case, the usual medical approach is to assume the patient may have preexisting coronary disease. Unless contraindicated, beta blockers should be used to treat such patients. Ideally, beta blockers should be started days to several weeks before surgery, titrating the dose to achieve a target heart rate of 50 to 60 beats a minute.[17] The clinical status, electrocardiographic findings, and hemodynamics of these patients should be monitored carefully after surgery.

For determination of perioperative risk, the first issue to address is whether the patient has had a recent coronary revascularization. If the patient has had coronary bypass surgery within the past 6 years and no subsequent coronary symptoms, the risk of perioperative events is relatively low. A second issue is whether the patient has had a recent coronary evaluation. Further preoperative testing is not usually required for patients whose recent stress test or coronary angiogram indicates minimal or no coronary disease, particularly if the evaluation was performed within the previous 2 years and the patient has undergone no change in status.

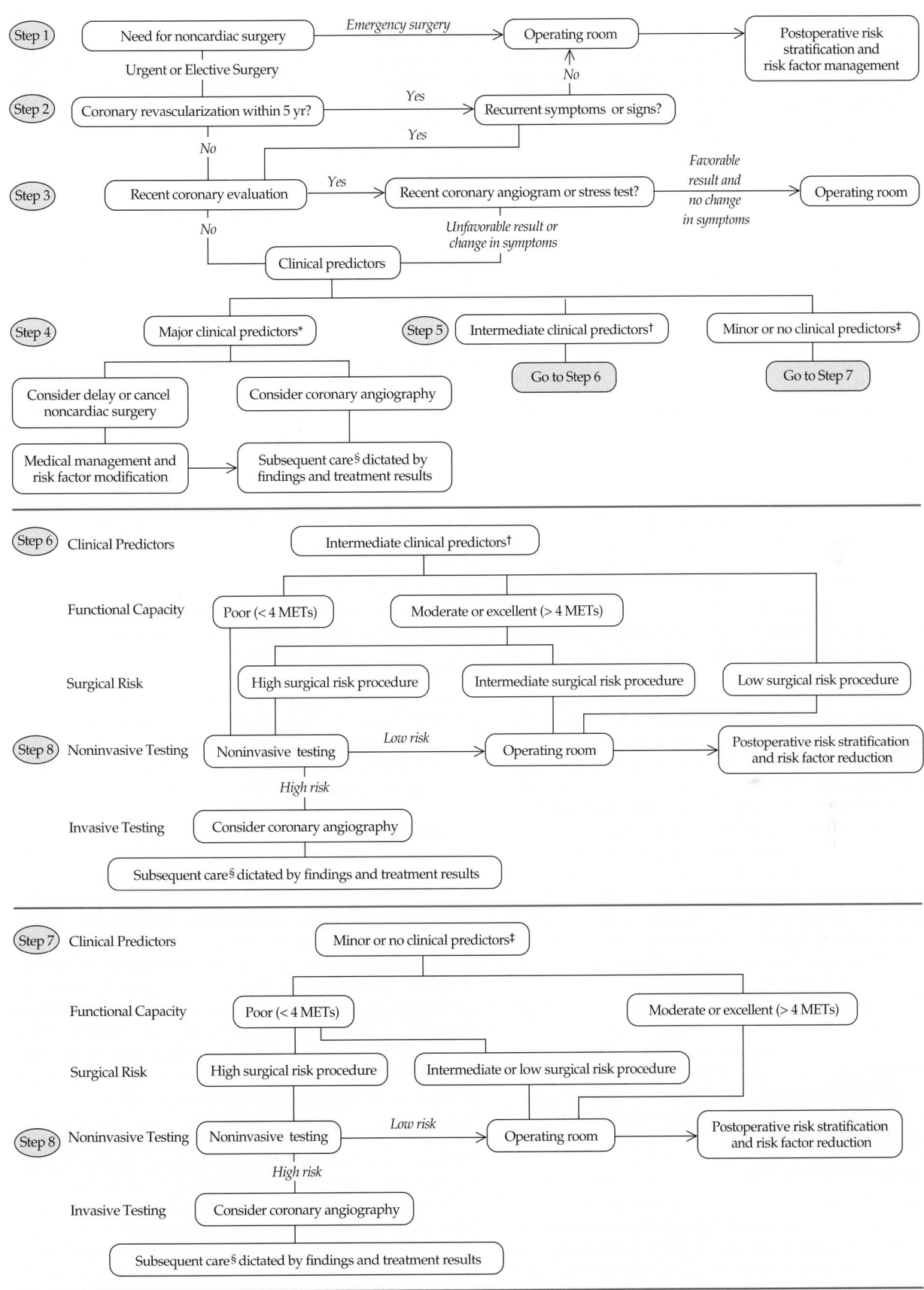

* Major clinical predictors: unstable coronary syndrome, decompensated CHF, significant arrhythmias, severe valvular disease.
† Intermediate clinical predictors: mild angina pectoris, prior MI, compensated or prior CHF, diabetes mellitus.
‡ Minor clinical predictors: advanced age, abnormal ECG, rhythm other than sinus, low functional capacity, history of stroke, uncontrolled systemic hypertension.
§ Subsequent care of patient may include cancellation or delay of surgery, coronary revascularization followed by surgery, or intensified care.

Figure 1 **Stepwise approach to cardiac assessment. (CHF—congestive heart failure; METs—metabolic equivalents; MI—myocardial infarction)**

Other patients with known prior coronary disease (prior myocardial infarction [MI] or angina), diabetes, or prior congestive heart failure should be more thoroughly evaluated. If such patients have poor functional capacity and have not undergone recent coronary evaluation, they should undergo a preoperative stress test to evaluate the severity of coronary disease and to determine the status of left ventricular function. When possible, exercise is generally the preferred method of stress testing[18] and appears to be safe in most patients. For patients who are unable to exercise, pharmacologic stress testing with either dobutamine echocardiography or adenosine thallium imaging is appropriate. Risk of cardiac events is directly related to the presence and extent of left ventricular (LV) dysfunction and ischemia.

The relative risk of perioperative cardiac morbidity or mortality is low (1% to 5%) in patients with no inducible ischemia and without evidence of fixed perfusion defects or wall motion abnormalities. In patients with extensive areas of ischemia or prior infarction detected during preoperative testing, perioperative event rates (death and MI) may be as high as 20% to 40%. Such patients should probably undergo coronary angiography and possibly coronary revascularization before undergoing major operative procedures.

Although the indications for coronary bypass surgery or percutaneous coronary interventions are generally the same for the preoperative patient and the general population, evaluation for potential heart disease before aneurysm resection may be the patient's first such evaluation. Coronary artery disease must be treated to the fullest extent before undertaking a potentially stressful noncardiac operation on the aorta.

Postoperative modification of risk factors A frequently forgotten issue in the management of patients undergoing abdominal aortic aneurysm resection is long-term modification of cardiovascular risk factors. The preoperative period represents an excellent opportunity to identify and treat hypertension, diabetes, hypercholesterolemia, smoking, obesity, and poor functional status. All patients identified as having vascular disease should take aspirin daily to prevent long-term cardiovascular events. Often, beta blockers are prescribed for patients with coronary artery disease, and the cholesterol profiles of such patients should be routinely assessed. Studies suggest that secondary prevention of vascular disease is enhanced by aggressive treatment of hypercholesterolemia, particularly in persons with a low-density lipoprotein cholesterol level exceeding 100 mg/dl. Currently, the best evidence suggests that the broad class of statin drugs (3-hydroxy-3-methylglutaryl coenzyme A [HMG-CoA] reductase inhibitors) are effective. Beta blockers have been championed as therapy both to reduce risk of MI and to potentially reduce the risk of expansion of aneurysms that may develop or be present elsewhere in patients who previously had significant aneurysms.

THORACIC AORTIC ANEURYSMS

Thoracic aortic aneurysms are less common than abdominal aneurysms. They are classified according to the involvement of the ascending aorta, the descending aorta, or a combination of the two. Aneurysms of the descending aorta are the most common. The etiology of thoracic aneurysms correlates with their location. Aneurysms of the ascending aorta are usually associated with cystic medial necrosis. This association is particularly common in patients with Marfan syndrome, Ehlers-Danlos syndrome, and annuloaortic ectasia, which represents the loss of

elastic tensile strength in the aorta. Descending thoracic aortic aneurysms are often seen in hypertensive patients with extensive atherosclerosis. They usually originate beyond the left subclavian artery and may be either fusiform or saccular. Aneurysms of the arch are often contiguous with aneurysms of the ascending or descending thoracic aorta.

Clinical Presentation

More than half of thoracic aortic aneurysms are symptomatic; the rest are discovered only incidentally, often after a routine chest x-ray. Symptoms usually reflect pressure on a contiguous structure or consequences such as concomitant aortic insufficiency. Local mass effects may include a superior vena cava syndrome, caused by obstruction of the superior vena cava; pressure on the trachea, leading to cough or wheezing; and, occasionally, dramatic hemoptysis, resulting from fistula formation between the aneurysm and a major airway. Pressure on the esophagus may produce dysphagia. Pressure on the recurrent laryngeal nerve may result in hoarseness from vocal chord paralysis. Chest pain is usually caused by direct pressure of the aneurysm on an intrathoracic structure or by erosion of a bony structure. Normally, this pain is steady and often severe. Rarely, aortitis may first present as an aortic aneurysm.[19]

A leaking or ruptured aneurysm usually presents with dramatic symptoms. Most such aneurysms leak or rupture into the left pleural space or pericardial space, resulting in hypotension and sudden onset of severe pain. Aortoesophageal fistulas may produce life-threatening gastrointestinal bleeding.

Diagnostic Evaluation

Physical examination The thoracic aorta is generally not palpable unless there is a significant pathologic process. Most often, this pathologic process consists of an ascending aortic arch aneurysm, and the aortic impulse can be palpated just above the sternum or at the right upper sternal border.

Imaging studies The diagnosis of thoracic aortic aneurysms is rarely suspected on physical examination. It is more often initially suspected on chest x-ray and then confirmed with noninvasive or invasive imaging. On chest x-ray, most aneurysms appear as a widening of the mediastinal silhouette. Small aneurysms may not be detected. MRI and spiral CT scanning are the most commonly used methods for delineating the size and extent of thoracic aneurysms. Transthoracic echocardiography (TTE) and transesophageal echocardiography (TEE) are also used to diagnose, measure, and monitor ascending aortic aneurysms. TTE can evaluate only the proximal 3 to 5 cm of the ascending aorta, and neither TTE nor TEE is useful for evaluating aneurysms below the diaphragm.

Management to Reduce Risk of Aneurysm Rupture

The natural history of a thoracic aneurysm can shed light on the disease process that has led to the aneurysm, on the risk factors that may affect the rate of aneurysm expansion, and on the concomitant presence of other vascular disease, including peripheral and coronary disease, that might affect long-term survival. Because size is a critical issue in terms of the risk of rupture, the initial size and potential growth of an aneurysm are important factors in the decision whether to operate on asymptomatic aneurysms. Aneurysms that are invading local structures or creating a marked vascular effect should usually be resected. Careful control of blood pressure is crucial for all patients and may require medical therapy, particularly with beta blockers, which may also slow the rate of aneurysm growth.[20]

The initial size of a thoracic aneurysm is an important predictor of subsequent growth. In general, small aneurysms tend to grow slowly, whereas large aneurysms have a higher probability of expansion and rupture. On average, thoracic aneurysms grow at 0.4 cm/yr, but the growth rate varies greatly.[21] Small aneurysms (i.e., < 5 cm in diameter) grow at about 0.1 cm/yr. Large aneurysms (i.e., > 5 cm) grow at about 0.5 to 1.0 cm/yr. Although these average growth rates are reassuring, it should be emphasized that rapid expansion can occur and can dramatically affect the natural history and management. In general, thoracic aneurysms smaller than 5 cm in diameter are unlikely to rupture, whereas those larger than 7 cm are at high risk for rupture. Currently, most thoracic centers recommend surgery for aneurysms that exceed 5.5 to 6 cm in an otherwise reasonable surgical candidate.[22,23] Because of their relatively young age, absence of associated disease, and low surgical risk of elective repair, patients with Marfan syndrome should undergo surgery when aneurysms reach 5 cm, particularly if the aneurysm is expanding. Some centers wait until aneurysms reach 6.5 or 7 cm before operating on high-risk surgical candidates. As in the case of treatment of abdominal aneurysm, the use of percutaneously placed aortic stent grafts may emerge as an attractive option in some patients with thoracic aneurysms.[24]

Surgical Treatment

The surgical approach to thoracic aortic aneurysms depends on the site. For ascending aortic aneurysms, the major issue is whether the aortic valve is competent and whether reimplantation of the coronary arteries will be necessary. With the availability of aortic homografts and stentless valves, surgical approaches to thoracic aortic aneurysm are undergoing rapid evolution. Individual patient characteristics and surgical preferences have a great deal to do with a given surgical approach.

Postoperative Complications

Neurologic sequelae are the most serious of potential postoperative complications. Currently, the risk of stroke after thoracic aneurysm resection ranges from 3% to 7%.[25] Efforts to reduce diffuse brain injury caused by prolonged periods of aortic cross clamping include hypothermic arrest and the use of retrograde cerebral perfusion by way of a superior vena cava cannula.[26] Efforts to reduce CNS embolic events focus on meticulous surgical technique to avoid dislodging atheroemboli present in the aortic margins and to avoid air embolism during surgery. The above issues are especially pertinent in aneurysms of the ascending aorta and the arch. Surgery on the posterior thoracic aorta carries a different neurologic risk—namely, postoperative paraplegia as a result of interrupting the supply of arterial blood to the spinal cord—and occurs in more than 5% of patients. Several methods have been devised to deal with this risk, but no definitive solution has yet emerged. Some centers have suggested that reattaching critical intercostal arteries leads to improved outcome,[27] whether or not the spinal cord is treated under epidural cooling during surgery.[28]

Aortic Dissection

The incidence of recognized aortic dissection in the United States is estimated to be 10 to 20 per million population, or about 5,000 cases a year. We stress, however, that the incidence of MI is greater than 500,000 cases annually; that is, MI is at least 100 times more common than aortic dissection. For most patients, dissection entails a tear in the intima, with the subsequent development of a propagating hematoma between the intima and the adventitia. Approximately two thirds of aortic dissections are initiated by a tear in the intima just above the aortic valve. Most of the remaining cases develop in the descending aorta at the attachment of the ligamentum arteriosum. Often, multiple communication sites are present between the true lumen and the false lumen. The dissection often spirals as it courses retrograde or antegrade along the aorta. Approximately 10% to 15% of aortic dissections are caused by intramural hematoma, which is spontaneous rupture of the vaso vasorum within the media, creating a hematoma in the media. This hematoma may extend a variable distance and may eventually rupture into the lumen, resulting in a more typical dissection.

CLASSIFICATION

Aortic dissections are classified as acute or chronic and according to their location. Dissections are termed acute when they are diagnosed within 2 weeks after the onset of symptoms; dissections diagnosed after 2 weeks of symptom onset are termed chronic. A key feature for classification is involvement of the ascending aorta, regardless of where the dissection began. Ascending aortic dissections are also called type A dissections. Dissections not involving the ascending aorta are typically classified as distal, or type B, dissections. Ascending aortic involvement identifies a patient population with high mortality if not treated surgically. A subset of patients with isolated aortic arch dissection has also been described. Normally, the life-threatening condition is caused by communication of the ascending aorta with the pericardial space, creating cardiac tamponade, or by spontaneous rupture or hemorrhage, leading to shock.

The predisposing factors for type A and type B dissections differ somewhat. Disorders of the media that result in cystic medial necrosis are a common precursor of type A dissection. Affected patients may include those with Marfan syndrome or other heritable disorders, such as Ehlers-Danlos syndrome, Noonan syndrome, and Turner syndrome. Another risk factor for ascending aortic dissection is aortic valve disease, such as bicuspid valve disease or prosthetic aortic valve disease. Although these conditions are classically associated with aortic dissection, over 90% of patients with acute aortic dissection do not have any recognized substrate for dissection. Distal, or type B, aortic dissection is most often seen in patients with long-standing hypertension. Patients with type B dissection are older on average than patients with type A dissection. An unexplained relation between aortic dissection and pregnancy also exists, perhaps because of changes in cardiac output, blood pressure, or blood volume or the effects of pregnancy on the aortic wall itself.[29] Aortic dissection after inhalation of crack cocaine has also been reported.

CLINICAL PRESENTATION

The most common distinguishing clinical feature of aortic dissection is the abrupt onset of pain.[30] The abruptness of onset is one of the clinical features reliably distinguishing the pain of aortic dissection from that accompanying other cardiovascular pathology (e.g., myocardial ischemia). This instantaneous pain may begin in the chest or back and may migrate to involve the neck, head, back, and legs as the dissection propagates. The classic combination of abrupt tearing pain, with pulse deficits and apparent aortic insufficiency, is seldom observed in actual practice.[30,31] Other presentations of type A dissection are sudden syncope or hypotension, resulting from dissection into the pericardial space; stroke, resulting from interruption of the blood supply to one or both internal carotid arteries; and, in rare instances, isolated congestive heart failure, when the dissection involves the ascending aorta and interrupts aortic valve function.

The most typical presentation of type B dissection is onset of severe interscapular pain, which may radiate down the back toward the legs. Type B dissection is frequently accompanied by hypertension, whereas type A dissection more often occurs in the presence of normal or low blood pressure.[30] Spinal cord ischemia, ischemic extremities, and mesenteric ischemia are most frequently encountered in type A dissection that has extended to involve the descending aorta. Whereas aortic insufficiency is noted on auscultation in 35% to 50% of the cases of ascending aortic dissection, it is rather unusual in cases of type B dissection. Pulse deficits are seen in about 25% of patients with type A dissection and in perhaps 5% to 10% of patients with type B dissection.[31]

Acute dissection remains a highly lethal entity. Mortality is commonly quoted as 1% per hour for the first 24 hours. Advanced age, hypotension, and limb and visceral ischemia are all predictors of greater mortality.[32,33] A published review of 500 patients with acute type A dissection identified a number of clinical factors that are predictors of death [see Figure 2]. Mortality in the study cohort ranged from 10% to 18%, depending on the number of adverse risk factors.[29]

DIAGNOSTIC EVALUATION

Because acute aortic dissection is a life-threatening emergency, rapid and accurate diagnosis is crucial to patient survival. Therefore, sophisticated imaging modalities may be required. Routine ECG in patients with suspected aortic dissection usually reveals only nonspecific abnormalities. Although type A dissection will affect one of the coronary arteries and lead to a transmural MI in 1% to 2% of patients, most patients have nonspecific ST-T wave changes or a finding of left ventricular hypertrophy related to long-standing hypertension.

The typical chest x-ray reveals widening of the mediastinal silhouette and may also demonstrate evidence of a pleural effusion, cardiomegaly, or congestive failure if severe aortic regurgitation is present. A normal-appearing chest x-ray is seen in more than 10% of documented acute aortic dissections.[30] Other laboratory abnormalities are generally nonspecific. An increase of smooth muscle myosin is present in more than 85% of patients presenting within 3 hours after onset of acute aortic dissection.[34] This serum assay, if further developed, may become a useful adjunctive tool to early assessment of suspected aortic dissection.

After a careful history and physical examination, the key to diagnosis is rapid identification of the aortic dissection, ascertainment of whether the ascending aorta is involved, and urgent cardiac surgery if proximal aortic dissection is diagnosed. The importance of rapid diagnosis and institution of definitive therapy for aortic dissection cannot be overemphasized. Given the 1% to 2% mortality per hour in the first 24 hours after presentation, even brief delays to achieve diagnostic imaging are unacceptable.[30,35]

Currently, four diagnostic tools are used to evaluate patients with suspected dissection[36]: CT scanning, echocardiography, MRI, and aortography. In general, the choice of which imaging modality to initially employ will depend on local expertise and availability. In most hospitals, the choice is either CT or TEE.

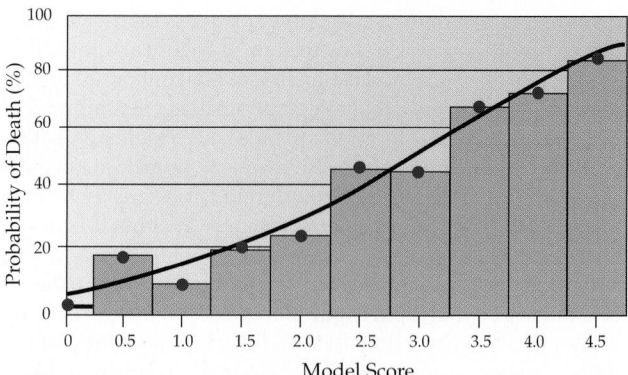

Figure 2 **Graphic demonstration of the increasing mortality in type A dissection when multiple risk factors are present. There is an observed increase in mortality in type A dissection that parallels that of the predictive model. The total risk score was the sum of individual risk factors that was determined from regression analysis to be significantly linked to outcome. The individual factors and their individual scores (in parentheses) were as follows: renal failure (1.6), hypotension/shock/tamponade (1.1), abrupt onset of pain (1.0), pulse deficit (0.7), abnormal ECG (0.6), age ≥ 70 (0.5), female (0.3). (bars—observed findings; line—model probabilities)**

CT scanning is widely available in most community and tertiary care hospitals. Spiral or ultrafast CT scanning gives even greater resolution than the older scanners and has a reported sensitivity and specificity for aortic dissection exceeding 95%.[37] TEE offers significant advantages in diagnosis [see Figures 3 and 4].[38] The primary attractiveness of TEE is its portability, making it suitable for performance in the emergency department, intensive care unit, or operating room. Thus, imaging can be achieved substantially faster with TEE than with other modalities.[39] Second, TEE is highly sensitive for the identification of type A dissection. TEE is also potentially useful when involvement of the aortic valve and the status of the left ventricle, pericardial space, and right and left coronary artery ostia are unknown.[40]

TEE can be very useful in detecting the mechanism of aortic insufficiency and detecting the feasibility of repair.[41,42] Valves in which aortic insufficiency is the result of sinotubular dilatation or extension of the dissection into the sinus are often candidates for repair. Patients with intrinsic disease of the aortic valve leaflets are less optimal candidates for repair.

MRI is less commonly used unless the MRI scanner is part of the emergency department. For most hospitals, however, the delay required in getting a patient into the MRI suite and completing the study makes this technology less efficient than TEE or chest CT.

Finally, although aortography is still used in some hospitals, it is seldom the initial test for aortic dissection. The reported false negative rate for aortography is in the range of 5% to 15%.[43] Aortography frequently misses lesions such as an intramural hematoma. In addition, the time required to get a patient to an angiography suite and complete the study is generally considerably longer than that for TEE. Our medical center and many others follow an algorithmic approach to evaluation and treatment of a suspected aortic dissection [see Figure 5].

TREATMENT

The treatment of aortic dissection includes aggressive medical therapy for all patients and definitive surgical therapy in selected patients. The decision to perform surgery depends first and foremost on the site of the aortic dissection [see Figure 5].

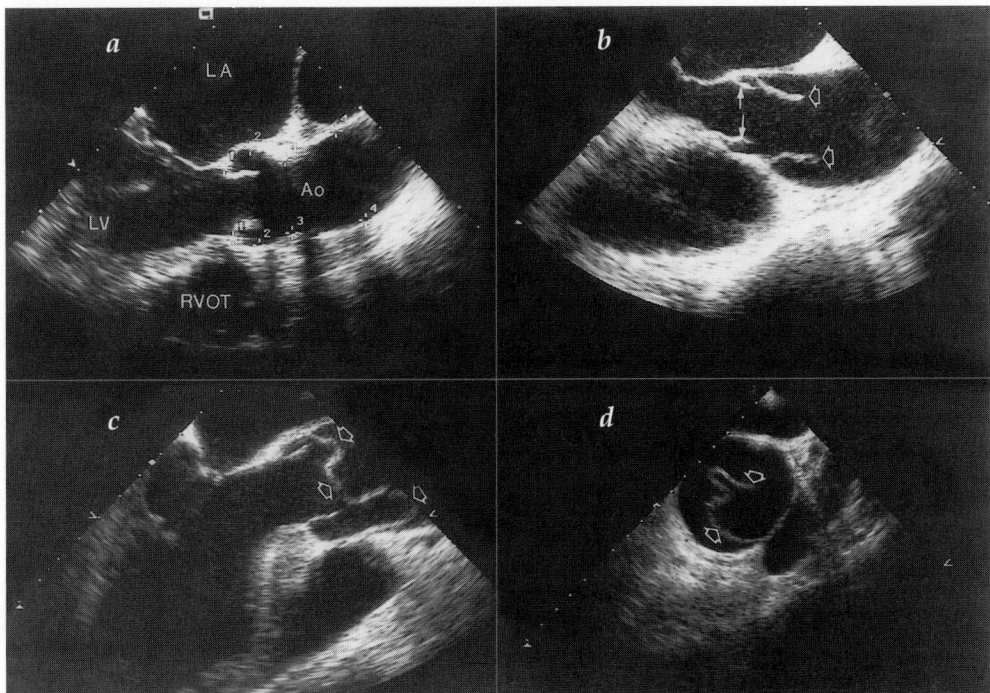

Figure 3   **Transesophageal echocardiograms from a patient with a normal ascending aorta (panel A) and three different ascending aortic dissections (panels B through D). In the normal ascending aorta, the cardiac chambers are noted. The ascending aorta is well visualized, including its annulus (point 1), the coronary sinuses (point 2), the sinotubular junction (point 3), and the true ascending aorta (point 4). Note that the aorta dilates at the level of the sinuses, narrows at the sinotubular junction to a dimension equivalent to that of the annulus, and then slightly dilates further in the ascending aorta. Shown is a normal aortic valve in its open position. Panel B was recorded in a patient with a proximal aortic dissection. The orientation is identical to that in panel A. The solid arrows denote the position of an open aortic valve leaflet. The open arrows represent the margins of a dissection that originated at the sinotubular junction and extended distally. Panel C was recorded in a patient with an ascending aortic dissection (orientation identical to that in panels A and B), and the aortic valve is open. In this instance, a convoluted intimal flap (open arrows) is clearly visualized in the proximal ascending aorta. Panel D was recorded in the short axis of the aorta in a patient with an aortic dissection. In the circular ascending aorta, multiple convolutions of an intimal flap are clearly visualized (open arrows). Note that a communication point (between the downward pointing arrow and the wall of the aorta) allows free communication of flow between the two lumens. (LA—left atrium; Ao—ascending aorta; RVOT—right ventricular outflow tract; LV—left ventricle)**

Surgical Repair

Type A aortic dissection   Any involvement of the ascending aorta carries with it a much greater risk of rupture into the pericardial space; development of coronary or cerebral ischemia, aortic regurgitation, and congestive heart failure; or free rupture of the aorta into the thorax. Thus, definitive surgical repair is carried out as quickly as possible for patients with proximal or type A aortic dissection who are appropriate candidates for the procedure.

For patients with type A dissection complicated by malperfusion, medical therapy plus percutaneous reperfusion utilizing aortic stenting or fenestration, or both, and selective branch stenting may allow stabilization and reduce risk associated with the operation. After a period of recovery, repair of the patient's ascending aorta may be undertaken.[44,45]

Definitive aortic repair includes resection of the dissected aorta and insertion of a conduit. The procedure often includes implanting a prosthetic aortic valve. Repair and resuspension of the aortic valve have proved feasible in many patients. For most patients, repair includes reimplantation of the coronary arteries. In some patients, this repair includes resection and placement of a graft to the aortic arch. Even in the best of cen-

ters, surgical mortality will range from 10% to 35%, depending on comorbidity.[30,32,46]

Type B aortic dissection   Surgery for type B dissection is indicated for patients with life-threatening complications that require a surgical approach. Examples include patients who experience ischemia of both kidneys, leading to reversible renal failure; development of ischemic bowel; ischemia involving one of the legs or arms; development of a progressive aneurysm; impending rupture; and recurrent extension of the dissection. In some centers, percutaneous insertion of aortic stents has been used to stabilize dissections of the descending aorta. This strategy may be preferable to surgery in some candidates.[47-49] In particular, stenting may promote thrombosis of the false channel and thereby reduce the long-term risk of aneurysm formation and aortic rupture. Surgical placement of an endoprosthesis, or so-called elephant trunk, has also been advocated as a preferred strategy for operative type B dissection.[50,51]

Postoperative Complications

In the management of aortic dissection, surgical complica-

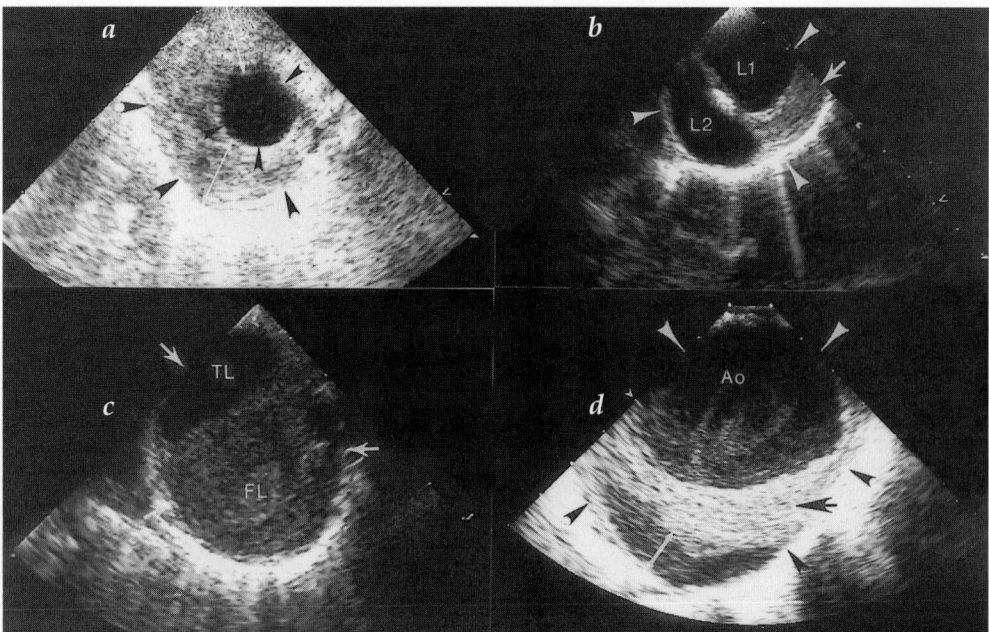

Figure 4   Panels A through D represent four transesophageal echocardiograms recorded in a short-axis view of the descending thoracic aorta in patients with aortic pathology. Panel A was recorded in a patient with an ascending aortic aneurysm and a large periaortic (adventitial) hematoma extending distally along the thoracic aorta. The smaller black arrows denote the boundaries of the normal-diameter descending thoracic aorta. The larger black arrows pointing inward mark the full dimension of the periaortic hematoma; the full dimension is also noted by the double-headed white arrows. In this instance, the intima of the descending thoracic aorta was not involved in the dissection process. However, a large periadventitial hematoma ruptured along the course of the descending thoracic aorta. Panel B was recorded in a patient with an aortic dissection localized to the descending thoracic aorta. The maximum external dimensions of the aorta are noted by the large white arrowheads. The white arrow notes an area of atherosclerosis and thrombus within the aorta. Two distinct lumens (L1 and L2) can be seen at this level. Panel C was recorded in a patient with an aortic dissection extending from the aortic valve to the bifurcation of the aorta. The large white arrows denote the outer dimension of the aorta. There is an echo-free lumen, or true lumen (TL), and a false lumen (FL) with early thrombus formation. Note the vague echo densities within the false lumen. Panel D was recorded in a patient with a large descending thoracic aortic aneurysm and intramural hematoma. The large arrowheads (black and white) denote the outer dimensions of the aorta. The dilated aortic lumen (Ao) is also noted. The black arrow denotes an area of marked atherosclerosis within the aorta, and the double-headed white arrow denotes an area of intramural hemorrhage, characterized by a lower echo density than the atherosclerotic components. Note also the low-density echoes, which represent stagnant blood flow within the aorta.

tions can be divided into the sequelae of operations involving the ascending aorta and those of operations involving the arch or descending aorta. Because some period of circulatory arrest is often required to approach the ascending aorta or arch, the most severe complication of surgery in this region is cerebral anoxia, with postoperative neurologic dysfunction. Currently, most aortic centers of excellence perform this operation under conditions of deep hypothermia and circulatory arrest, along with retrograde cerebral perfusion by way of the jugular veins. This technique has dramatically diminished the incidence of severe neurologic injury after aortic surgery.

For surgery on the descending thoracic aorta, the most serious complication is interruption of the blood supply to the spinal cord, with resultant paraplegia. Procedures to reduce this complication include the use of shunts and the careful isolation of ostia of the spinal arteries with reimplantation. This complication remains the one most feared in descending-aorta surgery. Additional risks are acute renal failure, mesenteric ischemia, distal atheroembolic events, and pulmonary complications.

Medical Therapy

All patients with aortic dissection receive aggressive medical therapy. This treatment is first directed at controlling the blood pressure. For hypertensive patients, administration of intravenous beta blockers followed by oral beta blockers, along with the concomitant administration of intravenous or oral vasodilators, is imperative. Patients who are normotensive should maintain a low-normal blood pressure and a low heart rate. The likelihood for propagation of dissection is believed to be in part related to acceleration of flow in the aorta—that is, the force of the aortic jet per unit time (i.e., dp/dt). Accordingly, beta blockers have been the most important therapy for the medical treatment of aortic dissection. Such therapy should maintain heart rates at or below 60 beats/min and keep blood pressure as low as possible while allowing perfusion of the brain, kidneys, and other vital organs. Also important are careful measurements of urine output and filling pressures of the heart.

Long-term management of aortic dissection requires aggressive medical therapy and careful surveillance. Patients who retain patency in the false channel of the aorta after either medical treatment or surgical repair have a significant risk of aneurysm formation and rupture of the false channel, especially in the first 6 months after initial therapy.[52] Expansion, rupture, or both are more common in patients who are older and have poorly controlled hypertension and chronic obstructive pulmonary disease.[53] Aggressive treatment of blood pressure and heart rate and careful monitoring of the patient's status with physical examination and noninvasive imaging are essential. At many centers, either CT scanning or MRI is performed on a regular basis after initial treatment of the dissection. For instance, the patient might be seen at 2 to 4 weeks after admission for adjustment of dosages of antihypertensive medications and beta blockers. At our center, spiral CT scanning is repeated 3 to 6 months after surgery to screen for the development of aneurysm in the false channel or at the margins of a surgical repair. After this, patients undergo aortic imaging annually, and scrupulous attention is directed to antihypertensive therapy.

Atypical Aortic Dissection

AORTIC DISSECTION WITHOUT INTIMAL TEAR

About 10% to 15% of patients presenting with symptoms suggestive of aortic dissection actually have aortic dissection without an intimal tear (intramural hematoma).[54] This hemorrhage into the medial layer of the aorta may produce a localized or discrete hematoma or may extend for a various distance by dissecting along the plane of the aortic media. Clinically, this hemorrhage mirrors aortic dissection in terms of both its risk factors and its presentation. Intramural hematoma is generally not identified on aortography. It is most easily diagnosed with ultrafast CT scanning. With noncontrast imaging, the hematoma appears as a crescent-shaped high-attenuation area along the aortic wall; moreover, this region cannot be enhanced with contrast imaging. MRI reveals the same crescent-shaped high-intensity area [see Figure 4], whereas on TEE, intramural hematoma may appear as a circular or crescentic thickening.[55]

Studies of the natural history of the intramural hematoma suggest that the outcome is similar to that of classic aortic dissection,[56,57] although some recent studies have suggested a more benign prognosis.[58] By 30 days, the rate of aortic expansion or death in patients with medically treated ascending aortic intramural hematoma approaches 50%. Patients with aneurysmal aortas—that is, those with aortas measuring more than 5 cm in diameter—are at particular risk.[59] By contrast, the mortality for intramural hematoma in the descending aorta appears to be between 10% and 15%, a rate similar to that for type B aortic dissection.

PENETRATING ATHEROSCLEROTIC ULCER

A second form of aortic disease that may have an acute pre-

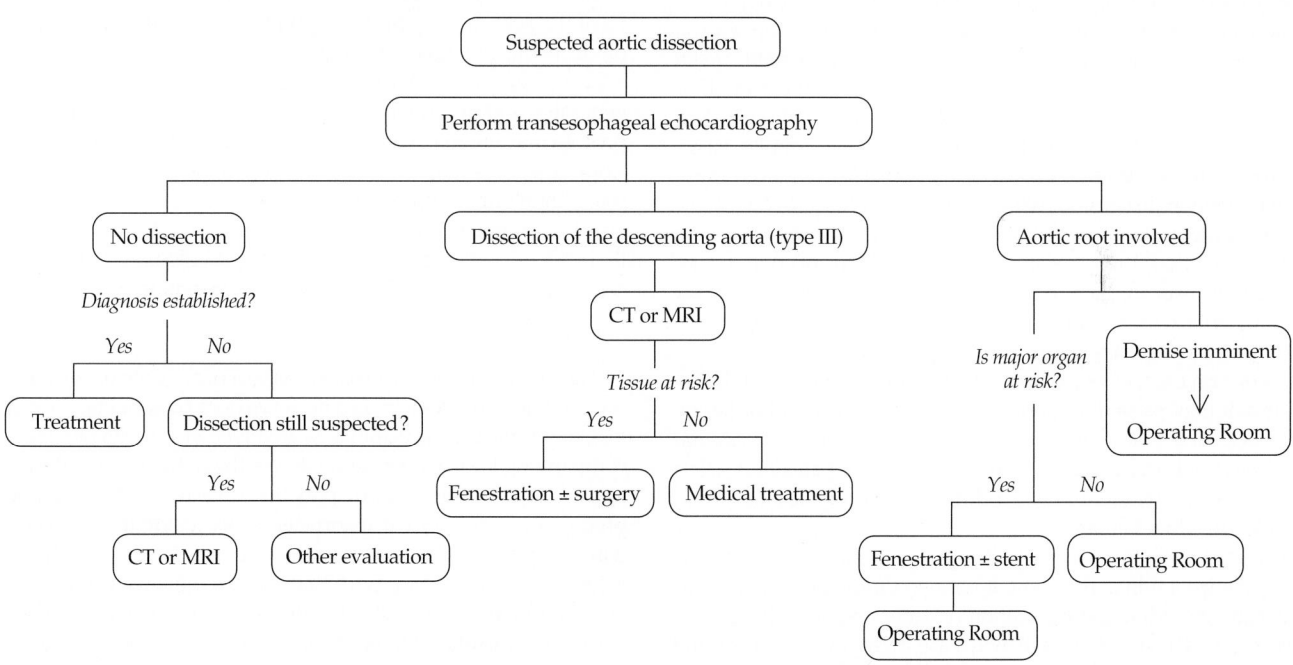

Indications for Surgical Intervention in Aortic Dissection

Ascending Aorta Only	Ascending and Descending Aorta	Descending Aorta Only
Emergent repair in appropriate candidates	Emergent repair if any of following are present: Aortic insufficiency with CHF Hypotension Pericardial effusion with compromise If ischemia in kidney, CNS, bowel, or major limb, attempt stabilization with stent or fenestration before surgery	Emergent repair if any of following are present: Rupture Impending rupture Uncontrolled pain Major organ at risk (stabilization with stent or fenestration not feasible)

Figure 5 **Decision algorithm for evaluation and treatment of a suspected aortic dissection. Type III dissection originates in the descending aorta and extends distally down the aorta or, in rare instances, retrograde into the aortic arch and ascending aorta. (CHF—congestive heart failure)**

sentation is a penetrating atherosclerotic ulcer.[60] Penetrating ulcers result from erosion of the intima of the aorta, usually because of extensive atherosclerosis. Ulcer formation may produce a hematoma in the media that extends several centimeters from its origin up or down the aorta. Occasionally, pseudo-aneurysms are created that may extend into the adventitia and, in rare instances, may rupture. This aortic process develops gradually in elderly patients with extensive atherosclerosis and often is heralded by chest pain or back pain and hypertension. Because it usually presents as a localized process, it is seldom associated with other symptoms of aortic dissection, such as pulse deficit, aortic valve regurgitation, or neurologic defects. Symptomatic penetrating atherosclerotic ulcer rarely requires surgery. Asymptomatic patients who experience progressive enlargement or recurrent atheroemboli may require surgical therapy. For most patients, however, medical therapy suffices and entails aggressive treatment of atherosclerotic risk factors, including cessation of smoking, control of hypertension, lipid-lowering therapy, and careful surveillance. The role of antiplatelet or anticoagulant therapy for this condition is not clear.

Aortic Atheromatous Emboli

Atherosclerosis of the aorta may be so extensive that it leads to overlying thrombosis and subsequent dislodgment of thrombi, cholesterol particles, or fibrinous material into the cerebrovascular or peripheral circulation. Risk factors are hypertension, diabetes, hyperlipidemia, advanced age, and other vascular diseases. Atheromatous disease is most common in the distal aorta but may also occur in the ascending aorta and arch. Evidence of ulceration of atherosclerotic plaques is an independent risk factor for stroke, as is the identification of a mobile, large, protruding aortic atheroma detected with TEE.[60] Plaques more than 4mm in dimension (whereas diameter is used to define the size of the aorta, dimension refers to the maximum size of the atheroma that protrudes into the lumen of the aorta) in the ascending aorta are particularly associated with an increased risk of ischemic stroke.[61] Atheroemboli or cholesterol-particle emboli may also involve the peripheral extremities, leading to ischemic lesions on the feet or toes (so-called blue-toe syndrome). These emboli may present as abdominal pain as a result of ischemic bowel. Acute nonoliguric renal failure is another occasional manifestation, as is gastrointestinal bleeding or pancreatitis. Cutaneous involvement may produce a characteristic skin lesion called livedo reticularis.

Cholesterol embolism syndrome is particularly common after manipulation of the aorta. It is most common in patients undergoing cardiac catheterization or other angiographic procedures in which catheters or wires are manipulated within the aorta. Because the occurrence of atheroemboli may be delayed after aortic manipulation, the relation between the two may not be apparent when the patient is first examined. If cutaneous manifestations are present, a biopsy of the lesions will often identify needle-shaped clefts in the arteriolar lumen characteristic of cholesterol embolization.

Treatment of cholesterol embolism syndrome begins with avoidance of further aortic manipulation (e.g., cardiac catheterization), if this has been a precipitant. Aggressive treatment of hypercholesterolemia is warranted. A search for an aortic aneurysm or protruding mobile atheromas is appropriate in patients for whom the syndrome develops without a concomitant iatrogenic source. Occasionally, recurrent emboli warrant the

resection of an aneurysm or of a severely diseased segment of atheromatous aorta.[62] The role of anticoagulant and antiplatelet drugs in this syndrome is uncertain.

Takayasu Arteritis and Giant Cell Arteritis

TAKAYASU ARTERITIS

Takayasu arteritis is a rare inflammatory condition that affects the aorta and its major branches. Other names include aortic arch syndrome, pulseless disease, and young female arteritis.[63] Although Takayasu arteritis is seen throughout the world, most cases occur in Asia and Africa. A specific etiologic agent has yet to be identified, but current evidence favors an autoimmune mechanism. Some studies suggest it may be linked to rheumatic fever, streptococcal infections, certain HLA subtypes, rheumatoid arthritis, and other collagen vascular diseases. Takayasu arteritis is more prevalent in women than in men. By definition, most patients are young, with an average age of 29 years. Takayasu arteritis has been divided into three types.[64] Type I involves the aortic arch and its branches, type II involves the distal aorta and spares the arch, and type III may affect both the ascending aorta and the descending aorta. A suggested fourth category involves the pulmonary arteries.

Pathophysiology

Takayasu arteritis generally involves a granulomatous arteritis of the aorta and its branches, with subsequent involvement of the media and adventitia. Later, the disease may progress to a sclerotic stage in which the intima is hyperplastic, the media degenerates, and the adventitia develops fibrosis. This late fibrotic process may encroach on the lumen of the aorta or its branches. Common areas of involvement are the main aorta and branch points of its major branch vessels. The pulmonary artery may also be involved. The coronary arteries are affected in fewer than 10% of patients. In some patients, involvement of the ascending aorta may lead to aortic valve regurgitation.

Clinical Presentation

The initial symptoms are often typical of an acute or systemic inflammatory process, including fever, loss of appetite, weight loss, night sweats, and arthralgias. Involved vessels may have accompanying localized tenderness over them. By the time the diagnosis is established, most patients have reached a sclerotic phase, in which vascular insufficiency is causing the predominant symptoms. It may involve the upper or lower extremities. Hypertension occurs in more than half of patients. Congestive heart failure occurs in 25% of patients because of hypertension, aortic valve insufficiency, or involvement of the coronary arteries.

Diagnostic Evaluation

Laboratory findings in patients with Takayasu arteritis generally include an elevated erythrocyte sedimentation rate, mild anemia, and a slightly increased white blood cell count. The chest x-ray may demonstrate a rim of calcification around the involved vessels. Aortography often shows an irregular intimal surface with stenoses of the aorta or its branch arteries. Poststenotic dilatation or frank arterial aneurysms may be visible. Similar diagnostic features can also be detected by TEE and MRI.[65] Among the established criteria for the clinical diagnosis of Takayasu arteritis is that patients must be no older than 40 years.

Treatment

The management of Takayasu arteritis begins with high-dose glucocorticoid therapy, which usually leads to abatement of constitutional symptoms and the laboratory signs of inflammation. Serial sedimentation rates are useful for monitoring the benefits of treatment. For patients who fail to respond to steroid therapy, cyclophosphamide at a dosage of 2 mg/kg/day has been used. Alternatively, low-dose methotrexate may enhance the efficacy of steroids or allow steroid tapering. Surgery may be necessary to treat unremitting peripheral ischemia or aortic valve disease or to treat renal artery stenosis that causes severe hypertension. For patients with involvement of the coronary ostia, bypass surgery may be indicated as well.[66] Percutaneously placed arterial stents have successfully treated segmental disease in a variety of vessels in patients with this syndrome.

GIANT CELL ARTERITIS

Giant cell arteritis is another form of aortoarteritis. In contrast to Takayasu arteritis, this illness is more commonly seen in Europe and the United States and in patients older than 50 years (the mean age at onset of disease is 67 years).

Pathophysiology

This form of arteritis often affects the branches of the proximal aorta, particularly the branches supplying the head and neck, the extracranial structures (including the temporal arteries), and the upper extremities. Aortic involvement often coexists with temporal arteritis and polymyalgia rheumatica. Unlike Takayasu arteritis, giant cell arteritis seldom has a sclerotic phase progressing to occlusion of vessels. However, giant cell arteritis may lead to aneurysm formation, aortic regurgitation, or aortic dissection.[67,68]

Clinical Presentation

The classic presentation of giant cell arteritis consists of headache, tenderness over involved arteries in the scalp or the temporal region, jaw claudication, difficulty combing one's hair, and constitutional symptoms. Fever is common, and the blood vessels involved are thick and tender. Pulses may be diminished, and bruits may be present. Occasionally, signs of aortic valve regurgitation are present.

A serious complication of this syndrome is blindness, which results when arteritis affects the ophthalmic artery. The progression to total blindness may be rapid. Visual symptoms of some type occur in as many as 50% of patients. An initial high dose followed by prolonged therapy with corticosteroids remains the treatment of choice.[69] In rare instances, giant cell arteritis may lead to reduced upper extremity pulses and blood pressure along with arm or leg claudication. It also may cause coronary ischemia or abdominal angina in rare cases. Unlike Takayasu arteritis, giant cell arteritis virtually never affects the kidneys. Aortic aneurysms occur in 15% of patients with giant cell arteritis, most commonly involving the ascending aorta. Such aneurysms may develop late in the disease, leading to rupture, aortic dissection, or severe aortic valve regurgitation.

Diagnostic Evaluation

An above normal erythrocyte sedimentation rate is characteristic of this disease, and the diagnosis is confirmed by biopsy of an involved artery, usually the temporal artery. Clinicians need to be aware, however, that temporal artery biopsy may be negative in as many as 15% of patients with confirmed disease; therefore, a second biopsy may be necessary in patients with a high likelihood of temporal arteritis.

Treatment

Standard therapy for giant cell arteritis is high-dose glucocorticoid therapy (e.g., prednisone, 40 to 60 mg/day). Methotrexate may be used to reduce the need for steroids or to treat patients who respond inadequately to steroids. Cyclophosphamide may also be useful for reducing the need for glucocorticoids. Surgery is typically reserved for patients who experience progressive ischemic symptoms or aortic aneurysms.

Traumatic Disease of the Aorta

Finally, a relatively common form of aortic pathology is partial or complete transection as a result of major blunt thoracic trauma, most commonly as a result of a high-speed motor vehicle accident. Most patients with complete aortic transection do not survive long enough for hospital evaluation. If rapidly diagnosed, patients with partial transection may survive long enough to undergo surgical correction. Evidence of aortic trauma is often obscured by other major organ trauma. Patients with aortic transection are typically in shock and may have diminished lower extremity pulses. The transection is usually located at the distal arch, immediately after the origin of the left subclavian artery.

Rapid diagnosis is the key to the survival of patients with aortic transection. The routine chest x-ray typically reveals a widened mediastinum, often with pleural effusions. The gold standard for diagnosis of this disorder remains aortography, but TEE,[60,70] CT,[71] and MRI have also been used successfully.[72] Successful treatment requires vigorous fluid and blood resuscitation and surgical repair of the aortic transsection.

Kim A. Eagle, M.D., has received grant and research support from Pfizer, Inc., and Aventis and is a consultant for COR Therapeutics, Inc.

William F. Armstrong, M.D., has served as an advisor or consultant to AstraZeneca Pharmaceuticals LP and St. Jude Medical, Inc.

References

1. Rodin MB, Daviglus ML, Wong GC, et al: Middle age cardiovascular risk factors and abdominal aortic aneurysm in older age. Hypertension 42:61, 2003

2. Crawford ES, Cohen ES: Aortic aneurysm: a multifocal disease. Arch Surg 117:1393, 1982

3. Ashton HA, Buxton MJ, Day NE, et al: The Multicentre Aneurysm Screening Study (MASS) into the effect of abdominal aortic aneurysm screening on mortality in men: a randomised controlled trial. Lancet 360:1531, 2002

4. Frame PS, Fryback DG, Patterson C: Screening for abdominal aortic aneurysm in men ages 60 to 80 years: a cost-effectiveness analysis. Ann Intern Med 119:411, 1993

5. Ernst CB: Abdominal aortic aneurysm. N Engl J Med 328:1167, 1993

6. Lederle FA, Wilson SE, Johnson GR, et al: Variability in measurements of abdominal aortic aneurysms. J Vasc Surg 21:945, 1995

7. Petersen MJ, Cambria RP, Kaufman JA, et al: Magnetic resonance angiography in the preoperative evaluation of abdominal aortic aneurysms. J Vasc Surg 21:891, 1995

8. Gadowski GR, Pilcher DB, Ricci MA: Abdominal aortic aneurysm expansion rate: effect of size and beta-adrenergic blockade. J Vasc Surg 19:727, 1994

9. Hollier LD, Taylor LM, Ochsner J: Recommended indications for operative treatment of abdominal aortic aneurysms: report of a subcommittee of the Joint Council of the Society for Vascular Surgery and of the North American Chapter of the International Society for Cardiovascular Surgery. J Vasc Surg 15:1046, 1992

10. Lederle FA, Wilson SE, Johnson GR, et al: Immediate repair compared with surveillance of small abdominal aortic aneurysms. N Engl J Med 346:1437, 2002

11. Lederle FA, Johnson GR, Wilson SE, et al: Rupture rate of large abdominal aortic aneurysms in patients refusing or unfit for elective repair. JAMA 287:2968, 2002

12. Mortality results for randomised controlled trial of early elective surgery or ultrasonographic surveillance for small abdominal aortic aneurysms. The UK Small Aneurysm Trial Participants. Lancet 352:1649, 1998

13. Ballard DJ, Fowkes FG, Powell JT: Surgery for small asymptomatic abdominal aortic aneurysms. Cochrane Database Syst Rev (2):CD001835, 2000

14. Wolf YG, Fogarty TJ, Olcott C, et al: Endovascular repair of abdominal aortic aneurysms: eligibility rate and impact on the rate of open repair. J Vasc Surg 32:519, 2000

15. Faries PL, Brener BJ, Connelly TL, et al: A multicenter experience with the Talent endovascular graft for the treatment of abdominal aortic aneurysms. J Vasc Surg 35:1123, 2002

16. Eagle KA, Brundage BH, Chaitman BR, et al: Guidelines for perioperative cardiovascular evaluation for noncardiac surgery. Report of the American College of Cardiology/ American Heart Association Task Force on Practice Guidelines. Committee on Perioperative Cardiovascular Evaluation for Noncardiac Surgery. Circulation 93:1278, 1996

17. Poldermans D, Boersma E, Bax JJ, et al: The effect of bisoprolol on perioperative mortality and myocardial infarction in high-risk patients undergoing vascular surgery. Dutch Echocardiographic Cardiac Risk Evaluation Applying Stress Echocardiography Study Group. N Engl J Med 341:1789, 1999

18. Best PJ, Tajik AJ, Gibbons RJ, et al: The safety of treadmill exercise stress testing in patients with abdominal aortic aneurysms. Ann Intern Med 129:628, 1998

19. Rojo-Leyva F, Ratliff NB, Cosgrove DM 3rd, et al: Study of 52 patients with idiopathic aortitis from a cohort of 1,204 surgical cases. Arthritis Rheum 43:901, 2000

20. Shores J, Berger KR, Murphy EA, et al: Progression of aortic dilatation and the benefit of long-term beta-adrenergic blockade in Marfan's syndrome. N Engl J Med 330:1335, 1994

21. Dapunt OE, Galla JD, Sadeghi AM, et al: The natural history of thoracic aortic aneurysms. J Thorac Cardiovasc Surg 107:1323, 1994

22. Elefteriades JA: Natural history of thoracic aortic aneurysms: indications for surgery, and surgical versus nonsurgical risks. Ann Thorac Surg 74:S1877, 2002

23. Coady MA, Rizzo JA, Hammond GL, et al: What is the appropriate size criterion for resection of thoracic aortic aneurysm? J Thorac Cardiovasc Surg 113:476, 1997

24. Mitchell RS, Miller DC, Dake MD, et al: Thoracic aortic aneurysm repair with an endovascular stent graft: the "first generation." Ann Thorac Surg 67:1971, 1999

25. Okita Y, Takamoto S, Ando M, et al: Mortality and cerebral outcome in patients who underwent aortic arch operations using deep hypothermic circulatory arrest with retrograde cerebral perfusion: no relation of early death, stroke, and delirium to the duration of circulatory arrest. J Thorac Cardiovasc Surg 115:129, 1998

26. Coselli JS, Buket S, Djukanovic B: Aortic arch operation: current treatment and results. Ann Thorac Surg 59:19, 1995

27. Coselli JA, LeMaire SA, deFigueiredo LP, et al: Paraplegia after thoracoabdominal aortic aneurysm repair: is dissection a risk factor? Ann Thorac Surg 63:28, 1997

28. Cambria RP, Davison JK, Zannetti S, et al: Clinical experience with epidural cooling for spinal cord protection during thoracic and thoracoabdominal aneurysm repair. J Vasc Surg 25:234, 1997

29. Elkayam U, Ostzega E, Shotan A, et al: Cardiovascular problems in pregnant women with the Marfan syndrome. Ann Intern Med 123:177, 1995

30. Hagan PG, Nienaber CA, Isselbacher EM, et al: The international registry of aortic dissection (IRAD): new insights into an old disease. JAMA 283:897, 2000

31. Armstrong WF, Bach DS, Carey LM, et al: Clinical and echocardiographic findings in patients with suspected acute aortic dissection. Am Heart J 136:1051, 1998

32. Mehta RH, Suzuki T, Hagan PG, et al: Predicting death in patients with acute type A aortic dissection. Circulation 105:200, 2002

33. Mehta RH, O'Gara PT, Bossone E, et al: Acute type A aortic dissection in the elderly: Clinical characteristics, management, and outcomes in the current era. J Am Coll Cardiol 40:685, 2002

34. Suzuki T, Katoh H, Tsuchio Y, et al: Diagnostic implications of elevated levels of smooth-muscle myosin heavy-chain protein in acute aortic dissection. The smooth muscle myosin heavy chain study. Ann Intern Med 133:537, 2000

35. Suzuki T, Katoh H, Kurabayashi M, et al: Biochemical diagnosis of aortic dissection by raised concentrations of creatine kinase BB-isozyme. Lancet 350:784, 1997

36. Nienaber CA, vonKodolitsch Y, Nicolas V, et al: The diagnosis of thoracic aortic dissection by noninvasive imaging procedures. N Engl J Med 328:1, 1993

37. Zeman RK, Berman PM, Silverman PM, et al: Diagnosis of aortic dissection: value of helical CT with multiplanar reformation and three-dimensional rendering. AJR Am J Roentgenol 164:1375, 1995

38. Evangelista A, Garcia-del-Castillo H, Gonzales-Alujas T, et al: Diagnosis of ascending aortic dissection by transesophageal echocardiography: utility of M-mode in recognizing artifacts. J Am Coll Cardiol 27:102, 1996

39. Banning AP, Ruttley MST, Musumeci F, et al: Acute dissection of the thoracic aorta: transesophageal echocardiography is the investigation of choice. BMJ 310:72, 1995

40. Armstrong WF, Bach DS, Carey L, et al: Spectrum of acute dissection of the ascending aorta: a transesophageal echocardiographic study. J Am Soc Echocardiogr 9:646, 1996

41. Movsowitz H, Levine RA, Hilgenberg AD, et al: Transesophageal echocardiographic description of the mechanisms of aortic regurgitation in acute type A aortic dissection: implications for aortic valve repair. J Am Coll Cardiol 36:884, 2000

42. Keane MG, Wiegers SE, Yang E, et al: Structural determinants of aortic regurgitation in type A dissection and the role of ventricular resuspension as determined by intraoperative transesophageal echocardiography. Am J Cardiol 85:604, 2000

43. Bansal RC, Chandrasekaran K, Ayala J, et al: Frequency and explanation of false negative diagnosis of aortic dissection by aortography and transesophageal echocardiography. J Am Coll Cardiol 25:1393, 1995

44. Deeb GM, William DM, Bolling SF, et al: Surgical delay for acute type A dissection with malperfusion. Ann Thorac Surg 64:1669, 1997

45. Bavaria JE, Brinster DR, Gorman RC, et al: Advances in the treatment of acute type A dissection: an integrated approach. Ann Thorac Surg 74:S1848, 2002

46. Fann JI, Smith JA, Miller C, et al: Surgical management of aortic dissection during a 30-year period. Circulation 92:II113, 1995

47. Nienaber CA, Fattori R, Lund G, et al: Nonsurgical reconstruction of thoracic aortic dissection by stent-graft placement. N Engl J Med 340:1539, 1999

48. Dake MD, Kato N, Mitchell RS, et al: Endovascular stent-graft placement for the treatment of acute aortic dissection. N Engl J Med 340:1546, 1999

49. Kato M, Matsuda T, Kaneko M, et al: Outcomes of stent-graft treatment of false lumen in aortic dissection. Circulation 98:II305, 1998

50. Palma JH, Almeida DR, Carvalho AC, et al: Surgical treatment of acute type B aortic dissection using an endoprosthesis (elephant trunk). Ann Thorac Surg 63:1081, 1997

51. Umana JP, Miller DC, Mitchell RS: What is the best treatment for patients with acute type B aortic dissections—medical, surgical, or endovascular stent-grafting? Ann Thorac Surg 74:S1840, 2002

52. Yamashita C, Okada M, Ataka K, et al: Cerebral complications and distal false lumen in the repair of aortic dissection with retrograde cerebral perfusion. J Cardiovasc Surg 38:581, 1997

53. Juvonen T, Ergin MA, Galla JD, et al: Risk factors for rupture of chronic type B dissections. J Thorac Cardiovasc Surg 117:776, 1999

54. Nienaber CA, von Kodolitsch Y, Petersen B, et al: Intramural hemorrhage of the thoracic aorta: diagnostic and therapeutic implications. Circulation 92:1465, 1995

55. Vilacosta I, San Roman JA, Ferreiros J, et al: Natural history and serial morphology of aortic intramural hematoma: a novel variant of aortic dissection. Am Heart J 134:495, 1997

56. Maraj R, Rerkpattanapipat P, Jacobs LE, et al: Meta-analysis of 143 reported cases of aortic intramural hematoma. Am J Cardiol 86:664, 2000

57. von Kodolitsch Y, Csosz SK, Koschyk DH, et al: Intramural hematoma of the aorta: predictors of progression to dissection and rupture. Circulation 107:1158, 2003

58. Song JK, Kim HS, Song JM, et al: Outcomes of medically treated patients with aortic intramural hematoma. Am J Med 113:181, 2002

59. Kaji S, Nishigama K, Akasada T, et al: Prediction of progression or regression of type A aortic intramural hematoma by computed tomography. Circulation 100:II281, 1999

60. Vilacosta I, San Román JA, Aragoncillo P, et al: Penetrating atherosclerotic aortic ulcer: documentation by transesophageal echocardiography. J Am Coll Cardiol 32:83, 1998

61. Willens HJ, Kessler KM: Transesophageal echocardiography in the diagnosis of diseases of the thoracic aorta: part II—atherosclerotic and traumatic diseases of the aorta. Chest 117:233, 2000

62. Bojar RM, Payne DD, Murphy RE, et al: Surgical treatment of systemic atheroembolism from the thoracic aorta. Ann Thorac Surg 61:1389, 1996

63. Numano F, Kobayashi Y: Takayasu arteritis—beyond pulselessness. Intern Med 38: 226, 1999

64. Ishikawa K: Diagnostic approach and proposed criteria for the clinical diagnosis of Takayasu's arteriopathy. J Am Coll Cardiol 12:964, 1988

65. Matsunaga N, Hayaski K, Sakamoto I, et al: Takayasu arteritis: MR manifestations and diagnosis of acute and chronic phase. J Magn Reson Imaging 8:406, 1998

66. Endo M, Tomizawa Y, Nishida H, et al: Angiographic findings and surgical treatments of coronary artery involvement in Takayasu arteritis. J Thorac Cardiovasc Surg 125:570, 2003

67. Evans JM, O'Fallon WM, Hunder GG: Increased incidence of aortic aneurysm and dissection in giant cell (temporal) arteritis: a population-based study. Ann Intern Med 122:502, 1995

68. Gravanis MB: Giant cell arteritis and Takayasu aortitis: morphologic, pathogenetic and etiologic factors. Int J Cardiol 75:S21, 2000

69. Hayreh SS, Zimmerman B: Management of giant cell arteritis: our 27-year clinical study: new light on old controversies. Ophthalmologica 217:239, 2003

70. Smith MD, Cassidy JM, Souther S, et al: Transesophageal echocardiography in the diagnosis of traumatic rupture of the aorta. N Engl J Med 332:356, 1995

71. Demetriades D, Gomez H, Velmahos CG, et al: Routine helical computed tomographic evaluation of the mediastinum in high-risk blunt trauma patients. Arch Surg 133:1084, 1998

72. Patel NH, Stephens KE Jr, Mirvis SE, et al: Imaging of acute thoracic aortic injury due to blunt trauma: a review. Radiology 209:335, 1998

29 Diseases of the Pericardium, Cardiac Tumors, and Cardiac Trauma

E. William Hancock, M.D., F.A.C.P.

Diseases of the Pericardium

The pericardium provides a protective sac around the heart. The sac contains a thin layer of fluid that permits the heart to move with minimal friction during the cardiac cycle. Neither the sac nor the fluid appears to be necessary for normal function. When one or more of the cardiac chambers dilate acutely, the pericardium restrains the heart. In chronic dilatation of the heart, however, the pericardium stretches and therefore does not exert a restraining effect, except during exercise or other acute stresses.

Pericardial disease results from diverse causes, many of which lead to responses to injury that are pathologically and clinically similar. There are three clinicopathologic responses to injury: acute pericarditis, pericardial effusion, and constrictive pericarditis.

ACUTE PERICARDITIS

Viral infection is usually assumed to be the cause of acute pericarditis that occurs as an apparently primary illness. Because most cases follow a brief and uncomplicated natural course, the syndrome is often termed acute benign pericarditis. Cases resulting from other conditions or treatments, such as rheumatic disease or radiotherapy, often exhibit clinical features similar to those of acute benign pericarditis.

Diagnosis

Clinical manifestations   The clinical diagnosis of acute pericarditis rests primarily on the findings of chest pain, pericardial friction rub, and electrocardiographic changes. The chest pain of acute pericarditis typically develops suddenly and is severe and constant over the anterior chest. In acute pericarditis, the pain worsens with inspiration—a response that helps distinguish acute pericarditis from myocardial infarction. Low-grade fever and sinus tachycardia also are usually present.

A pericardial friction rub can be detected in most patients when symptoms are acute. Pericardial friction rubs are typically triphasic: systolic and early diastolic components are followed in later diastole by a third component associated with atrial contraction.

ECG findings   Electrocardiographic changes are common in most forms of acute pericarditis, particularly those of an infectious etiology in which the associated inflammation in the superficial layer of myocardium is prominent. The characteristic change is an elevation in the ST segment in diffuse leads. The diffuse distribution and the absence of reciprocal ST segment depression distinguish the characteristic pattern of acute pericarditis from acute myocardial infarction. However, the normal variant pattern of ST segment elevation often complicates the differential diagnosis [*see Figure 1*]. Depression of the PR segment, which reflects superficial injury of the atrial myocardium, is as frequent and specific as ST segment elevation and is often the earliest electrocardiographic manifestation.[1]

Treatment

Analgesic agents, such as codeine (15 to 30 mg taken orally

every 4 to 6 hours) or hydrocodone (5 to 10 mg taken orally every 4 to 6 hours), are usually effective in providing symptomatic relief. Salicylates given at an initial dosage of 4 to 6 g a day or a nonsteroidal anti-inflammatory drug (NSAID) such as ibuprofen given at an initial dosage of 800 mg three times daily is often effective in reducing pericardial inflammation.[2] Corticosteroids such as prednisone given at an initial dosage of 40 to 60 mg/day often greatly relieve symptoms; however, steroid therapy should be reserved for severe cases that are unresponsive to other therapy, because symptoms may recur after steroid withdrawal. The corticosteroid dose should be reduced as soon as a clinical response is observed and should be tapered to zero over a period of 2 to 4 weeks.

Other Forms of Acute Pericarditis

Relapsing pericarditis   Acute pericarditis of any etiology may follow a recurrent or chronic relapsing course. In many instances, subjective manifestations (e.g., weakness, fatigue, or headache) are present in addition to the chest discomfort. Analgesic agents provide symptomatic relief, and a very slow tapering of the dose of a corticosteroid usually resolves the relapsing course eventually. Treatment with 1 mg of colchicine daily, methylprednisolone in 1 g pulses daily for 3 days, or an immunosuppressant such as prednisone (60 to 100 mg daily) or azathioprine (50 to 100 mg daily) has proved successful in patients with relapsing pericarditis, particularly in patients whose symptoms are mainly related to withdrawal of prednisone.[2,3]

Progression to constriction   In a few instances, acute pericarditis progresses to subacute or chronic constrictive pericarditis. In such cases, the pericarditis may be idiopathic or have a bacterial, viral, rheumatoid, radiation-induced, or dialysis-related origin. These patients usually have subacute rather than acute pericarditis initially; pericardial effusion is present at onset, usually with some degree of cardiac tamponade. Acute benign pericarditis unaccompanied by tamponade or substantial pericardial effusion in the acute phase rarely progresses to constrictive pericarditis.

PERICARDIAL EFFUSION AND CARDIAC TAMPONADE

Fluid may accumulate in the pericardial cavity in virtually any form of pericardial disease. The fluid may be a transudate or an exudate and is often serosanguineous in neoplastic, idiopathic, dialysis-related, radiation-induced, and tuberculous cases. The fluid is serosanguineous or frankly bloody in cases of coagulopathy, trauma, rupture of acute myocardial infarction, and aortic dissection. Chylopericardium and pneumopericardium also can occur, although rarely.[4] Cardiac tamponade or compression of the heart by effusion is the most important complication of pericardial effusion.

Pathophysiology

The physiologic effect of the accumulation of pericardial fluid depends on whether the fluid is under increased pressure.[5] If ef-

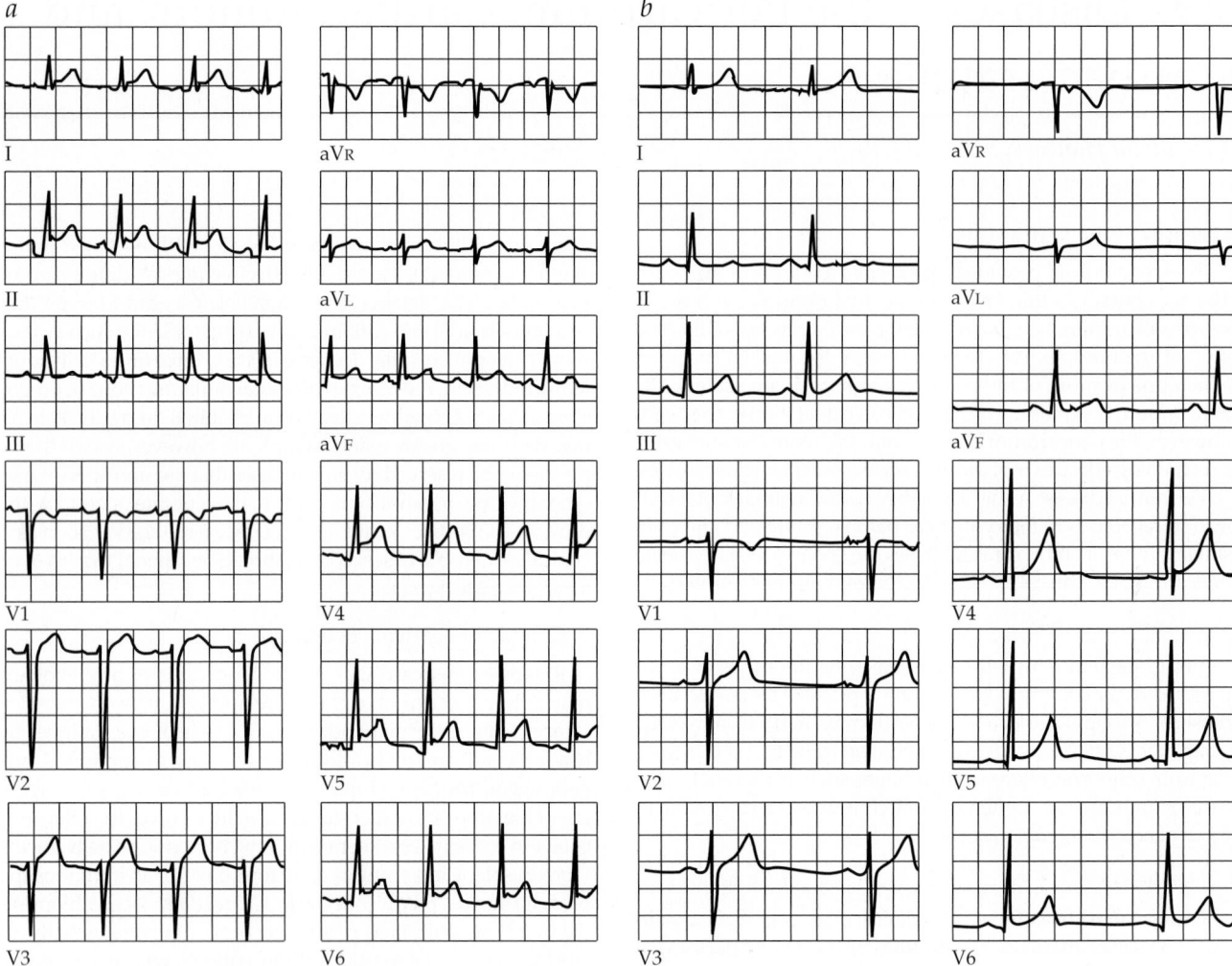

Figure 1 Electrocardiograms contrast the pattern of ST segment elevation characteristic of acute pericarditis (*a*) with the normal variant (early repolarization) pattern of ST segment elevation (*b*). The normal variant pattern is associated with a normal or slow heart rate and has relatively tall R waves and T waves in V4, V5, and V6. The ST segment elevation is less than 25% of the T wave amplitude. In contrast, the acute pericarditis has PR depression and lower T wave amplitude.

fusion develops gradually, the pericardium stretches enough to accommodate volumes that may exceed 2,000 ml. However, if the effusion develops acutely, as little as 200 ml of accumulated fluid may raise the intrapericardial pressure and cause cardiac tamponade.

As the pericardial fluid pressure rises, the right atrial and central venous pressures increase correspondingly. Thus, reading the central venous pressure gives an accurate reflection of the intrapericardial pressure.

Cardiac tamponade should be viewed as a spectrum of hemodynamic abnormalities of various severities rather than an all-or-none phenomenon. Depending on the severity of the tamponade, the blood pressure may be lowered or maintained near the normal range; in patients with preexisting hypertension, it may even be increased. The central venous pressure is almost always increased, except in the rare instances of low-pressure cardiac tamponade, which may occur when intravascular volume is depleted.

As a rule, paradoxical pulse—a marked decrease in arterial pressure during inspiration—is present in patients with cardiac tamponade, although it may not be easy to detect on clinical ex-

amination [*see Figure 2*]. The arbitrary value of 10 mm Hg is commonly used to indicate the upper limit of the normal decrease in arterial pressure with inspiration.

The inspiratory drop in arterial pressure reflects a selective impairment of diastolic filling of the left ventricle, probably the combined effects of two factors. First, when the filling of the right ventricle is augmented in inspiration, the simultaneous filling of the left ventricle is limited because the entire heart is enclosed in a fixed volume. Second, during inspiration, blood is sequestered in the lungs and pulmonary veins as a result of impaired transmission of changes in intrapleural pressure to the left atrium and to the intrapericardial portions of the pulmonary veins.

Diagnosis

Pericardial effusion Echocardiography is the most accurate and easily applied method for the clinical detection of pericardial effusion [*see Figure 3*]. Echocardiograms detect effusions as small as 20 ml and show characteristic findings with effusions larger than 100 ml. Computed tomography is also a reliable method for detecting both pericardial effusion and pericardial thickening. Magnetic resonance imaging provides information similar to that provided by CT [*see Figure 4*].[6]

Electrocardiograms usually show low voltage in patients with large pericardial effusions, but this finding is nonspecific. Electrical alternans occurs occasionally when the pericardial effusion is large and permits a beat-to-beat oscillation of the heart from one position to another within the pericardial sac [*see Figure 5*]. Electrical alternans is most common with effusion caused by neoplasm. This type of electrical alternans must be differentiated from other types, such as that occurring in supraventricular tachycardias or alternating intraventricular conduction defects.

Cardiac tamponade   The diagnosis of cardiac tamponade is often difficult.[7] The diagnosis is one of the most common important diagnoses made at autopsy but not during life.[8] This diagnosis should be based on a synthesis of various clinical findings, because no single finding is pathognomonic or necessarily present. Echocardiography, although essentially definitive for the demonstration of pericardial effusion, is not as certain a method of assessing tamponade. Several echocardiographic features are helpful, however, particularly the observation of an early diastolic inward motion (so-called collapse) of the right atrial wall or right ventricular wall, indicating similarity of intracavitary and intrapericardial pressures.[9] Another useful sign is an exaggerated respiratory variation in the velocity of flow through the mitral and tricuspid valves or in the left ventricular ejection, as detected in pulsed Doppler recordings [*see Figure 6*]. This phenomenon has the same significance as paradoxical pulse. A third sign suggestive of cardiac tamponade is plethora of the inferior vena cava, which occurs in the more severe cases and is a better guide to the need for pericardiocentesis than the other echocardiographic features.[10]

Loculated pericardial effusions may selectively compress one or more chambers of the heart, producing regional cardiac tamponade. This condition is seen most frequently after cardiac

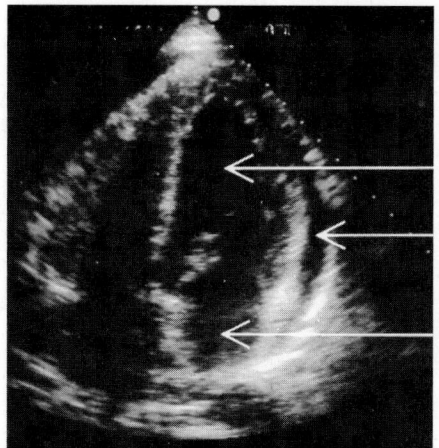

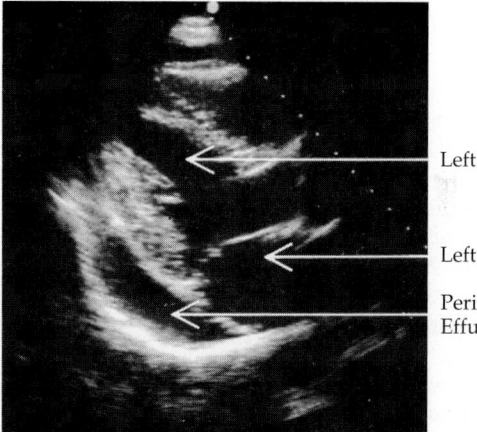

Figure 3   **Pericardial effusion is seen in the two-dimensional echocardiogram as an echo-free space outside the cardiac chambers. Two characteristic sites are lateral to the left ventricle in the apical four-chamber view (top) and posterior to the left ventricle in the parasternal long-axis view (bottom).**

surgery, when bloody fluid accumulates behind the sternum and selectively compresses the right atrium and right ventricle[11]; less often, the left ventricle and left atrium are compressed locally. Similar conditions may occur after closed chest trauma. Fluid accumulations in the mediastinum can compress the heart even when they are not truly within the pericardial space. Transesophageal echocardiography is superior to transthoracic echocardiography in demonstrating such local fluid accumulations, particularly those along the right heart border.

Treatment

Pericardial effusion   Occasionally, a syndrome of idiopathic chronic large pericardial effusion is seen, usually without tamponade. Colchicine may be effective in such cases.[12]

In patients with pericardial effusion but no tamponade, pericardiocentesis is rarely performed for the sole purpose of providing diagnostic studies of the fluid, because such specific diagnoses are uncommon in those patients, at least in regions of the world where tuberculous pericarditis has become rare.[13] Pericardial biopsy can be obtained by any of the usual surgical methods. However, pericardiocentesis can be useful in diagnosing infection or neoplastic disease. In addition, pericardioscopy can be

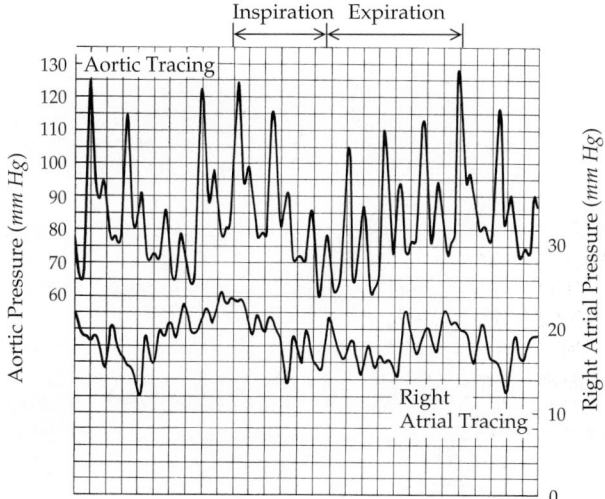

Figure 2   **The aortic pressure and right atrial pressure are recorded during quiet breathing in a patient with cardiac tamponade. The marked fall in arterial pressure that occurs during inspiration is a paradoxical pulse. The decrease in pulse pressure, defined as the difference between systolic and diastolic pressures, that accompanies the fall in systolic pressure indicates that left ventricular stroke volume decreases during inspiration. Central venous pressure, as indicated by the right atrial pressure, also falls during inspiration.**

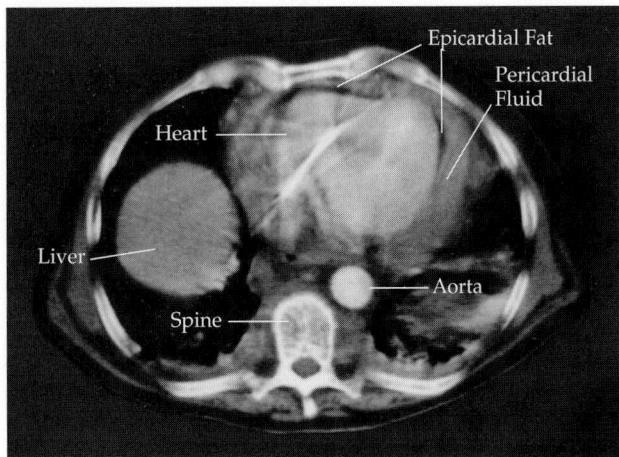

Figure 4 **In a CT scan of the chest of a patient with pericardial effusion, pericardial fluid appears less dense than the heart and is separated from the myocardium by epicardial fat in some areas.**

performed in association with subxiphoid pericardiostomy; biopsy under direct vision may permit the diagnosis of tuberculosis or neoplasm in some instances in which studies of the fluid alone might be inconclusive.[14] Surgery is usually not necessary in chronic idiopathic pericardial effusion in the absence of tamponade and effusive-constrictive disease.[15]

Cardiac tamponade Mild cardiac tamponade may be managed conservatively in some cases, but removal of the fluid is required for definitive treatment and should be carried out in most instances when the central venous pressure is increased. Pericardial fluid may be removed by needle pericardiocentesis or by a surgical technique (subxiphoid pericardiostomy, thoracoscopic pericardiostomy, or thoracotomy).[16,17]

The most acute forms of cardiac tamponade, such as hemopericardium secondary to aortic dissection, penetrating cardiac trauma, or rupture of acute myocardial infarction, require immediate surgery. Tamponade caused by cardiac perforation during invasive intravascular procedures can usually be managed by pericardiocentesis.[18] Pericardiocentesis is effective in most subacute forms of tamponade, such as those associated with idiopathic or viral acute pericarditis, rheumatic diseases, dialysis, or neoplasm.

Thoracoscopy and thoracotomy are usually reserved for patients with recurrent tamponade after an initial pericardiocentesis or subxiphoid pericardiostomy, usually for neoplastic disease. Pericardiostomy by means of a balloon catheter as part of a pericardiocentesis is another alternative for such cases.[19]

SPECIAL ETIOLOGIC FORMS OF ACUTE PERICARDITIS
AND PERICARDIAL EFFUSION

Pericarditis Related to Renal Failure and Dialysis

Acute pericarditis with pericardial effusion occurs in patients with end-stage renal disease and in patients who are on chronic dialysis [*see Chapter 166*]. In dialysis patients, conservative management with more intensive dialysis and NSAIDs is usually successful. An unexpected decrease in blood pressure during a dialysis session may be the clue to the presence of tamponade. Pericardiocentesis is occasionally necessary for the relief of tamponade, although fluid overload and left ventricular failure are

often important factors associated with causing increased central venous pressure. Cardiac catheterization in combination with pericardiocentesis is often useful in assessing the hemodynamic significance of those factors that contribute to an increase of pulmonary and systemic venous pressure in dialysis patients.

Radiation-Induced Pericardial Effusion

Pericardial effusion develops relatively frequently in patients with Hodgkin disease, other lymphomas, or breast carcinoma who survive for long periods after receiving large doses of radiation to the mediastinum. Radiation-induced effusion may evolve into chronic constrictive pericarditis after many years, usually with other forms of myocardial, coronary arterial, valvular, and pulmonary damage.[20]

Neoplastic Pericardial Effusion

Neoplastic pericardial effusion accounts for about one half of the cases of cardiac tamponade in patients who are seen in an internal medicine setting [*see Chapter 194*]. Lung cancer and breast cancer account for the majority of the cases of neoplastic pericardial effusion; lymphoma and leukemia account for most of the remainder.[21] In most cases, the primary neoplasm has been previously diagnosed; patients in whom pericardial effusion is the first manifestation of the disease usually have primary cancer of the lung. Cytologic examination of the pericardial fluid is highly accurate in diagnosing common carcinomas but less accurate in diagnosing other neoplasms, especially the

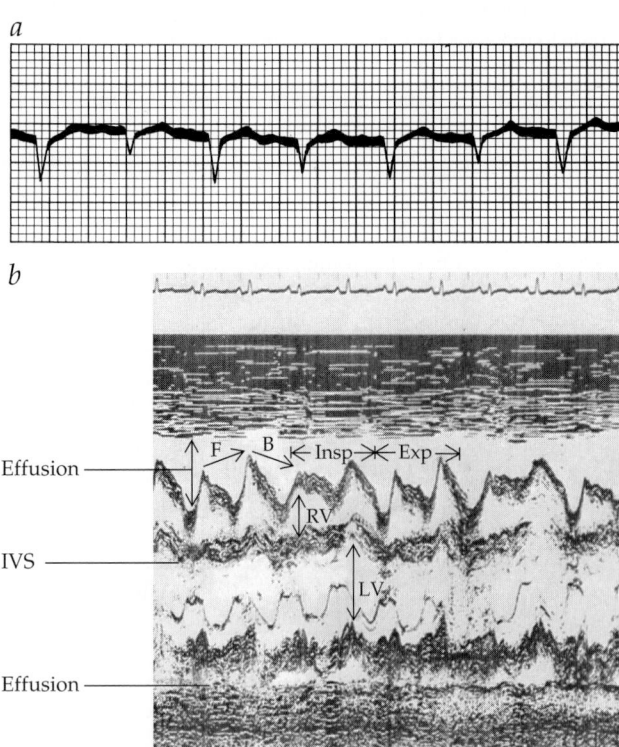

Figure 5 **The electrocardiogram (V2 lead) from a patient with pericardial effusion caused by malignant melanoma reveals a low voltage and electrical alternans (*a*). The echocardiogram (*b*) demonstrates that the heart moves forward (F) and backward (B) within the effusion on alternate beats, thus producing the alternation of the QRS axis characteristic of electrical alternans. The heart also moves with inspiration (Insp) and expiration (Exp), which accounts for a change in anterior wall motion with every two cardiac cycles.**

lymphomas and leukemias.[22]

Neoplastic pericardial effusion often can be managed conservatively when no symptoms directly related to the pericardial effusion are present. Symptomatic tamponade can be managed palliatively with pericardiocentesis, although recurrent effusion is more likely to form in such cases than in many other types of pericardial effusion. Subxiphoid pericardiostomy is often the preferred procedure, leading to a pericardial reaction that produces adhesion of the parietal and visceral layers of pericardium and thus prevents recurrent effusion. Balloon pericardiostomy is an alternative. Chemotherapy or radiotherapy may be of value, depending on the nature of the primary neoplasm. Intrapericardial instillation of chemotherapeutic agents has often been used with apparent success, but no results from controlled trials are available. Few patients survive longer than a year, and whether pericardiocentesis has a major effect on their longevity is difficult to determine, even when tamponade is relieved.[23]

Purulent Pericarditis

Tamponade is usually present in purulent bacterial pericarditis; after pericardiocentesis, the effusion is highly likely to recur rapidly and progress to constrictive pericarditis. Purulent pericarditis therefore usually requires a surgical drainage procedure; a partial pericardiectomy by a limited left lateral thoracotomy is often the best choice. Surgery may not be required for patients in whom tamponade or constriction does not develop, because antibiotics enter the pericardial cavity in effective concentrations. Active tuberculous pericarditis with effusion is particularly likely to progress to constriction and to require pericardiectomy in addition to antituberculous chemotherapy.[24,25] AIDS is a common cause of large pericardial effusions, the majority of which are not caused by identifiable opportunistic infective agents.[26] However, the incidence of tuberculous and other forms of bacterial pericarditis has increased in the United States as a result of AIDS.

Drug-Induced Pericarditis

Several drugs have been implicated in the etiology of pericardial disease, including procainamide, which leads to a lupuslike syndrome; minoxidil, which has been linked to pericardial effusion; and methysergide, which may lead to constrictive pericarditis.

Pericarditis after Cardiac Surgery

The postcardiotomy syndrome presents primarily as acute pericarditis. Whether it has an infective or autoimmune cause is unclear. A similar condition occurs after blunt or penetrating trauma, hemopericardium from other causes, or epicardial pacemaker implantation. Cardiac tamponade and constrictive pericarditis occur occasionally.

Pericardial Complications of Invasive Procedures

Cardiac tamponade occurs as a complication of various invasive procedures in the cardiac catheterization laboratory and in the intensive care unit. Particularly important, and usually preventable, is the perforation of the heart by central venous catheters that have been allowed to lie in the right atrium rather than in the superior vena cava.[27] The use of newer devices (e.g., stents) and procedures (e.g., rotational atherectomy) has increased the incidence of percutaneous coronary interventions with cardiac tamponade complications.[28] Most of these cases are managed successfully by pericardiocentesis.[18]

CONSTRICTIVE PERICARDITIS

Constrictive pericarditis was formerly widely considered to be primarily a tuberculous lesion and is still so regarded in many areas of the world. Most cases now seen in the United States are idiopathic or are related to previous cardiac surgery or radiotherapy.[29,30] Fewer cases result from purulent pericarditis, rheumatic diseases, dialysis, and various rarer conditions.

In the classic form of chronic constrictive pericarditis, fibrous scarring and adhesion of both pericardial layers obliterate the pericardial cavity. The resulting fibrotic lesion has been likened to a rigid shell around the heart, particularly when there is considerable calcification of the pericardium, a feature seen in longstanding cases. The subacute form of constrictive pericarditis is now more common than the chronic calcific type. In the subacute variant, the constriction is rather fibroelastic and may be produced by fibrous contracture of the visceral pericardial layer (epicardium) alone. The fibroelastic constriction may also exist in combination with persisting loculated or totally free pericardial effusion; this form is termed effusive-constrictive pericarditis, and it can be documented by measuring pericardial and central venous pressures before and after removal of the fluid.

Pathophysiology

The pathophysiology of constrictive pericarditis is similar to that of tamponade in that both conditions impede diastolic filling of the heart and lead to increased venous pressure and ultimately to reduced cardiac output. Differences exist in the diagnostic signs, however. Paradoxical pulse is a regular feature of cardiac tamponade but may be inconspicuous or absent in constrictive pericarditis. The Kussmaul sign (an increase in venous pressure with inspiration) is seen in some patients with constrictive pericarditis but not in patients with pure cardiac tamponade. When tamponade is present, the venous pulse shows a predominant systolic dip, whereas in constrictive pericarditis, the early diastolic dip is the more prominent deflection [see Figure 6].

An early diastolic sound (pericardial knock) is often heard in constrictive pericarditis but not in tamponade; this sound is directly related to the extent to which ventricular filling is restricted to early diastole, being abruptly checked at the peak of early filling when the heart reaches the fixed volume imposed by the constricting shell surrounding it.

Diagnosis

ECG and imaging studies Constrictive pericarditis is difficult to diagnose, frequently being misdiagnosed for prolonged periods as liver disease or idiopathic pleural effusion. Clinical diagnosis of constrictive pericarditis depends on the recognition of increased venous pressure in a patient who may not have other obvious signs or symptoms of heart disease. The heart size and lung fields often appear normal in the chest radiograph, and the ECG shows only minor nonspecific abnormalities. Echocardiography is also nondiagnostic in many instances, although the appearance of abnormal septal motion and pericardial thickening often provide clues. Transesophageal echocardiography and chest CT are superior to echocardiography for the demonstration of pericardial thickening [see Figure 7]; however, the pericardium is not measurably thicker than normal in noninvasive imaging studies in some patients with constriction.[31]

As in cardiac tamponade, pulsed wave Doppler studies show exaggerated respiratory variation in the mitral and tricuspid diastolic flow velocity in most cases of constrictive pericarditis. Doing the study in the upright position improves the sensitivity of

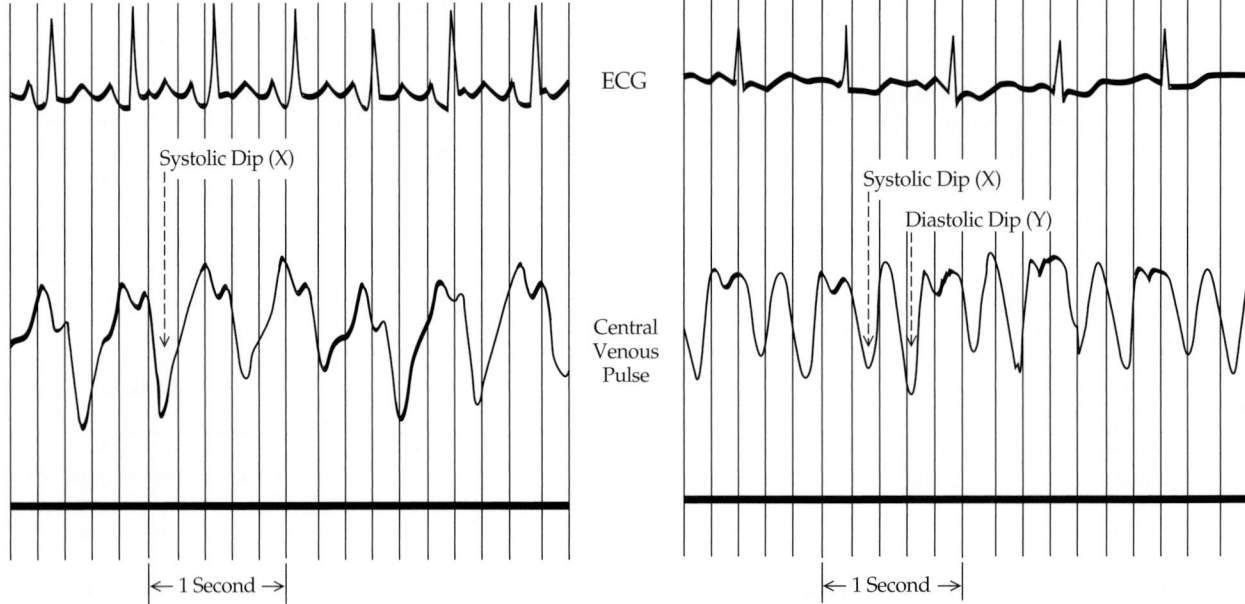

ECG

Systolic Dip (X)

Central
Venous
Pulse

Systolic Dip (X)

Diastolic Dip (Y)

|← 1 Second →|

|← 1 Second →|

Figure 6 **Differences between the central venous pulse contours characteristic of cardiac tamponade (left) and chronic constrictive pericarditis (right) provide the basis for differential diagnosis. The pressure contour in a patient with pericardial effusion and tamponade has a prominent systolic dip (X) but little or no diastolic deflection. The central venous pulse pattern in a patient with chronic constrictive pericarditis displays an M or W contour consisting of both systolic dip (X) and diastolic dip (Y), with the Y descent being more prominent.**

this test.[32] False positive results occur in patients with chronic obstructive pulmonary disease, but that can be recognized by performing Doppler studies of flow velocity in the superior vena cava; the changes in velocity with respiration are much greater in pulmonary disease than in constrictive pericarditis.[33]

Cardiac catheterization   Cardiac catheterization shows characteristic abnormalities, with increased central venous pressure, nondilated and normally contracting right and left ventricles, and near equilibration of the cardiac filling pressures of the right and left sides. These features may also be present in idiopathic restrictive cardiomyopathy or in specific myocardial diseases, especially cardiac amyloidosis; in such cases, the demonstration of pericardial thickness by CT or MRI and the use of endomyocardial biopsy are helpful.[34] Many other clues can assist in this differential diagnosis [*see Table 1*]. The increased interdependence

of the two ventricles in constrictive pericarditis causes the right and left ventricular systolic pressures to vary out of phase with each other in respiration; in conditions other than constrictive pericarditis, the two systolic pressures increase and decrease together with respiration. This is perhaps the most useful information yielded by cardiac catheterization in patients with suspected constrictive pericarditis.[35]

Treatment

Constrictive pericarditis occasionally resolves spontaneously when it develops as a complication of acute pericarditis.[35] In nearly all instances, however, relief of constrictive pericarditis requires surgical stripping and removal of both layers of the adherent, constricting pericardium. This operation is far more difficult to perform than the operation for relief of pericardial effusion. The operation must be thorough, which carries the risk of hemorrhage from perforations in the wall of the heart. Inadequate long-term relief after surgical removal of the pericardium may reflect the presence of associated myocardial disease, particularly in instances of radiation-induced pericardial disease.[36] In most other forms of constrictive pericarditis, however, myocardial function is normal.

Cardiac Tumors

Cardiac tumors may be either primary or secondary, and they may be either benign or malignant. Metastatic cardiac involvement occurs 20 to 40 times more frequently than primary tumors. However, primary tumors are often benign and curable by surgery.

METASTATIC TUMORS

About 10% of patients who die of malignant disease have metastatic cardiac involvement, but the metastases produce symptoms in only 5% to 10% of the affected patients. Neoplasms

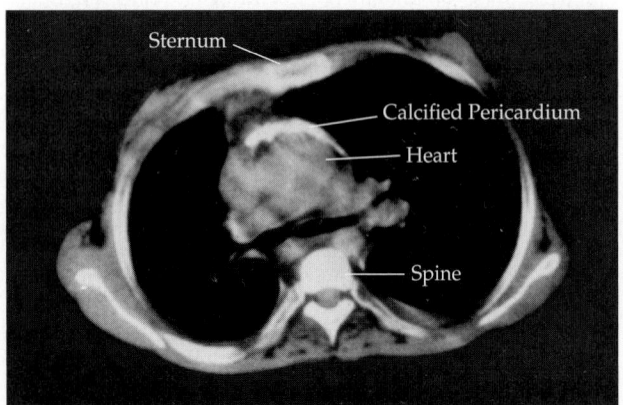

Sternum

Calcified Pericardium

Heart

Spine

Figure 7 **In this CT scan of the chest of a patient with chronic constrictive pericarditis, the dense layer on the anterior surface of the heart represents thickened and partially calcified pericardium.**

Table 1 Clinical Features That Differentiate Constrictive Pericarditis from Amyloidosis and Idiopathic Restrictive Cardiomyopathy

Clinical Feature	*Constrictive Pericarditis*	*Cardiac Amyloidosis*	*Idiopathic Restrictive Cardiomyopathy*
Early diastolic sound (S$_3$ or pericardial knock)	Frequent	Occasional	Occasional
Late diastolic sound (S$_4$)	Rare	Frequent	Frequent
Atrial enlargement	Mild or absent	Marked	Marked
Atrioventricular or intraventricular conduction defect	Rare	Frequent	Frequent
QRS voltage	Normal or low	Low	Normal or high
Mitral or tricuspid regurgitation	Rare	Frequent	Frequent
Paradoxical pulse	Frequent but usually mild	Rare	Rare
Exaggerated variation in mitral and tricuspid flow velocity with respiration, out of phase	Usual	Rare	Rare

particularly likely to metastasize to the heart are cancers of the lung or breast, melanoma, leukemia, and lymphoma.[37]

The most frequent clinical manifestation is pericardial effusion with cardiac tamponade. In such cases, the mass of the tumor is often relatively small. Extensive solid tumor in and around the heart is less common but may resemble constrictive pericarditis or effusive-constrictive pericarditis. Invasion of the myocardium most often manifests clinically as arrhythmias; atrial flutter and atrial fibrillation are particularly common.

Usually, the only effective treatment in metastatic involvement of the heart is relief of cardiac tamponade. Otherwise, treatment depends on the nature of the primary tumor.

PRIMARY BENIGN TUMORS

Eighty percent of all primary cardiac tumors are benign; myxomas account for more than half of these in adults, whereas rhabdomyomas and fibromas are the most common benign car-

diac tumors in children.[38-40] Cardiac rhabdomyomas in infancy and childhood have a high incidence of spontaneous regression; although they are sometimes responsible for a remarkable syndrome of paroxysmal ventricular tachycardia in infancy, this syndrome can be cured by surgical removal of the tumor. Echocardiography and MRI are both excellent methods for demonstrating intracardiac tumors [*see Figures 8 and 9*].

Myxoma Myxomas consist of scattered stellate cells embedded in a mucinous matrix. They are found in the cavities of the heart, attached to the endocardial wall (or, in rare cases, attached to one of the heart valves) by either a narrow stalk or a broader pedicle. The tumor often shows considerable movement within the cardiac chamber during the cardiac cycle [*see Figure 8*]. About 70% of myxomas are in the left atrium; the rest are mostly in the right atrium. Echocardiography is a reliable method with which to predict tumor size and morphology.[41]

a
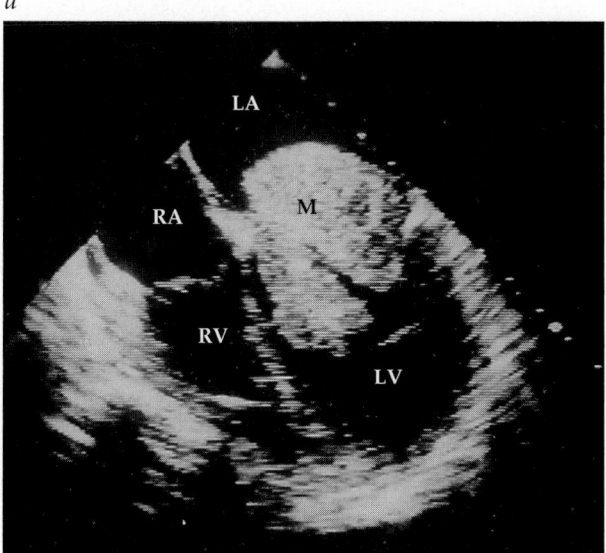

b
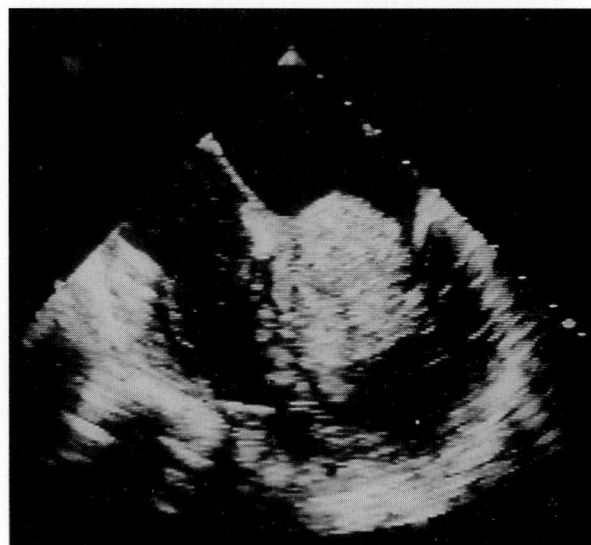

Figure 8 This transesophageal echocardiogram demonstrates a large myxoma (M) in the left atrium (LA) of a 23-year-old man. The picture on the left (*a*) was taken during early systole, and the picture on the right (*b*) was taken during early diastole. The marked mobility of the tumor is evident as it moves from the left atrium to the left ventricle (LV). The right atrium (RA) and right ventricle (RV) are also visible.

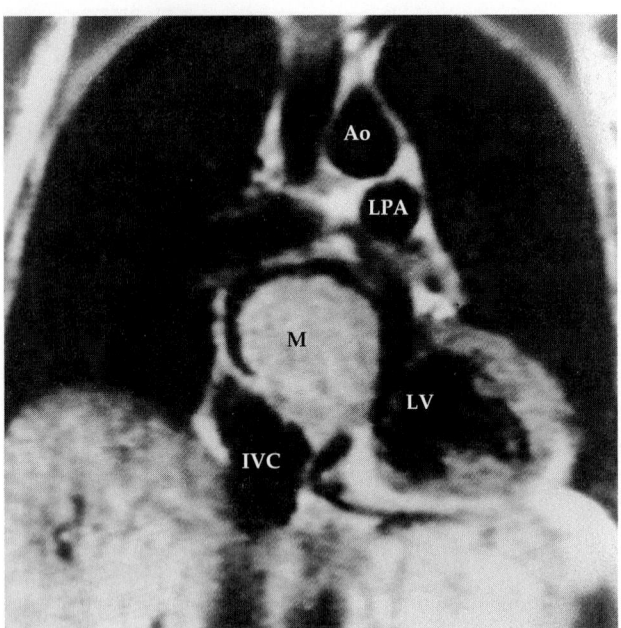

Figure 9 This magnetic resonance image, coronal view, shows a large left atrial myxoma (M). The left ventricle (LV), aorta (Ao), left pulmonary artery (LPA), and inferior vena cava (IVC) are also visible.

Myxomas are most often manifested clinically by mechanical hemodynamic effects, which often simulate mitral or tricuspid stenoses when they obstruct the valve orifice. They may simulate mitral or tricuspid regurgitation when they interfere with valve closure or cause a so-called wrecking-ball type of trauma to the mitral or tricuspid valve. Intermittent obstruction of the valve orifice can lead to such dramatic symptoms as syncope or to remarkable changes in physical signs that are sometimes related to changes in body position.

Myxomas also cause thromboembolic complications when portions of the tumor or thrombi from the surface of the tumor are detached. Another manifestation is a constitutional disturbance consisting of fatigue, fever, erythematous rash, myalgias, and weight loss, accompanied by anemia and an increased erythrocyte sedimentation rate. The constitutional symptoms may be caused by production of interleukin-6 by the myxoma.[42]

About 5% of cases of cardiac myxoma are familial, multicentric, or associated with a genetic syndrome that includes cutaneous lentiginosis, cutaneous myxomas, myxoid fibroadenomas of the breast, pituitary adenomas, adrenocortical micronodular hyperplasia with Cushing syndrome, and Sertoli cell tumors of the testis. These cases are referred to as complex myxoma, myxoma syndrome, or the Carney complex. A genetic mutation underlying this syndrome has been identified.[43]

Surgical treatment of cardiac myxomas is usually curative, particularly if the resection includes the portion of the atrial septum or atrial free wall from which the tumor has arisen. Recurrence and distant metastases are rare except in myxoma syndrome.[44]

Papillary fibroelastoma Papillary fibroelastomas are small tumors, usually attached to cardiac valves, that can be a cause of cardioembolic stroke. They have been recognized with increasing frequency since echocardiography has come into more widespread use.[45] Surgery may be indicated, especially if embolism recurs.

PRIMARY MALIGNANT TUMORS

Most malignant tumors of the heart are sarcomas, of either the spindle cell or the round cell type. Spindle cell tumors include fibrosarcomas, hemangiosarcomas, leiomyosarcomas, rhabdomyosarcomas, and fibromyxosarcomas. Round cell tumors include lymphosarcomas or reticulum cell sarcomas. Primary lymphoma of the heart, which is usually seen only in immune-compromised patients, is increasing in incidence.[46]

Malignant tumors are more apt to occur in the right side of the heart than in the left, being about equally frequent in the right atrium and the right ventricle. Signs and symptoms usually stem from intracavitary growth of the tumor, causing obstructive phenomena that simulate congestive heart failure. Pericardial effusion and tamponade are also common.

Malignant pericardial mesothelioma usually presents as pericardial effusion with tamponade or as subacute constrictive pericarditis.

Although surgical excision of malignant cardiac tumors is often attempted, cure is only rarely achieved. The tumors are usually unresponsive to radiation or chemotherapy, and most are fatal within a few months.

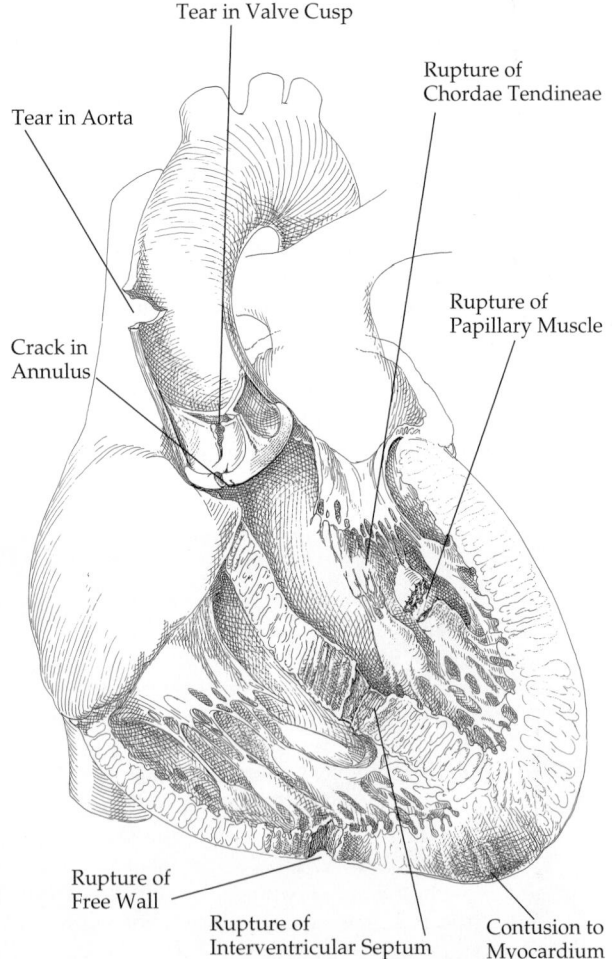

Figure 10 Blunt trauma, such as that caused by the impact of the chest against the steering wheel in an automobile accident, may injure various cardiac structures. Myocardial contusion is the most frequent injury, but rupture may occur at several sites, including the interventricular septum, the walls of the cardiac chambers, the papillary muscles, and the chordae tendineae. The shearing forces that accompany abrupt deceleration may also cause tearing of the aorta and the valve cusps and cracking of the annulus.

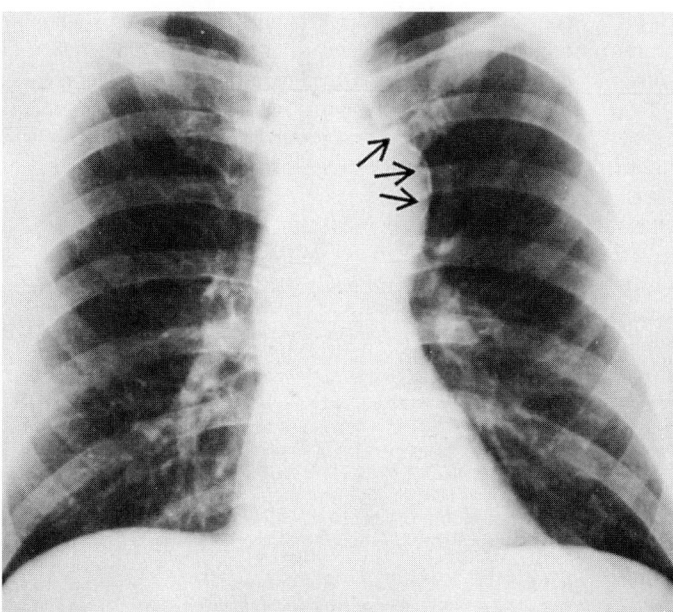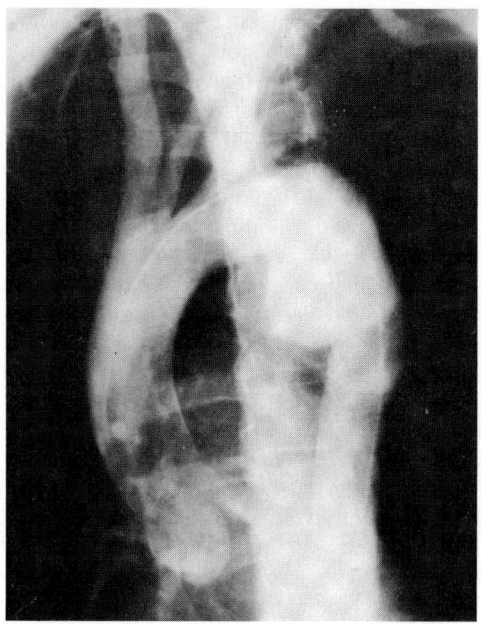

Figure 11 **A posteroanterior chest x-ray (left) reveals a posttraumatic aortic aneurysm at the aortic isthmus. Calcification (arrows) is evident in the wall of the aneurysm, which arose in a 45-year-old policeman who had sustained chest injuries in a motorcycle accident 24 years earlier. The lesion had gradually enlarged during a 10-year period of observation after its discovery. The aneurysm, outlined by angiography (right), was successfully excised.**

Cardiovascular Trauma

Cardiovascular injury may be either blunt (i.e., nonpenetrating) or penetrating.[47] Automobile accidents are the most common cause of blunt cardiovascular trauma; gunshots and stabbings are the most common causes of penetrating trauma. Both types of injury can damage the myocardium, the valves, the coronary arteries, the pericardium, and the great vessels, especially the aorta [*see Figure 10*]. Diagnosis in such instances is often difficult because the associated injuries can mask the cardiovascular trauma; cardiac trauma should therefore be suspected in all patients with chest injuries or severe generalized trauma.

BLUNT CARDIAC TRAUMA

Myocardial Contusion

Myocardial contusion is the most common blunt injury.[48] The right ventricle, because of its immediately substernal location, is the chamber most often involved. The pathologic changes in myocardial contusion consist of myocardial necrosis with hemorrhage, which may range in severity from scattered petechiae to intramural extravasations with associated transmural necrosis. In some instances, coronary arterial occlusion with secondary myocardial infarction is present. Seemingly innocuous blows to the chest by missiles such as baseballs or hockey pucks may cause sudden arrhythmic death, probably when they strike directly over the heart during the vulnerable portion of the T wave and induce ventricular fibrillation.[49]

The most important complication of myocardial contusion is cardiac arrhythmia. Hypotension, intracardiac thrombus, congestive heart failure, and cardiac tamponade occur occasionally.

Myocardial contusion is best recognized clinically by echocardiography, which shows localized areas of impaired wall motion. Transesophageal echocardiography is often superior to the transthoracic evaluation.[50] The abnormalities of wall motion usually resolve within a few days. Increases in the concentrations of creatine kinase (CK) and its MB fraction (CK-MB) in the blood are difficult to interpret because of the release of CK from injured skeletal muscle. Cardiac troponin-I is a more specific marker.[51] Diffuse nonspecific ST-T abnormalities in the electrocardiogram are common in injured patients, even in the absence of echocardiographically detected abnormalities in wall motion. However, localized changes, especially ST segment elevation, are more specific for contusion. Patients with Q wave infarct patterns and irreversible wall motion defects are likely to have a coronary arterial occlusion secondary to trauma with myocardial infarction. Severe contusions may also lead to the formation of traumatic left ventricular aneurysms or pseudoaneurysms that are sometimes detected months or years after the initial trauma. Management of myocardial contusion is conservative unless one or more specific complications (e.g., arrhythmia, tamponade, aneurysm, or perforation) are present.

Valvular Injury

Blunt trauma may injure any of the cardiac valves and lead to valvular regurgitation. Traumatic valvular regurgitation is more likely to be recognized after the patient has recovered from the acute injuries; it is less likely to play a major role in the early postinjury course.[52]

Aortic Injury

Injuries of the aorta result from abrupt deceleration in violent thoracic trauma and are relatively common. The most common injury results from a tear in the wall of the aorta at a point just distal to the left subclavian artery, where the aorta is fixed to the dorsal thoracic cage. Usually, complete transection of the aorta is quickly fatal. Less extensive tears can result in a localized hematoma or a localized false aneurysm. Such aneurysms may be recognized months or years after the initial injury, when they cause symptoms by gradually enlarging, or may be discovered incidentally by chest radiography [*see Figure 11*].

A widened mediastinal shadow in the chest radiograph is often the first clue to the presence of a traumatic aortic rupture. The chest CT and the transesophageal echocardiogram are useful aids in making the diagnosis.

At least 50% of patients with aortic rupture die before they reach a hospital, often of injuries unrelated to the aortic trauma. Surgical therapy should be undertaken as soon as possible, even if the bleeding from the ruptured aorta has stabilized; such therapy results in survival of about 80% of those patients who are still alive when they reach a medical facility. Resection of the injured segment and replacement with a prosthetic graft are usually required.

Usually, false aneurysms that are diagnosed long after the initial injury should be resected electively. Their natural history in most instances is to enlarge gradually and eventually rupture.

PENETRATING TRAUMA

Penetrating injuries of the heart and great vessels are caused either by stab wounds or by gunshot wounds. Any of the cardiac chambers or great vessels may be punctured, and injury of multiple structures is common. The most common sites of involvement, in order of decreasing frequency, are the right ventricle, the left ventricle, the right atrium, and the left atrium.

Stab wounds and, especially, bullet wounds of the heart often are immediately fatal. However, if the penetrating wound is relatively small, cardiac tamponade can occur, and the buildup of pressure in the pericardial sac may help reduce the severity of bleeding and thus increase the chance of survival.

Other sequelae of penetrating trauma include laceration of the aorta or the pulmonary artery; defects in the ventricular or atrial septum; fistulas between the great vessels and between the coronary arteries and the cardiac chambers; coronary arterial fistulas; puncture of any of the heart valves; and atrioventricular block as a result of disruption of the conduction system. Occasionally, a missile that lodges in a cardiac chamber or in one of the great arteries will embolize to a distal site, whereas missiles that initially lodge in distal sites may work their way through the veins to lodge in the chambers of the heart or the pulmonary artery.

The existence of intracardiac shunts, fistulas between the heart and great vessels, coronary arterial fistulas, or valve disruption is usually suggested by the presence of new murmurs. Echocardiography and Doppler studies generally allow precise definition, localization, and quantitation of the lesions.

Penetrating cardiac trauma usually requires prompt surgical intervention, even performance of a thoracotomy in the emergency department. The immediate availability of echocardiography in the emergency department or trauma unit is extremely valuable in management of penetrating wounds of the heart. The survival rate of patients who reach the hospital alive is about 50% for those with knife wounds of the heart and 30% for patients with gunshot wounds.[53]

ELECTRICAL INJURY

Electrical injury, a special type of cardiac trauma, is produced by a direct electrical effect on the tissues, the generation of heat from the passage of current from a high-voltage source through tissue with high electrical resistance, extreme release of catecholamines, or extreme autonomic stimulation. Sudden cardiac arrest occurs with exposure to either household AC current or a lightning strike. Lightning strikes also cause myocardial injury, which may be extensive; in such cases, ECG patterns change,

concentrations of cardiac enzymes increase, and wall motion exhibits abnormalities. Pericarditis and pericardial effusion also occur. The abnormalities usually resolve within several weeks.[54]

The author has no commercial relationships with manufacturers of products or providers of services discussed in this chapter.

References

1. Baljepally R, Spodick DH: PR-segment deviation as the initial electrocardiographic response in acute pericarditis. Am J Cardiol 81:1505, 1998

2. Spodick DH: Acute pericarditis: current concepts and practice. JAMA 289:1150, 2003

3. Adler Y, Finkelstein J, Guindo A, et al: Colchicine treatment for recurrent pericarditis: a decade of experience. Circulation 97:2183, 1998

4. Akashi H, Tayama K, Ishihara K: Isolated primary chylopericardium. Jpn Circ J 63:59, 1999

5. Spodick DH: Pathophysiology of cardiac tamponade. Chest 113:1372, 1998

6. Smith WH, Beacock DJ, Goddard AJ, et al: Magnetic resonance evaluation of the pericardium. Br J Radiol 74:384, 2002

7. Larose E, Ducharme A, Mercier LA, et al: Prolonged distress and clinical deterioration before pericardial drainage in patients with cardiac tamponade. Can J Cardiol 16:331, 2000

8. Roosen J, Frans E, Wilmer A, et al: Comparison of premortem clinical diagnoses in critically ill patients and subsequent autopsy findings. Mayo Clin Proc 75:562, 2000

9. Mercé J, Sagrista-Sauleda J, Permanyer-Miralda G, et al: Correlation between clinical and Doppler echocardiographic findings in patients with moderate and large pericardial effusion: implications for the diagnosis of cardiac tamponade. Am Heart J 138:759, 1999

10. Shaver JA, Reddy PS, Curtiss EI, et al: Noninvasive/invasive correlates of exaggerated ventricular interdependence in cardiac tamponade. J Cardiol 37:71, 2001

11. Beppu S, Tanaka N, Nakatani S, et al: Pericardial clot after open heart surgery: its specific localization and haemodynamics. Eur Heart J 14:230, 1993

12. Sagristà-Sauleda J, Angel J, Permanyer-Miralda G, et al: Long-term follow-up of idiopathic chronic pericardial effusion. N Engl J Med 341:2054, 1999

13. Soler-Soler J, Sagrista-Sauleda J, Permanyer-Miralda G: Management of pericardial effusion. Heart 86:235, 2001

14. Nugue O, Millaire A, Porte H, et al: Pericardioscopy in the etiologic diagnosis of pericardial effusion in 141 consecutive patients. Circulation 94:1635, 1996

15. Tsang TS, Barnes ME, Gersh BJ, et al: Outcomes of clinically significant idiopathic pericardial effusion requiring intervention. Am J Cardiol 91:704, 2003

16. Allen KB, Faber LP, Warren WH, et al: Pericardial effusion: subxiphoid pericardiostomy versus percutaneous catheter drainage: Ann Thorac Surg 67:437, 1999

17. Flores RM, Jaklitsch MT, DeCamp MM Jr, et al: Video-assisted thoracic surgery pericardial resection for effusive disease. Chest Surg Clin N Am 8:835, 1998

18. Tsang T, Enriquez-Sarano M, Freeman WK, et al: Consecutive 1127 therapeutic echocardiographically guided pericardiocenteses: clinical profile, practice patterns, and outcomes spanning 21 years. Mayo Clin Proc 77:429, 2002

19. Ziskind AA, Pearce AC, Lemmon CC, et al: Percutaneous balloon pericardiotomy for the treatment of cardiac tamponade and large pericardial effusions: description of technique and report of the first 50 cases. J Am Coll Cardiol 21:1, 1993

20. Piovaccari G, Ferretti RM, Prati F, et al: Cardiac disease after chest irradiation for Hodgkin's disease: incidence in 108 patients with long followup. Int J Cardiol 49:39, 1995

21. Wilkes JD, Fidias P, Vaickus L, et al: Malignancy-related pericardial effusion. 127 cases from the Roswell Park Cancer Institute. Cancer 76:1377, 1995

22. Bardales RH, Stanley MW, Schaefer RF, et al: Secondary pericardial malignancies: a critical appraisal of the role of cytology, pericardial biopsy, and DNA ploidy analysis. Am J Clin Pathol 106:29, 1996

23. Laham RJ, Cohen DJ, Kuntz RE, et al: Pericardial effusion in patients with cancer: outcome with contemporary management strategies. Heart 75:67, 1996

24. Trautner BW, Darouiche RO. Tuberculous pericarditis: optimal diagnosis and management. Clin Infect Dis 33:954, 2001

25. Mayosi BM, Ntsekhe M, Volmink JA, et al: Interventions for treating tuberculous pericarditis. Cochrane Database Syst Rev (4):CD000526, 2002

26. Rerkpattanapipat P, Wongpraparut N, Jacobs LE: Cardiac manifestations of acquired immunodeficiency syndrome. Arch Intern Med 160:602, 2000

27. Fletcher SL, Bodenham AR: Safe placement of central venous catheters: where should the tip of the catheter lie? (editorial). Br J Anaesth 85:188, 2000

28. Von Sohsten R, Kopistansky C, Cohen M, et al: Cardiac tamponade in the "new device" era: evaluation of 6999 consecutive percutaneous coronary interventions. Am Heart J 140:279, 2000

29. Dardas P, Tsikaderis D, Ioannides E, et al: Constrictive pericarditis after coronary artery bypass surgery as a cause of unexplained dyspnea: a report of five cases. Clin Cardiol 21:691, 1998

30. Veeragandham RS, Goldin MD: Surgical management of radiation-induced heart disease. Ann Thorac Surg 65:1014, 1998

31. Ling L, Oh J, Tei C, et al: Pericardial thickness measured with transesophageal echocardiography: feasibility and potential clinical usefulness. J Am Coll Cardiol

29:1317, 1997

32. Oh JK, Tajik AJ, Appleton CP, et al: Preload reduction to unmask the characteristic Doppler features of constrictive pericarditis: a new observation. Circulation 95:796, 1997

33. Boonyaratavej S, Oh JK, Tajik AJ, et al: Comparison of mitral inflow and superior vena cava Doppler velocities in chronic obstructive pulmonary disease and constrictive pericarditis. J Am Coll Cardiol 32:2043, 1998

34. Hancock EW: Differential diagnosis of restrictive cardiomyopathy and constrictive pericarditis. Heart 86:343, 2001

35. Nishimura RA. Constrictive pericarditis in the modern era: a diagnostic dilemma. Heart 86:619, 2001

36. Ling LH, Oh JK, Schaff HV, et al: Constrictive pericarditis in the modern era: evolving clinical spectrum and impact on outcome after pericardiectomy. Circulation 100:1380, 1999

37. Silvestri F, Bussani R, Pavletic N, et al: Metastases of the heart and pericardium. G Ital Cardiol 27:1252, 1997

38. Shapiro LM: Cardiac tumours: diagnosis and management. Heart 85:218 2001

39. Meng Q, Lai H, Lima J, et al: Echocardiographic and pathologic characteristics of primary cardiac tumors: a study of 149 cases. Int J Card 84:69, 2002

40. Stiller BB, Hetzer R, Meyer R, et al: Primary cardiac tumours: when is surgery necessary? Eur J Cardiovasc Surg 20:1002, 2001

41. Acebo E, Val-Bernal JF, Gomez-Roman JJ, et al: Clinicopathologic study and DNA analysis of 37 cardiac myxomas: a 28-year experience. Chest 123:1379, 2003

42. Pinede L, Duhaut P, Loire R: Clinical presentation of left atrial cardiac myxoma: a series of 112 consecutive cases. Medicine (Baltimore) 80:159, 2001

43. Matyakhina L, Pack S, Kirschner LS, et al: Chromosome 2 (2p16) abnormalities in Carney complex tumors. J Med Genet 40:268, 20032000

44. Bhan A, Mehrotra R, Choudhary SK, et al: Surgical experience with intracardiac myxomas: long-term follow-up. Ann Thorac Surg 66:810, 1998

45. Sun JP, Asher CR, Yang XS, et al: Clinical and echocardiographic characteristics of papillary fibroelastomas: a retrospective and prospective study in 162 patients. Circulation 103:2687, 2001

46. Rolla G, Bertero MT, Pastena G, et al: Primary lymphoma of the heart. A case report and review of the literature. Leuk Res 26:117, 2002

47. Baum VC: The patient with cardiac trauma. J Cardiothorac Vasc Anesth 14:71, 2000

48. Pretre R, Chilcott M: Blunt trauma to the heart and great vessels. N Engl J Med 336:626, 1997

49. Maron BJ, Gohman TE, Kyle SB, et al: Clinical profile and spectrum of commotio cordis. JAMA 287:1142, 2002

50. Lindstaedt M, Germing A, Lawo T, et al: Acute and long-term clinical significance of myocardial contusion following blunt thoracic trauma: results of a prospective study. J Trauma 52:479, 2002

51. Collins JN, Cole FJ, Weireter LJ, et al: The usefulness of serum troponin levels in evaluating cardiac injury. Am Surg 67:821, 2001

52. Wall MJJ, Soltero ER: Trauma to cardiac valves. Curr Opin Cardiol 17:188, 2002

53. Tyburski JG, Astra L, Wilson RF, et al: Factors affecting prognosis with penetrating wounds of the heart. J Trauma 48:587, 2000

54. Muehlberger T, Voft PM, Munster A: The long-term consequences of lightning injuries. Burns 27:829, 2001

30 Congenital Heart Disease

Larry T. Mahoney, M.D., and David J. Skorton, M.D.

Congenital diseases of the heart and vasculature are the most common birth defects, occurring in approximately eight per 1,000 live births. Some patients with congenital heart defects (CHDs) remain asymptomatic for many years; others survive to adulthood, thanks to the impressive progress in medical and surgical management made in recent decades. This relatively high incidence, coupled with improved management, has resulted in a large adult population of these patients: it has been estimated that almost one million adults with CHDs are currently living in the United States.[1] A broad range of clinicians must now become more knowledgeable about the care of these patients,[2] including issues such as endocarditis prophylaxis[3] [*see Sidebar* Selected Internet Resources for Congenital Heart Disease]. This chapter reviews CHDs most likely to be encountered in adult patients.

Acyanotic Disorders—Shunts

ATRIAL SEPTAL DEFECTS

Atrial septal defects (ASDs) occur in three main locations [*see Figure 1*]: the region of the fossa ovalis (such defects are termed ostium secundum ASDs); the superior portion of the atrial septum near the junction with the superior vena cava (SVC) (sinus venosus ASDs); and the inferior portion of the atrial septum near the tricuspid valve annulus (ostium primum ASDs). The ostium primum ASDs are considered to be part of the spectrum of atrioventricular septal defects (AVSDs) [*see* Atrioventricular Septal Defects, *below*].

Ostium secundum ASDs are the most common variety, accounting for over half of ASDs. A frequent accompanying defect is mitral valve prolapse. Relatively less prevalent is the sinus venosus defect. Anomalous pulmonary venous return is a common associated abnormality. The proximity of the sinoatrial node to the ASD may lead to sinoatrial node dysfunction and atrial arrhythmias.

Pathophysiology

ASDs are associated with left-to-right shunts of varying degrees. The main determinants of the direction and magnitude of shunt flow are the size of the defect and the relative compliances of the left ventricle (LV) and right ventricle (RV).[4]

Clinical Presentation

Most patients with ostium secundum or sinus venosus ASD are asymptomatic through young adulthood. As the patient reaches middle age, compliance of the LV may decrease, increasing the magnitude of left-to-right shunting. Long-standing atrial dilatation may lead to a variety of atrial arrhythmias, including premature atrial contractions, supraventricular tachycardia, and atrial fibrillation. A substantial number of middle-aged patients will report dyspnea, particularly with exertion, even if they do not have pulmonary hypertension. Approximately 10% of patients with ostium secundum ASDs will progress to pulmonary hypertension associated with pulmonary vascular obstructive disease (Eisenmenger syndrome) [*see* Eisenmenger Syndrome, *below*]. As the pulmonary pressure

rises, the left-to-right shunt will diminish and eventually be replaced by a right-to-left shunt; cyanosis and pulmonary hypertension will develop.

The hallmark of the physical examination in ASD is the wide and fixed splitting of the second heart sound. A systolic murmur (from increased pulmonary flow) is common, and if a large left-to-right shunt is present, the additional flow across the tricuspid valve may lead to a diastolic rumble reminiscent of tricuspid stenosis.

Laboratory Tests

All patients with suspected ASD should have an electrocardiogram, a chest x-ray, and an echocardiogram.

Electrocardiography The QRS axis usually is normal in ostium secundum ASD but may be slightly rightward, and an rSR' pattern is common in the right precordial leads. In sinus venosus ASD, the axis may be normal or relatively horizontal (less than 30°). Ectopic atrial rhythms or other evidence of sinoatrial node dysfunction may be seen.

Radiologic studies The chest x-ray reveals enlargement of the right atrium (RA), the RV, and the main pulmonary artery. The pulmonary vessels exhibit diffuse enlargement because of increased pulmonary blood flow. Magnetic resonance imaging, magnetic resonance angiography (MRA), or cardiac catheterization will identify anomalous pulmonary veins; these modalities should be considered when there is suspicion of this associated abnormality in patients with sinus venosus ASD.

The patient with secundum ASD who has pulmonary hypertension may benefit from right-sided heart catheterization to ascertain the level of pulmonary arterial pressure and resistance.

Echocardiography Echocardiography can confirm the presence of an ASD, determine its size, permit calculation of shunt flow through it, and identify any associated anomalies.

> ## Selected Internet Resources for Congenital Heart Disease
>
> International Society for Adult Congenital Cardiac Disease (ISACCD)
> **http://www.isaccd.org**
> Professional resources, patient information, and newsletter.
>
> Canadian Adult Congenital Heart Network and the Toronto Congenital Cardiac Centre for Adults at the University of Toronto (CACHNET)
> **http://www.cachnet.org**
> Information for physicians and patients.
>
> Grown Up Congenital Heart Patients Association (GUCH)
> **http://www.guch.org.uk**
> A United Kingdom site providing information and support for patients and their families.
>
> PediHeart
> **http://www.pediheart.org**
> Practitioner and patient information; mailing list.

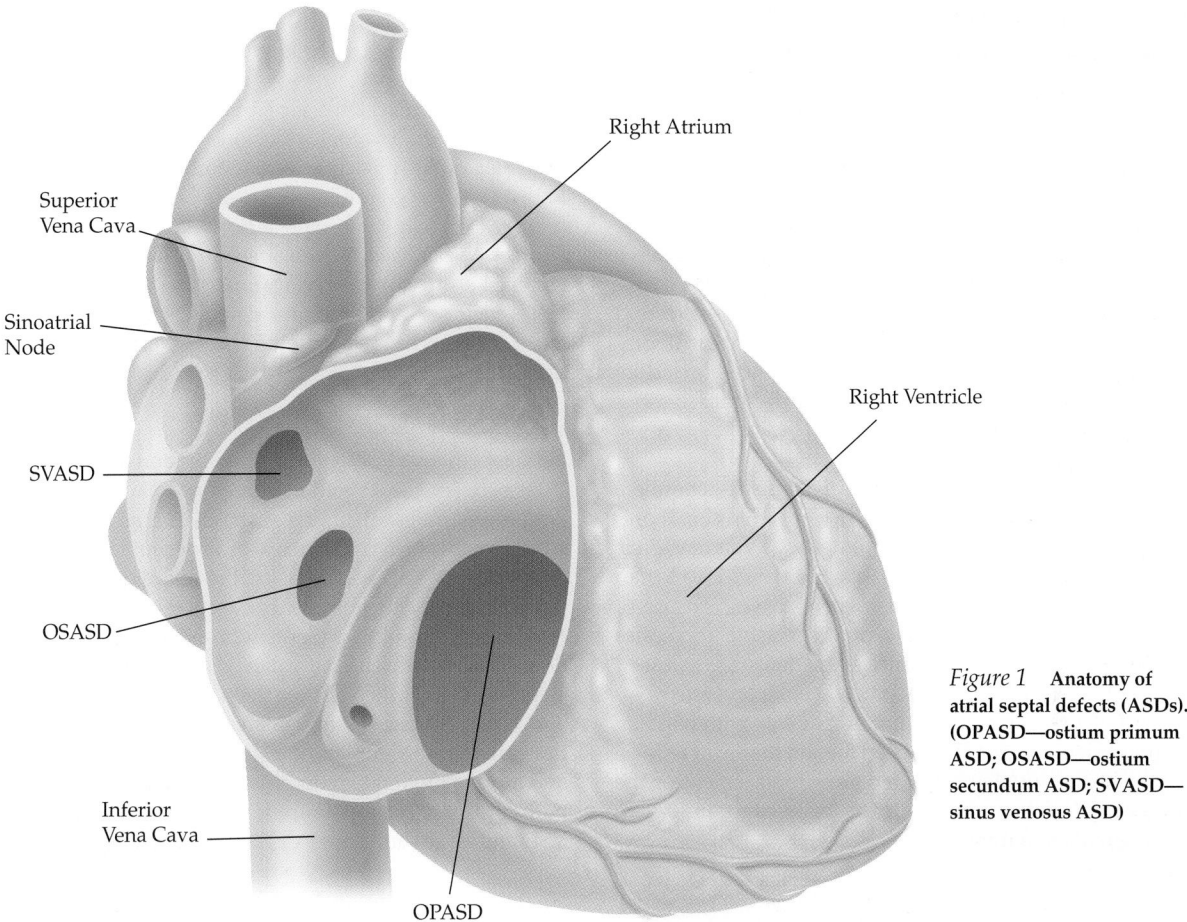

Superior
Vena Cava

Sinoatrial
Node

SVASD

OSASD

Inferior
Vena Cava

OPASD

Right Atrium

Right Ventricle

Figure 1 **Anatomy of atrial septal defects (ASDs). (OPASD—ostium primum ASD; OSASD—ostium secundum ASD; SVASD—sinus venosus ASD)**

Management

Large ASDs (defined as those with a pulmonary-to-systemic flow ratio [Qp:Qs] of over 1.5:1) should be closed to prevent the development of pulmonary hypertension and reduce the risk of paradoxical emboli. Direct surgical closure has been the method used, but devices are now available that permit catheterization-based closure of many defects.[5] Postclosure management includes periodic assessment for the development of atrial arrhythmias.[6] The need for endocarditis prophylaxis varies.

ATRIOVENTRICULAR SEPTAL DEFECTS

The septal leaflet of the tricuspid valve normally inserts into the septum slightly closer to the apex than does the septal leaflet of the mitral valve [*see Figure 2*]. Thus, the small portion of septal tissue superior to the tricuspid septal leaflet insertion separates the RA from the LV and so is called the atrioventricular septum. The term AVSD refers to a complex spectrum of disorders involving abnormalities of the atrioventricular septum and, frequently, the atrioventricular valves. Nomenclature for this spectrum of disorders has varied; synonymous terms include atrioventricular canal defect and endocardial cushion defect.

Pathophysiology

The spectrum of AVSDs ranges from a simple ostium primum ASD to a complete AVSD, which allows free communication among all four cardiac chambers. Variations of the anatomy of the anterior leaflet of the mitral valve and the septal leaflet of the tricuspid valve include a cleft or other abnormality in either or both of these leaflets; accessory chordae that attach in anomalous locations and alter function of the valve leaflets; or a com-

mon atrioventricular valve leaflet that bridges the septal defect. Physiologic consequences vary according to the extent of the anomaly; for example, the addition of a cleft mitral valve anterior leaflet adds varying degrees of mitral regurgitation (MR). Larger defects that also involve the ventricular septum, as well as complete AVSDs, can be associated with torrential left-to-right shunts or an admixture of venous and arterial blood.

Patients with an unrepaired complete AVSD are at risk for developing pulmonary hypertension. Eisenmenger syndrome is particularly common in AVSD patients who also have Down syndrome (trisomy 21).[7]

Clinical Presentation

Patients with isolated ostium primum ASDs may be asymptomatic until adulthood and then may present with fatigue, dyspnea, or symptoms related to atrial arrhythmias. Severe regurgitation of either atrioventricular valve can produce symptoms of heart failure or arrhythmias. Symptoms related to pulmonary hypertension occur in those patients who develop Eisenmenger syndrome.

Patients with only an ostium primum ASD will have clinical findings similar to those of patients with an ostium secundum ASD. The presence of a cleft in either atrioventricular valve will be associated with a pansystolic murmur. Finally, an additional pansystolic murmur can be found in patients with a complete AVSD.

Laboratory Tests

Electrocardiography Left axis deviation is present in the majority of patients. The combination of physical findings of

ASD along with left axis deviation on the ECG suggests the presence of an AVSD. RV conduction delay may be present as well.

Radiologic studies   The chest x-ray shows cardiomegaly and pulmonary vascular engorgement because of the left-to-right shunt.

Echocardiography   Echocardiography defines the specific anatomy and functional importance of the defects. Preoperative echocardiographic assessment includes estimation of the severity of atrioventricular valve regurgitation, the Qp:Qs ratio, and pulmonary arterial pressures. Postoperatively, echocardiography is used to identify and assess the significance of residual atrioventricular valve regurgitation or residual shunt.

Management

The rare patient who presents in adulthood with complete AVSD should be evaluated for pulmonary hypertension. If pulmonary pressures are normal or if pulmonary hypertension is not prohibitive (i.e., pulmonary vascular resistance is less than 50% of systemic vascular resistance), then surgical closure of the defect and repair of the atrioventricular valve anomalies should be undertaken. Postoperatively, patients are assessed for the adequacy of atrioventricular valve repair and are monitored for evidence of residual shunt. In patients with residual MR, management focuses on the need for and timing of reoperation, which may involve either repair or replacement of the mitral valve. The patient should also be followed for the development of atrial arrhythmias.

VENTRICULAR SEPTAL DEFECTS

VSDs are among the most common congenital cardiac disorders seen at birth but are less frequently seen as isolated lesions in adulthood. This is because most VSDs in infants either (1) are large and nonrestrictive (i.e., they permit equilibration of

pressures between the ventricles) and therefore lead to heart failure, necessitating early surgical closure, or (2) are small and close spontaneously.

Classification systems for VSD vary but usually are referenced to the embryologic divisions of the ventricular septum into inlet, outlet, muscular, and membranous portions [*see Figure 3*]. The most common defects are perimembranous defects. Inlet VSDs, located more posteriorly, may be part of the spectrum of AVSDs (see above). Single or multiple defects may occur in the muscular septum (muscular VSD). Finally, outlet VSDs include subpulmonary defects, which may allow prolapse of an aortic cusp, leading to associated aortic regurgitation (AR).

Pathophysiology

Nonrestrictive VSDs permit equilibration of ventricular pressures between the RV and LV, whereas small defects produce a large pressure gradient across the defect, so right heart pressures remain normal. The magnitude of shunt flow across moderate or large VSDs depends on the relative resistances of the systemic versus the pulmonary vascular bed. Rarely, clinicians may encounter adult patients who have large, nonrestrictive defects in the absence of other lesions. Moderate pulmonic stenosis at either the valve or the subvalvular level may create increased resistance to right ventricular outflow sufficient to reduce the left-to-right shunt; consequently, patients with VSD and mild to moderate pulmonic stenosis may reach adulthood without experiencing symptoms. Adults with long-standing VSD and large shunts may develop Eisenmenger syndrome.

Clinical Presentation

With the exception of those patients who contract infective endocarditis or those with Eisenmenger syndrome, adults with VSD are asymptomatic.

The classic physical finding of a restrictive VSD is a harsh, fre-

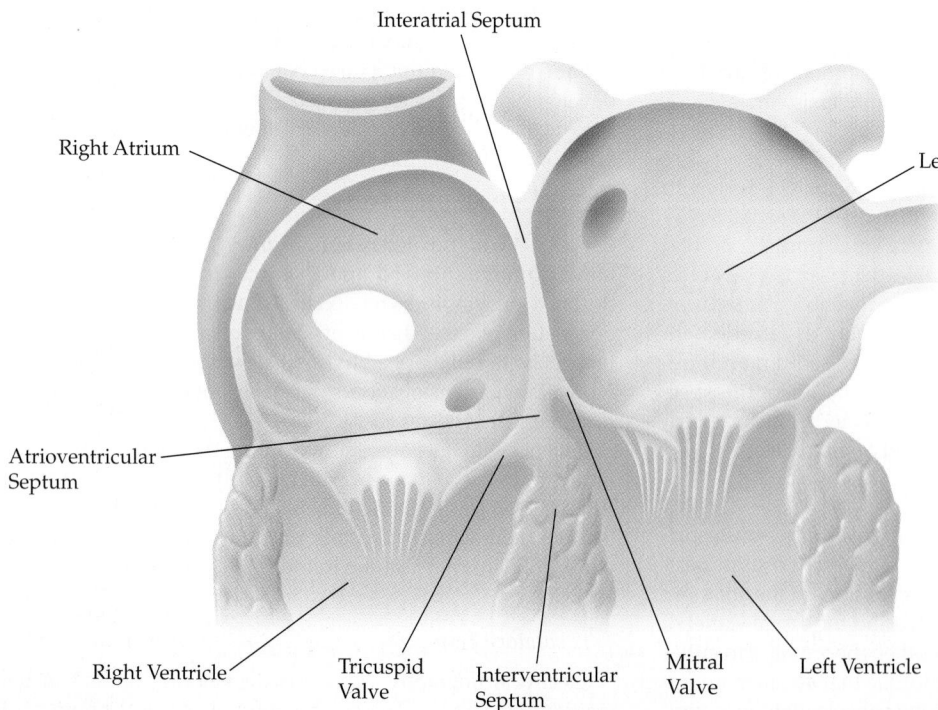

Interatrial Septum

Right Atrium

Left Atrium

Atrioventricular Septum

Right Ventricle

Tricuspid Valve

Interventricular Septum

Mitral Valve

Left Ventricle

Figure 2   **Anatomic cross-section showing the atrioventricular septum (AVS). Note that the septal leaflet of the tricuspid valve inserts closer to the apex than does the septal leaflet of the mitral valve; thus, the AVS separates the right atrium from the left ventricle.**

quently palpable, pansystolic murmur heard best at the left lower sternal border. Patients who have large defects that allow equilibration of ventricular pressures may present with less impressive murmurs than patients with small defects; the reason is that with small defects, there is a large gradient between the LV and the RV, which results in severe turbulence across the defect. When aortic cusp prolapse occurs, the murmur of AR will be audible.

Laboratory Tests

Electrocardiography The ECG may be normal or show evidence of left ventricular hypertrophy (LVH) and a pattern of so-called diastolic overload, featuring prominent Q waves in left precordial leads V5 and V6 and in leads I and aVL.

Radiologic studies The chest x-ray may be normal or show left ventricular enlargement and pulmonary arterial engorgement. Patients who have evidence of pulmonary hypertension should undergo right heart catheterization to determine the degree of pulmonary hypertension and the level of pulmonary resistance.

Echocardiography Echocardiography is the procedure of choice for identifying the location, size, and hemodynamic significance of a VSD; the interventricular gradient should be determined (to estimate RV pressure), and an assessment should be made of increased pulmonary blood flow.

Management

Patients with ventricular septal defects in which the Qp:Qs ratio is greater than 1.5:1 should be considered for surgical closure. Patients with pulmonary hypertension may undergo closure if pulmonary resistance is no more than about 50% of systemic resistance. Aortic cusp prolapse with resultant AR may diminish the shunt magnitude, but the presence of a prolapse constitutes an additional potential indication for closure.

Early VSD operative closures were performed through a right ventriculotomy, but now, many defects—particularly those in the perimembranous septum—are closed through a transatrial approach; such an approach leads to fewer problems with RV dysfunction and arrhythmias. Continual progress is being made in the deployment of transcatheter closure devices. Currently, however, surgical closure of VSD is still the most common approach. Postclosure management involves assessment for residual or recurrent VSD and atrial or ventricular arrhythmias, as well as assessment of RV function.

PATENT DUCTUS ARTERIOSUS

During fetal life, the ductus arteriosus connects the pulmonary artery to the aorta. Soon after birth, as a result of changes in circulating prostaglandin levels and arterial oxygen saturation, the ductus constricts; later, it closes permanently. Failure of the ductus to close leads to the condition termed patent ductus arteriosus (PDA).

Pathophysiology

The shunt from aorta to pulmonary artery increases pulmonary blood flow and return to the left heart. The size of the defect and the relative resistances of the pulmonary and systemic vascular beds determine the degree of shunting. Adults who have PDAs commonly present either with a small lesion without a large left-to-right shunt or with larger lesions and Eisenmenger syndrome.

Clinical Presentation

Except for patients with Eisenmenger syndrome, most adults with small to moderate PDAs will be asymptomatic, unless endarteritis supervenes.

The pathognomonic physical finding of PDA is the continuous murmur. A continuous murmur is one that is audible throughout systole and into diastole to any extent. The classic PDA murmur is machinelike and extends through systole and to variable degrees into diastole, peaking in intensity at the time of S_2. The runoff of blood into the pulmonary artery in diastole will produce a wide pulse pressure because of low aortic diastolic pressure.

Laboratory Tests

Electrocardiography The ECG in patients with PDA may be normal or may show evidence of LVH.

Radiologic studies If the shunt is small, the chest x-ray may be normal. Patients with larger shunts will have associated cardiomegaly and increased vascular markings. In adults, calcium may be noted within the wall of the ductus.

Echocardiography Echocardiography will identify the PDA and permit quantification of the Qp:Qs ratio.

Management

With the advent of reliable means of transcatheter closure of PDAs,[8] common practice is to recommend that most PDAs be closed. In rare cases, the ductus may need to be closed surgically if transcatheter closure is not successful. Postoperative management includes assessment for the need of a residual shunt, although this is uncommon. Patients who develop pulmonary hypertension are managed in the same way as those with Eisenmenger syndrome [see Eisenmenger Syndrome, *below*].

Acyanotic Disorders—Valvular Lesions

BICUSPID AORTIC VALVE AND OTHER CAUSES OF AORTIC STENOSIS

Abnormalities of the left ventricular outflow tract are common congenital cardiac disorders. In particular, as much as 2% of the population have congenitally bicuspid aortic valves. A bicuspid aortic valve may present as an incidental finding on physical examination or echocardiography done for other reasons; as significant aortic stenosis (AS) or AR; or when it results in infective endocarditis.

Pathophysiology

A stenotic bicuspid aortic valve will produce pressure overload of the LV, which leads to LVH and eventually to heart failure, angina pectoris, or sudden death from tachyarrhythmias. Similarly, the patient with an incompetent bicuspid aortic valve will exhibit LV dilatation, initially with normal systolic function; the condition will later progress to heart failure.

Clinical Presentation

On physical examination, the cardinal sign of a bicuspid aortic valve is an early systolic ejection click. If no significant hemodynamic abnormality is present, either no murmur or a soft ejection murmur may be heard; a very mild murmur of AR is not uncommon, even with hemodynamically insignificant bi-

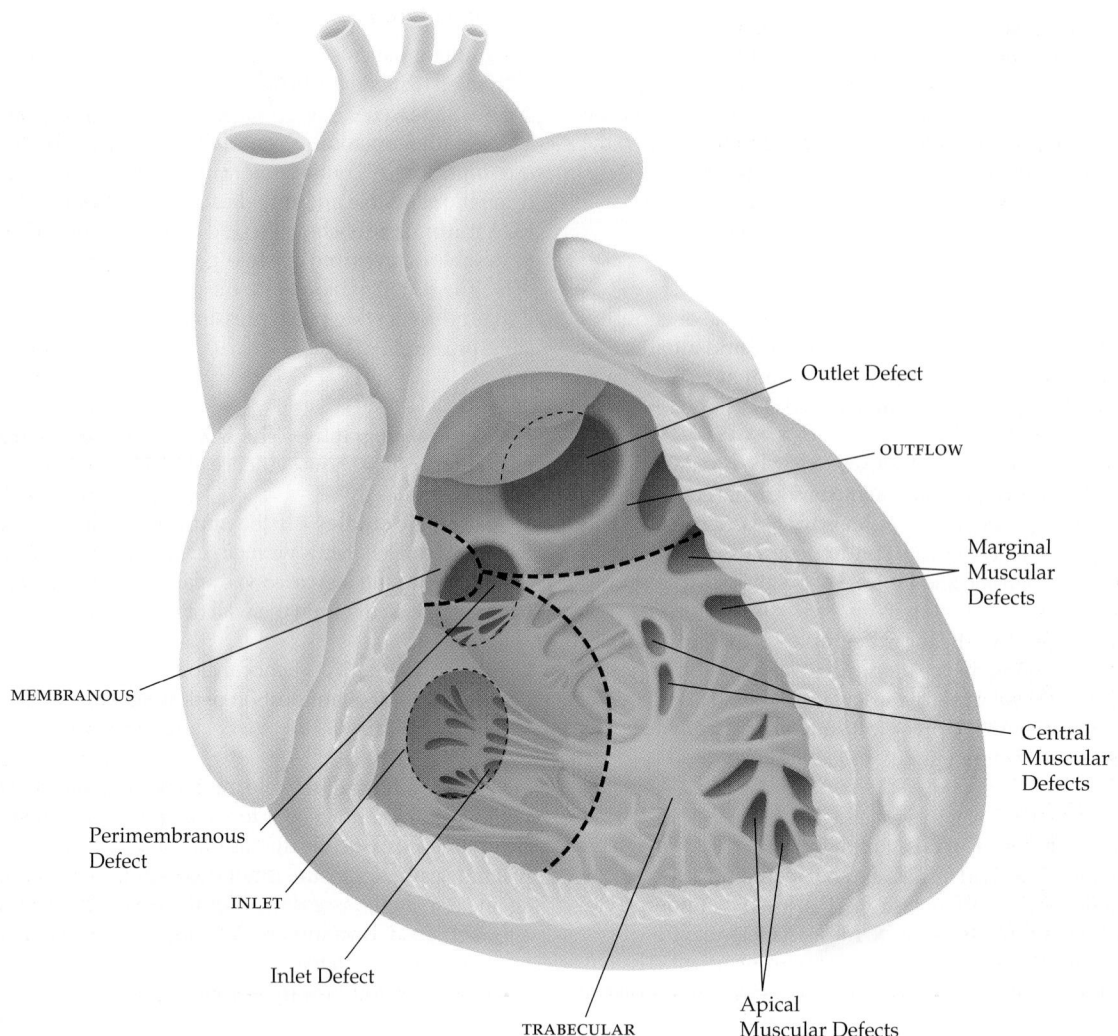

Figure 3 **Anatomic positions of ventricular septal defects. The major anatomic subdivisions of the ventricular septum are the membranous, outflow, inlet, and trabecular portions. Typical VSDs: outlet defect, perimembranous defect, marginal muscular defects, central muscular defects, inlet defect, apical muscular defects.**

cuspid aortic valves. More significant AS or AR will produce findings similar to those in patients with other disorders that cause these lesions.

Laboratory Tests

Electrocardiography   The ECG will be normal unless hemodynamically significant stenosis or regurgitation is present, in which case it will show LVH.

Radiologic studies   Chest x-ray findings in patients with hemodynamically significant bicuspid aortic valves are similar to those in patients with AS and AR from other etiologies. These may include LV dilatation in AR or in AS progressing to heart failure; the latter will also produce pulmonary congestion.

Echocardiography   Both the presence of a bicuspid aortic valve and its hemodynamic significance can be determined by echocardiography. Serial studies are useful in following the progression of the lesion.

Management

All patients with bicuspid aortic valves—even those patients with no significant stenosis or regurgitation—should be given instructions regarding endocarditis prophylaxis. Patients with AR from a bicuspid valve who are asymptomatic and have normal systolic function are followed with echocardiograms and history and physical examinations at regular intervals. If they begin to show evidence of decreasing systolic function, symptoms of heart failure, or progressive dilation of the LV, surgical replacement of the aortic valve is indicated.

Surgical or balloon valvuloplasty (in younger patients) should be considered in a patient with AS who has heart failure, syncope, or chest discomfort. A variety of surgical procedures are available, including direct repair of the valve; replacement with a bioprosthesis or mechanical prosthesis; replacement of the valve and proximal aortic root with a cadaver homograft; and the Ross procedure, in which the abnormal bicuspid valve is removed surgically and replaced with the patient's native pulmonic valve, which in turn is replaced with a cadaver homograft. The Ross procedure eliminates the need for a prosthetic valve in the aortic position. Postoperative management focuses on assessment for recurrent stenosis or progressive AR.

PULMONIC STENOSIS

Patients with pulmonic stenosis (PS) commonly have a malformed valve, with fusion of one or more of the commissures resulting in a dome-shaped valve. Most of these valves are thin and pliable. However, some patients have thickened valves, termed dysplastic.

Pathophysiology

The stenotic pulmonary valve imposes a pressure load on the ventricle, leading to right ventricular hypertrophy (RVH) and, in a subset of patients, RV failure. In patients with severely hypertrophic right ventricles, imbalance of myocardial oxygen supply and demand may lead to ischemia with attendant anginal chest discomfort and arrhythmias.

Clinical Presentation

Patients with PS of even a moderately severe degree may be asymptomatic for decades. Eventual symptoms may include chest discomfort reminiscent of angina pectoris from coronary artery disease, shortness of breath, fatigability, and symptoms of RV failure. Progression of disease and symptoms beyond adolescence is unusual.

The cardinal physical finding of PS is a systolic crescendo-decrescendo murmur of turbulence through the narrowed valve, preceded by a pulmonic ejection click. The behavior of the pulmonic ejection click during respiration may serve to differentiate it from the click of the bicuspid aortic valve. The pulmonic ejection click will exhibit a selective decrease in intensity with normal inspiration and may even disappear entirely with inspiration; in contrast, the bicuspid aortic valve click will exhibit no such selective decrease.

Laboratory Tests

All patients with suspected PS should have an ECG, a chest x-ray, and an echocardiogram.

Electrocardiography The ECG will be normal in patients with mild to moderate PS. Severe stenosis leads to RVH.

Radiologic studies In patients with mild to moderate degrees of PS, the chest x-ray may show no changes except mild poststenotic dilatation of the proximal pulmonary trunk.

Echocardiography Echocardiography is extremely accurate in identifying and diagnosing the severity of PS. It can also differentiate pliable from dysplastic pulmonary valves. Finally, the echocardiogram can assess RV systolic function.

Management

Early approaches to PS consisted of closed or open surgical valvotomy. In the past 20 years, the advent of reliable methods of balloon pulmonary valvuloplasty has brought a major change in the approach to these cases.[9] Particularly in patients with pliable-dome valves, the initial approach is to perform balloon valvuloplasty in cases of significant stenosis (defined by a right ventricular outflow tract gradient greater than 50 mm Hg). Some dysplastic valves are difficult to treat adequately by balloon valvuloplasty and require surgical repair or replacement. Postoperative management includes surveillance for recurrent stenosis or progressive regurgitation.

Acyanotic Disorders—Aortic Defects

COARCTATION OF THE AORTA

Coarctation of the aorta is a relatively common congenital heart defect that can be seen alone, in association with other defects (especially VSD), and in patients with Turner syndrome. A bicuspid aortic valve is a common associated lesion. Coarctation is a common cause of secondary hypertension and should be sought in all patients presenting with hypertension.

Pathophysiology

The essential pathology in coarctation of the aorta is a narrowing of the aortic lumen, usually in the vicinity of the ligamentum arteriosum, just distal to the take-off of the left subclavian artery. The narrowing of the aorta at the site of the coarctation divides the systemic circulation into a high-pressure zone proximal to the coarctation and a low-pressure zone distal to it. Hypertension may accelerate the development of atherosclerotic coronary artery disease and lead to stroke; stroke is a particular risk when aneurysms of the circle of Willis are present, as occurs with increased incidence in patients with coarctation.

Clinical Presentation

Although lower-extremity claudication may occur, even patients with significant coarctation of the aorta may be entirely asymptomatic. The cardinal feature on physical examination is the difference in pulses and blood pressures above versus below the coarctation. Palpation of the radial and femoral arteries in a normal patient will reveal simultaneous arrival or, perhaps, slightly earlier arrival of the pulse at the femoral artery. In coarctation of the aorta, the femoral pulse will occur later than the radial and is often lower in amplitude. Blood pressure should be evaluated in both arms and either leg when seeking coarctation of the aorta, because of variations in anatomy. When the coarctation is distal to the origin of the left subclavian artery, both arms will be in the high-pressure zone and both legs in the low-pressure zone. However, some coarctations are proximal to the left subclavian. Thus, the left arm and both legs will be in the low-pressure zone, and the diagnosis may be missed if only the left arm is used for measuring blood pressure. More rarely, there may be an anomalous origin of the right subclavian artery; the artery may arise directly from the aorta distal to the left subclavian instead of from the brachiocephalic (innominate) artery. In addition to differential blood pressures, physical examination may also reveal a murmur across the coarctation that can be best heard in the left infrascapular area.

Laboratory Tests

Electrocardiography The ECG in patients with coarctation will show varying degrees of LVH, depending on the severity of the narrowing.

Radiologic studies Dilatation of the aorta proximal and distal to the coarctation site may lead to a so-called 3 sign on chest x-ray. Rib notching is often present; this term refers to apparent effacement, or so-called scalloping, of the lower edges of ribs (usually the third through ninth ribs) because of large, high-flow intercostal collateral vessels that develop as a compensatory mechanism to bypass the narrowing at the coarctation site. Absence of rib notching does not rule out coarctation of the aorta, however.

MRI with MRA can be used effectively to identify coarctation and the collateral circulation. It is also useful for postrepair detection of aneurysms or restenosis at the site of repair.

Echocardiography Echocardiography is extremely helpful in identifying the site of the coarctation by direct visualization, as well as in measuring the pressure gradient across the coarctation site. Echocardiography can also identify bicuspid aortic valves, which frequently accompany coarctation of the aorta.

Management

Coarctation that is sufficient to produce hypertension should always be treated, either surgically or by balloon angioplasty with stent placement. The longest experience is with surgical excision of the coarctation and either end-to-end anastomosis or graft interposition. In recent years, balloon angioplasty has increasingly proved to be a viable alternative for both initial treatment of coarctation and for treatment of restenosis at the coarctation site that develops after repair or angioplasty.[10]

Both before and after correction of coarctation, patients are at risk for infective endarteritis in the vicinity of the coarctation or distal to it and should be treated with prophylactic antibiotics before procedures of risk.

Cyanotic Disorders

DEFINITION AND MECHANISMS

Central cyanosis is caused by an intracardiac shunt or an intrapulmonary right-to-left shunt. Cyanosis becomes evident when reduced (unoxygenated) capillary hemoglobin reaches about 5 g/dl, although this depends on the total hemoglobin concentration: cyanosis is more readily apparent in a patient with polycythemia and is less apparent in a patient with anemia. Mild cyanosis is difficult to detect. Generally, cyanosis does not become clinically apparent until the oxygen saturation falls below 85% (assuming a normal hemoglobin level). Patients with long-standing arterial desaturation will develop clubbing of the fingernails and toenails. Clubbing is characterized by thickening and widening of the nailbeds and loss of the angle between the nail and nail bed, producing a convex nail.

It is helpful to categorize cyanotic CHDs in terms of their effect on pulmonary blood flow. Defects producing decreased pulmonary blood flow include tetralogy of Fallot, tricuspid atresia, Ebstein anomaly, and pulmonary atresia. Defects associated with increased pulmonary blood flow include persistent truncus arteriosus, transposition of the great arteries with or without VSD or PDA, total anomalous venous return, a single or common ventricle, and hypoplastic left heart syndrome. Acyanotic patients with large left-to-right shunts may develop pulmonary vascular occlusive disease (Eisenmenger syndrome).

Adult patients with cyanotic CHD are at increased risk for hyperviscosity secondary to erythrocytosis. The erythrocytosis develops as a compensatory mechanism for red cell oxygen desaturation: a significantly increased red cell mass is necessary to deliver an adequate volume of oxygen to peripheral tissues, given the sometimes severe degree of desaturation. Venous and arterial thrombosis with secondary cerebrovascular accidents have been well documented in cyanotic CHD and have been attributed both to the increased red blood cell mass and to associated iron deficiency anemia, which also increases blood viscosity. This risk is increased in the presence of hypertension or atrial fibrilla-

tion and in patients with a history of phlebotomy and microcytosis, suggesting the need for a more conservative approach to phlebotomy and aggressive treatment of iron deficiency.

EISENMENGER SYNDROME

A serious complication of long-standing left-to-right shunts in the atria, ventricles, or great arteries is the development of severe, irreversible pulmonary hypertension, which is termed Eisenmenger syndrome.

Pathophysiology

Normally, the pulmonary vascular resistance is substantially lower than systemic vascular resistance; thus, large intracardiac or great artery communications tend to produce left-to-right shunting. As pulmonary vascular resistance rises, resistance to flow into the pulmonary circulation will eventually exceed that into the systemic circulation, and right-to-left shunting will occur. This will result in varying degrees of cyanosis as well as other physical findings of pulmonary hypertension. Unlike patients with polycythemia vera or polycythemia from chronic obstructive pulmonary disease, patients with Eisenmenger syndrome will often require hematocrits in the 60s, or even low 70s, to deliver sufficient oxygen to tissues to avoid ischemic symptoms.

Clinical Presentation

Patients with Eisenmenger syndrome may be asymptomatic except for cyanosis. Eventually, many patients will note decreased exercise tolerance and chest discomfort, often reminiscent of angina pectoris. If secondary erythrocytosis reaches severe levels, patients may develop symptoms of hyperviscosity, including visual disturbances, headaches, and other complaints.

Physical examination of a patient with Eisenmenger syndrome will reveal manifestations of pulmonary hypertension, including a loud pulmonary component of the second heart sound and the high-pitched diastolic murmur of high-pressure pulmonary regurgitation (the Graham Steell murmur). Additional findings include cyanosis, clubbing, and RV lift or heave.

Laboratory Tests

Electrocardiography The ECG shows right axis deviation and RVH, exhibited as tall R waves and ST-T abnormalities in V1 through V3.

Radiologic studies The chest x-ray will show enlarged central pulmonary arteries with peripheral arterial pruning. Cardiomegaly with specific chamber enlargement will reflect the underlying defect. Right-sided cardiac catheterization often is needed to assess pulmonary arterial pressure and resistance.

Echocardiography Echocardiography can identify and quantify the underlying cardiac shunt and provide an estimate of right heart pressures.

Management

Patients with Eisenmenger syndrome may live for decades after the diagnosis is made.[11] Alternatively, sudden death from ventricular arrhythmias may occur. Because pulmonary resistance is high and fixed in these patients, care needs to be taken to avoid situations that may lead to sudden decreases in systemic vascular resistance, which would exacerbate the right-to-left shunting, sometimes in a life-threatening manner. This would include avoidance of overly hot environments and dehydration; in addition, care should be taken during anesthesia or when using vasodilator drugs. Pregnancy is another state in which systemic vascular resistance falls; thus, pregnancy is extremely dangerous for a mother with pulmonary hypertension, as well as for her fetus. Iron deficiency should be treated if present. Only rarely will phlebotomy be required to relieve symptoms of hyperviscosity. A relatively recent therapeutic option for Eisenmenger syndrome is the use of prostacyclin[12] or endothelin-related drugs[13] to lower pulmonary vascular resistance. Heart-lung or lung transplantation has been successfully performed in some patients with Eisenmenger syndrome.[14]

TETRALOGY OF FALLOT

Pathophysiology

Tetralogy of Fallot is the most common form of cyanotic congenital heart disease. Classically, the syndrome includes pulmonary stenosis (subvalvar, valvar, supravalvar, or a combination of all of these), RVH, subaortic VSD, and dextropositioning of the aorta so that it overrides the interventricular septum. Associated anomalies include right aortic arch (25%), atrial septal defect (10%), and coronary artery anomalies (10%).[15] Approximately 15% of patients with tetralogy of Fallot have a deletion of chromosome 22q11 (CATCH 22 syndrome: cardiac anomalies, abnormal facies, thymic hypoplasia, cleft palate, hypocalcemia, and 22q11 deletion).[16]

Surgical Repair in Childhood

Current surgical practice warrants early repair, usually in the first year of life. Without surgery, survival beyond 20 years of age is uncommon.

Surgical repair consists of patch closure of the VSD and alleviation of the RV outflow tract obstruction by one or more of the following methods: infundibular muscle resection, pulmonary valvotomy, outflow tract or transannular patch augmentation, and patch augmentation of the main or proximal branch pulmonary arteries. In some cases, it is necessary to place a conduit from the RV to the pulmonary artery. The conduit may be valved or nonvalved, and it may be bioprosthetic or a homograft.

When pulmonary blood flow is inadequate, surgical repair includes a shunt from the systemic circulation to the pulmonary artery to provide additional pulmonary flow. This may consist of a Blalock-Taussig shunt, a Potts shunt, or a Waterston shunt. The classic Blalock-Taussig shunt connects the subclavian artery to the pulmonary artery; the modified form comprises an interposed tube graft, usually of expanded polytetrafluoroethylene [Gore-Tex]. A Potts shunt connects the descending aorta to the left pulmonary artery. A Waterston shunt connects the ascending aorta to the right pulmonary artery [see Figure 4].

Clinical Presentation after Repair

In patients who have undergone surgical repair of tetralogy of Fallot, the examination focuses on residual defects. Not uncommonly, these patients have murmurs related to residual outflow tract obstruction and mild to severe pulmonary regurgitation (PR), which produces a to-and-fro murmur. The severity of RV outflow tract obstruction directly determines the presence and degree of cyanosis. Systolic ejection murmurs are inversely related to the severity of the obstruction: a short, soft murmur suggests severe obstruction with a large right-to-left ventricular level shunt and minimal forward flow in the pul-

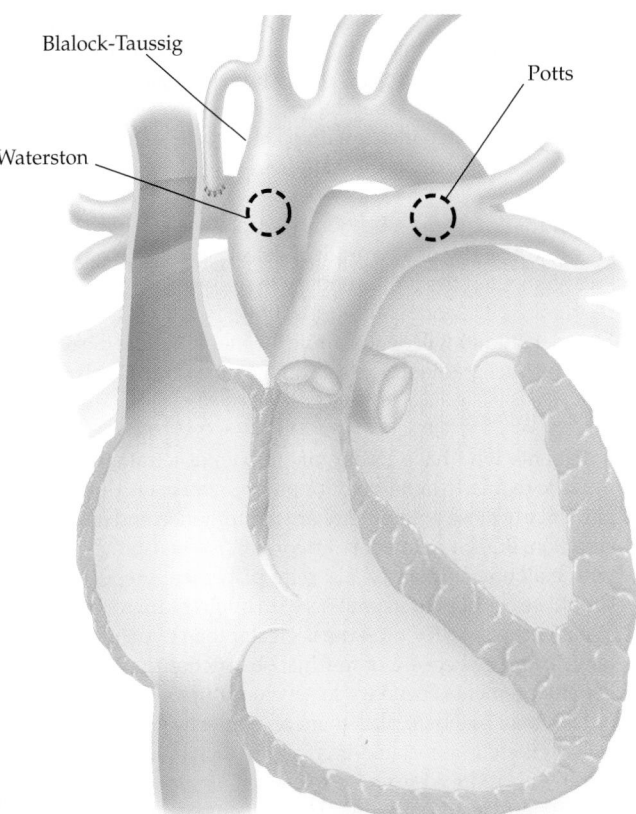

Figure 4 **Systemic artery–to–pulmonary artery shunts. The Blalock-Taussig shunt connects the subclavian artery to a pulmonary artery; the Waterston shunt connects the ascending aorta to the right pulmonary artery; and the Potts shunt connects the descending aorta to the left pulmonary artery.**

monary artery, whereas a long, harsh murmur suggests minimal obstruction.

Patent shunts will produce a continuous murmur. The degree of cyanosis will depend on the adequacy of pulmonary blood flow provided by the shunt.

A residual VSD may be detected. With increasing RV volume overload, the patient may experience exercise intolerance, right heart failure, and arrhythmias.

Laboratory Data

Electrocardiography   In patients who have undergone operative repair of tetralogy of Fallot, the ECG typically shows sinus rhythm, right axis deviation, and RVH; most of these patients also have right bundle branch block. Atrial and ventricular arrhythmias may be detected, especially on a 24-hour monitoring study.

Radiologic studies   The findings on chest x-ray vary with the surgical history. A right aortic arch may be noted. The pulmonary artery segment is concave because of the variable degree of pulmonary artery hypoplasia, and the RVH results in an upturned apex; together, these produce the classic finding of a boot-shaped heart. Surgical intervention may result in significant pulmonary regurgitation that eventually will lead to volume overload of the heart, producing cardiomegaly. Over time, patch augmentation of the outflow tract may become aneurysmal, which may be indicated by an enlarged pulmonary artery segment. Asymmetrical pulmonary blood flow suggests significant branch pulmonary artery obstruction and can be best quantitated by a pulmonary flow study. MRI with MRA is very useful to identify residual defects and assess ventricular function, especially in patients with poor acoustic windows and inadequate echocardiographic studies.

Echocardiography Echocardiography will establish the presence and severity of any residual defects, including progressive enlargement of the RV secondary to pulmonic regurgitation, a residual VSD, and continuous flow in a palliative shunt. Doppler studies will demonstrate the magnitude of the residual outflow tract gradient. The ascending aorta often is enlarged.

Management

Patients who have undergone repair of tetralogy of Fallot must be regularly monitored for progression of residual defects, particularly those with pulmonary regurgitation and conduit obstruction. Branch pulmonary artery stenosis may be approached with balloon angioplasty and stent placement. Repeat surgery should be considered in patients with a significant residual VSD; in patients whose RV pressure is greater than two thirds the systemic pressure because of residual obstruction; in patients with RV enlargement secondary to severe pulmonary regurgitation (which may mandate placement of a bioprosthetic valve, especially if there is associated tricuspid regurgitation [TR]); and in those with reduced exercise tolerance.[17] Reoperation in adults can be performed with low risk. Aortic valve or aortic root replacement is occasionally required because of progressive root dilatation and AR.[18] Ventricular arrhythmias, which are detected in 40% to 50% of patients, have been associated with older age at primary repair, RV volume overload, and QRS prolongation. Marked widening of the QRS to more than 180 msec and LV dysfunction have been identified as risk factors for sudden cardiac death. In such cases, consideration should be given to prophylactic placement of an implantable cardiac defibrillator.[19] Patients should be counseled to follow endocarditis prophylaxis during procedures that place them at risk.

DEXTROTRANSPOSITION OF THE GREAT ARTERIES

Pathophysiology

In the most common form of transposition of the great arteries (TGA), dextro-TGA (D-TGA), the aorta arises in an anterior position from the RV, and the pulmonary artery arises posteriorly from the LV. There is complete separation of the pulmonary and systemic circulations: systemic blood flow traverses the right heart and enters the aorta, whereas pulmonary blood flow traverses the left heart and enters the pulmonary artery. Most surviving patients have a patent ductus arteriosus and foramen ovale, permitting mixing of the two circulations. About one third have associated anomalies, including ASD and VSD. Left ventricular outflow tract obstruction is not uncommon. Unless intracardiac mixing is improved, survival beyond the first year is unusual.

Surgical Repair in Childhood

Initial treatment of D-TGA includes infusion of prostaglandin E to maintain patency of the ductus arteriosus and balloon septostomy (Rashkind procedure) to permit better mixing at the atrial level. Surgery initially consisted of redirecting the systemic venous return to the LV and the pulmonary venous return to the RV. These so-called atrial switch operations (Mus-

tard or Senning procedures), which used a baffle within the atria, restored physiologic circulation but required the RV to function as the systemic ventricle. The arterial switch operation has replaced the atrial switch operation, at least in patients who have normal function of both semilunar valves. In the arterial switch operation, the pulmonary artery and aorta are first transected above the semilunar valves and coronary arteries, and then they are switched. The aorta is connected to the neoaortic valve (formerly the pulmonic valve) arising from the LV, and the pulmonary artery is connected to the neopulmonary valve (formerly the aortic valve) arising from the RV. The coronary arteries are relocated to the neoaorta.

Patients with D-TGA and a large VSD may undergo the Rastelli procedure. The pulmonary artery is divided and oversewn. Flow from the LV must pass through the septal defect and is directed by a baffle to the aortic valve. A conduit from the RV to the pulmonary artery allows egress from the ventricle to the pulmonary circulation.

Clinical Presentation after Repair

Physical findings relate to the presence of associated anomalies (i.e., murmurs of VSD, PS, or PDA). Similarly, the larger the septal defect, the less severe the cyanosis.

Laboratory Tests

Electrocardiography The ECG in patients with the atrial switch shows right axis deviation and RVH. In patients with the arterial switch, the ECG may be normal, provided coronary blood flow is not compromised.

Radiologic studies Patients who have had the atrial switch procedure generally have cardiomegaly from a dilated RV, and the pulmonary artery may show preferential flow to the right lung. Patients with the arterial switch repair are likely to have normal heart size.

Echocardiography Echocardiography is used to assess associated residual defects: depressed RV function, progressive TR, left ventricular outflow tract obstruction, residual VSD, or coronary artery perfusion abnormalities.

Management

The long-term outlook after the atrial switch is quite good, with actuarial survival of 80% at 28 years and 76% of survivors having no symptoms.[20] However, these patients must be monitored for progressive RV enlargement and TR leading to ventricular dysfunction. Although this complication occurs in only 3% of cases, such patients may require cardiac transplantation if medical therapy is ineffective. Atrial arrhythmias, including sick sinus syndrome, are common. The atrial baffle may cause either systemic or pulmonary venous obstruction, which is addressed either by reoperation or by balloon angioplasty and stent placement.

The long-term prognosis of patients with the arterial switch is less well known, but arrhythmias are thought to be less frequent and to occur secondary to imperfections in the operative procedure.[21] Patients should undergo nuclear medicine studies or stress testing to monitor for inadequate coronary perfusion secondary to coronary artery reimplantation abnormalities. Stenosis of the pulmonary artery (the most common complication) or stenosis at aortic anastomosis sites may occur. Complications of the Rastelli procedure include subaortic obstruction (baffle or VSD obstruction), conduit stenosis (with or without regurgitation), baffle leak, and branch pulmonary artery stenosis. Significant residual defects require reoperation.[17]

THE UNIVENTRICULAR HEART

Pathophysiology

A functional single ventricle may result from hypoplastic left heart syndrome (aortic atresia, mitral atresia, or both), tricuspid atresia, pulmonary atresia with intact ventricular septum, or an unbalanced AVSD resulting in hypoplasia of either the RV or LV.

Surgical Repair in Childhood

The initial presentation of univentricular heart in childhood may include severe cyanosis associated with a marked decrease in pulmonary blood flow, mild cyanosis and heart failure associated with intracardiac admixture of circulations and excessive pulmonary blood flow, or nearly balanced systemic and pul-

monary blood flows and mild cyanosis. Patients who survive to adulthood generally have undergone one or more palliative surgical procedures; these include the Norwood, Glenn, and Fontan procedures.

Norwood The Norwood operation establishes a single outlet from the single ventricle by anastomosing the hypoplastic ascending aorta to the main pulmonary artery, producing a so-called neoaorta and connecting the distal pulmonary artery to a systemic shunt, usually a modified Blalock-Taussig shunt [*see Figure 5a*]. Often, an atrial septectomy is required to allow complete mixing at the atrial level.

Glenn The bidirectional Glenn procedure involves anastomosis of the SVC to the pulmonary artery. It includes takedown of a previously placed shunt and repair of any branch pulmonary artery stenosis [*see Figure 5b*]. The term bidirectional refers to the fact that the right pulmonary artery remains in con-

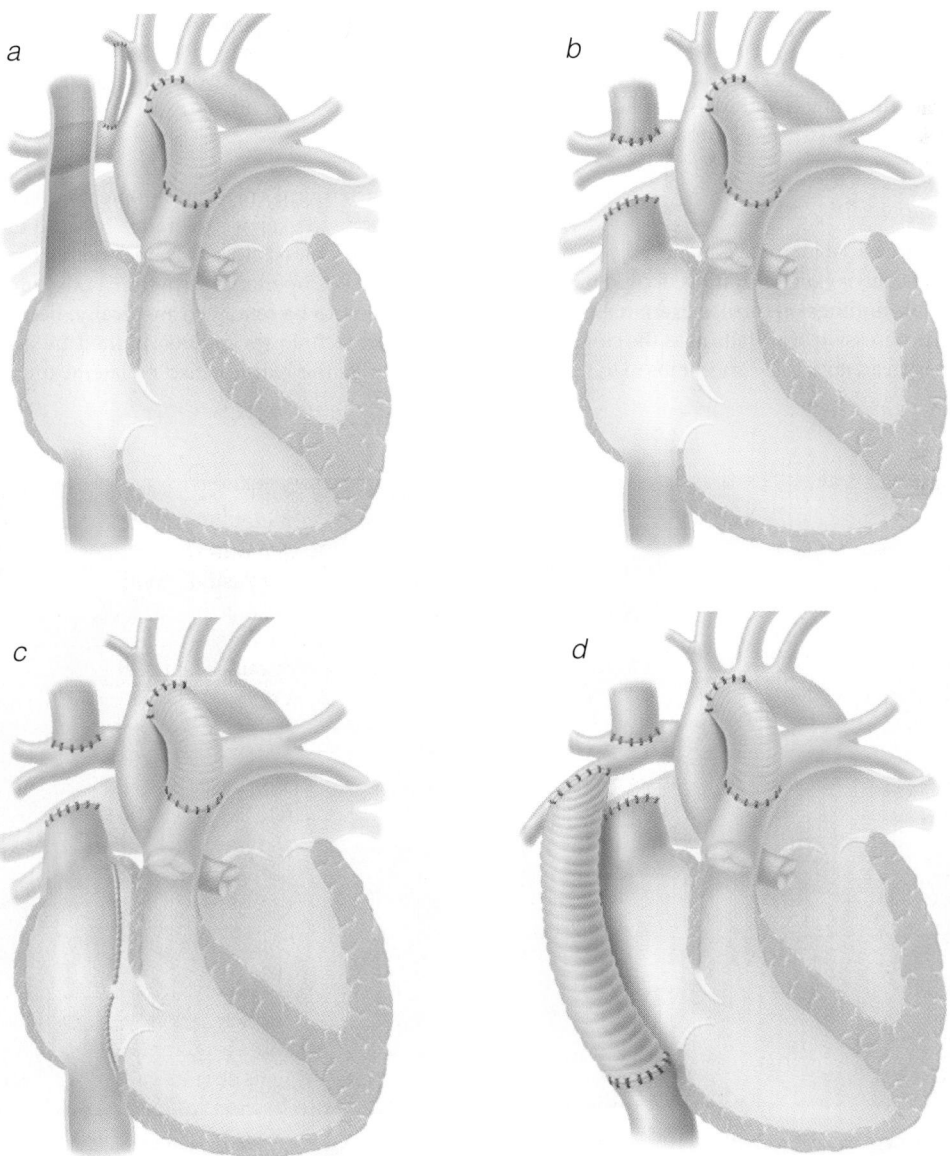

Figure 5 **Stages in the repair of functional single ventricles (see text for details). (*a*) Norwood; (*b*) bidirectional Glenn; (*c*) lateral tunnel; (*d*) extracardiac conduit.**

tinuity with the left pulmonary artery; this contrasts with the classic Glenn procedure, which involves anastomosis of the SVC to a right pulmonary artery that has been disconnected from the main and left pulmonary arteries. The bidirectional Glenn procedure is now done at 4 to 6 months of age.

Fontan   The Fontan procedure is the final palliative procedure, providing direct connection of flow from the SVC and inferior vena cava (IVC) to the pulmonary circuit. Initially, this was a one-stage procedure that involved attaching the RA to the pulmonary artery or RV outflow tract and was performed in patients older than 4 years. Current practice is to stage the anastomosis of SVC and IVC to the pulmonary circuit, with the final stage, total cavopulmonary artery anastomosis, occurring at 2 to 3 years of age. The IVC is connected to the pulmonary artery either by a lateral tunnel placed in the RA to direct blood from the IVC to the proximal SVC stump, which is then attached to the pulmonary artery [*see Figure 5c*], or by an extracardiac conduit connecting the IVC to the pulmonary artery directly [*see Figure 5d*]. With any of these routes of flow, a small communication (fenestration) may be made between the caval blood flow conduit and the functional left atrium. Pulmonary blood flow is achieved by passive venous return without assistance of a ventricular pumping chamber. Any mild alteration of pulmonary pressure or resistance will impair adequacy of pulmonary blood flow.

Clinical Presentation after Repair

Clinical features are variable. Some patients may be well palliated, with near-normal oxygen saturation, acceptable activity levels, and negligible findings on cardiac examination. Others will demonstrate progressive heart failure as the single ventricle (especially if it is an anatomic RV) succumbs to the increased pressure and volume overload secondary to progressive atrioventricular valve regurgitation and myocardial dysfunction. Both atrial and ventricular arrhythmias are common. The sluggish pulmonary blood flow may predispose to in situ thrombosis and pulmonary embolism, which in turn will impede pulmonary blood flow by raising pulmonary arterial pressure.

Laboratory Tests

Electrocardiography   ECG findings are quite variable and may include atrial or ventricular enlargement, axis deviation, conduction abnormalities, and arrhythmias.

Radiologic studies   The chest x-ray may show progressive cardiomegaly. Pulmonary vascular markings may be unequal, indicating stenosis of one or more pulmonary artery branches. MRI with MRA may show areas of branch pulmonary artery stenosis and progressive changes in chamber size and ventricular function.

Echocardiography   Echocardiographic studies are aimed at following the progression of atrioventricular valve regurgitation, ventricular enlargement, and dysfunction, as well as detecting so-called smoke or clots in the systemic venous–to–pulmonary artery circuit.

Management

After surgical correction, patients demonstrate significant limitations in exercise tolerance because they rely on passive pulmonary blood flow that does not increase maximally with exertion. Postoperative arrhythmias are common. Arrhythmias may need to be managed medically, because radiofrequency ablation techniques may be limited by access problems secondary to the extracardiac or lateral tunnel connections be-

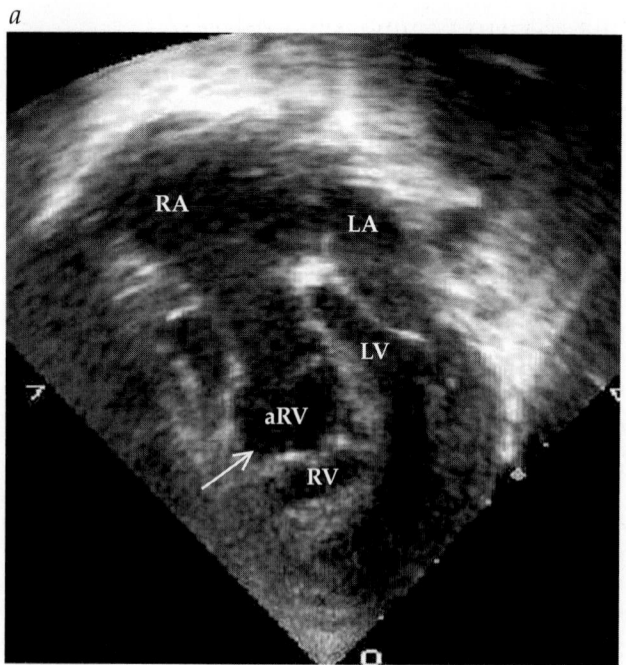
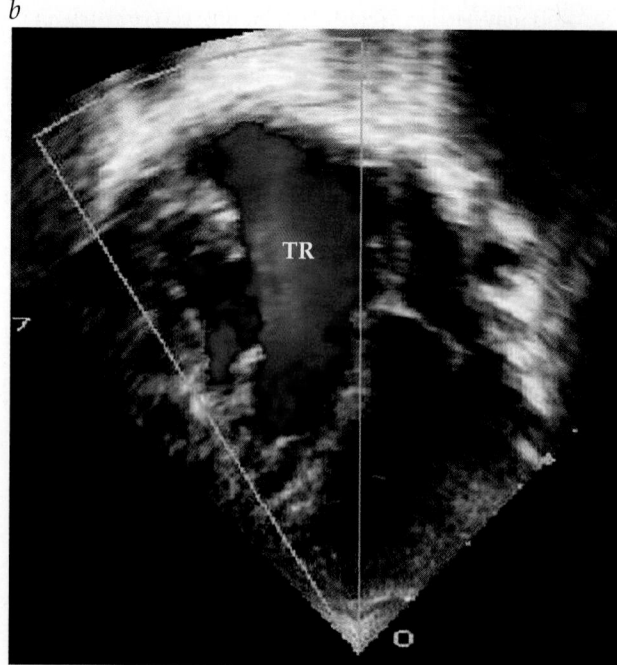

Figure 6   Echocardiograms of a patient with Ebstein anomaly. (*a*) Apical four-chamber view. The arrow indicates apical displacement of tricuspid leaflet. (*b*) Color Doppler flow image demonstrating severe tricuspid regurgitation (TR), originating deep in the right ventricle from the displaced tricuspid valve leaflet. (ARV—atrialized right ventricle; LA—left atrium; LV—left ventricle; RA—right atrium; RV—right ventricle)

tween the venous circulation and the pulmonary artery. The need for reoperation after the Fontan procedure is infrequent, with the most common indication being placement of a mechanical pacemaker. Protein-losing enteropathy (PLE) is a serious problem after the Fontan operation. Its cause is not known but probably relates to increased systemic venous and thoracic duct pressures. There may also be a local autoimmune or allergic component in the intestinal wall. PLE is characterized by peripheral edema, malabsorption, and a low serum protein level. Complications have become less frequent with staged surgery and provision of an atrial fenestration. Some older patients may benefit from conversion of classic Fontan to a total cavopulmonary artery anastomosis. Cardiac transplantation may be necessary for systemic ventricular failure or intractable PLE.[17]

EBSTEIN ANOMALY OF THE TRICUSPID VALVE

Pathophysiology

This uncommon anomaly of the tricuspid valve consists of adherence of the posterior and septal leaflets to the myocardium—causing a downward displacement of the functional annulus toward the RV apex—and enlargement of the anterior leaflet. The end result is an atrialization of the RV with resultant TR. In patients who present early in life, Ebstein anomaly is often found in association with other defects, including ASD and PS. Accessory pathways and clinical evidence of preexcitation are not uncommon, and arrhythmias are the most common presenting features in adults. There is an association with maternal lithium administration.

Clinical Presentation

Ebstein anomaly can become clinically evident at any age; the natural history of this lesion ranges from death in early life to adult survival without surgery, depending on the degree of regurgitation and whether significant arrhythmias are present. Cyanosis may occur, in neonates or adults, secondary to right-to-left shunting at the atrial level. Adult patients may complain of fatigue, shortness of breath, palpitations, or syncope. On auscultation, a murmur of TR is apparent and is often associated with a gallop rhythm, multiple systolic ejection sounds, and a widely split second sound.

Laboratory Tests

Electrocardiography   ECG findings are quite variable. The PR interval may be normal; short, with preexcitation; or prolonged. The axis may be superior or rightward, with or without a right bundle branch block. There may be evidence of RA enlargement. Arrhythmias are detected in 43% of adolescents and adults.[22]

Radiologic studies   The chest x-ray may show cardiomegaly with RA enlargement. Cardiac catheterization is not necessary unless there is concern regarding coronary artery disease or need for electrophysiologic assessment and possible radiofrequency ablation.

Echocardiography   Echocardiography can confirm the diagnosis and the degree of the tricuspid valve displacement (which may vary from mild tethering of the septal leaflet to severe apical displacement) and characterize the severity of TR [see Figure 6]. The anterior leaflet is large and sail-like and may

produce RV outflow obstruction. The atrial septum should be assessed for size of defect and magnitude of shunting.

Management

Surgery is recommended for patients with symptomatic heart failure and cardiomegaly, cyanosis, or arrhythmias; tricuspid valvuloplasty is preferred over valve replacement.[15] Surgery is not recommended for asymptomatic patients,[22] although some authors have advocated surgery if significant cardiomegaly is present, because this may be a better predictor of sudden death than functional status.[23]

The authors have no commercial relationships with manufacturers of products or providers of services discussed in this chapter.

References

1. Perloff JK, Miner PD: Specialized facilities for the comprehensive care of adults with congenital heart disease. Congenital Heart Disease in Adults, 2nd ed. Perloff JK, Child JS, Eds. Philadelphia, WB Saunders Co, 1998, p 9

2. Driscoll D, Allen HD, Atkins DL, et al: Guidelines for evaluation and management of common congenital cardiac problems in infants, children, and adolescents: a statement for healthcare professionals from the Committee on Congenital Cardiac Defects of the Council on Cardiovascular Disease in the Young, American Heart Association. Circulation 90:2180, 1994

3. Dajani AS, Taubert KA, Wilson W, et al: Prevention of bacterial endocarditis: recommendations by the American Heart Association. J Am Dent Assoc 128:1142, 1997

4. Driscoll DJ: Left-to-right shunt lesions. Pediatr Clin North Am 46:355, 1999

5. Berger F, Ewert P, Bjornstad PG, et al: Transcatheter closure as standard treatment for most interatrial defects: experience in 200 patients treated with the Amplatzer Septal Occluder. Cardiol Young 9:468, 1999

6. Gatzoulis MA, Freeman MA, Siu SC, et al: Atrial arrhythmia after surgical closure of atrial septal defects in adults. N Engl J Med 340:839, 1999

7. Suzuki K, Yamaki S, Mimori S, et al: Pulmonary vascular disease in Down's syndrome with complete atrioventricular septal defect. Am J Cardiol 86:434, 2000

8. Goyal VS, Fulwani MC, Ramakantan R, et al: Follow-up after coil closure of patent ductus arteriosus. Am J Cardiol 83:463, 1999

9. Stanger P, Cassidy SC, Girod DA, et al: Balloon pulmonary valvuloplasty: results of the Valvuloplasty and Angioplasty of Congenital Anomalies Registry. Am J Cardiol 65:775, 1990

10. Magee AG, Brzezinska-Rajszys G, Qureshi SA, et al: Stent implantation for aortic coarctation and recoarctation. Heart 82:600, 1999

11. Cantor WJ, Harrison DA, Moussadji JS, et al: Determinants of survival and length of survival in adults with Eisenmenger syndrome. Am J Cardiol 84:677, 1999

12. Rosenzweig EB, Kerstein D, Barst RJ: Long-term prostacyclin for pulmonary hypertension with associated congenital heart defects. Circulation 99:1858, 1999

13. Prendergast B, Newby DE, Wilson LE, et al: Early therapeutic experience with the endothelin antagonist BQ-123 in pulmonary hypertension after congenital heart surgery. Heart 82:505, 1999

14. Ueno T, Smith JA, Snell GI, et al: Bilateral sequential single lung transplantation for pulmonary hypertension and Eisenmenger's syndrome. Ann Thorac Surg 69:381, 2000

15. Brickner M, Hillis LD, Lange RA: Congenital heart disease in adults: second of two parts. N Engl J Med 342:334, 2000

16. Goldmuntz E, Clark BJ, Mitchell, et al: Frequency of 22q11 deletion in patients with conotruncal defects. J Am Coll Cardiol 32:492, 1998

17. Connelly MS, Webb GD, Somerville J, et al: Canadian consensus conference on adult congenital heart disease—1996. Can J Cardiol 14:399, 1998

18. Niwa K, Siu SC, Webb GD, et al: Progressive aortic root dilation in adults late after repair of tetralogy of Fallot. Circulation 106:1374, 2002

19. Ghai A, Silversides C, Harris L, et al: Left ventricular dysfunction is a risk factor for sudden cardiac death in adults late after repair of tetralogy of Fallot. J Am Coll Cardiol 40:1675, 2002

20. Wilson NJ, Clarkson PM, Barratt-Boyes BG, et al: Long-term outcome after the Mustard repair for simple transposition of the great arteries. J Am Coll Cardiol 32:758, 1998

21. Hunter PA, Kreb DL, Mantel SF: Twenty-five years' experience with the arterial switch operation. J Thorac Cardiovasc Surg 124:790, 2002

22. Celermajer DS, Bull C, Till JA, et al: Ebstein's anomaly: presentation and outcome from fetus to adult. J Am Coll Cardiol 23:170, 1994

23. Gentles TL, Calder L, Clarkson PM: Predictors of long-term survival with Ebstein's anomaly of the tricuspid valve. Am J Cardiol 53:332, 1992

Acknowledgment

Figures 1 through 5   Alice Y. Chen.

31 Peripheral Arterial Disease

Mark A. Creager, M.D.

Peripheral arterial diseases comprise those disorders that compromise blood flow to the limbs. Causes of limb artery obstruction include atherosclerosis, thrombus, embolism, vasculitis, arterial entrapment, adventitial cysts, fibromuscular dysplasia, arterial dissection, trauma, and vasospasm.

Peripheral Atherosclerosis

The most frequently encountered cause of peripheral arterial disease is atherosclerosis. The pathology of atherosclerosis that affects the limbs is similar to that of atherosclerosis of the aorta, coronary arteries, and extracranial cerebral arteries. Of patients who present with symptoms of peripheral atherosclerosis, approximately 80% have femoropopliteal artery stenoses, 30% have lesions in the aorta or iliac arteries, and 40% have tibioperoneal artery stenoses. Most patients have multiple stenoses.

EPIDEMIOLOGY

The prevalence of peripheral atherosclerosis, both asymptomatic and symptomatic, increases with age, ranging from 3% in persons younger than 60 years to greater than 20% in persons 75 years of age and older.[1-3] An epidemiologic study in Germany found that the overall prevalence of peripheral arterial disease in patients older than 65 years was 20% in men and 17% in women.[4] A community-based survey in primary physicians' offices in the United States found that of patients who were between the ages of 50 and 69 years who had diabetes mellitus or smoked cigarettes or who were older than 70 years, 29% had peripheral arterial disease.[5]

The prevalence of claudication ranges from 1% to 5%.[1] The peak incidence of claudication occurs between the sixth and seventh decades and develops later in women than in men. Each year, approximately 2% to 4% of all patients with intermittent claudication develop critical limb ischemia.[6]

Long-term survival is reduced in patients with peripheral atherosclerosis. The risk of death in populations with peripheral atherosclerosis is increased twofold to fourfold. Most patients die as a consequence of myocardial infarction or stroke.[7] Patients with claudication have a 5-year survival rate of approximately 15% to 30%, and patients with critical limb ischemia have a 1-year survival rate of approximately 25%.[1,2,6-8] Overall, there is an inverse relationship between the severity of peripheral arterial disease and survival.

RISK FACTORS

The risk factors associated with the development of peripheral atherosclerosis are similar to those associated with coronary atherosclerosis. These include cigarette smoking, diabetes mellitus, dyslipidemia, hypertension, a family history of premature atherosclerosis, and hyperhomocysteinemia. The risk of developing intermittent claudication is twofold to fivefold higher in smokers than in nonsmokers.[9,10] Moreover, continued cigarette smoking greatly increases the risk of progression from stable claudication to severe limb ischemia and amputation. Diabetes mellitus is associated with a threefold to fourfold increase in the risk of peripheral arterial disease.[9,11] Peripheral atherosclerosis is often more severe and extensive in diabetic patients than in non-

diabetic patients with atherosclerosis; in addition, the tibial and peroneal arteries are involved more frequently in diabetic patients than in nondiabetic patients. Prognosis is poor for patients with diabetes who have claudication: 30% to 40% develop critical limb ischemia over a 6-year period. The risk of amputation in diabetic patients is sevenfold to 15-fold higher than in nondiabetic patients with peripheral arterial disease.[2,12] Dyslipidemia, particularly hypercholesterolemia, is present in 40% of patients with peripheral atherosclerosis. The relative risk of peripheral arterial disease is 1.2 to 1.4 for each 40 to 50 mg/dl increase in total cholesterol.[10] Hypertriglyceridemia and an elevated plasma concentration of lipoprotein(a) each increase the risk of developing peripheral arterial disease. Hypertension increases the risk of claudication by at least twofold in men and by fourfold in women.[10] Hyperhomocysteinemia has emerged as an important risk factor for atherosclerosis and increases the risk of peripheral atherosclerosis by twofold to threefold.[13] Elevations in markers of inflammation, including levels of C-reactive protein and soluble intercellular adhesion molecule–1, are also independent predictors of the development of symptomatic peripheral arterial disease in otherwise healthy men.[14,15]

DIAGNOSIS

Clinical Presentation

The two principal symptoms of peripheral atherosclerosis are intermittent claudication and rest pain. However, many patients with peripheral arterial disease are asymptomatic, have symptoms that do not fit the typical pattern of intermittent claudication, or have symptoms from comorbid conditions (e.g., arthritis) that blur the presentation.[16]

Intermittent claudication is described as discomfort, pain, fatigue, or heaviness that is felt in the affected extremity during walking and resolves within a few minutes of resting. Intermittent claudication occurs when the metabolic demand of an exercising muscle exceeds supply. A hemodynamically significant stenosis prevents blood-flow augmentation during exercise. The increased pressure gradient that develops across the stenosis compromises perfusion pressure to the exercising muscle. As ischemia develops, autoregulatory mechanisms cause local vasodilatation and a further reduction in perfusion pressure, and extravascular forces created by the exercising muscle reduce perfusion pressure even further. The location of the symptom depends on the site of stenosis. Thigh, hip, or buttock claudication may develop in cases of proximal arterial occlusive disease involving the aorta or iliac arteries. Involvement of the femoral and popliteal arteries typically causes calf claudication. Tibial and peroneal artery stenoses may cause pedal claudication.

Rest pain occurs when the blood supply does not adequately meet the basic nutritional requirements of the tissues of the affected extremity. Pain typically occurs in the toes or foot. Initially, the pain is worse at night when the patient is lying in bed with the legs in a neutral position. Sitting up and dangling the leg may alleviate the discomfort, because this maneuver increases perfusion pressure via gravitational forces. Conversely, leg elevation worsens the pain. With persistent severe ischemia, skin breakdown occurs, leading to ulceration, necrosis, and gan-

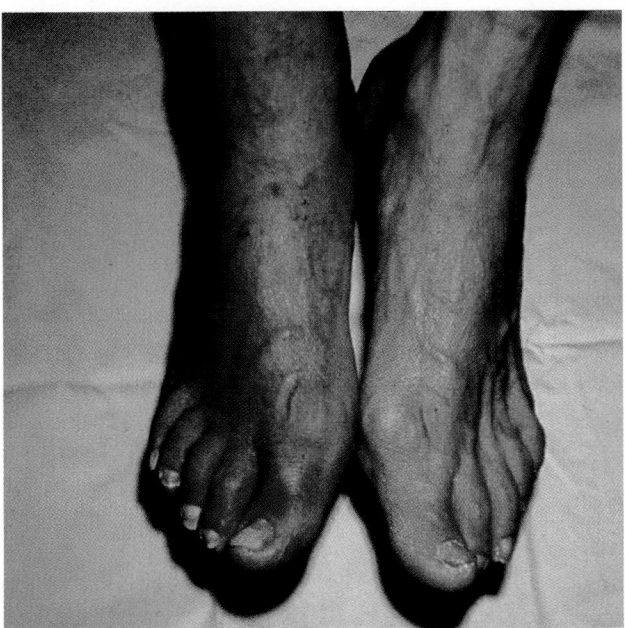

Figure 1 **Photograph shows an ischemic right foot demonstrating dependent rubor.**

grene. Even minor trauma to an ischemic foot may produce a skin lesion that fails to heal.

The most reliable physical finding in patients with peripheral arterial disease is decreased or absent pulses. Examination of femoral, popliteal, posterior tibial, and dorsalis pedis pulses may indicate sites of stenosis. Bruits auscultated in the abdomen, pelvis, and inguinal areas also may indicate the presence of arterial stenosis. Foot pallor may be observed at rest, with leg elevation, or after exercise of the calf muscles. Signs of chronic limb ischemia include subcutaneous atrophy; hair loss; coolness; pallor; and cyanosis, dependent rubor, or both [see Figure 1]. Additional signs of critical limb ischemia include petechiae, fissures, ulceration, and gangrene. Ulcers often involve the tips of the toes or the heel of the foot and occur at sites of trauma or pressure caused by poor-fitting footwear. Arterial ulcers have pale bases and irregular borders and are usually quite painful.

Several classifications have been proposed to characterize the severity of limb ischemia in patients with peripheral arterial disease. The most widely recognized classification was developed by René Fontaine [see Table 1]. A contemporary classification scheme takes into consideration symptoms, physical findings, perfusion pressure, and exercise capacity; the classification scheme comprises four grades and seven categories [see Table 2].[17]

Table 1   Fontaine Classification
of Chronic Limb Ischemia

Stage	Symptoms
I	Asymptomatic
II	Intermittent claudication
IIa	Pain-free; claudication walking > 200 m
IIb	Pain-free; claudication walking < 200 m
III	Rest pain and nocturnal pain
IV	Necrosis, gangrene

Table 2   Clinical Categories
of Chronic Limb Ischemia[75]

Grade	Category	Clinical Description
I	0	Asymptomatic, not hemodynamically significant
	1	Mild claudication
	2	Moderate claudication
	3	Severe claudication
II	4	Ischemic rest pain
	5	Minor tissue loss; nonhealing ulcer; focal gangrene with diffuse pedal ischemia
III	6	Major tissue loss extending above transmetatarsal level; foot no longer salvageable

Noninvasive Diagnostic Tests

Several noninvasive diagnostic tests can be used to evaluate patients with peripheral arterial disease. Segmental blood pressure measurement of the extremity is a quantitative means to assess the presence and severity of arterial stenoses [see Table 3]. Pneumatic cuffs are positioned along the leg and are inflated to suprasystolic pressures. During cuff deflation, the onset of flow (i.e., systolic blood pressure) is assessed by use of a Doppler probe placed over the dorsalis pedis or the posterior tibial arteries. Normally, the systolic blood pressure in the leg is the same as that in the arm. However, because of reflected waves, systolic blood pressure in the leg may be slightly higher than that in the arm. The normal ankle:brachial systolic blood pressure ratio (i.e., the ankle:brachial index) is therefore 1.0 or slightly greater. Taking into consideration the variability in blood pressure measurements, an ankle:brachial index less than 0.95 is considered abnormal. Patients with leg claudication typically have an ankle:brachial index less than 0.8; in patients with ischemia at rest, the ankle:brachial index is frequently less than 0.4 [see Table 3].

Measurement of the ankle:brachial index can be performed in a medical office. It is a sensitive indicator of peripheral arterial disease; it is more closely associated with leg function in patients with peripheral arterial disease than is intermittent claudication or other leg symptoms.[18] Because atherosclerosis is a systemic problem, a decreased ankle:brachial index suggests that the burden of disease is increased throughout the body, including the coronary arteries; for that reason, the lower the ankle:brachial index, the higher the risk of a cardiovascular event.[19,20]

In patients with peripheral arterial disease, the pressure gradient across a stenosis increases during exercise, as vascular resistance in the exercising muscle decreases. The exercise-induced increase in systemic pressure (i.e., brachial artery pressure) is not accompanied by a comparable increase in ankle pressure. Thus, the ankle:brachial index will be lower immediately after the patient has exercised than when the patient is at rest.

Plethysmographic devices are used to record the change in limb artery volume that occurs with each pulse (pulse volume recordings). The pulse volume waveform comprises a systolic upstroke with a sharp peak, a dicrotic wave, and a downsloping component. Distal to the site of an arterial stenosis, the amplitude of the pulse volume waveform is diminished, and the dicrotic wave disappears. In the presence of severe ischemia, the waveform may be entirely absent [see Figure 2].

Doppler ultrasonography can identify vessels with stenotic lesions. A Doppler probe is positioned at various sites along the limb's arteries. The Doppler waveform has three components, which correspond to three phases of blood flow: high-velocity antegrade flow during systole, transient flow reversal during early diastole, and low-velocity antegrade flow during late diastole. When stenosis is present, this triphasic waveform is altered distal to the stenosis: the amplitude is decreased, the rate of rise is delayed, and the reverse-flow component disappears. Duplex ultrasound scanning is a direct, noninvasive test that combines B-mode ultrasonography and pulsed Doppler ultrasonography to assess peripheral arterial stenoses. A B-mode scan identifies areas of intimal thickening, plaque formation, and calcification. Color Doppler imaging detects blood-flow abnormalities caused by arterial stenoses. An increase of greater than twofold in the systolic velocity is indicative of a hemodynamically significant stenosis, usually one that exceeds 50% of the artery diameter.

Transcutaneous oximetry, which measures the transcutaneous oxygen tension with oxygen-sensing electrodes placed at various sites on the legs, is used to assess the severity of skin ischemia in patients with peripheral arterial disease. Normally, the transcutaneous oxygen tension of the resting foot is approximately 60 mm Hg; it is often less than 40 mm Hg in patients with ischemia.

Angiography

Magnetic resonance angiography (MRA) and CT angiography can be used to evaluate the location and severity of peripheral atherosclerosis[21]; thus, these modalities can help determine whether a patient is a candidate for an endovascular intervention. In addition, they are free of the risks of conventional angiography. MRA is more widely used, although it is somewhat slower than CT angiography. The current generation of CT angiography machines can provide highly detailed images within minutes; however, CT angiography requires iodinated contrast and radiation exposure, which makes it less suitable for patients with renal insufficiency or contrast allergy.

In most patients, clinical evaluation and noninvasive testing are sufficient for confirming the diagnosis of peripheral arterial disease. Conventional catheter-based angiography is typically performed only when a diagnosis is in doubt or as a prelude to endovascular interventions or surgical reconstruction [see Figure 3]. Digital subtraction angiography is a computer-enhancing technique that is used to improve resolution; it is particularly useful in conjunction with the intra-arterial administration of radiographic contrast agent.

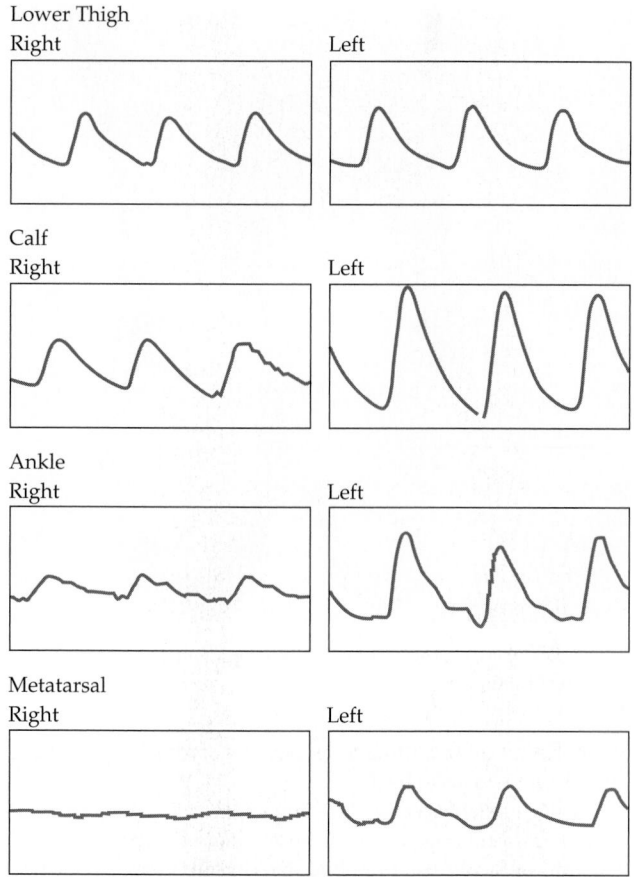

Lower Thigh
Right   Left

Calf
Right   Left

Ankle
Right   Left

Metatarsal
Right   Left

Figure 2 **Pulse volume recordings provide a qualitative assessment of blood flow to the extremity. In this example from a patient with right calf claudication and right foot pain, the pulse volume recordings are abnormal in the right calf, right ankle, and right metatarsal segments. In the right calf and ankle, the amplitude of the pulse is diminished and the rate of rise is delayed. No pulse volume can be recorded in the right metatarsal segment. The pulse volume recordings in the left leg are normal.**

TREATMENT

Risk Factor Modification and Antiplatelet Therapy

Risk factors for atherosclerosis should be identified and treated; this reduces the likelihood of progression of atherosclerosis and also helps to prevent adverse cardiovascular events in patients with peripheral arterial disease.[22,23] Patients who stop smoking cigarettes have a more favorable prognosis than those who continue to smoke. Aggressive lipid-lowering therapy reduces progression of peripheral atherosclerosis, but it has not been established that it prevents progression of symptoms from claudication to critical limb ischemia. Cholesterol-lowering therapy with statin drugs reduces adverse cardiovascular events in patients with atherosclerosis and may improve walking ability.[24-27]

Antihypertensive agents should be tailored to bring blood pressure into a normotensive range to reduce the risk of adverse events such as stroke, congestive heart failure, and renal insufficiency.[2,28] Occasionally, marked reduction of blood pressure may reduce perfusion pressure to an ischemic extremity and potentially aggravate symptoms. Angiotensin-converting enzyme inhibitors are effective antihypertensive drugs that may also reduce the risk of adverse cardiovascular events in patients with atherosclerosis, including those with peripheral arterial disease.[29]

Table 3   Leg Segmental Pressure Measurements in Patient with Right Calf Claudication and Right Foot Pain*

	Right	*Left*
Brachial	158	158
Upper thigh	160	162
Lower thigh	94	154
Calf	62	116
Ankle	42	116
Ankle:brachial ratio	0.27	0.68

*Findings are consistent with femoropopliteal and tibioperoneal artery stenoses in the right leg. The right ankle:brachial ratio indicates ischemia. Systolic pressure gradients between the lower thigh and calf and between the calf and ankle in the left leg are consistent with distal femoropopliteal artery and tibioperoneal artery stenoses. The left ankle:brachial ratio is consistent with symptoms of claudication.

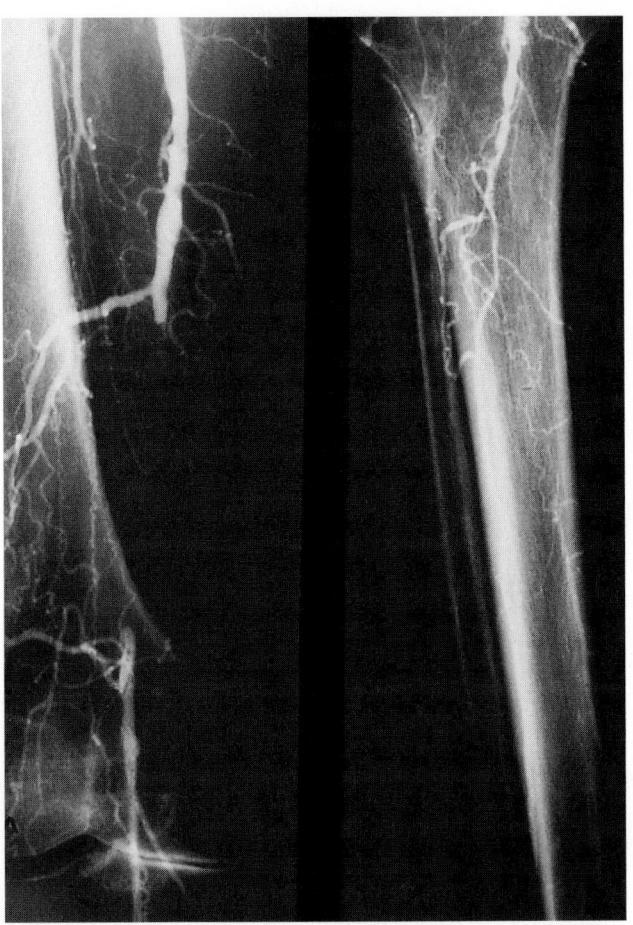

Figure 3 **Arteriogram of a patient with critical ischemia of the right foot. The left panel shows a long, total occlusion of the right superficial femoral artery. The popliteal artery reconstitutes via collaterals. The right panel reveals evidence of anterior tibial, posterior tibial, and peroneal artery occlusions with poor runoff.**

Beta blockers do not worsen intermittent claudication but may cause reflex peripheral cutaneous vasoconstriction and exacerbate critical limb ischemia.[30] Beta blockers are indicated to reduce the risk of myocardial infarction and death in patients with coronary artery disease—a condition that frequently coexists with peripheral arterial disease.

Aggressive treatment of diabetes mellitus reduces microangiopathic complications such as retinopathy and nephropathy.[2,28,31] It is not known whether aggressive treatment of diabetes reduces progression of atherosclerosis or prevents critical limb ischemia or foot ulceration. B-complex vitamins, such as folic acid, cobalamin, and pyridoxine, may lower homocysteine levels, but it is not yet known whether such therapy reduces cardiovascular events or prevents progression of peripheral atherosclerosis.

There is little information regarding the efficacy of platelet inhibition in treating symptoms of peripheral arterial disease. In one study, primary prevention with aspirin was shown to reduce the need for surgical revascularization in patients with peripheral arterial disease.[32] Small angiography trials have suggested that platelet inhibitors reduce the risk of acute peripheral arterial occlusion.[33] These agents may prevent thrombosis after plaque rupture in the peripheral arteries, as they do in coronary arteries. Antiplatelet therapy has been shown to reduce the risk

of adverse cardiac events such as nonfatal myocardial infarction and stroke and has been shown to reduce cardiovascular mortality in patients with atherosclerosis.[2,23,34] In one study, clopidogrel was more effective than aspirin in reducing the risk of adverse cardiovascular events, particularly in patients with peripheral arterial disease.[35]

Hygiene and Physical Therapy

Local measures are used to prevent skin ulceration and foot infection, particularly in patients with critical limb ischemia. The feet should be kept clean, and moisturizing cream should be applied to prevent drying and fissuring. The skin of the feet should be inspected frequently, and minor abrasions should be treated promptly. Stockings should be made of natural, absorbent fibers. Elastic hose are contraindicated because they restrict skin blood flow. Shoes should be carefully fitted to reduce the possibility of pressure-induced skin breakdown. In patients with critical limb ischemia, the limbs should be maintained in a dependent position to increase perfusion pressure. This can be achieved by angling the mattress so that the affected limb is below heart level. Cotton wicks placed between the toes absorb moisture and reduce friction. Sheepskin placed beneath the heels of the feet reduces pressure and necrosis. A warm environment is recommended to reduce vasoconstriction. Ulcerations and necrotic areas should be kept dry and covered with dry, nonadhesive material. Infections should be drained. Local antibiotics should be avoided. Pain should be treated with analgesics.

Supervised exercise training programs improve walking capacity in patients with peripheral arterial disease.[2,36] Among the most likely factors that account for the improvement are more efficient skeletal muscle metabolic function and changes in ergonomics.[37] Most studies have not found that exercise training improves blood flow to the exercising extremity, but investigations into the potential angiogenic effects of exercise are ongoing. Training programs should be individualized for each patient. Because supervised settings provide structure and guidance, patients have achieved the most success with supervised training. Programs typically involve treadmill exercise for approximately 1 hour three times a week for at least 3 months. Patients are encouraged to walk independently outside the supervised program.

Pharmacotherapy of Claudication and Critical Limb Ischemia

Drug therapy has generally not been successful in improving symptoms of claudication or reducing the complications of critical limb ischemia.[22] Although arterioles dilate in response to the metabolic demands of exercise, blood-flow augmentation is limited by critical stenoses. Thus, perfusion pressure distal to a stenosis falls further during exercise. Pharmacologic vasodilators may not reduce resistance to blood flow any more than endogenous vasodilators released during exercise. However, vasodilator drugs may increase blood flow to unaffected regions and thereby steal blood away from the ischemic limb.

Two drugs are approved by the Food and Drug Administration for the treatment of intermittent claudication: pentoxifylline and cilostazol. Pentoxifylline is a xanthine derivative with hemorrheologic properties. It has been reported to improve red cell flexibility and decrease blood viscosity. Pentoxifylline improved patients' exercise capacity in several but not all clinical trials.[30,38]

Cilostazol is a quinolinone derivative that inhibits phosphodiesterase III and thereby prevents the degradation of cyclic adenosine monophosphate. It has vasodilatory and platelet inhibitory properties, but its precise mechanism of action in patients with peripheral arterial disease is not known. Several trials have found that cilostazol leads to an increase in the distance walked before onset of claudication and also in the maximal walking distance in patients with peripheral arterial disease.[39-42]

Metal-chelating compounds, such as ethylenediaminetetraacetic acid (EDTA), are not useful in the treatment of patients with peripheral arterial disease.[43]

Several classes of drugs are currently undergoing investigation for use in the treatment of claudication, critical limb ischemia, or both. Some drug treatments are designed to increase the efficiency of substrate utilization, which enhances cellular energetics. L-Carnitine and its analogue, propionyl-L-carnitine, may decrease the ratio of acetyl coenzyme A (acetyl CoA) to CoA via the action of CoA:carnitine acetyltransferase and thereby stimulate glucose oxidation and energy production. Small placebo-controlled trials have found that treatment with L-carnitine or propionyl-L-carnitine improves exercise capacity in patients with intermittent claudication.[44,45]

In one study, L-arginine, the precursor of nitric oxide, improved endothelium-dependent vasodilatation and increased claudication distance after 3 weeks of intensive therapy.[46] Initial trials of prostaglandin E_1 (PGE_1) and prostacyclin (PGI_2) or their synthetic analogues suggested that these agents could increase the distance walked before onset of claudication, but subsequent definitive trials failed to show improvement in symptoms.[47,48] Angiogenic growth factors, such as vascular endothelial growth factor (VEGF) and basic fibroblast growth factor (bFGF), are undergoing intensive investigation for their potential efficacy in patients with peripheral arterial disease. These angiogenic factors may be delivered parenterally as recombinant proteins or through gene transfer using intra-arterial catheter techniques or intramuscular injection. Both VEGF and bFGF increase collateral blood vessel development and improve blood flow in experimental models of hindlimb ischemia. The efficacy of angiogenic growth factors in patients with intermittent claudication or critical limb ischemia is an active area of investigation. Several placebo-controlled trials in patients with claudication have been reported. In one trial, intra-arterial infusion of recombinant FGF-2 resulted in a significant increase in peak walking time at 90 days.[49] In another study, intramuscular administration of VEGF did not improve exercise performance.[50]

Autologous implantation of bone marrow mononuclear cells is a promising area of study. These cells have the potential to promote angiogenesis, because they can supply endothelial progenitor cells and they secrete angiogenic factors.[51]

Revascularization

Revascularization procedures are indicated for patients with disabling claudication, ischemic rest pain, or impending limb loss. Revascularization can be achieved by catheter-based endovascular interventions [*see Figure 4*] or surgical reconstruction.

Percutaneous transluminal angioplasty (PTA) of iliac arteries has an initial success rate of 90%.[52,53] Patency rates after 4 to 5 years are approximately 60% to 80% and are even higher with implantation of a stent.[54-56] The success rate of PTA of femoral and popliteal arteries is lower than that of PTA of iliac arteries. Patency rates at 1, 3, and 5 years are approximately 60%, 50%, and 45%, respectively.[54] The patency rate is better when PTA is performed for relief of claudication rather than for limb salvage and is also better in patients with good runoff (i.e., in patients with open distal vessels). Stents have not been shown to improve the patency rates of femoral and popliteal arteries over PTA alone. PTA of tibial and peroneal arteries is associated with poorer outcome than PTA of more proximal lesions and is usually performed in patients with critical limb ischemia who are considered at high risk for vascular surgery. Limb salvage rates of 1 to 2 years range from 50% to 75%. Thrombolytic therapy is not used routinely for the treatment of peripheral atherosclerosis but may be effective in restoring patency of native arteries and bypass grafts after acute arterial occlusion [*see* Acute Arterial Occlusion, *below*].

a

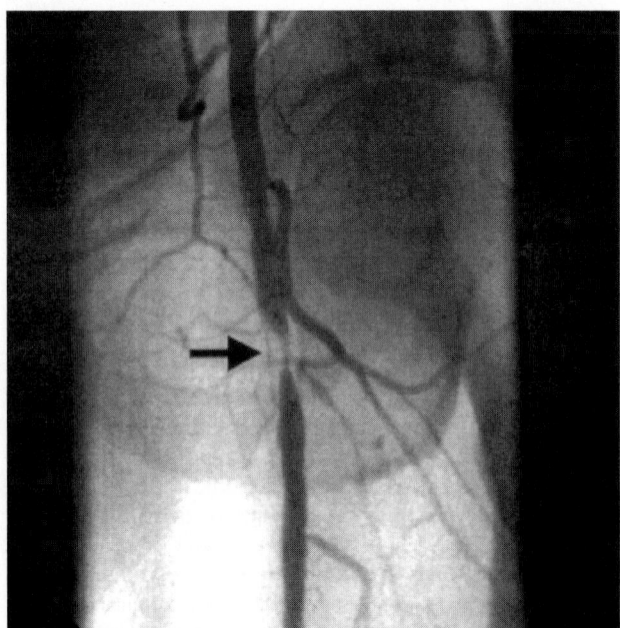

b

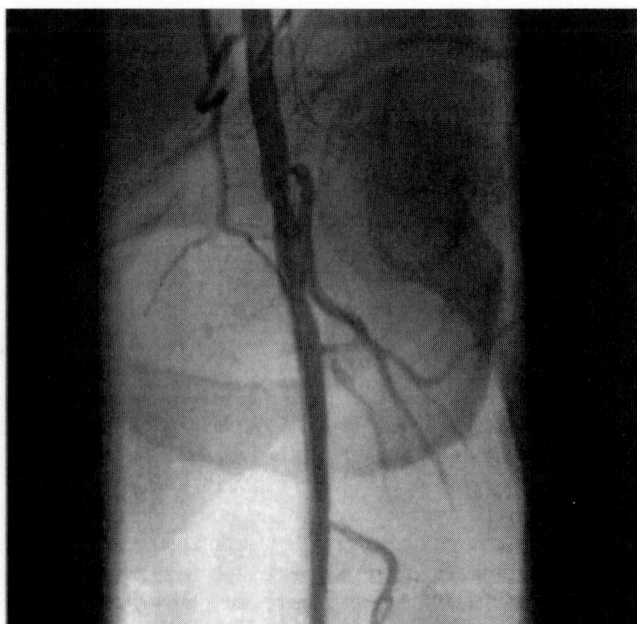

Figure 4 Arteriograms of a patient with disabling claudication of the left leg. A focal stenosis (arrow) of the superficial femoral artery is apparent (*a*). After percutaneous transluminal angioplasty, patency is restored (*b*).

The operative procedures used in vascular reconstruction depend on the location and severity of the arterial stenoses. Aortobifemoral bypass with a bifurcated Dacron or polytetrafluoroethylene prosthetic graft is the standard treatment for aortoiliac disease. Operative mortality ranges from 1% to 3% at centers with expertise in this technique. Long-term patency and relief of symptoms exceed 80% over 10 years.[57] Intra-abdominal aortoiliac reconstructive surgery is not feasible in patients whose comorbid conditions pose excessive surgical risk. Axillobifemoral bypass can circumvent the abdominal aorta and achieve revascularization of both legs. Femorofemoral bypass can be performed with the patient under regional anesthesia and is appropriate in cases of unilateral iliac artery obstruction.

Infrainguinal bypass procedures include femoral-popliteal and femoral-tibioperoneal reconstruction. Two techniques are generally used: the in situ saphenous vein bypass graft and the reversed autologous saphenous vein bypass graft. Femoralpopliteal reconstruction is most successful when the distal anastomosis is constructed proximal to the knee. The 5-year patency rate for all saphenous vein infrainguinal bypass grafts, including grafts that have undergone revision, is approximately 75% to 80%.[54,58] Patency rates are higher in claudicants than in patients with critical limb ischemia. Synthetic grafts made of polytetrafluoroethylene are used when veins are not available.[59] The patency of prosthetic grafts is inferior to those composed of veins, particularly because of early thrombotic occlusion. Synthetic grafts inserted below the knee have a very low patency rate and are typically not used for tibioperoneal reconstruction. Operative mortality for infrainguinal vascular reconstruction is 1% to 2%.[58] Antiplatelet agents should be administered to maintain graft patency after bypass grafts.[2,23,33]

Lumbar sympathectomy is used rarely to treat patients with critical limb ischemia. The pathophysiology of limb ischemia suggests that ischemic vessels are maximally vasodilated; thus, lumbar sympathectomy may not increase blood flow.

Amputation is a surgical alternative for patients with advanced limb ischemia in whom revascularization procedures are not possible or have failed. It is a final alternative for patients with unremitting rest pain or gangrene. Selection of the amputation level requires assessment of perfusion. Transphalangeal amputation causes minimal disability. Transmetatarsal amputation of the forefoot may affect balance, but patients are usually able to ambulate after rehabilitation. Patients who undergo below-theknee amputation and subsequently use a prosthesis expend 10% to 40% more energy to walk on a horizontal surface than a person who has use of both legs. Patients who undergo amputations above the knee and use a prosthetic device expend 65% more energy to walk than a person who has use of both legs. Overall prognosis after major leg amputation is poor, usually because of coexisting coronary and cerebrovascular disease.

Acute Arterial Occlusion

Acute arterial occlusion is to be distinguished from the gradual development of limb artery obstruction caused by peripheral atherosclerosis. The causes of acute arterial occlusion include embolism, thrombosis, dissection, and trauma. The most common cause is arterial embolism. The majority of systemic emboli arise from cardiac sources, including atrial fibrillation, valvular heart disease, congestive heart failure, left ventricular aneurysm, acute myocardial infarction, and cardiac tumors (e.g., left atrial myxomas). Noncardiac sources of embolism include aneurysms

of the aorta and aneurysms of the iliac, femoral, and popliteal arteries. A deep vein thrombus may enter the systemic circulation via an intracardiac shunt, resulting in what is termed paradoxical embolism. Thrombosis in situ may develop in peripheral atherosclerotic arteries at a site of plaque rupture and in bypass grafts. Thrombus may also develop in otherwise normal vessels of patients with procoagulant disorders such as hyperhomocysteinemia (including homocysteinuria), antiphospholipid antibody syndrome, and heparin-induced thrombocytopenia. Arterial thrombus formation is uncommon in patients with resistance to activated protein C and in patients deficient in protein C, protein S, or antithrombin. Aortic dissection and trauma may acutely occlude arteries by disrupting the integrity of the vessel lumen.

Acute arterial occlusion may cause severe limb ischemia, resulting in pain, paresthesia, and motor weakness distal to the site of occlusion. There is loss of peripheral pulses, cool skin, and pallor or cyanosis distal to the obstruction site. Noninvasive tests can provide additional evidence of peripheral arterial occlusion and may reveal the severity of ischemia, but definitive treatment should not be delayed. Arteriography is used to define the site of acute arterial occlusion and may distinguish thrombus in an atherosclerotic vessel from an arterial embolism. Once the diagnosis is made, anticoagulation with heparin should be initiated to prevent propagation of the thrombus.

Acute severe limb ischemia requires urgent revascularization. Catheter-directed intra-arterial thrombolysis with agents such as recombinant human tissue plasminogen activator may restore patency in acutely occluded arteries and bypass grafts. An embolectomy catheter can be used to remove arterial emboli. Surgical reconstruction to bypass the occlusion is considered if embolectomy is unsuccessful or not possible. The decision to utilize thrombolysis or surgery for acute arterial occlusion depends in part on the severity of ischemia and urgency of revascularization.[60,61]

Atheroembolism

Atherothrombotic debris from friable plaques in the aorta or other large arteries may dislodge and embolize to small distal limb arteries. Atheroembolism occurs spontaneously, although it occasionally occurs as a complication of arterial catheterization.[62] Violaceous discoloration, petechiae, and livedo reticularis appear when emboli occlude small vessels. Occlusion of digital vessels causes painful cyanotic toes (the blue toe syndrome), despite the presence of palpable pedal arteries [see Figure 5]. Embolic occlusion of intramuscular vessels causes pain and tenderness. Abnormal laboratory findings include an elevated eosinophil count and an increased erythrocyte sedimentation rate. Anemia, thrombocytopenia, and hypocomplementemia may also occur. Azotemia may occur if there is concurrent atheroembolism to the kidneys. Sites of shaggy atheroma may be identified by imaging the aorta with transesophageal echocardiography or MRA.[63] Confirmation of the diagnosis is made by skin or muscle biopsy. Tissue examination will reveal elongated needle-shaped clefts in small arteries that are associated with intimal thickening, perivascular fibrosis, inflammatory cells, and lipid-laden giant cells.

The risk of recurrence of atheroembolism is high. Platelet inhibitors have been used in this disorder, although it has not been established that these agents prevent recurrent atheroemboli. The role of warfarin is even less clear. Some investigators have found that warfarin reduces the likelihood of atheroembolism in patients with mobile atheromas, whereas others have suggested that warfarin may contribute to the development of atheroemboli in persons with a predisposition to the disease.[64-66] Surgical bypass of occluded vessels usually is not possible, because the emboli typically lodge in small distal arteries. If a proximal source, such as an aneurysm, is identified, bypass surgery and removal of the source from the circulation may reduce the risk of recurrence. Risk-factor modification—in particular, lipid-lowering therapy—can serve to stabilize atheromatous plaques and may reduce the risk of cardiovascular events; it is not known whether lipid-lowering therapy can prevent atheroembolism.[66]

Popliteal Artery Entrapment

Popliteal artery entrapment is caused by a congenital anomaly in which the medial head of the gastrocnemius muscle compresses or displaces the popliteal artery. In young patients who present with symptoms of intermittent claudication or rest pain, popliteal artery entrapment should be considered a possible diagnosis. It occurs more frequently in men than in women and is unilateral in two thirds of cases.[67]

The diagnosis is made by measuring ankle pressures before and after exercising the calf muscle, because contraction of the gastrocnemius muscle compresses the popliteal artery. Duplex ultrasonography can demonstrate popliteal artery compression and cessation of blood flow during gastrocnemius contraction. Angiography is used to confirm the diagnosis by delineating the altered course of the popliteal artery and may reveal a popliteal artery thrombus and poststenotic dilatation.

Popliteal artery entrapment should be treated surgically, preferably by relieving compression of the popliteal artery. Occasionally, thrombectomy or bypass grafting is required.

Thromboangiitis Obliterans

Thromboangiitis obliterans is a vasculitis that is also known as Buerger disease.[68] In the United States, the prevalence is approximately 1 per 10,000 population. It occurs throughout the world but is most prevalent in Asia, portions of Eastern Europe, and Israel. Thromboangiitis obliterans affects men primarily but may also occur in women. Onset of the disease usually occurs before

45 years of age. The most important predisposing factor is tobacco use.

Thromboangiitis obliterans affects small and middle-sized arteries and veins in the extremities. Inflammatory cells, particularly polymorphonuclear leukocytes, infiltrate the intima, media, and adventitia; thrombi typically occlude the lumen. Leukocytes and multinucleated giant cells may be found within or surrounding the thrombus. The internal elastic lamina and media remain intact.

Involvement of limb arteries causes forearm, calf, or foot claudication. Severe ischemia of the hand and foot causes rest pain, ulcerations, and skin necrosis. Raynaud phenomenon, which is indicative of digital artery obstruction, occurs in approximately 45% of patients. Migratory superficial vein thrombosis develops in approximately 40% of patients.

There are no specific serologic laboratory tests to diagnose thromboangiitis obliterans; however, serologic tests are used to exclude other causes of vasculitis. Serum immunologic markers such as antinuclear antibodies, rheumatoid factor, and antiphospholipid antibodies should not be present, and acute-phase reactants are usually normal. The diagnosis can be supported by arteriography, which reveals interspersed affected and normal segments of blood vessels. Collateral vessels circumventing sites of occlusion are often present. Biopsy of affected vessels should reveal the typical pathologic findings described above but is rarely indicated.

The most effective treatment for patients with thromboangiitis obliterans is smoking cessation. The risk of progression to critical limb ischemia and amputation is greater in patients who continue to smoke. Surgical revascularization is not usually an option because of involvement of small distal vessels. There is no established pharmacologic intervention. The use of vasodilator prostaglandins may be beneficial in some patients. Intramuscular administration of naked plasmid DNA encoding the 165 amino acid isoform of human vascular endothelial growth factor [phVEGF (165)] was reported to heal ulcers and relieve pain in some patients with thromboangiitis obliterans.[69] The efficacy of platelet inhibitors, anticoagulants, and thrombolytic therapy has not been established.

Raynaud Phenomenon

Raynaud phenomenon is episodic vasospastic ischemia of the digits. It is characterized by digital blanching, cyanosis, and rubor after exposure to cold and rewarming and can also be induced by emotional stress. Although many patients describe a triphasic color response, most experience only one or two color changes. The digital discoloration is confined primarily to the fingers or toes. Occasionally, the tongue, tip of the nose, or earlobes are affected. Blanching represents the ischemic phase of the phenomenon, caused by digital vasospasm. Cyanosis results from deoxygenated blood in capillaries and venules. With rewarming and resolution of the digital vasospasm, a hyperemic phase ensues, causing the digits to appear red.[70]

Raynaud phenomenon is categorized as primary or secondary [see Table 4]. The primary form of Raynaud phenomenon is also called Raynaud disease. Diagnostic criteria for Raynaud disease include episodic digital ischemia, absence of arterial occlusion, bilateral distribution, absence of symptoms or signs of other diseases that also cause Raynaud phenomenon, and duration of symptoms for 2 years or longer. Most people with Raynaud disease develop symptoms before they reach 40 years of

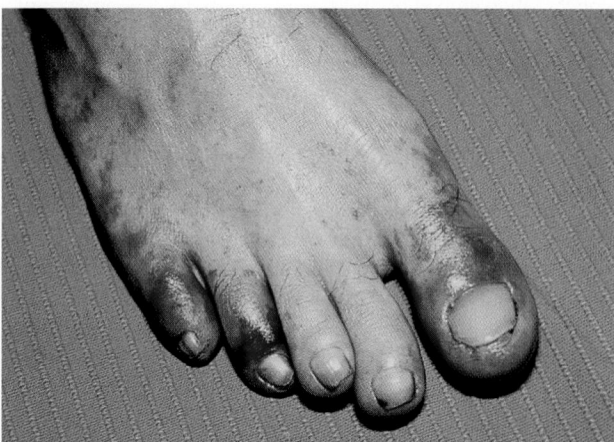

Figure 5 Ischemia of the toes of the right foot caused by atheroemboli. There is fixed violaceous discoloration of several toes and the lateral aspect of the right foot.

Table 4 Secondary Causes
of Raynaud Phenomenon

Connective tissue diseases
 Scleroderma
 Systemic lupus
  erythematosus
 Rheumatoid arthritis
 Dermatomyositis
 Mixed connective tissue
  disease
 Sjögren syndrome

Peripheral arterial occlusive
 diseases
 Atherosclerosis
 Thromboangiitis obliterans
 Thromboembolism
 Thoracic outlet syndrome

Neurologic disorders
 Carpal tunnel syndrome
 Reflex sympathetic dystrophy
 Stroke
 Intervertebral disk disease
 Spinal cord tumors
 Syringomyelia

Blood dyscrasias
 Hyperviscosity syndromes
 Myeloproliferative disorders

Cold agglutinin disease
Cryoglobulinemia

Trauma
 Thermal injury
  Frostbite
 Percussive injury
  Exposure to vibrating tools
  Hypothenar hammer
   syndrome

Drugs
 Antimetabolites
  Vinblastine
  Bleomycin
  Cisplatin
 Beta-adrenergic blockers
 Ergot alkaloids
  Ergotamine
  Bromocriptine
 Tricyclic antidepressants
  Imipramine
  Amphetamines

Miscellaneous conditions
 Primary pulmonary
  hypertension
 Hypothyroidism

age. It can occur in young children. Raynaud disease affects women three to five times more frequently than men. The prevalence is lower in warm climates than in cold climates.

ETIOLOGY

The mechanisms postulated to cause Raynaud phenomenon include increased sympathetic nervous system activity, heightened digital vascular reactivity to vasoconstrictive stimuli, circulating vasoactive hormones, and decreased intravascular pressure. The sympathetic nervous system mediates the digital vasoconstrictive response to cold exposure and emotional stress, but sympathetic nervous system activity has been discounted as a primary causal mechanism. Some investigators have suggested that increased sensitivity, increased numbers of postsynaptic alpha$_2$-adrenergic receptors, or both enhance the vasoconstrictive reactivity to sympathetic stimulation.[71] In some cases of Raynaud phenomenon, endogenous vasoactive substances (e.g., angiotensin II, serotonin, and thromboxane A$_2$) and exogenous vasoconstrictors (e.g., ergot alkaloids and sympathomimetic drugs) may cause digital vasospasm. Many patients with Raynaud phenomenon have low blood pressure. Decreased digital vascular pressure caused by proximal arterial occlusive disease or by digital vascular obstruction may increase the likelihood of digital vasospasm when vasoconstrictive stimuli occur.

DIAGNOSIS

Noninvasive vascular tests that are occasionally used to evaluate patients with Raynaud phenomenon include digital pulse volume recordings and measurement of digital systolic blood pressure and digital blood flow. Nail-fold capillary microscopy is normal in patients with Raynaud disease, whereas deformed capillary loops and avascular areas are present in patients with

connective tissue disorders or other conditions that cause digital vascular occlusion.[72] Determinations of the erythrocyte sedimentation rate and titers of antinuclear antibody, rheumatoid factor, cryoglobulins, and cold agglutinins are useful in excluding specific secondary causes of Raynaud phenomenon. Angiography is not necessary to diagnose Raynaud phenomenon but may be indicated in patients with persistent digital ischemia secondary to atherosclerosis, thromboembolism, or thromboangiitis obliterans to identify a cause that may be treated effectively with a revascularization procedure.

TREATMENT

Patients with Raynaud phenomenon should avoid unnecessary exposure to cold and should wear warm clothing. The hands, feet, trunk, and head should be kept warm to avoid reflex vasoconstriction. Pharmacologic intervention is indicated in patients who do not respond satisfactorily to conservative measures. Calcium channel blockers, such as nifedipine, and sympathetic nervous system inhibitors, such as prazosin and its longer-acting analogues, can be used to treat Raynaud phenomenon. Intravenous infusion of vasodilator prostaglandins, including PGE$_1$, PGI$_2$, and their analogues, has been reported to facilitate healing of digital ulcers in patients with scleroderma.[73] In patients with persistent severe digital ischemia, selective digital sympathectomy and microarteriolysis may facilitate ulcer healing and improve symptoms. Cervical and limb sympathectomy may also be considered in persons with severe Raynaud phenomenon, but long-term efficacy is not ensured.

Acrocyanosis

Raynaud phenomenon should be distinguished from acrocyanosis, a condition in which there is persistent bluish discoloration of the hands or feet.[74] Like Raynaud phenomenon, cyanotic discoloration intensifies during cold exposure, and rubor may appear with rewarming. Acrocyanosis affects both men and women; the age at onset is usually between 20 and 45 years. The prognosis of patients with idiopathic acrocyanosis is good, and loss of digital tissue is uncommon. Patients should avoid exposure to cold and should dress warmly. Pharmacologic intervention usually is not necessary. Alpha-adrenergic blocking agents and calcium channel blockers may be effective in some patients with acrocyanosis.

The author has received grant or research support from the Bristol-Myers Squibb–Sanofi-Aventis Partnership; he has served as a consultant for ARYx, Bristol-Myers Squibb–Sanofi-Aventis, Genzyme, Sigma Tau, Vasogen, and Wyeth; and he has participated in the speakers' bureau for Bristol-Myers Squibb–Sanofi-Aventis.

References

1. Dormandy JA, Rutherford RB: Management of peripheral arterial disease (PAD). TASC Working Group. J Vasc Surg 31:S1, 2000

2. Hirsch AT, Haskal ZJ, Hertzer NR, et al: ACC/AHA guidelines for the management of patients with peripheral arterial disease (lower extremity, renal, mesenteric, and abdominal aortic). J Am Coll Cardiol (in press)

3. Selvin E, Erlinger TP: Prevalence of and risk factors for peripheral arterial disease in the United States: results from the National Health and Nutrition Examination Survey, 1999–2000. Circulation 110:738, 2004

4. Diehm C, Schuster A, Allenberg JR, et al: High prevalence of peripheral arterial disease and co-morbidity in 6880 primary care patients: cross-sectional study. Atherosclerosis 172:95, 2004

5. Hirsch A, Criqui MH, Treat-Jacobson D, et al: Peripheral arterial disease detection, awareness, and treatment in primary care. JAMA 286:1317, 2001

6. Leng GC, Lee AJ, Fowkes FG, et al: Incidence, natural history and cardiovascular events in symptomatic and asymptomatic peripheral arterial disease in the general population. Int J Epidemiol 25:1172, 1996

7. Criqui M, Langer RD, Fronek A, et al: Mortality over a period of 10 years in patients with peripheral arterial disease. N Engl J Med 326:381, 1992

8. Dormandy J, Heeck L, Vig S: The fate of patients with critical leg ischemia. Semin Vasc Surg 12:142, 1999

9. Fowkes FG, Housley E, Riemersma RA, et al: Smoking, lipids, glucose intolerance, and blood pressure as risk factors for peripheral atherosclerosis compared with ischemic heart disease in the Edinburgh Artery Study. Am J Epidemiol 135:331, 1992

10. Murabito JM, D'Agostino RB, Silbershatz H, et al: Intermittent claudication: a risk profile from the Framingham Heart Study. Circulation 96:44, 1997

11. Hiatt WR, Hoag S, Hamman RF: Effect of diagnostic criteria on the prevalence of peripheral arterial disease. The San Luis Valley Diabetes Study. Circulation 91:1472, 1995

12. Diabetes-related amputations of lower extremities in the Medicare population—Minnesota, 1993–1995. MMWR Morb Mortal Wkly Rep 47:649, 1998

13. Graham IM, Daly LE, Refsum HM, et al: Plasma homocysteine as a risk factor for vascular disease. The European Concerted Action Project. JAMA 277:1775, 1997

14. Ridker PM, Stampfer MJ, Rifai N: Novel risk factors for systemic atherosclerosis: a comparison of C-reactive protein, fibrinogen, homocysteine, lipoprotein(a), and standard cholesterol screening as predictors of peripheral arterial disease. JAMA 285:2481, 2001

15. Pradhan AD, Rifai N, Ridker PM: Soluble intercellular adhesion molecule–1, soluble vascular adhesion molecule–1, and the development of symptomatic peripheral arterial disease in men. Circulation 106:820, 2002

16. McDermott MM, Greenland P, Liu K, et al: Leg symptoms in peripheral arterial disease: associated clinical characteristics and functional impairment. JAMA 286:1599, 2001

17. Rutherford RB, Baker JD, Ernst C, et al: Recommended standards for reports dealing with lower extremity ischemia: revised version. J Vasc Surg 26:517, 1997

18. McDermott MM, Greenland P, Liu K, et al: The ankle brachial index is associated with leg function and physical activity: the Walking and Leg Circulation Study. Ann Intern Med 136:873, 2002

19. Newman AB, Siscovick DS, Manolio TA, et al: Ankle-arm index as a marker of atherosclerosis in the Cardiovascular Health Study. Cardiovascular Heart Study (CHS) Collaborative Research Group. Circulation 88:837, 1993

20. Leng GC, Fowkes FG, Lee AJ, et al: Use of ankle brachial pressure index to predict cardiovascular events and death: a cohort study. BMJ 313:1440, 1996

21. Koelemay MJ, Lijmer JG, Stoker J, et al: Magnetic resonance angiography for the evaluation of lower extremity arterial disease: a meta-analysis. JAMA 285:1338, 2001

22. Hiatt WR: Medical treatment of peripheral arterial disease and claudication. N Engl J Med 344:1608, 2001

23. Collaborative meta-analysis of randomised trials of antiplatelet therapy for prevention of death, myocardial infarction, and stroke in high risk patients. Antiplatelet Trialists' Collaboration. BMJ 324:21, 2002

24. Mondillo S, Ballo P, Barbati R, et al: Effects of simvastatin on walking performance and symptoms of intermittent claudication in hypercholesterolemic patients with peripheral vascular disease. Am J Med 114:359, 2003

25. Mohler ER 3rd, Hiatt WR, Creager MA: Cholesterol reduction with atorvastatin improves walking distance in patients with peripheral arterial disease. Circulation 108:1481, 2003

26. Schillinger M, Exner M, Mlekusch W, et al: Statin therapy improves cardiovascular outcome of patients with peripheral artery disease. Eur Heart J 25:742, 2004

27. MRC/BHF Heart Protection Study of cholesterol lowering with simvastatin in 20,536 high-risk individuals: a randomised placebo-controlled trial. Lancet 360:7, 2002

28. Mehler PS, Coll JR, Estacio R, et al: Intensive blood pressure control reduces the risk of cardiovascular events in patients with peripheral arterial disease and type 2 diabetes. Circulation 107:753, 2003

29. Yusuf S, Sleight P, Pogue J, et al: Effects of an angiotensin-converting-enzyme inhibitor, ramipril, on cardiovascular events in high-risk patients. The Heart Outcomes Prevention Evaluation Study Investigators. N Engl J Med 342:145, 2000

30. Radack K, Deck C: Beta-adrenergic blocker therapy does not worsen intermittent claudication in subjects with peripheral arterial disease: a meta-analysis of randomized controlled trials. Arch Intern Med 151:1769, 1991

31. Intensive blood-glucose control with sulphonylureas or insulin compared with conventional treatment and risk of complications in patients with type 2 diabetes (UKPDS 33). UK Prospective Diabetes Study (UKPDS) Group. Lancet 352:837, 1998

32. Goldhaber SZ, Manson JE, Stampfer MJ, et al: Low-dose aspirin and subsequent peripheral arterial surgery in the Physicians' Health Study. Lancet 340:143, 1992

33. Collaborative overview of randomised trials of antiplatelet therapy. II: Maintenance of vascular graft or arterial patency by antiplatelet therapy. Antiplatelet Trialists' Collaboration. BMJ 308:159, 1994

34. Clagett GP, Sobel M, Jackson MR, et al: Antithrombotic therapy in peripheral arterial occlusive disease: the Seventh ACCP Conference on Antithrombotic and Thrombolytic Therapy. Chest 126(3 suppl):609S, 2004

35. A randomised, blinded trial of clopidogrel versus aspirin in patients at risk of ischaemic events (CAPRIE). CAPRIE Steering Committee. Lancet 348:1329, 1996

36. Gardner AW, Poehlman ET: Exercise rehabilitation programs for the treatment of claudication pain: a meta-analysis. JAMA 274:975, 1995

37. Stewart KJ, Hiatt WR, Regensteiner JG, et al: Exercise training for claudication. N Engl J Med 347:1941, 2002

38. Lindgarde F, Labs KH, Rossner M: The pentoxifylline experience: exercise testing reconsidered. Vasc Med 1:145, 1996

39. Beebe HG, Dawson DL, Cutler BS, et al: A new pharmacological treatment for intermittent claudication: results of a randomized, multicenter trial. Arch Intern Med 159:2041, 1999

40. Dawson DL, Cutler BS, Hiatt WR, et al: A comparison of cilostazol and pentoxifylline for treating intermittent claudication. Am J Med 109:523, 2000

41. Thompson PD, Zimet R, Forbes WP, et al: Meta-analysis of results from eight randomized, placebo-controlled trials on the effect of cilostazol on patients with intermittent claudication. Am J Cardiol 90:1314, 2002

42. Regensteiner J, Ware JE Jr, McCarthy WJ, et al: Effect of cilostazol on treadmill walking, community-based walking ability, and health-related quality of life in patients with intermittent claudication due to peripheral arterial disease: meta-analysis of six randomized controlled trials. J Am Geriatr Soc 50:1939, 2002

43. van Rij AM, Solomon C, Packer SG, et al: Chelation therapy for intermittent claudication: a double-blind, randomized, controlled trial. Circulation 90:1194, 1994

44. Brevetti G, Diehm C, Lambert D: European multicenter study on propionyl-L-carnitine in intermittent claudication. J Am Coll Cardiol 34:1618, 1999

45. Hiatt WR, Regensteiner JG, Creager MA, et al: Propionyl-L-carnitine improves exercise performance and functional status in patients with claudication. Am J Med 110:616, 2001

46. Boger RH, Bode-Boger SM, Thiele W, et al: Restoring vascular nitric oxide formation by L-arginine improves the symptoms of intermittent claudication in patients with peripheral arterial occlusive disease. J Am Coll Cardiol 32:1336, 1998

47. Lievre M, Morand S, Besse B, et al: Oral beraprost sodium, a prostaglandin I(2) analogue, for intermittent claudication: a double-blind, randomized, multicenter controlled trial. Beraprost et Claudication Intermittente (BERCI) Research Group. Circulation 102:426, 2000

48. Mohler ER 3rd, Hiatt WR, Olin JW, et al: Treatment of intermittent claudication with beraprost sodium, an orally active prostaglandin I2 analogue: a double-blinded, randomized, controlled trial. J Am Coll Cardiol 41:1679, 2003

49. Lederman RJ, Mendelsohn FO, Anderson RD, et al: Therapeutic angiogenesis with recombinant fibroblast growth factor–2 for intermittent claudication (the TRAFFIC study): a randomised trial. Lancet 359:2053, 2002

50. Rajagopalan S, Mohler ER 3rd, Lederman RJ, et al: Regional angiogenesis with vascular endothelial growth factor in peripheral arterial disease: a phase II randomized, double-blind, controlled study of adenoviral delivery of vascular endothelial growth factor 121 in patients with disabling intermittent claudication. Circulation 108:1933, 2003

51. Tateishi-Yuyama E, Matsubara H, Murohara T, et al: Therapeutic angiogenesis for patients with limb ischaemia by autologous transplantation of bone-marrow cells: a pilot study and a randomised controlled trial. Lancet 360:427, 2002

52. Kandarpa K, Becker GJ, Hunink MG, et al: Transcatheter interventions for the treatment of peripheral atherosclerotic lesions: part I. J Vasc Interv Radiol 12:683, 2001

53. Kanani RS, Garasic JM: Lower extremity arterial occlusive disease: role of percutaneous revascularization. Curr Treat Options Cardiovasc Med 7:99, 2005

54. Hunink MG, Wong JB, Donaldson MC, et al: Revascularization for femoropopliteal disease: a decision and cost-effectiveness analysis. JAMA 274:165, 1995

55. Bosch JL, Hunink MG: Meta-analysis of the results of percutaneous transluminal angioplasty and stent placement for aortoiliac occlusive disease. Radiology 204:87, 1997

56. Tetteroo E, van der Graaf Y, Bosch JL, et al: Randomised comparison of primary stent placement versus primary angioplasty followed by selective stent placement in patients with iliac-artery occlusive disease. Dutch Iliac Stent Trial Study Group. Lancet 351:1153, 1998

57. de Vries SO, Hunink MG: Results of aortic bifurcation grafts for aortoiliac occlusive disease: a meta-analysis. J Vasc Surg 26:558, 1997

58. Belkin M, Knox J, Donaldson MC, et al: Infrainguinal arterial reconstruction with nonreversed greater saphenous vein. J Vasc Surg 24:957, 1996

59. Abbott WM, Green RM, Matsumoto T, et al: Prosthetic above-knee femoropopliteal bypass grafting: results of a multicenter randomized prospective trial. Above-Knee Femoropopliteal Study Group. J Vasc Surg 25:19, 1997

60. Ouriel K, Veith FJ, Sasahara AA: A comparison of recombinant urokinase with vascular surgery as initial treatment for acute arterial occlusion of the legs. Thrombolysis or Peripheral Arterial Surgery (TOPAS) Investigators. N Engl J Med 338:1105, 1998

61. Results of a prospective randomized trial evaluating surgery versus thrombolysis for ischemia of the lower extremity. The STILE trial. Ann Surg 220:251, 1994

62. Fukumoto Y, Tsutsui H, Tsuchihashi M, et al: The incidence and risk factors of cholesterol embolization syndrome, a complication of cardiac catheterization: a prospective study. J Am Coll Cardiol 42:211, 2003

63. Atherosclerotic disease of the aortic arch as a risk factor for recurrent ischemic stroke. The French Study of Aortic Plaques in Stroke Group. N Engl J Med 334:1216, 1996

64. Transesophageal echocardiographic correlates of thromboembolism in high-risk patients with nonvalvular atrial fibrillation. The Stroke Prevention in Atrial Fibrillation Investigators Committee on Echocardiography. Ann Intern Med 128:639, 1998

65. Ferrari E, Vidal R, Chevallier T, et al: Atherosclerosis of the thoracic aorta and aortic debris as a marker of poor prognosis: benefit of oral anticoagulants. J Am Coll Cardiol 33:1317, 1999

66. Tunick PA, Kronzon I: Embolism from the aorta: atheroemboli and thromboemboli. Curr Treat Options Cardiovasc Med 3:181, 2001

67. Persky JM, Kempczinski RF, Fowl RJ: Entrapment of the popliteal artery. Surg Gynecol Obstet 173:84, 1991

68. Olin JW: Thromboangiitis obliterans (Buerger's disease). N Engl J Med 343:864, 2000

69. Isner JM, Baumgartner I, Rauh G, et al: Treatment of thromboangiitis obliterans (Buerger's disease) by intramuscular gene transfer of vascular endothelial growth factor: preliminary clinical results. J Vasc Surg 28:964, 1998

70. Wigley FM: Clinical practice. Raynaud's phenomenon. N Engl J Med 347:1001, 2002

71. Freedman RR, Baer RP, Mayes MD: Blockade of vasospastic attacks by alpha 2-adrenergic but not alpha 1-adrenergic antagonists in idiopathic Raynaud's disease. Circulation 92:1448, 1995

72. Anderson ME, Allen PD, Moore T, et al: Computerized nailfold video capillaroscopy: a new tool for assessment of Raynaud's phenomenon. J Rheumatol 32:841, 2005

73. Wigley FM, Wise RA, Seibold JR, et al: Intravenous iloprost infusion in patients with Raynaud phenomenon secondary to systemic sclerosis: a multicenter, placebo-controlled, double-blind study. Ann Intern Med 120:199, 1994

74. Nousari HC, Kimyai-Asadi A, Anhalt GJ: Chronic idiopathic acrocyanosis. J Am Acad Dermatol 45(6 suppl):S207, 2001

75. Rutherford RB: Standards for evaluating results of interventional therapy for peripheral vascular disease. Circulation 83(suppl I):1-6, 1991

32 Venous Thromboembolism

Clive Kearon, M.B., PH.D., and Jack Hirsh, M.D., F.A.C.P.

Venous thromboembolism (VTE), a term that encompasses both deep vein thrombosis (DVT) and pulmonary embolism (PE), is a leading cause of morbidity and mortality in hospitalized and nonhospitalized patients.[1-3]

Risk Factors and Etiology

Most patients with VTE have one or more clinical risk factors. The most common risk factors in hospitalized patients are recent surgery, previous VTE, trauma, and immobility, as well as serious illness, including malignancy, chronic heart failure, stroke, chronic lung disease, acute infections, and inflammatory bowel disease.[2,4] The common risk factors in outpatients include hospital admission within the past 3 months, malignancy, previous VTE, cancer chemotherapy, estrogen therapy, presence of an antiphospholipid antibody, and familial thrombophilia.[2,3,5] Less common risk factors are paroxysmal nocturnal hemoglobinuria, nephrotic syndrome, and polycythemia vera.

Classification

Although venous thrombosis can occur in any vein in the body, it usually involves superficial or deep veins of the legs. Thrombosis in a superficial vein of the leg is generally benign and self-limiting but can be serious if it extends from the long saphenous vein into the common femoral vein. Superficial thrombophlebitis is recognized by the presence of a tender vein surrounded by an area of erythema, heat, and edema. A thrombus can often be palpated in the affected vein. Superficial thrombophlebitis may be associated with DVT, which typically is clinically silent. Thrombosis involving the deep veins of the leg may be confined to calf veins or may extend into the popliteal or more proximal veins. Thrombi confined to calf veins are usually small, often asymptomatic, and are rarely associated with symptomatic PE. About 25% of calf vein thrombi, however, extend into the popliteal vein and beyond, where they can cause serious complications.[6] About 50% of patients with symptomatic proximal vein thrombosis also have clinically silent PE, and about 70% of patients with symptomatic PE have DVT, which is usually clinically silent.

Pulmonary embolism is the most serious and most feared complication of venous thrombosis, but the postthrombotic syndrome is responsible for greater morbidity. The postthrombotic syndrome occurs as a long-term complication in about 25% (and is severe in about 10%) of patients with symptomatic proximal vein thrombosis, with most cases developing within 2 years of the acute event.[4,7] Clinically, the postthrombotic syndrome typically presents as chronic leg pain that is associated with edema and worsens at the end of the day. Some patients also have stasis pigmentation, induration, and skin ulceration; a smaller number of patients have venous claudication on walking, caused by persistent obstruction of the iliac veins. In some cases, the onset of symptoms can be rapid and may mimic recurrent acute venous thrombosis.

Pathophysiology

Venous thrombi are composed predominantly of fibrin and red blood cells.[8] They usually arise at sites of vessel damage, the large venous sinuses of the calves, or the valve cusp pockets in the deep veins of the calves. Thrombosis occurs when blood coagulation overwhelms the natural anticoagulant mechanisms and the fibrinolytic system. Coagulation is usually triggered when blood is exposed to tissue factor on the surface of activated monocytes that are attracted to sites of tissue damage or vascular trauma. Clinical risk factors that activate blood coagulation include extensive surgery, trauma, burns, malignant disease, myocardial infarction, cancer chemotherapy, and local hypoxia produced by venous stasis. Malignant cells are rich in tissue factor that activates factor VII and initiates blood coagulation. Venous stasis and damage to the vessel wall increase the thrombogenic effect of blood coagulation. Venous stasis is produced by immobility, obstruction or dilatation of veins, increased venous pressure, and increased blood viscosity. The critical role of stasis in the pathogenesis of venous thrombosis is exemplified by the observation that thrombosis occurs with equal frequency in the two legs in paraplegic patients but occurs with much greater frequency in the paralyzed limb than in the nonparalyzed limb in stroke patients.[8]

Tissue damage also results in impaired fibrinolysis, triggered by the release of inflammatory cytokines in response to the damage. These cytokines induce endothelial cell synthesis of plasminogen activator inhibitor-1 (PAI-1). In addition, they reduce the protective effect of the vascular endothelium by downregulating the endothelial-bound anticoagulant thrombomodulin.

Increased central venous pressure, which produces venous stasis in the extremities, may explain the high incidence of VTE in patients with heart failure. Stasis resulting from venous dilatation occurs in elderly patients, in patients with varicose veins, and in women who are pregnant or using supplemental estrogen, and may contribute to the increased incidence of thrombosis in these persons. Venous obstruction contributes to the risk of venous thrombosis in patients with pelvic tumors. Increased blood viscosity, which also causes stasis, may explain the risk of thrombosis in patients with polycythemia vera, hypergammaglobulinemia, or chronic inflammatory disorders. Direct venous damage may lead to venous thrombosis in patients undergoing hip surgery, knee surgery, or varicose vein stripping and in patients with severe burns or trauma to the lower extremities.

Blood coagulation is modulated by circulating inhibitors or by endothelial cell–bound inhibitors. The most important circulating inhibitors of coagulation are antithrombin, protein C, and protein S.[9,10] An inherited deficiency of one of these three proteins is found in about 20% of patients who have a family history of VTE and whose first episode of VTE occurs before 41 years of age.[11] Some types of congenital dysfibrinogenemias can also predispose to thrombosis, as can a congenital deficiency of plasminogen. An inherited thrombophilic defect known as activated protein C (APC) resistance, or factor V Leiden, is the most common cause of inherited thrombophilia. It occurs in about 5% of whites who do not have a family history of VTE and in about 20% of patients with a first episode of VTE.[12,13] The second most common thrombophilic defect is a mutation (G20210A) in the 3' untranslated region of the prothrombin gene that results in about a 25% increase in prothrombin levels.[14] This mutation is found in about 2% of whites who have no family history of VTE and in about 5% of patients with a first episode of VTE. Elevated levels of clotting factors VIII and XI also predispose patients to thrombosis. The risk of thrombosis in patients with thrombophilic defects is increased through the use of estrogen-containing oral contraceptives.[15] Randomized trials have shown that the administration of estrogens in the doses used for postmenopausal hormone replacement therapy increases the risk of a first or recurrent thromboembolism about threefold, with the highest risk occurring within the first six months of starting therapy.[16-18]

Natural History and Prognosis

Most venous thrombi produce no symptoms and are confined to the intramuscular and deep veins of the calf. Many calf-vein thrombi undergo spontaneous lysis, but some extend into the popliteal and more proximal veins.[6] Complete lysis of proximal vein thrombi is less common. Most symptomatic pulmonary emboli and virtually all fatal emboli arise from thrombi in the proximal veins of the legs. Extensive venous thrombosis causes local valvular damage, which is thought to lead to the postthrombotic syndrome.[7] Patients with a history of VTE are more likely to experience additional episodes, particularly if they are exposed to high-risk situations.[2,6]

Untreated or inadequately treated VTE is associated with a high rate of complications. About 25% of untreated calf-vein thrombi extend into the popliteal vein, and about 50% of untreated proximal-vein thrombi also undergo extension. Patients with proximal-vein thrombosis who are inadequately treated have a recurrence rate of about 40%,[19] and patients with symptomatic calf-vein thrombosis treated with a 5-day course of intermittent intravenous heparin without continuation of oral anticoagulant therapy had a recurrence rate greater than 20% over the following 3 months.[20]

Table 1 Model for Determining Clinical Suspicion of Deep Vein Thrombosis[47]

Variables	Points*
Active cancer (treatment ongoing or within previous 6 months or palliative)	1
Paralysis, paresis, or recent plaster immobilization of the lower extremities	1
Recently bedridden for more than 3 days, or major surgery within the past 4 weeks	1
Localized tenderness along the distribution of the deep venous system	1
Entire leg swollen	1
Affected calf 3 cm greater than asymptomatic calf (measured 10 cm below tibial tuberosity)	1
Pitting edema confined to the symptomatic leg	1
Dilated superficial veins (nonvaricose)	1
Alternative diagnosis is at least as likely as that of DVT	-2
Total points	

*Pretest probability is calculated as follows: total points ≤ 0, low probability; 1 to 2, moderate probability; ≥ 3, high probability.
DVT—deep vein thrombosis

Complications can be markedly decreased by adequate anticoagulant therapy. Fewer than 3% of patients who have proximal-vein thrombosis experience a clinically detectable recurrence during the initial period of treatment with high-dose heparin or low molecular weight heparin (LMWH), and fewer than 3% of patients experience a recurrence during the subsequent 3 months if they are receiving oral anticoagulant therapy or moderate-dose subcutaneous heparin therapy.[21] After 3 months of anticoagulant therapy, patients have a risk of recurrence of about 3% in the first year after stopping treatment if their thrombosis developed after a reversible provocation, such as surgery; the recurrence risk is as high as 15% in the first year if the thrombosis was unprovoked or was associated with ongoing conditions, such as prolonged immobilization or cancer.[6,13,22-27] The recurrence rate is significantly higher after a 4- or 6-week course of warfarin treatment, compared with a 3- or 6-month course.[23,25,28] Additional risk factors for recurrent VTE include proximal versus isolated distal thrombosis; an antiphospholipid antibody; and male gender.[6,29,30] Hereditary thrombophilias appear to be weak risk factors for recurrent VTE.[13,22,31-33]

Diagnosis

DEEP VENOUS THROMBOSIS

Clinical Features

The clinical features of DVT, such as localized swelling, redness, tenderness, and distal edema, are nonspecific, and the diagnosis should always be confirmed by objective tests.

About 85% of ambulatory patients with clinically suspected DVT have another cause for their symptoms. The conditions that are most likely to simulate DVT are ruptured Baker cyst, cellulitis, muscle tear, muscle cramp, muscle hematoma, external venous compression, superficial thrombophlebitis, and the postthrombotic syndrome. Of the patients who actually have DVT, about 85% have proximal vein thrombosis; for the rest, thrombosis is confined to the calf.[6,34]

Although clinical features cannot unequivocally confirm or exclude a diagnosis of DVT, clinical assessment can stratify the probability of DVT as high (prevalence of thrombosis ~ 60%), intermediate (prevalence ~ 25%), or low (prevalence ~ 5%) on the basis of the following: (1) the presence or absence of risk factors (e.g., recent immobilization, hospitalization within the past month, or malignancy); (2) whether the clinical manifestations at presentation are typical or atypical, and their severity; and (3) whether there is an alternative explanation for the symptoms that is at least as likely as DVT [*see Table 1*].[35]

Diagnostic Testing

Four objective tests have been well validated for the diagnosis of DVT: venography, impedance plethysmography (now rarely used), venous ultrasonography, and D-dimer testing.[34,36] Magnetic resonance imaging and computed tomography also appear to be accurate tests, but they have not been as thoroughly evaluated.

Venography Venography, which involves the injection of a radiocontrast agent into a distal vein, is the reference standard for the diagnosis of DVT [*see Figure 1*]. Venography detects both proximal-vein thrombosis and calf-vein thrombosis. However, this test is technically difficult and expensive, can be

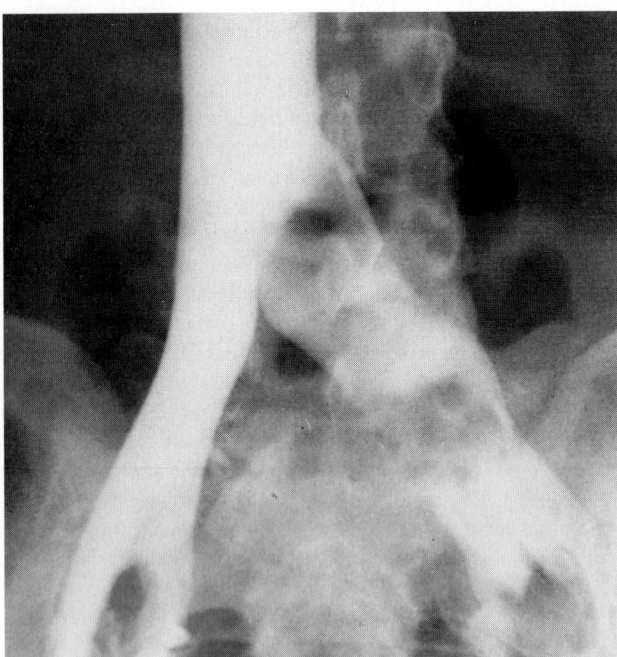

Figure 1 **Filling defects in the left iliac vein, apparent in this venogram, reveal the presence of thrombi.**

painful, and requires injection of radiographic contrast, which can cause allergic reactions or renal impairment. For these reasons, venography is usually reserved for resolution of any discrepancies between the findings on venous ultrasonography and the clinical assessment of the probability of DVT, or when venous ultrasonography is nondiagnostic (as often occurs in patients with a history of DVT).

Venous ultrasonography Venous ultrasonography is the noninvasive imaging method of choice for diagnosing DVT.[34] It is not painful and is easy to perform. The common femoral vein, superficial femoral vein, popliteal vein, and calf-vein trifurcation (i.e., very proximal deep-calf veins) are imaged in real time and compressed with the transducer probe. Inability to fully compress or obliterate the vein is diagnostic of DVT. Duplex ultrasonography, which combines real-time imaging with pulsed Doppler and color-coded Doppler technology, facilitates the identification of veins.

Venous ultrasonography is highly accurate for the detection of proximal-vein thrombosis in symptomatic patients, with reported sensitivity and specificity approaching 95%. The sensitivity for symptomatic calf-vein thrombosis is considerably lower and appears to be highly operator dependent. For this reason, many centers do not examine the deep veins of the calf with ultrasonography. Instead, if an initial test result excludes proximal DVT and clinical assessment for DVT is moderate or high, the test is repeated in 7 days to detect the small number of calf-vein thrombi that extend to the proximal veins after the initial presentation. If the test remains negative after 7 days, the risk that a thrombus is present and will subsequently extend to the proximal veins is negligible, and it is safe to withhold treatment.[34]

Ultrasonography is accurate when its results are concordant with clinical assessment; its accuracy drops if the results of these two assessments do not agree. Therefore, if the clinical suspicion for DVT is low and the ultrasound shows a localized abnormali-

ty (i.e., less convincing findings), or if clinical suspicion is high and the ultrasound is normal, venography should be considered. In about one quarter of such cases, the results of venography differ from those of the ultrasound. Because the prevalence of DVT is only about 2% (most of which is distal), a follow-up test is not necessary when the clinical suspicion of thrombosis is low and the result of an initial proximal venous ultrasound scan is normal [*see Table 2*]. In asymptomatic patients who have had elective hip or knee replacement, the sensitivity of ultrasonography for proximal DVT is only about 60%[34]; such screening is not recommended.

D-dimer blood testing D-dimer is formed when cross-linked fibrin in thrombi is broken down by plasmin; thus, low levels of D-dimer can be used to exclude DVT and PE. A variety of D-dimer assays are available, and they vary markedly in their accuracy as diagnostic tests for venous thromboembolism.[36,37]

All D-dimer assays have low specificity for DVT; an abnormal result is associated with a low positive predictive value and cannot be used to diagnose DVT. D-dimer assays that are used for the diagnosis of VTE can be divided into two groups on the basis of their sensitivity and specificity. Very highly sensitive D-dimer assays (e.g., sensitivity ≥ 98%; specificity ~ 40%) have a sufficiently high negative predictive value (≥ 98%) that a normal result can be used to exclude VTE without the need to perform additional diagnostic testing.[36-38] By contrast, a negative result on one of the moderate to highly sensitive D-dimer assays (sensitivity 85% to 97%; specificity 50% to 70%) needs to be combined with another assessment that identifies patients as having a lower likelihood of VTE in order to exclude DVT or PE. Management studies have shown that it is safe to withhold anticoagulant therapy and not necessary to repeat testing after 1 week to detect extending DVT in patients who have a normal result on a moderately sensitive D-dimer test in combination with (1) a low clinical suspicion for DVT or (2) a normal result on venous ultrasonography of the proximal veins [*see Table 2*].[36,37,39,40] D-dimer testing is much less specific and, therefore, has less clinical utility (i.e., fewer negative tests among those without venous thrombosis) in postoperative and hospitalized patients and the elderly. Also, D-dimer testing has less clinical utility in patients in whom there is a high clinical suspicion of VTE, because negative results are rarely obtained and because the predictive value of a negative test is lower in this group—both factors attributable to the high prevalence of disease in such cases.

RECURRENT DEEP VENOUS THROMBOSIS

The diagnosis of acute recurrent DVT can be difficult.[34] A negative D-dimer test can exclude recurrent DVT, although the safety of this approach in recurrent disease has been less well evaluated than for first episodes of DVT.[41] If D-dimer testing is positive, or has not been done, venous ultrasonography is performed. If the result is normal, the test should be repeated twice over the next 7 to 10 days. If the result on retesting is positive in the popliteal or common femoral vein segments and the result of the previous test was negative at the same site, a recurrence is diagnosed. Recurrence can also be diagnosed if venous ultrasonography shows other convincing evidence of more extensive thrombosis than was seen on previous examination (e.g., an increase in thrombus diameter of > 4 mm at the inguinal ligament or the midpopliteal fossa; or an unequivocal extension within the femoral vein of the thigh).[34,42]

Table 2   Test Results That Effectively Confirm or Exclude Deep Vein Thrombosis

Purpose	Test	Significant Result
Diagnostic for first DVT	Venography	Intraluminal filling defect
	Venous ultrasonography	Noncompressible proximal veins at two or more of the common femoral, popliteal, and calf trifurcation sites*
Excludes first DVT	Venography	All deep veins seen, and no intraluminal filling defects
	D-dimer	Normal value on a test that has at least a moderately high sensitivity (≥ 85%) and specificity (≥ 70%) and (1) normal results on venous ultrasonography of the proximal veins or (2) low clinical suspicion of DVT at presentation Negative result on a test that has a high sensitivity (≥ 98%)
	Venous ultrasonography	Normal proximal veins and (1) low clinical suspicion for DVT at presentation, (2) normal D-dimer test at presentation, or (3) normal second test after 7 days Normal proximal and distal veins*
Diagnostic for recurrent DVT	Venography	Intraluminal filling defect
	Venous ultrasonography	(1) A new noncompressible common femoral or popliteal vein segment or (2) a ≥ 4.0 mm increase in diameter of the common femoral or popliteal vein since a previous test†
Excludes recurrent DVT	Venography	All deep veins seen and no intraluminal filling defects
	Venous ultrasonography	Normal or ≤ 1 mm increase in diameter of the common femoral or popliteal veins on venous ultrasound since a previous test and continuing normal results (no progression on venous ultrasound) at 2 and 7 days
	D-dimer	Results as described as for a first episode of DVT; however, these criteria are less well evaluated for diagnosis of recurrence

*The diagnostic accuracy of isolated distal vein abnormalities that are detected on ultrasound—and the need to treat such abnormalities— is uncertain. For this reason, and because examination of the calf veins is difficult to perform, many centers confine the examination to the proximal veins.

†If other evidence is not consistent with recurrent DVT (e.g., clinical assessment or D-dimer), venography should be considered.

DVT—deep vein thrombosis

If findings on venous ultrasonography are equivocal, as compared with a previous scan, or a previous scan is not available for comparison, either venography should be performed or the ultrasound examination repeated twice over the next 7 to 10 days to detect extension of thrombosis. If the venogram shows a new intraluminal filling defect or evidence of thrombus extension since a previous venogram, recurrent DVT is diagnosed. If the venogram outlines all of the deep veins and does not show an intraluminal filling defect, recurrent DVT is excluded. If the venogram is nondiagnostic (i.e., nonfilling of segments of the deep veins), the patient can be followed with repeat venous ultrasonography (as described above), or recurrent DVT can be diagnosed on the basis of the results of all assessments, including clinical features [see Table 2].

PULMONARY EMBOLISM

Clinical Features

Dyspnea is the most common symptom of PE. Chest pain is also common; it is usually pleuritic but can be substernal and compressive. Tachycardia is relatively common, while hemoptysis is less frequent. Although most patients with PE also have DVT, fewer than 25% have clinical features of thrombosis.[43-45] However, the clinical features of PE, like those of DVT, are nonspecific, and in only about one quarter of symptomatic patients is the diagnosis confirmed by objective tests.

In the past, clinical assessment of the probability of PE was not standardized; physicians made the assessment informally on the basis of their experience and the results of initial routine tests (e.g., chest x-ray and electrocardiogram).[43,45] Two groups have published explicit criteria for determining the clinical probability of PE.[46-49] The model created by Wells and colleagues incorporates an assessment of symptoms and signs, the presence of an alternative diagnosis to account for the patient's condition, and the presence of risk factors for VTE.[47-49] Using this model, it is possible to categorize the clinical probability of PE in a particular patient as low or unlikely (prevalence < 10%), moderate (prevalence ~ 25%), or high (prevalence of 60%) [see Table 3].[47-49]

Diagnostic Tests

Chest radiography and electrocardiography   In patients with PE, chest x-rays show either normal or nonspecific findings. Chest radiography, however, is useful for exclusion of pneumothorax and other conditions that can simulate PE. The ECG also frequently shows normal or nonspecific findings, but it is valuable for excluding acute myocardial infarction. In the appropriate clinical setting, ECG evidence of right ventricular strain suggests PE.

Ventilation-perfusion lung scanning   In the past, ventilation-perfusion lung scanning was the most important test for diagnosing PE [see Figure 2].[43] More recently, however, computed tomographic pulmonary angiography (CTPA) has supplanted lung scanning, although lung scanning is still used, particularly when CTPA is contraindicated because of renal failure or associated radiation exposure to the chest (e.g., in young women). A normal perfusion scan excludes a diagnosis of PE. However, a normal result is obtained in only about 25% of consecutive patients (this percentage is higher in patients who are young, who do not have chronic lung disease, or who have an abnormal chest radiograph at presentation). An abnormal perfusion scan is nonspecific [see Table 4].

Table 3 Model for Determining a Clinical Suspicion of Pulmonary Embolism[47]

Variables	Points*
Clinical signs and symptoms of deep vein thrombosis (minimum leg swelling and pain with palpation of the deep veins)	3.0
An alternative diagnosis is less likely than pulmonary embolism	3.0
Heart rate > 100 beats/min	1.5
Immobilization or surgery in the previous 4 weeks	1.5
Previous deep vein thrombosis/pulmonary embolism	1.5
Hemoptysis	1.0
Malignancy (treatment ongoing or within previous 6 months or palliative)	1.0
Total points	

*Pretest probability is calculated as follows: a total score of ≤ 4 indicates a low probability (also termed "unlikely"); a score of 4.5 to 6 indicates moderate probability; and a score of > 6 indicates high probability.

Ventilation imaging improves the specificity of perfusion scanning for the diagnosis of PE, particularly when the ventilation scan is normal at the site of a large or segmental perfusion defect, a finding that is associated with an 85% or higher likelihood of PE (termed a high-probability lung scan).[43] About half of patients who have PE have a high-probability lung scan. Therefore, among consecutive patients who are investigated for PE, about 25% have a normal perfusion scan and can have the diagnosis excluded, about 15% have a high-probability scan and can be diagnosed with PE (provided the clinical probability is not low), and about 60% have an abnormal but nondiagnostic lung scan that requires further diagnostic testing.[43]

Computed tomographic pulmonary angiography Computed tomographic pulmonary angiography (CTPA), performed using helical CT (also known as spiral or continuous-volume CT), can directly visualize the pulmonary arteries [*see Figure 3*]. Helical CT technology has rapidly advanced from the use of single-detector scanners to the use of progressively larger numbers of detectors (termed multidetector CT) that allow more detailed examination of the pulmonary arteries.

Current evidence from the PIOPED II study suggests that CTPA is nondiagnostic in 6% of patients, and that among adequate examinations, the sensitivity for PE is 83%, specificity is 96%, positive predictive value is 86%, and negative predictive value is 95%.[50] Accuracy varies according to the size of the largest pulmonary artery involved: the positive predictive value was 97% for pulmonary emboli in the main or lobar artery, 68% for emboli in segmental arteries, and 25% for those in subsegmental arteries (4% of pulmonary emboli in this study). Predictive values were also influenced by clinical assessment of the probability of PE. The positive predictive value of CTPA was 96% when the clinical probability was high, 92% when it was intermediate, and 58% when the probability was low (8% of patients). The negative predictive value was 96% when the clinical probability was low, 89% when it was intermediate, and 60% when it was high (3% of patients).

The ability of CTPA to exclude PE has also been evaluated in management studies in which anticoagulant therapy was withheld in patients with negative CTPA. More recent studies suggest that fewer than 2% of patients with a negative CTPA for PE will return with symptomatic VTE during follow-up.[49,51,52] Taken together, these observations suggest the following conclusions [*see Figure 4*]:

(1) An intraluminal filling defect in a lobar or larger pulmonary artery is generally diagnostic for PE. However, if the clinical

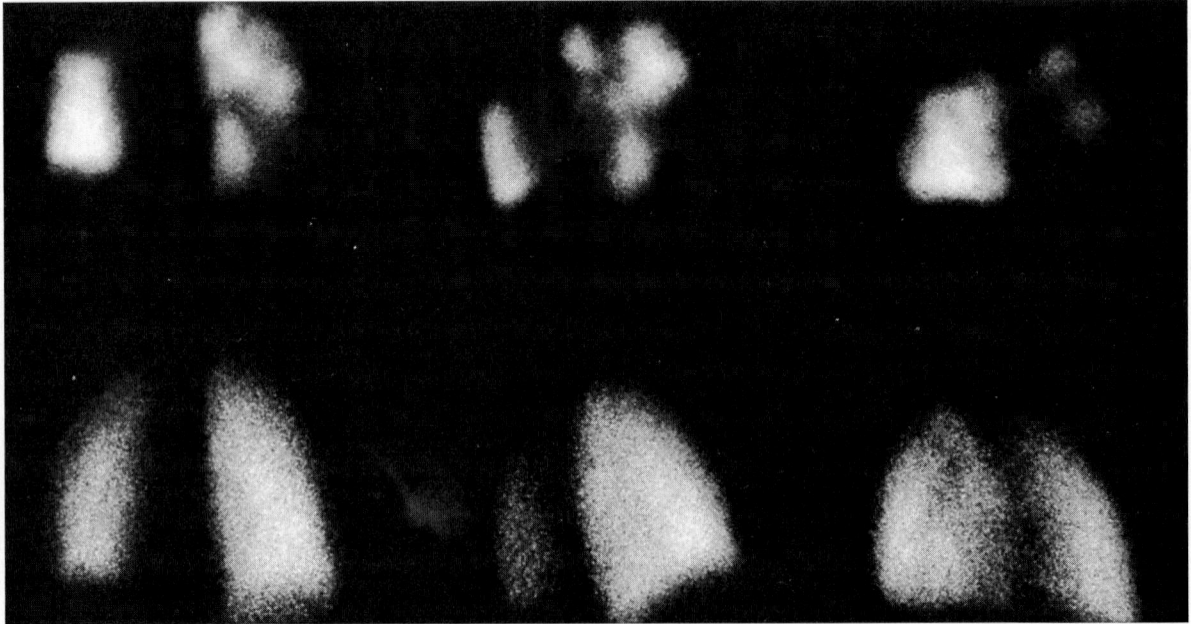

Figure 2 Posterior, right posterior oblique, and left posterior oblique perfusion scans (top), which were developed by using radiopharmaceutical technetium-99m (^{99m}Tc) microspheres of albumin, show multiple large perfusion defects, particularly involving the right lung. Ventilation scans (bottom) of the same projections, made with the patient breathing krypton-81m (^{81m}Kr), show that ventilation was well maintained compared to perfusion. The presence of multiple segmental perfusion defects with associated normal ventilation (best seen in the right lung) indicated a "high probability" lung scan and is diagnostic for pulmonary embolism.

Table 4 Test Results that Effectively Confirm or Exclude Pulmonary Embolism[43]

Conclusion	Test	Result
Diagnostic for PE	Pulmonary angiography	Intraluminal filling defect
	CT pulmonary angiography	Intraluminal filling defect in a segmental, lobar, or main pulmonary artery
	Ventilation-perfusion scan	High-probability scan and moderate/high clinical probability
	Tests for DVT*	Evidence of acute DVT with nondiagnostic ventilation-perfusion scan or CT pulmonary angiogram
Excludes PE	Pulmonary angiography	Normal
	CT pulmonary angiography	Negative†
	Lung perfusion scan	Normal
	High-sensitivity D-dimer test‡	Negative
	Moderate-sensitivity D-dimer test§	Negative, plus (1) low clinical suspicion of PE or (2) normal alveolar dead space fraction or (3) nondiagnostic lung scan and negative ultrasonography of proximal leg veins
	Combination of clinical assessment, ventilation-perfusion scan, ultrasonography of proximal leg veins	Low clinical suspicion, nondiagnostic scan, and negative ultrasonography

*See *Table 2*.
†If clinical suspicion is high, supplemental bilateral ultrasonography of the proximal leg veins is recommended.
‡D-dimer assay with very high sensitivity (i.e., 98%) and at least moderate specificity (i.e., 40%).
§D-dimer assay with at least moderately high sensitivity (i.e., 85%) and specificity (i.e., 70%).
DVT—deep vein thrombosis   PE—pulmonary embolism

probability is low and if there are additional findings that undermine a diagnosis of PE (e.g., a technically suboptimal study or a negative D-dimer test), further diagnostic testing should be considered (e.g., venous ultrasonography, ventilation-perfusion scanning, repeat CTPA, or conventional pulmonary angiography).

(2) A good-quality negative CTPA excludes PE provided there is not a high clinical suspicion for PE. If clinical suspicion is high or if the CTPA is suboptimal, imaging of the proximal deep veins of the legs should be performed to exclude DVT.

(3) Intraluminal filling defects that are confined to segmental pulmonary arteries are generally diagnostic for PE if the clinical suspicion is moderate or high, but they should be considered nondiagnostic if the clinical suspicion is lower or if there are additional findings that undermine a diagnosis of PE (see above).

(4) Intraluminal defects that are confined to subsegmental pulmonary arteries are generally nondiagnostic and require further investigation.

Magnetic resonance imaging (MRI) Magnetic resonance imaging is less well evaluated than helical CT for the diagnosis of PE but is expected to be less accurate. Both helical CT and MRI have the advantage of being able to identify alternative pulmonary diagnoses. MRI does not expose the patient to radiation or radiographic contrast media. Both MRI and helical CT can be extended to look for concomitant DVT.

D-dimer blood testing D-dimer testing is also a valuable test for the exclusion of PE, either when used alone (very sensitive D-dimer assay) or when combined with other assessments that indicate a reduced likelihood of PE [see Figure 4].[48,51-53]

Compression ultrasonography Compression ultrasonography to evaluate the proximal deep veins of the legs can aid in the diagnosis of PE. Demonstration of DVT, which occurs in about 5% of patients with nondiagnostic ventilation-perfusion lung scans, can serve as indirect evidence of PE. Exclusion of proximal DVT does not rule out PE in a patient with a nondiagnostic ventilation-perfusion scan, although it somewhat reduces the probability of that diagnosis. However, if there are no proximal deep vein thrombi on the day of presentation and if none are detected on two subsequent examinations one and

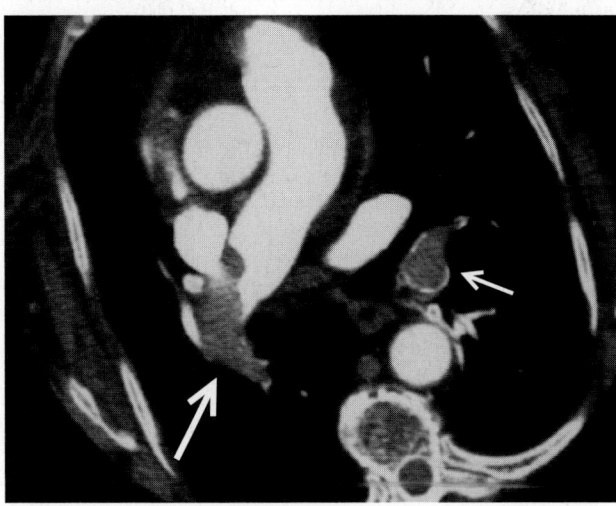

Figure 3 Computed tomographic pulmonary angiography (CTPA) demonstrates intraluminal filling defects caused by pulmonary embolism in the lobar artery of the left lower lobe (small arrow) and the main artery of the right lung (large arrow) in a patient with a chest deformity.

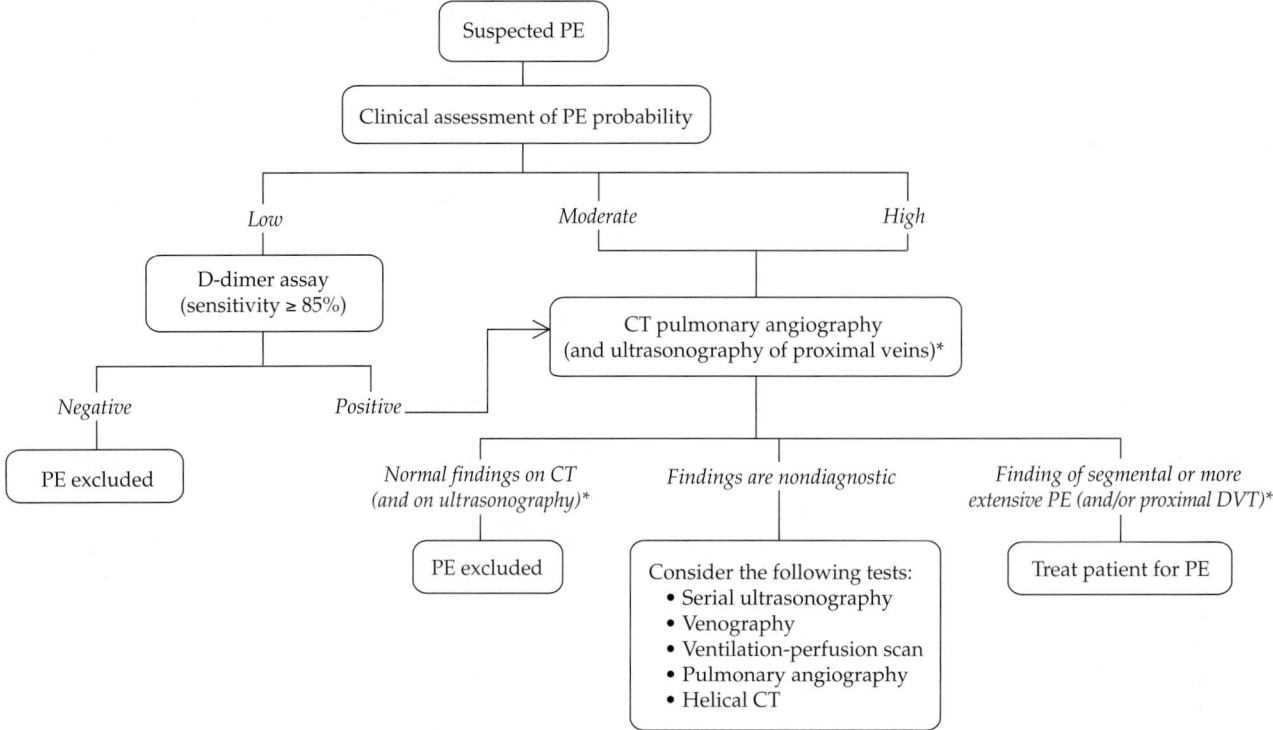

Figure 4 Algorithm outlines a diagnostic approach to pulmonary embolism. Use of a very sensitive D-dimer assay can obviate clinical assessment: A negative result excludes PE regardless of the results of the clinical assessment. However, the yield from D-dimer testing is low in patients in whom there is a high clinical suspicion of pulmonary embolism. A positive finding on the D-dimer assay can be followed by CT pulmonary angiography (CTPA). If the D-dimer assay is expected to be positive in the absence of PE (e.g., in a postoperative patient), CTPA can be performed as the initial objective test.
*Ultrasonography of the proximal deep veins of both legs is recommended to detect asymptomatic DVT if the clinical assessment indicates a high probability of PE. (DVT—deep vein thrombosis; PE—pulmonary embolism; VTE—venous thromboembolism)

two weeks later (DVT is diagnosed during serial testing in ~2% of patients), anticoagulant therapy can be withheld with a very low risk that patients will return with VTE (less than 2% during 3 months of follow-up).[52-54]

Earlier studies that evaluated CTPA suggested that a negative result did not exclude PE and, therefore, this exam should be followed by bilateral ultrasonography of the proximal veins. However, more recent studies of CTPA—conducted primarily with multidetector scanners—do not support the need for routine ultrasonography of the proximal deep veins in patients with a negative CTPA.[49,51] Instead, it appears to be reasonable to perform ultrasonography of the proximal deep veins only if clinical suspicion for PE is high. As for patients with nondiagnostic ventilation-perfusion lung scans, withholding of anticoagulant therapy and performance of serial ultrasonography is a reasonable approach to the management of those patients who have a CTPA that is suspicious for isolated subsegmental pulmonary embolism.

Pulmonary angiography Pulmonary angiography had been considered the reference standard for the diagnosis of PE but is now rarely performed because it is invasive and can usually be replaced by CTPA. Pulmonary angiography can be complicated by arrhythmias, cardiac perforation, cardiac arrest, and hypersensitivity to the contrast medium. Complications occur in 3% to 4% of patients undergoing pulmonary angiography. Various combinations of test results can be used to either confirm or exclude a diagnosis of PE [*see Table 4*].

Prophylaxis and Treatment

PHARMACOLOGY OF ANTICOAGULANT AGENTS

A less intense anticoagulant effect is required for the prevention of VTE than is required for its treatment. The anticoagulants in clinical use are heparin, LMWH, and fondaparinux, which are administered subcutaneously or intravenously; and coumarin compounds, which are given orally. Thrombolytic agents that are most commonly used for treatment of VTE are streptokinase and recombinant tissue plasminogen activator (rt-PA).

Heparin and LMWH Heparin is a highly sulfated glycosaminoglycan that produces its anticoagulant effect by binding to antithrombin, markedly accelerating the ability of the naturally occurring anticoagulant to inactivate thrombin, activated factor X (factor Xa), and activated factor IX (factor IXa).[55] At therapeutic concentrations, intravenous heparin has a half-life of about 60 minutes. Its clearance is dose dependent. Heparin has decreased bioavailability when administered subcutaneously in low doses but has approximately 90% bioavailability when administered in high therapeutic doses.

Heparin binds to a number of plasma proteins, a phenomenon that reduces the anticoagulant effect of heparin by limiting its accessibility to antithrombin. The concentration of heparin-binding proteins increases during illness, contributing to the variability in anticoagulant response in patients with thromboembolism.[55] Because of this variability, response to heparin should be monitored with the activated partial thromboplastin time (aPTT). The dose should be adjusted as necessary to achieve a therapeutic range, which for many aPTT reagents corresponds to an aPTT ratio of 1.8 to 2.5. A recent study showed that fixed, weight-adjusted, subcutaneous heparin was as effective and safe as LMWHs in patients with acute VTE.[56] This finding questions the need for laboratory monitoring of heparin when the anticoagulant is given subcutaneously in currently recommended weight-adjusted doses.

LMWHs are effective in the prevention and treatment of VTE. They are derived from standard commercial-grade heparin by chemical depolymerization to yield fragments approximately one third the size of heparin.[55] Depolymerization of heparin results in a change in its anticoagulant profile, bioavailability, and pharmacokinetics and in a lower incidence of heparin-induced thrombocytopenia and of osteopenia.[55] The plasma recoveries and pharmacokinetics of LMWHs differ from those of heparin because LMWHs bind much less avidly to heparin-binding proteins than does heparin. This property of LMWHs contributes to their superior bioavailability at low doses and their more predictable anticoagulant response. LMWHs also exhibit less binding to macrophages and endothelial cells than does heparin, a property that accounts for their longer plasma half-life (approximately 3 hours) and their dose-independent clearance. These potential advantages over heparin permit once-daily administration of LMWHs without laboratory monitoring and have led to the successful treatment of DVT, and of selected patients with PE, outside the hospital setting. The published research on LMWHs, which includes over 5,000 patients treated with either once-daily or twice-daily subcutaneous doses, has established this class of anticoagulants as safe, effective, and convenient for treating DVT and PE.[21,57] LMWH, given once daily, has been shown to be more effective than warfarin for the first 3 to 6 months of treatment of VTE in patients with cancer.[58,59]

Fondaparinux   Fondaparinux is a new parenteral synthetic anticoagulant composed of the five saccharide units that make up the active site of heparin that binds antithrombin.[60] The fondaparinux-antithrombin complex inhibits factor Xa but has no direct activity against thrombin. Fondaparinux is rapidly absorbed and is 100% bioavailable when administered subcutaneously. It is not metabolized, is renally excreted, and has a dose-independent elimination half-life of 15 hours, which makes it suitable for once-daily administration. Fondaparinux has been shown to be effective for prevention and treatment of VTE.[61-63]

Vitamin K antagonists   Oral anticoagulants such as coumarin compounds, the most common of which is warfarin, achieve their anticoagulant effect by producing hemostatically defective, vitamin K-dependent coagulant proteins (prothrombin, factor VII, factor IX, and factor X).[64]

The dose of warfarin must be monitored closely because the anticoagulant response varies widely among individuals. Laboratory monitoring is performed by measuring the prothrombin time (PT), a test responsive to depression of three of the four vitamin K-dependent clotting factors (prothrombin and factors VII and X). Commercial PT reagents vary markedly in their responsiveness to warfarin-induced reduction in clotting factors, but this variability problem has been overcome by the introduction of the international normalized ratio (INR).[64]

The starting dose of warfarin has traditionally been 10 mg, with an average maintenance dose of about 5 mg. However, the dose required varies widely among individuals. For example, el-

derly patients and women have been shown, on average, to require lower doses. A starting dose of 5 mg rather than 10 mg is preferable in most inpatients. Warfarin therapy is difficult to manage in some patients because of unexpected fluctuations in dose response, which may reflect changes in diet, inaccuracy in PT testing, undisclosed drug use, poor compliance, or surreptitious self-medication. Certain over-the-counter and prescription drugs can augment or inhibit the anticoagulant effect of coumarin compounds or prolong hemostasis by interfering with platelet function [see Table 5].

Patients receiving coumarin compounds are also sensitive to fluctuating levels of dietary vitamin K, which is obtained predominantly from leafy green vegetables. The effect of coumarins can be potentiated in sick patients with poor vitamin K intake, particularly if they are treated with antibiotics and intravenous feeding without vitamin K supplementation, and in states of fat malabsorption.

New anticoagulants   Direct thrombin inhibitors (e.g., bivalirudin, hirudin, ximelagatran) have been shown to be effective for prevention and treatment of VTE.[60,65] Ximelagatran, however, is associated with liver toxicity, which has prevented its use in clinical practice, and bivalirudin is being marketed for percutaneous coronary intervention. Hirudin and another direct thrombin inhibitor, called argatraban, are indicated for heparin-induced thrombocytopenia. A number of new compounds, including new direct antithrombins and inhibitors of other clotting factors, are at advanced stages of development.[60]

Complications of Antithrombotic Agents

Bleeding is the main complication of antithrombotic therapy.[66] With all antithrombotic agents, the risk of bleeding is influenced by the dose and by patient-related factors, the most important of which is recent surgery or trauma. Other patient characteristics that increase the risk of bleeding are older age, recent stroke, generalized hemostatic defect, a history of gastrointestinal hemorrhage, renal failure, and other serious comorbid conditions.

With heparin, the incidence of bleeding is influenced by dosage; independently of dosage, there is no clear relationship between bleeding and the aPTT.[55,66] Bleeding rates appear to be lower with LMWH than with intravenous heparin.[21]

Bleeding associated with coumarin anticoagulants is influenced by the intensity of anticoagulant therapy, particularly with progressive increases of the INR above 3.0.[66] A study that compared long-term treatment of VTE with warfarin targeted to an INR of 1.75 versus an INR of 2.5 found no difference in the bleeding rates, suggesting that differences in the INR between 1.5 and 3.0 are not associated with clinically important differences in bleeding risk.[67] Both heparin-induced bleeding and warfarin-induced bleeding are increased by concomitant use of aspirin, which impairs platelet function and produces gastric erosions. When the INR is less than 3.0, coumarin-associated bleeding frequently has an obvious underlying cause or is from an occult gastrointestinal or renal lesion.

Nonhemorrhagic side effects of heparin include: (1) urticaria at sites of subcutaneous injection; (2) thrombocytopenia, which occurs in about 1% of patients treated with high-dose heparin and is complicated by arterial or venous thrombosis in about 0.2% of treated patients [see Chapter 99]; (3) osteoporosis, which occurs with prolonged high-dose heparin use; and, rarely, (4) alopecia, adrenal insufficiency, and skin necrosis. The incidence

Table 5   Drug and Food Interactions with Warfarin by Strength of Supporting Evidence and Direction of Interaction[105]

Level of Causation	Anti-Infectives	Cardiovascular Drugs	Analgesics, Anti-inflammatories and Immunologics	CNS Drugs	GI Drugs and Food	Herbal Supplements	Other Drugs
Potentiation* Highly probable	Ciprofloxacin, cotrimoxazole, erythromycin, fluconazole, isoniazid, metronidazole, miconazole (oral), miconazole (vaginal), voriconazole	Amiodarone, clofibrate, diltiazem, fenofibrate, propafenone, propranolol, sulfinpyrazone	Phenylbutazone, piroxicam	Alcohol (with liver disease), citalopram, entacapone, sertraline	Cimetidine, fish oil, mango, omeprazole	Boldo-fenugreek, quilinggao	Anabolic steroids, zileuton
Probable	Amoxicillin-clavulanate, azithromycin, clarithromycin, itraconazole, levofloxacin, ritonavir, tetracycline	Acetylsalicylic acid, fluvastatin, quinidine, ropinirole, simvastatin	Acetaminophen, acetylsalicylic acid, celecoxib, dextropropoxyphene, interferon, tramadol	Chloral hydrate, disulfiram, fluvoxamine, phenytoin	Grapefruit juice	Danshen, dong quai, *Lycium barbarum*, PC-SPES	Fluorouracil, gemcitabine, levamisole/fluorouracil, paclitaxel, tamoxifen, tolterodine
Inhibition* Highly probable	Griseofulvin, nafcillin, ribavirin, rifampin	Cholestyramine	Mesalamine	Barbiturates, carbamazepine	High vitamin K foods/enteral feeds, avocado	—	Mercaptopurine
Probable	Dicloxacillin, ritonavir	Bosentan	Azathioprine	Chlordiazepoxide	Soy milk, sucralfate	Ginseng	Chelation therapy, influenza vaccine, multivitamin supplement, raloxifene hydrochloride

*Interactions for which there is "possible" supporting evidence are not included in this table. Although there is strong evidence that some drugs and foods do not interact with warfarin,[105] in general, caution and a higher frequency of INR monitoring is recommended whenever patients on warfarin start (or stop) a new medication.

of thrombocytopenia is lower with LMWH than with heparin. Similarly, there is evidence that the risk of osteopenia is lower with LMWH than with heparin.[55]

The most important nonhemorrhagic side effect of coumarin anticoagulants is skin necrosis, an uncommon complication usually observed on the third to eighth day of therapy. Skin necrosis is caused by extensive thrombosis of the venules and capillaries within the subcutaneous fat. An association has been reported between coumarin-induced skin necrosis and protein C deficiency—and, less commonly, protein S deficiency—but this complication can also occur in patients without these deficiencies.

PRIMARY PROPHYLAXIS

The most effective way to reduce the mortality associated with PE and the morbidity associated with the postthrombotic syndrome is to institute primary prophylaxis in patients at risk for VTE. On the basis of well-defined clinical criteria, patients can be classified as being at low, moderate, or high risk for VTE, and the choice of prophylaxis should be tailored to the patient's risk [see Table 6]. In the absence of prophylaxis, the frequency of fatal postoperative PE ranges from 0.1% to 0.4% in patients undergoing elective general surgery and from 0.4% to 5% in patients undergoing elective hip or knee surgery, emergency hip surgery or surgery for major trauma or spinal cord injury. Prophylaxis is cost-effective for most high-risk groups.[68]

Prophylaxis is achieved either by modulating activation of blood coagulation or by preventing venous stasis by using the following proven approaches: low-dose subcutaneous heparin,

intermittent pneumatic compression of the legs, coumarin anticoagulants, adjusted doses of subcutaneous heparin, graduated compression stockings, LMWHs, or fondaparinux.[61,68] Antiplatelet agents, such as aspirin, also prevent VTE but are less effective than the previously stated methods.[68,69]

Low-dose heparin is given subcutaneously at a dose of 5,000 units (U) 2 hours before surgery and 5,000 U every 8 or 12 hours after surgery. In patients undergoing major orthopedic surgical procedures, low-dose heparin is less effective than warfarin,

Table 6   Risk Categories for Venous Thromboembolism and Recommendations for Prophylaxis

	High Risk	Moderate Risk
Calf vein thrombosis	20%–50%	10%–20%
Proximal vein thrombosis	5%–20%	2%–5%
Fatal pulmonary embolism	0.4%–5%	0.1%–0.4%
Recommended prophylaxis	Low-molecular-weight heparin, oral anticoagulants, or fondaparinux (can be combined with graduated compression stockings or pneumatic compression)	Low-dose heparin, external pneumatic compression, or graduated compression stockings

LMWH, or fondaparinux. Intermittent pneumatic compression of the legs enhances blood flow in the deep veins and increases blood fibrinolytic activity. This method of prophylaxis is free of clinically important side effects and is particularly useful in patients who have a high risk of serious bleeding. It is the method of choice for preventing venous thrombosis in patients undergoing neurosurgery, is effective in patients undergoing major knee surgery, and is as effective as low-dose heparin in patients undergoing abdominal surgery.

Graduated compression stockings reduce venous stasis and prevent postoperative venous thrombosis in general surgical patients and in medical or surgical patients with neurologic disorders, including paralysis of the lower limbs.[68] In surgical patients, the combined use of graduated compression stockings and low-dose heparin is more effective than use of low-dose heparin alone. Graduated compression stockings are relatively inexpensive and should be considered in all high-risk surgical patients, even if other forms of prophylaxis are used.

Moderate-dose warfarin (INR = 2.0 to 3.0) is effective for preventing postoperative VTE in patients in all risk categories.[68] Warfarin therapy can be started at the time of surgery or in the early postoperative period. Although the anticoagulant effect is not achieved until the third or fourth postoperative day, warfarin is effective in patients at very high risk, including patients with hip fractures and those who undergo joint replacement. Prophylaxis with warfarin is less convenient than that with low-dose heparin, LMWHs, or fondaparinux because careful laboratory monitoring is necessary.

LMWH is a safe and effective form of prophylaxis in high-risk patients undergoing elective hip surgery, major general surgery, or major knee surgery, as well as in patients who have experienced hip fracture, spinal injury, or acute medical illness. LMWH is more effective than standard low-dose heparin in general surgical patients, patients undergoing elective hip surgery, and patients with spinal injury.

In patients who undergo hip or major knee surgery, LMWH is more effective than warfarin but is also associated with more frequent bleeding; both of these properties may be attributable to the more rapid onset of anticoagulation with postoperatively initiated LMWH than with warfarin. It is uncertain whether the superior efficacy of LMWH over warfarin in the prevention of venographically detectable DVT is mirrored by fewer symptomatic episodes of VTE.

Fondaparinux was shown to reduce the frequency of venographically detected DVT by 50% but to cause a small increase in bleeding compared with LMWH in a series of large trials in orthopedic surgical patients.[61]

Indications for Prophylaxis

General surgery and medicine Low-dose-heparin or LMWH prophylaxis is the method of choice for moderate-risk general surgical and medical patients. Both approaches are simple, inexpensive, convenient, and safe, and each reduces the risk of VTE by 50% to 70%.[68] If anticoagulants are contraindicated because of an unusually high risk of bleeding, graduated compression stockings, intermittent pneumatic compression of the legs, or both should be used. Fondaparinux has also been shown to be effective in these patients.

Major orthopedic surgery LMWH, fondaparinux, or oral anticoagulants provide effective prophylaxis for VTE in patients who have undergone hip surgery. Aspirin has also been shown to reduce the frequency of symptomatic VTE and fatal PE after hip fracture.[69] The relative efficacy and safety of aspirin versus LMWH, fondaparinux, or oral anticoagulants in patients who have a hip fracture or have undergone hip or knee arthroplasty is uncertain. However, because studies have shown that aspirin is much less effective than LMWH or oral anticoagulants at preventing venographically detectable DVT, aspirin is not recommended as the sole agent for postoperative prophylaxis.[68]

LMWH, warfarin, fondaparinux, and intermittent pneumatic compression are effective in preventing VTE in patients undergoing major knee surgery.

Extended prophylaxis with LWMH or warfarin for an additional 3 weeks after hospital discharge should be considered after major orthopedic surgery. Extended prophylaxis is strongly recommended for high-risk patients (e.g., those with previous VTE or active cancer).[68,70]

Genitourinary surgery, neurosurgery, and ocular surgery Intermittent pneumatic compression, with or without graduated compression stockings, is an effective prophylaxis for VTE and does not increase the risk of bleeding.

TREATMENT

The objectives of treating patients with VTE are to prevent PE, the postthrombotic syndrome, thromboembolic pulmonary hypertension, and recurrent VTE and to alleviate the discomfort of the acute event.

Superficial venous thrombosis usually can be treated conservatively with anti-inflammatory drugs. If superficial phlebitis is extensive or very symptomatic, a 1 to 2 week course of heparin or LMWH therapy can be used. In patients with DVT, anticoagulants can effectively reduce morbidity and mortality from PE.[59] Vena caval interruption, which is usually achieved with an inferior vena caval filter, is also effective but is more complicated, expensive, and invasive and is associated with a doubling of the frequency of recurrent DVT during long-term follow-up.[71] For these reasons, it is generally used only if anticoagulant therapy has failed or is contraindicated because of the risk of serious hemorrhage.[59]

Thrombolytic therapy is more effective than heparin in achieving early lysis of venous thromboemboli and is better than heparin for preventing death in patients with massive PE associated with shock.[59] Thrombolytic therapy is therefore the treatment of choice for patients with life-threatening PE. A regimen of 100 mg of recombinant tissue plasminogen activator (rt-PA) administered over 2 hours is generally recommended. The role of thrombolytic therapy in the treatment of DVT is uncertain. Systemic thrombolytic therapy increases lysis of DVT, particularly when employed early in the course of treatment, and may reduce the risk of developing the postthrombotic syndrome. However, systemic thrombolytic therapy increases the frequency of major bleeding, including intracranial hemorrhage. Catheter-directed thrombolytic therapy, often combined with mechanical disruption of thrombus and stent insertion if there is residual thrombosis, may be associated with a lower risk of bleeding.[59]

Thromboendarterectomy is effective treatment in selected cases of chronic thromboembolic pulmonary hypertension involving proximal pulmonary arterial obstruction.[72]

Routine early use of graduated compression stockings for 2 years has been reported to reduce the incidence of the postthrombotic syndrome by about 50% in some studies.[73,74] However, lingering doubts about their efficacy remains, and further evaluation is being performed.

Administration and Dosage Guidelines

Anticoagulant therapy Anticoagulants are the mainstay of treatment for most patients with VTE. In the past, the treatment of choice was heparin administered by continuous intravenous infusion or subcutaneous injection, in doses sufficient to produce an adequate anticoagulant response. Now many patients are treated with LMWH administered by subcutaneous injection without laboratory monitoring since this class of anticoagulant is as effective and safe as heparin.[28]

Fondaparinux is as effective and safe as LMWH for the treatment of DVT and as effective and safe as heparin for the treatment of PE.

The anticoagulant effect of intravenous heparin is immediate. With subcutaneous injection, the anticoagulant effect of heparin, LMWH, and fondaparinux is delayed for about an hour; peak levels occur at about 4 hours. The anticoagulant effect of subcutaneous heparin is maintained for about 12 hours with therapeutic doses. LMWH and fondaparinux are effective when administered subcutaneously once daily.[21]

Heparin therapy is usually monitored by the aPTT and less frequently by heparin assays, which measure the ability of heparin to accelerate the inactivation of factor Xa or thrombin by antithrombin. The starting dose of intravenous heparin is a bolus of 80 U/kg (or a set dose of 5,000 U) followed by an initial infusion of 18 U/kg/hr (or a set dose of about 1,300 U/hr). The anticoagulant effect should be monitored every 6 hours until the aPTT is in the therapeutic range, and then daily. The therapeutic range of aPTT is equivalent to a heparin level between 0.35 and 0.7 U/ml as measured by an anti-factor Xa assay. For many aPTT reagents, this range is an aPTT ratio of 1.8 to 2.5 times the mean of the normal laboratory control value.

A recent study showed that acute VTE can be treated with subcutaneous, weight-adjusted heparin without laboratory monitoring of coagulation (initial dose of 333 U/kg followed by 250 U/kg every 12 hours).[56]

LMWH is administered subcutaneously on a weight-adjusted basis at a dosage of either 100 anti-Xa U/kg every 12 hours or 150 to 200 anti-Xa units once daily.[59] Monitoring is not required.

Treatment with heparin or LMWH is usually continued for 5 to 6 days; warfarin therapy is started on the first or second day, overlapping the heparin therapy (or LMWH) for 4 or 5 days, and is continued until an INR of 2.0 is maintained for at least 24 hours. A 4- to 5-day period of overlap is necessary because the antithrombotic effects of oral anticoagulants are delayed. The initial course of heparin should be followed by warfarin for at least 3 months.[59] In patients with unprovoked VTE, administration of low-intensity warfarin (INR = 1.5 to 2.0) after the first 6 months of anticoagulant therapy reduces the risk of recurrent VTE by two thirds; however, low-intensity warfarin is less effective than conventional-intensity warfarin therapy (INR = 2.0 to 3.0) and has not been shown to reduce bleeding.[13,75] Low-intensity warfarin therapy has been used with less frequent monitoring of the INR (i.e., about every 2 months). Intermediate to full-dose LMWH can also be used in place of warfarin in the outpatient setting and is preferred to warfarin in patients with active cancer.[58,59]

Duration of anticoagulant therapy During the past decade, a series of well-designed studies has helped to define the optimal duration of anticoagulation. The findings of these studies can be summarized as follows:

- Shortening the duration of anticoagulation from 3[23,28] or 6[25] months to 4[23,28,76] or 6[25] weeks results in a doubling of the frequency of recurrent VTE during 1[23,28,76] to 2[25] years of follow-up.
- Patients with VTE provoked by a transient risk factor have a lower (about one third) risk of recurrence than those with an unprovoked VTE or a persistent risk factor.[22,23,25,28,77,78]
- Three months of anticoagulation is adequate treatment for VTE provoked by a transient risk factor; subsequent risk of recurrence is about 3% in the first year of follow-up.[22-24,28,78,79]
- Three months of anticoagulation may not be adequate treatment for an unprovoked (idiopathic) episode of proximal DVT or PE; subsequent early risk of recurrence is about 10% to 15% in the first year of follow-up.[13,22,24-27]
- After 6 months of anticoagulation, recurrent DVT is at least as likely to affect the contralateral leg; this suggests that systemic rather than local (including inadequate treatment) factors are responsible for recurrences after 6 months of treatment.[80]
- There is a persistently elevated risk of recurrent VTE after a first episode of VTE; this appears to be about 10% in the first year, and about 30% in the first 5 years, after 6 or more months of treatment for an unprovoked proximal DVT or PE.[22,24-27]
- Extending duration of anticoagulation beyond 3 to 6 or 12 months may delay, but ultimately not reduce, the risk of recurrence if therapy is then stopped.[26,27]
- After 3 months of initial treatment of unprovoked VTE with oral anticoagulants targeted at an INR of 2.5 (INR range 2.0 to 3.0), continuing treatment with:
  - Oral anticoagulants targeted at an INR of ~2.5 reduces the risk of recurrent VTE by over 90%.[13,81]
  - Oral anticoagulants targeted at an INR of ~1.75 reduces the risk of recurrent VTE by about 75%.[75]
  - Oral anticoagulants targeted at an INR of ~2.5 are more effective than using an INR target of ~1.75, without evidence of increased bleeding.[67]
- A second episode of VTE predicts a higher risk of recurrence but not necessarily high enough to justify indefinite anticoagulation.[82-84]
- Risk of recurrence is lower (about half) following an isolated calf (distal) DVT than after proximal DVT or PE, and this favors a shorter duration of treatment.[24,25]
- Risk of recurrence in patients who discontinue treatment is similar after an episode of either proximal DVT or PE.[25,82,85,86]
- About 5% of recurrent episodes of VTE are expected to be fatal.[82,85]
- Recurrent VTE is usually (about 60% of episodes) a PE after an initial PE, and usually (about 80% of episodes) a DVT after an initial DVT[82,85,87,88]; this effect is expected to increase mortality from recurrent VTE by 2- to 3-fold following a PE compared with that following a DVT.[89]
- Risk of recurrence is about 3-fold higher in patients with active cancers.[77,86,90]
- Long-term treatment with LMWH is more effective than warfarin in patients with VTE associated with cancer and may be a preferred option for such patients.[91]
- Estrogen therapy is an important risk factor for first[17,92] and recurrent[18] episodes of VTE; consequently, if VTE occurred while on estrogen therapy, the risk of recurrent VTE is expected to be lowered by stopping estrogens.[86]
- Risk of recurrence appears to be higher in patients with antiphospholipid antibodies (anticardiolipin antibodies, lupus anticoagulants, or both).[13,83,88]

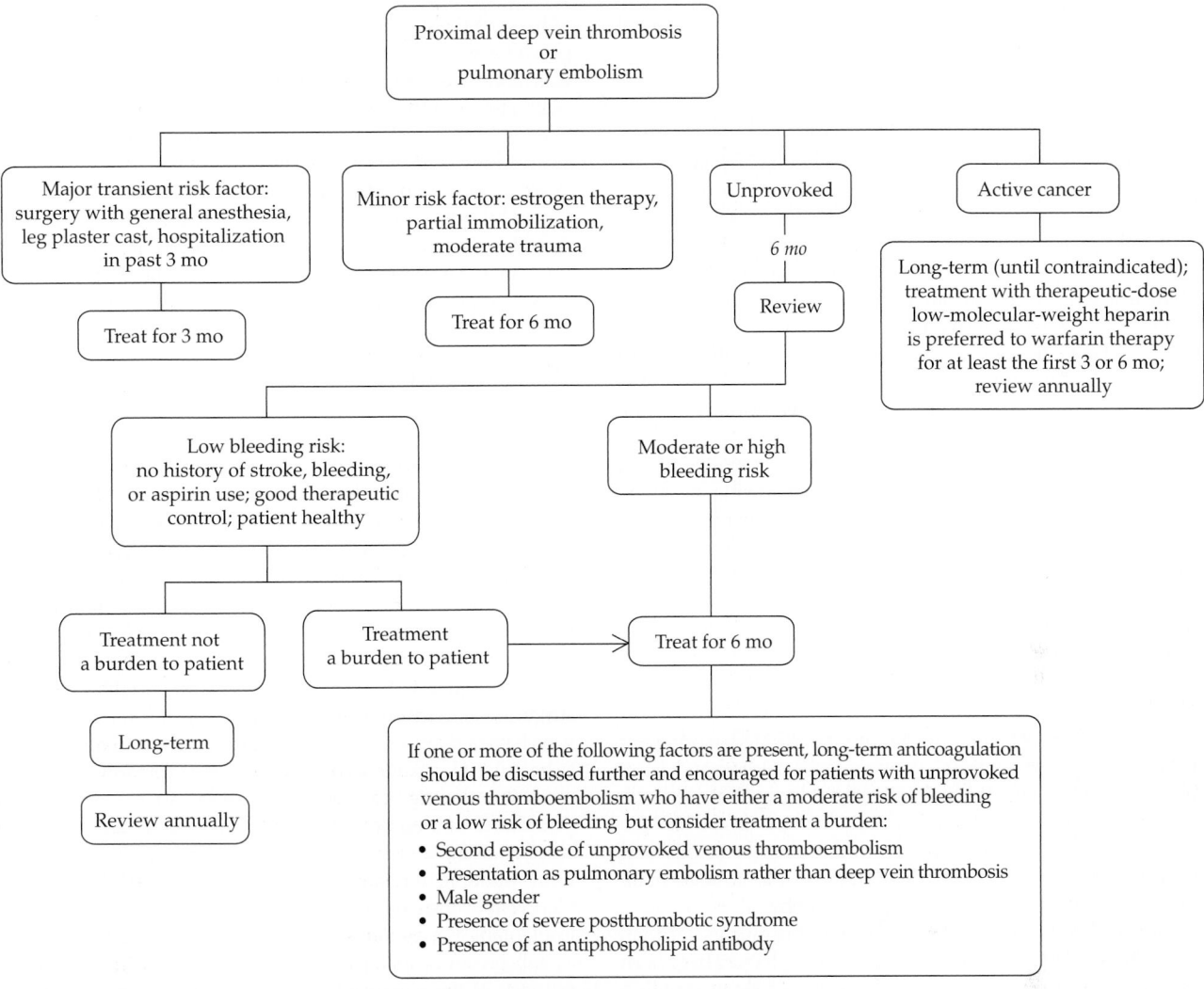

Figure 5 **Algorithm outlines the steps for selecting the duration of anticoagulation for patients with venous thromboembolism.**

- Hereditary thrombophilias, including heterozygous Factor V Leiden and the G20210A prothrombin gene mutations, double heterozygous states for these two genes, homozygous factor V Leiden, homozygous prothrombin gene G20210A, or deficiency of protein C, protein S, or antithrombin, appear to be weak risk factors for recurrent VTE.[22,31-33,93-95]
- Males appear to have about a 50% higher risk of recurrent VTE than females.[30]
- Other risk factors for recurrences may include advanced age; elevated levels of clotting factors VIII, IX, XI, and homocysteine; elevated D-dimer levels after stopping anticoagulant therapy; vena caval filters; and residual DVT on ultrasound; currently, these factors do not have clear implications for duration of treatment.[89]
- The risk of anticoagulant-induced bleeding is highest during the first 3 months of treatment and stabilizes after the first year.[96]
- Risk of bleeding differs markedly among patients depending on the prevalence of risk factors (e.g., advanced age, previous bleeding or stroke, renal failure. anemia, antiplatelet therapy, malignancy, poor anticoagulant control).[67,96,97]
- About 10% of episodes of major bleeding are fatal.[98]

- The risk of major bleeding in younger patients (e.g., those younger than 60 years) who do not have risk factors for bleeding and have good anticoagulant control (target INR 2.0 to 3.0) is about 1% per year.[67,96,99] The risk of major bleeding is expected to be at least 10-fold higher in patients with multiple risk factors for bleeding.[97]

These findings permit the construction of an algorithm for selecting duration of anticoagulation for VTE [*see Figure 5*]. Whether anticoagulant therapy (INR of 2.0 to 3.0) is recommended for 3 months, 6 months, or an indefinite period (with annual review) depends primarily on the presence of a provoking risk factor for VTE (i.e., major or minor transient risk factor, no risk factor, or cancer), risk factors for bleeding, and patient preference (i.e., burden associated with treatment). Secondary considerations include such factors as whether the patient has had a previous unprovoked VTE, whether the VTE presented as DVT or as PE, and whether the patient has biochemical risk factors for recurrent VTE.

Venous Thromboembolism in Pregnancy

The management of VTE during pregnancy is complicated because clinical diagnosis is unreliable, some of the objective diagnostic tests are potentially harmful to the fetus, and treatment may cause teratogenicity or fetal bleeding.[100,101]

DIAGNOSIS

In pregnant patients suspected of having DVT, venous ultrasonography of the proximal veins, including the iliac vein, should be used as the initial test.[34,101] If the result is unequivocally abnormal, a diagnosis of DVT is made and the patient is treated with anticoagulants. If the test result is normal, either a limited venogram can be performed with abdominal shielding to exclude isolated calf vein thrombosis, or serial compression ultrasonography can be performed on two occasions over the next 14 days. MRI may also be considered if there is continuing concern about iliac vein thrombosis. D-dimer testing may also be used as previously described, although false positive results are more common with this test, particularly in late pregnancy.

The diagnostic approach to PE in pregnancy is similar to that used in nonpregnant patients, but with the following modifications. Ultrasonography of the proximal deep veins can be performed first. If DVT is present, the patient is started on anticoagulant therapy without the need for further diagnostic testing. If DVT is not diagnosed, lung scanning or CTPA can be performed, but the techniques should be modified to reduce exposure of the fetus to radiation.[101]

TREATMENT

The treatment of VTE is much more complicated in pregnant patients because oral anticoagulants cross the placenta and, if administered during the first trimester, can cause warfarin embryopathy, which is characterized by nasal hypoplasia and skeletal abnormalities.[100] Warfarin administered during the second and third trimesters can cause dorsal midline dysplasia, abnormalities of the ventricular system, and optic atrophy.

Heparin does not cross the placenta and is much safer than oral anticoagulants during pregnancy. Although there have been reports associating heparin therapy during pregnancy with a high incidence of stillbirth or prematurity, most of these complications occurred in mothers receiving heparin for disorders that are known to be associated with a high rate of fetal loss. Other studies have shown that heparin is safe for the fetus but, when used on a long-term basis during pregnancy, can produce osteoporosis in the mother. The incidence of heparin-induced osteopenia diagnosed by dual-photon absorption x-ray or by conventional x-ray may be as high as 30%, but overt fractures are uncommon, occurring in fewer than 5% of patients. Heparin-induced bleeding is not a common problem during pregnancy, provided that heparin therapy is monitored carefully. The anticoagulant response to heparin can be prolonged if the drug is administered in high doses just before parturition, so there is the potential for local bleeding during and immediately after delivery.

In pregnant patients with acute VTE, continuous intravenous heparin or twice-daily LMWH should be administered for 4 to 7 days. This is followed for the remainder of the pregnancy by subcutaneous heparin, adjusted to achieve aPTT values or heparin levels that are in the therapeutic range midway between injections, or by continued use of LMWH.[89] An unwanted anticoagulant effect during delivery can be avoided by discontinuing subcutaneous heparin therapy 24 hours before elective induction of labor.

If there is no evidence of excessive postpartum bleeding, heparin therapy can be resumed within 12 hours of delivery and continued until oral anticoagulation is established. The intensity of heparin therapy will depend on the amount of time that has passed since the diagnosis of VTE was made: if the diagnosis was made less than 1 month ago, therapeutic doses may be used (with stepwise increases in subcutaneous or intravenous doses over 24 hours); if the diagnosis was made more than 1 month ago, prophylactic or intermediate doses of heparin may be used. Warfarin is started at the same time as heparin and is continued for a minimum of 6 weeks and preferably until patients have received a minimum of 3 months of anticoagulation. Warfarin does not enter breast milk and therefore can be administered to nursing mothers.[87,88]

Miscellaneous Thromboembolic Disorders

THROMBOSIS IN UNUSUAL SITES

Subclavian or Axillary Veins

Thrombosis of the subclavian or axillary veins may be idiopathic or may occur as a complication of local vascular damage.[102] It is now most frequently seen as a complication of chronic indwelling catheter use, but it also occurs as a complication after mastectomy and local radiotherapy for breast cancer. Idiopathic subclavian or axillary vein thrombosis often occurs in young muscular individuals and may be preceded by repetitive, strenuous activity involving the affected arm. Some of these persons have a fixed stenosis of the subclavian vein that is thought to be caused by external compression of the vein as it courses behind the clavicle. Occasionally, subclavian or axillary vein thrombosis can occur in patients with congenital deficiency of antithrombin, protein C, or protein S or in patients with antiphospholipid antibodies. Thrombosis of the axillary or subclavian vein or the superior vena cava is a rare complication of an implantable perivenous endocardial pacing system.

Subclavian or axillary thrombosis causes pain, edema, and cyanosis of the arm. In rare cases, the thrombosis extends into the superior vena cava and causes edema and cyanosis of the face and neck. Definitive diagnosis is made by venography, venous ultrasonography, CT, or MRI.[103] Subclavian or axillary vein thrombosis is usually treated with anticoagulants. Regional or systemic thrombolytic therapy may be considered in young patients without contraindications, because a substantial number of these patients experience aching and swelling when they exert the affected arm.

Mesenteric Vein

An uncommon disorder, mesenteric vein thrombosis usually occurs in the sixth or seventh decade of life. It generally involves segments of the small bowel, leading to hemorrhagic infarction.[104,105] Affected patients often have associated disorders, such as inflammatory bowel disease, malignancy, portal hypertension, or familial thrombophilia or polycythemia vera, or they may have a history of recent abdominal surgery. In about 20% of cases, no underlying cause is found.

The clinical manifestations of mesenteric vein thrombosis include intermittent abdominal pain, abdominal distention, vomiting, diarrhea, and melena. Blunt, semiopaque indentations of the bowel lumen ("thumbprinting") due to mucosal edema; gas in the wall of the bowel or the portal vein; or free peritoneal air may occur secondary to bowel infarction. CT, which shows an intraluminal filling defect in the mesenteric vein, is the diagnostic test of choice, and both Doppler ultrasonography and MRI are also helpful. Management includes acute and long-term anticoagulation, supportive care, and surgery if bowel resection is being considered. Mortality is about 30%, and up to 30% of patients experience a recurrence.

Renal Vein

Renal vein thrombosis can be idiopathic, or it may occur as a complication of the nephrotic syndrome. Patients may be asymptomatic or may present with abdominal, back, or flank pain and tenderness. PE is a relatively common complication of renal vein thrombosis. Anticoagulant therapy results in a gradual improvement in renal function, but patients may have long-standing proteinuria. Thrombolytic agents have been used, but the data are inadequate for critical appraisal of this form of treatment.

THROMBOPHILIA

The term thrombophilia denotes any increased tendency to thrombosis, whether inherited or acquired.[9,10] Thrombophilia is discussed in detail elsewhere [see Chapter 99].

Clive Kearon, M.B., Ph.D., is an advisor to Boehringer Ingelheim and GlaxoSmithKline.

Jack Hirsh, M.D., F.A.C.P., participates in the speakers' bureaus for AstraZeneca Pharmaceuticals LP and Sanofi-Synthelabo Inc.

References

1. White RH: The epidemiology of venous thromboembolism. Circulation 107:I4, 2003
2. Anderson FA Jr, Spencer FA: Risk factors for venous thromboembolism. Circulation 107:I9, 2003
3. Heit JA, Silverstein MD, Mohr DN, et al: Risk factors for deep vein thrombosis and pulmonary embolism: a population-based case-control study. Arch Intern Med 160:809, 2000
4. Anderson FA, Wheeler HB, Goldberg RJ, et al: The prevalence of risk factors for venous thromboembolism among hospital patients. Arch Intern Med 152:1660, 1992
5. Cogo A, Bernardi E, Prandoni P, et al: Acquired risk factors for deep-vein thrombosis in symptomatic outpatients. Arch Intern Med 154:164, 1994
6. Kearon C: Natural history of venous thromboembolism. Circulation 107:I22, 2003
7. Kahn SR, Ginsberg JS: Relationship between deep venous thrombosis and the post-thrombotic syndrome. Arch Intern Med 164:17, 2004
8. Kearon C, Salzman E, Hirsh J: Epidemiology, pathogenesis, and natural history of venous thrombosis. Hemostasis and Thrombosis, 4th ed. Colman R, Hirsh J, Marder JV, Eds. Lippincott Williams & Wilkins, Philadelphia, 2001.
9. Lane DA, Mannucci PM, Bauer KA, et al: Inherited thrombophilia: Part 1. Thromb Haemost 76:651, 1996
10. Lane DA, Mannucci PM, Bauer KA, et al: Inherited thrombophilia: Part 2. Thromb Haemost 76:824, 1996
11. Heijboer H, Brandjes PM, Buller HR, et al: Deficiencies of coagulation-inhibiting and fibrinolytic proteins in outpatients with deep-vein thrombosis. N Engl J Med 323:1512, 1990
12. Kearon C, Crowther M, Hirsh J: Management of patients with hereditary hypercoagulable disorders. Ann Rev Med 51:169, 2000
13. Kearon C, Gent M, Hirsh J, et al: A comparison of three months of anticoagulation with extended anticoagulation for a first episode of idiopathic venous thromboembolism. N Engl J Med 340:901, 1999
14. Poort SR, Rosendaal FR, Reitsma PH, et al: A common genetic variation in the 3'-untranslated region of the prothrombin gene is associated with elevated plasma prothrombin levels and an increase in venous thrombosis. Blood 88:3698, 1996
15. Vandenbroucke JP, Koster T, Briet E, et al: Increased risk of venous thrombosis in oral-contraceptive users who are carriers of factor V leiden mutation. Lancet 344:1453, 1994
16. Grady D, Herrington D, Bittner V, et al: Cardiovascular disease outcomes during 6.8 years of hormone therapy: Heart and Estrogen/progestin Replacement Study follow-up (HERS II). JAMA 288:49, 2002
17. Rossouw JE, Anderson GL, Prentice RL, et al: Risks and benefits of estrogen plus progestin in healthy postmenopausal women: principal results from the Women's Health Initiative randomized controlled trial. JAMA 288:321, 2002
18. Hoibraaten E, Qvigstad E, Arnesen H, et al: Increased risk of recurrent venous thromboembolism during hormone replacement therapy—results of the randomized, double-blind, placebo-controlled Estrogen in Venous Thromboembolism Trial (EVTET). Thromb Haemost 84:961, 2000.
19. Hull R, Delmore T, Genton E, et al: Warfarin sodium versus low-dose heparin in the long-term treatment of venous thrombosis. N Engl J Med 301:855, 1979

20. Lagerstedt CI, Olsson CG, Fagher BO, et al: Need for long-term anticoagulant treatment in symptomatic calf-vein thrombosis. Lancet 2:515, 1985
21. van Dongen CJJ, van der Belt AGM, Prins MH, et al: Fixed dose subcutaneous low molecular weight heparins versus adjusted dose unfractionated heparin for venous thromboembolism. Cochrane Database Syst Rev 4:CD001100, 2004
22. Baglin T, Luddington R, Brown K, et al: Incidence of recurrent venous thromboembolism in relation to clinical and thrombophilic risk factors: prospective cohort study. Lancet 362:523, 2003
23. Levine MN, Hirsh J, Gent M, et al: Optimal duration of oral anticoagulant therapy: a randomized trial comparing four weeks with three months of warfarin in patients with proximal deep vein thrombosis. Thromb Haemost 74:606, 1995
24. Pinede L, Ninet J, Duhaut P, et al: Comparison of 3 and 6 months of oral anticoagulant therapy after a first episode of proximal deep vein thrombosis or pulmonary embolism and comparison of 6 and 12 weeks of therapy after isolated calf deep vein thrombosis. Circulation 103:2453, 2001
25. Schulman S, Rhedin A-S, Lindmarker P, et al: A comparison of six weeks with six months of oral anticoagulant therapy after a first episode of venous thromboembolism. N Engl J Med 332:1661, 1995
26. Agnelli G, Prandoni P, Santamaria MG, et al: Three months versus one year of oral anticoagulant therapy for idiopathic deep vein thrombosis. N Engl J Med 345:165, 2001
27. Agnelli G, Prandoni P, Becattini C, et al: Extended oral anticoagulant therapy after a first episode of pulmonary embolism. Ann Intern Med 139:19, 2003
28. Research Committee of the British Thoracic Society: Optimum duration of anticoagulation for deep-vein thrombosis and pulmonary embolism. Lancet 340:873, 1992
29. Lim W, Crowther MA, Eikelboom JW: Management of antiphospholipid antibody syndrome: a systematic review. JAMA 295:1050, 2006
30. McRae S, Tran H, Schulman S, et al: Effect of patient's sex on risk of recurrent venous thromboembolism: a meta-analysis. Lancet 368:371, 2006
31. Ho WK, Hankey GJ, Quinlan DJ, et al: Risk of recurrent venous thromboembolism in patients with common thrombophilia: a systematic review. Arch Intern Med 166:729, 2006
32. Palareti G, Legnani C, Cosmi B, et al: Predictive value of D-dimer test for recurrent venous thromboembolism after anticoagulation withdrawal in subjects with a previous idiopathic event and in carriers of congenital thrombophilia. Circulation 108:313, 2003
33. Christiansen SC, Cannegieter SC, Koster T, et al: Thrombophilia, clinical factors, and recurrent venous thrombotic events. JAMA 293:2352, 2005
34. Kearon C, Julian JA, Newman TE, Ginsberg JS, for the McMaster Diagnostic Imaging Practice Guidelines Initiative: Non-invasive diagnosis of deep vein thrombosis. Ann Intern Med 128:663, 1998
35. Wells PS, Owen C, Doucette S, Fergusson D, Tran H: Does this patient have deep vein thrombosis? JAMA 295:199, 2006
36. Stein PD, Hull RD, Patel KC, et al: D-dimer for the exclusion of acute venous thrombosis and pulmonary embolism: a systematic review. Ann Intern Med 140:589, 2004
37. Kelly J, Rudd A, Lewis RR, Hunt BJ: Plasma D-dimers in the diagnosis of venous thromboembolism. Arch Intern Med 162:747, 2002
38. Perrier A, Desmarais S, Miron MJ, et al: Non-invasive diagnosis of venous thromboembolism in outpatients. Lancet 353:190, 1999
39. Wells PS, Anderson DR, Rodger M, et al: Evaluation of D-dimer in the diagnosis of suspected deep-vein thrombosis. N Engl J Med 349:1227, 2003
40. Kearon C, Ginsberg JS, Douketis J, et al: A randomized trial of diagnostic strategies after normal proximal vein ultrasonography for suspected deep venous thrombosis: D-dimer testing compared with repeated ultrasonography. Ann Intern Med 142:490, 2005
41. Rathbun SW, Whitsett TL, Raskob GE: Negative D-dimer result to exclude recurrent deep venous thrombosis: a management trial. Ann Intern Med 141:839, 2004
42. Linkins L, Pasquale P, Paterson S, et al: Change in thrombus length on venous ultrasound and recurrent deep vein thrombosis. Arch Intern Med 164:1793, 2004
43. Kearon C: Diagnosis of pulmonary embolism. CMAJ 168:183, 2003
44. Simonneau G, Sors H, Charbonnier B, et al: A comparison of low-molecular-weight heparin with unfractionated heparin for acute pulmonary embolism. N Engl J Med 337:663, 1997
45. Chunilal SD, Eikelboom JW, Attia J, et al: Does this patient have pulmonary embolism? JAMA 290:2849, 2003
46. Le Gal G, Righini M, Roy PM, et al: Prediction of pulmonary embolism in the emergency department: the revised Geneva score. Ann Intern Med 144:165, 2006
47. Wells PS, Anderson DR, Rodger M, et al: Derivation of a simple clinical model to categorize patients probability of pulmonary embolism: increasing the models utility with the SimpliRED D-dimer. Thromb Haemost 83:416, 2000
48. Kearon C, Ginsberg JS, Douketis J, et al: An evaluation of D-dimer in the diagnosis of pulmonary embolism: a randomized trial. Ann Intern Med 144:812, 2006
49. van Belle A, Buller HR, Huisman MV, et al: Effectiveness of managing suspected pulmonary embolism using an algorithm combining clinical probability, D-dimer testing, and computed tomography. JAMA 295:172, 2006
50. Stein PD, Fowler SE, Goodman LR, et al: Multidetector computed tomography for acute pulmonary embolism. N Engl J Med 354:2317, 2006
51. Quiroz R, Kucher N, Zou KH, et al: Clinical validity of a negative computed tomography scan in patients with suspected pulmonary embolism: a systematic review. JAMA 293:2012, 2005
52. Roy PM, Colombet I, Durieux P, et al: Systematic review and meta-analysis of strategies for the diagnosis of suspected pulmonary embolism. Br Med J 331:259, 2005
53. Kruip MJ, Leclercq MG, van der HC, et al: Diagnostic strategies for excluding pulmonary embolism in clinical outcome studies: A systematic review. Ann Intern Med 138:941, 2003

54. Wells PS, Ginsberg JS, Anderson DR, et al: Use of a clinical model for safe management of patients with suspected pulmonary embolism. Ann Intern Med 129:997, 1998

55. Hirsh J, Raschke R: Heparin and low-molecular-weight heparin: the Seventh ACCP Conference on Antithrombotic and Thrombolytic Therapy. Chest 126:188S, 2004

56. Kearon C, Ginsberg JS, Julian JA, et al: Comparison of fixed-dose weight-adjusted unfractionated heparin and low-molecular-weight heparin for acute venous thromboembolism. JAMA 296:935, 2006

57. Quinlan DJ, McQuillan A, Eikelboom JW: Low-molecular-weight heparin compared with intravenous unfractionated heparin for treatment of pulmonary embolism: a meta-analysis of randomized, controlled trials. Ann Intern Med 140:175, 2004

58. Lee AY, Levine MN, Baker RI, et al: Low-molecular-weight heparin versus a coumarin for the prevention of recurrent venous thromboembolism in patients with cancer. N Engl J Med 349:146, 2003

59. Buller HR, Agnelli G, Hull RD, et al: Antithrombotic therapy for venous thromboembolic disease: the Seventh ACCP Conference on Antithrombotic and Thrombolytic Therapy. Chest 126:401S, 2004.

60. Weitz JI, Hirsh J, Samama MM: New anticoagulant drugs: the Seventh ACCP Conference on Antithrombotic and Thrombolytic Therapy. Chest 126:265S, 2004

61. Turpie AG, Bauer KA, Eriksson BI, et al: Fondaparinux vs enoxaparin for the prevention of venous thromboembolism in major orthopedic surgery: a meta-analysis of 4 randomized double-blind studies. Arch Intern Med 162:1833, 2002

62. Buller HR, Davidson BL, Decousus H, et al: Subcutaneous fondaparinux versus intravenous unfractionated heparin in the initial treatment of pulmonary embolism. N Engl J Med 349:1695, 2003

63. Buller HR, Davidson BL, Decousus H, et al: Fondaparinux or enoxaparin for the initial treatment of symptomatic deep venous thrombosis: a randomized trial. Ann Intern Med 140:867, 2004

64. Ansell J, Hirsh J, Poller L, et al: The pharmacology and management of the vitamin K antagonists: the Seventh ACCP Conference on Antithrombotic and Thrombolytic Therapy. Chest 126:204S, 2004

65. Fiessinger JN, Huisman MV, Davidson BL, et al: Ximelagatran vs low-molecular-weight heparin and warfarin for the treatment of deep vein thrombosis: a randomized trial. JAMA 293:681, 2005.

66. Levine MN, Raskob G, Beyth RJ, et al: Hemorrhagic complications of anticoagulant treatment: the Seventh ACCP Conference on Antithrombotic and Thrombolytic Therapy. Chest 126:287S, 2004

67. Kearon C, Ginsberg JS, Kovacs MJ, et al: Comparison of low-intensity warfarin therapy with conventional-intensity warfarin therapy for long-term prevention of recurrent venous thromboembolism. N Engl J Med 349:631, 2003

68. Geerts WH, Pineo GF, Heit JA, et al: Prevention of venous thromboembolism: the Seventh ACCP Conference on Antithrombotic and Thrombolytic Therapy. Chest 126:338S, 2004

69. Prevention of pulmonary embolism and deep vein thrombosis with low dose aspirin: Pulmonary Embolism Prevention (PEP) trial [see comments]. Lancet 355:1295, 2000

70. Eikelboom JW, Quinlan DJ, Douketis JD: Extended-duration prophylaxis against venous thromboembolism after total hip or knee replacement: a meta-analysis of the randomised trials. Lancet 358:9, 2001

71. Decousus H, Leizorovicz A, Parent F, et al: A clinical trial of vena caval filters in the prevention of pulmonary embolism in patients with proximal deep-vein thrombosis. N Engl J Med 338:409, 1998

72. Fedullo PF, Auger WR, Kerr KM, et al: Chronic thromboembolic pulmonary hypertension. N Engl J Med 345:1465, 2001

73. Brandjes DPM, Büller HR, Heijboer H, Huisman MV, de Rijk M, Jagt H et al: Randomised trial of effect of compression stockings in patients with symptomatic proximal-vein thrombosis. Lancet 349:759, 1997

74. Prandoni P, Lensing AW, Prins MH, et al: Below-knee elastic compression stockings to prevent the post-thrombotic syndrome: a randomized, controlled trial. Ann Intern Med 141:249, 2004

75. Ridker PM, Goldhaber SZ, Danielson E, et al: Long-term, low-intensity warfarin therapy for prevention of recurrent venous thromboembolism. N Engl J Med. 348:1425, 2003

76. Kearon C, Ginsberg JS, Anderson DR, et al: Comparison of 1 month with 3 months of anticoagulation for a first episode of venous thromboembolism associated with a transient risk factor. J Thromb Haemost 2:743, 2004

77. Prandoni P, Lensing AWA, Cogo A, M et al: The long-term clinical course of acute deep venous thrombosis. Ann Intern Med 125:1, 1996

78. Pini M, Aiello S, Manotti C, et al: Low molecular weight heparin versus warfarin for the prevention of recurrence after deep vein thrombosis. Thromb Haemost 72:191, 1994

79. Pinede L, Duhaut P, Cucherat M, et al: Comparison of long versus short duration of anticoagulant therapy after a first episode of venous thromboembolism: a meta-analysis of randomized, controlled trials. J Intern Med 247:553, 2000

80. Lindmarker P, Schulman S: The risk of ipsilateral versus contralateral recurrent deep vein thrombosis in the leg: The DURAC Trial Study Group. J Intern Med 247:601, 2000

81. Schulman S, Granqvist S, Holmstrom M, P et al: The duration of oral anticoagulant therapy after a second episode of venous thromboembolism. N Engl J Med 336:393, 1997

82. Murin S, Romano PS, White RH: Comparison of outcomes after hospitalization for deep vein thrombosis or pulmonary embolism. Thromb Haemost 88:407, 2002

83. Schulman S, Svenungsson E, Granqvist S: Anticardiolipin antibodies predict early recurrence of thromboembolism and death among patients with venous thromboembolism following anticoagulant therapy. Am J Med 104:332, 1998

84. Schulman S, Wahlander K, Lundström T, Clason SB, Eriksson H, for the THRIVE III Investigators: Secondary prevention of venous thromboembolism with the oral direct thrombin inhibitor ximelagatran. N Engl J Med 349:1713, 2003

85. Douketis JD, Kearon C, Bates S, Duku EK, Ginsberg JS: Risk of fatal pulmonary embolism in patients with treated venous thromboembolism. JAMA 279:458, 1998

86. Heit JA, Mohr DN, Silverstein MD, et al: Predictors of recurrence after deep vein thrombosis and pulmonary embolism: a population-based cohort study. Arch Intern Med 160:761, 2000

87. Kniffin WD Jr, Baron JA, Barrett J, et al: The epidemiology of diagnosed pulmonary embolism and deep venous thrombosis in the elderly. Arch Intern Med 154:861, 1994

88. Schulman S, Lindmarker P, Holmstrom M, et al: Post-thrombotic syndrome, recurrence, and death 10 years after the first episode of venous thromboembolism treated with warfarin for 6 weeks or 6 months. J Thromb Haemost 4:724, 2006

89. Kearon C: Duration of therapy for acute venous thromboembolism. Clin Chest Med 24:63, 2003

90. Palareti G, Legnani C, Cosmi B, et al: Risk of venous thromboembolism recurrence: high negative predictive value of D-dimer performed after oral anticoagulation is stopped. Thromb Haemost 87:7, 2002

91. Lee AYY, Levine MN, Baker RI, et al: Low-molecular-weight heparin versus a coumarin for the prevention of recurrent venous thromboembolism in patients with cancer. N Engl J Med 349:146, 2003

92. Grady D, Wenger NK, Herrington D, et al: Postmenopausal hormone therapy increases risk for venous thromboembolic disease: the Heart and Estrogen/progestin Replacement Study. Ann Intern Med 132:689, 2000

93. Lindmarker P, Schulman S, Sten-Linder M, et al: The risk of recurrent venous thromboembolism in carriers and non-carriers of the G1691A allele in the coagulation factor V gene and the G20210A allele in the prothrombin gene. Thromb Haemost 81:684, 1999

94. Eichinger S, Pabinger I, Stumpflen A, et al: The risk of recurrent venous thromboembolism in patients with and without factor V Leiden. Thromb Haemost 77:624, 1997

95. Kearon C: Long-term management of patients after venous thromboembolism. Circulation 110 (suppl I):I10, 2004

96. Levine MN, Raskob G, Landefeld S, et al: Hemorrhagic complications of anticoagulant treatment. Chest 119:108S, 2001

97. Beyth RJ, Quinn LM, Landefeld S: Prospective evaluation of an index for predicting the risk of major bleeding in outpatients treated with warfarin. Am J Med 105:91, 1998

98. Linkins L, Choi PT, Douketis JD: Clinical impact of bleeding in patients taking oral anticoagulant therapy for venous thromboembolism: a meta-analysis. Ann Intern Med 139:893, 2003

99. Ansell J, Hirsh J, Dalen J, et al: Managing oral anticoagulant therapy. Chest 119:22S, 2001

100. Bates SM, Greer IA, Hirsh J, et al: Use of antithrombotic agents during pregnancy: the Seventh ACCP Conference on Antithrombotic and Thrombolytic Therapy. Chest 126:627S, 2004

101. Bates SM, Ginsberg JS: How we manage venous thromboembolism during pregnancy. Blood 100:3470, 2002

102. Baarslag HJ, van Beek EJ, Koopman MM, et al: Prospective study of color duplex ultrasonography compared with contrast venography in patients suspected of having deep venous thrombosis of the upper extremities. Ann Intern Med 136:865, 2002

103. Kumar S, Sarr MG, Kamath PS: Mesenteric venous thrombosis. N Engl J Med 345:1683, 2001

104. Oldenburg WA, Lau LL, Rodenberg TJ, et al: Acute mesenteric ischemia: a clinical review. Arch Intern Med 164:1054, 2004

105. Holbrook AM, Pereira JA, Labiris R, et al: Systematic overview of warfarin and its drug and food interactions. Arch Intern Med 165:1095, 2005

33 Approach to the Diagnosis of Skin Disease

Robert T. Brodell, M.D., and Stephen E. Helms, M.D.

Patients frequently see their primary care physician for skin disease[1]; however, compared with dermatologists, primary care physicians treat substantially fewer patients with common skin conditions, and the types of cutaneous disease they treat tend to be few in number.[2,3] One study reported that dermatologists had 728 and 352 office visits a year for acne and contact dermatitis, respectively; by contrast, internists averaged three and nine visits, a year, respectively, and family physicians averaged eight and 27 visits a year.[2] The relative inexperience with cutaneous presentations gives rise to possible error in the dermatologic care offered by nondermatologists. Some studies have reported that nondermatologists perform poorly in the diagnosis and treatment of skin disease.[4] One area of concern is the apparent low proficiency among nondermatologists in the diagnosis of skin cancer.[5,6] The root of most problems encountered by primary care physicians in the treatment of skin disease rests in establishing the accurate diagnosis of cutaneous presentations.

Diagnosis of a cutaneous disease is most reliably achieved by a stepwise approach to patient evaluation, beginning with an examination of the morphologic features of the skin lesions and frequently culminating in diagnostic testing. This chapter reviews the primary skin lesions that allow categorization of dermatologic disease (e.g., papulosquamous diseases, blistering diseases, nonscaling erythematous and infiltrative diseases, and tumors) and presents a method by which the physician can narrow the possible causes of a specific presentation and arrive at a diagnosis in a cost-effective manner.

Approach to the Patient with a Dermatologic Lesion

Dermatology is a visual specialty, and physical examination is primarily oriented toward observing the skin. Dermatologists approach skin disease in a manner that has been tested over time and perpetuated in the training of medical students and residents. A simple diagnostic evaluation based on the approach preferred by dermatologists allows primary care physicians to narrow the possible causes of a cutaneous presentation and arrive at an accurate diagnosis.

DIAGNOSTIC EVALUATION

Diagnostic evaluation of a cutaneous presentation begins with a brief patient history that is directed at the nature of the chief complaint and its onset; factors that aggravate and alleviate symptoms; and responses to over-the-counter or prescription medications. This is followed by careful inspection of the skin. In examining a patient with a rash, the first step is to try to identify primary lesions (i.e., lesions that appear early in the disease process) [see Morphologic Classification of Skin Disorders, Primary Lesions, *below*]); these lesions help to categorize the disease and provide the basis for diagnosis. Information derived from the identification of primary lesions is augmented by an examination of primary lesions that have undergone change. Secondary changes to primary lesions may occur naturally or after trauma, such as scratching [see Morphologic Classification of Skin Disorders, Secondary Changes, *below*]. The location, distri-

bution, and configuration of primary lesions and their secondary changes are analyzed, and the findings are categorized to promote the development of a differential diagnosis.

After an examination of the lesions, a more complete patient history is obtained, including the patient's family history, social history, and medical history. The expanded patient history is followed by a focused general medical examination. In the context of a detailed patient history, the general medical examination often provides diagnostic clues that further narrow the differential diagnosis.

The final step in a dermatologic examination comprises various forms of testing (e.g., dermatologic testing, skin biopsy, and laboratory tests) [see Arriving at a Diagnosis, *below*] to confirm the diagnosis or sufficiently narrow the differential diagnosis to permit selection of the most appropriate treatment. If the diagnosis remains uncertain after testing, consultation with a dermatologist may be useful in establishing the diagnosis. The patient is typically scheduled for a follow-up visit after initiation of treatment. The purpose of the follow-up visit is to assess the response to therapy and to confirm that the proper diagnosis was rendered.

SUBOPTIMAL METHODS OF DIAGNOSIS AND MANAGEMENT

Errors in dermatologic diagnosis can be classified into several categories. It is worth exploring these problems to avoid falling into predictable traps.

Treating Symptoms Rather than Diseases

Establishing the underlying cause of symptoms is a guiding principle in medicine; however, the treatment of dermatologic presentations frequently focuses on symptom management without addressing the underlying cause. This approach is seldom an efficient or effective form of management. For example, treatment of pruritus with antihistamines is a poor substitute for establishing a definitive diagnosis of the underlying condition that is the cause of the symptom. In the case of a patient with severe itching associated with dermatitis herpetiformis, treatment with a topical corticosteroid may give temporary relief from pruritus; however, a careful examination would most likely reveal grouped papulovesicles on the extensor surfaces of the extremities, and a biopsy would confirm the diagnosis of dermatitis herpetiformis. Treatment of dermatitis herpetiformis with a gluten-free diet and oral dapsone would lead to dramatic, long-lasting remission.

Snapshot Approach to Diagnosis

A snapshot diagnosis is rendered on the basis of physical appearance of a rash or other form of lesion in the absence of any other data. This method of examination is quick; however, it can lead to inaccurate diagnosis and imprecise and inadequate treatment. For example, a patient with widespread scaling, erythema, lichenification, and excoriations may appear to have eczema. On careful examination, the finger webs disclose burrows. The patient reports that itching is more severe at night, and that family members are also experiencing itching. A scabies preparation test discloses the presence of mites, confirming the diagnosis as

Table 1   Primary Lesions: Consensus Definitions
of Dermatologic Morphologic Terms[7]

Morphologic Term	DLP Proposed Definition
Bulla	A fluid-filled blister greater than 0.5 cm in diameter; fluid can be clear, serous, hemorrhagic, or pus-filled
Comedo	An enlarged hair follicular infundibulum primarily containing keratin and lipids and having a plugged, dilated follicular opening (blackhead) or a clinically unapparent follicular opening (whitehead)
Macule	A flat area of skin or mucous membranes having a color different from the surrounding tissue and a diameter generally less than 0.5 cm; macules may have nonpalpable, fine scales
Nodule	A dermal or subcutaneous firm, well-defined lesion usually greater than 0.5 cm in diameter
Papule	A discrete, solid, elevated body usually less than 0.5 cm in diameter; papules are further classified by shape, size, color, and surface change
Patch	A flat area of skin or mucous membranes having a color different from the surrounding tissue and a diameter generally greater than 0.5 cm; patches may have non-palpable, fine scales
Plaque	A discrete, solid, elevated body usually broader than it is thick and measuring more than 0.5 cm in diameter; plaques may be further classified by shape, size, color, and surface change
Pustule	A circumscribed elevation that contains pus; pustules are usually less than 0.5 cm in diameter
Vesicle	Fluid-filled cavity or elevation less than 0.5 cm in diameter; fluid may be clear, serous, hemorrhagic, or pus-filled
Wheal	An edematous, transitory papule or plaque

DLP—Dermatology Lexicon Project

scabies infestation. A snap diagnosis of eczema and treatment with topical steroids would have been inappropriate.

Scattershot Management

A suboptimal approach to the management of a dermatologic presentation is touted by physicians who delude themselves into believing that all rashes look alike. This leads to the scattershot approach to management, which advocates increasing the potential for successful treatment of an unknown skin disease by treating all possible causes. For example, the use of a topical steroid/antifungal preparation for a papulosquamous process may seem a prudent treatment of two possible disorders—namely, eczema and superficial fungal infection; however, if the patient has a dermatophyte-induced fungal infection, the topical steroid may decrease local immunity and slow the healing process. This management strategy is expensive, increases the risk of iatrogenic disease, and delays appropriate diagnosis and treatment.

A scattershot approach may also be used in diagnostic evaluation; such an approach entails the ordering of a broad battery of tests in the hope of stumbling upon the correct diagnosis. This inefficient method can lead to false positive results that confuse rather than confirm the diagnosis.

All rashes present physical diagnostic clues that are useful in establishing a diagnosis. A careful evaluation of the lesions' morphologic characteristics, coupled with a thorough patient history and examination, will most likely provide an accurate diagnosis. If the diagnosis remains uncertain, the morphologic condition of the lesion will suggest which specific tests are appropriate for arriving at the diagnosis.

Morphologic Classification of Skin Disorders

PRIMARY LESIONS

The first step in the diagnosis of a rash is to identify primary lesions [*see Table 1*]. Primary lesions are those physical characteristics of skin disease that appear initially and are most useful in developing a differential diagnosis. The characterizing features of primary lesions include whether they are flat or raised, solid or fluid filled, dark or light in color, large or small, smooth or rough. Lesions may be few or numerous, localized or widespread. The newly erupted and undisturbed lesions are most often helpful in categorizing skin conditions in a manner that leads to a correct diagnosis.

Primary skin lesions can be defined simply. Flat lesions are referred to as macules when they are smaller than 0.5 cm and as patches when they are greater than 0.5 cm in diameter [*see Figure 1*].

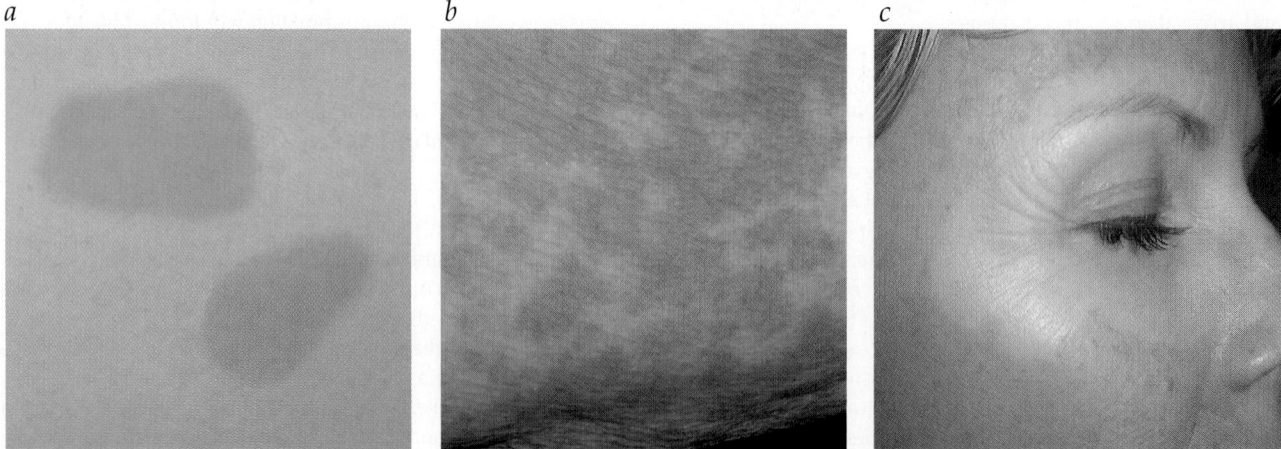

Figure 1   (*a*) **Schematic drawing of macules (lesions < 0.5 cm) or patches (lesions > 0.5 cm). Macules and patches are flat areas of skin for which the color and texture differ from that of the surrounding tissue. (*b*) Nonblanching erythematous macules and patches are present in a patient with a drug eruption. (*c*) Depigmented macules are noted on the face of a patient with vitiligo.**

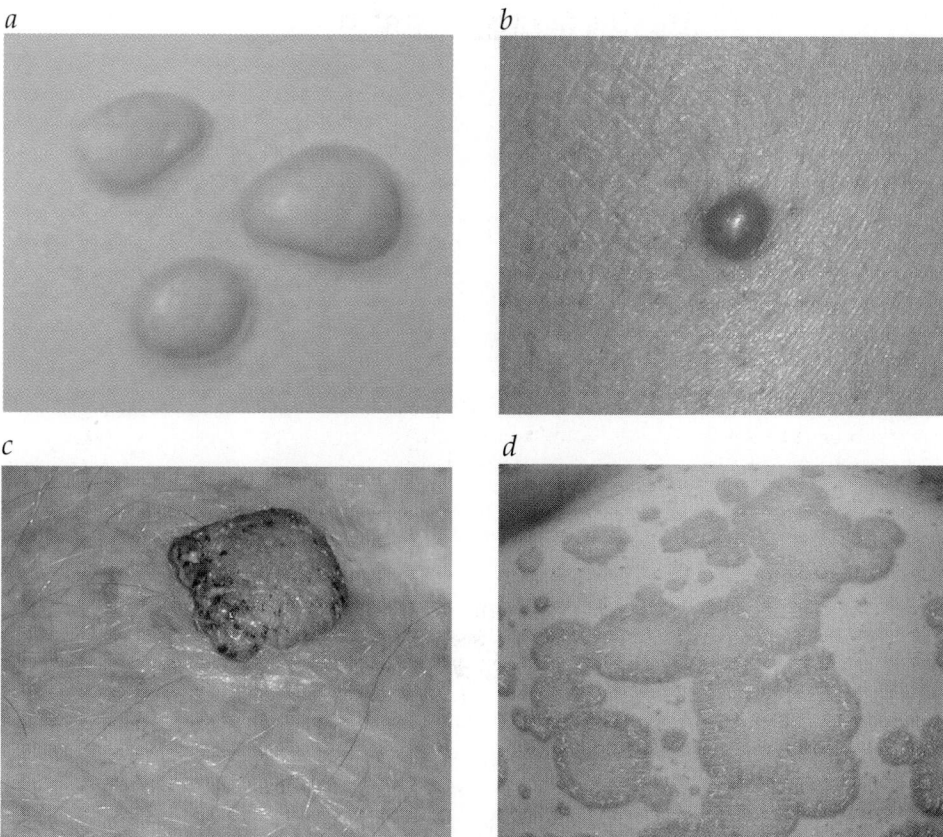

Figure 2 (*a*) **Schematic drawing of papules (lesions < 0.5 cm) or nodules (lesions > 0.5 cm). Papules and nodules are discrete, solid, elevated lesions. (*b*) A raised, dome-shaped, erythematous papule is seen in a case of dermatofibroma. (*c*) A raised, flat-topped, erythematous, and hyperkeratotic nodule with scalloped edges is present in a patient with squamous cell carcinoma. (*d*) Large, erythematous plaques of psoriasis have an annular appearance, owing to their elevated margins.**

Small raised bumps are referred to as papules [*see Figures 2a and b*], and large lesions of this type are referred to as nodules; nodules typically have a deeper dermal component [*see Figure 2c*]. Discrete, broad, raised eruptions are referred to as plaques [*see Figure 2d*]. Raised lesions containing fluid (commonly known as blisters) are referred to as vesicles when smaller than 0.5 cm [*see Figures 3a and b*] and as bullae when larger than 0.5 cm in diameter [*see Figure 3c*]. Vesicles and bullae are usually clear but may be turbid. White or yellow fluid-filled lesions are called pustules. Atrophic lesions exhibit a thinned epidermis that is often depressed; they have a scaly, shiny surface that has the texture of cigarette paper. An edematous transitory papule or plaque is called a wheal [*see Figure 4*].

The shape of primary lesions often provides diagnostic clues. Primary lesions may be round, oval, angular, or irregular; flat-topped or domed; or umbilicated or verrucous. The borders of primary lesions may be well circumscribed or poorly defined; the presence or absence of an elevated border may be a useful finding.

SECONDARY CHANGES

Secondary changes to lesions provide valuable diagnostic information; however, they are not as useful as primary lesions in arriving at a specific diagnosis [*see Table 2*]. Secondary changes may represent a late stage in the natural history of primary lesions, or they may be the result of trauma such as from scratching or rubbing of the skin. Secondary changes to lesions include the following:

- Scales: small flakes of superficial skin.
- Scale crusts: scales combined with serous exudate.
- Excoriations: abrasions resulting from the scratching of elevated lesions.
- Erosions: localized loss of epithelium.
- Ulcers: denuded areas of epidermis and some portion of dermis. Ulcers may be open or covered with a black eschar [*see Figure 5*].
- Scars: raised or depressed fibrous lesions caused by trauma or disease.
- Cutaneous horns: keratotic projections extending from a skin lesion.
- Fissures: cracks that extend through the epidermis into the dermis.

Numerous additional terms are helpful in characterizing the morphologic presentation of skin lesions [*see Table 3*]. It is critical that exacting definitions of descriptive terms be used by all clinicians if a reproducible method of diagnosis is to be promulgated. The Dermatology Lexicon Project (DLP) has provided an expert consensus of definitions for dermatologic terms [*see Tables 1 through 3*].[7]

MORPHOLOGIC PATTERNS OF PRESENTATION

Once the patient has been examined for primary and secondary lesions, the diagnostician must consider the overall presentation of the rash and determine its location, distribution, and configuration—three factors essential in determining a diagnosis.

a *b* *c*

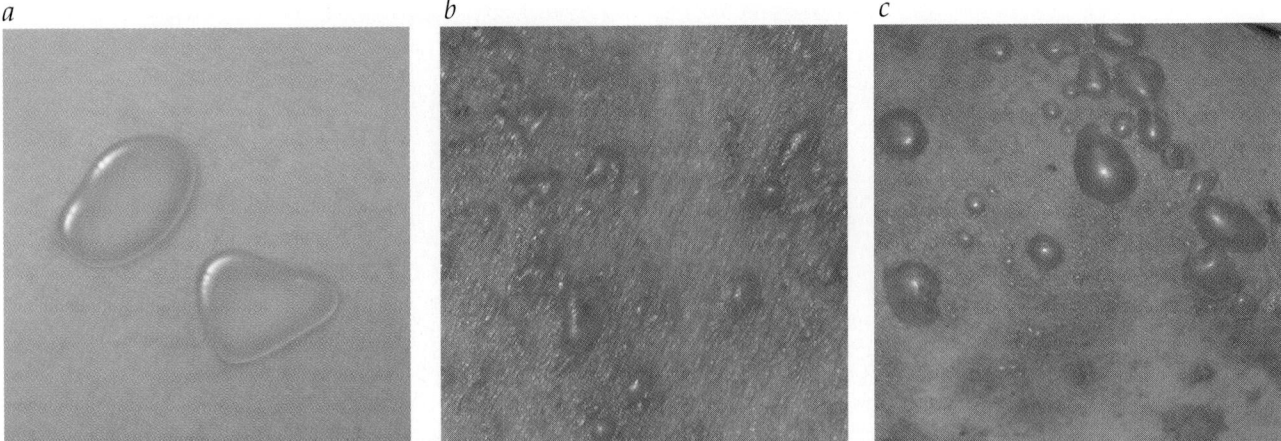

Figure 3 (*a*) Schematic drawing of a vesicle (lesions < 0.5 cm) or bulla (lesions > 0.5 cm). Vesicles, bullae, and pustules are fluid-filled elevations or cavities in the skin. Vesicles and bullae are clear; pustules are turbid and pus filled. (*b*) Small, clear, fluid-filled vesicles on an erythematous base are present in a patient who has herpes zoster. (*c*) Large, clear, fluid-filled bullae are present in a patient with bullous pemphigoid. The bullae are associated with erythematous patches.

Location

The location refers to the particular site where the lesion or lesions are found. The location should be carefully defined because some skin diseases target specific anatomic areas. Notation of involved anatomic sites should be as specific as possible, listing not only the involved sites but the affected aspects of those sites. For example, facial lesions may occur in the periorbital or perioral areas; hand lesions may occur on the fingers or palm; and foot lesions may occur on the toes or sole. Lesions might also be found on the upper arm or the forearm, the lower leg or the thigh, and the trunk. It is important to further describe the affected areas as being on the right or left side and on the proximal or distal, medial or lateral, dorsal or ventral, and flexural or extensor surfaces of the involved anatomic sites.

Distribution

The distribution of lesions describes the overall pattern of an eruption in relation to the entire cutaneous surface. The rash may be localized to one area of the body, may involve several areas, or may extend over much of the body surface. Rashes may be symmetrical or asymmetrical, and they may be present primarily on the trunk or on the extremities. Rashes may be present on exposed skin (i.e., skin that is not covered by clothing) or unexposed skin. These characteristics should be carefully noted because a particular distribution will narrow the differential diagnosis.

Configuration

The configuration of lesions refers to the pattern exhibited by multiple lesions within a defined area. Because the configuration of lesions may vary according to the disorder, any detectable pattern may be helpful in arriving at a definitive diagnosis. Some of the more common configurations include the following:

- Grouped or herpetiform configuration: multiple small lesions appearing within a small, defined area [*see Figure 6*].
- Zosteriform configuration: lesions occurring within a dermatone.
- Linear configuration: lesions oriented along a line [*see Figure 7*].
- Annular configuration: lesions appearing in a ringlike pattern.
- Target (iris) configuration: lesions appearing in concentric rings.

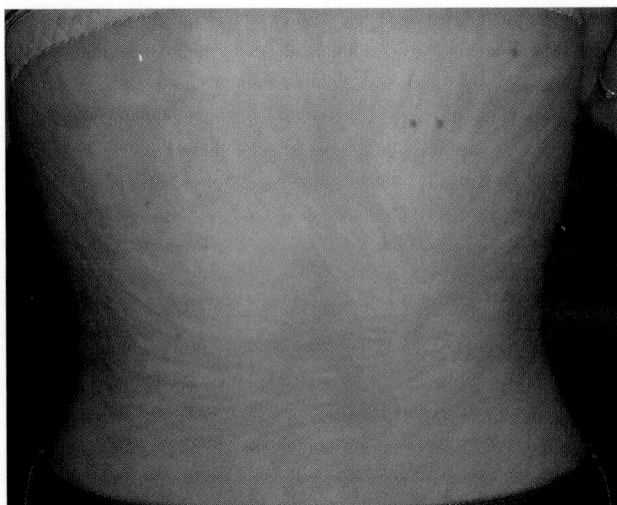

Figure 4 Multiple linear, erythematous wheals secondary to scratching are noted on the back of a patient with chronic urticaria and dermatographism.

Table 2 Selected Secondary Lesions: Consensus Definitions of Dermatologic Morphologic Terms[7]

Morphologic Term	DLP Proposed Definition
Horn	Abnormally keratinized cutaneous projection taller than it is broad
Erosion	A localized loss of the epidermal or mucosal epithelium
Fissure	A linear crack or cleavage within the skin usually found with thickened skin
Ulcer	A circumscribed loss of the epidermis and at least the upper dermis; ulcers are further classified by their depth, border/shape, edge, and tissue at their base

a

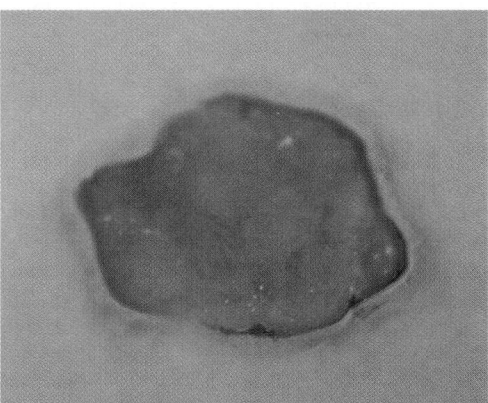

b

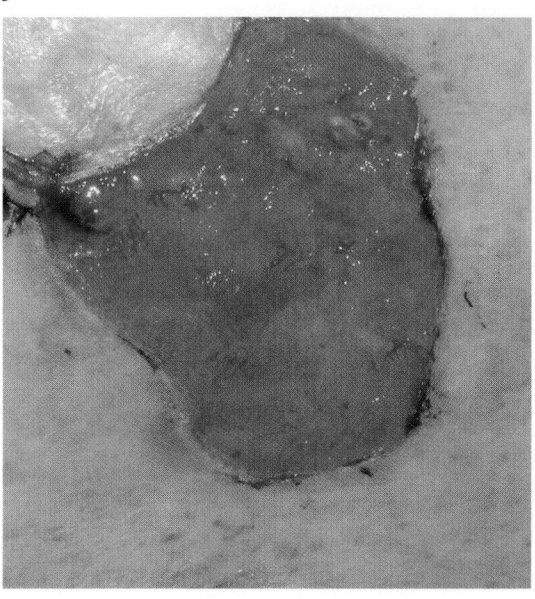

Figure 5 (*a*) **Schematic drawing of a skin ulceration. A skin ulceration is a circumscribed lesion denuded of epidermis and at least some dermis. (*b*) A well-defined 3.5 by 4.0 cm ulceration with an erythematous granulating base is present in a patient who has early evolving pyoderma gangrenosum.**

- Arcuate configuration: lesions appearing in a semicircular pattern.
- Polycyclic configuration: lesions appearing as interlocking rings.
- Serpiginous configuration: lesions appearing in snakelike whorls.
- Digitate configuration: lesions resembling the size and shape of a fingertip.

When lesions coalesce over large areas, they are termed confluent. Erythroderma describes a widespread confluence of rash covering nearly all of the cutaneous surface.

Color

The color of cutaneous lesions also provides important diagnostic clues. Lesions may be flesh-colored, hyperpigmented or hypopigmented, erythematous, or virtually any color of the rainbow. Purpuric rashes caused by the extravasation of red blood cells show no blanching on diascopy (i.e., a test in which a glass slide or lens is pressed against the skin).

Categories of Skin Diseases

The appearance of individual lesions on the skin (e.g., primary lesions and their secondary changes) classifies a rash or growth within a major category of skin disease. The most common skin diseases and many important rare conditions can be classified into one of five disease categories on the basis of their characteristic lesions. Once the category is determined, the diseases within that category are considered in the differential diagnosis of the presenting disorder [*see Table 4*].

As a clinician's dermatologic knowledge becomes more sophisticated, additional categories can be mastered, including (but not limited to) diseases of the hair, nails, or mucous membranes; photosensitivity diseases; diseases of vascular reactivity; ulcerative skin conditions; and conditions typical of specific distributions, such as diseases of the genitalia, feet and hands, and eyelids. Manuals of differential diagnosis based on the morphology of lesions and other physical features are plentiful and can be quite helpful in determining a diagnosis.

Table 3 Other Important Morphologic Terms: Consensus Definitions of Dermatologic Morphologic Terms[7]

Morphologic Term	DLP Proposed Definition
Abscess	A localized accumulation of pus in the dermis or subcutaneous tissue; frequently red, warm, and tender
Atrophy	A thinning of tissue defined by the location (e.g., epidermal atrophy, dermal atrophy, or subcutaneous atrophy)
Burrow	A threadlike linear or serpiginous tunnel in the skin typically made by a parasite
Carbuncle	An inflammatory nodule composed of coalescing furuncles
Ecchymosis	A discoloration of the skin or mucous membranes resulting from extravasation of blood that exhibits color change over time; the characteristic transition is from blue-black to brown-yellow to green
Erythema	Localized, blanchable redness of the skin or mucous membranes
Exfoliation	Desquamation of the superficial epidermis appearing as a fine scaling or as peeling sheets
Furuncle	A follicle-centered nodule caused by a suppurative infection characterized by pain, redness, and perhaps visible pus; usually greater than 1 cm in diameter
Induration	Hardening of the skin beneath the epidermis, usually caused by edema, dermal sclerosis, inflammation, or infiltration
Petechiae	Purpuric nonblanchable macules resulting from tiny hemorrhages, initially measuring 1 to 2 mm
Poikiloderma	An area of variegated pigmentation, atrophy, and telangiectasia
Purpura	Hemorrhaging into skin or mucous membranes that varies in size, color, and duration; types of purpura include palpable purpura, ecchymosis, and petechiae
Telangiectasia	Visible, persistent dilation of small, superficial cutaneous blood vessels

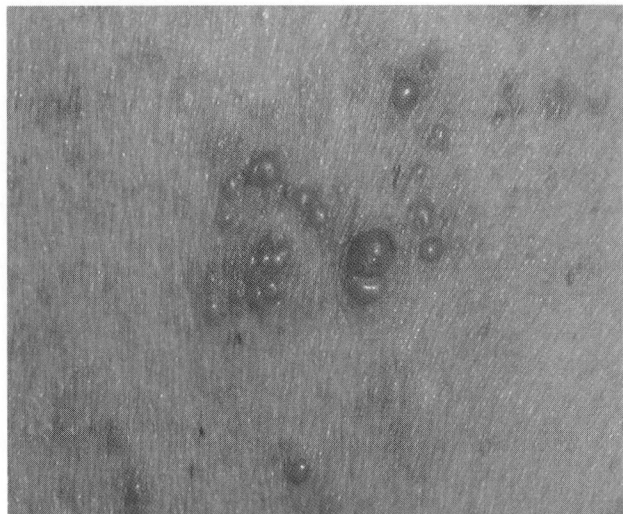

Figure 6 **Close-up view of a herpetiform pattern of vesicles on an erythematous base within a dermatome in a patient with herpes zoster.**

Arriving at a Diagnosis

It is important to begin the assessment of a skin condition with a broad differential diagnosis, noting the presentation as characteristic of one of the categories of skin disease [*see Table 4*]. Using physical findings, patient history, and diagnostic testing, the differential diagnosis is gradually narrowed until a diagnosis is determined. For example, scaling conditions, including rashes composed of both papules and plaques, are characterized as papulosquamous skin diseases; each papulosquamous condition [*see Table 4*] should be considered in the differential diagnosis of a scaling rash. The specific features of each of the papulosquamous conditions are compared with the patient's lesions to systematically identify the disorder. It is critical that the initial differential diagnosis be broadly determined. Jumping to an early conclusion and not systematically considering all of the possible papulosquamous disorders can result in an incorrect diagnosis. In fact, if the actual diagnosis is not among the diseases initially considered, it is much more difficult to determine the correct diagnosis.

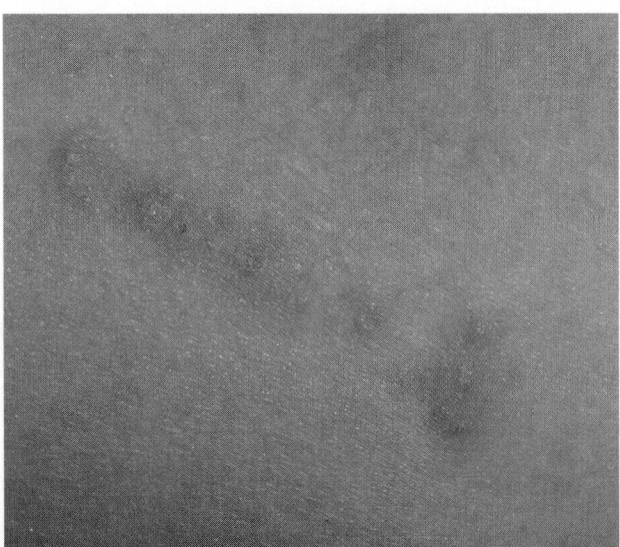

Figure 7 **Linear arrangement of papules in a patient with contact dermatitis caused by poison ivy.**

Table 4 Categories of Skin Disease

Papulosquamous diseases (discrete papules or plaques with scaling)	Psoriasis vulgaris Chronic atopic dermatitis Lichen planus Pityriasis rosea Fungal infections Secondary syphilis Mycosis fungoides
Blistering diseases (vesicles, bullae, pustules)	Acute allergic contact dermatitis Bullous pemphigoid Pemphigus vulgaris Dermatitis herpetiformis Herpesvirus infections Bacterial folliculitis
Nonscaling erythematous (macules, patches, wheals) and infiltrative diseases (plaques)	Urticaria Morbilliform drug eruptions Viral exanthems Sarcoidosis Leukemia and lymphoma cutis Amyloidosis
Diseases of pigmentation (macules or patches of various colors)	Vitiligo Tinea versicolor Pityriasis alba Café au lait macules Lentigines
Benign and premalignant tumors (macules, papules, nodules, tumors)	Actinic keratosis Basal cell carcinoma Squamous cell carcinoma Melanoma Acrochordons Dermatofibroma Neurofibroma Melanocytic nevi Adnexal tumors

Diagnosis is almost always more difficult than treatment. Consultation with a dermatologist is recommended when the diagnosis is uncertain, particularly in cases in which treatment may fail or may lead to iatrogenic disease. The dermatologist may help define the primary lesions that permit the accurate categorization of the disease process and, in turn, suggest the diagnosis.

If a diagnosis remains in doubt, a follow-up visit with the patient should be scheduled because, as the disease progresses, the development of primary lesions and lesion distribution may make the diagnosis more apparent. In addition, single, confirmatory tests often prove helpful in the diagnosis of cutaneous presentations; tests used to confirm a diagnosis include a Wood light examination, potassium hydroxide (KOH) preparation, sampling for fungal culture, scabies preparation, Tzanck preparation, patch testing, skin biopsy, dark-field microscopic examination, microscopic hair-shaft analysis, Gram stain, and viral or bacterial cultures.

A Wood light examination is performed by shining a black light on the skin in a dimly lit room. Epidermal pigmentation (e.g., lentigines) is highlighted by this examination, whereas dermal pigmentation (e.g., Mongolian spot) disappears. A search for depigmented spots such as ash-leaf macules in babies with tuberous sclerosis is also aided by the Wood lamp.

A KOH test for fungal infections involves applying KOH to scales of skin or hair shafts to clear the keratin so that fungal hyphae and spores can be identified. For example, scales can be lightly scraped onto a glass slide after placing the slide on the advancing margin of an annular plaque with central clearing. After a coverslip is applied, 2.5% KOH preparation is applied to the slide next to the coverslip. The KOH preparation spreads under the coverslip by capillary action. After gentle heating, excess KOH is blotted away, and the specimen is examined under a microscope. Fungal infections can also be confirmed by obtaining scales by lightly scraping papulosquamous lesions and sprinkling the scales onto Sabouraud dextrose agar. This agar preparation is then incubated at room temperature for several weeks, after which it is analyzed for colony growth, color, and morphology.

A scabies preparation test involves applying oil to excoriated lesions—frequently found on wrists and finger webs—and lightly scraping the burrows to obtain their contents. The scrapings are placed on a slide with coverslip; the test is positive if scabies mites, eggs, or feces are visible on microscopic examination.

Tzanck preparations are smears obtained from the base of intact vesicles and stained with one of a variety of nuclear stains. A finding of multinucleated giant cells suggests a diagnosis of herpes simplex or herpes zoster infection.

Patch testing is performed to objectively elucidate the specific cause of an allergic contact dermatitis. Standard allergens are applied under patches for 24 hours, and the reactions are read 48 hours and 1 week later.

Skin biopsies are helpful in confirming the diagnosis of a variety of inflammatory and neoplastic diseases. Dark-field microscopic examination of serous fluid from genital ulcers identifies spirochetes in lesions of primary syphilis. Hair-shaft analysis is helpful when alopecia is caused by hair-shaft abnormalities. Finally, viral and bacterial cultures using specific swabs can provide laboratory confirmation of a variety of viral and bacterial diseases.

The authors have no commercial relationships with manufacturers of products or providers of services discussed in this chapter.

References

1. Lowell BA, Froelich CW, Federman DG, et al: Dermatology in primary care: prevalence and patient disposition. J Am Acad Dermatol 45:250, 2001
2. Fleischer AB Jr, Herbert CR, Feldman SR, et al: Diagnosis of skin disease by nondermatologists. Am J Manag Care 6:1149, 2000
3. Feldman SR, Fleischer AB Jr, McConnell RC: Most common dermatologic problems identified by internists, 1990–1994. Arch Intern Med 158:1952, 1998
4. Federman D, Hogan D, Taylor JR, et al: A comparison of diagnosis, evaluation, and treatment of patients with dermatologic disorders. J Am Acad Dermatol 32:726, 1995
5. Whited JD, Hall RP, Simel DL, et al: Primary care clinicians' performance for detecting actinic keratoses and skin cancer. Arch Intern Med 157:985, 1997
6. Gerbert B, Maurer T, Berger T, et al: Primary care physicians as gatekeepers in managed care: primary care physicians' and dermatologists' skills at secondary prevention of skin cancer. Arch Dermatol 132:1030, 1996
7. Morphologic terminology. Dermatology Lexicon Project, 2002 http://www.dermatologylexicon.org

Reviews

Ashton R, Leppard B: Differential Diagnosis in Dermatology. Radcliffe Medical Press, Oxford, 1993
Ghatan HEY: Dermatological Differential Diagnosis and Pearls, 2nd ed. CRC Press, New York, 2002
Kusch SL: Clinical Dermatology: A Manual of Differential Diagnosis, 3rd ed. TaroPharma, 2003 http://www.taropharmadermatology.com
Lawrence CM, Cox NH: Physical Signs in Dermatology: Color Atlas and Text, 2nd ed. Mosby-Wolfe, London, 2001
Lazarus GS, Goldsmith LA: Diagnosis of Skin Disease. FA Davis Co, Princeton, 1980
Pocket Guide to Cutaneous Medicine and Surgery. Dover JS, Ed. Harcourt Brace, Philadelphia, 1996
White GM: Color Atlas of Regional Dermatology. Mosby, London, 1997

Acknowledgment

Figures 1a, 2a, 3a, and 5a Dragonfly Media Group.

34 Cutaneous Manifestations of Systemic Diseases

Mark Lebwohl, M.D.

The cutaneous manifestations of systemic diseases are so numerous and varied that a single chapter could not cover them all, even in a cursory way. Instead, this chapter reviews key cutaneous manifestations of systemic diseases that should be recognized by most physicians, and it highlights recent developments in the diagnosis and management of such disorders. For fuller discussions of specific diseases, including their cutaneous manifestations, readers are referred to the chapters devoted to these conditions.

In many of the disorders presented in this chapter, workup and therapy of the underlying systemic condition are essential to a favorable outcome. A finding of cutaneous sarcoidosis, for example, should prompt a search for systemic sarcoidosis. In other conditions—for example, recessive dystrophic epidermolysis bullosa—treatment of the skin disorder is key to the management of the systemic disease.

Cardiopulmonary and Vascular Diseases

SARCOIDOSIS

The cutaneous manifestations of sarcoidosis are as varied as its systemic manifestations [*see Chapter 219*]. Papules around the eyes or nose are the most characteristic cutaneous manifestations. The term lupus pernio refers to noncaseating granulomas that result in translucent, violaceous plaques of the ears, cheeks, and nose [*see Figure 1*]. Involvement of underlying bone can occur. Diagnosis is made by skin biopsy. Treatment with intralesional corticosteroids is traditional, and oral antimalarials and methotrexate have been used with success. More recently, infliximab has been successfully used for the treatment of sarcoidosis.[1] Other tumor necrosis factor–α (TNF-α) blockers such as etanercept have been used to successfully treat arthritis and skin lesions associated with sarcoidosis.[2] Infliximab has also been used to treat lupus pernio.[3]

There has been an increase in the use of interferon for the treatment of hepatitis C and multiple sclerosis, and a number of reports of sarcoidosis have been attributed to this treatment. Infliximab therapy has been found to effect a response in these cases.[4]

In some patients with sarcoidosis, erythema nodosum, characterized by deep, tender erythematous nodules, occurs on the lower extremities. Lupus pernio is associated with a more chronic course of sarcoidosis, whereas erythema nodosum indicates a more acute and benign disease.[5]

GRANULOMATOUS VASCULITIS

Wegener Granulomatosis

Wegener granulomatosis is associated with both distinctive and nonspecific mucocutaneous signs. Palpable purpura is one of the most common skin findings, but ulcers, papules, nodules, and bullae have also been described. In addition to upper and lower pulmonary symptoms [*see Chapter 218*], saddle-nose deformity, nasal ulcerations, and septal perforation should suggest the diagnosis of Wegener granulomatosis. Definitive diagnosis is made by demonstrating a necrotizing granulomatous vasculitis in a patient with upper and lower respiratory tract disease and glomerulonephritis. Cytoplasmic antineutrophil cytoplasmic autoantibodies (c-ANCA) are often present. Standard therapy is with cyclophosphamide and corticosteroids. TNF-α blockers have proved to be effective for some patients with refractory Wegener granulomatosis.[6]

Lymphomatoid Granulomatosis

Lymphomatoid granulomatosis is a rare, destructive, angiocentric disorder that results from Epstein-Barr virus–associated B cell lymphoproliferative disease.[7] This condition can be associated with skin lesions. Typically, patients develop erythematous papules or nodules that may or may not ulcerate.[8] This disorder is clinically distinguishable from Wegener granulomatosis by the absence of upper respiratory tract involvement. Diagnosis is established by demonstrating a granulomatous necrotizing infiltrate with atypical lymphoid cells around blood vessels. Lymphomatoid granulomatosis is usually fatal; however, rituximab has been used successfully to treat this condition.[9]

Churg-Strauss Syndrome

Churg-Strauss syndrome, or allergic granulomatous angiitis, most commonly presents as asthma and eosinophilia; however, related skin lesions develop in up to 40% of patients. Symmetrical, palpable purpura and petechiae of the lower extremities are the most common findings; these lesions show a leukocytoclastic vasculitis on skin biopsy. Cutaneous nodules caused by extravascular necrotizing granulomas and papules of the elbows also occur.[10] One of the clues to the diagnosis of this disorder is the presence of perinuclear antineutrophil cytoplasmic antibodies (p-ANCA).[11]

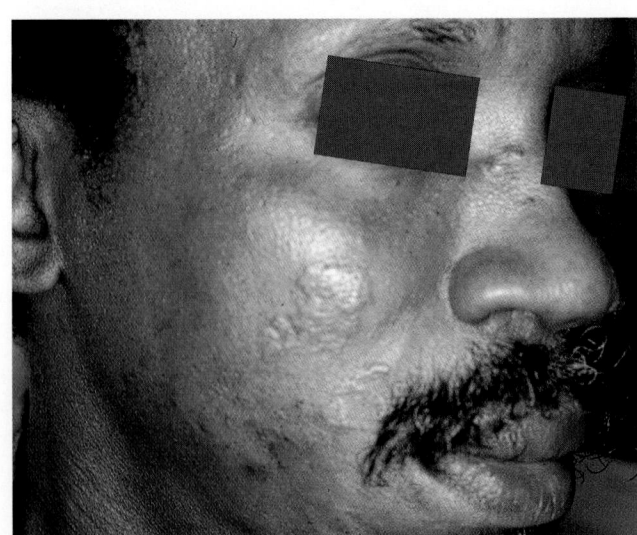

Figure 1   **Characteristic facial lesions of sarcoidosis, called lupus pernio, are shown.**

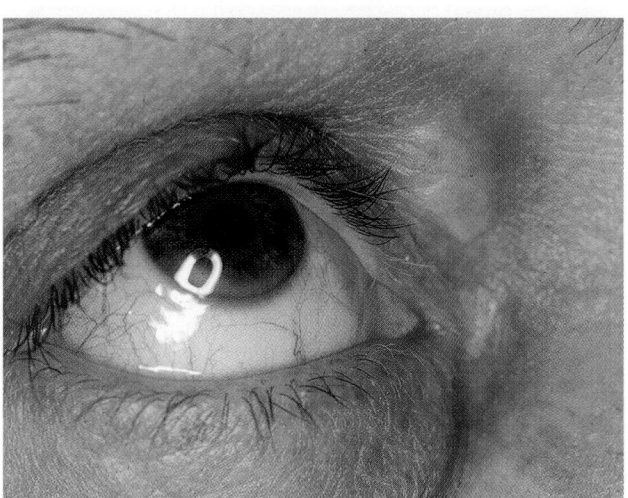

Figure 2 Xanthelasma and arcus senilis are shown in a patient with hypercholesterolemia.

HYPERLIPOPROTEINEMIA

Xanthomas are cutaneous manifestations of hyperlipoproteinemias. Several types of xanthomas occur with different lipid abnormalities. Xanthelasmas of the eyelids [*see Figure 2*] are the most common manifestations of familial hypercholesterolemia; however, in at least half the people who have eyelid lesions, plasma lipid levels are normal. Planar xanthomas are flat yellow plaques that can involve the palms, soles, neck, and chest. They can occur in patients with primary biliary cirrhosis or multiple myeloma. Tuberous xanthomas are large yellow or red nodules that appear on the extensor surfaces of joints, such as on the elbows and hands, but are not attached to underlying tendons. They can occur in patients with elevated triglyceride or cholesterol levels. In contrast, tendinous xanthomas, which can appear in patients with familial hypercholesterolemia, are fixed to underlying tendons of the elbows, ankles, knees, and hands. Eruptive xanthomas occur when plasma triglyceride levels suddenly become elevated. Skin lesions consist of small yellow papules that often resolve with lowering of triglyceride levels.

KAWASAKI DISEASE

Kawasaki disease, also called mucocutaneous lymph node syndrome [*see Chapter 117*], is a disorder in children that can be complicated by coronary artery occlusion and myocardial infarction, coronary artery aneurysms, ECG abnormalities, cardiac arrhythmias, or myocarditis.[12] It has been suggested that a toxin secreted by *Staphylococcus aureus* is responsible for this disease, but proof of the precise cause remains elusive.[13] Diagnosis is based on clinical criteria that include fever, conjunctivitis, lymphadenopathy, and rash. In addition to a generalized erythematous eruption, abnormalities of the oral mucosa, as well as swelling and erythema of the hands and feet, may develop. Striking desquamation of the palms and soles ultimately occurs. Perianal and scrotal erythema and scaling are common as well. Thrombocytosis is a late finding, with platelet counts increasing to more than one million over 2 weeks after the onset of the disease. Approximately 15% to 25% of untreated children develop coronary artery aneurysms that may lead to sudden death.[14] Treatment with intravenous immunoglobulin reduces the frequency of coronary artery abnormalities.[15]

PSEUDOXANTHOMA ELASTICUM

Pseudoxanthoma elasticum (PXE) is an autosomal recessively inherited disorder of elastic tissue caused by mutations in the ABCC6 transporter protein.[16] PXE is associated with a wide array of systemic manifestations. Angioid streaks, the ocular hallmark of PXE, are breaks in the Bruch membrane. Retinal bleeding and vision loss commonly occur. Calcification of the internal elastic laminae of arteries can result in bleeding or occlusion of these vessels. As a result, patients develop intermittent claudication on walking and occlusive coronary artery disease at an early age. Cardiac valvular abnormalities have also been described.[17] Skin lesions consist of yellow xanthomalike macules, papules, or redundant folds of skin in flexural areas, particularly the neck and axillae [*see Figure 3*]. Some patients may have systemic manifestations of PXE without clinically apparent skin lesions.[18] Diagnosis is established by biopsy of scar or normal-appearing flexural skin.[19] There is no therapy for the skin lesions associated with PXE.

RHEUMATIC FEVER

The two cutaneous manifestations of rheumatic fever are erythema marginatum and subcutaneous nodules. Erythema marginatum is a transient faint annular erythematous rash that often develops over joints [*see Figure 4*]. The subcutaneous nodules that appear with rheumatic fever are nontender, freely movable nodules measuring approximately 1 cm in diameter; they occur on the extensor surfaces of elbows, hands, or feet.

YELLOW NAIL SYNDROME

Yellow nail syndrome is caused by an abnormality of lymphatics [*see Figure 5*]. Affected patients develop lymphedema, usually of the legs, and pleural effusions. Pulmonary symptoms such as recurrent bronchitis are also common. Diagnosis is made by finding evidence of abnormal lymphatic function associated with yellow nails without other causes of nail pathology. Increased microvascular permeability with leakage of proteins may play a role in the development of the yellow nail syndrome.[20]

Endocrinologic Diseases

DIABETES MELLITUS

There are numerous cutaneous manifestations of diabetes mellitus. Acanthosis nigricans can occur in patients with diabetes and other endocrinopathies, such as Cushing syndrome, acromegaly, polycystic ovary syndrome, and thyroid disease. Insulin resistance is an underlying factor in several of the aforementioned endocrinopathies; it also may play a role in the development of acanthosis nigricans. Skin lesions consist of brown velvety patches in intertriginous areas, especially the neck and axillae [*see Figure 6*], and occur more commonly in obese patients with diabetes.[21] Acanthosis nigricans has also been associated with internal malignancies, particularly gastric adenocarcinoma or other gastrointestinal adenocarcinomas.

Necrobiosis lipoidica is a specific cutaneous manifestation of diabetes. Lesions consist of chronic atrophic patches with enlarging erythematous borders. The legs are most commonly affected. The centers of the lesions appear yellow because of subcutaneous fat that is visible through the atrophic dermis and epidermis. Occasionally, the lesions ulcerate. Necrobiosis lipoidica is often associated with diabetic nephropathy or retinopathy.[22]

Scleredema, another manifestation of diabetes, consists of induration of the skin of the back and posterior neck in obese pa-

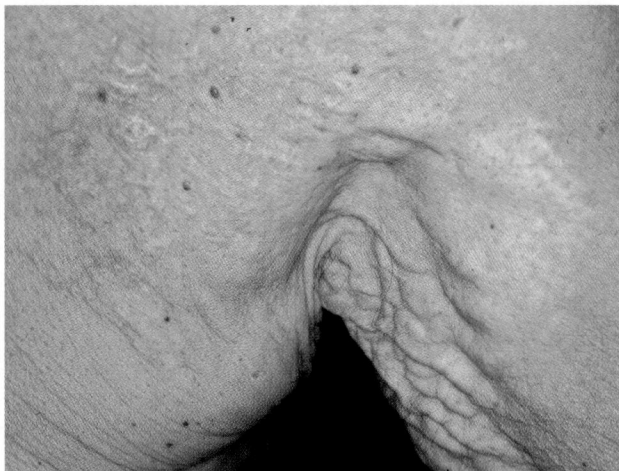

Figure 3   Xanthomalike papules are characteristic of pseudoxanthoma elasticum. The neck and axillae are the most common sites of involvement.

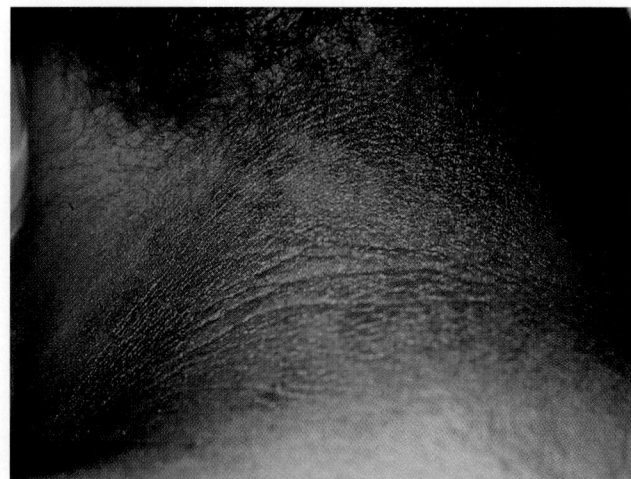

Figure 6   Acanthosis nigricans, a dark velvety acanthosis that can occur in patients with diabetes mellitus and other endocrine disorders, often appears on the neck.

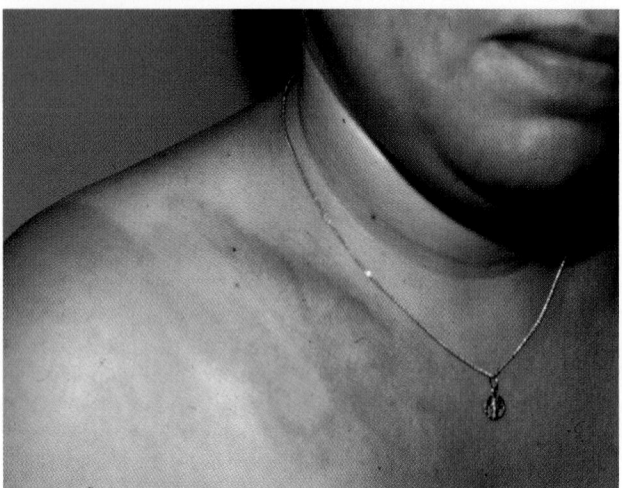

Figure 4   Transient annular erythematous rashes (erythema marginatum) typically occur in patients with rheumatic fever.

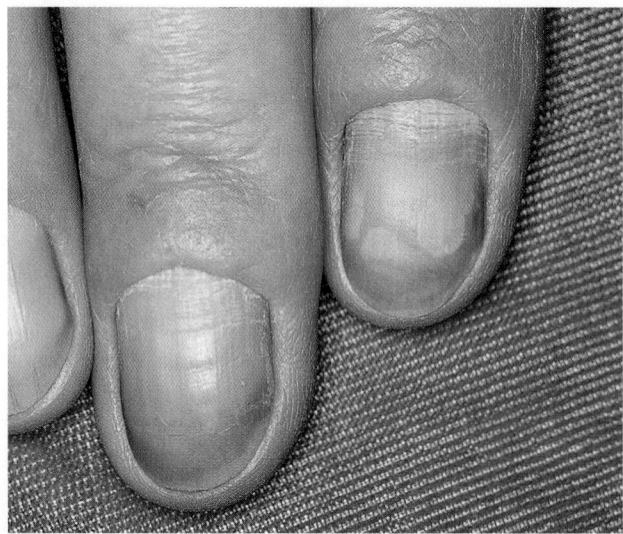

Figure 5   Yellow nails are a sign of underlying disease of the lymphatics in patients with yellow nail syndrome.

tients with type 2 (non–insulin-dependent) diabetes. Scleredema may improve if diabetes is controlled.[23] Less commonly, scleredema occurs in nondiabetic patients after streptococcal pharyngitis; in such patients, the disease is self-limited, resolving within 2 years of onset. High-dose corticosteroids,[24] radiation,[25] and ultraviolet-A1 irradiation (UVA1)[26] have all been used to treat scleredema.

Diabetic bullae, neuropathic ulcers, and so-called waxy skin and stiff joints occur in patients with diabetes. In the last condition mentioned, scleroderma-like induration of the skin over the dorsal aspect of the hands prevents full flexion or extension of the proximal interphalangeal joints.

Diabetic patients are prone to a number of infections, including erythrasma, a corynebacterial infection resulting in asymptomatic reddish-brown patches in intertriginous sites, especially the groin and axillae. Patients are also prone to staphylococcal infections and frequently develop furuncles and carbuncles. Candidal infections are another risk, particularly when blood glucose levels are poorly controlled.

GRAVES DISEASE

Graves disease consists of a triad of exophthalmos, hyperthyroidism, and pretibial myxedema [*see Chapter 50*]. Pretibial myxedema presents as skin-colored nodules and plaques that extend from the pretibial area down to the dorsa of the feet. Lesions often develop after treatment of hyperthyroidism, although they can occur at any stage in the evolution of Graves disease.

Onycholysis, the separation of the nail plate from the nail bed, occurs in many patients with hyperthyroidism. Other autoimmune skin diseases, such as vitiligo and alopecia areata, are increased in patients with Graves disease. Manifestations of thyroid disease include the stigmata of hypothyroidism. Patients can develop alopecia; specifically, they can lose the lateral third of the eyebrows. Edematous thickening of the lips, tongue, and nose occur as well.

Gastrointestinal Diseases

Patients with any of a number of gastrointestinal diseases may present with cutaneous manifestations; similarly, patients

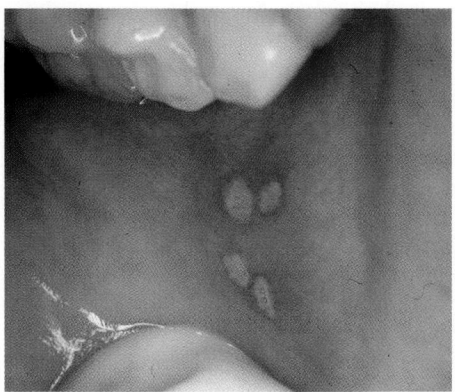

Figure 7 **Aphthous stomatitis is a common finding in patients with ulcerative colitis.**

Figure 8 **Pyoderma gangrenosum is characterized by ulcers that begin with craterlike holes draining pus.**

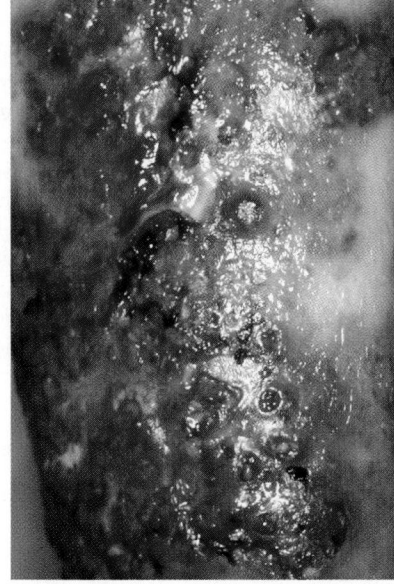

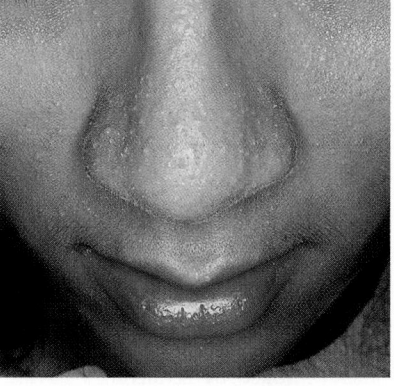

Figure 9 **The patient's nose and cheeks are covered with small papules called trichilemmomas, which represent the cutaneous hallmark of Cowden disease.**

with certain cutaneous diseases can develop gastrointestinal complications.

CARCINOID SYNDROME

The carcinoid syndrome is characterized by episodic flushing that can be associated with abdominal pain, diarrhea, and wheezing. Ninety percent of carcinoid tumors originate in the gastrointestinal tract; however, bronchial carcinoids occur occasionally. Less common cutaneous manifestations of carcinoid tumors include sclerodermatous changes. Cutaneous metastases present as deep nodules; hyperkeratosis may occur; and the patient may experience pigmentation changes similar to those seen in pellagra.

INFLAMMATORY BOWEL DISEASE

There are several specific and nonspecific cutaneous manifestations of inflammatory bowel disease [see Chapter 63]. In both Crohn disease and ulcerative colitis, disease can progress to a hypercoagulable stage, causing venous and arterial thromboses that can lead to loss of digits and limbs. Aphthous stomatitis is another nonspecific manifestation of inflammatory bowel dis-

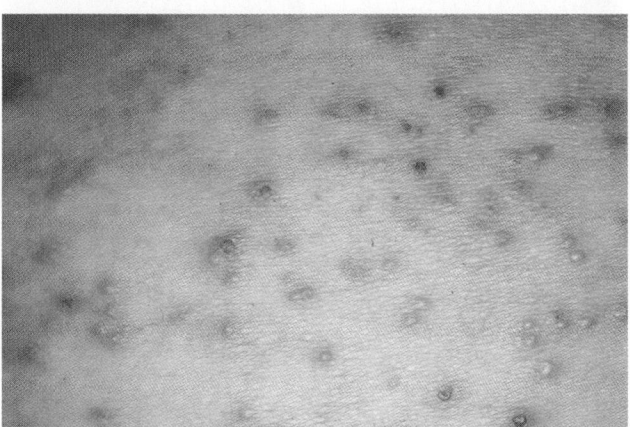

Figure 10 **The primary lesions of herpetiformis are vesicles that quickly break to form crusts and erosions.**

ease [see Figure 7]. In patients with Crohn disease, the lesions may appear as noncaseating granulomas, whereas in patients with ulcerative colitis, they may be indistinguishable from canker sores.

Pyoderma gangrenosum occurs in patients with Crohn disease and ulcerative colitis and has also been reported in patients with chronic active hepatitis, rheumatoid arthritis, and a number of myeloproliferative disorders. The lesions are distinguishable from other ulcers by the presence of craterlike holes, pustules, and purulent drainage [see Figure 8]. Pyoderma gangrenosum may occur at sites of trauma. Treatment with intralesionally injected or systemic corticosteroids may be required. Immunosuppressive agents such as cyclosporine have proved to be dramatically effective; in refractory cases, thalidomide has been shown to be beneficial.[27] Infliximab has proved to be highly effective in the treatment of refractory pyoderma gangrenosum.[28]

Erythema nodosum is a septal panniculitis that is associated with a number of conditions, including Crohn disease, ulcerative colitis, Behçet syndrome, sarcoidosis, infection, and the ingestion of estrogens and other drugs. Other manifestations of Crohn disease include inguinal abscesses and sinuses and anal fistulas.

METASTATIC CROHN DISEASE

The term metastatic Crohn disease refers to histologically proven noncaseating granulomas that are remote from the gastrointestinal tract in patients with Crohn disease. The clinical presentation can be quite variable, and the diagnosis of this disorder is frequently missed. In some cases, patients present with marked swelling of the scrotum or vulva.

CUTANEOUS CONDITIONS WITH GASTROINTESTINAL COMPLICATIONS

Cowden Disease

Cowden disease is an autosomal dominant disorder in which gastrointestinal polyps develop along with numerous skin lesions. This disease has been attributed to mutations of the tumor suppressor gene *PTEN*.[29] Wartlike papules known as trichilemmomas occur, particularly around the nose, mouth, and ears but also on the hands and feet [*see Figure 9*]. Small papules can also develop on the gingival mucosa, creating a cobblestone appearance. Hemangiomas and lipomas can occur.[30] A distinctive nodule of the scalp known as Cowden fibroma has been described. Up to 50% of women with Cowden disease develop breast cancer, a finding that has been associated independently with the *PTEN* mutation.[31] Thyroid carcinomas, thyroid adenomas, and thyroid goiters can occur as well.

Dermatitis Herpetiformis

Dermatitis herpetiformis is an immunobullous disease that is associated with a gluten-sensitive enteropathy [*see Chapter 43*]. Skin lesions begin as vesicles that are so pruritic that they are quickly broken by scratching, leaving only excoriations and crusts [*see Figure 10*]. Like patients with celiac disease who are not on a gluten-free diet, patients with dermatitis herpetiformis have an increased risk of gastrointestinal lymphoma.[32]

Peutz-Jegher Syndrome

In Peutz-Jegher syndrome, patients develop hamartomatous polyps of the small intestine; these polyps are associated with pigmented macules of the lips and oral mucosa [*see Chapter 45*]. Also, pigmented macules can develop on the palms, fingers, soles, and toes and in areas around the mouth, nose, and rectum. The disease is inherited as an autosomal dominant trait, and a significant proportion of cases are associated with mutations in the serine/threonine protein kinase I1/LKB1 (*STKI1/LKB1*) gene, although mutations in this gene do not account for all cases.[33]

Recessive Dystrophic Epidermolysis Bullosa

Recessive dystrophic epidermolysis bullosa is a congenital bullous disease with recurrent blistering and scarring, particularly on the hands and feet [*see Chapter 43*]. The scarring results in pseudosyndactyly, giving rise to mittenlike hands. Ingestion of coarse food can result in mucosal bullae of the esophagus, which heal with scarring and stricture formation. Dysphagia is a frequent complaint. Scarring of the esophagus can lead to squamous cell carcinoma, which is a leading cause of death in this disorder.[34] Gastroenterologists and dermatologists must play key roles in the management of these patients. Liquid and pureed diets and appropriate skin care are essential to the survival of patients with this debilitating disorder. Prenatal diagnosis can be made by sampling DNA from the chorionic villus.[35] All forms of dystrophic epidermolysis bullosa have been attributed to mutations in the type VII collagen gene.[36] Recently, through the use of a self-inactivating minimal lentivirus-based vector, the type VII collagen gene has been delivered and type VII collagen expressed in immunodeficient mice, suggesting the possibility that, in the future, gene therapy may be available to successfully treat this devastating disorder.[37]

Hematologic Diseases

AMYLOIDOSIS

There are several forms of local and systemic amyloidosis [*see Chapter 206*]. In a form associated with multiple myeloma, amyloid fibrils consisting of immunoglobulin light chains are deposited in the skin. Shiny translucent papules develop, particularly on the eyelids. Because of amyloid deposits in blood ves-

sels, spontaneous bleeding occurs. Minimal trauma results in petechiae and purpura. Macroglossia also occurs in some patients with myeloma-associated amyloidosis and in some with primary systemic amyloidosis. The systemic manifestations of myeloma-associated amyloidosis and primary systemic amyloidosis are quite varied. Hepatomegaly develops in 50% of patients with these disorders. Amyloid can affect the heart, resulting in heart failure or myocardial infarction. Survival of patients who undergo heart transplantations for cardiac amyloidosis is lower than survival after cardiac transplantation for other indications.[38] Amyloidosis of the gastrointestinal tract can result in malabsorption and protein-losing enteropathy. Treatment with thalidomide (up to 400 mg daily) and intermittent dexamethasone is rapidly effective in some patients, but side effects are frequent.[39]

MASTOCYTOSIS

Mastocytosis is caused by the infiltration of mast cells into the skin and other organs [*see Chapter 65*]. Urticaria pigmentosa refers to the skin lesions that occur in most patients with mastocytosis. Reddish-brown macules and papules resembling nevi are characteristic of mastocytosis [*see Figure 11*]. Stroking of individual lesions results in urticarial wheals—a phenomenon known as the Darier sign. Pruritus, flushing, abdominal pain, nausea, vomiting, and diarrhea are common complaints.

Most patients with mastocytosis have an indolent form of the disease, even when mast cells have infiltrated the bone marrow.[40] Malignant or aggressive systemic mast cell disease can involve the spleen, liver, and lymph nodes in addition to the skin and bone marrow. Histologically, infiltrates contain atypical nonmetachromatic mast cells that are monoclonal in some patients.[41] Children with urticaria pigmentosa usually have a better prognosis than adults with the disease.[42]

The diagnosis of mastocytosis is made by the demonstration of mast cells on skin biopsy. Because mast cells easily degranulate, making them difficult to identify, biopsies should be performed with a minimum of tissue manipulation.

PORPHYRIAS

The porphyrias result from defective hemoglobin synthesis, leading to excess porphyrins in the blood and in body tissues [*see Chapter 60*].

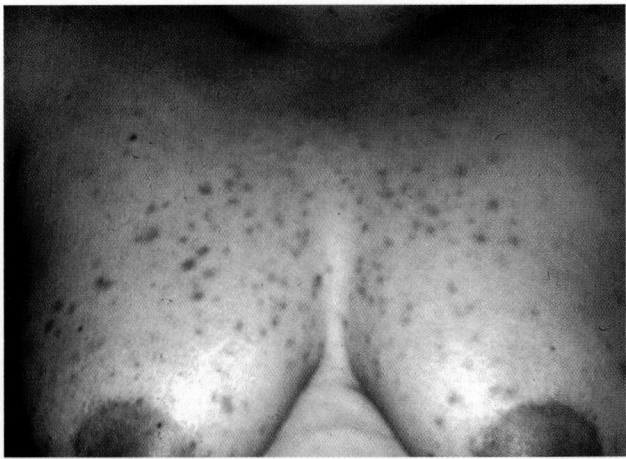

Figure 11 **Multiple brown macules resembling nevi occur in patients with urticaria pigmentosa.**

Congenital Erythropoietic Porphyria

Congenital erythropoietic porphyria is a rare autosomal recessive disorder that has been attributed to mutations in the gene for uroporphyrinogen III synthase.[43] This condition is characterized by severe photosensitivity. Vesicles and bullae develop after sun exposure; these lesions heal with scar formation. Erythrodontia (red-stained teeth) is a characteristic feature [*see Figure 12*]. Digit, ear, and nose loss is common in patients who manage to survive to adulthood [*see Figure 13*]. Hypertrichosis is another frequent complication. Formation of gallstones, splenomegaly, and hemolytic anemia are also associated with this condition.

Porphyria Cutanea Tarda

Porphyria cutanea tarda is characterized by photosensitivity, vesicle formation (especially on the dorsa of the hands) [*see Figure 14*], and hypertrichosis. The condition may be associated with ingestion of alcohol or medications such as estrogens. Diagnosis of the porphyrias can be established by elevated urinary porphyrin levels. Examination of the urine with a Wood lamp will often reveal pink-red fluorescence attributable to the high level of urinary porphyrins. Porphyria cutanea tarda can be associated with hepatitis C. Phlebotomy is effective therapy.

Immunodeficiency Diseases

AIDS

AIDS may result in cutaneous infections and neoplasms that are often dramatic in their extent and severity. This section of the chapter focuses on selected cutaneous manifestations of infections and other diseases associated with AIDS. (For a more comprehensive discussion of disorders associated with HIV infection, see Chapter 153 and other chapters devoted to specific conditions.)

Opportunistic Infections

Viral infections   Banal viral infections, such as molluscum contagiosum, that are ordinarily self-limited and easily curable have become widespread, chronic, and enormous problems in patients with AIDS. These umbilicated white papules, ordinarily only a few millimeters in diameter, can reach diameters of 1 to 2 cm in patients with AIDS. Similarly, condyloma acuminatum, caused by human papillomavirus (HPV) infection, is often difficult to treat in patients with AIDS.

Herpes simplex virus infections become chronic and erosive, forming large, nonhealing ulcers [*see Chapter 148*]. Acyclovir-resistant strains of herpes simplex virus have been reported in some patients with AIDS[44]; these patients require other antiviral agents, such as foscarnet. Mutations in thymidine kinase and DNA polymerase genes of herpes simplex viruses can render them resistant to acyclovir and foscarnet.[45] Topical cidofovir gel has been reported to be beneficial for herpes infections in patients infected with HIV.[46]

Herpes zoster infections are a common sign of HIV infection. In the non–HIV-infected host, herpes zoster is characterized by grouped vesicles in a dermatomal distribution. The eruption is self-limited, resolving within 1 to 2 weeks. In contrast, herpes zoster infection can develop into a disseminated vesicular eruption in patients with AIDS; and in some AIDS patients, chronic herpetic lesions develop and last for months.

Fungal infections   Fungal infections are common in patients

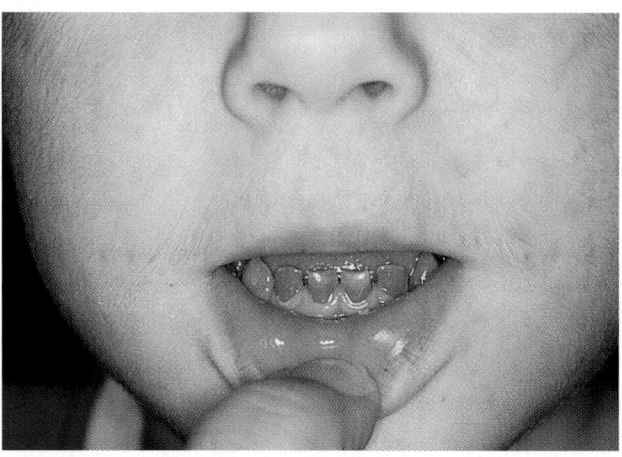

Figure 12   **A reddish pigmentation (erythrodontia) occurs when porphyrins are deposited in the teeth in congenital erythropoietic porphyria.**

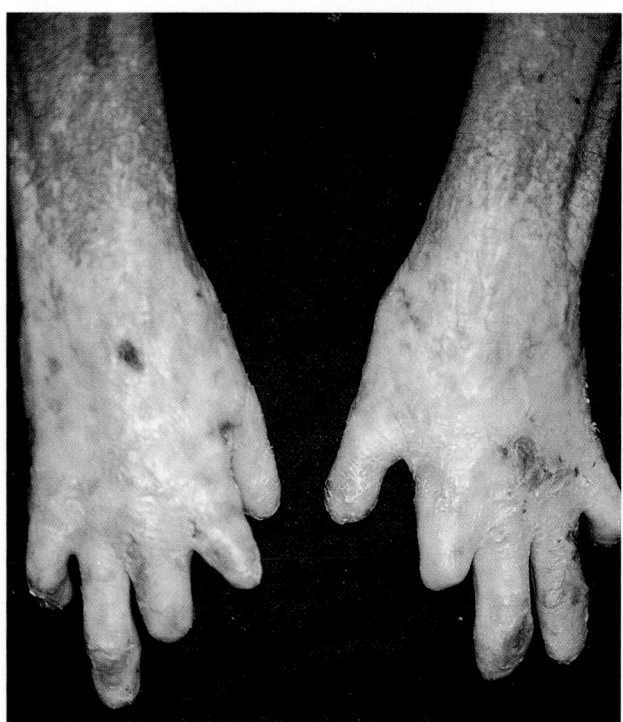

Figure 13   **Skin changes in congenital erythropoietic porphyria can be severe; scarring and loss of digits are common in older patients.**

with HIV infection. Monilial infections include oral thrush and candidiasis of the groin. Several fungal infections that rarely cause widespread infection in patients with normal immune systems (e.g., cryptococcosis, histoplasmosis, aspergillosis, and sporotrichosis) have emerged as serious pathogens in patients with AIDS.

Bacterial infections   Bacterial infections are more frequent and severe in patients with AIDS than in patients with normal immune systems. Bacillary angiomatosis, caused by *Bartonella henselae,* presents as purple papules and nodules that can be mistaken for Kaposi sarcoma (see below). Chronic fever and chills can occur, as can bone lesions. Epidemiologic evidence suggests that cats may be the source of human infection.[47] Diagnosis by use of serologic testing has been commonly used, but in the future, polymerase chain reaction may offer a more rapid and convenient way of establishing this diagnosis.[48] The condition resolves upon treatment with oral antibiotics [*see Chapter 141*].

Scabies and other pruritic eruptions Scabies, a severely pruritic eruption, has a predilection for the buttocks, the genitals, the periumbilical area, and the webs between the fingers. Norwegian scabies, a thickly crusted psoriasislike form of the parasitic disease, has been described in patients with Down syndrome and in other immunosuppressed persons. In recent years, Norwegian scabies has been reported most commonly in patients with AIDS. The scales of Norwegian scabies contain thousands of mites that are easily seen with the microscope. Burrows form linear lesions up to 1 cm long. The causative mite, *Sarcoptes scabiei*, can be identified by microscopic examination of scrapings from the burrows.

Eosinophilic pustular folliculitis and papular eruption of AIDS are pruritic rashes that affect patients with HIV infection. It has been suggested that pruritic papular eruption in patients with HIV infection may represent a reaction to arthropod bites.[49]

Both eosinophilic pustular folliculitis and papular eruption of AIDS are characterized by severe itching, and skin-colored papules and excoriations are common in both. Patients with eosinophilic pustular folliculitis can develop pustules and erythematous papules. Both conditions respond to treatment with ultraviolet B.

Kaposi Sarcoma

Kaposi sarcoma, a slowly progressive vascular neoplasm, was originally described in elderly Italian and Jewish men [*see Chapter 45*]. Subsequently, a more rapidly progressive form of the disorder was described in immunosuppressed patients with lymphomas and in kidney transplant patients on immunosuppressive drugs. An aggressive form has been described in patients with AIDS [*see Figure 15*]. Classic Kaposi sarcoma typically affects the lower extremities and only gradually progresses to other sites. In contrast, AIDS-related Kaposi sarcoma can occur on any surface of the body, including mucous membranes. Human herpesvirus type 8 has been implicated in both classic and AIDS-related Kaposi sarcoma.[50] Treatments include radiation therapy, cryotherapy, and intralesional injection with vinblastine; systemic chemotherapy can also be effective. In patients with AIDS, Kaposi sarcoma is best treated with antiretroviral regimens.

Oral Hairy Leukoplakia

Oral hairy leukoplakia, another condition that has been described in HIV-infected patients, consists of linear white papules on the lateral surfaces of the tongue that result in the so-called hairy appearance. Oral hairy leukoplakia can be distinguished from oral thrush in that the lesions cannot be rubbed off, as they can be in thrush.

Thanks to the development of effective antiretroviral therapy, the frequency of opportunistic infections in patients with HIV infection has diminished markedly.

OTHER IMMUNODEFICIENT STATES

Other inherited or acquired immunodeficiency states share a number of clinical features. Susceptibility to monilial infections or bacterial infections is increased in disorders such as chronic granulomatous disease and chemotherapy-induced neutropenia. Oral ulcers similarly occur in cyclic neutropenia and in chemotherapy-induced immunosuppression.

Some immunosuppressive drugs have characteristic cutaneous effects. Corticosteroids, when used long-term, cause vascular fragility, resulting in steroid purpura. They can also cause cutaneous atrophy, formation of striae, and acneiform eruptions. Cyclosporine is associated with hypertrichosis. Aphthous stomatitis is a characteristic effect of numerous immunosuppressive drugs, particularly agents that suppress bone marrow function. Chronic immunosuppression can lead to the development of lymphoma and nonmelanoma skin cancer. Avoidance of excessive exposure to sunlight may prevent development of the latter.

Infectious Diseases

Cutaneous manifestations can be major features of a number of systemic infections; for example, patients with overwhelming septicemia can develop disseminated intravascular coagulation (DIC), which results in cutaneous infarcts and hemorrhage into the skin. Key cutaneous features of selected systemic infections follow.

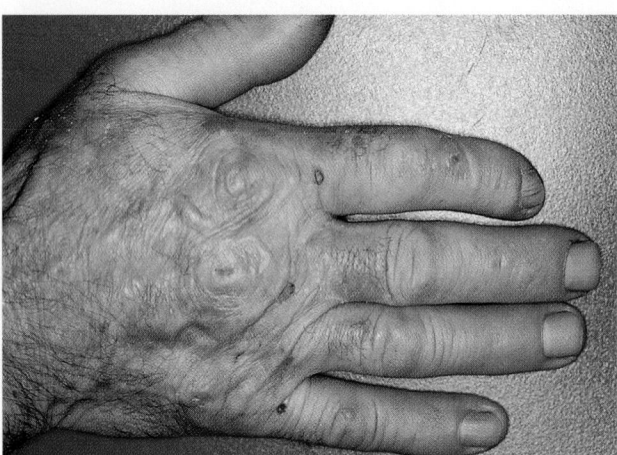

Figure 14 **Crusting and scarring follow the appearance of vesicles and bullae in porphyria cutanea tarda.**

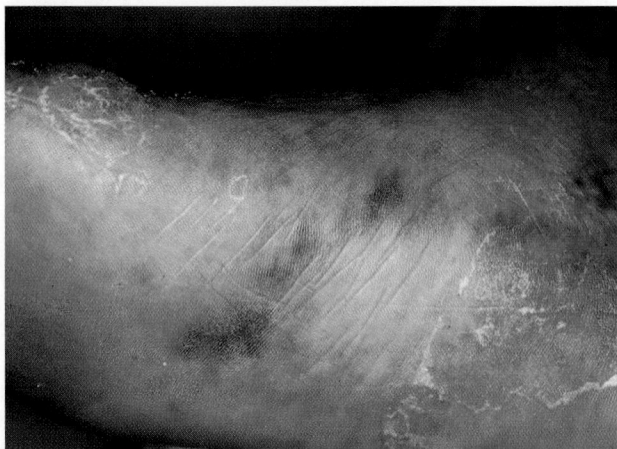

Figure 15 **Kaposi sarcoma is the most common malignancy of AIDS patients. It often presents as purple patches, plaques, or papules. Purple macules on the foot can be seen in patients with classic Kaposi sarcoma but are seen here in a patient with AIDS-related Kaposi sarcoma.**

INFECTIVE ENDOCARDITIS

The cutaneous manifestations of infective endocarditis include petechiae, splinter hemorrhages (linear red streaks under the nail), Osler nodes (tender purpuric nodules on the finger pads and toes), and Janeway lesions (nontender purpuric macules of the palms and soles). Skin lesions are caused by either septic emboli or vasculitis. Treatment of the underlying infection results in resolution of the cutaneous manifestations [*see Chapter 127*].

STAPHYLOCOCCAL TOXIC-SHOCK SYNDROME

Staphylococcal toxic-shock syndrome was first recognized in menstruating women who used superabsorbent tampons [*see Chapter 134*]. It is caused by an exotoxin produced by certain strains of *S. aureus*.[51] Staphylococcal infections in bone, soft tissue, and other sites have been implicated. Patients develop diffuse sunburnlike erythema, with swelling of the hands and feet; these symptoms are followed by desquamation of the palms and soles. Erythema of mucous membranes, fever, and hypotension also occur. Gastrointestinal symptoms, impaired renal function, elevated liver function values, thrombocytopenia, and myositis can develop.

STAPHYLOCOCCAL SCALDED SKIN SYNDROME

Staphylococcal scalded skin syndrome (SSSS) is caused by a circulating exfoliative toxin produced by *S. aureus* phage group 11. Generalized bulla formation with large areas of desquamation is characteristic of the disorder. Along with tenderness, erythema, and exfoliation of skin, patients have fever. The source of the staphylococcal infection is not always apparent; occasionally, the infection arises in a wound or in an occult abscess. Because the staphylococcal infection is usually remote from the affected skin, culture of the skin does not grow *S. aureus*.

SSSS must be differentiated from toxic epidermal necrolysis. Toxic epidermal necrolysis commonly affects adults and involves mucous membranes; SSSS usually affects children and spares mucous membranes. In addition, toxic epidermal necrolysis can last for several weeks and has a high mortality, whereas SSSS lasts a few days and usually has a good outcome. Histologically, SSSS shows bulla formation in the upper epidermis, and the bulla cavity contains free-floating, normal-appearing, acantholytic cells. In toxic epidermal necrolysis, bulla formation occurs at the basal layer of the epidermis, and the epidermal cells are necrotic. Treatment with antibiotics effective against *S. aureus* eliminates the underlying cause of SSSS.

NECROTIZING FASCIITIS

Necrotizing fasciitis is caused by a mixed anaerobic infection of an ulcer or a surgical or traumatic wound. The affected skin is erythematous, warm, and tender and develops hemorrhagic bullae that rupture to form rapidly enlarging areas of gangrene that extend down to the fascia. Surgical debridement is essential for this life-threatening infection.[52]

MENINGOCOCCEMIA

Acute meningococcemia can occur either in epidemics or in isolated cases [*see Chapter 137*]. Fever, headache, and a hemorrhagic rash develop. If untreated, patients develop DIC, with extensive hemorrhage, hypotension, and ultimately death. The causative organism, *Neisseria meningitidis*, is usually identified in cerebrospinal fluid but can also be identified by smear or cultures of skin lesions or by blood cultures. Treat-

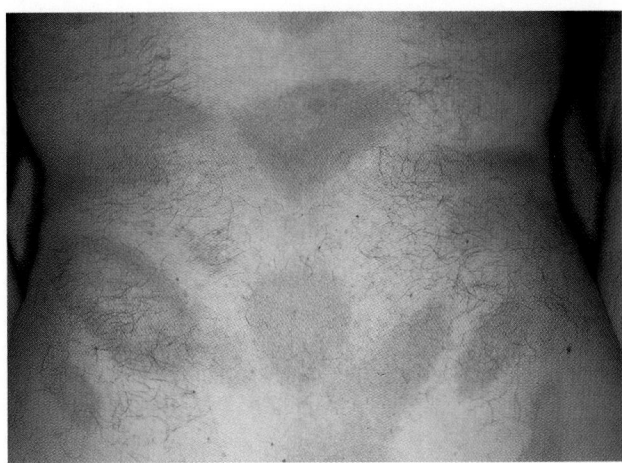

Figure 16   **Several weeks after primary infection with Lyme disease, hematogenous dissemination of spirochetes results in multiple patches of erythema chronicum migrans.**

ment with antibiotics and supportive care are essential aspects of therapy.

SCARLET FEVER

Scarlet fever begins with pharyngitis caused by group A *Streptococcus* [*see Chapter 134*]. A generalized rash develops 1 to 2 days after onset of the pharyngitis. The rash is characterized by pinpoint erythematous papules that may be easier to palpate than to see. Other characteristic lesions include a white strawberry tongue and linear petechial macules occurring in body folds (Pastia lines). As the rash fades, desquamation of the palms and soles appears. Treatment with penicillin results in rapid resolution of all symptoms.

VIBRIO INFECTION

Vibrio vulnificus infection arises from minor trauma sustained while swimming in lakes or the ocean or while cleaning seafood. Cellulitis occurs, with lymphangitis and bacteremia. In patients with hepatic cirrhosis, infection can occur after eating raw oysters. These patients develop hemorrhagic bullae, with leukopenia and DIC.[53] Treatment with antibiotics is necessary; management of complications may require intensive supportive care.

LYME DISEASE

Lyme disease is caused by the spirochete *Borrelia burgdorferi* and is transmitted primarily by the tick *Ixodes scapularis* [*see Chapter 139*]. The characteristic skin lesion, erythema chronicum migrans, begins as an erythematous macule or papule at the site of the tick bite. Over days and weeks, the erythematous lesion expands to form a red ring, often with central clearing. If left untreated, lesions last weeks or months. Hematogenous dissemination of spirochetes occurs after several weeks; dissemination results in multiple annular patches of erythema chronicum migrans [*see Figure 16*]. Systemic complications include an acute arthritis involving one or a few large joints a few weeks after the onset of symptoms. A chronic erosive arthritis develops in approximately 10% of patients. Neurologic symptoms, including Bell palsy, can occur, as can cardiac complications, including heart failure and cardiac conduction abnormalities.

Lyme disease can be prevented by the removal of ticks within 18 hours of attachment. Once symptoms have developed, oral antibiotics are effective at destroying *B. burgdorferi*. A vaccine containing a genetically engineered protein from the surface of the bacteria was found to prevent infection in most vaccinated people[54]; however, for a number of reasons, including lack of demand, the vaccine has been discontinued.[55]

ROCKY MOUNTAIN SPOTTED FEVER

Rocky Mountain spotted fever (RMSF) is a tick-borne illness caused by *Rickettsia rickettsii* [*see Chapter 145*]. It is characterized by the sudden onset of fevers, chills, and headache. Approximately 4 days later, a characteristic erythematous rash develops on the wrists and ankles and becomes purpuric. The rash then spreads centrally to involve the extremities, trunk, and face.

Because the mortality of RMSF is high, patients should be treated immediately with intravenous chloramphenicol or tetracycline if RMSF is suspected. Diagnosis can then be established by skin biopsy: immunofluorescence with antibodies against *R. rickettsii* shows the organism in the walls of cutaneous blood vessels. Serologic tests, such as the Weil-Felix reaction, can confirm the diagnosis after the acute phase of the illness.

Neurologic Diseases

BASAL CELL NEVUS SYNDROME

The basal cell nevus syndrome is an autosomal dominant disorder attributed to mutational inactivation of the *PTCH* gene[56]; patients with this disorder develop basal cell carcinomas at an early age [*see Chapter 45*]. Multiple skeletal abnormalities are associated with the syndrome, and affected individuals may also develop jaw cysts. Lamellar calcification of the falx cerebri occurs, as well as other neurologic abnormalities, including medulloblastomas.

EPIDERMAL NEVUS SYNDROME

The epidermal nevus syndrome is characterized by systemic manifestations, such as seizures, mental retardation, blindness, and skeletal abnormalities in association with large epidermal nevi. The nevi consist of long pigmented streaks that are linear or whirled and involve large areas of the body [*see Figure 17*].

INCONTINENTIA PIGMENTI

Incontinentia pigmenti is an inherited syndrome that affects the skin and nervous system. Mutations in the *NEMO* gene, an essential component of the nuclear factor–κB signaling cascade, account for 85% of cases.[57] The inheritance pattern is X-linked dominant and is lethal in male fetuses. The first skin manifestations begin within weeks after birth, occasionally occurring in utero, and consist of linear patterns of vesiculobullous lesions. Within weeks, these lesions evolve into verrucous papules and, eventually, into pigmented whirls. Apart from neurologic symptoms, patients may have ocular abnormalities, scarring alopecia, and skeletal malformations.

Hypomelanosis of Ito

Hypomelanosis of Ito, also called incontinentia pigmenti achromians, consists of whirls of hypopigmentation that are associated with neurologic symptoms in 50% of patients. Skin lesions are present at birth or develop in early childhood. In addition to seizures and mental retardation, skeletal and ocular abnormalities occur.

NEUROFIBROMATOSIS

Neurofibromatosis is a common autosomal dominant disorder involving the skin and nervous system [*see Chapter 44*]. Skin lesions include cutaneous neurofibromas, which are soft, skin-colored nodules that are often pedunculated [*see Figure 18*]. Café au lait macules are flat, evenly pigmented patches up to several centimeters in diameter. Six or more café au lait macules greater than 1.5 cm in diameter are found in most patients with neurofibromatosis type 1 (also called von Recklinghausen disease). Plexiform neuromas are larger, deeper tumors that are associated with hypertrophy of bony and soft tissues. In a small proportion of tumors, neurofibrosarcomas will arise. On skin biopsy, café au lait macules are found to contain macromelanosomes—giant granules of pigment in melanocytes and keratinocytes. Axillary and inguinal freckling also appear as pigmented macules that resemble small café au lait spots in intertriginous sites. Lisch nodules—pigmented iris hamartomas—are also found in most patients with neurofibromatosis.

Several variants of neurofibromatosis exist, including segmental neurofibromatosis, in which patients develop a segmental distribution of café au lait spots and cutaneous neurofibromas, and neurofibromatosis type 2, which consists of acoustic neuromas, schwannomas, and meningiomas without Lisch nodules and with fewer café au lait macules than appear in type 1. Patients with neurofibromatosis type 2 may have some cutaneous neurofibromas as well. Neurofibromatosis types 1 and 2 are caused by different genetic defects. Neurofibromatosis type 1 is caused by mutations in the *NF1* gene for neurofibromin on chromosome 17.[58] Neurofibromatosis type 2 has been attributed to inactivating mutations in the *NF2* tumor suppressor gene whose product, merlin, plays a number of roles in tumorigenesis.[59]

SNEDDON SYNDROME

Sneddon syndrome is a disease of the skin and nervous system caused by occlusion of small to medium-sized arteries in persons younger than 45 years. The skin lesions resemble livedo reticularis and have been called livedo racemosa. Transient ischemic attacks or strokes are common. Definitive diagnosis is made by demonstrating characteristic vascular changes on skin biopsy of patients with associated neurologic findings.

TUBEROUS SCLEROSIS

Tuberous sclerosis is an autosomal dominant disease that affects the skin and nervous system. Mutations that inactivate the *TSC1* or *TSC2* tumor suppressor genes affect the respective gene products, hamartin and tuberin, leading to tuberous sclerosis.[60] Affected patients can develop seizures, mental retardation, and brain lesions called tubers, which can be seen on CT scans. Adenoma sebaceum, the most characteristic cutaneous manifestation of tuberous sclerosis, consists of skin-colored papules of the face [*see Figure 19a*]. Other skin lesions are hypopigmented macules referred to as ash-leaf macules [*see Figure 19b*], smaller hypopigmented lesions called confetti macules, periungual and subungual fibromas (skin-colored nodules that arise around the fingers and toenails) [*see Figure 19c*], and the shagreen patch (a skin-colored plaque made of thick dermal connective tissue).

Renal Diseases

FABRY DISEASE

Fabry disease is caused by an abnormality of α-galactosidase

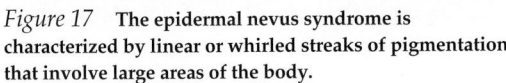

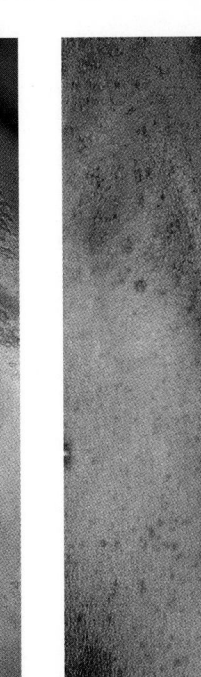

Figure 17   The epidermal nevus syndrome is characterized by linear or whirled streaks of pigmentation that involve large areas of the body.

Figure 18   Axillary freckling, café au lait spots, and neurofibromas are evident in a patient with neurofibromatosis type 1.

A, resulting in deposition of glycosphingolipids in body tissues. The disorder is inherited as an X-linked recessive trait. A variety of different mutations in the gene for α-galactosidase A have been found in unrelated families with Fabry disease.[61] Affected males often complain of severe pain in the extremities, with burning of the palms and soles. Episodes of pain are transient, but patients complain of persistent paresthesias in the hands and feet.

Skin lesions consist of angiokeratomas, which are pinpoint red or purple papules that resemble cherry hemangiomas [*see Figure 20*]. Angiokeratomas are most commonly found in the periumbilical area but can also occur on the palms, soles, trunk, extremities, and mucous membranes. In adults, glycosphingolipids become deposited in blood vessels and organs, affecting the heart, heart valves, coronary arteries, and kidneys. Re-

placement therapy with recombinant human α-galactosidase A can improve cutaneous, gastrointestinal, neurologic, and psychiatric symptoms; it has been shown to be safe and can eliminate substrate storage of glycosphingolipids, but questions remain regarding optimal dosing.[62]

POLYARTERITIS NODOSA

Polyarteritis nodosa is an inflammatory condition that affects muscular arteries [*see Chapter 117*]. Aneurysms form in many arteries, including those leading to the kidneys and subcutaneous tissue. Diagnosis of the systemic form of polyarteritis can be made by demonstrating aneurysms of the renal arteries on renal arteriograms.

A localized cutaneous form of polyarteritis nodosa most commonly presents as painful nodules of the lower extremi-

a

b

c

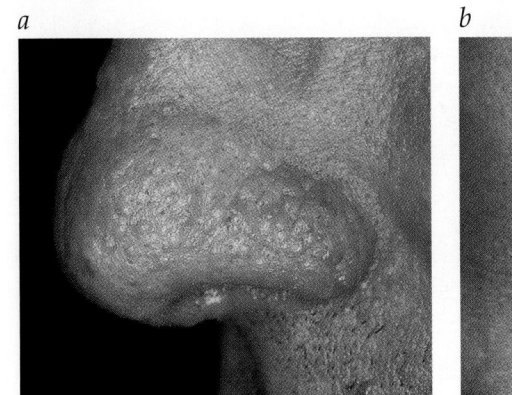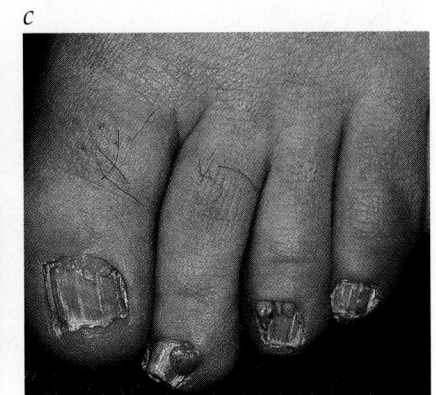

Figure 19   Several of the characteristic cutaneous findings of tuberous sclerosis are shown: adenoma sebaceum (*a*); ash-leaf macule (*b*); and periungual fibromas (*c*).

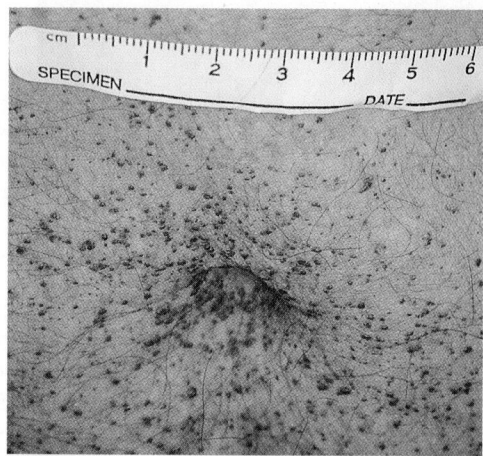

Figure 20 Angiokeratomas are particularly common in the periumbilical area of patients with Fabry disease.

ties.[63] In mild cases, patients may only have livedo reticularis; but in severe cases, skin lesions can ulcerate. A polyneuropathy may be associated with the disorder. Patients with classic polyarteritis and microaneurysms have an increased incidence of hepatitis B antigenemia; in contrast to patients with other vasculitides, they usually do not have antineutrophil cytoplasmic antibodies.[64]

PERFORATING DISORDERS

Perforating disorders include several conditions characterized by extrusion of dermal material through the epidermis. These lesions often develop in association with renal failure and diabetes mellitus.[65] Skin lesions are characterized by hyperkeratotic papules with central white craters that histologically can be shown to contain dermal material. Reactive perforating collagenosis, perforating folliculitis, and Kyrle disease are all examples of perforating disorders associated with renal failure.

CALCIPHYLAXIS

Calciphylaxis, also known as calcific uremic arteriolopathy, is a condition of patients with renal failure in which localized areas of skin become necrotic as a result of vascular calcification. Calciphylaxis begins with painful purpuric patches that may be reticulated, resembling livedo reticularis. These patches progress to

indurated plaques that may ulcerate, becoming necrotic [*see Figure 21*]. Calciphylaxis often eventuates in amputation or death. Parathyroidectomy may result in healing of affected skin without amputation.[66]

Rheumatologic Diseases

DERMATOMYOSITIS

The best-known cutaneous manifestations of dermatomyositis, an inflammatory disorder of muscle and skin, are Gottron papules and heliotrope erythema. Gottron papules are erythematous scaling macules and papules that occur on the dorsa of the knuckles [*see Figure 22*]. Heliotrope erythema consists of periorbital erythema and edema. Scalp lesions, which can be associated with alopecia, have been described.[67] The lesions are often misdiagnosed as seborrheic dermatitis or psoriasis.

The association between dermatomyositis and malignancy has been established[68,69]; one epidemiologic study indicates patients with dermatomyositis are at particular risk for ovarian and lung cancer.[69]

Classifications of dermatomyositis include a juvenile variant characterized by calcification of skin or muscle. A vasculitic form in children is complicated by cutaneous infarcts and ulceration and by gastrointestinal vasculitis with abdominal pain, bleeding, or perforation. The vasculitic form carries a poor prognosis, with many of the patients dying of this disease.

SCLERODERMA AND SCLERODERMA-LIKE DISEASES

The sclerodermas include a number of distinct syndromes that share a common feature, induration of the skin [*see Chapter 115*].

Progressive Systemic Sclerosis and CREST Syndrome

Progressive systemic sclerosis, also known as systemic scleroderma, is a frequently fatal disease in which patients present with Raynaud phenomenon and sclerodactyly (induration of the skin of the digits) [*see Figure 23*]. Cutaneous induration can become widespread. Involvement of the face can lead to a characteristic appearance with pursed lips and bound-down skin of the nose that creates a beaklike appearance. Patients with antibodies to Scl-70 have a poor prognosis, often succumbing to renal disease and malignant hypertension. Pulmonary fibrosis can

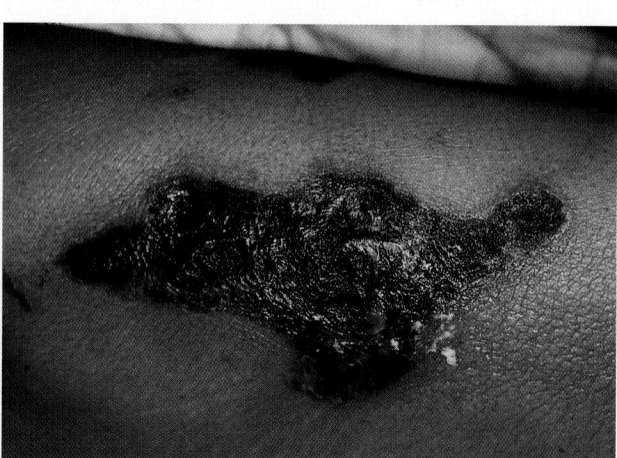

Figure 21 Calcification of arteries in patients with renal failure results in calciphylaxis. Affected skin forms a black, necrotic eschar.

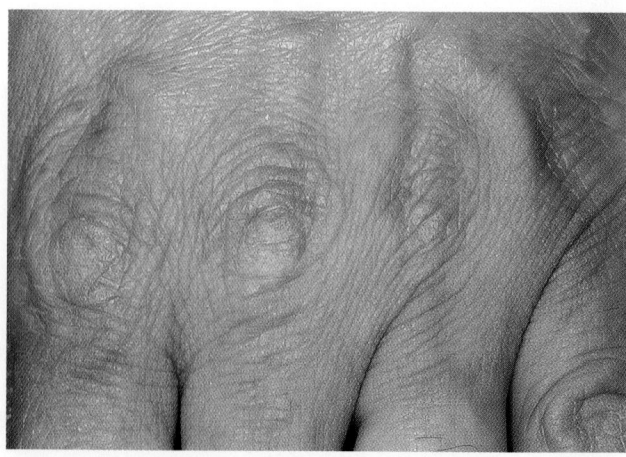

Figure 22 Erythematous scaling papules on the dorsal aspects of the knuckles (Gottron papules) are a sign of dermatomyositis.

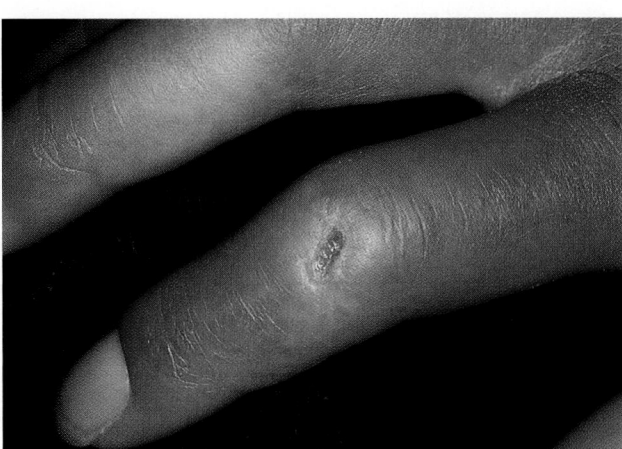

Figure 23 **Sclerodactyly with a nonhealing digital ulcer commonly occurs in progressive systemic sclerosis.**

occur. Patients with anticentromere antibodies have a more slowly progressive variant of scleroderma known as the CREST syndrome, which is characterized by cutaneous calcinosis, Raynaud phenomenon, esophageal dysmotility, sclerodactyly, and telangiectasia. With time, pulmonary hypertension and right-sided heart failure develop.

Morphea

Morphea, also called localized scleroderma, is characterized by sharply demarcated patches of indurated skin that can become generalized. It is distinguished from progressive systemic sclerosis by the absence of Raynaud phenomenon, sclerodactyly, or the systemic complications of scleroderma. There have been innovations in the treatment of both progressive systemic sclerosis and morphea. Exposure to psoralen and longwave ultraviolet light (PUVA) has been reported to improve progressive systemic sclerosis and morphea dramatically,[70] and exposure to UVA1 (the longer UVA spectrum, from 340 to 400 nm) has been reported to benefit patients with localized scleroderma.[71] Anecdotal evidence suggests that topical calcipotriene is an effective treatment for morphea.[72] Further studies must be done to confirm the efficacy of these treatments. Anecdotal reports have indicated that minocycline may benefit patients with progressive systemic sclerosis, but controlled trials are needed.[73]

Graft versus Host Disease

As organ transplantation becomes more common, another scleroderma-like illness, graft versus host disease, increases in frequency, particularly after bone marrow transplantation [*see Chapters 100 and 101*]. There are two stages of graft versus host disease. The first stage, acute graft versus host disease, develops 10 to 40 days after transplantation. Acute graft versus host disease consists of an erythematous macular and papular rash that is often associated with fever, hepatomegaly, lymphadenopathy, or gastrointestinal symptoms. Chronic graft versus host disease usually develops 3 months after transplantation but can occur later; it consists of purple papules resembling lichen planus [*see Figure 24*]. Sclerodermatous skin changes with telangiectasia, reticulated hyperpigmentation, and alopecia are most characteristic. Both cyclosporine and PUVA have proved to be useful in the prevention and treatment of graft versus host disease.[74,75] Infliximab has been used very successfully to treat acute graft versus host disease.[76]

Eosinophilic Fasciitis

Scleroderma-like hardening of the skin also occurs in eosinophilic fasciitis. Puckering of the skin on the extremities typically develops and is associated with pain. In contrast to progressive systemic sclerosis, Raynaud phenomenon does not occur. Definitive diagnosis requires biopsy of skin and fascia overlying the affected muscle. In some cases of eosinophilic fasciitis, hematologic abnormalities develop, including aplastic anemia, thrombocytopenia, Hodgkin disease, and leukemias.[77]

SYSTEMIC LUPUS ERYTHEMATOSUS

There are many cutaneous manifestations of systemic lupus erythematosus (SLE), including nonspecific manifestations such as Raynaud phenomenon, photosensitivity, alopecia, and mucosal ulcers. More specific cutaneous manifestations of SLE include so-called discoid lupus (characterized by round scarred skin lesions with central hypopigmentation and a rim of hyperpigmentation) and malar erythema [*see Chapter 114*]. As we learn more about lupus, the spectrum of skin diseases associated with this disorder continues to expand. Subacute cutaneous lupus, a variant characterized serologically by anti-Ro and anti-La antibodies, is associated with annular or psoriasiform skin lesions [*see Figure 25*].

Anticardiolipin Antibody Syndrome

The anticardiolipin antibody syndrome, which can occur in patients with SLE, has been described in patients who suffer re-

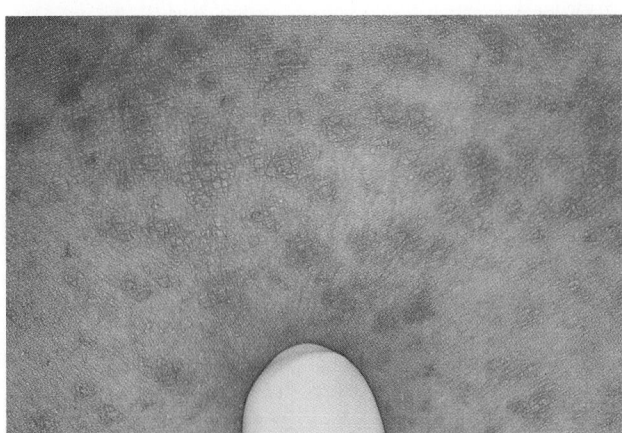

Figure 24 **Flat-topped papules are seen in this chronic lichenoid graft versus host reaction.**

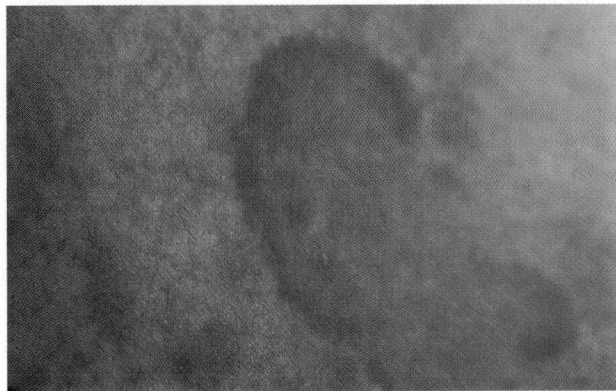

Figure 25 **Annular scaling erythematous patches are characteristic of subacute cutaneous lupus erythematosus.**

peated episodes of phlebitis, arterial thromboses, and repeated miscarriages. Cutaneous infarcts are common manifestations, and livedo reticularis can occur. Patients may have false positive serologies for syphilis and have a circulating lupus anticoagulant. Circulating antiphospholipid antibodies are the serologic hallmark of this syndrome; however, many asymptomatic persons have antiphospholipid antibodies,[78] and antiphospholipid antibody tests can have false negative results. In some patients, a battery of tests may be needed to establish diagnosis; the dilute Russell viper venom time, an assay for circulating lupus anticoagulant, has been found to be among the more sensitive tests.[79]

Livedo Vasculitis

Livedo vasculitis, another disorder that has been associated with lupus, is characterized by painful recurrent ulcers over the lower legs and ankles. The ulcers heal, leaving white sclerotic scars. Affected patients often have livedo reticularis. This condition, also known as atrophie blanche, has been attributed to thrombotic processes rather than immune complex deposition or leukocytoclastic vasculitis.[80]

Neonatal Lupus

Neonatal lupus is a distinct syndrome of annular, erythematous macules and papules occurring on the face of newborn infants. The disorder has been attributed to transplacental passage of anti-Ro and occasionally anti-La antibodies. Mothers are often asymptomatic, but some may have lupus or Sjögren syndrome. Congenital heart block is the most serious complication of this disorder.[81]

The author has served as an investigator, consultant, or speaker for the following companies: Abbott Laboratories, Inc., Allergen, Inc., Amgen, Inc., Biogen, Inc., Centocor, Inc., Connetics Corporation, Fujisawa Healthcare, Inc., Galderma Laboratories, L.P., Genentech, Inc., Leo Pharmaceuticals, and Warner-Chilcott Pharmaceuticals.

The FDA has not approved the following drugs for specific uses described in this chapter: infliximab and TNF-α blockers for the treatment of sarcoidosis and Wegener granulomatosis; rituximab for the treatment of lymphomatoid granulomatosis; and calcipotriene for the treatment of morphea.

References

1. Sorrentino D, Avellini C, Zearo E: Colonic sarcoidosis, infliximab, and tuberculosis: a cautionary tale. Inflamm Bowel Dis 10:438, 2004
2. Khanna D, Liebling MR, Louie JS: Etanercept ameliorates sarcoidosis arthritis and skin disease. J Rheumatol 30:1864, 2003
3. Haley H, Cantrell W, Smith K: Infliximab therapy for sarcoidosis (lupus pernio). Br J Dermatol 150:146, 2004
4. Menon Y, Cucurull E, Reisin EE, et al: Interferon-alpha-associated sarcoidosis responsive to infliximab therapy. Am J Med Sci 328:173, 2004
5. English JC 3rd, Patel PJ, Greer KE: Sarcoidosis. J Am Acad Dermatol 44:725, 2001
6. Kleinert J, Lorenz M, Kostler W, et al: Refractory Wegener's granulomatosis responds to tumor necrosis factor blockage. Wien Klin Wochenschr 116:334, 2004
7. Sebire NJ, Haselden S, Malone M, et al: Isolated EBV lymphoproliferative disease in a child with Wiskott-Aldrich syndrome manifesting as cutaneous lymphomatoid granulomatosis and responsive to anti-CD20 immunotherapy. J Clin Pathol 56:555, 2003
8. Beaty MW, Toro J, Sorbara L, et al: Cutaneous lymphomatoid granulomatosis: correlation of clinical and biologic features. Am J Surg Pathol 25:1111, 2001
9. Zaidi A, Kampalath B, Peltier WL, et al: Successful treatment of systemic and central nervous system lymphomatoid granulomatosis with rituximab. Leuk Lymphoma 45:777, 2004
10. Davis MD, Daoud MS, McEvoy MT, et al: Cutaneous manifestations of Churg-Strauss syndrome: a clinicopathologic correlation. J Am Acad Dermatol 37:199, 1997
11. Seo P, Stone JH: The antineutrophil cytoplasmic antibody–associated vasculitides. Am J Med 117:39, 2004
12. Gong F, Shiraishi H, Momoi MY: Follow-up of coronary artery lesions caused by Kawasaki disease and the value of coronary angiography. Clin Med J (Engl) 115:681, 2002

13. Curtis N: Kawasaki disease and toxic shock syndrome: at last the etiology is clear? Adv Exp Med Biol 549:191, 2004
14. Newburger JW, Takahashi M, Gerber MA, et al: Diagnosis, treatment, and long-term management of Kawasaki disease: a statement for health professionals from the Committee on Rheumatic Fever, Endocarditis and Kawasaki Disease, Council on Cardiovascular Disease in the Young, American Heart Association. Circulation 110:2747, 2004
15. Oates-Whitehead RM, Baumer JH, Haines L, et al: Intravenous immunoglobulin for the treatment of Kawasaki disease in children. Cochrane Database Syst Rev (4):CD004000, 2003
16. Ringpfeil F, Lebwohl MG, Christiano AM, et al: Pseudoxanthoma elasticum: mutations in the MRP6 gene encoding a transmembrane ATP-binding cassette (ABC) transporter. Proc Natl Acad Sci USA 97:6001, 2000
17. Lebwohl MG, DiStefano D, Prioleau PG, et al: Pseudoxanthoma elasticum and mitral valve prolapse. N Engl J Med 307:228, 1982
18. Lebwohl M, Halperin J, Phelps RG: Brief report: occult pseudoxanthoma elasticum in patients with premature cardiovascular disease. N Engl J Med 329:1237, 1993
19. Lebwohl M, Phelps RG, Yannuzzi L, et al: Diagnosis of pseudo-xanthoma elasticum by scar biopsy in patients without characteristic skin lesions. N Engl J Med 317:347, 1987
20. D'Alessandro A, Muzi G, Monaco A, et al: Yellow nail syndrome: does protein leakage play a role? Eur Respir J 17:149, 2001
21. Litonjua P, Pinero-Pilona A, Aviles-Santa L, et al: Prevalence of acanthosis nigricans in newly-diagnosed type 2 diabetes. Endocr Pract 10:101, 2004
22. Verrotti A, Chiarelli F, Amerio P, et al: Necrobiosis lipoidica diabeticorum in children and adolescents: a clue for underlying renal and retinal disease. Pediatr Dermatol 12:220, 1995
23. Rho YW, Suhr KB, Lee JH, et al: A clinical observation of scleredema adultorum and its relationship to diabetes. J Dermatol 25:103, 1998
24. Dogra S, Handa S, Kanwar AJ: Dexamethasone pulse therapy for scleredema. Pediatr Dermatol 21:280, 2004
25. Bowen AR, Smith L, Zone JJ: Scleredema adultorum of Buschke treated with radiation. Arch Dermatol 139:780, 2003
26. Janiga JJ, Ward DH, Lim HW: UVA-1 as a treatment for scleredema. Photodermatol Photoimmunol Photomed 20:210, 2004
27. Hecker MS, Lebwohl MG: Recalcitrant pyoderma gangrenosum: treatment with thalidomide. J Am Acad Dermatol 38:490, 1998
28. Tan MH, Gordon M, Lebwohl O, et al: Improvement of pyoderma gangrenosum and psoriasis associated with Crohn disease with anti–tumor necrosis factor alpha monoclonal antibody. Arch Dermatol 137:930, 2001
29. Kanaseki T, Torigoe T, Hiroshashi Y, et al: Identification of germline mutation of PTEN gene and analysis of apoptosis resistance of the lymphocytes in a patient with Cowden disease. Pathobiology 70:34, 2002
30. Barax CN, Lebwohl M, Phelps RG: Multiple hamartoma syndrome. J Am Acad Dermatol 17:342, 1987
31. Garcia JM, Silva J, Pena C, et al: Promoter methylation of the PTEN gene is a common molecular change in breast cancer. Genes Chromosomes Cancer 41:117, 2004
32. Collin P, Pukkala E, Reunala T: Malignancy and survival in dermatitis herpetiformis: a comparison with coeliac disease. Gut 38:528, 1996
33. Scott RJ, Crooks R, Meldrum CJ, et al: Mutation analysis of the STK11/LKB1 gene and clinical characteristics of an Australian series of Peutz-Jeghers syndrome patients. Clin Genet 62:282, 2002
34. Mallipeddi R: Epidermolysis bullosa and cancer. Clin Exp Dermatol 27:616, 2002
35. Christiano AM, LaForgia S, Paller AS, et al: Prenatal diagnosis for recessive dystrophic epidermolysis bullosa in 10 families by mutation and haplotype analysis in the type VII collagen gene (COL7A1). Mol Med 2:59, 1996
36. Gardella R, Castiglia D, Posteraro P, et al: Genotype-phenotype correlation in Italian patients with dystrophic epidermolysis bullosa. J Invest Dermatol 119:1456, 2002
37. Chen M, Kasahara N, Keene DR, et al: Restoration of type VII collagen expression and function in dystrophic epidermolysis bullosa. Nat Genet 32:670, 2002
38. Dubrey SW, Burke MM, Hawkins PN, et al: Cardiac transplantation for amyloid heart disease: the United Kingdom experience. J Heart Lung Transplant 23:1142, 2004
39. Palladini G, Perfetti V, Perlini S, et al: The association of thalidomide and intermediate-dose dexamethasone is an effective but toxic treatment for patients with AL (primary) amyloidosis. Blood Nov 30, 2004 [epub ahead of print]
40. Topar G, Staudacher C, Geisen F, et al: Urticaria pigmentosa: a clinical, hematopathologic, and serologic study of 30 adults. Am J Clin Pathol 109:279, 1998
41. Horny HP, Ruck P, Krober S, et al: Systemic mast cell disease (mastocytosis): general aspects and histopathological diagnosis. Histol Histopathol 12:1081, 1997
42. Kiszewski AE, Duran-Mckinster C, Orozco-Covarrubias L, et al: Cutaneous mastocytosis in children: a clinical analysis of 71 cases. J Eur Acad Dermatol Venereol 18:285, 2004
43. Shady AA, Colby BR, Cunha LF, et al: Congenital erythropoietic porphyria: identification and expression of eight novel mutations in the uroporphyrinogen III synthase gene. Br J Haematol 117:980, 2002
44. Pottage JC Jr, Kessler HA: Herpes simplex virus resistance to acyclovir: clinical relevance. Infect Agents Dis 4:115, 1995
45. Chibo D, Mijch A, Doherty R, et al: Novel mutations in the thymidine kinase and DNA polymerase genes of acyclovir and foscarnet resistant herpes simplex viruses infecting an immunocompromised patient. J Clin Virol 25:165, 2002
46. Lalezari J, Schacker T, Feinberg J, et al: A randomized, double-blind, placebo-controlled trial of cidofovir gel for the treatment of acyclovir-unresponsive mucocutaneous herpes simplex virus infection in patients with AIDS. J Infect Dis 176:892, 1997

47. Chang CC, Chomel BB, Kasten RW, et al: Molecular epidemiology of *Bartonella henselae* infection in human immunodeficiency virus-infected patients and their cat contacts, using pulsed-field gel electrophoresis and genotyping. J Infect Dis 186:1733, 2002

48. Agan BK, Dolan MJ: Laboratory diagnosis of *Bartonella* infections. Clin Lab Med 22:937, 2002

49. Resnick JS Jr, Van Beek M, Furmanski L, et al: Etiology of pruritic popular eruption with HIV infection in Uganda. JAMA 292:2614, 2004

50. Albrecht D, Meyer T, Lorenzen T, et al: Epidemiology of HHV-8 infection in HIV-positive patients with and without Kaposi sarcoma: diagnostic relevance of serology and PCR. J Clin Virol 30:145, 2004

51. Parsonnet J: Nonmenstrual toxic shock syndrome: new insights into diagnosis, pathogenesis, and treatment. Curr Clin Top Infect Dis 16:1, 1996

52. Childers BJ, Potyondy LD, Nachreiner R, et al: Necrotizing fasciitis: a fourteen-year retrospective study of 163 consecutive patients. Am Surg 68:109, 2002

53. Nakafusa J, Misago N, Miura Y, et al: The importance of serum creatine phosphokinase level in the early diagnosis, and as a prognostic factor, of *Vibrio vulnificus* infection. Br J Dermatol 145:280, 2001

54. Steere AC, Sikand VK, Meurice F, et al: Vaccination against Lyme disease with recombinant *Borrelia burgdorferi* outer-surface lipoprotein A with adjuvant. Lyme Disease Vaccine Study Group. N Engl J Med 339:209, 1998

55. Lymerix: lack of demand kills Lyme disease vaccine. Nursing 32:18, 2002

56. Lam CW, Leung CY, Lee KC, et al: Novel mutations in the PATCHED gene in basal cell nevus syndrome. Mol Genet Metab 76:57, 2002

57. Smahi A, Courtois G, Rabia SH, et al: The NF-kappaB signalling pathway in human diseases: from incontinentia pigmenti to ectodermal dysplasias and immune-deficiency syndromes. Hum Mol Genet 11:2371, 2002

58. Dasgupta B, Dugan LL, Gutmann DH: The neurofibromatosis 1 gene product neurofibromin regulates pituitary adenylate cyclase-activating polypeptide-mediated signaling in astrocytes. J Neurosci 23:8949, 2003

59. Xiao GH, Chernoff J, Testa JR: NF2: the wizardry of Merlin. Genes Chromosomes Cancer 38:389, 2003

60. Nellist M, Sancak O, Goedbloed MA, et al: Distinct effects of single amino-acid changes to tuberin on the function of the tuberin-hamartin complex. Eur J Hum Genet 2004

61. Germain DP, Shabbeer J, Cotigny S, et al: Fabry disease: twenty novel alpha-galactosidase A mutations and genotype-phenotype correlations in classical and variant phenotypes. Mol Med 8:306, 2002

62. Desnick RJ, Brady R, Barranger J, et al: Fabry disease, an under-recognized multisystemic disorder: expert recommendations for diagnosis, management, and enzyme replacement therapy. Ann Intern Med 138:338, 2003

63. Daoud MS, Hutton KP, Gibson LE: Cutaneous periarteritis nodosa: a clinicopathological study of 79 cases. Br J Dermatol 136:706, 1997

64. Guillevin L, Lhote F, Amouroux J, et al: Antineutrophil cytoplasmic antibodies, abnormal angiograms and pathological findings in polyarteritis nodosa and Churg-Strauss syndrome: indications for the classification of vasculitides of the polyarteritis nodosa group. Br J Rheumatol 35:958, 1996

65. Poliak S, Lebwohl MG, Parris A, et al: Reactive perforating collagenosis associated with diabetes mellitus. N Engl J Med 306:81, 1982

66. Arch-Ferrer JE, Beenken SW, Rue LW, et al: Therapy for calciphylaxis: an outcome analysis. Surgery 134:941, 2003

67. Kasteler JS, Callen JP: Scalp involvement in dermatomyositis: often overlooked or misdiagnosed. JAMA 272:1939, 1994

68. Buchbinder R, Forbes A, Hall S, et al: Incidence of malignant disease in biopsy-proven inflammatory myopathy: a population-based cohort study. Ann Intern Med 134:1087, 2001

69. Hill CL, Zhang Y, Sigurgeirsson B, et al: Frequency of specific cancer types in dermatomyositis and polymyositis: a population based study. Lancet 357:96, 2001

70. Kanekura T, Fukumaru S, Matsushita S, et al: Successful treatment of scleroderma with PUVA therapy. J Dermatol 23:455, 1996

71. Kerscher M, Volkenandt M, Gruss C, et al: Low-dose UVA phototherapy for treatment of localized scleroderma. J Am Acad Dermatol 38:21, 1998

72. Tay YK: Topical calcipotriol ointment in the treatment of morphea. J Dermatolog Treat 14:219, 2003

73. Le CH, Morales A, Trentham DE: Minocycline in early diffuse scleroderma. Lancet 352:1755, 1998

74. Zikos P, van Lint MT, Frasoni F, et al: Low transplant mortality in allogeneic bone marrow transplantation for acute myeloid leukemia: a randomized study of low-dose cyclosporin versus low-dose cyclosporin and low-dose methotrexate. Blood 91:3503, 1998

75. Vogelsang GB, Wolff D, Altomonte V, et al: Treatment of chronic graft-versus-host disease with ultraviolet irradiation and psoralen (PUVA). Bone Marrow Transplant 17:1061, 1996

76. Yamane T, Yamamura R, Aoyama Y, et al: Infliximab for the treatment of severe steroid refractory acute graft-versus-host disease in three patients after allogeneic hematopoietic transplantation. Leuk Lymphoma 44:2095, 2003

77. Kim SW, Rice L, Champlin R, et al: Aplastic anemia in eosinophilic fasciitis: responses to immunosuppression and marrow transplantation. Haematologia (Budap) 28:131, 1997

78. Tektonidou MG, Sotsiou F, Nakopoulou L, et al: Antiphospholipid syndrome nephropathy in patients with systemic lupus erythematosus and antiphospholipid antibodies: prevalence, clinical associations, and long-term outcome. Arthritis Rheum 50:2569, 2004

79. Proven A, Bartlett RP, Moder KG, et al: Clinical importance of positive test results for lupus anticoagulant and anticardiolipin antibodies. Mayo Clin Proc 79:467, 2004

80. McCalmont CS, McCalmont TH, Jorizzo JL, et al: Livedo vasculitis: vasculitis or thrombotic vasculopathy? Clin Exp Dermatol 17:4, 1992

81. Brucato A, Franceschini F, Buyon JP: Neonatal lupus: long-term outcomes of mothers and children and recurrence rate. Clin Exp Rheumatol 15:467, 1997

35 Acne Vulgaris and Related Disorders

Mark Lebwohl, M.D.

Acne and its clinical variants are among the most common causes of patient visits to the physician for cutaneous disorders. Severe forms of these disorders can be disfiguring and debilitating; and because the face is the primary site of involvement, patients will often seek therapy for even mild forms. Therapeutic approaches will therefore be stressed in this chapter.

Epidemiology and Etiology

Acne vulgaris is the most common dermatologic problem of adolescent years; it usually begins in puberty. Age of onset and severity of disease are affected by sex, genetics, and external factors such as cosmetics and medications. Acne is usually more severe in males than in females and often begins earlier (i.e., in early adolescence) in males. Acne often subsides after the teenage years, but the disease can remain a problem for adults in the third and fourth decades and beyond. A significant portion of women experience premenstrual flares of acne; this phenomenon may be more common in older women.[1]

Genetic factors clearly play a role in severe acne. A family history of severe acne can often be elicited during the workup of affected patients. Various external factors, such as occlusive cosmetics, can contribute to acne, and certain medications (e.g., corticosteroids, adrenocorticotropic hormone [ACTH], phenytoin sodium, isoniazid, lithium, progestins, potassium iodide, bromides, and actinomycin D) can cause acnelike lesions [*see* Chapter 40].

Pathogenesis

Multiple factors contribute to the development of acne in susceptible persons. Among the most significant are alterations in keratinization, accumulation of sebum, and inflammation. Androgenic influences may contribute to some of these factors.

Modified keratinization of the follicular infundibulum leads to proliferation and increased cohesiveness of keratinocytes, which causes plugs to form. These plugs block follicular outlets, allowing cellular debris in sebum to form comedones (the noninflammatory lesions of acne that are the precursor lesions of inflammatory acne).

The composition of sebum does not appear to be altered in patients with acne; however, sebaceous glands are often larger and sebum production is often greater in persons affected with acne than in unaffected persons.[2] Sebum is comedogenic and inflammatory, which may account for its role in acne.[3] Inflammation in acne has also been attributed to the anaerobic diphtheroid *Propionibacterium acnes*. The presence of *P. acnes* correlates with the occurrence of acne in adolescents.[4] The microbe's role in inflammation has been attributed to lipases, proteases, and hyaluronidases, as well as to chemotactic factors. For example, *P. acnes* may activate Toll-like receptor 2 and thereby trigger inflammatory cytokine responses.[5]

Androgens play a role in the development of acne, as evidenced by increased levels of dehydroepiandrosterone sulfate (DHEAS) in girls with acne[6] and an association of acne with endocrinopathies characterized by increased levels of circulating androgens. For example, the occurrence of acne is increased in patients with congenital adrenal hyperplasia, polycystic ovaries, and some ovarian and adrenal tumors. Androgens act to increase sebum production and enlarge sebaceous glands; they may also contribute to the follicular hyperkeratinization that leads to acne. However, serum androgen levels are usually within the normal range in patients with acne. Some researchers have postulated that local production of androgens in the skin can lead to acne. Skin biopsies from patients with acne show increases in 5α-reductase activity.[7] This increased androgenic activity may result in the conversion of testosterone to dihydrotestosterone in the skin, leading to the development of acne.

Diagnosis

CLINICAL FEATURES

The characteristic skin lesions of acne include open and closed comedones, erythematous papules, pustules, nodules, cysts, and scars. The most commonly affected site is the face, but in more severely affected individuals, the back and chest can be involved as well.

Comedonal Acne

Comedones consist of keratinized cells and sebum. Comedonal acne consists of a predominance of open and closed comedones. Open comedones (blackheads) are black papules measuring 0.1 to 2 mm that are easily extruded with gentle pressure. The material that is removed is greasy and has a gray-white color. Contrary to popular belief, the dark color of open comedones is caused by melanin, not by dirt or oxidized fatty acids. Closed comedones (whiteheads) consist of white papules measuring 0.1 to 2 mm; unless extracted, they persist somewhat longer than open comedones, often for weeks to months.

Inflammatory Acne

Erythematous papules, pustules, nodules, and cysts are the predominant lesions in inflammatory acne [*see* Figure 1]. Erythematous papules range in size from 3 to 10 mm and can develop into pustules or resolve into an erythematous macule that fades. Postinflammatory hyperpigmentation can occur. Pustules are superficial and usually dry in a few days. Nodules, which are 1 cm or larger, are erythematous and tender. They can be firm at onset but often become fluctuant. In severely affected individuals, these lesions form fluctuant sinuses that open to the surface through multiple tracts. Postinflammatory pigmentary changes and scarring commonly occur.

Clinical Variants of Acne

Acne conglobata Acne conglobata is a severe, scarring form of acne in which large cysts and abscesses become confluent to form draining sinus tracts. Scarring is often severe. Topical acne therapy and oral antibiotics are frequently ineffective; patients may require treatment with oral isotretinoin [*see* Treatment, below]. Intralesional injection of corticosteroids and drainage of abscesses are temporarily helpful.

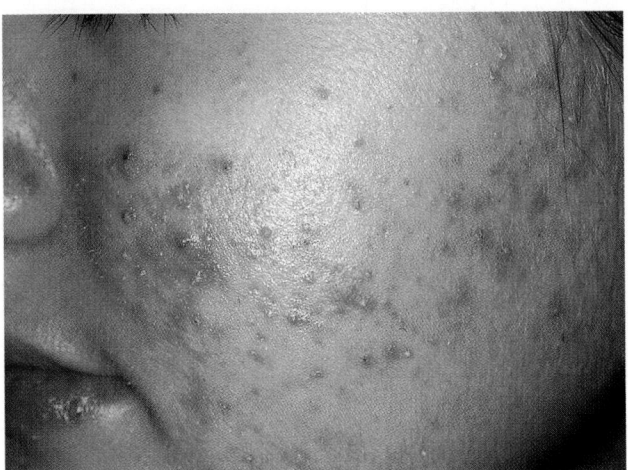

Figure 1 Inflammatory acne is characterized by erythematous papules and pustules.

Acne cosmetica A persistent, low-grade form of acne can result from the use of greasy, occlusive cosmetics, moisturizers, and sunscreens. Women are most commonly affected.

Acne excoriée Picking of minor acne lesions can cause large ulcers and erosions that heal with scarring. Young women are most typically affected.

Acne mechanica An acneiform eruption can result from repeated trauma associated with the wearing of sports helmets, shoulder pads, and bras and from the chin rests of violins and violas (so-called fiddler's neck).

Pomade acne A form of acne results from the use of thick oils in the hair. Comedones, papules, and pustules are usually found close to the hairline. Black men and women are most commonly affected.

Acne in neonates and children Neonatal acne has been attributed to maternal androgens, as well as androgens secreted by the neonatal adrenal gland. Erythematous papules and pustules may last for 2 to 3 months after birth but usually resolve spontaneously.

Infantile acne develops between 3 and 6 months after birth. This condition is characterized by inflamed papules and pustules; it signals early secretion of androgens by the gonads, particularly in boys. This condition may last until age 5. It has been suggested that affected infants may be predisposed to severe acne later in life.

LABORATORY TESTS

The clinical features of acne are so commonly recognized that laboratory investigation is usually not necessary. Laboratory tests should be considered, however, for female patients who have other signs of hyperandrogenism, such as hirsutism or irregular menses. Serum for determining DHEAS and free testosterone levels and for determining the ratio of luteinizing hormone to follicle-stimulating hormone (LH:FSH) should be obtained 2 weeks before the onset of menses [*see Table 1*]. Tests should also be undertaken in patients whose conditions do not respond to adequate doses of isotretinoin, the most potent treatment available for acne [*see Treatment, below*].

Differential Diagnosis

Clinical features of acne are sufficiently distinctive that diagnosis is usually obvious. Nevertheless, a number of disorders can be mistaken for acne.

Folliculitis The perifollicular pustules of folliculitis can be distinguished from the lesions of acne by their distribution. Folliculitis can affect the trunk and extremities and is not limited to the usual sites of acne (i.e., the face, back, and chest). Malassezia folliculitis is characterized by erythematous acneiform papules that do not respond to typical acne therapies. Gram stain of pus from the lesions reveals gram-positive budding yeast [*see Chapter 41*].

Gram-negative folliculitis In patients on long-term antibiotics, superficial pustules or nodules can develop at the anterior nares and spread outward on the face. This condition responds promptly to oral ampicillin; however, isotretinoin has become the treatment of choice.[8]

Milia Milia are white pinpoint cysts that resemble closed comedones. They frequently occur around the eyes but can develop anywhere on the face. If untreated, they last for months or years. Milia can be opened with a small surgical blade and their contents easily drained.

Perioral dermatitis Long-term use of topical corticosteroids on the face can result in acneiform, erythematous, inflamed papules on the chin and cheeks. Despite the name, the area immediately around the mouth is typically spared in perioral dermatitis. A similar eruption can occur in patients who have not used corticosteroids.

Chloracne Cysts and closed comedones that resemble acne lesions can be caused by exposure to halogenated hydrocarbons.

Hidradenitis suppurativa Hidradenitis suppurativa is a chronic condition in which inflamed cysts in the axillae and groin form fluctuant sinuses with draining tracts.

Favre-Racouchot disease Numerous open and closed comedones can appear around the eyes of elderly patients, especially men who have worked outdoors for much of their lives. This condition has been attributed to a lifetime of sun exposure.

Table 1 Laboratory Evaluation for Women with Acne and Signs of Hyperandrogenism

Finding	Suspected Condition

DHEAS
  4,000–8,000 ng/ml
  > 8,000 ng/ml
	Congenital adrenal hyperplasia
	Adrenal tumor

LH:FSH ratio > 2.0	Polycystic ovary disease

Testosterone (unbound)
  20–40 yr, > 107.5 pmol/L
  41–60 yr, > 86.7 pmol/L
  61–80 yr, > 69.3 pmol/L
	Polycystic ovary disease; ovarian tumor
	Polycystic ovary disease; ovarian tumor
	Polycystic ovary disease; ovarian tumor

DHEAS—dehydroepiandrosterone sulfate FSH—follicle-stimulating hormone
LH—luteinizing hormone

Rosacea Rosacea is a common condition that usually begins after 30 years of age. It is so similar to acne in some individuals that it has been called acne rosacea. Skin lesions consist of erythematous papules, pustules, and telangiectasia [see Figure 2]. Facial flushing is a common feature. In patients with a predominance of inflamed papules and pustules, differentiation from acne can be difficult. Presence of telangiectasia and the occurrence of flushing help distinguish rosacea from acne, as does the absence of comedones.

Common triggers of rosacea include alcohol, exercise, extremes of temperature, and hot or spicy foods. With long-standing disease, hypertrophy of sebaceous glands, swelling, erythema, and scarring of the nose lead to rhinophyma. Ocular involvement is common in rosacea and can include blepharitis and conjunctival hyperemia or, less commonly, iritis, episcleritis, superficial punctuate keratopathy, and corneal neovascularization.[9]

Helicobacter pylori may play a role in the pathogenesis of rosacea.[10] Further work must be done, however, to confirm the contribution of *H. pylori* to this antibiotic-responsive condition. An immunologic reaction to the mite *Demodex folliculorum* has been suggested, but not proved, as a contributing factor.

Treatment

Treatment of acne depends on the type and severity of lesions and on the patient's response to treatment. Comedonal acne is usually best managed with topical retinoids and acne surgery; inflammatory acne is treated with a range of topical therapies and may require oral therapy in moderate to severe cases. Because nodules and cysts are more likely than comedones to cause scarring, they are treated more quickly with oral antibiotics and, if necessary, isotretinoin (see below). Intralesional corticosteroids administered by dermatologists can prevent scarring from cysts. Incision and drainage of infected cysts may be necessary but can contribute to scarring. Unroofing of sinus tracts and other surgical procedures are best performed by physicians with expertise in dermatologic surgery [see Table 2]. Scars can be treated with dermabrasion or laser abrasion. The appearance of depressed scars can be improved by chemical peels and other resurfacing procedures, as well as by the injection of filler substances such as injectable collagen.[11]

Numerous over-the-counter cleansing agents are available to help patients remove seborrhea and oily debris from the skin, re-

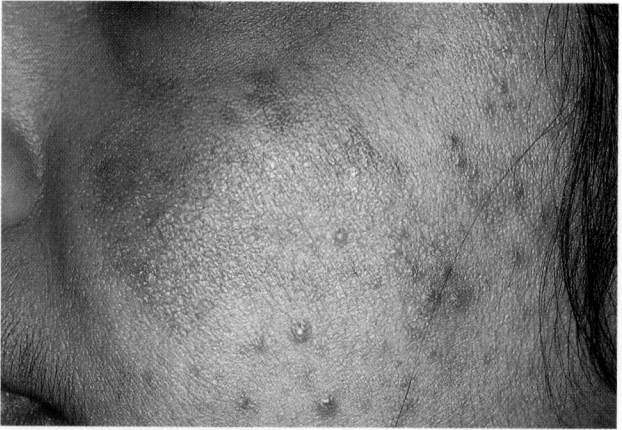

Figure 2 **Erythematous papules, pustules, telangiectasia, and flushing are features of rosacea.**

Table 2 Surgical Treatments for Acne Lesions and Acne Scars

Lesions	Extraction of comedones Drainage of pustules and cysts Intralesional injection of corticosteroids in cysts Excision and unroofing of sinus tracts and cysts
Scars	Dermabrasion Laser abrasion Acid peels Injection of filling materials (e.g., collagen) Excision Punch autografts

sulting in subjective improvements. Overmanipulation of lesions by picking, squeezing, or excessive washing can lead to exacerbation of lesions and even scarring.

Topical preparations, including sunscreens, soaps, and cosmetics, should be oil-free and noncomedogenic. Many over-the-counter oil-free, noncomedogenic moisturizers are available for persons who have dry skin and acne.

There is no role for dietary change in the management of acne. Previous beliefs that chocolate or oily foods cause acne have been disproved.

TOPICAL THERAPY

Comedonal Acne

Topical retinoids are among the most effective therapies for comedonal acne; these preparations unplug follicles and allow penetration of topical antibiotics and benzoyl peroxide. Retinoids can be used in combination with antibacterial agents and are also effective in the management of inflammatory acne.[12] They are often irritating when first applied; patients can reduce the irritation by reducing the frequency of application. Significant improvement is evident within 6 weeks and can continue for 3 to 4 months, at which time the frequency of application can be reduced, depending on the patient's response.

Newer formulations of retinoids that are purportedly less irritating include a tretinoin microsponge vehicle and adapalene, but few comparative studies examining irritation have been performed.[13,14] Tazarotene, a topical retinoid used for acne and psoriasis, can be used effectively in a short-contact method, in which it is applied for seconds to minutes.[15]

Inflammatory Acne

Topical antibiotics are not as effective as retinoids or benzoyl peroxide for inflammatory acne, but they are less irritating and better tolerated. The resistance of *P. acnes* to antibiotics has been well documented; such resistance threatens the efficacy of this form of acne therapy in the future.[16,17] It is therefore useful to prescribe antibiotics in combination with benzoyl peroxide, which does not induce resistance. A combined formulation of clindamycin 1% and benzoyl peroxide 5% has been found to produce faster and greater reductions in *P. acnes* than formulations containing clindamycin alone.[18] Moreover, the combination of benzoyl peroxide and clindamycin resulted in greater improvement in acne than either of its individual components alone.[19]

A commonly used regimen includes the combined antibiotic–benzoyl peroxide gel in the morning and topical retinoid in the evening. Azelaic acid, an anticomedonal and antibacterial

Table 3 Topical Therapies for Acne

Medication	Formulation	Frequency of Application	Primary Mechanism of Action	Adverse Effects
Azelaic acid	20% cream	b.i.d.	Anticomedonal, antibacterial	Stinging, irritation
Benzoyl peroxide	2.5%, 5%, 10% creams, gels, lotions, washes	b.i.d.	Antibacterial	Dryness, irritation, allergic contact dermatitis
Antibiotics				
Clindamycin	1% solutions, lotions, gels	b.i.d.	Antibacterial	Antibiotic resistance
Erythromycin	2% solutions, creams, gels, pledgets, wipes	b.i.d.	Antibacterial	Antibiotic resistance
Erythromycin–benzoyl peroxide	3% erythromycin–5% benzoyl peroxide gel	b.i.d.	Antibacterial	Dryness, irritation, allergic contact dermatitis; deteriorates if not refrigerated
Sodium sulfacetamide–sulfur	10% sodium sulfacetamide, 5% sulfur lotions	b.i.d.	Antibacterial	Dryness, irritation, allergic contact dermatitis
Retinoids				
Adapalene	0.1% gels	q.d.	Comedolytic	Dryness, irritation, photosensitivity
Tazarotene	0.05%, 0.1% gels	q.d.	Comedolytic	Dryness, irritation, photosensitivity
Tretinoin	0.025%, 0.05%, 0.1% creams; 0.01%, 0.025% gels; 0.05% solutions	q.d.	Comedolytic	Dryness, irritation, photosensitivity
Sulfur and resorcinol	2% resorcinol, 8% sulfur lotions, creams	q.d., b.i.d.	Comedolytic	Dryness, peeling, allergic contact dermatitis
Salicylic acid	0.5%–2% gels, pads, soaps	q.d., b.i.d.	Comedolytic	Dryness, irritation

agent, offers yet another choice for the topical treatment of acne. It, too, can be used in combination with topical retinoids, benzoyl peroxide, or topical antibiotics.[20] Salicylic acid, an over-the-counter comedolytic agent, plays a minor role in the treatment of acne. Skin-colored sulfur-resorcinol lotions are available; these very effective drying and peeling agents can be useful for treating individual lesions [see Table 3].

SYSTEMIC THERAPY

Systemic agents are warranted for patients with nodulocystic acne or inflammatory acne that is not responsive to topical therapy. Oral antibiotics are usually the first line of systemic treatment. Isotretinoin has generally been reserved for patients whose acne is refractory to antibiotics. Isotretinoin may be used as initial therapy in patients with particularly severe acne to prevent scarring and in patients with a history of antibiotic intolerance.

Antibiotics

Antibiotics have both antibacterial and anti-inflammatory effects that are beneficial in treating acne. The antibiotics most commonly used for acne are doxycycline, erythromycin, minocycline, tetracycline, and trimethoprim-sulfamethoxazole [see Table 4]. Because antibiotic resistance is a major problem with many of the older antibiotics, minocycline has been prescribed for many acne patients even though it is considerably more expensive. Strains of P. acnes that are resistant to minocycline have begun to emerge, however, and this may limit the usefulness of this drug in the future.[21] The duration of treatment with oral antibiotics depends on patient response. Azithromycin given at a dosage of 500 mg/day for 4 days, repeated at 10-day intervals for four cycles, is as effective as minocycline given at a dosage of 100 mg/day for 6 weeks.[22] Further refinements of regimens with these newer antibiotics will undoubtedly be performed before they achieve more widespread usage.

A lupuslike syndrome has been reported in patients taking oral minocycline. Synovitis, the presence of antinuclear antibodies, and elevations in hepatic transaminase levels were reported, but renal disease and central nervous system disease do not occur.[23] Upon discontinuance of minocycline, symptoms resolve, but upon retreatment, the syndrome recurs.

Controversy about the long-term use of antibiotics for the treatment of acne was raised by a 2004 study that suggested a correlation between antibiotic use and breast cancer risk. The study found that an increase in the cumulative number of days of antibiotic use—including use of tetracyclines and macrolides, which are prescribed for acne—was associated with greater breast cancer risk.[24] Although the results of this study have been questioned because of the way the study was performed and other shortcomings of the study, the possibility of increased risk remains a concern.

Isotretinoin

Oral isotretinoin is the most effective agent available for the treatment of acne. It results in long-lasting remissions or cures in the majority of patients treated. Because of its serious potential adverse effects, however, isotretinoin is not generally used as first-line therapy except for unusual cases.

Most of the side effects of isotretinoin are dose related and affect a majority of patients treated. For example, cheilitis uniformly occurs in patients treated with significant doses. Myalgias, dryness of mucous membranes, dry eczematous skin changes, and hyperlipidemia frequently occur. Total serum cholesterol levels can rise in patients taking isotretinoin, and triglyceride levels can rise sufficiently to cause pancreatitis.

Teratogenicity occurs with the administration of even a single dose of isotretinoin to pregnant women. Birth control counseling is an essential part of the management of women for whom isotretinoin is prescribed. The use of two forms of contraception is advised. Despite major educational efforts, pregnancies in women receiving isotretinoin continue to occur, resulting in severe birth defects.[25] With the introduction of generic isotretinoin, concern over teratogenicity increased. In response, the manufacturers of isotre-

Table 4 Commonly Prescribed Systemic Therapies for Acne

Medication	Dosage	Advantages	Adverse Effects
Antibiotics			
Doxycycline	50–100 mg p.o., b.i.d.	Inexpensive	Photosensitivity, GI symptoms, candidiasis
Erythromycin	250–500 mg p.o., b.i.d.	Alternative to tetracyclines	GI symptoms, candidiasis
Minocycline	50 mg p.o., q.d.–100 mg p.o., b.i.d.	Highly effective; antibiotic resistance rare at 200 mg/day	GI symptoms, candidiasis, vertigo, lupuslike syndrome (rare), autoimmune hepatitis (rare)
Tetracycline	250 mg p.o., q.d.–500 mg p.o., q.i.d. (b.i.d. dosing preferred)	Inexpensive	Photosensitivity, GI symptoms, candidiasis
Trimethoprim-sulfamethoxazole	160 mg trimethoprim–800 mg sulfamethoxazole b.i.d.	Alternative to tetracyclines and erythromycin	Bone marrow suppression, drug eruption
Other Agents			
Isotretinoin	0.5–2.0 mg/kg/day, in two divided doses	Most effective treatment; long-lasting remissions	Teratogenicity, hyperlipidemia, cheilitis, alopecia, pyogenic granulomas, dry eyes, epistaxis, rare pseudotumor cerebri (especially with concomitant antibiotics)
Norgestimate–ethinyl estradiol	0.18 mg norgestimate, 0.035 mg ethinyl estradiol p.o., q.d., for 21 days; repeat every 4 wk	Alternative to antibiotics and isotretinoin; less androgenic activity than progestins in other contraceptives	Thromboembolic disorders; ?antibiotic interaction; ?increased breast carcinoma; gallbladder disease; reduced glucose tolerance; headache; fluid retention; hypertension; breakthrough bleeding; breast swelling and tenderness
Drospirenone–ethinyl estradiol	3 mg drospirenone and 0.3 mg ethinyl estradiol p.o., q.d., for 21 days, followed by 7 days of inert pills; repeat monthly	Alternative to antibiotics and isotretinoin; less androgenic activity than progestins in other contraceptives	Thromboembolic disorders; ?antibiotic interaction; ?increased breast carcinoma; gallbladder disease; reduced glucose tolerance; headaches; fluid retention; hypertension; breakthrough bleeding; breast swelling and tenderness
Estrophasic contraceptive	1 mg norethindrone acetate and increasing doses of ethinyl estradiol: 20 µg, days 1–5; 30 µg, days 6–12; 35 µg, days 13–21; then 1 wk of inert tablet; repeat cycle every 4 wk	Alternative to antibiotics and isotretinoin; less androgenic activity than progestins in other contraceptives	Thromboembolic disorders; ?antibiotic interaction; ?increased breast carcinoma; gallbladder disease; reduced glucose tolerance; headaches; fluid retention; hypertension; breakthrough bleeding; breast swelling and tenderness

tinoin started a program in which physicians and pharmacists who prescribe and administer isotretinoin must register and agree to require that patients receiving isotretinoin undergo pregnancy testing on a regular basis.[26] Unfortunately, this program failed to eliminate pregnancies in women treated with isotretinoin. Attempts to enforce guidelines on the safe use of isotretinoin[27] have been deemed inadequate, and as a result, more stringent barriers to the prescription of isotretinoin are being instituted.[28]

There have been several instances of suicide and depression occurring in patients receiving oral isotretinoin.[29,30] Teenagers with severe acne may be at increased risk for suicide, regardless of the treatment they are using. A study compared the risk of depression, psychotic symptoms, suicide, and attempted suicide in acne patients receiving isotretinoin with the risk in acne patients being treated with oral antibiotics. The relative risk of depression or psychosis for isotretinoin-treated patients was 1.0, and the relative risk of suicide and attempted suicide was 0.9, suggesting that isotretinoin does not cause depression.[31] A study of pharmacy prescriptions yielded similar results. Prescriptions for antidepressants were quantified in 2,821 patients who filled isotretinoin prescriptions for the first time, and they were again quantified for patients filling isotretinoin prescriptions for a second time. The ratio of antidepressant use with the first prescription of isotretinoin to antidepressant use with the second prescription was not significantly different from 1.0—a finding that does not support an association between the use of isotretinoin and the onset of depression.[32]

Pseudotumor cerebri is a rare side effect of isotretinoin. It occurs more commonly in patients who are concomitantly given oral antibiotics.

Extensive counseling and monitoring—including complete blood counts, chemistry screens, and pregnancy tests when appropriate—should be done before treatment with isotretinoin; such counseling and monitoring should continue at 2-week intervals during the first month of treatment and monthly thereafter. Depending on patient response, treatment with 0.5 to 1.0 mg/kg/day in two divided doses should be continued to a cumulative dose of 120 to 150 mg/kg. Some clinicians have continued low-dose isotretinoin therapy for more than 6 months. Rarely, a second course of therapy is indicated when acne recurs.

Hormone Therapy

Estrogens in the form of oral contraceptives can be beneficial for patients with acne; progestins, however, can exacerbate the condition. The newer progestins—desogestrel, norgestimate, and gestodene—have less androgenic activity and therefore are less likely to exacerbate acne. A combination of ethinyl estradiol and norgestimate has been shown to be beneficial in the treatment of acne.[33] An oral contraceptive containing ethinyl estradiol in graduated doses, along with stable doses of norethindrone acetate, has been shown to have minimal androgenic activity and is also used for the treatment of acne.[34] A combined oral contraceptive containing ethinyl estradiol and drospirenone has also been found to effectively treat acne.[35] These agents are ideal for women who are seeking birth control methods and for women who are not candidates for, or who have not responded to, oral antibiotics or isotretinoin. Oral contraceptives can be particularly helpful to women with polycystic ovary syndrome. It is noteworthy that the beneficial effects of combined oral contraceptives are diminished in patients who are obese.[36]

Some concerns have been raised about the concomitant use of antibiotics and oral contraceptives because some antibiotics may interfere with contraceptive activity. Reviews of large numbers of patients treated concomitantly with oral contraceptives and antibiotics have not revealed significant increases in pregnancies.[37] Nevertheless, caution is advisable when a patient uses an antibiotic and an oral contraceptive together, especially one of the newer contraceptives that contain low doses of estrogen.

PHOTOTHERAPY

A number of light sources have been tested for the treatment of acne. Photodynamic therapy using topical δ-aminolevulinic acid has demonstrated efficacy for acne. Photodynamic therapy did not reduce *P. acnes* numbers or sebum excretion, so the mechanism by which it works is not entirely known.[38] A blue light administered twice weekly for 4 consecutive weeks has demonstrated efficacy for acne but not for nodulocystic lesions.[39] The 1,064 nm Q-switched neodymium:yttrium-aluminum-garnet (Nd:YAG) laser has proved useful for the treatment of acne scarring.[40]

TREATMENT OF ROSACEA

Avoidance of triggers such as alcohol, hot or spicy foods, and heat are an important part of the therapeutic regimen offered to patients with rosacea. Sunscreens are likewise important. Telangiectasia can be treated with laser therapy. Papules and pustules respond to the same topical and oral antibiotics used for acne, although benzoyl peroxide is less commonly used for rosacea. Flushing is difficult to treat. Azelaic acid may offer some benefit for the erythema associated with rosacea.[41]

Additional Information

Additional information about acne and its related disorders is available from the American Academy of Dermatology (http://www.aad.org) and the National Rosacea Society (http://www.rosacea.org).

The author has received grants from Allergan, Inc., Connetics Corp., Medicis, and Ortho-McNeil Pharmaceutical, Inc.

References

1. Stoll S, Shalita AR, Webster GF, et al: The effect of the menstrual cycle on acne. J Am Acad Dermatol 45:957, 2001

2. Harris HH, Downing DT, Stewart ME, et al: Sustainable rates of sebum secretion in acne patients and matched normal control subjects. J Invest Dermatol 8:200, 1983

3. Tucker SB, Rogers RS III, Winkelmann RK, et al: Inflammation in acne vulgaris: leukocyte attraction and cytotoxicity by comedonal material. J Invest Dermatol 74:21, 1980

4. Leyden JJ, McGinley KJ, Mills OH, et al: *Propionibacterium* levels in patients with and without acne vulgaris. J Invest Dermatol 65:382, 1975

5. Kim J, Ochoa MT, Krutzik SR, et al: Activation of toll-like receptor 2 in acne triggers inflammatory cytokine responses. J Immunol 169:1535, 2002

6. Lucky AW, Biro FM, Huster GA, et al: Acne vulgaris in premenarchal girls: an early sign of puberty associated with rising levels of dehydroepiandrosterone. Arch Dermatol 130:308, 1994

7. Sansone G, Reisner RM: Differential rates of conversion of testosterone to dihydrotestosterone in acne and in normal human skin: a possible pathogenic factor in acne. J Invest Dermatol 56:366, 1971

8. Boni R, Nehrhoff B: Treatment of gram-negative folliculitis in patients with acne. Am J Clin Dermatol 4:273, 2003

9. Stone DU, Chodosh J: Ocular rosacea: an update on pathogenesis and therapy. Curr Opin Ophthalmol 15:499, 2004

10. Utas S, Ozbakir O, Turasan A, et al: *Helicobacter pylori* eradication treatment reduces the severity of rosacea. J Am Acad Dermatol 40:433, 1999

11. Hirsch RJ, Lewis AB: Treatment of acne scarring. Semin Cutan Med Surg 20:190, 2001

12. Leyden JJ, Shalita A, Thiboutot D, et al: Topical retinoids in inflammatory acne: a retrospective, investigator-blinded, vehicle-controlled, photographic assessment. Clin Ther 27:216, 2005

13. Leyden J, Grove GL: Randomized facial tolerability studies comparing gel formulations of retinoids used to treat acne vulgaris. Cutis 67(6 suppl):17, 2001

14. Dunlap FE, Baker MD, Plott RT, et al: Adapalene 0.1% gel has low skin irritation potential even when applied immediately after washing. Br J Dermatol 139(suppl):52, 1998

15. Bershad S, Kranjac Singer G, Parente JE, et al: Successful treatment of acne vulgaris using a new method: results of a randomized vehicle-controlled trial of short-contact therapy with 0.1% tazarotene gel. Arch Dermatol 138:481, 2002

16. Leyden JJ: The evolving role of *Propionibacterium acnes* in acne. Semin Cutan Med Surg 20:139, 2001

17. Dreno B, Reynaud A, Moyse D, et al: Erythromycin-resistance of cutaneous bacterial flora in acne. Eur J Dermatol 11:549, 2001

18. Leyden J, Kaidbey K, Levy SF: The combination formulation of clindamycin 1% plus benzoyl peroxide 5% versus 3 different formulations of topical clindamycin alone in the reduction of *Propionibacterium acnes*: an in vivo comparative study. Am J Clin Dermatol 2:263, 2001

19. Leyden JJ, Berger RS, Dunlap FE, et al: Comparison of the efficacy and safety of a combination topical gel formulation of benzoyl peroxide and clindamycin with benzoyl peroxide, clindamycin and vehicle gel in the treatments of acne vulgaris. Am J Clin Dermatol 2:33, 2001

20. Webster G: Combination azelaic acid therapy for acne vulgaris. J Am Acad Dermatol 43(2 pt 3):S47, 2000

21. Ross JI, Snelling AM, Eady EA, et al: Phenotypic and genotypic characterization of antibiotic-resistant *Propionibacterium acnes* isolated from acne patients attending dermatology clinics in Europe, the U.S.A., Japan and Australia. Br J Dermatol 144:339, 2001

22. Gruber F, Grubisic-Greblo H, Kastelan M, et al: Azithromycin compared with minocycline in the treatment of acne comedonica and papulo-pustulosa. J Chemother 10:469, 1998

23. Lawson TM, Amos N, Bulgen D, et al: Minocycline-induced lupus: clinical features and response to rechallenge. Rheumatology (Oxford) 40:329, 2001

24. Velicer CM, Heckbert SR, Lampe JW, et al: Antibiotic use in relation to the risk of breast cancer. JAMA 291:827, 2004

25. Honein MA, Paulozzi LJ, Erickson JD: Continued occurrence of Accutane-exposed pregnancies. Teratology 64:142, 2001

26. Honein MA, Moore CA, Erickson JD: Can we ensure the safe use of known human teratogens? Introduction of generic isotretinoin in the US as an example. Drug Saf 27:1069, 2004

27. Goldsmith LA, Bolognia JL, Callen JP, et al: American Academy of Dermatology Consensus Conference on the safe and optimal use of isotretinoin: summary and recommendations. J Am Acad Dermatol 50:900, 2004 [erratum, J Am Acad Dermatol 51:348, 2004]

28. FDA announces enhancement to isotretinoin risk management program. US Food and Drug Administration, November 23, 2004 http://www.fda.gov/bbs/topics/ANSWERS/2004/ANS01328.html

29. Wysowski DK, Pitts M, Beitz J: An analysis of reports of depression and suicide in patients treated with isotretinoin. J Am Acad Dermatol 45:515, 2001

30. Ng CH, Tam MM, Hook SJ: Acne, isotretinoin treatment and acute depression. World J Biol Psychiatry 2:159, 2001

31. Jick SS, Kremers HM, Vasilakis-Scaramozza C: Isotretinoin use and risk of depression, psychotic symptoms, suicide, and attempted suicide. Arch Dermatol 136:1231, 2000

32. Hersom K, Neary MP, Levaux HP, et al: Isotretinoin and antidepressant pharmacotherapy: a prescription sequence symmetry analysis. J Am Acad Dermatol 49:424, 2003

33. Lucky AW, Henderson TA, Olson WH, et al: Effectiveness of norgestimate and ethinyl estradiol in treating moderate acne vulgaris. J Am Acad Dermatol 37:746, 1997

34. Boyd RA, Zegarac EA, Posvar EL, et al: Minimal androgenic activity of a new oral contraceptive containing norethindrone acetate and graduated doses of ethinyl estradiol. Contraception 63:71, 2001

35. Thorneycroft H, Gollnick H, Schellschmidt I: Superiority of a combined contraceptive containing drospirenone to a triphasic preparation containing norgestimate in acne treatment. Cutis 74:123, 2004

36. Cibula D, Hill M, Fanta M, et al: Does obesity diminish the positive effect of oral contraceptive treatment on hyperandrogenism in women with polycystic ovarian syndrome? Hum Reprod 16:940, 2001

37. London BM, Lookingbill DP: Frequency of pregnancy in acne patients taking oral antibiotics and oral contraceptives. Arch Dermatol 130:392, 1994

38. Pollock B, Turner D, Stringer MR, et al: Topical aminolaevulinic acid–photodynamic therapy for the treatment of acne vulgaris: a study of clinical efficacy and mechanism of action. Br J Dermatol 151:616, 2004

39. Tzung TY, Wu KH, Huang ML: Blue light phototherapy in the treatment of acne. Photodermatol Photoimmunol Photomed 20:266, 2004

40. Friedman PM, Jih MH, Skover GR, et al: Treatment of atrophic facial acne scars with the 1064-nm Q-switched Nd:YAG laser: six-month follow-up study. Arch Dermatol 140:1337, 2004

41. Elewski BE, Fleischer AB Jr, Pariser DM: A comparison of 15% azelaic acid gel and 0.75% metronidazole gel in the topical treatment of papulopustular rosacea: results of a randomized trial. Arch Dermatol 139:1444, 2003

Reviews

Feldman S, Careccia RE, Barham KL, et al: Diagnosis and treatment of acne. Am Fam Physician 69:2123, 2004

James WD: Clinical practice. Acne. N Engl J Med 352:1463, 2005

Webster GF: Acne vulgaris. BMJ 325:475, 2002

36 Papulosquamous Disorders

Elizabeth A. Abel, M.D.

Papulosquamous disorders comprise a group of dermatoses that have distinct morphologic features.[1] The characteristic primary lesion of these disorders is a papule, usually erythematous, that has a variable amount of scaling on the surface. Plaques or patches form through coalescence of the primary lesions. Some common papulosquamous dermatoses are pityriasis rosea, lichen planus, seborrheic dermatitis, tinea corporis, pityriasis rubra pilaris, psoriasis [*see Chapter 37*], and parapsoriasis. Drug eruptions, tinea corporis, and secondary syphilis may also have a papulosquamous morphology. Some papulosquamous disorders may be a cutaneous manifestation of AIDS.[2]

Pityriasis Rosea

Pityriasis rosea is a relatively common, self-limited, exanthematous disease characterized by oval papulosquamous lesions on the trunk and proximal areas of the extremities. Pityriasis rosea typically appears during the spring and fall in temperate climates[3]; its incidence is highest in persons between 10 and 35 years of age.[4]

A population-based 10-year epidemiologic survey identified 939 patients with pityriasis rosea, about one third of whom had antecedent acute infection or atopy.[5] It also showed that peak incidence occurred at 20 to 24 years of age, that the incidence was higher in colder months, and that recurrences were rare. Occurrences among household contacts are uncommon. This study also noted that the incidence of disease had appeared to decline.

ETIOLOGY

A viral etiology has been suggested for pityriasis rosea on the basis of immunologic and histologic data. The superficial dermis contains aggregates of CD4+ helper T cells in perivascular locations and increased numbers of Langerhans cells. It has been postulated that IgM antibodies to keratinocytes cause the secondary form of the eruption. An association between human herpesvirus type 7 (HHV-7) and pityriasis rosea was initially reported in 1997.[6] Studies using polymerase chain reaction and immunohistochemical analyses of tissue samples to detect HHV-7 DNA sequences and antigens have provided inconclusive evidence of a causal relationship between HHV-7 and pityriasis rosea. In a retrospective study of 13 patients and 14 control subjects, the prevalence of HHV-7 was lower in lesional skin of patients with pityriasis rosea than in control subjects.[7] A subsequent seroepidemiologic study of HHV-6 and HHV-7 was conducted in 44 patients with pityriasis rosea and in 25 patients with other skin eruptions. Although in this study several patients with pityriasis rosea had antibody titers consistent with active infection, the overall prevalence of HHV-6 and HHV-7 was no greater in patients with pityriasis rosea than in control subjects.[8] A meta-analysis reviewed the data from 13 studies and found insufficient evidence to support a causal relationship between HHV-7 infection and pityriasis rosea.[9] A viral etiology of pityriasis rosea thus remains elusive. Certain drugs that cause a pityriasis rosea–like eruption have been implicated in the etiology of this disorder. These drugs include the antihypertensive agent captopril, metronidazole, isotretinoin (13-*cis*-retinoic acid), peni-

cillamine, arsenic, gold, bismuth, barbiturates, and clonidine.[4]

DIAGNOSIS

The primary lesion, called a herald patch, appears first as a slightly raised, salmon-colored oval patch with a fine, wrinkled scale resembling cigarette paper. Typically, 7 to 10 days after the appearance of the herald patch, there occurs a bilaterally symmetrical eruption of smaller lesions; this secondary eruption occurs mainly on the trunk and upper extremities [*see Figure 1*]. Secondary lesions tend to follow cleavage lines (Langer lines) in a so-called fir tree distribution. A V-shaped formation on the upper chest and upper back, a circumferential pattern around the shoulders and hips, and a transverse pattern on the lower anterior trunk and lower back are seen in most patients.[10] The lesions are occasionally pruritic. The secondary rash is frequently more helpful in making a diagnosis than the initial herald patch, which is often misdiagnosed.[10] Atypical manifestations occur in 20% of persons affected. Such manifestations include a purpuric form of pityriasis rosea that resembles vasculitis, as well as papular, vesicular, pustular, and urticarial forms. An inverse variant of pityriasis rosea, more common in children than in adults, is characterized by lesions on the face and extremities, with relatively few lesions appearing on the trunk.[4]

DIFFERENTIAL DIAGNOSIS

Because lesions of pityriasis rosea may closely resemble those of secondary syphilis, a serologic test for syphilis may be indicated. Lesions may also resemble tinea corporis or tinea versicolor and should be examined by fungal scrapings and potassium hydroxide (KOH) wet mounts. A careful drug history must be obtained to exclude the possibility of a drug eruption.

TREATMENT

Pityriasis rosea lesions resolve spontaneously after 6 to 8 weeks. The patient should be reassured that the disorder is benign and self-limited; such reassurance, together with educating the pa-

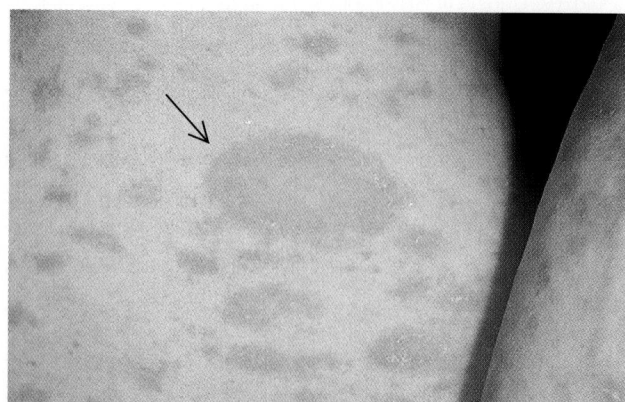

Figure 1 Pityriasis rosea commonly presents as a single, large salmon-colored plaque called a herald patch (arrow). Appearance of the isolated lesion is followed in a week to 10 days by a bilaterally symmetrical papulosquamous eruption, mainly on the trunk and upper extremities.

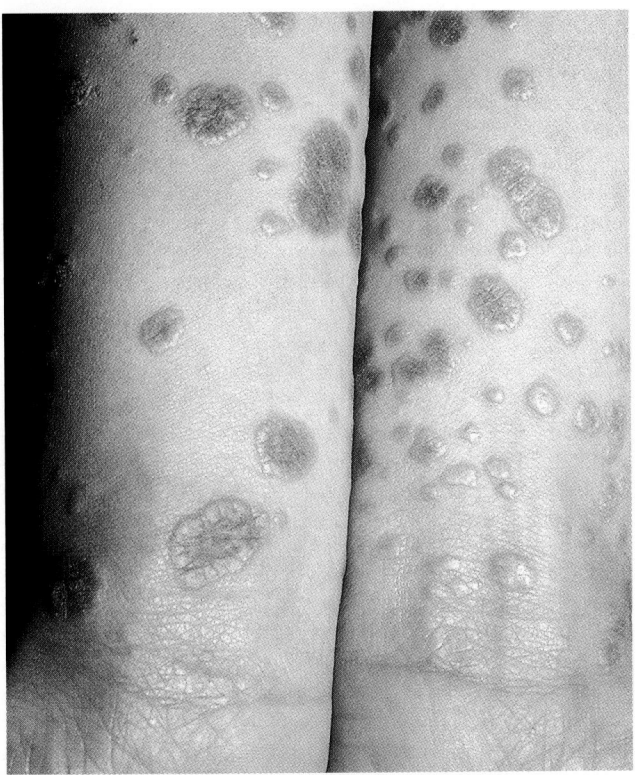

Figure 2   **Violaceous, flat-topped, polygonal papules are typical of lichen planus. A common location is the flexor aspect of the wrists and forearms.**

tient about the disease, is the most important aspect of treatment. Lesions are variably pruritic. Symptoms should be treated with bland emollients or systemic antipruritics. Sun exposure may accelerate clearing. Irradiation with ultraviolet B (UVB) sunlamps is beneficial in decreasing the severity of disease, especially when treatment is initiated within the first week of the eruption. One study found that 10 erythemogenic exposures of UVB substantially decreased the extent of pityriasis rosea, although it neither altered the duration of the disorder nor improved the itching.[11] Other evidence suggests that UVB therapy may hasten resolution of the rash but may cause hyperpigmentation.[12]

In a double-blind, placebo-controlled study in India, oral erythromycin administered in divided doses for 14 days was effective in treating patients with pityriasis rosea.[13] In this cohort, upper respiratory tract infections preceded the skin eruption in 68.8% of the 90 patients. A complete response, with complete resolution of skin lesions occurring within 2 weeks, was reported in 33% of the treatment group, as compared with 0% in the placebo group. The duration of disease was comparable for the two groups of patients. Although not all patients with pityriasis rosea benefit from erythromycin therapy, a trial of erythromycin is a safe treatment approach.

Lichen Planus

Lichen planus is a localized or generalized eruption with violaceous, flat-topped, polygonal papules and little or no observable scaling [see Figure 2]. It is often localized to the oral mucosa; 25% of patients with oral lichen planus have skin involvement as well.[14] The incidence is highest in young to middle-aged persons.

Lichen planus usually appears in the fifth or sixth decade and affects women more often than men.

ETIOLOGY

The etiology of lichen planus is unknown. An alteration in basal keratinocytes that induces humoral and cell-mediated immune responses has been postulated as a possible causal mechanism. Skin and mucous membrane lesions resembling lichen planus have been observed in patients with graft versus host disease (GVHD) [see Chapter 40]. Lichen planus has also been associated with other immune-mediated diseases, including ulcerative colitis, bullous pemphigoid, myasthenia gravis with thymoma, primary biliary cirrhosis, and chronic active hepatitis.[15]

There is an increased prevalence of viral hepatitis, especially hepatitis C, in patients with lichen planus. In a multicenter study of 303 sequential patients with lichen planus, the prevalence of hepatitis C virus (HCV) was 19.1%, compared with 3.2% in control subjects.[16] The role of HCV in the pathogenesis of lichen planus is not clearly understood; some investigators suggest that the cause of lichen planus may be related to the pattern of immune dysregulation induced by HCV.[17] There are a number of reports of lichen planus occurring after administration of different types of hepatitis B vaccine.[18] This is a rare occurrence, considering the widespread use of this vaccine; several cases have been reported from France and Italy, and one case has been reported from the Middle East. An immunologic mechanism has been postulated as the cause. The latency period ranges from several days to 3 months after any one of the three usual injections of vaccine.

A variety of drugs have been reported to cause lichenoid reactions in the skin, usually sparing the mucous membranes. Such drugs include beta blockers, methyldopa, penicillamine, quinidine, and quinine. Other drugs that have been implicated but for which causal evidence is insufficient include angiotensin-converting enzyme inhibitors, sulfonylurea agents, carbamazepine, gold, and lithium.[19] In one study, the administration of penicillamine for primary biliary cirrhosis was followed by the development of lichen planus in 17 of 24 patients[20]; in addition, after treatment with penicillamine, the skin eruption became worse in three of seven patients with biliary cirrhosis and preexisting lichen planus. Nonsteroidal anti-inflammatory drugs have been documented to cause a lichenoid drug eruption; these drugs include naproxen, indomethacin, diflunisal, ibuprofen, acetylsalicylic acid, and salsalate.[21] Although the latency period is highly variable, symptoms usually develop within a few months after drug initiation and resolve within weeks to months after discontinuance of the offending agent.

DIAGNOSIS

Lichen planus appears as flat-topped, shiny, violaceous papules, often with a fine, reticulated scale on the surface. Common sites of involvement include the skin, nails, mucous membranes, vulva, and penis. Wickham striae—white, lacy patterns on the papule surface—are apparent on magnification with a hand lens.[22] The occurrence of papules along a scratch line, as in linear lichen planus, is referred to as the Koebner phenomenon [see Figure 3]. In the hypertrophic form of the disease, papules coalesce to form thick plaques or nodules that are often found on the lower extremities. Pruritus may be severe, particularly in the generalized or hypertrophic forms of the disease. Common sites of involvement are the flexor surfaces of the wrists, the sacrum, the mucous membranes of the mouth, the medial thighs, and the genitalia. Mucous membrane lesions show a white, reticulated mosaic pattern [see Figure 4]. A severe erosive form of lichen planus can involve the oral mucous membranes. In rare cases, lesions occur in the esophagus, causing esophageal stricture and dysphagia.[23]

A follicular form known as lichen planopilaris may result in scarring alopecia. Variants of lichen planus with distinct morphologic features include actinic, annular, bullous, hypertrophic, linear, ulcerative, and zosteriform forms. The nails may also be involved [see Chapter 47]. The clinical features of some forms of lichen planus may resemble those of lupus erythematosus.[22]

Skin biopsy confirms the clinical diagnosis of lichen planus. Typically, the epidermis shows hyperkeratosis, a prominent granular layer, liquefaction degeneration of the basal cell layer, and an intense upper dermal inflammatory infiltrate. Immunoperoxidase studies using monoclonal antibodies to cell surface antigens have shown that most cells in the infiltrate are of the helper-inducer T cell subset. Colloid bodies (Civatte bodies) coated with immunoglobulin are frequently seen in the dermal papillae. On ultrastructural examination, numerous Langerhans cells can be observed at the dermoepidermal junction.

TREATMENT

Limited data exist for making evidence-based recommendations regarding treatment of lichen planus.[24,25] Definitive clinical trials have not been performed, and information on the efficacy of treatments is derived from small trials and anecdotal evidence.

Body Lesions

Emollients, topical glucocorticoids, a short course of systemic corticosteroids, and systemic antipruritics have been used to treat cutaneous lichen planus. Most experts recommend medium- to high-potency topical corticosteroids as first-line treatment for localized cutaneous lichen planus. Oral corticosteroids may be used for generalized cutaneous lichen planus. As an alternative to systemic corticosteroids, systemic retinoids, such as acitretin, are beneficial in some patients with cutaneous forms of lichen planus.[26] Azathioprine has been used for its steroid-sparing effect in erosive and generalized lichen planus.[27]

Other therapies that have been reported to have efficacy in the treatment of cutaneous lichen planus include phototherapy (psoralen plus ultraviolet A [PUVA]), cyclosporine, and hydroxychloroquine.[24] In a trial of oral psoralen photochemotherapy for widespread recalcitrant lichen planus, clinical remission occurred in six of seven patients and correlated with the disappearance of the upper dermal infiltrate.[28] Oral cyclosporine has also been effective, but potential renal toxicity and hypertension limit its long-term use.[22] Recombinant interferon alfa–2b, administered subcutaneously every other day, was successful in the treatment of generalized lichen planus in three patients with no evidence of hepatitis, further supporting the cell-mediated immunologic etiology of this disease.[29]

Mouth Lesions

For lichen planus that is localized to the oral mucosa, a high-potency corticosteroid such as clobetasol in a vehicle that is adherent to the mucosal surface (Orabase) is helpful.[24,29] Intralesional injections of corticosteroids may be used to treat localized, recalcitrant lesions. Use of miconazole gel in combination with chlorhexidine mouth rinses is effective for prophylaxis against oral candidiasis.[30] Topical isotretinoin gel is an effective alternative to corticosteroids, although relapses often occur after discontinuance of this medication.[31] In a double-blind, placebo-controlled study of 22 patients with biopsy-proven oral lichen planus, an 8-week course of 0.1% isotretinoin gel was found to be effective.[31] Cyclosporine mouth rinses have been helpful for some patients. A 6-month course of hydroxychloroquine, 200 to 400 mg daily, was successful in nine of 10 patients with oral lichen planus; ulcers healed and pain decreased after 1 to 2 months.[32] Topical tacrolimus, a macrolide that suppresses T cell activation, was used to treat erosive mucosal lichen planus in 19 patients whose conditions were resistant to conventional treatment. Therapeutic levels of tacrolimus were demonstrated in eight patients, and areas of ulceration showed a mean decrease of 73.3% over the 8-week study period; however, 13 of 17 patients suffered a relapse after cessation of therapy.[33] Topical pimecrolimus cream is being evaluated as a treatment for oral erosive lichen planus.[34] The role of these agents in the treatment of lichen planus must be further investigated, particularly in view of the alert by the Food and Drug Administration issued in 2005 regarding a possible link between use of topical tacrolimus and pimecrolimus and cases of lymphoma and skin cancer.

Genital and Perianal Lesions

Mild, nonerosive disease can be controlled with topical corticosteroids; erosive disease, although more difficult to treat, may

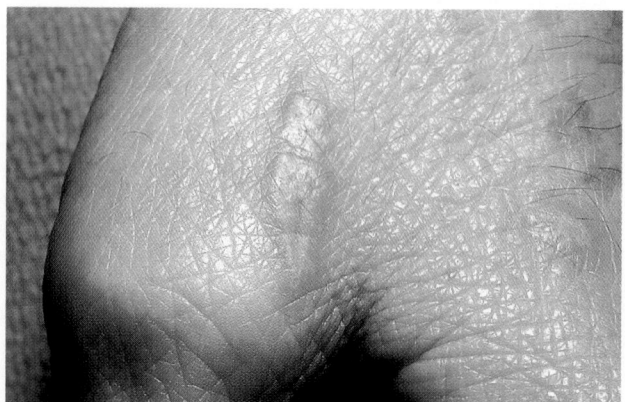

Figure 3 The Koebner phenomenon—the appearance of lesions along a scratch line—may be seen in patients with lichen planus.

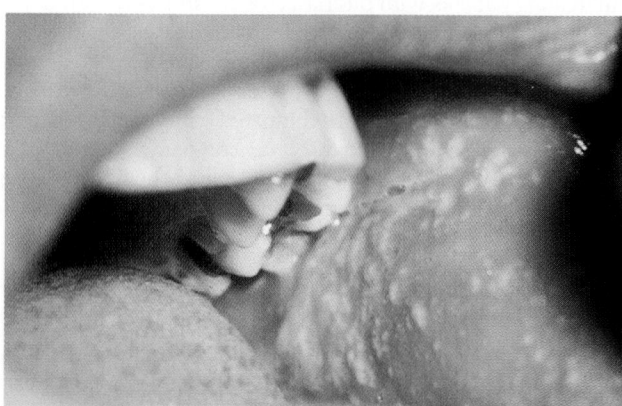

Figure 4 Lichen planus of the mucous membrane assumes a white, reticulated mosaic pattern, as seen above on the buccal mucosa.

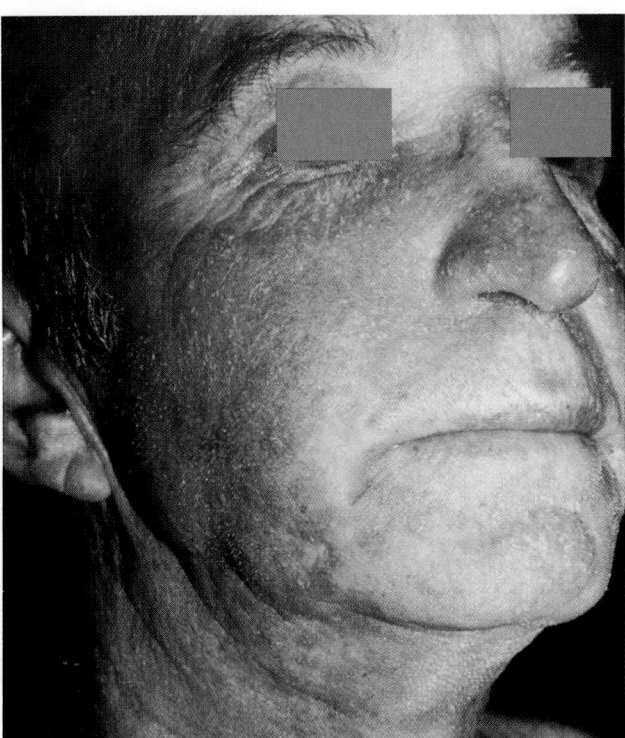

Figure 5   Seborrheic dermatitis seen on the face of this patient involves sites of sebaceous gland activity.

be treated with topical corticosteroids in combination with other topical or systemic medications.[35] Topical tacrolimus[36,37] and topical pimecrolimus[38] may be useful in the treatment of recalcitrant cases that have failed to respond to other therapies.

PROGNOSIS

Patients who experience an acute outbreak of lichen planus have a good prognosis; in most cases, the papules clear within several months to a year. The chronic form, however, may last for 10 years or longer. In a study following the long-term course of lichen planus in 214 patients for 8 to 12 years, lichen planus cleared in two thirds of the patients within 1 year. The recurrence rate was 49%, which was higher than recurrence rates reported in previous studies; the authors attributed the high rate of recurrence to treatment with potent topical corticosteroids.[39]

Seborrheic Dermatitis

Seborrheic dermatitis is a papulosquamous condition that is often associated with excessive oiliness or seborrhea, dandruff, and well-defined red, scaly patches on the face, trunk, and intertriginous areas.[40] Some cases may progress to a severe exfoliative erythroderma. Seborrheic dermatitis is a common skin disorder that occurs in otherwise healthy adults. It is increasingly prevalent in middle-aged and elderly persons. Seborrheic dermatitis does not occur before puberty except during infancy (usually between 2 and 12 weeks of age), at which time transplacentally derived maternal hormones are present. The prognosis in adults is one of lifelong recurrence, with each episode lasting weeks to months.

ETIOLOGY

The cause of seborrheic dermatitis is unknown. An occasional association with neurologic abnormalities, especially parkinson-

ism, has been observed. Genetic predisposition, emotional stress, diet, hormones, and climatic factors may also influence this disorder. It is thought that an association exists between the yeast-like organism *Pityrosporum* and seborrheic dermatitis. Seborrheic dermatitis may, in part, be the result of an abnormal or inflammatory immune response to this yeast, or it may be caused by an epidermal hyperproliferation of this organism.[41]

Patients with classic seborrheic dermatitis may have normal or reduced rates of sebum excretion; therefore, seborrhea is not essential for the development of this disorder.[42] However, seborrhea may play a role in the seborrheic dermatitis present in certain patients, such as those with parkinsonism. Reduction of seborrhea with improvement of the dermatitis has been observed after a favorable neurologic response to levodopa treatment for parkinsonism.

DIAGNOSIS

The scale associated with seborrheic dermatitis may be yellowish and either dry or greasy. Sites of predilection are the areas of sebaceous gland activity [*see Figure 5*], such as the scalp, eyebrows, eyelids, forehead, nasolabial folds, and presternal or interscapular regions. Blepharitis involves granular inflammation of the lid margin, with scaling and shedding of debris into the eye, which may cause conjunctivitis. Seborrheic dermatitis is the most common cause of otitis externa. When the scalp is involved, lesions often extend along the frontal hairline, forming a band of erythema. The postauricular area is a common site of involvement. Lesions of the trunk may consist of erythematous follicular papules covered by greasy scales, which may coalesce to form large plaques or circinate patches. Seborrheic dermatitis can be seen in areas of male pattern baldness, but it is not a cause of hair loss unless there has been a severe intervening secondary infection resulting in a scarring alopecia.

DIFFERENTIAL DIAGNOSIS

Seborrheic dermatitis should be considered in the differential diagnosis of chronic eczematous dermatitis and in that of papulosquamous disorders, particularly psoriasis. The clinical features of seborrheic dermatitis limited to the scalp and face may resemble those associated with psoriasis, giving rise to the term sebopsoriasis. Histologic features range from psoriasiform changes of acanthosis and parakeratosis to the spongiosis of eczema. Seborrheic dermatitis of the face may resemble the facial lesions found in lupus erythematosus or other photosensitivity dermatoses. Lesions on the trunk may be confused with tinea versicolor, but the latter is easily excluded by skin scraping and KOH preparation or Wood light examination. Atopic dermatitis and psoriasis, especially when partially treated, are also included in the differential diagnosis.

SEBORRHEIC DERMATITIS ASSOCIATED WITH AIDS

Severe seborrheic dermatitis can be one of the most common and earliest manifestations of AIDS. From 30% to 80% of patients with AIDS have seborrheic dermatitis, compared with 3% to 5% of HIV-negative young adults.[43] Lesions may be explosive in onset and are often resistant to therapy. Clinical features include a predominantly inflammatory papular eruption on the face, with a tendency to spare the scalp, in contrast to the mild erythema and scaling of the scalp typical of seborrheic dermatitis in persons without AIDS. Truncal involvement in seborrheic areas is common in AIDS patients, and the lesions may resemble psoriasis. Although the cause of the association of seborrheic dermatitis with AIDS is unknown, immunologic dysfunction may lead to an overgrowth of the yeast *P. orbiculare* in seborrheic areas.

Skin biopsy specimens from AIDS patients with seborrheic dermatitis have distinct histologic features, including keratinocyte necrosis, leukoexocytosis, a superficial perivascular infiltrate of plasma cells, and, frequently, neutrophils.[44]

TREATMENT

The condition on the scalp usually responds well to frequent—as often as daily—shampooing with a preparation containing 3% to 5% sulfur and 2% to 3% salicylic acid. Good response has also been reported with use of ciclopirox 1% shampoo once or twice weekly.[45] For the face and nonhairy areas, a mild cream containing precipitated 3% sulfur and 3% salicylic acid is effective. Involved areas also respond well to low-potency topical glucocorticoids, such as 1% hydrocortisone cream or desonide cream. Caution, however, must be exercised in the use of high-potency fluorinated steroid preparations, especially on the face and in skin folds; prolonged application may lead to chronic skin changes, such as atrophy and telangiectasia. Wet dressings followed by a topical antibiotic preparation are helpful in treating intertriginous areas, in which maceration and superficial secondary infection may occur.

Topical antifungal agents have been used in the treatment of seborrheic dermatitis. In addition to their antifungal properties, certain azoles (e.g., bifonazole, itraconazole, and ketoconazole) have demonstrated anti-inflammatory activity, which may be beneficial in alleviating symptoms.[46] In one study, 575 patients with seborrheic dermatitis underwent twice-weekly treatments with 2% ketoconazole shampoo; an excellent response was seen in 88% of the patients.[47] Continued prophylactic treatment once weekly over 6 months was helpful in preventing relapse of the disorder in a significant number of patients.

In a trial of 38 patients with seborrheic dermatitis, 1% metronidazole gel was found to be effective. Improvement was noted after 2 weeks, and marked improvement or complete clearing was noted at 8 weeks[48]; however, in a randomized, controlled trial, metronidazole 0.75% gel and placebo were found to have similar efficacy.[49] In a small randomized, open-label clinical trial, pimecrolimus 1% cream and betamethasone 1% cream were both found to be effective in reducing symptoms of seborrheic dermatitis, but relapses were observed more frequently with betamethasone.[50] A multicenter, randomized, controlled trial found oral terbinafine (an antimycotic allylamine compound) to be effective in patients with moderate to severe seborrheic dermatitis.[51]

Seborrheic blepharitis may be treated by applying baby shampoo with a cotton-tipped applicator to debride scales. If topical corticosteroids are required, the patient should be referred to an ophthalmologist to monitor potential side effects to the eye, such as increased intraocular pressure, glaucoma, cataracts, and activation of latent herpes infection.[1]

Treatment of HIV-associated seborrheic dermatitis is similar to that of seborrheic dermatitis in general, although HIV-associated seborrheic dermatitis is apt to be recalcitrant, requiring intensive, prolonged therapy. Treatment of the underlying HIV infection may lead to improvement of the associated seborrheic dermatitis.

Pityriasis Rubra Pilaris

Pityriasis rubra pilaris is a relatively uncommon chronic inflammatory dermatosis that is considered to be a disorder of ker-

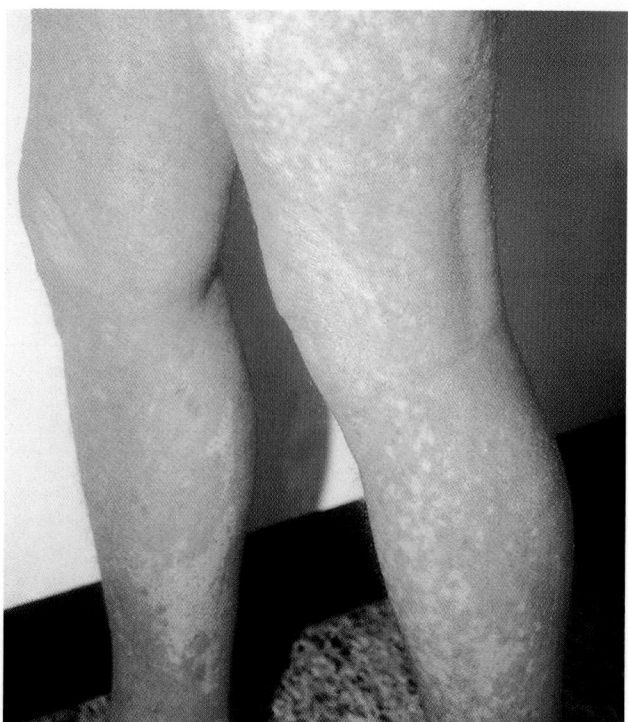

Figure 6 **Islands of spared skin within a background of diffuse erythema are present on the legs of this patient with pityriasis rubra pilaris.**

atinization. The age distribution is bimodal, occurring either in childhood or in the fifth decade; the clinical course is variable. An autosomal dominant inheritance has been postulated for the juvenile form of the disease.[52] Patients with the classic adult form of the disease have the best prognosis; resolution usually occurs over a 3-year period.

DIAGNOSIS

Typically, pityriasis rubra pilaris initially manifests itself as a seborrheic dermatitis–like eruption that occurs on sun-exposed areas of the body; this eruption is followed by the development of follicular papules that coalesce into psoriasiform patches on the trunk and extremities, with progression to erythroderma. Generalized involvement is characterized by yellow-orange erythema with desquamation. Diffuse areas of involvement generally show islands of spared skin [*see Figure 6*]. Additional features are palmoplantar hyperkeratosis [*see Figure 7*] and prominent follicular plugging over the dorsal aspects of the fingers. Pruritus is usually mild or absent. A pityriasis rubra pilaris–like eruption with follicular hyperkeratosis is a little known but distinctive cutaneous manifestation of dermatomyositis.[53]

TREATMENT

The response of patients with pityriasis rubra pilaris to conventional antipsoriatic therapies, such as topical corticosteroids, tars, and oral methotrexate, is often unsatisfactory; some patients, however, have shown a favorable response to topical calcipotriene (known outside the United States as calcipotriol).[54] UVB phototherapy may exacerbate the disease.[55] High-dose vitamin A in excess of 200,000 IU daily has been used but can cause liver or central nervous system toxicity. An oral retinoid such as acitretin or isotretinoin is indicated for the treatment of pityriasis rubra pilaris in men and postmenopausal women. In an early study in-

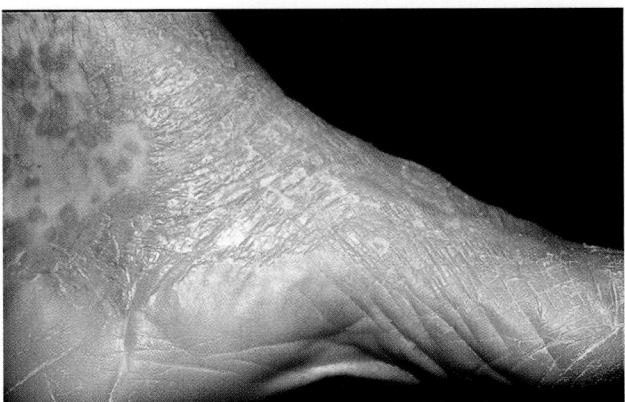

Figure 7 **Plantar hyperkeratosis and confluent erythematous follicular papules typical of pityriasis rubra pilaris are seen on the ankle and foot of this patient.**

volving 45 patients with pityriasis rubra pilaris, isotretinoin produced definite improvement in 50% of the patients after 4 weeks of therapy.[56] Remission of up to 6 months was sustained in some patients after the drug was withdrawn. Long-term use of this drug in patients with keratinizing disorders has been associated with irreversible skeletal toxicity. Because teratogenicity is a concern, women of childbearing age must use effective birth control with either agent.

In a study of patients with pediatric pityriasis rubra pilaris, isotretinoin achieved the best response among a range of therapies including steroids, systemic retinoids, and methotrexate; five of six patients treated with isotretinoin showed 90% to 100% clearing of lesions within 6 months of initiation of treatment.[57] Cyclosporine, 5 mg/kg/day, was effective in the treatment of three adult patients with pityriasis rubra pilaris, with a favorable response being noted within 2 to 4 weeks of initiation of therapy; however, relapse occurred when the dose was decreased to 1.2 mg/kg/day.[58]

Numerous reports have suggested that infliximab, a monoclonal antibody that binds to tumor necrosis factor–α, may be useful in the treatment of cutaneous inflammatory diseases, such as pityriasis rubra pilaris.[59] The drug is currently approved by the FDA for the treatment of rheumatoid arthritis and Crohn disease; further investigation is required to determine its efficacy for cutaneous dermatoses.

Parapsoriasis

Parapsoriasis encompasses a variety of relatively uncommon chronic inflammatory dermatoses of unknown etiology that are resistant to conventional treatment. Despite the designation parapsoriasis, the clinical appearance of the noninfiltrated scaly patches or plaques is distinct from that of psoriatic lesions. Classification of these disorders is controversial and is further complicated by the use of several terms to denote a single entity and by the use of various systems of nomenclature. A proposed standard nomenclature divides parapsoriasis into two distinct subgroups: pityriasis lichenoides, which may be acute or chronic, and small- and large-plaque parapsoriasis.[60]

PITYRIASIS LICHENOIDES

Diagnosis

The acute form of pityriasis lichenoides, also known as pityriasis lichenoides et varioliformis acuta (PLEVA) or Mucha-Haber-

mann disease, is characterized by the abrupt onset of a generalized eruption of reddish-brown maculopapules that evolve during a period of weeks to months. Lesions are typically present at all stages of evolution and may be vesicular, hemorrhagic, crusted, or necrotic [*see Figure 8*]. Healing with varioliform scarring is common. Nonspecific histologic features include intraepidermal lymphocytes and erythrocytes, dermal hemorrhage, and a lymphocytic vasculitis.[61] Skin lesions of PLEVA may resemble those of lymphomatoid papulosis, which has immunohistologic features of a CD30+ cutaneous T cell lymphoma.[62] Lymphomatoid papulosis occurs as a chronic, recurrent, self-healing papulonodular eruption; an association with mycosis fungoides has been observed in some patients. T cell clonality has been documented by PCR in 20 patients with PLEVA; similar findings have been made in patients with lymphomatoid papulosis.[63] Investigators have suggested that PLEVA is a lymphoproliferative process rather than an inflammatory reaction to various trigger factors, such as infectious agents. One case report demonstrated that pityriasis lichenoides lesions evolved concomitantly with a known Epstein-Barr virus (EBV)–mediated disease (i.e., acute infectious mononucleosis), suggesting that pityriasis lichenoides may be caused by EBV infection.[64]

A chronic form of pityriasis lichenoides, pityriasis lichenoides chronica, shows milder skin changes without necrosis. Lesions evolve during a period of weeks and may recur over many years.

Treatment

Treatment of both acute and chronic forms of pityriasis lichenoides is generally unsatisfactory. Topical corticosteroids, tars, and systemically administered methotrexate have all been tried, with variable success. Ultraviolet radiation from sunlamps[65] and oral psoralen photochemotherapy[66] may have a beneficial effect on the course of disease. High-dose tetracycline, 2 g/day for 1 month or more,[67] and minocycline, 100 mg once or twice daily, have also

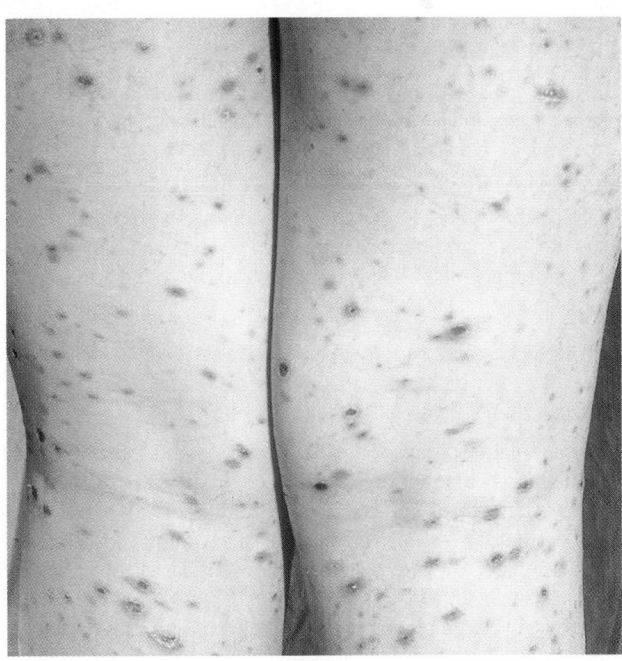

Figure 8 **Hemorrhagic brown-crusted varioliform papules are present on the lower legs of this patient with the acute form of pityriasis lichenoides.**

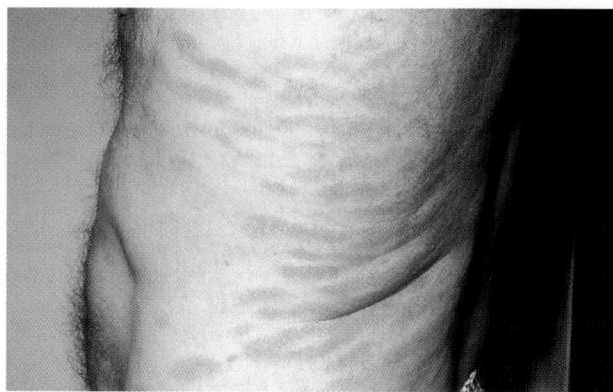

Figure 9 **The digitate variant of small-plaque parapsoriasis is seen in this patient.**

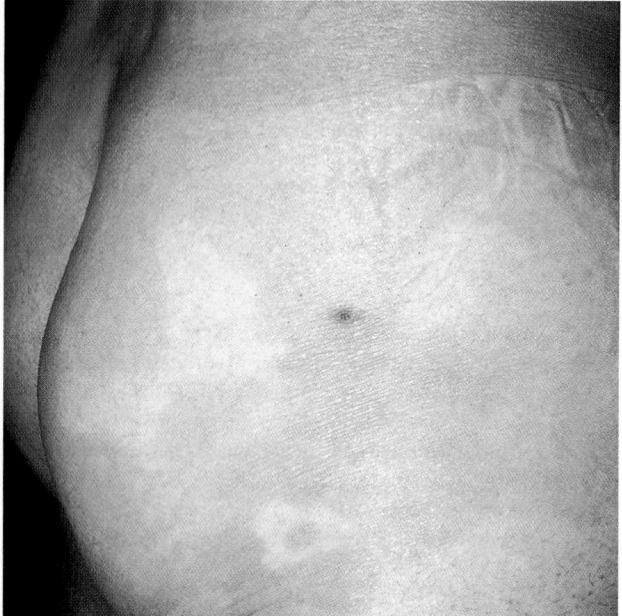

Figure 10 **Large-plaque parapsoriasis as seen on the buttocks of this patient may eventuate in cutaneous T cell lymphoma.**

been shown to be effective treatments. A rare type of Mucha-Habermann disease known as Degos disease (also called malignant atrophic papulosis), characterized by fever and hemorrhagic and papulonecrotic lesions, responds rapidly to the administration of methotrexate [*see Chapter 117*].[68]

SMALL- AND LARGE-PLAQUE PARAPSORIASIS

Diagnosis

Small-plaque parapsoriasis consists of slightly scaly, thin, oval erythematous plaques of less than 5 cm in diameter, commonly located on the trunk and proximal extremities. The variant—digitate dermatosis—shows elongated lesions falling along lines of skin cleavage. The two diseases follow similar chronic, benign courses [*see Figure 9*].

Clinically, large-plaque parapsoriasis consists of slightly thickened, red-brown, scaly plaques that are more than 10 cm in diameter and have ill-defined borders; such lesions are present mainly on the proximal extremities and the buttocks and on the breasts of women [*see Figure 10*]. Frequently, there is a compo-

nent of poikiloderma, which includes mottled hyperpigmentation and hypopigmentation, atrophy, and telangiectasia. Early lesions may show a nonspecific histology; late lesions show atypical lymphocytes within the epidermis.

It is important to differentiate large-plaque parapsoriasis from the small-plaque form because about 10% of cases of large-plaque parapsoriasis result in a cutaneous T cell lymphoma (mycosis fungoides).[60] Large-plaque lesions may be present for many years before malignant transformation is recognized histologically. The malignant change is suggested clinically by increased pruritus and progressive induration of lesions. The retiform variant may show prominent poikiloderma with atrophy and has a greater potential for malignant transformation.[69] Studies of T cell subsets using monoclonal antibodies to membrane markers have shown a variable predominance of helper T cells in the cutaneous infiltrates in atrophic parapsoriasis; such findings suggest a similarity to lesions of mycosis fungoides, although epidermotropism is absent.[70] Patients with this form of the disease should be evaluated with repeated biopsies of untreated lesions. Once a definitive diagnosis of mycosis fungoides has been established, specific treatment of this disease may be instituted.

Treatment

Treatment of large- and small-plaque parapsoriasis is similar to that of pityriasis lichenoides chronica [*see* Pityriasis Lichenoides, *above*].

Erythroderma

Papulosquamous and psoriasiform eczematous dermatitis may progress to generalized skin involvement with erythema and scaling, known as exfoliative erythroderma. Other causes of eryth-

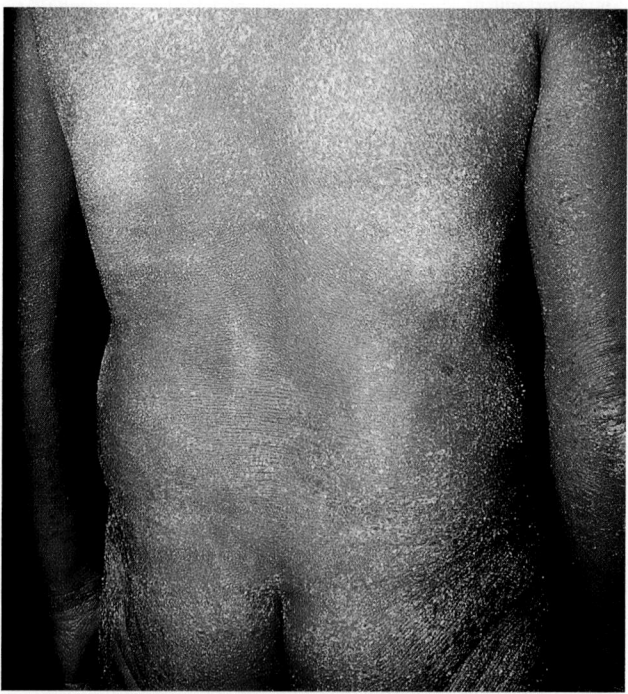

Figure 11 **Erythroderma, which appears as total skin erythema and scaling, can occur as a result of papulosquamous and eczematous disorders caused by a variety of diseases. Cutaneous T cell lymphoma, as seen in this patient with Sézary syndrome, can result in erythroderma.**

roderma include drug eruption, contact dermatitis, and pityriasis rubra pilaris. Eyrthroderma is a rare skin disorder that occurs more often as an exacerbation of a preexisting skin disorder; less commonly, it is idiopathic. There are no accurate studies on the incidence of erythroderma. On the basis of a survey of all dermatologists in the Netherlands, however, the annual incidence was estimated to be one to two patients per 100,000 inhabitants.[71]

DIAGNOSIS

Most cases of exfoliative erythroderma are associated with exacerbation of an underlying dermatosis, such as psoriasis, pityriasis rubra pilaris, seborrheic dermatitis, drug eruptions, atopic dermatitis, or contact dermatitis.[72] Some patients have idiopathic erythroderma, also called red man syndrome.[69] Common associated skin findings include palmoplantar keratoderma, alopecia, and nail dystrophy. Skin biopsy usually shows nonspecific inflammation. Lymph node biopsy may reveal dermatopathic lymphadenopathy. In some patients, idiopathic erythroderma may progress to cutaneous T cell lymphoma (e.g., erythrodermic mycosis fungoides and Sézary syndrome) [see Figure 11] [see Chapter 45].

Systemic symptoms associated with erythroderma include fever and chills, dehydration from transepidermal water loss, and high-output cardiac failure.

TREATMENT

Nonspecific treatment of exfoliative erythroderma includes restoration of fluid and electrolyte balance and supportive measures such as administration of antipruritics, application of cool compresses and mild topical corticosteroids, and bed rest. Antibiotics may be required for treatment of secondary bacterial infection. Generally, more aggressive topical and systemic therapies are avoided until the inflammation subsides. More specific treatment depends on the underlying diagnosis and cause of the erythroderma. For example, in patients with erythroderma that is secondary to Sézary syndrome, treatment would be directed toward the underlying cutaneous T cell lymphoma [see Chapter 45]. For erythroderma caused by a drug eruption, the offending drug must be discontinued. Systemic agents such as acitretin and methotrexate may be used to treat psoriatic erythroderma [see Chapter 37]. Drug-induced erythroderma may have the best prognosis.[72]

The author has served as advisor or consultant to Abbott Laboratories, Amgen, Inc., Biogen Idec, Inc., and Genentech, Inc.

References

1. Fox BJ, Odom RB: Papulosquamous diseases: a review. J Am Acad Dermatol 12:597, 1985

2. Sadick NS, McNutt NS, Kaplan MH: Papulosquamous dermatoses of AIDS. J Am Acad Dermatol 22:1270, 1990

3. Chuh AA, Molinari N, Sciallis G, et al: Temporal case clustering in pityriasis rosea: a regression analysis on 1379 patients in Minnesota, Kuwait, and Diyarbakir, Turkey. Arch Dermatol 141:767, 2005

4. Chuang T-Y, Ilstrup DM, Perry HO, et al: Pityriasis rosea in Rochester, Minnesota, 1969 to 1978: a 10-year epidemiologic study. J Am Acad Dermatol 7:80, 1982

5. Parsons JM: Pityriasis rosea update: 1986. J Am Acad Dermatol 15:159, 1986

6. Drago F, Ranieri E, Malaguti F, et al: Human herpesvirus 7 in 7 patients with pityriasis rosea. Dermatology 195:374, 1997

7. Kempf W, Adams V, Kleinhans M, et al: Pityriasis rosea is not associated with human herpesvirus 7. Arch Dermatol 135:1070, 1999

8. Kosuge H, Tanaka-Taya K, Miyoshi H, et al: Epidemiological study of human herpesvirus-6 and human herpesvirus-7 in pityriasis rosea. Br J Dermatol 143:795, 2000

9. Chuh AA, Chan HH, Zawar V: Is human herpesvirus 7 the causative agent of pityria-

sis rosea? Int J Dermatol 43:870, 2004

10. Chuh AA: Rash orientation in pityriasis rosea: a qualitative study. Eur J Dermatol 12:253, 2002

11. Leenutaphong V, Jiamton S: UVB phototherapy for pityriasis rosea: a bilateral comparison study. J Am Acad Dermatol 33:996, 1995

12. Stulberg DL, Wolfrey J: Pityriasis rosea. Am Fam Physician 69:87, 2004

13. Sharma PK, Yadav TP, Gautam RK, et al: Erythromycin in pityriasis rosea: a double-blind placebo-controlled clinical trial. J Am Acad Dermatol 42:241, 2000

14. Eisen D: The clinical features, malignant potential, and systemic associations of oral lichen planus: a study of 723 patients. J Am Acad Dermatol 46:207, 2002

15. Shai A, Halevy S: Lichen planus and lichen planus–like eruptions: pathogenesis and associated diseases. Int J Dermatol 31:379, 1992

16. Lodi G, Giuliani M, Majorana A, et al: Lichen planus and hepatitis C virus: a multicentre study of patients with oral lesions and a systematic review. Br J Dermatol 151:1172, 2004

17. Harden D, Skelton H, Smith KJ: Lichen planus associated with hepatitis C virus: no viral transcripts are found in the lichen planus, and effective therapy for hepatitis C virus does not clear lichen planus. J Am Acad Dermatol 49:847, 2003

18. Callista D, Morri M: Lichen planus induced by hepatitis B vaccination: a new case and a review of the literature. Int J Dermatol 43:562, 2004

19. Thompson DF, Skaehill PA: Drug-induced lichen planus. Pharmacotherapy 14:561, 1994

20. Powell FC, Rogers RS III, Dickson ER: Primary biliary cirrhosis and lichen planus. J Am Acad Dermatol 9:540, 1983

21. Powell ML, Ehrlich A, Belsito DV: Lichenoid drug eruption to salsalate. J Am Acad Dermatol 45:616, 2001

22. Boyd AS, Neldner KH: Lichen planus. J Am Acad Dermatol 25:593, 1991

23. Abraham SC, Ravich WJ, Anhalt GJ, et al: Esophageal lichen planus: case report and review of the literature. Am J Surg Pathol 24:1678, 2000

24. Cribier B, Frances C, Chosidow O: Treatment of lichen planus: an evidence-based medicine analysis of efficacy. Arch Dermatol 134:1521, 1998

25. Zakrzewska JM, Chan ES, Thronhill MH: A systematic review of placebo-controlled randomized clinical trials of treatments used in oral lichen planus. Br J Dermatol 153:336, 2005

26. Laurberg G, Geiger JM, Hjorth N, et al: Treatment of lichen planus with acitretin: a double-blind placebo-controlled study in 65 patients. J Am Acad Dermatol 24:434, 1991

27. Lear JT, English JS: Erosive and generalized lichen planus responsive to azathioprine. Clin Exp Dermatol 21:56, 1996

28. Ortonne JP, Thivolet J, Sannwald C: Oral photochemotherapy in the treatment of lichen planus (LP): clinical results, histological and ultrastructural observations. Br J Dermatol 99:77, 1978

29. Hildebrand A, Kolde G, Luger TA, et al: Successful treatment of generalized lichen planus with recombinant interferon alfa-2b. J Am Acad Dermatol 33:880, 1995

30. Carbone M, Conrotto D, Carrozzo M, et al: Topical corticosteroids in association with miconazole and chlorhexidine in the long-term management of atrophic-erosive oral lichen planus: a placebo-controlled and comparative study between clobetasol and fluocinonide. Oral Dis 5:44, 1999

31. Giustina TA, Stewart JB, Ellis CN, et al: Topical application of oral isotretinoin gel improves oral lichen planus: a double-blind study. Arch Dermatol 122:534, 1986

32. Eisen D: Hydroxychloroquine sulfate (Plaquenil) improves oral lichen planus: an open trial. J Am Acad Dermatol 28:609, 1993

33. Kaliakatsou F, Hodgson TA, Lewsey JD, et al: Management of recalcitrant ulcerative oral lichen planus with topical tacrolimus. J Am Acad Dermatol 46:35, 2002

34. Swift JC, Rees TD, Plemons JM, et al: The effectiveness of 1% pimecrolimus cream in the treatment of oral erosive lichen planus. J Periodontol 76:627, 2005

35. Moyal-Barracco M, Edwards L: Diagnosis and therapy of anogenital lichen planus. Dermatol Ther 17:38, 2004

36. Byrd JA, Davis MD, Rogers RS 3rd: Recalcitrant symptomatic vulvar lichen planus: response to topical tacrolimus. Arch Dermatol 140:715, 2004

37. Watsky KL: Erosive perianal lichen planus responsive to tacrolimus. Int J Dermatol 42:217, 2003

38. Lonsdale-Eccles AA, Velangi S: Topical pimecrolimus in the treatment of genital lichen planus: a prospective case series. Br J Dermatol 153:390, 2005

39. Irvine C, Irvine F, Champion RH: Long-term follow-up of lichen planus. Acta Derm Venereol 71:242, 1991

40. Plewig G: Seborrheic dermatitis. Dermatology in General Medicine, 4th ed, Vol 1. Fitzpatrick TB, Eisen AZ, Wolff K, et al, Eds. McGraw-Hill Book Co, New York, 1993, p 1569

41. Gupta AK, Madzia SE, Batra R: Etiology and management of seborrheic dermatitis. Dermatology 208:89, 2004

42. Burton JL, Pye RJ: Seborrhoea is not a feature of seborrhoeic dermatitis. Br Med J 26:1169, 1983

43. Odom RB: Common superficial fungal infections in immunosuppressed patients. J Am Acad Dermatol 31:S56, 1994

44. Soeprono FF, Schinella RA, Cockerell CJ, et al: Seborrheic-like dermatitis of acquired immunodeficiency syndrome: a clinicopathologic study. J Am Acad Dermatol 14:242, 1986

45. Shuster S, Meynadier J, Kerl H, et al: Treatment and prophylaxis of seborrheic dermatitis of the scalp with antipityrosporal 1% ciclopirox shampoo. Arch Dermatol 41:47, 2005

46. Gupta AK, Nicol K, Batra R: Role of antifungal agents in the treatment of seborrheic dermatitis. Am J Clin Dermatol 5:417, 2004

47. Peter RU, Richarz-Barthauer U: Successful treatment and prophylaxis of scalp seborrhoeic dermatitis and dandruff with 2% ketoconazole shampoo: results of a multicentre, double-blind, placebo-controlled trial. Br J Dermatol 132:441, 1995

48. Parsad D, Pandhi R, Negi KS, et al: Topical metronidazole in seborrheic dermatitis—a double-blind study. Dermatology 202:35, 2001

49. Koca R, Altinyazar HC, Esturk E: Is topical metronidazole effective in seborrheic dermatitis? A double-blind study. Int J Dermatol 42:632, 2003

50. Rigopoulos D, Ioannides D, Kalogeromitros D, et al: Pimecrolimus cream 1% vs. betamethasone 17-valerate 0.1% cream in the treatment of seborrhoeic dermatitis: a randomized open-label clinical trial. Br J Dermatol 151:1071, 2004

51. Scapparo E, Quadri G, Virno G, et al: Evaluation of the efficacy and tolerability of oral terbinafine (Daskil) in patients with seborrhoeic dermatitis: a multicentre, randomized, investigator-blinded, placebo-controlled trial. Br J Dermatol 144:854, 2001

52. Dicken CH: Treatment of classic pityriasis rubra pilaris. J Am Acad Dermatol 31:997, 1994

53. Requena L, Grilli R, Soriano L, et al: Dermatomyositis with a pityriasis rubra pilaris-like eruption: a little-known distinctive cutaneous manifestation of dermatomyositis. Br J Dermatol 136:768, 1997

54. Van de Kerkfho PC, Steijlen PM: Topical treatment of pityriasis rubra pilaris with calcipotriol. Br J Dermatol 130:675, 1994

55. Yaniv R, Barzilai A, Trau H: Pityriasis rubra pilaris exacerbated by ultraviolet B phototherapy (letter). Dermatology 189:313, 1994

56. Goldsmith LA, Weinrich AE, Shupack J: Pityriasis rubra pilaris response to 13-cis-retinoic acid (isotretinoin). J Am Acad Dermatol 6:710, 1982

57. Allison DS, El-Azhary RA, Calobrisis SD, et al: Pityriasis rubra pilaris in children. J Am Acad Dermatol 47:386, 2002

58. Usuki K, Sekiyama M, Shimada S, et al: Three cases of pityriasis rubra pilaris successfully treated with cyclosporin A. Dermatology 200:324, 2000

59. Gupta AK, Skinner AR: A review of the use of infliximab to manage cutaneous dermatoses. J Cutan Med Surg 8:77, 2004

60. Lambert WC, Everett MA: The nosology of parapsoriasis. J Am Acad Dermatol 5:373, 1981

61. Hood AF, Mark EJ: Histopathologic diagnosis of pityriasis lichenoides et varioliformis acuta and its clinical correlation. Arch Dermatol 118:478, 1982

62. El Shabrawi-Caelan L, Kerl H, Cerroni L: Lymphomatoid papulosis: reappraisal of clinicopathologic presentation and classification into subtypes A, B, and C. Arch Dermatol 140:441, 2004

63. Klein PA, Jones EC, Nelson JL, et al: Infectious causes of pityriasis lichenoides: a case of fulminant infectious mononucleosis. J Am Acad Dermatol 49:S151, 2003

64. Wenzel J, Gutgemann I, Distelmaier M, et al: The role of cytotoxic skin-homing CD8+ lymphocytes in cutaneous cytotoxic T-cell lymphoma and pityriasis lichenoides. J Am Acad Dermatol 53:422, 2005

65. LeVine MJ: Phototherapy of pityriasis lichenoides. Arch Dermatol 119:378, 1983

66. Satra KH, DeLeo VA: PUVA for photosensitivity and other skin diseases. Photochemotherapy in Dermatology. Abel EA, Ed. Igaku-Shoin Medical Publishers, New York, 1991, p 159

67. Humbert P, Treffel P, Chapuis J-F, et al: The tetracyclines in dermatology. J Am Acad Dermatol 25:691, 1991

68. Fink-Puches R, Soyer HP, Kerl H: Febrile ulceronecrotic pityriasis lichenoides et varioliformis acuta. J Am Acad Dermatol 30:261, 1994

69. Kikuchi A, Naka W, Harada T, et al: Parapsoriasis en plaques: its potential for progression to malignant lymphoma. J Am Acad Dermatol 29:419, 1993

70. Thestrup-Pedersen K, Halkier-Sorensen L, Sogaard H, et al: The red man syndrome: exfoliative dermatitis of unknown etiology: a description and follow-up of 38 patients. J Am Acad Dermatol 18:1307, 1988

71. Sigurdsson V, Steegmans PH, van Vloten WA: The incidence of erythroderma: a survey among all dermatologists in the Netherlands. J Am Acad Dermatol 45:675, 2001

72. Akhyani M, Ghodsi ZS, Toosi S, et al: Erythroderma: a clinical study of 97 cases. BMC Dermatol 5:5, 2005

37 Psoriasis

Elizabeth A. Abel, M.D., and Mark Lebwohl, M.D.

Psoriasis is an immune-mediated inflammatory cutaneous disorder characterized by chronic, scaling, erythematous patches and plaques of skin. It can begin at any age and can vary in severity. Psoriasis can manifest itself in several different forms, including pustular and erythrodermic forms. In addition to involving the skin, psoriasis frequently involves the nails, and some patients may experience inflammation of the joints (psoriatic arthritis). Because of its highly visible nature, psoriasis can compromise both the personal and the working lives of its victims.

Breakthroughs in the treatment of psoriasis have led to a better understanding of its pathogenesis. This chapter reviews current knowledge of the genetics, pathogenesis, and treatment of psoriasis.

Epidemiology

The estimated prevalence of psoriasis ranges from 0.5% to 4.6% worldwide. The reasons for the geographic variation in prevalence are unknown, but climate and genetics may play a role. Psoriasis is uncommon in blacks in tropical zones, but it is more often seen in blacks in temperate zones. It occurs commonly in Japanese persons but rarely in persons native to North and South America. In the United States, studies have variously reported that 4.5 million adults[1] or 7 million adults and children[2] have psoriasis.

Psoriasis can occur at any age, with some cases being reported at birth and others being reported in patients older than 100 years. In Farber and Nall's pioneer study of 5,600 patients, the average age of onset of psoriasis was 27.8 years; in 35% of patients, onset occurred before 20 years of age, and in 10%, onset occurred before 10 years of age.[3] Psoriasis occurs with equal frequency in men and women, but in Farber and Nall's study, onset occurred later in men. In populations in which there is a high prevalence of psoriasis, onset tends to occur at an earlier age. In the Faroe Islands, for example, the prevalence is 3%, and the average age of onset is 12.5 years. The average age of onset is 23 years in the United States. In persons with earlier age of onset, psoriasis is more likely to be severe, with involvement of a large area of skin surface.

Pathogenesis

Psoriasis was once thought to be caused by an abnormality in epidermal cell kinetics; it is now thought that an abnormality in the immune system triggers epidermal proliferation. The role of activated lymphocytes in the development of psoriasis was first proved through investigations of DAB389 interleukin-2 (IL-2), a fusion protein consisting of molecules of IL-2 fused to diphtheria toxin. This fusion protein binds to high-affinity IL-2 receptors on activated T cells, destroying those cells. In a study of DAB389 IL-2 treatment in 10 patients, four patients showed dramatic clinical improvement and four others showed moderate improvement.[4] Unfortunately, the side effects of DAB389 IL-2 have precluded its approval for the treatment of psoriasis.[5]

The skin of patients with lesional psoriasis has higher numbers of antigen-presenting cells that can activate T cells. For T cell activation to occur, antigen-presenting cells must deliver at least two signals to resting T cells. The first signal occurs when major histocompatibility complex (MHC) class II molecules of the antigen-presenting cells present antigens to the T cells. A second costimulatory signal must be delivered through the interaction of ligands on the surface of the antigen-presenting cells with receptors on the surface of T cells. Examples of this process include the interaction of B7 molecules with CD28 on the surface of resting T cells and the interaction of lymphocyte function–associated antigen 3 (LFA-3) with CD2 or intercellular adhesion molecule–1 (ICAM-1) with LFA-1 on the surface of T cells.[6,7] Blockade of any of these steps results in clearing of psoriasis.[8,9] Upon activation, T cells release Th1 (T helper type 1) cytokines, IL-2, and interferon gamma, which together induce proliferation of keratinocytes and further stimulation of T cells. Inflammatory cytokines such as tumor necrosis factor–α (TNF-α) are found in psoriatic skin lesions and joints, and treatment with TNF-α blockers results in clearing of psoriasis and of psoriatic arthritis.[10]

Etiology

GENETIC FACTORS

Several lines of evidence suggest that psoriasis has a genetic etiology. One third of persons affected have a positive family history. Studies have found a higher concordance rate in monozygotic twins than in dizygotic twins or siblings (70% versus 23%).[11]

Current evidence suggests genetic heterogeneity. Both autosomal dominant inheritance with incomplete penetrance and polygenic or multifactorial inheritance have been described. The most important psoriasis susceptibility gene appears to be *PSORS1*, which has been mapped to the region on chromosome 6p21 that codes for the MHC; seven other *PSORS* genes have been found on other chromosomes.[12] Psoriasis is also associated with a single-nucleotide polymorphism on chromosome 17q25 that impairs binding of a runt-related protein (RUNX1).[13]

CONTRIBUTING FACTORS

The course and severity of psoriasis can be affected by a number of endogenous and exogenous factors, including stress, climate, concurrent infections, and medications.

Psychological Stress

Many patients believe that anxiety or psychological stress has an adverse effect on the course of their psoriasis. The etiologic significance of stress in psoriasis is difficult to evaluate, however, because of the subjective nature of the evidence used in many of the investigations into this question.[14] In a prospective study, a multivariate statistical method revealed a positive correlation between severity of psoriasis symptoms and psychological stress related to adverse life events.[15] Psoriasis itself can be a source of stress: the effects of psoriasis on physical and mental function have been compared with the effects of cancer, heart disease, diabetes, and depression.[16]

Climate

It has long been known that psoriasis improves when patients are exposed to sunny climates and to regions of lower latitude. In northern latitudes, exacerbation of psoriasis commonly occurs during the fall and winter.

Infection

Viral or bacterial infections, especially streptococcal pharyngitis or tonsillitis, may precipitate the onset or exacerbation of psoriasis.[17] Guttate psoriasis, in particular, is often attributed to a previous streptococcal infection. Attempts to reverse psoriasis by treatment with oral antibiotics have not proved effective in double-blind trials.[18] Nevertheless, some investigators advocate antibiotic therapy for psoriasis.[19]

Infection with HIV has also been associated with psoriasis. In some patients with HIV infection, preexisting psoriasis becomes exacerbated; in other patients, psoriasis develops within a few years after HIV infection. Often, HIV-infected patients present with symptoms similar to those of Reiter syndrome.[20]

Drugs

Numerous drugs can worsen psoriasis.[21] Antimalarial agents such as chloroquine can cause exfoliative erythroderma or pustular psoriasis. Up to 31% of patients experience new onset or worsening of psoriasis as a result of antimalarial therapy. Lithium and beta blockers such as propranolol may precipitate the onset of psoriasis or cause exacerbations of psoriasis.[22] Some nonsteroidal anti-inflammatory drugs (NSAIDs) also exacerbate psoriasis, although this effect is sufficiently minor to allow NSAIDs to be used in the treatment of psoriatic arthritis.[23] Flares of pustular psoriasis may be precipitated by withdrawal from systemic corticosteroids or withdrawal from high-potency topical corticosteroids. Interferon therapy has been associated with development or exacerbation of psoriasis, presumably because of the Th1 effects of this therapy.[24]

Other Factors

Trauma to the clinically uninvolved skin of patients with psoriasis can cause a lesion to appear at the exact site of injury; this phenomenon is known as the Köbner response. Cuts, abrasions, injections, burns resulting from phototherapy, and other forms of trauma can elicit this reaction.

Smoking may be an exacerbating factor in psoriasis.[25] Alcohol use has also been implicated in the exacerbation of psoriasis.[26]

Surveys have suggested that diet plays a role in the development of psoriasis, and attempts have been made to affect the clinical course of psoriasis through modification of diet.[27] Double-blind studies, however, have failed to show that diet has either a beneficial or a detrimental effect on the severity of psoriasis.

Diagnosis

The diagnosis of psoriasis is usually made on clinical grounds. If unusual features are present, biopsy of affected skin can be done to confirm the diagnosis.

CLINICAL VARIANTS

Nearly 90% of patients with psoriasis have plaque type, a form that is characterized by sharply demarcated, erythematous, scaling plaques. The elbows [see Figure 1], knees, and scalp [see Figure 2] are the most commonly affected sites. The intergluteal cleft [see Figure 3], palms [see Figure 4], soles [see Figure 5], and genitals are also commonly affected, but psoriasis can involve any part of the body. Lesions frequently occur in a symmetrical pattern of distribution.

Many patients have only one or a few lesions that persist for years and that occasionally resolve after exposure to sunlight. Other patients can be covered with plaques that become confluent, affecting nearly 100% of the body surface area. Nail involvement is common, particularly in patients with severe disease.

The second most common form of psoriasis, guttate psoriasis, affects fewer than 10% of patients and is characterized by the development of small, scaling, erythematous papules on the trunk and the extremities [see Figure 6]. This form of psoriasis often follows streptococcal infection. Patients with plaque-type psoriasis can develop guttate psoriasis. Conversely, patients with guttate psoriasis frequently develop plaque-type psoriasis. Occasionally, guttate lesions enlarge and become confluent, resulting in the formation of plaques.

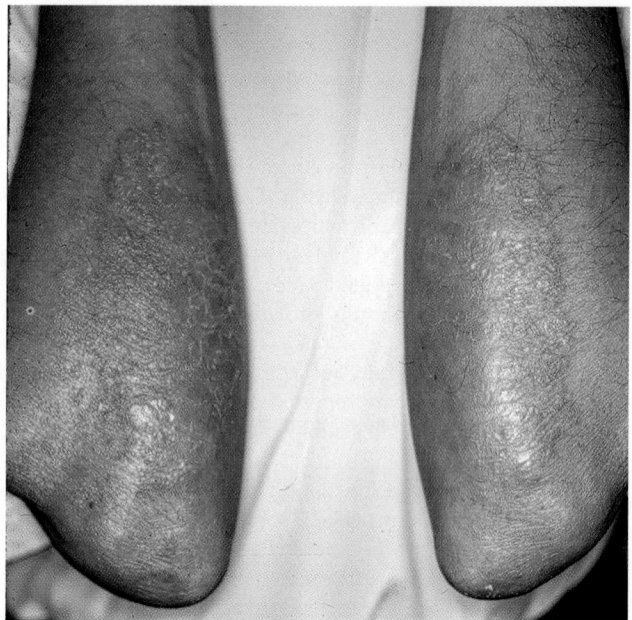

Figure 1   **Involvement of the elbows is characteristic of plaque psoriasis.**

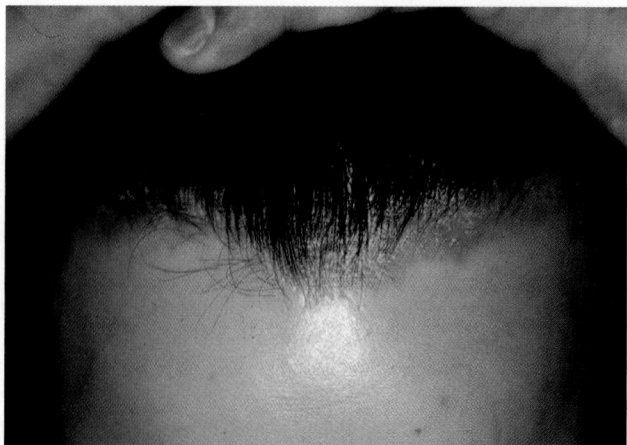

Figure 2   **The scalp is affected in the majority of patients with plaque psoriasis.**

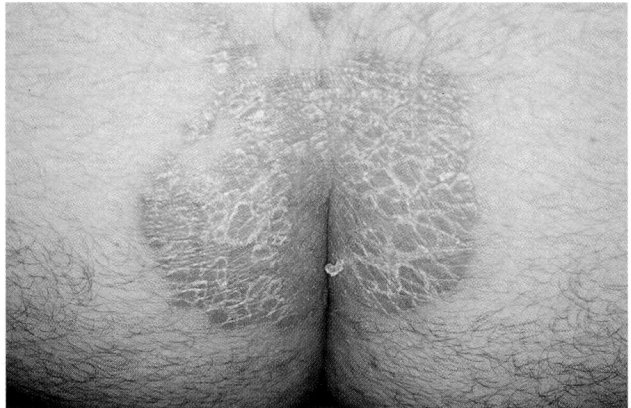

Figure 3 The intergluteal cleft is a common site of involvement in patients with plaque psoriasis.

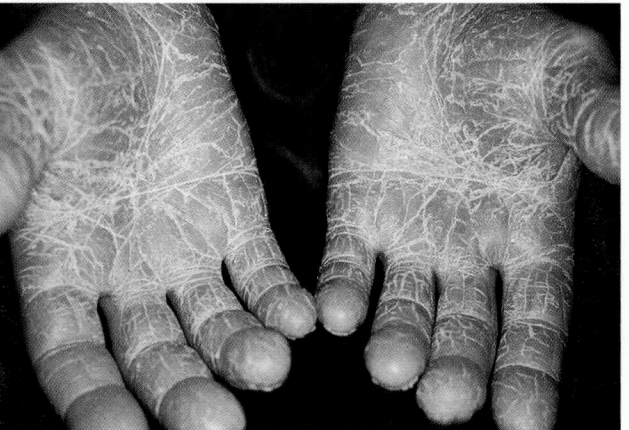

Figure 4 Psoriasis of the palms is shown in this patient.

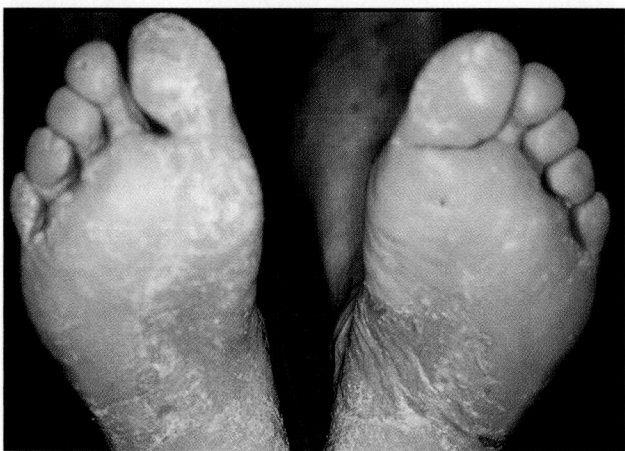

Figure 5 Sharply demarcated, erythematous, scaling plaques on the feet are apparent in this patient with psoriasis of the soles.

Erythrodermic psoriasis is a severe form of psoriasis that often affects the entire cutaneous surface. Patients present with an exfoliative erythroderma in which the skin is very red and inflamed and is constantly scaling [*see Figure 7*]. Patients are acutely ill, their skin having lost all protective function. Loss of temperature control, loss of fluids and nutrients through the impaired skin, and susceptibility to infection make this a potentially life-threatening condition.

Erythrodermic psoriasis can develop de novo or evolve from typical plaque-type or guttate psoriasis. Erythrodermic psoriasis can occur after withdrawal of systemic corticosteroids, after phototherapy burns, as a result of antimalarial treatment, as a result of a drug-induced hypersensitivity reaction, or for no apparent reason. Cutaneous T cell lymphoma may also present as erythroderma and needs to be differentiated from erythrodermic psoriasis.

Pustular psoriasis, another severe form of the disease, can occur in patients with preexisting psoriasis or can arise de novo. Pustular psoriasis can be generalized (von Zumbusch type) or localized to the palms and soles [*see Figure 8*]. In either case, the condition is severe and debilitating. In generalized

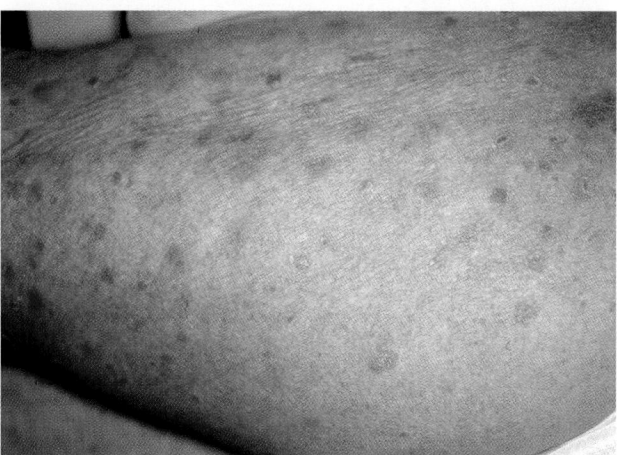

Figure 6 Guttate psoriasis is characterized by small scaly papules and plaques.

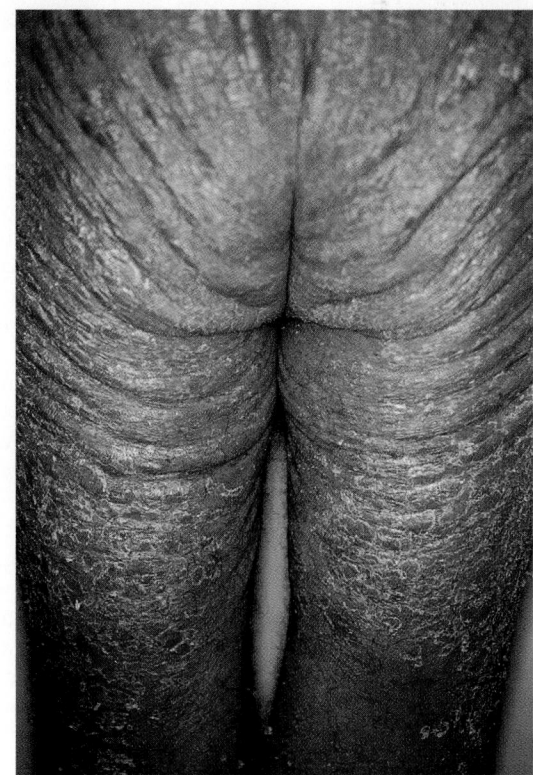

Figure 7 Erythrodermic psoriasis is characterized by generalized erythema and desquamation.

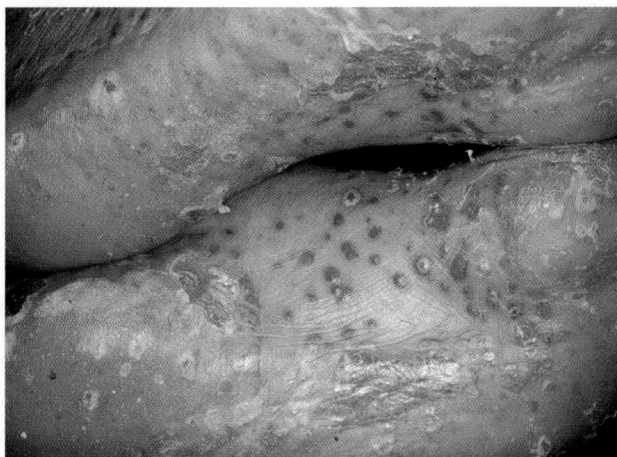

Figure 8 Pustular psoriasis can be localized to the palms and soles or generalized.

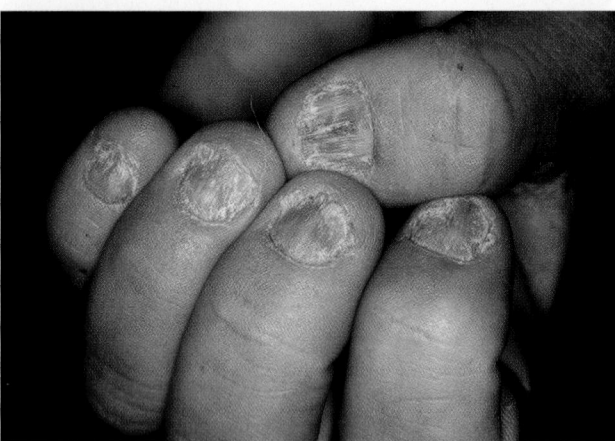

Figure 9 Involvement of the nails is common in psoriasis.

pustular psoriasis, the body is covered with sterile pustules. As with erythrodermic psoriasis, the protective functions of the skin are lost, and patients may succumb to infection or hypovolemia and electrolyte imbalance caused by loss of fluid through the skin. Although fever and leukocytosis are common features in pustular psoriasis, the possibility of infection should not be overlooked; patients with pustular psoriasis have died of staphylococcal sepsis.[28]

As with erythrodermic psoriasis, pustular psoriasis is most commonly precipitated by withdrawal of systemic corticosteroids. However, it can also result from therapy with antimalarial drugs or lithium, and it can develop spontaneously.

Nail Psoriasis

Nail changes can be of immeasurable value when the diagnosis is in doubt [*see Figure 9*]. In one study, 55% of patients with psoriasis experienced such changes.[29] The most common change consists of the appearance of tiny pits, as might be made with an ice pick, which often occur in groups. This characteristic pitting of the nails is highly specific for psoriasis, although a few isolated pits may be seen in healthy nails or as a result of past trauma. Yellowish discoloration is common in psoriatic toenails and may appear in fingernails as well. Onycholysis, or distal separation of the nail plate from its bed, frequently occurs.

Other changes include subungual hyperkeratosis—an accumulation of keratinous debris under the nail—as well as transverse and longitudinal ridging. These findings, however, are much less specific because they also occur secondary to dermatitis, fungal infection, vascular insufficiency, and other conditions. Occasionally, a patient shows typical psoriatic nail changes without any other cutaneous signs at initial examination; all such patients are probably psoriatic and may eventually manifest psoriatic lesions.

Psoriatic Arthritis

Psoriatic arthritis has been estimated to occur in 7% to 42% of patients with psoriasis.[30] Joint inflammation in psoriatic arthritis is chronic, with occasional remissions.[31] There are five classic subtypes. The most common presentation is an oligoarthritis in which one or a few joints are affected. This form accounts for approximately 70% of cases of psoriatic arthritis. Skin lesions of psoriasis usually precede articular disease by 5 to 10 years, but joint inflammation develops before skin lesions in some patients. If a diagnosis of psoriatic arthritis is suspected, the physician should carefully examine the scalp, nails, intergluteal cleft, external ear canal, and genital region for psoriasis lesions.

The second most common type of psoriatic arthritis is virtually identical to rheumatoid arthritis. This form is characterized by symmetrical involvement of the joints with ulnar deviation and typical deformities, such as swan-neck deformity and boutonnière deformity. The only distinguishing features are the presence of psoriasis and the absence of circulating rheumatoid factor.

Arthritis mutilans is a rare, severely destructive form of psoriatic arthritis in which the interphalangeal joints of the hands and feet are destroyed, resulting in deformed digits. Ankylosing spondylitis accounts for 5% of cases of psoriatic arthritis. As in other forms of ankylosing spondylitis, the genetic marker HLA-B27 is usually present.

Distal interphalangeal joint involvement is the most characteristic form of psoriatic arthritis. It is usually associated with nail involvement.

HISTOPATHOLOGY

The classic microscopic features of a psoriatic plaque include the following:
- A markedly thickened stratum corneum, with layered zones of parakeratosis (retention of nuclei).
- A moderately to markedly hyperplastic epidermis, with broadening of rete projections and elongation to a uniform depth in the dermis.
- Increased mitotic activity in the lower epidermis.
- Epidermal thinning over the dermal papillae.
- A scant amount of inflammatory infiltrate from mononuclear cells in the superficial dermis.
- Intracorneal or subcorneal collections of polymorphonuclear leukocytes (Munro microabscesses)

Differential Diagnosis

The differential diagnosis of psoriasis includes other scaling dermatoses [*see Chapter 36*]. Such dermatoses include the following:
- Seborrheic dermatitis that involves the scalp, nasolabial folds, and retroauricular folds.
- Pityriasis rosea, which begins with a herald patch and is self-limited.

- Lichen simplex chronicus, which is caused by repeated rubbing or scratching.
- Parapsoriasis, which is characterized by atrophy, telangiectasia, and pigmentary abnormalities.
- Pityriasis rubra pilaris, which is characterized by psoriasiform patches that often begin in sun-exposed areas.
- Other conditions (e.g., discoid eczema or secondary syphilis) that can be differentiated by clinical and pathologic criteria.

Treatment

More treatments are available for psoriasis than perhaps for any other dermatologic disease. New topical therapies, new systemic therapies, and new forms of phototherapy have been introduced, and additional treatments are in development. Biologic therapies that target specific molecules are likely to change the treatment of psoriasis in the future. Topical therapy will continue to be used by most patients, however.

TOPICAL THERAPY

The 1990s saw the development of many new therapies for psoriasis.[32] Topical therapy is the mainstay of treatment for most patients, particularly those with mild disease. Topical corticosteroids are the most commonly prescribed class of medication, but they are now often used together with topical calcipotriene, a vitamin D_3 analogue, or topical tazarotene, a retinoid; both calcipotriene and tazarotene have approval by the Food and Drug Administration for the treatment of psoriasis.[33] Tar and salicylic acid are available by prescription and as over-the-counter products. Use of anthralin has declined as effective nonsteroidal agents have become available.

Emollients are an important part of any topical regimen for psoriasis. Application of petrolatum alone may be sufficient therapy for some patients. More elegant creams and lotions are helpful but are somewhat less effective than greasy ointments. Tar and salicylic acid shampoos are valuable in the treatment of patients with scalp involvement. These preparations are available without prescription.

Corticosteroids

Topical corticosteroids are indicated for limited plaques of psoriasis. Because of their ease of use and their wide availability, topical corticosteroids are the most commonly prescribed medication for treatment of psoriasis. They have anti-inflammatory, antiproliferative, and antipruritic effects. Corticosteroids are more potent when they are applied under occlusion, which increases their percutaneous penetration. Unfortunately, occlusion also increases side effects.

Topical steroids have been ranked in seven categories in decreasing order of potency, with potency determined by a vasoconstriction assay [see Table 1]. Superpotent corticosteroids are in group I, and weak over-the-counter topical corticosteroids are in group VII.[34]

Side effects The most commonly encountered side effects of topical corticosteroids are local cutaneous reactions. Development of cutaneous atrophy, telangiectasia, and irreversible striae are the most common side effects. Perioral dermatitis, which is characterized by erythematous papules and pustules on the face, is caused by chronic use of topical corticosteroids. Tachyphylaxis, with habituation to topical corticosteroids and

loss of response to them, is noted by most patients. Flare or rebound of psoriasis upon sudden withdrawal of topical corticosteroids can occur. Finally, suppression of the hypothalamic-pituitary-adrenal axis can occur, especially with use of superpotent topical corticosteroids, the widespread application of corticosteroids, occlusion, or chronic use. Because of concern over side effects, the package inserts for some superpotent corticosteroids suggest that use be limited to 2 weeks' duration. A number of regimens have been developed in which, after the initial weeks of continuous treatment with superpotent topical corticosteroids, psoriasis plaques are subsequently treated only on weekends.[35]

Vitamin D Analogues

Calcipotriene The first topical vitamin D analogue to receive FDA approval for use in the United States, calcipotriene has rapidly gained acceptance, despite the fact that it is not as effective as superpotent topical corticosteroids. Calcipotriene is available in ointment and cream form and as a solution. The primary reason for its success is its freedom from any corticosteroid side effects—namely, cutaneous atrophy, telangiectasia, striae, or suppression of the hypothalamic-pituitary-adrenal axis. Calcipotriene is comparable in efficacy to a group II corticosteroid. It is applied twice daily.

Calcipotriene has been used very successfully in combination with several other medications. It is most effective when used in combination with a superpotent topical corticosteroid. A regimen of calcipotriene ointment and halobetasol propionate ointment, each applied once daily, has been found to be more effective than monotherapy with either calcipotriene twice daily or halobetasol propionate twice daily.[36] Up to 90% of patients achieve marked improvement within 2 weeks of combination therapy with once-daily calcipotriene and once-daily halobetasol propionate ointment. For long-term maintenance of remission, a regimen has been developed in which halobetasol propionate is applied only on weekends and calcipotriene is applied on weekdays.[37] Using this regimen, 76% of patients achieved marked improvement for at least 6 months; this level of improvement was achieved in only 40% of patients receiving halobetasol propionate ointment on weekends only. Calcipotriene has also been shown to improve the response to ultraviolet B light (UVB)[38] and to psoralen plus ultraviolet A light (PUVA).[39]

Caution must be used when combining calcipotriene ointment with other medications, because it is easily inactivated. Salicylic acid, for example, completely inactivates calcipotriene on contact. Several other topical medications, including topical corticosteroids, can inactivate calcipotriene. In contrast, halobetasol propionate ointment is compatible with calcipotriene even when one medication is applied on top of the other.[40] UVA has been shown to inactivate calcipotriene,[41] so calcipotriene should be applied after PUVA therapy, not before. Use of calcipotriene should be limited to a maximum of 120 g a week because of isolated reports of hypercalcemia.[42]

A combination product containing calcipotriene and betamethasone dipropionate is now available in Europe and Canada. It appears to be more effective than the individual medications applied separately.[43]

Other vitamin D analogues Several new vitamin D analogues are under investigation in the United States or are in use elsewhere. Tacalcitol and maxacalcitol are promising medications for the treatment of psoriasis. The only common side effect

Table 1 Ranking of Topical Steroids for Psoriasis in Order of High to Low Potency

Group	Generic Name	Trade Name	Strength (%)
I	Betamethasone dipropionate in optimized vehicle	Diprolene ointment	0.05
	Clobetasol propionate	Temovate cream, ointment	0.05
	Diflorasone diacetate	Psorcon ointment	0.05
II	Amcinonide	Cyclocort ointment	0.1
	Betamethasone dipropionate, augmented	Diprolene AF cream	0.05
	Betamethasone dipropionate	Diprosone ointment	0.05
	Mometasone furoate	Elocon ointment	0.1
	Diflorasone diacetate	Florone ointment, Maxiflor ointment	0.05
	Halcinonide	Halog cream	0.1
	Fluocinonide	Lidex cream, ointment; Topsyn gel	0.05
	Desoximetasone	Topicort cream, ointment	0.25
III	Triamcinolone acetonide	Aristocort cream (HP)	0.5
	Betamethasone dipropionate	Diprosone cream	0.05
	Diflorasone diacetate	Florone cream, Maxiflor cream	0.05
	Betamethasone valerate	Valisone ointment	0.1
IV	Triamcinolone acetonide	Aristocort ointment, Kenalog ointment	0.1
	Betamethasone benzoate	Benisone ointment	0.025
	Flurandrenolide	Cordran ointment	0.05
	Mometasone furoate	Elocon cream	0.1
	Fluocinolone acetonide	Synalar-HP cream	0.2
		Synalar ointment	0.025
V	Betamethasone benzoate	Benisone cream	0.025
	Flurandrenolide	Cordran cream	0.05
	Fluticasone propionate	Cutivate cream	0.05
	Betamethasone dipropionate	Diprosone lotion	0.02
	Triamcinolone acetonide	Kenalog cream, lotion	0.1
	Hydrocortisone butyrate	Locoid cream	0.1
	Fluocinolone acetonide	Synalar cream	0.025
	Betamethasone valerate	Valisone cream, lotion	0.1
	Hydrocortisone valerate	Westcort cream	0.2
VI	Alclometasone dipropionate	Aclovate cream	0.05
	Desonide	Tridesilon cream, ointment; DesOwen cream, ointment	0.05
	Flumethasone pivalate	Locorten cream	0.03
	Fluocinolone acetonide	Synalar solution	0.01
VII	Hydrocortisone	Hytone cream, lotion, ointment	2.5
		Hytone, Penecort, Synacort, Cort-Dome, Nutracort	1.0

is irritation, which occurs in up to 20% of patients, most often on the face and in intertriginous areas. Topical calcitriol has FDA approval for the treatment of psoriasis in several countries around the world[44]; it may be less irritating than calcipotriene in intertriginous sites.

Tazarotene

Tazarotene is a retinoid that has been developed for the treatment of psoriasis. It is available in 0.05% and 0.1% gels and in cream formulations. Tazarotene is comparable in efficacy to a group II corticosteroid cream. Patients receiving tazarotene 0.1% gel experience longer periods of remission after discontinuance of therapy than patients receiving corticosteroids.

Tazarotene has several advantages over the corticosteroids. First, it is not associated with cutaneous atrophy, telangiectasia, or the development of striae. In fact, tazarotene, like other retinoids, may actually prevent corticosteroid atrophy. Tazarotene has been shown to enhance the efficacy of UVB phototherapy.[45] It does, however, increase the ability of ultraviolet light to induce erythema.[46] Doses of UVB and UVA should therefore be reduced in patients who are also receiving tazarotene.

Side effects The main side effect of tazarotene is local irritation, which has caused many patients to discontinue its use. The combination of tazarotene and a topical corticosteroid reduces irritation and enhances the efficacy of both agents.

Tars

Tar has been used since the 19th century to treat psoriasis. Crude coal tar, a complex mixture of thousands of hydrocarbon compounds, affects psoriatic epidermal cells through enzyme inhibition and antimitotic action.[47] Crude coal tar is messy to apply, has a strong odor, and stains skin and clothing. It is applied in conjunction with UVB phototherapy in the Goeckerman regimen [see Phototherapy, below]. More refined tar preparations, which are cosmetically acceptable, are available by prescription and over the counter in the form of gels, creams, bath oils, shampoos, and solutions (liquor carbonis detergens). Tar is often used in combination therapies and as maintenance therapy after psoriasis plaques have resolved.

Anthralin

Anthralin (dithranol) has been used to treat psoriasis since

1916.[48] It is an extremely effective topical agent for psoriasis, probably because it inhibits enzyme metabolism and reduces epidermal mitotic turnover.[48]

Indications Because of the staining and irritation associated with the use of anthralin, this agent is usually prescribed for patients who do not respond to other topical therapies.

Formulations and regimens A modified Ingram regimen combines the daily application of anthralin in a stiff paste with tar baths and with exposure to ultraviolet light. This therapy involves application of progressively higher concentrations of anthralin for 6 to 8 hours at a time; it was introduced in the United States for hospitalized psoriatic patients[44] and for ambulatory patients in a psoriasis day care center.[49]

Modified anthralin formulations have been used to minimize the staining from anthralin, to decrease irritation, and to promote home use of the medication. Short-contact therapy consists of the application of anthralin to localized plaques for 30 minutes to 2 hours, after which time the anthralin must be thoroughly removed to minimize irritation of the surrounding skin.[50] Anthralin in a cream base, which can be removed by washing with water, is suitable for home use; it is available in 1% and 0.5% concentrations, for application to localized lesions on the skin and the scalp.

A formulation of 1% anthralin cream, composed of microencapsulated lipid crystals that release anthralin for absorption at skin temperature, is available. When used as short-contact therapy, this preparation carries a low risk of staining and irritation.[51]

Anthralin is most effective therapeutically when it is compounded in the form of a hard paste containing paraffin; this form is most commonly used in ambulatory psoriasis treatment centers. Anthralin ointment is less effective than anthralin paste, and anthralin cream is even less effective. With regard to patient compliance, this order is reversed. The end point of treatment is resolution of plaques to a macular state; this is usually associated with residual postinflammatory hyperpigmentation and temporary staining from anthralin. Resolution of symptoms usually occurs within 2 to 3 weeks after a modified Ingram regimen; remissions last for weeks to months.

Side effects Staining of skin, clothing, and the home is common with anthralin, as is irritation at the site of application.

SUNLIGHT

Ultraviolet radiation has a beneficial effect on psoriasis. Sunbathing for 2 to 4 weeks lessens the morbidity associated with the disorder, and climatotherapy at the Dead Sea is an effective alternative therapy for psoriasis for those who can travel to that part of the world. Because of its unique geographic location, 300 m below sea level, patients are exposed to naturally filtered ultraviolet light, which results in significant improvement or complete resolution of symptoms in 83% of patients over several weeks.[52] The sunlight at the Dead Sea accounts for most of the response, with little additional improvement resulting from bathing in the Dead Sea. Not surprisingly, patients treated at the Dead Sea have higher rates of nonmelanoma skin cancer.[53]

PHOTOTHERAPY

Phototherapy with UVB is an important therapeutic option for patients with extensive psoriasis. UVB irradiation can be used alone, but it has traditionally been combined with topical application of tar. Daily in-hospital application of crude coal tar and exposure to ultraviolet light (the Goeckerman regimen) can lead to a resolution of symptoms in widespread psoriasis within 3 or 4 weeks and can effect remissions that last for weeks to months.

In a reevaluation of the Goeckerman regimen, application of a 1% tar preparation was found to be as effective as a 6% preparation. Furthermore, application of the tar preparation for 2 hours before irradiation was equivalent to longer periods of application.[54] Contraindications to the use of the Goeckerman regimen include the presence of severely excoriated or inflamed psoriasis, erythrodermic and pustular forms of the disease, folliculitis, and a history of photosensitivity.

Newer regimens, which are more convenient and aesthetically acceptable, combine UVB with emollients. The emollient or vehicle decreases reflectance of the psoriatic scale, thereby increasing light transmission. According to a report by Lowe and colleagues, results with emollients are equivalent to those with tar, when used in regimens that utilize UVB in doses sufficient to cause erythema (erythemogenic); however, tar may have an additive effect when combined with a less aggressive regimen of suberythemogenic UVB.[55]

In a comparison study, outpatient UVB phototherapy was administered three times weekly, along with the application of either a tar oil or an emollient twice a day. This approach led to clearing of psoriatic lesions in 78% of patients [see Figure 10]. No difference in response was observed between the tar oil and the emollient.[56] Although the Lowe study had shown an additive effect for tar combined with UVB irradiation when patients were evaluated after 3 to 4 weeks (before their lesions had cleared),[57] this comparison study showed no such advantage in patients who were evaluated at the time of lesion clearing. Remission lasted longer in patients who received maintenance UVB phototherapy twice weekly for 1 to 2 months and then once weekly for up to 4 months than in patients who stopped receiving UVB phototherapy after the initial clearing.

Narrow-Band UVB

Narrow-band UVB, which comprises wavelengths of approximately 311 nm (as opposed to the 295 to 320 nm range of broadband UVB), is a newer approach that is more effective than broad-band UVB.[58] Like other forms of phototherapy, narrowband UVB works through local effects; therefore, covered areas, such as the scalp, do not respond.[59]

PHOTOCHEMOTHERAPY

Photochemotherapy with PUVA is indicated for patients with extensive, disabling psoriasis that has failed to respond to conventional forms of therapy, including conventional or narrowband UVB phototherapy. PUVA therapy entails the administration of the photosensitizing drug methoxsalen (8-methoxypsoralen)—in an oral dose or by soaking in a tub containing methoxsalen or applying topical methoxsalen—followed by exposure of the patient to high-intensity longwave ultraviolet light in a walk-in irradiation chamber. The initial UVA dose (in joules/cm^2) is based on the patient's skin type and calculated in accordance with established protocols.[60]

Although its therapeutic effect is local, PUVA is a systemic treatment in which photoactivated methoxsalen binds to epidermal DNA, forming monofunctional and bifunctional adducts. It has been postulated that the resulting interference with epider-

a *b*

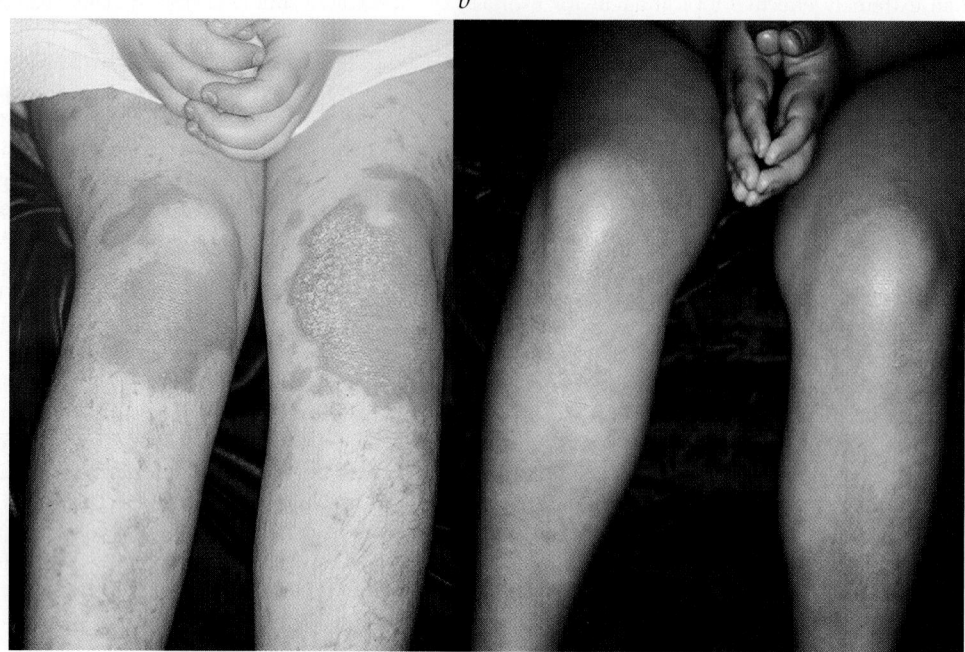

Figure 10   **Psoriasis in a child before (*a*) and after (*b*) phototherapy.**

mal mitosis is one of the mechanisms of action of PUVA therapy for psoriasis, although effects on immune function in the skin play an important role.

The efficacy of oral PUVA therapy has been established by several multicenter clinical trials.[61] A course of PUVA therapy administered two or three times weekly resulted in significant clearing of psoriasis lesions in approximately 90% of patients within a mean of 25 total treatments. After the initial course, a tapering maintenance regimen is instituted, and PUVA therapy is eventually discontinued. In most patients, psoriasis recurs months to years after PUVA is discontinued, indicating that this therapy is palliative rather than curative.

Side Effects

Acute side effects caused by phototoxicity, such as erythema and blistering, are dose related and can therefore be controlled. Pruritus, usually associated with dryness of the skin, is fairly common and can be alleviated by the use of emollients and oral antihistamines. Nausea may follow ingestion of methoxsalen. Of greater concern are the potential long-term side effects, particularly carcinogenicity. Although the FDA has approved the use of PUVA to treat psoriasis, patients must be closely monitored for long-term side effects. A multicenter study of more than 1,300 PUVA-treated patients in the United States who were evaluated after 1 to 3 years of follow-up revealed a significant increase in the number of squamous cell carcinomas (SCCs) in those patients with a history of exposure to ionizing radiation or a history of skin cancer.[62] A higher-than-expected ratio of SCCs to basal cell epitheliomas and an excess of SCCs in areas of the body that were not exposed to the sun were significant findings of the study. A 5.7-year follow-up study of the original cohort group revealed a dose-dependent increase in the risk of SCC.[63] There was only a slight increase in the risk of basal cell carcinoma in these patients. The risk of SCC was almost 13-fold higher in patients who had received high cumulative doses of PUVA than in patients who received low-dose therapy.

A follow-up study of the surviving members of that cohort, at least 15 years after original treatment, again assessed the risk of skin cancers. Of great concern was a small but statistically significant increase in the incidence of malignant melanoma.[64] Because that increase did not become apparent until after a period of at least 15 years, there is great concern that high rates of melanoma will occur in patients who began PUVA therapy years ago. Fortunately, this has not happened thus far.

Studies in animals suggest that PUVA may have ocular side effects. Methoxsalen has been detected in the lenses of rats after they have ingested the drug; subsequent exposure to UVA enhances such ultraviolet-induced changes as cataracts.[65] The risk of ocular toxicity and possible retinal damage is of particular concern in young persons, whose lenses transmit more UVA than the more opaque lenses of older persons, and in aphakic persons, in whom lenses are absent.[66] The use of UVA-opaque goggles during PUVA treatment sessions is extremely important. Glasses that block UVA must be worn from the time that methoxsalen is administered throughout the rest of the day. Some investigators advise protection of the eyes the day after therapy. Thus far, studies of patients treated with PUVA have not revealed an increase in the incidence of cataracts.

SYSTEMIC THERAPY

Methotrexate

Short-term use of the antimetabolite methotrexate can be an extremely effective treatment for psoriasis. Methotrexate is indicated for patients who do not respond adequately to phototherapy and for patients with psoriatic arthritis.

The source of methotrexate's efficacy against psoriasis was once thought to be its antimitotic effect on proliferating keratinocytes. However, tissue culture studies have suggested that activated lymphoid cells in the lymph nodes, blood, and skin are a likely target of methotrexate; proliferating macrophages and T cells are 100 times more sensitive to methotrexate than are proliferating epithelial cells.[67] These findings may be relevant to the mechanism of action of methotrexate in other immunologically based disorders, including psoriatic arthritis, rheumatoid arthritis, and Crohn disease.

Dosage Methotrexate is best given in a single weekly oral dose of up to 30 mg or in three divided doses at 12-hour intervals during a 24-hour period (e.g., at 8:00 A.M., at 8:00 P.M., and again at 8:00 A.M.).

Hepatoxicity and liver biopsy The use of liver biopsy has been advocated for monitoring patients with psoriasis who are receiving methotrexate. This recommendation is controversial, however; critics point out that liver biopsies are not routinely performed in patients with rheumatoid arthritis who are undergoing treatment with methotrexate.[68] Nevertheless, a review of the literature clearly shows that patients with psoriasis who are treated with methotrexate are more likely to develop hepatic fibrosis, possibly because of their underlying disease or because of the concomitant treatments they are given.

Current guidelines call for the use of liver biopsy in patients with psoriasis who have received a cumulative dose of 1 to 1.5 g of methotrexate and who do not have a history of liver disease or alcoholism. Biopsy should be performed early in the course of treatment in patients with a history of hepatitis C, alcoholism, or other liver disease. Other risk factors for hepatotoxicity are obesity, diabetes, and abnormalities on liver function testing.

Pathologic liver changes caused by methotrexate therapy have been graded as follows: grade I, normal liver histology or mild fatty infiltration; grade II, moderate to severe fatty infiltration with portal tract inflammation and necrosis; grade IIIA, mild fibrosis; grade IIIB, moderate to severe fibrosis; and grade IV, cirrhosis. Methotrexate should be discontinued in patients with grade IIIB or IV pathologic liver changes. The importance of strict adherence to current guidelines for the administration of methotrexate is emphasized by the occurrence of methotrexate-induced cirrhosis necessitating liver transplantation in three patients with long-term psoriasis who did not undergo serial liver biopsies.[69]

Other side effects In addition to hepatotoxicity, other side effects of methotrexate therapy include bone marrow suppression, nausea, diarrhea, and stomatitis. Methotrexate is teratogenic and can cause reversible oligospermia. Pneumonitis can occur early in the course of treatment if methotrexate is administered in oncologic doses. Evaluation by tests of liver function, renal function, and blood elements must be made before and throughout the course of methotrexate therapy.

Certain drugs increase the toxicity of methotrexate by reducing renal tubular secretion; these drugs include salicylates, sulfonamides, probenecid, and penicillins. Other drugs increase toxicity by displacing methotrexate from its binding sites on plasma proteins; these drugs include salicylates, probenecid, barbiturates, and phenytoin. Many of the NSAIDs and trimethoprim-sulfamethoxazole enhance methotrexate toxicity.[68] Cases of pancytopenia after low-dose methotrexate therapy underscore the hazards of using this drug in patients with renal insufficiency or in patients who are concomitantly receiving drugs that increase methotrexate toxicity.[70]

Contraindications to treatment with methotrexate and indications for stopping treatment should be heeded. Constant medical supervision is necessary, and therapy must be stopped at once if toxicity develops.

Acitretin

Indications and dosage Acitretin, an oral retinoid, has FDA approval for the treatment of plaque psoriasis. It is highly effective in the treatment of pustular psoriasis and can be very effective as monotherapy for erythrodermic psoriasis. For plaque-type and guttate psoriasis, however, acitretin is most useful in combination with other treatments, particularly UVB and PUVA phototherapy.[71,72] Acitretin is initiated 1 to 2 weeks before UVB or PUVA therapy is started. With combination treatment, symptoms resolve much more quickly. Doses of only 10 to 25 mg daily are effective, thus minimizing retinoid side effects.[71,72] When used as monotherapy, acitretin is prescribed in doses of 25 mg daily, which can be increased to 50 mg a day or higher.

Side effects Acitretin side effects are dose related and are common with doses above 25 mg daily. Hair loss, cheilitis, desquamation of the palms and soles, sun sensitivity, and periungual pyogenic granulomas are among the mucocutaneous side effects. Hyperlipidemia is common but is easily controlled with lipid-lowering agents. Elevations in liver enzyme levels can occur, and enzyme levels must be monitored. Serial liver biopsies have not demonstrated hepatic fibrosis in patients treated with oral retinoids.[73]

Acitretin poses a significant risk of teratogenicity. Characteristic retinoid birth defects occur in a high proportion of fetuses exposed to even small amounts of the drug in utero. Acitretin is eliminated from the body much more quickly than its prodrug etretinate. In the presence of alcohol, however, acitretin is converted back to etretinate,[74] raising concerns that women of childbearing age who take acitretin and who later become pregnant would then be at risk for exposing their fetus to acitretin's teratogenic effects. The FDA therefore requires that acitretin not be given to women planning a pregnancy within 3 years.

Long-term side effects of oral retinoids include calcification of ligaments and tendons and osteoporosis.[75,76] The long-term safety of etretinate, acitretin's prodrug, was examined in a 5-year prospective study of 956 patients with psoriasis. The investigators concluded that with appropriate patient selection and monitoring, there was no substantially increased risk of side effects related to cardiovascular disease, cancer, diabetes, cataracts, and inflammatory bowel disease. Although joint symptoms improved in some patients, more patients had joint problems associated with etretinate. Etretinate also caused short-term changes in liver enzyme levels in some patients and, in rare cases, caused acute hepatitis. The long-term risk of liver disease and cirrhosis with etretinate, however, was less than that associated with comparable periods of methotrexate.[77]

Cyclosporine

Cyclosporine in a microemulsion formulation was approved by the FDA for the treatment of psoriasis after extensive worldwide experience. In dosages of 2.5 to 5 mg/kg/day, cyclosporine is highly effective for psoriasis. Even at such doses, however, it may be associated with significant side effects, which have limited its use in patients with severe or refractory disease.

Indications and dosage Cyclosporine is indicated for patients in whom phototherapy or methotrexate therapy has failed. The microemulsion formulation of cyclosporine is better absorbed than earlier formulations. It is available in gel capsules of 25 and 100 mg and is most commonly taken in divided doses twice daily. At dosages of 5 mg/kg/day, a response is usually seen within 4 weeks, and some patients respond as quickly as 1 week. It should be noted that in the United States, the package insert for cyclosporine recommends an upper dosage limit of 4 mg/kg/day, although worldwide experience regarding the efficacy and safety of this drug has established an upper limit of 5 mg/kg/day.[78] In the United States, the maximum FDA-approved duration of treatment of cyclosporine is 1 year.

Side effects Cyclosporine is associated with a number of side effects that are easily managed; other side effects are of greater concern. Hypertrichosis, tremors, paresthesias, headache, gingival hyperplasia, joint pain, and fatigue can occur. Elevations in serum lipid levels and minor elevations in liver enzyme levels are also common. Hypomagnesemia may require magnesium supplementation. The most serious common side effects are hypertension and nephrotoxicity. Hypertension can be managed by lowering the dose or by instituting treatment with calcium channel blockers such as amlodipine besylate. There is some evidence that in normotensive patients receiving cyclosporine, amlodipine therapy may prevent some of the nephrotoxicity that has been associated with this potent psoriasis treatment.[79]

Renal interstitial fibrosis and renal tubular atrophy are common in patients on long-term therapy with cyclosporine.[80] Consequently, serum creatinine levels must be monitored on a regular basis. If the serum creatinine level rises more than 30% above baseline (or more than 25%, according to the United States package insert), the dosage may have to be reduced.[78]

Organ transplant patients taking cyclosporine, as well as other immunosuppressive drugs, to prevent rejection have experienced an increase in lymphoproliferative diseases and skin cancers.[81,82] It is hoped that the lower doses and intermittent usage of cyclosporine in psoriasis patients will not be associated with an increase in malignancies, but caution must be exercised. In one study, no increase in lymphoproliferative disorders was found in rheumatoid arthritis patients who were treated with cyclosporine for a short period (median, 1.6 years), compared with a parallel group of rheumatoid patients who were not treated with cyclosporine.[83] Nevertheless, caution must be used with this powerful new psoriasis treatment.

Tacrolimus

Although tacrolimus does not have FDA approval for use in psoriasis, it is a potent immunosuppressive agent that may be substituted for cyclosporine in patients who cannot tolerate the hypertrichosis associated with this agent. Tacrolimus has proved to be effective in the treatment of psoriasis. In a double-blind trial, 50 patients with severe recalcitrant psoriasis were given either oral tacrolimus or placebo.[84] In the tacrolimus group, starting dosages were 0.5 mg/kg/day, and the dosages could be increased to 0.10 mg/kg at week 3 or 6 if patient response was judged to be insufficient. After 9 weeks of treatment, patients receiving tacrolimus had an 84% reduction in Psoriasis Area and Severity Index (PASI) scores.

As with cyclosporine, there are concerns about hypertension, nephrotoxicity, and immunosuppression with tacrolimus. The use of this drug must be balanced against a risk of lymphoma and skin cancer.[85] Tacrolimus has not been studied as extensively as cyclosporine for psoriasis, and further investigations are warranted for this very effective antipsoriatic agent.

Hydroxyurea

Hydroxyurea may be considered for the treatment of psoriasis in patients with hepatic disease, because hepatotoxicity is uncommon with this agent.[86] Response is slower and less complete than with methotrexate, however, and resistance to hydroxyurea may develop more frequently. Hydroxyurea is administered orally at a dosage of 1 to 2 g/day. Careful monitoring of blood counts is necessary during therapy.

Sulfasalazine

Sulfasalazine does not have FDA approval for the treatment of psoriasis but is highly effective in selected patients. It is typically given in dosages of 3 to 4 g daily. In one study, over 25% of patients given sulfasalazine stopped the treatment because of side effects (cutaneous eruptions or nausea). In clinical practice, results have been less promising than in studies.[87]

Combination Therapy

Combinations of various psoriasis treatments have proved to be superior in efficacy to monotherapy. Acitretin is routinely used with UVB and PUVA, a combination that allows the use of smaller doses and minimizes toxicities of both retinoid therapy and phototherapy.[71,72] The combination of methotrexate and acitretin has been used successfully despite some concern that both drugs are hepatotoxic.[88] Careful monitoring of liver enzyme levels is essential. Methotrexate and cyclosporine can be used together, and their concurrent administration in small doses can result in greater efficacy and less toxicity than that which can be achieved with higher doses of either agent used alone.[89] Methotrexate has also been used very successfully in combination with UVB[90] and PUVA,[91] although there is some concern that methotrexate may potentiate the carcinogenic effect of PUVA.[92] Because cyclosporine has been associated with skin cancers, it is not routinely used in combination with PUVA. It can be used in combination with retinoids and mycophenolate mofetil.

Other Systemic Therapies

Mycophenolate mofetil, a drug that has FDA approval for the prevention of organ transplant rejection, is highly effective for some patients with psoriasis.[93] Mycophenolate mofetil is the prodrug of mycophenolic acid, a medication that was tested for psoriasis in the 1970s.[94] Although mycophenolic acid was found to be highly effective in the treatment of psoriasis, the manufacturers did not pursue FDA approval for that indication because of its side effects, which included gastrointestinal toxicity and an immunosuppressive effect that resulted in herpes zoster infections in more than 10% of treated patients.

6-Thioguanine is another anticancer chemotherapeutic agent that is highly effective for psoriasis. Unfortunately, it has been associated with bone marrow suppression in approximately 50% of patients.[95] Bone marrow toxicity from 6-thioguanine can be reduced by administering the drug two to three times a week rather than daily.[96]

Biologic Therapies

The ability to create molecules that target specific steps in the pathogenesis of psoriasis has led to the development of biologic agents that can treat psoriasis without the nephrotoxicity associated with cyclosporine and without the bone marrow and liver toxicities associated with methotrexate. Biologic agents are immunosuppressive, and their long-term toxicity is not known. As with other immunosuppressive agents, there is concern about the potential to predispose patients to infections or malignancies. Several biologic agents have FDA approval for use in psoriasis—namely, alefacept, efalizumab, and etanercept. Others have been approved for use in other diseases but are undergoing clinical trials for use in psoriasis—namely, adalimumab and infliximab. Still other agents, such as onercept, a TNF-α blocking agent, and anti–IL-12, are at earlier stages of development.

Alefacept Alefacept is a fusion protein consisting of LFA-3 fused to the Fc portion of human IgG1. The LFA-3 portion of the molecule attaches to its naturally occurring receptor, CD2, on the surface of a resting T cell, thereby blocking T cell activation. The Fc portion of the molecule attaches to Fc receptors on natural killer cells and macrophages, resulting in apoptosis of the bound T cell.[97]

Alefacept originally received FDA approval as intravenous and intramuscular formulations, but it is now available only in the intramuscular form. Alefacept is administered weekly for 12 weeks in a dose of 15 mg. In one study, by 14 weeks after the start of therapy, 21% of patients achieved PASI 75 (75% reduction in disease from baseline) and 42% of patients achieved PASI 50 (50% reduction in disease from baseline). Improvement typically progresses after the completion of treatment, with maximal disease reduction 8 weeks after a second course of therapy; in one study, 33% of patients achieved PASI 75 and 57% achieved PASI 50 by this point.[98] The most striking benefit of alefacept therapy is the long duration of remission achieved in a subgroup of patients. In patients who achieved PASI 75, the median time to recurrence of psoriasis (as defined by maintenance of PASI 50) was 7 months after a single 12-week course of therapy and more than a year after two courses of therapy.[99]

Drawbacks of alefacept therapy include the high cost of the drug and the need for weekly CD4+ T cell counts because the drug tends to reduce the number of these cells. The onset of action of alefacept is slow, with many patients achieving maximal response weeks after completing the 12-week course. Moreover, only a proportion of patients achieve a satisfactory response.

Efalizumab Efalizumab is a humanized monoclonal antibody directed against the CD11a portion of LFA-1. Efalizumab blocks the interaction between LFA-1 and ICAM-1, an interaction that is responsible for T cell activation and trafficking of T cells into inflamed skin. After a conditioning dose of 0.7 mg/kg the first week, patients self-administer subcutaneous injections of efalizumab at a dose of 1 mg/kg weekly. In double-blind, placebo-controlled trials, 22% to 39% of patients treated with weekly efalizumab for 12 weeks achieved PASI 75,[100-102] and nearly 60% of patients achieved PASI 50. With longer therapy, higher proportions of patients achieve greater degrees of improvement. Like the other biologic agents, efalizumab does not cause the nephrotoxicity associated with cyclosporine or the bone marrow or liver toxicity associated with methotrexate. The drug is fairly expensive, however, and flulike symptoms may develop after the first or second injection; a serious concern is the development of psoriasis rebound (defined as a worsening of psoriasis over baseline), which occurs in up to 15% of patients. To avoid psoriasis rebound, efalizumab should not be stopped abruptly but, rather, slowly converted to alternative therapies.

Etanercept Etanercept is a recombinant fusion protein that includes the p75 TNF receptor that binds to TNF-α, blocking its interaction with cell surface receptors. Etanercept originally received FDA approval for a dosage of 25 mg administered subcutaneously by the patient at home twice weekly for the treatment of psoriatic arthritis. Subsequently, etanercept received approval for the treatment of psoriasis at a dosage of 50 mg administered subcutaneously twice weekly for 3 months and then once weekly. In a double-blind, placebo-controlled, four-arm trial comparing placebo with three dosage regimens, analysis after 12 weeks of treatment showed that PASI 75 was achieved in 14% of patients who received 25 mg once a week, in 34% who received 25 mg twice a week, and in 49% who received 50 mg twice a week. Response rates were even higher at 24 weeks of therapy.[103]

The drawbacks of etanercept include its cost and the need to self-inject the medication on a long-term basis. Injection-site reactions, although common, are almost always minor and seldom require any treatment other than temporarily using a different site for injections. There is evidence that TNF-α blockers can cause an exacerbation of multiple sclerosis, so the drug should be avoided in patients with a personal or family history of demyelinating disease. Some controversy exists as to whether TNF-α blockers exacerbate chronic heart failure, and there is concern that the immunosuppressive effects of TNF-α blockers may contribute to an increase in the development of lymphoproliferative diseases.[104] Antinuclear antibodies also develop in etanercept-treated patients, but they are of questionable physiologic significance.

Infliximab Infliximab is a chimeric monoclonal antibody directed against TNF-α. In the short term (12 weeks), it is the most effective treatment for psoriasis, but it does not yet have FDA approval for this indication. It is administered by slow intravenous infusion at baseline, at weeks 2 and 6, and then every 8 weeks thereafter. In a double-blind, placebo-controlled trial evaluating patients at week 10, after only three infusions, 82% of patients achieved PASI 75.[105] Moreover, 55% of patients maintained PASI 50 or higher during 6 months of follow-up.

Like the other TNF-α blockers, infliximab is associated with worsening of chronic heart failure, multiple sclerosis, and lymphoproliferative diseases. In addition, infusion reactions develop in a significant proportion of patients; these appear to be related to the development of human antichimeric antibodies. Although infusion reactions are mild in the majority of patients, they can be severe, resulting in chest pain and hypotension. Pretreating patients with antibiotics is beneficial. TNF-α blocking plays a significant role in the control of mycobacterial infection, and an increase in reactivation of latent tuberculosis has been observed in patients treated with infliximab. Consequently, patients should undergo tuberculosis testing before starting on this medication.[106]

Adalimumab Adalimumab is a fully human monoclonal antibody against TNF-α. It has FDA approval for the treatment of rheumatoid arthritis and has been successfully tested for psoriasis.[107] Like the other biologics, adalimumab is not toxic to kidneys, liver, or bone marrow; however, also like the other biologic agents, it is quite expensive. The same concerns about heart failure, multiple sclerosis, and lymphoproliferative diseases that exist with etanercept and infliximab are also described in adalimumab's package insert. In a three-arm, placebo-controlled trial, PASI 75 was achieved by 53% of patients who received adalimumab every other week and by 80% of patients who received it weekly. An even greater number of patients achieved PASI 50. Adalimumab, 40 mg, is given by subcutaneous injection.

Prognosis

Psoriasis is usually lifelong, but the severity of the disease may vary, with periodic exacerbations and relative remissions in some patients. Although pustular psoriasis and erythrodermic psoriasis can be life-threatening, even stable plaque psoriasis can have a negative impact on overall health, possibly because of comorbid conditions such as psoriatic arthritis or obesity or because of complications of therapy.

Severe exacerbation of psoriasis taxes the ingenuity of even the most skilled clinician. Fortunately, because of the wide range of psoriasis therapies now available, clinicians are able to successfully treat almost all patients with psoriasis. The goal of therapy must be to minimize toxicity while achieving satisfactory improvement both in physical signs and symptoms and in patients' quality of life.

Elizabeth A. Abel, M.D., has been an investigator, consultant, or speaker for Abbott Laboratories, Allergan, Inc., Amgen, Inc., Biogen, Inc., Centocor, Inc., Connetics Corp., Genentech, Inc., and 3M.

Mark Lebwohl, M.D., has been an investigator, consultant, or speaker for Abbott Laboratories, Allergan, Inc., Amgen, Inc., Biogen, Inc., Centocor, Inc., Connetics Corp., Fujisawa Healthcare, Inc., Galderma Laboratories, Genentech, Inc., Novartis AG., and Warner Chilcott.

References

1. Stern RS, Nijsten T, Feldman SR, et al: Psoriasis is common, carries a substantial burden even when not extensive, and is associated with widespread treatment dissatisfaction. J Invest Dermatol Symp Proc 9:136, 2004

2. Koo J: Population-based epidemiologic study of psoriasis with emphasis on quality of life assessment. Dermatol Clin 14:485, 1996

3. Farber EM, Nall ML: The natural history of psoriasis in 5,600 patients. Dermatologica 148:1, 1974

4. Gottlieb SL, Gilleaudeau P, Johnson R, et al: Response of psoriasis to a lymphocyte-selective toxin (DAB389IL-2) suggests a primary immune, but not keratinocyte, pathogenic basis. Nat Med 1:442, 1995

5. Bagel J, Garland WT, Breneman D, et al: Administration of DAB389IL-2 to patients with recalcitrant psoriasis: a double-blind, phase II multicenter trial. J Am Acad Dermatol 38:938, 1998

6. Abrams JR, Lebwohl MG, Guzzo CA, et al: CTLA4Ig-mediated blockage of T-cell costimulation in patients with psoriasis vulgaris. J Clin Invest 103:1243, 1999

7. Griffiths CE: T-cell-targeted biologicals for psoriasis. Curr Drug Targets Inflamm Allergy 3:157, 2004

8. Lebwohl M, Tyring SK, Hamilton TK, et al: A novel targeted T-cell modulator, efalizumab, for plaque psoriasis. Efalizumab Study Group. N Engl J Med 349:2004, 2003

9. Lebwohl M, Christophers E, Langley R, et al: An international, randomized, double-blind, placebo-controlled phase 3 trial of intramuscular alefacept in patients with chronic plaque psoriasis. Alefacept Clinical Study Group. Arch Dermatol 139:719, 2003

10. Victor FC, Gottlieb AB, Menter A: Changing paradigms in dermatology: tumor necrosis factor alpha (TNF-alpha) blockade in psoriasis and psoriatic arthritis. Clin Dermatol 21:392, 2003

11. Farber EM, Nall ML, Watson W: Natural history of psoriasis in 61 twin pairs. Arch Dermatol 109:207, 1974

12. Capon F, Trembath RC, Barker JN: An update on the genetics of psoriasis. Dermatol Clin 22:339, 2004

13. Helms C, Cao L, Krueger JG, et al: A putative RUNX1 binding site variant between SLC9A3R1 and NAT9 is associated with susceptibility to psoriasis. Nat Genet 35:349, 2003

14. Lebwohl M, Tan MH: Psoriasis and stress. Lancet 351:82, 1998

15. Gaston L, Lassonde M, Bernier-Buzzanga J, et al: Psoriasis and stress: a prospective study. J Am Acad Dermatol 17:82, 1987

16. Rapp SR, Feldman SR, Exum ML, et al: Psoriasis causes as much disability as other major medical diseases. J Am Acad Dermatol 41:401, 1999

17. Telfer NR, Chalmers RG, Whale K, et al: The role of streptococcal infection in the initiation of guttate psoriasis. Arch Dermatol 128:39, 1992

18. Vincent F, Ross JB, Dalton M, et al: A therapeutic trial of the use of penicillin V or erythromycin with or without rifampin in the treatment of psoriasis. J Am Acad Dermatol 26:458, 1992

19. Rosenberg EW, Noah PW, Zanolli MD, et al: Use of rifampin with penicillin and erythromycin in the treatment of psoriasis: preliminary report. J Am Acad Dermatol 14:761, 1986

20. Obuch ML, Maurer TA, Becker B, et al: Psoriasis and human immunodeficiency virus infection. J Am Acad Dermatol 27:667, 1992

21. Abel EA: Diagnosis of drug-induced psoriasis. Semin Dermatol 11:269, 1992

22. Krueger GG: Psoriasis: current concepts of its etiology and pathogenesis. Yearbook of Dermatology. Dobson RL, Thiers BH, Eds. Year Book Medical Publishers, Chicago, 1982, p 13

23. Katayama H, Kawada A: Exacerbation of psoriasis induced by indomethacin. J Dermatol (Tokyo) 8:323, 1981

24. Magliocco MA, Gottlieb AB: Etanercept therapy for patients with psoriatic arthritis and concurrent hepatitis C virus infection: report of 3 cases. J Am Acad Dermatol 51:580, 2004

25. Gupta MA, Gupta AK, Watteel GN: Cigarette smoking in men may be a risk factor for increased severity of psoriasis of the extremities. Br J Dermatol 135:859, 1996

26. Naldi L, Peli L, Parazzini F: Association of early-stage psoriasis with smoking and male alcohol consumption: evidence from an Italian case-control study. Arch Dermatol 135:1479, 1999

27. Naldi L, Parazzini F, Peli L, et al: Dietary factors and the risk of psoriasis: results of an Italian case control study. Br J Dermatol 134:101, 1996

28. Green MS, Prystowsky JH, Cohen SR, et al: Infectious complications of erythrodermic psoriasis. J Am Acad Dermatol 34:911, 1996

29. Calvert HT, Smith MA, Wells RS: Psoriasis and the nails. Br J Dermatol 75:415, 1963

30. Mease PJ: Recent advances in the management of psoriatic arthritis. Curr Opin Rheumatol 16:366, 2004

31. Gladman DD, Hing EN, Schentag CT, et al: Remission in psoriatic arthritis. J Rheumatol 28:1045, 2001

32. Lebwohl M: Advances in psoriasis therapy. Dermatol Clin 18:13, 2000

33. Feldman SR, Fleischer AB, Cooper JZ: New topical treatments change the pattern of treatment of psoriasis: dermatologists remain the primary providers of this care. Int J Dermatol 39:41, 2000

34. Cornell RC, Stoughton RB: Correlation of the vasoconstriction assay and clinical activity in psoriasis. Arch Dermatol 121:63, 1985

35. Katz HI, Prawer SE, Medansky RS, et al: Intermittent corticosteroid maintenance treatment of psoriasis: a double-blind multicenter trial of augmented betamethasone dipropionate ointment in a pulse dose treatment regimen. Dermatologica 183:269, 1991

36. Lebwohl M, Siskin SB, Epinette W, et al: A multicenter trial of calcipotriene ointment and halobetasol ointment to either agent alone for the treatment of psoriasis. J Am Acad Dermatol 35:268, 1996

37. Lebwohl M, Yoles A, Lombardi K, et al: Calcipotriene ointment and halobetasol ointment in the long-term treatment of psoriasis: effects on the duration of improvement. J Am Acad Dermatol 39:447, 1998

38. Ramsay CA, Schwartz BE, Lowson D, et al: Calcipotriol cream combined with twice weekly broad-band UVB phototherapy: a safe, effective and UVB-sparing antipsoriatic combination treatment. The Canadian Calcipotriol and UVB Study Group. Dermatology 200:17, 2000

39. Speight EL, Farr PM: Calcipotriol improves the response of psoriasis to PUVA. Br J Dermatol 130:79, 1994

40. Patel B, Siskin S, Krazmien BA, et al: Compatibility of calcipotriene with other topical medications. J Am Acad Dermatol 38:1010, 1998

41. Lebwohl M, Hecker D, Martinez J, et al: Interactions between calcipotriene and ultraviolet light. J Am Acad Dermatol 37:93, 1997

42. Georgiou S, Tsambaos D: Hypercalcaemia and hypercalciuria after topical treatment of psoriasis with excessive amounts of calcipotriol. Acta Derm Venereol 79:86, 1999

43. Guenther LC: Fixed-dose combination therapy for psoriasis. Am J Clin Dermatol 5:71, 2004

44. Franssen ME, de Jongh GJ, van Erp PE, et al: A left/right comparison of twice-daily calcipotriol ointment and calcitriol ointment in patients with psoriasis: the effect on keratinocyte subpopulations. Acta Derm Venereol 84:195, 2004

45. Koo JY: Tazarotene in combination with phototherapy. J Am Acad Dermatol 39:S144, 1998

46. Hecker D, Worsley J, Yueh G, et al: Interactions between tazarotene and ultraviolet light. J Am Acad Dermatol 41:927, 1999

47. Lowe NJ, Breeding J, Wortzman MS: The pharmacological variability of crude coal tar. Br J Dermatol 126:608, 1992

48. Fiore M: Practical aspects of anthralin therapy. Cutis 46:351, 1990

49. Abel EA, O'Connell BM, Farber EM: Psoriasis Day Care Center treatment at Stanford: part-time and full-time programs. Int J Dermatol 26:500, 1987

50. Schaefer H, Farber EM, Goldberg L, et al: Limited application period for dithranol in psoriasis: preliminary report on penetration and clinical efficacy. Br J Dermatol 102:571, 1980

51. Volden G, Bjornberg A, Tegner E, et al: Short-contact treatment at home with micanol. Acta Derm Venereol Suppl (Stockh) 172:20, 1992

52. Even-Paz Z, Gumon R, Kipnis V, et al: Dead Sea sun vs. Dead Sea water in the treatment of psoriasis. Dermatol Treat 7:83, 1996

53. Frentz G, Olsen JH, Avrach WW: Malignant tumours and psoriasis: climatotherapy

at the Dead Sea. Br J Dermatol 141:1088, 1999

54. Petrozzi JW, Barton JO, Kaidbey KH, et al: Updating the Goeckerman regimen for psoriasis. Br J Dermatol 98:437, 1978

55. Lowe NJ, Wortzman MS, Breeding J, et al: Coal tar phototherapy for psoriasis reevaluated: erythemogenic versus suberythemogenic ultraviolet with a tar extract in oil and crude coal tar. J Am Acad Dermatol 8:781, 1983

56. Stern RS, Gange RW, Parrish JA, et al: Contribution of topical tar oil to ultra-violet B phototherapy for psoriasis. J Am Acad Dermatol 14:742, 1986

57. Lowe NJ, Stern RS: Contribution of topical tar oil to ultraviolet B phototherapy for psoriasis. J Am Acad Dermatol 15:1053, 1986

58. Barbagallo J, Spann CT, Tutrone WD, et al: Narrowband UVB phototherapy for the treatment of psoriasis: a review and update. Cutis 68:345, 2001

59. Dawe RS, Cameron H, Yule S, et al: UV-B phototherapy clears psoriasis through local effects. Arch Dermatol 138:1071, 2002

60. Abel EA: Administration of PUVA therapy: protocols, indications, and cautions. Photochemotherapy in Dermatology. Abel EA, Ed. Igaku-Shoin Medical Publishers, New York, 1992, p 75

61. Stern RS, Laird N: The carcinogenic risk of treatments for severe psoriasis. Cancer 73:2759, 1994

62. Stern RS, Thibodeau LA, Kleinerman RA, et al: Risk of cutaneous carcinoma in patients treated with oral methoxsalen photochemotherapy for psoriasis. N Engl J Med 300:809, 1979

63. Stern RS, Laird N, Melski J, et al: Cutaneous squamous-cell carcinoma in patients treated with PUVA. N Engl J Med 310:1156, 1984

64. Stern RS, Nichols KT, Vakeva LH: Malignant melanoma in patients treated for psoriasis with methoxsalen (psoralen) and ultraviolet A radiation (PUVA). The PUVA Follow-Up Study.N Engl J Med 336:1041, 1997

65. Lerman S, Borkman RF: A method for detecting 8-methoxypsoralen in the ocular lens. Science 197:1287, 1997

66. Lerman S: Ocular phototoxicity and psoralen plus ultraviolet radiation (320–400 nm) therapy: an experimental and clinical evaluation. J Natl Cancer Inst 69:287, 1982

67. Jeffes EB III, McCullough JL, Pittelkow MR, et al: Methotrexate therapy of psoriasis: differential sensitivity of proliferating lymphoid and epithelial cells to the cytotoxic and growth-inhibitory effects of methotrexate. J Invest Dermatol 104:183, 1995

68. Roenigk HH Jr, Auerbach R, Maibach H, et al: Methotrexate in psoriasis: consensus conference. J Am Acad Dermatol 38:478, 1996

69. Gilbert SC, Lintmalm G, Menter A, et al: Methotrexate-induced cirrhosis requiring liver transplantation in three patients with psoriasis: a word of caution in light of the expanding use of this "steroid-sparing" agent. Arch Intern Med 150:889, 1990

70. Al-Awadhi A, Dale P, McKendry RJ: Pancytopenia associated with low dose methotrexate therapy: a regional survey. J Rheumatol 20:1121, 1993

71. Lebwohl M: Acitretin in combination with UVB or PUVA. J Am Acad Dermatol 4:S22, 1999

72. Lebwohl M, Drake L, Menter A, et al: Consensus conference: acitretin in combination with UVB or PUVA in the treatment of psoriasis. J Am Acad Dermatol 45:544, 2001

73. Roenigk HH Jr, Callen JP, Guzzo CA, et al: Effects of acitretin on the liver. J Am Acad Dermatol 41:585, 1999

74. Larsen FG, Jakobsen P, Knudsen J, et al: Conversion of acitretin to etretinate in psoriatic patients is influenced by ethanol. J Invest Dermatol 100:623, 1993

75. DiGiovanna JJ, Sollitto RB, Abangan DL, et al: Osteoporosis is a toxic effect of long-term etretinate therapy. Arch Dermatol 131:1263, 1995

76. Wilson DJ, Kay V, Charig M, et al: Skeletal hyperostosis and extraosseous calcification in patients receiving long-term etretinate (Tigason). Br J Dermatol 119:597, 1988

77. Stern RS, Fitzgerald E, Ellis CN, et al: The safety of etretinate as long-term therapy for psoriasis: results of the Etretinate Follow-Up Study. J Am Acad Dermatol 33:44, 1995

78. Lebwohl M, Ellis C, Gottlieb A, et al: Cyclosporine consensus conference: with emphasis on the treatment of psoriasis. J Am Acad Dermatol 39:464, 1998

79. Raman GV, Campbell SK, Farrer A, et al: Modifying effects of amlodipine on cyclosporin A–induced changes in renal function in patients with psoriasis. J Hypertens Suppl 16:S39, 1998

80. Zachariae H, Kragballe K, Hansen HE, et al: Renal biopsy findings in long-term cyclosporin treatment of psoriasis. Br J Dermatol 136:531, 1997

81. Jensen P, Hansen S, Moller B, et al: Skin cancer in kidney and heart transplant recipients and different long-term immunosuppressive therapy regimens. J Am Acad Dermatol 40:177, 1999

82. Srivastava T, Zwick DL, Rothberg PG, et al: Posttransplant lymphoproliferative disorder in pediatric renal transplantation. Pediatr Nephrol 13:748, 1999

83. van den Borne BE, Landewe RB, Houkes I, et al: No increased risk of malignancies and mortality in cyclosporin A–treated patients with rheumatoid arthritis. Arthritis Rheum 41:1930, 1998

84. Systemic tacrolimus (FK 506) is effective for the treatment of psoriasis in a double-blind, placebo-controlled study. The European FK 506 Multicenter Psoriasis Study Group. Arch Dermatol 132:419, 1996

85. FDA issues public health advisory informing health care providers of safety concerns associated with the user of two eczema drugs, Elidel and Protopic. FDA Talk Paper. U.S. Food and Drug Administration. March 10, 2005

86. Smith CH: Use of hydroxyurea in psoriasis. Clin Exp Dermatol 24:2, 1999

87. Gupta AK, Ellis CN, Siegel MT, et al: Sulfasalazine improves psoriasis: a double-blind analysis. Arch Dermatol 126:487, 1990

88. Roenigk HH Jr: Acitretin combination therapy. J Am Acad Dermatol 41:S18, 1999

89. Wong KC, Georgouras K: Low dose cyclosporin A and methotrexate in the treatment of psoriasis. Acta Derm Venereol 79:87, 1999

90. Paul BS, Momtaz K, Stern RS, et al: Combined methotrexate–ultraviolet B therapy in the treatment of psoriasis. J Am Acad Dermatol 7:758, 1982

91. Morison WL, Momtaz K, Parrish JA, et al: Combined methotrexate–PUVA therapy in the treatment of psoriasis. J Am Acad Dermatol 6:46, 1982

92. Stern RS, Laird N: The carcinogenic risk of treatments for severe psoriasis. Photochemotherapy Follow-up Study. Cancer 73:2759, 1994

93. Kirby B, Yates VM: Mycophenolate mofetil for psoriasis. Br J Dermatol 139:357, 1998

94. Epinette WW, Parker CM, Jones EL, et al: Mycophenolic acid for psoriasis: a review of pharmacology, long-term efficacy, and safety. J Am Acad Dermatol 17:962, 1987

95. Zackheim HS, Glogau RG, Fisher DA, et al: 6-Thioguanine treatment of psoriasis: experience in 81 patients. J Am Acad Dermatol 30:452, 1994

96. Silvis NG, Levine N: Pulse dosing of thioguanine in recalcitrant psoriasis. Arch Dermatol 135:433, 1999

97. Krueger GG: Selective targeting of T cell subsets: focus on alefacept: a remittive therapy for psoriasis. Expert Opin Biol Ther 2:431, 2002

98. Hodak E, David M: Alefacept: a review of the literature and practical guidelines for management. Dermatol Ther 17:383, 2004

99. Gordon KB, Langley RG: Remittive effects of intramuscular alefacept in psoriasis. J Drugs Dermatol 2:624, 2003

100. Lebwohl M, Tyring SK, Hamilton TK, et al: A novel targeted T-cell modulator, efalizumab, for plaque psoriasis. Efalizumab Study Group. N Engl J Med 349:2004, 2003

101. Leonardi CL: Efalizumab in the treatment of psoriasis. Dermatol Ther 17:393, 2004

102. Gordon KB, Papp KA, Hamilton TK, et al: Efalizumab for patients with moderate to severe plaque psoriasis: a randomized controlled trial. Efalizumab Study Group. JAMA 290:3073, 2003

103. Leonardi CL, Powers JL, Matheson RT, et al: Etanercept as monotherapy in patients with psoriasis. Etanercept Psoriasis Study Group. N Engl J Med 349:2014, 2003

104. Brown SL, Greene MH, Gershon SK, et al: Tumor necrosis factor antagonist therapy and lymphoma development: twenty-six cases reported to the Food and Drug Administration. Arthritis Rheum 46:3151, 2002

105. Chaudhari U, Romano P, Mulcahy LD, et al: Efficacy and safety of infliximab monotherapy for plaque-type psoriasis: a randomized trial. Lancet 357:1842, 2001

106. Keane J, Gershon S, Wise RP, et al: Tuberculosis associated with infliximab, a tumor necrosis factor alpha-neutralizing agent. N Engl J Med 345:1098, 2001

107. Patel T, Gordon KB: Adalimumab: efficacy and safety in psoriasis and rheumatoid arthritis. Dermatol Ther 17:427, 2004

38 Eczematous Disorders, Atopic Dermatitis, and Ichthyoses

Seth R. Stevens, M.D.

Eczematous Disorders

Eczematous dermatitis, or eczema, is a skin disease that is characterized by erythematous vesicular, weeping, and crusting patches. Although the term eczema is often used as a diagnosis, it can in fact be used appropriately to describe lesions seen in several diseases. Itching is a characteristic symptom, and epidermal intercellular edema (spongiosis) is a characteristic histopathologic finding of eczematous conditions. The term eczema is also commonly used to describe atopic dermatitis [*see* Atopic Dermatitis, *below*].

CONTACT DERMATITIS

Contact dermatitis, a paradigmatic example of an eczematous disorder, is common and well studied [*see Chapter 39*]. Contact dermatitis can be either allergic or irritant in etiology. Allergic contact dermatitis differs from other eczematous disorders in that determination of the offending contactant is an important part of the evaluation. If the patient's history does not provide the answer, the body site of the lesion may (e.g., head involvement in allergy to paraphenylenediamine in hair dye). Patch testing may be required to confirm the diagnosis.[1]

The manifestations of irritant contact dermatitis are similar to those of allergic contact dermatitis[2]; in the irritant form, however, the mechanism is not immunologic. Given sufficient concentration and duration of contact, offending agents will induce irritation in anyone's skin. Detergents, acids, alkalis, solvents, formaldehyde, and fiberglass are common causes.

SEBORRHEIC DERMATITIS

Seborrheic dermatitis is another common eczematous condition [*see Chapter 36*]. Clinically, seborrheic dermatitis may exist without vesicle formation. Lesional morphology is usually a greasy scale on erythematous patches; however, the scale may be dry and the patches may have an orange hue. Scalp, eyebrows, mustache area, nasolabial folds, and chest are typical areas of involvement. Psoriasis may be part of the differential diagnosis. Treatment is with shampoos containing selenium sulfide, zinc pyrithione, tar, or ketoconazole; emollients; and mild (nonfluorinated) topical steroids. Antimicrobial therapy directed at the commensal yeast *Pityrosporum ovale* can be effective, although a causative role of the organism remains unproved.

OTHER ECZEMATOUS DERMATITIDES

Two other eczematous dermatitides are nummular eczema and dyshidrotic eczema (pompholyx). Nummular eczema describes well-demarcated, coin-shaped eczematous patches that are usually 2 to 4 cm (rarely more than 10 cm) in diameter. The lesions are quite pruritic and require potent topical steroids, antihistamines, and, occasionally, intralesional or systemic corticosteroids for treatment. Dyshidrotic eczema presents as a vesicular eruption of the hands and feet, accompanied on rare occasions by hyperhidrosis. Typically, 1 to 2 mm vesicles appear on the sides of fingers, although more extensive involvement can occur. Treatment is with compresses and soaks, antipruritics,

topical steroids, and, in severe recalcitrant cases, systemic corticosteroids. Photochemotherapy with topical psoralen and ultraviolet A irradiation (PUVA) may also be effective.

Atopic Dermatitis

Atopic dermatitis (AD) is a common chronic inflammatory dermatosis that generally begins in infancy. The term atopy was coined in the early 1920s to describe the associated triad of asthma, allergic rhinitis, and dermatitis.[3] Children with AD are at increased high risk of developing asthma and allergic rhinitis, and the risk is further increased for patients with a family history of atopy.[4] The role of reaginic antibodies and allergies in the etiology of AD is controversial; in 80% of patients with AD, however, serum immunoglobulin IgE is elevated, sometimes markedly.

ETIOLOGY AND PATHOGENESIS

The expression of AD is a complex integration of environmental and genetic factors. The lifetime prevalence is estimated to be 30% of the population,[5-7] possibly because of increasing contact with causative agents in the environment. Epidemiologic data suggest a genetic influence—25% of dizygotic twins and 75% of monozygotic twins are concordant for AD.[8] The condition develops in 60% of children who have one affected parent and in 80% of children with two affected parents.[9] The defect is likely carried in the immune system, because both antigen-specific IgE reactivity and AD have been transplanted from an AD-affected bone marrow donor to a previously unaffected recipient.[10] Candidate genes continue to be investigated.[11]

AD can be quickly exacerbated by environmental trigger factors.[12] Wool, lanolin, and harsh detergents are particularly irritating. Emotional stress can also lead to flares, which are characterized by increased itch, erythema, vesiculation, and excoriation, as well as expanded area of involvement. The role of airborne and foodborne allergens is difficult to assess. Although patients with AD frequently have circulating dust mite antigen-specific IgE and Th2 CD4+ T cells,[13] hyposensitization infrequently results in improvement. Contact urticaria to food occurs in AD,[14] but generalized exacerbation after eating is rare. In the absence of a strong supporting history, elimination diets are rarely effective in treating AD. A role has been frequently suggested for cow's milk in inducing AD; however, studies examining the association of AD and early feeding with cow's milk have shown varying results.[15,16] Meta-analyses indicate that exclusive breast-feeding during the first 3 months of life is associated with lower incidence rates of atopic dermatitis during childhood in children with a family history of atopy.[17]

Gut microflora may be a natural source of immune modulation that prevents atopic dermatitis. In a double-blind, randomized, placebo-controlled trial, a probiotic containing a strain of *Lactobacillus* was administered prenatally to mothers who had at least one first-degree relative with atopy and 6 months postnatally to their infants; the frequency of AD in the group receiving *Lactobacillus* was half that of the placebo group.[18] These findings suggest that impairment of the intestinal mucosal barrier may be involved in the pathogenesis of AD, and strengthening of the mucosal barrier with probiotic bacteria may help prevent AD in high-risk infants. Although intriguing, these results await confirmation.

Mechanisms have been proposed to explain a link between *Staphylococcus aureus* and exacerbations of AD,[19] including effects of cell wall constituents to increase expression of IgE, IgE receptor, and enterotoxin B, a superantigen that activates T cells in an antigen-independent fashion.[20]

The apparent paradox of reduced cell-mediated immunity[21,22] and hyperimmunoglobulinemia E seen in AD is addressed by the so-called Th1/Th2 model of helper T cells. In this model of the murine immune system, CD4[+] T cells are divided into two mutually exclusive classes on the basis of cytokine secretion: Th1 cells, which secrete cytokines that promote cell-mediated immunity (e.g., interleukin-2 [IL-2], interferon gamma), and Th2 cells, which secrete cytokines that promote humoral immunity and eosinophil function (e.g., IL-4 and IL-5). Atopy, including AD, has been seen as the paradigmatic condition of a so-called Th1-deficient state. Refinements have shown a heterogeneity of responses within different AD lesions, however. The current model is that blood and acute lesions of AD patients are more often dominated by Th2 cells, whereas chronic lesions are more often dominated by Th1 cells.[23]

Hyperstimulatory dendritic antigen-presenting cells (Langerhans cells) are present in patients with AD.[24] One proposed mechanism for the augmented function of Langerhans cells in AD is the binding of antigen-specific IgE and antigen to the IgE receptors on Langerhans cells as a means of antigen focusing.[25] Another antigen-presenting cell, the monocyte, also manifests altered function in AD. Cyclic adenosine monophosphate (cAMP) phosphodiesterase has increased activity in monocytes of patients with AD—leading to hyperproduction of prostaglandin E_2, among other effects. Increased cAMP phosphodiesterase in AD may explain aberrant adrenergic responses, and the increased prostaglandin E_2 leads to diminished interferon-gamma production. Additionally, monocytes secrete IL-10 in AD, which further augments the so-called Th2 responses.[26] Altered cyclic nucleotide metabolism leads to excessive release of histamine by basophils and, potentially, to mast cell degranulation. High levels of cAMP phosphodiesterase are found in the umbilical cord blood of infants of AD-affected parents.[27] This finding may indicate an early, if not primary, defect in the disease that may become the basis of a diagnostic laboratory test.

Because IL-5 is a critical eosinophil growth factor and activating cytokine, blood eosinophilia may be expected to occur in a Th2 disease such as AD[28]; tissue eosinophilia, however, is variable. Cutaneous endothelial cells are also activated in AD, leading to increased expression of adhesion molecules and recruitment of leukocytes into the skin (i.e., dermatitis).

DIAGNOSIS

AD remains a clinical diagnosis. Major diagnostic criteria are (1) personal or family history of atopy (AD, allergic rhinitis, allergic conjunctivitis, allergic blepharitis, or asthma); (2) characteristic morphology and distribution of lesions; (3) pruritus; and (4) chronic or chronically recurring dermatosis. Several minor features can be added [*see Table 1*].[14] Pruritus is a consistent feature of AD. The lack of itching or of another major diagnostic criterion should prompt consideration of alternative diagnoses [*see Differential Diagnosis, below*]. Cutaneous signs can vary, depending on the age of the lesions.

Acute lesions of AD are eczematous—erythematous, scaling, and papulovesicular. Weeping and crusted lesions may develop [*see Figure 1*]. Scratching results acutely in linear excoriations, presenting as erosions or a hemorrhagic crust. In extremely severe cases, exfoliative dermatitis (erythroderma) may occur, with generalized redness, scaling, weeping, and crusting. There may be accompanying systemic toxicity, sepsis, lymphadenopathy, altered thermoregulation (either hyperthermia or hypothermia), and high-output cardiac failure. Erythroderma is a potentially life-threatening condition.

Chronic lesions tend not to be eczematous (thus, atopic eczema is not an ideal synonym for AD). Instead, lichenified plaques [*see Figure 2*] or nodules predominate. Lichenification denotes areas of thickened skin divided by deep linear furrows. Lichenified plaques result from repeated rubbing or scratching and thus often occur in areas of predilection, such as the popliteal and antecubital fossae. As is typical of lesions in AD, lichenification is poorly demarcated. There may be accompanying acute signs. Lichenified lesions are very difficult to treat; once established, they may persist for months even with adequate therapy and avoidance of rubbing or scratching.

Clinical expression of AD also varies with the age of the patient. The infantile stage of AD occurs up to approximately 2 years of age. Of all cases of AD, approximately 90% arise before

---

Table 1 Diagnostic Criteria for Atopic Dermatitis[14]

Major criteria
  Personal or family history of atopy (atopic dermatitis, allergic rhinitis, allergic conjunctivitis, allergic blepharitis, or asthma)
  Characteristic morphology and distribution of lesions
  Pruritus
  Chronic or chronically recurring dermatosis
Minor features
  Hyperimmunoglobulinemia E
  Food intolerance
  Intolerance to wool and lipid solvents
  Recurrent skin infections
  Xerosis
  Sweat-induced pruritus
  White (not red) dermatographism
  Ichthyosis
  Chronically scaling scalp
  Accentuation of hair follicles
  Recurrent conjunctivitis
  Anterior subcapsular cataracts and keratoconus
  Morgan line, or Dennie sign (single or double creases in the lower eyelids)
  Periorbital darkening (allergic shiner)
  Pityriasis alba (hypopigmented, scaling patches, typically on the cheeks)
  Cheilitis
  Anterior neck folds
  Keratosis pilaris (perifollicular papules with keratotic plugs, typically on the arms and thighs)
  Nipple eczema
  Hyperlinear palms (increased folds, typically on the thenar or hypothenar eminence)
  Recurrent hand and foot dermatitis
  Exacerbation of symptoms by environmental or emotional factors

the fifth year and 60% in the first year of life; onset before 2 months of age is unusual, however.[8] During infancy, ill-defined, erythematous scaling patches and confluent, edematous papules and vesicles are typical. These lesions may become crusted and exudative. Intense pruritus leads to scratching, which induces linear excoriations and, with time, lichenification. Before the infant begins to crawl, the scalp and face are most often involved [see Figure 3], although lesions may be seen anywhere. After the child begins crawling, the extensor surfaces—particularly the knees—become involved. Involvement of fingers can be severe if the child sucks them frequently. Intense pruritus can lead to sleep disturbances of child and parents. Other features may arise [see Table 1]. Perifollicular accentuation and papules are commonly seen at any point in the life of an atopic patient, particularly in persons of Asian or African ancestry.

During childhood, the clinical features evolve into those seen in adults. Lesions tend to become less eczematous and drier, with increasing flexural and neck involvement. Scaling, fissured, and crusted hands may become especially troublesome. Infraorbital folds (sometimes called Morgan lines or the Dennie sign) and pityriasis alba can appear. Chronic or chronically relapsing pruritic, erythematous, papulovesicular eruptions that progress to scaling, lichenified dermatitis in a flexural distribution typify adult AD. Extensive areas of skin may be involved, including the face, chest, neck, flanks, and hands. Areas of dyspigmentation may result from repeated skin trauma. Approximately 10% to 15% of childhood AD persists after puberty.[8]

AD that begins after 20 years of age has been termed adult-onset atopic dermatitis.[29] This condition should be considered in patients with characteristic features of AD.

There are many associated features of AD. Asthma and allergic rhinitis, the major and minor criteria, respectively, have already been mentioned. Another important association, cutaneous infection, is related to diminished cutaneous cell-mediated immunity and defective chemotaxis. S. aureus is usually found on AD skin, and its density correlates with lesion severity.[30] Although such observations have implicated S. aureus as a cause of AD,[19,31] it is also clear that reduction in AD lesions reduces bacterial colonization.[32] Regardless, the high bacterial counts in lesional skin and the relative ease of their reduction suggest the desirability of extra efforts (e.g., use of topical steroids) to reduce the presence of S. aureus before elective procedures are performed through involved skin. Frank infection also occurs more commonly in AD, which results in pustules and oozing, crusted lesions.

Cutaneous fungal and viral infections also occur frequently and with increased severity in patients with AD. Eczema herpeticum, an extensive eruption of 2 to 3 mm vesicles, pustules, and punched-out erosions caused by herpes simplex virus, may coalesce into extensive areas of eroded skin. Frequently, the condition is most severe on the face (where it often arises from a herpetic lesion) and diminishes as it progresses to the trunk and extremities. Secondary bacterial infection is common. Lymphadenopathy, fever, and malaise may develop. Antiviral and antibiotic therapy can be lifesaving and should be started empirically upon presentation. Tzanck test, viral culture, and direct fluorescent antibody detection of viral antigens can confirm the diagnosis.

Molluscum contagiosum and common warts are also problematic in patients with AD, as are dermatophyte infections. Because of similar appearance, foot eczema must be distinguished from tinea pedis by potassium hydroxide preparation or fungal culture.

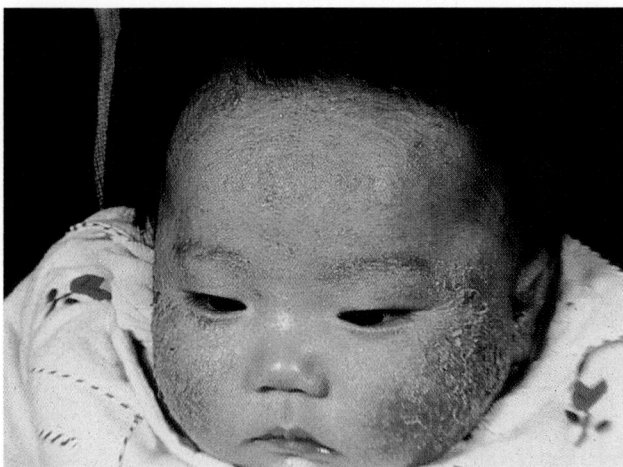

Figure 1 Extensive, severe, weeping, crusted acute eczematous patches on the face of this infant are characteristic of patients in this age group.

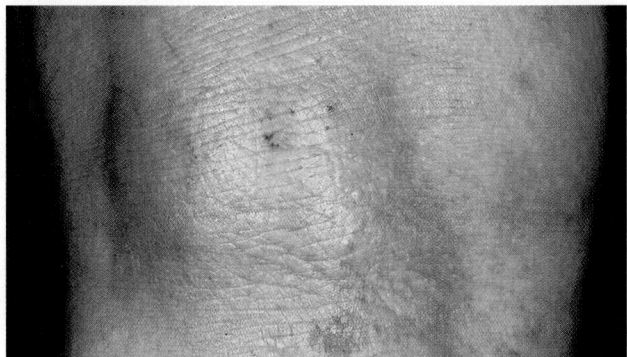

Figure 2 Lichenified patches appear after chronic rubbing of eczematous patches. These lesions are characteristic of chronic allergic contact dermatitis and atopic dermatitis.

Numerous ocular complications of AD exist.[33] These include anterior subcapsular cataracts, retinal detachment, keratoconus, blepharitis, conjunctivitis, and iritis.

DIFFERENTIAL DIAGNOSIS

The differential diagnosis of AD includes the eczematous conditions and ichthyoses described in this chapter and other immunologic, metabolic, neoplastic, and rheumatologic disorders [see Table 2]. Because 80% to 85% of patients with occupational hand dermatitis have AD, the possibility of coexisting AD and contact dermatitis needs to be considered. Another important element of the differential diagnosis is cutaneous T cell lymphoma. Cutaneous T cell lymphoma can arise clinically as scaling, erythematous patches or exfoliative erythroderma. The classic distribution—near axillae, buttocks, and groin—is distinct from that of AD, and patches are frequently well demarcated. There is often sufficient clinical overlap between the two conditions, however, to necessitate further investigation, including histology, immunophenotyping, and gene-rearrangement analysis of T cell receptors. Cutaneous T cell lymphoma can arise in patients with AD, and the lack of conclusive clinical or laboratory tests for either disease can make distinction difficult. Reassessment from time to time in such cases is recommended.[34]

TREATMENT

Reduction of Trigger Factors

Reduction of trigger factors (e.g., harsh chemicals, detergents, and wool) and avoidance of occupations that require contact with trigger factors (e.g., hairdressing, nursing, and construction) can be helpful.[35] Appropriate behaviors should be taught to patients and parents early during life, when habits are more easily formed.[36,37]

Bland Emollients

The use of mild, nonalkali soaps and frequent use of emollients are important elements in the long-term management of AD. Because moisture evaporating off the skin can trigger flares, bathing is sometimes discouraged. A better approach is the prompt application of an emollient such as petrolatum (finishing within 3 minutes of the end of the bath), which can serve to seal the moisture from the bath. Lotions and creams containing high amounts of water are usually inadequate, however, and can actually worsen AD. Products containing hydroxy acids, phenol, or urea can reduce dryness and scaling, but these can sting inflamed skin and should therefore be used with caution. Because of a specific reduction of ceramides in AD, a lotion that provides excess ceramides relative to other lipids has been shown to have a therapeutic advantage in AD.[38] Bubble baths and scented salts and oils can be irritating. Scalp care should include a bland shampoo. Topical tar products, such as shampoos and bath solutions, and topical creams and lotions containing 5% to 10% liquor carbonis detergens can help. Baths, soaks, and compresses with Burow solution can ameliorate crusted, infected, eczematous patches. Cotton clothing, washed to remove finishing (which often releases formaldehyde), is preferable to wool or synthetics.

Corticosteroids

Topical corticosteroids are another mainstay of therapy. Application immediately after bathing improves cutaneous pene-

tration. Lowering the risk of side effects with less potent preparations must be balanced against gaining control of a flare quickly with more potent preparations. Long-term use of inadequately potent topical corticosteroids may pose a greater risk of adverse effects than brief use of more potent agents followed by a rapid taper to bland emollients. Because steroid-induced cutaneous atrophy is a greater risk on the face, in intertriginous areas (e.g., groin, axillae, and inframammary folds), and under diapers, less potent steroids (e.g., hydrocortisone and desonide) should be used in these areas, and they should be used with particular caution. For the remainder of the body, midpotency preparations, such as 0.1% triamcinolone acetonide, are helpful. More potent ointments, such as fluocinonide and desoximetasone, are useful for lichenified plaques. Flurandrenolide tape is useful for nodular prurigo (so-called picker's nodules) because it also physically protects the area from manipulation. For the scalp, solutions are preferred.

Systemic corticosteroids (e.g., prednisone, 20 to 80 mg/day orally) may be useful to treat severe, acute flares. Because of the risks of gastrointestinal, endocrine, skeletal, central nervous system, and cardiovascular complications, however, they should not be used more than twice yearly.

Calcineurin Inhibitors

The steroid-free topical calcineurin inhibitors, tacrolimus ointment and pimecrolimus cream, are effective alternatives to topical corticosteroids. These agents do not cause the skin atrophy associated with prolonged use of topical corticosteroids and, therefore, are useful for treating skin on the face and neck.

The macrolide antibiotic tacrolimus (formerly FK506) has been found to be effective in treating moderate to severe atopic dermatitis. The efficacy of tacrolimus has been shown in several randomized, controlled trials.[39-41] The most common adverse side effects are skin burning, flulike symptoms, skin erythema, and headache.[41] Topical tacrolimus is available in 0.1% and 0.03% concentrations. In children with moderate and severe AD, treatment with tacrolimus ointment (0.03%) was shown to be superior to conventional 1% hydrocortisone acetate.[42]

The ascomycin derivative pimecrolimus (ASM 981) cream is a cell-selective cytokine inhibitor that was specifically developed for treatment of inflammatory skin diseases. Its mechanism of action is similar to that of topical tacrolimus. Two independent randomized, multicenter studies found pimecrolimus to be effective in infants and children with AD.[43] Another randomized, multicenter study found that pimecrolimus was effective in preventing AD flares, which reduced the need for topical corticosteroids.[44] In adults, pimecrolimus was found to be effective and well tolerated, and it reduced the incidence of AD flare.[45]

A meta-analysis of 16 trials involving more than 5,300 patients showed success rates of tacrolimus and pimecrolimus to be statistically similar; however, tacrolimus success rates were numerically higher than those of pimecrolimus, and tacrolimus was used in patients with more severe disease.[46] The efficacy of these drugs must be balanced against a potential cancer risk. The Food and Drug Administration recently issued a warning that these drugs should be used only as directed and only after other eczema treatments have failed to work.[47]

Other Therapies

Antihistamines can sometimes be helpful in breaking the itch-scratch cycle in AD. Sedating antihistamines, such as hydroxyzine and diphenhydramine, are particularly useful—especially

Table 2 Differential Diagnosis of Atopic Dermatitis

Type	Disorders
Dermatitides	Allergic contact dermatitis Dermatitis herpetiformis Irritant contact dermatitis (may be concomitant with atopic dermatitis) Nummular eczema Seborrheic dermatitis
Ichthyoses	Ichthyosis vulgaris
Immunologic disorders	Graft versus host disease HIV-associated dermatosis Hyperimmunoglobulinemia E syndrome Wiskott-Aldrich syndrome
Infectious diseases	Scabies Dermatophytosis
Metabolic disorders	Zinc deficiency Various inborn errors of metabolism
Neoplastic disorders	Cutaneous T cell lymphoma
Rheumatologic disorders	Dermatomyositis

when itching prevents sleep[48]; however, the sedative properties of antihistamines may limit their use in AD. Cetirizine, a sedating antihistamine, appears to be well tolerated in infants. A multinational, randomized, placebo-controlled trial examined the effects of long-term treatment with cetirizine on infants with AD; the drug proved to be safe, and it reduced the need for topical corticosteroids in patients with more severe disease.[49] Nonsedating antihistamines such as fexofenadine and loratadine are less useful. Doxepin, a tricyclic antidepressant known to have antihistaminic effects, can be beneficial when applied topically in a 5% cream.[50]

Virtually every phototherapy regimen has been reported to ameliorate AD. Some patients cannot tolerate the heat generated by the equipment, however—particularly that used in UVB irradiation. In addition to UVB, the following can be beneficial: UVA, longwave UVA1, narrow-band UVB, UVA-UVB, and PUVA. Extracorporeal photochemotherapy (photopheresis) is reported to be effective therapy for recalcitrant disease.[51] Phototherapies are expensive, and prolonged use of PUVA has been linked to an increased risk of melanoma.[52] Although some patients may benefit from natural sunlight, the risk of sunburn and induction of malignancy by ultraviolet light must be considered.

Antimicrobials are obviously important for patients with infection. Less clear is whether antimicrobial agents can directly treat AD by reducing bacterial products thought to exacerbate the condition. Antistaphylococcal therapy has been advocated for use in patients with AD; however, a double-blind, placebo-controlled study of flucloxacillin did not show improvement in AD despite reduced bacterial counts.[53] Ketoconazole, likewise, has been used; its success, however, may be the result of anti-inflammatory, rather than antifungal, effects.

More advanced therapeutic options exist for severe, recalcitrant AD. The altered expression of cytokines in AD [see Etiology and Pathogenesis, above] has led investigators to explore the use of interferon gamma. Clinical trials have demonstrated that for some patients, daily subcutaneous administration of interferon gamma is effective in reducing both signs and symptoms of AD[54,55] and that long-term treatment can maintain the benefit.[56] However, moderate results and high costs make interferon gamma less viable as a treatment option.

Oral cyclosporine (2.5 to 5 mg/kg/day orally),[57,58] methotrexate (15 to 25 mg/wk orally), and azathioprine (100 to 200 mg/day orally) can be used in severe,[59] recalcitrant disease provided that patients are monitored for adverse effects specific to those agents.

Traditional Chinese herbal medicine has been found to be effective in the treatment of AD, both in children[60] and in adults,[61] although the efficacy of this treatment remains controversial.[62] The mechanisms of action of these preparations are unclear. A small, randomized, placebo-controlled study found topical treatment with St. John's wort to be significantly superior to placebo in patients with moderate AD.[63] Although evening primrose oil has for many years been proposed to be effective in AD, a well-controlled study failed to show any benefit to patients taking either evening primrose oil or a combination of evening primrose oil and fish oil, as compared with those receiving placebo.[64] Patients should be cautioned that herbal remedies are not risk free and may carry a potential for hepatotoxicity, cardiomyopathy, and other adverse effects; such remedies should be monitored, as should any other treatment. To avoid potential adverse drug reactions, physicians should identify any herbal remedies used by patients.[65]

Topical vitamin B_{12} was found to be significantly superior to placebo in reducing the extent and severity of AD in a randomized, multicenter phase III study[66]; however, larger trials are needed to establish the efficacy of this therapy. The cAMP phosphodiesterase inhibitor cipamfylline in cream form has been shown to be more effective than placebo but significantly less effective than hydrocortisone cream in the treatment of AD.[67] The importance of well-controlled studies to assess efficacy of treatments must be stressed because AD patients on the placebo arms of most controlled studies tend to show benefit, sometimes marked.

Ichthyoses

The ichthyoses are a group of diseases of cornification that are characterized by excessive scaling.[68] Etiologies of the ichthyoses are diverse, including genetic defects of structural proteins and enzymes, as well as acquired forms. Only the major clinical variants will be discussed here.

MAJOR VARIANTS

Ichthyosis Vulgaris

Ichthyosis vulgaris, the most common form of ichthyosis, is found in approximately one in 300 births. This autosomal dominant condition presents as dry skin with fine scaling. The extensor surfaces of extremities are the most commonly affected areas. Ichthyosis vulgaris can occur concomitantly with keratosis pilaris and can also be associated with AD. Age at onset is typically between 3 months and 12 months. Implicated etiologic factors include reduced filaggrin (filament-aggregating protein) and its precursor profilaggrin, whose normal functions are to allow for aggregation of keratin filaments and to serve as sources of compounds that hydrate the skin. The clinical severity of ichthyosis vulgaris correlates with the degree of reduction in filaggrin and profilaggrin. Another possible etiologic factor is the reduced activity of proteases that normally lead to dissociation of keratinocytes.[69]

X-Linked Ichthyosis

Recessive X-linked ichthyosis occurs in approximately one in 2,000 to one in 6,000 male infants. Although collodion membrane may be present at birth, the skin is usually normal, with fine scaling beginning at 1 to 3 weeks of life. Typically, the scales are thick and dark, giving the skin a dirty appearance. Extensor distribution—combined with involvement of the sides of the neck and preauricular skin and sparing the flexural areas—is typical. Steroid sulfatase deficiency is an etiologic factor, causing an increase in cholesterol sulfate and a decrease in cholesterol in the stratum corneum.[70] The accumulated cholesterol sulfate may inhibit proteolysis—a process similar to the inhibition seen in ichthyosis vulgaris. Prenatal diagnosis is available, and gene therapy may be on the horizon.

Lamellar Ichthyosis

Lamellar ichthyosis occurs in one in 300,000 births. It is inherited in an autosomal recessive pattern. Collodion membrane may be present at birth but is then shed, revealing characteristic large, platelike scales. Erythroderma may be present, albeit difficult to discern because of the thickness of the scales. Ectropion is present in most patients and can give rise to ophthalmic complications. Lamellar ichthyosis is often caused by mutations in the gene encoding the enzyme transglutaminase 1.[71]

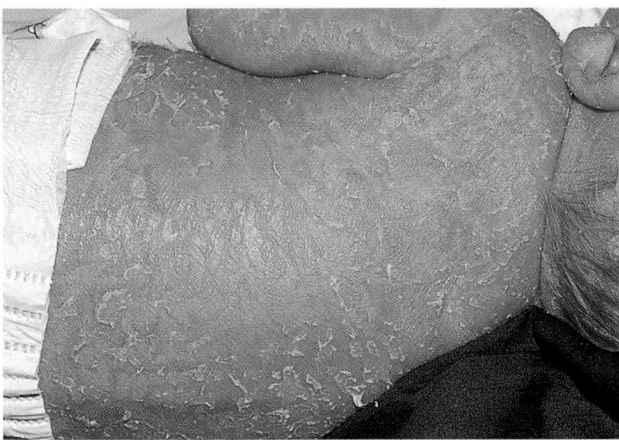

Figure 3   **Erythroderma (total body erythema) and extensive scaling are seen in this infant with congenital ichthyosiform erythroderma.**

Congenital Ichthyosiform Erythroderma

Formerly, congenital ichthyosiform erythroderma [*see Figure 3*] was considered to be a variant of lamellar ichthyosis. Both are inherited as autosomal recessive traits, and collodion membrane may be present at birth in both conditions. Ectropion, eclabion (eversion of the lip), and erythroderma can also occur. Like patients with lamellar ichthyosis, patients with congenital ichthyosiform erythroderma may have platelike scales on the lower extremities, but scales are fine and white on other parts of the body. Also in contrast to lamellar ichthyosis, X-linked ichthyosis, and ichthyosis vulgaris—whose lesions are scaly because of an abnormal ability to desquamate (so-called retention hyperkeratoses)—the lesions of congenital ichthyosiform erythroderma are scaly because of increased production of keratinocytes (so-called hyperproliferative ichthyosis).

Epidermolytic Hyperkeratosis

Epidermolytic hyperkeratosis (formerly called bullous congenital ichthyosiform erythroderma) is autosomal dominant in inheritance. The combinations of large blisters and erythema with denuded skin that appear at birth may be confused with epidermolysis bullosa, staphylococcal scalded skin syndrome, or toxic epidermal necrolysis. Several months to 1 year after

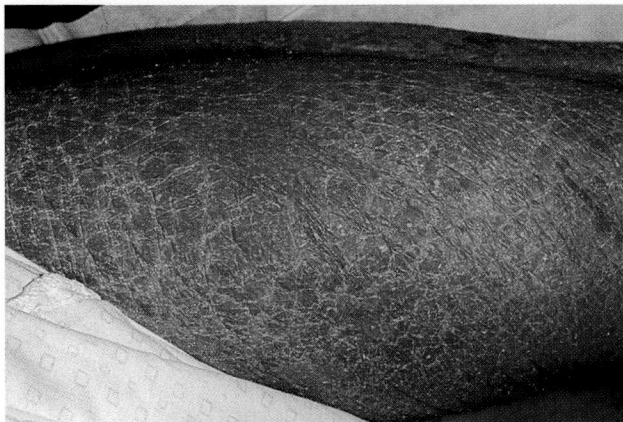

Figure 4   **This patient developed marked scaling (acquired ichthyosis) over a 6-month period. Investigation revealed non-Hodgkin lymphoma.**

birth, the blisters become less prominent, and thick, verrucous plaques comprising rows of hyperkeratotic ridges develop. Flexural skin is usually involved, but the disease can be more extensive. Bacterial colonization leads to a clinically significant foul odor. Abnormal keratin gene expression is the etiologic basis of this condition.[71]

Acquired Ichthyosis

Acquired ichthyoses have been associated with numerous systemic diseases and medications. Although the onset of scaling is commonly a manifestation of dryness or ichthyosis vulgaris, patients with unusual manifestations or with severe or recalcitrant disease warrant further investigation. Endocrinopathies (e.g., thyroid disease), autoimmune diseases, infectious diseases (e.g., HIV), and malignancies such as lymphomas [*see Figure 4*] and other carcinomas have been associated with the onset of ichthyosiform dermatosis.

TREATMENT

The standard therapy for the ichthyoses is emollients (e.g., petrolatum) and keratolytics (e.g., lactic acid with or without propylene glycol).[72] Lactic acid should be used cautiously in neonates to avoid causing excess absorption. Oral retinoids (which require lipid monitoring) can be helpful, particularly in the management of X-linked ichthyosis, congenital ichthyosiform erythroderma, and lamellar ichthyosis. Epidermolytic hyperkeratosis is the most difficult of these conditions to treat because of the risk of blistering induced by therapeutic agents. Antimicrobial agents can be useful to reduce the odor caused by bacterial colonization.

The author has no commercial relationships with manufacturers of products or providers of services discussed in this chapter.

References

1. Marks JG Jr, Belsito DV, DeLeo VA, et al: North American Contact Dermatitis patch-test results, 1998-2000. Am J Contact Dermat 14:59, 2003

2. Denig NI, Hoke AW, Maibach HI: Irritant contact dermatitis: clues to causes, clinical characteristics, and control. Postgrad Med 103:199, 1998

3. Coca AF, Cooke RA: On the classification of the phenomena of hypersensitiveness. J Immunol 8:163, 1922

4. Gustafsson D, Sjoberg O, Foucard T: Development of allergies and asthma in infants and young people with atopic dermatitis: a prospective follow-up to 7 years of age. Allergy 55:240, 2000

5. Worldwide variation in prevalence of symptoms of asthma, allergic rhinoconjunctivitis, and atopic eczema: The International Study of Asthma and Allergies in Childhood (ISAAC) Steering Committee. Lancet 351:1225, 1998

6. Laughter D, Istvan JA, Tofte SJ, et al: The prevalence of atopic dermatitis in Oregon schoolchildren. J Am Acad Dermatol 43:649, 2000

7. Foley P, Zuo Y, Plunkett A, et al: The frequency of common skin conditions in preschool-age children in Australia: atopic dermatitis. Arch Dermatol 137:293, 2001

8. Levy RM, Gelfand JM, Yan AC: The epidemiology of atopic dermatitis. Clin Dermatol 21:109, 2003

9. Uehara M, Kimura C: Descendant family history of atopic dermatitis. Acta Derm Venereol 73:62, 1993

10. Agosti JM, Sprenger JD, Lum LG, et al: Transfer of allergen-specific IgE-mediated hypersensitivity with allogeneic bone marrow transplantation. N Engl J Med 319:1623, 1998

11. Haagerup A, Bjerke T, Schiotz PO, et al: Atopic dermatitis: a total genome-scan for susceptibility genes. Acta Derm Venereol 84:346, 2004

12. Leung DY, Boguniewicz M, Howell MD, et al: New insights into atopic dermatitis. J Clin Invest 113:651, 2004

13. Bos JD, Wierenga EA, Sillevis Smitt JH, et al: Immune dysregulation in atopic eczema. Arch Dermatol 128:1509, 1992

14. Hanifin JM, Rajka G: Diagnostic features of atopic dermatitis. Acta Derm Venereol Suppl (Stockh) 92:44, 1980

15. Saarinen KM, Juntunen-Backman K, Jarvenpaa AL, et al: Breast-feeding and the development of cows' milk protein allergy. Adv Exp Med Biol 478:121, 2000

16. Gustafsson D, Lowhagen T, Andersson K: Risk of developing atopic disease after early feeding with cows' milk based formula. Arch Dis Child 67:1008, 1992

17. Halken S: Prevention of allergic disease in childhood: clinical and epidemiological aspects of primary and secondary allergy prevention. Pediatr Allergy Immunol 15(suppl 16):4, 2004

18. Kalliomaki M, Salminen S, Poussa T, et al: Probiotics and prevention of atopic disease: 4-year follow-up of randomized placebo-controlled trial. Lancet 361:1869, 2003

19. Zoller TM, Wichelhaus TA, Hartung A, et al: Colonization with superantigens producing *Staphylococcus aureus* is associated with increased severity of atopic dermatitis. Clin Exp Allergy 30:994, 2000

20. Herz U, Bunikowski R, Renz H: Role of T cells in atopic dermatitis: new aspects on the dynamics of cytokine production and the contribution of bacterial superantigens. Int Arch Allergy Immunol 115:170, 1998

21. Rees J, Friedmann PS, Matthews JN: Contact sensitivity to dinitrochlorobenzene is impaired in atopic subjects. Arch Dermatol 126:1173, 1990

22. Akdis CA, Akdis M, Trautmann A, et al: Immune regulation in atopic dermatitis. Curr Opin Immunol 12:641, 2000

23. Grewe M, Bruijnzeel-Koomen CAFM, Schöpf E, et al: A role for Th1 and Th2 cells in the immunopathogenesis of atopic dermatitis. Immunol Today 19:359, 1998

24. Taylor RS, Baadsgaard O, Hammerberg C, et al: Hyperstimulatory CD1a+CD1b+CD36+ Langerhans cells are responsible for increased autologous T lymphocyte reactivity to lesional epidermal cells of patients with atopic dermatitis. J Immunol 147:3794, 1991

25. Stingl G, Maurer D: IgE-mediated allergen presentation via Fc epsilon RI on antigen-presenting cells. Int Arch Allergy Immunol 113:24, 1997

26. Hanifin JM, Chan SC: Monocyte phosphodiesterase abnormalities and dysregulation of lymphocyte function in atopic dermatitis. J Invest Dermatol 105(1 suppl):84S, 1995

27. Heskel NS, Chan SC, Thiel ML, et al: Elevated umbilical cord blood leukocyte cyclic adenosine monophosphate-phosphodiesterase activity in children with atopic parents. J Am Acad Dermatol 11:422, 1984

28. Uehara M, Izukura R, Sawai T: Blood eosinophilia in atopic dermatitis. Clin Exp Dermatol 15:264, 1990

29. Bannister MJ, Freeman S: Adult-onset atopic dermatitis. Australas J Dermatol 41:225, 2000

30. Roll A, Cozzio A, Fisher B, et al: Microbial colonization and atopic dermatitis. Curr Opin Allergy Clin Immunol 4:373, 2004

31. Hofer MF, Lester MR, Schlievert PM, et al: Upregulation of IgE synthesis by staphylococcal toxic shock syndrome toxin-1 in peripheral blood mononuclear cells from patients with atopic dermatitis. Clin Exp Allergy 25:1218, 1995

32. Nilsson EJ, Henning CG, Magnusson J: Topical corticosteroids and *Staphylococcus aureus* in atopic dermatitis. J Am Acad Dermatol 27:29, 1992

33. Rich LF, Hanifin JM: Ocular complications of atopic dermatitis and other eczemas. Int Ophthalmol Clin 25:61, 1985

34. Fletcher CL, Orchard GE, Hubbard V, et al: CD30(+) cutaneous lymphoma in association with atopic eczema. Arch Dermatol 140:449, 2004

35. Ellis C, Luger T, Abeck D, et al: International consensus conference on atopic dermatitis II (ICCAD II): clinical update and current treatment strategies. Br J Dermatol 148(suppl 63):3, 2003

36. McHenry PM, Williams HC, Bingham EA: Management of atopic eczema. Joint Workshop of the British Association of Dermatologists and the Research Unit of the Royal College of Physicians of London. BMJ 310:843, 1995

37. Hanifin JM, Cooper KD, Ho VC, et al: Guidelines of care for atopic dermatitis, developed in accordance with the American Academy of Dermatology (AAD)/American Academy of Dermatology Association "Administrative Regulations for Evidence-Based Clinical Practice Guidelines." J Am Acad Dermatol 50:391, 2004

38. Chamlin SL, Fao J, Frieden IJ, et al: Ceramide-dominant barrier repair lipids alleviate childhood atopic dermatitis: changes in barrier function provide a sensitive indicator of disease activity. J Am Acad Dermatol 47:198, 2002

39. Paller A, Eichenfield LF, Leung DY, et al: A 12-week study of tacrolimus ointment for the treatment of atopic dermatitis in pediatric patients. J Am Acad Dermatol 44(suppl 1):S47, 2001

40. Hanifin JM, Ling MR, Langley R, et al: Tacrolimus ointment for the treatment of atopic dermatitis in adult patients: part I, efficacy. J Am Acad Dermatol 44(suppl 1):S28, 2001

41. Soter NA, Fleisher AB Jr, Webster GF, et al: Tacrolimus ointment for the treatment of atopic dermatitis in adult patients: part II, safety. J Am Acad Dermatol 44(suppl 1):S39, 2001

42. Reitamo S, Harper J, Bos JD, et al: 0.03% Tacrolimus ointment applied once or twice daily is more efficacious than 1% hydrocortisone acetate in children with moderate to severe atopic dermatitis: results of a randomized double-blind controlled trial. Br J Dermatol 150:554, 2004

43. Eichenfield LF, Lucky AW, Boguniewicz M, et al: Safety and efficacy of pimecrolimus (ASM 981) cream 1% in the treatment of mild and moderate atopic dermatitis in children and adolescents. J Am Acad Dermatol 46:495, 2002

44. Wahn U, Bos JD, Goodfield M, et al: Efficacy and safety of pimecrolimus cream in the long-term management of atopic dermatitis in children. Pediatrics 110:e2, 2002

45. Meurer M, Fartasch M, Albrecht G, et al: Long-term efficacy and safety of pimecrolimus cream 1% in adults with moderate atopic dermatitis. Dermatology 208:365, 2004

46. Iskedjian M, Piwko C, Shear NH, et al: Topical calcineurin inhibitors in the treatment of atopic dermatitis: a meta-analysis of current evidence. Am J Clin Dermatol 5:267, 2004

47. FDA issues public health advisory informing health care providers of safety concerns associated with the user of two eczema drugs, Elidel and Protopic. FDA Talk Paper. U.S. Food and Drug Administration. March 10, 2005
http://www.fda.gov/bbs/topics/answers/2005/ANS01343.html

48. Klein PA, Clark RA: An evidence-based review of the efficacy of antihistamines in relieving pruritus in atopic dermatitis. Arch Dermatol 135:1522, 1999

49. Diepgen TL: Long-term treatment with cetirizine of infants with atopic dermatitis: a multi-country, double-blind, randomized, placebo-controlled trial (the ETAC trial) over 18 months. Early Treatment of the Atopic Child Study Group. Pediatr Allergy Immunol 13:278, 2002

50. Groene D, Martus P, Heyer G: Doxepin affects acetylcholine induced cutaneous reactions in atopic eczema. Exp Dermatol 10:110, 2001

51. Richter HI, Billmann-Eberwein C, Grewe M, et al: Successful monotherapy of severe and intractable atopic dermatitis by photopheresis. J Am Acad Dermatol 38:585, 1998

52. Stern RS: The risk of melanoma in association with long-term exposure to PUVA. J Am Acad Dermatol 44:755, 2001

53. Ewing CI, Ashcroft C, Gibbs AC, et al: Flucloxacillin in the treatment of atopic dermatitis. Br J Dermatol 138:1022, 1998

54. Hanifin JM, Schneider LC, Leung DY, et al: Recombinant interferon gamma therapy for atopic dermatitis. J Am Acad Dermatol 28:189, 1993

55. Ellis CN, Stevens SR, Blok BK, et al: Interferon-gamma therapy reduces blood leukocyte levels in patients with atopic dermatitis: correction with clinical improvement. Clin Immunol 92:49, 1999

56. Stevens SR, Hanifin JM, Hamilton T, et al: Long-term effectiveness and safety of recombinant human interferon gamma therapy for atopic dermatitis despite unchanged serum IgE levels. Arch Dermatol 134:799, 1998

57. Berth-Jones J, Graham-Brown RA, Marks R, et al: Long-term efficacy and safety of cyclosporin in severe adult atopic dermatitis. Br J Dermatol 136:76, 1997

58. Harper JI, Ahmed I, Barclay G, et al: Cyclosporin for severe childhood atopic dermatitis: short course versus continuous therapy. Br J Dermatol 142:52, 2000

59. Berth-Jones J, Takwale A, Tan E, et al: Azathioprine in severe adult atopic dermatitis: a double-blind, placebo-controlled, crossover trial. Br J Dermatol 147:324, 2002

60. Sheehan MP, Atherton DJ: A controlled trial of traditional Chinese medicinal plants in widespread non-exudative atopic eczema. Br J Dermatol 126:179, 1992

61. Sheehan MP, Atherton DJ: One-year follow up of children treated with Chinese medicinal herbs for atopic dermatitis. Br J Dermatol 130:488, 1994

62. Fung AY, Look PC, Chong LY, et al: A controlled trial of traditional Chinese herbal medicine in Chinese patients with recalcitrant atopic dermatitis. Int J Dermatol 38:387, 1999

63. Schempp CM, Windeck T, Hezel S, et al: Topical treatment of atopic dermatitis with St. John's wort cream: a randomized, placebo controlled, double blind half-side comparison. Phytomedicine 10(suppl 4):31, 2003

64. Berth Jones J, Graham Brown RA: Placebo-controlled trial of essential fatty acid supplementation in atopic dermatitis. Lancet 341:1557, 1993

65. Simpson EL, Basco M, Hanifin J: A cross-sectional survey of complementary and alternative medicine use in patients with atopic dermatitis. Am J Contact Dermat 14:144, 2003

66. Stucker M, Pieck C, Stoerb C, et al: Topical vitamin B_{12}: a new therapeutic approach in atopic dermatitis: evaluation of efficacy and tolerability in a randomized, placebo-controlled multicentre clinical trial. Br J Dermatol 150:977, 2004

67. Griffiths CE, Van Leent EJ, Gilbert M, et al: Randomized comparison of the type 4 phosphodiesterase inhibitor cipamfylline cream, cream vehicle and hydrocortisone 17-butyrate cream for the treatment of atopic dermatitis. Br J Dermatol 147:299, 2002

68. Shwayder T: Disorders of keratinization: diagnosis and management. Am J Clin Dermatol 5:17, 2004

69. Rabinowitz LG, Esterly NB: Atopic dermatitis and ichthyosis vulgaris. Pediatr Rev 15:220, 1994

70. Paller AS: Laboratory tests for ichthyosis. Dermatol Clin 12:99, 1994

71. DiGiovanna JJ, Robinson-Bostom L: Ichthyosis: etiology, diagnosis, and management. Am J Clin Dermatol 4:81, 2003

72. Fleckman P: Management of the ichthyoses. Skin Therapy Lett 8:3, 2003

39 Contact Dermatitis and Related Disorders

James S. Taylor, M.D.

Contact dermatitis is an acute or chronic skin inflammation resulting from interaction with a chemical, biologic, or physical agent.[1] It is one of the most common conditions seen by physicians, accounting for more than 6.5 million physician visits a year and 95% of all reported occupational skin diseases.[2] Substances that produce contact dermatitis after a single exposure or multiple exposures may be irritant or allergenic. Direct tissue damage results from contact with irritants. Tissue damage by allergic substances is mediated through immunologic mechanisms. Eczema or dermatitis is the most common clinical expression of this induced inflammation. Of the more than 85,000 chemicals in our environment, most can be irritants, depending on the circumstances of exposure.[1] More than 3,700 substances have been identified as contact allergens.[3] The potential for these substances to cause contact dermatitis varies greatly, and the severity of the dermatitis ranges from a mild, short-lived condition to a severe, persistent, job-threatening, and possibly life-threatening disease.

Major Types of Contact Dermatitis

IRRITANT CONTACT DERMATITIS

Irritants cause as much as 80% of cases of contact dermatitis, act by direct nonimmunologic chemical or physical action on the skin, and are divided into marginal and acute types. Marginal irritants are the most common. Repeated daily exposures to low-grade irritants such as soap, detergents, surfactants, organic solvents, and oils may not cause clinical changes for days or months. Dryness of the skin with a glazed, parched appearance are often the initial signs; erythema, hyperkeratosis, and fissuring may supervene.

In contrast, acute irritants cause a more immediate reaction. Some irritants, such as strong acids and alkalis, aromatic amines, phosphorus, and metallic salts, produce a marked observable effect within minutes.[4,5] Others, such as hydrofluoric acid, ethylene oxide, podophyllin, and anthralin, produce a reaction within 8 to 24 hours after exposure.[4] Acute irritant contact dermatitis (ICD) is usually easily diagnosed by the patient history and often results from occupational accidents. The clinical appearance varies depending on the irritant and ranges from burns and deep-red ulcerations with sharp circumspection of the dermatitis, sometimes with a gravitational, dripping effect, to a vesicular dermatitis that is indistinguishable from acute allergic contact dermatitis.

Almost any substance can be an irritant, depending on the conditions of exposure [*see Figure 1*]. The nature of the irritant (i.e., its pH, solubility, physical state, and concentration), the duration of contact, and the nature of the vehicle affect disease severity. Host factors that predispose to ICD include preexisting dermatitis, skin dryness, sweating, and decreased thickness or breaks in the stratum corneum; environmental factors include high temperature, low humidity, friction, and pressure.

ICD provoked by work materials is believed to be a frequent cause of occupational skin disease. In one large population-based study, the highest annual incidence rates of ICD were re-

ported for hairdressers (46.9 per 10,000 workers per year), bakers (23.5 per 10,000 workers per year), and pastry cooks (16.9 per 10,000 workers per year).[6] The causative factors of ICD are complex and usually involve exposure to a combination of irritants. The sentinel event for irritant hand eczema in hairdressers is dermatitis developing in moist areas that are difficult to rinse and dry, such as under rings and in the web spaces of the fingers.[7] Dermatitis may spread to the dorsum of the hand, where the skin is thinner and less resistant than on the palms.

No universally accepted test exists for diagnosing ICD, which is often diagnosed by excluding allergic contact dermatitis (ACD). Because of the clinical similarities between allergic and irritant contact dermatitis, it is important that patients who are thought to have either disorder undergo patch testing, the results of which are positive with ACD and negative with ICD.

ICD may become chronic if it is not treated early [*see Treatment of Irritant and Allergic Contact Dermatitis, below*]. Even when the skin appears to be healed, its protective capacity remains impaired for weeks or months. Additionally, ICD impairs the barrier function of the skin, allowing penetration of potential contact allergens. Individuals who had childhood atopic eczema are more likely than others to develop ICD of the hands when their jobs involve wet work.

ALLERGIC CONTACT DERMATITIS

Allergic contact dermatitis is a type 4, T cell–mediated, delayed hypersensitivity reaction in the skin. The disorder affects

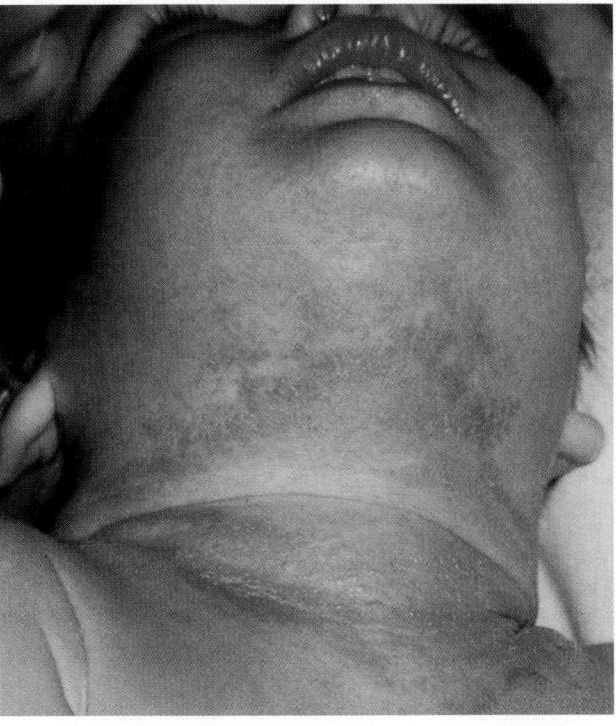

Figure 1 **Wearing a plastic bib resulted in irritant dermatitis in an 18-month-old child.**

Table 1   Body Sites Often Affected by 10 Common Contact Allergens

Allergen	*Common Uses*	*Localization Site*
Nickel	Costume jewelry	Earlobes, neck, fingers, wrists, abdomen
Neomycin	Topical antibiotics (dermatologic; ophthalmologic; ear, nose, throat)	Face, neck, trunk, extremities
Balsam of Peru	Fragrances, cosmetics, medications, flavorings	Face, trunk, extremities, perianal area
Fragrance mix	Toothpaste, fragrances, toiletries, cosmetics	Same as for balsam of Peru
Thimerosal	Topical antiseptic, contact lens solutions, eye cosmetics, nasal sprays	Eyelids, face, neck (relevance hard to prove)
Gold	Jewelry	Eyelids, earlobes, wrists, fingers
Formaldehyde	Cosmetics (preservative), shampoos, nail enamel	Eyelids, face, neck, trunk (especially intertriginous areas)
Quaternium-15	Cosmetics (preservative), shampoos, soaps, lotions	Face, trunk, extremities, hands
Cobalt	Metal-plated objects, jewelry	Earlobes, neck, fingers, wrists
Bacitracin	Topical antibiotics (dermatologic; ophthalmologic; ear, nose, throat)	Face, neck, trunk, extremities

only certain sensitized individuals, typically after two or more exposures, and accounts for about 20% of contact dermatitis cases.

Predisposing Factors

Immunologic status   Predisposing factors to ACD include the patient's immunologic status, which in turn is influenced by genetics, age, gender, and the presence of systemic disease. Patients with AIDS, severe combined immunodeficiency, advanced lymphoma or other malignancy, sarcoidosis, lepromatous leprosy, cachexia, and atopic dermatitis may have impaired cell-mediated immunity or anergy.[8] However, contact allergy should not be excluded in these individuals, especially those with atopic eczema. In experimental models, agents that affect the immune system, such as ultraviolet light (ultraviolet B or psoralen and ultraviolet A [PUVA]), glucocorticoids, cyclosporine, and various other drugs, may downregulate ACD.[8] Administration of systemic corticosteroids below certain dosages (e.g., prednisone, 20 mg or less daily), however, does not inhibit strong patch-test reactions.[9]

In patients with occupational dermatitis, a form of natural hyporeactivity termed hardening may occur with diminished but continued exposure to chemical irritants. The process is inducible and is not localized.[10] This acquired state of unresponsiveness, when describing adaptation to allergens, is called tolerance.[8]

Environment   The chemical environment in which we live defines opportunities for exposure to various allergens. A patient's age, gender, occupation, avocation, habits, and nationality are among the factors that determine the environment and thus the chemicals to which an individual is exposed. The most common source of contact allergy in the United States is *Toxicodendron*, a plant genus that includes poison ivy, poison oak, and poison sumac. In addition to *Toxicodendron*, 10 sources of contact allergens are commonly encountered in North America [*see Table 1*],[11] and numerous other allergens are known to cause contact reactions.[3]

Other cutaneous disorders   Skin that is infected, inflamed, burned, or eczematous predisposes a patient to ACD. Patients with stasis, hand and foot eczema, or chronic actinic dermatitis are at high risk for ACD. ACD occasionally occurs with other skin disorders, including seborrheic dermatitis, psoriasis, prurigo nodularis, and benign familial pemphigus (Hailey-Hailey disease).[12] Noneczematous contact reactions have also been reported: purpuric reactions caused by black rubber; lichen planus–like eruptions caused by color-film developers, gold, and other dental metals (oral mucosa); and granulomas caused by beryllium and zirconium.[12]

Pathogenesis

Some inflammatory immune reactions in ACD are the same as those in ICD—specifically, the two disorders have similar cytokine activity (tumor necrosis factor–α and interferon gamma) and accessory molecule activity (HLA-DR and intercellular adhesion molecule–1) producing the cascade of inflammation. However, there is no memory T cell function in ICD,[13] and the extent of reaction is directly related to the amount of irritant and duration of exposure.[14] In contrast, even small amounts of an allergen can trigger the T cell reaction in ACD. Minor variations in an allergen's physical and chemical properties may affect its ability to induce sensitization.[8] Most environmental allergens are haptens–that is, they are small (< 500 daltons) molecules that penetrate the skin and undergo in vivo conjugation with tissue, or carrier, protein. Once the complex forms, the carrier protein is no longer recognized by the immune system as self. ACD represents a delayed-type hypersensitivity reaction to this complex.

During the sensitization phase, which usually takes a minimum of 5 to 21 days, an individual acquires a specific hypersensitivity to a particular contact allergen. Sensitization not only can evoke a type 4 delayed hypersensitivity response (mediated by lymphocytes) but also can produce a type 1 immediate hypersensitivity reaction (mediated by circulating antibodies).

On reexposure to an allergen, a hapten-carrier complex capable of eliciting a specific reaction re-forms. The reaction time—the time required for a previously sensitized individual to manifest a clinical dermatitis after reexposure to the antigen—is usually 12 to 48 hours but may range from 8 to 120 hours.

A spontaneous flare may occur within 10 to 21 days without reexposure, possibly because enough allergen remains at the site to cause a reaction once the sensitization phase has occurred.

Cross-sensitization occurs when a patient who is allergic to one chemical also reacts to structurally related chemicals. Examples include *Toxicodendron* antigens (poison ivy, oak and sumac Japanese lacquer, mango, and cashew nutshell oil), aromatic amines (*p*-phenylenediamine, procaine, benzocaine, and *p*-aminobenzoic acid), and perfumes or flavors (balsam of Peru, benzoin, cinnamates, and vanilla). This phenomenon may explain persistence or reactivation of dermatitis when such exposures are unknown.[8,12,15]

Diagnosis

Diagnosis of ACD is based on the patient history; on the appearance, periodicity, and localization of the eruption; and on the clinical course. The history is especially important in cases of chronic dermatitis and putative occupational contact dermatitis. The history alone may be accurate only 50% of the time, on average, ranging from 80% accuracy for nickel to 50% accuracy for moderately common allergens to about 10% accuracy for less common allergens. Even with causes that are considered obvious, the specific allergen may not be known, and ACD that is caused by other chemicals may also be present. Skillful history taking is required to differentiate ACD from contact urticaria and ICD, with differentiation being especially difficult in chronic cases [*see Table 2*].[16] Also important is detailed questioning of the patient about all topical medications (over-the-counter and prescription), systemic medication, cosmetics, other lotions and creams, occupation, hobbies, travel, and clothing. A history of hypersensitivity to one or more of the major contact allergens (e.g., nickel, rubber, topical medications, and cosmetics [fragrances, preservatives, and dyes]) or obvious occupational or avocational exposures to certain substances or chemicals (e.g., chrome, epoxy, acrylics, latex gloves, clothing, first-aid creams, preservatives, and plants) may point to the diagnosis of ACD in an otherwise unexplained eruption.[16]

Clinical features In the acute stage, papules, oozing vesicles, and crusting lesions that are surrounded by inflammation predominate. These clinical features may occur anywhere, but they are best visualized on the palms, sides of the fingers, periungual areas, and soles of the feet. Frequently occurring or persistent episodes of ACD often become chronic; lesions associated with chronic ACD may appear thickened and exhibit lichenification, scaling, and fissuring [*see Figures 2 and 3*]. Post-inflammatory hyperpigmentation or hypopigmentation may occur. In the subacute stage of ACD, features characteristic of both acute and chronic ACD may be present. All forms of contact dermatitis frequently cause pruritus. The onset of ACD is often subtle. A low-grade, subacute to chronic eczema may appear as primarily a scaly or chapped eruption, especially on the face or on the dorsa of the hands.[12,16]

The distribution of dermatitis is often the single most important clue to the diagnosis of ACD. The area of most intense dermatitis usually corresponds to the site of most intense contact with the allergen. Exceptions occur, such as nail-polish allergy, which typically appears on ectopic sites, especially the eyelids, face, and neck. In addition to the transfer of allergens to distant sites, volatile airborne chemicals may cause dermatitis on exposed body areas. Regional differences in susceptibility to contact allergens exist. Thinner eyelid and genital skin is more susceptible to both allergic and irritant contact dermatitis. Because head hair is often protective of the scalp, allergic reactions to hair cosmetics frequently involve the upper face, eyelids, postauricular area, and neck. Other areas of the body have higher or lower

Table 2 Common Misconceptions about ACD[49]

Fallacy	Truth
Rash quickly follows contact	Rash is often delayed 1 to 2 days and may not appear for 1 wk after contact
Allergy develops only to new substances	Allergy can develop years after contact; an induction period may last virtually a lifetime
Allergy is dose-dependent	Allergy is not, within a wide range, dose-dependent
If changes in medications or cosmetics do not lead to clearing of the rash, those products are not the cause	Many products contain the same or cross-reacting allergens; also, the composition of the product may be altered without a change in the trade name of the product
Contact allergy occurs only at the site of exposure to the offending agent	Contact allergy can spread by direct or indirect contact, airborne exposure, connubial contact, or autoeczematization
Expensive products are not allergenic	Allergy is not related to cost
Negative prick or scratch test or RAST excludes ACD	Only patch testing is diagnostic of ACD
ACD is always bilateral if allergen exposure is bilateral	Shoe and glove allergy are often bilateral but may be unilateral
ACD is of the same intensity at all areas of exposure	Body sites may differ in responsiveness to allergens; ACD may be patchy (e.g., hand dermatitis from gloves)
ACD does not affect the palms and soles	ACD may occur on the palms and soles (e.g., from gloves, topical medicaments, shoes)

ACD—allergic contact dermatitis   RAST—radioallergosorbent test

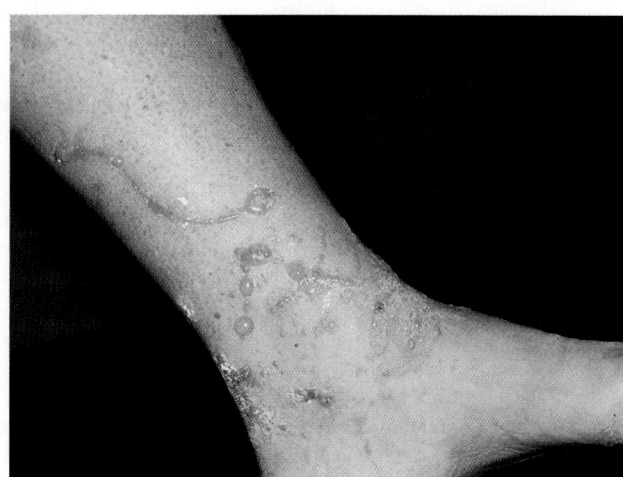

Figure 2   Exposure to poison oak produced this acute *Toxicodendron* dermatitis with erythema, edema, and linear vesicles and bullae.

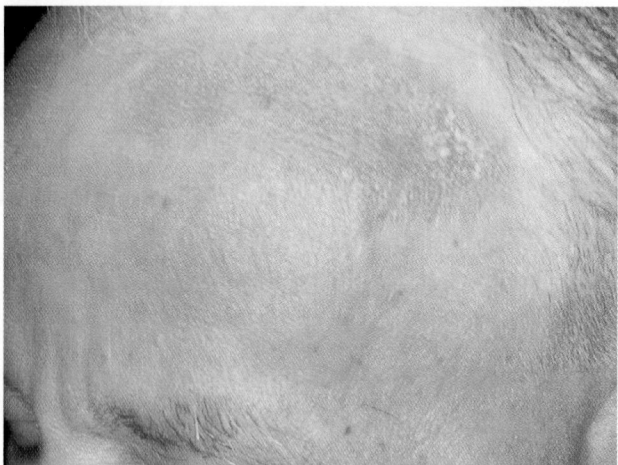

Figure 3   Chronic eczematous dermatitis, with scaling, lichenification, and hyperpigmentation, was caused by an allergy to leather components in a hatband.

Histopathology   Biopsies are of limited help in diagnosing contact dermatitis. Microscopic findings vary according to the stage of the process: acute, subacute, or chronic. The hallmark of eczema is spongiosis, or intercellular edema, associated with spongiotic vesicles. Intracellular edema may cause reticular degeneration of the epidermis with multilocular bullae formation. Most types of eczema show similar pathologic changes and cannot be distinguished with certainty.[17]

Patch test   The patch test is the only useful and reliable method—the gold standard—for the diagnosis of ACD. The proper performance and interpretation of this bioassay require

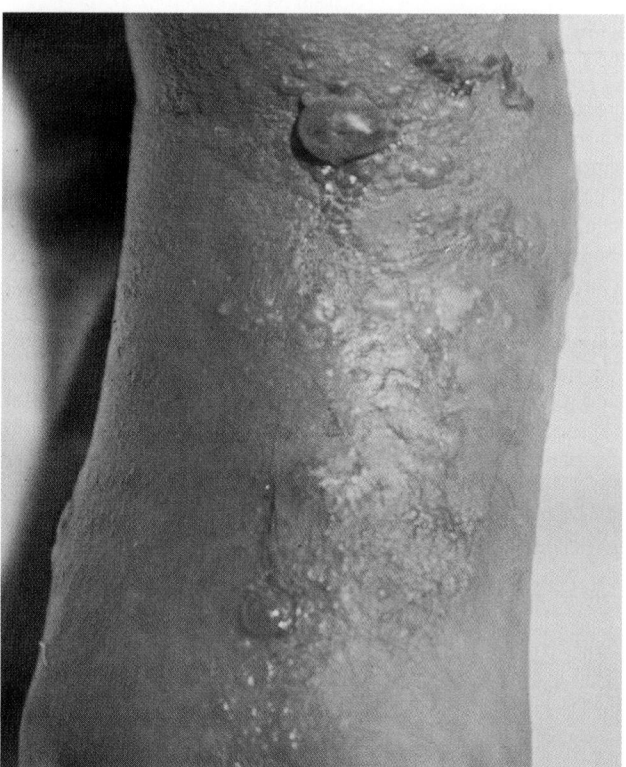

Figure 4   Acute contact dermatitis caused by wearing sandals typically involves the dorsal surface of the feet.

exposures to various allergens; these exposures are not always clear and are reflected in unusual distributions of dermatitis. Allergens in lotions and creams applied all over the body sometimes produce reactions in skin folds and intertriginous areas, where the chemicals tend to concentrate. Recognition of ACD on the basis of the physical examination alone may be only partially accurate. Linear vesicular streaks are commonly seen in poison ivy, poison oak, and poison sumac dermatitis, but contact with other plants can give a similar picture. Contact with liquids may also produce linear vesicles. Failure to examine the entire skin surface may result in misdiagnosis. Eczema on the trunk and arms may in fact represent autoeczematization from contact or stasis dermatitis of the legs. Significant regional variations are associated with contact dermatitis, and knowledge of substances that cause dermatitis of specific body sites facilitates the diagnosis. Three such areas are the hands, face and neck, and feet [*see Figures 4 through 7*].

If the history and clinical presentation reveal one or more risk factors for ACD, a patch test is indicated [*see Table 3* and Patch Test, *below*]. The differential diagnosis of ACD is extensive, and a list of key points can be useful in establishing an accurate diagnosis [*see Table 4*].

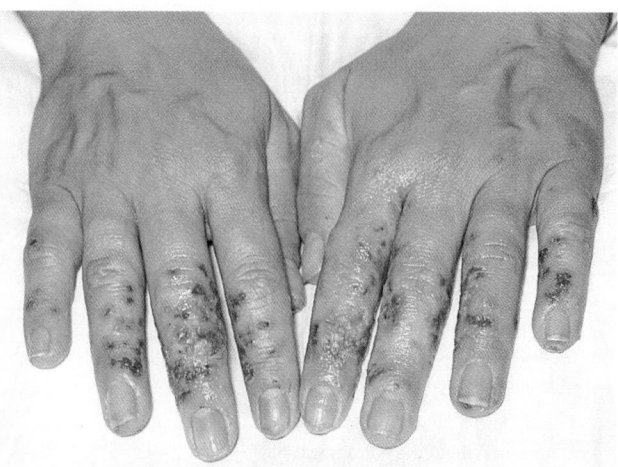

Figure 5   Hairdresser with acute allergic contact dermatitis of the hands, caused by glyceryl thioglycolate.

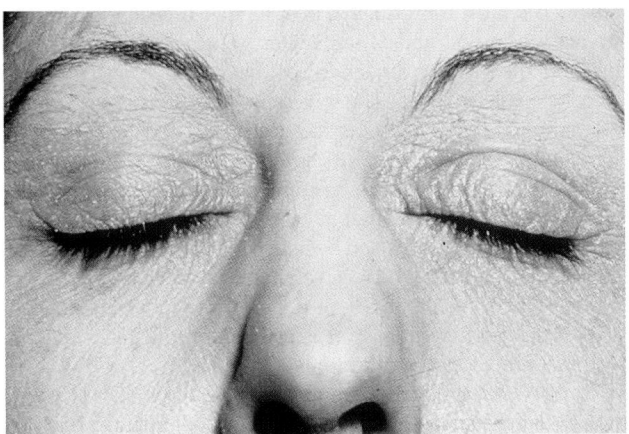

Figure 6 **Ectopic allergic contact dermatitis of the eyelids from tosylamide formaldehyde resin in nail polish.**

available patch-test system in the United States is the thin-layer rapid-use epicutaneous (T.R.U.E.) test. The T.R.U.E. test contains 23 preloaded allergens that are crystallized, micronized, or emulsified into gels that are affixed to paper tape.

With both systems, the tests are applied to the upper back or midback, which must be free of dermatitis. The patches are left in place and kept dry. When removed at 48 hours, the first reading is performed after 20 to 30 minutes, which allows time for pressure erythema to resolve. It is important to perform a second reading between 4 and 7 days after the patches are initially applied; otherwise, almost 20% of positive reactions will be missed. Neomycin, formaldehyde and formaldehyde-releasing preservatives, and tixocortol pivolate are often late reactors. Results at both readings are graded according to intensity of the reaction covering at least 50% of the patch-test site on a scale of 0 to 3+, as follows:

    0 = no reaction
    ? (doubtful) = weak erythema only
    1+ = erythema and edema
    2+ = erythema, edema, and papules
    3+ = vesicles or bullae

considerable experience. Because the procedure is subject to patient variability and observer error, the technique has been standardized by the North American Contact Dermatitis Group. First, the allergen is diluted in petrolatum or water to a concentration that does not produce active sensitization or irritation. A widely used patch-test system consists of strips of paper tape, onto which are fixed aluminum disks 8 mm in diameter (Finn Chambers on Scanpor tape). A small amount of allergen is placed within these disks, covering slightly more than one half of its diameter [*see Figure 8*]. Currently, the only commercially

Both false positive and false negative reactions can result. Thus, patch testing is best done by physicians who are familiar with the intricacies of the procedure and who have been trained to advise patients about allergen substitution, relevance of the test, and prognosis. Reading test results and interpreting relevance are as important as performing the test. Any reaction must be evaluated with regard to the individual patient. Thus,

a

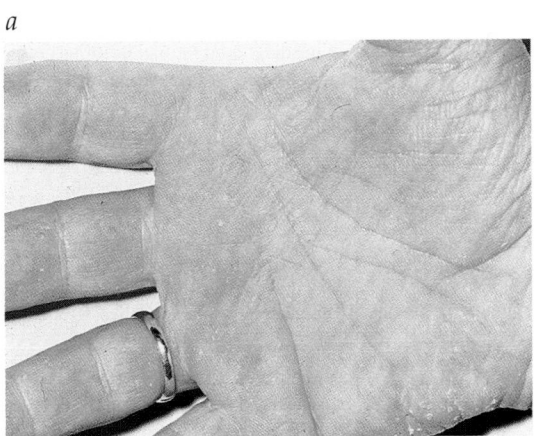

c

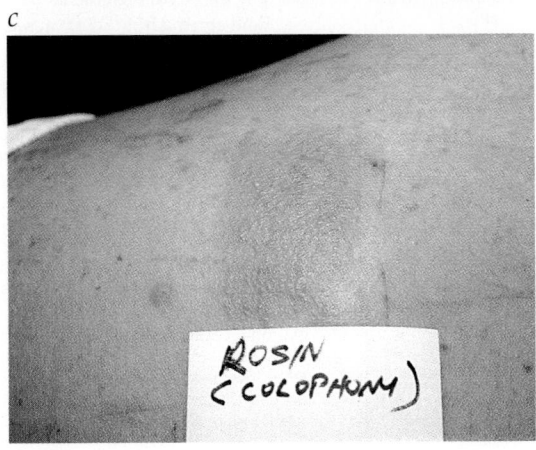

b

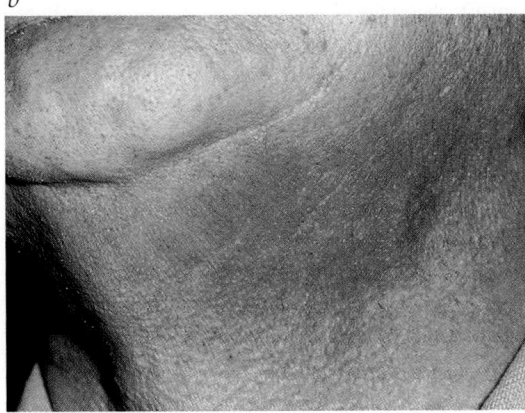

Figure 7 **Allergic contact dermatitis of the hands (*a*) and neck (*b*), with a positive patch test to rosin (colophony) (*c*).**

Table 3   Criteria* for Determining Which Patients with Putative ACD Should Be Patch Tested[49]

Presence of a specific type of eczema that places patient at higher risk for ACD (stasis, hand, foot, or chronic)

Patient is in a high-risk occupation
  Health care worker
  Cosmetologist (hairdresser)
  Rubber compounder
  Plastics processor
  Chemical worker
  Printer
  Machinist
  Woodworker

Specific allergen or substance is suspected

Patient has a highly suggestive history or distribution of dermatitis

Dermatitis flares or does not respond to treatment

Patient has previously undiagnosed dermatoses and erythroderma

Patient has putative occupational dermatitis

Special situation applies, such as photosensitivity or systemic contact dermatitis

*Test is ordered if any one of the risk factors is present.

---

small. The most reproducible positive patch tests were for fragrance mix, nickel, and balsam of Peru. Formaldehyde and lanolin were the least reproducible positive reactors, both of which may be weak irritants.[20] The sensitivity, specificity, and validity of a standard screening series has been estimated at about 70%,[21] indicating that about 30% of these patch-test results were not valid. The patients whose screening results were negative later had positive results to other allergens. It was assumed that the earlier screening results had been false negative. A study of 500 consecutive patients who received identical patch testing reported discordant results in 5% of patients; the investigators concluded that patch testing is a reasonably reproducible procedure as long as methodological error is minimized.[22]

The positive predictive value of a diagnosis of ACD is a function of the prevalence of ACD in the population and a function of the sensitivity and specificity of the patch test.[23] A large dose-response study that tested the impact of seasonal variation on the irritant susceptibility of skin identified a stronger reaction to irritants in winter.[24]

when an allergen is found to be positive, it cannot always be assumed to be the cause of ACD.[8,12,15] The relevance of positive reactions to present or past episodes of ACD ranges from a low of 7.2% for thimerosal to 93.4% for dimethylol-dimethylhydantoin (DMDM hydantoin) and diazolidinyl urea [see Table 5]. Thus, relevance is determined by correlating the patch-test results with chemicals, products, and processes encountered in the environment. Occasionally, when patients are allergic to chemicals in products they use, the allergen may be present in only minimal amounts and may not be responsible for the dermatitis.[8] In these cases, repeat open application testing (ROAT), in which the patient applies the commercial product to normal skin twice daily for several days, can be helpful. ROAT is typically used with products that are left on rather than washed off after application.

In the United States, patch testing for ACD is often initially performed using the T.R.U.E. test; however, because there are over 3,700 environmental contact allergens and this test screens for only 23 allergens, testing with additional chemicals is imperative for a thorough evaluation. In one study, the T.R.U.E. test series of 23 allergens would have completely identified all allergens in only 25.5% of patients and clinically relevant allergens in 28% of patients.[18] Additional substances can be obtained from chemical suppliers and prepared by a compounding pharmacist in appropriate concentrations, as detailed in a standard text, for testing with the Finn Chamber system. As an alternative, many centers in the United States use individual patch-test chemicals or series (e.g., corticosteroid, plastics and glues, acrylic, dental, machinist, hairdresser) that are available in Europe but have not been approved in the United States.[11,19]

Reproducibility and validity of patch testing   In a study in which 383 patients received simultaneous duplicate patch tests on opposite sides of the upper back, 8% of patients had completely discordant results: positive on one side of the back and negative on the other.[20] The intensity of the reactions was not disclosed, and clinical relevance of this problem was considered

---

Table 4   Key Points in the Diagnosis of ACD

Key Points	Examples
ACD may be identical to another disease	Tinea pedis misdiagnosed as ACD; a positive potassium hydroxide preparation made the diagnosis
	Psoriasis of the soles misdiagnosed as ACD caused by shoes; patch tests were negative
	Factitial eczema of the dorsal hand misdiagnosed as ACD; cured with an Unna Boot occlusive dressing
	ACD caused by fragrances and preservatives; misdiagnosed for 5 yr as lupus erythematosus
	ACD caused by hair tonic; misdiagnosed as seborrheic dermatitis
	ACD caused by sunscreen; misdiagnosed as sunburn
ACD may be concurrent with another disorder	ACD caused by neomycin; misdiagnosed as worsening atopic eczema
	Chronic actinic dermatitis of the face can be present with ACD caused by a fragrance
	Morphea of the leg can be present with ACD caused by a topical corticosteroid cream
ACD may be caused by an occult exposure to an allergen	Keys in pants pocket caused ACD of the lateral thigh in a man allergic to nickel
	ACD caused by the preservative imidazolidinyl urea, present in a sunscreen with a label that listed only the active ingredients
	Chronic hand eczema from ACD caused by red dye in window curtains
Diagnosis of ACD may be elusive because of inadequate or deceptive history	Patient allergic to neomycin had periorbital contact eczema caused by an ophthalmic ointment that contained tobramycin, which was not recognized as a cross-reacting allergen
	Chronic eczema worsened by use of a topical cream (doxepin) identified only from a pharmacy prescription list
Initial patch-testing may not provide accurate diagnosis	Occupational contact dermatitis of the hands attributed to a false positive irritant-patch-test reaction to a cleanser
	Occupational contact dermatitis of the hands with a false negative patch-test reaction to latex surgical gloves; further patch testing indicated an allergy to thiurams, which were present as accelerators in the gloves

a

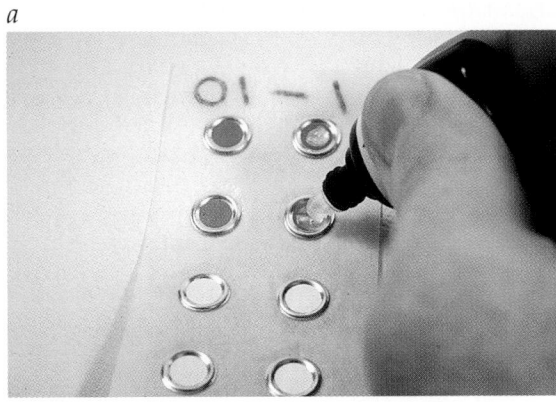

b

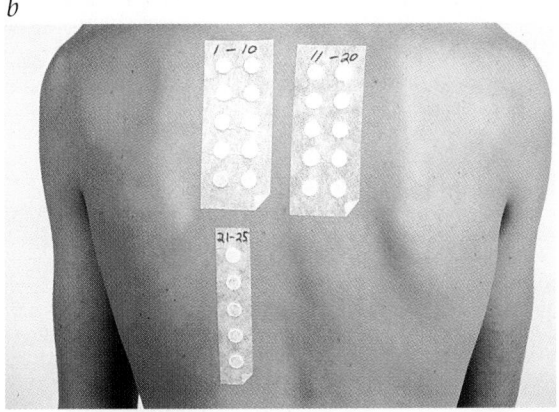

Figure 8 Patch-test allergens to be tested, usually in petrolatum and occasionally aqueous, are placed on Finn Chambers on Scanpor tape (*a*) for application to the patient's back (*b*) for 48 hours. See patch testing in text and Figure 7c for a positive patch test.

TREATMENT OF IRRITANT AND ALLERGIC CONTACT DERMATITIS

Most cases of contact dermatitis can be effectively treated and controlled once the offending irritant or allergen is identified and eliminated. Identifying hidden sources of allergens is important, and patients who have positive patch-test results are given exposure lists identifying various names of allergens, cross-reacting substances, lists of potential products and processes containing the allergen, and nonsensitizing substitutes. Standard texts should be consulted for detailed information[12,17]; the Internet is also a source of information on treatment of contact dermatitis [*see Sidebar* Internet Resources on Contact Dermatitis]. Examples of allergen alternatives include topical erythromycin or mupirocin ointments as substitutes for neomycin.[25] Neomycin may cross-react with gentamicin and tobramycin. Bacitracin should generally be avoided for neomycin-sensitive patients because of coreactivity.

Reasons for persistence of ACD include unidentified sources of allergens or irritants at home or at work, exposure to cross-reacting allergens, presence of underlying endogenous (e.g., atopic) eczema, and adverse reactions to therapy [*see* Topical-Medication Allergy, *below*].

Reduction of Trigger Factors

In the case of hand dermatitis, practical management must include protective measures, topical corticosteroids, and lubrication. The use of vinyl gloves with cotton liners to avoid the accumulation of moisture that often occurs during activities involv-

ing exposure to household or other irritants and foods (e.g., peeling or chopping fruits or vegetables) may be helpful. However, it is important to have the patient confirm that gloves are safe to use in the workplace around machinery before recommending them. Protective devices themselves may introduce new allergic or irritant hazards in the form of rubber in gloves and solvents in waterless cleansers. Barrier creams are generally the last resort and are probably best for workers who do not have dermatitis.[26] Hand alcohol may be a superior disinfectant to soap and water in occupations that require extensive wet-work exposure.[27] A barrier agent containing quaternium-18 bentonite has been shown to be effective with exposure to a specific allergen, such as poison ivy.[28] Principles of treatment of atopic dermatitis may also be applied to treatment of contact dermatitis [*see Chapter 38*].

Topical Therapy

Treatment of contact dermatitis depends on the severity of the dermatitis. When acute serous oozing is present, cool, wet compresses should be applied for 15 minutes two or three times a day. Isotonic saline or Domeboro powder dissolved in tap water to make a 1:40 dilution (aluminum acetate) may be used. A soft cloth, such as Kerlex gauze or a towel, is immersed in the solution. The cloth is wrung slightly and applied to the affected area of the skin. The solution should not be poured directly on the dressing. Lukewarm to cool water baths or sitz baths are antipruritic and anti-inflammatory; they also aid in cleansing and removing crusts and medications. Oatmeal in the form of Aveeno Oilated Bath Treatment (colloidal powdered oatmeal with oils) may be added to the bath for its antipruritic and drying effects.

In acute vesicular dermatitis such as that caused by poison ivy, treatment with compresses and baths should be followed by the application of a topical corticosteroid spray (either triamcinolone acetonide [Kenalog aerosol] or betamethasone dipropionate [Diprosone aerosol]). A spray of 2 or 3 seconds' duration on each affected area supplies sufficient coverage, providing the container is held 6 in. from the skin. In cases in which the dermatitis is extensive or less vesicular, one of the many topical corticosteroid creams may be used. Corticosteroid creams range in potency from extremely potent (e.g., clobetasol propionate [Temovate]), to potent (e.g., betamethasone dipropionate [Diprosone topical cream]), to midstrength formulations. In addition, a lotion of camphor, menthol, and hydrocortisone (Sarnol-HC) is soothing, drying, and antipruritic. Pramoxine, a topical anesthetic in a lotion base (Prax), may also relieve pruritus.

In the subacute and chronic stages of contact dermatitis, an emollient lotion (Eucerin) or ointment (Aquaphor) may be applied to moist skin after bathing for lubrication. Oil-in-water emulsions that contain perfluoropolyethers have been shown to significantly inhibit ICD caused by a wide variety of hydrophilic and lipophilic irritants.[29] A potent or midstrength topical glucocorticosteroid cream or ointment is often used in the treatment of subacute and chronic contact dermatitis. Hydrocortisone 1% is only occasionally effective. Fluorinated corticosteroids should be used with discretion; frequent and prolonged use of these agents in skin-fold areas may cause atrophy, telangiectasia, or striae, and their use on the face may cause steroid rosacea. For patients with chronic dermatitis, crude coal tar preparations may be used to control eczema. Topical PUVA treatment may be effective for contact dermatitis of the palms and soles.[30]

Table 5   Patch-Test Results in North America from 2001 through 2002[11]

Test Substance*	T.R.U.E. Test Allergen	Use	Frequency of Positive Reactions (%)	Relevance of Patient (%)†
Nickel sulfate 2.5%	TT	Metal	16.7	49.4
Neomycin sulfate 20%	TT	Antibiotic	11.6	32.3
Balsam of Peru (Myroxylon pereirae) 25%	TT	Fragrance	11.6	80.7
Fragrance mix 8%	TT	Fragrance	10.4	83.5
Thimerosal 0.1%	TT	Preservative	10.2	7.2
Gold sodium thiosulfate 0.5%		Metal	10.2	37.3
Quaternium-15 2%	TT	Preservative	9.3	84.3
Formaldehyde 1% aq	TT	Preservative	8.4	69.6
Bacitracin 20%		Antibiotic	7.9	42.6
Cobalt chloride 1%	TT	Metal	7.4	43.8
Methyldibromaglutaronitrile/phenoxyethanol 2.5%		Preservative	5.8	61.1
Carba mix 30%	TT	Rubber accelerator	4.9	76.6
p-Phenylenediamine 1%	TT	Hair dye	4.8	49.6
Thiuram 1%	TT	Rubber accelerator	4.5	78.9
Potassium dichromate 0.25%	TT	Metal	4.3	55.4
Benzalkonium chloride 0.1% aq		Preservative	4.3	26.9
Propylene glycol 30% aq		Medicine/cosmetic solvent	4.2	89.2
2-Bromo-2-nitropropane-1,3-diol 0.5%		Preservative	3.3	70.1
Diazolidinyl urea 1% aq		Preservative	3.2	91.1
Diazolidinyl urea 1%		Preservative	3.1	93.4
Imidazolidinyl urea 2%		Preservative	3.2	91.9
Tixocortol-21-pivalate 1%		Corticosteroid	3.0	86.9
Disperse blue 106 1%		Fabric dye	3.0	55.8
Ethylenediamine dihydrochloride 1%	TT	Medicine/cosmetic stabilizer	2.8	28.2
DMDM hydantoin 1%		Preservative	2.8	93.4
Cocamidopropyl betaine 1% aq		Cleanser/cosmetic solvent	2.8	89.2
Methyldibromoglutaronitrile/phenoxyethanol 4%		Preservative	2.7	70.9
Colophony (rosin) 20%	TT	Adhesive, etc.	2.6	46.1
Epoxy resin 1%	TT	Industrial coating/adhesive	2.3	60.5
Methylchloroisothiazolinone/methylisothiazolinone 100 ppm aq	TT	Preservative	2.9	83.3
Amidoamine 0.1% aq		By-product in manufacturing of cocamidopropyl betaine	2.3	83.2
Ethyleneurea melamine-formaldehyde resin 5%		Fabric-finish resin	2.3	67.6
Lanolin 30%	TT	Cosmetic emollient	2.2	82.1
DMDM hydantoin 1% aq		Preservative	2.2	88.2

(continued

Table 5   (continued)

Test Substance*	T.R.U.E. Test Allergen	Use	Frequency of Positive Reactions (%)	Relevance of Patient (%)†
p-tert-Butylphenol formaldehyde resin 1%	TT	Adhesives	1.9	47.4
Glyceryl thioglycolate 1%		Permanent-wave chemical	1.9	39
Imidazolidinyl urea 2% aq		Preservative	1.8	90.8
Benzocaine 5%	TT	Anesthetic	1.7	39
Tosylamide formaldehyde resin 10%		Nail-polish resin	1.6	70.2
Methyl methacrylate 2%		Resin/adhesive	1.4	57.8
Glutaraldehyde 1%		Antibacterial	1.4	49.3
Ethyl acrylate 0.1%		Acrylic nails/resin	1.3	59.4
Cocamidopropyl betaine 0.5%		Cleanser/cosmetic solvent	1.3	74.6
DL α-Tocopherol		Vitamin E	1.1	75
Budesonide 0.1%		Corticosteroid	1.1	86.5
Dimethylol dihydroxyethylene urea 4.5%		Textile resin	1.1	61.1
Ylang ylang oil 2%		Fragrance	1.1	85.4
Black rubber mix 0.6%		Rubber accelerator	1.0	43.1
Compositae mix 6%		Plant group used in food and cosmetics	1.0	66.7
Mercaptobenzothiazole 1%	TT	Rubber accelerator	0.9	77.8
Dibucaine 2.5%	TT	Anesthetic	0.9	15.2
Thioureas 1%		Rubber accelerator	0.8	78.9
Jasmine Abs 2%		Fragrance	0.7	87.5
Mercapto mix 1%	TT	Rubber accelerator	0.7	81.8
Lidocaine 15%		Anesthetic	0.7	26.5
Paraben mix 1%	TT	Preservative	0.6	79.2
Sesquiterpene lactone mix 0.1%		Plant oleoresins	0.7	44.8
Benzophenone 3%		Sunscreen	0.6	79.3
p-Chloro-m-xylenol 1%		Antibacterial	0.6	71.4
Tetracaine 1%	TT	Anesthetic	0.6	21.5
Hydrocortisone-17-butyrate 1%		Corticosteroid	0.5	81.8
DL α-Tocopherol acetate		Vitamin E	0.5	72
Iodopropynyl butylcarbamate 0.1%		Preservative	0.3	61.5
Phenoxyethanol 1%		Preservative	0.2	63.6
Prilocaine 2.5%		Anesthetic	0.1	50

*Allergens in petrolatum unless noted aqueous (aq).

†Definite, probable, or possible reactions detected in percentage testing population.

TT—T.R.U.E. (thin-layer rapid-use epicutaneous) test

Systemic Therapy

Intense itching may be relieved with sedating antihistamines such as diphenhydramine hydrochloride (Benadryl), hydroxyzine hydrochloride (Atarax), and doxepin hydrochloride (Sinequan), administered at night. Most cases of ICD and ACD are effectively managed without the use of systemic corticosteroids. However, short courses of systemic corticosteroids are indicated for patients with severe vesiculobullous eruptions of the hands and feet or the face [*see Figure 9*] or with severe disseminated ACD, such as poison ivy. Strategies to reduce the side effects of corticosteroid use are especially important in patients who have diabetes, hypertension, glaucoma, latent or active tuberculosis (as indicated by a positive skin-test reaction to purified protein derivative), and diseases that could be affected by steroid therapy. Attempts at desensitization have generally been unsuccessful.[8] Secondary infection sometimes arises as a complication of ICD and ACD; in such cases, systemic antibiotics may be indicated.[29]

Specific Etiologic Forms of Contact Dermatitis

TOPICAL-MEDICATION ALLERGY

Reactions to topically applied medications include allergic and irritant contact dermatitis, photosensitivity, airborne contact dermatitis, and contact urticaria and anaphylaxis. ACD is the most common skin reaction to topically applied drugs. The three most important contact allergens are topical antibiotics, anesthetics, and antihistamines. Neomycin and bacitracin are among the most frequently prescribed medications and are common causes of ACD.[15] Mupirocin ointment infrequently causes ACD.[25] Benzocaine, the most common topical anesthetic allergen, is still widely used in topical agents, and there have been a number of reports of contact allergy to topical doxepin.[31,32]

ACD from topical corticosteroids is most often caused by the steroid itself rather than the vehicle. Studies indicate that in patients screened for contact dermatitis, the prevalence of allergy to one or more corticosteroids ranges from 0.55% to 5.98%.[33,34] Patch testing for allergy to the corticosteroid markers tixocortol pivolate and budesonide detects a great majority of cases of ACD caused by topical corticosteroids.[34] Further patch or ROAT testing using commercial preparations from the major cross-reacting classes may identify additional allergenic steroids or, alternatively, nonreacting steroids. Delayed readings are important at 5 to 7 days, because without a late reading, up to 30% of cases of contact allergy to corticosteroid markers can be missed.[34] Allergy to inhaled corticosteroids may present as perinasal or perioral itching or dermatitis, mimicking impetigo and herpes simplex or worsening asthma or allergic rhinitis. In such cases, prior sensitization by the cutaneous route is the usual occurrence, although allergy occasionally develops in response to corticosteroid inhalation.[35]

Topical-drug allergy is particularly common in patients with other forms of dermatitis, especially stasis dermatitis [*see Figure 10*]. In patients with stasis dermatitis, allergy to topical drugs often presents as a nonhealing dermatitis, which can mask the underlying cause of the eruption. A detailed history is important and should include the patient's use of nonprescription preparations, topical agents meant for animal use, medicated bandages, borrowed medications, transdermal devices, and herbal medicines. Patch testing with the standard screening tray and the patient's topical medications is invaluable in diagnosing ACD caused by topical medications.

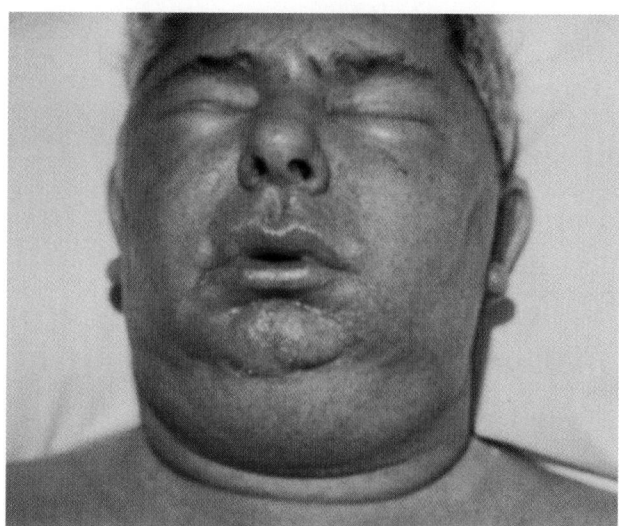

Figure 9 For this patient with allergic contact dermatitis with marked facial edema, a short course of therapy with systemic corticosteroids is indicated.

SYSTEMIC CONTACT DERMATITIS

Systemic contact dermatitis occurs in individuals with contact allergy to a hapten when they are exposed systemically to the hapten via the oral, subcutaneous, transcutaneous, intravenous, inhalational, intra-articular, or intravesicular route. The disorder has been caused by a number of medications, metals, and other allergens, including food components, but occurs infrequently compared with allergic and irritant contact dermatitis. Systemic contact dermatitis presents with the following clinically characteristic features[36,37]:

1. Flare-up of previous dermatitis or of prior positive-patch-test sites.
2. Skin disorders in previously unaffected skin, such as vesicular hand eczema, dermatitis in the elbow and knee flexures, nonspecific maculopapular eruption, vasculitis with palpable purpura, and the so-called baboon syndrome. This syndrome includes a pink–to–dark-violet eruption that is well demarcated on the buttocks and the genital area and is V-shaped on the inner thighs. It may occupy the whole area or only part of it.
3. General symptoms of headache, malaise, arthralgia, diarrhea, and vomiting.

Systemic contact dermatitis may start a few hours or 1 to 2 days after experimental provocation, suggesting that more than one type of immunologic reaction is involved. Documentation rests on patch testing and investigational oral-challenge studies. Well-controlled oral-challenge studies in sensitized individuals have been performed with medications but are more difficult to perform with ubiquitous contact allergens, such as metals and natural flavors. A relatively high dose of hapten is usually needed. Other variables include route of administration, bioavailability, individual sensitivity to the allergen, and interaction with amino acids and other allergens.[36] These variables can have dramatic effects on test results. For example, when 12 leg-ulcer patients with neomycin allergy were challenged with an oral dose of the hapten, 10 reacted.[37] However, of 29 patients with confirmed localized ACD caused by transdermal clonidine, only one had a skin reaction to oral clonidine.[38]

CLOTHING AND TEXTILE DERMATITIS

ACD from clothing is usually not caused by the fibers but rather by the dyes used to color the garments or by formalin finish resins added to make them wrinkle-resistant, shrink-proof, or wash-and-wear. Disperse blue dyes (especially blue 106 and blue 124) are highly valuable screening agents for diagnosing an important cause of textile dermatitis.[39] In a study in which 4,913 patients were patch tested using 65 allergens, disperse blue dye resulted in positive reactions in 3% of the study population [see Table 5].[11]

The distribution of dermatitis corresponds to areas where garments fit snugly, such as the upper and inner anterior thighs, popliteal fossae, buttocks, and waistband areas. Other areas include, in men, the parts of the neck that come in contact with stiff collars and, in women, the anterior or posterior axillary folds, vulva, and suprapubic area. Diagnosis is confirmed by patch testing with disperse dyes (especially blue 106 and blue 124) and formaldehyde-releasing fabric-finish resins (e.g., dimethyloldihydroxyethyleneurea and ethyleneurea melamine formaldehyde). Patch testing with the clothing (particularly acetate and polyester liners) of patients with dye allergy may yield positive results.[40]

Textile-dye dermatitis can be managed in the following ways[41]:

1. Avoiding clothes with the offending dye (especially 100% acetate or 100% polyester liners).

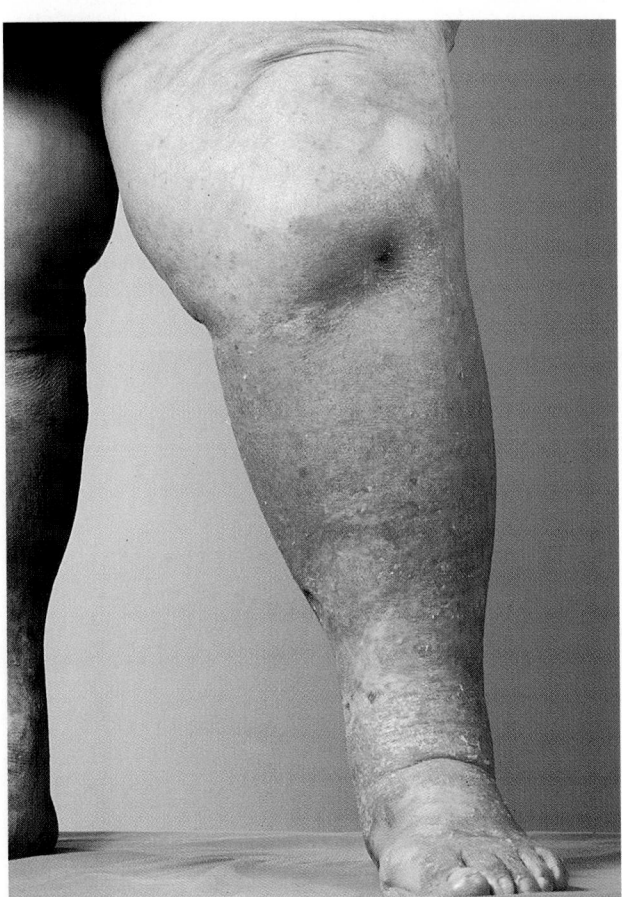

Figure 10 **Patients with stasis dermatitis are at high risk for allergic contact dermatitis, especially from topical medications. Bacitracin was the cause in this case.**

2. Avoiding nylon hose (especially beige tones) and tight synthetic spandex/Lycra exercise clothing.
3. Wearing 100% natural fabrics (i.e., cotton, linen, silk, wool) or 100% silk long-sleeved undershirts and slip pants.
4. Wearing loose-fitting clothing that has been washed (three times) before wearing.[42]

Many of these principles also apply to managing fabric-finish allergy, especially avoiding wrinkle-resistant, shrinkproof, and wash-and-wear clothing.

OCCUPATIONAL CONTACT DERMATITIS

Contact dermatitis, particularly of the hands, is one of the most common types of occupational skin disorders. Special issues associated with these disorders include the following:

1. Objective information on exposure history (a factory visit is ideal) is important. Direct exposure to chemicals can occur because of spills or routine work levels; indirect exposure can come from contaminated tools, rags, and gloves; and airborne exposures can result from mists, droplets, and sprays.
2. The skin is an important portal of entry for a number of toxic chemicals that may or may not have a direct effect on skin. These chemicals include aniline, carbon disulfide, ethylene glycol ethers, certain pesticides, tetrachloroethylene, and toluene.
3. Patch testing with industrial chemicals should be performed very carefully. Irritants should not be tested, and many require dilution to nonirritating concentrations. Testing with individual chemical components of mixtures is preferable in many cases.
4. Establishing occupational causation for ACD is often a challenge, and recommendations have been published.

Prevention and treatment of occupational contact dermatitis is the same as for ACD.[16]

Subtypes of Contact Dermatitis

PHOTOSENSITIVITY

Photosensitivity refers to a condition in which ultraviolet light in combination with endogenous or exogenous substances, usually drugs or chemicals, evokes an eruption on sun-exposed skin. Most cases are evoked by ultraviolet A, but on occasion, eruptions are caused by ultraviolet B (sunburn irradiation) or by visible light. The most common causes are systemic exposure to photosensitizing drugs [see Table 6] or cutaneous exposure, usually accidental, to psoralen in plants.

Photosensitivity reactions are of two types: phototoxicity and photoallergy. Many substances that are photoallergic at low concentrations may be phototoxic at high concentrations.[43]

Phototoxicity

Phototoxicity is analogous to irritation and occurs in any individual after one exposure to sufficient amounts of chemical and light. Phototoxicity has been likened to an exaggerated sunburn response, consisting of delayed erythema and edema followed by pigmentation and desquamation. Asphalt workers and roofers working with pitch develop the so-called smarts when exposed to sufficient sunlight. Phytophotodermatitis, or meadow dermatitis, is a particularly striking phototoxicity characterized by streaky bullae after contact, sometimes while sunbathing, with psoralen containing umbelliferones. Berloque der-

Table 6 Topical and Systemic Photosensitizers[17,44]

Agent	PT/PA	Common Sources/Forms
Topical photosensitizers		
Psoralens	PT	Plants and drugs
Pitch, creosote, and coal tar derivatives	PT	Medications/industrial products
Halogenated salicylanilides (e.g., bithionol, dibromo-salicylanilide)	PA	Antibacterials in soaps and detergents
Musk ambrette	PA	Fragrance
Oxybenzone/padimate O	PA	Sunscreens
Phenothiazines	PA	Topical drugs
Ketoprofen	PA	Nonsteroidal anti-inflammatory drugs
Systemic photosensitizers		
Thiazides	PT	Diuretics
Phenothiazines	PT	Tranquilizers
Dimethylchlorotetracycline	PT	Antibiotic
Griseofulvin	PT	Antifungal
Nalidixic acid	PT	Antibiotic
Sulfonamides	PT	Antibiotic
Psoralens	PT	Photosensitizing drug
Piroxicam	PT?	Nonsteroidal anti-inflammatory drugs, especially in thimerosal-sensitive patients

PA—photoallergenic reaction   PT—phototoxic reaction

matitis is a phototoxic dermatitis characterized by the appearance of hyperpigmented, droplike patches on the neck, face, and breast. This reaction is caused by exposure to 5-methoxypsoralen present in perfumes or colognes containing oil of bergamot, and the hyperpigmentation may persist for many months. Photo-onycholysis has been reported with tetracyclines, psoralen, and other phototoxic drugs. Not all cases exhibit obvious skin phototoxicity.[43] Most cases of phototoxicity are caused by administration of phototoxic systemic drugs [see Table 6].

Photoallergy

Photoallergy is analogous to ACD and is an immunologic reaction in which exposure of the photosensitizing compound to UV light plays a role in formation of a complete antigen. A delayed eruption, usually eczematous, appears in sun-exposed body areas, usually the face and dorsal hands, typically sparing the submental and retroauricular areas [see Figure 11]; shaded areas and covered areas remain relatively clear but occasionally are involved. Most cases are caused by topical photoallergens [see Table 6], and the most common photocontact allergens are sunscreen chemicals, which act by absorbing ultraviolet light. Oxybenzone is a common allergen; however, other sunscreen chemicals, such as padimate O and the dibenzoylmethanes, have also been reported to cause photoallergic contact dermatitis.[43]

Photoallergic contact dermatitis is reproduced and diagnosed by photopatch testing, a procedure in which ultraviolet light (usually ultraviolet A) is combined with patch testing. This form of testing is particularly helpful in differentiating eruptions caused by polymorphous light from photoallergic contact dermatitis. Photopatch testing is not indicated in phototoxic drug eruptions. In some persons, photoallergic reactions can persist as chronic actinic dermatitis (CAD), which can be difficult to treat (see below). Patients with photoallergic contact dermatitis often have contact allergy and should also be patch tested.

Treatment of Phototoxicity and Photoallergy

Elimination of exposure to the photoallergen or phototoxic agent is effective for most patients, except for a few with CAD. Broad-spectrum sunscreens or sunblocks, especially those containing micronized titanium, along with sun-protective clothing, may be helpful. Topical corticosteroids are helpful for mildly affected patients, but severely affected patients with CAD may require azathioprine, with or without systemic corticosteroids; psoralen ultraviolet A therapy and cyclosporine have also been used in some severe cases.[17]

LATEX ALLERGY

Latex allergy is an IgE-mediated hypersensitivity to one or more of a number of proteins present in raw or uncured natural rubber latex (NRL). The paradigm for immunologic contact urticaria is latex allergy, which, over the past decade, has become a significant medical and occupational health problem.

Populations at Risk

Individuals at highest risk are patients with spina bifida (30% to 65% prevalence), health care workers, and other workers with significant NRL exposure.[44] Most reported series of occupational cases of latex allergy involve health care workers; 5% to 11% of those studied are affected.[45] Studies of populations of non–health care workers are infrequent; however, evidence indicates that sensitization to NRL is more common in food handlers, construction workers, painters, hairdressers, cleaners, and miscellaneous other occupations in which NRL is utilized.[46] Children with chronic renal failure appear to be at increased risk for latex sensitization.[47]

Risk Factors and Etiology

Predisposing risk factors are hand eczema, allergic rhinitis, allergic conjunctivitis, or asthma in individuals who frequently wear NRL gloves; mucosal exposure to NRL; and multiple surgical procedures.[44,45] The majority of cases of latex allergy involve reactions from wearing NRL gloves or being examined by individuals wearing NRL gloves. Reactions from other medical and

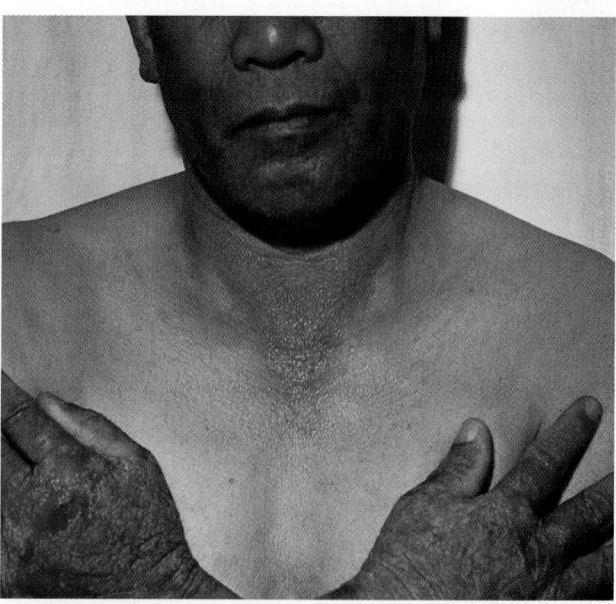

Figure 11 Photocontact dermatitis characteristically involves areas exposed to the sun.

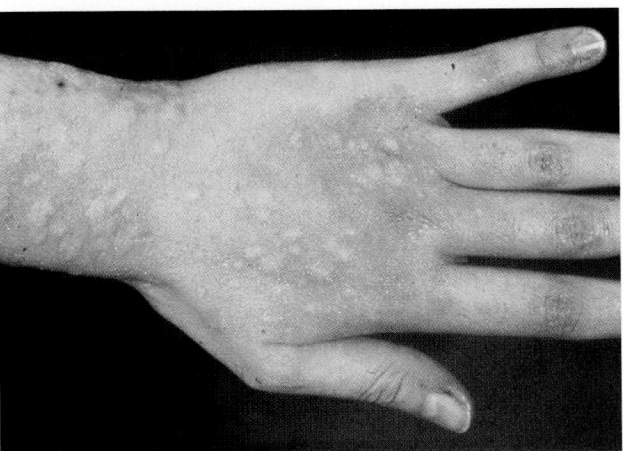

Figure 12 **Contact urticaria of the hands in a nurse allergic to her powdered natural rubber latex gloves (latex allergy). She also experienced allergic rhinitis and asthma while at work. Urticaria is often short-lived after gloves are used and may be absent at the time of examination.**

nonmedical NRL devices have occurred; these include balloons, rubber bands, condoms, vibrators, dental dams, anesthesia equipment, and toys for animals or children.

The route of exposure to NRL proteins includes direct contact with intact or inflamed skin and mucosal exposure, such as inhalation of powder from NRL gloves, especially in medical facilities and in operating rooms.[47] Most immediate-type NRL reactions result from exposure to dipped NRL products (e.g., gloves, condoms, balloons, and tourniquets). Dry-molded rubber products (e.g., syringes, plungers, vial stoppers, and baby-bottle nipples) contain lower residual protein levels or have less easily extracted proteins than do dipped NRL products.

NRL allergy is sometimes associated with allergic reactions to fruit (especially bananas, kiwi, and avocados) and to chestnuts. This allergic reaction results from cross-reactivity between proteins in NRL and those found in some fruits and nuts. Symptoms range from oral itching and angioedema to asthma, gastrointestinal upset, and anaphylaxis. Cross-reactivity to NRL may be a factor in other skin eruptions. One report suggests that the use of commercially available black henna tattoos may cause hypersensitivity to NRL.[48]

Internet Resources on Contact Dermatitis

Contact Dermatitis

American Contact Dermatitis Society
http://www.contactderm.org

American Academy of Dermatology
http://www.aad.org

Occupational Contact Dermatitis

National Institute for Occupational Safety and Health
http://www.cdc.gov/NIOSH

Canadian Centre for Occupational Health and Safety
http://www.ccohs.ca/oshanswers/diseases/allergic_derm.html

Latex Allergy

A.L.E.R.T. Inc.
http://www.latexallergyresources.org

Spina Bifida Association of America
http://www.sbaa.org

Diagnosis

Clinical signs of NRL allergy include contact urticaria [*see Figure 12*], generalized urticaria, allergic rhinitis, allergic conjunctivitis, angioedema, asthma, and anaphylaxis.[45] More than 600 serious reactions to NRL, including 16 fatal anaphylactic reactions, were reported to the Food and Drug Administration by the early 1990s.

Diagnosis of NRL allergy is strongly suggested by a history of angioedema of the lips when inflating balloons and by a history of itching, burning, urticaria, or anaphylaxis when donning gloves; when undergoing surgical, medical, and dental procedures; or after exposure to condoms or other NRL devices. Diagnosis is confirmed by a positive wear or use test with NRL gloves, a valid positive intracutaneous prick test with NRL, or a positive serum radioallergosorbent test with NRL.[44] Severe allergic reactions have occurred from prick and wear tests; epinephrine latex-safe resuscitation equipment free of NRL should be available during these procedures.[45]

Treatment and Risk Reduction

Hyposensitization to NRL is not yet feasible, and NRL avoidance and substitution are imperative. Because many patients with NRL allergy have hand eczema, have immediate allergic symptoms, or both, the most important issues for physicians are accurate diagnosis, appropriate treatment, and counseling.

Preventive measures have significantly reduced the prevalence of reported reactions to NRL.[45] Risk reduction and control of NRL allergy include latex avoidance in health care settings for affected workers and patients. Synthetic non-NRL gloves should be available to replace latex gloves. Also, in many cases, low-allergen NRL gloves should be worn by coworkers so as to minimize symptoms and decrease induction of NRL allergy in those allergic to NRL. Allergen content of gloves should be requested from manufacturers and suppliers; lists of glove allergen levels have also been published. Patients with NRL allergy should wear Medic-Alert bracelets identifying them as NRL sensitive, and they should inform health care providers of their sensitivity. These patients should be given lists of substitute gloves, other non-NRL devices, potentially allergenic fruits, latex-safe anesthesia protocols, occult sources of NRL exposure such as toys (for animals and children), and dental prophylaxis cups. Some of this information is available in published sources, government agencies, and latex-allergy support groups that publish newsletters and other relevant information. Some sources have Web sites [*see Sidebar* Internet Resources on Contact Dermatitis].

The author receives grants for clinical research from Guidant Corp. and Mekos Laboratories AS and serves as a consultant for ConvaTec and Procter & Gamble.

References

1. Rietschel RR, Adams RM, Daily AD, et al: Guidelines of care for contact dermatitis. J Am Acad Dermatol 32:109, 1995

2. Schappert SM: National Ambulatory Medical Care Survey: 1994 Summary. Adv Data 273:1, 1996

3. De Groot AC: Patch Testing: Test Concentrations and Vehicles for 3700 Chemicals, 2nd ed. Elsevier, Amsterdam, 1994

4. Wigger-Alberti W, Elsner P: Contact dermatitis due to irritation. Handbook of Occupational Dermatology. Kanerva L, Elsner P, Wahlberg JE, et al, Eds. Springer Verlag, Berlin, 2000, p 99

5. Iliev D, Elsner P: Clinical irritant contact dermatitis syndromes. Immunol Allergy Clin North Am 17:365, 1997

6. Dickel H, Kuss O, Schmidt A, et al: Importance of irritant dermatitis in occupational skin disease. Am J Clin Dermatol 3:283, 2002

7. Schwanitz HJ, Uter W: Interdigital dermatitis: sentinel skin damage in hairdressers.

Br J Dermatol 142:1011, 2000

8. Belsito DV: Allergic contact dermatitis. Fitzpatrick's Dermatology in General Medicine, 6th ed. Freedberg IM, Eisen AZ, Wolff, K, et al, Eds. McGraw-Hill, New York, 2003, p 1447

9. Condie MW, Adams RM: Influence of oral prednisone on patch test reaction to Rhus antigen. Arch Dermatol 107:540, 1973

10. Wulfhorst B: Skin hardening in occupational dermatology. Handbook of Occupational Dermatology. Kanerva L, Elsner P, Wahlberg J, et al, Eds. Springer Verlag, New York, 2000, p 115

11. Pratt MD, Belsito DV, DeLeo VA, et al: North American Contact Dermatitis Group patch-test results, 2001–2002 study period. Dermatitis 15:176, 2004

12. Rietschel RL, Fowler JF: Fisher's Contact Dermatitis, 5th ed. Williams & Wilkins, Baltimore, 2000

13. Gaspari AA: The role of keratinocytes in the pathophysiology of contact dermatitis. Immunol Allergy Clin North Am 17:377, 1997

14. Corsini E, Galli CL: Cytokines and irritant contact dermatitis. Toxicol Lett 102:277, 1998

15. Krob HA, Fleischer AB Jr, D'Agostino R Jr, et al: Prevalence and relevance of contact dermatitis allergens: a meta-analysis of 15 years of published T.R.U.E. test data. J Am Acad Dermatol 51:349, 2004

16. Taylor JS: Recognizing allergic contact dermatitis. Practical Contact Dermatitis. Guin JD, Ed. McGraw Hill, New York, 1995, p 31

17. Beck MH, Wilkinson SM: Contact dermatitis: allergic. Rook's Textbook of Dermatology, 7th ed. Burns T, Griffiths CE, Kinghorn BP, et al, Eds. Blackwell Science, London, 2004, p 20-1

18. Saripalli YV, Achen F, Belsito DV: The detection of clinically relevant contact allergens using a standard screening tray of twenty-three allergens. J Am Acad Dermatol 49:65, 2003

19. Rietschel RL: Experience with supplemental allergens in the diagnosis of contact dermatitis. Cutis 65:27, 2000

20. Bourke JF, Batta K, Prais L, et al: The reproducibility of patch tests. Br J Dermatol 140:102, 1999

21. Nethercott JR, Holness DL: Validity of patch test screening trays in the evaluation of patients with allergic contact dermatitis. J Am Acad Dermatol 21:568, 1989

22. Ale SI, Maibach HI: Reproducibility of patch test results: a concurrent right-versus-left study using TRUE Test. Contact Dermatitis 50:304, 2004

23. Diepgen TL, Coenraads PJ: Sensitivity, specificity and positive predictive value of patch testing: the more you test, the more you get? Contact Dermatitis 42:315, 2000

24. Basketter DA, Griffiths HA, Wang XM, et al: Individual, ethnic, and seasonal variation in irritant susceptibility of skin: the implications for a predictive human patch test. Contact Dermatitis 35:208, 1996

25. Zappi E, Brancaccio RR: Allergic contact dermatitis from mupirocin ointment. J Acad Derm 36:266, 1977

26. Wigger-Alberti W, Elsner P: Preventive measures in contact dermatitis. Clin Dermatol 15:661, 1997

27. Jungbauer FH, van der Harst JJ, et al: Skin protection in nursing work: promoting the use of gloves and hand alcohol. Contact Dermatitis 51:135, 2004

28. Marks JG Jr, Fowler JF Jr, Sherertz EF, et al: Prevention of poison ivy and poison oak allergic contact dermatitis by quaternium-18 bentonite. J Am Acad Dermatol 33:212, 1995

29. Elsner P, Wiggerti-Alberti W, Pantini G: Perfluoropolyethers in the prevention of irritant contact dermatitis. Dermatology 197:141, 1998

30. Taylor JS: Occupational dermatoses. Conn's Current Therapy. Rakel RE, Ed. WB Saunders, Philadelphia, 1996, p 823

31. Taylor JS, Praditsuwan P, Handel D, et al: Allergic contact dermatitis from doxepin cream: a one-year patch test clinic experience. Arch Dermatol 132:515, 1996

32. Bonnel RA, La Grenade L, Karwoski CB, et al: Allergic contact dermatitis from topical doxepin: Food and Drug Administration's postmarketing surveillance experience. J Am Acad Dermatol 48:294, 2003

33. Keegel T, Saunders H, Milne R, et al: Topical corticosteroid allergy in an urban Australian center. Contact Dermatitis 50:6, 2004

34. Isaksson M, Andersen KE, Brandao FM, et al: Patch testing with corticosteroid mixes in Europe: a multicentre study of the EECDRG. Contact Dermatitis 42:27, 2000

35. Isaksson M, Bruze M: Allergic contact dermatitis in response to budesonide reactivated by inhalation of the allergen. J Am Acad Dermatol 46:880, 2002

36. Veien NK: Ingested food in systemic contact dermatitis. Clin Dermatol 15:547, 1997

37. Menne T, Veien N, Sjolin K-E, et al: Systemic contact dermatitis. Am J Contact Dermatitis 5:1, 1994

38. Maibach HI: Oral substitution in patients sensitized by transdermal clonidine treatment. Contact Dermatitis 16:1, 1987

39. Seidenari S, Giusti F, Massone F, et al: Sensitization to disperse dyes in a patch test population over a five-year period. Am J Contact Dermatitis 13:101, 2002

40. Hatch KL, Motschi H, Maibach HI: Disperse dyes in fabrics of patients patch-test-positive to disperse dyes. Am J Contact Dermatitis 14:205, 2003

41. Mathias CGT: Contact dermatitis and worker's compensation: criteria for establishing occupational causation and aggravation. J Am Acad Dermatol 20:842, 1989

42. Pratt M, Taraska V: Disperse blue dyes 106 and 124 are common causes of textile dermatitis and should serve as screening allergens for this condition. Am J Contact Dermatitis 11:30, 2000

43. Isaksson M, Bruze M: Photocontact dermatitis: photopatch testing. Clin Dermatol 15:615, 1997

44. Taylor JS, Wattanakrai P, Charous L, et al: Latex allergy. 1999 Yearbook of Dermatology and Dermatologic Surgery. Thiers BH, Lang PG, Eds. Mosby, St. Louis, 1999, p 1

45. Taylor JS, Erkek E: Latex allergy: diagnosis and management. Dermatol Ther 17:289, 2004

46. Valks R, Conde-Salazar L, Cuevas M: Allergic contact urticaria from natural rubber latex in healthcare and non-healthcare workers. Contact Dermatitis 50:222, 2004

47. Sparta G, Kemper MJ, Gerber AC, et al: Latex allergy in children with urological malformation and renal failure. J Urol 171:1647, 2004

48. Martin JA, Hughes TM, Stone NM: 'Black henna' tattoos: an occult source of natural rubber latex allergy? Contact Dermatitis 52:145, 2005

49. Marks JG, DeLeo V: Contact and Occupational Dermatology, 2nd ed. Mosby, St. Louis, 1997

Acknowledgments

Figure 7   Courtesy of James R. Nethercott, M.D. (deceased), Department of Dermatology, University of Maryland, Baltimore.

Figure 11   Courtesy of Kristina Turjanmaa, M.D., and Arto Lahti, M.D., Tampere and Oulu, Finland.

40 Cutaneous Adverse Drug Reactions

Neil H. Shear, M.D., F.A.C.P., Sandra Knowles, B.Sc. Phm., and Lori Shapiro, M.D.

An adverse drug reaction (ADR) is defined as any noxious, unintended, and undesired effect of a drug that occurs at doses used in humans for prophylaxis, diagnosis, or therapy.[1] An ADR may range from a cutaneous eruption to severe syndromes (e.g., drug hypersensitivity syndrome, Stevens-Johnson syndrome [SJS], toxic epidermal necrolysis [TEN], and serum sickness–like reaction). Over the past 25 years, a dramatic shift has occurred in the understanding of drug-induced cutaneous eruptions. It is now believed that many severe cutaneous adverse drug reactions are caused by the formation of reactive oxidative metabolites and perhaps the formation of antibodies to drug-protein complexes and skin proteins, or both. The predisposition to drug-induced eruptions may be genetic, and family counseling and in vitro testing are being used in certain centers to manage patients and their families. This chapter reviews the pathophysiology and clinical manifestations that are important for correct diagnosis and treatment of cutaneous ADRs.

Epidemiology

Epidemiologic studies have shown that ADRs occur in 6.7% of all hospitalized patients,[2] and 3% to 6% of all hospital admissions are the result of ADRs.[3] In the Boston Collaborative Drug Surveillance Program,[4] the prevalence of cutaneous ADRs in hospitalized patients was 2.2%. Antibiotics were responsible for 75% of detected reactions. In the Harvard Medical Practice Study, approximately 14% of ADRs in hospital patients were cutaneous or allergic in nature.[5] The cost of drug-related morbidity and mortality has been estimated at $30 billion a year,[6] and ADRs are thought to be between the fourth and sixth leading cause of death in the United States.[2,6]

Etiology

Cutaneous reactions to drugs often occur in complicated clinical scenarios that may include exposure to multiple agents. New drugs started within the preceding 6 weeks are potential causative agents, as are drugs that have been used intermittently, including over-the-counter preparations and herbal and naturopathic remedies.

Diagnosis

CLINICAL MANIFESTATIONS

The morphology of cutaneous eruptions may be exanthematous, urticarial, blistering, or pustular. The extent of the reaction is variable. For example, once the morphology of the reaction has been documented, a specific diagnosis (e.g., fixed drug eruption or acute generalized exanthematous pustulosis) can be made. The reaction may also present as a syndrome (e.g., serum sickness–like reaction or hypersensitivity syndrome reaction). Fever is associated with the more serious cutaneous ADRs.

DIFFERENTIAL DIAGNOSIS

Differential diagnoses can include viral exanthems (e.g., infectious mononucleosis and parvovirus B19 infection), bacterial infections, Kawasaki syndrome, collagen vascular disease, and neoplasia.

LABORATORY TESTS

Penicillin skin testing with major and minor determinants is useful for confirmation of an IgE-mediated immediate hypersensitivity reaction to penicillin. Skin tests are performed 6 weeks to 6 months after complete healing of the cutaneous drug reaction.[7] Oral rechallenges may be useful in the diagnosis of ADRs; however, they should not be used in patients who experienced a serious reaction, such as SJS or TEN. Patch testing may be helpful in the diagnosis of fixed drug eruptions or contact dermatitis.[8]

Exanthematous Eruptions

SIMPLE ERUPTIONS

Exanthematous eruptions, also known as morbilliform, maculopapular, or scarlatiniform eruptions, are the most common cutaneous ADRs.[4] Simple exanthems are erythematous changes in the skin without blistering or pustulation.

Many drugs can cause exanthematous eruptions, including the penicillins, sulfonamides, barbiturates, antiepileptic medications, nonnucleoside reverse transcriptase inhibitors (e.g., nevirapine), and antimalarials.[4] Exanthematous eruptions occur in 3% to 7% of patients receiving such aminopenicillins as ampicillin and amoxicillin. However, these eruptions may occur in 60% to 100% of patients taking ampicillin or amoxicillin who are receiving concurrent allopurinol therapy or who have concomitant lymphocytic leukemia, infectious mononucleosis, cytomegalovirus infection, or hyperuricemia.[9]

Studies suggest that some exanthematous eruptions represent cell-mediated hypersensitivity.[10] The etiology of the ampicillin rash concurrent with a viral infection is unknown, but the rash does not appear to be IgE mediated, and patients can tolerate all β-lactam antibiotics, including ampicillin, once the infectious process has resolved. Similar reactions are seen in 50% of HIV-infected patients exposed to sulfonamide antibiotics.[11] Drug-specific T cells play a major role in exanthematous, bullous, and pustular drug reactions.[12]

Simple exanthems are symmetrical and often become generalized. Pruritus is the most frequently associated symptom. Fever is not associated with simple exanthematous eruptions. These eruptions usually occur within 1 week after the start of therapy and generally resolve within 7 to 14 days.[13] A change in color of the exanthem from bright red to brownish red signifies resolution. Resolution may be followed by scaling or desquamation. Some patients with ampicillin- or amoxicillin-induced exanthematous eruptions may have a positive result on a patch test or on a delayed intradermal test.[9] In general, however, skin testing is not considered helpful in the diagnosis of an exanthematous eruption.

The differential diagnosis of drug-induced exanthematous eruption includes viral exanthem (patients should be tested for

Table 1   Clinical Features of Hypersensitivity Syndrome Reaction and Serum Sickness–like Reaction

	Rash	Fever	Internal Organ Involvement	Arthralgia	Lymphadenopathy
Hypersensitivity syndrome reaction	Exanthem Exfoliative dermatitis Pustular eruptions Erythema multiforme Stevens-Johnson syndrome Toxic epidermal necrolysis	Present	Present	Absent	Present
Serum sickness–like reaction	Urticaria Exanthem	Present	Absent	Present	Present

mononucleosis), collagen vascular disease, bacterial infection, and rickettsial infection. Hypersensitivity syndrome should be considered in the differential diagnosis.

The treatment of simple exanthematous eruptions is generally supportive. For example, oral antihistamines used in conjunction with soothing baths may help relieve pruritus. Topical corticosteroids are indicated when antihistamines do not provide relief. Systemic corticosteroids are used only in severe cases. Discontinuance of the offending agent is recommended in most cases.

COMPLEX ERUPTIONS

Hypersensitivity Syndrome Reaction

Hypersensitivity syndrome reaction is a complex drug reaction that affects various organ systems. A triad of fever, skin eruption, and internal organ involvement signals this potentially life-threatening syndrome. It occurs in approximately one in 3,000 exposures to such agents as aromatic anticonvulsants (e.g., phenytoin, phenobarbital, and carbamazepine), lamotrigine, sulfonamide antibiotics, dapsone, nitrofurantoin, nevirapine, minocycline, and allopurinol.

It has been suggested that the metabolism of aromatic anticonvulsants by cytochrome P-450 plays a pivotal role in the development of the hypersensitivity syndrome reaction with these drugs.[14] In most people, the chemically reactive metabolites that are produced are detoxified by epoxide hydroxylases. If detoxification is defective, however, one of the metabolites may act as a hapten and initiate an immune response, stimulate apoptosis, or cause cell necrosis directly. There also appears to be an association between human herpesvirus type 6 (HHV-6) infection (either initial infection or reactivation) and severe hypersensitivity syndrome. Viral infections may act as, or generate the production of, danger signals that lead to damaging immune responses to drugs, rather than to immune tolerance.[15,16]

In one study, 75% of patients with hypersensitivity syndrome reactions to one aromatic anticonvulsant showed in vitro cross-reactivity to the other two aromatic anticonvulsants.[14] In addition, in vitro testing has shown that there is a familial occurrence of hypersensitivity to anticonvulsants.[14] Although lamotrigine is not an aromatic anticonvulsant, it too can cause a hypersensitivity syndrome reaction.[17] There is no evidence that lamotrigine cross-reacts with the aromatic anticonvulsants. Lamotrigine and other anticonvulsants are also associated with more severe reactions (e.g., SJS and TEN) [*see* Complex Eruptions, *below*].

Sulfonamide antibiotics can cause hypersensitivity syndrome reactions in susceptible persons. The primary metabolic pathway for sulfonamides involves acetylation of the drug to a nontoxic metabolite and renal excretion. An alternative metabolic pathway, quantitatively more important in patients who are slow acetylators, engages the cytochrome P-450 mixed-function oxidase system. These enzymes transform the parent compound to reactive metabolites—namely, hydroxylamines and nitroso compounds, which produce cytotoxicity independently of preformed drug-specific antibody. In most people, detoxification of the metabolite occurs. However, hypersensitivity syndrome reactions may occur in patients who are unable to detoxify this metabolite (e.g., those who are glutathione deficient).[18] Although the detoxification defect is present in 2% of the population, only one in 10,000 persons will manifest a hypersensitivity syndrome reaction in response to sulfonamide antibiotics. Siblings and other first-degree relatives of patients with the detoxification defect are at increased risk (perhaps one in four) for having a similar defect.

Other aromatic amines, such as procainamide, dapsone, and acebutolol, are also metabolized to chemically reactive compounds. We recommend that patients who develop symptoms compatible with a sulfonamide hypersensitivity syndrome reaction avoid these aromatic amines, because the potential exists for cross-reactivity. However, cross-reactivity should not occur between sulfonamides and drugs that are not aromatic amines (e.g., sulfonylureas, thiazide diuretics, furosemide, and acetazolamide).[19]

Allopurinol is associated with the development of serious drug reactions, including hypersensitivity syndrome reaction. In a review of 13 patients with allopurinol adverse reactions, fever and rash were the most common presenting symptoms. Other associated abnormalities included leukocytosis (62%), eosinophilia (54%), renal impairment (54%), and liver dysfunction (69%).[20] Reactivation of HHV-6 infection has been reported in a patient who developed an allopurinol-induced hypersensitivity syndrome reaction with hepatitis, as documented by polymerase chain reaction analysis showing HHV-6 DNA in his blood; HHV-6 DNA was also detected in the cerebrospinal fluid.[21]

Allopurinol-induced adverse reactions, including hypersensitivity syndrome reaction, SJS, and TEN, have been strongly associated with a genetic predisposition in Han Chinese; the HLA-B*5801 allele is an important genetic risk factor.[22] Susceptibility to nevirapine hypersensitivity may be enhanced by the presence of the HLA-DRB1*0101 allele but inhibited by low CD4+ T cell counts.[23] Abacavir is also associated with a potentially life-threatening adverse reaction in approximately 8% of patients given this drug. Studies have shown a strong predictive association between abacavir hypersensitivity syndrome reaction and HLA-B*5701.[24]

Hypersensitivity syndrome reaction occurs most frequently on first exposure to the drug, with initial symptoms starting 1 to 6 weeks after exposure [see Table 1]. Fever and malaise, which can be accompanied by pharyngitis and cervical lymphadenopathy, are the presenting symptoms in most patients. This is often followed by edema and swelling of the face, especially upon rising in the morning. Atypical lymphocytosis, with subsequent eosinophilia, may occur during the initial phases of the reaction in some patients. A cutaneous eruption, which occurs in approximately 85% of patients, can range from an exanthematous eruption [see Figure 1] to the more serious SJS or TEN. The liver is often involved, resulting in hepatitis, although other internal organs may be affected, such as the kidney (e.g., interstitial nephritis and vasculitis), the central nervous system (e.g., encephalitis and aseptic meningitis), and the lungs (e.g., interstitial pneumonitis, respiratory distress syndrome, and vasculitis). A subgroup of patients may become hypothyroid as part of an autoimmune thyroiditis within 2 months after the initiation of symptoms.[25] This condition is characterized by a low thyroxine level, an elevated level of thyroid-stimulating hormone, and the presence of thyroid autoantibodies, including antimicrosomal antibodies.

After the occurrence of a hypersensitivity syndrome reaction has been recognized from the symptom complex of fever, rash, and lymphadenopathy, some laboratory tests can be used to evaluate internal organ involvement, which may be asymptomatic. A complete blood count, urinalysis, and measurements of liver transaminase and serum creatinine levels should be performed. In addition, the clinician should be guided by symptoms that may suggest specific internal organ involvement (e.g., respiratory symptoms). Thyroid function should be evaluated on presentation of hypersensitivity syndrome reaction and then 2 to 3 months after presentation. A skin biopsy may help confirm the diagnosis when the patient has a blistering or a pustular eruption. Unfortunately, diagnostic or confirmatory tests are not readily available. An in vitro test employing a mouse hepatic microsomal system is used for research purposes to characterize patients who develop hypersensitivity syndrome reaction.[14,26] Because of the severity of the reaction, oral rechallenges are not recommended. In fact, in patients with a history of hypersensitivity

syndrome reaction, reexposure to the offending agent may cause the development of symptoms within 1 day.

Although the role of corticosteroids is controversial, most clinicians begin a regimen of prednisone at a dosage of 1 to 2 mg/kg/day when symptoms are severe. There are reports of successful treatment with cyclosporine[27] or intravenous immunoglobulin (IVIg).[28] Antihistamines, topical corticosteroids, or both can be used to alleviate symptoms. Because the risk of hypersensitivity syndrome reaction in first-degree relatives of patients who have had reactions is substantially higher than in the general population, family members should receive counseling about their risk of hypersensitivity syndrome reaction.

Urticarial Eruptions

SIMPLE ERUPTIONS

Urticaria and Angioedema

Urticaria is characterized by pruritic red wheals of varying sizes that can occur with any medication. When deep dermal and subcutaneous tissues are also swollen, the reaction is known as angioedema[29] [see Chapter 107]. Urticaria and angioedema usually result from a type I immediate hypersensitivity reaction. This mechanism is typified by immediate reactions to penicillin and other antibiotics. Binding of the drug or its metabolite to IgE bound to the surfaces of cutaneous mast cells leads to activation, degranulation, and release of vasoactive mediators such as histamine, leukotrienes, and prostaglandins.[30]

Urticarial reactions may also result from nonimmunologic activation of inflammatory mediators. Drugs such as acetylsalicylic acid and nonsteroidal anti-inflammatory drugs (NSAIDs),[31] radiocontrast media, and narcotic analgesics may directly cause the release of histamine from mast cells, independently of IgE. Angiotensin-converting enzyme (ACE) inhibitors are frequent causes of angioedema.[32] The mechanism of this reaction is unclear but may relate to the accumulation of bradykinin or activation of the complement system.

Although medications tend to cause urticaria, angioedema, or both, other causal agents are food [see Chapter 109], physical factors (e.g., dermatographism and cholinergic urticaria) [see Chapter 107], and idiopathic factors. Certain foods containing proteins that can cross-react with latex proteins, such as bananas, kiwifruit, avocados, and chestnuts, can cause oral itching and swelling, hives, or wheezing after ingestion. The risk of latex allergy is especially high in children with spina bifida and health care workers.[33,34] Latex allergy can present as contact urticaria at sites of latex exposure; such reactions include lip swelling in a person who has blown up a balloon or in an infant who has sucked on a pacifier. Contact with aerosolized powder from latex gloves to which the latex protein has adhered may cause mucosal symptoms, such as itchy, swollen eyes; runny nose; sneezing; or wheezing. Anaphylaxis may also occur.

Signs and symptoms of IgE-mediated allergic reactions are typically pruritus, urticaria, cutaneous flushing, angioedema, nausea, vomiting, diarrhea, abdominal pain, nasal congestion, rhinorrhea, laryngeal edema, and bronchospasm or hypotension or both. Fever is not associated with urticaria or angioedema reactions. In general, individual lesions of urticaria last for less than 24 hours, although new lesions can continually develop. Adverse reactions to ACE inhibitors usually begin within hours of starting the drug but can occur as late as 1 week to several

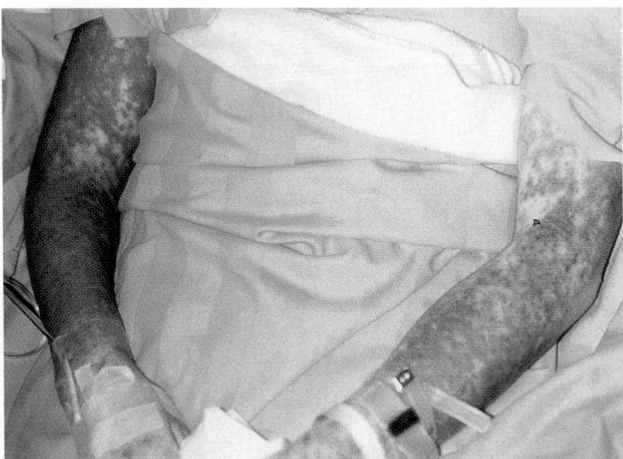

Figure 1 This 35-year-old woman developed hypersensitivity syndrome reaction, characterized by fever, rash, and hepatitis, 14 days after starting trimethoprim-sulfamethoxazole therapy. The rash is an extensive, symmetrical, red edematous eruption.

months into therapy.[35] With treatment, the resulting angioedema usually resolves within 48 hours.

Skin testing may be helpful in cases of IgE-mediated urticaria. For example, penicillin skin testing with the major and minor determinants identifies approximately 99% of patients who have had an IgE-mediated reaction to penicillin. A latex skin test is a sensitive indicator of IgE sensitization. Positive immediate skin-test reactions identify patients at risk for IgE-mediated reactions from large-molecular-weight agents, such as insulin, neutral protamine Hagedorn (NPH) insulin,[36] and egg-containing vaccines.

Withdrawal of the causative agent is recommended. When angioedema or anaphylaxis occurs, immediate therapy with epinephrine and systemic steroids may be needed. Symptomatic relief can generally be achieved with antihistamines (H$_1$ receptor blockers). The safety of angiotensin II receptor antagonists in patients with a history of angioedema with ACE inhibitors is not yet known.[37]

Differential diagnosis Allergic urticaria must be differentiated from urticaria caused by physical factors. Cold urticaria, for example, is precipitated by exposure to cold, occurring within minutes after immersion of hands or body in cold water or after exposure to cold air. In severe cases, patients may experience systemic symptoms, including wheezing and syncope. A rare familial form of cold urticaria that is autosomal dominant has been linked to chromosome 1q44.[38]

Cold urticaria can be differentiated from other forms of urticaria by eliciting an urticarial reaction with an ice cube applied to the skin for 5 to 10 minutes. Other physical urticarias also have distinguishing causes or features. Solar urticaria occurs within minutes of exposure to sunlight and can be produced by exposing limited areas of skin to sunlight or to appropriate wavelengths of ultraviolet light in a phototherapy response to physical pressure. Cholinergic urticaria, which is characterized by small urticarial papules, can be induced by exposure to heat or by exercise.

Histologically, all the urticarias are characterized by an increase in mast cells in the dermis. Edema, vascular changes, and mononuclear infiltrates are more striking in the dermis of patients with cold urticaria. Mononuclear infiltrates are also more prominent in the deep dermis of patients with delayed pressure urticaria.[39]

As with drug-induced urticaria, first-line therapy of most urticarias consists of oral antihistamines and avoidance of precipitating factors. Psoralen plus ultraviolet A (PUVA) has been used successfully to treat patients with solar urticaria. Montelukast has been used successfully to treat delayed pressure urticaria,[40] and cyclosporine is promising for cases of severe refractory chronic urticaria.[41]

COMPLEX ERUPTIONS

Serum Sickness–like Reactions

Serum sickness–like reactions are defined by fever, rash (usually urticarial), and arthralgias occurring 1 to 3 weeks after drug initiation. Other symptoms, such as lymphadenopathy and eosinophilia, may also be present. In contrast to true serum sickness, serum sickness–like reactions are without immune complexes, hypocomplementemia, vasculitis, and renal lesions [see Table 1].

Epidemiologic studies in children suggest that the risk of serum sickness–like reactions is greater with cefaclor than with other antibiotics, including other cephalosporins.[42,43] The overall incidence of cefaclor serum sickness–like reactions has been estimated to be 0.024% to 0.2% per course of cefaclor.

Although the pathogenesis is unknown, it has been postulated that in genetically susceptible hosts, metabolism of cefaclor produces a reactive metabolite that may bind to tissue proteins and elicit an inflammatory response that manifests as a serum sickness–like reaction.[43]

Other drugs that have been implicated in serum sickness–like reactions are cefprozil,[44] bupropion,[45] minocycline,[46] rituximab,[47] and infliximab.[48] The incidence of serum sickness–like reactions caused by these drugs is unknown.

Discontinuance of the culprit drug and symptomatic treatment with antihistamines and topical corticosteroids are recommended for patients with serum sickness–like reactions. A short course of oral corticosteroids may be required for patients with more severe symptoms. The drug that caused the serum sickness–like reaction should be avoided. For cefaclor and cefprozil, the risk of cross-reaction with β-lactam antibiotics is small, and the administration of another cephalosporin is usually well tolerated.[49] However, some clinicians recommend that patients who experience serum sickness–like reactions from cefaclor avoid all β-lactam drugs.[50]

Blistering Eruptions

SIMPLE ERUPTIONS

Fixed Drug Eruptions

Fixed drug eruptions usually appear as solitary pruritic, erythematous, bright-red or dusky-red macules that may evolve into an edematous plaque [see Figure 2]. In some patients, multiple lesions may be present. Blistering and erosion may occur on mucosal surfaces. Fixed drug eruptions recur in the same skin area after readministration of the causative medication.

Many drugs have been implicated in fixed drug eruptions, including phenolphthalein, naproxen, ibuprofen, sulfonamides, tetracyclines, and barbiturates.[51] The pathogenesis of fixed drug eruptions has not been fully elucidated. A haplotype linkage in the setting of trimethoprim-sulfamethoxazole–induced fixed drug eruptions has been documented.[52]

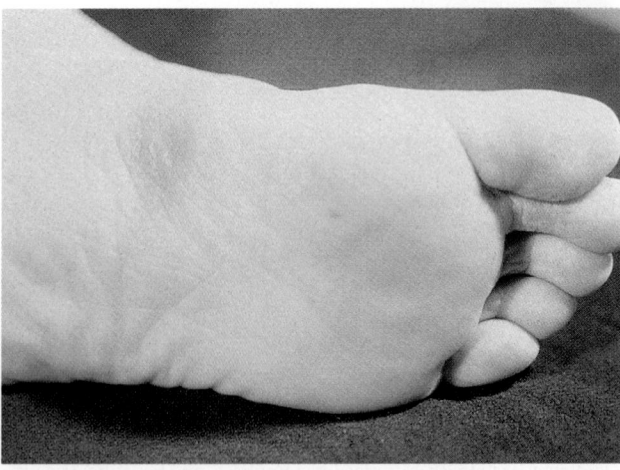

Figure 2   This 28-year-old man taking tetracycline for acne vulgaris developed a fixed drug eruption.

Fixed drug eruptions are most common on the genitalia and in the perianal area, although they can occur anywhere on the skin surface. The onset of a fixed drug eruption can be sudden, developing within 30 minutes to 8 to 16 hours after ingestion of the medication. In patients who continue to take the offending drug, the number of eruption sites may gradually increase.[52]

After the initial acute phase, which lasts days to weeks, residual hyperpigmentation develops. Some patients may complain of burning or stinging on the affected skin sites. Systemic manifestations, which are present in approximately 25% of cases, can include fever, malaise, and abdominal symptoms.[52]

No conclusive diagnostic tests are available, but a challenge or provocation test with the suspected drug may be useful in confirming the diagnosis. Patch testing at the site of a previous lesion yields a positive response in up to 43% of patients. Prick and intradermal skin tests are reported to yield positive reactions in 24% and 67% of patients, respectively, but results vary with different drugs and reaction patterns. Patients with maculopapular rashes are more likely to have positive patch tests than patients with urticarial rashes.[53]

Treatment includes discontinuance of the causative agent and symptomatic therapy (e.g., topical corticosteroids).

Pseudoporphyria

Pseudoporphyria is a cutaneous phototoxic disorder that can resemble either porphyria cutanea tarda (PCT) or erythropoietic protoporphyria (EPP). Tetracycline, furosemide, and naproxen have been implicated in PCT- and EPP-pseudoporphyria.[54] The eruption may begin within 1 day after initiation of therapy or may be delayed for as long as 1 year. PCT-pseudoporphyria is characterized by skin fragility, blister formation, and scarring in areas exposed to sunlight; it occurs with normal porphyrin metabolism. The second clinical pattern mimics EPP and presents as cutaneous burning, erythema, vesiculation, angular scars, and waxy thickening of the skin.

Because of the risk of permanent facial scarring, the implicated drug should be discontinued when skin fragility, blistering, or scarring occurs. In addition, broad-spectrum sunscreen and protective clothing should be recommended to the patient.

COMPLEX ERUPTIONS

Drug-Induced Linear IgA Disease

Linear IgA disease is an autoimmune bullous dermatosis that is identified on the basis of the linear deposition of IgA at the basement membrane zone.[55] This disease can be induced by such drugs as vancomycin, lithium, diclofenac, and amiodarone. The drug-induced disease probably represents an immunologic response to the offending drug.

Drug-induced linear IgA disease is heterogeneous in clinical presentation. Cases have shown morphologies resembling erythema multiforme, bullous pemphigoid, and dermatitis herpetiformis. Drug-induced disease cannot be distinguished from the idiopathic variety either clinically, histologically, or immunologically; however, the clinical courses of these presentations differ. In drug-induced disease, spontaneous remission occurs once the offending agent is withdrawn; in idiopathic linear IgA disease, immune deposits disappear from the skin once the lesions resolve. Steroids and dapsone do not influence the healing process in drug-induced disease, whereas these agents have proved effective in the treatment of idiopathic linear IgA disease.[56]

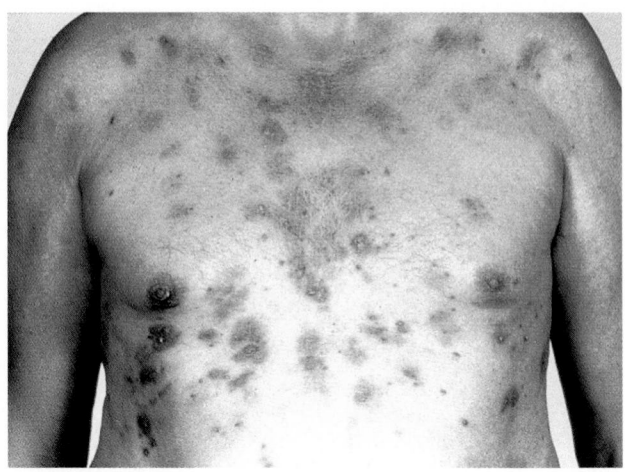

Figure 3 Pemphigus foliaceus developed in this 64-year-old man taking enalapril.

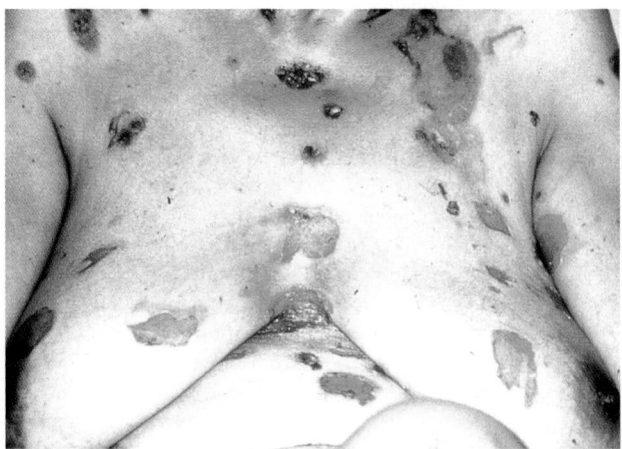

Figure 4 Pemphigus vulgaris developed in this 59-year-old woman who took penicillamine as treatment for rheumatoid arthritis.

Drug-Induced Pemphigus

Pemphigus may be drug induced or drug triggered (i.e., the latent disease is unmasked by the drug exposure).

Drugs that cause pemphigus are penicillin, rifampin, phenylbutazone, propranolol, progesterone, piroxicam, interferon beta, interleukin-2, and levodopa.[53] An active amide group found in masked thiol drugs such as penicillin and cephalosporins and in nonthiol drugs such as enalapril may contribute to the pathogenesis of pemphigus.[57,58] Pemphigus foliaceus [see Figure 3] caused by penicillamine and other thiol drugs tends to resolve spontaneously in 35% to 50% of cases.[57] The average interval to onset is 1 year. Antinuclear antibodies are detected in 25% of affected patients.

Nonthiol drug–induced pemphigus manifests clinical, histologic, immunologic, and evolutionary aspects similar to those of idiopathic pemphigus vulgaris [see Figure 4]. Drug-induced pemphigus is associated with mucosal involvement. Spontaneous recovery after drug withdrawal occurs in 15% of affected patients.

Treatment of drug-induced pemphigus begins with drug withdrawal. Systemic corticosteroids are often required until all symptoms of active disease disappear. Vigilant follow-up is required after remission for an early relapse to be detected. The patient's serum should be monitored regularly for autoantibodies.[57]

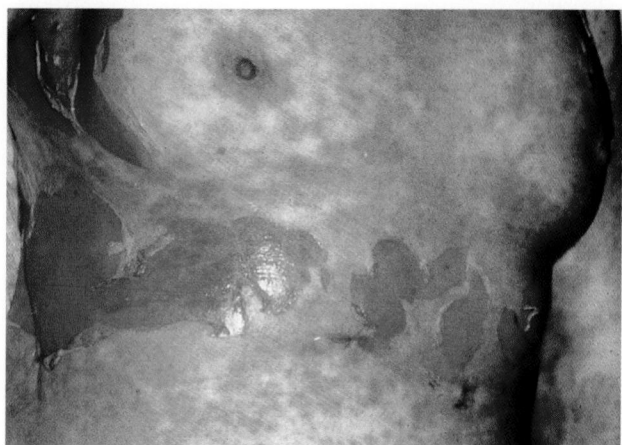

Figure 5 **This 50-year-old woman developed toxic epidermal necrolysis 17 days after starting phenytoin therapy.**

Erythema Multiforme, Stevens-Johnson Syndrome, and Toxic Epidermal Necrolysis

The eruptions of erythema multiforme (EM), SJS, and TEN may represent variants of the same disease process. Reactions encompass a spectrum ranging from the less serious eruptions seen in EM to more serious reactions seen in SJS and TEN [*see Figure 5*].

A large percentage of EM and SJS cases are not drug related; these disorders may develop after a variety of predisposing factors, including infections, neoplasia, and autoimmune diseases. The drugs most frequently cited as causes of EM, SJS, and TEN are anticonvulsants, antibiotics (e.g., sulfonamides), allopurinol, and NSAIDs (e.g., piroxicam).[59] With anticonvulsants, risk appears to be greatest during the first 8 weeks of therapy.[60]

The pathogenesis of severe cutaneous ADRs is unknown, although a metabolic basis has been hypothesized.[61] Sulfonamides and anticonvulsants, the two groups of drugs most frequently associated with SJS and TEN, are metabolized to toxic metabolites that are subsequently detoxified in most persons. However, in predisposed patients with a genetic defect, the metabolite may bind covalently to proteins. In some of these patients, the metabolite-protein adducts may trigger an immune response that leads to a cutaneous ADR.[62] In addition, the detection of drug-specific T cell proliferation provides evidence that T cells are involved in severe skin rashes. Drug-specific major histocompatibility complex (MHC) class I–restricted perforin- and granzyme-mediated cytotoxicity may have a primary role in the development of TEN.[63] Clinically, the reaction patterns of EM, SJS, and TEN are characterized by the triad of mucous membrane erosions, target lesions, and epidermal necrosis with skin detachment. SJS is characterized by mucous membrane erosions and blisters on less than 10% of the total body surface area, whereas TEN involves more than 30% of the total body surface area.[64] The more severe the reaction, the more likely it is that it was drug-induced. Cases of severe cutaneous ADRs to lamotrigine (e.g., SJS and TEN) have been reported.[65] The prevalence of severe cutaneous ADRs associated with lamotrigine has been reported to be as high as one in 1,000 in adults and higher in children. The risk is increased in the presence of valproic acid.

Complete blood counts, liver enzyme measurements, and chest x-rays should be performed to rule out concurrent internal organ involvement.

Treatment of EM, SJS, and TEN includes discontinuance of a suspected drug and such supportive measures as careful wound care, hydration, and nutritional support.[66] The use of corticosteroids in SJS and TEN is controversial.[67] IVIg (0.4 to 1.0 g/kg/day for 2 to 4 days), which contains naturally occurring Fas ligand (FasL)–blocking antibodies, has been shown in most reports to halt progression of TEN, especially when IVIg is started early.[68] However, other studies did not find an improved outcome in patients with TEN who were treated with IVIg.[69] Patients who have developed a severe cutaneous ADR (i.e., EM, SJS, or TEN) should not be rechallenged with the drug or undergo desensitization with the medication.

Pustular Eruptions

SIMPLE ERUPTIONS

Acneiform Eruptions

Eruptions morphologically mimicking acne vulgaris may be associated with drug ingestion. Iodides, bromides, adrenocorticotropic hormone, corticosteroids, isoniazid, androgens, lithium, dactinomycin, and phenytoin are reported to induce acne-like lesions.[70] Acne fulminans was induced by testosterone in 1% to 2% of adolescent boys who were treated for excessively tall stature.[71]

Drug-induced acne often appears on the face and back, but it may appear in atypical areas, such as arms and legs, and is usually monomorphous. Comedones are usually absent. Fever is absent. Acneiform eruptions do not affect prepubertal children, indicating that previous hormonal priming is a prerequisite. Topical tretinoin may be useful when the drug cannot be stopped.

COMPLEX ERUPTIONS

Acute Generalized Exanthematous Pustulosis

Acute generalized exanthematous pustulosis is characterized by acute onset, fever, and a cutaneous eruption with nonfollicular sterile pustules on an edematous erythema, generally starting within days of drug ingestion[72] [*see Figure 6*]; leukocytosis is another common finding. Generalized desquamation occurs 2 weeks later. Differential diagnosis includes pustular psoriasis, subcorneal pustular dermatosis (Sneddon-Wilkinson disease),

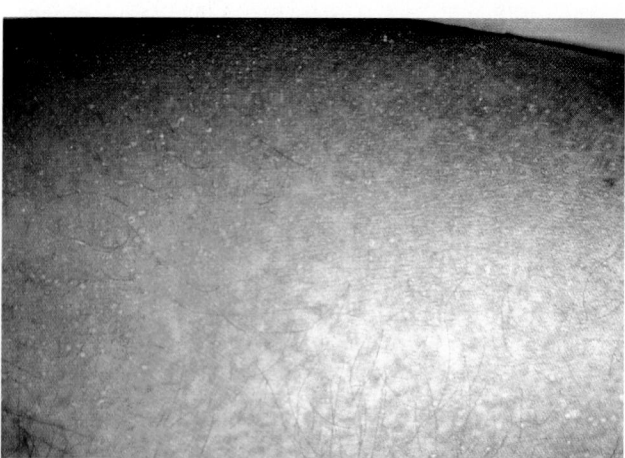

Figure 6 **Acute generalized exanthematous pustulosis (small nonfollicular pustules on a red base) in a 70-year-old man who took cloxacillin as treatment for cellulitis.**

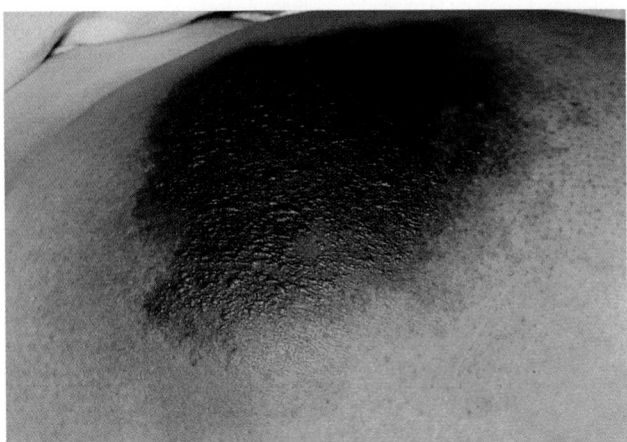

Figure 7 **Coumarin-induced skin necrosis in a 57-year-old woman who was given coumarin as treatment for atrial fibrillation.**

hypersensitivity syndrome reaction with pustulation, and pustular eruptions of infancy.

Acute generalized exanthematous pustulosis is most commonly associated with β-lactam and macrolide antibiotic usage. Many other drugs have been implicated, however, including calcium channel blockers and analgesics. The estimated incidence is approximately one to five cases per million patients per year.[73] Discontinuance of therapy is usually the extent of treatment necessary in most patients, although some patients may require the use of corticosteroids. Patch testing to the putative drug is often positive, resulting in a localized pustular reaction. Positive patch tests and lymphocyte transformation tests suggest involvement of T cells in acute generalized exanthematous pustulosis. Drug-specific CD4+ and CD8+ T cells have been isolated from patch test sites and blood from patients with a history of this disorder.[74]

Other Eruptions

ANTICOAGULANT-INDUCED SKIN NECROSIS

Anticoagulant drugs may induce hypercoagulable states with subsequent vascular infarction and cutaneous necrosis [*see Figure 7*]. Both coumarin and heparin (unfractionated and low-molecular-weight) can induce skin necrosis. Clinical pearls that can help differentiate these reactions involve the location, timing, platelet count, and primary diagnosis [*see Table 2*].

The pathogenesis of coumarin-induced skin necrosis is the paradoxical development of occlusive thrombi in cutaneous and subcutaneous venules caused by a transient hypercoagulable state. This condition results from the suppression of the natural anticoagulant protein C at a greater rate than natural procoagulant factors. Coumarin-induced skin necrosis is associated with

protein C and protein S deficiency, but pretreatment screening is not warranted. An association with heterozygosity for the factor V Leiden mutation has been reported.[75]

It is estimated that one in 10,000 persons who take coumarin are at risk for this adverse event.[76] The prevalence is four times higher in women than in men. In both sexes, the peak incidence occurs in the sixth and seventh decades of life. Afflicted patients tend to be obese.

Coumarin-induced skin necrosis begins 3 to 5 days after initiation of treatment. Painful red plaques develop in adipose-rich sites such as breasts, buttocks, and hips. These plaques may blister, ulcerate, or develop into necrotic areas. An accompanying infection, such as pneumonia, viral infection, or erysipelas, may occur in as many as 25% of patients. Purple-toe syndrome occurs 3 to 8 weeks after initiation of coumarin therapy.

Treatment entails the discontinuance of coumarin, administration of vitamin K, and infusion of heparin at therapeutic doses. Fresh frozen plasma and purified protein C concentrates have been used.[77] Supportive measures for the skin are recommended. Plastic surgery for remediation is necessary in 60% of affected patients.

DRUG-INDUCED LICHENOID ERUPTIONS

The lesions of drug-induced lichen planus are clinically and histologically indistinguishable from those of idiopathic lichen planus. Many drugs, including beta blockers, penicillamine, NSAIDs, gold, and ACE inhibitors, especially captopril, have been reported to produce this reaction.

The latent period between the start of administration of the drug and appearance of the eruption is variable. The mean latent period is between 2 months and 3 years for penicillamine, approximately 1 year for beta blockers, and 3 to 6 months for ACE inhibitors. The latent period may be shorter if the patient was previously exposed to the drug.[78] In general, resolution usually occurs within 2 to 4 months.

Rechallenge with the culprit drug has been attempted in a few patients, with reactivation of symptoms within 4 to 15 days.[79] Patch testing has not proved helpful in most cases of drug-induced lichen planus. However, results of patch tests performed with contact inducers of lichen drug eruptions (e.g., color-film developers and dental restorative materials) are usually positive.[78]

DRUG-INDUCED VASCULITIS

Drug-induced vasculitis represents approximately 10% of the acute cutaneous vasculitides; it usually affects small vessels [*see Figure 8*].[80] Drug-induced vasculitis should be considered in any patient with small vessel vasculitis that is confined to the skin.[81] Drugs that are most frequently associated with vasculitis include propylthiouracil, hydralazine, granulocyte colony-stimulating

Table 2   Clinical Pearls to Identify Anticoagulant-Induced Skin Necrosis

	Interval to Onset	*Location*	*Other*
Coumarin-induced skin necrosis	3–5 days	Adipose-rich sites	—
Heparin-induced thrombocytopenia and thrombosis	4–14 days	Extremities	Thrombocytopenia occurs concurrently
Purple-toe syndrome	3–8 wk	Acral location	Often occurs after angiography

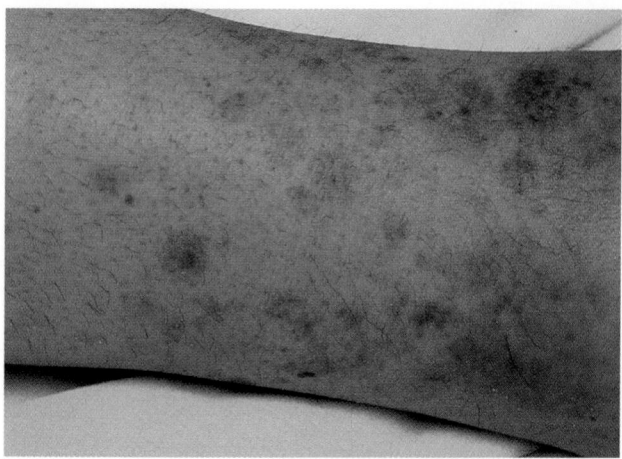

Figure 8   **Leukocytoclastic vasculitis developed in this 47-year-old woman taking hydrochlorothiazide.**

factor (G-CSF), granulocyte-macrophage CSF (GM-CSF), allopurinol, cefaclor, minocycline, penicillamine, phenytoin, and isotretinoin.[79] The average interval to onset of drug-induced vasculitis is 7 to 21 days.[82]

The clinical hallmark of cutaneous vasculitis is palpable purpura, classically found on the lower extremities, although any cutaneous site may be affected. Urticaria can be a manifestation of small vessel vasculitis. Unlike nonvasculitic allergic urticaria, vasculitic urticaria lasts longer than 1 day, may evolve into purpuric lesions, and may be accompanied by hypocomplementemia.[83] Other features are hemorrhagic bullae, urticaria, ulcers, nodules, Raynaud disease, and digital necrosis. The same vasculitic process may also affect internal organs, such as the liver, kidney, gut, and CNS, and is potentially life-threatening.[84]

Histologically, the small blood vessels of the dermis display fibrinoid necrosis, polymorphonuclear infiltration into the blood vessel wall, extravasation of red blood cells, and nuclear dust. Direct immunofluorescence may show deposits of IgM and C3 in the blood vessel walls. Therefore, these reactions are immune complex–dependent drug reactions. The immune complexes may be composed of antibodies directed against drug-related haptens, but this has not been proved.

Drug-induced vasculitis can be difficult to diagnose, and diagnosis is often one of exclusion. Alternative causes of cutaneous vasculitis, such as infection or autoimmune disease, must be eliminated. Tissue eosinophilia may be an indicator of drug induction in cutaneous small vessel vasculitis.[85]

Treatment consists of drug withdrawal. Therapy for patients with severe manifestations includes hemodialysis, pulse corticosteroids, cyclophosphamide, and plasmapheresis.[79]

Neil H. Shear, M.D., has received grants for clinical research or educational purposes and served as advisor for Roche, Galderma SA, Genesoft Co. Ltd., GlaxoSmithKline, Novartis AG, and Fujisawa Healthcare Inc.

Sandra Knowles, B.Sc. Phm., and Lori Shapiro, M.D., have no commercial relationships with manufacturers of products or providers of services discussed in this chapter.

References

1. Karch FE, Lasagna L: Adverse drug reactions: a critical review. JAMA 234:1236, 1975

2. Lazarou J, Pomeranz BH, Corey PN: Incidence of adverse drug reactions in hospitalized patients: a meta-analysis of prospective studies. JAMA 279:1200, 1998

3. Lakshmanan M, Hershey C, Breslau D: Hospital admissions caused by iatrogenic disease. Arch Intern Med 146:1391, 1986

4. Bigby M, Jick S, Jick H, et al: Drug-induced cutaneous reactions: a report from the Boston Collaborative Drug Surveillance Program on 15,438 consecutive inpatients, 1975 to 1982. JAMA 256:3358, 1986

5. Leape LL, Brennan TA, Laird N, et al: The nature of adverse events in hospitalized patients: results of the Harvard Medical Practice Study II. N Engl J Med 324:377, 1991

6. Classen DC, Pestotnik SL, Evans RS, et al: Adverse drug events in hospitalized patients: excess length of stay, extra costs and attributable mortality. JAMA 277:301, 1997

7. Barbaud A, Goncalo M, Bruynzeel D, et al: Guidelines for performing skin tests with drugs in the investigation of cutaneous adverse drug reactions. Contact Derm 45:321, 2001

8. Barbaud A: Drug patch testing in systemic cutaneous drug allergy. Toxicology 209:209, 2005

9. Romano A, Quaratino D, DiFonso M, et al: A diagnostic protocol for evaluating nonimmediate reactions to aminopenicillins. J Allergy Clin Immunol 103:1186, 1999

10. Romano A, Quaratino D, Papa G, et al: Aminopenicillin allergy. Arch Dis Child 76:513, 1997

11. Coopman S, Johnson R, Platt R, et al: Cutaneous disease and drug reactions in HIV infection. N Engl J Med 328:1670, 1993

12. Pichler W, Yawalkar N, Schmid S, et al: Pathogenesis of drug-induced exanthems. Allergy 57:884, 2002

13. Nigen S, Knowles SR, Shear NH: Drug eruptions: approaching the diagnosis of drug-induced skin diseases. J Drugs Dermatol 2:278, 2003

14. Shear NH, Spielberg SP: Anticonvulsant hypersensitivity syndrome: in vitro assessment of risk. J Clin Invest 82:1826, 1988

15. Kano Y, Inaoka M, Shiohara T: Association between anticonvulsant hypersensitivity syndrome and human herpesvirus 6 reactivation and hypogammaglobulinemia. Arch Dermatol 140:183, 2004

16. Wong G, Shear N: Is a drug alone sufficient to cause the drug hypersensitivity syndrome? Arch Dermatol 140:226, 2004

17. Wadelius M, Karlsson T, Wadelius C, et al: Lamotrigine and toxic epidermal necrolysis. Lancet 348:1041, 1996

18. Shear NH, Spielberg SP, Grant DM, et al: Differences in metabolism of sulfonamides predisposing to idiosyncratic toxicity. Ann Intern Med 105:179, 1986

19. Knowles S, Shapiro L, Shear N: Should celecoxib be contraindicated in patients who are allergic to sulfonamides? Revisiting the meaning of "sulfa" allergy. Drug Safety 24:239, 2001

20. Khoo B, Leow Y: A review of inpatients with adverse drug reactions to allopurinol. Singapore Med J 41:156, 2000

21. Masaki T, Fukunaga A, Tohyama M, et al: Human herpes virus 6 encephalitis in allopurinol-induced hypersensitivity syndrome. Acta Derm Venereol 83:128, 2003

22. Hung S, Chung W, Liou L, et al: HLA-B*5801 allele as a genetic marker for severe cutaneous adverse reactions caused by allopurinol. Proc Natl Acad Sci USA 102:4134, 2005

23. Martin A, Nolan D, James I, et al: Predisposition to nevirapine hypersensitivity associated with HLA-DRB1*0101 and abrogated by low CD4 T-cell counts. AIDS 19:97, 2005

24. Martin AM, Krueger R, Almeida CA, et al: A sensitive and rapid alternative to HLA typing as a genetic screening test for abacavir hypersensitivity syndrome. Pharmacogenet Genomics 16:353, 2006

25. Gupta A, Eggo M, Uetrecht J, et al: Drug-induced hypothyroidism: the thyroid as a target organ in hypersensitivity reactions to anticonvulsants and sulfonamides. Clin Pharmacol Ther 51:56, 1992

26. Rieder MJ: In vivo and in vitro testing for adverse drug reactions. Pediatr Clin North Am 44:93, 1997

27. Harman K, Morris S, Higgins E: Persistent anticonvulsant hypersensitivity syndrome responding to ciclosporin. Clin Exp Dermatol 28:364, 2003

28. Kano Y, Inaoka M, Sakuma K, et al: Virus reactivation and intravenous immunoglobulin (IVIG) therapy of drug-induced hypersensitivity syndromes. Toxicology 209:165, 2005

29. Tan EK, Grattan CE: Drug-induced urticaria. Expert Opin Drug Saf 3:471, 2004

30. Anderson J: Allergic reactions to drugs and biologic agents. JAMA 268:2845, 1992

31. Simon RA, Namazy J: Adverse reactions to aspirin and nonsteroidal anti-inflammatory drugs (NSAIDs). Clin Rev Allergy Immunol 24:239, 2003

32. Dykewicz MS: Cough and angioedema from angiotensin-converting enzyme inhibitors: new insights into mechanisms and management. Curr Opin Allergy Clin Immunol 4:267, 2004

33. Mazon A, Nieto A, Linana JJ, et al: Latex sensitization in children with spina bifida: follow-up comparative study after two years. Ann Allergy Asthma Immunol 84:207, 2000

34. Taylor JS, Erkek E: Latex allergy: diagnosis and management. Dermatol Ther 17:289, 2004

35. Pavletic AJ: Late angioedema in patients taking angiotensin-converting-enzyme inhibitors. Lancet 360:493, 2002

36. Dykewicz M, Kim HW, Orfan N, et al: Immunologic analysis of anaphylaxis to protamine component in neutral protamine Hagedorn human insulin. J Allergy Clin Immunol 93:117, 1994

37. Tan EK, Grattan CE: Drug-induced urticaria. Expert Opin Drug Saf 3:471, 2004

38. Hoffman HM, Wright FA, Broide DH, et al: Identification of a locus on chromosome

1q44 for familial cold urticaria. Am J Hum Genet 66:1693, 2000

39. Haas N, Toppe E, Henz BE: Microscopic morphology of different types of urticaria. Arch Dermatol 134:41, 1998

40. Erbagci Z: The leukotriene receptor antagonist montelukast in the treatment of chronic idiopathic urticaria: a single-blind, placebo-controlled, cross-over clinical study. J Allergy Clin Immunol 110:484, 2002

41. Ilter N, Gurer MA, Akkoca MA: Short-term oral cyclosporine for chronic idiopathic urticaria. J Eur Acad Dermatol Venereol 12:67, 1999

42. Heckbert SR, Stryker WS, Coltin KL, et al: Serum sickness in children after antibiotic exposure: estimates of occurrence and morbidity in a health maintenance organization population. Am J Epidemiol 132:336, 1990

43. Kearns GL, Wheeler JG, Childress SH, et al: Serum sickness–like reactions to cefaclor: role of hepatic metabolism and individual susceptibility. J Pediatr 125:805, 1994

44. Lowery N, Kearns GL, Young RA, et al: Serum sickness–like reactions associated with cefprozil therapy. J Pediatr 125:325, 1994

45. McCollom RA, Elbe DH, Ritchie AH: Bupropion-induced serum sickness–like reaction. Ann Pharmacother 34:471, 2000

46. Shapiro LE, Knowles SR, Shear NH: Comparative safety and risk management of tetracycline, doxycycline and minocycline. Arch Dermatol 133:1224, 1997

47. Hellerstedt B, Ahmed A: Delayed-type hypersensitivity reaction or serum sickness after rituximab treatment. Ann Oncol 14:1792, 2003

48. Gamarra RM, McGraw SD, Drelichman VS, et al: Serum sickness-like reactions in patients receiving intravenous infliximab. J Emerg Med 30:41, 2006

49. Vial T, Pont J, Pham E, et al: Cefaclor-associated serum sickness–like disease: eight cases and review of the literature. Ann Pharmacother 26:910, 1992

50. Grammer LC: Cefaclor serum sickness. JAMA 275:1152, 1996

51. Lee AY: Fixed drug eruptions: incidence, recognition and avoidance. Am J Clin Dermatol 1:277, 2000

52. Ozkaya-Bayazit E, Akar U: Fixed drug eruption induced by trimethoprim-sulfamethoxazole: evidence for a link to HLA-A30 B13 Cw6 haplotype. J Am Acad Dermatol 45:712, 2001

53. Barbaud A, Reichert-Penetrat S, Trechot P, et al: The use of skin testing in the investigation of cutaneous adverse drug reactions. Br J Dermatol 139:49, 1998

54. Al-Khenaizan S, Schecter JF, Sasseville D: Pseudoporphyria induced by propionic acid derivatives. J Cutan Med Surg 3:162, 1999

55. Kuechle MK, Stegemeir E, Maynard B, et al: Drug-induced linear IgA bullous dermatosis: report of six cases and review of the literature. J Am Acad Dermatol 30:187, 1994

56. Neughebauer BI, Negron G, Pelton S, et al: Bullous skin disease: an unusual allergic reaction to vancomycin. Am J Med Sci 323:273, 2002

57. Brenner S, Bialy-Gohan A, Ruocco V: Drug-induced pemphigus. Clin Dermatol 16:393, 1998

58. Wolf R, Brenner S: An active amide group in the molecule of drugs that induce pemphigus: a casual or causal relationship? Dermatology 189:1, 1994

59. Roujeau JC, Kelly JP, Naldi L, et al: Medication use and the risk of Stevens-Johnson syndrome or toxic epidermal necrolysis. N Engl J Med 333:1600, 1995

60. Rzany B, Correia O, Kelly JP, et al: Risk of Stevens-Johnson syndrome and toxic epidermal necrolysis during first weeks of antiepileptic therapy: a case-control study. Study Group of the International Case Control Study on Severe Cutaneous Adverse Reactions. Lancet 353:2190, 1999

61. Chave TA, Mortimer NJ, Sladden MJ, et al: Toxic epidermal necrolysis: current evidence, practical management and future directions. Br J Dermatol 153:241, 2005

62. Wolkenstein P, Charue D, Bagot M, et al: Metabolic predisposition to cutaneous adverse drug reactions. Arch Dermatol 131:544, 1995

63. Nassif A, Bensussan A, Boumsell L, et al: Toxic epidermal necrolysis: effector cells are drug-specific cytotoxic T cells. J Allergy Clin Immunol 114:1209, 2004

64. Bastuji-Garin S, Rzany B, Stern RS, et al: Clinical classification of cases of toxic epidermal necrolysis, Stevens-Johnson syndrome, and erythema multiforme. Arch Dermatol 129:92, 1993

65. Schlienger RG, Shapiro LE, Shear NH: Lamotrigine-induced severe cutaneous adverse reactions. Epilepsia 39:S22, 1998

66. Garcia-Doval I, LeCleach L, Bocquet H, et al: Toxic epidermal necrolysis and Stevens-Johnson syndrome: does early withdrawal of causative drugs decrease the risk of death? Arch Dermatol 136:323, 2000

67. Patterson R, Miller M, Kaplan M, et al: Effectiveness of early therapy with corticosteroids in Stevens-Johnson syndrome: experience with 41 cases and a hypothesis regarding pathogenesis. Ann Allergy 73:27, 1994

68. French LE, Trent JT, Kerdel FA: Use of intravenous immunoglobulin in toxic epidermal necrolysis and Stevens-Johnson syndrome: our current understanding. Int Immunopharmacol 6:543, 2006

69. Shortt R, Gomez M, Mittmann N, et al: Intravenous immunoglobulin does not improve outcome in toxic epidermal necrolysis. J Burn Care Rehabil 25:246, 2004

70. Remmer H, Falk W: Successful treatment of lithium-induced acne. J Clin Psychiatry 47:48, 1986

71. Traupe H, von Muhlendahl K, Bramswig J, et al: Acne of the fulminans type following testosterone therapy in three excessively tall boys. Arch Dermatol 124:414, 1988

72. Beylot C, Doutre MS, Beylot-Barry M: Acute generalized exanthematous pustulosis. Semin Cutaneous Med Surg 15:244, 1996

73. Sidoroff A, Halevy S, Bavinck JN, et al: Acute generalized exanthematous pustulosis (AGEP): a clinical reaction pattern. J Cutan Pathol 28:113, 2001

74. Britschgi M, Pichler W: Acute generalized exanthematous pustulosis, a clue to neutrophil-mediated inflammatory processes orchestrated by T cells. Curr Opin Allergy Clin Immunol 2:325, 2002

75. Freeman BD, Schmieg RE, McGrath S, et al: Factor V Leiden mutation in a patient with warfarin-associated skin necrosis. Surgery 127:595, 2000

76. Bauer KA: Coumarin-induced skin necrosis. Arch Dermatol 129:766, 1993

77. Schramm W, Spannagel M, Bauer KA, et al: Treatment of coumarin-induced skin necrosis with a monoclonal antibody purified protein C concentrate. Arch Dermatol 19:753, 1993

78. Thompson DF, Skaehill A: Drug-induced lichen planus. Pharmacotherapy 14:561, 1994

79. ten Holder SM, Joy MS, Falk RJ: Cutaneous and systemic manifestations of drug-induced vasculitis. Ann Pharmcother 36:130, 2002

80. Sanchez NP, Van Hale HM, Su WP: Clinical and histopathologic spectrum of necrotizing vasculitis: reports of findings in 101 cases. Arch Dermatol 121:220, 1985

81. Jennette J, Falk K: Small-vessel vasculitis. N Engl J Med 337:1512, 1997

82. Merkel PA: Drugs associated with vasculitis. Curr Opin Rheumatol 10:45, 1998

83. Mehregan D, Hall M, Gibson E: Urticarial vasculitis: a histopathologic and clinical review of 72 cases. J Am Acad Dermatol 26:441, 1992

84. Wiik A: Clinical and laboratory characteristics of drug-induced vasculitis syndromes. Arthritis Res Ther 7:191, 2005

85. Bahrami S, Malone JC, Webb KG, et al: Tissue eosinophilia as an indicator of drug-induced cutaneous small-vessel vasculitis. Arch Dermatol 142:155, 2006

41 Fungal, Bacterial, and Viral Infections of the Skin

Jan V. Hirschmann, M.D.

Despite its large surface area and constant exposure to the environment, the skin resists infection well. The most important protective factor is an intact stratum corneum, the tough barrier of protein and lipid formed on the cutaneous surface by the underlying epidermis.[1] This barricade impedes invasion by environmental pathogens, and its dryness discourages colonization and growth of the many organisms that require moisture to survive, such as gram-negative bacilli. Furthermore, the constant shedding of cells of the epidermis impedes most microbes from establishing permanent residence.

Some organisms, however, can attach to skin cells and reproduce there; the normal cutaneous flora comprises primarily aerobic, gram-positive cocci and bacilli in densities ranging from about 10^2 organisms/cm^2 on dry skin to 10^7 organisms/cm^2 in moist areas, such as the axilla.[2] This resident population inhibits harmful organisms from colonizing the skin by occupying binding sites on the epidermal cells, competing for nutrients, producing antimicrobial substances, and maintaining the skin surface at a low pH (about 5.5). Anaerobes are sparse except in areas with abundant sebaceous glands, such as the face and chest; in the deeper portions of these sites, as well as in hair follicles, anaerobes reach concentrations of 10^4 to 10^6 organisms/cm^2.

Cutaneous infections occur when the skin's protective mechanisms fail, especially when trauma, inflammation, maceration from excessive moisture, or other factors disrupt the stratum corneum. The organisms causing infection may originate from the victim's own resident flora, either on the skin or on adjacent mucous membranes, but many come from other people, animals, or the environment.

Dermatophyte Infections

Dermatophytes are fungi (molds) that can infect the skin, hair, and nails. These organisms, which include *Trichophyton, Microsporum,* and *Epidermophyton* species, are classified as anthropophilic, zoophilic, or geophilic, depending on whether their primary source is humans, animals, or the soil, respectively.[3] Geophilic dermatophyte infections occur sporadically, primarily among gardeners and farm workers. Zoophilic dermatophytes (*Trichophyton* and *Microsporum* species) may have a restricted range of hosts (e.g., *M. persicolor* infects only voles) or may afflict many different animals (e.g., *T. mentagrophytes* can infect mice and other rodents, dogs, cats, and horses). Human infections with zoophilic species have occurred after exposure to dogs, cats, horses, cattle, pigs, rodents, poultry, hedgehogs, and voles. Anthropophilic dermatophytes are the most common cause of fungal skin infections in humans. Transmission of these infections occurs from direct contact between people or from exposure to desquamated skin cells present in the environment—arthrospores can survive for months. Direct inoculation of the spores through breaks in the skin can lead to germination and subsequent invasion of the superficial cutaneous layers.

Dermatophyte infections occur more frequently in certain ethnic groups and in people with impaired cell-mediated immunity. Many of the anthropophilic dermatophyte infections occur more often in one gender or age group.[4]

Infection of the scalp, for example, is primarily a disease of children. Involvement of the feet and groin is most common in adolescents and young adults, especially males, but is unusual in children. Nail infection is more frequent in both men and women of advancing age. The reasons for these differences are unknown.

The anthropophilic dermatophytes also have unique geographic distribution patterns. The most common cause of scalp infection in the United States, for example, is *T. tonsurans*, but in Southeast Asia and the Middle East, it is *T. violaceum*. These differences may relate to climatic or racial factors.

The various forms of dermatophytosis, also called ringworm, are named according to the site involved. These infections include tinea capitis (scalp), tinea corporis (body), tinea barbae (beard area of men), tinea faciei (face), tinea cruris (groin), tinea pedis (feet), tinea unguium (nails), and tinea manuum (hands). The characteristic skin lesion is an annular scaly patch [*see Figure 1*], though the clinical appearance varies not only with the site involved but also with the host's immune status and the type of infecting organism. In general, anthropophilic species elicit little inflammation and cause chronic infections. Zoophilic and geophilic species, however, often provoke intense inflammation, which sometimes leads to eradication of the organisms and healing without treatment.

CLINICAL PRESENTATIONS

Tinea Capitis

Tinea capitis occurs primarily in children but may develop in adults—especially the elderly, those who are unkempt, and the impoverished. Transmission can occur between humans by the sharing of combs, brushes, or headgear. Only *Microsporum* and *Trichophyton* species cause tinea capitis. Infection begins with invasion of the stratum corneum of the scalp skin. The hairs then become infected, in one of three microscopic patterns: ectothrix, endothrix, or favus. In ectothrix, the spores are outside the hair shaft and destroy the cuticle; in endothrix, they lie within the hair and do not affect the cuticle; and in favus, broad hyphae and air spaces

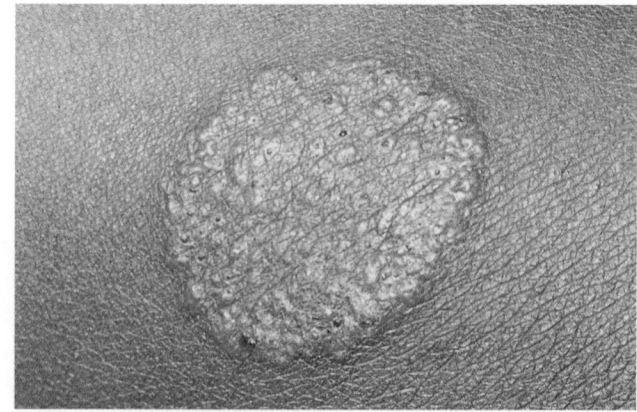

Figure 1 Classic annular lesion of tinea corporis shows a raised or vesicular margin with central clearing.

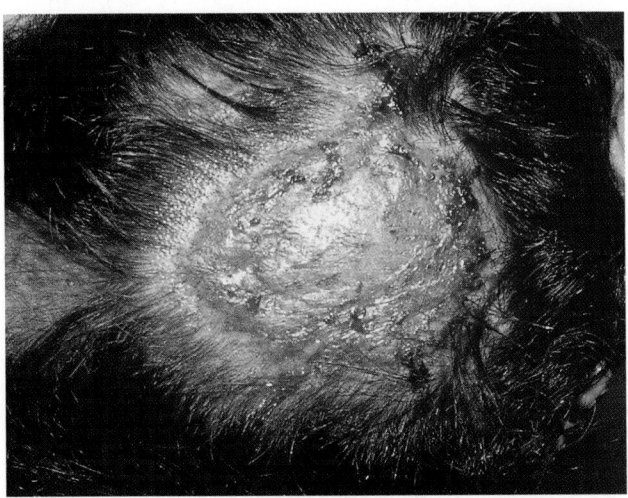

Figure 2 **A typical kerion presenting as a zoophilic *Microsporum canis* infection of the scalp (tinea capitis).**

form within the hair, but spores are absent. In all three types, scaling, hair loss, and inflammation of varying degrees are present.[5]

T. tonsurans, the major cause of tinea capitis in adults, characteristically produces a noninflammatory infection with either well-demarcated or irregular and diffuse areas of scaling and alopecia. Because the swollen hairs may fracture at or just below the scalp epidermis, the scalp sometimes appears to be marked by small black dots. As with all *Trichophyton* infections, these scalp lesions do not fluoresce under a Wood light.

T. schoenleinii causes favus, characterized by an inflammatory crust (scutulum) in which hair appears to be matted in the dried,

yellow exudate. Hair shedding late in the infection is common because the hair shaft is not damaged until the infection is well advanced.

M. audouinii, which causes an ectothrix infection, produces well-delineated, noninflammatory patches of alopecia in which the hair breaks at the epidermal surface and is often dull gray because of the presence of numerous spores on the surface of the hair shaft. As in all *Microsporum* infections, these lesions fluoresce under a Wood light. The most severe inflammation, usually from a zoophilic species, results in a kerion, a painful, boggy mass in which follicles may discharge pus and in which sinus tracts form [*see Figure 2*]. Crusting and matting of adjacent hairs are common, and cervical lymph nodes may enlarge.

Tinea Corporis

Tinea corporis typically appears as a single lesion or multiple circular lesions with scaling, well-delineated margins and a raised, erythematous edge. Often, the lesions have an area of central clearing. The amount of inflammation varies; when the inflammation is intense, pustules, vesicles, and even bullae may occur. Sometimes, involvement of the hair follicles in the middle of a patch of scaling erythema leads to perifollicular nodules, a condition called Majocchi granuloma. This infection usually occurs on the legs of patients infected with *T. rubrum;* it can be precipitated by topical corticosteroid therapy. In immunocompromised hosts, subcutaneous abscesses may develop.

Tinea Barbae

Tinea barbae occurs in adult men and involves the skin and coarse hairs of the beard and mustache area. The usual cause is a zoophilic species, primarily *T. verrucosum* or *T. mentagrophytes;* these species commonly infect cattle and horses. Patients are

a

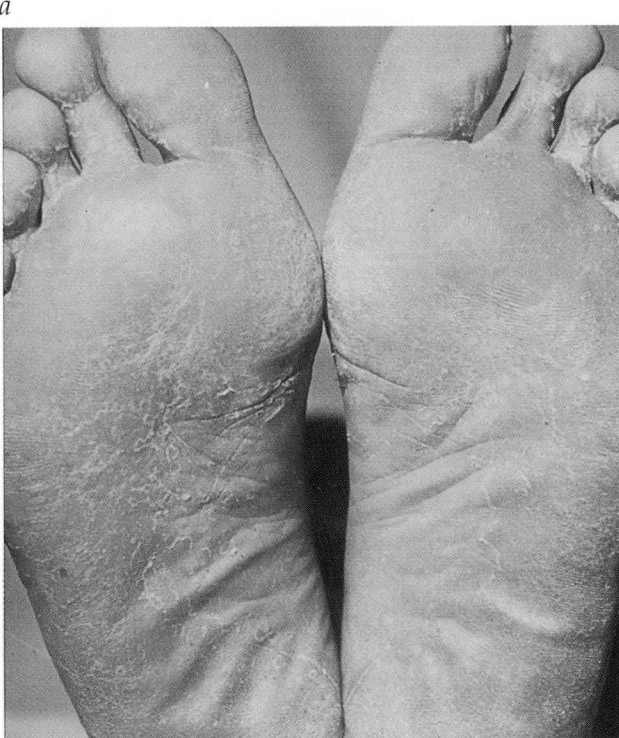

b

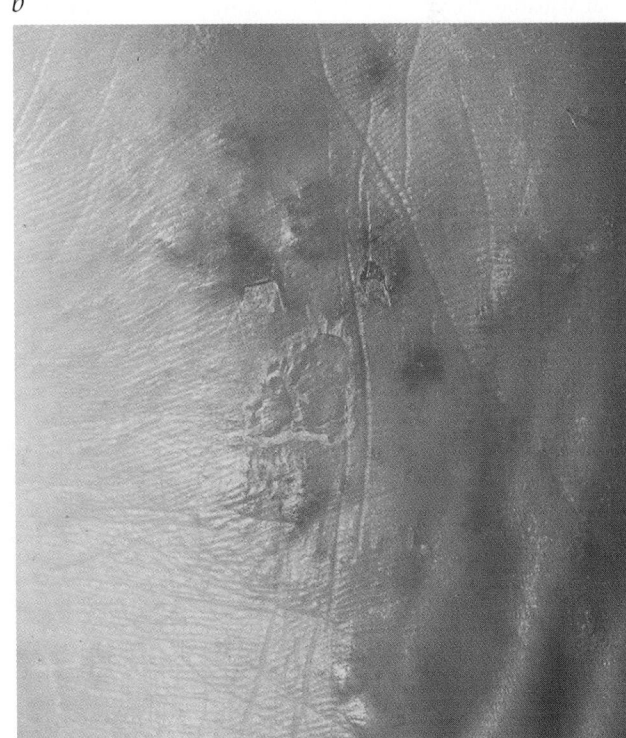

Figure 3 (*a*) **The scaling of tinea pedis appears between and under the toes and on the plantar surface. (*b*) Tinea pedis may also present as vesicles.**

generally farm workers, and the infection usually causes erythema, scaling, and follicular pustules. Many hairs become loose and are easily removed with a forceps.

Tinea Faciei

Tinea faciei occurs as an infection of the face in women and children and infection of the area outside the mustache and beard in men. The usual causes are *T. rubrum* and *T. mentagrophytes;* these organisms reach the face through direct inoculation or by spreading from another site of infection on the body. Patients often complain of itching and burning, and symptoms may worsen after exposure to sunlight. The lesions may be scaly, annular erythematous patches, but often they are indistinct red areas with little or no scaling.

Tinea Cruris

Tinea cruris, infection of the groin, is much more common in men than women and is often associated with infection of the feet. *T. rubrum* and *E. floccosum* are the most common causes. The lesions are usually red, scaling, sharply demarcated areas with raised, erythematous borders. The infection, which affects the medial portion of the upper thighs but consistently spares the scrotum, may extend to the buttocks, abdomen, and lower back. Vesicles, nodules, pustules, and maceration may be present.

Tinea Pedis

Tinea pedis is most frequently caused by *T. rubrum, E. floccosum,* and *T. mentagrophytes.* The most common form consists of fissuring, scaling, and maceration in the interdigital spaces, especially between the fourth and fifth toes. A second type involves scaling, hyperkeratosis, and erythema of the soles, heels, and sides of the feet. In this kind of tinea pedis, the lesions occur in a so-called moccasin distribution pattern [*see Figure 3a*]. The plantar skin may become very thick and scaly. A third form demonstrates an inflammatory pattern characterized by vesicles, pustules, or even bullae, usually on the soles [*see Figure 3b*].

An important complication of tinea pedis is streptococcal cellulitis of the lower leg. Streptococci do not ordinarily survive on normal skin, but the presence of interdigital fissuring, scaling, or maceration from fungal disease or other causes apparently permits streptococci of various groups, including A, B, C, and G, to colonize the toe webs.[6] From this location, these bacteria may invade the skin damaged by the tinea pedis or migrate to locations higher up the leg and enter the skin through any defects.

Tinea Unguium

Nail involvement usually occurs from adjacent fungal infection of the hands or feet. The organisms typically invade the nail from the distal or lateral borders, and infection spreads proximally. The nails are thickened, opaque, and yellowish to brownish. They may crack or crumble, and often, subungual hyperkeratosis lifts the nail plate from the underlying bed (a condition known as onycholysis) [*see Figure 4*]. Splinter hemorrhages are common.

Tinea Manuum

Tinea manuum is an infection of the hands. Most cases have accompanying involvement of the feet; inexplicably, usually only one hand is affected (so-called two-feet, one-hand disease). The most common finding is scaling or hyperkeratosis of the palms and fingers. Occasionally, vesicles, papules, or follicular nodules form on the dorsal surface of the hands.

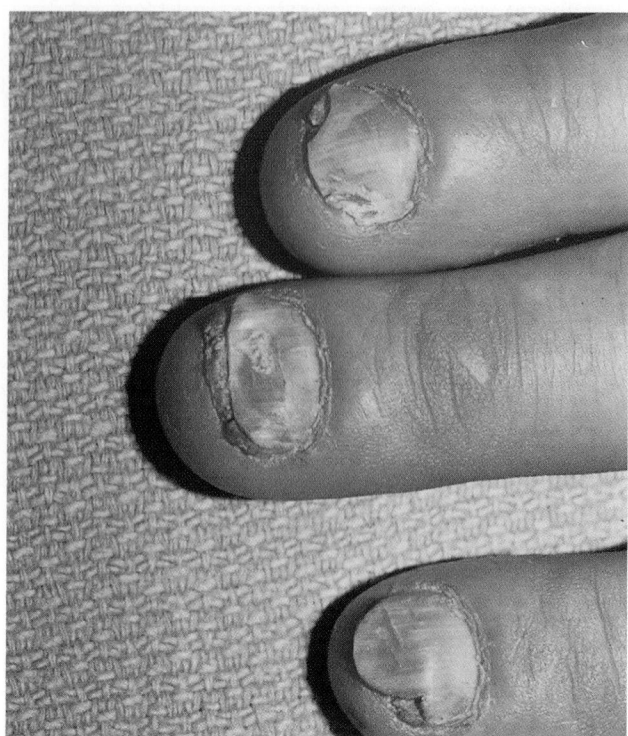

Figure 4 Nails are usually thickened, cracked, and crumbly in tinea unguium; subungual debris may be present, as shown.

DIAGNOSIS

Clinicians should suspect dermatophyte infection in patients with any scaling, erythematous eruption and in patients whose nails exhibit the characteristics of tinea unguium (see above). The diagnosis can be confirmed by microscopy or culture of properly obtained specimens. The optimal method of obtaining specimens from the skin is by scraping the scaly lesions; specimens from the nails are best obtained by taking fragments of subungual debris.

The specimen is prepared for microscopic examination by first placing it on a glass slide and treating it with potassium hydroxide (KOH), which digests the keratin of the skin, nails, and hair, and then heating it to hasten the process. The basic culture medium for isolating dermatophytes is an agar containing Sabouraud medium, often combined with antibiotics to eliminate bacteria and with cycloheximide to inhibit saprophytic fungi. Growth is usually apparent in 3 to 14 days. A dermatophyte test medium culture can be used in the office and is both accurate and inexpensive.[7] When both KOH preparations and cultures are negative, a biopsy may be useful in identifying the infecting organism, usually by special tissue stains such as periodic acid–Schiff or Gomori methenamine-silver stains. As an alternative to cultures, a biopsy may be used as the primary method for establishing the diagnosis.

TREATMENT

Tinea corporis, tinea cruris, tinea pedis, and tinea faciei respond to topical agents applied once or twice daily to the affected area, usually for 2 to 4 weeks. Good choices include azoles (e.g., miconazole, econazole, or clotrimazole) or terbinafine. The cost of the preparation can dictate which agent to recommend; many are available without prescription. Tinea pedis often recurs after effective therapy, especially in cases of the moccasin form of the disease. When infection reappears, the previous therapy can be resumed without loss of effectiveness.

Oral therapy is necessary for extensive lesions, for infection involving the hair or hair follicles (e.g., tinea capitis and tinea barbae), for tinea unguium, and, often, for tinea manuum and various forms of dermatophytoses in immunocompromised hosts. Five oral agents are currently available: griseofulvin, ketoconazole, itraconazole, fluconazole, and terbinafine. Griseofulvin, a fungistatic agent, is the oldest oral treatment available and is still useful, primarily in infections not involving the nails. Griseofulvin reduces the serum levels of barbiturates and warfarin. Some patients receiving griseofulvin note a diminished tolerance to alcohol.

The azoles include ketoconazole, itraconazole, and fluconazole; like griseofulvin, they are fungistatic. Ketoconazole is usually well tolerated, but hepatotoxicity occurs in about 1 in 10,000 patients, typically after several weeks of use. Fluconazole and itraconazole provide protracted levels of antibiotic in the nails, allowing short or intermittent courses of therapy for tinea unguium. Both fluconazole and itraconazole can cause gastrointestinal disorders, rashes, and, occasionally, hepatotoxicity and can have serious interactions with several medications, including cyclosporine, digoxin, and quinidine. Ketoconazole, itraconazole, and fluconazole can interact with other medications; pharmacologic sources should be consulted for potential interactions.

Terbinafine, an allylamine, is fungicidal, unlike both griseofulvin and the azoles, which are fungistatic. High levels of terbinafine penetrate the nails, and the drug persists for many weeks to exert antifungal effects long after discontinuance. Its few side effects include gastrointestinal reactions and, occasionally, skin rashes. Hepatotoxicity and hematologic abnormalities are rare, and drug interactions are uncommon. These oral antifungals are quite effective for tinea capitis. The adult dosage for griseofulvin is 500 mg twice daily for 8 weeks. The other agents are effective when given for 1 to 3 weeks. Daily doses are as follows: itraconazole, 200 mg; fluconazole, 200 mg; and terbinafine, 250 mg. Of these, griseofulvin is the least expensive, but some *T. tonsurans* isolates are resistant to it. All these medications are effective in cases of tinea barbae; Majocchi granuloma; extensive tinea corporis; and tinea manuum that is unresponsive to topical agents. Griseofulvin and terbinafine appear to be superior to fluconazole and itraconazole for the treatment of tinea capitis.[8]

Tinea unguium is difficult to eradicate, particularly in the toenails. The most effective agent is terbinafine, administered at a dosage of 250 mg daily for 6 weeks for fingernail infections and for 12 weeks for toenail involvement.[9] The terbinafine regimens produce short-term eradication of infection in about 70% to 90% of patients with fingernail infection and in about 50% to 80% of patients with toenail infection. Relapse is common, and patients often require a second course of treatment. About 75% of patients who receive one or more courses of terbinafine will have a clinical cure 5 years later. This medication is expensive, and clinicians must decide in each case whether its use is warranted.

Yeast Infections

Yeasts are unicellular fungi that reproduce by budding. They may form filamentous projections, which, unlike the hyphae of molds, do not contain separate cells. Accordingly, they are called pseudohyphae. *Candida* species are not part of the normal skin flora, but they commonly reside in the oropharynx, vagina, and colon. From these locations, they may cause infections in adjacent traumatized skin. Alternatively, with reduction in the other flora or with impaired host defense mechanisms, these yeasts may proliferate in large numbers to produce lesions on the mucosal surfaces of the mouth and vagina.

Malassezia furfur (also called *Pityrosporum orbiculare* or *P. ovale*) is a yeast that requires lipids for growth. It normally colonizes the skin of adults, especially the scalp and upper trunk, where the presence of sebum is highest. For unknown reasons, these organisms, which are ordinarily commensals, can become pathogenic and cause tinea versicolor (also known as pityriasis versicolor) or folliculitis. Cogent evidence suggests that these organisms also cause seborrheic dermatitis and dandruff.

CANDIDIASIS

Clinical Presentations

Oral candidiasis One form of oral candidiasis, thrush, appears as white to gray patches (pseudomembranes) on the tongue, soft palate, gingiva, oropharynx, and buccal mucosa. Removing the material from the mucosal surface reveals an underlying erythematous base. Predisposing factors in adults include diabetes mellitus, use of systemic or local corticosteroids, use of broad-spectrum antibiotics, use of radiotherapy or chemotherapy, and impaired cell-mediated immunity, especially from HIV infection. Acute atrophic candidiasis especially follows antibiotic therapy and causes painful, red, denuded lesions of the mucous membranes; the tongue may have erythematous areas with atrophic filiform papillae. In chronic atrophic candidiasis, contamination of dentures with *Candida* causes painful, red, and sometimes edematous lesions with a shiny, atrophic epithelium and well-demarcated borders where the dentures contact the mucous membranes. Poor dental hygiene and prolonged use of dentures are common predisposing factors. Some patients with these predisposing factors have angular cheilitis (perleche), characterized by erythema and fissuring of the corners of the mouth. Other contributing conditions are maceration from excessive salivation or licking, poorly fitting dentures, and a larger fold from diminished alveolar ridge height. *Candida* is present in most, but not all, patients with this disorder.

Chronic hyperplastic candidiasis (candidal leukoplakia) consists of irregular, white, persistent plaques on the tongue or mucous membranes that are difficult to remove; this form of candidiasis occurs especially in male smokers. Soreness, burning, and roughness of the affected areas are the usual symptoms. Candidiasis of the tongue can also take the form of median rhomboid glossitis, a diamond-shaped area of atrophic papillae in the central portion of the lingual surface.

Candidal intertrigo *Candida* infection may occur in any skin fold, causing soreness and itching. Obese patients are especially vulnerable. Commonly affected areas include the groin, inframammary regions, and folds of the abdominal pannus. The lesions are patches of bright erythema accompanied by maceration and an irregular, scalloped border, beyond which papules and pustules (satellite lesions) commonly form [*see Figure 5*].

Candidal vulvovaginitis and balanitis Most women with candidal vulvovaginitis have no underlying disease, but candidal vulvovaginitis may accompany diabetes mellitus and HIV infection. It also occurs as a complication of therapy with certain antibiotics. Candidal vulvovaginitis causes white plaques on a swollen, red vaginal mucosa; a creamy vaginal discharge; and erythema, sometimes with pustules, on the vulvar skin. Soreness and burning are common symptoms. Male sexual partners of women with candidal vulvovaginitis—especially male sexual partners who are uncircumcised—may develop balanitis, characterized by erythema, pustules, and erosions on the glans of the penis. Balanitis may occur spontaneously as well.

Candidal paronychia and nail infection   Maceration of the tissue surrounding the nail, typically caused by excessive moisture, may cause paronychia, which is characterized by erythema, swelling, and pain of the nail fold with loss of the cuticle [*see Figure 6*]. *Candida* organisms often colonize the area but are probably pathogenic only when pus forms. With chronic colonization, nail involvement may occur, producing yellowish discoloration and separation of the nail plate from the nail bed (onycholysis). For chronic paronychia without purulence, topical corticosteroids, such as triamcinolone cream applied twice daily for 3 weeks, are the best therapy.[10]

Diagnosis

Scrapings from cutaneous or mucous membrane lesions may be mixed with KOH solution and examined under the microscope to identify budding yeasts with pseudohyphae. Gram stains of the same specimen are easier to evaluate because they disclose very large, oval, gram-positive organisms that may demonstrate budding or pseudohyphal formation. These yeasts are much larger than bacteria and are much easier to see on Gram stain than on KOH preparations. Culture of specimens may be useful if the microscopy is normal or ambiguous. These organisms grow rapidly on both fungal and conventional bacterial media.

Treatment

Oral candidiasis   For oral candidiasis, topical nystatin suspension, 200,000 to 400,000 units three to five times a day, is usu-

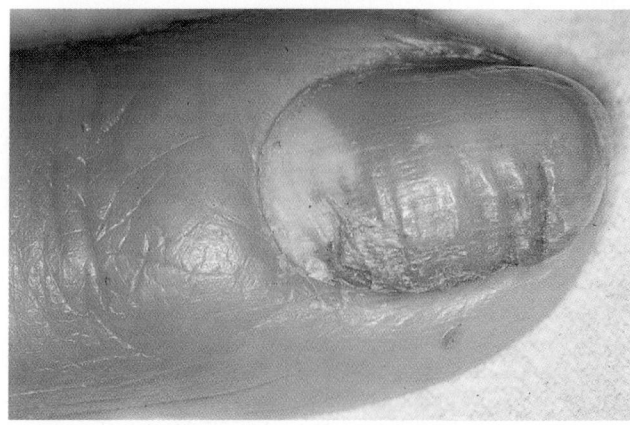

Figure 6   In a *Candida* paronychia, seen on this patient's thumb, the nail fold becomes red, swollen, and painful. Nail dystrophy is also seen.

ally effective; an alternative treatment is clotrimazole troches. For patients in whom topical treatment is ineffective or poorly tolerated, systemic therapies include ketoconazole (200 mg/day), fluconazole (100 mg/day), and itraconazole (100 mg twice a day). Angular cheilitis usually responds to an azole cream, such as miconazole or clotrimazole. Dentures should be cleaned carefully with an effective disinfectant, such as chlorhexidine.

Candidal intertrigo and balanitis   Candidal intertrigo and balanitis respond to a topical azole cream, such as miconazole or clotrimazole.

Candidal vulvovaginitis   Treatment of vulvovaginitis includes a topical azole in the form of a cream, suppository, or ointment, administered intravaginally, typically once daily for 7 days. A cream may be used for vulvar involvement. An alternative to suppositories is treatment with a single oral dose (150 mg) of fluconazole, which is at least as effective as topical therapy and is often preferred by patients.

Candidal paronychia   Patients with candidal paronychia should keep their fingers dry; when wet work is unavoidable, patients should use cotton liners under rubber gloves. Prolonged topical therapy with creams or solutions of various azole preparations, such as clotrimazole, is often necessary to eradicate the infection.

MALASSEZIA INFECTIONS

Clinical Presentations

Tinea versicolor (pityriasis versicolor)   Because the term tinea traditionally refers to dermatophyte infection, some clinicians prefer the term pityriasis, which means scaling, for this yeast infection. Usually asymptomatic, tinea versicolor may cause itching or skin irritation. The lesions are small, discrete macules that tend to be darker than the surrounding skin in light-skinned patients and hypopigmented in patients with dark skin. They often coalesce to form large patches of various colors (versicolor) ranging from white to tan [*see Figure 7*]. Scratching the lesions produces a fine scale. This infection most commonly involves the upper trunk, but the arms, axillae, abdomen, and groin may also be affected. Most lesions fluoresce a yellowish color under a Wood light.

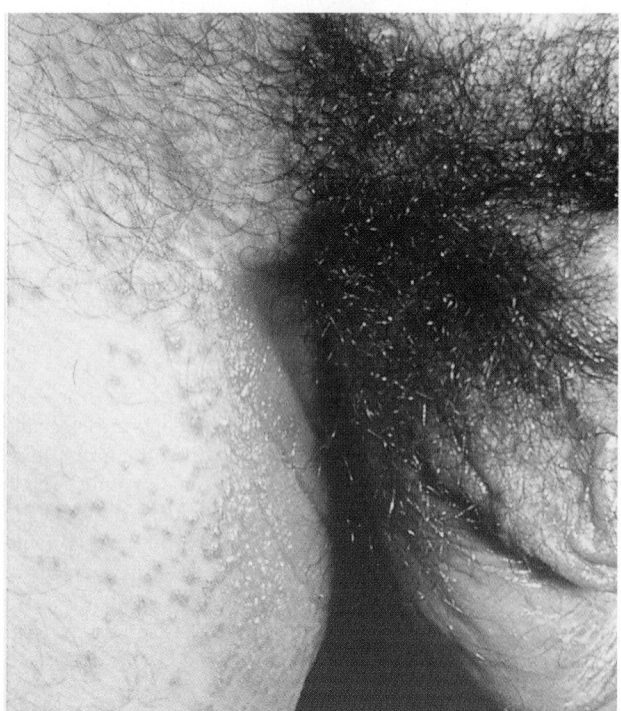

Figure 5   Prominent satellite lesions of discrete vesicles are seen in a patient with candidiasis.

Malassezia folliculitis (Pityrosporum folliculitis) In folliculitis, inflammation of the hair follicle causes red papules and pustules that surround individual hairs. One cause of folliculitis is various *Malassezia* species. Lesions appear predominantly on the trunk but occasionally occur on the arms as well. The lack of comedones distinguishes the lesion from acne. Pruritus and stinging may be present.

Diagnosis

In patients with tinea versicolor, KOH preparations of scrapings from the lesions demonstrate pseudohyphae and yeasts, which resemble spaghetti and meatballs. This finding is sufficient to establish the diagnosis. The yeast form prevails in folliculitis and is easily seen on Gram stain of purulent material from a pustule, appearing as a large, oval, gram-positive organism that is much larger than bacteria. Biopsies of these lesions show yeasts around and within the hair follicle, with accompanying neutrophilic inflammation. The yeasts are best seen with periodic acid–Schiff or Gomori methenamine-silver stain. Because these yeasts form part of the normal cutaneous flora, growth of the organism on cultures from scrapings of the skin surface is not very helpful diagnostically. Culture of the yeast from the pus of folliculitis is definitive; however, it requires special media, such as Sabouraud agar with olive oil, to provide the necessary lipids for growth. Growth typically occurs in 3 to 5 days.

Treatment

Simple treatment of tinea versicolor and *Malassezia* folliculitis involves applying selenium sulfide shampoo from the chin to the waist and from the shoulders to the wrist, allowing the shampoo to dry, and then washing it off after 10 to 15 minutes. Repeating this regimen after 1 week is usually effective; reapplication once every few weeks as necessary should prevent relapses, which are otherwise common. With tinea versicolor, scaling resolves promptly, but the pigmentary changes may take weeks to months to disappear. Topical azoles, such as ketoconazole, miconazole, and clotrimazole, are also effective, but they are more expensive. For patients who have difficulty applying a topical agent because of physical disabilities or other factors, oral ketoconazole or fluconazole in a single 400 mg dose is an effective alternative. This oral program can be repeated for recurrences.

Bacterial Infections

SKIN INFECTIONS CAUSED BY STREPTOCOCCI, STAPHYLOCOCCI, OR BOTH

Impetigo

Initially a vesicular infection of the skin, nonbullous impetigo rapidly evolves into pustules that rupture, with the dried discharge forming honey-colored crusts on an erythematous base [see Figure 8]. The lesions are often itchy. Nonbullous impetigo characteristically occurs on skin damaged by previous trauma, such as abrasions or cuts. Exposed areas are most commonly involved, typically the extremities or the areas around the mouth and nose. Nonbullous impetigo is usually a disease of young children and is more frequent in hot, humid climates than in temperate ones.

The usual cause of nonbullous impetigo is *Staphylococcus aureus*, but sometimes, *Streptococcus pyogenes* (group A streptococci) is also present; occasionally, *S. pyogenes* is the sole organism

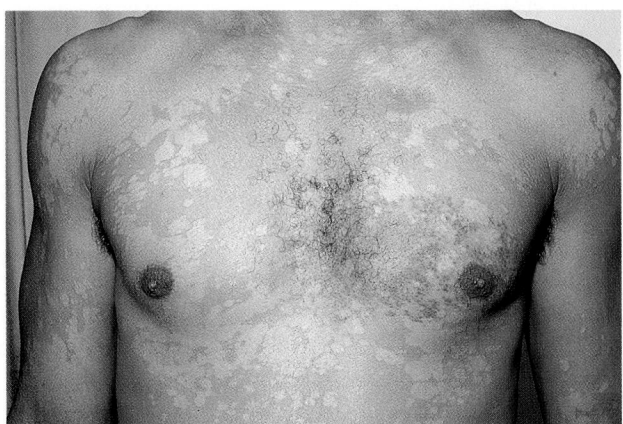

Figure 7 **Tinea versicolor appears on the chest of this patient as oval, hypopigmented, finely scaling macules.**

cultured.[11] Some strains of *S. aureus* elaborate a toxin that causes a split in the epidermis and the development of thin-roofed bullae. In this disorder, known as bullous impetigo, superficial, fragile, and flaccid vesiculopustules form and then rupture, with the exudate drying into a thin, brown, varnishlike crust. Sometimes, the vesiculopustules are not apparent, and erythematous erosions, often surrounded by a collar of remnants from the roof of the ruptured bulla, are the only evident disturbance. Gram-positive cocci in clusters are usually evident on a Gram stain of the fluid or pus from the bullae or from the surface of the erosions. Culturing *S. aureus* from these specimens establishes the diagnosis of bullous impetigo. Growth of *S. aureus, S. pyogenes*, or both from the skin lesions of nonbullous impetigo confirms the diagnosis of nonbullous impetigo, but cultures are unnecessary in characteristic cases. For treatment of sparse, nonbullous lesions, topical mupirocin ointment applied three times daily for 7 days is as effective as oral antimicrobials. Systemic antibiotics active against both *S. aureus* and *S. pyogenes*, such as cephalexin or dicloxacillin (250 mg orally four times a day for 7 days), represent an alternative to topical treatment. For extensive lesions, these antibiotics are preferred to topical therapy, and they are the treatment of choice for bullous impetigo. Because of the superficial nature of these infections, the lesions heal without scarring.

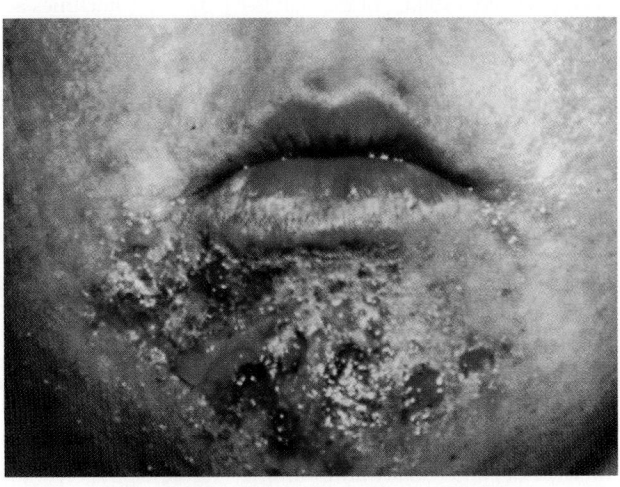

Figure 8 **Vesicopustules or bullae of impetigo rupture quickly and leave an erythematous base covered with a thin, seropurulent exudate. The exudate dries, forming layers of honey-colored crusts.**

Ecthyma

Ecthyma is a deeper infection than impetigo. As with nonbullous impetigo, *S. aureus*, *S. pyogenes*, or both may be the cause. Ecthyma commonly occurs in patients with poor hygiene or malnutrition or patients who have had skin trauma. The lesions, which are often multiple and are most common on the lower extremities, begin as vesicles that rupture, creating circular, erythematous lesions with adherent crusts. Beneath the scabs, which may spontaneously slough, are ulcers that leave a scar when healing occurs. Culture of the ulcer base yields the causative organisms. Treatment should be with an oral antistaphylococcal agent, such as dicloxacillin or cephalexin (250 mg orally four times a day for 7 days).

SKIN INFECTIONS CAUSED BY STREPTOCOCCI

Cellulitis and Erysipelas

Cellulitis and erysipelas are acute, spreading infections of the skin caused by streptococci of various groups, including A, B, C, and G. Erysipelas involves the superficial dermis, especially the dermal lymphatics, and cellulitis affects the deeper dermis and subcutaneous fat. Erysipelas has an elevated, sharply demarcated border, but differences in the clinical appearances of erysipelas and cellulitis are unimportant and often unclear. The most common sites of infection are the face and lower extremities. The causative organisms may enter the skin at obvious areas, such as traumatic wounds and leg ulcers, or through cutaneous inflammation (e.g., eczema); often, however, no point of entry is apparent. Edema from any cause, including venous insufficiency, hypoalbuminemia, and lymphatic damage, is a predisposing factor. Infection commonly occurs on skin that has been permanently damaged by burns, trauma, radiotherapy, or surgery. For example, cellulitis may occur at the site of a saphenous vein removal for cardiac or vascular surgery months to years after the procedure.[12] An important predisposing factor in patients with cellulitis or erysipelas is toe intertrigo (fissuring and maceration between the toes); streptococci that colonize these areas can invade the skin between the toes or can migrate to more proximal locations on the leg and enter through abnormal skin. Obesity is also a predisposing condition.[13]

Diagnosis Cutaneous findings include rapidly expanding erythema and swelling of the skin [*see Figure 9*], sometimes accompanied by proximal streaks of redness, representing lymphangitis, and tender, enlarged regional lymph nodes. Vesicles, bullae, petechiae, and ecchymoses may occur. The cutaneous surface may resemble the skin of an orange (peau d'orange) because the hair follicles remain tethered to the deeper structures, keeping their openings below the surrounding superficial edema and creating the characteristic dimpling of the skin. On the face, the typical location is on one or both cheeks, with a butterfly pattern of erythema and swelling. Extension to the eyelids, ears, or neck is common. Systemic symptoms, such as fever, headache, and confusion, can accompany these infections; sometimes, such symptoms precede by hours any cutaneous findings on examination. Other patients have no systemic features despite severe skin abnormalities.

The diagnosis is largely clinical; in a typical case, cultures are unnecessary and usually unrewarding. Needle aspiration of the lesion yields an isolate in about 5% to 20% of specimens. Blood cultures in febrile patients are positive in fewer than 5%. Because of their low yield, blood cultures are unnecessary in typical cases

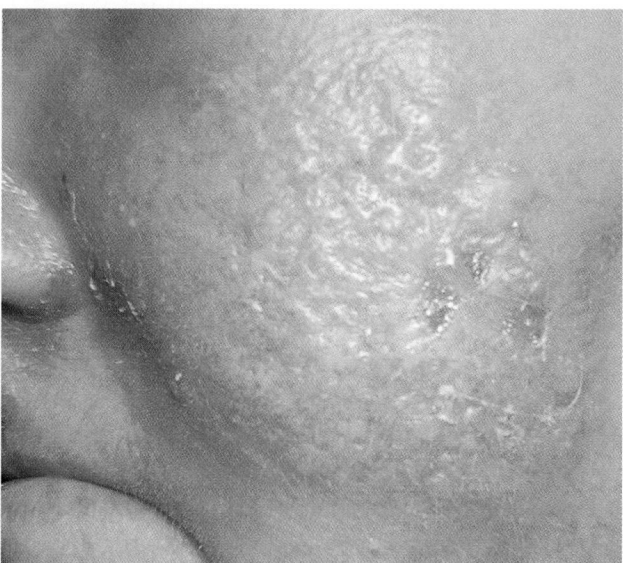

Figure 9 **Erythema, edema, and sharp demarcation of the lesion from the normal surrounding skin characterize facial erysipelas.**

of cellulitis.[14] Punch biopsies of the skin are culture-positive in about 20% of cases.[15] These results, together with serum antibody tests for streptococci[16] and immunofluorescent studies of skin biopsies,[17] indicate that streptococci cause the vast majority (probably about 90%) of cases of cellulitis and erysipelas. *S. aureus* is often suspected but rarely implicated in cellulitis in the absence of an abscess or penetrating injury, including needle sticks from the injection of illicit drugs. Additional circumstances in which organisms other than streptococci are likely to be responsible for cases of cellulitis include immunodeficiency, penetrating trauma, immersion injuries in freshwater or saltwater, granulocytopenia, and animal bites or scratches. Cultures are appropriate in these situations.

Treatment Treatment consists of elevation of the affected area to help reduce edema and administration of systemic antibiotic therapy. For patients who do not have serious systemic illness, oral treatment is satisfactory. Penicillin is the drug of choice for streptococcal infections; for outpatients who may not take an oral medication as prescribed, I.M. benzathine penicillin G in an adult dose of 1.2 million units provides a complete course. Instead of penicillin, many clinicians prescribe an antistaphylococcal agent—either a first-generation cephalosporin or a penicillinase-resistant penicillin—because of concerns about *S. aureus*. Patients often get worse shortly after therapy, with further extension of the cellulitis, higher fever, greater toxicity, and increased white blood cell counts, presumably because rapid killing of the organisms releases potent enzymes, such as streptokinase and hyaluronidase, that cause many of the clinical features. One study showed that oral prednisolone, taken for 8 days in doses of 30 mg, 15 mg, 10 mg, and 5 mg, with each dose taken for 2 days, decreases the duration of cellulitis and shortens hospital stay; it is a reasonable treatment for those with no contraindications to systemic corticosteroids.[18]

In patients with leg cellulitis, treatment of tinea pedis is useful in preventing further episodes, which are likely to cause permanent lymphatic damage and can lead to lymphedema and further risk of infection. Other measures to diminish the frequency of future attacks, which occur in about 5% to 10% of patients annually, include control of edema by diuretics or mechanical means, such as elastic stockings, and, for those with frequent episodes, prophylactic antibiotics. The easiest approach is the administration of oral penicillin or erythromycin, 250 mg twice daily.[19,20]

INFECTIONS DUE TO *STAPHYLOCOCCUS AUREUS*

Furunculosis

A furuncle (or boil) is a deep-seated inflammatory nodule with a pustular center that develops around a hair follicle [*see Figure 10*]. With involvement of several adjacent follicles, a mass called a carbuncle may form, with pus discharging from multiple follicular orifices. This infection typically develops on the back of the neck and appears more commonly in patients with diabetes than in the general population. Moist heat is usually adequate for small furuncles, which ordinarily drain spontaneously. Incision and drainage are appropriate for large or multiple furuncles and for all carbuncles. Systemic antibiotics are unnecessary unless there is fever or substantial surrounding cellulitis.

Recently, in many areas throughout the world, methicillin-resistant *Staphylococcus aureus* (MRSA) has emerged as a major cause of community-acquired skin and soft-tissue infections.[21] These organisms differ from hospital-associated MRSA in molecular biology, clinical manifestations of infection, and antimicrobial resistance. Most isolates have genes that cause production of Panton-Valentine leukocidin, a toxin that destroys neutrophils and produces tissue necrosis. Many of the reported infections have occurred in outbreaks among groups living together or having close physical contact (e.g., soldiers or sporting teams), but isolated cases are common.

Most of the cases involve furuncles or cutaneous abscesses that often begin as painful red papules, with variable surrounding erythema, that develop purulent or necrotic centers. Many patients interpret the lesions as spider bites. The appropriate therapy is incision and drainage, which often yields minimal pus and primarily necrotic material. Antimicrobials are usually unnecessary. Some patients continue to develop new lesions, even without evidence of staphylococcal nasal carriage. In these patients, the organisms may remain on various skin sites, and antimicrobial therapy may be useful in terminating the recurrences. Oral agents to which most isolates are susceptible include doxycycline (100 mg orally two times a day), clindamycin (150 mg orally four times a day), sulfamethoxazole-trimethoprim (1 double-strength tablet two times a day), and fluoroquinolones (e.g., ciprofloxacin, 500 mg two times a day).

Some patients have recurrent episodes of furunculosis. Although a few patients have definable abnormalities in host defenses, such as neutrophil disorders, most are otherwise healthy people who, like 20% to 40% of the population, carry *S. aureus* in the anterior nares. From this site or occasionally from the perineum or axilla, organisms can spread and enter the skin, presumably through minor, usually inapparent, trauma. Successful prevention of recurrent infection requires eradication of these bacteria from their site of residence, but most systemic antibiotics do not achieve adequate levels of drug in the anterior nares. An exception is clindamycin, which, when given as a single daily dose of 150 mg for 3 months, is very effective in preventing subsequent episodes.[22] A less effective alternative is mupirocin ointment, applied in the anterior nares twice daily for 5 days each month.[23]

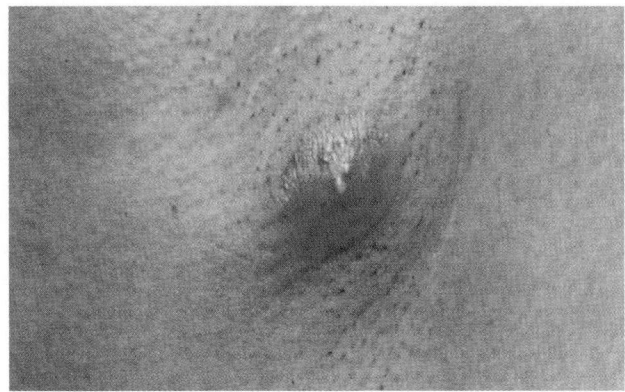

Figure 10 **A furuncle, or boil, occurs as an acute, painful, localized staphylococcal abscess surrounding a hair follicle.**

SKIN INFECTIONS CAUSED BY THE RESIDENT CUTANEOUS FLORA

The normal cutaneous flora helps prevent infection by other organisms through the mechanisms mentioned above: occupying available sites of residence, competition for nutrients, establishment of a low pH, and the elaboration of antibacterial substances. Occasionally, however, the resident skin flora causes cutaneous infections, especially with trauma or alterations in the stratum corneum. Examples are erythrasma, pitted keratolysis, trichomycosis axillaris, and most cases of cutaneous abscesses.

Cutaneous Abscesses

Cutaneous abscesses are collections of pus within the dermis and deeper skin tissues. They probably occur as a result of trauma. Sites of trauma associated with cutaneous abscesses may be apparent, as with sites of injections in illicit-drug users,[24] or they may be minor and unnoticed. *S. aureus*, usually in pure culture, causes about 25% of cutaneous abscesses, especially in the axillae, on the hand, and on the breasts of women after childbirth.[25] In other sites, however, the predominant organisms are anaerobes. Anaerobes occur either alone or in the mixture of anaerobes and aerobes that constitutes the normal regional flora; they are sometimes accompanied by microbes from adjacent mucous membranes. In anogenital infections, such as scrotal, inguinal, vaginal, buttock, and perirectal abscesses, the organisms are commonly fecal bacteria, including streptococci, anaerobic gram-positive cocci, and anaerobic gram-negative bacilli, such as *Bacteroides fragilis*. On the extremities, trunk, neck, and head, the usual microbes include coagulase-negative staphylococci, anaerobic gram-positive cocci, and *Propionibacterium acnes*, an anaerobic gram-positive bacillus. These organisms ordinarily possess little virulence, but when introduced into the dermis or subcutaneous tissue by trauma or through a disrupted cutaneous surface, they may become pathogenic.

Cutaneous abscesses usually cause a painful, fluctuant, red, tender swelling, on which may rest a pustule. Treatment is incision and drainage of the area. Gram stain and culture of the pus are ordinarily unnecessary, as are topical antimicrobials. Systemic antibiotics are reserved for patients with extensive surrounding cellulitis, neutropenia, cutaneous gangrene, or systemic manifestations of infection, such as high fever.

Erythrasma

Porphyrin-producing coryneform bacteria, which are gram-positive bacilli that constitute part of the normal cutaneous flora, cause a superficial, usually asymptomatic, skin disorder called erythrasma. One particular species, *Corynebacterium minutissimum*, has often been cited as the sole cause of this infection, but its precise role, if any, remains unclear. The most common site of erythrasma is between the toes, especially in the fourth interdigital space, where it causes fissuring, maceration, and scaling, resembling tinea pedis. Other locations are intertriginous areas, such as the axillae, groin, submammary area, and intergluteal cleft. In these regions, the lesions are usually scaly, brownish-red, sharply circumscribed patches. In hot, humid climates, more extensive disease may occur. The definitive diagnostic technique is examination of the skin with a Wood light, which, because the organisms produce porphyrins, reveals a coral-red fluorescence. Culture of the lesions, which requires special media, is unnecessary. Because they possess some activity against gram-positive bacteria, topical azoles, such as miconazole and clotrimazole, are effective in the treatment of this infection. Topical erythromycin or clindamycin is also effective. Oral erythromycin (250 mg q.i.d. for 2 weeks) is an alternative.[26]

Pitted Keratolysis

Coryneform bacteria, *Kytococcus sedentarius* (a gram-positive coccus), and *Dermatophilus congolensis* (a gram-positive bacillus) together or individually cause a disorder called pitted keratolysis that affects the soles—typically in pressure-bearing areas—or, occasionally, the palms.[27] Pitted keratolysis consists of small pitted erosions about 0.7 to 7 mm in diameter that may be present on reddened plaques and are often more apparent after soaking in water for a few minutes. This infection occurs with increased moisture, such as caused by excessive sweating, occlusive footwear, or frequent contact with water. It appears more commonly in hot, humid climates than in more temperate ones. An impressive malodor of the feet is often apparent, presumably from the production of sulfur-compound by-products. Although the disorder may cause no symptoms, some patients complain of itching, tenderness, or sliminess of the feet, which often results in the feet sticking to socks. As in erythrasma, topical azoles, such as clotrimazole and miconazole, are effective, as are topical erythromycin, clindamycin, and mupirocin. With treatment, the problem usually clears within 3 to 4 weeks.

Trichomycosis axillaris

Trichomycosis axillaris is characterized by colored concretions of axillary hair that result from infection of the hair shafts by large colonies of various species of *Corynebacterium*. The nodules may be yellow, black, or red; and because the organisms may invade the cuticle, the hair can become brittle. The same process occasionally affects the facial or pubic hair.[28] Excessive sweating, poor hygiene, and failure to use an axillary deodorant are predisposing factors. Shaving the hair is effective treatment; other options include topical erythromycin or clindamycin.

INFECTIONS DUE TO OTHER BACTERIA

Necrotizing Fasciitis

Necrotizing fasciitis, a necrotizing infection of the subcutaneous tissue, can be caused by streptococci; more often, however, the responsible organisms are a combination of aerobic bacteria—such as gram-negative enteric organisms (e.g., *Escherichia coli*) and gram-positive cocci—and anaerobes, including *B. fragilis*.[29] Occasionally, cases have occurred from infection with community-acquired MRSA.[30] Necrotizing fasciitis often occurs after a penetrat-

ing wound to the extremities. The injury is typically deep, but sometimes, infection occurs after apparently trivial trauma, such as abrasions or lacerations. The necrotizing process may develop from extension of an adjacent infection, especially in the second most common location, the anogenital area. There, infection typically arises from a perianal abscess; as an extension of a periurethral gland infection, especially in men with urethral strictures; through retroperitoneal suppuration from perforated abdominal viscera; or as a complication of a preceding surgery. Necrotizing infection involving the genitalia is called Fournier gangrene.

These infections typically begin with fever, systemic toxicity, severe pain in the affected site, and the development of a painful, red swelling that rapidly progresses to necrosis of the subcutaneous tissue and overlying skin. Early on, the pain may appear disproportionate to the clinical findings. In some cases involving *S. pyogenes* infection, the characteristics of the streptococcal toxic-shock syndrome may appear[31] [*see Chapter 134*]. When anaerobes or certain aerobic gram-negative bacilli cause the infection, gas may form in tissues, evident as crepitus on physical examination or visible on radiographic studies. Although the disease may resemble uncomplicated cellulitis, the following signs and symptoms should suggest the presence of a necrotizing subcutaneous infection: edema extending beyond the erythematous border; rapid development of bullae and ecchymoses; cutaneous gangrene; fluctuance; crepitus; loss of sensation in the affected area; and radiographically visible gas. Computed tomography or magnetic resonance imaging may be helpful in some cases in detecting the infection and defining its extent. Aspiration of the affected tissue may yield purulent fluid, which on Gram stain demonstrates only gram-positive cocci in chains when *S. pyogenes* is responsible, gram-positive cocci in clumps when *S. aureus* causes the infection, or a variety of many different organisms when a mixed infection is present. The findings on Gram stain and culture of the pus should dictate antibiotic choice, but a good initial program is ampicillin-sulbactam (3 g intravenously every 6 hours) combined with clindamycin (600 mg intravenously every 8 hours). For patients with severe penicillin allergies, an alternative to ampicillin-sulbactam is a fluoroquinolone, such as ciprofloxacin (400 mg intravenously every 6 to 8 hours). Vancomycin (1 g intravenously every 12 hours) is appropriate when *S. aureus* infection is suspected. Most important is incision and drainage of the affected area, which should include removal of any necrotic tissue. Often, the amount of disease revealed at surgery is much greater than was apparent on the preoperative clinical examination, because the infection typically extends far beyond the borders of cutaneous inflammation. Repeat operation after 24 hours is typically prudent to drain new areas of infection and remove necrotic tissue.

Folliculitis

Folliculitis is an inflammation at the opening of the hair follicle that causes erythematous papules and pustules surrounding individual hairs [*see Figure 11*]. The most common location is the trunk. The initiating factor seems to be occlusion of the opening of the follicle, which may occur from contact with chemicals, such as oils or cosmetics; overhydration of the skin from excessive moisture; or repetitive trauma, such as friction from tight-fitting clothing, which elicits hyperkeratosis and follicular plugging. Subsequently, inflammation develops, which may be provoked by bacteria, yeast, or other nonmicrobial substances trapped beneath the occluded ostium.

a

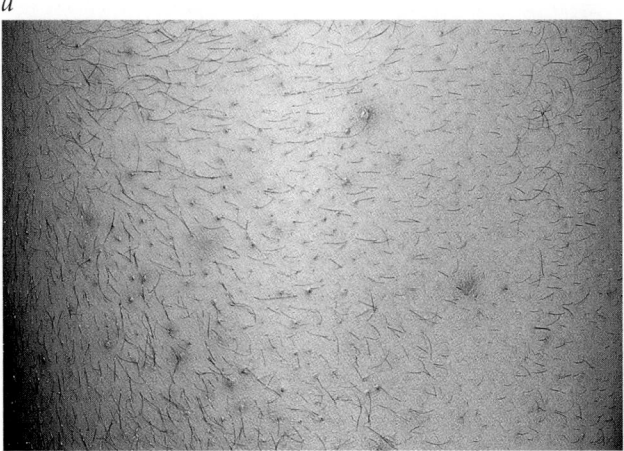

b

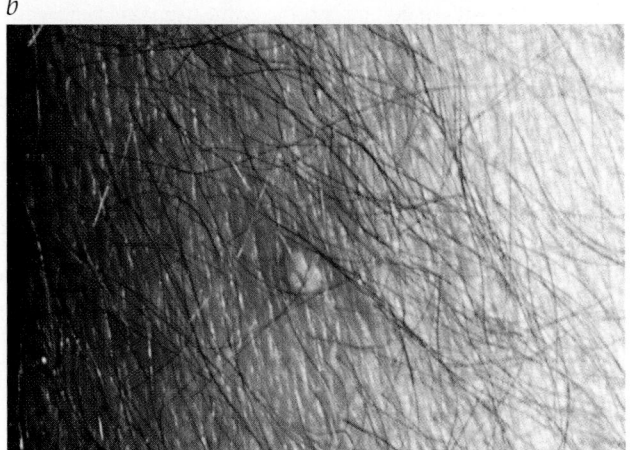

Figure 11 **Folliculitis is a superficial or deep inflammation of the hair follicles, appearing at follicular openings as small pustules surrounded by erythema (*a*). Folliculitis may also occur as an isolated lesion (*b*).**

Among bacteria, *S. aureus* is often suspected but rarely found, except in cases of folliculitis of the nasal hairs. When bacteria are present in the pustules, Gram stain and culture usually reveal normal skin flora. In these patients, doxycycline (100 mg orally two times a day) may be effective in eradicating the lesions. Another cause is *Malassezia* species; *Malassezia* are yeasts that normally reside on the skin. In Gram stain of pus, these yeasts are visible as large gram-positive oval organisms that can bud [*see Malassezia* Folliculitis, *above*]. In some patients, Gram stain and culture of the pus reveal no organisms, and the avoidance of oily substances on the skin or tight clothing leads to resolution of the problem.

Occasionally, *Pseudomonas aeruginosa* causes folliculitis, as a consequence of inadequate disinfection of hot tubs, swimming pools, or whirlpools.[32] This gram-negative bacillus grows well in hot water. Outbreaks occur an average of 48 hours after exposure, with a range of several hours to several days. Erythematous, pruritic papules, often with a pinpoint central pustule, appear in areas exposed to the contaminated water; papules are particularly numerous in regions occluded by tight-fitting swimming suits. The lesions disappear spontaneously over several days, leaving no scars; ordinarily, no topical or systemic therapy is necessary. Some patients have sore throat, rhinitis, earache, and headache, but fever or bacteremia is very rare. Cultures of the skin lesions and the contaminated water usually yield the or-

ganism. Adequate disinfection of the source of the contaminated water is critical in preventing recurrences.

Cutaneous Anthrax

Spores of *Bacillus anthracis* sent through the mail in the fall of 2001 as an act of bioterrorism caused cases of inhalational and cutaneous anthrax in several states. Otherwise, anthrax has been very rare in the United States over the past few decades. Ordinarily, this bacterium resides in the soil, where it forms spores that can persist for years. When ingested—primarily by herbivores (e.g., cattle, horses, sheep, and goats) grazing on contaminated land—these spores may cause infection. This veterinary disease is most frequent in tropical and subtropical areas, but extensive vaccination of livestock can markedly diminish its frequency.

Except for cases associated with bioterrorism [*see Chapter 13*], humans usually develop anthrax from exposure to affected animals or their products, such as hides. Occasional laboratory-acquired cases also occur. The cutaneous form develops when spores enter the skin through abrasions and then transform into bacilli, which produce toxins that cause local tissue edema and necrosis. Macrophages can transport spores to regional lymph nodes, but bacteremia is uncommon. After an incubation period of about 1 to 7 days, a painless, pruritic papule forms at the entry site, most commonly the head, neck, and extremities. Over the next few hours, the lesion enlarges, and a ring of erythema may form around it. In 1 to 2 days, vesicles appear, surrounding the papule and containing numerous bacteria but few neutrophils. Painless, gelatinous, nonpitting edema then encircles the lesion, often spreading extensively to adjacent skin and soft tissue [*see Figure 12*]. This pronounced edema is especially characteristic of anthrax. After enlarging, the vesicles become hemorrhagic and rupture. In the depressed center of the lesion, a black eschar forms and sloughs within 1 to 2 weeks, leaving a shallow ulcer that heals with minimal, if any, scarring. In the early days of illness, patients commonly have headache, malaise, and fever. Regional lymph nodes often enlarge, causing pain and tenderness.

Diagnosis *B. anthracis*, a broad, encapsulated gram-positive rod, is visible on Gram stains of material from a skin lesion as single organisms or chains of two or three bacilli. It grows readily at 37° C on blood agar media. Skin biopsies reveal necrosis, hemorrhage, and massive edema. Organisms are demonstrable with tissue Gram stain or immunohistochemical staining for the

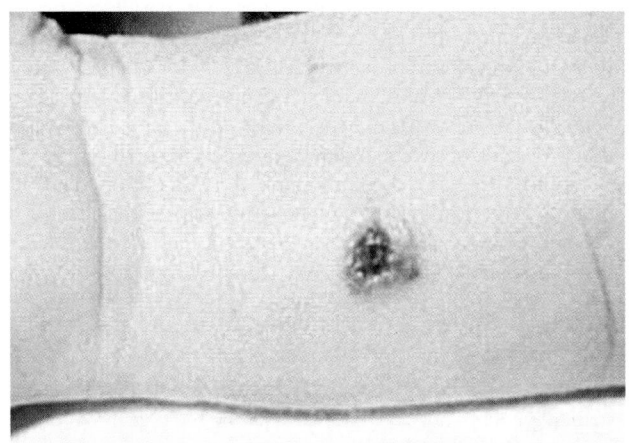

Figure 12 **Cutaneous anthrax lesion, seen on the seventh day after infection.**

bacteria's cell wall antigen. Because it requires acute and convalescent blood specimens, serologic testing for antibodies to *B. anthracis* is unhelpful for immediate diagnosis but may establish a retrospective diagnosis of suspected but unconfirmed cases.

Treatment The treatment of cutaneous anthrax that is not associated with bioterrorism is penicillin V (500 mg q.i.d. orally) or amoxicillin (500 mg t.i.d. orally) for mild cases and, for more severe disease, penicillin G (6 to 8 million units I.V. daily). For penicillin-allergic patients or cases arising from bioterrorism, the recommended therapy is oral ciprofloxacin (500 mg b.i.d.) or doxycycline (100 mg b.i.d). Antibiotic therapy does not alter the course of eschar formation and healing, but it does decrease the risk of systemic disease. Ordinarily, the duration of therapy is 7 to 10 days, but the recommended regimen for cases associated with bioterrorism is 60 days because of the possibility of simultaneous aerosol exposure.[33]

Viral Infections

WARTS

Warts, or verrucae, are caused by human papillomaviruses (HPVs), a subgroup of DNA-containing papovaviruses, of which there are numerous types. Humans are the only known reservoir; transmission probably occurs from close contact with infected people or possibly from exposure to sloughed, infected epidermal cells. The virus presumably enters through small breaks in the skin. The incubation period is difficult to discern but is probably several months. Autoinoculation from one portion of the body to another also occurs. Cell-mediated immunity appears important in controlling these infections, which can be very extensive and refractory to treatment in immunocompromised patients.

Verrucae vary according to location. They include the common, elevated wart (verruca vulgaris), typically appearing on the hands; the flat wart (verruca plana), on the face and legs; the moist wart (condyloma acuminatum), in the anogenital area; and the callus-covered plantar wart (verruca plantaris), on the sole of the foot. A histologic feature that distinguishes a wart from other papillomas is the presence in the upper epidermis of large, vacuolated cells that contain numerous viral particles.

Verruca Vulgaris

The common wart consists of single or multiple skin-colored papules, which often have a hyperkeratotic, papillary surface. They are commonly present on the fingers. The estimated nationwide prevalence of hand warts is 3.5% for people 18 to 64 years of age; the greatest frequency (5.5%) occurs in men 18 to 24 years of age. The warts may be filiform, with a small base and a thin projection of several millimeters, especially on the face.

Liquid nitrogen is a common initial treatment of choice for many warts. Administered with a cotton-tipped applicator or cryospray device, liquid nitrogen freezes the lesion, causing it to blister and subsequently dissolve. More than one application at 2- to 3-week intervals may be necessary for large or periungual warts. Electrodesiccation and curettage or laser surgery is effective for persistent or recurrent lesions. Use of duct tape is an alternative, patient-conducted treatment that involves application of the tape for 6 days, its removal, soaking the area in water, debridement of the wart with an emery board or pumice stone, and reapplication of the tape for 6 day-intervals. One randomized study demonstrated results superior to cryotherapy.[34]

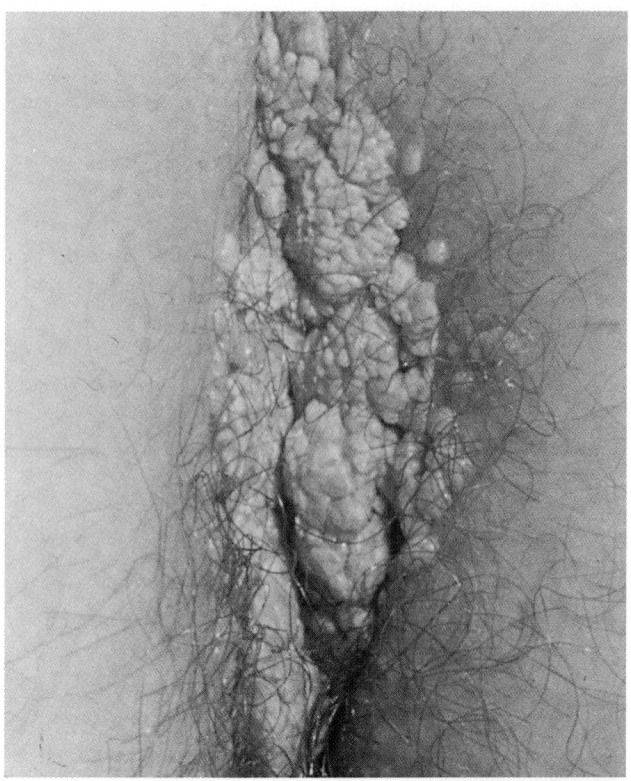

Figure 13 **Condyloma acuminatum may appear as a large cauliflower-like mass that resembles a malignant tumor.**

Verruca Plana

The flat wart is a skin-colored or light-brown, slightly elevated, smooth papule commonly seen on the face and the dorsum of the hand. These may be difficult to treat, but freezing with liquid nitrogen, application of trichloroacetic acid, or painting the lesions with 10% salicylic acid and 10% lactic acid in flexible collodion may be effective.

Verruca Plantaris

The plantar wart is often painful and disabling. A mosaic wart, a variant of verruca plantaris, consists of multiple discrete or confluent superficial lesions and is often difficult to treat. A plantar wart that is covered by a callus can be distinguished from an ordinary callus by paring off the surface keratin; multiple, pinpoint dots, representing thrombosed vessels, or bleeding points from surface capillaries will become apparent if it is a wart. Paring of the wart can be followed by immediate treatment with liquid nitrogen, the application of strong acid (50% trichloroacetic acid), or the nightly administration of salicylic acid in plasters, an acrylic vehicle, or collodion.

Condyloma Acuminatum

Anogenital warts consist of skin-colored or gray, discrete or confluent cauliflower-like excrescences that may cause no symptoms or produce itching, burning, pain, or tenderness [see *Figure 13*]. The incidence is highest in young adults; most often, it is a sexually transmitted disease, though some anogenital warts may develop from autoinoculation or may be acquired in other ways.[35]

Infection with some types of HPV predisposes to malignancy. Most cases of squamous carcinoma of the cervix are caused by HPV, especially HPV-16 and HPV-18, but fortunately, these

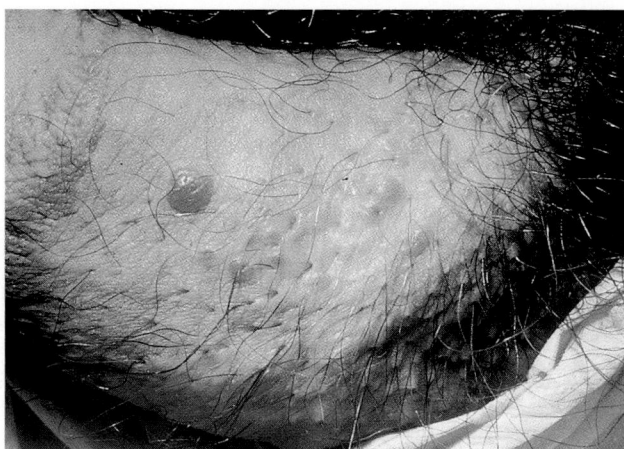

Figure 14   **Benign lesions of bowenoid papulosis, as seen on the shaft of the penis, may histologically resemble carcinoma in situ.**

types represent only a small percentage of the isolates from anogenital warts. Genital verrucous carcinoma, also called giant condyloma acuminatum of Buschke-Löwenstein, is a low-grade genital malignancy caused by HPV-6 and HPV-11. Squamous carcinoma of the anus is associated primarily with HPV-16. The Food and Drug Administration recently approved an HPV vaccine (Gardasil), which is reported to be 95% to 100% effective against HPV-6, HPV-11, HPV-16, and HPV-18.[36] The vaccine is approved for use by girls and women 9 to 26 years of age; it is recommended that the vaccine be administered before the start of sexual activity. More studies are needed to determine the period of protection offered by the vaccine.

Anogenital warts may be difficult to eradicate, and several treatments are often necessary.[35] Therapies administered by clinicians include liquid nitrogen, podophyllin resin, trichloroacetic or bichloroacetic acid, surgical removal, laser therapy, or intralesional interferon. Patient-applied treatments are podophyllotoxin, which the patient applies twice daily for 3 days, or imiquimod cream, used at bedtime three times a week for up to 16 weeks. Another approach involves fluorouracil (5-FU) cream administered twice daily for 1 to 3 weeks. This medication is particularly suitable for large wart plaques and warts of the urethral meatus, but side effects, including discomfort and painful erosions, are common.

Bowenoid Papulosis

Bowenoid papulosis consists of benign-appearing erythematous or pigmented papules in the anogenital area that histologically resemble Bowen disease (squamous cell carcinoma in situ) [*see Figure 14*]. Its course, however, is not aggressive, and the papules should be treated as anogenital warts (see above). HPV-16 is a common cause, however, and malignancy does occasionally develop, especially in women.

The author has no commercial relationships with manufacturers of products or providers of services discussed in this chapter.

References

1. Roth RR, James WD: Microbiology of the skin: resident flora, ecology, infection. J Am Acad Dermatol 20:367, 1989

2. Leyden JJ, McGinley KJ, Nordstrom KM, et al: Skin microflora. J Invest Dermatol 88(suppl):65s, 1987

3. Macura AB: Dermatophyte infections. Int J Dermatol 32:313, 1993

4. DeVroey C: Epidemiology of ringworm. Semin Dermatol 4:185, 1985

5. Elewski BE: Tinea capitis: a current perspective. J Am Acad Dermatol 45:320, 2001

6. Semel JD, Goldin H: Association of athlete's foot with cellulitis of the lower extremities: diagnostic value of bacterial cultures of ipsilateral interdigital space samples. Clin Infect Dis 23:1162, 1996

7. Elewski BE, Leyden J, Rinaldi MG, et al: Office practice–based confirmation of onychomycosis: a US nationwide prospective survey. Arch Intern Med 162:2133, 2002

8. Gupta AK, Adam P, Dlova N, et al: Therapeutic options for the treatment of tinea capitis caused by *Trichophyton* species: griseofulvin versus the new oral antifungal agents terbinafine, itraconazole, and fluconazole. Pediatr Dermatol 18:433, 2001

9. Evans EV, Sigurgeirsson B: Double blind, randomized study of continuous terbinafine compared with intermittent itraconazole in treatment of toenail onychomycosis. The LION Study Group. BMJ 318:1031, 1999

10. Tosti A, Piraccini BM, Ghetti E, et al: Topical steroids versus systemic antifungals in the treatment of chronic paronychia: an open, randomized double-blind and double dummy study. J Am Acad Dermatol 47:73, 2002

11. Demidovich CW, Wittler RR, Ruff ME, et al: Impetigo: current etiology and comparison of penicillin, erythromycin, and cephalexin therapies. Am J Dis Child 144:1313, 1990

12. Dan M, Heller K, Shapira I, et al: Incidence of erysipelas following venectomy for coronary artery bypass surgery. Infection 15:107, 1987

13. Dupuy A, Benchikhi H, Roujeau JC, et al: Risk factors for erysipelas of the leg (cellulitis): case-control study. BMJ 318:1591, 1999

14. Perl B, Gottehrer NP, Raveh D, et al: Cost-effectiveness of blood cultures for adult patients with cellulitis. Clin Infect Dis 29:1483, 1999

15. Hook EW, Hooton TM, Horton CA, et al: Microbiologic evaluation of cutaneous cellulitis in adults. Arch Intern Med 146:295, 1986

16. Eriksson B, Jorup-Rönstrom C, Karkkonen K, et al: Erysipelas: clinical and bacteriologic spectrum and serological aspects. Clin Infect Dis 23:1091, 1996

17. Bernard P, Bedane C, Mounier M, et al: Streptococcal cause of erysipelas and cellulitis in adults: a microscopic study using a direct immunofluorescence technique. Arch Dermatol 125:779, 1989

18. Bergkvist PI, Sjöbeck K: Antibiotic and prednisolone therapy of erysipelas: a randomized, double blind placebo-controlled study. Scand J Infect Dis 29:377, 1997

19. Kremer M, Zuckerman R, Avraham Z, et al: Long-term antimicrobial therapy in the prevention of recurrent soft-tissue infections. J Infect 22:37, 1991

20. Hirschmann JV: Antimicrobial prophylaxis in dermatology. Semin Cutan Med Surg 19:2, 2000

21. Maltezou HC, Giamarellou H: Community-acquired methicillin-resistant *Staphylococcus aureus* infections. Int J Antimicrob Agents 27:87, 2006

22. Klempner MS, Styrt B: Prevention of recurrent staphylococcal skin infections with low-dose oral clindamycin therapy. JAMA 260:2682, 1988

23. Raz R, Miron D, Colodner R, et al: A 1-year trial of nasal mupirocin in the prevention of recurrent staphylococcal nasal colonization and skin infection. Arch Intern Med 156:1109, 1996

24. Ebright JR, Pieper B: Skin and soft tissue infections in injection drug users. Infect Dis Clin North Am 16:697, 2002

25. Meislin HW, Lerner SA, Graves MH, et al: Cutaneous abscesses: anaerobic and aerobic bacteriology and outpatient management. Ann Intern Med 87:145, 1977

26. Holdiness MR: Management of cutaneous erythrasma. Drugs 62:1131, 2002

27. Takama H, Tamada Y, Yano K, et al: Pitted keratolysis: clinical manifestations in 53 cases. Br J Dermatol 137:282, 1997

28. White SW, Smith J: Trichomycosis pubis. Arch Dermatol 115:444, 1979

29. Stone DR, Gorbach SL: Necrotizing fasciitis: the changing spectrum. Dermatol Clin 15:213, 1997

30. Miller LG, Perdreau-Remington F, Rieg G, et al: Necrotizing fasciitis caused by community-associated methicillin-resistant *Staphylococcus aureus* in Los Angeles. N Engl J Med 352:1445, 2005

31. Dahl PR, Perniciaro C, Holmkvist KA, et al: Fulminant group A streptococcal necrotizing fasciitis: clinical and pathologic findings in 7 patients. J Am Acad Dermatol 47:489, 2002

32. Agger WA, Mardan A: *Pseudomonas aeruginosa* infections of intact skin. Clin Infect Dis 20:302, 1995

33. Inglesby TV, O'Toole T, Henderson DA, et al: Anthrax as a biological weapon, 2002. Updated recommendations for management. JAMA 287:2236, 2002

34. Focht DR 3rd, Spicer C, Fairchok MP: The efficacy of duct tape vs cryotherapy in the treatment of verruca vulgaris (the common wart). Arch Pediatr Adolesc Med 156:971, 2002

35. Von Krogh G, Gross G: Anogenital warts. Clin Dermatol 15:355, 1997

36. Human papillomavirus (HPV) vaccines for cervical cancer. National Cancer Institute. U.S. National Institutes of Health (accessed 7/06) http://www.cancer.gov/cancertopics/hpv-vaccines

Acknowledgment

Figure 12   Centers for Disease Control and Prevention Public Health Image Library.

42 Parasitic Infestations

Elizabeth A. Abel, M.D.

Ectoparasites may cause severely pruritic infectious diseases of the skin. With early detection and treatment, parasitic infestations can be cured and their spread to other persons prevented. The most common parasitic diseases of the skin that occur in nontropical environments are scabies, which is caused by itch mites, and pediculosis capitis, pediculosis corporis, and pediculosis pubis, which are caused by bloodsucking lice.

An increase in international travel, including vacation travel to tropical destinations and immigration from such areas, has led to the occurrence of parasitic disorders endemic to tropical regions in persons living in temperate climates. The differential diagnosis of skin disorders in patients treated at a tropical disease clinic in Paris over a 2-year period included cutaneous larva migrans, pyodermas, arthropod-reactive dermatitis, myiasis, tungiasis, urticaria, and cutaneous leishmaniasis.[1] The prevalence of ectoparasitoses in the general population is usually low, but it can be high in vulnerable groups. Management of some infestations (e.g., scabies and head lice) can be complicated because resistance to insecticides is spreading and unpredictable.[2]

Scabies

Scabies is caused by infestation with *Sarcoptes scabiei*, an ectoparasite that bores into the corneal layer of human skin, forming burrows in which it deposits its eggs. The incubation period is 2 to 6 weeks in a person who has not been previously exposed. During this time, the host develops delayed hypersensitivity to mite antigens. Upon reinfestation, symptoms occur in sensitized persons within 24 to 48 hours after exposure.[3]

The scabies mite does not survive for more than 48 hours away from the host. Therefore, most infestations are transmitted through direct personal skin-to-skin and sexual contact.[3] However, transfer of organisms can occur by exposure to fomites such as contaminated bedding, clothing, or furniture and is a common cause of epidemics of scabies in nursing homes and other institutions.[3,4]

DIAGNOSIS

Clinical Features

Scabies causes severe itching, which is usually worse at night. Characteristic sites of infestation are the webs of the fingers, the flexor aspects of the wrists, the axillae, the buttocks, the umbilicus, the penis and scrotum of males, and the breasts and nipples of females. The disease is more generalized in infants and children than in adults.

The burrow of the female *Sarcoptes* may be seen as an irregular zigzag line in the stratum corneum, with a black dot at one end that indicates the presence of the mite [*see Figure 1*]. Secondary lesions represent immunologic reactions to the mites and usually appear as small erythematous papules and vesicles with surrounding edema and scratch marks [*see Figure 2*]. The type and number of lesions depend predominantly on the immune status of the host. Occasionally, nodular lesions, which may resemble lesions of histiocytosis X (Langerhans cell granulomatosis) or lymphoma, occur as a hypersensitivity reaction to re-

tained mite parts. Fewer lesions occur in people who practice good hygiene, and the condition may be masked in those who are using topical steroids. Secondary bacterial infection with impetiginization is common, especially in children and in elderly patients who actively excoriate their lesions.

Atypical presentations of scabies have been described in immunosuppressed persons, including organ transplant recipients, patients with lymphoma or leukemia, and patients with AIDS. Itching and scratching, with elimination of mites and burrows, may be minimal in patients who lack an immunologic host response, allowing for thousands of mites to reproduce and thrive.[3] Crusted scabies, which was originally described in Norway, is associated with widespread hyperkeratotic lesions and deep fissures in the skin. Crusted scabies can develop in patients with malnutrition or severe mental deficiency and in institutionalized patients. The condition is highly contagious because of the large number of mites present in the exfoliating skin.

A severe form of scabies with unusual clinical features consisting of crusted lesions and a widespread pruritic papular dermatitis has been described in HIV-infected patients.[3,5] In these patients, multiple treatment applications may be needed because of the large mite population and the patients' impaired immunologic response.

Skin Scrapings

A skin scraping that demonstrates the presence of mite eggs or mite products can confirm a diagnosis of scabies. A No. 15 surgical blade is used to scrape across one or more burrows. Saline solution or mineral oil is used to remove scrapings from the blade. The scrapings are then placed on a glass slide with a coverslip and examined under a microscope at low-power magnification. The scraping is positive if the gravid female, eggs, or scybala (fecal pellets) are seen [*see Figure 3*]. The yield is greatest in burrows that are not yet excoriated, which may be difficult to find. For this reason, if the scraping is negative but the clinical suspicion of scabies is high, the patient should be treated empirically. Histopathologic examination of a skin biopsy sample is also diagnostic if it reveals the mite or the superficial skin bur-

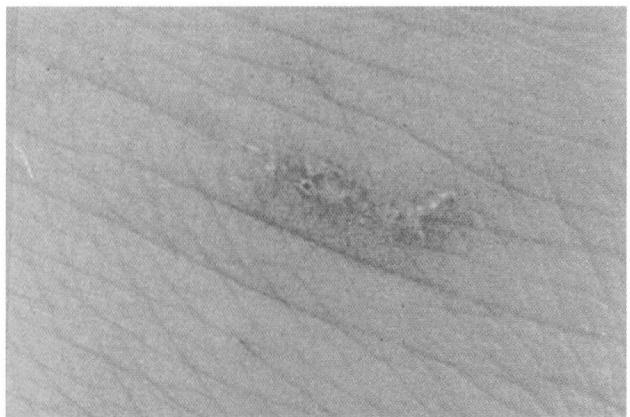

Figure 1   **Typical scabies lesions are small erythematous papules and vesicles with surrounding edema.**

row and its contents.[6] In atypical or subtle cases of scabies, epiluminescence microscopy (ELM) or polymerase chain reaction may be useful in confirming the diagnosis.[7,8] ELM, which allows visualization of the skin down to the superficial papillary dermis, is able to detect the presence of scabies within minutes, with no discomfort to the patient. PCR can amplify *S. scabiei* DNA when the number of mites is so few that diagnosis by standard means is inconclusive.

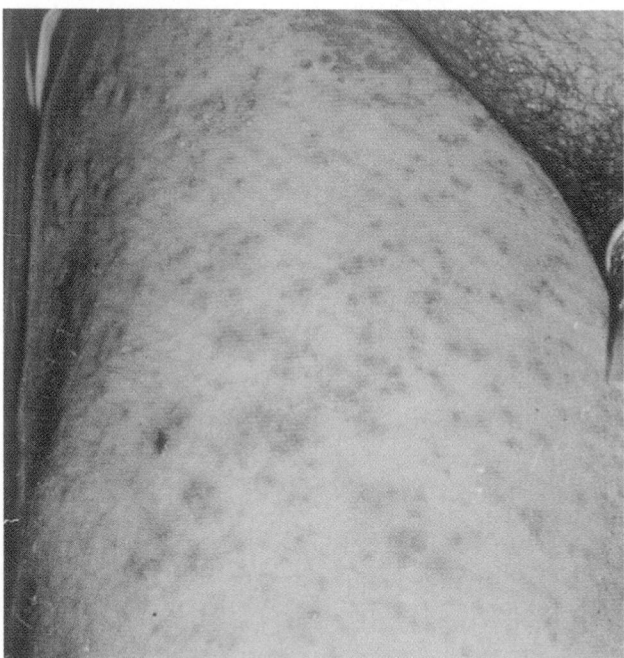

Figure 2   The burrow of the female *Sarcoptes* frequently appears as an irregular line several millimeters to a few centimeters long in the stratum corneum.

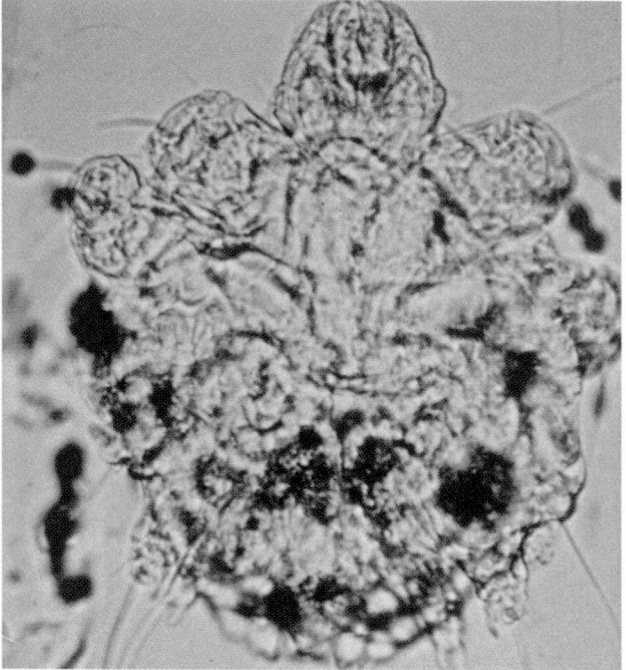

Figure 3   Observation of the *Sarcoptes scabiei* or its eggs and feces confirms the diagnosis of scabies. Magnification is 400 times.

DIFFERENTIAL DIAGNOSIS

Clinical differential diagnosis includes drug eruption, papular urticaria, folliculitis, atopic dermatitis, dermatitis herpetiformis, and contact dermatitis, particularly from fiberglass. Crusted scabies may be mistaken for eczema. Papular urticaria is an intensely itchy eruption caused by a hypersensitivity reaction to bites from such insects as fleas, bedbugs, and animal scabies. Lesions occur as small papules that may have a central punctum, often occurring in groups on exposed skin.

TREATMENT

Initial Treatment

After a cleansing bath or shower, the patient should allow the skin to dry and cool and then apply a scabicide over the entire body, excluding the face and scalp. Care must be taken to include skin folds such as toe webs and the skin under the nails. The medication is left in place for 8 to 12 hours, usually overnight. In the morning, the patient showers and changes clothes. All clothing worn within 2 days before treatment, in addition to towels and bed linens, is laundered in hot water or dry-cleaned. Chairs and mattresses should be vacuumed.

First-line treatment for uncomplicated scabies is permethrin 5% cream (Elimite, Acticin); other available scabicides include 1% lindane, or gamma benzene hexachloride, lotion or cream (Kwell, Gamene); 10% to 20% benzyl benzoate lotion; crotamiton cream (Eurax); and 6% precipitated sulfur ointment [*see Table 1*]. Ivermectin, although not approved by the Food and Drug Administration as a scabicide, has shown promising results in several trials.

Permethrin, a synthetic pyrethroid with low toxicity, has proved to be safe and effective for use in infants, children, and pregnant women.[9] Natural pyrethrins, which are derived from chrysanthemum flowers, have greater toxicity and less insecticidal activity than the synthetic pyrethroids. The low toxicity of the drug is a result of its rapid breakdown into inactive metabolites. Permethrin cream can be safely used in children and infants older than 2 months and in the elderly. Acticin is a form of permethrin in a base that has a lower viscosity to promote ease of application. Alternative scabicides that can be used for young children and pregnant or lactating women include crotamiton cream and sulfur ointment. Six-percent precipitated sulfur ointment is applied three times: at diagnosis, after 24 hours, and at 1 week. Crotamiton cream is applied for 2 or more consecutive days but is less effective than permethrin. Permethrin appears to be more effective than crotamiton in clinical and parasitic cure rates.[9]

Lindane is lipophilic and can accumulate in fat and bind to brain tissue. Toxic reactions may occur in patients who have increased absorption; infants and young children, who have a higher ratio of skin surface to body volume than do adults, are especially susceptible. Excessive treatment with lindane has been reported to cause central nervous system toxicity resulting in convulsions and seizures.[10] In 2003, the FDA issued a label change for lindane emphasizing its use as second-line therapy; treatment with lindane should be considered only if other medications have failed or cannot be tolerated (information on lindane can be found on the Internet, at http://www.fda.gov/cder/drug/infopage/lindane/default.htm). Lindane lotion should be used with caution in persons weighing less than 110 lb; its use in infants is not recommended.[11] Nevertheless, low cost, ease of application, and experience with the drug have made lindane one of

Table 1 Drug Therapy for Scabies Infestations

Route	Drug	Dosage	Relative Efficacy	Comments
Topical	Permethrin 5% cream	Single total-body application left on for 8–12 hr	First-line therapy	Effective and safe for use in infants older than 2 mo, pregnant women, and elderly patients; for a treatment failure, a second application is given 1 wk later
	Crotamiton cream	Total-body applications on 2 or more consecutive days	Alternative first-line therapy	Safe for infants and pregnant women but less effective than permethrin
	Precipitated 6% sulfur ointment	3 total-body applications: at diagnosis, 24 hr, and 1 wk	Alternative first-line therapy	Safe for infants and young children; must be compounded
	Lindane 1% lotion[†]	Apply for 8 hr once weekly for 2 wk	Second-line therapy; consider after failure of first-line therapy	Associated with neurotoxicity; indicated if other medications have failed or cannot be tolerated; should be used with caution in persons weighing < 110 lb; use in infants is not recommended
Oral	Ivermectin[*]	Single dose, 200 µg/kg	Alternative first-line therapy for uncomplicated scabies	Safe and effective in children 6 mo of age or older; advantage of oral medication is ease of use and increased compliance
		200 µg/kg initially and 2 wk later	First-line therapy for resistant scabies	Effective for treatment of crusted and resistant scabies in HIV patients; successfully used to treat outbreaks in institutional settings

[*]Not approved by the Food and Drug Administration for use as a scabicide.
[†]Gamma benzene hexachloride.

the most commonly prescribed scabicides; the FDA considers the benefits of lindane to outweigh the risks when the medication is used as directed.

Oral ivermectin is another treatment option that has been found to be safe and effective in children as young as 6 months[12] and in HIV-positive patients. A single oral dose of 200 µg/kg of ivermectin was used to treat uncomplicated scabies in 11 otherwise healthy patients and in 11 patients with HIV infection.[13] Clearing was documented by negative skin scrapings at 2 weeks and 4 weeks after treatment, and cure was achieved in all of the otherwise healthy patients and in eight of the HIV-infected patients. Advantages of an oral medication are its ease of use, lack of treatment-associated dermatitis, and increased compliance. In a comparative study of oral ivermectin and topical permethrin, a single application of permethrin was found to be superior to a single dose of ivermectin. Two doses of ivermectin were required for eradication of scabies. The lack of ovicidal activity of ivermectin may explain the difference in effectiveness between the two drugs.[14] Ivermectin is toxic to invertebrate nerve and muscle cells but may not be effective against younger stages of the parasite that do not have a developed nervous system. Permethrin acts at early stages of the life cycle of the parasite, and topical application ensures adequate drug concentration in the skin.[14]

Oral ivermectin has been used successfully to control outbreaks of scabies infestations in institutional settings[4,15]; it may prove to be the treatment of choice in nursing homes and other institutions in which topical therapy is impractical.

Topical ivermectin has also been investigated for treatment of scabies. A total of 75 patients were found to be cured, on the basis of clinical and parasitologic examinations, within 48 hours after a single application of ivermectin. Postscabies itching, which persisted in 50% of the patients, was effectively treated by a second application of ivermectin within 5 days.[16]

Postscabies Itch

Postscabies itch is thought to represent a hypersensitivity reaction to the mite or mite products and is not caused by active in-

festation. The pruritus may persist for weeks to months and can be treated with an antipruritic or anti-inflammatory agent, such as a low-potency to midpotency corticosteroid cream, in addition to oral antihistamines. Overtreatment with the scabicide may result in a primary irritant dermatitis that may be confused with persistent infestation. The use of bland emollients and a corticosteroid cream and avoidance of skin irritants may reduce the dermatitis. Patients should be evaluated at 4 weeks, which is the time required for viable eggs to mature to the adult stage, to determine the efficacy of treatment. If lesions are healed and no new outbreaks have occurred, the patient is considered cured.[3]

Resistant Scabies

Overuse and misuse of certain scabicides, notably lindane, have decreased their efficacy. Differing resistance patterns have been identified within a single city; more commonly, resistance corresponds to local or regional patterns.[2] If treatment failure occurs with one scabicide, the use of a different scabicide may be indicated. For example, treatment failure with topical permethrin may prompt the consideration of lindane as a second-line therapy. Pyrethroids are effective in cases of lindane-resistant scabies.[17] Treatment failures can also occur in cases involving impetiginized or crusted scabies. In these cases, treatment with the appropriate oral antibiotic is initiated along with application of the scabicide and is followed within a week by a second application of the scabicide. Keratolytics are useful as an aid in removal of the crusts.

Oral ivermectin has been used to treat resistant scabies.[18] Although it has not been approved by the FDA for this purpose, oral ivermectin is rapidly gaining acceptance as an effective therapy for resistant scabies. Combination treatment with one or two doses of ivermectin 8 days apart, in addition to permethrin and mechanical removal of subungual debris, has been advocated for outbreaks of crusted scabies in the geriatric population.[19]

In Europe, combination therapy with oral ivermectin, 200 mg/kg, and benzylbenzoate, 15% solution applied twice daily for 3 days, was found to be more effective than either agent alone for the treatment of crusted scabies in patients with HIV.[20]

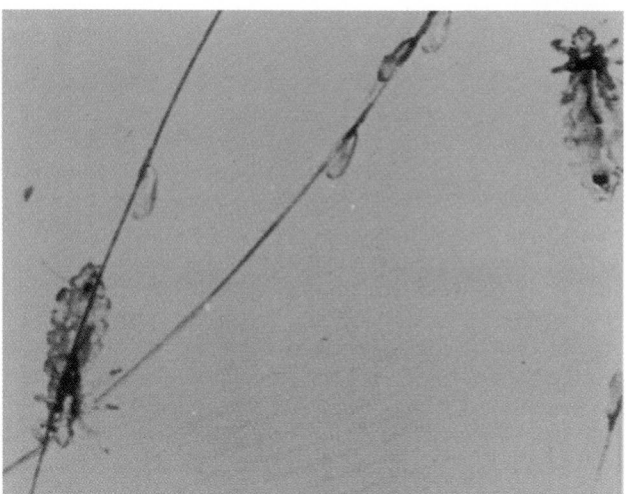

Figure 4 **Pediculosis capitis is caused by infestation of the scalp with** *Pediculus humanus* **var.** *capitis*. **Magnification is 10 times.**

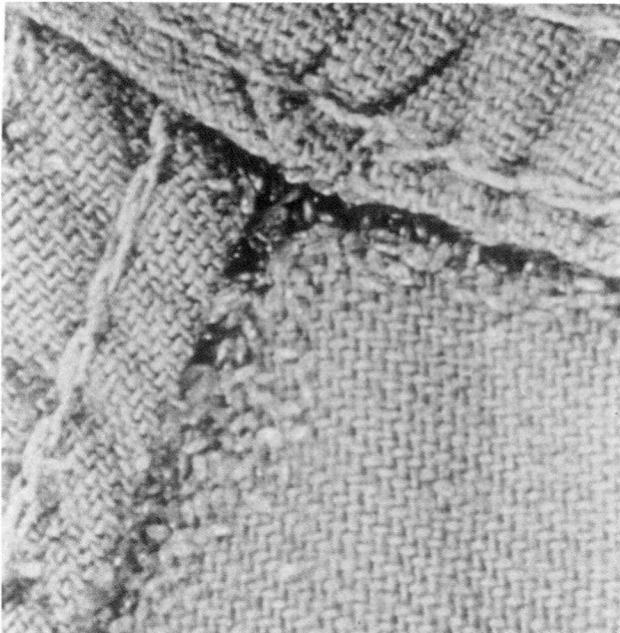

Figure 5 **Pediculosis corporis is caused by infestation with** *Pediculus humanus* **var.** *corporis* **organisms, which live in the seams of clothing.**

In the United States, a combination of oral ivermectin, total body therapy with permethrin cream, and keratolytic agents to hasten removal of crusts was used successfully to treat crusted scabies in patients with HIV.[21]

Cases of apparent resistant scabies may be the result of reinfestation. Therefore, family members and sexual partners of persons with scabies should be treated because they may be asymptomatic carriers. Scabies occurring in patients and personnel in long-term health care facilities may be difficult to diagnose and manage. In this setting, it is extremely important to treat all nursing contacts, as well as family members and other visitors of affected patients. In addition to the patients with scabies, other patients in the facility need to be assessed, and care must be coordinated to treat all affected persons simultaneously. In cases of crusted scabies, the head and neck must be treated, as well as subungual areas, which may also harbor the mites.[4]

ANIMAL SCABIES

Animal scabies is a common disorder in farm animals and domestic animals—especially dogs, in which the external ear is frequently infested with a species-specific mite. In persons who handle affected animals, an extremely pruritic papular eruption can develop that differs from ordinary scabies in several ways: distribution of lesions is proximal, with involvement of the thighs, abdomen, and forearms. Burrows are usually absent. The course is self-limited, provided there is no reexposure. Other persons in the household do not have to be treated, because human-to-human transmission of animal scabies does not occur.

The *Cheyletiella* mite is an ectoparasite that resides in the fur of dogs, cats, and rabbits. Persons who hold infested house pets, especially cats, are susceptible to a dermatitis from the mite bites. However, the mites do not live on humans, so diagnosis requires a high index of suspicion. Lesions may appear as urticarial papules, vesicles, or bullae on the arms, trunk, and legs. Cases most commonly occur in the fall or winter. An important part of the overall treatment of *Cheyletiella* infestation is treatment of the household pets by a veterinarian.[22]

Pediculosis

The three types of bloodsucking lice that cause pediculosis are *Pediculus humanus* var. *capitis* (head louse), *Pediculus humanus* var. *corporis* (body louse), and *Phthirus pubis* (pubic, or crab, louse). The first two types are closely related. The third is a separate genus and is distinctive not only in appearance and location on the body but also in its characteristic attachment to the skin for long periods. Any form of pediculosis causes intense pruritus, which is aggravated by scratching and is often complicated by secondary bacterial infection.[23]

The most common infestation is pediculosis capitis. Infestations of *P. captitis* have been reported worldwide, and an estimated 12 million cases occur annually in the United States alone.[23] Pediculosis corporis, which is usually less prevalent than pediculosis captitis, becomes widespread under conditions of overcrowding and poor sanitation or in wartime. In pediculosis capitis and pediculosis corporis, the lice may be transmitted directly from person to person or indirectly through contact with contaminated personal objects such as combs and brushes, clothing, and bedding. Pediculosis pubis (also called crabs) is usually transmitted sexually; only occasionally are the lice transmitted through contact with fomites such as contaminated bedding or toilet seats. Epidemiologic data indicate that *P. capitis* infestations are more frequent in the warmer months, whereas *P. pubis* infestations occur more frequently in the cooler months.[24]

The natural history of lice is important because it suggests specific preventive measures. The life expectancy of the organism is about 1 month. Eggs live up to 10 days but need the body heat of the host to hatch. Eggs ordinarily hatch in 7 to 8 days, and organisms reach adulthood and attain sexual reproductive capacity in 3 to 4 weeks. Lice can survive 48 hours without a blood meal.

DIAGNOSIS

Pediculosis capitis is confined to the scalp and is most prevalent in women and children. Louse infestation may present as scalp pruritus, excoriations, cervical lymphadenopathy, or conjunctivitis.[23] Examination of the itchy scalp may reveal the lice, which look like tiny black dots that are barely visible to the

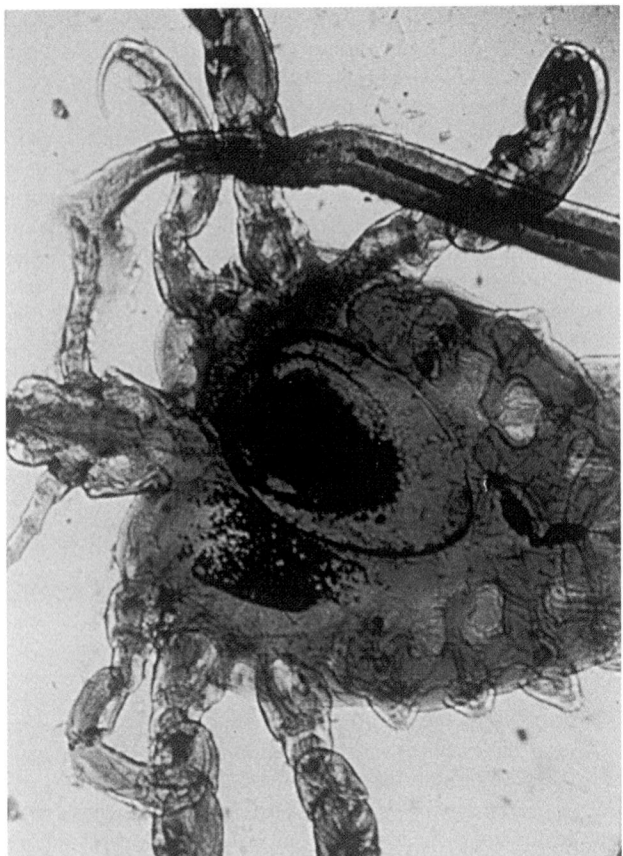

Figure 6 **Pediculosis pubis, also called crabs, is caused by infestation with *Phthirus pubis*. Magnification is 100 times.**

naked eye, and lice eggs (nits), which are white and are attached to the hair shafts [*see Figure 4*]. Except in conditions of increased warmth and high humidity, viable nits are attached close to the scalp. Those that occur several millimeters away from the surface on hairs that have grown out are empty egg cases. The hair may become matted because of exudation and secondary infection of lesions. Visual examination may not detect infestation; the use of a louse comb is recommended because it is four times more efficient than visual examination alone in the diagnosis of active pediculosis capitis.[25]

Pediculosis corporis, also called vagabond disease, affects areas of the body covered by clothing. Body lice live in the seams of clothing, and they attach to the body only to feed [*see Figure 5*]. They may serve as vectors of infectious disease under conditions of overcrowding or poor hygiene, as in wartime or during natural disasters. Characteristic lesions include erythematous macules and wheals. Lesions are most common on the shoulders, buttocks, and abdomen; furunculosis is an occasional complication. Excoriations and secondary infection may result from intense scratching. After the eggs hatch, the organisms reach adulthood in 10 days and complete their life cycle in approximately 1 month. Adult lice lay about 10 eggs a day.

Pediculosis pubis, which is caused by infestation with *Phthirus pubis* [*see Figure 6*], tends to be limited to the pubic area but occasionally affects the axillae, eyelashes, or other hairy parts of the body. Examination will reveal lice attached to the skin and lice eggs attached to the hair shafts [*see Figure 7*]. Blue macules, which are caused by the lice's sucking blood from the dermis, may be seen on the thighs or pubic area.

TREATMENT

Pediculosis Capitis

Over-the-counter preparations available for the treatment of pediculosis capitis include synergized pyrethrin products, such as RID, R&C Spray, A-200, and a 1% permethrin cream rinse (Nix) [*see Table 2*]. These products are cosmetically acceptable and require only 10 minutes to apply but may not always be effective. Repeat treatment in 7 to 10 days is advisable because the initial treatment does not kill all the eggs. If pyrethrin or permethrin fails to eradicate the infestation, the treatment of choice is malathion.[26] Malathion, which was recently reintroduced in the United States as a prescription medication for head lice, is an effective, fast-acting pediculicide and ovicide; it has not been associated with treatment resistance or notable adverse effects.[27,28] In children, proper use of malathion is safe; however, serious side effects can occur with ingestion.[29]

One of the most widely used remedies for pediculosis capitis in the United States is 1% lindane (Kwell, Gamene). However, potentially serious adverse effects associated with lindane shampoo prompted the FDA to issue a label change for this medication; treatment with lindane is now indicated only if other medications have failed or cannot be tolerated.[11,27] For the treatment of pediculosis capitis, 2 tbsp (30 ml) of the shampoo is applied to affected and adjacent areas of the scalp for at least 4 minutes, followed by thorough rinsing and drying. Adherent nits may be removed with a fine-tooth comb. Distilled white vinegar can be used to soften the nit cementing material to aid in removal of the nits.

Resistance to lindane has emerged over the past 2 decades,[30] and treatment of lice infestation has been complicated by the development of resistance to permethrin.[28] Mechanical methods of removing head lice and nits[31] and application of occlusive oils or ointments[32] have been advocated for treatment of resistant head lice. Oral ivermectin has been administered as a single dose of 12 mg (2 to 6 mg tablets), followed by a second dose 7 to 10 days lat-

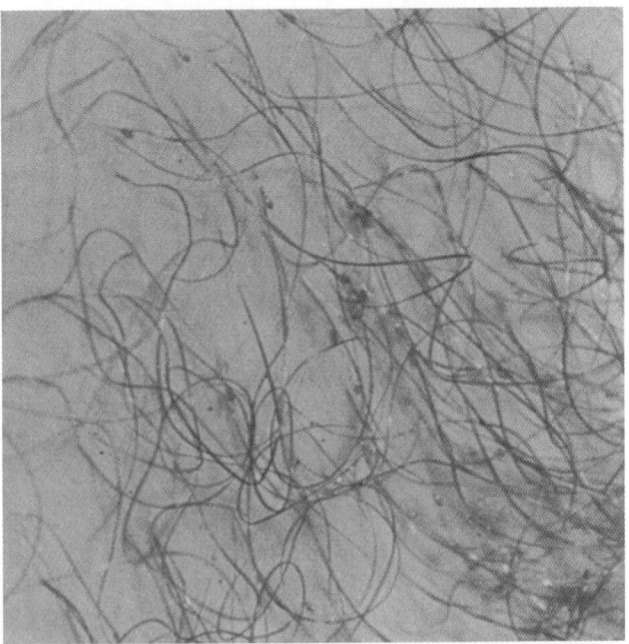

Figure 7 **Lice attached to the skin and lice eggs attached to the hair shafts can be seen on a patient with pediculosis pubis.**

Table 2   Drug Therapy for Pediculosis Infestations

Disease	Drug	Dosage	Relative Efficacy	Comments
Pediculosis capitis	Pyrethrin 0.3% shampoo and permethrin 1% cream rinse	Apply shampoo for 10 min and rinse; repeat in 7–10 days	First-line therapy	Effective and safe for use in children
	Malathion 0.5% lotion	Apply for 8–12 hr daily for 1 wk	First-line therapy; most effective therapy for resistant head lice	Safe and effective in children; potential serious adverse effects if ingested
	Lindane shampoo†	2 tbsp of shampoo applied to affected and adjacent areas of scalp and allowed to stand for at least 4 min	Second-line therapy	Associated with neurotoxicity; indicated if other medications have failed or cannot be tolerated; should be used with caution in persons weighing < 110 lb; use in infants is not recommended
	Ivermectin (oral)*	Single dose of 12 µg (2–6 tablets), followed by second dose 7–10 days later	Alternative first-line therapy	Safe and effective in children 6 mo of age or older; advantage of oral medication is ease of use and increased compliance
Pediculosis pubis, pediculosis corporis	Pyrethrin 0.3% shampoo or lotion	Apply shampoo or lotion for 10 min and rinse	First-line therapy	Resistance may occur
	Lindane lotion†	1 oz applied to affected areas	Second-line therapy	Associated with neurotoxicity; caution is advised in prescribing lindane for patients with conditions that increase risk of seizure

*Not approved by the Food and Drug Administration for use as a pediculicide.
†Gamma benzene hexachloride.

er.[23] Current evidence suggests that permethrin, pyrethrin, and malathion are equally effective in the treatment of head lice; the best choice of therapy depends on local resistance.[33]

Pediculosis Pubis and Pediculosis Corpis

To treat hairy areas of the body infested with *P. pubis*, a cleansing bath or shower should first be taken and the skin dried with a towel. One ounce of lindane cream or lotion is applied to the affected and surrounding areas and left on for 12 to 24 hours. To discourage percutaneous absorption, the lotion should be applied only after the skin has become cool and dry. Lotions containing pyrethrins and piperonyl butoxide are acceptable alternatives, and their use is preferred in select patients and children (see below).[11] After another bath or shower, freshly laundered clothing should be donned; bedsheets and towels should also be changed. Lindane may be applied a second time after 1 week if infestation continues. Lindane should not be applied to the face and eyelids, because it causes irritation; eyelash infestation may be treated by local application of 0.25% physostigmine ophthalmic ointment. An alternative treatment for eyelash infestation that is effective and nonirritating is the application of a thick layer of petrolatum twice a day, followed by mechanical removal of the nits.

Neurologic complications can ensue from absorption of lindane after extensive or prolonged topical application [*see* Scabies, *above*]; severe adverse reactions have also occurred after a single use (information on lindane can be found on the Internet, at http://www.fda.gov/cder/drug/infopage/lindane/default.htm). Careful consideration should be given before prescribing lindane to patients with conditions that increase the risk of seizure (e.g., HIV infection, history of past seizure, or severe hepatic cirrhosis) or whose concomitant medications include drugs that lower risk of seizure. Alternative treatments are indicated in infants (who are especially susceptible), young children, pregnant women, and the elderly.

A combination of pyrethrins with piperonyl butoxide (RID or A-200) has been shown to be considerably less toxic than lindane in animal experiments and in clinical experience. However, this combination irritates the eyes and mucous membranes and may also cause allergic contact dermatitis in susceptible people.

General Treatment Measures

All family members should be carefully examined for pediculosis and treated, if necessary, to avoid spread or reinfection of previously treated persons. In the case of pediculosis pubis, sexual contacts should be examined and treated. Because sexually transmitted diseases are frequently present in persons infested with *P. pubis*, a serologic test for syphilis and screening for HIV are usually done. To prevent spread of pediculosis, contaminated clothing and other articles, such as towels and bedding, should be boiled, machine washed in hot water, and placed in a dryer using a 20-minute hot cycle or should be dry-cleaned. Items such as combs and brushes may be cleaned with medicated shampoo or soaked in 5% Lysol. To eradicate *P. corporis*, the patient's clothing must be put through the same decontamination process as that used for *P. pubis*. A hot iron with pressure applied, especially to the seams of clothing, may also be used to kill *P. corporis*. Systemic antibiotics should be prescribed for concomitant secondary bacterial infections such as furunculosis and impetigo, both of which are commonly associated with pediculosis capitis.

Miscellaneous Infestations

FLEA INFESTATIONS

Fleas are small (approximately 3 mm), bloodsucking, wingless ectoparasites of the insect order Siphonaptera. Fleas are medically significant because they are vectors of infectious disease [*see* Chapters 141 and 145]. These external parasites can also cause considerable cutaneous symptoms, particularly if the symptoms are associated with an allergic hypersensitivity reaction, as seen in patients with papular urticaria. There are approximately 250 species of flea, 20 of which can infest humans. Two common species that infest cats and dogs are *Ctenocephalides felis* and *C. canis*. *C. felis* and *C. canis* are not host specific and can therefore infest humans as well. *Pulex irritans*, the house flea, primarily infests humans and in most places is not a problem for pets. Flea bites appear as erythematous edematous papules with hemorrhagic puncta in clusters or groups on the lower extremities, especially on the ankles. Occasionally, vesicles and bullae appear, as well as larger urticarial lesions. Secondary impetiginization may occur as a result of scratching.[34]

Fleas are difficult to eradicate because of their unpredictable life cycle, which consists of egg, larva, pupa, and adult stages. The eggs are laid on the host but can drop to the ground; onto carpets, pet bedding , and furniture; and into floor cracks. Eggs hatch in 2 to 21 days into larvae. A larva molts twice and, in the third larval stage, spins a cocoon, in which it becomes a pupa. Within 7 days to 1 year or more, the adult emerges, depending on various trigger factors (e.g., a vibration caused by a nearby pet or human). The life cycle from egg to adult generally ranges from 14 to 21 days but, under ideal conditions, can be as long as 20 months.[34]

Eradication of the fleas may require consultation with a veterinarian. Pets must be treated more than once with topical agents to kill the eggs, larvae, and pupae, as well as the residual fleas. Systemic agents are available to protect pets from reinfestation. A household flea spray should be combined with a fogger to fumigate the house. A proper extermination procedure includes vacuuming the furniture and vacuuming or steam cleaning carpets or rugs. The yard should be sprayed and cleared of organic debris. Treatment of flea bites consists of cool-water compresses, application of a corticosteroid cream and an antipruritic lotion, and oral antihistamines in the case of allergic hypersensitivity reaction. Systemic antibiotics are prescribed for secondary bacterial infection.

Tungiasis

Cutaneous infestation by the sandflea *Tunga penetrans* is endemic in Central and South America, parts of Mexico, tropical Africa, Pakistan, and the west coast of India. Isolated cases have been reported in the United States, Australia, and New Zealand. Tungiasis is more prevalent in poverty-stricken areas and is associated with domestic animals such as pigs, dogs, and cattle, which serve as intermediaries in the biologic life cycle.[35] The female adult sandflea exists in sandy soils and requires a warm-blooded host to complete its life cycle. The organism penetrates the stratum corneum, resulting in erythematous nodules with a central dark spot. Common sites of skin involvement are the soles of the feet, the web spaces between fingers and toes, the ankles, the perineal area, and the buttocks.

Infestation can be prevented by wearing shoes and proper clothing and by the use of insecticides.

MYIASIS

Myiasis is caused by the larvae (maggots) of feeding flies of the order Diptera. The larvae may invade the skin primarily[36] or become secondarily implanted in a preexisting skin wound.[37] Many species of the genus *Cuterebra* can cause myiasis, but in North America, *C. cuterebra* and *C. dermatobia* cause furuncular cutaneous infestations. Mosquitoes act as vectors by transporting fly eggs from infected animals to human hosts.[38] The skin lesions appear as nonhealing single or multiple nodules on the upper trunk, usually at the site of a painful bite wound. Skin lesions may be misdiagnosed as cellulitis, boils, or sebaceous cysts. Myiasis is commonly reported in travelers to endemic areas such as Central and South America and tropical and subtropical Africa. Preventive measures include the use of insect repellents, the wearing of protective clothing to prevent mosquito bites, and the avoidance of direct skin contact with sand that may be infested with eggs. Furuncular myiasis is effectively treated by removal of the larvae by incision and drainage with debridement. Antibiotics are prescribed for secondary bacterial infection. Occlusion with such agents as liquid paraffin, lubricating jelly, and even the fatty portion of raw bacon has been suggested to cause suffocation of the larvae or migration of the larvae from the wound.[39]

CUTANEOUS LARVA MIGRANS

Cutaneous larva migrans is caused by penetration and migration of larval hookworms (usually *Ancylostoma braziliense*) within the skin. Patients are usually travelers returning from seawater beaches in tropical areas and commonly present to the dermatologist with pruritic skin lesions. The abdomen or feet are most often involved, with a characteristic eruption consisting of one or several erythematous linear to serpiginous thin lines in the skin.

Optimal management is controversial, and most treatment trials have been of low quality; however, it is generally agreed that the most effective agents in treating cutaneous larva migrans are topical or oral anthelmintics, including albendazole, thiabendazole, and ivermectin. Regimens include topical thiabendazole (10% to 15% cream) three times daily for 5 to 10 days; oral albendazole, 400 mg daily for 3 to 5 days; oral ivermectin, single dose of 12 mg; and oral thiabendazole, 50 mg/kg weekly for 2 to 3 weeks. Topical thiabendazole (10% cream) is effective and safe in children,[40,41] but it is difficult to obtain. Systemic therapy, either with albendazole or ivermectin, may be preferable to topical therapies. Oral albendazole has a high cure rate and appears to be effective in cases of multiple lesions.[42,43] Oral ivermectin is effective and reportedly safe.[43] Oral thiabendazole has been reported to cure long-standing cutaneous larva migrans, but it may cause side effects such as headaches, nausea, and vomiting.[44]

SEABATHER'S ERUPTION

Seabather's eruption, also known as sea lice by laypersons, is an acute pruritic dermatitis that occurs within 24 hours of seawater exposure and resolves spontaneously after 3 to 5 days.[45] Lesions affect areas of the skin covered by swimwear, particularly those that are subjected to pressure or friction, such as the waistline, axillae, neck, and inner thighs [see Figure 8]. The larvae of the thimble jellyfish *Linuche unguiculata*, which are washed ashore by ocean currents, have been identified as the cause of seabather eruption in southern Florida and the Caribbean.[46] Similar outbreaks on Long Island, New York, are thought to be caused by larvae of the sea anemone *Edwardsiella lineata*.[47] Treatment is symptomatic and includes antihistamines, topical antipruritic agents, and steroids.

SWIMMER'S ITCH

Cercarial dermatitis, known as swimmer's itch, is caused by an avian schistosome, *Microbilharzia variglandis*. The skin eruption appears approximately 12 hours after contact with seawater as a pruritic papulovesicular dermatitis on exposed skin sites.[48] The inflammatory response is attributed to dermatologic penetration by cercariae, which are the free-swimming larvae of *M. variglandis* and other bird schistosomes.

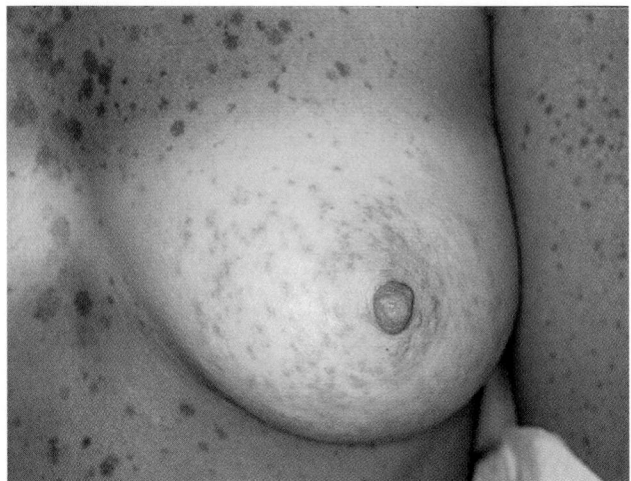

Figure 8 Seabather's eruption is characterized by the development of pruritic papules on areas covered by the patient's bathing suit.

Treatment of cercarial dermatitis is symptomatic and includes antihistamines, topical antipruritic agents, topical corticosteroids, and antibiotic treatment of superimposed bacterial infection.

CUTANEOUS AND MUCOCUTANEOUS LEISHMANIASIS

There are distinctive skin lesions associated with the cutaneous and mucocutaneous forms of leishmaniasis [see Figure 9]. Leishmaniasis is caused by an obligate intracellular parasite introduced by the *Phlebotomus* sandfly, which feeds on infected animals. *Leishmania braziliensis* and *L. mexicana* are the most common causes of American, or New World, leishmaniasis. *L. donovani* causes Old World leishmaniasis, which is endemic in Asia and West Africa [see Chapter 157]. Infection by *L. major* is the cause of cutaneous leishmaniasis in United States military personnel returning from Afghanistan and Iraq.[49]

Cutaneous leishmaniasis—the initial, or primary, form of the disease—appears as a localized, usually single, lesion involving the mouth and nose. A red-brown papule develops at the site of inoculation into a nodule that becomes verrucous or

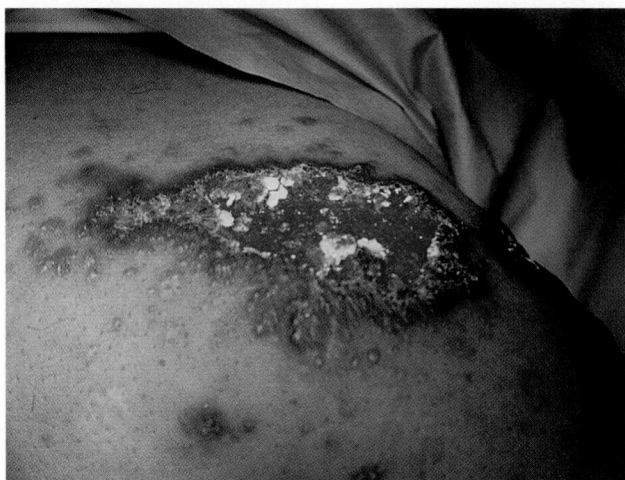

Figure 9 Leishmaniasis can present as chronic cutaneous ulcerations.

ulcerates, and satellite nodules may form. Spontaneous healing with an atrophic scar occurs in most cases. Old World leishmaniasis is usually limited to the skin, whereas New World leishmaniasis can cause mutilating mucocutaneous involvement.[50] After a period of months to years, the mucocutaneous, or secondary, form of the disease may develop, depending on host immunologic factors. Lesions in this stage range from edema of the lips and nose to perforation of the nasal cartilage. A rare form, disseminated cutaneous leishmaniasis, which has widespread nodules resembling lepromatous leprosy, may occur in immunosuppressed patients.

The differential diagnosis includes various inflammatory and neoplastic disorders, including squamous cell carcinoma. Diagnosis is made by skin biopsy with histopathologic examination. Cultures from skin biopsy may be inconclusive; PCR shows promise as a sensitive single diagnostic test.[51] Appropriate therapy depends on species identification. A pentavalent antimony compound, such as sodium stibogluconate, is the drug of choice for New World leishmaniasis, which tends to be more aggressive. Lesions acquired in the Middle East and North Africa may spontaneously involute or may respond to local therapy, including cryosurgery, heat therapy, or intralesional injection of antimonials.

Delusions of Parasitosis

Patients with delusions of parasitosis express the conviction that there are scabies, insects, lice, fleas, worms, or other vermin infesting their skin and producing a crawling, itching, or prickling sensation.[52] They may have excoriations or skin inflammation and erosions consistent with factitial dermatitis. Frequently, patients will bring small containers filled with lint, hairs, pieces of skin, fibers, or other debris for examination. Despite the lack of objective evidence for infestation—including negative results from clinical examination, microscopic examination of skin scrapings, and skin biopsy—the delusions persist. Associated underlying psychiatric disturbances may range from a phobic-obsessive state or anxiety reaction to a frank psychosis with either depression or paranoia. Not infrequently, the delusion is shared by the spouse or other family members, as in the classic folie à deux or folie à famille. The patient usually functions in a highly organized manner in other aspects of his or her life. Such patients typically resist seeking psychiatric evaluation.

Treatment with pimozide, a high-potency antipsychotic neuroleptic of the diphenylbutylpiperidine group, has been used successfully.[52] The effectiveness of the drug may be mediated by its ability to specifically block central dopamine receptors. As is characteristic of high-potency antipsychotic drugs, pimozide has fewer cardiovascular and anticholinergic effects but greater neurologic toxicity, especially with long-term use, than does low-potency antipsychotic drugs. Tardive dyskinesia, an extrapyramidal syndrome characterized by involuntary movements of facial muscles and extremities, may occur in 10% to 20% of patients on antipsychotic drugs. Other side effects may include skin discoloration, dermatitis, and blurred vision. Thorough medical and psychiatric evaluation should be obtained before antipsychotic medication is instituted.

The author has served as advisor or consultant to Amgen, Inc., Biogen Idec, Inc., Genentech, Inc., Abbott Laboratories, Ligand Pharmaceuticals, Inc., and 3M Co.

The drug ivermectin has not been approved by the FDA for uses described in this chapter.

References

1. Lucchina LC, Wilson ME, Drake LA: Dermatology and the recently returned traveler: infectious diseases with dermatologic manifestations. Int J Dermatol 36:167, 1997

2. Heukelbach J, Feldmeier H: Ectoparasites: the underestimated realm. Lancet 363:889, 2004

3. Chouela E, Abeldano A, Pellerano G, et al: Diagnosis and treatment of scabies: a practical guide. Am J Clin Dermatol 3:9, 2002

4. Scheinfeld N: Controlling scabies in institutional settings: a review of medications, treatment models, and implementation. Am J Clin Dermatol 5:31, 2004

5. Schlesinger I, Oelrich DM, Tyring SK: Crusted (Norwegian) scabies in patients with AIDS: the range of clinical presentations. South Med J 87:352, 1994

6. Head ES, Macdonald EM, Ewert A, et al: *Sarcoptes scabiei* in histopathologic sections of skin in human scabies. Arch Dermatol 126:1475, 1990

7. Argenziano G, Fabbrocini G, Delfino M: Epiluminescence microscopy: a new approach to in vivo detection of *Sarcoptes scabiei*. Arch Dermatol 133:751, 1997

8. Bezold G, Lange M, Schiener R, et al: Hidden scabies: diagnosis by polymerase chain reaction. Br J Dermatol 144:614, 2001

9. Walker GJ, Johnstone PW: Interventions for treating scabies. Cochrane Database Syst Rev (3):CD000320, 2000

10. Fischer TF: Lindane toxicity in a 24-year-old woman. Ann Emerg Med 24:972, 1994

11. Labeling changes for lindane. FDA Consum 37:6, 2003

12. Brooks PA, Grace RF: Ivermectin is better than benzyl benzoate for childhood scabies in developing countries. J Paediatr Child Health 38:401, 2002

13. Meinking TL, Taplin D, Hermida JL, et al: The treatment of scabies with ivermectin. N Engl J Med 333:26, 1995

14. Usha V, Gopalakrishnan Nair TV: A comparative study of oral ivermectin and topical permethrin cream in the treatment of scabies. J Am Acad Dermatol 42:236, 2000

15. Leppard B, Naburi AE: The use of ivermectin in controlling an outbreak of scabies in a prison. Br J Dermatol 143:520, 2000

16. Youssef MYM, Sadaka HAH, Eissa MM, et al: Topical application of ivermectin for human ectoparasites. Am J Trop Hyg 53:652, 1995

17. Purvis RS, Tyring SK: An outbreak of lindane-resistant scabies treated successfully with permethrin 5% cream. J Am Acad Dermatol 26(pt 1):1015, 1991

18. Cook AM, Romanelli F: Ivermectin for the treatment of resistant scabies. Ann Pharmacother 37:279, 2003

19. Paasch U, Haustein U-F: Management of endemic outbreaks of scabies with allethrin, permethrin, and ivermectin. Int J Dermatol 39:463, 2000

20. Alberici F, Pagani L, Ratti G, et al: Ivermectin alone or in combination with benzyl benzoate in the treatment of human immunodeficiency virus-associated scabies. Br J Dermatol 142:969, 2000

21. Taplin D, Meinking TL: Treatment of HIV-related scabies with emphasis on the efficacy of ivermectin. Semin Cutan Med Surg 16:235, 1997

22. Lee BW: *Cheyletiella* dermatitis: a report of fourteen cases. Cutis 47:111, 1991

23. Ko CJ, Elston DM: Pediculosis. J Am Acad Dermatol 50:1, 2004

24. Minouni D, Ankol OE, Gdalevich M, et al: Seasonality trends of *Pediculosis capitis* and *Phthirus pubis* in a young adult population: follow-up of 20 years. J Eur Acad Dermatol Venereol 16:257, 2002

25. Mumcuoglu KY, Friger M, Ioffe-Uspensky I, et al: Louse comb versus direct visual examination for the diagnosis of head louse infestations. Pediatr Dermatol 18:9, 2001

26. Jones KN, English JC 3rd: Review of common therapeutic options in the United States for the treatment of pediculosis capitis. Clin Infect Dis 36:1355, 2003

27. Burkhart CG: Relationship of treatment-resistant head lice to the safety and efficacy of pediculicides. Mayo Clin Proc 79:661, 2004

28. Yoon KS, Gao JR, Lee SH, et al: Permethrin-resistant human head lice, *Pediculus capitis*, and their treatment. Arch Dermatol 139:994, 2003

29. Frankowski BL: American Academy of Pediatrics guidelines for the prevention and treatment of head lice. Am J Manag Care 10:S269, 2004

30. Forrester MB, Sievert JS, Stanley SK: Epidemiology of lindane exposures for pediculosis reported to poison centers in Texas, 1998-2002. J Toxicol Clin Toxicol 42:55, 2004

31. Roberts RJ, Casey D, Morgan DA, et al: Comparison of wet combing with malathion for treatment of head lice in the UK: a pragmatic randomised controlled trial. Lancet 356:540, 2000

32. Mumcuoglu KY: Prevention and treatment of head lice in children. Paediatr Drugs 1:211, 1999

33. Dodd CS: Interventions for treating headlice. Cochrane Database Syst Rev (3)CD001165

34. Hutchins ME, Burnett JW: Fleas. Cutis 51:241, 1993

35. Campos Macias P, Mendez Sashida P: Cutaneous infestation by *Tunga penetrans*. Int J Dermatol 39:296, 2000

36. Jelinek T, Nothdurft HD, Rieder N, et al: Cutaneous myiasis: review of 13 cases in travelers from tropical countries. Int J Dermatol 34:624, 1995

37. Sherman RA: Wound myiasis in urban and suburban United States. Arch Intern Med 160:2004, 2000

38. Maier H, Honigsmann H: Furuncular myiasis caused by *Dermatobia hominis*, the human botfly. J Am Acad Dermatol 50:S26, 2004

39. Brewer TF, Wilson ME, Gonzalez MD, et al: Bacon therapy and furuncular myiasis. JAMA 270:2087, 1993

40. Jelinek T, Maiwald H, Nothdurft HD, et al: Cutaneous larva migrans in travelers: synopsis of histories, symptoms, and treatment of 98 patients. Clin Infect Dis 19:1062, 1994

41. Simon MW, Simon NP: Cutaneous larva migrans. Pediatr Emerg Care 19:350, 2003

42. Rizzitelli G, Scarabelli G, Veraldi S: Albendazole: a new therapeutic regimen in cutaneous larva migrans. Int J Dermatol 36:700, 1977

43. Caumes E, Carriere J, Datry A, et al: A randomized trial of ivermectin versus albendazole for the treatment of cutaneous larva migrans. Am J Trop Med Hyg 49:641, 1993

44. Richey TK, Gentry RH, Fitzpatrick JE, et al: Persistent cutaneous larva migrans due to *Ancylostoma* species. South Med J 89:609, 1996

45. Tomchik RS, Russell MT, Szmant AM, et al: Clinical perspectives on seabather's eruption, also known as "sea lice." JAMA 269:1669, 1993

46. Segura-Puertas L, Ramos ME, Aramburo C, et al: One *Linuche* mystery solved: all three stages of the coronate scyphomedusa *Linuche unguiculata* cause seabather's eruption. J Am Acad Dermatol 44:624, 2001

47. Freudenthal AR, Joseph PR: Seabather's eruption. N Engl J Med 329:542, 1993

48. Verbrugge LM, Rainey JJ, Reimink RL: Swimmer's itch: incidence and risk factors. Am J Public Health 94:738, 2004

49. Update: cutaneous leishmaniasis in U.S. military personnel: Southwest/Central Asia, 2002-2004. MMWR Morb Mortal Wkly Rep 53:264, 2004

50. Koff AB, Rosen T: Treatment of cutaneous leishmaniasis. J Am Acad Dermatol 31:693, 1994

51. Faber WR, Oskam L, van Gool T, et al: Value of diagnostic techniques for cutaneous leishmaniasis. J Am Acad Dermatol 49:70, 2003

52. Driscoll MS, Rothe MJ, Grant-Kels JM, et al: Delusional parasitosis: a dermatologic, psychiatric, and pharmacologic approach. J Am Acad Dermatol 29:1023, 1993

43 Vesiculobullous Diseases

Elizabeth A. Abel, M.D., and Jean-Claude Bystryn, M.D.

Vesiculobullous diseases, which number more than 50, are characterized by fluid-filled blisters in the skin. Blisters smaller than 0.5 cm are called vesicles, and larger ones are called bullae. Vesicles and bullae are reaction patterns of skin to injury and thus can be caused by a wide variety of conditions.

Most primary vesiculobullous diseases are either immunologic or genetic. They are caused by autoimmune reactions to components of skin, by allergic reactions to external agents in which the skin is the major organ system affected, and by genetic conditions in which some components of the skin are missing or abnormal. The final common pathway is disadhesion: one or more of the structures that hold the skin together separate, and a fluid-filled cavity appears. The different diseases are classified by the structure or structures affected and the mechanism or mechanisms by which disadhesion occurs [*see Table 1*]. In this subsection, several paradigmatic vesiculobullous diseases are discussed in the context of a general diagnostic approach to the patient with blistering lesions.

General Clinical Assessment

Diagnosis is based on clinical features, histologic findings, and immunologic findings. Clinical features of diagnostic importance include the following:

1. The history. Is the condition acute or chronic? Is it aggravated by sun or physical trauma?
2. The appearance of individual lesions [*see Table 2*]. Is the lesion a vesicle or bulla? Is it tense, flaccid, or umbilicated? Does the skin at the base of the blister appear normal, urticarial, or scarred? Is the border of each urticarial lesion annular or oval or is it irregular? Is the blister in the middle of urticarial plaques or on the periphery? Do more than one bulla arise from the same plaque?
3. The grouping of individual lesions. Are the lesions in closely spaced groups (as occurs in herpes simplex), or are they randomly distributed?
4. Sites of involvement. Are lesions on mucosal surfaces as well as on the skin? Are they predominantly on flexural or extensor surfaces; on the palms and soles or on the dorsa of the hands and feet; on the scalp, face, and upper torso; or on areas exposed to trauma?

The most important histologic finding in vesiculobullous disease is the layer of skin where the blister forms. If the blister forms in the epidermis, does it form immediately above the basal cell layer or higher up (beneath the stratum corneum)? If it forms in the basement membrane zone, is it within the lamina lucida or below the lamina densa? The precise location may be determined by immunofluorescence or by electron microscopic procedures.

The most important immunologic finding is the presence or absence of abnormal circulating or tissue-fixed antibodies to skin. These are usually detected by immunofluorescence techniques: (1) indirect immunofluorescence to detect circulating antibodies and (2) direct immunofluorescence on skin biopsy specimens to detect tissue-fixed antibodies. Recently, enzyme-linked immunosorbent assays (ELISAs) using purified antigens have become available to detect the antibodies that occur in some of the bullous diseases, such as pemphigus.

Pemphigus

DEFINITION AND PATHOGENESIS

Pemphigus is characterized by blisters that arise within the epidermis and by a loss of cohesion of the epidermal cells (acantholysis) that results in the formation of clefts above the basal cell layer. Autoantibodies directed against adhesion molecules cause epidermal keratinocytes to separate, resulting in intraepidermal bullae. There are two types of pemphigus: deep (e.g., pemphigus vulgaris) and superficial (e.g., pemphigus foliaceus). They differ in the epidermal layers that are injured, in the clinical manifestations of the diseases, and in the associated immunologic abnormalities.[1] In the deep forms, the blisters form immediately above the basal cell layer and are associated with autoantibodies to desmoglein 3; about half the cases are associated with antibodies to desmoglein 1 glycoprotein keratinocyte adhesion molecules.[2] In the superficial forms, the bullae form immediately below the stratum corneum. The superficial forms of pemphigus are associated with antibodies to desmoglein 1.

CLINICAL FEATURES

Pemphigus Vulgaris

Pemphigus vulgaris is the most common form of pemphigus. It can develop at any age but usually occurs in persons between 30 and 60 years old. The disorder tends to affect persons of Mediterranean ancestry but can occur in persons of any ethnicity. Pemphigus is more common in persons with certain HLA allotypes. The occurrence of the disease in first-degree relatives, although rare, suggests an inherited susceptibility transferred as a dominant trait. However, other unknown factors are required for expression of the disorder in predisposed persons.[3] Studies of HLA class II alleles in Japanese patients as well as in other ethnic groups show an association with HLA-DRB1*04 and HLA-DRB1*14 in patients with pemphigus vulgaris across racial lines.[4]

Pemphigus vulgaris usually, but not invariably, begins with chronic, painful, nonhealing ulcerations in the oral cavity [*see Figure 1*]. Bullae are rarely seen because they rupture easily, leaving ulcerated bases. The ulcerations are usually multiple, superficial, and irregular in shape. Any oral mucosal surface can be involved, but the most common sites are the buccal and labial mucosae, the palate, and the gingiva. The occurrence of multiple ulcerations differentiates these lesions from ulcerated malignant tumors of the oral cavity, which are usually single. A diagnosis of pemphigus is usually considered only after lesions have been present for weeks to months.

Skin lesions can also be the initial manifestation, beginning as small fluid-filled bullae on otherwise normal-looking skin. The blisters are usually flaccid because the thin overlying epidermis cannot sustain much pressure. Bullae therefore rupture rapidly, usually in several days, and may be absent when a patient is examined. Sharply outlined, coin-sized, superficial erosions with a collarette of loose epidermis around the periphery of the erosions may appear instead. The upper chest, back, scalp, and face are common sites of involvement, but lesions can occur on any part of the body. The condition progresses over weeks to months [see Figure 2]. Sites often overlooked include the periungual areas (manifested as painful, erythematous, paronychial swelling), the pharynx and larynx (pain on swallowing and hoarseness), and the nasal cavity (nasal con-

Table 1 Differentiating Features and Standard Therapy for Selected Blistering Diseases

	Disease	Features	Therapy
Epidermal	Pemphigus vulgaris	Chronic, painful ulcerations in the oral cavity; small, flaccid bullae *or* coin-sized superficial erosions arising from normal skin; positive Nikolsky sign; IgG and C3 at intercellular spaces; serum antidesmoglein 1 or 3 antibodies	*Localized:* Intralesional or topical corticosteroids, low-dose systemic corticosteroids
	Pemphigus vegetans	Hypertrophic proliferation of epidermis in intertriginous areas; IgG and C3 at intercellular spaces; serum antidesmoglein 3 antibodies	*Extensive or rapidly progressive disease:* corticosteroids, adjuvant therapy with cytotoxic and immunosuppressive agents *Refractory disease:* plasmapheresis, IVIg, pulse therapy with megadoses of I.V. methylprednisolone
	Pemphigus foliaceus	Small, pruritic, crusted lesions on upper torso, face, or scalp; chronic superficial erosions; rare oral involvement; immunopathology higher in epidermis	*Localized:* Intralesional or topical corticosteroids, low-dose systemic corticosteroids
	Pemphigus erythematosus	Erythematous scaly to crusted eruption on face and upper chest; lupuslike immunologic abnormalities (granular deposits of IgG and C3 at epidermal-dermal junction)	*Extensive or rapidly progressive disease:* corticosteroids, adjuvant therapy with cytotoxic and immunosuppressive agents
	Fogo selvagem	Features similar to pemphigus foliaceus (primarily affects persons < 30 yr in rural areas of Brazil, Colombia, Tunisia)	
	Paraneoplastic mixed bullous disease (paraneoplastic pemphigus)	Large, tense bullae; target lesions on skin; oral erosions; keratinocyte necrosis; clinical features overlap between pemphigus and erythema multiforme; subepidermal separation; IC and BMZ antibodies on direct IF	Difficult (standard treatments for autoimmune blistering diseases fail in most patients)
	Hailey-Hailey disease	Multiple vesicles on inflammatory bases in intertriginous areas and other areas subject to friction or pressure; loss of bridges between epidermal cells; no circulating or tissue-fixed autoantibodies	Involved areas kept dry and free of friction; administration of topical and systemic antibiotics; topical, intralesional corticosteroids; ablation of involved areas
Subepidermal	Bullous pemphigoid	Crops of large, tense blisters recurring from urticarial plaques on torso and flexures; negative Nikolsky sign; oral lesions (10%–25% of patients); circulating BMZ antibodies; IgG and C3 at BMZ in a linear pattern on direct IF	Administration of systemic corticosteroids at doses lower than those used for pemphigus (≤ 80 mg/day prednisone) [see also Bullous Pemphigoid, Treatment, *in text*]
	Cicatricial pemphigoid	Blisters on mucosal surfaces (oral cavity, esophagus, eyes) that heal with scarring, often occurring repeatedly at same site; diffuse, painful erythema and atrophy of the gingival mucosa; IgG and C3 at BMZ in a linear pattern on direct IF	Combination therapy with systemic corticosteroids and dapsone or azathioprine; long-term therapy with systemic corticosteroids, sometimes combined with immunosuppressive agents; intralesional corticosteroids
	Herpes gestationis	Pruritic urticarial plaques occurring in pregnancy (beginning around the umbilicus, spreading to abdomen and thighs); laminal blisters with linear deposits of C3 or IgG at the epidermal-dermal junction; circulating complement-fixing BMZ antibodies on indirect IF	Normally clears after delivery
	Dermatitis herpetiformis	Clusters of intensely pruritic, small, polymorphic vesicles on elbows, knees, buttocks, scapular area, and scalp; accumulations of neutrophils and eosinophils in dermal papillae; granular deposits of IgA in BMZ; no circulating antibodies to normal skin components	Administration of sulfones (dapsone, 100–200 mg/day; sulfapyridine, 1–3 g/day in divided doses; or sulfamethoxypyridazine); reduction of gluten intake
	Linear IgA dermatosis	Blisters resembling those of dermatitis herpetiformis or erythema multiforme; linear deposition of IgA in BMZ on direct IF	Administration of sulfones
	Erythema multiforme	Sudden eruption of crops of lesions on elbows, knees, hands, and feet; target papule or vesicle with halo of erythema; subepidermal edema, deep perivascular inflammatory infiltrate	Elimination of underlying causes (e.g., infectious agents, drugs); *in mild cases,* topical glucocorticoids, anti-inflammatories, antipruritics, antibiotics; *in severe cases,* prednisone 40–120 mg/day in divided doses
	Toxic epidermal necrolysis	Rapidly progressive painful denudation of epithelium (usually a drug reaction); full-thickness epidermal necrosis; absence of immune reactants within skin blood vessels; little dermal inflammation	Meticulous wound care with debridement of necrotic tissue, fluid and electrolyte replacement, and prevention of sepsis; IVIg[56]
	Staphylococcal scalded skin syndrome	Scarlatiniform eruption accompanied by skin tenderness, fever, and irritability; lack of mucous membrane involvement or target lesions	Intravenous penicillinase-resistant penicillins
	Epidermolysis bullosa	[See Epidermolysis Bullosa, *in text*]	Supportive therapy; counseling; promotion of wound healing; prevention of complications

BMZ—basal membrane zone IC—intercellular IF—immunofluorescence IVIg—intravenous immunoglobulin

Table 2   Pathologic Typology of Blisters[57]

Blister Type	Mode of Formation	Site of Formation	Disease
Subcorneal blister	Detachment of horny layer	Epidermis (subcorneal layer)	Miliaria crystallina Impetigo
Blister due to intracellular degeneration	Separation of cells from one another	Upper epidermis	Friction blisters
Spongiotic blister	Intercellular edema	Epidermis	Dermatitis (eczema) Miliaria rubra
Acantholytic blister	Dissolution of intercellular bridges	Epidermis (suprabasal layer)	Keratosis follicularis (Darier disease) Pemphigus vulgaris
		Epidermis (subcorneal layer)	Pemphigus foliaceus
Viral blister	Ballooning degeneration leading to acantholysis	Epidermis	Herpes simplex Herpes zoster Varicella
Blister due to degeneration of basal cells	Cytolysis of basal cells	Basal cell layer	Epidermolysis bullosa simplex Erythema multiforme (epidermal type)
	Loss of dermal contact by damaged basal cells	Basal cell layer	Lichen planus Lupus erythematosus
Blister due to degeneration of basement membrane zone	Damage in the structures that cause coherence of basal cells	Basement membrane zone	Bullous pemphigoid Dermatitis herpetiformis Erythema multiforme (dermal type)
Dermolytic blister	Anchoring fibrils are decreased and rudimentary	Dermis	Dystrophic epidermolysis bullosa Acquired epidermolysis bullosa

gestion and a bloody mucous discharge, particularly noticeable upon blowing the nose in the morning).

A characteristic feature of all severe active forms of pemphigus is the Nikolsky sign, in which sliding firm pressure on normal-appearing skin causes the epidermis to separate from the dermis. The Nikolsky sign is elicited most easily on clinically uninvolved skin adjacent to an active lesion.

If left untreated, the erosions and bullae of pemphigus vulgaris gradually spread, involving an increasing surface area, and can become complicated by severe infections and metabolic disturbances. Before the advent of corticosteroids, pemphigus was almost invariably fatal—approximately 75% of patients died within a year.[5] However, as better techniques have permitted the diagnosis of earlier, milder forms of the disease, the prognosis has improved significantly.[6] Mild forms may regress spontaneously, and the progression of even the most severe forms can be reversed in most cases. With treatment (see below), lesions normally heal without scarring. Most patients treated for pemphigus will enter a partial remission within 2 to 5 years. They can then be maintained lesion-free with minimal doses of corticosteroids (approximately 15 mg of prednisone daily). In a longitudinal study of outcome in 40 patients with pemphigus vulgaris, 45% entered a complete and long-term remission after 5 years and 71% after 10 years. Patients in remission remained lesion-free without any therapy.[7] The hyperpigmentation that is commonly associated with pemphigus usually resolves after several months.

In pregnancy, pemphigus appears to be associated with an increased incidence of premature delivery and fetal death.[8] The lesions of pemphigus can appear on the skin of the neonate; however, they normally resolve spontaneously in several weeks.

Pemphigus Foliaceus

Pemphigus foliaceus is the second most common form of pemphigus. It usually begins with small (approximately 1 cm), pruritic, crusted lesions resembling corn flakes on the upper torso and face. The crusts are easily removed, leaving chronic, superficial erosions.

Over weeks to months, the condition progresses, with an increasing number of lesions appearing on the upper torso, face, and scalp. In extensive cases, lesions develop over the entire body, become confluent, and can progress to an exfoliative erythroderma. In contrast to the deep forms of pemphigus, oral involvement in pemphigus foliaceus is very rare.

The prognosis of untreated pemphigus foliaceus is more favorable than that of pemphigus vulgaris. The lesions of pemphi-

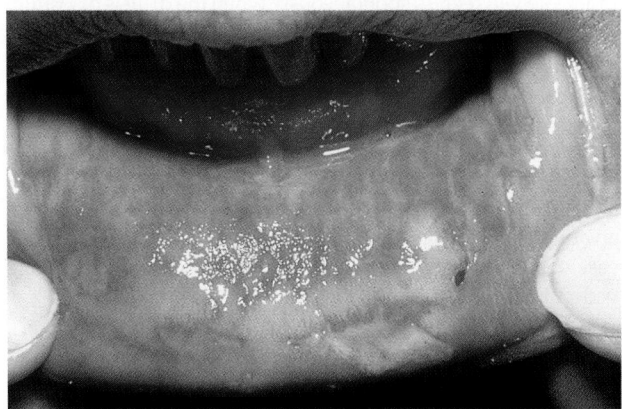

Figure 1   **Painful ulcerations or erosions in the mouth may be present many months before the onset of generalized pemphigus vulgaris.**

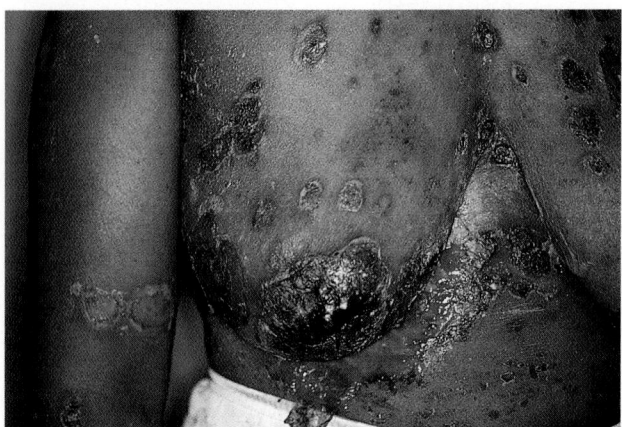

Figure 2 Flaccid bullae of pemphigus vulgaris have broken down to form erosions and crusts, particularly under the breasts.

gus foliaceus are not as deep, and there is less chance for infection, fluid loss, and metabolic disturbance. Although pemphigus foliaceus is less severe, the doses of medications required for control are similar to those used for pemphigus vulgaris. There are two clinical variants: pemphigus erythematosus and fogo selvagem. Pemphigus erythematosus (also known as Senear-Usher syndrome) has features of lupus erythematosus. Fogo selvagem (Portuguese for "wild fire"; also known as endemic pemphigus and Brazilian pemphigus) [*see Table 1*] may be triggered by exposure to one or more environmental antigens.[9]

Drug-Related Pemphigus

Both pemphigus vulgaris and pemphigus foliaceus can be either induced or triggered (i.e., latent disease unmasked) by certain drugs. Pemphigus that continues after a patient stops using a drug is referred to as triggered, whereas lesions that clear soon after withdrawal are referred to as induced. Although drug-related pemphigus is uncommon, its possibility must be excluded in all patients with newly diagnosed disease. The clinical, histologic,[10] and immunofluorescence abnormalities[11] of drug-induced pemphigus are similar to those of the idiopathic variety. However, pemphigus caused by drugs containing a sulfhydryl radical (thiol drugs) is clinically distinct from pemphigus caused by nonthiol drugs. The presence or absence of a sulfhydryl radical appears to influence both the type of pemphigus that is expressed and the prognosis of the drug-induced condition. Thiol drugs are more likely to induce pemphigus foliaceus, which is more likely to regress spontaneously when the drug is discontinued [*see Chapter 40*]. Nonthiol drugs are more likely to trigger pemphigus vulgaris, which can persist even after the drug is stopped. The most commonly implicated agents are thiol drugs such as penicillamine and captopril. Other responsible drugs include sulfur-containing drugs such as penicillins and cephalosporins. These undergo metabolic changes to form thiol groups and are termed masked thiol drugs. Nonthiol drugs that contain an amide group (e.g., dipyrone and enalapril) can provoke a disease that is indistinguishable from spontaneously occurring pemphigus vulgaris.[11]

Endemic Pemphigus

Epidemiologic features of fogo selvagem in rural areas of Brazil suggest that the production of pathologic antibodies to desmoglein 1 is linked to exposure to one or more environmental antigens.[9]

Paraneoplastic Mixed Bullous Disease

Paraneoplastic pemphigus is an autoimmune disease of the skin and oral mucosa that develops in patients with an underlying neoplasm. It is characterized by large, tense bullae. Unfortunately, standard treatments for autoimmune blistering diseases fail in most cases. Paraneoplastic pemphigus shares clinical features of both pemphigus and severe erythema multiforme.[12]

Hailey-Hailey Disease

Familial benign chronic pemphigus, or Hailey-Hailey disease, is an autosomal dominant disorder marked by multiple vesicles on inflammatory bases in skin subject to friction or pressure, such as intertriginous areas. In addition to pharmacologic treatment (see below), therapy includes keeping involved areas dry and free of friction.

HISTOLOGIC AND IMMUNOLOGIC FINDINGS

The diagnosis should always be confirmed by histopathologic examination and immunofluorescence studies.[13] Biopsies for pemphigus and all other bullous diseases should be performed at the edge of a lesion, so as to include clinically uninvolved adjacent skin. Acantholysis (the separation of keratinocytes from each other) is the fundamental abnormality in all forms of pemphigus.

All forms of pemphigus are associated with circulating and tissue-fixed intercellular (IC) autoantibodies that react against cell-surface keratinocyte antigens. The detection of these antibodies is very helpful in establishing the diagnosis, because they rarely appear in other conditions. Circulating IC autoantibodies are detected by indirect immunofluorescence assays on serum, and tissue-fixed IC autoantibodies are detected by direct immunofluorescence on skin biopsies. In both cases, they cause a lacelike pattern of fluorescence within the epidermis. Low titers of IC autoantibodies may also be present in burns, fungal infections, and allergic drug reactions. Antibodies against ABO blood group antigens, which are present in approximately 5% of the normal population, are the most common cause of false positive tests for IC autoantibodies. Tissue-fixed IC autoantibodies are present in lesions and adjacent normal skin in approximately 90% of patients with pemphigus and are more sensitive and specific for the diagnosis of pemphigus than are circulating IC autoantibodies. The most common autoantibodies are IgG, but IgM and IgA (with or without C3) may also be deposited.

TREATMENT

Initial Therapy

Initial therapy is determined by the extent and rate of progression of lesions. Localized, slowly progressive disease can be treated with intralesional injections of corticosteroids (triamcinolone acetonide, 10 to 20 mg/ml) or topical application of high-potency corticosteroids. New lesions that continue to appear in increasing numbers can be controlled in some cases with low-dose systemic corticosteroids (prednisone, 20 mg/day). Patients with extensive or rapidly progressive disease are treated with moderately high doses of corticosteroids (prednisone, 70 to 90 mg/day). This dose is rapidly escalated every 4 to 14 days in 50% increments until disease activity is controlled, as evidenced by an absence of new lesions and the disappearance of skin pain or itching. If the disease remains active despite high doses of corticosteroids (e.g., 120 to 160 mg/day of prednisone), one of the following approaches should be considered for rapid control:

1. Plasmapheresis, normally performed three times a week for removal of 1 to 2 L of plasma per procedure.[14]
2. Intravenous immunoglobulin (IVIg), usually given at a dosage of 400 mg/kg/day for 5 days or in higher doses for 3 days.[15] The procedure may need to be repeated every 2 to 3 weeks for several cycles. It is very expensive. The use of IVIg for the treatment of skin diseases has recently been reviewed.[16] With both IVIg and plasmapheresis it is important to concurrently administer an immunosuppressive agent such as cyclophosphamide or azathioprine to minimize rebound in the level of pemphigus antibodies,[14] and it is also important to monitor the level of these antibodies to ensure that the patient is responding to treatment.
3. Pulse therapy with megadoses of intravenous methylprednisolone, given at a dosage of 1 g/day for 5 days.[17]

No comparative studies have yet evaluated the relative effectiveness of these procedures. On the basis of such limited experience, IVIg may be preferred because it has fewer side effects than the other procedures and is associated with a significantly higher response rate. Once disease activity is controlled, the patient is maintained on the type and dose of medications required to establish control until approximately 80% of lesions are healed. Therapy should not be tapered while new lesions are appearing.

Rituximab, an anti-CD20 chimeric monoclonal antibody, is approved for use in non-Hodgkin lymphoma. However, there is a case report of partial remission from recalcitrant, life-threatening pemphigus vulgaris after treatment with rituximab.[18]

Adjuvant Therapy

The role of adjuvants in the treatment of pemphigus remains controversial. Because of a lack of controlled studies, it is not known whether the potential benefits of adjuvants outweigh the additional toxicities.[5] Indications for adjuvant therapy include the presence of relative contraindications to systemic corticosteroids, development of serious corticosteroid side effects, and repeated flares of disease activity that make it undesirable to reduce corticosteroid doses.[7] Because they require 4 to 6 weeks to become effective, adjuvants are not used to control active, rapidly progressive disease.

Adjuvant treatments for pemphigus include a variety of cytotoxic and immunosuppressive agents (e.g., cyclophosphamide, azathioprine, cyclosporine, methotrexate, and mycophenolate mofetil[19]); dapsone; anti-inflammatory agents (e.g., gold); antimalarials; and certain antibiotics (e.g., tetracycline and minocycline).

Bullous Pemphigoid

PATHOGENESIS

The immediate cause of bullous pemphigoid (BP) appears to be an autoantibody response to the 180 kd (BP180) and 230 kd (BP230) basement membrane zone antigens.[20] Passive transfer of these antibodies into animals can cause lesions of the disease[21]; anti-BP180 autoantibodies have been found to be a poor prognostic factor in a study of 94 elderly patients.[22]

CLINICAL FEATURES

BP is a nonscarring, subepidermal blistering disease that is characterized by recurrent crops of large, tense blisters arising from urticarial bases. Lesions normally appear on the torso and flexures, particularly on the inner thighs. Blisters can range in size from a few millimeters to several centimeters [see Figure 3]. They

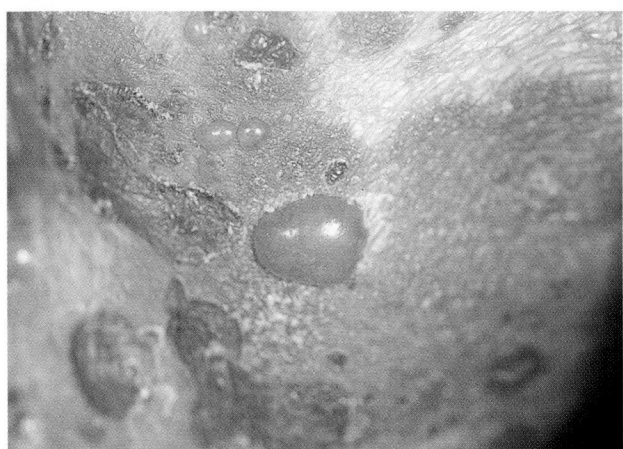

Figure 3   Tense bullae characteristically occur in bullous pemphigoid.

are usually filled with a clear fluid, but they can be hemorrhagic. Erosions are much less common than in pemphigus, and the Nikolsky sign is negative. A characteristic feature is that multiple bullae usually arise from large (palm-sized or larger), irregular, urticarial plaques. This is in contrast to the bullae of erythema multiforme (see below); in erythema multiforme, a single bulla arises from the center of a smaller (coin-sized) urticarial base.

In acute flares of BP, bullae may arise from normal-appearing skin. Oral lesions occur in 10% to 25% of patients; ocular involvement, however, is rare. Without treatment, the disease may become very extensive.

BP is a sporadic disease that occurs mainly in the elderly but can occur at any age and in any race. It has been reported in a 2-month-old infant.[23] Precipitating factors include trauma, burns, ionizing radiation, ultraviolet light, and certain drugs. In a case-control study of 116 incident cases, neuroleptics and diuretics—particularly aldosterone antagonists—were more commonly used by patients who developed BP than by control subjects.[24] There is still controversy as to whether BP is associated with an increased incidence of cancer[25]; however, correlations between flare in disease activity and recurrence of underlying cancer suggest such an association in individual patients.

BP is characterized by spontaneous remissions followed by flares in disease activity that can persist for years. Even without therapy, BP is often self-limited, resolving after a period of many months to years. The disease is nonetheless serious, particularly in older patients who have been treated with high doses of oral corticosteroids.[26] Mortality is low in younger persons but is significant in the elderly. In one study of patients older than 68 years, nearly a third died of the disease or complications (mainly sepsis and cardiovascular disease) within 1 year.[22]

HISTOLOGIC AND IMMUNOLOGIC FINDINGS

The earliest lesion of BP is a blister arising in the lamina lucida, between the basal membrane of keratinocytes and the lamina densa. This is associated with loss of anchoring filaments and hemidesmosomes. Histologically, there is a superficial inflammatory cell infiltrate and a subepidermal blister without necrotic keratinocytes. The infiltrate consists of lymphocytes and histiocytes and is particularly rich in eosinophils. There is no scarring.

Approximately 70% to 80% of patients with active BP have circulating antibodies to one or more basement membrane zone antigens. On direct immunofluorescence, the antibodies are deposited in a thin linear pattern; and on immune electron microscopy, they are present in the lamina lucida. By contrast, the antibodies to basement membrane zone antigens that are present in the skin of patients with systemic lupus erythematosus are deposited in a granular pattern.

Two less common subepidermal blistering diseases that are closely related to BP are cicatricial mucous membrane pemphigoid and herpes gestationis [see Table 1]. The differential diagnosis also includes dermatitis herpetiformis and acquired epidermolysis bullosa (see below). Scar formation in mucous membrane pemphigoid and acquired epidemolysis bullosa can lead to major disability.[27]

TREATMENT

Treatment of BP is generally similar to that of pemphigus.[28] The differences are as follows: (1) BP normally, but not invariably, responds to lower doses of systemic corticosteroids (alone or combined with other oral or topical agents), with most patients improving on prednisone at a dosage of 80 mg/day or less; (2) in an open prospective study of 18 cases, low-dose methotrexate was shown to be effective for maintenance of clinical remission induced by initial short-term use of potent topical steroids[29]; and (3) BP is more likely to respond to dapsone[30] or to the combination of tetracycline and niacinamide.[31,32] Considering that the prognosis of untreated BP is better than that of pemphigus, side effects of treatment are of greater concern. Two small studies of severe ocular mucous membrane pemphigoid suggest that this condition responds more favorably to treatment with cyclophosphamide combined with prednisone, whereas dapsone suppresses some cases of mild to moderate disease.[27]

Dermatitis Herpetiformis

Dermatitis herpetiformis (DH) is a rare vesiculobullous disease characterized by intensely pruritic, small vesicles that are

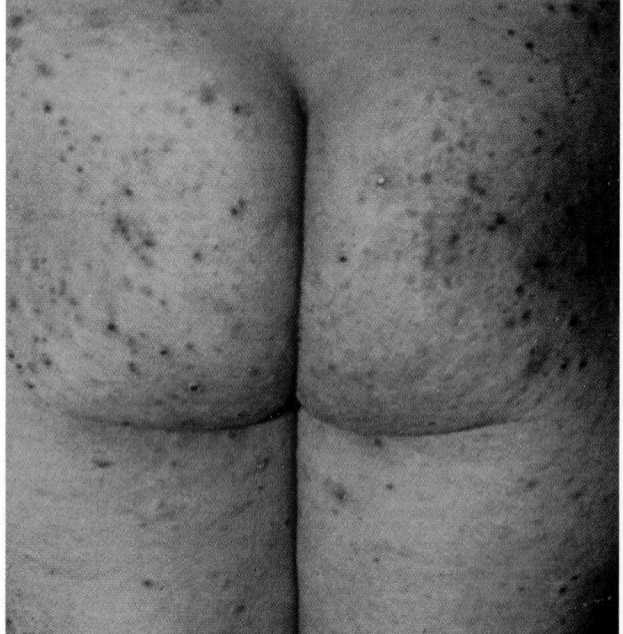

Figure 4 **Dermatitis herpetiformis, an extremely pruritic eruption, commonly presents as excoriated, grouped papulovesicles, often in a symmetrical distribution.**

grouped in small clusters and typically appear on the extensor aspects of the extremities and on the buttocks, scalp, and back. The condition is believed to be an immune-mediated disorder and is associated with abnormal granular deposits of IgA at the basement membrane zone and with asymptomatic, gluten-sensitive, spruelike enteropathy. The disease is chronic, with periods of exacerbation and remission. Lesions may clear if patients follow a strict gluten-free diet. Linear IgA dermatosis [see Table 1] is an uncommon subepidermal blistering disease that may clinically resemble DH or erythema multiforme (see below).

PATHOGENESIS

The cause of DH is unknown. It may be related to gluten-sensitive celiac disease; there is a strong association between the two conditions, and they share a similar genetic basis (both are associated with HLA-B8 and HLA-DR3). DH is thought to result from an abnormal IgA immune response to an unidentified antigen (possibly found in gluten) that contacts the gut. Skin lesions may result from deposition of immune complexes against this antigen in skin.

CLINICAL FEATURES

Skin lesions of DH are polymorphic. They usually begin as small, very pruritic urticarial papules or vesicles that are grouped in a herpetiform pattern [see Figure 4]. Actual vesicles or other primary lesions are rarely seen because they are excoriated by patients' scratching. The distribution of lesions is characteristic: they occur most commonly on the elbows, knees, buttocks, scapular area, and scalp. Sometimes, lesions are scattered over the entire body. The lesions tend to appear suddenly and symmetrically, sometimes after ingestion of large amounts of gluten. Lesions heal, leaving hyperpigmentation; scarring may result from scratching or secondary infection. Involvement of mucous membranes is rare.

The disease is twice as common in men as in women. It predominantly affects persons between the ages of 20 and 50 years. There may be an associated patchy duodenal and jejunal atrophy that resembles the gluten-sensitive enteropathy of adult celiac disease.[33,34] The enteropathy is usually asymptomatic and, like celiac disease, responds to gluten restriction. Because celiac disease is associated with gastrointestinal lymphoma, there is concern that the same may be true for DH. However, although lymphomas of the small intestine have been reported in DH,[35] the association appears to be rare.

HISTOLOGIC AND IMMUNOLOGIC FINDINGS

Two characteristic laboratory features of DH are used for diagnosis. First, the disease is characterized histologically by accumulations of neutrophils and eosinophils in microabscesses at the tips of dermal papillae. In more severe cases, edema appears and can progress to subepidermal blisters appearing just below the lamina densa. Secondly, granular deposits of IgA are found at the basement membrane zone in almost all patients. These are often associated with granular deposits of C3 and, occasionally, of IgG and IgM. When found alone, IgA is one of the most sensitive and specific diagnostic markers for DH. When IgA is found with deposits of IgG, IgM, or C3, immune complex vasculitis and systemic lupus erythematosus are added to the differential diagnosis. Although basement membrane zone deposits of IgA alone also occur in linear IgA disease,[36] the deposits in that condition are linear rather than granular. There are no circulating antibodies to normal skin components in DH.

TREATMENT

DH responds rapidly and dramatically to sulfones. Dapsone at a dosage of 100 to 200 mg/day is most commonly used for treatment. Glucose-6-phosphate dehydrogenase (G6PD) deficiency must be excluded before starting therapy, because lack of this enzyme can result in severe drug-induced anemia. Sulfapyridine at a dosage of 1 to 3 g/day in divided doses (or sulfamethoxypyridazine) can be used in patients who cannot tolerate dapsone. Doses of these drugs are gradually reduced to the lowest amount that will suppress pruritus and development of new lesions. As indicated, patients also respond to a gluten-free diet; however, such diets are difficult to follow. Nevertheless, even a partial decrease in gluten intake will result in a decreased requirement for sulfones and should therefore be encouraged.

Erythema Multiforme

Erythema multiforme is an acute, recurrent, self-limiting disease that affects all age groups and races. It is characterized by the sudden eruption of crops of lesions, which represent a cell-mediated hypersensitivity reaction of the skin and mucous membranes to a variety of precipitating factors, including infectious agents and drugs [see Table 3].[37] Recent or recurrent infection with herpes simplex virus is a principal risk factor for erythema multiforme.[38]

CLINICAL FEATURES

Lesions may be localized or widespread and may affect both the skin and the mucous membranes. The eruption often occurs bilaterally and symmetrically on the extensor surfaces of the extremities and on both the dorsal and the volar areas of the hands and feet. Lesions vary from well-defined, red or purple, edematous macules and papules to vesicular or bullous lesions that may ulcerate, encrust, erode, and become infected. A target lesion consisting of a papule or vesicle surrounded by a region of normal skin and a halo of erythema at the periphery [see Figure 5] is characteristic.

Stevens-Johnson syndrome is a severe form of erythema multiforme that is usually disseminated, fulminant, and multisystemic [see Figure 6]. The syndrome may be accompanied by high fever, malaise, chills, headache, tachycardia, tachypnea, and prostration. Drugs are more commonly the underlying etiologic agent than infection. Some of these include long-acting sulfonamides (particularly trimethoprim-sulfamethoxazole), anticonvulsants, barbiturates, and nonsteroidal anti-inflammatory drugs. The mucous membranes in the mouth, the anus, and the vagina contain round or oval erythematous macules that form vesicles, bullae, and ulcers. Ocular lesions are bilateral yellowish-gray papules that often ulcerate and become secondarily infected, resulting in conjunctivitis. Ocular involvement has produced blindness.

Toxic epidermal necrolysis (TEN) has a potentially fatal outcome because of detachment of large areas of epidermis. TEN is considered by some to be a form of erythema multiforme, usually a reaction to medication. However, the absence of immune reactants within the blood vessels in the skin and the paucity of dermal inflammation have led other researchers to consider TEN a separate disease.

Staphylococcal scalded skin syndrome also causes large areas of epidermal necrosis. This syndrome, which results from toxins produced by Staphylococcus aureus,[39] is sometimes confused with TEN [see Table 1].

Table 3 Precipitating Factors in Erythema Multiforme

Viral diseases	Herpes simplex Hepatitis Influenza A Vaccinia Mumps
Fungal diseases	Dermatophytoses Histoplasmosis Coccidioidomycosis
Bacterial diseases	Hemolytic streptococcal infections Tuberculosis Leprosy Typhoid
Collagen vascular disorders	Rheumatoid arthritis Systemic lupus erythematosus Dermatomyositis Allergic vasculitis Polyarteritis nodosa
Malignant tumors	Carcinoma Lymphoma after radiation therapy
Hormonal changes	Pregnancy Menstruation
Drugs	Penicillins Sulfonamides Barbiturates Salicylates Halogens Phenolphthalein
Miscellaneous	Rhus dermatitis Dental extractions Mycoplasma pneumoniae infection

HISTOLOGIC AND IMMUNOLOGIC FINDINGS

Characteristic cutaneous histologic findings of erythema multiforme include subepidermal edema, bulla formation, epidermal cell necrosis, and a deep perivascular inflammatory infiltrate composed of mononuclear cells involving vessels in the upper dermis. The chemokine profile, with dominance of lymphocytic attractant chemokines at the dermoepidermal junction, is a feature of the interface dermatitis.[40] There are no specific immunofluorescence findings and no circulating antibodies, although direct immunofluorescence may show granular deposits of C3 and fibrin at the dermoepidermal junction and deposits of IgM, C3, and fibrin in the dermal blood vessels.

In vitro studies suggest that different immunopathogenic processes may be involved in herpes-mediated erythema multiforme and the drug-mediated forms of the disease.[41]

TREATMENT

Erythema multiforme eruptions may recur without warning, despite preventive measures. It is therefore important to identify and eliminate underlying causes. Mild cases are treated symptomatically with topical glucocorticoids and topical anti-inflammatory, antipruritic, or antibiotic preparations. Oral acyclovir may be effective in the prophylaxis of recurrent postherpetic erythema multiforme. In more severe cases, treatment with prednisone, 40 to 120 mg/day in divided doses, is indicated. If the eyes

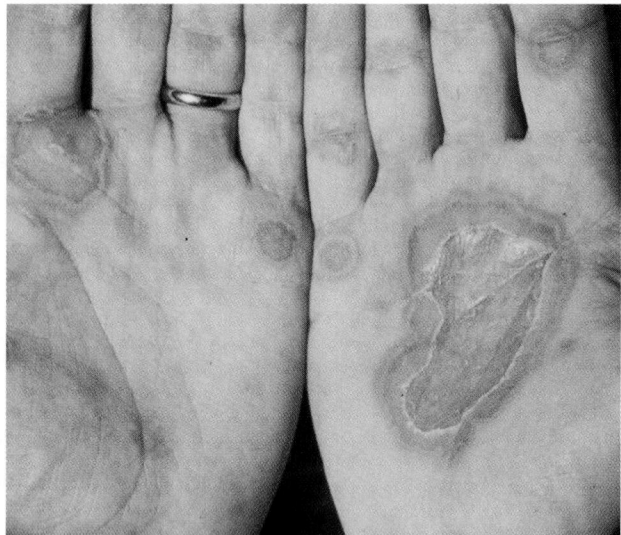

Figure 5   Target lesions are characteristic of erythema multiforme.

are involved, prompt ophthalmologic consultation should be obtained. Patients with large areas of epidermal necrosis (e.g., those with Stevens-Johnson syndrome) may require specialized intensive care, such as in a burn unit.

Early treatment with high-dose IVIg has been reported to be safe and effective in improving survival of patients with TEN.[42] However, there is no standard treatment of TEN that can be used as a basis for comparative studies.[43]

Epidermolysis Bullosa

Epidermolysis bullosa (EB) comprises a group of genetically based disorders with a prevalence of approximately one in 500,000 persons. There are more than 20 different phenotypes of EB, which may be inherited as an autosomal recessive trait. These disorders are characterized by blistering and erosions that arise after minor skin trauma or friction and heal with or without scarring. Extent of involvement ranges from localized blisters (e.g., on the palms and soles) to severe widespread sloughing of the skin, with a risk of severe morbidity and mortality from secondary infection, fluid and electrolyte imbalance, anemia, or other complications.

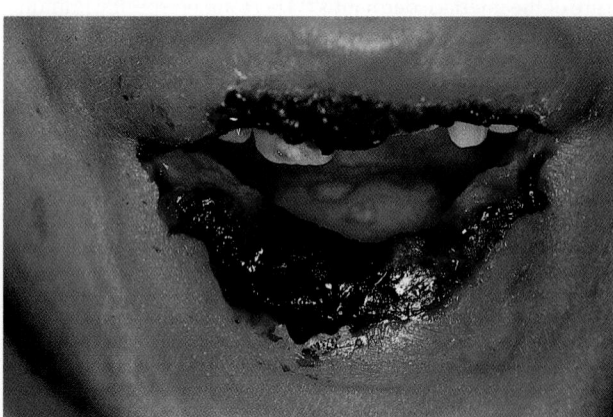

Figure 6   Stevens-Johnson syndrome is a fulminating form of erythema multiforme associated with marked mucocutaneous involvement, eye involvement, and severe constitutional symptoms.

EB is classified primarily on the basis of an ultrastructural level of skin cleavage in the basement membrane zone [*see Figure 7*]. Three major subtypes include EB simplex or epidermolytic (intraepidermal), junctional EB (intra–lamina lucida), and dystrophic or dermolytic EB (sub–lamina densa). Electron microscopy examination localizes the lesions to a specific layer.[44] Because this technology may not be widely available, immunofluorescence mapping with monoclonal antibodies can be used to target components of the basement membrane layers such as BP antigen (basal cell layer), laminin (lamina lucida), and type IV collagen (lamina densa).[45] The prenatal diagnosis may be made by immunocytochemical probes for antigenic components of the basement membrane in fetal skin biopsy, such as in the junctional EB pyloric atresia syndrome.[46]

EPIDERMOLYSIS BULLOSA SIMPLEX

There are three major forms of EB simplex.[47] The most common type is a mild autosomal dominant form that appears at birth or shortly thereafter as either localized or generalized blisters that do not usually result in scarring. A second type is Weber-Cockayne disease, which can be either localized or generalized. In the localized form, blisters appear acrally on the palms and soles during childhood or adolescence. In the generalized form, disease activity is usually greater in a warm climate.

The Dowling-Meara variant (EB herpetiformis) is a less common form of EB simplex that presents as severe generalized blistering in infancy; it resembles recessive junctional and dystrophic EB. EB herpetiformis becomes less severe with age.

JUNCTIONAL EPIDERMOLYSIS BULLOSA

Junctional EB is a recessively inherited group of disorders that exhibit a decreased number of hemidesmosomes and hypoplasia of hemidesmosomes, as revealed by electron microscopy, and separation at the level of the lamina lucida. Mucosal involvement and dystrophic nails are common. The most severe form, EB letalis, occurs within the first few days or months of life and has a high mortality. Patients with EB letalis have a high incidence of respiratory arrest at an early age because of laryngeal and tracheal involvement. Less severe forms of junctional EB exhibit severe generalized blistering at birth that gradually improves. Esophageal strictures may develop.

DYSTROPHIC EPIDERMOLYSIS BULLOSA

There are two forms of dystrophic EB that are inherited in an autosomal dominant fashion. Hyperplastic EB dystrophica (Cockayne-Touraine syndrome) appears in early infancy or childhood as serosanguineous blisters, predominantly on extensor aspects of the lower extremities, in association with nail dystrophy. The albopapuloid type of EB dystrophica is characterized by white papules that develop during adolescence on the trunk or extremities; however, blistering is present in the perinatal period. In both forms, ultrastructural examination reveals sublaminal dermal separation, with abnormalities in anchoring fibrils or a decrease in their number.

Recessive forms of EB dystrophica appear during the neonatal period as severe serosanguineous blistering that is either localized to sites of skin trauma or generalized. Milium formation is uncommon, but lesional scarring may result. Other complications include dental abnormalities, nail dystrophy or loss, digital fusion, flexion contractures, and esophageal strictures [*see Figure 8*]. Growth retardation, malnutrition, and chronic anemia also occur. Patients with recessive EB dystrophica are at increased

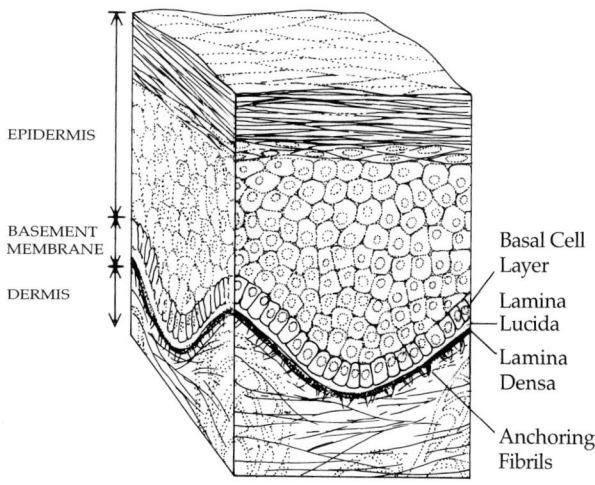

Figure 7 **Three major forms of epidermolysis bullosa (EB) have been recognized: EB simplex, in which a split occurs within the basal cell layer; junctional EB, which is characterized by separation within the lamina lucida; and dystrophic EB, in which separation occurs below the basement membrane zone.**

risk for squamous cell carcinoma, with a high incidence of fatal metastases.

Prenatal diagnosis of recessive dystrophic EB may be made by fetoscopy and skin biopsy; ultrastructural analysis of the tissue reveals dermolytic blister formation. An alternative method for prenatal diagnosis of recessive dystrophic EB involves testing of chorionic villus samples for mutation and haplotype analysis in the type VII collagen gene.[48]

Supportive treatment of EB is directed toward promotion of wound healing and prevention of complications. Daily skin care may include wet dressings or whirlpool baths, antibiotic ointment, and nonadhesive dressings, such as fine-mesh gauze (N-terface). A multidisciplinary approach that includes genetic counseling, psychological or psychiatric counseling, and support systems for the patient and family is essential, particularly for managing the severe forms of the disease.

A national registry has been established by the Dystrophic Epidermolysis Bullosa Research Association of America (http://www.debra.org) to collect epidemiologic data, to assess economic and social aspects of EB, and to register patients willing to participate in various research protocols.

ACQUIRED EPIDERMOLYSIS BULLOSA

Acquired epidermolysis bullosa, or epidermolysis bullosa acquisita (EBA), is a trauma-induced blistering disorder in adults who have no genetic basis for disease. Both circulating and tissue-bound IgG anti–basement membrane zone antibodies may be demonstrated by immunohistology. The blisters develop below the epidermis and heal with atrophic scars and malformation. They are usually confined to the extremities at sites of mechanical trauma. Oral lesions and nail dystrophy may be associated with EBA. Underlying malignant, autoimmune, and inflammatory diseases may be associated with this condition. The presence of ulcerative colitis or Crohn disease in approximately 30% of cases suggests that EBA should be included among the extraintestinal manifestations of inflammatory bowel disease.[49]

The diagnosis is made by excluding other bullous disorders, particularly BP (see above) and porphyria cutanea tarda. Immunoelectron microscopy may be used as an additional diagnostic aid, although this technique may not be widely available. Direct immunofluorescence with the use of salt-split skin to separate the lamina lucida aids in the differential diagnosis. With this method, the IgG antibodies appear on the dermal side of the split specimens in EBA and on the epidermal side in pemphigoid.[50] The antigen of EBA has been identified as the globular carboxyl terminus of type VII procollagen,[51] a major constituent of anchoring fibrils.[12] EBA may also be triggered by certain drugs, such as penicillin, cephalosporins, diclofenac, and captopril.[52]

Differential Diagnosis of Vesiculobullous Disorders

The major forms of bullous diseases occurring on an autoimmune or inherited basis have been discussed. The differential diagnosis includes a number of additional conditions in which vesicles or bullae are less common or appear secondary to other disease processes.

Acantholytic blisters occur in keratosis follicularis (Darier disease) as well as in pemphigus. Such blisters are a histologic rather than a clinical finding. Darier disease is an autosomal dominant disorder that manifests as greasy papules and plaques on seborrheic areas and in the flexures; almost all patients have nail abnormalities. Unlike pemphigus vulgaris, Darier disease is most effectively treated with oral retinoids.[53]

A fixed drug eruption may produce localized bullae that appear after ingestion of a particular drug [*see Chapter 40*]. Eczematous dermatitis results in spongiotic vesicles caused by intercellular edema [*see Chapter 38*]. This is manifested clinically by large bullae in acute allergic contact dermatitis triggered by poison ivy or poison oak. Systemic lupus erythematosus [*see Chapter 114*] occasionally produces bullae by causing degeneration of basal cells.

A bullous eruption on the dorsa of the hands and other sun-exposed sites in patients receiving long-term hemodialysis may resemble porphyria cutanea tarda [*see Chapter 60*].[54] Porphyrin levels are usually within normal limits. Intraepidermal or subepidermal bullae, primarily on the extremities, may be a cutaneous sign of diabetes mellitus.[55] Bacterial infections of the skin, such as impetigo, may be associated with subcorneal bulla formation. Bullae may occur on the feet in patients with severe dermatophytosis.

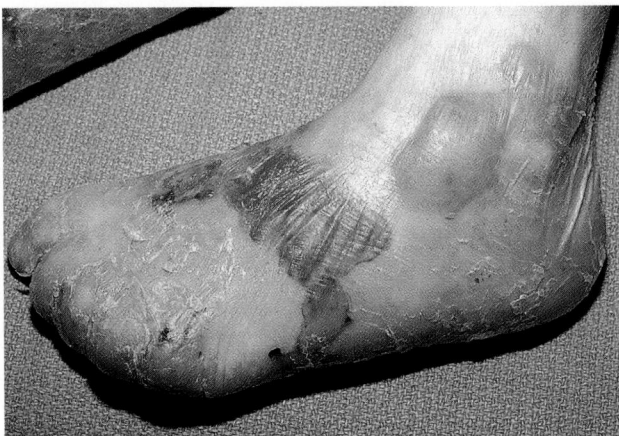

Figure 8 **Recessive dystrophic epidermolysis bullosa may cause severe scarring and syndactyly.**

Various viral infections, including varicella (chickenpox), herpes simplex, and herpes zoster, also must be considered in the differential diagnosis [see Chapters 41, 132, and 148]. Lastly, blisters from physical trauma, burns, or cold must also be considered.

Elizabeth A. Abel, M.D., has received research support from Allergan Inc. and is a consultant for Centocor, Inc.

Jean-Claude Bystryn, M.D., has no commercial relationships with manufacturers of products or providers of services discussed in this chapter.

References

1. Korman NJ, Eyre RW, Klaus-Kovtun V, et al: Demonstration of an adhering-junction molecule (plakoglobin) in the autoantigens of pemphigus foliaceus and pemphigus vulgaris. N Engl J Med 321:631, 1989

2. Amagai M: Desmoglein as a target in autoimmunity and infection. J Am Acad Dermatol 48:244, 2003

3. Starzycki Z, Chorzelski TP, Jablonska S: Familial pemphigus vulgaris in mother and daughter. Int J Dermatol 37:211, 1998

4. Miyagawa S, Higashimine I, Iida T, et al: HLA-DRB1*04 and DRB1*14 alleles are associated with susceptibility to pemphigus among Japanese. J Invest Dermatol 109:615, 1997

5. Bystryn JC, Steinmen NM: The adjuvant therapy of pemphigus: an update. Arch Dermatol 132:203, 1996

6. Ljubojevic S, Lipozencic J, Brenner S, et al: Pemphigus vulgaris: a review of treatment over a 19-year period. J Eur Acad Dermatol Venereol 16:599, 2002

7. Herbst A, Bystryn JC: Remissions in pemphigus. J Invest Dermatol 106:850, 1996

8. Ruach M, Ohel G, Rahav D, et al: Pemphigus vulgaris and pregnancy. Obstet Gynecol Surv 50:755, 1995

9. Warren SJ, Lin MS, Giudice GJ, et al: The prevalence of antibodies against desmoglein 1 in endemic pemphigus foliaceus in Brazil. N Engl J Med 343:23, 2000

10. Landau M, Brenner S: Histopathologic findings in drug-induced pemphigus. Am J Dermatopathol 19:411, 1997

11. Brenner S, Bialy-Golan A, Anhalt GJ: Recognition of pemphigus antigens in drug-induced pemphigus vulgaris and pemphigus foliaceus. J Am Acad Dermatol 36:919, 1997

12. Anhalt GJ, Kim SC, Stanley JR, et al: Paraneoplastic pemphigus: an autoimmune mucocutaneous disease associated with neoplasia. N Engl J Med 323:1729, 1990

13. Mutasim DF, Adams BB: Immunofluorescence in dermatology. J Am Acad Dermatol 45:803, 2001

14. Turner MS, Sutton D, Sauder DN: The use of plasmapheresis and immunosuppression in the treatment of pemphigus vulgaris. J Am Acad Dermatol 43:1058, 2000

15. Bystryn JC, Jiao D, Natow S: Treatment of pemphigus with intravenous immunoglobulin. J Am Acad Dermatol 47:358, 2002

16. Dahl MV, Bridges AG: Intravenous immune globulin: fighting antibodies with antibodies. J Am Acad Dermatol 45:690, 2001

17. Werth VP: Treatment of pemphigus vulgaris with brief, high-dose intravenous glucocorticoids. Arch Dermatol 132:1435, 1996

18. Salopek TG, Logsetty S, Tredget EE: Anti-CD20 chimeric monoclonal antibody (rituximab) for the treatment of recalcitrant, life-threatening pemphigus vulgaris with implications in the pathogenesis of the disorder. J Am Acad Dermatol 47:785, 2002

19. Chams-Davatchi C, Nonahal Azar R, Daneshpazooh M, et al: Open trial of mycophenolate mofetil in the treatment of resistant pemphigus vulgaris. Ann Dermatol Venereol 129:23, 2002

20. Moll R, Moll I: Epidermal adhesion molecules and basement membrane components as target structures of autoimmunity. Virchows Arch 432:487, 1998

21. Lin MS, Mascaro JM Jr, Liu Z, et al: The desmosome and hemidesmosome in cutaneous autoimmunity. Clin Exp Immunol 107(suppl 1):9, 1997

22. Bernard P, Bedane C, Bonnetblanc JM: Anti-BP180 autoantibodies as a marker of poor prognosis in bullous pemphigoid: a cohort analysis of 94 elderly patients. Br J Dermatol 138:694, 1997

23. Cunha PR, Thomazeski PV, Hipolito E, et al: Bullous pemphigoid in a 2-month-old infant. Int J Dermatol 37:935, 1998

24. Bastuji-Garin S, Joly P, Picard-Dahan C, et al: Drugs associated with bullous pemphigoid: a case-control study. Arch Dermatol 132:272, 1996

25. Ogawa H, Sakuma M, Morioka S, et al: The incidence of internal malignancies in pemphigus and bullous pemphigoid in Japan. J Dermatol Sci 9:136, 1995

26. Joly P, Roujeau JC, Benichou J, et al: A comparison of oral and topical corticosteroids in patients with bullous pemphigoid. N Engl J Med 346:321, 2002

27. Kirtschig G, Murrell D, Wojnarowska F, et al: Interventions for mucous membrane

28. Yancey KB, Egan CA: Pemphigoid: Clinical, histologic, immunopathologic, and therapeutic considerations. JAMA 284:350, 2000

29. Dereure O, Bessis D, Guillot B, et al: Treatment of bullous pemphigoid by low-dose methotrexate associated with short-term potent topical steroids: an open prospective study of 18 cases. Arch Dermatol 138:1255, 2002

30. Bouscarat F, Chosidow O, Picard-Dahan C, et al: Treatment of bullous pemphigoid with dapsone: retrospective study of thirty-six cases. J Am Acad Dermatol 34:683, 1996

31. Hornschuh B, Hamm H, Wever S, et al: Treatment of 16 patients with bullous pemphigoid with oral tetracycline and niacinamide and topical clobetasol. J Am Acad Dermatol 36:101, 1997

32. Thornfeldt CR, Menkes AW: Bullous pemphigoid controlled by tetracycline. J Am Acad Dermatol 16:305, 1987

33. Brow JR, Parker F, Weinstein WM, et al: The small intestinal mucosa in dermatitis herpetiformis: I. Severity and distribution of the small intestinal lesion and associated malabsorption. Gastroenterology 60:355, 1971

34. Katz SI, Hall RP III, Lawley TJ, et al: Dermatitis herpetiformis: the skin and the gut. Ann Intern Med 93:857, 1980

35. Jenkins D, Lynde CW, Stewart WD: Histiocytic lymphoma occurring in a patient with dermatitis herpetiformis. J Am Acad Dermatol 9:252, 1983

36. Guide SV, Marinkovich MP: Linear IgA bullous dermatosis. Clin Dermatol 19:719, 2001

37. Fine JD: Management of acquired bullous skin diseases. N Engl J Med 333:1475, 1995

38. Auquier-Dunant A, Mockenhaupt M, Naldi L, et al: Correlations between clinical patterns and causes or erythema multiforme majus, Stevens-Johnson syndrome, and toxic epidermal necrolysis: results of an international prospective study. Arch Dermatol 138:1019, 2002

39. Manders SM: Toxin-mediated streptococcal and staphylococcal disease. J Am Acad Dermatol 39:383, 1998

40. Spandau U, Brocher EB, Kampgen E, et al: CC and CXC chemokines are differentially expressed in erythema multiforme in vivo. Arch Dermatol 138:1027, 2002

41. Kokuba H, Aurelian L, Burnett J: Herpes simplex virus associated erythema multiforme (HAEM) is mechanistically distinct from drug-induced erythema multiforme: interferon V is expressed in HAEM lesions and tumor necrosis factor–alpha in drug-induced erythema multiforme lesions. J Invest Dermatol 113:808, 1999

42. Prins C, Kerdel FA, Padilla RS, et al: Treatment of toxic epidermal necrolysis with high-dose intravenous immunoglobulins: multicenter retrospective analysis of 48 consecutive cases. Arch Dermatol 139:26, 2003

43. Wolff K, Tappeiner G: Treatment of toxic epidermal necrolysis. Arch Dermatol 139:85, 2003

44. Fine JD, Eady RA, Bauer EA, et al: Revised classification system for inherited epidermolysis bullosa: report of the Second International Consensus Meeting on diagnosis and classification of epidermolysis bullosa. J Am Acad Dermatol 42:1051, 2000

45. Hintner H, Stingl G, Schuler G, et al: Immunofluorescence mapping of antigenic determinants within the dermal-epidermal junction in the mechanobullous diseases. J Invest Dermatol 76:113, 1981

46. Shimizu H, Fine JD, Suzumori K, et al: Prenatal exclusion of pyloric atresia-junctional epidermolysis bullosa syndrome. J Am Acad Dermatol 31:429, 1994

47. Okulicz JF, Kihiczak NI, Janniger CK: Epidermolysis bullosa simplex. Cutis 70:19, 2002

48. Christiano AM, LaForgia S, Paller AS, et al: Prenatal diagnosis for recessive dystrophic epidermolysis bullosa in 10 families by mutation and haplotype analysis in the type VII collagen gene (COL7A1). Mol Med 2:59, 1996

49. Raab B, Fretzin DF, Bronson DM, et al: Epidermolysis bullosa acquisita and inflammatory bowel disease. JAMA 250:1746, 1983

50. Vaillant L, Bernard P, Joly P, et al: Evaluation of clinical criteria for diagnosis of bullous pemphigoid. Arch Dermatol 134:1075, 1998

51. Woodley DT, Burgeson RE, Lunstrum G, et al: The epidermolysis bullosa acquisita antigen is the globular carboxyl terminus of type VII procollagen. J Clin Invest 81:683, 1988

52. Delbaldo C, Chen M, Friedli A, et al: Drug-induced epidermolysis bullous acquisita with antibodies to type VII collagen. J Am Acad Dermatol 46(5 suppl):S161, 2002

53. Cooper SM, Burge SM: Darier's disease: epidemiology, pathophysiology, and management. Am J Clin Dermatol 4:97, 2003

54. Glynne P, Deacon A, Goldsmith D, et al: Bullous dermatoses in end-stage renal failure: porphyria or pseudoporphyria? Am J Kidney Dis 34:155, 1999

55. Perez MI, Kohn SR: Cutaneous manifestations of diabetes mellitus. J Am Acad Dermatol 30:519, 1994

56. Viard I, Wehrli P, Bullani R, et al: Inhibition of toxic epidermal necrolysis by blockade of CD95 with human intravenous immunoglobulin. Science 282:490, 1998

57. Elder D, Elenitsas R, Jaworsky C, et al: Lever's Histopathology of the Skin, 8th ed. Lippincott-Raven, Philadelphia, 1997

44 Benign Cutaneous Tumors

Elizabeth A. Abel, M.D.

General Considerations

CLASSIFICATION

Tumors of the cutaneous surface may arise from the epidermis, dermis, or subcutaneous tissue or from any of the specialized cell types in the skin or its appendages. Broad categories include tumors derived from epithelial, melanocytic, or connective tissue structures. Within each location or cell type, lesions are classified as benign, malignant, or, in certain cases, premalignant.[1,2]

Benign epithelial tumors include tumors of the surface epidermis that form keratin; tumors of the epidermal appendages; and cysts of the skin.

Melanocytic, or pigment-forming, lesions are very common. One of the most frequently encountered forms is the nevus cell nevus. The term nevus has two meanings: a malformation commonly involving the entire skin layer (tissue nevus) and a benign growth of melanocytic cells (nevus cells).

Nevus cells are closely related to melanocytes and may be defined as modified neuroectodermal melanin-producing elements. The word mole, often used as a synonym for nevus, is an imprecise term because it refers to birthmarks that may or may not contain nevus cells. Neural tumors, such as neurofibromas, are related to melanocytic tumors because both are of neuroectodermal origin.

Tumors that are derived from connective tissue include the following: fibromas, histiocytomas, lipomas, leiomyomas, and hemangiomas.

HISTOLOGIC EVALUATION

For cases in which it is not possible to distinguish clinically between benign and malignant cutaneous tumors, histopathologic examination is extremely important. The type of biopsy performed depends on the location, size, and nature of the lesion and on cosmetic considerations. In all cases, the clinical features must be correlated with the distinctive microscopic appearance of the tumor to confirm or exclude the diagnosis on the basis of physical examination.

Epithelial Tumors

SEBORRHEIC KERATOSIS

Diagnosis

Seborrheic keratosis (seborrheic wart) consists of a sharply circumscribed, rough or smooth papule or plaque that is 1 mm to several centimeters in size and dirty yellow or light to dark brown in color. The lesions often have the appearance of being stuck on and are characterized by prominent follicular plugging. They are most common in light-skinned races, first appearing in adults on the face and upper trunk and occurring more frequently with increasing age [*see Figure 1*].

Transient eruptive seborrheic keratoses have been associated with inflammatory skin conditions, including erythroderma associated with psoriasis and drug eruptions. These keratoses tend to resolve when the skin inflammation clears.[3] These transient keratoses should be distinguished from eruptive seborrheic keratoses—the sign of Leser-Trelat—which are associated with internal malignancy, particularly adenocarcinoma. The true value of the sign of Leser-Trelat as a marker of underlying malignancy is a subject of debate. Dermatosis papulosa nigra is similar to seborrheic keratosis, but it is seen in dark-skinned races; it usually appears on the face and presents at an earlier age than seborrheic keratosis [*see Figure 2*].

Differential Diagnosis

The differential diagnosis of seborrheic keratosis and dermatosis papulosa nigra includes lentigo, wart, and nevus cell nevus. A biopsy may be required to rule out a pigmented basal cell carcinoma or, in the case of an inflamed seborrheic keratosis, squamous cell carcinoma or malignant melanoma. A shave biopsy that includes the base of the lesion may be performed before treatment with curettage. Seborrheic keratosis with basal clear cells can microscopically mimic melanoma in situ; however, careful conventional microscopy combined with a panel of immunostains allows for an accurate diagnosis.[4]

Treatment

Curettage is a satisfactory treatment. When multiple lesions are present, anesthesia may be achieved by freezing the affected area with an ethyl chloride spray before performing curettage. For larger lesions, electrodesiccation is unnecessary and may cause scarring. Smaller lesions may be successfully treated with electrodesiccation, cryotherapy, or topical application of 50% trichloroacetic acid.

EPIDERMAL NEVUS

Diagnosis

Epidermal nevus consists of closely set, skin-colored or hyperpigmented papules that either may be localized to one side of the body and arranged in linear fashion or may be widespread. When localized, the condition is termed nevus

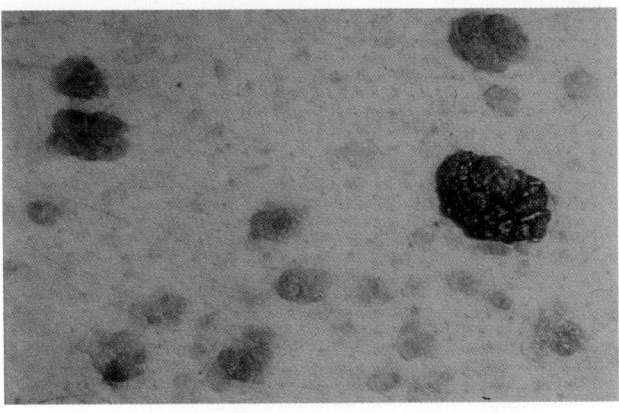

Figure 1 **Verrucous, hyperpigmented lesions of seborrheic keratosis with a stuck-on appearance are present on the trunk of this patient.**

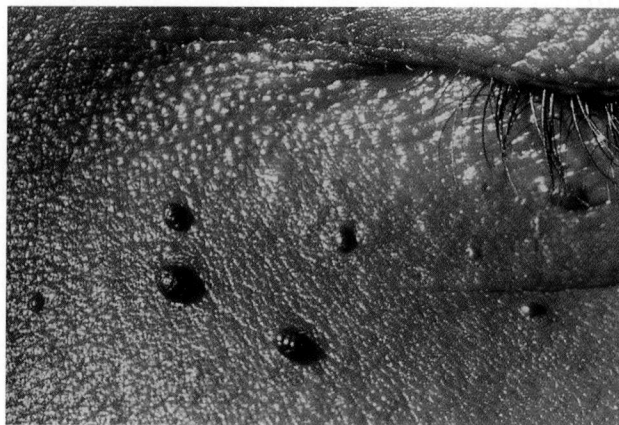

Figure 2 Dermatosis papulosa nigra, as seen on the face, appears in dark-skinned races at a younger age than seborrheic keratosis.

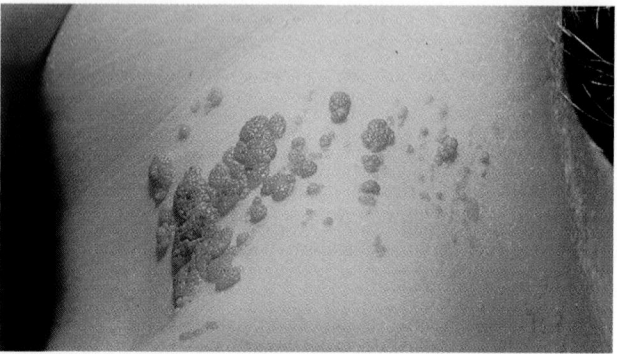

Figure 3 Epidermal nevus with discrete and confluent brown papillomas is present in a somewhat linear arrangement.

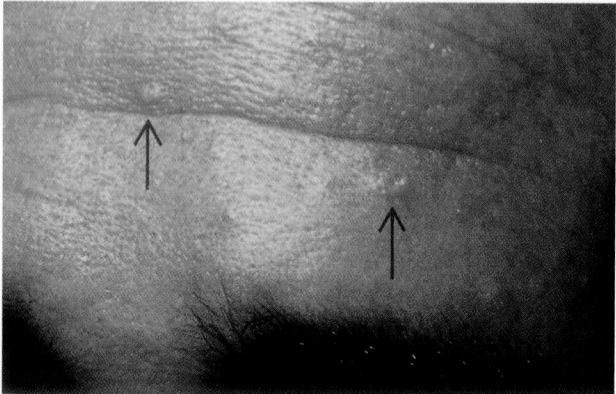

Figure 4 Skin-colored or yellowish, often umbilicated papules of sebaceous hyperplasia, as seen on the forehead, may clinically resemble basal cell carcinomas.

unius lateris [*see Figure 3*]. When widespread, it is called systematized nevus. Lesions affect about one in 1,000 people; they are present at birth or appear in early childhood. The lesions have no malignant potential but may constitute a serious cosmetic problem.

Histologically, epidermal nevi exhibit hyperplasia of the epidermis; the structure or maturation of these lesions is not significantly different from that of normal epidermis. One variant, the inflammatory linear verrucous epidermal nevus, shows psoriasiform hyperplasia. Another variant, which is common in systematized nevi, shows granular degeneration of epidermolytic hyperkeratosis histologically. This type of epidermal nevus is a mosaic genetic disorder of suprabasal keratin. Mutations in the *K10* gene are associated with lesions of the skin, whereas the normal gene is found in unaffected skin.[5]

Variants

The epidermal nevus syndrome involves a spectrum of different types of epidermal nevi associated with manifestations in the skeletal, urogenital, cardiovascular, and nervous systems that are caused by genomic mosaicism.[6] This rare syndrome is apparent at birth; the presence of widespread epidermal nevi should trigger a search for associated anomalies.

Nevus comedonicus is a variant of an epidermal nevus affecting the pilosebaceous structures; it occurs as clusters of comedonelike papules, usually in a linear pattern on the face, neck, upper arms, and trunk.[6]

Nevus sebaceous is a benign tumor that shows sebaceous differentiation. The lesion has a yellow hue and a granular surface and occurs in a linear pattern on the face or scalp. At puberty, nevus sebaceous may become more elevated; in adulthood, there is an associated risk of basal cell carcinoma.

Treatment

Treatment of epidermal nevi with electrodesiccation and curettage is often unsuccessful and may cause scarring. Surgical or laser removal may be indicated for localized lesions. Cryotherapy with curettage is useful for thinner lesions. Epidermal nevus syndromes involving other organ systems (e.g., Proteus syndrome, CHILD [congenital hemidysplasia with ichthyosiform erythroderma and limb defects] syndrome, Becker nevus syndrome) must be evaluated and managed appropriately through a multidisciplinary approach.

Tumors of the Epidermal Appendages

There are a large number of benign tumors of the hair follicles, the sebaceous glands, and the apocrine and eccrine glands. Solitary skin tumors of these epidermal appendages are typically nonhereditary, whereas multiple neoplasms may show an autosomal dominant inheritance pattern.[7]

SEBACEOUS HYPERPLASIA

Sebaceous hyperplasia is a common clinical condition that appears as multiple skin-colored or yellowish, often umbilicated papules or plaques, usually on the forehead, nose, or cheeks of persons after the fifth decade of life. These lesions consist of enlarged sebaceous gland lobules with a central dilated duct. Sebaceous hyperplasia may respond to electrodesiccation, cryotherapy with liquid nitrogen, or the application of a dilute solution of trichloroacetic or bichloroacetic acid. Individual lesions may be excised. Photodynamic therapy using topical 5-aminolevulinic acid and pulsed–dye laser irradiation has resulted in clinical improvement of sebaceous hyperplasia.[8] Lesions may sometimes be confused clinically with basal cell carcinoma [*see Figure 4*]. In the familial form of this disorder, onset occurs in puberty; with the passage of time, the lesions increase in extent over the face, neck, and upper thorax. This condition must be distinguished from acne vulgaris, rosacea, and the angiofibromas of tuberous sclerosis.

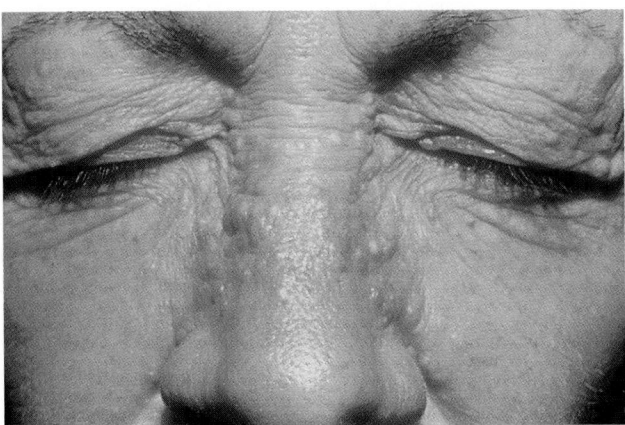

Figure 5 **Symmetrical papules of trichoepithelioma appear on the eyelids and nasolabial areas and may be inherited as an autosomal dominant trait.**

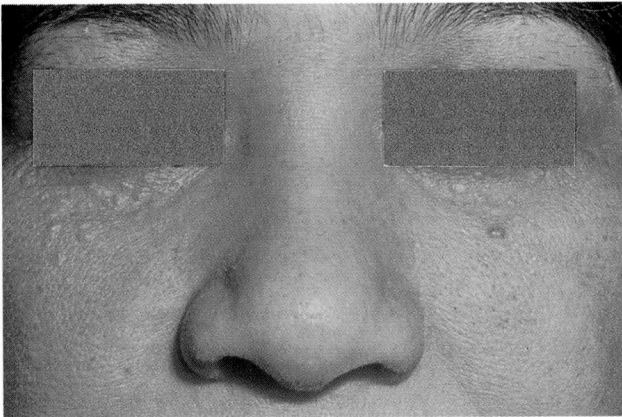

Figure 6 **Syringomas—benign tumors of eccrine ducts—are commonly seen on the face, especially on the lower eyelids.**

TRICHOEPITHELIOMAS

Trichoepitheliomas usually present as multiple yellowish-pink, translucent papules distributed symmetrically on the cheeks, eyelids, and nasolabial areas [*see Figure 5*]. Often inherited as an autosomal dominant trait, the papules first appear at puberty and grow slowly for years. The gene for multiple familial trichoepitheliomas has been mapped to chromosome 9p21.[9] Lesions may be confused both clinically and histologically with basal cell carcinoma, though trichoepithelioma usually shows differentiation toward the formation of hair. A single or localized trichoepithelioma may be removed by electrodesiccation and curettage. Multiple lesions are difficult to treat and may be a cosmetic problem. Treatment of multiple trichoepitheliomas with topical imiquimod and tretinoin has been reported to clear lesions without scarring; however, more evidence is required to assess the usefulness of this therapy.[10]

SYRINGOMAS

Syringomas usually present in groups of multiple small papules that are distributed symmetrically over the face, especially on the lower eyelids [*see Figure 6*]. Eruptive syringoma, a rare condition, is characterized by widespread lesions. Histologically, there is a benign proliferation of the eccrine ducts.

EPIDERMOID CYST

Diagnosis

Commonly called wens, epidermoid cysts have a lining that resembles the epidermis. Several types of cyst exist, but they are usually clinically indistinguishable from one another. On histologic examination, most of these cysts appear to be derived from hair follicles.

The epidermoid cyst is commonly located on the back and consists of one or more slow-growing, elevated, firm nodules, often with a central pore [*see Figure 7*]. The diameters of the lesions vary from 0.2 to 5.0 cm.

Treatment

Small, stable epidermoid cysts may be asymptomatic and not require treatment. The epidermoid cyst, when inflamed, may be incised with a pointed scalpel to express its wall and contents, which consist of a thick keratinous material. If the cyst wall is not completely removed, there may be a recurrence of the lesion. Occasionally, the entire cyst has to be excised. Preliminary treatment with a systemic antibiotic, such as erythromycin, and warm-water compresses applied three or four times daily may be instituted if the cyst is inflamed and infected. When the inflammation and infection resolve, the residual lesion can be removed. Repeated episodes of infection may cause fibrosis, after which the cyst may have to be surgically excised.

Other Cysts

The pilar cyst, which is less common, has a wall that contains keratin similar to that found in hair. The contents of these cysts are semifluid and often have a rancid odor. A milium is similar to an epidermoid cyst but differs mainly in size. Milia are white, hard subepidermal keratin cysts, 1 to 2 mm in diameter, that commonly arise spontaneously on the face [*see Figure 8*]. They may also arise secondarily in scars or in association with certain bullous diseases. Incision and expression of contents with a comedo extractor may be performed.

Familial Tumor Syndromes

Multiple cutaneous neoplasms may be a feature of familial tumor syndromes that are thought to be mediated by inactivation of tumor suppressor genes. It is important to recog-

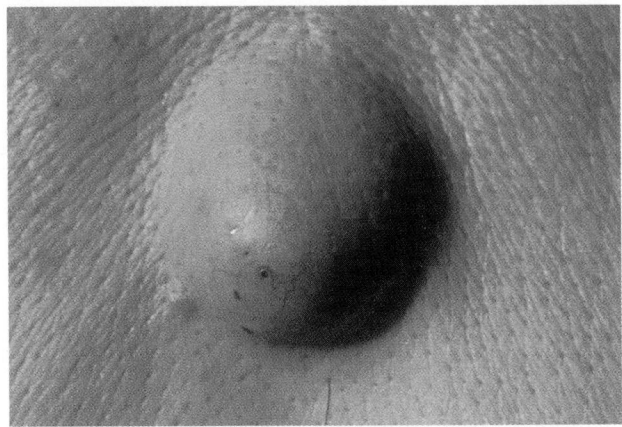

Figure 7 **This large epidermoid cyst has a central pore, contains thick keratinous material, and has a lining that resembles the epidermis.**

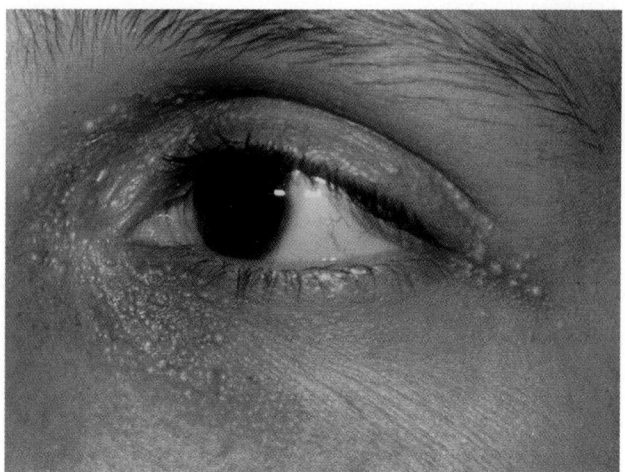

Figure 8   Milia, which are multiple small subepidermal inclusion cysts, can be observed in the periorbital area of this patient.

nize these syndromes because they may be associated with underlying malignancies.

MUIR-TORRE SYNDROME

Muir-Torre syndrome (MTS), previously known as Torre syndrome, is an autosomal-dominant disorder characterized by the presence of sebaceous gland neoplasms that are associated with visceral carcinoma and that arise from colonic epithelium. Sebaceous gland tumors may include, in decreasing order of frequency, adenomas, epitheliomas, and carcinomas.[11] Keratoacanthomas and sebaceous hyperplasia are also seen in patients with MTS. Colorectal cancer develops in 51% of patients with MTS a decade earlier than it develops in the general population. Genitourinary cancer develops in 24% of MTS patients. A germline mutation in the DNA mismatch repair gene *hMSH2* has been identified in patients with MTS. Predictive diagnosis in family members should be preceded by careful genetic counseling.[11]

GARDNER SYNDROME

Gardner syndrome consists of the triad of intestinal polyposis, bony tumors, and soft tissue lesions; it has an autosomal dominant inheritance. The colonic polyps eventually become malignant if left untreated. Soft tissue lesions include epidermoid cysts, sebaceous cysts, desmoid tumors, and scattered lentigines on the head and extremities.[12]

COWDEN SYNDROME

Cowden syndrome is characterized by facial trichilemmomas and acral fibromas, and it is associated with an increased risk of cancer of the breast, thyroid, and gastrointestinal tract. This rare genodermatosis, which is also known as multiple hamartoma syndrome, is inherited as an autosomal dominant trait. It is important to make a prompt diagnosis of this syndrome because of the high risk of malignancy, particularly cancer of the breast in women.[13]

BIRT-HOGG-DUBÉ SYNDROME

Birt-Hogg-Dubé syndrome (BHDS) is an autosomal dominant multisystem disorder characterized by the cutaneous triad of fibrofolliculomas, trichodiscomas, and acrochordons; the development of spontaneous pneumothorax

in association with lung cysts; and a predisposition to renal neoplasms.[14] Fibrofolliculomas, which are the characteristic skin lesions of BHDS, are benign tumors of the hair follicle; they are firm, pink or skin-colored papules measuring 1 to 3 mm that appear on the face, particularly the nose, earlobes, and forehead. In the original kindred described by Birt (a dermatologist), Hogg (a pathologist), and Dubé (a pathologist), family members were afflicted with medullary carcinoma of the thyroid. Subsequently, there appeared reports of patients with BHDS who had intestinal polyps, adenocarcinoma of the colon, parathyroid adenomas, and renal cell carcinoma. The skin tumors begin in early adulthood; systemic tumors appear years later. In families with recognized renal cell carcinoma, BHDS may account for 6% of the cases.[15]

Melanocytic (Pigment-Forming) Tumors

Benign tumors of pigment-forming cells, including those containing nevus cells (melanocytic nevi) and those of epidermal or dermal melanocytes, are of neuroectodermal origin.

MELANOCYTIC NEVUS

Melanocytic nevus, also called nevus cell nevus, has a characteristic life history of evolution and involution. Melanocytic nevi are the most common of all skin tumors; each young adult has an average of 20 to 40 of them. Their incidence increases with age up to the second or third decade of life, after which they occur less commonly.

Risk Factors for Melanoma

An increase in the total number of melanocytic nevi is a risk factor for melanoma.[16] In a study of 716 patients with newly diagnosed melanoma, an increased number of small nevi (25 to 49) was associated with a twofold increase in risk of melanoma, greater numbers of nevi were associated with further increased risk.[17] The presence of one clinically dysplastic nevus was associated with a twofold increase in risk of melanoma, and 10 or more, with a 12-fold increase in risk. Criteria for dysplastic nevi included large size (over 5 mm), flatness (entirely macular or having a macular component), and at least two of the following: irregular pigmentation, asymmetry, and indistinct borders [*see Chapter 45*]. The presence of freckling conferred additional risk of melanoma for all types of nevi.

The relation between sun exposure and melanocytic nevi has been investigated to determine what environmental factors influence melanoma and to facilitate preventive measures. Studies suggest that melanocytic nevi are more common on sun-exposed skin sites and reach a peak incidence earlier in age on these sites than on covered areas of the body.[16,18] A study of Australian schoolchildren showed an increasing prevalence of nevi with decreasing latitude, particularly in children 6 and 9 years of age.[19] Sun exposure during childhood was considered to be a factor in the development of melanocytic nevi and an associated risk factor for melanoma.[19,20] In Australia, however, sun exposure may be sufficient to maximally induce nevi regardless of latitude. Further studies need to be performed on persons living at higher latitudes to see whether the relation between sun exposure and nevi continues into adulthood.

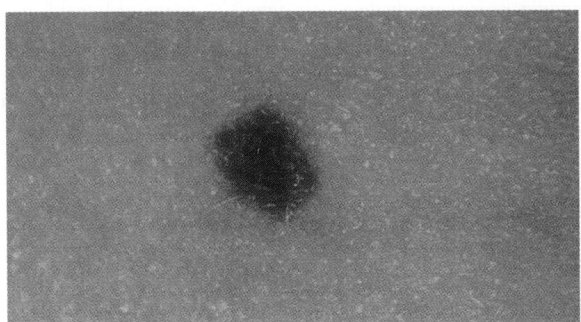

Figure 9 **A flat junctional nevus with dark pigmentation is seen in this patient.**

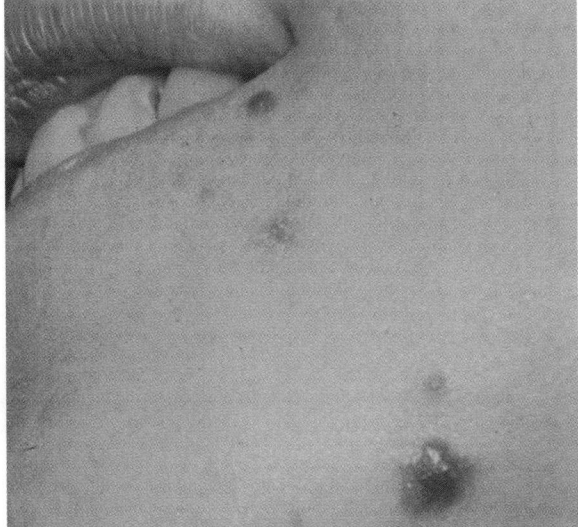

Figure 10 **This slightly raised compound nevus typically has less pigmentation than a junctional nevus.**

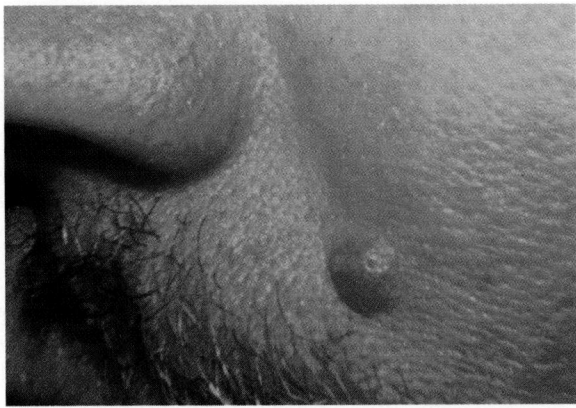

Figure 11 **A skin-colored intradermal nevus with a dome-shaped configuration is seen on the face.**

Because melanomas form on skin not exposed to the sun, investigators are exploring what other factors besides sun exposure increase the risk of melanocytic nevi. Maldonado and colleagues studied the distribution of *BRAF* gene mutations in 115 patients with invasive primary melanomas; their findings indicated that *BRAF* mutations were significantly more common in melanomas occurring on intermittently sun-exposed skin and rare on chronically sun-

damaged skin.[21] These findings strongly suggest that distinct genetic pathways lead to melanoma.

Diagnosis

A melanocytic nevus that is present at birth or appears during the first year of life is considered to be congenital. Certain syndromes are associated with congenital nevi, including epidermal (linear sebaceous) nevus syndrome, neurocutaneous melanosis, premature-aging syndrome, and occult spinal dysraphism or tethered cord syndrome.[22] Various neuroectodermal defects and multisystem abnormalities may also be present. Giant congenital melanocytic nevi are associated with an increased risk of melanoma (see below).

Acquired melanocytic nevi vary considerably in form, ranging from flat to pedunculate. They may be hairy or hairless and may be skin colored, dark brown, or even black. Nevi that are flat and darkly pigmented are called junctional nevi. Slightly raised nevi are often compound; that is, they contain both epidermal and dermal components. Nevi that are predominantly intradermal are usually more elevated and contain less pigment than compound or junctional nevi. Nevi that are papillomatous, dome shaped, or pedunculate are usually intradermal [*see Figures 9 through 11*].

Differential Diagnosis

The differential diagnosis of benign melanocytic nevi includes ephelis (freckle), lentigo, café au lait spot (see below), wart, seborrheic keratosis, and skin tag (a small pedunculate protrusion of skin that does not contain nevus cells). Ephelis is a tan macule, commonly seen in children after sun exposure; it often disappears in the winter. Lentigo, also called senile lentigo or liver spot, is a tan or brown macule commonly seen on exposed skin areas, such as the face, the backs of the hands, and the neck. The labial melanotic macule is a distinct entity that appears in adults as a well-defined brown or black-pigmented macule on the lip. In a study of 79 patients, the majority of melanocytic lesions (94%) were on the central third of the lower lip, suggesting that exposure to ultraviolet light has a causative role.[23] Patients followed for up to 13 years had no adverse developments, a finding indicative of the benign nature of this lesion.

Treatment

No treatment is required for melanocytic nevi. However, shave biopsy or excisional biopsy may be performed for cosmetic reasons or when a nevus is subject to irritation because of pressure from clothing or because it is located in an intertriginous area. Patients should be followed with serial photographs. Biopsy should be performed for nevi that appear prone to malignant transformation; nevi that show severe dysplasia should be removed. Removal of mildly or moderately dysplastic nevi is advocated by some but not all experts [*see Chapter 45*].

CAFÉ AU LAIT SPOTS

Café au lait spots are common benign congenital or acquired birthmarks. They are tan, round to oval macules ranging in size from several millimeters to 10 to 20 cm. They can occur on any area of the body but are more common on the trunk, buttocks, and lower extremities. The presence in a prepubertal child of five or more café au lait spots larger than 0.5 cm may be a marker for neurofibromatosis-1 (NF-1) (see below).[24]

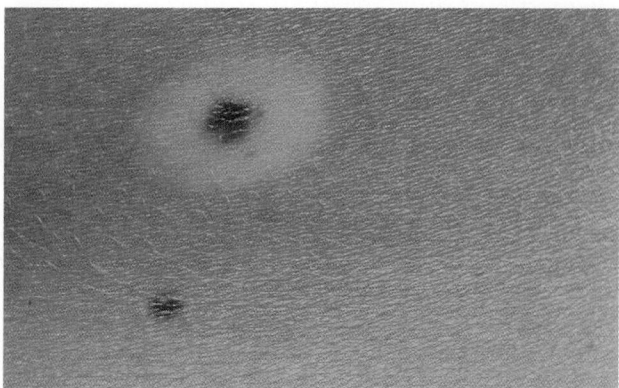

Figure 12 **The halo nevus may represent an autoimmune phenomenon; a zone of hypopigmentation may appear around a nevus, with subsequent involution of the pigmented tumor.**

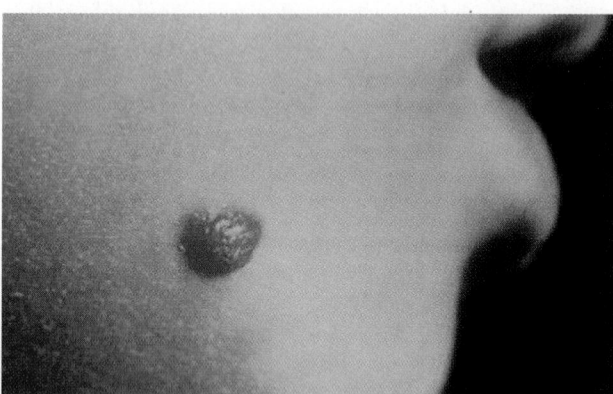

Figure 13 **The spindle cell nevus is an active compound nevus that may be difficult to distinguish histologically from a melanoma.**

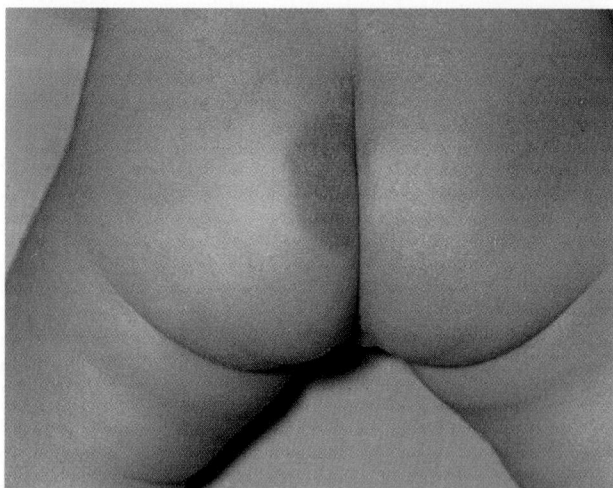

Figure 14 **The bluish pigmentation of a mongolian spot is seen in the lumbosacral area and is caused by the persistence of dermal melanocytes.**

Histologically, café au lait spots show an increased number of dihydroxyphenylalanine (DOPA)-positive melanocytes that produce an increased concentration of melanosomes. The café au lait spots that are seen in Albright hereditary osteodystrophy are usually unilateral and show jagged rather than smooth margins. Some reports suggest that an

association of juvenile xanthogranulomas with café au lait macules carries an increased risk of underlying systemic disorders, including leukemia[25]; however, other studies have reported no evidence of hematologic malignancy in these patients.[26]

HALO NEVUS

A halo nevus consists of an acquired zone of hypopigmentation surrounding a pigmented tumor, most commonly a compound nevus [*see Figure 12*]; other tumors, even malignant melanoma, may also be surrounded by a depigmented halo. The halo lesion typically involutes during a period of months in the absence of clinical signs of inflammation. Histologically, a chronic lymphocytic infiltrate surrounds the nevus cells, which may represent an autoimmune phenomenon.

SPINDLE CELL NEVUS

Formerly called benign juvenile melanoma, spindle cell nevus usually arises in childhood as a pink or reddish-brown, smooth or slightly scaly, firm papule with a predilection for the face, especially the cheeks [*see Figure 13*].[27] Although benign, spindle cell nevus may closely resemble a malignant melanoma. Excisional biopsy is therefore advisable in many cases.

MONGOLIAN SPOT

The mongolian spot is a bluish macule that is seen in newborns of dark-skinned races. The discoloration is caused by persistence of dermal melanocytes, often in the lumbosacral region [*see Figure 14*]. The lesion usually disappears by 3 or 4 years of age.

BLUE NEVUS

The common blue nevus occurs as a solitary, sharply circumscribed, blue-black papule [*see Figure 15*]. This malformation consists of a group of melanocytes with long, thin surface projections in the middle and lower thirds of the dermis and in subcutaneous fat. The common blue nevus does not show a tendency toward malignant transformation. The cellular blue nevus, which appears as a blue-black nodule or an indurated plaque, contains two types of cells: spindle shaped and rounded. The cellular blue nevus may in rare instances become malignant.

NEVUS OF OTA

The nevus of Ota occurs in infancy or appears in adolescence as a blue-gray macule in the distribution of the trigeminal nerve. The lesion is unilateral in 90% of cases. Asian females are most commonly affected. Histologically, a benign dendritic melanocytosis is present in the papillary and upper reticular dermis. High-energy fluences of the Q-switched ruby laser results in lightening of the lesion, without scarring, after a few treatments.[28] A combination of the Q-switched 532 nm neodymium:yttrium-aluminum-garnet (Nd:YAG) laser and a Q-switched 1,064 nm Nd:YAG laser has been reported to be more effective than the 1.064 nm laser alone for the treatment of nevus of Ota.[29]

BECKER NEVUS

A malformation of epidermal melanocytes, Becker nevus occurs as a large area of hyperpigmentation and increased hair growth and is usually located on one shoulder. It appears most

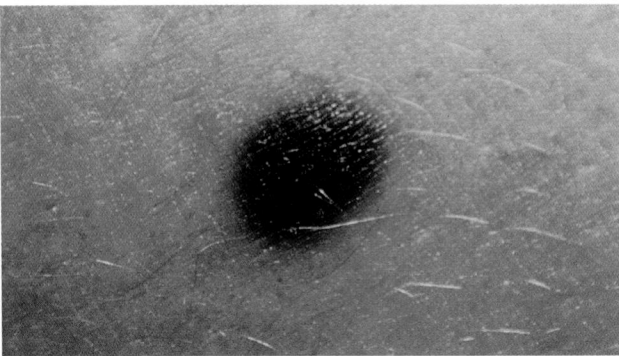

Figure 15 **The presence of melanocytes in the middle and lower dermis is responsible for the color of the blue nevus.**

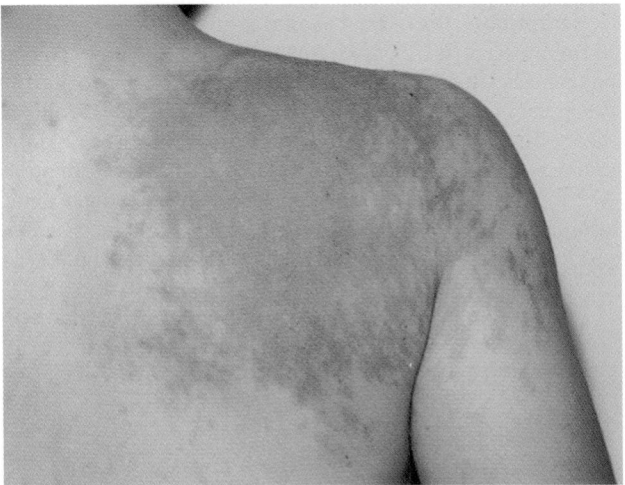

Figure 16 **Becker nevus, an acquired localized malformation of epidermal melanocytes that may be associated with hypertrichosis, is seen on the shoulder.**

commonly in males during adolescence [*see Figure 16*]; however, cases with associated lipoatrophy are more frequently reported in women. Reports of atypical Becker nevus indicate that the clinical spectrum of Becker nevus may be greater than commonly thought.[30] Underlying bony and soft tissue abnormalities may be associated with this disorder.[31]

Light microscopy reveals hyperpigmentation of the basal layer of the epidermis, with melanin-containing phagocytes in the dermis but no nevus cells.

CONGENITAL PIGMENTED NEVUS

Giant pigmented nevus is an uncommon birthmark appearing sporadically in one in 20,000 live births. Its features are different from those of an ordinary, acquired nevus. Lesions are often darkly pigmented, hairy, and slightly infiltrated, eventually becoming verrucous or nodular. They tend to occur in the distribution of a dermatome and may be quite extensive, as in bathing trunk nevus [*see Figure 17*]. Satellite lesions may be present. The condition not only is of cosmetic concern but also has a high association with malignant melanoma, with a reported 10% to 15% of nevus patients developing melanoma.[32] Histologic features of an ordinary compound nevus, an intradermal nevus, a neural nevus, or a blue nevus may be present.[1] Treatment consists of multiple operations to excise as much of the lesion as possible.

NEUROCUTANEOUS MELANOSIS

Lesions on the scalp and neck may be associated with neurocutaneous melanosis of the leptomeninges that can be complicated by epilepsy, mental retardation, or central nervous system melanoma. Large congenital melanocytic nevi (LCMN) carry a poor prognosis in the presence of CNS signs or symptoms such as abnormal reflexes, hydrocephalus, and papilledema. Posterior axial LCMN, especially in association with satellite nevi, is a risk factor for CNS melanosis. Magnetic resonance imaging should be considered in the evaluation of newborns with these findings. In one study, CNS involvement occurred in 33 of 289 patients with LCMN. All the patients with CNS involvement had nevi in the posterior axial location. Satellite nevi were present in 31 of the 33 patients.[33] These findings suggest that melanocytic malformation occurs during the migration of neural crest cells that give rise to cutaneous leptomeningeal melanocytes. Malformation resulting in LCMN on the extremities occurs after migration from the neural crest and is not associated with CNS melanosis.

Neural Tumors

Neural tumors, such as neurofibromas, are of neuroectodermal origin, as are melanocytic tumors. Neurilemmomas (also called schwannomas) are benign nerve sheath tumors that extend subcutaneously adjacent to a peripheral nerve. They usually occur in solitary form but may occur as multiple lesions in the syndrome of neurilemmomatosis.[34] These tumors are usually painful and may be associated with nerve compression. Other benign tumors that must be considered in the differential diagnosis of painful skin nodules are neuromas, angiolipomas and angiomyolipomas, leiomyomas,

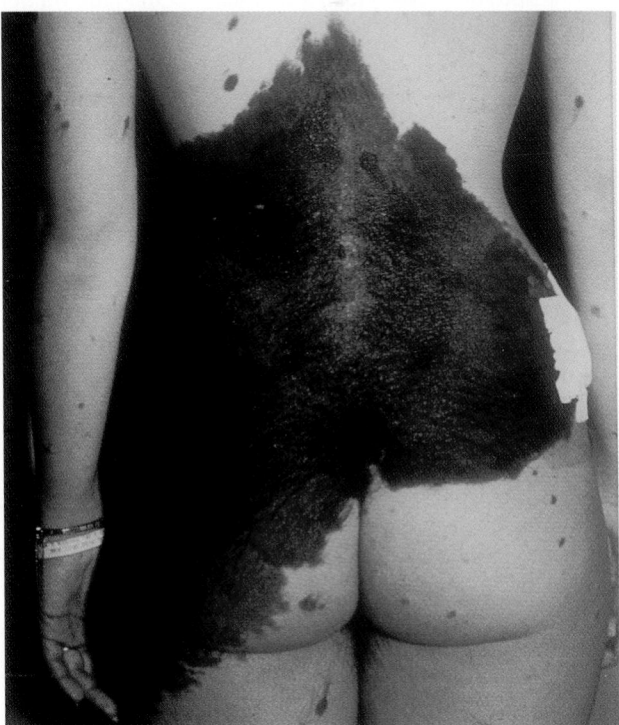

Figure 17 **This form of congenital giant pigmented hairy nevus is associated with an increased risk of malignant melanoma, which develops within the lesion.**

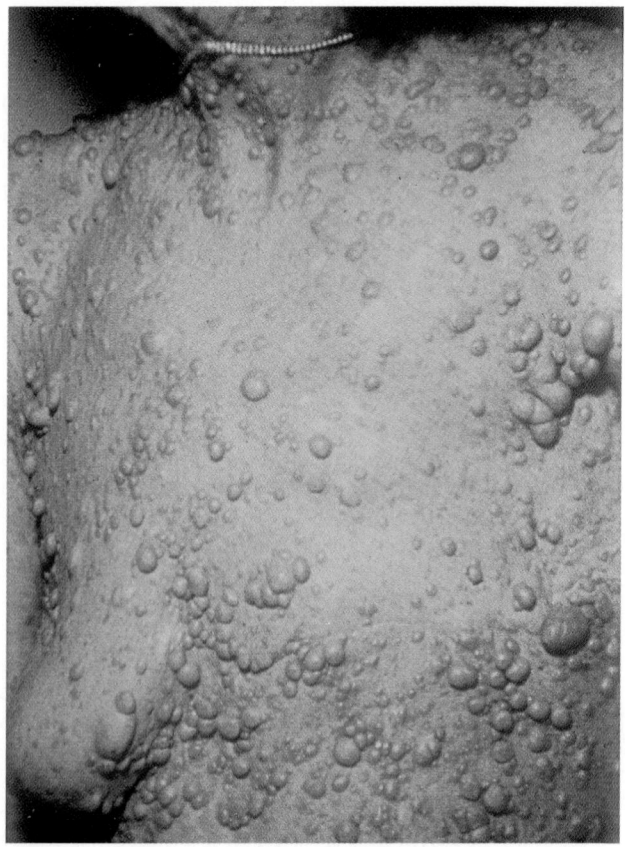

Figure 18 Multiple neurofibromas, as seen in von Recklinghausen disease, usually appear in late childhood and increase in size and number with age.

eccrine spiradenomas, glomus tumors, and the blue rubber bleb nevus.

NEUROFIBROMATOSIS

Neurofibromatosis represents a spectrum of disorders involving the skin, central and peripheral nervous systems, bones, and blood vessels. This neurocutaneous syndrome is transmitted via an autosomal dominant gene at an estimated frequency of one in 3,000 persons with almost complete penetrance.[35]

Diagnosis

Two distinct forms of neurofibromatosis are recognized, but variant forms also exist.

Neurofibromatosis-1 The most common form (occurring in 85% to 90% of all cases) is NF-1, or von Recklinghausen disease [*see Figure 18*]. This is a common autosomal disorder, with an incidence of one in 2,600 to one in 3,000 persons.[36] Mutations in the *NF1* gene result in loss of functional protein, causing the wide spectrum of clinical findings, including *NF1*-associated tumors. NF-1 is characterized by the presence of café au lait spots, intertriginous freckling, multiple spinal and peripheral neurofibromas, plexiform neuromas, bilateral iris hamartomas (also known as Lisch nodules), neurologic impairment, and bone abnormalities. The disease is progressive and is associated with a predisposition to a malignant state.

Sarcomatous degeneration of skin lesions is rare but may

occur in extracutaneous tumors. Café au lait spots of NF-1 may be present at birth and may be best visualized under a Wood light. Neurofibromas begin to appear at puberty as soft, globoid, and pedunculated tumors that are skin colored or violaceous. Lesions may be large and numerous, causing complications resulting from impingement on surrounding structures.

A diagnosis of NF-1 can be established in most patients by the age of 6 years on the basis of routine physical examination, with special attention given to the disease-associated cutaneous features.[36] Patients with NF-1 develop both benign and malignant tumors at increased frequency throughout life.[37] Optic pathway gliomas are the predominant type of intracranial neoplasms; however, other central CNS and non-CNS tumors can occur.

Neurofibromatosis-2 A second form of the disease, neurofibromatosis-2 (NF-2), is characterized by bilateral acoustic neuromas, which are Schwann cell tumors that arise from vestibular nerves.[38] Associated features may include meningiomas, gliomas, paraspinal neurofibromas, and subcapsular cataracts. Skin tumors and café au lait spots are less commonly seen in NF-2 than in NF-1. NF-2 has been attributed to inactivating mutations in the *NF2* tumor suppressor gene, whose product, merlin, plays a number of roles in tumorigenesis.[39]

Variants Other forms of neurofibromatosis include seg-

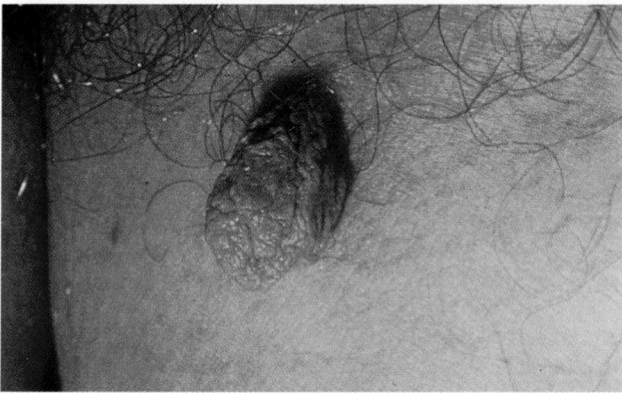

Figure 19 Skin tags, also called acrochordons or soft fibromas, are skin-colored or tan papules. They are commonly seen in such intertriginous areas as the groin or axillae.

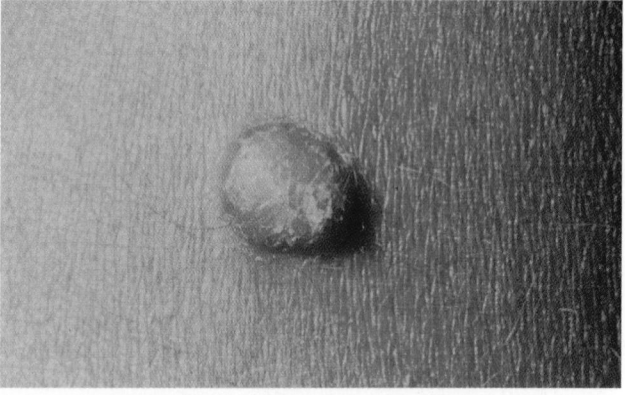

Figure 20 Dermatofibroma appears as a firm skin-colored or reddish-brown papule and may arise spontaneously or follow minor trauma to the skin.

mental cases in which café au lait spots or neurofibromas are localized to a single dermatome.

Genetic Counseling

Patients with either NF-1 or NF-2 should seek genetic counseling because there is a 50% risk that their offspring will also be affected with neurofibromatosis. In NF-1, optic glioma can appear in early childhood; patients with NF-1 may also have scoliosis. In NF-2, bilateral acoustic neuromas can cause deafness. The genes for the two distinct forms of neurofibromatosis have been located on two separate chromosomes. This finding may lead to improved diagnosis, which would facilitate genetic counseling and enable prenatal testing.[38]

Treatment

For treatment of selected neurofibromas, surgery, radiation, and, in rare instances, chemotherapy are the major treatment modalities employed. Surgical excision is more successful than scalpel removal or electrodesiccation and curettage.[40] For patients who are not candidates for surgical resection or in whom only a partial resection is possible, fractionated radiation therapy or stereotactic radiosurgery may be used to treat tumors.

The bilateral acoustic neuromas of NF-2 may be visualized by computed tomography or MRI. Hearing loss is an early symptom that may begin in the second or third decade of life; it can be detected by an audiologic study with brain stem auditory-evoked response. Unilateral acoustic neuromas that are not associated with neurofibromatosis and that are not inherited are more common in older persons and pose fewer management problems.[38] Surgical removal of small acoustic neuromas may improve neurologic or audiologic status.

Connective Tissue Tumors

Fibroma of the skin comprises multiple conditions that may represent reactions to hemorrhage, infection, or chronic irritation.

SKIN TAG

Skin tag, also called acrochordon, commonly occurs as multiple skin-colored or tan, filiform or smooth-surfaced papules that are 2 to 3 mm in diameter. Lesions are often located on the neck or axillae but may also appear in the groin or on the extremities, often as isolated larger polypoid growths [see Figure 19]. The fibrous stalk consists of loose connective tissue with dilated capillaries. Lesions may become inflamed if they are irritated or are traumatized from twisting of the stalk. Biopsy is performed if the clinical diagnosis is uncertain. Skin tags may be removed for cosmetic reasons by using scissors to clip the pedunculate lesions at the base.

DERMATOFIBROMA

Dermatofibroma, also called histiocytoma, is a firm, skin-colored or reddish-brown sessile papule or nodule that arises spontaneously or after minor trauma, usually in adults [see Figure 20]. A dermatofibromatous lesion may occur, for example, after an insect bite on an extremity. A solitary lesion is most common, though multiple or eruptive histiocytomas have been reported. It may be necessary to perform a biopsy when the diagnosis is uncertain. Treatment is necessary only for cosmetic reasons.

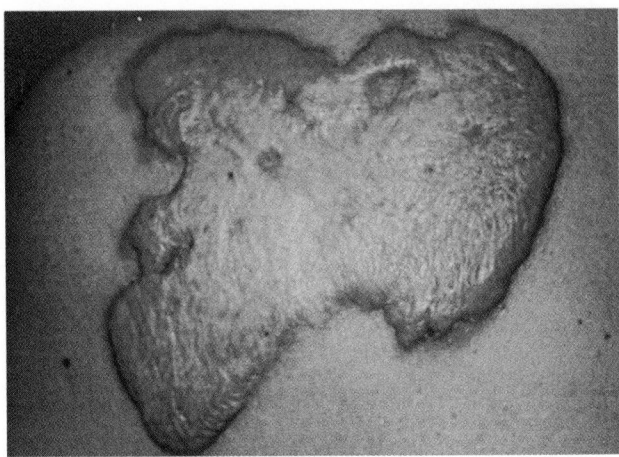

Figure 21 **The proliferation of scar tissue in a keloid may extend beyond the original site of injury.**

KELOID AND HYPERTROPHIC SCAR

Normal wound healing in response to tissue injury involves several integrated processes: inflammation, production of granulation tissue, formation of the extracellular matrix, wound contraction, and, finally, scar formation. In the final phases of wound healing, fibroblasts degrade and produce bundles of collagen fibers. These bundles become thicker and are aligned along the lines of tension to which the tissues are exposed. As a result of these changes, wound tensile strength gradually increases. The resulting scar is relatively acellular and has fewer macrophages, blood vessels, and fibroblasts than the unwounded tissue.

Diagnosis

Scars may be normotrophic, atrophic, hypertrophic, or keloidal. Both hypertrophic and keloidal scars are abnormal responses to tissue injury. Hypertrophic scars mature and flatten over time, usually after 6 months. The keloid appears as a shiny, smooth, raised proliferation of scar tissue with typical crablike extensions beyond the site of the original injury [see Figure 21]. Keloids differ from hypertrophic scars in that their development is delayed, sometimes occurring months after tissue injury. Keloids do not regress, and they frequently cause pain, itching, and burning. Keloids are more common in African Americans, Hispanics, and persons with a personal or family history of keloids. Other factors associated with the development of keloids include wound tension, especially in skin sites such as the chest, shoulders, and back; ear piercing; healing by second intention; pregnancy; young age; and deep laceration.[41]

In atrophic scars, there is thinning of the skin and loss of normal architecture. Striae distensae, a so-called stretch mark, is a common dermal atrophic scar that tends to appear during periods of rapid weight gain and in the presence of excess glucocorticoid, as well as late in gestation.

Treatment

Treatment with intralesional corticosteroids, 10 to 40 mg/ml once a month for up to 6 months, can effectively flatten keloid and hypertrophic scars. A systematic review found that injection of intralesional corticosteroid resulted in flattening of keloids in up to 70% of patients, although the recurrence rate was high in some studies.[42] Potential side effects of intralesional corticosteroid treatment include atrophy, depigmentation, telangiectasia, ulceration, and dose-related systemic effects.

Cryotherapy (a 30-second application once a month for 3 months) has been found to be safe and effective[43]; it may prove particularly useful in combination with intralesional corticosteroid injection.[44] Topical silicone gel sheeting, which was first used for burn scars, has been used in the treatment of keloids and hypertrophic scars; however, a meta-analysis of 13 trials found that there was weak evidence that silicon gel sheeting provides benefit as treatment for hypertrophic and keloid scarring.[45] Medical treatment for keloid and hypertrophic scarring includes corticosteroids, 5-fluorouracil, and imiquimod.[46]

Vascular Birthmarks

Vascular proliferations are broadly classified as hyperplasias that show a tendency to regress or as benign vascular tumors that persist.[47,48] Vascular hyperplasias include pyogenic granuloma and pseudo-Kaposi sarcoma. Vascular hemangiomas are proliferating vascular tumors that are not necessarily present at birth [see Hemangiomas, below]. Hemangiomas can be subdivided according to their histologic cell of origin (endothelial cell, pericyte, glomus cell), depth of tissue involvement (superficial or deep), and size of involved vessels (capillaries, venules, arterioles, veins, or arteries). Vascular birthmarks such as nevus flammeus and salmon patch may resemble angiomas but are nonproliferative malformations that usually do not involve [see Vascular Malformations, below].

EPIDEMIOLOGY

Hemangiomas occur in a female-to-male ratio of 5:1, whereas vascular malformations occur with equal frequency in males and females. A rare familial occurrence of hemangiomas, vascular malformations, or both has been reported in six kindreds, suggesting autosomal dominant inheritance in these cases.[49] Vascular malformations are congenital developmental defects that are generally of unknown etiology. Port-wine stains are the most common vascular malformations, occurring in one in 1,000 people. Most port-wine stains are isolated anomalies, but they may be associated with developmental defects, such as the Klippel-Trenaunay and Sturge-Weber syndromes.

PATHOGENESIS

The etiopathogenesis of hemangiomas and vascular malformations is not well understood. Hemangiomas arise in response to an angiogenic stimulus that may begin in utero. Through use of immunohistochemical techniques, infantile hemangiomas and placental microvessels were found to coexpress the vascular antigens GLUT-1 and Lewis Y antigen (LeY).[50] These antigens are not present in other vascular tumors, such as pyogenic granulomas, or in vascular malformations. A pathogenic link involving aberrant differentiation of vascular precursor cells or embolization of placental cells to fetal tissue has been hypothesized.[50] These antigens are also absent in congenital nonprogressive hemangioma, a distinctive hemangioma consisting of lesions that are fully formed at birth and that either remain static or rapidly involute.[51]

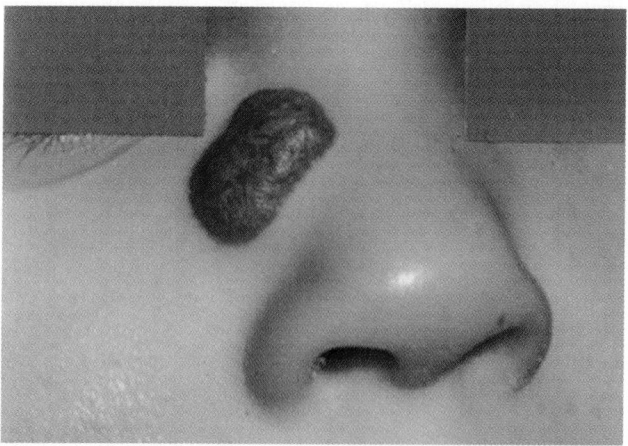

Figure 22 **The strawberry, or capillary, hemangioma appears between the second and fifth weeks of life and undergoes spontaneous involution over a period of several years.**

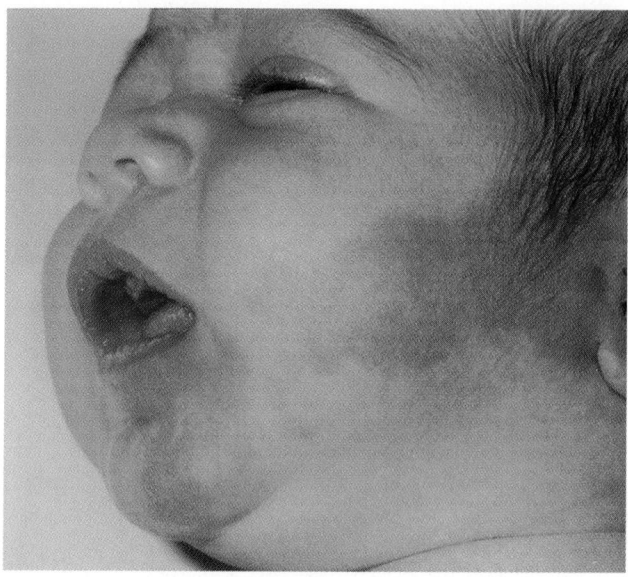

Figure 23 **A nevus flammeus is present at birth as a reddish or violaceous macular discoloration, often in a unilateral and segmental distribution; it shows little tendency to involute later in life.**

OVERVIEW OF MANAGEMENT

Evaluation and management of hemangiomas and malformations require a multidisciplinary approach. Specific diagnosis may be aided by imaging techniques such as CT and MRI to assess depth of involvement and extension to adjacent structures and to evaluate associated abnormalities. Laboratory evaluation for associated systemic disease may be required in addition to ophthalmologic, neurologic, and cardiologic assessment for complications of vascular tumors and dysmorphic syndromes.

HEMANGIOMAS

The biologic classification of hemangiomas is very different from that of vascular malformations. Vascular tumors can be classified according to their cell of origin, the size of the involved vessels, and the depth of involvement. Such classifications have led to refinement in terminology.[52] The terms strawberry hemangioma and cavernous hemangioma are descriptive clinical terms that do not specify the type of vessels that are involved.

Diagnosis

The vascular lesion may appear in neonates as a faint pink patch that subsequently undergoes rapid proliferation over a period of months to years before the lesion stabilizes and regresses.

Capillary hemangioma, also known as strawberry hemangioma, appears as a single vascular lesion or multiple lesions during the second to the fifth week of life. Infantile hemangiomas are bright-red, soft, lobulated tumors that increase in size for a period of months [*see Figure 22*]. Lesions spontaneously involute, sometimes with fibrosis, over a period of several years.[47] Histologically, the capillary hemangioma shows a proliferation of endothelial cells that form many new small vessels.

Treatment

It is important to realize that most hemangiomas are uncomplicated and regress without treatment early in life with minimal residual scarring. Parents may require considerable reassurance that the best course is to refrain from treatment.[53] Care must be taken to prevent trauma and infection, which may lead to scarring.

There is considerable controversy as to when to intervene in the treatment of complicated hemangiomas because of potential side effects, such as scarring. The ideal time to treat would be at the beginning of the period of rapid growth, but this is difficult to predict. Indications for treatment include involvement of a vital orifice, infection, ulceration, ocular involvement, and severe cosmetic deformity.

Medical options for the treatment of hemangiomas include intralesional or systemic corticosteroids, the latter at a dose of 1 to 3 mg/kg/day. Antimetabolites have been used for their antiproliferative effect. Interferon alfa has been used to treat severe hemangiomatosis, but its use is associated with systemic side effects and the potential risk of spastic diplegia. Laser surgery with 585 nm pulsed dye laser may be used to treat the superficial proliferative component of the hemangioma; however, early therapeutic intervention with laser therapy may not prevent proliferative growth of the deeper or subcutaneous component.[54]

Radiation therapy may lead to scarring. In addition, radiation therapy is discouraged in children because of long-term radiation effects, including risk of malignancy. Interventional techniques involving embolization of vessels may be required in cases involving airway obstruction or other life-threatening complications. A multidisciplinary team approach involving the dermatologist, a pediatrician, a radiologist, a surgeon, and other specialists is needed for optimal management of complicated cases.[55]

VASCULAR MALFORMATIONS

Vascular malformations are usually present at birth. They are permanent or progress in the form of ectasias but do not proliferate. Vascular malformations may be subdivided into the following groups: venous, lymphatic, combined arteriovenous, and capillary (such as port-wine stain).[56] Dysmorphic syndromes such as Sturge-Weber and Klippel-Trénaunay syndromes are more commonly associated with vascular malformations than with hemangiomas.

Diagnosis

Salmon patch The salmon patch, one of the most common vascular birthmarks, is a dull-pink macule that appears on the nape of the neck, central forehead, or eyelids. Although the salmon patch is sometimes classified as a nevus flammeus, it is distinguished from the latter by its tendency to fade in early life. The salmon patch is caused by the persistence of fetal capillary ectasia in the dermis.[47]

Port-wine stain Port-wine stain, also called nevus flammeus, appears at birth as a reddish or violaceous macular discoloration, usually in a unilateral, segmental distribution [*see Figure 23*]. Mature dilated capillaries are present in the dermis. After puberty, nevus flammeus lesions may become thickened and nodular or papular. There is little tendency toward involution. Nevus flammeus lesions may be associated with abnormalities of the larger vessels and with neurologic manifestations.

Sturge-Weber syndrome A facial port-wine stain that involves the skin innervated by the first branch of the trigeminal nerve is a feature of the Sturge-Weber syndrome, a rare congenital vascular disorder (also known as encephalotrigeminal angiomatosis). Other features of the Sturge-Weber syndrome include ipsilateral congenital glaucoma and contralateral seizures caused by leptomeningeal angiomatosis. Ophthalmologic and neurologic evaluation may be warranted in patients with the Sturge-Weber syndrome.

Klippel-Trénaunay syndrome The triad of findings seen in Klippel-Trénaunay syndrome includes a port-wine stain, usually in a patchy distribution on the involved extremity; varicose veins; and soft tissue or bony hypertrophy. The most common site of involvement is the lower leg; the next most common sites of involvement are the arms and trunk.[51] One study indicated that the morphologic characteristics of port-wine stains may have importance in identifying lymphatic disease and risk of complications in patients with Klippel-Trénaunay syndrome.[57] Patients with sharply demarcated geographic stains had greater evidence of lymphatic disease and increased risk of complications than patients with blotchy, poorly demarcated stains.

Venous malformation Formerly referred to as cavernous hemangiomas, vascular malformation consists of a collection of abnormal veins and venous pouches that commonly occur around the head and neck but can occur anywhere on the body. They are frequently multiple or have satellite lesions. Superficially, they appear as a subcutaneous swelling with a bluish hue on the skin surface or mucous membrane. Deeper components may be invisible on clinical examination. Lesions enlarge for several months, become stationary for an indefinite period, and spontaneously resolve.

Treatment

Because vascular malformations do not proliferate, treatment may be cosmetic and can be postponed to later in life. However, a multidisciplinary approach is needed to treat potential complications of vascular malformations associated with dysmorphic syndromes. Salmon patch tends to fade in early life and usually requires no treatment.

Treatment of port-wine stains by excision, tattooing,

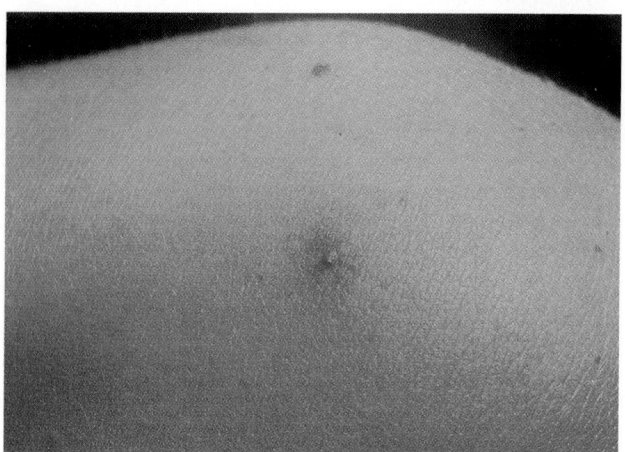

Figure 24   **A spider angioma, which has a central arteriole from which fine vessels radiate, blanches with pressure.**

ionizing radiation, cryosurgery, or dermabrasion is largely unsatisfactory. Use of the argon laser has resulted in lightening of vascular lesions; however, there is wide variability in the response to argon laser therapy. The effectiveness of this treatment results from the selective absorption of the monochromatic 585 nm laser light by red hemoglobin pigment, which produces thermal energy with resultant photocoagulation of tissue.[58] Thinner lesions are more responsive than thicker lesions that have undergone progressive vascular ectasia. In a study of 100 patients of different age groups who had port-wine stains of the head and neck and who were treated with a flashlamp pulsed dye laser, treatment was no more effective when given in early childhood than when given at a later date.[59]

Acquired Vascular Disorders

DIAGNOSIS

Spider Angioma

Spider angioma, also called spider nevus or arterial spider, appears as a central red punctum from which fine vessels radiate; the appearance of the lesion is suggestive of a red spider [*see Figure 24*]. The central arteriole may be pulsatile. These telangiectasias (dilated capillaries) are commonly seen on the face, neck, trunk, and upper extremities and occur most commonly in middle-aged or elderly persons. They may arise spontaneously or in association with pregnancy or hepatic dysfunction.[56] Spider angiomas may be treated with laser therapy for cosmetic purposes.

Unilateral Telangiectasia

Acquired unilateral telangiectatic nevi are uncommon; those that have been reported resulted from mechanical or physical trauma, including sun damage.[60]

Cherry Angioma

Cherry angioma, also called senile angioma, appears as multiple bright-red, soft, dome-shaped papules on the trunk of middle-aged or older persons. Trauma produces slight bleeding. Electrodesiccation may be performed for cosmetic purposes.

Pyogenic Granuloma and Other Vascular Tumors

The pyogenic granuloma is a soft red lesion that is solitary, raised, and nonpulsatile; it often appears after minor skin trauma, such as a puncture wound. Other predisposing factors include hormonal effects, infection, viral oncogenes, microscopic arteriovenous anastomoses, and growth factors.[61] Epulis gravidarum is a variant of a pyogenic granuloma. The lesion was formerly believed to be caused by a pyogenic infection of a small wound; histologically, however, an early lesion resembles a capillary hemangioma. The thin, sometimes verrucous epidermis is friable and apt to become eroded or ulcerated. Lesions rapidly reach a size of 1 to 2 cm and then remain static. Common sites of involvement are the fingers, feet, and face [*see Figure 25*]. Biopsy is performed to rule out malignant tumors, such as Kaposi sarcoma and amelanotic melanoma.

Other benign tumors with a vascular component include angiofibroma, angioleiomyoma, and angiolipoma. Some of these can be painful. The differential diagnosis of painful skin tumors includes glomus tumor, angiolipoma, angioleiomyoma, neuromas, and eccrine spiradenoma.[48] Lesions are usually easily removed by electrodesiccation and curettage. If

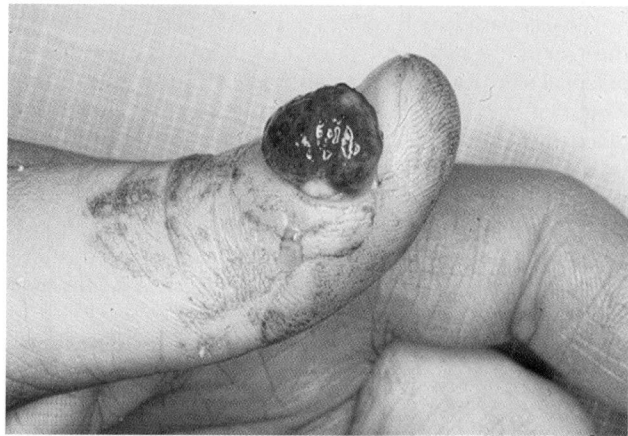

Figure 25   **The pyogenic granuloma, which may show a smooth, verrucous, eroded, or friable surface, may be confused with a malignant tumor.**

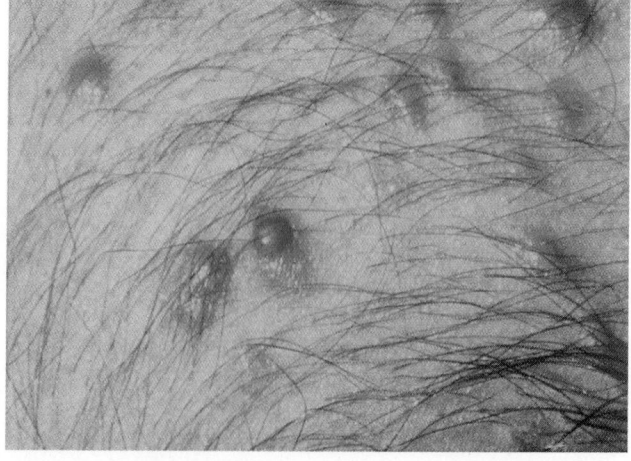

Figure 26   **Leiomyomas are sometimes painful papules that arise from smooth muscle of blood vessels or the arrector pili.**

they recur or if satellite lesions appear after such treatment, excisional biopsy is recommended.

Kimura Disease

Kimura disease and angiolymphoid hyperplasia with eosinophilia are rare tumors of unknown cause that occur mainly on the head and neck in young adults and may resemble pyogenic granuloma.[62] Kimura disease, which was first reported in Korea, is most common in Asians. It appears as a granulomatous proliferation of lymphoid tissue that may be accompanied by peripheral eosinophilia and contiguous lymphadenopathy. Lesions may occasionally be seen on the trunk, extremities, and genitalia in addition to the head and neck. Angiolymphoid hyperplasia with eosinophilia, which may or may not represent a different disease, appears as localized single or multiple nodules. Infectious, allergic, hormonal, and traumatic mechanisms have been postulated. Immunodermatopathologic studies suggest an unusual distribution of adhesion molecules, IgE, and CD23 in these angioproliferating tumors.[63]

Lipoma

The lipoma, which is a soft, rounded to lobulated subcutaneous tumor of mature fat cells, is commonly seen on the trunk, neck, or forearms. Lesions are rubbery in consistency and are freely movable under the overlying skin, which appears normal. There may be a single lesion or multiple lesions, and they are usually asymptomatic unless they impinge on a nerve. Lipomas are of variable size and grow slowly. Histologically, the tumors are usually encapsulated and show fat cells that are indistinguishable from normal adipose tissue. Admixture of other tissue components may result in fibrolipomas (fibrous tissue), angiolipomas (blood vessels), and myolipomas (smooth muscle). Excision may be performed for cosmetic reasons. If a lesion grows rapidly, biopsy should be performed, though lipomas rarely become malignant.

Leiomyoma

The leiomyoma is an uncommon tumor of smooth muscle that appears as a single brownish-red papule or as multiple papules or small nodules, which are sometimes painful [see Figure 26]. Leiomyomas may arise from the arrector pili (the smooth muscle attached to the hair follicle sheath) or from the smooth muscle surrounding cutaneous blood vessels (angioleiomyoma). Painful lesions can be excised.

Lymphangioma Circumscriptum

Lymphangioma circumscriptum is characterized by groups of persistent localized or diffuse translucent vesicles. Indications for treatment include severe cosmetic problems, persistent leakage of lymphatic fluid or blood, and recurrent infection. The vesicles frequently recur after surgery, radiotherapy, electrocautery, or cryosurgery because of the persistence of deep lymphatic cisterns. Carbon dioxide laser in a vaporization mode has been used to ablate superficial cutaneous lesions in patients with lymphangioma circumscriptum.[64] The major advantage of this technique is that it may reduce the frequency of recurrences because it seals the communicating channels to the deeper cisterns by vaporizing the superficial lymphatics. Sclerotherapy has been reported as useful in the treatment of cutaneous lesions in patients with lymphangioma circumscriptum.[65]

The author serves as an adviser for Amgen, Inc., Biogen Idec, Inc., Abbott Laboratories, Inc., Genentech, Inc., and Novartis Pharmaceuticals Corp.

References

1. Lever's Histopathology of the Skin, 9th ed. Elder D, Elenitsas R, Jaworsky C, et al, Eds. Lippincott-Williams and Wilkins, Philadelphia, 2004

2. Fitzpatrick's Dermatology in General Medicine, 6th ed. Freedberg IM, Eisen AZ, Wolff K, et al, Eds. McGraw-Hill Book Co, New York, 1993

3. Flugman SL, McClain SA, Clark RF: Transient eruptive seborrheic keratoses associated with erythrodermic psoriasis and erythrodermic drug eruption: report of two cases. J Am Acad Dermatol 45:S212, 2001

4. Neuhaus IM, LeBoit PE, McCalmont TM: Seborrheic keratosis with basal clear cells: a distinctive microscopic mimic of melanoma in situ. J Am Acad Dermatol 54:132, 2006

5. Paller AS, Syder AJ, Chan YM, et al: Genetic and clinical mosaicism in a type of epidermal nevus. N Engl J Med 331:1408, 1994

6. Sugarman JL: Epidermal nevus syndrome. Semin Cutan Med Surg 23:145, 2004

7. Ricks M, Elston DM, Sartori CR: Multiple basaloid follicular hamartomas associated with acrochordons, seborrhoeic keratoses and chondrosarcoma. Br J Dermatol 146:1068, 2002

8. Alster TS, Tanzi EL: Photodynamic therapy with topical aminolevulinic acid and pulsed dye laser irradiation for sebaceous hyperplasia. J Drugs Dermatol 2:501, 2003

9. Sidhu SK, Wakelin SH, Wilkinson JD: Multiple familial trichoepitheliomas. Cutis 63:239, 1999

10. Urquhart JL, Weston WL: Treatment of multiple trichoepitheliomas with topical imiquimod and tretinoin. Pediatr Dermatol 22:67, 2005

11. Ponti G, Losi L, Di Gregorio C, et al: Identification of Muir-Torre syndrome among patients with sebaceous tumors and keratoacanthomas: role of clinical features, microsatellite instability, and immunohistochemistry. Cancer 103:1018, 2005

12. Parks ET, Caldemeyer KS, Mirowski GW: Radiologic images in dermatology: Gardner syndrome. J Am Acad Dermatol 45:940, 2001

13. Fistarol SK, Anliker MD, Itin PH: Cowden disease or multiple hamartoma syndrome: cutaneous clue to internal malignancy. Eur J Dermatol 12:411, 2002

14. Zbar B, Alvord WG, Glenn G, et al: Risk of renal and colonic neoplasms and spontaneous pneumothorax in the Birt-Hogg-Dube syndrome. Cancer Epidemiol Biomarkers Prev 11:393, 2002

15. Lindor NM, Hand J, Burch PA, et al: Birt-Hogg-Dube syndrome: an autosomal dominant disorder with predisposition to cancers of the kidney, fibrofolliculomas, and focal cutaneous mucinosis. Int J Dermatol 40:653, 2001

16. Baur J, Buttner P, Wiecker TS, et al: Risk factors of incident melanocytic nevi: a longitudinal study of a cohort of 1,232 young German children. Int J Cancer 115:121, 2005

17. Tucker MA, Halpern A, Holly EA, et al: Clinically recognized dysplastic nevi: a central risk factor for cutaneous melanoma. JAMA 277:1439, 1997

18. Augustsson A, Stierner U, Rosdahl I, et al: Melanocytic naevi in sun-exposed and protected skin in melanoma patients and controls. Acta Derm Venereol (Stockh) 71:512, 1991

19. Kelly JW, Rivers JK, MacLennan R, et al: Sunlight: a major factor associated with the development of melanocytic nevi in Australian schoolchildren. J Am Acad Dermatol 30:40, 1994

20. English DR, Milne E, Simpson JA: Sun protection and the development of melanocytic nevi in children. Cancer Epidemiol Biomarkers Prev 14:2873, 2005

21. Maldonado JL, Fridlyand J, Patel H, et al: Determinants of BRAF mutations in primary melanomas. J Natl Cancer Inst 95:1878, 2003

22. Marghoob AA, Orlow SJ, Kopf AW: Syndromes associated with melanocyti nevi. J Am Acad Dermatol 29:373, 1993

23. Gupta G, Williams REA, Mackie RM: The labial melanotic macule: a review of 79 cases. Br J Dermatol 136:772, 1997

24. Cohen JB, Janniger CK, Schwartz RA: Café-au-lait spots. Cutis 66:22, 2000

25. Thami GP, Kaur S, Kanwar A: Association of juvenile xanthogranuloma with café-au-lait macules. Int J Dermatol 40:281, 2001

26. Cambiaghi S, Restano L, Caputo R: Juvenile xanthogranuloma associated with neurofibromatosis 1: 14 patients without evidence of hematologic malignancies. Pediatr Dermatol 21:97, 2004

27. Mooney MA, Barr RJ, Buxton MG: Halo nevus or halo phenomenon: a study of 142 cases. J Cutan Pathol 22:342, 1995

28. Lowe NJ, Wieder JM, Sawcer D, et al: Nevus of Ota: treatment with high energy fluences of the Q-switched ruby laser. J Am Acad Dermatol 29:997, 1993

29. Ee HL, Goh CL, Khoo LS, et al: Treatment of acquired bilateral nevus of Ota-like macules (Hori's nevus) with a combination of the 532 nm Q-switched Nd:YAG laser followed by the 1,064 nm Q-switched Nd:YAG is more effective: prospective study. Dermatol Surg 32:34, 2006

30. Alfadley A, Hainau B, Al Robace A, et al: Becker's melanosis: a report of 12 cases with atypical presentation. Int J Dermatol 44:20, 2005

31. Glinick SE, Alper JC, Bogaars H, et al: Becker's melanosis: associated abnormalities. J Am Acad Dermatol 9:509, 1983

32. Zaal LH, Mooi WJ, Klip H, et al: Risk of malignant transformation of congenital melanocytic nevi: a retrospective nationwide study from the Netherlands. Plast Reconstr Surg 116:1902, 2005

33. DeDavid M, Orlow SJ, Provost N, et al: Neurocutaneous melanosis: clinical features of large congenital melanocytic nevi in patients with manifest central nervous system melanosis. J Am Acad Dermatol 35:529, 1996

34. Buenger KM, Porter NC, Dozier SE, et al: Localized multiple neurilemmomas of the lower extremity. Cutis 51:36, 1993

35. Riccardi VM: Von Recklinghausen neurofibromatosis. N Engl J Med 305:1617, 1981

36. Lammert M, Friedman JM, Kluwe L, et al: Prevalence of neurofibromatosis 1 in German children at elementary school enrollment. Arch Dermatol 141:71, 2005

37. Airewele GE, Sigurdson AJ, Wiley KJ, et al: Neoplasms in neurofibromatosis I are related to gender but not to family history of cancer. Genet Epidemiol 20:75, 2001

38. Martuza RL, Eldridge R: Neurofibromatosis 2 (bilateral acoustic neurofibromatosis). N Engl J Med 318:684, 1988

39. Xiao GH, Chernoff J, Testa JR: NF2: the wizardry of merlin. Genes Chromosomes Cancer 38:389, 2003

40. Mrugala MM, Batchelor TT, Plotkin SR: Peripheral and cranial nerve sheath tumors. Curr Opin Neurol 18:604, 2005

41. Sahl WJ, Clever H: Cutaneous scars: part I. Int J Dermatol 33:681, 1994

42. Shaffer JJ, Taylor SC, Cook-Bolden F: Keloidal scars: a review with a critical look at therapeutic options. J Am Acad Dermatol 46:S63, 2002

43. Zouboulis CC, Blume U, Buttner P, et al: Outcomes of cryosurgery in keloids and hypertrophic scars: a prospective consecutive trial of case series. Arch Dermatol 129:1146, 1993

44. Yosipovitch G, Widijanti Sugeng M, Goon A, et al: A comparison of the combined effect of cryotherapy and corticosteroid injections versus corticosteroids and cryotherapy alone on keloids: a controlled study. J Dermatolog Treat 12:87, 2001

45. O'Brien L, Pandit A: Silicon gel sheeting for preventing and treating hypertrophic and keloid scars. Cochrane Database Syst Rev (1):CD003826, 2006

46. Kelly AP: Medical and surgical therapies for keloids. Dermatol Ther 17:212, 2004

47. Requena L, Sangueza OP: Cutaneous vascular proliferations. Part II: hyperplasias and benign neoplasms. J Am Acad Dermatol 37:887, 1997

48. Requena L, Sangueza OP: Cutaneous vascular proliferations. Part III: malignant neoplasms, other cutaneous neoplasms with significant vascular component, and disorders erroneously considered as vascular neoplasms. J Am Acad Dermatol 38:143, 1998

49. Blei F, Walter J, Orlow SJ, et al: Familial segregation of hemangiomas and vascular malformations as an autosomal dominant trait. Arch Dermatol 134:718, 1998

50. North PE, Waner M, Mizeracki A, et al: A unique microvascular phenotype shared by juvenile hemangiomas and human placenta. Arch Dermatol 137:559, 2001

51. North PE, Waner M, James CA, et al: Congenital nonprogressive hemangioma: a distinct clinicopathologic entity unlike infantile hemangioma. Arch Dermatol 137:1607, 2001

52. Marler JJ, Mulliken JB: Current management of hemangiomas and vascular malformations. Clin Plast Surg 32:99, 2005

53. Frieden IJ, Eichenfield LF, Esterly NB, et al: Guidelines of care for hemangiomas of infancy. American Academy of Dermatology Guidelines, Outcomes Committee. J Am Acad Dermatol 37:631, 1997

54. Poetke M, Philipp C, Berlien HP: Flashlamp-pumped pulsed dye laser for hemangiomas in infancy: treatment of superficial versus mixed hemangiomas. Arch Dermatol 136:628, 2000

55. Mathes EF, Haggstrom AN, Dowd C, et al: Clinical characteristics and management of vascular anomalies: findings of a multidisciplinary vascular anomalies clinic. Arch Dermatol 140:979, 2004

56. Requena L, Sangueza OP: Cutaneous vascular anomalies. Part I: hamartomas, malformations, and dilatation of preexisting vessels. J Am Acad Dermatol 37:523, 1997

57. Maari C, Frieden IJ: Klippel-Trenaunay syndrome: the importance of "geographic stains" in identifying lymphatic disease and risk of complications. J Am Acad Dermatol 51:391, 2004

58. Railan D, Parlette EC, Uebelhoer NS, et al: Laser treatment of vascular lesions. Clin Dermatol 24:8, 2006

59. van der Horst CM, Koster PL, de Borgie CM, et al: Effect of the timing of treatment of port-wine stains with the flash-lamp–pumped pulsed-dye laser. N Engl J Med 338:1028, 1998

60. Pasyk KA: Acquired lateral telangiectatic nevus: port-wine stain or nevus flammeus. Cutis 51:281, 1993

61. Mooney MA, Janniger CK: Pyogenic granuloma. Pediatr Dermatol 55:133, 1995

62. Chun SI, Ji HG: Kimura's disease and angiolymphoid hyperplasia with eosinophilia: clinical and histopathologic differences. J Am Acad Dermatol 27:954, 1992

63. von den Driesch P, Gruschwitz M, Schell H, et al: Distribution of adhesion molecules, IgE, and CD23 in a case of angiolymphoid hyperplasia with eosinophilia. J Am Acad Dermatol 26:799, 1992

64. Bailin PL, Kantor GR, Wheeland RG: Carbon dioxide laser vaporization of lymphangioma circumscriptum. J Am Acad Dermatol 14:257, 1986

65. Park CO, Lee MJ, Chung KY: Treatment of unusual vascular lesions: usefulness of sclerotherapy in lymphangioma circumscriptum and acquired digital arteriovenous malformation. Dermatol Surg 31:1451, 2005

45 Malignant Cutaneous Tumors

Allan C. Halpern, M.D., and Patricia L. Myskowski, M.D.

Malignant tumors can arise from cells of any layer of the skin—keratinocytes, melanocytes, fibroblasts, endothelial cells, or adipocytes—as well as from cells such as lymphocytes, which normally transit through the skin. Cutaneous metastases may also arise from other primary sites. In this chapter, we review the most common malignant cutaneous tumors in their order of frequency.

Malignant Tumors of the Epidermis

Epidermal skin cancers are the most common cancers in humans. They arise in the keratinocytes and the melanocytes of the epidermis. Epidermal skin cancers present a unique opportunity for effective intervention with both early detection and primary prevention. They are amenable to clinical diagnosis by simple visual inspection and to pathologic diagnosis by minimally invasive biopsy.

Basal cell carcinoma (BCC) and squamous cell carcinoma (SCC) originate from the keratinocytes of the epidermis. Because these two cancers share many features, they are often lumped together under the term nonmelanoma skin cancer (NMSC).

Malignant melanoma is a malignancy arising from a melanocyte. Although malignant melanomas can arise in any melanocyte of the body, including the eye, the vast majority occur in the skin. Cutaneous malignant melanoma has been categorized into four major histogenetic types: lentigo maligna melanoma, superficial spreading melanoma, nodular melanoma, and acral lentiginous melanoma.

SUN EXPOSURE AND SKIN CANCER

Several lines of evidence implicate ultraviolet (UV) radiation in the pathogenesis of all three of the major epidermal skin cancers.[1] Epidemiologic data implicate long-term cumulative sun exposure in the development of SCC and intense intermittent sun exposure in the development of BCC and melanoma. Laboratory studies indicate that both UVA (320 nm to 400 nm) and UVB (290 nm to 320 nm) radiation from sunlight can damage DNA both directly and through oxidative damage. In addition, UV radiation can suppress the cutaneous immune system.[2] The association of some SCCs with chemical carcinogens and the occurrence of acral lentiginous and mucosal melanomas in unexposed areas of the body underscore the need for studies to identify additional etiologic agents.

Recognition of the important role of sunlight in the etiology of skin cancer affords an opportunity for primary prevention through the use of sun protection. Unfortunately, the exact timing and doses of UV exposure involved in the development of skin cancer in humans are not known and likely vary among the types of skin cancer. Accordingly, patients should be educated about the deleterious effects of sun exposure and tanning. Sun-protection efforts should be geared to an overall reduction of sun exposure through the avoidance of sun-seeking behavior and the use of sun-protective clothing. Broad-spectrum sunscreens with a sun protection factor (SPF) of 15 or greater are a useful adjunct to sun protection, but they should not be used to increase the amount of time spent in direct sunlight.[3] The use of tanning beds should be avoided. The use of sunless tanning agents is

safe, but the darkening of the skin that results from the use of these agents does not offer significant UV protection. For individuals who are assiduous in their sun protection efforts, attention should be given to adequate vitamin D intake through diet or supplements.[4]

NONMELANOMA SKIN CANCER

NMSC typically occurs as pink lesions on the sun-exposed skin surface. Any pink skin lesion that persists or recurs in the same location, especially if easily irritated by minor trauma, should raise the suspicion of NMSC. Some forms of NMSC will fade with changes in season (i.e., with reduced sun exposure) or with the application of topical steroids, and the clinician should advise patients that any lesion that recurs warrants further attention.

Basal Cell Carcinoma

BCC is a malignant cutaneous tumor arising from the basal keratinocytes of the epidermis.

Epidemiology BCC is the most common skin cancer. The reported incidence ranges from 3.4 per 100,000 per year in African Americans to over 1,100 per 100,000 per year in Townsville, Queensland, Australia.[5,6] Although rare, metastases and death from BCC do occur.

Etiology and risk factors UV radiation—specifically, intense intermittent sun exposure—appears to play an important role in the development of BCC. Studies of basal cell nevus syndrome (Gorlin syndrome) have yielded dramatic insights into the genetics of BCC. The patched gene, which was first recognized as a developmental gene in the fruit fly *Drosophila*, has been identified as playing a critical role in the development of BCC. Almost all patients with basal cell nevus syndrome appear to inherit a mutated copy of the patched gene, and studies of sporadic BCC suggest that mutations in the patched gene pathway (i.e., the sonic hedgehog pathway) are a necessary and often sufficient step in the development of most BCCs.[7]

Diagnosis The majority of BCCs occur on the head and neck. They occur in nodular and superficial forms, as well as in a variety of less common forms.

Nodular BCC appears as a raised, pearly, translucent, pink bump on the skin surface. It is often easily irritated, fragile, and associated with episodes of superficial ulceration or hemorrhage. When ulceration is prominent, it can lead to the appearance of a so-called rodent ulcer, in which the pearly translucent border is barely appreciable. Some nodular BCC lesions appear more white than pink and, on close observation, often demonstrate small telangiectasias. They tend to have a smoother, shinier surface and a firmer texture than common dermal nevi [see Figure 1].

Superficial BCC appears as a pink patch of skin. On close inspection, most superficial BCCs demonstrate a thready, translucent border, with areas of seemingly normal or slightly fibrotic skin within the lesion. Superficial BCC is usually found on the upper trunk, arms, and legs.

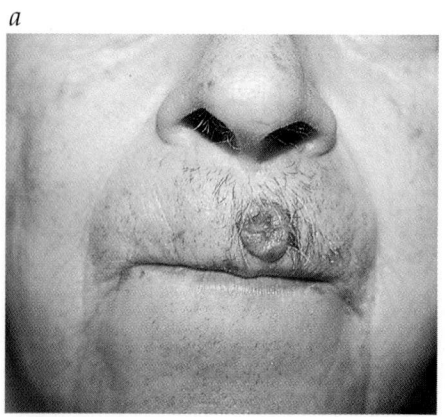
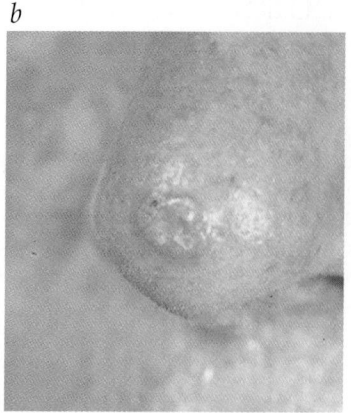
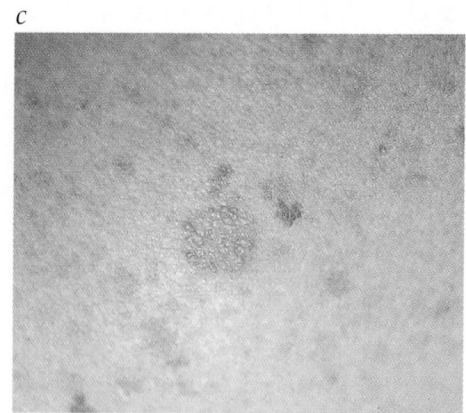

a   *b*   *c*

Figure 1   Nodular basal cell carcinoma—shown here above a patient's lip, with a so-called rodent's ulcer (*a*)—commonly presents as a raised, pearly, translucent pink bump on the skin surface (*b*). A superficial form appears as a pink patch of skin (*c*).

Less common clinical variants of BCC include morpheaform, pigmented, and cystic lesions. Morpheaform BCCs have an infiltrative pattern that histologically and clinically resembles a scar. Pigmented BCCs typically contain specks of blue-black pigment, but they may be deeply pigmented throughout. Pigmented lesions are most commonly a variant of nodular BCC. Cystic BCCs tend to be softer than typical nodular BCCs and may have a clear to blue-gray appearance.

Patient history plays a critical role in the diagnosis of BCC. When questioned about lesions that become easily irritated or bleed from minor trauma, patients can often alert the clinician to early lesions that would otherwise elude detection. With the patient under local anesthesia, a biopsy should be obtained of any suspicious lesion.

Differential diagnosis   Nodular BCC can be confused with angiofibromas, dermal nevi, amelanotic melanoma, cutaneous metastases, dermatofibroma, and a host of benign adnexal tumors (e.g., trichoepithelioma). Superficial BCCs mimic several inflammatory dermatoses (e.g., eczema and tinea) and share several clinical features with actinic keratoses. Pigmented BCC can easily be confused with a primary melanocytic neoplasm. Cystic BCCs can be confused with cystic adnexal tumors and inflammatory lesions.

Treatment   The goal of therapy is to adequately eradicate the lesion and ensure the best cosmetic and functional outcome. Multiple factors—such as the size, location, and histologic subtype of the lesions and attributes of the patient, including age, general health, skin color, and skin laxity—should be taken into consideration in choosing an optimal therapy.

The vast majority of BCCs are amenable to surgical treatment. The primary options include curettage and electrodesiccation, excision, and Mohs micrographic surgery. A small but significant subset of BCCs can be treated effectively with Mohs micrographic surgery, which entails microscopic examination of frozen sections of the entire undersurface of the excised specimen at the time of surgery. The technique may be indicated for recurrent lesions and lesions that have a high likelihood of recurrence. Such lesions include ill-defined lesions, large lesions (> 2 cm), lesions with a high-risk histology (i.e., aggressive growth pattern, sclerosing pattern, or perineural involvement), and lesions overlying embryonal fusion planes (e.g., ocular canthi or

nasofacial sulcus). The cure rate of Mohs micrographic technique is significantly higher than the cure rates of other treatments of these high-risk lesions.[8]

Radiation therapy can be an effective, painless, and well-tolerated alternative that is typically reserved for older patients who are poor surgical candidates. Radiation therapy should be avoided, however, in patients with basal cell nevus syndrome. Cryotherapy is another therapeutic option for BCC in patients who are poor surgical candidates.

Topical therapy combined with pharmacotherapy using the immune response modifier imiquimod five times weekly for 6 weeks has been approved by the Food and Drug Administration for the treatment of superficial BCC of the trunk and extremities. One packet (250 mg) of imiquimod 5% cream is applied to 25 cm^2 of affected skin.

Experimental therapies under investigation include intralesional chemotherapy, next-generation topical immune modulators, and photodynamic therapy.

All patients treated for BCC are at risk for local recurrence, and they are at significant risk for the development of additional skin cancers. Patients should be instructed in the self-examination of their skin, as well as in methods of sun protection. In addition, they should receive routine professional follow-up.

Prognosis   The risk of local recurrence relates to the lesion's size, location, and histology. Metastases are very rare: a prevalence of 0.0028% was reported in a series of 50,000 Australians.[9] Metastases occur through both the lymphatic and the hematogenous routes; risk factors include basal cell nevus syndrome, immunosuppression, and previous exposure to ionizing radiation. Metastases that are not amenable to surgical management are associated with a poor outcome.

Squamous Cell Carcinoma

Like BCC, cutaneous SCC arises from the keratinocytes of the epidermis. Histologically, the cells of well-differentiated SCC resemble the cells of the superior portion of the epidermis.

Epidemiology   An estimated 150,000 to 250,000 new cases of cutaneous SCC were diagnosed in the United States in 1994.[10] The estimated mortality from SCC in the United States in 1988 was approximately 0.5 per 100,000. Several lines of data suggest significant increases in SCC incidence. In Australia, for example,

a 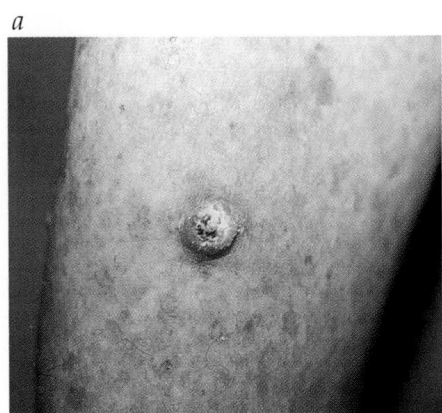 *b*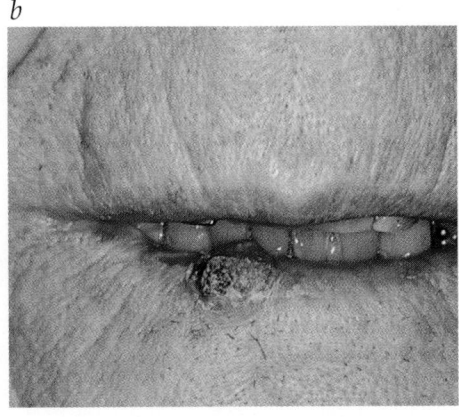

Figure 2 **A squamous cell carcinoma is shown on an arm (*a*) and lower lip (*b*).**

the incidence of SCC increased by 51% between the years 1985 and 1990.[11] In the United States, some of the highest rates of NMSC have been detected in the southwest. A population-based survey in New Mexico found the incidence of SCC doubled in both males and females between 1978 and 1999.[12]

Etiology and risk factors In addition to sunlight, other known etiologic agents that contribute to the development of cutaneous SCC are ionizing radiation, chemical carcinogens, thermal burns, and chronic nonhealing wounds. Sun-related SCCs demonstrate a lower risk of metastases and death than SCCs related to other exposures. Factors involved in predisposition to SCC from sun exposure include light skin color, a tendency to burn, and an inability to tan.

Pathophysiology and pathogenesis Sun-related SCC is often associated with a precursor lesion called an actinic keratosis. Such lesions occur on the scalp, the face, the extensor surfaces of the forearms, and the backs of the hands. They tend to be rough-surfaced, irregularly shaped, and pink. They are often more readily felt than seen. The majority of patients with actinic keratoses have multiple lesions. The risk of SCC in these individuals has been estimated to be as high as 20%.[13] SCC may also appear on normal-looking skin.

SCC of the oral or genital mucosa may arise in precursor lesions termed leukoplakia or erythroplakia. Mucosal SCCs are associated with a significant risk of metastases. Immune surveillance affects the progression of SCC. Immunosuppression, as occurs in transplant recipients and patients with lymphoma, is associated with a high incidence of SCC.[14] In these patients, infection with human papillomavirus appears to play an etiologic role in conjunction with sun exposure. SCCs tend to be more aggressive in immunosuppressed persons.

Diagnosis Most lesions occur in areas of the body that are usually exposed to the sun. The lesions are pinkish, firm plaques that often have a rough, scaly surface [*see Figure 2*]. Biopsy is required for definitive diagnosis.

Differential diagnosis The differential diagnosis of SCC includes keratoacanthoma, Bowen disease, verrucous carcinoma, BCC, hypertrophic actinic keratosis, and common warts.

Keratoacanthomas share many features with SCC, both clinically and histologically. They arise de novo on normal-looking skin and grow very rapidly. They are typically pink, dome-shaped, shiny bumps with a central crateriform keratotic plug that occur on the surface of the skin. They may become very

large. Although keratoacanthomas are not associated with a risk of metastasis, they can be locally destructive. Spontaneous regression of keratoacanthoma over the course of months has been well documented.

Bowen disease is SCC that is confined to the epidermis. It appears as red, scaly, minimally elevated plaques with well-defined, irregular borders. The reported association of Bowen disease with internal malignancy has not held up to closer scrutiny.[15]

SCCs that lack a scaly keratotic surface can be confused with a host of other adnexal and dermal skin tumors.

Treatment Small SCCs evolving from an actinic keratosis can be adequately treated with simple curettage and electrodesiccation. Larger actinic lesions, as well as lesions arising in non–sun-exposed areas of skin, are best treated with definitive surgical excision with confirmation of negative margins. High-risk, ill-defined lesions, especially those occurring in the surgically sensitive areas of the face, genitalia, hands, and feet, are often best treated by Mohs micrographic surgery.

Fractionated radiation therapy is an alternative treatment of primary SCC in older patients who are poor surgical candidates. The benefits of adjuvant radiation therapy are less clear, as are the benefits of sentinel lymph node biopsy and elective lymph node dissection (ELND) for patients with high-risk SCC of the head and neck.

Cytotoxic chemotherapy and biologic response modifiers have been used in patients who have advanced SCC; this therapeutic approach has been reported to have complete response rates of up to 68%, but there are few long-term survivors.[16] Actinic keratoses are treated with cryotherapy, curettage, topical therapies (e.g., fluorouracil, imiquimod, or diclofenac), photodynamic therapy, and laser resurfacing to prevent progression to SCC.[17] Regularly updated guidelines for the treatment of SCC and BCC are available through the National Comprehensive Cancer Network (NCCN).[18]

Prognosis Regardless of the therapy employed, high-risk lesions have a significant rate of local recurrence at 5 years. High-risk SCCs include those in specific anatomic sites (e.g., ears, lips, genitalia, and other non–sun-exposed areas), those greater than 2 cm in diameter, those with aggressive histologic features (depth > 4 mm, Clark level IV and above, and poorly differentiated histology), and those in immunosuppressed patients.[19] The primary route of SCC metastasis is via lymphatic spread to regional lymph nodes. Reported rates of metastasis vary from as low as 0.3% in small, sun-derived lesions to 33% in larger, poorly differentiated lesions.[19] Reported overall 5-

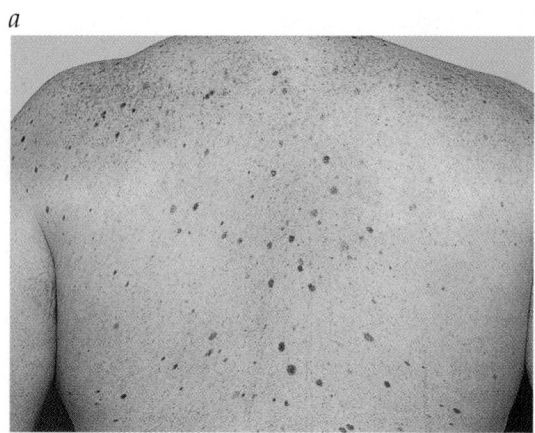
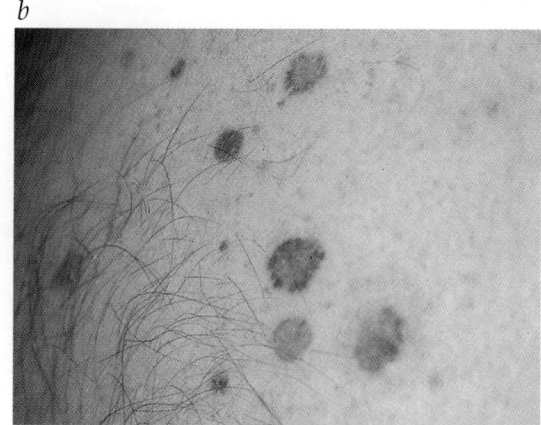

Figure 3 Dysplastic nevi typically are larger than common moles (*a*) and have variegate pigmentation and ill-defined borders (*b*).

year survival rates for patients with regionally metastatic SCC have ranged from 25% to 47%.[19]

MALIGNANT MELANOMA

Epidemiology

In the United States, a person's lifetime risk for developing melanoma is about 1 in 75 (1.3%).[20] Between 1973 and 1994, the incidence of melanoma rose by 121%, and the mortality rose by 39%.[21] Encouraging trends include a shift toward the detection of earlier disease, as well as a stabilization of incidence rates in some segments of the population. In terms of both morbidity and mortality, however, the burden of melanoma-related disease continues to increase. Although melanoma can occur in anyone, it is primarily a disease of whites. Melanomas occurring in blacks are more commonly of the acral lentiginous variety.

Table 1 Adjusted Estimated Relative Risks of Melanoma by Nevus Type and Number[25]

Type	Number	Adjusted Relative Risk*
Nevi > 2 mm and < 5 mm	0–24	1.0
	25–49	1.8 (1.3–2.5)
	50–99	3.0 (2.1–4.4)
	≥ 100	3.4 (2.0–5.7)
Nondysplastic nevi > 5 mm	0	1.0
	1	0.9 (0.7–1.3)
	2–4	1.3 (1.0–1.8)
	5–9	1.7 (1.0–2.7)
	≥ 10	2.3 (1.2–4.3)
Dysplastic nevi	None	1.0
	Indeterminate	1.0 (0.7–1.6)
	1	2.3 (1.4–3.6)
	2–4	7.3 (4.6–12.0)
	5–9	4.9 (2.5–9.8)
	≥ 10	12.0 (4.4–31.0)

*Mutually adjusted and adjusted for age, sex, center, referral pattern, morphologic dysplastic nevi < 5 mm, sunburns, freckles, solar damage, scars, nevus excisions, and family history of melanoma (confidence interval = 95%).

Etiology and Risk Factors

Sun exposure Although strong epidemiologic and basic-science evidence supports an association between melanoma and sun exposure, the relationship appears to be complex.[22] Lentigo maligna melanoma is associated with long-term cumulative sun exposure. Superficial spreading melanoma and nodular melanoma appear to be associated with intense intermittent sun exposure, especially in youth. Acral lentiginous melanoma has no apparent association with sun exposure. Basic-science studies and animal models have implicated different wavelengths of UV in melanoma carcinogenesis; UV wavelength may vary among types of melanoma.

Skin color Melanoma can occur in all racial/ethnic groups but is much more common in lighter-skinned individuals. Among whites, several additional risk factors have been identified, such as fair complexion, a tendency to burn, an inability to tan, freckling, and a family history of melanoma.[22] Screening of the family members of patients with melanoma (particularly multiple melanomas) may be a useful preventive and diagnostic measure.[23]

Moles and dysplastic nevi The strongest phenotypic markers of melanoma risk are moles (nevi)—more specifically, increased numbers of moles and the presence of atypical moles (dysplastic nevi). Melanoma can arise in a preexisting mole or may arise de novo on normal-appearing skin.

Several epidemiologic studies have correlated dysplastic nevi with melanoma risk. Clinically, dysplastic nevi are large (> 5 mm) moles with variegate pigmentation and ill-defined borders [*see Figure 3*]. Histologically, dysplastic nevi are characterized by the presence of architectural atypia and random cytologic atypia. The degree of melanoma risk associated with dysplastic nevi depends on the genetic context. In families with familial melanoma–dysplastic nevus syndrome, the abnormal mole phenotype appears to be inherited in an autosomal dominant fashion. Members of these families with dysplastic nevi have a lifetime melanoma risk that approaches 100%.[24] Outside the context of familial melanoma, dysplastic nevi occur in approximately 5% to 15% of whites. In this general population, dysplastic nevi are markers of increased melanoma risk [*see Table 1*].[25]

Genetic Factors

Approximately 5% of patients with melanomas have a family history of melanoma. Mutations in the cell-cycle regulatory gene *p16* (cyclin-dependent kinase inhibitor–2a) are associated with melanoma in approximately 40% of familial-melanoma families, with linkage of the gene to chromosome 9p.[26] A highly specific activating somatic mutation in the *BRAF* proto-oncogene (a member of the RAF family of kinases) is found in the majority of melanomas and benign nevi, suggesting a pivotal role for this genetic pathway in melanocytic tumor progression.[27] Genomic analyses are beginning to distinguish biologically distinct subsets of melanoma.[28]

Diagnosis

As a pigmented lesion occurring on the surface of the skin, melanoma is amenable to early detection by simple visual inspection at an easily curable stage. Left untreated, melanoma is among the deadliest and most therapeutically unresponsive forms of cancer.

Physical examination Early recognition of melanoma requires attention to pigmented lesions on all body surfaces. Despite the strong association of melanoma with sun exposure, melanomas can occur anywhere on the skin or mucosa. Patients' self-examination, as well as physician examination, must therefore include all skin surfaces, including the scalp, genitalia, and soles of the feet. Any pigmented skin lesion with recent change or with features described by the ABCD mnemonic (asymmetry, border irregularity, color variation, diameter > 6 mm) warrants

consideration of the possibility of melanoma. Although any mole may change gradually over time, any that change color, shape, or size relative to a patient's other moles deserve special attention [*see Figure 4*].[29] Dysplastic nevi present both opportunity and challenge in melanoma detection. On one hand, their recognition allows efficient targeting of a high-risk group. On the other, they can complicate attempts at melanoma detection by clinically mimicking early melanomas. Although some dysplastic nevi may progress to melanoma, the overwhelming majority remain benign. Furthermore, not all melanomas arising in patients with dysplastic nevi develop in a preexisting mole. Wholesale removal of dysplastic nevi is an impractical approach to melanoma prevention. In patients with dysplastic nevi, melanoma detection is predicated on specialized visual examination aided by self-examination and professional follow-up to identify changing lesions.[30]

Diagnostic aids Several specialized aids to the diagnosis of melanoma in patients with dysplastic nevi are under development. Dermoscopy entails the use of a handheld otoscope-like device to magnify a pigmented lesion while applying pressure and oil to the surface. The technique allows the visualization of pigment patterns and features not apparent with simple visual inspection. With experience and training, dermoscopy can be a useful aid in distinguishing melanoma from benign pigmented lesions; however, when used inexpertly, dermoscopy may actually decrease diagnostic accuracy.[30,31] Another aid to melanoma detection in high-risk individuals is photographically assisted follow-up.[32] A baseline set of whole-

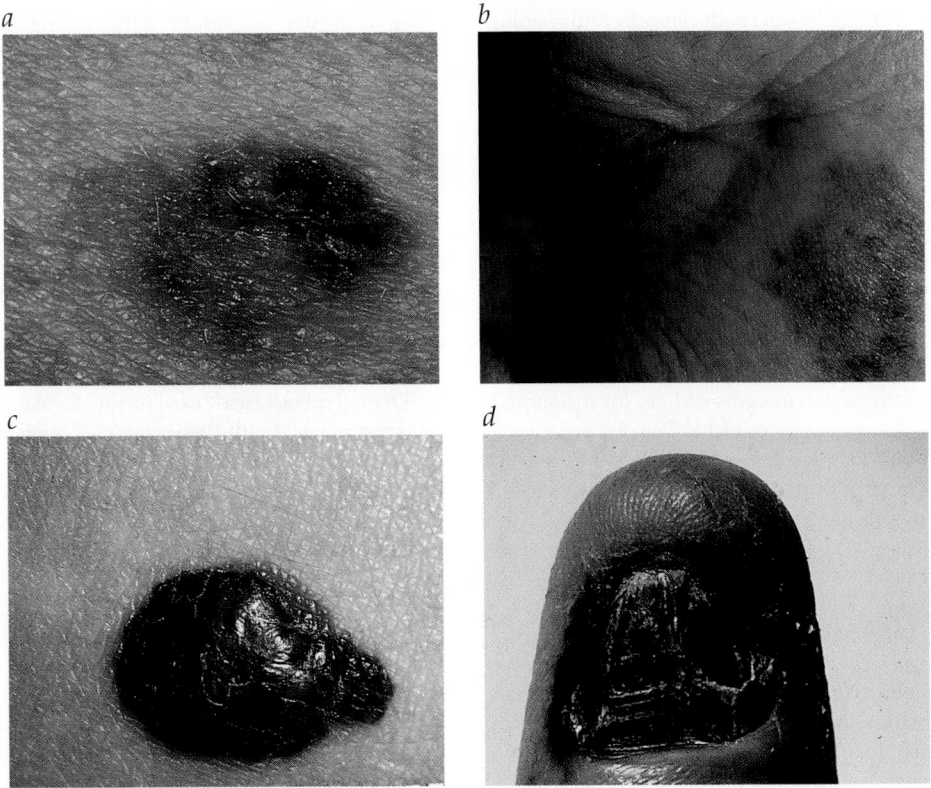

Figure 4 Superficial spreading malignant melanoma begins as a small, irregular brown lesion (*a*). Variation in color and contour is characteristic of lentigo maligna melanoma (*b*). Nodular melanoma often grows more in thickness than in diameter (*c*). Acral lentiginous melanoma can resemble a hematoma under the nail (*d*).

body photographs of the skin are used during self-examination and professional follow-up examination to assess change in the lesions. This procedure helps to prevent unnecessary excision of stable lesions and improves the sensitivity of examinations in detecting change. New imaging technologies such as in vivo confocal scanning laser microscopy hold promise for future improvements in the noninvasive diagnosis of melanoma.[33]

Full-thickness excision and biopsy Any lesion that raises a clinical suspicion of melanoma requires definitive diagnosis. Full-thickness excision is the preferred technique for biopsy of a suspicious pigmented lesion. Partial biopsy can lead to misdiagnosis through sampling error or by depriving the pathologist of a view of the overall architecture and cytology of the lesion. Incisional biopsies with good clinicopathologic correlation may be appropriate, however, in the assessment of large lesions and of lesions occurring in surgically sensitive areas. There is no evidence to suggest that incisional biopsy increases the risk of metastasis.

Differential Diagnosis

Dysplastic nevi share many features with early superficial spreading melanoma. Other common lesions that may mimic melanoma include lentigines, sunburn freckles, traumatized nevi, thrombosed angiomas, pigmented BCCs, pigmented Bowen disease, dermatofibromas, and atypical seborrheic keratoses. Two other challenges in the differential diagnosis of melanoma deserve special mention. Amelanotic melanomas (melanomas without pigment) present as pink lesions that may be misdiagnosed as BCCs or Spitz nevi. Spitz nevi can be difficult to differentiate from melanoma both clinically and histologically. Spitz nevi occur most commonly in children, but they also occur in adults. Like nodular melanomas, Spitz nevi tend to appear suddenly and range in color from red to reddish brown.

Treatment

Primary site Primary cutaneous melanoma is managed surgically with definitive reexcision. The wide excisions of the past have given way to resections with more modest margins. Multiple prospective, randomized trials have investigated the surgical resection of primary cutaneous melanoma utilizing different margins of resection; these studies have focused on varied and overlapping patient populations. On the basis of these data, the NCCN recommends resection margins of 1 cm for melanomas less than 1 mm in thickness, margins of 1 to 2 cm for melanomas between 1 and 2 mm in thickness, and margins of 2 cm for melanomas greater than 2 mm in thickness.[34,35] Primary closure and reconstructive flaps are preferable, cosmetically and functionally, to skin grafts and should be used instead of grafts whenever possible.

Lymph nodes Patients with clinically evident regional lymph node disease are treated with therapeutic lymph node dissection.[34] Elective lymph node dissection in patients with primary melanoma and who have no clinical evidence of lymph node involvement has been abandoned on the basis of the failure of multiple randomized trials to demonstrate an overall survival benefit with this procedure.

Sentinel lymph node biopsy is being increasingly used in patients with primary cutaneous melanoma. This technique utilizes lymphoscintigraphy to identify the draining regional lymph node basins for the skin at the site of the primary melanoma. At the time of definitive reexcision of the melanoma, a blue dye and radioisotope are injected into the dermis around the melanoma site. A small incision is made over the spot that has been identified on lymphoscintigraphy as the proximal area of drainage of the regional lymph node basin. The first lymph node identified as taking up the blue dye and radioisotope (i.e., the sentinel node) is then excised.

The sentinel node is then histologically evaluated, often with the use of immunohistochemical techniques and occasionally with the use of polymerase chain reaction, which is more sensitive. The absence of melanoma in the sentinel node is highly sensitive for ruling out the presence of metastases in the remainder of the lymph node basin when the procedure is performed by an experienced team. When the sentinel node is found to be positive for melanoma, a "completion" lymph node dissection of the affected basin is typically performed. Prospective studies have demonstrated sentinel node status to be strongly correlated with 5-year survival.[36] Patients with positive sentinel nodes are appropriate candidates for consideration of adjuvant therapy [see Adjuvant Therapy, below]. Several multicenter trials are currently under way to assess the clinical utility of this procedure.[37] Initial reports from the first of these trials have failed to indicate an overall survival advantage associated with the procedure.[38]

In-transit metastases In-transit metastases are metastases that establish tumors within regional dermal and subcutaneous lymphatics before reaching the regional lymph nodes. In-transit metastases can remain confined to a single limb for prolonged periods. Amputation does not appear to provide a long-term survival benefit in this setting.[34] Slow-growing individual in-transit metastases can be managed surgically. More extensive disease can be treated with sensitization therapy with dinitrochlorobenzene (DNCB), intralesional interferon, or topical agents for modifying the immune response. For extensive in-transit metastases confined to an extremity, limb perfusion therapy can result in dramatic palliation and limb salvage. The procedure entails isolation of the vasculature of the involved extremity from the systemic vasculature and perfusion of the isolated limb with chemotherapeutic agents, biologic agents, or both at doses that could not be tolerated if given systemically.[39]

Distant metastases Despite the development of several novel approaches to the treatment of patients with metastatic melanoma, including multiagent chemotherapy, biologic therapy, immunotherapy, and combinations of these treatments, no regimens have demonstrated a clear survival advantage over single-agent chemotherapy. Monotherapy with dacarbazine (2 to 4.5 mg/kg daily for 10 days, repeated every 4 weeks) or recombinant interleukin-2 (IL-2) (600,000 IU/kg every 8 hours for up to 14 doses) are the only treatment regimens approved by the FDA for the treatment of metastatic melanoma. Objective responses to dacarbazine are seen in approximately 5% to 20% of patients; durable complete responses are rare.[40] Objective responses to IL-2, a significantly more toxic agent, are seen in approximately 15% of patients; durable responses are seen in about 5%. Radiation therapy can play an important palliative role. In the absence of more effective clinically proven therapy, patients with distant metastases should be offered the opportunity to participate in clinical trials of experimental therapy. Many current experimental therapies are

Table 2   AJCC TNM Classification[45]

TNM Classification	Tumor Thickness, Node Number, Metastases Site	Subclassification
T classification T1	≤ 1.0 mm	a: Without ulceration and Clark level II or III b: With ulceration or Clark level IV or V
T2	1.01–2.0 mm	a: Without ulceration b: With ulceration
T3	2.01–4.0 mm	a: Without ulceration b: With ulceration
T4	> 4.0 mm	a: Without ulceration b: With ulceration
N classification N1	One lymph node	a: Micrometastasis* b. Macrometastasis†
N2	2–3 lymph nodes	a: Micrometastasis* b. Macrometastasis† c: In-transit met(s)/satellites(s) without metastatic lymph nodes
N3	4 or more metastatic lymph nodes, matted lymph nodes, or combination of in-transit met(s)/satellite(s) with metastatic lymph nodes	—
M classification M1a	Distant skin, subcutaneous, or lymph node mets	Normal LDH
M1b	Lung mets	Normal LDH
M1c	All other visceral mets Any distant mets	Normal LDH Elevated LDH with any M

*Micrometastases are diagnosed after sentinel or elective lymphadenectomy.
†Macrometastases are defined as clinically detectable nodal metastases confirmed by therapeutic lymphadenectomy; the term also applies to nodal metastases that exhibit gross extracapsular extension.
AJCC—American Joint Committee on Cancer   LD—lactic dehydrogenase   mets—metastases

predicated on decades of experience with immunotherapy of melanoma, as well as the recent availability of pharmacologic inhibitors of elements of the Ras signaling pathway that are implicated in melanoma pathogenesis.[40]

Adjuvant therapy   Patients with cutaneous or regional disease who have been surgically rendered disease free but who are at high risk for recurrence or metastasis are potential candidates for adjuvant therapy.[41] Various adjuvant therapies have been used in melanoma, including immunostimulants such as bacillus Calmette-Guérin, *Corynebacterium parvum,* and levamisole. Several chemotherapeutic agents have been tried as well. More recently, immunotherapies with cytokines, such as interferons, and active immunization with vaccines have been studied. A high-dose regimen of interferon alfa (20 million units/m² I.V. daily for 1 month followed by 10 million units/m² S.C. three times a week for 48 weeks) has been approved by the FDA for use as adjuvant therapy for melanoma. Two studies have demonstrated a small but statistically significant improvement in overall survival with this regimen. Multiple studies have failed to demonstrate improved long-term overall survival with the use of adjuvant interferon in intermediate-dose or low-dose regimens.[42,43]

A host of novel strategies, including active immunization, passive immunization, and myriad biologic therapies, are currently being studied and may provide opportunities for patients who are appropriate candidates for trials.[44]

Prognosis

Stage   The single strongest prognostic factor for melanoma is stage of disease. Various staging classifications have been used over the years. All staging systems for melanoma take into account the classic TNM classification of tumor size (T), lymph node involvement (N), and distant metastases (M). The differences across staging systems relate largely to the staging of the primary site. New staging systems attempt to use the attributes of the primary tumor that strongly correlate with outcome. These attributes include thickness, ulceration, and, in the case of thin melanomas measuring less than 1 mm thick, the Clark level of invasion. The advent of sentinel node biopsy has led to the inclusion of microstaging of lymph nodes in the staging system [*see Tables 2 and 3*].[45,46]

Attributes of the primary tumor   Several attributes of the primary tumor have been identified as predictors of outcome from primary cutaneous melanoma. A strong predictor of outcome is the Breslow tumor thickness, which is measured in millimeters from the granular layer of the epidermis to the deepest tumor cell. Other important histologic parameters are the Clark level of tumor invasion, the presence or absence of ulceration, the rate of mitosis, the presence of tumor-infiltrating lymphocytes, and vascular invasion. For thin primary melanomas, one of the strongest predictors of outcome is growth phase.[47] Radial-growth-phase melanoma does not appear to metastasize, whereas vertical-growth-phase melanoma (characterized by the for-

Table 3 AJCC Staging System and Survival Rate[45]

Pathologic Stage	TNM	5-Year Survival	10-Year Survival
IA	T1a	95.3 ± 0.4	87.9 ± 1.0
IB	T1b	90.9 ± 1.0	83.1 ± 1.5
	T2a	89.0 ± 0.7	79.2 ± 1.1
IIA	T2b	77.4 ± 1.7	64.4 ± 2.2
	T3a	78.7 ± 1.2	63.8 ± 1.7
IIB	T3b	63.0 ± 1.5	50.8 ± 1.7
	T4a	67.4 ± 2.4	53.9 ± 3.3
IIC	T4b	45.1 ± 1.9	32.3 ± 2.1
IIIA	N1a	69.5 ± 3.7	63.0 ± 4.4
	N2a	63.3 ± 5.6	56.9 ± 6.8
IIIB	N1a	52.8 ± 4.1	37.8 ± 4.8
	N2a	49.6 ± 5.7	35.9 ± 7.2
	N1b	59.0 ± 4.8	47.7 ± 5.8
	N2b	46.3 ± 5.5	39.2 ± 5.8
IIIC	N1b	29.0 ± 5.1	24.4 ± 5.3
	N2b	24.0 ± 4.4	15.0 ± 3.9
	N3	26.7 ± 2.5	18.4 ± 2.5
IV	M1a	18.8 ± 3.0	15.7 ± 2.9
	M1b	6.7 ± 2.0	2.5 ± 1.5
	M1c	9.5 ± 1.1	6.0 ± 0.9

AJCC—American Joint Committee on Cancer

mation of a tumor nodule in the dermis) is associated with significant risk of metastasis even in lesions less than 1 mm thick.[48] Patient characteristics associated with improved survival from melanoma include young age (< 60 years), female sex, and location of the melanoma on an extremity other than the palms or soles. Multivariable models for predicting outcome from melanoma have been developed [*see Table 4*].[49]

Malignant Tumors of the Dermis

METASTATIC TUMORS

Cutaneous metastases occur in approximately 5% of patients with solid tumors and are usually associated with widespread disease. The relative frequency of skin metastases is gender specific, reflecting the rates of the primary cancers.[50] In women, two thirds of metastases are from breast cancer, but lung cancer, colorectal cancer, melanoma, and ovarian cancer are also frequent. In men, lung cancer is most common, followed by cancer of the large intestine, melanoma, SCC of the head and neck, and cancer of the kidneys.[50] The anatomic distribution of skin metastases is not random. Cutaneous metastases from breast cancer often involve the chest wall and may appear as nodules, lymphedema, or cellulitis. The scalp is a common site for metastasis, especially of cancer from the lung and kidney (in men) and breast (in women). Head and neck cancers may invade the skin by local extension, giving rise to a firm, dusky-red edema of the skin that resembles cellulitis. Abdominal wall metastases, often called Sister Joseph's nodules, may occur with gastrointestinal or ovarian malignancies.[50] Clinically, cutaneous metastases are often minimally symptomatic dermal papules or nodules and are flesh-col-

ored or pink; dissemination occurs via lymphatic or vascular pathways. Cutaneous metastases may clinically reflect the histology of the primary tumor (e.g., black, brown, or gray nodules with metastatic melanoma, and vascular nodules with renal cell or thyroid carcinoma).

PRIMARY TUMORS

Primary malignancies of the dermis may develop from any of the myriad structures of the skin, including sebaceous glands (sebaceous carcinoma), connective tissue (dermatofibrosarcoma protuberans), smooth muscle (leiomyosarcoma), and other adnexal tissue (eccrine carcinoma). Most of these primary dermal neoplasms are rare; they may exhibit aggressive biologic behavior. Although these neoplasms are quite varied histologically, many share a common clinical presentation of a rapidly growing flesh-colored to pink or red subcutaneous nodule that occasionally resembles a sebaceous cyst.

Merkel cell carcinoma This neoplasm is a dermal malignancy of neuroendocrine origin. It usually appears as a red to violaceous dermal papule or nodule on the head and neck of elderly patients, although all age groups are affected. The treatment of choice is wide local excision with or without lymphadenectomy. Sentinel node biopsy has been proposed by some for evaluation of the regional lymph nodes. Adjuvant radiation therapy can be considered. Local recurrences are frequent, and distant metastases occur in more than one third of patients. Chemotherapy of metastases is generally disappointing.[51,52]

Paget disease A rare malignancy of the skin associated with an underlying adenocarcinoma,[50,51] Paget disease usually presents as an erythematous, often weeping unilateral dermatitis of the breast that involves the nipple and areola. The differential diagnosis includes eczema, psoriasis, contact dermatitis, and impetigo. For this reason, biopsy of an inflammatory, nonresolving dermatitis of the nipple or areola is imperative. In Paget disease, the biopsy will reveal typical pale-staining Paget cells in the epidermis. Appropriate surgical resection of the cutaneous and underlying neoplasm is the treatment of choice; lymph node metastases often occur.[51]

Extramammary Paget disease Extramammary Paget disease is even more uncommon than Paget disease. It typically presents as red, often ulcerated, plaques in the perineal areas of elderly persons.[50,51] Lesions may be pruritic or asymptomatic, are often long-standing, and may have been misdiagnosed as psoriasis, contact dermatitis, or chronic fungal infection. Underlying associated tumors include rectal and genitourinary carcinomas. Even without an associated internal malignancy, extramammary Paget disease is difficult to treat, and it is associated with a high local recurrence rate.[51]

Angiosarcoma A rare, often highly aggressive vascular malignancy,[51] angiosarcoma may appear as multicentric reddish-purple patches or nodules in a lymphedematous limb, such as on a lymphedematous arm after a mastectomy (Stewart-Treves syndrome). Another presentation is violaceous patches or plaques on the head or neck (especially scalp) of elderly persons. Patients with angiosarcoma have a poor prognosis, with pulmonary metastases frequently developing despite surgery or radiation.[51]

Dermatofibrosarcoma protuberans Dermatofibrosarcoma protuberans is a slow-growing, locally aggressive malignancy that rarely metastasizes but often recurs. Lesions typically present as firm reddish-brown or purple nodules, usually on the trunk or non–sun-exposed extremities. The differential diagnosis includes keloids and benign dermatofibroma. Young adults are most often affected, although the tumor may occur at any age. Wide local excision with or without Mohs micrographic surgery offers the best chance of cure.[51]

KAPOSI SARCOMA

Kaposi sarcoma (KS) is a multicentric cutaneous neoplasm that has four distinct clinical variants.[53-56] In spite of its name, KS is not a true sarcoma. Although the cell of origin has not been clearly established,[53,54] KS cells share phenotypic markers with lymphatic endothelium, as well as vascular smooth muscle cells, suggesting a vascular or pluripotent mesenchymal cell origin.[56] In its classic form, KS is an indolent disease of elderly men of Mediterranean or eastern European origin, in which violaceous nodules and plaques develop on the lower extremities.[53-55] A second variant, lymphadenopathic KS, is endemic to some areas of Africa. African KS, which typically affects young adults and children, pursues a more aggressive course than classic KS, with frequent bone, lymph node, and visceral involvement.[53-55] A third variant of KS occurs in iatrogenically immunosuppressed patients, especially organ transplant recipients.[57] In this variant, men are affected slightly more often than women.[53-55] The fourth variant is an aggressive epidemic KS that occurs in AIDS patients.

Epidemiology

Before the advent of AIDS, KS was rare in the United States, with an age-adjusted annual incidence of 0.29 per 100,000 population in men and 0.07 per 100,000 population in women.[54] KS was an AIDS-defining illness for 30% to 40% of patients in the earliest years of the HIV epidemic.[53] During that period, the incidence of KS in HIV-infected homosexual men was 73,000-fold higher than in the general United States population; in HIV-in-

fected women and HIV-infected nonhomosexual men, the incidence was 10,000-fold higher.[52,53] The incidence has significantly declined since the introduction of highly active antiretroviral therapy (HAART). For example, in a large European-based study of HIV-infected patients, there was an estimated 39% annual reduction in the incidence of KS between 1994 and 2003, such that the incidence of KS in 2003 was 10% less than that reported in 1994.[58]

Etiology and Risk Factors

Human herpesvirus type 8 The epidemiology of KS has long suggested a transmissible infectious agent or cofactor.[53-55] Kaposi sarcoma–associated herpesvirus (KSHV), also known as human herpesvirus type 8 (HHV-8), has been detected in all variants of KS.[59] HHV-8 has also been found in patients with body cavity–based lymphoma, Castleman disease, and angioblastic lymphadenopathy, as well as in certain skin lesions of organ transplant recipients.[53] The mechanism by which HHV-8 infection leads to KS tumorigenesis is unclear but probably involves a complex combination of inflammation, angiogenesis, and neoplastic proliferation.[53,54] The prevalence of KS largely parallels the rate of HHV-8 infection in various populations.[54] Although the incidence of HHV-8 infection may be as high as 2% to 10% in the general population, the incidence of KS is very low, suggesting that the majority of infections are subclinical.[53,54]

Host factors Host factors, particularly immunosuppression, are crucial in some populations with KS.[47,48,50] HIV may play an indirect role in the development of KS through CD4+ T cell depletion and stimulated production of growth factors and cytokines such as IL-1 and IL-6.[53,54,56] Immunosuppressive drugs, especially cyclosporine, azathioprine, and prednisone, increase the risk of developing KS, primarily in kidney and liver transplant recipients.[49]

Despite the prevalence of KS in some ethnic groups, the role of any possible genetic factors is unclear. An increased incidence of HLA-DR5 in patients with classic KS has been debated.[54] Fa-

Table 4 Estimated Probability of 10-Year Survival in Patients with Primary Cutaneous Melanoma[47]

Tumor Thickness/Age of Patient	Probability of 10-Year Survival*			
	Tumor with Extremity Location		Tumor with Axis Location†	
	Female Patients	Male Patients	Female Patients	Male Patients
< 0.76 mm				
≤ 60 yr	0.99 (0.98–1.0)	0.98 (0.95–0.99)	0.97 (0.93–0.99)	0.94 (0.88–0.97)
> 60 yr	0.98 (0.95–0.99)	0.96 (0.89–0.98)	0.92 (0.82–0.96)	0.84 (0.70–0.93)
0.76–1.69 mm				
≤ 60 yr	0.96 (0.92–0.98)	0.93 (0.85–0.97)	0.86 (0.76–0.92)	0.75 (0.62–0.84)
> 60 yr	0.90 (0.80–0.95)	0.81 (0.64–0.91)	0.67 (0.50–0.81)	0.50 (0.33–0.67)
1.70–3.60 mm				
≤ 60 yr	0.89 (0.80–0.94)	0.80 (0.65–0.89)	0.65 (0.50–0.77)	0.48 (0.35–0.61)
> 60 yr	0.73 (0.57–0.85)	0.57 (0.38–0.75)	0.38 (0.24–0.55)	0.24 (0.14–0.37)
> 3.60 mm				
≤ 60 yr	0.74 (0.53–0.87)	0.58 (0.36–0.77)	0.39 (0.21–0.60)	0.24 (0.13–0.40)
> 60 yr	0.48 (0.28–0.69)	0.32 (0.16–0.53)	0.18 (0.08–0.35)	0.10 (0.04–0.20)

*Confidence interval = 95%.
†Axis location includes the trunk, head, neck, and volar and subungual sites.

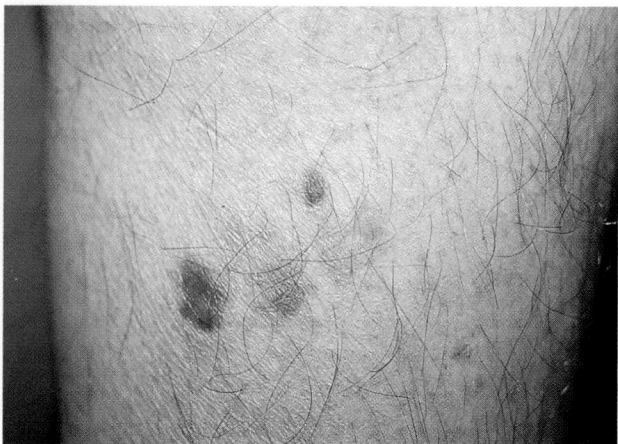

Figure 5 HIV-associated Kaposi sarcoma lesions vary from pink patches (shown) to deep-purple plaques.

milial KS is extremely rare, suggesting that genetic factors alone are not responsible.

Finally, gender appears to be a significant risk factor, especially in classic KS, in which the male-to-female ratio may range from 3:1 to 10:1.[53,54] The reasons for this male predominance remain unclear.[48,49]

Diagnosis

Clinical manifestations The clinical manifestations of KS differ among the variants of the disorder.[53-55] In classic KS, faint reddish-purple macules or patches or purple nodules first appear on the feet, especially the soles. Lymphadenopathy (especially inguinal) is present on rare occasions. Lesions may also occasionally develop on the arms and genital areas. As the disease progresses, the lesions coalesce into violaceous plaques.

HIV-associated KS usually presents as cutaneous lesions, but the first lesions may appear in the oral mucosa or lymph nodes. In contrast to classic KS lesions, HIV-associated KS lesions often begin on the upper body (face, trunk, or arms). Most typically, HIV-associated KS lesions are purple-red, often oval, papules that follow a pityriasis rosea–like distribution [*see Chapter 36*].[53-55] Lesions vary from pink macules to deep-purple plaques [*see Figure 5*] or may resemble ecchymoses, especially in patients with low CD4[+] T cell counts. Oral lesions are typically red-purple plaques or nodules on the palate, gingiva, or buccal mucosa. Patients with darker skin may have dark-purple to black lesions or hyperpigmented plaques.[54]

As HIV-associated KS progresses, lymphedema may develop in the feet, scrotum, genitalia, and periorbital regions, and lymphadenopathy (especially inguinal) may occur. Gastrointestinal lesions are usually submucosal and asymptomatic but may result in gastrointestinal hemorrhage. Pulmonary KS carries a poor prognosis.[54]

Laboratory studies Laboratory workup of patients with KS should include HIV antibody testing, complete blood count, fecal occult blood testing, and chest radiograph. CD4[+] T cell counts are indicated in HIV-positive patients. A complete medical history and physical examination should be performed, with special attention paid to the presence of opportunistic infections in HIV-infected or otherwise immunosuppressed patients. Skin biopsy should be obtained in patients with suspected KS. The histopathology of KS is characterized by the presence of spindle-

shaped cells in the dermis, with extravasated red blood cells present in slits between irregular vascular spaces.[55]

Differential Diagnosis

The clinical differential diagnosis of KS includes dermatofibroma, purpura, pyogenic granuloma, bacillary angiomatosis, metastatic melanoma, and BCC. Other histopathologic entities that may resemble KS include angiosarcoma and stasis dermatitis.[55]

Treatment

Classic Kaposi sarcoma The therapy for KS is palliative. In classic KS, where the disease is indolent and the patients are elderly, aggressive systemic therapy is rarely warranted.[53,54] Instead, radiation therapy is the treatment of choice.[54,60] KS is very radiosensitive: single doses of 800 cGy have been used for rapid palliation in patients with poor prognoses. Total doses of 800 to 3,500 cGy have yielded 50% complete responses and 46% partial responses, with more than half of patients needing no follow-up treatment for as long as 13 years.[60] A treatment regimen equivalent to 3,000 cGy in 10 fractions over 2 weeks has been advocated.[60]

For patients with classic KS who have only one or two papules, excisional biopsy may be sufficient for both diagnosis and treatment. Cryotherapy with liquid nitrogen may be useful for isolated papules. Systemic therapy for classic KS may be indicated in cases of extensive cutaneous disease or visceral involvement. Single-agent chemotherapy with vinca alkaloids (i.e., vincristine or vinblastine) is commonly used. Low-dose recombinant interferon alfa may also be effective in classic KS; however, side effects (e.g., fever, chills, myalgias, and fatigue) may not be well tolerated by elderly patients.[53,54]

Transplant-associated Kaposi sarcoma Spontaneous KS regression has been observed in transplant recipients after withdrawal of cyclosporine and corticosteroids.[54] Sirolimus (rapamycin), an immunosuppressive drug with antineoplastic and antiangiogenic properties, was successfully used in 15 renal transplant recipients who developed KS. After KS was diagnosed, cyclosporine and mycophenolate mofetil were discontinued and sirolimus was started. Cutaneous KS resolved in all patients, without episodes of acute rejection or changes in renal graft function.[58]

HIV-associated Kaposi sarcoma Although KS is more aggressive in HIV-infected patients, the extent of immune suppression and the presence of opportunistic infections or other systemic illnesses may be of equal importance in staging, determining prognosis, and choosing appropriate therapy.[53,54] Clinical features that were traditionally associated with a more favorable outcome included a CD4[+] T cell count higher than 200 cells/mm[3], a lack of systemic illness, KS limited to the skin or lymph nodes, and minimal (i.e., not nodular) oral KS; poor risk factors included a CD4[+] T cell count below 200 cells/mm[3], KS-associated lymphedema, visceral KS, ulcerated KS, nodular oral KS, and opportunistic infection.[61] With the advent of HAART, however, physicians treating patients with HIV-associated KS now have the opportunity to influence and even reverse immune suppression by affecting both HIV viral load and the CD4[+] T cell count. Regression of KS has been observed after initiation of HAART, often during the first few months of therapy[56,62]; consequently, this is often first-line therapy for patients with limited cutaneous HIV-associated KS.[54]

Local therapy is a reasonable approach in KS patients with limited disease, those with infectious complications, and those who cannot tolerate systemic therapy.[62] Radiation therapy is effective in HIV-associated KS in doses similar to those used for classic KS (see above). Responses in HIV-associated KS are generally short-lived, however.[54] Topical alitretinoin (9-*cis*-retinoic acid) gel may be effective in HIV-associated KS and has been approved by the FDA for this use.[62] Intralesional injections of vinblastine or interferon have also been useful in selected lesions.[53,54] Cryotherapy with liquid nitrogen is effective for small lesions[62]; however, cryotherapy is contraindicated in dark-skinned patients in whom posttreatment hypopigmentation may appear much worse cosmetically than the original KS lesion.

Systemic therapy has included conventional chemotherapy and biologic response modifiers. For patients with slowly progressive, limited cutaneous KS (< 25 lesions), systemic antitumor therapy may not be necessary; HAART with or without local therapy may be sufficient.[51] However, HAART alone has not been demonstrated to be the treatment of choice for advanced HIV-associated KS.[63] Liposomal anthracyclines (e.g., doxorubicin, daunomycin) are approved by the FDA as first-line therapy of HIV-associated KS.[64-66] A reasonable approach to the treatment of advanced HIV-associated KS is the use of a combination of HAART and liposomal anthracyclines, followed by a combination of HAART plus paclitaxel if response to the first regimen is inadequate.[56,63,65] Promising investigational approaches for HIV-associated KS include antiangiogenic compounds, thalidomide, matrix metalloproteinase inhibitors, and retinoids. Prevention of HIV-associated KS may also be achieved through antiviral therapy of HHV-8.[62]

Complications

Bacterial infections and sepsis are common in patients with KS and may be associated with ulcerated tumors of the legs and feet. Opportunistic infections may intervene, especially in patients with very low $CD4^+$ T cell counts.

Prognosis

The total $CD4^+$ T cell count is the most important predictor of survival in HIV-associated KS.[61] Large tumor burdens, lymphedema, and pulmonary KS are also predictive of poorer outcomes.[61,65]

Cutaneous Lymphoma

Lymphomas may be of B cell or T cell lineage and may involve the skin primarily or secondarily [*see Chapter 193*]. B cell lymphomas, particularly non-Hodgkin lymphomas, may involve the skin secondarily in advanced disease. They typically appear as reddish-purple subcutaneous plaques or nodules. Primary B cell lymphomas of the skin are even rarer. They appear as reddish nodules that often remain localized to the skin but may progress to systemic disease. The vast majority of primary cutaneous lymphomas fall into the spectrum of cutaneous T cell lymphoma (CTCL).

CTCL includes mycosis fungoides (MF) and Sézary syndrome, which is a leukemic variant of MF.[66,67] MF is the largest subset of CTCL; the two terms, however, sometimes are used interchangeably. Another variant of CTCL is associated with human T cell lymphotropic virus type I (HTLV-I) and is part of the spectra of adult T cell lymphoma/leukemia and peripheral T cell lymphoma.[66]

EPIDEMIOLOGY

CTCL is a rare disorder. In the United States, approximately 1,000 new cases of CTCL are diagnosed annually.[66] From 1973 to 1984, the incidence of CTCL rose from 0.19 per 100,000 population to 0.42 per 100,000 population. CTCL primarily affects middle-aged adults; the median age at presentation is 50 years.[68] The male-to-female ratio is approximately 2:1; blacks are twice as likely as whites to develop CTCL.[68]

ETIOLOGY

Host susceptibility and an environmental antigen, perhaps viral, are hypothesized as playing important roles in the pathogenesis of CTCL.[66] Genetic factors may be related to major histocompatibility antigens, such as an increase in HLA-DRB1*11 (formerly HLA-DR5) and HLA-DQB1*03.[69] Chronic antigenic stimulation (e.g., infection) may play an etiologic role.[66] For example, HTLV-I infection may be an etiologic factor in the development of the peripheral T cell lymphoma variant.[66]

DIAGNOSIS

Clinical Manifestations

The clinical manifestations of MF typically evolve over many months to years. In one classic study, the mean duration of symptoms before diagnosis was 7.5 years.[70] Flat, erythematous patches, often scaling and occasionally atrophic, begin most commonly on the trunk and thighs, especially in a so-called bathing-trunk distribution [*see Figure 6*]. Lesions are asymptomatic or mildly pruritic and may spontaneously remit or respond to topical corticosteroid therapy. Patients may also report improvement after sun exposure. As MF progresses, patches tend to enlarge and thicken into plaques. The color may become dark red; in dark-skinned persons, the lesions may initially be hyperpigmented or hypopigmented and may acquire an erythematous or violaceous hue. In advanced MF, tumors may develop or transform to a large-cell lymphoma.[66,67,71]

In approximately 10% of cases, tumors are the initial presentation of CTCL (tumor d'emblée). Generalized erythroderma with circulating atypical T cells (in Sézary syndrome) is the presentation in 5% of CTCL patients.[66,67]

Physical examination of patients with suspected CTCL includes complete skin examination, including classification of lesions (patch, plaque, or tumor) and extent of body surface area involved. Lymph nodes, the liver, and the spleen should be palpated.

Skin Biopsy

Skin biopsy is necessary for the definitive diagnosis of CTCL. The presence of atypical lymphoid cells with hyperconvoluted cerebriform nuclei in clusters in the epidermis (Pautrier microabscesses) and a bandlike lymphocytic infiltrate in the upper dermis are diagnostic of CTCL.[66,67] The malignant cell is a T cell, with most of the cells expressing the pan–T cell markers CD2, CD3, and CD5, as well as frequent deletion of CD7, CD26, or both.[66,67,72] The use of T cell receptor gene rearrangement studies to confirm clonality in early disease may be an aid to diagnosis.[66] Neither immunophenotypic studies nor electron microscopy may be considered to be definitively diagnostic of CTCL; clinicopathologic correlation is necessary.

a

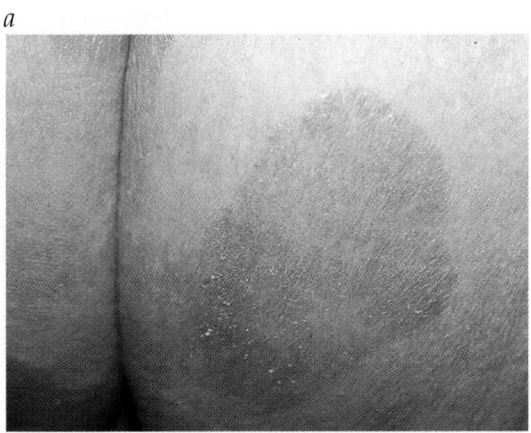

b

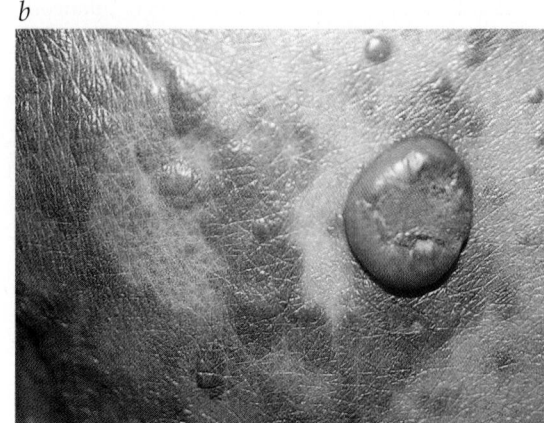

Figure 6   Cutaneous T cell lymphoma is shown in the large-patch stage (*a*) and as tumor-stage mycosis fungoides (*b*).

Laboratory Studies

The laboratory evaluation for CTCL includes complete blood count, eosinophil count, Sézary cell count, lactic dehydrogenase level, and liver function tests. Bone marrow biopsy is unnecessary in the absence of circulating leukemic cells. HTLV-I testing should be considered for patients with risk factors or atypical presentations. Lymph node biopsy should be considered for palpable nodes, especially those larger than 2 cm. Abdominal computed tomography or chest radiography may be important in patients with tumors or suspected visceral involvement.

DIFFERENTIAL DIAGNOSIS

In its early stages, CTCL may resemble any of a number of benign inflammatory disorders (e.g., drug reaction, eczema, psoriasis, or contact dermatitis). These disorders should be ruled out before contemplating therapy.

STAGING

The staging of CTCL is based on an evaluation of the type and extent of skin lesions and the extent of lymph node, peripheral blood, and visceral involvement.[70,71] Early disease is characterized by limited patch or plaque disease (stage IA) or generalized patch or plaque disease without evidence of extracutaneous involvement (stages IB and IIA); more advanced disease is characterized by cutaneous tumors (stage IIB), extracutaneous disease (stage III), and extracutaneous disease involving either lymph nodes (stage IVA) or viscera (stage IVB).

TREATMENT

Topical Therapy

Topical therapy is the mainstay of the treatment of early disease (stage IA, IB, and IIA). Early aggressive therapy with radiation and chemotherapy has not proved to be superior to local approaches in controlling disease or improving survival in patients with limited disease.[66,67] A rational approach for treating early limited (or histologically equivocal) disease is topical corticosteroids.[73] Topical nitrogen mustard (mechlorethamine), in either aqueous or ointment form, is the most frequently used topical chemotherapy. In one series, the overall response rate to nitrogen mustard was 83%, with a complete response rate of 50%, after a median treatment time of 12 months.[74] Median time to relapse was also 12 months.[74]

Carmustine (BCNU) solution, applied daily to lesions, is another useful regimen. Treatment generally lasts 8 to 16 weeks but has been continued for up to 6 months. Because systemic absorption can result in bone marrow suppression, complete blood counts must be monitored.[62] Bexarotene, a topical retinoid, has been shown to be effective in CTCL; it is approved by the FDA for use in CTCL.[75]

Ultraviolet Radiation

Radiation therapy for CTCL takes several forms, from ultraviolet light to ionizing radiation. UVB is useful in stage I disease. In a retrospective study of 21 patients with stage I disease, narrowband UVB led to complete remission in 81% of patients and to partial remission in 19%; the mean relapse-free interval was 24.5 months.[76]

Another effective approach to treatment of CTCL is the combination of psoralen and UVA (PUVA). In one study, 65% of patients with stage I CTCL had complete clinical clearing, with a mean relapse-free interval of 43 months; the disease-free survival rates at 5 and 10 years for stage IA were 56% and 30%, respectively.[77] In another study, complete remission was observed in 71% of early-stage patients; in this study, the mean relapse-free interval was 22.8 months.[76]

Radiation Therapy

Total skin electron beam (TSEB) radiation delivers radiotherapy to the skin surface without a significant internal dose. It is especially useful with plaque disease. Typical doses are 2,400 to 3,600 cGy, fractionated over several weeks with 4 to 9 MeV electron beam radiation.[78] Treatment responses are related to CTCL stage[79]; early-stage (stage IA) patients have a 95% response rate, but 50% will experience relapse within 10 years. TSEB may also be useful in stage IB disease (90% remission rate), but two thirds of patients treated with this modality will experience relapse within 5 years.[73] Patients with tumor-stage (stage IIB) CTCL may receive effective palliation from TSEB, especially in combination with other therapies.[79]

Systemic Therapy

Systemic therapy has been undertaken as primary therapy in advanced CTCL (stages III through IVB); in early-stage disease, systemic therapy is used as part of sequential therapy to promote more durable responses.[66,67]

Oral bexarotene has yielded response rates of up to 45% in advanced CTCL, and it is approved by the FDA for use in this disease.[80] Another systemic therapy used in the treatment of advanced CTCL is denileukin diftitox [DAB(389) IL-2].[81] This receptor-targeted cytotoxic fusion protein binds to the IL-2 receptor on T cells; it achieved a 30% response rate in heavily-pretreated patients.[81]

Extracorporeal photopheresis, which is an accepted therapy for advanced CTCL, appears most useful in erythrodermic CTCL and Sézary syndrome.[66,67] In this treatment, the patient is given a photoactivating drug (8-methoxypsoralen), the patient's white blood cells are collected via leukapheresis and irradiated with UVA, and the irradiated cells are returned to the patient intravenously. Advanced CTCL characterized by cutaneous tumors (stage III) or visceral involvement (stage IV) has also been treated with single-agent and combination chemotherapy using methotrexate, adenosine analogues, interferon alfa, and retinoids.[66,67,82]

Combination Therapy

Early aggressive treatment using TSEB followed by combination chemotherapy provides no survival advantage over sequential topical therapy.[83,84] In a randomized controlled trial, 103 patients with MF received TSEB followed by either parenteral chemotherapy with cylophosphamide, doxorubicin, etoposide, and vincristine or sequential topical treatment. Patients receiving combined therapy had a significantly higher rate of complete response than those receiving sequential topical therapy; however, there was no difference in the rates of disease-free and overall survival between the two groups after a mean follow-up of 75 months.[83] In an uncontrolled study, multimodality therapy was examined in patients with early and advanced disease. In this study, 95 CTCL patients received in consecutive phases of therapy interferon alfa and oral isotretinoin, TSEB, and maintenance therapy consisting of topical nitrogen mustard and interferon alfa. Patients with advanced disease also received six cycles of combination chemotherapy before TSEB. Although multimodality therapy resulted in high response rates (85% response, 60% complete response), the study provided no evidence that this form of combination therapy could improve the overall survival rates currently achieved with sequential topical therapy.[80] In general, the heterogeneity of reported combination therapy regimens in CTCL makes it virtually impossible to compare results.

Future Directions

A number of experimental approaches are being investigated in CTCL, including allogeneic bone marrow transplantation, histone deacetylase inhibitors, monoclonal antibodies, and fusion toxins.[67] Other investigative modalities include cytokines such as recombinant IL-12 and IL-2.[66]

COMPLICATIONS

The most serious complications of CTCL are infections. Sepsis from ulcerated cutaneous tumors is a common cause of death. Visceral CTCL may occur, as may transformation to large cell lymphoma in some CTCL patients (39% probability after 12 years).[71] In long-term survivors with early disease, local therapies (e.g., TSEB or PUVA) may contribute to the development of other skin cancers (e.g., BCC or SCC) and cataracts.[85]

PROGNOSIS

Many different attempts have been made to classify CTCL into useful prognostic groups. An early and still valid study that used the TNM system identified three major groups: good-risk patients (stages IA, IB, and IIA, with plaque-only skin disease and no lymph node, blood, or visceral involvement [median survival, > 12 years]); intermediate-risk patients (stages IIB, III, and IVA, with cutaneous tumors, erythroderma, or plaque disease and node or blood involvement but no visceral disease or node effacement [median survival, 5 years]); and poor-risk patients (stage IVB, with visceral involvement or node effacement [median survival, 2.5 years]).[70]

Eosinophilia is also associated with shortened survival.[70] Other long-term studies have revealed that stage IA patients do not have a reduced life expectancy and that fewer than 10% of these patients experience disease progression to more advanced stages.[86] Survival of patients with generalized patch/plaque MF (stage IB or IIA), at a median of 11.7 years, is significantly worse than that of a race-, age-, and sex-matched control population.[87] Gender and race appear to have no effect on survival, but older patients (> 58 years) have shorter disease-specific survivals.[68]

Allan C. Halpern, M.D., has no commercial relationships with manufacturers of products or providers of services discussed in this chapter.

Patricia L. Myskowski, M.D., has received grant or research support from Merck & Co., Inc., and is a consultant for Ligand Pharmaceuticals Inc.

Topical corticosteroids, topical nitrogen mustard, and carmustine have not been approved by the FDA for treatment of cutaneous T cell lymphoma; interferon alfa, sirolimus, and HAART have not been approved by the FDA for treatment of Kaposi sarcoma.

References

1. Green A, Whiteman D, Frost C, et al: Sun exposure, skin cancers and related skin conditions. J Epidemiol 9(6 suppl):S7, 1999

2. Ullrich S: Mechanisms underlying UV-induced immune suppression. Mutat Res 571:185, 2005

3. Dummer R, Maier T: UV protection and skin cancer. Recent Results Cancer Res 160:7, 2002

4. Scarlett WL: Ultraviolet radiation: sun exposure, tanning beds, and vitamin D levels. What you need to know and how to decrease the risk of skin cancer. J Am Osteopath Assoc 103: 371, 2003

5. Buettner PG, Raasch BA: Incidence rates of skin cancer in Townsville, Australia. Int J Cancer 78:587, 1998

6. Serrano H, Scotto J, Shornick G, et al: Incidence of nonmelanoma skin cancer in New Hampshire and Vermont. J Am Acad Dermatol 24:574, 1991

7. High A, Zedan W: Basal cell nevus syndrome. Curr Opin Oncol 17:160, 2005

8. Shriner DL, McCoy DK, Goldberg DJ, et al: Mohs micrographic surgery. J Am Acad Dermatol 39:79, 1998

9. Paver K, Poyzer K, Burry N, et al: Letter: the incidence of basal cell carcinoma and their metastases in Australia and New Zealand. Australas J Dermatol 14:53, 1973

10. Miller DL, Weinstock MA: Nonmelanoma skin cancer in the United States: incidence. J Am Acad Dermatol 30:774, 1994

11. Staples M, Marks R, Giles G: Trends in the incidence of non-melanocytic skin cancer (NMSC) treated in Australia 1985–1995: are primary prevention programs starting to have an effect? Int J Cancer 78:144, 1998

12. Athas WF, Hunt WC, Key CR: Changes in nonmelanoma skin cancer incidence between 1977–1978 and 1998–1999 in Northcentral New Mexico. Cancer Epidemiol Biomarkers Prev 12:1105, 2003

13. Kirkham N: Tumors and cysts of the epidermis. Lever's Histophathology of the Skin, 9th ed. Elder DE, Murphy GF, Johnson BL, et al, Eds., Lippincott Williams & Wilkins, Philadelphia, 2004, p 805

14. Lindelof B, Sigurgeirsson B, Gabel H, et al: Incidence of skin cancer in 5356 patients following organ transplantation. Br J Dermatol 143:513, 2000

15. Sarmiento JM, Wolff BG, Burgart LJ, et al: Perianal Bowen's disease: associated tumors, human papillomavirus, surgery, and other controversies. Dis Colon Rectum 40:912, 1997

16. Guthrie TH Jr, Porubsky ES, Luxenberg MN, et al: Cisplatin-based chemotherapy in advanced basal and squamous cell carcinomas of the skin: results in 28 patients including 13 patients receiving multimodality therapy. J Clin Oncol 8:342, 1990

17. Jorizzo JL: Current and novel treatment options for actinic keratosis. J Cutan Med Surg 8(suppl 3):13, 2004

18. Basal Cell and Squamous Cell Skin Cancers. Clinical Practice Guidelines in Oncology, Version 2.2005. National Comprehensive Cancer Network, Jenkintown, Pennsylvania, 2005
http://www.nccn.org/professionals/physician_gls/PDF/nmsc.pdf

19. Rowe DE, Carroll RJ, Day CL Jr: Prognostic factors for local recurrence, metastasis,

and survival rates in squamous cell carcinoma of the skin, ear, and lip. Implications for treatment modality selection. J Am Acad Dermatol 26:976, 1992

20. Jemal A, Murray T, Ward E, et al: Cancer statistics, 2005. CA Cancer J Clin 55:10, 2005

21. Hall HI, Miller DR, Rogers JD: Update on the incidence and mortality from melanoma in the United States. J Am Acad Dermatol 40:35,1999

22. Jemal A, Devesa SS, Hartge P, et al: Recent trends in cutaneous melanoma incidence among whites in the United States. J Natl Inst 93:678, 2001

23. Blackwood MA, Holmes R, Synnestvedt M, et al: Multiple primary melanoma revisited. Cancer 94:2248, 2002

24. Carey WP Jr, Thompson CJ, Synnestvedt M, et al: Dysplastic nevi as a melanoma risk factor in patients with familial melanoma. Cancer 74:3118, 1994

25. Elder DE, Clark WH Jr, Elenitsas R, et al: The early and intermediate precursor lesions of tumor progression in the melanocytic system: common acquired nevi and atypical (dysplastic) nevi. Semin Diagn Pathol 10:18, 1993

26. Haluska FG, Hodi FS: Molecular genetics of familial cutaneous melanoma. J Clin Oncol 16:670,1998

27. Tuveson DA, Weber BL, Herlyn M: BRAF as a potential therapeutic target in melanoma and other malignancies. Cancer Cell 4:95, 2003

28. Bastian BC: Understanding the progression of melanocytic neoplasia using genomic analysis: from fields to cancer. Oncogene 22:3081, 2003

29. Abbasi NR, Shaw HM, Rigel DS, et al: Early diagnosis of cutaneous melanoma: revisiting the ABCD criteria. JAMA 292:2771, 2004

30. Naeyaert JM, Brochez L: Clinical practice. Dysplastic nevi. N Engl J Med 349:2233, 2003

31. Braun RP, Rabinovitz HS, Oliviero M, et al: Dermoscopy of pigmented skin lesions. J Am Acad Dermatol 52:109, 2005

32. Halpern AC: The use of whole body photography in a pigmented lesion clinic. Dermatol Surg 26:1175, 2000

33. Marghoob AA, Swindle LD, Moricz CZ, et al: Instruments and new technologies for the in vivo diagnosis of melanoma. J Am Acad Dermatol 49:777, 2003

34. Melanoma. Clinical Practice Guidelines in Oncology, Version 2.2005. National Comprehensive Cancer Network, Jenkintown, Pennsylvania, 2005

http://www.nccn.org/professionals/physician_gls/PDF/melanoma.pdf

35. Cook J: Surgical margins for resection of primary cutaneous melanoma. Clin Dermatol 22:228, 2004

36. Roberts AA, Cochran AJ: Pathologic analysis of sentinel lymph nodes in melanoma patients: current and future trends. J Surg Oncol 85:152, 2004

37. Reintgen D, Pendas S, Jakub J, et al: National trials involving lymphatic mapping for melanoma: the Multicenter Selective Lymphadenectomy Trial, the Sunbelt Melanoma Trial, and the Florida Melanoma Trial. Semin Oncol 31:363, 2004

38. Morton DL, Thompson JF, Cochran AJ, et al: Interim results of the Multicenter Selective Lymphadenectomy Trial (MSLT-I) in clinical stage I melanoma. Proceedings of the American Society of Clinical Oncology Annual Meeting, abstract 7500. New Orleans, Jan. 20 to 22, 2005

39. Fraker DL: Management of in-transit melanoma of the extremity with isolated limb perfusion. Curr Treat Options Oncol 5:173, 2004

40. Buzaid AC: Management of metastatic cutaneous melanoma. Oncology (Williston Park) 18:1443, 2004

41. Agarwala SS, Kirkwood JM: Adjuvant interferon treatment for melanoma. Hematol Oncol Clin North Am 12:823, 1998

42. Kirkwood JM, Strawderman MH, Ernstoff MS, et al: Interferon alfa-2b adjuvant therapy of high-risk resected cutaneous melanoma: the Eastern Cooperative Oncology Group Trial EST 1684. J Clin Oncol 14:7, 1996

43. Kirkwood JM, Ibrahim JG, Sosman JA, et al: High-dose interferon alfa-2b significantly prolongs relapse-free and overall survival compared with the GM2-KLH/QS-21 vaccine in patients with resected stage IIB-III melanoma: results of intergroup trial E1694/S9512/C509801. J Clin Oncol 19:2370, 2001

44. Hersey P: Adjuvant therapy for high-risk primary and resected metastatic melanoma. Int Med J 33:33, 2003

45. Balch CM, Soong SJ, Atkins, MB, et al: An evidence-based staging system for cutaneous melanoma. CA Cancer J Clin 54:131, 2004

http://caonline.amcancersoc.org/cgi/content/full/54/3/131

46. Balch CM, Soong SJ, Gershenwald JE, et al: Prognostic factors analysis of 17,600 melanoma patients: validation of the American Joint Committee on Cancer melanoma staging system. J Clin Oncol 19:3622, 2001

47. Guerry D 4th, Synnestvedt M, Elder DE, et al: Lessons from tumor progression: the invasive radial growth phase of melanoma is common, incapable of metastasis, and indolent. J Invest Dermatol 100:342S, 1993

48. Elder DE, Van Belle P, Elenitsas R, et al: Neoplastic progression and prognosis in melanoma. Semin Cutan Med Surg 15:336, 1996

49. Schuchter L, Schultz DJ, Synnestvedt M, et al: A prognostic model for predicting 10-year survival in patients with primary melanoma. The Pigmented Lesion Group. Ann Intern Med 125:369, 1996

50. Schwartz RA: Cutaneous metastatic disease. J Am Acad Dermatol 33:161, 1995

51. Demetrius RW, Randle HW: High-risk nonmelanoma skin cancers. Dermatol Surg 24:1272, 1998

52. Allen PJ, Bowne WB, Jaques DP, et al: Merkel cell carcinoma: prognosis and treatment of patients from a single institution. J Clin Oncol 23:2300, 2005

53. Antman K, Chang Y: Kaposi's sarcoma. N Engl J Med 342:1027, 2000

54. Myskowski P, Krown S: Kaposi's sarcoma. Skin Cancer. Sober AJ, Haluska FG, Eds. American Cancer Society Atlas of Clinical Oncology series. BC Decker, Philadelphia, 2001

55. Schwartz RA: Kaposi's sarcoma: an update. J Surg Oncol 87:146, 2004

56. Cheung TW: AIDS-related cancer in the era of highly active antiretroviral therapy (HAART): a model of the interplay of the immune system, virus, and cancer. "On the offensive—the Trojan Horse is being destroyed." Part A: Kaposi's sarcoma. Cancer Invest 22:774, 2004

57. Stallone G, Schena A, Infante B, et al: Sirolimus for Kaposi's sarcoma in renal-transplant recipients. N Engl J Med 352:1317, 2005

58. Mocroft A, Kirk O, Clumeck N, et al: The changing pattern of Kaposi sarcoma in patients with HIV, 1994–2003: the EuroSIDA Study. Cancer 100:2644, 2004

59. Moore PS, Chang Y: Detection of herpesvirus-like DNA sequences in Kaposi's sarcoma in patients with and without HIV infection. N Engl J Med 332:1181, 1995

60. Cooper JS, Sacco J, Newall J: The duration of local control of classic (non–AIDS-associated) Kaposi's sarcoma by radiotherapy. J Am Acad Dermatol 19:59, 1988

61. Krown SE, Testa MA, Huang J: AIDS-related Kaposi's sarcoma: prospective validation of the AIDS Clinical Trials Group staging classification. AIDS Clinical Trials Group Oncology Committee. J Clin Oncol 15:3085, 1997

62. Cattelan AM, Trevenzoli M, Aversa SM: Novel pharmacological therapies for the treatment of AIDS-related Kaposi's sarcoma. Expert Opin Investig Drugs 13:501, 2004

63. Krown SE: Highly active antiretroviral therapy in AIDS-associated Kaposi's sarcoma: implications for the design of therapeutic trials in patients with advanced, symptomatic Kaposi's sarcoma. J Clin Oncol 22:399, 2004

64. Northfelt DW, Dezube BJ, Thommes JA, et al: Pegylated-liposomal doxorubicin versus doxorubicin, bleomycin, and vincristine in the treatment of AIDS-related Kaposi's sarcoma: results of a randomized phase III clinical trial. J Clin Oncol 16:2445, 1998

65. Welles L, Saville MW, Lietzau J, et al: Phase II trial with dose titration of paclitaxel for the therapy of human immunodeficiency virus–associated Kaposi's sarcoma. J Clin Oncol 16:1112, 1998

66. Pichardo DA, Querfeld C, Guitart J, et al: Cutaneous T-cell lymphoma: a paradigm for biological therapies. Leuk Lymphoma 45:1755, 2004

67. Foss F: Mycosis fungoides and the Sézary syndrome. Curr Opin Oncol 16:421, 2004

68. Weinstock MA, Reynes JF: The changing survival of patients with mycosis fungoides: a population-based assessment of trends in the United States. Cancer 85:208, 1999

69. Hodak E, Klein T, Gabay B, et al: Familial mycosis fungoides: report of 6 kindreds and a study of the HLA system. J Am Acad Dermatol 52:393, 2005

70. Sausville EA, Eddy JL, Makuch RW, et al: Histopathologic staging at initial diagnosis of mycosis fungoides and the Sézary syndrome: definition of three distinctive prognostic groups. Ann Intern Med 109:372, 1988

71. Diamandidou E, Colome-Grimmer M, Fayad L, et al: Transformation of mycosis fungoides/Sézary syndrome: clinical characteristics and prognosis. Blood 92:1150, 1998

72. Kim EJ, Hess S, Richardson SK, et al: Immunopathogenesis and therapy of cutaneous T cell lymphoma. J Clin Invest 115:798, 2005

73. Zackheim HS, Kashani-Sabet M, Amin S: Topical corticosteroids for mycosis fungoides. Experience in 79 patients. Arch Dermatol 134: 949, 1998

74. Kim YH, Martinez G, Varghese A, et al: Topical nitrogen mustard in the management of mycosis fungoides: update of the Stanford experience. Arch Dermatol 139:165, 2003

75. Breneman D, Duvic M, Kuzel T, et al: Phase 1 and 2 trial of bexarotene gel for skin-directed treatment of patients with cutaneous T-cell lymphoma. Arch Dermatol 138:325, 2002

76. Diederen PV, van Weelden H, Sanders CJ, et al: Narrowband UVB and psoralen-UVA in the treatment of early-stage mycosis fungoides: a retrospective study. J Am Acad Dermatol 48:215, 2003

77. Querfeld C, Rosen ST, Kuzel TM, et al: Long-term follow-up of patients with early-stage cutaneous T-cell lymphoma who achieved complete remission with psoralen plus UV-A monotherapy. Arch Dermatol 141:305, 2005

78. Jones GW, Kacinski BM, Wilson LD, et al: Total skin electron radiation in the management of mycosis fungoides: consensus of the European Organization for Research and Treatment of Cancer (EORTC) Cutaneous Lymphoma Project Group. J Am Acad Dermatol 47:364, 2002

79. Duvic M, Apisarnthanarax N, Cohen DS, et al: Analysis of long-term outcomes of combined modality therapy for cutaneous T-cell lymphoma. J Am Acad Dermatol 49:35, 2003

80. Duvic M, Hymes K, Heald P, et al: Bexarotene is effective and safe for treatment of refractory advanced-stage cutaneous T-cell lymphoma: multinational phase II-III trial results. J Clin Oncol 19:2456, 2001

81. Olsen E, Duvic M, Frankel A, et al: Pivotal phase III trial of two dose levels of denileukin diftitox for the treatment of cutaneous T-cell lymphoma. J Clin Oncol 19:376, 2001

82. Zackheim HS, Kashani-Sabet M, McMillan A: Low-dose methotrexate to treat mycosis fungoides: a retrospective study of 69 patients. J Am Acad Dermatol 49:873, 2003

83. Kaye FJ, Bunn PA Jr, Steinberg SM, et al: A randomized trial comparing combination electron-beam radiation and chemotherapy with topical therapy in the initial treatment of mycosis fungoides. N Engl J Med 321:1784, 1989

84. Apisarnthanarax N, Talpur R, Duvic M: Treatment of cutaneous T cell lymphoma: current status and future directions. Am J Clin Dermatol 3:193, 2002

85. van Praag MC, Tseng LN, Mommaas AM, et al: Minimising the risks of PUVA treatment. Drug Saf 8:340, 1993

86. Kim YH, Jensen RA, Watanabe GL, et al: Clinical stage IA (limited patch and plaque) mycosis fungoides: a long-term outcome analysis. Arch Dermatol 132:1309, 1996

87. Kim YH, Chow S, Varghese A, et al: Clinical characteristics and long-term outcome of patients with generalized patch and/or plaque (T2) mycosis fungoides. Arch Dermatol 135:26, 1999

46 Disorders of Hair

David A. Whiting, M.D., F.A.C.P.

Physiology and Evaluation of Hair Growth

A basic knowledge of the hair growth cycle is needed to evaluate disorders of hair growth.[1,2] Scalp hair follicles cycle independently of one another. At any given time, approximately 90% of scalp hairs are in the anagen (growing) phase and 10% are in the telogen (resting) phase. Anagen lasts an average of 3 years, with a range of 1 to 7 years. Telogen usually lasts 3 months, after which the resting hairs are shed and new hairs grow in. The average rate of scalp hair growth is approximately 0.35 mm/day, or 1 cm/month (1 in. every 2 to 3 months).

The scalp typically has about 100,000 hairs. An average loss of 100 hairs a day is normal, with larger numbers of hairs being lost on shampoo days. When obtaining a history, it is important to determine whether shedding is abnormal and whether the shed hairs break off or come out by the roots.[3] Hair normally comes out by the roots; however, trauma or excessive fragility may cause hair to break.

Examination of the patient should include a routine examination for broken-off hairs and the performance of hair-pull tests on the top, sides, and back of the scalp. The hair-pull test is performed by grasping groups of 10 to 20 hairs between the index finger and thumb and pulling steadily.[4,5] Extraction of more than 20% of the grasped hairs indicates a potential for abnormal shedding, usually involving telogen hairs (club hairs). Telogen hairs are easily recognized by their whitish club-shaped bulbs and by the lack of root sheaths. Anagen hairs are normally difficult to detach and have blackish, indented roots with intact root sheaths.

Androgenetic Alopecia

Androgenetic alopecia is the common type of nonscarring hair loss affecting the crown. It results from a genetically determined end-organ sensitivity to androgens. It is often referred to as common baldness, male-pattern alopecia, and female-pattern alopecia.

EPIDEMIOLOGY AND PATHOGENESIS

Androgenetic alopecia affects at least 50% of men by 50 years of age and 40% to 50% of women by 60 years of age.[6] Males have more androgen than females and therefore are usually affected earlier and more severely. Male-pattern alopecia often starts between 15 and 25 years of age. Male-pattern alopecia has two characteristic components, bitemporal recession and vertex balding [*see Figure 1*], which in pronounced cases can progress to complete balding of the crown.[6] Female-pattern alopecia is more likely to start between 25 and 30 years of age (or sometimes later, after menopause). It is characterized by an intact frontal hairline and an oval area of diffuse thinning over the crown [*see Figure 2*]. Bitemporal recession in women is much less obvious than it typically is in men, or it can be nonexistent. In general, androgenetic alopecia in women progresses to mild, moderate, or severe thinning but not to complete baldness. The best predictor of outcome is the degree of progression in affected relatives.

Androgenetic alopecia is an autosomal dominant disorder with variable penetrance. Susceptible hairs on the crown are predisposed to miniaturize under the influence of androgens, notably dihydrotestosterone. In both sexes, miniaturization results from a shortening of the anagen cycle, from years to months or weeks. Miniaturized hairs are characterized by reduced length and diameter; this accounts for the appearance of hair loss.[7] Androgenetic alopecia largely spares the back and sides of the scalp.

DIAGNOSIS

The diagnosis of androgenetic alopecia is usually obvious from the clinical pattern of hair loss from the top of the head.[8] In some men, a female pattern of alopecia (see above) causes diagnostic confusion but has no other significance. In women, a male pattern of alopecia (i.e., bitemporal recession and vertex balding) occurring with menstrual irregularities, acne, hirsutism, and a deep voice is significant. The virilism indicates significant hyperandrogenism, the cause of which must be identified and treated [*see Chapters 55 and 79*].

Scalp biopsies are rarely necessary to diagnose androgenetic alopecia. Biopsies cut horizontally are sometimes useful, however, in differentiating female-pattern alopecia from chronic telogen effluvium (see below).

TREATMENT

Depending on the severity of the condition, management of androgenetic alopecia ranges from watchful inactivity to medical and surgical treatment; a hairpiece or wig may be used in the most refractory cases.

Topical Therapy

The Food and Drug Administration approved topical 2% minoxidil for use in men in 1987 and in women in 1989. Minoxidil is applied twice daily with a dropper, spread over the top of the scalp, and gently rubbed in. The drug should be tried for at least a year. Minoxidil acts by initiating and prolonging anagen. It produces visible hair growth in approximately one third of male and female patients, fine-hair growth in approximately

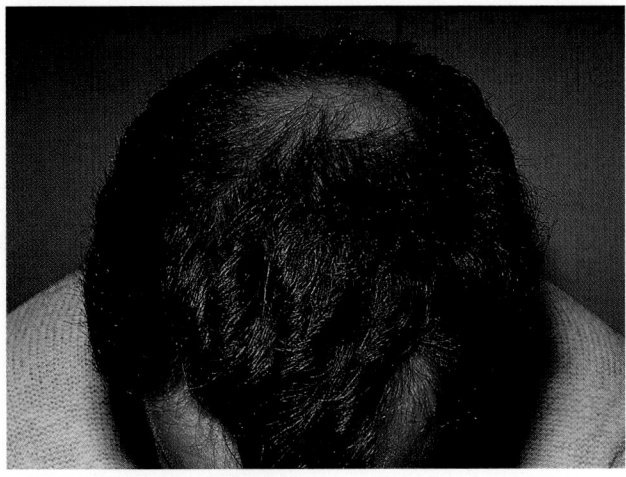

Figure 1 **Bitemporal recession and vertex balding are present in this patient with male-pattern androgenetic alopecia.**

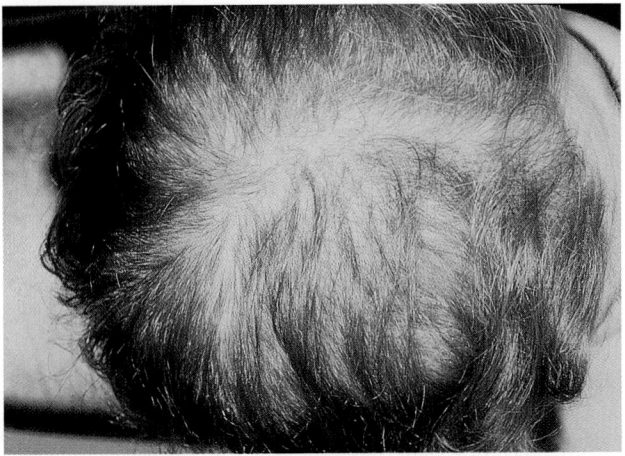

Figure 2 Intact frontal hairline and diffuse thinning over the crown are characteristic of female-pattern androgenetic alopecia.

one third, and no growth in approximately one third. It is more effective as a preventive agent, retarding hair loss in approximately 80% of patients.[6]

Topical 5% minoxidil, which was approved for use in men in 1997, produces visible hair growth in 45% of patients in less time than the 2% solution. Both concentrations are available over the counter. Side effects are not significant and include scalp irritation and increased facial hair.[9] The medication has to be continued indefinitely.[10] Topical 5% minoxidil foam, which is less irritating and easier to apply than standard minoxidil in propylene glycol, gained FDA approval for use in men in 2006.

Systemic Therapy

Oral finasteride, at a dosage of 1 mg/day, was approved by the FDA for the treatment of male-pattern alopecia in 1997. Finasteride is a powerful type II 5α-reductase inhibitor that prevents formation of dihydrotestosterone in the prostate gland and in the hair follicle. It reduces circulating dihydrotestosterone by 65% to 70%. When administered at a dosage of 1 mg/day for 2 years to men with androgenetic alopecia who were between 18 and 41 years of age, finasteride resulted in the growth of visible hair in 66% of patients and prevented further hair loss in 83%.[11] The efficacy of finasteride was maintained in a 5-year study.[12] Hair-weight studies have shown that finasteride increases hair length and diameter, producing better coverage from existing hairs.[13]

Side effects in men are minimal and include lack of libido, lack of potency, and a mild reduction in semen in approximately 0.5% of patients. These effects are reversed when the drug is stopped and often disappear as the drug is continued. A 1-year trial of finasteride at a dosage of 1 mg/day in postmenopausal women failed to show any positive effects.[14]

Because of the likelihood of finasteride to cause severe side effects in the male fetus, the drug is contraindicated in fertile, premenopausal women.

Therapy for Hair Loss in Women

Topical minoxidil is currently the best available treatment for androgenetic alopecia in women.[9,15] However, various antiandrogenic drugs have been used. Oral contraceptives (e.g., ethinyl estradiol–ethynodiol diacetate [Demulen], desogestrel–ethinyl estradiol [Desogen], ethinyl estradiol–norgestimate

[Ortho Tri-Cyclen], and ethinyl estradiol-drospirenone [Yasmin]) can reduce hair loss and occasionally lead to slight hair growth.[6] Oral spironolactone in dosages of 75 to 200 mg/day can produce androgen blockade. Dexamethasone in dosages of 0.125 to 0.5 mg/day can suppress adrenal overactivity. Cyproterone acetate, which is not available in the United States, is not as effective as minoxidil in female-pattern hair loss unless other signs of hyperandrogenism are present.[16]

Therapy for Refractory Cases

In patients who do not respond to pharmacologic treatment, the next step may be hair transplantation. Micrografts and minigrafts can produce a good cosmetic appearance in patients who have a sufficient reserve of hair on the back and sides of the scalp.[17] If all therapies fail, a hairpiece may be an option.

Diffuse Alopecia

Diffuse alopecia is generalized hair loss over the entire scalp. Because the loss is so diffuse, it is often unnoticeable until 30% to 50% of scalp hair is shed. Causes of diffuse alopecia include telogen effluvium, anagen arrest, drug reactions, and a number of systemic and nonsystemic conditions [*see Table 1*].[18,19]

TELOGEN EFFLUVIUM

Telogen effluvium is the most common form of diffuse alopecia.[20] It presents as a generalized shedding of telogen hairs from normal resting follicles. The basic cause of telogen effluvium is a premature interruption of anagen, leading to an increase in the number of hairs cycling into telogen. When the 3-month telogen period ends, new anagen hairs grow in and numerous telogen hairs fall out. Patients may need reassurance that this apparent loss of hair is actually a sign of regrowth.

Acute telogen effluvium can be caused by childbirth, febrile illnesses, surgery, chronic systemic diseases, crash diets, traction, severe emotional stress, and drug reactions [*see Table 2*]. It can also be a physiologic reaction in neonates.[21]

During acute telogen effluvium, pull tests are positive all over the scalp, yielding two to 10 club hairs. Telogen effluvium is often accompanied by bitemporal recession; this is a useful diagnostic sign in women [*see Figure 3*]. The acute form usually ends within 3 to 6 months. The diagnosis is usually made on the basis of the history of an initiating event 3 months before the onset of shedding. Chronic telogen effluvium has a long, fluctuating course of 6 months to 7 years or more.[22] By definition, no identifiable cause can be found.

Table 1 Causes of Diffuse Alopecia[18]

Telogen effluvium (acute and chronic)
Anagen arrest
Reactions to drugs and other chemicals
Thyroid disorder
Iron deficiency and other nutritional deficiencies
Malabsorption
Renal failure
Hepatic failure
Systemic disease
Miscellaneous causes (e.g., diffuse alopecia areata, congenital hypotrichosis) and idiopathic causes

Table 2 Categories of Drugs
That Can Cause Alopecia[18]

Category	Selected Agents
Alpha blockers	Doxazosin, prazosin, terazosin
Angiotensin-converting enzyme inhibitors	Captopril, enalapril
Anticancer drugs	Bleomycin, cyclophosphamide, cytarabine, dactinomycin, daunorubicin, doxorubicin, etoposide, floxuridine, fluorouracil, methotrexate, mitomycin, mitoxantrone, procarbazine, thioguanine, vinblastine, vincristine
Anticoagulant drugs	Dicumarol, heparin, warfarin
Anticonvulsant drugs	Ethotoin, mephenytoin, paramethadione, phenytoin, trimethadione, valproate sodium
Antithyroid drugs	Carbimazole, methylthiouracil, methimazole, propylthiouracil
Beta blockers	Acebutolol, atenolol, labetalol, metoprolol, nadolol, pindolol, propranolol, timolol
Calcium channel blockers	Diltiazem, verapamil
Cholesterol reducers	Clofibrate, lovastatin
H_2 receptor blockers	Cimetidine, famotidine, ranitidine
Nonsteroidal anti-inflammatory drugs	Fenoprofen, ibuprofen, indomethacin, ketoprofen, meclomen, naproxen, piroxicam, sulindac
Retinoids and retinol	Acitretin, etretinate, isotretinoin, vitamin A overdose
Tricyclic antidepressants	Amitriptyline, amoxapine, desipramine, doxepin, imipramine, nortriptyline, protriptyline, trimipramine

Diagnosis

The diagnosis of telogen effluvium is usually clinical; biopsies may be necessary to distinguish telogen effluvium from an acute onset of widespread androgenetic alopecia or from diffuse alopecia areata.[22] Other causes of hair loss should be excluded by a careful drug history and tests for iron deficiency, syphilis, and disorders of the thyroid, kidney, and liver.

Treatment

No treatment is needed for acute telogen effluvium because the hair invariably regrows within a short time. In chronic telogen effluvium, topical minoxidil in a 2% or 5% solution may be indicated. The patient should be reassured that telogen effluvium rarely causes permanent baldness.

ANAGEN ARREST (ANAGEN EFFLUVIUM)

So-called anagen effluvium represents a diffuse loss of anagen hairs from growing follicles.[23] The term anagen effluvium is a misnomer. Normally, hairs pass through a brief transition phase (catagen) between the anagen and telogen phases before falling out by the roots. In anagen arrest, inhibition of cell division in the hair bulb matrix leads to a progressive narrowing of the hair shaft and sometimes failure of hair formation. As the growing hair narrows near the skin surface, it may break off. The resultant shedding can occur within a few weeks, unlike in telogen effluvium, in which shedding takes 3 months to occur.

Causes of anagen arrest include reactions to cytostatic drugs and other toxic agents, radiation therapy, endocrine diseases, alopecia areata, cicatricial alopecia, trauma and pressure, and severe protein calorie malnutrition. Because 90% of scalp hairs are in anagen at any given time, this condition causes obvious and severe baldness [see Figure 4].

Diagnosis

The diagnosis of anagen arrest is easily made by the history, evidence of extensive hair loss, and hair-pull tests that yield easily broken hairs with proximal tapering.

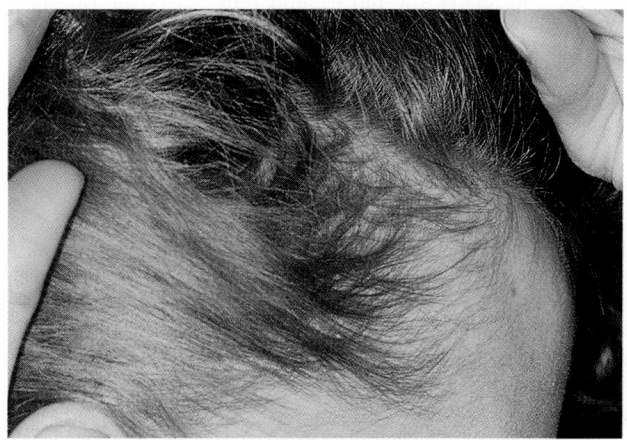

Figure 3 **In women, marked bitemporal recession is often a sign of telogen effluvium.**

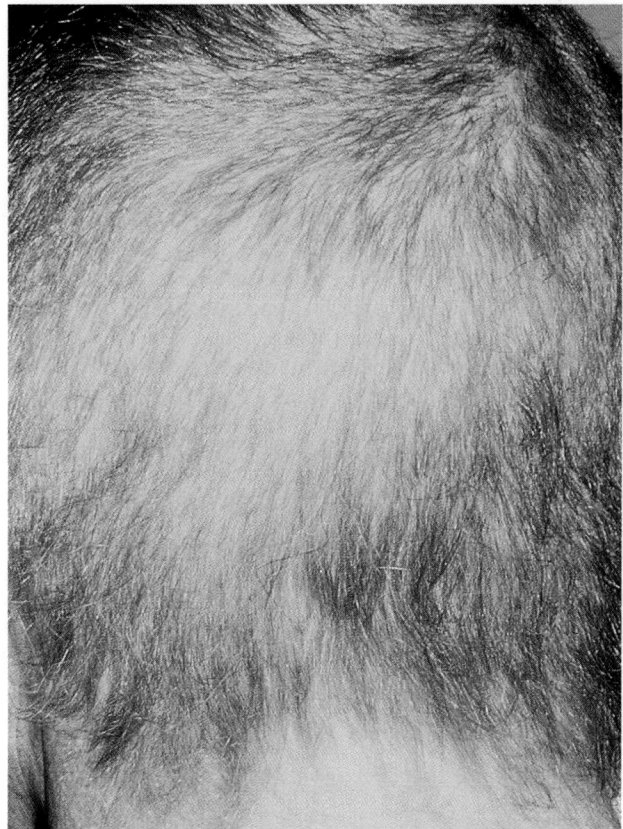

Figure 4 **Anagen arrest causes severe, diffuse hair loss.**

Treatment

Treatment of anagen arrest lies in elimination of the underlying cause. Once the antimitotic influence is removed, the anagen hair will regrow promptly with a normally tapering shaft. Unbroken hairs that regrow often show the Pohl-Pinkus deformity (i.e., a constriction that results in a dumbbell shape).

ALOPECIA CAUSED BY DRUGS AND CHEMICALS

Substance-induced alopecia is relatively common but is often hard to diagnose because of the large number of drugs and chemicals that can cause hair loss [*see Tables 2 and 3*]. Identification of the underlying cause often requires a time-consuming process of trial and error: many patients are exposed to several alopecia-inducing substances, and removal of the causative agent may not result in immediate regrowth of hair.

OTHER CAUSES OF DIFFUSE ALOPECIA

Hypothyroidism and iron deficiency should be excluded in patients with diffuse hair loss [*see Table 1*]. Appropriate treatment may lead to hair regrowth.

Alopecia Areata

Alopecia areata is typically characterized by patchy hair loss; however, involvement can vary from a single patch on the scalp or elsewhere to total body baldness (alopecia universalis).[24]

EPIDEMIOLOGY AND PATHOGENESIS

In the United States, alopecia areata affects 1.7% of the population younger than 50 years.[25] From 70% to 75% of cases are not associated with any other disease. In these patients, the onset of alopecia areata occurs when patients are in their 20s or 30s, although it can occur at any age. In only about 6% of these patients with alopecia areata does the disease progress to total loss of scalp hair. Even total alopecia can reverse itself.

Alopecia areata is currently regarded as an autoimmune disease. There is a genetic predisposition to alopecia areata, as indicated by the fact that 20% of alopecia areata patients have a positive family history for the condition. Certain HLA groups have been associated with mild or severe cases of alopecia areata.[26] Although the exact cause is unknown, many researchers presume that an infectious agent such as a virus has an etiologic role. Stress, seasonal factors, and infection are among the factors that trigger active episodes of hair loss.

In approximately 5% of alopecia areata cases—usually those occurring in middle-aged patients—there is a history of autoimmune disease (e.g., thyroiditis) in the patient or in the patient's family. Approximately 10% of these patients will experience loss of all scalp hair in the course of the disorder. Approximately 20% to 25% of cases—often those occurring in childhood—may be associated with atopic disease (e.g., hay fever, asthma, or eczema). The incidence of complete scalp hair loss is much higher in these patients.

Despite its long course, often recurring over many years, the prognosis of alopecia areata is often favorable. Most patients will regrow hair at one time or another. In cases of extensive alopecia areata, alopecia totalis, and alopecia universalis, however, hair loss may be permanent.

DIAGNOSIS

Active alopecia areata is characterized by a spreading, annular area of hair loss; a smooth, depressed area of scalp that is

Table 3 Miscellaneous Chemicals That Can Cause Alopecia[40]

Chemical	*Common Source*
Abrin	Plant source (*Abrus precatorius* [rosary pea, jequirity bean, or precatory bean])
Arsenic	Pesticides
Bismuth	Old treatment for syphilis
Boric acid	Mouthwashes, occupational exposure
Chloroprene dimers	Occupational exposure (synthetic-rubber manufacturing)
Lead	Paints
Mercury	Cosmetics, teething powders, antiseptics
Mimosine	Plant source (*Leucaena glauca*)
Selenocystothione	Plant source (*Lecythis* species)
Thallium salts	Rodenticides

slick to the touch is surrounded by hairs that often include so-called exclamation-point hairs (i.e., broken hairs 3 to 4 mm long, usually with an expanded tip and a telogen bulb). These hairs are not always seen but are diagnostic when present. They delineate the active spreading margin of alopecia areata. The bald patches generally affect the scalp but can also involve eyebrows, eyelashes, beard hair, and body hair. Spontaneous regrowth is common.

This condition is extremely unpredictable, often fluctuating without any obvious reason. However, seasonal outbreaks are noted in many patients. The initial patch may enlarge, or additional patches may develop and become confluent [*see Figure 5*]. The condition can progress to large irregular areas of baldness. In severe cases, patients lose all scalp hair or all body hair.

Ophiasis is a chronic and difficult to treat form of alopecia areata in which a band of baldness circles the scalp, very often around the inferior margin. This slowly extending lesion is often present for several years before any regrowth occurs. Permanent hair loss may result in some areas.

A scalp biopsy may be needed to confirm the diagnosis of alopecia areata.[27]

TREATMENT

The treatment of alopecia areata depends on the severity of the disease.[28] Small patches of alopecia areata often resolve spontaneously. If regrowth of hair does not occur, such patches usually respond to medium- or high-potency topical corticosteroids or to intralesional injections of triamcinolone acetonide at a concentration of 5 mg/ml.

In more severe cases, intralesional corticosteroids may be tried; however, this approach may not be feasible in patients with extensive hair loss. Daily, short-contact topical therapy with 0.25% to 1% anthralin cream for up to an hour at a time may help and is suitable for children and adults. Psoralen and ultraviolet A (PUVA) therapy has also been used with some success.

Topical 5% minoxidil can be tried to speed hair regrowth and lengthen existing hairs. Minoxidil has no effect on the course of the disease but may improve hair coverage. It has few side effects and is often used in older children; however, the

FDA has approved minoxidil for use only in persons 18 years of age and older. Systemic steroids are effective; however, they have shown a potential for side effects and do not prevent future recurrences. Prednisone (20 to 40 mg daily in the morning for 1 or 2 months, followed by slow tapering) has controlled the disease in adults; a change to alternate-day therapy is advisable whenever possible.

Topical immunotherapy with the sensitizing chemical diphencyprone has been used in some centers; it has a response rate comparable to that of systemic corticosteroids.[29] Success with this treatment usually requires supervision in a specialized clinic. Sulfasalazine has been reported to have a 23% success rate in the treatment of severe alopecia areata.[30] Other immunosuppressive drugs, such as oral cyclosporine, have been used experimentally. Such therapies are risky and expensive, however, and have not been approved in the United States for alopecia areata.

TRAUMATIC ALOPECIA

Traumatic alopecia may be caused by a variety of physical or chemical injuries to the hair and scalp. These injuries may be deliberate or accidental, inflicted by self or others, and acute or repetitive. The cause may be obvious or unclear.[31] Potential causes include trichotillomania, habit tics, pruritic dermatoses, traction, pressure and friction, heat, radiation, and chemicals. In most cases of traumatic alopecia, management consists of removal of the underlying cause. In areas with permanent damage, hair transplantation may be necessary.

TRICHOTILLOMANIA

Trichotillomania is a compulsion to pull out one's hair. It is characterized by an increasing sense of tension before, and a sense of relief after, the hair is pulled. Trichotillomania is now classified as a specific disorder of impulse control.[31,32] It is more common in children, in whom it is often caused by insecurity resulting from sibling rivalry, lack of attention, divorce of parents, learning disabilities, or unhappiness or teasing at school. In adolescents and adults, trichotillomania may be accompanied by mood disorders, anxiety disorders, or mental retardation and is often harder to treat than in children.

The diagnosis is based on the presence of irregular, broken-off hairs in patches on the scalp [see Figure 6]. The hairs are irregular in length because they are broken off at different times. The scalp itself is normal. Occasionally, biopsies are necessary to confirm the diagnosis. The best treatment is to explain cause and remedy to the patient in a nonconfrontational manner; usually, reassurance and understanding go a long way in the treatment of this condition. In more difficult cases, psychiatric consultation may be indicated.[33] If habit tics or head rolling and banging are found to be causing traumatic hair loss, those behaviors should be treated.

OTHER CAUSES OF TRAUMATIC ALOPECIA

Pruritic Dermatoses

Pruritic dermatoses such as acne necrotica, folliculitis, lichen simplex chronicus, pediculosis capitis, prurigo nodularis, psoriasis, seborrheic dermatitis, and neurotic excoriations can lead to hair loss from excoriation. They need to be identified and treated.

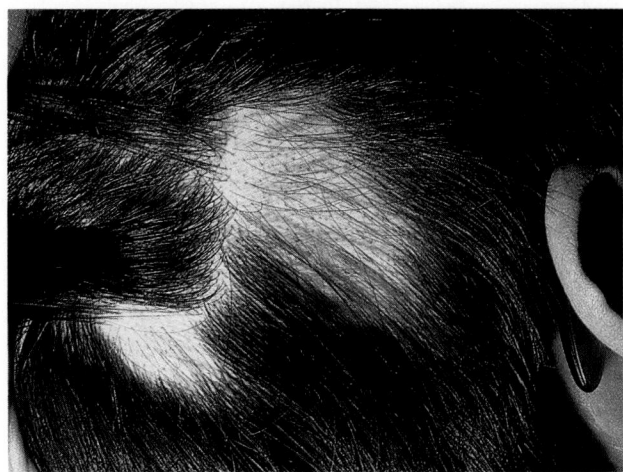

Figure 5 **Circumscribed patches of hair loss are present in alopecia areata.**

Traction Alopecia and Loose Anagen Syndrome

Traction alopecia may be acute (caused by accidental or deliberate avulsion of the scalp) or may arise from a familial condition, the loose anagen syndrome. Common causes of traction alopecia are excessive brushing and combing; backcombing and pulling the hair into braids, cornrows, and ponytails; weaving; and application of rollers.[31]

Loose anagen syndrome is usually seen in fair-haired children 2 to 5 years of age.[34] It often presents as patchy hair loss following an incident of hair tugging. Prompt hair regrowth is the rule. The condition becomes asymptomatic with gentle hair care. Diagnosis is made on the basis of positive hair-pull tests showing many anagen hairs.

Alopecia Caused by Pressure and Friction

Prolonged pressure on a localized area of the scalp in immobilized neonates or patients under anesthesia, in coma, or with debilitating illness may result in ischemia leading to pressure alopecia. The hair usually regrows with time, but if the damage is severe, permanent hair loss and scarring may result.[31] Alopecia caused by friction from vigorous massage has been described but is easily remedied.

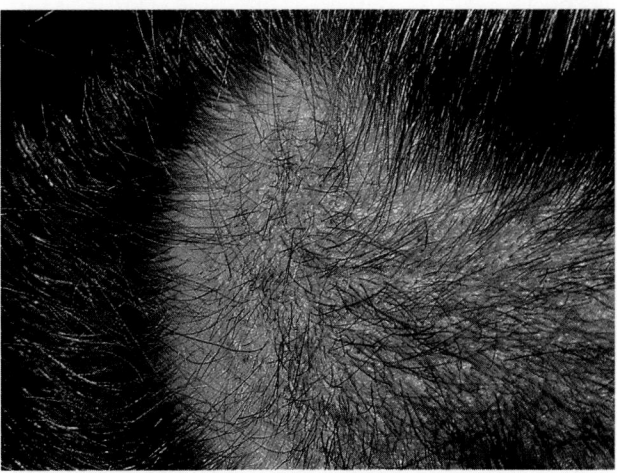

Figure 6 **Irregular, broken-off hairs are seen in trichotillomania.**

Alopecia Caused by Heat, Radiation, and Chemicals

Excessive heat from hot oils and pomades, hot combs, and hot rollers is a common cause of chronic hair loss. Overheated hair dryers frequently cause the fluid droplets in wet hair shafts to expand, leading to the formation of bubble hairs.[35] These brittle hairs are a frequent cause of follicle damage. The source of the overheating needs to be identified and removed.

Radiation dermatitis can cause hair loss. Permanent scarring alopecia is still seen in patients who were overtreated with x-rays for tinea capitis before oral antifungal agents became available.

Many chemicals can cause hair loss; the list includes hair dyes, moisturizers, oils and pomades, permanent waves, relaxers and straighteners, setting lotions, certain cationic and detergent shampoos, and saltwater.[36] A careful history of hair care and grooming is needed to uncover these causes.

Cicatricial Alopecia

Cicatricial alopecia results from permanent scarring of the hair follicles. It may be widespread or localized and is sometimes difficult to identify. The causes of cicatricial alopecia may be primary or secondary and include hereditary or congenital conditions, infections, injuries, neoplasms, and dermatoses [*see Table 4*].[37]

DIAGNOSIS

On clinical examination, scarring is detected by the absence of follicular orifices and a pearly or scarred appearance of the skin. The scar may be depressed or hypertrophic. Associated lesions such as folliculitis, follicular plugs, scales, and telangiectasias may be found, along with broken, twisted, or easily extractable hairs. Other lesions may be present on skin or mucous membranes. If the disease is active, a specific diagnosis may be possible; in inactive cases, the initial cause is often inapparent.

Clinical Variants

The common variants of primary cicatricial alopecia of the scalp include central centrifugal cicatricial alopecia, discoid lupus erythematosus, lichen planopilaris, folliculitis decalvans, and nonspecific cicatricial alopecia (pseudopelade).[38-40] The end phases of these conditions are similar; they are characterized by a lack of pores and by inflammation in white, scarred areas. For an accurate diagnosis, an early biopsy from an area of activity might show the identifying pathology. In the final scarring stage, it is usually not possible to identify the original cause.

Central centrifugal cicatricial alopecia This condition usually affects middle-aged, African-American women, but it can occur in other races and in men. Central centrifugal cicatricial alopecia usually starts in the central vertex area of the scalp and gradually extends forward, assuming the outlines of a female-pattern alopecia. It is destructive and progressive. It is sometimes familial and is becoming more common. It may be aggravated by physical and chemical trauma—hence, its old name of hotcomb alopecia.

Discoid lupus erythematosus The lesions of discoid lupus erythematosus are often itchy at onset and lead to erythema, scaling, telangiectasia, follicular spines, and atrophy [*see Figure* 7]. They often occur centrally in bare patches of scarring with an inactive border [*see Chapter 114*].

Table 4   Causes of Cicatricial Alopecia[40]

Dermatoses	Cicatricial pemphigoid, dermatomyositis, folliculitis decalvans, lichen planopilaris, lupus erythematosus, neurotic excoriations, pseudopelade, scleroderma
Hereditary and congenital disorders	Aplasia cutis, epidermal nevi, epidermolysis bullosa
Infections	
Bacterial	Acne keloidalis, dissecting cellulitis, folliculitis, syphilis
Fungal	Favus (tinea capitis), kerion, mycetoma
Protozoan	Leishmaniasis
Viral	Herpes zoster, varicella
Injuries	Burns, mechanical trauma, radiodermatitis
Neoplasms	Angiosarcoma, basal cell epithelioma, lymphoma, melanoma, metastatic tumors, squamous cell carcinoma

Lichen planopilaris Central scarring characterizes these lesions. The condition generally starts with bare, white patches that bud out from one another like pseudopods. Prominent follicular hyperkeratosis is present around the residual terminal hairs at the edges of the lesion, and varying degrees of erythema, scaling, and telangiectasia may occur. Itching may be present.

Folliculitis decalvans Crops of follicular pustules surrounding multiple, slowly expanding, and round or oval areas of alopecia characterize this condition. It may involve large areas of the skin. Secondary infection may be severe, with crusting and oozing. Eventually this condition gradually becomes less active and looks like other forms of chronic cicatricial alopecia.

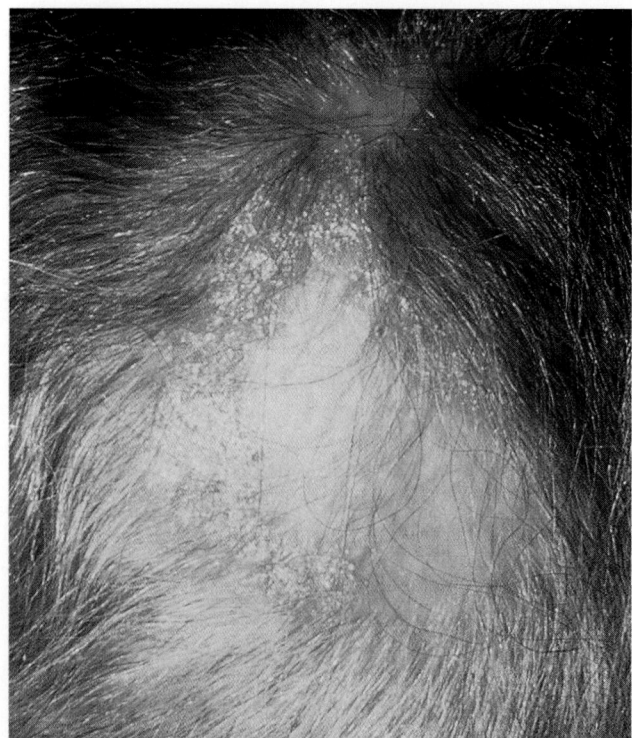

Figure 7   **Atrophic scarring with erythema, scaling, telangiectasia, and follicular spines are characteristic of discoid lupus erythematosus.**

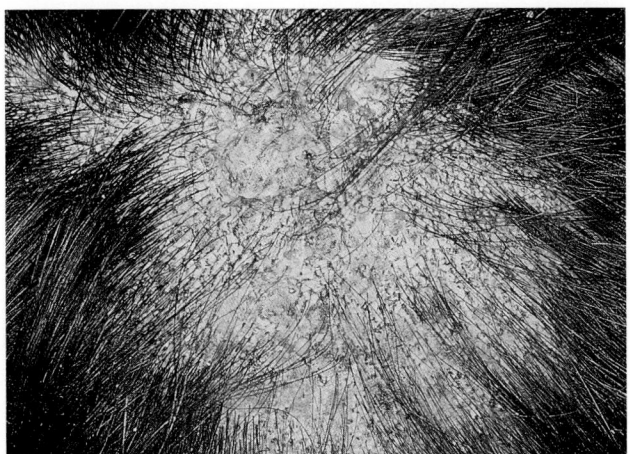

Figure 8 In endothrix tinea capitis, black dots represent brittle, infected hairs snapped off flush with the scalp.

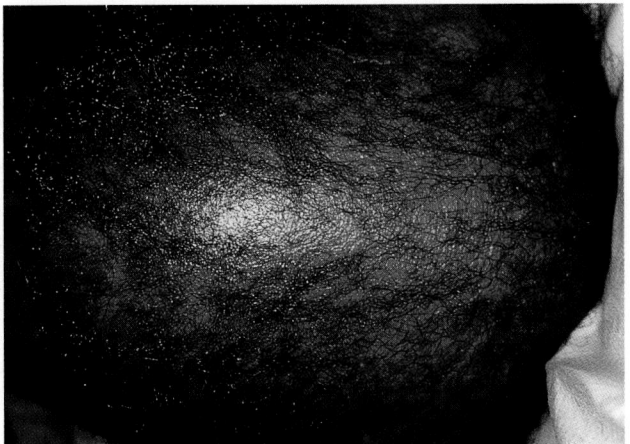

Figure 9 The characteristic irregular, so-called moth-eaten diffuse alopecia caused by syphilis is seen here.

Nonspecific cicatricial alopecia (pseudopelade) The majority of cases previously classified as pseudopelade are in fact cases of nonspecific cicatricial alopecia in which the initial cause has not been established. In general, there is an insidious spread of a scarring process, which is apparently noninflammatory. It often involves the crown and occurs mainly in middle-aged women. It may represent the end result of lichen planopilaris or, less commonly, discoid lupus erythematosus or other disorders. It is characterized by patchy areas of alopecia with irregular extensions. The affected skin is smooth, white, and devoid of erythema, scaling, or pores; hence the descriptive term footprints in the snow. The course is variable and may last for a few years or several decades.

The original cases were described as a specific entity in the late 19th century and were reported as pseudopelade of Brocq. This eponym is rarely used currently, except perhaps for a small cohort of cases with no inflammatory phase at all, particularly occurring in children.

TREATMENT

Treatment of cicatricial alopecia depends on the level of activity of the underlying disease. Central centrifugal cicatricial alopecia, discoid lupus erythematosus, and lichen planopilaris may respond to topical, intralesional, or systemic steroids; oral chloro-

quine therapy; or immunosuppressive agents such as mycophenolate mofetil or cyclosporine. Topical minoxidil is sometimes helpful in regrowing any surviving hairs, which may be normal, dystrophic, or in a resting stage. The application of a 2% or 5% solution twice daily should be tried for at least a year on scarred areas that show some hair. Folliculitis decalvans may respond to treatment with long-term antibiotics such as tetracycline (500 mg daily), minocycline (100 mg), erythromycin (250 mg), ciprofloxacin (750 mg), cephalexin (500 mg), trimethoprim-sulfamethoxazole (regular strength), or rifampin (300 mg, with regular-strength trimethoprim-sulfamethoxazole, given twice daily for at least 3 months). When the conditions have burned themselves out, either scalp reduction (i.e., surgical removal of a bald area of scalp and stretching of adjacent scalp over the removed area) or hair transplants may be helpful.

Miscellaneous Causes of Hair Loss

As mentioned earlier, less common causes of hair loss include infections (e.g., tinea capitis),[41] infestations, hair shaft abnormalities, hereditary and congenital conditions, and various dermatoses involving the scalp.

In the United States, tinea capitis is now largely caused by *Trichophyton tonsurans*, an endothrix that infects the inside of the hair shaft. This makes the shaft brittle, which causes it to snap off flush with the skin, leaving a characteristic black dot of hair [*see Figure 8*]. The clinical diagnosis depends on this finding of black dots in patchy areas of hair loss. Removing the black dot with a small scalpel blade and dissolving it in potassium hydroxide (KOH) should reveal many spores packed inside the affected hair shaft. Ectothrix ringworm caused by *Microsporum canis* and *M. audouinii* is much less common; it can usually be diagnosed by Wood light or by a finding of fungal spores around the hair shaft with KOH. Suitable oral antifungal treatments include griseofulvin, itraconazole, terbinafine, and fluconazole.

Secondary syphilis can cause a somewhat nondescript, moth-eaten type of diffuse alopecia [*see Figure 9*]. In such cases, a routine serologic test for syphilis is indicated.

Scalp lice should always be sought in cases of hair loss accompanied by pruritus. Lice are most likely to be found around and behind the ears and on the nape of the neck. Lymphadenopathy may also be present. Suitable treatment with permethrin shampoo or 0.5% malathion can be given. Ivermectine tablets may be useful in resistant cases.

Hair shaft abnormalities frequently present as broken-off hairs. Structural abnormalities of the hair shaft include fractures, irregularities, coiling and twisting, and extraneous matter.[42,43] They can often be diagnosed by light microscopy.

There are many different types of congenital and inherited hair loss.[44] These include congenital hypotrichosis with or without associated defects, congenital triangular alopecia, and many ectodermal dysplasias that affect the hair, teeth, nails, and sweat glands. One major form of congenital hypotrichosis is the Marie-Unna syndrome, which affects large families that have a dominant gene.[45] Minor forms of hypotrichosis can occur in patients with other hereditary syndromes and chromosomal abnormalities. In most of these conditions, a reduction of hair follicles accounts for the hair loss. Some patients have surviving hairs that are often in telogen and may benefit from topical minoxidil.

The author is a consultant and participates in the speakers' bureaus for Pharmacia & Upjohn, Merck & Co., Inc., and GlaxoSmithKline.

Oral contraceptives and antiandrogens discussed in this chapter have not been approved by the FDA for use in androgenetic alopecia; topical minoxidil discussed in this chapter has not been approved by the FDA for use in chronic telogen effluvium and cicatricial alopecia; diphencyprone, sulfasalazine, and cyclosporine discussed in this chapter have not been approved by the FDA for use in alopecia areata; and rifampin discussed in this chapter has not been approved by the FDA for use in folliculitis decalvans.

References

1. Cotsarelis G, Millar SE, Chan EF: Embryology and anatomy of the hair follicle. Disorders of Hair Growth: Diagnosis and Treatment, 2nd ed. Olsen EA, Ed. McGraw-Hill, New York, 2003, p 1

2. Krause K, Foitzik K: Biology of the hair follicle: the basics. Semin Cutan Med Surg 25:2, 2006

3. Olsen EA: Clinical tools for assessing hair loss. Disorders of Hair Growth: Diagnosis and Treatment, 2nd ed. Olsen EA, Ed. McGraw-Hill, New York, 2003, p 75

4. Rietschel RL: A simplified approach to the diagnosis of alopecia. Dermatol Clin 14:691, 1996

5. Whiting DA, Howsden FL: Assessment of patient with hair loss. Color Atlas of Differential Diagnosis of Hair Loss, rev. Whiting DA, Howsden FL, Eds. Canfield Publishing, Fairfield, New Jersey, 1998, p 8

6. Olsen EA: Pattern hair loss in men and women. Disorders of Hair Growth: Diagnosis and Treatment, 2nd ed. Olsen EA, Ed. McGraw-Hill, New York, 2003, p 321

7. Birch MP, Messenger JF, Messenger AG: Hair density, hair diameter and the prevalence of female pattern hair loss. Br J Dermatol 144:297, 2001

8. Whiting DA, Howsden FL: Androgenetic alopecia. Color Atlas of Differential Diagnosis of Hair Loss, rev. Whiting DA, Howsden FL, Eds. Canfield Publishing, Fairfield, New Jersey, 1998, p 18

9. Shapiro J, Price VH: Hair regrowth: therapeutic agents. Dermatol Clin 16:341, 1998

10. Olsen EA, DeLong ER, Weiner MS: Long-term follow-up of men with male pattern baldness treated with topical minoxidil. J Am Acad Dermatol 16:688, 1987

11. Kaufman KD, Olsen EA, Whiting DA, et al: Finasteride in the treatment of men with androgenetic alopecia. Finasteride Male Pattern Hair Loss Study Group. J Am Acad Dermatol 39:578, 1998

12. Kaufman KD: Long-term (5-year) multinational experience with finasteride 1 mg in the treatment of men with androgenetic alopecia. Eur J Dermatol 12:38, 2002

13. Price VH, Menefee E, Sanchez M, et al: Changes in hair weight and hair count in men with androgenetic alopecia after treatment with finasteride, 1 mg, daily. J Am Acad Dermatol 46:517, 2002

14. Olsen EA, Messenger AG, Shapiro J, et al: Evaluation and treatment of male and female pattern hair loss. J Am Acad Dermatol 52:301, 2005

15. Whiting DA, Olsen EA, Savin R, et al: Efficacy and tolerability of finasteride 1mg in men aged 41–60 years with male pattern hair loss. Eur J Dermatol 13:150, 2003

16. Vexiau P, Chaspoux C, Boudou P, et al: Effects of minoxidil 2% vs. cyproterone acetate treatment on female androgenetic alopecia: a controlled, 12-month randomized trial. Br J Dermatol 146:992, 2002

17. Avram MR: Hair transplantation for men and women. Semin Cutan Med Surg 25:60, 2006

18. Fiedler VC, Gray AC: Diffuse alopecia: telogen hair loss. Disorders of Hair Growth: Diagnosis and Treatment, 2nd ed. Olsen EA, Ed. McGraw-Hill, New York, 2003, p 303

19. Sinclair R: Diffuse hair loss. Int J Dermatol 38(suppl 1):8, 1999

20. Headington JE: Telogen effluvium: new concepts and review. Arch Dermatol 129:356, 1993

21. Kligman AM: Pathologic dynamics of human hair loss 1: telogen effluvium. Arch Dermatol 83:175, 1961

22. Whiting DA: Chronic telogen effluvium: increased scalp hair shedding in middle-aged women. J Am Acad Dermatol 35:899, 1996

23. Sinclair R, Grossman KL, Kvedar JC: Anagen hair loss. Disorders of Hair Growth: Diagnosis and Treatment, 2nd ed. Olsen EA, Ed. McGraw-Hill, New York, 2003, p 275

24. Hordinsky MK: Alopecia areata. Disorders of Hair Growth: Diagnosis and Treatment, 2nd ed. Olsen EA, Ed. McGraw-Hill, New York, 2003, p 239

25. Safavi KH, Muller SA, Suman VJ, et al: Incidence of alopecia areata in Olmsted County, Minnesota, 1975 through 1989. Mayo Clin Proc 70:628, 1995

26. Price VH, Colombe BW: Heritable factors distinguish two types of alopecia areata. Dermatol Clin 14:679, 1996

27. Whiting DA: Histopathological features of alopecia areata: a new look. Arch Dermatol 139:1555, 2003

28. Hordinsky MK: Medical treatment of noncicatricial alopecia. Semin Cutan Med Surg 25:51, 2006

29. Madani S, Shapiro J: Alopecia areata update. J Am Acad Dermatol 42:549, 2000

30. Ellis CN, Brown MF, Voorhees JJ: Sulfasalazine for alopecia areata. J Am Acad Dermatol 46:541, 2002

31. Whiting DA: Traumatic alopecia. Int J Dermatol 38(suppl 1):34, 1999

32. Walsh KH, McDougle CJ: Trichotillomania: presentation, etiology, diagnosis and therapy. Am J Clin Dermatol 2:327, 2001

33. Hautmann G, Hercogova J, Lotti T: Trichotillomania. J Am Acad Dermatol 46:807, 2002

34. Price VH, Gummer CL: Loose anagen syndrome. J Am Acad Dermatol 20:249, 1989

35. Detwiler SP, Carson JL, Woosley JT, et al: Bubble hair: case caused by overheating hair dryer and reproducibility in normal hair with heat. J Am Acad Dermatol 30:54, 1994

36. Wilborn WS: Disorders of hair growth in African Americans. Disorders of Hair Growth: Diagnosis and Treatment, 2nd ed. Olsen EA, Ed. McGraw-Hill, New York, 2003, p 497

37. Amato L, Mei S, Massi D, et al: Cicatricial alopecia: a dermatopathologic and immunopathologic study of 33 patients (pseudopelade of Brocq is not a specific clinicopathologic entity). Int J Dermatol 41:8, 2002

38. Price VH: The medical treatment of cicatricial alopecia. Semin Cutan Med Surg 25:56, 2006

39. Whiting DA: Cicatricial alopecia: clinico-pathological findings and treatment. Clin Dermatol 19:211, 2001

40. Bergfeld WF, Elston DM: Cicatricial alopecia. Disorders of hair Growth: Diagnosis and Treatment, 2nd ed. Olsen EA, Ed. McGraw-Hill, New York, 2003, p 363

41. Roberts JL, DeVillez RL: Infectious, physical and inflammatory causes of hair and scalp abnormalities. Disorders of Hair Growth: Diagnosis and Treatment, 2nd ed. Olsen EA, Ed. McGraw-Hill, New York, 2003, p 87

42. Whiting DA: Hair shaft defects. Disorders of Hair Growth: Diagnosis and Treatment 2nd ed. Olsen EA, Ed. McGraw-Hill, New York, 2003, p 123

43. Whiting DA, Dy LC: Office diagnosis of hair shaft defects. Semin Cutan Med Surg 25: 24, 2006

44. Olsen EA: Hair loss in childhood. Disorders of Hair Growth: Diagnosis and Treatment, 2nd ed. Olsen EA, Ed. McGraw-Hill, New York, 2003, p 177

45. Roberts JL, Whiting DA, Henry D, et al: Marie Unna congenital hypotrichosis: clinical description, histopathology, scanning electron microscopy of a previously unreported large pedigree. J Invest Dermatol Symp Proc 4:261, 1999

Acknowledgments

Figures 2, 4, 7, and 8   D. A. Whiting and F. L. Howsden: *Color Atlas of Differential Diagnosis of Hair Loss, rev.* Canfield Publishing, Fairfield, New Jersey, 1998. Used with permission.

47 Disorders of the Nail

James Q. Del Rosso, D.O., and C. Ralph Daniel III, M.D.

The human nail is a complex unit composed of five major modified cutaneous structures: the nail matrix, nail bed, nail plate, nail folds, and cuticle (eponychium).[1] These components are structurally supported by specialized mesenchyme, which provides a ligamentlike function, anchoring the soft tissue structures of the nail to the underlying phalangeal bone. The primary function of the human nail is to provide protection for the distal digits. Nails also assist in performance of fine touch and digital dexterity. For many individuals, nails serve as an important aesthetic symbol of optimal appearance, enhanced self-image, or individuality; several cosmetic techniques are available to modify the appearance of the nail plate. The basic anatomic components of the nail unit are diagrammed [*see Figure 1*].

Nail Structure, Function, and Pathophysiology

NAIL MATRIX

The nail matrix is the dynamic, germinative portion of the nail unit that produces the nail plate.[2-4] The lunula is the visible portion of the nail matrix, appearing under the proximal nail plate as a gray-white half moon projecting just distal to the proximal nail-fold cuticle. That lunula decreases with age in approximately 20% of persons.[5]

Nails are usually devoid of pigmentation because of the relatively sparse number of melanocytes present in matrix epithelium.[1,2] Because nail-matrix or nail-bed melanocytes tend to be more numerous in blacks, Asians, and Hispanics, persons of these racial backgrounds may present more commonly with diffuse or banded nail-plate or nail-bed hyperpigmentation.

Pathophysiology Affecting the Nail Matrix

Because of the diagonal orientation of the ventral nail matrix, the proximal portion of the nail matrix produces the superior portion of the nail plate.[6] As a result, disorders of the proximal matrix produce surface abnormalities of the nail plate. A characteristic example is nail-plate pitting secondary to psoriasis. Diseases of the distal nail matrix result in abnormalities of the undersurface of the nail plate, changes that are visible at the free edge of the nail, or both. Permanent damage to the matrix as the result of trauma, surgical intervention, or disease may result in permanent nail-plate dystrophy.

NAIL BED

The nail bed is a layer of epithelium lying between the lunula and the hyponychium (the distal epithelium at the free edge of the nail). The surface epithelium of the nail bed is longitudinally ridged, with small superficially oriented vessels coursing along the same axis, interdigitating with a complementary array of ridges on the undersurface of the nail plate.[3] This anatomic feature explains the longitudinal linearity of splinter hemorrhages, which are foci of extravasation wedged between the bed and the plate. As outgrowth of the nail plate occurs, splinter hemorrhages progress distally.

Pathophysiology Affecting the Nail Bed

The epidermis of the nail bed is thin and minimally keratinized, without a granular layer. If there is prolonged loss of nail plate as a result of disease or surgical intervention, in-

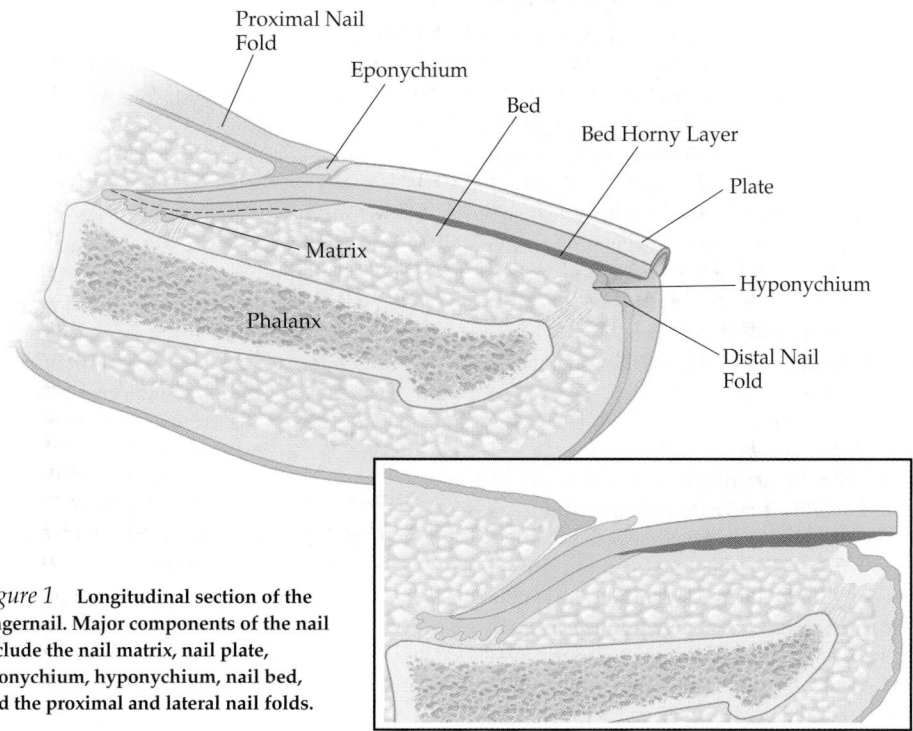

Figure 1 **Longitudinal section of the fingernail. Major components of the nail include the nail matrix, nail plate, eponychium, hyponychium, nail bed, and the proximal and lateral nail folds.**

creased nail-bed keratinization with development of a granular layer prevents the firm attachment of the ingrowing nail plate to the underlying nail bed. Melanocytes are more sparsely distributed in nail-bed epithelium than in the nail matrix [see Nail Matrix, above]. The dermal layer of the nail bed is very thin and is supported by very sparse subcutaneous tissue; it is firmly attached to the underlying bony phalanx.

NAIL PLATE

The nail plate, which is composed of densely compacted keratinized epithelial cells, is produced by the matrix and progesses distally toward the free edge of the nail as newly formed plate slowly pushes forward in a distal direction. Formation and outgrowth of the nail plate is a continual process. A fully formed nail plate extends from below the proximal nail-fold cuticle to beyond the hyponychium and extends laterally below the cuticle of the lateral nail folds. Nail-plate abnormalities frequently occur secondary to changes or disorders affecting function of the nail matrix; infections such as onychomycosis; or trauma.

Age-Related Nail-Plate Findings

The growth rate of an adult fingernail plate is approximately 3 mm/mo, with marked variability among individuals.[2] Toenail plate growth occurs at one third to one half the rate of fingernail growth. A general rule is that adult fingernails take approximately 6 months to grow out fully; adult toenails, 12 to 18 months. Nail-plate growth is faster in children, peaking between 10 and 14 years of age; there is a slowly progressive decline after the second decade of life.[2] Linear nail-plate growth decreases by 50 % over a lifetime, with periods of slow decline alternating with periods of rapid decline in approximate 7-year increments.[7] Nail-plate growth increases during pregnancy and decreases during lactation, after use of chemotherapeutic agents, and in conditions characterized by limb paralysis, persistently diminished circulation, or malnutrition.[2,3,8] Yellow nail syndrome is characterized by very slow or absent growth of nail plate; it usually affects both fingernails and toenails and is seen in association with several underlying conditions, such as lymphedema, respiratory disorders (e.g., bronchiectasis and pleural effusions), and nephrotic syndrome.[9]

Constitutional age-related findings in the nail plate include changes in nail color and luster, longitudinal ridging, changes in convexity, and brittle nails.[8,10] Nail plates, especially of toenails, often develop a yellow or gray color with a dull, opaque appearance. Longitudinal ridging may affect some or all nails and may present as slightly indented grooves or projection ridges or as beading. Over time, the surface of the nail plate may become flattened (platyonychia) or spooned (koilonychia). Temporary koilonychia, especially of the toenails, is also seen in infants.[6]

Pathophysiology Affecting the Nail Plate

Brittle nails is a common complaint; its incidence is 20% in the overall population (27% in female patients) and increases with advancing age.[10] When nail water content falls below 16%, nail plates become brittle; when the water content rises above 25%, nail plates become soft. The most common cause of brittle nails is dehydration, which can be caused or exacerbated by external factors such as use of nail-polish remover or exposure to dry climate. Onychoschizia, which presents as a layered, superficial splitting of the nail plate, may increase in incidence with

age. This condition is seen much more frequently in female patients. It is likely related to recurrent exposures to water or irritants, such as during nail-care procedures.

Fingernails demonstrate a tendency to become thinner and more fragile over time. Toenails usually become thicker and harder. Onychogryphosis is a marked thickening, usually of the large toenail, resulting in a compacted mass of heaped-up dystrophic nail plate.[8] Contributing factors appear to be advanced age, poor nail care, chronic trauma, decreased peripheral circulation, and neuropathy. Poor-fitting shoewear causes long-term exposure to lateral pressure and friction, resulting in gryphotic changes (marked thickening or heaping of nail plate), usually of the first and fifth toenails.

NAIL FOLDS

The nail folds are the cutaneous soft tissue that houses the nail unit, invaginating proximally and laterally to encompass the emerging nail plate. The proximal nail fold, with the exception of the lunula, covers the underlying matrix and is devoid of sebaceous glands and dermatoglyphic skin markings.[11] The term paronychia describes inflammation of the nail folds. Paronychia may be acute or chronic and may occur secondary to a variety of conditions, including contact dermatitis, psoriasis, bacterial infection, and fungal infection.[12,13] The cuticle (eponychium) is a thin, keratinized membrane of modified stratum corneum that extends from the distal portion of the nail fold, reflecting onto the nail-plate surface. Intact cuticle serves as a seal that protects the space between the nail folds and the nail plate from exposure to external irritants, allergens, and pathogens. Loss of cuticle allows for exposure and trapping of these deleterious external agents, providing an environment in which either inflammatory or infectious paronychia can develop.

Nail Findings Associated with Disease States

Several nail findings have been associated with both underlying systemic and dermatologic conditions. The following is a review of selected, recognized associations. Diagnosis is based on proper evaluation of clinical findings; treatment is based on a confirmed etiology or the recognition of an underlying systemic association.

Special care must be taken when performing biopsy of the nail bed or matrix to avoid trauma to the tissue specimen and surrounding structures upon specimen removal. The most appropriate plane of dissection during nail-bed or nail-matrix biopsy is subdermal. The sampled tissue should be manipulated very gently throughout the biopsy procedure to avoid crush artifact, which may interfere significantly with histopathologic evaluation. It is also important to carefully dissect along the undersurface of the specimen, ensuring nontraumatic separation of the biopsy tissue from its underlying firm attachment to bone.

SPLINTER HEMORRHAGES

Splinter hemorrhages may be secondary to trauma, high altitude, primary dermatoses (i.e., psoriasis), or several underlying conditions (e.g., arterial emboli, collagen vascular disease, or thromboangiitis obliterans). The simultaneous appearance of splinter hemorrhages in several nails should raise suspicion of a possible underlying systemic disorder, especially in female patients.[14]

KOILONYCHIA

Koilonychia may be found in association with other conditions, including congenital conditions, iron deficiency anemia, cardiac disease, endocrinopathy, occupational exposures, and trauma.[3,15]

TRANSVERSE NAIL-PLATE DEPRESSIONS (BEAU LINES)

Beau lines present as well-delineated, transverse depressions in the nail plate. They are believed to occur secondary to temporary growth arrest of the nail matrix. The grooves become evident weeks after the occurrence of an abrupt, stressful event, such as an acute febrile illness. The width of the groove reflects the duration of interrupted nail-matrix function. When limited to one or a few digits, Beau lines may be associated with trauma, carpal tunnel syndrome, or Raynaud disease, or they may occur subsequent to tourniquet application during hand surgery.[15] Approximately 1 to 2 months after birth, infants may demonstrate physiologic Beau lines, which mark the transition from intrauterine to extrauterine life.[16] Multiple transverse grooves (stepladder appearance) may be seen in as-

sociation with repeated cycles of chemotherapy, or they may be related to zinc deficiency. Multiple Beau lines should not be confused with the multiple transverse depressions that are stacked longitudinally along the central nail plate (washboard nails), resulting from the obsessive habit of repeatedly pushing back the cuticle or picking at the proximal nailfold margin (habit-tic deformity) [see Figure 2].[15,17] There is no specific treatment for Beau lines. They grow out over time after resolution of the growth-arrest period.

ONYCHOLYSIS

Onycholyis is defined as the separation of the nail plate from the nail bed. In most cases, onycholysis begins distally; it is often related to acute or chronic trauma that produces a lever effect, lifting the nail plate upward and away from its bed. Other causes of onycholysis are chemical exposure (allergic or irritant dermatitis), onychomycosis, and primary dermatoses (e.g., psoriasis or lichen planus).[13] Associations with underlying systemic disease (e.g., thyroid disease) have been sporadically reported but are less commonly encountered in clinical practice. When moisture accumulates under onycholytic nail plate, bacterial proliferation may occur. This can cause a green discoloration of the nail plate as a result of a pigment produced by certain organisms (e.g., *Pseudomonas aeruginosa*) [see Figure 3].

Treatment requires avoidance of precipating factors for onycholysis, debridement of separated nail plate, and the twice-daily topical application of diluted acetic acid solution (consisting of equal parts white vinegar and water), gentamicin, or the combination of polymyxin B and bacitracin.[18]

LEUKONYCHIA

Leukonychia, a white discoloration of the nail plate or subungual tissue, has multiple presentations. Small 1 to 3 mm white spots (punctate leukonychia) or irregular transverse streaks (leukonychia variegata) of the nail plate are the most common varieties.[15] These two presentations are generally secondary to repeated microtrauma to the matrix, growing out distally with outgrowth of the nail plate. Mee lines specifically refer to transverse 1 to 2 mm white bands, which usually are demonstrated at the same site in multiple nails and reported in association with arsenic intoxication, Hodgkin disease, sickle cell anemia, renal failure, and cardiac insufficiency. Leukonychia is also associated with systemic infection and chemotherapy.[19-21]

Half-and-half nails (Lindsay nails) present as a diffuse, dull whitening of the proximal nail bed that obscures the lunula and as a distal region of pink or reddish-brown discoloration that occupies from 20% to 60% of the nail length.[15,22] The most commonly reported association with half-and-half nails is chronic renal failure. When the distal brown band of discoloration constitutes less than 20% of the total nail length, the anomaly is known as Terry nails, which occurs in association with chronic congestive heart failure, hepatic cirrhosis, type 2 (non–insulin-dependent) diabetes mellitus, and advanced age. In both half-and-half nails and Terry nails, the proximal portion of the nail bed may be light pink, exhibiting a more normal appearance, rather than white.

Muehrcke nails present as paired, white, narrow transverse bands of the nail bed, separated by normal-appearing thin pink bands.[15,22] Muehrcke nails have been associated with chronic hypoalbuminemia. Resolution of this nail finding correlates with normalization of serum albumin levels.[15]

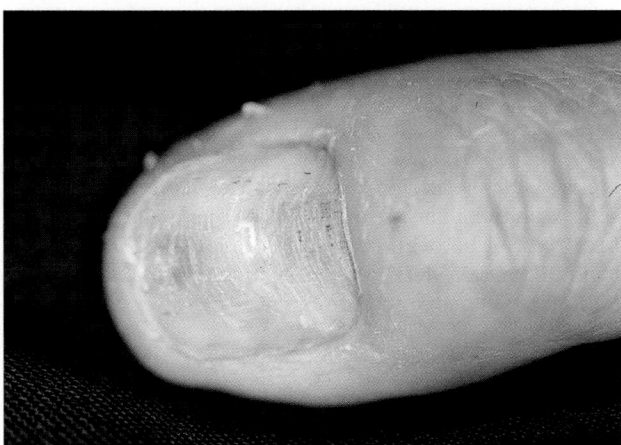

Figure 2   Stacking of transverse linear grooves traversing the entire length of the central nail plate, resulting from the repeated picking of the proximal nail fold margin (habit-tic deformity). Note the marked hypertrophy of the lunula, which is typical of this disorder.

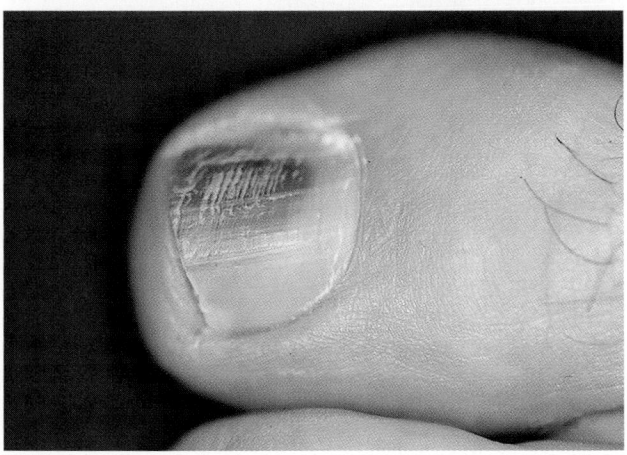

Figure 3   Colonization of the closed space between the nail bed and nail plate with *Pseudomonas aeruginosa*, causing a green nail. Moisture trapped in the onycholytic space provides an optimal environment for proliferation of this bacterium.

CLUBBING

When the normal angle between the proximal nail fold and the nail plate exceeds 180°, digital clubbing is present. The morphologic changes of clubbing typically include hypertrophy of the surrounding soft tissue of the nail folds as a result of hyperplasia of dermal fibrovasculature and edematous infiltration of the pulp tip.[21] Radiologic changes are identified in fewer than 20% of cases.[15]

Clubbing may be hereditary, or it may be seen in association with several underlying disease states, such as hypertrophic pulmonary osteoarthropathy, chronic congestive heart failure, congenital heart disease associated with cyanosis, polycythemias associated with hypoxia, Graves disease, chronic hepatic cirrhosis, lung cancer, Crohn disease, and irritable bowel disease.[15,22,23] When clubbing is unilateral, consideration should be given to underlying causes of obstructed circulation, such as aneurysm, arteriovenous fistula, and a pulmonary sulcus tumor (Pancoast tumor); disorders producing soft tissue edema; and diseases causing localized changes in underlying digital bone (e.g., sarcoidosis). Unilateral clubbing can also be found in cases of hemiplegia,[24] and a case of subungual perineurioma caused by unilateral clubbing has been reported.[25] Paronychia and distal phalangeal resorption may cause changes that simulate true clubbing (pseudoclubbing).

NAIL-PLATE PITTING

Nail-plate pitting (onychia punctata) develops as a result of focal defects in nail-plate formation from the proximal nail matrix. The number, size, and shape of the superficial depressions may vary.[15] The extent and duration of involvement with nail pitting correlates with the duration of nail-matrix abnormality. Psoriasis, the most common association with nail pitting, may produce a random array of shallow or deep pitted indentations, usually affecting one or more fingernails.[26,27]

Psoriasis of the nails often responds poorly to treatment, and it tends to recur. Topical corticosteroids, topical tazarotene, and intralesional corticosteroid injection may help in some cases.[28,29] It is a common misconception that nail pitting is pathognomonic for psoriasis.[27] Nail pitting may also be seen in association with alopecia areata, punctate keratoderma, idiopathic trachyonychia, occasionally in normal nails, and rarely in association with collagen vascular disease or syphilis. Fingernail pitting occurs in one third of children with alopecia areata; mild disease involving only a few nails is observed in approximately 20% of cases.[27] Compared to psoriasis, nail pitting seen in alopecia areata is typically more uniform and patterned, often presenting as orderly rows of shallow pitted depressions. Currently, there is no available treatment for this type of nail pitting.

LONGITUDINAL PIGMENTED BANDS

Longitudinal pigmented bands (melanonychia striata), also referred to as longitudinal melanonychia, is the presence of single or multiple longitudinally oriented brown or black bands [see Figure 4]. Homogeneous longitudinal bands occur in approximately 75% of African Americans older than 20 years. It usually affects the thumb and index finger.[30,31] Melanonychia striata is also commonly seen in Hispanics, may be found in up to 20% of Japanese, and is rare in whites.[30]

The deposition of melanin in the nail plate may result from increased melanin synthesis by matrix melanocytes that are usually nonfunctional; it may also occur as a result of a prolif-

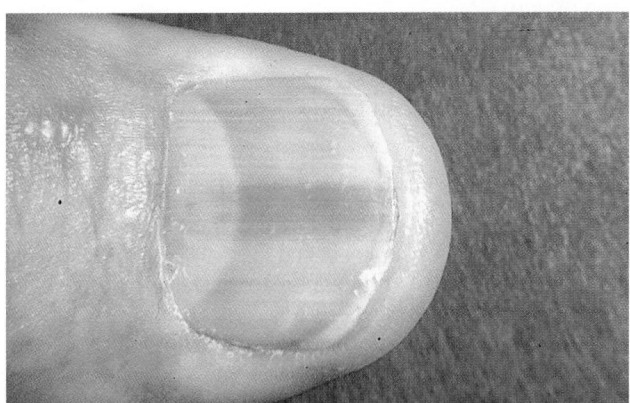

Figure 4 Melanonychia striata (longitudinal pigmented band) produced by a melanocytic nevus of the nail matrix. A high index of suspicion for subungual melanoma is very important when a longitudinal pigmented band of the nail is identified.

eration of matrix melanocytes.[30] Melanonychia striata affecting a single nail may result from a benign melanocytic nevus or a subungual melanoma. Thus, it is important to distinguish between a benign cause and a malignant cause of a longitudinal pigmented band. Factors suggesting the presence of melanoma or an atypical melanocytic proliferation are (1) single digit involvement; (2) periungual spread of pigment onto the nail-fold region (Hutchinson sign); (3) border irregularity or variegated color within the linear streak; and (4) changes in appearance (e.g., color or borders) involving an established longitudinal band.[32] Because of the severity of subungual melanoma and the importance of making a prompt diagnosis, the index of suspicion must be high. A simple biopsy of the nail plate is not satisfactory in establishing the diagnosis, because it will only demonstrate the presence of melanin. An appropriate biopsy inclusive of the nail matrix, as well as the nail bed if clinically indicated, should be performed by a surgeon who is familiar with the intricacies of performing a nail biopsy.[33] Because of limited experience and the difficulties that are commonly con-

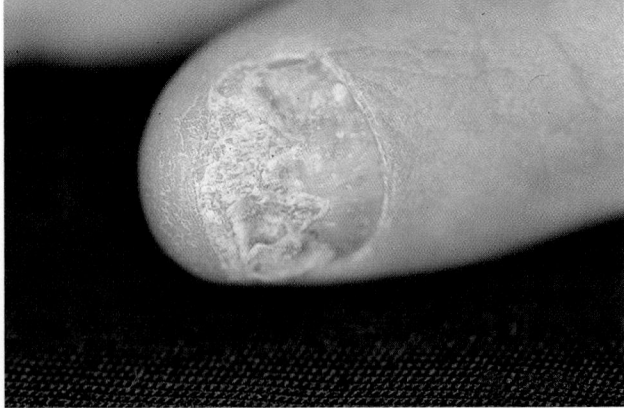

Figure 5 Psoriasis of the nail, characterized by subungual hyperkeratosis and loss of distal onycholytic nail plate. This patient was unsuccessfully treated with oral antifungal therapy after an erroneous diagnosis of onychomycosis was made on the basis of clinical diagnosis alone. Careful examination of the proximal intact nail plate reveals pitting, a feature characteristic for psoriasis and not onychomycosis.

a 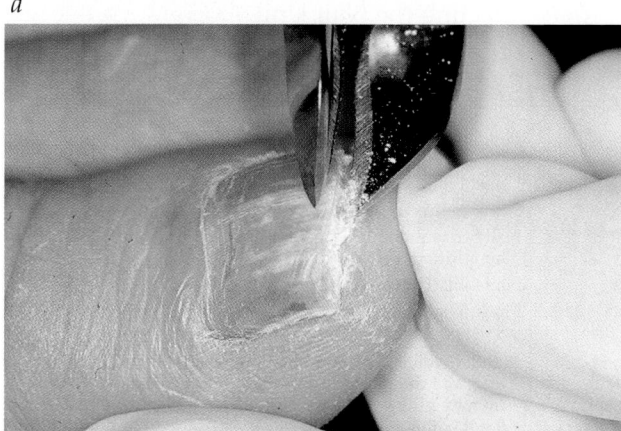 *b*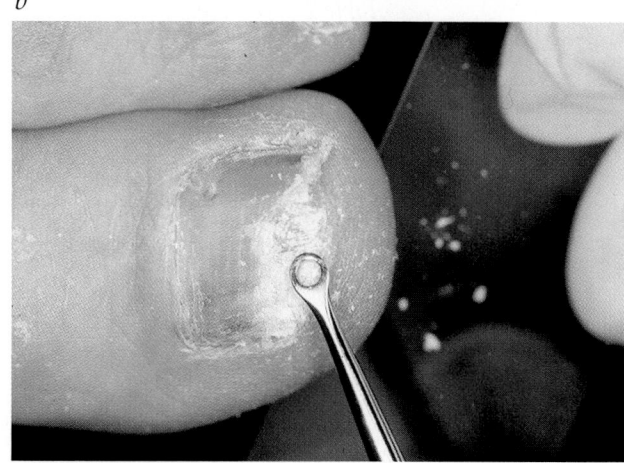

Figure 6 (*a*) **When obtaining a nail specimen for potassium hydroxide (KOH) preparation, it is important to expose the affected nail bed by first trimming away and discarding the distal, separated (onycholytic) nail plate. (*b*) Small specimen fragments of subungual hyperkeratosis of the nail bed and exposed undersurface of the nail plate are effectively obtained using a small curette. The smaller fragments are more easily dissolved by KOH, allowing for more accurate microscopic visualization, and can be easily plated on fungal culture medium.**

fronted in the histologic interpretation of nail specimens, biopsies of melanonychia striata are best interpreted by a dermatopathologist.[34]

When nail-bed pigmentation is noted, other causes such as systemic drugs (e.g., antimalarials, zidovudine, bleomycin, doxorubicin, minocycline, and hydroxyuria) or systemic disease (e.g., Addison disease and HIV infection) must be considered; however, these causes usually result in a broader, more diffuse pigmentation, often involving multiple nails.[35] Another reported association with melanonychia striata is systemic lupus erythematosus.[36] Frictional melanonychia resulting from trauma from athletic activities or poorly fitting shoewear may cause nail pigmentation, including pigmentation of the nail fold, especially in dark-skinned persons (pseudo-Hutchinson sign).[32]

Bacterial and Fungal Nail Infections

BACTERIAL PARONYCHIA

Bacterial infection of the nail folds (bacterial paronychia) is usually acute in nature. It is is characterized by swelling, erythema, discomfort, and sometimes purulence. The most common etiologic pathogen is *Staphylococcus aureus*. Treatment requires drainage of a focal abscess, if present, and oral antibiotic therapy.[37]

CHRONIC PARONYCHIA

Chronic paronychia results from persistent or frequently recurrent nail-fold inflammation, which is usually the result of chronic irritant dermatitis and loss of cuticle from trauma or nail-care practices. Secondary candidal infection may occur.[29,38]

Table 1 Oral Antifungal for Toenail Onychomycosis*[46]

Drug	*Dosage*	*Comments*
Griseofulvin tablets or liquid	500 mg – 1 g daily × 12 – 18 mo	Generally not recommended because of limited efficacy and because more effective agents are available; only active against dermatophyte organisms
Itraconazole capsules	Pulse therapy†: 200 mg twice daily × 1 wk/mo for 3 consecutive mo Continuous therapy: 200 mg daily × 3 mo	Contraindications include specific drug interactions and congestive heart failure; potential hepatotoxicity (rare); effective for dermatophytes, *Candida* species, and some nondermatophytic molds; should be administered with food; absorption may be decreased by increased gastric pH (as might result from use of H₂ blockers, antacids, proton pump inhibitors); blood clearance in 1 – 2 wk; therapeutic nail levels 9 mo posttherapy
Terbinafine tablets	250 mg daily × 3 mo	Most active for dermatophytes; some efficacy for certain nondermatophytic molds; limited activity against most *Candida* species; potential hepatotoxicity (rare); sporadic reports of blood dyscrasias (rare); reversible change or loss of taste (< 2%); blood clearance in 1 – 2 mo; therapeutic nail levels 9 mo posttherapy
Fluconazole tablets‡	150 – 300 mg × 9 – 12 mo	Effective against dermatophytes and *Candida* species; potential hepatotoxicity (rare); some significant drug interactions; limited therapeutic drug reservoir in nail posttherapy

*Topical ciclopirox 8% nail lacquer is FDA approved for onychomycosis caused by *Trichophyton rubrum*. Treatment involves application once daily for 12 mo (or until outgrowth of clear nail occurs), combined with debridement/trimming of onycholytic nail plate. Efficacy is lower than that seen with newer oral agents (e.g., itraconazole, terbinafine). No oral or topical agent is currently FDA approved for nondermatophytic onychomycosis (e.g., *Candida* species, molds).
†Pulse itraconazole is FDA approved for fingernail tinea unguium; established efficacy has been demonstrated for toenail disease.
‡Fluconazole is not FDA approved for onychomycosis; established efficacy has been demonstrated for tinea unguium.

Table 2   Selected Dermatologic Disorders Affecting the Nail Unit

Disease State	Disease Features	Nail Findings
Inflammatory diseases		
Psoriasis	Nail findings in 10% – 50% of patients; 39% of children with psoriasis with nail changes (usually pitting); nail disease present in 50% – 85% of patients with psoriatic arthritis	Proximal matrix involvement: pitting, transverse grooving, deeply ridged plate surface (onychorrhexis) Distal matrix involvement: plate thinning, lunula erythema Nail bed: subungual hyperkeratosis, oil drop sign, splinter hemorrhages Nail folds: cutaneous lesions of psoriasis Phalangeal/joint involvement: psoriatic arthritis
Lichen planus	Nail changes occur in up to 10% of patients with lichen planus; may occur in childhood or adulthood; nail involvement may be present with or without skin or mucosal disease; potentially reversible in early inflammatory stage; irreversible in cicatricial (later stage) of disease; may present as ridged, rough-surfaced, lusterless plates (trachyonychia) or 20-nail dystrophy in children	Matrix involvement: combination of nail-plate ridging, splitting, and progressive uniform thinning; distal-edge splitting, fragility, crumbling, brittleness, nail-plate shedding (onychomadesis) Focal matrix scarring: pterygium formation (scarring bridge between proximal nail fold and subungual epidermis with focal loss of nail plate) Nail-bed involvement: subungual hyperkeratosis, onycholysis Diffuse matrix/nail-bed disease: total nail-plate loss, atrophy, scarring
Alopecia areata	Nail changes in 10% of patints with alopecia areata; nail changes in over 40% of children with alopecia areata; fingernail involvement most common; may present in children as 20-nail dystrophy	Matrix involvement: orderly nail pitting arranged in a cross-hatched pattern (glen-plaid sign); roughened nail-plate surface (trachyonychia); fragility; splitting; longitudinal ridging; spotted or red lunula (erythema); nail-plate shedding (onychomadesis)
Nail tumors		
Glomus tumor	75% occur on the hand, usually subungual (nail bed); a benign vascular hamartoma	Visible through plate as a light-red, reddish-blue spot; rarely exceeds 1 cm in size; characteristic symptom of intense or pulsatile pain; pain is spontaneous or provoked by slight trauma or pressure
Digital myxoid (mucus) cyst	A form of focal mucinosis; not a true cyst (no epithelial lining); contains clear, viscous, jellylike fluid; usually seen in adults	Soft, domed, translucent, pink or skin-colored, shiny, soft neoplasm of proximal nail fold or overlying distal interphalangeal joint; those over fold may compress matrix, producing flattening of plate; those over joint may connect to underlying joint space
Subungual exostoses	Outgrowths of calcified cartilage or normal bone; most seen on great toe; most frequent in adolescents and young adults; benign lesions	Emerge from the dorsal digit at distal phalanx; may erode through plate or project from under distal or lateral edge of plate; often painful; may become eroded
Periungual angiofibromas	Arise out of nail fold; often multiple; seen in 50% of cases of tuberous sclerosis (Borneville-Pringle disease); usually arise in early teenage years; benign neoplasm	Small, round, flesh-colored or pink, firm papules with shiny, smooth surface arising from nail-fold region; may partially cover nail plate; usually asymptomatic

ONYCHOMYCOSIS

Onychomycosis, the most common infection of the nail, is a fungal infection characterized by nail-bed and plate involvement. Dermatophyte onychomycosis (tinea unguium) is the most common type of fungal nail infection.[39] It is seen far more commonly in adults than in children and most frequently affects one or more toenails. The mode of fungal invasion usually presents as distal-lateral subungual onychomycosis, occurring as dermatophyte organisms migrate from pedal skin to below the nail plate and invade nail-bed tissue.[40] Tinea pedis and onychomycosis frequently coexist in a patient.[41,42]

The dermatophytes that most commonly cause onychomycosis are *Trichophyton rubrum* and *T. mentagrophytes*.[43] The tendency to harbor dermatophytes (especially *T. rubrum*), predominantly on pedal skin, has been noted in some kindreds. As a result, patients with such a tendency are prone to tinea pedis, tinea unguium, tinea cruris, and diffuse tinea corporis. They may present with dermatophyte infections earlier in life than usually seen and often experience recurrence of dermatophyte infection after completion of initially effective therapy.

The most characteristic clinical features of dermatophyte onychomycosis are distal onycholysis, subungual hyperkeratosis, and a dystrophic, discolored nail plate.[42] Because this combination of features is also seen in persons with nail psoriasis, accurate diagnosis may require performance of a potassium hydroxide (KOH) preparation and fungal culture [*see Figure 5*]. It is important that specimens be obtained from the nail bed [*see Figure 6*] and that culture specimens be transported and plated appropriately, because different culture media are required for identification of dermatophyte and nondermatophyte fungal nail pathogens.[42] Dermatophyte test medium (DTM) may be used as an in-office culture technique that has no special incubation requirements. DTM is inexpensive and accurate in the diagnosis of dermatophyte onychomycosis.[44] The clinical presentation of proximal white subungual onychomycosis, another presentation of dermatophyte onychomycosis, has been reported in association with systemic immunosuppression, including HIV disease.[45]

Candida onychomycosis is far less common than dermatophyte onychomycosis. *Candida* onychomycosis is often associated with immunosuppression (e.g., HIV disease and chronic mucocutaneous candidiasis). The *Candida* organisms may invade the nail as a secondary pathogen, and they more frequently affect the fingernails.[42] Nondermatophyte molds, including *Aspergillus* species, *Scopulariopsis brevicaulis*, *Fusarium* species, *Scytalidium hyalinum,* and *Scytalidium dimidiatum,* have been reported to cause fingernail or toenail infection; however, such infections are relatively uncommon.[42,46] Associated paronychia may be seen when nondermatophytic fungi cause onychomycosis. Effective therapy for onychomycosis includes the use of an oral antifungal agent [*see Table 1*].[47] Because nails grow slowly, clinical response is delayed.[46] Infections with *Scytalidium* species are rare in the United States, and such infections respond poorly to currently available antifungal agents.

DERMATOLOGIC DISORDERS AFFECTING THE NAIL

Complete reviews of dermatologic, systemic, neoplastic, and exogenous disorders affecting the nail are beyond the scope of this chapter. An overview of selected dermatologic disorders affecting the nail unit and their associated clinical findings is provided [*see Table 2*].

James Q. Del Rosso, D.O., participates in the speakers' bureaus and is a consultant for Allergan, Inc., Janssen Pharmaceutica Products, L.P., Dermik Laboratories, Inc., Novartis Pharmaceuticals Corp., and Medicis Co.

C. Ralph Daniel III, M.D., has no commercial relationships with manufacturers of products or providers of services discussed in this chapter.

References

1. Gonzalez-Serva A: Structure and function. Nails: Therapy, Diagnosis, Surgery. Scher RK, Daniel CR, Eds. WB Saunders Co, Philadelphia, 1997, p 12

2. Fleckman P: Basic science of the nail unit. Nails: Therapy, Diagnosis, Surgery. Scher RK, Daniel CR, Eds. WB Saunders Co, Philadelphia, 1997, p 44

3. Dawber RPR, De Berker DAR, Baran R: Science of the nail apparatus. Diseases of the Nails and Their Management. Baran R, Dawber RPR, Eds. Blackwell Science, Oxford, England, 1994, p 5

4. Fleckman P, Allan C: Surgical anatomy of the nail unit. Dermatol Surg 27:257, 2001

5. Cohen PR: The lunula. J Am Acad Dermatol 34:943, 1996

6. Tosti A, Peluso AP, Piraccini BM: Nail diseases in children. Adv Dermatol 13:353, 1998

7. Orentreich N, Markofsky J, Vogelman JH: The effect of aging on the rate of linear nail growth. J Invest Dermatol 73:126, 1979

8. Cohen PR, Scher RK: Geriatric nail disorders: diagnosis and treatment. J Am Acad Dermatol 26:521, 1992

9. Tosti A, Baran R, Dawber RPR: The nails in systemic disease and drug-induced changes: yellow nail syndrome. Diseases of the Nails and Their Management. Baran R, Dawber RPR, Eds. Blackwell Science, Oxford, England, 1994, p 185

10. Lubach D, Cohrs W, Wurzinger R: Incidence of brittle nails. Dermatologica 172:144, 1986

11. Baran R, Dawber RPR, Tosti A: Science of the nail apparatus and relationship to foot function. A Text Atlas of Nail Disorders. Baran R, Dawber RPR, Tosti A, Eds. Martin Dunitz, London, 1996, p 3

12. Daniel CR III, Daniel MO, Gupta AK: Nonfungal infections and paronychia. Nails: Therapy, Diagnosis, Surgery. Scher RK, Daniel CR, Eds. WB Saunders Co, Philadelphia, 1997, p 165

13. Kern D: Occupational disease. Nails: Therapy, Diagnosis, Surgery. Scher RK, Daniel CR, Eds. WB Saunders Co, Philadelphia, 1997, p 285

14. Tosti A, Baran R, Dawber RPR: The nails in systemic disease and drug-induced changes: splinter hemorrhages. Diseases of the Nails and Their Management. Baran R, Dawber RPR, Eds. Blackwell Science, Oxford, England, 1994, p 183

15. Baran R, Dawber RPR: Physical signs. Diseases of the Nails and Their Management. Baran R, Dawber RPR, Eds. Blackwell Science, Oxford, England, 1994, p 35

16. Baran R, Dawber RPR: Physical signs: Beau's lines and transverse grooves. Diseases of the Nails and Their Management. Baran R, Dawber RPR, Eds. Blackwell Science, Oxford, 1994, p 50

17. Habif TP: Nail diseases: habit-tic deformity. Clinical Dermatology. Habif TP, Ed. Mosby, St Louis, 1996, p 774

18. Daniel CR III, Daniel MO, Gupta AK: Appendix 2. Nails: Therapy, Diagnosis, Surgery. Scher RK, Daniel CR, Eds. WB Saunders Co, Philadelphia, 1997, p 368

19. Naumann R, Wozel G: Transverse leukonychia following chemotherapy in a patient with Hodgkin's disease. Eur J Dermatol 19:392, 2000

20. Cribier B, Mena ML, Rey D, et al: Nail changes in patients infected with human immunodeficiency virus: a prospective controlled study. Arch Dermatol 134:1216, 1998

21. Mautner GH, Lu I, Ort RJ, et al: Transverse leukonychia with systemic infection. Cutis 65:318, 2000

22. Daniel CR III, Sams WM, Scher RK: Nails in systemic disease. Nails: Therapy, Diagnosis, Surgery. Scher RK, Daniel CR, Eds. WB Saunders Co, Philadelphia, 1997, p 219

23. Myers KA, Farquhar DR: The rational clinical examination: does this patient have clubbing? JAMA 286:341, 2001

24. Siragusa M, Schepis C, Cosentino FI, et al: Nail pathology in patients with hemiplegia. Br J Dermatol 144:557, 2001

25. Baran R, Perrin C: Subungual perineurioma: a peculiar location. Br J Dermatol 146:125, 2002

26. Farber EM, Nall ML: Nail psoriasis. Cutis 50:174, 1992

27. Del Rosso JQ, Basuk P, Scher RK, et al: Dermatologic diseases of the nail unit. Nails: Therapy, Diagnosis, Surgery. Scher RK, Daniel CR, Eds. WB Saunders Co, Philadelphia, 1997, p 172

28. Scher RK, Stiller M, Zhu YI: Tazarotene 0.1% gel in the treatment of fingernail psoriasis: a double-blind, randomized, vehicle-controlled study. Cutis 68:355, 2001

29. Tosti A, Piraccini BM: Treatment of common nail disorders. Dermatol Clin 18:339, 2000

30. Baran R, Haneke E: Tumors of the nail apparatus and adjacent tissues: longitudinal melanonychia. Diseases of the Nails and Their Management. Baran R, Dawber RPR, Eds. Blackwell Science, Oxford, England, 1994, p 485

31. Haneke E, Baran R: Longitudinal melanonychia. Dermatol Surg 27:580, 2001

32. Baran R, Dawber RPR, Tosti A: Nail colour changes (chromonychia). A Text Atlas of Nail Disorders. Baran R, Dawber RPR, Tosti A, Eds. Martin Dunitz, London, 1996, p 147

33. Salasche SJ: Surgery. Dermatologic diseases of the nail unit. Nails: Therapy, Diagnosis, Surgery. Scher RK, Daniel CR, Eds. WB Saunders Co, Philadelphia, 1997, p 335

34. Fleckman P, Omura EF: Histopathology of the nail. Adv Dermatol 17:385, 2001

35. Aste N, Fumo G, Contu F, et al: Nail pigmentation caused by hydroxyurea: report of 9 cases. J Am Acad Dermatol 47:146, 2002

36. Skowron F, Combemale P, Faisant M, et al: Functional melanonychia due to involvement of the nail matrix in systemic lupus erythematosus. J Am Acad Dermatol 47(suppl):S187, 2002

37. Habif T: Nail diseases: acute paronychia. Clinical Dermatology. Habif TP, Ed. Mosby, St. Louis, 1996, p 763

38. Van Laborde S, Scher RK: Developments in the treatment of nail psoriasis, melanonychia striata, and onychomycosis: a review of the literature. Dermatol Clin 18:37, 2000

39. Gupta AK, Taborda P, Taborda V, et al: Epidemiology and prevalence of onychomycosis in HIV-positive individuals. Int J Dermatol 39:746, 2000

40. Elewski BE: Onychomycosis: treatment, quality of life, and economic issues. Am J Clin Dermatol 1:19, 2000

41. Lauritz B: Dermatoses of the feet. Am J Clin Dermatol 1:181, 2000

42. Elewski BE, Charif MA, Daniel CR III: Onychomycosis. Nails: Therapy, Diagnosis, Surgery. Scher RK, Daniel CR, Eds. WB Saunders Co, Philadelphia, 1997, p 152

43. Jennings MB, Weinberg JM, Koestenblatt EK, et al: Study of clinically suspected onychomycosis in a podiatric population. J Am Podiatr Med Assoc 92:327, 2002

44. Pariser D, Opper C: An in-office diagnostic procedure to detect dermatophytes in a nationwide study of onychomycosis patients. Manag Care 11:43, 2002

45. Baran R, Dawber RPR, Tosti A: Onychomycosis and its treatment. A Text Atlas of Nail Disorders. Baran R, Dawber RPR, Tosti A, Eds. Martin Dunitz, London, 1996, p 157

46. Del Rosso JQ: Current management of onychomycosis and dermatomycoses. Curr Infect Dis Rep 2:438, 2000

47. Crawford F, Young P, Godfrey C, et al: Oral treatments for toenail onychomycosis: a systematic review. Arch Dermatol 138:811, 2002

Acknowledgment

Figure 1 Tom Moore.

48 Disorders of Pigmentation

Pearl E. Grimes, M.D.

Disorders of Hyperpigmentation

MELASMA

Definition

Melasma is a common acquired symmetrical hypermelanosis characterized by irregular light-brown to gray-brown macules involving the face. There is a predilection for the cheeks, forehead, upper lips, nose, and chin [*see Figure 1*]. Lesions may occasionally occur in other sun-exposed areas, including the forearms and back.[1-3]

Epidemiology

Melasma is most commonly observed in females. Men constitute only 10% of the cases but usually demonstrate the same clinicopathologic features as women do. The condition affects all racial and ethnic groups but is most prevalent in persons with darker complexions (skin types IV through VI). It is also more common in geographic areas with intense ultraviolet radiation (sunlight), such as tropical and subtropical regions.

Etiology and Pathogenesis

Although the precise cause of melasma is unknown, multiple factors have been implicated in the etiology and pathogenesis of this condition. These factors include genetic influences, intense ultraviolet radiation exposure, pregnancy, oral contraceptive use, hormone replacement therapy, cosmetics, and phototoxic and antiseizure medications.[1]

Endocrinologic studies of patients with melasma have shown varying results. Although a detailed study of nine women with melasma showed significantly increased levels of luteinizing hormone (LH) and low levels of estradiol, suggesting a role for subclinical mild ovarian dysfunction, a study of 26 women found no difference in LH, follicle-stimulating hormone (FSH), and α-melanocyte–stimulating hormone (α-MSH) levels between patients with melasma and control subjects.[3] Another study reported increased expression of α-MSH in the affected skin areas of 10 women with melasma. α-MSH stimulates tyrosinase and melanin synthesis.[4]

Clinically, the light-brown patches are commonly evident on the malar prominences, forehead, chin, nose, and upper lip. The patches may have a malar, centrofacial, or mandibular distribution. Histologically, an epidermal, epidermal-dermal, or dermal pattern of increased pigmentation occurs. Histologic studies document an increase in epidermal pigmentation, increased numbers of melanocytes, and increased activity of melanogenic enzymes.[5] A Wood-light examination enhances the epidermal pattern of pigment deposition. Such epidermal lesions are most amenable to treatment.

The differential diagnosis of melasma includes other conditions that cause facial hyperpigmentation, such as postinflammatory hyperpigmentation, drug-induced hyperpigmentation, lichen planus actinicus, and photosensitivity disorders.

Treatment

Current treatments for melasma include broad-spectrum sunscreens, 2% (over the counter) and 4% (prescription) hydroquinone formulations, azelaic acid, kojic acid formulations, α-hydroxyacid products, retinoic acid, retinol, superficial chemical peels, and microdermabrasion.[1,6-9] A triple-combination product containing 4% hydroquinone, 0.01% fluocinolone, and 0.05% retinoic acid has enhanced efficacy. This product was previously compounded by pharmacists, but it is now available as a commercial preparation (Tri-Luma cream, Galderma Laboratories) that has been approved by the Food and Drug Administration for treatment of melasma. Because the combination contains a fluorinated steroid, treatment should be limited to 8 weeks. Laser therapy offers minimal long-term success and, instead, may worsen the condition. Intense pulsed light therapy may offer some improvement in patients with melasma.[10,11]

Although all of these therapies reduce the severity of melasma, none are curative. Hence, it is essential for patients to rigidly adhere to a regimen of daily sun protection (e.g., using sunscreen or wearing protective clothing) to control the progression of melasma.

POSTINFLAMMATORY HYPERPIGMENTATION

Definition

Postinflammatory hyperpigmentation is characterized by an acquired increase in cutaneous pigmentation secondary to an inflammatory process [*see Figure 2*]. Excess pigment deposition may occur in the epidermis or in both the epidermis and the dermis.

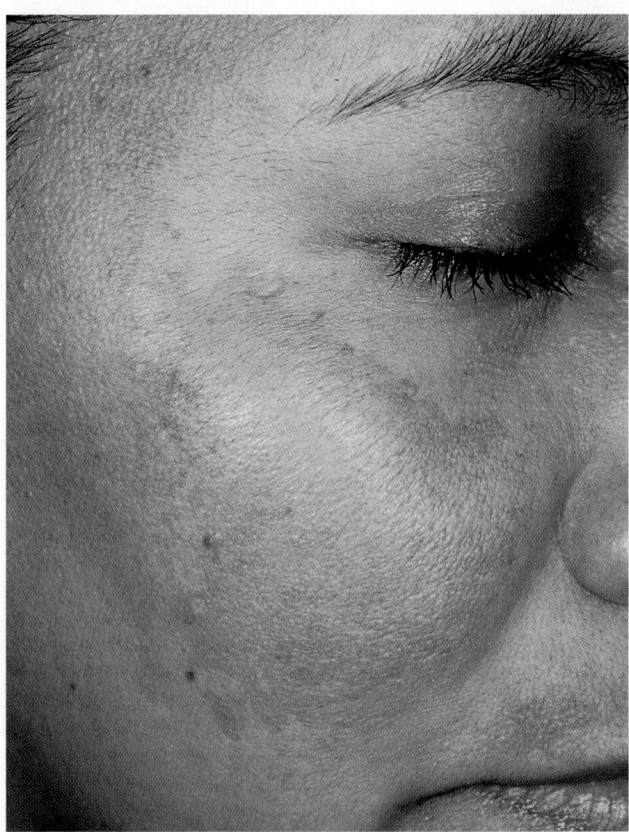

Figure 1 **Melasma is characterized by hyperpigmentation of the cheek, forehead, and upper lip.**

Epidemiology

All racial and ethnic groups are susceptible to postinflammatory hyperpigmentation, but the incidence of the condition is higher in persons with darker complexions. In a diagnostic survey of 2,000 African-American patients seeking dermatologic care, the third most common diagnosis was pigmentary disorders, of which postinflammatory hyperpigmentation was the most prevalent.[1]

Etiology and Pathogenesis

Pigmentary changes may be a result of production of inflammatory mediators and altered cytokine production.[12,13] Such changes may lead to an increase in the number and size of epidermal melanocytes. In addition, hyperpigmentation may be a consequence of pigmentary incontinence, with deposition of pigment in the upper dermis. Postinflammatory hyperpigmentation may be a sequela of conditions such as acne, allergic reactions, drug eruptions, papulosquamous disorders, eczematoid disorders, and vesiculobullous disorders.[14]

Diagnosis

Clinically, postinflammatory pigmentary changes may be localized, circumscribed, or generalized. Lesions range in color from brown to black to ashen gray and usually follow the distribution of the primary dermatosis.

Treatment

Therapies for postinflammatory hyperpigmentation include over-the-counter and prescription hydroquinone preparations. Higher concentrations are indicated for moderate to severe involvement. Other treatments include azelaic acid, kojic acid, retinoic acid [see Melasma, above], and adapalene.[15]

DRUG-INDUCED HYPERPIGMENTATION

Medications are a common cause of cutaneous hyperpigmentation. Lesions may be localized or generalized. Medications can also cause hyperpigmentation of the oral mucosa and nails. There may be some improvement upon withdrawal of the offending agent; however, drug-induced hyperpigmentation can persist for many years.

Medications causing drug-induced hyperpigmentation include oral contraceptives, hormone replacement therapies, antibiotics, antidepressants, antiviral agents, antimalarials, antihypertensives, and chemotherapeutic agents. Such medications include progesterone, estrogen, zidovudine (AZT), minocycline, tetracycline, bleomycin, hydrochlorothiazide, hydantoin, amiodarone, chlorpromazine, quinacrine, hydroxychloroquine, chloroquine, imipramine, amitriptyline, diltiazem, citalopram, hydroxyurea, doxorubicin, busulfan, daunorubicin, cisplatin, cyclophosphamide, thiotepa, vinblastine, and vincristine.[16-23]

Heavy-metal preparations can also cause hyperpigmentation. These preparations include arsenic, gold, silver, mercury, and bismuth.

Treatment with the Q-switched alexandrite laser has proven to be an effective treatment for drug-induced pigmentation.[19,24]

ERYTHEMA DYSCHROMICUM PERSTANS

Definition

Erythema dyschromicum perstans (EDP, or ashy dermatosis) is an acquired benign condition characterized by slate-gray to violaceous macules. It was first described in 1957.

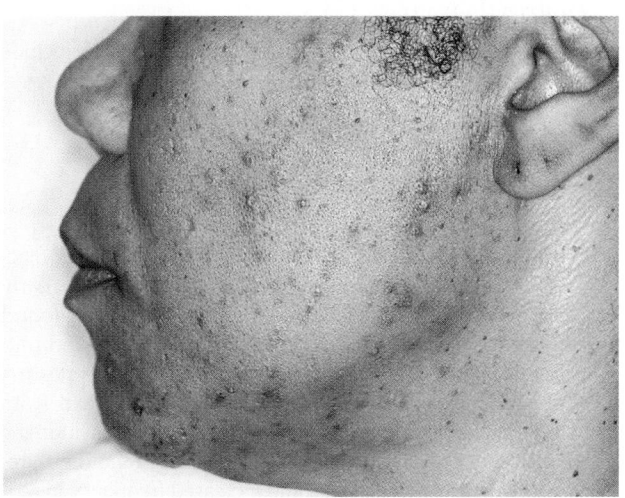

Figure 2 **Postinflammatory hyperpigmentation of the face may be secondary to acne vulgaris.**

Epidemiology

EDP is reported most commonly in dark-skinned persons. However, cases have been reported globally and in all skin types. The disease appears to have a relatively equal frequency in men and women. It has also been reported in children.

Etiology and Pathogenesis

The precise cause of EDP is unknown. Studies suggest that pollutants, pesticides, hair dyes, chemicals, and drug exposure may play a role in the pathogenesis.[23-28] Findings in light microscopic, ultrastructural, and immunofluorescent studies of EDP have been similar to those in studies of lichen planus, leading some investigators to postulate that EDP may be a variant of lichen planus. Other studies suggest that EDP is a distinct entity. Expression of intercellular adhesion molecule–I (ICAM-I) and major histocompatibility complex (MHC) class II molecules (HLA-DR) has been reported.[29] These findings suggest that aberrant cell-mediated immunity may be involved in the pathogenesis of EDP.

Diagnosis

Clinically, the macules of EDP are ashen and may have an erythematous, slightly raised border during the early stages of the disease. Erythematous macules have also been described during the early stages. Areas of erythema eventually resolve, leaving slate-gray areas of pigmentation. The lesions are usually symmetrically distributed and vary in size from small macules to very large patches. Common sites of involvement include the face, neck, trunk, and upper extremities. Mucous membranes, palms, soles, and nails are usually spared. Light microscopic findings are slight epidermal atrophic changes, spongiosis, lymphocytic exocytosis, and basal vacuolopathy in the epidermis, as well as lymphohistiocytic, lichenoid dermal infiltrates. In later stages, the lesions lack the epidermal changes and show increased deposition of dermal pigment.

Postinflammatory hyperpigmentation, idiopathic eruptive macular pigmentation, pityriasis rosea, lichen planus, fixed drug eruption, Addison disease, pinta, syphilis, macular amyloidosis, hemochromatosis, and argyria must be distinguished from EDP.

Treatment

Therapies for EDP have been minimally effective. They include sunscreens, hydroquinone, topical corticosteroids, systemic steroids, griseofulvin, clofazamine, antibiotics, and antimalarials.[30]

LENTIGINES

Definition

A lentigo is a well-circumscribed, brown to brown-black macule, usually less than 1 cm in size, that appears at birth or in early childhood. Lentigines occur in all skin types and may be found on any cutaneous surface, including the palms, soles, and mucous membranes. They do not darken with sun exposure. Lentigines can be localized and must be distinguished from freckles (ephelides). Clinical differentiating features include the later appearance of freckles (at 4 to 6 years of age) and their predominance on sun-exposed skin and increased frequency in redheads and fair-skinned persons. Freckles also tend to fade in winter and with advancing age.

Epidemiology

Multiple lentigines have been reported in 18.5% of black newborns and 0.04% of white newborns. Solar lentigines have been reported in 90% of whites older than 60 years.

Diagnosis

Several types of lentigines are recognized, including lentigo simplex, solar lentigines, nevus spilus, lentigines induced by psoralens plus ultraviolet A (PUVA), generalized lentiginosis, and syndrome-related lentiginosis.

Lentigo simplex lesions may occur as solitary localized macules or may be numerous and widespread. They often occur during the first decade of life and can be found on any cutaneous surface.

Solar (senile) lentigines, or so-called liver spots, are brown macules that appear late in adult life on chronically sun-exposed skin. These lesions are present in 90% of whites older than 70 years and occur in response to solar exposure. Solar lentigines correlate with the tendency to freckle and with two or more sunburns after 20 years of age.

Nevus spilus, or speckled lentiginous nevus, is a congenital brown patch on which dotted brown macules develop during childhood. Histologically, the brown patch has features of a lentigo, whereas the dotted brown macules most often reveal features of junctional nevi. Zosteriform patterns have also been described. Generalized lentiginosis is characterized by innumerable lentigines unassociated with other abnormalities.

Syndromes characterized by multiple lentiginosis include multiple lentigines (LEOPARD [multiple lentigines, electrocardiographic conduction abnormalities, ocular hypertelorism, pulmonary stenosis, abnormal genitalia, retardation of growth, sensorineural deafness]) syndrome, Moynahan syndrome, centrofacial lentiginosis, Carney complex, Laugier-Hunziker disease, Peutz-Jeghers syndrome, and Bannayan-Ruvalcaba-Riley syndrome.[31,32]

The histopathology of lentiginosis shows elongated rete ridges, increased numbers of basal melanocytes, and increased basal melanization. In contrast, freckles result from hypermelanization of basal melanocytes without a concomitant increase in number.

Lentigo must be distinguished from other flat, pigmented lesions, including freckles, junctional nevi, postinflammatory hyperpigmentation, and pigmented actinic keratoses.

Treatment

The treatment of lentigines includes hydroquinone-containing bleaching agents, cryotherapy, Q-switched neodymium:yttrium-aluminum-garnet (Nd:YAG) laser, and intense pulsed light.[33,34]

CONFLUENT AND RETICULATED PAPILLOMATOSIS OF GOUGEROT AND CARTEAUD

Definition

The eruption of confluent and reticulated papillomatosis was initially described by Gougerot and Carteaud in 1927 and 1932. The condition consists of 2 to 5 mm hyperpigmented papules that have a predilection for the sternal area and midline of the back and neck.

Epidemiology

Confluent and reticulated papillomatosis occurs in equal frequency in men and women and shows no racial or ethnic predilections. The disease usually begins during the third decade of life.

Etiology and Pathogenesis

The precise cause of confluent and reticulated papillomatosis is unknown. Abnormal host response to *Pityrosporum orbiculare* (*Malassezia furfur;* the fungus that causes tinea versicolor), abnormal response to colonization by follicular bacteria, and genetically determined defects of keratinization have been suggested.[35,36] The disease has been associated with Cushing syndrome, diabetes, hypopigmentation, and thyroid disorders.

Diagnosis

Patients present with 2 to 5 mm hyperpigmented, slightly verrucoid papules that have a predilection for the back, scapula, and inframammary areas. The papules become confluent near the midline and possess a reticulated pattern near the periphery. The lesions do not form a true scale but, rather, a mealy deposit that can be easily removed with the fingertips.

Histologically, studies show hyperkeratosis, decreased granular cell layers, papillomatosis, absence of sweat glands, and fragmentation of elastic fibers. Electron microscopic studies have shown increased numbers of transitional cells between the stratum granulosum and stratum corneum. This finding suggests premature keratinization. In addition, increased expression of keratin 16 has been reported, suggesting abnormal proliferation, differentiation, or both.[36]

Other conditions that simulate confluent and reticulated papillomatosis are tinea versicolor and acanthosis nigricans.

Treatment

Minocycline is reportedly beneficial.[37] Other treatments that have shown some efficacy include selenium sulfide shampoo, salicylic acid, urea, vitamin A, corticosteroids, calcipotriol, tetracycline, erythromycin, doxycycline, retinoids, and PUVA.[38-41]

DOWLING-DEGOS DISEASE

Definition

Dowling-Degos disease, or reticulated pigmented anomaly of the flexures, is an autosomal dominant disorder with variable penetrance characterized by brownish-black macules of the flexures that develop in a reticulated pattern. It may be caused by an underlying defect in follicular epithelial proliferation.

Diagnosis

Dowling-Degos disease presents as symmetrical, reticulated hyperpigmentation of the groin, axilla, antecubital area, inframammary areas, and neck.[42] The lesions begin as 1 to 3 mm macules that gradually become confluent, assuming a reticulated lacelike pattern. In addition, perinasal and facial involvement is common. Pigmented pinhead-sized comedones are frequently observed in the affected areas, and perinasal, pitted acneiform scars can occur around the mouth.

Lesions of Dowling-Degos disease begin in early adult life and are slowly progressive. The condition has been reported in association with reticulated acropigmentation of Kitamura and hidradenitis suppurativa,[43] suggesting an underlying defect in follicular epithelial proliferation. In addition, the disease has been reported in a large kindred with reticulate acropigmentation of Kitamura and acropigmentation of Dohi, suggesting an association between and overlap of these conditions.[44] Histologically, thin, pigmented epithelial strands of downgrowth extend from the epidermis and follicular wall in a filiform pattern resembling adenoid seborrheic keratoses.[42,45]

Treatment

In general, there is no effective treatment for Dowling-Degos disease. Adapalene and the erbium:YAG laser have been reported to offer some benefit.[46]

Disorders of Hypopigmentation

VITILIGO

Definition

Vitiligo is a common acquired, idiopathic skin disorder characterized by one or more patches of depigmented skin. The depigmentation results from loss of cutaneous melanocytes. These lesions are cosmetically disfiguring and usually cause emotional trauma in both children and adults [*see Figure 3*].

Epidemiology

Vitiligo affects 1% to 2% of the population. Onset may begin at any age, but peak incidence is in the second or third decade of life. The disease shows no racial or ethnic predilection, but because of the stark contrast between depigmented and darker skin tones, it is more cosmetically disfiguring in darker racial and ethnic groups. Females are affected more often than males. The disease has a familial incidence of 25% to 30%. Genetic studies suggest a polygenic inheritance pattern.

HLA studies have reported increases in a variety of haplotypes of class I and class II antigens in patients with vitiligo. However, results vary significantly by race and ethnicity of the population studied. The reported HLA associations include increased frequencies of HLA A30, CW6, CW7, DR1, DR3, DR4, and DQW3.[47]

Etiology and Pathogenesis

The precise cause of vitiligo is unknown. Multiple theories have been proposed, including genetic, autoimmune, neural, biochemical, and viral mechanisms. Reviews addressing the etiology of vitiligo suggest that vitiligo is probably a heterogeneous disease encompassing multiple etiologies.[47,48]

An immune-mediated pathogenesis is the most popular theory. This theory is predicated on the increased frequency of a

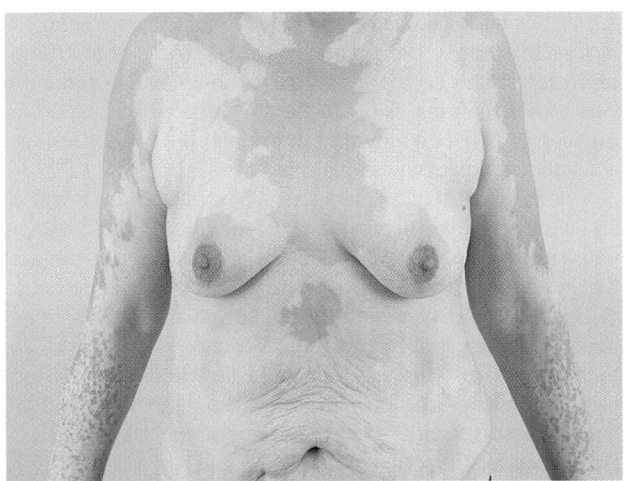

Figure 3 **Vitiligo is indicated by generalized patches of depigmentation of the trunk.**

plethora of immunologic diseases in patients with vitiligo, including hypothyroidism (Hashimoto thyroiditis), Graves disease, pernicious anemia, diabetes mellitus, and alopecia areata. Thyroid diseases are the most common associated diseases. Other disorders reported in association with vitiligo include Addison disease, atopic dermatitis, asthma, lichen planus, morphea, lichen sclerosus et atrophicus, mucocutaneous candidiasis, biliary cirrhosis, myasthenia gravis, Down syndrome, AIDS, and cutaneous T cell lymphoma.

Humoral and cell-mediated immunologic defects are a common phenomenon in vitiligo.[47,48] Numerous studies have documented an increased frequency of organ-specific autoantibodies. Antithyroid, gastric antiparietal cell, and antinuclear antibodies are most commonly demonstrated. Patients with positive organ-specific autoantibodies unassociated with autoimmune disease have an increased risk of subsequent subclinical or overt autoimmune disease.

Antimelanocyte antibodies, often demonstrated in the sera of patients with vitiligo, induce the destruction of cultured melanocytes by complement-mediated lysis and antibody-dependent cellular cytotoxicity. The presence and titer of antimelanocyte antibodies correlate with the severity and activity of vitiligo. These antibodies are directed against melanocyte cell surface antigens with molecular weights of 25, 35 to 40, 75, 90, and 150 kd. Studies suggest that the antimelanocyte antibody may mediate the destruction of melanocytes in vitiligo. Tyrosinase antibodies have also been reported in patients with localized and generalized disease.[49]

Cellular immune-mediated defects include diminished contact sensitization and quantitative and qualitative alterations in T cells and natural-killer cells. Skin-homing cytotoxic T cells have also been implicated in the destruction of melanocytes. Immunohistochemical studies have demonstrated abnormal expression of MHC class II and ICAM-I by melanocytes in vitiligo, which may contribute to the aberrant cellular immune response. In addition, there is increased expression of the antiadhesive matrix component tenasin in perilesional and lesional vitiliginous skin. Increased tenasin expression may be a consequence of elevated cytokine production and cellular infiltrates in vitiligo.[47] Studies have documented alterations in cytokine production in patients with vitiligo. Studies of affected skin showed a significantly lower expression of granulocyte-macrophage colony-stimulating factor

(GM-CSF), basic fibroblast growth factor (bFGF), and stem cell factor.[50] In contrast, expression of interleukin 6 (IL-6) and tumor necrosis factor–α (TNF-α) was greater in lesional skin than in perilesional or normal skin. Another study reported increased expression of TNF-α, interferon gamma, and IL-10 in the lesional and adjacent skin of vitiligo patients.[51]

Cytomegalovirus DNA has been demonstrated in the involved and uninvolved skin of patients with vitiligo. No viral DNA was detected in matched control subjects.[52] These findings suggest that in some cases, vitiligo may be triggered by a viral infection.

The neural theory is supported by several clinical, biochemical, and ultrastructural observations. These observations include the occurrence of segmental vitiligo; the demonstration of lesional autonomic dysfunction, such as increased sweating; and the demonstration of nerve ending–melanocyte contact. The last observation is rare in normal skin.

Several studies suggest that oxidative stress may be the initial event in the destruction of melanocytes.[53,54] Defective recycling of tetrahydrobiopterin, increased production of hydrogen peroxide, and decreased catalase have been demonstrated in the skin of patients with vitiligo.[55,56] In addition, lesional catecholamine biosynthesis and release are increased. Thus, abnormal release of catecholamines from autonomic nerve endings and oxidative stress may damage melanocytes by altering the free radical defense of the epidermis.

The self-destruction hypothesis proposes that melanocytes may be destroyed by phenolic compounds formed during the synthesis of melanin. In vivo and in vitro studies have demonstrated the destruction of melanocytes by phenols and catechols. In addition, industrial workers who are exposed to catechols and phenols may experience depigmentation of areas of skin.

A variety of environmentally ubiquitous compounds containing catechols, phenols, and sulfhydryls can induce hypopigmentation, depigmentation, or both. These compounds are most often encountered in industrial chemicals and cleaning agents. Possible mechanisms for altered pigment production by these compounds include melanocyte destruction via free radical formation, inhibition of tyrosinase activity, and interference with the production or transfer of melanosomes.

Diagnosis

Clinical manifestations Vitiliginous lesions are typically asymptomatic depigmented macules without clinical signs of inflammation. However, inflammatory vitiligo with erythematous borders has been reported. Hypopigmented lesions may coexist with depigmented lesions. The patches are occasionally pruritic. Macules frequently begin on sun-exposed or perioral facial skin and either remain localized or disseminate to other cutaneous sites. Areas of depigmentation vary in size from a few millimeters to many centimeters, and their borders are usually distinct. Trichrome lesions are most often observed in darker-complexioned persons. These lesions are characterized by zones of white, light-brown, and normal skin color. Depigmented hairs are often present in lesional skin and do not preclude repigmentation of a lesion. In addition, there is a high incidence of premature graying of scalp hair in patients with vitiligo and in their families. Vitiliginous lesions can remain stable or can slowly progress for years. In some instances, patients undergo almost complete spontaneous depigmentation over a few years.

Vitiligo is subclassified into different types on the basis of the distribution of skin lesions. These subclassifications include the generalized or vulgaris, acral or acrofacial, localized, and seg-

mented types. The generalized pattern is characterized by symmetrical macules or patches occurring in a random distribution. Acral or acrofacial vitiligo consists of depigmented macules confined to the extremities or to the face and extremities, respectively. A subcategory of the acrofacial type is the lip-tip variety, in which lesions are confined to the lips and the tips of the digits. The generalized and acrofacial varieties are the most common. Segmental vitiligo occurs in a dermatomal or quasidermatomal distribution; lesions rarely spread beyond the affected dermatome. This type is the less common variety of vitiligo and most often occurs along the distribution of the trigeminal nerve.

Melanocytes of the eye, ear, and leptomeninges may also be involved in vitiligo. Depigmented areas of the retinal pigment epithelium and choroid have been reported in 39% of patients studied. These lesions usually do not interfere with vision. Vitiligo is also a manifestation of the Vogt-Koyanagi-Harada syndrome, which is characterized by poliosis, chronic uveitis, alopecia, dysacusis, vitiligo, and signs of meningeal irritation. It usually begins in the third decade of life, and although no race is spared, the disease tends to be more severe in darker-complexioned races, especially Asians.

The syndrome has been divided into stages. The first, or meningeal, stage, is associated with headache, nausea, vomiting, fever, confusion, cranial nerve palsies, hemiparesis, and cerebrospinal fluid pleocytosis. Usually, there are a few neurologic sequelae. In the second stage, ophthalmic and auditory changes predominate, including photophobia, ocular pain, visual loss, anterior or posterior uveitis, and sometimes retinal detachment, tinnitus, and dysacusis. Cutaneous lesions are dominant in the third, or convalescent, stage, occurring as the uveitis begins to subside. Common features are vitiligo, which frequently involves the eyelids and periorbital region [*see Figure 4*]; poliosis of the scalp, hair, eyelashes, and eyebrows; and diffuse or patchy alopecia.

Patients with malignant melanoma frequently experience a vitiligolike depigmentation surrounding melanoma lesions and at distant sites. The presence of depigmentation in melanoma patients portends a longer survival.

Laboratory findings Histologically, the predominant finding in vitiligo is an absence of melanocytes in lesional skin. Light microscopy and ultrastructural studies have also revealed vacuolar degeneration of basal and parabasal keratinocytes and revealed epidermal and dermal lymphohistiocytic cell infiltrates.

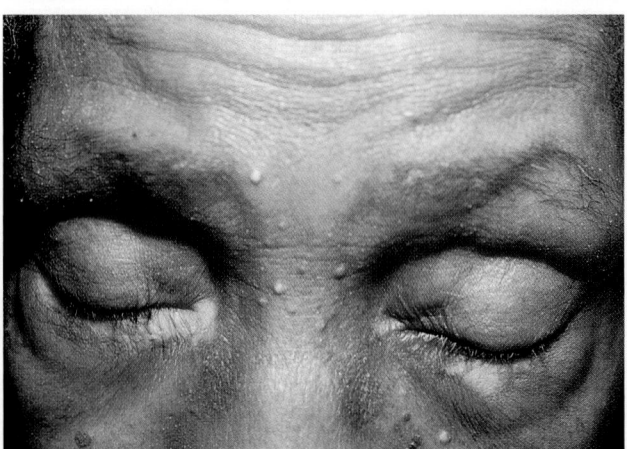

Figure 4 **A patient with Vogt-Koyanagi-Harada syndrome shows periorbital depigmentation.**

Immunohistochemical staining has confirmed the presence of a predominantly T cell infiltrate in vitiliginous and adjacent skin.

In view of the association of vitiligo with myriad other autoimmune diseases, the routine baseline evaluation of a patient should include a thorough history and physical examination. Recommended laboratory tests include a complete blood count; sedimentation rate; comprehensive metabolic panel, including liver function tests; and autoantibody tests (antinuclear antibody, thyroid peroxidase, and parietal cell antibodies).

Differential Diagnosis

Other disorders characterized by depigmentation may occasionally mimic vitiligo clinically. These include piebaldism, nevus depigmentosus, nevus anemicus, postinflammatory depigmentation or hypopigmentation, pityriasis alba, tinea versicolor, discoid lupus erythematosus, scleroderma, hypopigmented mycosis fungoides, and sarcoidosis. Therefore, in some instances, a skin biopsy may be necessary to substantiate a diagnosis of vitiligo.

Treatment Selection

Therapeutic objectives in vitiligo should include both stabilization of the disease and repigmentation of vitiliginous skin lesions. Repigmentation can be accomplished medically[57-59] or, in patients with localized stable lesions, surgically.[60] The choice of repigmentation therapies should be predicated on the age of the patient, extent of cutaneous surface involvement (severity), and activity or progression of the disease. The disease can be divided into four stages: limited (less than 10% involvement), moderate (10% to 25% involvement), moderately severe (26% to 50% involvement), and severe (greater than 50% involvement) [see Table 1].

Medical Treatment

Medical therapies for vitiligo include topical and systemic steroids, topical and systemic PUVA, narrow-band ultraviolet light therapy (UVB), excimer laser therapy, nutritional vitamin supplementation, immunomodulators, calcipotriol, phenylalanine, and khellin.[57-59]

Steroids Mid- to high-potency steroids are indicated in patients with limited involvement. Low-potency topical steroids are usually ineffective. Topical mid- to high-potency steroids can be used safely for 2 to 3 months, then interrupted for 1 month or tapered to low-potency preparations. Patients must be closely monitored for topical steroid side effects, which include skin atrophy, telangiectasias, hypertrichosis, and acneiform eruptions. Since the introduction of topical immunomodulators (tacrolimus and pimecrolimus), topical steroids are used less often in vitiligo patients.

Short courses of oral prednisone for 1 to 2 weeks or intramuscular triamcinolone acetonide injections, 40 mg/month for 2 to 3 months, are often extremely helpful for stabilizing rapidly progressive vitiligo. However, prolonged use of systemic steroids is not indicated.[57-59]

Photochemotherapy Until recently, topical and systemic PUVA therapies were the mainstay for repigmenting vitiliginous lesions.[57,58] However, in the past several years, these therapies have been overshadowed by new ones, including narrow-band UVB phototherapy, lasers, and topical immunomodulators.

Topical photochemotherapy can be administered in the office or outside the office in combination with sunlight. The choice of topical PUVA is predicated on the severity of vitiligo, patient

Table 1 Therapeutic Approaches for Vitiligo

Stages I and II disease*	Topical steroids
	Topical photochemotherapy
	  PUVA-sol
	  In-office PUVA
	Bath photochemotherapy
	Pseudocatalase/UVB
	UVB phototherapy
	  Narrow band
	  Broad band
	Excimer laser
	Topical immunomodulators
	  Tacrolimus
	  Pimecrolimus
	L-phenylalanine/UV
	Topical khellin/UVA
	Melagenina
	Calcipotriol/PUVA
	Tar emulsions
	Vitamin supplementation
	Autologous melanocyte grafting
	  (stable lesions)

Stages III and IV disease*	Oral photochemotherapy
	Systemic steroids (oral, I.M.) (for
	  stabilization)
	Bath photochemotherapy
	UVB phototherapy
	  Narrow band
	  Broad band
	Oral khellin/UVA
	L-phenylalanine/UV
	Immunomodulators
	  Isoprinosine
	  Levamasole
	Immunosuppressives
	  Cyclosporine
	  Cyclophosphamide
	  Nitrogen mustard
	Depigmentation (severe, recalcitrant
	  lesions)

*Stage I, < 10% involvement; stage II, 10%–25% involvement; stage III, 26%–50% involvement; stage IV, > 50% involvement.
PUVA—psoralens plus ultraviolet A   UV—ultraviolet   UVA—ultraviolet A
UVB—ultraviolet B

lifestyle, and convenience for the patient. Topical in-office PUVA is appropriate for patients with less than 20% cutaneous surface involvement. A thin coat of 0.01% to 0.1% methoxsalen ointment is applied to affected areas 30 minutes before UVA exposure. Treatments are weekly or twice weekly. For patients with less than 10% involvement, an alternative approach involves the use of 0.001% methoxsalen ointment applied 30 minutes before sunlight exposure. Patients are allowed to expose the affected areas for 10 minutes, gradually increasing exposure time to 30 minutes. Treatments are daily or every other day.

Oral photochemotherapy is indicated in patients with greater than 20% to 25% cutaneous surface involvement. The standard dose of 8-methoxypsoralen (8-MOP) is usually 0.3 to 0.4 mg/kg ingested 1.5 hours before UVA exposure. The treatments are administered twice weekly. Broad-spectrum sunscreen protection is essential after PUVA treatments. In addition, because of the ocular pharmacokinetics of 8-MOP, protective UVA sunglasses should be worn indoors and outdoors for 18 to 24 hours after ingestion of 8-MOP.

Contraindications to oral PUVA treatment include liver disease and photosensitivity disorders. Side effects include headaches, nausea, vomiting, xerosis, pruritus, photoaging, diffuse hyperpigmentation, and hypertrichosis. Compared with topical PUVA, the major advantages of oral PUVA include its effectiveness in controlling the progression of active disease and its lower frequency of blistering reactions. Oral PUVA therapy has been associated with an increase in nonmelanoma and melanoma skin cancer in patients with psoriasis. However, similar documentation has not been reported in patients with vitiligo.

Factors that portend enhanced PUVA-induced repigmentation include young age (children), patient motivation, maintenance of adequate lesional phototoxicity, and location of lesions. Maximal repigmentation occurs on the face and neck, and minimal responses occur in the hands and feet. Overall, mean repigmentation of 60% to 65% of the affected areas can be achieved.[58]

Narrow-band UVB   Recent studies have reported the benefits of narrow-band UVB phototherapy (NB-UVB).[61] NB-UVB treatment was shown to be as effective as topical PUVA, with fewer side effects. In a study of NB-UVB phototherapy versus oral PUVA, 56% of the UVB group had greater than 25% repigmentation, compared with 63% of the oral PUVA group. The difference was not statistically significant. Because of its efficacy and safety profile, NB-UVB has emerged as the therapy of choice for patients with moderate to severe disease.

NB-UVB phototherapy offers several advantages over oral psoralen photochemotherapy, including ease of treatment, lack of need for posttreatment ocular protection, lack of the side effects (e.g., nausea, headaches, and gastritis) associated with oral methoxsalen, and minimal phototoxic reactions. Furthermore, NB-UVB phototherapy can be used to treat young children who have extensive, progressive vitiligo. Disadvantages include the need for more treatments for maximal efficacy (three times weekly for NB-UVB, compared with twice weekly for PUVA) and the lack of data concerning the possible long-term carcinogenic effects of NB-UVB phototherapy.

Dermatologists continue to treat patients with PUVA, and it remains the gold standard despite its inherent difficulties. Patients whose vitiligo does not respond to NB-UVB phototherapy are often switched to oral PUVA.

Repigmentation occurs gradually and requires many treatments: 16 to 24 treatments are usually needed for new pigment to become evident. In general, maximal repigmentation involves 6 to 12 months of NB-UVB or PUVA therapy.

Laser therapy   The excimer laser (308 nm UVB), recently approved by the FDA for treatment of psoriasis, also shows promise as a therapy for vitiligo.[62,63] This laser can be used as monotherapy or in combination with other modalities. Laser therapy targets the lesional area and theoretically reduces UV exposure. In addition, because the laser provides a focused, high-intensity dose of NB-UVB, treatment duration, in theory, may be reduced. Long-term, controlled studies are needed to further define the efficacy, risks, and benefits of the excimer laser for treatment of vitiligo.

Pseudocatalase   The beneficial effects of pseudocatalase and calcium applied twice daily and UVB exposure twice weekly have also been reported. The rationale for this therapy is derived from previous studies that demonstrated aberrant catalase and calcium homeostasis in patients.[64]

Vitamins   Preliminary open-label studies have documented stabilization and repigmentation in vitiligo patients treated with high-dose vitamin supplementation, including daily doses of ascorbic acid (1,000 mg), vitamin B_{12} (1,000 μg), and folic acid (1 to 5 mg).[57]

Topical immunomodulators   Abnormalities of both humoral and cell-mediated immunity have been well documented in patients with vitiligo,[47-52] which explains the apparent efficacy of several immunomodulators for this disease. Preliminary investigations have reported repigmentation of vitiliginous lesions with isoprinosine, levamisole, suplatast tosilate, and cyclosporine.[57]

Tacrolimus ointment is a novel topical immunomodulatory drug for treatment of adult and pediatric atopic dermatitis. Tacrolimus exerts its therapeutic effect via inhibition of the production of proinflammatory cytokines. Moderate to excellent repigmentation was reported in five of six patients treated with tacrolimus. Patients ranged in age from 6 to 32 years. Repigmentation responses did not correlate with disease duration.[58, 65]

Calcipotriol   Several studies have documented the efficacy of calcipotriol for repigmentation of vitiligo. Used in combination with UV exposure, calcipotriol was well tolerated and effective in both children and adults.[58] Melanocytes are thought to express $1\alpha,25$-dihydroxyvitamin D_3 receptors, which may play a role in stimulating melanogenesis.

Depigmentation   Since the 1950s, monobenzylether of hydroquinone (MBEH, or monobenzene) has been used as a depigmenting agent for patients with extensive vitiligo. In general, MBEH causes permanent destruction of melanocytes and induces depigmentation locally and remotely from the sites of application. Hence, the use of MBEH for other disorders of pigmentation is contraindicated.

Depigmentation is a viable therapeutic alternative in patients with greater than 50% cutaneous depigmentation who have demonstrated recalcitrance to repigmentation or in patients with extensive vitiligo who have no desire to undergo repigmentation therapies.[55,58] The major side effects of MBEH therapy are dermatitis and pruritus, which usually respond to topical and systemic steroids. Other side effects include severe xerosis, alopecia, premature graying, and suppression of lymphoproliferative responses.

Surgical Treatment

Surgical treatment is appropriate for patients with localized, stable areas of vitiligo that have been recalcitrant to medical treatment.[60] Such approaches are contraindicated in patients with keloids or hypertrophic scars. Techniques for surgical grafting include suction blister grafts, punch grafts, sheet grafts, pure melanocyte cultures, and cocultures of melanocytes and keratinocytes. These techniques are indeed beneficial for localized lesions.

Micropigmentation is often associated with the induction of koebnerization; therefore, its use should be limited to treatment of mucous membrane lesions.

ALBINISM

Definition

Albinism is an uncommon, complex congenital disorder characterized by hypopigmentation of the hair, eyes, and skin. Albinism is generally subclassified as oculocutaneous albinism (OCA) and ocular albinism (OA); in the latter, reduction of melanin is limited to the eye.[66-71] Sometimes, different mutations in the same gene can cause OCA or OA.

Epidemiology

OCA has been reported by investigators in all mammalian orders and in all human ethnic groups. It is one of the most widely distributed genetic abnormalities in the animal kingdom. Human albinism has been noted throughout history. OCA is the most common inherited disorder of generalized hypopigmentation.

Etiology and Pathogenesis

Albinism may result from primary defects that are specific for the melanin synthetic pathway or from defects that are not specific for melanin synthesis. Mutations in seven genes have been reported to cause OCA or OA.[67,68] They include the tyrosinase gene (OCA1 on chromosome 12q1), the oculocutaneous albinism gene (OCA2, a missed mutation of the P gene on 15q11), the tyrosinase-related protein 1 gene (OCA3), the HPS gene (Hermansky-Pudlak syndrome at 10q23 and mutations of the β3A-adaptin gene), the CHS gene (Chédiak-Higashi syndrome), and the OA1 gene (X-linked ocular albinism).

Diagnosis

Clinically, the most severe disease is observed in OCA1A, which is OCA resulting from mutations in the tyrosinase gene. It is characterized by absent tyrosinase activity, which results in complete absence of melanin in the eyes, skin, and hair. There is no improvement with age. Affected individuals have marked photophobia, nystagmus, and profound sun sensitivity because of the inability to tan.

OCA1B, or yellow albinism, is less severe. Tyrosinase activity is low or absent, and pigmentation of the hair and skin improves with age. In contrast to OCA1A, pigmented freckles and lentigines develop with age.

OCA1-MP, or minimal-pigment OCA, is characterized by white skin and hair at birth. Iris pigment is present at birth, or it appears during the first decade of life. All reported cases have been in white persons. The tyrosinase gene mutation produces a less active enzyme.

Temperature-sensitive OCA (OCA1-TS) is characterized by white skin and hair and blue eyes at birth and by development of patterned pigmentation by puberty. Darker hair develops in cooler areas (extremities), and white hair is retained in warmer areas (axilla and scalp). The pattern results from a tyrosinase mutation that causes a temperature-sensitive enzyme.

OCA2, tyrosinase-positive OCA with normal tyrosinase activity, is the most common variety. The hair darkens with age, but the skin remains white. Pigmented nevi, lentigines, and freckles develop and are especially pronounced in sun-exposed areas. This type has recently been ascribed to mutation of the P gene, which encodes the tyrosinase-transporting membrane protein. The P gene is on chromosome 15q.

OCA3 encompasses the Rufous variety and some cases of brown albinism. Clinically, there is minimal pigment reduction in the hair, eyes, and skin.

The secondary varieties of albinism in which the primary defect is not specific for the melanin synthetic pathway include Hermansky-Pudlak syndrome,[71] Chédiak-Higashi syndrome, Cross-McKusick-Breen syndrome, Prader-Willi syndrome, and Angelman syndrome.

The autosomal recessive Hermansky-Pudlak syndrome is characterized by low to absent tyrosinase activity. The HPS gene has been mapped to chromosome 10q23.[71-73] Skin and hair color varies from white to light brown. Freckles and lentigines develop

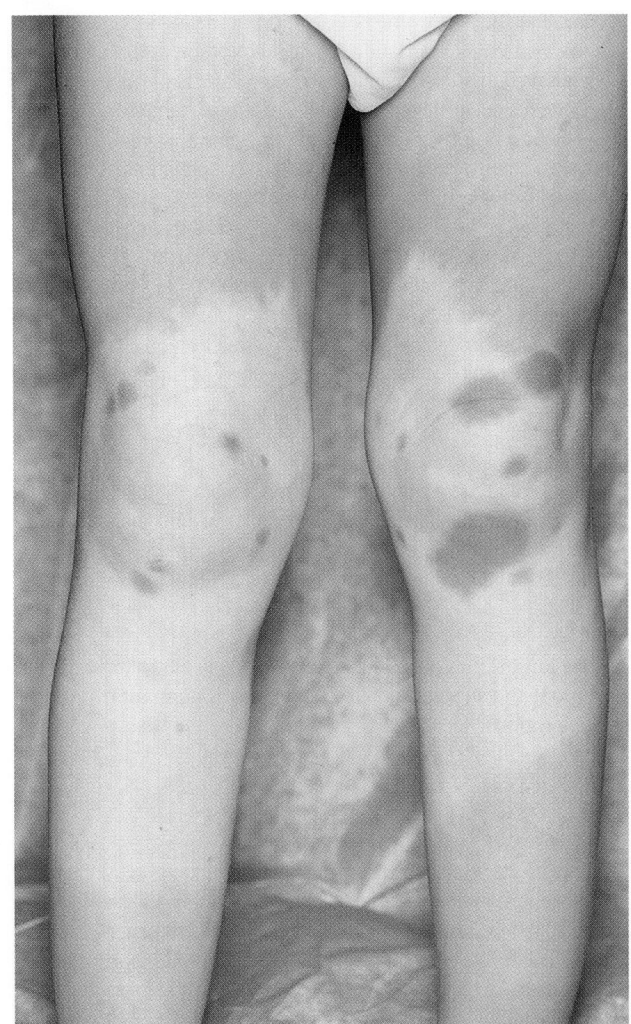

Figure 5 A patient with piebaldism has the classic midextremity areas of depigmentation with islands of hyperpigmentation.

with age. Iris pigment correlates with hair and skin pigmentation. Affected individuals experience a hemorrhagic diathesis secondary to a platelet-storage-pool deficiency. Their platelets lack storage granules (i.e., sites of storage for serotonin, calcium, and adenine nucleotides). Ceroidlike deposits are present in macrophages of the bone marrow, lungs, liver, spleen, and gastrointestinal tract. These patients bruise easily and are subject to epistaxis and gingival bleeding. Pulmonary fibrosis and granulomatous colitis develop as a consequence of the ceroid deposits.

Chédiak-Higashi syndrome consists of hypopigmentation, recurrent sinopulmonary bacterial infections, peripheral neuropathy, and giant lysosomal granules, with death occurring at an early age as a result of lymphoreticular malignancies. The CHS gene locus is on chromosome 1q29. Chédiak-Higashi syndrome must be distinguished from Griscelli syndrome, which is characterized by partial albinism, lymphohistiocytosis, immunodeficiency, neutropenia, and thrombocytopenia. Griscelli syndrome has been mapped to chromosome15q21, around the myosin-Va gene. However, the presence of giant lysosomal granules is pathognomonic for Chédiak-Higashi syndrome.[74,75]

Cross-McKusick-Breen syndrome includes hypopigmentation, microphthalmia, nystagmus, and severe mental and physical retardation.

Prader-Willi syndrome is a developmental syndrome characterized by mental retardation, neonatal hypotonia, and poor feeding, followed by hyperphagia and obesity later in life. Short stature, hypogonadism, and inappropriate emotional behavior constitute the syndrome. Fifty percent of patients have a deletion on the long arm of chromosome 15. Patients have ocular abnormalities and skin and hair hypopigmentation consistent with OCA.

Mutation of the *P* gene has been reported in Angelman syndrome and is also characterized by mental retardation, abnormal behavior, and hypopigmentation. The pattern of hypopigmentation is similar to that in Prader-Willi syndrome. In addition, Angelman syndrome is associated with a deletion on chromosome 15. However, in contrast to Prader-Willi syndrome, the deletion occurs on the maternal chromosome.

Treatment

The management of patients with albinism should include genetic counseling and patient education regarding the use of sunscreens and clothing for protection against ultraviolet radiation–induced damage. Magnifiers are beneficial for ocular symptoms.

Complications

The long-term consequences of albinism are solar keratoses and basal and squamous cell carcinomas. Malignant melanoma is uncommon.

PIEBALDISM

Definition

Piebaldism is a rare autosomal dominant congenital disorder of pigmentation. It is a stable leukoderma and is characterized by patches of white skin and white hair. The affected areas are principally the frontal scalp, forehead, ventral chest, abdomen, and extremities. A white forelock occurs in 80% to 90% of patients.

Epidemiology

Although rare, piebaldism occurs in all ethnic groups worldwide. Its estimated occurrence is one in 100,000 persons. It is found with equal frequency in males and females.

Etiology and Pathogenesis

Molecular genetics studies have shown that piebaldism results from mutations of the *KIT* proto-oncogene, which encodes the cell surface receptor tyrosine kinase for mast cell or stem cell factor located on chromosome segment 4q12. Mutations occur in the highly conserved tyrosinase domain of *KIT*. A number of different mutations in the *KIT* gene can cause piebaldism.[76-80] The locations of the *KIT* gene mutation correlates with severity of disease. Mutations of the intracellular tyrosine kinase domain are associated with the most severe phenotypes.[77] Reduced *KIT* function arrests the migration of melanocytes into affected hair follicles and epidermis during embryonal development.[76-78]

In general, patients with piebaldism are healthy and do not have associated systemic abnormalities. However, the disorder occasionally has been associated with heterochromia irides, mental retardation, osteopathia striata, Woolf syndrome, and Hirschsprung disease.

Diagnosis

Cutaneous depigmentation is the only manifestation of piebaldism in 10% to 20% of cases. Amelanotic macules are usually present on the ventral surface of the thorax and abdomen and extend to the back but spare the midline. Characteristic extremity lesions extend from midarm to wrist and occur on the midleg [*see Figure 5*]. White patches of the mucous membranes have also been reported. Hyperpigmented macules may appear within the areas of depigmentation.

Light and electron microscopic studies of the white macules have typically revealed an absence of melanocytes. However, melanocytes have been demonstrated in the white forelock and amelanotic skin of three patients studied.

Differential Diagnosis

Piebaldism is sometimes confused with vitiligo, but in piebaldism, the leukodermic patches are both congenital and relatively static in shape and size.

Treatment

The lesions of piebaldism are usually stable throughout life, although some patients have reported spontaneous repigmentation. In general, therapeutic approaches, including psoralen photochemotherapy and grafting, are unsatisfactory. Autologous melanocyte grafting procedures may offer some benefit for localized or limited areas of involvement.

IDIOPATHIC GUTTATE HYPOMELANOSIS

Definition

Idiopathic guttate hypomelanosis (IGH) is a common asymptomatic disorder characterized by hypopigmentation and depigmented polygonal macules ranging from approximately 2 to 8 mm in diameter.

Epidemiology

IGH appears to be a very common, benign dermatosis. It occurs in all races, with a frequency ranging from 46% to 70%, but is more prevalent in darker-skinned racial and ethnic groups. Macules may begin to appear during the third or fourth decade of life and gradually increase in number thereafter.

Etiology and Pathogenesis

The precise pathogenesis has not been established for IGH. Long-term sun exposure, trauma, genetic influences, and aging, with a gradual loss of melanocytes, have been implicated in the pathogenesis of this disorder.[81]

Diagnosis

The lesions of IGH are macules that are punctate to polygonal in shape, 2 to 8 mm in diameter, and hypopigmented to depigmented. They are most commonly observed on the lower extremities. There is no atrophy or change in the overlying skin. Histologic evaluation of lesions reveals hyperkeratosis, epidermal atrophy, and decreased epidermal melanin. Melanocytes may be normal or decreased. Immunoperoxidase studies show a markedly reduced number of melanocytes. Melanocyte differentiation appears to be unaffected.[82]

Differential Diagnosis

IGH must be differentiated from other hypopigmentary disorders, such as vitiligo, scleroderma, leukodermic guttate parapsoriasis, tinea versicolor, hypopigmented sarcoidosis, pityriasis alba, chemical depigmentation, and postinflammatory hypopigmentation.

Treatment

No definitive treatment is currently available. Patients often need reassurance regarding the banality of lesions. For patients concerned about the cosmetic appearance of lesions, clinicians have used camouflage, intralesional steroids, and topical photochemotherapy. Localized superficial dermabrasion may offer some improvement.[83]

The author has received grants for clinical research from Allergan Inc., Fujisawa Healthcare, Inc., and Galderma Laborotories, L.P.

References

1. Grimes PE: Melasma: etiologic and therapeutic considerations. Arch Dermatol 131:1453, 1995

2. O'Brien TJ, Dyall-Smith D, Hall AP: Melasma of the forearms. Australas J Dermatol 38:35, 1997

3. Boissy RE, Nordlund JJ: Molecular basis of congenital hyperpigmentary disorders in humans: a review. Pigment Cell Res 10:12, 1997

4. Im S, Kim J, On WY, et al: Increased expression of alpha-melanocyte-stimulating hormone in the lesional skin of melasma. Br J Dermatol 146:165, 2002

5. Kang WH, Yoon KH, Lee ES, et al: Melasma: histopathological characteristics in 56 Korean patients. Br J Dermatol 146:228, 2002

6. Piamphongsant T: Treatment of melasma: a review with personal experience. Int J Dermatol 37:897, 1998

7. Grimes PE: The safety and efficacy of salicylic acid peels in darker-racial ethnic groups. Dermatol Surg 25:18, 1999

8. Grimes PE: Agents for ethnic skin peeling. Dermatol Ther 13:159, 2000

9. Rajan P, Grimes PE: Skin barrier changes induced by aluminum oxide and sodium chloride microdermabrasion. Dermatol Surg 28:390, 2002

10. Negishi K, Tezuka Y, Kushikata N: Photorejuvenation for Asian skin by intense pulsed light. Dermatol Surg 27:627, 2001

11. Gerardo A, Arias M, Ferrando J: Intense pulsed light for melanocytic lesions. Dermatol Surg 27:397, 2001

12. McKenzie RC, Sauder DN: The role of keratinocyte cytokines in inflammation and immunity. J Invest Dermatol 95(6 suppl):1055, 1990

13. Kinbauer R, Kock A, Neuner P, et al: Regulation of epidermal cell interleukin-6 production by UV light and corticosteroids. J Invest Dermatol 96:484, 1991

14. Ruiz-Maldonado R, Orozco-Covarrubias ML: Postinflammatory hypopigmentation and hyperpigmentation. Semin Cutan Med Surg 16:36, 1997

15. Jacyk WK: Adapalene in the treatment of African patients. J Eur Acad Dermatol Venereol 15(suppl 3):37, 2001

16. Granstein R, Sober AJ: Drug- and heavy metal–induced hyperpigmentation. J Am Acad Dermatol 5:1, 1981

17. Lerner EA, Sober AJ: Chemical and pharmacologic agents that cause hyperpigmentation or hypopigmentation of the skin. Dermatol Clin 6:327, 1988

18. Ozog DM, Gogstetter DS, Scott G, et al: Minocycline-induced hyperpigmentation in patients with pemphigus and pemphigoid. Arch Dermatol 136:1133, 2000

19. Green D, Friedman KJ: Treatment of minocycline-induced cutaneous pigmentation with the Q-switched Alexandrite laser and a review of the literature. J Am Acad Dermatol 44(2 suppl):342, 2001

20. Mineg ME, Bhawan J, Stefanato CM, et al: Imipramine-induced hyperpigmentation: four cases and a review of the literature. J Am Acad Dermatol 40:159, 1999

21. Koppel RA, Boh EE: Cutaneous reactions to chemotherapeutic agents. Am J Med Sci 321:327, 2001

22. Alley E, Green R, Schuchter L: Cutaneous toxicities of cancer therapy. Curr Opin Oncol 14:212, 2002

23. Scherschun L, Lee MW, Lim HW: Diltiazem-associated photodistributed hyperpigmentation: a review of 4 cases. Arch Dermatol 137:179, 2001

24. Atkin DH, Fitzpatrick RE: Laser treatment of imipramine-induced hyperpigmentation. J Am Acad Dermatol 43:77, 2000

25. Combemale P, Faisant M, Guennoc B, et al: Erythema dyschromicum perstans: report of a new case and critical review of the literature. J Dermatol 25:747, 1998

26. Dominguez-Soto L, Hojyo-Tomoka T, Vega-Memije E, et al: Pigmentary problems in the tropics. Dermatol Clin 12:777, 1994

27. Penagos H, Jimenez V, Fallas V, et al: Chlorethalanil: a possible cause of erythema dyschromicum perstans (ashy dermatitis). Contact Derm 35:214, 1996

28. Spiewak R: Pesticides as a cause of occupational skin diseases in farmers. Ann Agric Environ Med 8:1, 2001

29. Baranda L, Torres-Alvarez B, Cortes-Franco R, et al: Involvement of cell adhesion and activation molecules in the pathogenesis of erythema dyschromicum perstans (ashy dermatitis): the effect of clofazimine therapy. Arch Dermatol 133:32, 1997

30. Osswald SS, Proffer LH, Sartori CR: Erythema dyschromicum perstans: a case report and review. Cutis 68:25, 2001

31. Stratakis CA: Genetics of Peutz-Jeghers syndrome, Carney complex, and other familial lentiginoses. Horm Res 54:334, 2000

32. Abdelmalek NF, Gerber TL, Menter A: Cardiocutaneous syndromes and associations. J Am Acad Dermatol 46:161, 2002

33. Todd M, Rallis TM, Gerwels JW, et al: A comparison of 3 lasers and liquid nitrogen in the treatment of solar lentigines: a randomized, controlled, comparative trial. Arch Dermatol 136:841, 2000

34. Kawada A, Shiraishi H, Asai M, et al: Clinical improvement of solar lentigines and ephelides with an intense pulsed light source. Dermatol Surg 28:504, 2002

35. Lee MP, Stiller MJ, McClain SA, et al: Confluent and reticulated papillomatosis: response to high-dose oral isotretinoin therapy and reassessment of epidemiologic data. J Am Acad Dermatol 31:327, 1994

36. Inaloz H, Patel GK, Knight AG: Familial confluent and reticulated papillomatosis. Arch Dermatol 138:276, 2002

37. Purg L, de Moragas JM: Confluent and reticulated papillomatosis of Gougerot and Carteaud: minocycline deserves trial before etretinate. Arch Dermatol 131:109, 1995

38. Angeli-Besson C, Koeppel MC, Jacquart SP, et al: Confluent and reticulated papillomatosis (Gougerot-Carteaud) treated with tetracyclines. Int J Dermatol 34:567, 1995

39. Carrozzo AM, Gatti S, Ferranti G, et al: Calcipotriol treatment of confluent and reticulated papillomatosis (Gougerot-Carteaud syndrome). J Eur Acad Dermatol Venereol 14:131, 2000

40. Gulec AT, Seckin D: Confluent and reticulated papillomatosis: treatment with topical calcipotriol. Br J Dermatol 141:1150, 1999

41. Schwartzburg J, Schwartzburg H: Response of confluent and reticulated papillomatosis of Gougerot and Carteaud to topical tretinoin. Cutis 66:291, 2000

42. Kim YC, Davis MD, Schanbacher CF, et al: Dowling-Degos disease (reticulate pigmented anomaly of the flexures): a clinical and histopathologic study of 6 cases. J Am Acad Dermatol 40:462, 1999

43. Lestringant GG, Masouye I, Frossard PM, et al: Co-existence of leukoderma with features of Dowling-Degos disease and reticulate acropigmentation Kitamura spectrum in five unrelated patients. Dermatology 195:337, 1997

44. Thami GP, Jaswal R, Kanwar AJ, et al: Overlap of reticulate acropigmentation of Kitamura, acropigmentation of Dohi and Dowling-Degos disease in four generations. Dermatology 196:350, 1998

45. Kim YC, Davis MD, Schanbacher CF, et al: Dowling-Degos disease (reticulate pigmented anomaly of the flexures): a clinical and histopathological study of 6 cases. J Am Acad Dermatol 40:462, 1999

46. Wenzel J, Tappe K, Gerdsen R, et al: Successful treatment of Dowling-Degos disease with Er:YAG laser. Dermatol Surg 28:748, 2002

47. Kovacs SO: Vitiligo. J Am Acad Dermatol 38:647, 1998

48. Le Poole C, Boissy RE: Vitiligo. Semin Cutan Med Surg 16:3, 1997

49. Baharav E, Merimski O, Shoenfeld Y, et al: Tyrosinase as an autoantigen in patients with vitiligo. Clin Exp Immunol 105:84, 1996

50. Moretti S, Spallanzani A, Amato L, et al: New insights into the pathogenesis of vitiligo: imbalance of epidermal cytokines at sites of lesions. Pigment Cell Res 15:87, 2002

51. Grimes PE, Wojdani A, Loeb LJ, et al: The effects of isoprinosine treatment on repigmentation and immunologic aberrations in vitiligo (abstr). J Invest Dermatol 98:534, 1992

52. Grimes PE, Sevall JS, Wojdani A: Cytomegalovirus DNA identified in skin biopsy specimens of patients with vitiligo. J Am Acad Dermatol 35:21, 1996

53. Dell'Anna M, Maresca V, Briganti S, et al: Mitochondrial impairment in peripheral blood mononuclear cells during the active phase of vitiligo. J Invest Dermatol 117:908, 2001

54. Picardo M, Grammatico P, Roccella F, et al: Imbalance in the antioxidant pool in melanoma cells and normal melanocytes from patients with melanoma. J Invest Dermatol 107:322, 1996

55. Schallreuter KU, Wood JM, Berger J: Low catalase levels in the epidermis of patients with vitiligo. J Invest Dermatol 97:1081, 1991

56. Schallreuter KU, Wood JM, Pittelkow MR, et al: Regulation of melanin biosynthesis in the human epidermis by tetrahydrobiopterin. Science 263:1444, 1994

57. Grimes PE: Therapies for vitiligo. Drug Therapy in Dermatology. Millikan L, Ed. Marcel Dekker, New York, 2000

58. Grimes PE: Psoralen photochemotherapy for vitiligo. Clin Dermatol 15:921, 1997

59. Jimbow K: Vitiligo: therapeutic advances. Dermatol Clin 16:399, 1998

60. Falabella R: Surgical therapies for vitiligo. Clin Dermatol 15:927, 1997

61. Westerhof W, Nieuweboer-Krobotova L: Treatment of vitiligo with UV-B radiation vs topical psoralen plus UV-A. Arch Dermatol 133:1525, 1997

62. Grimes PE: Therapeutic trends for the treatment of vitiligo. Cosmet Derm 15:21, 2002

63. Spencer JM, Nossa R, Ajmeri J: Treatment of vitiligo with the 308-nm excimer laser: a pilot study. J Am Acad Dermatol 46:727, 2002

64. Schallreuter KU, Wood JM, Lemke KR, et al: Treatment of vitiligo with a topical application of pseudocatalase and calcium in combination with short-term UVB exposure: a case study on 33 patients. Dermatology 190:223, 1995

65. Grimes PE, Soriano T, Dytoc M: The efficacy and safety of tacrolimus ointment. J Am Acad Dermatol (in press)

66. Lyle WM, Sangster JO, Williams TD: Albinism: an update and review of the literature. J Am Optom Assoc 68:623, 1997

67. Oetting WS, King RA: Molecular basis of albinism: mutations and polymorphism or pigmentation genes associated with albinism. Hum Mutat 13:99, 1999

68. Orlow SJ: Albinism: an update. Semin Cutan Med Surg 16:24, 1997

69. Sarangarajan R, Boissy RE: Tyrp 1 and oculocutaneous albinism type 3. Pigment Cell Res 14:437, 2001

70. Oetting WS: The tyrosinase gene and oculocutaneous albinism type 1 (OCA1): a model for understanding the molecular biology of melanin formation. Pigment Cell Res 13:320, 2000

71. Shotelersuk V, Gahl WA: Hermansky-Pudlak syndrome: models for intracellular vesicle formulation. Molec Genet Metab 65:85, 1998

72. Spritz RA: Hermansky-Pudlak syndrome and pale ear: melanosome-making for the new millennium. Pigment Cell Res 13:15, 2000

73. Turner M, Gahl WA, Toro J: Dermatologic manifestations of Hermansky-Pudlak syndrome in patients with and without a 16-base pair duplication in the HPS 1 gene. Arch Dermatol 135:774, 1999

74. Klein C, Philippe N, Le Deist F, et al: Partial albinism with immunodeficiency (Griscelli syndrome). J Pediatr 125:886, 1994

75. Pastural E, Barrat FJ, Dufourcq-Lagelouse R, et al: Griscelli disease maps to chromosome 15q21 and is associated with mutations in the myosin-Va gene. Nat Genet 16:289, 1997

76. Spritz RA, Holmes SA, Itin P, et al: Novel mutations of the KIT (mast/stem cell growth factor receptor) proto-oncogene in human piebaldism. J Invest Dermatol 101:22, 1993

77. Richards KA, Fukai K, Osio N, et al: A novel KIT mutation results in piebaldism with progressive depigmentation. J Am Acad Dermatol 44:288, 2001

78. Syrris P, Malik N, Murday VA, et al: Three novel mutations of the proto-oncogene KIT cause human piebaldism. Am J Med Genet 95:79, 2000

79. Spritz RA: Piebaldism, Waardenburg syndrome and related disorders of melanocyte development. Semin Cutan Med Surg 16:15, 1997

80. Spritz RA, Hearing VJ Jr: Genetic disorders of pigmentation. Adv Hum Genet 22:1, 1994

81. Falabella R: Idiopathic guttate hypomelanosis. Dermatol Clin 6:241, 1988

82. Wallace ML, Grichnik JM, Prieto VG, et al: Numbers and differentiation status of melanocytes in idiopathic guttate hypomelanosis. J Cutan Pathol 25:375, 1998

83. Hexsel DM: Treatment of idiopathic guttate hypomelanosis by localized superficial dermabrasion. Dermatol Surg 25:917, 1999

49 Pituitary

Shlomo Melmed, M.D., F.A.C.P.

Functional Anatomy of the Pituitary

The pituitary gland regulates the critical hormonal functions of growth, development, reproduction, stress homeostasis, and metabolic control. Because of its prominent role in these processes, the pituitary has been termed the master gland.

The pituitary is situated within the sella turcica at the base of the brain and weighs about 600 mg. It comprises functionally distinct anterior and posterior lobes. The blood supply to the anterior pituitary is predominantly derived from the hypothalamic-pituitary portal vessels. The posterior lobe is supplied directly by the systemic inferior hypophyseal arteries.

Anatomically and functionally, the pituitary is closely linked with the hypothalamus [*see Figure 1 and Table 1*]. Neural cell bodies in the hypothalamus synthesize releasing and inhibiting hormones that control pituitary hormone secretion. These hypothalamic hormones are secreted into the portal vessels of the pituitary stalk and are transported to the anterior pituitary cell surface receptors.

The anterior pituitary synthesizes and secretes adrenocorticotropic hormone (ACTH), growth hormone (GH), prolactin (PRL), thyroid-stimulating hormone (TSH), follicle-stimulating hormone (FSH), and luteinizing hormone (LH).[1,2] The posterior pituitary secretes vasopressin (also known as antidiuretic hormone [ADH]) and oxytocin, both of which are synthesized in the hypothalamus.

Pituitary tropic hormones elicit responses from their respec-

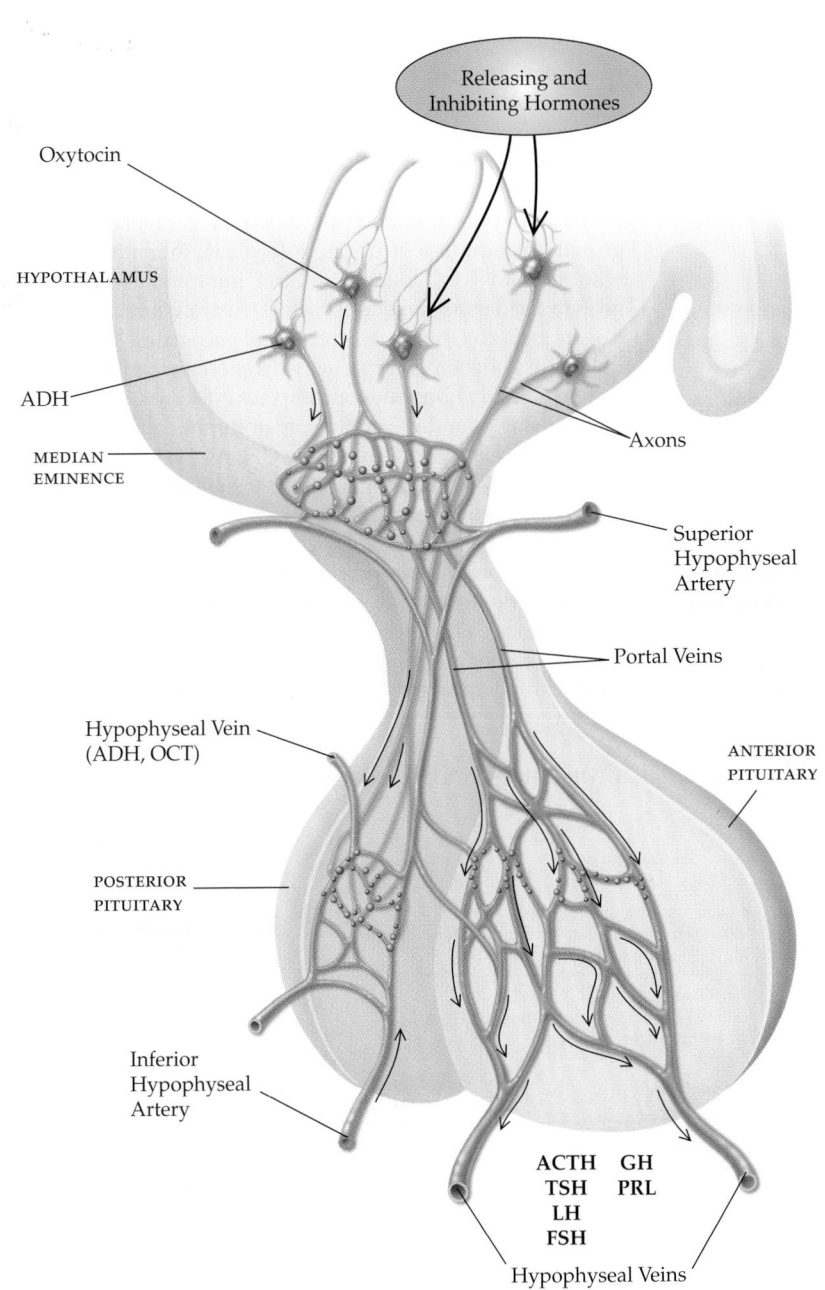

Figure 1 **The anterior pituitary and the hypothalamus are connected by the hypophyseal portal vasculature. Releasing or inhibiting hormones secreted by hypothalamic neurons enter the primary plexus of the hypophyseal portal vasculature. They flow down the long portal veins in the pituitary stalk to the secondary plexus, a capillary network that enmeshes the cells of the anterior pituitary. The anterior pituitary cells secrete their hormones in response to the releasing hormones. Because neither the hypothalamus nor the anterior pituitary is isolated by the blood-brain barrier, feedback signals have direct access to both sites of regulation. The posterior pituitary is made up of the terminal portions of neurons whose origin is the hypothalamus. (ACTH—adrenocorticotropic hormone; ADH—antidiuretic hormone; FSH—follicle-stimulating hormone; GH—growth hormone; LH—luteinizing hormone; PRL—prolactin; TSH—thyroid-stimulating hormone)**

Table 1 Hypothalamic and Related Pituitary Hormones

Hypothalamic Hormones	Pituitary Hormones
Growth hormone–releasing hormone	Growth hormone (GH)
Growth hormone release–inhibiting hormone (somatostatin)	GH
Prolactin release inhibitory factor (dopamine)	Prolactin
Gonadotropin-releasing hormone	Follicle-stimulating hormone Luteinizing hormone
Corticotropin-releasing hormone Vasopressin (arginine vasopressin; antidiuretic hormone)	Adrenocorticotropic hormone (corticotropin)
Thyrotropin-releasing hormone	Thyrotropin (thyroid-stimulating hormone)

tive target glands; the latter secrete endocrine hormones that activate specific tissue receptors. Circulating levels of these peripheral hormones influence secretion of their respective pituitary tropic hormone by negative feedback [*see Table 2*].

Pituitary Masses

LOCAL MASS EFFECTS

Pituitary masses can cause symptoms by secreting hormones, by impinging on adjacent structures, or both. These masses may also compress adjacent normal pituitary tissue, leading to pituitary failure. Expanding intrasellar lesions can exert significant compressive effects on surrounding vascular and neurologic structures, including the cavernous sinuses, cranial nerves, and optic chiasm. Intrasellar lesions may invade contiguous local structures and may compress central structures, depending on their anatomic location [*see Figure 2*]. The sellar roof presents the least resistance to soft tissue expansion from within the confines of the bony sella; this accounts for the vulnerability of the optic chiasm to sellar mass expansion. Small changes in intrasellar pressure may stretch the dural plate and cause headache, the severity of which does not necessarily correlate with mass size

or extension. Chiasmic pressure can result in bilateral or unilateral visual defects. Pituitary stalk compression encroaches on the portal vessels, with resultant hyperprolactinemia and concurrent failure of other pituitary tropic hormones. Cavernous sinus invasion may lead to palsies of the third, fourth, and sixth cranial nerves, as well as lesions of the ophthalmic and maxillary branches of the fifth cranial nerve. Inferior extension through the bony sellar floor involves the sphenoid sinus; further extension into the palate roof may result in nasopharyngeal invasion and, rarely, cerebrospinal fluid leakage. Tumor invasion of the temporal or frontal lobe can cause seizures and personality disorders. Hypothalamic encroachment by an invasive pituitary mass may have metabolic sequelae, including precocious puberty or hypogonadism, diabetes insipidus, dysthermia, appetite disorders, and sleep disturbances.

PITUITARY TUMORS

Pituitary Adenomas

Pituitary adenomas account for about 15% of all intracranial neoplasms. They arise from one of the specific anterior pituitary cell types as benign monoclonal expansions. Loss of heterozygosity of regions of chromosome 11q13, 13, and 9 occurs in up to 20% of larger sporadic pituitary tumors, suggesting the presence of tumor suppressor genes at these loci. Other factors involved in initiation and promotion of pituitary adenoma growth include loss of negative feedback inhibition, as seen with thyroidal or gonadal failure; intrapituitary paracrine growth factors (angiogenesis factors), mainly mediated by estrogen; and activation of any of several oncogenes.

Pituitary adenomas are usually diagnosed when they hypersecrete pituitary hormones or compress adjacent structures. Tumors arising from lactotroph, somatotroph, corticotroph, and thyrotroph cells hypersecrete PRL, GH, ACTH, or TSH, respectively [*see Table 3*]. Functional tumors exhibit autonomous tropic hormone secretion, leading to hyperprolactinemia, acromegaly, Cushing disease, or, rarely, TSH hypersecretion. Plurihormonal tumors may produce mixed clinical features. About one third of adenomas do not actively secrete hormones and are clinically nonfunctional. On autopsy, up to one quarter of patients are found to harbor an unsuspected microadenoma (diameter < 10 mm) with no apparent clinical sequelae. Rarely, ectopic secre-

Table 2 Pituitary Hormones, Their Mediators, and Their Effects

Pituitary Hormones	Stimulators	Inhibitors	Target Glands	Tropic Effects
Gonadotropins: follicle-stimulating hormone, luteinizing hormone	Gonadotropin-releasing hormone	Sex steroids, inhibin	Ovary, testis	Sex steroid production, reproductive activity
Thyroid-stimulating hormone	Thyrotropin-releasing hormone (TRH)	Triiodothyronine (T_3), thyroxine (T_4), dopamine, somatostatin, glucocorticoids	Thyroid	T_3, T_4 synthesis and secretion
Prolactin	Estrogen, TRH	Dopamine	Breast, other tissues	Milk production
Growth hormone (GH)	GH-releasing hormone, GH secretagogue	Somatostatin, insulinlike growth factor (IGF)	Liver, bones, other tissues	IGF-1 production, growth induction, insulin antagonism
Adrenocorticotropic hormone	Corticotropin-releasing hormone, vasopressin, cytokines	Glucocorticoids	Adrenal	Steroid production

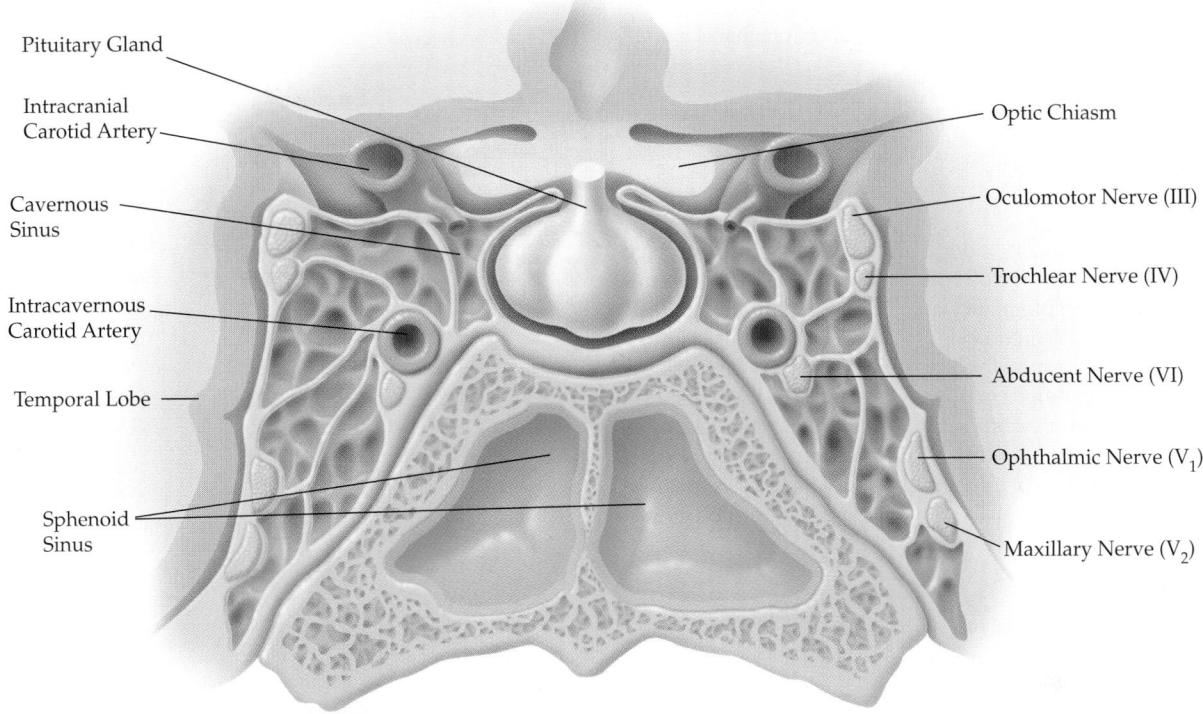

Figure 2 **Cross section of the pituitary gland and adjacent structures.**

tion of GH-releasing hormone (GHRH) or corticotropin-releasing hormone (CRH) elaborated by abdominal or chest tumors results in hyperplasia of the cells that secrete GH or ACTH; these patients may present with pituitary hyperplasia and acromegaly or Cushing syndrome.

Genetic Syndromes Associated with Pituitary Adenomas

Multiple endocrine neoplasia type I Multiple endocrine neoplasia type I (MEN I) is an autosomal dominant syndrome caused by an inactivating mutation in the coding region of *menin*, a tumor suppressor gene located at the q13 locus of chromosome 11. The syndrome comprises parathyroid, pancreatic, and pituitary adenomas, including prolactinomas, and may present as acromegaly or Cushing syndrome.

Carney syndrome Carney syndrome is an autosomal dominant syndrome associated with activated protein kinase activity. It comprises spotty skin pigmentation; myxomas; and testicular, adrenal, and pituitary adenomas.

McCune-Albright syndrome The McCune-Albright syndrome is associated with chromosome 20q13.2 mosaicism and constitutive activation of cyclic adenosine monophosphate (cAMP). This syndrome manifests as polyostotic fibrous dysplasia (cancellous bone is replaced with immature woven bone and fibrous tissue), pigmented skin patches, precocious puberty, and acromegaly.

Familial acromegaly Affected persons with this rare syn-

Table 3 Effects of Pituitary Adenomas

General Effect	Adenoma Cell Origin	Hormone Product	Clinical Syndrome
Hormone hypersecretion	Lactotroph	PRL	Hypogonadism, galactorrhea
	Somatotroph	GH	Acromegaly/gigantism
	Corticotroph	ACTH	Cushing disease
	Mixed growth hormone and prolactin cell	GH, PRL	Acromegaly, hypogonadism, galactorrhea
	Acidophil stem cell, mammosomatotroph	PRL, GH	Hypogonadism, acromegaly
	Thyrotroph	TSH	Hyperthyrotoxinemia
	Other plurihormonal cell	Any	Mixed
Hypopituitarism	Gonadotroph	FSH, LH, subunits	Silent or hypogonadism
	Null cell	None	Pituitary failure from mass effect
	Oncocytoma	None	Pituitary failure from mass effect

Note: all tumors may cause local pressure effects, including visual disturbances, cranial nerve palsy, and headache.
ACTH—adrenocorticotropic hormone FSH—follicle-stimulating hormone GH—growth hormone LH—luteinizing hormone PRL—prolactin
TSH—thyroid-stimulating hormone

drome have acromegaly or gigantism and exhibit loss of heterozygosity at an 11q13 chromosomal locus distinct from that of *menin*.

Anterior Pituitary Hormones and Associated Disorders

PROLACTIN

Synthesis

Lactotrophs comprise about 20% of the anterior pituitary cells. Estrogen causes lactotroph cell hyperplasia, which occurs transiently during pregnancy and lactation. Central inhibitory control of PRL secretion is mediated predominantly by dopamine from the hypothalamus. Physiologic, pharmacologic, or pathologic alterations in dopamine availability or action disrupt PRL regulation. For example, if the hypophyseal-portal system is disrupted by pituitary compression or pituitary stalk damage and the flow of hypothalamic dopamine to the anterior pituitary is compromised, the resulting loss of lactotroph inhibition leads to PRL hypersecretion.[3]

Secretion

Normal serum PRL levels are 10 to 25 µg/L. The PRL level rises approximately 10-fold during pregnancy, as does the estrogen level. The PRL level declines rapidly within 2 weeks after delivery and returns to normal during the subsequent 3 months. Basal levels remain elevated during breastfeeding, and suckling induces a transient (approximately 30 minutes) reflex rise in PRL level.

Actions

PRL induces and maintains puerperal lactation. It also attenuates reproductive function, thus helping to ensure that lactation is not interrupted by pregnancy. In the primed puerperal breast, integration of multihormonal signals—from PRL, placental lactogens, progesterone, and local paracrine growth factors—leads to lactation. PRL also enhances milk production by improving calcium absorption and mobilization.

Hyperprolactinemia

Etiology Hyperprolactinemia has many possible causes; it may be physiologic, pathologic, or iatrogenic in origin [*see Table 4*]. Pregnancy, lactation, nipple stimulation, and chest wall lesions (including surgical incisions and herpes zoster) are associated with hyperprolactinemia. PRL-secreting pituitary adenomas (prolactinomas) produce the highest elevations of serum PRL levels [*see Prolactinomas, below*]. Medications, compromised pituitary stalk function, hypothyroidism, and renal failure typically produce lesser elevations in PRL level [*see Table 1*]. Hypothalamic dopamine delivery may be disrupted by hypothalamic tumors, cysts, infiltrations, and radiation-induced damage. Plurihormonal tumors commonly hypersecrete PRL, and clinically nonfunctioning pituitary tumors may also compromise stalk integrity and cause hyperprolactinemia.

Diagnosis The clinical features of hyperprolactinemia vary by the sex of the patient. In males, PRL attenuates LH secretion, leading to low testosterone levels. Men with hyperprolactinemia present with diminished libido and diminished sexual potency, oligospermia, and lowered ejaculate volume; up to about 30% may have galactorrhea. In women, hyperprolactinemia leads to loss of pulsatile LH secretion, blunting of the LH peak, hypoestrogenism, and anovulation [*see Figure 3*]. Women with

Table 4   Causes of Hyperprolactinemia[39]

Physiologic hypersecretion	Pregnancy Lactation Chest wall lesions Sleep Stress

Hypothalamic-pituitary damage	Masses
	  Craniopharyngioma
	  Suprasellar pituitary mass extension
	  Rathke cyst
	  Meningioma
	  Dysgerminoma
	  Metastases
	Granulomas
	Infiltration
	  Lymphocytic hypophysitis
	Trauma
	  Pituitary stalk section
	  Suprasellar surgery
	  Cranial irradiation

Pituitary hypersecretion	Prolactinoma Acromegaly Empty sella syndrome
Systemic disorders	Chronic renal failure Hypothyroidism Cirrhosis Epileptic seizures

Drug-induced hypersecretion	Dopamine receptor blockers
	  Phenothiazines (e.g., chlorpromazine, perphenazine)
	  Butyrophenones (e.g., haloperidol)
	  Thioxanthenes
	  Metoclopramide
	Dopamine synthesis inhibitor
	  α-Methyldopa
	Catecholamine depletor
	  Reserpine
	Opiates
	H$_2$ antagonists (e.g., cimetidine, ranitidine)
	Imipramines
	  Amitriptyline, amoxapine
	Selective serotonin reuptake inhibitors (e.g., fluoxetine)
	Calcium channel blockers (e.g., verapamil)
	Hormones
	  Estrogens
	  Antiandrogens

hyperprolactinemia develop oligomenorrhea and amenorrhea. Anovulation and estrogen deprivation result in vaginal dryness, dyspareunia, loss of libido, and infertility. Hyperprolactinemia is also associated with enhanced risk of bone loss, which is further exacerbated by associated hypoestrogenemia.

In patients with clinical complaints consistent with hyperprolactinemia, a careful history and physical examination may reveal the source of the problem. Laboratory studies are indicated to exclude hypothyroidism, which can cause hyperprolactin-

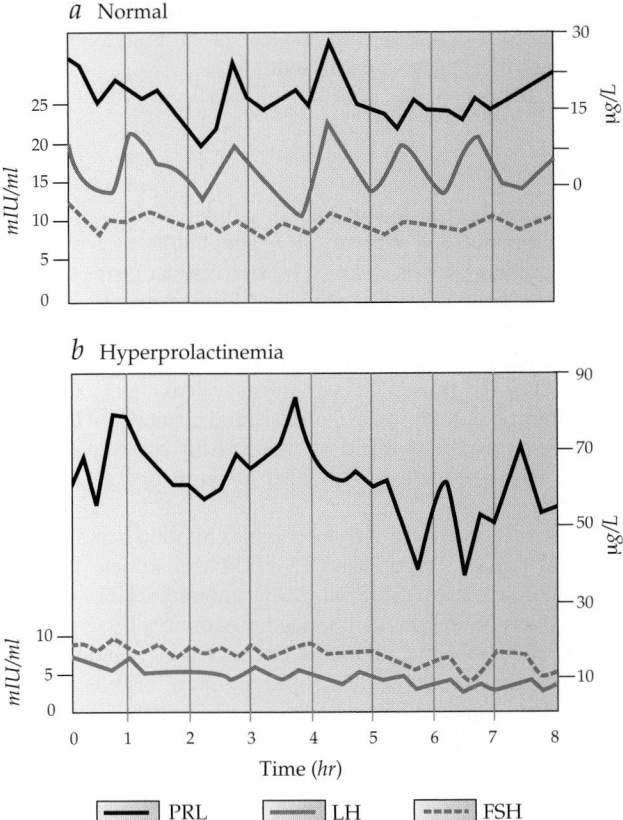

a Normal

b Hyperprolactinemia

| PRL | LH | FSH |

Figure 3 In women, hyperprolactinemia results in loss of pulsatile luteinizing hormone (LH) secretion and lowering of follicle-stimulating hormone (FSH) levels.[39] (PRL—prolactin)

emia. Alternatively, hypothyroidism and hyperprolactinemia can result from pituitary disease.

The degree of PRL elevation may offer a clue to the source of the prolactinemia. Prolactinomas account for most elevations of prolactin level higher than 100 μg/L; serum prolactin levels greater than 200 μg/L almost invariably indicate a prolactinoma.

All patients with symptoms of hyperprolactinemia and PRL levels above 30 μg/L should undergo MRI imaging of the pituitary. Small microadenomas (< 2 mm), which are undetectable on MRI scanning, may account for most cases of idiopathic hyperprolactinemia.

Treatment Treatment of hyperprolactinemia is aimed at normalizing PRL levels, alleviating gonadal dysfunction and galactorrhea, and preserving bone mineral density. Medications known to alter PRL levels should be discontinued, if possible. Dose titration of critical neuroleptic drugs with a dopamine agonist can normalize serum PRL levels and alleviate reproductive dysfunction. Hyperprolactinemia usually resolves after thyroid hormone replacement in hypothyroid patients and after renal transplantation in patients with chronic renal failure who are on dialysis. Hypothalamic or nonadenomatous sellar mass lesions should be removed surgically. Spontaneous resolution of hyperprolactinemia occurs in up to 30% of patients, whether or not they have a visible pituitary microadenoma.

Prolactinoma

Prolactinomas arising from lactotrophs are the most common functional pituitary tumors, with an annual incidence of about

three per 100,000 population. Microadenomas are less than 1 cm in diameter and do not invade the parasellar region. Macroadenomas are more than 1 cm in diameter, are locally invasive, and may compress vital structures, leading to symptoms such as headaches and visual defects. Microprolactinomas have a female preponderance (20:1). Macroadenomas occur equally in both sexes, although men usually present with larger tumors. Tumor size correlates with PRL concentrations—serum PRL values above 200 μg/L are invariably associated with larger adenomas.

Diagnosis Prolactinoma should be suspected in patients with clinical signs of hyperprolactinemia (see above) and high random PRL levels. Men with prolactinomas tend to have relatively higher PRL levels than do women with prolactinomas. Diagnosis is confirmed by visualizing a pituitary adenoma on MRI.

Treatment Prolactinomas can be treated medically, with cabergoline or bromocriptine [*see Table 5*], or, rarely, surgically.

Cabergoline is a long-acting dopamine agonist that suppresses prolactin for more than 14 days after a single oral dose and shrinks prolactinomas in most patients.[4] The dosage is 0.5 to 1.0 mg twice weekly. Normal serum prolactin levels are achieved in about 80% of patients with microadenomas; normal gonadal function is restored and galactorrhea improves or resolves in 90% of patients. In patients with macroadenomas, cabergoline normalizes prolactin levels and shrinks the tumor in about 70% of cases. Cabergoline may be more effective in patients resistant to bromocriptine. Adverse effects and drug intolerance are less commonly encountered with cabergoline than with bromocriptine.

Bromocriptine mesylate is a D_2 dopamine receptor agonist that normalizes prolactin secretion in up to 70% of patients with microadenomas; it decreases tumor size and restores gonadal function. Prolactin levels normalize in 70% of patients with macroadenomas, and tumor mass shrinkage of 50% or more is achieved in about 50% of patients. Headaches and visual disorders usually improve or resolve within days, and sexual function improves. Therapy is initiated with 0.625 to 1.25 mg given at bedtime with a

Table 5 Dopamine Agonists in the Treatment of Prolactinomas

Treatment Response	Bromocriptine Patient Response (%)*	Cabergoline Patient Response (%)†
Microadenomas		
Prolactin level normalized	70	80
Menses resumed	70	80
Macroadenomas		
Prolactin level normalized	65	70
Menses resumed	85	80
Tumor shrinkage		
≥ 50%	40	25
< 50%	40	55
None	20	20
Visual-field improvement	90	70
Drug intolerance	15	5

*2.5–7.5 mg/day; bromocriptine is preferred for infertility because it is short acting and can be discontinued immediately on pregnancy confirmation.
†0.5–1 mg twice weekly; cabergoline offers better compliance because it is long acting and has fewer gastrointestinal side effects.

snack, and the dosage is gradually increased. Successful control is usually achieved with a daily dose of less than 7.5 mg (i.e., 2.5 mg t.i.d.). About 20% of patients are resistant to the drug.

Side effects of dopamine agonists include transient nausea, vomiting, and postural hypotension with faintness; these symptoms occur in about 25% of patients. Other side effects include reversible constipation, nasal stuffiness, nightmares, and insomnia. For women who cannot tolerate orally administered agonists, intravaginal administration of bromocriptine tablets is often effective.

Indications for surgical resection of prolactinomas include resistance to or intolerance of pharmacologic treatment and the presence of an invasive macroadenoma that causes compromised vision and that fails to rapidly improve with dopamine agonists.[5] Initial attempts at resection lead to normalization of prolactin levels in about 70% of patients with microprolactinomas but only 30% of patients with macroadenomas. Prolactinomas recur in up to 20% of patients within the first year after surgery; long-term recurrence rates for macroadenomas exceed 50%.

Therapeutic goals in patients with prolactinomas include control of hyperprolactinemia; reduction of tumor size; resolution of galactorrhea; and restoration of menses, fertility, or both [see Figure 4].[6] Dopamine agonists suppress PRL secretion and synthesis and lactotroph cell proliferation. Patients are monitored with measurement of serum PRL levels, pituitary MRI scans, and visual field examinations. Once controlled, PRL levels can be measured every 6 months and MRI can be performed every 2 years. Medication doses are titrated to the lowest levels required to normalize PRL levels, restore reproductive function, and shrink the tumor mass.

If fertility is not desired, no treatment of microprolactinoma may be needed. Such patients should be monitored through regular serial PRL measurements, pituitary MRI scans, and assessment of bone mineral density. For patients with macroadenomas, visual field testing is performed before initiating dopamine agonists. MRI results and visual fields should be assessed serially until the mass shrinks, and annually thereafter. Reduction in PRL levels invariably precedes radiographically evident tumor shrinkage, and failure to lower PRL levels usually portends lack of tumor shrinkage. Radiotherapy is reserved for the rare patients with aggressive tumors that do not respond to maximally tolerated dopamine agonists or surgery.

Prolactinomas and pregnancy   Women with prolactinomas who wish to become pregnant should receive bromocriptine and use barrier methods of contraception until they have had regular menses for 3 months; this will permit accurate conception dating. Contraception may then be discontinued. When pregnancy is confirmed, bromocriptine should be discontinued and PRL levels followed serially. The patient should be carefully monitored for headaches or visual field disturbance. Cabergoline is not approved for restoration of fertility.

During pregnancy, the pituitary swells and there is an increased risk of prolactinoma growth; in particular, up to 30% of macroadenomas may grow during pregnancy. In women harboring macroadenomas, bromocriptine is restarted if visual field defects develop. Although pituitary MRI is considered safe during pregnancy, it is reserved for patients who develop severe headache or documented visual field defects. In the rare cases in which vision is threatened during the third trimester, surgical decompression may be indicated. Bromocriptine can be safely restarted during pregnancy. Comprehensive surveillance

data do not indicate an adverse impact on the fetus; nevertheless, this approach should be undertaken cautiously, and only with the patient's informed consent.

GROWTH HORMONE

Synthesis and Secretion

GH is the most abundant anterior pituitary hormone; GH-secreting somatotroph cells constitute about 50% of the pituitary cell population. GH is encoded by five distinct genes situated on chromosome 17q22. The pituitary GH gene gives rise to a circulating form of GH that is 22 kilodaltons in size, and to a less abundant, cleaved 20-kd GH molecule. Placental syncytiotrophoblast cells express a GH variant, as well as chorionic somatotrophin. Somatotroph development and pituitary GH expression are largely determined by the Pit-1 nuclear transcription factor, whose mutations may also account for rare cases of hereditary pituitary failure.

GH secretion is controlled by complex hypothalamic and peripheral factors. Hypothalamic GHRH and somatostatin release-inhibitor factor (SRIF) stimulate and inhibit GH secretion, respectively. Ghrelin is synthesized predominantly in the gastrointestinal tract and stimulates GH secretion by binding to a specific pituitary GH secretagogue receptor.[7] SRIF is also expressed in extrahypothalamic tissues, including the GI tract and the pancreas. SRIF binds to five distinct receptor subtypes (SSTR1 to SSTR5), of which SSTR2 and SSTR5 are expressed on the surface membranes of pituitary cells. Signaling through the SSTR2 and SSTR5 subtypes preferentially suppresses secretion of GH (and also TSH). Insulinlike growth factor–1 (IGF-1), the peripheral target hormone for GH, inhibits GH via negative feedback.

GH secretion occurs in pulsatile peaks, interspersed by periods during which GH may be undetectable.[8] GH secretion peaks during puberty and declines by middle age, in parallel with age-related decline in muscle mass. Mean integrated nocturnal GH levels are at least twice that of daytime levels. GH levels rise within 1 hour after onset of deep sleep, as well as after exercise and trauma. GH secretion is low in the elderly and the obese and is higher in women; GH secretion is enhanced by estrogen replacement therapy. Increased GH pulse frequency and peak amplitudes occur with chronic malnutrition and prolonged fasting. Glucose loading suppresses GH to below 0.7 μg/L in women and below 0.07 μg/L in men. A complex interaction of nutritional factors and hypothalamic appetite-regulating peptides, including leptin, mediate GH secretion. Therefore, random measurements of GH levels do not readily identify adult patients with GH deficiency.[9] Differences in linear growth patterns in males and females may reflect differences in GH pulsatility. Higher GH pulses observed in males, as compared with the relatively continuous GH secretion patterns in females, may determine liver enzyme induction and postreceptor activity levels of GH-signaling molecules.

Actions

Peripheral GH receptors are most abundant in the liver. The extracellular domain of GH receptors is a soluble form—GH binding protein (GHBP)—which circulates in the blood. Binding of GH to its receptor induces intracellular signaling that is mediated by a phosphorylation cascade involving the Janus kinase-signal transducer and activator of transcription (JAK/STAT) pathway.[10]

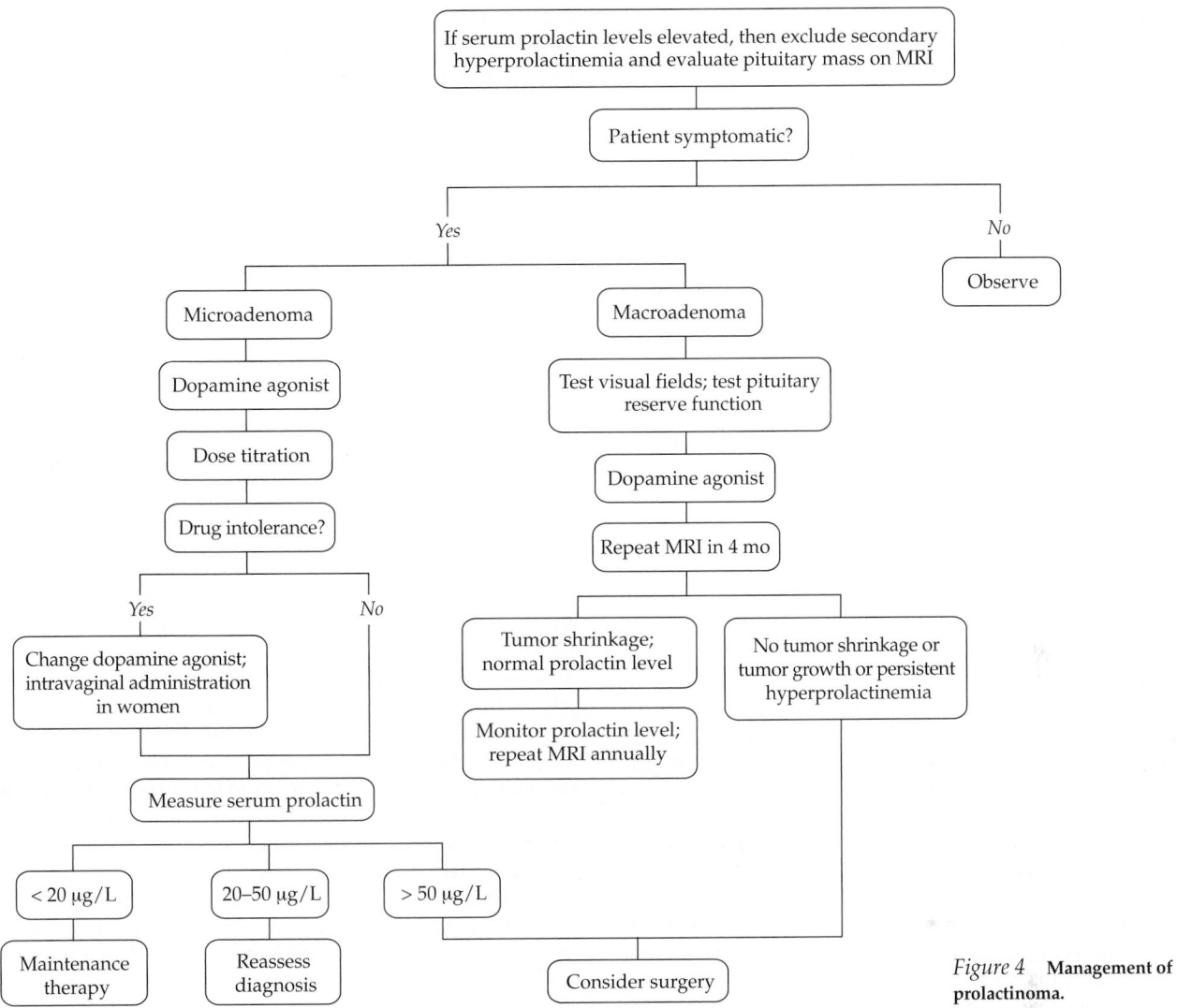

Figure 4 **Management of prolactinoma.**

In children and adolescents, GH stimulates the differentiation of epiphyseal prechondrocytes into IGF-1–responsive cells. GH also induces local IGF-1 and chondrocyte expansion. Linear growth is maintained by complex endocrine and paracrine mechanisms. In persons of all ages, GH antagonizes insulin action, impairs glucose tolerance, induces protein synthesis, enhances lipolysis, and increases lipid oxidation.

Insulinlike growth factors The IGF family of polypeptide growth factors comprises IGF-1, IGF-2, and proinsulin. IGF-1 in peripheral tissue exerts local paracrine actions, which are both GH dependent and independent. GH induces increases in circulating levels and tissue levels of IGF-1. Both IGF-1 and IGF-2 are bound to one of six high-affinity circulating IGF binding proteins (IGFBPs) that also regulate IGF bioactivity. IGFBP3 is GH dependent and is the major carrier protein for circulating IGF-1. GH deficiency, GH insensitivity, and malnutrition are associated with low IGFBP3 levels. Serum IGF-1 levels increase throughout puberty, peak at 16 years of age, and decline thereafter. Concentrations are higher in female subjects, especially during puberty. IGF-1 levels are lower in patients with GH deficiency, cachexia, malnutrition, or sepsis; they are invariably high in patients with acromegaly.

Adult GH Deficiency

Somatotroph damage and the subsequent development of pituitary tropic hormone deficiency follows a sequential pattern in which loss of adequate GH reserve usually foreshadows subsequent deficits of other pituitary hormones. The presence of central hypogonadism, hypothyroidism, or hypoadrenalism invariably implies concomitant GH deficiency. About half of all patients with pituitary insufficiency will already manifest GH deficiency if specifically tested.

Diagnosis Clinically, GH deficiency in adults is marked by impaired quality of life, body composition changes, and decreased exercise capacity [*see Table 6*]. Cardiovascular risk factors increase in patients with GH deficiency; indeed, the increase in mortality associated with adult hypopituitarism, and, possibly, GH deficiency in particular, is primarily from cardiovascular and cerebrovascular disease.[11] Because adult GH deficiency is rare and its symptoms are largely nonspecific, patients should be carefully selected for evaluation on the basis of well-defined risk criteria. These criteria include a history of pituitary surgery; pituitary or hypothalamic mass lesions; cranial irradiation; the need for GH replacement therapy in childhood, or the finding of a low IGF-1 level, as compared to the age- and sex-

Table 6 Findings in Adult Growth Hormone Deficiency[39]

Clinical Manifestations
Impaired quality of life
   Decreased energy and drive
   Poor concentration
   Low self-esteem
   Social isolation
Body-composition changes
   Increased body fat mass
   Abdominal fat
   Increased waist-hip ratio
   Decreased lean body mass
Imaging Studies
Pituitary: mass or structural damage
Bone: reduced density
Abdomen: excess omental adiposity

Laboratory Tests
Evoked GH level < 3 ng/ml
IGF-1 and IGFBP3 levels low or normal
Lipid disorders
Concomitant deficits in gonadotropin, TSH, or ACTH reserve
Reduced Exercise Capacity
Reduced maximum O$_2$ uptake
Impaired cardiac function
Reduced muscle mass
Cardiovascular Risk Factors
Impaired cardiac structure and function
Abnormal lipid profile
Decreased fibrinolytic activity
Atherosclerosis
Omental obesity

ACTH—adrenocorticotropic hormone   GH—growth hormone
IGF—insulinlike growth factor   TSH—thyroid-stimulating hormone

matched population.[12] A subnormal evoked GH response (i.e., < 3 μg/ml) to a standard GH stimulation test establishes the diagnosis of adult GH deficiency. If other pituitary tropic hormone deficits are present, GH deficiency will be an inevitable concomitant finding; for that reason, some experts have recommended that GH testing not be required in this setting.[13] About 25% of GH-deficient adults have normal IGF-1 levels.

Treatment   GH replacement is indicated for adult patients with unequivocal GH deficiency.[14] The decision to treat is also determined by informed patient perception of therapeutic benefits, including prevention of future ischemic heart disease and skeletal fractures, improved exercise capacity and energy levels, and enriched quality of life. For replacement therapy, GH is started at a dosage of 0.15 to 0.2 mg/day and titrated to a maximum of 1.25 mg/day, to maintain midrange age- and sex-matched IGF-1 levels. Women require higher GH doses than men, and elderly patients require lower doses.[15]

Contraindications to therapy include the presence of an active neoplasm or both uncontrolled diabetes and retinopathy. The risks of pituitary tumor regrowth are currently being assessed in long-term surveillance studies.

The side effects of GH replacement include reversible dose-related fluid retention, joint pain, and myalgia and parethesia associated with carpal tunnel syndrome. These side effects occur in up to 30% of patients.[16] Patients with type 2 (non–insulin-dependent) diabetes mellitus will initially experience increased insulin resistance. However, glycemic control may improve in association with sustained loss of abdominal fat during long-term GH replacement.

If after 6 months there is no clinical response to GH replacement, treatment should be discontinued. In patients who show a response, GH replacement is continued in conjunction with regular monitoring of IGF-1 levels, lipids, and bone density.

GH is not indicated for adults with intact pituitary function, except for those with AIDS-related cachexia. The hormone should not be used for nonapproved indications, because the risk of side effects—especially glucose intolerance and fluid retention—outweigh potential benefits ascribed to improved muscle energy and anti-aging properties. Results of prospective controlled trials for these potential indications are not yet at hand.

Acromegaly

Etiology   GH hypersecretion usually results from a GH-secreting pituitary adenoma [*see Table 7*]. Occasionally, patients with partially empty sella may harbor a small GH-secreting adenoma within the compressed rim of pituitary tissue. Rarely, GH is secreted ectopically by abdominal or chest tumors. GHRH may be elaborated by hypothalamic tumors or carcinoid tumors in the chest or abdomen, causing acromegaly through chronic somatotroph overstimulation.

Diagnosis   The manifestations of GH and IGF-1 hypersecretion are protean and develop slowly; they are often not diagnosed for 10 years or more [*see Table 8*]. Acral bony overgrowth results in frontal bossing, increased hand and foot size, and mandibular enlargement with prognathism and a widening of incisor spaces. GH hypersecretion that occurs before epiphyseal long-bone closure causes pituitary gigantism. Soft tissue swelling results in coarse facial features; increased heel pad thickness; and enlargement of the feet and hands, evidenced by increased shoe or glove size and ring tightening. Hyperhidrosis; oily skin; a deepening of the voice; arthropathy; kyphosis; carpal tunnel syndrome; proximal muscle weakness and fatigue; skin tags; and visceromegaly, including macroglossia, cardiomegaly, thyroid, and salivary gland enlargement, may be encountered. About 30% of patients develop coronary artery disease, cardiomyopathy with arrhythmias, left ventricular hypertrophy, decreased diastolic function, or hypertension. Sleep apnea, caused by soft tissue laryngeal airway obstruction or central sleep dysfunction, is an important comorbidity. Diabetes develops in 25% of patients, because GH is a potent insulin an-

Table 7 Causes of Acromegaly

Excess growth hormone (GH) secretion
   Pituitary (~98% of cases)
      GH cell adenoma
      Mixed GH cell and prolactin cell adenoma
      Mammosomatotroph cell adenoma
      Plurihormonal adenoma
      GH cell carcinoma or metastases
      Multiple endocrine neoplasia type 1 (GH cell adenoma)
      McCune-Albright syndrome (rarely, adenoma)
      Ectopic sphenoid or parapharyngeal sinus pituitary adenoma
   Extrapituitary tumor (< 1% of cases)
      Pancreatic islet cell tumor
Excess GH-releasing hormone secretion
   Central (< 1% of cases)
      Hypothalamic hamartoma, choristoma, ganglioneuroma
   Peripheral (~1% of cases)
      Bronchial carcinoid
      Pancreatic islet cell tumor
      Small cell lung cancer
      Adrenal adenoma
      Medullary thyroid carcinoma
      Pheochromocytoma

Table 8 Features of Acromegaly

Enlarged hands and feet	Profuse sweating/hot
Coarsening of facial features/prognathism	Headache
	Carpal tunnel syndrome
Bite problems	Arthritis/arthralgias
Skin tags	Hypertension and heart disease
Frontal bossing	Sleep apnea and snoring
Cystic acne	Glucose intolerance
Colonic polyps	Hyperprolactinemia
Deepening of voice	Visual problems
Oily skin	Sexual dysfunction

tagonist; most patients with elevated GH levels are intolerant of glucose. Colon polyps are present in up to one third of patients. Overall mortality is enhanced about threefold, primarily as a result of cardiovascular and cerebrovascular disorders and respiratory disease. Unless GH levels are tightly controlled, survival is reduced by an average of 10 years compared with an age-matched control population.

Measurement of serum IGF-1 can be used for case finding in patients with possible acromegaly; in patients with GH hypersecretion, IGF-1 levels are invariably elevated, as compared with the levels in the age- and sex-matched population. Single random GH measurements are not useful for diagnosis. Instead, diagnosis is confirmed by demonstrating a failure to suppress GH levels to below 1 µg/L within 1 to 2 hours after an oral glucose load (75 g); about 20% of patients exhibit a paradoxical glucose-induced rise in GH. PRL levels are elevated in about 25% of patients. Thyroid function studies and assays of gonadotropin and sex steroid levels may show attenuation, which is the result of the compressive effects of an expanding pituitary mass.

Treatment   Control of acromegaly can be achieved by a judicious application of multimodal therapeutic approaches.[17,18] Therapeutic interventions include surgery, somatostatin analogues, and dopamine agonists. Transsphenoidal surgical resection by an experienced surgeon is indicated for both microadenomas and macroadenomas. Resection results in control of disease in about 70% of patients with microadenomas but in less than 50% of patients with macroadenomas. GH levels fall rapidly after tumor resection, and IGF-1 levels return to normal within 3 to 4 days. The disorder recurs in about 10% of patients, and pituitary failure develops in up to 15% of patients after surgery. Persistent postoperative GH hypersecretion necessitates adjuvant therapy, typically with somatostatin analogues.

Octreotide acetate is an 8–amino acid synthetic somatostatin analogue that binds mainly to SSTR2 receptors and effectively controls GH hypersecretion.[19] Octreotide is given in a dosage of 50 to 400 µg subcutaneously every 8 hours. Within an hour of receiving an injection, most patients experience an 80% reduction in GH level. About 10% of patients show no response. Rapid relief of headache and soft tissue swelling occurs, with amelioration of excessive perspiration, obstructive apnea, and cardiac failure. Significant pituitary tumor shrinkage occurs in about 40% of patients.[20] A long-acting octreotide formulation, Sandostatin LAR Depot, provides sustained GH suppression, with effects lasting for up to 6 weeks after a 30 mg intramuscular injection. Long-term treatment with monthly injections of 20 to 40 mg maintains GH and IGF-1 suppression in about 70% of

patients, and pituitary tumor size is controlled. Because it is effective, and well tolerated and is less inconvenient for the patient than subcutaneous preparations, the long-acting formulation is the medical treatment choice for these patients.[21,22]

Side effects of somatostatin analogues are typically minor and transient; they are mostly related to suppression of GI motility and secretion. Nausea, abdominal discomfort, diarrhea, and flatulence occur in one third of patients but usually remit within 2 weeks. In the United States, up to 30% of patients receiving long-term treatment develop echogenic gallbladder sludge or asymptomatic cholesterol gallstones. Mild glucose intolerance, hypothyroxinemia, asymptomatic bradycardia, and local pain at the injection site have been reported.

Bromocriptine may suppress GH secretion in some patients. High doses (i.e., 20 mg/day or more) are usually required. About 10% of patients receiving bromocriptine have normalized IGF-1 levels. Cabergoline suppresses GH when given at a relatively high dosage (i.e., 0.5 mg/day). Combination treatment with octreotide plus cabergoline offers additive biochemical control compared with either drug alone.

GH antagonists have been developed. These new GH analogues antagonize GH action by blocking peripheral GH receptor binding. Pegvisomant, administered in daily subcutaneous injections, lowers serum IGF-1 levels and so may block the deleterious peripheral effects of GH. GH levels may remain elevated, but the excess hormone is effectively inactive. Long-term monitoring of pituitary adenoma size and liver function testing are suggested. The drug is particularly useful in those patients with persistently elevated IGF-1 levels and controlled GH levels.

External radiation therapy or high-energy radiosurgery suppresses GH levels to below 5 µg/L, although 50% of patients require at least 8 years of therapy for this outcome.[23] Interim medical therapy is required in the years before patients attain maximal radiation benefits. Most patients also develop gonadotropin, ACTH, or TSH deficiency within 10 years of therapy. Rarely, visual deficits, brain necrosis, or new tumor formation are encountered. Stereotactic ablation of GH-secreting adenomas by gamma-knife radiosurgery is promising, but compelling long-term results are not yet available, and long-term side-effect profiles have not been established.

The initial treatment option for well-circumscribed GH-secreting tumors is surgical resection. Somatostatin analogues reduce GH hypersecretion and are used for preoperative shrinkage of large, invasive macroadenomas; for immediate relief of debilitating symptoms in frail patients experiencing morbidity; for patients who decline surgery; and for patients in whom surgery fails to result in biochemical control, as is inevitable in cases of invasive adenoma.[24] Irradiation or repeat surgery is indicated for patients for whom medical therapy fails. The main disadvantages of radiotherapy are the slow rate of biochemical response (i.e., 5 to 15 years) and the high rate of hypopituitarism. Comorbid features of acromegaly, including cardiovascular disease, diabetes, and arthritis, should be aggressively treated. Maxillofacial surgery may be indicated for mandibular repair.

Adrenocorticotropic Hormone Synthesis

Up to 20% of the pituitary consists of ACTH-secreting corticotroph cells. These cells express products of the *POMC* (pro-opiomelanocortin) gene, which include 1-39 ACTH, β-lipotropin, and endorphins. β-Lipotropin gives rise to α-lipotropin and β-endorphin; the latter contains the sequence for met-enkephalin. The *POMC* gene, located on chromosome 2, possesses different promoter regions that determine pituitary-specific and peripheral tissue–specific POMC expression, respectively. Ectopic ACTH/POMC transcripts are expressed in gonads, placenta, GI tissues, kidney, adrenal medulla, lung, and lymphocytes; POMC products also arise from peripheral neuroendocrine tumors.

Secretion ACTH synthesis and release are stimulated by CRH. In addition, ACTH release is induced by vasopressin, cytokines, physical stress, exercise, acute illness, and hypoglycemia.

ACTH secretion is pulsatile and follows a circadian rhythm that is highest in early morning and declines at night. This rhythm is paralleled by a diurnal pattern of adrenal glucocorticoid secretion. ACTH levels peak at 6 A.M., with values ranging from 8 to 25 pg/ml; peak values are approximately fourfold higher than the nadir levels measured between 11 P.M. and 3 A.M. Glucocorticoids suppress CRH and ACTH release. The loss of cortisol inhibition that occurs with primary adrenal failure results in extremely high compensatory ACTH levels.

Actions

The hypothalamic-pituitary-adrenal (HPA) axis maintains metabolic homeostasis and mediates the neuroendocrine stress response. The pituitary affects the pattern and quantity of adrenal cortisol secretion by integrating peripheral and central signals. The neuroendocrine stress response reflects the net result of sensitively integrated hypothalamic, intrapituitary, and peripheral hormone and cytokine signals, resulting in cortisol production. The HPA axis is triggered by acute inflammatory or septic insults that mediate release of inflammatory cytokines, bacterial toxins, and neural signals. ACTH stimulates steroidogenesis by maintaining adrenal cell proliferation and function. Cortisol elevation curtails the inflammatory response and provides host protection.

Pro-opiomelanocortin peptides and appetite control Several lines of experimental and clinical evidence implicate the POMC system in appetite control. The melanocortin receptor family comprises important regulators of central appetite control. Inactivation of MC-2 receptors leads to obesity, hypoadrenalism, and red hair pigmentation. Disruption of MC4 receptors is associated with childhood obesity and elevations in the level of circulating leptins; disruption is also genetically linked to the POMC gene locus [see Chapter 58].

HPA Axis Testing

Insulin-induced hypoglycemia and cortisol levels Intravenous administration of insulin (0.05 to 0.3 U/kg) lowers blood glucose levels to 50% of baseline within 30 minutes. This evokes plasma cortisol increases of 7 mg/dl or greater; peak cortisol levels of at least 20 µg/dl are evoked within 30 to 45 minutes of nadir blood glucose levels and indicate intact pituitary ACTH reserve production.

Metyrapone The pituitary response to a decrease in the serum cortisol level can be assessed with metyrapone testing. A 3 g oral dose of metyrapone administered at 11 P.M. with a snack blocks conversion of the cortisol precursor 11-deoxycortisol (compound S) to cortisol. The resulting fall in serum cortisol level normally stimulates ACTH secretion, raising the compound S level to above 8 µg/dl at 8 A.M. the next morning. Cortisol inhibition by metyrapone can be confirmed by finding that the plasma cortisol level is less than 5 µg/dl.

Synthetic ACTH Injection of synthetic ACTH (Cortrosyn) at a dose of 250 µg intravenously or intramuscularly evokes adrenal cortisol reserve after 30 and 60 minutes. Cortisol levels should rise to at least twice the baseline value, rise at least 7 µg/dl, or peak at above 20 µg/dl; any one of those three reactions indicates normal reserve. Blunted cortisol responses to ACTH reflect compromised pituitary ACTH reserve, primary adrenal failure, or steroid ingestion.

CRH Intravenous CRH, 1 µg/kg, directly stimulates ACTH secretion during the 60 minutes after injection. Pituitary damage prevents an evoked response. Patients with Cushing disease associated with an ACTH-secreting corticotroph cell adenoma often have exaggerated ACTH responses to CRH. CRH injection does not stimulate a further rise in ACTH secretion by ectopic ACTH-secreting tumors.

ACTH Deficiency

Diagnosis Clinically, pituitary ACTH deficiency results in secondary hypocortisolism with tiredness, weakness, anorexia, nausea, and vomiting; occasionally, hypoglycemia results from diminished counterregulation of insulin. Stressful acute illness may unmask the presence of partial ACTH deficiency and cause life-threatening hypocortisolism.

On laboratory testing, ACTH deficiency is characterized by inappropriately low ACTH levels in conjunction with low cortisol levels. Low basal serum cortisol levels or blunted cortisol responses to provocative ACTH stimulation reflect diminished adrenal reserve caused by prolonged insufficient ACTH tropic action on the adrenal cortex.

Treatment Hydrocortisone replacement reverses most clinical and biochemical features of cortisol deficiency. Hydrocortisone is given two or three times daily. The total daily dose should usually not exceed 20 mg. Doses should be increased severalfold during periods of acute illness or stress.

ACTH-Secreting Adenoma (Cushing Disease)

ACTH-producing adenomas account for about 10% to 15% of all pituitary adenomas and are usually well-differentiated microadenomas. Cushing syndrome is also caused by ectopic ACTH production by tumors, including small-cell lung carcinomas and bronchial and thymic carcinoids. In contrast to ACTH secretion by pituitary tumors, which can be suppressed by high-dose glucocorticoids, ectopic ACTH secretion by neoplasms is usually not suppressible, a fact that highlights the unrestrained malignant gene expression.

Diagnosis Unrestrained ACTH secretion causes hypercortisolemia, which results in thin, brittle skin; central obesity; hypertension; plethoric moon facies; purple striae and susceptibility to bruising; glucose intolerance or diabetes; gonadal dysfunction; osteoporosis; proximal muscle weakness; acne; hirsutism; and labile depression, mania, or psychosis [see Table 9]. Leukocytosis, lymphopenia, and eosinopenia also may develop. In young women, osteoporosis may be particularly prominent. Cardiovascular disease is the primary cause of death.

The differential diagnosis of ACTH-secreting pituitary tumor includes other causes of hypercortisolism: iatrogenic glucocorticoid administration, ectopic ACTH-secreting tumor, and cortisol-secreting adrenal tumor. In ectopic Cushing syndrome, manifestations usually develop acutely: patients present with

Table 9 Clinical Features of Cushing Syndrome[40]

Symptoms and Signs	Frequency (%)
Obesity or weight gain (>115% ideal body weight)	80
Thin skin	80
Moon facies	75
Hypertension	75
Purple skin striae	65
Hirsutism	65
Abnormal glucose tolerance	55
Impotence	55
Menstrual disorders (usually amenorrhea)	60
Proximal muscle weakness	50
Truncal obesity	50
Acne	45
Bruising	45
Mental changes	45
Osteoporosis	40
Edema of lower extremities	30
Hyperpigmentation	20
Hypokalemic alkalosis	15
Diabetes	15

Note: manifestations seen in patients of all ages.

florid skin hyperpigmentation, severe myopathy, hypertension, hypokalemic alkalosis, glucose intolerance, and edema. Serum potassium levels are below 3.3 mmol/L in most patients with ectopic ACTH secretion.

The diagnosis of pituitary Cushing disease requires documentation of hypercortisolism in the presence of pituitary-derived ACTH elevation. Reproducible markers for hypercortisolism include the failure to experience suppression of the cortisol level after a dose of dexamethasone and an elevation in 24-hour urinary free cortisol level. Urinary cortisol levels greater than 300 µg/day indicate the presence of Cushing syndrome. Urinary 17-hydroxysteroid levels reflect secretion of cortisol metabolites.

In general, ACTH-secreting pituitary tumors retain feedback responsiveness to circulating glucocorticoids. Basal ACTH levels are usually about eightfold higher in patients with ectopic ACTH secretion, but considerable overlap with pituitary adenoma–derived ACTH may preclude an accurate biochemical distinction of the two disorders. In patients with endogenous (adrenal) or exogenous (iatrogenic) Cushing syndrome, ACTH levels are suppressed. Elevated concentrations of circulating ACTH and cortisol measured at midnight usually indicate the presence of Cushing syndrome.

Dynamic testing should be undertaken when hypercortisolemia has been rigorously documented.[25] Dexamethasone suppression of ACTH and ultimately of cortisol levels is the standard test for diagnosis of ACTH-dependent Cushing disease. Ingestion of 1 mg oral dexamethasone at 11 P.M. should result in suppression of serum cortisol levels to below 7 µg/dl at 8 A.M. the next morning, unless obesity, chronic depression, or alcoholism is present. In patients with ACTH-secreting pituitary adenomas or ectopic tumors, overnight dexamethasone does not suppress plasma ACTH or serum cortisol levels, and longer-term dexamethasone suppression testing is required. Baseline pretesting of 24-hour urinary free cortisol and 17-ketosteroids or 17-hydroxysteroid values is followed by administration of low-dose dexamethasone (0.5 mg every 6 hours) for 2

days. Plasma ACTH, serum cortisol, and 24-hour urinary free cortisol levels remain elevated in patients with Cushing disease. High-dose dexamethasone (2 mg every 6 hours) for the subsequent 2 days will usually suppress 17-hydroxysteroid levels by 50% or less and suppress urinary free cortisol to less than 90% of baseline in patients with pituitary ACTH-secreting tumors, but this result will be seen in only 10% of those patients with ectopic ACTH secretion.

MRI scanning is indicated for patients with documented hypercortisolemia and nonsuppressed ACTH levels. If a pituitary mass is clearly visible on MRI, transsphenoidal surgical resection should be undertaken after rigorous biochemical confirmation of pituitary-derived ACTH hypersecretion. However, most ACTH-secreting tumors are less than 5 mm in diameter; about half are less than 2 mm in diameter, and so are undetectable even by sensitive MRI. Therefore, MRI has only limited ability to visualize ACTH-secreting pituitary tumors. Bilateral inferior petrosal sinus ACTH sampling before and after CRH administration may distinguish pituitary from ectopic ACTH hypersecretion.[26] Because most ectopic ACTH-secreting tumors are located in the chest or abdomen, imaging studies of those areas are indicated for diagnosis. The diagnosis of ectopic ACTH secretion is ultimately confirmed by four measures: (1) rigorous exclusion of a pituitary lesion; (2) demonstration of an arteriovenous ACTH gradient over the tumor bed; (3) resolution of hypercortisolism with excision of the tumor; and (4) confirmation of *POMC* gene expression in excised tumor tissue.

Adrenal imaging is indicated when suppressed ACTH levels point to an adrenal origin of hypercorticolism. Bilateral adrenal hyperplasia with cortical thickening usually indicates tropic effects of ACTH hypersecretion. Adrenal adenomas causing Cushing syndrome are usually clearly visible, and adrenal carcinomas are larger than adenomas (> 2 cm). The contralateral gland may be normal or atrophic. Adrenal nodularity may occur unilaterally or bilaterally, with approximately 50% of glands appearing normal [*see Chapter 55*].

Treatment Selective transsphenoidal resection after careful preoperative localization is the preferred treatment for ACTH-secreting pituitary adenomas.[27] Remission rates are about 80% for microadenomas but less than 50% for the less common ACTH-secreting macroadenomas. After successful surgery, patients may experience a period of compensatory adrenal insufficiency for up to 6 months and may require low-dose cortisol replacement during that time. Within 5 years of the operation, approximately 5% of patients in whom surgery was initially successful will experience biochemical recurrence.

Patients with ACTH hypersecretion that is not controlled by surgery require pituitary irradiation. Cortisol-lowering agents (i.e., mitotane, ketoconazole, or aminoglutethimide) are administered after irradiation to achieve earlier biochemical remission. Rarely, all these measures fail, and bilateral adrenalectomy is required.

FOLLICLE-STIMULATING HORMONE AND LUTEINIZING HORMONE

Synthesis

Gonadotroph cells comprise up to 10% of anterior pituitary cells. The gonadotropins FSH and LH (along with TSH and human chorionic gonadotropin) are glycoprotein hormones comprising a common α and a specific β subunit. Gonadotroph cells exhibit cytoplasmic immunostaining for both FSH and LH β subunits, as well as for the common α subunit. Primary gonadal failure, resulting from gonadal damage, is associated with hyperplastic gonadotroph cells with accumulation of hormone secretory granules, reflecting loss of negative feedback by peripheral sex steroids.

Hypothalamic gonadotropin-releasing hormone (GnRH) regulates both LH and FSH secretion. GnRH, under positive feedback control by peripheral estrogens, is secreted in a pulsatile fashion every 60 to 120 minutes; it regulates the complex reproductive cycles. Activins also induce gonadotropins, whereas inhibins suppress their secretion.

ACTIONS

Gonadotropins interact with their respective cell surface receptors on the ovary and testis, thereby controlling the development and maturation of germ cells and the synthesis of steroid hormones. In women, LH mediates ovulation and the maintenance of the corpus luteum, and FSH mediates ovarian follicle development and induces ovarian estrogen production. In men, LH induces testosterone secretion by the Leydig cells, and FSH regulates seminiferous tubule development and stimulates spermatogenesis.

Gonadotropin Deficiency

Gonadotropin secretion is sensitive to pituitary damage, and hypogonadism is the most common presenting feature of adult hypopituitarism. Congenital or acquired central hypogonadotropic hypogonadism results from a pituitary or hypothalamic disorder that disrupts GnRH availability. Hypothalamic defects causing hypogonadism include Kallmann syndrome and a mutation in the *DAX-1* gene that is associated with deficient GnRH and pituitary gonadotropin synthesis. Inactivating mutations in the LH and FSH β-subunit gene cause hypogonadism by disrupting gonadotropin formation and function.

Diagnosis Clinical features of hypogonadism depend on the age at onset of the disorder. Primary amenorrhea, immature internal and external genitalia, absent secondary sex characteristics, and eunuchoidal body proportions occur in adolescent girls. In premenopausal women, decreased ovarian function presents as oligomenorrhea or amenorrhea, infertility, decreased vaginal secretions, decreased libido, breast atrophy, and hot flushes. The onset of hypogonadotropism during male adolescence results in sexual infantilism, with a smooth scrotum and small penis, diminished or absent postpubertal sex drive, absent secondary sexual characteracteristics, central obesity, eunuchoid proportions, delayed epiphyseal closure, and a characteristic high-pitched prepubertal voice. In men, testicular failure is associated with decreased libido and potency, infertility, decreased muscle mass with weakness, attenuated beard and body hair growth, soft testes, and fine facial wrinkles [*see Chapter 56*]. Prolonged hypogonadism results in osteoporosis in both females and males.

Central hypogonadism is diagnosed by a finding of low-normal or low serum gonadotropin levels and low sex hormone concentrations (testosterone in males, estradiol in females). Male patients have abnormal results on semen analysis. Normal values for circulating FSH and LH in menstruating women are 4 to 20 mIU/ml, depending on the menstrual phase; levels rise considerably with menopause. FSH and LH levels in men are 1 to 12 mIU/ml. Normal total testosterone levels in men are above 280 ng/100 ml; the serum testosterone concentration

should be measured at about 8 A.M., when it is at its peak [*see Chapter 56*]. In women, circulating estradiol levels vary with the menstrual cycle.

Pituitary gonadotropin deficiency can sometimes be confirmed with GnRH stimulation testing. Gonadotrophs are stimulated by intravenous injection of 100 μg GnRH; evoked LH levels peak within 30 minutes, and FSH plateaus during the subsequent 60 minutes. Normal responses vary with the age and sex of the subject and, in women, the menstrual cycle stage. However, a robust gonadotropin response does not necessarily exclude pituitary gonadotroph damage, and the absence of a response does not reliably distinguish pituitary from hypothalamic causes of hypogonadism. In patients with documented central hypogonadism, pituitary MRI and pituitary function testing are required.

Treatment In premenopausal women, estrogen and progesterone replacement therapy results in the maintaining of secondary sexual characteristics and genitourinary tract integrity; in addition, it prevents osteoporosis. Gonadotropin therapy is used for ovulation induction. Pulsatile GnRH is effective for treating hypothalamic hypogonadism. In women who exercise vigorously and maintain a low body mass index (e.g., athletes and ballet dancers), caloric replacement may restore menses. In males, testosterone replacement therapy will result in the attaining and maintaining of growth and development of the external genitalia and secondary sexual characteristics, and patients will maintain libido, muscle mass, and bone density [*see Chapter 56*].

Nonfunctioning Pituitary Adenomas

So-called nonsecreting adenomas arising from gonadotroph cells are the most common pituitary adenomas. Because these adenomas are clinically nonfunctional, they usually produce no distinct hypersecretory syndrome.[28] Some adenomas express gonadotropin α-subunits but not intact FSH or LH molecules, and administration of thyrotropin-releasing hormone (TRH) may inappropriately evoke gonadotropins or subunit secretion. Clinically inactive, asymptomatic pituitary microadenomas are commonly encountered as incidental findings on MRI; these are termed pituitary incidentalomas.

Diagnosis Nonsecreting adenomas may be incidentally discovered on an MRI performed for another indication. Mass effects, including optic chiasm pressure and other neurologic symptoms, are the usual initial presenting symptoms of large tumors. Gradual onset of visual defects with progressive bitemporal field defects, scotoma, or impaired acuity may occur. Compression of surrounding pituitary tissue by an adenoma may disrupt gonadotropin secretion, resulting in hypogonadism. Amenorrhea and infertility occur in women, whereas men present with progressively decreased potency and low testosterone levels. Rarely, excess FSH or LH secretion results in ovarian hyperstimulation or the downregulation of the reproductive axis.

On laboratory testing, circulating gonadotropin α-subunit levels are elevated in about 15% of male patients. TRH administration evokes LH β-subunit levels in most patients of both sexes. The serum prolactin level should be measured: an elevation suggests a prolactinoma; a PRL level below 100 μg/L in a hypogonadal patient harboring a pituitary mass suggests pituitary stalk compression by a nonfunctioning adenoma. In postmenopausal women, physiologic elevations of FSH concentrations may be difficult to distinguish from tumor-derived FSH elevations. Primary ovarian or testicular failure may lead to compensatory gonadotroph cell hyperplasia and uniformly elevated LH and FSH levels.

Treatment Nonfunctioning microadenomas have a benign natural history. They are slow-growing and can safely be followed with annual imaging and visual testing, as long as the patient remains asymptomatic. Nonfunctioning pituitary masses greater than 1 cm in diameter should be resected. These larger masses should be distinguished from nonadenomatous lesions by MRI characteristics and histologic evaluation of resected tissue.[29] After resection, the tissue diagnosis of a clinically nonsecreting gonadotroph adenoma should be confirmed.[30] Visual improvement occurs in 70% of patients with preoperative visual field defects. Hypopituitarism resulting from compression of normal pituitary tissue improves and may resolve completely. Early complications of surgery include diabetes insipidus, inappropriate antidiuretic hormone secretion, or both. Approximately 15% of tumors recur within 5 to 6 years after initially successful surgical resection.[31] Adjuvant pituitary radiotherapy after transsphenoidal surgery has been advocated to prevent future tumor regrowth in patients with residual adenoma tissue.[32]

THYROID-STIMULATING HORMONE

Synthesis

TSH-secreting thyrotroph cells constitute 5% of the anterior pituitary cell population. Hypothalamic TRH stimulates TSH synthesis and secretion. TRH also stimulates lactotroph cells to secrete PRL. Thyroid hormones, dopamine, SRIF, and glucocorticoids suppress TSH and override TRH induction. Thyroid damage, including surgical thyroidectomy, radiation-induced hypothyroidism, chronic thyroiditis, or prolonged goitrogen exposure are associated with reversible thyrotroph hypertrophy and hyperplasia with prominent TSH secretory granules and sellar enlargement. Thyrotroph cells regress with thyroid hormone treatment and hormone-mediated TSH suppression.

TSH Deficiency

Hypothyroidism from TSH deficiency has the same clinical features as primary hypothyroidism [*see Chapter 50*]. On thyroid function testing, however, patients with pituitary hypothyroidism have low levels of both TSH and thyroxine (T_4). Patients with hypothyroidism of hypothalamic origin have normal, low, or slightly elevated TSH levels and low T_4 values.

Testing of TSH reserve is used to confirm the diagnosis of central hypothyroidism. Twofold to threefold increases in TSH levels occur within 30 minutes of an intravenous injection of TRH (200 µg) in normal patients. Primary hypothyroidism is associated with an exaggerated TSH response to TRH because of release of the thyrotroph from negative feedback inhibition. Hyperthyroidism, exogenously administered thyroid hormone, and pituitary damage result in blunted TSH responses to TRH.

Thyrotropin-Secreting Adenomas

TSH-producing pituitary adenomas are very rare. Patients with these tumors usually present with a goiter and mild or frank hyperthyroidism.[33] The diagnosis is made by demonstrating elevated serum T_4 levels, inappropriately high TSH or α-subunit secretion, and evidence of a pituitary adenoma on MRI. These tumors are usually large and locally invasive. Adminis-

tration of thyroid hormone fails to suppress TSH secretion, wheras administration of TRH evokes a blunted TSH response. In such cases, it is important to exclude thyroid hormone resistance, which can produce abnormalities in TSH and T_4 levels identical to those seen with TSH-producing adenomas.

Treatment TSH-producing pituitary adenomas are debulked surgically. Total resection is often not achieved because most of these tumors are large and locally invasive. Postoperative treatment with a somatostatin analogue controls residual TSH and α-subunit hypersecretion, shrinks the tumor mass in approximately 50% of patients, and improves visual fields in about 75% of patients.

Posterior Pituitary Hormones and Associated Disorders

Vasopressin and oxytocin are stored in the posterior pituitary and released in response to appropriate stimuli. Serum vasopressin levels (and, thus, urinary concentrations) vary in response to changes in serum osmolality. The sensitivity and, to a lesser extent, the threshold of vasopressin response to a change in tonicity show considerable variability from one person to another; at least part of this variation is hereditary. Chronic heart failure lowers the osmotic threshold for vasopressin release, whereas aging and other factors reduce sensitivity of vasopressin release (i.e., the rate of vasopressin release per unit change in osmolality). Shifts in blood volume and pressure of greater than 10% affect vasopressin release significantly. Hypotension and hypovolemia stimulate vasopressin release by lowering the osmotic threshold; hypertension and hypervolemia inhibit release by raising the threshold. These influences are mediated by baroreceptor pathways that have left atrial afferents.

Nausea, but not vomiting, is a powerful stimulus to vasopressin release; it raises the serum vasopressin up to 1,000 times the level required for maximal antidiuresis. Pain, however, is not an important stimulant of vasopressin release. Many neural pathways influence vasopressin release in response to nonosmotic stimuli. In general, alpha-adrenergic pathways stimulate and beta-adrenergic pathways inhibit vasopressin release.

The principal disorders of vasopressin secretion consist of partial or complete deficiency (diabetes insipidus) and the syndrome of inappropriate antidiuretic hormone (SIADH) excess [*see Chapter 162*].

DIABETES INSIPIDUS

Polyuria is a common clinical problem. A patient passing large quantities of urine generally has one of three abnormalities: an osmotic diuresis (e.g., from glycosuria), resistance to vasopressin, or deficient vasopressin secretion. Resistance to vasopressin (i.e., nephrogenic diabetes insipidus) is discussed elsewhere [*see Chapter 162*]. Deficiency of vasopressin (i.e., neurogenic diabetes insipidus) reflects either functional or structural disease of the supraoptic hypothalamic neurons that secrete the hormone. Brain tumors, craniopharyngiomas, metastatic cancer, hypothalamic-pituitary surgery or trauma, pituitary stalk damage, histiocytosis, and lymphocytic hypophysitis are the conditions that account for most cases of vasopressin deficiency. Rare familial polyuric syndromes may also present as hypothalamic diabetes insipidus.

Diagnosis

Two clinical clues suggest vasopressin deficiency: sudden

onset of polyuria and a preference for iced beverages. However, neurogenic diabetes insipidus must be distinguished from primary polydipsia, because overdrinking also results in polyuria and suppressed vasopressin secretion.

Neurogenic and nephrogenic diabetes insipidus can usually be differentiated by means of clinical testing. After confirmation that the blood glucose level is normal, the patient is deprived of water until 3% to 5% of body weight is lost and the serum tonicity is higher than 295 mOsm/kg. If polyuria disappears and the urine concentration rises above 500 mOsm/kg, vasopressin secretion is adequate. If polyuria and dilute urine (< 300 mOsm/kg) persist, then 20 mg desmopressin acetate (DDAVP), a synthetic vasopressin analogue, is given intranasally; alternatively, 300 µU of DDAVP can be administered intravenously. If urine flow decreases and urine concentration rises, vasopressin deficiency can be inferred. If, however, the serum becomes concentrated and the urine remains dilute despite administration of DDAVP, the patient has nephrogenic diabetes insipidus.

Some cautions should be kept in mind when conducting dehydration tests. First, the term partial diabetes insipidus describes a patient who, when deprived of water, achieves a urine concentration greater than the serum osmolality but less than that obtained after administration of vasopressin. Functional testing can be misleading in patients with neurogenic or nephrogenic partial diabetes insipidus. In such patients, who have a urine concentration between 300 and 500 mOsm/kg, measurement of the serum vasopressin level can be extremely helpful. A high vasopressin level in the presence of concentrated serum and relatively dilute urine points to nephrogenic diabetes insipidus; a low value points to hormone deficiency. Conversely, partial resistance to vasopressin can result from chronic overdrinking, with secondary dilution of the medullary concentration in the kidney. If such patients control their excess water intake, they recover a normal renal medullary concentration and, at the same rate, a normal response to vasopressin. Finally, water deprivation appears to produce less thirst in older men than in younger men. Men older than 80 years must be watched carefully after testing to ensure that they resume appropriate water intake.

Granulomas, trauma, infection, and other infiltrations can all produce diabetes insipidus. Metastatic tumor seldom produces insufficiency in other endocrine glands, but secondary tumors arising from lung, breast, and other organs can all produce insufficiency in the posterior pituitary. The sensitivity of MRI has considerably refined the approach to the diagnosis of diabetes insipidus.

Diabetes insipidus can develop suddenly after neurosurgery or external trauma. Cases that develop after neurosurgery may be marked by a triphasic sequence of vasopressin deficiency, vasopressin excess, and vasopressin deficiency. In postoperative or posttraumatic diabetes insipidus, a dilute polyuria with a serum sodium level greater than 145 mEq/L allows a presumptive diagnosis, and parenteral DDAVP should be given immediately. Conversely, hyponatremia from increased vasopressin secretion after transsphenoidal surgery should also be anticipated by following serum sodium levels. Explosive and fatal central diabetes mellitus and diabetes insipidus have been reported in young women with postoperative hyponatremia that was not aggressively treated. The pathogenesis of the disorder is not understood, but the pathologic sequence included cerebral edema and herniation, compression of the third cranial nerve, hypoxic infarction of the pituitary and hypothalamus, respiratory arrest, and coma. The rapidity of deterioration in these patients indicates that the hyponatremia in such cases should be promptly corrected, even though fixed pupillary dilatation, secondary to compression of the oculomotor nerve, may suggest brain death.

Treatment

There are several approaches to the treatment of diabetes insipidus. If the polyuria is mild and does not interfere with sleep, no treatment may be needed. Chlorpropamide potentiates the effect of vasopressin on renal concentrating ability and can be used to treat partial diabetes insipidus. It is given in a dosage of 250 to 375 mg once a day and usually does not produce hypoglycemia in normal persons. However, if patients do not eat regularly or if they have unsuspected anterior pituitary insufficiency, chlorpropamide can be hazardous.

For patients with severe diabetes insipidus, intranasal or oral DDAVP provides excellent control of polyuria and polydipsia. Intranasal DDAVP is effective, nontoxic, and nonirritating. Tablets of DDAVP are given in a dose of 0.1 or 0.2 mg, taken one to three times daily. All patients with diabetes insipidus should be warned that in circumstances of extreme water loss or unconsciousness, they are exposed to added risk unless they are under the care of a physician who is aware of the diagnosis.

Pituitary Failure

Attenuated pituitary secretory reserve can develop as a result of impingement and compression of an expanding mass on adjacent functioning pituitary cells or because of acquired or inherited pituitary cell damage.[34] Tropic hormone failure associated with pituitary compression or destruction usually occurs sequentially, with GH; then FSH, LH, and TSH; and finally ACTH. In childhood, growth retardation is often the presenting feature; in adults, hypogonadism is the earliest symptom. Pressure effects may impair synthesis or secretion of hypothalamic hormones, with pituitary failure [see Table 10].

DEVELOPMENTAL PITUITARY DYSFUNCTION

Developmental pituitary dysfunction occurs with aplastic, hypoplastic, or ectopic pituitary gland development. Midline craniofacial disorders may be associated with structural pituitary dysplasia. Birth trauma—including cranial hemorrhage, asphyxia, and breech delivery—can cause acquired pituitary failure in the newborn.

Transcription Factor Mutations

Tissue-specific transcription factors, including Pit-1 and PROP-1, determine tissue-specific development and expression of pituitary hormones and are critical for maintaining anterior pituitary cell function. Hereditary transcription factor mutations may result in disruption of pituitary function, which may manifest during infancy, childhood, puberty, or early adulthood. Autosomal dominant or recessive Pit-1 mutations result in combined deficiency of GH, PRL, and TSH. Pituitary imaging may reveal a normal or hypoplastic gland. PROP-1 is an early transcription factor that appears to be necessary for Pit-1 function. PROP-1 mutations result in combined deficiency of GH, TSH, gonadotropins, and sometimes ACTH. Most afflicted patients have growth retardation and do not enter puberty spontaneously. By adulthood, most patients are deficient in TSH and gonadotropins, and some have an enlarged pituitary gland. T-Pit mutations result in isolated ACTH deficiency.

Dysgenesis of the septum pellucidum or corpus callosum

Table 10 Causes of Pituitary Failure[39]

Development/ structural	Transcription factor defect Pituitary dysplasia/aplasia Congenital central nervous system masses, encephalocele Primary empty sella Congenital hypothalamic disorders (e.g., septo-optic dysplasia, Prader-Willi syndrome, Laurence-Moon-Biedl syndrome, Kallmann syndrome)
Traumatic	Surgical resection Radiation damage Accidental
Neoplastic	Pituitary adenoma Parasellar mass (meningioma, germinoma, ependymoma, glioma) Rathke cyst Craniopharyngioma Hypothalamic hamartoma, gangliocytoma Pituitary metastases Lymphoma and leukemia Meningioma
Infiltrative/ inflammatory	Lymphocytic hypophysitis Sarcoidosis Histiocytosis X Hemachromatosis Granulomatous hypophysitis
Vascular	Pituitary apoplexy Pregnancy-related infarction Sickle cell disease Arteritis
Infections	Fungal (histoplasmosis) Parasitic (toxoplasmosis) Tuberculosis *Pneumocystis carinii*

may lead to hypothalamic dysfunction and hypopituitarism, with manifestations that include diabetes insipidus, GH deficiency, and, occasionally, TSH deficiency. Affected children harbor a mutation in the *HESX-1* gene. Clinical features include cleft palate, syndactyly, ear deformities, and hypertelorism.

ACQUIRED PITUITARY FAILURE

Rarely, infiltration of the hypothalamus by diseases such as sarcoidosis, histiocytosis X, amyloidosis, or hemachromatosis may disrupt hypothalamic and pituitary function.[35] This hypothalamic infiltration may result in diabetes insipidus and, if GH attenuation occurs before pubertal bone closure, in growth retardation. Hypogonadotropic hypogonadism and, rarely, hyperprolactinemia occur with disrupted gonadotropin secretion. Pituitary damage may be directly caused by accidental or neurosurgical trauma; pituitary or hypothalamic neoplasms, including pituitary adenomas, craniopharyngioma, Rathke cysts, chordomas, or metastatic deposits; inflammatory disease, such as lymphocytic hypophysitis; or pituitary irradiation. Tuberculosis, opportunistic fungal infections associated with HIV infection, and tertiary syphilis may destroy pituitary tissue.

Cranial Irradiation

Cranial irradiation results in long-term compromise of hypothalamic and pituitary function. Children and adolescents who

have undergone therapeutic irradiation of the brain or head and neck are at especially high risk. The resulting hormonal abnormalities correlate strongly with radiation dosage, as well as the time elapsed since completion of radiotherapy. By 10 to 15 years after therapy, GH deficiency invariably occurs, whereas central hypogonadism and ACTH deficiency less commonly occur. Anterior pituitary function should be tested in previously irradiated patients, and replacement therapy instituted when required.

Lymphocytic Hypophysitis

Lymphocytic hypophysitis usually occurs in pregnant or postpartum women. It presents as hyperprolactinemia and a pituitary mass resembling an adenoma on MRI; PRL levels are often mildly elevated.[36] Transient pituitary failure and symptoms of progressive sellar compression, such as headache and visual disturbance, may occur, and the erythrocyte sedimentation rate may be elevated. Because its appearance on MRI may be indistinguishable from that of a pituitary adenoma, lymphocytic hypophysitis should be excluded in a postpartum woman with a newly diagnosed pituitary mass. Pituitary surgery is unnecessary in such cases: glucocorticoid treatment usually restores pituitary function within 6 months, and the mass invariably resolves.

Pituitary Apoplexy

Acute intrapituitary hemorrhage may result in catastrophic vascular compression of parasellar structures.[37] Hemorrhage may occur in a preexisting adenoma, often in association with diabetes or hypertension, or in the postpartum period (Sheehan syndrome). During pregnancy, swelling of the pituitary increases the risk of intrapituitary hemorrhage and infarction. Hypoglycemia, hypotension, shock, apoplexy, and death may follow. Severe headache with signs of meningeal irritation, visual loss, dynamically changing ophthalmoplegia, cardiovascular collapse, and loss of consciousness portend acutely progressive intrasellar bleeding. Pituitary imaging may reveal signs of intratumoral or sellar hemorrhage, with deviation of vital structures, including compression of noninvolved pituitary tissue. If vision is intact and consciousness is unimpaired, patients can be treated conservatively with observation and high-dose steroid infusions. Visual loss or decreased consciousness is an indication for urgent surgical decompression. Subsequent pituitary hormone replacement will be required for the inevitable pituitary damage.

Empty Sella Syndrome

Clinically silent pituitary mass infarction may result in development of a partially or totally empty sella. CSF fills the dural herniation. Pituitary function often remains intact, because the surrounding tissue is fully functional. Hypopituitarism may develop insidiously, however. A partially or apparently totally empty sella is usually an incidental MRI finding. Rarely, small functional pituitary adenomas may arise within the rim.

DIAGNOSIS

Pituitary failure is characterized by the clinical impact of single or multiple tropic hormone loss. Growth disorders and abnormal body composition result from GH loss in children and adults, respectively; menstrual disorders and infertility in women and decreased sexual function, infertility, and loss of secondary sexual characteristics in men are caused by gonadotropin deficits; hypothyroidism is caused by TSH loss; hypocortisolism with hypoglycemia is caused by ACTH loss; and failed lactation is caused by PRL loss. Polyuria and poly-

Table 11 Replacement Therapy for Hypopituitarism in Adults

Tropic Hormone Deficit	Hormone Replacement
ACTH	Hydrocortisone, 10–15 mg q. A.M., 5 mg q. P.M. Cortisone acetate, 25 mg q. A.M., 12.5 mg q. P.M.
TSH	Levothyroxine, 0.075–0.15 mg daily

FSH/LH	Males
	  Testosterone enanthate, 200 mg I.M. q. 2 wk
	  Testosterone skin patch, 5–7.5 mg/day
	Females
	  Conjugated estrogen, 0.65–1.25 mg daily for 25 days
	  Ethinyl estradiol, 0.02–0.05 mg
	  Progesterone on days 16–25 to facilitate uterine shedding
	  Estradiol skin patch, 4–8 mg, twice weekly

GH	Somatotropin, 0.15–1.0 mg S.C. daily

Vasopressin	Desmopressin
	  Intranasal: 5–20 µg, b.i.d.
	  Oral: 300–600 µg, q.d.

Note: Doses should be individualized and should be reassessed during stress, surgery, or pregnancy. Treatment for infertility (gonadotropins or gonadotropin-releasing hormone) should be individualized.
ACTH—adrenocorticotropic hormone   FSH—follicle-stimulating hormone
GH—growth hormone   LH—luteinizing hormone   TSH—thyroid-stimulating hormone

dipsia reflect loss of ADH secretion. These features may occur selectively or may be sequential and ultimately result in panhypopituitarism. Enhanced mortality in patients with long-standing pituitary damage is caused mainly by increased cardiovascular and cerebrovascular disease.[38]

On laboratory tests, patients with pituitary insufficiency demonstrate lack of normal hormonal feedback responses, with low tropic hormone levels in conjunction with low target hormone concentrations. Provocative tests confirm lack of pituitary hormone reserve.

TREATMENT

Replacement of pituitary hormones or their respective target hormones usually results in clinical homeostasis with few side effects [*see Table 11*]. Hormone replacement therapy for pituitary failure includes glucocorticoids, thyroid hormone, sex steroids, GH, and vasopressin. Rational replacement regimens ensure a normal and safe quality of life. Patients receiving glucocorticoid replacement require dose increases during stressful events, including dental procedures, trauma, and hospitalizations for acute illness.

The author has received research support and been a scientific consultant for Eli Lilly and Co. and Novartis Pharmaceuticals Corp. for the past 12 months.

References

1. Prezant TR, Melmed S: Molecular pathogenesis of pituitary disorders. Curr Opin Endocrinol Diabetes 9:61, 2002
2. Faglia G, Spada A: Genesis of pituitary adenomas: state of the art. J Neurooncol 54:95, 2001
3. Goffin V, Binart N, Touraine P, et al: Prolactin: the new biology of an old hormone. Annu Rev Physiol 64:47, 2002
4. Verhelst J, Abs R, Maiter D, et al: Cabergoline in the treatment of hyperprolactinemia: a study in 455 patients. J Clin Endocrinol Metab 84:2518, 1999
5. Losa M, Mortini P, Barzaghi R, et al: Surgical treatment of prolactin-secreting pituitary adenomas: early results and long-term outcome. J Clin Endocrinol Metab 87:3180, 2002
6. Colao A, di Sarno A, Pivonello R, et al: Dopamine receptor agonists for treating prolactinomas. Expert Opin Investig Drugs 11:787, 2002
7. Cunha SR, Mayo KE: Ghrelin and growth hormone (GH) secretagogues potentiate GH-releasing hormone (GHRH)-induced cyclic adenosine 3′,5′-monophosphate production in cells expressing transfected GHRH and GH secretagogue receptors. Endocrinology 143:4570, 2002
8. Giustina A, Veldhuis JD: Pathophysiology of the neuroregulation of growth hormone secretion in experimental animals and the human. Endocr Rev 19:717, 1998
9. Biller BM, Samuels MH, Zagar A, et al: Sensitivity and specificity of six tests for the diagnosis of adult GH deficiency. J Clin Endocrinol Metab 87:2067, 2002
10. Herrington J, Carter-Su C: Signaling pathways activated by the growth hormone receptor. Trends Endocrinol Metab 12:252, 2001
11. Colao A, Cuocolo A, Di Somma C, et al: Impaired cardiac performance in elderly patients with growth hormone deficiency. J Clin Endocrinol Metab 84:3950, 1999
12. Shalet SM, Toogood A, Rahim A, et al: The diagnosis of growth hormone deficiency in children and adults. Endocr Rev 19:203, 1998
13. Hartman ML, Crowe BJ, Biller BM, et al: Which patients do not require a GH stimulation test for the diagnosis of adult GH deficiency? J Clin Endocrinol Metab 87:477, 2002
14. Gibney J, Wallace JD, Spinks T, et al: The effects of 10 years of recombinant human growth hormone (GH) in adult GH-deficient patients. J Clin Endocrinol Metab 84:2596, 1999
15. Carroll PV, Christ ER, Sonksen PH: Growth hormone replacement in adults with growth hormone deficiency: assessment of current knowledge. Trends Endocrinol Metab 11:231, 2000
16. Attanasio AF, Bates PC, Ho KK, et al: Human growth hormone replacement in adult hypopituitary patients: long-term effects on body composition and lipid status—3-year results from the HypoCCS Database. J Clin Endocrinol Metab 87:1600, 2002
17. Friend KE: Acromegaly: a new therapy. Cancer Control 9:232, 2002
18. Melmed S, Casanueva FF, Cavagnini F, et al: Guidelines for acromegaly management. J Clin Endocrinol Metab 87:4054, 2002
19. Lamberts SW, Reubi JC, Krenning EP: Somatostatin analogs in the treatment of acromegaly. Endocrinol Metab Clin North Am 21:737, 1992
20. Colao A, Ferone D, Marzullo P, et al: Long-term effects of depot long-acting somatostatin analog octreotide on hormone levels and tumor mass in acromegaly. J Clin Endocrinol Metab 86:2779, 2001
21. Caron P, Beckers A, Cullen DR, et al: Efficacy of the new long-acting formulation of lanreotide (lanreotide Autogel) in the management of acromegaly. J Clin Endocrinol Metab 87:99, 2002
22. Davies PH, Stewart SE, Lancranjan L, et al: Long-term therapy with long-acting octreotide (Sandostatin-LAR) for the management of acromegaly. Clin Endocrinol (Oxf) 48:311, 1998
23. Chon BH, Loeffler JS: Efficacy and risk for radiotherapy for pituitary tumors. Endocrinologist 12:525, 2002
24. Melmed S, Jackson I, Kleinberg D, et al: Current treatment guidelines for acromegaly. J Clin Endocrinol Metab 83:2646, 2002
25. Ruff H, Kindling F: A physiologic approach to diagnosis of the Cushing syndrome. Ann Intern Med 138:980, 2003
26. Nieman LK: Diagnostic tests for Cushing's syndrome. Ann N Y Acad Sci 970:112, 2002
27. Swearingen B, Biller BM, Barker FG II, et al: Long-term mortality after transsphenoidal surgery for Cushing disease. Ann Intern Med 130:821, 1999
28. Greenman Y, Melmed S: Diagnosis and management of nonfunctioning pituitary tumors. Annu Rev Med 47:95, 1996
29. King JT Jr, Justice AC, Aron DC: Management of incidental pituitary microadenomas: a cost-effectiveness analysis. J Clin Endocrinol Metab 82:3625, 1997
30. Wilson CB: Surgical management of pituitary tumors. J Clin Endocrinol Metab 82:2381, 1997
31. Cappabianca P, Cavallo LM, Colao A: Surgical complications associated with the endoscopic endonasal transsphenoidal approach for pituitary adenomas. J Neurosurg 97:293, 2002
32. Gittoes NJ, Bates AS, Tse W, et al: Radiotherapy for non-function pituitary tumours. Clin Endocrinol (Oxf) 48:331, 1998
33. Beck-Peccoz P, Brucker-Davis F, Persani L, et al: Thyrotropin-secreting pituitary tumors. Endocr Rev 17:610, 1996
34. Vance ML: Hypopituitarism. N Engl J Med 330:1651, 1994
35. Saeger W: Tumor-like lesions of the pituitary and sellar region. Endocrinologist 12:300, 2002
36. Cheung CC, Ezzat S, Smyth HS, et al: The spectrum and significance of primary hypophysitis. J Clin Endocrinol Metab 86:1048, 2001
37. Randeva HS, Schoebel J, Byrne J, et al: Classical pituitary apoplexy: clinical features, management and outcome. Clin Endocrinol (Oxf) 51:181, 1999
38. Association between premature mortality and hypopituitarism. West Midlands Prospective Hypopituitary Study Group. Lancet 357:425, 2001
39. Tolis G: Prolactin: physiology and pathology. Hosp Pract 15:85, 1980
40. Melmed S: Disorders of the anterior pituitary and hypothalamus. Harrison's Textbook of Medicine, 15th ed, Braunwald E, Fauci AS, Kasper DL, et al, Eds. McGraw-Hill, New York, 2001, p 2029

Acknowledgment

Figures 1 and 2   Alice Y. Chen.

50 Thyroid

Paul W. Ladenson, M.D., F.A.C.P.

Thyroid disorders are the most common endocrine conditions encountered in clinical practice. Persons of either sex and any age can be affected, although almost all forms of thyroid disease are more frequent in women than in men, and many thyroid ailments increase in frequency with age. The presentation of thyroid conditions can range from clinically obvious to clinically silent. Their consequences can be widespread and serious, even life-threatening. With proper testing, the diagnosis and differential diagnosis can be established with certainty, and effective treatments can be instituted for almost all patients.

Definitions

States of thyroid dysfunction include hypothyroidism and thyrotoxicosis, both of which have ubiquitous metabolic and organ-specific consequences that result in a wide variety of clinical presentations and complications. Thyrotoxicosis is sometimes referred to as hyperthyroidism, but the latter term is more properly limited to forms of thyrotoxicosis in which there is an overproduction of thyroid hormones by the gland.

Both categories of thyroid dysfunction are further classified as overt or mild. In overt thyroid dysfunction, the concentrations of thyrotropin (thyroid-stimulating hormone [TSH]) and one or both thyroid hormones are outside of their normal ranges. In mild thyroid dysfunction, the serum TSH level is abnormal, but the serum thyroid hormone concentrations remain within their reference ranges. Although the terms clinical and subclinical are often used in reference to overt and mild thyroid dysfunction, respectively, these states are actually defined on the basis of biochemical criteria, not of clinical manifestations.

Epidemiology

In the third National Health and Nutrition Survey (NHANES III), thyroid function tests were assessed in a group of 17,353 persons 12 years of age or older whose makeup reflected the geographic and ethnic diversity of the United States population.[1] Hypothyroidism was identified in 4.6% (0.3% overt and 4.3% mild), and thyrotoxicosis was found in 1.3% (0.5% overt and 0.7% mild) [*see Figure 1*].

THYROID NODULES

Thyroid nodules (masses within the gland) are relatively common in adults. In the Framingham Study, 6% of women and 2% of men had palpable thyroid nodules.[2] The prevalence of nonpalpable thyroid nodules incidentally detected by imaging studies such as sonography and CT has been reported to be as high as 27% in adults.[3] Diffuse thyroid gland enlargement (goiter) is declining in prevalence—a tendency that reflects the increase in levels of dietary iodine in the United States. Whereas goiter was identified in 3% of persons in a 10-state United States survey in the 1970s, it was self-reported by less than 0.5% of persons in the more recent NHANES III.[4,5]

THYROID CANCER

Thyroid cancer is the 14th most common malignancy in the United States, with an estimated annual incidence of 23,600 new cases and a female-to-male ratio of 3 to 1.[6] However, the epidemiology of thyroid cancer is more important than this incidence ranking would imply, for two reasons. First, thyroid cancer is currently the malignancy with the fastest rising incidence in the United States, with increases of 3.8% annually from 1992 to 2001. Second, because treatment is highly effective, with 95% or more of patients surviving, there may be about 300,000 thyroid cancer survivors in the United States, all of whom require monitoring for recurrent disease.

Hypothyroidism

EPIDEMIOLOGY

Hypothyroidism is a common disorder that occurs more commonly in women than in men; in both sexes, the incidence increases during and after middle life.[7] In the NHANES III, 2% of persons 65 years and older had overt hypothyroidism, and 14% had mild hypothyroidism.[1] Prevalences of thyroid dysfunction were also higher in whites and Mexican Americans than in blacks (5%, 4%, and 2%, respectively).

Certain individuals are at higher risk for developing hypothyroidism, including those with a family history of autoimmune thyroid disorders[8]; postpartum women[9]; those with a history of head and neck or thyroid irradiation or surgery; those with certain other autoimmune endocrine conditions[10] (e.g., type 1 diabetes mellitus, adrenal insufficiency, and ovarian failure); and those with certain nonendocrine autoimmune disorders (e.g., celiac disease, vitiligo, pernicious anemia, and Sjögren syndrome). Hypothyroidism also develops more frequently in persons with Down syndrome or Turner syndrome.

ETIOLOGY AND GENETICS

The causes of hypothyroidism vary, depending on whether the disease is congenital or acquired. In addition, the causes of primary hypothyroidism (i.e., disease of the thyroid gland itself) differ from those of secondary (central) hypothyroidism, which involves deranged hypothalamic-pituitary control of the gland.

Congenital Hypothyroidism

Endemic iodine deficiency remains an important cause of congenital hypothyroidism in certain regions of the world. Even with sufficient dietary iodine, congenital hypothyroidism affects one in 4,000 infants because of thyroid gland dysgenesis (as related, for example, to mutant *PAX8* and *TTF1* genes) or inherited defects in thyroid hormone synthesis (e.g., mutations in the genes that code for thyroid peroxidase, sodium-iodide symporter, and thyroglobulin). Absent or ineffective TSH responsiveness can be the result of mutations in the genes affecting pituitary thyrotrope differentiation (e.g., *POU1F1* and *PROP1*) or the structures of the thyrotropin-releasing hormone (TRH) receptor, the TSH β chain, and the TSH receptor. A mutation in the gene for $G_s\alpha$, which mediates adenylate cyclase activation in thyroid cells, causes hypothyroidism in pseudohypoparathyroidism. Inherited resistance to thyroid hormone can be caused by mutations in the β isoform of the nuclear triiodothyronine (T_3) receptor.

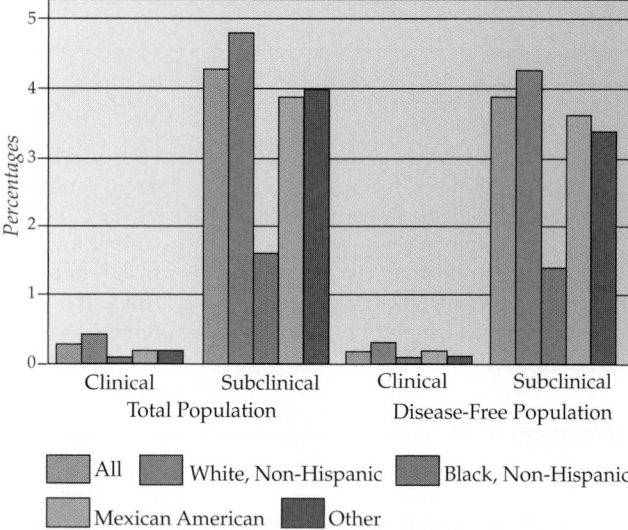

Figure 1   **Prevalences of abnormalities on thyroid function tests in different populations in the third National Health and Nutrition Examination Survey.**

Acquired Hypothyroidism

Autoimmune thyroiditis   Autoimmune thyroiditis, also called Hashimoto disease, is far and away the leading cause of hypothyroidism.[11] Its autoimmune pathogenesis is evidenced by the lymphocytic infiltration of the thyroid, the presence of circulating thyroid autoantibodies and activated CD4$^+$ T cells specific for thyroid antigens, and the expression of antigen-presenting major histocompatibility complex (MHC) class II proteins by thyrocytes. There is a genetic predisposition to autoimmune thyroiditis, and a polygenic basis for this predisposition is suggested by linkage to several genetic loci in affected kindreds.[12] Because autoimmune thyroiditis is more common in populations with higher dietary-iodine content, it has been postulated that high levels of dietary iodine cause an increase in thyroglobulin antigenicity. Thyroid autoimmunity can be initiated by interferon-alfa therapy and can cause either hypothyroidism or hyperthyroidism.[13] Discontinuance of immunomodulatory therapy often reverses this effect.

Other causes of thyroid injury   Thyroid surgery or thyroid irradiation—whether in the form of radioactive iodine therapy for thyrotoxicosis or external-beam radiotherapy for head and neck malignancies[14]—commonly results in hypothyroidism. In hemochromatosis, iron infiltration of the gland can cause thyroid failure. Transient primary hypothyroidism also occurs with lymphocytic thyroiditis (also known as postpartum or painless thyroiditis) and subacute thyroiditis.

Drug and toxins causing hypothyroidism   Long-term administration of iodine in pharmacologic quantities, such as with amiodarone[15] or iodine-containing expectorants, can inhibit thyroid hormone production, particularly in patients with underlying autoimmune thyroiditis. Lithium carbonate interferes with hormone release from the thyroid gland, resulting in transient TSH elevation in one third of patients and sustained hypothyroidism in 10%; those with autoimmune thyroiditis are especially vulnerable.[16] The antiretroviral agent stavudine and the drugs aminoglutethimide and thalidomide have also been reported to cause hypothyroidism. Industrial exposure to polybrominated

and polychlorinated biphenyls and resorcinol have been reported to produce hypothyroidism in workers. Although perchlorate is capable of inhibiting thyroid hormone synthesis, this chemical has not been shown to cause hypothyroidism at concentrations reported in contaminated drinking water.[17]

Central (secondary) hypothyroidism   Diseases that interfere with TRH production by the hypothalamus or that impair pituitary TSH production can produce central hypothyroidism. The most common causes are pituitary adenomas and the surgical procedures or radiotherapy used to treat them.[18] In addition, tumors impinging on the hypothalamus or pituitary stalk, traumatic transection of the pituitary stalk,[19] and certain infiltrative diseases (e.g., sarcoidosis, hemochromatosis, and Langerhans cell histiocystosis) can interfere with hypothalamic TRH production or delivery. Pituitary thyrotrope dysfunction can be caused by lymphocytic hypophysitis; infection; metastatic disease; apoplexy (e.g., Sheehan syndrome or tumor infarction); and bexarotene, a retinoid X receptor–selective ligand used to treat cutaneous T cell lymphoma.[20]

PATHOGENESIS

Clinical hypothyroidism reflects a widespread lack of thyroid hormone actions at the genomic level in target tissues, where T_3 binds to receptors that are members of the nuclear receptor superfamily.[21] These T_3 receptors are in turn bound to thyroid-response elements located in the regulatory regions of certain genes that increase or decrease their transcription in response to thyroid hormone. Some biochemical and clinical manifestations of hypothyroidism can be explained on the basis of specific deficiencies in molecular actions. For example, reduced expression of the hepatic low-density lipoprotein (LDL) receptor gene decreases LDL cholesterol clearance, causing hypercholesterolemia; decreased expressions of the myocardial α-myosin heavy-chain genes and the sarcoplasmic reticulum adenosine triphosphatase genes impair myocardial systolic and diastolic performance, respectively. Many other clinical aspects of hypothyroidism are not yet understood in terms of specific genomic actions. Some of these may result from putative nongenomic thyroid hormone actions on G protein–coupled membrane receptors and mitochondria.[22]

DIAGNOSIS

Clinical Manifestations

Classic symptoms of hypothyroidism include fatigue, lethargy, cold intolerance, weight gain, constipation, dry skin, hoarseness, slowed mentation, and depressed mood. In a study of patients with short-term hypothyroidism, 38% to 58% of patients had one or more of these clinical findings.[23] However, the diagnostic accuracy of such symptoms is low. Of newly diagnosed hypothyroid patients in a case-control study by Canaris and colleagues, only 30% had any symptoms, and 17% of euthyroid control subjects had one or more of the same nonspecific complaints.[24] As a result, individual symptoms had a positive predictive value of only 8% to 12%.

Inaccuracy in clinical diagnosis of hypothyroidism is attributable to various factors, including the fact that many other disorders produce similar symptoms; the typically gradual onset of thyroid hormone deficiency; and, sometimes, the impaired insight that hypothyroidism produces in some patients. Symptoms that are new or that occur in combination are more likely to represent hypothyroidism. In the Canaris study, patients with seven or more new symptoms were almost ninefold more likely to be hypothyroid than those with fewer new symptoms. In addition, more hypothyroid patients than euthyroid patients reported that their symptoms had changed from the previous year.[24]

Hypothyroidism can be associated with cognitive deficits, particularly memory problems.[25] Although hypothyroidism is in the differential diagnosis of dementia and is not uncommonly detected in demented elderly patients, thyroid hormone treatment rarely reverses dementia in these patients.[26] Other neurologic findings in hypothyroid patients can include depression, psychosis, ataxia, seizures, and coma. Hypothyroidism is a potentially reversible cause of sleep apnea. It can also cause decreases in the senses of hearing, taste, and smell.

Other special manifestations of hypothyroidism have been reported in children and adolescents. Thyroid hormone deficiency can cause growth failure, delayed or precocious puberty, muscle pseudohypertrophy, and galactorrhea.

Physical Examination

Classic physical signs of hypothyroidism include bradycardia, diastolic hypertension, and hypothermia; coarse, cool, and pale skin; loss of scalp and eyebrow hair; hoarse, slow, and dysarthric speech; distant heart tones; diffuse nonpitting edema; and slowed deep tendon reflexes, particularly during the relaxation phase. However, none of these findings is sufficiently sensitive or specific for diagnosis. Additional signs may be identified when hypothyroid patients present with other unusual features, such as chronic heart failure, pericardial and pleural effusions, ileus and intestinal pseudo-obstruction, or coagulopathy.

In patients with autoimmune thyroiditis, which is the most common type of hypothyroidism, the thyroid gland can be nonpalpable, normal in size, or diffusely enlarged with an irregular contour, firm consistency, and palpable pyramidal lobe. The gland is only rarely painful and tender. There may be signs related to the other endocrine deficiency states associated with the polyendocrine failure syndromes: type 1, which includes hypoparathyroidism (Chvostek and Trousseau signs), adrenal insufficiency (hyperpigmentation), and chronic mucocutaneous candidiasis; and type 2, which includes adrenal insufficiency, type 1 diabetes mellitus, and primary ovarian failure. There can also be evidence of other associated nonendocrine autoimmune disorders, including vitiligo, atrophic gastritis, pernicious anemia, systemic sclerosis, and Sjögren syndrome.

Laboratory Tests

Routine laboratory tests Abnormalities in routine laboratory tests can be the first diagnostic clue suggesting hypothyroidism. Hypercholesterolemia and hyperhomocysteinemia are especially common in hypothyroid patients.[27] In addition, hyponatremia, hyperprolactinemia, hypoglycemia, and elevations in levels of creatine phosphokinase (predominantly MM band) can all be caused by thyroid hormone deficiency.

Serum thyroid function tests Whether it is prompted by clinical or routine laboratory test findings or performed for patient or population screening, measurement of serum TSH should usually be the first test in the diagnosis of hypothyroidism. An elevated serum TSH level identifies patients with primary hypothyroidism regardless of its cause or severity, even those with mild thyroid hormone deficiency and a serum free thyroxine (T_4) concentration within the reference range. Normal serum TSH levels

---

Table 1   Causes of Elevated Serum TSH Levels

Primary hypothyroidism
Central hypothyroidism*
Recovery after nonthyroidal illnesses
Renal insufficiency
Adrenal insufficiency
Drugs
  Metoclopramide
  Phenothiazines?
Analytic problems
  Anti-TSH antibodies
  Anti–mouse immunoglobulin antibodies

*Attributable to TSH with reduced biologic-to-immunologic activity ratio.

---

in disease-free populations are typically 0.4 to 4.0 µU/L. However, values are not normally distributed; the mean TSH concentration, 1.5 µU/L, is in the lower half of the reference range.[1] Even a high-normal serum TSH level (e.g., 3.0 µU/L) may reflect very mild thyroid dysfunction, particularly in a patient who has other clinical or laboratory features of autoimmune thyroiditis. As a result, some authorities have recommended lowering the TSH assay's upper limit of normal to 2.5 µU/L.[28]

When an elevation in serum TSH is detected in a potentially hypothyroid patient, the test should be repeated, and the serum free T_4 concentration should be measured. This further testing confirms the diagnosis of hypothyroidism—an important step, because such patients will typically be committed to lifelong thyroid hormone therapy—and more fully defines the severity of hypothyroidism. The serum T_3 concentration has limited sensitivity and specificity and therefore is a poor test for hypothyroidism.

The TSH assay may fail to detect hypothyroidism in a few settings. In patients with central hypothyroidism, the serum TSH level can be low, normal, or even modestly elevated.[29] The absence of an elevation in the TSH level in a patient with a low free T_4 level is attributable to the synthesis of a TSH molecule that has a decreased ratio of biologic to immunologic activity.[30] Central hypothyroidism should be suspected in the absence of TSH elevation if the patient has clinical features of hypothyroidism; has clinical findings suggesting a sellar mass lesion or other anterior pituitary hormone deficiencies; or has a history of head trauma or conditions known to cause hypopituitarism, such as sarcoidosis. In these settings, both the serum free T_4 and TSH concentrations should be measured. Detection of a low serum free T_4 concentration, regardless of the TSH level, indicates the need for further testing, which may include cranial imaging, performance of a TRH stimulation test to assess TSH responsiveness, and other pituitary function testing.

There are also circumstances in which an elevated serum TSH level may not reflect hypothyroidism [see Table 1]. Euthyroid patients with renal or adrenal insufficiency may have modest TSH elevations (e.g., levels of 5 to 10 µU/L). Two rare forms of TSH-mediated hyperthyroidism that may present as clinical and biochemical hyperthyroidism with an inappropriately normal or elevated serum TSH are TSH-secreting pituitary tumors[31] and isolated pituitary resistance to thyroid hormone.[32] However, the elevation in levels of serum free T_4, T_3, or both in these patients provides a clue to the diagnosis. Circulating anti-TSH antibodies can yield falsely elevated TSH immunoassay readings.

Effects of nonthyroid illnesses and drugs Distinguishing central hypothyroidism from the thyroid function abnormalities that often accompany severe nonthyroid illnesses can be challenging. Cytokine-mediated TSH suppression can mask mild primary hypothyroidism. Furthermore, certain drugs used to treat severe illness (e.g., glucocorticoids, dopamine, and dobutamine) can normalize elevated serum TSH concentrations in patients with overt primary hypothyroidism. Conversely, false positive transient TSH elevation can be seen in patients recovering from critical illness.[33] Consequently, with severely ill patients, it is best to limit thyroid function testing to those in whom there is a significant clinical suspicion of hypothyroidism; otherwise, abnormal results are much more likely to represent false positive than true positive findings. Similarly, the antiseizure medications phenytoin and carbamazepine can cause decreases in the levels of serum total T_4, free T_4 (as measured by immunoassay), and TSH; these findings can be confused with those of central hypothyroidism.[34] In some patients who are severely ill or who are taking these antiseizure medications, free T_4 measurement by equilibrium dialysis and pituitary imaging may be required to diagnose or exclude central hypothyroidism.

DIFFERENTIAL DIAGNOSIS

Given that the clinical manifestations of hypothyroidism are quite nonspecific and can be caused by myriad other medical conditions and life circumstances, the key to diagnosis is simply for the physician to keep this condition in mind. Once the possibility of hypothyroidism is entertained, serum TSH measurement can confirm or exclude the diagnosis in almost all cases. In a survey of 1,721 primary care physicians, 80% to 90% appreciated the fact that a middle-aged woman presenting with fatigue, impaired memory, or depression might have hypothyroidism and therefore would order a serum TSH concentration for such a patient; however, only half of these physicians would screen for hypothyroidism in a hypercholesterolemic patient.[35]

The cause of primary hypothyroidism may be evident from the history alone; for example, the patient may have previously undergone thyroid surgery or radiation therapy or may currently be taking medications known to cause hypothyroidism. When the history provides no clue, sustained primary hypothyroidism can usually be assumed to be caused by autoimmune thyroiditis. Confirmatory laboratory tests are seldom required. Nonetheless, it is sometimes helpful to confirm this diagnosis by detection of thyroid autoantibodies. Anti–thyroid peroxidase antibody assay is the most sensitive test to confirm the diagnosis of autoimmune thyroiditis. Thyroid autoantibody testing can also be useful in predicting the development of hypothyroidism in patients with mild hypothyroidism and in pregnant and postpartum women.[36-38]

MANAGEMENT

Thyroid Hormone Therapy

Levothyroxine sodium (thyroxine) is the treatment of choice for patients with hypothyroidism. Thyroxine is well absorbed by the proximal small bowel. Thyroxine circulates with a 7-day half-life because of plasma protein binding, and it is metabolized in target tissues, in part by deiodination to T_3. Its long half-life permits a single daily dose; its conversion to T_3 in target tissues mimics normal physiology. The multiple dose strengths available in North America facilitate precise dose titration. Nonetheless, thyroxine and other thyroid hormone preparations have narrow therapeutic indexes and hence have the potential for ad-

verse reactions with even modest overtreatment. Several studies examining the adequacy of thyroid hormone therapy in large populations and in patients in generalist and specialty practices have found that one fifth of patients with treated hypothyroidism are receiving an inadequate dose and one fifth an excessive dose.[39]

Dosing considerations and drug interactions The optimal thyroxine dosage for hypothyroid patients is related to body weight. In adults, this is approximately 1.8 µg/kg/day.[40] Elderly patients, whose metabolic clearance of thyroxine is reduced, have a lower dosage requirement of 0.5 µg/kg/day. The thyroxine dose is usually higher in patients who have undergone thyroidectomy than in patients with autoimmune thyroiditis, who often have residual functioning thyroid tissue. Thyroxine absorption can be decreased in patients with malabsorption from gastrointestinal disorders or previous small bowel bypass surgery. Several mineral supplements, medications, and dietary constituents can interfere with thyroxine absorption; these include iron, calcium carbonate, cholestyramine, aluminum hydroxide gel, sucralfate, soy, and perhaps dietary fiber. Metabolism of thyroxine is accelerated in the nephrotic syndrome, in other severe systemic illnesses, and with the use of phenobarbital, phenytoin, carbamazepine, and rifampin. In 75% of pregnant women, the thyroxine dose requirement is increased by 50% to 100%.[41] Postmenopausal hormone replacement therapy increases the required thyroxine dose in 35% of women.[42]

Patient noncompliance is the most common cause of inadequate thyroxine therapy. Several observations should raise suspicion that a patient is not taking thyroxine faithfully: the apparent thyroxine dose requirement is higher than expected; thyroid function test results vary without correlation with prescribed thyroxine doses; and the serum TSH concentration is elevated, yet the serum free T_4 level is in the mid- to high-normal range, reflecting improved compliance immediately before testing.

Thyroxine treatment should typically start with a dosage at the lower end of the anticipated requirement (e.g., 125 µg/day in a 70 kg adult). In otherwise healthy younger patients, there is no need to titrate the dose upward from a very low starting dose. Laboratory monitoring of treated hypothyroid patients should be performed 4 to 6 weeks after starting a new thyroxine dose or tablet formulation; thereafter, it should be performed annually. It should also be performed whenever a patient's symptoms suggest thyroid hormone deficiency or excess. The goal for most patients is to restore the TSH level to the lower half of the normal range (i.e., 1.0 to 2.0 µU/L). In patients with central hypothyroidism, the serum free T_4 concentration must be monitored; treatment should usually be targeted for a concentration in the upper half of the normal range.

Metabolism of certain other drugs can be affected by the hypothyroid state and by the initiation of thyroxine treatment. Hypothyroid patients may have increased sensitivity to anesthetic and sedative agents. Reduced digoxin clearance and drug distribution volume may predispose patients to toxicity. Sensitivity to warfarin may be decreased because of slowed metabolism of vitamin K–dependent clotting factors, and restoring euthyroidism can increase the required warfarin dose.

Adverse reactions to thyroid hormone therapy Adverse reactions to thyroxine overtreatment include symptomatic thyrotoxicosis and subclinical thyrotoxicosis with increased risks of bone loss and atrial tachyarrhythmias.[43,44] The predisposition to osteoporosis is principally in postmenopausal women. Atrial fibrillation is more common in patients 60 years of age or older. Both of these complications have been shown to occur when the serum TSH concentration is suppressed to less than 0.1 µU/L.

Complications can also arise from restoring euthyroidism, particularly in patients with underlying ischemic heart disease[45] (see below) and borderline adrenal cortical insufficiency. Concomitant thyroid and adrenal gland failure can occur in hypopituitarism and in the type 2 polyendocrine failure syndrome (Schmidt syndrome), which is marked by autoimmune thyroiditis and idiopathic adrenal insufficiency.

A few patients experience acute sympathomimetic symptoms soon after institution of thyroxine treatment. This syndrome is poorly understood; it can be circumvented by reducing the thyroxine dose to a very low level and advancing it slowly.

Transient scalp hair loss may occur during first few weeks of thyroxine replacement therapy. Patients can be assured that this phenomenon is temporary. Treatment of hypothyroidism sometimes reveals an underlying urticarial disorder, but true allergy to thyroxine formulations has not been well documented.

Special Therapeutic Issues

Hypothyroid patients with ischemic heart disease Because thyroid hormone has positive inotropic and chronotropic effects, thyroid hormone therapy can exacerbate myocardial ischemia in hypothyroid patients with underlying coronary artery disease. In such patients, thyroxine therapy should be initiated at a low dosage (e.g., 25 µg/day) and titrated upward in increments of 12.5 to 25 µg every 4 to 6 weeks. Patients should be monitored vigilantly with clinical assessments and electrocardiography. Deliberate suboptimal dosing, which was previously advocated to limit myocardial oxygen demand, has been shown to actually increase the risk of progressive coronary atherosclerosis. Beta-blocker therapy should sometimes be initiated or intensified when thyroxine therapy is initiated. Hypothyroid patients who experience worsening myocardial ischemia despite these precautions can undergo coronary angioplasty and even surgical bypass grafting with minimal or no increased perioperative risk.[46,47]

Mild hypothyroidism Whether to identify and treat patients with mild hypothyroidism, defined by an elevated serum TSH level with a normal free T_4 level, is controversial. There is agreement that mild hypothyroidism is highly prevalent, particularly in older women, and that clinical diagnosis is inaccurate. Diagnostic serum TSH testing and thyroxine treatment of mild hypothyroidism are clearly effective and are relatively safe and inexpensive. The outstanding issue is whether mild hypothyroidism causes clinical consequences that are important enough to justify widespread screening and therapy.[48] Proponents of detection and treatment argue that it prevents progression to overt hypothyroidism in affected patients, particularly those whose serum TSH concentration is greater than 10 µU/L, who are 65 years of age or older, or who have thyroid autoantibodies, indicating underlying autoimmune thyroiditis. Advocates believe that treatment of mild hypothyroidism may reduce the risk of future atherosclerotic cardiovascular disease. They hold this view on the basis of the following observations: affected patients have higher mean cholesterol levels; most studies have shown that TSH-normalizing thyroxine therapy lowers serum total cholesterol and LDL cholesterol concentrations[49]; and some epidemiologic studies have found that persons with mild hypothy-

roidism have a higher risk of atherosclerotic cardiovascular disease.[50] Some proponents are persuaded by four small, controlled, double-blind trials that showed that thyroxine therapy was more effective than placebo in improving symptoms and neuropsychologic performance in patients with mild hypothyroidism.[51] On the basis of these studies, two decision and cost-effectiveness models suggested that the cost-effectiveness of screening for and treating mild hypothyroidism is comparable to that of other widely accepted preventive medicine strategies.[52,53] On the other hand, opponents of screening and treatment of mild hypothyroidism point out that these putative benefits have not been rigorously confirmed by large, randomized, controlled trials.[54] When physicians do recommend treatment for patients with mild hypothyroidism, the thyroxine dosage is typically lower than that for overt hypothyroidism—0.5 µg/kg/day.

Residual hypothyroid symptoms and T_3 therapy Compared with euthyroid patients, hypothyroid patients more often have constitutional and neuropsychological complaints, even when serum TSH measurements suggest adequate treatment.[55] This observation may represent only ascertainment bias (i.e., symptomatic patients seeking medical care are more likely to be diagnosed and treated for hypothyroidism). However, it has been postulated that the presence of residual symptoms in thyroxine-treated patients reflects a failure to replace the small amount of T_3 normally secreted by the thyroid gland. Four clinical trials in which a fraction of the thyroxine dose was replaced with a small dose of T_3 failed to confirm an earlier report of significant improvement with combination thyroxine/T_3 therapy.[56] Combination therapy has the disadvantages of a fluctuating and supraphysiologic T_3 level, a greater risk of iatrogenic thyrotoxicosis, and increased complexity and expense. Treatment with desiccated thyroid, a biologic preparation that also contains both T_4 and T_3, has the same disadvantages.

COMPLICATIONS

Severe hypothyroidism (myxedema) can become complicated by multiple organ system failure when it is profound and prolonged, especially in elderly patients who have other cardiac, pulmonary, neurologic, renal, and infectious diseases. Myxedema coma, the most severe expression of hypothyroidism, is associated with substantial mortality. Such complications of thyroid hormone deficiency can be prevented with sustained thyroxine therapy. In newly diagnosed patients, preventive measures also include giving special attention to other potentially provocative medical conditions (e.g., heart failure, renal failure, pneumonia) and medications—particularly sedative, anesthetic, and analgesic medications that suppress ventilatory drive and other central nervous system functions.

Treatment of complicated hypothyroidism includes thyroid hormone replacement and aggressive management of organ system complications that can be present. Two thyroid hormone regimens have proven efficacy for myxedema coma: (1) thyroxine in a full replacement dose (1.8 µg/kg/day), with or without a 500 µg loading dose to replete the normal body thyroxine pool[57]; and (2) T_3 in divided doses, advocated because of the impaired T_4-to-T_3 conversion that occurs in critically ill patients. No trial has rigorously compared these regimens, but one small retrospective study found a higher mortality in T_3-treated patients.[58]

PROGNOSIS

The prognosis for hypothyroid patients who are properly

treated with thyroxine should be excellent. However, discontinuance of thyroid hormone therapy predictably leads to recurrent hypothyroidism, with its potential for serious complications in the elderly. This occurs most often in settings of social neglect, poor access to health care, and associated neuropsychological impairment. Lesser degrees of suboptimal therapy are also associated with long-term risks. Inadequately treated patients may have increased risk of atherosclerotic cardiovascular disease, and iatrogenic thyrotoxicosis can predispose patients to osteoporosis and atrial tachyarrhythmias.

Patients with autoimmune thyroiditis, the most common cause of hypothyroidism, are at risk for certain associated conditions, for which they should be monitored. Pernicious anemia and gastric achlorhydria with consequent iron and calcium malabsorption affect 3% and 25% of autoimmune thyroiditis patients, respectively. Much less commonly, other autoimmune diseases (e.g., Sjögren syndrome and systemic sclerosis), endocrine deficiency states (adrenal insufficiency, type 1 diabetes, hypoparathyroidism, and hypogonadism), and primary thyroid lymphoma can occur.

Thyrotoxicosis

EPIDEMIOLOGY

The alert clinician will diagnose thyrotoxicosis several times each year. NHANES III found thyrotoxicosis in 0.5% of a surveyed cohort that reflected the demographics of the United States adult population.[1] Three disorders account for the majority of cases: diffuse toxic goiter (Graves disease), toxic nodular goiter, and iatrogenic thyrotoxicosis in thyroid hormone–treated patients. The incidence of Graves disease in one United Kingdom community survey was one to two cases per 1,000 population annually; 2.7% of women and 0.2% of men had Graves disease or a history of Graves disease.[59] The highest incidence of Graves disease is in women 30 to 60 years of age, but the disease can affect persons of virtually any age, from neonates to the very elderly. Toxic adenoma and toxic multinodular goiter are more common causes of thyrotoxicosis than Graves disease in regions where dietary iodine deficiency is prevalent; in women; and in older patients.[60] Iatrogenic thyrotoxicosis has been reported in approximately 20% of thyroid hormone–treated patients.[1,39,61]

ETIOLOGY, GENETICS, AND PATHOGENESIS

Thyrotoxicosis can be divided into three etiologic categories: abnormal stimulation of the thyroid gland, thyroid gland autonomy, and gland inflammation with unregulated thyroid hormone release. Each of these categories includes several diseases [see Table 2].

Graves Disease (Diffuse Toxic Goiter)

There is compelling evidence that there is a genetic predisposition to Graves disease, that the incidence is higher in women, that unknown environmental factors are involved in its initiation, and that gland stimulation by antibodies against the TSH receptor is the immediate precipitant of the condition. Identical twins and some families show increased incidences of Graves disease.[62] The condition has been genetically linked to certain MHC components (e.g., HLA-B8 and HLA-DR3), which are on the surface of cells that present antigenic peptide epitopes to T cell receptors. One theory is that certain HLA-DR molecules may be better able to present TSH receptor epitopes, inciting autoimmunity. Anoth-

Table 2 Etiologic Classification of Thyrotoxicosis

Cause	Individual Diseases
Abnormal stimulation of the thyroid gland	Graves disease hCG-mediated thyrotoxicosis TSH-mediated thyrotoxicosis
Thyroid gland autonomy	Toxic adenoma Toxic multinodular goiter Congenital thyrotoxicosis Iodine-induced hyperthyroidism Thyroid cancer–related thyrotoxicosis
Gland inflammation with unregulated thyroid hormone release	Subacute (de Quervain) thyroiditis Lymphocytic thyroiditis Amiodarone-induced thyrotoxicosis, type 2 Acute thyroiditis

hCG—human chorionic gonadotropin

er hypothesis is that these HLA-DR recognition sequences are involved in aberrant thymic T cell selection for tolerance. Graves disease has also been linked to polymorphisms in the gene encoding CTLA-4, a T cell receptor important for interaction with antigen-presenting cells.[63] In whites, a susceptibility locus for Graves disease has been identified on chromosome 20q11.

Several environmental factors have been implicated in the initiation of Graves disease. These include stressful life events, smoking, large amounts of dietary iodine, and preceding infection with certain bacterial agents that have been postulated to induce molecular mimicry. Radiation injury to the thyroid gland may increase the risk of the condition, possibly because of increased TSH receptor exposure and immunoreactivity.

Whatever the underlying genetic and environmental factors, the vast majority of Graves disease patients have detectable antibodies that are directed against the TSH receptor and are capable of stimulating it[64] [see Figure 2]. Assays using thyroid cells or their membranes can detect circulating TSH receptor autoantibody species in 70% to 90% of patients with Graves disease. These autoantibodies are capable of stimulating intracellular cyclic adenosine monophosphate production (thyroid-stimulating immunoglobulins [TSI]), inhibiting TSH receptor activation (TSH receptor inhibitory immunoglobulins), and inhibiting the binding of TSH to its receptor (TSH receptor–binding inhibitory immunoglobulins [TBII]).

Toxic Adenoma and Toxic Multinodular Goiter

Solitary and multiple thyroid adenomas and diffusely hyperplastic thyroid tissue possess a growth advantage, and their constituent thyrocytes sometimes produce thyroid hormones autonomously (i.e., without regard to TSH regulation). These hyperplastic and neoplastic conditions cause hyperthyroidism when the mass and efficiency of functioning thyroid tissue are great enough to generate hormone excess in target tissues, including suppression of endogenous pituitary TSH production and function of extranodular thyroid tissue.[65] Both genetic and environmental factors are involved in the development of this autonomous function. A twin study showed that genetic factors could account for 82% of the predisposition to nodular goiter, and familial multinodular goiter has been linked to a gene locus on chromosome 14q.[66] At the same time, environmental factors (e.g., dietary iodine deficiency, goitrogens, and radiation exposure) also clearly predispose to the development of autonomous-

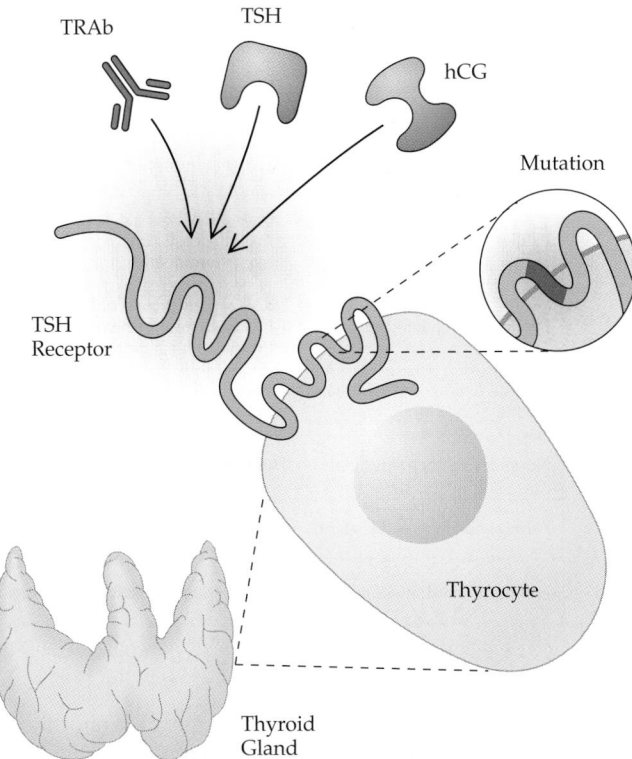

Figure 2   Certain forms of hyperthyroidism result from deranged physiologic activation of the thyroid-stimulating hormone (TSH) receptor. In Graves disease, TSH receptor autoantibodies (TRAb) bind the TSH receptor. In patients with TSH-secreting pituitary tumors, the autonomously secreted TSH overstimulates the receptor. In molar pregnancy and choriocarcinoma, high concentrations and aberrant forms of human chorionic gonadotropin (hCG) can activate the TSH receptor. In some patients with toxic adenomas, a constitutively activating somatic mutation of the TSH receptor results in autonomous secretion of thyroid hormone.

ly functioning thyroid tissue. Genetic and environment factors promote thyroid tissue growth by activating intraglandular growth factors (e.g., insulinlike growth factor and epidermal growth factor receptor)[67] and signaling pathway proteins (e.g., $G_s\alpha$ and ras). Constitutively activating somatic mutations of the TSH receptor and $G_s\alpha$ itself have been described in 25% to 80% of toxic adenomas, more commonly in patients from regions where dietary iodine deficiency is prevalent.[68]

Iodine-Induced Hyperthyroidism

Iodine is both a substrate and a physiologic regulator of thyroid hormone synthesis. Excessive iodine intake normally inhibits thyroid hormone production by reducing the trapping of inorganic iodide and its oxidation into an organic form (organification) and by thyroid hormone release. At the same time, exposure to pharmacologic amounts of iodine (typically 1,000-fold more than the physiologic requirement of 150 μg/day) can cause hyperthyroidism, a condition termed the Jod-Basedow effect. Patients with hyperplastic and benign neoplastic thyroid conditions and those with latent Graves disease are particularly vulnerable to iodine-induced hyperthyroidism. Epidemics of thyrotoxicosis have repeatedly been observed when iodine supplementation is instituted in regions of previous dietary iodine deficiency.[69] However, iodine-induced hyperthyroidism can also

occur in patients from iodine-sufficient environments whose thyroid glands are apparently normal, especially when excess iodine exposure is substantial and sustained, as it is with long-term amiodarone therapy.[70] The precise molecular and biochemical basis for iodine-induced hyperthyroidism is poorly understood. Iodine-induced hyperthyroidism is typically transient, lasting only a few weeks, but more prolonged thyroid dysfunction can occur when iodine exposure is prolonged, as occurs with the lipid-soluble drug amiodarone and with myelographic radiocontrast agents.

Thyroiditis

Inflammation of thyroid tissue caused by infectious diseases, autoimmune processes, or pharmacologic toxicity can cause thyrocyte death, disruption of follicular architecture, and unregulated leakage of thyroid hormones from the gland into the circulation, resulting in thyrotoxicosis[71] [*see Table 3*]. Thyroiditis-related thyrotoxicosis is typically self-limited, lasting 2 to 8 weeks, with spontaneous resolution once glandular stores of thyroid hormone are exhausted. A comparable period of transient hypothyroidism often follows because of lingering impairment of thyroid hormone synthesis, but most patients ultimately become euthyroid [*see Figure 3*].

Amiodarone-Induced Thyrotoxicosis

The iodine-containing antiarrhythmic agent amiodarone can cause thyrotoxicosis by two mechanisms.[72] Type 1 amiodarone-induced thyrotoxicosis is caused by iodine, whereas type 2 amiodarone-induced thyrotoxicosis is the result of gland inflammation. Both forms can be severe, prolonged, and life-threatening, particularly because affected patients have underlying cardiac disease.

Chorionic Gonadotropin–Mediated Hyperthyroidism

Human chorionic gonadotropin (hCG), which is structurally similar to TSH, can stimulate the TSH receptor and increase thyroid function when circulating in high concentration or when variant forms of either hCG or the TSH receptor increase the affinity of their hormone receptor interaction[73] [*see Figure 3*]. In fact, during the first trimester of normal pregnancy, when a marked physiologic elevation of hCG occurs, a modest rise in the serum free T_4 level and a decline in the serum TSH level are typically seen.[74] An exaggeration of this phenomenon can cause thyrotoxicosis, as can trophoblastic tumors.

Trophoblastic tumors   Women with hydatidiform mole and choriocarcinoma, as well as men with metastatic testicular choriocarcinoma, can develop hyperthyroidism as a result of very high concentrations of circulating hCG.[75] Furthermore, these tumors have been shown to produce a variant form of hCG with heightened TSH receptor stimulatory properties.

Gestational transient thyrotoxicosis   Mild transient thyrotoxicosis occurs late in the first trimester of pregnancy in 1% to 3% of white women and in as many as 11% of Asian women.[76] The serum hCG level is higher in affected pregnant women than in those who remain euthyroid. Furthermore, gestational thyrotoxicosis appears to be more common in women who have hyperemesis gravidarum or twin pregnancies, both of which are characterized by higher serum hCG concentrations. A rare form of familial gestational thyrotoxicosis has been reported in which a mother and daughter both had recurrent hy-

Table 3 Characteristic Features of Thyroiditis

Form of Thyroiditis	Presumed Etiology	Classic Pattern of Thyroid Dysfunction	Other Clinical Manifestations	Treatment
Autoimmune	T cell–mediated autoimmunity	Hypothyroidism	Firm small-to-medium goiter	Thyroxine for hypothyroidism
Lymphocytic (painless, silent, postpartum)	T cell–mediated autoimmunity?	Transient thyrotoxicosis followed by hypothyroidism	Painless small goiter	Observation, beta blockade for thyrotoxicosis, thyroxine for hypothyroidism
Subacute (de Quervain)	Viral infection?	Transient thyrotoxicosis followed by hypothyroidism	Painful and tender hard goiter	NSAID or glucocorticoid, beta blockade for thyrotoxicosis, thyroxine for hypothyroidism
Acute (suppurative)	Bacterial, fungal, and protozoal infections	Thyroid dysfunction (rare)	Painful, tender, and inflamed goiter	Antibiotic therapy, surgical drainage
Amiodarone-induced type 1	Iodine-induced hyperthyroidism	Thyrotoxicosis	Normal-size nontender gland	Thionamide antithyroid medication
Amiodarone-induced type 2	Inflammatory thyroiditis, precise cause unknown	Transient thyrotoxicosis	Normal-size nontender gland	Glucocorticoids
Riedel (invasive fibrous)	Idiopathic fibrosis?, autoimmune?	Hypothyroidism in one third of patients	Enlarging, hard, fixed mass	Surgery, glucocorticoids, tamoxifen

NSAID—nonsteroidal anti-inflammatory drug

perthyroidism during their pregnancies and were found to have a mutant TSH receptor with increased affinity and signaling responsiveness to hCG.[77]

TSH-Mediated (Central) Hyperthyroidism

Hyperthyroidism can be caused by excessive TSH secretion in two rare conditions: TSH-secreting pituitary adenoma and the syndrome of isolated central resistance to thyroid hormone.[78] Excessive and relatively autonomous TSH production by pituitary tumors predictably results in goitrous hyperthyroidism.[79] The TSH produced by TSH-secreting pituitary tumors has increased bioactivity, and normal inhibition of TSH release by dopamine has been shown to be defective in these patients. However, the fundamental cause of these tumors, which often cosecrete other pituitary hormones, is unknown.

Isolated central resistance to thyroid hormone is a rare inherited condition in which impaired negative feedback of thyroid hormone on pituitary thyrotropes leads to TSH hypersecretion and hyperthyroidism.[80] In one patient with isolated central resistance to thyroid hormone, a novel mutation in the thyroid hormone receptor–β gene was identified. In patients with this syndrome, unlike those with generalized resistance to thyroid hormone, other target tissues for thyroid hormone, such as the brain, heart, and liver, respond normally to the resulting thyrotoxicosis.

Exogenous Thyrotoxicosis

Iatrogenic thyrotoxicosis is relatively common, occurring in 20% of thyroid hormone–treated patients.[1,39,61] Possible explanations for this condition include improved patient compliance with therapy, decreased metabolic clearance of thyroid hor-

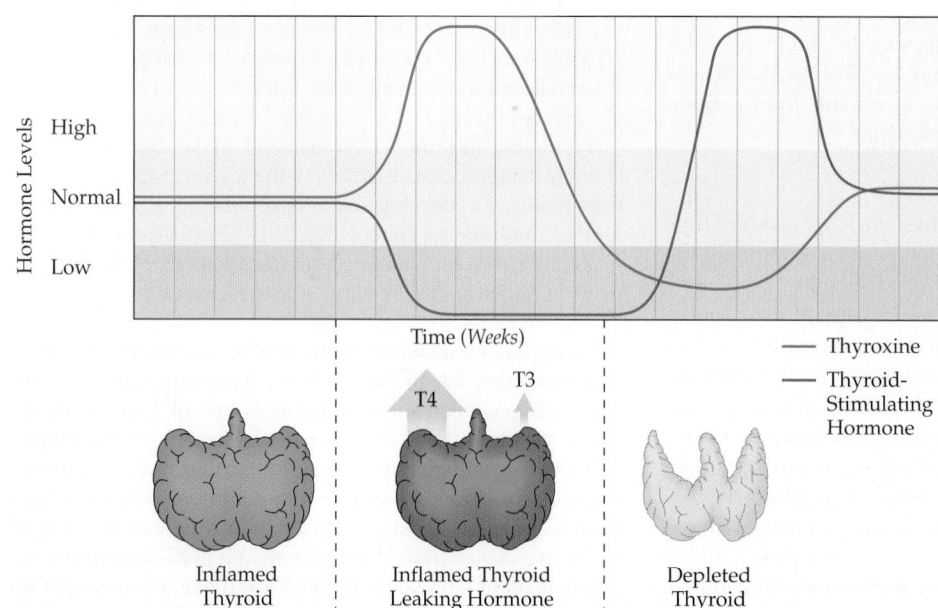

Figure 3 **In acute thyroiditis, inflammation of thyroid tissue leads to unregulated leakage of thyroid hormones from the gland into the circulation. The resulting thyrotoxicosis typically lasts 2 to 8 weeks and ends spontaneously as the glandular hormone stores are exhausted. A comparable period of hypothyroidism often follows, because of impaired thyroid hormone synthesis, but in most patients, the gland gradually returns to normal function.**

mones with aging, a substantial decrease in body weight, an increase in underlying gland function in patients with treated Graves disease or nodular goiter, and discontinuance of medications that interfere with thyroid hormone absorption or that accelerate its metabolism. Factitious thyrotoxicosis is sometimes prompted by a desire to enhance energy and weight loss; it can also occur through the complex psychopathology of Munchausen syndrome. Accidental or suicidal thyroid hormone intoxication can be life-threatening; its clinical manifestations may take 12 to 48 hours to become fully expressed, necessitating close observation even of asymptomatic patients, especially children.[81]

DIAGNOSIS

Clinical Manifestations

The classic symptoms of thyrotoxicosis are familiar to every third-year medical student—weight loss despite good appetite, heat intolerance, tremor, palpitations, and anxiety—yet even experienced clinicians are often slow to make the diagnosis, for several reasons. First, many common symptoms of thyroid hormone excess are nonspecific, such as fatigue, insomnia, dyspnea, and atypical chest pain. Second, patients can present with atypical chief complaints: weight gain; anorexia, nausea, and vomiting; muscle weakness; headache; urticaria; and, in elderly patients, apathy without sympathomimetic symptoms. Severe thyrotoxicosis may also present as heart failure, delirium, or an apparent febrile illness. Third, thyrotoxicosis can occur without the full complement of findings associated with Graves disease (e.g., prominent goiter and ocular findings). For example, thyrotoxicosis can be overlooked in a postpartum woman with weight loss and anxiety from acute lymphocytic thyroiditis, in a middle-aged man with bilateral earache reflecting radiation pain from subacute thyroiditis, and in the older patient with "failure to thrive" related to toxic nodular goiter. Fourth, new thyrotoxic complaints often arise in patients who have been otherwise entirely well and in whom the symptoms can potentially be discounted as a minor intercurrent illness or life stress. Finally, the spectrum of thyrotoxicosis includes entirely asymptomatic disease that nonetheless can have potential health consequences related to mild thyroid hormone excess.

A history of exposure to certain drugs, radiocontrast dye, homeopathic or traditional medicines, and dietary supplements can sometimes be the key to diagnosis. For example, a history of therapy with thyroid hormone, amiodarone, or interferon alfa suggests both the possibility and the likely cause of thyrotoxicosis. A history of recent radiocontrast studies or the recent ingestion of kelp may suggest iodine-induced hyperthyroidism. The family history is also often important in revealing a predisposition to autoimmune thyroid disease, nodular goiter, or, in rare cases, inherited forms of thyrotoxicosis.

Physical Examination

Physical signs related to thyrotoxicosis are often the key to diagnosis and differential diagnosis. Classic signs accompanying thyrotoxicosis can include an anxious, hyperactive demeanor and pressured speech; tachycardia, systolic hypertension, and widened pulse pressure; velvety, warm, and moist skin; onycholysis; flaxen, oily hair; staring gaze and lid lag; prominent apical impulse and systolic flow murmur; and proximal leg muscle weakness and tremor.

Certain findings on physical examination are characteristic of specific etiologies of thyrotoxicosis [see Table 3]. In Graves disease, patients typically have a symmetrical, rubbery goiter that is nontender and smooth or subtly lobulated; an audible bruit is sometimes noted. They may also have subtle or prominent eye findings, including episcleral injection, conjunctival swelling, periorbital edema, proptosis, limitation of extraocular motility, and impaired visual acuity or color vision. Less commonly, these patients may have pretibial myxedema, an orange peel–like thickening of the soft tissues of the anterior aspect of the lower leg from subcutaneous mucopolysacharide deposition; rarely, they may have clubbing of the fingers. Graves disease patients may also have physical signs of associated disorders, such as vitiligo and prematurely gray hair, which often escape detection without specific inquiry.

Other findings may suggest other etiologies for thyrotoxicosis. A solitary palpable thyroid nodule or multinodular goiter suggests the possibility of toxic adenoma or toxic multinodular goiter, respectively. Modest thyroid enlargement with an exquisitely tender, wood-hard gland may represent subacute thyroiditis. Thyrotoxic symptoms and signs in a pregnant woman may reflect hCG-related hyperthyroidism or, in a postpartum woman, acute lymphocytic thyroiditis. Signs of an expanding sellar mass lesion or other syndromes of pituitary hormone excess (e.g., acromegaly, Cushing syndrome, or galactorrhea) may suggest the presence of a TSH-secreting pituitary adenoma.

Laboratory Tests

Routine laboratory tests   Abnormalities on routine laboratory studies can be the first clue to thyrotoxicosis. Such abnormalities include hypercalcemia, an elevated serum alkaline phosphatase concentration, and a serum total or LDL cholesterol concentration that is either low or that is lower than previously documented for that patient. Serum ferritin, angiotensin-converting enzyme, and testosterone-binding globulin concentrations are all increased in thyrotoxicosis, and such increases may suggest the diagnosis. New significant atrial arrhythmias detected by electrocardiography, particularly atrial fibrillation, mandate testing for thyrotoxicosis.

Serum thyroid function tests   Serum TSH measurement is a highly sensitive way to diagnose or exclude all common forms and degrees of thyrotoxicosis.[82] Physiologic inhibition of pituitary thyrotrope function by thyroid hormones results in a serum TSH concentration that is low—almost invariably, less than $0.1 \mu U/L$ in patients with thyrotoxicosis. When the TSH assay is employed to diagnose thyrotoxicosis, it must have a detection limit low enough to distinguish normal from low values; a functional sensitivity to less than $0.02 \mu U/L$ has been recommended.[83] The serum TSH concentration is so sensitive in detecting thyroid hormone excess that it can be suppressed even when a patient's serum thyroid hormone concentration rises but remains within the reference range for that population—so-called subclinical thyrotoxicosis (see below).

In a few circumstances, however, TSH measurement can be inaccurate in the diagnosis of thyrotoxicosis. First, in patients with rare forms of TSH-mediated thyrotoxicosis (see above), the serum TSH concentration can be elevated, inappropriately normal, or only modestly decreased (i.e., 0.1 to $0.5 \mu U/L$). Second, spurious elevations of the measured TSH level, masking thyrotoxicosis, can occur with rare analytic problems, such as the presence of interfering anti-TSH autoantibodies. Third, there are other causes of a low serum TSH level, including central hypothyroidism and severe nonthyroidal illnesses. Whenever one of

Table 4   Causes of Elevated Serum
Total Thyroxine Level

Thyrotoxicosis
Increased serum protein binding
  Increased serum thyroxine-binding globulin concentrations
    Inherited
    Estrogen (pregnancy, exogenous, tumor produced)
    Hepatitis
    Hepatoma
    HIV infection
    Drugs (methadone, heroin, clofibrate, 5-fluorouracil)
  Familial dysalbuminemic hyperthyroxinemia
  Increased serum transthyretin binding or concentrations
    Inherited
    Carcinoma of the pancreas
    Hepatoma
Inhibition of T_4-to-T_3 conversion
  Medical illnesses
  Drugs (high-dose propranolol, amiodarone)
Test artifacts (assay interference from anti-T_4 immunoglobulins)

these circumstances is suspected, serum free T_4 and T_3 levels should be obtained to rule out thyrotoxicosis definitively.

Serum T_4 and T_3 measurements are useful to confirm the diagnosis of thyrotoxicosis, define its severity, and monitor the response to treatment. However, elevated serum total thyroid hormone concentrations are not specific for thyrotoxicosis[84] [*see Table 4*]. Because most of the circulating thyroid hormones are bound to plasma proteins (e.g., thyroxine-binding globulin, transthyretin [thyroxine-binding prealbumin], and albumin), conditions that increase the concentration or binding affinity of these proteins can cause euthyroid hyperthyroxinemia—an increase in the total serum T_4 level without elevation of the small fraction (0.03% for T_4) of biologically active free hormone. The most common such condition is the estrogen-induced increase in thyroxine-binding globulin level that occurs in women who are pregnant or who are taking estrogen preparations. Conversely, a decrease in binding of thyroid hormone by plasma proteins, such as occurs with nephrotic syndrome or androgen use, can mask the diagnosis of thyrotoxicosis on the basis of total T_4 measurement.

The serum free (or unbound) T_4 concentration can help distinguish thyrotoxicosis from euthyroid hyperthyroxinemia. Although equilibrium dialysis is the most accurate approach to free T_4 measurement, it is technically demanding and few laboratories perform it. Free T_4 immunoassays are now widely available and relatively inexpensive. They provide much the same information and have largely supplanted the free T_4 index, which provides an estimate of the unbound T_4 concentration on the basis of partition of radiolabeled thyroid hormone between plasma proteins and a binding resin. Both the free T_4 immunoassay and free T_4 index can reliably differentiate between the hyperthyroxinemia of thyrotoxicosis and that associated with thyroxine-binding globulin elevation.

Certain other conditions causing euthyroid hyperthyroxinemia still cannot be reliably differentiated from thyrotoxicosis with conventional methods of measuring free T_4. For example, free T_4 immunoassays often report falsely elevated values in patients with familial dysalbuminemic hyperthyroxinemia, in which a mutant albumin binds T_4 with increased affinity.[85] Similarly, increased transthyretin binding of thyroxine caused by a

mutant transthyretin gene or acquired transthyretin overproduction by hepatic or pancreatic neoplasms can yield deceptively elevated free T_4 immunoassay values.[86] T_4-binding autoantibodies, which occasionally develop in patients with autoimmune thyroiditis, can cause spurious serum T_4 elevation.[87] Hyperthyroxinemia can also occur with disorders and medications that reduce T_4 clearance, including acute systemic illnesses, psychosis, and treatment with amiodarone or high-dose propranolol. Finally, patients with the syndrome of generalized resistance to thyroid hormone typically have elevated serum total and free T_4 and T_3 concentrations.

In summary, hyperthyroxinemia is not pathognomonic of thyrotoxicosis. Clinical information—such as the presence of symptoms and signs of thyrotoxicosis or other conditions or the use of medications associated with hyperthyroxinemia—often permit a straightforward differentiation of thyrotoxicosis from euthyroid hyperthyroxinemia. Serum TSH measurement is invaluable in distinguishing all common forms of thyrotoxicosis, in which serum TSH is low, from euthyroid hyperthyroxinemia, in which serum TSH is usually normal.

Serum total and free T_3 concentrations are elevated in most patients with thyrotoxicosis caused by increased thyroid T_3 production and increased extrathyroid conversion of T_4 to T_3. Less than 5% of hyperthyroid patients have T_3 thyrotoxicosis (i.e., a high serum T_3 concentration and a normal serum T_4 concentration). An elevated serum total T_3 concentration is not entirely specific for thyrotoxicosis, because it can also occur with thyroxine-binding globulin excess, a rare form of familial dysalbuminemic hypertriiodothyroninemia, and anti-T_3 autoantibodies. Serum T_3 assays are useful clinically for fully defining the severity of certain forms of hyperthyroidism, particularly Graves disease; in addition, they are useful, along with the free T_4 concentration, for monitoring the response to treatment of thyrotoxicosis.

DIFFERENTIAL DIAGNOSIS

It is vital for the physician to establish the underlying cause of thyrotoxicosis, because the etiology determines the therapy. In many patients, the history and physical examination alone are sufficient for specific diagnosis. For example, a thyrotoxic woman with a diffuse goiter and exophthalmos almost certainly has Graves disease, whereas a febrile patient with an extremely tender, wood-hard thyroid gland probably has subacute thyroiditis. In other patients, however, the underlying cause may be less certain. For example, a woman with postpartum thyrotoxicosis could have painless (postpartum) thyroiditis, Graves disease, or even factitious thyrotoxicosis—each of which would be treated quite differently. In such patients, further laboratory or radionuclide studies are needed to define the cause and optimal treatment.

The relative degrees of serum T_3 and T_4 elevations can provide a clue to the form of thyrotoxicosis. Predominant T_3 overproduction is common in Graves hyperthyroidism and, to a lesser extent, in toxic nodular goiter (i.e., a serum T_3-to-T_4 [ng/dl:μg/dl] ratio greater than 20). In contrast, T_4-predominant thyrotoxicosis (i.e., a serum T_3-to-T_4 ratio less than 15) suggests thyroiditis (subacute or lymphocytic), iodine-induced thyrotoxicosis, or exogenous T_4 ingestion.

Determining the fractional thyroid uptake of radioactive iodine or pertechnetate and thyroid imaging are required for etiologic diagnosis in some patients. Hyperthyroidism from excessive thyroid hormone synthesis, as in Graves disease, is typically accompanied by increased fractional uptake of the tracer in functioning tissue. In contrast, thyrotoxicosis caused by thyroid inflammation, exogenous thyroid hormone ingestion, and iodine exposure are all associated with a low thyroid uptake. Radionuclide imaging of the thyroid gland often permits differentiation of Graves disease from toxic nodular goiter, because tracer distribution is homogeneous in the former and focal in the latter. Radionuclide imaging can also localize ectopic thyroid tissue that may be hyperfunctioning, such as substernal toxic multinodular goiter and struma ovarii, an ovarian teratoma in which a toxic adenoma can arise.

Anti–TSH receptor immunoglobulin assays have limited clinical uses in differential diagnosis and management.[83] They may be helpful in confirming the diagnosis of Graves disease in clinically and biochemically euthyroid patients who have ophthalmopathy or when differentiation of Graves disease from toxic multinodular goiter is otherwise difficult and important for treatment. In pregnant women with Graves disease, the level of thyroid-stimulating immunoglobulins can predict the likelihood of fetal and neonatal thyrotoxicosis.

Other tests may be helpful in diagnosing certain other causes of thyrotoxicosis. Patients with subacute thyroiditis usually have an elevated erythrocyte sedimentation rate (ESR) and C-reactive protein level, whereas patients with lymphocytic (silent) thyroiditis do not.[88] In patients with thyrotoxicosis caused by thyroid hypersecretion or inflammation, the serum thyroglobulin concentration is high, whereas it is low in patients with factitious thyrotoxicosis. Measurements of the serum glycoprotein hormone α subunit may be useful to confirm the diagnosis of TSH-secreting pituitary adenoma, in which the molar ratio of the α subunit to intact TSH is higher than normal.

Differentiating the two causes of amiodarone-induced thyrotoxicosis is often very difficult, if not impossible. Both the iodine-induced type (type 1) and the inflammatory type (type 2) can be severe; both can be T_4 predominant, and both can be associated with a low thyroid radioiodine uptake. Early reports of higher interleukin-2 levels in the inflammatory form have not been confirmed. Glandular blood flow, as defined by Doppler sonography, is decreased in some patients with the inflammatory form, but this has also proved to be an imperfect distinguishing feature in many affected patients.

MANAGEMENT

Optimal treatment of patients with thyrotoxicosis depends on the underlying cause and severity of their condition and sometimes on the presence of complications that result from hyperthyroidism itself or the patient's other medical disorders. Transient thyrotoxicosis (e.g., exogenous and thyroiditis-related thyrotoxicosis) may require only symptomatic therapy with a beta-adrenergic blocking agent while awaiting spontaneous restoration of euthyroidism. Hyperthyroid Graves disease can be treated with antithyroid medication, radioiodine, or surgery; most of these patients ultimately require an ablative treatment. The hyperthyroidism caused by a toxic adenoma or toxic multinodular goiter will also respond to thionamides (e.g., methimazole and propylthiouracil [PTU]), but it almost never remits spontaneously, so radioiodine or surgery is always required. Fortunately, these three most commonly required therapies are quite comparable with regard to cost-effectiveness, and the vast majority of patients are satisfied with the treatment that they have chosen. Certain special forms of thyrotoxicosis, such as TSH-secreting pituitary adenoma and thyroid hormone intoxication, require other modes of treatment tailored to the responsible cause.

Beta-Adrenergic Blocking Agents

Beta blockers provide prompt relief from some symptoms of thyrotoxicosis, including tremor, palpitations, and anxiety. However, constitutional complaints, such as fatigue and weakness, and hypermetabolic manifestations, such as heat intolerance and weight loss, are unrelieved by beta-adrenergic blockade. These drugs are often valuable for temporary control of symptoms while awaiting a response to more definitive therapies or spontaneous remission of thyrotoxicosis. Beta blockers can be used—optimally, in combination with other drugs—to prepare patients with thyrotoxicosis for surgery. They are also useful for ventricular rate control in patients with thyrotoxic atrial fibrillation (see below). When used judiciously, beta blockers can be a component of treatment for some patients with thyrotoxic heart failure. Some beta blockers, such as propranolol, also partially inhibit extrathyroid T_4-to-T_3 conversion, but these agents do not otherwise address the underlying pathogenesis of thyrotoxicosis.

Antithyroid Drugs

The thionamide antithyroid drugs inhibit iodination and coupling, which are key steps in thyroid hormonogenesis.[89] Consequently, methimazole and PTU are effective treatments for forms of hyperthyroidism caused by excess thyroid hormone production by the gland, such as Graves disease. However, they are ineffective when thyrotoxicosis is caused by unregulated release of hormone from an inflamed gland, such as that which occurs in subacute thyroiditis. Overtreatment with thionamides causes hypothyroidism, so the dose must be titrated or thionamide use must be accompanied by thyroxine replacement. Compared with ablative therapies, antithyroid drugs have the advantage of lowering the long-term incidence of hypothyroidism. However, Graves disease is associated with a 25% long-term incidence of hypothyroidism, which results from the destructive effects of gland inflammation and occurs even with prolonged antithyroid drug treatment.

Thionamide treatment is an appropriate choice for patients with mild Graves disease, in whom the absence of severe manifestations (e.g., a large goiter, a very elevated serum T_4 level, or ophthalmopathy) predicts a higher spontaneous remission rate. Typically, antithyroid drugs are prescribed for 6 to 24 months, after which the dose is tapered to determine whether a remission has occurred. The antithyroid drugs are also useful in four other circumstances: (1) for temporary treatment of patients with Graves disease who are unwilling to accept definitive radioiodine therapy immediately, (2) for preliminary control of hyperthyroidism before definitive radioiodine or surgical treatment, (3) for the management of pregnant women with hyperthyroidism and neonatal Graves disease, and (4) to determine whether nonspecific symptoms are in fact related to mild thyrotoxicosis.

The antithyroid drugs have several limitations. First, they typically take 3 to 8 weeks to restore euthyroidism. Although they inhibit new thyroid hormone synthesis, they do not block the gland's release of existing hormone stores, which can be plentiful in patients with goitrous Graves disease, toxic nodular goiter, and amiodarone-induced thyrotoxicosis. Second, the antithyroid drugs' actions end when the drug is discontinued. As a result, virtually all patients with toxic nodular goiter and the majority of those with Graves disease will experience relapse when the medication is stopped. Third, antithyroid drugs have potential side effects. In addition to hypothyroidism resulting from overtreatment, they cause rash, pruritus, and fever in approximately 5% of treated patients. Much less commonly, severe adverse reactions can occur, including potentially fatal granulocytosis, vasculitis, or, with PTU, hepatic failure. All thionamide-treated patients must be warned of the symptoms and signs of these problems and be advised that if such manifestations occur, they should report the manifestations and immediately discontinue the medication. The likelihood of another adverse reaction occurring if a patient is switched from one thionamide to another is poorly documented, but such cross-reactivity does occur. Consequently, it is generally advisable in this circumstance to recommend radioiodine or surgery.

For most hyperthyroid patients, methimazole, 10 to 30 mg a day, is more effective and safer than PTU. Methimazole's longer half-life permits a single daily dose, which improves compliance; in contrast, PTU must be given three times daily for sustained effect. Methimazole at dosages of less than 40 mg a day is less likely than PTU to cause agranulocytosis and is not associated with hepatic failure. In certain circumstances, however, PTU, 100 to 200 mg a day in divided doses, may be preferred. In patients with severe and complicated thyrotoxicosis (see below), PTU has the advantage of also blocking extrathyroid T_4-to-T_3 conversion; a benefit in pregnant women is that PTU crosses the placenta less readily than methimazole and therefore has less of an effect on fetal thyroid function.

Radioiodine

Iodine-131 (^{131}I) is a highly effective, safe, and convenient treatment for hyperthyroid patients with hyperthyroid Graves disease, toxic multinodular goiter, and toxic adenoma. This radioisotope of iodine is preferentially concentrated in thyrocytes, where it emits beta particles (electrons) with a short path-length that limits the field of its destructive effects to the thyroid gland. With dosing regimens that are based on estimated gland size and preliminary thyroid radioiodine fractional uptake determinations, or even with empirical doses, a single dose will provide effective treatment for approximately 75% of Graves disease patients and 50% of patients with toxic nodular goiter. Almost all of the remaining patients are cured with a second radioiodine treatment, which is usually best held until the initial dose has proved ineffective after 6 months. For patients with toxic multinodular goiter, there is limited experience with the use of recombinant thyrotropin to increase thyroid uptake of radioiodine—a strategy that might be expected to improve the cure rate and permit a reduction in the administered dose of radioiodine.

Radioiodine has limitations. It takes 1 to 2 months before irradiated thyrocytes die and hyperthyroidism resolves; during this time, patients must often be treated with adjunctive beta-adrenergic blockade, antithyroid drugs, or stable iodide (see below). Approximately 25% of patients develop a transient worsening of thyrotoxicosis 2 to 4 weeks after treatment because of radiation thyroiditis, which can also cause mild and short-lived gland discomfort. The principal side effect of radioiodine is postablative hypothyroidism, which occurs within 3 months in more than half of radioiodine-treated Graves disease patients. Furthermore, in Graves disease patients who remain euthyroid, gland failure continues to occur at a rate of 3% annually, so lifelong follow-up of their thyroid function is essential. In patients with hyperthyroidism resulting from toxic multinodular goiter and toxic adenoma, the incidence of postablative hypothyroidism is lower (approximately 25%) because the suppressed normal extranodular tissue receives much less irradiation. During the more than 65 years that radioiodine has been used to treat hyperthyroidism,

the preponderance of evidence has shown no higher long-term incidence of thyroid or other malignancies. In radioiodine-treated women, no higher incidences of subsequent infertility or spontaneous abortion has been found, nor has there been a higher incidence of teratogenesis in their children. In one large follow-up study, radioiodine treatment of children and adolescents was associated with a higher subsequent incidence of benign thyroid nodules. As a result, many experts prefer to treat pediatric patients with antithyroid drugs for several years before resorting to radioiodine. However, radioiodine should not be withheld from children when hyperthyroidism is poorly controlled or side effects occur with thionamide therapy.

Radioiodine is inappropriate in several circumstances. It is absolutely contraindicated in pregnant women. All women of childbearing age should be advised to avoid pregnancy until euthyroidism is restored; this typically requires 3 to 6 months. Radioiodine is not indicated in transient forms of thyrotoxicosis, such as subacute and lymphocytic thyroiditis. Furthermore, it is ineffective in these and other forms of thyrotoxicosis in which the thyroid uptake of radioiodine is decreased, including amiodarone-induced thyrotoxicosis.

Surgery

Thyroidectomy by an experienced surgeon who has a demonstrated low incidence of complications is a highly effective, prompt, and relatively safe alternative. However, transient pain and scarring are universal after thyroidectomy, and postanesthetic symptoms are common. Partial thyroidectomy has an unacceptably high rate of residual hyperthyroidism; thus, gland resection that is extensive enough to ensure success can be expected to result in postsurgical hypothyroidism. Even in the most skilled surgical hands, there is a small risk (approximately 2% to 5%) of hypoparathyroidism or injury to the recurrent laryngeal nerve. Finally, for most patients, surgery is less convenient and entails greater interruption of life commitments than does radioiodine therapy.

Despite its drawbacks, surgery is the best choice in several settings. Pregnant women with severe thionamide side effects have no alternative. In some hyperthyroid patients, other aspects of their condition may make neck surgery necessary (e.g., the patient may have a cytologically suspicious thyroid nodule or hyperparathyroidism). Amiodarone-induced thyrotoxicosis can require surgery when medical treatment is ineffective and the patient's cardiovascular and metabolic status is deteriorating. For some patients, such as those planning prolonged travel in the near future and those who cannot or will not take medications reliably, surgery is attractive because it provides prompt and certain cure. Thyroidectomy is also preferred in countries that require prolonged hospitalization for even low-dose radioiodine therapy.

Other surgical procedures play a role in the treatment of certain rare forms of hyperthyroidism. Transsphenoidal pituitary adenomectomy is typically the first step in treatment of patients with TSH-secreting adenomas, but it is curative in only one third of patients.[90] Oophorectomy is appropriate when hyperthyroidism results from a toxic adenoma arising in teratomatous ovarian tissue in a patient with struma ovarii.

Other Agents

Stable iodide, given as either potassium iodide or Lugol solution in pharmacologic amounts (i.e., 30 mg or more a day), blocks thyroid hormone release from the gland and inhibits organification of iodide in patients with Graves disease. When combined with antithyroid drug therapy, iodide can accelerate the decline in circulating thyroid hormone concentrations. However, its effects are only temporary, dissipating after 10 to 14 days, after which hyperthyroidism recurs. Consequently, it is useful in only two settings. First, it can be employed as a short-term measure to prepare patients for thyroidectomy. Second, it can be started several days after radioiodine treatment to accelerate restoration of euthyroidism. In such patients, the irradiated gland is incapable of escaping from iodide's inhibitory effects. Iodide has infrequent side effects of rash, gastritis, and sialadenitis.

Iodinated radiocontrast agents, such as sodium iopanoate, can have two salutary effects in patients with severe thyrotoxicosis. First, they are an abundant source of iodide. Second, they inhibit T_4-to-T_3 conversion.

Lithium carbonate also inhibits hormone release from the thyroid gland. It is used in rare cases to accelerate recovery from severe thyrotoxicosis, as an adjunct to antithyroid medication in type 1 amiodarone-induced thyrotoxicosis, or as a short-term treatment for patients who have experienced severe thionamide side effects. Potassium perchlorate, which blocks iodide uptake by the thyroid, is a rarely used treatment of type 1 amiodarone-induced thyrotoxicosis.

Nonsteroidal anti-inflammatory drugs (NSAIDs) such as aspirin and ibuprofen are first-line agents for controlling thyroid pain and constitutional symptoms in subacute thyroiditis. They do not, however, accelerate recovery of normal thyroid function.

Glucocorticoids (e.g., prednisone, 40 mg/day) can be used to treat thyrotoxicosis under a few specific circumstances. When subacute thyroiditis is resistant to NSAID therapy, steroids are almost invariably effective. However, their side effects and the fact that they may prolong the overall course of subacute thyroiditis make them second-line agents. Glucocorticoid therapy is also useful in the treatment of type 2 amiodarone-induced thyrotoxicosis. Finally, when combined with high-dose antithyroid medication and iodinated radiocontrast agents, glucocorticoids can often be effective in controlling even severe thyrotoxic Graves disease within 1 week after initiation of therapy.

Other agents are employed to treat rare causes of thyrotoxicosis. Cholestyramine can be an adjunct in the treatment of patients with exogenous thyroid hormone intoxication; it interrupts the enterohepatic circulation of thyroid hormones and increases their fecal disposal. Somatostatin analogues are useful in the medical management of patients with inoperable TSH-secreting pituitary tumors or of patients whose tumors were incompletely resected.[91]

COMPLICATIONS

Atrial Fibrillation

Atrial tachyarrhythmias can occur with even mild thyrotoxicosis. Atrial fibrillation is the most common and potentially the most serious of these dysrhythmias; atrial flutter and paroxysmal atrial tachycardia also occur. Thyrotoxic atrial fibrillation occurs more often in older persons and men, as well as in persons with intrinsic cardiac diseases, particularly when these diseases cause left atrial enlargement. Thyrotoxic atrial fibrillation can be complicated by heart failure and thromboembolism. Beta blockers are useful for ventricular rate control; they are less likely to cause hypotension than calcium channel blockers, which remain an alternative. Anticoagulation is generally advisable. Exceptions are in patients in whom thyrotoxic atrial fibrillation has

been of short duration and rapidly reverts to sinus rhythm or in those with contraindications to anticoagulation. Cardioversion should generally be deferred until the patient is euthyroid. It should be attempted if spontaneous reversion to sinus rhythm does not occur by 3 months after euthyroidism has been restored[92] [*see Chapter 19*].

Thyrotoxic Heart Failure

When thyrotoxicosis is severe and prolonged or when the patient has intrinsic cardiac disease, heart failure can occur.[93] Contributing factors can include atrial fibrillation; ventricular hypertrophy and dilatation with impaired diastolic function; failure of mitral valve leaflet apposition and resulting regurgitation; and tachycardia-induced cardiomyopathy. Typically, one or more of these factors occurs in the context of increased peripheral tissue demands, vasodilatation, and an expanded blood volume. The left ventricular ejection fraction may be normal at rest but deteriorates with exertion. Therapy includes aggressive treatment of thyrotoxicosis, ventricular rate control, restoration of sinus rhythm when possible, and optimization of blood volume and ventricular filling pressures.

Thyroid Crisis

Thyroid crisis—so-called thyroid storm—refers to the life-threatening constellation of fever; heart failure, often with atrial fibrillation; delirium or psychosis; and fluid and electrolyte depletion resulting from poor oral intake and gastrointestinal losses caused by vomiting or diarrhea.[94] Patients with severe hyperthyroidism, underlying cardiac disease or superimposed infection, and poor access to health care are at increased risk for these complications.[95] Treatment entails medical management of each individual complication and aggressive therapy for thyrotoxicosis, typically with multiple agents appropriate for the underlying cause. Because Graves disease is the most common cause of thyroid storm, treatment typically includes PTU, sodium iopanoate, and glucocorticoids.

Graves Orbitopathy

For some patients with Graves disease, ocular and orbital involvement represents the most disabling aspect of their condition. Exposure keratitis resulting from proptosis, eyelid retraction, and lagophthalmos (inability to close the eye) causes symptoms and can be complicated by infection and ulceration. Treatment includes moistening eyedrops and lubricant ointments, sunglasses, taping the eyelids shut for sleeping, and sometimes blepharoplasty, orbital decompression surgery, and irradiation. Extraocular muscle swelling and fibrosis can cause diplopia, which can require prisms and sometimes corrective surgery. Optic nerve compression can threaten vision; it is treated acutely with high-dose glucocorticoids and definitively by orbital decompression surgery.

PROGNOSIS

Although the short-term morbidity of thyrotoxicosis can be disabling, the long-term outlook is generally bright, given accurate etiologic diagnosis and appropriate therapy targeted to the specific cause. However, many patients with Graves disease ultimately require lifelong treatment of postablative hypothyroidism, and their ophthalmopathy may be an ongoing source of discomfort, cosmetic concern, and, rarely, visual impairment. Mortality and severe long-term disability are rare events that typically result from either cardiovascular complications of thyrotoxicosis or side effects of antithyroid medication or thyroid surgery.

Thyroiditis

There are several types of thyroiditis, each of which has distinct causes, clinical manifestations, and treatments [see Table 3]. Some types cause thyroid dysfunction. When thyrotoxicosis occurs in these conditions, it is a transient result of the unregulated release of hormone from the gland, whereas hypothyroidism can be transient or permanent. Goiter occurs in some of these disorders (e.g., autoimmune thyroiditis and Reidel thyroiditis), whereas it is not a prominent feature of others. Pain is characteristic of subacute thyroiditis but is an uncommon feature of the other types.

AUTOIMMUNE THYROIDITIS

Autoimmune thyroiditis (Hashimoto disease) is a common condition, particularly in women, who are affected over 10 times more often than men. Its incidence increases with age; during and after middle life, approximately 20% of women have serologic evidence of the condition (i.e., thyroid autoantibodies), and 10% to 15% have an elevated serum TSH level secondary to thyroid hormone insufficiency. Its etiology, genetics, and pathogenesis are discussed elsewhere [see Hypothyroidism, above].

Clinical manifestations of autoimmune thyroiditis, when present, include hypothyroidism and a goiter. However, most affected patients have either no symptoms or only nonspecific ones, and they do not have significant gland enlargement. When present, the goiter is typically diffuse, modest in size, nontender, and firm with a roughened contour. Patients with the fibrous variant can have more substantial gland enlargement. Pain and tenderness are rarely present.

The presence of thyroid autoantibodies confirms the diagnosis, which can often be established on clinical grounds alone. Immunoassay for antithyroid peroxidase antibodies, which are present in 90% of patients, is the most sensitive single test[96]; antithyroglobulin antibodies are present in only 60% of patients. An elevated serum TSH concentration indicates associated primary hypothyroidism. The differential diagnosis of diffuse goiter includes simple euthyroid goiter, Graves disease, iodine-deficiency goiter, and, rarely, diffusely infiltrating malignancies (i.e., lymphoma, papillary cancer, and anaplastic cancer).

The management of patients with autoimmune thyroiditis includes thyroid hormone replacement for those who are hypothyroid and periodic thyroid function testing for those who are euthyroid but remain at risk for the development of hypothyroidism later in life. Women who have experienced transient hypothyroidism are particularly at risk. Associated goiter rarely requires any treatment, but thyroid hormone replacement sometimes results in partial gland shrinkage. The rare patient with thyroid pain may benefit from NSAIDs. The prognosis for properly treated and monitored patients is excellent. Certain other autoimmune disorders occur more often in affected patients; these can include vitiligo, pernicious anemia, adrenal insufficiency, Sjögren syndrome, and systemic sclerosis. Thyroid lymphoma is more common as well, but it is still a very rare event.

LYMPHOCYTIC THYROIDITIS

Lymphocytic thyroiditis (also known as painless thyroiditis, silent thyroiditis, or postpartum thyroiditis) is believed to be caused by cell-mediated autoimmunity. This belief is based on the fact that the gland is infiltrated with lymphocytes and the condition's incidence is highest postpartum—a time when autoimmune disorders are more common.[97] The condition is relatively common in the postpartum period, affecting approximately 6% of women between 2 and 12 months after delivery or abortion. Women with thyroid autoantibodies, previous episodes of postpartum thyroiditis, or type 1 diabetes mellitus are at markedly increased risk. The condition also occurs during treatment with immunomodulatory agents (see below). Rarely, lymphocytic thyroiditis may present in women or men at other times.

Lymphocytic thyroiditis can cause several patterns of transient thyroid dysfunction: thyrotoxicosis alone, thyrotoxicosis followed by hypothyroidism, hypothyroidism alone, or, rarely, hypothyroidism followed by thyrotoxicosis. The pathogenesis of these derangements is described elsewhere [see Thyrotoxicosis, above]. In postpartum women, symptoms of thyroid dysfunction can often be overlooked or mistaken for depression. Affected patients have a modest goiter or no goiter.

Serum TSH measurement is the best first-line test to detect thyroid dysfunction in patients with lymphocytic thyroiditis. In thyrotoxic patients, the condition can be differentiated from Graves disease, which can also present postpartum, by the absence of significant goiter or eye involvement; by relatively greater concentration of serum T_4 than of serum T_3 (ratio > 20:1 in μg/dl:ng/dl); and by a low thyroid radioisotope uptake. In hypothyroid patients, postpartum thyroiditis can best be distinguished from autoimmune thyroiditis by whether it remits spontaneously or not. Thyroid autoantibodies are detected in many postpartum thyroiditis patients.

Management can often be expectant, without drug treatment. Symptomatic thyrotoxicosis and hypothyroidism can be treated with temporary beta-adrenergic blockade and thyroxine, respectively. One quarter of affected patients go on to develop typical autoimmune thyroiditis and permanent hypothyroidism.

SUBACUTE THYROIDITIS (DE QUERVAIN OR GRANULOMATOUS THYROIDITIS)

Subacute thyroiditis is believed to be the result of a viral infection, because of its association with prodromal symptoms, the presence of circulating viral antibody titers, and electron microscopic evidence of viral particles. Classically, episodes of subacute thyroiditis have three clinical components. First are the systemic manifestations: symptoms suggesting a viral upper respiratory tract infection, followed by malaise, fever, and chills. The second is a painful goiter, which is characteristically moderate in size, wood-hard, and extremely tender. The third is transient thyrotoxicosis, which can be quite severe. The thyrotoxicosis lasts for 2 to 8 weeks and is typically followed by transient hypothyroidism. Although the clinical features of subacute thyroiditis are usually sufficient to suggest the diagnosis, constitutional symptoms (especially high fever) can mimic other infections, and thyroid pain radiating to the ears can be confused with otitis. Thyrotoxicosis is confirmed by a low serum TSH and a high serum T_4 concentration. Marked elevation of the ESR is detectable during the acute phase of the illness. Other causes of painful thyroid enlargement include hemorrhage into a thyroid nodule, which is usually asymmetrical; acute thyroiditis (see below); thyroid lymphoma or anaplastic thyroid cancer; and, very rarely, autoimmune thyroiditis or Graves disease.

Management of subacute thyroiditis entails prescription of an NSAID in high dosage. In approximately 20% of patients, this provides inadequate relief of pain and constitutional symptoms;

these patients can be treated with glucocorticoid therapy (e.g., prednisone, 40 mg/day with a slow taper over 3 to 8 weeks). Transient thyrotoxic symptoms are treated with beta blockers; transient hypothyroid symptoms are treated with thyroxine. In more than 80% of cases, normal thyroid function returns and the condition does not recur.

ACUTE THYROIDITIS (SUPPURATIVE THYROIDITIS)

Acute or suppurative thyroiditis is a rare condition caused by either untreated bacterial infections of the upper respiratory tract or cervical soft tissues or by opportunistic agents in immuno-compromised hosts. Hematogenous spread to the thyroid of fungal, mycobacterial, and parasitic infections have all been reported. Piriform sinus fistula, multinodular goiter, or autoimmune thyroiditis may predispose patients to acute thyroiditis.

Patients with suppurative infections typically are extremely ill, with high fever; a painful, tender, swollen thyroid gland; and erythema and warmth of overlying soft tissues. Glands infected with opportunistic pathogens (e.g., *Pneumocystis jiroveci*) may have more subtle signs of gland infection. Treatment requires aggressive, often parenteral, antibiotic therapy and sometimes surgical drainage.

DRUG-INDUCED THYROIDITIS

Several drugs have been associated with painless thyroiditis and thyroid dysfunction, including amiodarone (see above). Treatment of hepatitis C with interferon alfa and interleukin-2 causes thyroid dysfunction in as many as 15% of patients; such dysfunction includes transient thyrotoxicosis with or without subsequent hypothyroidism, as well as persistent hypothyroidism and persistent hyperthyroidism (i.e., Graves disease). Lithium carbonate can exacerbate thyroid dysfunction and cause hypothyroidism in patients with underlying autoimmune thyroiditis. Rarely, pharmacologic doses of iodide can cause transient thyroiditis.

REIDEL THYROIDITIS

Reidel thyroiditis is an extremely rare form of invasive fibrous thyroiditis that can cause substantial goiter with compression and infiltration of adjacent structures. Some patients with this idiopathic disorder also develop hypothyroidism. It may be encountered in patients with retroperitoneal and mediastinal fibrosis. Treatment options are limited. Surgery is challenging and is limited to palliation of obstructive complications. There are reports of effective drug treatment with glucocorticoids and tamoxifen.[98]

Goiter, Thyroid Nodules, and Thyroid Cancer

GOITER

Epidemiology

The prevalence of goiter in populations varies inversely with dietary iodine intake. There are estimated to be 100 million persons with dietary iodine deficiency and one billion with borderline iodine sufficiency. Consequently, in some regions, goiter is almost universal, particularly in women, whereas in regions with an adequate iodine intake, goiter affects less than 5% of the population.

Etiology and Pathogenesis

Worldwide, dietary iodine deficiency is the most common cause of thyroid gland enlargement. In addition, populations have been described in which exposure to goitrogens in drinking water or dietary substances has caused endemic goiter.[99] Although modest thyroid gland enlargement occurs during pregnancy, the so-called goiter of pregnancy is largely restricted to women with associated dietary iodine deficiency. Tobacco smoking has been associated with goiter development, especially in populations without ample dietary iodine. Mutations in genes encoding key proteins involved in thyroid hormone synthesis (e.g., thyroglobulin and thyroid peroxidase), can result in a compensatory goiter. Activation of the TSH receptor by TSH predictably causes diffuse goiter, as occurs in a variety of conditions, including primary hypothyroidism from autoimmune thyroiditis or drugs, TSH-secreting pituitary adenoma, and resistance to thyroid hormone. The TSH receptor can be aberrantly stimulated when thyroid-stimulating immunoglobulins or high levels of hCG bind to it or when a mutation in the TSH receptor gene itself leads to constitutive activation. For the majority of patients with hyperplastic thyroid glands arising despite sufficient dietary iodine—a condition that is sometimes apparently inherited and sometimes sporadic—the precise molecular cause remains unknown. Activation of the biochemical pathways signaling thyrocyte growth or abnormal local levels or activity of intrathyroid growth factors seems likely to be involved. Goiter can also be the result of gland infiltration with inflammatory cells (e.g., leukocytes and multinucleated giant cells in subacute thyroiditis) or tumor cells (e.g., anaplastic or diffusely infiltrating papillary thyroid cancers).

In summary, goiter can be associated with hypothyroidism, euthyroidism (nontoxic goiter), or hyperthyroidism (toxic goiter). It can be a manifestation of benign hyperplastic or neoplastic conditions, malignancy, and inflammation. In many of these disorders, thyroid gland enlargement is initially diffuse, but with time, the thyroid becomes multinodular, and it may become asymmetrical.

Diagnosis and Differential Diagnosis

For the clinician evaluating a patient with a goiter, three pragmatic questions are typically more important than the specific etiologic diagnosis. First, is the enlarged thyroid gland producing pain or other local symptoms as a result of obstruction or invasion of adjacent structures, or is it so large as to be unsightly? Second, is the goiter a manifestation of a disorder causing hypothyroidism or hyperthyroidism that requires treatment? Third, is the gland enlarged because of malignancy?

Clinical manifestations Symptoms related to a goiter reflect gland impingement on adjacent structures. A sensation of cervical fullness, tightness, or pain can occur when the enlarging gland stretches its capsule, which has sensory innervation, and compresses adjacent tissues and structures. Thyroid pain can radiate to the jaw or ears. Tracheal compression can cause cough and difficulty clearing mucus; tracheal invasion from thyroid malignancy can cause hemoptysis. Esophageal compression can produce dysphagia and, rarely, odynophagia. Compression of the recurrent laryngeal nerve results in hoarseness, a weak voice, and dysphagia for fluids; bilateral nerve dysfunction can also cause dyspnea from airway obstruction.

Physical examination Inspection during deglutition often provides the first clue to the presence of a goiter. In addition, it helps distinguish true enlargement of the thyroid, which moves cephalad with swallowing, whereas subcutaneous fat does not.

Any tracheal deviation, cervical vein engorgement, or visible adenopathy should also be noted. On palpation, the dimensions of the gland and its symmetry, contour, consistency, mobility, and tenderness should all be noted.

Other physical findings can provide important information. A bruit suggests either a hypervascular Graves disease gland or compression of cervical blood vessels. Venous engorgement and facial plethora that develops when the patient touches the hands together above the head (Pemberton sign) implies near obstruction of the thoracic outlet by a goiter. Signs of hypothyroidism or hyperthyroidism should, of course, be sought.

Laboratory tests and imaging studies In all patients with goiter, the serum TSH and free T_4 concentrations should be measured to assess gland function. Serologic testing for thyroid autoantibodies, especially anti–thyroid peroxidase antibody, can help establish the diagnosis of autoimmune thyroiditis, the most common cause of diffuse goiter in populations with sufficient dietary iodine.

Ultrasonography can be useful in confirming that a neck mass is, in fact, a goiter. It can define the gland size; determine whether there is diffuse heterogeneity typical of autoimmune thyroiditis or discrete nodules; and identify potentially related cervical adenopathy. A chest and lower cervical x-ray can show tracheal deviation and suggest mediastinal extension of a goiter, but computed tomography or magnetic resonance imaging provides a fuller depiction of the gland's substernal extent and its relationship to the trachea and intrathoracic structures. The decision whether or not to use iodinated radiocontrast agents with CT imaging should be thoughtfully addressed, because these agents can precipitate hyperthyroidism in patients with multinodular goiter and can interfere with subsequent postoperative radioiodine therapy in patients who prove to have thyroid cancer. Radionuclide imaging is seldom required in the initial assessment of patients with goiter, but it can confirm that a superior or mediastinal mass concentrating radioiodine is thyroidal in origin. Radioiodine fractional uptakes and imaging can be useful in the differential diagnosis of goitrous thyrotoxicosis (see above). Assessment of ventilatory flow-volume loops can be useful in determining whether dyspnea in a patient with goitrous tracheal compression is caused by the thyroid condition. Although cytologic evaluation plays a central role in the differential diagnosis of thyroid nodules, it is required in only a small minority of patients with diffuse goiters that cannot be readily characterized with clinical, laboratory, and imaging findings.

Management

Management of goiter addresses three key clinical issues: size, function, and potential malignancy. Treatment for thyroid dysfunction or thyroid cancer is the same as in patients without goiter. Large nontoxic, multinodular goiters causing obstructive symptoms or cosmetic concerns can be surgically excised or, if obstruction is not severe, treated with radioiodine.[100] Surgery provides more prompt relief and excludes cancer with certainty, but it is associated with greater short-term morbidity than radioiodine therapy. Even goiters with substantial substernal extension can often be removed through a cervical incision. Recombinant thyrotropin can successfully augment ^{131}I concentration by nodular goiters, which typically have only a normal fractional radioiodine uptake.[101] TSH-suppressive thyroxine therapy has limited value in the treatment of most patients with goiters of significant dimensions. Published experience shows that no more than half

of patients have a response, which is often only partial.[102] Furthermore, long-term TSH suppression is associated with risks of bone loss and atrial fibrillation.

Complications and Prognosis

The type and probability of complications in patients with goiter depend on the underlying cause. Most patients with gland enlargement of benign cause never suffer local compressive symptoms and require treatment only if they have associated thyroid dysfunction (i.e., hypothyroidism in patients with autoimmune thyroiditis or hyperthyroidism in patients with multinodular goiter). However, large multinodular goiters can cause dyspnea from tracheal narrowing or dysphagia from esophageal compression. Recurrent laryngeal nerve impingement and dysfunction is very unusual and should raise concern of malignancy. Rarely, thyroid substernal goiter extension can cause superior vena cava obstruction. Goiter from papillary or anaplastic thyroid cancer or lymphoma can cause all of the complications associated with goiters from benign causes, as well as pain from invasion of adjacent structures, hemoptysis from tracheal invasion, and vocal cord paresis from recurrent laryngeal nerve involvement.

THYROID NODULES

Epidemiology and Etiology

Thyroid nodules are palpable in 6% of women and 2% of men.[2] Nonpalpable thyroid nodules can be detected by sonography in one third of women. The prevalence of nodules increases with age. The genetic and environmental factors associated with thyroid nodule development are essentially the same as those for goiter. Nodules may represent solid tissue composed of thyroid cells or colloid or represent cysts from accumulated serous fluid or blood, often from hemorrhage within a solid nodule in the gland. The majority of thyroid nodules are benign; in adults, 5% to 10% of thyroid nodules are cancerous.

Diagnosis

Three clinical issues must be addressed in patients with thyroid nodules: the nodule's size and the resulting potential for local complications, the possibility of associated thyroid dysfunction, and malignancy.[103] The same principles and approach apply to palpable thyroid nodules as to incidentally detected nodules (so-called thyroid incidentalomas) that are greater than 1.0 to 1.5 cm in diameter.[104] After proper assessment, the majority of patients will be found to have none of these three problems, and they can be monitored conservatively.

Clinical Manifestations

Thyroid nodules are usually detected incidentally by asymptomatic patients themselves or by their physicians. Rapidly enlarging or invasive nodules may cause pain in the anterior neck, jaw, or ear. Tracheal or esophageal compression can cause cough or dysphagia, respectively. Invasion of the trachea or recurrent laryngeal nerve by tumor can produce the worrisome symptoms of hemoptysis or hoarseness, respectively. Symptoms of thyrotoxicosis suggest the possibility of toxic adenoma, whereas complaints consistent with hypothyroidism may reflect autoimmune thyroiditis and an asymmetrical goiter that is mimicking a true nodule.

The presence of pulmonary, skeletal, or neurologic symptoms suggesting metastatic disease increases concern about a primary thyroid cancer. An increased risk of thyroid cancer is also suggested by a history of childhood or adolescent irradiation; irradiation was employed until the early 1950s for thymic enlargement, tonsillitis, adenoiditis, cutaneous hemangiomas, and acne. A family history of thyroid cancer is also an indication for thorough assessment, especially if the familial disease is medullary or papillary thyroid cancer. A history of hyperparathyroidism or pheochromocytoma raises the possibility of the multiple endocrine neoplasia type II (MEN II) syndrome, which includes these disorders and medullary thyroid cancer.[105] Hypercalcitoninemia in patients with metastatic medullary thyroid cancer can cause flushing, pruritus, and diarrhea.

Physical Examination

Nodules that are fixed or associated with ipsilateral cervical adenopathy are worrisome for thyroid cancer. Nodule size and consistency are not reliable features for distinguishing benign from malignant lesions. Although multiple thyroid nodules are typical of benign multinodular goiter, a nodule that is larger, that is growing more rapidly, or that is more symptomatic than others in the gland requires the same assessment as a solitary thyroid nodule. Signs of hyperthyroidism or hypothyroidism suggest toxic adenoma or autoimmune thyroiditis, respectively. Patients with the MEN IIB (or MEN III) syndrome, which includes medullary thyroid cancer and pheochromocytoma, can have a Marfanoid body habitus and submucosal neuromas that are visible as lumps beneath the buccal mucosa and conjunctivae.

Laboratory Tests

The serum TSH concentration should be measured: a low serum TSH suggests a possible toxic adenoma; a high TSH, autoimmune thyroiditis. Antithyroid antibody screening can corroborate the diagnosis of autoimmune thyroiditis in patients who actually have diffuse but asymmetrical thyroid gland enlargement. Serum calcitonin should be measured in patients with clinical features that suggest hypercalcitoninemia or the MEN II syndrome. The serum thyroglobulin assay is not helpful in distinguishing benign from malignant thyroid nodules.

For most thyroid nodules, the definitive diagnostic procedure is fine-needle aspiration to provide cytologic material for examination by an experienced pathologist. Sonographic guidance of aspiration can be useful when nodules are poorly localized by palpation or for the assessment of lesions that have a cystic component; in addition, it can sometimes be useful in identifying additional nonpalpable nodules requiring assessment.[106] Radionuclide imaging currently has only a secondary role in thyroid nodule assessment. In thyroid nodule patients whose serum TSH concentration is low, a iodine-123 or technetium-99m pertechnetate scan that indicates that the nodule is "hot" (i.e., that shows a concentration of tracer in the nodule, with suppression of uptake in the remainder of the gland) provides assurance that the nodule is benign. CT and MRI have no role in the evaluation of the typical patient with a thyroid nodule unless there is substernal extension of a nodular goiter.

Differential Diagnosis

Clinical features of thyroid nodules are sometimes helpful but seldom provide definitive diagnosis. Sonography can confirm that an ambiguous neck mass is thyroidal. Radionuclide imaging should be limited to patients with a suppressed serum TSH concentration. The sensitivity and specificity of cytologic assessment of thyroid nodules are 97% and 95%, respectively. However, approximately 20% of nodules are cytologically indeterminate, among which approximately 15% are malignant.[107] Some thyroid nodules can ultimately be definitively diagnosed only by surgical excision and histopathologic examination.

Management, Complications, and Prognosis

Most cytologically benign thyroid nodules can be managed with observation only, unless the lesion is so large as to cause discomfort, other local compressive complications, or cosmetic concern. Because cytology is not 100% sensitive for cancer exclusion, patients should be followed up for 12 to 24 months. For palpable lesions, follow-up should consist of physical examination; for nonpalpable lesions, sonography is usually advisable. Toxic adenomas diagnosed on the basis of a low serum TSH level and radionuclide confirmation of hot-nodule status can usually be assumed to be benign; treatment of associated thyrotoxicosis is, of course, indicated. Patients with cytologically malignant nodules should undergo thyroidectomy unless their general medical condition contraindicates it. Most patients with cytologically indeterminate nodules require surgery for definitive diagnosis, although if the suspicion of cancer is low, thyroid lobectomy may be worth considering. A subset of patients with cytologically indeterminate thyroid nodules (e.g., older women with multinodular goiter and no clinical features suggesting malignancy) can be followed with sonographic monitoring of the nodules' dimensions.

THYROID CANCER

Epidemiology

Thyroid cancers represent approximately 2% of clinically detected malignancies.[108] The most common tumor types, arising from follicular epithelium (i.e., papillary, follicular, and Hürthle cell cancers), occur three times more often in women and increase in incidence with age. Medullary thyroid cancer arising from parafollicular C cells represents less than 10% of all thyroid cancers but has special importance because of its common familial occurrence. In the United States, the reported incidence of thyroid cancer is rising, perhaps because these tumors are being detected more easily with contemporary diagnostic tools.[109]

Etiology and Pathogenesis

The cause of most thyroid cancers is unknown. Genetic predisposition to papillary thyroid cancer is seen in the familial syndromes of familial adenomatous polyposis (*APC* gene mutation) and Cowden syndrome (*PTEN* gene mutations). It can also occur as familial isolated papillary thyroid cancer. Overall, however, familial cases represent less than 10% of all thyroid cancers.[110] Thyroid irradiation from external sources and accidental radioiodine exposure predisposes to the development of malignant and benign thyroid tumors, as has been observed after radiotherapy (e.g., for recurrent tonsillitis and lymphoma) and after exposure to radioactive iodine fallout from a nuclear-weapon detonation or nuclear-reactor accident. Radioiodine exposure has been shown to produce a characteristic chromosomal rearrangement that creates the *RET/PTC* oncogene.

Progression and clinical aggressiveness of thyroid malignancies have been associated with a sequence of molecular events, including *BRAF* gene mutation and loss of the *p53* tumor suppressor gene.[111] Controversy surrounds evidence relating the development of thyroid cancer to preexisting benign thyroid conditions; to parity and estrogen therapy in women; to previous therapeutic radioiodine exposure; and to dietary factors, including iodine intake. Dietary iodine does clearly influence the distribution of thyroid cancer types, with more papillary cancers in populations with generous dietary iodine content.

Diagnosis

Clinical manifestations and physical examination Most thyroid cancers present as a thyroid nodule in an otherwise asymptomatic and euthyroid patient. Enlargement of the mass over weeks or months is more suspicious for cancer than long-standing stable size or very rapid appearance, which can represent hemorrhage into a preexisting benign nodule. Less commonly, patients develop complaints related to local invasion (e.g., pain, hoarseness, or hemoptysis) or distant metastatic disease (e.g., dyspnea, bone pain, or neurologic symptoms). On physical examination, nodule fixation or ipsilateral cervical adenopathy suggests thyroid cancer.

Laboratory tests Cytologic diagnosis of thyroid cancer can often be established from material obtained by fine-needle aspiration of suspicious thyroid nodules [*see* Thyroid Nodules, *above*]. Patients with cytologically indeterminate lesions usually require surgery for definitive diagnosis. Novel molecular markers, such as *BRAF* in papillary thyroid cancers, may in the future permit more accurate preoperative diagnosis and exclusion of cancer in these lesions. In thyroid cancer patients who present with metastatic disease in cervical nodes, lungs, bone, and other sites, biopsy of the identified lesion often establishes the diagnosis, which can be confirmed by thyroglobulin immunostaining. Subsequent careful examination and sonographic imaging of the thyroid gland typically reveal a nodule that can then itself be subject to biopsy.

Management

The therapeutic modalities commonly employed to treat patients with epithelial thyroid cancers are surgical thyroidectomy, radioiodine, and TSH-suppressive thyroid hormone therapy. Physicians and surgeons face the challenge of determining how aggressively these treatments should be applied to these patients, who exhibit a wide spectrum of disease behavior.[112]

When the diagnosis has been made preoperatively, total or near-total thyroidectomy is the procedure of choice. The rationale for bilateral thyroid excision is that papillary cancer, the most common thyroid malignancy, is often multifocal, involving the contralateral lobe in at least 20% of cases. Bilateral surgery has been shown to be associated with a lower papillary cancer recurrence rate.[113] In addition, removal of all, or nearly all, normal thyroid tissue positions patients for more accurate long-term monitoring with serum thyroglobulin measurement and radioiodine imaging. When thyroid cancer is unexpectedly diagnosed after lobectomy, these potential benefits must be balanced against the risks and inconvenience of completion thyroidectomy. For patients with microscopic papillary and minimally invasive follicular cancers, unilateral surgery may be deemed to have been adequate.[114] Unless regional node metastases are recognized before thyroidectomy, selective central neck compartment node excision is generally advisable, although modified radical neck dissection is justifiable when extensive nodal involvement is identified before or at the time of initial surgery.

Postoperatively, ^{131}I is often recommended for patients with epithelial thyroid cancers, with the rationale of eradicating residual disease and ablating remnant thyroid tissue that will otherwise limit the accuracy of long-term monitoring with serum thyroglobulin and radioiodine scans. The value of adjunctive radioiodine treatment to reduce risk of tumor recurrence has been shown in retrospective and observational trials for patients with more advanced stages of disease.[115] The principal factors related to an increased risk of recurrence are older patient age, larger tumor size, extrathyroidal invasion, incomplete tumor resection, and extensive and nodal metastases. In addition, certain histologic subtypes of thyroid cancer are more likely to recur, including the tall cell, columnar cell, and insular variants of papillary thyroid cancer, as well as follicular cancers with vascular invasion. Traditionally, patients have been withdrawn from thyroid hormone therapy postoperatively to effect a rise in endogenous TSH and to facilitate radioiodine uptake by residual thyroid tissue. This is effective but predictably causes clinical hypothyroidism. It has now been shown that radioiodine therapy can also be effective in euthyroid patients who are given recombinant thyrotropin.[116]

Patients with epithelial thyroid carcinoma require long-term thyroxine therapy both to replace thyroid hormone and to suppress TSH to reduce the risk of tumor recurrence. Typically, the thyroxine dose is increased until the lowest dosage capable of suppressing the serum TSH concentration to less than 0.1 μU/L is identified. In patients with symptoms of thyrotoxicosis or patients at low risk for tumor recurrence, the target TSH concentration may adjusted to the 0.1 to 0.5 μU/L range.

Patients treated for epithelial thyroid cancers require long-term follow-up to detect recurrent disease, which can present years after initial therapy. Serum thyroglobulin measurement has become the first-line choice for tumor detection.[117] This thyroid-specific protein should be undetectable in the blood of patients who have no residual thyroid cancer and who have undergone complete ablation of normal thyroid tissue. When circulating thyroglobulin is detected—whether during thyroid hormone therapy or after TSH stimulation by either thyroid hormone withdrawal or recombinant TSH administration—imaging techniques should be employed to localize the residual disease. Cervical sonography and fine-needle aspiration of suspicious adenopathy is the most productive initial step, followed by CT of the chest and, in patients with a serum thyroglobulin concentration greater than 10 ng/ml, 18-fluorodeoxyglucose positron emission tomography. Radioiodine scanning with ^{123}I or ^{131}I is another monitoring technique that is particularly helpful in identifying residual normal thyroid tissue as the source of circulating thyroglobulin and in localizing iodine-avid residual cancer tissue that may be amenable to radioiodine therapy. Radioiodine imaging also requires TSH stimulation by thyroid hormone withdrawal or recombinant TSH administration.[118]

Additional treatment modalities may be required for patients with advanced epithelial thyroid cancers.[119] Radioiodine can be employed for iodine-avid metastatic disease that is nonresectable, such as pulmonary metastases in younger patients with papillary thyroid cancer and metastatic follicular thyroid cancer in older patients. Repeat surgery may be indicated to excise recurrent cervical disease and, occasionally, other distant metastatic lesions that are solitary or that threaten to cause complications. External-beam radiotherapy can be used to treat nonresectable cervical disease, painful bone lesions, or pulmonary metastases causing airway obstruction or hemoptysis. Chemotherapy for these tumors has only a partial response rate; moreover, the response rate is relatively low, and the risk of side effects is significant. Nonetheless, chemotherapy may be offered when other alternatives have been exhausted.

Less common and more aggressive thyroid malignancies are managed with some of the same therapeutic modalities. Medullary thyroid cancer is treated with initial thyroidectomy.[120] Thyroid hormone therapy for replacement, but not TSH suppression, is then prescribed. Patients are followed with serial calcitonin and carcinoembryonic antigen measurements. Repeat surgery, external-beam radiotherapy, and chemotherapy (which is relatively ineffective) are sometimes employed. Thyroid lymphoma, which is primary to the thyroid gland in half of cases, is diagnosable with tissue biopsy and is treated, sometimes rather effectively, with combined chemotherapy and radiation therapy. Anaplastic thyroid cancer is typically nonresectable and is also treated with combined external-beam radiotherapy and chemotherapy.[121] Only in exceptional cases, however, do these interventions significantly alter the grim prognosis.

Complications

Complications can occur in thyroid cancer patients as a result of the malignancy or its treatment. Local cervical invasion of the recurrent laryngeal nerve can cause temporary or permanent hoarseness, dysphagia, and dyspnea. Progression of tumor in the neck can lead to strangulation or esophageal obstruction and malnutrition. Pulmonary failure can occur with pulmonary metastases, fractures with bony involvement, paraparesis with paraspinal lesions, and other neurologic consequences with brain dissemination. Functioning metastases can cause thyrotoxicosis in patients with follicular cancer and, rarely, in patients with papillary carcinoma.

Thyroidectomy may be complicated by recurrent laryngeal nerve injury or hypoparathyroidism. Radioiodine treatment can cause gastritis with short-term symptoms, and it can cause sialadenitis, whose symptoms are dry mouth, loss of taste, and dental caries. High cumulative doses of therapeutic ^{131}I have been associated with an increase in the risk of leukemia. External-beam radiotherapy and chemotherapy have their usual potential for adverse reactions.

Prognosis

The indolent growth of most thyroid tumors and the efficacy of available therapies result in a low mortality, with survival rates of 98% for papillary, 92% for follicular, and 80% for medullary cancers.[122] Clinical recurrence is common, however; for example, almost one third of papillary thyroid cancers recur. Extracervical medullary cancer is incurable but generally follows a slowly progressive course. Poorly differentiated epithelial cell thyroid cancers and anaplastic thyroid cancers unfortunately can be among the most aggressive and treatment-resistant malignancies known.

The author has received grants for clinical research or educational activities from or served as advisor or consultant to Abbott Laboratories and Genzyme Corporation during the past year.

Recombinant thyroid-stimulating hormone has not been approved by the FDA for treatment of nodular goiter and postoperative ablation of thyroid gland remnant tissue.

References

1. Hollowell JG, Staehling NW, Flanders WD, et al: Serum TSH, T(4), and thyroid antibodies in the United States population (1988 to 1994): National Health and Nutrition Examination Survey (NHANES III). J Clin Endocrinol Metab 87:489, 2002

2. Vander JB, Gaston EA, Dawber TR: The significance of nontoxic thyroid nodules: final report of a 15 year study of the incidence of thyroid malignancy. Ann Intern Med 69:537, 1968

3. Brander AE, Viikinkoski VP, Nickels JI, et al: Importance of thyroid abnormalities detected at US screening: a 5-year follow-up. Radiology 215:801, 2000

4. Trowbridge FL, Hand KE, Nichaman MZ: Findings relating to goiter and iodine in the Ten-State Nutrition Survey. Am J Clin Nutr 28:712, 1975

5. Soldin OP, Soldin SJ, Pezzullo JC: Urinary iodine percentile ranges in the United States. Clin Chim Acta 328:185, 2003

6. NCI Fact Book. National Cancer Institute, Washington DC, 2004, p C-2 http://www3.cancer.gov/admin/fmb/03Factbk.pdf

7. Roberts C, Ladenson PW: Hypothyroidism. Lancet 363:793, 2004

8. Chopra IJ, Solomon DH, Chopra U, et al: Abnormalities in thyroid function in relatives of patients with Graves disease and Hashimoto's thyroiditis: lack of correlation with inheritance of HLA-B8. J Clin Endocrinol Metab 45:45, 1977

9. Muller AF, Drexhage HA, Berghout A: Postpartum thyroiditis and autoimmune thyroiditis in women of childbearing age: recent insights and consequences for antenatal and postnatal care. Endocr Rev 22:605, 2001

10. Falorni A, Laureti S, Santeusanio F: Autoantibodies in autoimmune polyendocrine syndrome type II. Endocrinol Metab Clin North Am 31:369, 2002

11. Dayan CM, Daniels GH: Chronic autoimmune thyroiditis. N Engl J Med 335:99, 1996

12. Allen EM, Hsueh W-C, Sabra M, et al: A genome-wide scan for autoimmune thyroid disease in the Old Order Amish: replication of loci on chromosomes 5q11.2-q14.3 and 18p11.31 and modest evidence for linkage in four other regions. J Clin Endocrinol Metab 88:1292, 2003

13. Koh LK, Greenspan FS, Yeo PP: Interferon-alpha induced thyroid dysfunction: three clinical presentations and a review of the literature. Thyroid 7:891, 1997

14. Sklar C, Whitton J, Mertens A, et al: Abnormalities of the thyroid in survivors of Hodgkin's disease: data from the Childhood Cancer Survivor Study. J Clin Endocrinol Metab 85:3227, 2000

15. Martino E, Safran M, Aghini-Lombardi F, et al: Environmental iodine intake and thyroid dysfunction during chronic amiodarone therapy. Ann Intern Med 101:28, 1984

16. Lazarus JH: The effects of lithium therapy on thyroid and thyrotropin-releasing hormone. Thyroid 8:909, 1998

17. Li FX, Squartsoff L, Lamm SH: Prevalence of thyroid diseases in Nevada counties with respect to perchlorate in drinking water. J Occup Environ Med 43:630, 2001

18. Rose SR: Cranial irradiation and central hypothyroidism. Trends Endocrinol Metab 12:97, 2001

19. Segal-Lieberman G, Karasik A, Shimon I: Hypopituitarism following closed head injury. Pituitary 3:181, 2000

20. Sherman SI: Etiology, diagnosis, and treatment recommendations for central hypothyroidism associated with bexarotene therapy for cutaneous T-cell lymphoma. Clin Lymphoma 3:249, 2003

21. Yen PM: Physiological and molecular basis of thyroid hormone action. Physiol Rev 81:1097, 2001

22. Davis PJ, Davis FB: Nongenomic actions of thyroid hormone. Thyroid 6:497, 1996

23. Ladenson PW, Braverman LE, Mazzaferri EL, et al: Comparison of administration of recombinant human thyrotropin with withdrawal of thyroid hormone for radioactive iodine scanning in patients with thyroid carcinoma. N Engl J Med 337:888, 1997

24. Canaris GJ, Steiner JF, Ridgway EC: Do traditional symptoms of hypothyroidism correlate with biochemical disease? J Gen Intern Med 12:544, 1997

25. Nickel SN, Frame B: Neurological manifestations of myxedema. Neurology 8:511, 1958

26. Clarnette RM, Patterson CJ: Hypothyroidism: does treatment cure dementia? J Geriatr Psychiatry Neurol 7:23, 1994

27. Morris MS, Bostom AG, Jacques PF, et al: Hyperhomocysteinemia and hypercholesterolemia associated with hypothyroidism in the Third US National Health and Nutrition Examination Survey. Atherosclerosis 155:195, 2001

28. Demers LM, Spencer CA: Laboratory support for the diagnosis and monitoring of thyroid disease. The National Academy of Clinical Biochemistry Laboratory Medicine Practice Guidelines. National Academy of Clinical Biochemistry, Washington DC, 2002 http://www.nacb.org/lmpg/thyroid_lmpg_pub.stm

29. Faglia G, Bitensky L, Pinchera A, et al: Thyrotropin secretion in patients with central hypothyroidism: evidence for reduced biological activity of immunoreactive thyrotropin. J Clin Endocrinol Metab 48:989, 1979

30. Beck-Peccoz P, Amr S, Menezes-Ferreira MM, et al: Decreased receptor binding of biologically inactive thyrotropin in central hypothyroidism: effect of treatment with thyrotropin-releasing hormone. N Engl J Med 312:1085, 1985

31. Beck-Peccoz P, Brucker-Davis F, Persani L, et al: Thyrotropin-secreting pituitary tumors. Endocr Rev 17:610, 1996

32. Beck-Peccoz P, Chatterjee VK: The variable clinical phenotype in thyroid hormone resistance syndrome. Thyroid 4:225, 1994

33. Hamblin PS, Dyer SA, Mohr VS, et al: Relationship between thyrotropin and thyroxine changes during recovery from severe hypothyroxinemia of critical illness. J Clin Endocrinol Metab 62:717, 1986

34. Smith PJ, Surks MI: Multiple effects of 5,5'-diphenylhydantoin on the thyroid hormone system. Endocr Rev 5:514, 1984

35. Meyer CM, Ladenson PW, Scharfstein JA, et al: Evaluation of common problems in primary care: effects of physician, practice, and financial characteristics. Am J Manag Care 6:457, 2000

36. Vanderpump MP, Tunbridge WM, French JM, et al: The incidence of thyroid disorders in the community: a twenty-year follow-up of the Whickham Survey. Clin Endocrinol (Oxf) 43:55, 1995

37. Glinoer D, Riahi M, Grun JP, et al: Risk of subclinical hypothyroidism in pregnant

women with asymptomatic autoimmune thyroid disorders. J Clin Endocrinol Metab 79:197, 1994

38. Premawardhana LD, Parkes AB, John R, et al: Thyroid peroxidase antibodies in early pregnancy: utility for prediction of postpartum thyroid dysfunction and implications for screening. Thyroid 14:610, 2004

39. Parle JV, Franklyn JA, Cross KW, et al: Thyroxine prescription in the community: serum thyroid stimulating hormone level assays as an indicator of undertreatment or overtreatment. Br J Gen Pract 43:107, 1993

40. Fish LH, Schwartz HL, Cavanaugh J, et al: Replacement dose, metabolism, and bioavailability of levothyroxine in the treatment of hypothyroidism: role of triiodothyronine in pituitary feedback in humans. N Engl J Med 316:764, 1987

41. Alexander EK, Marqusee E, Lawrence J, et al: Timing and magnitude of increases in levothyroxine requirements during pregnancy in women with hypothyroidism. N Engl J Med 351:241, 2004

42. Arafah BM: Increased need for thyroxine in women with hypothyroidism during estrogen therapy. N Engl J Med 344:1743, 2001

43. Quan ML, Pasieka JL, Rorstad O: Bone mineral density in well-differentiated thyroid cancer patients treated with suppressive thyroxine: a systematic overview of the literature. J Surg Oncol 79:62, 2002

44. Sawin CT, Geller A, Wolf PA, et al: Low serum thyrotropin concentrations as a risk factor for atrial fibrillation in older persons. N Engl J Med 331:1249, 1994

45. Keating FR Jr, Parkin TW, Selby JB, et al: Treatment of heart disease associated with myxedema. Prog Cardiovasc Dis 3:364, 1961

46. Sherman SI, Ladenson PW: Percutaneous transluminal angioplasty in hypothyroidism. Am J Med 90:367, 1991

47. Ladenson PW, Levin AA, Ridgway EC, et al: Complications of surgery in hypothyroid patients. Am J Med 77:261, 1984

48. Surks MI, Ortiz E, Daniels GH, et al: Subclinical thyroid disease: scientific review and guidelines for diagnosis and management. JAMA 291:228, 2004

49. Danese MD, Ladenson PW, Meinert CL, et al: Effect of thyroxine therapy on serum lipoproteins in patients with mild thyroid failure: a quantitative review of the literature. J Clin Endocrinol Metab 85:2993, 2000

50. Hak AE, Pols HAP, Visser TJ, et al: Subclinical hypothyroidism is an independent risk factor for atherosclerosis and myocardial infarction in elderly women: the Rotterdam Study. Ann Intern Med 132:270, 2000

51. Nystrom E, Caidahl K, Fager G, et al: A double-blind crossover 12-month study of L-thyroxine treatment of women with "subclinical" hypothyroidism. Clin Endocrinol (Oxf) 29:62, 1988

52. Danese MD, Powe NR, Sawin CT, et al: Screening for mild thyroid failure at the periodic health examination: a decision and cost-effectiveness analysis. JAMA 276:285, 1996

53. Bona M, Santini F, Rivolta G, et al: Cost effectiveness of screening for subclinical hypothyroidism in the elderly: a decision-analytical model. Pharmacoeconomics 14:209, 1998

54. Screening for thyroid disease: recommendation statement. U.S. Preventive Services Task Force. Ann Intern Med 140:125, 2004

55. Saravanan P, Chau WF, Roberts N, et al: Psychological well-being in patients on "adequate" doses of L-thyroxine: results of a large, controlled community-based questionnaire study. Clin Endocrinol (Oxf) 57:577, 2002

56. Walsh JP, Shiels L, Lim EM, et al: Combined thyroxine/liothyronine treatment does not improve well-being, quality of life, or cognitive function compared to thyroxine alone: a randomized controlled trial in patients with primary hypothyroidism. J Clin Endocrinol Metab 88:4543, 2003

57. Holvey DN, Goodner CJ, Nicoloff JT, et al: Treatment of myxedema coma with intravenous thyroxine. Arch Intern Med 113:89, 1964

58. Yamamoto T, Fukuyama J, Fujiyoshi A: Factors associated with mortality of myxedema coma: report of eight cases and literature survey. Thyroid 9:1167, 1999

59. Tunbridge WM, Evered DE, Hall R, et al: The spectrum of thyroid disease in a community: the Wickham Survey. Clin Endocrinol 7:481, 1977

60. Laurberg P, Pedersen KM, Vestergaard H, et al: High incidence of multinodular toxic goitre in the elderly population in a low iodine intake area vs. high incidence of Graves' disease in the young in a high iodine intake area: comparative surveys of thyrotoxicosis epidemiology in East-Jutland Denmark and Iceland. J Intern Med 229:415, 1991

61. Canaris GJ, Manowitz NR, Mayor G, et al: The Colorado thyroid disease prevalence study. Arch Intern Med 160:526, 2000

62. Brix TH, Christensen K, Holm NV, et al: A population-based study of Graves' disease in Danish twins. Clin Endocrinol (Oxf) 48:397, 1998

63. Yanagawa T, Hidaka Y, Guimaraes V, et al: CTLA-4 gene polymorphism associated with Graves' disease in a Caucasian population. J Clin Endocrinol Metab 80:41, 1995

64. Saravanan P, Dayan CM: Thyroid autoantibodies. Endocrinol Metab Clin North Am 30:315, 2001

65. Derwahl M, Studer H: Hyperplasia versus adenoma in endocrine tissues: are they different? Trends Endocrinol Metab 13:23, 2002

66. Brix TH, Kyvik KO, Hegedus L: Major role of genes in the etiology of simple goiter in females: a population-based twin study. J Clin Endocrinol Metab 84:3071, 1999

67. Bidey SP, Hill DJ, Eggo MC: Growth factors and goitrogenesis. J Endocrinol 160:321, 1999

68. Parma J, Duprez L, Van Sande J, et al: Diversity and prevalence of somatic mutations in the thyrotropin receptor and Gs alpha genes as a cause of toxic thyroid adenomas. J Clin Endocrinol Metab 82:2695, 1997

69. Stanbury JB, Ermans AE, Bourdoux P, et al: Iodine-induced hyperthyroidism: occurrence and epidemiology. Thyroid 8:83, 1998

70. Roti E, Uberti ED: Iodine excess and hyperthyroidism. Thyroid 11:493, 2001

71. Pearce EN, Farwell AP, Braverman LE: Thyroiditis. N Engl J Med 348:2646, 2003; erratum in N Engl J Med 349:620, 2003

72. Bartalena L, Wiersinga WM, Tanda ML, et al: Diagnosis and management of amiodarone-induced thyrotoxicosis in Europe: results of an international survey among members of the European Thyroid Association. Clin Endocrinol (Oxf) 61:494, 2004

73. Hershman JM: Physiological and pathological aspects of the effect of human chorionic gonadotropin on the thyroid. Best Pract Res Clin Endocrinol Metab 18:249, 2004

74. Glinoer D: The regulation of thyroid function in pregnancy: pathways of endocrine adaptation from physiology to pathology. Endocr Rev 18:404, 1997

75. Hershman JM: Human chorionic gonadotropin and the thyroid: hyperemesis gravidarum and trophoblastic tumours. Thyroid 9:653, 1999

76. Yeo CP, Khoo DH, Eng PH, et al: Prevalence of gestational thyrotoxicosis in Asian women evaluated in the 8th to 14th weeks of pregnancy: correlations with total and free beta human chorionic gonadotrophin. Clin Endocrinol (Oxf) 55:391, 2001

77. Rodien P, Bremont C, Sanson ML, et al: Familial gestational hyperthyroidism caused by a mutant thyrotropin receptor hypersensitive to human chorionic gonadotropin. N Engl J Med 339:1823, 1998

78. McDermott MT, Ridgway EC: Central hyperthyroidism. Endocrinol Metab Clin North Am 27:187, 1998

79. Brucker-Davis F, Oldfield EH, Skarulis MC, et al: Thyrotropin-secreting pituitary tumors: diagnostic criteria, thyroid hormone sensitivity, and treatment outcome in 25 patients followed at the National Institutes of Health. J Clin Endocrinol Metab 84:476, 1999

80. Gershengorn MC, Weintraub BD: Thyrotropin-induced hyperthyroidism caused by selective pituitary resistence to thyroid hormone. J Clin Invest 56:633,1975

81. White JD, Ladenson PW: Thyroid hormone overdose. Clinical Management of Poisoning and Drug Overdose. Haddad LM, Winchester JE, Eds. WB Saunders Co, Philadelphia, 1988

82. Ladenson PW: Diagnosis of hyperthyroidism. The Thyroid, 9th ed. Braverman LE, Utiger RD, Eds. JB Lippincott, Philadelphia (in press)

83. Laboratory medicine practice guidelines: laboratory support for the diagnosis and monitoring of thyroid disease. National Academy of Clinical Biochemistry Guidelines Committee. Thyroid 13:3, 2003

84. Borst GC, Eil C, Burman KD: Euthyroid hyperthyroxinemia. Ann Intern Med 98:366, 1983

85. Rushbrook JI, Becker E, Schussler GC, et al: Identification of a human serum albumin species associated with familial dysalbuminemic hyperthyroxinemia. J Clin Endocrinol Metab 80:461, 1995

86. Moses AC, Rosen HN, Moller DE, et al: A point mutation in transthyretin increases affinity for thyroxine and produces euthyroid hyperthyroxinemia. J Clin Invest 86:2025, 1990

87. Sakata S: Autoimmunity against thyroid hormones. Crit Rev Immunol 14:157, 1994

88. Pearce EN, Bogazzi F, Martino E, et al: The prevalence of elevated serum C-reactive protein levels in inflammatory and noninflammatory thyroid disease. Thyroid 13:643, 2003

89. Cooper DS: Antithyroid drugs for the treatment of hyperthyroidism caused by Graves' disease. Endocrinol Metab Clin North Am 27:225, 2003

90. Brucker-Davis F, Oldfield EH, Skarulis MC, et al: Thyrotropin-secreting pituitary tumors: diagnostic criteria, thyroid hormone sensitivity, and treatment outcome in 25 patients followed at the National Institutes of Health. J Clin Endocrinol Metab 84:476, 1999

91. Beck-Peccoz P, Persani L: Medical management of thyrotropin-secreting pituitary adenomas. Pituitary 5:83, 2002

92. Nakazawa HK, Sakurai K, Hamada N, et al: Management of atrial fibrillation in the post-thyrotoxic state. Am J Med 72:903, 1982

93. Kahaly GJ, Dillmann WH: Thyroid hormone action in the heart. Endocr Rev Jan 4, 2005 [Epub ahead of print]

94. Dillmann WH: Thyroid storm. Curr Ther Endocrinol Metab 6:81, 1997

95. Sherman SI, Simonson L, Ladenson PW: Clinical and socioeconomic predispositions to complicated thyrotoxicosis: a predictable and preventable syndrome. Am J Med 101:192, 1996

96. Knobel M, Barca MF, Pedrinola F, et al: Prevalence of anti-thyroid peroxidase antibodies in autoimmune and nonautoimmune thyroid disorders in a relatively low-iodine environment. J Endocrinol Invest 17:837, 1994

97. Muller AF, Drexhage HA, Berghout A: Postpartum thyroiditis and autoimmune thyroiditis in women of childbearing age: recent insights and consequences for antenatal and postnatal care. Endocr Rev 22:605, 2001

98. Yasmeen T, Khan S, Patel SG, et al: Clinical case seminar: Riedel's thyroiditis: report of a case complicated by spontaneous hypoparathyroidism, recurrent laryngeal nerve injury, and Horner's syndrome. J Clin Endocrinol Metab 87:3543, 2002

99. Gaitan E: Goitrogens in food and water. Annu Rev Nutr 10:21, 1990

100. Hegedus L, Bonnema SJ, Bennedbaek FN: Management of simple nodular goiter: current status and future perspectives. Endocr Rev 24:102, 2003

101. Huysmans DA, Nieuwlaat WA, Hermus AR: Towards larger volume reduction of nodular goitres by radioiodine therapy: a role for pretreatment with recombinant human thyrotropin? Clin Endocrinol (Oxf) 60:297, 2004

102. Castro MR, Caraballo PJ, Morris JC: Effectiveness of thyroid hormone suppressive therapy in benign solitary thyroid nodules: a meta-analysis. J Clin Endocrinol Metab 87:4154, 2002

103. Hegedus L: Clinical practice: the thyroid nodule. N Engl J Med 351:1764, 2004

104. Tan GH, Gharib H: Thyroid incidentalomas: management approaches to nonpalpable nodules discovered incidentally on thyroid imaging. Ann Intern Med 126:226, 1997

105. Gertner ME, Kebebew E: Multiple endocrine neoplasia type 2. Curr Treat Options

Oncol 5:315, 2004

106. Mandel SJ: Diagnostic use of ultrasonography in patients with nodular thyroid disease. Endocr Pract 10:246, 2004

107. Chow LS, Gharib H, Goellner JR, et al: Nondiagnostic thyroid fine-needle aspiration cytology: management dilemmas. Thyroid 11:1147, 2001

108. Sherman SI: Thyroid carcinoma. Lancet 361:501, 2003

109. Schneider AB, Ron E: Carcinoma of the follicular epithelium: epidemiology and pathogenesis. The Thyroid, 9th ed. Braverman LE, Utiger RD, Eds. JB Lippincott, Philadelphia, 2005, p 889

110. Jemal A, Tiwari RC, Murray T, et al: Cancer statistics, 2004. CA Cancer J Clin 54:8, 2004

111. Fagin JA: Challenging dogma in thyroid cancer molecular genetics: role of RET/PTC and BRAF in tumor initiation. J Clin Endocrinol Metab 89:4264, 2004

112. Ringel MD, Ladenson, PW: Controversies in the follow-up and management of well-differentiated thyroid cancer. Endocr Relat Cancer 11:97, 2004

113. Hay ID, Grant CS, Bergstralh EJ, et al: Unilateral total lobectomy: is it sufficient surgical treatment for patients with AMES low-risk papillary thyroid carcinoma? Surgery 124:958, 1998

114. Pearce EN, Braverman LE: Papillary thyroid microcarcinoma outcomes and implications for treatment. J Clin Endocrinol Metab 89:3710, 2004

115. Mazzaferri EL, Jhiang SM: Long-term impact of initial surgical and medical therapy on papillary and follicular thyroid cancer. Am J Med 97:418, 1994; erratum in Am J Med 98:215, 1995

116. Lippi F, Capezzone M, Angelini F, et al: Radioiodine treatment of metastatic differentiated thyroid cancer in patients on L-thyroxine, using recombinant human TSH. Eur J Endocrinol 144:5, 2001

117. Mazzaferri EL, Robbins RJ, Spencer CA, et al: A consensus report of the role of serum thyroglobulin as a monitoring method for low-risk patients with papillary thyroid carcinoma. J Clin Endocrinol Metab 88:1433, 2003

118. Haugen BR, Pacini F, Reiners C, et al: A comparison of recombinant human thyrotropin and thyroid hormone withdrawal for the detection of thyroid remnant or cancer. J Clin Endocrinol Metab 84:3877, 1999

119. Wilson PC, Millar BM, Brierley JD: The management of advanced thyroid cancer. Clin Oncol (R Coll Radiol) 16:561, 2004

120. Massoll N, Mazzaferri EL: Diagnosis and management of medullary thyroid carcinoma. Clin Lab Med 24:49, 2004

121. De Crevoisier R, Baudin E, Bachelot A, et al: Combined treatment of anaplastic thyroid carcinoma with surgery, chemotherapy, and hyperfractionated accelerated external radiotherapy. Int J Radiat Oncol Biol Phys 60:1137, 2004

122. Gilliland D, Hunt WC, Morris DM, et al: Prognostic factors for thyroid carcinoma: a population-based study of 15,698 cases from the Surveillance, Epidemiology and End Results (SEER) program 1973–1991. Cancer 79:564, 1997

Acknowledgment

Figures 2 and 3   Seward Hung.

51 Hypoglycemia

F. John Service, M.D., PH.D., F.A.C.P.

Definition

Hypoglycemia is a clinical syndrome of diverse etiologies characterized by episodes of low blood glucose. These episodes are typically marked by autonomic manifestations such as trembling, sweating, nausea, and, in more severe episodes, central nervous system manifestations (neuroglycopenia) such as dizziness, confusion, and headache.

Classification

Hypoglycemic disorders have long been categorized as fasting or postprandial (reactive). This classification lacks practical value. Insulinoma, which is the archetypal cause of fasting hypoglycemia, may produce symptoms postprandially and, indeed, in some cases solely postprandially. Patients with factitious hypoglycemia evince symptoms irrespective of meals.

A more useful approach for the practitioner is a classification based on the patient's clinical characteristics. Persons who appear otherwise healthy have hypoglycemic disorders different from those of persons who are ill.

HYPOGLYCEMIA IN APPARENTLY HEALTHY PATIENTS

In apparently healthy persons, single episodes of hypoglycemia may result from accidental drug ingestion (e.g., ethanol in children). In addition to ethanol, salicylates and quinine can lower blood glucose levels; the combined effects of ethanol and quinine are responsible for so-called gin-and-tonic hypoglycemia. The healthy-appearing adult patient with a history of repeated episodes of neuroglycopenia usually has a disorder involving excessive insulin production, such as insulinoma; rarely, the hypoglycemia is factitious, caused by surreptitious or inadvertent use of a hypoglycemic agent (e.g., insulin or a sulfonylurea) [see Conditions That Cause Hypoglycemia, *below*].

Hypoglycemia may occur in patients who have coexistent disease but whose disease is being controlled with medical treatment. Typically, the hypoglycemia in these cases is a side effect of the medication being used to treat the coexistent disease, or it results from the mistaken dispensing of a sulfonylurea instead of the prescribed drug.

HYPOGLYCEMIA IN ILL PATIENTS

Illness can lead to hypoglycemia through a variety of mechanisms, only some of which involve insulin and not all of which are known. Many illnesses (e.g., renal failure and sepsis) are known to pose the risk of low blood glucose levels [see Table 1]; hypoglycemia in a patient with one of these illnesses requires little if any investigation of its cause. However, not all patients with a disease that has a proclivity to generate hypoglycemia actually experience low blood glucose levels. Why only some ill patients experience hypoglycemia is unknown.

Hospitalized patients are at increased risk for hypoglycemia, often from iatrogenic factors. In any inpatient with hypoglycemia, medication should be considered a potential cause.

Low blood glucose levels may be found on laboratory testing of ill patients who have no symptoms of hypoglycemia. In patients with leukemia or severe hemolysis, the hypoglycemia may be an artifact resulting from consumption of glucose in the blood collection tube by large numbers of leukocytes or by nucleated red blood cells, respectively.[1,2] Patients with glycogen storage disease may be asymptomatic because they have adapted to lifelong hypoglycemia from their disease.[3]

Diagnosis

Although the diagnosis of hypoglycemia requires the measurement of blood glucose, such measurement often is not feasible when symptoms arise during activities of ordinary life. Under these circumstances, the physician must take a detailed history to determine whether to proceed with further evaluation. The history should include a full description of the patient's symptoms and the circumstances under which they occur.

A medication history is also an important aspect of the evaluation in a patient with clinical manifestations of hypoglycemia, especially if the onset coincides with the filling of a new prescription. Because of the potential for drug error, all medications taken by the patient should be identified by a medical professional, such as a physician or pharmacist.

CLINICAL MANIFESTATIONS

The symptoms of hypoglycemia have been classified into two major groups: autonomic and neuroglycopenic. In a study of experimentally induced hypoglycemia in diabetic and nondiabetic persons, a principal-components analysis assigned sweating, trembling, feelings of warmth, anxiety, and nausea to the autonomic group and dizziness, confusion, tiredness, difficulty in speaking, headache, and inability to concentrate to the neuroglycopenic group. Hunger, blurred vision, drowsiness, and weakness could not be confidently assigned to either group.[4] In a retrospective analysis of 60 patients with insulinomas, 85% had various combinations of diplopia, blurred vision, sweating, palpitations, and weakness; 80% had confusion or abnormal behavior; 53% had amnesia or went into coma during the episode; and 12% had generalized seizures.[5]

The symptoms of hypoglycemia differ between persons but are nevertheless consistent from episode to episode in any one person.[6,7] There is no consistent chronologic order to the evolution of symptoms; autonomic symptoms do not always precede neuroglycopenic ones. In many patients, neuroglycopenic symptoms are the only ones observed.[7] Patients who have autonomic symptoms only are unlikely to have a hypoglycemic disorder. An additional factor that influences the generation of symptoms in hypoglycemia is their blunting by earlier hypoglycemic episodes.

PHYSICAL EXAMINATION

In patients who appear healthy, with or without coexistent compensated disease, the physical examination is normal or reveals only minor abnormalities that are unlikely to be germane to the underlying hypoglycemic disorder. In patients suspected of having factitious hypoglycemia from injection of insulin, a search for needle-puncture sites is fruitless. In ill patients with a primary disorder that can cause hypoglycemia, the results of physical examination will reflect that disease. For the patient observed while hypoglycemic, findings may include diaphoresis,

Table 1 Causes of Hypoglycemia

Drugs	Disopyramide Ethanol Haloperidol Quinine Salicylates
Drugs in specific illnesses	Pentamidine in *Pneumocystis* pneumonia Propoxyphene in renal failure Quinine in malaria Trimethoprim-sulfamethoxazole in renal failure Topical salicylates in renal failure

Endogenous hyperinsulinism	Insulinoma
	Islet hyperplasia/nesidioblastosis
	  Persistent hyperinsulinemic hypoglycemia
	   of infancy
	  Noninsulinoma pancreatogenous
	   hypoglycemia syndrome
	Insulin autoimmune hypoglycemia

Conditions that predispose to hypoglycemia	Neonatal
	  Infant small for gestational age
	  Erythroblastosis fetalis
	  Infant of diabetic mother
	  Cyanotic congenital heart disease
	  Beckwith-Wiedemann syndrome
	Inherited
	  Defects in amino acid and fatty acid
	   metabolism
	  Glycogen storage disease
	  Hereditary fructose intolerance
	  Isolated adrenocorticotropic hormone (ACTH)
	   deficiency
	  Isolated growth hormone deficiency
	Acquired
	  Addison disease
	  Carnitine deficiency
	  Intense exercise
	  Hypopituitarism
	  Heart failure
	  Lactic acidosis
	  Severe liver disease
	  Postoperative status
	  Renal failure
	  Reye syndrome
	  Sepsis
	  Shock
	  Spinal muscular atrophy
	  Starvation
	   Anorexia nervosa
	  Large mesenchymal tumors (fibroma, sarcoma,
	   small cell carcinoma, mesothelioma)

widened pulse pressure, and neurologic abnormalities ranging from slowed mentation or withdrawal from spontaneous communication to more overt confusion, erratic behavior, coma, seizure, and hypothermia.

LABORATORY TESTS

Serum Glucose

Studies of acute insulin-induced hypoglycemia in healthy persons have shown that the threshold for the development of symptoms is a serum glucose concentration of approximately 60 mg/dl; the threshold for impairment of brain function is approx-

imately 50 mg/dl.[8,9] These measurements were taken from arterialized venous blood (i.e., blood drawn from a vein in a heated hand [the application of heat shunts arterial blood into the venous system]); comparable levels in venous blood would probably be about 3 mg/dl lower. The rate of decrease in the serum glucose level does not influence the occurrence of the symptoms and signs of hypoglycemia.

Because symptoms of hypoglycemia are nonspecific, it is necessary to verify their origin. This is accomplished by applying a set of criteria first proposed by Whipple in 1938. The Whipple triad comprises spontaneous symptoms consistent with hypoglycemia, a low serum glucose concentration at the time the symptoms occur, and relief of the symptoms through normalization of the glucose level.[10]

A normal serum glucose concentration, reliably obtained during the occurrence of spontaneous symptoms, eliminates the possibility of a hypoglycemic disorder. Capillary glucose measurements that patients take themselves with a blood glucose meter during the occurrence of spontaneous symptoms are often unreliable, because nondiabetic patients usually are not experienced in this technique and because the measurements are obtained under adverse circumstances. Patients with a confirmed low serum glucose level (< 50 mg/dl) or a history of neuroglycopenic symptoms should undergo further testing. This is best accomplished with a prolonged fast.

The Prolonged (72-Hour) Fast

The prolonged (72-hour) fast is the classic diagnostic test for hypoglycemia. It should be conducted in a standardized manner [*see Table 2*]. The fast may be undertaken to demonstrate the Whipple triad and thereby establish that hypoglycemia is the basis for the patient's symptoms. If the Whipple triad has already been documented, the fast may be conducted for the purpose of determining the mechanism of the hypoglycemia, through measurement of beta cell polypeptide and plasma sulfonylurea levels. In the latter case, the fast can be terminated when the serum glucose level drops to 55 mg/dl or less (or, better yet, ≤ 50 mg/dl), which is the concentration at which beta cell polypeptides should be suppressed. Not all patients will need the full 72 hours to accomplish the purpose for the fast. In a study of 170 patients with surgically proven insulinomas, termination of the fast occurred within 12 hours in 33% of patients, within 24 hours in 65%, within 36 hours in 84%, within 48 hours in 93%, and within 72 hours in 99%.[11] Truncation of the fast at 48 hours, if hypoglycemia has not occurred by then, risks misdiagnosis.

Starting the fast overnight has allowed 40% of patients (including those with insulinoma and other causes of hypoglycemia) to conclude their fast in the outpatient endocrine-testing unit. Patients whose fast is not completed by the end of the business day are admitted to the hospital to complete the fast.

The decision whether to end the fast may not be easy to make when the Whipple triad is the goal. Because of delays in the availability of glucose measurements, the bedside glucose meter may have to serve as a guide. Some patients have slightly depressed glycemic levels without symptoms or signs of hypoglycemia. In other patients, fasting evokes the symptoms they experience in ordinary life but their serum glucose levels are not in the hypoglycemic range. In such instances, symptoms cannot be attributed to hypoglycemia. To complicate matters, young, lean, healthy women—and, to a lesser degree, some men—may have serum glucose concentrations in the range of 40 mg/dl or even lower during prolonged fasting.[12] Careful examination and testing for subtle signs or symptoms of hypoglycemia should therefore be conducted repeatedly when the patient's serum glucose level is near or in the hypoglycemic range. To end the fast solely on the basis of a low serum glucose level, in the absence of symptoms or signs of hypoglycemia, may jeopardize accurate diagnosis. On the other hand, failing to appreciate the manifestations of neuroglycopenia and, hence, concluding that the results of the fast are negative is an equally egregious error. It is essential to monitor patients closely during the fast and to be vigilant for subtle signs of neuroglycopenia.

Beta Cell Polypeptides and Their Surrogates

Concentrations of beta cell polypeptides (insulin, C-peptide, and proinsulin) are interpreted in the context of the concomitant serum glucose concentration. The normal overnight fasting ranges for these polypeptides do not apply when the serum glucose level is low. When immunochemiluminometric assays (ICMA) are used, the criteria for endogenous hyperinsulinemia are as follows: serum insulin, 3 µU/ml or greater; C-peptide, 200 pmol/L or greater; and proinsulin, 5 pmol/L or greater [see Figure 1].[13]

Insulin concentrations rarely exceed 100 µU/ml in patients with insulinomas. Values above this level suggest recent insulin administration or the presence of insulin antibodies.

Ratios of glucose to insulin, and vice versa, have no diagnostic utility [see Figure 1]. The molar ratio of insulin to C-peptide is the same for patients with insulinomas and healthy persons (approximately 0.2). The molar ratio of proinsulin to insulin appears to be higher in persons with insulinoma, but it provides poor diagnostic utility.

Because insulin has an antiketogenic effect, serum levels of the ketone body β-hydroxybutyrate can be used as a surrogate for measurement of insulin. The serum β-hydroxybutyrate level is low—2.7 mmol/L or less—in patients with insulin-mediated hypoglycemia; normal persons and those with non–insulin-mediated hypoglycemia have higher levels [see Figure 1].[13]

At the end of the fast, the patient is given an intravenous dose of 1 mg of glucagon, and the subsequent glucose response is measured. Because insulin is glycogenic and antiglycogenolytic, the glucagon injection results in an increase in the serum glucose level of 25 mg/dl or greater in patients with insulin-mediated hypoglycemia, whereas normal persons or those with non–in-

sulin-mediated hypoglycemia have lesser increases [see Figure 1].[13] An exuberant serum insulin response to intravenous glucagon has been considered an indication of insulinomas, but unfortunately, no normative data have been generated for this test. Measurement of beta cell polypeptides and insulin surrogates (β-hydroxybutyrate and glucose response to intravenous glucagon) has diagnostic utility only when the serum glucose level is 60 mg/dl or lower at the end of the fast.

Sulfonylureas and Meglitinides

Persons with hypoglycemia from inappropriate use of sulfonylureas or meglitinides (e.g., repaglinide) have concentrations of beta cell polypeptides that are identical to those observed in persons with insulinoma. Consequently, plasma assays for these drugs is an essential aspect of the evaluation. I use a highly sensitive and accurate liquid chromatographic tandem mass spectroscopy method to identify these drugs. A positive assay suggests either covert or inadvertent usage.

Insulin Antibodies

An assay for insulin antibodies should be done in every patient with clear evidence of hypoglycemia. The detection of insulin antibodies in a nondiabetic patient was once considered to be firm evidence of insulin factitious hypoglycemia, especially when animal insulin was the only commercially available type. Currently, most patients with factitious hypoglycemia have no detectable insulin antibodies, possibly because of the use of human insulin, which is less antigenic than beef or pork insulin. Rather, the presence of insulin antibodies, especially in high titers, is diagnostic of insulin autoimmune hypoglycemia (IAH) (see below).[13] Very low titers of insulin antibodies may sometimes be detected in persons without hypoglycemia[14] and, in rare instances, in patients with insulinomas.

Glycated Hemoglobin

Measurement of glycated hemoglobin is not a standard aspect of the clinical evaluation of hypoglycemia. Concentrations of glycated hemoglobin are statistically significantly lower in patients with insulinomas than in normal persons, but there is too much overlap between the two groups for this test to provide a diagnostic criterion.[6]

Oral Glucose Tolerance Test

The oral glucose tolerance test should not be used for the evaluation of hypoglycemia, because it is fraught with risk of misdiagnosis. At least 10% of healthy persons have serum glucose nadirs below 50 mg/dl, and the results of the test do not correlate with serum glucose responses to a mixed meal (i.e., a meal containing a balance of proteins, carbohydrates, and fat).

Mixed-Meal Test

For persons with a history of neuroglycopenic symptoms within 5 hours after food ingestion, a mixed-meal test may be conducted. The test is considered to be positive if the patient experiences neuroglycopenic symptoms when a concomitant serum glucose level measures 50 mg/dl or less. A positive mixed-meal test does not provide a diagnosis, only biochemical confirmation of the history.

C-Peptide Suppression Test

C-peptide is formed during the conversion of proinsulin to insulin by the pancreatic beta cells. In the C-peptide suppression

---

Table 2 Protocol for Prolonged Supervised Fast

1. Date the onset of the fast as of the last ingestion of calories. Discontinue all nonessential medications.
2. Allow the patient to drink calorie-free and caffeine-free beverages.
3. Ensure that the patient is active during waking hours.
4. Measure plasma glucose, insulin, C-peptide, and, if an assay is available, proinsulin in the same specimen. Repeat measurements every 6 hr until the plasma glucose drops below 60 mg/dl; then repeat the measurements every 1–2 hr.
5. When the plasma glucose is less than 45 mg/dl and the patient has symptoms or signs of hypoglycemia, measure plasma glucose, insulin, C-peptide, proinsulin, β-hydroxybutyrate, and sulfonylurea in the same specimen; then inject 1 mg of glucagon I.V. and measure plasma glucose after 10, 20, and 30 min.
6. Feed the patient.

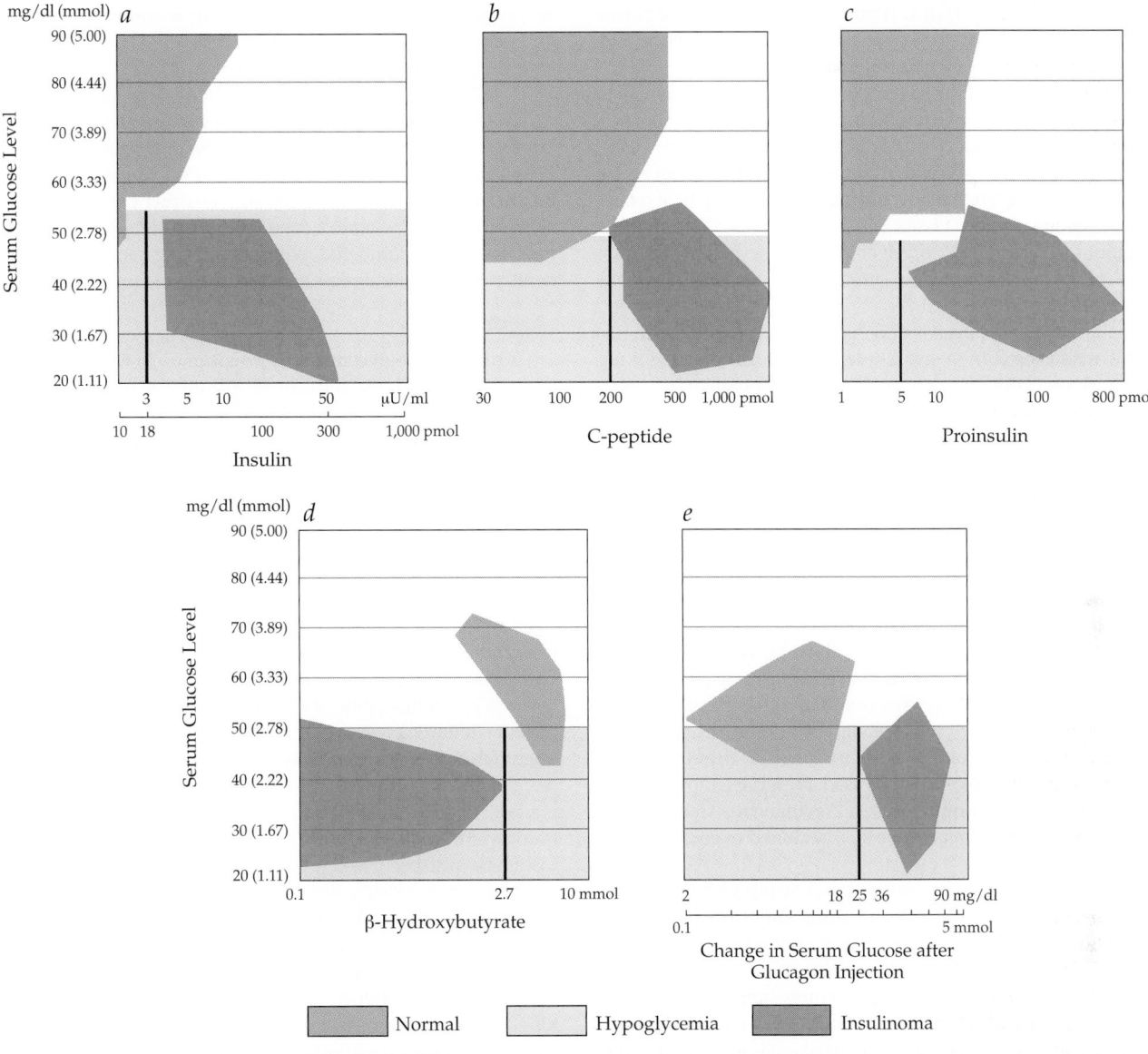

Figure 1   **During the 72-hour fast, levels of serum glucose are compared with serum levels of insulin (*a*), C-peptide (*b*), proinsulin (*c*), and β-hydroxybutyrate (*d*). At the end of the fast, 1 mg of glucagon is injected intravenously, and its effect on glucose levels is measured (*e*). Normal patients may have glucose levels that drop into the hypoglycemic range, so careful documentation of hypoglycemic symptoms is necessary.**

test, the patient fasts overnight and then receives an hour-long intravenous infusion of insulin, during which levels of serum glucose and C-peptide are measured. In normal patients, hypoglycemia from the exogenous insulin results in suppression of C-peptide production; patients with insulinomas have higher levels of C-peptide. When the likelihood of a hypoglycemic disorder is not high, a normal result on the C-peptide suppression test may preclude the need for a 72-hour fast. Interpretation of the C-peptide suppression test requires normative data appropriately adjusted for the patient's body mass index and age.[7]

Intravenous Tolbutamide Test

In the past, serum glucose response to an intravenous injection of tolbutamide was used in the diagnosis of insulinoma. This test is potentially dangerous and is less accurate than other tests for insulinoma and, therefore, has been rarely used in recent years.

Conditions That Cause Hypoglycemia

The causes of hypoglycemia in healthy-appearing adults encompass the following conditions: insulinoma, factitious hypoglycemia from insulin or sulfonylurea, noninsulinoma pancreatogenous hypoglycemia syndrome (NIPHS), and insulin autoimmune hypoglycemia.

INSULINOMA

Epidemiology

Between 1927 and 1986, 224 hypoglycemic patients underwent their first pancreatic exploration at the Mayo Clinic and were found to have insulinoma. Because of the relatively large number of cases of insulinoma treated at the Mayo Clinic, in comparison with other medical centers, and the comprehensive epidemiologic database that the Mayo Clinic maintains for Olmsted County, Minnesota, it was possible to determine the population-based incidence of insulinoma, the risk of recurrence, and the survival in patients with insulinoma.[15]

The median age of the Mayo Clinic insulinoma patients was 47 years, with a range of 8 to 82 years; 59% were female. The incidence in Olmsted County was 4 cases per 1 million person-years. Of the 224 patients, 7.6% had multiple endocrine neoplasia type I (MEN I) and 5.8% had malignant insulinoma. The risk of recurrence was greater in patients with MEN I (21%) than in those without this condition (7%). Over a 45-year period, overall survival of the total cohort was similar to the expected survival (78% versus 81%).

Insulinomas have been found in pregnant patients and in patients with type 2 (non–insulin-dependent) diabetes mellitus. One case of insulinoma in type 1 (insulin-dependent) diabetes mellitus has been reported.[16]

Diagnosis

Laboratory tests   Insulinoma is characterized by hypoglycemia caused by elevated levels of endogenous insulin. Confirmation of the diagnosis requires exclusion of hypoglycemia from exogenous sources.

Localization   Once a biochemical diagnosis of insulinoma has been made, the next step is localization. Success with the various modalities reflects local skill and experience. Great success has been seen with transabdominal ultrasonography and triple-phase spiral computed tomography. Magnetic resonance imaging and scintigraphy with indium-111 (In-111)–pentetreotide (OctreoScan) can also be used. I reserve endoscopic ultrasonography for complex cases. Percutaneous transhepatic portal venous sampling has been abandoned even by its former proponents.

In patients whose tumor is not found by ultrasonography or CT, the selective arterial calcium stimulation test provides a means to both regionalize and confirm endogenous hyperinsulinemia. This test involves serial injections of calcium into the splenic, gastroduodenal, and superior mesenteric arteries. Subsequent doubling of serum insulin concentrations in the right hepatic vein indicates hyperfunctioning beta cells in the part of the pancreas served by that artery.

There is general agreement that the best localization of insulinomas is achieved with intraoperative ultrasonography and careful mobilization and palpation of the pancreas by a surgeon experienced with insulinoma surgery. This approach has seen a 98% success rate in the identification of insulinoma. After this test, these patients go straight to surgery.

Management

The treatment of choice for insulinomas is surgical removal. Depending on the lesion, the surgery required may range from enucleation of the insulinoma to subtotal pancreatectomy. It is advisable for the surgery to be performed at an institution with expertise in the management of insulinoma.

Medical therapy is less effective than tumor resection, but the former can be used in patients who are not candidates for surgery, who refuse surgery, or whose surgery is unsuccessful. The most effective medication for controlling symptomatic hypoglycemia in these patients is diazoxide, which lowers insulin secretion. Diazoxide is given in divided doses of up to 1,200 mg daily. Side effects include edema, which may require high doses of loop diuretics, and hirsutism. Other medications for insulinomas include verapamil, phenytoin, and octreotide.

FACTITIOUS HYPOGLYCEMIA

The term factitious (or factitial) has been used in medical parlance to imply covert patient activity. The consideration of such a possibility often changes the patient-physician relationship, leading the physician to feel deceived and the patient to feel mistrusted. However, the pejorative connotation with which factitious illness has been encumbered requires softening because some patients with factitious disease suffer through no fault of their own.

Epidemiology

Factitious hypoglycemia is more common in women and occurs most often in the third or fourth decade of life. Many of these patients work in health-related occupations.

Factitious hypoglycemia in patients with diabetes is probably more common than the incidence noted in published series.[17] Confirmation of the diagnosis in these cases can be very difficult. When deprived of access to hypoglycemic agents, diabetic patients with factitious hypoglycemia become hyperglycemic.

Etiology

Factitious hypoglycemia results from the use of insulin or the use of sulfonylureas or meglitinides that stimulate insulin secretion. The most common form of factitious hypoglycemia is the covert self-administration of a hypoglycemic drug or insulin by a patient without diabetes or the inappropriate manipulation of hypoglycemic drugs or insulin by a patient with diabetes. Less often, a parent may administer a hypoglycemic agent to a child; this is a form of child abuse.[18] In all reported cases, the alleged perpetrator was the patient's mother, who had ready access to insulin. Insulin has also been used to attempt suicide or homicide.[19]

There are increasing numbers of patients who, by taking a prescribed medication in good faith, incur hypoglycemia because a sulfonylurea was mistakenly dispensed.[20] In most instances, confusion in dispensing the drug arose because of similarity in spelling between the intended medication and the sulfonylurea. In some cases, however, the dispensing error was a result of negligence. On occasion, cases have arisen in which a nondiabetic person mistakenly takes hypoglycemic medication belonging to another member of the household.

Diagnosis

The possibility of factitious hypoglycemia should be considered in every patient undergoing evaluation for a hypoglycemic disorder, especially when the hypoglycemia has a chaotic occurrence—that is, when it has no relation at all to meals or fasting. All medications should be identified; the assistance of a pharmacist is desirable. The practice of searching personal effects and labeling insulin with a traceable substance that can be detected in blood or urine is probably unacceptable in the current climate of patients' rights.

The diagnosis of factitious hypoglycemia can usually be established by measuring serum insulin, sulfonylurea, and C-peptide when the patient is hypoglycemic. If a spontaneous episode of hypoglycemia is not observed, the patient should undergo a 72-hour fast. The results of the fast may be negative, however, should the patient not take the offending agent.

In a patient whose hypoglycemia results from covert use of a hypoglycemic agent, the agent will be present in the blood. A sensitive method such as liquid chromatography linked to mass spectroscopy should be used for the detection of sulfonylureas and meglitinides.

In insulin-related factitious hypoglycemia, the serum insulin level is high and the C-peptide level is suppressed, usually being close to the lower limit of detection. This observation applies both to nondiabetic patients and to those with type 2 diabetes. Patients with type 1 diabetes are characteristically severely insulin deficient and have low or undetectable serum concentrations of C-peptide. Although the C-peptide values in these patients cannot be further suppressed, confirmation that the values are low during a hypoglycemic episode eliminates any consideration of endogenous hyperinsulinism.

Management

Treatment of factitious hypoglycemia is simple: the patient stops taking the offending medication. The difficulty involved when medication is taken in error is identification of the drug. In the case of deliberate covert use, psychiatric referral is indicated.

NONINSULINOMA PANCREATOGENOUS HYPOGLYCEMIA SYNDROME

There have been cases of adults who do not have insulinomas but have hypoglycemia resulting from postprandial hypersecretion of insulin by pancreatic beta cells. Because of the unique clinical, diagnostic, radiologic, surgical, and histologic features of this disorder, it warrants designation as a new syndrome. We have termed it noninsulinoma pancreatogenous hypoglycemia syndrome, or NIPHS.[21]

Epidemiology

Like insulinoma, NIPHS affects patients across a broad age range—16 to 78 years, in one series—and causes severe neuroglycopenia, with loss of consciousness and, in some cases, generalized seizures. Unlike insulinoma, NIPHS occurs predominantly in males (70%).

Pathophysiology and Pathogenesis

Histologic analysis of pancreatic tissue from patients with NIPHS shows cells budding off ducts, which is best seen by chromogranin A and insulin immunohistochemical staining. Islet cell hypertrophy is also evident. No gross or microscopic tumor has been identified on hematoxylin-eosin–stained sections in any NIPHS patients.

Whether islet hypertrophy, nesidioblastosis, or both are pathogenic in these patients is open to question, as is the case with persistent hyperinsulinemic hypoglycemia of infancy (PHHI). However, a role for some form of diffuse islet cell dysfunction appears well established in these cases. Whatever the pathologic process may be, it is nonfocal, yet it does not necessarily involve the entire pancreas uniformly.

The histologic findings in NIPHS are similar to those in PHHI. Although familial forms of PHHI may be associated with mutations in the *Kir6.2* and *SUR1* genes, analysis of these genes in NIPHS patients has not shown such mutations.[22] However, these patients may have common mutations at another, as yet unspecified, locus.

Diagnosis

Clinical manifestations Symptoms of NIPHS occur primarily in the postprandial state 2 to 4 hours after eating. Although insulinoma patients may experience symptoms postprandially, they also have symptoms during food deprivation. It is extremely rare for insulinoma patients to have symptoms solely in the postprandial state.

Laboratory tests Patients with NIPHS have low serum glucose levels and elevated serum insulin levels in the postprandial period. Because of the short half-life of insulin, the criteria for hyperinsulinemia used in the fasting state appear to apply in the postprandial state, as long as the low glucose level occurs more than 30 minutes from the peak postprandial insulin level. Supervised 72-hour fasts have shown normal results in patients with NIPHS, whereas a negative 72-hour fast in a patient with insulinoma is a rare occurrence.

The selective arterial calcium stimulation test has shown positive results for patients with NIPHS.[23,24] All radiologic localizing studies in patients with NIPHS (transabdominal ultrasonography, triple-phase CT, celiac axis angiography, and intraoperative ultrasonography) have been negative for insulinoma.

Management

Gradient-guided partial pancreatectomy has been effective in relieving symptoms in patients with NIPHS. The pancreas is resected to the left of the superior mesenteric vein when results of the selective arterial calcium stimulation test are positive only for the splenic artery, and the pancreas is resected to the right of the superior mesenteric vein when the test is positive for an additional artery. Fortunately, gradient-guided debulking of the pancreas can ameliorate the symptoms of NIPHS even in patients whose disease would appear to have involved the whole pancreas. In rats, the mechanism for this effect may be related to decreased insulin secretion, attributed to reduced glucose transporter GLUT2, in remnant pancreas after partial pancreatectomy.[25] Unfortunately, recurrence of hypoglycemia after a few symptom-free years has developed in a few of the NIPHS patients.

INSULIN AUTOIMMUNE HYPOGLYCEMIA

Epidemiology

IAH is an extraordinarily rare disorder that is observed primarily, although not exclusively, in persons of Japanese and Korean ethnicity. The disorder may occur at any age. IAH tends to be self-limited in Asians, but it may be persistent in whites. There is no gender predilection. Many patients have an ongoing autoimmune disorder or a history of treatment with a sulfhydryl-containing drug such as antithyroid medication. No patients have had a history of exposure to insulin.[14]

Pathogenesis

IAH is characterized by the presence of autoantibodies to insulin or the insulin receptor. There is speculation that meal ingestion in these patients may result in the unbinding of insulin from these antibodies. However, measurements of total insulin and free insulin have shown no postprandial alteration in their relative concentrations. The mechanism for the generation of insulin antibodies is unknown but may involve enhanced immunogenicity resulting from an effect of the disulfide bond in drugs with a sulfhydryl component.

Diagnosis

Clinical manifestations Patients with IAH typically experience postprandial hypoglycemia resulting in neuroglycopenia. The symptomatic severity of IAS appears to vary greatly. Whites may become more seriously debilitated than Asians.

Laboratory tests Serum insulin levels are markedly elevated in IAH, because the insulin antibodies interfere with this assay. Values can be as high as 1,000 μU/ml. Oddly, C-peptide levels are usually not suppressed. Insulin antibody titers are very high, higher than those seen in insulin-treated diabetic patients. The antibodies may bind only to human insulin or to both human insulin and beef and pork insulin. The antibodies may be polyclonal or monoclonal, and they usually have characteristics similar to those that occur in patients with type 1 diabetes mellitus. It should be noted that very low titers of insulin antibodies may also be observed in healthy persons without hypoglycemia and occasionally in persons with insulinoma.

Management

Supportive treatment, such as frequent small meals, may be effective in IAH, especially for mild cases. For more severely affected patients, a variety of approaches have been tried, including glucocorticoids, immunosuppressants, plasmapheresis, octreotide, and diazoxide. Unfortunately, all these treatments usually fail. Use of partial pancreatectomy and splenectomy has led to amelioration but not complete resolution of symptoms.

The author has no commercial relationships with manufacturers of products or providers of services discussed in this chapter.

References

1. Goodenow TJ, Malarkey WB: Leukocytosis and artifactual hypoglycemia. JAMA 237:1961, 1977

2. Macaron CI, Kadri A, Macaron Z: Nucleated red blood cells and artifactual hypoglycemia. Diabetes Care 4:113, 1981

3. Service FJ, Veneziale CM, Nelson RA, et al: Combined deficiency of glucose-6-phosphate and fructose-1,6-diphosphate: studies of glucagon secretion and fuel utilization. Am J Med 64:698, 1978

4. Hepburn DA, Deary IJ, Frier BM, et al: Symptoms of acute insulin-induced hypoglycemia in humans with and without IDDM: factor-analysis approach. Diabetes Care 14:949, 1991

5. Service FJ, Dale AJD, Elveback LR, et al: Insulinoma: clinical and diagnostic features of 60 consecutive cases. Mayo Clin Proc 51:417, 1976

6. Hassoun AAK, Service FJ, O'Brien PC: Glycated hemoglobin in insulinoma. Endocr Pract 4:181, 1998

7. Service FJ, O'Brien PC, Kao PC, et al: C-peptide suppression test: effects of gender, age and body mass index: implications for the diagnosis of insulinoma. J Clin Endocrinol Metab 74:204, 1992

8. Schwartz NS, Clutter WE, Shah SD, et al: Glycemic thresholds for activation of glucose counterregulatory systems are higher than the threshold for symptoms. J Clin Invest 79:777, 1987

9. Mitrakou A, Ryan C, Veneman T, et al: Hierarchy of glycemic thresholds for counterregulatory hormone secretion, symptoms and cerebral dysfunction. Am J Physiol 260:E57, 1991

10. Whipple AE: The surgical therapy of hyperinsulinism. J Int Chir 3:237, 1938

11. Service FJ, Natt N: Clinical perspective: the prolonged fast. J Clin Endocrinol Metab 85:3973, 2000

12. Merimee TJ, Fineberg SE: Homeostasis during fasting: II. Hormone substrate differences between men and women. J Clin Endocrinol Metab 37:698, 1973

13. Service FJ: Diagnostic approach to adults with hypoglycemic disorders. Endocrinol Metab Clin North Am 28:519, 1999

14. Redmon JB, Nuttall FQ: Autoimmune hypoglycemia. Hypoglycemic Disorders 28:603, 1999

15. Service FJ, McMahon MM, O'Brien PC, et al: Functioning insulinoma—incidence, recurrence, and long-term survival of patients: a 60-year study. Mayo Clin Proc 66:711, 1991

16. Svartberg J, Stridsberg M, Wilander E, et al: Tumour-induced hypoglycaemia in a patient with insulin-dependent diabetes mellitus. J Intern Med 239:181, 1996

17. Tattersall RB, Gregory R, Selby C, et al: Course of brittle diabetes: 12 year follow up. BMJ 302:1240, 1991

18. Mayefsky JH, Sarnaik AP, Postellon DC: Factitious hypoglycemia. Pediatrics 69:804, 1982

19. Marks V, Teale JD: Hypoglycemia: factitious and felonious. Endocrinol Metab Clin North Am 28:579, 1999.

20. Hooper PL, Tello RJ, Burstein PH, et al: Pseudoinsulinoma: the Diamox-Diabinese switch. N Engl J Med 323:448, 1990

21. Service FJ, Natt N, Thompson GB, et al: Noninsulinoma pancreatogenous hypoglycemia: a novel syndrome of hyperinsulinemic hypoglycemia in adults independent of mutations in *Kir6.2* and *SUR1* genes. J Clin Endocrinol Metab 84:1582, 1999

22. Thomas PM, Cote GJ, Wohlik N, et al: Mutations in the sulfonylurea receptor gene in familial hyperinsulinemic hypoglycemia of infancy. Science 268:426, 1995

23. Doppman JL, Chang R, Fraker DL, et al: Localization of insulinomas to regions of the pancreas by intraarterial stimulation by calcium. Ann Intern Med 123:269, 1995

24. O'Shea D, Rohrer-Theus A, Lynn JA, et al: Localization of insulinomas by selective intraarterial calcium injection. J Clin Endocrinol Metab 81:1623, 1996

25. Zangen DH, Bonner-Weir S, Lee CH, et al: Reduced insulin, GLUT2, and IDX-1 in beta-cells after partial pancreatectomy. Diabetes 46:258, 1997

52 Type 1 Diabetes Mellitus

Saul Genuth, M.D., F.A.C.P.

Definition and Classification

Type 1 diabetes mellitus is a metabolic disease characterized by destruction of the pancreatic beta cells, resulting in an absolute deficiency of insulin secretion, with subsequent hyperglycemia.[1] Destruction of the beta cells typically results from an autoimmune process. The unusual cases of type 1 diabetes in which there is no evidence of autoimmune activity and for which no other causes for beta cell destruction (e.g., cystic fibrosis) can be found are classified as type 1 idiopathic.[1]

The current classification of diabetes mellitus was revised by a task force of the American Diabetes Association (ADA) that included representation from Europe.[1] Major etiologic classes of the disease, along with more esoteric examples, have been categorized [see Table 1]. Type 1 constitutes 5% to 10% of all diabetes cases; type 2 accounts for most of the remainder.

Type 1 and 2 diabetes were formerly known as insulin-dependent diabetes mellitus (IDDM) and non–insulin-dependent diabetes mellitus (NIDDM), respectively. This classification was abandoned largely because it was difficult to distinguish patients with IDDM from patients with NIDDM who eventually required insulin treatment to mitigate hyperglycemia. The current classification, which is based on etiology rather than mode of treatment, puts a greater emphasis on the history and characteristics of the patients to determine the probable etiology and type.

Epidemiology

Available studies, though not up-to-date, suggest that the prevalence of type 1 diabetes mellitus in the United States is 1.7 per 1,000 in individuals younger than 19 years and 2.1 per 1,000 in adults.[2] A total prevalence of approximately 500,000 is estimated. Current estimates of annual incidence are 18 per 100,000 population in the 0- to 19-year age range and 9 per 100,000 population in those older than 20 years.[2] The peak incidence is at 11 years of age, but new cases can occasionally appear in the elderly. Approximately 30,000 cases of type 1 diabetes mellitus are estimated to occur yearly in the United States, and it is more common in whites than in African Americans. Worldwide, the highest annual incidence of type 1 diabetes mellitus is found in Finland (45 cases per 100,000) and the lowest is found in Korea (< 1 per 100,000). The incidence of type 1 diabetes is increasing at a rate of approximately 3% a year; by 2010, the annual incidence in many populations is expected to exceed 30 per 100,000.[3]

Hormonal Regulation of Metabolism

Diabetes involves the most fundamental aspects of human metabolism. The hormonal abnormalities of diabetes affect all of the following: energy production and expenditure; the proportioning of carbohydrate, fat, and protein as energy sources; the storage of energy as carbohydrate and fat; and the balance between protein synthesis (anabolism) and degradation (catabolism). To understand the pathogenesis of diabetes, it is useful to start with a brief review of normal metabolism.[4]

A proper balance between insulin and glucagon is one crucial hormonal regulator of basal metabolic homeostasis. Insulin primarily facilitates storage of glucose as glycogen, free fatty acids

in triglycerides, and amino acids in protein, and it inhibits glycogenolysis, lipolysis, ketogenesis, proteolysis, and gluconeogenesis [see Figure 1]. Glucagon stimulates mobilization of glucose, free fatty acids, and glycerol, as well as the hepatic uptake of amino acids and the conversion of their carbon skeletons to

---

Table 1   Etiologic Classification of Diabetes

Type 1 diabetes mellitus* (β cell destruction, usually leading to absolute insulin deficiency)
  Immune mediated
  Idiopathic

Type 2 diabetes mellitus* (may range from predominantly insulin resistance with relative insulin deficiency to a predominantly insulin secretory defect with insulin resistance)

Other specific types of diabetes
  Genetic defects of β cell function
    Chromosome 12, HNF-1α (formerly MODY3)
    Chromosome 7, glucokinase (formerly MODY2)
    Chromosome 20, HNF-4α (formerly MODY2)
    Mitochondrial DNA defects
  Genetic defects in insulin action
    Type A insulin resistance
  Disease of the exocrine pancreas
    Pancreatitis
    Trauma/pancreatectomy
    Neoplasia
    Cystic fibrosis
    Hemochromatosis
  Endocrinopathies
    Acromegaly
    Cushing syndrome
    Glucagonoma
    Pheochromocytoma
  Drug- or chemical-induced
    Nicotinic acid
    Glucocorticoids
    Thiazides
    Pentamidine
    α-Interferon
  Infections
    Congenital rubella
    Cytomegalovirus
  Uncommon forms of immune-mediated diabetes
    Stiff-man syndrome
    Anti-insulin receptor antibodies
  Other genetic syndromes associated with diabetes
    Down syndrome
    Turner syndrome
    Friedreich ataxia
    Myotonic dystrophy

Gestational diabetes mellitus (GDM)

Note: The list of other specific types of diabetes is not comprehensive. There are many other such syndromes, especially genetic syndromes of beta cell function and genetic syndromes associated with diabetes.

*Patients with any form of diabetes may require insulin treatment at some stage of their disease. Such use of insulin does not, of itself, classify the patient.

633

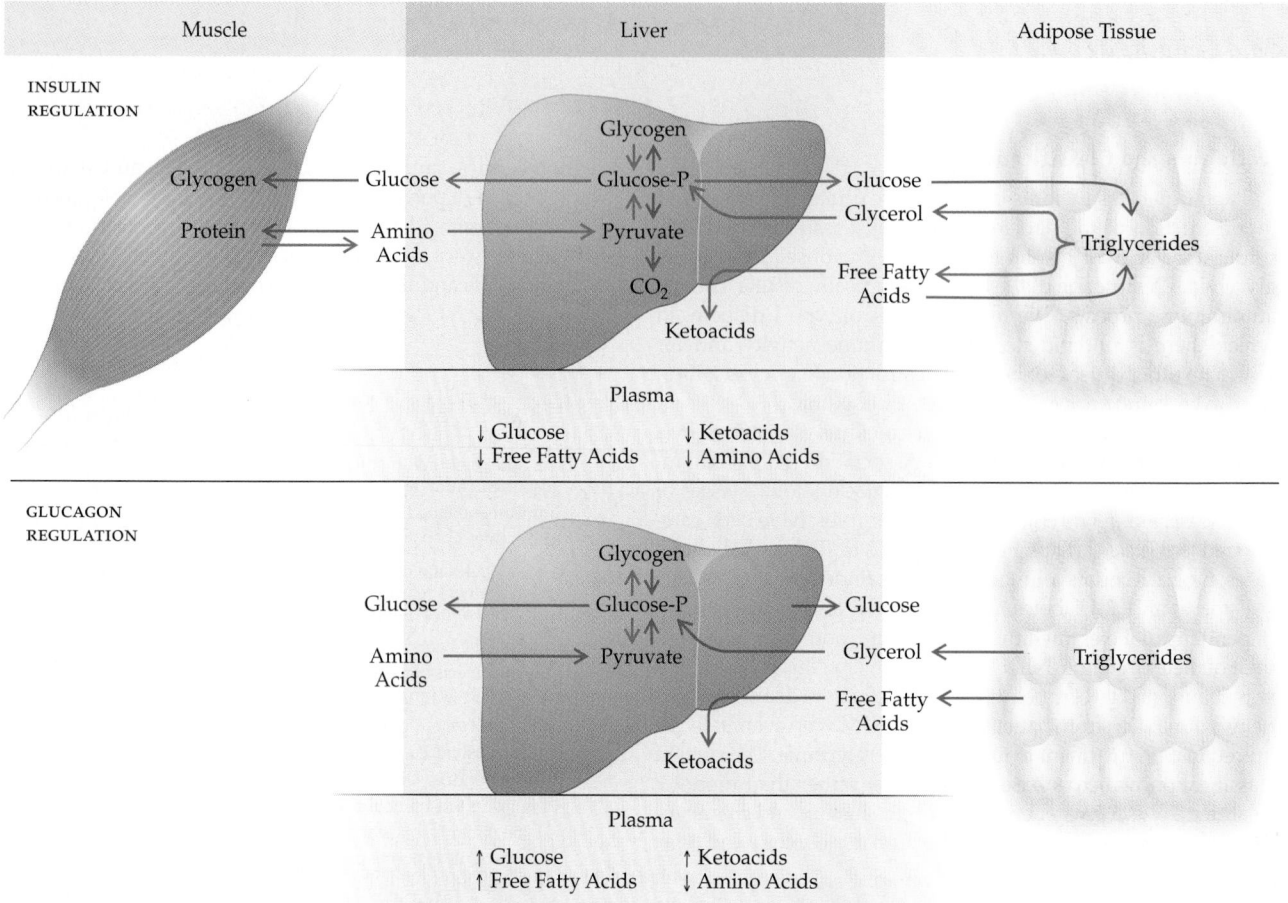

Muscle	Liver	Adipose Tissue

INSULIN
REGULATION

Plasma

↓ Glucose   ↓ Ketoacids
↓ Free Fatty Acids ↓ Amino Acids

GLUCAGON
REGULATION

Plasma

↑ Glucose   ↑ Ketoacids
↑ Free Fatty Acids ↓ Amino Acids

Figure 1 **The opposing actions of insulin and glucagon, particularly within the liver, on substrate flow and plasma levels are seen here. The two hormones have directly opposite effects on key enzymes, such as glycogen synthase and phosphorylase. Thus, stimulatory effects of glucagons on glucose and ketoacid production are magnified when insulin is deficient, as in type 1 diabetes mellitus. Red arrows indicate stimulation. Blue arrows indicate inhibition.**

glucose. Glucagon also stimulates ketogenesis from free fatty acids [*see Figure 1*]. The normal steady-state levels of insulin and glucagon help maintain the overnight fasting plasma glucose level at 60 to 110 mg/dl, free fatty acid levels at less than 0.7 mmol/L, ketoacids at less than 0.2 mmol/L, and each amino acid at its unique level. After a mixed meal, plasma insulin rises sharply [*see Figure 2*] and, with it, the insulin-glucagon ratio. This condition reverses all the previously described processes of energy mobilization and glucose synthesis. Dietary carbohydrate is stored in muscle and liver glycogen, free fatty acids are reesterified and stored as triglycerides in adipose tissue, and protein metabolism shifts back toward anabolism. When all the nutrients have been assimilated and plasma glucose returns to its basal preprandial level, plasma insulin [*see Figure 2*] and the insulin-glucagon ratio promptly return to basal levels, preventing an overshooting of insulin action that would cause hypoglycemia. Thus, an immediate rise, an early peak, and a prompt fall in insulin secretion are requisite to normal postprandial metabolism [*see Figure 2*].

Insulin is synthesized in pancreatic islet beta cells from a larger molecule called proinsulin, which is then split to yield insulin and an intramolecular connecting peptide called C-peptide [*see Figure 3*]. The two molecules are stored in the same granules and are secreted in an equimolar ratio when the beta cell is stimulat-

ed. Thus, plasma C-peptide levels are a faithful marker of beta cell function [*see Figure 3*].

Insulin acts via a plasma insulin receptor that leads to the generation of multiple mediators of insulin's numerous intracellular cytoplasmic and nuclear effects [*see Figure 4*]. Insulin regulates both the activities and syntheses of target enzymes. The sensitivity of target tissues to insulin is the other major determinant of insulin action [*see Figure 5*]. A feedback loop exists between insulin responsiveness in target tissues and insulin secretion by beta cells. This relation operates to increase insulin secretion in individuals relatively resistant to insulin action—for example, obese persons [*see Figure 2*]—and to decrease insulin release in individuals very sensitive to insulin action [*see Figure 5*]. The result is one critical mechanism for maintaining fasting and postprandial plasma glucose levels within narrow normal ranges.

Pathogenesis

Type 1 diabetes mellitus is characterized by absolute insulin deficiency, making patients dependent on exogenous insulin replacement for survival.[1,5] Insulin deficiency results from the destruction or disappearance of the insulin-producing beta cells that constitute 60% to 70% of the pancreatic islets of Langerhans.

When 90% of the beta cells have been eliminated, clinical diabetes occurs [*see Figure 6*].

AUTOIMMUNE FACTORS

There is strong evidence that a cell-mediated autoimmune process is involved in the destruction of beta cells in the majority

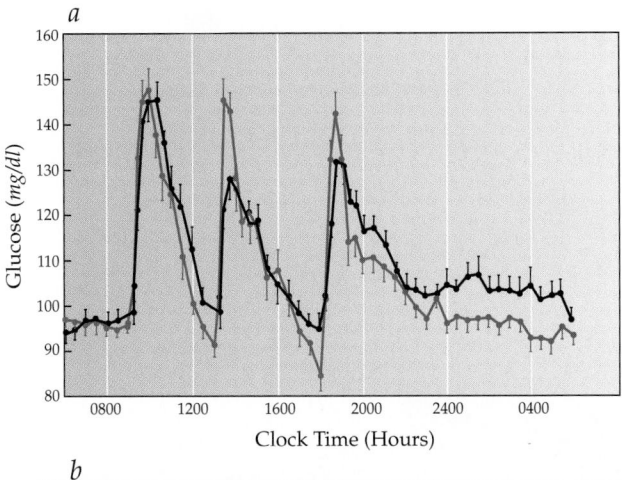

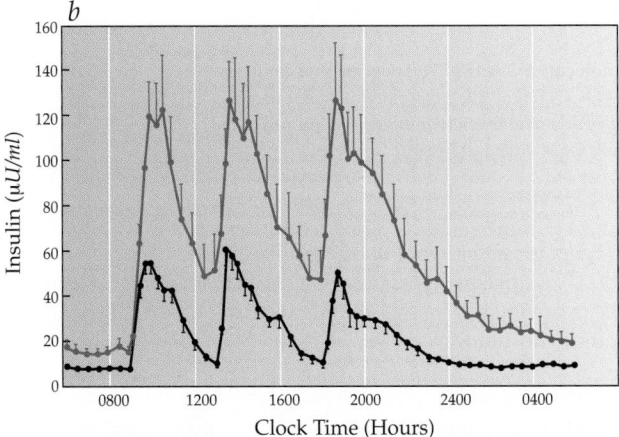

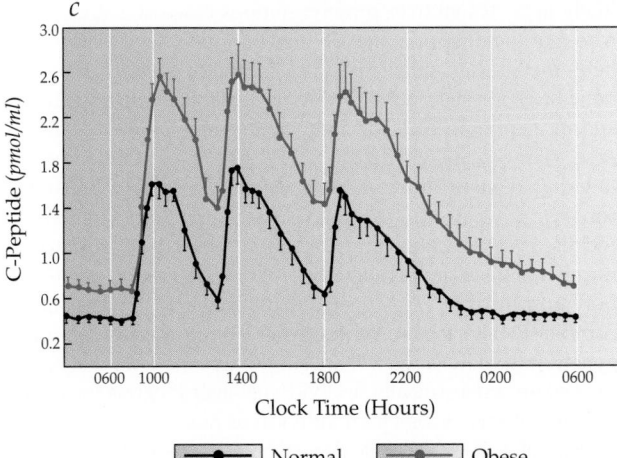

Figure 2 **Plasma glucose (*a*) is normally kept within a narrow range throughout the day, largely because of beta cell function. Plasma insulin (*b*) and plasma C-peptide (*c*) rise sharply from their basal levels with each meal and, after reaching peaks, return promptly to basal levels, which are maintained throughout the night. Note also that plasma insulin and C-peptide levels are elevated in obese persons who are insulin resistant.**

of cases of type 1 diabetes mellitus.[6-8] In a number of cases in which death occurred from an accident or from an illness other than diabetes shortly after the patient was diagnosed as having type 1 diabetes mellitus, a mononuclear lymphocytic infiltrate was found in the islets. T cell distribution in such cases is marked by an increase in CD8+ suppressor-inducer T cells and a decrease in CD4+ helper-inducer T cells.[6] A similar immunocellular response has been found in animal models of spontaneous insulin-deficient diabetes.[8] In some instances, experimental manipulations that prevent T cell lymphocytic responses also prevent the development of diabetes. Furthermore, the transfer of diabetes from affected animals to nonaffected animals by lymphocytes has also been described. Interleukins and other cytokines have been shown to exhibit toxic effects on the beta cells and to inhibit insulin secretion.

Autoantibodies to a variety of beta cell and islet autoantigens are present in the sera of patients with type 1 diabetes mellitus at the time of diagnosis.[9-11] The autoantigens include the enzymes glutamic acid decarboxylase (GAD), carboxypeptidase H, a protein tyrosine phosphatase labeled ICA512 or IA-2, and insulin itself.[9-11] Some studies have shown that islet autoantibodies are capable of inhibiting insulin secretion in vitro or even causing lysis of beta cells. Other evidence supports the importance of autoimmune phenomena in the pathogenesis of type 1 diabetes mellitus. For example, studies in identical twins who are discordant for type 1 diabetes mellitus have shown that, in the absence of immunosuppressive therapy, the diabetic identical twin will reject a pancreas transplant from the nondiabetic twin; presumably, the recipient's autoantibodies recognize antigens in the donor twin's pancreatic islets, which are identical to the recipient's antigens. If treatment of type 1 diabetes mellitus with the immunosuppressive agent cyclosporine is initiated within 2 to 6 weeks after the clinical onset of diabetes, dependency upon insulin can be eliminated or insulin doses markedly reduced, but only as long as immunosuppression is maintained.[12,13] The toxicity associated with cyclosporine and other immunosuppressive agents has precluded use of this form of therapy in clinical practice.

It is now clear that the autoimmune phenomena begin long before the clinical onset of the disease. Islet or beta cell autoantibodies can be found in 2% to 4% of first-degree relatives of patients with type 1 diabetes mellitus, which is 10 to 20 times the prevalence in control subjects. Longitudinal studies have shown that type 1 diabetes mellitus is much more likely to develop in clinically unaffected relatives with high autoantibody titers than in relatives without such antibodies, and that the disease will develop in such patients within a few years.[14-16] Longitudinal serial testing of plasma insulin responses to intravenous glucose injection demonstrates progressively declining beta cell function in autoantibody-positive relatives before the clinical onset of diabetes.[17]

ENVIRONMENTAL FACTORS

Because only 30% to 50% of unaffected identical twins of patients with type 1 diabetes mellitus will eventually develop the disease, it is likely that an environmental factor may be required to trigger the autoimmune destructive process.[18] In addition, individuals with genotypes that place them at high risk for diabetes make up a lower percentage of the diabetic population than in the past—a fact that suggests an environmental cause for the increasing incidence of type 1 diabetes.[19]

A number of viral candidates have been proposed.[18] The only certain association is that the offspring of women who are infect-

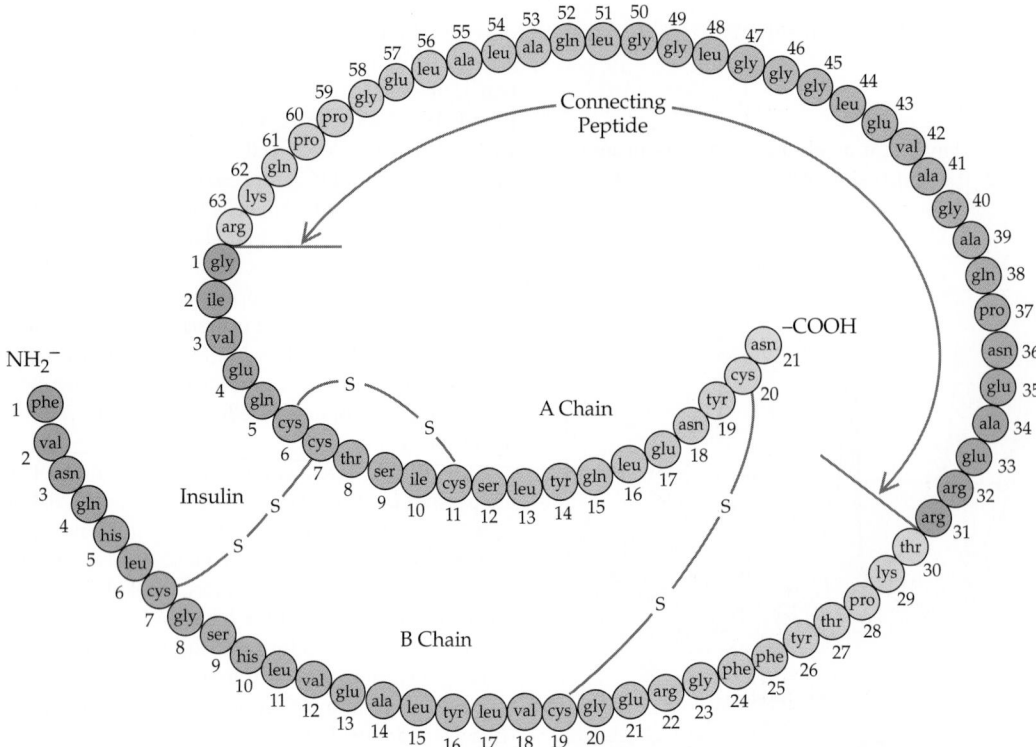

Figure 3 The structure of human proinsulin, the precursor molecule to insulin. The peptide that connects the amino terminus (NH₂⁻) of the A chain to the carboxyl terminus (–COOH) of the B chain is called connecting peptide (C-peptide). Proinsulin is converted to insulin and C-peptide, and these two molecules are packaged together in the secretory granule. On stimulation of the beta cell, C-peptide and insulin are secreted in equimolar proportions. Thus, C-peptide levels reflect beta cell functional capacity.

ed with rubella during pregnancy are at increased risk for type 1 diabetes mellitus. In addition, a small amount of indirect evidence associates coxsackievirus B with type 1 diabetes mellitus.[20] Toxins in the environment or diet might also initiate the destruction of genetically vulnerable beta cells. An international consortium has been established to follow persons with high-risk human leukocyte antigen (HLA) genotypes (*see* Genetic Factors, *below*) from birth through adolescence, in an effort to identify infectious agents, dietary factors, or other environmental factors that can trigger islet autoimmunity in this genetically susceptible population.[21]

TEMPORAL SEQUENCE OF BETA CELL DESTRUCTION

At the time of the clinical onset of type 1 diabetes mellitus, at least a small number of beta cells are still potentially capable of functioning.[22,23] After several weeks of exogenous insulin treatment, particularly if exemplary metabolic control has been established,[24] dependency on exogenous insulin decreases or ceases entirely for weeks to months in some patients. This temporary so-called honeymoon remission phase is marked by an increase in serum C-peptide levels, which indicates an increase in endogenous insulin secretion [*see Figure 6*].[23] However, within 5 years after diagnosis of childhood type 1 diabetes mellitus, C-peptide virtually disappears from the serum.[25]

Type 1 diabetes mellitus does not develop in all autoantibody-positive individuals. Moreover, the latency period between the initiation of beta cell destruction and the appearance of the clinical disorder may be many years[26]; the disease does not appear in some patients until considerably later in life. This condition has been termed latent autoimmune diabetes in adults (LADA).[27]

The gradual, indolent nature of the disease in these autoantibody-positive patients is also suggested by the fact that some can be treated with beta cell–stimulating drugs before absolutely requiring insulin.[28]

GENETIC FACTORS

Although a family history of type 1 diabetes mellitus is more likely to be absent than present in index cases, it is nonetheless true that the offspring and siblings of patients with type 1 diabetes mellitus are at increased risk for the disease. There is a genetic basis for susceptibility to type 1 diabetes mellitus, but no specific genotype leads inevitably to the development of the disease.[29] The disease will develop in 5% to 10% of first-degree relatives of patients with type 1 diabetes mellitus and in 20% of persons who have two first-degree relatives (e.g., both parents) with the disease. Association and linkage studies have incriminated a number of genes involved in the risk of type 1 diabetes mellitus. Polymorphism of HLA genes in the major histocompatibility complex (MHC) locus on chromosome 6 accounts for 50% of the genetic risk.[29] DR3 and DR4 are susceptibility alleles that appear to operate synergistically. Individuals heterozygous for DR3 or DR4 are at greater risk than individuals homozygous for either DR3 or DR4. The DR2 allele decreases the risk and dominates the susceptibility effect of DR3 or DR4 when either is accompanied by DR2. The HLA-DQ locus also is associated with an increased risk of diabetes.[30] Substitution of alanine, valine, or serine for the more usual aspartic acid at position 57 of DQ β chain or the presence of arginine at position 52 of DQ α chain increases the risk of type 1 diabetes mellitus. A number of mechanisms have been suggested to explain how HLA class II molecules might predis-

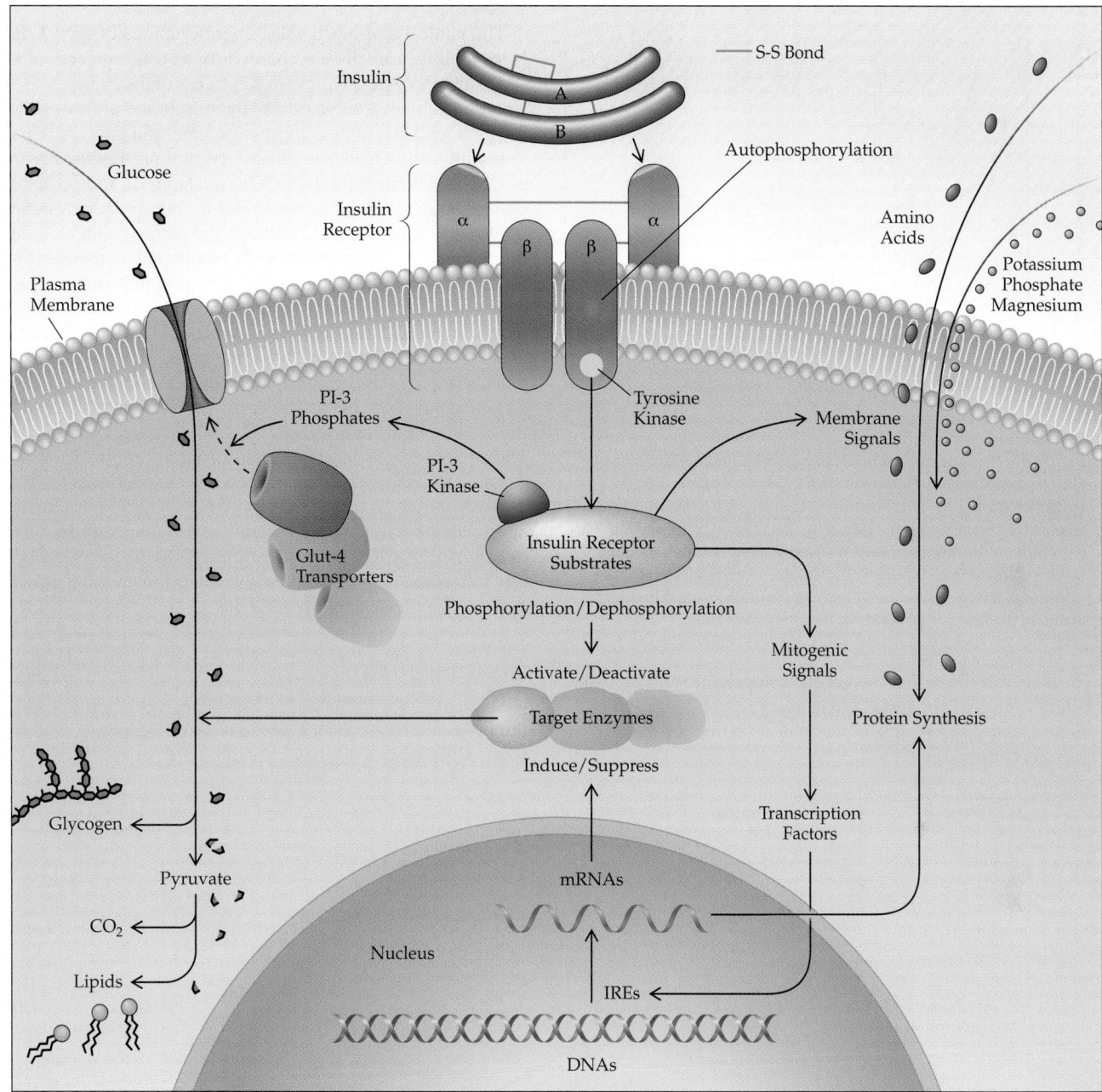

Figure 4   **The cellular actions of insulin begin with binding to its plasma membrane receptor. As a result, certain tyrosine molecules in the intracellular portion of the transmembrane receptor are autophosphorylated, creating tyrosine kinase activity in the receptor. Several intracellular insulin receptor substrates (IRS) are then tyrosine phosphorylated by the receptor. Phosphorylated IRS docks and either activates or inactivates numerous enzymes (e.g., phosphatidylinositol-3-kinase [PI-3 kinase]) and other mediating molecules. Among the chief effects of these insulin-stimulated cascades are translocation of glucose (Glut-4) transporters to the plasma membrane, where they facilitate glucose diffusion into the cell; shifting of intracellular glucose metabolism toward storage as glycogen by activating glycogen synthase; stimulation of cellular uptake of amino acids, phosphate, potassium, and magnesium; stimulation of protein synthesis and inhibition of proteolysis; and regulation of gene expression via insulin regulatory elements (IRE) in target DNA molecules. Numerous intermediates in these various pathways, along with the molecules mentioned above, are products of candidate genes whose mutation could produce the state of insulin resistance characteristic of type 2 diabetes mellitus. Red connectors between insulin chains A and B and among insulin receptor subunits α and β indicate S-S bonds. The A chain also has an intramolecular S-S bond.**

pose to or protect against the disease.[31] Despite the accumulation of considerable knowledge, the development of type 1 diabetes mellitus still cannot be predicted with complete certainty.[32]

Type 1 diabetes mellitus is associated with at least 15 additional loci on nine other chromosomes.[32] Of particular interest is that a variable number of tandem repeats in the promoter region of the insulin gene has been associated with the disease. However, the insulin molecule itself is apparently normal in structure in patients with type 1 diabetes mellitus. With the human genome sequenced and advanced genetic technology becoming cost-

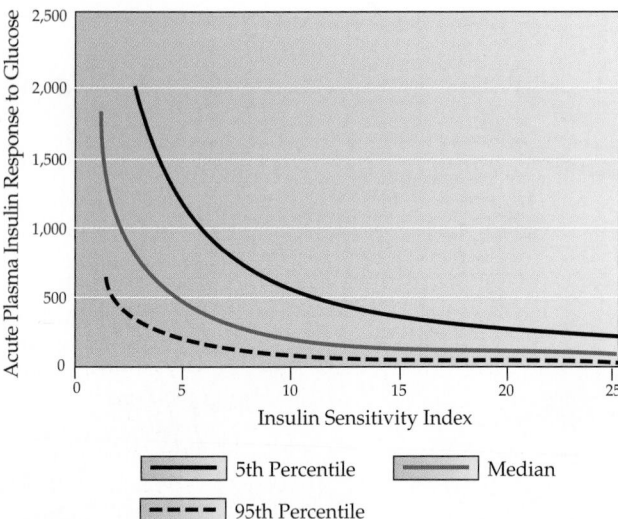

Figure 5 Measurement of insulin levels after the administration of glucose provides an indication of both insulin sensitivity (i.e., the uptake of glucose by peripheral tissues in response to insulin) and responsiveness of pancreatic beta cells. The median, 95th, and 5th percentiles of insulin sensitivity are shown. Note that the amount of insulin secreted in response to glucose administration increases as insulin sensitivity decreases. This feedback mechanism helps to maintain plasma glucose levels in the physiologic range.

effective, it is likely that the genetic components of type 1 diabetes mellitus will be sorted out in a way that will make it possible to identify susceptible individuals who might benefit from preventive therapies.

INSULIN DEFICIENCY

The clinical and biochemical manifestations of type 1 diabetes mellitus can all be accounted for as consequences of insulin deficiency [*see Figures 1 and 7*].[33] Loss of the stimulating effect of insulin on glucose uptake by muscle and adipose tissue coupled with loss of the suppressive effect of insulin on hepatic glucose output lead to severe hyperglycemia. Fasting plasma glucose levels rise typically to 300 to 400 mg/dl, and postprandial glucose levels rise to 500 to 600 mg/dl in patients before treatment.[33] This increase results in the presentation of a high filtered load of glucose to the renal tubules and consequently a severe osmotic diuresis, manifested by polyuria and compensatory polydipsia. Loss of the lipogenic and antilipolytic effects of insulin on adipose tissue leads to high plasma levels and increased hepatic uptake of free fatty acids. This condition enhances ketogenesis, and ultimately, high plasma ketoacid levels cause metabolic acidosis. Protein breakdown is favored in the absence of the anticatabolic and anabolic actions of insulin. The proteolysis of muscle protein provides amino acids that sustain high rates of gluconeogenesis. These processes result in the loss of both fat and lean body mass; weight loss is further aggravated by an increase in basal energy expenditure.[34] The negative nitrogen balance, accompanied by losses of potassium, magnesium, and phosphate in the urine, impairs growth and development in children.

Prevention

Serologic evidence, as well as genetic markers, can often identify persons who are at increased risk for developing type 1 diabetes. At the time of diagnosis, about 90% of patients with type 1

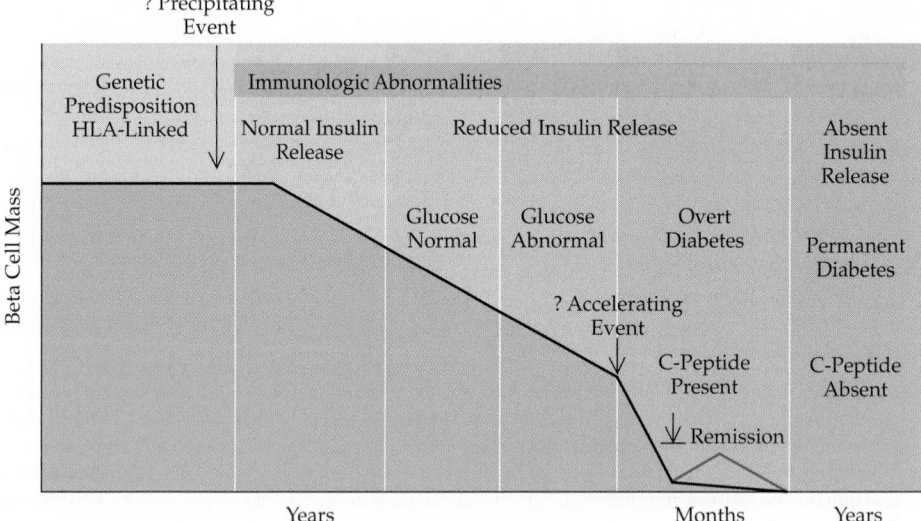

Figure 6 Current view of the pathogenesis of type 1 autoimmune diabetes mellitus. In some individuals, HLA-linked genes set in motion an autoimmune attack on islet cells, predominantly beta cells. In other individuals, HLA-linked genes protect against the autoimmune destructive response. An initiating event, such as exposure to a virus with an antigenic epitope that resembles a beta cell antigen or to a toxin, may start the process of self-destruction. Disappearance of the beta cells may occur because the viral antigen accelerates the normal rate of apoptosis (programmed cell death). As time passes, insulin production and secretion diminish, despite increasing hyperglycemia. When insulin release falls to trivial amounts or stops altogether, diabetic ketoacidosis results. Another external event may trigger this final beta cell catastrophe. A few beta cells may survive, because after this, a brief period of remission marked by reappearance of C-peptide in plasma may ensue if plasma glucose levels are controlled very tightly with exogenous insulin. Eventually, all beta cell function ceases, leading to metabolic instability.

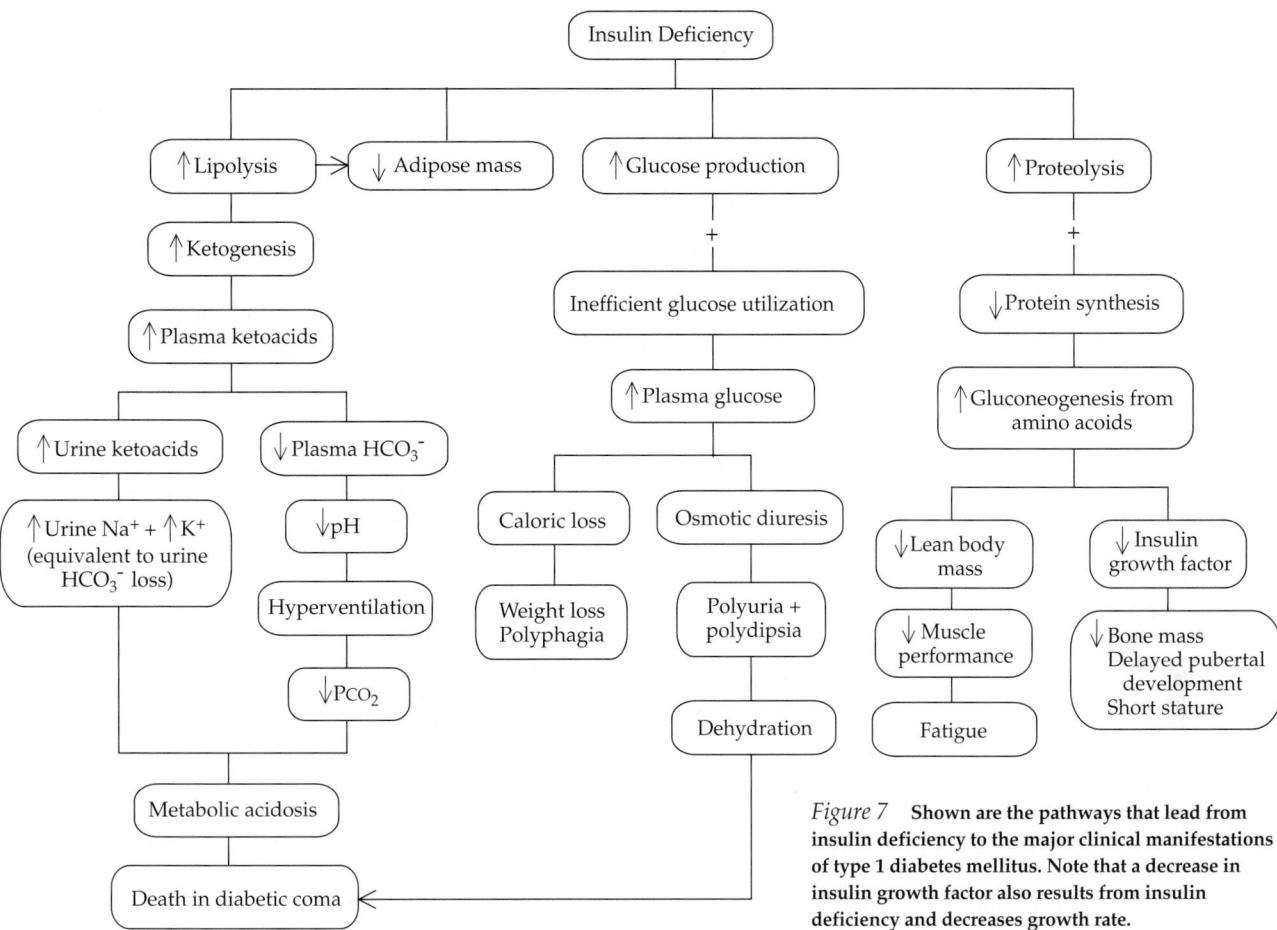

Figure 7 **Shown are the pathways that lead from insulin deficiency to the major clinical manifestations of type 1 diabetes mellitus. Note that a decrease in insulin growth factor also results from insulin deficiency and decreases growth rate.**

diabetes mellitus have autoantibodies to GAD, IA-2, or insulin, alone or in combination. The presence of islet cell autoantibodies predicts the development of autoimmune diabetes in first-degree relatives, whereas in the general population, the presence of two or more autoantibodies is highly predictive of future diabetes; IA-2 antibodies indicate very high risk.[35] The existence of such markers, as well as the long period between their appearance and the development of clinical disease, has inspired research into the possibility of intervention to prevent clinical diabetes.

A trial sponsored by the National Institute of Diabetes and Digestive and Kidney Diseases unfortunately found no evidence that type 1 diabetes mellitus can be prevented by inducing immune tolerance to exogenous human insulin given subcutaneously or orally to relatives of patients with high titers of islet autoantibodies. A hypothesis-generating analysis suggested, however, that study patients with high levels of insulin autoantibodies who received oral insulin may have experienced a delay and perhaps a reduction in the incidence of type 1 diabetes.[36]

Early studies showed that treatment with cyclosporine offered an effective, albeit impractical, method for suppressing type 1 diabetes [*see* Pathogenesis, Autoimmune Factors, *above*]. In recent studies, the use of anti-CD3 monoclonal antibodies for targeting T cells showed some promise for protecting beta cells from destruction.[37-39]

Diagnosis

The diagnosis of type 1 diabetes mellitus is still almost always made on the basis of symptom history; the diagnosis is con-

firmed by finding of a blood or plasma glucose level greater than 200 mg/dl, along with glucosuria and, often, ketonuria. The classic symptoms are polyuria, polydipsia, weight loss despite normal or even increased food intake, fatigue, and blurred vision. These symptoms are commonly present 4 to 12 weeks before medical attention is sought. In the future, however, diagnosis in advance of clinical onset may be possible through serologic methods, complemented by beta cell function tests.

Management

Of all chronic diseases, diabetes is unique in that its therapy involves daily self-management by the patient and a host of lifestyle adaptations. For optimal metabolic control, patients must prick their fingers to test the blood glucose level at least four times daily, inject insulin at least three times daily, pay regular attention to the timing and content of their meals, and try to follow a scheduled exercise program. The patient is truly at the center of his or her care. Patient self-management requires intensive education with regard to the skills of injection and blood glucose monitoring, urine ketone testing on sick days, meal planning, detection and treatment of hypoglycemia, and management of intercurrent illness. Family members and close associates of the patient need to be included as is appropriate, particularly with regard to the recognition and treatment of hypoglycemia. Ideally, the patient should understand the pathophysiology of diabetes and its long-term complications almost as well as health care professionals. Some aspects of care require periodic educational reinforcement, which is often stimulated by some therapeutic mishap, such as a preventable episode of severe hypoglycemia or ketoacidosis.

The clinical goals of treatment include (1) decreasing plasma glucose levels and urine glucose excretion to eliminate polyuria, polydipsia, polyphagia, caloric loss, and adverse effects such as blurred vision from lens swelling and susceptibility to infection, particularly vaginitis in women, (2) abolishing ketosis, (3) inducing positive nitrogen balance to restore lean body mass and physical capability and to maintain normal growth, development, and life functioning, and (4) preventing or greatly minimizing the late complications of diabetes.

THE DIABETES CONTROL AND COMPLICATIONS TRIAL

The introduction of insulin therapy in 1922 allowed patients with type 1 diabetes mellitus to live long enough to experience the distinctive microvascular complications of diabetes—retinopathy and nephropathy—as well as neuropathy. The appearance of these complications in the 1930s generated a 50-year debate about whether diabetic retinopathy, nephropathy, and neuropathy were the direct result of the metabolic abnormalities, most notably hyperglycemia, or whether they were a parallel independent consequence of diabetes that had formerly been usually preempted by death from extreme metabolic disequilibrium (i.e., diabetic coma). The debate was not merely academic, because it was reflected in quite different approaches to treatment. A belief that complications were caused by hyperglycemia impelled the physician to work with inadequate means to help the patient achieve as close to normal blood glucose levels as possible. Conversely, a belief that complications occurred independently of hyperglycemia encouraged a somewhat more laissez-faire approach, in which the physician attempted primarily to eliminate the immediate symptoms, such as polyuria, that occurred when plasma glucose levels exceeded the renal threshold (> 180 mg/dl). Furthermore, the risk of hypoglycemia associated with the more aggressive approach to hyperglycemia reinforced the arguments of the conservative practitioners. A large body of evidence was eventually built up that supported but did not prove the so-called glucose hypothesis (i.e., the hypothesis that treatment that normalizes glucose levels will prevent or delay the long-term complications of diabetes mellitus). The Diabetes Control and Complications Trial (DCCT) ended this debate for type 1 diabetes.

The DCCT was a randomized clinical trial that tested the glucose hypothesis in patients with type 1 diabetes mellitus.[40] Half of the patients with diabetes of 1 to 5 years' duration participated in a primary prevention trial that excluded all patients with retinopathy or microalbuminuria, and half of the patients with diabetes of 1 to 15 years' duration participated in a secondary intervention trial that included only patients who already had mild to moderate nonproliferative diabetic retinopathy but less than 200 mg/day of urinary albumin excretion. In both of these DCCT trials, patients were randomly assigned either to receive conventional treatment (no more than two insulin injections a day) or to receive intensive treatment (three to four insulin injections a day or use of a continuous subcutaneous insulin infusion [CSII] pump; self-monitoring of blood glucose levels at least four times a day; premeal target blood glucose levels of 70 to 120 mg/dl; a glycosylated hemoglobin [HbA_{1c}] goal of less than 6.05%; and very frequent contacts between patient and treatment team). An HbA_{1c} difference of 1.8% (8.9% versus 7.1%), corresponding to a mean blood glucose difference of around 75 mg/dl, was maintained between the two treatment groups.[41]

Over a mean follow-up of 6.5 years, intensive treatment produced substantial benefits. The risk of de novo development of retinopathy (i.e., the appearance of microaneurysms) was reduced by 27%, whereas the risk of progression of retinopathy was reduced 76%; the development of microalbuminuria was reduced by 35%; macroalbuminuria (i.e., proteinuria) was reduced by 56%; and development of clinical neuropathy, confirmed by abnormal nerve conduction velocities or autonomic nervous system function tests, was reduced by 60%.[40] Patients in the primary prevention cohort, with a mean diabetes duration of 2.5 years, had a somewhat greater overall response to intensive treatment than did patients in the secondary prevention cohort, with a mean diabetes duration of 8.5 years.

The main adverse effect of intensive treatment was a threefold increase in the risk of severe hypoglycemic episodes, defined as episodes requiring the assistance of others to treat and reverse.[40,42] At least one such event per year was experienced by 25% of the intensively treated patients, and 50% experienced more than one such episode by the end of the study; 14% experienced 10 or more episodes. About 25% of all episodes of severe hypoglycemia resulted in coma or convulsions. The overall rate of severe hypoglycemia was 62 events per 100 patient-years for those patients receiving intensive treatment, compared with 19 events per 100 patient-years for those receiving conventional treatment. Further analysis of the data, however, showed no association between multiple episodes of severe hypoglycemia and cognitive decrements, and no effect of intensive treatment on neuropsychological performance.[43]

In addition to hypoglycemic episodes, intensive treatment caused greater weight gain; one third of the patients exceeded 120% of ideal body weight (approximate body mass index [BMI], 27) by the end of the study.[40] Intensive treatment was also more expensive than conventional treatment.[44] However, the cost was partly offset by a projected decrease in costs associated with a lower rate of complications[45]; the estimated cost per year of quality life gained was $28,661, a figure thought to represent a good value.

The DCCT provided clinical trial proof (i.e., grade A evidence) that microvascular and neuropathic complications could be prevented or at least substantially delayed by maintaining blood glucose levels as near to normal as treatment techniques would safely allow. The DCCT could not prove that hyperglycemia caused microvascular complications, but it provided strong support for that hypothesis. The risk of retinopathy was shown to be related to the mean HbA_{1c} level in a similar exponential fashion in each DCCT treatment group.[46] The risk of retinopathy decreased 44% for each proportional 10% decrease in HbA_{1c} (e.g., a decrease in HbA1c from 9.0% to 8.1%). The relationships between HbA_{1c} levels and the risks of developing microalbuminuria or neuropathy were similar. Moreover, the DCCT analyses did not indicate any glycemic threshold below which there was no further risk of microvascular complications.[47] This observation means that normoglycemia should be the ideal goal of treating type 1 diabetes mellitus. Furthermore, the benefits of previous intensive treatment (or the adverse effects of previous conventional treatment) were still demonstrable years after the DCCT was completed. Follow-up of the DCCT cohort, reported in the Epidemiology of Diabetes Interventions and Complications (EDIC) study, showed that the HbA_{1c} levels of the intensive-therapy and conventional-therapy groups converged within 2 years after the DCCT ended. Nonetheless, compared with participants who received conventional therapy, those who received intensive insulin therapy during the DCCT experienced less progression of retinopathy, nephropathy, and neuropathy for 11 years afterward.[48-51] Moreover, for patients who received intensive treatment, the risks of cardiovascular disease events were reduced over the mean 17 years of follow-up in the DCCT plus the EDIC study,[52] as was the risk of the progression of atherosclerosis (measured as the increment in carotid artery intimal-medial thickness).[53]

Thus, sustained periods of glycemic exposure have long-term consequences. A level of hyperglycemia that would now be considered unacceptable continues to have adverse effects even after some improvement in metabolic control has occurred, and a prolonged marked reduction in hyperglycemia with intensive treatment early in the course of type 1 diabetes continues to have beneficial effects even after some worsening in metabolic control. Of note, intensive treatment during the DCCT led to no long-term decrease in cognitive function assessed 10 years after the end of the DCCT.[54]

GLYCEMIC GOALS

Current ADA standards of care reflect the DCCT results [*see Table 2*].[55] These standards include the following goals: (1) maintaining preprandial capillary plasma glucose levels at 90 to 130 mg/dl (5.0 to 7.2 mmol/L) and peak postprandial capillary plasma glucose levels (i.e., levels 1 to 2 hours after the beginning of the meal) at less than 180 mg/dl (< 10.0 mmol/L), and (2) maintaining HbA_{1c} levels of less than 7.0% (relative to a nondiabetic DCCT range of approximately 4.0% to 6.0%). Realistically, current therapeutic tools make it difficult to achieve these stringent goals in many patients with type 1 diabetes mellitus, particularly those with absolutely no endogenous insulin secretion. The exponential relation between the risk of microvascular complications and HbA_{1c} predicts that only normal HbA_{1c} levels would completely prevent the complications. However, maintaining the HbA_{1c} level below 7.0% will remove much of the absolute risk from most patients. Efforts to achieve an HbA_{1c} value of less than 7.0% should be started as soon as is safely possible and should continue as long as hypoglycemia can be minimized.

MONITORING OF GLYCEMIC CONTROL

Glucose Meters

Current blood glucose meters are small, use little blood, may permit the use of the forearm as well as the fingertips as puncture sites, are relatively invulnerable to inaccuracy because of patient errors, and have memory programs that allow the patient or caregiver to assess the pattern of blood glucose control over the previous 2 months, largely eliminating the problem of incorrect or fabricated written transcriptions of results. Continuous glucose monitoring systems, which use subcutaneous sensors to record average glucose levels every 5 minutes for up to 72 hours, have been approved by the Food and Drug Administration. Although the recorded profile can provide only a small window into a lifetime of blood glucose fluctuation, such a profile can guide periodic adjustments of the regimen by identifying glycemic instability (e.g., nocturnal hyperglycemia or excessive postprandial hyperglycemia) that might escape detection by HbA_{1c} or intermittent glucose meter testing.

Blood glucose testing before each meal or large snack is essential if the patient is to adjust each dose of rapid-action insulin to the level of blood glucose before the meal and to the amount of carbohydrate about to be ingested. Blood glucose levels also

Table 2 American Diabetes Association Standards* for Glycemic Control in Diabetes Mellitus[55]

Measurement	Normal	Goal
Preprandial capillary plasma glucose	< 100 mg/dl (< 5.5 mmol/L)	90–130 mg/dl (5.0–7.2 mmol/L)
Peak postprandial capillary plasma glucose[†]	< 140 mg/dl (< 7.7 mmol/L)	< 180 mg/dl (< 10.0 mmol/L)
Hemoglobin A_{1c} (%)	< 6	< 7

*The values shown in this table are by necessity generalized to the entire population of patients with diabetes. Goals should be individualized: patients with comorbid diseases, the very young, older adults, and patients with unusual conditions or circumstances may warrant different treatment goals. These values are for nonpregnant adults. Less intensive glycemic goals may be indicated in patients with severe or frequent hypoglycemia; more stringent glycemic goals (i.e., reducing hemoglobin A_{1c} levels to normal [< 6%]) may further reduce complications, but at the cost of increased risk of hypoglycemia. Hemoglobin A_{1c} is the primary target for glycemic control; postprandial glucose may be targeted if hemoglobin A_{1c} goals are not met despite reaching preprandial glucose goals. Additional suggested actions depend on individual patient circumstances. Such actions may include enhanced diabetes self-management education, comanagement with a diabetes team, referral to an endocrinologist, change in pharmacologic therapy, initiation of or increase in self-monitored blood glucose testing, or more frequent contact with the patient. Hemoglobin A_{1c} is referenced to a nondiabetic range of 4.0% to 6.0% (mean, 5.0%; standard deviation, 0.5%).
†Postprandial glucose measurements should be made 1–2 hr after the beginning of the meal.

need to be periodically checked after meals to ensure that undue postprandial hyperglycemia is not occurring. Patients should also check blood glucose levels before or after intensive exercise to prevent or abort hypoglycemia. Because severe hypoglycemia can have adverse effects on drivers' judgment and reaction times, which can contribute to accidents, it is very important to check blood glucose levels before driving.[56]

Occasional 3 A.M. blood glucose readings are useful in monitoring for otherwise unrecognized frequent nocturnal hypoglycemia. Most important, during intercurrent illnesses, especially those accompanied by nausea, vomiting, and a reduction in fluid and caloric intake, patients must test blood frequently to

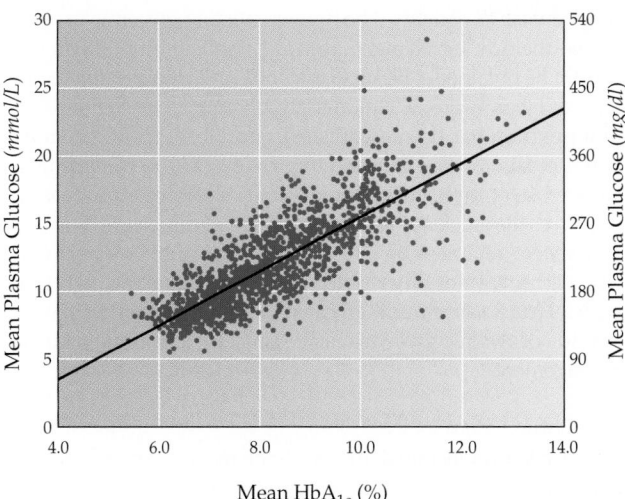

Figure 8 The 12-month mean value of all seven-sample-a-day blood glucose profile values measured quarterly in the Diabetes Control and Complications Trial central biochemistry laboratory is plotted against the 12-month mean of quarterly hemoglobin A_{1c} (HbA_{1c}) values in the same patients (r = 0.82, P < 0.001). The black line indicates the regression line.

Table 3   Insulin Preparations

Insulin Type	Onset	Duration (hr)	Time to Peak (hr)
Rapid acting			
Regular insulin	30–60 min	6–8	2–4
Inhaled insulin	15–30 min	6–8	2–4
Very rapid acting			
Lispro	5–15 min	4–6	1–2
Aspart	5–15 min	4–6	1–2
Glulisine	5–15 min	4–6	1–2
Intermediate acting			
Neutral protamine Hagedorn (NPH)	1–2 hr	10–14	4–8
Long acting			
Detemir	2–3 hr	9–24	No peak
Glargine	1.5–3 hr	20–24	No peak

guide insulin treatment. In addition, the risk of ketoacidosis under these circumstances mandates the testing of urine or blood for ketoacids. The presence of significant levels of ketoacids is a signal to call the caregiver immediately and establish frequent contact for instructions regarding insulin doses and carbohydrate intake.

Glycosylated Hemoglobin Measurement

To monitor overall glycemic control and the risk of later complications, HbA_{1c} is measured in the physician's office. This product of nonenzymatic glycation of hemoglobin provides an excellent index of average blood glucose levels for approximately the preceding 2 months [*see Figure 8*].[57,58] In at least one study, patients whose HbA_{1c} level was measured periodically had a better health status, lower glycemic levels, and fewer hospitalizations than a randomly selected group of patients whose HbA_{1c} level remained unknown to both the patient and the physician.[59]

Current ADA recommendations call for measuring HbA_{1c} at least twice a year in patients who are meeting treatment goals and have stable glycemic control, and measuring HbA_{1c} four times a year in patients who are not meeting glycemic goals or whose therapy has changed; during pregnancy, monthly levels should be obtained.[55] Because methods and results have varied among laboratories, a national glycohemoglobin standardization program has been established, and HbA_{1c} should be measured in laboratories certified to provide DCCT-equivalent results.[58] Use of rapid-turnaround, point-of-service HbA_{1c} assays improves the efficiency with which diabetes caregivers can modify patients' regimens on office visits and can improve treatment results.[60] Assays of other products of nonenzymatic glycation, such as fructosamine and glycated albumin, that reflect shorter periods of chronic glycemia, are less useful in routine diabetes management.[58]

INSULIN TYPES AND DELIVERY

Correction of insulin deficiency is the most critical component in managing type 1 diabetes mellitus. Before the availability of insulin, patients with type 1 diabetes mellitus and complete insulin deficiency inevitably followed a predictable downhill course [*see Figure 7*] and died either in diabetic coma or essentially of starvation and inanition. Insulin extracted from beef and pork pancreas and purified to increasingly high levels was the mainstay of therapy until recombinant DNA technology made it

possible to produce authentic human insulin in large quantities. Although animal insulins are therapeutically bioequivalent to human insulin, they disappeared from the market as manufacturers switched over to making only human insulin. In rare instances of local allergy to human insulin, rapid-action insulin (e.g., insulin lispro; see below) can be substituted. In emergency situations, patients with systemic allergy to human insulin can be desensitized by administering extremely small amounts and gradually increasing the dose over 6 to 24 hours until the patient is tolerant and responsive to human insulin.

The basic principle of insulin replacement is to provide a slow, long acting, continuous supply that mimics the nighttime and interprandial basal secretion by normal beta cells.[61-63] In addition, a rapid and relatively short-acting form of insulin delivered before meals mimics the normal meal-stimulated burst of insulin secretion [*see Figure 2*]. A number of insulin preparations for subcutaneous administration are currently available [*see Table 3*]. It is important to recognize that there is considerable variability in the pharmacokinetic characteristics of these different forms of insulin between patients and in an individual patient from day to day. Rates of insulin absorption from the skin vary with the injection site, the depth and angle of injection, ambient temperature, and exercise of an injected limb. Injection into the subcutaneous tissue of the abdomen produces the least variable results. The expected therapeutic action can also be affected by fluctuations in the patient's sensitivity to insulin from time to time. Despite the variability of results, certain average patterns can be expected from the multiple daily injection regimens in common use [*see Figure 9*]. CSII by use of an external pump provides smooth basal delivery and somewhat more predictable acute increases in plasma insulin for meals. Only rapid-action insulin (i.e., insulin lispro, aspart, or glulisine) or regular insulin should be used in such pumps, which is one reason for their greater consistency of effect.

Synthetic Insulin Analogues

Rapid-action insulin   Several insulin analogues have been created to provide pharmacokinetics that more closely mimic physiologic insulin secretion and needs.[64] One of the features of natural (or synthetic) human insulin is that six molecules associate with a zinc molecule to form hexamers. Insulin hexamers must disassociate to monomers before they can be absorbed from subcutaneous injection sites. This requirement is the main

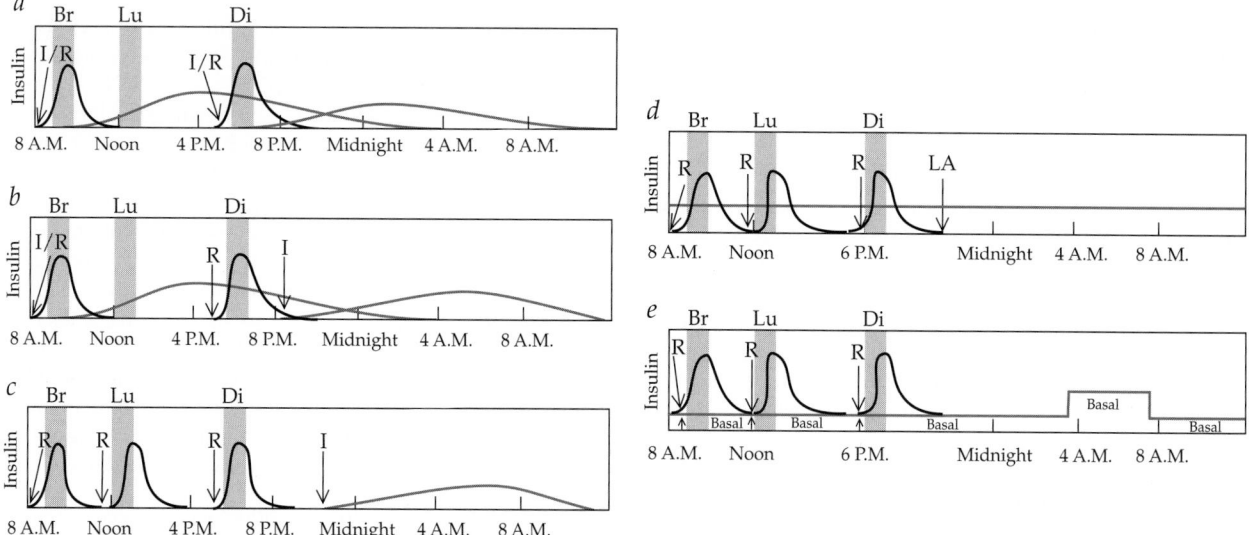

Figure 9 Different combinations of various insulin preparations can be employed in establishing glycemic control in type 1 diabetes mellitus (and in those patients with type 2 diabetes mellitus who eventually reach an equivalent degree of insulin deficiency). Arrows indicate time of injection. Black curves represent rapid-action or regular (R) insulin. Blue curves represent intermediate-acting (I) neutral protamine Hagedorn (NPH) insulin or long-acting (LA) insulin (e.g., detemir or glargine). (*a*) A mixed injection of I and R insulin is administered before breakfast and dinner in this nonintensive regimen. In addition to the risk of hypoglycemia before lunch and in the late afternoon, the predinner administration of I insulin predisposes patients to hypoglycemia from 2:00 A.M. to 4:00 A.M. (*b*) In this safer regimen, the patient receives three injections: a mixed injection before breakfast, R insulin before dinner, and I insulin before bed. The risk of nocturnal hypoglycemia is lower with this regimen, and fasting blood glucose is better controlled. (*c*) This intensive regimen combines three preprandial injections of R insulin with one injection of I insulin before bed. Preprandial doses of R insulin are adjusted according to glucose levels and meal size. (*d*) This intensive regimen uses long-acting insulin at bedtime to replace basal insulin secretion. In some patients, injections of long-acting insulin have to be given to improve blood glucose levels before lunch and dinner. Preprandial doses of R insulin are adjusted according to blood glucose levels and anticipated meal carbohydrate content. (*e*) This intensive regimen provides only R insulin as regular or rapid-action insulin. A pump-driven continuous subcutaneous infusion of R insulin (blue line) replaces basal insulin secretion. Basal rates can be varied during different times of day or activities. For example, the basal rate can be lowered or even suspended during periods of intensive aerobic exercise. The nocturnal basal rate can be increased 1.5 to 2.0 times from 3:00 A.M. to 4:00 A.M. until breakfast to accommodate the rising early morning insulin requirement known as the dawn phenomenon. Preprandial bolus doses are individually dialed in and rapidly pumped in, adjusted according to blood glucose levels and anticipated meal carbohydrate content. (Br = breakfast, Lu = lunch, Di = dinner)

reason that crystalline zinc insulin (regular insulin) has a peak action 2 to 4 hours after injection and must be taken 30 to 60 minutes before eating to have any chance of limiting postprandial hyperglycemia.

Pharmaceutical companies have developed a variety of insulin analogues to prevent hexamer formation and create a monomer that is rapidly absorbed from an injection site. In these analogues, different amino acids are substituted for amino acids in the B chain of the insulin molecule. With insulin lispro, the first rapid-action insulin analogue developed, lysine and proline are exchanged at positions 28 and 29 of the B chain [*see Figure 3*]. With insulin aspart, aspartic acid is substituted for proline at position 28.[65] With insulin glulisine, lysine replaces asparagine at position 3 and glutamic acid replaces lysine at position 29.[66] Onset of action with these insulin analogues begins within 15 minutes, the peak effect is reached at 1 to 2 hours, and the duration of action is only 4 to 6 hours. Thus, rapid-action insulin injected just before a meal provides a postprandial plasma insulin profile similar to that of normal human insulin secretion [*see Figure 2*]. The chief benefits of using rapid-action insulin are to reduce postprandial blood glucose peaks and to somewhat decrease the hypoglycemia that can result from the late rise in regular insulin action.[67,68] However, loss of that late action can lead to recurrent hyperglycemia before the next meal. Hence, patients who are switched from regular insulin to a rapid-action insulin may have

no reduction in HbA_{1c} unless they receive an increase in their doses of basal insulin (neutral protamine Hagedorn [NPH], insulin glargine, or insulin detemir or the basal rate in CSII).[69] It may even prove useful to combine a rapid-action insulin with regular insulin in a single injection to optimize postprandial control.

Inhaled insulin Inhaled insulin was approved by the FDA in January 2006. The pharmacokinetic properties of inhaled insulin resemble those of rapid-action insulins, so inhaled insulin is suitable for preprandial use, but it must be given in conjunction with an injected basal insulin. Use of inhaled insulin has been associated with improved patient satisfaction and quality of life, presumably because of the reduced number of injections.[70] In clinical trials, however, HbA_{1c} levels achieved with inhaled insulin have not been lower than those achieved with injected insulin.

In clinical trials, decreases in pulmonary function have occurred in the first several weeks of treatment with inhaled insulin; for that reason, the use of inhaled insulin is not recommended in patients who have underlying lung disease or who smoke, and all patients being considered for inhaled insulin treatment should undergo spirometry and perhaps measurement of carbon monoxide diffusing capacity [*see Chapter 214*].[71] Pulmonary function testing should be repeated after the first 6 months of inhaled insulin treatment, and annually thereafter, even if the patient has no pulmonary symptoms.

Long-acting insulin Two long-acting insulin analogues, glargine and detemir, have been synthesized for use as a basal insulin.[72-74] These long-acting analogues have no discernible peak and a longer duration of action than Ultralente insulin, which was withdrawn from the market in July 2005. Glargine has two additional arginines at the carboxyl terminus of the insulin B chain, B31 and B32, and it has a glycine for arginine substitution at position A21; detemir was created by omitting threonine in position B30 and adding a C14 fatty acid chain at position B29 [see Figure 3]. Detemir has a long duration of action because it reversibly binds to plasma albumin, which slows its exit rate from plasma and decreases access to target cells. Detemir has a lower affinity for insulin receptors than human insulin, which necessitates the use of higher doses. Reduction in body weight is an additional advantage of detemir.

Glargine and detemir are usually given as a single bedtime injection to provide basal insulin for 24 hours with less nocturnal hypoglycemia.[73,74] Occasionally, morning and evening injections are required for optimal glycemic control.

INSULIN REGIMENS

Intensive treatment regimens are the preferred form of therapy for patients with type 1 diabetes, including children, although glycemic targets may have to be somewhat higher in children to avoid severe hypoglycemia. Different combinations of insulin preparations can be used to approximate (but never reliably reproduce) normal plasma insulin profiles [see Figure 9]. Type 1 diabetes mellitus can almost never be satisfactorily controlled on less than two injections a day of intermediate-acting insulin or one or two injections a day of long-acting insulin combined with premeal rapid-action insulin. Only in patients experiencing a honeymoon remission or in patients with late-onset autoimmune type 1 diabetes mellitus can satisfactory metabolic control be maintained for a time with a single injection of insulin daily. Such success is made possible only by the presence of some normally regulated endogenous insulin secretion.

The average total daily dose of insulin is 0.6 to 0.7 units per kilogram of body weight.[41] This average rises to 1.0 U/kg during adolescence, when insulin resistance increases temporarily. As a rule of thumb, a basal insulin injection and a mealtime insulin injection each constitutes approximately 50% of the average total daily dose. The dose of rapid-action or regular insulin before each meal is chosen by the patient on the basis of the blood glucose level, the estimated amount of carbohydrate to be eaten, or both. A typical regimen would call for 1 to 2 extra units of insulin for each 50 mg/dl increment in blood glucose above the dose called for by the preprandial target of 80 to 120 mg/dl, or 1 U for every 10 to 15 g of extra carbohydrate to be ingested above the usual amount of carbohydrate prescribed by the nutrition plan. Very sophisticated patients can combine both guidelines.

Fixed-dose mixtures of insulin are not physiologically very suitable for patients with type 1 diabetes mellitus. However, for patients who can or will implement only such conventional treatment, a typical regimen might be a total daily dose of 0.6 to 0.7 U/kg. Two thirds to three fourths of the dose would be given before breakfast and the remainder before supper; the ratio of intermediate-acting insulin to rapid-action insulin might be 2:1 to 4:1 before breakfast and 1:1 before supper. Because giving NPH or long-acting insulin before supper increases the risk of hypoglycemia between 2 and 4 A.M., patients on conventional treatment should be urged to switch to a three-injection regimen, taking intermediate- or long-acting insulin at bedtime to avoid nocturnal hypoglycemia and to better control the prebreakfast blood glucose level. Glargine or detemir insulin may also be helpful in minimizing nocturnal hypoglycemia.[73,74]

Insulin requirements are increased by greater caloric and especially carbohydrate intake, by weight gain of both lean body mass and fat mass, by the onset of puberty, by infections and other medical or surgical stresses, by glucocorticoid administration, and sometimes by the physiologic changes that precede the onset of menses. During acute illnesses, patients will require extra doses of rapid-action insulin when hyperglycemia accelerates and especially if ketosis occurs. Frequent telephone contact with caregivers allows timely professional guidance of the extra insulin doses, nutrient intake to prevent hypoglycemia, and fluid intake to prevent dehydration. Rapid-action insulin analogues are especially useful in these circumstances because the effect of an overdose is short lived and hypoglycemia is less likely.

Diabetes Mellitus during Pregnancy

Women with type 1 diabetes who are in their reproductive years should be instructed to inform their physicians when they have decided to have a child. Conception when diabetes control is inadequate markedly increases the risk of major congenital abnormalities in the fetus. This risk can be reduced to the nondiabetic background rate when glycemic control is excellent.[75,76] Therefore, the patient's HbA$_{1c}$ level should be brought as close to normal as possible before conception with intensive treatment, and it should be kept there throughout pregnancy. The average of preprandial and postprandial home blood glucose test results should be less than 126 mg/dl.[76]

Throughout pregnancy, normoglycemia (relative to the normal pregnant state) is required to prevent intrauterine death and perinatal morbidity and mortality. Preprandial blood glucose targets during pregnancy are 60 to 90 mg/dl; postprandial targets are 120 to 140 mg/dl.[77,78] Insulin requirements may drop in the first trimester but then rise to above the prepregnancy doses in the third trimester, when insulin resistance increases markedly. No insulin is needed during labor; in fact, glucose infusion may be required during active labor to prevent maternal hypoglycemia.[79] During the first 48 hours after delivery, as well, insulin requirements may be strikingly lower than those of the third trimester, but they soon return to the usual for that patient.

Insulin Pumps

CSII has improved considerably since its introduction in the 1970s.[80] Modern insulin infusion pumps permit programming with multiple basal rates, allowing flexibility during the day, as well as automatic adjustment of doses while sleeping at night. Frequently, the basal rate needs to be lower in the first half of the night and then increased to accommodate the so-called dawn phenomenon [see Figure 9]. The latter is a slow rise in the plasma glucose level before the patient awakens; it is demonstrable in normal persons but is exaggerated in persons with type 1 diabetes mellitus who cannot limit it by increasing endogenous insulin secretion. On the other hand, interruption of insulin delivery from a pump for as little as 8 hours can result in extreme hyperglycemia, diabetic ketoacidosis (DKA), and hyperkalemia. In the DCCT, patients who used an insulin pump had a slightly but significantly higher DKA event rate (1.8 per 100 patient-years) than patients on multiple daily injection regimens (0.8 per 100 patient-years).[41] There was no difference in risk of severe hypoglycemia between patients treated with insulin pumps and patients treated with multiple daily injections, although episodes resulting in coma or seizure were more common in CSII-treated patients.[41] The rate of infection at catheter sites was kept very low by frequent change of catheters and preemptive use of antibiotics at the first visible signs of infection. Pump use has grown exponentially in the past 10 years; it is estimated that 200,000 patients or more now use pumps. Pumps can be used to good effect in adolescents,[81] a group whose diabetes is especially hard to control, for physiologic, behavioral, and social reasons.

Implantable pumps, which deliver insulin into the peritoneal cavity and result in a more physiologic first pass of insulin through the liver, have provided acceptable HbA_{1c} levels with a lower frequency of severe hypoglycemia.[82] Difficulties with obstruction of insulin delivery and infection have occurred, and implantable pumps are not yet approved for commercial use. Completely closed–loop insulin delivery—in which blood glucose levels are monitored continuously and the results automatically drive insulin delivery rates—is under development but will not have practical utility until researchers have devised an implantable glucose sensor with a realistically long operational lifespan.

PRAMLINTIDE

Insulin is not the only hormone that regulates plasma glucose levels. Amylin, which is produced by pancreatic beta cells, contributes to postprandial lowering of glucose levels; like insulin, it is absent or deficient in persons with diabetes mellitus.

Pramlintide, a synthetic analogue of amylin, was approved by the FDA in 2005 as an adjunct treatment for patients with diabetes mellitus who fail to achieve desired glucose control despite optimal mealtime insulin therapy. When added to a preexisting insulin regimen, pramlintide lowered HbA_{1c} levels 0.5% to 0.7% from baseline.[83] Pramlintide is injected subcutaneously just before major meals, in a different syringe from that used for insulin injections. When starting pramlintide, patients should initially reduce their preprandial doses of rapid-action or regular insulin by 50%. To minimize nausea and vomiting, pramlintide is started at a low dose (15 µg) and titrated upward as necessary, at intervals of at least 3 days, to a maintenance dose of 30 to 60 µg.[84]

PANCREAS TRANSPLANTATION

Pancreas transplantation remains controversial as a routine form of insulin replacement therapy.[85] Over the period of 1994 to 1997, 1-year graft survival rates were 82% when a pancreas was transplanted with a needed kidney transplantation and 62% when a pancreas was transplanted alone.[86] Successful pancreas transplants provide nondiabetic HbA_{1c} levels and free the patient from the rigors of diet, blood glucose testing, and insulin injection, and they virtually eliminate episodes of hypoglycemia.[86] Quality of life is usually improved. On the negative side, the patient incurs the risk of operative mortality and morbidity and must remain on immunosuppressive therapy with its attendant risks of infection and malignant disease.[85] Length of stay, readmission rates, morbidity, and the number of acute rejection episodes are higher for patients undergoing pancreas transplantation than for patients undergoing kidney transplantation. From 1994 to 1996, the 1-year pancreas transplantation survival rate was 81%, compared with a kidney transplantation survival rate of 88%.[85] The large majority of pancreas transplantations are still performed as an option in conjunction with a necessary kidney transplantation.

Transplantation of isolated islets can be accomplished without major surgery. Furthermore, the ability to immunomodulate isolated islets in the laboratory (by masking or removing cell surface antigens) may someday allow transplantation with little or no immunosuppression. Alternatively, islets can be placed in semipermeable hollow tubes that allow glucose to enter and insulin to leave but that shield the islets from inflammatory reactions to a foreign body. Islet transplantation in which function lasts at least 1 year has been achieved in less than 10% of attempts worldwide.

Initial reports of islet transplantation using a protocol developed in Edmonton, Canada, suggested a high success rate.[87] In the Edmonton protocol, purified islets from the pancreases of as many as five cadaveric donors are infused into the recipient's portal vein. The protocol does not use glucocorticoids for immunosuppression; instead, induction therapy with interleukin-2 is followed by immunosuppression with sirolimus and low-dose tacrolimus.

However, a 5-year follow-up of 65 patients who underwent islet transplantation with the Edmonton protocol showed that although 80% had maintained C-peptide secretion, only about 10% were still insulin independent.[88] Complications included toxicity from immunosuppressive therapy, as well as increased requirements of multiple antihypertensive medications and statins.

A modification of the Edmonton protocol using islets from single cadaver donors and induction immunosuppression with antithymocyte globulin, daclizumab, and etanercept has been studied.[89] Five of the eight patients maintained insulin independence for longer than 1 year. Clearly, challenges remain to be overcome before islet transplantation can deliver insulin physiologically for extended periods of life in insulin-deficient patients.[90]

NUTRITION AND EXERCISE

Nutrition

Insulin treatment will produce unsatisfactory results unless it is correlated with nutrient intake. To facilitate the matching of insulin doses to meals and to prevent hypoglycemia, patients with type 1 diabetes mellitus should eat consistent, regular meals with about 50% of the calories being carbohydrates. Although the premeal insulin dose is largely determined by the absolute carbohydrate content of the meal, patients should also pay attention to total energy intake from protein and fat. From 60% to 70% of energy intake should be in the form of carbohydrate and monounsaturated fat. Less than 10% of energy intake should be in the form of saturated fats, and cholesterol intake should be less than 300 mg a day.[91] In patients with low-density lipoprotein cholesterol levels of 100 mg/dl or greater, lowering dietary levels of saturated fat below 7% and cholesterol below 200 mg daily may be beneficial. Various methods of teaching patients how to assess amounts of foods and their nutrient and caloric content have been utilized. These methods include exchange lists that place foods into six categories; each category has approximately the same quantity of carbohydrate, protein, and calories per serving. These exchange categories are bread, meat, milk, fruit, fat, and vegetable. Another approach is to focus only on the carbohydrate content of foods because carbohydrates cause most of the postprandial hyperglycemia. Because different carbohydrates are digested and absorbed at different rates and therefore have different effects on plasma glucose levels, glycemic indices have been developed for common foods that take into account their different effects.[92] Numerous studies have disproved the myth that sucrose raises blood glucose more than equivalent amounts of other carbohydrates.[91] For optimal instruction and reinforcement of diet therapy, a dietitian should be part of the diabetes care team.

Exercise

Exercise is another important component of diabetes care because it helps maintain cardiovascular conditioning, insulin sensitivity, and general well-being. However, patients must learn how their glucose levels respond to different forms of exercise, and they must be instructed as to how to adjust their meals, their insulin doses and timing, or both, to prevent hypoglycemia during, immediately after, or even 6 to 12 hours after exercise as muscle glycogen stores are replenished from plasma glucose.[93]

In general, patients should avoid physical activity if their fasting glucose levels are 250 mg/dl or higher and they have ketosis, and they should use caution if glucose levels are above 300 mg/dl and no ketosis is present.[94] They should ingest additional carbohydrates before exercise if their glucose levels are below 100 mg/dl. They should monitor blood glucose before and after moderate to strenuous physical activity and have carbohydrate-based food readily available during and afterwards.

High-impact sports are contraindicated for patients with advanced retinopathy who are at risk for vitreous hemorrhage, as well as for patients with peripheral neuropathy or vascular disease who are at risk for foot trauma.

DIABETIC EMERGENCIES IN TYPE 1 DIABETES MELLITUS

Diabetic Ketoacidosis

DKA is the ultimate result of insulin deficiency[94] [see Figure 6]; it is aggravated by stress-induced elevations of glucagon, cortisol, growth hormone, epinephrine, and norepinephrine that add a component of insulin resistance.[95] Each year, DKA occurs in 2% to 5% of patients with type 1 diabetes mellitus. In the closely followed DCCT patients, overall event rates were 2.0 per 100 patient-years in the intensively treated group and 1.8 per 100 patients-years in the conventionally treated group.[42] Reported mortality varies worldwide from as low as 0% to as high as 10%. Most cases occur in patients already diagnosed with type 1 diabetes mellitus, but DKA still can be the first manifestation of diabetes, especially in children. Self-monitoring of blood glucose and urine ketone levels and close contact with the diabetes care team should facilitate recognition and abortion of evolving DKA by early and aggressive treatment with extra insulin and fluids at home. Approximately half the cases of DKA are precipitated by infection. Sepsis, myocardial infarction, and other major comorbid illnesses are more often the cause of death than the metabolic disequilibrium itself. In children, cerebral edema is a rare, serious complication. It usually appears 6 to 12 hours after treatment is initiated when biochemical improvement is manifest; yet it is often fatal.

Presenting features Patients experiencing DKA present with signs and symptoms of dehydration secondary to osmotic diuresis and vomiting and, sometimes, to diarrhea caused by concurrent gastroenteritis; of compensatory hyperventilation to eliminate CO_2; and of various degrees of depressed mentation or decreased consciousness. Seizures are notably not a result of DKA. Complete coma almost certainly indicates a long period of DKA before the patient received medical attention. DKA yields a number of characteristic laboratory findings [see Table 4]. The metabolic acidosis represents an anion gap secondary to elevated levels of acetoacetate and betahydroxybutyrate, with small contributions from lactate and free fatty acids. Although serum potassium and phosphate levels are usually normal or even high initially, this finding masks a total body depletion of these electrolytes, as well as depletion of magnesium. If serum levels are low on admission, the depletion is profound. Deviations from the customary pattern create pitfalls in diagnosis. Ketones, which current common tests detect only as acetoacetate or acetone, may be absent from the serum if the redox potential of the patient is very high and the equilibrium of the ketoacids is shifted toward betahydroxybutyrate (as may occur in alcohol intoxication). Rapid blood tests for betahydroxybutyrate are currently available in many hospital laboratories for confirming the diagnosis of DKA. Serum bicarbonate levels may be normal if there is coexisting respiratory acidosis. Arterial blood pH may be normal if there is coexistent metabolic alkalosis caused by diuretic ingestion or pernicious vomiting. Occasionally, plasma glucose levels are less than 250 mg/dl because of fasting,[96] high alcohol intake, profound inanition, or pregnancy.

Treatment Treatment of DKA requires careful monitoring of the patient [see Table 4].[94,97,98] Volume repletion is as important as insulin therapy.[99] Intravenous 0.9% saline should be started even before the diagnosis is established. After administration of an initial liter over 30 to 60 minutes, fluid therapy should contin-

Table 4 Typical Laboratory Findings and Monitoring in Diabetic Ketoacidosis

Test	Average	Range
Plasma glucose	600 mg/dl (33 mmol/L)	200–2,000 mg/dl (11–110 mmol/L)
Plasma ketones (positive)	1:16	1:2–1:64
Blood betahydroxybutyrate (mmol/L)	—	3–25
Plasma HCO_3 (mEq/L)	10	4–15
Blood pH	7.15	6.80–7.30
Pco_2 (mm Hg)	20	14–30
Plasma anion gap ($Na^+ - [Cl + HCO_3]$) (mEq/L)	23	16–30

Perform complete blood count, serum urea nitrogen measurement, serum creatinine measurement, urinalysis, appropriate cultures, and chest radiography.

1. Weigh on admission and every 12 hr.
2. Record cumulatively intake and output every 1 to 2 hr (Foley catheter if incontinent).
3. Check blood pressure, pulse, respiration, mental status every 1 to 2 hr and temperature every 8 hr.
4. Check blood (fingerstick) or plasma (laboratory) glucose every 1 to 2 hr.
5. Check serum potassium every 2 to 4 hr; check other electrolytes and serum ketones or betahydroxybutyrate every 4 hr.
6. Check arterial blood pH and gases on admission (in children, venous pH may be substituted; add 0.1 to result). If pH < 7.0 on admission, recheck as required until pH exceeds 7.1.
7. Check serum phosphate, magnesium, and calcium levels on admission. If low, repeat every 4 hr; otherwise, every 8 to 12 hr.
8. Spot-check voidings for ketones and glucose.
9. Perform ECG on admission; repeat if follow-up serum potassium level is abnormal or unavailable.

Note: 1–9 should be carried out until the patient is stable, glucose levels have reached and are maintained at 250 mg/dl, and acidosis is largely reversed (plasma HCO_3 > 15–18, plasma anion gap < 16). An intensive care setting is preferred.

ue aggressively until the circulating volume is replenished, as indicated by an increase in blood pressure to normal and a reduction in compensatory tachycardia. Subsequent total volume repletion is carried out more slowly at 150 to 500 ml/hr with 0.45% saline, switching to 5% glucose-containing solutions once plasma glucose has decreased to 250 mg/dl. Typical fluid deficits range from 50 to 100 mEq/kg. Average sodium deficits are 7 mEq/kg, and most important, potassium deficits may be as high as 7 mEq/kg. The effective depletion of total body bicarbonate through loss of the strong organic acids acetoacetate and betahydroxybutyrate as their cation neutralized salts in the urine is revealed later, when a hyperchloremic metabolic acidosis often ensues. Potassium repletion (10 to 40 mEq/hr) should begin promptly after insulin administration and as soon as hyperkalemia and oliguria or anuria have been ruled out. Otherwise, serious hypokalemia will result as insulin stimulates potassium uptake by cells [see Figure 4]. If the serum potassium level is less than 4.0 mEq/L on admission, a very large deficit exists and repletion should be at a faster rate to maintain a level no lower than 3.5 to 4.0 mEq/L. Insulin should be withheld in such circumstances until the serum potassium level reaches 4.0 mEq/L. Hypokalemia is the most tragic cause of death resulting from therapeutic misjudgment.

Subcutaneous injection of a rapid-action insulin analogue is a simple and effective route for insulin administration for the treatment of DKA.[100] This important new approach can be employed on a general medical ward. In this regimen, a rapid-action insulin (e.g., insulin lispro) is given in a dosage of 0.15 U/kg every 2 hours.

An older approach is to give regular or rapid-action insulin intravenously, starting with a bolus of 10 U or 0.1 U/kg, followed by the same dose given hourly by infusion, preferably with a pump and through its own intravenous line. This approach requires admission to an intensive care unit, where close monitoring and quick responses to changing clinical circumstances and laboratory results offer greater security. For the sicker patient, this setting should be preferred.

Routine addition of sodium bicarbonate or potassium phosphate has not been found to hasten recovery in ordinary cases of DKA.[94] Possible indications for administration of sodium bicarbonate (50 to 200 mEq) include arterial pH less than 7.0, electrocardiogaphic changes indicative of hyperkalemia, hypotension that does not respond to rapid infusion of 0.9% saline, and left ventricular failure. If bicarbonate therapy is given, serum potassium and arterial pH should be monitored hourly and extra potassium given to prevent hypokalemia. Rhabdomyolysis, hemolysis, and central nervous system deterioration can be caused by severe hypophosphatemia (< 1.5 mg/dl); these conditions call for the intravenous administration of potassium phosphate, 60 mmol (approximately 2 g), over 6 hours. Once the anion gap has decreased to near normal, the betahydroxybutyrate level has decreased to below 3 mmol/L, and the bicarbonate level has risen to 15 to 18 mEq/L, the insulin infusion rate can be decreased to 2 U/hr. In general, it is best to maintain the insulin infusion at 1 to 2 U/hr with accompanying 5% or 10% glucose infusion, with the aim being to keep the plasma glucose level at around 150 mg/dl until the following morning, at which time a subcutaneous mixed insulin regimen can be started or resumed along with a diet.

Persistent vomiting calls for gastric intubation, and the airway of an obtunded patient should be protected to prevent aspiration. Any suspicion of sepsis mandates treatment with broad-spectrum antibiotics, an antifungal agent, or both, when appropriate.

Hypoglycemia

Hypoglycemia is a more common emergency than DKA and is potentially as dangerous. Clinical hypoglycemia can range from annoying symptoms accompanying a biochemically low blood glucose level (< 50 to 60 mg/dl) to confusion, seizures, or coma. Any episode that requires intervention by another person to reverse is categorized as severe hypoglycemia. Severe hypoglycemia can have disastrous consequences, particularly if the patient is driving any sort of vehicle, working at heights, or operating potentially dangerous machinery.

The most common causes of hypoglycemia are missed meals and snacks,[101] insulin dosage errors, exercise, alcohol, and drugs such as beta blockers. During the DCCT, 55% of hypoglycemic episodes occurred during sleep.[101] Such episodes often go undetected.[102]

Glucagon and epinephrine are the major counterregulatory hormones that are secreted in response to hypoglycemia.[103] Both restore glucose levels by increasing hepatic glucose output, and epinephrine also decreases the sensitivity of muscles to insulin. Furthermore, catecholamine secretion alerts the patient to treat the episode because it produces the sympathoadrenal symptoms noted below. Cortisol and growth hormone are also secreted in response to hypoglycemia and play a role in maintaining glucose levels but not in rapid recovery from hypoglycemia.

Presenting features The most common symptoms of early mild hypoglycemia are adrenergic and include palpitations (from tachycardia), tremulousness, anxiety, and sweating.[104] Sweating requires sympathetic activation of cholinergic nerves that innervate the sweat glands. Blurred vision and dizziness can also occur.

Factors affecting severity of hypoglycemic episodes The development of primary or secondary adrenal insufficiency, hypopituitarism, and hypothyroidism may increase the risk of hypoglycemia by increasing sensitivity to insulin, decreasing appetite, or both. Stress, exercise, or the use of alcohol or illicit drugs may blunt or prevent recognition of hypoglycemia. Patients who recognize incipient hypoglycemia but who consciously do not respond expeditiously (for example, they may wait for a meal in a restaurant or continue to drive after symptoms first appear) are also at increased risk for severe hypoglycemia. Moreover, some risk factors for hypoglycemia have multiple effects that can precipitate, prolong, or worsen the severity of hypoglycemia. Alcohol, for instance, impairs judgment and inhibits gluconeogenesis and hepatic glucose output, thereby delaying recovery. When hypoglycemia is inadequately treated, more severe hypoglycemia often ensues.

Finally, because glucagon and epinephrine are the major defense hormones against prolonged hypoglycemia, their absence promotes longer and more severe episodes by two mechanisms: (1) compensatory hepatic glucose output is decreased when not stimulated by glucagon or epinephrine and (2) the familiar adrenergic symptoms may cease in the absence of epinephrine, resulting in failure to recognize the episode. The glucagon response to hypoglycemia often wanes in patients after they have had type 1 diabetes mellitus for a few years. In the absence of glucagon, epinephrine secretion still provides adequate counterregulatory defense; however, epinephrine response can also be lost eventually, sometimes in association with other autonomic neuropathies and sometimes selectively. Many patients lose the ability to counterregulate effectively against hypoglycemia during the first 10 years that they have type 1 diabetes mellitus.

Given the importance of intensive regimens to prevent microvascular complications from hyperglycemia, it is most unfortunate that a lowered glucose threshold for the release of glucagon and epinephrine in response to hypoglycemia has been observed, particularly in patients undergoing intensive insulin therapy.[105] The lowered glucose level needed to stimulate counterregulation narrows the safety margin of therapy. For instance, the first symptom of hypoglycemia may occur only at glucose levels as low as 35 mg/dl (as opposed to 55 to 60 mg/dl) and may consist of confusion or loss of judgment, which interferes with self-treatment. Some evidence suggests that unawareness of hypoglycemia is self-generating, because each episode may lower the threshold at which autonomic counterregulation begins in subsequent episodes.[106] The converse of this is that a period free of hypoglycemia, produced by daily therapeutic contact with caregivers, may restore hypoglycemia awareness,[106,107] though it may not restore normal counterregulatory responses.[106] Increased uptake of glucose by the brain in the presence of hypoglycemia[108,109] is a likely explanation for the relative infrequency of clinical hypoglycemic catastrophes.

Treatment   Patients recognize most episodes of hypoglycemia quickly and can effectively treat themselves with an oral carbohydrate capable of being absorbed promptly. Approximately 15 g of carbohydrate is usually sufficient to restore blood glucose levels to normal. This amount is provided by approximately 6 oz of orange juice, 4 oz of a cola drink (regular, not "diet"), 3 to 4 tsp of table sugar, five Life Savers, or three glucose tablets (each containing 5 g of glucose). The use of complex carbohydrates and foods with a high fat content, such as chocolate, may delay digestion and absorption of the glucose; these foods are not first choices for the treatment of hypoglycemia. If the patient cannot swallow or is incapable of self-treatment, a gel containing glucose and simple carbohydrates can be administered by mouth; such a gel is applied between the gums and cheeks, from where it slowly and generally safely trickles down into the stomach. Glucagon (1 mg administered subcutaneously or intramuscularly) will also usually raise blood glucose levels sufficiently within 15 to 30 minutes, at which time the patient can then take oral carbohydrates. Glucagon comes in emergency kits, and it should always be on hand for patients with a history of severe hypoglycemic episodes. Glucagon may cause nausea, vomiting, and headache, especially in children. When all else fails, intravenous glucose must be given by emergency medical service personnel or in the emergency department, whichever is quicker. When the timing of an episode suggests it was caused by intermediate- or long-acting insulin or by prior exercise, the blood glucose level may fall to hypoglycemic levels again, and re-treatment may be necessary. Thus, a patient who has required assistance from others in reversing hypoglycemia should be kept under surveillance for some time thereafter.

Patients with severe hypoglycemia usually respond rapidly to treatment, although patients who are postictal or in a prolonged coma may require days to regain normal mental status and cognitive function. Quite often, patients experience amnesia for extended episodes, including a period preceding the onset of hypoglycemia. In rare instances, neurologic deficits can be permanent. In general, however, long-term consequences of hypoglycemia have not been detected in adults.[43,110,111] In children 5 years and younger, repeated episodes of hypoglycemia may be associated with cognitive deficits later in childhood.[112,113] In view of the potential consequences of prolonged episodes, hypoglycemia should always be treated immediately.

Prevention   Patients should be instructed to treat themselves as though they have hypoglycemia whenever they suspect it, even if they are unable to do a confirmatory blood glucose test at the time. The threshold for symptoms of hypoglycemia varies from person to person and even varies in the same person on different occasions. Therefore, whenever possible, a confirmatory blood glucose test should be done to help the patient discriminate nonspecific symptoms from true hypoglycemia. Patients at increased risk for severe hypoglycemia should monitor their blood glucose levels more frequently.

Complications

The complications of type 1 diabetes mellitus are discussed in detail elsewhere [*see Chapter 54*].

The author has no commercial relationships with manufacturers of products or providers of services discussed in this chapter.

References

1. Diagnosis and classification of diabetes mellitus. American Diabetes Association. Diabetes Care 29:S43, 2006

2. LaPorte RE, Matsushima M, Chang YF: Prevalence and incidence of insulin-dependent diabetes. Diabetes in America, 2nd ed. NIDDK NIH Publication No. 95-1468, 1995 http://diabetes.niddk.nih.gov/dm/pubs/america/pdf/chapter3.pdf

3. Onkamo P, Vaananen S, Karvonen M, et al: Worldwide increase in incidence of type I diabetes: the analysis of the data on published incidence trends. Diabetologia 42:1395, 1999

4. Genuth S: Hormones of the pancreatic islets. Physiology, 4th ed. Berne RM, Levy MN, Eds. Mosby, St. Louis, 1998, p 822

5. Haller MJ, Atkinson MA, Schatz D: Type 1 diabetes mellitus: etiology, presentation, and management. Pediatr Clin North Am 52:1553, 2005

6. Eisenbarth GS: Type 1 diabetes mellitus: a chronic autoimmune disease. N Engl J Med 314:1360, 1986

7. Foulis AK, McGill M, Farquharson MA: Insulitis in type 1 (insulin-dependent) diabetes mellitus in man: macrophages, lymphocytes, and interferon-gamma containing cells. J Pathol 165:97, 1991

8. Rossini AA, Greiner DL, Friedman HP, et al: Immunopathogenesis of diabetes mellitus. Diabetes Reviews 1:43, 1993

9. Littorin B, Sundkvist G, Hagopian W, et al: Islet cell and glutamic acid decarboxylase antibodies present at diagnosis of diabetes predict the need for insulin treatment. Diabetes Care 22:409, 1999

10. Falorni A, Lernmark A: Humoral autoimmunity. Diabetes Mellitus: A Fundamental and Clinical Text, 1st ed. LeRoith D, Taylor SI, Olefsky JM, Eds. Lippincott-Raven Publishers, Philadelphia, 1996, p 298

11. Palmer JP, Asplin CM, Clemons P, et al: Insulin antibodies in insulin-dependent diabetics before insulin treatment. Science 222:1337, 1983

12. Feutren G, Papoz L, Assan R, et al: Cyclosporin increases the rate and length of remissions in insulin-dependent diabetes of recent onset: results of a multicentre double-blind trial. Lancet 2:119, 1986

13. Bougneres PF, Landais P, Boisson C, et al: Limited duration of remission of insulin dependency in children with recent overt type 1 diabetes treated with low-dose cyclosporin. Diabetes 39:1264, 1990

14. Riley WJ, Maclaren NK, Krischer J, et al: A prospective study of the development of diabetes in relatives of patients with insulin-dependent diabetes. N Engl J Med 323:1167, 1990

15. Tarn AC, Thomas JM, Dean BM, et al: Predicting insulin-dependent diabetes. Lancet 1:845, 1988

16. Ziegler AG, Herskowitz RD, Jackson RA, et al: Predicting type 1 diabetes. Diabetes Care 13:762, 1990

17. Srikanta S, Ganda OP, Gleason RE, et al: Pre-type 1 diabetes: linear loss of beta cell response to intravenous glucose. Diabetes 33:717, 1984

18. Rayfield EJ, Ishimura K: Environmental factors and insulin-dependent diabetes mellitus. Diabetes Metab Rev 3:925, 1987

19. Gillespie KM, Bain SC, Barnett AH, et al: The rising incidence of childhood type 1 diabetes and reduced contribution of high-risk HLA haplotypes. Lancet 364:1699, 2004

20. Jones DB, Armstrong NW: Coxsackie virus and diabetes revisited. Nat Med 1:284, 1995

21. The Environmental Determinants of Diabetes in the Young (TEDDY) Consortium. National Institute of Diabetes and Digestive and Kidney Diseases, National Institutes of Health, Bethesda, Maryland, 2006 http://www.niddk.nih.gov/patient/TEDDY/TEDDY.htm

22. Agner T, Damm P, Binder C: Remission in IDDM: prospective study of basal C-peptide and insulin dose in 268 consecutive patients. Diabetes Care 10:164, 1987

23. Heinze E, Beischer W, Keller L, et al: C-peptide secretion during the remission phase of juvenile diabetes. Diabetes 27:670, 1978

24. Shah SC, Malone JI, Simpson NE: A randomized trial of intensive insulin therapy in newly diagnosed insulin-dependent diabetes mellitus. N Engl J Med 320:550, 1989

25. Effects of age, duration and treatment of insulin-dependent diabetes mellitus on residual beta-cell function: observations during eligibility testing for the Diabetes Control and Complications Trial (DCCT). Diabetes Control and Complications Trial Research Group. J Clin Endocrinol Metab 65:30, 1987

26. Gorsuch AN, Spencer KM, Lister J, et al: Evidence for a long prediabetic period in type I (insulin-dependent) diabetes mellitus. Lancet 2:1363, 1981

27. Groop LC, Bottazzo GF, Doniach D: Islet cell antibodies identify latent type 1 diabetes in patients aged 35–75 years at diagnosis. Diabetes 35:237, 1986

28. Karjalainen J, Salmela P, Ilonen J, et al: A comparison of childhood and adult type I diabetes mellitus. N Engl J Med 320:881, 1989

29. Pugliese A: Unraveling the genetics of insulin-dependent type 1A diabetes: the search must go on. Diabetes Reviews 7:39, 1999

30. Baisch JM, Weeks T, Giles R, et al: Analysis of HLA-DQ genotypes and susceptibility in insulin-dependent diabetes mellitus. N Engl J Med 322:1836, 1990

31. Nepom GT: Immunogenetics and IDDM. Diabetes Reviews 1:93, 1993

32. Palmer JP: Predicting IDDM: use of humoral immune markers. Diabetes Reviews 1:104, 1993

33. Genuth SM: Plasma insulin and glucose profiles in normal, obese, and diabetic persons. Ann Intern Med 79:812, 1973

34. Nair KS, Halliday D, Garrow JS: Increased energy expenditure in poorly controlled type I (insulin-dependent) diabetic patients. Diabetologia 27:13, 1984

35. Gillespie KM: Type 1 diabetes: pathogenesis and prevention. CMAJ 175:165, 2006

36. Skyler JS, Krischer JP, Wolfsdorf J, et al: Effects of oral insulin in relatives of patients with type 1 diabetes: the Diabetes Prevention Trial–Type 1. Diabetes Care 28:1068, 2005

37. Herold KC, Gitelman SE, Masharani U, et al: A single course of anti-CD3 monoclonal antibody hOKT3gamma1(Ala-Ala) results in improvement in C-peptide responses and clinical parameters for at least 2 years after onset of type 1 diabetes. Diabetes 54:1763, 2005

38. Keymeulen B, Vandemeulebroucke E, Ziegler AG, et al: Insulin needs after CD3-antibody therapy in new-onset type 1 diabetes. N Engl J Med 352:2598, 2005

39. Bisikirska B, Colgan J, Luban J, et al: TCR stimulation with modified anti-CD3 mAb expands CD8+ T cell population and induces CD8+CD25+ Tregs. J Clin Invest 115:2904, 2005

40. The effect of intensive treatment of diabetes on the development and progression of long-term complications in insulin-dependent diabetes mellitus. Diabetes Control and Complications Trial Research Group. N Engl J Med 329:977, 1993

41. Implementation of treatment protocols in the Diabetes Control and Complications Trial. Diabetes Control and Complications Trial Research Group. Diabetes Care 18:361, 1995

42. Adverse events and their association with treatment regimens in the Diabetes Control and Complications Trial. Diabetes Control and Complications Trial Research Group. Diabetes Care 18:1415, 1995

43. Effects of intensive diabetes therapy on neuropsychological function in adults in the Diabetes Control and Complications Trial. Diabetes Control and Complications Trial Research Group. Ann Intern Med 124:379, 1996

44. Resource utilization and costs of care in the Diabetes Control and Complications Trial. Diabetes Control and Complications Trial Research Group. Diabetes Care 18:1468, 1995

45. Lifetime benefits and costs of intensive therapy as practiced in the Diabetes Control and Complications Trial. Diabetes Control and Complications Trial Research Group. JAMA 276:1409, 1996

46. The relationship of glycemic exposure (HbA$_{1c}$) to the risk of development and progression of retinopathy in the Diabetes Control and Complications Trial. Diabetes Control and Complications Trial Research Group. Diabetes 44:968, 1995

47. The absence of a glycemic threshold for the development of long-term complications: the perspective of the Diabetes Control and Complications Trial. Diabetes Control and Complications Trial Research Group. Diabetes 45:1289, 1996

48. Martin CL, Albers J, Herman WH, et al: Neuropathy among the diabetes control and complications trial cohort 8 years after trial completion. Diabetes Care 29:340, 2006

49. Sustained effect of intensive treatment of type 1 diabetes mellitus on development and progression of diabetic nephropathy: the Epidemiology of Diabetes Interventions and Complications (EDIC) study. Diabetes Control and Complications Trial (DCCT)/Epidemiology of Diabetes Interventions and Complications (EDIC) Research Group. JAMA 290:2159, 2003

50. Genuth S: Insights from the diabetes control and complications trial/epidemiology of diabetes interventions and complications study on the use of intensive glycemic treatment to reduce the risk of complications of type 1 diabetes. Endocr Pract 12(suppl 1):34, 2006

51. Effect of intensive therapy on the microvascular complications of type 1 diabetes mellitus. DCCT Research Group and EDIC Research Group. JAMA 287:2563, 2002

52. Nathan DM, Cleary PA, Backlund JY, et al: Intensive diabetes treatment and cardiovascular disease in patients with type 1 diabetes. N Engl J Med 353:2643, 2005

53. The effect of intensive diabetes therapy on carotid atherosclerosis in type 1 diabetes mellitus. DCCT Research Group and EDIC Research Group. N Engl J Med 348:2294, 2003

54. Kerr M: Repeated bouts of severe hypoglycemia have no adverse effect on cognition. Medscape Diabetes & Endocrinology. Accessed August 25, 2006 http://www.medscape.com/viewarticle/536285

55. Standards of medical care in diabetes. American Diabetes Association. Diabetes Care 29:S4, 2006

56. Stork ADM, van Haeften TW, Veneman TF: Diabetes and driving: desired data, research methods and their pitfalls, current knowledge, and future research. Diabetes Care 29:1942, 2006

57. Rohlfing DL, Wiedmeyer HM, Little RR, et al: Defining the relationship between plasma glucose and HbA(1c): analysis of glucose profiles and HbA(1c) in the Diabetes Control and Complications Trial. Diabetes Care 25:275, 2002

58. Goldstein DE, Little RR, Lorenz RA, et al: Tests of glycemia in diabetes. Diabetes Care 27:1761, 2004

59. Larsen ML, Horder M, Mogensen EF: Effect of long-term monitoring of glycosylated hemoglobin levels in insulin-dependent diabetes mellitus. N Engl J Med 323:1021, 1990

60. Cagliero E, Levina EV, Nathan DM: Immediate feedback of HbA$_{1c}$ levels improves glycemic control in type 1 and insulin-treated type 2 diabetic patients. Diabetes Care 22:1785, 1999

61. Skyler JS: Insulin treatment. Therapy for Diabetes Mellitus and Related Disorders, 3rd ed. Lebovitz HE, Ed. American Diabetes Association, Alexandria, Virginia, 1998, p 186

62. Mooradian AD, Bernbaum M, Albert SG: Narrative review: a rational approach to starting insulin therapy. Ann Intern Med 145:125, 2006

63. Hirsch IB: Type 1 diabetes mellitus and the use of flexible insulin regimens. Am Fam Physician 60:2343, 1999

64. Hirsch IB: Insulin analogues. N Engl J Med 352:174, 2005

65. Raskin P, Guthrie RA, Leiter L, et al: Use of insulin aspart, a fast-acting insulin analog, as the mealtime insulin in the management of patients with type 1 diabetes. Diabetes Care 23:583, 2000

66. Robinson DM, Wellington K: Insulin glulisine. Drugs 66:861, 2006

67. Garg SK, Carmain JA, Braddy KC, et al: Pre-meal insulin analogue insulin lispro vs Humulin R insulin treatment in young subjects with type 1 diabetes. Diabet Med 13:47, 1996

68. Anderson JH Jr, Brunelle RL, Koivisto VA, et al: Reduction of postprandial hyperglycemia and frequency of hypoglycemia in IDDM patients on insulin-analog treatment. Diabetes 46:265, 1997

69. Del Sindaco P, Ciofetta M, Lalli C, et al: Use of the short-acting insulin analogue lispro in intensive treatment of type 1 diabetes mellitus: importance of appropriate replacement of basal insulin and time-interval injection-meal. Diabet Med 15:592, 1998

70. Royle P, Waugh N, McAuley L, et al: Inhaled insulin in diabetes mellitus. Cochrane Database Syst Rev (3):CD003890, 2004

71. Dunn C, Curran MP: Inhaled human insulin (Exubera): a review of its use in adult patients with diabetes mellitus. Drugs 66:1013, 2006

72. Heinemann L, Linkeschova R, Rave K, et al: Time-action profile of the long-acting insulin analog insulin glargine (HOE901) in comparison with those of NPH insulin and placebo. Diabetes Care 23:644, 2000

73. Rosenstock J, Park G, Zimmerman J: Basal insulin glargine (HOE 901) versus NPH insulin in patients with type 1 diabetes on multiple daily insulin regimens. Diabetes Care 23:1137, 2000

74. Insulin detemir (levemir), a new long-acting insulin. Med Lett Drugs Ther 48:54, 2006

75. Jovanovic L, Nakai Y: Successful pregnancy in women with type 1 diabetes: from preconception through postpartum care. Endocrinol Metab Clin North Am 35:79, 2006

76. Langer O: Is normoglycemia the correct threshold to prevent complications in the pregnant diabetic patient? Diabetes Reviews 4:2, 1996

77. de Veciana M, Major CA, Morgan MA, et al: Postprandial versus preprandial blood glucose monitoring in women with gestational diabetes mellitus requiring insulin therapy. N Engl J Med 333:1237, 1995

78. Kjos SL, Buchanan TA: Gestational diabetes mellitus. N Engl J Med 341:1749, 1999

79. Jovanovic L: Glucose and insulin requirements during labor and delivery: the case for normoglycemia in pregnancies complicated by diabetes. Endocr Pract 10(suppl 2):40, 2004

80. Mecklenburg RS: Insulin-pump therapy. Therapy for Diabetes Mellitus and Related Disorders, 3rd ed. Lebovitz HE, Ed. American Diabetes Association, Alexandria, Virginia, 1998, p 204

81. Boland EA, Grey M, Oesterle A, et al: Continuous subcutaneous insulin infusion: a new way to lower risk of severe hypoglycemia, improve metabolic control, and enhance coping in adolescents with type 1 diabetes. Diabetes Care 22:1779, 1999

82. Dunn FL, Nathan DM, Scavini M, et al: Long-term therapy of IDDM with an implantable insulin pump. Diabetes Care 20:59, 1997

83. Whitehouse F, Kruger DF, Fineman M, et al: A randomized study and open-label extension evaluating the long-term efficacy of pramlintide as an adjunct to insulin therapy in type 1 diabetes. Diabetes Care 25:724, 2002

84. Lebovitz HE: Therapeutic options in development for management of diabetes: pharmacologic agents and new technologies. Endocr Pract 12(suppl 1):142, 2006

85. Robertson RP, Holohan TV, Genuth S: Therapeutic controversy: pancreas transplantation for type I diabetes. J Clin Endocrinol Metab 83:1868, 1998

86. Robertson RP, Davis C, Larsen J, et al: Pancreas and islet transplantation for patients with diabetes. Diabetes Care 23:112, 2000

87. Shapiro J, Lakey JR, Ryan EA, et al: Islet transplantation in seven patients with type 1 diabetes mellitus using a glucocorticoid-free immunosuppressive regimen. N Engl J Med 343:230, 2000

88. Ryan EA, Paty BW, Senior PA, et al: Five-year follow-up after clinical islet transplantation. Diabetes 54:2060, 2005

89. Hering BJ, Kandaswamy R, Ansite JD, et al: Single-donor, marginal-dose islet transplantation in patients with type 1 diabetes. JAMA 293:830, 2005

90. Rother KI, Harlan DM: Challenges facing islet transplantation for the treatment of type 1 diabetes mellitus. J Clin Invest 114:877, 2004

91. Franz MJ, Bantle JP, Beebe CA, et al: Nutrition principles and recommendations in diabetes. American Diabetes Association. Diabetes Care 27:S36, 2004

92. Jenkins DJ, Wolever TM, Taylor RH, et al: Glycemic index of foods: a physiological basis for carbohydrate exchange. Am J Clin Nutr 34:362, 1981

93. Zinman B, Ruderman N, Campaigne BN, et al: Physical activity/exercise and diabetes. American Diabetes Association. Diabetes Care 27:S58, 2004

94. Umpierrez GE, Kitabchi AE: Diabetic ketoacidosis: risk factors and management strategies. Treat Endocrinol 2:95, 2003

95. Barrett EJ, DeFronzo RA, Bevilacqua S, et al: Insulin resistance in diabetic ketoacidosis. Diabetes 31:923, 1982

96. Burge MR, Hardy KJ, Schade DS: Short-term fasting is a mechanism for the development of euglycemic ketoacidosis during periods of insulin deficiency. J Clin Endocrinol Metab 76:1192, 1993

97. DeFronzo RA, Matsuda M, Barrett EJ: Diabetic ketoacidosis: a combined metabolic-nephrologic approach to therapy. Diabetes Reviews 2:209, 1994

98. Trachtenbarg DE: Diabetic ketoacidosis. Am Fam Physician 71:1705, 2005

99. Waldhausl W, Kleinberger G, Korn A, et al: Severe hyperglycemia: effects of rehydration on endocrine derangements and blood glucose concentration. Diabetes 28:577, 1979

100. Della Manna T, Steinmetz L, Campos PR, et al: Subcutaneous use of a fast-acting insulin analog: an alternative treatment for pediatric patients with diabetic ketoacidosis. Diabetes Care 28:1856, 2005

101. Epidemiology of severe hypoglycemia in the Diabetes Control and Complications Trial. The DCCT Research Group. Am J Med 90:450, 1991

102. Gale EA, Tattersall RB: Unrecognised nocturnal hypoglycaemia in insulin-treated diabetics. Lancet 1:1049, 1979

103. Cryer PE, Davis SN, Shamoon H: Hypoglycemia in diabetes. Diabetes Care 26:1902, 2003

104. Heller SR, Macdonald IA, Herbert M, et al: Influence of sympathetic nervous system on hypoglycaemic warning symptoms. Lancet 2:359, 1987

105. Mokan M, Mitrakou A, Veneman T, et al: Hypoglycemia unawareness in IDDM. Diabetes Care 17:1397, 1994

106. Dagogo-Jack S: Hypoglycemia in type 1 diabetes mellitus: pathophysiology and prevention. Treat Endocrinol 3:91, 2004

107. Fanelli C, Pampanelli S, Epifano L, et al: Long-term recovery from unawareness, deficient counterregulation and lack of cognitive dysfunction during hypoglycaemia, following institution of rational, intensive insulin therapy in IDDM. Diabetologia 37:1265, 1994

108. Boyle PJ, Kempers SF, O'Connor AM, et al: Brain glucose uptake and unawareness of hypoglycemia in patients with insulin-dependent diabetes mellitus. N Engl J Med 333:1726, 1995

109. Criego AB, Tkac I, Kumar A, et al: Brain glucose concentrations in healthy humans subjected to recurrent hypoglycemia. J Neurosci Res 82:525, 2005

110. Effects of intensive diabetes therapy on neuropsychological function in adults in the Diabetes Control and Complications Trial. Diabetes Control and Complications Trial Research Group. Ann Intern Med 124:379, 1996

111. Kramer L, Fasching P, Madl C, et al: Previous episodes of hypoglycemic coma are not associated with permanent cognitive brain dysfunction in IDDM patients on intensive insulin treatment. Diabetes 47:1909, 1998

112. Ryan C, Vega A, Drash A: Cognitive deficits in adolescents who developed diabetes early in life. Pediatrics 75:921, 1985

113. Bjorgraas M, Gimse R, Vik T, et al: Cognitive function in type 1 diabetic children with and without episodes of severe hypoglycaemia. Acta Paediatr 86:148, 1997

Acknowledgments

I am grateful to the previous author of this chapter, Dr. David Nathan, for providing such an excellent template and for generously permitting me to retain certain sections that required only minor updating. I also wish to thank Eileen Campbell and Molly Genuth for skilled assistance in preparing the manuscript.

Figures 1 and 4   Seward Hung.

53 Type 2 Diabetes Mellitus

Matthew C. Riddle, M.D., and Saul Genuth, M.D., F.A.C.P.

Type 2 diabetes mellitus is similar to type 1 and other forms of diabetes in that it is defined by high levels of plasma glucose and is associated with many long-term complications caused or enhanced by hyperglycemia and related metabolic abnormalities. It differs from other types of diabetes in its very high prevalence, gradual onset and progression, complex underlying physiologic defects, and significance as a major public health problem. Current estimates are that of the approximately 21 million persons with diabetes in the United States, up to 90% have type 2 diabetes. About a third of those, or 7 million persons, are not yet diagnosed and therefore are not being treated. Moreover, both the incidence and prevalence of type 2 diabetes are increasing.

Although type 2 diabetes is strongly determined by inheritable factors, it is likely polygenic, and the specific genetic mechanisms remain poorly understood. The underlying defects include abnormalities of the insulin-producing beta cells of the pancreatic islets; diminished sensitivity of muscle, adipose tissue, and liver to the effects of insulin; and alterations of normal mechanisms controlling carbohydrate and lipid metabolism after ingestion of nutrients. These abnormalities, especially loss of normal sensitivity to insulin, are affected by various behavioral and environmental factors—notably, decreased physical activity and increased calorie intake leading to obesity.

In addition to high levels of glucose in plasma, type 2 diabetes is characterized by high levels of free fatty acids and abnormal lipoprotein patterns, as well as by changes of various hormonal and neural regulatory mechanisms affecting all tissues of the body. The consequences of these abnormalities include impairment or loss of vision, renal insufficiency, various forms of neuropathy and cognitive impairment, and greatly increased risks of heart disease, stroke, and peripheral vascular disease. Although the short-term effects of hyperglycemia and other metabolic abnormalities of type 2 diabetes are often minimal and even tolerable, the cumulative burden of disability and early mortality is very significant. Early diagnosis and effective treatment of hyperglycemia, associated cardiovascular risk factors, and the various complications of diabetes are essential to relieve these long-term burdens.

Definitions

DIABETES

Diabetes is defined by the glycemic threshold at which retinopathy begins to occur, as documented in population-based studies.[1] Levels of fasting plasma glucose (FPG), plasma glucose 2 hours after ingestion of 75 g of glucose, and hemoglobin A_{1c} (HbA_{1c}) predict retinopathy equally well. The American Diabetes Association (ADA) glycemic criteria for type 2 diabetes mellitus are FPG values of 126 mg/dl (7 mmol/L) or higher, or 2-hour glucose challenge test results of 200 mg/dl (11.1 mmol/L) or higher [*see Table 1*]. HbA_{1c} levels above 6% correlate similarly with the appearance of retinopathy; however, because the assay has not been standardized worldwide, results can be confounded by hematologic variants or the presence of hematologic disorders. In addition, HbA_{1c} measurement is more expensive than glucose measurement. For these reasons, this test has not been endorsed for diagnosis. Nevertheless, HbA_{1c} can be measured during acute illness to assess the patient's glycemic history; values over 7% are routinely associated with glucose values in the diabetic range. Also, because of its convenience as a measure of chronic hyperglycemia, HbA_{1c} is used as an indicator of medical risk in research studies and to measure the success of glycemic therapies in clinical practice.

PREDIABETES

Less pronounced hyperglycemia, intermediate between normal glucose levels and diabetes, is called prediabetes and is divided into two categories: impaired fasting glucose (IFG) and impaired glucose tolerance (IGT) [*see Table 1*].[1] Normal glucose levels are defined as less than 100 mg/dl (5.5 mmol/L) after fasting overnight, and less than 140 mg/dl (7.8 mmol/L) 2 hours after ingestion of 75 g of glucose. IFG is defined by overnight plasma glucose values of 100 to 125 mg/dl (5.6 to 6.9 mmol/L), and IGT by 2-hour glucose challenge test values of 140 to 199 mg/dl (7.8 to 11.1 mmol/L). Both conditions are associated with a high future risk of diabetes, but they may not result from the same dominant pathogenetic mechanism, and they coexist in only about one third of persons with prediabetes. Persons with IFG or, especially, IGT are also at increased risk for cardiovascular disease, at least partly because of associated risk factors such as obesity, central adiposity, hypertension, and abnormal lipoprotein patterns. In addition, epidemiologic analyses suggest that even modest elevations of glucose (or associated lipid or hormonal changes) may have harmful effects on vascular tissue. Whether normalization of glycemia can reduce cardiovascular risks in this setting is still unknown, however.[2] Both IFG and IGT are common and are usually not recognized.

Epidemiology

Surveys in the United States show a progressive increase of the prevalence of diabetes, most of which is type 2 diabetes.[3] In 1990, 4.9% of persons 18 years of age or older in the United States reported having diagnosed diabetes. By 2001, this proportion had increased to 7.9%. The frequency of known diabetes by self-report in 2001 was somewhat higher in women than men (8.9% versus 6.8%), and it was higher in African Americans (11.2%) and Hispanics (9.0%) than in whites (7.2%). These figures must be lower than the actual prevalence of diabetes, because earlier studies have shown that up to a third of persons with diabetes do not know they have the disease.[4] The same 2001 figures show a strong association of known diabetes with increasing age: the prevalence climbs from 2.1% in persons 18 to 29 years of age to 15.5% in persons 70 and older [*see Figure 1*]. Obesity is also strongly associated with diabetes, with a prevalence of 14.9% in persons with class II obesity (defined as a body mass index [BMI] of 35.0 to 39.9 kg/m²) and 25.6% in persons with class III obesity (BMI ≥ 40), compared with 4.1% in persons of normal weight.

From data of this kind, supplemented by information on demographic trends, the future prevalence of diabetes in the United States population has been projected.[5] The mathematical model

Table 1   American Diabetes Association Diagnostic Criteria for
Glycemic Abnormalities

Diagnosis	Plasma Glucose (mg/dl)		
	Fasting ≥ 8 hr	2 hr after 75 mg Oral Glucose	Random Test
Normal	< 100	< 140	—
Impaired fasting glucose	100–125	—	—
Impaired glucose tolerance	—	140–199	—
Diabetes mellitus	≥ 126	≥ 200	≥ 200 plus symptoms of diabetes

predicts that a male born in the year 2000 has a 33% chance of developing diabetes in his lifetime; if he does develop diabetes, his lifespan is likely to be 9 years shorter than that of a person without diabetes. A female is predicted to have a 39% lifetime risk and to lose 12 years of life if she develops the disease.

Risk Factors

Much of the increase in diabetes rates is related to the increased prevalence of obesity in the United States and elsewhere in the world.[6] This so-called epidemic of obesity is presumed to stem from lower levels of physical activity and a shift from traditional eating patterns toward diets of high fat content and high caloric density[7] [*see Chapter 58*].

Family history is also an important risk factor. An extraordinary example is found among the Pima Indians on the Gila River reservation in Arizona, where 50% of the adult population has type 2 diabetes mellitus. A strong hereditary influence is also demonstrated in monozygotic twins, in which diabetes, if present in one of the twins, nearly always develops in the other twin as well. Offspring and siblings of diabetic patients are at high risk for the disease.

No HLA markers have been identified for type 2 diabetes mellitus, in contrast to type 1 diabetes mellitus [*see Chapter 52*]. The common forms of type 2 diabetes mellitus seem to represent a complex multigenic disorder.[8] Examination of known pathophysiologic mechanisms suggests many logical candidate genes. Study of a variety of genes associated with the cellular actions of insulin has thus far failed to provide clear answers.[9] Genes that could cause obesity or that could impair growth or survival of beta cells are under active investigation. One promising candidate gene is a variant of transcription factor 7–like–2 (*TCF7L2*) that may contribute to regulation of proglucagon gene expression in gut endocrine cells. This variant has been proposed to account for 21% of the risk of type 2 diabetes in Icelandic, Danish, and United States populations.[10]

The Metabolic Syndrome

The metabolic syndrome (also known as syndrome X, insulin resistance syndrome, Reaven syndrome, and the cardiometabolic syndrome) is defined by the clustering of multiple cardiovascular risk factors.[11] Among these are elevated BMI; increased abdominal girth or waist-hip ratio; hypertension; high serum triglyceride levels; low serum high-density lipoprotein (HDL) concentrations; microalbuminuria; and IFG, IGT, or type 2 diabetes [*see Chapter 58*].

The choice of diagnostic criteria for the metabolic syndrome has been controversial. Other questions raised are whether there is a single characteristic (such as a specific form of insulin resistance) unifying the various risk factors, and how the concept can be clinically useful. Because the majority of persons with IFG, IGT, and type 2 diabetes have some of these additional risk factors, and because many persons without glycemic abnormalities but with these other risk factors eventually develop diabetes, these issues are relevant to the management of diabetes.

The INTERHEART study provides guidance on the relationship between the metabolic syndrome, diabetes, and cardiovascular disease.[12] This study evaluated over 15,000 myocardial infarction (MI) patients in 52 countries, and a similar number of persons without MI. Four lifestyle-related risk factors (smoking, eating fruits and vegetables, exercise, and drinking alcohol) and five other cardiovascular risk predictors (diabetes, hypertension, abdominal obesity, apoprotein B/apoprotein A ratio, and a psychosocial index) were measured. Diabetes itself conferred a 4.3-fold increased risk of MI in women and 2.7-fold increase in men and accounted for about 15% of the overall (adjusted) risk of MI in the population. In comparison, abdominal obesity increased risk 2.2-fold and accounted for almost 35% of overall risk, and hypertension increased risk 2.5-fold and accounted for

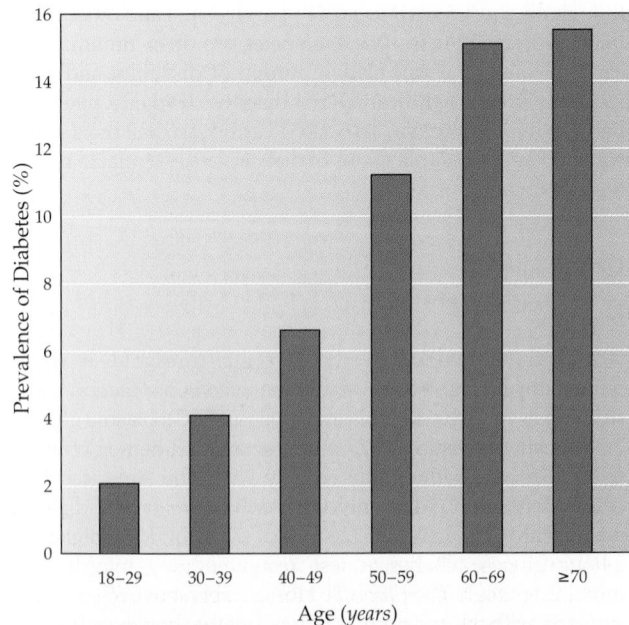

Figure 1   **Age-related prevalence of diabetes mellitus in the United States.[3] Cross-sectional data from a telephone survey shows a high frequency of self-reported diabetes in older age groups.**

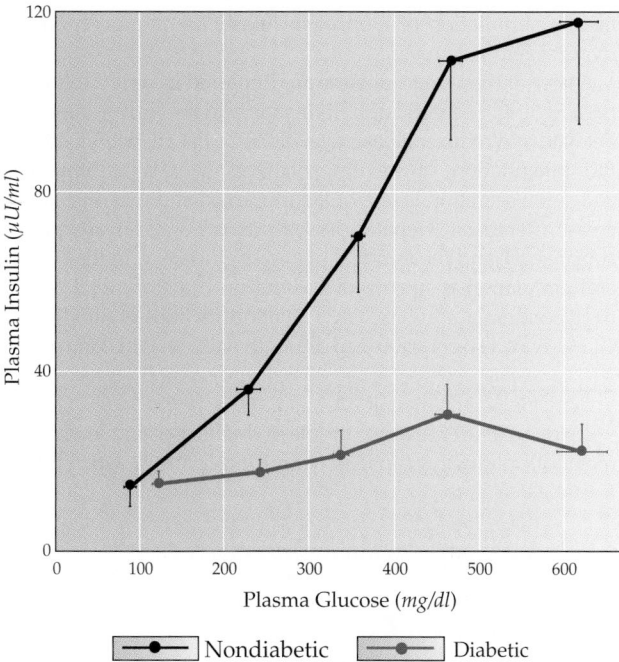

Figure 2 The insulin response to a graded infusion of glucose, producing progressively higher basal glucose levels, is diminished in type 2 diabetes.[14] Eight adults with type 2 diabetes and eight healthy persons of similar age and weight had plasma insulin measured while plasma glucose was maintained at various levels by glucose infusion. Basal insulin levels normally rise sharply to defend against rising basal glucose, but this response is markedly diminished in diabetes.

somewhat less than 30% of overall risk. However, over 90% of the total risk in the population was accounted for by the combined effects of the nine easily measured and potentially modifiable risk factors. These findings confirm that identifying other cardiovascular risk factors in patients with diabetes or prediabetes is essential. They also support the view that treating individual risk factors separately may be sufficient, without invoking additional unique risks linked to an overarching syndrome. Moreover, there is at present no single intervention that can reverse or blunt all aspects of the metabolic syndrome and that has been proven to reduce the associated risk of cardiovascular disease.

Pathophysiology

The alterations of metabolism in patients with type 2 diabetes partially overlap with those alterations of metabolism seen in patients with type 1 diabetes. Absolute or relative deficiency of insulin is common to both disorders, as is a severe disturbance of the patterns of glucose and lipid levels in plasma. However, the fluctuations of plasma glucose are less extreme in type 2 diabetes than in type 1 diabetes, and the exaggerated catabolic state of severe insulin deficiency often seen in type 1 is uncommon in type 2. Rather than being lean and likely to lose weight during periods of hyperglycemia, patients with type 2 diabetes are characteristically overweight or obese and often are gaining weight when diagnosed. The pathophysiologic abnormalities of type 2 diabetes are best understood when divided into three components: relative insulin deficiency, diminished sensitivity of tissues to the effects of insulin, and abnormal metabolic responses to eating.

INSULIN DEFICIENCY

Although the microscopic appearance of insulin-producing beta cells of the pancreatic islets may be relatively normal early in the course of type 2 diabetes, insulin secretion is always abnormal.[13] The most characteristic abnormality is a reduction of the rapid (acute-phase) secretion that normally occurs after the beta cell is stimulated by the rapid intravenous injection of glucose. Diminished early secretion of insulin is also seen after oral ingestion of glucose. The insulin response to a graded infusion of glucose, producing progressively higher basal glucose levels, is diminished as well[14] [*see Figure 2*]. Under normal conditions, the secretion of insulin in response to an acute stimulus is enhanced by an elevation of basal glucose levels, an effect known as glucose potentiation, but this is diminished in patients with type 2 diabetes. Normal rhythmic oscillations of insulin secretion and pulses of insulin secretion in response to endogenous pulses of plasma glucose are also altered, reflecting a fundamental abnormality of beta cell regulatory mechanisms. Because of these abnormalities, the beta cells fail to secrete insulin in the finely tuned manner that normally keeps glucose concentrations between 70 and 130 mg/dl.

After 10 or more years of type 2 diabetes, insulin secretion is markedly reduced. Beta cells are visibly fewer in number and also contain accumulations of amyloid protein derived from condensation of molecules of another beta cell peptide hormone, amylin.[15] Whether islet amyloid injures beta cells or is a marker of other destructive processes is not clear. The mechanisms responsible for the reduced survival of beta cells—for example, enhanced programmed cell death (apoptosis)—and the impaired differentiation of islet precursor cells into new beta cells is currently under study.[16]

INSULIN RESISTANCE

The gold standard for testing the insulin sensitivity of tissues is with a euglycemic glucose insulin clamp. Insulin is infused at a constant rate; the rate of glucose infusion necessary to maintain plasma glucose at a constant basal level is considered a measure of peripheral insulin sensitivity. Because muscle and adipose tissue are the main sites of disposal of glucose given intravenously, this method mainly defines the ability of these tissues to remove glucose from plasma. The mass of muscle tissue, the perfusion of this tissue, and the responsiveness of individual cells to insulin all contribute to this measure of insulin sensitivity. In type 2 diabetes, this measure is routinely diminished, and the patient is said to be insulin resistant[17,18] [*see Figure 3*].

Another important site of insulin action is the liver, which is the main source of glucose production during fasting. Although hepatic sensitivity to insulin is more difficult to measure, it too is routinely diminished in patients with type 2 diabetes.[18]

The cellular mechanisms underlying insulin resistance in muscle, adipose tissue, and liver are complex and incompletely understood. They include changes of insulin signaling pathways [*see Chapter 52*]; increases in the amounts of intracellular fat; elevated levels of circulating free fatty acids (FFA) and other adipose tissue products; and effects of increased glucagon, cortisol, epinephrine, and norepinephrine. The relationships between excessive intra-abdominal adipose tissue and diminished insulin sensitivity of muscle and liver are under intensive study. Among the mediators are high circulating concentrations of FFA, tumor necrosis factor–α, and the adipokine resistin, which reduce insulin sensitivity; and reduced concentrations of the adipose cell hormone adiponectin, which normally increases the

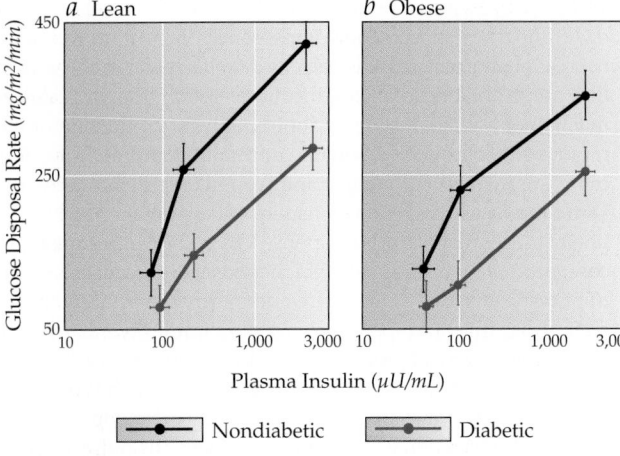

Figure 3 **Diminished uptake of glucose by tissues at different levels of stable plasma insulin in type 2 diabetes.**[18] **Adults with type 2 diabetes and healthy persons of similar age and weight had glucose infused intravenously to maintain constant plasma glucose while plasma insulin levels were clamped at various stable levels. Glucose uptake by tissues was lower in diabetic patients than healthy persons at similar insulin levels, reflecting insulin resistance. In both healthy persons and those with diabetes, glucose uptake was higher in lean persons (***a***) than in obese ones (***b***).**

insulin sensitivity of tissues.[19] In a person without diabetes, as weight and adiposity increase, beta cells compensate for the resulting decline in insulin sensitivity by increasing insulin output. This poorly understood adaptive response is increasingly ineffective in patients with type 2 diabetes, leading to increasing hyperglycemia.[20]

METABOLIC RESPONSES TO EATING

Most of the glucose cleared from the peripheral circulation during fasting is taken up at a constant rate by the CNS and other tissues that do not require insulin for glucose uptake. Thus, the rate of hepatic glucose production determines fasting glucose concentrations. The main factors regulating hepatic glucose production are the portal insulin and glucagon concentrations and the sensitivity of the liver to insulin. Regulation of postprandial plasma glucose and other metabolic pathways involves additional mechanisms.[21,22] Rapid, large increases in insulin secretion result in the suppression of hepatic glucose production (by reducing both gluconeogenesis and glycogenolysis); the level of insulin in peripheral plasma becomes high enough to increase the uptake of glucose by muscle and adipose tissue. The ingestion of food leads to the secretion of other hormones that affect glucose regulation. Amylin is secreted by the beta cell with insulin. Amylin's actions include slowing of gastric emptying, suppression of glucagon secretion, and an increase in the sense of satiety, limiting food intake. Glucagon-like peptide-1 (GLP-1) and glucose-dependent insulinotropic polypeptide (GIP) are secreted from the intestinal mucosa after eating. Both GLP-1 and GIP potentiate prandial insulin secretion and slow gastric emptying; GLP-1, like amylin, suppresses glucagon secretion and increases satiety. These changes limit food intake, prolong the time during which nutrients are absorbed, reduce glucose production, promote the uptake of glucose by the liver, and enhance peripheral uptake of the portion of ingested carbohydrate that passes through the liver. Thus, little postprandial hyperglycemia occurs. Uptake of ingested fat by adipose tissue is enhanced by

insulin stimulation of ipoprotein lipase, limiting postprandial hypertriglyceridemia.

Many of these mechanisms are impaired in type 2 diabetes[23] [*see Figure 4*]. Secretion of both insulin and amylin after meals is delayed and reduced. Plasma levels of GLP-1 are decreased, and the potentiation of insulin secretion by GIP is impaired. Glucagon secretion is not well suppressed and may instead increase after meals. Hepatic glucose production is not adequately suppressed, and the removal of excess glucose from the peripheral circulation is impaired. Fasting and postprandial hypertriglyceridemia may appear. The abnormalities of amylin and GLP-1 may also contribute to difficulty with weight control.

GLUCOSE TOXICITY

Inadequate regulation of plasma glucose and associated metabolic pathways can lead to a vicious cycle in which hyper-

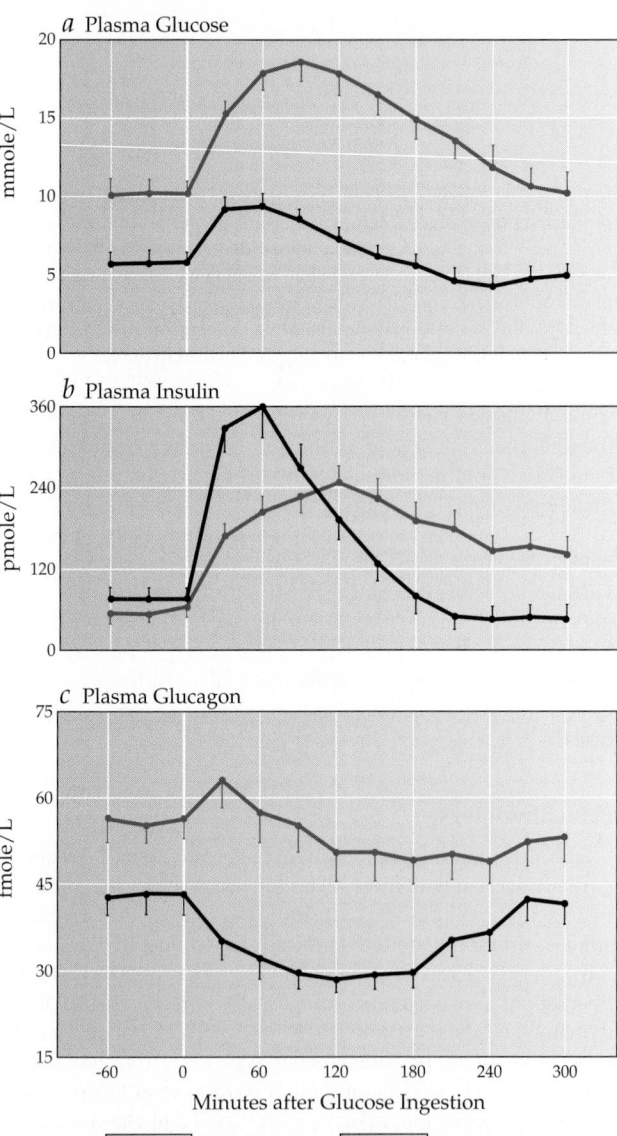

Figure 4 **On glucose tolerance testing in 10 patients with type 2 diabetes and 10 healthy persons of similar age and weight, patients with diabetes had (***a***) excessive and prolonged elevation of plasma glucose, (***b***) delayed and diminished increase of plasma insulin, and (***c***) lack of suppression of plasma glucagon.**[23]

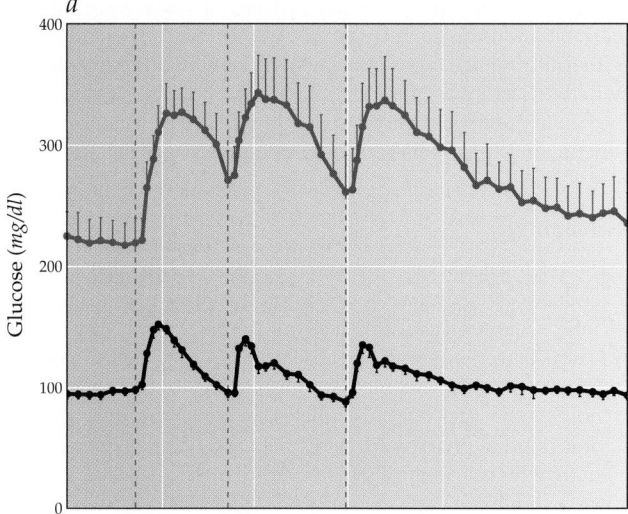

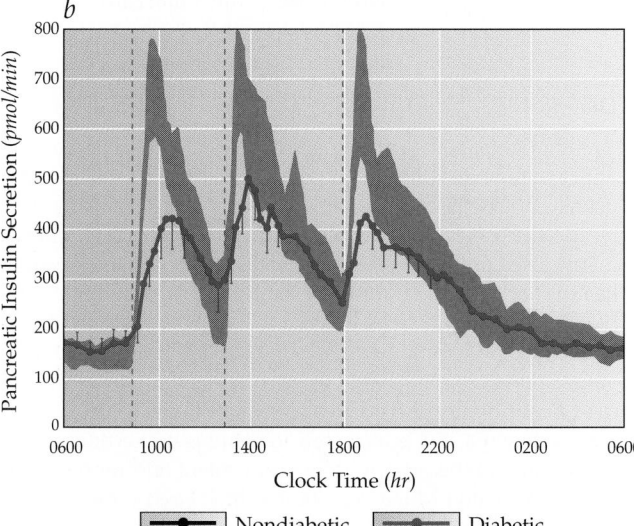

Figure 5 **Typical 24-hour glucose and insulin patterns in untreated patients with type 2 diabetes.**[25] **(*a*) Compared with healthy persons, patients with diabetes have high basal (fasting) glucose with further elevation after each meal (*b*). Nocturnal insulin secretion in abnormal patients with diabetes is normal, but increases after meals are smaller than in healthy persons (shaded area).**

glycemia and high levels of FFAs reduce both insulin secretion and insulin action.[24] This process has been termed glucose toxicity (or glucolipotoxicity). Onset of glucose toxicity may occur after a period of stable or gradually progressing hyperglycemia; more rapid deterioration may be caused either by the addition of a new factor (e.g., a viral illness or glucocorticoid treatment) or attainment of a critical level of hyperglycemia. The diagnosis of diabetes is often made at this time. Initiation of successful treatment with any modality can break the cycle of glucose toxicity; this leads to an improvement in insulin secretion and a reversal in insulin resistance to a greater degree than the direct effects of the treatment alone. After vigorous initial treatment, much simpler and less intensive efforts may maintain glycemic control.

GLYCEMIC PROFILES

The net effect of the underlying abnormalities on typical 24-hour glucose and insulin patterns in untreated patients with type 2 diabetes is shown [*see Figure 5*].[25] The FPG level is elevated, with further incremental increases in the postprandial glucose level occurring during the day. The fasting plasma insulin level is not greatly altered from the level seen in weight-matched persons without diabetes, but postprandial increments in insulin are moderately delayed and reduced in magnitude. This relationship between glucose and insulin reflects a reduction in insulin response to rising FPG levels; the FPG level is continuously elevated and just enough insulin is secreted to prevent further increase. In effect, in a person with untreated type 2 diabetes, the glucose regulatory system is reset so as to maintain a higher FPG level. This higher level can be quite stable, in the absence of treatment, for long periods.

A notable feature of the glycemic profile is that when control is relatively poor, most of the excess glycemic exposure of tissues results from basal hyperglycemia (i.e., elevated fasting and preprandial glucose levels) rather than postprandial hyperglycemia.[26] Because current treatments are principally effective in decreasing FPG levels, patients whose hyperglycemia is well controlled with medications frequently have lower FPG levels but less improvement in elevations in postprandial glucose levels.

Pathogenesis

Because there is a strong genetic predisposition for type 2 diabetes that becomes clinically manifest in the presence of environmental factors, hyperglycemia typically appears intermittently or gradually over a period of years. When a woman with genetic vulnerability becomes pregnant, gestational diabetes may occur as an early transitory manifestation of type 2 diabetes; the diabetes goes into remission after delivery but returns years later as permanent type 2 diabetes. Acute illness or therapy with glucocorticoids may also precipitate hyperglycemia and lead to the diagnosis. However, it is also common for asymptomatic, gradually progressive hyperglycemia to occur in the absence of any medical condition other than obesity, and thus escape detection for years. An analysis of two populations, one in the United States and one in Australia, has shown that retinopathy, an easily identified (but, in its early stages, silent) complication of hyperglycemia, is often present when type 2 diabetes is diagnosed and then increases in prevalence linearly [*see Figure 6*].[27] Projection of the prevalence slope backward, to a period preceding the diagnosis, showed that hyperglycemia was likely to have been present in these populations for at least 4 to 7 years before diagnosis.[27] Similarly, in the United Kingdom Prospective Diabetes Study (UKPDS), many patients with newly diagnosed type 2 diabetes were found to have retinopathy visible on retinal examination (21%), an abnormal electrocardiogram (18%), absent pedal pulses (13%), or an abnormal vibration threshold in the feet (7%).[28]

Prevention

In patients with multiple risk factors for developing type 2 diabetes, an effort to prevent the emergence of overt disease is highly desirable. Randomized clinical trials have shown that the risk of progression from IGT to diabetes can be reduced by lifestyle changes or pharmacologic interventions. The Diabetes Prevention Program (DPP),[29] the Finnish Diabetes Prevention Study,[30] and the Da Qing IGT and Diabetes Study[31] showed that intensive diet and exercise therapy reduced the progression from IGT to diabetes over 3 to 6 years by 42% to 58%. The weight

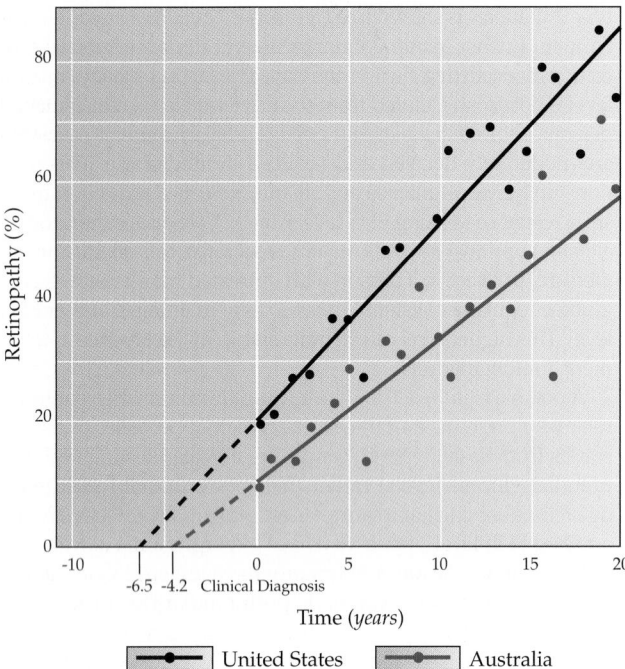

Retinopathy (%)

Time (*years*)

United States   Australia

Figure 6   **Retinopathy is often present before type 2 diabetes is diagnosed and then increases in prevalence linearly.**[27] **This graph shows the prevalence of visible retinopathy at various durations of known type 2 diabetes in 1,166 patients in the United States and 904 in Australia. In each population, some patients had retinopathy at the time of diagnosis; the slope of the lines indicates that retinopathy began to appear 4 to 6 years before diagnosis.**

loss achieved and the amount of exercise performed were modest—5.6 kg (7% of body weight) and 150 minutes of brisk walking a week in the DPP.

The DPP also included a placebo-controlled metformin treatment arm. In this arm, taking 850 mg of metformin twice daily was associated with a 31% reduction of progression to diabetes. Most of this effect persisted after a 1-week washout from metformin. Lifestyle intervention was particularly effective in older persons, whereas metformin was about as effective for middle-aged or younger persons. In the STOP-NIDDM trial, 100 mg of acarbose three times daily, compared with placebo, reduced progression to diabetes by 25%.[32] In a group of Hispanic women with previous gestational diabetes, daily treatment with 400 mg of troglitazone (a thiazolidinedione no longer commercially available), compared with placebo, reduced the development of diabetes.[33] This benefit was still present after an 8-month drug washout.

The largest diabetes prevention trial to date, the international DREAM (Diabetes REduction Assessment with ramipril and rosiglitazone Medication) trial, followed 5,269 patients with prediabetes over a median of 3 years.[34] In this trial, progression to type 2 diabetes occurred in 10.6% of patients who received 8 mg of rosiglitazone daily, compared with 25% of placebo recipients—a risk reduction of 62%. Heart failure was reported in 0.5% of study subjects taking rosiglitazone, compared with 0.1% of placebo recipients.

Despite these results, preventive drug therapy needs further testing. Lifestyle intervention, however, is strongly encouraged in all persons at risk for type 2 diabetes.[35] Although the efficacy, safety, and consistency of lifestyle interventions are impressive,

long-term follow-up is needed to determine how long patients can maintain this therapy and how durable the benefits from either lifestyle changes or drugs will be. Equally important is whether cardiovascular events will eventually be reduced. A secondary analysis from the STOP-NIDDM trial suggests a reduction in MI and total cardiovascular disease events.[36]

Screening

Screening for diabetes by measurement of FPG is recommended for persons without symptoms who are older than 45 years of age, especially if they are overweight (BMI of 25 or greater). Screening should be repeated at 3-year intervals. Earlier or more frequent screening should be considered for patients who have had gestational diabetes; who belong to a high-risk ethnic population (e.g., African, Hispanic, Native American, or Asian); who have a family history of diabetes; or who have hypertension, hypertriglyceridemia, or other risk factors for diabetes or cardiovascular disease.[37] It is also reasonable to screen for diabetes in patients who present with a first cardiovascular event.

Diagnosis

Although patients with type 2 diabetes mellitus may present with symptoms as florid as those of type 1 diabetes mellitus (but usually not with spontaneous ketonuria), most patients with type 2 disease have relatively mild polyuria and polydipsia; many cases are diagnosed only by office screening or other health checks. The diagnosis is established by a randomly sampled (not fasting) plasma glucose value above 200 mg/dl, accompanied by symptoms suggesting hyperglycemia, or an FPG value above 126 mg/dl, with or without symptoms. In either case, a confirmatory second test is required.[1] Oral glucose tolerance testing (OGTT) is more sensitive but is not recommended for routine use because it is less convenient and reproducible and more costly. Moreover, the treatment recommended for most overweight or obese patients would be the same regardless of OGTT results: a combined regimen of nutritional therapy, exercise, and weight loss.

Treatment

GOALS OF THERAPY

In general, the goals of treatment of type 2 diabetes are the same as for type 1. For a typical patient, these include an HbA_{1c} level of less than 7%, fasting and preprandial glucose levels between 90 and 130 mg/dl, and peak postprandial glucose values below 180 mg/dl.[38] It is generally advisable to lower FPG into the target range first, as this is the floor above which all other blood glucose tests of the day will rise. Less stringent glycemic targets should be selected for older patients and patients with severe or complex associated medical conditions, or social or behavioral barriers to self-care. All patients with diagnosed diabetes should learn about the disorder itself, its natural history and complications, and the range of therapies available. All should learn about self-measurement of blood glucose (SMBG) and obtain the necessary equipment.

The major risk factors for cardiovascular disease—hypertension, dyslipidemia, and smoking—should be assessed and treated if present. Basic instruction on medical nutrition therapy should be provided, and the patient should try to reduce weight or at least prevent further weight gain.

NUTRITION AND PHYSICAL ACTIVITY

Better eating and exercise behavior can markedly reduce the progression from prediabetes to diabetes [see Prevention, above]. Once type 2 diabetes has developed, achieving glycemic targets with lifestyle modification is more challenging. All patients in the UKPDS study entered an intensive 3-month dietary program as initial therapy.[39] Only 16% of those enrolled achieved excellent glycemic control, defined as an FPG of 108 mg/dl or less, with dietary treatment alone. At the end of 1 year, only about 9% of the starting group maintained this level of control. This experience confirms what is obvious in clinical practice: even motivated patients, with support from medical providers, have difficulty controlling overt diabetes with nutritional efforts and exercise alone.

Nevertheless, much evidence confirms that patients who are able to follow excellent dietary regimens obtain profound benefit, and most patients will obtain some benefit from their efforts.[36,40] With the help of a dietitian, patients should be provided with individualized, culturally appropriate instructions to reduce intake by at least 250 to 500 calories a day. Such a decrease generally leads to an overall weight loss of 0.5 to 1 lb a week. Alternatively, the patient can be instructed to reduce daily caloric intake to below the basal metabolic rate, which can be estimated at 10 calories per pound (20 cal/kg) of ideal body weight. This will decrease energy intake to less than energy expenditure. Consensus guidelines recommend that the diet consist of less than 30% total fat, less than 10% saturated fat, less than 10% polyunsaturated fat, 10% to 15% monounsaturated fat, 10% to 20% protein, and 50% to 55% carbohydrate.[41] Table sugar and other concentrated forms of carbohydrates are allowable in small portions at any one time (e.g., 5 g or 1 tsp of table sugar). Adding high-fiber foods can also lower plasma glucose modestly.[42] Learning to count the contemplated grams of carbohydrate before each meal helps some patients limit postprandial glucose increases. Periodic reinforcement of nutritional recommendations by the dietitian and physician is essential.

Weight losses of 5% to 10% (10 to 20 lb) produce significant decreases in FPG and HbA$_{1c}$ over 1 to 3 months.[40] In the UKPDS, mean HbA$_{1c}$ fell from 9% to 7% during the 3-month dietary run-in period.[39] However, the group randomized to receive nutritional treatment alone showed significant weight gain and gradual worsening of glycemic control in the first 2 years. For patients such as these, several drugs may be considered to assist with weight control. These include orlistat,[43] a gastrointestinal lipase inhibitor that causes malabsorption of fat calories; sibutramine,[44] an inhibitor of dopamine, norepinephrine, and serotonin reuptake; and rimonabant,[45] an agent that blocks endocanabinnoid receptors. Even after the addition of a weight-loss drug, nutritional efforts remain essential. Surgical procedures altering gastric volume or intestinal pathways[46,47] can effectively control both weight and type 2 diabetes and are gaining acceptance for very obese patients (BMI > 35) who are unresponsive to other therapy [see Chapter 58]. These procedures may work in part by altering the concentrations of gastrointestinal hormones that regulate appetite or satiety.

Additional benefits accrue from gradually increased exercise aimed at achieving at least 60% of maximal heart rate (220 minus age), such as walking 45 minutes at a brisk pace (approximately 3 to 5 miles an hour) three to five times a week.[48] Exercise decreases insulin resistance and glycemia, contributes modestly to weight loss, reduces the risk of future cardiovascular disease, improves prognosis should an MI occur, and enhances the patient's sense of well-being and physical fitness. Conversely, physical inactivity predicts mortality in men with type 2 diabetes mellitus.[49] In the presence of known coronary artery disease (CAD), the exercise should be prescribed with input from the patient's cardiologist. If the patient has had type 2 diabetes mellitus for 5 to 10 years or longer or already has peripheral vascular or cerebral vascular disease, autonomic neuropathy, microalbuminuria, dyslipidemia, or a history of smoking, an ECG is essential and an ECG exercise tolerance test is prudent before starting a formal exercise program.

ANTIHYPERGLYCEMIC DRUGS

A wide array of pharmacologic agents is available for treatment of type 2 diabetes [see Tables 2 through 4]. The effects of various drugs on HbA$_{1c}$ are fairly similar, ranging from about 0.5% to 2.0% (absolute) reduction from the starting value [see Table 3] (except for insulin, which can achieve greater reductions). With all agents, the reduction of HbA$_{1c}$ is generally greater when starting from a higher baseline level, but most patients whose initial HbA$_{1c}$ is above 9% will not be able to reach the 7% target with a single oral agent. Because each class has a different mode of action, their effects are generally additive, and it is possible to combine agents from different classes for optimal results.

Sulfonylureas

Sulfonylureas (SUs) are the oldest oral antihyperglycemic drugs and continue to have an important place in treatment. Their primary mechanism of action is to close adenosine triphosphate–sensitive potassium (K$_{ATP}$) channels in the membrane of beta cells (and other cells). In the beta cell, this causes an influx of calcium and stimulation of exocytosis of insulin granules. SUs are most effective in patients who have had diabetes for less than 10 years and can still secrete considerable amounts of insulin. Although initial doses of SUs directly stimulate secretion of insulin, long-term treatment mainly potentiates the effects of glucose (and other stimuli such as amino acids) on insulin secretion, allowing adequate insulin levels at lower glucose levels. The result is a predominant reduction of FPG, typically 50 to 70 mg/dl, with very little effect on postprandial increments.[50] Fasting plasma insulin levels remain about the same, and postmeal increments of insulin are modestly greater than before starting treatment. These changes of glucose lead to a reduction of HbA$_{1c}$ by 1% to 2%.[51]

For most patients, SU treatment is initiated with the lowest recommended dose, and the dose is increased every 1 to 2 weeks until target blood glucose levels are attained or a practical maximal dose is reached. Modern SUs (e.g., extended-release glipizide, glimepiride) are usually taken in a single daily dose but occasionally are more effective when taken twice daily. Symptomatic patients with an FPG greater than 250 mg/dl may begin with half the maximal recommended dose; the rapid glycemic improvement usually seen is one of the advantages of SUs for such patients.

Hypoglycemia, in particular, and weight gain are adverse effects of SUs. Hypoglycemia is especially frequent and severe in elderly patients who live alone and lack involved family or friends.[52,53] Concern about an increased rate of cardiovascular mortality associated with SUs has persisted since publication of

Table 2 Formulations of Oral Drugs Commonly Used for Type 2 Diabetes

Drug Class	Agent	Lowest Usual Dosage	Maximum Effective Dosage	Generic Available
Sulfonylureas (SUs)	Glyburide	1.25 mg q.d.	5 mg b.i.d.	Yes
	Glipizide	2.5 mg q.d.	10 mg b.i.d.	Yes
	Glipizide extended release	2.5 mg q.d.	5 mg q.d.	Yes
	Glimepiride	1 mg q.d.	4 mg q.d.	Yes
Non-SU secretagogues	Repaglinide	0.5 mg q.d.	4 mg t.i.d.	No
	Nateglinide	60 mg q.d.	120 mg t.i.d.	No
α-Glucosidase inhibitors	Acarbose	25 mg t.i.d.	100 mg t.i.d.	No
	Miglitol	25 mg t.i.d.	100 mg t.i.d.	No
Biguanides	Metformin	500 mg q.d.	1,000 mg b.i.d.	Yes
	Metformin extended release	500 mg q.d.	1,000 mg b.i.d.	Yes
Thiazolidinediones	Pioglitazone	15 mg q.d.	45 mg q.d.	No
	Rosiglitazone	2 mg q.d.	4 mg b.i.d.	No

results from the University Group Diabetes Program in 1970.[54] This study showed an excess of cardiovascular and total mortality associated with tolbutamide. Reassuringly, the UKPDS did not show any trend toward increased cardiovascular events or mortality with SUs.[55] Tolbutamide is no longer widely used, but glyburide (called glibenclamide in Europe), which remains in common use, has been shown to interfere with ischemic preconditioning, a cardioprotective mechanism related to K_{ATP} channels in myocardial cells.[56] Whether this effect indeed causes increased cardiovascular risk has not been fully proven or disproven, and probably never will be because the introduction of newer SUs has rendered the issue moot. Glimepiride, glipizide, and gliclazide appear to lack glyburide's unwanted effect on the myocardium and should be preferred for this reason. These SUs also are less dependent on normal renal function for clearance and cause less hypoglycemia.[57] SUs are contraindicated in patients with hepatic insufficiency and are dangerous when combined with heavy use of alcohol. Patients with hypoglycemia caused by SUs, particularly those with long half-lives, need close monitoring until they demonstrate the ability to maintain normal plasma glucose levels without carbohydrate supplementation.

Other Beta Cell Stimulants

Repaglinide and nateglinide are newer beta cell stimulants that differ in structure and timing of action from SUs.[58] Like SUs, they bind to K_{ATP} channels in beta cells,[59] but they are more rapidly absorbed and cleared. Nateglinide has an especially rapid and transitory effect, peaking at about an hour and lasting about 4 hours. This pattern leads to greater reduction of postprandial increments of glucose but less effect on FPG than is seen with SUs. As monotherapy, repaglinide and nateglinide are most logically used early in type 2 diabetes, when FPG is not greatly elevated. Because of their short half-lives they are less likely than SUs to cause prolonged hypoglycemia.[58] To avoid hypoglycemia, these agents should be taken only with meals, ideally 10 to 15 minutes before the patient starts to eat. Like SUs, they can cause weight gain.

α-Glucosidase Inhibitors

The α-glucosidase inhibitors (AGIs) available in the United States are acarbose and miglitol. These agents are poorly absorbed but act within the gut to inhibit the digestion of complex carbohydrates, leading to a delay of glucose absorption.

Table 3 Properties of Oral Drugs Commonly Used for Type 2 Diabetes

Drug or Drug Class	Mechanism of Action	+Hemoglobin A_{1c} Reduction (%)	Adverse Effects	Possible Nonglycemic Benefits
Sulfonylureas	Potentiate insulin secretion	1–2	Hypoglycemia, weight gain	—
Repaglinide	Potentiates insulin secretion	1–1.5	Hypoglycemia, weight gain	—
Nateglinide	Potentiates insulin secretion	0.5–1	Hypoglycemia, weight gain	—
α-Glucosidase inhibitors	Block carbohydrate digestion	0.5–0.8	Flatulence, diarrhea	Weight control, lower CV risk
Metformin	Reduces hepatic insulin resistance	1–2	Nausea, diarrhea, rare lactic acidosis	Lower CV risk
Thiazolidinediones	Reduce insulin resistance in muscle, adipose tissue, liver	0.5–1.4	Weight gain, edema, uncommonly heart failure	Lower CV risk

CV—cardiovascular

Glycemic increments after meals are typically reduced by 30 to 50 mg/dl, and FPG is reduced by 15 to 20 mg/dl; HbA_{1c} generally falls 0.5% to 0.8%.[60] These agents have no statistically significant effect on lipid levels or body weight.[61] AGIs are mostly useful as monotherapy for patients whose principal problem is postprandial hyperglycemia. They must be taken at the start of a meal. Flatulence, abdominal cramping, and diarrhea are frequent side effects, resulting from undigested carbohydrate reaching bacteria in the lower bowel. These symptoms often limit patient acceptance of treatment with AGIs. Treatment should start with 25 mg, and doses should be increased very gradually to enhance tolerance. Except for rare elevations of alanine aminotransferase (ALT) and aspartate aminotransferase (AST) levels, AGIs are nontoxic. Although hypoglycemia does not occur with monotherapy, it can result when an AGI is added to an SU, nateglinide or repaglinide, or insulin. Should hypoglycemia occur, patients must be warned to treat it only with pure glucose (e.g., glucose tablets) because absorption of starches and sucrose is delayed by the therapeutic actions of AGIs.

Metformin

Metformin is the only member of the biguanide drug class used in the United States.[62] Metformin decreases hepatic glucose production, mostly through inhibiting gluconeogenesis.[63,64] Because it requires the presence of insulin to be effective and because plasma insulin levels decrease during its use, metformin may be considered an hepatic insulin sensitizer. Metformin can reduce FPG by 50 to 70 mg/dl; it has less effect on postprandial increments, resulting in reduction of HbA_{1c} by 1% to 2%.[65] Weight is unchanged or may decline.[62]

Hypoglycemia almost never occurs with metformin monotherapy. Metformin also decreases plasma triglyceride and low-density lipoprotein (LDL) cholesterol levels, and it sometimes increases HDL cholesterol levels. In addition, plasma plasminogen activator inhibitor–1 (PAI-1) activity declines.[66] These effects on cardiovascular risk factors may explain one of the most interesting observations in the UKPDS. Compared with conventional diet treatment, metformin monotherapy substantially decreased the incidence of MI, diabetes-related death, and all-cause mortality in obese patients.[67] Although metformin monotherapy has similar glycemic effects in both normal-weight and obese patients with type 2 diabetes mellitus, obese patients especially benefit because of the absence of weight gain.

The most common side effects of metformin therapy are diarrhea (which can be severe), nausea, and abdominal cramps. To reduce the likelihood of these symptoms, the starting dosage should not exceed 500 mg twice a day, and the drug should be used only with special caution by patients with inflammatory gastrointestinal disease. The maximum effective dosage is 2,000 mg/day.[68] The most feared adverse effect associated with metformin is lactic acidosis.[69] Whether this association is caused by metformin (as was clearly the case with phenformin, an older biguanide) or is coincidentally occurring in individuals at risk for lactic acidosis for other reasons has never been firmly determined. Given this uncertainty, metformin, which is entirely dependent on renal clearance, should not be used by patients with renal insufficiency or in patients at risk for developing it. The following are contraindications to the use of metformin: serum creatinine level greater than 1.4 mg/dl in women and greater than 1.5 mg/dl in men; intravenous administration of radiographic iodinated contrast media; acute MI; heart failure; and any ischemic condition. Nausea, vomiting, tachypnea, and change in mental status call for measurements of serum electrolytes and lactate to rule out lactic acidosis.

Thiazolidinediones

Thiazolidinediones (TZDs), the newest class of oral drugs, include pioglitazone and rosiglitazone.[70] TZDs act by binding to

Table 4 Insulin and Other Parenteral Drugs Used for Type 2 Diabetes

Category	Drug	Onset (min)	Peak (hr)	Duration (hr)	Comment
Injected insulin	Long-acting Glargine	60–120	Minimal	24+	Glargine cannot be mixed in syringe with other drugs

	Intermediate-acting
	  Detemir
	  NPH
		60–120
		60
			4–10
			4–8
				12–20
				10–16	

	Short-acting
	  Human regular
	  Aspart
	  Glulisine
	  Lispro
		30–60
		15–30
		15–30
		15–30
			2–4
			1–2
			1–2
			1–2
				6–8
				4–6
				4–6
				4–6	

	Mixtures
	  Human 70/30 (regular/NPH)
	  Aspart 70/30 (protamine aspart/aspart)
	  Lispro 75/25 (protamine lispro/lispro)
		30–60
		15–30
		
		15–30
			4–6
			4–6
			
			4–6
				10–16
				10–16
				
				10–16
					Single action peak
					Single action peak
					
					Single action peak

Inhaled insulin	Exubera	15–30	1–3	6–8	Contraindicated in smokers
GI peptide hormone receptor agonists	Pramlintide	15–30	0.5–1.0	2–3	Use with basal bolus insulin
	Exenatide	15–30	0.5–1.0	6–8	Use with SU, metformin, or both

GI—gastrointestinal NPH—neutral protamine Hagedorn SU—sulfonylurea

the peroxisome proliferator–activated receptor gamma (PPARγ), thereby regulating the expression of multiple genes.[71] They improve insulin sensitivity in muscle and adipose tissue, and they improve hepatic insulin sensitivity and reduce hepatic glucose production as well. Some of these effects stem from suppression of FFA release and enhancement of adiponectin secretion from adipose tissue.

Like metformin, TZDs require the presence of insulin, and thus they may be ineffective in slender, insulin-deficient patients. Although their glycemic effects are greater in obese patients, some obese persons respond less well than others. Typically, TZDs decrease FPG by 40 to 60 mg/dl, with a moderate additional reduction of postprandial increments.[70] HbA$_{1c}$ decreases by about 1% to 1.5%. Plasma insulin levels also decrease. In patients with marked elevations of FPG, it is appropriate to begin TZDs at a midrange dose (e.g., 4 mg rosiglitazone or 30 mg pioglitazone). Otherwise, the lowest dose is appropriate. Because the clinical effects develop slowly (over 4 to 12 weeks), the dosage should not be increased at intervals shorter than 12 weeks.

TZDs often cause weight gain, consisting partly of adipose tissue and partly of extracellular fluid, sometimes of 40 lb or more.[72] The accumulation of fluid presents as peripheral edema, which can be troublesome in itself, and less often as congestive heart failure in persons with underlying heart disease. For that reason, TZDs should not be used by patients with previous congestive failure or known impairment of myocardial function. The hemoglobin level and hematocrit may decline, perhaps in part from hemodilution. The adipose tissue gain is largely subcutaneous rather than visceral.

The first TZD to be marketed, troglitazone, was withdrawn from use because of its association with rare severe hepatic toxicity, in some cases leading to liver transplantation or death. In clinical studies, neither rosiglitazone nor pioglitazone caused AST and ALT elevations in excess of those caused by placebo, and subsequent evaluations have not confirmed an excess of hepatic failure. However, liver function studies must be performed before and during TZD treatment; the Food and Drug Administration warns that rosiglitazone and pioglitazone should not be prescribed if the ALT level is greater than 2.5 times the upper limit of normal, and the drugs should be stopped if such levels are reached on periodic follow-up testing.

TZDs have nonglycemic effects, which are postulated to reduce cardiovascular risk.[73] These effects include reduction of serum triglyceride and increase of serum HDL cholesterol levels. An increase of LDL cholesterol can occur, but this has been reported to be associated with a shift of the LDL spectrum from small, dense atherogenic particles to larger, more buoyant, less atherogenic particles.[74] Other cardiovascular risk factors that may improve include blood pressure, fibrinolytic status, and endothelial function.[75,76] Whether TZDs will decrease rates of cardiovascular events through such actions remains to be seen. A large study (PROactive) in which either pioglitazone or placebo was added to other therapies had inconclusive results.[77] The primary composite cardiovascular endpoint showed no statistically significant benefit of pioglitazone, but a secondary composite endpoint showed a 16% treatment effect. A 0.5% reduction of HbA$_{1c}$ and small improvements in blood pressure probably contributed to this benefit. Hospital admissions for congestive heart failure were significantly increased with pioglitazone, even in this population from which known congestive heart failure was excluded. The net long-term cardiovascular risks versus benefits of TZDs require further study.

Because of the associated risk of heart failure, the American Heart Association and the ADA recommend assessing for risk factors for heart failure before starting diabetic patients on a TZD; using these agents cautiously (i.e., starting at low doses and titrating upward slowly and carefully while monitoring for symptoms) in patients who have such risk factors or who have asymptomatic or mildly symptomatic heart failure; and avoiding TZDs in patients with New York Heart Association class III or IV heart failure.[78]

Insulin

About 40% of patients with known type 2 diabetes in the United States use insulin. Some of them actually have late-onset type 1 diabetes and need insulin very soon after diagnosis. Insulin should be considered as initial therapy for patients of any age who have a sudden onset of diabetes, hyperglycemia over 300 mg/dl, significant recent weight loss, and increased urine volume accompanied by thirst. Some of these patients will be found to have type 1 diabetes and will require insulin permanently. Those with type 2 diabetes may recover a degree of insulin secretion and sensitivity through reversal of glucose toxicity, in which case control with oral agents alone may be possible after a tapering of insulin dosage.[79]

In the more common situation, the progression of type 2 diabetes is gradual and insulin becomes necessary only after years of successful treatment with diet, exercise, and oral therapies. Use of insulin in this setting differs from insulin therapy for type 1 diabetes in several ways. First, beta cell function is markedly reduced but not absent, so insulin therapy is a supplement rather than a complete replacement, at least when first started. As a result, type 2 patients can take insulin with less exact dosing and timing than is possible in type 1 diabetes. Second, the dosage needed may be much higher than in type 1 diabetes, as a result of insulin resistance. Daily requirements of up to 1 U/kg are common, and some very obese patients may need 400 U a day or more. Third, concern about potential adverse effects of insulin has provoked much discussion and in some cases reluctance to use insulin for type 2 diabetes. Epidemiologic studies in persons without diabetes or with prediabetes show a correlation between plasma insulin levels and cardiovascular risk,[80] leading to concern that treatment with insulin might further increase this risk by further increasing insulin levels and causing weight gain as well. Fortunately, administering metformin along with insulin greatly reduces the tendency to gain weight.[81] Moreover, treatment with insulin in the UKPDS did not increase cardiovascular events.[82] Long-term follow-up of type 1 patients from the Diabetes Control and Complications Trial (DCCT) has provided further reassurance, showing about 50% reduction of cardiovascular events in patients who had received intensive insulin treatment, compared with less intensive insulin treatment.[82] In addition, insulin treatment can improve physiologic markers of cardiovascular risk, and insulin has anti-inflammatory properties.[83] Finally, although insulin can cause serious hypoglycemia, the frequency and severity of events is much lower in type 2 than in type 1 diabetes. Although hypoglycemia should always be kept to a minimum, it rarely prevents patients with type 2 diabetes from maintaining good glycemic control through the skilful use of insulin. Ongoing trials should clarify both the risks and benefits of insulin therapy for type 2 diabetes, but the balance of current evidence suggests that fears about potential hazards of insulin in patients with type 2 diabetes have been excessive.

All the formulations of insulin used for type 1 diabetes may be used for type 2 diabetes [*see Table 4 and Chapter 52*]. In addition, premixed insulins can be used effectively by some patients with type 2 diabetes, whereas they are rarely indicated in type 1 diabetes. Mixtures commonly available consist of 70% neutral protamine Hagedorn (NPH) and 30% regular human insulin, 70% protamine aspart and 30% unmodified aspart, or 75% protamine lispro and 25% unmodified lispro.

Gastrointestinal Hormone Agents

Two injectable agents that mimic the agonist effects of GI peptide hormones have become available for treating diabetes.[84] Pramlintide, which is an analogue of the hormone amylin, is indicated for use in patients who have not achieved optimal glycemic control despite taking both basal and preprandial injections of insulin and whose HbA_{1c} level is below 9.0%. It adds to postprandial control by slowing gastric emptying and suppressing glucagon levels, and it frequently leads to reductions in food intake and weight. HbA_{1c} is typically reduced by about 0.5%. Insulin can easily cause postprandial hypoglycemia when pramlintide is added, so the dose of preprandial insulin should be reduced by half when pramlintide is started. Because pramlintide can cause nausea and vomiting, especially at the initiation of treatment, it should be started at low dosage (e.g., 30 to 60 μg) with slow titration to full dosage, usually 120 μg with each meal. Careful patient education is necessary because pramlintide doses, which are expressed in micrograms, must be converted to insulin unit equivalents for injection with a U-100 insulin syringe.

Exendin is a naturally occurring peptide that is derived from the saliva of the Gila monster. Its effects are very similar to those of GLP-1. Synthetically produced exendin-4, called exenatide, is approved for use in patients taking a sulfonylurea, metformin, or both. It is given by injection twice daily. Like pramlintide, it slows gastric emptying, suppresses glucagon, and favors weight loss, but, unlike pramlintide, exenatide potentiates insulin secretion. A 1% reduction of HbA_{1c} is typically seen. To minimize nausea and vomiting, exenatide should be started at 5 μg twice daily and increased to 10 μg after a month. Hypoglycemia can occur if an SU is used concurrently. Another GLP-1 receptor agonist, liraglutide, is in clinical trials.

Animal studies show that exenatide (and probably other agents that mimic or potentiate the effect of GLP-1) may improve the survival or regeneration of beta cells, and it is hoped a similar effect will occur in humans. Should this prove true, the clinical value of these agents would greatly increase. GLP-1 and other peptide hormones have very short half-lives because they are rapidly inactivated by the plasma enzyme dipeptidyl peptidase IV (DPP-IV). Orally administered agents that block DPP-IV have been developed. The DPP-IV inhibitors vildagliptin and sitagliptin are less effective than exenatide or pramlintide in limiting postprandial hyperglycemia; they do not cause weight loss, but they do reduce HbA_{1c} levels about as effectively as exenatide, and they may also protect beta cells. Sitagliptin was approved by the FDA in October 2006 for use as monotherapy and as combination therapy with metformin or a thiazolidinedione. Vildagliptin is being tested in clinical trials. The long-term roles of all the agents related to GI hormones will depend on the results of ongoing studies.

PRINCIPLES OF PHARMACOTHERAPY

Because type 2 diabetes is a chronic, progressive disorder, it requires a long-term strategy.[85,86] Several basic principles have emerged. Standard, evidence-based methods of treatment should be used whenever possible. However, because of the heterogeneity of this disorder and the variability of daily living patterns, some patients require individualized methods that are not fully validated by specific studies. A definite target for glycemic control should always be established, and treatment should be systematically intensified to attain this target. The usual evidence-based target is an HbA_{1c} level of 7%. Because multiple physiologic defects underlie type 2 diabetes, several agents with different mechanisms of action (combination therapy) will be needed in most cases. Combination therapy should begin with the simplest regimen and lead to more complex combinations.

Oral Monotherapy

It is something of a misnomer to describe therapy consisting of a single oral agent as monotherapy, because nutritional treatment and exercise should always be employed when an oral agent is started. For this reason, treatment with a single drug may be regarded as the simplest form of combination therapy.

Because the evidence of benefit from therapy with metformin and the SUs is most complete and because these drugs have been used the longest, they are the standard initial oral treatments. Metformin leads to weight loss rather than gain; in addition, when used as a single-agent therapy, it does not cause hypoglycemia. In general, patients with initial HbA_{1c} levels below 9% are best started on metformin, especially if they are obese. The ADA and the European Association for the Study of Diabetes recommend metformin treatment, along with lifestyle interventions, as the first step in the treatment of type 2 diabetes.[85]

SUs are equally effective as metformin, however, and have advantages in some settings. SUs act more rapidly than metformin and can be taken once daily. In general, patients with HbA_{1c} above 9% should start with an SU.

Patients whose FPG level is barely elevated but who have especially prominent postprandial hyperglycemia may be candidates for an AGI or nateglinide as the initial agent. Should future studies verify either a unique cardiovascular benefit or a beta cell protective effect of TZDs, an agent from this class may be considered for initial therapy. At present, however, evidence does not support this as a routine practice.

Oral Combination Therapy

Improved understanding of the pathogenesis of hyperglycemia in type 2 diabetes mellitus and longer experience with oral therapies have greatly increased interest in and the popularity of combinations of oral drugs.[86,87] In patients with severe hyperglycemia, none of the current drugs reliably reduces HbA_{1c} to 7% when used alone, probably because they act primarily by correcting single abnormalities. Moreover, all forms of monotherapy (including insulin used conventionally, but possibly not TZDs) become less effective after a number of years.

The need to advance from monotherapy to combination therapy was best shown by the UKPDS experience.[55,88] Combinations attack two or more different causes of hyperglycemia simultaneously—for example, metformin can reduce insulin resistance in the liver while an SU increases basal insulin secretion.[65]

Moreover, when monotherapy fails after initial success, switching to a drug from a different drug class has not been effective (except for insulin). By contrast, addition of either metformin[65] or a TZD[89] to an SU did lower HbA_{1c} significantly. The combinations of metformin with repaglinide,[90] metformin with a TZD,[64] and repaglinide with a TZD[91] have also been more effective than any of these agents given alone. AGIs complement the different actions of each of the other drugs, including insulin.[92] All other oral drugs are effective when added to SUs, except probably repaglinide or nateglinide, for which data are still lacking. Metformin and a TZD also work in triple combination with an SU, repaglinide, or nateglinide. Combinations of oral drugs may at least postpone having to initiate insulin therapy.

Pharmaceutical companies have responded to these considerations by marketing combination pills containing two agents in a fixed-dose combination. The proposal that these formulations might improve adherence is plausible but has not been rigorously tested. It is also possible that the multiplicity of formulations, dosages, and names might increase the risk of medication errors, and that the inability to titrate dosages separately might lead to either excessive side effects or inadequate titration. Objective comparisons of separately given or combined antihyperglycemic agents are mostly lacking.

Insulin Treatment

Addition of insulin to oral agents The simplest way to introduce insulin to the regimen in patients who have been using oral antihyperglycemic agents is to add a single injection of longer-acting (basal) insulin while continuing the other agents at the same dosages.[86] The transition is easily understood by patients, permits starting with a low dose, and requires only a single daily fasting (prebreakfast) glucose test to guide adjustment of the dose. Both hypoglycemia and worsening hyperglycemia are very uncommon with this tactic, in contrast to what may occur when oral agents are stopped and a more complex insulin regimen is started abruptly. The usual insulin preparations for this purpose are NPH, glargine, and, more recently, detemir. NPH is started at bedtime, and detemir is started in the evening or at bedtime. Both NPH and detemir have to be taken twice daily for optimal results in some patients. Glargine is taken at bedtime, in the morning, or before dinner and only rarely needs to be taken twice daily. Common starting doses are 10 units or 0.1 to 0.15 units/kg. Titration of insulin doses should be done systematically, on the basis of the patient's SMBG values before breakfast. One approach is to increase by 2 units once or twice a week until the FPG level is less than 120 mg/dl.[93] Another strategy, used in the Treat-to-Target Trial,[94] is to increase the dose weekly, in increments of 6 to 8 units, until the FPG declines to 140 mg/dl or less; this typically takes 4 to 6 weeks. The insulin dose is then increased in increments of 2 to 4 units. With this approach, target FPG levels are typically achieved within 12 weeks.

When the FPG level is adequately controlled on the oral drug regimen but postprandial glucose is not, an alternative approach is to add a dose of regular or rapid-acting insulin before each meal. If regular insulin is used, the dose should be taken at least 30 minutes before eating. If a rapid-action insulin analogue is used, it can be taken just before the meal or just afterward. Titration schedules for this approach are less well tested than for basal insulin, and whether to use glucose measurements for both efficacy and safety before the next meal (or at bedtime), as opposed to 1 to 2 hours after the meal to guide changes, has also not been studied adequately. This lack of clear algorithms, together with the need for frequent dosing and glucose testing, has limited the use of this approach. The introduction of an inhalable insulin formulation may make the approach more appealing.[95]

Adding premixed insulin in two daily doses is also an option. In such cases, it is usual to begin by administering equal doses (e.g., 5 to 10 units) before breakfast and dinner, with SMBG performed before breakfast and before dinner and doses systematically titrated on the basis of those results. This method is widely used, and can be effective, but studies show that midday hypoglycemia and significant weight gain may occur with it.[96]

Whether to continue oral therapies after insulin therapy proves successful has been debated. In general, continuation of one or more oral agents improves the success of insulin treatment in patients with type 2 diabetes, though it adds complexity and cost. Oral therapy with any type of agent may improve the glycemic control achieved, but metformin has the additional benefit of limiting weight gain. The combination of a TZD with insulin increases the concern regarding congestive heart failure. When multiple injections of insulin are needed because of a decline in endogenous insulin secretion, SUs usually contribute little if any to glycemic control and may be stopped. Eventually—especially after having diabetes for many years—patients may need full basal-bolus insulin therapy, much like patients with type 1 diabetes.

The best way to use injections of pramlintide or exenatide is not yet well defined. Pramlintide may help some patients who are taking both basal and mealtime insulin but who cannot obtain good postprandial glycemic control without gaining too much weight. Exenatide may postpone the need for insulin in some patients for whom oral agents are no longer effective, and it has the advantage of causing weight loss rather than weight gain. Whether exenatide will prove psychologically more acceptable as injection therapy than insulin in general use remains to be seen. Moreover, the long-term balance between the desired effects and the unwanted effects of these agents is not fully tested. The potential safety and effectiveness of combining exenatide with a TZD or insulin is also not established.

MONITORING GLYCEMIC OUTCOMES

Self-Measurement of Blood Glucose

Patients with type 2 diabetes need to test their blood glucose levels regularly. Relatively frequent SMBG may be desirable in patients with newly diagnosed diabetes, because the results can teach these patients about their daily patterns of glucose and the effect of meals, exercise, stress, and hypoglycemic drugs on these patterns. Seeing the effect of specific food choices on SMBG readings contributes powerfully to learning. Once treatment is established, some patients with type 2 diabetes may be able to reduce the frequency of SMBG, particularly if they have stable glycemic patterns and are taking agents that pose only modest risk of hypoglycemia. For example, a patient with stable control on one or two oral agents may need to test glucose once daily, or even less often. On the other hand, patients who start insulin should perform SMBG at least as many times a day as they inject insulin. Specifically, a patient who is taking a single bedtime dose of NPH or glargine insulin should test once daily before breakfast—and occasionally at 3 A.M., if nocturnal hypoglycemia is suspected—whereas a patient who takes twice-daily injections of premixed insulin may need to test both before breakfast and before the evening meal. Postprandial tests help guide therapy with rapid-action or regular insulin and with acute beta cell stimulants. All patients should also test glucose whenever they have symptoms they believe might be caused by hypoglycemia, in order to confirm this suspicion, guide treatment for the present event, and gain information that can be used to prevent a recurrence. Patients using full basal-bolus treatment should test at least three times a day and possibly up to six times a day, as do patients with type 1 diabetes who use this regimen.

Measurement of Hemoglobin A$_{1c}$

Monitoring of HbA$_{1c}$ is a critical supplement to SMBG. This product of nonenzymatic glycation provides an excellent index of average blood glucose levels for the preceding 2 to 3 months.[96,97] Whereas SMBG promotes success in reaching short-term glycemic goals and identifies glycemic patterns, HbA$_{1c}$ can measure long-term success in reaching targeted levels of control that will reduce the risk of long-term complications. The typical patient with type 2 diabetes should have HbA$_{1c}$ tested at least every 6 months. Use of rapid-turnaround, point-of-service HbA$_{1c}$ assays improves the efficiency with which diabetes caregivers can modify regimens during office visits and improves treatment results.[98-100] Assays of other products of nonenzymatic glycation (such as fructosamine and glycated albumin) that reflect shorter periods of chronic hyperglycemia are generally less useful.[99]

MANAGEMENT OF HYPERGLYCEMIA DURING ACUTE ILLNESS

Hyperosmolar Hyperglycemic Nonketotic Coma

Type 2 diabetes mellitus seldom gives rise to diabetic ketoacidosis unless the patient experiences a severe medical stress. On the other hand, hyperosmolar hyperglycemic nonketotic coma (HHNC) is an infrequent but feared acute complication of type 2 diabetes. It is characterized by extreme hyperglycemia (over 600 mg/dl) and serum hyperosmolarity (over 320 mOsm/L) but with little or no ketosis.[101,102] The main clinical effect of extreme hyperosmolarity is somnolence or confusion, which can progress to coma, but focal or generalized seizures or transitory focal neurologic deficits may occur as well. The absence of severe ketonemia is usually attributed to residual insulin secretion that is sufficient to restrain lipolysis, although other factors may contribute. HHNC is marked by extreme dehydration, with both a marked deficit of free water and serious compromise of intravascular volume and tissue perfusion. Thus, most patients with HHNC have hypotension, extremely dry skin and mucous membranes, and gross elevation of hematocrit, urea nitrogen, creatinine, and albumin levels. Secondary lactic acidosis is not uncommon, with a low serum bicarbonate level and an increased anion gap.[101] Increased viscosity and coagulability of the blood predisposes to thrombotic events in the cerebral and coronary artery circulations or elsewhere. Conversely, stroke and myocardial infarction may precipitate HHNC, as may pancreatitis, sepsis, and drugs such as hydrochlorothiazide, phenytoin, and glucocorticoids. Elderly patients living in nursing homes are particularly vulnerable because their thirst mechanisms are less sensitive to a rising serum osmolality and because dementia, decreased alertness, or institutional conditions may combine to reduce water intake to less than urinary and insensible water losses. At presentation of HHNC, serum sodium is usually elevated or normal in the face of extreme hyperglycemia (i.e., the expected pseudohyponatremia is absent). Whatever the presenting level of serum sodium, it will rise, sometimes markedly, when glucose levels decline with insulin treatment.

Fluid replacement is the most important component of therapy for HHNC. Restoration of circulating volume is an urgent first priority and is accomplished by rapid intravenous infusion of 1 to 2 liters of 0.9% saline, followed by 0.45% saline. Later, when plasma glucose levels have declined to 250 to 300 mg/dl, 5% glucose in water or in 0.2% saline is given. Total fluid deficits of as much as 12 liters may have to be replaced. Insulin treatment, as for diabetic ketoacidosis, is started immediately after administration of isotonic saline. Potassium must be added to intravenous fluids to prevent hypokalemia caused by insulin action, but it should not be started until urine flow is verified or hypokalemia is proven, because potassium levels can be high initially. The patient may require days of fluid replacement, the tonicity of which must be carefully adjusted to achieve a gradual steady decrease in serum osmolality and sodium levels, before central nervous system function returns to normal or at least to baseline. The mortality from HHNC is still high. Infection, especially of the urinary tract, even if only suspected, should be treated with broad-spectrum antibiotics. Papillary necrosis may be seen. Patients with a history of arterial or venous thrombosis can benefit from low-dose prophylactic heparin administration.

Other Illness in Hospitalized Patients

Patients with type 2 diabetes who are hospitalized for other conditions are at high risk for complications, in part because of the frequent presence of vascular and neural disorders, which may not have been previously identified. Oral antihyperglycemic agents usually should be discontinued in patients admitted to hospital with acute illness, both because these agents are relatively ineffective during acute illness and because their side effects may be especially problematic in this setting. Insulin is the preferred treatment of hyperglycemia in the hospital; it is most effective when given by continuous intravenous infusion. Studies have shown significant reductions of morbidity and mortality among patients in intensive care units when plasma glucose is kept below approximately 120 mg/dl with insulin infusions.[103] The transition from infused insulin to subcutaneous regimens may be complicated by variable oral and parenteral intake of nutrients and the use of glucocorticoids. The best results are achieved when an experienced team follows the patient through this process and when multiple daily injections of insulin are given according to a predefined plan rather than as a so-called sliding-scale reaction to excessively high glucose levels. Hospitalization offers the opportunity for reinforced patient education by a diabetes nurse educator and, if the admission HbA$_{1c}$ is well above target, for establishment of a new home treatment regimen.

COMPLICATIONS

The complications of diabetes mellitus are discussed in detail elsewhere [*see Chapter 54*].

Matthew C. Riddle, M.D., has received honoraria for consulting or speaking, or research grant support from Amylin, GlaxoSmithKline, Lilly, Novo-Nordisk, Sanofi-Aventis, and Pfizer.

Saul Genuth, M.D., F.A.C.P., has no commercial relationships with manufacturers of products or providers of services discussed in this chapter.

References

1. Diagnosis and classification of diabetes mellitus. American Diabetes Association. Diabetes Care 29:S43, 2006
2. Gerstein HC: Preventing cardiovascular diseases in people with diabetes. Can J Cardiol 15 (suppl G):65G, 1999
3. Mokdad AH, Ford ES, Bowman BA, et al: Prevalence of obesity, diabetes, and obesity-related health risk factors, 2001. JAMA 289:76, 2003
4. Harris MI, Flegal KM, Cowie CC, et al: Prevalence of diabetes, impaired fasting glucose, and impaired glucose tolerance in U.S. adults: the Third National Health and Nutrition Examination Survey, 1988–1994. Diabetes Care 21:518, 1998
5. Narayan KM, Boyle JP, Thompson TJ, et al: Lifetime risk for diabetes mellitus in the United States. JAMA 290:1884, 2003
6. Mokdad AH, Serdula MK, Dietz WH, et al: The spread of the obesity epidemic in the United States, 1991–1998. JAMA 282:1519, 1999

7. Silventoinen K, Sans S, Tolonen H, et al: Trends in obesity and energy supply in the WHO MONICA Project. Int J Obes Relat Metab Disord 28:710, 2004

8. Malecki MT: Genetics of type 2 diabetes mellitus. Diabetes Res Clin Pract 68(suppl 1):S10, 2005

9. Stern MP: Strategies and prospects for finding insulin resistance genes. J Clin Invest 106:323, 2000

10. Grant SF: Variant of transcription factor 7–like 2 (TCF7L2) gene confers risk of type 2 diabetes. Nat Genet 38:320, 2006

11. Kahn R, Buse J, Ferrannini E, et al: The metabolic syndrome: time for a critical appraisal: joint statement from the American Diabetes Association and the European Association for the Study of Diabetes. Diabetes Care 28:2289, 2005

12. Yusuf S, Hawken S, Ounpuu S, et al: Effect of potentially modifiable risk factors associated with myocardial infarction in 52 countries (the INTERHEART study): case-control study. Lancet 364:937, 2004

13. Polonsky KS, Sturis J, Bell GI: Non–insulin-dependent diabetes mellitus: a genetically programmed failure of the beta cell to compensate for insulin resistance. Seminars in Medicine of the Beth Israel Hospital, Boston. N Engl J Med 334:777, 1996

14. Ward WK, Beard JC, Halter JB, et al: Pathophysiology of insulin secretion in non–insulin-dependent diabetes mellitus. Diabetes Care 7:491, 1984

15. Kahn SE, Andrikopoulos S, Verchere CB: Islet amyloid: a long-recognized but underappreciated pathological feature of type 2 diabetes. Diabetes 48:241, 1999

16. Butler AE, Janson J, Soeller WC, et al: Increased beta-cell apoptosis prevents adaptive increase in beta-cell mass in mouse model of type 2 diabetes: evidence for role of islet amyloid formation rather than direct action of amyloid. Diabetes 52:2304 2003

17. Unwin N, Shaw J, Zimmet P, et al: Impaired glucose tolerance and impaired fasting glycemia: the current status on definition and intervention. Diabet Med 19:708, 2002

18. Firth R, Bell P, Rizza R: Insulin action in non–insulin-dependent diabetes mellitus: the relationship between hepatic and extrahepatic insulin resistance and obesity. Metabolism 36:1091, 1987

19. Chandran M, Phillips SA, Ciaraldi T, et al: Adiponectin: more than just another fat cell hormone? Diabetes Care 26:2442, 2003

20. Weyer C, Bogardus C, Mott DM, et al: The natural history of insulin secretory dysfunction and insulin resistance in the pathogenesis of type 2 diabetes mellitus. J Clin Invest 104:787, 1999

21. Dinneen S, Gerich J, Rizza R: Carbohydrate metabolism in non–insulin-dependent diabetes mellitus. N Engl J Med 327:707, 1992

22. Leiter LA, Ceriello A, Davidson JA, et al: Postprandial glucose regulation: new data and new implications. Clin Ther 27(suppl 2):S42, 2005

23. Mitrakou A: Pathogenesis of hyperglycaemia in type 2 diabetes. Diabetes Obes Metab 4:249, 2002

24. Poitout V, Robertson RP: Minireview: secondary beta-cell failure in type 2 diabetes—a convergence of glucotoxicity and lipotoxicity. Endocrinology 143:339, 2002

25. Polonsky KS, Given BD, Hirsch LJ, et al: Abnormal patterns of insulin secretion in non–insulin-dependent diabetes mellitus. N Engl J Med 318:1231, 1988

26. Monnier L, Colette C, Monnier L, et al: Contributions of fasting and postprandial glucose to hemoglobin A1c. Endocr Pract 12(suppl 1):42, 2006

27. Harris MI, Klein R, Welborn TA, et al: Onset of NIDDM occurs at least 4–7 yr before clinical diagnosis. Diabetes Care 15:815, 1992

28. UK Prospective Diabetes Study 6: complications in newly diagnosed type 2 diabetic patients and their association with different clinical and biochemical risk factors. UK Prospective Diabetes Study Group. Diabetes Res 13:1, 1990

29. Knowler WC, Barrett-Connor E, Fowler SE, et al: Reduction in the incidence of type 2 diabetes with lifestyle intervention or metformin. Diabetes Prevention Program Research Group. N Engl J Med 346:393, 2002

30. Tuomilheto J, Lindstrom J, Ericksson JG, et al: Prevention of type 2 diabetes mellitus by changes in lifestyle among subjects with impaired glucose tolerance. Finnish Diabetes Prevention Study Group. N Engl J Med 344:1343, 2001

31. Pan XR, Li GW, Hu YH, et al: Effects of diet and exercise in preventing NIDDM in people with impaired glucose tolerance: the Da Qing IGT and diabetes study. Diabetes Care 20:537, 1997

32. Acarbose for prevention of type 2 diabetes mellitus: the STOP-NIDDM randomized trial. STOP-NIDDM Trial Research Group. Lancet 359:2072, 2002

33. Buchanan TA, Xiang AH, Peters RK, et al: Preservation of pancreatic b-cell function and prevention of type 2 diabetes by pharmacological treatment of insulin resistance in high-risk Hispanic women. Diabetes 51:2796, 2002

34. Effect of rosiglitazone on the frequency of diabetes in patients with impaired glucose tolerance or impaired fasting glucose: a randomized controlled trial. The DREAM (Diabetes Reduction Assessment with ramipril and rosiglitazone Medication) Trial Investigators. Lancet 368:666, 2006

35. Standards of medical care in diabetes. IV. Prevention/delay of type 2 diabetes. Diabetes Care 29(suppl 1):S7, 2006

36. Acarbose treatment and the risk of cardiovascular disease and hypertension in patients with impaired glucose tolerance: the STOP-NIDDM Trial. STOP-NIDDM Trial Research Group. JAMA 290:486, 2003

37. Screening for type 2 diabetes. American Diabetes Association. Diabetes Care 26:S21, 2003

38. Standards of medical care in diabetes. V. Diabetes care. American Diabetes Association. Diabetes Care 29(suppl 1):S8, 2006

39. UK Prospective Diabetes Study 7: response of fasting plasma glucose to diet therapy in newly presenting type II diabetic patients. UKPDS Group. Metabolism 39:905, 1990

40. Bosello O, Armellini F, Zamboni M, et al: The benefits of modest weight loss in type II diabetes. Int J Obes Relat Metab Disord 21(suppl 1):S10, 1997

41. Franz MJ, Bantle JP, Beebe CA, et al: Nutrition principles and recommendations in diabetes. Diabetes Care 27(suppl 1):S36, 2004

42. Chandalia M, Garg A, Lutjohann D, et al: Beneficial effects of high dietary fiber intake in patients with type 2 diabetes mellitus. N Engl J Med 342:1392, 2000

43. Kelley DE, Jneidi M: Orlistat in the treatment of type 2 diabetes mellitus. Expert Opin Pharmacother 3:599, 2002

44. Wirth A, Krause J: Long-term weight loss with sibutramine: a randomized controlled trial. JAMA 286:1331, 2001

45. Pi-Sunyer FX, Aronne LJ, Heshmati HM, et al: Effect of rimonabant, a cannabinoid-1 receptor blocker, on weight and cardiometabolic risk factors in overweight or obese patients: RIO-North America: a randomized controlled trial. JAMA 295:761, 2006 (erratum in JAMA 295:1252, 2006)

46. Sjöström L, Lindroos AK, Peltonen M, et al: Lifestyle, diabetes, and cardiovascular risk factors 10 years after bariatric surgery. N Engl J Med 351:2683, 2004

47. Chapman AE, Kiroff G, Game P, et al: Laparoscopic adjustable gastric banding in the treatment of obesity: a systematic literature review. Surgery 135:326, 2004

48. Zinman B, Ruderman N, Campaigne BN, et al: Physical activity/exercise and diabetes mellitus. Diabetes Care 26(suppl 1):S73, 2003

49. Wei M, Gibbons LW, Kampert JB, et al: Low cardiorespiratory fitness and physical inactivity as predictors of mortality in men with type 2 diabetes. Ann Intern Med 132:605, 2000

50. Del Prato S, Pulizzi N: The place of sulfonylureas in the therapy for type 2 diabetes mellitus. Metabolism 55(5 suppl 1):S20, 2006

51. Ashcroft FM: Mechanisms of the glycaemic effects of sulfonylureas. Horm Metab Res 28:456, 1996

52. Shorr RI, Ray WA, Daugherty JR, et al: Individual sulfonylureas and serious hypoglycemia in older people. J Am Geriatr Soc 44:751, 1996

53. Shorr RI, Ray WA, Daugherty JR, et al: Incidence and risk factors for serious hypoglycemia in older persons using insulin or sulfonylureas. Arch Intern Med 157:1681, 1997

54. A study of the effects of hypoglycemic agents on vascular complications in patients with adult-onset diabetes. I: Design, methods and baseline results. II: Mortality results. University Group Diabetes Program. Diabetes 19:747, 1970

55. Intensive blood-glucose control with sulphonylureas or insulin compared with conventional treatment and risk of complications in patients with type 2 diabetes (UKPDS 33). UK Prospective Diabetes Study (UKPDS) Group. Lancet 352:837, 1998

56. Brady PA, Terzic A: The sulfonylurea controversy: more questions from the heart. J Am Coll Cardiol 31:950, 1998

57. Schwartz TB, Meinert CL: The UGDP controversy: thirty-four years of contentious ambuigity laid to rest. Perspect Biol Med 47:564, 2004

58. Lebovitz HE: Insulin secretagogues: old and new. Diabetes Reviews 7:139, 1999

59. Malaisse WJ: Pharmacology of the meglitinide analogs: new treatment options for type 2 diabetes mellitus. Treat Endocrinol 2:401, 2003

60. Coniff RF, Shapiro JA, Robbins D, et al: Reduction of glycosylated hemoglobin and postprandial hyperglycemia by acarbose in patients with NIDDM: a placebo-controlled dose-comparison study. Diabetes Care 18:817, 1995

61. Van de Laar FA, Lucassen PL, Akkermans RP, et al: Alpha-glucosidase inhibitors for type 2 diabetes mellitus. Cochrane Database Syst Rev (2):CD003639, 2005

62. Kirpichnikov D, McFarlane SI, Sowers JR: Metformin: an update. Ann Intern Med 137:25, 2002

63. Stumvoll N, Nurjhan N, Perriello G, et al: Metabolic effects of metformin in non–insulin-dependent diabetes mellitus. N Engl J Med 333:550, 1995

64. Inzucchi SE, Maggs DG, Spollett GR, et al: Efficacy and metabolic effects of metformin and troglitazone in type II diabetes mellitus. N Engl J Med 338:867, 1998

65. Efficacy of metformin in patients with non–insulin-dependent diabetes mellitus. Multicenter Metformin Study Group. N Engl J Med 333:541, 1995

66. Lebovitz HE: Effects of oral antihyperglycemic agents in modifying macrovascular risk factors in type 2 diabetes. Diabetes Care 22(suppl 3):S41, 1999

67. Effect of intensive blood-glucose control with metformin on complications in overweight patients with type 2 diabetes (UKPDS 34). UK Prospective Diabetes Study (UKPDS) Group. Lancet 352:854, 1998

68. Garber AJ, Duncan TG, Goodman AM, et al: Efficacy of metformin in type II diabetes: results of a double-blind, placebo-controlled, dose-response trial. Am J Med 102:491, 1997

69. Salpeter SR, Greyber E, Pasternak GA, et al: Risk of fatal and nonfatal lactic acidosis with metformin use in type 2 diabetes mellitus: systematic review and meta-analysis. Arch Intern Med 163:2594, 2003

70. Yki-Jarvinen H: Thiazolidinediones. N Engl J Med 351:1106, 2004

71. Olefsky JM: Treatment of insulin resistance with peroxisome proliferator-activated receptor γ agonists. J Clin Invest 106:467, 2000

72. Fonseca V: Effect of thiazolidinediones on body weight in patients with diabetes mellitus. Am J Med 115(suppl 8A):42S, 2003

73. Chiquette E, Ramirez G, Defronzo R: A meta-analysis comparing the effect of thiazolidinediones on cardiovascular risk factors. Arch Intern Med 164:2097, 2004

74. Tack CJJ, Smits P, Demacker PN, et al: Troglitazone decreases the proportion of small, dense LDL and increases the resistance of LDL to oxidation in obese subjects. Diabetes Care 21:796, 1998

75. Parulkar AA, Pendergrass ML, Granda-Ayala R, et al: Nonhypoglycemic effects of thiazolidinediones. Ann Intern Med 134:61, 2001 (erratum in Ann Intern Med 135:307, 2001)

76. Haffner SM, Greenberg AS, Weston WM, et al: Effect of rosiglitazone treatment on nontraditional markers of cardiovascular disease in patients with type 2 diabetes melli-

tus. Circulation 106:679, 2002

77. Dormandy JA, Charbonnel B, Eckland DJ, et al: Secondary prevention of macrovascular events in patients with type 2 diabetes in the PROactive Study (PROspective pioglitAzone Clinical Trial In macroVascular Events): a randomised controlled trial. Lancet 366:1279, 2005

78. Nesto RW, Bell D, Bonwow RO, et al: Thiazolidinedione use, fluid retention, and congestive heart failure: a consensus statement from the American Heart Association and American Diabetes Association. Circulation 108:2941, 2003

79. Ilkova H, Glaser B, Tunckale A, et al: Induction of long-term glycemic control in newly diagnosed type 2 diabetic patients by transient intensive insulin treatment. Diabetes Care 20:1353, 1997

80. Elliott TG, Viberti G: Relationship between insulin resistance and coronary heart disease in diabetes mellitus and the general population: a critical appraisal. Baillieres Clin Endocrinol Metab 7:1079, 1993

81. Wulffele MG, Kooy A, Lehert P, et al: Combination of insulin and metformin in the treatment of type 2 diabetes. Diabetes Care 25:2133, 2002

82. Nathan DM, Cleary PA, Backlund JY, et al: Intensive diabetes treatment and cardiovascular disease in patients with type 1 diabetes. N Engl J Med 353:2643, 2005

83. Dandona P, Aljada A, Dhindsa S, et al: Insulin as an anti-inflammatory and antiatherosclerotic hormone. Clin Cornerstone suppl 4:S13, 2003

84. Riddle MC, Drucker DJ: Emerging therapies mimicking the effects of amylin and glucagon-like peptide 1. Diabetes Care 29:435, 2006

85. Nathan DM, Buse JB, Davidson MB, et al: Management of hyperglycemia in type 2 diabetes: a consensus algorithm for the initiation and adjustment of therapy: a consensus statement from the American Diabetes Association and the European Association for the Study of Diabetes. Diabetes Care 29:1963, 2006

86. Riddle MC: Glycemic management of type 2 diabetes: an emerging strategy with oral agents, insulins, and combinations. Endocrinol Metab Clin North Am 34:77, 2005

87. Yki-Jarvinen H: Combination therapies with insulin in type 2 diabetes. Diabetes Care 24:758, 2001

88. Turner RC, Cull CA, Frighi V, et al: Glycemic control with diet, sulfonylurea, metformin, or insulin in patients with type 2 diabetes mellitus. JAMA 281:2005, 1999

89. Horton ES, Whitehouse F, Ghazzi MN, et al: Troglitazone in combination with sulfonylurea restores glycemic control in patients with type 2 diabetes. Diabetes Care 21:1462, 1998

90. Moses R, Slobodniuk R, Boyages S, et al: Effect of repaglinide addition to metformin monotherapy on glycemic control in patients with type 2 diabetes. Diabetes Care 22:119, 1999

91. Raskin P, Jovanovic L, Berger S, et al: Repaglinide/troglitazone combination therapy: improved glycemic control in type 2 diabetes. Diabetes Care 23:979, 2000

92. Lebovitz HE: Alpha-glucosidase inhibitors. Current Therapies for Diabetes 26:539, 1997

93. Yki-Jarvinen H, Kauppinen-Makelin R, Tiikkainen M, et al: Insulin glargine or NPH combined with metformin in type 2 diabetes: the LANMET study. Diabetologia 49:442, 2006

94. Riddle MC, Rosenstock J, Gerich J, et al: The treat-to-target trial: randomized addition of glargine or human NPH insulin to oral therapy of type 2 diabetic patients. Diabetes Care 26:3080, 2003

95. Royle P, Waugh N, McAuley L, et al: Inhaled insulin in diabetes mellitus. Cochrane Database Syst Rev (3):CD003890, 2004

96. Diabetes Control and Complications Trial (DCCT): results of feasibility study. The DCCT Research Group. Diabetes Care 10:1, 1987

97. Goldstein DE, Little RR, Lorenz RA, et al: Tests of glycemia in diabetes. Diabetes Care 27:1761, 2004

98. Larsen ML, Horder M, Mogensen EF: Effect of long-term monitoring of glycosylated hemoglobin levels in insulin-dependent diabetes mellitus. N Engl J Med 323:1021, 1990

99. Cagliero E, Levina EV, Nathan DM: Immediate feedback of HbA1c levels improves glycemic control in type 1 and insulin-treated type 2 diabetic patients. Diabetes Care 22:1785, 1999

100. Skyler JS: Insulin treatment. Therapy for Diabetes Mellitus and Related Disorders, 3rd ed. Lebovitz HE, Ed. American Diabetes Association, Alexandria, Virginia, 1998, p 186

101. Genuth SM: Diabetic ketoacidosis and hyperglycemic hyperosmolar coma. Current Therapy in Endocrinology and Metabolism, 6th ed. Bardin CW, Ed. Mosby–Year Book, St. Louis, 1997, p 438

102. Nugent BW: Hyperosmolar hyperglycemic state. Emerg Med Clin North Am 23:629, 2005

103. Van den Berghe G, Wilmer A, Hermans G, et al: Intensive insulin therapy in the medical ICU. N Engl J Med 354:449, 2006

54 Complications of Diabetes Mellitus

Mark E. Molitch, M.D., F.A.C.P., and Saul Genuth, M.D., F.A.C.P.

The long-term complications of diabetes mellitus include retinopathy, nephropathy, and neuropathy. These distinctive features of diabetes, which are specifically related to hyperglycemia, can have devastating consequences: retinopathy can result in loss of vision; nephropathy may lead to end-stage renal disease (ESRD); and neuropathy poses the risk of foot ulcers, amputation, Charcot joints, sexual dysfunction, and potentially disabling dysfunction of the stomach, bowel, and bladder. Hyperglycemia sufficient to cause pathologic and functional changes in target tissues may be present for some time before clinical symptoms lead to a diagnosis of diabetes, especially in patients with type 2 diabetes. Diabetic patients are also at increased risk for atherosclerotic cardiovascular, peripheral vascular, and cerebrovascular disease. These conditions may be related to hyperglycemia, as well as to the hypertension and abnormal lipoprotein profiles that are often found in diabetic patients. Prevention of these complications is a major goal of current therapeutic policy and recommendations for all but transient forms of diabetes [*see Table 1*].

Pathogenesis

RELATION OF MICROVASCULAR COMPLICATIONS TO GLYCEMIA

The microvascular complications of diabetes were not recognized until the introduction of insulin therapy in 1922 allowed patients with type 1 diabetes mellitus to live long enough to experience these complications. Although controversy once existed regarding the relationship of hyperglycemia and its treatment to the microvascular complications, the clear results from the Diabetes Control and Complications Trial (DCCT) and United Kingdom Prospective Diabetes Study (UKPDS) ended this debate for type 1 and type 2 diabetes mellitus, respectively, in the 1990s.

The DCCT was a randomized clinical trial in which 1,441 patients 13 to 39 years of age who had type 1 diabetes were randomly assigned either to receive conventional treatment (i.e., no more than two insulin injections a day) or intensive treatment. Patients in the intensive treatment arm of the study either received three or four insulin injections a day, or they received insulin via a continuous subcutaneous infusion pump. Intensive treatment involved self-monitoring of blood glucose levels at least four times a day. For patients in the intensive treatment group, the premeal target blood glucose levels were 70 to 120 mg/dl; the goal for the glycated hemoglobin (HbA$_{1c}$) level was less than 6.05%. In addition, patients in the intensive treatment group had very frequent contact with members of the treatment team.

A comparison of HbA$_{1c}$ values for patients in the two treatment groups found a difference of 1.8% (8.9% for the conventional-treatment group, as compared with 7.1% in the intensive-treatment group); this difference was maintained between the two treatment groups for up to 9 years. Over a mean follow-up period of 6.5 years, intensive treatment resulted in a risk reduc-

tion for the initial development or progression of retinopathy of 27% to 76%; a risk reduction for the development of microalbuminuria (defined as a urinary albumin level of 30 to 299 mg/24 hours) of 35% and of albuminuria (defined as a urinary albumin level of ≥ 300 mg/24 hours) of 56%; and a risk reduction for the development of clinical neuropathy, confirmed by abnormal nerve conduction velocities or autonomic nervous system function tests, of 60%.[1,2] The main adverse effect of intensive treatment was a threefold increase in the risk of severe hypoglycemic episodes characterized by coma, seizures, or the required assistance of others to treat and reverse the episode.[1,2] However, detailed cognitive function testing showed no permanent damage from such episodes of hypoglycemia.[2]

After the completion of the DCCT, 1,349 of the study patients were followed in the observational Epidemiology of Diabetes Interventions and Complications (EDIC) study. The previous difference in HbA$_{1c}$ values between the original intensive-treatment group and the conventional-treatment group disappeared within 2 years, and both groups then maintained mean HbA$_{1c}$ values around 8.0% over the subsequent years. Despite closure of the gap in glycemic control, early intensive control appeared to provide a sustained protective effect against all complications, including a 75% risk reduction for the progression of retinopathy, a 59% risk reduction in the development of new microalbuminuria, an 84% risk reduction in development of albuminuria, a 51% reduction in neuropathic symptoms, and a 43% reduction in neuropathic signs; these findings suggest the presence of a so-called metabolic memory effect and emphasize the importance of early intervention.[3-5]

The UKPDS[6,7] enrolled 5,102 patients with newly diagnosed type 2 diabetes mellitus; the mean age of the patients was 53 years, and the mean body mass index (BMI) was 28. After a 3-month dietary run-in, 1,138 patients were randomly assigned to a continuation of diet treatment only as long as their fasting plasma glucose (FPG) level remained below 270 mg/dl and they had no hyperglycemic symptoms. In the study, 2,729 patients were randomly assigned to intensive treatment, 1,573 to receive one of three sulfonylurea drugs, and 1,156 to receive insulin; 342 patients were also randomized to receive intensive treatment with metformin. The goal of intensive treatment was an FPG level of less than 108 mg/dl. Of the conventional-treatment patients, 80% ultimately required drugs to maintain their treatment goals of an FPG level of less than 270 mg/dl and freedom from symptoms, although nearly 60% of their total treatment time was spent on diet therapy alone. Likewise, in the intensive-treatment groups, metformin therapy had to be added to sulfonylurea therapy, and insulin had to be substituted for, or added to, oral drug therapy to maintain the stringent treatment goal. Despite these drug crossovers, after 10 years of follow-up, patients who received intensive treatment showed a 25% lower risk of serious microvascular complications (i.e., vitreous hemorrhage, need for laser treatment, and renal failure), compared with patients given conventional treatment.[6] This important benefit was associated

Table 1   Screening for Diabetes Complications in Adults[25]

Complication	Screening Method	Frequency	Goals
CVD	Blood pressure measurement	Every routine visit	< 130/80 mm Hg
Dyslipidemia	LDL, HDL, and triglyceride measurement	Annually; every 2 yr in patients with values at goal who are not receiving treatment and who have no CVD	Patients without overt CVD: LDL < 100 mg/dl Patients with overt CVD: consider LDL < 70 mg/dl; HDL > 40 mg/dl in men, > 50 mg/dl in women; triglycerides < 150 mg/dl
Nephropathy	Urine microalbumin	Annually*	Normal albumin < 30 mg/24 hr or albumin-creatinine ratio < 30 mg/g in a random urine specimen
	Serum creatinine, for estimation of GFR	Annually	Normal GFR > 90 ml/min/1.72m²
Retinopathy	Dilated and comprehensive eye examination	Type 1: 3–5 yr after onset; type 2, shortly after diagnosis; repeat annually, more often if retinopathy is progressing or during pregnancy	Prevention of irreversible damage and vision loss
Neuropathy	Examination for DPN	At diagnosis and annually	Early detection
	Assessment for autonomic neuropathy	Type 1: 5 yr after diagnosis Type 2: at diagnosis	Early detection
	Inspection of insensate feet	Every visit	Intact skin
	Comprehensive foot examination	Annually	Normal examination

*In type 1 diabetic patients who have had diabetes for ≥ 5 yr and in all type 2 diabetic patients starting at diagnosis and during pregnancy.
CVD—cardiovascular disease   DPN—distal symmetrical polyneuropathy   GFR—glomerular filtration rate   HDL—high-density lipoprotein   LDL—low-density lipoprotein

with an HbA$_{1c}$ difference of 0.9% (7.9% for conventional therapy; 7.0% for intensive therapy). Serious hypoglycemia occurred in 3% of insulin-treated patients each year and in 1% to 2% of sulfonylurea-treated patients. These rates of hypoglycemia were much lower than the rates seen with intensive treatment in patients with type 1 diabetes mellitus in the DCCT.

The DCCT and the UKPDS provided experimental proof that microvascular and neuropathic complications can be prevented, or at least substantially delayed, by maintaining blood glucose levels as near to normal as treatment techniques safely allow. In the DCCT, the risk of retinopathy was directly related to the preceding mean HbA$_{1c}$ difference in a similar exponential fashion in each of the two treatment groups.[8] The risk of retinopathy was decreased by about 44% for each proportional 10% decrease in HbA$_{1c}$ (e.g., a decrease in HbA$_{1c}$ from 10% to 9.0%). Microalbuminuria and neuropathy showed risk relations similar to those of glycemia. Similarly, in the UKPDS, the risk of microvascular complications decreased by about 37% for every absolute decrease of 1% in HbA$_{1c}$.[9] These similarities suggest that similar biologic processes are at work. Neither the UKPDS nor the DCCT analyses indicated any glycemic threshold in the diabetic range of HbA$_{1c}$ below which there was no further risk of microvascular complications.[9,10] This observation sets normoglycemia as the ultimate goal of the treatment of type 1 and type 2 diabetes mellitus. Furthermore, the EDIC study showed that the benefits of previous intensive treatment (or the adverse effects of previous conventional treatment) were still being felt years after the DCCT was completed, during which time the mean HbA$_{1c}$ concentrations in both groups were nearly identical (approximately 8.0%).[3-5] Thus, sustained periods of glycemic exposure are associated with prolonged consequences. An unacceptable level of hyperglycemia continues to have adverse effects even after some improvement in metabolic control, and a marked reduction in hyperglycemia with intensive treatment continues to have beneficial effects even after some worsening in metabolic control.

From a management perspective, it is important to note that HbA$_{1c}$ levels are determined principally by mean blood glucose levels, rather than by glycemic instability (i.e., wide swings in blood glucose levels)[11] and that HbA$_{1c}$ levels better reflect the risk of the development of complications than do blood glucose levels.[12] Thus, evidence from the DCCT/EDIC and the UKDPS supports an HbA$_{1c}$ goal of 7% or less, although many have advocated even lower goals. However, the rates of development of hypoglycemia increase substantially as HBA$_{1c}$ levels decrease below 8%, so the benefit of preventing complications must always be balanced against the risk of hypoglycemia.

MECHANISMS OF MICROVASCULAR COMPLICATIONS

Increased glucose concentrations may cause damage to the retina, kidney, and nerves by multiple mechanisms [*see Figure 1*].[13] First, advanced glycation end products (AGEs) form from glucose-derived dicarbonyl precursors (glyoxal, methylglyoxal, 3-deoxyglucosone) generated intracellularly in proportion to intracellular hyperglycemia and react with free amino groups in N-terminal amino acids and lysine residues of proteins. HbA$_{1c}$ is one such molecule. Proteins modified by AGEs have altered function; this is true of intracellular proteins, extracellular matrix proteins, and plasma proteins, which bind to endothelial cells, mesangial cells, and macrophages. These actions induce reactive oxygen species, with activation of transcription factor nuclear factor–κB, thereby causing changes in gene expression of various cytokines and growth factors. Near the end of the DCCT, concentrations of long-lived AGEs in skin collagen were higher in conventionally treated patients than in intensively treated patients.[14] AGEs correlated with HbA$_{1c}$ and, independently of HbA$_{1c}$, with the presence of retinopathy, nephropathy, and neuropathy.[14] The glycated collagen level and the AGE carboxymethyl-lysine level predicted the subsequent 10-year progression of retinopathy and nephropathy during the EDIC study.[15]

A second mechanism is that hyperglycemia can secondarily produce oxidative stress in tissues, with depletion of glutathione and formation of reactive oxygen species and free radicals.[13] Third, when glucose is insufficiently metabolized by insulin-stimulated routes, it can overflow into the sorbitol (polyol) pathway via the enzymes aldose reductase and sorbitol dehydrogenase. The major effect of activation of the polyol pathway is to decrease the amount of intracellular glutathione, thereby exacerbating intracellular oxidative stress.[13] Fourth, elevated glucose levels increase levels of protein kinase C, an enzyme that can influence numerous cellular processes with potentially damaging effect; such effects include stimulating neovascularization and epithelial cell proliferation; increasing collagen synthesis; increasing vascular permeability; increasing apoptosis (programmed cell death); increasing oxidative stress; and mediating the actions of vascular endothelial growth factor (VEGF), which stimulates angiogenesis, and of transforming growth factor–β.[16] Fifth, elevated glucose levels cause an increase in the production of VEGF. VEGF is present in high concentrations in human diabetic ocular tissues and in the kidneys of animals with experimentally induced diabetes. VEGF is a logical candidate to mediate development of proliferative retinopathy.[17] Sixth, hyperglycemia stimulates nitric oxide synthase to produce nitric oxide, a molecule that itself generates damaging free radicals.[13] Finally, excess blood glucose overflows into the hexosamine pathway, resulting in deleterious products.[13] A single mitochondrial defect that leads to the overproduction of reactive oxygen species can result in at least three of the above-mentioned mechanisms; such a defect has been proposed as the primary culprit in hyperglycemic damage. In addition, a number of these pathways are mutually reinforcing, setting up vicious cycles that can accelerate tissue damage.[13]

The therapeutic importance of elucidating the mechanistic links between hyperglycemia and the resulting microvascular

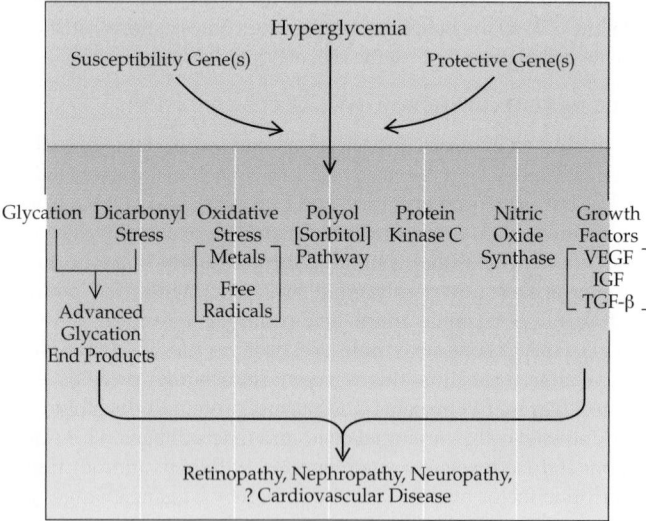

Figure 1 **Multiple pathways have been described that may link high blood glucose levels to the microvascular and neuropathic complications of diabetes (see text). There are good reasons to believe that genetic factors, possibly operating through such pathways, may explain the observation that some individuals with consistently high blood glucose levels do not experience complications, whereas other individuals with near-normal blood glucose levels do experience complications. (IGF—insulinlike growth factor; TGF-β—transforming growth factor-β; VEGF—vascular endothelial growth factor)**

and neuropathic complications lies in our current inability to normalize blood glucose consistently. Therefore, drug therapies that intercept pathogenetic processes after hyperglycemia has developed hold promise for preventing these complications. An inhibitor of AGE formation, aminoguanidine, has been successful in animal experiments, but human trials have revealed unacceptable toxicity. Several inhibitors of aldose reductase, which catalyzes the first step in the polyol pathway, have been studied in clinical trials, but none have shown sufficient clinical benefit or an acceptable adverse-effect profile to warrant approval in the United States. In clinical trials, the use of antioxidants such as vitamin E has not proved successful, but a relatively nontoxic oral inhibitor of protein kinase C, ruboxastaurin, has shown some benefit in early studies of retinopathy and nephropathy.[16] Antagonists to VEGF and other growth factors, administered by systemic or local injection, are undergoing trials.[17] A thiamine analogue, bentotiamine, reduces mitochondrial overproduction of reactive oxygen species from glucose (see above) and prevents retinopathy and nephropathy in experimental diabetic animals.[18,19]

GENETICS OF MICROVASCULAR COMPLICATIONS

There is considerable evidence from several studies that diabetic nephropathy and severe retinopathy cluster in families.[20,21] Thus, either genetic susceptibility or genetic protection is likely to explain the fact that nephropathy develops in only 35% to 40% of patients with diabetes. There is conflicting evidence as to whether the gene for angiotensin-converting enzyme (ACE) or the gene for angiotensinogen has a role in determining a person's risks of nephropathy and retinopathy. A number of other candidate genes are also currently being evaluated.

Retinopathy

Given a long enough duration, retinopathy occurs in almost all patients with type 1 diabetes mellitus and in most patients with type 2 diabetes mellitus who receive conventional treatment but whose glycemic levels remain significantly elevated.[22,23] The most common form of retinopathy is nonproliferative retinopathy (also termed background retinopathy) [*see Table 2*]. It begins with loss of capillary pericytes, the supporting cells of the retinal vasculature; such loss leads to capillary dilatations (microaneurysms) [*see Figure 2a*]. Microaneurysms tend to cluster near the macula, the area responsible for central vision and visual acuity. Small dot hemorrhages form when microaneurysms leak blood. Hard lipid exudates form as a result of the leakage of serum [*see Figure 2a*]. These lesions are usually benign unless they occur quite close to the macula and in sufficient number to cause clinically significant macular edema. The latter is a feared complication that can decrease central vision and acuity. The 10-year incidence of clinically significant macular edema is 20% in patients with type 1 diabetes and 14% in those with type 2 diabetes.[23]

In the phase of preproliferative retinopathy, capillaries become obstructed, causing retinal ischemia. Infarctions of the retinal nerve layer appear as soft (cotton wool) exudates. The retina responds to further ischemia with proliferation of new blood vessels from its surface [*see Figure 2b*]. In this phase of proliferative retinopathy, the ischemic retina releases VEGF, which stimulates the formation of new vessels. These new vessels grow forward into the vitreous. They are extremely fragile and can bleed into the vitreous, causing temporary loss of vision until the blood is reabsorbed. If no reabsorption occurs, blindness can re-

Table 2   Diabetic Retinopathy

Stage*	Pathologic Process	Manifestations
Background	Loss of capillary integrity Leakage, exudation, diapedesis Early capillary closure	Microaneurysms Dot hemorrhages Hard exudates Macular edema
Preproliferative	Capillary closure Microinfarcts Ischemia	Blot hemorrhages Soft exudates Intraretinal microvascular abnormalities Venous beading Macular edema
Proliferative	Forward growth of new large vessels Fibrosis Traction on retina or vitreous	Preretinal hemorrhage Vitreous hemorrhage Retinal detachment Macular edema

*Loss of visual acuity may occur from macular edema at any stage. Blindness may occur from severe macular edema, vitreous hemorrhage, or retinal detachment.

sult unless successful vitrectomy is carried out. Even after reabsorption of the vitreous blood, fibrous scars can cause traction on the retina and can lead to retinal detachment, another cause of profound and often permanent loss of vision.

SCREENING

The role of the internist and ophthalmologist is to detect retinopathy significant enough to require laser therapy before irreversible damage and loss of vision occur. The ability of internists and endocrinologists to detect progressive retinopathy with a standard fundoscopic examination, even using dilation, is limited.[24] Therefore, regular dilated eye examinations should be performed yearly by an experienced eye care specialist, usually an ophthalmologist.[22,24,25] Furthermore, a complete ophthalmologic examination can detect other conditions such as cataracts, glaucoma, and macular edema. In patients with type 1 diabetes mellitus, significant retinopathy (beyond microaneurysms) seldom occurs within 5 years of disease onset, so regular yearly ophthalmologic examinations do not need to commence until then. By contrast, 20% to 40% of patients with type 2 diabetes mellitus already have detectable retinopathy at the time of diagnosis.[26] Therefore, yearly ophthalmologic examinations should begin at the time of diagnosis.[19] Pregnancy is a recognized risk factor for progression of retinopathy in type 1 diabetes mellitus,[27] and ophthalmologic examinations should be performed at the beginning of pregnancy and thereafter with a frequency dependent on the findings of the first examination. This increased risk from pregnancy continues into the year after delivery.[27]

TREATMENT

Laser treatment of high-risk proliferative retinopathy and of macular edema has been demonstrated to preserve vision.[28] For proliferative retinopathy, panretinal scatter photocoagulation is performed to ablate ischemic retina in the periphery capable of producing VEGF. For macular edema, finely focused laser treatment is performed to close visibly leaking perimacular vessels that are demonstrated by fluorescein angiography. For patients with vitreous hemorrhage that does not clear or with significant vitreous scarring and debris, vitrectomy can be performed. Fibroproliferative scars can be excised, and a detached retina can be reattached. The vitreous is replaced with a salt solution.

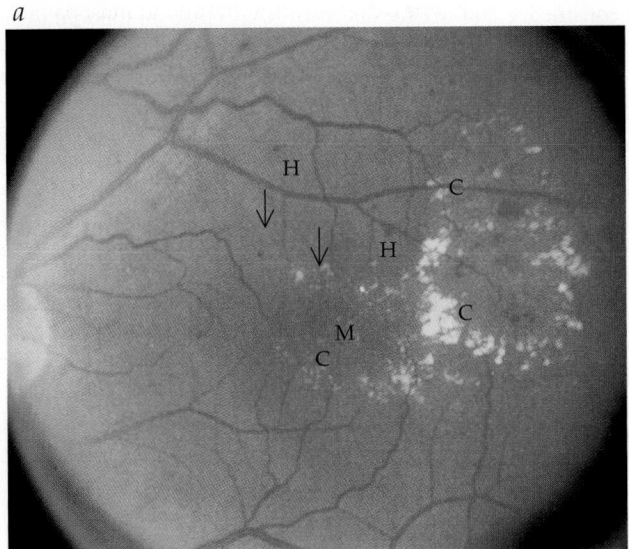
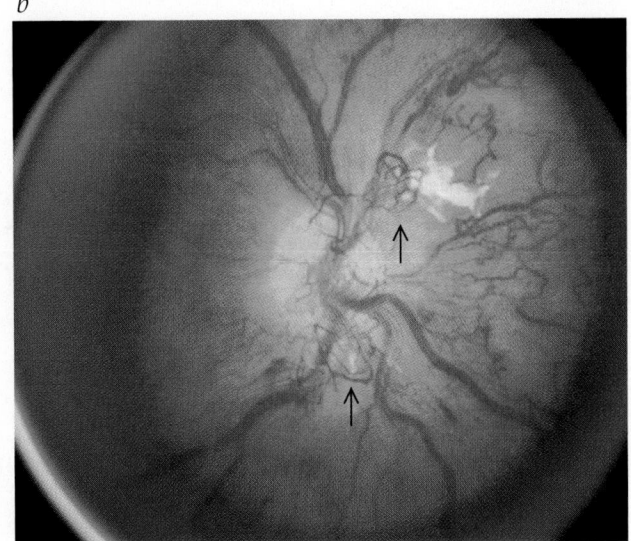

Figure 2   (*a*) This fundus photograph reveals nonproliferative (or background) retinopathy in a diabetic patient. Microaneurysms (arrows) occur at end capillaries. Punctate (or dot-and-blot) hemorrhages (H) and hard exudates (C) can also be seen. The hard exudates form three distinct circles (termed circinate retinopathy), which indicate leakage of plasma proteins from abnormal vessels located in the centers of the three circles. Lesions in the area of the macula (M) are potentially more dangerous, as they may lead to macular edema requiring laser therapy. (*b*) In proliferative retinopathy, new vessels grow from the retina into the vitreous. This fundus photograph reveals fine, tangled, new vessels originating from several areas of the disk (arrows). The vessels often form arcades and characteristically have thin walls and are fragile. They tend to bleed into the vitreous; the scars that form can cause retinal detachment and loss of vision. Proliferation within one disk diameter of the disk (termed neovascularization of the disk) is particularly dangerous, because these vessels are especially prone to bleed and form traction scars.

Nephropathy

From 35% to 45% of patients with type 1 diabetes mellitus and a somewhat smaller percentage of patients with type 2 diabetes mellitus experience significant nephropathy.[4,29-32] Histologically, the earliest change is thickening of the capillary basement membrane; subsequently, mesangial matrix material accumulates in the glomerulus. Ultimately, there is loss of podocytes and development of peritubular fibrosis. Excretion of low but abnormal levels of albumin in the urine is a marker of the incipient phase of nephropathy.[31,32] Over time, albuminuria increases, and eventually the glomerular filtration rate (GFR) begins to fall [see Figure 3]. Microalbuminuria is defined as excretion of 30 to 299 mg of albumin a day or an albumin-creatinine ratio of 30 to 299 mg/g in a random urine specimen.[31,32] Albuminuria is defined as the excretion of 300 mg/24 hour or more of albumin or an albumin-creatinine ratio of 300 mg/g or higher. The nephrotic syndrome may also eventually occur. However, 30% to 50% of persons with diabetes may have a fall in GFR even without any increase in urinary albumin excretion, albeit the presence of albuminuria appears to carry a worse prognosis with respect to the rate of fall of GFR.[33]

Coincident with or shortly after the development of microalbuminuria, hypertension often appears.[34,35] Hypertension in turn further aggravates diabetic nephropathy and is an important component in the progression to renal failure.[36]

The risk of cardiovascular disease (CVD) is far higher in diabetic patients who have evidence of nephropathy than in those without evidence of nephropathy, even at the early stage, when only microalbuminuria is present[30,37-40]; the risk increases as the kidney disease progresses to albuminuria and the GFR subsequently decreases.[30,41] Data from the UKPDS show that once patients with type 2 diabetes develop albuminuria, their annual risk of dying of CVD is greater than their risk of progressing to a stage of nephropathy characterized by a decrease in GFR.[30]

SCREENING

Screening for nephropathy is recommended annually,[25] with measurements of urinary albumin and serum creatinine and then calculation of the GFR from the creatinine concentration, using one of the standard formulas such as that from the Modification of Diet in Renal Disease study.[37] Unlike the risk of retinopathy, the risk of nephropathy does not continue to rise with increasing duration of diabetes. The incidence of nephropathy peaks at approximately 15 to 17 years and declines somewhat thereafter.[29] The prevalence of nephropathy remains approximately constant after that time.

PREVENTION AND TREATMENT

The best preventive approach for diabetic nephropathy in both type 1 and type 2 diabetes mellitus is the maintenance of near-normal glycemic levels, which can markedly reduce the initial development of microalbuminuria and the progression to albuminuria (see above). Data demonstrating that glycemic control slows the progressive decline in GFR is meager; however, in the EDIC, the rate of disease progression, as defined by a serum creatinine concentration above 2 mg/dl, was decreased in those patients who had undergone intensive treatment.[4]

Good blood pressure (BP) control is of paramount importance. The UKPDS showed that a decrease in systolic BP of 10 mm Hg and in diastolic BP of 5 mm Hg results in a relative risk reduction of 29% for the initial development of microalbuminuria and 39% for the development of albuminuria.[42] Once GFR begins to fall, maintaining BP below 130/80 mm Hg markedly decreases the rate at which GFR declines.[36] A retrospective analysis of the Irbesartan Diabetic Nephropathy Trial showed that lowering the systolic BP to 120 mm Hg was associated with improved patient survival and renoprotection.[43]

Antihypertensive agents that block the renin-angiotensin-aldosterone system (RAAS) appear to have additional beneficial effects on the progression of nephropathy above and beyond their BP-lowering effects.[31,44] These agents appear to do this by decreasing intraglomerular pressure and by blocking the vasoconstrictive and trophic effects of RAAS that are thought to be important factors in the pathogenesis of vascular injury in diabetes.[31,44] Studies have shown ACE inhibitors to be superior to

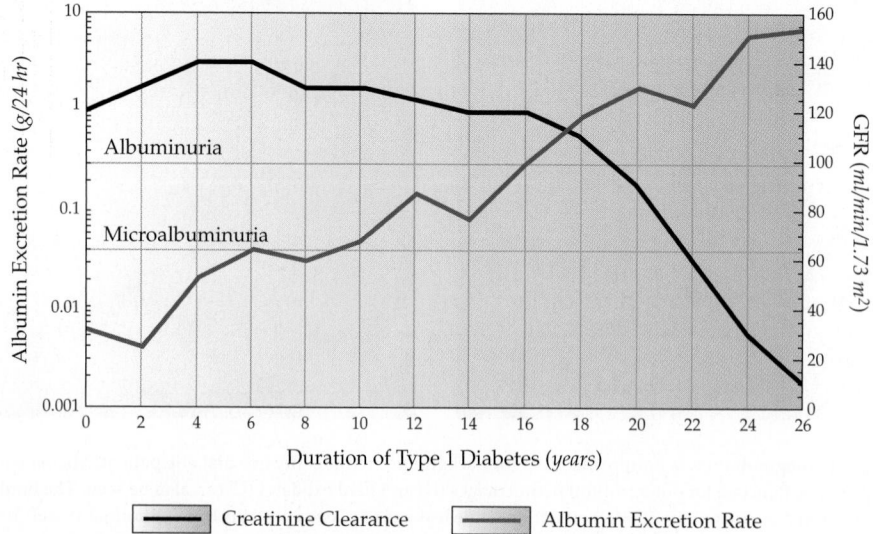

Figure 3   **Natural history of nephropathy in type 1 diabetes. In the 30% to 35% of patients who develop nephropathy, microalbuminuria generally develops between 5 and 15 years after the onset of diabetes. Over approximately the next 10 years, there is a greater than 40% chance of progression to albuminuria. Some time after the onset of albuminuria, the glomerular filtration rate (GFR) begins to fall.[140]**

other classes of antihypertensive agents in decreasing the development of microalbuminuria and albuminuria in patients with type 1 diabetes, including those without hypertension.[45,46] ACE inhibitors also decrease the rate at which GFR declines.[45] Currently, there are no data regarding the effects of angiotensin receptor blockers (ARBs) on nephropathy in patients with type 1 diabetes, but the efficacy and superiority of ACE inhibitors have generally been extrapolated to ARBs.

Both ACE inhibitors and ARBs appear to be effective in type 2 diabetes. The Microalbuminuria, Cardiovascular, and Renal Outcomes–Heart Outcomes Prevention Evaluation (MICRO-HOPE) study involved 3,577 patients, most of whom had type 2 diabetes; ramipril showed a statistically significant benefit over placebo in preventing the progression from microalbuminuria to overt nephropathy (24% risk reduction), as well as a nonsignificant decrease in the rate of development of new microalbuminuria.[47] The Bergamo Nephrologic Diabetes Complications Trial (BENEDICT) showed similar benefits with trandolapril.[48] Studies of ARBs, such as the Reduction in Endpoints in Non–Insulin Dependent Diabetes Mellitus with the Angiotensin II Antagonist Losartan (RENAAL) study and the Irbesartan Diabetic Nephropathy Trial (IDNT), showed that ARBs are beneficial in decreasing the rate at which GFR declines in patients with modestly decreased GFR and with albuminuria[49,50]; other studies in patients with hypertension and microalbuminuria showed that irbesartan was able to decrease the rate of progression of microalbuminuria to albuminuria.[51,52] It should be noted that in women who wish to become pregnant, the use of ACE inhibitors in the first trimester has been associated with an increased risk of major congenital malformations.[53] Therefore, this class of drugs should not be used in women who wish to become pregnant. Whether such a risk extends to ARBs is unknown.

Usually, three or more drugs are required to control hypertension in patients with advancing nephropathy, with either an ACE inhibitor or an ARB used as the first drug of the three-drug regimen.[36] Hypertension in such patients almost always has a volume component, so a diuretic should generally be used as a second agent; dietary sodium should be restricted as well. If an ARB was used as the first drug, then an ACE inhibitor should be used as the third drug. If an ACE inhibitor was used as the first drug, then an ARB should be used as the third drug. Calcium channel blockers and drugs of other classes can also be used. Beta blockers should be used with caution in patients with type 1 diabetes who are undergoing intensive insulin treatment, because these agents may mask the symptoms associated with hypoglycemia and may also impair the ability of released epinephrine to raise glucose levels.

If the GFR continues to fall despite excellent glycemic and BP control, protein restriction may be of some benefit. The consensus recommendation is to prescribe a protein intake of approximately the adult Recommended Dietary Allowance (RDA) of 0.8 g/kg/day (approximately 10% of daily calories) in the patient with nephropathy. However, it has been suggested that once the GFR begins to fall, further restriction to 0.6 g/kg/day may prove useful in slowing the decline of GFR in selected patients.[54]

With all forms of therapy for ESRD, mortality is higher in diabetic patients than nondiabetic patients, largely because of cardiovascular complications.[55] Renal transplantation is the preferred replacement therapy, because long-term outcomes are considerably better for patients who undergo renal transplantation than for patients on dialysis.[56] For patients with type 1 diabetes, the possibility of combined kidney-pancreas transplantation allows for considerably better outcomes.[57] However, the immunosuppressive regimens themselves may impair insulin secretion and action, causing either so-called transplantation diabetes or worsening of glycemic control in patients not receiving a kidney transplant.[58]

Neuropathy

Diabetic neuropathy may be, in part, another microvascular complication, but the pathogenesis is still not completely understood.[59,60] Abnormal neural regulation of arteriolar blood flow can lead to decreased blood flow in the vasa nervorum, causing further neural damage. Demyelinization of nerves is manifested by decreases in motor and sensory nerve conduction velocities. Axonal degeneration is reflected in decreased amplitudes of action potentials. Histologically, swelling is seen at the axonal nodes. An inflammatory component to diabetic neuropathy has also been suggested.[59]

The most common type of diabetic neuropathy is peripheral, symmetrical, sensorimotor neuropathy, which affects up to 50% of patients.[61] Early symptoms of numbness or tingling in the toes and feet are only mildly disturbing and require no specific treatment. These symptoms may even abate over time as neuropathy becomes more severe and hypoesthesia or anesthesia takes the place of paresthesias and dysesthesias. Ultimately, insensate feet become very vulnerable to trauma; neuropathic foot ulcers are frequent causes of hospitalization and even amputation.[62] Regular screening for neuropathy with examination of the feet is therefore recommended for diabetic patients [*see Tables 1 and 3*].[25] The best tests for the detection of early neuropathy include testing for vibration sensation using a 128 mHz tuning fork and testing of Achilles tendon reflexes.[61] Testing sensation with a 10 g nylon (Semmes-Weinstein) monofilament is an effective way to identify patients at high risk for foot ulcers.[61] Patients who cannot detect the pressure of the nylon filament have a 30- to 40-fold increased risk of foot ulcer.[59]

In some instances, neuropathy is manifested by severe pain that can interfere with sleep and normal daily activities.[61] The distribution of pain can suggest mononeuropathy and radiculopathy.

Abrupt onset of cranial neuropathies that most commonly give rise to extraocular muscle weakness and diplopia has been attributed to microinfarcts caused by thrombosis of nutrient blood vessels.[60] Carpal tunnel syndrome and other entrapment syndromes are more frequent in diabetic patients than in nondiabetic patients.[60]

Involvement of the autonomic nervous system is also common and can become debilitating. Manifestations include male impotence; female anorgasmia; difficulty voiding and urinary retention; impaired gastric emptying with early satiety and emesis; diarrhea or constipation; orthostatic hypotension; and decreased sweating and vasomotor tone in the lower extremities.[60] The combination of decreased sympathetic tone and loss of vagal control of the heart rate can produce persistent resting sinus tachycardia; sudden death is associated with the presence of cardiac autonomic neuropathy.[63]

A form of diabetic neuropathy called amyotrophy occurs mostly in elderly men with diabetes. It first manifests as severe, unremitting pain and weakness in the thigh muscles. Severe depression, cachexia, and weight loss may mark the 1- to 2-year course of this form of neuropathy. Rarely, muscle infarcts occur; such infarcts are usually in the thigh muscles, are marked by the abrupt onset of severe pain that lasts several months, and are

Table 3 Foot Care Recommendations
for Patients with Diabetes[25]

Provide patient education on self-care, including daily self-examination of the feet.

Assess feet at each patient visit.

Perform a comprehensive foot examination and provide foot self-care education annually for patients with diabetes to identify risk factors predictive of ulcers and amputation.

The foot examination should include the use of 10 g monofilament for sensation, a 128 mHz tuning fork for vibration sensation, palpation, and a visual examination.

A multidisciplinary approach is recommended for patients with foot ulcers and high-risk feet, especially those with a history of ulcer or amputation.

Refer patients who smoke or who previously had lower-extremity complications to foot care specialists for ongoing preventive care and lifelong monitoring.

Initial screening for peripheral arterial disease should include a history for claudication and an assessment of the pedal pulses. Consider obtaining an ankle-brachial index (ABI), because many diabetic patients with peripheral arterial disease are asymptomatic.

Refer patients with significant claudication or an abnormal ABI for further vascular assessment; consider exercise, medications, and surgical options.

sometimes confused with painful neuropathy. Magnetic resonance imaging of the affected area can demonstrate the presence of necrosis.

The only intervention capable of altering the development and course of neuropathy is better glycemic control.[5] Otherwise, the management of diabetic neuropathy is still largely symptomatic and often inadequate. Duloxetine, a serotonin-norepinephrine reuptake inhibitor antidepressant, and pregabalin, an analogue of the neurotransmitter γ-aminobutyric acid, have been shown to be effective in decreasing pain in double-blind, prospective, randomized studies[64] and are approved by the Food and Drug Administration for this use. Other studies have shown variable benefit for venlafaxine, another serotonin-norepinephrine reuptake inhibitor, as well as for gabapentin, lamotrigine, and topiramate. Several older studies showed that tricyclic antidepressants and topical capsaicin are useful for the relief of pain and dysesthesias.[64] A Consensus Advisory Board recommended that duloxetine, pregabalin, and tricyclic antidepressants be considered first-tier therapy, on the basis of evidence from two or more randomized, controlled studies of these agents.[64] Second-tier therapy includes carbamazepine, gabapentin, lamotrigine, tramadol, and venlafaxine[64] [*see Chapter 183*]. Intensive blood glucose control may benefit patients with diabetic amyotrophy and radiculopathy.[60]

Prevention of foot ulcers remains very important; patient self-examination of the feet daily and physician-nurse examination at each office visit unequivocally reduce the risk of foot ulcer and amputation.[65] When a foot ulcer does occur, it should be treated aggressively with broad-spectrum antibiotics effective against staphylococci and anaerobes, vigorous debridement as necessary, and radiographic examination for osteomyelitis; special weight-offloading casts can also be used.[65] The use of locally applied growth factors appears promising for reducing healing time.[66] Peripheral vascular disease usually accompanies neuropathy and contributes to the susceptibility to and poor healing of ulcers. The aggravating effects of ischemia may be alleviated by revascularization of the leg when it is still possible to abort

gangrene.[65] Appropriate specialists should be consulted early for achievement of the best outcomes.

Management of autonomic neuropathy is especially challenging. Patients with gastroparesis can benefit from frequent small feedings and either parenteral or liquid oral preparations of metoclopramide.[60] Cisapride and domperidone can be of considerable benefit in improving stomach emptying, but these drugs have been associated with cardiac arrhythmias and are not available in the United States. Gastric pacing using an inserted pacemaker and injection of botulinum toxin into the pyloric muscle are experimental approaches that have met with some success in difficult cases. A feeding jejunostomy can be considered for intractable cases. Diarrhea sometimes responds to tetracycline antibiotics; clonidine and occasionally somatostatin are effective.[60] Bladder dysfunction may be improved through the use of oral bethanechol, the Credé maneuver to compress the bladder, and regular timed voiding, but self-catheterization is necessary in severe cases of atony.[60] Use of indwelling catheters should be minimized because of the danger of bacterial or fungal infection. For patients with orthostatic hypotension, compression stockings, ample sodium intake, and fludrocortisone are beneficial. The use of midodrine is limited by the risks of excessive hypotension or urinary retention.[60] Phosphodiesterase V inhibitors (e.g., sildenafil) are effective for diabetic impotence[67] but may be dangerous in diabetic men with established or unsuspected coronary disease. Other less satisfactory approaches include penile injection or urethral insertion of alprostadil, vacuum pumps or, increasingly rarely, by implantation of a penile prosthesis.[60]

Cardiovascular Complications of Diabetes Mellitus

Diabetes is an independent risk factor for CVD, especially in women; the risk of CVD in women with diabetes is as high as that in men overall.[68,69] The risk of a first myocardial infarction (MI) in patients with diabetes is equal to that of a second MI in nondiabetic persons.[70] Furthermore, acute and subsequent mortality is greater with diabetic-related MIs than with nondiabetic MIs.[71] Cardiovascular complications are the most prominent cause of morbidity and the most frequent cause of mortality in patients with type 2 diabetes mellitus.[72-74] The decline in heart disease mortality noted in recent years in the United States was less in diabetic persons than in nondiabetic persons, and mortality even increased in women with diabetes.[75] The same common CVD risk factors important in nondiabetic individuals are frequently seen in individuals with type 2 diabetes mellitus as part of the metabolic syndrome[74] [*see Chapter 58*]. The pathologic picture of atherosclerosis in diabetic persons is similar to that in nondiabetic persons, and the same processes lead to ischemic events, but diabetes appears to accelerate the course of CVD.[71] Data from several populations[76-79] and the UKPDS[9] have shown that HbA$_{1c}$ elevation is a risk factor for cardiovascular events and death.

Intensive treatment of type 1 or type 2 diabetes mellitus that results in near-normal glycemia reduces the incidence of cardiovascular complications. In the UKPDS, intensive treatment with insulin or a sulfonylurea decreased MI by 16% ($P = 0.052$).[6] Long-term follow-up of the DCCT patients in the EDIC study showed that prior intensive therapy ultimately resulted in a 42% reduction in first macrovascular events and a 57% reduction in non-fatal MI, stroke, and cardiovascular death [*see Figure 4*].[80] However, because we still cannot always eliminate whatever risk is incurred from hyperglycemia or insulin resistance per se, we must work assiduously to minimize or negate the adverse effects of

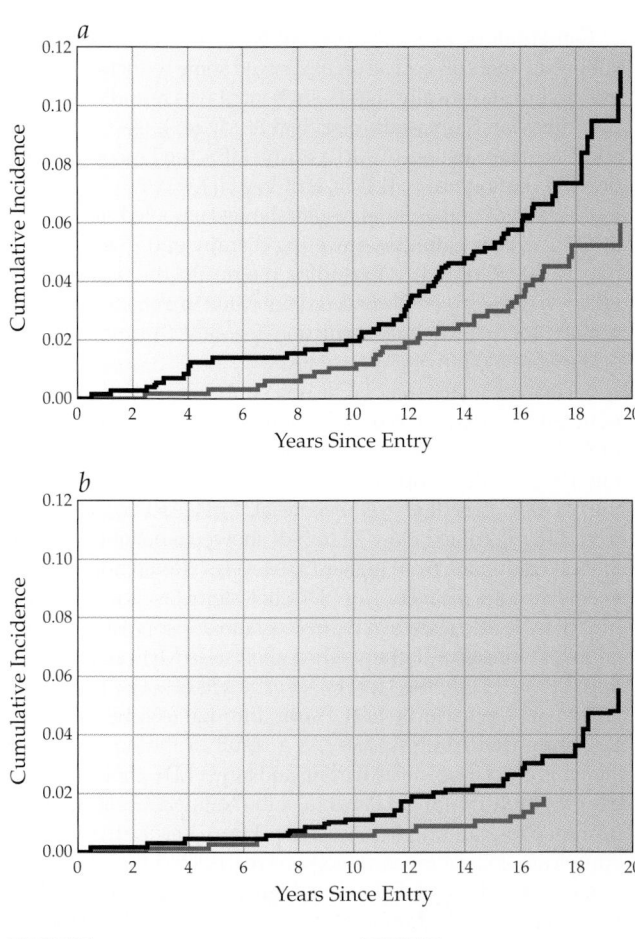

Figure 4 (*a*) Cumulative incidence of the first cardiovascular event that included clinical findings or the need for revascularization and (*b*) cumulative incidence of the first occurrence of nonfatal myocardial infarction, stroke, or death from cardiovascular disease in patients with type 1 diabetes enrolled in the Diabetes Control and Complications Trial/Epidemiology of Diabetes Interventions and Complications.[80]

hypertension, dyslipidemia, smoking, obesity, and physical inactivity on the cardiovascular system.

HYPERTENSION

Early observational studies suggested that BP control could reduce mortality in patients with type 1 diabetes.[81-83] Epidemiologic data demonstrated that for each incremental increase in BP of 20/10 mm Hg above 115/75 mm Hg, the risk of CVD doubles,[81] whereas for every 10 mm Hg reduction in systolic BP, there is a 12% risk reduction in the incidence of any diabetes-related complication.[84] Several large, randomized, prospective trials have confirmed the significant benefits of controlling BP in diabetic patients; again, patients with diabetes have been found to derive even greater benefit than those without diabetes in terms of a reduction in cardiovascular endpoints.[81-83] In the UKPDS, of 1,148 subjects with type 2 diabetes who had hypertension, those randomized to achieve tight BP control (goal < 150/85 mm Hg) experienced reductions in the risks of diabetes-related deaths (32%), all diabetes complications (24%), stroke (44%), heart failure (56%), and retinopathy (34%), as compared with patients whose BP was controlled only to a goal of less than

180/105 mm Hg.[85] The final BPs achieved in these two groups were 144/82 mm Hg and 154/87 mm Hg, respectively—a difference of 10/5 mm Hg.[85]

The Hypertension Optimal Treatment (HOT) study included over 18,000 patients; the 1,501 patients with diabetes whose target diastolic BP was 80 mm Hg or lower had 50% less risk of cardiovascular events than those targeted to 90 mm Hg or lower.[86] The Appropriate Blood Pressure Control in Diabetes (ABCD) trial randomized 470 patients with diabetes and hypertension to receive either intensive BP control (target diastolic BP, 75 mm Hg) or moderate BP control (target diastolic BP, 80 to 90 mm Hg); it demonstrated a difference in total mortality for the two groups of patients (5.5% versus 10.7%, respectively).[87] In another arm of the ABCD study, 480 subjects with diabetes were classified as normotensive; in these patients, intensive BP control (i.e., a lowering of BP to 10 mm Hg below the baseline diastolic BP) decreased the progression of diabetic retinopathy and nephropathy, as well as the incidence of stroke.[88]

As a result of these and other trials, the American Diabetes Association, the American Heart Association, and the American College of Cardiology have recommended a target BP of 130/80 mm Hg or lower in patients with diabetes.[25,89] A secondary analysis of data from the large (22,576 patients) International Verapamil-Trandolapril Study (INVEST) supports this goal; in addition, INVEST showed that the statistical relationship between diastolic BP and all-cause mortality/total MI was J-shaped, with the risk of adverse events decreasing as diastolic BP fell from hypertensive levels, but then increasing as diastolic BP fell below 70 mm Hg.[90]

In addition to its effects on nephropathy, ACE inhibitor therapy has been shown to have beneficial effects on CVD in patients with diabetes (primarily type 2). The MICRO-HOPE study of 3,577 diabetic patients (97% of them type 2) showed an impressive 25% reduction in primary outcome (composite of MI, stroke, and cardiovascular death) with ramipril.[47] The Captopril Prevention Project (CAPPP; captopril versus diuretics or beta blockers or both),[91] the ABCD trial (enalapril versus nisoldipine),[92] the Fosinopril versus Amlopidine Cardiovascular Events Trial (FACET),[93] the Swedish Trial of Old Patients with Hypertension–2 (STOP-2),[94] and the Second Australian National Blood Pressure Study Group trial (ANBP2; ACE inhibitor versus diuretic)[95] all provided evidence for the superiority of ACE inhibitors in reducing the incidence of various cardiovascular endpoints. However, the UKPDS showed similar reductions in macrovascular endpoints whether treatment was with captopril or atenolol.[96] Moreover, the Antihypertensive and Lipid Lowering Treatment to Prevent Heart Attack Trial (ALLHAT), which is the largest such study to date, showed no advantage of lisinopril over the thiazide diuretic chlorthalidone or the calcium channel blocker amlodipine with regard to various cardiovascular endpoints in either the total study population or the diabetic subgroup.[97] The ARB losartan also decreased CVD events more than did the beta blocker atenolol in the Losartan Intervention for Endpoint Reduction in Hypertension Study (LIFE).[98] However, a meta-analysis by the Blood Pressure Lowering Treatment Trialists' Collaboration (BPLTTC) failed to show any consistent cardiovascular benefit of one class of drugs compared with another when given as single agents for the treatment of hypertension in diabetic and nondiabetic patients.[99]

The primary objective, therefore, is to achieve the BP goal of less than 130/80 mm Hg, which generally requires adding successive medications. ACE inhibitors and ARBs are typically used as first-line treatment because of the cardiovascular benefit shown in some studies, as well as their renal benefits (see above). Because of the volume component of the hypertension, a diuretic is generally added as a second agent. At present, calcium channel blockers are probably best used as third agents if ACE inhibitors, diuretics, and possibly beta blockers fail to achieve the target BP, although ARBs and ACE inhibitors can also be used together. Central alpha$_2$ agonists (e.g., clonidine), alpha$_1$ antagonists (e.g., prazosin, terazosin, and doxazosin), and combined alpha and beta antagonists (e.g., labetalol) also can be used, although orthostatic hypotension may limit their utility, particularly in patients with autonomic neuropathy.[83] It is important to realize that for many patients with diabetes and hypertension, three or more drugs may well be necessary to achieve BP targets.[83]

Special caution is needed for older patients, in whom lowering elevated systolic blood pressures may be very difficult. Often, four or more drugs are needed, and the risk of orthostatic hypotension, which may result in falls, increases substantially. Clinical judgment must always be employed in caring for such potentially fragile patients.

DYSPLIPIDEMIA

Type 1 diabetes is usually associated with normal levels of low-density lipoprotein (LDL) and high-density lipoprotein (HDL) cholesterol and high triglyceride levels, the last primarily because of poor glycemic control.[100] Poor control with inadequate provision of insulin leads to a reduction in the activity of lipoprotein lipase and, consequently, an inability to clear chylomicrons and very low density lipoprotein (VLDL).[100] When control is very poor, HDL cholesterol levels may also be decreased and LDL cholesterol levels elevated.[100] Type 2 diabetes is generally associated with reduced HDL cholesterol levels, elevated triglyceride levels, and normal LDL cholesterol levels, albeit there is a shift in the LDL particle size to that of the more atherogenic small, dense LDL particles.[101]

Several large, prospective, randomized studies have demonstrated marked cardiovascular benefits with the treatment of dyslipidemia in patients with and without diabetes. Generally, the first priority is to decrease LDL cholesterol levels, with lowering of triglyceride levels and raising of HDL cholesterol levels being of secondary priority. Most of the studies examining these treatment effects on patients with diabetes utilized subset analyses of this group that were part of the original study design, and all but two studies used statins as the intervention; the Helsinki Heart Study (HHS)[102] and the Veterans Administration High-Density Lipoprotein Cholesterol Intervention Trial (VA-HIT)[103] used gemfibrozil.

Of primary prevention trials in which diabetes subgroup analyses were performed, five of six showed benefit with regard to CVD, but statistically significant benefit was found only in the very large Heart Protection Study (HPS) and the Anglo-Scandinavian Cardiac Outcomes Trial–Lipid-Lowering Arm (ASCOT-LLA).[102,104-109] In a formal meta-analysis of these trial results, the pooled relative risk of CVD events in diabetic patients with lipid-lowering therapy was 0.78 (confidence interval, 0.67 to 0.89).[110] The Collaborative Atorvastatin Diabetes Study (CARDS) was a more recent primary prevention placebo-controlled study that was limited to patients with type 2 diabetes.[111] CARDS showed that in 2,838 patients, those randomized to receive atorvastatin (10 mg daily) had a relative risk reduction of 37% for cardiovascular events, a reduction in stroke of 48%, and a 27% reduction in total mortality.[111]

Eight trials of secondary prevention have included a diabetes subgroup analysis, and all eight showed some reduction of CVD events, but statistically significant benefit was found only in the Scandinavian Simvastatin Survival Study (4S), the Cholesterol and Recurrent Events (CARE) study, HPS, the Lescol Intervention Prevention Study (LIPS), and VA-HIT.[102,106-108,112-116] A formal meta-analysis of these trial results showed a pooled relative risk of CVD events with lipid-lowering therapy of 0.76 (confidence interval, 0.59 to 0.93).[110] Excluding the results of HHS and VA-HIT, which used gemfibrozil, did not result in a change in the estimates for relative risk reduction for either primary or secondary prevention of CVD events.[110]

Secondary analyses of HPS showed that in both diabetic and nondiabetic patients, risk reductions for CVD occurred when LDL cholesterol levels were lowered from 116 mg/dl to below 77 mg/dl[103]; for the entire study cohort, even reductions from 97 mg/dl to 65 mg/dl proved beneficial.[104] In CARDS, a reduction from 118 mg/dl to below 70 mg/dl showed a benefit similar to that of a reduction from higher LDL levels.[111] Reductions in CVD events through a lowering of LDL cholesterol levels to around 70 mg/dl were also shown in the Pravastatin or Atorvastatin Evaluation and Infection Therapy–Thrombolysis in Myocardial Infarction (PROVE-IT),[117] the Treat to New Targets (TNT),[118] and the Incremental Decrease in End Points through Aggressive Lipid Lowering (IDEAL)[119] studies. As a result of these newer trials showing efficacy at lower starting and target LDL cholesterol levels, the Adult Treatment Panel III of the National Cholesterol Education Program and the American Heart Association and the American College of Cardiology have updated their treatment guidelines, indicating that in very high risk patients, such as those with diabetes and additional proven vascular disease or those at risk for vascular disease, an LDL cholesterol goal of less than 70 mg/dl is reasonable, even in patients whose starting levels are below 100 mg/dl.[89,120]

Severe hypertriglyceridemia may complicate diabetic ketoacidosis in type 1 diabetes mellitus, but it clears rapidly with insulin treatment. Restriction of saturated fat and calories, elimination of excess weight, exercise, and improved glycemic control reduce triglyceride levels and increase HDL levels.[100] When these measures are insufficient, gemfibrozil or fenofibrate should be prescribed with the intent of decreasing triglyceride levels to less than 150 mg/dl and increasing HDL levels to greater than 35 mg/dl in men and greater than 45 mg/dl in women. When prescribing statins and fibrates, physicians should take care to measure the creatine phosphokinase level if the patient experiences excessive muscle discomfort, because this symptom signals the risk of rhabdomyolysis and subsequent renal failure.[120] Niacin, in the form of a delayed-release preparation (Niaspan), may also be useful in raising HDL levels, as well as lowering LDL levels.[120]

SMOKING

Referral to successful smoking-cessation programs and use of oral or dermal nicotine preparations during withdrawal from tobacco should be employed as needed to rid patients of this serious risk factor for CVD. Success appears to be directly related to the amount of counseling and support provided by physicians or other professionals.[121] Newer pharmacologic agents, such as rimonabant and varenicline, are on the horizon and may also prove useful.

ASPIRIN

In the Early Treatment of Diabetic Retinopathy Study (ET-

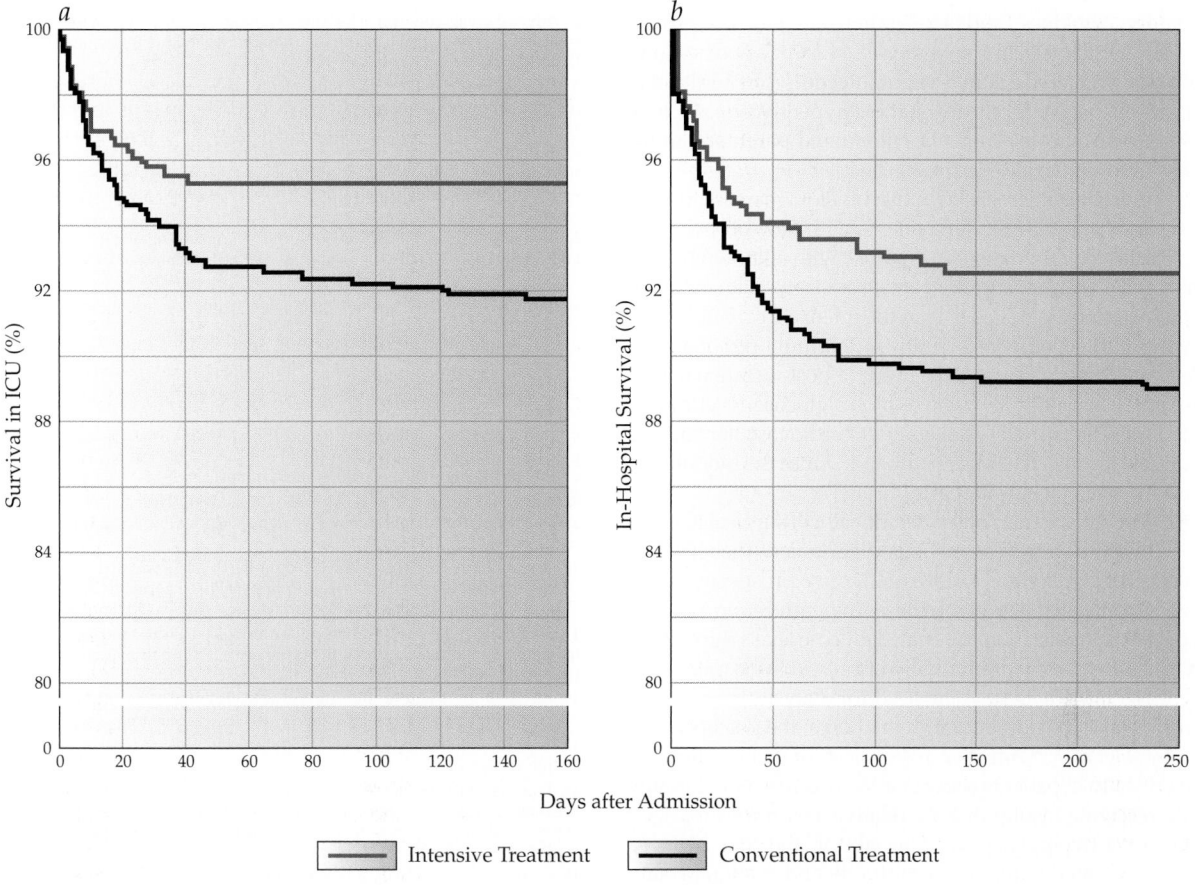

Figure 5   **Kaplan-Meier curves from a study of patients who received intensive insulin treatment or conventional treatment in the intensive care unit show improved cumulative survival to (*a*) discharge from the ICU, and (*b*) discharge from the hospital.**[134]

DRS), administration of 650 mg of aspirin a day resulted in a statistically significant 17% reduction in the combined risk of fatal or nonfatal MIs.[122] All-cause mortality and CVD mortality tended to decrease, whereas strokes tended to increase, but none of these differences were statistically significant. Preventive use of aspirin is now recommended by the American Diabetes Association for patients who already have CVD or who have other risk factors for CVD in addition to diabetes.[123]

MANAGEMENT OF CORONARY ARTERY DISEASE

Stress testing has been recommended for diabetic patients who meet any one of the following criteria: (1) typical or atypical cardiac symptoms; (2) a resting electrocardiogram suggestive of ischemia or infarction; (3) peripheral or carotid occlusive vascular disease; (4) sedentary lifestyle, age 35 years or older, and plans to begin a vigorous exercise program; or (5) more than two of the following risk factors: total cholesterol 240 mg/dl or higher, LDL cholesterol 160 mg/dl or higher, or HDL cholesterol below 35 mg/dl; hypertension; smoking; family history of premature coronary artery disease; or albuminuria (microscopic or macroscopic).[124] A review of stress testing in 116 patients who met these criteria (primarily criteria 3 and 5) found that 39 (33.6%) had abnormal results; of the 32 of these 39 who underwent cardiac catheterization, 23 demonstrated significant coronary artery disease.[125] Thus, these criteria seem reasonable ones to determine appropriate candidates for screening for coronary artery disease with stress testing.

Beta blockers, nitrates, and calcium channel blockers can all be used as in nondiabetic patients,[126] with the proviso that when beta blockers are prescribed for patients receiving intensive insulin therapy, the patient should be cautioned that these agents may mask the symptoms of hypoglycemia. When a revascularization procedure has been deemed necessary, coronary artery bypass surgery has been reported to be superior to angioplasty in 5-year survival and recurrent MI rates in patients receiving pharmacologic treatment of type 2 diabetes mellitus.[127] In patients without mandatory indications for immediate surgical intervention, such as significant left main coronary artery stenosis, a clinical research trial (Bypass Angioplasty Revascularization Investigation 2 Diabetes [BARI 2D]) is currently attempting to determine whether a prompt revascularization procedure with aggressive medical therapy is superior to aggressive medical therapy alone.[128]

Intensive Insulin Therapy in the Hospital

Hyperglycemia is common in the hospitalized patient, with a prevalence of approximately 25%, and is an independent risk factor for poor clinical outcome in multiple patient populations.[129,130] Critical illness causes an impairment of insulin secretion and insulin action, resulting in hyperglycemia even in normal individuals and a worsening of the hyperglycemia in patients with diabetes.[131] In severe illness and other states of physical stress, hyperglycemia results from a myriad of factors, including increases in counterregulatory hormones, release of inflammatory cytokines, and accelerations in fat and protein breakdown with net effects of muscle wasting, poor wound healing, and impaired ability to fight infection.[131] In addition to stress, factors that contribute to inpatient hyperglycemia include the use of pharmacologic agents, enteral and parenteral nutrition, and glucocorticoid therapy.

Hyperglycemia is associated with a ninefold increase in mortality during hospitalization in patients with new-onset hyperglycemia and a twofold increase in those with a known history of diabetes.[129] In cardiac surgery patients, diabetes is an independent predictor of prolonged stay in the intensive care unit, sternal wound infection, postoperative delirium, perioperative stroke, renal dysfunction, and the need for postoperative reintubation.[132] Patients with an average blood glucose level higher than 150 mg/dl during the 3 days after cardiovascular surgery have double the infection rate and up to 13 times the mortality of their normoglycemic counterparts.[133]

In a 2001 Belgian study of septic, critically ill surgical ICU patients who did not have a previous diagnosis of diabetes, the prevalence of hyperglycemia was 50%.[134] A prospective, randomized, controlled study of these hyperglycemic patients showed that normalization of elevated glucose levels through intensive insulin therapy dramatically improved in-hospital mortality, sepsis rates, ICU stay, the need for dialysis, the need for transfusion, and the duration of ventilation in the postoperative setting [see Figure 5].[134] A meta-analysis of studies of insulin therapy in critically ill patients showed a 15% decrease in mortality in those receiving insulin therapy relative to control subjects.[135] Postoperative hyperglycemia, especially in the first 24 to 48 hours, is associated with greater mortality and is an important predictor of serious postoperative infectious complications. In retrospective analyses, 3 days of I.V. insulin treatment with maintenance of glucose levels below 150 mg/dl after coronary artery bypass grafting resulted in a marked decrease in postoperative mortality and deep sternal wound infections in diabetic patients.[133] However, in a prospective, randomized study of medical ICU patients, maintenance of glucose levels below 110 mg/dl with insulin infusions had no effect on overall mortality or infections, but it did reduce newly acquired renal insufficiency, accelerate weaning from mechanical ventilation, and reduce length of stay.[136]

At present, intensive insulin therapy for diabetes using insulin infusions in the ICU and a combination of basal and bolus subcutaneous insulin outside of the ICU is becoming the standard of care on surgical services and some medical services.[137,138] A number of protocols have been published that allow for individualization of insulin doses.[137-139] Crucial to the use of such protocols is an experienced clinician who can adjust the protocols as needed to the changing clinical scenario of the critically ill patient and who has both the responsibility and authority to do so promptly.[139]

Mark E. Molitch, M.D., F.A.C.P., has received research support from Sanofi-Aventis, Inc., Eli Lilly & Co., Novo-Nordisk, Inc., and Pfizer, Inc., and has served as a consultant to Sanofi-Aventis, Inc., Novo-Nordisk, Inc., and Abbott Laboratories.

Saul Genuth, M.D., F.A.C.P., has no commercial relationships with manufacturers of products or providers of services discussed in this chapter.

References

1. The effect of intensive treatment of diabetes on the development and progression of long-term complications in insulin-dependent diabetes mellitus. The Diabetes Control and Complications Trial Research Group. N Engl J Med 329:977, 1993

2. Adverse events and their association with treatment regimens in the Diabetes Control and Complications Trial. The Diabetes Control and Complications Trial Research Group. Diabetes Care 18:1415, 1995

3. Effect of intensive therapy on the microvascular complications of type 1 diabetes mellitus. Diabetes Control and Complications Trial/Epidemiology of Diabetes Interventions and Complications Research Group. JAMA 287:2563, 2002

4. Sustained effects of intensive treatment of type 1 diabetes mellitus on the development and progression of diabetic nephropathy. Epidemiology of Diabetes Interventions and Complications (EDIC)/Diabetes Control and Complications Trial (DCCT) Study Group. JAMA 290:2159, 2003

5. Martin CL, Albers J, Herman WH, et al: Neuropathy among the Diabetes Control and Complications Trial Cohort 8 years after trial completion. Diabetes Care 29:340, 2006

6. Intensive blood-glucose control with sulphonylureas or insulin compared with conventional treatment and risk of complications in patients with type 2 diabetes (UKPDS 33). UK Prospective Diabetes Study (UKPDS) Group. Lancet 352:837, 1998

7. Effect of intensive blood-glucose control with metformin on complications in overweight patients with type 2 diabetes (UKPDS 34). UK Prospective Diabetes Study (UKPDS) Group. Lancet 352:854, 1998

8. The relationship of glycemic exposure (HbA$_{1c}$) to the risk of development and progression of retinopathy in the Diabetes Control and Complications Trial. The Diabetes Control and Complications Trial Research Group. Diabetes 44:968, 1995

9. Stratton IM, Adler AI, Neil HA, et al: Association of glycaemia with macrovascular and microvascular complications of type 2 diabetes (UKPDS 35): prospective observational study. BMJ 321:405, 2000

10. The absence of a glycemic threshold for the development of long-term complications: the perspective of the Diabetes Control and Complications Trial. The Diabetes Control and Complications Trial Research Group. Diabetes 45:1289, 1996

11. McCarter RJ, Hempe JM, Chalew SA: Mean blood glucose and biological variation have greater influence on HbA$_{1c}$ than glucose instability: an analysis of data from the Diabetes Control and Complications Trial. Diabetes Care 29:352, 2006

12. McCarter RJ, Hempe JM, Gomez R, et al: Biological variation in HbA$_{1c}$ predicts risk of retinopathy and nephropathy in type 1 diabetes. Diabetes Care 27:1259, 2004

13. Brownlee M: Biochemistry and molecular cell biology of diabetic complications. Nature 414:813, 2001

14. Monnier VM, Bautista O, Kenny D, et al: Skin collagen glycation, glycoxidation, and crosslinking are lower in subjects with long-term intensive versus conventional therapy of type 1 diabetes: relevance of glycated collagen products versus HbA$_{1c}$ as markers of diabetic complications. Diabetes 48:870, 1999

15. Genuth S, Sun W, Cleary P, et al: Glycation and carboxymethyllysine levels in skin collagen predict the risk of future 10-year progression of diabetic retinopathy and nephropathy in the Diabetes Control and Complications Trial and epidemiology of diabetes interventions and complications participants with type 1 diabetes. Diabetes 54:3103, 2005

16. Vinik A: The protein kinase C-β inhibitor, ruboxistaurin, for the treatment of diabetic microvascular complications. Expert Opin Investig Drugs 14:1547, 2005

17. Aiello LP: The molecular biology of diabetic retinopathy: opportunities for therapeutic intervention. Adv Stud Ophthalmol 3:8, 2006

18. Hammes HP, Du X, Edelstein D, et al: Benfotiamine blocks three major pathways of hyperglycemic damage and prevents experimental diabetic retinopathy. Nat Med 9:294, 2003

19. Babaei-Jadidi R, Karachalias N, Ahmed N, et al: Prevention of incipient diabetic nephropathy by high-dose thiamine and benfotiamine. Diabetes 52:2110, 2003

20. Quinn M, Angelico MC, Warram JH, et al: Familial factors determine the development of diabetic nephropathy in patients with IDDM. Diabetologia 39:940, 1996

21. Clustering of long-term complications in families with diabetes in the Diabetes Control and Complications Trial. The Diabetes Control and Complications Trial Research Group. Diabetes 46:1829, 1997

22. Fong DS, Aiello L, Gardner TW, et al: Diabetic retinopathy. Diabetes Care 26:226, 2003

23. Williams R, Airey M, Baxter H, et al: Epidemiology of diabetic retinopathy and macular edema: a systematic review. Eye 18:963, 2004

24. Willams GA: Diabetes care: the ophthalmology connection. Adv Stud Ophthalmol 3:13, 2006

25. American Diabetes Association: Standards of medical care in diabetes—2006. Diabetes Care 29(suppl 1):S4, 2006

26. Harris MI, Klein R, Welborn TA, et al: Onset of NIDDM occurs at least 4–7 yr before clinical diagnosis. Diabetes Care 15:815, 1992

27. Effect of pregnancy on microvascular complications in the diabetes control and complications trial. The Diabetes Control and Complications Trial Research Group. Diabetes Care 23:1084, 2000

28. Ferris FL III, Davis MD, Aiello LM: Treatment of diabetic retinopathy. Drug Therapy 341:667, 1999

29. Andersen AR, Christiansen JS, Andersen JK, et al: Diabetic nephropathy in type 1 (insulin-dependent) diabetes: an epidemiological study. Diabetologia 25:496, 1983

30. Adler AI, Stevens RJ, Manley SE, et al: Development and progression of nephropathy in type 2 diabetes: the United Kingdom Prospective Diabetes Study (UKPDS 64). Kidney Int 63:225, 2003

31. Mogensen CE, Cooper ME: Diabetic renal disease: from recent studies to improved clinical practice. Diabet Med 21:4, 2004

32. Gross JL, Canani LH, de Azevedo MJ, et al: Diabetic nephropathy: diagnosis, prevention, and treatment. Diabetes Care 28:176, 2005

33. Kramer HJ, Nguyen QD, Curhan G, et al: Renal insufficiency in the absence of albuminuria and retinopathy among adults with type 2 diabetes mellitus. JAMA 289:3273, 2003

34. Levey A, Bosch J, Breyer Lewis J, et al: A more accurate method to estimate glomerular filtration rate from serum creatinine. Ann Intern Med 139:461, 1999

35. Thomas W, Shen Y, Molitch ME, et al: Rise in albuminuria and blood pressure in patients who progressed to diabetic nephropathy in the Diabetes Control and Complications Trial. J Am Soc Nephrol 12:333, 2001

36. Bakris GL, Williams M, Dworkin L, et al: Preserving renal function in adults with hypertension and diabetes: a consensus approach. Am J Kidney Dis 36:646, 2000

37. Borch-Johnsen K, Andersen PK, Deckert T: The effect of proteinuria on relative mortality in type 1 (insulin-dependent) diabetes mellitus. Diabetologia 28:590, 1985

38. Jensen T, Borch-Johnsen K, Kofoed-Enevoldsen A, et al: Coronary heart disease in young type 1 (insulin-dependent) diabetic patients with and without diabetic nephropathy: incidence and risk factors. Diabetologia 30:144, 1987

39. Dinneen SF, Gerstein HC: The association of microalbuminuria and mortality in non–insulin-dependent diabetes mellitus: a systematic overview of the literature. Arch Intern Med 157:1413, 1997

40. Valmadrid CT, Klein R, Moss SE, et al: The risk of cardiovascular disease mortality associated with microalbuminuria and gross proteinuria in persons with older-onset diabetes mellitus. Arch Intern Med 160:1093, 2000

41. Tonelli M, Keech A, Shepherd J, et al: Effect of pravastatin in people with diabetes and chronic kidney disease. J Am Soc Nephrol 16:3748, 2005

42. Tight blood pressure control and risk of macrovascular and microvascular complications in type 2 diabetes: UKPDS 38. UK Prospective Diabetes Study Group. BMJ 317:703, 1998

43. Pohl MA, Blumenthal S, Cordonnier DJ, et al: Independent and additive impact of blood pressure control and angiotensin II receptor blockade on renal outcomes in the Irbesartan Diabetic Nephropathy Trial: clinical implications and limitations. J Am Soc Nephrol 16:3027, 2005

44. Karalliedde J, Viberti G: Evidence for renoprotection by blockade of the renin-angiotensin-aldosterone system in hypertension and diabetes. J Hum Hypertens 20:239, 2006

45. Lewis EJ, Hunsicker LG, Bain RP, et al: The effect of angiotensin-converting-enzyme inhibition on diabetic nephropathy. N Engl J Med 329:145, 1993

46. Should all patients with type 1 diabetes mellitus and microalbuminuria receive angiotensin-converting enzyme inhibitors? A meta-analysis of individual patient data. ACE Inhibitors in Diabetic Nephropathy Trialist Group. Ann Intern Med 134:370, 2001

47. Effects of ramipril on cardiovascular and microvascular outcomes in people with diabetes mellitus: results of the HOPE study and MICRO-HOPE substudy. Heart Outcomes Prevention Evaluation Study Investigators. Lancet 355:253, 2000

48. Ruggenenti P, Fassi A, Ilieva AP, et al: Preventing microalbuminuria in type 2 diabetes. N Engl J Med 351:1941, 2004

49. Brenner BM, Cooper ME, de Zeeuw D, et al: Effects of losartan on renal and cardiovascular outcomes in patients with type 2 diabetes and nephropathy. N Engl J Med 345:861, 2001

50. Lewis EJ, Hunsicker LG, Clarke WR, et al: Renoprotective effect of the angiotensin-receptor antagonist irbesartan in patients with nephropathy due to type 2 diabetes. N Engl J Med 345:851, 2001

51. Parving HH, Lehnert H, Brochner-Mortensen J, et al: The effect of irbesartan on the development of diabetic nephropathy in patients with type 2 diabetes. N Engl J Med 345:870, 2001

52. Viberti G, Wheeldon NM: Microalbuminuria reduction with valsartan in patients with type 2 diabetes mellitus: a blood pressure–independent effect. MicroAlbuminuria Reduction With VALsartan (MARVAL) Study Investigators. Circulation 106:672, 2002

53. Cooper WO, Hernandez-Diaz S, Arbogast PG, et al: Major congenital malformations after first-trimester exposure to ACE inhibitors. N Engl J Med 354:2443, 2006

54. Pedrini M, Levey A, Lau J, et al: The effect of dietary protein restriction on the progression of diabetic and nondiabetic renal diseases: a meta-analysis. Ann Intern Med 124:627, 1996

55. Foley RN, Murray AM, Li S, et al: Chronic kidney disease and the risk for cardiovascular disease, renal replacement, and death in the United States Medicare population, 1998 to 1999. J Am Soc Nephrol 16:489, 2005

56. Wolfe RA, Ashby VB, Milford El, et al: Comparison of mortality in all patients on dialysis, patients on dialysis awaiting transplantation, and recipients of a first cadaveric transplant. N Engl J Med 341:1725, 1999

57. Becker BN, Brazy PC, Becker YT, et al: Simultaneous pancreas-kidney transplantation reduces excess mortality in type-1 diabetic patients with end-stage renal disease. Kidney Int 57:2129, 2000

58. Markell M: New-onset diabetes mellitus in transplant patients: pathogenesis, complications and management. Am J Kidney Dis 43:953, 2004

59. Eaton S, Tesfaye S: Clinical manifestations and measurement of somatic neuropathy. Diabetes Rev 7:312, 1999

60. Vinik AI: Diabetic neuropathy: pathogenesis and therapy. Am J Med 107(suppl 2B):17S, 1999

61. Argoff CE, Cole BE, Fishbain DA: Diabetic peripheral neuropathic pain: clinical and quality-of-life issues. Mayo Clin Proc 81(suppl 4):S3, 2006

62. Boulton AJ, Vileikyte L, Ragnarson-Tennvall G, et al: The global burden of diabetic foot disease. Lancet 366:1719, 2005

63. Maser RE, Mitchell BD, Vinik AI, et al: The association between cardiovascular autonomic neuropathy and mortality in individuals with diabetes: a meta-analysis. Diabetes Care 26:1895, 2003

64. Argoff CE, Backonja MM, Belgrade MJ, et al: Consensus Guidelines: treatment planning and options. Mayo Clin Proc 81(suppl 4):S12, 2006

65. Cavanagh PR, Lipsky BA, Bradbury AW, et al: Treatment for diabetic foot ulcers. Lancet 366:1725, 2005

66. Falanga V: Wound healing and its impairment in the diabetic foot. Lancet 366:1736, 2005

67. Stuckey BG, Jadzinsky MN, Murphy LJ, et al: Sildenafil citrate for treatment of erectile dysfunction in men with type 1 diabetes: results of a randomized controlled trial. Diabetes Care 26:279, 2003

68. Stamler J, Vaccaro O, Neaton JD, et al: Diabetes, other risk factors, and 12-yr cardiovascular mortality for men screened in the Multiple Risk Factor Intervention Trial. Diabetes Care 16:434, 1993

69. Barrett-Connor EL, Cohn BA, Wingard DL, et al: Why is diabetes mellitus a stronger risk factor for fatal ischemic heart disease in women than in men? The Rancho Bernardo Study. JAMA 265:627, 1991

70. Haffner SM, Lehto S, Rönnemaa T, et al: Mortality from coronary heart disease in subjects with type 2 diabetes and in nondiabetic subjects with and without prior myocardial infarction. N Engl J Med 339:229, 1998

71. Nesto RW: Correlation between cardiovascular disease and diabetes mellitus: current concepts. Am J Med 116:11S, 2004

72. Grundy SM, Benjamin IJ, Burke GL, et al: Diabetes and cardiovascular disease: a statement for healthcare professionals from the American Heart Association. Circulation 100:1134, 1999

73. Gu K, Cowie CC, Harris MI: Mortality in adults with and without diabetes in a national cohort of the U.S. population, 1971–1993. Diabetes Care 21:1138, 1998

74. Bonow RO, Gheorghiade M: The diabetes epidemic: a national and global crisis. Am J Med 116:2S, 2004

75. Gu K, Cowie CC, Harris MI: Diabetes and decline in heart disease mortality in US adults. JAMA 281:1291, 1999

76. Moss SE, Klein R, Klein BE, et al: The association of glycemia and cause-specific mortality in a diabetic population. Arch Intern Med 154:2473, 1994

77. Kuusisto J, Mykkänen L, Pyörälä K, et al: NIDDM and its metabolic control predict coronary heart disease in elderly subjects. Diabetes 43:960, 1994

78. Andersson DK, Svärdsudd K: Long-term glycemic control relates to mortality in type II diabetes. Diabetes Care 18:1534, 1995

79. Wei M, Gaskill SP, Haffner SM, et al: Effects of diabetes and level of glycemia on all-cause and cardiovascular mortality: the San Antonio Heart Study. Diabetes Care 21:1167, 1998

80. Nathan DM, Cleary PA, Backlund JY, et al: Intensive diabetes treatment and cardiovascular disease in patients with type 1 diabetes. Diabetes Control and Complications Trial/Epidemiology of Diabetes Interventions and Complications (DCCT/EDIC) Study Research Group. N Engl J Med 353:2643, 2005

81. Chobanian AV, Bakris GL, Black HR, et al: The Seventh Report of the Joint National Committee on Prevention, Detection, Evaluation, and Treatment of High Blood Pressure: the JNC 7 report. JAMA 289:2560, 2003

82. Snow V, Weiss KB, Mottur-Pilson C: The evidence base for tight blood pressure control in the management of type 2 diabetes mellitus. Ann Intern Med 138:587, 2003

83. Bakris GL: The importance of blood pressure control in the patient with diabetes. Am J Med 116:30S, 2004

84. Adler AI, Stratton IM, Neil HA, et al: Association of systolic blood pressure with macrovascular and microvascular complications of type 2 diabetes (UKPDS 36): prospective observational study. BMJ 321:412, 2000

85. Tight blood pressure control and risk of macrovascular and microvascular complications in type 2 diabetes: UKPDS 38. UK Prospective Diabetes Study Group. BMJ 317:703, 1998

86. Hansson L, Zanchetti A, Carruthers SG, et al: Effects of intensive blood-pressure lowering and low-dose aspirin in patients with hypertension: principal results of the Hypertension Optimal Treatment (HOT) randomised trial. Lancet 351:1755, 1998

87. Estacio RO, Jeffers BW, Gifford N, et al: Effect of blood pressure control on diabetic microvascular complications in patients with hypertension and type 2 diabetes. Diabetes Care 23:B54, 2000

88. Schrier RW, Estacio RO, Esler A, et al: Effects of aggressive blood pressure control in normotensive type 2 diabetic patients on albuminuria, retinopathy and strokes. Kidney Int 61:1086, 2002

89. Smith SC Jr, Allen R, Blair SN, et al: AHA/ACC guidelines for secondary prevention for patients with coronary and other atherosclerotic vascular disease: 2006 update. J Am Coll Cardiol 47:2130, 2006

90. Messerli FH, Mancia G, Conti CR, et al: Dogma disputed: can aggressively lowering blood pressure in hypertensive patients with coronary artery disease be dangerous? Ann Intern Med 144:884, 2006

91. Niskanen L, Hedner T, Hansson L, et al: Reduced cardiovascular morbidity and mortality in hypertensive diabetic patients on first-line therapy with an ACE inhibitor compared with a diuretic/beta-blocker–based treatment regimen: a subanalysis of the Captopril Prevention Project. Diabetes Care 24:2091, 2001

92. Estacio RO, Jeffers BW, Hiatt WR, et al: The effect of nisoldipine as compared with enalapril on cardiovascular outcomes in patients with non–insulin-dependent diabetes and hypertension. N Engl J Med 338:645, 1998

93. Tatti P, Pahor M, Byington RP, et al: Outcome results of the Fosinopril versus Amlodipine Cardiovascular Events Randomized Trial (FACET) in patients with hypertension and NIDDM. Diabetes Care 21:597, 1998

94. Hansson L, Lindholm LH, Ekbom T, et al: Randomised trial of old and new antihypertensive drugs in elderly patients: cardiovascular mortality and morbidity: the

Swedish Trial in Old Patients with Hypertension–2 study. Lancet 354:1751, 1999

95. Wing LM, Reid CM, Ryan P, et al: A comparison of outcomes with angiotensin-converting–enzyme inhibitors and diuretics for hypertension in the elderly. N Engl J Med 348:583, 2003

96. Efficacy of atenolol and captopril in reducing risk of macrovascular and microvascular complications in type 2 diabetes: UKPDS 39. UK Prospective Diabetes Study Group. BMJ 317:713, 1998

97. Major outcomes in high-risk hypertensive patients randomized to angiotensin-converting enzyme inhibitor or calcium channel blocker vs diuretic: the Antihypertensive and Lipid-Lowering Treatment to Prevent Heart Attack Trial (ALLHAT). ALLHAT Collaborative Research Group. JAMA 288:2981, 2002

98. Lindholm L, Ibsen H, Dahlof B, et al: Cardiovascular morbidity and mortality in patients with diabetes in the Losartan Intervention For Endpoint reduction in hypertension study (LIFE): a randomized trial against atenolol. LIFE Study Group. Lancet 359:1004, 2002

99. Turnbull F, Neal B, Algert C, et al: Effects of different blood pressure-lowering regimens on major cardiovascular events in individuals with and without diabetes mellitus. Blood Pressure Lowering Treatment Trialists' Collaboration. Arch Intern Med 165:1410, 2005

100. O'Brien T, Nguyen TT, Zimmerman BR: Hyperlipidemia and diabetes mellitus. Mayo Clin Proc 73:969, 1998

101. Ginsburg HN: Efficacy and mechanism of action of statins in the treatment of diabetic dyslipidemia. J Clin Endocrinol Metab 91:383, 2006

102. Koskinen P, Manttari M, Manninen V, et al: Coronary heart disease incidence in NIDDM patients in the Helsinki Heart Study. Diabetes Care 15:820, 1992

103. Rubins HB, Robins SJ, Collins D, et al: Diabetes, plasma insulin, and cardiovascular disease: subgroup analysis from the Department of Veterans Affairs high-density lipoprotein intervention trial (VA-HIT). Arch Intern Med 162:2597, 2002

104. Downs JR, Clearfield M, Weis S, et al: Primary prevention of acute coronary events with lovastatin in men and women with average cholesterol levels: results of AFCAPS/TexCAPS. Air Force/Texas Coronary Atherosclerosis Prevention Study. JAMA 279:1615, 1998

105. Major outcomes in moderately hypercholesterolemic, hypertensive patients randomized to pravastatin vs. usual care: the Antihypertensive and Lipid-Lowering Treatment to Prevent Heart Attack Trial (ALLHAT-LLT). ALLHAT Collaborative Research Group. JAMA 288:2998, 2002

106. MRC/BHF Heart Protection Study of cholesterol-lowering with simvastatin in 20,536 high-risk individuals: a randomised placebo-controlled trial. Heart Protection Study Collaborative Group. Lancet 360:7, 2002

107. MRC/BHF Heart Protection Study of cholesterol-lowering with simvastatin in 5963 people with diabetes: a randomised placebo-controlled trial. Heart Protection Study Collaborative Group. Lancet 361:2005, 2003

108. Shepherd J, Blauw GJ, Murphy MB, et al: Pravastatin in elderly individuals at risk of vascular disease (PROSPER): a randomised controlled trial. PROSPER Study Group. Lancet 360:1623, 2002

109. Sever PS, Poulter NR, Dahlöf B, et al: Reduction in cardiovascular events with atorvastatin in 2,532 patients with type 2 diabetes: Anglo-Scandinavian Cardiac Outcomes Trial – Lipid-Lowering Arm (ASCOT-LLA). ASCOT Investigators. Diabetes Care 28:1151, 2005

110. Vijan S, Hayward RA: Pharmacologic lipid-lowering therapy in type 2 diabetes mellitus: background paper for the American College of Physicians. Ann Intern Med 140:650, 2004

111. Colhoun HM, Betteridge DJ, Durrington PN, et al: Primary prevention of cardiovascular disease with atorvastatin in type 2 diabetes in the Collaborative Atorvastatin Diabetes Study (CARDS): multicenter randomized placebo-controlled trial. CARDS Investigators. Lancet 364:685, 2004

112. Pyorala K, Pedersen TR, Kjekshus J, et al: Cholesterol lowering with simvastatin improves prognosis of diabetic patients with coronary heart disease: a subgroup analysis of the Scandinavian Simvastatin Survival Study (4S). Diabetes Care 20:614, 1997

113. Goldberg RB, Mellies MJ, Sacks FM, et al: Cardiovascular events and their reduction with pravastatin in diabetic and glucose intolerant myocardial infarction survivors with average cholesterol levels: subgroup analysis in the Cholesterol and Recurrent Events (CARE) trial. Care Investigators. Circulation 98:2513, 1998

114. Keech A, Colquhoun D, Best J, et al: Secondary prevention of cardiovascular events with long-term pravastatin in patients with diabetes or impaired fasting glucose. LIPID Study Group. Diabetes Care 26:2713, 2003

115. Serruys PW, de Feyter P, Macaya C, et al: Fluvastatin for prevention of cardiac events flowing successful first percutaneous coronary intervention: a randomized controlled trial. Lescol Intervention Prevention Study (LIPS) Investigators. JAMA 287:3215, 2002

116. Hoogwerf BJ, Waness A, Cressman M, et al: Effects of aggressive cholesterol lowering and low-dose anticoagulation on clinical and angiographic outcomes in patients with diabetes: the Post Coronary Artery Bypass Graft Trial. Diabetes 48:1289, 1999

117. Cannon CP, Braunwald E, McCabe CH, et al: Intensive versus moderate lipid lowering with statins after acute coronary syndromes. Pravastatin or Atorvastatin Evaluation and Infection Therapy—Thrombosis in Myocardial Infarction 22 Investigators. N Engl J Med 350:1495, 2004

118. LaRosa JC, Grundy SM, Waters DD, et al: Intensive lipid lowering with atorvastatin in patients with stable coronary disease. Treating to New Targets (TNT) Investigators. N Engl J Med 352:1425, 2005

119. Pedersen TR, Faergeman O, Kastelein JJ, et al: High-dose atorvastatin vs. usual-dose simvastatin for secondary prevention after myocardial infarction: the IDEAL study: a randomized controlled trial. Incremental Decrease in End Points Through Aggressive Lipid Lowering (IDEAL) Study Group. JAMA 294:2437, 2005

120. Grundy SM, Cleeman JI, Merz CN, et al: Implications of recent clinical trials for the National Cholesterol Education Program Adult Treatment Panel III Guidelines. Coordinating Committee of the National Cholesterol Education Program. J Am Coll Cardiol 44:720, 2004

121. Haire-Joshu D, Glasgow RE, Tibbs TL: Smoking and diabetes. Diabetes Care 22:1887, 1999

122. Aspirin effects on mortality and morbidity in patients with diabetes mellitus: Early Treatment Diabetic Retinopathy Study report 14. ETDRS Investigators. JAMA 268:1292, 1992

123. Aspirin therapy in diabetes. American Diabetes Association. Diabetes Care 27(suppl 1):S72, 2004

124. Consensus development conference on the diagnosis of coronary heart disease in people with diabetes. American Diabetes Association. Diabetes Care 21:1551, 1998

125. Kharlip J, Naglieri R, Mitchell BD, et al: Screening for silent coronary heart disease in type 2 diabetes: clinical application of American Diabetes Association guidelines. Diabetes Care 29:692, 2006

126. Klein L, Gheorghiade M: Management of the patient with diabetes mellitus and myocardial infarction: clinical trials update. Am J Med 116:47S, 2004

127. Comparison of coronary bypass surgery with angioplasty in patients with multivessel disease. Bypass Angioplasty Revascularization Investigation (BARI) Investigators. N Engl J Med 335:217, 1996

128. Brooks MM, Frye RL, Genuth S, et al: Hypotheses, design, and methods for the Bypass Angioplasty Revascularization Investigation 2 Diabetes (BARI 2D) Trial. Am J Cardiol 97:9G, 2006

129. Umpierrez GE, Isaacs SD, Barzagan N, et al: Hyperglycemia: an independent marker of in-hospital mortality in patients with undiagnosed diabetes. J Clin Endocrinol Metab 87:978, 2002

130. Capes SE, Hunt D, Malmberg K, et al: Stress hyperglycemia and prognosis of stroke in nondiabetic and diabetic patients: a systematic overview. Stroke 32:2426, 2001

131. McCowen KC, Malhotra A, Bistrian BR: Stress-induced hyperglycemia. Crit Care Clin 17:07, 2001

132. Bucerius J, Gummert J, Walther T, et al: Impact of diabetes mellitus on cardiac surgery outcome. Thorac Cardiovasc Surg 51:11, 2003

133. Furnary AP, Wu Y, Bookin SO: Effect of hyperglycemia and continuous intravenous insulin infusions on outcomes of cardiac surgical procedures: the Portland Diabetic Project. Endocr Pract 10(suppl 2):21, 2004

134. Van den Berghe G, Wouters P, Weekers F, et al: Intensive insulin therapy in critically ill patients. N Engl J Med 345:1359, 2001

135. Pittas AG, Siegel RD, Lau J: Insulin therapy for critically ill hospitalized patients. Arch Intern Med 164:2005, 2004

136. Van den Berghe G, Wilmer A, Hermans G, et al: Intensive insulin therapy in the medical ICU. N Engl J Med 354:449, 2006

137. Clement S, Braithwaite SS, Magee MF, et al: Management of diabetes and hyperglycemia in hospitals. Diabetes Care 27:553, 2004

138. Moghissi E, Hirsch I: Hospital management of diabetes. Inpatient Diabetes and Metabolic Control Task Force, American Association of Clinical Endocrinologists. Endocrinol Metab Clin North Am 34:99, 2005

139. DeSantis A, Schmeltz L, Schmidt K, et al: Inpatient management of diabetes: the Northwestern experience. Endocr Pract (in press)

140. Molitch ME: ACE inhibitors and diabetic nephropathy. Diabetes Care 17:456, 1994

55 The Adrenal

D. Lynn Loriaux, M.D., PH.D., M.A.C.P.

Anatomy

There are two adrenal glands, which are adjacent to the rostral pole of each kidney. The glands weigh 3 to 5 g each and are about 5 cm in largest dimension. They are the shape of a flattened sphere, with one side invaginated. Hence, on tomographic views, the gland has an upside-down Y shape, with a trunk and two limbs [*see Figure 1*]. The thickness of the gland in a given person should be no greater than that of the ipsilateral crus of the diaphragm.

Histologically, the adrenal gland is composed of a cortex and a medulla. The cortex has three zones [*see Figure 2*]. From the capsule inward, these zones are the glomerulosa, the fasciculata, and the reticularis. The glomerulosa is a thin, discontinuous zone in which the cells are arranged in a fashion similar to that of glomeruli. In the process of fixation, lipid is lost from these cells disproportionately; as a result, they are histologically clear. The glomerulosa accounts for about 5% of the cortical volume. The cells of the fasciculata are arranged in linear fashion, vertically, similar to that of the fascicles of pages in the spine of a book. The fasciculata accounts for about 70% of the volume of the adrenal cortex. The reticularis is intensely eosinophilic, with cells arranged in a poorly organized netlike fashion. This zone of the cortex is referred to as the x-zone in fetal life, when it accounts for most of the cortical volume. The reticularis disappears in childhood and then reappears at the time of adrenarche, which usually takes place 2 to 3 years before the onset of puberty. In the mature adrenal cortex, the reticularis accounts for 10% to 20% of the volume of the gland. The innermost zone of the adrenal gland is the medulla. Its structure is analogous to that of a sympathetic ganglion, being composed of chromaffin cells innervated by presynaptic sympathetic axons.

Physiology

The adrenal gland makes three principal hormones: hydrocortisone, or cortisol, which is necessary for life; aldosterone, which promotes salt retention and thereby permits maintenance of salt balance in a salt-poor environment; and adrenaline, or epinephrine, which features prominently in the fight-or-flight response (etymologically, the two terms are identical, with the former deriving from the Latin *ad renal* and the latter from the Greek *epi nephros*). Additionally, the adrenal gland secretes small amounts of estrogen and androgen, as well as two androgen precursor steroids, androstenedione and dehydroepiandrosterone (DHEA). These hormones and prohormones are products of distinct zones of the gland: aldosterone from the glomerulosa, cortisol from the fasciculata, DHEA from the reticularis, and epinephrine from the medulla.

Cortisol levels are regulated by a feedback loop [*see Figure 3*]. The synthesis and secretion of cortisol are stimulated by adrenocorticotropic hormone (ACTH) from the pituitary gland. Once in the bloodstream, cortisol levels rapidly regulate the synthesis and secretion of ACTH by the pituitary. ACTH release is also dependent on corticotropin-releasing hormone (CRH) from the hypothalamus. CRH is also regulated by cortisol, but at a much slower tempo.

Aldosterone levels are also regulated by feedback loops [*see Figure 3*]. Renin, a polypeptide hormone secreted by the juxta-glomerular cells of the kidney, is converted to angiotensin II, notably in the lungs, and stimulates adrenal aldosterone synthesis and secretion. Aldosterone acts on the thick ascending limb of the loop of Henle to enhance salt retention and thus expand vascular volume. The juxtaglomerular cells monitor vascular volume in the afferent artery of the glomerulosa and decrease renin secretion in response to expanded volume. DHEA and epinephrine have no known feedback regulation. All the adrenal hormones can now be measured specifically and accurately by radioimmunoassay, greatly facilitating the study of adrenal physiology and pathophysiology.

Diseases of the adrenal gland can be conveniently categorized as conditions associated with increased or decreased activity of the key hormones: hypercortisolism and hypocortisolism, hyperaldosteronism and hypoaldosteronism, virilization and feminization from sex hormone secretion, and catecholamine excess or deficiency.

Hypercortisolism (Cushing syndrome)

Cortisol is normally secreted at a rate of 6.5 mg/m²/day.[1] Secretion of cortisol in excess of this rate can, with time, lead to Cushing syndrome. Harvey Cushing described this syndrome in his book *The Pituitary Body and Its Disorders*, published in 1919.[2] The classic clinical presentation of Cushing syndrome includes central obesity, striae, moon facies, supraclavicular fat pads, diabetes mellitus, hypertension, hirsutism and oligomenorrhea in women, and erectile dysfunction in men [*see Table 1*].[3]

The causes of cortisol excess can best be categorized as ACTH dependent or ACTH independent. The two categories can be distinguished by the measurement of ACTH in the blood. ACTH-dependent causes account for about 90% of cases of noniatrogenic Cushing syndrome, and they most often result from

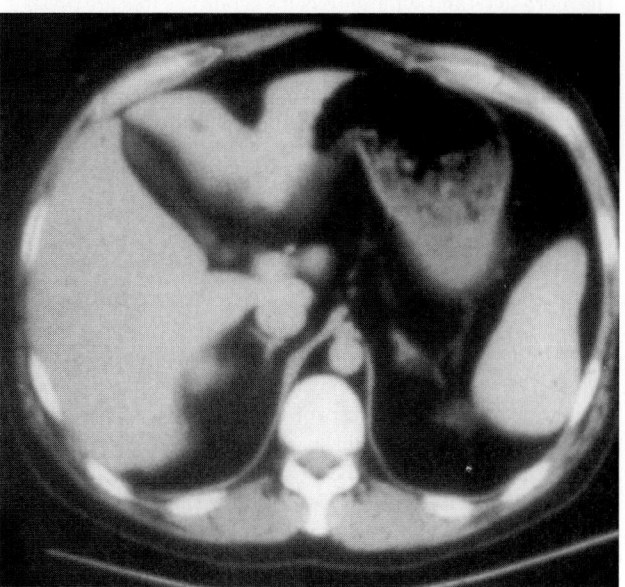

Figure 1 **A computed tomographic image shows a normal adrenal gland.**

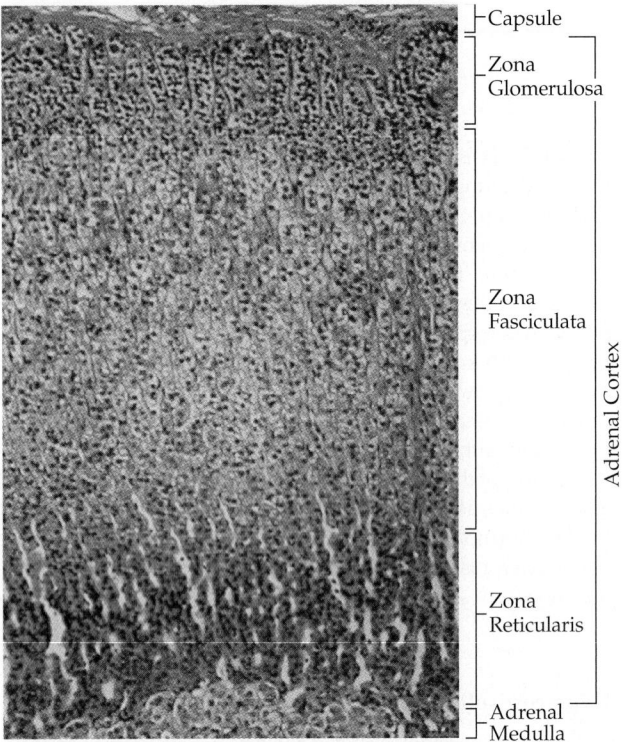

Figure 2   **Hematoxylin and eosin staining distinguishes the zones of the adrenal cortex.**

The labels on the figure read: Capsule; Zona Glomerulosa; Zona Fasciculata; Adrenal Cortex; Zona Reticularis; Adrenal Medulla.

ACTH secretion by a pituitary microadenoma that is relatively insensitive to the feedback effects of cortisol (i.e., Cushing disease). The most common cause of ACTH-independent Cushing syndrome is iatrogenic long-term glucocorticoid administration. The most common naturally occurring cause of ACTH-independent Cushing syndrome is cortisol secretion from a benign adrenal adenoma [*see Table 2*].

DIAGNOSIS

The diagnosis of Cushing syndrome is principally clinical. The more signs and symptoms of the syndrome that are present, the more confident of the diagnosis the physician can be. The firmer the clinical diagnosis, the less important is biochemical confirmation. Typically, patients will have some, but not all, of the clinical manifestations of Cushing syndrome, and the diagnosis will require confirmation by demonstrating an elevated urinary free cortisol excretion on 24-hour urine testing, which is the single best biochemical marker of Cushing syndrome. The upper limit of the normal range of urinary free cortisol in unstressed persons is generally agreed to be about 100 µg/day as measured in commercial laboratories. If the patient has florid signs of Cushing syndrome, the diagnosis can be made even in the absence of convincing biochemical confirmation. On the other hand, if the patient has few clinical signs of Cushing syndrome, the urinary free cortisol must be greater than 300 µg/day to permit the diagnosis on that basis alone.

Taken together, the number of clinical manifestations and the level of urinary free cortisol define three general categories of Cushing disease: atypical, anorexia-associated, and classic [*see Figure 4*]. Atypical Cushing syndrome is characterized by low levels of urinary free cortisol but many clinical manifestations. Anorexia-associated Cushing syndrome is characterized by high levels of urinary free cortisol and few clinical manifesta-

tions. Classic Cushing syndrome is characterized by high levels of urinary free cortisol and many clinical manifestations.

Each of these general categories of Cushing syndrome has an associated differential diagnosis. The most common cause of atypical Cushing syndrome is glucocorticoid use, whether iatrogenic or factitious, and that of anorexia-associated Cushing syndrome is small cell carcinoma of the lung. The most powerful tool in the identification of these less common causes of Cushing syndrome is the clinical history.

In patients with classic Cushing syndrome, a search for the cause should not be undertaken unless the diagnosis is secure. Once that is accomplished, the first step in the differential diagnosis is to determine whether the condition is ACTH dependent or ACTH independent. This is most easily done by measuring the level of circulating plasma ACTH. There is no need to perform dexamethasone suppression testing.[4]

Although an ACTH level greater than 10 pg/ml indicates ACTH dependence, this threshold will fail to identify 5% of ACTH-dependent cases. Consequently, patients with a random plasma ACTH level of less than 10 pg/ml should undergo a CRH challenge. In this test, ACTH levels are measured 10 to 30 minutes after injection of an intravenous bolus of CRH.[5] If the plasma ACTH is less than 10 pg/ml after a CRH challenge and if the urinary free cortisol level is normal or high, the disorder is adrenal in origin; in other words, it is ACTH independent. Either CT or MRI scans will reveal these lesions with a high degree of accuracy. If no tumor is found on adrenal imaging studies, micronodular adrenal dysplasia should be suspected.[6] The familial form of micronodular adrenal dysplasia, Carney syndrome, is an autosomal dominant disorder characterized by pigmented lentigines, blue nevi, and multiple tumors.

ACTH-secreting pituitary microadenomas are often too small to be visible on MRI scans [*see Chapter 49*]. Consequently, patients with ACTH-dependent Cushing syndrome and a normal pituitary MRI should undergo an inferior petrosal sampling procedure to search for a gradient in ACTH levels between blood draining the pituitary gland (inferior petrosal sinus blood) and peripheral antecubital blood. An ACTH gradient greater than 3 between simultaneously sampled central and peripheral blood confirms a pituitary etiology for Cushing syndrome.[7] If the gradient is less than 3, the search for an ectopic source of ACTH should be undertaken. Chest CT and MRI scans (with CT scans typically performed first) are central to this investigation, because 95% of these tumors are intrathoracic. The most common offending tumor is a bronchial carcinoid.

TREATMENT

Except for atypical Cushing syndrome, in which the treatment is to discontinue exogenous glucocorticoid, all treatments for Cushing syndrome are surgical. ACTH-independent cases should be treated with adrenal tumor resection or, in the case of micronodular adrenal dysplasia, bilateral adrenalectomy. ACTH-dependent cases should be treated with transsphenoidal microadenomectomy or ablation of the ectopic ACTH-secreting tumor. When an ectopic source for ACTH cannot be identified, the patient can be treated temporarily with a cortisol synthesis inhibitor, most commonly ketoconazole, until the lesion is found. If it is not found within 18 to 24 months, bilateral adrenalectomy should be performed.

Effective surgery for an ACTH-secreting tumor renders the patient adrenally insufficient. This is documented by measurement of the plasma cortisol level on the morning after surgery. If the

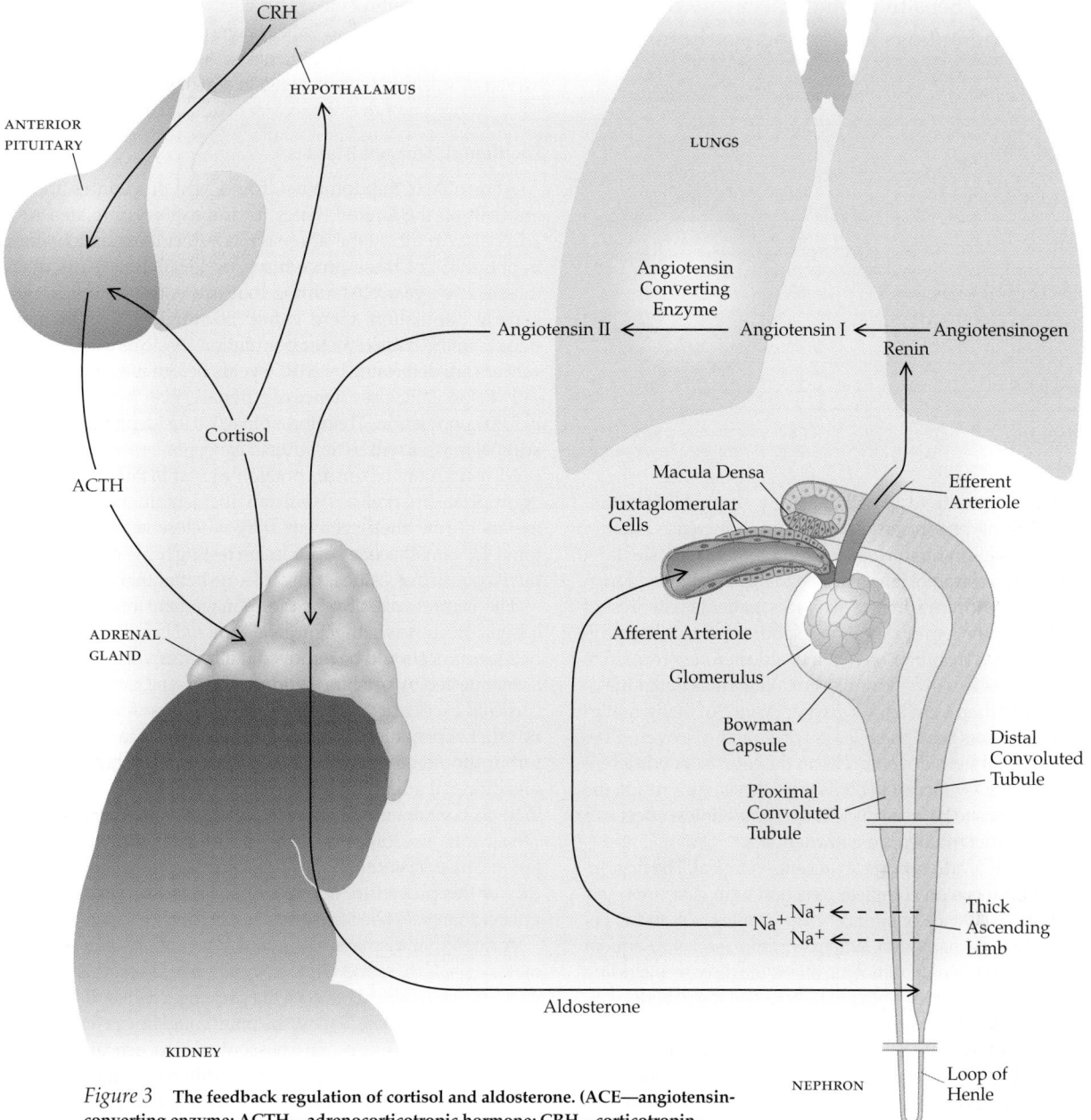

Figure 3 **The feedback regulation of cortisol and aldosterone. (ACE—angiotensin-converting enzyme; ACTH—adrenocorticotropic hormone; CRH—corticotropin-releasing hormone)**

level is greater than 20 μg/dl, the operation has not been successful and no cortisol therapy is indicated. If the plasma cortisol level is below the normal range (i.e., less than 5 μg/dl), the operation has been successful, and steroid replacement therapy will be required until the hypothalamic-pituitary-adrenal (HPA) axis can recover—possibly 1 year or longer. During this period, the patient should be treated with hydrocortisone at a rate of 12 mg/m² in a single daily dose with breakfast. Adrenal function is tested with a synthetic ACTH (cosyntropin) stimulation test at 3-month intervals. In patients with cortisol values between 5 and 20 μg/dl after cosyntropin stimulation, cortisol replacement therapy can be withdrawn; but 3-month testing should continue, and cortisol replacement therapy should be reinstituted if signs and symptoms of adrenal insufficiency appear. As soon as the cortisol level reaches 20 μg/dl or greater after cosyntropin stimulation, discontinuance of cortisol replacement without continued testing is safe.

If the operation has not been curative, Cushing syndrome will reappear with time. In addition to cortisol replacement, patients who have undergone bilateral adrenal resection will also require aldosterone replacement in the form of fludrocortisone, 0.1 mg each morning.

Without treatment, Cushing syndrome is fatal. Except for adrenal cancer, however, all causes of Cushing syndrome can be cured. Successful treatment restores normal life expectancy.

Adrenal Cancer

Adrenocortical cancer is a rare disease, with an annual incidence of 1 in 600,000.[8] Thus, about 500 new cases are diagnosed in the United States each year. This disease usually presents clinically as a combination of steroid hormone excess syndromes, the most common being Cushing syndrome with virilization.

Table 1 Sensitivity and Specificity of Selected Findings in Cushing Syndrome

Finding	Sensitivity (%)	Specificity (%)
Central obesity	90	71
Glucose intolerance	88	23
Plethora	82	69
Proximal muscle weakness	65	93
Striae	40	78
Hyperkalemia	25	96
Osteoporosis	64	97

Differential diagnostic tests will generally show ACTH-independent Cushing syndrome associated with increased serum testosterone levels in hirsute or virilized women. Occasionally, increased serum estradiol levels will be found in feminized men with Cushing syndrome. In rare instances, patients will present with virilization or feminization only, and some will have hypertension caused by tumor secretion of aldosterone precursors. CT or MRI scans usually show a large unilateral adrenal mass. Masses greater than 6 cm have a greater chance of being malignant. These tumors tend to be large when first discovered because the adrenal steroidogenic cells, in the course of dedifferentiation, become less efficient in cortisol synthesis. As a result, the tumor burden has to be large to yield the same clinical effect as a small, highly differentiated, benign adenoma.

The treatment of adrenocortical cancers is surgical. The first operation should focus on complete resection with clear margins. However, the incidence of surgical cure is unknown and is believed to be low, perhaps zero. With recurrence, each subsequent operation should focus on removing all visible disease, including accessible metastases. If left untreated, about half the patients with adrenocortical cancer will die in a few months. With aggressive surgery, their survival can be extended to about 48 months. When surgery is no longer feasible, treatment with steroid hormone synthesis blockers is indicated. Ketoconazole is typically used for this purpose. In addition, ortho,para'-DDD (mitotane) can be considered. At full dosages (> 2 g/day in divided doses), mitotane can produce remission in about 25% of patients. The average remission is 7 months long. Lengthened life span has not been demonstrated, and mitotane has severe side effects—nausea, vomiting, lethargy, and vertigo—so some physicians argue that the cost-to-benefit ratio (quality of life versus days of life gained) does not justify the use of this drug. Other chemotherapeutic regimens are under development, and patients with this rare disease are best served by referral to a center engaged in this research.[9]

Incidental Adrenal Masses

About 300,000 abdominal CT and MRI procedures are done annually in the United States for indications unrelated to the adrenals. An incidental adrenal mass (incidentaloma) is found in about 4% of these procedures, or 12,000 newly discovered masses each year.[10] Assuming that this is the incidence in the general population, there would be roughly 12 million such masses in the United States population. Assuming that adrenal cancers are detectable by MRI 6 years before they become clinically evident, the prevalence of adrenal cancer would be about 1 in 3,000 population. Therefore, 1 in 4,000 incidentally discovered adrenal masses will be an adrenal cancer.

Measurement of serum potassium and bicarbonate levels is appropriate in patients with an incidentaloma. Plasma free metanephrine measurement may disclose a pheochromocytoma. Dexamethasone suppression testing has been advocated,[10] but its predictive value is only 0.5—no better than tossing a coin.

The central question in the management of the incidental adrenal mass is whether surgical removal is indicated. Certainly, the tumor should be removed if it is metabolically functional, as manifested by Cushing syndrome, the syndrome of mineralocorticoid excess, or virilization or feminization for which there is no other explanation. If there is no evidence of functionality, the tumor should be studied with a CT contrast washout study. Benign adrenal adenomas are lipid rich, whereas malignant ones tend to contain much more cellular and intercellular water. Thus, water-soluble contrast agents tend to wash out of benign lesions much faster than they do from malignant ones. The accuracy of this procedure in experienced hands is very high, with greater than 90% specificity and sensitivity.[11,12]

A mass that displays slow washout can be assumed to be a metastasis. If the patient has a known malignancy, the adrenal mass can be treated as part of the primary process. If there is no known primary malignancy, the mass could be the first manifestation of metastasis or a rare nascent adrenocortical carcinoma. Percutaneous needle biopsy can readily differentiate between these two possibilities, but it does involve risks, such as pneumothorax and tumor seeding. Alternatively, the mass can be removed laparoscopically and a pathologic analysis done.

In most series, 5% to 6% of incidental adrenal masses are pheochromocytomas.[13] This possibility should be excluded before biopsy or operation so as to avoid the hypertensive crises that can be associated with surgery. The safest course is to assume that the lesion is a pheochromocytoma and to prepare all such patients for surgery with adequate alpha blockade [*see* Pheochromocytoma, *below*].

Adrenal Insufficiency

Adrenal insufficiency (Addison disease) is categorized as primary or secondary. Primary adrenal insufficiency results from destruction of the adrenal cortex. There is a long list of causes of primary adrenal insufficiency [*see Table 3*]; worldwide, tuberculosis is the most common cause, and in the industrialized nations, idiopathic or autoimmune adrenal destruction is the most common cause. Secondary adrenal insufficiency results from disruption of

Table 2 Differential Diagnosis of Cushing Syndrome

ACTH-dependent causes	Pituitary ACTH-producing tumor Ectopic ACTH-producing tumor
ACTH-independent causes	Glucocorticoid use (factitious or iatrogenic) Adrenal adenoma Adrenal carcinoma Micronodular adrenal disease

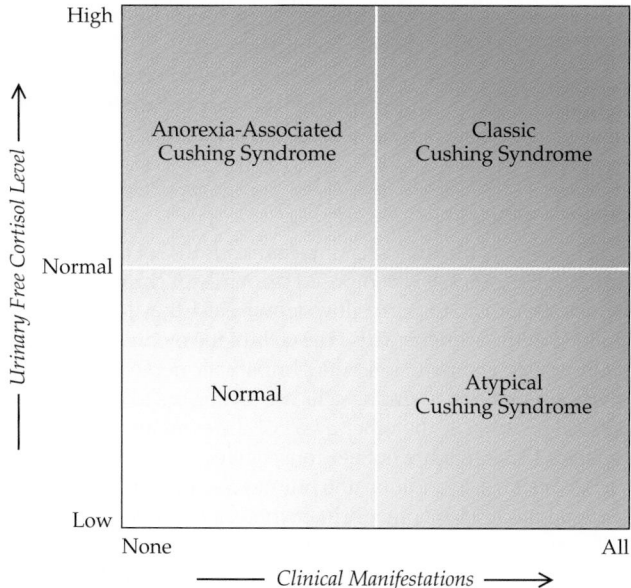

Figure 4 **The severity of the clinical manifestations and the level of urinary free cortisol can be used to define three categories of Cushing syndrome: classic, atypical, and anorexia associated.**

pituitary secretion of ACTH, which by far is most commonly caused by prolonged treatment with exogenous glucocorticoids. With time, doses of exogenous glucocorticoids sufficient to suppress ACTH secretion will lead to dysfunction of CRH-secreting neurons and attendant ACTH deficiency; subsequent withdrawal of glucocorticoids, for whatever reason, will then unmask the deficiency. Recovery of function may require a year or more. A far less common cause of disrupted ACTH secretion is destructive lesions in and around the pituitary gland and hypothalamus [*see Table 4*].

The symptoms and signs of adrenal insufficiency can be grouped into chronic and acute syndromes. The chronic syndrome is characterized by anorexia, weight loss, fatigue, and orthostatic hypotension. In patients with primary disease, the predominant signs are weight loss and hyperpigmentation of the skin, especially of the sun-exposed areas and extensor surfaces. The acute syndrome is closely analogous to cardiogenic or septic shock, with reduced cardiac output into a dilated and unresponsive vascular system. Symptoms include prostration and all of

---

Table 3   Causes of Primary
Adrenal Insufficiency

Autoimmunity (70% of cases)
  Polyendocrine deficiency syndrome
Tuberculosis (20% of cases)
Other (10% of cases)
  Fungal infection
  Adrenal hemorrhage
  Adrenomyeloneuropathy
  Adrenoleukodystrophy
  Sarcoidosis
  Amyloidosis
  Congenital adrenal hyperplasia
  Congenital unresponsiveness to ACTH
  Metastatic cancer
  AIDS

Table 4   Causes of Secondary
Adrenal Insufficiency

Iatrogenic suppression of the hypothalamic-pituitary-adrenal
  axis (90% of cases)
Other (10% of cases)
  Hypophysectomy
  Pituitary irradiation
  Head trauma
  Hypophysitis
  Hemochromatosis
  Infection
    Actinomycosis
    Nocardiosis
  Intracranial tumor
  Pituitary tumor

---

the signs and symptoms of the shock syndrome. Shock in this setting tends to be unresponsive to volume replacement and vasoconstrictor therapy.

With both chronic and acute syndromes, the diagnosis should be suspected on clinical grounds, but it requires laboratory confirmation. The critical test for the diagnosis of chronic adrenal insufficiency is the cosyntropin stimulation test. Synthetic ACTH (cosyntropin) is administered in a 250 µg intravenous bolus, and plasma cortisol levels are then measured after 45 and 60 minutes. Values greater than 20 µg/dl exclude adrenal insufficiency as a cause of the clinical findings. Values less than 20 µg/dl suggest that adrenal compromise could be a contributing factor. In this situation, treatment with glucocorticoids is mandatory until the clinical situation is clarified with more precision.

In acute adrenal insufficiency, the most useful test is measurement of the plasma cortisol level. Cosyntropin stimulation testing is not necessary; the illness, which is sufficiently severe to merit admission to an intensive care unit, represents an endogenous source of maximal physiologic stress. Plasma cortisol levels in patients with acute stress are greater than 20 µg/dl, with the only exception being in patients who have a low plasma albumin concentration, which lowers the total cortisol concentration.[14] Unfortunately, there are no published data on the interpretation of plasma cortisol values in patients with low albumin concentrations, so most clinicians adhere to the 20 µg/dl standard. Currently, if the cortisol value is less than 20 µg/dl, it should be confirmed with a standard cosyntropin stimulation test.

The differential diagnosis of adrenal insufficiency requires the discrimination of primary and secondary causes; the most useful test is measurement of the circulating plasma ACTH level. ACTH levels greater than normal define primary disease; values in the normal range or below define secondary disease.

Patients with primary adrenal disease should have the adrenal glands imaged with CT or MRI. Infectious, malignant, and vascular causes of adrenal insufficiency all result in enlargement of the adrenal glands. In idiopathic or autoimmune adrenal insufficiency, the glands are normal or small in size. Patients with secondary adrenal insufficiency should first be assessed for exogenous glucocorticoid use. If that can be eliminated as a cause, they should undergo CT or MRI scanning of the hypothalamus and pituitary gland to exclude destructive lesions in this area.

TREATMENT

The goal in treating adrenal insufficiency is to replace the

Table 5 Differential Diagnosis
of Pheochromocytoma

Panic attacks
Thyrotoxicosis
Amphetamine use
Cocaine use
Over-the-counter cold medicines containing phenylephrine or pseudoephedrine
Monoamine oxidase inhibitors
Hypoglycemia
Insulin reaction
Brain tumor
Subarachnoid hemorrhage
Menopausal hot flashes
Toxemia of pregnancy
Selective serotonin reuptake inhibitors

---

missing hydrocortisone and aldosterone in quantities calibrated to the clinical situation. Hydrocortisone can be replaced with oral or intravenous hydrocortisone. Aldosterone is replaced with oral fludrocortisone. Exogenous hydrocortisone and fludrocortisone are both equipotent with the endogenously secreted hormone. Unstressed persons secrete hydrocortisone at a rate of 6.5 mg/m^2 daily. In the face of stress, such as a surgical procedure or serious trauma, hydrocortisone secretion can rise more than 10-fold. The secretion rate of aldosterone is 100 μg/day in persons consuming large amounts of sodium (i.e., a typical United States diet).

Primary chronic adrenal insufficiency is treated with oral hydrocortisone, 12 to 15 mg/m^2/day. This is roughly double the amount of hydrocortisone that is normally secreted; the added amount is needed to compensate for first-pass hepatic metabolism. Hydrocortisone is best given as a single daily dose with breakfast. Fludrocortisone is given at a dose of 0.1 mg/day. When moderate stress is anticipated (e.g., a root canal procedure), the dose of hydrocortisone is temporarily doubled, beginning the day before the stress and continuing until 2 days afterward. It is not necessary to alter the fludrocortisone dose. With anticipated major stress (e.g., appendectomy with general anesthesia), the hydrocortisone dosage is increased to 100 mg every 6 hours from the day before the procedure until 2 days afterward. Hydrocortisone dosage increases are not required for periods of psychological stress, such as major depression, psychosis, or grief.

These replacement regimens roughly reproduce the patterns of cortisol and aldosterone secretion in persons with normal adrenal function. The need for these temporary dosage increases has not been clearly established, on either clinical or biologic grounds, but this has become the standard of practice and is not likely to change. Chronic secondary adrenal insufficiency is treated in the same way as chronic primary disease but with replacement of hydrocortisone only, not aldosterone.

Patients with acute adrenal insufficiency are treated in the same fashion as those with chronic adrenal insufficiency who are experiencing major stress. Treatment is monitored clinically. Signs of Cushing syndrome indicate overtreatment; hyponatremia, orthostasis, and anorexia indicate undertreatment. There is no good clinical evidence to suggest that the dosage regimens ever need to be exceeded. If a patient on recommended replacement doses of hydrocortisone and fludrocortisone

fails to do as well as expected, the reason is something other than the adrenal replacement regimen.

All patients with adrenal insufficiency should wear a medical-alert bracelet imprinted with the words "adrenal insufficiency" and carry a similar wallet card at all times.

Pheochromocytoma

The adrenal medulla accounts for about 10% of the weight of the adrenal gland. It is composed primarily of chromaffin cells, which are named for the yellow-brown color they take on when stained with chromatic salts. The cells of the medulla are directly innervated by preganglionic sympathetic nerve cells. Hence, these epinephrine-secreting cells are analogous to the postganglionic neurons in the other areas of the sympathetic nervous system. These cells are not neurons, however, and have no dendrites or axons. In addition, the primary secretory product of the adrenal medulla is epinephrine, whereas the remainder of the sympathetic nervous system employs norepinephrine as the neurotransmitter. The reason for this difference is that the blood supply to the adrenal medulla is derived from the capillary plexus draining the adrenal cortex. This capillary blood is extremely rich in cortisol—perhaps the highest concentration of cortisol in the human body is in the adrenal medulla—and cortisol induces catechol-O-methyl transferase, the enzyme that converts norepinephrine to epinephrine. The primary disease of the adrenal medulla is pheochromocytoma; 90% of pheochromocytomas occur in the adrenal medulla. Extra-adrenal tumors of the chromaffin cell are known as paraganglions or chemodectomas, depending on the location. All have similar clinical presentations, and all are treated in the same way (see below).

The main clinical manifestation of pheochromocytomas is hypertension. The hypertension can be sustained or episodic; the two forms occur with equal frequency. Paroxysmal hypertension is associated with tachycardia, diaphoresis, anxiety, and a sense of foreboding. Patients also complain of nausea and abdominal pain. The association of headache, palpitations, and sweating with hypertension has a high (> 90%) sensitivity and specificity for pheochromocytoma. The differential diagnosis for pheochromocytoma is extensive and includes anxiety and panic attacks, thyrotoxicosis, amphetamine and cocaine use, and use of over-the-counter cold medicines that depend upon catecholamines for effect, such as atomizers for nasal congestion [see Table 5]. Pheochromocytomas are usually benign (90%) and usually unilateral (90%). The incidence of pheochromocytoma is markedly increased in several genetic syndromes: multiple endocrine neoplasia types 2a and 2b and the phakomatoses, including neurofibromatosis, cerebelloretinal hemangioblastosis, tuberous sclerosis, and Sturge-Weber syndrome.

DIAGNOSIS

The traditional tests for diagnosing pheochromocytoma are measurements of the urinary fractionated catecholamines and urinary metanephrine excretion in 24-hour urine samples. Total catecholamine excretion is normally less than 100 μg/day, with no more than 25% being epinephrine. Urinary metanephrine excretion is normally less than 1.3 mg/day. The urine for these tests must be collected in an acid medium (laboratories typically provide appropriate containers) and need not be refrigerated. Creatinine should also be measured, as an indicator of completeness of collection. The patient should be taken off all medications when possible. If the hypertension must be treated, diuretics, vasodila-

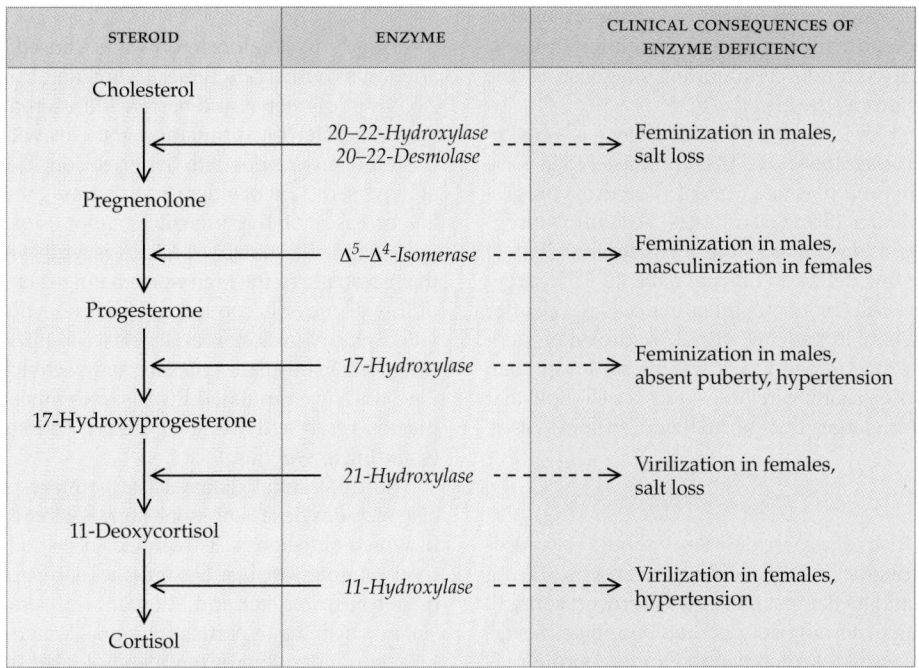

STEROID	ENZYME	CLINICAL CONSEQUENCES OF ENZYME DEFICIENCY
Cholesterol ↓	20–22-Hydroxylase 20–22-Desmolase	Feminization in males, salt loss
Pregnenolone ↓	Δ^5–Δ^4-Isomerase	Feminization in males, masculinization in females
Progesterone ↓	17-Hydroxylase	Feminization in males, absent puberty, hypertension
17-Hydroxyprogesterone ↓	21-Hydroxylase	Virilization in females, salt loss
11-Deoxycortisol ↓	11-Hydroxylase	Virilization in females, hypertension
Cortisol		

Figure 5 Congenital adrenal hyperplasia may result from mutations that inactivate any of the six enzymatic steps in the biosynthesis of cortisol from cholesterol. The clinical manifestations of the disorder vary with the enzyme deficiency.

tors, calcium channel blockers, and angiotensin-converting enzyme (ACE) inhibitors interfere minimally with the assays. When there is concordance between the clinical picture and the biochemical tests, CT or MRI scans should be employed to localize the tumor. MRI is particularly useful because these tumors almost always "brighten" with T_2-weighted images. If CT and MRI fail to reveal an adrenal tumor, radiolabeled meta-iodobenzylguanidine (MIBG) can be a useful scanning technique for locating tumors outside of the adrenal gland, such as those in the carotid body, heart, urinary bladder, and the organ of Zuckerkandl.

TREATMENT

The treatment of pheochromocytoma is surgical. The surgery should be undertaken only by a team experienced and skilled in the management of pheochromocytoma. Before the surgical procedure, complete alpha blockade should be induced to avoid intraoperative hypertensive crisis. Preparation should begin 7 days before the planned procedure, using phenoxybenzamine at an initial dosage of 10 mg by mouth twice daily. The dose should be increased daily, and by the seventh day, the patient should be taking at least 1 mg/kg/day in three divided doses. Adequate blockade is associated with reduced blood pressure and reduced orthostatic hypotension as the vascular volume is restored.

Malignant pheochromocytoma should be treated with surgical debulking, ongoing alpha blockade with phenoxybenzamine, and comanagement with an oncologist. Radiation therapy is useful for bone pain, and some success has been achieved with combination chemotherapy, including cyclophosphamide, vincristine, and dacarbazine.

Congenital Adrenal Hyperplasia

There are six enzymatic steps in the biosynthesis of cortisol from cholesterol, and all can be affected by inactivating mutations [see Figure 5]. Because cortisol is essential for life, cortisol concentrations are maintained in the normal range at the expense of adrenal hypertrophy and increased adrenal secretion of the steroid biosynthetic intermediate in the step immediately before the affected enzyme. Depending on which enzyme is blocked, the increased concentrations of the steroid biosynthetic intermediate can lead to virilization in females and to hypertension. In some cases, primarily because of reduced androgen secretion in utero—a time when there is no feedback regulation of testosterone—male fetuses can be feminized.

The most common underlying disorder in congenital adrenal hyperplasia is 21-hydroxylase deficiency. The virilizing form of this disease is thought to be the most common autosomal recessive disorder.

21-Hydroxylase deficiency is categorized according to two clinical distinctions: (1) the classic form, which can be salt losing or non–salt losing, and (2) the nonclassic form.

The degree to which a person with 21-hydroxylase deficiency loses salt in a salt-poor environment correlates with the degree of expression of the enzyme defect in the zona glomerulosa. In persons with mild expression, salt loss is sufficiently minimal that a standard United States diet will maintain a normal salt balance.

The classic form of the disease is usually diagnosed in the neonatal period and is characterized by failure to thrive as a result of the salt loss and by male pseudohermaphroditism in female infants. The nonclassic form of the disease, which is sometimes referred to as adult onset or attenuated, usually becomes clinically apparent in adolescence. It is manifested by a slightly earlier age at puberty (approximately 1 year) and, in females, oligomenorrhea and androgen-mediated hirsutism. Adults who present with the classic form of 21-hydroxylase deficiency usually have a well-documented diagnosis since infancy, have a gender assignment, and have completed a series of genital reconstructive plastic surgical procedures. The usual clinical questions are whether ongoing treatment is necessary and, if so, whether the current regimen is appropriate.

The typical adult patient with the nonclassic or attenuated form is a young woman with oligomenorrhea, infertility, and hirsutism. The most common confounding diagnosis is the polycystic ovary syndrome [see Chapter 79].

The diagnostic test for 21-hydroxylase deficiency is a cosyntropin stimulation test: synthetic ACTH is administered in a 250 μg intravenous bolus, and plasma levels of 17-hydroxyprogesterone are measured after 45 and 60 minutes. 17-Hydroxyprogesterone is the steroid biosynthetic intermediate immediately proximal to the enzyme defect. In normal patients, 17-hydroxyprogesterone levels will rise to no higher than 340 ng/dl after cosyntropin stimulation; in patients with 21-hydroxylase deficiency, 17-hydroxyprogesterone levels will be no lower than 1,000 ng/dl. CT or MRI scanning in these patients will show that the adrenal glands are larger than normal and, in some cases, nodular.

TREATMENT

All patients with 21-hydroxylase deficiency should be considered to have some degree of salt loss. Fludrocortisone, 0.2 mg every morning, should be the first therapy. Hydrocortisone, 12 to 15 mg/m² as a single morning dose, should be initiated several days later. After 2 weeks of combined therapy, a morning 17-hydroxyprogesterone level should be measured. If the target level of 400 to 600 ng/dl is achieved, the fludrocortisone dose can be reduced by half. Two weeks later, the 17-hydroxyprogesterone should be measured again; if it is still below 600 ng/dl, that establishes the fludrocortisone dose as the patient's maintenance dose. If the 17-hydroxyprogesterone level has risen above 600 ng/dl, the fludrocortisone dose should be restored to the initial 0.2 mg/day, which likely will be the maintenance dose. Reduction of 17-hydroxyprogesterone levels to within the normal range is not recommended. Achieving this level often requires doses of fludrocortisone that produce adrenal suppression and lead to Cushing syndrome.

Lifelong treatment is required in patients with 21-hydroxylase deficiency to prevent the appearance of adrenal rest tumors, which are nodules of ectopic adrenal tissue that become hypertrophic because of ongoing ACTH stimulation. These tumors are usually found in the broad ligament in women and in the testes in men. In women, hemorrhage or necrosis of adrenal rest tumors occasionally necessitates emergency pelvic surgery; in men, these tumors can result in testicular pain, testicular masses, and infertility. Testicular pain may be so severe and intractable that castration is required.

Hyperaldosteronism

Hyperaldosteronism can be primary or secondary. In primary hyperaldosteronism, there is disordered function of the renin-aldosterone feedback axis; in secondary hyperaldosteronism, the renin-aldosterone axis is responding normally to chronic intravascular volume deficiency, which may result from such conditions as heart failure or ascites associated with cirrhosis of the liver.

Aldosterone acts on the epithelial cells of the renal collecting tubule to promote reabsorption of sodium and excretion of potassium and hydrogen. Other tissues similarly affected include sweat glands, salivary glands, and intestinal epithelium. Clinically, the result of excess aldosterone is the so-called mineralocorticoid excess syndrome, characterized by hypokalemia, metabolic alkalosis, and, sometimes, hypertension.

Primary hyperaldosteronism is caused by benign adrenal adenomas, which are typically unilateral, are usually less than 2.5 cm in diameter, and secrete aldosterone independently of renin-angiotensin stimulation. Patients with primary hyperaldosteronism present with hypertension; in fact, primary adrenal hypersecretion of aldosterone is thought to account for about 2% of cases of hypertension. Laboratory testing shows hypokalemia and metabolic alkalosis, with a serum sodium level that is usually in the high-normal range [see Figure 6]. Diagnosis of this disorder is confirmed by demonstrating normal or elevated plasma aldosterone levels (> 14 ng/dl) along with suppression of stimulated plasma renin activity (PRA) to less than 2 ng/ml/hr. Stimulated PRA is determined by measuring the plasma renin activity level after 2 hours of upright posture (standing or walking).

The differential diagnosis of primary hyperaldosteronism also includes dexamethasone-suppressible hyperaldosteronism, in which aldosterone is secreted in response to ACTH rather than angiotensin [see Dexamethasone-Suppressible Hyperaldosteronism, below], and idiopathic bilateral adrenal hyperplasia, in which the hypertrophic zona glomerulosa secretes aldosterone independent of renin-angiotensin stimulation [see Idiopathic Bilateral Adrenal Hyperplasia, below]. Dexamethasone-suppressible hyperaldosteronism is confirmed by the suppression of aldosterone levels with dexamethasone administration, 2 mg/day in divided doses for 7 days. In most cases, aldosterone levels decrease by the third day of treatment. If dexamethasone fails to suppress plasma aldosterone levels and to ameliorate the associated hypertension, CT or MRI should be employed to search for an adrenal adenoma. If an adenoma is not found by CT or MRI, simultaneous adrenal venous sampling for the measurement of aldosterone and cortisol will be needed to define the source of aldosterone secretion.[15] If the venous sampling identifies unilateral aldosterone secretion, the patient should be treated as if primary adrenal hypoaldosteronism is present, despite the absence of a visible adenoma. The surgeon, at the time of operation, can define unilateral versus bilateral disease.

The treatment of primary adrenal hyperaldosteronism is unilateral adrenalectomy, preferably by a laparoscopic procedure. The cure rate, defined as correction of hyperaldosteronism and hypertension, is about 75%.[16] Patients whose blood pressure remains elevated postoperatively will require ongoing antihypertensive therapy, which is managed as if essential hypertension were present.

Idiopathic Bilateral Adrenal Hyperplasia

The clinical presentation of idiopathic bilateral adrenal hyperplasia is indistinguishable from that of primary hyperaldosteronism caused by an adrenal adenoma. However, patients with idiopathic bilateral adrenal hyperplasia have no dominant adrenal adenoma, and aldosterone secretion from both adrenal glands can be documented by bilateral adrenal venous sampling. Adrenalectomy in these patients does not correct the hypertension. Thus, treatment is directed at the hypertension. Interestingly, antagonizing aldosterone activity with spironolactone is usually ineffective. Calcium channel blockers, however, are effective antihypertensive agents in these patients, as are ACE inhibitors. If hypokalemia persists during the treatment of hypertension, it can usually be managed by the addition of a potassium-sparing diuretic.

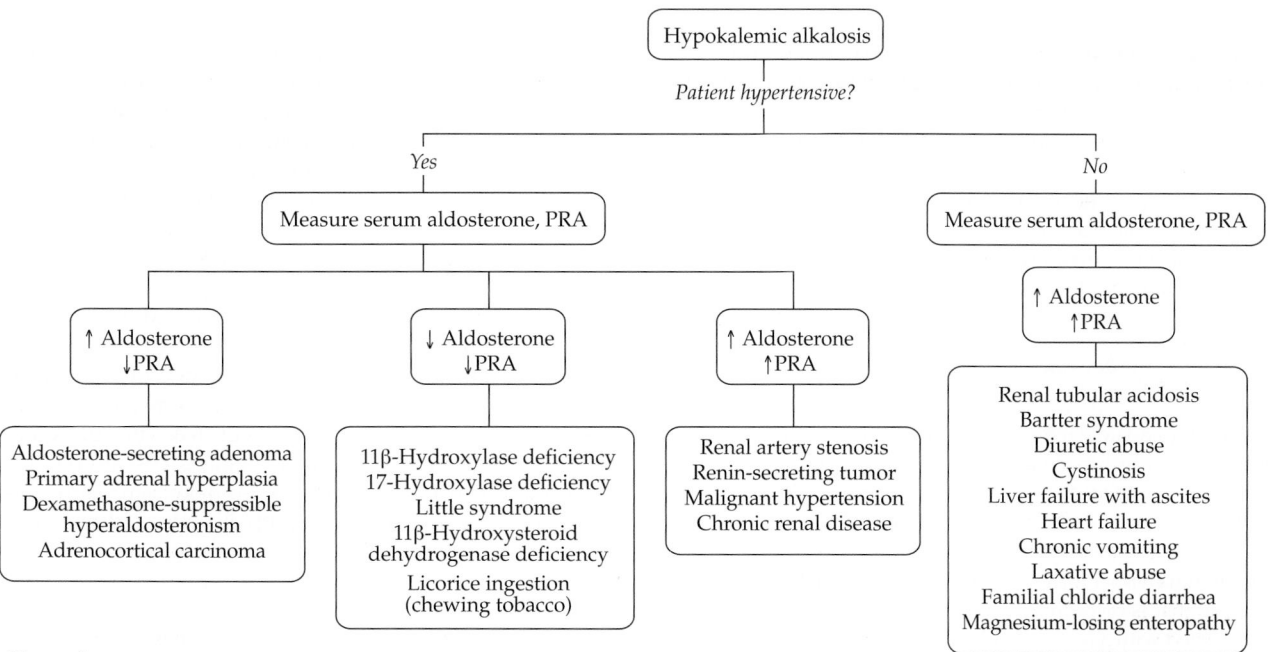

Figure 6   **Differential diagnosis of primary hypoaldosteronism. (PRA—plasma renin activity)**

Dexamethasone-Suppressible Hyperaldosteronism

Dexamethasone-suppressible hyperaldosteronism is a rare familial cause of hyperaldosteronism and is transmitted as an autosomal dominant trait. The cause of the disorder is a fusion gene in which the coding region for ACTH-responsive regulation of 11-β hydrolase is coupled with the coding region for aldosterone synthase. Thus, aldosterone secretion becomes entrained to ACTH secretion and is "blind" to renin-angiotensin levels. Because ACTH secretion is not modulated by aldosterone, aldosterone secretion becomes independent of salt balance, blood potassium levels, and vascular volume.

Treatment for this disorder starts with the use of a potassium-sparing diuretic such as amiloride or triamterene. This regimen has the advantage of not suppressing the HPA axis. If it is unsuccessful, ACTH secretion can be suppressed with dexamethasone, usually 0.5 mg in a single daily dose.

SECONDARY HYPERALDOSTERONISM

Secondary hyperaldosteronism may or may not be associated with hypertension. Patients with hypertension usually have underlying renal pathology, including renal artery stenosis, renin-secreting tumors, and chronic renal failure. Both plasma renin activity and aldosterone are elevated in such cases. Treatment should be directed at the underlying cause.

Secondary hyperaldosteronism that is not associated with hypertension occurs in disorders characterized by decreased vascular volume. Renal causes include chronic nephritis, renal tubular acidosis, and calcium- and magnesium-losing nephropathies. Chronic diuretic abuse also is a cause. Gastrointestinal causes include chronic vomiting, laxative abuse, and chronic diarrhea of any kind. Probably the most common causes are chronic heart failure and cirrhosis of the liver with ascites. Again, treatment is best directed at the underlying disorder.

Finally, there are two forms of congenital adrenal hyperplasia in which overproduction of mineralocorticoids other than aldosterone leads to the syndrome of mineralocorticoid excess. These two disorders are 11-hydroxylase deficiency and 17-hydroxy-

lase deficiency. Both renin and aldosterone levels are low in these disorders. Treatment is the same as that for 21-hydroxylase deficiency (see above), but without fludrocortisone.

Bartter syndrome is associated with hypokalemic alkalosis, hyperreninemia, and hyperaldosteronism; in patients with Bartter syndrome, blood pressure is normal. This pattern can be seen in a number of disorders causing secondary hyperaldosteronism. Bartter syndrome is caused by a deficit in chloride transport in the thick ascending limb of the loop of Henle. Diagnosis of this disorder is difficult because the pattern of electrolyte abnormalities mimics that seen in diuretic abuse. A more detailed discussion of Bartter syndrome is provided elsewhere [*see Chapter 163*].

Hypoaldosteronism

PRIMARY HYPOALDOSTERONISM

Primary hypoaldosteronism is defined as aldosterone deficiency of adrenal cause. Hypoaldosteronism manifests as an inability to conserve sodium, leading to a negative salt balance in a salt-poor environment. This leads to hypotension, hyperkalemia, dehydration, and volume depletion associated with a mild metabolic acidosis. The disorder can be corrected by a high-salt diet or by replacement of aldosterone with fludrocortisone.

Primary adrenal insufficiency is the most common cause of primary hypoaldosteronism. Diagnosis and treatment are the same as those for adrenal insufficiency (see above). Two rare autosomal recessive disorders, corticosterone methyl oxidase (CMO) deficiency types I and II, can result in markedly reduced adrenal secretion of aldosterone. CMO deficiency type I is recognized by the syndrome of mineralocorticoid deficiency and low aldosterone levels associated with high plasma corticosterone concentration. CMO deficiency type II is similar, except that high levels of 18-hydroxycorticosterone will be associated with low levels of aldosterone. These are primarily diseases of childhood, becoming less severe with age and free access to salt.

SECONDARY HYPOALDOSTERONISM

The syndrome of hyporeninemic hypoaldosteronism is the most common form of secondary hypoaldosteronism. The disorder is often referred to as renal tubular acidosis type 4. It has been described in almost every disorder of renal function. Chronic renal disease is present in 80% of patients with the disorder. The clinical picture is that of hyperkalemia, hyponatremia, and metabolic acidosis in association with a low plasma renin activity and a low plasma aldosterone level. The most direct and rational therapy for this syndrome is replacement of aldosterone with fludrocortisone at a dosage of 0.1 to 0.2 mg/day.

PSEUDOHYPOALDOSTERONISM (MINERALOCORTICOID RESISTANCE)

Pseudohypoaldosteronism type I and type II are syndromes of end-organ resistance to the effects of aldosterone. Type I is caused by an inactivating mutation in the mineralocorticoid receptor, and type 2 is ascribed to an ill-defined defect in aldosterone action distal to its binding to the mineralocorticoid receptor. Pseudohypoaldosteronism type 1 is characterized by salt wasting that is resistant to mineralocorticoid replacement. It is best treated with a high-salt diet, 10 to 40 mEq/kg/day. Pseudohypoaldosteronism type II (Gordon syndrome) is a non–salt-wasting disorder that can be associated with hypertension, metabolic acidosis, and hyperkalemia. Plasma renin activity and aldosterone are both low, and administration of mineralocorticoid fails to correct the hyperkalemia and acidosis. The basic defect is thought to be a chloride shunt disorder in the nephron. Treatment is with a potassium-wasting diuretic; hydrochlorothiazide and furosemide are most often used.

Glucocorticoid Therapy

Glucocorticoids can be valuable, even lifesaving, in the treatment of many inflammatory and neoplastic diseases. Although cortisol accounts for about half of the mineralocorticoid effect produced by the adrenal gland, the synthetic steroids that are customarily used for glucocorticoid therapy (e.g., prednisone and dexamethasone) have virtually no salt-retaining activity and, therefore, do not cause unacceptable salt retention. On the other hand, their glucocorticoid effect is far more powerful than that of cortisol. Gram for gram, prednisone has four times the glucocorticoid potency of cortisol; dexamethasone has about 25 times the potency.

The target tissues in glucocorticoid-responsive diseases are glucocorticoid resistant. The basis for this resistance remains unknown, but the prevailing hypothesis is that the chaperone proteins produced in stressed cells, particularly the heat shock proteins, in some way attenuate glucocorticoid action. Overcoming glucocorticoid resistance may require dosages of prednisone as high as 100 mg/day and dosages of dexamethasone as high as 20 mg/day. These high doses expose the rest of the tissues in the patient's body, which have normal responsiveness to glucocorticoid, to an extremely enhanced glucocorticoid effect. Over time, this leads to Cushing syndrome, whose potentially lethal effects may force the tapering or even discontinuance of glucocorticoid therapy.

An invariable aspect of Cushing syndrome induced by exogenous glucocorticoid is suppression of ACTH secretion. In contrast to the recovery of pituitary secretion of other hormones, such as thyroid-stimulating hormone or luteinizing hormone and follicle-stimulating hormone, recovery of ACTH secretion is very slow; the return to normal may require a year or more. Thus, the physician must ensure that the HPA axis is intact before completely withdrawing long-term glucocorticoids.

Pharmacologic glucocorticoid therapy is typically initiated at a high dose (e.g., prednisone, 60 mg daily in divided doses). As soon as the disease process is controlled, the dose is reduced in 5% increments weekly in an attempt to find the lowest effective dose as quickly as possible. The ultimate goal is to taper to normal replacement doses of the glucocorticoid. When the glucocorticoid dose approximates the replacement level, the preparation is changed to an equivalent dose of hydrocortisone given at a dosage of 12 mg/m² once a day in the morning. This dose remains unchanged until it is safe to withdraw glucocorticoid therapy completely or until the disease reactivates, in which case the process is begun anew. Patients receiving hydrocortisone at the replacement dose should undergo cosyntropin stimulation testing every 3 months. When the plasma cortisol response to cosyntropin exceeds 20 μg/dl, hydrocortisone can be discontinued safely. In the event that the dose cannot be lowered to replacement levels because of recurrent disease activity, alternative and adjunctive non–glucocorticoid-based therapies must be aggressively pursued in the hope that they might permit tapering of the glucocorticoid to replacement dose before the ravages of Cushing syndrome demand cessation of glucocorticoid treatment in the setting of an uncontrolled inflammatory or neoplastic illness.

The author has no commercial relationships with manufacturers of products or providers of services discussed in this chapter.

References

1. Esteban NV, Loughlin T, Yergey AL, et al: Daily cortisol production rate in men determined by stable isotope dilution/mass spectrometry. J Clin Endocr Metab 72:39, 1991

2. Cushing H: The Pituitary Body and Its Disorders. JB Lippincott, Philadelphia, 1912

3. Danese RD, Aron DC: Principles of clinical epidemiology and their application to the diagnosis of Cushing's syndrome: Rev. Bayes meets Dr. Cushing. Endocrinologist 4:339, 1994

4. Reimondo G, Paccotti P, Minetto M, et al: The corticotrophin-releasing hormone test is the most reliable noninvasive method to differentiate pituitary from ectopic ACTH secretion in Cushing's syndrome. Clin Endocrinol (Oxf) 58:718, 2003

5. Nieman LK, Loriaux DL: Corticotropin releasing hormone: clinical applications. Annu Rev Med 40:331, 1989

6. Hodge BO, Froesch TA: Familial Cushing's syndrome: micronodular adrenocortical dysplasia. Arch Intern Med 148:1133, 1988

7. Oldfield EH, Chrousos GP, Schulte HM, et al: Preoperative lateralization of ACTH secreting pituitary microadenomas by bilateral and simultaneous inferior petrosal sinus sampling. N Engl J Med 312:100, 1985

8. Ng L, Libertino JM: Adrenocortical carcinoma: diagnosis, evaluation and treatment. J Urol 169:5, 2003

9. Schteingart DE: Current perspective in the diagnosis and treatment of adrenocortical carcinoma. Rev Endocr Metab Disord 2:323, 2001

10. NIH state-of-the-science statement on management of the clinically inapparent adrenal mass ("incidentaloma"). NIH Consens State Sci Statements 19:1, 2002

11. Pena CS, Boland GW, Hahn PF, et al: Characterization of intermediate (lipid poor) adrenal masses: use of washout characteristics of contrast-enhanced CT. Radiology 217:798, 2000

12. Dunnick NR, Korobkin M: Imaging of adrenal incidentalomas: current status. AJR Am J Roentgenol 179:559, 2002

13. A survey on adrenal incidentaloma in Italy. Study Group on Adrenal Tumors of the Italian Society of Endocrinology. J Clin Endocrinol Metab 85:637, 2000

14. Hamrahian AH, Oseni TS, Arafah BM: Measurement of serum free cortisol in critically ill patients. N Engl J Med 350:1629, 2004

15. Dunnick NR, Doppman JL, Gill JR Jr, et al: Localization of functional adrenal tumors by computed tomography and venous sampling. Radiology 142:429, 1982

16. Young WF Jr, Horgan MJ, Klee GG, et al: Primary aldosteronism: diagnosis and treatment. Mayo Clin Proc 65:96, 1990

Acknowledgment

Figures 3, 4, and 5 Seward Hung.

56 Testes and Testicular Disorders

Peter J. Snyder, M.D.

The testes begin to function early in utero and continue to function into senescence, but the consequences of their function differ at different stages of life. Diseases that affect testicular function, therefore, also have different consequences at different stages of life. Testicular function can be affected by diseases of the hypothalamus and pituitary, as well as by diseases of the testes themselves. The diseases may be either congenital or acquired [see Tables 1 and 2].

Normal Testicular Function

The testes have two functions, the secretion of testosterone by the Leydig cells and the production of sperm by the seminiferous tubules. The cumulative effect of testosterone is to produce and maintain a phenotypic male. Testicular function is stimulated by the gonadotropins, follicle-stimulating hormone (FSH) and luteinizing hormone (LH), which are secreted by the gonadotroph cells of the pituitary gland, which in turn are stimulated by gonadotropin-releasing hormone (GnRH) from the hypothalamus.

GONADOTROPIN SYNTHESIS AND SECRETION

GnRH is a decapeptide cleaved from a larger precursor peptide that is synthesized in the arcuate nucleus of the hypothalamus. FSH and LH are synthesized in the gonadotroph cells of the pituitary. Each is a heterodimeric glycopeptide consisting of a common α subunit and a unique β subunit.

GnRH travels via the hypothalamic-pituitary portal circulation to the pituitary, where it binds to G protein–coupled receptors on the surface of the gonadotroph cell. This triggers a cascade of intracellular signaling pathways and stimulates LH and FSH release. Although GnRH cannot be measured readily in the portal or peripheral circulation of humans, its secretion is thought to be pulsatile, because LH secretion is pulsatile. In addition, administration of GnRH to men who have GnRH deficiency increases LH secretion to normal only if GnRH is administered in pulses.[1]

TESTOSTERONE

Synthesis and Secretion

LH stimulates testosterone synthesis by binding to a surface receptor on the Leydig cells and activating a cyclic adenosine monophosphate–mediated mechanism that increases cholesterol side-chain cleavage and conversion to pregnenolone and eventually to testosterone. Testosterone is synthesized at a rate of 5 to 7 mg a day. Testosterone secretion is episodic, like that of LH, and follows a diurnal pattern. In normal young men, the highest concentrations of testosterone occur at about 8 A.M.; the lowest, at about 8 P.M.[2]

Plasma Binding

Circulating testosterone is 98% to 99% bound. About 40% is bound to sex hormone–binding globulin (SHBG) with high affinity; 60% is bound to albumin with low affinity. Testosterone bound to SHBG is not available to tissues, but that bound to albumin probably is available. SHBG synthesis is stimulated by estrogens and decreased by androgens and obesity.

Actions

Testosterone has many different effects in many different tissues, at least partly because it can act on a cellular level as three

Table 1   Causes of Primary Hypogonadism

Congenital	Chromosomal abnormalities 　Klinefelter syndrome 　46 XX male 　Microdeletions of the long arm of the Y chromosome Cryptorchidism Disorders of androgen biosynthesis Myotonic dystrophy
Acquired	Orchitis (e.g., mumps) Ionizing radiation Drugs 　Alkylating agents 　Ketoconazole 　Alcohol Trauma Testicular torsion Autoimmune damage AIDS

Table 2   Causes of Secondary Hypogonadism

Congenital	Isolated gonadotropin deficiency 　Isolated gonadotropin-releasing hormone (GnRH) 　　deficiency 　　　With anosmia (Kallmann syndrome) 　　　With other abnormalities (Prader-Willi, 　　　　Lawrence-Moon-Biedl syndromes) 　　　Without other abnormalities 　　Mutations of the GnRH receptor, *LH*β, or *DAX-1* genes Multiple hypothalamic and pituitary hormone 　deficiencies
Acquired	Benign tumors and cysts 　Pituitary adenomas 　Craniopharyngiomas, dysgerminomas, Rathke 　　pouch cysts Malignant tumors 　Metastases from lung, breast, and other malignancies 　Meningiomas, gliomas 　Lymphomas Infiltrative diseases (e.g., sarcoidosis, Langerhans cell 　histiocytosis, hemochromatosis Infectious diseases (e.g., tuberculosis, histoplasmosis) Infarction of the pituitary (e.g., Sheehan syndrome) Lymphocytic hypophysitis Trauma Surgery Radiation Systemic illness (starvation, anorexia, acute and 　chronic illness) Medications (glucocorticoids, megestrol acetate, suramin) Drugs of abuse (alcohol, opiates) Hyperprolactinemia Isolated acquired GnRH deficiency

distinct hormones: testosterone itself and its two metabolites, dihydrotestosterone (DHT) and estradiol. Both testosterone and DHT act by binding to the androgen receptor, which is encoded by a gene that is located on the X chromosome and belongs to the steroid-retinoid-thyroid hormone superfamily of receptors.[3] Although there is only one androgen receptor, the presence of coactivators or corepressors of transcription in certain types of cells could explain why the effects of testosterone vary in different tissues.[4]

The direct effect of testosterone on cells is mediated by its passive diffusion into cells, its binding to the androgen receptor, the binding of the testosterone–androgen receptor complex to DNA, and subsequent stimulation of messenger RNA (mRNA) and protein synthesis. This mechanism appears to be responsible for testosterone's stimulation of the wolffian ducts to become the male internal genitalia during embryonic development[5] and for testosterone's inhibition of gonadotropin secretion. Testosterone has a probable role in the stimulation of erythropoiesis; the growth of muscle; an increase in linear bone growth; and, to some degree, an increase in bone mineral density.

In tissues that express the enzyme 5α-reductase, testosterone is irreversibly converted to DHT in the target cell cytoplasm. Two forms of 5α-reductase have been identified: type 1, which is found predominantly in nongenital skin and the liver; and type 2, which is found predominantly in urogenital tissue in both men and women. DHT binds to the androgen receptor with greater affinity than does testosterone and so has a greater effect than testosterone. After DHT binds to the androgen receptor, the DHT-receptor complex binds to DNA, stimulating mRNA and protein synthesis. This mechanism appears to be responsible for male differentiation of the external genitalia in utero,[5] enlargement of the male external genitalia during puberty, and the development of sexual hair during puberty.

In tissues that express the enzyme complex aromatase—especially some hypothalamic nuclei, adipose tissue, liver, and perhaps bone—testosterone is converted to estradiol, which binds to an estrogen receptor. This mechanism appears to mediate several effects of testosterone. One effect is on bone: in males who have mutations of the gene coding for the estrogen receptor[6] or the aromatase enzyme,[7] the epiphyses do not close and the bones are osteoporotic. Another effect is on libido, as suggested by the case report of a man who lacked aromatase and had poor libido until he was treated with estradiol.[8] Aromatase appears to partially mediate the inhibition of LH secretion by testosterone and to entirely mediate the inhibition of FSH secretion by testosterone.[9]

SPERMATOGENESIS

Spermatogenesis occurs in the seminiferous tubules, stimulated principally by testosterone. The concentration of testosterone within the testes is 100 times that in the peripheral circulation. This high concentration, which is essential for spermatogenesis, probably results from both the LH-stimulated production of testosterone in the nearby Leydig cells and the FSH-stimulated binding of testosterone by androgen-binding protein, produced by the Sertoli cells of the seminiferous tubules. FSH also stimulates the Sertoli cells to secrete activin, which stimulates spermatogenesis. In addition, the Sertoli cells secrete inhibin, which inhibits FSH secretion by the pituitary.

Spermatogenesis takes approximately 3 months. Maturation of a spermatogonium to a mature spermatozoon takes approxi-

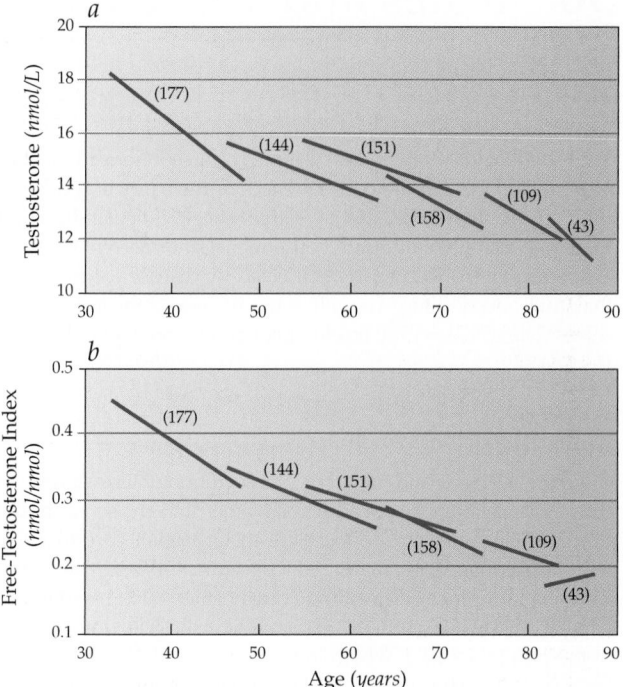

Figure 1 **Serum concentration of testosterone (*a*) and the free-testosterone index (*b*) versus age in healthy men who were followed longitudinally.[12] Each line represents the mean for a cohort of men, and the numbers in parentheses represent the number of men in each cohort.**

mately 75 days; passage through the epididymis, where motility is acquired, takes another 14 days.

TESTICULAR FUNCTION THROUGHOUT LIFE

Testicular function begins in utero, increases briefly in the first few months of infancy, develops fully during puberty, and declines gradually during adulthood.

In Utero

Sexual differentiation occurs during the first trimester in utero.[10] In the presence of the *SRY* gene, which is the sex-determining region of the Y chromosome, the undifferentiated gonads become testes. The Sertoli cells of the testes secrete antimüllerian hormone, which suppresses the müllerian ducts, thereby preventing the development of female internal genitalia.[11] Human chorionic gonadotropin (hCG) from the placenta stimulates the Leydig cells of the testes to secrete testosterone, which in turn stimulates the nearby wolffian ducts to become the male internal genitalia—the vas deferens and seminal vesicles. In addition, testosterone is converted to DHT by the anlage of the external genitalia, and DHT influences the anlage to become the penis, scrotum, and prostate. During the third trimester, LH from the fetal pituitary stimulates the fetal testes to secrete testosterone, which results in penile growth. During the first few months post partum, there is a third testosterone elevation, to levels approximating that of a midpubertal boy. The consequences of this elevation are not known. Thereafter, the serum testosterone concentration falls to relatively low values until puberty.

Puberty

Puberty in boys begins with an increase in the secretion of LH and FSH by the pituitary, which is presumably stimulated by an increase in GnRH secretion by the hypothalamus. This takes place at a mean age of 11.4 years (with a standard deviation of ± 1.1 years). The initial consequence is an increase in testicular volume, from 2 ml toward its adult volume of 20 to 25 ml. Rising levels of circulating testosterone cause an increase in the size of the phallus and promote the growth of pubic, axillary, and eventually body and facial hair, along with regression of temporal scalp hair. Testosterone also causes an increase in long bone growth and body height, thickening of the vocal cords and lowering of the voice, and an increase in hemoglobin concentration. Most of these changes are completed within 4 to 5 years, but full development of body hair and beard may take several more years, and temporal scalp hair regression continues for decades.

Senescence

As men age, their serum total testosterone concentration decreases [see Figure 1].[12-14] The decrease in the serum concentration of total testosterone is very gradual and of relatively small magnitude. SHBG, however, increases with increasing age, so the free-testosterone concentration decreases to a greater degree than the total. By 80 years of age, according to cross-sectional studies, the free-testosterone concentration is one half to one third that at 20 years of age.[15,16] The decrease in testosterone appears to result from both decreased LH secretion and decreased responsiveness of the Leydig cells.[17] The parallels between male senescence and male hypogonadism—both of which are marked by decreases in libido, energy, muscle mass and strength, and bone mineral density—suggest that testosterone deficiency could be a cause of the changes in male senescence.[17] Serum estradiol concentration also decreases with increasing age, however. Several studies show a better correlation of some consequences of aging, such as the decrease in bone mineral density, with the estradiol level than with the testosterone level. Nevertheless, there is preliminary evidence that increasing the serum testosterone concentration of elderly men to that of young men increases bone mineral density[18] and muscle mass and decreases fat mass,[19] which supports the notion that the decrease in testosterone does have adverse consequences.

Male Hypogonadism

ETIOLOGY

Male hypogonadism can occur as a consequence of a disease of the testes (primary hypogonadism) or as a consequence of a disease of the pituitary or hypothalamus (secondary hypogonadism). Certain clinical findings suggest hypogonadism, but these are usually nonspecific, so the diagnosis must be confirmed by laboratory tests.

DIAGNOSIS

Clinical Findings

The clinical findings of hypogonadism result from either decreased spermatogenesis or decreased testosterone secretion. The sole clinical finding of decreased spermatogenesis is infertility. In contrast, decreased testosterone secretion causes a wide variety of clinical findings; specific findings depend on the stage of life in which the deficiency occurs. When testosterone defi-

ciency occurs in the first trimester in utero, male sexual differentiation is incomplete. Complete lack of testosterone during this period results in female external genitalia (i.e., clitoris and labia). Incomplete testosterone deficiency causes partial virilization, ranging from posterior labial fusion when testosterone deficiency is severe to hypospadias when testosterone deficiency is mild. Testosterone deficiency that begins in the third trimester in utero results in normal male sexual differentiation but microphallus at birth. When testosterone deficiency occurs in childhood but before puberty, the result is incomplete puberty. When testosterone deficiency develops after puberty, some pubertal changes regress; such changes usually occur slowly, and the effects can occur at different rates. Energy and libido diminish within days to weeks of the fall in testosterone, and the hemoglobin concentration and hematocrit decline within a few months. Decreases in sexual hair, muscle mass, and bone mineral density are usually not recognized for several years.

Physical Examination

The physical examination focuses primarily on whether sexual development is consistent with the patient's age. If the patient is an adult, he should have facial, chest, and other body hair; temporal scalp hair should be receding appropriately for the patient's age and family pattern; and pubic hair should be dense and in a diamond pattern. The voice should be appropriately deep. Musculature should be normal for a man. Subcutaneous fat should be less than that of a boy or a woman. The testes should be 4 to 7 cm in length (20 to 25 ml in volume). If the patient is an adolescent, development should be appropriate for his age. If the patient is a child, the testes should be descended, and no hypospadias should be present.

The physical examination should also include evaluation for possible eunuchoid proportions and gynecomastia. An adult male usually has an upper body segment approximately equal to his lower segment and an arm span equal to his height. The absence of testosterone and the continued presence of growth hormone during puberty, as occurs in primary hypogonadism and isolated secondary hypogonadism, causes a delay in epiphyseal closure and an increase in the length of the long bones. In such patients, the lower body segment becomes longer than the upper and the arms become longer than the legs—a relationship known as eunuchoid proportions. This relationship persists even after testosterone treatment. Consequently, a man of any age who has a heel-to-pubis measurement more than 2 cm longer than his pubis-to-crown measurement and an arm span more than 2 cm longer than his height was probably hypogonadal during adolescence. Gynecomastia often occurs in hypogonadism; it is especially common in patients with primary hypogonadism.

Laboratory Findings

Once the diagnosis of hypogonadism has been suspected on the basis of symptoms and signs, the diagnosis must be confirmed by documenting decreased production of sperm or testosterone. If hypogonadism is confirmed, the next step is to measure LH and FSH. Elevated serum concentrations of LH and FSH indicate primary hypogonadism, whereas subnormal or normal values indicate secondary hypogonadism.

Spermatogenesis Sperm production can be assessed most readily by counting the sperm in an ejaculated semen specimen. Generally accepted normal values for ejaculated sperm are a density of greater than 20×10^6 sperm/ml of ejaculate and a total count of more than 40×10^6 sperm/ejaculate. More than 60% of the sperm should be motile, and more than 30% should be normal in morphology. A study of the male partners in 765 infertile couples and 696 fertile couples showed that fertility was associated with a sperm density of greater than 48×10^6 sperm/ml, sperm motility of greater than 63%, and normal morphology in more than 12% of sperm.[20] Low fertility was associated with a sperm density of less than 13.5×10^6 sperm/ml, sperm motility of less than 32%, and normal morphology in less than 9%. Indeterminate fertility was associated with intermediate values. A severely subnormal sperm count (e.g., $< 5 \times 10^6$ sperm/specimen) can result from either primary or secondary hypogonadism. A normal or mildly subnormal sperm count (e.g., 35×10^6 sperm/specimen) associated with markedly abnormal sperm motility more likely indicates a primary spermatogenic abnormality and less likely indicates secondary hypogonadism.

Testicular biopsy usually provides no more information about spermatogenesis than a semen analysis, because the variety of histologic responses to testicular injury is very limited. Testicular biopsy is likely to be helpful only when the ejaculated semen contains no sperm but the testicular size is normal and the serum concentrations of testosterone, LH, and FSH are normal. Such a patient may have obstruction of the ejaculatory outflow, or he may have suffered damage to the seminiferous tubules sufficient to impair spermatogenesis but not sufficient to cause an elevation in the serum FSH concentration. A testicular biopsy showing normal seminiferous tubules would favor the former diagnosis.

Testosterone concentration   Testosterone secretion is best evaluated by measuring the serum concentration of total testosterone, because the total testosterone level is usually an accurate reflection of the free-testosterone level. Also, most of the current assay techniques for free testosterone are not as accurate as those for total testosterone. Testosterone is secreted into the circulation episodically, in a diurnal pattern; the serum testosterone concentration is highest at about 8 A.M. and lowest at about 8 P.M.[2] Therefore, the serum testosterone concentration should be measured at 8 A.M. If the result is low or borderline, the test should be repeated. Measurement of free testosterone and SHBG may be helpful in situations in which the total testosterone level does not accurately reflect the free-testosterone level, such as would be the case with obese patients. If free testosterone is measured, the assay method should be equilibrium dialysis.

Gonadotropins   If the testosterone concentration is low, serum LH and FSH concentrations should be measured. If those values are high, the patient has primary hypogonadism; otherwise, he has secondary hypogonadism. In a patient with a distinctly subnormal sperm count but a normal serum testosterone concentration, the combination of an elevated FSH concentration and a normal LH concentration indicates that there has been damage to the seminiferous tubules but that the Leydig cells have not been affected.

In patients with secondary hypogonadism, magnetic resonance imaging of the sellar region is indicated. The MRI scan will show whether the patient has a mass lesion and, if so, whether it is in the pituitary, the hypothalamus, or the parasellar region. Pituitary and hypothalamic lesions cannot be distinguished on the basis of the LH response to a single dose of exogenous GnRH. Administration of repeated doses of exogenous GnRH, however, will result in a normal LH response to an individual dose of GnRH in patients who have hypothalamic disease, but not in patients who have pituitary disease. In patients with hypothalamic disease, the length of time required for LH response to become normal varies widely.

DISEASES THAT CAUSE HYPOGONADISM

Overall, primary hypogonadism [*see Table 1*] is more common than secondary hypogonadism [*see Table 2*]. Once a patient's hypogonadism has been identified as primary or secondary, the specific etiology can be sought.

Primary Hypogonadism

Primary hypogonadism may be congenital or acquired. Many cases of primary hypogonadism have no identifiable cause, however. Presumably, many causes are yet unknown.

Congenital   Of the congenital abnormalities that cause primary hypogonadism, the most common is Klinefelter syndrome,[21] which occurs in approximately 0.2% of newborns. It is the phenotypic presentation of a male with more than one X chromosome. The most common genotype is 47 XXY, but additional X chromosomes (e.g., 48 XXXY) and mosaics (e.g., 46 XY/47 XXY) have also been reported. The 47 XXY genotype results from nondisjunction of the sex chromosomes of either parent during meiotic division. Mosaicism probably results from nondisjunctive mitotic division after conception. The severity of the phenotypic consequences usually increases with the number of extra X chromosomes. The gonadal consequences are usually severe damage to the seminiferous tubules and variable damage (minimal to severe) to the Leydig cells. Consequently, men with Klinefelter syndrome usually have very small testes, no sperm in their ejaculate, infertility, and markedly high serum FSH concentrations. Their serum testosterone concentrations vary from normal to subnormal; correspondingly, their virilization varies from normal to low and their serum LH concentrations vary from normal to elevated. Klinefelter syndrome is also usually marked by abnormalities of behavior and of the long bones. These abnormalities are not directly related to the gonadal abnormalities. The behavioral abnormality is manifested as difficulty in social interactions that is recognized in childhood, and it leads to problems in school and eventually in work. The long-bone abnormality is increased length of the legs but not the arms; this abnormality occurs independently of increased length of both the arms and legs as a result of testosterone deficiency.

The diagnosis of Klinefelter syndrome can usually be made by determining the karyotype of the peripheral leukocytes. Testosterone deficiency, if present, can be treated with testosterone replacement (see below). The behavioral abnormality cannot be treated satisfactorily, but a support group can be helpful for the patient's family, and school counselors should be advised of the diagnosis.

Cryptorchidism, or undescended testes, is also associated with damage to the testes and with greater damage to the seminiferous tubules than to the Leydig cells. More than one mechanism may be involved: testosterone deficiency in utero may inhibit descent, and the heat of the abdomen may cause further damage to the undescended testis. The clinical consequences depend partly on whether one or both testes are undescended. If only one testis is undescended, there is a 25% to 33% likelihood that the sperm count will be subnormal and the serum FSH level slightly high.[22] If both testes are undescended, the sperm count will likely be severely subnormal and the patient infertile; the serum testosterone concentration may be subnormal, and the patient may be undervirilized as well. Neoplasms are two to five times more likely to develop in cryptorchid testes.[23] The diagnosis is made in patients younger than 1 year by failure to palpate a testis that either is within the scrotum or can be manipulated manually from the inguinal canal into the scrotum.

Varicocele—a varicosity of the venous plexus within the scrotum—has for decades been considered a possible cause of infertility. The proposed mechanism is that varicocele causes an increase in blood flow, which impairs spermatogenesis by raising scrotal temperature above normal. However, scrotal temperatures are similar in infertile men with and without varicoceles, and varicoceles are not much more common in infertile than fertile men, so it is not certain that varicocele can cause infertility. More important, in a randomized trial of the surgical treatment of varicocele in men who were infertile, fertility was not found to be improved as a result of treatment.[24] Therefore, surgical treatment of a varicocele cannot be recommended as a means of improving fertility.

Congenital deficiency of testosterone production can also result from mutations of genes that encode enzymes necessary for androgen biosynthesis. These disorders are rare. The cholesterol side-chain cleavage enzymes 3β-hydroxysteroid dehydrogenase and 17α-hydroxylase occur in the adrenal as well as in the testes, so deficiencies of either of these enzymes lead to deficient cortisol secretion as well. Deficiency of 17β-hydroxysteroid oxidoreductase affects only the testes. All of these disorders result in deficient testosterone secretion, beginning in the first trimester in utero, and subsequent incomplete virilization. The degree of incompleteness, especially of phallic development, influences whether these babies are raised as boys or girls. The testosterone deficiency itself can be treated in the same way as testosterone deficiency from any other cause.

Deletions on the long arm of the Y chromosome appear to be associated with infertility. Azoospermia is more common than oligospermia in such cases.[25]

Acquired Many acquired illnesses can cause primary hypogonadism. These include infections—notably, mumps orchitis. Orchitis is an uncommon complication of mumps and may be unilateral. In bilateral cases, both testes initially become markedly swollen and severely painful, then gradually atrophy. Diminished sperm production is common; decreased testosterone secretion is less common. The diagnosis is made by eliciting a history of painful swelling of the testes during systemic mumps infection.

Treatment of neoplasms with chemotherapeutic drugs (especially alkylating agents) or with radiation therapy to the inguinal lymph nodes often damages the seminiferous tubules; less often, it damages the Leydig cells. Radiation causes damage despite shielding of the testes, because of radiation scatter. The degree of damage is usually proportionate to the radiation dose. In cases of less extensive treatment, the damage may be reversible. No specific remedy for such damage is available, however.

Medications and drugs of abuse can produce hypogonadism. The antifungal agent ketoconazole impairs testosterone production. Heavy alcohol ingestion damages the testes.

HIV infection and AIDS wasting are commonly associated with hypogonadism.[26] Several mechanisms appear to be involved in these cases. Some men with HIV infection and subnormal serum testosterone concentrations have inappropriately low serum concentrations of LH. This may be the result of conditions such as malnutrition, opiate abuse, and megestrol acetate administration, all of which are known to cause secondary hypogonadism. Other men with HIV infection lack known risk factors for secondary hypogonadism but have elevated serum concentrations of LH, indicating primary hypogonadism. Hypogonadism in HIV-infected men has been observed less commonly since the introduction of retroviral therapy.

Testicular torsion can cause permanent damage if not treated promptly. Trauma to the testes can sometimes be sufficiently severe to damage them.

Hypogonadism may be induced (surgically or chemically) as a therapeutic strategy in cases of advanced prostate cancer [see Chapter 201]. Bilateral orchiectomy is used as a treatment for bilateral testicular cancer. In testicular cancer patients, however—unlike those treated with castration for prostate cancer—there is no reason to withhold testosterone replacement.

Secondary Hypogonadism

Like primary hypogonadism, secondary hypogonadism (also called hypogonadotropic hypogonadism) has both congenital and acquired causes in men [see Table 2]. Unlike primary hypogonadism, secondary hypogonadism often has a cause that is amenable to specific treatment. For that reason, finding the cause carries particular importance. Pituitary adenomas, other benign tumors and cysts of the sellar area, and malignancies that arise in the sellar region or metastasize there can usually be detected by MRI. Infiltrative diseases (e.g., sarcoidosis, hemochromatosis) usually produce manifestations in other organ systems that suggest the diagnosis. Tumors, cysts, and infiltrative lesions are often accompanied by deficiencies of other hypothalamic or pituitary hormones.

Some cases of secondary hypogonadism are not associated with any other hormonal abnormalities and are called isolated. Some cases appear to be caused by a deficiency of GnRH secretion by the hypothalamus; such cases can be congenital or acquired. When congenital, they may or may not be a part of Kallmann syndrome.[27] Patients with Kallmann syndrome have deficient GnRH secretion, variably associated with anosmia, cryptorchidism, red-green color blindness, and long-bone and urogenital tract abnormalities. Kallmann syndrome may occur sporadically or in families; familial cases can be inherited in an autosomal dominant pattern, with expression mostly limited to males, or in an X-linked recessive pattern. The genetic defect responsible both for the deficiency in GnRH secretion and for anosmia in some patients who have the X-linked recessive form of Kallmann syndrome is a mutation in the *KAL-1* gene, which encodes a neural cell adhesion protein, anosmin. When this protein is not present during embryogenesis, GnRH-secreting neurons do not migrate from the olfactory placode to the olfactory bulb and then to the hypothalamus, resulting in both anosmia and hypogonadotropic hypogonadism.

Another cause of isolated secondary hypogonadism is a mutation of the GnRH receptor. In these cases, GnRH is secreted by the hypothalamus but does not stimulate LH secretion by the pituitary. A third cause is a mutation of the *DAX-1* gene, which leads to hypogonadotropic hypogonadism and to adrenal hypoplasia congenita.

Gonadotropin secretion can be reversibly inhibited by any systemic illness or by hyperprolactinemia. Inhibition from medications, such as glucocorticoids, suramin, and opiates, is also reversible. Since the introduction and widespread use of controlled-release forms of opioids for chronic-pain management, hypogonadism from these medications has become more common.[28] Heroin addicts may experience hypogonadism by the same mechanism. Damage to the pituitary from surgery or radiation, in contrast, usually results in permanent inhibition of gonadotropin secretion.

Delayed puberty is diagnosed in any boy whose pubertal development does not begin by more than two standard deviations past the mean age. In some cases, this delay represents a normal variant; these patients eventually enter puberty spontaneously. In other cases, the delay is caused by secondary hypogonadism. Distinguishing a normal variant from pathologic delay can be difficult. The degree of hypogonadism is usually not helpful in making this distinction, nor is any biochemical test. A family history of delayed puberty or constitutional short stature increases the likelihood of physiologic delayed puberty. Anosmia, symptoms of a chiasmal lesion, or other signs of a specific hypothalamic or pituitary disease increase the likelihood of an organic lesion as the cause. In many cases, the diagnosis can be made only by continued observation.

In an otherwise healthy elderly man, an unequivocally subnormal serum testosterone concentration, along with an LH concentration that is not elevated, can be considered a form of secondary hypogonadism.

TREATMENT

Testosterone Replacement

Testosterone can be replaced whether the hypogonadism is primary or secondary. Unlike estrogen, testosterone itself is not suitable for oral replacement, because it is catabolized rapidly during its first pass through the liver. Derivatives of testosterone that are alkylated in the 17α position do not undergo this rapid hepatic catabolism; however, these agents appear to lack the full virilizing effect of testosterone, and they may cause hepatic toxicity, including cholestatic jaundice, a cystic condition of the liver called peliosis, and, possibly, hepatocellular carcinoma. Consequently, the 17α-alkylated androgens should not be used to treat testosterone deficiency.

Currently, replacement therapy is delivered by the intramuscular or transdermal route. The intramuscular formulations, testosterone enanthate and testosterone cypionate, are long-acting esters of testosterone produced by esterifying the hydroxyl group in the 17β position with a fatty acid. These do produce full virilization. They are usually administered in doses of 150 to 200 mg by deep intramuscular injection every 2 weeks. With this regimen, serum testosterone values peak within 1 to 2 days after the injection and fall to a nadir just before the next injection [*see Figure 2*].[29] These fluctuations are noticed by some patients as fluctuations in energy, mood, and libido.

Transdermal testosterone is available in both patch[30] and gel[31] form [*see Figure 2*]. In most hypogonadal men, these preparations usually produce serum testosterone concentrations that are within the normal range and that fluctuate no more than physiologically, resulting in reasonable stability of energy, mood, and libido. The relatively physiologic pattern of serum testosterone concentrations and the infrequency of side effects make transdermal preparations the best means of testosterone replacement for most hypogonadal men.

During replacement therapy, clinicians should monitor patients for the efficacy and side effects of testosterone. Efficacy is determined by measurement of the serum testosterone concentration, which should be in the middle of the normal range mid-

way between injections of testosterone esters and at any time after application of a transdermal preparation. Serum testosterone concentrations can vary with any of these preparations, however, so testosterone should be measured more than once to determine whether the initial dose is optimal. Serum testosterone should be measured again after a dose is changed and then once or twice a year. If the serum testosterone concentration is maintained within the normal range, the patient should experience reversal of the consequences of testosterone deficiency. Specifically, energy, libido, hemoglobin concentration, muscle mass, and bone density will increase.[32]

Men older than 40 years who are receiving testosterone replacement should be monitored for testosterone-dependent diseases, such as prostate cancer, benign prostatic hyperplasia, and erythrocytosis. However, there is as yet no evidence that exogenous testosterone is more likely to exacerbate any of these conditions than is endogenous testosterone.

Stimulation of Spermatogenesis

When sperm production is impaired by damage to the seminiferous tubules, no treatment can improve fertility. However, if some mature sperm are produced, they may be used for in vitro fertilization. When the sperm count is low because of pituitary or hypothalamic disease, sperm production can often be stimulated to within the normal range by administration of exogenous gonadotropins. If the hypogonadism occurred postpubertally, usually only LH need be replaced. If the hypogonadism occurred prepubertally, usually both LH and FSH need to be replaced.[33] In hypogonadism secondary to hypothalamic disease, spermatogenesis can also be stimulated by pulsatile administration of GnRH.

Androgen Insensitivity

Generalized tissue insensitivity to the action of androgens results in abnormalities similar to those of testosterone deficiency. Such insensitivity can be caused by abnormalities of either the androgen receptor[34] or 5α-reductase type 2 enzyme.[35] Both conditions result from genetic mutations, both are rare, and both result in incomplete virilization of the external genitalia.

Many different mutations of the androgen receptor gene have been described. Some of these mutations interfere with binding of androgen to the receptor, and others interfere with binding of the androgen-receptor complex to the DNA of the androgen-responsive cell.

The clinical presentations of the different receptor abnormalities also vary. In the most severe clinical presentation, called complete androgen insensitivity, the affected person is born with testes in the inguinal canals, no internal genitalia, and female external genitalia. At puberty, the serum testosterone concentration increases to a high-normal or slightly above-normal value, but sexual hair does not develop. Breasts do develop, because testosterone can still be converted to estradiol. In incomplete androgen insensitivity, there is variable partial fusion of the labial folds: a lesser degree of fusion results in genitalia that are still more female than male, and a greater degree results in genitalia that are more, but still incompletely, male. The least severe form of androgen resistance is manifested only by infertility and sometimes gynecomastia. Serum testosterone and LH concentrations are high normal to slightly high in all of these forms of androgen resistance.

Kennedy disease consists of a relatively mild form of androgen insensitivity but progressively severe spinal bulbar neuropa-

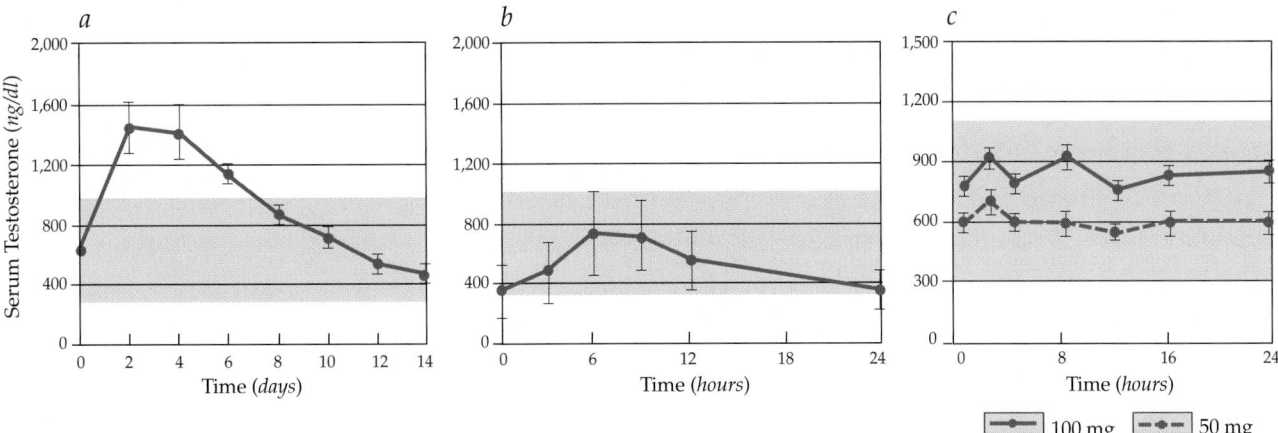

Figure 2 **Serum testosterone concentrations during the course of chronic administration of three different testosterone preparations to hypogonadal men. (*a*) Concentrations during 14 days after the injection of 200 mg of testosterone enanthate.[29] (*b*) Concentrations during the 24 hours after application of a testosterone patch that delivers approximately 5 mg of testosterone.[41] (*c*) Concentrations during the 24 hours after application of a testosterone gel containing 50 or 100 mg of testosterone.[31]**

thy. It is caused by a mutation leading to doubling of the number of N-terminal glutamines in the androgen receptor.

Other mutations of the androgen receptor have been described in metastatic prostate cancer that has become resistant to androgen deprivation. These mutations may allow ligands other than testosterone to bind to the receptor and stimulate receptor-dependent functions even in the absence of testosterone.

Mutations of the 5α-reductase type 2 gene also lead to incomplete virilization of the external genitalia because virilization requires conversion of testosterone to DHT by this enzyme.[35] At birth, most males with 5α-reductase type 2 deficiency have external genitalia that are predominantly female, so the sex of rearing is usually female. At puberty, the serum testosterone concentration increases and overcomes the lack of DHT to some degree; binding of testosterone to the androgen receptor causes phallic enlargement and hair growth in an adult male pattern. If the patient is being raised as a female, the testes can be removed before puberty to prevent these events.

Gynecomastia

Gynecomastia is the development of glandular breast tissue in a man. In most cases of gynecomastia, the stimulation of glandular tissue appears to result from an increased ratio of estrogen to androgen.

EPIDEMIOLOGY

Gynecomastia is common at all ages of life but is more common in infancy, puberty, and from middle age on. In most large series, gynecomastia can be detected in 10% to 20% of midpubertal boys and in more than 50% of men older than 50 years. These high rates probably reflect the hormonal changes that typically occur at those ages and do not represent disease.

ETIOLOGY AND PATHOGENESIS

The common mechanism for gynecomastia appears to be an increased estrogen-to-androgen effect on the breast. This may involve an increase in estrogen effect or a decrease in androgen effect, or both, and may result from changes in hormonal production or in hormonal action at the cellular level. Normally, most of the estrogen in the peripheral circulation in men is produced by the conversion of testosterone to estradiol or of androstenedione to estrone by the enzyme complex aromatase, which is concentrated in adipose tissue and the liver.

Exposure to Exogenous Estrogen

Gynecomastia from exogenous estrogens is uncommon. Reported cases have involved exposure to a partner's vaginal cream, application of antibalding creams, dietary intake, and occupational exposure.

Increased Estrogen Secretion

The most common cause of increased endogenous estrogen secretion is increased gonadotropin stimulation of the testes, which increases intratesticular aromatase levels and thereby increases the amount of estradiol secreted relative to testosterone. This is the likely mechanism by which gynecomastia occurs in normal males during puberty; with refeeding after starvation; and after successful treatment of severe illness, such as chronic cardiac, hepatic, or renal disease. In these situations, a period of secondary hypogonadism is followed by normal gonadotropin secretion. Increased gonadotropin (specifically, LH) secretion is also the cause of gynecomastia in primary hypogonadism. Increased secretion of hCG is the cause in patients who have tumors of the testes or liver. Administration of hCG therapeutically (e.g., to stimulate spermatogenesis) acts similarly, especially when the dose is excessive.

Increased Peripheral Conversion of Androgens to Estrogens

Increased peripheral conversion of testosterone to estradiol or of androstenedione to estrone can occur via several mechanisms: (1) an increased rate of conversion, as in hyperthyroidism or cirrhosis of the liver; (2) an increase in the amount of aromatase, as occurs in obesity; and (3) an increased substrate for aromatization, as occurs when an adrenal carcinoma secretes large amounts of androstenedione or when an aromatizable androgen, such as a long-acting testosterone ester, is administered in excessive doses.

Inhibition of Androgen Binding

Many drugs that cause gynecomastia appear to do so by binding to the androgen receptor and thereby blocking endogenous testosterone. As a consequence, endogenous androgens have less androgenic action but are still converted to estrogens. Drugs that can block the androgen receptor include spironolactone, cimetidine, flutamide, bicalutamide, and cyproterone acetate. Inherited disorders of the androgen receptor produce similar results, although in these cases, the inhibition of binding is, of course, irreversible.

DIAGNOSIS

The diagnosis of gynecomastia is confirmed by physical examination. The examiner places a spread thumb and forefinger above and below the patient's nipple and draws them together, like calipers, toward the nipple, hugging the chest wall. Subcutaneous tissue feels soft as the fingers are drawn together, whereas gynecomastia feels firm. The diameter of the gynecomastia can be measured with a ruler. Mammography is usually unnecessary. Gynecomastia is generally bilateral, although it is occasionally unilateral. It is often asymmetrical. If the tissue is tender, the gynecomastia is more likely to be of recent origin.

Having confirmed that gynecomastia exists, the clinician then needs to find the cause. This involves inquiring about medications and searching for diseases known to cause gynecomastia [see Etiology and Pathogenesis, above].

DIFFERENTIAL DIAGNOSIS

Gynecomastia must be distinguished from carcinoma of the male breast, which is rare, and from adiposity, which is common. Breast cancer should be suspected when the breast enlargement is unilateral, nontender, not centered directly under the nipple, and hard. The diagnosis can be confirmed by mammography. Breast adiposity is bilateral and can usually be distinguished from gynecomastia by the absence of palpable glandular tissue on physical examination.

TREATMENT

Gynecomastia is not physically harmful, and it usually regresses once the cause has been removed, although regression may take many years. Therefore, treatment is indicated only if the gynecomastia is causing psychological distress. The only accepted treatment is surgical removal, which is best performed by a plastic surgeon. Small series suggest that the antiestrogen drug tamoxifen and the aromatase inhibitor testolactone can reduce gynecomastia. Anastrozole is a more potent aromatase inhibitor than testolactone, but a double-blind trial of anastrozole treatment for pubertal gynecomastia failed to show any beneficial effect over placebo.[36]

Erectile Dysfunction

Erectile dysfunction is the inability to achieve or maintain an erection sufficient for intercourse. Although occasional erectile dysfunction does not indicate disease, its occurrence on most attempts to engage in sexual activity may indicate disease and is usually very troubling to the patient and his partner. Erectile dysfunction is not the same as a decrease in libido, which is decreased sexual interest. The two usually have different causes and, therefore, different treatments.

EPIDEMIOLOGY

In a cross-sectional survey of noninstitutionalized men 40 to 70 years of age, all degrees of erectile dysfunction, from minimal to complete, occurred in 50% of men. Older men were more commonly affected, however. For example, impotence occurred in 5% of 40-year-old men and in 15% of 70-year-old men.[37] When men from the same population were followed longitudinally, the incidence of new cases was 2.5% a year.[38]

PATHOPHYSIOLOGY

Development of an erection requires intact psychological, neurologic, and vascular mechanisms.[39,40] Erotic stimuli result in neural impulses that are carried from the cerebral cortex to the penis via the spinal cord, and stimulation of the penis results in neural impulses that loop to the spinal cord and back to the penis via parasympathetic nerves. These stimuli trigger blood flow into the corpora cavernosa. The inflow of blood is mediated by relaxation of arteriolar smooth muscle under the influence of nitric oxide, the production of which is catalyzed by the enzyme nitric oxide synthetase. Nitric oxide, in turn, promotes the production of cyclic guanosine monophosphate (cGMP), which also relaxes arteriolar smooth muscle and increases blood flow. Outflow of blood from the engorged corpora cavernosa is impeded by an increase in venous resistance.

Disruption of any of these steps can lead to erectile dysfunction. The neural mechanisms can be disrupted mechanically (such as by radical prostatectomy, surgery for an abdominal aortic aneurysm, or spinal cord trauma) or pathologically (such as by diabetic autonomic neuropathy or autonomic insufficiency syndromes). They also can be disrupted functionally, such as by drugs. The vascular mechanism can be disrupted by large vessel (atherosclerotic) or small vessel (diabetic) disease. The mechanism by which hyperprolactinemia causes impotence is not known, although it does not appear to be via hypogonadism.

DIAGNOSIS

History, physical examination, and laboratory testing all contribute to finding the cause of erectile dysfunction. From the history, the physician can determine whether the patient is taking a drug or has a disease associated with this disorder. Several drugs that are used to treat hypertension may occasionally cause erectile dysfunction; these include thiazide diuretics and alpha- and beta-blocking agents. Other drugs include tranquilizers and antidepressants. Excessive alcohol ingestion can also cause erectile dysfunction. The physician should ask about a history of diabetes of long duration, including other manifestations of diabetic neuropathy, and explore psychogenic factors, including depression, anxiety, fatigue, interpersonal stresses, and chronic illness. It is useful to ask whether the patient can obtain an erection under any circumstances. If the patient has an erection on awakening in the morning or can get an erection on some occasions but not others, the cause is more likely to be psychogenic than organic.

On physical examination, the absence of peripheral pulses and the presence of femoral bruits indicate vascular disease. Neurologic disease is indicated by diminished touch sensation and proprioception and a diminished cremasteric reflex (retraction of the testis on stroking of the ipsilateral inner thigh).

Laboratory evaluation should include measurement of the serum prolactin concentration, because hyperprolactinemia can be detected in no other way. The serum testosterone concentration should be measured in a man who has decreased libido as well as erectile dysfunction, but it will rarely be helpful in a man who has erectile dysfunction but normal libido.

DIFFERENTIAL DIAGNOSIS

Erectile dysfunction should be differentiated from decreased libido, if possible, because they often have different causes and different treatments. The two conditions may occur together, however. Decreased libido is decreased sexual interest, of which the principal hormonal cause is hypogonadism. Hypogonadism does not by itself impair erectile ability. A man who has a normal libido but has difficulty getting an erection probably does not have hypogonadism, whereas a man who has decreased libido and potency should be evaluated for hypogonadism as well as erectile dysfunction.

TREATMENT

Treatment of erectile dysfunction depends on the cause. If a medication is the source of the problem, it may be possible to substitute a drug that does not affect erectile function. For example, if the patient is being treated for hypertension with a thiazide diuretic, it might be replaced with an angiotensin-converting enzyme inhibitor or a calcium channel blocker—agents that do not seem to interfere with erectile function.

Underlying disorders should be corrected whenever possible. Hyperprolactinemia can be treated with a dopamine agonist (e.g., cabergoline).

The most effective treatment for erectile dysfunction of psychogenic, vascular, or neurologic origin is sildenafil, vardenafil, or tadalafil. These agents inhibit phosphodiesterase, the enzyme that degrades cGMP, and therefore enhance smooth muscle relaxation in the corpora cavernosa, increasing arteriolar blood flow and promoting erection. In one randomized study of 329 men with erectile dysfunction who received either sildenafil or placebo, the men who took sildenafil were eventually able to get an erection on 69% of attempts, compared with 22% of attempts in men who received placebo.[39,40]

Other treatments include intraurethral instillation of alprostadil, intracavernous injection of alprostadil or prostaglandin E_1, and application of a vacuum pump to the penis. These are more cumbersome and therefore less popular than sildenafil, even when they are effective.

The author has received research support from, and has been a consultant to, Solvay Pharmaceuticals, Inc.

References

1. Crowley WF Jr, Filicori M, Spratt DI, et al: The physiology of gonadotropin-releasing hormone (GnRH) secretion in men and women. Recent Prog Horm Res 41:473, 1985

2. Bremner WJ, Vitiello V, Prinz PN: Loss of circadian rhythmicity in blood testosterone levels with aging in normal men. J Clin Endocrinol Metab 56:1278, 1983

3. Zhou ZX, Wong CI, Sar M, et al: The androgen receptor: an overview. Recent Prog Horm Res 49:249, 1994

4. Heinlein CA, Chang C: Androgen receptor (AR) coregulators: an overview. Endocr Rev 23:175, 2002

5. Wilson JD, Griffin JE, Leshin M, et al: Role of gonadal hormones in development of the sexual phenotypes. Hum Genet 58:78, 1981

6. Smith EP, Boyd J, Frank GR: Estrogen resistance caused by a mutation in the estrogen-receptor gene in a man. N Engl J Med 331:1056, 1994

7. Bilezikian JP, Morishima A, Bell J, et al: Increased bone mass as a result of estrogen therapy in a man with aromatase deficiency. N Engl J Med 339:599, 1998

8. Carani C, Rochira V, Faustini-Fustini M, et al: Role of oestrogen in male sexual behaviour: insights from the natural model of aromatase deficiency. Clin Endocrinol (Oxford) 51:517, 1999

9. Hayes FJ, DeCruz S, Seminara SB, et al: Differential regulation of gonadotropin secretion by testosterone in the human male: absence of a negative feedback effect of testosterone on follicle-stimulating hormone secretion. J Clin Endocrinol Metab 86:53, 2001

10. Parker KL, Schedl A, Schimmer BP: Gene interactions in gonadal development. Annu Rev Physiol 61:417, 1999

11. Lee MM, Donahoe PK: Mullerian inhibiting substance: a gonadal hormone with multiple functions. Endocr Rev 14:152, 1993

12. Longitudinal effects of aging on serum total and free testosterone levels in healthy men. Baltimore Longitudinal Study of Aging. J Clin Endocrinol Metab 86:724, 2001

13. Morley JE, Kaiser FE, Perry HM 3rd, et al: Longitudinal changes in testosterone, luteinizing hormone, and follicle-stimulating hormone in healthy older men. Metabolism 46:410, 1997

14. Feldman HA, Longcope C, Derby CA, et al: Age trends in the level of serum testosterone and other hormones in middle-aged men: longitudinal results from the Massachusetts male aging study. J Clin Endocrinol Metab 87:589, 2002

15. Deslypere JP, Vermeulen A: Leydig cell function in normal men: effect of age, lifestyle, residence, diet, and activity. J Clin Endocrinol Metab 59:955, 1984

16. Purifoy FE, Koopmans LH, Mayes DM: Age differences in serum androgen levels in normal adult males. Hum Biol 53:499, 1981

17. Snyder PJ: Effects of age on testicular function and consequences of testosterone treatment. J Clin Endocrinol Metab 86:2369, 2001

18. Snyder PJ, Peachey H, Hannoush P, et al: Effect of testosterone treatment on bone mineral density in men over 65 years of age. J Clin Endocrinol Metab 84:1966, 1999

19. Snyder PJ, Peachey H, Hannoush P, et al: Effect of testosterone treatment on body composition and muscle strength in men over 65 years of age. J Clin Endocrinol Metab 84:2647, 1999

20. Guzick DS, Overstreet JW, Factor-Litvak P, et al: Sperm morphology, motility, and concentration in fertile and infertile men. N Engl J Med 345:1388, 2001

21. Smyth CM, Bremner WJ: Klinefelter syndrome. Arch Intern Med 158:1309, 1998

22. Lipshultz LI, Caminos-Torres R, Greenspan CS, et al: Testicular function after orchiopexy for unilaterally undescended testis. N Engl J Med 295:15, 1976

23. Stang A, Ahrens W, Bromen K, et al: Undescended testis and the risk of testicular cancer: importance of source and classification of exposure information. Int J Epidemiol 30:1050, 2001

24. De Kretser DM, Baker HW: Infertility in men: recent advances and continuing controversies. J Clin Endocrinol Metab 84:3443, 1999

25. Foresta C, Moro E, Ferlin A: Y chromosome microdeletions and alterations of spermatogenesis. Endocr Rev 22:226, 2001

26. Sellmeye DE, Grunfeld C: Endocrine and metabolic disturbances in human immunodeficiency virus infection and acquired immunodeficiency syndrome. Endo Rev 17:518, 1996

27. Seminara SB, Hayes FJ, Crowley WF Jr: Gonadotropin-releasing hormone deficiency in the human (idiopathic hypogonadotropic hypogonadism and Kallmann's syndrome): pathophysiological and genetic considerations. Endocr Rev 19:521, 1998

28. Abs R, Verhelst J, Maeyaert J, et al: Endocrine consequences of long-term intrathecal administration of opioids. J Clin Endocrinol Metab 85:2215, 2000

29. Snyder PJ, Lawrence DA: Treatment of male hypogonadism with testosterone enanthate. J Clin Endocrinol Metab 51:1535, 1980

30. Findlay JC, Place VA, Snyder PJ: Treatment of primary hypogonadism in men by the transdermal administration of testosterone. J Clin Endocrinol Metab 68:369, 1989

31. Swerdloff RS, Wang C, Cunningham G, et al: Long-term pharmacokinetics of transdermal testosterone gel in hypogonadal men. J Clin Endocrinol Metab 85:4500, 2000

32. Snyder PJ, Peachey H, Berlin JA, et al: Effects of testosterone replacement in hypogonadal men. J Clin Endocrinol Metab 85:2670, 2000

33. Finkel DM, Phillips JL, Snyder PJ: Stimulation of spermatogenesis by gonadotropins in men with hypogonadotropic hypogonadism. N Engl J Med 313:651, 1985

34. McPhaul MJ: Molecular defects of the androgen receptor. Recent Prog Horm Res 57:181, 2002

35. Wilson JD, Griffin JE, Russell DW: Steroid 5 alpha-reductase 2 deficiency. Endocr Rev 14:577, 1993

36. Plourde PV, Reiter EO, Jou HC, et al: Safety and efficacy of anastrozole for the treatment of pubertal gynecomastia: a randomized, double-blind, placebo-controlled trial. J Clin Endocrinol Metab 89:4428, 2004

37. Feldman HA, Goldstein I, Hatzichristou DG, et al: Impotence and its medical and psychosocial correlates: results of the Massachusetts Male Aging Study. J Urol 151:54, 1994

38. Johannes CB, Araujo AB, Feldman HA, et al: Incidence of erectile dysfunction in men 40 to 69 years old: longitudinal results from the Massachusetts male aging study. J Urol 163:460, 2000

39. Lue TF: Erectile dysfunction. N Engl J Med 342:1802, 2000

40. Oral sildenafil in the treatment of erectile dysfunction. Sildenafil Study Group. N Engl J Med 338:1397, 1998

41. Dobs AS, Meikle AW, Arver S, et al: Pharmacokinetics, efficacy, and safety of a permeation-enhanced testosterone transdermal system in comparison with bi-weekly injections of testosterone enanthate for the treatment of hypogonadal men. J Clin Endocrinol Metab 84:3469, 1999

57 Diseases of Calcium Metabolism and Metabolic Bone Disease

Elizabeth H. Holt, M.D., PH.D., *and Silvio E. Inzucchi*, M.D.

Calcium Metabolism

The precise regulation of body calcium stores and of the calcium concentration in both extracellular and intracellular compartments is critically important, for the following reasons: calcium is the chief mineral component of the skeleton; calcium serves major roles in neurologic transmission, muscle contraction, and blood coagulation; and it is a ubiquitous intracellular signal. A typical laboratory range for serum calcium concentration is between 8.8 and 10.5 mg/dl; 50% to 60% of the calcium in the blood is bound to plasma proteins or is complexed with citrate and phosphate. The remaining ionized (free) calcium controls physiologic actions. The body regulates not only ionized calcium concentrations but also the entry and exit of calcium into its main storage site, bone, through the activity of para-

thyroid hormone (PTH) and 1,25-dihydroxyvitamin D_3 (1,25-$(OH)_2D_3$) [*see Figure 1*]. PTH, secreted by the parathyroid glands, is an 84–amino acid peptide with a very short plasma half-life (2 to 4 minutes). Cholecalciferol (vitamin D_3) is generated by the skin, upon exposure to ultraviolet light; it is also supplied by dietary sources (chiefly fortified liquid milk products). In the liver, vitamin D_3 is hydroxylated to 25-$(OH)D_3$, which is in turn hydroxylated in the kidney to 1,25-$(OH)_2D_3$ (calcitriol), markedly increasing its potency. In concert, this hormonal system expresses its action at the level of the gastrointestinal tract, bone, and the kidney and maintains circulating ionized calcium concentrations under extremely tight control (variation < 0.1 mg/dl), despite significant variations in calcium supply.

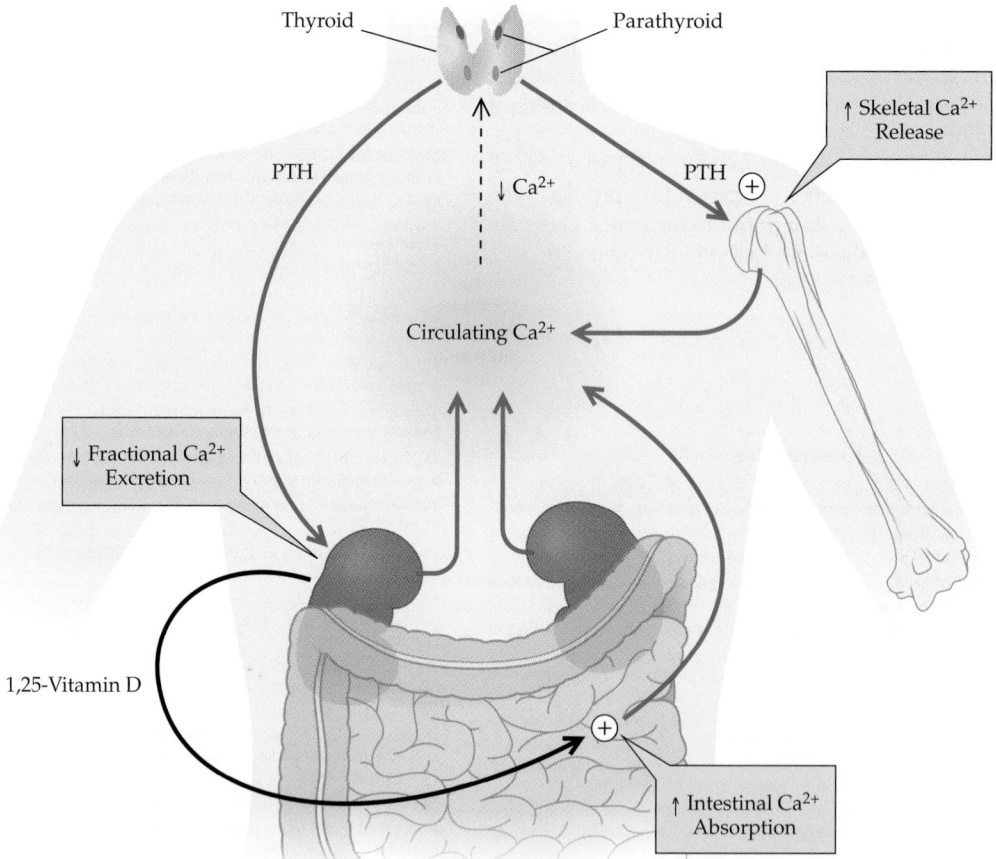

Figure 1 Circulating concentrations of ionized calcium are maintained under extremely tight control by parathyroid hormone (PTH) and the vitamin D axis. Absorption of dietary calcium by the gastrointestinal tract, reduction of calcium excretion by the kidneys, and release of stored calcium from bones serve as sources for circulating calcium. Decreases in circulating calcium trigger the release of PTH, which promotes release of calcium into the extracellular space by increasing bone resorption; the release of PTH also causes an increase in calcium reabsorption in the distal nephron, resulting in a decrease in urinary calcium loss. PTH also augments renal production of 1,25-dihydroxyvitamin D, which secondarily increases calcium absorption in the gut.

Under normal conditions, despite ranges in dietary calcium consumption that can vary from 400 to 2,000 mg daily, net calcium absorption from the GI tract averages about 150 to 200 mg/day. In steady state, this equals the amount of calcium excreted by the kidneys. Ongoing remodeling of bone results in the consumption and release of approximately 500 mg of calcium a day. Through humoral regulation, this calcium reservoir can be exploited to maintain extracellular calcium levels in a narrow range despite increased physiologic need or decreased intake, such as results from severe curtailment of the dietary calcium supply or from impairment of intestinal calcium absorption.

Changes in the extracellular ionized calcium concentration are registered by parathyroid cells via the cell surface calcium-sensing receptor (CaSR).[1] Interaction of calcium ions with the extracellular domain of the CaSR triggers a series of intracellular signaling events, which ultimately govern PTH secretion. As circulating concentrations of calcium fall, PTH secretion rises, and vice versa.

PTH increases bone resorption and distal nephron calcium reabsorption, the former promoting calcium release into the extracellular space and the latter decreasing urinary calcium loss-es. PTH also augments renal production of calcitriol, which then increases fractional calcium absorption in the gut. If calcium intake increases beyond the body's needs, PTH secretion decreases, leading to decreased calcitriol production and decreased calcium absorption by the gut. If calcium is absorbed in excess of requirements, it will be promptly excreted. In this elegant manner, circulating ionized calcium concentration is guarded closely, albeit sometimes at the expense of skeletal calcium stores. Disturbances of PTH, vitamin D action, or both are most often manifested by altered serum calcium or phosphate concentration and by abnormal bone turnover. In some cases, bone mineral density (BMD) is decreased.

Measurement of Calcium

Diagnosis of a calcium disorder depends first on accurate measurement of serum or ionized calcium or both. Serum measurements are usually performed by spectrophotometry or by atomic absorption spectrophotometry, which yields more accurate measurements. Spurious readings may occur with tourniquet stasis (i.e., if the tourniquet is in place too long before the

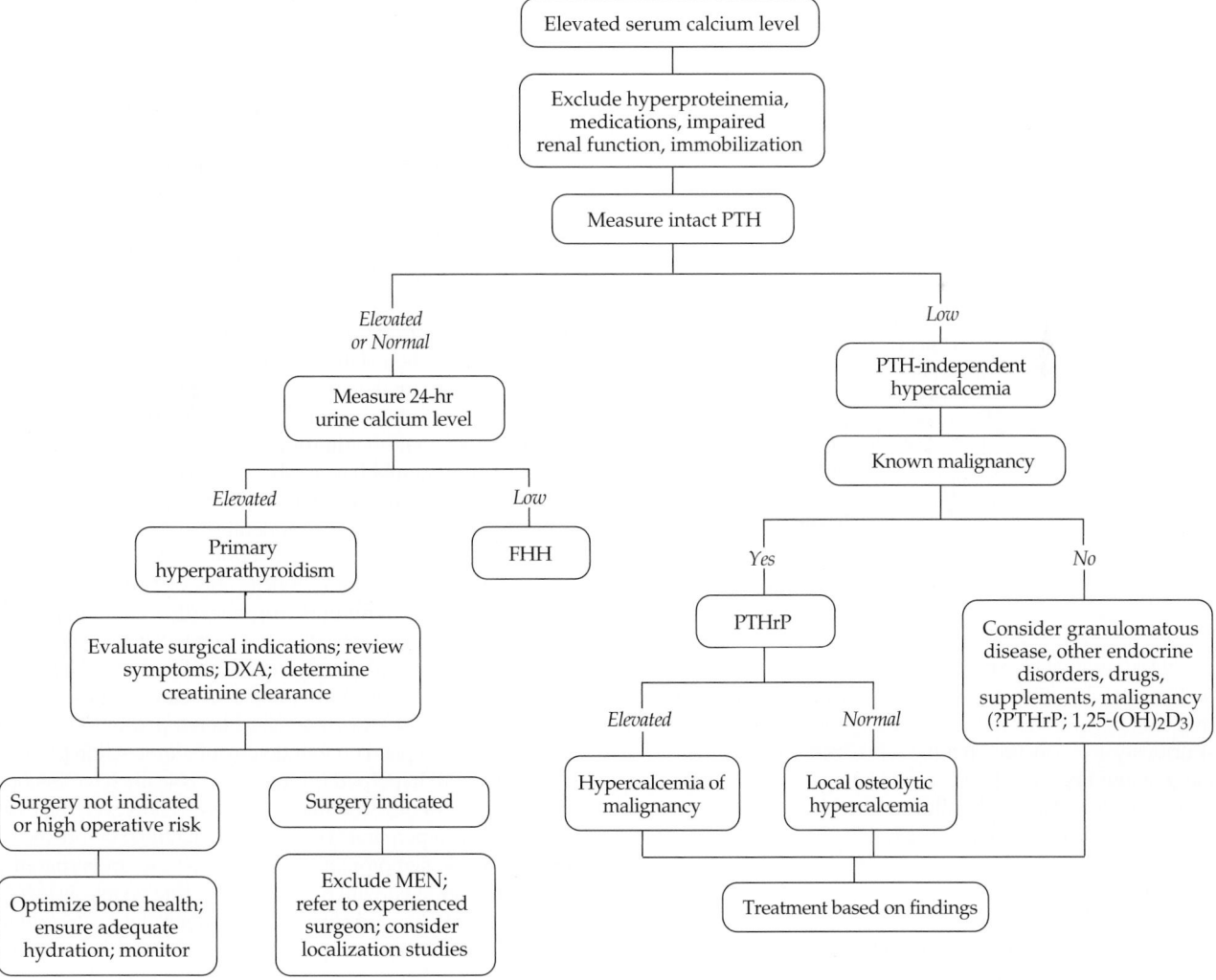

Figure 2 **Evaluation and management of hypercalcemia. (DXA—dual-energy x-ray absorptiometry; FHH—familial hypocalciuric hypercalcemia; MEN—multiple endocrine neoplasia; PTH—parathyroid hormone; PTHrP— parathyroid hormone–related protein)**

Table 1   Differential Diagnosis of Hypercalcemia

Parathyroid hormone–mediated hypercalcemia	Primary hyperparathyroidism
	  Parathyroid adenoma
	  Parathyroid hyperplasia
	  Parathyroid carcinoma
	Tertiary hyperparathyroidism

Parathyroid hormone–independent hypercalcemia	Humoral hypercalcemia of malignancy
	  Parathyroid hormone–related protein mediated
	    Squamous cell carcinoma of the lung
	    Carcinoma of the oropharynx, nasopharynx, larynx, and esophagus
	    Cervical carcinoma
	    Ovarian carcinoma
	    Renal cell carcinoma
	    Transitional cell carcinoma of the bladder
	    Pheochromocytoma
	    Islet cell neoplasms of the pancreas
	    T cell lymphoma
	    Others
	  1,25-$(OH)_2$ D_3 mediated
	    B cell lymphoma
	Local osteolytic hypercalcemia
	  Multiple myeloma
	  Breast carcinoma
	  Lymphoma
	  Others
	Medications/supplements
	  Vitamin D
	  Vitamin A
	  Lithium
	  Thiazides
	  Calcium antacids (milk-alkali syndrome)
	Granulomatous diseases
	  Sarcoidosis
	  Tuberculosis
	  Histoplasmosis
	  Leprosy
	Other conditions
	  Increased plasma protein levels (factitious hypercalcemia)
	  Acute renal failure
	  Thyrotoxicosis
	  Adrenal insufficiency
	  Immobilization
	  Familial hypocalciuric hypocalcemia (benign familial hypercalcemia)

blood is drawn), which can elevate serum calcium values by up to 1 mg/dl. Dilution of blood by drawing samples from indwelling intravenous catheters is a common error that leads to spuriously low calcium readings. Ionized calcium measurements should be considered accurate only when performed on samples collected anaerobically (i.e., in a blood gas syringe) and placed on ice, with immediate analysis.

Hypercalcemia

Hypercalcemia is a common metabolic abnormality. Signs and symptoms of hypercalcemia vary significantly from patient to patient and correlate somewhat with the degree of calcium elevation and its rate of change. The diagnostic workup of hypercalcemia is straightforward [*see Figure 2*].[2] The etiology of hyper-

calcemia is usually discovered after a comprehensive history, physical examination, focused laboratory assessment, and, occasionally, diagnostic imaging studies.[3]

CLINICAL MANIFESTATIONS

Most patients with mild hypercalcemia (serum calcium level < 11 mg/dl) are asymptomatic, although some may experience mild fatigue, vague changes in cognitive function, depression, or polyuria and polydipsia (from decreased urine concentrating ability caused by a high calcium level). Those with moderate hypercalcemia (serum calcium levels of 11 to 14 mg/dl) are more likely to be symptomatic. The likelihood of classic manifestations of hypercalcemia increases sharply when calcium levels rise to 12 to 14 mg/dl. These symptoms include anorexia, nausea, vomiting, abdominal pain, constipation, muscle weakness, and altered mental status. Severe hypercalcemia (i.e., serum calcium levels greater than 14 mg/dl) may cause progressive lethargy, disorientation, and even coma.

In addition to the degree of elevation, the rate of increase in serum calcium may influence the clinical picture. Chronically hypercalcemic patients can function and feel reasonably well with serum calcium values even as high as 15 to 16 mg/dl. In contrast, patients whose calcium level has risen abruptly will often experience symptoms at lesser calcium elevations. Elderly or debilitated patients are also more likely to be symptomatic.

HISTORY AND PHYSICAL EXAMINATION

The history and physical examination are directed at uncovering signs or symptoms of hypercalcemia, as well as signs of the most common causes of hypercalcemia: hyperparathyroidism, malignancy, granulomatous diseases, and certain endocrinopathies. Evidence of any related condition, such as osteoporosis or urinary tract stones, should also be sought. The medical record should be reviewed to determine the duration of the hypercalcemia. The most common cause of hypercalcemia, primary hyperparathyroidism, presents as stable or gradually progressive elevation of the serum calcium level over a period of years. In contrast, malignancy typically causes a more acute rise in serum calcium. All recent medications, foods, and nutritional supplements should be thoroughly reviewed for possible culprits. A careful family history should be performed to identify disorders of calcium metabolism; renal stones; fragility fractures; and any related endocrinopathies, such as diseases of the pituitary, adrenal, thyroid, or endocrine pancreas.

Aside from mental status deficits and signs of dehydration, physical examination findings are generally normal in patients with hypercalcemia, especially if calcium levels are only mildly to moderately elevated. Rarely, severe and prolonged hypercalcemia results in a visible horizontal calcium deposit on the cornea, a condition known as band keratopathy. Other signs and symptoms depend on the etiology of the elevation [*see Table 1*]. Patients with hyperparathyroidism classically have osteopenia, bone pain, or nephrolithiasis. Currently, however, most cases of primary hyperparathyroidism are identified before the patient becomes symptomatic. Patients whose hyperparathyroidism is associated with multiple endocrine neoplasia (MEN) syndromes may have specific manifestations of the other conditions that are part of these syndromes. Patients with sarcoidosis may present with fever, lymphadenopathy, skin rashes, or pulmonary symptoms. Hypercalcemia of malignancy develops only when a substantial tumor burden is present; consequently, most of these patients have an established cancer diagnosis and clinical features associated with the specific tumor type and extent of disease.

LABORATORY STUDIES

The first step in the laboratory assessment is to exclude factitious hypercalcemia, which may result from an increase in circulating concentrations of plasma proteins. About 50% to 60% of circulating calcium is bound to these proteins, so elevation in their concentrations (as occurs in HIV infection, chronic viral hepatitis, and multiple myeloma) will produce a proportionate rise in the total calcium concentration. The ionized calcium concentration, however, remains normal. To adjust for elevations in plasma protein, the serum calcium level should be lowered by 0.8 mg/dl for every 1 g/dl of albumin (or protein) above the normal range. When performed correctly, ionized calcium measurement is more accurate than adjusted total calcium. Because acute renal failure may occasionally lead to hypercalcemia, renal function should also be assessed.

Once hypercalcemia is confirmed, the next step is measurement of the serum PTH concentration. This is the most important test for determining the cause of hypercalcemia.[3] Several PTH assays are commercially available. The most commonly utilized is the two-site immunochemiluminometric assay (ICMA, or so-called bio-intact PTH). Earlier assays could not distinguish between full-length PTH and inactive molecular fragments that circulate in significant concentrations. The ICMA measures only the intact PTH molecule and is therefore the preferred test in most instances, especially in patients whose serum creatinine level is elevated.

Other helpful tests include measurement of serum creatinine and alkaline phosphatase, as well as inorganic phosphorus assays and an electrolyte panel. Assessment of 24-hour urinary calcium excretion is usually performed. Serum creatinine may be elevated in patients with nephrocalcinosis secondary to prolonged hypercalcemia. The alkaline phosphatase level may be elevated in patients with hypercalcemic states involving increased bone turnover. Patients with hypercalcemia caused by malignancy may demonstrate biochemical or hematologic findings consistent with the site of neoplasia and the degree of its dissemination. Most causes of hypercalcemia are also accompanied by hypercalciuria (24-hour urinary calcium excretion > 4 mg/kg/day), which may lead to nephrocalcinosis or renal stone formation. A serum calcium × phosphate product greater than 70 suggests the patient is at risk for calciphylaxis, and efforts to lower the serum phosphate level (e.g., with phosphate binders) should accompany the interventions to lower serum calcium.

Other diagnostic studies may be dictated by clinical circumstances. Electrocardiographic abnormalities of severe hypercalcemia include shortening of the QT_c interval and, rarely, atrioventricular blocks. In addition, many hypercalcemic conditions cause a decrease in BMD, which may be noted on plain x-rays but is best quantified by measurement of bone density (see below). Abdominal x-rays may identify renal stones or nephrocalcinosis. Specific bone radiographic findings are few, and in primary hyperaparathyroidism, specific bony abnormalities are now rare, thanks to early detection of hypercalcemia.

DIFFERENTIAL DIAGNOSIS

The results of PTH measurement indicate whether hypercalcemia is or is not mediated by PTH and thus provide a broad indication of the cause of hypercalcemia [see Table 1]. When PTH levels are high or, in some cases, inappropriately normal, the hypercalcemia is PTH mediated; this is commonly referred to as hyperparathyroidism. When PTH levels are suppressed, the hypercalcemia is said to be non–PTH mediated, or PTH independent. In turn, this distinction guides subsequent patient assessment.

HYPERPARATHYROIDISM (PTH-MEDIATED HYPERCALCEMIA)

Classification

Primary hyperparathyroidism   Primary hyperparathyroidism is the most common cause of hypercalcemia in outpatients. Current estimates place the annual incidence at approximately four per 100,000 population; the incidence peaks in the fifth to sixth decade of life, and there is a female-to-male ratio of 3:2.[4] The most common clinical presentation is that of asymptomatic mild hypercalcemia. Pathologically, a solitary parathyroid adenoma is present in 80% to 85% of cases; hyperplasia involving multiple glands is found in 15% to 20% of cases, and parathyroid carcinoma is found in less than 1%. Occasionally, double adenomas are found. Patients with type I MEN (MEN I) or MEN II usually have parathyroid hyperplasia.[5]

Lithium therapy can change the set point for the calcium-sensing receptor such that a higher serum calcium concentration is needed to inhibit PTH secretion. This can lead to biochemical abnormalities (e.g., high levels of calcium and high-normal to elevated PTH levels) that mimic primary hyperparathyroidism. Patients on lithium will often have very low urinary calcium excretion.

Secondary hyperparathyroidism   Conditions that tend to decrease serum calcium increase PTH secretion as a corrective measure. This increase of PTH secretion is termed secondary hyperparathyroidism. Once circulating PTH is elevated, the serum calcium may return to normal or remain low. Common causes of secondary hyperparathyroidism include chronic renal insufficiency, vitamin D deficiency, intestinal malabsorption, renal calcium losses, and severe dietary inadequacy. Correction of the underlying calcium abnormality will return serum PTH concentrations to normal.

Familial hypocalciuric hypercalcemia   Familial hypocalciuric hypercalcemia (FHH), also referred to as benign familial hypercalcemia, is a rare inherited condition caused by various inactivating mutations in the CaSR. This results in inappropriately increased PTH secretion and a higher set point for the extracellular ionized calcium concentration. Patients with FHH have chronic asymptomatic hypercalcemia associated with relatively depressed urinary calcium excretion.

Tertiary hyperparathyroidism   In some patients with prolonged secondary hyperparathyroidism, hyperplasia or neoplasia of the parathyroid glands develops. These parathyroids no longer respond appropriately to serum calcium; instead, they produce excess PTH at all times, leading to chronic hypercalcemia. This is most often seen in patients with chronic kidney disease. More than one parathyroid gland is usually affected.

Diagnosis

Clinical manifestations   The clinical manifestations of hyperparathyroidism depend, in part, on the severity of the hypercalcemia. When hyperparathyroidism was first described more than 50 years ago, most patients presented with late-stage complications of prolonged and severe hypercalcemia, such as abnormalities of bone (osteitis fibrosa cystica)[6] or kidneys (nephrocalcinosis, renal failure). Since the development more than 30 years ago of laboratory equipment for measuring serum chemistry, hyperparathyroidism is often diagnosed by routine blood testing, before the development of symptoms. It also may be uncovered during the evaluation of osteoporosis or during the workup of renal stone disease.

When symptomatic, patients with hyperparathyroidism demonstrate clinical manifestations of hypercalcemia (see above).

Physical examination   In general, parathyroid tumors are too small to be palpable. Indeed, a palpable parathyroid tumor should be suspected as a malignancy until proved otherwise. Evidence of the consequences of hyperparathyroidism should be sought, such as osteoporosis (kyphosis) or nephrolithiasis (costovertebral angle tenderness).

Laboratory tests   Currently, most patients with hyperparathyroidism have a serum calcium concentration of less than 12 mg/dl (unless coexisting volume contraction is present), and they may have mild to moderate hypophosphatemia and a non–anion gap metabolic acidosis (from renal tubular acidosis). Urinary calcium excretion is often increased; in these patients, the reduction of fractional calcium excretion by PTH is overcome by the high filtered calcium load. This may result in nephrocalcinosis or nephrolithiasis.

Renal stones in patients with hyperparathyroidism are usually composed of calcium oxalate and tend to occur bilaterally, especially when urinary calcium excretion is high. Rarely, nephrocalcinosis and azotemia develop, usually in those with the most severe and protracted hypercalcemia, especially if dehydration or other renal insult is superimposed. Because PTH increases both osteoclast and osteoblast activity, there are increases in serum and urinary concentrations of biochemical markers of bone turnover, including bone alkaline phosphatase.

Elevation of both the serum calcium and the PTH concentrations (in the absence of low urinary calcium excretion) supports a diagnosis of primary hyperparathyroidism. PTH levels are usually increased to less than five times the upper limit of normal. In certain mild cases, the calcium level is only slightly high, and the PTH is minimally elevated or inappropriately normal. Rarely, patients with primary hyperparathyroidism have serum calcium levels in only the high-normal range. In fact, most such patients have elevated serum ionized calcium values and therefore are not actually normocalcemic. The diagnosis in such patients can be extremely challenging.

When the PTH level is normal or mildly elevated and the 24-hour urinary calcium level is low, consideration should be given to the possibility of FHH.[7] The relatively low urinary calcium output seen in FHH may help distinguish this condition from primary hyperparathyroidism, although low urinary calcium excretion may also occur in hyperparathyroidism.

The possibility of FHH is raised when there is a strong family history of symptomatic, stable hypercalcemia, especially in patients younger than 40 years; when family members have undergone unsuccessful parathyroid surgery; or when the patient's urinary calcium output is unexpectedly low. When this diagnosis is suspected, further evaluation is necessary, such as the screening of other family members. Unfortunately, specific genetic testing is not currently widely available from commercial laboratories. In some cases, FHH cannot be distinguished

confidently from primary hyperparathyroidism. However, in most such patients, expectant management is safe and avoids unnecessary parathyroid exploration. When there is trouble distinguishing between primary hyperparathyroidism and FHH, parathyroid imaging is sometimes useful. In primary hyperparathyroidism, enlarged parathyroid glands are easily found, whereas parathyroid size is usually normal in FHH.

Once the diagnosis of primary hyperparathyroidism is secured, it will usually already be apparent whether the patient is a candidate for parathyroidectomy. If the patient does not meet criteria for surgery on the basis of age, renal function, urinary calcium excretion, history of fractures, or renal stones/nephrocalcinosis, then measurement of bone density with a dual-energy x-ray absorptiometry (DXA) scan may be useful. In addition to the standard left hip and lumbar spine measurements, assessment at the distal radius may be particularly helpful, because hyperparathyroidism may affect this predominantly cortical site more than the other locations, which have a greater percentage of trabecular bone.[6]

Other diagnostic studies are usually not necessary. Consideration should also be given to the possibility of one of the MEN syndromes, particularly if the patient is young or has a personal or family history of a related endocrinopathy.[5] This information will be helpful to the surgeon, because the patient with primary hyperparathyroidism in the setting of a MEN syndrome usually has multigland parathyroid hyperplasia, and in such patients a surgical procedure beyond a single parathyroidectomy is necessary. If MEN II is suspected, medullary thyroid cancer should be considered, and pheochromocytoma must be excluded before the patient goes to surgery.

Treatment

Previous controversy over which patients with hyperparathyroidism require surgical intervention has been largely resolved. Those without symptoms or complications clearly related to hyperparathyroidism can be followed safely for long periods. Treatment of the patient with primary hyperparathyroidism must take into account the degree of the hypercalcemia, the presence of symptoms, and the severity of any end-organ damage.[8] Understandably, it is widely agreed that patients with symptoms clearly attributable to hypercalcemia should undergo surgery.

Guidelines for surgical intervention in patients with primary hyperparathyroidism were developed at a National Institutes of Health workshop in 2002.[9] The indications for surgical intervention are as follows:

1. Significant bone, renal, gastrointestinal, or neuromuscular symptoms typical of primary hyperparathyroidism.
2. Elevation of serum calcium by 1 mg/dl or more above the normal range (i.e., ≥ 11.5 mg/dl in most laboratories).
3. Marked elevation of 24-hour urine calcium excretion (e.g., > 400 mg).
4. Decreased creatinine clearance (i.e., reduced by ≥ 30% compared with age-matched normal persons.
5. Significant reduction in bone density (i.e., > 2.5 standard deviations below peak bone mass [T score < –2.5 at the lumbar spine, proximal femur, or distal radius]).
6. Consistent follow-up is not possible or is undesirable because of coexisting medical conditions.
7. Age younger than 50 years.

Those patients with mild hypercalcemia who are truly asymptomatic can be followed clinically for the subsequent development of surgical indications. Most will likely remain asymptomatic and will not require intervention.[9]

Preoperative localization Imaging studies to locate parathyroid adenomas have become more widely used, particularly as more centers have started offering minimally invasive surgery with intraoperative PTH assays (see below).[10,11] In most cases of adenoma in a single gland, precise knowledge of the location of the adenoma may decrease operative time by allowing the surgeon to direct attention to the area of suspicion. It is important to remember, however, that in good hands, parathyroidectomy for primary hyperparathyroidism has a cure rate in the range of 90% to 95%, even without such localization studies. Thus, it is unlikely that preoperative localization will ever be demonstrated to improve overall surgical outcomes. Localization studies are mandatory before minimally invasive parathyroidectomy, in the setting of a second neck exploration for persistent or recurrent hyperparathyroidism, or if previous thyroid surgery has been performed. The localization test of choice is technetium-99m sestamibi scintigraphy.[12,13] This is often followed by a neck ultrasound of the region demonstrating scintigraphic activity to confirm the location of an enlarged parathyroid gland. An additional benefit of ultrasound at this stage in the evaluation is to provide the opportunity for any coexisting thyroid abnormalities to be addressed.

Surgical management The surgical procedure required in patients with hyperparathyroidism resulting from a solitary parathyroid adenoma is resection of that gland. If intraoperative PTH assays show a drop in the PTH level by more than 50% a few minutes after resection, no further neck exploration is required. Intraoperative measurement of PTH is considered by some experts to be critical in the case of ectopic parathyroid adenoma (which would not be easily found during routine neck exploration) and in reoperations. If an intraoperative PTH assay is not used, the other three glands must be directly inspected to ensure that a second adenoma or generalized hyperplasia is not present.[14] If a second adenoma is found, it too should be excised. If hyperplasia is encountered, the surgeon performs a subtotal parathyroidectomy: removal of approximately three to three and one half glands. In some centers, this is followed by autotransplantation of remaining parathyroid tissue to the forearm, which may simplify follow-up surgical exploration in the event of recurrent hypercalcemia. Additional parathyroid tissue may be frozen in case future need develops. Parathyroid autotransplantation is a controversial treatment, because some patients experience aggressive regrowth of parathyroid tissue within the forearm muscles. This can require challenging and disfiguring surgery to correct.

At certain centers, so-called minimally invasive parathyroidectomy is being offered in conjunction with intraoperative PTH measurements.[11] This approach is best suited for a good surgical candidate in whom both history and preoperative imaging studies suggest a single adenoma (which is, in fact, the most common situation in primary hyperparathyroidism). With information from scintigraphy and ultrasound already in hand, the diseased gland can be excised through a smaller, unilateral incision, under local nerve block, in an ambulatory setting. Success is gauged by the drop in PTH levels intraoperatively. This approach usually provides a better cosmetic result, quicker recovery time, and a lower incidence of postoperative hypocalcemia. Minimally invasive surgery may not be appropriate in

Table 2   2002 NIH Working Group Recommendations Regarding Follow-up Testing for Patients with Primary Hyperparathyroidism Who Do Not Undergo Surgery[9]

Measurement	*Frequency*
Serum calcium	Biannually
24-hour urine calcium	At initial evaluation only
Creatinine clearance	At initial evaluation only
Serum creatinine	Annually*
Bone mineral density	Annually (lumbar spine, femur, and forearm)
Abdominal radiograph (or ultrasound)	At initial evaluation only

* If the serum creatinine suggests a change in renal function, measurement of creatinine clearance is recommended.

suboptimal surgical candidates, in patients who may have multigland disease, and in reoperative cases. However, it is quite likely that the majority of parathyroidectomies will be performed in this fashion in the future.

Hyperparathyroidism occasionally persists after operative intervention, usually because of failure to identify the culprit gland, occasionally because of undiagnosed multigland hyperplasia, and rarely because of undiagnosed parathyroid carcinoma.[15-17] Scar tissue and the sometimes unexpected location of remaining pathologic parathyroid tissue make second surgeries notoriously more challenging and prone to complications. Consequently, preoperative imaging studies are invaluable in patients undergoing repeat surgery for persistent hyperparathyroidism. Catheterization studies with venous sampling may also be helpful in certain difficult cases. The identity of putative parathyroid glands can be confirmed by fine-needle aspiration with real-time PTH assay.

Nonsurgical management Although there is as yet no recognized medical therapy for primary hyperparathyroidism, patients who do not meet the criteria for surgical intervention or who refuse surgery can be followed expectantly. This involves periodic monitoring of serum and urine calcium levels, renal function, and BMD, as well as evaluation for nephrocalcinosis or nephrolithiasis. The extent and frequency of this monitoring should be tailored to the individual patient's disease and comorbidities. [*see Table 2*].[9] Drugs that have a tendency to raise serum calcium levels, such as thiazides and lithium, should be avoided. Calcium and excessive vitamin D supplementation should generally be avoided. Dietary calcium should not be restricted, because such restriction may lead to further elevation of PTH and may possibly have detrimental effects on bone mass. Vitamin D deficiency should be identified and treated with gradual supplementation, because vitamin D deficiency will enhance the adverse effects of hyperparathyroidism on bone. Good hydration should be maintained at all times to avoid the development of renal insufficiency and renal stones, especially in patients with hypercalciuria. In patients with low BMD, a bisphosphonate will help to slow bone loss. In patients who are very hypercalcemic but cannot or will not have surgery, calcimimetic agents have been used to control hypercalcemia, although they are not approved by the Food and Drug Administration for use in this particular setting. For example, the calcimimetic agent cinacalcet is approved for the treatment of secondary hyperparathyroidism in patients with chronic kidney disease who are on dialysis, as well as for the treatment of hypercalcemia in patients with parathyroid cancer. Calcimimetic agents activate the CaSR and thus diminish PTH production. The high cost of these agents and the relative ease of parathyroid surgery make their widespread use in the future unlikely.[18]

PTH-INDEPENDENT HYPERCALCEMIA

Cancer remains the most common cause of PTH-independent, persistent, substantial hypercalcemia and is most frequently to blame when an acutely elevated calcium level is discovered in a hospitalized patient. Other causes include sarcoidosis, certain endocrine disorders, and various drugs and supplements.

Etiology

Malignancy Malignancy-associated hypercalcemia has two forms: humoral hypercalcemia of malignancy (HHM) and local osteolytic hypercalcemia (LOH).

HHM results from the elaboration by the tumor of a circulating factor that has systemic effects on skeletal calcium release, renal calcium handling, or GI calcium absorption. Rarely, it can be caused by the unregulated production of calcitriol (usually by B cell lymphomas). However, the best-recognized mediator responsible for HHM is parathyroid hormone–related protein (PTHrP).[19] Normally, PTHrP appears to serve as a paracrine factor in a variety of tissues (e.g., bone, skin, breast, uterus, and blood vessels); it is involved in cellular calcium handling, smooth muscle contraction, and growth and development. The amino terminus of PTHrP is homologous with that of PTH, and they share a common receptor. When PTHrP circulates in supraphysiologic concentrations, it induces most of the metabolic effects of PTH, such as osteoclast activation, decreased renal calcium output, and increased renal phosphate clearance.

Tumors that produce HHM by secreting PTHrP are usually squamous cell carcinomas (e.g., lung, esophageal, laryngeal, oropharyngeal, nasopharyngeal, or cervical carcinomas).[20] Other tumor types that occasionally produce PTHrP include adenocarcinoma of the breast and ovary, renal cell carcinoma, transitional cell carcinoma of the bladder, islet cell tumors of the pancreas, T cell lymphomas, and pheochromocytoma. All tumors that elaborate PTHrP do so in relatively small amounts; thus, the syndrome typically develops in patients with a large tumor burden. It is also unusual for HHM to be the presenting feature of the cancer.

LOH occurs when a tumor growing within bone itself causes the local release of calcium through the production of cytokines that activate osteoclasts; there is no production of a systemic factor in these cases. The classic tumor associated with this syndrome is multiple myeloma, although other neoplasms, such as adenocarcinoma of the breast and various lymphomas, may also cause LOH. Local factors produced by bone cells may further enhance the growth of such tumors; this results in the skeleton inadvertently working in concert with the tumor to promote progressive bone resorption and calcium release and further advancement of the cancer. (This is the basis of the success of bisphosphonates in the treatment of multiple myeloma.)

Other causes PTH-independent hypercalcemia may be caused by sarcoidosis and other granulomatous diseases, such as tuberculosis, in which granulomas produce calcitriol. Endocrine conditions that may occasionally lead to hypercalcemia include hyperthyroidism (which stimulates bone turnover) and Addison disease (in which volume contraction reduces calcium clearance). Immobilization may increase calcium levels, usually in persons with active bone turnover, such as adolescents or those with previously unrecognized hyperparathyroidism or Paget disease of bone (see below). Use of drugs and dietary supplements (e.g., vitamin D and vitamin A) may be associated with hypercalcemia. The association of thiazides with hypercalcemia is now thought to occur when a thiazide-induced reduction in calcium excretion unmasks previously unrecognized primary hyperparathyroidism. Although only rarely encountered today, the so-called milk-alkali syndrome results from the long-term consumption of large quantities of milk and antacids; milk and antacids were the standard treatment of peptic ulcers in the days before the development of H_2 receptor blockers and proton pump inhibitors.

Diagnosis

If the serum calcium concentration is elevated but the PTH level is very low, the patient has PTH-independent hypercalcemia. Possible causes include malignancy, granulomatous disease, thyrotoxicosis, and vitamin D intoxication. These cases require further laboratory assessment, with the choice of tests depending on the clinical situation.

In malignancy-associated hypercalcemia, the degree of calcium elevation is usually moderate or severe. Evidence of significant volume depletion and generalized debility may dominate the clinical picture, along with other cancer-related symptoms. Typically, the diagnosis of malignancy has already been established. The diagnosis of malignancy-associated hypercalcemia should be suspected in cancer patients with hypercalcemia who have abnormally low PTH concentrations. In patients with tumors associated with HHM, measurement of PTHrP is indicated. Radioimmunoassays for PTHrP are commercially available; an elevation of PTHrP concentration will essentially confirm the diagnosis of most cases of HHM. Special care should be taken to ensure that blood for PTHrP levels is drawn and handled correctly to avoid spuriously low results. In HHM from B cell lymphomas, circulating plasma concentrations of calcitriol are increased. In local osteolytic disease, PTHrP and calcitriol are within normal ranges, and there is definitive evidence of bony metastases.

When the PTH is low and the patient is not known to have a malignancy, diagnostic possibilities include granulomatous diseases, other endocrine disorders, drugs or dietary supplements, and immobilization. Possible laboratory studies in such patients might include measurement of vitamin D metabolites, thyroid hormone levels, or 24-hour urine calcium excretion. If investigation of these diagnoses proves unrewarding, the very rare possibility of unrecognized malignancy may be considered, especially if measurement of PTHrP is performed and shows elevated values. Further imaging studies are indicated in such cases, including a plain chest radiograph or a computed tomographic scan of the thorax as the initial study. If the results are negative, consideration should be given to a comprehensive otolaryngoscopic examination, esophagoscopy, or CT of the abdomen. Should such further assessment be unrevealing, radiographic or endoscopic assessment of the genitourinary tract should be considered.

Treatment

Acute hypercalcemia A nonparathyroid disorder, often a malignancy, is responsible for most cases of acute hypercalcemia [*see Table 1*]. When the serum calcium level is substantially elevated, treatment includes attempts to increase renal calcium excretion while simultaneously attenuating either bone resorption or intestinal calcium absorption, depending on which is the primary source of calcium. Because most patients have at least moderate volume contraction, which further exacerbates their ability to excrete calcium, the initial intervention should be expansion of the intravascular volume with an intravenous infusion of normal saline [*see Table 3*]. This will augment the delivery of sodium and water to the distal nephron, both of which will, in turn, increase urinary calcium excretion. Once the intravascular volume is repleted, adding a loop diuretic such as furosemide will allow continued aggressive saline hydration and may further increase calcium excretion. If the serum calcium concentration does not normalize quickly with intravenous fluid and diuresis, pharmacologic therapy is indicated.[21] Because almost all causes of severe hypercalcemia involve some degree of increased osteoclast activation, drugs that decrease bone turnover are favored. The treatment of choice is a bisphosphonate, such as pamidronate or zoledronic acid, both of which are available for intravenous infusion. Pamidronate is given in a dosage of 60 to 90 mg intravenously over several hours; it is generally well tolerated. Typically, serum calcium levels begin to decrease within 24 to 48 hours of the infusion, although the peak effect may not occur for several days. The action of pamidronate may persist for up to several weeks; treatment can be repeated as needed if renal function will allow. Zoledronic acid is given at a dosage of 4 mg intravenously over no less than 15 minutes. It appears to have a higher potency and an even longer duration of action than pamidronate. A repeat dose may be provided after 7 days. Use of intravenous bisphophonates, especially zoledronic acid, is often associated with an acute-phase response after the first dose, with flulike symptoms. Caution should be employed with these agents in the setting of renal dysfunction. In addition, if parathyroidectomy is planned, use of bisphosphonates should be considered carefully, because they may make postoperative hypocalcemia management more difficult. When more rapid action is desired, subcutaneous injection of calcitonin can be tried, either alone or in conjunction with a bisphosphonate. Calcitonin is given at a dosage of 4 IU/kg twice daily. Calcitonin is a relatively weak hypocalcemic agent; tachyphylaxis to the effects of calcitonin is common and limits its use to a few days. Other possible therapies are plicamycin and gallium nitrate, although certain toxicities limit their use as first-line agents. In severe or refractory cases, hemodialysis against a low-calcium bath may also be undertaken.

In the more unusual situation of hypercalcemia resulting from an increase in gut calcium absorption, such as in vitamin D intoxication or granulomatous diseases, glucocorticoid therapy may have an integral role. Glucocorticoids directly impede intestinal calcium transport and also decrease renal or granulomatous 1α-hydroxylase activity, which results in a decrease in concentrations of calcitriol. In patients with lymphoma, steroids may also have an antineoplastic effect.

Contributing factors to hypercalcemia, such as the use of oral calcium or vitamin D supplements, diuretic therapy, or immobilization, should be corrected, if possible.

In malignancy-associated hypercalcemia, effective surgery, chemotherapy, or radiotherapy targeted at the tumor itself will

---

Table 3 Therapy for Acute Hypercalcemia

Fluids
    0.9% NaCl I.V.
    Loop diuretic (forced diuresis)
Medications
    Bisphosphonates
        Pamidronate (60–90 mg I.V.)
        Zolendronic acid (4 mg I.V.)
    Calcitonin (4 IU/kg S.C. q. 12 hr)
    Plicamycin (15–25 µg/kg I.V.)
    Gallium nitrate (200 mg/m² /day continuous infusion for 5 days)
    Glucocorticoids (20–100 mg of prednisone a day)
Other
    Primary therapy directed at tumor
        Surgery
        Chemotherapy
        Radiation
    Decrease calcium and vitamin D intake
    Maintain adequate hydration
    Mobilize patient

---

reduce the hypercalcemia. However, because hypercalcemia is often an end-stage complication, further chemotherapy or radiotherapy may be neither possible nor desired.

Hypocalcemia

Hypocalcemia is defined as a serum calcium level below the reference range for the laboratory. As with hypercalcemia, an ionized calcium determination on a correctly collected sample is the best way to confirm hypocalcemia.

ETIOLOGY

An abnormally low level of serum calcium on laboratory testing is most often factitious, resulting from a decrease in plasma protein concentration secondary to decreased protein synthesis or hemodilution. Because circulating calcium is so highly protein bound, decreases in serum albumin concentrations—such as occurs with malnourishment, liver disease, or nephrotic syndrome—produce proportionate reductions in total serum calcium. In such situations, the serum calcium level may be corrected by adding 0.8 mg/dl for each 1 g/dl reduction in the serum albumin level below 4 g/dl. An accurate ionized calcium measurement will circumvent many of these pitfalls.

True hypocalcemia is most often related to vitamin D deficiency or impaired parathyroid gland function. Removal of or vascular injury to the parathyroids during neck surgery can result in hypoparathyroidism, which is manifested by hypocalcemia, hyperphosphatemia, and inappropriately low concentrations of PTH. However, unless all four parathyroids are removed or their blood supply is severely impaired, hypocalcemia after parathyroidectomy is usually a transient phenomenon. Normal parathyroid function typically returns after a period of several days to weeks. Patients who experience prolonged, severe primary hyperparathyroidism and significant bone resorption before undergoing parathyroidectomy may experience protracted hypocalcemia and hypophosphatemia after surgery, as a result of the deposition of large quantities of mineral into the skeleton. This is referred to as the "hungry bone syndrome."

Autoimmune destruction of the parathyroid glands may be

seen in certain conditions, including autoimmune polyglandular syndrome type 1, a condition marked by hypoparathyroidism, premature ovarian failure, Addison disease, and mucocutaneous candidiasis.[22] Certain infiltrative diseases, such as hemochromatosis, may also adversely affect parathyroid function, as may external-beam irradiation of the neck. Functional hypoparathyroidism may also result from hypomagnesemia, because magnesium is necessary for both PTH release and PTH action. This is often seen in hospitalized alcoholic patients. Pseudohypoparathyroidism is caused by inherited PTH resistance, which results in hypocalcemia and secondary marked elevations of PTH levels.

Because vitamin D ultimately regulates intestinal calcium absorption, disorders of its supply, production, or activity may lead to hypocalcemia. In such conditions, serum calcium concentrations are usually not severely affected, thanks to compensatory increases in PTH levels. Indeed, the primary clinical manifestations are in the skeleton (e.g., rickets in children and osteomalacia in adults). Dietary vitamin D deficiency in the elderly is common, but it is often overlooked.[23] At-risk adults include the elderly and darker-skinned persons with poor dietary habits who avoid liquid milk products and have little sun exposure, particularly in northern climates. However, recent reports suggest that vitamin D deficiency may be more frequent than traditionally considered, even in persons not previously thought to be at risk.[24]

Hypocalcemia may occur in patients with acute pancreatitis, when fatty acids released through the action of pancreatic lipase complex with calcium. The complexing of phosphate with calcium also occurs in severely hyperphosphatemic states, such as acute renal failure, rhabdomyolysis, and the tumor lysis syndrome, and it may result in a decrease in serum calcium concentrations. Hypocalcemia may also be caused by large-volume blood transfusions using red blood cells to which calcium chelators have been added to prevent clotting.

DIAGNOSIS

Chronic mild to moderate hypocalcemia is usually well tolerated. However, when the serum calcium level falls below 7.5 to 8 mg/dl (assuming that plasma protein levels are normal), the patient may develop symptoms of neuromuscular irritability, such as tremor, muscle spasms, or paresthesias. On examination, Chvostek and Trousseau signs may be present. If the serum calcium level drops further, tetany or seizures may result. Prolongation of the QT_C interval may also occur, predisposing the patient to cardiac arrhythmias.

As with hypercalcemia, the cause of hypocalcemia can usually be discerned after a careful history (including a review of medications, previous surgeries, and dietary and social habits) and by the measurement of the circulating concentrations of calcium, phosphorus, PTH, and $25-(OH)D_3$. The differential diagnosis consists principally of conditions that result in an abnormal supply or the abnormal action of PTH or vitamin D, but the use of medications or supplements and the presence of other conditions must be considered [see Table 4].

TREATMENT

In patients with symptoms of marked hypocalcemia (e.g., neuromuscular irritability), calcium should be infused slowly (e.g., as calcium gluconate) to raise the serum calcium level until symptoms are relieved. Individual boluses of intravenous calcium will not achieve this effect. Concurrently, any deficiency in magnesium stores should be corrected. In severe cases, hypocalcemia may recur quickly after discontinuance of calcium infusion, so oral calcium should be administered concurrently. In less severe cases, calcium can be administered orally as calcium carbonate or calcium citrate in doses of 1,000 to 2,000 mg of elemental calcium daily in divided doses. If appropriate, vitamin D should also be provided. If dietary deficiency of vitamin D is suspected, cholecalciferol (vitamin D_3) or, if cholecalciferol is unavailable, ergocalciferol (vitamin D_2), may be adequate. Because hydroxylation of cholecalciferol may take several days, however, a brief course of calcitriol may also be necessary. In cases of hypoparathyroidism, long-term administration of calcitriol is needed, because renal 1α-hydroxylase may not be active in the absence of PTH. In hypoparathyroid patients, it is important to not fully normalize the serum calcium level, because this often results in hypercalciuria and hyperphosphaturia, increasing the risk of nephrocalcinosis or renal stones. Instead, serum calcium should be kept around the lower limit of the normal range, at a level sufficient to relieve symptoms and reverse tetanic signs (e.g., Trousseau sign). Periodic monitoring for nephrocalcinosis in these patients may be appropriate.

Table 4   Differential Diagnosis of Hypocalcemia

Abnormal supply or action of parathyroid hormone	Hypoparathyroidism
	  Surgical
	  External-beam irradiation (to neck)
	  Autoimmune
	    Polyendocrine syndromes
	  Congenital
	  Infiltrative
	    Hemochromatosis
	    Thalassemia
	    Wilson disease
	  Magnesium deficiency
	  DiGeorge syndrome
	PTH resistance
	  Pseudohypoparathyroidism

Abnormal supply or action of vitamin D	Vitamin D–dependent rickets (VDDR)/
	  osteomalacia
	  Nutritional deficiency
	  Malabsorption
	  Altered vitamin D metabolism
	    Cirrhosis
	    Renal failure
	    Anticonvulsant medications
	Vitamin D pseudodeficiency (VDDR I)
	Abnormal vitamin D receptor (VDDR II)
	Vitamin D–resistant hypophosphatemic
	  rickets/osteomalacia
	  Oncogenic osteomalacia

Medications/ supplements	Phosphate Calcitonin Bisphosphonates Plicamycin

Other conditions	Hypoalbuminemia (factitious)
	Acute pancreatitis
	Rhabdomyolysis
	Calcium malabsorption
	Hyperphosphatemia
	Large transfusions of citrate-containing
	  blood products
	Osteoblastic metastases (prostatic or breast
	  carcinoma)

Metabolic Bone Disease

OSTEOPOROSIS

Osteoporosis is defined as a loss of bone mass, including loss of trabecular bone microarchitecture and connectivity and a thinning of cortical bone, leading to an increased risk of fracture. Clinically, osteoporosis is usually diagnosed by measuring BMD, which reflects the bone calcium content and is a surrogate for bone mass. The diagnostic criteria of the World Health Organization are based on the results of standardized bone density measurements: osteoporosis is present when the BMD is more than 2.5 standard deviations (SDs) below that of a normal, young adult control population (in whom bone density is at its peak). Osteopenia is present when the BMD falls between –1.0 and –2.5 SDs from peak bone density.

Epidemiology

Peak bone mass occurs in persons who are in their late 20s or early 30s; after this age, bone density decreases slowly. Consequently, the incidence of osteoporosis increases with age, becoming most common in persons older than 60 years. Because peak bone mass is lower in women than in men, women generally have lower bone density at each succeeding stage of life.[25] Therefore, women experience higher rates of fracture. The most common sites of so-called fragility fractures are the hip, the distal forearm, and vertebrae.

The lifetime risk of experiencing any fragility fracture for white women is 40%, whereas for white men it is 13%. By site, the respective risks for women and men are as follows: 18% and 6% for hip fracture, 16% and 3% for distal radius fracture, and 18% and 6% for vertebral fracture.[26] The incidence of hip fracture in women and men aged 65 years is approximately 300 and 150 per 100,000 person-years, respectively. These rates increase to approximately 3,000 and 2,000 per 100,000, respectively, by 85 years of age.[25] African Americans generally have higher BMD and are at lower risk for fracture than their white, Hispanic, or Asian counterparts.

Osteoporosis produces enormous burdens, both for patients and for society at large. In the United States, the direct costs of treatment of osteoporotic fractures alone are estimated to be $10 billion to $15 billion annually. Hip fracture carries the highest morbidity and mortality of all fractures. Deaths may occur from associated complications, such as pulmonary embolism or pneumonia. Only one third of patients with hip fracture return to their previous level of functioning. Of the remainder, one third will be placed in long-term nursing care facilities. Rates of depression and anxiety also increase after osteoporotic fracture.[10] Because of the high cost to patients and the insurance system, prevention of hip fracture has been a major focus of osteoporosis prevention and treatment.

Pathogenesis

Bone remodeling occurs continuously in adults; at any given time, as much as 5% to 10% of the skeleton is in a state of turnover. The cells involved in this remodeling process are the osteoclasts, which resorb bone, and the osteoblasts, which form new bone. A cycle of bone remodeling begins with the recruitment of osteoclasts. Osteoclast-mediated resorption of bone from the site releases mineral and collagen breakdown products into the circulation. Through local osteoclast-derived cytokine signals, osteoblasts are then recruited to the site and create new bone matrix to fill the resorption pit left behind by the osteo-

clasts. The matrix is then mineralized through the physiochemical crystallization of hydroxyapatite. Each bone turnover cycle lasts approximately 3 months.

Through the process of bone remodeling, the skeleton is constantly rejuvenated. In an accelerated form, the bone remodeling process allows for the healing of fractures. In addition, the massive mineral stores of the skeleton are continuously made available to the body for systemic needs, especially during times of decreased calcium supply.

With advancing age, slightly less bone is formed than was resorbed during each remodeling cycle, presumably because of a gradual decline in osteoblast activity. As a result, net bone loss occurs with each cycle, resulting in the gradual decline in bone mass with aging. Therefore, bone loss is to some degree linked to the rate of bone turnover. Any process that increases bone resorption without increasing bone formation will result in a decrease in bone mass and in a concomitant increase in the risk of fracture.

Bone mass accumulates during the first 2 decades of life, achieves its peak in the late third or early fourth decade, stabilizes during the next 1 or 2 decades, and then declines slowly. The age-related decline in bone mass occurs at a rate of approximately 0.1% to 0.5% a year in both sexes. In women, however, the rate of bone loss accelerates during the relatively abrupt loss of gonadal steroids during menopause, especially just before and during the first 6 or 7 years after the cessation of menses. During this period, bone mass may actually fall by up to 4% a year. Thus, by the end of this period, a woman may have lost one quarter to one third of her total skeletal mass.[26,27] Subsequently, bone loss tends to slow to a rate similar to that seen in aging men.

Risk Factors and Pathologic Causes

The most important risk factors for decreased bone density and osteoporotic fracture are advanced age, female gender, postmenopausal status, white or Asian race, personal or family history of fragility fracture, and low body weight.[28,29] These risk factors assist in identifying patients who are at increased risk for bone loss and consequent fracture. Those patients warrant prophylactic measures to help maintain bone mass, and they may benefit from formal bone density measurement to more precisely quantify risk. Other factors contributing to bone loss include cigarette smoking, ethanol abuse, insufficient dietary calcium, and lack of physical exercise.

Diseases or conditions associated with low bone density include Cushing syndrome, glucocorticoid therapy, thyrotoxicosis, excessive thyroid hormone replacement, primary hyperparathyroidism, hypogonadism, intestinal malabsorption, chronic obstructive pulmonary disease, chronic renal or hepatic failure, multiple myeloma and other malignancies, hypopituitarism (growth hormone deficiency), rheumatoid arthritis and other connective tissue diseases, and organ transplantation.

Diagnosis

Although risk-factor analysis assists in determining which patients are at greatest risk for osteoporosis and fracture, the measurement of bone density remains an essential tool to assess risk. Several modalities for measuring bone density are currently in use, including DXA, quantitative CT (QCT), and ultrasound. QCT is not yet widely used clinically. Ultrasound is used for screening purposes, but selected patients must be followed with central DXA measurements. DXA has the highest accuracy and precision of any densitometric method and is currently the diagnostic tool preferred by most authorities.[30,31] It is also the method most widely employed in large clinical trials of osteoporosis treatment regimens and is both widely available and safe. DXA should therefore be used for the initial screening and follow-up.

In a typical DXA report, the bone density measurements (expressed in g/cm²) are converted to T scores and Z scores. The T score is the number of SDs the patient's BMD falls above or below the mean value for young, healthy persons at peak bone density. The Z score represents the number of SDs the patient's BMD falls above or below the average value for persons of the patient's age and sex. The T score is the best indicator of fracture risk. Bone density reference databases are currently available only for whites and African Americans; this limits the value of the results obtained for other ethnic groups. The most common sites measured by DXA are the proximal femur and lumbar spine, although the distal nondominant radius can also be assessed. Pitfalls in the interpretation of DXA scans include incorrect patient positioning and improper selection of the region of interest for analysis. Degenerative disease or scoliosis in the lumbar spine can make the bones appear denser, leading to falsely reassuring results. Each SD below peak bone mass represents a loss of 10% to 12% of bone mineral content and corresponds to an approximate twofold to 2.5-fold increase in fracture risk at that site. It should be noted, however, that factors other than bone density play important roles in the risk of fracture. Recent attention has been directed to so-called bone quality, which refers to the microarchitecture and fracture resistance of the bone, and which may not correspond to BMD as measured by DXA.[32] In elderly persons, in particular, additional factors that increase the risk of fractures include low visual acuity, impaired neuromuscular function, decreased mobility, cognitive decline, sedative drug use, and residence in a nursing home.[33] In a review of the risk of fracture in almost 8,000 women enrolled in a longitudinal study of osteoporosis, the clinical factors found to be most important for risk of fracture included a history of fracture after 50 years of age, maternal history of hip fracture, weight less than 125 lb, current cigarette smoking, and the inability to raise oneself from the seated position without use of the arms. By combining these factors with the T score at the hip, these researchers were able to create a fracture risk index that predicted the patient's likelihood of hip fracture over the subsequent 5 years with greater accuracy than seen with the bone density result alone.[34]

In 1998, the National Osteoporosis Foundation recommended that DXA be used as a screening modality in women with established osteoporotic fractures (to establish a baseline for follow-up measurements) and in women without established osteoporotic fractures who are 65 years of age or older or who are younger than 65 years but have one or more accepted risk factors for fragility fracture. These risk factors include low body weight (< 128 lb); current smoking; and personal history of, or a first-degree family relative with, a low-trauma fracture.[29] Indications for bone density measurement in any patient include fracture from mild or moderate trauma, evidence of osteopenia on plain radiography, pending organ transplant, and ongoing or anticipated long-term corticosteroid therapy. Bone density measurements are also useful in the evaluation of patients with conditions that might adversely affect bone mass (e.g., hyperparathyroidism) and for monitoring patients who are receiving therapy for osteoporosis. When follow-up bone density studies

are performed, it is important that they be done in a reproducible fashion, so that an accurate comparison can be made. It is best to use the same densitometer at the same facility from one year to the next. Identical patient positioning for each scan will also help eliminate error.

Once the diagnosis of osteoporosis or osteopenia is made, the clinician may wish to undertake a selective evaluation to exclude causes of secondary osteoporosis (other than estrogen deficiency). In a premenopausal woman or a man with decreased bone density, such investigations are imperative. A comprehensive history and physical examination will reveal many of the causes of secondary bone loss. The evaluation should explore symptoms of chronic illness, hyperthyroidism, hyperparathyroidism, intestinal disease, and glucocorticoid use.[35] Lifelong calcium and vitamin D intake should be reviewed. In women, the menstrual history should also be discussed, because even relatively short periods of amenorrhea (reflecting estrogen deficiency) in the past may have a detrimental effect on bone mass.[36] Lifestyle factors such as physical activity level, eating disorders, cigarette smoking, and alcohol abuse should also be addressed. In men, osteoporosis is more often associated with a secondary cause, the more common ones being alcoholism, steroid use, and hypogonadism.[37] However, in about half of men with osteoporosis, the disorder is idiopathic.

An extensive biochemical assessment of the patient, other than that indicated by the clinical evaluation, is not necessary. It is reasonable, however, to perform routine blood chemistry studies, including measurement of levels of serum calcium and phosphorus, serum creatinine, and alkaline phosphatase along with a complete blood count. Immunofixation electrophoresis can also be performed to rule out early myeloma if there is any suspicion of malignancy. Subclinical hyperthyroidism can be ruled out with a thyroid-stimulating hormone determination. Measurement of PTH and vitamin D levels is often helpful, because asymptomatic disease is common. Measurement of 24-hour urinary calcium excretion will evaluate for calcium malabsorption or excessive renal losses of calcium.

Treatment

Modifiable risk factors Lifestyle modification is the first step in the prevention or treatment of osteoporosis. Smoking cessation and moderation of alcohol consumption are important first steps. Exercise is an important aspect of osteoporosis management. Weight-bearing physical activity attenuates bone loss; exercise also helps maintain the proximal muscle strength and balance necessary to avoid falls.[38] A physical therapy evaluation is appropriate for patients considered at high risk for falls. Physical therapists can conduct home safety evaluations to identify and address conditions that might promote falls (e.g., trailing electric cords, throw rugs). Physical therapy can also improve strength and gait stability, thus decreasing fall risk. For frail elderly patients, it is prudent to review medication lists and try to eliminate medications that may cause dizziness or sedation and thus predispose patients to falls. Hip protectors have been shown in some, but not all, studies to prevent hip fracture if a patient falls.[39]

Nutritional therapy Any patient being treated for bone loss must consume adequate amounts of both calcium and vitamin D. The recommended daily dietary intake of elemental calcium is 1,000 to 1,500 mg, depending on age and menopausal status [see Table 5],[40] and recommended vitamin D intake ranges from

Table 5 Dietary Reference Intakes for Calcium[*76]

Population	Age (yr)	DRI (mg)
Children	1–3	500
	4–8	800
Males and females	9–18	1,300
	19–50	1,000
	> 50	1,200
Pregnant/lactating women	≤ 18	1,300
	≥ 19	1,000

*Recommended Daily Allowances (RDA) are being replaced with dietary reference intakes (DRI).

400 to 800 IU a day. Patients taking medications that increase vitamin D metabolism (e.g., phenytoin) may need higher vitamin D doses. Substantial and prolonged deficiencies in calcium intake may lead to secondary hyperparathyroidism with reduction of bone mass, as bone is resorbed to release calcium for systemic requirements. Several investigators have demonstrated that calcium and vitamin D supplementation has a beneficial effect on postmenopausal bone loss, although the effects are not as dramatic as those seen with antiresorptive or anabolic therapies.[41] In addition, vitamin D supplementation in the elderly appears to be associated with as much as a 22% decreased risk of falls.[42] Skeletal muscle has vitamin D receptors, and it is thought that vitamin D sufficiency is necessary for optimal muscle strength.

Preferably, calcium and vitamin D should be from dietary sources.[40] Unless milk products are a major component of the diet, however, achieving adequate intake may be difficult; therefore, commercially available supplements should be used. In patients who are elderly, in patients who are taking proton pump inhibitors or H$_2$-blockers, or in patients who have pernicious anemia, calcium citrate may be better absorbed than calcium carbonate. In all major clinical trials of osteoporosis therapies, participants were also provided basal calcium and vitamin D supplements. Thus, the efficacy of currently available pharmacologic agents for osteoporosis generally has been demonstrated only in persons with adequate calcium and vitamin D intake.

Antiresorptive therapy Osteoporosis is most often treated with antiresorptive agents. FDA-approved agents for the treatment of established osteoporosis include the bisphosphonates (e.g., alendronate, risedronate), selective estrogen receptor modulators (SERMs) (e.g., raloxifene), calcitonin,[28] and estrogen.[43-46] All of these agents reduce vertebral and nonvertebral fracture rates (on the order of 30% to 60%) over 2 to 3 years,[28,37,40,43,44,47-53] but only estrogen[54] and the bisphosphonates have been shown to reduce hip fracture risk.[47-49] All of these agents tend to be more effective for increasing bone density and lowering fracture risk at the spine than at the hip. Estrogen is less widely used for prevention of postmenopausal bone loss since the publication of the Women's Health Initiative (WHI) results. The WHI studies showed an increased risk of cardiovascular disease, breast cancer, stroke, and pulmonary embolism in patients treated with estrogen in combination with progestin,[55] as well as an increase in stroke risk for women treated with estrogen alone.[56]

Antiresorptive therapy should be considered for postmenopausal women for the prevention of osteoporosis, particularly in those with established fracture and those who are at high risk for fracture. For the prevention of osteoporosis, the antiresorptives currently approved by the FDA are alendronate, risedronate, raloxifene, and estrogen. These agents increase BMD at both the hip and the spine during the first 2 to 3 years of use, with subsequent stabilization.

Bisphosphonates Given their demonstrated safety record and their ability to prevent hip fractures, the bisphosphonates should be considered for initial prevention and treatment of osteoporosis. Bisphosphonates bind to skeletal hydroxyapatite and decrease osteoclast activity, thus slowing bone resorption while new bone formation continues. Over a period of 2 to 3 years, they produce a 6% increase in bone density and a 30% to 50% reduction in fracture risk at both vertebral and nonvertebral sites, with greater effectiveness at the former.[48-51] Alendronate is dosed at 70 mg once weekly for osteoporosis treatment and at 35 mg once weekly for osteoporosis prevention.[57] Risedronate is given at 35 mg once weekly for prevention or treatment of osteoporosis.[58] Risks of bisphosphonate therapy include esophagitis; these agents are contraindicated in patients with active esophagitis, achalasia, or esophageal stricture, and they should be used with caution in anyone with a history of esophagitis or gastroesophageal reflux disease. Caution should be taken in prescribing these agents for women of childbearing age: they persist in bone matrix and can be measured in the blood for years after discontinuance, so there is a risk of passage to the fetus even in patients no longer taking them.

Because they are poorly absorbed, bisphosphonates should be taken on an empty stomach immediately upon awakening in the morning. After taking the agent, the patient should remain upright and should not consume food for at least 1 hour. How long bisphosphonate therapy should be provided is an area of active interest in osteoporosis research. Alendronate use for up to 10 years provides a sustained benefit and is well tolerated.[59] The bone-preserving effects of alendronate may persist for up to 2 years after the drug is discontinued, presumably because it remains in bone matrix. There has been concern that prolonged therapy with bisphosphonates might lead to adynamic bone, a condition associated with low bone turnover, microfractures, and chronic pain. It may be appropriate to consider a 1- to 2-year drug holiday after 5 to 10 years of bisphosphonate therapy to avoid these theoretical risks, although no guidelines currently exist for duration of bisphosphonate therapy for osteoporosis.

Raloxifene Raloxifene, a SERM, can be used for osteoporosis prevention or treatment.[60] Raloxifene acts as an estrogen agonist in bone, but it acts as an estrogen antagonist in breast and uterus. Thus, its use is not associated with endometrial hyperplasia, and concurrent treatment with progestins is not required. Raloxifene also does not increase the risk of breast cancer. In fact, it is under active investigation for its potential role in preventing breast cancer in high-risk patients.[61] Raloxifene increases bone density by only about 1% over 12 to 24 months, but data on vertebral fracture are comparable to those of estrogen replacement therapy (ERT) or bisphosphonate therapy. Raloxifene has not been shown to reduce the incidence of hip fracture. It is generally well tolerated but may exacerbate menopausal hot flashes. Patients should be advised that raloxifene carries a threefold increased risk of thromboembolic disease, which is similar to that seen with estrogen. Preliminary reports suggest no detrimental effect on cardiovascular risk.[62] Raloxifene is a good choice for patients who have bone loss primarily in the spine, for women with relatively low risk of hip fracture, and for patients who are unable to tolerate oral bisphosphonates. Raloxifene is not approved for use in premenopausal women or men.

Calcitonin Calcitonin has much less potent effects on BMD and fracture than do the bisphosphonates, raloxifene, or estrogen.[63] This hormone, which is normally produced by the parafollicular cells (C cells) of the thyroid, typically circulates in low concentration in humans. The precise role of calcitonin in the body is not fully understood, but it appears to be a weak regulator of serum calcium concentrations and bone turnover. Commercially available products include calcitonin injections and nasal spray. Both are approved for the treatment of established osteoporosis but not for its prevention. In most of the calcitonin trials, the average increase in bone density was only 1% to 2% over 2 years. Calcitonin has been primarily shown to prevent vertebral fractures and has not been shown to prevent nonvertebral or hip fractures.[52] Calcitonin is generally safe; occasional flushing, headaches, anosmia, or nasal irritation is observed with the nasal spray. There is a concern about tachyphylaxis, or decreased effectiveness over time, with calcitonin use. Because of the availability of other safe and more potent drugs for osteoporosis, calcitonin is rarely used except when other options are lacking.

Estrogen Until recently, ERT was widely recommended as first-line therapy for both the prevention and treatment of osteoporosis, although it is approved by the FDA for prevention only.[43] Advocates argued that estrogen directly corrected the chief pathophysiologic defect of the menopause: estrogen deficiency. However, use of ERT to maintain bone health has fallen out of favor because of data indicating that it may actually increase the risk of cardiovascular disease, as well as the risk of breast cancer and ovarian cancer. The multicenter WHI was created to study the effects of hormone replacement therapy in healthy postmenopausal women. Women receiving estrogen in combination with progestin had a lower incidence of fracture, but this arm of the study was stopped prematurely because of a 26% increase in the risk of breast cancer and a lack of overall benefit in this treatment group. The WHI also found that, compared with women taking a placebo, women taking the combination of estrogen and progestin had a 29% increase in myocardial infarction, a 41% increase in stroke, and a doubling of thromboembolic events. For hysterectomized women taking estrogen without progestin, the risk of stroke was increased compared with the group receiving placebo. As a result of the WHI findings, estrogen should probably no longer be considered the optimal first-line preventive or therapeutic agent for bone loss in postmenopausal women.[55] On the basis of these data, the use of estrogen for osteoporosis prevention or treatment should be limited to women who require its beneficial effects for menopausal symptoms. For other women, there are equally effective and probably safer alternatives. When used, ERT should be accompanied by a comprehensive screening program consisting of regular lipid profiles, breast examinations, mammography, and gynecologic assessments.[64]

Anabolic therapy with recombinant human PTH (1-34)
Currently, PTH (1-34)—teriparatide—is the only available anabolic agent for osteoporosis in the United States, although other anabolic agents have been developed [*see* Future Therapies, *below*]. Teriparatide was approved by the FDA in late 2002 for use

in osteoporosis. Although chronic elevation in PTH results in bone loss, brief increases in PTH have anabolic effects on bone. A daily injection of recombinant human PTH (hPTH) provides a brief rise in PTH, resulting in increased BMD. To date, teriparatide is the anabolic agent with the most potent effects on BMD. Its effects are particularly dramatic in the spine: in one study comparing teriparatide and alendronate treatment, at the end of 14 months, alendronate-treated patients had a 5.6% increase in lumbar spine BMD, whereas teriparatide-treated patients had a 12.2% increase.[65] It should be noted, however, that teriparatide has not been demonstrated to prevent hip fracture, and it does not have FDA approval for that purpose.

Teriparatide is administered nightly in a standard subcutaneous dose by a pen delivery system. Side effects include flushing, hypercalcemia, and hypercalciuria. Patients must be monitored with measurement of serum calcium and 24-hour urine calcium levels, and calcium intake must be adjusted as needed to keep urine and serum calcium in a normal range. Teriparatide comes with a black-box warning from the FDA concerning an association with risk of sarcomas, based on its effects in rats. For this reason, it is administered for no longer than 2 years, and its use is contraindicated in patients with active malignancy. Unfortunately, the high cost of teriparatide has limited its use, because much of its target population is on Medicare and does not have prescription drug coverage.

Selection of patients for this costly and potent drug should be done with care. Osteoporosis experts have developed a consensus opinion, published in the spring of 2004, to help clinicians identify appropriate patients for teriparatide therapy. Indications for its use were as follows: (1) history of vertebral fracture, T score –3.0 or below, or age greater than 69 years; (2) fracture or unexplained bone loss in patients on antiresorptive therapy; and (3) intolerance of oral bisphosphonate therapy. Contraindications listed include hypercalcemia, Paget disease, history of irradiation to the skeleton, sarcoma, or malignancy involving bone.[66]

Combining teriparatide and bisphosphonates Simultaneous administration of teriparatide and oral bisphosphonates impairs the anabolic effects of teriparatide.[67] When these agents are given sequentially, however, the increase in BMD seen with initial teriparatide therapy is followed by additional gain during subsequent bisphosphonate treatment.[68] This increase in BMD in the setting of bisphosphonate use is thought to reflect mineralization of bone matrix laid down during the teriparatide treatment. Interestingly, when teriparatide is administered to patients who have previously been treated with bisphosphonate, their response to teriparatide is blunted.[69] This finding is of concern, because many patients currently being considered for teriparatide therapy have already been treated with bisphosphonates.

National Osteoporosis Foundation guidelines The most comprehensive set of guidelines for the management of osteoporosis comes from the National Osteoporosis Foundation (NOF).[70] These guidelines, which were updated in 2004, recommend that any postmenopausal women with a prior vertebral or hip fracture should receive pharmacologic therapy to reduce fracture risk. Therapy should also be initiated in women with a hip T score lower than –1.5 and one or more of the following risk factors for osteoporotic fracture: (1) a family history of osteoporosis in a first-degree relative, (2) a personal history of any fracture as an adult, (3) low body weight (< 127 lb), (4) current smoking, or (5) use of oral corticosteroid therapy for more than 3 months. Women with no risk factors for osteoporotic fracture (other than age, gender, and menopausal status) should be treated if the hip T score is below –2.0. In the NOF guidelines, the choice of antiosteoporotic therapy follows current FDA indications, without specific recommendations of one agent over another [see Table 6 for other sources of information].

Follow-up For purposes of monitoring, a follow-up bone density study is indicated no sooner than 1 to 2 years after the initial determination, depending on the results and whether any therapy is initiated. Subsequent measurements may be made at similar or longer intervals, depending on the patient's progress and any further therapeutic alterations. For more precise comparison, follow-up studies should be performed using the same DXA unit, if possible. It should be borne in mind that with many of these therapies, the expected increase in BMD seen on follow-up DXA studies will be minimal in comparison with the improvement in fracture risk. However, patients who continue to lose bone despite ongoing antiresorptive therapy should be evaluated for previously unrecognized causes of secondary osteoporosis. Biochemical bone turnover markers (e.g., N-telopeptide, pyridinoline cross-links) may be helpful to document patient response to antiresorptive therapy, but they show significant variability within individuals, and therefore large changes are necessary for proper interpretation. In addition, their concentrations may be influenced by timing of collection, diet, and other factors. Accordingly, widespread consensus is lacking on their precise role in osteoporosis management.

Future therapies Recombinant hPTH (1-84) is currently in phase III trials and appears to have effects similar to those of hPTH (1-34) (see above). Additional agents in the SERM class include lasofoxifene (currently being evaluated for FDA approval) and bazedoxifene (in phase III trials). Strontium ranelate is an anabolic agent that appears to act on the CaSR to induce osteoblast differentiation. It enhances both bone resorption and formation, with an emphasis on formation, resulting in significantly decreased risk of vertebral fracture.[71] It was approved for use in Europe in late 2004. Preclinical studies of the anabolic effects of vitamin D on bone are under way[72] and may lead to the development of vitamin D analogues for osteoporosis therapy.

OSTEOMALACIA

Osteomalacia is a condition in which the bone matrix is normal in quantity but is weakened by insufficient mineral content. Osteomalacia in the growing skeleton is termed rickets. Causes of osteomalacia include nutritional deficiencies of calcium, phosphate, or vitamin D; intestinal disease affecting the absorption of these substances; abnormalities in vitamin D metabolism, such as occurs in liver disease, renal failure, or through the use of antiepileptic drugs; vitamin D resistance; renal phosphate leak; and oncogenic osteomalacia (a humoral syndrome of increased urinary phosphate loss associated with rare tumors of mesenchymal origin).[73] In adults, severe osteomalacia presents as fatigue, proximal muscle weakness, and diffuse or focal skeletal pain. Mild osteomalacia is common and often asymptomatic.[74] Decreased or low-normal concentrations of both calcium and phosphorus are noted on biochemical testing, and the alkaline phosphatase concentration is elevated. Depending on the cause, decreased levels of either 25-(OH)D$_3$ or calcitriol may be seen. Plain films may demonstrate osteopenia and pseudofrac-

tures. When necessary, the diagnosis can be confirmed with bone biopsy processed and analyzed by an experienced bone pathologist. The treatment of osteomalacia depends on the pathogenesis of the condition. For the majority of cases in which the problem is dietary insufficiency or malabsorption of vitamin D, administration of high doses of cholecalciferol and calcium will rapidly correct deficits and heal the bone. Underlying conditions such as celiac disease (which may be asymptomatic) should be identified and treated. Other conditions, such as tumor-induced osteomalacia, represent special cases and require a different approach (e.g., phosphate supplementation).

PAGET DISEASE OF BONE

Paget disease is a relatively common condition in which abnormal osteoclast function leads to accelerated and disordered bone remodeling, producing highly disorganized bone microarchitecture in affected areas. This sometimes leads to deformity of affected bones, increased vascularity, nerve impingement syndromes, and a propensity to fracture. Paget disease is commonly seen in the elderly and may be familial. The precise etiology is not yet known, although a viral origin is suspected. Many persons with Paget disease are asymptomatic. The sole manifestation may be increased serum alkaline phosphatase activity, detected incidentally on blood testing. If the disease is severe or extensive, pain syndromes may result. Very often, the discomfort originates not from bone itself but from arthritic changes in adjacent joints caused by altered biomechanics. The skull may be enlarged, or there may be significant bowing of the long bones of the legs. Bony overgrowth may lead to local impingement on spinal nerve roots, with pain or neurologic deficits; overgrowth in the inner ear can lead to sensorineural hearing loss. Rare complications include high-output chronic heart failure (from multiple vascular shunts in bone) and transformation to osteosarcoma.

Diagnosis

The diagnosis of Paget disease is typically made after finding isolated elevation of the serum alkaline phosphatase level without evidence of liver disease. (Fractionation of alkaline phosphatase isoenzymes can confirm bone as the source). A nuclear bone scan is performed next to identify involved areas. The results of the bone scan will identify which bones should be evaluated by plain x-ray to exclude signs of metastatic disease and confirm pagetic findings.

Treatment

Treatment of Paget disease is indicated for patients with bone pain; it is also indicated, regardless of symptoms, if there is involvement of a weight-bearing bone or a joint. Antiresorptive

Table 6 Internet Resources for Osteoporosis and Bone Metabolism

American Dietetic Association Nutrition Resources
http://www.eatright.org
American Society for Bone and Mineral Research
http://www.asbmr.org
BoneKEY-Osteovision Site of the International Bone and Mineral Society (IBMS)
http://www.bonekey-ibms.org
International Osteoporosis Foundation
http://www.iofbonehealth.org

agents, such as high-dose oral or injectable bisphosphonates (see above) or injectable calcitonin, can be used to treat this disorder.[75] Treatment of any vitamin D deficiency is essential before starting intravenous bisphosphonate therapy to avoid hypocalcemia. Disease activity and response to therapy are assessed with serial measurement of alkaline phosphatase or other bone turnover markers. The goal of treatment is normalization of alkaline phosphatase. Re-treatment is indicated if the alkaline phosphatase level begins to rise above normal. Patients with skull involvement should have periodic audiometry to exclude hearing loss.

Elizabeth H. Holt, M.D., Ph.D., has no commercial relationships with manufacturers of products or providers of services discussed in this chapter.

Silvio E. Inzucchi, M.D., has received research funding from Eli Lilly Co. and speakers' honoraria from Merck & Co., Inc.

References

1. Brown EM: Physiology and pathophysiology of the extracellular calcium–sensing receptor. Am J Med 106:238, 1999

2. Marx SJ: Hyperparathyroid and hypoparathyroid disorders. N Engl J Med 343:1863, 2000

3. Inzucchi SE: Management of hypercalcemia: diagnostic workup, therapeutic options for hyperparathyroidism and other common causes. Postgrad Med 115:27, 2004

4. Wermers RA, Khosla S, Atkinson EJ, et al: The rise and fall of primary hyperparathyroidism: a population-based study in Rochester, Minnesota, 1965–1992. Ann Intern Med 126:433, 1997

5. Brandi ML, Gagel RF, Angeli A, et al: Guidelines for diagnosis and therapy of MEN type 1 and type 2. J Clin Endocrinol Metab 86:5658, 2001

6. Khan A, Bilezikian J: Primary hyperparathyroidism: pathophysiology and impact on bone. CMAJ 163:184, 2000

7. Brown EM: Familial hypocalciuric hypercalcemia and other disorders with resistance to extracellular calcium. Endocrinol Clin North Am 29:503, 2000

8. Silverberg SJ, Shane E, Jacobs TP, et al: A 10-year prospective study of primary hyperparathyroidism with or without parathyroid surgery. N Engl J Med 341:1249, 1999

9. Bilezikian JP, Potts JT Jr, Fuleihan Gel-H, et al: Summary statement from a workshop on asymptomatic primary hyperparathyroidism: a perspective for the 21st century. J Bone Miner Res 17(suppl 2):N2, 2002

10. Westerdahl J, Lindblom P, Bergenfelz A: Measurement of intraoperative parathyroid hormone predicts long-term operative success. Arch Surg 137:186, 2002

11. Monchik JM, Barellini L, Langer P, et al: Minimally invasive parathyroid surgery in 103 patients with local/regional anesthesia, without exclusion criteria. Surgery 131:502, 2002

12. Civelek AC, Ozalp E, Donovan P, et al: Prospective evaluation of delayed technetium-99m sestamibi SPECT scintigraphy for preoperative localization of primary hyperparathyroidism. Surgery 131:149, 2002

13. Dackiw AP, Sussman JJ, Fritsche HA Jr, et al: Relative contributions of technetium Tc 99m sestamibi scintigraphy, intraoperative gamma probe detection, and the rapid parathyroid hormone assay to the surgical management of hyperparathyroidism. Arch Surg 135:550, 2000

14. Irvin GL 3rd, Carneiro DM: Management changes in primary hyperparathyroidism. JAMA 284:934, 2000

15. Udelsman R: Six hundred fifty-six consecutive explorations for primary hyperparathyroidism. Ann Surg 235:665, 2002

16. Kearns AE, Thompson GB: Medical and surgical management of hyperparathyroidism. Mayo Clin Proc 77:87, 2002

17. Shepherd JJ, Burgess JR, Greenaway TM, et al: Preoperative sestamibi scanning and surgical findings at bilateral, unilateral, or minimal reoperation for recurrent hyperparathyroidism after subtotal parathyroidectomy in patients with multiple endocrine neoplasia type 1. Arch Surg 135:844, 2000

18. Peacock M, Bilezikian JP, Klassen, PS, et al: Cinacalcet hydrochloride maintains long-term normocalcemia in patients with primary hyperparathyroidism. J Clin Endocrinol Metab 90:135, 2005

19. Dunbar ME, Wysolmerski JJ, Broadus AE: Parathyroid hormone–related protein: from hypercalcemia of malignancy to developmental regulatory molecule. Am J Med Sci 312:287, 1996

20. Rankin W, Grill V, Martin TJ: Parathyroid hormone–related protein and hypercalcemia. Cancer 80(8 suppl):1564, 1997

21. Ziegler R: Hypercalcemic crisis. J Am Soc Nephrol 12(suppl 17):S3, 2001

22. Betterle C, Greggio NA, Volpato M: Clinical review 93: autoimmune polyglandular syndrome type 1. J Clin Endocrinol Metab 83:1049, 1998

23. Thomas MK, Lloyd-Jones DM, Thadhani RI, et al: Hypovitaminosis D in medical inpatients. N Engl J Med 338:777, 1998

24. Meyer C: Scientists probe role of vitamin D: deficiency a significant problem, experts say. JAMA. 292:1416, 2004

25. Cummings SR, Melton LJ: Epidemiology and outcomes of osteoporotic fractures. Lancet 359:1761, 2002

26. Seeman E: Pathogenesis of bone fragility in women and men. Lancet 359:1841, 2002

27. Melton LJ III, Thamer M, Ray NF, et al: Fractures attributable to osteoporosis: report from the National Osteoporosis Foundation. J Bone Miner Res 12:16, 1997

28. Heinemann DF: Osteoporosis: an overview of the National Osteoporosis Foundation clinical practice guide. Geriatrics 55:31, 2000

29. Fitzpatrick LA: Secondary causes of osteoporosis. Mayo Clin Proc 77:453, 2002

30. Kanis JA: Diagnosis of osteoporosis and assessment of fracture risk. Lancet 359:1929, 2002

31. Miller PD, Zapalowski C, Kulak CA, et al: Bone densitometry: the best way to detect osteoporosis and to monitor therapy. J Clin Endocrinol Metab 84:1867, 1999

32. Ammann P, Rizzoli R: Bone strength and its determinants. Osteoporo Int 14(S3):S13, 2003

33. Slemenda C: Prevention of hip fractures: risk factor modification. Am J Med 103(2A):65S, 1997

34. Black DM, Steinbach M, Palermo L, et al: An assessment tool for predicting fracture risk in postmenopausal women. Osteoporos Int 12:519, 2001

35. Canalis E, Giustina A: Glucocorticoid-induced osteoporosis: summary of a workshop. J Endocrinol Metab 86:5681, 2001

36. Miller KK, Klibanski A: Clinical review 106: amenorrheic bone loss. J Endocrinol Metab 84:1775, 1999

37. Bilezikian JP: Osteoporosis in men. J Endocrinol Metab 84:3431, 1999

38. Messinger-Rapport BJ, Thacker HL: Prevention for the older woman: a practical guide to prevention and treatment of osteoporosis. Geriatrics 57:16, 2002

39. Kannus P, Parkkari J, Niemi S, et al: Prevention of hip fracture in elderly people with use of a hip protector. N Engl J Med 343:1506, 2000

40. Weaver CM: Calcium requirements of physically active people. Am J Clin Nutr 72(2 suppl):579S, 2000

41. Atkinson SA, Ward WE: Clinical nutrition: 2. The role of nutrition in the prevention and treatment of adult osteoporosis. CMAJ 165:1511, 2001

42. Bischoff-Ferrari HA, Dawson-Hughes B, Willett WC, et al: The effect of vitamin D on falls: a meta-analysis. JAMA 291:1999, 2004

43. Manson JE, Martin KA: Clinical practice: postmenopausal hormone-replacement therapy. N Engl J Med 345:34, 2001

44. Altkorn D, Vokes T: Treatment of postmenopausal osteoporosis. JAMA 285:1415, 2001

45. Delmas PD: Treatment of postmenopausal osteoporosis. Lancet 359:2018, 2002

46. NIH Consensus Development Panel on Osteoporosis Prevention, Diagnosis, and Therapy. JAMA 285:785, 2001

47. Liberman UA, Weiss SR, Broll J, et al: Effect of oral alendronate on bone mineral density and the incidence of fractures in postmenopausal osteoporosis. N Engl J Med 333:1437, 1995

48. Hosking D, Chilvers CED, Christiansen C, et al: Prevention of bone loss with alendronate in postmenopausal women under 60 years of age. N Engl J Med 338:485, 1998

49. Fracture risk reduction with alendronate in women with osteoporosis: the Fracture Intervention Trial. FIT Research Group. J Clin Endocrinol Metab 85:4118, 2000

50. Randomized trial of the effects of risedronate on vertebral fractures in women with established postmenopausal osteoporosis. Vertebral Efficacy with Risedronate Therapy (VERT) Study Group. Osteoporos Int 11:83, 2000

51. Effect of risedronate on the risk of hip fracture in elderly women. Hip Intervention Program Study Group. N Engl J Med 344:333, 2001

52. Rico H, Revilla M, Hernandez ER, et al: Total and regional bone mineral content and fracture rate in postmenopausal osteoporosis treated with salmon calcitonin: a prospective study. Calcif Tissue Int 56:181, 1995

53. Maricic M, Adachi JD, Sarkar S, et al: Early effects of raloxifene on clinical vertebral fractures at 12 months in postmenopausal women with osteoporosis. Arch Intern Med 162:1140, 2002

54. Effects of hormone therapy on bone mineral density: results from the postmenopausal estrogen/progestin interventions (PEPI) trial. PEPI Writing Group. JAMA 276:1389, 1996

55. Rossouw JE, Anderson GL, Prentice RL, et al: Risks and benefits of estrogen plus progestin in healthy post-menopausal women: principal results from the Women's Health Initiative randomized controlled trial. JAMA 288:321, 2002

56. Anderson GL, Limacher M, Assaf AR, et al: Effects of conjugated equine estrogen in postmenopausal women with hysterectomy: the Women's Health Initiative randomized controlled trial. JAMA 291:1701, 2004

57. Vasikaran SD: Bisphosphonates: an overview with special reference to alendronate. Ann Clin Biochem 38(pt 6):608, 2001

58. Crandall C: Risedronate: a clinical review. Arch Intern Med 161:353, 2001

59. Bone HG, Hosking D, Devogelaer JP, et al: Ten years' experience with alendronate for osteoporosis in postmenopausal women. N Engl J Med 350:1189, 2004

60. Khovidhunkit W, Shoback DM: Clinical effects of raloxifene hydrochloride in women. Ann Intern Med 130:431, 1999

61. Continued breast cancer risk reduction in postmenopausal women treated with raloxifene: 4-year results from the MORE trial. Multiple Outcomes of Raloxifene Evaluation. Breast Cancer Res Treat 65:125, 2001

62. Barrett-Connor E, Grady D, Sashegyi A, et al: Raloxifene and cardiovascular events in osteoporotic postmenopausal women: four-year results from the MORE (Multiple

Outcomes of Raloxifene Evaluation) randomized trial. JAMA 287:847, 2002

63. Downs RW Jr, Bell NH, Ettinger MP, et al: Comparison of alendronate and intranasal calcitonin for treatment of osteoporosis in postmenopausal women. J Clin Endocrinol Metab 85:1783, 2000

64. Burkman RT, Collins JA, Greene RA: Current perspectives on benefits and risks of hormone replacement therapy. Am J Obstet Gynecol 185(2 suppl):S13, 2001

65. Body JJ, Gaitch GA, Scheele WH, et al: A randomized double-blind trial to compare the efficacy of teriparatide [recombinant human parathyroid hormone (1-34)] with alendronate in postmenopausal women with osteoporosis. J Clin Endocrinol Metab 87:4528, 2002

66. Miller PD, Bilezikian JP, Deal C, et al: Clinical use of teriparatide in the real world: initial insights. Endocr Practice 10:139, 2004

67. Finkelstein JS, Hayes A, Hunzelman JL, et al: The effects of parathyroid hormone, alendronate, or both in men with osteoporosis. N Engl J Med 349:1216, 2003

68. Rittmaster RS, Bolognese M, Ettinger MP, et al: Enhancement of bone mass in osteoporotic women with parathyroid hormone followed by alendronate. J Clin Endocrinol Metab 85:2129, 2000

69. Ettinger B, San Martin J, Crans G, et al: Differential effects of teriparatide on BMD after treatment with raloxifene or alendronate. J Bone Miner Res 19:745, 2004

70. Physician's Guide to Prevention and Treatment of Osteoporosis. National Osteoporosis Foundation, Washington, DC, 2003

www.nof.org/physguide

71. Meunier PJ, Roux C, Seeman E, et al: The effects of strontium ranelate on the risk of vertebral fracture in women with postmenopausal osteoporosis. N Engl J Med 350:459, 2004

72. Gardiner EM, Baldock PA, Thomas GP, et al: Increased formation and decreased resorption of bone in mice with elevated vitamin D receptor in mature cells of the osteoblast lineage. FASEB J 14:1908, 2000

73. Drezner MK: Tumor-induced osteomalacia. Rev Endocrinol Metab Disord 2:175, 2001

74. Reginato AJ, Falasca GF, Pappu R, et al: Musculoskeletal manifestations of osteomalacia: report of 26 cases and literature review. Semin Arthr Rheum 28:287, 1999

75. Lyles KW, Siris ES, Singer FR, et al: A clinical approach to diagnosis and management of Paget's disease of bone. J Bone Miner Res 16:1379, 2001

76. Dietary Reference Intakes (DRI) and Recommended Dietary Allowances (RDA). Food and Nutrition Information Center, USDA/ARS/National Agriculture Library, Beltsville, Maryland, December 2002
http://www.nal.usda.gov/fnic/etext/000105.html

Acknowledgment

Figure 1   Seward Hung.

58 Obesity

Jonathan Q. Purnell, M.D.

Obesity and its associated disorders are leading causes of morbidity and premature mortality around the world. Obese persons are also vulnerable to low self-esteem and depression because of the psychological and social stigmata that can be associated with obesity. Despite societal prejudicial perceptions that obesity develops because of deficient self-control, research has provided insight into the physiology behind unwanted weight gain. Indeed, during the past decade, the field of body-weight regulation (the study of the homeostatic mechanisms controlling body weight and fat content and the pathophysiology leading to unwanted weight gain or weight loss) has undergone an explosion in research, particularly in the area of neuroendocrine control of appetite and energy expenditure. As with other leading diseases in developed countries, such as hypertension and diabetes, obesity is recognized as a chronic condition resulting from an interaction between environmental influences and an individual's genetic predisposition to weight gain.

The initial evaluation of overweight and obese patients begins with the exclusion of secondary causes of weight gain and the identification of comorbid disorders such as hypertension, diabetes, heart disease, and sleep apnea. Once screening is completed, the approach to the treatment of overweight and obesity is similar to that of other chronic diseases: begin with lifestyle improvements, and then consider medical and surgical options. Although the weight loss that accompanies current therapeutic options is modest on average, the future promises better diagnostic and treatment options for obesity that are based on research into the mechanisms of weight regulation and their role in unwanted weight gain and maintenance of the obese state.

Definition of Obesity

Obesity is an abnormal accumulation of body fat in proportion to body size. Overweight persons have a body-fat proportion that is intermediate between normal and obese. Ideally, an obesity classification system would be based on a practical measurement of body fat that could be performed in the office, would accurately predict disease risk, and would apply to patients from diverse ethnic backgrounds. The most direct measures of body fat, such as underwater weighing or dual-energy x-ray absorptiometry (DXA) scanning, are impractical for use in a clinical setting. Indirect estimates of body fat are clinically more practical.

Classification of Obesity

BODY MASS INDEX

Body mass index (BMI), which is calculated by dividing the body weight in kilograms by height in meters squared, is a classification system that attempts to allow comparison of weights independent of stature across populations. Except in persons who have increased lean weight as a result of intense exercise (e.g., bodybuilders), BMI does correlate with percentage of body fat, but this relationship is independently influenced by sex, age, and race.[1] In the United States, data from the second National Health and Nutrition Examination Survey (NHANES II) were used to define obesity in adults as a BMI of 27.3 kg/m² or more for women and a BMI of 27.8 kg/m² or more for men.[2] These de-

finitions were based on the gender-specific 85th-percentile values of BMI for persons 20 to 29 years of age. In 1998, however, the National Institutes of Health (NIH) Expert Panel on the Identification, Evaluation, and Treatment of Overweight and Obesity in Adults adopted the World Health Organization (WHO) classification for overweight and obesity.[3] The WHO classification, which predominantly applies to people of European ancestry, assigns an increasing risk for comorbid conditions—including hypertension, type 2 diabetes mellitus, and cardiovascular disease—to persons with higher BMIs [*see Table 1*] relative to persons of normal weight (i.e., those with a BMI between 18.5 kg/m² and 25 kg/m²). Asian populations, however, are known to be at increased risk for diabetes and hypertension at lower BMI ranges than those for non-Asian groups.[4] Consequently, the WHO has suggested lower cutoff points for consideration of therapeutic intervention in Asians: a BMI of 18.5 to 23 kg/m² represents acceptable risk, 23 to 27.5 kg/m² represents increased risk, and 27.5 kg/m² or higher represents high risk.[5]

FAT DISTRIBUTION

In addition to an increase in total body fat, a proportionally greater amount of fat in the abdomen or trunk compared with fat in the lower extremities or hips has been associated with increased risk for diabetes, hypertension, and heart disease in both men and women.[6] Abdominal obesity is commonly reported as a waist-to-hip ratio, but it is most easily quantified by a single circumferential measurement obtained at the level of the superior iliac crest.[3] Current guidelines categorize men at increased relative risk for coronary artery disease, diabetes, and hypertension if they have a waist circumference greater than 40 inches (102 cm); women are at increased risk if their waist circumference exceeds 35 inches (88 cm) [*see Table 1*]. Thus, an overweight person with abnormal fat patterning may be at high risk for these diseases even if that person is not obese by BMI criteria. In those of Asian descent, abdominal (central) obesity is recognized to be a better predictor of comorbidity than BMI.[7] Therefore, the WHO has recommended lower waist circumference cutoffs to assign increased risk for comorbidities in this population: 36 inches (90 cm) or more in men and 32 inches (80 cm) or more in women.[4]

Table 1 Classification of Weight and Risk for Comorbid Conditions[2]

Classification	Body Mass Index (kg/m²)	Risk for Diabetes, Hypertension, and Cardiovascular Disease	
		Normal Waist Circumference*	Increased Waist Circumference*
Underweight	< 18.5	Average	Average
Normal	18.5–24.9	Average	Average
Overweight	25–29.9	↑	↑↑
Obese	30–34.9	↑↑	↑↑↑
	35–39.9	↑↑↑	↑↑↑
	≥ 40	↑↑↑↑	↑↑↑↑

*Normal waist circumference is ≤ 102 cm (40 in) in men, ≤ 88 cm (35 in) in women.

Epidemiology

In the United States, the prevalence of overweight has been increasing over the past several decades [*see Figure 1*]. In the most recently published United States data (1999 to 2002), 65% of adults are overweight (BMI 25 to 30 kg/m²), 30% of the total population are obese (BMI 30 to 40 kg/m²), and 5% have a BMI of 40 kg/m² or higher.[8,9] The prevalence of obesity has also risen in some minority populations, with the highest rates found in some Native American groups, Hispanics, and African Americans; the lowest rates have been found in populations of Asian ancestry [*see Figure 2*].[9-12] Prevalence rates for obesity in the United States are also highest in populations with less education and lower income levels.[12] Internationally, obesity rates are generally lower than those in the United States.[13] However, even in societies that traditionally had the lowest prevalence of overweight and obesity, the rates of weight gain are beginning to meet or exceed those of Western societies.[14]

The age at which obesity is most prevalent has also increased. Until NHANES III (1988 through 1994), obesity in the United States peaked between the ages of 40 and 59 years, then declined in the older-age groups.[9] According to the most recent NHANES data (1999 to 2002), the prevalence of obesity now remains high past the age of 60 years, reaching 30.5% in men and 34.7% in women.[9] In studies that have measured body composition in unselected populations, fat mass also peaks just past middle age in men and women, but percent body fat continues to increase past this age, particularly in men, because of a proportionally greater loss in lean mass.[15-17] The menopausal period has also been associated with an increase in percent body fat and propensity for central fat distribution, even though total body weight changes very little during this time.[18] A propensity for greater abdominal adiposity has also been demonstrated in men,[19] in older individuals,[20] and in persons with impaired glucose tolerance or type 2 diabetes.[21]

Etiology and Genetics

Studies of populations, families, adoptions, and twins have established a strong genetic role in determining body weight. Estimates of the genetic contribution to the variance of relative body weight and adiposity range from a low of approximately 20% to a high of 90%.[22] The largest study to date to address the contribution of nature versus nurture to body weight, which used a dataset that included over 25,000 twin pairs and 50,000 biologic and adoptive family members, found that genetic factors accounted for 67% of the variance in adiposity in men and women.[22] Rarely, childhood-onset obesity will manifest itself as a result of a single-gene obesity syndrome, such as Prader-Willi syndrome or Bartlett-Biedel syndrome, or from a mutation in one of the genes encoding proteins involved with body-weight regulation, such as the pro-opiomelanocortin (*POMC*) gene, which makes α-melanocortin–stimulating hormone (α-MSH); the melanocortin receptor (MC4); leptin; the leptin receptor; and prohormone convertase enzymes.[23]

Although the genetics explaining the tendency toward overweight and obesity in the majority of the population remains to be elucidated, over 600 genetic markers have been described in association with obesity-related variables in humans (e.g., BMI, skin-fold thickness, waist-to-hip ratio, fat mass, and percent fat mass).[23] With time, discoveries of specific gene products, the role that these proteins play in the pathophysiology of weight regulation, and their interaction with the environment in the expression of unwanted weight gain should lead to more specific pharmacologic treatments for overweight and obese patients who fail to respond adequately to lifestyle measures alone.

Epidemiologic studies have identified several environmental factors that contribute to the continued weight gain documented over the past several decades in westernized countries. The foremost among these factors are an increasingly sedentary lifestyle (e.g., increased car use, community and work environments that discourage activity, and more time spent watching television) and the availability of energy-dense (high-fat, concentrated-sugar), low-fiber foods.[24-28] In children, the increased consumption of sugar-added beverages and reduction of dairy intake have also been associated with greater weight gain in prospective studies.[29,30] Similar environmental predictors of weight gain have been described in societies adopting Western lifestyles in the transition to First World economies.[14,31] Additional societal trends that are thought to have contributed to the increasing weight gain in the United States include smoking cessation (cigarette smoking is known to reduce body weight)[25,32] and eating a greater proportion of food away from home, particularly at fast-food restaurants, where food is typically very calorically dense.[28,33]

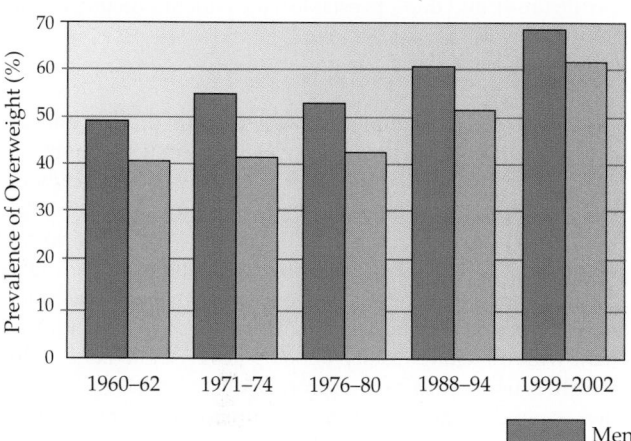

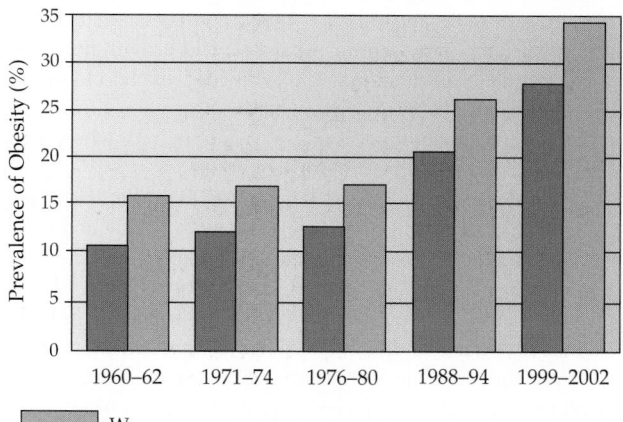

Figure 1   **Time trends of age-adjusted prevalence of overweight (BMI ≥ 25 kg/m²) and obesity (BMI ≥ 30 kg/m²) in United States men and women who are 20 years of age and older.**[8]

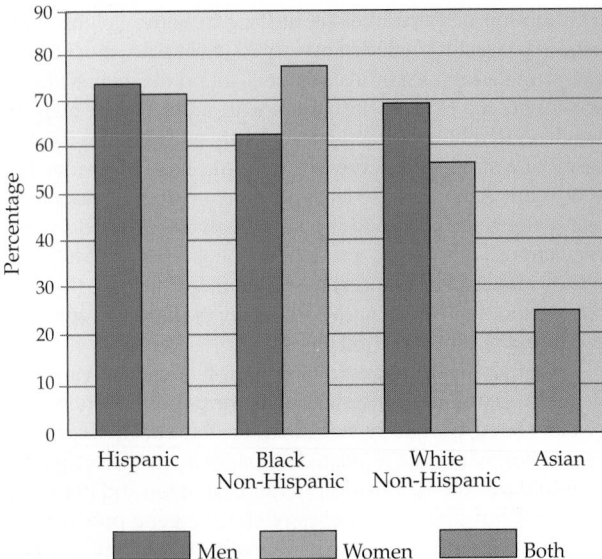

Figure 2   **Age-adjusted percentage of United States adults who were overweight (BMI ≥ 25 kg/m²), by sex and race/ethnicity, 1999–2002.**[8] **Data for Asians include both men and women in 2003.**[11]

Pathophysiology and Pathogenesis

Arguably the most significant recent advances in the science of obesity have been in the area of neuroendocrine control of energy homeostasis, including the understanding of the mechanisms that lead to unwanted weight gain and the counterregulatory systems that restore weight lost after caloric restriction. At its most basic level, body weight is the end result of a balance between energy taken in and energy expended. Weight gain ensues when more energy is consumed than expended. Weight loss occurs through restriction of energy intake, increased energy output, or both. However, this simple model fails to incorporate what are now known to be complex homeostatic systems that counteract voluntary energy perturbations, whether they be forced overfeeding or caloric restriction.

A homeostatic model of weight regulation is conceptually identical to other tightly regulated systems in the body. For example, blood glucose levels reflect input from meals and hepatic stores balanced against clearance through uptake by peripheral tissues and excretion by the kidneys. Glucose levels are kept within a normal range by complex, integrated responses from insulin, glucagon, and other so-called counterregulatory hormones such as catecholamines, cortisol, and growth hormone, which regulate production and clearance. Elevated blood glucose levels and diabetes result when the secretion of primary regulators (i.e., insulin and glucagon) is impaired, when resistance to insulin signaling develops, or both.

Like glucose, body weight is regulated at multiple levels to maintain a normal range or set point through an interaction between systems that control meal-to-meal intake (satiety) and those that control relative fat mass (adiposity) [*see Figure 3*].[34] Although short-term (meal-to-meal) signals such as cholecystokinin have been studied for decades, a long-term afferent signal from the fat tissue, leptin, was not discovered until 1994.[35] Leptin is a hormone that is secreted by fat cells in direct proportion to total fat mass, is transported across the blood-brain barrier, and has receptors in hypothalamic nuclei that control appetite and energy expenditure.[34] When leptin levels decline with

weight loss from caloric restriction or when they increase with overfeeding, altered signaling in central hypothalamic centers become integrated with other input signals (e.g., insulin and ghrelin) to set in motion systems that restore body weight to baseline. Therefore, most obese patients fail to sustain long-term weight loss with calorie restriction alone because of activation of these counterregulatory systems and their promotion of a positive energy balance. In this feedback-loop model of weight regulation, primary obesity results when leptin signaling to central centers is reduced (leptin resistance),[34] resulting in uncompensated weight gain that eventually reestablishes energy homeostasis at a higher body-weight set point and blood level of leptin, analogous to insulin levels rising in compensation for acquired insulin resistance.

Although this model oversimplifies the complex nature of body-weight regulation, it nonetheless provides a starting point for clinicians in their education of patients about the pathophysiology of obesity and in the rationale for medical management. To achieve sustained weight reduction in overweight and obese patients, interventions must prevent activation of counterregulatory systems that act to restore lost weight by increasing appetite or reducing energy expenditure. Future medical therapies will be based on an understanding of the body's weight regulatory system and will have greater promise for success in maintaining weight loss.

With aging, dysregulation of a number of hypothalamic-pituitary systems may contribute to increased fat mass and sarcopenia. For example, growth hormone secretion diminishes with age.[36] Prospective trials in older adults that involved replacing growth hormone and targeting levels of insulinlike growth factor–1 (IGF-1) to the midnormal to upper-normal range have demonstrated improved body composition (less fat, more lean tissue) and, in some studies, reduced central fat.[36-38] In addition, the decline in testosterone levels in men, the drop in estrogen levels in women at menopause, and increased levels of cortisol in both sexes may also contribute to reduced muscle mass, central fat distribution, or both.[18,39-41]

Diagnosis

The history, physical examination, and laboratory evaluation of overweight and obese patients are directed toward three goals: first, to identify secondary causes of obesity [*see Differential Diagnosis, below*]; second, to identify comorbid conditions [*see Figure 4*]; and third, to establish the patient's dietary and activity habits.

HISTORY

A number of the symptoms associated with diseases that can cause or contribute to unwanted weight gain, such as hypothyroidism or Cushing disease, occur frequently in overweight patients. These include fatigue, aches, cold intolerance, constipation, poor exercise tolerance, central obesity, loss of libido, and depression. Deciding when to screen a patient for secondary causes of obesity, therefore, can be a challenge for the practitioner. Establishing a pattern of weight gain may be helpful. A patient with a lifelong history of being heavy and a stable adult weight is unlikely to have a secondary cause of obesity. A sudden or rapid weight gain over a few months or years, however, especially when accompanied by onset of comorbid conditions, may correspond to the prescription of medications that contribute to excess weight gain (especially steroids and newer an-

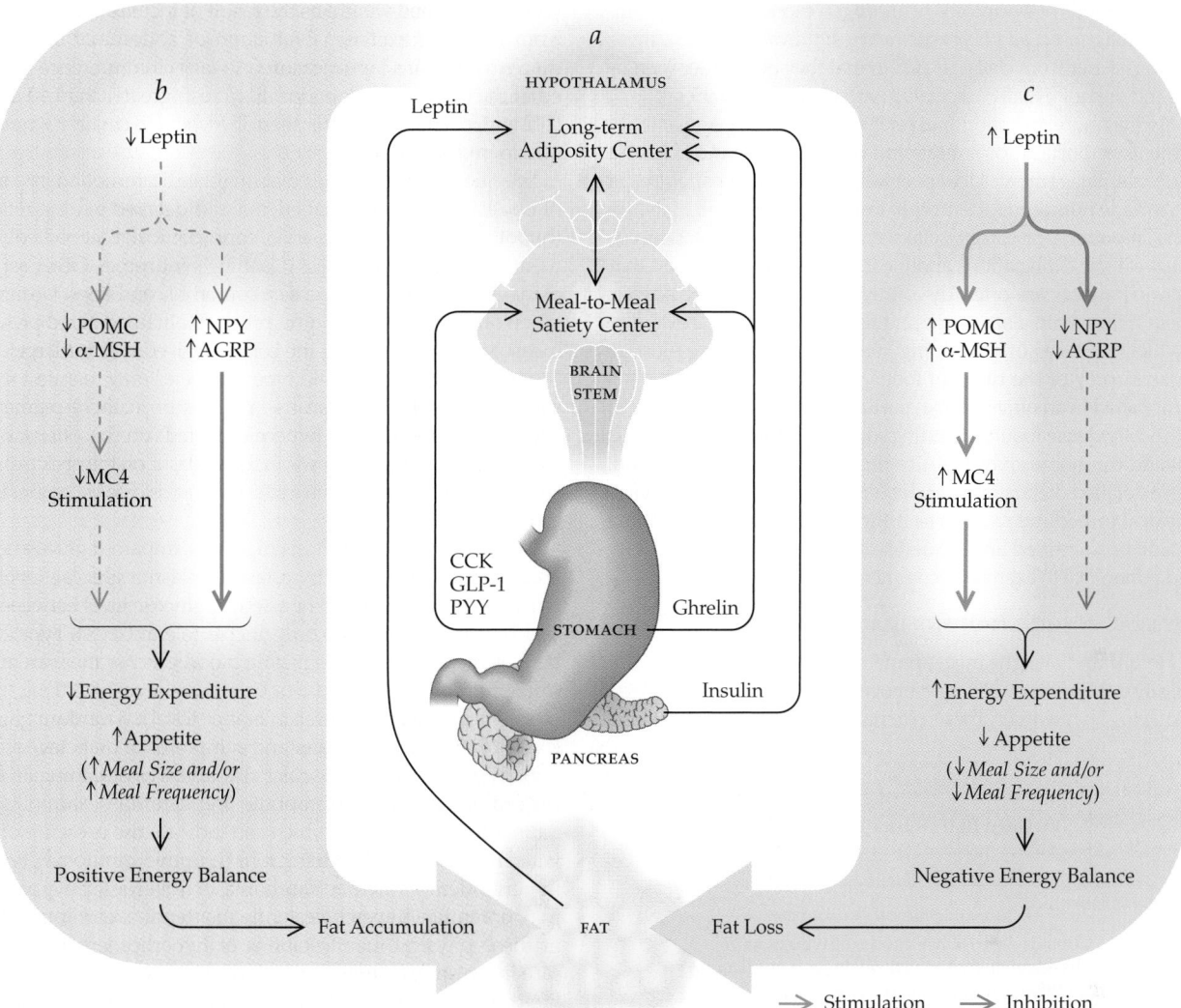

Figure 3 (*a*) **A feedback model for body-weight regulation in humans based on data from animal models.**[34] **Hypothalamic centers that control long-term energy homeostasis sense fat stores through circulating levels of leptin and insulin. Satiety signals (short-term or meal-to-meal regulators) from the gut are relayed through the brain stem to the hypothalamus, where they are integrated with signals reflecting fat stores. These integrated signals then affect appetite and energy expenditure so as to maintain body weight within a set point range. (*b*) Leptin controls appetite and energy expenditure in the hypothalamus by alternatively stimulating production of pro-opiomelanocortin (POMC) and α-melanocortin (α-MSH) and inhibiting production of neuropeptide-Y (NPY) and agouti-related protein (AGRP). α-MSH binds to the melanocortin-4 receptor (MC4), which inhibits appetite and increases energy expenditure. NPY and AGRP stimulate appetite while decreasing energy expenditure. Reduced leptin secretion, such as that which occurs after voluntary caloric restriction,[59,146] leads to enhanced NPY/AGRP signaling, diminished MC4 signaling, and positive energy balance once caloric restriction ceases.[147,148] On the other hand, overfeeding leads to increased fat mass and leptin secretion,[149] reduced NPY/AGRP signaling, increased MC4 signaling, and negative energy balance[148,150] until body weight is restored to baseline. (CCK—cholecystokinin; GLP-1—glucagonlike peptide–1; PYY—peptide YY)**

tipsychotics) or indicate onset of an illness that requires further evaluation.

The history should include questions about diseases for which overweight and obese patients are at higher risk, including hypertension, impaired glucose tolerance or diabetes, hyperlipidemia, heart disease, pulmonary disease, and sleep apnea. These conditions may cause minimal or no symptoms and therefore may be present for months or years before a diagnosis is made. Sleep apnea in particular is a common cause of fatigue and poor concentration or work performance in obese patients; these symptoms are often mistakenly ascribed to an abnormally functioning thyroid gland (despite normal results on thyroid function tests) or a so-called altered metabolism. This diagnosis may be missed unless the clinician specifically asks about characteristic symptoms: restless sleep at night, snoring or observed apnea, fatigue or headache upon awakening and during the daytime, and spontaneous daytime sleep when inactive or while driving. In severely obese patients, increasing peripheral edema, orthopnea, and worsening exercise tolerance may be symptoms of congestive heart failure or pulmonary hypertension and right-sided heart failure from severe sleep apnea. New-onset headaches may indicate normal-pressure hydrocephalus. Gastroesophageal reflux disease usually results in heartburn or an acid taste in the throat. During a period of weight gain, women may develop irregular periods or symptoms of androgen excess. Although commonly diagnosed as polycystic ovary syndrome (PCOS), these findings differ from classic PCOS in that they occur after menarche and are not usually associated with polycystic ovaries.

Finally, inquiring about past and present dietary and activity habits is important for subsequent discussions of medical and surgical management. Most overweight and obese patients will have made numerous attempts to lose weight, through diets, exercise regimens, or commercial weight-loss programs. Because of unrealistic expectations and the inevitable weight regain that occurs, patients are often discouraged or leery of new advice. These failures can also compound feelings of guilt or inadequacy, fueling cycles of worsening self-image and depression. A broad survey of the types of foods people eat can often be accomplished in an office visit; in particular, asking about intake of calorically dense foods, including sodas, and frequency of meals outside the home may identify habits that can be improved. More detailed dietary analysis requires a visit with a nutritionist. Physical impediments such as arthritis, back pain, and asthma should be identified and treated so as to optimize daily activity and adherence to exercise recommendations.

PHYSICAL EXAMINATION AND LABORATORY TESTS

Height and weight measurements in the office are used to classify patients as overweight or obese according to BMI criteria [see Table 1]; however, these criteria may not apply to patients

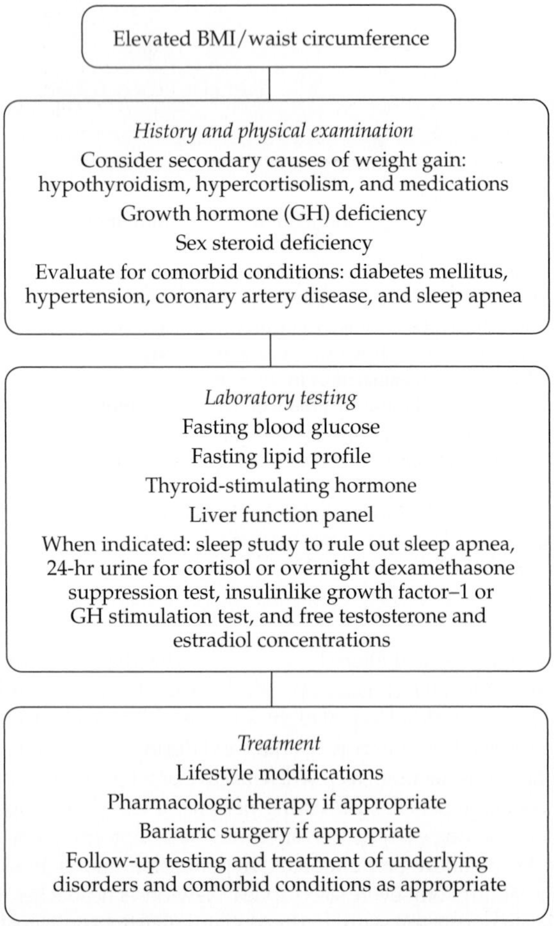

Figure 4   Evaluation, laboratory testing, and treatment of overweight and obese patients.

who have gained weight as the result of increased muscle mass from intensive exercise. Evaluation of abdominal obesity requires the use of a tape measure. A waist circumference (obtained at the level of the superior iliac crest) greater than 40 inches (102 cm) in a man or greater than 35 inches (88 cm) in a woman is considered abnormal.

Specific physical findings that might indicate secondary causes of obesity include pretibial edema and delayed tendon reflexes (hypothyroidism), purple striae, supraclavicular fat pad enlargement, and muscle weakness (Cushing syndrome). Other aspects of the clinical evaluation focus on comorbid conditions. Documentation of hypertension requires properly obtained blood pressure measurements (i.e., using the correctly sized cuff for larger persons). Insulin resistance and type 2 diabetes may manifest themselves as acanthosis nigricans—patches of feathery-pigmented skin (hyperkeratotic and hyperpigmented) on the extensor surfaces of the hands and elbows, in the axilla, or on the neck [see Chapter 34]. Hepatomegaly can indicate hepatosteatosis, especially in centrally obese subjects.

With or without acanthosis nigricans, impaired glucose tolerance may be diagnosed by a fasting plasma glucose level between 100 and 125 mg/dl or a 2-hour glucose level between 140 and 200 mg/dl during an oral glucose tolerance test. Type 2 diabetes is diagnosed by two fasting blood glucose measurements of 126 mg/dl or greater, a 2-hour glucose level of 200 mg/dl or more during an oral glucose tolerance test, or a random glucose level of 200 mg/dl or greater and symptoms of diabetes.

Screening for macrovascular risk involves obtaining an electrocardiogram when appropriate and carefully examining the patient for xanthomata, which can indicate the presence of elevated blood levels of chylomicrons (eruptive xanthoma), type III hyperlipidemia (palmar xanthoma or tuberoeruptive xanthoma), or familial hypercholesterolemia (tendon xanthoma). Each of these physical manifestations of hyperlipidemia, although rare in a primary care practice, indicates a severe or potentially life-threatening condition that requires urgent diagnosis and treatment. A fasting lipid profile should be obtained to complete the cardiovascular risk assessment, and if necessary, treatment should be instituted according to guidelines from the National Cholesterol Education Program Expert Panel.[42] This panel also incorporated several nonlipid risk factors for cardiovascular disease into its recommendations for clinical care by defining criteria for a condition that has become known as the metabolic syndrome (also called syndrome X, the deadly quartet, and the insulin-resistance syndrome). The metabolic syndrome includes the most common abnormalities of lipid and glucose metabolism that accompany abdominal obesity [see Table 2]. Identifying these abnormalities in a patient allows the practitioner to better assign that patient's risk for diabetes and coronary artery disease.[43] Similar criteria are now recognized by the Centers for Disease Control and Prevention (CDC) as the dysmetabolic syndrome X and have been assigned a diagnosis code (277.7) in the International Classification of Diseases, 9th Revision (ICD-9). Screening laboratory tests for hepatosteotosis include a liver panel. In addition, all overweight patients should have documentation of normal thyroid function with a thyroid-stimulating hormone level.

Although obesity is associated with abnormal levels of a number of hormones and cytokines, including leptin, ghrelin, interleukins, and tumor necrosis factor, measurement of these variables should be limited to research protocols and are not currently recommended for general clinical practice.

Table 2 Criteria for Metabolic Syndrome[42,151]

Any Three of the Following:

Increased waist circumference
  Men: > 102 cm (40 in)
  Women: > 88 cm (35 in)

Fasting plasma glucose ≥ 100 mg/dl

Elevated blood pressure
  Systolic ≥ 130 mm Hg
  Diastolic ≥ 85 mm Hg

Serum triglyceride level ≥ 150 mg/dl

Decreased high-density lipoprotein (HDL) cholesterol level
  Men < 40 mg/dl
  Women < 50 mg/dl

Differential Diagnosis

It is important for clinicians to be alert for secondary medical causes of obesity but also to be aware that, in most cases, treatment of these coexisting diseases rarely leads to complete reversal of the obese state. As an example, hypothyroidism is relatively common in the general population and may be present in an obese patient, but the weight loss that might be expected with thyroid hormone replacement is limited and variable.

Hypercortisolemia of Cushing syndrome is a rare cause of unwanted weight gain, but clinicians should have a low threshold for screening for this disease when patients experience large amounts of weight gain in a short period, especially when the weight gain is accompanied by hypertension, diabetes, or muscle weakness. Deficiencies of growth hormone or gonadal steroids are also associated with modest increases in body adiposity. Growth hormone deficiency can lead to reduced muscle mass and increased fat mass, which is improved with hormone replacement therapy.[44] Similar changes in body composition have been described in hypogonadal men[45] and in postmenopausal women.[18] Unfortunately, obesity is often accompanied by low levels of IGF-1 and, in men, low testosterone levels because of low sex-hormone–binding globulin levels. To distinguish obesity-associated low testosterone from a true deficiency state, free testosterone levels can be measured. In addition, weight loss will increase both IGF-1 and total testosterone levels in obese patients but not in patients with true deficiencies.

A number of medications can lead to unwanted weight gain and obesity; if possible, such patients should be switched to alternative agents [*see Table 3*]. Drug-related weight gain occurs most commonly during long-term glucocorticoid treatment of inflammatory conditions (e.g., asthma and inflammatory arthritis), with immunosuppression after transplantation, and with cancer chemotherapy. When possible, reducing or discontinuing a glucocorticoid in favor of an alternative medication can reverse this weight gain. Patients with type 1 or type 2 diabetes often gain weight after starting therapy; this weight gain is proportional to the degree of improved glycemic control and results from a reduction in glucosuria and improvement in metabolic efficiency.[46] Long-term studies have shown that intensive insulin treatment of type 1 diabetes can result in excessive weight gain and obesity in up to 25% of patients; in type 2 diabetes, intensive glycemic control with insulin, a sulfonylurea, or one of the thiazolidinediones may also result in greater weight gain than that predicted by improved glycemic control alone.[47] Therapy with metformin plus nighttime long-acting insulin may reduce or prevent this extra weight gain,[48] and newer diabetes medications, such as pramlintide and exenatide, can improve glycemic control in both type 1 and type 2 diabetes with a modest weight loss.[47] Neuropsychotropic drugs, particularly newer antipsychotic and antiseizure medications, have been associated with weight gain (sometimes massive), obesity, and diabetes.[49,50]

Table 3 Medications Commonly Associated with Weight Gain and Obesity, with Possible Alternative Agents[47,49,152]

Medication Class	Agents	Alternatives
Steroids	Glucocorticoids	Asthma: inhalers Cancer chemotherapy: non–glucocorticoid-based regimens Rheumatoid arthritis: methotrexate and remitting agents
Antidiabetic drugs	Insulin Sulfonylureas Thiazolidinediones	Metformin, acarbose, pramlintide, exenatide
Antiepileptic drugs	Gabapentin Valproic acid	Lamotrigine Topiramate Zonisamide
Antipsychotic agents	Clozapine Olanzapine Quetiapine Risperidone Sertindole	Aripiprazole Haloperidol Ziprasidone
Antidepressants	Tricyclic antidepressants Monoamine oxidase inhibitors Mirtazapine	Bupropion Nefazodone Selective serotonin reuptake inhibitors Venlafaxine

Treatment

As a first step in the management of obesity, appropriate follow-up testing and treatment should be provided for any secondary causes of obesity and comorbid conditions identified during screening. Then, the approach to the treatment of obesity is similar to that of other chronic conditions, such as hypertension, hypercholesterolemia, and diabetes. Intervention starts with lifestyle measures for 3 to 6 months. For obesity, these lifestyle interventions include improved diet and increased activity. For patients whose weight does not change with lifestyle intervention alone or whose weight loss is insufficient to lower their long-term health risk, consideration is then given to pharmacologic or surgical management. An NIH expert panel has suggested that patients whose BMI is 30 or more or who have a BMI of 27 or more plus obesity-related risk factors (i.e., diabetes, hypertension, or hyperlipidemia) could be considered for pharmacologic therapy.[3] Patients with a BMI of 40 or more or a BMI of 35 or more plus obesity-related risk factors could be considered for surgical therapy.

The weight-loss goal for the treatment of obesity is sustained weight loss of 5% or more of initial body weight. Although this goal does not result in attainment of a normal body weight (BMI of 19 to 25) in the majority of patients, it still represents a weight loss that can be achieved with available intervention modalities and that has been associated with lower morbidity, including reductions in risk for diabetes and heart disease.[51,52]

For some patients who are experiencing a period of weight gain, weight stability may be their primary goal. This is especially common in patients who have just completed a low-calorie weight-loss program and are struggling to remain below their initial weight.

NONMEDICAL (LIFESTYLE) THERAPY

Diet Modification

Caloric restriction Hypocaloric diets have been a mainstay recommendation by the medical community for obese patients. These diets range from a moderate reduction in daily intake (200 to 500 fewer calories a day) to more stringent, very low calorie diets (600 to 800 total calories a day), which require careful follow-up by a nutritionist and a physician to avoid life-threatening electrolyte disorders and symptomatic cholelithiasis. Although it is possible to achieve short-term weight loss with these strategies, long-term weight loss is poor even when behavior-modification weight-maintenance programs are continued. Analyses of published data on long-term weight-loss maintenance showed that approximately 50% of the initial lost body weight is regained within the first 1 to 2 years, and 95% or more is regained by 5 years after the completion of the calorie-restriction phase.[53,54] This restoration of lost body weight after a period of calorie-restriction–induced weight loss can be explained by the reduction of fat-dependent feedback signals to the brain, such as leptin, which then activate counterregulatory systems to restore body weight to baseline [see Pathophysiology and Pathogenesis, above].

The long-term failure to maintain weight loss after caloric restriction also indicates that the central set point for body weight is not reset at a lower body weight with the passage of time. Another important implication of these data is that obesity treatments lacking mechanisms that interfere with this counterregulatory system will likely fail to allow long-term weight-loss maintenance. Some existing therapies do result in limited weight loss

without activation of appetite (see below) and can be combined with caloric restriction for improved long-term weight-loss maintenance; these include a low-fat diet,[55,56] exercise,[56] and pharmacologic treatments.[57,58]

Dietary-fat restriction An increase in dietary-fat intake leads to obesity in animal studies and has been associated with a higher prevalence of overweight and obesity in many human-population studies.[25] Prospectively randomizing overweight and obese persons to ad libitum feeding (eating until one feels full, then stopping) of a fat-restricted diet results in a spontaneous reduction in caloric intake and subsequent modest weight loss, compared with results in persons on a diet that contains a higher amount of fat typical of Western societies.[59] This calorie reduction occurs despite a concomitant fall in leptin levels, in contrast to the increase in appetite that follows a fall in leptin levels with weight loss from caloric restriction.[59-61] By implication, an increase in dietary fat results in a state of central leptin resistance, requiring a higher level of body fat and leptin levels to attain a new body-weight equilibrium,[62] whereas dietary-fat restriction leads to partial improvement in leptin signaling, resulting in spontaneous reduction in appetite and body weight.

The average amount of weight loss attributable to a low-fat diet in these studies, however, is only on the order of 3 to 4 kg (6.6 to 8.8 lb).[59] In addition, the weight-loss responses of persons to a low-fat diet can vary tremendously, with some individuals losing 13 kg (28.7 lb) or more and others losing no weight or even gaining weight.[63] This variable response to a lifestyle intervention, such as a change in a specific diet component, is common in chronic diseases whose expression results from an interaction between a genetic predisposition and environmental influence. In patients with hypertension, for example, blood pressure reductions in response to restriction of dietary salt are also heterogeneous.

An apparent paradox has been reported in that the average percent fat content of the American diet is dropping, yet the weight of the American population keeps increasing. Although it is true that the average percentage of total calories from fat in the American diet has declined over the past several decades (from 36% to 34%, according to the most recent NHANES data),[64] this did not occur because Americans have been eating less fat (daily dietary fat intake was 81.9 g in 1972 and increased to 85.5 g in 1990) but, rather, because total calories increased, leading to a lower fat percentage.[65] In contrast, studies that documented weight loss with a lower fat intake did so by lowering the absolute amount of fat in the diet. It is worth noting that the levels of fat restriction leading to weight loss in these studies were not severe. Severe fat restriction (< 20% of total calories) may not be sustainable for many patients because of limited food options and palatability.

Dietary-carbohydrate changes Increasing dietary-carbohydrate intake while lowering total fat intake results in modest spontaneous reduction in caloric intake and weight loss in overweight and obese persons. In the studies that documented this effect, the additional carbohydrates were derived from fruits, vegetables, and grain products, and the resulting increase in dietary fiber also may have played a role in greater satiety and weight loss. In society (especially in young people), however, dietary carbohydrates have increasingly been consumed in the form of processed foods sweetened with sucrose or fructose. These simple carbohydrates (especially fructose) may potentially have deleterious effects on insulin resistance, lipid levels, and body weight when consumed in large amounts.[29,66]

Paradoxically, severe carbohydrate restriction (< 30 g/day) may also lead to modest spontaneous weight loss without initial activation of appetite. Such severe carbohydrate restriction initially mobilizes glycogen stores in the liver and induces ketogenesis, and the resulting diuresis accounts for some of this weight loss.[67] At one time, the ability to draw meaningful conclusions about the longer-term safety and efficacy of low-carbohydrate diets was impeded by the paucity of controlled studies and the variability of carbohydrate restriction from study to study (from < 20 to ≥ 200 g/day).[68] Although methodological issues remain, randomized, controlled studies have now shown that during the first 6 months of diet treatment, persons placed on a low-carbohydrate diet lose weight more rapidly than those placed on a low-calorie, low-fat diet.[69-71] Subsequently, however, individuals on the low-carbohydrate diet either stop losing weight or regain weight, and by 1 year, weight loss is the same with the two diets.[70-72] The average 1-year weight loss ranged from 2.5 to 5.1 kg in these studies, and both diets had a high dropout rate, of approximately 30% to 40%.[70-72] Contrary to popular beliefs about the potential adverse effects of consuming diets high in fat or carbohydrates, lipid levels and glucose metabolism improved with both diets in proportion to weight loss.[69-73]

Dietary-protein changes Increasing dietary-protein intake has also been associated with weight loss. In one of the few prospective, randomized studies of an ad libitum high-protein diet (fat restricted), obese patients experienced significantly greater weight loss than obese control subjects who followed a regular diet or a low-fat, high-carbohydrate diet over a period of 6 months.[74] After 12 months, however, total weight loss on the high-protein diet was attenuated and no longer differed from that seen with the high-carbohydrate diet.[74]

Most nutrition societies recommend limiting protein intake to approximately 10% to 15 % of daily calories because of concerns regarding long-term health consequences of high intake of protein (especially animal protein). These concerns include the possible association of increased protein intake with intestinal cancers, bone disease, and renal disease. To date, prospective studies have shown that increasing dietary protein increases the glomerular filtration rate,[75] which may be harmful to patients with existing renal disease or diabetes, but the long-term effect of increased glomerular filtration rate in otherwise healthy persons is not known.

Dietary fiber Increased dietary fiber has been shown to improve body weight and cardiovascular risk factors.[76,77] Typical high-fiber foods include fruits, vegetables, oat and wheat bran, and legumes, which are also low in fat. Even after controlling for low-fat content, however, diets higher in fiber result in reduced intake and a weight loss of approximately 2 kg.[76] Although it is possible to increase fiber through the use of supplements such as psyllium or methylcellulose, the current intake of fiber in the United States of about 15 g/day could be increased to 25 to 30 g/day by avoiding calorically dense, refined-sugar foods and increasing consumption of fruits, vegetables, and whole-grain products.

Summary of dietary recommendations Overall, an initial recommendation to lower dietary-fat intake and increase dietary-fiber intake for weight loss is reasonable and supported by the scientific literature. Long-term studies of greater than 1 year have not been conducted to show that this weight loss is sustained. Nevertheless, animal models of obesity, population studies, and prospective studies of 1 year or less of low-fat, high-fiber diets versus high-fat diets have documented that a high-fat diet is detrimental to body weight and that restriction of dietary fat to 25% to 30% of calories and an increase of 10 to 15 g of fiber a day result in a significant, albeit limited, weight loss for the average patient.

It is important that clinicians discourage unrealistic expectations about weight loss from a low-fat, high-fiber diet so that patients do not become disillusioned with this therapy. Also, patients should be informed that low-fat, high-fiber diets have been shown to reduce numerous health risks, especially when instituted as part of an overall lifestyle change that includes exercise.[50,78] For this dietary advice to be effective, however, it is often necessary to refer patients to a nutritionist for evaluation and follow-up.

A low-fat diet can be achieved by substituting either carbohydrate or protein for fat; this allows tailoring of the diet to the individual patient. Some patients may respond better to a high-carbohydrate diet in terms of food preferences and weight loss, whereas others might have better responses to a high-protein diet, although all these diet variations have shown only moderate weight loss.[72] A low-carbohydrate diet cannot currently be recommended for clinical practice, because it has not been shown to be superior to other diets[70,72]; the long-term health outcomes of sustained ketosis are uncertain; and increased intake of saturated fat and *trans*-fatty acids may negate the benefit of weight loss by increasing serum cholesterol and triglyceride levels in some patients.[72,73] Many questions concerning the effects of a higher protein intake (up to 30% of total calories) on patients' renal function remain unanswered. For this reason, high-protein diets should be avoided in patients with existing renal disease and diabetes.

Exercise

Increasing energy expenditure through exercise has been another mainstay of obesity therapy. Without counterregulation (alteration in appetite or non–exercise-based energy expenditure), an increase in activity should lead to continued and sustained weight loss. Prospective intervention studies have shown, however, that the average amount of weight loss attributable to exercise alone (no caloric restriction in addition to the exercise) is small, ranging from 1 to 4 kg (2.2 to 8.8 lb).[79,80] Further weight loss presumably is limited by alterations in nonexercise energy expenditure that compensate for the increase in exercise-induced energy expenditure; increased appetite can be discounted as the source of counterregulation, because most studies show little change in energy intake.[81]

Current recommendations are to participate in 3 to 5 hours of moderate to vigorous activity per week. For many patients, especially those with limited mobility, simply increasing activity may be an initial goal. As with alterations in the macronutrient content of the diet, exercise leads to variable degrees of weight loss, ranging from little or none to a substantial amount. Even with moderate weight loss, which is typical, patients should be encouraged to continue with increased activity because of the numerous health benefits attributable to being fit.[82,83]

Combined Diet and Exercise

A number of studies have prospectively examined the effect of combined diet and exercise interventions on health outcomes.

Sustained weight loss with caloric restriction can be improved with a low-fat diet[84,85] or regular exercise.[79,86] In a national survey seeking to determine the characteristics of persons who have been able to sustain a weight loss of at least 13.6 kg (30 lb) for 1 year, responders reported that on average, they followed a diet consisting of approximately 24% fat[87] and expended an average of 2,827 kcal/wk in exercise (roughly the equivalent of walking 28 miles/wk).[88] This level of activity is nearly three times more than the 1,000 kcal/wk recommended by the American College of Sports Medicine for the minimum weekly exercise for the purposes of reducing body weight.[88] Prospective studies of dietary-fat restriction and exercise have also demonstrated reduced progression, or even reversal, of heart disease in patients with known cardiovascular disease[78] and up to a 58% reduction in the incidence of type 2 diabetes in overweight patients with impaired glucose tolerance.[50]

Because of the overall health benefits, the initial treatment of overweight and obese patients should include increased activity in addition to dietary-fat restriction and increased dietary fiber. If caloric restriction is recommended, the likelihood of long-term weight-loss maintenance may be improved by the addition of these interventions. Dietary and activity advice should be implemented using individualized, sustainable behavioral and lifestyle changes. Again, it is important for both clinicians and patients not to have unreasonable expectations for weight loss from diet and exercise. For some patients, the best that may be achieved through lifestyle improvements is prevention of further weight gain. Patients who fail to meet unreasonable goals may become frustrated and return to a less healthy lifestyle. Even when little or no weight loss ensues, these lifestyle changes offer many health benefits, including improved lipid levels, increased insulin sensitivity, and reduced risk for progression of cardiovascular disease and for onset of type 2 diabetes.[89] After institution of lifestyle measures, if a patient's body weight remains above the guideline cutoff points, medical and surgical treatment options remain.[90]

Prevention

Once patients have become overweight or obese, lifestyle interventions play an important role in reducing comorbidities, but they typically have modest effects on body weight (see above). These patients will then require lifelong medical or surgical management to achieve more meaningful weight loss (see below). This failure of the body-weight set point to remain at a lower level in the average patient greatly increases the importance of prevention of unwanted weight gain. Prevention requires targeted improvements in food choices for pregnant mothers and children and, more importantly, a reversal of the societal trend toward reduced activity levels.

The hurdles for implementing these simple recommendations are, however, considerable. Increasing intake of healthy foods includes not only overcoming personal and cultural preferences for higher-fat foods but also consideration of the economic costs of food at home and at schools (calorically dense foods are often cheaper than fruits and vegetables) and the impact of family and work demands on ability to eat at home or purchase prepared foods.[91] Increasing activity does not necessarily require going to a gym on a regular basis. Rather, it includes maintaining physical activity in routine daily events, such as physical education in schools, designing work spaces and buildings to promote walking and stair use, planning urban environments to promote more pedestrian activity (e.g., safer streets, more sidewalks, in-

creased density of commercial and residential properties), and overcoming a cultural reliance on automobiles for routine travel.[92] Even with immediate institution of lifestyle improvements, though, it is likely that reversing the current decades-long trend in weight gain will take several generations.

PHARMACOLOGIC THERAPY

The Food and Drug Administration has approved several prescription medications for the treatment of obesity [*see Table 4*].[90] These medications fall into two categories: centrally acting drugs, which suppress appetite, and peripherally acting drugs, which reduce fat absorption. For example, phentermine and sibutramine act centrally, reducing appetite by promoting the release of norepinephrine from presynaptic terminals (phentermine) and inhibiting the uptake of both norepinephrine and serotonin (sibutramine) in central nuclei. Orlistat acts peripherally, inhibiting the action of lipases in the brush border of the intestine and thereby reducing lipid absorption.

Clinicians who treat obese patients with medical therapy should keep in mind four important principles. First, most studies have included an initial treatment phase in which patients are placed on a hypocaloric diet (usually, daily caloric intake is reduced by 500 to 1,000 kcal) at the time of randomization or just before drug treatment. Second, the weight loss with obesity agents varies considerably: some patients lose a dramatic amount of weight; others lose only a little weight; and still others lose some weight only to regain it despite continuation of the medication. In any case, average weight loss with currently approved medications does not usually exceed 10% of the baseline weight. Third, weight loss is greatest during the first 3 to 6 months, followed by a plateau at a new lower weight even with continuation of the therapy. Intermittent therapy (i.e., 3 months on therapy followed by 3 months off, 3 months on, etc.) does not increase weight loss[93,94] and has been associated with increased side effects (e.g., dry mouth).[93] Finally, every drug-treatment study that has included posttreatment follow-up has shown rapid weight regain toward baseline after discontinuance of the medication. The plateauing of weight after initial weight loss and the regaining of weight after medication discontinuance have been interpreted to indicate that the medication became ineffective with time or failed because weight loss was neither sufficient nor sustained after cessation of the treatment. However, pharmacologic therapy for obesity is no different from therapy for other common chronic diseases. For instance, patients with hypertension often have a variable response to a first-line agent. In some cases, blood pressure lowering may be insufficient and may require the addition of a second medication, and hypertension returns when the medication is discontinued. Once a person begins receiving medical therapy for obesity, continued efficacy is evidenced by sustained weight-loss maintenance. Treatment should therefore be continued indefinitely unless the weight is regained or significant side effects develop.

Agents Approved for Short-Term Use

Benzphetamine, phendimetrazine, diethylpropion, mazindol, and phentermine are approved by the FDA for the short-term treatment of obesity (weeks). All but phentermine are rarely, if ever, used in clinical practice today. Benzphetamine and phendimetrazine are both Drug Enforcement Administration (DEA) schedule III drugs, with higher abuse potential than the others. Diethylpropion and mazindol have indications and side effects identical to those of phentermine (all are DEA schedule IV), but

Table 4 Pharmacologic Agents Approved by the Food and Drug Administration
for the Treatment of Obesity

Duration of Treatment	Drug (Trade Name)	Dose	Average Weight Loss	Comments
Short term	Phentermine	30 mg resin; 15 or 37.5 mg tablets	8.7 kg	—
Long term*	Orlistat (Xenical)	250 mg with each meal (two or three times a day)	7–13 kg	Patients must already be on a low-fat diet (< 30% of total calories from fat); supplemental multivitamins are needed to prevent reduction in fat-soluble vitamins
	Sibutramine (Meridia)	5 mg 10 mg 15 mg	3.7 kg 5.7 kg 7.0 kg	On average, blood pressure and pulse rise slightly with treatment; contraindicated in patients with untreated hypertension and coronary artery disease

*Data are for treatment duration of 6 mo to 1 yr when combined with a low-calorie diet.

they are less well studied and have not had the same acceptance in clinical practice as phentermine; consequently, diethylpropion and mazindol are not extensively discussed in this chapter.

Phentermine Phentermine inhibits appetite and causes an average weight loss of 8.7 kg (19.2 lb) (net weight loss of 5.1 kg [11.2 lb] when compared with placebo).[95] The agent is available as a 30 mg resin and in 15 mg and 37.5 mg tablets. Doses in excess of 37.5 mg are not recommended because of unacceptable side effects.

Little information is available about subsequent improvement in health outcomes with phentermine treatment alone, because studies of this drug have historically been short term, and the drug was frequently used in combination with fenfluramine. A group of postmenopausal women treated with phentermine and a low-calorie diet experienced a 14% weight loss, along with reduction in low-density lipoprotein (LDL) cholesterol and triglyceride levels and an increase in high-density lipoprotein (HDL) cholesterol levels over 9 months.[96] In patients with diabetes, despite a net loss of 3.8 kg (8.4 lb) compared with placebo over 6 months, use of phentermine produced no improvement in glycemic control or glycosuria and no significant reduction in hypoglycemic drug use.[97]

As a result of central nervous system activation by phentermine, patients may experience anxiousness, insomnia, palpitations, and dry mouth. In case reports, phentermine treatment has been associated with vasospasm, psychosis, and ischemic events,[98-100] although in a larger cohort study, phentermine was not associated with stroke.[101]

Agents Approved for Long-Term Use

Sibutramine The FDA approved sibutramine for the medical treatment of obesity in 1997. The recommended duration for therapy was 1 year, but treatment may be continued beyond that time if no significant side effects occur and sustained weight loss is documented.

The average weight loss on the highest currently approved dose, 15 mg, is 7.0 kg (15.4 lb) (net weight loss of 5.7 kg [12.6 lb] when compared with placebo).[102] In a 2-year study of sibutramine therapy, a weight loss of 10.2 kg (22.5 lb) (net weight loss of 5.5 kg [12.1 lb] when compared with placebo) persisted for up to 18 months, at which time a slight upward trend became evident.[57] With placebo, in contrast, patients began to regain weight immediately after completion of the hypocaloric phase, which

was at 6 months. After 2 years, significantly greater proportions of patients taking sibutramine, compared with control subjects, had maintained 5% and 10% weight loss. These results may have limited applicability, however, because only persons who completed the initial 6-month weight-loss phase and lost at least 5% of their initial body weight by caloric restriction were subsequently randomized to placebo or continued sibutramine therapy. This represents a 23% dropout rate before randomization to drug therapy. In addition, approximately 30% of the patients treated with sibutramine and 50% of the patients given placebo withdrew from the study. A higher pretreatment body weight[103] and weight loss of at least 1.8 kg (4 lb) during the first month of therapy[102] have been shown to predict continued weight-loss response with longer treatment.

Sibutramine treatment is also associated with improvements in lipid levels, including lower triglyceride levels and higher HDL levels.[57,94,104] Sibutramine has been safely used in patients with type 2 diabetes, with improvements in lipid levels being similar to those reported in nondiabetic patients.[105] Glycemic control also improves in diabetic patients on sibutramine therapy, with the greatest reductions in hemoglobin A_{1c} occurring in those patients who lose more than 10% of their initial body weight.[105] Common side effects of sibutramine treatment include dry mouth, constipation, insomnia, palpitations, and headache. Sibutramine consistently raises average blood pressures slightly and pulse rate more so, even with weight loss.[57,102] In populations not selected for hypertension, studies have documented increases in average diastolic pressure of 0 to 3.4 mm Hg, increases in systolic blood pressure of 0 to 2.7 mm Hg, and increases of average pulse rate of 4.1 to 6 beats/min.[57,94,102] Similar results with sibutramine have been shown for hypertensive patients receiving a variety of antihypertensive medications.[106,107] Therefore, sibutramine treatment can be used if blood pressure is controlled, but blood pressure and pulse rate should be monitored routinely.[108] However, because of the potential for added cardiovascular demand, sibutramine should not be used in patients with a diagnosis of cardiovascular disease, heart failure, arrhythmia, or stroke. To date, sibutramine has not been associated with either valvular disease or pulmonary hypertension.

Orlistat Orlistat inhibits lipases in the gastrointestinal lumen, thereby antagonizing triglyceride hydrolysis and reducing fat absorption by roughly 30%. Because orlistat is not absorbed to any significant extent, its primary mechanism of action is thought to be through providing what is in effect a low-fat diet, thereby promoting lower caloric intake and weight loss [see Dietary-Fat Restriction, above], as well as improved weight-loss maintenance, when combined with a low-calorie diet.[109] As with sibutramine, orlistat treatment should be continued as long as the patient maintains weight loss and avoids significant side effects.

To minimize side effects related to fat malabsorption, candidates for orlistat treatment are first placed on a diet containing only 30% of calories from fat. When combined with a calorie-restricted diet, orlistat treatment (120 mg with each meal) results in an average weight loss of 7.2 to 13 kg (16 to 28.7 lb) (net weight loss of 1.3 to 5.6 kg [2.9 to 12.3 lb] when compared with placebo). After 1 year, patients taking orlistat maintain greater weight loss than those taking placebo [see Table 4].[58,110,111] During continued follow-up for another year, regaining of weight is seen but remains less than that in patients given placebo.[57,110,111]

Patients who lose weight with orlistat also experience a significant reduction in levels of total and LDL cholesterol (approximately 4% to 8%, which is significantly lower than reductions in patients given placebo).[110,111] Levels of triglycerides and HDL cholesterol are either reduced or left unchanged; these results are not different from those in the placebo group. Blood pressure and insulin levels also decrease with weight loss in patients on orlistat therapy.[58,110,111] Similar improvements in lipid levels, along with improvements in glycemic control, have been documented in obese persons with type 2 diabetes who lose weight with orlistat.[112]

Gastrointestinal side effects may occur in up to 80% of patients when they begin therapy with orlistat (such side effects are also seen in 50% to 60% of patients given placebo), but this incidence diminishes with time. Symptoms include abdominal discomfort, flatus, fecal urgency, oily spotting, and fecal incontinence. When administered to patients who adhere to a low-fat diet, orlistat is generally well tolerated. The fat malabsorption that accompanies orlistat treatment can also lead to reductions in fat-soluble vitamins, but in prospective studies, the average levels for vitamins A, D, E, and β-carotene remained in the normal range.[58,110,113] In one study, only 2.4% of orlistat-treated patients had documented below-normal levels of β-carotene; only 3.1%, below-normal levels of vitamin D; and only 1.6%, below-normal levels of vitamin E.[110] Nevertheless, orlistat should not be given to patients with existing malabsorptive states, and it is recommended that patients take a daily multivitamin supplement during therapy.

Non–FDA-Approved Medical Therapy for Obesity

Observational data from studies of patients with depression suggested that treatment with selective serotonin reuptake inhibitors (SSRIs) may result in weight loss, but this effect is slight and short-lived. Moreover, in prospective studies, SSRI treatment is sometimes associated with mild weight gain.[49] Bupropion is currently approved as an antidepressant and for smoking cessation. The mechanism of action of bupropion is not precisely known, but it includes weak inhibition of norepinephrine and dopamine reuptake. Combining bupropion (300 to 400 mg/day) with moderate daily caloric restriction has been shown to result in greater weight loss than placebo (net weight loss of 3 to 4 kg [6.6 to 8.8 lb], on average) after 6 months in obese patients with no symptoms or mild symptoms of depression.[114-116] Bupropion is contraindicated in patients with seizures, anorexia nervosa, and bulimia.

Deficiencies of growth hormone and sex steroids have been associated with higher body-fat content and greater central obe-sity. Replacing growth hormone reduces fat mass, increases lean mass, and reduces central obesity. Similar improvements in body composition have been reported with testosterone replacement in hypogonadal men. Although obese persons have documented abnormalities in the hypothalamic-pituitary-gonadal and somatotropic axes, treatment of overweight or centrally obese persons with growth hormone, sex steroids, or both has not been shown to produce clear improvements in body composition, fat distribution, or comorbid conditions.

Surgical Therapy

With improved safety from technical advances and demonstrated efficacy, bariatric (obesity) operations clearly have a role in the current management of severely obese patients.[90] The mechanisms whereby these operations result in sustained weight loss are poorly understood, but they likely include alterations in the gut-derived hormonal and neural inputs to the central nervous system.[117] In general, these procedures can be classified into one of three types: restriction of food passage, malabsorption of nutrients, or a combination of the two [see Table 5]. As an example of a purely restrictive procedure, vertical-banded gastroplasty involves the formation of a small stoma for the passage of food. The rationale behind this procedure is to increase a sense of fullness and reduce food intake. Procedures resulting in malabsorption typically involve bypassing sections of small or large intestine. Early procedures in which large sections, or even the entire length, of the small intestine were bypassed often resulted in severe malabsorption and sometimes hepatic failure and death. Subsequent modifications have led to bypass of shorter sections and lower morbidity. Patients must understand that bypass surgery is anatomically irreversible in most cases and has a potentially high postoperative complication rate.

Several large-scale studies have demonstrated the efficacy of various bariatric procedures in severely obese patients. One study of gastric bypass reported sustained loss of approximately 50% of baseline body weight (at 5- to 10-year follow-up).[118] In the ongoing Swedish Obesity Subjects (SOS) Intervention Study of 1,157 severely obese persons (average BMI of 42 kg/m²), weight loss in the first postoperative year ranged from 21% after gastric banding to 38% after gastric bypass.[119] Some weight regain was found on 10-year follow-up, but the gastric banding patients remained 13% below and the gastric bypass patients 25% below their initial body weight.[119]

A more recent technique known as laparoscopic gastric banding, in which a restrictive band is placed around the upper stomach, has also shown efficacy in sustained weight loss in studies up to 4 years. The weight loss with laparoscopic gastric banding is generally felt to be similar to that with vertical-banded gastroplasty but not as great as that with gastric bypass.[120]

An important benefit of bariatric surgery is that the large weight losses bring improvements in the comorbid conditions that accompany obesity,[121,122] including lowering of lipid levels and blood pressure and reduced rates of diabetes, progression to diabetes, and sleep apnea.[119,122] Moreover, cohort and population-based studies have demonstrated that weight loss after bariatric surgery is associated with both reduced mortality and reduced use of health care resources.[123]

Complication rates for bariatric surgery will vary by surgeon, site, and technique. The most common operative-related complications, occurring in up to 30% of patients, are wound infections, atelectasis or pneumonia, and hernia.[118,124-127] Serious but rare complications include anastomotic stenosis or leakage, throm-

Table 5   Most Commonly Used Bariatric Procedures[118,153,154]

Type of Surgery	Procedure	Average Weight Loss	Medical Complications	Management
Restrictive	Vertical-banded gastroplasty	~17% (5 yr)	Nausea, vomiting Gastric distention	Reversal of procedure if complications unacceptable
	Laparoscopic adjustable gastric banding	17%–21% (3 yr)	Nausea, vomiting Slippage Erosion and leakage	Adjustment of band to minimize nausea; reversal of procedure if necessary
Malabsorptive	Biliopancreatic diversion	~27% (5 yr)	Diarrhea, fatty stools Protein-calorie malnutrition Anemia (low iron) Deficiency of vitamin D (and other fat-soluble vitamins) Hypocalcemia Hyperparathyroidism Metabolic bone disease Vitamin B_{12} deficiency, Wernicke encephalopathy (rare)	Monitoring of levels and replacement of nutritional deficiencies; patients often require high oral or parenteral doses
Combination	Gastric bypass	~27% (5 yr)	Dumping syndrome Reductions in levels of iron, vitamin B_{12}, folate, calcium, vitamin D Nesidioblastosis (rare)	Small, frequent meals; monitoring of nutrient levels and oral supplementation with iron tablets (325 mg), vitamin B_{12} (500 µg), folate (1 mg), calcium (500–1,000 mg), and vitamin D

boembolism, and bowel obstruction. Perioperative death rates have ranged from 0.2% to 1.3%.[118,125-127] The laparoscopic techniques offer greater safety than open procedures without sacrificing efficacy.[128,129] Nesidioblastosis has been described in a small series of obese patients after gastric bypass operations.[130] These patients experienced serious or life-threatening postprandial hypoglycemic episodes. A number of questions remain, however, regarding the frequency of this finding, the validity of the link between the gastric bypass and beta cell hypertrophy, and how to best do a workup of patients who may have this condition. Nevertheless, clinicians should include nesidioblastosis in the differential diagnosis of gastric bypass patients who complain of symptoms that have heretofore been ascribed to the so-called dumping syndrome (i.e., rapid transit of food into the small intestine associated with rapid increases in blood volume to the gut and insulin secretion): weakness, dizziness, palpitations, and near-syncope.

Because of the potential for rapid weight loss after bariatric surgery, follow-up by a nutritionist and physician is important to ensure that patients preserve lean mass and maintain hydration and to monitor for symptomatic cholelithiasis. Lifelong alteration of dietary habits may be required to ensure the continued success of the surgery, and dietary supplements may be needed to prevent nutritional deficiencies [see Table 5].

Surgical therapy for obesity results in significant, sustained weight loss in a majority of patients with severe obesity.[121,122] With regard to total weight loss and improved disease outcomes, the gastric bypass procedure has the greatest support from published studies,[121,122] whereas the gastric banding procedure has the lowest published rates of morbidity (11%) and mortality (0.05%).[120] With the considerable improvements in comorbidity and quality of life that result from this weight loss, bariatric surgery is not only efficacious but also cost-effective in the management of severe obesity.[122,123,131]

Complications of Obesity

Persons who are overweight or obese and have central adiposity are at increased risk for hyperlipidemia, hypertension, and cardiovascular disease mortality.[6,132-135] In addition, obesity and central adiposity are both strong risk factors for the development of type 2 diabetes.[11,136] Other diseases with a higher incidence in obese persons include gallstones, high uric acid levels and gout, hepatic steatosis, osteoarthritis, obesity hypoventilation, atrial fibrillation, nephrolithiasis, and certain cancers.[137,138] Sleep apnea is likely underdiagnosed in overweight and obese patients[139] and should be strongly considered in patients with complaints of fatigue, daytime somnolence, snoring, restless sleep, and morning headaches. People who are overweight and obese also carry a significant psychosocial burden. Obesity is accompanied by lower self-esteem in children[140] and prospectively predicts depression in adults.[141] Young adults who were overweight as adolescents are less likely to marry, will complete less schooling, and have lower incomes than nonoverweight peers.[142] The economic costs of the treatment of obesity and its comorbidities are high: estimates from 1995 United States data put the costs at $99.2 billion, and of this, $52 billion, or 5.7% of the United States national health expenditure, went to pay direct medical costs.[143]

Prognosis

Mortality increases when men and women become overweight or obese, in large part because of comorbid conditions (see above). This impact of obesity on mortality is greatest in younger age groups and diminishes with age[144,145] and may be significantly influenced by the patient's fitness status. Prospective observational studies suggest that mortality and risk associated with coronary artery disease are highest in the least fit and lowest in the most fit, independent of body weight.[82,83] Evidence of lower mortality after specific lifestyle, medical, or surgical interventions for obesity is currently lacking. Instead, decreased severity of a number of diseases and cardiovascular risk factors associated with increased mortality have been demonstrated after even modest weight loss.[89] Insulin resistance, hyperlipidemia, hypertension, sleep apnea, diabetes, and cardiovascular disease have all been shown to improve with weight loss that follows intensive lifestyle interventions (e.g., low-fat, high-fiber diet and exercise) and medical therapy.[51,52,58,78,89,104,105] With the greater weight loss that accompanies bariatric surgery, resolution of diseases such as diabetes and sleep apnea[119,123] and increased survival[124] have been reported. Optimal therapy for obesity, however, remains elusive. Simple caloric restriction alone results in short-term weight loss (months to years), but without additional interventions such as a low-fat diet, exercise, pharmacologic therapy, or a combination of these, 95% or more of the weight initially lost will be regained within 5 years.[54] Lifestyle interventions alone, including a low-fat, high fiber diet and increased activity, have only small effects on body weight but result in significant improvements in obesity-related morbidity.[51] Current pharmacologic therapy is effective in achieving weight loss of up to 10% of initial body weight for at least up to 2 years.[57,110] Bariatric surgery has been shown to increase weight loss to up to 50% of initial weight for at least 10 years,[118,119] but it carries the risks of surgery and, with most operations, irreversible anatomic modification. Nonetheless, for patients with severe obesity who are at high risk for morbidity and mortality, bariatric surgery can offer hope for improved survival while more effective medical therapies are being developed.

The author has served as a consultant for Amylin Pharmaceuticals, Inc.

The drug bupropion, which is discussed in this chapter, has not been approved by the FDA for use in obesity.

References

1. Jackson AS, Stanforth PR, Gagnon J, et al: The effect of sex, age and race on estimating percentage body fat from body mass index: the Heritage Family Study. Int J Obes Relat Metab Disord 26:789, 2002

2. Najjar MF, Rowland M: Anthropometric reference data and prevalence of overweight, United States, 1976–80. Vital Health Stat 11(238):1, 1987

3. Clinical guidelines on the identification, evaluation, and treatment of overweight and obesity in adults—The Evidence Report. National Institutes of Health. Obes Res 6(suppl 2):51S, 1998

4. The Asia-Pacific Perspective: Redefining Obesity and Its Treatment. World Health Organization, Western Pacific Region; International Association for the Study of Obesity; International Obesity Task Force, 2000

5. Appropriate body-mass index for Asian populations and its implications for policy and intervention strategies. WHO Expert Consultation. Lancet 363:157, 2004

6. Janssen I, Katzmarzyk PT, Ross R: Waist circumference and not body mass index explains obesity-related health risk. Am J Clin Nutr 79:379, 2004

7. Fujimoto WY, Bergstrom RW, Boyko EJ, et al: Susceptibility to development of central adiposity among populations. Obes Res 3(suppl 2):179S, 1995

8. Health, United States, 2004. National Center for Health Statistics, Hyattsville, Maryland, 2004, p 241
http://www.cdc.gov/nchs/data/hus/hus04.pdf

9. Hedley AA, Ogden CL, Johnson CL, et al: Prevalence of overweight and obesity among US children, adolescents, and adults, 1999–2002. JAMA 291:2847, 2004

10. Knowler WC, Pettitt DJ, Saad MF, et al: Obesity in the Pima Indians: its magnitude and relationship with diabetes. Am J Clin Nutr 53(6 suppl):1543S, 1991

11. Lethbridge-Çejku M, Vickerie J: Summary health statistics for U.S. adults: National Health Interview Survey, 2003. National Center for Health Statistics. Vital Health Stat 10(225):1, 2005

12. Paeratakul S, Lovejoy JC, Ryan DH, et al: The relation of gender, race and socioeconomic status to obesity and obesity comorbidities in a sample of US adults. Int J Obes Relat Metab Disord 26:1205, 2002

13. York DA, Rossner S, Caterson I, et al: American Heart Association. Prevention Conference VII: Obesity, a worldwide epidemic related to heart disease and stroke: Group I: worldwide demographics of obesity. Circulation 110:e463, 2004

14. Popkin BM, Horton S, Kim S, et al: Trends in diet, nutritional status, and diet-related noncommunicable diseases in China and India: the economic costs of the nutrition transition. Nutr Rev 59:379, 2001

15. Mott JW, Wang J, Thornton JC, et al: Relation between body fat and age in 4 ethnic groups. Am J Clin Nutr 69:1007, 1999

16. Gallagher D, Ruts E, Visser M, et al: Weight stability masks sarcopenia in elderly men and women. Am J Physiol Endocrinol Metab 279:E366, 2000

17. Hughes VA, Frontera WR, Roubenoff R, et al: Longitudinal changes in body composition in older men and women: role of body weight change and physical activity. Am J Clin Nutr 76:473, 2002

18. Trémollieres FA, Pouilles JM, Ribot CA: Relative influence of age and menopause on total and regional body composition changes in postmenopausal women. Am J Obstet Gynecol 175:1594, 1996

19. Lemieux S, Prud'homme D, Bouchard C, et al: Sex differences in the relation of visceral adipose tissue accumulation to total body fatness. Am J Clin Nutr 58:463, 1993

20. Matsuzawa Y, Shimomura I, Nakamura T, et al: Pathophysiology and pathogenesis of visceral fat obesity. Obes Res 3(suppl 2):187S, 1995

21. Shuman WP, Morris LL, Leonetti DL, et al: Abnormal body fat distribution detected by computed tomography in diabetic men. Invest Radiol 21:483, 1986

22. Maes HH, Neale MC, Eaves LJ: Genetic and environmental factors in relative body weight and human adiposity. Behav Genet 27:325, 1997

23. Perusse L, Rankinen T, Zuberi A, et al: The human obesity gene map: the 2004 update. Obes Res 13:381, 2005

24. Bray GA, Popkin BM: Dietary fat intake does affect obesity! Am J Clin Nutr 68:1157, 1998

25. Coakley EH, Rimm EB, Colditz G, et al: Predictors of weight change in men: results from the Health Professionals Follow-up Study. Int J Obes Relat Metab Disord 22:89, 1998

26. Ludwig DS, Pereira MA, Kroenke CH, et al: Dietary fiber, weight gain, and cardiovascular disease risk factors in young adults. JAMA 282:1539, 1999

27. Gordon-Larsen P, Adair LS, Popkin BM: Ethnic differences in physical activity and inactivity patterns and overweight status. Obes Res 10:141, 2002

28. Drewnowski A, Specter SE: Poverty and obesity: the role of energy density and energy costs. Am J Clin Nutr 79:6, 2004

29. Ludwig DS, Peterson KE, Gortmaker SL: Relation between consumption of sugar-sweetened drinks and childhood obesity: a prospective, observational analysis. Lancet 357:505, 2001

30. Pereira MA, Jacobs DR Jr, Van Horn L, et al: Dairy consumption, obesity, and the insulin resistance syndrome in young adults: the CARDIA Study. JAMA 287:2081, 2002

31. Stookey JD, Adair L, Stevens J, et al: Patterns of long-term change in body composition are associated with diet, activity, income and urban residence among older adults in China. J Nutr 131:2433S, 2001

32. Flegal KM, Troiano RP, Pamuk ER, et al: The influence of smoking cessation on the prevalence of overweight in the United States. N Engl J Med 333:1165, 1995

33. Pereira MA, Kartashov AI, Ebbeling CB, et al: Fast-food habits, weight gain, and insulin resistance (the CARDIA study): 15-year prospective analysis. Lancet 365:36, 2005

34. Schwartz MW, Woods SC, Porte D Jr, et al: Central nervous system control of food intake. Nature 404:661, 2000

35. Zhang Y, Proenca R, Maffei M, et al: Positional cloning of the mouse obese gene and its human homologue. Nature 372:425, 1994

36. Lamberts SW, van den Beld AW, van der Lely AJ: The endocrinology of aging. Science 278:419, 1997

37. Munzer T, Harman SM, Hees P, et al: Effects of GH and/or sex steroid administration on abdominal subcutaneous and visceral fat in healthy aged women and men. J Clin Endocrinol Metab 86:3604, 2001

38. Blackman MR, Sorkin JD, Munzer T, et al: Growth hormone and sex steroid administration in healthy aged women and men: a randomized controlled trial. JAMA 288:2282, 2002

39. Van Cauter E, Leproult R, Kupfer DJ: Effects of gender and age on the levels and circadian rhythmicity of plasma cortisol. J Clin Endocrinol Metab 81:2468, 1996

40. Anawalt BD, Merriam GR: Neuroendocrine aging in men: andropause and somatopause. Endocrinol Metab Clin North Am 30:647, 2001

41. Purnell JQ, Brandon DD, Isabelle LM, et al: Association of 24-hour cortisol production rates, cortisol-binding globulin, and plasma-free cortisol levels with body composition, leptin levels, and aging in adult men and women. J Clin Endocrinol Metab 89:281, 2004

42. Executive summary of the third report of the National Cholesterol Education Program (NCEP) Expert Panel on Detection, Evaluation, and Treatment of High Blood Cholesterol in Adults (Adult Treatment Panel III). JAMA 285:2486, 2001

43. Eckel RH, Grundy SM, Zimmet PZ: The metabolic syndrome. Lancet 365:1415, 2005

44. Carroll PV, Christ ER, Sonksen PH: Growth hormone replacement in adults with growth hormone deficiency: assessment of current knowledge. Trends Endocrinol Metab 11:231, 2000

45. Wang C, Swerdloff RS, Iranmanesh A, et al: Transdermal testosterone gel improves sexual function, mood, muscle strength, and body composition parameters in hypogonadal men. Testosterone Gel Study Group. J Clin Endocrinol Metab 85:2839, 2000

46. Makimattila S, Nikkila K, Yki-Jarvinen H: Causes of weight gain during insulin therapy with and without metformin in patients with type II diabetes mellitus. Diabetologia 42:406, 1999

47. Purnell JQ, Weyer C: Bodyweight effects of current and experimental drugs for diabetes mellitus. Treat Endocrinol 2:33, 2003

48. Yki-Jarvinen H: Combination therapies with insulin in type 2 diabetes. Diabetes Care 24:758, 2001

49. Vanina Y, Podolskaya A, Sedky K, et al: Body weight changes associated with psychopharmacology. Psychiatr Serv 53:842, 2002

50. Casey DE: Metabolic issues and cardiovascular disease in patients with psychiatric disorders. Am J Med 118(suppl 2):15S, 2005

51. Knowler WC, Barrett-Connor E, Fowler SE, et al: Reduction in the incidence of type 2 diabetes with lifestyle intervention or metformin. N Engl J Med 346:393, 2002

52. Blackburn G: Effect of degree of weight loss on health benefits. Obes Res 3(suppl 2):211s, 1995

53. Tsai AG, Wadden TA: Systematic review: an evaluation of major commercial weight loss programs in the United States. Ann Intern Med 142:56, 2005

54. Safer DJ: Diet, behavior modification, and exercise: a review of obesity treatments from a long-term perspective. South Med J 84:1470, 1991

55. Toubro S, Astrup A: Randomised comparison of diets for maintaining obese subjects' weight after major weight loss: ad lib, low fat, high carbohydrate diet v fixed energy intake. BMJ 314:29, 1997

56. Wing RR, Hill JO: Successful weight loss maintenance. Annu Rev Nutr 21:323, 2001

57. James WP, Astrup A, Finer N, et al: Effect of sibutramine on weight maintenance after weight loss: a randomised trial. STORM Study Group. Sibutramine Trial of Obesity Reduction and Maintenance. Lancet 356:2119, 2000

58. Davidson MH, Hauptman J, DiGirolamo M, et al: Weight control and risk factor reduction in obese subjects treated for 2 years with orlistat: a randomized controlled trial. JAMA 281:235, 1999

59. Astrup A, Grunwald GK, Melanson EL, et al: The role of low-fat diets in body weight control: a meta-analysis of ad libitum dietary intervention studies. Int J Obes Relat Metab Disord 24:1545, 2000

60. Weigle DS, Cummings DE, Newby PD, et al: Roles of leptin and ghrelin in the loss of body weight caused by a low fat, high carbohydrate diet. J Clin Endocrinol Metab 88:1577, 2003

61. Weigle DS, Breen PA, Matthys CC, et al: A high-protein diet induces sustained reductions in appetite, ad libitum caloric intake, and body weight despite compensatory changes in diurnal plasma leptin and ghrelin concentrations. Am J Clin Nutr 82:41, 2005

62. El-Haschimi K, Pierroz DD, Hileman SM, et al: Two defects contribute to hypothalamic leptin resistance in mice with diet-induced obesity. J Clin Invest 105:1827, 2000

63. Schaefer EJ, Lichtenstein AH, Lamon-Fava S, et al: Body weight and low-density lipoprotein cholesterol changes after consumption of a low-fat ad libitum diet. JAMA 274:1450, 1995

64. Daily dietary fat and total food-energy intakes—Third National Health and Nutrition Examination Survey, Phase 1, 1988–91. MMWR Morb Mortal Wkly Rep 43:116, 1994

65. Ernst ND, Sempos CT, Briefel RR, et al: Consistency between US dietary fat intake and serum total cholesterol concentrations: the National Health and Nutrition Examination Surveys. Am J Clin Nutr 66(4 suppl):965S, 1997

66. Elliott SS, Keim NL, Stern JS, et al: Fructose, weight gain, and the insulin resistance syndrome. Am J Clin Nutr 76:911, 2002

67. Freedman MR, King J, Kennedy E: Popular diets: a scientific review. Obes Res 9(suppl 1):1S, 2001

68. Bravata DM, Sanders L, Huang J, et al: Efficacy and safety of low-carbohydrate diets: a systematic review. JAMA 289:1837, 2003

69. Brehm BJ, Seeley RJ, Daniels SR, et al: A randomized trial comparing a very low carbohydrate diet and a calorie-restricted low fat diet on body weight and cardiovascular risk factors in healthy women. J Clin Endocrinol Metab 88:1617, 2003

70. Foster GD, Wyatt HR, Hill JO, et al: A randomized trial of a low-carbohydrate diet for obesity. N Engl J Med 348:2082, 2003

71. Stern L, Iqbal N, Seshadri P, et al: The effects of low-carbohydrate versus conventional weight loss diets in severely obese adults: one-year follow-up of a randomized trial. Ann Intern Med 140:778, 2004

72. Dansinger ML, Gleason JA, Griffith JL, et al: Comparison of the Atkins, Ornish, Weight Watchers, and Zone diets for weight loss and heart disease risk reduction: a randomized trial. JAMA 293:43, 2005

73. Yancy WS Jr, Olsen MK, Guyton JR, et al: A low-carbohydrate, ketogenic diet versus a low-fat diet to treat obesity and hyperlipidemia: a randomized, controlled trial. Ann Intern Med 140:769, 2004

74. Due A, Toubro S, Skov AR, et al: Effect of normal-fat diets, either medium or high in protein, on body weight in overweight subjects: a randomised 1-year trial. Int J Obes Relat Metab Disord 28:1283, 2004

75. Skov AR, Toubro S, Bulow J, et al: Changes in renal function during weight loss induced by high vs low-protein low-fat diets in overweight subjects. Int J Obes Relat Metab Disord 23:1170, 1999

76. Howarth NC, Saltzman E, Roberts SB: Dietary fiber and weight regulation. Nutr Rev 59:129, 2001

77. Davy BM, Melby CL: The effect of fiber-rich carbohydrates on features of syndrome X. J Am Diet Assoc 103:86, 2003

78. Ornish D, Scherwitz LW, Billings JH, et al: Intensive lifestyle changes for reversal of coronary heart disease. JAMA 280:2001, 1998

79. Wing RR: Physical activity in the treatment of the adulthood overweight and obesity: current evidence and research issues. Med Sci Sports Exerc 31(11 suppl):S547, 1999

80. Votruba SB, Horvitz MA, Schoeller DA: The role of exercise in the treatment of obesity. Nutrition 16:179, 2000

81. Blundell JE, King NA: Exercise, appetite control, and energy balance. Nutrition 16:519, 2000

82. Wei M, Kampert JB, Barlow CE, et al: Relationship between low cardiorespiratory fitness and mortality in normal-weight, overweight, and obese men. JAMA 282:1547, 1999

83. Farrell SW, Braun L, Barlow CE, et al: The relation of body mass index, cardiorespiratory fitness, and all-cause mortality in women. Obes Res 10:417, 2002

84. Pascale RW, Wing RR, Butler BA, et al: Effects of a behavioral weight loss program stressing calorie restriction versus calorie plus fat restriction in obese individuals with NIDDM or a family history of diabetes. Diabetes Care 18:1241, 1995

85. Toubro S, Astrup A: Randomised comparison of diets for maintaining obese subjects' weight after major weight loss: ad lib, low fat, high carbohydrate diet v fixed energy intake. BMJ 314:29, 1997

86. Jakicic JM, Winters C, Lang W, et al: Effects of intermittent exercise and use of home exercise equipment on adherence, weight loss, and fitness in overweight women: a randomized trial. JAMA 282:1554, 1999

87. Shick SM, Wing RR, Klem ML, et al: Persons successful at long-term weight loss and maintenance continue to consume a low-energy, low-fat diet. J Am Diet Assoc 98:408, 1998

88. Klem ML, Wing RR, McGuire MT, et al: A descriptive study of individuals successful at long-term maintenance of substantial weight loss. Am J Clin Nutr 66:239, 1997

89. Pi-Sunyer FX: A review of long-term studies evaluating the efficacy of weight loss in ameliorating disorders associated with obesity. Clin Ther 18:1006, 1996

90. Snow V, Barry P, Fitterman N, et al: Pharmacologic and surgical management of obesity in primary care: a clinical practice guideline from the American College of Physicians. Ann Intern Med 142:525, 2005

91. Drewnowski A, Darmon NR: The economics of obesity: dietary energy density and energy cost. Am J Clin Nutr 82(1 suppl):265S, 2005

92. Booth KM, Pinkston MM, Poston WS: Obesity and the built environment. J Am Diet Assoc 105(5 suppl 1):S110, 2005

93. Weintraub M, Sundaresan PR, Schuster B, et al: Long-term weight control study. II (weeks 34 to 104): an open-label study of continuous fenfluramine plus phentermine versus targeted intermittent medication as adjuncts to behavior modification, caloric restriction, and exercise. Clin Pharmacol Ther 51:595, 1992

94. Wirth A, Krause J: Long-term weight loss with sibutramine: a randomized controlled trial. JAMA 286:1331, 2001

95. Bray GA: Use and abuse of appetite-suppressant drugs in the treatment of obesity. Ann Intern Med 119:707, 1993

96. Cordero-MacIntyre ZR, Lohman TG, Rosen J, et al: Weight loss is correlated with an improved lipoprotein profile in obese postmenopausal women. J Am Coll Nutr 19:275, 2000

97. Campbell CJ, Bhalla IP, Steel JM, et al: A controlled trial of phentermine in obese diabetic patients. Practitioner 218:851, 1977

98. Kim I, Whitsett TL: Acute vasospasm associated with anorexiant use. J Okla State Med Assoc 81:395, 1988

99 Devan GS: Phentermine and psychosis. Br J Psychiatry 156:442, 1990

100. Kokkinos J, Levine SR: Possible association of ischemic stroke with phentermine. Stroke 24:310, 1993

101. Derby LE, Myers MW, Jick H: Use of dexfenfluramine, fenfluramine and phentermine and the risk of stroke. Br J Clin Pharmacol 47:565, 1999

102. Bray GA, Blackburn GL, Ferguson JM, et al: Sibutramine produces dose-related weight loss. Obes Res 7:189, 1999

103. Hansen D, Astrup A, Toubro S, et al: Predictors of weight loss and maintenance during 2 years of treatment by sibutramine in obesity: results from the European multicentre STORM trial. Sibutramine Trial of Obesity Reduction and Maintenance. Int J Obes Relat Metab Disord 25:496, 2001

104. Dujovne CA, Zavoral JH, Rowe E, et al: Effects of sibutramine on body weight and serum lipids: a double-blind, randomized, placebo-controlled study in 322 overweight and obese patients with dyslipidemia. Am Heart J 142:489, 2001

105. Finer N, Bloom SR, Frost GS, et al: Sibutramine is effective for weight loss and diabetic control in obesity with type 2 diabetes: a randomised, double-blind, placebo-controlled study. Diabetes Obes Metab 2:105, 2000

106. Bray GA: Sibutramine and blood pressure: a therapeutic dilemma. J Hum Hypertens 16:1, 2002

107. Sramek JJ, Leibowitz MT, Weinstein SP, et al: Efficacy and safety of sibutramine for weight loss in obese patients with hypertension well controlled by beta-adrenergic blocking agents: a placebo-controlled, double-blind, randomised trial. J Hum Hypertens 16:13, 2002

108. Jordan J, Scholze K, Matiba B, et al: Influence of sibutramine on blood pressure: evidence from placebo-controlled trials. Int J Obes Relat Metab Disord 29:509, 2005

1090. Hutton B, Fergusson D: Changes in body weight and serum lipid profile in obese patients treated with orlistat in addition to a hypocaloric diet: a systematic review of randomized clinical trials. Am J Clin Nutr 80:1461, 2004

110. Randomised placebo-controlled trial of orlistat for weight loss and prevention of weight regain in obese patients. European Multicentre Orlistat Study Group. Lancet 352:167, 1998

111. Weight loss, weight maintenance, and improved cardiovascular risk factors after 2 years treatment with orlistat for obesity. European Orlistat Obesity Study Group. Obes Res 8:49, 2000

112. Kelley DE, Jneidi M: Orlistat in the treatment of type 2 diabetes mellitus. Expert Opin Pharmacother 3:599, 2002

113. Efficacy and tolerability of orlistat in the treatment of obesity: a 6-month dose-ranging study. Orlistat Dose-Ranging Study Group. Eur J Clin Pharmacol 54:125, 1998

114. Gadde KM, Parker CB, Maner LG, et al: Bupropion for weight loss: an investigation of efficacy and tolerability in overweight and obese women. Obes Res 9:544, 2001

115. Jain AK, Kaplan RA, Gadde KM, et al: Bupropion SR vs. placebo for weight loss in obese patients with depressive symptoms. Obes Res 10:1049, 2002

116. Anderson JW, Greenway FL, Fujioka K, et al: Bupropion SR enhances weight loss: a 48-week double-blind, placebo-controlled trial. Obes Res 10:633, 2002

117. Cummings DE, Overduin J, Foster-Schubert KE: Gastric bypass for obesity: mechanisms of weight loss and diabetes resolution. J Clin Endocrinol Metab 89:2608, 2004

118. Pories WJ, MacDonald KG Jr, Morgan EJ, et al: Surgical treatment of obesity and its effect on diabetes: 10-y follow-up. Am J Clin Nutr 55(2 suppl):582S, 1992

119. Sjöström L, Lindroos AK, Peltonen M, et al: Lifestyle, diabetes, and cardiovascular risk factors 10 years after bariatric surgery. N Engl J Med 351:2683, 2004

120. Chapman AE, Kiroff G, Game P, et al: Laparoscopic adjustable gastric banding in the treatment of obesity: a systematic literature review. Surgery 135:326, 2004

121. Brolin RE: Bariatric surgery and long-term control of morbid obesity. JAMA 288:2793, 2002

122. Buchwald H, Avidor Y, Braunwald E, et al: Bariatric surgery: a systematic review and meta-analysis. JAMA 292:1724, 2004 (erratum in JAMA 293:1728, 2005)

123. Christou NV, Sampalis JS, Liberman M, et al: Surgery decreases long-term mortality, morbidity, and health care use in morbidly obese patients. Ann Surg 240:416, 2004

124. Flum DR, Dellinger EP: Impact of gastric bypass operation on survival: a population-based analysis. J Am Coll Surg 199:543, 2004

125. Wolf AM, Kortner B, Kuhlmann HW: Results of bariatric surgery. Int J Obes Relat Metab Disord 25(suppl 1):S113, 2001

126. Schauer PR, Ikramuddin S, Gourash W, et al: Outcomes after laparoscopic Roux-en-Y gastric bypass for morbid obesity. Ann Surg 232:515, 2000

127. Podnos YD, Jimenez JC, Wilson SE, et al: Complications after laparoscopic gastric bypass: a review of 3464 cases. Arch Surg 138:957, 2003

128. Lujan JA, Frutos MD, Hernandez Q, et al: Laparoscopic versus open gastric bypass in the treatment of morbid obesity: a randomized prospective study. Ann Surg 239:433, 2004

129. Nguyen NT, Goldman C, Rosenquist CJ, et al: Laparoscopic versus open gastric bypass: a randomized study of outcomes, quality of life, and costs. Ann Surg 234:279, 2001

130. Service GJ, Thompson GB, Service FJ, et al: Hyperinsulinemic hypoglycemia with nesidioblastosis after gastric-bypass surgery. N Engl J Med 353:249, 2005

131. Clegg A, Colquitt J, Sidhu M, et al: Clinical and cost effectiveness of surgery for morbid obesity: a systematic review and economic evaluation. Int J Obes Relat Metab Disord 27:1167, 2003

132. Rimm EB, Stampfer MJ, Giovannucci E, et al: Body size and fat distribution as predictors of coronary heart disease among middle-aged and older US men. Am J Epidemiol 141:1117, 1995

133. Manson JE, Willett WC, Stampfer MJ, et al: Body weight and mortality among women. N Engl J Med 333:677, 1995

134. Lakka HM, Laaksonen DE, Lakka TA, et al: The metabolic syndrome and total and cardiovascular disease mortality in middle-aged men. JAMA 288:2709, 2002

135. Jonsson S, Hedblad B, Engstrom G, et al: Influence of obesity on cardiovascular risk: twenty-three-year follow-up of 22,025 men from an urban Swedish population. Int J Obes Relat Metab Disord 26:1046, 2002

136. Mokdad AH, Ford ES, Bowman BA, et al: Prevalence of obesity, diabetes, and obesity-related health risk factors, 2001. JAMA 289:76, 2003

137. Bray GA: Medical consequences of obesity. J Clin Endocrinol Metab 89:2583, 2004

138. Must A, Spadano J, Coakley EH, et al: The disease burden associated with overweight and obesity. JAMA 282:1523, 1999

139. Peppard PE, Young T, Palta M, et al: Longitudinal study of moderate weight change and sleep-disordered breathing. JAMA 284:3015, 2000

140. Strauss RS: Childhood obesity and self-esteem. Pediatrics 105:e15, 2000

141. Roberts RE, Kaplan GA, Shema SJ, et al: Are the obese at greater risk for depression? Am J Epidemiol 152:163, 2000

142. Gortmaker SL, Must A, Perrin JM, et al: Social and economic consequences of overweight in adolescence and young adulthood. N Engl J Med 329:1008, 1993

143. Wolf AM, Colditz GA: Current estimates of the economic cost of obesity in the United States. Obes Res 6:97, 1998

144. Bender R, Jockel KH, Trautner C, et al: Effect of age on excess mortality in obesity. JAMA 281:1498, 1999

145. Fontaine KR, Redden DT, Wang C, et al: Years of life lost due to obesity. JAMA 289:187, 2003

146. Kolaczynski JW, Considine RV, Ohannesian J, et al: Responses of leptin to short-term fasting and refeeding in humans: a link with ketogenesis but not ketones themselves. Diabetes 45:1511, 1996

147. Keim NL, Stern JS, Havel PJ: Relation between circulating leptin concentrations and appetite during a prolonged, moderate energy deficit in women. Am J Clin Nutr 68:794, 1998

148. Leibel RL, Rosenbaum M, Hirsch J: Changes in energy expenditure resulting from altered body weight. N Engl J Med 332:621, 1995

149. Kolaczynski JW, Ohannesian JP, Considine RV, et al: Response of leptin to short-term and prolonged overfeeding in humans. J Clin Endocrinol Metab 81:4162, 1996

150. Sims EA, Danforth E Jr, Horton ES, et al: Endocrine and metabolic effects of experimental obesity in man. Recent Prog Horm Res 29:457, 1973

151. Diagnosis and classification of diabetes mellitus. American Diabetes Association. Diabetes Care 27(suppl 1):S5, 2004

152. Gadde KM, Franciscy DM, Wagner HR 2nd, et al: Zonisamide for weight loss in obese adults: a randomized controlled trial. JAMA 289:1820, 2003

153. Ren CJ, Horgan S, Ponce J: US experience with the LAP-BAND system. Am J Surg 184:46S, 2002

154. Anthone GJ, Lord RV, DeMeester TR, et al: The duodenal switch operation for the treatment of morbid obesity. Ann Surg 238:618, 2003

Acknowledgment

Figure 3   Seward Hung.

59 Diagnosis and Treatment of Dyslipidemia

John D. Brunzell, M.D., F.A.C.P., and R. Alan Failor, M.D.

Disorders of lipoprotein metabolism, in conjunction with the prevalence of high-fat diets, obesity, and physical inactivity, have resulted in an epidemic of atherosclerotic disease in the United States and other developed countries. The interaction of common genetic and acquired disorders of lipoproteins with these adverse environmental factors leads to the premature development of atherosclerosis. In the United States, mortality from coronary artery disease (CAD), particularly in persons younger than 60 years, has been declining since 1970; however, atherosclerotic cardiovascular disease remains the most common cause of death among both men and women.

Formerly, hyperlipidemia was defined as elevation of a lipoprotein level in the population. The recognition that a low level of high-density lipoprotein (HDL) and the presence of small, dense low-density lipoprotein (LDL) particles are clinically important in the pathophysiology of lipid disorders has led to the use of the term dyslipidemia to describe a range of disorders that include both abnormally high and low lipoprotein levels, as well as abnormalities in the composition of these particles. Dyslipidemias are clinically important, principally because of their contribution to atherogenesis. Pancreatitis and fatty liver disease are less common but clinically significant manifestations of lipid disorders.

Lipoprotein Physiology

LIPOPROTEIN COMPOSITION AND METABOLISM

Lipoproteins are spherical macromolecular complexes of lipid and protein [*see Figure 1*]. Clinically important lipids in the blood include cholesterol (both unesterified and esterified) and triglyceride (molecules consisting of three fatty acids attached to a glycerol backbone). Cholesterol has three primary functions: it plays a role in the structure of cell membranes, in the synthesis of steroid hormones, and in the formation of bile acids. The major functions of triglyceride are energy storage (in fat) and energy use (by muscle). Because fat cannot readily dissolve in plasma, cholesterol and triglyceride are made miscible by incorporation into lipoproteins (e.g., very low density lipoprotein [VLDL], LDL, and HDL). Apolipoproteins are the protein component of lipoproteins; they aid in the lipid transport and delivery process in three ways: they serve as structural elements, as ligands for receptors, and as regulatory cofactors [*see Table 1*].

LIPOPROTEIN STRUCTURE AND CLASSIFICATION

A mature lipoprotein particle is a sphere consisting of a central core of lipids (triglyceride and cholesteryl ester) surrounded by a monolayer surface of phospholipid, unesterified cholesterol, and apolipoproteins [*see Figure 1*]. Operationally, the lipoproteins can be described on the basis of their size and buoyancy characteristics [*see Figure 2*].

Chylomicron Chylomicrons are the largest of the lipoprotein particles. The major structural protein is apolipoprotein B-48 (apo B-48). The bulk (~ 80%) of the lipid core consists of triglyceride. Synthesized in and secreted from the intestine, chylomi-

crons transport exogenous cholesterol, fatty acids, and fat-soluble vitamins absorbed from digested food [*see Exogenous Pathway, below*].

VLDL This triglyceride-rich particle (~ 80% of the lipid core consists of triglyceride) is synthesized in the liver, delivers triglyceride to the periphery, and is the precursor for intermediate-density lipoproteins (IDLs) and LDL. The major structural protein of this lipoprotein is apo B-100 [*see Endogenous Pathway, below*].

IDL The remnant of VLDL is of IDL density. It is formed after triglyceride in VLDL is hydrolyzed by lipoprotein lipase. The core is roughly 50% triglyceride and 50% cholesteryl ester. Approximately half of the body's IDL particles are cleared from the plasma into the liver; the other half are further processed to form LDL [*see Endogenous Pathway, below*]. In clinical practice, assessment of LDL levels includes the determination of cholesterol in both IDL and LDL fractions.

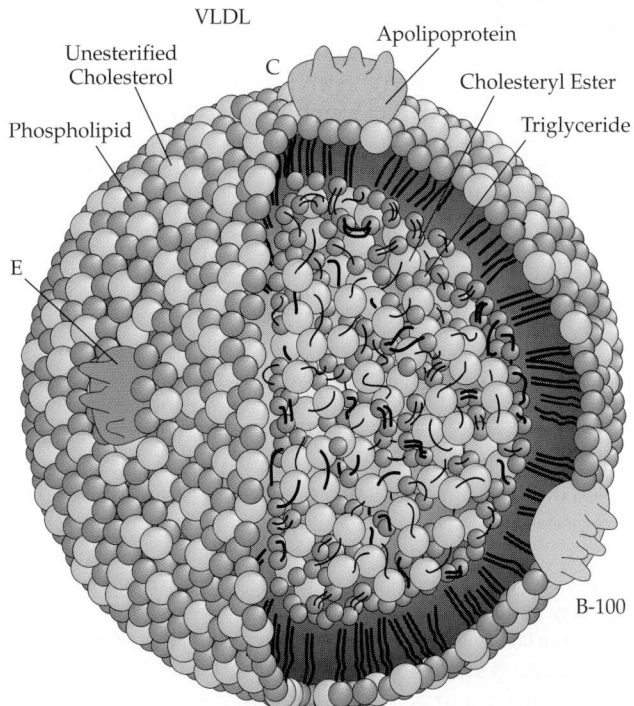

Figure 1 **Lipoproteins transport water-insoluble triglyceride and cholesterol through the bloodstream. All apo B–containing lipoproteins have a structure similar to that shown for very low density lipoproteins (VLDLs). The core is composed of triglyceride and cholesteryl ester, whereas the monolayer surface is composed of phospholipid, unesterified cholesterol, and protein in the form of apolipoproteins. VLDL contains apolipoproteins B-100, C-I, C-II, and E. Low-density lipoprotein (LDL), which transports most of the cholesterol found in blood, contains primarily apo B-100.**

Table 1   Major Apolipoproteins and
Their Functions

Apolipoprotein	Function
Apo A-I	Structural protein of HDL; activates lecithin-cholesterol acyltransferase
Apo A-II	Structural protein of HDL
Apo B-48	Structural protein of chylomicron
Apo B-100	Structural protein of VLDL, IDL, and LDL; ligand for LDL receptor
Apo C-II	Activator of LPL
Apo C-III	Potential inhibitor of apo C-II and apo E functions
Apo E	Ligand for chylomicron remnant receptor and LDL receptor
Apo(a)	Function unknown; antagonizes plasminogen

HDL—high-density lipoprotein   IDL—intermediate-density lipoprotein
LDL—low-density lipoprotein   LPL—lipoprotein lipase   VLDL—very low
density lipoprotein

LDL   This lipoprotein results from the hepatic processing of VLDL remnants. The core is rich in cholesteryl ester and accounts for the majority of cholesterol circulating in the blood. LDL plays a major role in the development of atherosclerosis [*see* LDL Catabolism, *below*].

HDL   HDL forms from the unesterified cholesterol and phospholipid removed from peripheral tissues and the surface of triglyceride-rich proteins [*see* Function and Regulation of HDL, *below*]. The major structural protein is apo A-I; the core is predominantly cholesteryl ester. HDL mediates the return of lipoprotein and tissue cholesterol to the liver for excretion in the process referred to as reverse cholesterol transport. Another function of HDL is to shuttle apo E and apo C-II to and from chylomicrons and VLDL.

LIPOPROTEIN ASSEMBLY AND CATABOLISM

Exogenous Pathway

After a meal, intestinal cells absorb fatty acids and cholesterol, esterify them into triglyceride and cholesteryl ester, and incorporate them into the core of chylomicrons.[1] Triglyceride greatly predominates over cholesterol ester in the chylomicron core. The chylomicrons are secreted into plasma, where apo C-II on the chylomicron surface activates endothelial-bound lipoprotein lipase (LPL). LPL in turn hydrolyzes the chylomicron's core triglyceride and releases free fatty acids, which are taken up by adipose tissue for storage and by muscle for energy. During lipolysis, the chylomicron decreases in size, and some surface components are transferred to HDL; the remaining particle is the chylomicron remnant particle. This chylomicron remnant next acquires apo E from HDL and is subsequently taken up by the liver after binding to sites that recognize apo E. It is then degraded, thereby delivering dietary cholesterol to the liver.

Endogenous Pathway

The liver secretes triglyceride-rich VLDL into plasma, where they too acquire apo C-II from HDL. As with chylomicrons, VLDL interacts with LPL on the capillary endothelium, and the core triglyceride is hydrolyzed to provide fatty acids to adipose

and muscle tissues.[1] About half of the catabolized VLDL remnants (IDL density) are taken up by hepatic receptors that bind to apo E for degradation; the other half—apo B-100 particles, depleted of triglyceride relative to cholesteryl ester—are converted by the liver to cholesteryl ester–rich LDL. As IDL is converted to LDL, apo E becomes detached, leaving only one apolipoprotein, apo B-100. Each particle in this cascade from VLDL to LDL contains one molecule of apo B-100.

In the metabolism of both chylomicrons and VLDL, apo C-II permits the hydrolysis of triglyceride by lipoprotein lipase, and apo E prompts hepatic uptake of remnants. A major difference in the metabolism of these particles is that chylomicrons contain a truncated form of apo B (i.e., apo B-48), whereas VLDL contains the complete form (i.e., apo B-100). Another difference is that chylomicron remnants are degraded after they are absorbed by the liver, whereas many of the VLDL remnants are most likely processed in the hepatic sinusoids to become LDL.

REGULATION OF LIPOPROTEIN METABOLISM

There are four major clinically significant physiologic steps in the lipoprotein cascade from VLDL to LDL—namely, VLDL assembly, hydrolysis by LPL, remnant catabolism, and LDL catabolism [*see Figure 3*].[1,2] Defects at any step in the cascade can lead to hyperlipidemia. These defects can be genetic or acquired (i.e., secondary to disease or the effects of drugs) or the result of an interaction of genetic and acquired factors.

Lipoprotein Assembly

Apo B-100 is synthesized constitutively in the endoplasmic reticulum of the hepatocyte, and much of it is degraded in the endoplasmic reticulum. Triglyceride is added to the surviving apo B that will be secreted as VLDL. It is transported to the Golgi complex, where it acquires additional core lipid, forming the nascent VLDL particle. This particle is secreted into plasma, where it acquires apolipoproteins (e.g., apo C-II and apo E) from HDL.[1]

Abnormalities in VLDL secretion can occur in two genetic forms of hyperlipidemia: familial hypertriglyceridemia (FHTG)

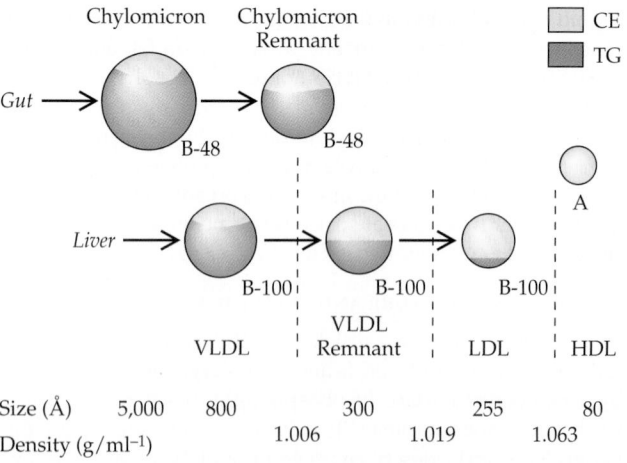

Size (Å)   5,000   800   300   255   80
Density (g/ml⁻¹) 1.006 1.019 1.063

Figure 2   **Size and buoyancy characteristics of lipoproteins. Chylomicrons, which are composed largely of triglyceride, are the largest and most buoyant of the lipoproteins. High-density lipoprotein (HDL) particles are substantially smaller and denser and are composed mostly of cholesteryl ester. (CE—cholesteryl ester; TG—triglyceride)**

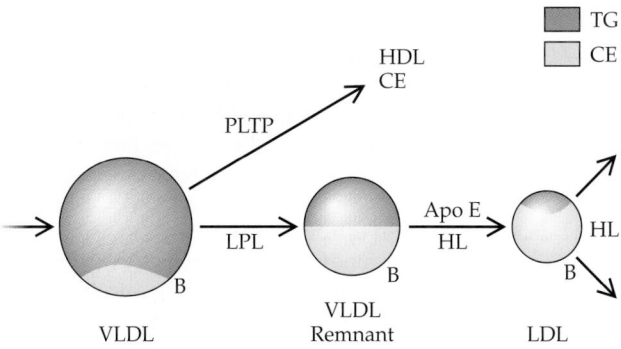

Figure 3 **The apolipoprotein B-100 (apo B-100) cascade. VLDL is secreted from the liver with one apo B on the surface and triglyceride and cholesteryl ester in the core. Core triglyceride is hydrolyzed by lipoprotein lipase and becomes a remnant lipoprotein that is recognized by the liver—in part, by apo E. The remnant lipoprotein is further processed to form LDL, which has a cholesterol-rich core and an intact apo B on its surface. The LDL particle can be removed by peripheral or hepatic LDL receptors. As the VLDL core is hydrolyzed, the unesterified cholesterol and phospholipid are transferred to HDL by phospholipid transfer protein to become the cholesteryl ester of HDL. (CE—cholesteryl ester; HL— hepatic lipase; LPL—lipoprotein lipase; PLTP—phospholipid transfer protein; TG—triglyceride)**

and familial combined hyperlipidemia (FCHL). FHTG is characterized by the overproduction of triglyceride contained within a normal number of VLDL particles; this results in each particle's having an excessive amount of triglyceride. In FCHL, an excessive amount of apo B-100 is secreted into VLDL or LDL particles; these particles tend to be smaller than normal.[3]

The metabolic syndrome, which is a common condition in the general population, is a component of most cases of FCHL and also contributes to the residual dyslipidemia seen in patients with type 2 diabetes mellitus who have been treated with insulin or insulin secretagogues. The molecular basis of the hepatic triglyceride or apo B oversecretion in these disorders is unknown.

A deficiency in lipoproteins containing apo B is referred to as hypobetalipoproteinemia; an absence of apo B is termed abetalipoproteinemia. Abetalipoproteinemia may occur because of a defect involving both apo B genes that prevents the production of apo B. It also may occur in individuals who are homozygous for mutations in the microsomal triglyceride transport protein, which is critical for apo B transport in the endoplasmic reticulum. Homozygous hypobetalipoproteinemia and abetalipoproteinemia lead to deficiencies in fat-soluble vitamins because each of these conditions results in a shortage of apo B–containing lipoproteins, which are needed to transport fat-soluble vitamins. Hypobetalipoproteinemia, which is characterized by apo B levels that are 50% of normal, can be caused by a defect in a single apo B gene.[4]

Lipoprotein(a) Lipoprotein(a) [Lp(a)] is a specific class of lipoprotein particles that are synthesized in the liver and that have a lipid composition similar to that of LDL. Lp(a) differs from LDL by the presence of apolipoprotein(a) [apo(a)], a protein whose structure is homologous to plasminogen.[5] The apo(a) protein is bound by a disulfide linkage to apo B-100 to form Lp(a). High levels of Lp(a) are both prothrombotic and atherogenic.[5] Levels of Lp(a) in plasma are almost completely determined by genetic variation in the *Lp(a)* gene.

Lipoprotein Catabolism

Lipoprotein lipase–mediated triglyceride removal LPL is synthesized in adipose tissue and muscle and then transported to the luminal surface of the endothelial lining of the adjacent capillary, where it acts on triglyceride-rich lipoproteins. The fatty acids that are released during the processing of triglyceride-rich particles (i.e., chylomicrons and VLDL) can be used for energy by muscle, or they can be reesterified into triglyceride and stored in adipocytes for later use.[6] Apo C-II, the LPL activator, is carried on the triglyceride-rich lipoproteins—chylomicrons and VLDL.

Genetic defects that result in impaired lipoprotein lipase synthesis or function are rare autosomal recessive causes of hyperlipidemia. Usually, these mutations present in neonates or infants as severe hypertriglyceridemia. Heterozygote parents of these children often have mild hypertriglyceridemia. Acquired defects of LPL, such as untreated diabetes or uremia, are more common causes of hyperlipidemia. When an acquired defect of LPL is associated with a disorder characterized by excessive input of VLDL, marked hypertriglyceridemia can ensue. The coexistence of two or more disorders that independently increase the level of triglycerides in plasma (e.g., FHTG or FCHL coexistent with untreated diabetes) can lead to marked hypertriglyceridemia.[6]

Remnant catabolism Both chylomicron and VLDL remnants acquire apo E from HDL before they can bind to hepatic receptors for either uptake and degradation or further processing to LDL. Three alleles of the *APOE* gene (i.e., *APOE*E2*, *APOE*E3*, and *APOE*E4*) result in six possible combinations. The *APOE*E4* allele product has the greatest affinity for hepatic receptors, followed by the *APOE*E3* allele product; the *APOE*E2* allele product has markedly reduced receptor affinity.

Individuals who are homozygous for the *APOE*E2* allele (E2/E2) have marked impairment of hepatic remnant lipoprotein uptake, which results in the accumulation of these remnants in the plasma and in very low levels or the absence of LDL. Interestingly, individuals with E2/E2 typically have either normal or low cholesterol levels because of the paucity of LDL particles characteristic of this disorder.[7] If, however, an individual who is homozygous for the *APOE*E2* allele (E2/E2) has a defect—either inherited or acquired—that causes excessive input of VLDL, then excessive accumulation of VLDL remnants and hyperlipidemia occur. This results in remnant removal disease. Because chylomicron and VLDL remnants contain roughly equal amounts of triglyceride and cholesterol, the hyperlipidemia of remnant removal disease is characterized by both hypercholesterolemia and hypertriglyceridemia.[7]

LDL catabolism The final step at which a defect in lipoprotein metabolism can occur is in LDL catabolism. Apo B-100 on the surface of LDL binds to its receptor on the cell surface; LDL is then absorbed into the cell, where it is catabolized [*see Figure 4*]. After hydrolysis of the core lipids, unesterified cholesterol is used by cells for synthesis of membranes, bile acids, and steroid hormones and for various regulatory actions that prevent overaccumulation of cholesterol within the cell. The vast majority of LDL particles in plasma are taken up by the liver by means of the LDL receptor.

Mutations of the LDL receptor (as found in familial hypercholesterolemia [FH]) or, less commonly, mutations in the apo B-100 molecule (as found in familial defective apo B-100) lead to an impairment in the interaction of LDL with its receptor; this can re-

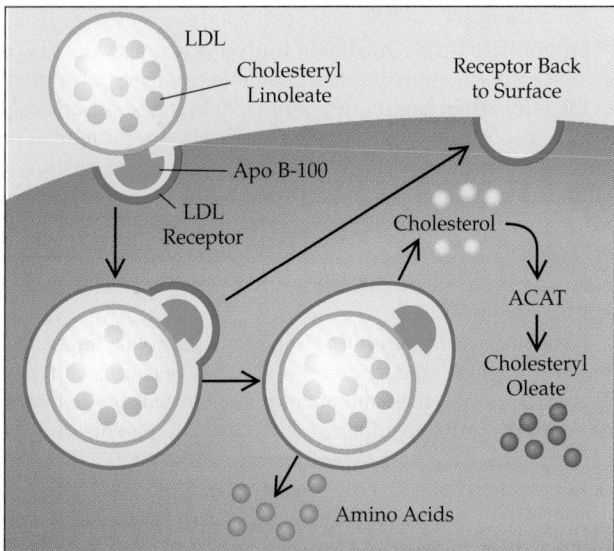

Figure 4 **LDL is absorbed by cells through the LDL receptor. This receptor recognizes apo B-100, the apolipoprotein on the surface of LDL. Once internalized, the lipoprotein is catabolized, releasing cholesterol and amino acids. The free cholesterol is converted to cholesteryl oleate by the enzyme acyl–coenzyme A: cholesterol acyltransferase (ACAT). The LDL receptor is recycled back to the cell surface.**

sult in elevated LDL levels. LDL levels also can be influenced by dietary factors. For example, dietary cholesterol delivered to the liver by chylomicron remnants can suppress hepatic LDL receptors, leading to impaired LDL removal from plasma. Dietary saturated fats also may reduce LDL receptor activity and may increase LDL production. Hypothyroidism can also be associated with defective LDL receptor–mediated cholesterol removal.[8]

Function and Regulation of HDL

The major HDL apolipoproteins are apo A-I and apo A-II, which are formed in the liver and small intestine.[9] Apo A-I is secreted with phospholipid in a disklike structure called nascent HDL. Most of the apolipoproteins and phospholipid destined to become nascent HDL are initially secreted on the surface of chylomicrons and VLDL. After LPL hydrolyzes triglyceride in chylomicrons and VLDL, the core lipid content in these lipoprotein particles becomes smaller, and redundancies of unesterified cholesterol and phospholipid occur in the surface layer. These redundant surface components are transferred to HDL by phospholipid transfer protein. Nascent HDL particles also pick up excess unesterified cholesterol and phospholipid from peripheral tissues via the transporter ABCA1. This HDL cholesterol then undergoes esterification by the plasma enzyme lecithin-cholesterol acyltransferase (LCAT). LCAT is activated by apo A-I on the HDL surface to esterify free cholesterol into cholesteryl ester, causing it to move into the core. In this process, the particle becomes the larger, more buoyant HDL_3 particle and progresses to the even larger HDL_2 particle.[9,10] At some point, apo A-II may be added to the HDL_2 particle, which then is directed to deliver cholesteryl ester to the liver by cholesteryl ester transfer protein (CETP). Hepatic lipase activity on the liver surface hydrolyzes the phospholipid and triglyceride in the HDL_2 particle, promoting the decrease in size and density to HDL_3 and then to even smaller HDL particles.[10] Recycling of some of the apo A-I causes the process to repeat itself [*see Figure 5*].

Abnormally high or low levels of HDL cholesterol may be caused, rarely, by genetic defects. Elevations in the HDL cholesterol level may result from genetic hyperalphalipoproteinemia or CETP deficiency. Markedly reduced HDL cholesterol levels may be caused by apo A-I structural mutation; homozygosity for mutations in ABCA1,[11] leading to Tangier disease; or homozygosity for mutations in the enzyme LCAT, leading to LCAT deficiency and fish-eye disease. Factors associated with an increase in HDL levels include female sex, aerobic exercise, weight reduction, high-fat diets, and certain drugs (e.g., alcohol, estrogens, fibrates, and nicotinic acid) [*see Table 2*]. Factors associated with a decrease in HDL levels include male sex, central obesity, cigarette smoking, low-fat diets, hypertriglyceridemia, uremia, being heterozygous for Tangier disease, and certain drugs (e.g., androgens, progestins, and some antihypertensive agents) [*see Table 2*]. Low HDL particle number is commonly associated with increased triglyceride levels, as seen in the metabolic syndrome.

Function of Hepatic Lipase

Hepatic lipase is synthesized in the hepatocyte, binds to endothelial surfaces in the liver sinusoids, and acts on lipoproteins.[10] After triglyceride-rich VLDL particles exchange triglyceride for the cholesteryl ester in LDL and HDL, hepatic lipase can hydrolyze the phospholipid and triglyceride in LDL and HDL [*see Figure 6*]. This process leads to the formation of small, dense LDL and converts HDL_2 to HDL_3. This process may be driven by the presence of excessive levels of triglyceride-rich VLDL in the presence of normal hepatic lipase activity or by increases in the level of hepatic lipase. Factors such as male sex and the accumulation of intra-abdominal fat predispose to increased hepatic lipase levels and are associated with an increase in small, dense LDL levels and a decrease in HDL_2 levels. Increased hepatic lipase activity is an important factor in the dyslipidemia of the metabolic syndrome.[10,12] Hepatic lipase also may facilitate hepatic recognition and uptake of chylomicron and VLDL remnant lipoproteins.

Clinical Manifestations of Dyslipidemia

The main clinical consequences of hyperlipidemia are premature atherosclerosis; pancreatitis, which is usually associated with the chylomicronemia syndrome; and nonalcoholic fatty liver disease. Atherosclerosis is most clearly associated with elevated levels of LDL cholesterol and reduced levels of HDL cholesterol. In both pancreatitis and fatty liver disease, the underlying lipid disorder is hypertriglyceridemia.

DYSLIPIDEMIA IN ATHEROSCLEROSIS

There is consensus that elevated plasma LDL levels and reduced HDL levels are associated with an increased risk of atherosclerosis. The role of hypertriglyceridemia as a cardiovascular risk factor is more complex. Hypertriglyceridemia may be a marker for other lipoprotein abnormalities (e.g., increased levels of small, dense LDL particles; low levels of HDL; or remnant accumulation) that are part of the dyslipidemic pattern associated with FCHL, type 2 diabetes mellitus, and the metabolic syndrome. In these settings, hypertriglyceridemia is a predictor of increased premature cardiovascular risk. However, other forms of hypertriglyceridemia may not be associated with premature cardiovascular disease [*see Familial Hypertriglyceridemia, below*]. The precise mechanisms by which elevated LDL levels result in increased atherosclerotic risk are unclear. Very high levels of large, buoyant LDL particles, such as occur in FH and familial defective apo B-100, as well as the presence of more moderate numbers of small, dense LDL particles are associated with an increased risk of cardiovascular disease. Accumulating evidence suggests that LDL needs to be modified before it becomes atherogenic.[13] Oxidation of LDL may increase its atherogenicity. Oxidized LDL has many biologic properties that may cause it to become atherogenic. The atherogenicity of small, dense LDL particles may result from the ability of LDL to enter the arterial intima, where it is retained by matrix molecules and undergoes oxidation more readily than larger, more buoyant LDL particles. The antiatherogenic properties of HDL are probably related to its role in reverse cholesterol transport, and HDL may have anti-inflammatory and antioxidant effects.

DYSLIPIDEMIA IN THE CHYLOMICRONEMIA SYNDROME

Pancreatitis is associated with chylomicronemia, usually with elevated levels of VLDL. The mechanism by which chylomicronemia causes pancreatitis is unclear. Pancreatitis is believed to result from the release of more free fatty acids and lysolecithin from chylomicrons than can be bound by pancreatic lipase in the pancreatic capillaries.

The chylomicronemia syndrome occasionally occurs when LPL is defective as a result of genetic variation in the enzyme or its cofactor, apo C-II. Much more commonly, chylomicronemia is caused by the coexistence of a genetic form of hypertriglyc-

eridemia combined with an acquired disorder of plasma triglyceride metabolism, the most common being untreated diabetes. Other conditions may be implicated (e.g., hypothyroidism and nephrotic syndrome), as may the use of drugs that raise triglyceride levels.

The chylomicronemia syndrome is associated with abdominal pain, eruptive xanthomas, and transient memory loss. Eruptive xanthomas occur most frequently on the buttocks and the extensor surfaces of the upper limb. A reversible loss of memory, particularly for recent events, and peripheral neuropathy, which sometimes mimics the carpal tunnel syndrome, also may occur. The retinal vessels occasionally demonstrate lipemia retinalis. If the chylomicronemia syndrome is not corrected, it may lead to acute pancreatitis. Acute pancreatitis can be fatal and is often recurrent until low triglyceride levels are maintained. The risk of pancreatitis caused by severe hypertriglyceridemia markedly increases with triglyceride levels over 2,000 mg/dl.

DYSLIPIDEMIA IN NONALCOHOLIC FATTY LIVER DISEASE

Fatty liver disease seems to occur in both genetic and acquired hypertriglyceridemia. It usually is caused by the synthesis of hepatic triglyceride in amounts that are excessive relative to the amount of apo B that is synthesized; this leads to accumulation of triglyceride in the liver, rather than the hepatic secretion of VLDL triglyceride. Fatty liver disease also may occur in het-

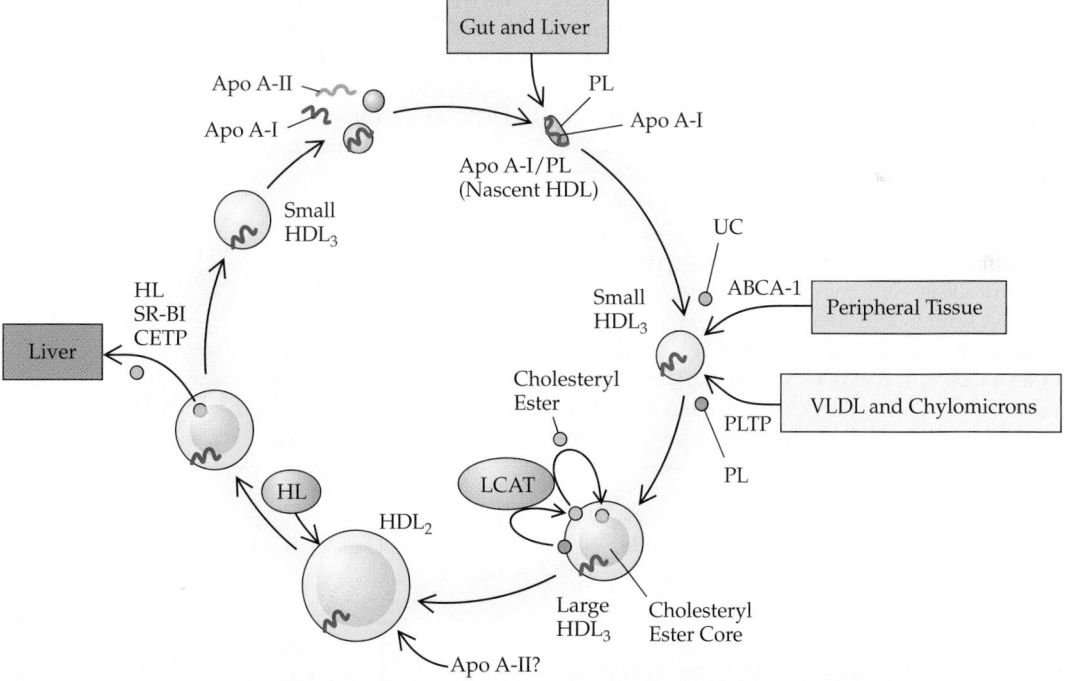

Figure 5 **The circular pathway of HDL formation and degradation.[11] HDL begins as an apo A-1 phospholipid complex. Unesterified cholesterol and phospholipid are added to the nascent HDL via adenosine triphosphate–binding cassette transporter A-1 and phospholipid transfer protein to begin the formation of the smaller HDL_3 particle. LCAT transfers a fatty acid from phospholipid to unesterified cholesterol to cholesteryl ester, which moves to the HDL core. In this process, the HDL particle becomes the larger, more buoyant HDL_3 particle and progresses to the even larger HDL_2 particle. Cholesteryl ester transfer protein contributes to the transfer of cholesteryl ester from HDL_2 to the liver and various lipoproteins; with this loss of cholesteryl ester, the HDL particle shrinks in size. Hepatic lipase hydrolyzes the phospholipid and triglyceride in the HDL_2 particle, promoting the decrease in size and density to HDL_3 and then to even smaller HDL particles, including apo A-1. Recycling of some of the apo A-I causes the process to repeat itself. The role of apo A-II in this process in humans is not clear. (ABCA1—ATP-binding cassette transporter A1; CETP—cholesteryl ester transfer protein; LCAT—lecithin-cholesterol acyltransferase; LPL—lipoprotein lipase; PL—phospholipid; PLTP—phospholipid transfer protein; SR-BI—scavenger receptor BI; UC—unesterified cholesterol)**

Table 2 ATP-III Classification of Total Cholesterol, LDL Cholesterol, HDL Cholesterol, and Triglyceride Levels[15]

Total cholesterol (mg/dl)*	
< 200	Desirable
200–239	Borderline high
≥ 240	High
LDL cholesterol (mg/dl)	
< 100	Optimal
100–129	Near or above optimal
130–159	Borderline high
160–189	High
≥ 190	Very high
HDL cholesterol (mg/dl)	
< 40	Low
≥ 60	High
Triglycerides (mg/dl)	
< 150	Normal
150–199	Borderline high
200–499	High
≥ 500	Very high

*Elevation of total cholesterol can reflect increased LDL, increased HDL, or both. Increased LDL is proatherosclerotic, whereas elevated HDL is antiatherosclerotic.

erozygous familial hypobetalipoproteinemia because of the decreased synthesis of hepatic apo B associated with this disorder. Alcoholic fatty liver disease also occurs with increased hepatic triglyceride synthesis in the face of impaired apo B synthesis.[14] Fatty liver disease has been associated with the metabolic syndrome,[12] which is related to central obesity, insulin resistance, and hypertriglyceridemia.

Any severe form of hypertriglyceridemia with defective VLDL catabolism also can be associated with fatty liver and hepatosplenomegaly. In fact, familial LPL deficiency—a form of hypertriglyceridemia caused entirely by an extrahepatic defect in triglyceride hydrolysis—is commonly associated with fatty liver disease; in this setting, fatty liver disease regresses rapidly with restriction of dietary fat. In some patients, fatty liver disease progresses to steatohepatitis that is associated with fibrosis and necrosis; the reasons for such a progression are not clear. Perhaps a second insult is needed for these patients to develop nonalcoholic steatohepatitis and then progress to cirrhosis.

Approach to the Patient with Abnormal Lipid Levels

PATIENTS WITH ISOLATED ELEVATION OF LDL CHOLESTEROL LEVELS

A patient's LDL cholesterol level is said to be "borderline high" in an individual with low atherosclerotic risk if the LDL cholesterol level exceeds 130 mg/dl. High LDL levels are those above 160 mg/dl [*see Table 2*]. The patient's triglyceride level is by definition normal,[15] and the HDL cholesterol level is variable but is often normal. The lipid disorders in these patients are usually discovered through routine cholesterol screening. Although some observers question the cost-effectiveness of screening men and women older than 20 years, the high prevalence of elevated LDL cholesterol in the United States warrants population screening, as recommended by the National Cholesterol Education Program (NCEP) and other authorities.

Severely elevated cholesterol levels are an indication of FH. The ability to diagnose FH is valuable because affected individuals will require drug therapy from a relatively young age [*see* Familial Hypercholesterolemia, *below*].

Isolated hypercholesterolemia may be present intermittently in patients with FCHL. A family history that is strongly positive for premature cardiovascular disease, or the presence of any of the other criteria for FCHL, should provide clues to the diagnosis of this disorder [*see* Familial Combined Hyperlipidemia, *below*]. Not all cases of mild isolated hypercholesterolemia are indicative of FH or FCHL; such cases may result from interactions of acquired and environmental factors, particularly dietary factors, with unknown genetic factors that confer susceptibility to hypercholesterolemia.

Most current treatment guidelines are based primarily on LDL cholesterol levels, because reduction of LDL has been shown to reduce cardiovascular disease by as much as 50%.[16] Reduction in the consumption of dietary saturated fat and cholesterol usually leads to a modest reduction in LDL cholesterol levels; such a reduction depends in part on the baseline diet [*see Chapter 4*]. Lifestyle changes, including diet and weight loss, will suffice in some individuals for reducing LDL cholesterol levels to an acceptable range. However, this approach is unlikely to suffice in patients with familial forms of dyslipidemia, such as FH or FCHL.

In patients with familial forms of the disease or in patients for whom lifestyle measures alone fail to bring LDL cholesterol levels within guideline goals, cholesterol-lowering drugs should be added to the treatment regimen [*see* Drug Therapy in Dyslipidemia, *below*]. Diet therapy can reduce LDL cholesterol levels an additional 5% to 15% beyond reductions achieved with drugs.[17] Diet therapy can therefore lead to a reduction in the dosages of required drugs and should be used in combination with drug

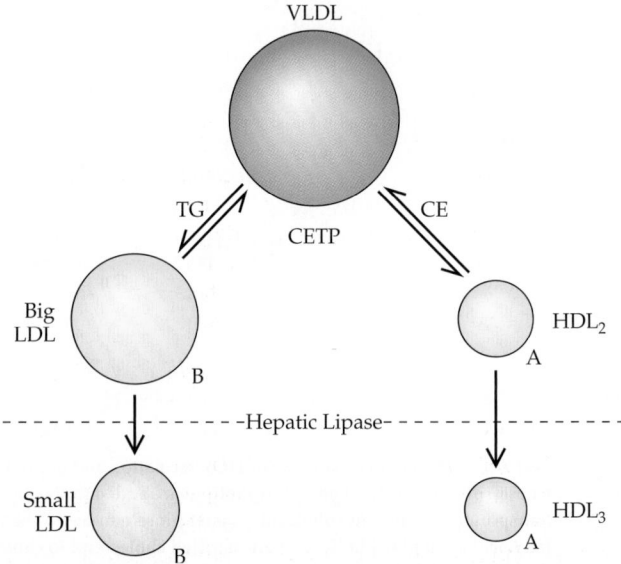

Figure 6 **Dyslipidemia in the metabolic syndrome. Triglyceride-rich VLDL exchanges triglyceride for the cholesteryl ester in LDL and HDL particles. This change in lipoprotein composition is initiated by cholesteryl ester transfer protein. Hepatic lipase hydrolyzes the triglyceride and phospholipid in large LDL and HDL particles, decreasing the size of each particle. (CE—cholesteryl ester; CETP—cholesterol ester transfer protein; TG—triglyceride)**

therapy. The major class of drugs used to reduce LDL cholesterol is the statins. However, bile acid–binding resins and drugs that block cholesterol absorption are of value in patients who do not respond adequately to statins alone, and they can be used in combination with statins and other drugs.

PATIENTS WITH ISOLATED ELEVATION OF TRIGLYCERIDE LEVELS

An isolated elevation in triglyceride levels may be caused by a primary disorder of lipid metabolism (e.g., FHTG or FCHL); it may arise secondary to the use of therapeutic drugs; or it may be a component of the metabolic syndrome or type 2 diabetes mellitus. Unlike with cholesterol levels, it has been difficult to determine the level of triglyceride at which the risk of CAD increases or decreases. It is valuable to ascertain the cause of the hypertriglyceridemia, because the therapeutic approaches may differ.

For example, it is important to distinguish FHTG, which confers no risk of premature CAD, from FCHL, which is associated with a high incidence of premature atherosclerosis.[17] However, it can be difficult to distinguish these disorders when FCHL is associated with hypertriglyceridemia. A positive personal or family history of premature atherosclerosis suggests FCHL. In addition, patients with FCHL frequently have nonlipid cardiovascular risk factors (i.e., central obesity, hypertension, insulin resistance, impaired glucose tolerance, increased levels of plasminogen activator inhibitor–1 (PAI-1), and increased levels of circulating inflammatory markers). Hypertriglyceridemia present in FCHL indicates the presence of increased numbers of small, dense LDL particles and confers an increased risk of premature cardiovascular disease.[12] Similarly, hypertriglyceridemia associated with type 2 diabetes mellitus and the metabolic syndrome is an important cardiovascular risk factor. Other cardiovascular risk factors are usually present in patients with type 2 diabetes mellitus, the metabolic syndrome, or FCHL. Therefore, the therapeutic strategy must consider factors beyond the lipid disorder.

Patients with FHTG do not appear to be at significantly increased risk for the premature development of CAD. However, they are at increased risk for the development of the chylomicronemia syndrome when secondary forms of hypertriglyceridemia are present, such as the hypertriglyceridemia caused by the use of triglyceride-raising drugs [see Table 3]. The chylomicronemia syndrome occurs in FCHL in combination with other causes of hypertriglyceridemia as well. In patients with pancreatitis caused by hypertriglyceridemia, triglyceride levels exceed 2,000 mg/dl and can be much higher. It is recommended that plasma triglyceride levels be maintained below 2,000 mg/dl to prevent recurrent acute pancreatitis. A safe goal would be a level of less than 1,000 mg/dl.

PATIENTS WITH ELEVATIONS IN CHOLESTEROL AND TRIGLYCERIDE LEVELS

Patients with elevations in the levels of both total plasma cholesterol and triglyceride fall into three categories. In the first category, there is an elevation in VLDL and in LDL, as seen in FCHL. In the second category, there is an elevation in VLDL remnants and chylomicron remnants, as in remnant removal disease. The third category consists of patients with very high triglyceride levels in whom the increase in total cholesterol is a result of the cholesterol in VLDL and chylomicrons.

In patients with FCHL, an increase in triglycerides and in LDL cholesterol is often seen. These patients have elevated apo B levels and small, dense LDL particles. Therapy for these individuals often requires several drugs, one aimed at lowering the triglyceride level and one aimed at reducing the amount of small, dense LDL particles [see Drug Therapy in Dyslipidemia, below].

In patients with remnant removal disease, the levels of plasma cholesterol and triglyceride are often equal. It is important to consider remnant removal disease in these circumstances. Therapy is directed at decreasing hepatic lipoprotein secretion with statins, fibrates, or niacin.

In patients with severe hypertriglyceridemia, the increase in total plasma cholesterol is a result of the cholesterol in VLDL and chylomicrons. Fibrates are often the drug of choice. However, it is very important to determine the etiology of the severe hypertriglyceridemia and remove any offending drug [see Table 3] or treat any secondary cause for the hypertriglyceridemia.

PATIENTS WITH LOW HDL CHOLESTEROL LEVELS

Many if not most patients with hypertriglyceridemia have a concomitant reduction in HDL cholesterol levels. Therefore, the management of low HDL cholesterol levels should be considered in the context of the management of the underlying disorder (e.g., FCHL or type 2 diabetes mellitus) [see Patients with Isolated Elevation of Triglyceride Levels, above]. Isolated low HDL cholesterol levels of 20 to 30 mg/dl without concomitant hypertriglyceridemia or other changes in lipid and lipoprotein levels are rare, but such low levels are a risk factor for cardiovascular disease.[9] In the past, these reductions in HDL levels were often not identified; the screening strategies that were employed were based on the assessment of total cholesterol levels, and total cholesterol levels often are not elevated in patients with isolated reductions in HDL. Specific measurement of HDL cholesterol is required to identify these patients. The treatment of the rare patients with isolated low levels of HDL cholesterol remains somewhat controversial. There are no currently available drugs that effectively increase HDL cholesterol levels only.[18] Gemfibrozil, a fibrate that decreases VLDL triglyceride levels, also raises HDL cholesterol levels. Many studies of fibrate therapy for

Table 3 Effects of Selected Drugs on Lipoprotein Levels

Drug	VLDL	LDL	HDL
Alcohol*	+	0	+
Estrogens, estradiol*	+	–	+
Androgens, testosterone	+	+	–
Progestins	–	+	–
Glucocorticoids*	+	0	+
Cyclosporines	+	+	+
Tacrolimus	+	+	+
Thiazide diuretics*	+	+	–
Beta blockers*	+	0	–
Sertraline*	Possible+	+	0
Protease inhibitors*	+	0	0
Valproate and related drugs	+	0	0
Isotretinoin*	+	0	–

*Can cause severe hypertriglyceridemia and chylomicronemia syndrome in patients with a familial form of hypertriglyceridemia or type 2 diabetes mellitus.

atherosclerosis have been inconclusive. However, the Veterans Affairs High-Density Lipoprotein Cholesterol Intervention Trial (VA-HIT) demonstrated a reduction in cardiovascular events.[19] Nicotinic acid, which acts at many metabolic sites, also raises HDL cholesterol. It decreased cardiovascular death in the Coronary Drug Project of the 1970s.[20] A more recent trial showed that adding extended-release niacin to statin therapy slowed the progression of atherosclerosis in people with known CAD and low HDL cholesterol levels.[21] Few other studies have evaluated the effect of niacin on atherosclerotic events.

On rare occasions, a middle-aged patient with established atherosclerosis is seen to have no detectable lipid or lipoprotein abnormality. In addition to the standard lipid profile, measurement of apo B and Lp(a) will often reveal subtle lipoprotein abnormalities, such as increased numbers of small, dense LDL particles, in these patients. Assessment of nonlipoprotein risk factors (e.g., homocysteine and inflammatory markers such as C-reactive protein [CRP]) also may be of value in assessing cardiovascular risk. Although the levels of some of these risk factors can be reduced by various strategies (e.g., homocysteine by folate therapy), the use of statins in all categories of high-risk individuals, particularly those who have established vascular disease, has been shown to be of benefit, even if lipid levels are apparently normal.

Genetic Disorders of Lipoprotein Metabolism

Primary disorders of lipoprotein metabolism are those that arise from genetic defects in the metabolic pathways of lipoproteins (i.e., familial disorders caused by increased hepatic secretion of lipoproteins or by catabolic defects). The disorders that cause increased lipoprotein secretion are the metabolic syndrome, familial combined hyperlipidemia, type 2 diabetes mellitus, and FHTG; elevations of Lp(a) can also cause increased lipoprotein secretion. Disorders of LDL catabolism are FH and familial defective apo B-100. Remnant removal disease is a defect in remnant catabolism.

METABOLIC SYNDROME

The metabolic syndrome consists of a central distribution of adiposity or visceral obesity; insulin resistance; elevations in plasma free fatty acid levels; impaired glucose tolerance; hypertension; dyslipidemia; and an abnormal procoagulant state. Many features of this syndrome are known to predispose men and women to premature CAD.[12]

Etiology and Risk Factors

An accumulation of visceral rather than subcutaneous fat has been observed in individuals with the central body fat distribution characteristic of the metabolic syndrome. Men have more visceral fat than premenopausal women, even when matched for body mass index. It has been suggested that these differences in visceral fat and the associated changes in lipoproteins and blood pressure could account, in part, for the difference in risk of premature CAD between men and premenopausal women.[22] Increased visceral fat is associated with insulin resistance, hyperinsulinemia, low plasma adiponectin levels, and elevations in plasma free fatty acid levels.[23] It has been suggested that the accumulation of visceral fat precedes and causes insulin resistance and the resultant hyperinsulinemia, because insulin sensitivity increases and free fatty acid levels fall when visceral fat is decreased after caloric restriction.[24]

The levels of insulin, glucose, triglyceride, HDL cholesterol, blood pressure, PAI-1, and other inflammatory markers are increased above the mean normal in patients with the metabolic syndrome. Although these variables are usually shifted to high levels, some of these variables are in the high-normal range in some affected individuals. HDL levels tend to be lower than mean normal. Genetic and environmental factors appear to affect the distribution of these variables in both normal persons and those with the metabolic syndrome. Because the metabolic syndrome is associated with multiple cardiovascular risk factors, individuals with the metabolic syndrome are at increased risk for CAD. Whether all individuals who meet the NCEP guidelines for the metabolic syndrome[25] [*see* Diagnosis, *below*] are at increased risk for premature CAD is unknown. However, type 2 diabetes mellitus and FCHL are specific disorders of which the metabolic syndrome is a component.[12] These two disorders account for at least 40% to 50% of premature CAD and need to be considered in the context of the metabolic syndrome.

The risk of abdominal fat patterning, dyslipidemia, impaired glucose metabolism, and hypertension—the sentinel symptoms of the metabolic syndrome—increases with age.[26] Central obesity associated with the metabolic syndrome may be evident in young adults after completion of adolescent growth; however, it is more typical for central obesity and insulin resistance to manifest in midlife. Whereas elevations in LDL cholesterol levels may not predict the onset of atherosclerosis in the elderly, central obesity, hypertension, and insulin resistance are risk factors for atherosclerosis, and their prevalence increases with age,[26-30] possibly because of the metabolic syndrome.

Pathophysiology

Although the association of central obesity and insulin resistance with dyslipidemia is well established, the underlying cause remains unclear. One mechanism that would explain the association of central obesity and insulin resistance with dyslipidemia is an increase in the level of portal vein long-chain free fatty acids. Such an increase would inhibit hepatic apo B from undergoing degradation in the endoplasmic reticulum and would increase the likelihood of apo B undergoing hepatic secretion as triglyceride-containing lipoproteins. This would account for the increased levels of triglyceride and the increased number of VLDL and LDL particles seen in patients in insulin-resistant states.[31] Another effect of long-chain free fatty acids is to increase hepatic lipase on the surface of hepatic cells. Hepatic lipase hydrolyzes triglyceride and phospholipid in LDL and HDL, decreasing the size of each particle [*see Figure 6*].[12] However, CETP also contributes to this lipoprotein remodeling process; whether hepatic lipase or CETP has the predominant effect on the size and density of LDL and HDL particles depends on the triglyceride content of VLDL and the secretion rate of VLDL. The differences in LDL particle size and HDL_2 levels between men and premenopausal women can largely be accounted for by differences in visceral fat in men and women.

Diagnosis

The National Cholesterol Education Program Adult Treatment Panel III (NCEP ATP-III) has suggested five clinical variables as diagnostic criteria for the metabolic syndrome: (1) increased waist circumference, (2) increased triglyceride level, (3) decreased HDL cholesterol level, (4) increased blood pressure,

Table 4 Clinical Features of the
Metabolic Syndrome[15]

The presence of three or more variables indicates a diagnosis of
    metabolic syndrome:
Abdominal obesity: waist circumference > 35 in (women) or
    > 40 in (men)
Triglycerides ≥ 150 mg/dl
HDL cholesterol < 50 mg/dl (women) or < 40 mg/dl (men)
Blood pressure ≥ 130/85 mm Hg
Fasting plasma glucose ≥ 110 mg/dl

and (5) elevated level of fasting plasma glucose [*see Table 4*].[15] A diagnosis of the metabolic syndrome is made when three or more of these clinical variables are present. When these five variables were assessed in a survey of 8,814 adult men and women, approximately 24% of those surveyed met the diagnostic criteria for diagnosis of the metabolic syndrome.[32,33] The World Health Organization (WHO) also has criteria for the metabolic syndrome. An attempt to harmonize the two sets of criteria is in progress.

Visceral obesity and insulin resistance are major contributors to the dyslipidemia associated with the metabolic syndrome. The following lipid abnormalities are associated with the metabolic syndrome: increased levels of triglyceride; increased numbers of small, dense LDL particles; increased apo B levels; and decreased levels of HDL cholesterol. However, in normal, randomly selected populations, isolated visceral obesity and insulin resistance were associated with only a slight increase in triglyceride levels and only a slight decrease in HDL cholesterol levels.[23] In contrast, visceral obesity and insulin resistance can contribute to a more severe dyslipidemia when associated with type 2 diabetes mellitus and FCHL.[12]

The dyslipidemia of the metabolic syndrome can be diagnosed by demonstrating mild to moderate increases in plasma triglyceride and apo B levels, decreased levels of HDL cholesterol, and normal levels of LDL cholesterol. Although the LDL cholesterol level is normal in patients with this disorder, the number of LDL particles is generally increased; the predominant form is small, dense LDL particles, which are cholesterol poor relative to large, buoyant LDL particles. The presence of small, dense LDL particles can be determined by direct measurement of LDL size or density. The routine measurement of plasma apo B levels in clinical practice is not necessary for the diagnosis of this disorder; however, measurement of plasma apo B levels can indicate the presence of increased numbers of small, dense LDL particles. Similarly, total HDL levels reflect changes in the HDL_2 values, indicating that HDL subfractions do not need to be measured.[34]

Treatment

Aerobic exercise and a diet low in saturated fat are indicated as therapy for most people with the metabolic syndrome. If the metabolic syndrome is severe or FCHL or type 2 diabetes mellitus is present, more aggressive therapy is indicated [*see Chapter 4* and *see* Drug Therapy in Dyslipidemia, *below*].

FAMILIAL COMBINED HYPERLIPIDEMIA

FCHL is an autosomal dominant disorder that accounts for up to half of the familial causes of CAD[35]; it was first described in families of survivors of myocardial infarction (MI).[36-38] FCHL is characterized by elevations in triglyceride or cholesterol levels,

or both, in affected relatives. In addition to increases in triglyceride and cholesterol levels, patients with FCHL characteristically have elevations in apo B levels and increased numbers of small, dense LDL particles.[39]

Genetic linkage analysis suggests that the inheritance of the lipid phenotype in FCHL involves separate gene effects[40] for the elevation in apo B levels[41] and the increased numbers of small, dense LDL particles that are present in FCHL families. Further evidence for genetic heterogeneity comes from studies that found that in one third of individuals with FCHL, the activity level of LPL in postheparin plasma was reduced by half.[42] Visceral obesity and insulin resistance contribute to the dyslipidemia seen in FCHL but cannot account for the elevation in apo B levels.[43]

In the Familial Atherosclerosis Treatment Study (FATS), intensive lipid-lowering therapy with nicotinic acid or lovastatin in combination with colestipol led to decreased hepatic lipase activity; decreased numbers of small, dense LDL particles; and elevated levels of HDL_2 cholesterol, with subsequent regression of CAD, as evidenced by angiography.[44] Intensive lipid lowering resulted in subsequent regression of atherosclerosis, particularly in individuals with small, dense LDL particles who had FCHL or who had elevated Lp(a) levels at baseline.

An aggressive approach to modify reversible cardiovascular risk factors should be undertaken in individuals affected by this disorder. Diet therapy and therapeutic lifestyle modification that includes physical activity should be undertaken [*see Chapter 4*], together with lipid-lowering drug therapy [*see* Drug Therapy in Dyslipidemia, *below*][18] and management of other cardiovascular risk factors. Which lipid-lowering drug to use depends to some extent on whether the primary lipid manifestation is hypercholesterolemia, hypertriglyceridemia, or combined elevations of cholesterol and triglyceride. If hypercholesterolemia is the primary manifestation, the approach should be the same as that for the hypercholesterolemic patient [*see* Patients with Isolated Elevation of LDL Cholesterol Levels, *above*]. If hypertriglyceridemia is the major abnormality, the initial approach might be that used for patients with isolated hypertriglyceridemia. However, most patients will have elevations in both triglyceride and LDL levels and will require combination therapy; regimens may combine a statin and niacin, fibrate, or ezetimibe [*see* Drug Therapy in Dyslipidemia, *below*].

TYPE 2 DIABETES MELLITUS

Patients undergoing treatment of type 2 diabetes mellitus characteristically have visceral obesity and insulin resistance. A defect in insulin secretion is present in insulin-resistant individuals who develop hyperglycemia. First-degree relatives of individuals with type 2 diabetes mellitus may be centrally obese and have insulin resistance, or they may experience decreased insulin secretion in response to glucose; first-degree relatives who are both centrally obese and have a defect in insulin secretion invariably develop type 2 diabetes mellitus. Although the genes contributing to central obesity, insulin resistance, and defective insulin secretion are mostly unknown, type 2 diabetes mellitus is a classic example of an oligogenic disorder. Determining all of the genes involved will require careful phenotypic characterization of subsets of individuals with type 2 diabetes mellitus.

The dyslipidemia of untreated diabetes mellitus and hyperglycemia is discussed later in this chapter [*see* Endocrine Disorders That Cause Dyslipidemia, *below*]. The dyslipidemia of treated type 2 diabetes mellitus is similar to that of the metabolic syndrome and FCHL; it is characterized by a mild increase in triglyceride levels, decreased HDL_2 cholesterol levels, and increased numbers of small, dense LDL particles. Treatment entails diet therapy, increased physical activity, and lipid-lowering drug therapy [see Drug Therapy in Dyslipidemia, below].[45]

FAMILIAL HYPERTRIGLYCERIDEMIA

FHTG is a common inherited disorder, thought to be autosomal dominant, that affects about 1% of the population. FHTG is characterized by an increase in triglyceride synthesis resulting in VLDL particles enriched with triglyceride secreted in normal quantities. Affected people have elevated VLDL levels but low levels of LDL and HDL and are generally asymptomatic unless severe hypertriglyceridemia (i.e., chylomicronemia syndrome) develops. FHTG does not appear to be associated with an increased risk of premature CAD.[17]

A diagnosis is made by family history and examination of fasting lipoprotein profiles of the patient and relatives. The triglyceride level ranges from 250 to 1,000 mg/dl in approximately one half of first-degree relatives; a strong family history of premature CAD usually is lacking; and elevated LDL levels should not be present.

Patients with FHTG should lose weight if necessary, exercise regularly, and reduce their intake of saturated fatty acids and cholesterol. Alcohol, exogenous estrogens, and other drugs that increase VLDL levels might need to be restricted. Diabetes, if present, should be well controlled. Hypertriglyceridemia in patients with FHTG often responds to these measures. If triglyceride levels exceed 500 mg/dl after 6 months of nonpharmacologic therapy, drug therapy with a fibrate should be considered[19]; at levels above 1,000 mg/dl, drug therapy should be instituted.

Fibrates are the drugs of choice to reduce elevated triglyceride levels in patients with familial hypertriglyceridemia [see Drug Therapy in Dyslipidemia, below]. In familial combined hyperlipidemia, niacin can be very useful. Niacin has several additional beneficial effects on blood lipids—it increases HDL cholesterol levels, it reduces levels of small, dense LDL particles, and it may reduce Lp(a) levels. Despite having a less dramatic effect on triglycerides than fibrates, statins have been shown to be of value in high-risk patients with moderate hypertriglyceridemia and increased levels of small, dense LDL particles, such as occur in patients with type 2 diabetes mellitus and FCHL.

FAMILIAL HYPERCHOLESTEROLEMIA

FH is an autosomal dominant disorder caused by a mutation in the gene encoding the LDL receptor protein. The extremely rare homozygote with FH has two mutant alleles at the LDL receptor locus, leaving the person with an absolute or nearly absolute inability to clear LDL from the circulation by the LDL receptor.[8] Heterozygotes with FH possess one normal allele, giving them approximately one half of the normal receptor activity. Because the LDL receptor contributes to VLDL remnant clearance from the plasma, a deficiency of LDL receptors may lead to some accumulation of remnant lipoproteins. High concentrations of LDL result in nonreceptor-mediated uptake of LDL by the extracellular matrix, including that of the arterial wall, which leads to the formation of xanthomas and atherosclerosis. The heterozygous form of this disorder has a prevalence of about one in 500 people, making it one of the more common genetic diseases.[8]

Diagnosis

Hypercholesterolemia can be detected at birth in umbilical cord blood. If FH is not detected at birth, various associated conditions may suggest the diagnosis later in life. Tendon xanthomas are a highly specific sign of FH; typically, they begin to appear by 20 years of age and may be present in up to 70% of older patients. Occasionally, xanthomas are seen on the patellar tendon. Because xanthomas are subtle, careful examination of the dorsal hand tendons and Achilles tendon is required for their detection. Xanthelasma (cutaneous xanthomas on the palpebra) and corneal arcus are common in patients with FH after 30 years of age; however, they also occur in normocholesterolemic persons. Early corneal arcus is seen superiorly and inferiorly in the eyes and later becomes totally circumferential.

CAD develops early, with symptoms often manifesting in men in the fourth or fifth decade. Approximately 5% of all cases of premature MI occur in patients with heterozygous FH.[8] Before the development of statin therapy, at least 50% of men with heterozygous FH experienced MI by 60 years of age; in women, symptoms tend to develop about 10 years later. The total cholesterol level in heterozygous patients generally ranges from 350 to 550 mg/dl. The triglyceride level may be mildly elevated, and the HDL cholesterol level is reduced in about 10% of heterozygotes. LDL receptor function can be measured only in special laboratories.

Heterozygous FH should be suspected when severe hypercholesterolemia from elevated LDL is detected. If tendon xanthomas are present, the diagnosis is virtually certain. If tendon xanthomas are absent, secondary causes of hypercholesterolemia (e.g., hypothyroidism) should be sought, but the diagnosis of familial hypercholesterolemia is not excluded. A comprehensive family history should reveal a strong history of premature CAD and hypercholesterolemia without hypertriglyceridemia; the disorder affects approximately one half of first-degree relatives. The presence of hypercholesterolemia and tendon xanthomas in a parent or sibling is virtually diagnostic, as is hypercholesterolemia in a child in the family. Careful screening of family members is mandatory, because 50% of first-degree relatives will be affected and will require aggressive lipid-lowering therapy.[18,46]

Treatment

Management of FH requires both dietary intervention and drug therapy. The goal of therapy is to lower the LDL cholesterol level to less than 130 mg/dl, or even lower if the patient exhibits CAD. In patients with heterozygous FH, effective treatment is possible with combinations of statins, intestinally active drugs, and nicotinic acid. Because LDL cholesterol levels tend to be very high, combination therapy with two drugs is often required, and three drugs may be necessary [see Drug Therapy in Dyslipidemia, below]. Although diet therapy alone is not sufficient for patients with heterozygous FH, reducing saturated fatty acid and cholesterol intake will lower LDL levels and reduce the amount of medication required. This is particularly important in children and adolescents before initiation of drug therapy. Tendon xanthomas have been shown to regress when LDL levels are maintained in a desirable range. Aggressive reduction of LDL cholesterol in men and women who have heterozygous FH may cause a regression of coronary atherosclerosis.

FAMILIAL DEFECTIVE APOLIPOPROTEIN B-100

A mutation in apo B-100 that inhibits its binding to the LDL receptor is another genetic cause of elevations in the LDL level. The prevalence of this disorder is unknown but is estimated to be 5% to 10% that of FH. LDL receptor structure and function are normal. A full-length apo B-100 molecule is produced with a single amino acid substitution; this results in apo B that binds poorly to LDL receptors, leading to LDL accumulation in the plasma.

Affected individuals are clinically indistinguishable from patients with heterozygous FH: they may present with severe hypercholesterolemia, tendon xanthomas, and premature atherosclerosis. Treatment with statins appears to lower LDL cholesterol levels in patients with this disorder. Specialized tests available only in selected research laboratories are required to distinguish affected people with defective apo B from those with defective LDL receptors.

INCREASED LEVELS OF LIPOPROTEIN(A)

Lp(a) is a specific class of lipoprotein particles synthesized in the liver.[5] An important component of Lp(a) is apo(a), which has a structure homologous with plasminogen, a key protein in the coagulation cascade. Plasma concentrations of Lp(a) vary markedly among individuals, ranging from undetectable to 200 mg/dl. Lp(a) plasma concentration is strongly controlled by genetic factors.

Most epidemiologic studies suggest that Lp(a) is a risk factor for CAD and stroke. If Lp(a) is atherogenic, it may be because of its LDL-like properties: Lp(a) has been shown to undergo endothelial uptake and oxidative modification and to promote foam cell formation. Because Lp(a) has a high degree of homology with plasminogen, it may play a role in thrombosis by interfering with the binding of plasminogen to fibrin. Elevated Lp(a) levels appear to increase the atherogenicity of other cardiovascular risk factors, with earlier onset of cardiovascular events.

Data suggest that reducing LDL cholesterol levels in patients with high levels of Lp(a) may be an effective strategy to slow the progression of atherosclerosis and to prevent coronary events. The Lp(a) level itself can be reduced with high-dose niacin, estrogen, or tamoxifen, as well as with LDL apheresis. Insufficient data exist regarding the efficacy of lowering the Lp(a) level per se to inhibit atherosclerosis or to prevent coronary events.[5]

REMNANT REMOVAL DISEASE

Remnant removal disease, also called type III hyperlipoproteinemia, dysbetalipoproteinemia, and broad-beta disease, is defined as the presence of VLDL particles that migrate in the beta position on electrophoresis (normal VLDL particles migrate in the pre-beta location). Beta-VLDL particles are chylomicron and VLDL remnants.

Remnant removal disease is caused in part by a mutation in the *APOE* gene[7] [*see* Regulation of Lipoprotein Catabolism, *above*]; this mutation leads to an impairment in the hepatic uptake of apo E–containing lipoproteins and stops the conversion of VLDL and IDL to LDL. Without the presence of additional genetic, hormonal, or environmental factors, remnants do not accumulate to a degree sufficient to cause hyperlipidemia, because they are cleared by hepatic receptors that also bind, with less avidity, to apo B-48 and apo B-100. Remnant removal disease results when an apo E defect (almost always the E2/E2 genotype) occurs in conjunction with a second genetic or acquired defect that causes either overproduction of VLDL (such as occurs with FCHL) or a reduction in LDL receptor activity (such as occurs in heterozygous FH or hypothyroidism). The E2/E2 genotype is found in 1% of the white population and in virtually all persons with remnant removal disease.

Diagnosis

Persons with remnant removal disease have elevations in both cholesterol and triglyceride levels and are likely to develop premature CAD. For reasons that are not understood, these patients are at particularly increased risk for peripheral vascular disease. Hyperlipidemia usually does not develop before adulthood. Palmar xanthomas (xanthoma striata palmaris)—orange-yellow discolorations of the palmar creases—are pathognomonic for genetic remnant removal disease, but they are not always present. Palmar xanthomas may be difficult to see and should be carefully sought using good lighting. Tuboeruptive xanthomas are occasionally found at pressure sites, particularly the elbows, buttocks, and knees.

The diagnosis of remnant removal disease should be suspected in a person with elevated total cholesterol and triglyceride levels, elevated VLDL and IDL cholesterol levels, and reduced LDL and HDL cholesterol levels. Cholesterol and triglyceride levels range from 300 to 1,000 mg/dl and are roughly equal, except during an acute exacerbation, at which time hypertriglyceridemia tends to predominate. Beta-migrating VLDL is present on electrophoresis, although this test is seldom used today. Ultracentrifugation demonstrates that the ratio of VLDL cholesterol to total plasma triglyceride is greater than 0.3. Definitive diagnosis is made by detecting the E2/E2 phenotype by isoelectric focusing of plasma lipoproteins or the genotype by gene analysis.

Treatment

Generally, therapy for remnant removal disease is the same as that for other forms of hypertriglyceridemia. A low-fat diet, weight loss, and exercise can have a major effect on lipid levels. Fibrates, statins, and nicotinic acid have been used successfully in this disorder. However, drugs that increase triglyceride levels, such as bile acid-binding resins, must be avoided.

RARE DISORDERS

Severe hypertriglyceridemia can present in childhood as a result of LPL deficiency or, extremely rarely, as apo C-II deficiency. These patients are at risk for acute pancreatitis with severe hypertriglyceridemia and must be treated with moderate to severe dietary-fat restriction until plasma triglyceride levels are below 1,000 to 2,000 mg/dl.

Homozygous FH is extremely rare and leads to severe hypercholesterolemia, atherosclerosis, and death, often in the first two decades of life. Patients with homozygous FH may benefit from LDL apheresis. At the other extreme, the absence of apo B-containing lipoproteins can result from defects in the synthesis of apo B (e.g., homozygous hypobetalipoproteinemia) or from defects in the transport of apo B into the hepatic endoplasmic reticulum. Individuals with very low apo B levels are not at risk for atherosclerosis.

The absence of HDL can occur in persons with homozygosity for defects in the cholesterol and phospholipid transporter ABCA-1. The heterozygous state is an uncommon cause of isolated low-HDL cholesterolemia[11] (i.e., hypoalphalipoproteinemia).

MISCELLANEOUS COMMON DYSLIPIDEMIAS

Polygenic hypercholesterolemia was once thought to be common. The term polygenic hypercholesterolemia used to refer to the occurrence of mild elevations in LDL cholesterol in the apparent absence of a familial form of dyslipidemia or of dyslipidemia of secondary cause. This category of dyslipidemia continues to shrink as LDL variants such as Lp(a) and small, dense LDL particles are discovered.

Mild to moderate hypertriglyceridemia may occur in the presence of modest defects in LPL. Typically, it presents as an increase in VLDL cholesterol levels in conjunction with a decrease in HDL cholesterol levels. It is seen in the obligate heterozygote parents of children with LPL deficiency. This defect may predispose to premature CAD.

Secondary Disorders of Lipoprotein Metabolism

Secondary dyslipoproteinemias are caused by acquired defects in lipoprotein metabolism that result in hypercholesterolemia, hypertriglyceridemia, or combined hyperlipidemia; the HDL level may or may not be low. Secondary hypertriglyceridemia in conjunction with a common genetic form of hypertriglyceridemia may be severe enough to cause chylomicronemia with pancreatitits. Dyslipoproteinemia may also be caused by selected medications.

ENDOCRINE DISORDERS THAT CAUSE DYSLIPIDEMIA

Untreated Hyperglycemia

Untreated hyperglycemia in patients with diabetes mellitus causes an increase in VLDL synthesis, a reduction in VLDL catabolism with an accompanying reduction in LPL activity, or both. These abnormalities result in hypertriglyceridemia and a reduction in the level of HDL. The LDL level usually is normal. Fasting chylomicronemia occurs when there is a coexisting primary form of hypertriglyceridemia. VLDL and chylomicrons compete to interact with LPL, and both lipoproteins may accumulate. A low HDL level results from impaired lipolysis of triglyceride-rich lipoproteins, which supply lipid components for HDL development. These defects occur in both untreated type 1 and untreated type 2 diabetes mellitus. Lipid levels should approach normal with comprehensive treatment of diabetes; if they fail to do so, additional causes should be sought [see Genetic Disorders of Lipoprotein Metabolism, above]. In diabetic patients with persistent moderate to severe hypertriglyceridemia, a fibric acid is suitable because it reduces the secretion of VLDL and enhances the activity of LPL. Nicotinic acid may be used, but with care, particularly in patients with type 2 diabetes mellitus, because it may exacerbate hyperglycemia.[47] Statins are effective in reducing the incidence of coronary events in diabetic patients.[45]

Hypothyroidism

Hypothyroidism may cause a severe elevation of LDL levels because of reduced LDL receptor activity; in addition, it frequently causes hypertriglyceridemia and an associated reduction in the HDL level as a result of reduced LPL activity. Remnants of chylomicrons and VLDL may also accumulate and unmask remnant removal disease. The dyslipoproteinemia that occurs with hypothyroidism is corrected by thyroid hormone replacement.

Dyslipidemia Secondary to Estrogen and Progestin Therapy

Oral contraceptives that contain a combination of estrogen and progestin can have variable effects on lipoproteins, depending on the specific combination used. Estrogen tends to raise VLDL and HDL levels and lower LDL levels. Progestins tend to lower VLDL and HDL levels and raise LDL levels, but the effect varies considerably. Postmenopausal estrogen replacement ther-

apy lowers LDL levels and raises HDL levels; the addition of progesterone to protect the uterus lessens these effects but does not eliminate them.[48] Estrogen may increase triglycerides to severe levels in women who have an underlying primary triglyceride disorder, leading to pancreatitis; therefore, triglyceride levels should be closely monitored in these patients.[6] Oral combination therapy with estrogen and progesterone was associated with a mild increase in CAD[43] in the Women's Health Initiative Study. In this randomized study of 16,608 women, use of oral hormone replacement therapy also was associated with an excess rate of breast cancer. In women who have undergone hysterectomies, estrogen therapy has been shown to increase the risk of stroke [see Managing Dysplipidemia in Women, below].[49] These studies have led to a decrease in the use of postmenopausal hormone replacement therapy.

RENAL DISORDERS THAT CAUSE DYSLIPIDEMIA

Nephrotic Syndrome

The nephrotic syndrome causes enhanced hepatic secretion of apo B-100–containing lipoproteins (i.e., VLDL) in response to the loss of albumin and other proteins in the urine. Hepatic synthesis of cholesterol is also increased. The LDL level is typically elevated, and it may be severely elevated. The VLDL level elevation may be associated with a reduction in the HDL level as lipolysis becomes impaired.[50] Patients with the nephrotic syndrome are at increased risk for CAD, and the lipid disorder should be treated aggressively. Dietary change, weight loss, and exercise may improve lipoprotein levels, but pharmacologic therapy is necessary to achieve desirable lipoprotein levels. Nicotinic acid should be effective in the treatment of this disorder because it inhibits hepatic secretion of apo B-100–containing lipoproteins; however, it has not been studied extensively for this use. The statins are useful in lowering LDL cholesterol levels in patients with the nephrotic syndrome. Combination drug therapy with statins, nicotinic acid, fibrates, or ezetimibe may be necessary for the reduction of LDL cholesterol and triglyceride levels [see Drug Therapy in Dyslipidemia, below]. Studies are needed to evaluate the effects of various drug combinations on cardiovascular outcomes.

Chronic Renal Failure

Chronic renal failure produces hypertriglyceridemia as a result of a decrease in LPL and hepatic triglyceride lipase.[50] Triglyceride levels typically range from 150 to 750 mg/dl, and the HDL level is usually low; the risk of CAD is increased. Dietary measures should be initiated while drug treatment is being considered. Gemfibrozil, a drug that enhances LPL activity, is effective in lowering triglyceride levels in patients with renal insufficiency.[51] Gemfibrozil is preferred over other fibrates (e.g., fenofibrate and clofibrate) in this setting because gemfibrozil is partly cleared by the liver; as such, it carries a lower risk of drug-induced myopathy than do fibrates that are cleared by the kidneys. Nonetheless, because gemfibrozil is partially excreted renally, the drug should be administered in the lowest effective dose. Nicotinic acid and statins have been less well studied in this condition. Combination therapy with nicotinic acid, statins, or gemfibrozil may be necessary to attain the therapeutic goal.

GASTROINTESTINAL DISORDERS THAT CAUSE DYSLIPIDEMIA

Primary biliary cirrhosis is the most significant gastrointestinal cause of dyslipidemia. In the early stages of primary biliary cirrhosis, when some hepatocellular function remains, mild elevations of VLDL and LDL levels occur because of elevations in the levels of remnant lipoproteins and HDL. Terminal liver disease with cirrhosis results in severe elevation in cholesterol levels because of increased production of lipoprotein X—an abnormal lipoprotein particle containing albumin and other plasma components that is rich in free cholesterol and phospholipid. Treatment of this terminal disorder requires liver transplantation.

OTHER CAUSES OF SECONDARY DYSLIPIDEMIA

Many commonly used drugs have adverse effects on lipoproteins [see Table 3]. Discontinuance of the drug often will improve lipid levels. An increase in VLDL, LDL, and HDL cholesterol levels can result from the use of drugs for the prevention of rejection after organ transplantation. Pravastatin is the drug of choice for lowering LDL levels in such cases because of its unique catabolic pathways. Immunosuppressive agents such as cyclosporine compete with atorvastatin and simvastatin for the cytochrome P-450 3A4 system. The use of antifungal agents also can interfere with the metabolism of these statins. The predominant dyslipidemia that is seen in patients with AIDS is similar to the dyslipidemia that occurs in patients with the metabolic syndrome; mild hypertriglyceridemia is common, and low HDL cholesterol is seen in some patients.[52] In others, extreme hypertriglyceridemia can result from the use of HIV drugs, and the resultant hypertriglyceridemia may be associated with pancreatitis. The etiology of dyslipidemia in AIDS is complex: excessive free fatty acid mobilization is seen, along with the development of lipodystrophy and insulin resistance. In addition, AIDS patients typically use dyslipidemia-causing drugs. The specific therapy needs to be individualized for each patient.

Prevention and Treatment of Coronary Artery Disease

PRIMARY PREVENTION

The treatment of lipid disorders in individuals who do not have clinical evidence of CAD is considered primary prevention. Primary prevention is based on the assumption that modification of lipid risk factors will alter the natural history of the untreated condition—the so-called lipid hypothesis. An association between cholesterol and CAD has been known since the early 1950s; however, it was not until the publication of the Lipid Research Clinics Coronary Primary Prevention Trial (LRC-CPPT) in 1984 that there were data to support the lipid hypothesis.

The LRC-CPPT enrolled almost 4,000 men with moderate hypercholesterolemia; patients were followed for 7 years. The treatment group was prescribed cholestyramine, which resulted in LDL cholesterol levels being 12.6% lower than those of the control subjects, who were given placebo. The cholestyramine group had a 19% reduction in CAD deaths and nonfatal myocardial infarcts ($P < 0.05$), although no decrease in total mortality was observed.[53] Further analysis demonstrated that the extent of benefit depended upon the achieved reduction in serum cholesterol (reflecting drug compliance). Use of a proportional hazards model indicated that a 25% decrease in total cholesterol or a 35% decrease in LDL cholesterol would be expected to decrease the risk of a CAD event by 50%.[54]

The Helsinki Heart Study used the fibrate gemfibrozil to treat dyslipidemic men without CAD. After 6 years of follow-up, a 34% reduction in CAD events was seen in the treatment group, compared with the group receiving placebo.[55] Again, no decrease in CAD mortality was demonstrated.

In both the Helsinki Heart Study and the LRC-CPPT, the sample size was calculated on the basis of the power of the study to detect CAD events, not on fatal outcomes alone. As such, the lack of an effect on mortality was not surprising, but an increase (not statistically significant) in noncoronary death in the treatment groups of both these studies was troublesome and confounded the recommendations for primary preventive therapy in hypercholesterolemic patients.[53-55] These concerns were not completely addressed until 1995, when results of the West of Scotland Coronary Prevention Study (WOSCOPS) were published.[56]

The WOSCOPS trial evaluated the effect of 5 years of treatment with pravastatin on the incidence of nonfatal MI and CAD deaths in 6,595 men. The men were middle-aged (45 to 64 years of age) and moderately hypercholesterolemic (LDL cholesterol level above 155 mg/dl). The treatment group manifested a 20% reduction in total cholesterol, a 26% reduction in LDL cholesterol, a 12% decrease in triglycerides, and a 5% increase in HDL cholesterol, as compared with the control group. On the basis of intention-to-treat principles, these changes were associated with a 31% risk reduction in nonfatal MI or CAD deaths ($P < 0.001$), a 32% risk reduction in all cardiovascular deaths ($P = 0.033$), and a 22% risk reduction in total mortality ($P = 0.051$). In addition, coronary interventions (i.e., angiography, angioplasty, and coronary artery bypass surgery) were reduced 31% to 37% ($P < 0.01$).

The reduction in clinical events began within 6 months of randomization and was independent of other risk factors, such as diabetes, smoking, blood pressure, family history of CAD, and the ratio of total cholesterol to HDL cholesterol.[57] Although there was no risk reduction without a decrease in LDL cholesterol, a decrease in LDL cholesterol of approximately 24% was adequate to realize the full benefit of statin treatment. Thus, LDL reduction alone did not account for all the benefits of treatment with pravastatin.[58] Importantly, there was no increase in noncoronary deaths, as had been reported in earlier primary preventive trials with other drugs.

The Air Force/Texas Coronary Atherosclerosis Prevention Study (AFCAPS/TexCAPS) was the first large primary intervention trial to study the effects of cholesterol lowering in individuals with average cholesterol levels.[59] That is, the mean total cholesterol level and the mean LDL cholesterol level were nearer the average values for the general population (221 mg/dl and 150 mg/dl, respectively). In addition, AFCAPS/TexCAPS was the first large study to include women (997 of a total of 6,605 patients). Lovastatin was the treatment agent in this randomized, placebo-controlled trial. LDL cholesterol was reduced by 25%; the average follow-up was 5.2 years. The total absolute benefit was 2%, meaning that 50 patients had to be treated for 5 years to prevent one event. The treatment group had a 28% reduction in cardiovascular hospitalizations, a 23% decrease in angioplasty, and a 32% reduction in coronary bypass surgery. An analysis of the cost-effectiveness of lovastatin treatment demonstrated a 27% ($524 per patient) reduction in cardiovascular health care costs for the lovastatin group, as compared with the group that received placebo.[60]

Persons with average cholesterol levels were also evaluated in the Anglo-Scandinavian Cardiac Outcomes Trial–Lipid Lowering Arm (ASCOT-LLA).[61] Nearly 20,000 hypertensive patients were randomized to one of two antihypertensive regimens. In the lipid-lowering arm of this study, 10,305 patients with total cholesterol levels of 251 mg/dl or lower were randomized to receive either treatment with atorvastatin or a placebo. The study was halted early because a significant benefit was observed in the treatment group. The median follow-up was 3.3 years. The study did not demonstrate statistically significant reductions in cardiovascular or all-cause mortality; however, significant reductions were seen in total coronary events, total cardiovascular events and procedures, and stroke.[61]

The effect of atorvastatin (10 mg/day) on the primary prevention of cardiovascular disease in diabetic patients was examined in the Collaborative Atorvastatin Diabetes Study (CARDS).[45] CARDS randomized almost 3,000 diabetic patients with LDL levels of 160 mg/dl or lower, triglyceride levels of 600 mg/dl or lower, and at least one of the following: retinopathy, albuminuria, smoking habit, or hypertension. The trial was stopped 2 years early because predetermined criteria had been met. The atorvastatin group demonstrated a 36% reduction in coronary events, a 31% reduction in coronary revascularization procedures, a 48% decrease in stroke, and a 27% reduction in all-cause deaths, as compared with the placebo group.

These studies support lipid-lowering therapy as primary prevention for patients with both high and average LDL values. There are virtually no data on primary prevention in patients with other lipid abnormalities, such as isolated low HDL cholesterol levels or elevated triglyceride levels.

SECONDARY PREVENTION

Lipid-lowering therapy in patients with documented CAD is considered secondary prevention. Lipid levels have a significant influence on CAD death rates in those with and without CAD; however, the impact is significantly greater in patients with established CAD.[62]

Several trials have investigated the effect of aggressive lifestyle intervention in patients with CAD. The Saint Thomas Atherosclerosis Regression Study (STARS) randomized men with CAD and total cholesterol levels above 232 mg/dl to receive either conventional care or a low-fat, low-cholesterol diet. Despite relatively modest changes in lipid levels (in the intervention group, the average LDL cholesterol level was 162 mg/dl), the progression of CAD decreased and the rate of regression increased in the intervention group. Angina symptoms also improved.[63]

The effects of a Mediterranean diet (increased α-linoleic acid) were compared with those of a prudent Western diet in the Lyon Diet Heart Study.[64] All study participants had had a first MI. Those consuming the Mediterranean diet had lower rates of primary (death and MI) and secondary (unstable angina, stroke, heart failure) end points than those on the prudent Western diet at 27 months. This effect persisted after 4 years of follow-up. The group on the Mediterranean diet had a rate of combined primary and secondary end points of 2.59 events per 100 patients per year, compared with 9.03 events per 100 patients per year in the group on the prudent diet.[65]

A variety of pharmacologic agents have been used alone and in combination in secondary prevention trials. Some trials have used angiographic end points in assessing progression or regression of CAD, whereas others have used clinical end points. The Familial Atherosclerosis Treatment Study (FATS) examined the effect of several lipid-reducing regimens in men with elevated apo B levels. The two most aggressive regimens (nicotinic acid–colestipol and lovastatin-colestipol) were equally effective; both regimens were associated with delayed progression (21% and 25%, respectively, versus 46% in the placebo-colestipol group) and an increased likelihood of regression of coronary artery stenoses (32% and 39%, respectively, versus 11% in the

placebo-colestipol group). Clinical end points (death, MI, worsening angina, and revascularization) were also reduced in the more aggressively treated groups (4.2% and 6.5%, respectively, versus 19% in the placebo-colestipol group).[44] This was the first major study to document the regression of CAD with aggressive lipid-lowering therapy. A subsequent analysis of these patients correlated the change in CAD severity with therapy-induced changes in LDL buoyancy and hepatic lipase activity.[66]

The Scandinavian Simvastatin Survival Study (4S) evaluated 4,444 patients with known CAD and moderate to severe hypercholesterolemia at baseline (total cholesterol concentration ranging from 212 to 309 mg/dl).[67] Patients were randomized to a regimen of diet plus simvastatin or diet plus placebo. At 5.4 years, there was a significant reduction in total mortality (8% with simvastatin versus 12% with placebo), major coronary events (19% versus 28%), CAD deaths (42% reduction), and cerebrovascular events (2.7% versus 4.3%). The reduction in cardiovascular events correlated with total cholesterol and LDL cholesterol levels and with changes from baseline.[68]

The Long-Term Intervention with Pravastatin in Ischaemic Disease (LIPID) trial randomized approximately 9,000 men and women with a history of recent MI or unstable angina to receive either placebo or pravastatin.[69] The study was stopped prematurely at 60 months because of a significant benefit associated with pravastatin therapy. CAD death was reduced in the treatment arm of the study (6.4% versus 8.3%), as were total mortality (11% versus 14%), stroke (20% relative decrease), need for bypass surgery (8.9% versus 11.3%), and MI (7.4% versus 10.1%). The benefit was primarily related to changes in lipid levels and was seen in all predefined subgroups. The greatest reduction in coronary events was seen in those patients thought to be at highest risk, as assessed by concomitant risk factors.[70]

The Cholesterol and Recurrent Events (CARE) trial evaluated 4,159 patients with relatively low lipid levels. The average total cholesterol level was 209 mg/dl, and the average LDL cholesterol level was 139 mg/dl. Treatment with pravastatin over 5 years resulted in significant reductions in coronary death or nonfatal myocardial infarction (10.2% versus 13.2% for placebo), need for revascularization (14.1% versus 18.8%), and frequency of stroke (2.6% versus 3.8%).[71] However, in contrast to the results seen with 4S and LIPID, the absolute or percentage reductions in LDL had little relationship to coronary events.[72] The benefits were seen only in patients whose baseline LDL levels were above 125 mg/dl.[72]

The Heart Protection Study enrolled over 20,000 persons with a history of cardiovascular disease (coronary, cerebrovascular, or peripheral vascular disease), diabetes, or treated hypertension.[73] As such, it was a mixture of primary and secondary intervention. One third of the individuals had baseline LDL cholesterol levels below 116 mg/dl, and 25% had initial LDL levels ranging from 116 to 135 mg/dl. Participants were randomized to receive simvastatin or placebo. After an average follow-up of 5.5 years, the lipid-lowering group showed a 24% reduction in major cardiovascular events, an 18% reduction in cardiovascular deaths, and a 13% reduction in all-cause mortality, as compared with the placebo group. The percentage reductions in events were similar in all three tertiles of baseline LDL cholesterol levels and in patients with LDL cholesterol levels below 100 mg/dl at baseline. These results differ from those reported in the CARE study, but they are consistent with results from the 4S and LIPID trials. The results of the Heart Protection Study also suggest that there may not be a threshold beyond which increased LDL-lowering therapy ceases to improve outcome, at least in patients at high risk for recurrent coronary events.

Aggressive LDL-lowering therapy appears to be more effective than standard lipid-lowering treatment. The Pravastatin or Atorvastatin Evaluation and Infection Therapy (PROVE-IT) trial compared standard LDL-lowering treatment (pravastatin, 40 mg daily) with intensive LDL-lowering treatment (atorvastatin, 80 mg daily) in more than 4,000 patients recently hospitalized with an acute coronary syndrome.[74] The average follow-up was 24 months. The median LDL cholesterol level achieved with atorvastatin was 62 mg/dl, compared with 96 mg/dl in the group treated with pravastatin. The primary composite end point was death from any cause, MI, unstable angina not requiring hospitalization, coronary revascularization, and stroke. The rate of reaching the primary end point was 22.4% in the atorvastatin group and 26.3% in the pravastatin group. The benefit of aggressive therapy with atorvastatin was apparent as early as 30 days after initiating therapy and was consistent over time.

The Reversal of Atherosclerosis with Aggressive Lipid Lowering (REVERSAL) trial also compared moderate LDL-lowering therapy (pravastatin, 40 mg daily) with more intensive LDL-lowering therapy (atorvastatin, 80 mg daily).[75] The study used coronary intravascular ultrasound, a sensitive means of measuring plaque volume, as a baseline measurement and primary end point. The median percentage change in atheroma volume was –0.4% in the atorvastatin group, compared with +2.7% in the pravastatin group. This finding correlated with mean LDL cholesterol levels of 79 mg/dl in the atorvastatin group and 110 mg/dl in the pravastatin group. These results gave further support to the view that aggressive LDL-lowering therapy is superior to standard LDL-lowering therapy.

Few studies have examined the benefit of raising HDL cholesterol levels in the secondary prevention of CAD. The VA-HIT trial enrolled 2,531 patients with known CAD and with LDL cholesterol levels below 140 mg/dl, HDL cholesterol levels of 40 mg/dl or above, and triglyceride levels of 300 mg/dl or below.[19] The patients were randomized to receive gemfibrozil or placebo. The subsequent mean HDL cholesterol level in the gemfibrozil group was 6% higher than that in the placebo group, and the mean triglyceride level in the gemfibrozil group was 31% lower. The mean LDL cholesterol levels were 113 mg/dl in both groups. The combined primary end point of cardiac death and nonfatal myocardial infarction was 17% in the gemfibrozil group and 22% in the placebo group (relative risk reduction, 22%). The beneficial effect of gemfibrozil did not become apparent until 2 years after randomization.

Combination therapy using a statin to lower LDL cholesterol levels and niacin to raise HDL cholesterol levels has been shown to provide increased cardioprotection. In one study, patients were randomized to one of four groups: simvastatin plus niacin, vitamins, simvastatin-niacin plus antioxidants, or placebos. At entry, the HDL cholesterol level was below 35 mg/dl, and the LDL cholesterol level was below 145 mg/dl. The mean LDL and HDL cholesterol levels were unaltered in the antioxidant and placebo groups but were changed significantly in the simvastatin plus niacin groups (mean LDL cholesterol level reduced by 42% and mean HDL cholesterol level raised by 26%). At 3 years, the reduction of clinical events in the simvastatin and niacin groups was greater than that which is usually reported in studies of statins alone (relative risk, 0.1 to 0.4 compared with placebo), suggesting that a benefit may be associated with the elevation of HDL cholesterol levels. The antioxidants provided no additional benefit and may even have attenuated the benefits of combination therapy.[76]

RISK STRATIFICATION

CAD risk factors seldom occur in isolation, and the risk associated with each varies widely in combination with other risk factors. The variability in risk prompted the NCEP ATP-III to standardize guidelines for risk assessment of CAD. Over time, the guidelines were revised to recommend more aggressive lipid-lowering targets as a means of reducing CAD risk [see Tables 5 and 6]. This evolution in guidelines is the result of consistently emerging data that extend our understanding of dyslipidemia, associated risk factors and their relationship to CAD, and the utility of new therapeutic options.

The ATP guidelines focus primarily on LDL cholesterol levels as the major lipid risk factor. More recently, low HDL levels have become a factor in risk assessment. In ATP-III, the metabolic syndrome was added as a risk factor in an attempt to assess risk for CAD in centrally obese patients who have modest elevations in triglyceride levels, low HDL cholesterol levels, and small, dense LDL particles, as well as type 2 diabetes mellitus or FCHL. In an effort to better identify those at highest risk for CAD

Table 5 ATP-III LDL-C Goals and Cutpoints for Therapeutic Lifestyle Changes and Drug Therapy in Different Risk Categories[83]

Risk Category	LDL-C Goal	Initiate Therapeutic Lifestyle Changes	Consider Drug Therapy
High risk: CAD or CAD risk equivalents (noncoronary atherosclerotic disease, diabetes, and 2+ CAD risk factors with 10-year risk for CAD > 20%)*	< 100 mg/dl (optional goal: < 70 mg/dl)	≥ 100 mg/dl	≥ 100 mg/dl (< 100 mg/dl: consider drug options)
Moderately high risk: 2+ CAD risk factors [see Table 6] with 10-year risk for CAD 10%–20%*	< 130 mg/dl (optional goal: < 100 mg/dl)	≥ 130 mg/dl	≥ 130 mg/dl (100–129 mg/dl: consider drug options)
Moderate risk: 2+ CAD risk factors with 10-year risk for CAD < 10%*	< 130 mg/dl	≥ 130 mg/dl	≥ 160 mg/dl
Low risk: 0–1 CAD risk factor with 10-year risk for CAD < 10%	< 160 mg/dl	≥ 160 mg/dl	≥ 190 mg/dl (160–189 mg/dl: LDL-lowering drug optional)

*Online 10-year risk calculators: www.nhlbi.nih.gov/guidelines/cholesterol.
CAD—coronary artery disease LDL-C—low-density lipoprotein cholesterol

Table 6 ATP-III Major Risk Factors (Exclusive of LDL Cholesterol) That Modify LDL Goals*[15]

Cigarette smoking
Hypertension (blood pressure ≥ 140/90 mm Hg or on antihypertensive medication)
Low HDL cholesterol (< 40 mg/dl)[†]
Family history of premature CAD (CAD in male first-degree relative < 55 yr; CAD in female first-degree relative < 65 yr)
Age (men ≥ 45 yr; women ≥ 55 yr)

*Diabetes is regarded as a CAD risk equivalent.
[†]HDL cholesterol > 60 mg/dl counts as a negative risk factor; its presence removes one risk factor from the total count.
CAD—coronary artery disease   HDL—high-density lipoprotein

events, the NCEP recognizes several CAD equivalents. They include diabetes mellitus, peripheral arterial disease, abdominal aortic aneurysm, symptomatic carotid artery disease, and multiple risk factors that confer a 10-year risk of CAD greater than 20%.[15] The presence of these CAD equivalents requires a level of therapeutic aggressiveness equal to that recommended for patients with established CAD.

The American College of Physicians (ACP) has adopted a somewhat less aggressive recommendation for treatment of individuals with type 1 diabetes mellitus. The ACP reserves the use of statins for patients with type 2 diabetes and other CAD risk factors.[77] The ATP-III guidelines do not differentiate between the risk of CAD in patients with type 1 diabetes and that in patients with type 2 diabetes. An argument can be made that the CAD risk is greater in patients with type 2 diabetes and that treatment guidelines should differentiate between these entities.

The ATP-III guidelines use the Framingham scoring system for estimating the 10-year risk of CAD. Some studies indicate that the Framingham score overestimates risk in Japanese-American and Hispanic men, Native-American women, and some European and Asian populations.[78-80] It also has been suggested that the Framingham score weights age too heavily as a risk factor. The Pravastatin in Elderly Individuals at Risk of Vascular Disease (PROSPER) study, which is the only prospective study to assess statin therapy in men and women older than 70 years, demonstrated that statin therapy was of no benefit in those without preexisting atherosclerosis.[81] Any age bias present in the Framingham scoring system is eliminated when the system is used to predict risk in nonelderly patients.

A multicenter, international study confirmed the validity of risk stratification. In this study of over 15,000 patients with acute MI from 52 countries, over 90% of the population-attributable risk could be accounted for by nine potentially modifiable risk factors.[82] Most of the risk is accounted for by an elevated apo B to apo A1 ratio, smoking, hypertension, and diabetes. These risk factors were more important in younger than in older individuals. As such, principles of cardiovascular disease prevention are similar worldwide and have the potential to have a major impact.

DRUG THERAPY IN DYSLIPIDEMIA

Drugs Used to Lower LDL Cholesterol Levels

Several classes of drugs can lower LDL cholesterol levels [*see Table 7*].[16] Before the introduction of statins in the mid-1980s, the major drugs used for this purpose were the bile-acid sequestrants and niacin. The introduction of statins, with their powerful effects on LDL cholesterol, their tolerability, and their relative

Table 7 Drug Treatment of Lipid Disorders

Drug	Dosage	Cost (per Month)	Comment
Bile acid–binding resins	Start with one packet (2 g for colestipol tabs) b.i.d., increase over 1–2 wk to desired dose		For elevated LDL, normal triglycerides; take other drugs 1 hr before or 4 hr after; may be used with nicotinic acid, statins, or fibrates
Cholestyramine	Maximum 24 g/day b.i.d. or t.i.d.	$70	
Colestipol powder	Maximum 30 g/day b.i.d. or t.i.d.	$339	t.i.d. more effective
Colestipol tablets	Maximum 16 g/day	$297	
Colesevelam	Six 625 mg tablets per day, taken with meals either as a single dose or divided into two doses; maximum seven tablets/day	$172	Better tolerated than other resins
Ezetimibe	10 mg/day	$88	Can reduce LDL cholesterol by ~20% without increasing plasma triglyceride levels
Fenofibrate	145 or 200 mg/day	$97	For elevated triglycerides and patients in whom both LDL and triglycerides are elevated; may be used with bile acid–binding resins or nicotinic acid; decrease dose with severe renal disease
Gemfibrozil	600 mg b.i.d.	$16	
Niacin			
Crystalline	Start with 250 mg q.d. after dinner; increase to 0.5 g t.i.d. to q.i.d.; maximum 6 g/day	$7	For elevated LDL, triglycerides, or both; may be used with bile acid–binding resins, statins or fibrates
Controlled release	1.5 g at bedtime	$169	
Statins [*see Table 8*]	—	—	For elevated LDL; possibly useful for patients in whom both LDL and triglycerides are elevated; may be used with bile acid–binding resins or nicotinic acid

lack of toxicity, provided a significant advance in the management of patients with hypercholesterolemia. The introduction of intestinally active drugs has provided additional approaches both for monotherapy—especially for individuals who are unable to tolerate statins—and, more particularly, for combination therapy. Drug therapy should be sufficient to produce a reduction in LDL cholesterol levels of at least 30% to 40%.[83]

Statins Several statins are now available, and new ones continue to be introduced. To date, statins have been highly effective in clinical trials in reducing clinical events, including stroke. Although some of the benefits of statins have been attributed to the so-called pleiotropic effects (e.g., anti-inflammatory effects) of this class of drugs, the extent of reduction in LDL cholesterol levels nonetheless appears to be the major determinant of risk reduction [see Table 8].

Intestinally active compounds Bile-acid sequestrants were among the earliest drugs to become available for the treatment of hypercholesterolemia, and they were the first class of drugs to demonstrate that the reduction of LDL cholesterol was associated with a reduced risk of CAD; however, their use was limited by their very poor tolerability and their modest effect in reducing LDL cholesterol. Moreover, triglyceride levels tend to increase with their use in patients with high baseline plasma triglyceride levels. The introduction of a more tolerable bile-acid sequestrant, colesevelam, resulted in improved compliance with this class of drugs, especially when used in combination therapy in patients with very high LDL cholesterol levels (e.g., for patients with FH).

Unlike bile-acid sequestrants, the intestinally active drug ezetimibe directly inhibits cholesterol absorption. Although clinical data are limited, it appears ezetimibe is able to reduce LDL cholesterol by approximately 20%, whether used as monotherapy or in combination with other lipid-lowering agents.[84] In addition, ezetimibe does not cause an increase in plasma triglyceride levels, as occurs with bile-acid sequestrants. Ezetimibe has not yet been evaluated in clinical trials with cardiovascular end points.

Drugs Used Primarily to Lower Triglyceride Levels

The preferred drugs for the treatment of hypertriglyceridemia are the fibrates and niacin. Niacin is the best drug currently available for raising HDL cholesterol levels. It also produces modest reductions in LDL and lowers apo B levels, but because it worsens insulin sensitivity, its use in patients with type 2 diabetes mellitus is limited. Fibrates are the drugs of choice for patients with marked hypertriglyceridemia, for whom the primary goal of therapy is the prevention of pancreatitis and other features of the chylomicronemia syndrome. They also are of use in hypertriglyceridemic states (e.g., patients with the familial forms of hypertriglyceridemia and some patients with diabetic dyslipidemia), especially when triglyceride levels are more than mildly elevated. Fibrates also have a modestly beneficial effect on HDL cholesterol levels. Both fibrates and niacin are useful in combination therapy, primarily with statins.

Omega-3 fatty acids (e.g., those found in marine oils) have been used for the treatment of hypertriglyceridemia, especially when other modalities of therapy have failed to reduce markedly elevated levels of triglycerides.

Combination Therapy

Combinations of drugs often need to be used when both LDL cholesterol and triglyceride levels are elevated. Combination therapy also is of use when monotherapy, especially with statins, fails to achieve target lipid and lipoprotein levels, especially LDL cholesterol levels. Commonly used combinations include statins and fibrates—although little is known of their additive benefit in reducing clinical events—and statins and niacin. Statins and bile-acid sequestrants also are a useful combination, and the use of the new cholesterol absorption inhibitors with other classes of drugs, particularly statins, is likely to be of value. In some cases, triple therapy (e.g., statins, niacin, and an intestinally active agent) is required.

Special Issues in the Management of Dyslipidemia

SCREENING FOR HYPERCHOLESTEROLEMIA IN CHILDREN

Numerous autopsy studies demonstrate that coronary atherosclerosis begins in childhood and adolescence and that lipoprotein levels are consistently associated with the extent of such atherosclerosis. Children in families with FH and early CAD have higher cholesterol levels, and childhood cholesterol levels are significant predictors of adult levels. However, a significant proportion of children and adolescents who have mildly elevated cholesterol levels will not as adults develop cholesterol levels high enough to warrant intervention; screening all children for high cholesterol would risk labeling many young people as diseased. All children older than 2 years would benefit from a diet that is low in saturated fat; this goal should be a part of any population strategy for controlling epidemic atherosclerosis. However, the safety and efficacy of long-term drug therapy have not been established in this age group, and treatment must be approached cautiously.

Considering these and other issues, the recommendations of the NCEP's Expert Panel on Blood Cholesterol Levels in Children and Adolescents seem appropriate.[85] Physicians should advise patients younger than 55 years who have known CAD or a lipid disorder that their children or grandchildren should undergo regular cholesterol testing, and patients with a genetically well-defined lipid disorder should obtain appropriate genetic counseling. Physicians who care for patients younger than 20 years who have markedly elevated LDL levels should exhaust all lifestyle interventions before considering medications. If such measures are ineffective, bile-acid sequestrants should be used, and referral to a specialty clinic should be considered.

Treatment of young adults with elevated cholesterol levels is controversial. The strategy of matching the intensity of interven-

Table 8 Doses of Statins Required To Achieve an Approximate 30% to 40% Reduction of LDL-C Levels[83]

Drug	Dose (mg/day)	LDL Reduction (%)	Cost (per month)
Atorvastatin	10	39	$75
Lovastatin	40	31	$35
Pravastatin	40	34	$132
Simvastatin	20–40	35–41	$125
Fluvastatin	40–80	25–35	$69–138
Rosuvastatin	5–10	39–45	$93–94
Ezetimibe plus simvastatin	10/10–10/40	33–41	$91–93

tion with the level of risk of atherosclerosis has been proposed, but for young adults, a short-term (e.g., 10-year) risk assessment may be inadequate for estimating the potential benefit of cholesterol lowering. It is incorrect to argue that all treatment can be safely deferred to later life or until the occurrence of an atherosclerotic event. Population-level prevention and lifestyle interventions should still be favored for young adults, but advances in technology that better enable the identification of asymptomatic patients (of any age) who should take steps to reduce risk are greatly needed. Such advances may make it possible to reliably identify or quantify vulnerable plaques; markers of inflammation; or noninvasive measurements of endothelial dysfunction.

MANAGING DYSLIPIDEMIA IN WOMEN

Before menopause, women have a lower incidence of CAD than men of the same age. Although rare, CAD does occur in premenopausal women, usually in association with multiple genetic and environmental risk factors, such as in patients with familial forms of dyslipidemia or in diabetic patients who smoke cigarettes.

After menopause, some women develop the metabolic syndrome, characterized by visceral obesity, insulin resistance, hypertension, and dyslipidemia.[21] There is some evidence that estrogen replacement therapy can reverse these findings. However, the Women's Health Initiative Study demonstrated that combined oral estrogen and progesterone did not protect women from CAD and that it in fact had adverse effects.[86] The estrogen-alone component of the Women's Health Initiative Study indicated that estrogen therapy carried a modest risk of CAD (i.e., MI or CAD death); the study was halted prematurely because of increased risk of stroke.[49]

MANAGING DYSLIPIDEMIA IN OLDER PATIENTS

Age is the most significant risk factor for the development of atherosclerosis. CAD is currently a major cause of disability and mortality in older populations; however, the relative risk associated with any single coronary risk factor decreases with age because of the comorbid conditions and noncardiovascular mortality that affect an aging population. One implication of the complex relationships between risk factors and comorbid conditions in the pathogenesis of coronary-related events in the elderly is represented by the multiple effects of treatment of single risk factors, such as the decrease in LDL cholesterol levels and inflammation markers yielded by statins. A growing body of evidence from clinical trials indicates that statin therapy is effective in the elderly; lipid-lowering therapy is probably indicated in this population in persons who are at high risk for atherosclerosis or who have preexisting atherosclerosis.[73,81] Primary intervention with drug therapy in persons not at high risk for atherosclerosis is controversial. In the PROSPER trial of persons older than 70 years, no benefit was seen with statin therapy in those who did not have preexisting clinical atherosclerosis. Indeed, there was a suggestion of increased gastrointestinal cancer with statin therapy in these elderly patients.[81] Attention to other concomitant diseases and the nutritional state, as well as to capabilities of the elderly, are important considerations in the management of older patients with dyslipidemia.[87]

John D. Brunzell, M.D., F.A.C.P., has served as a consultant for GlaxoSmith-Kline, Merck, Abbott Laboratories, and Novartis Pharmaceuticals Corp.

R. Alan Failor, M.D., has served as a consultant for GlaxoSmithKline.

References

1. Havel R, Kane J: Introduction: structure and metabolism of plasma lipoproteins. The Metabolic and Molecular Bases of Inherited Disease, 8th ed. Scriver CR, Beaudet AL, Sly WS, et al, Eds. McGraw-Hill Book Co, New York, 2001, p 2705

2. Brunzell JD, Chait A, Bierman EL: Pathophysiology of lipoprotein transport. Metabolism 27:1109, 1978

3. Brunzell JD, Albers JJ, Chait A, et al: Plasma lipoproteins in familial combined hyperlipidemia and monogenic familial hypertriglyceridemia. J Lipid Res 24:147, 1983

4. Kane JP, Havel RJ: Disorders of the biogenesis and secretion of lipoproteins containing the B apolipoproteins. The Metabolic and Molecular Bases of Inherited Disease, 8th ed. Scriver CR, Beaudet AL, Sly WS, et al, Eds. McGraw-Hill Book Co, New York, 2001

5. Utermann G: Lipoprotein (a). The Metabolic and Molecular Bases of Inherited Disease, 8th ed. Scriver CS, Beaudet AL, Sly WS, et al, Eds. McGraw-Hill Book Co, New York, 2001, p 2753

6. Brunzell J, Deeb S: Familial lipoprotein lipase deficiency, apo CII deficiency, and hepatic lipase deficiency. The Metabolic and Molecular Bases of Inherited Disease, 8th ed. Scriver CR, Beaudet AL, Sly WS, et al, Eds. McGraw-Hill Book Co, New York, 2001, p 2789

7. Mahley R, Rall S: Type III hyperlipoproteinemia (dysbetalipoproteinemia): the role of apolipoprotein E in normal and abnormal lipoprotein metabolism. The Metabolic and Molecular Bases of Inherited Disease, 8th ed. Scriver CR, Beaudet AL, Sly WS, et al, Eds. McGraw-Hill Book Co, New York, 2001, p 2835

8. Goldstein JL, Hobbs HH, Brown MS: Familial hypercholesterolemia. The Metabolic and Molecular Bases of Inherited Disease, 8th ed. Scriver CS, Beaudet AL, Sly WS, et al, Eds. McGraw-Hill Book Co, New York, 2001, p 2863

9. Tall A, Breslow J, Rubin E: Genetic disorders affecting plasma high-density lipoproteins. The Metabolic and Molecular Bases of Inherited Disease, 8th ed. Scriver CS, Beaudet AL, Sly WS, et al, Eds. McGraw-Hill Book Co, New York, 2001, p 2915

10. Deeb SS, Zambon A, Carr MC, et al: Hepatic lipase and dyslipidemia: interactions among genetic variants, obesity, gender, and diet. J Lipid Res 44:1279, 2003

11. Frikke-Schmidt R, Nordestgaard BG, Jensen GB, et al: Genetic variation in ABC transporter A1 contributes to HDL cholesterol in the general population. J Clin Invest 114:1343, 2004

12. Carr MC, Brunzell JD: Abdominal obesity and dyslipidemia in the metabolic syndrome: importance of type 2 diabetes and familial combined hyperlipidemia in coronary artery disease risk. J Clin Endocrinol Metab 89:2601, 2004

13. Griffin BA: Lipoprotein atherogenicity: an overview of current mechanisms. Proc Nutr Soc 58:163, 1999

14. Steinberg D, Pearson TA, Kuller LH: Alcohol and atherosclerosis. Ann Intern Med 114:967, 1991

15. Executive summary of the third report of the National Cholesterol Education Program (NCEP) expert panel on detection, evaluation, and treatment of high blood cholesterol in adults (adult treatment panel III). Expert Panel on Detection, Evaluation, and Treatment of High Blood Cholesterol in Adults. JAMA 285:2486, 2001 www.nhlbi.nih.gov/guidelines/cholesterol/atp_iii.htm

16. Brown CD, Higgins M, Donato KA, et al: Body mass index and the prevalence of hypertension and dyslipidemia. Obes Res 8:605, 2000

17. Austin MA, McKnight B, Edwards KL, et al: Cardiovascular disease mortality in familial forms of hypertriglyceridemia: a 20-year prospective study. Circulation 101:2777, 2000

18. Knopp RH: Drug treatment of lipid disorders. N Engl J Med 341:498, 1999

19. Rubins HB, Robins SJ, Collins D, et al: Gemfibrozil for the secondary prevention of coronary heart disease in men with low levels of high-density lipoprotein cholesterol. Veterans Affairs High-Density Lipoprotein Cholesterol Intervention Trial Study Group. N Engl J Med 341:410, 1999

20. Clofibrate and niacin in coronary heart disease. Coronary Drug Project Research Group. JAMA 231:360, 1975

21. Taylor AJ, Sullenberger, LE, Lee HJ, et al: Arterial Biology for the Investigation of the Treatment Effects of Reducing Cholesterol (ARBITER) 2: A double-blind, placebo-controlled study of extended-release niacin on atherosclerosis progression in secondary prevention patients treated with statins. Circulation 110:3512, 2004

22. Carr MC: The emergence of the metabolic syndrome with menopause. J Clin Endocrinol Metab 88:2404, 2003

23. Nieves D, Cnop M, Retzlaff B, et al: The atherogenic lipoprotein profile associated with obesity and insulin resistance is largely attributable to intra-abdominal fat. Diabetes 52:172, 2003

24. Purnell JQ, Kahn SE, Albers JJ, et al: Effect of weight loss with reduction of intra-abdominal fat on lipid metabolism in older men. J Clin Endocrinol Metab 85:977, 2000

25. Grundy SM: Approach to lipoprotein management in 2001 National Cholesterol Guidelines. Am J Cardiol 90:11i, 2002

26. Cefalu WT, Wang ZQ, Werbel S, et al: Contribution of visceral fat mass to the insulin resistance of aging. Metabolism 44:954, 1995

27. Bermudez OI, Tucker KL: Total and central obesity among elderly Hispanics and the association with type 2 diabetes. Obes Res 9:443, 2001

28. Lempiainen P, Mykkanen L, Pyorala K, et al: Insulin resistance syndrome predicts coronary heart disease events in elderly nondiabetic men. Circulation 100:123, 1999

29. Mykkanen L, Kuusisto J, Haffner SM, et al: Hyperinsulinemia predicts multiple atherogenic changes in lipoproteins in elderly subjects. Arterioscler Thromb 14:518, 1994

30. Cefalu WT, Werbel S, Bell-Farrow AD, et al: Insulin resistance and fat patterning with aging: relationship to metabolic risk factors for cardiovascular disease. Metabolism 47:401, 1998

31. Ginsberg HN: Insulin resistance and cardiovascular disease. J Clin Invest 106:453, 2000

32. Ford E, Giles W, Dietz W: Prevalence of the metabolic syndrome among US adults: findings from the third National Health and Nutrition Examination Survey. JAMA 287:356, 2002

33. Alexander CM, Landsman PB, Teutsch SM, et al: NCEP-defined metabolic syndrome, diabetes, and prevalence of coronary heart disease among NHANES III participants age 50 years and older. Diabetes 52:1210, 2003

34. Lamarche B, Moorjani S, Cantin B, et al: Associations of HDL2 and HDL3 subfractions with ischemic heart disease in men. Arterioscler Thromb Vasc Biol 17:1098, 1997

35. Williams RR, Hopkins PN, Hunt SC, et al: Population-based frequency of dyslipidemia syndromes in coronary-prone families in Utah. Arch Intern Med 150:582, 1990

36. Goldstein JL, Hazzard WR, Schrott HG, et al: Hyperlipidemia in coronary heart disease. I. Lipid levels in 500 survivors of myocardial infarction. J Clin Invest 52:1533, 1973

37. Goldstein JL, Schrott HG, Hazzard WR, et al: Hyperlipidemia in coronary heart disease. II. Genetic analysis of lipid levels in 176 families and delineation of a new inherited disorder, combined hyperlipidemia. J Clin Invest 52:1544, 1973

38. Hazzard WR, Goldstein JL, Schrott MG, et al: Hyperlipidemia in coronary heart disease. III. Evaluation of lipoprotein phenotypes of 156 genetically defined survivors of myocardial infarction. J Clin Invest 52:1569, 1973

39. Ayyobi AF, McGladdery SH, McNeely MJ, et al: Small, dense LDL and elevated apolipoprotein B are the common characteristics for the three major lipid phenotypes of familial combined hyperlipidemia. Arterioscler Thromb Vasc Biol 23:1289, 2003

40. Jarvik GP, Brunzell JD, Austin MA, et al: Genetic predictors of FCHL in four large pedigrees: influence of ApoB level major locus predicted genotype and LDL subclass phenotype. Arterioscler Thromb 14:1687, 1994

41. Austin MA, Horowitz H, Wijsman E, et al: Bimodality of plasma apolipoprotein B levels in familial combined hyperlipidemia. Atherosclerosis 92:67, 1992

42. Babirak SP, Brown BG, Brunzell JD, et al: Familial combined hyperlipidemia and abnormal lipoprotein lipase. Arterioscler Thromb 12:1176, 1992

43. Purnell JQ, Kahn SE, Schwartz RS, et al: Relationship of insulin sensitivity and apoB levels to intra-abdominal fat in subjects with familial combined hyperlipidemia. Arterioscler Thromb Vasc Biol 21:567, 2001

44. Brown G, Albers JJ, Fisher LD, et al: Regression of coronary artery disease as a result of intensive lipid-lowering therapy in men with high levels of apolipoprotein B. N Engl J Med 323:1289, 1990

45. Colhoun HM, Betteridge DJ, Durrington PN, et al: Primary prevention of cardiovascular disease with atorvastatin in type 2 diabetes in the Collaborative Atorvastatin Diabetes Study (CARDS): multicentre randomised placebo-controlled trial. Lancet 364:685, 2004

46. Marks D, Thorogood M, Neil HA, et al: A review on the diagnosis, natural history, and treatment of familial hypercholesterolaemia. Atherosclerosis 168:1, 2003

47. Grundy SM, Vega GL, McGovern ME: Efficacy, safety, and tolerability of once-daily niacin for the treatment of dyslipidemia associated with type 2 diabetes: results of the assessment of diabetes control and evaluation of the efficacy of Niaspan trial. Arch Intern Med 162:1568, 2002

48. Effects of estrogen or estrogen/progestin regimens on heart disease risk factors in postmenopausal women: the Postmenopausal Estrogen/Progestin Interventions (PEPI) trial. The Writing Group for the PEPI trial. JAMA 273:199, 1995

49. Anderson GL, Limacher M, Assaf AR, et al: Effects of conjugated equine estrogen in postmenopausal women with hysterectomy: the Women's Health Initiative randomized controlled trial. JAMA 291:1701, 2004

50. Joven J, Villabona C, Vilella E, et al: Abnormalities of lipoprotein metabolism in patients with the nephrotic syndrome. N Engl J Med 323:579, 1990

51. Samuelsson O, Attman PO, Knight-Gibson C, et al: Effect of gemfibrozil on lipoprotein abnormalities in chronic renal insufficiency: a controlled study in human chronic renal disease. Nephron 75:286, 1997

52. Khovidhunkit W, Memon RA, Feingold KR, et al: Infection and inflammation-induced proatherogenic changes of lipoproteins. J Infect Dis 181:S462, 2000

53. The Lipid Research Clinics Coronary Primary Prevention Trial results. I. Reduction in incidence of coronary heart disease. JAMA 251:351, 1984

54. The Lipid Research Clinics Coronary Primary Prevention Trial results. II. The relationship of reduction in incidence of coronary heart disease to cholesterol lowering. JAMA 251:365, 1984

55. Frick MH, Elo O, Haapa K, et al: Helsinki Heart Study: primary-prevention trial with gemfibrozil in middle-aged men with dyslipidemia: safety of treatment, changes in risk factors, and incidence of coronary heart disease. N Engl J Med 317:1237, 1987

56. Shepherd J, Cobbe SM, Ford I, et al: Prevention of coronary heart disease with pravastatin in men with hypercholesterolemia. West of Scotland Coronary Prevention Study Group. N Engl J Med 333:1301, 1995

57. Baseline risk factors and their association with outcome in the West of Scotland Coronary Prevention Study. The West of Scotland Coronary Prevention Study Group. Am J Cardiol 79:756, 1997

58. Influence of pravastatin and plasma lipids on clinical events in the West of Scotland Coronary Prevention Study (WOSCOPS). Circulation 97:1440, 1998

59. Downs JR, Clearfield M, Weis S, et al: Primary prevention of acute coronary events with lovastatin in men and women with average cholesterol levels: results of AFCAPS/TexCAPS. Air Force/Texas Coronary Atherosclerosis Prevention Study. JAMA 279:1615, 1998

60. Gotto AM Jr, Boccuzzi SJ, Cook JR, et al: Effect of lovastatin on cardiovascular resource utilization and costs in the Air Force/Texas Coronary Atherosclerosis Prevention Study (AFCAPS/TexCAPS). AFCAPS/TexCAPS Research Group. Am J Cardiol 86:1176, 2000

61. Sever PS, Dahlof B, Poulter NR, et al: Prevention of coronary and stroke events with atorvastatin in hypertensive patients who have average or lower-than-average cholesterol concentrations, in the Anglo-Scandinavian Cardiac Outcomes Trial—Lipid Lowering Arm (ASCOT-LLA): a multicentre randomised controlled trial. Lancet 361:1149, 2003

62. Pekkanen J, Linn S, Heiss G, et al: Ten-year mortality from cardiovascular disease in relation to cholesterol level among men with and without preexisting cardiovascular disease. N Engl J Med 322:1700, 1990

63. Watts GF, Lewis B, Brunt JN, et al: Effects on coronary artery disease of lipid-lowering diet, or diet plus cholestyramine, in the St Thomas' Atherosclerosis Regression Study (STARS). Lancet 339:563, 1992

64. de Lorgeril M, Salen P, Martin JL, et al: Effect of a Mediterranean type of diet on the rate of cardiovascular complications in patients with coronary artery disease: insights into the cardioprotective effect of certain nutriments. J Am Coll Cardiol 28:1103, 1996

65. de Lorgeril M, Salen P, Martin JL, et al: Mediterranean diet, traditional risk factors, and the rate of cardiovascular complications after myocardial infarction: final report of the Lyon Diet Heart Study. Circulation 99:779, 1999

66. Zambon A, Hokanson JE, Brown BG, et al: Evidence for a new pathophysiological mechanism for coronary artery disease regression: hepatic lipase-mediated changes in LDL density. Circulation 99:1959, 1999

67. Randomised trial of cholesterol lowering in 4444 patients with coronary heart disease: the Scandinavian Simvastatin Survival Study (4S). Lancet 344:1383, 1994

68. Pedersen TR, Olsson AG, Faergeman O, et al: Lipoprotein changes and reduction in the incidence of major coronary heart disease events in the Scandinavian Simvastatin Survival Study (4S). Circulation 97:1453, 1998

69. Prevention of cardiovascular events and death with pravastatin in patients with coronary heart disease and a broad range of initial cholesterol levels. The Long-Term Intervention with Pravastatin in Ischaemic Disease (LIPID) Study Group. N Engl J Med 339:1349, 1998

70. Simes RJ, Marschner IC, Hunt D, et al: Relationship between lipid levels and clinical outcomes in the Long-term Intervention with Pravastatin in Ischemic Disease (LIPID) trial: to what extent is the reduction in coronary events with pravastatin explained by on-study lipid levels? Circulation 05:1162, 2002

71. Sacks FM, Pfeffer MA, Moye LA, et al: The effect of pravastatin on coronary events after myocardial infarction in patients with average cholesterol levels. Cholesterol and Recurrent Events Trial investigators. N Engl J Med 335:1001, 1996

72. Sacks FM, Moye LA, Davis BR, et al: Relationship between plasma LDL concentrations during treatment with pravastatin and recurrent coronary events in the Cholesterol and Recurrent Events Trial. Circulation 97:1446, 1998

73. MCR/BHF Heart Protection Study of cholesterol lowering with simvastatin in 20,536 high-risk individuals: a randomised placebo-controlled trial. Heart Protection Study Collaborative Group. Lancet 360:7, 2002

74. Cannon CP, Braunwald E, McCabe CH, et al: Intensive versus moderate lipid lowering with statins after acute coronary syndromes. N Engl J Med 350:1495, 2004

75. Nissen SE, Tuzcu EM, Schoenhagen P, et al: Effect of intensive compared with moderate lipid-lowering therapy on progression of coronary atherosclerosis: a randomized controlled trial. JAMA 291:1071, 2004

76. Brown BG, Zhao XQ, Chait A, et al: Simvastatin and niacin, antioxidant vitamins, or the combination for the prevention of coronary disease. N Engl J Med 345:1583, 2001

77. Snow V, Aronson MD, Hornbake ER, et al: Lipid control in the management of type 2 diabetes mellitus: a clinical practice guideline from the American College of Physicians. Ann Intern Med 140:644, 2004

78. D'Agostino RB Sr, Grundy S, Sullivan LM, et al: Validation of the Framingham coronary heart disease prediction scores: results of a multiple ethnic groups investigation. JAMA 286:180, 2001

79. Liu J, Hong Y, D'Agostino RB Sr, et al: Predictive value for the Chinese population of the Framingham CHD risk assessment tool compared with the Chinese Multi-Provincial Cohort Study. JAMA 291:2591, 2004

80. Brindle P, Emberson J, Lampe F, et al: Predictive accuracy of the Framingham coronary risk score in British men: prospective cohort study. BMJ 327:1267, 2003

81. Shepherd J, Blauw GJ, Murphy MB, et al: Pravastatin in elderly individuals at risk of vascular disease (PROSPER): a randomised controlled trial. Lancet 360:1623, 2002

82. Yusuf S, Hawken S, Ounpuu S, et al: Effect of potentially modifiable risk factors associated with myocardial infarction in 52 countries (the INTERHEART study): case-control study. Lancet 364:937, 2004

83. Grundy SM, Cleeman JI, Merz CN, et al: Implications of recent clinical trials for the National Cholesterol Education Program Adult Treatment Panel III guidelines. Circulation 110:227, 2004

84. Davidson MH, McGarry T, Bettis R, et al: Ezetimibe coadministered with simvastatin in patients with primary hypercholesterolemia. J Am Coll Cardiol 40:2125, 2002

85. Cholesterol in childhood. American Academy of Pediatrics, Committee on Nutrition. Pediatrics 101:141, 1998

86. Rossouw JE, Anderson GL, Prentice RL, et al: Risks and benefits of estrogen plus progestin in healthy postmenopausal women: principal results from the Women's Health Initiative randomized controlled trial. JAMA 288:321, 2002

87. Carlsson CM, Carnes M, McBride PE, et al: Managing dyslipidemia in older adults. J Am Geriatr Soc 47:1458, 1999

Acknowledgments

Figures 1 and 4   Andy Christie.

Figures 2, 3, 5, and 6   Seward Hung.

60 The Porphyrias

Shigeru Sassa, M.D., PH.D, and Attallah Kappas, M.D., F.A.C.P.

The porphyrias are uncommon disorders caused by deficiencies in the activities of the enzymes of the heme biosynthetic pathway. The enzymatic defects that cause porphyrias may be either inherited or acquired, and there is significant interplay between the gene defect and acquired or environmental factors in the expression of clinical symptoms.

Acute forms of the porphyrias may be life threatening and may be misdiagnosed because of the nonspecific nature of the clinical presentations (e.g., acute abdominal pain, psychiatric disturbances, and polyneuropathies). The course of the acute forms of disease is characterized by long latent periods interrupted by acute attacks, which are associated with substantial morbidity and mortality.

Classification

Porphyrias may be classified as neurovisceral or photosensitive, depending on their prominent clinical characteristic, but some porphyrias have both symptoms [*see Figure 1*]. Alternatively, the porphyrias can be classified as hepatic or erythropoietic, depending on the principal site of expression of the specific enzymatic defect involved, but in some porphyrias the expressions overlap.

Pathophysiology

The porphyrias are best understood by the examination of the basic scheme of heme synthesis [*see Figure 2*]. The rate of synthesis is controlled by the mitochondrial enzyme δ-aminolevulinic acid (ALA) synthase. Subsequently, in the cytoplasm, the tetrapyrrole rings remain in the reduced state (porphyrinogens), but the number of carboxyl residues progressively decreases. The last three enzymatic reactions take place in the mitochondrion, resulting in heme, which represses the production of ALA in the liver, the initial and rate-limiting enzyme in this metabolic pathway. The loss of carboxyl groups makes each successive compound less water soluble.

The oxidation of porphyrinogen by the removal of hydrogen atoms results in a series of porphyrins that absorbs light with a wavelength of approximately 400 nm (the Soret band), accounting for the fluorescence characteristic of all porphyrins. Porphyrinogen intermediates oxidize spontaneously, especially in the presence of light. The resulting porphyrins are excreted in the urine, the stool, or both, depending on their relative water solubility.

Each specific abnormality in the pattern of excretion of porphyrins and porphyrin precursors is caused by a reduction in the activity of one of the enzymes from ALA dehydratase (ALAD) to ferrochelatase. The two major organs that are active in heme syn-

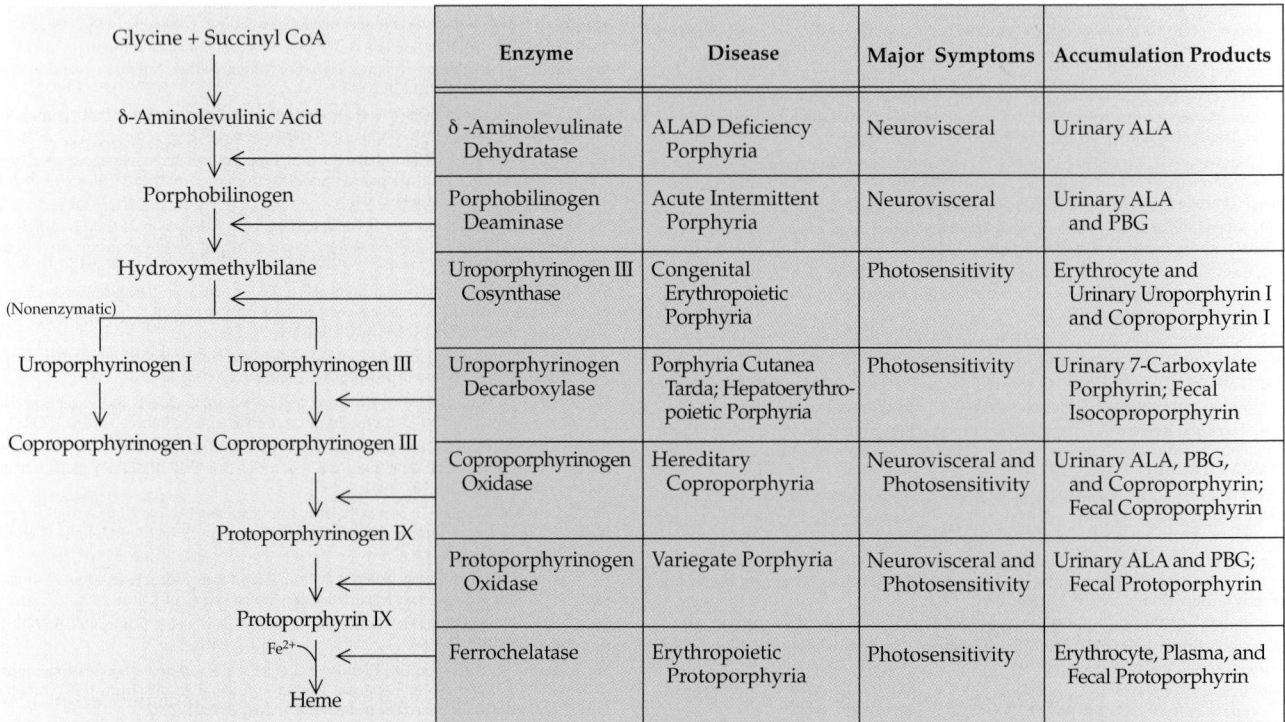

Enzyme	Disease	Major Symptoms	Accumulation Products
δ-Aminolevulinate Dehydratase	ALAD Deficiency Porphyria	Neurovisceral	Urinary ALA
Porphobilinogen Deaminase	Acute Intermittent Porphyria	Neurovisceral	Urinary ALA and PBG
Uroporphyrinogen III Cosynthase	Congenital Erythropoietic Porphyria	Photosensitivity	Erythrocyte and Urinary Uroporphyrin I and Coproporphyrin I
Uroporphyrinogen Decarboxylase	Porphyria Cutanea Tarda; Hepatoerythropoietic Porphyria	Photosensitivity	Urinary 7-Carboxylate Porphyrin; Fecal Isocoproporphyrin
Coproporphyrinogen Oxidase	Hereditary Coproporphyria	Neurovisceral and Photosensitivity	Urinary ALA, PBG, and Coproporphyrin; Fecal Coproporphyrin
Protoporphyrinogen Oxidase	Variegate Porphyria	Neurovisceral and Photosensitivity	Urinary ALA and PBG; Fecal Protoporphyrin
Ferrochelatase	Erythropoietic Protoporphyria	Photosensitivity	Erythrocyte, Plasma, and Fecal Protoporphyrin

Pathway (left side):
Glycine + Succinyl CoA → δ-Aminolevulinic Acid → Porphobilinogen → Hydroxymethylbilane → (Nonenzymatic) → Uroporphyrinogen I / Uroporphyrinogen III → Coproporphyrinogen I / Coproporphyrinogen III → Protoporphyrinogen IX → Protoporphyrin IX → (Fe^{2+}) → Heme

Figure 1 Classification and major symptoms of the porphyrias. δ-Aminolevulinate dehydratase deficiency and porphobilinogen deaminase deficiency are accompanied by acute hepatic porphyria, but not by photocutaneous porphyria, because their enzymatic blocks result in a decrease in porphyrin precursor synthesis. Enzymatic defects beyond uroporphyrinogen III cosynthase are all associated with photocutaneous porphyrias, because they produce excessive amounts of various porphyrins. Both hereditary coproporphyria and variegate porphyria are additionally associated with acute hepatic porphyria.

thesis are the liver and the erythroid bone marrow, and the consequences of inherited enzymatic defects in the porphyrias are mainly expressed in these tissues. There is significant tissue-specific regulation for some enzymes in the heme biosynthetic pathway.[1] For example, there are two genes for ALA synthase (ALAS)—namely, the erythroid-specific ALAS gene (ALAS2, also called ALAS-E) and the housekeeping ALAS gene (ALAS1, also called ALAS-N). Heme-mediated regulation of ALAS is also tissue specific—namely, ALAS1 expression in the liver is suppressed by heme, whereas ALAS2 in the erythroid bone marrow is not. Although deficiency of ALAS does not cause porphyria, ALAS2 gene defects are associated with X-linked sideroblastic anemia. Genetic deficiency of ALAS1 has not been described, suggesting that it may not be compatible with life. In addition, there are the erythroid-specific and housekeeping messenger RNAs (mRNAs) for ALAD, porphobilinogen deaminase (PBGD), and uroporphyrinogen cosynthase (UCS), as well as the erythroid-specific and housekeeping enzymes for ALAS and PBGD.

The presence of functional or nonfunctional enzyme proteins can be verified by cross-reaction with specific antibodies to the normal enzymatic protein (called cross-reacting immunologic material [CRIM]). Because individual mutations define differing protein structures, gradations of enzyme activities are encountered and can account for some of the differences in clinical severity.

Clinical Presentation of the Porphyrias

PORPHYRIAS ASSOCIATED WITH NEUROVISCERAL ATTACKS

Porphyrias associated with neurovisceral attacks are also called acute hepatic porphyrias; they include acute intermittent porphyria (AIP), variegate porphyria (VP), hereditary coproporphyria (HCP), and ALAD-deficiency porphyria (ADP). Along with having neurovisceral attacks, patients with HCP and VP may also present with photosensitivity [see Figure 1].

Acute Intermittent Porphyria

AIP is an autosomal dominant disorder resulting from a partial deficiency of PBGD.[2] In most patients, the deficient enzyme activity (i.e., approximately 50% of normal) is found in all tissues, including erythrocytes, whereas in 5% of patients, it is found in nonerythroid cells but not in erythrocytes. The cardinal pathobiologic defect of the disease is a neurologic dysfunction that may affect the peripheral, autonomic, and central nervous systems. The majority of persons with this inherited enzyme deficiency remain clinically normal throughout life. Clinical expression of the disease is usually linked to environmental or acquired factors (e.g., nutritional status, drugs, sex steroids, and other chemicals of endogenous or exogenous origin), indicating that there is a significant environmental effect on the clinical expression of the primary gene defect.

Epidemiology AIP is the severest form of the acute hepatic porphyrias and probably the most common of the genetic porphyrias. The highest incidence of AIP occurs in Lapland, Scandinavia, and the United Kingdom, although it has been reported in many population groups. The disorder is expressed clinically almost invariably after puberty and more often in women than in men.

Molecular defects and pathophysiology PBGD catalyzes the condensation of four molecules of PBG to yield hydroxy-

methylbilane [see Figure 2]. In the presence of the next enzyme, uroporphyrinogen III cosynthase, hydroxymethylbilane is converted to uroporphyrinogen III, which involves an intramolecular rearrangement of the D-ring pyrrole.[3] Both the hepatocyte and erythrocyte PBGD are derived from a gene containing 15 exons, but the mRNA is spliced differently in the two tissues, allowing heme synthesis to be regulated differently.[4] In the hepatocyte, transcription starts from exon 1 and encodes an enzyme slightly larger (i.e., 17 additional amino acids at the amino-terminal of the enzyme but otherwise identical) than the enzyme in the erythrocyte. In the erythrocyte, transcription starts at exon 2 rather than at exon 1.

More than 170 different point mutations of the human PBGD gene have been described in AIP. Patients with AIP can be classified into three subsets: type I, type II, and type III.

Patients with type I mutations are characterized by PBGD mutations that are negative for CRIM, and they exhibit 50% reduction in enzyme activity and PBGD protein. Mutations found in type I AIP are mostly single-base substitutions or deletions that lead to a single amino acid change or to truncated proteins, which result in the loss of expression of the enzyme protein.

Type II mutations are observed in fewer than 5% of AIP patients and are characterized by decreased PBGD activity in nonerythroid cells (e.g., liver cells) but normal erythroid PBGD activity. The mutations found in type II AIP are single-base substitutions that occur in the exon-intron boundary of exon 1, resulting in a splicing defect that affects the nonspecific form of PBGD but not the erythroid-specific PBGD.[5]

Patients with type III mutations are characterized by CRIM-positive mutations—that is, decreased enzyme activity and the presence of structurally abnormal enzyme protein.[6] Mutations characterizing type III AIP, which mostly occur in exons 10 and 12, are observed in the region that is essential for catalytic activity.

Diagnosis Abdominal pain is the most common symptom of AIP and is often the initial symptom of an acute attack. Other gastroenterologic features may include nausea, vomiting, constipation or diarrhea, abdominal distention, and ileus. Urinary retention, incontinence, and dysuria are frequently observed. Tachycardia, hypertension, and, less commonly, fever, sweating, restlessness, and tremor are also observed. Peripheral neuropathy and muscle weakness are common features of AIP. Muscular weakness can progress to quadriparesis and respiratory paralysis and arrest, which may resemble the Guillain-Barré syndrome.[7]

Acute attacks of AIP may be accompanied by seizures, especially in patients with hyponatremia caused by vomiting, inappropriate fluid therapy, or the syndrome of inappropriate antidiuretic hormone. No cutaneous manifestations are associated with this enzyme deficiency. Patients with clinically expressed AIP excrete increased amounts of ALA and PBG in the urine during attacks and sometimes between attacks. In severe cases, the urine develops a port-wine color from a high content of porphobilin, an auto-oxidation product of PBG.

In persons with latent disease, an acute attack may be precipitated by endogenous or exogenous environmental factors. Precipitating factors of AIP fall into five categories: (1) drugs that induce ALAS1 in the liver; (2) endocrine factors that facilitate ALAS1 induction; (3) reduced caloric intake that derepresses the synthesis of ALAS1; (4) drugs that induce hepatic cytochrome P-450, thereby driving heme synthesis; and (5) various oxidative stresses (e.g., infections and surgery) that induce heme oxygenase–1, which results in excessive heme catabolism and leads to the derepression of ALAS1. In women, relapses occur, particularly premenstrually. One study showed oral contraceptives precipitated acute attacks in 24% of the persons studied, whereas menopausal hormone replacement therapy only rarely affected the disorder.[8] Nevertheless, as a precaution, it is practical to restrict use of exogenous sex hormones in all women who have AIP.

The diagnosis of clinically expressed AIP requires demonstration of increased urinary excretion of PBG and ALA. A urine sample can be rapidly screened for PBG by the Watson-Schwartz or the Hoesch test, both of which utilize the Ehrlich reagent to detect a chromogen. Twenty-four-hour urine samples should be collected, placed in opaque containers, refrigerated, and delivered to a qualified laboratory for quantitative analysis of ALA, PBG, and porphyrins. Because the other hepatic porphyrias (i.e., VP, HCP, and ALAD deficiency) may produce identical neuropathic syndromes and may be marked by excess excretion of PBG, ALA, or both, definitive diagnosis should be sought by the erythrocyte PBGD assay. The diagnosis of AIP types I and III can be made by demonstrating decreased PBGD activity using an erythrocyte PBGD assay.

Treatment   The same treatment is applied to all acute hepatic porphyrias, including AIP. During latent periods, when clinical manifestations are absent, management of AIP comprises adequate nutritional intake, avoidance of drugs and chemicals known to exacerbate porphyria, and prompt treatment of concurrent diseases or infections. Drug treatment should be prescribed only after reviewing a drug list. Some drugs are generally agreed to be safe in acute porphyria; some are considered unsafe [see Table 1]. Reactions to a drug, however, may be variable depending on the individual patient.

Severe cases of AIP should be treated with I.V. administration of carbohydrate (dextrose) to provide a minimum of 300 g of carbohydrate a day.[9] Intravenous hematin (4 mg/kg every 12 hours) is probably most effective in reducing ALA and PBG excretion, as well as in curtailing acute attacks.[10]

Variegate Porphyria

VP, also known as South African genetic porphyria, is caused by a heterozygous deficiency in protoporphyrinogen oxidase (PPO) activity and is inherited as an autosomal dominant trait.[2] The disease is called variegate because patients with this disorder can present with neurovisceral symptoms, photosensitivity, or both.

Epidemiology   VP is rarer than AIP but has a substantially higher incidence in South Africa (three per 1,000 population) than elsewhere.[11] In 1980, it was estimated that there were 10,000 affected individuals in South Africa, and good evidence suggests that they were all descendants of a single union between two Dutch settlers in 1688.[12,13] With the exception of the incidence of disease in South Africa, VP probably has no racial or geographic predilection. Very rare forms of VP are seen with homozygous deficiency in PPO activity.[14]

Molecular defects and pathophysiology   VP is attributed to a 50% reduction of PPO activity. PPO catalyzes the oxidation of protoporphyrinogen to yield protoporphyrin [see Figure 2]. In homozygous VP patients, which are rare, PPO mutations are found that are usually not found in heterozygous VP patients,

suggesting that the PPO mutations in homozygotes are associated with residual activity.[15]

Diagnosis   Patients with VP can have neurovisceral symptoms, photosensitivity, or both. The neurovisceral findings in VP are identical to those observed in the other acute hepatic porphyrias (e.g, abdominal pain, gastroenterologic symptoms, peripheral neuropathy, and muscle weakness). Photosensitivity and the resulting lesions tend to be more chronic in VP than in hereditary coproporphyria. Typically, lesions appear in sun-exposed areas. Blisters, as well as superficial ulcers, are present in various stages of healing and scarring. Mechanical fragility is common, especially at sites of bony protuberances such as knuckles and ankles. Skin lesions and neuropathic lesions may occur separately or together. Because the skin lesions are identical to those seen in hereditary coproporphyria and porphyria cutanea tarda, VP must be differentiated from these two conditions. The presence of neuropathic lesions without cutaneous manifestations in VP necessitates differentiation from AIP. When both cutaneous and neuropathic lesions occur in a person or kindred, hereditary coproporphyria should be considered in the differential diagnosis.

PPO activity in most patients with VP is decreased by 50%. In very rare cases of homozygous VP, however, a virtual absence of PPO activity has been documented.[16]Symptoms in homozygous VP patients are severe photosensitivity, growth and mental retardation, and marked neurologic abnormalities. Onset of the homozygous disease is in childhood. Protoporphyrin is excreted by the liver and partially reabsorbed in the gut. It must be sought in plasma and feces, where increased levels of protoporphyrin are found in 95% of VP cases. Thus, the biochemical hallmark of VP is an elevated concentration of plasma and fecal protoporphyrin IX. Plasma porphyrin analysis is more sensitive than that of fecal porphyrin analysis.[17] Increased plasma porphyrin in VP is readily detected as a fluorescence emission maximum at 626 to 628 nm.

Treatment   The treatment of neurovisceral symptoms in VP is the same as that in AIP. Cutaneous lesions are limited to sun-exposed areas, but management of VP skin lesions remains inadequate. Protection from sunlight, therefore, is an important management consideration and may include wide-brimmed hats, protective clothing, and sunscreen.

Hereditary Coproporphyria

HCP is a disease caused by a heterozygous deficiency of coproporphyrinogen oxidase (CPO) activity that is inherited as an autosomal dominant trait.[2] Clinically, the disease is similar to AIP, although it is often milder; additionally, HCP may be associated with cutaneous photosensitivity. Very rarely, homozygous deficiency of CPO occurs and is associated with a more severe form of HCP.[18]

Molecular defects and pathophysiology   CPO is a mitochondrial enzyme that catalyzes the removal of the carboxyl group and two hydrogens from the propionic groups of pyrrole rings A and B of coproporphyrinogen to form vinyl groups at these positions [see Figure 2]. Molecular analysis of several families with HCP revealed a variety of mutations in the CPO gene. These include missense, nonsense, and splicing mutations, as well as insertions and deletions. CPO activity in HCP is typically reduced by about 50% in heterozygotes and by 90% to 98% in homozygotes, who are rare.[18]

Diagnosis Neurovisceral symptoms predominate in HCP and are essentially indistinguishable from those seen in other acute hepatic porphyrias. Abdominal pain, vomiting, constipation, neuropathies, and psychiatric manifestations are common. Cutaneous photosensitivity is a feature in about 30% of cases. Attacks can be precipitated by the same factors as those that are known to aggravate AIP.

The biochemical hallmark of HCP is hyperexcretion of coproporphyrin (predominantly type III) in urine and feces. Hyperexcretion of ALA, PBG, and coproporphyrin into the urine may accompany exacerbation of the disease; however, in contrast to such findings in AIP, these findings in HCP generally return to normal between attacks.

HCP should be suspected in patients with the signs, symptoms, and clinical course characteristic of the acute hepatic porphyrias but in whom PBGD activity is normal. Urinary excretion of heme precursors in HCP is similar to that in VP, but the predominant or exclusive presence of fecal coproporphyrin is highly suggestive of HCP. Fecal or urinary predominance of harderoporphyrin, with greatly reduced CPO activity, was reported in a case of harderoporphyria,[19] a variant form of HCP.

Treatment Treatment of and prophylaxis for HCP are the same as those for VP and AIP. The use of drugs in patients with HCP should be the same as that in patients with AIP [see Table 1].

ALAD-Deficiency Porphyria

ADP is the rarest of the porphyrias; only four cases have been reported as confirmed by molecular diagnosis. The symptomatology is similar to that seen in AIP, but ADP can be differentiated from AIP by the lack of PBG overproduction. Urinary ALA excretion is greatly increased, whereas urinary PBG excretion is within the normal range. Patients with ADP display markedly decreased activity of ALAD in erythrocytes, as well as in nonerythroid cells (less than 2% of normal), and their parents typically show 50% decreases in enzyme activity.

ADP results from a marked reduction in ALAD activity caused by a homozygous enzyme deficiency [see Figure 2].[2] ALAD catalyzes the reaction that converts two molecules of ALA to form a monopyrrole, PBG, by the removal of two molecules of water. The enzyme is a homo-octamer, with a subunit size of 36,274 daltons,[20] and requires an intact sulfhydryl group and one zinc atom per subunit for full activity.[21] The human ALAD genomic structure is 16 kb in length, with two promoter regions and two alternative noncoding exons, 1A and 1B, that generate housekeeping and erythroid-keeping transcripts, respectively.[22] The two transcripts encode the same amino acid sequence, because translation begins in exon 2. Lead displaces zinc from the enzyme, resulting in an inactive enzyme and neurologic disturbances, some of which resemble those of ADP.[23] The most potent inhibitor of the enzyme is succinylacetone, a structural analogue of ALA, which is found in urine and blood of patients with hereditary tyrosinemia, who frequently develop symptoms similar to those of ADP.[24,25]

All ALAD point mutations have been studied by bacterial expression. The studies have revealed that eight of nine different mutations are unique and have markedly decreased enzyme activity, indicating the highly heterogeneous nature of the enzyme phenotypes.[26]

The clinical management of ADP is essentially identical to that of AIP.

The porphyrias associated with cutaneous photosensitivity are porphyria cutanea tarda (PCT), hepatoerythropoietic porphyria (HEP), erythropoietic protoporphyria (EPP), and congenital erythropoietic porphyria (CEP) [see Figure 1]. CEP, HEP, and EPP are also called erythropoietic porphyrias.

Porphyria Cutanea Tarda

PCT refers to a heterogeneous group of cutaneous porphyric diseases caused by uroporphyrinogen decarboxylase (UROD) deficiency, which may be either inherited or, more commonly, acquired.[2,27]

Epidemiology PCT is probably the most common of all forms of the porphyrias, but its exact incidence is not clear. The disease is recognized worldwide, and there is no racial predilection except for the high incidence of hemochromatosis found in the Bantus in South Africa. PCT was once considered more common in men, possibly because of greater alcohol intake; however, the incidence in women has recently matched that of men, which may be explained by women's use of contraceptive steroids and postmenopausal estrogens and increased alcohol intake .

Molecular defects and pathophysiology UROD is a cytosolic enzyme that catalyzes the removal of the four carboxyl groups of the carboxymethyl side chains from uroporphyrinogen to yield coproporphyrinogen [see Figure 2]. In contrast to the unique erythroid-expression mechanism for the first four enzymes of the heme biosynthetic pathway, the UROD gene has only a single promoter, and the gene is transcribed as a single mRNA.[28] Both PCT and the much rarer HEP [see Hepatoerythropoietic Porphyria, below] are characterized by a partial and a nearly complete UROD deficiency, respectively. Inherited PCT is caused by heterozygous UROD deficiency, whereas HEP is caused by homozygous UROD deficiency. Both inherited and noninherited forms of PCT display reductions in hepatic UROD activity, but erythrocyte UROD activity may or may not be decreased, depending on the clinical subtype. There are three types of PCT. Type I PCT, which accounts for 80% to 90% of all cases, is an acquired disease that typically presents in adults as decreased hepatic UROD activity but not decreased erythroid UROD activity. The disease may occur spontaneously, but it more commonly occurs in conjunction with precipitating environmental factors, such as use of alcohol, estrogen, or drugs. Type II PCT is inherited as an autosomal dominant trait and is associated with decreased UROD activity in all tissues. Type III PCT is also inherited, but the defect is confined to the UROD activity in the liver and in erythrocytes, and its protein concentrations are normal.

A variety of UROD mutations causing type II familial PCT have been identified, including missense, nonsense, and splice-site mutations; several small and large deletions; and a small insertion. In contrast to genetic defects in type II PCT, UROD mutations are not found in type I PCT.[29]

The pathogenetic processes of PCT are not fully understood. Porphyrin-mediated activation of the complement system after irradiation is implicated as one of the possible mechanisms and has been demonstrated in patients with PCT; activation of the complement system is presumed to result from the generation of reactive oxygen species, most likely singlet oxygen.[30]

Diagnosis The pathognomonic clinical feature of PCT is the formation of vesicles on sun-exposed areas of the skin, particularly the dorsal aspects of the hands, as well as on the face, forearms, and legs. The vesicles are superseded by crusting, su-

perficial scarring, or milia formation and by residual pigmentation. Facial hypertrichosis may be present and is conspicuous in women. Iron, estrogens, alcohol, viral hepatitis, and chlorinated hydrocarbons can aggravate PCT.[31] Mild iron overload is nearly always present in patients with PCT. Iron plays a particularly important role in the symptomatology of PCT, in that phlebotomy to decrease hepatic iron overload is effective in treating PCT [see Treatment, below], whereas iron supplementation results in

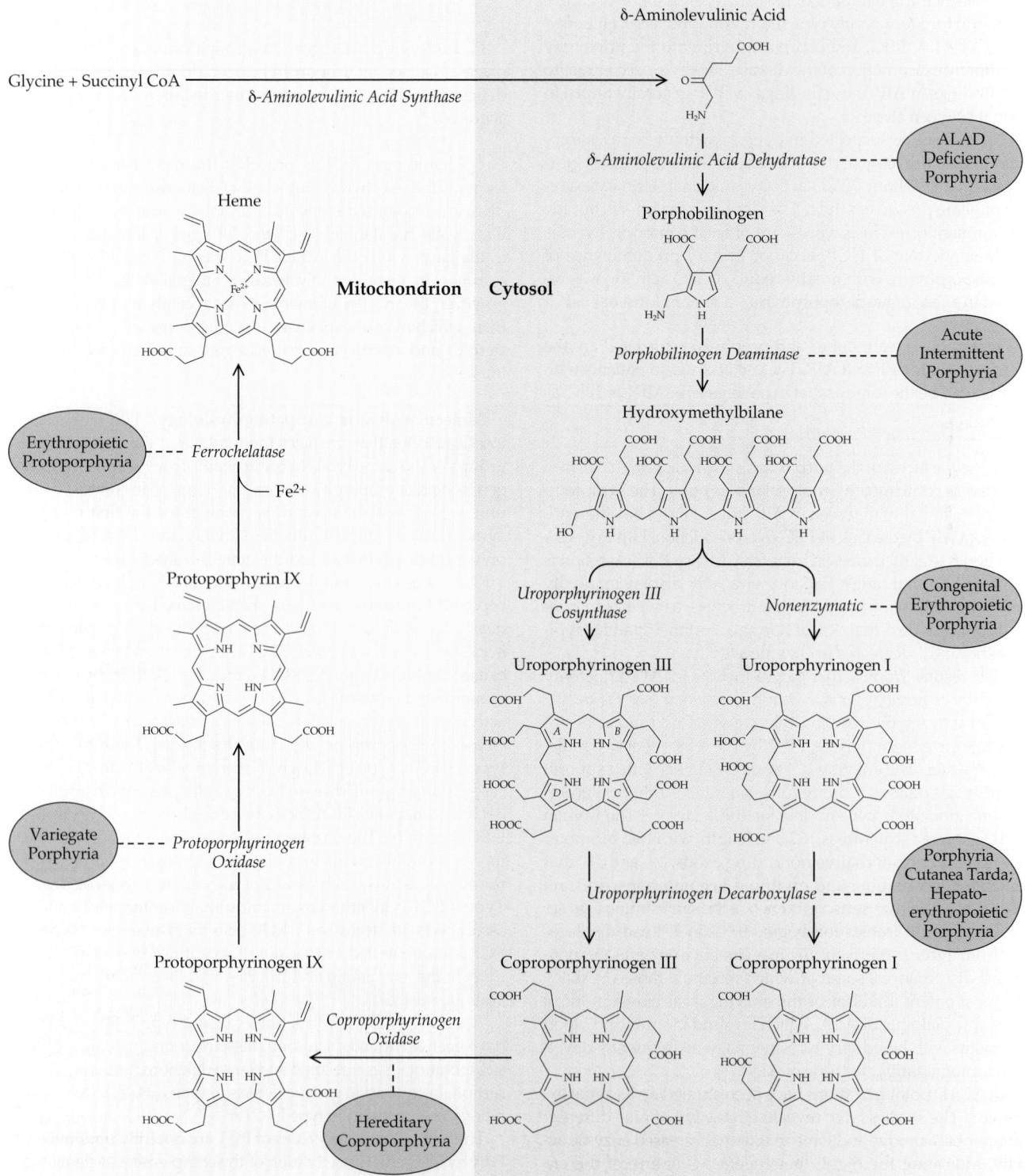

Table 1 Safe and Unsafe Drugs for Patients with Acute Intermittent Porphyria, Variegate Porphyria, Hereditary Coproporphyria, or ALA Dehydratase Deficiency Porphyria

Safe Drugs		Unsafe Drugs	
Acetaminophen	Heme arginate	Barbiturates[†]	Nifedipine
Acetazolamide	Heparin	Captopril	Oral contraceptives[‡]
Acyclovir	Insulin	Chloramphenicol[†]	Orphenadrine[†]
Allopurinol	Iron	Chlordiazepoxide[†]	Oxycodone
Amiloride		Chlorpropamide[†]	
Ampicillin	Lithium salts		Pentazocine[†]
Aspirin	Meperidine	Diazepam[‡]	Phenobarbital[†]
Atropine	Mequitazine	Diltiazem	Phenytoin[†]
	Metformin	Diphenhydramine	Piroxicam
Bumetanide	Metoprolol	Doxycycline	Pivampicillin[†]
Bupivacaine	Morphine		Progesterone[†]
Buprenorphine		Ergot compounds[†]	Pyrazinamide[†]
	Nadolol	Erythromycin	
Chlorothiazide*		Estrogen	Sodium valproate[‡]
Codeine phosphate	Oxytocin	Ethanol[†]	
Corticosteroids*			Terfenadine
	Penicillin	Furosemide[‡]	Tetracyclines[‡]
Deferoxamine	Procaine		Theophylline[†]
Demerol	Propofol	Griseofulvin[†]	Trimethoprim
Digoxin	Propylthiouracil		
		Hydralazine	Verapamil
Fentanyl	Quinine	Hydrochlorothiazide[‡]	
Follicle-stimulating hormone (FSH)	Ranitidine*	Imipramine[†]	
	Salbutamol	Lidocaine	
Gabapentin	Senna		
Gentamicin		Methyldopa[†]	
Glipizide	Temazepam	Metoclopramide[‡]	
	Thyroxine	Metronidazole	
Haloperidol	Warfarin		

Note: See also the American Porphyria Foundation Web site, at http://www.porphyriafoundation.com. The American Porphyria Foundation charges a nominal fee to access their site.
*Has produced conflicting results (occasionally positive but mainly negative) in experiments on porphyrinogenicity. None of the safe drugs listed has been associated with human porphyric attacks.
[†]Has been associated with acute attacks of porphyria.
[‡]Has produced conflicting results (some positive, some negative) in experiments on porphyrinogenicity.

relapse of PCT. A significant number of PCT patients have associated hemochromatosis gene (*HFE*) mutations.[32] Isocoproporphyrin, unique to PCT and HEP, may be detected in serum or in stool and is diagnostic of PCT. Plasma porphyrin levels are increased in PCT, HEP, and other photosensitizing porphyrias. In PCT, serum ferritin levels are also typically elevated.

Although many PCT patients have moderately excessive alcohol intake or hepatitis C infection, few have advanced liver disease at the time of initial presentation. However, liver abnormalities are seen even in patients without heavy alcohol intake or hepatitis C, indicating PCT itself is associated with liver damage. PCT appears to increase the risk for hepatocellular carcinoma in patients with chronic liver disease.[33]

Treatment The identification and avoidance of precipitating factors represent the first line of treatment, particularly for patients with type I PCT. Abstinence from alcohol ingestion should be recommended in all types of PCT.

Figure 2 **The initial rate-limiting step in the synthesis of heme is the synthesis of δ-aminolevulinic acid (ALA) from glycine and succinyl–coenzyme A (succinyl-CoA). This step is catalyzed by the intramitochondrial enzyme ALA synthase. The next step, which takes place in the cytosol, consists of the condensation of two molecules of ALA by the enzyme ALA dehydratase (ALAD) to form the ring pyrrole, porphobilinogen. Porphobilinogen contains two carboxyl residues, acetate (– CH_2COOH) and propionate (– CH_2CH_2COOH) and is water soluble. Porphobilinogen deaminase catalyzes the third step in the biosynthesis of heme, involving the sequential condensation of four molecules of porphobilinogen, yielding the first tetrapyrrole in the biosynthetic pathway, hydroxymethylbilane. In the presence of uroporphyrinogen III cosynthase, hydroxymethylbilane is rapidly converted to uroporphyrinogen III, the vital substrate for subsequent porphyrin and heme formation. In the absence of uroporphyrinogen III cosynthase, hydroxymethylbilane is converted nonenzymatically to the nonphysiologic porphyrin isomer, uroporphyrinogen I. Only uroporphyrinogen III is a precursor of heme. Partial decarboxylation of uroporphyrinogen III yields coproporphyrinogen III, which contains four carboxyl groups. Coproporphyrinogen III reenters the mitochondrion and is oxidized by coproporphyrinogen oxidase to form protoporphyrinogen IX, with a loss of two more propionate residues. The enzyme protoporphyrinogen oxidase catalyzes futher oxidation of the molecule, with a loss of six hydrogen atoms, to form protoporphyrin IX. Finally, the insertion of Fe^{2+} by the mitochondrial enzyme ferrochelatase completes the synthesis of heme. Heme may inhibit ALA-synthase activity directly but also acts to repress synthesis of the enzyme. The porphyrias are caused by inherited defects in specific enzymes in the heme synthetic pathway. A partial blockage at any step in the pathway, when combined with certain endogenous or exogenous factors, results in an overproduction of intermediates or of products normally produced only in small amounts and is associated with overt clinical disease.**

The cornerstone of therapy for all types of PCT is depletion of iron, even in patients lacking biochemical evidence of iron overload. Repeated phlebotomy of one unit of blood twice monthly for a total of 2.5 to 7.5 L, with treatment guided by the patient's hematocrit, serum transferrin saturation, and ferritin levels, decreases both uroporphyrin excretion and photosensitivity. Improvement occurs within several months to a year. Patients who are on hemodialysis, who are anemic, or who cannot tolerate phlebotomy should receive erythropoietin. Subcutaneous infusion of desferrioxamine by portable syringe pump (1.0 to 1.5 g in 8 to 10 ml of sterile water for 8 to 10 hours 5 nights a week for 2 to 5 months) is also effective.[34]

If phlebotomy is ineffective or contraindicated, low-dose chloroquine therapy may also be considered. Chloroquine, which forms complexes with uroporphyrin, has produced improvement over 3 to 6 months; however, hepatotoxicity may occur. Resolution of type 1 PCT has followed successful interferon therapy for HCV infection.[35] Recombinant erythropoietin administration is now the treatment of choice for PCT patients with end-stage renal disease, because it can correct anemia, mobilize iron, and support phlebotomy in this condition.

Hepatoerythropoietic Porphyria

HEP is a rare form of porphyria resulting from a homozygous deficiency of UROD.[36] Individuals in HEP families who have heterozygous UROD deficiency usually do not have clinical symptoms. HEP is characterized clinically by the childhood onset of severe photosensitivity and skin fragility and is indistinguishable from CEP. Some 20 cases have been reported.

Molecular defects and pathophysiology As in PCT, HEP is caused by a UROD deficiency [see Figure 2]. A variety of UROD mutations have been identified in HEP patients, indicating the molecular heterogeneity of the disease. Most UROD mutations in HEP have not been found in familial PCT and are associated with residual UROD activity.[29]

Diagnosis Clinical findings of HEP are very similar to those of CEP. Pink urine, severe photosensitivity leading to scarring and mutilation of sun-exposed areas of skin, sclerodermoid changes, hypertrichosis, erythrodontia, anemia (often hemolytic), and hepatosplenomegaly are characteristic features of HEP. In contrast to PCT, serum iron concentrations are usually normal, and phlebotomy has no beneficial effects in patients with HEP. Isocoproporphyrin concentrations are equal to or greater than concentrations of coproporphyrin found in urine and feces, and although the reasons are unclear, an elevated erythrocyte zinc protoporphyrin concentration is commonly observed.

Urinary fluorescence under ultraviolet light and quantitation and identification of isocoproporphyrin by thin-layer or high-performance liquid chromatography establish the diagnosis of HEP.

As in other photosensitizing porphyrias, plasma porphyrin levels are elevated in HEP. Fecal porphyrin levels are often elevated. The detection of isocoproporphyrin in feces is diagnostic of HEP and PCT. The diagnosis of HEP should be suspected in patients with severe photosensitivity and should especially be included in the differential diagnosis of CEP.

Treatment The identification and avoidance of precipitating factors represent the first line of treatment for PCT. In contrast to treatment for PCT, avoidance of the sun and the use of topical sun-

screens are essentially all that can be recommended to patients with HEP; phlebotomy, which is most useful for treatment of PCT, provides no beneficial response in patients with this disorder.

Erythropoietic Protoporphyria

EPP is due to a partial deficiency of ferrochelatase and is inherited as an autosomal dominant trait.[2] Biochemically, this defect results in massive accumulations of protoporphyrin in erythrocytes, plasma, and feces. Clinically, the disease is characterized by the childhood onset of cutaneous photosensitivity in light-exposed areas, but skin lesions are milder and less disfiguring than those in CEP. EPP is the most common form of the erythropoietic porphyrias. There is no racial or sexual predilection, and onset is typically in childhood.

Molecular defects and pathophysiology Ferrochelatase catalyzes the final reaction in heme biosynthesis—that is, the insertion of iron into protoporphyrin IX. Unlike other steps in the heme biosynthetic pathway, this mitochondrial enzyme utilizes protoporphyrin IX, rather than its reduced form (i.e., protoporphyrinogen IX), as substrate. However, the enzyme specifically requires the reduced form of iron (i.e., ferrous, not ferric, iron) [see Figure 2]. The gene for human ferrochelatase has been assigned to chromosome 18q21.3.

EPP patients have only 10% to 25% of normal ferrochelatase activity, whereas their asymptomatic family members typically have 50% ferrochelatase activity. A normal coding ferrochelatase sequence allele, expressed at a lower than normal level,[37] is present in about 10% of the white population. Inheritance of a ferrochelatase mutation in cis and the low expression allele in trans appears to account for the markedly low ferrochelatase activity and clinical expression of the disease.[37]

Light-excited porphyrins generate free radicals and singlet oxygen.[38] Such radicals, notably singlet oxygen, can lead to peroxidation of lipids and cross-linking of membrane proteins, which, in erythrocytes, can result in reduced deformability and thus hemolysis. Protoporphyrin IX, but not zinc protoporphyrin IX, can be released from erythrocytes after irradiation.[39] This finding explains why patients with EPP exhibit elevated levels of free protoporphyrin in plasma and manifest photosensitivity, whereas patients with lead intoxication and iron deficiency, who have elevated zinc protoporphyrin levels in erythrocytes, do not exhibit photosensitivity.[40]

Diagnosis Cutaneous photosensitivity of EPP is quite different from that of CEP or PCT. Stinging or painful burning sensations of the skin occur within 1 hour after exposure to the sun and are followed several hours later by erythema and edema. Petechiae or, more rarely, purpura, vesicles, and crusting may develop and may persist for several days after sun exposure. Symptoms are usually worse during spring and summer and occur in light-exposed skin. Excoriations secondary to scratching may be present. Recurrence of the lesions as a result of chronic sun exposure may result in onycholysis, scarring, altered pigmentation, lichenification, and premature aging of the skin. Gallstones, sometimes presenting at an early age, are fairly common in patients with EPP, and hepatic disease, although unusual, may be severe and associated with significant morbidity.

The biochemical hallmark of EPP is excessive concentrations of protoporphyrin in erythrocytes, plasma, bile, and feces—but not in urine, because of the poor solubility of protoporphyrin in water.

Photosensitivity should suggest the diagnosis of EPP, which can be confirmed by the demonstration of increased concentrations of free protoporphyrin in erythrocytes, plasma, and stool and normal levels of urinary porphyrins. The presence of protoporphyrin in both plasma and erythrocytes is a finding specific for EPP. Fluorescent reticulocytes on examination of peripheral blood smear also suggest the diagnosis.

Treatment Avoidance of the sun and use of topical sunscreen agents are helpful in the management of EPP. Oral administration of β-carotene can afford systemic photoprotection, resulting in improved, although highly variable, tolerance to the sun. The recommended serum β-carotene level of 600 to 800 μg/dl is usually achieved with oral dosages of 120 to 180 mg daily, and beneficial effects are typically seen 1 to 3 months after the therapy is begun. The mechanism of this beneficial effect of β-carotene probably involves quenching of activated oxygen radicals.[41]

Congenital Erythropoietic Porphyria

CEP, which is also referred to as Günther disease, is an autosomal recessive disorder caused by a homozygous deficiency of the cytosolic enzyme, uroporphyrinogen cosynthase (UCS). The enzymatic defect results in accumulation and hyperexcretion of predominantly type I porphyrins.[2] Fewer than 200 cases have been reported, and some of these cases may have been PCT or HEP. No clear racial or sexual predilection is apparent.[2]

Molecular defects and pathophysiology UCS catalyzes the formation of uroporphyrinogen III (UROIII) from hydroxymethylbilane (HMB). In the absence of UCS, HMB is converted nonenzymatically to uroporphyrin I, which is then enzymatically converted to coproporphyrin I [*see Figure* 2]. Excess porphyrin causes the staining of bones and teeth (erythrodontia), hemolysis, dark urine, and photosensitivity, all of which are usually identified early in infancy.

Similar to the *ALAD* and *PBGD* genes, the *UCS* gene has alternative promoters that generate housekeeping and erythroid transcripts.[39] A heterogeneity of mutations in the *UCS* gene is found in patients with CEP. A Cys[73] → Arg point mutation appears to occur more frequently than others, because it has been found in eight of 21 unrelated patients with CEP (about 21% of CEP alleles).[42]

Diagnosis The first clue suggesting the diagnosis of CEP at birth is pink to dark-brown staining of diapers, which is caused by large amounts of porphyrins in the urine. Early onset of cutaneous photosensitivity is characteristic and is exacerbated by exposure to sunlight. Subepidermal bullous lesions progress to crusted erosions that heal with scarring and either hyperpigmentation or, less commonly, hypopigmentation. Hypertrichosis and alopecia are frequent and erythrodontia (appearing as red fluorescence under ultraviolet light) is pathognomonic of CEP. Patients may display symptoms and signs of hemolytic anemia with splenomegaly and porphyrin-rich gallstones. Bone marrow shows erythroid hyperplasia, which may result in pathologic fractures or vertebral compression-collapse and shortness of stature. Urinary levels of uroporphyrins and coproporphyrins are always elevated (20- to 60-fold), with predominant elevations of type I isomers.

Pink urine or the onset of severe cutaneous photosensitivity in infancy (and rarely in adults) suggests the diagnosis of CEP.

Demonstration of increased levels of urinary, fecal, and erythrocyte porphyrins, together with elevated type I isomers of uroporphyrin and coproporphyrin, establish the diagnosis of CEP.

Treatment The avoidance of sunlight, trauma to the skin, and infections is the most important preventive measure. Topical sunscreens may be of some help, as may oral administration of β-carotene. Transfusions with packed erythrocytes transiently decrease hemolysis and its attendant drive to increased erythropoiesis and also decrease porphyrin excretion by suppressing erythropoiesis in the bone marrow. Bone marrow transplantation is curative.[43]

The authors have no commercial relationships with manufacturers of products or providers of services discussed in this chapter.

References

1. Sassa S: The hematological aspects of porphyrias. Williams Hematology. Beutler E, Lichtman MA, Coller BS, et al, Eds. McGraw-Hill, New York, 2001, p703

2. Kappas A, Sassa S, Galbraith RA, et al: The porphyrias. The Metabolic and Molecular Basis of Inherited Disease. Scriver CR, Beaudet AL, Sly WS, et al, Eds. McGraw-Hill, New York, 1995, p 2103

3. Grandchamp B, Beaumont C, de Verneuil H, et al: Genetic expression of porphobilinogen deaminase and uroporphyrinogen decarboxylase during the erythroid differentiation of mouse erythroleukemic cells. Porphyrins and Porphyrias. Nordmann Y, Ed. John Libbey & Company Ltd, London, 1986, p 35

4. Romeo PH, Chretien S, Dubart A, et al: Erythroid specific promoter of a housekeeping gene. Prog Clin Biol Res 251:55, 1987

5. Grandchamp B, Picat C, Mignotte V, et al: Tissue-specific splicing mutation in acute intermittent porphyria. Proc Natl Acad Sci USA 86:661, 1989

6. Grandchamp B, Picat C, de Rooij F, et al: A point mutation G → A in exon 12 of the porphobilinogen deaminase gene results in exon skipping and is responsible for acute intermittent porphyria. Nucl Acids Res 17:6637, 1989

7. Elder GH, Hift RT, Meissner PN: The acute porphyrias. Lancet 349:1613, 1997

8. Andersson C, Innala E, Backstrom T: Acute intermittent porphyria in women: clinical expression, use and experience of exogenous sex hormones: a population-based study in northern Sweden. J Intern Med 254:176, 2003

9. Sassa S: Diagnosis and therapy of acute intermittent porphyria. Blood Reviews 10:53, 1996

10. Mustajoki P, Tenhunen R, Pierach C, et al: Heme in the treatment of porphyrias and hematological disorders. Semin Hematol 26:1, 1989

11. Eales L, Day RS, Blekkenhorst G.H: The clinical and biochemical features of variegate porphyria: an analysis of 300 cases studied at Groote Schuur Hospital, Cape Town. Int J Biochem 12:837, 1980

12. Dean G.: The porphyrias: a study of inheritance and environment. Pitman Medical, London, 1971

13. Meissner PN, Dailey TA, Hift RJ, et al: A R59W mutation in human protoporphyrinogen oxidase results in decreased enzyme activity and is prevalent in South Africans with variegate porphyria. Nature 13:95, 1996

14. Roberts AG, Whatley SD, Daniels J, et al: Partial characterization and assignment of the gene for protoporphyrinogen oxidase and variegate porphyrias to human chromosome 1q23. Human Mol Genet 4:2387, 1995

15. Frank J, McGrath J, Lam H, et al: Homozygous variegate porphyria: identification of mutations on both alleles of the protoporphyrinogen oxidase gene in a severely affected proband. J Invest Dermatol 110:452, 1998

16. Kordac V, Martasek P, Zeman J, et al: Increased erythrocyte protoporphyrin in homozygous variegate porphyria. Photo-Dermatology 2:257, 1985

17. Hift RJ, Meissner D, Meissner PN: A systematic study of the clinical and biochemical expression of variegate porphyria in a large South African family. Br J Dermatol 151:465, 2004

18. Grandchamp B, Phung N, Nordmann Y: Homozygous case of hereditary coproporphyria. Lancet 2:1348, 1977

19. Nordmann Y, Grandchamp B, de Verneuil H, et al: Harderoporphyria: a variant hereditary coproporphyria. J Clin Invest 72:1139, 1983

20. Wetmur JG, Bishop DF, Ostasiewicz L, et al: Molecular cloning of a cDNA for human δ-aminolevulinate dehydratase. Gene 43:123, 1986

21. Sassa S: δ-Aminolevulinic acid dehydratase assay. Enzyme 28:133, 1982

22. Kaya AH, Plewinska M, Wong DM, et al: Human δ-aminolevulinate dehydratase (ALAD) gene: structure and alternative splicing of the erythroid and housekeeping mRNAs. Genomics 19:242, 1994

23. Granick JL, Sassa S, Kappas A: Some biochemical and clinical aspects of lead intoxication. Advances in Clinical Chemistry. Bodansky O, Latner AL, Eds. Academic Press, New York, 1978, p 287

24. Lindblad B, Lindstedt S, Steen G: On the genetic defects in hereditary tyrosinemia. Proc Natl Acad Sci USA 74:4641, 1977

25. Sassa S, Kappas A: Hereditary tyrosinemia and the heme biosynthetic pathway. Profound inhibition of δ-aminolevulinic acid dehydratase activity by succinylacetone. J Clin Invest 71:625, 1983

26. Maruno M, Furuyama K, Akagi R, et al: Highly heterogenous nature of δ-aminolevulinate dehydratase (ALAD) deficiencies in ALAD porphyria. Blood 97:2972, 2001

27. de Verneuil H, Nordmann Y, Phung N, et al: Familial and sporadic porphyria cutanea: two different diseases. Int J Biochem 9:927, 1978

28. Romeo PH, Raich N, Dubart A, et al: Molecular cloning and tissue-specific expression analysis of human porphobilinogen deaminase and uroporphyrinogen decarboxylase. Porphyrins and Porphyrias. Nordmann Y, Ed. John Libbey & Company Ltd, London, 1986, p 25

29. Elder GH: Porphyria cutanea tarda. Semin Liver Dis 18:67, 1998

30. Lim HW, Poh-Fitzpatrick MB, Gigli I: Activation of the complement system in patients with porphyrias after irradiation in vivo. J Clin Invest 74:1961, 1984

31. Blauvelt A, Harris HR, Hogan DJ, et al: Porphyria cutanea tarda and human immunodeficiency virus infection. Int J Dermatol 31:474, 1992

32. Bulaj ZJ, Phillips JD, Ajioka RS, et al: Hemochromatosis genes and other factors contributing to the pathogenesis of porphyria cutanea tarda. Blood 95:1565, 2000

33. Fracanzani AL, Taioli E, Sampietro M, et al: Liver cancer risk is increased in patients with porphyria cutanea tarda in comparison to matched control patients with chronic liver disease. J Hepatol 35:498, 2001

34. Gilbertini P, Rocchi E, Cassanelli A, et al: Advances in the treatment of porphyria cutanea tarda: effectiveness of slow subcutaneous desferrioxamine infusion. Liver 4:280, 1984

35. Sheikh MY, Wright RA, Burruss JB: Dramatic resolution of skin lesions associated with porphyria cutanea tarda after interferon-alpha therapy in a case of chronic hepatitis C. Dig Dis Sci 43:529, 1998

36. Elder GH, Smith SG, Herrero C, et al: Hepatoerythropoietic porphyria: a new uroporphyrinogen decarboxylase defect or homozygous porphyria cutanea tarda? Lancet 1:916, 1981

37. Gouya L, Puy H, Lamoril J, et al: Inheritance in erythropoietic protoporphyria: a common wild-type ferrochelatase allelic variant with low expression accounts for clinical manifestation. Blood 93:2105, 1999

38. Spikes JD: Porphyrins and related compounds as photodynamic sensitizers. Ann NY Acad Sci 244:496, 1975

39. Aizencang GI, Bishop DF, Forrest D, et al: Uroporphyrinogen III synthase. an alternative promoter controls erythroid-specific expression in the murine gene. J Biol Chem 275:2295, 2000

40. Sandberg S, Talstad I, Hovding G, et al: Light-induced release of protoporphyrin, but not of zinc protoporphyrin, from erythrocytes in a patient with greatly elevated erythropoietic protoporphyria. Blood 62:846, 1983

41. Mathews-Roth MM: Systemic photoprotection. Dermatol Clin 4:335, 1986

42. Solis C, Aizencang GI, Astrin KH, et al: Uroporphyrinogen III synthase erythroid promoter mutations in adjacent GATA1 and CP2 elements cause congenital erythropoietic porphyria. J Clin Invest 107:753, 2001

43. Harada FA, Shwayder TA, Desnick RJ, et al: Treatment of severe congenital erythropoietic porphyria by bone marrow transplantation. J Am Acad Dermatol 45:279, 2001

61 Esophageal Disorders

Stuart Jon Spechler, M.D.

Approach to the Patient with Dysphagia

The esophagus is susceptible to three types of diseases that cause dysphagia [*see Table 1*]: (1) mucosal (intrinsic) diseases that narrow the lumen of the esophagus through inflammation, fibrosis, or neoplasia; (2) mediastinal (extrinsic) diseases that encase and obstruct the esophagus by direct invasion or through lymph node enlargement; and (3) diseases affecting the esophageal muscle or its innervation (esophageal motility disorders) that disrupt peristalsis, interfere with sphincter relaxation, or both. The American Gastroenterological Association has endorsed algorithms summarizing the approach to the patient with dysphagia [*see Figures 1 through 4*].[1]

CLINICAL EVALUATION

History

On the basis of a careful history alone, the astute clinician can determine the cause of dysphagia in approximately 80% of patients.[2] Eight questions form the key elements of the history.

Is the dysphagia for solid foods, liquids, or both? Mucosal and mediastinal diseases that involve the esophagus cause dysphagia by narrowing the lumen. Such mechanical narrowing usually does not impede the passage of liquids, and consequently, such a disease causes dysphagia for solid foods only. Diseases that disrupt peristalsis, however, may cause dysphagia for both solids and liquids. Of the esophageal motility disorders, achalasia is the one most likely to cause dysphagia for liquids. In achalasia, chronic contraction of the lower esophageal sphincter (LES) causes complete mechanical obstruction of the esophagus that persists until either the sphincter relaxes or the hydrostatic pressure of the retained material exceeds the pressure generated by the sphincter muscle. Even in the absence of peristalsis, gravity often can empty the esophagus of liquid effectively, provided that the LES is relaxed. Therefore, patients who have disordered peristalsis with an LES that is profoundly hypotensive often experience no dysphagia or experience dysphagia only for solid foods.

Where does the patient perceive that ingested material sticks? Patients with esophageal strictures often perceive that swallowed material sticks at a point that is either above or at the level of the stricture.[3] It is uncommon for patients to perceive that swallowed material is stuck below the obstructing lesion. Thus, the history that a swallowed bolus sticks above the suprasternal notch is of little value in localizing the obstruction, because this sensation could be caused by a lesion located anywhere from the pharynx to the gastroesophageal junction. If the patient localizes the obstruction to a point below the suprasternal notch, however, then it is highly likely that the dysphagia is caused by an esophageal disorder.

Are there symptoms of oropharyngeal dysfunction? Oropharyngeal dysfunction often results from diseases that affect the striated muscles of the oropharynx or their innervation. Examples include muscular dystrophies, dermatomyositis,

myasthenia gravis, and cerebrovascular accidents.[4] Patients with these neuromuscular diseases may experience difficulty in initiating a swallow, and swallowing may be accompanied by nasopharyngeal regurgitation, pulmonary aspiration, and a sensation that residual material remains in the pharynx. If any of these symptoms are prominent, evaluation for oropharyngeal dysfunction (e.g., with videofluoroscopy) is appropriate.

Is the dysphagia intermittent or progressive? Patients who have a lower esophageal mucosal (Schatzki) ring (see below) typically complain of discrete episodes of dysphagia for solid foods that are intermittent and nonprogressive. The episodes often occur during meals in restaurants (hence the term steakhouse syndrome) or at social functions. Dysphagia episodes may be separated by a period of weeks, months, or years, and the patient typically experiences no swallowing difficulty between episodes. In contrast, esophageal strictures usually cause dysphagia that is progressive in frequency and severity. With benign strictures, the progression is typically slow and insidious (over a period of months to years), and weight loss is minimal. Malignant esophageal strictures usually cause dysphagia that progresses rapidly (over a period of weeks to months), and weight loss may be profound.

Is there a history of chronic heartburn? Heartburn is the cardinal symptom of gastroesophageal reflux disease (GERD). Thus, a history of chronic heartburn supports the possibility that dysphagia may result from a peptic esophageal stricture. However, up to 25% of patients with peptic strictures have no antecedent history of heartburn. Furthermore, the majority of patients with dysphagia from adenocarcinoma in Barrett esophagus have a history of long-standing heartburn. Also, around 30% of patients with achalasia complain of heartburn. Therefore, conclusions regarding the etiology of dysphagia should not be based primarily on the presence or absence of heartburn.

Has the patient taken medications likely to cause pill esophagitis? A number of medications taken in pill form are

Table 1   Diseases of the Esophagus That Cause Dysphagia

Mucosal diseases	Gastroesophageal reflux disease (peptic stricture)
	Esophageal rings
	Esophageal tumors
	Caustic injury (e.g., lye ingestion, pill esophagitis, sclerotherapy)
	Radiation injury
	Infectious esophagitis
Mediastinal diseases	Tumors (e.g., lung cancer, lymphoma)
	Infections (e.g., tuberculosis, histoplasmosis)
Diseases affecting smooth muscle and its innervation	Achalasia
	Scleroderma
	Other motility disorders

757

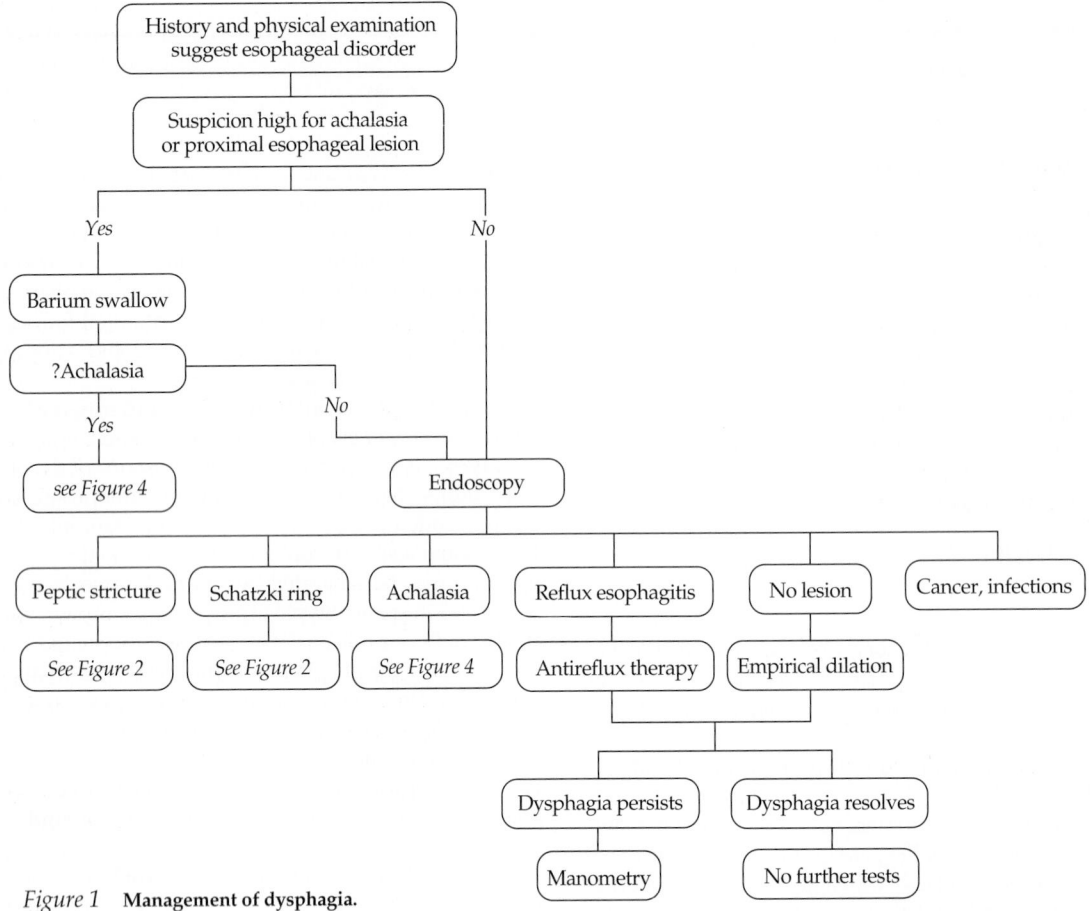

Figure 1 **Management of dysphagia.**

potentially caustic to the esophagus and can cause ulceration with stricture formation if they have prolonged contact with the esophageal mucosa. Although a large number of medications have been reported to cause pill esophagitis, most cases have been caused by antibiotics (e.g., doxycycline), potassium chloride preparations, nonsteroidal anti-inflammatory drugs (NSAIDs), and quinidine.

Is there a history of collagen vascular disease? Collagen vascular diseases such as scleroderma, rheumatoid arthritis, and systemic lupus erythematosus can cause disordered esophageal motility that is often associated with Raynaud phenomenon.[5] In scleroderma and related collagen vascular disorders, fibrosis and vascular obliteration in gut smooth muscle cause poor esophageal contractility and weakness of the lower esophageal sphincter that predisposes to severe GERD. Also, patients with collagen vascular disease often are treated with medications, such as NSAIDs, that can cause pill esophagitis. Consequently, dysphagia associated with collagen vascular disease may be the result of disordered esophageal motility, severe GERD, pill esophagitis, or some combination thereof.

Is the patient immunosuppressed? Infectious esophagitis occurs most often in patients whose immune system has been compromised by infection with HIV, by advanced malignancy, or by organ transplantation with the administration of potent immunosuppressive drugs. Odynophagia is usually the predominant symptom in infectious esophagitis, but most patients with this disease also experience dysphagia.[6] In rare cases, esophageal stricture can be a late complication of infectious esophagitis.

Physical Examination

The physical examination of the patient with dysphagia is important primarily for assessing the patient's nutritional status and ability to tolerate the invasive procedures that may be considered to treat the esophageal disorder. Only infrequently does the physical examination provide specific clues to the etiology of dysphagia. For patients with dysphagia caused by collagen vascular disease, physical examination may reveal characteristic features such as joint abnormalities, calcinosis, telangiectasias, sclerodactyly, proximal muscle weakness, and rashes. A palpable left supraclavicular (Virchow) lymph node suggests dysphagia from a malignancy in the abdomen (e.g., adenocarcinoma of the esophagogastric junction). Also, the physical examination may reveal evidence of a neuromuscular disorder that can interfere with swallowing (e.g., Parkinson disease).

DIAGNOSTIC TESTS

Testing in patients with dysphagia generally starts with barium swallow or endoscopy. If initial testing discloses an esophageal motility disorder, manometry may then be done. Videofluoroscopy, in which a motion recording is made while the patient swallows barium suspensions and barium-coated materials, is an excellent technique for assessing oropharyngeal function but generally is not needed for evaluating esophageal disorders.

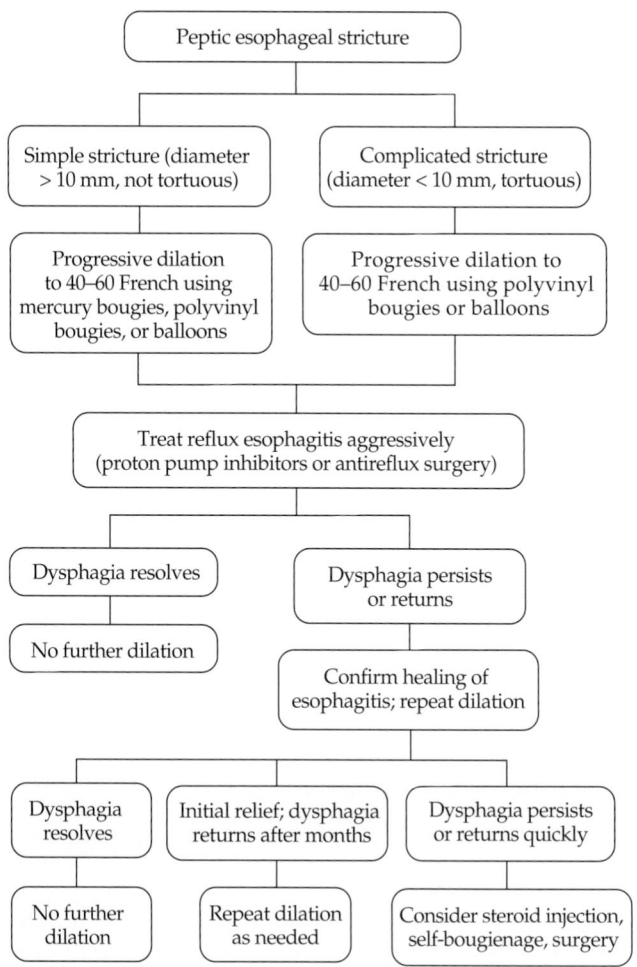

Figure 2 **Management of peptic esophageal stricture.**

There is an unresolved debate about whether to start the evaluation of dysphagia with a barium swallow or with esophageal endoscopy. Proponents of the latter approach argue that endoscopy is almost always required to evaluate dysphagia, for both diagnostic and therapeutic purposes, and that a barium swallow usually does not provide sufficient additional information to justify its expense and inconvenience. On the other side of the argument are those who contend that a barium swallow can provide valuable anatomic information about the esophagus that may help direct therapy and prevent procedural complications. In the absence of studies validating the cost-effectiveness of either approach, this debate continues.

Barium Swallow

A barium contrast examination can be more sensitive than endoscopy for detecting subtle narrowings of the esophagus (e.g., rings, peptic strictures greater than 10 mm in diameter) and for identifying esophageal dysmotility.[7] A barium swallow may be especially helpful in suggesting the diagnoses of achalasia and diffuse esophageal spasm, conditions that may be difficult to identify endoscopically. The early radiographic demonstration of achalasia may spare the patient repeat endoscopy, a situation that can occur because the endoscopist either did not recognize the disorder on the initial evaluation or was not prepared to perform endoscopic therapy at that time. A barium swallow can identify lesions that may pose potential

hazards or confuse the endoscopist, such as a large Zenker diverticulum or an epiphrenic diverticulum. For patients with an esophageal stricture, a barium swallow can provide information on the extent and severity of the lesion that may help in choosing the type of dilator to be used for treatment. Finally, an initial barium swallow provides an objective baseline record of the esophagus that can be useful in assessing the response to therapy or progression of disease.

Endoscopy

For virtually all patients with dysphagia of esophageal origin, endoscopy is recommended to establish or confirm a diagnosis, seek evidence of esophagitis and malignancy, and implement therapy when appropriate. The endoscopist can obtain biopsy and brush cytology specimens of esophageal lesions that may establish the diagnosis of neoplasms or specific infections. Endoscopy also is more sensitive than radiology for identifying subtle mucosal lesions of the esophagus (e.g., mild esophagitis).

Esophageal Manometry

Esophageal manometry is the gold standard test for esophageal motility disorders. Esophageal manometry has been shown to be especially useful for establishing the diagnoses of achalasia and diffuse esophageal spasm and for detecting esophageal motor abnormalities associated with collagen vascular diseases.[8]

For patients with dysphagia, the history and the results of the barium swallow or endoscopy can be used to decide whether esophageal manometry is indicated. An esophageal motility study usually is not needed for patients with mechanical causes of dysphagia, such as peptic strictures or rings, unless their dysphagia persists despite appropriate treatment. For patients thought to have dysphagia caused by motility abnormalities associated with collagen vascular diseases, manometry need not be performed routinely if dysphagia responds to treatment of any associated reflux esophagitis and esophageal stenoses. If the dysphagia persists despite such treatment, manometry can establish the nature of the motility problem.

Dysphagia from Benign Esophageal Strictures and Rings

BENIGN ESOPHAGEAL STRICTURES

Strictures develop from severe esophageal inflammation, usually associated with ulceration, that stimulates fibrous tissue production and collagen deposition. Approximately two thirds of all cases of benign esophageal stricture in the United States are caused by reflux esophagitis (so-called peptic strictures).[9] The remainder are the result of caustic ingestions (e.g., lye), pill esophagitis, infectious esophagitis, and radiation esophagitis.

Treatment

Benign esophageal strictures usually are treated with dilation [*see Figure 2*]. Three major types of esophageal dilating devices are used commonly: (1) mercury-filled bougies that are passed blindly through the mouth (e.g., tapered-tipped Maloney dilators, blunt-tipped Hurst dilators); (2) polyvinyl bougies that can be passed over a fine guide wire that is positioned in the stricture, under either fluoroscopic or endoscopic guidance (e.g., Savary dilators), and (3) balloon dilators that are passed either over a guide wire or through the endoscope (so-called through-the-scope [TTS] balloons). Usually, the physician passes a series of dilators of increasing diameter to stretch

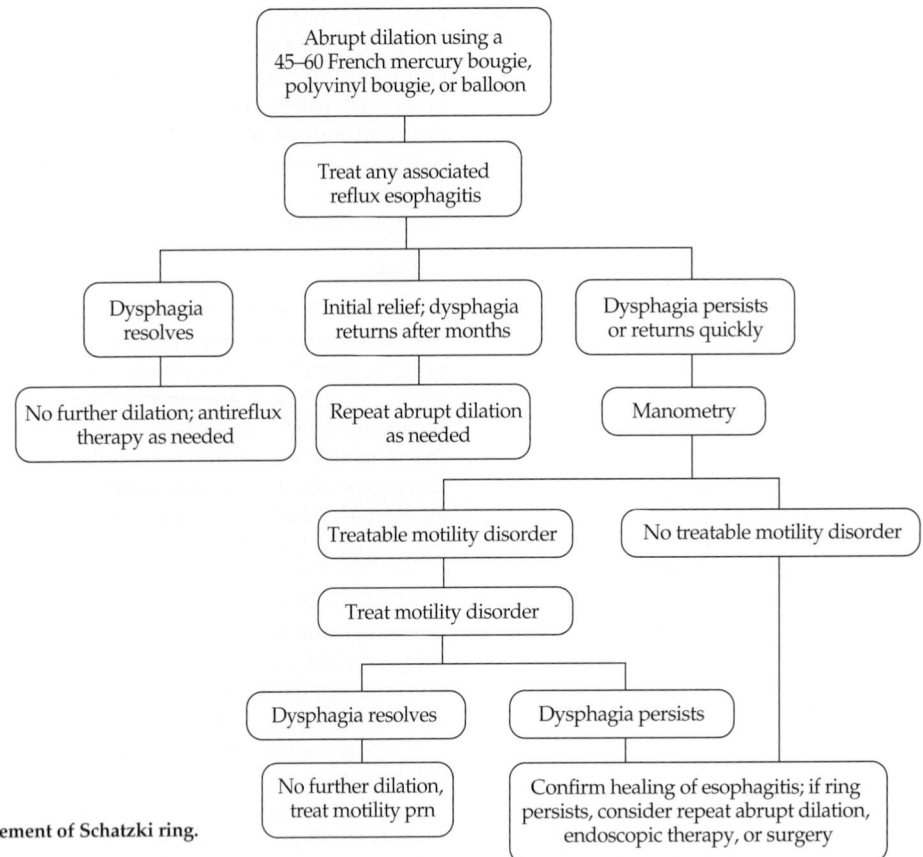

Figure 3   **Management of Schatzki ring.**

the stricture gradually. No study has established the superiority of one type of dilator over another. Serious complications such as perforation and bleeding occur in approximately 0.5% of all esophageal dilation procedures.[2]

For patients with peptic strictures caused by GERD, aggressive treatment with proton pump inhibitors both improves dysphagia and decreases the need for subsequent esophageal dilations.[10] Surgical therapy can be used for esophageal strictures that do not respond to dilation and antisecretory therapy. There are two major surgical approaches: (1) antireflux surgery with intraoperative stricture dilation for patients with peptic strictures or (2) resection of the stenotic esophagus with esophageal reconstruction (e.g., by interposing a loop of bowel between the remaining esophagus and the stomach).

LOWER ESOPHAGEAL (SCHATZKI) RINGS

The lower esophageal mucosal (Schatzki) ring is a thin, diaphragmlike, circumferential fold of mucosa that protrudes into the lumen of the distal esophagus, thereby posing a physical barrier to the passage of solid material.[11] Mucosal rings usually are located at the squamocolumnar junction and have squamous epithelium lining their upper surface and columnar epithelium lining the lower aspect. With careful radiologic technique aimed at distending the distal esophagus, a lower esophageal ring can be found in approximately 15% of all patients who have barium swallows. Only a minority of these rings cause dysphagia, however.

The pathogenesis of lower esophageal mucosal rings is disputed. It is not clear whether they are congenital or acquired structures. Lower esophageal mucosal rings often are associated with hiatal hernias and GERD, and some authorities have

suggested that the rings are in fact thin peptic strictures. Data on the role of GERD in the pathogenesis of Schatzki rings are inconclusive and contradictory, however.

Treatment

Dilation therapy is recommended for patients who have dysphagia from Schatzki rings [*see Figure 3*]. Traditionally, this involves the passage of a single large bougie or balloon (45 to 60 French) aimed at fracturing (rather than merely stretching) the mucosal fold. This approach differs from that for peptic strictures, which are treated by gradual stretching for fear of rupturing the fibrotic esophagus with a single, abrupt dilation. Most patients experience immediate relief of dysphagia after dilation, but recurrence is common and many patients require repeated dilations.

Esophageal Motility Abnormalities

Spechler and Castell have proposed a classification system for esophageal motility disorders. This system categorizes such disorders according to four major patterns of esophageal manometric abnormalities: inadequate LES relaxation, uncoordinated contraction, hypercontraction, and hypocontraction [*see Table 2*].[12] Most esophageal motility abnormalities fall predominantly into one of these four major categories, although there can be considerable overlap.

Processes that affect the inhibitory innervation of the LES (e.g., achalasia) can interfere with LES relaxation and thereby delay esophageal clearance. In the body of the esophagus, abnormal motility is characterized by uncoordinated contraction, hypercontraction, and hypocontraction. Uncoordinated esopha-

Table 2 Classification of Esophageal
Motility Abnormalities[12]

Inadequate relaxation of lower esophageal sphincter (LES)
    Classic achalasia
    Atypical disorders of LES relaxation
Uncoordinated contraction
    Diffuse esophageal spasm
Hypercontraction
    Nutcracker esophagus
    Isolated hypertensive LES
Hypocontraction
    Ineffective esophageal motility

geal contractions (i.e., contractions that are not peristaltic and directed toward the stomach) can delay esophageal clearance. Such uncoordinated contractions are the hallmark of diffuse esophageal spasm. Hypercontraction abnormalities are those that are characterized by contractions that are of high amplitude, long duration, or both. The putative disorders of hypercontraction (e.g., nutcracker esophagus, isolated hypertensive LES) are perhaps the most controversial of the abnormal esophageal motility patterns because it is not clear whether esophageal hypercontraction has any pathophysiologic significance. In contrast, hypocontraction abnormalities that result from weak (low-amplitude) muscle contractions can cause ineffective esophageal motility that delays esophageal clearance, and LES hypotension can result in GERD.

ACHALASIA

Primary achalasia is the best characterized of all the esophageal motility disorders.[13] In achalasia, there is degeneration of neurons in the wall of the esophagus, especially the nitric oxide–producing inhibitory neurons that effect the relaxation of esophageal smooth muscle necessary for opening of the LES and for coordinated esophageal contraction. Degenerative changes also may be found in brain stem ganglion cells and their efferent fibers, but the disordered motility appears to result primarily from the degeneration of intramural neurons. The loss of inhibitory innervation in the LES causes basal sphincter pressures to rise and interferes with sphincter relaxation. In the body of the esophagus, the loss of intramural neurons results in aperistalsis.

Primary achalasia has an annual incidence of approximately one case per 100,000 population. The disorder affects men and women equally and usually is diagnosed in patients who are between 25 and 60 years of age.

Secondary achalasia, or pseudoachalasia, which can be

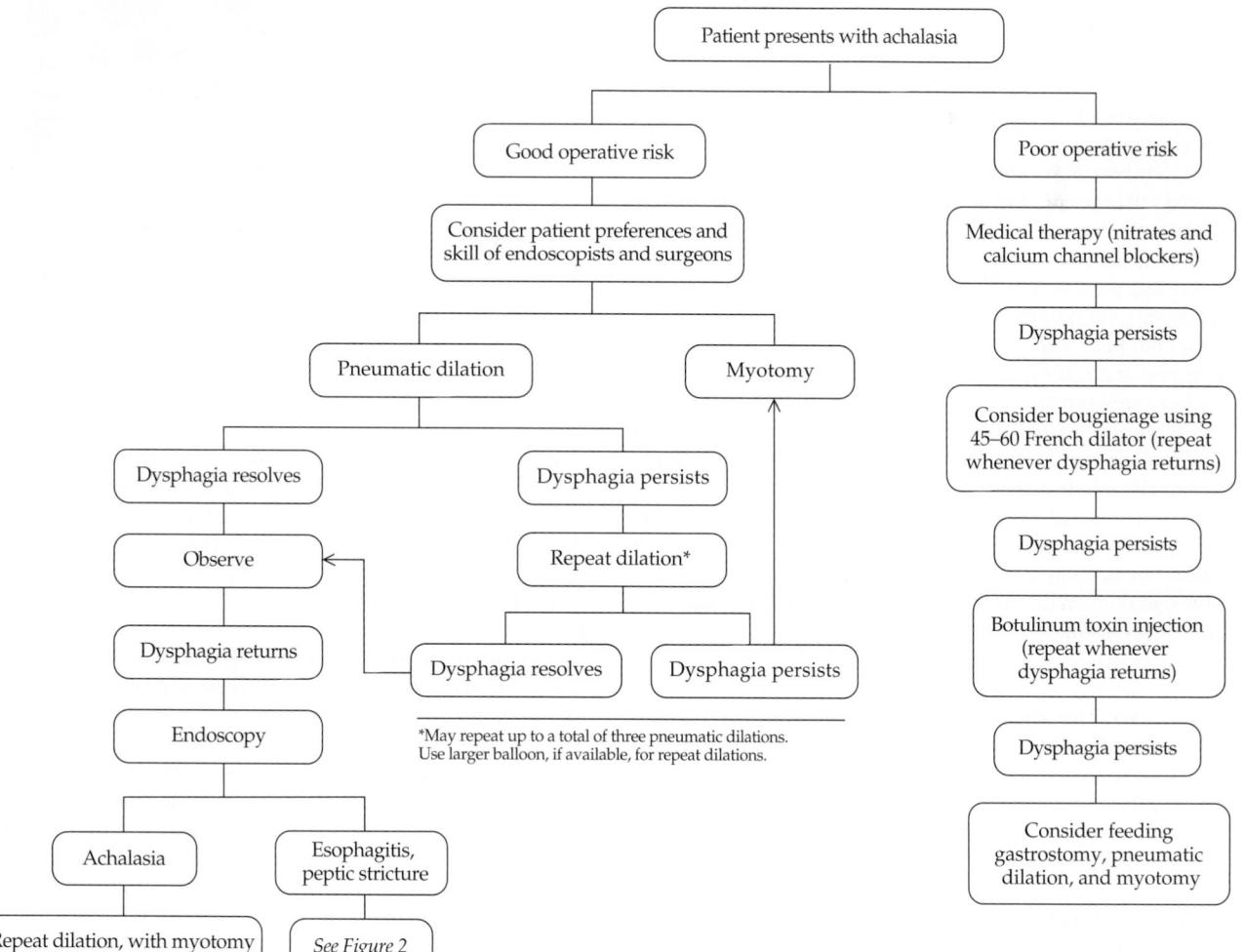

Figure 4 **Management of achalasia.**

*May repeat up to a total of three pneumatic dilations.
Use larger balloon, if available, for repeat dilations.

caused by certain diseases, exhibits esophageal motor abnormalities identical to those of primary achalasia. In Chagas disease, for example, esophageal infection with *Trypanosoma cruzi* can destroy intramural ganglion cells and cause aperistalsis with incomplete LES relaxation. Malignancies can cause pseudoachalasia by invading the esophageal neural plexuses directly or, very rarely, by releasing uncharacterized humoral factors that disrupt esophageal function as part of a paraneoplastic syndrome.

Diagnosis

Clinical features   Dysphagia for both solid foods and liquids is the primary symptom of achalasia. Moderate weight loss, regurgitation, and chest pain also are common clinical features. For reasons that are not clear, approximately one third of patients complain of heartburn, and achalasia occasionally can be confused with GERD. The symptoms of achalasia can be insidious in onset and gradual in progression, and patients frequently experience symptoms for years before seeking medical attention.

Diagnostic studies   Achalasia can be confirmed with radiographic, manometric, and endoscopic evaluation. Occasionally, the diagnosis is suggested on a plain radiograph of the chest that shows widening of the mediastinum from the dilated esophagus and reveals absence of the normal gastric air bubble, because LES contraction prevents swallowed air from entering the stomach. Barium swallow, which has a diagnostic accuracy for achalasia of 95%, typically shows a dilated esophagus that terminates in a beaklike narrowing caused by persistent contraction of the LES [*see Figure 5*].

Esophageal manometry is the gold standard for the diagnosis of achalasia. The requisite manometric features are (1) incomplete relaxation of the LES (defined as a mean swallow-induced fall in resting LES pressure to a nadir value more than 8 mm above gastric pressure) and (2) aperistalsis characterized either by simultaneous esophageal contractions with amplitudes less than 40 mm Hg or by no apparent esophageal contractions. Other common manometric features of classic achalasia include LES hypertension (resting pressure greater than 45 mm Hg) and resting pressure in the esophageal body that exceeds resting pressure in the stomach.

Diagnostic endoscopy is recommended for patients with achalasia, primarily to exclude malignancy at the esophagogastric junction. In primary achalasia, the endoscopist sees a dilated esophagus that often contains residual food. The LES does not open spontaneously, but in contrast to cases of obstruction caused by neoplasms or fibrotic strictures, the contracted LES of achalasia usually can be traversed easily with gentle pressure on the endoscope.

Treatment

Treatments for achalasia are aimed at decreasing the resting pressure in the LES to the point that the LES no longer impedes the passage of swallowed material [*see Figure 4*]. There is no therapy that can halt or reverse the degeneration of enteric neurons, and no treatment reliably restores peristaltic function in the body of the esophagus.

Pharmacotherapy   Nitrates and calcium channel blockers relax the smooth muscle of the LES, and these agents have been used to treat achalasia, with limited success. The drugs usually

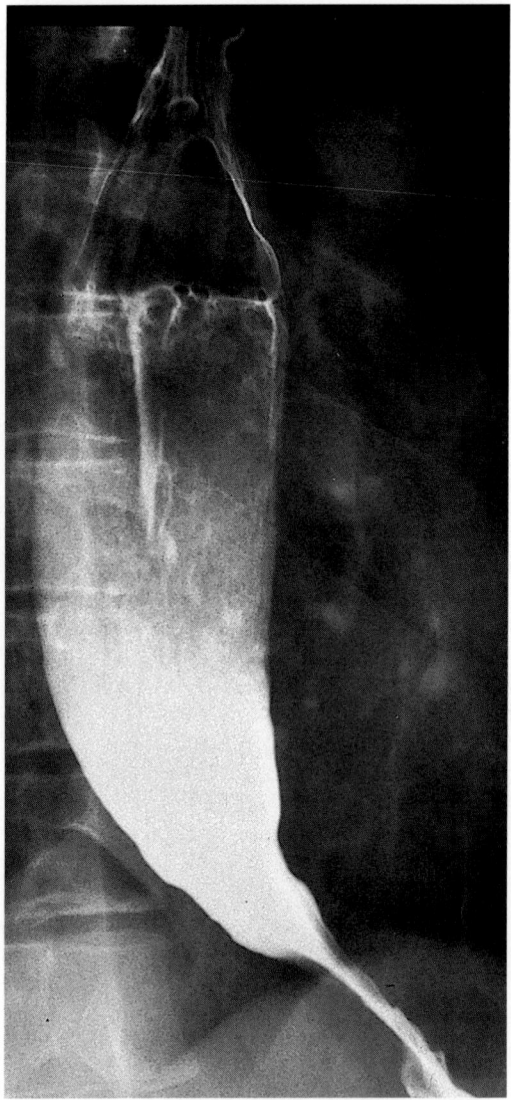

Figure 5   Barium swallow in a patient with achalasia shows dilatation of the esophagus with a beaklike narrowing at the esophagogastric junction.

are taken sublingually 10 to 30 minutes before meals. Unfortunately, pharmacotherapy for achalasia is inconvenient, often ineffective, and frequently associated with side effects (e.g., headache and hypotension) and tachyphylaxis. Consequently, pharmacotherapy is used primarily for patients who are unwilling or unable to tolerate invasive therapies.

Pneumatic dilation therapy   In pneumatic dilation therapy for achalasia, a large deflated balloon is passed through the mouth to the LES, where the balloon is inflated rapidly to tear the sphincter muscle and thereby weaken the LES.[14] Most studies describe good short-term relief of dysphagia in 60% to 85% of patients who are treated with a single session of pneumatic dilation. Esophageal perforation is the most common serious complication of the procedure, occurring in 2% to 6% of cases in most large series. Approximately 50% of patients who are treated with pneumatic dilation will require further therapy within 5 years, and subsequent pneumatic dilations are progressively less likely to result in a sustained remission.

Surgical therapy Achalasia also can be treated by surgical myotomy, in which the surgeon weakens the LES by cutting its muscle fibers. The procedure now can be performed laparoscopically, and good to excellent relief of symptoms has been described in 70% to 90% of patients. There are few serious complications, although reflux esophagitis develops postoperatively in approximately 10% of patients. Some surgeons recommend that an antireflux (fundoplication) procedure be performed at the time of myotomy to prevent this complication. The few long-term studies available suggest that surgical myotomy results in sustained remission rates of approximately 85% at 10 years and 65% at 20 years. In a prospective, randomized comparison of myotomy with pneumatic dilation, excellent results were found after median follow-up of approximately 5 years in 40 of 42 (95%) patients in the surgical group, compared with 24 of 37 (65%) patients who had pneumatic dilation.[15] Currently, the decision between pneumatic dilation and myotomy as initial therapy for achalasia should take into consideration the patient's preferences and the experience of available personnel.

Botulinum toxin therapy Endoscopic injection of botulinum toxin into the LES poisons the excitatory (acetylcholine-releasing) neurons that contribute to LES smooth muscle tone, thereby decreasing LES pressure and relieving achalasia.[16] The procedure is safe, and most patients treated with botulinum toxin injection experience immediate symptomatic improvement. Unfortunately, this effect usually is short lived. With repeated injections, approximately two thirds of patients with achalasia can be maintained in remission for 6 months. Of those patients in remission at 6 months, however, only about two thirds are still in remission at 1 year, despite repeated injections. Botulinum toxin injection is used primarily to treat patients with serious comorbidities, for whom pneumatic dilation and surgical myotomy pose inordinate risks.

DIFFUSE ESOPHAGEAL SPASM

Diffuse esophageal spasm is a rare condition of unknown etiology characterized by uncoordinated (spastic) motor activity in the smooth muscle portion of the esophagus. The esophageal spasms are manifested clinically by episodes of dysphagia and chest pain and on radiography and manometry by tertiary (nonperistaltic) contractions of the esophagus. The requisite manometric features of diffuse esophageal spasm are (1) simultaneous contractions associated with more than 10% of wet swallows and (2) a mean simultaneous contraction amplitude greater than 30 mm Hg.[12] A common manometric pattern is intermittent normal peristalsis alternating with periods of spontaneous, repetitive, and multiple-peaked contractions.

Diffuse esophageal spasm is treated with agents that relax esophageal smooth muscle, such as nitrates and calcium channel blockers, although few reports document the efficacy of this therapy. Psychotropic agents such as tricyclic antidepressants may help relieve the pain of diffuse esophageal spasm. Surgical treatment by long myotomy of the esophagus has been reported, but the efficacy of this operation is poorly documented.

NUTCRACKER ESOPHAGUS

In nutcracker esophagus, manometry reveals peristaltic waves in the distal esophagus that have mean amplitudes more than 2 standard deviations above normal values.[17] Although high-amplitude peristalsis is the most common motility abnormality observed in patients with noncardiac chest pain,[18] the clinical and physiologic importance of this manometric finding is disputed. It is not clear whether the hypercontraction of esophageal muscle is a cause of chest pain or is merely an epiphenomenon that is associated with the chest pain syndrome. The clinical response to smooth muscle–relaxing agents (nitrates and calcium channel blockers) is often disappointing. Treatment with psychotropic agents such as tricyclic antidepressants can be effective in controlling the chest pain.

ISOLATED HYPERTENSIVE LES

In patients with isolated hypertensive LES, esophageal motility is normal and the LES relaxes appropriately, but the mean resting LES pressure is abnormally high (i.e., > 45 mm Hg). Although this condition has been reported in patients with noncardiac chest pain, it is unlikely that the isolated hypertensive LES has any clinical consequences.

SCLERODERMA

In 80% of patients with scleroderma (progressive systemic sclerosis), fibrosis and ischemia damage the esophageal muscles and nerves. This damage causes manometric abnormalities, including weak contractions in the body of the esophagus and hypotension of the LES.[19] The LES hypotension can result in GERD. When the amplitude of peristaltic contractions falls below 30 mm Hg, esophageal clearance is compromised.

In addition to weak peristalsis, patients with scleroderma often exhibit abnormalities in the progression of peristalsis, including (1) failed peristalsis, in which the peristaltic wave progresses through the pharynx and proximal esophagus but fails to traverse the entire length of the distal esophagus; (2) simultaneous esophageal contractions; and (3) absent esophageal contractions.

The manometric features of scleroderma are not specific for the disorder. Identical manometric abnormalities can be found in patients with the CREST variant (limited scleroderma [calcinosis, Raynaud phenomenon, esophageal involvement, sclerodactyly, and telangiectasias]) and other collagen vascular disorders (e.g., mixed connective tissue disease, rheumatoid arthritis, and systemic lupus erythematosus) and certain nonrheumatic diseases (e.g., diabetes mellitus and amyloidosis). Furthermore, otherwise healthy patients who have GERD often exhibit scleroderma-like motility disturbances, yet such patients infrequently develop rheumatic diseases. For these reasons, some authorities discourage use of the term scleroderma esophagus and recommend use of the term ineffective esophageal motility to describe the constellation of manometric abnormalities typical of scleroderma.[20]

There is currently no effective treatment for ineffective esophageal motility. Proton pump inhibitors can treat and prevent complications from associated GERD. Prokinetic agents such as metoclopramide are often used but are rarely effective, especially when the disease is advanced.

Gastroesophageal Reflux Disease

In GERD, the reflux of gastric juice into the esophagus or oropharynx causes symptoms, tissue injury, or both. Approximately 20% of adults in the United States experience GERD symptoms such as heartburn and acid regurgitation at least once a week.[21] Severe GERD can result in ulceration of the esophagus, which can lead to fibrosis and esophageal stricture formation. In some cases, the ulcerated squamous epithelium of the distal esophagus is replaced by a metaplastic, intestinal-type mucosa (a condition called Barrett esophagus) that predisposes to cancer. Consequently, GERD is a strong risk factor for esophageal adenocarcinoma,[22] a tumor whose frequency has increased profoundly in western countries over the past 2 decades.

PATHOPHYSIOLOGY

The development of GERD is a multifactorial process involving dysfunction of the antireflux mechanisms that normally prevent gastric juice from entering the esophagus and of the clearance mechanisms that normally rid the esophagus of refluxed material.[23]

Antireflux Mechanisms

The normal barrier to gastroesophageal reflux comprises three major components: (1) the LES, (2) the crural diaphragm, and (3) anatomic features of the gastroesophageal junction.

Lower esophageal sphincter The LES normally prevents reflux by maintaining a resting pressure that is 10 to 30 mm Hg higher than ambient pressure in the stomach.[24] In the 1980s, Dodds showed that episodic collapse of LES pressure, a phenomenon called transient LES relaxation (TLESR), is the major mechanism for gastroesophageal reflux both in normal individuals and in patients with GERD.[25] Unlike the brief (2- to 8-second) LES relaxations that normally accompany primary (swallow-induced) peristalsis, TLESRs are not preceded by swallowing and last from 10 to 45 seconds.[26] When LES pressure becomes identical to gastric pressure during a TLESR, the sphincter can no longer function as a barrier to acid reflux.

TLESRs occur two to six times per hour in normal persons, especially after meals, and 40% to 50% of these TLESRs are accompanied by brief episodes of acid reflux. In patients with GERD, TLESRs occur three to eight times per hour, and 60% to 70% of these are associated with acid reflux. In severe GERD, approximately 70% of reflux episodes are the result of TLESRs; the remaining reflux episodes are from feeble basal LES pressure, swallow-induced LES relaxation, and sudden elevations in abdominal pressure.[24]

Gaseous distention of the stomach normally triggers a TLESR that allows the gas to escape into the esophagus (the belch reflex).[26] The nucleus tractus solitarius in the medulla mediates the belch reflex by integrating sensory information from the stomach and by controlling the neural circuits that induce the TLESR. Activation of medullary neurons with γ-aminobutyric acid B (GABA$_B$) receptors inhibits TLESRs, as does cholinergic blockade with atropine. The sphincter relaxation of the TLESR is effected by the activation of cholecystokinin-A receptors in LES muscle.

Crural diaphragm The right crus of the diaphragm normally encircles the distal esophagus. During inspiration, contraction of the diaphragmatic crura pinches the distal esophagus to prevent reflux. Crural contraction also helps minimize reflux during the sudden increases in abdominal pressure that accompany events such as coughing, sneezing, and straining. Thus, the crural muscle functions as an external esophageal sphincter that buttresses the LES.[27] TLESRs often are accompanied by relaxation of the crura, and studies in dogs have shown that gastroesophageal reflux does not occur during a TLESR unless the episode is attended by neural inhibition of the crural diaphragm.

Anatomic features of the gastroesophageal junction The acute angle formed by the junction of the esophagus and the stomach (the angle of His) can function as a one-way flap valve that stops reflux. Also, a portion of the distal esophagus normally is located within the abdomen, where the high ambient pressure pushes the esophageal walls together to prevent reflux.[27]

Disruption of the Antireflux Barrier by Hiatal Hernia

Most patients with severe GERD have a hiatal hernia in which the proximal portion of the stomach herniates into the chest through the diaphragmatic hiatus formed by the right crus of the diaphragm. With a large hiatal hernia, the LES muscle is completely dissociated from the crural diaphragm. In this situation, contraction of the crural diaphragm does not pinch the esophagus; rather, it creates an intrathoracic pouch of stomach whose contents may reflux readily into the esophagus.[28,29] With no buttressing of the internal sphincter by the crural diaphragm, sudden elevations in abdominal pressure caused by inspiration, coughing, and straining can far exceed LES pressure, resulting in reflux. Reduction of the angle of His and loss of the intra-abdominal portion of the esophagus also may compromise the antireflux barrier. Furthermore, patients with large hiatal hernias have an abnormally high frequency of TLESRs induced by gastric distention.[30]

Disruption of Esophageal Clearance

To injure the esophagus, caustic refluxed material must remain in contact with the mucosa for a sufficient period. The duration of this contact is determined by the efficacy of the esophageal clearance mechanisms, which include gravity, peristalsis, salivation, and bicarbonate secretion by the submucosal glands of the esophagus. When gastric juice refluxes into the esophagus, most of the material is cleared by the combined effects of gravity and peristalsis.[31] The small quantity of residual acidic material is neutralized by alkaline saliva and, to a lesser extent, by bicarbonate secreted by the submucosal glands.

Peristaltic abnormalities that can interfere with esophageal emptying (e.g., failed peristalsis, hypotensive peristalsis) have been found in 25% to 48% of patients with reflux esophagitis.[32] Patients with large hiatal hernias frequently have impaired esophageal clearance because of the retrograde flow of material from the hernia back into the esophagus. Cigarette smoking also has been shown to increase esophageal acid exposure both by increasing the frequency of acid reflux events and by decreasing salivary flow.[33]

Normal persons regularly experience brief episodes of acid reflux that do not cause esophageal injury. Most patients with reflux esophagitis have prolonged esophageal acid exposure that overwhelms the normal epithelial defenses. In some patients with reflux esophagitis, however, 24-hour pH monitoring studies demonstrate a normal daily duration of acid reflux. It is conceivable that these patients have uncharacterized defects that render the esophageal epithelium vulnerable to normal acid reflux.

ETIOLOGY

NSAIDs

There is evidence to suggest that aspirin and other NSAIDs may contribute to GERD.[34,35] Some NSAID preparations are caustic to the esophageal mucosa, and esophagitis can result if the tablet lingers in the esophagus (pill esophagitis). Patients with esophageal strictures may be especially susceptible to NSAID-induced esophageal injury.

Helicobacter pylori

Some studies suggest that gastric infection with *H. pylori* protects the esophagus from GERD and its complications.[36] In general endoscopy units, *H. pylori* infection has been found significantly less often in patients with reflux esophagitis than in control patients without GERD.[37] Reflux esophagitis has developed in some patients with duodenal ulcers after their *H. pylori* infections were eradicated with antibiotics.[38] There is a negative association between esophageal adenocarcinoma and *H. pylori* infections, particularly for infections with *cagA*-positive strains that may be especially likely to cause severe pangastritis.[39,40] Graham and others have proposed that *H. pylori* infections that cause pangastritis also cause a decrease in gastric acid production that may protect against GERD.[41] This issue remains highly controversial, however, and the role of *H. pylori* infection in GERD is not yet clear.

DIAGNOSIS

Clinical Features

Heartburn, the cardinal symptom of GERD, is an uncomfortable, burning sensation that is located behind the sternum. The sensation often originates in the epigastrium and radiates up the chest. Patients who describe heartburn often wave an open hand vertically over the sternum, whereas patients with angina pectoris typically hold a clenched fist stationary over the chest while describing their pain. Heartburn may be associated with the ingestion of foods that predispose to reflux by decreasing pressure in the LES, such as chocolate, onions, and fat. Spicy foods, citrus products, and tomato products may cause the sensation of heartburn by irritating the inflamed esophageal mucosa directly. Some patients experience heartburn when they bend over or exercise, presumably because these activities induce acid reflux by increasing intra-abdominal pressure. Characteristically, heartburn caused by gastroesophageal reflux is relieved immediately by antacids and can be eliminated by the administration of potent acid-suppressing agents.

When refluxed gastric juice reaches the oropharynx, patients may complain of regurgitation of sour (acid) or bitter-tasting (bilious) material. Dysphagia may result from a peptic stricture or from reflux esophagitis alone. With ulcerative esophagitis, patients may complain of odynophagia. Some patients experience water brash, in which the mouth suddenly fills with saliva as a result of reflex salivation stimulated by acid in the esophagus.

In addition to these typical symptoms, GERD can have a variety of so-called atypical manifestations.[42-45] Esophageal irritation by acid reflux may result in chest pain that can mimic ischemic heart disease. If gastric juice reaches the oropharynx, it can cause globus, sore throat, and burning tongue, and the acid can erode dental enamel. Laryngitis and pulmonary problems such as chronic cough and asthma can result from aspiration of material into the airway. Asthma may also be a consequence of acid in the esophagus that triggers reflex bronchoconstriction.

Diagnostic Studies

Patients who have a typical history of heartburn that disappears with antisecretory therapy can be assumed to have GERD, and diagnostic tests are not necessary merely to con-firm the diagnosis. Moreover, by definition, patients with GERD can have symptoms without objective evidence of esophageal damage, so normal test results often cannot exclude GERD as a cause of symptoms. However, diagnostic tests may be needed to evaluate atypical symptoms or to look for complications of GERD. For such patients, several options are available, such as radiography, endoscopy, biopsy, acid perfusion test, and pH monitoring.

Radiography Radiography has a limited role in the evaluation of GERD. A barium swallow can show signs of reflux esophagitis (e.g., thickening of the esophageal folds, erosions, and ulcerations) that support the diagnosis of GERD. A barium swallow can also identify peptic strictures. Radiography is considerably less sensitive than endoscopy for demonstrating esophagitis, however; and endoscopic examination has the added advantage of permitting biopsy of specimens from any abnormal areas.

Endoscopy An endoscopic examination is the most sensitive test for establishing the diagnosis of reflux esophagitis and Barrett esophagus. However, the clinician should appreciate that a normal endoscopic examination does not eliminate GERD as a cause of symptoms. Gastroesophageal reflux can cause disabling symptoms without causing visible esophageal damage.[46] Endoscopy shows reflux esophagitis in only 50% to 70% of patients who complain of frequent heartburn, and heartburn severity is not a reliable index for the severity of esophagitis.[47] Furthermore, the esophagus typically appears normal on endoscopy in patients who have only extraesophageal symptoms of GERD, such as chronic cough and laryngitis.

The Practice Parameters Committee of the American College of Gastroenterology recommends that endoscopy be reserved for patients with uncomplicated GERD in whom empirical therapy is unsuccessful. Endoscopic evaluation without an empirical trial of therapy is appropriate in patients who have symptoms suggesting complicated disease, including fever, anorexia, weight loss, dysphagia, odynophagia, and bleeding.[48] In patients with long-standing GERD symptoms, particularly those 50 years of age and older, endoscopy is indicated to look for Barrett esophagus.[49] It is important to appreciate that these guidelines are merely committee recommendations whose efficacy has not been established by clinical studies.

Biopsy Biopsy specimens of the squamous epithelium in the distal esophagus of patients with GERD frequently show the histologic abnormalities of reflux esophagitis, including lengthening of the papillae, hyperplasia of cells in the basal zone, and infiltration of the epithelium with eosinophils and polymorphonuclear cells. The importance of these histologic changes of GERD is disputed, however; and routine biopsy of the squamous epithelium to seek evidence of reflux esophagitis generally is not recommended for clinical purposes.

Acid perfusion test The acid perfusion (Bernstein) test has been used in patients who have atypical chest pain. The esophagus is perfused with 0.1N hydrochloric acid; reproduction of the chest pain implicates GERD as the etiology. This test has limited sensitivity and specificity, however, and has largely been replaced by ambulatory esophageal pH monitoring.

pH monitoring Ambulatory monitoring of esophageal

pH is used to document the pattern, frequency, and duration of acid reflux and to seek a correlation between reflux episodes and symptoms. In most ambulatory systems, an episode of acid reflux is defined as a drop in esophageal pH below 4. Esophageal pH monitoring records a number of different variables, such as the total number of reflux episodes, the number of episodes that last longer than 5 minutes, and the duration of the longest episode. The most useful variable appears to be the percentage of the monitoring period in which esophageal pH remains below 4 (in normal individuals, this is less than 4.5% of the 24-hour test). Ambulatory esophageal pH monitoring usually is not needed for patients with typical signs and symptoms of GERD. For patients with atypical or unresponsive symptoms, however, the test can be very useful in documenting an association between symptoms and acid reflux, as well as the efficacy of antisecretory therapy in reducing acid reflux.

TREATMENT

The efficacy of antireflux therapy is inversely related to the severity of the underlying reflux esophagitis.[50] A treatment that is highly effective for mild esophagitis may be virtually useless for patients with severe disease. Ulcerative esophagitis does not respond reliably to medical therapy with agents other than proton pump inhibitors (PPIs), the most effective antisecretory medications. For patients with mild or moderate esophagitis, some authorities advocate a step-up approach to therapy that begins with antireflux lifestyle modifications and progresses eventually to the most potent medications (i.e., PPIs) only when the disease does not respond to lesser treatments.[51] Others advocate a step-down approach that begins with the most effective therapy (PPIs).[52] The optimal approach remains disputed. However, for patients who are known to have severe, ulcerative reflux esophagitis, it is appropriate to begin therapy immediately with PPIs rather than proceeding stepwise through trials of agents unlikely to effect healing.

Lifestyle Modifications

A number of lifestyle modifications have been proposed to decrease esophageal acid exposure [*see Table 3*]. Few published data support the efficacy of these lifestyle modifications in controlling GERD, however, and it is unclear how many patients for whom such modifications are prescribed actually comply with them.

Antacids and Alginic Acid

Antacids and alginic acid can provide temporary relief of episodic heartburn. Despite the wide use of these over-the-counter products, surprisingly few data are available on their utility for healing reflux esophagitis or for the long-term management of GERD symptoms.

H_2 Receptor Blocking Agents

H_2 receptor antagonists are safe medications that relieve GERD symptoms and heal esophagitis within 12 weeks in approximately one half to two thirds of all patients.[50] The H_2 blockers are most useful for patients with GERD of mild to moderate severity, in whom the highest rates of healing can be anticipated. However, healing rates with these agents are poor in patients who have severe reflux esophagitis. High doses of H_2 receptor blockers (up to eight times the conventional dose) have been used effectively to treat esophagitis in severe cases of

---

Table 3   Lifestyle Modifications for Gastroesophageal Reflux Disease

Elevate the head of the bed on 4- to 6-in blocks
Weight loss for obese patients
Avoid recumbency for several hours after meals
Avoid bedtime snacks
Avoid fatty foods, chocolate, peppermint, onions, and garlic
Avoid cigarettes and alcohol
Avoid drugs that decrease lower esophageal sphincter pressure and delay gastric emptying, such as calcium channel blocking agents
Avoid nonsteroidal anti-inflammatory drugs

GERD, but this approach generally is not recommended. Few data document the long-term efficacy of H_2 receptor blockers used in any dosage, and many patients develop tolerance to the antisecretory effects of these agents. For patients with severe GERD, most authorities prescribe PPIs rather than high-dose H_2 receptor blocker therapy.

Prokinetic Agents

In theory, prokinetic agents may decrease gastroesophageal reflux by increasing LES pressure and by enhancing esophageal and gastric clearance. Currently, metoclopramide is the only prokinetic agent available in the United States for the treatment of GERD. Metoclopramide is a dopamine antagonist, and its use is limited by side effects such as agitation, restlessness, somnolence, and extrapyramidal symptoms, which occur in up to 30% of patients. Cisapride, a serotonin-4 (5-HT_4) receptor agonist, demonstrated efficacy in mild GERD, but this agent was withdrawn when it was found to cause lethal cardiac arrhythmias in patients with a number of predisposing conditions. Domperidone is as effective as metoclopramide, and it has an acceptable safety profile[48]; nonetheless, domperidone has not been marketed in the United States. Baclofen, a GABA receptor type B agonist, has been reported to reduce the number of reflux episodes after a single dose of 40 mg[53]; however, the CNS side effects of this agent restrict its use. There is ongoing intensive research to identifying a baclofenlike agent with a better side-effect profile.[48]

Proton Pump Inhibitors

The PPIs are substituted benzimidazoles that decrease gastric acid secretion through inhibition of H^+,K^+-ATPase, the proton pump of the parietal cell. These agents are clearly the most effective inhibitors of gastric acid secretion available. Five PPIs are used widely for the treatment of GERD: omeprazole, esomeprazole (the S-optical isomer of omeprazole), lansoprazole, pantoprazole, and rabeprazole. All of these preparations are similar in efficacy and side-effect profiles, although when used in conventional dosages, esomeprazole may effect marginally higher rates of healing of reflux esophagitis than lansoprazole.[54] Patients with mild to moderately severe reflux esophagitis who are treated with PPIs in conventional dosages achieve healing rates of 80% to 100% within 8 to 12 weeks.[50,55] Very severe reflux esophagitis may persist despite conventional-dose PPI therapy in up to 40% of cases, however.[56] In most of these resistant cases, the esophagitis usually can be healed by increasing the dose of the PPI.[57] Recent studies also have shown that aggressive acid suppression with PPIs improves dysphagia and decreases the need for esophageal dilation in patients who have peptic esophageal strictures.[10]

Most patients with severe GERD who respond to PPIs require maintenance therapy, because GERD recurs shortly after stopping the drug.[58] For most patients, the dose of PPI necessary to maintain remission is at least the dose required to heal the acute esophagitis. In some patients with severe GERD, furthermore, PPI maintenance-dose requirements may increase with time. One long-term study of patients with severe GERD who were given a maintenance dose of 20 mg of omeprazole daily found that relapses occurred at the rate of 1 per 9.4 treatment-years and that patients often required increasing doses of omeprazole (up to 120 mg/day) to maintain GERD in remission.[57]

The profound acid suppression that can be achieved with PPIs has raised theoretical concerns regarding their long-term safety.[53] Nevertheless, there are no reports of tumors or nutritional deficiencies clearly attributable to the use of PPIs after more than a decade of extensive clinical experience with these agents.

Antireflux Surgery

Antireflux operations share four fundamental features: (1) reduction of the hiatal hernia, (2) restoration of an intra-abdominal segment of esophagus, (3) approximation of the diaphragmatic crura, and (4) fundoplication, in which the surgeon wraps a portion of the gastric fundus around the distal esophagus. The operations differ primarily in the approach (e.g., transthoracic versus transabdominal) and in the extent of fundoplication.

The precise mechanisms whereby these operations prevent reflux are not clear, but a number of potential ones have been proposed.[59] The fundoplication may prevent the distention of the gastric fundus that ordinarily triggers TLESRs. Restoration of the distal esophagus to the positive pressure environment of the abdomen may prevent reflux, and the anatomic rearrangement of the gastroesophageal junction may create an antireflux flap-valve effect. Also, reduction of the hiatal hernia and approximation of the diaphragmatic crura may restore the normal antireflux function of the crural diaphragm.

Antireflux surgery can be performed laparoscopically.[60] The laparoscopic approach has become popular not because it is safer or produces a better functional result than the open procedure, but because it supposedly offers the advantages of less postoperative discomfort, shorter hospital stay, and better cosmetic outcome. Two recent randomized trials of laparoscopic versus open Nissen fundoplication found no significant differences in the functional results of the two procedures (i.e., relief of GERD symptoms and reduction in esophageal acid exposure).[61,62] However, one of the studies was terminated prematurely because an interim analysis showed an excess of adverse outcomes (primarily dysphagia) in the group treated laparoscopically.[62] At least one study has shown that the primary factor involved in overall patient satisfaction with antireflux surgery is the relief of GERD symptoms. These observations suggest that the primary decision for the clinician to make is whether the patient should have an antireflux operation, not how the operation should be performed.

Uncontrolled retrospective studies of antireflux surgery generally have described excellent results, with success rates exceeding 80%.[60] Few randomized trials have done direct comparisons of medical and surgical antireflux therapies, however. In the late 1980s (before the release of PPIs for clinical use in the United States), the Department of Veterans Affairs conducted a large cooperative study that prospectively compared the efficacy of medical therapy with that of surgical therapy in 247 patients with complicated GERD.[63] Patients were prescribed antireflux lifestyle modifications and randomly assigned to receive one of three types of treatment: (1) continuous medical therapy (antacid tablets and ranitidine taken on a daily basis regardless of symptoms, with metoclopramide and sucralfate added if necessary to control symptoms); (2) symptomatic medical therapy (the same drugs as in the continuous-medical-therapy group but used only when necessary for control of symptoms); or (3) surgical therapy (open Nissen fundoplication). All three groups showed significant improvements in the symptoms and endoscopic signs of GERD for up to 2 years. However, surgical therapy was significantly better than both medical therapies during that period, and surgical patients had higher overall satisfaction.

In the 1990s, a Scandinavian group conducted a randomized trial of omeprazole versus open antireflux surgery in 310 patients with erosive esophagitis.[64] In patients who received a fixed dose of 20 mg of omeprazole a day, antireflux surgery was superior in maintaining GERD in remission for the 3-year duration of the study. In clinical practice, however, the dose of a PPI is typically titrated to control symptoms. In this study, when the physician was permitted to titrate the PPI dose, there was no statistically significant difference between the medical group and the surgical group in maintaining remission for 3 years.

Relatively few reports have described the long-term outcome of antireflux surgery. Some uncontrolled studies have found success rates that exceed 90% at 10 to 20 years after open fundoplication,[65] whereas others have described breakdown of the operation and the return of reflux esophagitis in more than 50% of cases.[66] A follow-up study was conducted on the patients who participated in the VA cooperative study (see above).[67] During the follow-up period of 10 to 13 years, surgical patients were significantly less likely to have taken antireflux medications regularly, and when antireflux medications were discontinued, the GERD symptoms in these patients were significantly less severe than those in the medical group. However, 62% of the surgical patients took antireflux medications on a regular basis, and there were no significant differences between the groups in the rates of neoplastic and peptic complications of GERD, overall physical and mental well-being scores, and overall satisfaction with antireflux therapy. There were 79 deaths, involving 33 (40%) of the 82 surgical patients and 46 (28%) of the 165 medical patients ($P = 0.047$). For reasons that are not clear, the excess deaths in the surgical group were from heart disease. This and other studies suggest that antireflux surgery does not effect a permanent cure for GERD in the majority of patients and that surgery is no better than medication for preventing the peptic and neoplastic complications of GERD.

Endoscopic Antireflux Procedures

Two endoscopic therapies for GERD have been approved by the Food and Drug Administration. One system uses an endoscopic sewing-machine device to plicate the gastroesophageal junction; the other system delivers radiofrequency (microwave) energy to create thermal lesions in the LES muscle, which may narrow the lumen and destroy nerves that mediate TLESRs. A number of other endoscopic antireflux procedures are under investigation. Small studies describe promising results,[68,69] but the safety and efficacy of these procedures are not yet known, and their role in the treatment of GERD is not clear.

Barrett Esophagus

Barrett esophagus is a sequela of chronic GERD in which the stratified squamous epithelium that normally lines the distal esophagus is replaced by an abnormal columnar epithelium.[70] The abnormal columnar epithelium typical of Barrett esophagus is an incomplete form of intestinal metaplasia called specialized intestinal metaplasia. This metaplastic epithelium predisposes to esophageal adenocarcinoma, which develops in patients with Barrett esophagus at the rate of approximately 0.5% a year.

DIAGNOSIS

Endoscopy

The diagnosis of Barrett esophagus is established when the endoscopist sees columnar epithelium lining the distal esophagus. Columnar epithelium has a characteristic dull, reddish appearance that is readily distinguished from squamous epithelium, which is normally glossy and pale [see Figure 6]. The diagnosis is confirmed by esophageal biopsy specimens showing specialized intestinal metaplasia.

Barrett esophagus can be further categorized according to the extent of esophageal involvement. In traditional, or long-segment, Barrett esophagus (LSBE), specialized intestinal metaplasia extends for 3 cm or more into the distal esophagus. LSBE is usually found in patients who have severe GERD. Less than 3 cm of metaplasia constitutes short-segment Barrett esophagus (SSBE), a condition often associated with only mild GERD. It is not clear whether these two types of Barrett esophagus have the same pathogenesis and natural history, nor is it clear whether SSBE progresses to LSBE. Currently, however, SSBE and LSBE are managed similarly.

Regular endoscopic surveillance for esophageal cancer has been recommended in patients with Barrett esophagus. Retrospective studies have documented that cancers discovered during surveillance endoscopies tend to be less advanced than those detected during endoscopies performed because of cancer symptoms (e.g., dysphagia and weight loss). There is no direct proof that surveillance reduces cancer mortality in Barrett esophagus, however.

Biopsy

Esophageal biopsy specimens are taken during surveillance endoscopy primarily to identify dysplasia, a histologic diagnosis suggesting that one or more clones of epithelial cells have acquired genetic alterations rendering them neoplastic and predisposed to malignancy. Unfortunately, dysplasia is an imperfect predictor of malignancy in Barrett esophagus. The histologic abnormalities of low-grade dysplasia are not specific for neoplasia, and interobserver agreement for the diagnosis of low-grade dysplasia in Barrett esophagus may be less than 50%. For high-grade dysplasia, in contrast, interobserver agreement is approximately 85%. Dysplasia has no distinctive gross features, so endoscopists must rely on random biopsy sampling techniques to find it. Consequently, biopsy sampling error is a major problem. Of patients with Barrett esophagus whose biopsy specimens show high-grade dysplasia, approxi-

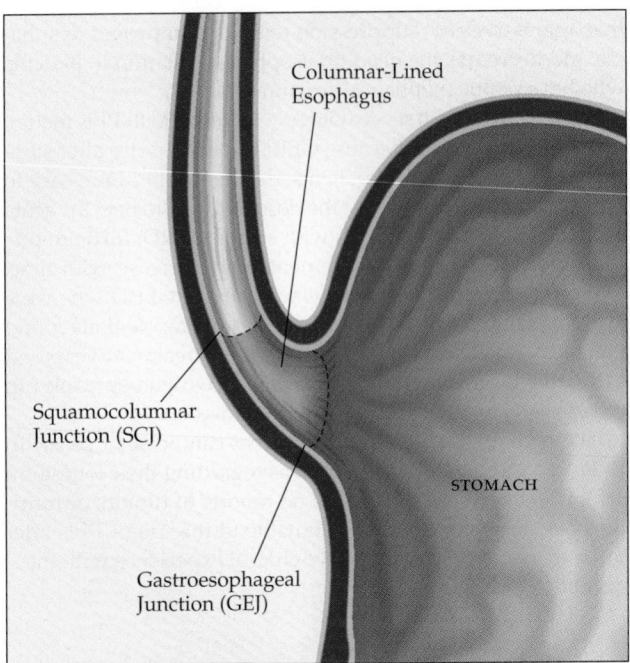

Figure 6   **In Barrett esophagus, columnar epithelium extends proximal to the gastroesophageal junction (the imaginary line at which the esophagus ends and the stomach begins, which corresponds to the most proximal extent of the gastric folds).**

mately one third already have an invasive cancer that was missed because of sampling error. Extensive biopsy sampling can reduce, but not eliminate, this problem. Finally, the natural history of dysplasia is not well defined.

Researchers have been searching for better alternatives to random biopsy sampling for dysplasia in Barrett esophagus. Other markers for malignant potential (e.g., flow cytometry and abnormalities in p53 expression) have been studied, as have endoscopic techniques to target dysplastic areas for biopsy. Despite some promising preliminary data, none of these tests and techniques has yet been shown to provide sufficient clinical information to justify its routine application in practice.

TREATMENT

Fit patients with verified high-grade dysplasia in Barrett esophagus have three management options: esophagectomy, endoscopic ablative therapy, and intensive surveillance (withholding invasive therapy until biopsy specimens show adenocarcinoma). Esophagectomy, the only therapy that clearly can prevent the progression from dysplasia to invasive cancer, is associated with operative mortality of 3% to 12% and with a 30% to 50% rate of serious operative complications. Endoscopic ablative therapies (e.g., laser photoablation and photodynamic therapy) use thermal or photochemical energy to destroy the metaplastic esophageal epithelium.[71] No study has shown that endoscopic ablation decreases the long-term risk for cancer development, so at present these therapies should be considered experimental. Although intensive surveillance for high-grade dysplasia (e.g., endoscopy every 3 months) has been endorsed as a management option by the American College of Gastroenterology, few published data directly support the safety and efficacy of the practice. The esophagus has an extensive lymphatic system and no confining serosa, features that can facilitate the spread of malignant cells and contribute to the dismal prognosis for patients with esophageal cancer. The concern about surveillance for high-grade dysplasia is that by the time biopsy specimens reveal adenocarcinoma, the tumor already may be incurable because of systemic metastases.

Management Recommendations

A management algorithm for patients with Barrett esophagus has been developed [*see Figure 7*].[70] This strategy assumes that patients have had an initial endoscopic examination in which four-quadrant biopsy specimens are taken at intervals of 2 cm or less throughout the columnar-lined esophagus. If biopsy sampling during the initial endoscopic procedure is not adequate or if there is any question regarding the degree of dysplasia, endoscopy should be repeated to resolve these issues. If inflammation interferes with the histologic assessment of dysplasia, the patient should be treated with intensive antireflux therapy (e.g., a PPI administered at least twice daily) for 8 to 12 weeks before repeating the endoscopy. Data regarding the safety of intensive endoscopic surveillance for patients with high-grade dysplasia are limited, and available studies have involved primarily older patients. The clinician should be especially cautious in applying the results of these studies to the management of high-grade dysplasia in younger patients. Intensive endoscopic surveillance may be a valid alternative to immediate esophagectomy for older patients with high-grade dysplasia who can comply with the program. For patients who are too old, infirm, or unwilling to assume the risks of esophagectomy, endoscopic ablative therapy may be a reasonable alternative if the procedure is performed as part of a study protocol. Finally, the clinician should bear in mind that these recommendations have not been validated by studies demonstrating that this strategy prolongs survival or enhances quality of life.

Infectious Esophagitis

Most esophageal infections are caused by *Candida*, herpes simplex virus (HSV), or cytomegalovirus (CMV), alone or in combination.[6] These organisms rarely infect the esophagus of normal persons, but they often cause esophagitis in patients whose immune system has been compromised by AIDS, advanced malignancy, or the immunosuppressive drugs used to prevent rejection of organ transplants. Immune dysfunction that can accompany diabetes mellitus, alcoholism, and advanced age also may predispose to esophageal infection, especially by *Candida*. Antibiotic therapy that alters the normal microbial flora of the oropharynx and esophagus and corticosteroid therapy that suppresses immune function also can result in candidal esophagitis, as can abnormalities that delay the clearance of *Candida* from the esophagus, such as progressive systemic sclerosis (scleroderma), achalasia, and esophageal strictures.

The clinical manifestations of esophageal infections are similar, regardless of the pathogen. Dysphagia and odynophagia are the presenting symptoms in 60% to 95% of patients with infectious esophagitis, and weight loss is reported by 35%.[6] CMV esophagitis often is only one component of a generalized CMV infection, and 20% to 40% of patients with CMV esophagitis have systemic symptoms [*see Cytomegalovirus Esophagitis, below*]. In contrast, *Candida* and HSV esophagitis usually are not associated with infection in other organs, and systemic symptoms are uncommon. However, oral lesions (e.g., thrush and focal ulcerations) are found frequently in patients who

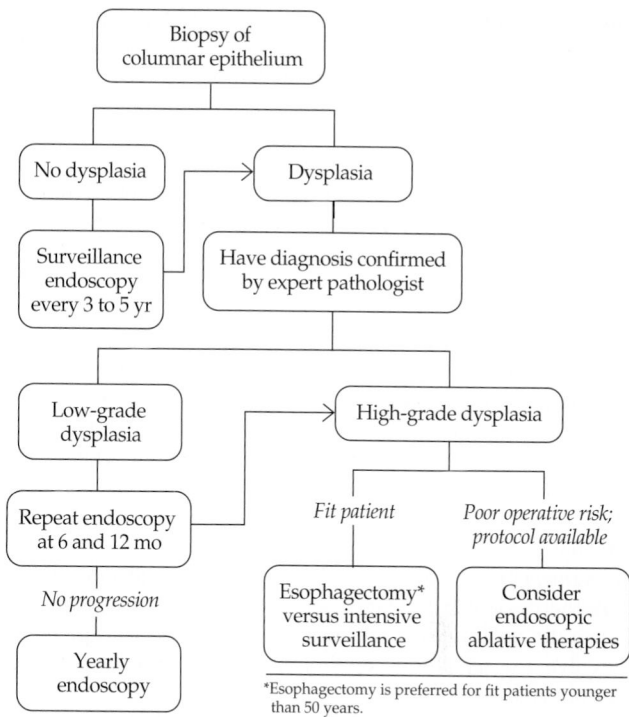

Figure 7 **Management of patients with Barrett esophagus.**[73]

have *Candida* and HSV esophagitis, but they are not found in patients with CMV esophagitis.

A surprising number of esophageal infections are asymptomatic. In published series, approximately one quarter of all cases of candidal esophagitis were discovered incidentally during radiographic or endoscopic examinations performed for the evaluation of extraesophageal symptoms.

CANDIDAL ESOPHAGITIS

Candida, a yeast that is part of normal oropharyngeal flora, is the most frequent cause of esophageal infections in immunocompromised patients. Most cases of candidal esophagitis are caused by *C. albicans*, although other candidal species, such as *C. tropicalis* and *C. glabrata*, occasionally infect the esophagus. Approximately 85% of patients with candidal esophagitis have oral thrush, and the combination of oral thrush and esophageal symptoms has a high positive predictive value for candidal esophagitis.

Typically, endoscopic evaluation of patients with candidal esophagitis reveals raised, white plaques that resemble cottage cheese clinging to the esophageal mucosa. On barium swallow, coating of the raised plaques and their interstices with barium gives the esophageal mucosa a characteristic irregular, shaggy appearance. Confirmation of the diagnosis requires the demonstration of budding yeast cells, hyphae, or pseudohyphae in brush cytology or biopsy specimens of the esophagus.

Several antifungal agents are available for the treatment of *Candida* infections. The decision regarding which agent to choose is influenced principally by the severity of the infection and the severity of the patient's immunocompromise. A patient who has a mild esophageal infection and minimal immunocompromise (e.g., a young patient who develops mild candidal esophagitis during a limited course of steroid therapy for asthma) often can be treated effectively with a topical antifungal agent such as clotrimazole. In contrast, a patient with moderately severe candidal esophagitis and substantial immunocompromise (e.g., a patient with troublesome odynophagia and AIDS) usually requires the oral administration of a systemic antifungal agent such as fluconazole. Patients who have severe infection and profound immunocompromise (e.g., disseminated candidiasis or candidal esophagitis in the setting of severe granulocytopenia) generally require treatment with intravenous amphotericin B [see Chapter 156].

HERPES SIMPLEX VIRUS ESOPHAGITIS

Primary HSV infections of the oropharynx are common in the general population, and they result when oral mucous membranes or breaks in the facial skin are exposed to secretions from a person with an active HSV infection. The virus enters the nerves that supply the infected epithelium, where it remains in latent form after healing of the primary infection. The latent virus in the neurons can be reactivated and spread to epithelial cells through the nerve fibers. In immunocompetent persons, HSV reactivation commonly causes cold sores of the lips (herpes labialis). When reactivation of latent virus occurs in the setting of immunodeficiency, however, HSV can spread to involve the squamous epithelium of the oropharynx and esophagus.

The endoscopic findings in persons with HSV esophagitis vary with the duration of infection.[72] The earliest lesions are small (1 to 3 mm), rounded vesicles that usually involve the middle to distal esophagus. Sloughing of the vesicles results in small, sharply demarcated ulcers that have raised margins and a yellowish base. In severe cases, the small ulcers coalesce to form large ulcers that can be covered with dense exudates resembling candidal plaques.

Histologic diagnosis is best accomplished by examining biopsy and brush cytology specimens from the squamous epithelium at the edges of ulcerated areas. Specimens obtained from the ulcer base often contain only nonspecific granulation tissue and exudates. Typical histologic changes in HSV infection include multinucleated giant cells and intranuclear Cowdry type A inclusion bodies.

In immunocompetent patients, HSV esophagitis usually is a short-lived illness that may require no therapy other than supportive care and expectant management. HSV esophagitis often does not resolve spontaneously in immunocompromised patients, however, so such patients should receive systemic antiviral therapy. Acyclovir currently is the drug of choice for HSV infections of the esophagus.

CYTOMEGALOVIRUS ESOPHAGITIS

CMV is a ubiquitous herpesvirus that usually is transmitted from person to person by exposure to infected secretions. The virus can also be transmitted through transfused blood that carries infected leukocytes or through transplanted infected organs. CMV can infect virtually any tissue in the body, and after recovery from the primary infection, evidence of latent CMV infection can be found in most organs. With the development of immunodeficiency, the latent virus can reactivate and cause esophagitis.[73] Immunocompromised patients can also develop CMV esophagitis during primary CMV infections. CMV esophagitis is extremely uncommon in immunocompetent persons.

Patients who have CMV esophagitis often have widespread CMV infection, with systemic symptoms such as fever, weight loss, nausea, vomiting, and diarrhea. CMV tends to cause discrete, shallow esophageal ulcerations that are very elongated (up to 15 cm in length) and surrounded by normal-appearing esophageal mucosa. Tissue sampling for histologic examination and culture is necessary to distinguish these giant CMV ulcerations from the giant idiopathic esophageal ulcerations that can be associated with HIV infection.

Histologic examination of cells infected with CMV reveals distinctive abnormalities that include cellular enlargement and inclusion bodies in both the nucleus and the cytoplasm. Although the virus is found most often in fibroblasts and endothelial cells, biopsy specimens from granulation tissue in the base of the esophageal ulcer have a higher yield on histology and culture than specimens from squamous epithelial cells at the edges of the ulcer. Unfortunately, no single test for CMV infection is highly sensitive. In a study of 14 bone marrow transplant recipients who developed CMV disease, for example, conventional and centrifugation cultures of endoscopic biopsy specimens identified the organism in only 57% of patients, and conventional histologic examination of the specimens revealed characteristic findings in only 30%.[74] For patients with negative test results, therefore, repeated diagnostic testing may be necessary if the suspicion of CMV infection is high. However, evidence of CMV infection is not proof of the presence of CMV disease. The mere identification of CMV in an inflamed esophagus does not establish that CMV is the cause of the inflammation.

CMV disease can respond to treatment with ganciclovir. Maintenance therapy with ganciclovir may be indicated for patients who have recurrences of CMV disease or who have a high risk of recurrence (e.g., patients with advanced AIDS). Prophylactic antiviral therapy is commonly recommended for recipients of solid-organ and bone marrow transplants.

ESOPHAGEAL DISEASE IN HIV INFECTION

Within 2 to 3 weeks after primary exposure to HIV, some patients develop a self-limited, infectious mononucleosis–like illness with malaise, fever, myalgias, pharyngitis, and rash. This acute HIV seroconversion syndrome can be complicated by the development of esophageal ulcerations that cause odynophagia.[75] Endoscopically, the ulcers are typically multiple, round, 3 to 15 mm in diameter, well demarcated, and surrounded by normal-appearing esophageal mucosa. Usually, the ulcers heal and the symptoms of the acute HIV seroconversion syndrome resolve spontaneously within 2 weeks. Patients then may remain asymptomatic for years until the development of AIDS.

Symptoms of esophageal disease occur in 30% to 40% of AIDS patients.[76] Although the symptoms are usually from infections with Candida, HSV, or CMV, these patients can also have large esophageal ulcerations in which no pathogenic microorganism can be identified by culture or by histologic and immunohistochemical tests. Radiographically and endoscopically, HIV-associated idiopathic ulcerations of the esophagus closely resemble the large esophageal ulcerations caused by CMV. HIV-associated idiopathic esophageal ulcerations can be found in approximately 10% of patients with AIDS who complain of esophageal symptoms and in up to 40% of such patients who have discrete esophageal ulcerations on endoscopic examination.

HIV-associated idiopathic ulcerations generally do not respond to therapy with antimicrobial agents. Rather, patients with these lesions usually experience symptomatic relief and ulcer healing during treatment with systemic corticosteroids. Although corticosteroid therapy entails substantial risk for patients who already are profoundly immunosuppressed, the treatment is surprisingly well tolerated in most cases. The injection of methylprednisolone through the endoscope directly into idiopathic ulcerations also has resulted in relief of esophageal symptoms in some cases, but experience with this treatment is limited. Finally, thalidomide, which has immunomodulatory effects, has been used successfully to treat idiopathic ulcerations.

Candida is by far the most common cause of esophageal infection in AIDS, and candidal esophagitis is found in more than 50% of AIDS patients who have esophageal symptoms. Although CMV and HSV esophagitis also occur commonly in AIDS patients, these viruses often are not the sole pathogens that can be identified in the inflamed esophagus. CMV usually is discovered in biopsy specimens from an esophagus that is also infected by *Candida,* and most patients with coexistent CMV and candidal esophagitis respond well to antifungal therapy alone. Consequently, authorities have recommended that patients with AIDS who have esophageal symptoms should be treated empirically with antifungal therapy, usually fluconazole; endoscopy is reserved for patients who fail to respond to empirical treatment.

Esophageal Cancer

EPIDEMIOLOGY

The two major histologic types of esophageal cancer, squamous cell carcinoma and adenocarcinoma, differ profoundly in their epidemiologic features.[77] Squamous cell carcinoma of the esophagus has a strong predilection for blacks and Asians, whereas esophageal adenocarcinoma is predominantly a disease of whites. In the United States, the incidence of squamous cell carcinoma of the esophagus is six times greater in African Americans than in whites, whereas esophageal adenocarcinoma is at least four times more frequent in whites than in African Americans. Worldwide, more than 90% of all esophageal cancers are squamous cell carcinomas; this tumor ranks among the world's 10 most frequent malignancies. Exceptionally high incidence rates of squamous cell carcinoma are found in the Transkei region of South Africa, in southern Brazil, in parts of northern France and Italy, and throughout an esophageal cancer belt that extends from the shores of the Caspian Sea of Iran across northern China. In the Henan province of China, the incidence of esophageal squamous cell carcinoma exceeds 100 per 100,000. In the United States, in contrast, the incidence of this tumor in the general population is less than 4 per 100,000. In most countries, cancer of the esophagus affects men two to four times more often than women.

RISK FACTORS

GERD and Barrett esophagus are the major risk factors for adenocarcinoma of the esophagus.[70] For squamous cell carcinoma, cigarette smoking and alcoholism are the major risk factors.[78] The combination of cigarette smoking and alcoholism appears to have a synergistic (rather than merely additive) effect in esophageal carcinogenesis, but the mechanism of this synergy is not known. Generalized malnutrition and a variety of specific nutritional deficiencies, including deficiencies in vitamin A, vitamin C, magnesium, selenium, and zinc, have been associated with squamous cell carcinoma. In contrast, obesity is

a risk factor for adenocarcinoma. Carcinogens such as *N*-nitroso compounds can be formed from the nitrates and amines in pickled vegetables and cured meats, and ingestion of these foods has been linked to esophageal cancer. Regional practices such as opium smoking and the long-term ingestion of very hot foods and beverages may contribute to the pathogenesis of squamous cell cancers. Also, some high-incidence areas for squamous cell carcinoma have soils that are deficient in certain elements, such as molybdenum and zinc.

Local differences in endemic microflora have been proposed as underlying reasons for some of the regional variations in the incidence of esophageal squamous cell carcinoma. For example, the food and water in some high-incidence areas are contaminated with fungi and bacteria that promote the formation of *N*-nitroso compounds from dietary nitrates. The human papillomavirus (HPV) can infect squamous epithelial cells, and HPV infection has been implicated in the development of squamous cell carcinoma of the esophagus. In high-incidence regions for esophageal cancer, such as China and South Africa, researchers have found HPV DNA in more than 20% of squamous cell carcinomas. In low-incidence areas, such as the United States, however, esophageal tumors generally do not show evidence of HPV infection.

A number of medical conditions predispose to the development of esophageal squamous cell carcinoma. Patients with tylosis, a rare heritable disorder characterized by hyperkeratosis of the palms and soles, are at very high risk for development of the esophageal tumor. These patients have mutations in the tylosis esophageal cancer gene, a putative tumor suppressor gene located on the long arm of chromosome 17. Achalasia, lye stricture of the esophagus, and Plummer-Vinson, or Paterson-Kelly, syndrome also are risk factors for squamous cell cancers, perhaps because these conditions are associated with stasis of esophageal contents that leads to chronic inflammation of the mucosa. Squamous cell cancer of the esophagus is strongly associated with malignancies of the head, neck, and lungs, probably because these tumors share the strong risk factor of cigarette smoking. Finally, celiac sprue has been associated with esophageal cancer, for reasons that are not clear.

DIAGNOSIS

Clinical Features

Most patients with cancer of the esophagus present with dysphagia and weight loss. The dysphagia usually involves solid foods only and progresses rapidly in severity (over a period of weeks to months). Approximately 60% of patients who have esophageal adenocarcinoma have a long-standing history of GERD symptoms. Proximal esophageal tumors can invade the recurrent laryngeal nerve, causing vocal cord paralysis with hoarseness. The development of coughing associated with swallowing may indicate that the tumor has invaded the airway and caused an esophagobronchial fistula. Ulcerated tumors can cause odynophagia, and tumor necrosis occasionally causes esophageal hemorrhage. Local tumor invasion can cause chest pain, and metastatic disease can cause bone pain. Symptoms of esophageal cancer generally develop only when the tumor has grown to the extent that it has narrowed the lumen of the esophagus substantially, has invaded local structures, or has metastasized. Therefore, the presence of symptoms usually indicates advanced disease and a poor prognosis.

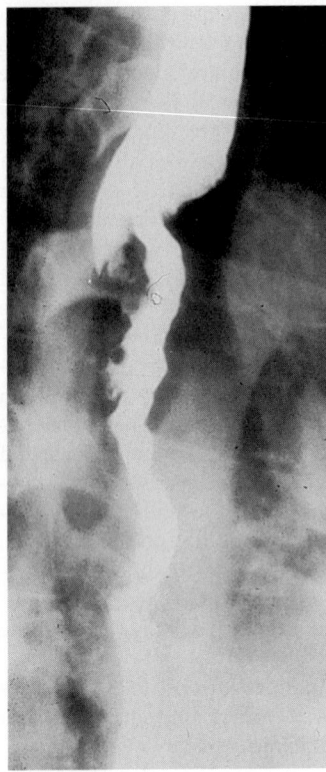
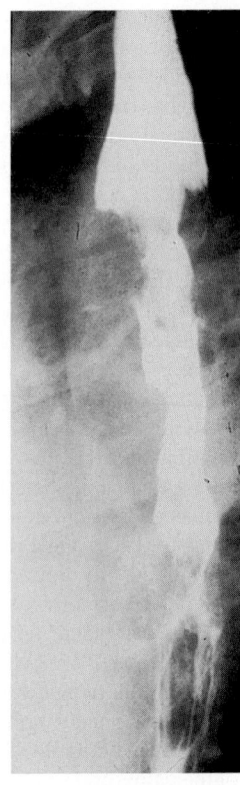

Figure 8   **Barium swallow showing an extensive cancer of the esophagus.**

Diagnostic Studies

Barium swallow and endoscopy   Both barium swallow and endoscopy are useful for the evaluation of patients with esophageal cancer. Radiographic features that suggest malignancy include irregular borders and sharp angles [*see Figure 8*]. Endoscopically, esophageal cancers typically appear as nodular lesions that protrude into the lumen of the esophagus [*see Figure 9*]. In Asian countries where there is a high incidence of esophageal cancer, endoscopists often recognize early esophageal cancers that cause either slight elevations or shallow depressions in the mucosal surface. Staining of the esophagus with vital dyes such as toluidine blue or Lugol iodine (chromoendoscopy) can be useful for finding such early lesions during endoscopic evaluation. These superficial esophageal cancers are diagnosed infrequently in western countries.

Imaging studies   Computed tomography of the chest and abdomen generally is recommended to assess the extent of disease within the chest and to look for metastases. However, the sensitivity and specificity of CT for determining the depth of esophageal tumor penetration (the T level) and the presence of regional lymph node metastases (the N status) are poor. Endoscopic ultrasonography (EUS) is superior to CT in this regard, accurately predicting the T level and N status in 70% to 80% of patients.

Invasive modalities   In addition to EUS, invasive diagnostic modalities sometimes used for the staging of esophageal cancer include bronchoscopy, laparoscopy, thoracotomy, and thoracoscopy. There is little consensus regarding the need for these procedures in the routine evaluation of patients with

esophageal cancer, and usage of the procedures varies widely among different institutions.

MANAGEMENT

Cancer of the esophagus usually is disseminated at the time of diagnosis, and because there is no treatment that reliably eradicates metastatic disease, cure is not possible in most cases. Furthermore, patients are often elderly, and many have severe comorbidities (e.g., malnutrition or pulmonary, cardiac, or liver disease) that further limit their treatment options. Initial treatment usually involves a choice between surgery, radiation therapy, chemotherapy, and some combination of these three modalities.[79,80] Squamous cell cancer and adenocarcinoma are treated similarly, with similarly poor survival rates. Despite recent advances in therapeutic options, overall cure rates for cancer of the esophagus remain below 10%.

Surgical therapy   Esophagectomy, with or without lymphadenectomy, can provide immediate palliation of symptoms and, arguably, the best potential for cure of esophageal cancer. Mortality for esophagectomy ranges from 3% to more than 12%, and serious complications of the operation (e.g., pneumonia, atelectasis, arrhythmias, myocardial infarction, heart failure, wound infections, and anastomotic leaks) can be expected in 30% to 50% of patients. Cure rates vary widely among institutions. Prognostic factors include tumor stage and the number of positive lymph nodes. Surgery generally is not recommended for patients who have metastatic disease.

Radiation therapy   The acute mortality of radiation therapy is low, and radiation can cover a wider treatment area than is practical with surgery (to eradicate local and regional disease). However, radiation therapy usually takes 2 to 8 weeks to complete; palliation can be delayed for weeks; there can be substantial radiation damage to surrounding normal tissues; and the overall cure rate is low. Trials of radiation therapy as the

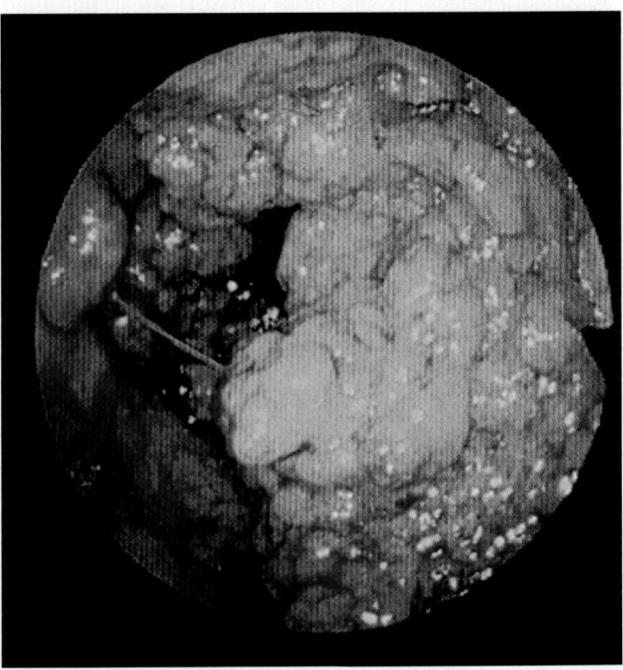

Figure 9   **Endoscopic photograph of an esophageal adenocarcinoma.**

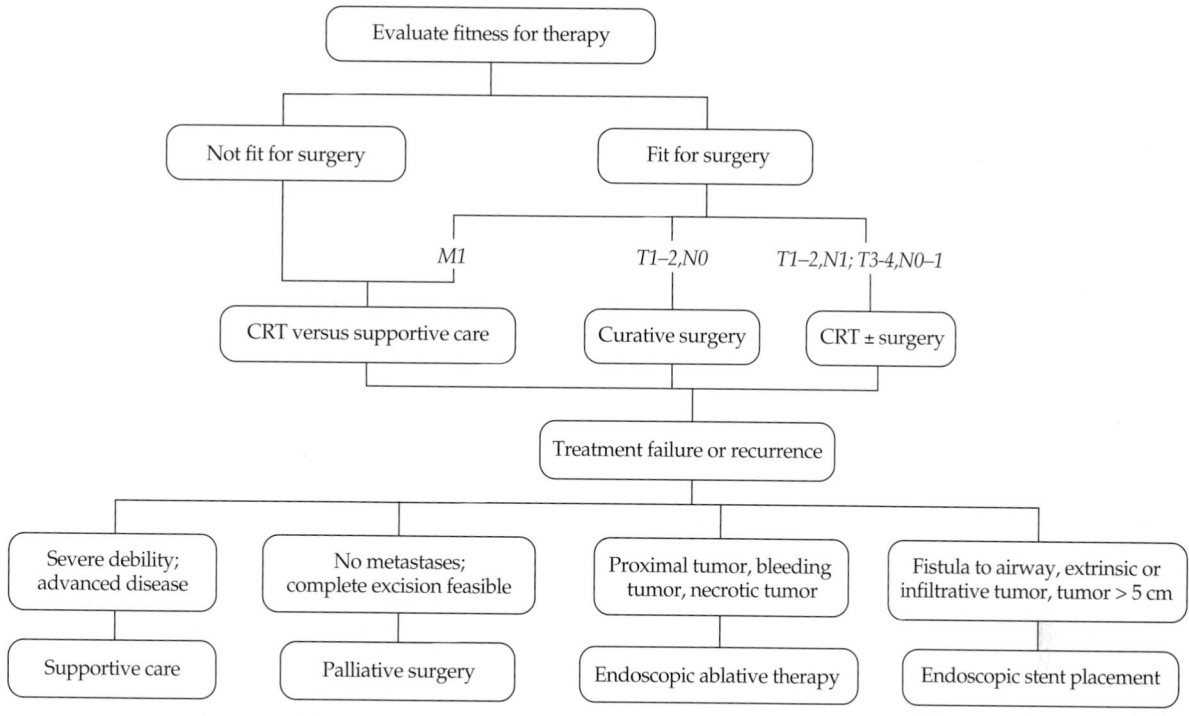

Figure 10 **Management of patients with cancer of the esophagus. (CRT—chemoradiotherapy)**

sole treatment modality for esophageal cancer have involved primarily patients with advanced squamous cell carcinomas that were deemed unresectable. Results appear to be comparable to surgery, but there are no randomized trials directly comparing radiation therapy alone with surgery alone.

Chemotherapy Chemotherapy has the potential to reach the disseminated disease that usually is present in symptomatic patients. Unfortunately, chemotherapy is associated with substantial morbidity and considerable mortality; it is often ineffective; and the tumor response, if any, is often brief. Studies of chemotherapy as the sole treatment modality have included primarily patients with unresectable tumors. Modern studies have used cisplatin-based regimens, and response rates appear to be better with combination regimens than with single agents. Chemotherapy alone does not appear to improve survival, however.

A number of studies have explored the role of radiation therapy or chemotherapy used either before (neoadjuvant) or after (adjuvant) definitive surgery for squamous cell carcinoma of the esophagus. Unfortunately, most randomized, controlled trials have shown no convincing benefit for neoadjuvant or adjuvant treatment with either radiation therapy or chemotherapy for patients with potentially resectable tumors. One recent trial showed a modest survival benefit for patients who received preoperative chemotherapy in a relatively low dose, however.[80]

Combination therapy Much recent interest has focused on the role of combining chemotherapy with radiation therapy (chemoradiotherapy) for esophageal cancer.[81] In some studies of patients treated with chemoradiotherapy followed by esophagectomy, complete histologic response (defined as no histologic evidence of tumor in the resected specimen) has been observed in almost 30% of cases. Complete histologic response is not tantamount to cure, however, and even complete

responders frequently succumb to recurrent disease. Furthermore, chemoradiotherapy is associated with serious toxicity. Some randomized trials of chemoradiotherapy for patients with potentially resectable tumors have shown significant improvements in survival, whereas others have not. Consequently, the role of chemoradiotherapy remains unclear. Preliminary studies suggest that patients who have locally advanced tumors might benefit from preoperative chemoradiotherapy.

Palliative therapy Purely palliative therapies include esophageal dilatation and the placement of intraluminal stents. There also are palliative techniques designed to ablate the portion of the neoplasm that obstructs the esophageal lumen. These ablative therapies include endoscopic laser irradiation, the application of tumor probes that burn the neoplasm directly, the injection of caustic chemicals directly into the tumor body, and photodynamic therapy that uses photochemical energy to destroy the tumor.

Given that the optimal treatment for cancer of the esophagus is not clear, patients should be treated according to well-designed, established research protocols whenever possible. If the initial use of research protocols is not feasible, management should be individualized [*see Figure 10*]. After staging of the tumor that includes at least EUS and a CT scan of the chest and abdomen, the next step is to decide whether the patient is fit enough to undergo surgery. If surgery is not a viable option because of advanced age or comorbidity, primary therapy might include chemoradiation or supportive care alone. In general, surgery is not indicated for patients with metastatic disease. For tumors that do not invade beyond the muscularis propria and do not involve local lymph nodes, surgery appears to offer the best hope for cure. For lesions that are more advanced (i.e., with lymph node involvement or invasion to the esophageal adventitia and beyond), the choices for primary therapy include chemoradiation with or without surgery.

If these primary treatments fail or if the tumor recurs, there are a number of palliative treatment options. For patients who are severely debilitated and have advanced disease, the most humane option may be supportive care only, with careful attention to pain control. If there are no apparent metastases and complete excision of the tumor is possible, surgery can be considered for palliation. The other options are ablative therapies or stents. Stents may not provide good palliation for patients with proximal tumors, bleeding tumors, and necrotic tumors; ablative therapy may be preferable in these circumstances. Alternatively, ablative therapy has little to offer for a patient with an esophagobronchial fistula or for a patient with a tumor that is extrinsic or infiltrative. Also, ablative therapy may be difficult and time-consuming for patients with very long tumors. Stenting may be preferable in these circumstances.

The author has received grants for clinical research or educational activities from AstraZeneca, Janssen Pharmaceutica Products LP, TAP Pharmaceuticals, Inc., and Wyeth-Ayerst.

References

1. Spechler SJ: American Gastroenterological Association medical position statement on treatment of patients with dysphagia caused by benign disorders of the distal esophagus. Gastroenterology 117:229, 1999

2. Castell DO, Knuff TE, Brown FC, et al: Dysphagia. Gastroenterology 76:1015, 1979

3. Wilcox CM, Alexander LN, Clark WS: Localization of an obstructing esophageal lesion: is the patient accurate? Dig Dis Sci 40:2192, 1995

4. Cook IJ, Kahrilas PJ: AGA technical review on management of oropharyngeal dysphagia. Gastroenterology 116:455, 1999

5. Lapadula G, Muolo P, Semeraro F, et al: Esophageal motility disorders in the rheumatic diseases: a review of 150 patients. Clin Exp Rheumatol 12:515, 1994

6. Baehr PH, McDonald GB: Esophageal infections: risk factors, presentation, diagnosis, and treatment. Gastroenterology 106:509, 1994

7. Ott DJ, Richter JE, Chen YM, et al: Esophageal radiography and manometry: correlation in 172 patients with dysphagia. AJR Am J Roentgenol 149:307, 1987

8. Kahrilas PJ, Clouse RE, Hogan WJ: American Gastroenterological Association technical review on the clinical use of esophageal manometry. Gastroenterology 107:1865, 1994

9. Marks RD, Shukla M: Diagnosis and management of peptic esophageal strictures. Gastroenterologist 4:223, 1996

10. A comparison of omeprazole and ranitidine in the prevention of recurrence of benign esophageal stricture. The Restore Investigator Group. Gastroenterology 107:1312, 1994

11. DeVault KR: Lower esophageal (Schatzki's) ring: pathogenesis, diagnosis, and therapy. Dig Dis 14:323, 1996

12. Spechler SJ, Castell DO: Classification of oesophageal motility abnormalities. Gut 49:145, 2001

13. Wong RKH, Maydonovitch CL: Achalasia. The Esophagus, 2nd ed. Castell DO, Ed. Little, Brown, Boston, 1995, p 219

14. Spiess AE, Kahrilas PJ: Treating achalasia: from whalebone to laparoscope. JAMA 280:638, 1998

15. Csendes A, Braghetto I, Henriquez A, et al: Late results of a prospective randomised study comparing forceful dilatation and oesophagomyotomy in patients with achalasia. Gut 30:299, 1989

16. Pasricha PJ, Rai R, Ravich WJ, et al: Botulinum toxin for achalasia: long-term outcome and predictors of response. Gastroenterology 110:1410, 1996

17. Dalton CB, Castell DO, Richter JE: The changing faces of the nutcracker esophagus. Am J Gastroenterol 83:623, 1988

18. Richter JE, Bradley LA, Castell DO: Esophageal chest pain: current controversies in pathogenesis, diagnosis, and therapy. Ann Intern Med 110:66, 1989

19. Lock G, Holstege A, Lang B, et al: Gastrointestinal manifestations of progressive systemic sclerosis. Am J Gastroenterol 92:763, 1997

20. Leite LP, Johnston BT, Barrett J, et al: Ineffective esophageal motility (IEM): the primary finding in patients with nonspecific esophageal motility disorder. Dig Dis Sci 42:1859, 1997

21. Locke GR III, Talley NJ, Fett SL, et al: Prevalence and clinical spectrum of gastroesophageal reflux: a population-based study in Olmsted County, Minnesota. Gastroenterology 112:1448, 1997

22. Lagergren J, Bergström R, Lindgren A, et al: Symptomatic gastroesophageal reflux as a risk factor for esophageal adenocarcinoma. N Engl J Med 340:825, 1999

23. Kahrilas PJ: Gastroesophageal reflux disease. JAMA 276:983, 1996

24. Holloway RH, Dent J: Pathophysiology of gastroesophageal reflux: lower esophageal sphincter dysfunction in gastroesophageal reflux disease. Gastroenterol Clin North Am 19:517, 1990

25. Dodds WJ, Dent J, Hogan WJ, et al: Mechanisms of gastroesophageal reflux in patients with reflux esophagitis. N Engl J Med 307:1547, 1982

26. Mittal RK, Holloway RH, Penagini R, et al: Transient lower esophageal sphincter relaxation. Gastroenterology 109:601, 1995

27. Mittal RK, Balaban DH: The esophagogastric junction. N Engl J Med 336:924, 1997

28. Sloan S, Rademaker AW, Kahrilas PJ: Determinants of gastroesophageal junction incompetence: hiatal hernia, lower esophageal sphincter, or both? Ann Intern Med 117:977, 1992

29. Kahrilas PJ, Lin S, Chen J, et al: The effect of hiatus hernia on gastro-oesophageal junction pressure. Gut 44:476, 1999

30. Kahrilas PJ, Shi G, Manka M, et al: Increased frequency of transient lower esophageal sphincter relaxation induced by gastric distention in reflux patients with hiatal hernia. Gastroenterology 118:688, 2000

31. Helm JF, Dodds WJ, Pele LR, et al: Effect of esophageal emptying and saliva on clearance of acid from the esophagus. N Engl J Med 310:284, 1984

32. Kahrilas PJ, Dodds WJ, Hogan WJ, et al: Esophageal peristaltic dysfunction in peptic esophagitis. Gastroenterology 91:897, 1986

33. Kahrilas PJ, Gupta RR: The effect of cigarette smoking on salivation and esophageal acid clearance. J Lab Clin Med 114:431, 1989

34. Lanas A, Hirschowitz BI: Significant role of aspirin use in patients with esophagitis. J Clin Gastroenterol 13:622, 1991

35. Cryer B, Spechler SJ: Effects of non-steroidal anti-inflammatory drugs (NSAIDs) on acid reflux in patients with gastroesophageal reflux disease (GERD). Gastroenterology 118:A862, 2000

36. O'Connor HJ: *Helicobacter pylori* and gastro-oesophageal reflux disease—clinical implications and management. Aliment Pharmacol Ther 13:117, 1999

37. Werdmuller BFM, Loffeld RJLF: *Helicobacter pylori* infection has no role in the pathogenesis of reflux esophagitis. Dig Dis Sci 42:103, 1997

38. Labenz J, Blum AL, Bayerdörffer E, et al: Curing *Helicobacter pylori* infection in patients with duodenal ulcer may provoke reflux esophagitis. Gastroenterology 112:1442, 1997

39. Chow WH, Blaser MJ, Blot WJ, et al: An inverse relation between *cagA*+ strains of *Helicobacter pylori* infection and risk of esophageal and gastric cardia adenocarcinoma. Cancer Res 58:588, 1998

40. Vicari JJ, Peek RM, Falk GW, et al: The seroprevalence of *cagA*-positive *Helicobacter pylori* strains in the spectrum of gastroesophageal reflux disease. Gastroenterology 115:50, 1998

41. Graham DY, Yamaoka Y: *H. pylori* and *cagA*: relationships with gastric cancer, duodenal ulcer, and reflux esophagitis and its complications. Helicobacter 3:145, 1998

42. Richter JE: Chest pain and gastroesophageal reflux disease. J Clin Gastroenterol 30 (3 suppl):S39, 2000

43. Jailwala JA, Shaker R: Oral and pharyngeal complications of gastroesophageal reflux disease: globus, dental erosions, and chronic sinusitis. J Clin Gastroenterol 30(3 suppl):S35, 2000

44. Harding SM, Richter JE: The role of gastroesophageal reflux in chronic cough and asthma. Chest 111:1389, 1997

45. Ormseth EJ, Wong RKH: Reflux laryngitis: pathophysiology, diagnosis and management. Am J Gastroenterol 94:2812, 1999

46. Richter JE, Peura D, Benjamin SB, et al: Efficacy of omeprazole for the treatment of symptomatic acid reflux disease without esophagitis. Arch Intern Med 160:1810, 2000

47. Spechler SJ: Epidemiology and natural history of gastro-oesophageal reflux disease. Digestion 51(suppl 1):24, 1992

48. DeVault KR, Castell DO: Updated guidelines for the diagnosis and treatment of gastroesophageal reflux disease. Am J Gastroenterol 100:190, 2005

49. DeVault KR, Castell DO: Guidelines for the diagnosis and treatment of gastroesophageal reflux disease. Arch Intern Med 155:2165, 1995

50. Eggleston A, Wigerinck A, Huijghebaert S, et al: Cost effectiveness of treatment for gastro-oesophageal reflux disease in clinical practice: a clinical database analysis. Gut 42:13, 1998

51. Inadomi JM, Jamal R, Murata GH, et al: Step-down management of gastroesophageal reflux disease. Gastroenterology 121:1095, 2001

52. Spechler SJ: Peptic ulcer disease and its complications. Sleisenger & Fordtran's Gastrointestinal and Liver Disease. Feldman M, Friedman LS, Sleisenger MH, Eds. WB Saunders Co, Philadelphia, 2002, p 747

53. Zhang Q, Lehmann A, Rigda R, et al: Control of transient lower esophageal sphincter relaxations and reflux by the GABA(B) agonist baclofen in patients with gastroesophageal reflux disease. Gut 50:19, 2002

54. Vakil N, Fennerty MB: Direct comparative trials of the efficacy of proton pump inhibitors in the management of gastro-oesophageal reflux disease and peptic ulcer disease. Aliment Pharmacol Ther 18:559, 2003

55. Hetzel DJ, Dent J, Reed WD, et al: Healing and relapse of severe peptic esophagitis after treatment with omeprazole. Gastroenterology 95:903, 1988

56. Long-term omeprazole treatment in resistant gastroesophageal reflux disease: efficacy, safety, and influence on gastric mucosa. Long-Term Study Group. Gastroenterology 118:661, 2000

57. Dent J, Yeomans ND, Mackinnon M, et al: Omeprazole v ranitidine for prevention of relapse in reflux oesophagitis: a controlled double blind trial of their efficacy and safety. Gut 35:590, 1994

58. Rydberg L, Ruth M, Lundell L: Mechanism of action of antireflux procedures. Br J

Surg 86:405, 1999

59. Hinder RA, Libbey JS, Gorecki P, et al: Antireflux surgery: indications, preoperative evaluation, and outcome. Gastroenterol Clin North Am 28:987, 1999

60. Laine S, Rantala A, Gullichsen R, et al: Laparoscopic vs conventional Nissen fundoplication: a prospective randomized study. Surg Endosc 11:441, 1997

61. Laparoscopic or conventional Nissen fundoplication for gastro-oesophageal reflux disease: randomised clinical trial. The Netherlands Antireflux Surgery Study Group. Lancet 355:170, 2000

62. Spechler SJ: Comparison of medical and surgical therapy for complicated gastroesophageal reflux disease in veterans. N Engl J Med 326:786, 1992

63. Long-term management of gastro-oesophageal reflux disease with omeprazole or open antireflux surgery: results of a prospective, randomized clinical trial. The Nordic GORD Study Group. Eur J Gastroenterol Hepatol 12:879, 2000

64. DeMeester TR, Bonavina L, Albertucci M: Nissen fundoplication for gastroesophageal reflux disease: evaluation of primary repair in 100 consecutive patients. Ann Surg 204:9, 1986

65. Brand DL, Eastwood IR, Martin D, et al: Esophageal symptoms, manometry, and histology before and after antireflux surgery: a long-term follow-up study. Gastroenterology 76:1393, 1979

66. Spechler SJ, Lee E, Ahnen D, et al: Long-term outcome of medical and surgical treatments for gastroesophageal reflux disease: follow-up of a randomized controlled trial. JAMA 285:2331, 2001

67. Filipi CJ, Lehman GA, Rothstein RI, et al: Transoral, flexible endoscopic suturing for treatment of GERD: a multicenter trial. Gastrointest Endosc 53:416, 2001

68. Triadafilopoulos G, DiBaise JK, Nostrant TT, et al: The Stretta procedure for the treatment of GERD: 6 and 12 month follow-up of the U.S. open label trial. Gastrointest Endosc 55:149, 2002

69. Spechler SJ: Barrett's esophagus. N Engl J Med 346:836, 2002

70. Van den Boogert J, van Hillegersberg R, Siersema PD, et al: Endoscopic ablation therapy for Barrett's esophagus with high-grade dysplasia: a review. Am J Gastroenterol 94:1153, 1999

71. McBane RD, Gross JB Jr: Herpes esophagitis: clinical syndrome, endoscopic appearance, and diagnosis in 23 patients. Gastrointest Endosc 37:600, 1991

72. Meyers JD: Prevention and treatment of cytomegalovirus infection. Ann Rev Med 42:179, 1991

73. Hackman RC, Wolford JL, Gleaves CA, et al: Recognition and rapid diagnosis of upper gastrointestinal cytomegalovirus infection in marrow transplant recipients: a comparison of seven virologic methods. Transplantation 57:231, 1994

74. Rabeneck L, Popovic M, Gartner S, et al: Acute HIV infection with painful swallowing and esophageal ulcers. JAMA 263:2318, 1990

75. Laine L, Bonacini M: Esophageal disease in human immunodeficiency virus infection. Arch Intern Med 154:1577, 1994

76. Blot WJ, McLaughlin JK: The changing epidemiology of esophageal cancer. Semin Oncol 26(suppl 15):2, 1999

77. Stoner G, Gupta A: Etiology and chemoprevention of esophageal squamous cell carcinoma. Carcinogenesis 22:1737, 2001

78. Siewert JR, Stein HJ, Sendler A, et al: Esophageal cancer: clinical management. Gastrointestinal Oncology: Principles and Practice. Kelsen D, Daly JM, Kern SE, et al, Eds. Lippincott Williams & Wilkins, Philadelphia, 2002, p 261

79. Surgical resection with or without preoperative chemotherapy in oesophageal cancer: a randomised controlled trial. Medical Research Council Oesophageal Cancer Working Group. Lancet 359:1727, 2002

80. Bosset JF, Gignoux M, Triboulet JP, et al: Chemoradiotherapy followed by surgery compared with surgery alone in squamous-cell cancer of the esophagus. N Engl J Med 337:161, 1997

81. Spechler SJ: The role of gastric carditis in metaplasia and neoplasia at the gastroesophageal junction. Gastroenterology 117:218, 1999

Acknowledgments

Figures 4, 8, and 9   American Gastroenterological Association.

Figure 6   Seward Hung.

62 Peptic Ulcer Diseases

Mark Feldman, M.D., F.A.C.P.

Definition

Peptic ulcers are holes in the inner lining of the gastrointestinal (GI) tract that are attributed to exposure of the mucosa to gastric acid and pepsin. Peptic ulcers extend through the mucosa and the muscularis mucosae, a thin layer of smooth muscle separating the mucosa from the deeper submucosa, muscularis propria, and serosa. Most peptic ulcers are round or oval, but some are linear, triangular, or irregular in shape. Ulcers have depth when viewed through an endoscope. Typically, only a single ulcer is present. An erosion is a focal loss of superficial epithelial cells and glands, without extension through the muscularis mucosae. On endoscopy, erosions appear as breaks in the mucosal lining without depth. At the other extreme, a peptic ulcer may burr itself entirely through the wall of the GI tract, thus connecting the GI lumen with the peritoneal cavity (perforated ulcer), a solid organ such as the pancreas (penetrating ulcer), or another hollow organ such as the intestine or bile duct (fistulizing ulcer).

Epidemiology

In the United States, peptic ulcer disease affects 10% of men and 4% of women at some time in their lives. The incidence is influenced by age (older persons are more susceptible than younger persons) and gender (males are more susceptible than females). Because ulcer disease is often recurrent, its prevalence exceeds its incidence. Eradication of *Helicobacter pylori* from the stomach markedly reduces recurrence of ulcer disease. With the widespread use of treatment regimens for *H. pylori*, the prevalence of peptic ulcer is decreasing in the United States. Reinfection with *H. pylori* remains an uncommon event in the United States (approximately one reinfection per 100 patients a year).

Pathogenesis and Etiologic Factors

The normal stomach and duodenum are able to resist autodigestion by acid-pepsin. However, high rates of acid-pepsin secretion or impaired mucosal resistance factors, such as prostaglandin deficiency, can predispose to duodenal ulcer formation (typically in the most proximal part of the duodenum, the bulb) or to gastric ulcer formation (typically in the most distal part of the stomach, the antrum).

On rare occasions, peptic ulcers occur in the second, third, or fourth portion of the duodenum (postbulbar ulcer) or even in the proximal jejunum. Ordinarily, alkaline secretions from the duodenum, biliary tract, and pancreas neutralize gastric acid in the duodenum, but high rates of gastric acid secretion (e.g., in Zollinger-Ellison syndrome) can overwhelm these endogenous alkaline secretions and lead to postbulbar or jejunal ulcerations.

In patients with pathologic amounts of gastroesophageal reflux of acid-pepsin and in many patients with gastric acid hypersecretion, erosions and ulcers may develop in the lower esophagus [*see Chapter 61*]. Peptic ulcers may also occur where acid and pepsin are secreted heterotopically, such as in a congenital ileal (Meckel) diverticulum.

Regardless of location and etiology, chronic peptic ulcers are similar pathologically. In addition to the focal loss of mucosal epithelial cells, these ulcers have four characteristic layers at their base: fibrinoid necrosis, exudate, granulation tissue, and a fibrous scar, the deepest layer. A layer of granulation tissue and fibrosis may be absent in acute ulcers that occur in settings of serious trauma or severe surgical or medical illnesses [*see Acute Stress Ulcers, below*].

Why a peptic ulcer is such a focal lesion is unclear. Although peptic ulcers require the presence of acid-pepsin, acid-pepsin alone is only rarely sufficient to produce an ulcer—such as in Zollinger-Ellison syndrome, in which marked gastric hypersecretion is present. In the majority of patients, there must be another predisposing factor, such as *H. pylori* infection of the stomach,[1,2] use of nonsteroidal anti-inflammatory drugs (NSAIDs), or stress [*see Figure 1*].

H. PYLORI ULCERS

The prevalence of *H. pylori* infection of the stomach is much higher in duodenal ulcer patients and, to a somewhat lesser extent, in gastric ulcer patients than in age-matched control subjects [*see Figure 2*].[3] In addition, cure of *H. pylori* infection with antimicrobial therapy markedly reduces recurrences of duodenal and gastric ulcers.[4,5] The correlation of *H. pylori* infection with peptic ulcers is not consistent, however. Duodenal ulcers develop in some infected persons and gastric ulcers in others, but most infected persons experience no ulcers at all. Patients with duodenal ulcers tend more often to be infected with *cagA*-positive strains than do *H. pylori*–infected patients without ulcer,[6] but how this is mediated is not clear.

The etiologic mechanism linking *H. pylori* infection with ulcer development is not yet absolutely established, for the following reasons: (1) voluntary ingestion of *H. pylori* led to gastric *H. pylori* infection and to gastritis but not to ulcers; (2) duodenal or gastric ulcers develop in only 10% to 20% of individuals with *H. pylori* gastritis, implying that only certain persons with additional genetic, anatomic, physiologic, or environmental risk factors are predisposed to ulcers or that only certain *H. pylori* strains are ulcerogenic; (3) *H. pylori* induces diffuse inflammation in the stomach, yet the strongest link between *H. pylori* and peptic ulcer is with focal duodenal bulbar ulcer; and (4) gastric *H. pylori* infection is as common in women as in men, yet duodenal ulcer is two to three times less common in women. Currently, *H. pylori* can be considered the most important risk factor for duodenal and gastric ulcers, but it is clear that the mere presence of *H. pylori* in the stomach is not sufficient to cause peptic ulcers [*see Figure 1a*].

NSAID ULCERS

The ulcerogenicity of NSAIDs has been established experimentally by exposing animals, human volunteers, and patients to these drugs. Experimental studies have been corroborated by numerous case-control studies and autopsy studies. Unlike *H. pylori*–related peptic ulcers, which more often occur in the duodenal bulb, NSAID ulcers typically occur in the stomach. A gastric or duodenal ulcer associated with NSAID use is classified as a peptic ulcer, and it usually heals with potent acid antisecretory therapy, even if NSAID use is continued. NSAIDs can also cause ulcers in the jejunum, ileum, or colon, areas where there is little

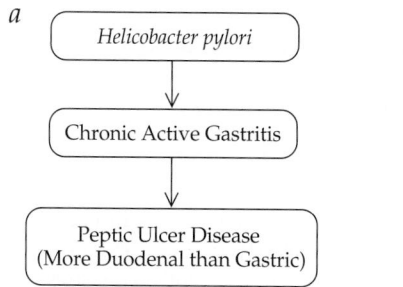

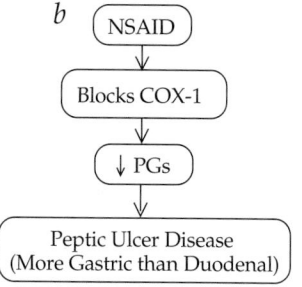

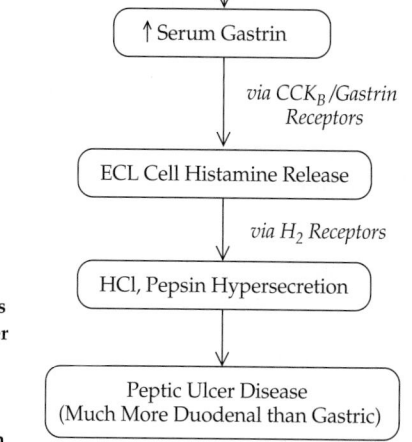

Figure 1 Etiopathogenesis of peptic ulcers. (*a*) *Helicobacter pylori* induces a diffuse, chronic, active superficial gastritis, usually throughout the stomach. Exactly how this infectious gastritis results in peptic ulcer disease is unknown. (*b*) Nonselective nonsteroidal anti-inflammatory drugs (NSAIDs) block cyclooxygenase-1 (COX-1) to reduce the amount of gastroduodenal prostaglandins (PGs) synthesized from their precursor, arachidonic acid. COX-2 selective NSAIDs produce a lesser reduction in prostaglandins and are associated with fewer peptic ulcers than nonselective COX-1– or COX-2–inhibiting NSAIDs. (*c*) Gastrinoma cells in the pancreas or duodenum secrete large amounts of gastrin into the circulation. Elevated serum gastrin levels promote the release of histamine by acting on receptors for cholecystokinin$_B$ (CCK$_B$) and for gastrin, which are located on gastric enterochromaffin-like (ECL) cells. Histamine acts on H$_2$ receptors on parietal and chief cells to augment hydrochloric acid (HCl) and pepsin secretion.

or no acid-pepsin. These ulcers are not actually peptic ulcers.

Although the pathogenesis of NSAID ulcers is multifactorial, by far the most important mechanism appears to be inhibition of cyclooxygenase-1 (COX-1), the rate-limiting enzyme in GI prostaglandin synthesis [*see Figure 1b*]. Prostaglandins normally protect the GI mucosa from damage by maintaining mucosal blood flow and increasing mucosal secretion of mucus and bicarbonate. Blockade of COX-1 activity by NSAIDs reduces prostaglandin synthesis and thus lowers GI mucosal blood flow and secretion of mucus and bicarbonate. Evidence continues to accumulate that in NSAID users, *H. pylori* gastritis produces about a twofold increase in the risk of gastroduodenal ulcer formation.[7] Moreover, clinically symptomatic peptic ulcers occur much less commonly if *H. pylori* gastritis is treated before the start of long-term NSAID therapy.[8] Clinically diagnosed peptic ulcers will develop in approximately 2% to 4% of persons taking NSAIDs per year of exposure. The extent to which the damaging effects of NSAIDs on the stomach are topical rather than systemic is unclear. Many NSAIDs, such as aspirin, are acidic and thus nonionized in the acidic stomach, where they can be absorbed and initiate gastric mucosal damage. However, NSAIDs (e.g., ketorolac) given by parenteral injection and aspirin given transdermally are ulcerogenic, as are so-called NSAID prodrugs, such as sulindac and nabumetone (neither drug inhibits gastric prostaglandins until it is metabolized to its active form after GI absorption). Evidence suggests that acute mucosal damage by NSAIDs (i.e., hemorrhages and erosions, but seldom ulcers) is mainly caused by the topical damaging effects of NSAIDs. Chronic ulcer formation, often with complications such as bleeding and perforation, is mainly the result of the systemic effect of NSAIDs on prostaglandin synthesis by the GI mucosa.

Epidemiologic studies suggest that NSAIDs vary in their ability to cause ulcers,[9] but this issue is complicated by the difficulty of comparing equipotent doses of NSAIDs. All prescription or over-the-counter NSAIDs should be considered ulcerogenic, with the risk of ulcer dependent on dosages and other patient-related factors, particularly advanced age and previous ulcer history. Even low doses of aspirin used for prophylaxis of cardiovascular disease (75 to 325 mg/day) are ulcerogenic.[10] Neither buffering of aspirin nor enteric coating appears to reduce

the incidence of clinically detected ulcer formation.[11] Nonacetylated salicylates such as salicylsalicylic acid (salsalate) do not block COX-1 and are not ulcerogenic. Epidemiologic studies indicate that the greatest risk of NSAID ulcers is early in the course of treatment (between day 7 and day 30 after initiation), with the risk decreasing thereafter.

Most NSAIDs, including aspirin, block both COX-1 and COX-2. Unlike COX-1, COX-2 is induced and expressed at inflammatory sites but not in the normal GI tract.[12] Selective COX-2 inhibitors (coxibs) such as celecoxib and valdecoxib

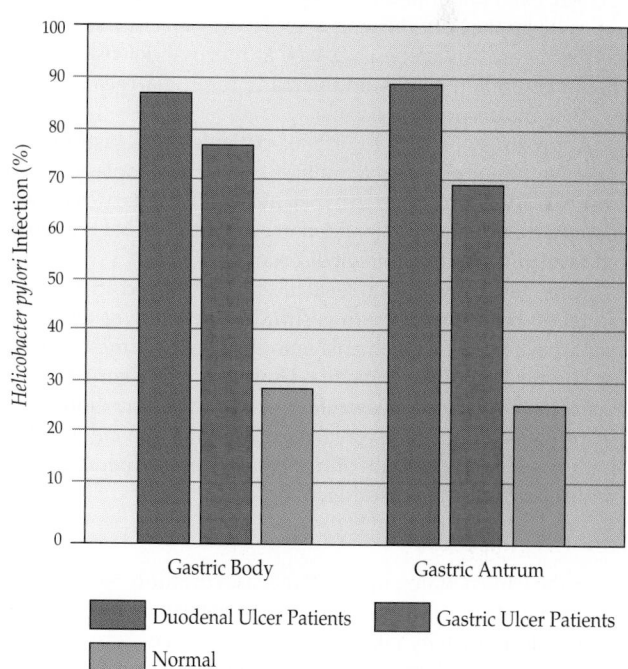

Figure 2 Prevalence of *H. pylori* infection in either the gastric body or the gastric antrum, as assessed by endoscopic biopsy and mucosal histology. Normal control subjects were matched by age and sex to patients with duodenal ulcers and to patients with gastric ulcers. None of the ulcer patients were receiving aspirin or NSAIDs.[3]

are analgesic and anti-inflammatory but seem to cause less GI ulcer formation than currently available cyclooxygenase inhibitors when used in recommended doses.[13] However, the cardiovascular risk associated with COX-2 inhibitors has diminished enthusiasm for their use.[14]

Corticosteroids, which block COX-2,[12] are not ulcerogenic when used alone, although they impair healing of preexisting ulcers. When corticosteroids are used in combination with NSAIDs, the risk of ulcer formation is much greater than when NSAIDs are used alone.

ULCERS IN GASTRINOMA OR OTHER HYPERSECRETORY STATES

A gastrinoma is an endocrine tumor of the pancreas or duodenum (usually malignant) consisting of gastrin (G) cells. Gastrinoma causes less than 1% of all peptic ulcers. Peptic ulcers develop in 95% of patients with gastrinoma (Zollinger-Ellison syndrome); ulcers occur most commonly in the duodenal bulb but are also seen in the postbulbar duodenum, jejunum, lower esophagus, and stomach. Multiple ulcers are present in up to 25% of cases of Zollinger-Ellison syndrome.

Patients with a gastrinoma have high circulating levels of gastrin [see Figure 1c], which acts on receptors for cholecystokinin$_B$ (CCK$_B$) and gastrin located on enterochromaffin-like (ECL) cells within the mucosa of the gastric body. ECL cells then release histamine, which acts on H$_2$ receptors present on the membrane of neighboring parietal cells to stimulate (via an adenylate cyclase–cyclic adenosine monophosphate [cAMP]–mediated pathway) the secretion of hydrochloric acid by a unique proton pump, the H$^+$,K$^+$–ATPase pump. Of less physiologic importance, gastrin also acts directly on CCK$_B$/gastrin receptors on parietal cells, increasing cytosol calcium levels in the parietal cells.

Hypergastrinemia in Zollinger-Ellison syndrome results in a continuous high rate of secretion of hydrochloric acid and pepsin, even under basal (fasting) conditions. These secretions overwhelm the buffering and neutralizing capacity of food and upper digestive secretions, as well as mucosal defense factors. Peptic ulceration results, and in many cases, diarrhea (with or without malabsorption) occurs.

Approximately 20% to 30% of patients with gastrinomas have features suggesting a multiple endocrine neoplasia type I (MEN I) syndrome, such as hypercalcemia secondary to hyperparathyroidism, a pituitary adenoma, or both. MEN I is inherited as an autosomal dominant disorder.

Some patients with duodenal ulcer have marked acid hypersecretion but normal serum gastrin levels. A few of these patients have hyperhistaminemia caused by systemic mastocytosis or chronic basophilic leukemia. However, the majority of patients have no known reason for the acid hypersecretion (idiopathic basal acid hypersecretion), although some are infected with *H. pylori*. Eradication of *H. pylori* in these individuals may reduce basal acid hypersecretion.

IDIOPATHIC ULCERS

In the United States, up to 20% of cases of chronic gastric and duodenal ulcers occur in patients who have no evidence of *H. pylori* infection, deny taking NSAIDs, and have normal serum gastrin concentrations. These ulcers are referred to as idiopathic peptic ulcers. Some patients with this disorder may be taking NSAIDs surreptitiously or are unaware that they are taking these drugs. In others, emotional stress, perhaps associated with gastric acid hypersecretion, may be a contributing factor.[15] Cigarette smoking is also a risk factor for peptic ulcers.

ACUTE STRESS ULCERS

Acute gastroduodenal erosions and ulcers are very common in patients with serious medical and surgical conditions.[16] Such conditions include severe head injury (Cushing ulcers); burn injury (Curling ulcers); major surgical procedures; and life-threatening illnesses such as septic shock, respiratory failure requiring mechanical ventilation, hepatic failure, renal failure, and multiorgan failure. Unlike peptic ulcers, stress ulcers are typically asymptomatic, rarely causing dyspepsia or epigastric pain. Approximately 10% to 25% of patients with acute stress ulcers experience painless upper GI bleeding of variable severity. Bleeding may manifest itself in the intensive care unit as a dark (socalled coffee-ground) or bloody nasogastric aspirate, as a declining hematocrit, as an increasing transfusion requirement, or as unexplained hypotension.

The pathogenesis of stress ulcers is not well understood. The common denominator seems to be tissue hypoxia and acidosis, precipitated by mucosal vasoconstriction and ischemia. Systemic hypoxia, metabolic acidosis, anemia, and reduced cardiac output often are contributing factors. Once mucosal hypoxia develops, mucosal defense factors are impaired and the cells lining the stomach and duodenum become vulnerable to damage by acidpepsin. Acute stress ulcers have become less common because of the routine use of effective prophylactic medications in patients at high risk for this condition (see below).

CAMERON ULCERS

Linear gastric erosions that occur in a hiatus hernia are known as Cameron ulcers.[16] The erosions are thought to be related either to traumatic injury of the stomach by the surrounding diaphragm or to mucosal ischemia at the point where the stomach herniates through the diaphragm. Like acute stress ulcers, Cameron ulcers tend to present as bleeding without dyspepsia. Both acute and chronic GI blood loss are possible outcomes of Cameron ulcers.

Diagnosis

CLINICAL MANIFESTATIONS

Peptic ulcers produce a variety of symptoms but none specific for the disease. Also, symptoms of duodenal ulcer are indistinguishable from those of gastric ulcer. Patients with uncomplicated ulcers typically experience mild to moderate abdominal pain, usually in the epigastrium. However, the pain may be localized to the left or right upper quadrant of the abdomen, to the lower chest (subxiphoid or substernal), the midabdomen, or the back. The pain is often gnawing or burning. It may occur in the middle of the night; rarely, it occurs upon first awakening in the morning. Discomfort is typically relieved by food or an antacid.

Severe pain or a rapid increase in pain suggests an ulcer complication (e.g., perforation or penetration) or another diagnosis (e.g., acute pancreatitis). Associated dyspeptic symptoms include nausea, bloating, heartburn, and belching. Although vomiting may occur with uncomplicated peptic ulcers and may temporarily relieve pain, repeated vomiting suggests an ulcer complication (e.g., gastric outlet obstruction) or another diagnosis (e.g., intestinal obstruction).

Peptic ulcers are the most common cause of acute upper GI bleeding. Therefore, hematemesis, melena, or both, even in a patient with no history of ulcer and no dyspeptic symptoms, should suggest the possibility of a bleeding peptic ulcer. Patients who develop ulcers while taking prescription or over-the-counter NSAIDs or low (cardiovascular) doses of aspirin often have no history of ulcerlike pain. Other patients with bleeding ulcers will have experienced dyspeptic symptoms for the preceding days or weeks, only to have these symptoms wane when bleeding ensues.

In addition to a review of the patient's symptoms and ulcer risk factors (particularly NSAID use and smoking), a family history should be obtained. A family history of ulcer can usually be attributed to within-family infection by *H. pylori*, to NSAID use, or to smoking. However, a family history of ulcer, hyperparathyroidism, kidney stones, or endocrine tumor should alert the physician to the possibility of gastrinoma (Zollinger-Ellison syndrome), with or without autosomal dominant MEN I syndrome.

PHYSICAL EXAMINATION FINDINGS

In uncomplicated peptic ulcer disease, the examination is generally normal. The presence of epigastric tenderness does not distinguish dyspepsia caused by peptic ulcer from other types of dyspepsia.

Patients who have complicated ulcers often have tachycardia and hypotension, which are exaggerated when the patient assumes an upright position. These findings may indicate a bleeding ulcer, a perforated ulcer with peritonitis, or an obstructing ulcer with protracted vomiting and volume depletion. Pulse and blood pressure measurements may give misleading information about the extent of volume contraction if the patient has preexisting hypertension, has cardiovascular disease, or is receiving medication that can affect these parameters (e.g., a beta-adrenergic blocker or a calcium channel blocker). Fever and tachypnea suggest ulcer perforation with peritonitis.

Special attention should be given to the patient's mental status, skin and mucous membranes, heart and lungs, and, of course, abdomen and rectum. Involuntary guarding, rigidity, rebound tenderness, and a paucity or absence of bowel sounds suggests ulcer perforation with peritonitis. These findings may be less prominent or even absent in the very young, the elderly, and patients on corticosteroids or analgesics. Abdominal distention suggests gastric outlet obstruction or ileus. In a patient who has not eaten in 6 hours, a splashing sound over the stomach when the body is shaken (succussion) suggests gastric outlet obstruction or delayed gastric emptying caused by ileus. Melena or a positive fecal occult blood test suggests ulcer bleeding. Hematochezia or maroon-colored stool may be present if bleeding is voluminous and intestinal transit is rapid. Detection of melena, hematochezia, or maroon-colored stool should prompt placement of a nasogastric tube to obtain an aspirate of gastric contents. If this aspirate is grossly bloody, the diagnosis of upper GI bleeding is confirmed and the likelihood of a bleeding ulcer is increased.

LABORATORY STUDIES

Laboratory results are normal in most patients with uncomplicated ulcer. A complete blood count should be done if blood loss or ulcer perforation is suspected; and serum electrolytes, blood urea nitrogen (BUN), and serum creatinine should be measured if the patient has poor oral intake, nausea, or vomiting. An elevated serum calcium level suggests the possibility of hyperparathyroidism and MEN I with Zollinger-Ellison syndrome, but the pretest probability of this condition is too low in patients presenting with ulcerlike symptoms to recommend routine measurement of serum calcium. If the patient has a

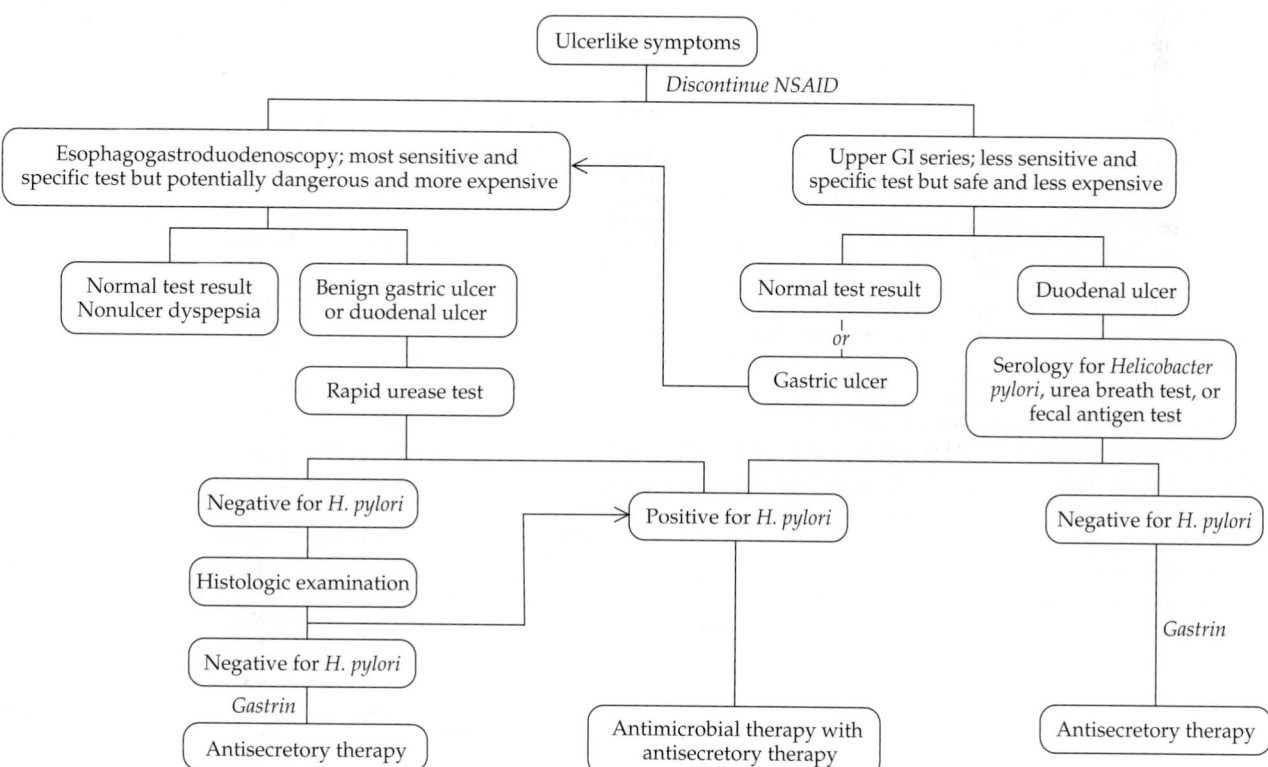

Figure 3 **Approach to a patient with new and undiagnosed ulcerlike symptoms refractory to a trial of antisecretory therapy with an H2 receptor blocker or a proton pump inhibitor at customary doses or a patient with recurrent ulcerlike symptoms when the antisecretory therapy is stopped.**

a

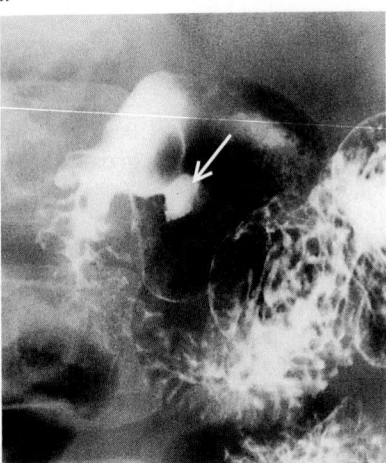

b

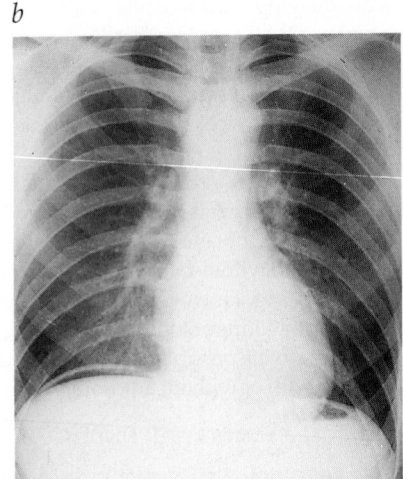

Figure 4 (*a*) Upper GI series in which double contrast (barium and air) is used, showing rounded collection of barium in an ulcer (arrow) in the duodenal bulb of a patient presenting with dyspepsia (uncomplicated duodenal ulcer). (*b*) Upright chest x-ray showing air beneath the right hemidiaphragm (pneumoperitoneum) of a patient presenting with an acute abdomen caused by a perforated duodenal ulcer.

strong family history of ulcer disease or of renal stones or has a personal history of renal stones, measurement of serum calcium is warranted, as is measurement of fasting serum gastrin once ulcer disease is confirmed and other causes of ulcer are excluded. If the calcium level is elevated, a serum parathyroid hormone measurement should be ordered.

Patients with complicated ulcers often have significant laboratory abnormalities, but these abnormalities are not specific for ulcer disease. Patients with bleeding ulcers have anemia and may have leukocytosis. The red cell indices (e.g., mean corpuscular volume) are typically normal. In the first several hours after an acute ulcer bleed, the hemoglobin concentration will not completely reflect the severity of the blood loss until compensatory hemodilution occurs or until intravenous fluids such as isotonic saline are administered. Thus, the pulse rate and blood pressure in the supine and upright positions are better initial indicators of extent of blood loss than are red cell counts. Patients with bleeding ulcers typically have azotemia, with ratios of BUN to serum creatinine concentrations exceeding 20:1, resulting from digestion and intestinal absorption of nitrogenous blood components in concert with reduced renal perfusion.

In patients with perforated ulcers and peritonitis, exudation of plasma into the peritoneal cavity (so-called third space) may result in an increased hemoglobin concentration from hemoconcentration. The presence of leukocytosis, elevated band forms, or leukopenia should raise suspicion of intra-abdominal sepsis. Lactic acidosis with an increased anion gap may ensue as a consequence of a sepsis syndrome or hypovolemia.

Patients with gastric outlet obstruction typically exhibit a hypokalemic, hypochloremic metabolic alkalosis. If volume loss is extreme, a coexistent metabolic lactic acidosis with an increased anion gap may be present, which may cause an elevated serum bicarbonate level to drop toward normal or even to low levels. Likewise, mild to moderate hyponatremia often develops in patients with vomiting from gastric outlet obstruction. Prerenal azotemia and a BUN–serum creatinine ratio greater than 20:1 are typical.

IMAGING STUDIES

Although ulcer disease can be suggested by history, physical examination, and laboratory studies, none of these has sufficient specificity to confirm the diagnosis. Ulcers are diagnosed endoscopically, radiologically, or surgically. Once an ulcer is diag-

nosed, additional studies can help in determining the cause of the ulcer (e.g., *H. pylori* infection, NSAID use, gastrinoma, or cancer masquerading as benign ulcer).

Endoscopy

Endoscopy is the most accurate way to diagnose a peptic ulcer [*see Figure 3*]. Most patients require local anesthesia of the pharynx and conscious sedation with an intravenous agent such as midazolam. The advantages of endoscopy are its nearly 100% specificity (rare false positives), greater than 90% sensitivity, portability (i.e., it can be performed in the intensive care unit, emergency department, or operating room), and ability to obtain tissue samples to help determine the etiology of the ulcer. The disadvantages of endoscopy are its cost and its potential for serious side effects. The most serious complications of endoscopy are respiratory depression and perforation of the GI tract. When a bleeding or obstructing ulcer is suspected, the stomach should be intubated and emptied with a large-bore tube before endoscopy to decrease the possibility of bronchopulmonary aspiration of gastric contents and to facilitate endoscopic visualization of mucosal lesions. Endoscopy is contraindicated in cases of suspected ulcer perforation.

Radiology

Despite having a lower sensitivity and specificity than endoscopy, an upper GI series using barium and air (double contrast) may be favored by primary care physicians and patients over referral for endoscopy for suspected uncomplicated ulcer. An upper GI series offers lower cost, wider availability, and fewer complications [*see Figure 3*]. However, for troublesome and undiagnosed dyspepsia, an upper GI series may be superfluous, because a normal result will often necessitate endoscopy (endoscopy is more sensitive than radiography) and because an upper GI series showing a gastric ulcer will also necessitate endoscopy for biopsy of the ulcer to exclude gastric malignancy. In many patients, only a finding of a duodenal bulbar ulcer on an upper GI series will preclude endoscopy [*see Figure 4*].

Plain films of the abdomen, abdominal sonography, and computed tomographic scans may be helpful in patients presenting with suspected complicated ulcers, particularly perforated or obstructing ulcers. Upright chest x-rays of a patient with a perforated ulcer may show free intraperitoneal air [*see Figure 4b*], typically beneath the right hemidiaphragm. When plain films are negative or equivocal, pneumoperitoneum may be diagnosed by abdominal sonography or CT scan. Such studies should be performed only if the diagnosis of perforation is unclear; if physical signs of peritonitis are obvious, the patient should be referred to a surgeon. Patients with gastric outlet obstruction may have an enlarged stomach with old food debris visible on plain film of the abdomen, upper GI series, abdominal sonography, or CT scan.

SURGICAL DIAGNOSIS

Certain patients will not have ulcers diagnosed until surgery is performed. Such patients include those presenting with an acute abdomen, in whom the diagnosis of perforated ulcer is made at exploratory laparotomy; those presenting with copious upper GI bleeding, in whom it is difficult for the endoscopist to visualize and treat the ulcer; and those with an obstructing ulcer who have a pinpoint pylorus or a duodenal stricture that prevents passage of the endoscope beyond the stenosis.

Tests to Establish the Etiology of the Ulcer

ENDOSCOPIC TESTS

The endoscopist can take a biopsy sample of the stomach of an ulcer patient to determine whether *H. pylori* organisms are present [*see Figure 5*]. *H. pylori* organisms contain abundant amounts of urease, which splits urea into carbon dioxide and ammonia. If the biopsy sample is placed on a urea-containing medium that also contains a pH-sensitive dye, a change in color indicates that ammonia is being produced. This so-called rapid urease test has a high sensitivity and specificity (> 90%) for *H. pylori*. If the rapid urease test is negative, a separate biopsy specimen should be sent to a pathology laboratory in formalin for histology. *H. pylori* can be detected with routine hematoxylin and eosin stains [*see Figure 5*] or, if necessary, by special stains. Moreover, the presence of diffuse, active, chronic gastritis is highly suggestive of *H. pylori* infection, and its absence excludes *H. pylori* infection.

Another useful endoscopic procedure is to obtain multiple biopsies from the edges and the base of the ulcer to exclude malignancy. This is routinely done in cases of gastric ulcer because 2% to 4% of benign-appearing gastric ulcers are in actuality an ulcer within a malignancy, usually an adenocarcinoma. Duode-

nal ulcers need not be biopsied unless the ulcer is located in a mass distal to the duodenal bulb.

Endoscopy may also demonstrate a neuroendocrine tumor, compatible with a gastrinoma on special stains. Such a tumor is usually located in the proximal duodenum.

In an ulcer patient with a negative rapid urease test and no *H. pylori*–related gastritis or gastric malignancy on histology, further history regarding NSAID use should be obtained from the patient or the patient's family. Many patients with NSAID-related ulcers have erosions, subepithelial hemorrhages, or both, which clue the endoscopist to the possibility of occult or surreptitious NSAID use; these lesions may occur with or without gastric or duodenal ulcers.[7]

SEROLOGIC TESTS

A number of serum antibody tests for *H. pylori* are available that have a greater than 90% sensitivity and specificity if the patient has not yet received therapy for *H. pylori*.[17] In patients with active ulcers diagnosed by radiology or surgery in whom gastric tissue is not available, *H. pylori* serology can confirm infection with high accuracy [*see Figure 3*].

In ulcer patients with no evidence of *H. pylori* infection or NSAID use, the fasting serum gastrin concentration should be measured [*see Figure 3*] to screen for gastrinoma (Zollinger-Ellison syndrome). If the serum gastrin concentration is greater than 1,000 pg/ml in a patient with duodenal ulcer, the diagnosis of gastrinoma is confirmed. A modest elevation in fasting serum gastrin concentration (> 150 pg/ml but < 1,000 pg/ml) is suggestive of gastrinoma, but a provocative test should be performed using intravenous secretin (2 IU/kg as a bolus).[18] A rise in serum gastrin concentration of more than 200 pg/ml after secretin administration has a greater than 90% sensitivity and specificity for gastrinoma. Because achlorhydria can produce marked hypergastrinemia as a result of the loss of negative feedback of gastric acid on gastrin release, basal acid output or pH should be measured to confirm that the stomach secretes acid in ulcer patients with fasting hypergastrinemia. The combination of achlorhydria, hypergastrinemia, and duodenal ulcer is exceedingly rare, whereas the combination of achlorhydria, hypergastrinemia, and gastric ulcer is sometimes encountered and should suggest gastric adenocarcinoma or NSAID use. A fasting gastric pH measurement will almost invariably distinguish gastrinoma (pH 1 to 2) from achlorhydria (pH 6 to 8), unless the pa-

a   *b*

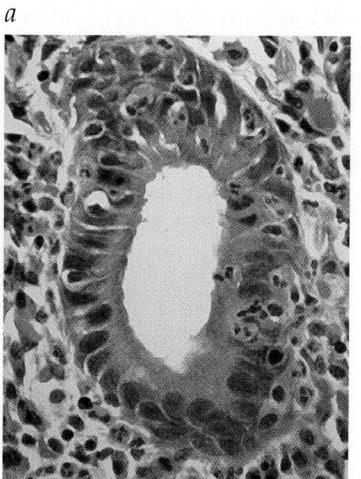 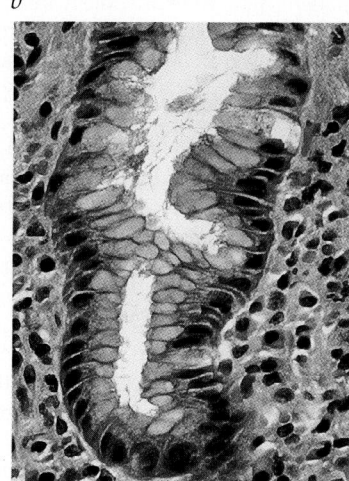

Figure 5   **Gastric biopsy samples stained with hematoxylin and eosin demonstrating (*a*) chronic active gastritis with a few *H. pylori* organisms faintly seen in the lumen of a gland and (*b*) chronic active gastritis with *H. pylori* organisms more abundant.**

Table 1 Differential Diagnosis
of Peptic Ulcer Disease

Presentation	Diagnosis
Suspected uncompli-cated ulcer	Nonulcer dyspepsia, gastroesophageal reflux, biliary colic, pancreatic disease, angina pectoris, gastric cancer
Bleeding ulcer	Varices, Mallory-Weiss tear, esophagitis, vascular lesion (arteriovenous malformation, Dieulafoy lesion, angiodysplasia)
Perforated ulcer	Appendicitis, pancreatitis, cholecystitis, spontaneous bacterial peritonitis, bowel ischemia or infarction, diverticulitis
Penetrating ulcer	Pancreatitis, muscle strain, herniated vertebral disk, ureteral stone
Fistulizing ulcer	Gallstones, GI malignancy, Crohn disease, intra-abdominal abscess

tient has received a potent acid antisecretory agent before pH measurement.

Measurement of serum thromboxane B_2 (platelet COX-1 activity) has been used in research laboratories to demonstrate occult or surreptitious NSAID use.[19] However, this assay is not widely available.

BREATH TESTS

A noninvasive method for detecting *H. pylori* in the stomach, the urea breath test, begins with oral ingestion of urea that has been labeled with carbon-13 (^{13}C) or carbon-14 (^{14}C). If *H. pylori*, with its abundant urease, is present in the stomach, the labeled urea will be rapidly converted to $^{13}CO_2$ or $^{14}CO_2$, which can be detected in breath samples collected during the first 30 to 60 minutes after urea ingestion. Sensitivity and specificity of the breath test are comparable to those of serology.[16] In a patient for whom there is no clinical indication for endoscopy, a urea breath test is an alternative to serology for documenting *H. pylori* infection [*see Figure 3*]. However, because proton pump inhibitors can suppress *H. pylori* without eradicating it, use of these drugs should be avoided for 2 weeks before the urea breath test is administered, to minimize false negative results.

Because serology is quicker, it is preferred to breath testing for initial diagnosis. Breath testing is more useful than serology in diagnosing failure of eradication of *H. pylori* or reinfection in patients who were previously treated for *H. pylori* infection, because the serology will usually remain positive for several months even after successful treatment.[20]

FECAL ANTIGEN TEST

Stool testing for *H. pylori* antigen compares favorably with urea breath tests.[21] Like breath testing, stool testing can distinguish current infection (antigen present in stool) from past infection (antigen not present in stool).

Differential Diagnosis

The most common disorder confused with uncomplicated peptic ulcer is nonulcer dyspepsia; the most serious GI disorder confused with uncomplicated peptic ulcer is gastric cancer [*see Chapter 199*].

Nonulcer, or functional, dyspepsia is a symptom complex similar to that experienced by patients with peptic ulcers. However, no ulcers or other lesions are visible on endoscopy. Nonulcer dyspepsia is a heterogeneous, poorly understood group of disorders. *H. pylori* gastritis probably causes dyspepsia in a few of these patients, and many physicians treat all dyspeptic patients who are infected with *H. pylori*. The cost-effectiveness of this approach has not been established, however; studies show that eradication of *H. pylori* is unlikely to relieve symptoms of nonulcer dyspepsia.[22-24] Many patients with nonulcer dyspepsia appear to suffer from a dysmotility of the upper GI tract that is akin to irritable bowel syndrome of the lower GI tract. Such individuals may complain of abdominal fullness, postprandial bloating, early satiety, and nausea, all suggestive of delayed gastric emptying. In some of these patients, gastric prokinetic agents such as domperidone or metoclopramide may help relieve symptoms.

Complicated ulcers may be confused with a variety of disorders. These include both intra-abdominal and musculoskeletal processes [*see Table 1*].

Treatment

The goals of ulcer therapy are rapid relief of symptoms; healing the ulcer; preventing ulcer recurrences; and reducing ulcer-related complications, morbidity (including the need for endoscopic therapy or surgery), and mortality. The general strategy in a patient with an ulcer should be to treat complications aggressively if present; to determine the etiology of the ulcer; to discontinue NSAID use if possible; to eradicate *H. pylori* infection if present or strongly suspected, even if other risk factors (e.g., NSAID use) are also present; and to use acid antisecretory therapy to heal the ulcer if *H. pylori* infection is not present. Smoking cessation should be encouraged. If duodenal ulcer is diagnosed by endoscopy, rapid urease testing of endoscopically obtained gastric biopsy samples, with or without histologic examination, should reliably establish the presence or absence of *H. pylori*. If duodenal ulcer is diagnosed by x-ray, then a serologic, urea breath, or fecal antigen test to diagnose *H. pylori* infection is recommended before treating the patient for *H. pylori*.

TREATMENT OF UNCOMPLICATED DUODENAL ULCERS

H. pylori–*Related Duodenal Ulcer*

Duodenal ulcer associated with *H. pylori* infection should be treated with antimicrobial therapy because successful therapy is associated with markedly reduced ulcer recurrences [*see Figure 6*][4,5] Antimicrobial therapy is usually empirical rather than based on results of culture and in vitro antimicrobial sensitivity testing. No single antimicrobial agent has an acceptably high success rate against *H. pylori*. Combinations of antimicrobial agents are required, and some regimens that have been approved by the Food and Drug Administration can be recommended [*see Table 2*].

H. pylori has adapted to the acidic stomach, and potent acid antisecretory agents facilitate eradication of *H. pylori* by antimicrobial agents. Bismuth compounds, like proton pump inhibitors, suppress the growth of *H. pylori* but usually do not by themselves eradicate it from the stomach. For this reason, they are frequently employed together with antibiotics.

Antimicrobial agents with activity against *H. pylori* include metronidazole, tetracycline, amoxicillin, and clarithromycin. Most popular are 10- to 14-day regimens, although 7-day courses

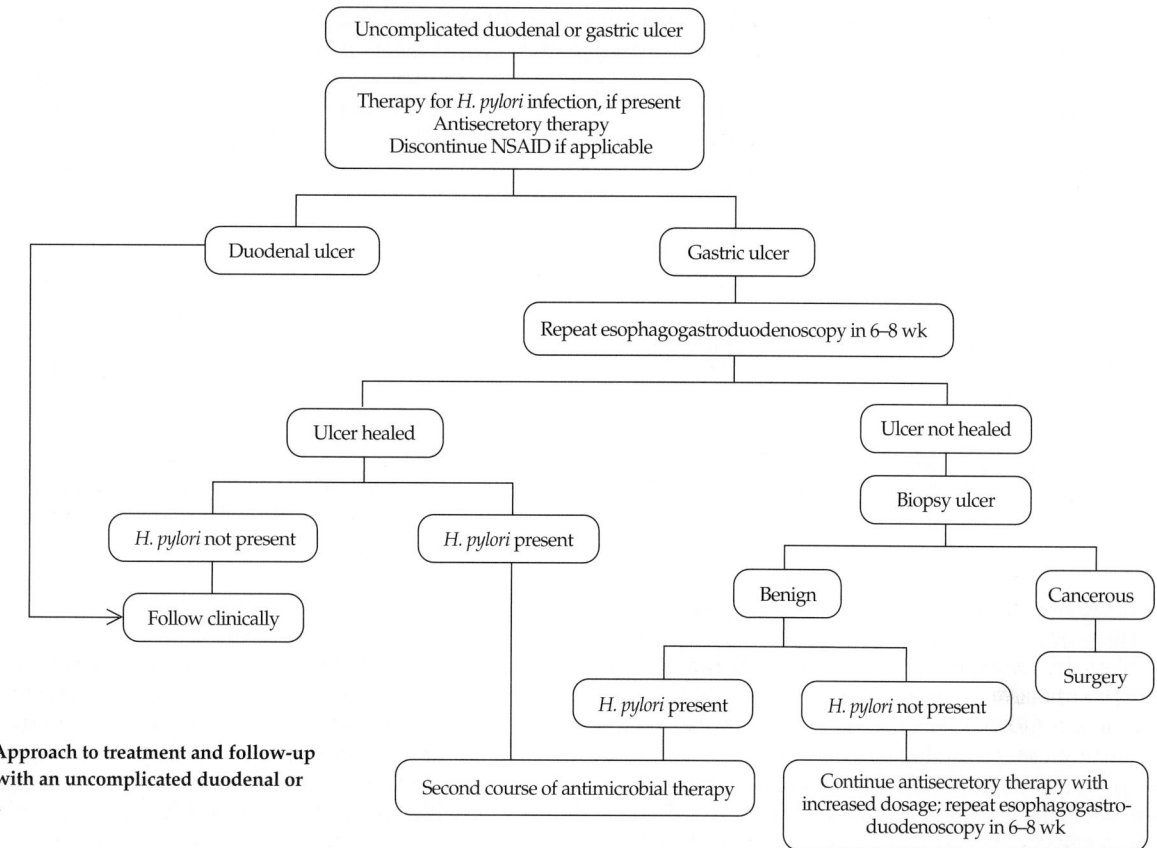

Figure 6 **Approach to treatment and follow-up of a patient with an uncomplicated duodenal or gastric ulcer.**

may be effective and are especially favored in Europe. A 2-week course of a three-drug regimen that includes a proton pump inhibitor, clarithromycin, and amoxicillin has a success rate approaching 90%. The major causes of treatment failure are poor compliance with the regimen and clarithromycin resistance; the latter occurs in around 10% of current strains and is increasing with more macrolide use in the population. Metronidazole resistance occurs in 30% to 40% of strains. However, unlike resistance to clarithromycin, which is usually absolute, resistance to metronidazole is relative and can be overcome in some patients.

If a patient carefully complies with one of the clarithromycin-based regimens yet the treatment fails, clarithromycin resistance is likely. In such cases, the retreatment regimen should not include clarithromycin. Most physicians choose a regimen consisting of metronidazole, tetracycline, bismuth (e.g., Pepto Bismol), and a proton pump inhibitor or H₂ receptor blocker. Because of the frequency of metronidazole resistance, other antimicrobials with activity against *H. pylori* are being used more often.[25-28] These agents include azithromycin, the quinolones norfloxacin and levofloxacin, and rifabutin [*see Table 3*]. In one study, a 7-day rescue treatment for persistent *H. pylori* infection using the proton pump inhibitor rabeprazole plus rifabutin and levofloxacin had a 95% success rate, as did a four-drug regimen consisting of rabeprazole, bismuth subcitrate, metronidazole, and tetracycline.[29]

It may also be possible to predict resistance to clarithromycin or to metronidazole by taking a careful history to look for prior exposure to these drugs. Such a history might help the physician choose a first-line regimen that will be more likely to be successful.

Side effects of *H. pylori*–directed therapy are not uncommon but are generally mild. Physicians should be aware of potential drug-drug interactions if the patient is receiving other medications. If the patient has an active, symptomatic ulcer, an antisecretory drug should be continued at a reduced (standard) dosage for 2 to 5 weeks after completion of antimicrobial agents.

After a patient has completed a course of ulcer therapy for an *H. pylori*–related uncomplicated duodenal ulcer, it is acceptable

Table 2 Selected Clarithromycin-Based Regimens to Eradicate *Helicobacter pylori*

Esomeprazole, amoxicillin, clarithromycin (EAC)
 Esomeprazole, 40 mg b.i.d. for 10 days; then 40 mg q.d. for 18 days if an active ulcer is present
 Amoxicillin, 1 g b.i.d. for 10 days
 Clarithromycin, 500 mg b.i.d. or t.i.d. for 10 days

Lansoprazole, amoxicillin, clarithromycin (LAC)
 Lansoprazole, 30 mg b.i.d. for 10–14 days; then 15 mg q.d. for 14–18 days if an active ulcer is present
 Amoxicillin, 1 g b.i.d. for 10–14 days
 Clarithromycin, 500 mg b.i.d. for 10–14 days

Omeprazole, amoxicillin, clarithromycin (OAC)
 Omeprazole, 20 mg b.i.d. for 10 days; then 20 mg q.d. for 18 days if an active ulcer is present
 Amoxicillin, 1 g b.i.d. for 10–14 days
 Clarithromycin, 500 mg b.i.d. for 10 days

Rabeprazole, amoxicillin, clarithromycin (RAC)
 Rabeprazole, 20 mg b.i.d. for 7 days; then 20 mg q.d. for 21 days if an active ulcer is present
 Amoxicillin, 1 g b.i.d. for 7 days
 Clarithromycin, 500 mg b.i.d. for 7 days

Table 3   Additional Antimicrobial Agents
with Activity against *Helicobacter pylori*

Agent*	Dosage	Comments
Azithromycin	500 mg q.d.	Combined with either amoxicillin or metronidazole, plus a proton pump inhibitor, for 3–7 days
Norfloxacin	400 mg b.i.d.	Combined with a proton pump inhibitor for 14 days
Levofloxacin	500 mg q.d.	Combined with either amoxicillin or metronidazole, plus a proton pump inhibitor, for 7 days
Rifabutin	300 mg q.d.	Combined with amoxicillin and a proton pump inhibitor for 7–10 days

*These agents are marketed in the United States, but they are not yet approved for *H. pylori* therapy.

to follow the patient clinically without confirming eradication, because most compliant patients will be successfully cured of their *H. pylori* infection [*see Figure 6*]. A patient with an *H. pylori*–related duodenal ulcer that does not recur symptomatically within 2 years after antimicrobial therapy is probably cured. Serology has often reverted to negative by this time.[20]

Those in whom recurrent ulcer symptoms develop during the first 2 years after therapy should be assessed either by endoscopy (for ulcer recurrence and for *H. pylori* persistence or reinfection) or by a urea breath test or fecal antigen test. The most common cause of recurrent ulceration in patients treated for *H. pylori*–related duodenal ulcer is failure to eradicate the organism. Retreatment of these patients is indicated [*see* Treatment of

Intractable Duodenal Ulcers or Gastric Ulcers, *below*]. Rarer causes of duodenal ulcer recurrence include an acid hypersecretory state (e.g., Zollinger-Ellison syndrome), NSAID use, and reinfection with *H. pylori*.

H. pylori–*Negative Duodenal Ulcer*

In a duodenal ulcer patient who is *H. pylori* negative, the physician should consider NSAID use and gastrinoma (Zollinger-Ellison syndrome).[30] Patients with duodenal ulcer who are taking NSAIDs should discontinue the NSAID, if possible. At the same time, an acid antisecretory drug should be administered for 4 to 8 weeks [*see Table 4*]. The anticipated healing rate with this regimen is 85% to 95%.

Table 4   FDA-Approved Antisecretory Drugs
for Active Peptic Ulcer Disease*

Class	Drugs	Dosage	Drug Interactions‡
H₂ receptor blockers†	Cimetidine	800 mg h.s. *or* 400 mg b.i.d.	Warfarin, theophylline, phenytoin, benzodiazepines, itraconazole, ketoconazole, atazanavir, cefpodoxime, cefditoren, gefitinib, memantine, metformin, and many others
	Ranitidine	300 mg h.s. *or* 150 mg b.i.d.	Warfarin, atazanavir, itraconazole, ketoconazole, cefpodoxime, cefditoren, enoxacin, gefitinib, memantine, metformin, tolazoline
	Nizatidine	300 mg h.s. *or* 150 mg b.i.d.	Atazanavir, itraconazole, ketoconazole, cefpodoxime, cefditoren
	Famotidine	40 mg h.s. *or* 20 mg b.i.d.	Atazanavir, itraconazole, ketoconazole, cefpodoxime, cefditoren
Proton pump inhibitors§	Omeprazole	20 mg q.d., a.c.	Benzodiazepines, ampicillin, atazanavir, digoxin, iron, itraconazole, ketoconazole, voriconazole, methotrexate, tacrolimus
	Lansoprazole	15 mg q.d., a.c.	Ampicillin, atazanavir, digoxin, iron, itraconazole, ketoconazole
	Esomeprazole	40 mg q.d., a.c.	Atazanavir, digoxin, iron, ketoconazole
	Rabeprazole	20 mg q.d., a.c.	Warfarin, ampicillin, atazanavir, digoxin, iron, itraconazole, ketoconazole
	Pantoprazole	40 mg q.d., a.c.	Ampicillin, atazanavir, iron, itraconazole, ketoconazole

*Patients with gastrinoma (Zollinger-Ellison syndrome) will usually require much higher dosages of antisecretory drugs than listed here.

†Use for 4–8 wk in the treatment of duodenal ulcer and 6–12 wk in the treatment of gastric ulcer. Duodenal ulcers that do not heal by 8 wk and gastric ulcers that do not heal by 12 wk are considered intractable. Dosage of H₂ receptor blockers should be reduced in patients with renal failure.

‡Micromedex Health Care Services. Most of these drug interactions are minor and not clinically relevant; nevertheless, caution is advised.

§Omeprazole and lansoprazole are approved for gastric ulcers; omeprazole, lansoprazole, and rabeprazole are approved for duodenal ulcers.

Table 5 Treatment and Prevention of Peptic Ulcers

Type of Ulcer	Treatment	Prevention	Comments
Helicobacter pylori–related ulcers	Antibiotics [*see Tables 2 and 3*] ± antisecretory agents [*see Table 4*]	None needed if *H. pylori* eradicated	Highly cost-effective; document healing in gastric ulcer; document *H. pylori* eradication in complicated duodenal or gastric ulcer and in intractable duodenal or gastric ulcer
NSAID-related ulcers	Antisecretory agents (proton pump inhibitors have greater efficacy than H_2 receptor blockers) [*see Table 4*] Discontinue NSAID use, if possible	Misoprostol (600–800 µg/day) or proton pump inhibitor (e.g., omeprazole, 20–40 mg q.d., or lansoprazole, 15–30 mg q.d.) along with an NSAID	Diarrhea may limit compliance in patients treated with misoprostol; avoid misoprostol during pregnancy (abortifacient); proton pump inhibitors are not yet approved by the FDA for prevention of NSAID-related ulcers
Ulcers associated with Zollinger-Ellison syndrome and other hypersecretory states	High-dose proton pump inhibitor	Proton pump inhibitor, adjusted to keep basal acid output < 5–10 mEq/hr	Consider exploratory laparotomy (guided by abdominal imaging studies) to remove easily resectable gastrinomas, if feasible; consider MEN I syndrome (present in 20%–30% of cases)[21]
Idiopathic ulcers	H_2 receptor blocker or proton pump inhibitor	Nocturnal H_2 receptor blocker or A.M. proton pump inhibitor	Parietal cell vagotomy for intractable duodenal ulcer and antrectomy for intractable gastric ulcer
Stress ulcers (ICU)	I.V. H_2 receptor blocker or proton pump inhibitor (e.g., pantoprazole) ?Angiography ?Surgery	I.V. H_2 receptor blocker or proton pump inhibitor; intragastric sucralfate; or intragastric antacid	Maintain pH above 4 with H_2 receptor blocker, proton pump inhibitor or antacid; continuous I.V. infusion is superior to I.V. boluses of antisecretory drug
Cameron ulcers (linear gastric erosions in a hiatal hernia)	Iron salts; packed red cell transfusions; endoscopic hemostasis ?Angiography ?Surgery	Hiatal hernia repair, laparoscopic or open	Roles of H_2 receptor blockers and proton pump inhibitors are unproved

MEN I—multiple endocrine neoplasia type I NSAID—nonsteroidal anti-inflammatory drug

Patients with duodenal ulcer as part of the Zollinger-Ellison syndrome should be managed initially with a high dose of a proton pump inhibitor, followed by a maintenance dose guided by gastric acid measurements. If there is no evidence of hepatic metastasis on abdominal CT scan, then exploratory laparotomy for gastrinoma resection, with or without parietal cell vagotomy, is warranted.[31] Radionuclide scintigraphy with octreotide, an analogue of somatostatin, is a highly sensitive and specific preoperative test for detecting and staging gastrinoma, as is endoscopic ultrasonography.

The vast majority of duodenal ulcers, regardless of cause, heal after 8 weeks of antisecretory therapy with a proton pump inhibitor or an H_2 receptor blocker. Antacids are often prescribed as needed to relieve ulcer symptoms.

In rare cases of idiopathic duodenal ulcer, it is prudent that, after the ulcer has been healed by an acid antisecretory agent, the patient be placed on a maintenance dose of an H_2 receptor blocker given at bedtime to reduce ulcer recurrences. Proton pump inhibitors are also effective in preventing duodenal ulcer recurrences. It is not necessary to confirm duodenal ulcer healing by endoscopy or x-ray before reducing the antisecretory drug dose to a maintenance level.

TREATMENT OF UNCOMPLICATED GASTRIC ULCERS

H. pylori–*Related Gastric Ulcer*

Gastric ulcer associated with *H. pylori* should be treated with antibiotics [*see Table 2*]. Because they are larger than duodenal ulcers, gastric ulcers take longer to heal. Thus, after antibiotic administration, the patient should be treated with an acid antise-

cretory agent [*see Tables 3 and 4*] for an additional 4 to 8 weeks. Patients with gastric ulcers should be followed endoscopically until complete healing has been achieved so that an ulcerated gastric cancer is not missed. Gastric biopsies should be obtained during follow-up endoscopy to determine whether eradication of *H. pylori* has occurred [*see Figure 6*]. Patients with a history of an uncomplicated gastric ulcer that is currently quiescent should be screened for *H. pylori* infection, and if the result is positive, they should be treated for *H. pylori* infection to prevent ulcer recurrences.

NSAID-Related Gastric Ulcer

The therapy for an active NSAID-related gastric ulcer is administration of a proton pump inhibitor [*see Tables 4 and 5*], as well as discontinuance of the NSAID. Healing rates with H_2 receptor blockers are nearly as high as with proton pump inhibitors if the NSAID can be stopped.

TREATMENT OF INTRACTABLE DUODENAL ULCERS OR GASTRIC ULCERS

Ulcers That Fail to Heal

Ulcers refractory to pharmacotherapy are rare, and in most cases, prolonging the course of the gastric antisecretory drug, increasing the dose, or taking both measures will lead to healing. The causes of nonhealing include poor compliance with medications, an acid hypersecretory state requiring higher-than-customary doses of antisecretory drugs, continued NSAID use, and persistent *H. pylori* infection. Often, combinations of these factors and others (e.g., smoking and stress) are present.

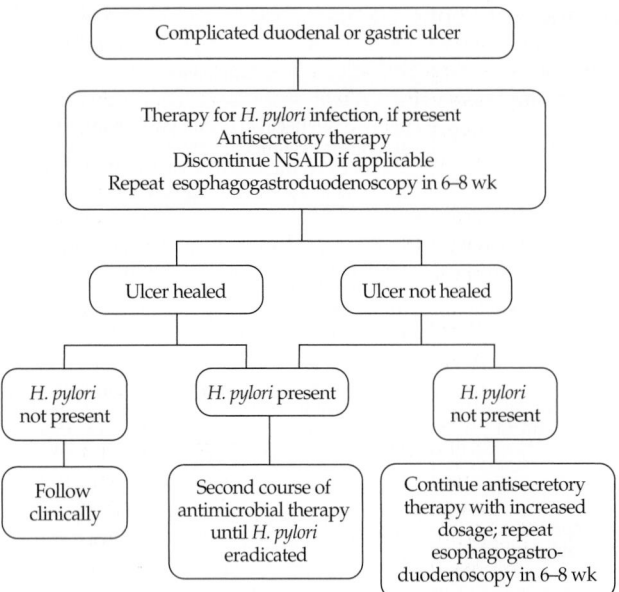

Figure 7 **Approach to treatment and follow-up of a patient with a complicated duodenal or gastric ulcer.**

Poor compliance with medications necessitates patient education and consideration of elective ulcer surgery. A fasting serum gastrin concentration can be used to screen for an acid hypersecretory state resulting from Zollinger-Ellison syndrome. Physicians should be aware that antisecretory drugs (especially proton pump inhibitors) can also raise serum gastrin levels modestly (to 150 to 600 pg/ml). Definitive documentation of an acid hypersecretory state requires quantitative gastric acid measurement (gastric analysis). NSAID use should be discontinued if at all possible. Persistent *H. pylori* infection is the result of poor compliance with medications or is caused by drug-resistant strains.[25-29] *H. pylori* has proved to be resistant to metronidazole in 30% to 40% of cases and to clarithromycin in 10% of cases; resistance to tetracycline or amoxicillin occurs in 1% of strains or less.[25] Combined resistance to macrolides (e.g., clarithromycin) and imidazoles (e.g., metronidazole) occurs in approximately 5% of patients, in whom infection may prove difficult to eradicate. Culture of gastric biopsy material for *H. pylori,* followed by antimicrobial drug-susceptibility testing when available, can guide retreatment. In the absence of this information, the patient should be retreated for 2 weeks with a proton pump inhibitor, with amoxicillin or tetracycline, and with either clarithromycin or metronidazole (whichever antimicrobial agent the patient did not receive initially). Some physicians use a bismuth preparation (e.g., colloidal bismuth subcitrate, bismuth subsalicylate, or ranitidine bismuth citrate) in place of a proton pump inhibitor [*see Table 2*]. Several other antibiotics have activity against *H. pylori* and may prove to be useful in rescue therapy for patients in whom treatments have failed; many such patients harbor antibiotic-resistant strains.[25-29] Agents that are available in the United States include the macrolide azithromycin, the quinolones norfloxacin and levofloxacin, and rifabutin [*see Table 3*].

Frequently Recurring Ulcers

Another type of intractability is frequent ulcer recurrences (at least three a year). This type of intractability occurs most often when *H. pylori* has not been eradicated (necessitating retreat-

ment) or, less often, when NSAID use is resumed or when an acid hypersecretory state is present. Some idiopathic ulcers recur frequently and require lifelong maintenance therapy with an H_2 receptor blocker or a proton pump inhibitor. Alternatively, patients may choose ulcer surgery (parietal cell vagotomy for duodenal ulcer or antrectomy for gastric ulcer) over lifelong medication.

TREATMENT OF COMPLICATED PEPTIC ULCERS

Bleeding Ulcers

The first priority in a patient with a suspected bleeding peptic ulcer is to stabilize the vital signs with volume resuscitation, ideally in an intensive care unit. Such an approach is associated with improved patient outcomes.[32] Hemodynamic monitoring may assist in fluid and blood replacement, particularly if the patient has significant (New York Heart Association class III or IV) cardiac disease.

After the patient becomes clinically stable, diagnostic upper GI endoscopy is performed [*see Figure 7*]. If an actively bleeding ulcer or an ulcer with a visible vessel is found, the lesion is treated endoscopically, by injection of epinephrine, by thermal application with a heater probe or a bipolar electrode, or by a combination of these methods. Endoscopic therapy is successful in controlling bleeding in approximately 90% of patients; the other 10% are referred for surgery if major bleeding continues. Random gastric biopsies are obtained at the time of endoscopy to detect *H. pylori* by rapid urease testing and, if necessary, gastric histology.

Once an ulcer is demonstrated, intravenous gastric antisecretory therapy, usually with a proton pump inhibitor (e.g., pantoprazole) can be started. Oral therapy with a proton pump inhibitor is superior to no therapy in reducing early rebleeding if endoscopic therapy is not attempted[33]; proton pump inhibitors also reduce ulcer rebleeding after endoscopic therapy.[34] The combination of endoscopic therapy and an intravenous proton pump inhibitor is superior to the proton pump inhibitor alone in patients with visible vessels or with clots adherent to the ulcer.[35] However, endoscopic therapy may fail, necessitating surgery, or result in a perforation.[35] Patients who have been on intravenous therapy should be switched to oral therapy with a proton pump inhibitor as soon as they resume oral intake. If the rapid urease test or gastric histology is positive for *H. pylori*, the patient should receive at least two effective antibiotics (e.g., clarithromycin and amoxicillin) for 14 days, along with a proton pump inhibitor [*see Figure 7*]. The proton pump inhibitor is continued at the same dosage until week 6 for duodenal ulcer or week 8 for gastric ulcer. If a subsequent endoscopy shows complete ulcer healing and disappearance of *H. pylori* by both rapid urease testing and gastric histology, the risk of rebleeding is low[34,36,37] and therapy can be stopped. Future use of NSAIDs or aspirin is almost always prohibited. Although the use of coxibs instead of an NSAID is attractive, freedom from rebleeding is not guaranteed. If an NSAID or low-dose aspirin is absolutely necessary, it should be coprescribed with the prostaglandin E_1 analogue misoprostol[38] or a proton pump inhibitor.[39] If the ulcer heals but *H. pylori* organisms are still present, the patient should be treated again for *H. pylori* or left on maintenance therapy with an H_2 receptor blocker or proton pump inhibitor. If the ulcer is not healed, persistent *H. pylori* infection is likely. Under such circumstances, gastric tissue can be cultured for *H. pylori*, if available facilities exist, so that antibiotic sensitivities can be determined before retreatment. Finally, if the ulcer has not healed even though *H. pylori* has been eradicated, then NSAID use, an acid hypersecretory state, or cancer should be considered. Biopsy samples of the ulcer should be obtained, especially if the ulcer is in the stomach.

A patient with a bleeding peptic ulcer that is negative for *H. pylori* by rapid urease testing and gastric histology usually has an NSAID-related ulcer. The NSAID is stopped if possible, and a high-dose proton pump inhibitor (e.g., 40 mg of omeprazole or 30 mg of lansoprazole) is prescribed for 8 weeks for gastric ulcer or 4 to 6 weeks for duodenal ulcer. Repeat endoscopy is usually indicated to assess healing of a gastric ulcer; if the ulcer has not healed, it is biopsied. Whether to perform a repeat endoscopy to assess healing 4 to 8 weeks after an NSAID-related bleeding duodenal ulcer is controversial. If the ulcer is shown to have healed after the patient is off the NSAID, no further therapy is required unless the patient is placed back on an NSAID or aspirin, even a low dose of aspirin. In such cases, misoprostol (200 μg q.i.d.) is modestly protective against subsequent bleeding.[38] There is also evidence that maintenance therapy with a proton pump inhibitor such as lansoprazole or omeprazole is associated with a low rate of NSAID-related ulcer rebleeding. In general, however, NSAIDs should be avoided in patients with ulcers that have bled. In a study of high-risk arthritis patients with prior ulcer bleeding, use of a coxib (celecoxib) proved to be as effective as the combination of a nonselective NSAID (diclofenac) and a proton pump inhibitor (omeprazole).[40] With either therapy, however, 5% to 6% of such patients rebled over the ensuing 6 months.[40]

Patients with bleeding ulcers that are idiopathic and that heal on an antisecretory drug should receive long-term maintenance therapy with an H_2 receptor blocker or proton pump inhibitor. There is evidence that maintenance therapy with the H_2 receptor blocker ranitidine is effective in preventing rebleeding from duodenal ulcers.[41]

Perforated Ulcers

When a perforated viscus is documented or strongly suspected, the patient is started on broad-spectrum intravenous antibiotics covering gram-negative aerobic bacilli, enterococci, and anaerobes such as *Bacteroides* species and is then taken to surgery for closure of the perforation with a patch of omentum. If the surgeon does not obtain an intraoperative gastric biopsy sample, the patient should undergo postoperative testing for *H. pylori* by serology, urea breath test, or fecal antigen test, and the infection should be treated if present.[42] Many perforated ulcers are associated with NSAID use rather than with *H. pylori* infection.[43] Regardless of the patient's *H. pylori* status, antisecretory drugs should be administered for 6 to 8 weeks postoperatively. Endoscopy is then performed to assess healing, and success of eradication of *H. pylori* is ascertained by gastric biopsy with rapid urease testing and histology.

Up to 10% of perforated gastric ulcers are in fact perforated gastric cancers. If no biopsy or resection of the ulcer is done at the time of repair of the perforation, postoperative endoscopy with biopsy is imperative before the patient is discharged from the hospital or soon thereafter.

The mortality in patients with perforated peptic ulcers is 5% to 10%. Factors associated with higher mortality include delayed diagnosis and treatment of perforation; advanced age; comorbid conditions, such as cardiac, pulmonary, or liver disease; immunodeficiency; and advanced malignancy.

A small number of patients with suspected or probable perforated peptic ulcer improve rapidly before surgery is performed. Others refuse surgery or are poor surgical candidates. An alternative to surgery in these situations is nonoperative therapy consisting of nothing by mouth; intravenous fluids and electrolytes; a broad-spectrum antibiotic such as ticarcillin–clavulanic acid or piperacillin-tazobactam; and nasogastric suction. Compared with surgical therapy, nonoperative therapy is associated with more abdominal complications (e.g., abscesses), fewer pulmonary complications (e.g., atelectasis), and similar mortality.[44]

Obstructing Ulcers

The patient with an obstructing ulcer is initially placed on nasogastric suction, intravenous fluids and electrolytes, and an intravenously administered proton pump inhibitor. If the obstruction is the result of edema associated with an active ulcer, the gastric outlet may open as edema subsides and the ulcer heals, over several days to weeks. If, on the other hand, obstruction is the result of scarring from previous ulcers, it will not resolve with these measures. In some patients, it is difficult to determine whether edema or fibrosis is the primary cause of gastric outlet obstruction. Because obstruction may resolve with time, early consideration should be given to parenteral hyperalimentation. This intervention prevents or minimizes tissue catabolism during the waiting period and also induces a positive nitrogen balance, which will be beneficial if the gastric outlet fails to open up and the patient requires surgery.

A saline load test can be used to guide management. Thirty minutes after 750 ml of isotonic saline is infused into the stomach through the nasogastric tube, gastric contents (saline plus secretions) are aspirated. A return of less than 200 ml indicates normal gastric emptying of liquids and a good prognosis; 200 to 400 ml is indeterminate; and more than 400 ml is suggestive of a high-grade obstruction that will likely require intervention. Repeating the saline load test every day or two may also provide information about whether the obstruction is resolving.

If the obstruction resolves within 3 to 7 days, the nasogastric tube is removed and the patient is fed and observed clinically. An oral proton pump inhibitor or H_2 receptor blocker is started as soon as it is feasible. Gastric prokinetic agents (e.g., metoclopramide) should not be used. At least 50% of patients whose obstruction resolves with conservative medical therapy will experience another obstruction in about a year. Whether routine treatment of *H. pylori* infection will reduce this high recurrence rate is unknown. Unlike bleeding or perforation, obstruction is usually a late complication of ulcer disease. Thus, *H. pylori* eradication in ulcer patients is more likely to be effective in primary prevention of obstruction than in secondary prevention. NSAIDs may cause gastric outlet obstruction as well and should therefore be avoided. Endoscopic therapy is an option for obstruction that does not resolve with conservative therapy.[45] Using inflatable balloons placed over guide wires, the endoscopist can dilate a stenotic pylorus or duodenum under fluoroscopic guidance, although complications such as perforation may occur. Endoscopic balloon dilatation, when feasible, is a temporizing measure and rarely obviates surgery. Thus, obstruction that recurs after medical therapy or after endoscopic therapy is an indication for surgery. Pyloroplasty, gastroenterostomy, and resection plus gastroenterostomy are the most popular operations for an obstructing ulcer. Pyloroplasty and gastroenterostomy are typically combined with a vagotomy to reduce the likelihood of recurrent ulceration.

Fistulizing Ulcers

Gastric or duodenal ulcers associated with fistulas must be biopsied to exclude malignancy. Initially, benign ulcers are treated as described for an uncomplicated ulcer [see Figure 6]. An antisecretory agent—ideally, a proton pump inhibitor—should be prescribed, along with antibiotics, if H. pylori organisms are present. Ulcer healing may be associated with closure of the fistula. If the fistula persists, surgical resection of the fistula is warranted only if significant symptoms are present (e.g., troublesome diarrhea in a patient with a gastrocolonic fistula or cholangitis in a patient with a duodenocholedochal fistula).

TREATMENT OF ACUTE STRESS ULCERS

Therapy for bleeding acute stress ulcers and erosions involves blood transfusion if necessary and attempts to treat the underlying disease state. The role of intravenous H_2 receptor blockers or proton pump inhibitors is unproved. Endoscopic therapy is not usually curative, because multiple bleeding lesions are often present. In rare cases, visceral angiography with embolization of the major bleeding site is attempted. Gastrectomy for continuous bleeding or significant rebleeding is used as a last resort and is associated with a very high mortality.

Because of the dire consequences of stress ulcers and the lack of an effective therapy, high-risk patients in intensive care units should be placed on stress ulcer prophylaxis.[46] The patients at highest risk for bleeding are those with multiorgan failure and those who receive ventilatory assistance for more than 24 hours. The incidence of significant bleeding in high-risk patients is reduced from about 10% to 25% to about 1% to 5% with the use of prophylactic intragastric or oral antacids or sucralfate or with the use of intravenous H_2 receptor blockers or proton pump inhibitors given by continuous infusion. I prefer intravenous antisecretory therapy because of ease of administration, the ability to monitor gastric pH to assess effectiveness (the goal is a pH > 4), and proven efficacy in clinical trials.

TREATMENT OF CAMERON ULCERS

Although acid secretory inhibitors are often used in the treatment of linear erosions in hiatal hernias (Cameron ulcers), their value is uncertain.[16] Standard therapy consists of packed red cell transfusions for acute bleeding, oral iron replacement for chronic bleeding, and laparoscopic or open repair of the hiatal hernia when medical therapy fails. Because many of the patients with Cameron ulcers are elderly or at high risk, surgery should be undertaken only when medical therapy fails or becomes cumbersome.

The author has no commercial relationships with manufacturers of products or providers of services discussed in this chapter.

References

1. Blaser MJ: The bacteria behind ulcers. Sci Am 274:104, 1996

2. Helicobacter pylori in peptic ulcer disease. NIH Consensus Development Panel on Helicobacter pylori in Peptic Ulcer Disease. JAMA 272:65, 1994

3. Cryer B, Faust TW, Goldschmiedt M, et al: Gastric and duodenal mucosal prostaglandin concentrations in gastric or duodenal ulcer disease: relationships with demographics, environmental, and histological factors, including Helicobacter pylori. Am J Gastroenterol 87:1747, 1992

4. Forbes GM, Glaser ME, Cullen DJE, et al: Duodenal ulcer treated with Helicobacter pylori eradication: seven-year follow-up. Lancet 343:258, 1994

5. Sung JJY, Chung SCS, Ling TKW, et al: Antibacterial treatment of gastric ulcers associated with Helicobacter pylori. N Engl J Med 332:139, 1995

6. Spechler SJ, Fischbach L, Feldman M: Clinical aspects of genetic variability in Heli-

cobacter pylori. JAMA 283:1264, 2000

7. Papatheodoridis GV, Papadelli D, Cholongitas E, et al: Effect of Helicobacter pylori infection on the risk of upper gastrointestinal bleeding in users of nonsteroidal anti-inflammatory drugs. Am J Med 116:601, 2004

8. Chan FLK, To KF, Wu JCY, et al: Eradication of Helicobacter pylori and risk of peptic ulcers in patients starting long-term treatment with non-steroidal anti-inflammatory drugs: a randomised trial. Lancet 359:9, 2002

9. Henry D, Lim LL, Rodriguez LAG, et al: Variability in risk of gastrointestinal complications with individual non-steroidal anti-inflammatory drugs: results of a collaborative meta-analysis. BMJ 312:1563, 1996

10. Cryer B, Feldman M: Effects of very low dose daily, long-term aspirin therapy on gastric, duodenal, and rectal prostaglandin levels and on mucosal injury in healthy humans. Gastroenterology 117:17, 1999

11. Kelly JP, Kaufman DW, Jurgelson JM, et al: Risk of aspirin-associated major upper-gastrointestinal bleeding with enteric-coated or buffered product. Lancet 348:1413, 1996

12. Cryer B, Feldman M: Cyclooxygenase-1 and cyclooxygenase-2 selectivity of widely used NSAIDs and other anti-inflammatory or analgesic drugs: studies in whole blood and gastric mucosa of healthy humans. Am J Med 104:413, 1998

13. Silverstein F, Faich G, Goldstein JL, et al: Gastrointestinal toxicity with celecoxib versus nonsteroidal anti-inflammatory drugs for osteoarthritis and rheumatoid arthritis: The CLASS Study: A Randomized Controlled Trial. JAMA 284:1247, 2000

14. COX-2 selective (includes Bextra, Celebrex, and Vioxx) and nonselective nonsteroidal anti-inflammatory drugs (NSAIDs). Center for Drug Evaluation and Research. U.S. Food and Drug Administration, July 18, 2005 www.fda.gov/cder/drug/infopage/cox2/

15. Aoyama N, Kinoshita Y, Fujimoto S, et al: Peptic ulcers after the Hanshin-Awaji earthquake: increased incidence of bleeding gastric ulcer. Am J Gastroenterol 93:311, 1998

16. Spechler SJ: Peptic ulcer disease and its complications. Gastrointestinal and Liver Disease, 7th ed. Feldman M, Friedman LF, Sleisenger MS, Eds. WB Saunders Co, Philadelphia, 2002, p 747

17. Cutler AF, Havstad S, Ma CK, et al: Accuracy of invasive and noninvasive tests to diagnose Helicobacter pylori infection. Gastroenterology 109:136, 1995

18. Metz DC, Buchanan M, Purich E, et al: A randomized controlled crossover study comparing synthetic porcine and human secretins with biologically derived porcine secretin to diagnose Zollinger-Ellison syndrome. Aliment Pharm Ther 15:669, 2001

19. Lanas A, Sekar MC, Hirschowitz BI: Objective evidence of aspirin use in both ulcer and nonulcer upper and lower gastrointestinal bleeding. Gastroenterology 103:862, 1992

20. Feldman M, Cryer B, Lee E, et al: Role of seroconversion in confirming cure of Helicobacter pylori infection. JAMA 280:363, 1998

21. Vaira D, Nimish V, Menegatti M, et al: The stool test for detection of Helicobacter pylori after eradication therapy. Ann Intern Med 136:280, 2002

22. Blum AL, Talley NJ, O'Morain C, et al: Lack of effect of treating Helicobacter pylori infection in patients with nonulcer dyspepsia. N Engl J Med 339:1875, 1998

23. McColl K, Murray L, El-Omar E, et al: Symptomatic benefit from eradicating Helicobacter pylori infection in patients with nonulcer dyspepsia. N Engl J Med 339:1869, 1998

24. Friedman LS: Helicobacter pylori and nonulcer dyspepsia. N Engl J Med 339:1928, 1998

25. Meyer JM, Silliman NP, Wang W, et al: Risk factors for Helicobacter pylori resistance in the United States: the surveillance of H. pylori antimicrobial resistance partnership study. Ann Intern Med 136:13, 2002

26. Guslandi M: Alternative antibacterial agents for Helicobacter pylori eradication. Aliment Pharmacol Ther 15:1543, 2001

27. Gisbert JP, Pajares JM: Helicobacter pylori 'rescue' regimen when proton pump inhibitor-based therapies fail. Aliment Pharmacol Ther 16:1047, 2002

28. Perri F, Festa V, Clemente R, et al: Randomized study of two 'rescue' therapies for Helicobacter pylori-infected patients after failure of standard triple therapies. Am J Gastroenterol 96:58, 2001

29. Wong WM, Gu Q, Lam SK, et al: Randomized controlled study of rabeprazole, levofloxacin and rifabutin triple therapy vs. quadruple therapy as a second-line treatment for Helicobacter pylori infection. Aliment Pharm Ther 17:553, 2003

30. McColl KEL, El-Nujumi AM, Chittajallu RS, et al: A study of pathogenesis of Helicobacter pylori negative chronic duodenal ulceration. Gut 34:762, 1993

31. McArthur KE, Richardson CT, Barnett CC, et al: Long-term outcome after exploratory laparotomy and proximal gastric vagotomy in Zollinger-Ellison syndrome. Am J Gastroenterol 91:1104, 1996

32. Baradarian R, Ramdhaney S, Chapalamadugu R, et al: Early intensive resuscitation of patients with upper gastrointestinal bleeding decreases mortality. Am J Gastroenterol 99:619, 2004

33. Khuroo M, Yattoo GN, Javid G, et al: A comparison of omeprazole and placebo for bleeding peptic ulcer. N Engl J Med 336:1054, 1997

34. Lau JW, Sung JJY, Lee KKC, et al: Effect of intravenous omeprazole on recurrent bleeding after endoscopic treatment of bleeding peptic ulcers. N Engl J Med 343:310, 2000

35. Sung JJY, Chan FKL, Lau JYW, et al: The effect of endoscopic therapy in patients receiving omeprazole for bleeding ulcers with nonbleeding visible vessels or adherent clots. Ann Intern Med 139:237, 2003

36. Rokkas T, Karameris A, Mavrogeorgis A, et al: Eradication of Helicobacter pylori reduces the possibility of rebleeding in peptic ulcer disease. Gastrointest Endosc 41:1, 1995

37. Macri G, Milani S, Surrenti E, et al: Eradication of Helicobacter pylori reduces the rate

of duodenal ulcer rebleeding: a long-term follow-up study. Am J Gastroenterol 93:925, 1998

38. Silverstein FE, Graham DY, Senior JR, et al: Misoprostol reduces serious gastrointestinal complications in patients with rheumatoid arthritis receiving nonsteroidal anti-inflammatory drugs: a randomized, double-blind, placebo-controlled trial. Ann Intern Med 123:241, 1995

39. Lai K, Lam SK, Chu KM, et al: Lansoprazole for the prevention of recurrences of ulcer complications from long-term low-dose aspirin use. N Engl J Med 346:2033, 2002

40. Chan FKL, Hung LCT, Suen BY, et al: Celecoxib versus diclofenac and omeprazole in reducing the risk of recurrent ulcer bleeding in patients with arthritis. N Engl J Med 347:2104, 2002

41. Jensen DM, Cheng S, Kovacs TOG, et al: A controlled study of ranitidine for the prevention of recurrent hemorrhage from duodenal ulcer. N Engl J Med 330:382, 1994

42. Ng EK, Lam YH, Sung JJ, et al: Eradication of *Helicobacter pylori* prevents recurrence of ulcer after simple closure of duodenal ulcer perforation: randomized controlled trial. Ann Surg 231:153, 2000

43. Reinbach DH, Cruickshank G, McColl KEL: Acute perforated duodenal ulcer is not associated with *Helicobacter pylori* infection. Gut 34:1344, 1993

44. Crofts TJ, Park KGM, Steele RJC, et al: A randomized trial of nonoperative treatment for perforated peptic ulcer. N Engl J Med 320:970, 1989

45. DiSario JA, Fennerty MB, Tietze CC, et al: Endoscopic balloon dilation for ulcer-induced gastric outlet obstruction. Am J Gastroenterol 89:868, 1994

46. Cook D, Guyatt G, Marshall J, et al: A comparison of sucralfate and ranitidine for prevention of upper gastrointestinal bleeding in patients requiring mechanical ventilation. N Engl J Med 338:791, 1998

Acknowledgments

Figures 1 and 3   Marcia Kammerer.

Figure 5   Courtesy of Edward Lee, M.D.

The author thanks Tracy Thornburg for help in preparing this chapter.

63 Inflammatory Bowel Diseases

Stephen B. Hanauer, M.D., F.A.C.P.

Ulcerative colitis (UC) and Crohn disease (CD) constitute the two major idiopathic inflammatory bowel diseases (IBDs). Gastroenterologists recognize that there is a spectrum of IBDs, encompassing varying types and degrees of intestinal inflammation, and that these idiopathic disorders must be distinguished from inflammation caused by infections, drugs (particularly nonsteroidal anti-inflammatory drugs [NSAIDs]), ischemia, and radiation. UC and CD are the most common and best understood IBDs, with a well-defined epidemiology and pathogenesis; their etiologies, however, remain elusive.[1]

Epidemiology

UC and CD share most epidemiologic characteristics.[2] These diseases are relatively common in developed nations and infrequent in countries with poor sanitation. In North America and Europe, the incidence is approximately five cases per 100,000 population for each disease, with a combined prevalence of approximately 100 per 100,000 population. The diseases can affect persons of any age, but onset most commonly occurs in the second and third decades of life. Much smaller, secondary peaks in incidence occur in the sixth and seventh decades. Males and females are affected equally. Risk of disease is higher in some ethnic groups than in others. Ashkenazi Jews have a higher risk of IBD than Africans, African Americans, and Asians; the incidence of IBD increases in these lower-risk groups, however, when they emigrate to developed nations or adopt Western culture and diet.

Etiology

The cause of IBD has yet to be established. IBD probably has multiple causes, involving an interplay between genetically mediated susceptibility, environmental factors, and aberrant immune function. These disorders may well prove to be a series of syndromes with overlapping features.[1] As yet, no dietary factor has been identified, despite case-control studies suggesting a possible association with the ingestion of large amounts of refined sugar and, perhaps, fat (essentially, the Western diet).[3] Extrapolation from animal models of IBD suggests that commensal (rather than pathogenic) flora can initiate inflammation in genetically susceptible individuals,[1,4] but no specific infectious agent has been identified as causative of either UC or CD.

There are two major clues to the etiology of IBDs. The first is the familial association of IBD, which suggests a genetic predisposition.[5] Both UC and CD are more common in families with an affected relative. Once a proband has been identified, the risk of the disease occurring in a second family member is approximately 20% (40% if the proband is a child). The risk is distributed throughout families, with an estimated risk for individuals of 3% to 5% spread among first-, second-, and third-degree relatives. If both parents have IBD, the risk of disease in an offspring is nearly 50%. There is a concordance for disease type (and subtype, in the case of CD) within families, although either UC or CD may be seen.[5] Risk of disease is highest in identi-

cal twins, with a concordance of 20% for UC and 60% for CD. This degree of risk suggests a polygenic causation with higher penetrance in CD.[6] Genetic loci for IBD have been found: for example, the *NOD2/CARD15* gene on chromosome 16 (*IBD1*) increases susceptibility to CD; other potential loci are being investigated.[5]

The second etiologic clue is the relationship between cigarette smoking and UC and CD.[7] Case-control studies from around the world have demonstrated that cigarette smokers are less likely to develop UC and more likely to develop CD. In contrast, ex-smokers are more likely to develop UC. Cigarette smoking also influences the course of IBD; for example, ex-smokers with UC are more likely to have refractory disease and to require surgery than are patients who have never smoked.[8] Cigarette smoking also protects against the development of primary sclerosing cholangitis associated with UC.[9] Conversely, current cigarette smokers with CD are more likely to have disease that is refractory to medical therapies and that recurs more rapidly after surgical resection; these effects can be reversed by smoking cessation.[10] It has not been established whether nicotine is the primary factor in the associations of cigarette smoking with UC and CD. Nicotine delivered by transdermal patch appears to have a modest therapeutic potential for UC,[11] although not as much as resumption of smoking.

Pathogenesis

There are numerous animal models for IBD, including the cotton-top tamarin, a New World monkey that, in captivity, develops a so-called spontaneous colitis with many features that are similar to those of human UC. These shared features include the development of antiepithelial antibodies, response to anti-inflammatory medications, and the development of dysplasia and adenocarcinoma.

Other animal models more closely mimic CD. These include genetically engineered transgenic rats that overexpress human HLA-B27 and β_2-microglobulin molecules and knock-out mice with targeted deletions of interleukin 2 (IL-2), IL-10, T cell receptor chains, and transforming growth factor–β. The transfer of enriched populations of functional T helper type 1 (Th1) lymphocytes into severe combined immunodeficient mice induces colitis and wasting that can be prevented by transfer of unfractionated CD4$^+$ T cells.[1]

Regardless of species or immune status, animals raised in germ-free environments do not develop intestinal inflammation.[12] The significantly higher rate of autoimmune diseases in developed versus developing countries suggests that infectious agents (bacterial, viral, and parasitic) act as antigenic triggers and that exposure to numerous microorganisms early in life may protect against autoimmunity later in life; this is the so-called hygiene hypothesis.[13] The loss of immune tolerance to specific (bacterial) antigenic triggers has been demonstrated in patients with CD.[14] Hypothetically, environmental factors interact with a genetically determined, defective innate immune response. The innate immune defects may involve dendritic cells[15] and Toll-like receptors[16]; in addition, bacterial invasion of the mucosa may be facilitated by impairment of the mucosal protection mediated by mucins, trefoil peptides, or defensins.[17] Subsequently, the onset of IBD symptoms may be triggered by acute infections (e.g., traveler's diarrhea or acute gastroenteritis), antibiotic exposure, or other environmental factors in genetically susceptible hosts. Whether a trigger (either specific or nonspecific) modifies the disease subtype cannot as yet be discerned.

Once intestinal inflammation begins, the primary difference between patients with IBD and unaffected persons is an impaired ability to downregulate mucosal inflammation.[1] Chronic inflammatory cells are normal in the intestinal mucosa; they comprise the gut component of the mucosa-associated lymphoid tract. The number of lymphoid elements in the mucosa is proportional to enteric exposure to bacteria. Persons raised in a sanitary environment (as is typical of developed countries) have less chronic inflammation than those raised in countries with poor sanitation. An extreme example is that of tropical sprue, in which mucosal inflammation is extensive and is associated with atrophy and ulceration of the small bowel villi.

In IBD, most immune elements (including tissue macrophages and mucosal T cells) respond to an exaggerated degree when triggered by an antigen. Activated macrophages and T cells are prominent in the recruitment of nonspecific inflammatory cells—primarily neutrophils, which are the final mediators of tissue damage.[1] The cytokine responses in UC and CD seem to differ, which may account for differences in disease phenotypes.[18] Many studies have demonstrated increases in levels of IL-1, IL-6, and tumor necrosis factor–α (TNF-α) in the mucosa of patients with UC and CD, although it is becoming apparent that the balance of cytokines may be different in the two diseases. CD is marked by a higher Th1 cytokine profile (interferon gamma, IL-2, IL-12, and TNF-α), whereas in UC, the balance is more consistent with a Th2 profile, with increased proportions of mucosal B cells, plasma cells, and antibodies.[1] In UC, increased production of both antineutrophil cytoplasmic antibodies and IgG antibodies reacting with a 40 kd tropomysin protein have been identified, although the pathogenic consequences of this interaction have not been defined.[19] Conversely, patients with CD have a greater likelihood of developing antibodies to a common brewer's yeast (Saccharomyces cerevisiae).[19]

A final pathway of tissue destruction is through the recruitment and activation of macrophages and neutrophils.[20] Activation of the arachidonic acid cascade leads to increased tissue levels of cyclooxygenase products (prostaglandins and thromboxanes), lipoxygenase products (primarily leukotriene B$_4$), and platelet activating factor. These compounds and other nonspecific mediators (e.g., nitric oxide, neutrophil tissue proteases, and reactive oxygen species) contribute to tissue destruction and can be targeted for specific and nonspecific anti-inflammatory therapy.[1,4]

Ulcerative Colitis

CLASSIFICATION

UC is marked by diffuse, superficial inflammation of the colonic mucosa, beginning in the rectum and extending proximally to involve any contiguous length of colon. The small intestine is not involved, except in the setting of extensive colitis, in which the most distal terminal ileum may exhibit similar superficial inflammation, termed backwash ileitis. Because the extent of colitis usually remains constant from the onset, the length of involved colon defines the classification of UC: proctitis (limited to the rectum), proctosigmoiditis or left-sided colitis (extending up to the splenic flexure), or pancolitis (extending into the transverse colon). Proximal extension occurs in approximately one third of patients with distal disease, and regression from pancolitis is also possible.[21,22] The extent of involvement does not necessarily imply severity but does pertain to prognosis (e.g., the risk of cancer) and to treatment selection. The symptoms and course of UC relate to both the extent and the severity of inflammation within the involved segment of colon.

DIAGNOSIS

The diagnosis of UC is made on the basis of clinical, endoscopic, and histologic findings. The presence of rectal bleeding or diarrhea should raise the suspicion of UC. Symptoms are often chronic, but they may also be intermittent or progressive. The easiest way to exclude UC is by direct examination of the rectosigmoid colon with a proctoscope or flexible sigmoidoscope. Radiography (barium enemas) has been almost completely replaced by more sensitive endoscopic examinations. Because UC always involves the rectum, inflammatory changes should be visible with a limited examination. In newly diagnosed patients, stool cultures are performed to rule out infectious diseases that may mimic or complicate UC, such as infection with Salmonella, Shigella, Campylobacter, hemorrhagic Escherichia coli, and Clostridium difficile.

Clinical Manifestations

The onset of UC typically is insidious rather than abrupt, although the disease occasionally presents acutely after infectious colitis or traveler's diarrhea.[23] Rectal bleeding is the most consistent feature. Bleeding may be gross or may be noted with evacuation of mucopus. Associated rectal urgency and tenesmus are related to diminished compliance of the rectum. Diarrhea, distinguished from the passage of mucopus without stool, relates to the extent of colonic involvement. Patients with proctitis often present with constipated bowel movements with interim passage of blood or mucus. Abdominal cramps preceding bowel movements are common, although abdominal pain or tenderness (related to transmural inflammation) signifies progressive, severe disease. In severe or fulminant colitis, systemic symptoms of night sweats, fever, nausea and vomiting, and weight loss accompany diarrhea. Extraintestinal manifestations can include inflammation of the eyes, skin, joints, and liver.

Ulcerative proctitis In the most common variant of UC, accounting for approximately 25% to 30% of cases and usually being the mildest, inflammation is limited to the distal 15 to 20 cm of rectum. Patients with ulcerative proctitis typically present with hematochezia, a sense of rectal urgency, and constipated bowel movements because of delayed transit of fecal material in the right colon. Systemic manifestations are uncommon, but skin or joint symptoms can occur.[24] The disease usually remains confined to the rectum but may advance proximally in as many as 30% to 40% of patients.[21]

Proctosigmoiditis Left-sided colitis is an intermediate syndrome of UC, accounting for about one third of cases. Patients present with either constipation or diarrhea accompanied by tenesmus, urgency, and rectal bleeding. Left lower quadrant cramping abdominal pain is more common than with proctitis, as are extraintestinal symptoms. The proximal disease margin usually remains fixed throughout the course but can spread more proximally or even retract distally.

Extensive colitis (pancolitis) In pancolitis, inflammation extends into the transverse or right colon. Patients are more likely to present with diarrhea because of diminished absorptive capacity of the colon, accompanied by rectal bleeding and urgency. Abdominal cramps may be diffuse or localized, and patients are more likely to have weight loss, systemic or extraintestinal symptoms, and anemia.

Toxic megacolon Toxic megacolon refers to the most severe manifestation of UC, which occurs when the inflammation extends from the superficial mucosa into the submucosa and muscular layers of the colon.[25] Toxic megacolon occurs more commonly with extensive colitis but can also occur with severe distal colitis. The colonic wall becomes tissue-paper thin as the colon dilates and becomes hypomotile; perforation may occur. The patient often has fever, prostration, severe cramps, abdominal distention, and abdominal tenderness; the tenderness may be localized, diffuse, or rebound.

Clinical Severity

The severity of UC depends on both the length of colon involved and the severity of colonic inflammation. The set of criteria most commonly used to define the severity of disease was created by Truelove and Witts.[26-28] Although the criteria were developed to assess improvement in clinical trials, they remain useful in classifying severity in clinical practice, and they have been modified to include fulminant colitis [*see Table 1*]. Severity criteria are as follows:

Mild In mild UC, patients have less than four bowel movements daily, with minimal cramps and urgency. Usually, most of the bowel movements occur early in the day; and after the morning evacuations, the patient is able to proceed with activities of daily life.

Moderate Patients with moderate UC have four to eight bowel movements daily, more frequent rectal urgency, and postprandial cramping and bowel movements. Blood is present in most stools, and nocturnal wakening for bowel movements is common. The disease can interfere with daily work or school activities and social life.

Severe Patients with severe UC have more than eight bowel movements daily, nocturnal bowel movements, severe urgency with or without incontinence, and systemic signs that include low-grade fever, night sweats, weakness, and weight loss. Abdominal tenderness, tachycardia, anemia, leukocytosis, and hypoalbuminemia are common.

Fulminant Patients with fulminant colitis have more than 10 bowel movements a day, nocturnal bowel movements, severe abdominal pain or relentless tenesmus, and rebound tenderness or distention with tympanic bowel sounds. They also have prostration, high fever, and hypotension. Radiographic studies show evidence of mucosal edema, intramural air (pneumatosis coli), colonic dilatation (toxic megacolon), or free abdominal air (perforation).

Physical Examination

In most patients with UC, the physical examination results are normal. There may be mild abdominal tenderness to deep palpation, particularly in the left colon, but significant abdominal findings are limited to patients with moderate to severe disease, in whom tenderness is more prominent. Surprisingly, despite the frequent diarrhea, perianal manifestations are absent. Any significant perianal findings (e.g., large hemorrhoids, skin tags, fissures, abscesses, or fistulas) suggest CD rather than UC.

Table 1 Classification of Ulcerative Colitis

Feature	Mild Disease	Moderate Disease	Severe Disease	Fulminant Disease
History				
Stools	< 4/day (usually early in the day); minimal abdominal cramps and urgency	4–8/day; abdominal cramps and urgency	> 8/day; nocturnal bowel movements; severe urgency with or without incontinence	> 10/day; nocturnal bowel movements; severe urgency; tenesmus; severe abdominal pain
Blood in stool	Intermittent	Frequent	Frequent	Continuous
Physical examination				
Abdominal findings	Nontender abdomen; normal bowel sounds	Nontender or minimally tender over sigmoid	Tender abdomen; no rebound tenderness	Distended abdomen; decreased bowel sounds; rebound tenderness
Temperature	Normal	Normal	> 37.5° C (99.5° F)	> 37.5° C
Pulse	Normal	Normal	> 90	> 90
Other physical findings	Normal	Pallor	Weakness, pallor, weight loss	Prostration, hypotension
Laboratory tests				
Hemoglobin	Normal	Mild anemia	< 75% of normal	Transfusion required
Erythrocyte sedimentation rate	< 30 mm/hr	< 30 mm/hr	> 30 mm/hr	> 30 mm/hr
Radiography	Normal gas pattern	Absent stool in involved segment	Edematous colon wall, thumbprinting	Dilated colon, mucosal edema, intramural air, free abdominal air

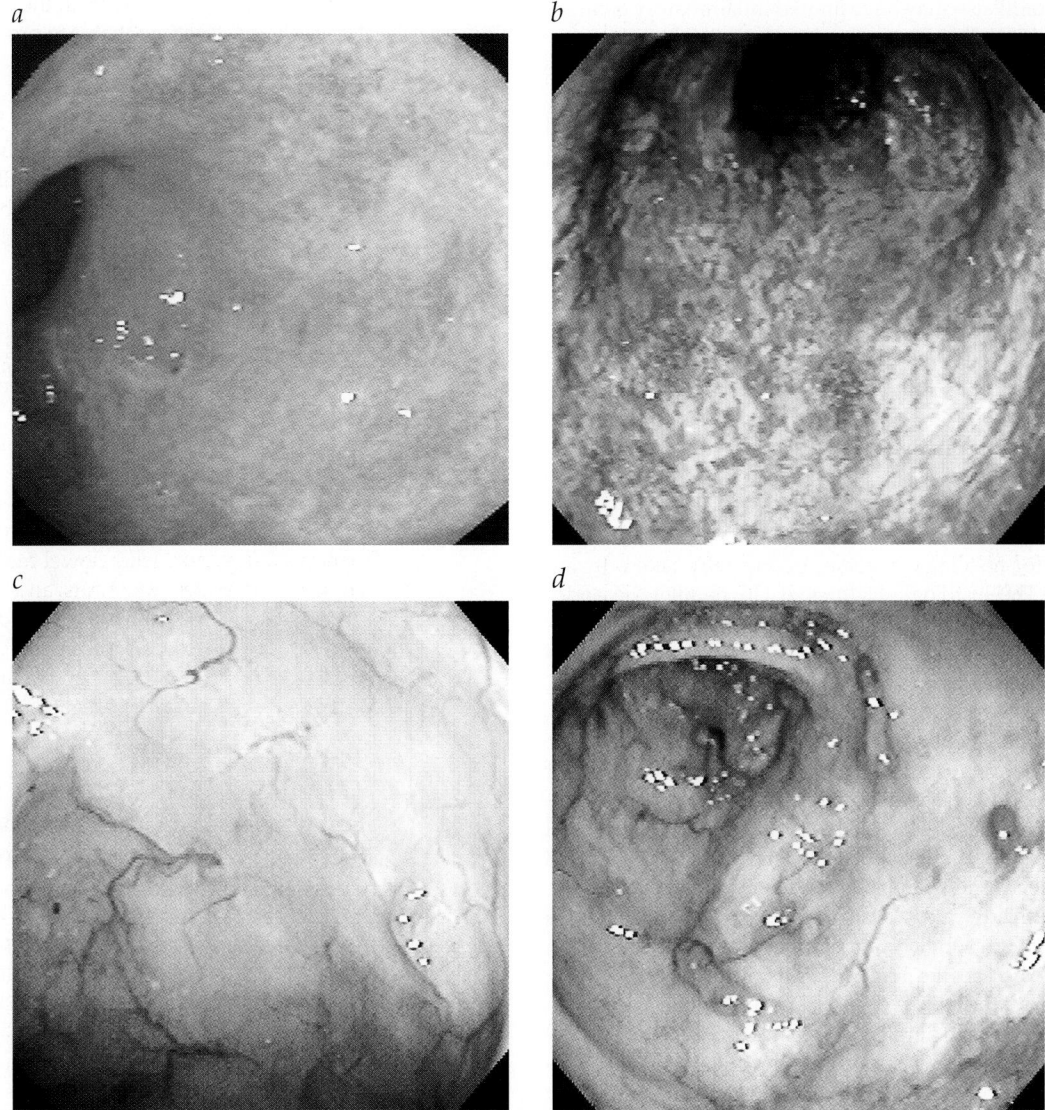

Figure 1 The endoscopic spectrum of ulcerative colitis includes (*a*) mucosal edema, erythema, loss of vasculature; (*b*) granular mucosa with pinpoint ulceration and friability; (*c*) regenerated (i.e., healed) mucosa with distorted mucosal vasculature; and (*d*) regenerated mucosa with typical postinflammatory pseudopolyps.

Conjunctival pallor is common because of anemia. Patients may present with ocular inflammation, erythema nodosum, pyoderma gangrenosum, or arthritis of larger joints.[29] Low back pain with diminished range of motion, or sacroiliac tenderness, is uncommon. Hepatomegaly, splenomegaly, or evidence of chronic liver disease is rare and limited to patients with end-stage primary sclerosing cholangitis.

Endoscopy

UC can almost always be diagnosed by endoscopic examination of the rectum and sigmoid colon.[30] The disease presents as diffuse and continuous inflammation beginning in the rectum, with proximal extension that varies among individual patients. In most cases, it is advisable to determine the proximal margin of disease, from the standpoints of prognosis[24] and therapy.[26,27] The initial examination should be performed without enema preparation, to avoid confusion with trauma or inflammation from administration of the enema. Patients with active colitis rarely have any fecal material in the involved lumen.

Healthy colonic mucosa is smooth and glistening, reflects light back from the scope, and demonstrates a branching mucosal vascular pattern. With inflammation, the mucosa becomes erythematous and more granular, which breaks apart the light reflection, and the vascular pattern becomes obscured by edema [*see Figure 1*]. The granularity of the mucosa may be fine or coarse. Coarse granularity represents microscopic or pinpoint ulcerations and is associated with friability (hemorrhage from the mucosa that may be spontaneous or induced by scope trauma). Exudates of mucopus are a common associated finding. Gross ulcerations represent more severe disease and, although usually shallow, can progress to a total denudation of the mucosa with exposure of the underlying circular musculature. These changes can be continuous up to a distinct margin where the mucosa appears normal, or they may extend diffusely to the cecum and, occasionally, into the distal ileum (backwash ileitis). In the setting of pancolitis, the ileocecal valve is usually wide open (patulous), allowing easy entry into the terminal ileum. Some patients with distal UC (involving the rectum or sigmoid) also may have limited inflammatory changes around the appendix in the cecum (cecal red patch).[31]

As ulcerative colitis heals, the mucosal changes may become more focal.[32] The colonic mucosa regenerates from ulceration to granularity, with gradual restitution of a distorted mucosal vascular pattern with less distinct branching or irregular, pruned-appearing vessels. In areas that had been more severely inflamed, granulation tissue may protrude and become reepithelialized as so-called pseudopolyps. These postinflammatory changes can arise in a variety of sizes and shapes and are more likely to become fingerlike projections, or even mucosal bridges, in areas that had severe, undermining ulcerations [see Figure 1]. Pseudopolyps have no neoplastic potential but can be difficult to differentiate from adenomatous polyps. When pseudopolyps are extensive, they can totally carpet the mucosa, making it impossible to discern distinct, potentially neoplastic polyps.

Histology

Samples for histologic analysis are typically taken during endoscopy. The histologic features of UC parallel the endoscopic appearance of diffuse, continuous mucosal inflammatory changes. The principal components are disruption of glandular architecture and an inflammatory infiltrate.[33] A hallmark distinction between chronic IBDs such as UC and acute self-limited (infectious) colitis is architectural distortion [see Figure 2]. In UC, the normal vertical (so-called test-tube) alignment of glands is distorted; the glands are separated by expanded lamina propria lymphocytes, plasma cells, and eosinophils, as well as by neutrophils, which normally are sparse. The glands themselves become irregular in shape and, often, branched. The neutrophil infiltrate is localized to the base of the glandular crypts and invades the crypts, producing crypt abscesses. In more severe disease, the epithelial lining is destroyed, leaving ulcerations over the lamina propria. The inflammatory changes are usually superficial, limited by the muscularis mucosae. Despite severe superficial changes, deeper inflammation is uncommon, except in the setting of fulminant colitis. In fulminant colitis, the muscular layers are breached by expanding inflammatory ulceration that can leave the bowel wall tissue-paper thin and protected only by the serosa.

As the mucosa heals, the glands may become atrophied or shortened and irregularly shaped, with a thinned-out lamina propria. Inflammatory polyps are composed of vascular granulation tissue with a thin colonic epithelium. In quiescent colitis, the architectural distortion is present but acute inflammation (neutrophils and crypt abscesses) is absent [see Figure 2].

Both acute inflammation and regeneration of the colonic epithelium produce cellular atypia that must be distinguished from epithelial dysplasia.[34] In regenerating mucosa, the glandular epithelium can become irregularly shaped and hyperchromatic, with depletion of normal apical mucus. Stratification of nuclei and loss of polarity are manifestations of neoplastic transformation (i.e., dysplasia).

Imaging Studies

Radiography Radiographs have largely been supplanted by endoscopic examinations for the diagnosis of UC, but radiography remains a valuable adjunct to endoscopy in specified clinical situations. Plain abdominal radiographs are useful in the setting of severe colitis. These examinations outline the air-filled colon and can demonstrate the presence or absence of

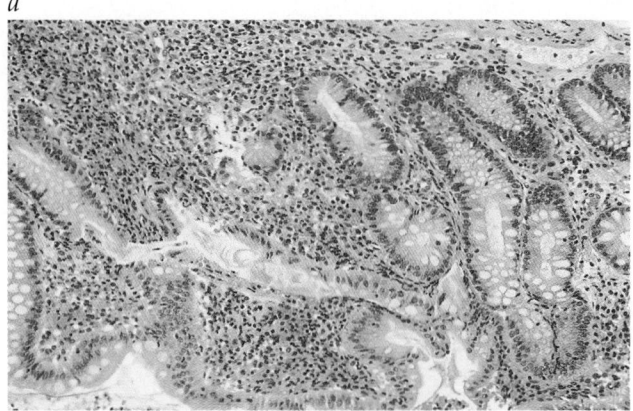

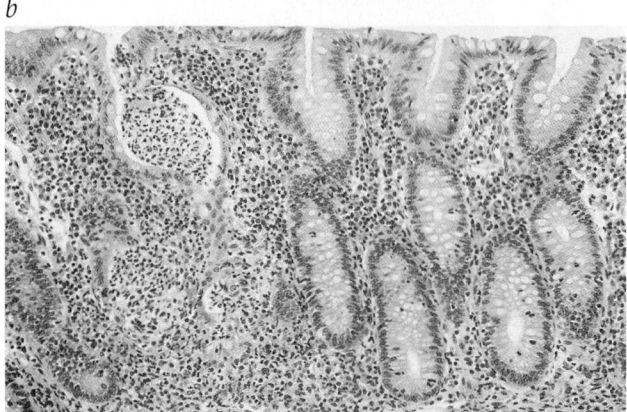

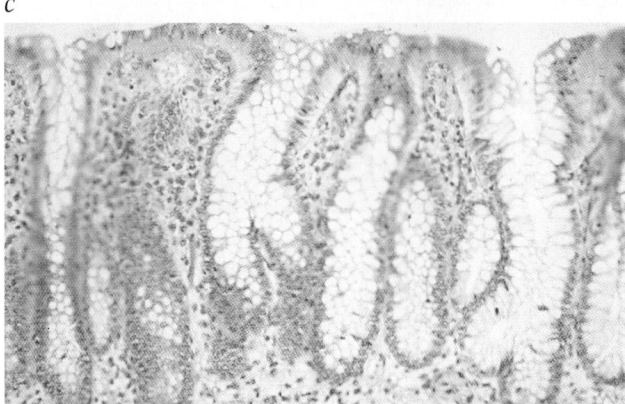

Figure 2 Pathologic changes in ulcerative colitis include (*a*) acute superficial inflammation with distortion of the normal crypt architecture, (*b*) crypt abscesses, and (*c*) quiescent colitis without acute inflammation but with distortions of crypt architecture (abnormal branched crypts).

haustrations or dilatation of the colon (to rule out toxic megacolon) [see Figure 3]. Extraluminal gas under the diaphragm (free air) and evidence of an ileus pattern are additional features of severe colitis. Plain abdominal radiographs also provide a view of the sacroiliac joints and lumbosacral spine as a gross assessment of sacroiliitis or ankylosing spondylitis for patients presenting with low back pain.

Contrast barium studies, once the primary diagnostic modality, are less commonly employed because endoscopic examinations provide higher diagnostic sensitivity and specificity and

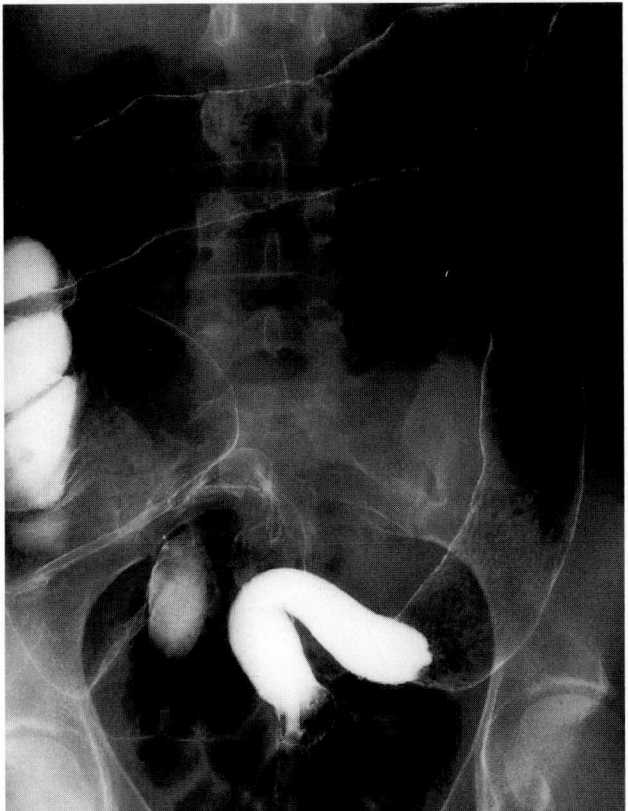

Figure 3 In this air-contrast radiograph of ulcerative colitis, the mucosal pattern is granular with loss of normal haustrations in a diffuse, continuous pattern.

permit histologic sampling.[26] Air-contrast barium enemas demonstrate the fine or coarse mucosal granularity of microscopic ulcerations or the diffuse, continuous, and symmetrical pattern of ulceration involving the rectum to the proximal extent of disease [*see Figure 3*]. Other features of UC that may be visible on barium enemas are the loss of haustration in inflamed segments, foreshortening of the colon, and an increase in the space between the sacrum and the rectum. Barium enema examin-

ations are contraindicated in severely ill patients because of the potential for perforation or the induction of a toxic megacolon.

Scintigraphy Scanning with indium-labeled or technetium-labeled leukocytes is occasionally indicated for severely ill adults or children when the extent of colitis is uncertain or when small bowel disease has not been excluded.[35] These studies provide relatively rapid determination of the extent, severity, and continuity of intestinal inflammation. Scintigraphy is noninvasive, is sensitive and specific for intestinal inflammation, and is occasionally helpful in discriminating UC from CD.

Crohn Disease

CD is manifested by focal, asymmetrical, and transmural inflammation of the digestive tract, at times accompanied by granuloma formation. In contrast to the inflammation of UC, which is diffuse, continuous, superficial (mucosal), and typically limited to the colon, the inflammation of CD is more patchy, may be transmural, and can involve any segment of the gastrointestinal tract from mouth to anus. Because the inflammation may be transmural, CD can lead to intestinal complications of stenoses (strictures) and fistulas. Although a hallmark of CD is the histologic finding of noncaseating granulomas, these granulomas are identified in only about 30% of patients and are not necessary to make the diagnosis.

Because CD may involve any segment of the gastrointestinal tract, the presentation is more heterogeneous than that of UC and is determined by the location, extent, severity of inflammation, and inflammatory pattern. The location and pattern tend to remain constant for each patient.[36] CD produces a spectrum of inflammatory patterns: from superficial inflammation similar to that of UC, to formation of fibrostenosing strictures, to penetration of the bowel wall and fistula formation accompanied by a mesenteric inflammatory mass or perienteric abscess. An attempt to classify CD on the basis of inflammatory patterns[37] has been compromised by the tendency of inflammatory patterns to progress to stenoses over time.[38] In contrast to UC, CD is usually not curable by surgery; intestinal resection and anastomosis are almost inevitably followed by recurrence of the disease involving the anastomotic site and proximal intestine.[39]

Table 2 Key Distinguishing Features of Ulcerative Colitis and Crohn Disease

Feature	Ulcerative Colitis	Crohn Disease
History Smoking status	Nonsmoker or ex-smoker	Smoker

Physical examination
  Symptoms
  Signs
	
	Rectal bleeding, cramps
	Normal perianal findings, no abdominal mass
		
		Diarrhea, abdominal pain, weight loss, nausea, vomiting
		Perianal skin tags, fistulas, abscesses; abdominal mass; clubbing of digits

Laboratory tests
  Endoscopy
 	
  Radiology
 	
  Histology
 	
  Serology
	
	Rectal involvement; continuous superficial inflammation with granular, friable mucosa; terminal ileum normal or showing backwash ileitis
	Diffuse, continuous superficial ulceration; ahaustral (lead-pipe) colon; backwash ileitis
	Diffuse, continuous, superficial inflammation; crypt architectural deformity
	Elevated p-ANCA (60%–80% of patients)
		
		Rectal sparing; local ulceration with normal intervening mucosa; aphthous, linear, or stellate ulcers; terminal ileum inflamed with aphthous or linear ulcers
		Focal, asymmetrical, transmural ulceration; strictures, inflammatory masses, fistulas; small bowel disease
		Focal inflammation, aphthous ulcers, lymphoid aggregates, transmural inflammation, granulomas (15%–30% of patients)
		Elevated ASCA (~ 30% of patients)

p-ANCA—perinuclear antineutrophil cytoplasmic antibody   ASCA—anti–*Saccharomyces cerevisiae* antibody

In clinical trials, the instrument most commonly used to quantify disease activity has been the CD Activity Index (CDAI).[40] However, because of its complex derivation and lack of discrimination between symptoms and inflammation, the CDAI is not used in clinical practice. Instead, patients require individualized assessments of the severity of disease according to inflammatory symptoms, obstruction, fistulization, abscess formation, systemic complications, and effect on the patient's quality of life.[41]

DIAGNOSIS

CD is diagnosed on the basis of clinical, radiographic, endoscopic, and histologic criteria. As with UC, there is no pathognomonic marker. The clinical presentation and key features of the history, physical examination, and laboratory studies determine the diagnostic workup and serve to differentiate CD from UC [see Table 2].

Clinical Manifestations

CD most commonly involves the terminal ileum and cecum. However, the pattern of CD can be quite varied [see Figure 4].

The presentation depends on the site, extent, severity, and complications of intestinal and extraintestinal disease.[42,43] Patients usually present with chronic disease, but CD can be acute, with severe abdominal pain, intestinal blockage, or hemorrhage. Abdominal pain is a more common feature of CD than of UC because the transmural extension of CD results in stimulation of pain receptors in the serosa and peritoneum. Abdominal cramping and postprandial pain are common symptoms that often are accompanied by diarrhea, rectal bleeding, nocturnal bowel movements, fevers, night sweats, and weight loss. Nausea and vomiting occur in the presence of intestinal strictures that produce partial or complete bowel obstructions. Transmural disease commonly manifests in the perianal region as skin tags or perirectal abscesses or fistulas,[44] but it also can present as an inflammatory mass in the right lower quadrant. In children and adolescents, the presentation often is more insidious, with weight loss, failure to grow or to develop secondary sex characteristics, arthritis, or fevers of undetermined origin. Skin lesions, primarily erythema nodosum, may precede intestinal symptoms.[45,46]

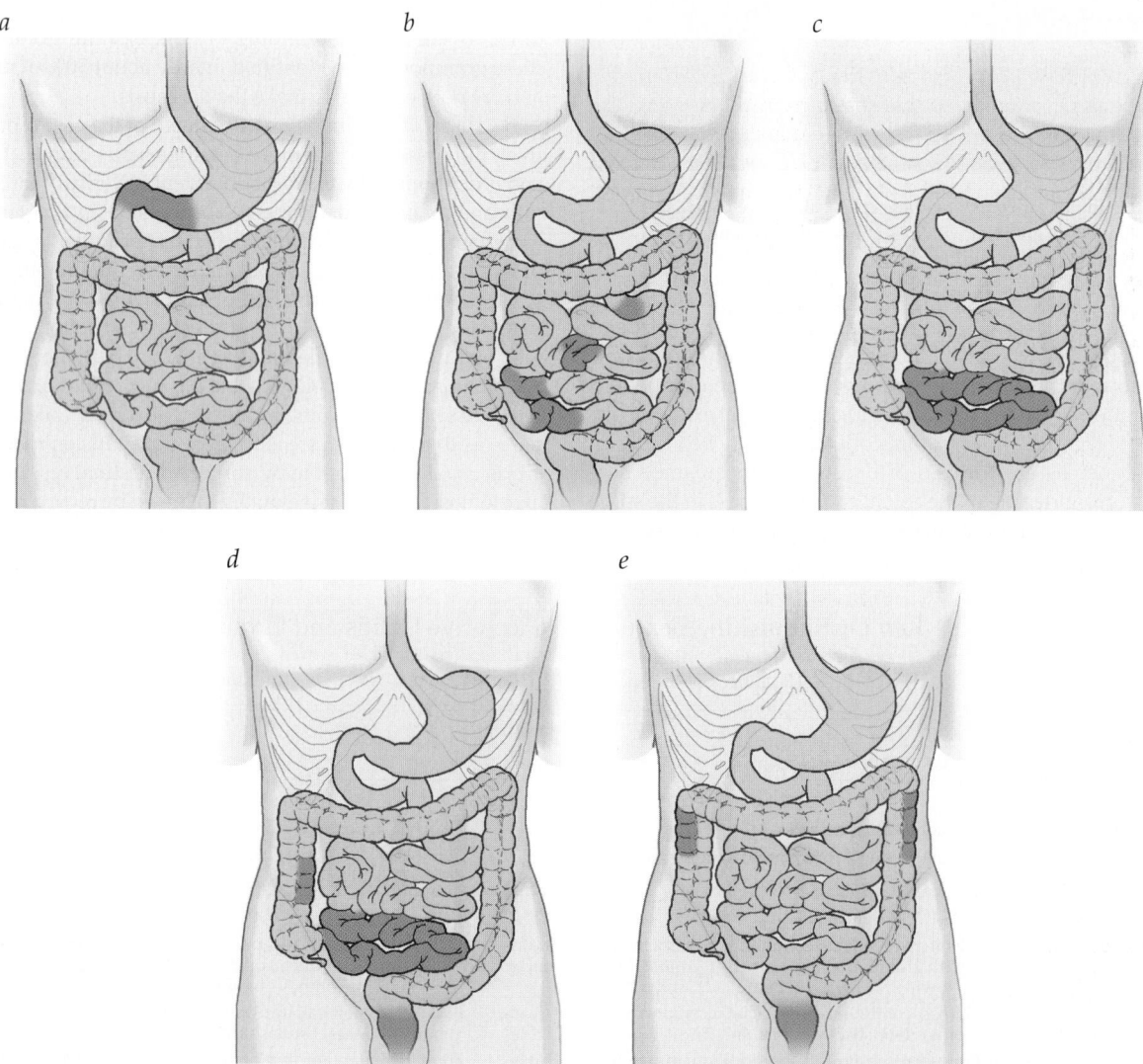

Figure 4   The spectrum of Crohn disease presentations includes (*a*) gastroduodenitis (7% of patients), (*b, c*) jejunoileitis and ileitis (33% of patients), (*d*) ileocolitis (45% of patients), and (*e*) colitis (15% of patients).

Crohn disease of the esophagus, stomach, and duodenum Infrequently, primary manifestations of CD mimic gastroesophageal reflux or peptic ulcer disease.[47,48] Heartburn, dysphagia, nausea, dyspepsia, epigastric pain, and early satiety or postprandial vomiting typically accompany other systemic inflammatory symptoms such as fever, night sweats, and rectal bleeding.

Jejunoileitis Another relatively uncommon presentation of CD, jejunoileitis most often presents with vomiting and diarrhea, cramping abdominal pain, and weight loss.[49] Patients describe borborygmi related to focal, segmental strictures compromising the passage of enteric contents. Diarrhea is multifactorial and can be secondary to malabsorption as a consequence of inflammation, protein-losing enteropathy, or stasis and small bowel bacterial overgrowth proximal to strictures.

Ileitis and ileocecal Crohn disease CD most commonly presents as right lower quadrant abdominal pain and tenderness (often accompanied by an inflammatory mass), diarrhea with or without rectal bleeding, weight loss, fevers, chills, and night sweats. An acute presentation may mimic appendicitis; occasionally, Crohn ileitis will be diagnosed at exploratory laparotomy for presumed appendicitis.

Crohn colitis Approximately 15% of CD cases are limited to the colon. Distinguishing these cases from UC can be difficult, because the clinical manifestations—diarrhea, rectal bleeding, and urgency—overlap with those of UC [*see Table 2*]. However, CD of the colon is more likely than UC to be accompanied by perianal manifestations (skin tags and perirectal abscess or fistulas), and the rectum often is spared, whereas UC always involves the rectum. In approximately 10% to 20% of patients presenting with colitis, the classification may be indeterminate in the setting of diffuse or severe inflammation or of questionable focal inflammation.[50]

Perianal Crohn disease Perianal involvement in CD most often accompanies colonic disease and begins within the anal crypts.[51] Small fistulas from the anorectal junction progress through or around the anal sphincter and present as perirectal abscesses or fistulas. Often, perianal tissue becomes hypertrophied, producing skin tags [*see Figure 5*]; these may be misdiagnosed as hemorrhoids. At times, perianal manifestations are the primary presentation, and in extreme situations, the anal sphincter and perineum can become grossly deformed.

Physical Examination

Key findings on physical examination of patients with CD include both abdominal and general systematic abnormalities. The abdominal examination may be significant for distension and abnormal bowel sounds in the presence of intestinal strictures producing partial intestinal obstruction. Tenderness in the area of involvement and the presence of an inflammatory mass are common. It is important to examine the perianal region and rectum for evidence of abscess, fistula, skin tags, or anal stricture.

Patients with CD often are chronically ill and can present with weight loss and pallor. The eye exam may demonstrate episcleritis or uveitis. Aphthous ulcerations in the mouth are common, and in extreme cases, patients may exhibit evidence of nutritional deficiencies (e.g., cheilosis or tongue atrophy). Examination of the musculoskeletal system may demonstrate

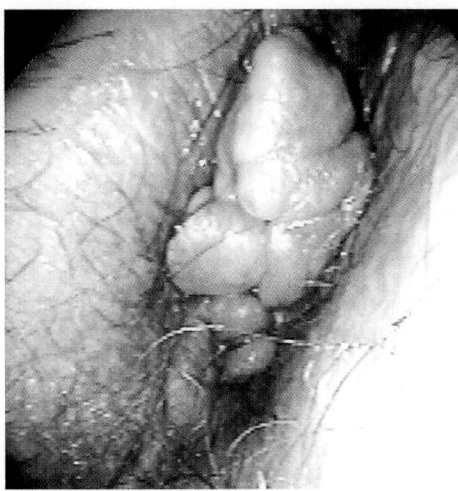

Figure 5 **The typical perianal skin tag of CD differs from the typical hemorrhoid tag.**

swelling or redness of large joints (e.g., knees, ankles, or wrists) or clubbing of the fingers. Skin examination can reveal erythema nodosum or, rarely, pyoderma gangrenosum.

Laboratory Studies

Anemia is common in CD. Anemia can result from deficiencies of iron, vitamin B_{12}, or folic acid or may be the anemia of chronic disease. Serum ferritin levels correlate better than iron and iron-binding protein levels with bone marrow iron stores in IBD.[52] Leukocytosis is common, depending on the severity of inflammation and the presence of suppurative complications. Thrombocytosis also is common and is related to inflammation or iron deficiency. Elevated erythrocyte sedimentation rates and C-reactive protein levels reflect nonspecific acute-phase reactions.[53] Electrolyte disturbances depend on the severity of diarrhea and dehydration. Serum albumin levels often are reduced as a result of malnutrition and enteric protein losses. Patients with severe weight loss may have prolonged clotting times because of vitamin K deficiency. Urinalysis commonly demonstrates calcium oxalate crystals.

Quantitative stool examinations are useful in the setting of diarrhea to assess fecal leukocytes (confirming inflammatory diarrhea), stool volume, and fecal fat. Quantification of either fecal calprotectin[54] or lactoferrin[55] is a surrogate for the presence of fecal leukocytes. The presence of the serologic markers anti–*Saccharomyces cerevisiae* antibody and an antibody to the outer core membrane of *E. coli* (OmpC) have high specificity for CD.[56]

Imaging Studies

Radiography Barium contrast studies are the most commonly used diagnostic tools to assess and confirm CD of the small intestine and are useful for assessing the upper digestive tract and colon. In colonic disease, barium studies can define intestinal complications (e.g., stricture formation or fistulas) that cannot be adequately assessed by endoscopy. Features of CD that are shown with barium examinations include mucosal edema, aphthous and linear ulcerations, asymmetrical narrowing or strictures, and separation of adjacent loops of bowel caused by mesenteric thickening. Abnormalities are focal and asymmetrical, with ulcerations most often involving the antimesenteric border. Cobblestoning of the mucosa represents networks of linear ulcerations outlining islands of residual normal mucosa. Pseudodiverticula formation or dilated loops of bowel are common proximal to strictures. There may be evidence of fistulas extending from any involved segment to an adjacent loop of bowel, the mesentery, or the urinary bladder or from the rectum to the vagina or perineum. CT scanning after direct injection of barium into the small bowel through a nasogastric tube (enteroclysis) provides excellent discrimination between intestinal and extra-intestinal disease.[57]

Other imaging studies Ultrasound examinations or CT scans are useful to assess for abscess in patients who have an inflammatory abdominal mass or who have fever, leukocytosis, or abdominal tenderness. Ultrasound or CT scan is also warranted to assess for hydronephrosis in the setting of an inflammatory mass in the right lower quadrant, because these have the potential to obstruct the right ureter. Transrectal ultrasound, CT scan, and MRI also are useful to assess the extent of

perianal and sphincter involvement in patients presenting with perianal or perirectal pain.[51] Scintigraphy using leukocytes labeled with indium or technetium can be helpful to define locations of intestinal inflammation when barium studies are not possible or the results are indeterminate.[35,58]

Endoscopy Colonoscopic examinations have become a primary means of diagnosing CD that involves the colon. Endoscopy in these patients typically reveals sparing of the rectum, with focal inflammatory changes in the more proximal colon and terminal ileum. Other typical features include the presence of aphthous, linear, or irregularly shaped ulcerations with normal intervening mucosa [see Figure 6]. Inflammatory strictures may preclude examination of proximal segments of bowel. Inflammatory pseudopolyps may be seen, as in UC. In some patients, polypoid or masslike inflammatory changes may be difficult to differentiate from neoplastic masses; biopsy and histologic analysis may be required. Similar endoscopic

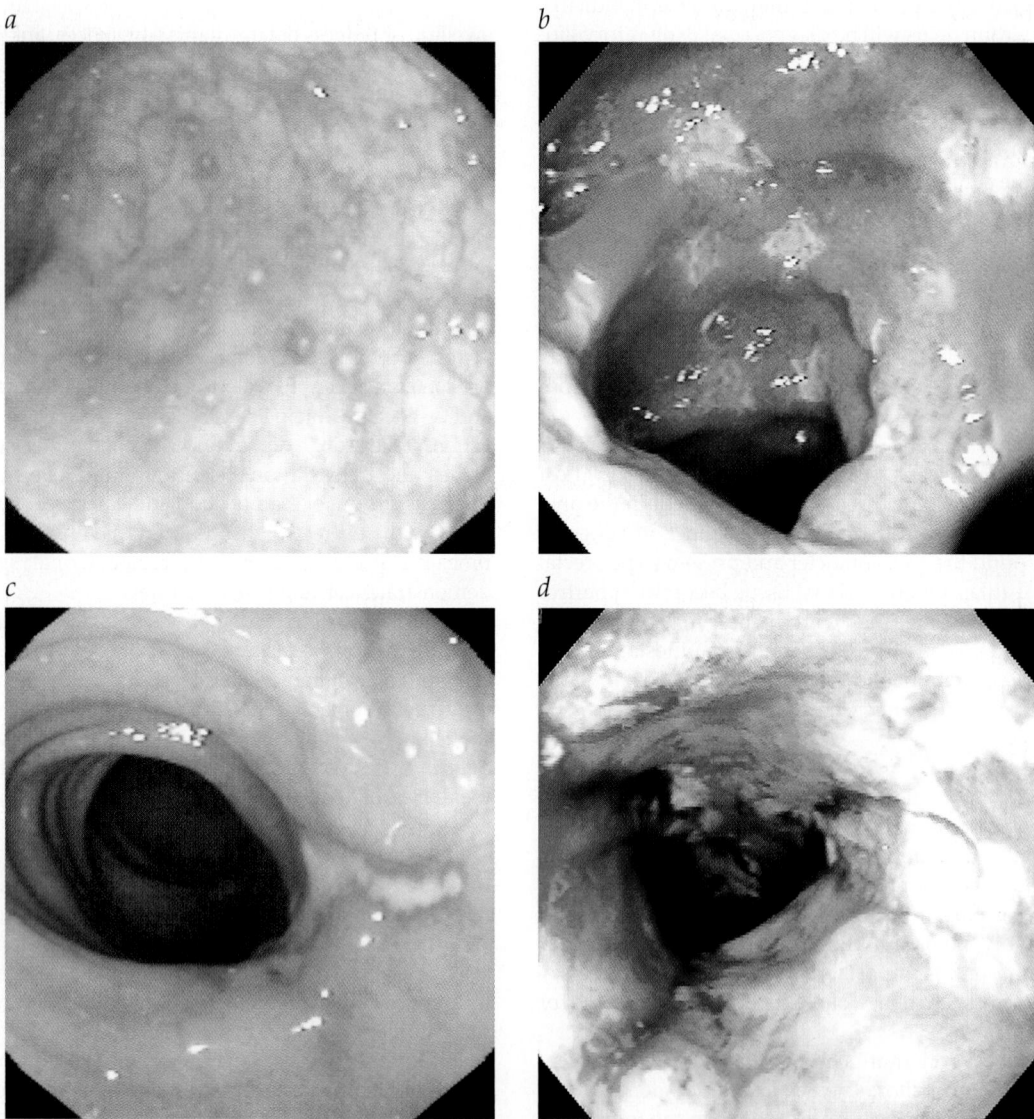

Figure 6 Endoscopic spectrum of Crohn disease includes (*a*) aphthous ulcerations amid normal colonic mucosal vasculature; (*b*) deeper, punched-out ulcers in ileal mucosa; (*c*) a single colonic linear ulcer; and (*d*) deep colonic ulcerations forming a stricture.

features may be present in the esophagus, stomach, or duodenum. An important aspect of endoscopic examinations is the ability to obtain samples for pathologic interpretation.

Wireless capsule endoscopy is now being used to diagnose CD. This technique offers access to parts of the small bowel that cannot be reached by standard endoscopy and may be more sensitive than conventional radiographic studies for identifying subtle lesions.[59]

Histology

Pathologic findings in CD reflect the gross pattern of focal and asymmetrical intestinal involvement.[32,33,50] The primary histologic lesion is an aphthous ulcer [*see Figure 7*]. These begin as erosions overlying lymphoid aggregates. As the minute ulceration extends, in either a linear or a transmural pattern, the microscopic and macroscopic changes that develop include a mixed acute and chronic inflammatory cell infiltrate composed of lymphocytes, plasma cells, and neutrophils. Crypt abscesses are common, and the inflammatory infiltrates often are located adjacent to normal epithelium. Noncaseating granulomas, which may be identified in mucosal biopsies or in resected specimens, are characteristic of CD; however, they are not necessary for confirming the diagnosis.

Granulomas may be found in mucosal specimens that appear grossly normal. Specimens from resected intestine demonstrate transmural inflammatory changes extending from the mucosa into the serosa (which is hyperemic, with creeping mesenteric fat). At times, there may be paradoxical involvement of the deeper layers of the bowel wall, with lymphoid aggregates overlying normal-appearing epithelium. Submucosal fibrosis, deep fissuring ulcerations, and fistulizing ulcerations communicate between loops of bowel or into the adjacent mesentery.

Differential Diagnosis

IBD should be considered in any patient who presents with rectal bleeding or diarrhea. Identification of fecal leukocytes is the simplest means of discerning an inflammatory process of the intestine. Other causes of rectal bleeding are either traumatic or neoplastic. Diarrhea is nonspecific and has a large differential schema [*see Chapter 66*]. The primary chronic diarrheal illness that requires differentiation from UC or CD is irritable bowel syndrome (IBS). IBS is never associated with rectal bleeding, and nocturnal symptoms are uncommon. The presence of occult blood or fecal leukocytes excludes IBS.

Patients with gross or occult blood in the stool require endoscopic evaluation. Colonic neoplasia is a prominent consideration for patients older than 50 years, whereas hemorrhoids or anal fissures are common in younger patients. NSAID-induced colitis is common and may contribute to ischemic colitis in persons in older age groups.[60] Ischemic colitis presents acutely in elderly patients after precipitating events such as dehydration or heart failure; in younger patients, the condition is associated with oral contraceptive use, vasculitis, and hypercoagulable states.[61] Endoscopic examination demonstrates focal hemorrhagic or ulcerated mucosa in the so-called watershed segments of the sigmoid colon or splenic flexure. Diverticular hemorrhage is typically profuse and painless. Some patients, however—particularly elderly persons taking NSAIDs—may present with less vigorous rectal bleeding from diverticulosis involving a segment of the sigmoid colon.[62]

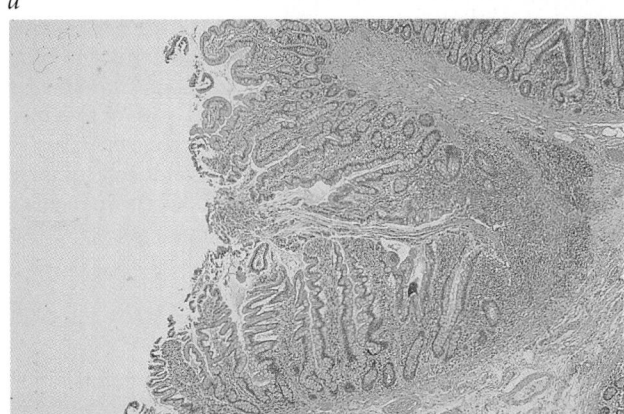

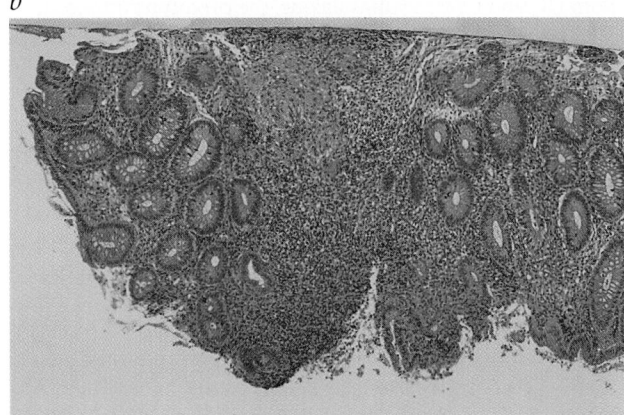

Figure 7 **Pathologic changes in Crohn disease include (*a*) ileal aphthous ulceration overlying a lymphoid aggregate and (*b*) focal colonic ulcer with noncaseating granuloma in lymphoid tissue.**

Inflammatory diarrhea can be either infectious or noninfectious.[63] The infectious colitides are caused by bacteria such as *Salmonella, Shigella, Campylobacter*, and hemorrhagic *E. coli*. Most of these diseases are acute and self-limited and need be considered only in patients who present with sudden onset of bloody diarrhea and fever. UC and CD develop insidiously, over a period of weeks. *C. difficile* colitis can also mimic ulcerative colitis and may be more chronic, lasting weeks [*see Chapter 136*]. In immunocompetent hosts, viral or parasitic infections rarely mimic UC. The exception is amebiasis, which may cause acute or subchronic symptoms. Amebiasis can often be distinguished from IBD by wet-mount examination of the stool for motile ameba and the more typical focal (so-called collar button) ulcerations in the colon [*see Chapter 157*]. Although most cases of infectious diarrhea are acute and self-limited, intercurrent infections and traveler's diarrhea can initiate flare-ups of IBD.[64] Consequently, patients presenting with new-onset IBD or acute exacerbations of IBD should be evaluated for a complicating enteric infection.

Management

The treatment of UC or CD is based on the location, extent, and severity of disease, as well as the patient's response to past therapy.[26,27] Factors that contribute to exacerbations of activity or refractoriness to therapy should be addressed. Such factors may include concomitant medications (e.g., NSAIDs or antibiotics), intercurrent infections (e.g., with *C. difficile*), menstruation, and dietary or lifestyle changes.

Treatment follows a sequential approach: induction of remission and, then, maintenance of remission. Clinicians can now choose from a variety of medication classes for treatment of IBD, and both medication selection and dosage may vary according to whether the therapeutic intent is induction or maintenance. Surgical treatment is indicated in selected patients to treat severe disease activity or specific complications.

ANTI-INFLAMMATORY AGENTS

Aminosalicylates

Aminosalicylates are the primary therapies for mild or moderate UC and CD.[26,27] These agents have a long history of clinical use and have been extensively studied in clinical trials for both UC and CD.[65,66] Sulfasalazine, the prototype aminosalicylate [*see Figure 8*], was developed with the intention of providing both an antibacterial agent (sulfapyridine) and an anti-inflammatory agent (5-aminosalicylic acid [5-ASA], mesalamine, or mesalazine) into the connective tissues. It was subsequently recognized that sulfasalazine remains intact through the stomach and small intestine, with minimal enteric absorption. On reaching the colon, the azo bond between sulfapyridine and 5-ASA is cleaved by colonic bacteria. Released sulfapyridine is almost completely absorbed from the colon and undergoes hepatic acetylation and subsequent renal excretion. In contrast, the 5-ASA released into the colon is poorly absorbed and is primarily eliminated in the feces.[67] Therefore, sulfasalazine primarily serves as a carrier for 5-ASA to the colon. The 5-ASA moiety accounts for the primary therapeutic benefits, whereas sulfapyridine causes the majority of side effects attributed to sulfasalazine. These attributes have led to the development of a series of sulfa-free aminosalicylates (e.g., olsalazine, balsalazide, and formulations of mesalamine) that can be targeted to specific sites along the gastrointestinal tract. A basic premise regarding the aminosalicylates is that the effects of 5-ASA are topical (mucosal), rather than systemic, and that the active moiety needs to be delivered to the site of intestinal inflammation.

Sulfasalazine and mesalamine have multiple anti-inflammatory effects, including inhibition of the arachidonic acid cascade along the cyclooxygenase, lipoxygenase, and platelet-activating factor pathways.[65,66] In addition, the aminosalicylates inhibit oxygen radical production and scavenge free radicals.[68] They inhibit lymphocyte and monocyte function and production of

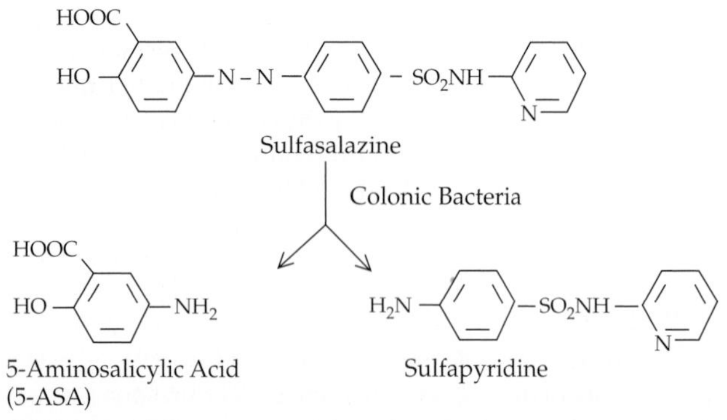

Figure 8 Sulfasalazine is composed of sulfapyridine and 5-aminosalicylic acid (mesalamine), linked by an azo bond.

immunoglobulin by plasma cells. Sulfasalazine also has been shown to inhibit production of IL-1 and nuclear factor κB.[69]

Adverse effects of sulfasalazine are common and are primarily related to plasma sulfapyridine concentrations; these concentrations depend on the rate of hepatic acetylation of sulfapyridine, which is genetically determined.[70] Intolerance side effects (i.e., nausea, vomiting, malaise, anorexia, dyspepsia, and headaches) are dose related. In contrast, hypersensitivity reactions (i.e., rash, fever, hemolytic anemia, agranulocytosis, hepatitis, hypersensitivity pneumonitis, pancreatitis, and worsening of colitis) are independent of dose. Reversible sperm abnormalities and folate malabsorption are unique complications related to sulfasalazine.

Mesalamine has relatively few side effects, and dose-related toxicities are unusual in patients taking up to 4.8 g/day of delayed-release formulations.[70,71] Rare idiosyncratic reactions, including pancreatitis, interstitial nephritis, and worsening of colitis, have been reported. Eighty percent of patients who are unable to tolerate sulfasalazine can tolerate a nonsulfa aminosalicylate containing mesalamine. One unique complication of olsalazine is dose-related diarrhea.

Sulfasalazine and the oral aminosalicylates are equally effective for treatment of mild to moderate UC.[26,27,72] Oral aminosalicylates are effective for both proximal and distal colitis. Mesalamine suppositories and enemas effectively treat distal colitis, provided the formulation reaches the proximal extent of disease.[73] A dose-response relationship for the oral aminosalicylates is well defined for up to 4.8 g/day of mesalamine, with higher doses being more effective for moderately active disease.

Prevention of relapse and the prolongation of remission have been primary indications for all of the aminosalicylates in UC.[26,27,74] All the nonsulfa formulations provide comparable efficacy to sulfasalazine for maintenance therapy.[74] In ulcerative proctitis and distal colitis, topical mesalamine is also effective at preventing relapse and is more effective than oral treatment when continued on a long-term basis.[73]

The efficacy of aminosalicylates in CD is less definitive than that in UC and is more dependent on location of disease activity.[27,66] In CD involving the colon, the efficacy of sulfasalazine is determined by the presence of the colonic bacteria needed to cleave the azo bond and liberate 5-ASA. Aminosalicylates are commonly used as maintenance therapy for patients with quiescent CD, despite differing interpretations of the clinical trials of this indication.[27,65] The specific release characteristics [*see Table 3*] should correspond to the disease location.

Corticosteroids

Corticosteroids are the primary therapy for moderate to severe and fulminant UC and moderate to severe active CD.[27,75] They are ineffective at maintaining remissions of UC and CD, however.[76] The mechanisms of action of corticosteroids in IBD are multifactorial and are similar to their mechanisms of action in other inflammatory diseases.[77] Like aminosalicylates, corticosteroids can be targeted to specific sites within the digestive tract. Newer glucocorticoids (e.g., budesonide) both enhance potency and minimize systemic exposure.[78]

Ulcerative colitis Oral corticosteroids are the primary treatment for outpatients with moderately severe UC.[26,27,79] Prednisone, 20 to 60 mg daily, is administered once or in divided doses. In general, 40 mg is the optimal dose; the modest benefits of higher doses are offset by increasing side effects.[80]

Table 3   Aminosalicylate Preparations for Management of Ulcerative Colitis and Crohn Disease

Preparation	Formulation	Delivery	Dosing
Oral Agents			
Azo bond			
Sulfasalazine (Azulfidine, 500 mg)	Sulfapyridine carrier	Colon	3–6 g/day (acute)
			2–4 g/day (maintenance)
Olsalazine (Dipentum, 250 mg)	5-Aminosalicylic acid dimer	Colon	1–3 g/day
Balsalazide (Colazal, 750 mg)	Aminobenzoyl-alanine carrier	Colon	6.75 g/day
Delayed Release			
Mesalamine (Asacol, 400 mg, 800 mg)	Eudragit S (pH, 7)	Distal ileum–colon	2.4–4.8 g/day (acute)
			0.8–4.8 g/day (maintenance)
(Claversal,* Mesasal,* Salofalk,*	Eudragit L (pH, 6)	Ileum-colon	1.5–3.0 g/day (acute)
250 mg, 500 mg)			0.75–3.0 g/day (maintenance)
Sustained Release			
Mesalamine	Ethylcellulose granules	Stomach-colon	2–4 g/day (acute)
(Pentasa, 250 mg, 500 mg, 1,000 mg*)			1.5–4.0 g/day (maintenance)
Rectal Agents			
Mesalamine suppository	—	Rectum	1.0–1.5 g/day (acute)
(Canasa, 400 mg,* 500 mg, 1,000 mg*)			500–1,000 mg/day (maintenance)
Mesalamine enema	60 ml, 100 ml suspension	Rectum–splenic flexure	1–4 g/day (acute)
(Rowasa, 1 g,* 4 g)			1 g q.d.–1 g t.i.w. (maintenance)

*Not available in the United States.

Rectal (i.e., topical) administration of systemically absorbed glucocorticoids (e.g., hydrocortisone) and of rapidly metabolized glucocorticoids (e.g., budesonide) is effective therapy for active distal colitis and has been incorporated into the treatment of severe colitis as an adjunct to parenteral steroids.[81]

Parenteral corticosteroids are the mainstay of therapy for hospitalized patients with severe or fulminant UC. Although controlled trial data are limited, there is consensus supporting the use of intravenous hydrocortisone, methylprednisolone, or prednisolone in dosages equivalent to 40 to 60 mg/day of prednisone; these agents may be given either in a continuous infusion or in divided doses.[26,27,79,80] There is no evidence supporting dosages higher than 60 mg of prednisone. Corticosteroids are not effective in preventing relapse of quiescent UC.[26,27,79,80]

Crohn disease   Corticosteroids are the primary therapy for moderate to severe CD.[27,82] Both uncontrolled and controlled trials demonstrate a response rate of approximately 75%. Parenteral steroids have not been formally assessed in the setting of severe CD, but there is a consensus that they are as effective in severe CD as in severe UC. As a first-line therapy for mild to moderate CD, enteric-coated, delayed-release formulations of budesonide can deliver topically active steroids to targeted sites (ileum and proximal colon).[78,83] However, as with corticosteroids in UC, neither conventional nor topically active steroids have proved effective for preventing relapse in CD.[76,82]

IMMUNOMODULATORY AGENTS

Immunomodulating therapies have had an expanding role in the treatment of IBD. These agents can be used either to induce or to maintain remission in UC and CD.

Azathioprine and 6-Mercaptopurine

Although azathioprine (AZA) and 6-mercaptopurine (6-MP) have been used to treat IBD for over 30 years, their mechanisms of action and optimal use remain incompletely known. AZA is rapidly absorbed and converted to 6-MP, which is metabolized to thioinosinic acid, an inhibitor of purine ribonucleotide synthesis and cell proliferation.[84] Although AZA is considered a purine antimetabolite, its exact mechanism of action has not been defined. Presumably, AZA inhibits some function of long-lived lymphocytes, which accounts for the 3- to 6-month delay in onset of action. There is increasing evidence that these agents promote apoptosis of T cells.[85] In addition, a genetic polymorphism has been recognized in the enzyme thiopurine methyltransferase, which metabolizes the purine analogues into 6-thioguanine.[84,86] One in 300 persons lacks this enzyme, and an additional 11% of the population has depressed levels of it. Homozygotes are susceptible to increased accumulation of 6-thioguanine nucleotides and bone marrow suppression.

AZA and 6-MP usually are well tolerated.[80] Pancreatitis occurs in 3% to 15% of patients, usually within the first few weeks of therapy, and resolves completely upon withdrawal of the drug. Other potential side effects include nausea, fever, rash, and hepatitis. Bone marrow suppression, particularly leukopenia, is dose related and may be delayed, necessitating long-term monitoring of blood counts. IBD patients treated with purine analogues may experience a slight increase in relative risk of neoplasia, but the absolute risk remains extremely small.[80,87] There is a growing consensus that these agents are effective and safe for use through pregnancy and lactation.[88]

Ulcerative colitis   Both controlled trials with AZA and uncontrolled series with 6-MP have supported the role of purine analogues for the long-term (maintenance) treatment of UC.[26,27,79] There have not been adequate comparative studies between AZA and 6-MP or dose-ranging trials for these agents, and to date, there are no standard guidelines for their use in UC.[26] Most authorities agree that if patients are to be started on full-dose therapy (i.e., 2.5 mg/kg/day of AZA or 1.5 mg/kg/day of 6-MP), activity of the enzyme thiopurine methyltransferase should be measured before therapy is initiated.[80,89] However, many clinicians start therapy at lower doses and monitor the white blood cell count. Alternatively, in the event of therapeutic unresponsiveness, elevated liver enzymes, or potential noncompliance, these clinicians measure levels of the thiopurine metabolites 6-methylmercaptopurine and 6-thioguanine.

Crohn disease AZA and 6-MP can induce remission in active CD, but prolonged therapy is necessary: 56% of patients with active CD respond after 4 months of treatment with either AZA (2.0 to 2.5 mg/kg/day) or 6-MP (1.0 to 1.5 mg/kg/day).[82,90] Because of their delayed onset of action, AZA and 6-MP are most often used to maintain remission or as steroid-sparing agents.[91] They can also be used to treat CD fistulas and perianal disease.[51]

Cyclosporine

Cyclosporine is a potent inhibitor of T cells, primarily via inhibition of IL-2 production by helper T cells, and inhibits recruitment of cytotoxic T cells and production of IL-3, IL-4, interferon gamma, and TNF-α. Treatment with cyclosporine can provide dramatic results in severe IBD, particularly in UC.[79,92] Cyclosporine has a much more rapid onset of action than AZA or 6-MP; its effects are usually evident within the first week. There is controversy regarding the long-term benefits of cyclosporine, however. Cyclosporine is metabolized by a cytochrome P-450 enzyme, and interactions with a number of drugs can increase or decrease cyclosporine levels.[80]

UC trials have used intravenous cyclosporine as a continuous infusion of 2 to 4 mg/kg/day.[93] However, a dosage of 2 mg/kg/day appears to be as effective as higher doses and may reduce toxicity.[94] Correlations between response and blood levels have not been defined; similarly, the correlation between blood levels and toxicity is poor.[80]

The narrow therapeutic margin and significant potential toxicity of cyclosporine remain obstacles for its use outside of centers with transplantation expertise. Major toxicities include nephrotoxicity and opportunistic infections. Nephrotoxicity can manifest as hypertension or elevations in blood urea nitrogen and creatinine levels. Because of the increased risk of opportunistic infections, including *Pneumocystis* pneumonia, prophylaxis with trimethoprim-sulfamethoxazole has been recommended for patients receiving cyclosporine in conjunction with high-dose steroids.

The primary use of cyclosporine for IBD is in hospitalized patients with severe UC in whom therapy with oral or intravenous steroids has failed[26,27]; 50% to 80% of such patients respond to short-term treatment with intravenous cyclosporine.[79] Duration of use is limited to 3 to 6 months. The long-term prognosis after cyclosporine therapy is controversial, but approximately 40% to 50% of responders to cyclosporine may avoid eventual surgical colectomy.[93] This response improves to greater than 60% when patients are transitioned to long-term therapy with AZA or 6-MP.[95]

Cyclosporine also has been successfully used for steroid-refractory and fistulizing CD.[96] Beneficial results are primarily achieved with intravenous cyclosporine. Oral cyclosporine has not been found to be effective for maintaining remission in CD, possibly because of poor and variable absorption.

Methotrexate

Only limited evidence supports the use of methotrexate in UC. Despite early optimism from uncontrolled clinical experience, methotrexate has not been effective therapy for UC in a small number of clinical trials.[97]

In studies of steroid-dependent CD patients, approximately 40% of patients were able to achieve clinical remission while tapering steroids during a 16-week trial of methotrexate, given parenterally (intramuscularly or subcutaneously) in a weekly dose of 25 mg.[82,98] In a subsequent study, approximately two thirds of patients who achieved remission and remained on parenteral methotrexate, at a dosage of 15 mg/wk, continued in remission for 40 weeks.[99]

Methotrexate is well tolerated in IBD patients. Toxicity, which includes bone marrow suppression and hepatic fibrosis, is uncommon provided that blood counts and liver enzyme levels are monitored.[97] Hypersensitivity pneumonitis is a rare but potentially irreversible complication. Methotrexate is a known teratogen and abortifacient, precluding its use in women anticipating pregnancy.

Other Immunomodulatory Agents

Tacrolimus has been used as therapy for refractory fistulas in CD[100] and as an oral therapy for refractory UC.[101] The indications for tacrolimus are very limited, however, now that infliximab has become available for CD [*see* Biologic Therapies, *below*].

ANTIBIOTICS

Antibiotic therapy has been used selectively in both UC and CD.[102] Although a specific therapeutic role for antibiotics in UC remains unproved, most centers continue to advocate broad-spectrum antibiotics as a component of the intensive intravenous therapy used in patients with fulminant colitis and toxic megacolon.[26,27] Antibiotics are also effective in the treatment of pouchitis after ileoanal anastomoses in patients with UC.[103]

In CD, the role for antibiotic therapy as a first-line agent for mild to moderate disease continues to be debated.[104-106] In mild to moderate CD, metronidazole has proved to be comparable to sulfasalazine and superior to placebo at doses of 20 mg/kg/day.[107] Metronidazole is also effective for the treatment of perianal CD[51] and can reduce the likelihood of relapse after intestinal resection.[108] Ciprofloxacin is comparable to mesalamine for mild to moderate CD and has been used successfully in combination with metronidazole for ileal disease and perianal CD.[109-111] Combinations of antimycobacterial therapies for CD have not had consistent results in the treatment of active CD or as maintenance therapies.[112]

BIOLOGIC THERAPIES

The introduction of biologic agents has opened a new era in the treatment of IBD. Current biologic agents target cellular messengers, including cytokines, chemokines, and adhesion molecules.

The first biologic agent approved by the Food and Drug Administration for CD was infliximab, a chimeric monoclonal antibody of the IgG1 subclass that targets TNF-α. In clinical trials, infliximab has been shown to induce and maintain clinical remissions in patients with moderate to severe active luminal or fistulizing CD refractory to therapy with aminosalicylates, corticosteroids, and immunomodulators.[113-115] Infliximab is administered intravenously in a dose of 5 mg/kg. After the initial dose, repeat doses are given 2 weeks and 6 weeks later and, then, every 8 weeks on average. Infliximab is similarly effective in UC. Two large trials that enrolled patients with moderately active UC that was refractory to aminosalicylates, corticosteroids, and immunomodulators also demonstrated positive results.[116]

Infliximab is generally well tolerated. The primary risk with infliximab therapy is infection with intracellular organisms (e.g., tuberculosis, histoplasmosis, or cryptococcosis) in exposed or endemic populations.[117] Pretreatment skin testing with purified protein derivative and chest x-rays is recommended, but false negative results are possible because many patients with CD are anergic.[118] For that reason, clinicians must exercise clinical judgment regarding potential tuberculosis exposure. Infliximab is contraindicated in patients with active infections.

Unique adverse events with infliximab include the development of antibodies to the drug that reduce the effectiveness of the agent and are associated with infusion reactions (e.g., acute infusion reactions and serum sickness–like reactions).[119] Additionally, antinuclear antibodies and anti-DNA antibodies develop in approximately 10% of patients with CD who are receiving infliximab therapy. Drug-induced lupus reactions have been reported but are uncommon. Delayed hypersensitivity (i.e., serum sickness–like reactions) has been observed in patients retreated after a long hiatus between doses (3 months to 4 years) but not in patients who have received continuous retreatment at 8-week intervals. A small increase in the risk of lymphomas has been observed with anti-TNF therapy in IBD,[120] but it is not clear whether the increase reflects a small underlying risk in patients with CD or is the result of immune suppression.[121] Other biologic therapies under development to treat IBD include inhibitors of so-called selective adhesion molecules[122]; anti–IL-12, anti–IL-2, and anti-CD3 monoclonal antibodies[123,124]; epidermal growth factor[125]; and granulocyte-macrophage colony-stimulating factor.[126]

MISCELLANEOUS THERAPIES

The recognition that cigarette smoking can protect against the development of UC has led to trials utilizing nicotine as adjunctive therapy. Although trials have demonstrated a role for nicotine in the symptomatic management of UC, nicotine therapy has not been shown to be effective at inducing remissions.[127] Currently, nicotine is not a proven therapy for UC, but it may be a useful adjunctive measure in patients with UC that develops after smoking cessation.

Omega-3 fatty acids inhibit synthesis of leukotriene B_4 and, at high doses, have shown a modest benefit in the treatment of active UC or as maintenance therapy.[128,129] An enteric-coated fish oil preparation has proved to be effective in reducing relapse rates in CD[130] and may eventually offer an alternative therapeutic option in IBD. However, current treatment guidelines do not include these agents.

Other novel therapeutic approaches to IBD that are currently under investigation include phosphodiesterase inhibitors,[131] small molecules targeting mitogen-activated protein kinases,[132] probiotics,[133] apheresis,[134] and targeting of costimulatory molecules.[135]

NUTRITIONAL THERAPIES

Hypotheses regarding dietary intraluminal antigens as important stimuli of the mucosal immune response have led to the investigation of nutritional therapies for IBD.[3,136] Dietary manipulations have not been effective in treating UC, but patients with active CD have responded to several nutritional approaches.[136,137] Bowel rest and total parenteral nutrition (TPN) are as effective as corticosteroids at inducing short-term remissions in active CD. In contrast, enteral nutrition in the form of elemental or liquid polymeric preparations has been shown to be less effective than corticosteroids.[138] It has been suggested that elemental diets may provide the small intestine with nutrients vital to cell growth (e.g., glutamine) while avoiding complications related to TPN. However, despite their efficacy in active CD, neither enteral nor parenteral nutrition is effective at maintaining remissions.[136]

Patients with IBD are susceptible to nutritional deficits as a consequence of blood loss, protein-losing enteropathy, small bowel bacterial overgrowth, surgical resections (in CD), or inanition. IBD does not increase the risk of lactose intolerance, but ingestion of lactose can contribute to diarrhea in IBD patients with an inflamed small bowel or impaired colonic absorptive capacity. Similarly, consumption of nonabsorbable carbohydrates (e.g., sorbitol) or fats (e.g., olestra) can lead to excess flatus, bloating, or diarrhea. Occasionally, patients with proctitis present with constipation that improves with additional dietary fiber.

SUPPORTIVE THERAPIES

Many symptoms of IBD are not related to active inflammation and can therefore be treated separately from the inflammation. The management of these symptoms, which include pain and diarrhea, is as important to the patient's well-being as the treatment of mucosal inflammation. Treatment should be individualized according to symptoms and clinical disease state.

IBS is as common in IBD patients as it is in the general population.[139] A dietary history is important to identify potentially aggravating components contributing to digestive symptoms. Although the stress of day-to-day living does not impact on the inflammatory activity of IBD, many patients identify stressful aspects in life as being associated with worsening of symptoms. IBS often responds to antispasmodics, antidiarrheals, fiber supplementation, or low doses of tricyclic antidepressants [see Chapter 67]. Antispasmodics, primarily anticholinergic agents (e.g., dicyclomine, clidinium bromide, hyoscyamine, propantheline, or belladonna alkaloids), can treat cramping abdominal discomfort or symptoms of IBS that accompany UC and CD. Similarly, antidiarrheal preparations (e.g., diphenoxylate, loperamide, or codeine) can be utilized in patients with mild or moderate IBD to reduce the frequency of bowel movements and rectal urgency. Antimotility agents should be avoided in patients with severe or fulminant IBD because of the risk of inducing toxic megacolon.

In women with IBD, flares of disease activity are often related to the menstrual cycle, occurring more often during the premenstrual and menstrual phases.[140] If menstrual cycles impact greatly on symptoms, ablation of the menstrual cycle with progesterone or leuprolide may be warranted. Pregnancy is associated with both exacerbations and remissions of IBD.[141]

There is no predisposing psychiatric personality profile in IBD, and there is no routine role for sedative, anxiolytic, antidepressant, or antipsychotic therapy. Psychopharmacologic therapies are reserved for individual patients as needed, usually after consultation with a psychiatrist.

Treatment of IBD patients with narcotic analgesia is rarely indicated. Pain in UC is related either to visceral hyperalgesia and muscle spasm or to transmural inflammation. The former condition is treated with antispasmodics and the latter with specific anti-inflammatory therapy. In CD, abdominal pain may be related to transmural inflammation or stenosis, but given the chronic nature of the disease, addictive analgesics should be avoided because of the risk of tolerance. Attempts should be made to reduce the inflammatory component of symptoms and to treat irritability with antispasmodics or nonaddictive analgesics.

NSAIDs (both nonspecific agents and cyclooxygenase-2 inhibitors) may exacerbate disease activity in IBD and can contribute to refractory disease.[139,142-144] Minor pain, fever, menstrual symptoms, or arthralgias should be treated with alternatives to NSAIDs. If these agents are used, it should be with great caution and continued observation for their potential to exacerbate IBD.

Approximately half of patients with IBD use complementary therapies.[145] Consequently, the history should include a careful review of nonprescription vitamins, health foods, homeopathic agents, or herbs, which may identify factors contributing to changes in bowel habits.

Patients with CD who have undergone bowel resection often have increased diarrhea, related to the length of bowel removed. Bile salt malabsorption may complicate resections of less than 100 cm; the diarrhea in these patients often responds to cholestyramine or alternative bile-salt sequestrants. Longer resections result in steatorrhea, which is managed with a low-fat diet.

MEDICAL TREATMENT OF ULCERATIVE COLITIS

Ulcerative Proctitis

Induction therapies Topical aminosalicylates are the most effective treatments for distal UC.[73] A daily dose of 1,000 to 4,000 mg is administered nightly as an enema or in divided doses as a suppository or foam. Topical corticosteroids (given via suppository, enema, or foam) are acceptable alternatives to mesalamine.[26,27] Foam preparations are easier to retain and are better tolerated, allowing maintenance of daily activities despite twice-daily administration.

Oral aminosalicylates can be used to treat mild to moderate symptoms of proctitis but are less effective than topical therapies.[146] Sulfasalazine, 2 to 6 g/day in divided doses, is the most cost-effective aminosalicylate, but sulfa intolerance, toxic reactions, or allergy can compromise therapy. Mesalamine, olsalazine, or balsalazide formulations are preferable for patients with a history of sulfa allergy or for patients who develop sulfa-related side effects.

Inductive therapy is continued until the patient is asymptomatic. Although improvement should begin within a week, a complete response may require 4 to 12 weeks. Clinicians should recognize that patients with treated UC are capable of, as well as expected to, achieve a clinical remission, which is defined by the resolution of all inflammatory symptoms and a regeneration of the colonic mucosa.

Maintenance therapies Maintenance therapy is indicated for the majority of patients with UC. In patients with proctitis, however, the limited nature of the disease permits treatment of any recurrent attacks on an as-needed basis.

Once remission has been achieved, the daily dose of mesalamine can be tapered according to the initial response; nevertheless, continuation of the inductive therapy, excluding steroids, is most effective for maintenance treatment. Mesalamine suppositories (or enemas) administered nightly, with gradual tapering to every other night and then every third night, will maintain remission in most patients. An oral aminosalicylate is added if patients continue to experience flares despite attempts to wean them from topical therapy; it may also be added after induction and then tapering of topical steroids.[133]

Left-Sided Colitis

Induction therapies Mesalamine enemas are the most effective therapy for left-sided colitis, with steroid enemas being an alternative.[73] Oral aminosalicylates also are effective, with improvement generally noted by 2 to 4 weeks.[147] The oral amnosalicylates are generally equivalent in their efficacy for distal colitis.[67,148]

Patients with moderate to severe disease and those in whom therapy with topical and oral aminosalicylates has failed are treated as outpatients with oral steroids to induce remission, in a manner similar to that for patients with extensive colitis (see below). As with extensive colitis (see below), severe left-sided colitis requires hospitalization and treatment with systemic steroids.

Maintenance therapies Inductive therapy is continued until the patient achieves clinical remission (normal bowel movements without bleeding, urgency, tenesmus, or inability to evacuate flatus). The transition to a maintenance regimen is then begun. Neither oral steroids nor topical steroids are effective at maintaining remissions. Patients who have responded to rectal mesalamine can continue with this therapy or switch to oral treatment.[26,148] The combination of oral and topical mesalamine has advantages over either therapy alone for maintenance therapy for left-sided UC.[149]

If patients who are taking an oral aminosalicylate experience relapse, the dose should be increased to up to 4.8 g of mesalamine. Maintenance of remission in such patients may require topical mesalamine. After inductive treatment with steroid enemas, patients should be transitioned to an oral aminosalicylate, with gradual tapering of the topical therapy. Those requiring systemic steroids should be maintained on an oral aminosalicylate, with or without topical mesalamine.

Extensive Colitis

Induction therapies Oral aminosalicylates are the primary therapy for outpatients with mild to moderate extensive colitis, but these agents may be supplemented with topical mesalamine or steroids.[26,27,108] The dose of the oral aminosalicylate is more important than the specific formulation.[67,72] Response rates of up to 80% can be anticipated with 4 to 6 g of sulfasalazine or 2 to 4.8 g of a mesalamine formulation given over 6 to 8 weeks. Therapy is continued as long as the patient is improving, to the point of clinical remission (i.e., normal bowel movements without blood or urgency). In the absence of a complete response, the dose of the aminosalicylate should be increased to a maximum of 4.8 g of mesalamine. An antispasmodic or antidiarrheal preparation may be added to treat abdominal cramping or mild diarrhea.

In patients who fail to improve or whose condition worsens, steroid therapy should be added in the form of prednisone, 40 to 60 mg/day.[75] Once the patient has achieved a clinical remission, which generally takes 2 to 4 weeks, steroids are tapered according to the time course to improvement. Prednisone can be tapered by approximately 5 mg every week down to 20 mg daily. Below 20 mg of prednisone, the daily dosage is reduced 2.5 to 5 mg every 1 to 2 weeks. Aminosalicylate therapy is continued as steroids are reduced.

Patients who respond to steroids but who are unable to completely taper without relapse despite optimal doses of an aminosalicylate should be started on AZA or 6-MP, which typically permits steroid withdrawal.[26,27] Achieving the therapeutic benefits of these agents requires 3 to 6 months, during which time steroids are maintained at the lowest dose needed to prevent recurrence of symptoms. Calcium and vitamin D supplementation is indicated during steroid therapy to prevent metabolic bone disease. Reduced bone density is an indication for additional therapy with a bisphosphonate, estrogen replacement in postmenopausal women, or calcitonin.[150]

Hospitalization is indicated for patients who have significant weight loss, fever, disabling extraintestinal manifestations, frequent nocturnal bowel movements, severe anemia, or progressive symptoms despite outpatient therapy with corticosteroids.[26,27] A low-residue diet is prescribed, to minimize abdominal cramps and bowel movements; the diet should contain sufficient protein and calories to counter the catabolic influence of active inflammation and steroids. Antispasmodics or antidiarrheals should be used with caution, and patients should be monitored for worsening symptoms.

Intravenous steroids are indicated for severely ill patients with fever, orthostasis, evidence of dehydration, more than 10 to 12 stools daily, rectal bleeding necessitating transfusion, protein depletion, or abdominal tenderness or distention. Prompt correction of fluid and electrolyte imbalances is critical. In patients with active bleeding, transfusions of packed red blood cells should be given to maintain the hematocrit above 30%. Anticholinergics, antidiarrheals, and narcotic analgesics are contraindicated because they can worsen colonic dilatation and mask peritoneal signs in debilitated, steroid-treated patients.

The intensive intravenous steroid regimen consists of prednisolone (40 to 60 mg/day), methylprednisolone (32 to 48 mg/day), or hydrocortisone (300 to 400 mg/day) administered in divided doses or as a continuous infusion. Steroid enemas (e.g., with 100 mg of hydrocortisone) can be used as adjunctive treatment to reduce rectal urgency or tenesmus. Oral aminosalicylates are discontinued because their anti-inflammatory effects are minor compared with those of high-dose steroids, as well as because of the potential for intolerance and the rare instances in which 5-ASA can worsen colitis.

When vital signs normalize, the hematocrit stabilizes, and the patient is able to tolerate a full (low-residue) diet with formed bowel movements without blood or urgency, treatment can be transitioned to an oral regimen. Full-dose therapy with an aminosalicylate is resumed and intravenous steroids are replaced with oral steroids.

If the patient is not improving after 5 to 7 days of intensive intravenous steroid therapy, the likelihood of improvement is small and the patient should be considered a candidate for cyclosporine therapy or surgery. Intravenous cyclosporine has been an important advance in the therapy of severe UC, but its use should be limited to clinicians experienced in the monitoring of immune suppression. A response is anticipated within 4 to 5 days, but if there is no significant improvement within 1 week, the patient should be referred for surgery. When clinical remission is achieved with intravenous cyclosporine, the regimen is replaced with both oral cyclosporine and prednisone. The daily dose of cyclosporine is doubled and administered in two divided doses (e.g., if the patient was receiving 200 mg daily, the oral dosing is 200 mg twice daily). Because of the high relapse rate after intravenous cyclosporine therapy, AZA or 6-MP is usually added to the oral regimen.[26,151] In addition, trimethoprim-sulfamethoxazole is given three times weekly as prophylaxis against *Pneumocystis* pneumonia.[26]

Outpatient monitoring of cyclosporine levels and other laboratory measures are repeated weekly for the first month and then less often. Steroids are tapered (see above), generally over 8 to 12 weeks; cyclosporine is gradually discontinued; and maintenance therapy is begun.

Maintenance therapy Maintenance therapy for extensive UC is determined by the intensity of therapy needed to induce remission. If aminosalicylate therapy has been sufficient to induce remission, continuation of the same dosage is optimal for maintenance. Patients treated with steroids require a more individualized approach, with the rate of steroid tapering determined by the rapidity of response as maximum doses of aminosalicylate are continued. Patients receiving AZA or 6-MP also are continued on maximum aminosalicylate therapy. The optimum doses of immunomodulators, as well as the doses that will cause leukopenia, have not been clarified.[26,89] Complete blood counts should be obtained on at least a quarterly basis to detect delayed bone marrow suppression.[152]

Fulminant Colitis and Toxic Megacolon

Fulminant colitis, with or without colonic dilatation (toxic megacolon), is a medical emergency that is best managed by an experienced team of gastroenterology specialists and surgeons. Management is similar to that for severe colitis but with several modifications. Patients take nothing by mouth until they show clinical improvement. In the presence of small bowel ileus, a nasogastric tube should be inserted and maneuvers undertaken to reduce colonic distention and to allow passage of colonic gas by rectum (i.e., by rolling the patient from side to side, inserting a rectal tube, or placing the patient in the knee-elbow position).[26] Intravenous steroids are continued and broad-spectrum antibiotic coverage is added for presumed transmural extension of disease, risk of microperforation, and systemic bacteremia. Cyclosporine in this setting is controversial but has been used in selected cases.

Aggressive medical management is successful in 40% to 50% of patients with fulminant colitis or toxic megacolon. Unfortunately, many patients are destined to develop complications or resistant disease, including recurrent toxic megacolon.[25] Persisting peritoneal signs, any deterioration, or failure to improve within 24 to 72 hours is an indication for immediate colectomy.

SURGICAL TREATMENT OF ULCERATIVE COLITIS

UC is cured by proctocolectomy, and the quality of life after such surgery is generally excellent. The advantages of surgery include the elimination of the drawbacks of medical treatment, which include continued morbidity, adverse reactions to therapy, and the risk of neoplasia.[26]

Indications for Surgery

Indications for colectomy in UC are emergent, urgent, or elective. Emergent indications include exsanguinating hemorrhage, perforation, and unresponsive fulminant colitis or toxic megacolon. Urgent indications are chronic refractory colitis and significant complications of the disease or medical therapy (e.g., hemolytic anemia, pyoderma gangrenosum, and steroid-induced psychosis).

Surgical indications are often less acute and allow preparation and education of the patient and family to optimize timing and minimize physical and emotional consequences. Patients with quiescent colitis but with dysplasia diagnosed during colonoscopic surveillance are often feeling well and must adjust to the need for a major operation.

The most common indications for surgery are medically intractable disease, poor quality of life, or chronic complications from colitis or medical therapy. Given the availability of a surgical cure, it is not acceptable for patients to suffer physical debility, psychosocial dysfunction, or intolerable side effects.

Surgical Procedures

Proctocolectomy   Removal of the colon with an end ileostomy cures UC. This is the standard procedure with which all other treatments must be compared. Proctocolectomy and ileostomy are usually performed in a single procedure, even in the most urgent of settings. This approach has the least likelihood of complications. The primary drawback is the need for a permanent stoma. Quality of life after proctocolectomy is usually good, although many patients have difficulty adjusting to the cosmetic and functional aspects of the ileostomy. An unanticipated complication of proctocolectomy has been reduced fecundity in women.[153]

Sphincter-saving procedures   Because UC is essentially limited to the colonic mucosa, alternative procedures have been developed that involve removing the proximal colon, stripping the rectal mucosa off the distal rectal musculature, and sparing the anal sphincter.[154] These so-called sphincter-saving procedures afford the opportunity of curing colitis and reestablishing continuity between the ileum and anus via an ileoanal anastomosis. Although a direct communication is technically feasible, it would result in intolerable postoperative diarrhea. Thus, these procedures include the provision of an ileal pouch to provide reservoir function. These J-, S-, or W-shaped pouches are created by folding the distal ileum and anastomosing the outlet to the anal canal.

Additional surgical modifications include the actual surgical stripping of the distal rectal mucosa or the stapling of the distal ileum to a short strip of residual rectal mucosa. In experienced surgical centers, the outcomes of stripping and stapling procedures are comparable.

Most often, sphincter-saving procedures are performed in stages: first, the surgeon removes the colon and performs an ileostomy, leaving the distal rectum as a Hartmann pouch; then, the surgeon creates the ileoanal anastomosis with a diverting ileostomy; and finally, the surgeon closes the ileostomy, which allows continuity of enteric flow through the pouch. Depending on surgeon preference and patient status, these procedures can be performed in one, two, or three stages.

Quality of life after an ileoanal anastomosis is excellent. Most patients describe full continence, with an average of six unformed (but not urgent) bowel movements daily.[155] Approximately 10% of patients develop small bowel obstructions, either between stages or after completion of the procedure. The most common complication after colectomy and ileoanal anastomosis is the development of so-called pouchitis, a superficial inflammation within the pouch that is similar to the inflammation of UC.[156] Pouchitis presents as increased urgency and evacuations that may be associated with bleeding and extraintestinal manifestations such as arthralgias, fever, and malaise. Most episodes of pouchitis respond to a course of an antibiotic, such as metronidazole or ciprofloxacin.[103] Approximately 15% of patients who develop pouchitis will have a more chronic course requiring long-term antibiotics or oral budesonide.[156] There is also evidence that high doses of the probiotic agent VSL#3 can prevent the onset of pouchitis or maintain remission of pouchitis after antibiotic therapy for recurrent or refractory pouchi-

tis.[157-159] As with proctocolectomy, ileoanal anastomoses have been associated with reduced fecundity in women.[153]

TREATMENT OF CROHN DISEASE

Gastroduodenal Crohn Disease

Dyspepsia, epigastric burning, or nausea in CD patients with gastroduodenal involvement usually responds to acid reduction therapy with an H_2 receptor antagonist or a proton pump inhibitor.[160,161] More profound nausea or vomiting responds to corticosteroids, followed by an immunomodulator for steroid-sparing effects. Gastric outlet obstruction that does not respond to steroids or immunomodulators, or both, is an indication for surgical decompression with a gastrojejunostomy.

Jejunoileitis

In patients with isolated proximal small bowel CD, diarrhea should be evaluated from a mechanistic standpoint. Malabsorption from short bowel syndrome or resection is treated with a low-fat diet, whereas small bowel bacterial overgrowth is managed with antibiotics. Patients presenting with prominent pain or small bowel obstruction are treated with short-term corticosteroids and then usually with AZA or 6-MP. Bowel obstructions that do not respond to short-term steroid therapy require surgical resection or, more commonly, stricturoplasty.

Ileitis, Ileocolitis, and Colitis

In patients with limited ileal or ileocolonic CD, therapy should be staged to alleviate presenting symptoms, then to maintain long-term well-being, while minimizing chronic complications related to the disease or therapy.

Mild to moderate disease   Outpatient therapy with anti-inflammatory agents, symptom-specific medications, and diet is utilized in patients who have abdominal pain and tenderness, diarrhea, low-grade fevers, weight loss without obstruction, painful mass, or severe malnutrition. Aminosalicylates, including sulfasalazine and mesalamine, have been effective at relatively higher doses than those that are used in UC. Sulfasalazine is effective in dosages of 3 to 6 g/day for ileocolonic and colonic CD but has not had significant benefits in limited small bowel disease.[27] In contrast, mesalamine, 4 g/day, provides modest benefits for small bowel and colonic involvement if the formulation releases the mesalamine at involved segments.[162] Benefits of sulfasalazine and mesalamine are modestly better than those achieved with placebo and less than those achieved with corticosteroids.[163] Enteric-coated, delayed-release budesonide, 9 mg daily, is an alternative first-line therapy for mild to moderate CD affecting the ileum, right colon, or both; it is more effective than mesalamine therapy.[163] Despite the limited potency of aminosalicylates, however, their potential long-term efficacy and absence of side effects make them first-line agents. As long as the patient continues to respond, the medication should be continued at the same dose used for induction. For patients with ileal or right colon disease who fail to respond within a short time (i.e., 2 to 4 weeks), budesonide therapy is a logical alternative.

Antibiotic therapy with metronidazole or ciprofloxacin, alone or in combination, is an alternative to aminosalicylates for ileocolonic and colonic CD.[27,102] Although there are no long-term data regarding antibiotic therapy for ileal or ileocolonic CD, clinical observations have suggested that maintenance therapy is likely to be necessary. Patients receiving long-term metronidazole therapy should be monitored for peripheral neuropathy.

Dietary and nutritional therapy should focus on reduction of symptoms, prevention or correction of nutritional deficits, and avoidance of long-term complications. Elemental diets have short-term efficacy but are not practical for the majority of adult patients.[27,138] The disease location, complications, and surgical history will direct attention to potential nutritional deficiencies. Calorie and protein requisites are the primary concern. Secondary considerations include maintenance of iron stores and levels of water-soluble vitamins in the setting of proximal small bowel disease, as well as levels of vitamins B_{12}, A, D, and E with ileal disease or resection. Adequate calcium and vitamin D intake are of particular importance to avoid metabolic bone disease.

Moderate to severe disease A different therapeutic approach is required in patients who fail to respond to aminosalicylates or steroids or who present with fever, greater than 10% weight loss, and abdominal pain accompanied by tenderness (without obstruction) but who are able to maintain oral intake. Corticosteroids are required to induce a clinical remission; however, clinicians must exclude perforating complications (i.e., abscesses) before starting corticosteroids. Oral treatment with prednisone, 0.5 to 1 mg/kg, reduces symptoms in most patients.[27,75] However, the clinical response usually does not persist after steroid tapering; approximately 70% of patients will have a relapse or become steroid dependent within 1 year.[164]

Prednisone is continued at the initial dose until the patient responds completely (i.e., resolution of inflammatory symptoms). The dose is then decreased according to the time course to response. Tapering can usually proceed by 5 to 10 mg/wk, until a daily dose of 20 mg is reached, and then by 2.5 to 5 mg/wk. Calcium and vitamin D supplements reduce the risk of accelerated osteoporosis; in patients with reduced bone density, bisphosphonate or calcitonin should also be considered.[150] Clinical monitoring is continued, with attention paid to relapse of inflammatory symptoms. Persisting noninflammatory symptoms (e.g., nonbloody diarrhea or abdominal cramps) can be treated with dietary modifications, antispasmodics, and antidiarrheals without intensifying anti-inflammatory therapy.

Severe disease Infliximab may be beneficial in CD patients whose symptoms persist despite use of oral corticosteroids.[119] A single infusion of 5 mg/kg provides significant improvement and clinical remission for patients who have not responded to aminosalicylates, antibiotics, steroids, or immune suppressants. However, a three-dose induction regimen followed by maintenance infusions given every 8 weeks affords a more optimal long-term approach. Concomitant treatment with an immune suppressant minimizes the risk of developing antibodies to infliximab that are associated with loss of response and infusion reactions.[119] Before receiving infliximab, patients should be interviewed regarding exposure to tuberculosis and should undergo skin testing and chest x-rays.

Patients presenting with dehydration, high fever, cachexia, GI bleeding, obstructive symptoms, rebound tenderness, or an abscess require hospitalization and resuscitation with intravenous fluids, electrolytes, or transfusion. Acute obstructive symptoms, in the absence of chronic symptoms, mandate assessment for a mechanical cause (i.e., adhesions) rather than an inflammatory narrowing. Parenteral nutritional support is indicated as a supplement for patients unable to tolerate sufficient caloric intake and is mandatory for patients with profound malnutrition and an inability to eat.

Intravenous corticosteroids are indicated for severe manifestations of CD, once an abscess has been ruled out.[27] Prednisolone (40 to 60 mg), hydrocortisone (200 to 300 mg), or methylprednisolone (32 to 48 mg) is given in an intermittent or continuous infusion and continued until the patient is free of pain and is passing flatus and stool or until the patient no longer has diarrhea. Oral steroids are then substituted at an equivalent dose. Failure to improve with intravenous steroids should cause consideration of surgical intervention, prolonged total parenteral nutrition and bowel rest, use of intravenous cyclosporine, or use of infliximab. Broad-spectrum antibiotics are added for febrile patients and those with abdominal tenderness or an inflammatory mass. These agents are continued until defervescence unless a specific pathogen has been identified and a narrow-spectrum agent can be substituted.

Maintenance Therapy

Maintenance therapy for CD was once discounted because of poor results from early studies that evaluated low-dose sulfasalazine and corticosteroids. However, it is now apparent that other forms of maintenance therapy can reduce the possibility of clinical relapse in certain patients.[165] As with UC, steroids are not effective and should not be routinely used as maintenance agents for CD.

The aminosalicylates are useful maintenance agents when continued after inductive therapy, but they have limited value after steroid-induced remissions.[27,66] In contrast, immunomodulators have been shown to have steroid-sparing and maintenance benefits. AZA and 6-MP are effective steroid-sparing agents for patients who cannot be weaned from steroids. Initial therapy is AZA, 2 to 2.5 mg/kg, or 6-MP, 1 to 1.5 mg/kg. The dosage is adjusted at 2-week intervals according to the leukocyte count, which must be maintained above leukopenic levels. The efficacy of these agents may not be evident until after 3 to 6 months of treatment, but benefits have been demonstrated to last for at least 4 years. To avoid unanticipated bone marrow suppression, monitoring of blood counts on a quarterly basis must continue once the patient is off steroids.

Maintenance therapy to delay postsurgical relapse has been evaluated according to different end-point criteria (e.g., endoscopic evidence of relapse, clinical symptoms, or repeat surgery).[39] There is evidence that mesalamine, 3 to 4 g/day, can prevent postoperative recurrence, particularly when therapy is initiated shortly after surgery[27]; conversely, postponing therapy for more than 3 months circumvents any benefits. In addition to mesalamine, metronidazole is effective for reducing postoperative recurrence when administered at high doses (20 mg/kg) for 3 months after resection. There are no data regarding lower doses of metronidazole, prolongation of therapy beyond 3 months, or the use of other antibiotics.[27,102] Finally, 6-MP at doses of 50 mg/day may reduce postoperative relapse for at least 2 years after resection.[166] In view of the negative impact of cigarette smoking on the postoperative course of CD, however, all patients who smoke should be advised to stop.[27]

Surgical Therapy

Unlike UC, CD is not cured by surgery, except in the case of CD confined to the colon, for which proctocolectomy and ileostomy provide similar likelihoods of cure; sphincter-saving procedures are not advocated because of the high likelihood of recurrence after anastomoses. With CD in other locations, disease recurrence at the anastomotic site is virtually inevitable. Therefore, surgery is undertaken to treat refractory disease or complications, rather than to cure the disease. Nevertheless, in view of the excellent quality of life after limited surgery and the evolving capability to reduce or delay recurrence, it is imperative that surgery not be deferred because of fear of recurrence.

Purulent complications (e.g., abscesses) require percutaneous or surgical drainage. Surgery in CD patients is also indicated for intractable hemorrhage, perforation, persisting or recurrent obstruction, or toxic megacolon. The most common indications for surgery are intractable disease, failure of medical therapy, or complications related to treatment (e.g., steroid dependence). Many of these indications are subjective, requiring experienced clinical judgment and cooperative consultation between medical and surgical specialists. Surgical resections should be limited to macroscopic disease, and in general, primary anastomoses should not be performed in the setting of uncontained purulent complications.[27]

IBD AND PREGNANCY

Fertility is usually normal in both men and women with IBD, although an increase in disease activity correlates with a decrease in libido and with menstrual irregularities.[167] Risk of early miscarriage is increased in women with active disease. When disease activity is controlled, the course and outcome of pregnancy do not differ substantially from those in the general population. Therefore, the best means of ensuring normal fetal outcome is to time conception when disease is under control, aggressively treat disease activity during pregnancy, and maintain the health of the mother.[27] Aminosalicylates, steroids, and immunomodulators are safe during pregnancy and lactation, but they should be added only when necessary to maintain maternal well-being.[88,168,169] Conversely, because of the risk of maternal worsening, neither acute nor maintenance therapy should be withdrawn during or after pregnancy. Attention to the mother's nutritional status is essential throughout pregnancy and during lactation. Neonates born to women on high doses of steroids should be monitored for adrenal suppression.

Complications

INTESTINAL COMPLICATIONS

The intestinal complications of IBD include hemorrhage, stricture, fistulas, toxic megacolon, and neoplasia. Chronic blood loss, with subsequent iron deficiency anemia, is common in both UC and CD. Profuse bleeding, however, is uncommon, particularly in UC, because the inflammation is superficial. Occasionally, patients with CD experience severe lower gastrointestinal bleeding when deep ulcerations erode into large vessels.

Strictures are more common in CD than in UC and result from transmural inflammation and fibrosis. These strictures remain fixed and lead to progressive bowel obstruction. In UC, narrowing of the lumen can occur from smooth muscle hypertrophy; the narrowing is related to disease activity and is reversible with treatment of acute inflammation. Fixed strictures in UC are almost always dysplastic or malignant. Toxic megacolon, although more common in UC, is not unique to UC and can occur in infectious colitis or CD.[170]

EXTRAINTESTINAL COMPLICATIONS

The extraintestinal complications of IBD can result from inflammation or from an HLA-related autoimmune process that underlies the intestinal disease.[171] Complications may also occur as a metabolic consequence of intestinal disease or its treatment.[29]

Mucocutaneous complications include eye changes of episcleritis or scleritis. These complications most commonly parallel colonic disease activity. Involvement of the anterior or posterior chambers with iritis or uveitis is related to HLA-B27 and follows a course that is independent of disease activity in the bowel.[172] Skin lesions of erythema nodosum and pyoderma gangrenosum usually accompany or herald the onset of colitis and respond to treatment of bowel inflammation.

Musculoskeletal lesions can either be independent of or correlate with intestinal disease activity. Peripheral arthralgias and arthritis commonly involve larger joints (e.g., the hips, knees, ankles, elbows, and wrists) in an asymmetrical pattern. The inflammation usually accompanies intestinal disease activity and is almost never deforming, progressive, or associated with rheumatoid nodules. In contrast, arthritis of the central spine, ankylosing spondylitis, and sacroiliitis are associated with HLA-B27 and progress independently of intestinal disease. Metabolic bone disease is most often a consequence of long-term steroid use and, in CD, can be accelerated by malabsorption or inadequate dietary supplementation with vitamin D or calcium.[150]

A spectrum of hepatobiliary involvement occurs in both UC and colonic CD.[173] Inflammation of the intrahepatic and extrahepatic bile ducts may take the form of a mild, periportal inflammatory infiltrate (pericholangitis or small-duct sclerosing cholangitis) that is asymptomatic, nonprogressive, and manifested only as mild elevations of γ-glutamyltransferase (GGT), alkaline phosphatase, and transaminases. At the other extreme, such inflammation may lead to full-blown sclerosing cholangitis with progressive secondary biliary cirrhosis. Of interest, cigarette smoking, which protects against UC, also protects against primary sclerosing cholangitis.[9] Hepatic steatosis commonly manifests as a mild elevation of biliary enzymes in the presence of malnutrition or steroid therapy. Patients with CD who have ileal involvement or have had ileal resections are at increased risk for gallstones because of reduced enterohepatic circulation of bile salts, which increases biliary cholesterol saturation.

Urinary tract complications are more common in CD than UC.[174] Kidney stones may reflect dehydration from diarrhea or an ileostomy.[175] In the setting of ileitis or after ileal resections, the mechanism of nephrolithiasis is hyperoxaluria caused by steatorrhea. Normally, oxalate in the diet binds to free calcium in the colonic lumen and is excreted in the feces as calcium oxalate crystals. In patients with steatorrhea, free luminal calcium preferentially binds to fatty acids, creating soaps that are similarly excreted in the feces. Lacking calcium to bind it, the free oxalate is instead absorbed by the colon and excreted by the kidneys in abnormally high amounts. In the urine, oxalate complexes with urinary calcium to form calcium oxalate crystals. Patients with CD are also more susceptible to nephrolithiasis because their kidneys excrete low amounts of citrate, which acts as a nonspecific solubilizer in the urine. Calcium oxalate stones may result from either hyperoxaluria or idiopathic hypercalciuria; the two conditions can be differentiated by measuring calcium and oxalate levels in a 24-hour urine sample. If hyperoxaluria is identified, the treatment is to reduce fat intake (to reduce steatorrhea) and increase calcium supplementation.

Hematologic complications of IBD include anemia and clotting abnormalities. Anemia is most often caused by iron loss from bleeding or, in CD, from impaired iron absorption because of proximal small bowel disease.[176] Folic acid deficiency is most often related to concurrent use of sulfasalazine, but occasionally, it is related to inadequate dietary consumption of folic acid or extensive jejunal disease. Vitamin B_{12} deficiency from extensive ileal disease or resection can lead to macrocytic anemia. Hypercoagulability is a nonspecific complication of active IBD that results from increased production of acute-phase reactants and that increases the risk of venous thrombosis.[177] Rarely, enteric losses of anticoagulant factors are a consequence of protein-losing enteropathy. In contrast, hypocoagulability may be a complication of vitamin K malabsorption or prolonged antibiotic administration.

Management of Extraintestinal Complications

Treatment of extraintestinal complications of IBD varies according to whether the manifestations are dependent or independent of intestinal (usually colonic) inflammation.[29,171] Peripheral arthritis, erythema nodosum, pyoderma gangrenosum, and episcleritis occur in the presence of active disease and require intensification of anti-inflammatory therapy.

In some patients, complications can be treated independently, along with therapy for intestinal inflammation. For example, inflamed joints can be drained or injected with steroids, and pyoderma gangrenosum can be approached with a combination of topical and systemic approaches. Infliximab therapy has been very effective for the treatment of pyoderma gangrenosum associated with CD.[178] Ocular complications should be evaluated by an ophthalmologist to prevent irreversible damage. Erythema nodosum usually responds to more aggressive therapy for colitis and should not be treated with NSAIDs. Peripheral articular manifestations of colitis can be treated with acetaminophen and increased doses of sulfasalazine; again, NSAIDs should be avoided.

Ankylosing spondylitis, sacroiliitis, and iritis (uveitis) are HLA-B27–associated manifestations that follow a course independent from colitis. The same is true of primary sclerosing cholangitis. Physical therapy is critical for patients with ankylosing spondylitis and sacroiliitis. Concurrent immunomodulatory therapy with methotrexate, hydroxychloroquine, or infliximab is indicated for inflammatory arthropathies.

NEOPLASIA

Adenocarcinoma of the intestines is a potential long-term complication of IBD, with features that are distinct from those of spontaneous adenocarcinomas in the general population.[179] The risks of colonic neoplasia are similar in UC and CD and historically have been related to the extent and duration of disease, age at onset, and stricture formation, with primary sclerosing cholangitis indicating an increased risk for cholangiocarcinoma. In addition, evidence now suggests that in UC, severity of inflammation is also a risk factor for development of neoplasia.[180] In contrast to colorectal cancer in the general population, which develops from adenomatous polyps, dysplasia is the precursor to cancer in IBD patients.[34] Dysplasia is a neoplasia and has been defined on a pathologic basis and categorized as indefinite, low grade, or high grade (carcinoma in situ).[34] Patients with dysplasia have an increased risk of cancer elsewhere in the colon if they have high-grade lesions (up to 50% of these patients have other colonic cancers) or low-grade

lesions that are multifocal or in a raised plaque (dysplasia-associated lesion or mass).[181]

The ability to identify histologic dysplasia in UC makes it possible to perform surveillance colonoscopic examinations. Despite the absence of prospective data regarding colonoscopic surveillance for dysplasia in UC, most North American centers recommend that, after 8 to 10 years of UC, patients who are at increased risk for adenocarcinoma be entered into a colonoscopic surveillance program.[26,181,182] Surveillance colonoscopies are recommended every 2 to 3 years for patients with 10 to 20 years of disease and every 1 to 2 years for patients with over 20 years of disease. The confirmation of low-grade dysplasia on surveillance colonoscopy strongly predicts progression to advanced neoplasia and warrants a recommendation for colectomy.[183] Patients with indefinite dysplasia are treated aggressively to control inflammation and should undergo repeat colonoscopy after 3 to 6 months.

The risk of cancer in CD is also related to the location and chronicity of inflammation and, thus, includes a risk for small bowel adenocarcinoma in long-standing small bowel disease.[184] However, because of the varied locations and segmental involvement in CD, there are no standardized guidelines for surveillance. Although there is no means of screening for small bowel dysplasia or cancer in CD, patients with colonic CD can be followed with colonoscopic surveillance in a manner similar to that used in patients with UC. Unfortunately, stricture formation in these patients often prevents visualization of the entire colon.

In addition to being associated with adenocarcinomas, IBD is associated with a small increase in the relative risk of lymphomas.[185] This increase may be associated with immunosuppressive therapy.[186-188] However, it is difficult to tease out any small increase in the relative risk from immunomodulatory therapy from the underlying risk associated with the chronic inflammatory disease and a potential association with Epstein-Barr virus infection.[189,190]

Prognosis and Conclusion

The diagnosis and treatment of IBD challenge the physician to guide patients through chronic illness. It is important to recognize the perceptions and concerns of the patient and family members confronted with a chronic, medically incurable, socially embarrassing, and potentially disfiguring condition.[27] Despite the absence of known causes, medical therapy is usually effective, and surgical techniques have improved to the point that both longevity and quality of life can be preserved. The life expectancy of patients without fulminant disease is the same as that of the general population. Patience, optimism, and empathy are required to balance the concerns and misinformation that surround the disease, as well as the guilt associated with misconceptions that IBD is a so-called neurotic, psychosomatic, or self-induced disorder.

Patient information and support groups constitute a valuable part of management in IBD. Resources for high-quality patient information and support are available through national organizations such as the Crohn's and Colitis Foundation of America (http://www.ccfa.org).

The author has received grant support from Centocor, Inc, The Procter & Gamble Company, and Prometheus Laboratories, Inc.; has been a consultant for Centocor, Inc., The Procter & Gamble Company, Prometheus Laboratories,

Inc., Salix Pharmaceuticals, Inc., and Shire Pharmaceuticals Group; and has participated in speakers' bureaus for Centocor, Inc., The Procter & Gamble Company, and Salix Pharmaceuticals, Inc.

References

1. Podolsky DK: Inflammatory bowel disease. N Engl J Med 347:417, 2002

2. Loftus EV Jr, Sandborn WJ: Epidemiology of inflammatory bowel disease. Gastroenterol Clin North Am 31:1, 2002

3. Cashman KD, Shanahan F: Is nutrition an aetiological factor for inflammatory bowel disease? Eur J Gastroenterol Hepatol 15:607, 2003

4. Hendrickson BA, Gokhale R, Cho JH: Clinical aspects and pathophysiology of inflammatory bowel disease. Clin Microbiol Rev 15:79, 2002

5. Mathew CG, Lewis CM: Genetics of inflammatory bowel disease: progress and prospects. Hum Mol Genet 13:R161, 2004

6. Halfvarson J, Bodin L, Tysk C, et al: Inflammatory bowel disease in a Swedish twin cohort: a long-term follow-up of concordance and clinical characteristics. Gastroenterology 124:1767, 2003

7. Cosnes J: Tobacco and IBD: relevance in the understanding of disease mechanisms and clinical practice. Best Pract Res Clin Gastroenterol 18:481, 2004

8. Beaugerie L, Massot N, Carbonnel F, et al: Impact of cessation of smoking on the course of ulcerative colitis. Am J Gastroenterol 96:2113, 2001

9. Loftus EV Jr, Sandborn WJ, Tremaine WJ, et al: Primary sclerosing cholangitis is associated with nonsmoking: a case-control study. Gastroenterology 110:1496, 1996

10. Cosnes J, Beaugerie L, Carbonnel F, et al: Smoking cessation and the course of Crohn's disease: an intervention study. Gastroenterology 120:1093, 2001

11. Sandborn WJ: Nicotine therapy for ulcerative colitis: a review of rationale, mechanisms, pharmacology, and clinical results. Am J Gastroenterol 94:1161, 1999

12. Shanahan F: The host-microbe interface within the gut. Best Pract Res Clin Gastroenterol 16:915, 2002

13. Danese S, Sans M, Fiocchi C: Inflammatory bowel disease: the role of environmental factors. Autoimmun Rev 3:394, 2004

14. Landers CJ, Cohavy O, Misra R, et al: Selected loss of tolerance evidenced by Crohn's disease–associated immune responses to auto- and microbial antigens. Gastroenterology 123:689, 2002

15. Stagg AJ, Hart AL, Knight SC, et al: The dendritic cell: its role in intestinal inflammation and relationship with gut bacteria. Gut 52:1522, 2003

16. Sartor RB: Innate immunity in the pathogenesis and therapy of IBD. J Gastroenterol 38(suppl 15):43, 2003

17. Fellermann K, Wehkamp J, Herrlinger KR, et al: Crohn's disease: a defensin deficiency syndrome? Eur J Gastroenterol Hepatol 15:627, 2003

18. Bouma G, Strober W: The immunological and genetic basis of inflammatory bowel disease. Nat Rev Immunol 3:521, 2003

19. Shanahan F: Inflammatory bowel disease: immunodiagnostics, immunotherapeutics, and ecotherapeutics. Gastroenterology 120:622, 2001

20. Papadakis KA, Targan SR: The role of chemokines and chemokine receptors in mucosal inflammation. Inflamm Bowel Dis 6:303, 2000

21. Langholz E, Munkholm P, Davidsen M, et al: Changes in extent of ulcerative colitis: a study on the course and prognostic factors. Scand J Gastroenterol 31:260, 1996

22. Moum B, Ekbom A, Vatn MH, et al: Change in the extent of colonoscopic and histological involvement in ulcerative colitis over time. Am J Gastroenterol 94:1564, 1999

23. Schumacher G, Sandstedt B, Kollberg B: A prospective study of first attacks of inflammatory bowel disease and infectious colitis: clinical findings and early diagnosis. Scand J Gastroenterol 29:265, 1994

24. Farmer RG, Easley KA, Rankin GB: Clinical patterns, natural history, and progression of ulcerative colitis: a long-term follow-up of 1116 patients. Dig Dis Sci 38:1137, 1993

25. Gan SI, Beck PL: A new look at toxic megacolon: an update and review of incidence, etiology, pathogenesis, and management. Am J Gastroenterol 98:2363, 2003

26. Kornbluth A, Sachar DB: Ulcerative colitis practice guidelines in adults (update): American College of Gastroenterology, Practice Parameters Committee. Am J Gastroenterol 99:1371, 2004

27. Carter MJ, Lobo AJ, Travis SP: Guidelines for the management of inflammatory bowel disease in adults. Gut 53(suppl 5):V1, 2004

28. Rizzello F, Gionchetti P, Venturi A, et al: Review article: monitoring activity in ulcerative colitis. Aliment Pharmacol Ther 16(suppl 4):3, 2002

29. Su CG, Judge TA, Lichtenstein GR: Extraintestinal manifestations of inflammatory bowel disease. Gastroenterol Clin North Am 31:307, 2002

30. Chutkan RK, Scherl E, Waye JD: Colonoscopy in inflammatory bowel disease. Gastrointest Endosc Clin N Am 12:463, 2002

31. D'Haens G, Geboes K, Peeters M, et al: Patchy cecal inflammation associated with distal ulcerative colitis: a prospective endoscopic study. Am J Gastroenterol 92:1275, 1997

32. Geboes K, Dalle I: Influence of treatment on morphological features of mucosal inflammation. Gut 50(suppl 3):III37, 2002

33. Tanaka M, Riddell RH, Saito H, et al: Morphologic criteria applicable to biopsy specimens for effective distinction of inflammatory bowel disease from other forms of colitis and of Crohn's disease from ulcerative colitis. Scand J Gastroenterol 34:55, 1999

34. Riddell RH, Goldman H, Ransohoff DF, et al: Dysplasia in inflammatory bowel disease: standardized classification with provisional clinical applications. Hum Pathol 14:931, 1983

35. Martin-Comin J, Prats E: Clinical applications of radiolabeled blood elements in inflammatory bowel disease. Q J Nucl Med 43:74, 1999

36. Farmer RG, Whelan G, Fazio VW: Long-term follow-up of patients with Crohn's disease: relationship between the clinical pattern and prognosis. Gastroenterology 88:1818, 1985

37. Gasche C, Scholmerich J, Brynskov J, et al: A simple classification of Crohn's disease: report of the Working Party for the World Congresses of Gastroenterology, Vienna 1998. Inflamm Bowel Dis 6:8, 2000

38. Cosnes J, Cattan S, Blain A, et al: Long-term evolution of disease behavior of Crohn's disease. Inflamm Bowel Dis 8:244, 2002

39. Lewis JD, Schoenfeld P, Lichtenstein GR: An evidence-based approach to studies of the natural history of gastrointestinal diseases: recurrence of symptomatic Crohn's disease after surgery. Clin Gastroenterol Hepatol 1:229, 2003

40. Hanauer SB: Measurement of disease activity. Inflammatory Bowel Disease: From Bench to Bedside, 1st ed. Targan SR, Shanahan F, Eds. Williams & Wilkins, Baltimore, 1994, p 429

41. Cohen RD: The quality of life in patients with Crohn's disease. Aliment Pharmacol Ther 16:1603, 2002

42. Bernstein CN, Blanchard JF, Rawsthorne P, et al: The prevalence of extraintestinal diseases in inflammatory bowel disease: a population-based study. Am J Gastroenterol 96:1116, 2001

43. Loftus EV Jr, Schoenfeld P, Sandborn WJ: The epidemiology and natural history of Crohn's disease in population-based patient cohorts from North America: a systematic review. Aliment Pharmacol Ther 16:51, 2002

44. Schwartz DA, Loftus EV Jr, Tremaine WJ, et al: The natural history of fistulizing Crohn's disease in Olmsted County, Minnesota. Gastroenterology 122:875, 2002

45. Langholz E, Munkholm P, Krasilnikoff PA, et al: Inflammatory bowel diseases with onset in childhood: clinical features, morbidity, and mortality in a regional cohort. Scand J Gastroenterol 32:139, 1997

46. Mamula P, Telega GW, Markowitz JE, et al: Inflammatory bowel disease in children 5 years of age and younger. Am J Gastroenterol 97:2005, 2002

47. Decker GA, Loftus EV Jr, Pasha TM, et al: Crohn's disease of the esophagus: clinical features and outcomes. Inflamm Bowel Dis 7:113, 2001

48. Wagtmans MJ, Verspaget HW, Lamers CB, et al: Clinical aspects of Crohn's disease of the upper gastrointestinal tract: a comparison with distal Crohn's disease. Am J Gastroenterol 92:1467, 1997

49. Higuero T, Merle C, Thiefin G, et al: Jejunoileal Crohn's disease: a case-control study. Gastroenterol Clin Biol 28:160, 2004

50. Guindi M, Riddell RH: Indeterminate colitis. J Clin Pathol 57:1233, 2004

51. Sandborn WJ, Fazio VW, Feagan BG, et al: AGA technical review on perianal Crohn's disease. Gastroenterology 125:1508, 2003

52. Oldenburg B, Koningsberger JC, Van Berge Henegouwen GP, et al: Iron and inflammatory bowel disease. Aliment Pharmacol Ther 15:429, 2001

53. Vermeire S, Van Assche G, Rutgeerts P: C-reactive protein as a marker for inflammatory bowel disease. Inflamm Bowel Dis 10:661, 2004

54. Wassell J, Dolwani S, Metzner M, et al: Faecal calprotectin: a new marker for Crohn's disease? Ann Clin Biochem 41:230, 2004

55. Kane SV, Sandborn WJ, Rufo PA, et al: Fecal lactoferrin is a sensitive and specific marker in identifying intestinal inflammation. Am J Gastroenterol 98:1309, 2003

56. Nakamura RM, Matsutani M, Barry M: Advances in clinical laboratory tests for inflammatory bowel disease. Clin Chim Acta 335:9, 2003

57. Zalis M, Singh AK: Imaging of inflammatory bowel disease: CT and MR. Dig Dis 22:56, 2004

58. Alberini JL, Badran A, Freneaux E, et al: Technetium-99m HMPAO-labeled leukocyte imaging compared with endoscopy, ultrasonography, and contrast radiology in children with inflammatory bowel disease. J Pediatr Gastroenterol Nutr 32:278, 2001

59. Kornbluth A, Legnani P, Lewis BS: Video capsule endoscopy in inflammatory bowel disease: past, present, and future. Inflamm Bowel Dis 10:278, 2004

60. Cipolla G, Crema F, Sacco S, et al: Nonsteroidal anti-inflammatory drugs and inflammatory bowel disease: current perspectives. Pharmacol Res 46:1, 2002

61. Alapati SV, Mihas AA: When to suspect ischemic colitis: why is this condition so often missed or misdiagnosed? Postgrad Med 105:177, 1999

62. Peppercorn MA: The overlap of inflammatory bowel disease and diverticular disease. J Clin Gastroenterol 38(5 suppl):S8, 2004

63. Sands BE: From symptom to diagnosis: clinical distinctions among various forms of intestinal inflammation. Gastroenterology 126:1518, 2004

64. Stallmach A, Carstens O: Role of infections in the manifestation or reactivation of inflammatory bowel diseases. Inflamm Bowel Dis 8:213, 2002

65. Gisbert JP, Gomollon F, Mate J, et al: Role of 5-aminosalicylic acid (5-ASA) in treatment of inflammatory bowel disease: a systematic review. Dig Dis Sci 47:471, 2002

66. Lim WC, Hanauer SB: Controversies with aminosalicylates in inflammatory bowel disease. Rev Gastroenterol Disord 4:104, 2004

67. Sandborn WJ, Hanauer SB: The pharmacokinetic profiles of oral mesalazine formulations and mesalazine pro-drugs used in the management of ulcerative colitis. Aliment Pharmacol Ther 17:29, 2003

68. Allgayer H: Review article: mechanisms of action of mesalazine in preventing colorectal carcinoma in inflammatory bowel disease. Aliment Pharmacol Ther 18(suppl 2):10, 2003

69. Wahl C, Liptay S, Adler G, et al: Sulfasalazine: a potent and specific inhibitor of nu-

clear factor kappa B. J Clin Invest 101:1163, 1998

70. Walker AM, Szneke P, Bianchi LA, et al: 5-Aminosalicylates, sulfasalazine, steroid use, and complications in patients with ulcerative colitis. Am J Gastroenterol 92:816, 1997

71. Cunliffe RN, Scott BB: Monitoring for drug side-effects in inflammatory bowel disease. Aliment Pharmacol Ther 16:647, 2002

72. Sutherland L, MacDonald JK: Oral 5-aminosalicylic acid for induction of remission in ulcerative colitis. Cochrane Database Syst Rev (3):CD000543, 2003

73. Cohen RD, Woseth DM, Thisted RA, et al: A meta-analysis and overview of the literature on treatment options for left-sided ulcerative colitis and ulcerative proctitis. Am J Gastroenterol 95:1263, 2000

74. Sutherland L, Roth D, Beck P, et al: Oral 5-aminosalicylic acid for maintenance of remission in ulcerative colitis. Cochrane Database Syst Rev (4):CD000544, 2002

75. Katz JA: Treatment of inflammatory bowel disease with corticosteroids. Gastroenterol Clin North Am 33:171, 2004

76. Steinhart AH, Ewe K, Griffiths AM, et al: Corticosteroids for maintenance of remission in Crohn's disease. Cochrane Database Syst Rev (4):CD000301, 2003

77. Farrell RJ, Kelleher D: Glucocorticoid resistance in inflammatory bowel disease. J Endocrinol 178:339, 2003

78. McKeage K, Goa KL: Budesonide (Entocort EC Capsules): a review of its therapeutic use in the management of active Crohn's disease in adults. Drugs 62:2263, 2002

79. Bebb JR, Scott BB: How effective are the usual treatments for ulcerative colitis? Aliment Pharmacol Ther 20:143, 2004

80. Ardizzone S, Porro GB: Comparative tolerability of therapies for ulcerative colitis. Drug Saf 25:561, 2002

81. Marshall JK, Irvine EJ: Rectal corticosteroids versus alternative treatments in ulcerative colitis: a meta-analysis. Gut 40:775, 1997

82. Bebb JR, Scott BB: How effective are the usual treatments for Crohn's disease? Aliment Pharmacol Ther 20:151, 2004

83. Kane SV, Schoenfeld P, Sandborn WJ, et al: The effectiveness of budesonide therapy for Crohn's disease. Aliment Pharmacol Ther 16:1509, 2002

84. Sandborn WJ: Azathioprine: state of the art in inflammatory bowel disease. Scand J Gastroenterol Suppl 225:92, 1998

85. Tiede I, Fritz G, Strand S, et al: CD28-dependent Rac1 activation is the molecular target of azathioprine in primary human CD4+ T lymphocytes. J Clin Invest 111:1133, 2003

86. Louis E, Belaiche J: Optimizing treatment with thioguanine derivatives in inflammatory bowel disease. Best Pract Res Clin Gastroenterol 17:37, 2003

87. Vial T, Descotes J: Immunosuppressive drugs and cancer. Toxicology 185:229, 2003

88. Polifka JE, Friedman JM: Teratogen update: azathioprine and 6-mercaptopurine. Teratology 65:240, 2002

89. Lichtenstein GR: Use of laboratory testing to guide 6-mercaptopurine/azathioprine therapy. Gastroenterology 127:1558, 2004

90. Sandborn W, Sutherland L, Pearson D, et al: Azathioprine or 6-mercaptopurine for inducing remission of Crohn's disease. Cochrane Database Syst Rev (2):CD000545, 2000

91. Pearson DC, May GR, Fick G, et al: Azathioprine for maintaining remission of Crohn's disease. Cochrane Database Syst Rev (2):CD000067, 2000

92. Loftus CG, Egan LJ, Sandborn WJ: Cyclosporine, tacrolimus, and mycophenolate mofetil in the treatment of inflammatory bowel disease. Gastroenterol Clin North Am 33:141, 2004

93. Hanauer SB: Medical therapy for ulcerative colitis 2004. Gastroenterology 126:1582, 2004

94. Van Assche G, D'Haens G, Noman M, et al: Randomized, double-blind comparison of 4 mg/kg versus 2 mg/kg intravenous cyclosporine in severe ulcerative colitis. Gastroenterology 125:1025, 2003

95. Sandborn WJ: Cyclosporine in ulcerative colitis: state of the art. Acta Gastroenterol Belg 64:201, 2001

96. Egan LJ, Sandborn WJ, Tremaine WJ: Clinical outcome following treatment of refractory inflammatory and fistulizing Crohn's disease with intravenous cyclosporine. Am J Gastroenterol 93:442, 1998

97. Feagan BG, Alfadhli A: Methotrexate in inflammatory bowel disease. Gastroenterol Clin North Am 33:407, 2004

98. Feagan BG, Rochon J, Fedorak RN, et al: Methotrexate for the treatment of Crohn's disease. The North American Crohn's Study Group Investigators. N Engl J Med 332:292 1995

99. Feagan BG, Fedorak RN, Irvine EJ, et al: A comparison of methotrexate with placebo for the maintenance of remission in Crohn's disease. North American Crohn's Study Group Investigators. N Engl J Med 342:1627, 2000

100. Sandborn WJ, Present DH, Isaacs KL, et al: Tacrolimus for the treatment of fistulas in patients with Crohn's disease: a randomized, placebo-controlled trial. Gastroenterology 125:380, 2003

101. Hogenauer C, Wenzl HH, Hinterleitner TA, et al: Effect of oral tacrolimus (FK 506) on steroid-refractory moderate/severe ulcerative colitis. Aliment Pharmacol Ther 18:415, 2003

102. Isaacs KL, Sartor RB: Treatment of inflammatory bowel disease with antibiotics. Gastroenterol Clin North Am 33:335, 2004

103. Sandborn W, McLeod R, Jewell D: Pharmacotherapy for inducing and maintaining remission in pouchitis. Cochrane Database Syst Rev (2):CD001176, 2000

104. Greenberg GR: Antibiotics should be used as first-line therapy for Crohn's disease. Inflamm Bowel Dis 10:318, 2004

105. Shanahan F, Bernstein CN: Antibiotics as a first-line therapy for Crohn's disease: is there any consensus? Inflamm Bowel Dis 10:324, 2004

106. Wild GE: The role of antibiotics in the management of Crohn's disease. Inflamm Bowel Dis 10:321, 2004

107. Hanauer SB, Sandborn W: Management of Crohn's disease in adults. Am J Gastroenterol 96:635, 2001

108. Achkar JP, Hanauer SB: Medical therapy to reduce postoperative Crohn's disease recurrence. Am J Gastroenterol 95:1139, 2000

109. Colombel JF, Lemann M, Cassagnou M, et al: A controlled trial comparing ciprofloxacin with mesalazine for the treatment of active Crohn's disease. Groupe d'Etudes Therapeutiques des Affections Inflammatoires Digestives (GETAID). Am J Gastroenterol 94:674, 1999

110. Prantera C, Zannoni F, Scribano ML, et al: An antibiotic regimen for the treatment of active Crohn's disease: a randomized, controlled clinical trial of metronidazole plus ciprofloxacin. Am J Gastroenterol 91:328, 1996

111. Greenbloom SL, Steinhart AH, Greenberg GR: Combination ciprofloxacin and metronidazole for active Crohn's disease. Can J Gastroenterol 12:53, 1998

112. Borgaonkar M, MacIntosh D, Fardy J, et al: Anti-tuberculous therapy for maintaining remission of Crohn's disease. Cochrane Database Syst Rev (2):CD000299, 2000

113. Akobeng AK, Zachos M: Tumor necrosis factor–alpha antibody for induction of remission in Crohn's disease. Cochrane Database Syst Rev (1):CD003574, 2004

114. Hanauer S, Lukas M, Macintosh D, et al: A randomized, double-blind, placebo-controlled trial of the human anti–TNF-alpha monoclonal antibody adalimumab for the induction of remission in patients with moderate to severely active Crohn's disease (abstr). Gastroenterology 127:332, 2004

115. Sands BE, Anderson FH, Bernstein CN, et al: Infliximab maintenance therapy for fistulizing Crohn's disease. N Engl J Med 350:876, 2004

116. Olson A: Personal communication, 2005

117. Colombel JF, Loftus EV Jr, Tremaine WJ, et al: The safety profile of infliximab in patients with Crohn's disease: the Mayo Clinic experience in 500 patients. Gastroenterology 126:19, 2004

118. Mow WS, Abreu-Martin MT, Papadakis KA, et al: High incidence of anergy in inflammatory bowel disease patients limits the usefulness of PPD screening before infliximab therapy. Clin Gastroenterol Hepatol 2:309, 2004

119. Rutgeerts P, Van Assche G, Vermeire S: Optimizing anti-TNF treatment in inflammatory bowel disease. Gastroenterology 126:1593, 2004

120. Khanna D, McMahon M, Furst DE: Safety of tumour necrosis factor–alpha antagonists. Drug Saf 27:307, 2004

121. Aithal GP, Mansfield JC: Review article: the risk of lymphoma associated with inflammatory bowel disease and immunosuppressive treatment. Aliment Pharmacol Ther 15:1101, 2001

122. Sandborn WJ, Yednock TA: Novel approaches to treating inflammatory bowel disease: targeting alpha-4 integrin. Am J Gastroenterol 98:2372, 2003

123. Mannon PJ, Fuss IJ, Mayer L, et al: Anti–interleukin-12 antibody for active Crohn's disease. N Engl J Med 351:2069, 2004

124. Lim WC, Hanauer SB: Emerging biologic therapies in inflammatory bowel disease. Rev Gastroenterol Disord 4:66, 2004

125. Sinha A, Nightingale J, West KP, et al: Epidermal growth factor enemas with oral mesalamine for mild-to-moderate left-sided ulcerative colitis or proctitis. N Engl J Med 349:350, 2003

126. Dieckgraefe BK, Korzenik JR: Treatment of active Crohn's disease with recombinant human granulocyte-macrophage colony-stimulating factor. Lancet 360:1478, 2002

127. McGrath J, McDonald J, Macdonald J: Transdermal nicotine for induction of remission in ulcerative colitis. Cochrane Database Syst Rev (4):CD004722, 2004

128. Aslan A, Triadafilopoulos G: Fish oil fatty acid supplementation in active ulcerative colitis: a double-blind, placebo-controlled, crossover study. Am J Gastroenterol 87:432, 1992

129. Loeschke K, Ueberschaer B, Pietsch A, et al: n-3 fatty acids only delay early relapse of ulcerative colitis in remission. Dig Dis Sci 41:2087, 1996

130. Belluzzi A, Brignola C, Campieri M, et al: Effect of an enteric-coated fish-oil preparation on relapses in Crohn's disease. N Engl J Med 334:1557, 1996

131. Banner KH, Trevethick MA: PDE4 inhibition: a novel approach for the treatment of inflammatory bowel disease. Trends Pharmacol Sci 25:430, 2004

132. van Deventer SJ: Small therapeutic molecules for the treatment of inflammatory bowel disease. Gut 50(suppl 3):III47, 2002

133. Shanahan F: Probiotics in inflammatory bowel disease—therapeutic rationale and role. Adv Drug Deliv Rev 56:809, 2004

134. Takazoe M, Tanaka T, Kondo K, et al: The present status and the recent development of the treatment for inflammatory bowel diseases: desirable effect of extracorporeal immunomodulation. Ther Apher 6:305, 2002

135. Danese S, Sans M, Fiocchi C: The CD40/CD40L costimulatory pathway in inflammatory bowel disease. Gut 53:1035, 2004

136. Graham TO, Kandil HM: Nutritional factors in inflammatory bowel disease. Gastroenterol Clin North Am 31:203, 2002

137. Gassull MA: Nutrition and inflammatory bowel disease: its relation to pathophysiology, outcome and therapy. Dig Dis 21:220, 2003

138. Zachos M, Tondeur M, Griffiths AM: Enteral nutritional therapy for inducing remission of Crohn's disease. Cochrane Database Syst Rev (3):CD000542, 2001

139. Miner PB Jr: Factors influencing the relapse of patients with inflammatory bowel disease. Am J Gastroenterol 92(12 suppl):1S, 1997

140. Kane SV, Sable K, Hanauer SB: The menstrual cycle and its effect on inflammatory bowel disease and irritable bowel syndrome: a prevalence study. Am J Gastroenterol 93:1867, 1998

141. Kane S, Kisiel J, Shih L, et al: HLA disparity determines disease activity through pregnancy in women with inflammatory bowel disease. Am J Gastroenterol 99:1523, 2004

142. Felder JB, Korelitz BI, Rajapakse R, et al: Effects of nonsteroidal antiinflammatory drugs on inflammatory bowel disease: a case-control study. Am J Gastroenterol 95:1949, 2000

143. Biancone L, Tosti C, Geremia A, et al: Rofecoxib and early relapse of inflammatory bowel disease: an open-label trial. Aliment Pharmacol Ther 19:755, 2004

144. Bonner GF: Exacerbation of inflammatory bowel disease associated with use of celecoxib. Am J Gastroenterol 96:1306, 2001

145. Hilsden RJ, Scott CM, Verhoef MJ: Complementary medicine use by patients with inflammatory bowel disease. Am J Gastroenterol 93:697, 1998

146. Gionchetti P, Rizzello F, Venturi A, et al: Comparison of oral with rectal mesalazine in the treatment of ulcerative proctitis. Dis Colon Rectum 41:93, 1998

147. Safdi M, DeMicco M, Sninsky C, et al: A double-blind comparison of oral versus rectal mesalamine versus combination therapy in the treatment of distal ulcerative colitis. Am J Gastroenterol 92:1867, 1997

148. Haghighi DB, Lashner BA: Left-sided ulcerative colitis. Gastroenterol Clin North Am 33:271, 2004

149. d'Albasio G, Pacini F, Camarri E, et al: Combined therapy with 5-aminosalicylic acid tablets and enemas for maintaining remission in ulcerative colitis: a randomized double-blind study. Am J Gastroenterol 92:1143, 1997

150. Bernstein CN, Leslie WD, Leboff MS: AGA technical review on osteoporosis in gastrointestinal diseases. Gastroenterology 124:795, 2003

151. Cohen RD, Stein R, Hanauer SB: Intravenous cyclosporin in ulcerative colitis: a five-year experience. Am J Gastroenterol 94:1587, 1999

152. Colombel JF, Ferrari N, Debuysere H, et al: Genotypic analysis of thiopurine S-methyltransferase in patients with Crohn's disease and severe myelosuppression during azathioprine therapy. Gastroenterology 118:1025, 2000

153. Ording Olsen K, Juul S, Berndtsson I, et al: Ulcerative colitis: female fecundity before diagnosis, during disease, and after surgery compared with a population sample. Gastroenterology 122:15, 2002

154. Larson DW, Pemberton JH: Current concepts and controversies in surgery for IBD. Gastroenterology 126:1611, 2004

155. Michelassi F, Lee J, Rubin M, et al: Long-term functional results after ileal pouch anal restorative proctocolectomy for ulcerative colitis: a prospective observational study. Ann Surg 238:433, 2003

156. Mahadevan U, Sandborn WJ: Diagnosis and management of pouchitis. Gastroenterology 124:1636, 2003

157. Gionchetti P, Rizzello F, Helwig U, et al: Prophylaxis of pouchitis onset with probiotic therapy: a double-blind, placebo-controlled trial. Gastroenterology 124:1202, 2003

158. Gionchetti P, Rizzello F, Venturi A, et al: Oral bacteriotherapy as maintenance treatment in patients with chronic pouchitis: a double-blind, placebo-controlled trial. Gastroenterology 119:305, 2000

159. Mimura T, Rizzello F, Helwig U, et al: Once daily high dose probiotic therapy (VSL#3) for maintaining remission in recurrent or refractory pouchitis. Gut 53:108, 2004

160. Tremaine WJ: Gastroduodenal Crohn's disease: medical management. Inflamm Bowel Dis 9:127, 2003

161. van Hogezand RA, Witte AM, Veenendaal RA, et al: Proximal Crohn's disease: review of the clinicopathologic features and therapy. Inflamm Bowel Dis 7:328, 2001

162. Hanauer SB, Stromberg U: Oral Pentasa in the treatment of active Crohn's disease: a meta-analysis of double-blind, placebo-controlled trials. Clin Gastroenterol Hepatol 2:379, 2004

163. Sandborn WJ, Feagan BG: Review article: mild to moderate Crohn's disease: defining the basis for a new treatment algorithm. Aliment Pharmacol Ther 18:263, 2003

164. Faubion WA Jr, Loftus EV Jr, Harmsen WS, et al: The natural history of corticosteroid therapy for inflammatory bowel disease: a population-based study. Gastroenterology 121:255, 2001

165. Brookes MJ, Green JR: Maintenance of remission in Crohn's disease: current and emerging therapeutic options. Drugs 64:1069, 2004

166. Hanauer SB, Korelitz BI, Rutgeerts P, et al: Postoperative maintenance of Crohn's

disease remission with 6-mercaptopurine, mesalamine, or placebo: a 2-year trial. Gastroenterology 127:723, 2004

167. Friedman S, Regueiro MD: Pregnancy and nursing in inflammatory bowel disease. Gastroenterol Clin North Am 31:265, 2002

168. Moskovitz DN, Bodian C, Chapman ML, et al: The effect on the fetus of medications used to treat pregnant inflammatory bowel-disease patients. Am J Gastroenterol 99:656, 2004

169. Norgard B, Pedersen L, Fonager K, et al: Azathioprine, mercaptopurine and birth outcome: a population-based cohort study. Aliment Pharmacol Ther 17:827, 2003

170. Stein R, Hanauer SB: Life-threatening complications of IBD: how to handle fulminant colitis and toxic megacolon. J Crit Illness 13:518, 1998

171. Orchard T: Extraintestinal complications of inflammatory bowel disease. Curr Gastroenterol Rep 5:512, 2003

172. Orchard TR, Chua CN, Ahmad T, et al: Uveitis and erythema nodosum in inflammatory bowel disease: clinical features and the role of HLA genes. Gastroenterology 123:714, 2002

173. Ahmad J, Slivka A: Hepatobiliary disease in inflammatory bowel disease. Gastroenterol Clin North Am 31:329, 2002

174. Pardi DS, Tremaine WJ, Sandborn WJ, et al: Renal and urologic complications of inflammatory bowel disease. Am J Gastroenterol 93:504, 1998

175. Worcester EM: Stones from bowel disease. Endocrinol Metab Clin North Am 31:979, 2002

176. Wilson A, Reyes E, Ofman J: Prevalence and outcomes of anemia in inflammatory bowel disease: a systematic review of the literature. Am J Med 116(suppl 7A):44S, 2004

177. van Bodegraven AA: Haemostasis in inflammatory bowel diseases: clinical relevance. Scand J Gastroenterol Suppl (239):51, 2003

178. Regueiro M, Valentine J, Plevy S, et al: Infliximab for treatment of pyoderma gangrenosum associated with inflammatory bowel disease. Am J Gastroenterol 98:1821, 2003

179. Itzkowitz SH, Yio X: Inflammation and cancer IV. Colorectal cancer in inflammatory bowel disease: the role of inflammation. Am J Physiol Gastrointest Liver Physiol 287:G7, 2004

180. Rutter M, Saunders B, Wilkinson K, et al: Severity of inflammation is a risk factor for colorectal neoplasia in ulcerative colitis. Gastroenterology 126:451, 2004

181. Itzkowitz SH: Cancer prevention in patients with inflammatory bowel disease. Gastroenterol Clin North Am 31:1133, 2002

182. Mpofu C, Watson AJ, Rhodes JM: Strategies for detecting colon cancer and/or dysplasia in patients with inflammatory bowel disease. Cochrane Database Syst Rev (2):CD000279, 2004

183. Ullman T, Croog V, Harpaz N, et al: Progression of flat low-grade dysplasia to advanced neoplasia in patients with ulcerative colitis. Gastroenterology 125:1311, 2003

184. Lichtenstein GR: Reduction of colorectal cancer risk in patients with Crohn's disease. Rev Gastroenterol Disord 2(suppl 2):S16, 2002

185. Loftus EV Jr, Tremaine WJ, Habermann TM, et al: Risk of lymphoma in inflammatory bowel disease. Am J Gastroenterol 95:2308, 2000

186. Bebb JR, Logan RP: Review article: does the use of immunosuppressive therapy in inflammatory bowel disease increase the risk of developing lymphoma? Aliment Pharmacol Ther 15:1843, 2001

187. Farrell RJ, Ang Y, Kileen P, et al: Increased incidence of non-Hodgkin's lymphoma in inflammatory bowel disease patients on immunosuppressive therapy but overall risk is low. Gut 47:514, 2000

188. Fraser AG, Orchard TR, Robinson EM, et al: Long-term risk of malignancy after treatment of inflammatory bowel disease with azathioprine. Aliment Pharmacol Ther 16:1225, 2002

189. Dayharsh GA, Loftus EV Jr, Sandborn WJ, et al: Epstein-Barr virus–positive lymphoma in patients with inflammatory bowel disease treated with azathioprine or 6-mercaptopurine. Gastroenterology 122:72, 2002

190. Loftus EV Jr, Sandborn WJ: Lymphoma risk in inflammatory bowel disease: influences of referral bias and therapy. Gastroenterology 121:1239, 2001

Acknowledgment

Figure 4   Tom Moore.

64 Diverticulosis, Diverticulitis, and Appendicitis

William V. Harford, M.D., F.A.C.P.

Colonic Diverticular Disease

Colonic diverticula are herniations of colonic mucosa and submucosa that extend through the muscularis propria. They occur where perforating arteries traverse the circular muscle layer and form parallel rows between the mesenteric and antimesenteric taenia. Diverticulosis describes the presence of diverticula, whereas diverticulitis refers to the inflammation of diverticula. Diverticulosis is a common condition; of persons with known diverticulosis, about 10% to 20% will develop diverticulitis or diverticular bleeding.[1]

DIVERTICULOSIS

Epidemiology

There are no population-based studies of the prevalence of diverticulosis. About 1% of the United States population reported having diverticulosis in the 1983–1987 National Health Interview Survey (NHIS). Women were two to three times more likely than men to report having diverticulosis, and whites were more likely than African Americans. The prevalence of self-reported diverticulosis increased with age. It was 0.1% at 45 years of age or younger and 4.4% at 75 years of age or older. Unrecognized diverticulosis is more common than known diverticulosis. It is estimated that 10% to 20% of persons older than 50 years have diverticulosis.[2] In Western countries, diverticula occur predominantly in the left colon, particularly the sigmoid colon, which is involved in 95% of cases. In the Orient, including Japan, diverticula occur predominantly in the right colon.[3,4]

About 85% of persons with self-reported diverticulosis in the NHIS were asymptomatic or reported no limitations resulting from diverticulosis. Patients who are asymptomatic at the time of diagnosis are unlikely to develop diverticulitis. In the First National Health and Nutrition Examination Survey (NHANES I) Epidemiologic Follow-up Study, a cohort of physicians with asymptomatic diverticulosis were followed for a 10-year period. The probability of hospitalization for diverticular disease was less than 1% for physicians who were 25 to 44 years of age at the beginning of the follow-up period and was about 5% for those who were 65 to 74 years of age.[2] In English and Finnish populations, the risk of acute diverticulitis was about four per 100,000 population per year.[5,6] The risk of diverticulitis increases with age and with the use of nonsteroidal anti-inflammatory drugs (NSAIDs), steroids, and opioids.[1,5,7]

Pathogenesis

Reduced colonic diameter and reduced colonic wall compliance are felt to predispose persons to diverticulosis. A reduced colonic diameter causes the formation of closed segments during colonic contractions, thereby increasing intraluminal pressure. Diverticulosis is common in countries where a low-fiber diet is consumed, because a low-fiber diet leads to reduced stool volume and colonic diameter, particularly in the sigmoid colon. A high-fiber diet reduces the risk of diverticular disease.[8,9] Patients with diverticulosis have an age-related increase in elastin deposition and collagen cross-linking.[10] Increased proline absorption from Western diets may be a factor contributing to increased elastin deposition.[11] Changes in elastin and collagen lead to thickening and shortening of the taenia and circular muscle layers (myochosis) in many patients with diverticulosis, increasing the possibility of segmentation. These elastin and collagen changes also result in reduced compliance of the colonic wall, so that for any colonic diameter, intraluminal pressure is higher than it is in patients with normal compliance.[12] Increased intraluminal pressure leads to herniation of mucosa through the defects in the muscularis of the colon associated with perforating arteries.

Only mucosa and submucosa separate the lumen of diverticula from the colonic serosa. Diverticulitis may result from abrasion of the mucosa by inspissated stool. Changes in bacterial colonic microflora have been reported in patients with diverticulosis. It has been proposed that these changes may lead to low-grade chronic inflammation, predisposing to the development of diverticulitis.[13,14] Chronic intermittent use of oral rifaximin, a poorly absorbed antibiotic, and mesalazine, an anti-inflammatory agent, appears to reduce the risk of diverticulitis.[15,16]

Diverticula form where medium-sized perforating arteries penetrate the muscularis propria to enter the submucosa. Pathologic examination has been reported to reveal evidence of chronic injury to the internal elastic lamina and media of these arteries. This injury can cause arterial rupture into the lumen of the colon. Diverticular bleeding is rarely associated with acute diverticulitis.

DIVERTICULITIS

Diagnosis

Diverticula are most often discovered incidentally during investigation of another condition. Diverticulitis varies in presentation and severity. The diagnosis of acute diverticulitis is often made on the basis of the history and physical examination, which includes abdominal, rectal, and pelvic examinations; imaging studies are used to confirm the diagnosis. Computed tomography has become the optimal method of investigation for patients suspected of having diverticulitis. The modified Hinchey classification, which takes into account both clinical and CT findings, is useful for prognosis and management [*see Table 1*].[17]

Clinical presentation Patients with mild diverticulitis (Hinchey stage 0 or 1a) have limited inflammation or phlegmon in the area of the involved diverticulum. They typically present with left-sided lower abdominal pain and localized tenderness, low-grade fever, anorexia, and nausea without vomiting. They may have mild leukocytosis. Patients with mild diverticulitis can often be managed without hospitalization.[4] Patients with more severe diverticulitis usually must be hospitalized. They often have a diverticular abscess (stage 1b or 2), which is usually contained in the pericolic fat, mesentery, or pelvis but may extend beyond the pelvis. Patients with an abscess (or large phlegmon) commonly have systemic toxicity, high fever, severe localized abdominal tenderness, and leukocytosis. The phlegmon or abscess may be palpable. Rupture of a diverticular abscess results in purulent peritonitis (stage 3), which usually leads to diffuse abdominal tenderness. Free perforation of a diverticulum with fecal soiling of the abdominal cavity leads to feculent peritonitis (stage 4). Feculent peritonitis causes severe acute generalized peritonitis and sepsis.

Colonic inflammation associated with diverticulitis may cause either diarrhea or constipation. Acute diverticulitis may lead to colonic or small bowel obstruction. Repeated episodes of diverticulitis with fibrosis may cause colonic stricture.

Diverticulitis may cause fistula formation, most commonly from the sigmoid colon to the bladder. Inflammation adjacent to the bladder may lead to dysuria even if no fistula is present. Overt lower gastrointestinal bleeding is rarely associated with acute diverticulitis. Other causes of bleeding (e.g., angiodysplasia, a neoplasm, or inflammatory bowel disease) must be excluded in patients with diverticulitis who present with overt bleeding or who have positive fecal occult blood tests.

In a large retrospective study of patients who required hospitalization for acute diverticulitis, 72% of patients had no abscess (Hinchey stage 0 or 1a); 19%, an abscess (Hinchey stage 1b or 2); 5%, prurulent peritonitis (Hinchey stage 3); 1%, feculent peritonitis (Hinchey stage 4); 1%, obstruction; and 2%, fistula. Overall, surgery was required in 26% of patients.[17] Comparable distribution of stages has been reported in other studies.[18-20]

Diverticulitis in areas other than the sigmoid colon is uncommon in Western countries. In such cases, clinical presentation may be atypical and confusing. Cases of right-sided colonic and cecal diverticulitis are often clinically indistinguishable from appendicitis.[21-23]

Diverticulitis may lead to episodic abdominal pain. In a study of patients previously hospitalized for acute diverticulitis, 70% subsequently experienced new, recurrent episodes of abdominal pain, usually lasting less than 4 hours.[24] After the first episode of diverticulitis, 30% to 50% of patients have subsequent episodes. About 20% to 25% of patients have subsequent episodes of complicated diverticulitis within the first several years of follow-up.[18,19] Patients who initially have a large diverticular abscess have an increased risk of recurrence of diverticulitis, even if the

Table 1   Modified Hinchey Classification of Acute Diverticulitis[17]

Stage	Characteristic Symptoms
0	Mild clinical diverticulitis (left lower quadrant abdominal pain, low-grade fever, leukocytosis, no imaging information)
1a	Confined pericolic inflammation, no abscess
1b	Confined pericolic abscess (abscess or phlegmon may be palpable; fever; severe, localized abdominal pain)
2	Pelvic, retroperitoneal, or distant intraperitoneal abscess (abscess or phlegmon may be palpable, fever, systemic toxicity)
3	Generalized purulent peritonitis, no communication with bowel lumen
4	Feculent peritonitis, open communication with bowel lumen
Complications	Fistula, obstruction (large bowel or small bowel)

abscess is treated by antibiotics and drainage by interventional radiology.[17]

Imaging studies   Patients with symptoms and signs of mild, uncomplicated diverticulitis who respond promptly to outpatient medical treatment do not necessarily require an imaging study immediately. Confirmation of the diagnosis can be delayed for 4 to 6 weeks, when active inflammation has resolved. If there is uncertainty about the diagnosis, outpatient CT is performed to exclude conditions that mimic diverticulitis [*see* Differential Diagnosis, *below*].

On CT, diverticula are seen as collections of gas or contrast measuring 5 to 10 mm and protruding from the wall of the colon. Symmetrical thickening of the colonic wall may be noted. In diverticulitis, a phlegmon is marked by streaky enhancement of pericolic or perirectal soft tissue and the mesentery [*see Figure 1*]. Perforation and fistula may be visualized by air or contrast. Abscess is seen as one or more discrete fluid collections.[25] If the abscess communicates with the colonic lumen, contrast may enter the abscess cavity. CT readily detects remote abscess. When abscess is detected, the feasibility of CT-guided drainage can be determined.[8,26,27]

Diagnostic tests   The objectives of diagnostic testing in suspected acute diverticulitis are to exclude other important conditions, to confirm the diagnosis of diverticulitis, to determine if complications have occurred, and to plan treatment.

Leukocytosis is usually present in acute diverticulitis. The urine may contain a modest number of white cells or red blood cells. Recurrent or polymicrobial urinary tract infections should suggest the possibility of a colovesical fistula. Plain abdominal x-rays are most useful to exclude other abdominal conditions, such as intestinal obstruction. Occasionally, an inflammatory mass with gas may be noted, confirming the presence of an abscess. Free air in the abdominal cavity is unusual in diverticulitis.

Colonoscopy is generally not required for diagnosis in suspected acute diverticulitis, and air insufflation caused by introduction of air may worsen a contained perforation. Colonoscopy can be performed with relative safety if no fluid or free air is noted on abdominal CT.[28] After treatment and resolution of an acute epsisode of diverticulitis, patients should have an elective examination either by colonoscopy or by fiberoptic sigmoidoscopy after barium enema ; the purpose of elective colonoscopy is to exclude the presence of colon cancer and inflammatory bowel disease.[29] Barium enema should be avoided in suspected acute diverticulitis because of the risk of barium contamination of the peritoneum if a perforation is present.

Differential Diagnosis

A number of conditions may mimic acute diverticulitis [*see Table 2*]; among the differential diagnoses less frequently considered are epiploic appendagitis and omental torsion/infarction, which may be distinguished from diverticulitis by CT. Epiploic appendices are small peritoneal pouches filled with fat that are situated along the margin of the colon. These structures can become inflamed, resulting in acute epiploic appendagitis, which may mimic diverticulitis or appendicitis. The clinical presentation consists of acute abdominal pain and tenderness. Peritoneal signs sometimes occur, as do low-grade fever and mild leukocytosis. On CT scan, epiploic appendagitis has a characteristic appearance: an oval, fatty mass surrounded by mesenteric stranding, and mural thickening of adjacent colon is typically present.[30-32]

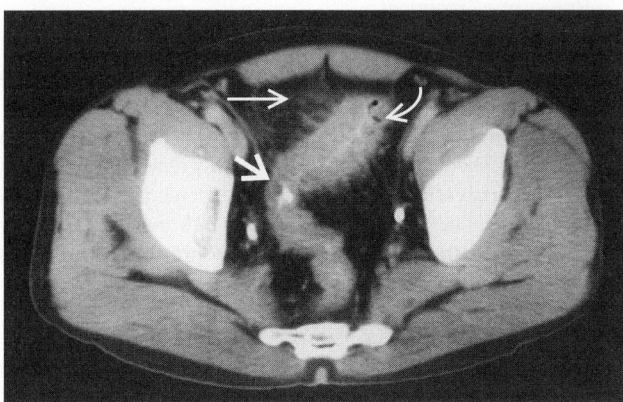

Figure 1 **CT diverticulitis. The wall of the sigmoid colon is thickened (broad arrow). Air is seen within a diverticulum (curved arrow). Streaky enhancement of pericolis fat (horizontal arrow) is caused by inflammation.**

In rare cases, the omentum may undergo spontaneous torsion, causing ischemia or infarction. The clinical presentation may mimic acute diverticulitis, appendicitis, or cholecystitis. The diagnosis of omental torsion may be determined preoperatively by the use of abdominal CT.[33,34]

Diverticulitis in Specific Patient Groups

Immunocompromised patients Immunocompromised patients, such as those on glucocorticoids or those who have had an organ transplant, may not manifest the usual signs of diverticulitis, and diagnosis in these patients may therefore be delayed. The severity of diverticulitis may also be underestimated. The threshold for diagnostic evaluation should be low in such patients.

Abdominal CT with rapid helical technique is the most useful diagnostic study when complicated acute diverticulitis is suspected or when the diagnosis is not clear. Specificity and sensitivity are reported to be over 95%.[35] The colon should be filled with water-soluble contrast given either orally (most commonly) or by gentle enema. CT can confirm the diagnosis, identify complications, and aid in planning of treatment. If the patient does not have acute diverticulitis, abdominal CT will usually lead to the correct diagnosis. Conditions other than diverticulitis are found in up to 25% of CT studies.[35]

Women suspected of gynecologic conditions Abdominal ultrasonography may be most useful for women when gynecologic conditions are part of the differential diagnosis. Abdominal ultrasonography may be an alternative test when CT is not readily available or is contraindicated. On ultrasound, diverticula are echogenic and produce acoustic shadowing. On a graded compression ultrasound, the colonic wall in diverticulitis is thickened, noncompressible, and hypoechoic. The involved segment is hypoperistaltic. A phlegmon causes irregular enhancement of pericolic soft tissue, whereas an abscess appears as a fluid collection, within which gas is readily appreciated, if present. When an abscess is identified on ultrasound, a CT scan should be performed to evaluate the potential for radiographic drainage.[26,36]

Magnetic resonance imaging has been reported to be useful in the diagnosis of acute diverticulitis in pregnant women. MRI has the advantage over CT of avoiding fetal exposure to radiation.[37]

TREATMENT

Outpatient Management

Fewer than 20% of patients with acute diverticulitis require hospitalization.[38] Patients who present with mild diverticulitis should be placed on a regimen of oral fluid/electrolyte solution (e.g., a sports drink) and oral antibiotics. Patients should eat no solid foods during this period. The antibiotic regimen should provide coverage against gram-negative and anaerobic bacteria. For example, amoxicillin–clavulanic acid at a dosage of 875/125 mg twice daily is acceptable monotherapy; a suitable combination therapy is a quinolone (e.g., levofloxacin, 750 mg once daily) combined with metronidazole (500 mg twice daily).[39] The patient should be instructed to report back at once if symptoms worsen. Reevaluation is scheduled for 48 to 72 hours after the office visit. If improvement is satisfactory, the diet is advanced to full liquids, antibiotics are continued, and another office visit is scheduled at 7 days. If improvement is evident at 7 days, the patient can resume a regular diet and discontinue antibiotics.[4] Patients whose symptoms worsen or who do not have a favorable response within 48 to 72 hours should be hospitalized. If there is uncertainty about the diagnosis, outpatient CT is performed. An elective colonoscopy or sigmoidoscopy and barium enema exam is scheduled for 6 weeks after the acute illness, unless such a study was performed within the past 5 years.

Inpatient Management

Patients should be hospitalized if there are signs of severe or complicated diverticulitis, such as systemic toxicity, temperature exceeding 101° F (38.3° C), vomiting, an abdominal mass, or signs of peritonitis; patients should also be hospitalized if they fail to respond within 2 to 3 days to outpatient management. Hospitalized patients should be placed on bowel rest and given intravenous fluids and antibiotics. Antibiotic coverage must include both aerobic and anaerobic gram-negative bacteria. An example of a suitable monotherapy regimen is ampicillin-sulbactam (1.5 to 3.0 g every 6 hours); an acceptable combination therapy regimen is levofloxacin (750 mg I.V. once daily) combined with metronidazole (1 g I.V. every 12 hours).[39] A surgical consultation should be obtained upon admission. CT scanning should be done promptly. If a phlegmon or small abscess (< 3 cm) is found, antibiotic treatment alone may suffice. Abscesses larger than 5 cm should be drained by interventional radiology, unless radiologic drainage is contraindicated by the location of the abscess or the presence of multiple abscesses.[27] Antibiotic treatment and radiologic abscess drainage often allow control of infection in cases of complicated diverticulitis. Control of infection im-

---

Table 2 Differential Diagnosis of Acute Diverticulitis

Inflammatory bowel disease: Crohn disease, ulcerative colitis
Perforated colon cancer
Ischemic colitis
Infectious colitis
Mesenteric appendagitis, omental torsion
Gynecologic conditions: pelvic inflammatory disease; ovarian torsion, ruptured follicle or cyst; endometriosis
Appendicitis (situs inversus)

proves the possibility of elective single-stage resection and re-anastomosis. Urgent surgery should be considered for patients with large abscesses that are not amenable to radiologic drainage or with multiple abscesses; for patients failing to respond within 48 to 72 hours; and for patients with evidence of free rupture of an abscess or a large perforation with fecal spillage. About 20% to 30% of patients hospitalized for the first time with acute diverticulitis require either urgent or elective surgery.[17]

Surgical Treatment

Open resection The optimal surgical treatment of acute diverticulitis involves resection of the involved segment at the initial operation whenever this is technically possible. Leaving the diseased colon in place and performing only a diverting colostomy is associated with a higher rate of complications than primary resection. Primary reanastomosis is generally possible.[40] If there is concern that the anastomosis is at undue risk of disruption, a temporary diverting ileostomy may be performed. Alternatively, the distal rectal segment can be closed (Hartmann procedure) and a descending colostomy created. Patients undergoing surgery for diverticulitis should be informed about the possibility that an ostomy, if created, may be permanent. Because of comorbidities and other issues, about 35% of ostomies performed for diverticulitis will still be in place 4 years after surgery.[41] In the case of sigmoid diverticulitis, it is important to extend the resection to the rectum—to include the entire segment involved with diverticula—because failure to do so markedly increases the probability of recurrent diverticulitis.[42,43]

Laparoscopic surgery Laparoscopic surgical techniques are increasingly being used for diverticular disease. Results of laparoscopic resection for diverticulitis are the same as those of open resection if the resection extends to the rectum and no sigmoid colon is left in place.[44,45] Laparoscopic resection is safe and effective; its advantages over open surgery include decreased blood loss, faster recovery of bowel function, and shorter hospital stay. There are no differences in operative time or mortality with the two procedures.[45] Less than 10% of cases require conversion from laparoscopic to open resection.[44]

Elective surgery Factors considered in the recommendation of elective surgery for diverticulitis include the general health of the patient, the number and severity of episodes, and the degree to which symptoms resolve between episodes. As mentioned, about 20% to 25% of patients will have a subsequent episode of complicated diverticulitis within several years after their first episode.[18,20] Surgery is often recommended after one episode of complicated diverticulitis or two episodes of uncomplicated diverticulitis; however, a decision analysis study suggested that the best overall outcome—taking into account mortality, morbidity, the number of surgical procedures, and the number of ostomies—may be achieved if elective colectomy is recommended after the fourth episode of uncomplicated diverticulitis, which is a more conservative recommendation than is generally practiced.[46]

Young, overweight men have been reported in some series to have a higher risk of complicated diverticulitis and recurrent diverticulitis than other patients. Some surgeons therefore recommend surgery after the first episode of diverticulitis in such patients[29,47,48]; however, this increased risk has not been confirmed in other series, and some surgeons have suggested that the recommendation for surgery after the first episode be tempered.[20,49,50]

Preventive Treatment

A diet high in insoluble fiber and low in fat and red meat appears to reduce the risk of diverticular disease. Higher levels of physical activity are also associated with reduced risk of diverticulitis.[8,9]

The intermittent use of rifaximin, a poorly absorbed oral antibiotic, has been reported to provide a greater reduction of symptoms of diverticular disease and risk of recurrence than the use of fiber alone.[15] Rifaximin is given in a dosage of 400 mg by mouth twice daily for 1 week of each month. Mesalamine has been used for the same purpose in a dosage of 800 mg by mouth twice daily for 1 week of each month. The combination of rifaximin and mesalamine has been reported to be more effective than mesalamine alone.[16]

It is prudent to advise patients with a history of diverticular disease to avoid NSAIDs if possible, as these medications have been associated with an increased risk of complications.[5,7]

COMPLICATIONS OF DIVERTICULAR DISEASE

Fistula

Fistula is the presenting complication in 10% to 15% of patients who require surgery for diverticular disease. There is often no history of acute diverticulitis. Patients may present with symptoms related primarily to the organ involved with the diverticular fistula, which is the bladder in most cases. Diverticular disease is the most common cause of colovesical fistula, followed by colon cancer and Crohn disease. Colovesical fistulas are much less common in women than in men, presumably because the uterus is interposed between the sigmoid colon and the bladder. Patients with colovesical fistulas usually present with recurrent polymicrobial bladder infections, pneumaturia, or both. Fistulas may also connect with other parts of the colon, the small bowel, the uterus, or the vagina. Colocutaneous fistulas are unusual and generally occur after surgery for diverticulitis.[51]

Colovesical fistulas are difficult to visualize. CT scanning may be the most useful single study. Even though fistulas are rarely directly visualized, CT is very sensitive for detection of air in the bladder, which is virtually diagnostic of an enterovesical fistula in the absence of prior bladder catheterization. CT demonstrates the presence of diverticula, and thickening of the bladder wall adjacent to an area of diverticulitis supports the diagnosis.[52] Colovesical fistulas are often not identified by a barium enema study, although secondary changes of diverticulitis are usually apparent. Cystoscopy often reveals focal mucosal inflammation in the area of a fistula, even though the opening is not apparent. Fistulas may be visualized by contrast cystography.[53] Colonoscopy should be done at some point to exclude cancer or inflammatory bowel disease, but it rarely reveals the fistula. CT, barium enema, cystoscopy, and colonoscopy are complementary studies for the evaluation of a suspected colovesical fistula.[52] Patients with a diverticular fistula should have elective surgical resection of the involved segment of colon once the acute inflammatory process has been controlled. In the case of colovesical fistulas, the adherent colon can usually be dissected off the bladder and the involved bladder oversewn, rather than resected.[54]

Obstruction and Stricture

Acute obstruction during an episode of diverticulitis is often self-limited. It may be caused by a large phlegmon or abscess. Secondary ileus may mimic obstruction. Chronic stricture is an uncommon presentation of diverticular disease. It usually occurs after repeated episodes of diverticulitis. A diverticular stricture may be difficult to distinguish from a malignant stricture, particularly by CT or a barium enema study. Colonoscopy with biopsies is the best means of making this distinction, although visualization may be limited even with colonoscopy.

Segmental Colitis Associated with Diverticular Disease

In about 1% of cases, chronic diverticular disease is associated with patchy mucosal hemorrhage, congestion, and granularity in the sigmoid colon. On microscopic examination, a lymphocytic infiltrate, lymphoglandular complexes, mucin depletion, mild cryptitis, crypt distortion, Paneth cell metaplasia, and ulceration can be seen. These changes may mimic Crohn colitis, ulcerative colitis, or ischemic colitis. However, in segmental colitis associated with diverticular disease (SCAD), the changes are limited to areas of diverticulosis.[55,56]

Risk of Colon Cancer in Diverticular Disease

Some studies have shown an increased risk of sigmoid colon cancer in patients with a history of diverticulitis, but other studies have not confirmed this finding.[57-59] In addition to the difficulty in distinguishing a diverticular stricture from a malignant stricture, perforated colon cancer can mimic acute diverticulitis accompanied by a phlegmon or abscess. Thus, it seems prudent to recommend elective colonoscopy to patients with diverticular disease.

DIVERTICULAR BLEEDING

Diverticular bleeding is less frequent than diverticulitis as a complication of diverticulosis. It is difficult to arrive at a firm estimate of what proportion of major lower gastrointestinal bleeding is caused by colonic diverticula. Estimates have ranged from 15% to 56%.[60-62] In many cases, the source is presumed to be diverticular when no other cause is found.

Diverticular bleeding is usually sudden and painless. Typically, moderate to large amounts of bright-red blood, clots, or maroon stool are passed. Bleeding stops spontaneously in 70% to 80% of cases; bleeding eventually recurs in 25% to 35% of cases.[63,64] Lower gastrointestinal bleeding (occult bleeding in particular) should not be attributed to diverticulosis unless other causes have been excluded. The most common causes of lower gastrointestinal bleeding in adults are diverticulosis, inflammatory bowel disease, neoplasm, angioectasias, benign anorectal disease, and upper gastrointestinal sources.[65]

Practice guidelines for the evaluation and management of lower gastrointestinal bleeding have been published.[64]

Emergent Management and Evaluation

The first priority in lower gastrointestinal bleeding is volume restoration with intravenous fluids and blood. During resuscitation, a directed history is taken and a physical examination is performed; the physical examination includes anoscopy and proctoscopy to exclude an anorectal source. A nasogastric aspirate should be obtained, because about 10% to 15% of apparent major lower gastrointestinal bleeding is, in actuality, from an upper gastrointestinal source.[61] Lack of blood in the nasogastric aspirate, however, is not conclusive proof of a lower gastrointestinal source. Bleeding from an upper gastrointestinal source may have stopped, and the stomach may have evacuated residual blood. Blood from a duodenal source may not reflux into the stomach. Some clinicians perform an upper gastrointestinal endoscopy before colonoscopy even if the nasogastric aspirate is negative for blood, particularly for apparent major lower gastrointestinal bleeding.

Colonoscopy Many clinicians consider colonoscopy to be the most useful initial study for the evaluation of patients presenting with major lower gastrointestinal bleeding of unknown cause.[66] Lower gastrointestinal bleeding is usually intermittent and often stops before hospital admission or shortly thereafter. Adequate colonic purging followed by colonoscopy is almost always possible even in spite of moderate active lower gastrointestinal bleeding.[61,66] The most important contribution of colonoscopy is to establish a presumptive diagnosis of diverticular bleeding by excluding other causes and to determine the distribution of diverticula, which is important if colonic resection becomes necessary. Some authors recommend urgent colonoscopy and report a high success rate in localizing and treating diverticula responsible for bleeding.[66] In another report, however, there was no correlation between the timing of colonoscopy and success in localizing the bleeding diverticulum over an interval of 7 to 29 hours.[67] If active bleeding or an adherent clot is found at the time of colonoscopy, endoscopic therapy can be performed with epinephrine injection, cautery, hemostatic clips, or banding.[68,69]

Labeled blood cell scintigraphy Technetium-99m (^{99m}Tc)–labeled red blood cell scintigraphy is another tool for the evaluation of acute lower gastrointestinal bleeding. After injection with ^{99m}Tc, imaging is done continuously for 60 to 120 minutes. Dynamic scans are viewed in a computer-generated cinematic format. Continuous scanning improves the probability of detecting intermittent bleeding.[70] The radioactive label remains active for over 24 hours; thus, if the scan is not positive initially, scanning can be repeated at any time during the first day if there are indications of recurrent bleeding. A scan is considered positive if there is a focus of increased activity that changes in location and intensity over time [see Figure 2]. ^{99m}Tc-labeled red blood cell scanning is the most sensitive study for detection of acute gastrointestinal bleeding. It can theoretically detect bleeding rates as low as 0.5 ml/min. Localization of bleeding to the small bowel, right colon, or left colon is generally possible, but reports of the accuracy of ^{99m}Tc-labeled red blood cell scanning have been inconsistent.[70-72] False positive readings may occur with vascular neoplasms, inflammatory conditions, vascular grafts, varices, splenosis, and bladder or penile activity.

^{99m}Tc scanning does not elucidate the cause of bleeding; rather, it demonstrates active bleeding and the approximate location of its source. Colonoscopy is still necessary to determine the presence of diverticula and exclude other potential colonic sources. Once diverticula have been established as the probable cause of bleeding, scanning has a role in detecting recurrent bleeding. A positive ^{99m}Tc scan also provides prognostic information; patients with positive scans are much more likely to have positive arteriograms and are more likely to require surgery than those with negative scans.[72]

Treatment

Visceral angiography and vasopressin infusion Visceral angiography may be useful in persistent moderate to severe lower gastrointestinal bleeding, particularly when the site has not been discovered by colonoscopy and upper gastrointestinal endoscopy or when colonoscopy is not feasible. Angiography can provide precise localization of bleeding in patients who have a positive bleeding scan. If active bleeding is detected and local-

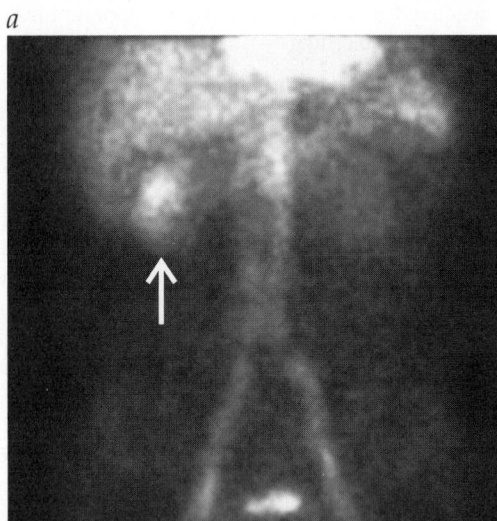 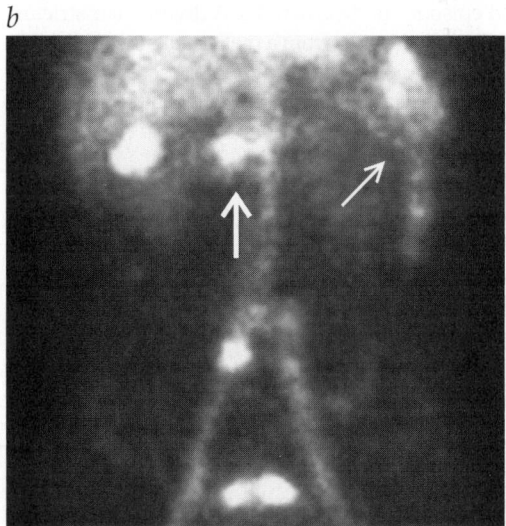

Figure 2 (*a*) Technetium-99m red cell scanning shows increased tracer activity in the area of the hepatic flexure (arrow). (*b*) Later, tracer activity has progressed to the transverse colon (broad arrow), as well as the splenic flexure and descending colon (small arrow), confirming that the right colon is the source of the bleeding.

ized, it may then be treated with intra-arterial vasopressin infusion. Rebleeding occurs in 25% of patients when the vasopressin infusion is stopped. Even temporary control may provide time to stabilize the patient and prepare for elective surgery.[64,71]

Arterial embolization Arterial embolization of the bleeding artery has been reported, but it is associated with a substantial risk of intestinal infarction, particularly if followed by vasopressin infusion.[71] Bowel or myocardial ischemia, as well as other complications inherent to contrast arteriography, may complicate both vasopressin infusion and embolization.

Surgery About 20% of patients hospitalized for diverticular bleeding require surgery during that hospitalization.[63] Patients who initially require four units or more of blood have a 50% risk of continued bleeding, as compared with a 2% risk of continued bleeding for patients who require two or more units of blood. Persistent instability despite aggressive resuscitation demands surgical intervention.[63]

Elective surgery for recurrent bleeding The risk of recurrent diverticular bleeding after the first episode is about 10% after 2 years and 25% after 4 years.[60] The risk is higher after a second episode. Elective surgery is usually recommended after two or more episodes of bleeding. If diverticula are limited to the left side of the colon, left hemicolectomy is appropriate. The decision regarding the extent of resection is more difficult when diverticula are distributed throughout the colon. If all previous episodes of diverticular bleeding have been localized to either the right or the left side by scintigraphy or angiography, some clinicians would advocate a corresponding hemicolectomy. The risk of recurrent bleeding from diverticula in the remaining colon is not known. Other clinicians would recommend a subtotal colectomy. Occasionally, persistent or recurrent severe lower gastrointestinal bleeding cannot be localized. Blind segmental resection is associated with an unacceptable recurrence rate, and subtotal colectomy is the favored procedure.[61]

Appendicitis

EPIDEMIOLOGY

The lifetime risk of appendicitis is about 9% for males and 7% for females.[73] Appendicitis rarely occurs in infants; it increases in frequency between the ages of 2 and 4; and it reaches a peak between the ages of 10 and 20. About 80% of cases occur before the age of 45. Nevertheless, there is a steady low incidence in older individuals. The mortality associated with acute appendicitis declined between 1945 and 1960, coincident with advances in antibiotic treatment. In 1990, the mortality associated with acute uncomplicated appendicitis was approximately equal to that associated with general anesthesia. However, the mortality associated with gangrenous appendicitis is about 0.5 %, and that of perforated appendicitis is 5%. Most deaths from acute appendicitis occur in persons older than 65 years.[73]

ANATOMY AND PATHOGENESIS

The adult appendix is a tubular structure that is 4 to 25 cm long and arises from the medial posterior wall of the cecum several centimeters below the ileocecal valve. Its location in the peritoneal cavity varies. Atypical locations, such as the pelvis, retrocecal area, and right upper quadrant, lead to atypical clinical presentations [*see* Atypical Presentations, *below*].

Appendicitis is generally caused by obstruction of the lumen of the appendix, followed by infection. The appendix has abundant lymphoid tissue. Appendicitis increases in frequency during the period of lymphoid hyperplasia in childhood. During periods of childhood enteric infection, lymphoid tissue may obstruct the appendiceal lumen. About one third of cases of appendicitis are associated with obstruction by fecaliths. Foreign bodies, tumor (e.g., carcinoid or cecal adenocarcinoma), barium, and adhesions may also cause obstruction. Obstruction leads to bacterial overgrowth. Mucus accumulates in the lumen proximal to the obstruction, and intraluminal pressure increases. Impairment of lymphatic and venous drainage leads to mucosal ulceration, bacterial invasion, transmural inflammation, and ischemia. During the first 24 hours after obstruction, most patients have only inflammation. The incidence of necrosis and perforation increases markedly after that. Patients who present with a history of symptoms for 48 hours should be strongly suspected of having perforation and abscess. Free perforation causes generalized peritonitis.

DIAGNOSIS

Clinical Presentation

Appendicitis usually causes a distinctive sequence of symptoms and signs. More than 90% of patients with appendicitis complain of pain. The pain of appendicitis is initially caused by obstruction of the appendiceal lumen. It has the qualities of midgut visceral pain and is referred to the periumbilical or epigastric areas. It may be cramping or aching in nature, but it is often difficult for patients to describe. Within 12 to 24 hours, inflammation becomes transmural, involving the adjacent parietal peritoneum. Pain then becomes somatic in quality: sharper and more localized. At this time, patients may note exacerbation of pain by coughing, sneezing, or movement.

Anorexia is present in 80% to 90% of patients. Vomiting, when it occurs, does not occur initially but follows the onset of pain. Prominent vomiting is unusual and suggests the possibility of another diagnosis, such as gastroenteritis or small bowel obstruction. Fever is usually low grade. High fever or rigors suggest perforation.

Tenderness in the right lower quadrant can be elicited in more than 90% of patients. Proximity of the inflammatory process to the retroperitoneal muscles produces the psoas and obturator signs. The psoas sign is present when pain occurs as the patient raises the right leg against resistance or, alternatively, when the physician passively extends the right hip with the patient lying on the left side. The obturator sign is present when pain occurs upon internal rotation of the hip. Local hyperesthesia of the skin in the right lower quadrant may be noted. Voluntary guarding progresses to involuntary muscle rigidity as the inflammatory process worsens. Diffuse abdominal tenderness and rigidity suggest perforation. An abdominal mass suggests phlegmon or abscess formation.

The presentation of appendicitis may mimic a broad range of diseases [see Table 3].

There is evidence that appendicitis may resolve spontaneously and recur. Occasionally, the patient history includes previous episodes of acute appendicitis that resolved without treatment. Examination of appendixes removed incidentally at surgery or at autopsy sometimes show fibrosis and obliteration of a portion of the lumen, suggesting previous episodes of appendicitis.[74,75]

Atypical presentations Atypical presentations of appendicitis are as common as the classic presentation. Atypical location of the appendix leads to atypical symptoms and signs. An inflamed retrocecal appendix is relatively shielded from the parietal peritoneum. Pain may be less severe and abdominal tenderness less pronounced. The characteristic shift in pain location to the right lower quadrant may be delayed. A pelvic appendix may cause symptoms resulting from inflammation of the bladder or rectum, such as dysuria or tenesmus. In such cases, tenderness may be best elicited on pelvic or rectal examination. Incomplete intestinal rotation and third-trimester pregnancy displace the appendix toward the right upper quadrant, causing confusion with cholecystitis or perforated peptic ulcer.

Tip appendicitis and stump appendicitis In appendicitis that involves only the tip of the appendix, inflammation may be less severe and may resolve spontaneously; cases of recurrent appendicitis may involve such a pathophysiology. Partial visualization of the appendix on CT may be mistaken for complete filling and lead to a false negative reading.[76] Appendicitis has been reported to occur in the stump of the appendix that is left behind after a previous appendectomy; this can lead to confusion and a delay in diagnosis.[77]

Appendicitis and appendiceal tumors Tumor of the appendix, such as carcinoids, may obstruct the lumen and lead to appendicitis. In elderly men with appendicitis, there is a relatively high incidence of appendiceal tumors.[13,69]

Appendicitis in special groups of patients The diagnosis of appendicitis is difficult in certain groups of patients. Young children, for example, often do not express their symptoms clearly; they may present with only lethargy, irritability, and anorexia.[78] Elderly patients may have a reduced inflammatory reaction; in such cases, pain may be vague, and there may be less fever or abdominal tenderness.[79] Consideration of other diagnoses, such as diverticulitis, may delay surgery. Delayed diagnosis of appendicitis contributes to an incidence of perforation that is close to 20% in the elderly and small children.[80]

In women of childbearing age, gynecologic conditions and pregnancy cause difficulty in diagnosing appendicitis.[81] In one study, the preoperative diagnosis was incorrect in 25% of cases.[82] Complications of pregnancy attributable to appendicitis are considerable. Appendicitis in pregnancy has been reported to result in fetal loss in 33% of first-trimester cases and 14% of second-trimester cases.[82]

Diagnosis of appendicitis may also be difficult in immunosuppressed patients; for example, patients on glucocorticoids often have attenuated symptoms, leading to delay in presentation and a high incidence of complications. In patients with AIDS, symptoms may be typical, but concerns about a multiplicity of other diagnoses may delay surgery.

Diagnostic Evaluation

In the management of suspected appendicitis, it is important to minimize the delay to surgery—and thus reduce the risk of perforation—while at the same time minimizing the number of

---

Table 3 Differential Diagnosis
of Appendicitis

Crohn disease
Gynecologic conditions: ovarian torsion (especially during pregnancy), ovarian vein thrombosis, endometriosis
Perforated right-sided colon cancer
Cecal diverticulitis
Foreign-body perforation of right colon
Meckel diverticulitis
Omental torsion
Epiploic appendagitis
Infections (particularly those involving the ileum): yersinosis, brucellosis, salmonellosis, tuberculosis, amebiasis
Vasculitis
Appendiceal tumors
Psoas abscess

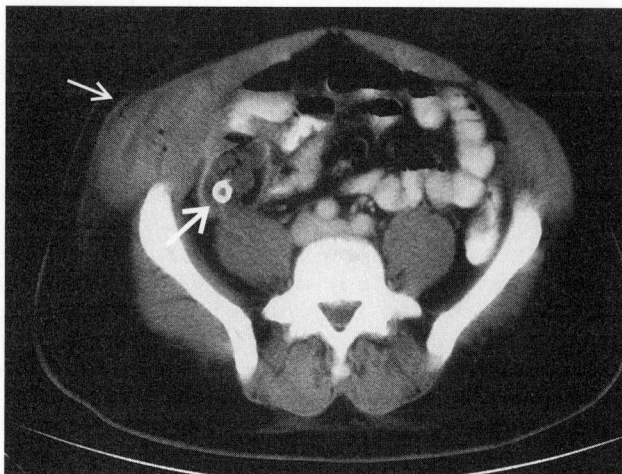

Figure 3   **CT of appendicitis. A calcified appendicolith is noted within a complex abscess containing fluid and air (broad arrow). The abscess involves the soft tissues of the abdominal wall (small arrow).**

unnecessary appendectomies. Taking into account the serious consequences of progression to perforation and the relatively low morbidity of appendectomy, most surgeons adopt a relatively aggressive approach to early surgery, accepting a 10% to 15% rate of negative appendectomies (i.e., negative exploration in patients with clinically suspected acute appendicitis).

Some factors that lead to a delay in diagnosis are not under physician control, such as a patient's delay in seeking medical care. Factors that are under physician control include decisions to perform additional diagnostic studies or to observe the patient for the purpose of improving diagnostic accuracy and reducing the number of unnecessary appendectomies. Clinical scoring systems have generally not been found to improve preoperative diagnostic accuracy.[83]

Abdominal examination   The abdominal examination is very important for the diagnosis of appendicitis. This has led some physicians to delay the administration of narcotic analgesics until a surgeon has had the opportunity to examine the patient. It has been proved that this practice is unnecessary: morphine does not change the physical examination in acute appendicitis, and early pain relief does not affect the decision for surgery in adults.[84,85]

Diagnostic Tests

The role of diagnostic studies for suspected appendicitis depends on the particular clinical presentation. In cases characterized by a classic presentation, it is standard practice to base the decision to operate primarily on the history and physical examination. A complete blood count, a urinalysis, and plain x-rays of the chest and abdomen may be obtained, but these serve the purpose of excluding other conditions rather than confirming the diagnosis of appendicitis. The total white blood cell count, the differential count, or both are abnormal in more than 90% of cases, but the decision to perform surgery should not be delayed if the white blood cell count is not elevated.[86]

In women of childbearing age, a pregnancy test is mandatory. In many cases, no further diagnostic studies are performed. Among women of childbearing age, the rate of negative appendectomy can be as high as 40%.[81] In other patients, particularly young children or the elderly, the presentation may be atypical

and the diagnosis uncertain. In such patients, additional diagnostic studies may be appropriate and helpful.

Abdominal ultrasound   Examination by transabdominal or transvaginal ultrasound or both is useful in pregnant and nonpregnant women of childbearing age to exclude a gynecologic cause of symptoms.[81,87] Ultrasound examination is also useful for evaluation of children in cases in which the diagnosis is doubtful. Sonography is widely available, fast, safe, and inexpensive.

On graded compression ultrasonography, the inflamed appendix is a noncompressible, aperistaltic tubular structure that is greater than 6 mm in diameter and located in the right lower quadrant. It has a target appearance, and the lumen is filled with anechoic or hyperechoic material. An appendicolith may be visualized in up to 30% of cases. Pericecal inflammation or phlegmon is seen as prominent fat; abscess appears as loculated fluid. In experienced hands, the sensitivity and specificity for the diagnosis of appendicitis are 85% and 95%, respectively.[88] Despite abdominal tenderness, most patients find the examination tolerable if it is performed gently. Marked peritonitis or abdominal gas may compromise the examination.

Abdominal ultrasound is not as accurate as CT for the diagnosis of appendicitis in adults and adolescents; in addition, it is not as useful as CT for the evaluation of phlegmon or abscess.[89]

Abdominal CT   Abdominal CT scanning can increase diagnostic accuracy in many cases of suspected appendicitis. The development of rapid scanning techniques has made CT readily available and practical even in emergency room settings. CT is useful when the diagnosis is unclear, as in elderly patients in whom diverticulitis and perforated colon cancer are important considerations. Abdominal CT may be helpful in women if pregnancy has been ruled out.[90] The routine use of appendiceal CT in the emergency room setting has been reported to reduce both the number of unnecessary appendectomies and delays before necessary appendectomies.[91] CT is helpful when an appendiceal abscess is suspected. It provides information about the size, location, and number of abscesses, as well as the feasibility of percutaneous drainage under radiologic guidance.[92]

CT for suspected appendicitis has been reported to have an accuracy of about 95%.[93,94] CT scan for appendicitis is best done using thin collimation helical scanning. The terminal ileum and cecum must be opacified with contrast that is administered by mouth or by rectum. Rectal administration of contrast has been reported to have advantages over oral contrast for assessing appendiceal filling.[84] The diagnosis of appendicitis is established when pericecal inflammation , phlegmon, or abscess is seen with either an appendicolith or an abnormal appendix. In appendicitis, the appendix is enlarged to more than 6 mm in diameter and fails to fill with contrast. If intravenous contrast has been given, the inflamed appendix will also show enhancement.[71] CT is useful for the evaluation of the degree and extent of periappendiceal inflammation [see *Figure 3*]. Inflammation may cause thickening of the adjacent cecum or ileum. Streakiness of periappendiceal fat is seen with phlegmon. Loculated fluid and, sometimes, gas bubbles are seen with abscess; if gas bubbles are not present, an air-fluid level may be apparent.

Barium enema   Since the advent of abdominal ultrasound and CT examination, barium enema has had little place in the evaluation of suspected appendicitis. Appendicitis is most likely to be discovered on barium enema exam when the study is done for determination of another diagnosis. In acute appendicitis, the appendix fails to fill with contrast on barium enema exam; this finding is more valuable in children than in adults, because the appendix fails to fill with contrast in 15% to 20% of normal adults. Partial filling of the appendix is often difficult to distinguish from complete filling, given the marked anatomic variations in the length of the appendix. Appendicitis may produce a mass effect or inflammatory changes in the adjacent cecum or ileum that can be appreciated by barium enema, but CT provides much more information than barium enema in this regard. Barium enema exam may be helpful in the evaluation of chronic or recurrent right lower quadrant abdominal conditions that mimic "chronic" appendicitis, such as Crohn disease.

TREATMENT

Preoperative Management

The treatment of appendicitis is prompt appendectomy. Preoperative preparation consists of intravenous volume repletion and antibiotics. For simple appendicitis, one dose of a broad-spectrum antibiotic given before surgery and one dose given postoperatively is sufficient.[95] One example of an appropriate regimen for adults is cefazolin (1.5 g I.V.) preoperatively and metronidazole (500 mg I.V.) postoperatively.[39]

If perforated appendicitis is suspected, antibiotic coverage should be broadened. An example of an acceptable regimen for adults is levofloxacin (750 mg I.V. once daily) combined with metronidazole (1 g I.V. every 12 hours).[39] If the presence of a phlegmon or abscess is confirmed, antibiotics are customarily continued for 7 to 14 days postoperatively. However, a prospective, randomized study found that adding a 7-day regimen of oral antibiotics after a course of intravenous antibiotics made no difference in outcome, either in complicated or uncomplicated appendicitis.[96]

Patients with free, unconfined perforation should have abdominal saline lavage during surgery. A prolonged ileus should be anticipated.

Appendectomy

Appendectomy can be performed by a traditional open incision or by laparoscopy. Compared to open appendectomy, laparoscopic appendectomy results in decreased wound infections but slightly increased intra-abdominal infections. Postoperative pain is reduced in laparoscopic appendectomy, and patients return to normal activity sooner. Overall, the benefits of laparoscopic appendectomy over open appendectomy are modest; the greatest benefits occur in women and obese patients.[97-99] The laparoscopic approach is useful in women because it allows for accurate diagnosis of gynecologic conditions if appendicitis is not responsible for the symptoms.[100,101]

Complications occur in fewer than 5% of cases of simple appendicitis but can be anticipated in 30% to 50% of cases of appendicitis after perforation. The most common complications are wound infections, intra-abdominal abscess, intestinal obstruction, and prolonged ileus. Postoperative abscesses are heralded by recurrent malaise, anorexia, and fever, and they are best evaluated by CT.

Interval Appendectomy

Some patients with a contained perforation can be managed by interval appendectomy after treatment with antibiotics or CT-guided percutaneous drainage. The information from preoperative CT or sonography is useful in planning therapy. If imaging shows a phlegmon or small abscess and the patient responds to antibiotic treatment within 48 hours, appendectomy may be postponed for 6 weeks, until the inflammatory process has subsided. If the abscess is large but well circumscribed and accessible, CT-guided percutaneous catheter drainage may be used to reduce the abscess before surgery. The catheter is placed in the abscess and left until drainage from the abscess becomes minimal.[92] If drainage is successful, appendectomy can be postponed for 6 weeks. However, if a patient with a contained perforation does not respond promptly to antibiotic treatment or drainage, surgery should not be delayed. Catheter drainage is not possible if imaging shows a poorly defined or multilocular abscess or if the abscess is not accessible to percutaneous drainage.

If a patient is operated on for suspected appendicitis and the appendix is found to be normal at surgery, it should be removed to prevent future confusion. The cecum and terminal ileum should be examined for evidence of Crohn disease or other acute inflammatory bowel disease, for tumor, or for Meckel diverticulitis. Lymph nodes in the area should be inspected for evidence of mesenteric adenitis, and biopsies should be performed if the lymph nodes appear abnormal. The gallbladder and duodenum should be palpated. If necessary, the incision should be extended to permit wider exposure. Before closing, the surgeon must feel confident that the cause of the clinical presentation has been explained and that there is no other acute abdominal condition.

Incidental Appendectomy

Incidental appendectomy, performed during surgery for another cause, may be justified in individuals younger than 30 years if the primary surgery would not be compromised. Appendectomy does not increase morbidity when performed under these circumstances.[102]

The author has no commercial relationships with manufacturers of products or providers of services discussed in this chapter.

References

1. Floch MH, Bina I: The natural history of diverticulitis: fact and theory. J Clin Gastroenterol 38(5 Suppl):S2, 2004

2. Mendeloff AI, Everhart JE: Diverticular disease of the colon. Digestive Diseases in the United States: Epidemiology and Impact. Everhart JE, Ed. National Institutes of Health, National Institute of Diabetes and Digestive and Kidney Diseases. Washington, DC, 1994, p 551

3. Nakada I, Ubukata H, Goto Y, et al: Diverticular disease of the colon at a regional general hospital in Japan. Dis Colon Rectum 38:755, 1995

4. Mizuki A, Nagata H, Tatemichi M, et al: The out-patient management of patients with acute mild-to-moderate colonic diverticulitis. Aliment Pharmacol Ther 21:889, 2005

5. Morris CR, Harvey IM, Stebbings WS, et al: Anti-inflammatory drugs, analgesics and the risk of perforated colonic diverticular disease. Br J Surg 90:1267, 2003

6. Makela J, Kiviniemi H, Laitinen S: Prevalence of perforated sigmoid diverticulitis is increasing. Dis Colon Rectum 45:955, 2002

7. Hart AR, Kennedy HJ, Stebbings WS, et al: How frequently do large bowel diverticula perforate? An incidence and cross-sectional study. Eur J Gastroenterol Hepatol 12:661, 2000

8. Ambrosetti P, Rober J, Witzig JA: Prognostic factors from computed tomography in acute left colonic diverticulitis. Br J Surg 79:117, 1992

9. Aldoori W, Ryan-Harshman M: Preventing diverticular disease. Review of recent evidence on high-fibre diets. Can Fam Physician 48:1632, 2002

10. Wess L, Eastwood MA, Wess TJ, et al: Cross linking of collagen is increased in colonic diverticulosis. Gut 37:91, 1995

11. Ludeman L, Warren BF, Shepherd NA: The pathology of diverticular disease. Best Pract Res Clin Gastroenterol 16:543, 2002

12. Whiteway J, Morson BC: Elastosis in diverticular disease of the sigmoid colon. Gut 26:258, 1985

13. Bucher P, Mathe Z, Demirag A, et al: Appendix tumors in the era of laparoscopic appendectomy. Surg Endosc 18:1063, 2004

14. Colecchia A, Sandri L, Capodicasa S, et al: Diverticular disease of the colon: new perspectives in symptom development and treatment. World J Gastroenterol 9:1385, 2003

15. Tursi A: Preventive therapy for complicated diverticular disease of the colon: looking for a correct therapeutic approach. Gastroenterology 127:1865, 2004

16. Tursi A, Brandimarte G, Daffina R: Long-term treatment with mesalazine and rifaximin versus rifaximin alone for patients with recurrent attacks of acute diverticulitis of colon. Dig Liver Dis 34:510, 2002

17. Kaiser AM, Jeng-Kae J, Lake JP, et al: The management of complicated diverticulitis and the role of computed tomography. Am J Gastroenterol 100:910, 2005

18. Macias LH, Haukoos JS, Dixon MR, et al: Diverticulitis: truly minimally invasive management. Am Surg 70:932, 2004

19. Bahadursingh AM, Virgo KS, Kaminski DL, et al: Spectrum of disease and outcome of complicated diverticular disease. Am J Surg 186:696, 2003

20. Biondo S, Pares D, Marti RJ, et al: Acute colonic diverticulitis in patients under 50 years of age. Br J Surg 89:1137, 2002

21. Lo CY, Chu KW: Acute diverticulitis of the right colon. Am J Surg 171:244,1996

22. Junge K, Marx A, Peiper C, et al: Caecal-diverticulitis: a rare differential diagnosis for right-sided lower abdominal pain. Colorectal Dis 5:241, 2003

23. Fang JF, Chen RJ, Lin BC, et al: Aggressive resection is indicated for cecal diverticulitis. Am J Surg 185:135, 2003

24. Simpson J, Neal KR, Scholefield JH, et al: Patterns of pain in diverticular disease and the influence of acute diverticulitis. Eur J Gastroenterol Hepatol 15:1005, 2003

25. Kircher MF, Rhea JT, Kihiczak D, et al: Frequency, sensitivity, and specificity of individual signs of diverticulitis on thin-section helical CT with colonic contrast material: experience with 312 cases. AJR Am J Roentgenol 178:1313, 2002

26. McKee RF, Deignan RW, Krukowski ZH: Radiological investigation in acute diverticulitis. Br J Surg 80:560, 1993

27. Kaiser AM, Jiang JK, Lake JP, et al: The management of complicated diverticulitis and the role of computed tomography. Am J Gastroenterol 100:910, 2005

28. Sakhnini E, Lahat A, Melzer E, et al: Early colonoscopy in patients with acute diverticulitis: results of a prospective pilot study. Endoscopy 36:504, 2004

29. Wong WD, Wexner SD, Lowry A, et al: Practice parameters for sigmoid diverticulitis-supporting documentation. The Standards Task Force. The American Society of Colon and Rectal Surgeons. Dis Colon Rectum 43:290, 2000

30. Zissin R, Hertz M, Osadchy A, et al: Acute epiploic appendagitis: CT findings in 33 cases. Emerg Radiol 9:262, 2002

31. Legome EL, Belton AL, Murray RE, et al: Epiploic appendagitis: the emergency department presentation. J Emerg Med 22:9, 2002

32. Blinder E, Ledbetter S, Rybicki F: Primary epiploic appendagitis. Emerg Radiol 9:231, 2002

33. Young TH, Lee HS, Tang HS: Primary torsion of the greater omentum. Int Surg 89:72, 2004

34. Abadir JS, Cohen AJ, Wilson SE: Accurate diagnosis of infarction of omentum and appendices epiploicae by computed tomography. Am Surg 70:854, 2004

35. Werner A, Diehl SJ, Farag-Soliman M, et al: Multi-slice spiral CT in routine diagnosis of suspected acute left-sided colonic diverticulitis: a prospective study of 120 patients. Eur Radiol 13:2596, 2003

36. Zielke A, Hasse C, Nies C, et al: Prospective evaluation of ultrasonography in acute colonic diverticulitis. Br J Surg 84:385,1997

37. Schreyer AG, Furst A, Agha A, et al: Magnetic resonance imaging based colonography for diagnosis and assessment of diverticulosis and diverticulitis. Int J Colorectal Dis 19:474, 2004

38. Schecter S, Mulvey J, Eisenstat TE: Management of uncomplicated acute diverticulitis. Dis Colon Rectum 42: 470, 1999

39. Sanford JP, Gilbert DN, Sande MA: The Sanford Guide to Antimicrobial Therapy. Antimicrobial Therapy, Inc., Hyde Park, Vermont, 2004

40. Wedell J, Banzhaf G, Chaoui R, et al: Surgical management of complicated colonic diverticulitis. Br J Surg 84:380, 1997

41. Maggard MA, Zingmond D, O'Connell JB, et al: What proportion of patients with an ostomy (for diverticulitis) get reversed? Am Surg 70:928, 2004

42. Thaler K, Weiss EG, Nogueras JJ, et al: Recurrence rates at minimum five-year follow-up: laparoscopic versus open sigmoid resection for uncomplicated diverticulitis. Acta Chir Iugosl 51:45, 2004

43. Thaler K, Baig MK, Berho M, et al: Determinants of recurrence after sigmoid resection for uncomplicated diverticulitis. Dis Colon Rectum 46:385, 2003

44. Schwandner O, Farke S, Bruch HP: Laparoscopic colectomy for diverticulitis is not associated with increased morbidity when compared to non-diverticular disease. Int J Colorectal Dis 20:165, 2005

45. Gonzalez R, Smith CD, Mattar SG, et al: Laparoscopic vs open resection for the treatment of diverticular disease. Surg Endosc 18:276, 2004

46. Salem L, Veenstra DL, Sullivan SD, et al: The timing of elective colectomy in diverticulitis: a decision analysis. J Am Coll Surg 199:904, 2004

47. Spivak H, Weinrauch S, Harvey JC: Acute colonic diverticulitis in the young. Dis Colon Rectum 40:570, 1997

48. Schauer PR, Ramos R, Ghiatas AA, et al: Virulent diverticular disease in young obese men. Am J Surg 164:443, 1992

49. Chautems RC, Ambrosetti P, Ludwig A, et al: Long-term follow-up after first acute episode of sigmoid diverticulitis: is surgery mandatory?: a prospective study of 118 patients. Dis Colon Rectum 45:962, 2002

50. Guzzo J, Hyman N: Diverticulitis in young patients: is resection after a single attack always warranted? Dis Colon Rectum 47:1187, 2004

51. Lavery IC: Colonic fistulas. Surg Clin North Am 76:1183, 1996

52. Jarrett TW, Vaughan ED Jr: Accuracy of computerized tomography in the diagnosis of colovesical fistula secondary to diverticular disease. J Urol 153:44, 1995

53. Kirsh GM, Hampel N, Shuck JM, et al: Diagnosis and management of vesicoenteric fistulas. Surg Gynecol Obstet 173:91, 1991

54. Wilson RG, Smith AN, Macintyre IM: Complications of diverticular disease and non-steroidal anti-inflammatory drugs: a prospective study. Br J Surg 77:1103, 1990

55. West AB, Losada M: The pathology of diverticulosis coli. J Clin Gastroenterol 38:S11, 2004

56. Ghorai S, Ulbright TM, Rex DK: Endoscopic findings of diverticular inflammation in colonoscopy patients without clinical acute diverticulitis: prevalence and endoscopic spectrum. Am J Gastroenterol 98:802, 2003

57. Stefansson T, Ekbom A, Sparen P, et al: Association between sigmoid diverticulitis and left-sided colon cancer: a nested, population-based, case control study. Scand J Gastroenterol 39:743, 2004

58. Krones CJ, Klinge U, Butz N, et al: The rare epidemiologic coincidence of diverticular disease and advanced colonic neoplasia. Int J Colorectal Dis 2005

59. Kieff BJ, Eckert GJ, Imperiale TF: Is diverticulosis associated with colorectal neoplasia? A cross-sectional colonoscopic study. Am J Gastroenterol 99:2007, 2004

60. Longstreth GF: Epidemiology and outcome of patients hospitalized with acute lower gastrointestinal hemorrhage: a population-based study. Am J Gastroenterol 92:419, 1997

61. Jensen DM, Machicado GA: Colonoscopy for diagnosis and treatment of severe lower gastrointestinal bleeding: routine outcomes and cost analysis. Gastrointest Endosc Clin North Am 7:477, 1997

62. Peura DA, Lanza FL, Gostout CJ: The American College of Gastroenterology bleeding registry: preliminary findings. Am J Gastroenterol 92:924, 1997

63. Bokhari M, Vernava AM, Ure T, et al: Diverticular hemorrhage in the elderly: is it well tolerated? Dis Colon Rectum 39:191, 1996

64. Zuccaro G: Management of the adult patient with acute lower gastrointestinal bleeding. Am J Gastroenterol 93:1202, 1998

65. Zuckerman GR, Prakash C: Acute lower intestinal bleeding: part II: etiology, therapy, and outcomes. Gastrointest Endosc 49:228, 1999

66. Jensen DM, Machicado GA, Jutahbha R, et al: Urgent colonoscopy for the diagnosis and treatment of severe diverticular hemorrhage. N Engl J Med 342:78, 2000

67. Smoot RL, Gostout CJ, Rajan E, et al: Is early colonoscopy after admission for acute diverticular bleeding needed? Am J Gastroenterol 98:1996, 2003

68. Farrell JJ, Graeme-Cook F, Kelsey PB: Treatment of bleeding colonic diverticula by endoscopic band ligation: an in-vivo and ex-vivo pilot study. Endoscopy 35:823, 2003.

69. Simpson PW, Nguyen MH, Lim JK, et al: Use of endoclips in the treatment of massive colonic diverticular bleeding. Gastrointest Endosc 59:433, 2004

70. Maurer AH: Gastrointestinal bleeding and cine-scintigraphy. Semin Nucl Med 26:43, 1996

71. O'Neill BB, Gosnell JE, Lull RJ, et al: Cinematic nuclear scintigraphy reliably directs surgical intervention for patients with gastrointestinal bleeding. Arch Surg 135:1076, 2000

72. Suzman MS, Talmor M, Jennis R, et al: Accurate localization and surgical management of active lower gastrointestinal hemorrhage with technetium-labeled erythrocyte scintigraphy. Ann Surg 224:29, 1996

73. Everhart JE, Mendeloff AI: Acute appendicitis. Digestive Diseases in the United States: Epidemiology and Impact. Everhart JE, Ed. National Institutes of Health, National Institute of Diabetes and Digestive and Kidney Diseases, Washington, DC, 1994, p 457

74. Barber MD, McLaren J, Rainey JB: Recurrent appendicitis. Br J Surg 84:110, 1997

75. Babb RR, Trollope ML: Recurrent appendicitis. uncommon, but it does occur. Postgrad Med 106:135, 1999

76. Levine CD, Aizenstein O, Wachsberg RH: Pitfalls in the CT diagnosis of appendicitis. Br J Radiol 77:792, 2004

77. Watkins BP, Kothari SN, Landercasper J: Stump appendicitis: case report and review. Surg Laparosc Endosc Percutan Tech 14:167, 2004

78. Mason JD: The evaluation of acute abdominal pain in children. Emerg Med Clin North Am 14:629, 1996

79. Franz MG, Norman J, Fabri P J: Increased morbidity of appendicitis with advancing age. Am Surg 61:40, 1995

80. Korner H, Sondenaa K, Soreida JA, et al: Incidence of acute nonperforated and perforated appendicitis: age-specific and sex-specific analysis. World J Surg 21:313, 1997

81. Rothrock SG, Green SM, Dobson M, et al: Misdiagnosis of appendicitis in nonpregnant women of childbearing age. J Emerg Med 13:1, 1995

82. Andersen B, Nielsen TF: Appendicitis in pregnancy: diagnosis, management and complications. Acta Obstet Gynecol Scand 78:758, 1999

83. Ohmann C, Yang Q, Franke C: Diagnostic scores for acute appendicitis. Abdominal Pain Study Group. Eur J Surg 161:273, 1995

84. Wolfe JM, Smithline HA, Phipen S, et al: Does morphine change the physical examination in patients with acute appendicitis? Am J Emerg Med 22:280, 2004

85. Vermeulen B, Morabia A, Unger PF, et al: Acute appendicitis: influence of early pain relief on the accuracy of clinical and US findings in the decision to operate—a randomized trial. Radiology 210:639, 1999

86. Cardall T, Glasser J, Guss DA: Clinical value of the total white blood cell count and temperature in the evaluation of patients with suspected appendicitis. Acad Emerg Med 11:1021, 2004

87. Barloon T J, Brown BP, Abu-Yousef MM, et al: Sonography of acute appendicitis in

pregnancy. Abdom Imaging 20:149, 1995

88. Kaiser S, Frenckner B, Jorulf HK: Suspected appendicitis in children: US and CT—a prospective randomized study. Radiology 223:633, 2002

89. Terasawa T, Blackmore CC, Bent S, et al: Systematic review: computed tomography and ultrasonography to detect acute appendicitis in adults and adolescents. Ann Intern Med 141:537, 2004

90. Antevil J, Rivera L, Langenberg B, et al: The influence of age and gender on the utility of computed tomography to diagnose acute appendicitis. Am Surg 70:850, 2004

91. Rao PM, Rhea JT, Novelline RA, et al: Effect of computed tomography of the appendix on treatment of patients and use of hospital resources. N Engl J Med 338:141, 1998

92. Jeffrey RB, Federle MP, Tolentino CS: Periappendiceal inflammatory masses: CT-directed management and clinical outcome in 70 patients. Radiology 167:13, 1988

93. Rao PM, Rhea JT, Novelline RA, et al: Helical CT combined with contrast material administered only through the colon for imaging of suspected appendicitis. AJR Am J Roentgenol 169:1275, 1997

94. Stroman DL, Bayouth CV, Kuhn JA, et al: The role of computed tomography in the diagnosis of acute appendicitis. Am J Surg 178:485,1999

95. Gorecki WJ, Grochowski JA. Are antibiotics necessary in nonperforated appendicitis in children? A double blind randomized controlled trial. Med Sci Monit 7:289, 2001

96. Taylor E, Berjis A, Bosch T, et al: The efficacy of postoperative oral antibiotics in appendicitis: a randomized prospective double-blinded study. Am Surg 70:858, 2004

97. Hellberg A, Rudberg C, Kullman E, et al: Prospective randomized multicentre study of laparoscopic versus open appendicectomy. Br J Surg 86:48, 1999

98. Pedersen AG, Petersen OB, Wara P, et al: Randomized clinical trial of laparoscopic versus open appendicectomy. Br J Surg 88:200, 2001

99. Sauerland S, Lefering R, Neugebauer E: Laparoscopic versus open surgery for suspected appendicitis. Cochrane Database Syst Rev 18:CD001546, 2004

100. Borgstein PJ, Gordjin RV, Eijsbouts QA, et al: Acute appendicitis: a clear-cut case in men, a guessing game in young women: a prospective study of the role of laparoscopy. Surg Endosc 11:923, 1997

101. Larsson PG, Henriksson G, Olsson M, et al: Laparoscopy reduces unnecessary appendicectomies and improves diagnosis in fertile women: a randomized study. Surg Endosc 15:200, 2001

102. Fisher KS, Ross DS: Guidelines for therapeutic decision in incidental appendectomy. Surg Gynecol Obstet 171:95, 1990

65 Diseases Producing Malabsorption and Maldigestion

Charles M. Mansbach II, M.D.

Definition

Malabsorption classically means the impaired absorption of fat (steatorrhea), because fat absorption is the best indicator of the normality of the overall process of nutrient absorption. Under certain conditions, however, fat absorption may be normal but other specific substances may be poorly absorbed, such as iron, calcium, bile salts, or, in certain hereditary conditions, specific amino acids, disaccharides, or monosaccharides.

Overview of Diseases Producing Malabsorption

ETIOLOGY

There are three principal causes of fat malabsorption: small bowel disease, liver or biliary tract disease, and pancreatic exocrine insufficiency [see Table 1].

Small Bowel Disease

Small bowel disease can result in moderate amounts of fat in the stool (7 to 30 g/day on a diet containing 100 g of fat). Patients with small bowel disease may leak protein (protein-losing enteropathy) through a diseased intestinal mucosa, which results in a reduced serum albumin concentration. Deficiencies of fat-soluble vitamins (i.e., vitamins A, D, E, and K) may occur in small bowel disease. Severe disease or surgical resection (usually over 60 cm) of the terminal ileum may result in malabsorption of vitamin B_{12}. Folic acid may also be malabsorbed, and hypocalcemia and hypomagnesemia may also be present.

Liver or Biliary Tract Disease

Patients with liver or biliary tract disease usually have only small increases in fat in the stool (7 to 15 g/day) and may also malabsorb fat-soluble vitamins. The association of cholestatic liver disease, especially primary biliary cirrhosis, with osteoporosis is well known. Osteoporosis may be the presenting symptom of the liver disease. Vitamin K deficiency, as manifested by a prolonged prothrombin time, may also occur. Administration of vitamin K corrects the clotting defect, provided that the liver disease is not severe enough to impede clotting factor synthesis.

Pancreatic Exocrine Insufficiency

Patients with pancreatic exocrine insufficiency may have up to 80 g of fat/day in the stool. Any fat absorption that does take place occurs through the action of gastric lipases. Gastric lipase is present in the chief cells of the human stomach[1] and is thought to account for any lipid absorbed in the setting of chronic pancreatitis, as exemplified by cystic fibrosis. Indeed, in cystic fibrosis, an increase in gastric lipase has been reported.[2]

CLINICAL MANIFESTATIONS

The symptoms of malabsorption are protean. In the most obvious case, the patient complains of weight loss despite a good appetite. In these cases, there is a clear change in the quality of the stool and usually an increase in stool number. Because of excess fat and gas,[3] the stool becomes softer in consistency, more malodorous, buoyant, and difficult to flush down the toilet. Oil drops or a lipid sheen may appear on the water. Depending on other dietary constituents that are malabsorbed, patients may experience a distended abdomen, borborygmi, abdominal cramps (lactose intolerance), easy bruising (vitamin K deficiency), osteopenia or tetany (vitamin D deficiency and calcium malabsorption), iron deficiency, or night blindness (vitamin A deficiency). The most challenging cases are those in which the possibility of malabsorption is not raised because the quality of the stools does not change.

The diarrhea of malabsorption is classified as osmotic and usually stops during fasting. In fat malabsorption, the diarrhea is caused not only by the excessive osmotically active particles but also by fatty acids, which stimulate cyclic adenosine monophosphate (cAMP)–dependent Cl^- secretion.

Specific physical findings of various diseases may accompany the malabsorptive state and assist in making the diagnosis. For example, the skin changes of scleroderma or dermatitis herpetiformis may be present. Signs of diabetic neuropathy may be disclosed. Although thyrotoxicosis may be associated with excessive fat in the stool, patients with thyrotoxicosis usually eat gluttonously but absorb a normal percentage of dietary fat eaten (95%) and therefore do not malabsorb in the true sense.

Table 1 Causes of Malabsorptive Syndromes

Diseases of the small intestine	Gluten-sensitive enteropathy
	Tropical sprue
	Collagenous sprue
	Eosinophilic enteritis
	Radiation enteritis
	Amyloidosis
	Mastocytosis
	Abetalipoproteinemia
	Whipple disease
	Intestinal lymphangiectasia
	Immunoproliferative small intestinal disease
	Ischemic bowel disease
	Giardia lamblia infection
	AIDS
	Short bowel syndrome
	Ileal resection
	Ileitis (e.g., Crohn disease)
Diseases of the liver and biliary tract	Cirrhosis/parenchymal liver disease
	Intrahepatic cholestasis syndrome
	Cholestasis due to extrahepatic obstruction
Diseases of the pancreas	Chronic pancreatitis
	Cystic fibrosis
	Cancer
Combined or multiple defects in digestion and absorption	Hyperthyroidism
	Diabetes mellitus
	Carcinoid syndrome
	Zollinger-Ellison syndrome
	Postgastrectomy (Billroth II type)

TESTS FOR SUSPECTED MALABSORPTION

The tests for malabsorption involve determining whether there is excessive fecal fat excretion [see Table 2]. Protein is produced in large quantities by the digestive tract, especially the pancreas, making creatorrhea difficult to interpret. Malabsorbed carbohydrate delivered to the colon may be metabolized by colonic bacteria to short-chain fatty acids, which are in part absorbed by the colon. Thus, the quantitative measurement of carbohydrate absorption is inaccurate, although a fall in stool pH occurs, which is indicative of excessive amounts of the short-chain fatty acids that are excreted under these conditions.

Measurement of Fecal Fat

Fecal fat can be measured qualitatively and quantitatively. The qualitative measurement of fecal fat using Sudan III staining and microscopy has been shown to be surprisingly accurate,[4] especially if clinically significant amounts of fat are being excreted. The skill of the microscopist is crucial to success. The quantitative measurement of fecal fat is the benchmark by which all other tests are ranked. It is important to remember that the stool must be collected for 3 days. Carmine dye–containing capsules are ingested at the start of the study and 3 days later. Stool collection is begun after the passage of the first red stool and stops when the second wave of red stool is passed. The test cannot be performed unless the patient is able to eat at least 80 g, preferably 100 g, of fat a day. An alternative is the acid steatocrit, in which homogenized stool is mixed with perchloric or hydrochloric acid and the percentage of stool occupied by the fatty layer after centrifugation is calculated. A newer method for measuring fecal fat, not widely available, is near infrared reflectance analysis (NIF).[5]

D-*Xylose Absorption Test*

The absorptive surface area of the intestine is measured by the ability of the patient to absorb the sugar xylose. Unlike glucose, xylose is not actively absorbed by the intestine but is absorbed by the slower process of passive diffusion. In the D-xylose absorption test, 25 g of D-xylose is given by mouth and the urine is collected for 5 hours. The normal urinary excretion of xylose is greater than 4 g over 5 hours. For an adequate urinary flow to be ensured, the patient should drink 500 ml of water after drinking the xylose. This intake should result in a urine volume of at least 300 ml during the collection period. Xylose excretion can be falsely low in patients with reduced renal function or in patients with ascites in which the xylose is diluted in the ascitic fluid. To avoid falsely low results, it is advisable to measure the concentration of xylose in blood [see Table 2]. Malabsorbed xylose reaches the colon and can be metabolized by the resident bacteria to hydrogen. Hydrogen may be quantitated in the breath; this test is reportedly as accurate as the measurement of xylose in the serum or urine.

Imaging Studies

A plain film or ultrasonogram of the abdomen is usually not helpful in most cases of malabsorption. However, 30% of patients with chronic pancreatitis have visible calcifications on an abdominal plain film. Detection of pancreatic calcification can be increased if computed tomography or ultrasonography is used. CT or ultrasonography also can identify dilated pancreatic ducts, another characteristic sign of chronic pancreatitis. Endoscopic retrograde pancreatography (ERP) can also be helpful when ductular changes indicative of chronic pancreatitis are seen [see Chapter 73] as can magnetic resonance cholangiopancreatography (MRCP).

Table 2 Tests of Digestive-Absorptive Function

	Characteristics	Clinical Use
Fecal fat analysis Qualitative	Simple microscopic study for increase in fat globules	A good screening test for moderate increase in stool fat, but quantitative fecal fat analysis is preferable
Quantitative	Chemical analysis for fat excretion during a 72 hr period by titration with NaOH; most sensitive test for malassimilation of fat; normal is < 6 g/day; does not distinguish between small intestine, pancreatic, or luminal abnormalities	The most important test to identify maldigestion or malabsorption; indicated in all patients suspected of having malassimilation
D-Xylose absorption	As a pentose not requiring luminal or intestinal surface digestion, xylose allows assessment of small intestine function; normally, > 4 g/5 hr is excreted in urine after ingestion of 25 g; plasma xylose should be 10–20 mg/dl/1.73 m² of body surface area at 60–75 min	Indicated whenever quantitative fecal fat is abnormal; not as sensitive as fat analysis but localizes the abnormality to the small intestine
Small intestine x-ray	Allows analysis of continuity of small intestine and identification of diverticula or alteration of mucosa; diseased pancreas may impinge on duodenum	Indicated when quantitative fecal fat excretion is increased
Small intestine peroral biopsy	Permits direct histologic examination of mucosa; characteristic alterations occur in several diseases producing malabsorption	Indicated when fecal fat excretion is increased, particularly if the xylose test or small intestine x-ray is abnormal; a portion of biopsy may be assayed for disaccharidases
Bile acid breath test	In small intestine bacterial overgrowth or ileal disease that produces malabsorption, ^{14}C–glycocholic acid (5 μCi) will be deconjugated, metabolized, and excreted via the lungs as ^{14}CO$_2$	Indicated in patients with documented steatorrhea caused by suspected bacterial overgrowth or ileal dysfunction
Bentiromide test	The peptide bond in this nonabsorbable arylamine is cleaved specifically by intraluminal chymotrypsin to yield PABA, which is then readily absorbed and excreted by the intestine	Indicated when fecal fat excretion is increased; less sensitive than quantitative fat analysis but, when positive, establishes insufficiency of intraduodenal pancreatic digestive enzyme levels Not available in U. S.

PABA—*p*-aminobenzoic acid

Radiographic studies of the small intestine after oral ingestion of barium can aid in the diagnosis of several abnormalities. The presence of diverticula of the small intestine or of impaired peristalsis, as seen in scleroderma or idiopathic intestinal dysmotility, can be an indicator of bacterial overgrowth. A careful examination of the terminal ileum can identify Crohn disease. Strictures may be identified in some patients with radiation injury or injury caused by nonsteroidal anti-inflammatory drugs. Hypoalbuminemia affecting the small intestine may lead to thickening of small bowel folds and the so-called stack-of-coins sign.

Small Bowel Biopsy

A biopsy sample of the small bowel, read by an experienced pathologist, may be helpful in determining the cause of malabsorption. Biopsy results can support the diagnoses of gluten-sensitive enteropathy (with or without dermatitis herpetiformis), hypogammaglobulinemic sprue, tropical sprue, Whipple disease, *Mycobacterium avium* complex disease, stasis (bacterial overgrowth) syndrome, amyloidosis, and intestinal lymphangiectasia.

Assessment of Pancreatic Exocrine Function

More than 90% of pancreatic exocrine function needs to be destroyed before symptomatic malabsorption results [see Chapter 73].[6] The most sensitive test of pancreatic exocrine function requires the passage of a double-lumen tube.[7] Cholecystokinin (CCK) or secretin is administered intravenously, and gastric and duodenal secretions are collected separately. However, secretin has been unavailable in the United States since 1999, when the manufacturer discontinued production. If CCK is given, lipase or trypsin activity is determined using appropriate substrates. When secretin is administered, duodenal fluid volume and bicarbonate concentration are measured.

The noninvasive bentiromide test is based on the action of trypsin on bentiromide to yield *p*-aminobenzoic acid (PABA) and benzoyl-tyrosine. PABA is readily absorbed by the intestine and excreted into the urine. In healthy persons, when 500 mg of bentiromide is ingested, 57% or more of the PABA appears in the urine within 6 hours. In patients with chronic pancreatitis, the absence of trypsin results in failure to cleave bentiromide, and consequently the amount of PABA excreted is significantly less, averaging 42%. Using the 57% excretion as a cutoff, the sensitivity is 67% to 80% and the specificity is 95%.[8] PABA may also be measured in the plasma 120 minutes after ingestion of bentiromide, which may enhance the sensitivity of the test.[9] Plasma measurements are helpful in patients with impaired renal excretion (e.g., some elderly patients). Because PABA is identified colorimetrically, the presence of other arylamines (e.g., acetaminophen, lidocaine, procainamide, sulfonamides, and thiazide diuretics) can interfere with its determination.[10] Impaired intestinal absorption, such as with sprue, may reduce the absorption of released PABA, leading to a falsely low urinary recovery (a false positive result). Unfortunately, the bentiromide test remains normal when less than 90% of the pancreatic gland is destroyed (a false negative result). Nevertheless, the test may be useful in the workup of a patient with steatorrhea, because steatorrhea does not develop until an equal amount of glandular destruction has occurred.

Although the vast majority of pancreatic proteases and lipases are stored in zymogen granules and are released from the apical portion of the pancreatic exocrine cell into the pancreatic duct, a small percentage leaks into the interstitium of the gland, is carried into the circulation, and can be measured (i.e., by the serum trypsinogen assay). Because the activation peptide of trypsin is not yet released and any active trypsin is quickly bound by α_1-antitrypsin, the free-circulating form of trypsin is trypsinogen. In patients who have chronic pancreatitis with exocrine insufficiency, the serum concentration of trypsinogen is lower than in healthy persons (2 to 18 ng/ml, compared with 29 to 79 ng/ml in healthy persons).[11] A low serum trypsinogen level appears to have a high degree of specificity for chronic pancreatitis but is only modestly sensitive. Measurement of the fecal concentration of pancreatic elastase 1 has a high degree of sensitivity (> 90 %) for patients with moderate to severe pancreatic exocrine function, as judged by the secretin-CCK test in both adults[12] and children.[13]

Bile Acid Absorption Tests

Bile acids are synthesized from cholesterol in the liver and require conjugation by either glycine or taurine before they are excreted into the intestine via the common bile duct. These bile acid conjugates solubilize the products of triacylglycerol hydrolysis into complex micelles, which facilitate the rapid absorption of dietary lipid. Bile acids are not absorbed in the proximal intestine with dietary lipid but, rather, are absorbed in the distal ileum. The bile acid pool recirculates six times a day. About 95% of bile acids are reabsorbed and recirculate in the enterohepatic circulation each day; approximately 0.5 g of bile acids appears in the stool daily, which equals the hepatic synthesis rate under steady-state conditions. If bile acids are not adequately absorbed, diarrhea results (choleretic enteropathy). In the complete absence of bile salts, fatty acids are less efficiently absorbed, with up to 25% to 50% of ingested lipid appearing in the stool. In patients with idiopathic diarrhea or with diarrhea after ileal resection (≥ 30 cm), the malabsorption of bile acids is an etiologic possibility. Also, children who have unexplained diarrhea may have a congenital defect of the sodium-dependent bile salt transporter in the terminal ileum.[14]

To test for the presence of bile acid malabsorption, two methods are available, although they are not widely used. The first is the ^{14}C-glycocholic acid breath test, and the second is the selenium-75–labeled homocholic acid–taurine (^{75}SeHCAT) absorption test. In the former test [see Figure 1], a trace amount of ^{14}C-glycocholic acid is given by mouth. Many bacteria are capable of hydrolyzing the amide bond and releasing the ^{14}C-glycine; either it is absorbed and $^{14}CO_2$ is produced in the liver, or it is further metabolized in the intestinal lumen to $^{14}CO_2$. In either event, the $^{14}CO_2$ appears in the breath in measurable amounts. The percentage of the ingested dose excreted in the breath increases if there is intestinal stasis, in which case the intestinal lumen contains more bacteria than normal, or ileal dysfunction, in which case an excess of bile acids is delivered to the colon. A gastric antisecretory drug may also increase the resident population of bacteria in the intestine to a level that results in an abnormal breath test.[15] The usefulness of this test as an indicator of bile acid malabsorption is therefore limited. The ^{75}SeHCAT test has more potential clinical usefulness because of its strong correlation with cholate excretion and the ease of measurement of ^{75}Se retention by the whole-body gamma camera. Normal persons retain greater than 19% of an orally administered dose of ^{75}Se after 7 days, whereas patients with significant ileal dysfunction or resection retain less than 12%.[16]

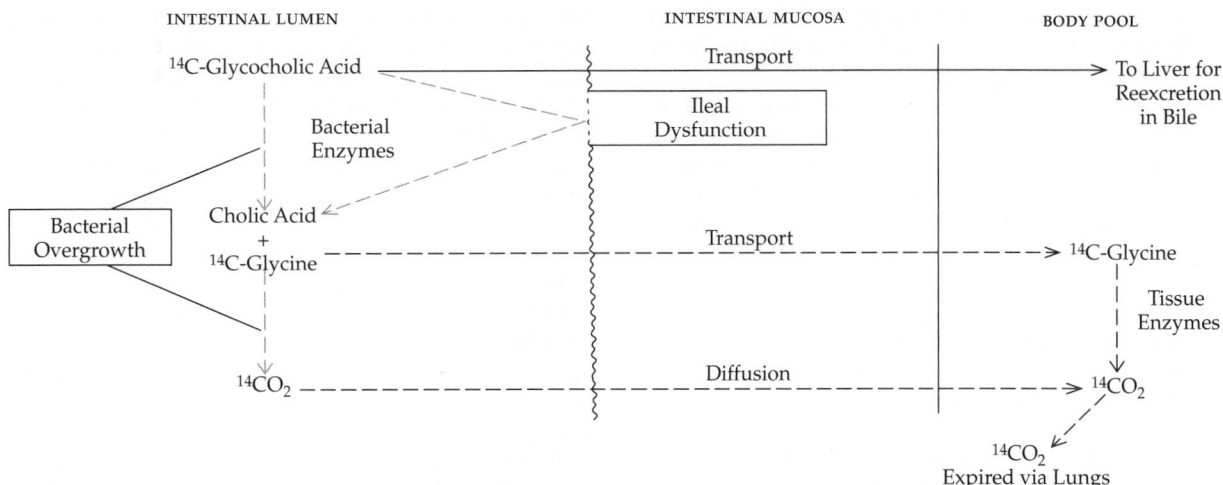

Figure 1 In the bile acid breath test, a small dose of ^{14}C–glycocholic acid is ingested and its fate determined by measurement of $^{14}CO_2$ excretion in breath. In a normal person, little of the ^{14}C–glycocholic acid is metabolized for excretion in breath because it passes intact to the ileum for absorption and return to the enterohepatic circulation. If there is either intestinal bacterial overgrowth or ileal dysfunction, however, bacterial enzymes will deconjugate the bile acid (broken blue lines), releasing cholic acid and ^{14}C-glycine. The radioactive glycine may be transported across the intestinal mucosa (upper broken gray line) and subsequently degraded to $^{14}CO_2$ by tissue enzymes; alternatively, the ^{14}C-glycine may be metabolized within the intestinal lumen to $^{14}CO_2$, which then diffuses (lower broken gray line) into the circulation and is carried to the lungs. Consequently, $^{14}CO_2$ excretion is 10 times greater in either intestinal bacterial overgrowth or ileal dysfunction than it is in the normal state.

Now that the human sodium-dependent bile acid transporter has been cloned, congenital defects are being discovered that lead to bile acid malabsorption resulting in diarrhea.[14] Such defects may be the cause of primary bile acid malabsorption.

Tests for Short Bowel Syndrome

The length of bowel remaining after intestinal resection can be measured at surgery or after a barium small bowel follow-through x-ray examination. Another method that predicts small bowel function (with 95 % positive predictive value) is the measurement of the nonprotein amino acid citrulline with a cutoff value of 20 µmol/L.[17]

Small Bowel Diseases Producing Malabsorption

GLUTEN-SENSITIVE ENTEROPATHY

Gluten-sensitive enteropathy (GSE) was once called celiac disease in children and idiopathic or nontropical sprue in adults. In 1960, it was recognized that the diseases are the same, caused by the major wheat protein gluten and, more specifically, its alcohol-soluble component, gliadin.[18] Current data from serum antibody testing in both adults and children suggest that the prevalence of GSE is much higher than originally thought (1:133 to 1:250),[19-21] although in many affected persons, there is no clinical expression.

Genetic and Etiologic Factors

GSE is associated with haplotypes HLA-DQ2 (DQA1*501, DQB1*201) and HLA-DQ8 (DQA1*031, DQB1*302). Another, unknown (nongenetic) factor appears to be important in disease causation, however, given that concordance for GSE in monozygotic twins is only about 70%. A 33–amino acid peptide part of gliadin has been shown to be poorly digested by proteases and to cause T cell activation in GSE patients.[22,23] This may be partly be-

cause of the impaired intracellular digestion of gliadin peptides by patients with active GSE but not those with treated GSE.[24]

Pathogenesis of Steatorrhea

The causes of steatorrhea in GSE are many. CCK cells are either reduced in number or so defective that the amount of CCK present in the duodenal mucosa is greatly reduced.[18] This CCK deficiency leads to a reduced amount of pancreatic lipase and bile acids delivered to the intestinal lumen in response to dietary lipid. The intestinal crypt cells are the major fluid-secreting cells of the intestine, via their cAMP-dependent Cl^- secretion with attendant water secretion. In GSE, the cryptal portion of the villous complex is greatly expanded, leading to increased water secretion. Because the villous tip cells, which normally absorb the water, are diseased and reduced in number, water and electrolyte absorption is impaired, and the intestine becomes secretory.[18] Thus, the concentration of bile acids in the intestinal lumen is reduced below that expected simply from the impaired CCK release. The ability of bile acids to solubilize the products of lipolysis depends on the presence of bile salts at a concentration greater than their critical micellar concentration (CMC) of 1.4 mM.[25] Normally, the intestine has a postprandial bile salt concentration of 10 mM.[26] The brush borders at the surface of mature enterocytes are severely affected in GSE. Further, the villous structures are flattened. These two conditions lead to a severely reduced surface area that limits lipid absorption. The amount of reduction in surface area can be estimated by the D-xylose absorption test. The enterocytes that are at the surface of the intestine are not as mature as normal enterocytes, because their turnover rate is greatly increased, which probably results in a reduced capacity to process absorbed lipid.

Diagnosis

Clinical manifestations Although GSE may start in childhood and respond to gluten withdrawal, children with the disease undergo a remission in their teenage years even if they ingest a diet containing gluten. As adults, these patients, 25% or more of whom were symptomatic in childhood, may present with a variety of complaints. Usually, weight loss, fatigue, abdominal cramps, distention, bloating, and diarrhea (steatorrhea) are prominent, although there may be no loss of appetite. In some patients, the disease is insidious in onset and the symptoms are mild. It is only after these patients have been treated that they realize, in retrospect, how ill they were. In population studies in which the presence of disease was determined by intestinal biopsy, patients whose biopsy result was consistent with GSE were often asymptomatic but sometimes of shorter stature than unaffected siblings. Because nothing specifically leads to the diagnosis, especially in the absence of clinically evident steatorrhea, the realization that the patient has GSE may be delayed. This problem is most likely to occur with patients who do not have steatorrhea but do have osteoporosis, easy bruising as a result of vitamin K deficiency, or unexplained iron deficiency anemia. Because the classic presenting symptoms of diarrhea, steatorrhea, and weight loss are much less common today than is the insidious onset of GSE, physicians should include GSE in the differential diagnosis in patients with osteoporosis or iron deficiency anemia without an obvious intestinal bleeding site.

Laboratory tests   In a patient in whom the likelihood of GSE is high—such as a first-degree relative of a known GSE patient; a patient who has a history of a childhood disease that caused diarrhea, was evaluated by a specialist, and was treated with a special diet; or a patient with malabsorption who is not an alcoholic and does not have another obvious reason for malabsorbing fat—a positive tissue transglutaminase antibody test makes the diagnosis almost certain [see Figure 2].[27] Alternatively, the diagnosis might rest on small bowel biopsy findings [see Figure 3]. Classic features include partial or complete villous atrophy, abnormal-appearing enterocytes at the villous tips, an increase in intraepithelial lymphocytes, a lamina propria infiltrate consisting predominantly of lymphocytes and macrophages, an increase in the size of the crypts both vertically and horizontally, and an increase in the number of mitotic figures.[18] These features, although typical, are not pathognomonic. For the diagnosis to be

definitive, the patient must respond to dietary therapy. Symptomatic improvement can be expected in 80% of patients within 1 month, but histologic improvement lags behind considerably. Another 10% of patients do not respond until 2 months have passed, and the remainder may take up to 2 years. Even with the strictest dietary control, the biopsy findings might not return to normal. Most often, the patients' diets remain under good control because of the symptomatic improvement while on the diet, but many patients will eventually either test whether they are cured or be in a situation that forces them to commit a dietary indiscretion. This lapse inevitably results in recurrence of symptoms, further securing the diagnosis.

Another helpful test is the identification of an antiendomysial antibody. This antibody is present in up to 95% of patients and is rarely present in control subjects.[28] Other tests of malabsorption, such as the D-xylose absorption test or stool fat studies, may be abnormal. Low levels of clotting factors, anemia caused by folate or iron deficiency, or osteoporosis may also be present. None of these conditions are specific for GSE, however.

Treatment

The treatment of GSE is a strict gluten-exclusion diet—no wheat, rye, or barley. Oats are thought to be safe but are usually avoided during the early stage, when the clinical response to the diet is being judged. Keeping the patient on the diet is sometimes difficult because many foods have hidden gluten content. In addition to its necessity for controlling symptoms, maintaining a gluten-exclusion diet is important because intestinal lymphomas are more likely to develop in patients who do not.[29] Support groups, such as those organized by the American Celiac Society, can be helpful, especially when the disease is newly diagnosed [see http://www.webmd.com/hw/raising_a_family/shc29cel.asp]. Information such as what to look for on package labels and recipes for gluten-free dishes can be instrumental in helping the patient maintain the gluten-exclusion diet. During the trial period, patients should not consume beer, ale, or whiskey, which may contain enough gluten to cause sensitization. After a clear dietary response has occurred, patients may try these drinks, if they wish, to determine whether they are sensitive. Other products that are not usually thought of as containing gluten, but often do, are ice

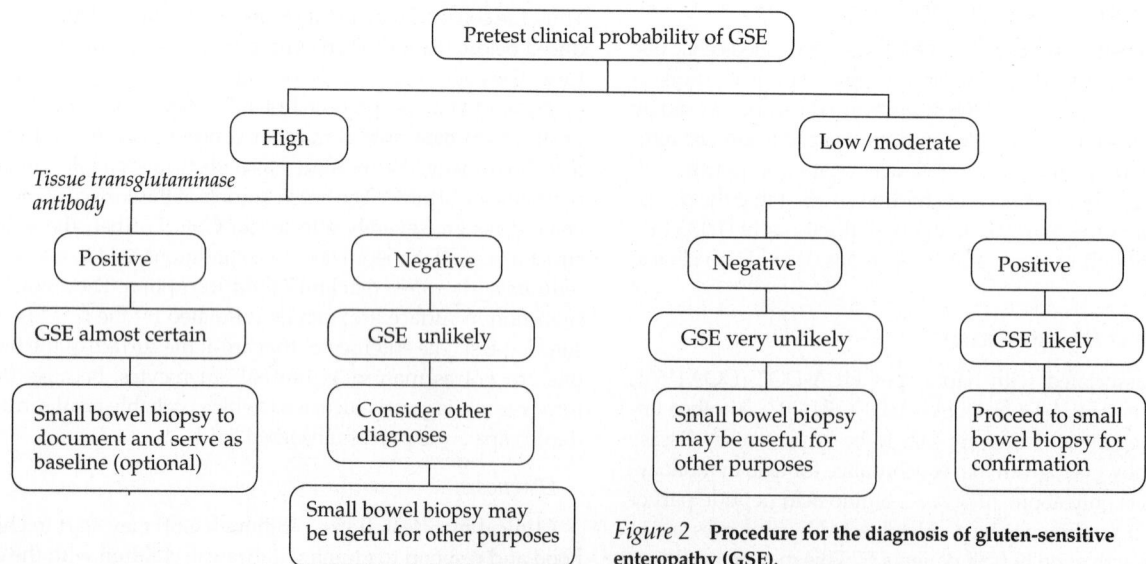

Figure 2   **Procedure for the diagnosis of gluten-sensitive enteropathy (GSE).**

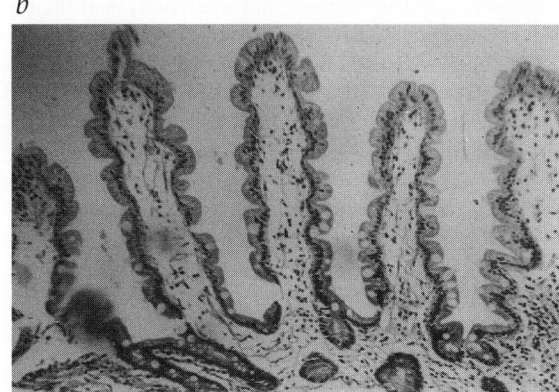

Figure 3 Biopsy specimen from the small intestine of a patient with untreated celiac sprue (*a*) demonstrates a flat surface with plasmocytic infiltration of the subepithelial region (magnified 400 times). In contrast, a biopsy sample taken from a patient with pancreatic exocrine insufficiency (*b*) is indistinguishable from a normal specimen and shows tall, scalloped villi and minimal subepithelial mononuclear infiltration (magnified 100 times).

cream, communion wafers, and even some drugs (as a filler). Despite the restrictions, many dietary options are open to the patient, including certain breakfast cereals, milk, cheese, eggs, meat, chicken, fish, chocolate, and products made from corn, rice, or potato flour. Patients may also wish to explore less well-known gluten-free grains, such as amaranth, millet, and quinoa.

If the patient does not respond, the most likely reason is failure to follow the diet fully. In such cases, it is helpful to have a dietitian carefully go over the patient's dietary history.[18] Less often, the patient will have an intestinal stasis syndrome or pancreatic insufficiency. When these subsidiary problems are diagnosed and successfully treated, the patient usually shows a response to the diet.

OTHER SPRUELIKE DISORDERS

Dermatitis Herpetiformis and GSE

Many patients with dermatitis herpetiformis will have GSE.[30] The intensely pruritic, blistering lesions of dermatitis herpetiformis appear on the knees, elbows, shoulders, and buttocks [*see Chapter 34*]. Skin biopsies of dermatitis herpetiformis lesions have characteristic immunoglobulin A (IgA) deposits. On a gluten-exclusion diet, both the dermatologic and the intestinal lesions improve, indicating a linkage between the two. However, the skin lesions respond to dapsone treatment and the intestinal lesions do not, which indicates that there are differences between the two diseases as well.

Tropical Sprue

Tropical sprue is a malabsorptive illness that appears in certain areas of the world, especially the tropics, among both the indigenous populations and tourists. In two carefully studied populations, 5% to 13% of North Americans living in Puerto Rico for 6 months or longer experienced symptoms of tropical sprue. Expatriates from the United States who return from the tropics or other areas endemic for tropical sprue may experience symptoms of tropical sprue more than 10 years after their return.[31] Peace Corps volunteers from the United States who spent time in Pakistan had demonstrable small bowel lesions and functional abnormalities that reverted to normal over several months after returning home.[32] Indians and Pakistanis living in the United States may take a longer time (up to 4 years) to excrete normal amounts of D-xylose.[33] Exactly what causes these changes in the small bowel is not clear, but the tropical sprue syndrome is thought to be caused by one or more species of coliform bacteria, such as *Klebsiella* species, 25 of which colonize the upper intestinal tract.

Diagnosis The symptoms of tropical sprue differ from those of GSE. Weight loss caused mostly by anorexia is very prominent, as is diarrhea. A sore tongue (70% of patients), pedal edema (25% of patients), folate and vitamin B[12] deficiency (75% to 100% of patients), or an abnormal result on the Schilling test (96% to 100% of patients) is much more common in tropical sprue than in nontropical sprue.[34] The symptoms can be quite severe, sometimes leading to death in endemic areas. However, the prognosis, in general, is excellent for treated patients, whether they remain in the tropics or return to the United States.

The diagnosis of tropical sprue is made by performing a small bowel biopsy in patients with a compatible clinical presentation and travel history. Villi are leaflike or blunt, and the lamina propria are packed with inflammatory cells [*see Figure 4*]. Thin villous structures are seen in North Americans and Europeans [*see Figure 3*]. In considering this disease, it should be noted that intestinal biopsy results in residents of endemic areas or in tourists who do not stay in mainstream hotels in endemic areas would be classified as abnormal in persons living in the United States or Europe.

Treatment Treatment of tropical sprue should begin with folic acid (5 mg/day).[34] This therapy is associated with rapid improvement in appetite, and it eliminates most of the clinical symptoms. In patients with a short duration of symptoms (less than 4 months), folate given for 6 months to 1 year may suffice. For patients with a longer duration of symptoms (more than 4 months), antibiotics, such as tetracycline (2 g/day for 1 year), should be added. Most patients returning to the United States gain weight quickly even if the results of absorption tests or intestinal biopsies do not return to normal.

Collagenous Sprue

Collagenous sprue is a rare, devastating disease in which there is a layer of collagen underneath the enterocytes of the small bowel. The relation of collagenous sprue to collagenous colitis is unclear, but the basic histologic feature of subepithelial collagen deposition is the same. The origin of collagenous colitis is unknown, but it develops in approximately half the patients who have refractory celiac disease (i.e., those unresponsive to the gluten-exclusion diet).[35]Although it is known that type 6 collagen is deposited in the more commonly diagnosed collagenous colitis, the type of collagen laid down in the small bowel in collagenous sprue is unknown. In collagenous colitis, the symptoms (primarily diarrhea) are usually modest, but in collagenous sprue, symptoms are more severe and include obvious malabsorption. This severity of symptoms is probably caused by the diffusion barrier presented by the collagen, which prevents nutrients from diffusing either into the portal capillaries or into the lymphatics.

Diagnosis The diagnosis of collagenous sprue is made by the classic histologic picture of villous atrophy and subepithelial collagen deposition. If the diagnosis is missed, however, and the patient is thought to have GSE on the basis of the flat villous structure, the patient will usually not respond to the gluten-free diet.

Treatment Therapy for collagenous sprue is uncertain. The most common problem is the osmotic diarrhea caused by the gross malabsorptive state induced by the disease process. In this event, the patient is treated as if he or she had the short bowel syndrome. Some patients respond to steroid therapy.[36] A few respond to steroids and a gluten-exclusion diet, with the patient's improved condition eventually making it possible to taper the steroid dosage.[37]

Hypogammaglobulinemic Sprue

The gastrointestinal tract is the largest lymphoid organ in the body. The environment to which this immune system is exposed is filled with foreign antigens that must be sorted, identified, and, if necessary, reacted to. Thus, it is not surprising that intestinal dysfunction may develop in patients who are immune deficient, particularly those with IgA deficiency, because IgA is the most important immunoglobulin of the intestine. Some patients who have one of the hypogammaglobulinemic syndromes experience malabsorption.[38] Patients with IgA deficiency also usually have a history of recurrent respiratory infections,[38] which further

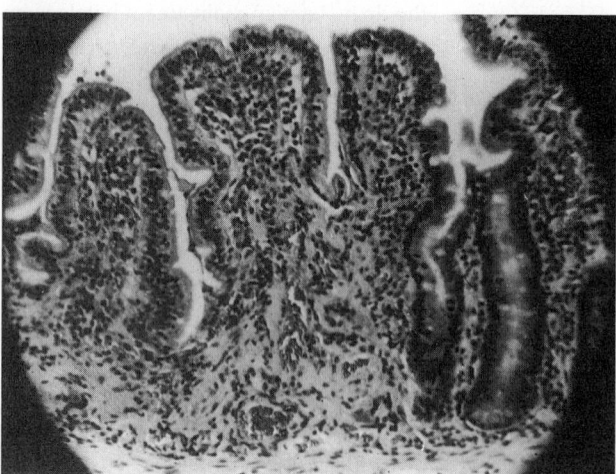

Figure 4 **In a biopsy specimen from the small intestine of a patient with tropical sprue, villi are broadened and shortened and the crypts are deepened; these changes yield a villus-to-crypt ratio of 1:1 (magnified 100 times).**

distinguishes them from patients who have GSE. The most common cause of malabsorption seen in this condition is giardiasis.

Diagnosis The diagnosis is suspected if the patient has signs and symptoms of malabsorption and low levels of serum immunoglobulins, especially IgA. Intestinal biopsy specimens lack plasma cells and thus are easily distinguishable from those of patients with GSE, in which plasma cell types are abundant. Plasma cells are readily seen in normal biopsy specimens as well. *Giardia lamblia* organisms may also be present in hypogammaglobulinemic sprue.

Treatment Frequently, the intestinal symptoms of hypogammaglobulinemic sprue improve if metronidazole is given at 750 mg/day for 10 days to treat giardiasis.

Malabsorption Secondary to Massive Small Bowel Resection

Massive small bowel resection is used to treat various diseases, including mesenteric ischemia, volvulus, and Crohn disease. Because the intestine requires a certain surface area over which absorption can occur, reducing the area below a critical value results in malabsorption. Depending on the amount of bowel resected, the results can range from mildly inconvenient to catastrophic. Retention of the ileocecal valve lessens symptoms. The ileum responds to jejunal resection by hyperplasia much more effectively than the jejunum responds to an ileal resection. There are also specialized mechanisms present in the ileum that are not available to the jejunum, such as bile salt and vitamin B transporters. The maintenance of an adequate bile acid pool is important for fat absorption because the reduced absorptive surface area in patients who have undergone bowel resection makes it necessary for fat absorption to be as efficient as possible. Alternatively, the ileum can perform most of the functions of the jejunum except for absorption of folic acid, Ca^{2+}, and Fe^{2+}. However, these can be replenished by appropriate supplementation.

Diagnosis The diagnosis is made by history of bowel resection in combination with barium x-ray evidence of a short bowel and clinical manifestations of the short bowel syndrome such as diarrhea, steatorrhea, weight loss, trace-element deficiencies, hyponatremia, and hypokalemia. A low blood citrulline concentration (< 20 μmol/L) is also helpful.[17]

Treatment Treatment in these patients is dependent on what part of the bowel and how much bowel has been resected. Protein requires the greatest surface area for absorption.[39] Thus, achieving adequate assimilation may become problematic, despite the water solubility of proteins and their hydrolytic products. Vitamins and minerals also need to be added to any therapeutic regimen, depending on what part of the bowel is missing. Treatment can include eating multiple small meals each day, eating quickly absorbed foods such as canned liquid nutritional supplements, having food finely chopped or ground, and eating foods containing medium-chain triglycerides, which can be absorbed in the absence of bile salts.[39] Foods rich in polyunsaturated fatty acids, such as vegetable oils, are more easily absorbed than meats, which have more saturated fat. Finally, completely hydrolyzed dietary supplements are rapidly absorbed. To slow bowel transit, diphenoxylate-atropine, loperamide, or deodorized tincture of opium can be used effectively. An alternative method is to have the patient drink a small amount of safflower oil just before a meal. The lipid quickly goes to the ileum (if present), the colon, or both[40] and elaborates peptide YY,[41] which is the putative ileal brake, slowing gastric emptying. Having patients try different diets will often enable them to ingest food orally rather than receive total parenteral nutrition, which is less desirable.

RADIATION ENTERITIS

Injury of the intestine is an all too common result of delivery of ionizing radiation as oncologic treatment. Injury to the small bowel is more common if the patient has had previous abdominal surgery, which may restrict the movement of the small bowel. The terminal ileum may become involved during pelvic irradiation.

WHIPPLE DISEASE

Whipple disease is a rare wasting disease caused by the bacterium *Tropheryma whippelii*.[42] Accurate diagnosis is imperative because mortality approaches 100% without antibiotic treatment.

Diagnosis

Clinical manifestations Classically, Whipple disease begins in a middle-aged man with a nondeforming arthritis that usually starts years before the onset of the intestinal symptoms. Other complaints include fever, abdominal distention, diarrhea, weight loss, lymphadenopathy, hyperpigmentation of the skin, and steatorrhea.[43] Many patients express the HLA-B27 isotype. Occasionally, intestinal symptoms are absent, even in some patients with central nervous system involvement.[44] In a well-documented but unusual case, intestinal involvement was not identified, even after extensive biopsies in two laboratories, despite the fact that the patient otherwise had typical symptoms of the disease.[45] Interestingly, as many as 35% of clinically normal persons may harbor *T. whippelii* DNA in their saliva[46]; for that reason, DNA evidence alone, without a clinical component, does not establish a diagnosis of Whipple disease.

Laboratory tests The recognition of Whipple disease in patients without intestinal symptoms or involvement by the disease is increasing with the advent of polymerase chain reaction (PCR) techniques that identify the unique 16S ribosomal RNA of *T. whippelii*.[47] The diagnosis rests on identifying the classic periodic acid–Schiff (PAS)–positive macrophages, which contain sickleform particles.[43] By far the most common site of biopsy that yields positive results is the intestine. The histologic lesion shows distended villi (so-called clubbed villi) filled with the foamy, PAS-positive macrophages and lymphatic dilatation. In extreme cases, the villous surface is flat. These findings need to be differentiated in the appropriate clinical setting from those of *M. avium* complex disease, in which PAS-positive macrophages are also found. A stain for acid-fast bacilli should differentiate between them. CNS involvement, occasionally associated with typical macrophages in the cerebrospinal fluid, as substantiated by the more sensitive PCR technique, may be present in the absence of neurologic symptoms.[48] Occasionally, a brain biopsy is required, which can be guided by magnetic resonance imaging. Cardiac and pulmonary involvement may also be found.[49]

Treatment

Because Whipple disease is so uncommon, a well-defined treatment plan is difficult to establish. The originally proposed treatment was penicillin (250 mg q.i.d.) and streptomycin (1 g I.M.) for 2 weeks, followed by tetracycline (1 g) for 1 year. Currently, the regimen typically used consists of trimethoprim-sulfamethoxazole (one double-strength tablet b.i.d.) given for 1 year; this may be preceded by 2 weeks of cephalosporins.[50] All antimicrobial agents are used in customary doses.

Although the intestinal and systemic symptoms respond readily to either treatment, the major concern is treatment of CNS manifestations. Usually, in those patients who do not have CNS involvement initially, CNS symptoms may appear a year or more after treatment of the systemic and intestinal symptoms, especially if the antibiotic used is one that does not cross the blood-brain barrier. The pathognomonic signs of CNS Whipple disease, when present, are oculomasticatory myorhythmia and oculofacial-skeletal myorhythmia; progressive dementia may also occur.[51] Antibiotics that cross the blood-brain barrier are therefore required. Interestingly, the short period of penicillin-streptomycin administration is enough to block CNS symptoms, whereas even long-term trimethoprim-sulfamethoxazole therapy occasionally fails to prevent CNS manifestations of Whipple disease.[52] Tetracycline alone does not eradicate CNS disease and should not be given by itself, even though it is effective in treating the intestinal and systemic symptoms. An important aspect to keep in mind is that in 50% of patients, the CSF may contain Whipple disease macrophages or PCR-positive material even in the absence of CNS symptoms.[48] Once CNS involvement occurs, treatment is usually not curative, although with treatment, some improvement may be noted and the disease may not progress.

IMMUNOPROLIFERATIVE SMALL INTESTINAL DISEASE

Immunoproliferative small intestinal disease (IPSID), previously known as primary intestinal lymphoma, is a condition in which the lamina propria of the small bowel is intensely infiltrated with lymphocytes and the overlying enterocytes are normal morphologically [*see Figure 5*]. In a series of Chinese patients, six of 45 patients with intestinal lymphoma had this condition.[53] These patients presented with severe malabsorption. Among lymphoma patients without IPSID, 65% had abdominal pain,

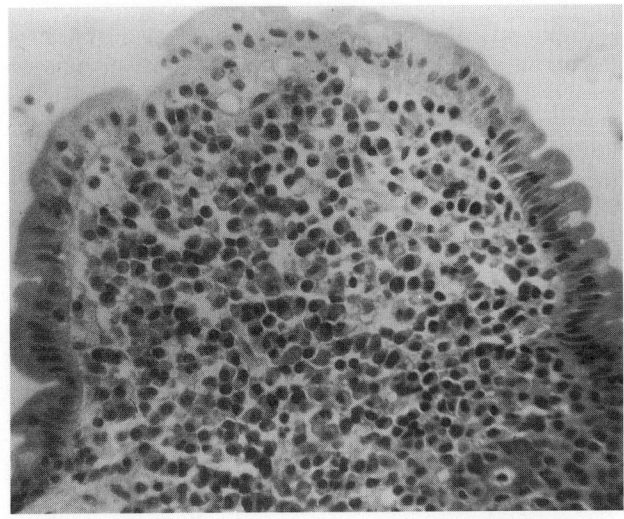

Figure 5 **Small intestinal biopsy specimen from a patient with primary intestinal lymphoma shows a single broadened villus (magnified 400 times). The epithelium is composed of normal columnar cells, but the lamina propria is packed with plasma cells and other mononuclear cells. Surgical biopsies in this patient revealed evidence of generalized subepithelial histiocytic lymphoma.**

weight loss, abdominal masses, obstruction, and perforation. IP-SID is associated with α heavy chains (from IgA), with parapro-tein present in the serum, urine, or jejunal fluid. The disease is rare in developed nations and more common in underprivileged populations, primarily in persons in the second and third decades of life, with a male predominance. It is a B cell disorder involving the mucosa-associated lymphoid tissue (MALT) and is one of the infectious pathogen–associated lymphomas. *Campylobacter jejuni* is the inciting agent.[54] Duodenography shows thick-ened folds and many nodular elevations without ulceration. The diagnosis may be made by small bowel biopsy in 85% of cases.[55] Early in the course of the disease, the condition appears to be treatable with antibiotics. If allowed to progress, however, it may develop into more aggressive forms of lymphoma.[56]

INTESTINAL LYMPHANGIECTASIA

Intestinal lymphangiectasia is often a congenital condition in which deformed lymphatics impair the transport of chylomicrons from the enterocytes to the mesenteric lymph duct. A similar pathophysiologic picture is acquired in certain cases of intestinal lymphomas, granulomatous enteritis, tuberculous enteritis, or Whipple disease in which normal lymphatic drainage is blocked.

Diagnosis

The blockage of lymphatic drainage may result in chylous as-cites, chyluria, or chylometrorrhea.[57] Protein-losing enteropathy and lymphopenia are prominent features. Modest steatorrhea is also present, with fat excretion commonly reaching 20 g/day. In the congenital form of the disease, lymphedema of the legs or of one leg and one arm is seen. On endoscopic examination, white villi, white nodules, and submucosal elevations may be noted.[58] The white appearance of the mucosa is undoubtedly caused by retained chylomicron triacylglycerol. Double-contrast barium x-ray examination shows smooth nodular protrusions and thick mucosal folds without ulceration.[59] On histologic examination, dilated lymphatics with club-shaped villi are seen, sometimes in asymptomatic patients, in whom the outcome is benign.

Treatment

Treatment is directed toward any identified causative process. In patients with the congenital condition, in whom improve-ment of the deranged lymphatics is not expected, a low-fat diet supplemented with medium-chain triglycerides is usually help-ful. Surgery can be used to remove isolated areas of lymphatic dysfunction, if these areas can be identified, or to anastomose a lymph duct to the venous system. Sometimes a peritoneovenous (LeVeen) shunt is helpful.

ABETALIPOPROTEINEMIA

Persons with the rare congenital condition of abetalipopro-teinemia do not have postprandial chylomicronemia, because they are unable to adequately couple apolipoprotein B to the de-veloping chylomicron. Because lipid and lipid-soluble vitamins are transported from the intestine in chylomicrons, the conse-quent reduction in lipid and lipid-soluble vitamin absorption re-sults in symptomatic steatorrhea, neurologic abnormalities, a variant of retinitis pigmentosa, and spiculated red cells. In con-trast to earlier theories about the etiology of this disease, these pa-tients have normally transcribed apolipoprotein B mRNA from which the protein is adequately translated. Nevertheless, apolipoprotein B is not secreted from the intestinal cell. The defect in this condition is in various mutations in the gene that encodes

the M component of microsomal triglyceride transport protein.[60] This chaperonelike protein complex, which consists of a 97 kd M component and a 55 kd component (protein disulfide isomerase), helps to translocate the apolipoprotein across the membrane of the endoplasmic reticulum.[61] Without this step, the apolipopro-tein is degraded by cytosolic and microsomal peptidases. The re-sult of this defect is that both the intestine and the liver are unable to produce and secrete their triacylglycerol-rich lipoproteins, chy-lomicrons, and very low density lipoproteins. Because chylomi-crons cannot transport the fat out of the enterocyte, it is pre-sumed, but not proved, that the surprisingly large amount of lipid that is absorbed (80%) is absorbed via the portal vein.[62]

Diagnosis

In addition to having intestinal symptoms, patients with abetalipoproteinemia have severe neurologic problems. These neurologic problems may be caused in part by essential fatty acid deficiency and in part by either the impaired delivery of lipid to nerves or an interference with the local synthesis of lipids. The result is a demyelinating condition resulting in a sen-sory ataxia caused by the loss of position and vibratory sensa-tions. The symptoms are similar to but less severe than those of Friedreich ataxia.[63] Patients may have muscle weakness and athetoid movements. Patients also experience retinitis pigmen-tosa, usually with mild loss of visual acuity but preservation of central vision. In addition to the neurologic abnormalities, pa-tients have acanthocytes in their blood. Acanthocytes are spicu-lated red cells that have a near-normal life span but that demon-strate an increased susceptibility to mechanical trauma on in vi-tro testing.

These patients have low plasma triacylglycerol and choles-terol levels. On histologic examination, the enterocytes are seen to be laden with fat. Despite this phenotype, the amount of steat-orrhea is modest (about 20 g/day).

Abetalipoproteinemia is usually discovered in childhood be-cause patients with the disease fail to thrive and have steator-rhea. In adults, the disease can be recognized by the combination of neurologic and ophthalmologic findings, the red cell mor-phology, the very low levels of plasma lipids, and the modest steatorrhea. On small bowel biopsy, the enterocytes are seen to be stuffed with lipid even after an overnight fast, indicating that the absorbed lipid cannot exit the enterocytes.[64]

Treatment

Treatment should include vitamin E as well as the other fat-soluble vitamins and medium-chain triglycerides to reduce the steatorrhea, if required.

EOSINOPHILIC GASTROENTERITIS

Eosinophilic gastroenteritis is a rare disease that is character-ized by the presence of eosinophilic infiltration of one or more portions of the GI tract, anywhere from the esophagus to the colon, in conjunction with gastrointestinal symptoms. Rarely, the pancreas is involved as well.[65] No identifiable cause of the eosinophilic infiltrate, such as parasitic infestation, is present. Many patients have an underlying allergic diathesis (e.g., hay fever, asthma, atopic dermatitis, or drug allergies).

It is not known why eosinophils congregate in the GI tract in this condition, but evidence suggests that eosinophils, once acti-vated, can produce cytokines that self-perpetuate the accumula-tion of additional eosinophils. These cytokines are interleukin-3 (IL-3), IL-5, and granulocyte-macrophage colony-stimulating factor (GM-CSF), which have been identified in eosinophils of patients but not in control subjects with irritable bowel syndrome. Local production of these cytokines is suggested by the finding that serum levels of IL-5 are normal in patients with eosinophilic gastroenteritis, in contrast to patients with the hypereosinophilic syndrome, who have increased levels of IL-5 in their blood.[66]

Diagnosis

Although eosinophils are a normal constituent of the GI tract, in eosinophilic gastroenteritis the eosinophils appear more numerous than normal and are more invasive. For example, eosinophilic invasion of the crypts in the small intestine is a hallmark of this condition. A peripheral eosinophilia is often seen but is not always present.

Eosinophilic gastroenteritis can be divided into two basic forms: a tumorous mass of eosinophils producing a granulomatous-type lesion and a more diffusely infiltrative form. In the former case, the lesions are most often in the distal stomach, which may produce obstructive symptoms, or the masses may be found in the more proximal stomach, small bowel, or colon. When lesions are in the small bowel or colon, the condition needs to be differentiated from a lymphoma or Crohn disease.[67] In the case of diffuse disease involving the small bowel, the infiltration can be mucosal, with symptoms of protein-losing enteropathy or malabsorption. If the infiltration is primarily in the muscle layers of the intestine, obstructive symptoms are common. Finally, the disease may be found in the subserosal area of the intestine, with resultant eosinophilic ascites.[68]

Treatment

Most patients respond to conservative measures and steroids. Surgery should be avoided unless it is needed to relieve persistent pyloric or small bowel obstruction.

Prednisone, 40 mg orally every morning and tapered slowly over 2 weeks, is the most effective therapy for patients with obstructive symptoms and ascites. If high-dose steroids are needed to maintain remission, azathioprine can be added for its steroid-sparing effect.

Diet elimination therapy may be beneficial in patients with mucosal layer involvement.

CROHN DISEASE

Crohn disease, a stenosing, fistulizing disease of the intestine, may impair intestinal absorption by at least two mechanisms, ileal dysfunction and the stasis syndrome [see Stasis (Bacterial Overgrowth) Syndrome, below]. In the case of either ileal resection or severe ileal involvement with Crohn disease, the ileum cannot absorb bile salts normally. In that event, postprandial bile salt deficiency occurs in the upper intestine; this condition may become more severe the later in the day a meal is eaten.[69] Postprandial bile salt deficiency occurs despite increased bile acid synthesis by the liver, in response to bile acid loss from the enterohepatic circulation. The increase in bile salt synthesis is not adequate because each time the gallbladder contracts in response to a meal, most of the bile salt pool is lost to the colon if significant amounts of the ileum have been resected.[70] Thus, the liver does not have time to generate enough replacement bile salts for the complete absorption of the meal just eaten or the next one. The colonic perfusion of bile acids may result in diarrhea. This condition has been termed choleretic enteropathy and may occur when more than 30 cm of the terminal ileum is resected. The excess fluid in the colon is caused by cAMP-driven Cl^- secretion, specifically by the dihydroxylated bile acids chenodeoxycholate and deoxycholate, not trihydroxylated cholic acid.[71]

Diagnosis

The loss of bile acids to the colon and thus to the enterohepatic circulation can be associated with no or minimal steatorrhea.[72]

With more extensive (100 cm or greater) ileal resection, however, the diarrhea is caused not only by bile acids but also by malabsorbed fatty acids (steatorrhea).[73] Thus, diarrhea in patients with Crohn disease may be caused not by active disease but rather by the results of ileal resection. This scenario is suggested by diarrhea that occurs when the patient first eats after surgery—a time when disease activity may be low secondary to active disease resection—or by the fact that the patient had no or minimal diarrhea before surgery, with diarrhea becoming more prominent afterward.

Because of the stenosis present in some patients with Crohn disease, the stasis syndrome can develop [see Stasis (Bacterial Overgrowth) Syndrome, below].

Treatment

When the diarrhea is caused by bile acid loss, the treatment is cholestyramine (4 g a.c. and h.s.).[73] This resin preferentially binds the dihydroxylated bile acids, reducing their aqueous concentration and reducing their proportion in the total bile acid pool. Both effects are beneficial. In the case of larger ileal resections in which steatorrhea is prominent, cholestyramine may actually provoke more diarrhea and malabsorption because it reduces the aqueous bile acid concentration in the upper intestine when taken before meals. In this case, medium-chain fatty acids are used as a replacement for the long-chain fatty acids. The results of this strategy are often not as good as desired. Vitamin B_{12} absorption should also be evaluated in all patients with ileal resection; if absorption is found to be abnormal, vitamin B_{12} should be given parenterally.

Some patients with severe Crohn disease undergo extensive intestinal resection, resulting effectively in short bowel syndrome. Similarly, patients who have numerous enteroenteric fistulas also have symptoms of short bowel syndrome because the fistulas cause the chyme to bypass large sections of the small intestine. Both types of patients should be treated as if they had short bowel syndrome.

STASIS (BACTERIAL OVERGROWTH) SYNDROME

The stasis (bacterial overgrowth) syndrome occurs when intestinal stasis allows bacteria to proliferate locally. This condition has a multiplicity of causes. The most prominent causes are diabetes; scleroderma; intestinal diverticulosis; afferent loop of a gastrojejunostomy; and intestinal obstruction caused by strictures, adhesions, or cancer. These disorders may be present years before the development of symptoms. Symptoms may appear in an otherwise stable patient because of the administration of a proton pump inhibitor, which reduces gastric acid production, allowing gastric and small bowel overgrowth; or the administration of an opiate that further reduces intestinal motility.

Pathophysiology

Intestinal dysfunction in the stasis syndrome is probably caused by bacterial glycosidases that hydrolyze the carbohydrate moieties that form the extensive glycosylation of the apical brush-border proteins.[74] Although bile acid deconjugation occurs in the stasis syndrome, which may theoretically lead to impaired solubilization of the products of triglyceride hydrolysis, studies have shown that in fact the fatty acid concentration in the aqueous phase of postprandial intestinal content is normal.[75] Electron micrographs, however, show that there is damage to the enterocytes, in that absorbed lipid collects in the endoplasmic reticulum and does not progress normally to the Golgi apparatus.[75]

Diagnosis

Clinical manifestations Symptoms of the stasis syndrome are similar to those of other malabsorptive states and include steatorrhea and anemia. The patient may have vitamin B_{12} deficiency, which has several causes, including binding of the vitamin to bacteria[76] and bacterial metabolism of the vitamin to metabolically ineffective metabolites. Folic acid levels are usually high, secondary to bacterial production of folate.[77] Serum albumin levels may be low secondary to protein-losing enteropathy and remain low for months after adequate treatment. The diagnosis is usually made in a patient with malabsorption in the appropriate clinical setting. Intestinal (usually jejunal) diverticulosis is usually unsuspected until a small bowel x-ray is performed.

Laboratory tests Establishing the diagnosis of the stasis syndrome is not simple. The most accurate way is to pass an aspiration tube into the intestine. The fluid must be quantitatively cultured both aerobically and especially anaerobically. In most cases, more than 10^5 anaerobes will be found. Alternatively, the noninvasive hydrogen breath test may be used. A high resting hydrogen level or a quick increase in the breath hydrogen in response to a fermentable substrate, such as glucose or lactulose, can be used. Another breath test is the 1 g (^{14}C)-D-xylose test, in which the breath $^{14}CO_2$ is measured.

Treatment

The first choice of treatment for the stasis syndrome is surgical correction of defects, such as an afferent loop that is harboring bacteria, or a jejunocolic fistula. If the surgical option is not available, then recurrent dosing of an antibiotic is required. Tetracycline, at a dosage of 1 to 2 g/day for a 7- to 10-day course, gives good results, or another antibiotic that is active against anaerobic bacteria may be used (e.g., trimethroprim-sulfamethoxazole, one double-strength tablet b.i.d.). The patient will need to be re-treated if clinical symptoms reappear, or the patient can receive treatment for 1 week every month.

AMYLOIDOSIS

The intestine is often involved in patients with systemic amyloidosis, especially if they have polyneuropathy. In patients older than 85 years, 36% have intestinal involvement with amyloidosis,[78] although most are asymptomatic. Endoscopically, mucosal erosion, friability, or polypoid protrusions can be seen.[79] The diagnosis is made by either full-thickness or peroral intestinal biopsies. If a peroral biopsy is performed, it must be deep enough to have arteries visible, so that amyloid, if present, can be demonstrated. Congo red–stained arterioles that become apple green under polarized light confirm the diagnosis. Small bowel follow-through x-rays may show swollen intestinal plicae, possibly with separated loops of bowel. If steatorrhea is present, it may be the result either of bacterial overgrowth caused by intestinal dysmotility or of impaired bile acid absorption.[80] No specific effective therapy is available. If bacterial overgrowth is present, then appropriate antibiotics should be given.

SYSTEMIC MASTOCYTOSIS

Systemic mastocytosis is a rare condition in which the skin (99% of cases), bones (9%), liver (12%), spleen (11%), lymph nodes, and GI tract are involved with proliferating mast cells. Diarrhea or abdominal pain or both (23% of cases), peptic ulceration (4%), and itching and flushing (36%) may be seen. Headache, fatigue, and malaise are seen in 12% of cases. There may also be cognitive dysfunction. Eosinophilia is seen in 12% to 50% of cases.[81] Many of these manifestations of the disease are secondary to histamine, which is released from the mast cells. Histamine release may be precipitated by alcohol, aspirin, narcotics, and nonsteroidal anti-inflammatory drugs, causing episodic disturbances of flushing, diarrhea, abdominal pain, and hypotension that may progress to syncope.[81]

Excess histamine is excreted into the urine in approximately 75% of patients with systemic mastocytosis, making this test useful for diagnostic purposes.[81] The urinary excretion of a metabolite of prostaglandin D_2 from mast cells may be an even better test.[82] X-ray studies of the small intestine may show thickened folds or nodulation. These findings are not diagnostic but may point to a diseased small bowel.

Histamine-mediated overproduction of gastric acid may lead to peptic ulceration. H_2 blockers or proton pump inhibitors are effective in controlling symptoms in such patients. In the skin, urticaria pigmentosa may be effectively treated with H_1 receptor antagonists such as diphenhydramine (25 mg every 6 to 8 hours). If diarrhea persists, cromolyn sodium may be given at a dosage of 100 mg orally four times a day.

Parasitic Infestations

Hookworm and *G. lamblia* infections can cause mild malabsorption that is rarely clinically important. Eradication of the parasites cures the absorptive defect. These issues are discussed more fully elsewhere [*see Chapter 157 and 158*].

Chronic Pancreatitis with Exocrine Insufficiency

Most cases of chronic pancreatitis are caused by alcoholism. In rare cases, the disease is inherited. Patients with chronic pancreatitis experience weight loss resulting from malabsorption of food. Malabsorption caused by pancreatitis is discussed elsewhere [*see Chapter 73*].

Combined or Multiple Defects in Digestion and Absorption

POSTGASTRECTOMY STEATORRHEA

One of the consequences of gastric surgery is steatorrhea, primarily in patients who have the Billroth II gastric resection with a gastrojejunostomy. In this operation, the antrum and a variable portion of the body of the stomach are resected, the stomach is sutured closed, and a gastrojejunostomy is created. Thus, food bypasses the duodenum and most proximal jejunum, the sites of maximal cholecystokinin and secretin concentrations and the active sites for folate, calcium, and iron absorption. Approximately one half of patients who have undergone the Billroth II procedure have steatorrhea of 10 to 15 g of fat/day. This condition is thought to result from food entering the jejunum without the hormone-sensitive sites in the duodenum receiving the appropriate signals for hormone release. Thus, there is poor gallbladder contraction and reduced release of pancreatic digestive enzymes to the intestine, resulting in poor admixing of the chyme with pancreatic enzymes and bile acids. The afferent loop, which drains the duodenum and proximal jejunum, may become blocked or atonic and harbor bacteria. The stasis syndrome may occur if enough bacteria are present. Because of their small stomachs, these patients cannot eat as much as they previously could. This decrease in food consumption, in combination with steatorrhea, causes many patients who undergo the Billroth II procedure to maintain a lower weight than they did before surgery. Osteopenia and iron deficiency anemia are also found. The constant loss of small amounts of blood from the gastric ostomy site, combined with impaired iron absorption, contribute to the iron-deficient state, which is the most common form of anemia. Folate deficiency secondary to the inability to generate absorbable monoglutamyl folate from nonabsorbable heptaglutamyl folate (the common form of folate found in the diet) is also found.[83] Least commonly seen is vitamin B_{12} deficiency caused by hypochlorhydria and resection of intrinsic factor–containing gastric parietal cells. Treatment of the steatorrhea is usually not necessary, because it is not clinically significant. Iron, calcium, or vitamin B_{12} and folic acid must be replaced as indicated. If the patient has early satiety, multiple small meals may be efficacious.

Symptoms of GSE may develop in patients after gastric surgery.[84] It is likely that these patients had clinically silent GSE before the operation. The operation itself causes modest steatorrhea (10 to 15 g of fat/day) in 50% of cases, even in patients whose intestine is otherwise normal. In the previously compensated GSE patient, however, surgery is enough to cause clinical symptoms. Therefore, an evaluation for GSE is warranted in postgastrectomy patients who exhibit excessive steatorrhea. Inflammatory bowel disease that develops in patients after gastrectomy may likewise be an indication of the presence of previously silent GSE.[85]

DIABETES MELLITUS AND MALABSORPTION

Diarrhea, which is one of the more common complications of diabetes, has multiple causes[86] and may result in malabsorption [see Chapter 66]. The most common causes are bacterial overgrowth, secondary to diabetic autonomic dysfunction that results in intestinal stasis, and GSE. In one study, screening with antiendomysial antibody assays identified GSE in three of 47 diabetic patients (6%), a much higher incidence than would be expected by chance.[87]

The author has no commercial relationships with manufacturers of products or providers of services discussed in this chapter.

References

1. Moreau H, Gargouri Y, Bernadal A, et al: Etude biochemique et physiologique des lipases préduodéales d'origines animale et humaine. Revue Française des Corps Gras 35:169, 1988

2. Roulet M, Weber A, Roy C: Perspectives in Cystic Fibrosis. Canada Cystic Fibrosis Foundation, Toronto, 1980, p 172

3. Levitt MD, Duane WC: Floating stools: flatus versus fat. N Engl J Med 286:973, 1972

4. Drummy GD, Benson JA Jr, Jones CM: Microscopical examination of the stool for steatorrhea. N Engl J Med 264:85, 1961

5. Neucker AV, Bijleveld CM, Wolthers BG, et al: Comparison of near infrared reflectance analysis of fecal fat, nitrogen and water with conventional methods, and fecal energy content. Clin Biochem 35:29, 2002

6. DiMagno EP, Go VLW, Summerskill WHJ: Relation between pancreatic enzyme outputs and malabsorption in severe pancreatic insufficiency. N Engl J Med 288:813, 1973

7. Dreiling DA, Janowitz HD: The measurement of pancreatic secretory function. The Exocrine Pancreas. De Reuck AVS, Cameron MP, Eds. Ciba Foundation Symposium. Little, Brown & Co, New York, 1961, p 225

8. Kato H, Nakao A, Kishimoto W, et al: 13C-labeled trioctanoin breath test for exocrine pancreatic function test in patients after pancreatoduodenectomy. Am J Gastroenterol 88:64, 1993

9. Lang C: Value of serum PABA as a pancreatic function test. Gut 25:508, 1984

10. Bando N, Ogawa T, Tsuji H: Enzymatic method for selective determination of 4 aminobenzoic acid in urine. Clin Chem 36:1937, 1990

11. Jacobson DG, Curlington C, Connery K, et al: Trypsin-like immunoreactivity as a test for pancreatic insufficiency. N Engl J Med 310:1307, 1984

12. Loser C, Mollgaard A, Folsch UR: Faecal elastase 1: a novel, highly sensitive, and specific tubeless pancreatic function test. Gut 39:580, 1996

13. Walkowiak J, Cichy WK, Herzig KH: Comparison of fecal elastase-1 determination with the secretin-cholecystokinin test in patients with cystic fibrosis. Scand J Gastroenterol 34:202, 1999

14. Oelkers P, Kirby LC, Heubi JE, et al: Primary bile acid malabsorption caused by mutations in the ileal sodium-dependent bile acid transporter gene. J Clin Invest 99:1880, 1997

15. Shindo K, Yamazaki R, Koide K, et al: Alteration of bile acid metabolism by cimetidine in healthy humans. J Investig Med 44:462, 1996

16. Nyhlin H, Merrick MV, Eastwood MA, et al: Evaluation of ileal function using 23-selena-25-homotaurocholate, a γ-labeled conjugated bile acid. Gastroenterology 84:63, 1983

17. Crenn P, Coudray-Lucas C, Thuillier F, et al: Postabsorptive plasma citrulline concentration is a marker of absorptive enterocyte mass and intestinal failure in humans. Gastroenterology 119:1496, 2000

18. Make M, Collin P: Coeliac disease. Lancet 349:1755, 1997

19. Not T, Horvath K, Hill ID, et al: Celiac disease risk in the USA: high prevalence of antiendomysium antibodies in healthy blood donors. Scand J Gastroenterol 33:494, 1998

20. Catassi C, Fabiani E, Ratsch IM, et al: The coeliac iceberg in Italy: a multicentre antigliadin antibodies screening for coeliac disease in school-age subjects. Acta Paediatr Suppl 412:29, 1996

21. Fasano A, Berti I, Gerarduzzi T, et al: Prevalence of celiac disease in at-risk and not-at-risk groups in the United States: a large multicenter study. Arch Intern Med 163:286, 2003

22. Anderson RP, Degano P, Godkin AJ, et al: In vivo antigen challenge in celiac disease identifies a single transglutaminase-modified peptide as the dominant α-gliadin T-cell epitope. Nat Med 6:337, 2000

23. Shan L, Molberg O, Parrot I, et al: Structural basis for gluten intolerance in celiac sprue. Science 297:2218, 2002

24. Matysiak-Budnik T, Candalh C, Dugave C, et al: Alterations of the intestinal transport and processing of gliadin peptides in celiac disease. Gastroenterology 125:696, 2003

25. Hofmann AF: The function of bile salts in fat absorption. Biochem J 89:57, 1963

26. Mansbach CM II, Cohen RS, Leff PB: Isolation and properties of the mixed micelles present in intestinal content during fat digestion in man. J Clin Invest 56:781, 1975

27. Dieterich W, Laag E, Schöpper H, et al: Autoantibodies to tissue transglutaminase as predictors of coeliac disease. Gastroenterology 115:1317, 1998

28. Volta V, Molinaro N, deFranceschi L, et al: IgA antiendomysial antibodies on human umbilical cord tissue for celiac disease screening. Dig Dis Sci 40:1902, 1995

29. Holmes GKT, Prior P, Lane MR, et al: Malignancy in coeliac disease: effect of a gluten-free diet. Gut 30:333, 1989

30. Gawkrodger DJ, Vestey JP, O'Mahouny S: Dermatitis herpetiformis and established coeliac disease. Br J Dermatol 129:694, 1993

31. Klipstein FA, Falaiye JM: Tropical sprue in expatriates from the tropics living in the continental United States. Medicine 48:475, 1969

32. Lindenbaum J, Gerson CD, Kent TH: Recovery of small intestinal structure and function after residence in the tropics: I. studies in Peace Corps volunteers. Ann Intern Med 74:218, 1971

33. Gerson CD, Kent TH, Saha JR, et al: Recovery of small intestinal structure and function after residence in the tropics: II. studies in Indians and Parkistanis living in New York City. Ann Intern Med 75:41, 1971

34. Haghighi P, Wolf PL: Tropical sprue and subclinical enteropathy: a vision for the nineties. Crit Rev Clin Lab Sci 34:313, 1997

35. Robert ME, Ament ME, Weinstein WM: The histologic spectrum and clinical outcome of refractory and unclassified sprue. Am J Surg Pathol 24:676, 2000

36. Freeman HJ: Collagenous mucosal inflammatory diseases of the gastrointestinal tract. Gastroenterology 129:338, 2005

37. McCashland TM, Donovan JP, Strobach RS, et al: Collagenous enterocolitis: a manifestation of gluten-sensitive enteropathy. J Clin Gastroenterol 15:45, 1992

38. Hermaszewski RA, Webster AD: Primary hypogammaglobulinaemia: a survey of clinical manifestations and complications. Q J Med 86:31, 1993

39. Ladefoged K, Hessov I, Jarnum S: Nutrition in short-bowel syndrome. Scand J Gastroenterol 216(suppl):122, 1996

40. Lin HC, Zhao XT, Wang L: Fat absorption is not complete by midgut but is dependent on load of fat. Am J Physiol 271(1 pt 1):G62, 1996

41. Lin HC, Zhao XT, Wong H: Fat-induced ileal brake in the dog depends on peptide YY. Gastroenterology 110:1491, 1996

42. Redman DA, Schmidt TM, McDermott RP, et al: Identification of the uncultured bacillus of Whipple's disease. N Engl J Med 327:393, 1992

43. Durand DV, Lecomte C, Cathebras P, et al: Whipple disease: clinical review of 52 cases. The SNFMI Research Group on Whipple Disease. Medicine (Baltimore) 76:170, 1997

44. Dobbins WO III: HLA antigens in Whipple's disease. Arthritis Rheum 30:102, 1987

45. Mansbach CM II, Shelburne J, Stevens RD, et al: Lymph node bacilliform bodies morphologically resembling those of Whipple's disease in a patient without intestinal involvement. Ann Intern Med 89:64, 1978

46. Street S, Donoghue HD, Neild GH: *Tropheryma whippelii* DNA in saliva of healthy people. Lancet 354:1178, 1999

47. Swartz MN: Whipple's disease: past, present and future. N Engl J Med 342:648, 2000

48. von Herbay A, Ditton HJ, Schumacher F, et al: Whipple's disease: staging and monitoring by cytology and polymerase chain reaction analysis of cerebrospinal fluid. Gastroenterology 113:434, 1997

49. Kelly CA, Egan M, Rawlinson J: Whipple's disease presenting with lung involvement. Thorax 51:343, 1996

50. Monkemuller K, Fry LC, Rickes S, et al: Whipple's disease. Curr Infect Dis Rep 8:96, 2006

51. Louis ED, Lynch T, Kaufmann P, et al: Diagnostic guidelines in central nervous system Whipple's disease. J Ann Neurol 40:561, 1996

52. Feurle GE, Marth T: An evaluation of antimicrobial treatment for Whipple's disease: tetracycline versus trimethoprim-sulfamethoxazole. Dig Dis Sci 39:1642, 1994

53. Shih LY, Liaw SJ, Dunn P, et al: Primary small-intestinal lymphomas in Taiwan: immunoproliferative small-intestinal disease and nonimmunoproliferative small-intestinal disease. J Clin Oncol 12:1375, 1994

54. Al-Saleem T, Al-Mondhiry H: Immunoproliferative small intestinal disease (IPSID): a model for mature B-cell neoplasms. Blood 105:2274, 2005

55. Halphen M, Najjar T, Jaafoura H, et al: Diagnostic value of upper intestinal fiber endoscopy in primary small intestinal lymphoma: a prospective study by the Tunisian-French Intestinal Lymphoma Group. Cancer 58:2140, 1986

56. Khojasteh A, Haghighi P: Immunoproliferative small intestinal disease: portrait of a potentially preventable cancer from the Third World. Am J Med 89:483, 1990

57. Fox C, Lucani G: Disorders of the intestinal mesenteric lymphatic system. Lymphology 26:61, 1993

58. Aoyagi K, Iida M, Yao T, et al: Characteristic endoscopic features of intestinal lymphangiectasia: correlation with histological findings. Hepatogastroenterology 44:133, 1997

59. Aoyagi K, Iida M, Yao T, et al: Intestinal lymphangiectasia: value of double-contrast radiographic study. Clin Radiol 49:814, 1994

60. Sharp D, Blinderman L, Combs KA, et al: Cloning and gene defects in microsomal triglyceride transfer protein associated with abetalipoproteinaemia. Nature 365:65, 1993

61. Gordon DA, Jamil H, Gregg RE, et al: Inhibition of the microsomal triglyceride transfer protein blocks the step of apolipoprotein B lipoprotein assembly but not the addition of bulk core lipids in the second step. J Biol Chem 271:33047, 1996

62. Mansbach CM II, Dowell RF, Pritchett D: Portal transport of absorbed lipids in the rat. Am J Physiol 261:G530, 1991

63. Isselbacher KJ, Scheig R, Plotkin GR, et al: Congenital β-lipoprotein deficiency: an hereditary disorder involving a defect in the absorption and transport of lipids. Medicine (Baltimore) 43:347, 1964

64. Ways PO, Parmentier CM, Kayden HJ, et al: Studies on the absorptive defect for triglyceride in abetalipoproteinemia. J Clin Invest 46:35, 1967

65. Lyngbaek S, Adamsen S, Aru A, et al: Recurrent acute pancreatitis due to eosinophilic gastroenteritis: case report and literature review. JOP 7:211, 2006

66. Desreumaux P, Blogot F, Seguy D, et al: Interleukin 3, granulocyte-macrophage colony-stimulating factor, and interleukin 5 in eosinophilic gastroenteritis. Gastroenterology 110:768, 1996

67. Salmon PR, Paulley JW: Eosinophilic granuloma of the gastrointestinal tract. Gut 8:8, 1967

68. Klein NC, Hargrove RL, Sleisenger MH, et al: Eosinophilic gastroenteritis. Medicine (Baltimore) 49:299, 1970

69. Van Deest BW, Fordtran JS, Morawski SG, et al: Bile salt and micellar fat concentration in proximal small bowel contents of ileectomy patients. J Clin Invest 47:1314, 1968

70. Low-Beer TS, Wilkins RM, Lack L, et al: Effect of one meal on enterohepatic circulation of bile salts. Gastroenterology 67:490, 1974

71. Merhjian HS, Phillips SF, Hofmann AF: Colonic secretion of water and electrolytes induced by bile acids: perfusion studies in man. J Clin Invest 50:1569, 1971

72. Mansbach CM II, Newton DF, Stevens RD: Fat digestion in patients with bile acid malabsorption but minimal steatorrhea. Dig Dis Sci 25:353, 1980

73. Hofmann AF, Poley JR: Role of bile acid malabsorption in pathogenesis of diarrhea and steatorrhea in patients with ileal resection: I. Response to cholestyramine or replacement of dietary long chain triglyceride by medium chain triglyceride. Gastroenterology 62:918, 1972

74. Riepe S, Goldstein J, Alpers DH: Effect of secreted *Bacteroides* proteases on human intestinal brush border hydrolases. J Clin Invest 66:314, 1980

75. Ament ME, Shimoda SS, Saunders DR, et al: Pathogenesis of steatorrhea in three cases of small intestinal stasis syndrome. Gastroenterology 63:728, 1972

76. Gianella RA, Broitman SA, Zamcheck N: Vitamin B_{12} uptake by intestinal microorganisms: mechanisms and relevance to syndromes of bacterial overgrowth. J Clin Invest 50:1100, 1971

77. Hoffbrand AV, Tabaqchali S, Booth CC, et al: Small intestinal bacterial flora and folate status in gastrointestinal disease. Gut 12:27, 1971

78. Rocken C, Saeger W, Linke RP: Gastrointestinal amyloid deposits in old age: report of 110 consecutive autopsical patients and 98 retrospective bioptic specimens. Pathol Res Pract 190:641, 1994

79. Tada S, Iida M, Yao KK, et al: Endoscopic features in amyloidosis of the small intestine: clinical and morphologic differences between chemical types of amyloid protein. Gastrointest Endosc 40:45, 1994

80. Suhr O, Danielsson A, Steen L: Bile acid malabsorption caused by gastrointestinal motility dysfunction? An investigation of gastrointestinal disturbances in familial amyloidosis with polyneuropathy. Scand J Gastroenterol 27:201, 1992

81. Golkar L, Bernhard JD: Mastocytosis. Lancet 349:1379, 1997

82. Morrow JD, Guzzo C, Lazarus G, et al: Improved diagnosis of mastocytosis by measurements of the major urinary metabolite of prostaglandin D_2. J Invest Dermatol 104:937, 1995

83. Rosenberg IH: Folate absorption and malabsorption. N Engl J Med 293:1303, 1975

84. Bai J, Moran C, Martinez C: Celiac sprue after surgery of the upper gastrointestinal tract: report of 10 patients with special attention to diagnosis, clinical behavior, and follow-up. J Clin Gastroenterol 13:521, 1991

85. Kitis G, Holmes GTK, Cooper BT: Association of coeliac disease and inflammatory bowel disease. Gut 21:636, 1980

86. Valdovinos MA, Camilleri M, Zimmerman BR: Chronic diarrhea in diabetes mellitus: mechanisms and an approach to diagnosis and treatment. Mayo Clin Proc 68:691, 1993

87. Rensch MJ, Merenich JA, Lieberman M, et al: Gluten-sensitive enteropathy in patients with insulin-dependent diabetes mellitus. Ann Intern Med 124:564, 1996

Acknowledgment

Figure 1   Dana Burns-Pizer.

66 Diarrheal Diseases

Lawrence R. Schiller, M.D., F.A.C.P.

The word diarrhea is derived from the Greek words for "flowing through." For most persons, diarrhea means the frequent passage of loose stools.[1] This definition includes two major components: loose-stool consistency (pourable stools) and increased stool frequency (more than two bowel movements daily). Physicians often include a third component: increased stool weight (> 200 g/24 hr), but patients are poor estimators of stool output. In addition, some patients report diarrhea when they have fecal incontinence, even if stools are solid; therefore, every patient complaining of diarrhea should be asked about incontinence.

Diarrhea is a universal human experience. Most persons have had acute infectious diarrhea at some time during their lives. The incidence of acute diarrhea is roughly 5% to 7% annually in the United States.[2] Infectious diarrhea is associated with contaminated food and water and typically is spread via fecal-oral transmission. Chronic diarrhea (i.e., lasting more than 4 weeks) is also common, with a prevalence of approximately 5% in the United States.[3] It is less likely to be caused by infection and more likely to be a symptom of other disorders, such as inflammatory bowel disease, celiac disease, or lactose intolerance.

Pathophysiology and Classification

Diarrhea results from excess water in the stool.[4] To understand the pathophysiology of diarrhea, it is necessary to briefly review how water is transported across the mucosa of the gastrointestinal tract. Water moves in response to osmotic gradients that are established by the absorption of salts (mainly sodium chloride but also potassium and bicarbonate salts) and nutrients (monosaccharides, amino acids, and fatty acids). Salts and nutrients move both passively in response to electrochemical gradients across the mucosa and actively in response to molecular pumps located in the enterocyte membranes.[5]

Each day, a typical person ingests about 2 L of fluid and produces 7 to 8 L of secretions (i.e., saliva, gastric juice, bile, pancreatic juice, and succus entericus). Thus, a total volume of 9 to 10 L enters the upper intestine daily. Most of the water is absorbed in the jejunum, along with nutrients. Absorption of residual nutrients and salts in the ileum results in a reduction of the volume of luminal contents entering the colon to only 1 to 1.5 L daily, a 90% reduction in the volume of fluid entering the intestine each day. The colonic mucosa can absorb salt against large electrochemical gradients and can reclaim 90% of the fluid passing the ileocecal valve each day, making the overall efficiency of small bowel and colonic water absorption about 99%.

Diarrhea develops if the overall efficiency of absorption declines by as little as 1%. This can occur under the following circumstances: the rate of intestinal nutrient and salt absorption decreases; net electrolyte secretion develops (an unusual circumstance except in cases of severe secretory diarrhea such as cholera, in which stool output can exceed 10 L/day); transit through the intestine speeds up, thereby limiting the time available for absorption; or poorly absorbable substances are ingested and increase intraluminal osmotic activity, causing the retention of water within the intestine.[6]

Common problems that primarily cause a reduction in the rate of intestinal nutrient and salt absorption include mucosal diseases, such as celiac disease; inflammatory diseases that disrupt the integrity of the intestinal mucosa (e.g., Crohn disease); and infections that cause diarrhea as the result of toxins that affect enterocyte function.

Isolated acceleration of intestinal transit is a poorly recognized mechanism of diarrhea, although historically, diarrhea was always attributed to it. Some patients with so-called functional diarrhea have rapid intestinal transit, which is likely to be important in the pathogenesis of their condition. Many patients with chronic idiopathic diarrhea have normal rates of fluid and electrolyte absorption when measured under perfusion conditions during which motility effects are neutralized, suggesting that motility must be playing a role in the pathogenesis of their diarrhea under ordinary circumstances.[7] Accelerated transit is also a major factor in diarrhea that is associated with some endocrine diarrheas (e.g., hyperthyroidism, carcinoid syndrome, and other peptide-secreting tumors) or with irritable bowel syndrome.

Poorly absorbed substances that can induce osmotic diarrhea include lactose in lactose-intolerant individuals. Osmotic diarrhea can also occur with ingestion of excess quantities of other poorly absorbed carbohydrates (e.g., fructose and the sugar alcohols mannitol and sorbitol) and ions such as magnesium, phosphate, and sulfate.

Mechanisms that reduce the overall efficiency of absorption may coexist in various disease states. For instance, in celiac disease, loss of intestinal villi results in reduced salt and water absorption, as well as reduced nutrient absorption. Thus, increased stool water in this condition results from both a reduced rate of electrolyte absorption and the increased intraluminal osmotic activity of poorly absorbed substances. Intestinal transit may accelerate in many diarrheal states because of stimulation of peristalsis by increased intraluminal volumes.

FECAL OSMOTIC GAP

As the rate of intestinal salt absorption decreases, the concentration of salts in stool rises to the point at which the concentration approaches plasma osmolality (290 mOsm/kg), which is defined as the osmolality that intestinal contents must maintain beyond the proximal jejunum. If the rate of salt absorption is unimpaired but either nutrients are malabsorbed or poorly absorbable substances are ingested, fecal salt concentrations decrease because most of the available osmotic space is occupied by the poorly absorbed substance. This is the basis for calculation of the fecal osmotic gap [see Figure 1].[8] In this calculation, the contribution of electrolytes to stool osmolality is estimated by doubling the concentration of sodium and potassium (the predominant cations in stool water) to account for unmeasured anions (mostly fatty anions, bicarbonate, or chloride). This value is then subtracted from 290 mOsm/kg (the putative osmolality of gut contents) to determine the contribution of nonelectrolytes to fecal osmolality. When electrolytes constitute most of luminal osmolality, the calculated fecal osmotic gap will be low (< 50 mOsm/kg). When poorly absorbable substances are present, the fecal osmotic gap will be large (> 100 mOsm/kg). Watery diarrhea with a low osmotic gap is classified as secretory diarrhea; diarrhea with a large fecal osmotic gap is classified as osmotic di-

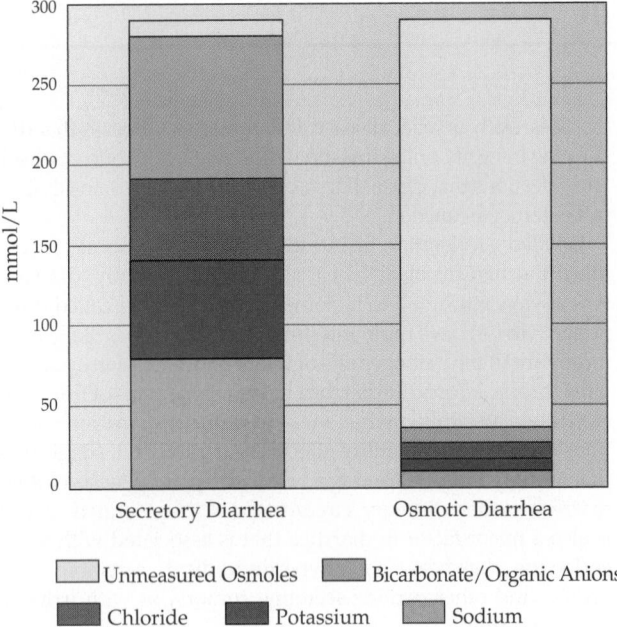

Unmeasured Osmoles Bicarbonate/Organic Anions
Chloride Potassium Sodium

Figure 1 Fecal electrolyte concentrations in secretory diarrhea (left column) and in osmotic diarrhea (right column). Note that most of the fecal osmolality can be attributed to fecal electrolytes in secretory diarrhea, whereas most of the osmolality in osmotic diarrhea results from the unmeasured (nonelectrolyte) osmoles. Calculation of the fecal osmotic gap allows an estimate of the contribution of unmeasured osmoles to fecal osmolality.[82]

arrhea. These categories are most helpful in the evaluation of patients with chronic diarrhea.

CLASSIFICATION OF DIARRHEA

For clinical purposes, diarrhea can be classified as either acute (< 4 weeks' duration) or chronic (> 4 weeks' duration). Chronic diarrhea is further divided into watery, inflammatory, and fatty on the basis of stool characteristics.[3] The value of this classification is that it allows the physician to direct evaluation and management more effectively, because diarrheal diseases can be distinguished by the duration of illness and the type of stools produced.

Acute Diarrhea

ETIOLOGY

Infectious Causes of Acute Diarrhea

Most forms of acute diarrhea (i.e., those lasting less than 4 weeks) are caused by infections and are self-limiting; the majority are caused by viruses (e.g., adenovirus, Norwalk agent, rotovirus), but some are caused by bacteria (e.g., *Salmonella*, *Shigella*, and *Escherichia coli*) and others by protozoa (e.g., *Giardia*, amebas) [*see Table 1*].[2] The disease course of most viral and bacterial diarrheas lasts less than 1 week; therefore, infectious diarrhea lasting more than 7 days is more likely to be caused by protozoa.[9]

The epidemiology of acute infectious diarrhea depends on the circumstances of the infection and where one contracts the infection. For example, a history of recent travel, particularly to developing countries, makes a diagnosis of traveler's diarrhea likely. Previous antibiotic use and residence in an institution where antibiotic use is common (e.g., hospitals and nursing homes) are risk factors for *Clostridium difficile* infection. Children in day care facilities and their contacts, people engaging in promiscuous sexual activity, and users of illicit intravenous drugs are all at increased risk of contracting infectious diarrhea. Consumption of potentially contaminated food and drink is another risk factor for infectious diarrhea. With the globalization of commerce and mass processing of food, esoteric infections from overseas and large outbreaks of diarrhea have become more common.[10]

Pathogenic infections cause diarrhea by one of four mechanisms: (1) enterotoxins that subvert the regulatory mechanisms of enterocytes, (2) cytotoxins that destroy enterocytes, (3) adherence to the mucosa by organisms (so-called enteroadherent organisms) that alter enterocyte function as a result of physical proximity to the mucosa, and (4) invasion of the mucosa by organisms that provoke an inflammatory response by the immune system.[11] In general, patients with cytotoxin-mediated diarrhea and those with invasive organisms experience more toxicity and have more abdominal pain than patients with enterotoxin-mediated diarrhea or enteroadherent infections.

Toxic Causes of Acute Diarrhea

Another mechanism for acute diarrhea is ingestion of a preformed toxin.[12] Several species of bacteria, such as *Staphylococcus aureus*, *Clostridium perfringens*, and *Bacillus cereus*, can produce toxins that in turn cause so-called food poisoning (i.e., vomiting and diarrhea within 4 hours after ingestion). In such cases, the bacteria do not need to establish an intraluminal infection; ingestion of the toxin alone can produce the disease. Symptoms subside after the toxin is cleared, usually by the next day, and evidence of toxicity (e.g., fever) is minimal.

Other Causes of Acute Diarrhea

Other potential causes of acute diarrhea include food allergies and medication reactions. Food allergies are rarely recognized as causes of diarrhea in adults in the United States unless the diarrhea is associated with urticaria or other allergic symptoms. Medications often produce diarrhea as a side effect; this association is typically recognized by the patient because of the temporal relation between drug ingestion and diarrhea.

Finally, acute diarrhea may represent the initial stages of chronic diarrhea. However, patients with chronic diarrhea often do not seek help during the initial weeks of their illness unless the diarrhea is severe or is complicated by dehydration, symptomatic electrolyte disorders, or fever.

DIAGNOSIS

Medical History

A careful medical history is the key to the diagnosis of diarrhea. The acuity and severity of the process should be determined. Frequency of defecation is the easiest parameter for patients to relate, but frequency does not necessarily correlate with stool weight, which is a more meaningful measure of the physiologic impact of diarrhea. Manifestations of dehydration or volume depletion, such as orthostasis, thirst, decreased urine output, and weakness, suggest voluminous diarrhea. Acute weight loss can also be a guide to the severity of diarrhea; voluminous diarrhea produces substantial weight loss if rehydration efforts are suboptimal.

Stool characteristics are also quite important. The presence of blood or pus in the stool raises the issue of inflammatory diarrhea, such as that from colitis or enteroinvasive bacteria. Watery

Table 1   Selected Infectious Diarrheas

Organism	Vehicle	Mechanism	Classic Characteristics	Complications
Campylobacter	Food (poultry); animal-to-person	Invasion; inflammation	Watery or bloody diarrhea; ileitis and/or colitis, ulceration	Guillain-Barré syndrome; reactive arthritis
Salmonella	Food (poultry, eggs, seafood); animal-to-person	Invasion; inflammation	Gastroenteritis, ileitis, colitis; enteric fever (*S. typhi*)	Endovascular infection; osteomyelitis; sepsis
Shigella	Food (poultry); day care centers	Cytotoxin; inflammation	Two phases: enteritis (fever, cramps, diarrhea), followed by colitis (ulcers, inflammation)	Seizures, encephalopathy; reactive arthritis
E. coli O157:H7	Food (beef); fruit juices	Cytotoxin	Hemorrhagic colitis	Hemolytic-uremic syndrome
Enteroinvasive *E. coli*	Food (various); water	Invasion; inflammation	Colitis	Fever, sepsis
Enterotoxigenic *E. coli*	Food (various); water	Enterotoxin	Watery diarrhea	Dehydration, shock
Enteropathogenic and enteroadherent *E. coli*	Food (various); water	Contact with brush border	Watery diarrhea; may be prolonged	Dehydration
Vibrio cholerae	Water, seafood	Enterotoxin	Voluminous watery diarrhea	Dehydration, shock
Clostridium difficile	Person-to-person	Cytotoxin	Nosocomial infection; antibiotic-associated diarrhea; toxicity	Toxic megacolon; protein-losing enteropathy
Aeromonas, Plesiomonas	Water	Enterotoxin	Watery diarrhea; may be prolonged	
Yersinia	Raw milk	Invasion; inflammation	Acute diarrhea or chronic ileo-colitis-like Crohn disease	Reactive arthritis, extraintestinal infection, Guillain-Barré syndrome
Bacillus cereus	Fried rice	Exotoxin	Acute gastroenteritis	Fulminant liver failure
Staphylococcus	Fatty foods	Exotoxin	Acute gastroenteritis	
Clostridium perfringens	Fatty foods	Exotoxin	Acute gastroenteritis	
Viruses	Person-to-person; water	Inflammation; ?toxins	Acute gastroenteritis; watery diarrhea	
Giardia	Person-to-person; animal-to-person; water; day care	Contact	Watery diarrhea, dyspepsia	
Cryptosporidium	Water; day care; animal-to-person	Contact	Watery diarrhea, may be prolonged; epidemics	
Cyclospora	Imported fruit	Inflammation	Watery diarrhea, flatulence, pain, fatigue; may be prolonged	
Entamoeba histolytica	Person-to-person	Invasion; inflammation	Variable: asymptomatic to dysentery; may mimic irritable bowel syndrome, inflammatory bowel disease	Liver abscess
Strongyloides	Larvae invade skin	Invasion; inflammation	Abdominal pain and diarrhea	Hyperinfection in immunosuppressed hosts

stools are more in keeping with a secretory process. The relationship of defecation to meals or fasting and the occurrence of nocturnal diarrhea, fecal urgency, or incontinence are other points of potential significance. Urgency and incontinence do not necessarily indicate voluminous diarrhea; more often, they reflect independent defects in the continence mechanisms. Additional symptoms of diarrhea that should be noted are abdominal pain or cramps; flatulence; bloating or distention; fever; and weight loss. A list of all prescription, over-the-counter, and herbal medications being taken by the patient should be compiled, and pre-vious surgeries or radiation therapy should be discussed. The patient's diet should be scrutinized, and epidemiologic features (e.g., family members or other contacts with diarrhea, recent travel, water source, occupation, sexual activity, and illicit drug use) should be investigated.

Physical Examination

The physical examination is more useful for judging the severity of diarrhea than for determining its cause. Volume status should be assessed by looking for orthostatic change in blood

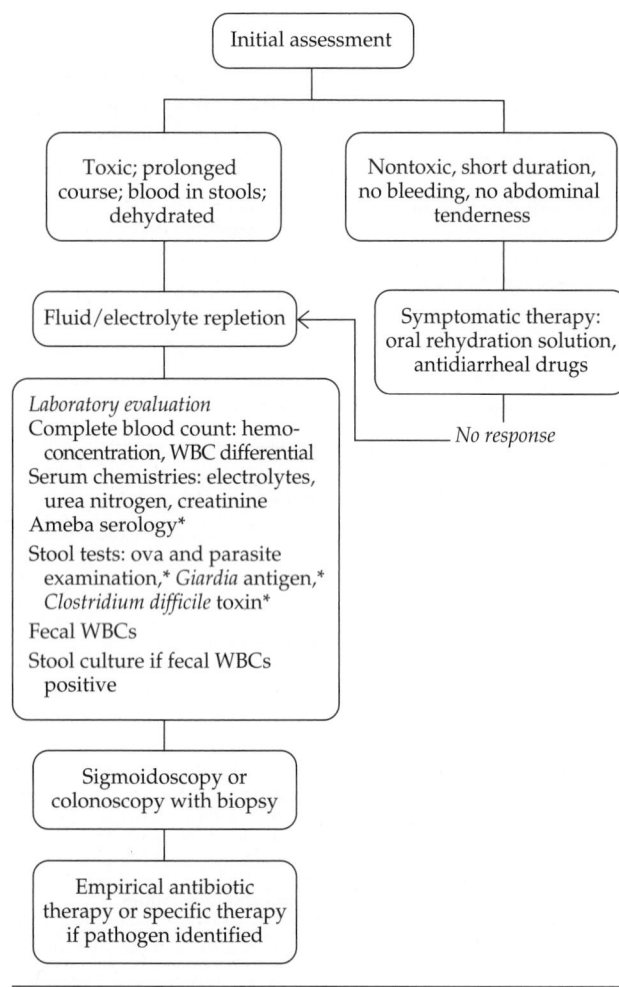

*In appropriate epidemiologic circumstances.

Figure 2   **Initial evaluation of acute diarrhea.**[83]

sive. Some experts recommend obtaining stool cultures only for patients who have leukocytes (or the leukocyte marker lactoferrin) in the stool, because the yield of pathogenic bacteria will be higher in this group.[13] Other researchers dispute this recommendation.[14] Laboratories routinely test for *Salmonella, Shigella, Campylobacter,* and *E. coli* serotype O157:H7. Special cultures for tuberculosis, *Yersinia, Aeromonas,* or *Plesiomonas* may need to be requested in appropriate patients. Polymerase chain reaction (PCR) testing with primers that are based on bacterial DNA is proving to be an accurate and sensitive technique for specific diagnosis.

Examination of stool for ova and parasites has variable utility, depending on the pretest probability of certain infections. For example, such testing might be very useful in a day care worker with diarrhea, but it would be of little help in a patient with hospital-acquired diarrhea. Enzyme-linked immunosorbent assay (ELISA) testing for giardiasis and serologic testing for amebiasis are more accurate tests for such specific infections in most settings. Patients who were treated with antibiotics during the 3 months before the onset of diarrhea or patients who develop diarrhea in institutional settings should have a stool sample analyzed for *C. difficile* toxin.

Imaging and Endoscopic Tests

In patients who have toxicity, blood in their stools, or persistent acute diarrhea, sigmoidoscopy or colonoscopy should be considered. In most patients without rectal bleeding, sigmoidoscopy is probably adequate as an initial evaluation, because most patients with colitis will have involvement of the left side of their colon. In patients with bleeding or those with AIDS and diarrhea, colonoscopy is preferable because some opportunistic infections and lymphomas are seen only in the right colon.[15] Mucosal biopsies should be obtained in either case, particularly if the colon is grossly inflamed, because the pathologist can readily distinguish self-limited colitis from chronic ulcerative colitis even early on in the course of the disease.[16] Patients with toxicity should undergo abdominal x-rays or computed tomography to confirm a diagnosis of colitis, to determine its extent, and to look for evidence of ileus or megacolon.

TREATMENT

Nonspecific Therapy

Because most cases of acute diarrhea are self-limited, most patients do not require specific therapy. Instead, judicious replacement of fluid and electrolyte losses is sufficient. This can be accomplished by intravenous fluids or oral rehydration solutions. Oral rehydration solutions are based on the concept that nutrient absorption accelerates sodium and fluid absorption by the jejunum.[17] Initially, rehydration formulas used glucose as the absorbable nutrient; more recently, cereal-based oral rehydration solutions have been found to be more efficient. Oral rehydration solution does not reduce fecal losses (it may actually increase stool output); instead, it increases net fluid and electrolyte absorption. These solutions cannot be used if vomiting precludes ingestion; in such situations, intravenous rehydration must be used. Sports drinks (e.g., Gatorade) are designed to offset fluid and electrolyte losses from sweating and do not contain sufficient amounts of sodium to replace fecal losses. Solutions that more closely approximate World Health Organization rehydration solution are now commercially available (e.g., Rehydralyte, Resol, Ricalyte).

pressure and pulse. Fever and other signs of toxicity should be recorded. A careful abdominal examination, with emphasis on bowel sounds and the presence of distention or tenderness, should be conducted.

Laboratory Testing

Blood tests   Extensive laboratory testing is not necessary for most patients with acute diarrhea; it should be reserved for those with toxicity, dehydrating diarrhea, or persistence of diarrhea for longer than would be expected, given its probable cause [*see Figure 2*]. In patients requiring extensive laboratory tests, a complete blood count should be obtained to assess for hemoconcentration, anemia, or leukocytosis. Patients with viral diarrhea typically have normal white blood cell (WBC) counts and differentials, although lymphocytosis may be seen. Invasive bacterial infections typically produce leukocytosis with many immature WBCs, but salmonellosis can induce leukopenia. Serum electrolytes and renal tests can define the metabolic impact of diarrhea.

Stool tests   Stool testing is of value for patients with blood in their stools, dehydrating diarrhea, prolonged diarrhea, or dysentery and for patients who present as part of an outbreak of diarrhea. Stool cultures are sensitive and specific, but they are expen-

Diet Most patients seek advice about altering their diets when suffering from diarrhea. Other than the provision of adequate water and salt, no specific instructions are needed. Some physicians routinely restrict dairy products in patients with diarrhea on the theory that these patients may have temporary lactase deficiency. This precaution is not necessary unless there is clinical evidence of lactose intolerance (e.g., exacerbation of diarrhea or flatus with ingestion of dairy products).

Antibiotics Empirical antibiotic therapy for acute diarrhea may be appropriate under certain circumstances (e.g., diarrhea in travelers, outbreaks of bacterial or protozoan diarrhea, patient frailty, and patient toxicity). However, experts discourage routine use of empirical antibiotic therapy because of its lack of demonstrable efficacy in many infections and because of concerns about precipitating complications, such as hemolytic-uremic syndrome in patients with E. coli serotype O157:H7.[18] A meta-analysis suggests that this latter point is not supported by the literature.[19] When indicated, fluoroquinolones or trimethoprim-sulfamethoxazole is commonly used as empirical therapy. Rifaximin, a nonabsorbable antibiotic with activity against most bacterial enteric pathogens, is useful in patients with infections that are limited to the lumen (e.g., traveler's diarrhea), but it may not be effective against invasive organisms.[20] In cases of persistent diarrhea in which protozoan infection is more likely, nitazoxanide, metronidazole, or tinidazole may be more appropriate.[21]

Nonspecific antidiarrheal agents, such as opiates, can reduce stool frequency and stool weight, and they may reduce associated symptoms, such as abdominal cramps.[22] Concerns about slowing the clearance of pathogens from the intestine by reducing peristalsis have largely not been borne out. Intraluminal agents, such as bismuth subsalicylate (Pepto-Bismol) and adsorbents (e.g., kaolin), are also sometimes used [see Table 2].

Therapy for Specific Infections and Syndromes

Campylobacter A frequent cause of acute ileocolitis in the United States,[23] Campylobacter is usually acquired by eating under-cooked chicken; it has an incubation period of up to 1 week. Ulceration of the colonic mucosa and bloody diarrhea may occur with this infection. Antibiotics, such as erythromycin, shorten the course of the illness if given within the first few days of symptoms.

Salmonella enteritidis and S. choleraesuis S. enteritidis and S. choleraesuis are spread via contaminated food or water and cause acute gastroenteritis, ileocolitis, or colitis characterized by watery diarrhea.[24] Antibiotic therapy with a fluoroquinolone, ampicillin, or trimethoprim-sulfamethoxazole should be reserved for severely ill patients or patients with compromised immunity (e.g., infants, elderly patients, pregnant women, and AIDS patients).[25]

Salmonella typhi S. typhi causes typhoid fever, a form of enteric fever.[26] The propensity of S. typhi to produce bacteremia distinguishes it from other enteric pathogens. When the infection is limited to the intestine of an otherwise healthy individual, no specific therapy is indicated, because antibiotics may paradoxically prolong excretion of the organism and increase relapses. When the infection becomes systemic and the patient is very ill, therapy is necessary, especially if the organism produces a metastatic endovascular infection. Fluoroquinolones are most often used. The diagnosis of a carrier state is made when stool cultures are positive for over 1 year.

Shigella Shigella species are invasive organisms, but they also produce an enterotoxin that reduces water and electrolyte absorption.[27] Shigellosis commonly causes a watery diarrhea initially (this watery diarrhea is most likely related to the enterotoxin). Watery diarrhea is followed by bloody diarrhea, which results from colitis produced by invasion of the colonic mucosa. Because of growing resistance to the fluoroquinolones in the United States, trimethoprim-sulfamethoxazole is the recommended initial treatment for most patients with shigellosis. Shigellosis contracted overseas is initially treated with fluoroquinolones, because those strains are more likely to be resistant to trimethoprim-sulfamethoxazole.

E. coli serotype O157:H7 The O157:H7 organism has become a common cause of food-borne infection in the United States.[28] It produces toxins similar to those produced by Shigella.[29] Infection with this organism causes a hemorrhagic segmental colitis. The disease often occurs in large outbreaks from contamination of widely distributed foods, such as hamburger meat. Patients can become quite ill; hemolytic-uremic syndrome is a well-recognized complication. Antibiotics do not seem to improve the course of the illness and may cause hemolytic-uremic syndrome in children, although this theory is controversial.[18,19]

Clostridium difficile C. difficile has become the most common cause of nosocomial diarrhea in many institutions.[30] In nonhospitalized adults, carriage rates for this organism are low, but it is spread easily from person to person by spores. Suppression of the normal bacterial flora of the colon can result in an overgrowth of C. difficile, if it is present. The organisms produce toxin A and toxin B; these cytotoxins inactivate small guanosine triphosphate (GTP)–binding proteins in the enterocytes, resulting in apoptosis.[31] In institutional settings, the organism can be distributed efficiently to a large pool of susceptible persons by health care workers who do not wash their hands. The disease produced can range from a simple, self-limited diarrhea to a fulminant colitis.

Table 2 Nonspecific Treatment of Diarrhea

Category	Treatment	Typical Adult Dose
Rehydration	Intravenous fluid	1–5 L/24 hr
	Oral rehydration solution	1–5 L/24 hr
Intraluminal agents	Adsorbents (kaolin-pectin)	15–60 ml q.i.d.
	Bismuth subsalicylate	30 ml q.i.d.
	Texture modifiers (psyllium)	18–30 g/24 hr
Drugs that inhibit transit	*Opiates*	
	Deodorized tincture of opium (10 mg morphine/ml)	5–20 drops q.i.d.
	Paregoric (0.4 mg morphine/ml)	5–10 ml q.i.d.
	Morphine sulfate (20 mg/ml)	2–10 drops q.i.d.
	Codeine phosphate or sulfate	15–60 mg q.i.d.
	Diphenoxylate with atropine	1–2 tablets q.i.d.
	Difenoxin with atropine	1–2 tablets q.i.d.
	Loperamide (2 mg)	1–2 tablets q.i.d.
	Others	
	Clonidine	0.1–0.3 mg t.i.d.
	Octreotide injection	50–200 mg t.i.d.

Treatment for 2 weeks with metronidazole, 250 mg four times daily, or vancomycin, 125 to 500 mg four times daily, is effective against *C. difficile*. Relapses occur in up to 25% of patients, probably because of residual spores.[32] Ingestion of probiotic bacteria or the nonpathogenic yeast *Saccharomyces boulardii* may reduce relapse rates.[33] In most instances of relapse, longer periods of antibiotic therapy are indicated.

Other nosocomial diarrheas Noninfectious causes of nosocomial diarrhea include medications (particularly elixirs that contain sorbitol or mannitol as noncaloric sweeteners and cancer chemotherapeutic drugs) and enteral feeding; in addition, nosocomial paradoxical diarrhea can occur in patients with fecal impaction. Infections with organisms other than *C. difficile* also occur in institutions, particularly extended-stay facilities. An important cohort of hospital patients that may develop infectious diarrhea are those who are immunocompromised by diseases such as AIDS or by drugs that are used to treat transplant rejection or inflammatory diseases. These patients are often infected with opportunistic pathogens, including viruses (e.g., cytomegalovirus and herpesvirus), bacteria (e.g., *Mycobacterium avium* complex), and parasites (e.g., *Cryptosporidium* and *Strongyloides*).[34,35] In addition, bone marrow transplant recepients may develop acute diarrhea from graft versus host disease.

Parasites Acute diarrhea in noninstitutionalized patients can be caused by parasites.[36] The likelihood of parasitic disease as a cause of acute diarrhea is profoundly influenced by geography and epidemiologic features. Giardiasis, for example, is a common infection in some areas but not others, probably because of variability in the effectiveness of water treatment. Ingestion of as few as a dozen cysts of *G. lamblia* may establish an infection, which accounts for the frequency of person-to-person transmission of this disease. ELISA for *Giardia* antigen is superior to microscopic inspection of stool (so-called ova and parasites testing) for the detection of giardiasis. Therapy with tinidazole, metronidazole, or nitazoxanide is effective in most patients, but reinfection can occur.[37]

Amebiasis is also common in some areas. Persons with amebiasis may be asymptomatic or may be extremely ill from invasion and spread of the organism to other organs, such as the liver.[38] Diagnosis is typically made by microscopic examination of fresh stools, but ELISA shows promise in distinguishing the pathogenic species, *Entamoeba histolytica*, from nonpathogenic amebas. The colonoscopic appearance of amebiasis is often distinctive, and the organism can be identified in colonic biopsy specimens.

Cryptosporidiosis is a common but unappreciated cause of diarrhea.[39] *Cryptosporidium* is resistant to chlorination, and it can cause large outbreaks when water supplies are contaminated. Microscopic inspection of stools has poor sensitivity for this organism, and many cases go undiagnosed. Treatment with nitazoxanide reduces the duration of diarrhea in children and adults with this infection.[39]

Other parasites that may cause acute diarrhea include *Isospora*, *Cyclospora*, *Trichuris trichiura* (whipworm), and *Strongyloides*. Special tests that may be necessary to identify these parasites include concentration of stool samples and mucosal biopsy. If these organisms are suspected, consultation with the laboratory staff allows use of the proper diagnostic tests.

Chronic Diarrhea

In contrast to acute diarrhea, in which infection is the overwhelmingly likely cause of illness, chronic diarrhea has an extensive and daunting list of possible causes [*see Table 3*].[3] The simplest approach to making a diagnosis is to classify chronic diar-

Table 3 Major Causes of Chronic Diarrhea

Osmotic diarrhea
  Osmotic laxative abuse
    Mg^{2+}, SO_4^{2-}, PO_4^{3-}, lactulose, mannitol, sorbitol, polyethylene glycol
  Carbohydrate malabsorption
    Lactose, fructose, others
Fatty diarrhea
  Malabsorption syndromes
    Mucosal diseases
    Short bowel syndrome
    Postresection diarrhea
    Small bowel bacterial overgrowth
    Mesenteric ischemia
  Maldigestion
    Pancreatic insufficiency
    Reduced luminal bile acid
Inflammatory diarrhea
  Inflammatory bowel disease
    Ulcerative colitis
    Crohn disease
    Diverticulitis
    Ulcerative jejunoileitis
  Infections
    Invasive bacterial infection
      Clostridium, E. coli, tuberculosis, others

    Ulcerating viral infection
      Cytomegalovirus
      Herpes simplex
    Invasive parasites
      Amebiasis
      Strongyloides
  Ischemic colitis
  Radiation enterocolitis
  Neoplasia
    Carcinoma of the colon
    Lymphoma
Secretory diarrhea
  Congenital chloridorrhea
  Chronic infections
  Inflammatory bowel disease
    Ulcerative colitis
    Crohn disease (ileum)
  Microscopic colitis
    Lymphocytic colitis
    Collagenous colitis
  Diverticulitis
Drugs and poisons
  Stimulant laxative abuse

  Disordered regulation
    Postvagotomy
    Postsympathectomy
    Diabetic neuropathy
    Irritable bowel syndrome
  Ileal bile acid malabsorption
  Endocrine diarrhea
    Hyperthyroidism
    Addison disease
  Neuroendocrine tumors
    Gastrinoma
    VIPoma
    Somatostatinoma
    Mastocytosis
    Carcinoid syndrome
    Medullary carcinoma of the thyroid
  Other neoplasia
    Colon carcinoma
    Lymphoma
    Villous adenoma
  Idiopathic secretory diarrhea
    Epidemic (Brainerd)
    Sporadic

rhea by the characteristics of the stools. Three categories of chronic diarrhea are recognized: watery, inflammatory, and fatty. Watery diarrhea can be subdivided further into osmotic and secretory diarrhea on the basis of stool analysis.

WATERY DIARRHEA

Osmotic Diarrhea

Osmotic diarrhea results from ingestion of an osmotically active, poorly absorbable substance that necessitates the retention of water intraluminally to maintain isosmotic conditions.[40] In practical terms, osmotic diarrhea is caused by ingestion of osmotic laxatives (magnesium, phosphate, and sulfate salts; sugar analogues, such as lactulose; sugar alcohols, such as mannitol or sorbitol; and polyethylene glycol) and carbohydrate malabsorption. The ingestion of osmotic laxatives may be purposeful [see Laxative Abuse, below] or accidental, as when excess magnesium is ingested as part of an antacid, mineral supplement, or multivitamin tablet. Carbohydrate malabsorption is most often the result of acquired lactase deficiency (a normal development in adult mammals) or mucosal disease, such as celiac sprue, that interferes with nutrient absorption.

Secretory Diarrhea

Secretory diarrhea has a much larger list of possible causes than does osmotic diarrhea [see Table 3].

Congenital chloridorrhea Rarely, congenital absence of a transporter mechanism results in diarrhea. This is the case in congenital chloridorrhea, in which the chloride-bicarbonate exchanger in the ileum is not active.[41] Under such conditions, chloride becomes poorly absorbable in the distal bowel and obligates water retention intraluminally.

Chronic infections Some bacterial infections can last long enough to produce chronic secretory diarrhea.[42] These include *Aeromonas*, *Plesiomonas*, enteropathogenic *E. coli*, *C. difficile*, *M. tuberculosis*, and *Yersinia enterocolitica*. A special situation is small bowel bacterial overgrowth syndrome, in which structural problems, such as jejunal diverticulosis, or motility problems, such as those seen in scleroderma, result in proliferation of bacteria in the jejunum.[43] Although this bacterial overgrowth disrupts digestive processes and may produce fatty diarrhea, it also may reduce water and salt absorption, producing secretory diarrhea. Infection with parasites, such as *G. lamblia*, *E. histolytica*, and *Cryptosporidium*, also can produce chronic diarrhea.[44]

Inflammatory bowel disease Typically, inflammatory bowel diseases (e.g., ulcerative colitis and Crohn disease) produce inflammatory diarrhea, with blood and pus in the stool. Watery diarrhea can occur, especially when the distal colon is not involved. One form of inflammatory bowel disease that typically produces a watery diarrhea is microscopic colitis syndrome (lymphocytic colitis and collagenous colitis), in which the mucosa is inflamed but not ulcerated.[45] Colonic diverticulitis is sometimes associated with a secretory diarrhea, which is probably mediated by inflammation-linked cytokines. Vasculitis and systemic inflammatory diseases may also be associated with secretory diarrhea.

Drugs Drug therapy is a key cause of secretory diarrhea.[46] Many drugs have diarrhea as a side effect. These include antibi-

otics; cardiovascular agents, such as beta-adrenergic antagonists, digitalis, and quinidine; cancer chemotherapy; nonsteroidal antiinflammatory drugs (NSAIDs); and colchicine. Thus, in taking the history of a patient with chronic diarrhea, it is critical to formulate a detailed drug list, including over-the-counter and alternative medications. A special category of drug-induced secretory diarrhea is surreptitious ingestion of stimulant laxatives.

Other causes Disordered motility or regulation can produce secretory diarrhea. Secretory diarrhea associated with disordered motility can occur in patients who have undergone vagotomy or sympathectomy, patients with autonomic neuropathy from diabetes or amyloidosis, and many patients with irritable bowel syndrome.[47,48] In the United States, irritable bowel syndrome is the most common diagnosis made in patients with chronic diarrhea. This diagnosis is often incorrect, however, and may delay accurate diagnosis and treatment.

Malabsorption of bile acid in the ileum occurs in many diarrheal diseases as a result of ileal disease or resection and may be secondary to other processes, such as vagotomy, cholecystectomy, and rapid transit past the ileum. In a relatively small group of patients, idiopathic bile acid malabsorption is the cause of diarrhea.[49]

Endocrine causes of secretory diarrhea include hyperthyroidism, Addison disease, and a group of rare tumors of the endocrine cells of the gut, including gastrinomas, carcinoid tumors, vasoactive intestinal peptide tumors (VIPomas), somatostatinomas, and medullary carcinoma of the thyroid.[50,51] These tumors produce peptides and other mediators that affect intestinal mucosal and muscle function and thereby produce diarrhea. In most cases, rapid intestinal transit seems to be the major mechanism producing diarrhea in these disorders, although this remains controversial.

Other tumors that produce secretory diarrhea include colon cancer (mechanism uncertain), villous adenoma of the rectum, lymphoma, and mastocytosis. Mastocytosis (and probably some lymphomas) produce diarrhea by release of histamine or other mediators that affect gut function. Infiltration of the mucosa also may play a role in some cases.

Secretory diarrhea can also be idiopathic.[52] Idiopathic secretory diarrhea occurs in both sporadic and epidemic forms and may be caused by an as-yet unidentified infection.

INFLAMMATORY DIARRHEA

Inflammatory diarrhea is characterized by the presence of blood and pus in the stools, which usually occurs as a result of ulceration of the mucosa. Inflammatory bowel diseases, such as Crohn disease and ulcerative colitis, are in this category [see Chapter 63]. Some patients with diverticulitis and diarrhea may have blood and pus in the stool, as do patients with the rare condition ulcerative jejunoileitis. Ulcerating infectious diseases may also produce inflammatory diarrhea. Such infections include pseudomembranous colitis from *C. difficile* infection; invasive bacterial infections, such as tuberculosis and yer-siniosis; ulcerating viral infections, such as those caused by cytomegalovirus or herpesvirus; and invasive parasitic infections, such as amebiasis and *Strongyloides*. Inflammatory diarrhea also may be seen with ischemic colitis and radiation colitis, as well as colon cancer and lymphoma.

FATTY DIARRHEA

Fatty diarrhea may be caused by fat malabsorption resulting from mucosal diseases, such as celiac disease or Whipple disease; short bowel syndrome secondary to extensive surgical resection of the small intestine; small bowel bacterial overgrowth syndrome; and mesenteric ischemia. Fatty diarrhea also may be the consequence of maldigestion of fat caused by pancreatic exocrine deficiency or inadequate luminal bile acid concentration [see Chapter 65].

Diagnosis

Medical history   An accurate medical history is even more important in cases of chronic diarrhea than in acute diarrhea. In addition to all the issues that should be discussed with patients who have acute diarrhea [see Acute Diarrhea, above], the history of patients with chronic diarrhea should include long-term trends in body weight, current appetite and food intake, review of previous medical problems and surgeries, potential secondary gains from illness, previous evaluations and treatments for diarrhea, and a detailed review of systems to look for clues to systemic illnesses [see Table 4].

A principal diagnostic distinction in chronic diarrhea is between diarrhea associated with irritable bowel syndrome and diarrhea associated with other functional or organic problems. Irritable bowel syndrome is characterized by abdominal pain associated with defecation and an altered bowel habit.[53] Variable stool consistency and intermittent constipation are common. Painless diarrhea should no longer be considered to be a type of irritable bowel syndrome; other causes of diarrhea should be sought in such cases.

Physical examination   The physical examination may provide clues to the diagnosis of chronic diarrhea. Characteristic skin changes may be seen in mastocytosis, glucagonoma, Addison disease, amyloidosis, carcinoid syndrome, Degos disease, and celiac disease. Amyloidosis may produce orthostatic hypotension and hepatosplenomegaly. Thyroid nodules or findings of hyperthyroidism may suggest medullary carcinoma of the thyroid or thyroid adenoma causing hyperthyroidism. Carcinoid syndrome may produce hepatosplenomegaly, edema, and a right-sided heart murmur in addition to flushing. Arthritis may be a clue to inflammatory bowel disease, Whipple disease, and some enteric infections. Lymphadenopathy could be present in patients with AIDS or lymphoma. The absence of peripheral arterial pulses or bruits suggests the possibility of mesenteric vascular disease. Rectal examination may disclose defective functioning of the anal sphincter or pelvic floor muscle, which could produce fecal incontinence. The physical findings that reflect the severity of diarrhea should also be recorded [see Acute Diarrhea, above].

Laboratory tests   As in acute diarrhea, routine laboratory testing is indicated to help determine the severity of chronic diarrhea [see Acute Diarrhea, above]. Unlike acute diarrhea, in which stool analysis is typically not used, stool analysis plays a key role in the assessment of chronic diarrhea by allowing adequate categorization of the type of diarrhea, thereby limiting the number of conditions to be considered.[3] The stool analysis can be obtained on either a random sample or a timed collection. The value of a timed collection is that it allows the physician to quantitate stool output accurately. However, stool analysis obtained on a random sample can still provide many diagnostic clues.

Table 4   Steps in the Evaluation and Classification of Chronic Diarrhea[3]

Step	Elements	Findings/Considerations
History	Onset	Congenital, abrupt, gradual
	Pattern	Continuous, intermittent
	Duration	—
	Epidemiologic features	Travel, food, water
	Stool characteristics	Watery, bloody, fatty
	Fecal incontinence	—
	Abdominal pain	Occurs in inflammatory bowel disease, irritable bowel syndrome, ischemia
	Weight loss	May be severe in malabsorption or neoplasm
	Aggravating factors	Diet, stress
	Mitigating factors	Diet, over-the-counter drugs, prescription drugs
	Previous medical evaluation	
	Iatrogenic diarrhea	From drugs, radiation, surgery
	Factitious diarrhea	Laxatives; may be surreptitious
	Systemic disease	Diarrhea may complicate hyperthyroidism, diabetes mellitus, collagen vascular disease, tumor syndromes, AIDS, immunoglobulin deficiencies
Routine laboratory tests	CBC	Anemia, leukocytosis
	Serum chemistry	Fluid/electrolyte status, nutritional status, serum protein/globulin
Stool analysis	Weight	—
	Electrolytes	For calculating fecal osmotic gap
	pH	Acid stools suggest carbohydrate malabsorption
	Stool leukocytes	Found in inflammatory diarrhea
	Fat output	Can be assessed by Sudan stain or quantitatively
	Laxative screen	
Categorization	Watery diarrhea (secretory or osmotic) Inflammatory diarrhea Fatty diarrhea	—

Stool tests Stool characteristics to measure include stool sodium and potassium concentrations, osmolality, and pH. Fecal occult blood testing and examination of stool for WBCs (or a surrogate chemical test, such as fecal lactoferrin concentration) should be conducted. Stool fat output should be measured quantitatively or assessed qualitatively with a Sudan stain of a fecal smear.

Measurement of stool electrolyte concentrations allows calculation of the fecal osmotic gap [*see* Fecal Osmotic Gap, *above*]. This can be used to identify watery diarrhea as being osmotic or secretory. Measurement of actual stool osmolality is only of value in detecting samples that have been contaminated with water or dilute urine and therefore have an osmolality less than 290 mOsm/kg. Stool osmolality rises rapidly in vitro because of bacterial fermentation, so the actual measurement should not be used to calculate the fecal osmotic gap. The pH of stool water can indicate whether or not carbohydrate malabsorption is present. Carbohydrates (or sugar alcohols) that are not absorbed in the small bowel and that reach the bacterial flora of the colon are fermented into short-chain fatty acids that reduce fecal pH, usually to less than 6. Thus, acid stools suggest carbohydrate malabsorption.[8]

Fatty diarrhea can be identified by measurement of stool fat, although careful interpretation of the results is sometimes necessary [*see* Steatorrhea, *below*]. When appropriate, a laxative screen should be obtained. Measurement of laxatives by chemical or chromatographic methods can detect surreptitious laxative ingestion.

Completion of the stool analysis allows the clinician to characterize chronic diarrhea as being watery (whether secretory or osmotic diarrhea), inflammatory, or fatty. The subsequent evaluation depends on this categorization.

Evaluation of Watery Secretory Diarrhea

Secretory diarrhea is associated with many disorders; a thorough evaluation is therefore needed to identify the underlying cause [*see Figure 3*].

Stool tests Infection should be excluded by stool culture for bacteria, stool assay for *C. difficile* toxin, and other tests for parasites, including ELISA for giardiasis. Biopsies of the small bowel or colon may be necessary to find the pathogens, especially in patients with AIDS or other immunodeficiencies. Small bowel aspirate for quantitative culture is the best test for detecting small bowel bacterial overgrowth.

Imaging and endoscopic tests Structural diseases (e.g., short bowel syndrome or fistula, mucosal diseases, inflammatory bowel disease, and tumors) should be sought by radiographic and endoscopic testing. Small bowel radiography remains an important test in such cases. CT scans can detect small bowel and colonic disease, as well as problems extrinsic to the gut that may cause diarrhea, such as endocrine tumors. Inspection of the colonic mucosa by colonoscopy or sigmoidoscopy is essential in patients with secretory diarrhea, both to evaluate for gross changes and to obtain biopsy samples to look for evidence of microscopic colitis syndrome. Biopsies should be obtained even if the gross appearance of the colon is normal, because of the prevalence of microscopic colitis syndrome in patients with chronic watery diarrhea. A long endoscope that can reach the jejunum to obtain biopsy samples and aspirates is a valuable adjunct when other studies are unrevealing. The role of capsule endoscopy in the evaluation of patients with chronic diarrhea is under investigation; studies suggest that it may be helpful in de-

tecting Crohn disease and, perhaps, celiac disease.[54-56] However, capsule endoscopy does not allow for biopsy of abnormalities that are visualized during the procedure, which limits its utility. Double-balloon enteroscopy offers the possibility of visualizing and obtaining biopsies from the entire small intestine; this technique may find a place in the evaluation of patients with watery secretory diarrhea.[57]

Serum peptide measurement Because diarrheagenic endocrine tumors are very rare, the measurement of serum peptides (e.g., gastrin, vasoactive intestinal polypeptide, calcitonin, and glucagons) or urinary excretion of secretagogue metabolites (e.g., 5-hydroxyindoleacetic acid or metanephrine) should be restricted to patients with symptoms consistent with tumor syndromes or those in whom a diagnosis remains elusive after initial testing.[58] More common endocrine problems, such as diabetes, hyperthyroidism, or Addison disease, should be excluded with appropriate blood tests.

Bile acid absorption measurement Ileal resection or ileal disease can result in the escape of sufficient bile acid into the colon to increase luminal bile acid concentrations above 3 to 5 mmol. At these concentrations, bile acids reduce colonic mucosal water and electrolyte absorption; alternatively, they stimulate secretion, resulting in increased stool water. In most circum-

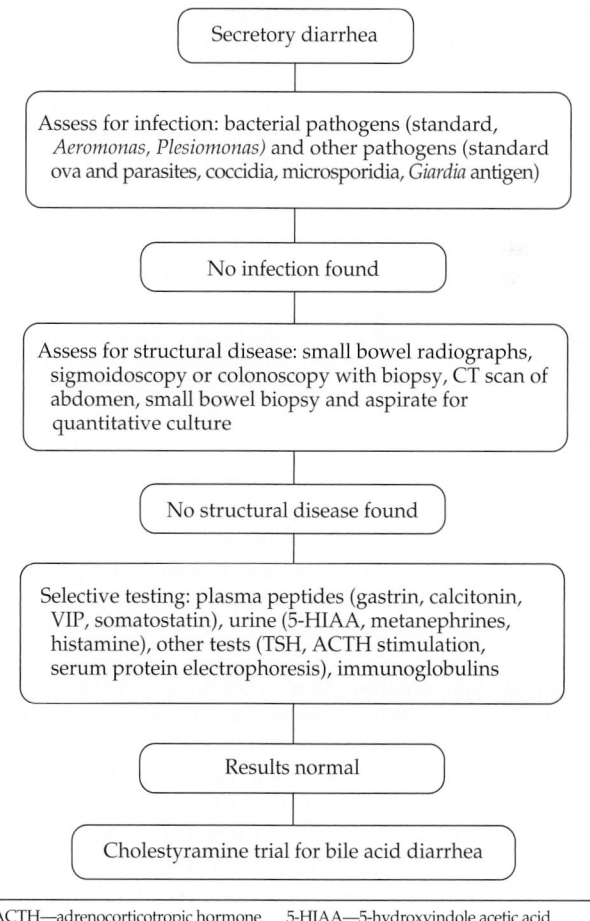

ACTH—adrenocorticotropic hormone   5-HIAA—5-hydroxyindole acetic acid
TSH—thyroid-stimulating hormone   VIP—vasoactive intestinal peptide

Figure 3 **Evaluation of chronic secretory diarrhea.[3] Every test does not need to be done for every patient.**

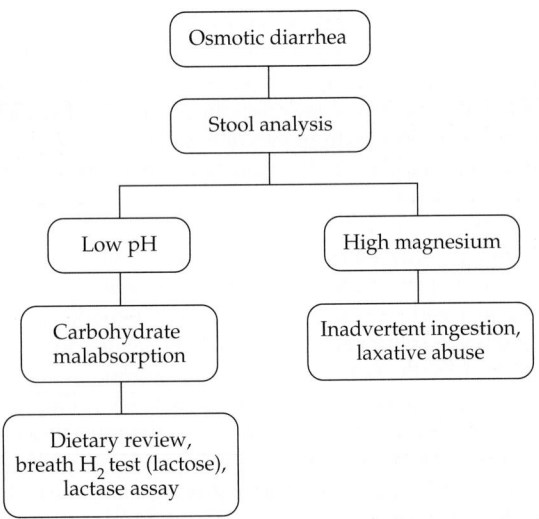

Figure 4 **Evaluation of chronic osmotic diarrhea.[3] Every test does not need to be done for every patient.**

stances, bile acid malabsorption can be inferred from a history of ileal resection or disease. More controversial is the concept that bile acid malabsorption occurring in the absence of ileal resection or obvious ileal disease is responsible for idiopathic secretory diarrhea.[59] Although bile acid malabsorption can be documented in many of these patients, administration of bile acid–binding resins does not always mitigate the diarrhea, casting doubts on bile acid malabsorption as the cause of the diarrhea.[49] Therefore, in patients with secretory diarrhea that appears to be idiopathic, it is more practical to give a therapeutic trial of bile acid–binding resins than to measure bile acid malabsorption directly.

Evaluation of Watery Osmotic Diarrhea

Because osmotic diarrhea has fewer potential causes than secretory diarrhea, the evaluation is simpler [*see Figure 4*]. If stool water has low electrolyte concentrations (and therefore a high fecal osmotic gap), some other substance is taking up the osmotic space and is holding water in the lumen. In practice, this substance is usually magnesium ingestion or carbohydrate malabsorption.

Magnesium ingestion Magnesium can be measured accurately in stool water. Excretion of more than 15 mmol (30 mEq) daily or concentrations greater than 45 mmol/L (90 mEq/L) strongly suggest magnesium-induced diarrhea.[60] This diarrhea may be intentional (surreptitious laxative ingestion) or accidental (magnesium-containing antacids or mineral supplements).

Carbohydrate malabsorption Carbohydrate malabsorption can occur from ingestion of poorly absorbable carbohydrates, such as lactose in someone with lactase deficiency, or from reduced carbohydrate absorption as a result of small bowel mucosal disease. In addition to ingestion of lactose, common causes of osmotic diarrhea include excessive ingestion of fructose (often used as a sweetener in commercial products),[61] ingestion of poorly absorbed sugar alcohols (such as mannitol and sorbitol, which are used as low-calorie sweeteners), and use of inhibitors of carbohydrate absorption, such as acarbose. Because malabsorbed carbohydrate is rapidly fermented by colonic bacteria, gas and bloating are frequent symptoms. Diagnosis is made on the basis

of a finding of low stool pH (typically less than 6) and a thorough dietary history.

Evaluation of Chronic Inflammatory Diarrhea

Patients with WBCs or blood in the stool are classified as having inflammatory diarrhea. Causes may include inflammatory bowel disease, infections, ischemia, radiation enteritis, and neoplasia [*see Table 3*]. Sometimes, these conditions produce a watery, secretory diarrhea without blood or pus in the stool; therefore, they must also be considered in the evaluation of that type of diarrhea [*see Evaluation of Watery Secretory Diarrhea, above*].

Imaging and endoscopic tests Evaluation of patients with chronic inflammatory diarrhea should start with radiographic and endoscopic tests to look for structural problems [*see Figure 5*]. Sigmoidoscopy or colonoscopy should be considered first, because colitis is a common cause of inflammatory diarrhea. Biopsies should be performed to properly categorize colitis. CT has proved useful in many patients with inflammatory diarrhea because of the ability of CT to visualize inflammatory changes in the small bowel and colon and to identify complications of inflammation, such as abscess.

Infections that may produce chronic diarrhea, such as *C. difficile*, cytomegalovirus, amebiasis, and tuberculosis, need to be excluded by culture, biopsy, or serologic testing. It is important to realize that infection may complicate the courses of established problems, such as ulcerative colitis or Crohn disease. Patients with AIDS need an especially careful search for opportunistic infections.

Evaluation of Chronic Fatty Diarrhea

Steatorrhea Excessive fat in the stool, or steatorrhea, implies a problem with fat solubilization, digestion, or absorption in the small intestine. Steatorrhea is usually defined as stool fat output of more than 7 g over 24 hours or daily output of more than 9% of the intake of fat. These criteria may not be valid in patients with diarrhea, however, because voluminous stools per se may increase fat excretion. In one study, artificially induced diarrhea produced mild steatorrhea of up to 14 g/24 hr in 35% of normal persons.[62] Thus, in patients with diarrhea, fecal fat excretion of up to 14 g/24 hr has a low specificity for the diagnosis of defective fat absorption. The threshold for the diagnosis of steatorrhea also should be corrected for fat intake, because some patients

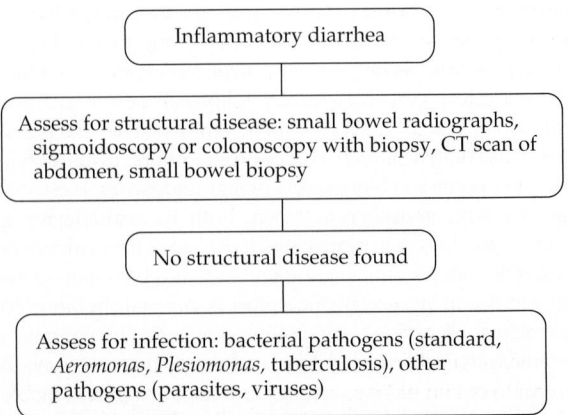

Figure 5 **Evaluation of chronic inflammatory diarrhea.[3] Every test does not need to be done for every patient.**

with diarrhea have anorexia and some patients with steatorrhea have hyperphagia. When possible, fat intake should be estimated from diet diaries that are maintained during the collection period. Finally, measurement of fat excretion can be compromised by ingestion of poorly absorbed fat substitutes, such as olestra.

Qualitative estimation of fat excretion by Sudan stain of a fecal smear can be used when a timed collection or quantitative analysis is not possible. Semiquantitative methods employing assessment of the number and size of fat globules correlate well with quantitative analysis of fat excretion.

The fecal fat concentration may provide a clue to the etiology of steatorrhea. The major causes of steatorrhea are mucosal diseases (e.g., celiac disease), pancreatic exocrine insufficiency (e.g., chronic pancreatitis), and lack of bile acids (e.g., advanced biliary cirrhosis). Mucosal diseases are often associated with reduced fluid and electrolyte absorption; as a result, fat is diluted by unabsorbed water. Furthermore, in mucosal disease, fat still can be digested to fatty acids, which can inhibit water absorption in the colon. In contrast, diseases that alter fat solubilization or digestion typically do not alter mucosal water and electrolyte absorption; as a result, unabsorbed fat is disbursed in a smaller stool volume. Fecal fat concentrations of more than 9.5 g/100 g strongly suggest pancreatic or biliary steatorrhea. Assessment of patients with chronic fatty diarrhea should therefore begin with measurement of fecal fat excretion and concentration [see Figure 6].

Imaging and endoscopic tests If the cause of steatorrhea is not obvious from the patient's history and the results of fecal fat assessment, the next step is evaluation of the absorptive surface of the small intestine by endoscopic, histologic, and radiographic tests. During endoscopy, small bowel biopsies should be obtained for histologic analysis, and small bowel contents should be aspirated for quantitative culture to assess for small bowel bacterial overgrowth. Indirect tests, such as measurement of antigluten (antiendomysial) antibodies or tissue transglutaminase antibodies for the diagnosis of celiac disease or breath tests for bacterial overgrowth, have not displaced endoscopic testing as the gold standard for diagnosis of these conditions. Such tests, however, may be useful in some cases. Small bowel radiography and CT are valuable adjuncts for structural assessment in patients with steatorrhea.

If the absorptive surface is normal, attention should shift to luminal problems with fat solubilization or digestion. Testing for pancreatic exocrine insufficiency is rarely done, because of unwillingness to use duodenal intubation tests. An indirect test, such as measurement of stool chymotrypsin activity, has limited sensitivity and specificity. The best test for pancreatic exocrine insufficiency may be a therapeutic trial of pancreatic enzyme supplementation. If this is done, a large dose of enzymes should be administered and objective measurement of fat excretion should be monitored to assess the response to therapy. Likewise, testing for the adequacy of bile salt solubilization of fat is rarely done. If necessary, duodenal bile salt concentration can be measured.

TREATMENT

Nonspecific Therapy

Nonspecific therapy is used in patients with chronic diarrhea in three situations: (1) as a temporizing or initial therapy before diagnostic testing, (2) after diagnostic testing has failed to result in a diagnosis, and (3) when a diagnosis has been made, but no specific treatment is available or specific treatment has failed.[22]

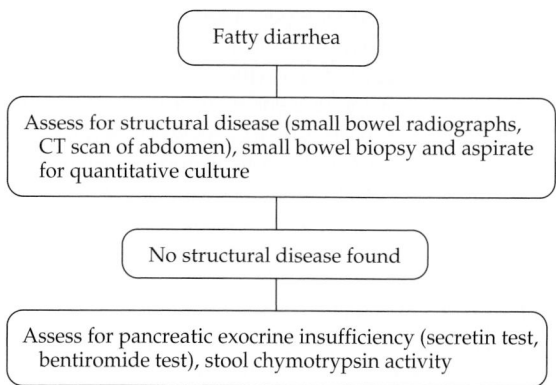

Figure 6 **Evaluation of chronic fatty diarrhea.[3] Every test does not need to be done for every patient.**

Antibiotic therapy Antibiotics are less useful in chronic diarrhea than in acute diarrhea because bacterial infection is less likely to be the cause of chronic diarrhea. Nevertheless, many clinicians try an empirical course of metronidazole or a fluoroquinolone before starting an extensive evaluation.

Symptomatic therapy with antidiarrheal drugs is often required in patients with chronic diarrhea [see Table 2]. Loperamide or diphenoxylate with atropine can be tried initially. In patients with chronic diarrhea, routine dosing (e.g., two tablets before each meal or at bedtime) is more effective than as-needed dosing after passing loose stools. More potent opiates, such as codeine, opium, and morphine, are underutilized in patients who do not respond to loperamide or diphenoxylate with atropine. Although these are controlled substances because of the possibility of abuse, abuse is unlikely in closely monitored patients with chronic diarrhea. Dosing should be started at a low level (e.g., codeine, 30 mg q.i.d.; deodorized tincture of opium, 3 drops q.i.d.; or morphine, 2 mg q.i.d.) and titrated up gradually to an effective dose. Stool-modifying agents, such as psyllium, can alter stool consistency but do not reduce stool weight. They may be of special help in patients with coexisting fecal incontinence.

Treatment of Specific Diseases and Syndromes

Osmotic diarrhea Osmotic diarrhea should abate with fasting or elimination of the offending agent from the diet. This response may be incomplete if other diarrhea-producing mechanisms are still active, such as short bowel syndrome or diseases of small bowel mucosa.

Irritable bowel syndrome and functional diarrhea Patients with chronic diarrhea in whom no other etiology is established are commonly diagnosed with irritable bowel syndrome or functional diarrhea. Irritable bowel syndrome is characterized chiefly by abdominal pain that is associated with altered bowel function, including constipation, diarrhea, or alternating diarrhea and constipation.[53] A diagnosis of functional diarrhea is made when patients do not have prominent abdominal pain and have no evidence of other specific causes of diarrhea. Obviously, these diagnoses are only as firm as the evaluation that is used to exclude other causes of diarrhea. For example, most cases of diarrhea from malabsorption of bile acid or carbohydrates are characterized as functional diarrhea or irritable bowel syndrome because specific testing for those malabsorption disorders is not done. Thus, careful consideration of alternative diagnoses should precede a diagnosis of irritable bowel syndrome or functional diarrhea in patients with chronic diarrhea.

Nevertheless, there are certain clues to the diagnosis of irritable bowel syndrome or functional diarrhea that should be sought by the physician. Features that suggest a diagnosis of irritable bowel syndrome include a long history of diarrhea dating back to adolescence or young adulthood; passage of mucus; and exacerbation of symptoms with stress. Historical points that argue against irritable bowel syndrome include recent onset of diarrhea, especially in older individuals; nocturnal diarrhea; weight loss; blood in stools; voluminous stools (> 400 g/24 hr); and blood tests indicating anemia, leukocytosis, a low serum albumin concentration, or a high erythrocyte sedimentation rate.

New treatments for irritable bowel syndrome are being developed[63] in response to current theories about the pathogenesis of this disorder; pathogenetic processes that may yield new treatment strategies include dysregulation by the enteric nervous system,[64] food allergies,[65] small bowel bacterial overgrowth,[66] and changes in the colonic bacterial flora.[67]

Microscopic colitis syndrome Microscopic colitis syndrome, which subsumes the diagnoses of lymphocytic colitis and collagenous colitis, is a frequent cause of chronic diarrhea.[45,68,69] This disorder is characterized by chronic watery diarrhea and microscopic evidence of mucosal inflammation in the presence of normal gross colonoscopic findings. Histologic findings in both lymphocytic colitis and collagenous colitis include intraepithelial lymphocytic infiltration and chronic inflammation in the lamina propria without crypt destruction. Collagenous colitis and lymphocytic colitis are distinguished by the presence or absence of a thickened subepithelial collagen layer.

The cause of microscopic colitis syndrome is uncertain. It is associated with many autoimmune disorders and immunologically mediated diseases, such as celiac disease, which suggests that immune dysregulation is important. Bacterial antigens within the colonic lumen may also play a role. NSAIDs have been implicated in some reports.

Women are more likely than men to have collagenous colitis; lymphocytic colitis is equally likely in men and women. Diarrhea is of moderate severity (typically, 500 to 1,000 g/24 hr) and is characteristically secretory in nature because it results from failure of the colonic mucosa to absorb water and salt. Diagnosis is made by obtaining biopsy material from normal-appearing mucosa at the time of sigmoidoscopy or colonoscopy.

Treatment options include budesonide, bismuth subsalicylate, 5-aminosalicylate drugs, prednisone, and azathioprine.[45,68,69] Bile acid–binding drugs also have been reported to be successful in reducing diarrhea.[70] Microscopic colitis can have a remitting and relapsing course, and symptomatic therapy with opiate antidiarrheal drugs may be all that is needed. There is no evidence that microscopic colitis is a risk factor for colon carcinoma, and no surveillance program is currently recommended.

Laxative abuse Although rarely suspected, laxative abuse occurs regularly in four groups of patients: (1) those with anorexia or bulimia, (2) those who obtain a secondary gain from illness (e.g., disability payments, attention from relatives), (3) those with Munchausen syndrome, and (4) those who are dependent on others for their health care and who are poisoned by their caregivers (caregivers who do this are usually motivated by the desire to demonstrate their devotion to the patients).[71] Physicians need to consider surreptitious laxative

abuse in patients who confound diagnosis and who are in one of the categories.

Detection of laxative abuse depends on having a high index of suspicion. Clues include the presence of hypokalemia in a patient who is able to eat (suggesting stimulant laxative abuse or concurrent ingestion of diuretics), melanosis coli (brownish pigmentation in the colonic mucosa caused by ingestion of anthraquinone laxatives) in a patient being evaluated for chronic diarrhea, or a large fecal osmotic gap (seen with magnesium ingestion). Most laxatives can be detected in stool water by chemical techniques. Adulteration of stool by added water or hypotonic urine can be detected by finding a low measured stool osmolality (< 280 mOsm/kg). The addition of hypertonic urine can be detected by impossibly high stool osmolality (> 600 mOsm/kg) and the presence of a negative fecal osmotic gap resulting from high urinary sodium or potassium concentrations. Negative fecal osmotic gaps may also be calculated in patients ingesting laxatives containing phosphate or sulfate.

Before patients are confronted with the diagnosis of laxative abuse, testing should be confirmed on another stool specimen, and appropriate psychiatric consultation should be available, because some of these patients become suicidal when confronted, and all of them need counseling. In cases of laxative poisoning by a caregiver, legal proceedings need to be instituted to separate the patient from the caregiver. Outcome studies in laxative-abuse patients are few. One study suggested that nearly half of the patients sought further medical attention elsewhere for chronic diarrhea.[72]

Postsurgical diarrhea Diarrhea can occur after several different kinds of operations. Peptic ulcer surgery is less common than it used to be, but new kinds of gastric operations, such as gastric bypass for obesity, produce similar complications. Dumping syndrome is the term used to describe a condition characterized by postprandial flushing, hypotension, diarrhea, and hypoglycemia.[73] This syndrome results from unregulated gastric emptying, osmotic shifts of fluid into the gut, and the rapid release of peptide hormones from the small intestine. Dumping syndrome can occur after vagotomy (intentional or accidental), pyloroplasty, gastrojejunostomy, and gastric resection. It can be treated with dietary modifications, antidiarrheal drugs [see Table 2], and the somatostatin analogue octreotide. Gastric surgery may also predispose patients to bacterial overgrowth in the small intestine, abnormally rapid intestinal transit, bile acid malabsorption, and pancreatic exocrine insufficiency from inadequate stimulation of the pancreas.

Bowel resection can result in loss of surface area sufficient to impair absorption of nutrients or water and salt. Lesser degrees of resection can result in diarrhea if an area of specialized function is removed.[74] For example, resection of the terminal ileum and right colon reduces bile acid absorption and the ability to absorb sodium against a large electrochemical gradient; these defects cannot be overcome by other areas of the intestine. With time, intestinal adaptation can overcome impaired electrolyte absorption, but intestinal adaptation cannot reverse loss of these specialized functions.

Ileostomy diarrhea is said to occur when stoma output exceeds 1,000 ml/24 hr. It may be caused by loss of absorptive surface area, if a substantial length of bowel has been resected; it may result from stomal stenosis, partial bowel obstruction, bacterial overgrowth, recurrent disease, medications, or intraperitoneal infection.[75] A special situation occurs in patients with ulcerative colitis who have had an ileoanal anastomosis with creation of an ileal reservoir pouch. These patients may develop inflammation of the pouch (so-called pouchitis) caused by bacterial overgrowth or recurrent inflammatory bowel disease.[76] Pouchitis can be treated with antibiotics such as metronidazole, anti-inflammatory drugs such as mesalamine, or ingestion of probiotic bacteria. Ordinary ileostomy diarrhea can be treated successfully with antidiarrheal opiate drugs.

Postcholecystectomy diarrhea occurs in as many as 20% of patients. It may be delayed in onset, and it is rarely severe. Diarrhea may occur as a result of ileal bile acid malabsorption at night, when the migrating motor complex may sweep bile acid past the absorptive sites in the terminal ileum, but some cases may have other causes.[77] Postcholecystectomy diarrhea is best treated with bile acid–binding agents given at bedtime. Opiate antidiarrheal drugs may be needed in refractory cases.

Diabetic diarrhea   Up to 30% of patients with long-standing diabetes mellitus may experience chronic diarrhea.[78] This diarrhea has been attributed to autonomic neuropathy and dysregulation of motility, but definitive evidence of neuropathy is not always evident. If steatorrhea is present, three conditions that occur with increased prevalence in diabetics should be considered: (1) small bowel bacterial overgrowth, (2) pancreatic exocrine insufficiency, and (3) celiac disease. Other causes that need to be considered are medications, such as acarbose, and ingestion of dietetic foods containing sugar alcohols (e.g., sorbitol or mannitol).

When watery diarrhea is present, treatment with clonidine, an alpha$_2$-adrenergic agonist drug, may have special value. When clonidine cannot be tolerated because of its hypotensive effect or when it is not effective, opiate antidiarrheal drugs may be used. Fecal incontinence related to diabetic sensorimotor neuropathy may complicate diarrhea; this form of diarrhea needs to be evaluated, because therapies to mitigate incontinence, such as biofeedback training, may have a dramatic effect on quality of life.[79]

Diarrhea in patients with AIDS   Diarrhea in AIDS patients is likely to result from opportunistic infections or lymphoma. A careful search for the cause of diarrhea can result in targeted therapy that may cure the diarrhea.[80] Colonoscopy is preferable to sigmoidoscopy because it allows visualization and biopsy of the right colon and ileum, which are often the sites of infection. It is possible that HIV-1 may directly produce diarrhea (so-called AIDS enteropathy), but in most cases, a specific infection can be identified.

Idiopathic secretory diarrhea   The diagnosis of idiopathic secretory diarrhea can be made when an exhaustive evaluation fails to reveal a cause of chronic secretory diarrhea. This condition often begins suddenly in previously normal individuals, and it is distinguished from the acute secretory diarrhea by its persistence for more than 4 weeks. It occurs in two forms, epidemic and sporadic.

Epidemic idiopathic secretory diarrhea occurs in outbreaks that are seemingly related to contaminated food or water.[81] The initial description of this condition involved an epidemic of chronic diarrhea in Brainerd, Minnesota, and the condition has consequently become known as Brainerd diarrhea. Several outbreaks have been described in detail since the initial epidemic, and although the epidemiology suggests an infectious cause, no organism has been isolated.

Sporadic idiopathic secretory diarrhea affects individuals in an identical fashion as the epidemic form, but it does not seem to be acquired easily by family members or others.[52] Many patients describe a history of travel to local lakes or recreational sites, but they are the only members of their parties that become ill.

Both forms of idiopathic secretory diarrhea begin abruptly and reach maximum intensity shortly thereafter. Fever is unusual. Weight loss of up to 20 lb characteristically occurs in the first few months of the illness, but it does not become progressive thereafter. Empirical trials of antibiotics and bile acid–binding drugs are ineffective, but nonspecific opiate antidiarrheal drugs provide some relief. Idiopathic secretory diarrhea is self-limited and usually disappears within 2 years of onset. The offset of diarrhea is gradual, occurring over 2 to 3 months.

Diarrhea of obscure origin   Diarrhea of obscure origin is said to be present when chronic diarrhea has evaded diagnosis in spite of an evaluation for structural problems. Patients are often referred commonly to centers interested in diarrheal diseases, where a specific cause for their diarrhea is often identified. Common diagnoses in these patients include fecal incontinence, drug-induced diarrhea, surreptitious laxative ingestion, microscopic colitis syndrome, bile acid–induced diarrhea, pancreatic exocrine insufficiency, carbohydrate malabsorption, sporadic chronic idiopathic secretory diarrhea, and, rarely, endocrine tumors. Most of these conditions can be recognized with a careful history, an appropriate index of suspicion, proper testing, or a well-conducted therapeutic trial. Failure to make a diagnosis is usually the result of not thinking through the differential diagnosis of chronic diarrhea and not appreciating the evidence at hand.

The author has received grants for educational activities from and served as an advisor for Novartis Pharmaceuticals Corp., GlaxoSmithKline, Romark Laboratories, Salix Pharmaceuticals, Inc., Santarus, Inc., and Takeda Pharmaceuticals North America, Inc.; has received grants for clinical research from Novartis Pharmaceuticals Corp. and GlaxoSmithKline; and has served as an advisor to TAP Pharmaceutical Products, Inc.

References

1. Talley NJ, Weaver AL, Zinsmeister AR, et al: Self-reported diarrhea: what does it mean? Am J Gastroenterol 89:1160, 1994

2. Thielman NM, Guerrant RL: Clinical practice. Acute infectious diarrhea. N Engl J Med 350:38, 2004

3. Fine KD, Schiller LR: AGA technical review on the evaluation and management of chronic diarrhea. Gastroenterology 116:1464, 1999

4. Wenzl HH, Fine KD, Schiller LR, et al: Determinants of decreased fecal consistency in patients with diarrhea. Gastroenterology 108:1729, 1995

5. Sellin JH: Intestinal electrolyte absorption and secretion. Gastrointestinal and Liver Disease: Pathophysiology/Diagnosis/Management, 7th ed. Feldman M, Friedman LS, Sleisenger MH, Eds. WB Saunders Co, Philadelphia, 2002, p 1693

6. Schiller LR, Sellin JH: Diarrhea. Gastrointestinal and Liver Disease: Pathophysiology/Diagnosis/Management, 7th ed. Feldman M, Friedman LS, Sleisenger MH, Eds. WB Saunders Co, Philadelphia, 2002, p 131

7. Fordtran JS: Pathophysiology of chronic diarrhoea: insights derived from intestinal perfusion studies in 31 patients. Clin Gastroenterol 15:477, 1986

8. Eherer AJ, Fordtran JS: Fecal osmotic gap and pH in experimental diarrhea of various causes. Gastroenterology 103:545, 1992

9. Guerrant RL, Van Gilder T, Steiner TS, et al: Practice guidelines for the management of infectious diarrhea. Clin Infect Dis 32:331, 2001

10. Brito GA, Alcantara C, Carneiro-Filho BA, et al: Pathophysiology and impact of enteric bacterial and protozoal infections: new approaches to therapy. Chemotherapy 51:23, 2005

11. Vazquez-Torres A, Fang FC: Cellular routes of invasion by enteropathogens. Curr Opin Microbiol 3:54, 2000

12. Crane JK: Preformed bacterial toxins. Clin Lab Med 19:583, 1999

13. Silletti RP, Lee G, Ailey E: Role of stool screening tests in the diagnosis of inflammatory bacterial enteritis and in selection of specimens likely to yield invasive enteric pathogens. J Clin Microbiol 34:1161, 1996

14. Savola KL, Baron EJ, Tompkins LS, et al: Fecal leukocyte stain has diagnostic value for outpatients but not inpatients. J Clin Microbiol 39:266, 2001

15. Bini EJ, Cohen J: Diagnostic yield and cost-effectiveness of endoscopy in chronic human immunodeficiency virus–related diarrhea. Gastrointest Endosc 48:354, 1998

16. Surawicz CM, Haggitt RC, Husseman M, et al: Mucosal biopsy diagnosis of colitis: acute, self-limited colitis and idiopathic inflammatory bowel disease. Gastroenterology 107:755, 1994

17. Desjeux JF, Briend A, Butzner JD: Oral rehydration solution in the year 2000: pathophysiology, efficacy and effectiveness. Baillieres Clin Gastroenterol 11:509, 1997

18. Wong CS, Jelacic S, Habeeb RL, et al: The risk of the hemolytic-uremic syndrome after antibiotic treatment of *Escherichia coli* O157:H7 infections. N Engl J Med 342:1930, 2000

19. Safdar N, Said A, Gangnon RE, et al: Risk of hemolytic-uremic syndrome after antibiotic treatment of *Escherichia coli* O157:H7 enteritis: a meta-analysis. JAMA 288:1014, 2002

20. Huang DB, DuPont HL: Rifaximin: a novel antimicrobial for enteric infections. J Infect 50:97, 2005

21. Cohen SA: Use of nitazoxanide as a new therapeutic option for persistent diarrhea: a pediatric perspective. Curr Med Res Opin 21:999, 2005

22. Schiller LR: Antidiarrhoeal pharmacology and therapeutics. Aliment Pharmacol Ther 9:87, 1995

23. Allos BM: *Campylobacter jejuni* infections: update on emerging issues and trends. Clin Infect Dis 32:1201, 2001

24. Edwards BH: *Salmonella* and *Shigella* species. Clin Lab Med 19:469, 1999

25. Oldfield EC 3rd, Wallace MR: The role of antibiotics in the treatment of infectious diarrhea. Gastroenterol Clin North Am 30:817, 2001

26. House D, Bishop A, Parry C, et al: Typhoid fever: pathogenesis and disease. Curr Opin Infect Dis 14:573, 2001

27. Sandvig K: Shiga toxins. Toxicon 39:1629, 2001

28. Tarr PI, Neill MA: *Escherichia coli* O157:H7. Gastroenterol Clin North Am 30:735, 2001

29. Nakao H, Takeda T: *Escherichia coli* Shiga toxin. J Nat Toxins 9:299, 2000

30. Moyenuddin M, Williamson JC, Ohl CA: *Clostridium difficile*–associated diarrhea: current strategies for diagnosis and therapy. Curr Gastroenterol Rep 4:279, 2002

31. Voth DE, Ballard JD: *Clostridium difficile* toxins: mechanisms of action and role in disease. Clin Microbiol Rev 18:247, 2005

32. Bricker E, Garg R, Nelson R, et al: Antibiotic treatment for *Clostridium difficile*–associated diarrhea in adults. Cochrane Database Syst Rev (1):CD004610, 2005

33. Cremonini F, Di Caro S, Nista EC, et al: Meta-analysis: the effect of probiotic administration on antibiotic-associated diarrhoea. Aliment Pharmacol Ther 16:1461, 2002

34. Monkemuller KE, Wilcox CM: Investigation of diarrhea in AIDS. Can J Gastroenterol 14:933, 2000

35. Ziring D, Tran R, Edelstein S, et al: Infectious enteritis after intestinal transplantation: incidence, timing, and outcome. Transplantation 79:702, 2005

36. Schuster H, Chiodini PL: Parasitic infections of the intestine. Curr Opin Infect Dis 14:587, 2001

37. Ali SA, Hill DR: *Giardia intestinalis.* Curr Opin Infect Dis 16:453, 2003

38. Stauffer W, Ravdin JI: *Entamoeba histolytica:* an update. Curr Opin Infect Dis 16:479, 2003

39. Chappell CL, Okhuysen PC: Cryptosporidiosis. Curr Opin Infect Dis 15:523, 2002

40. Hammer HF, Santa Ana CA, Schiller LR, et al: Studies of osmotic diarrhea induced in normal subjects by ingestion of polyethylene glycol and lactulose. J Clin Invest 84:1056, 1989

41. Canani RB, Terrin G, Cirillo P, et al: Butyrate as an effective treatment of congenital chloride diarrhea. Gastroenterology 127:630, 2004

42. Lee SD, Surawicz CM: Infectious causes of chronic diarrhea. Gastroenterol Clin North Am 30:679, 2001

43. Attar A, Flourie B, Rambaud JC, et al: Antibiotic efficacy in small intestinal bacterial overgrowth–related chronic diarrhea: a crossover, randomized trial. Gastroenterology 117:794, 1999

44. Thielman NM, Guerrant RL: Persistent diarrhea in the returned traveler. Infect Dis Clin North Am 12:489, 1998

45. Schiller LR: Microscopic colitis syndrome: lymphocytic colitis and collagenous colitis. Semin Gastrointest Dis 10:145, 1999

46. Cappell M: Colonic toxicity of administered drugs and chemicals. Am J Gastroenterol 99:1175, 2004

47. Sellin JH, Hart R: Glucose malabsorption associated with rapid intestinal transit. Am J Gastroenterol 87:584, 1992

48. Camilleri M: Motor function in irritable bowel syndrome. Can J Gastroenterol 13(suppl A):8A, 1999

49. Schiller LR, Bilhartz LE, Santa Ana CA, et al: Comparison of endogenous and radiolabeled bile acid excretion in patients with idiopathic chronic diarrhea. Gastroenterology 98:1036, 1990

50. Warner RR: Enteroendocrine tumors other than carcinoid: a review of clinically significant advances. Gastroenterology 128:1668, 2005

51. Modlin IM, Kidd M, Latich I, et al: Current status of gastrointestinal carcinoids. Gastroenterology 128:1717, 2005

52. Afzalpurkar RG, Schiller LR, Little KH, et al: The self-limited nature of chronic idiopathic diarrhea. N Engl J Med 327:1849, 1992

53. Thompson WG, Longstreth GF, Drossman DA, et al: Functional bowel disorders and functional abdominal pain. Gut 45(suppl 2):II43, 1999

54. Petroniene R, Dubcenco E, Baker JP, et al: Given capsule endoscopy in celiac disease: evaluation of diagnostic accuracy and interobserver agreement. Am J Gastroenterol 100:685, 2005

55. Kalantzis N, Papanikolaou IS, Giannakoulopoulou E, et al: Capsule endoscopy: the cumulative experience from its use in 193 patients with suspected small bowel disease. Hepatogastroenterology 52:414, 2005

56. Sturniolo GC, Di Leo V, Vettorato MG: Clinical relevance of small-bowel findings detected by wireless capsule endoscopy. Scand J Gastroenterol 40:725, 2005

57. Matsumoto T, Moriyama T, Esaki M, et al: Performance of antegrade double-balloon enteroscopy: comparison with push enteroscopy. Gastrointest Endosc 62:392, 2005

58. Schiller LR, Rivera LM, Santangelo WC, et al: Diagnostic value of fasting plasma peptide concentrations in patients with chronic diarrhea. Dig Dis Sci 39:2216, 1994

59. Brydon WG, Nyhlin H, Eastwood MA, et al: 7-Alpha-hydroxy-4-cholesten-3-one and selenohomocholyltaurine (SeHCAT) whole body retention in the assessment of bile acid induced diarrhoea. Eur J Gastroenterol Hepatol 8:117, 1996

60. Fine KD, Santa Ana CA, Fordtran JS: Diagnosis of magnesium-induced diarrhea. N Engl J Med 324:1012, 1991

61. Johlin FC Jr, Panther M, Kraft N: Dietary fructose intolerance: diet modification can impact self-rated health and symptom control. Nutr Clin Care 7:92, 2004

62. Fine KD, Fordtran JS: The effect of diarrhea on fecal fat excretion. Gastroenterology 102:1936, 1992

63. Schoenfeld P: Efficacy of current drug therapies in irritable bowel syndrome: what works and does not work. Gastroenterol Clin North Am 34:319, 2005

64. Gershon MD: Nerves, reflexes, and the enteric nervous system: pathogenesis of the irritable bowel syndrome. J Clin Gastroenterol 39(suppl 3):S184, 2005

65. Zar S, Benson MJ, Kumar D: Food-specific serum IgG4 and IgE titers to common food antigens in irritable bowel syndrome. Am J Gastroenterol 100:1550, 2005

66. Walters B, Vanner SJ: Detection of bacterial overgrowth in IBS using the lactulose H2 breath test: comparison with 14C-D-xylose and healthy controls. Am J Gastroenterol 100:1566, 2005

67. Malinen E, Rinttila T, Kajander K, et al: Analysis of the fecal microbiota of irritable bowel syndrome patients and healthy controls with real-time PCR. Am J Gastroenterol 100:373, 2005

68. Pardi DS: Microscopic colitis: an update. Inflamm Bowel Dis 10:860, 2004

69. Chande N, Driman DK, Reynolds RP: Collagenous colitis and lymphocytic colitis: patient characteristics and clinical presentation. Scand J Gastroenterol 40:343, 2005

70. Ung KA, Gillberg R, Kilander A, et al: Role of bile acids and bile acid binding agents in patients with collagenous colitis. Gut 46:170, 2000

71. Ewe K, Karbach U: Factitious diarrhea. Clin Gastroenterol 15:723, 1986

72. Slugg PH, Carey WD: Clinical features and follow-up of surreptitious laxative users. Cleveland Clin Q 51:167, 1984

73. Hasler WL: Dumping syndrome. Curr Treat Options Gastroenterol 5:139, 2002

74. Arrambide KA, Santa Ana CA, Schiller LR, et al: Loss of absorptive capacity for sodium chloride as a cause of diarrhea following partial ileal and right colon resection. Dig Dis Sci 34:193, 1989

75. Metcalf AM, Phillips SF: Ileostomy diarrhoea. Clin Gastroenterol 15:705, 1986

76. Heuschen UA, Allemeyer EH, Hinz U, et al: Diagnosing pouchitis: comparative validation of two scoring systems in routine follow-up. Dis Colon Rectum 45:776, 2002

77. Sauter GH, Moussavian AC, Meyer G, et al: Bowel habits and bile acid malabsorption in the months after cholecystectomy. Am J Gastroenterol 97:1732, 2002

78. Saslow SB, Camilleri M: Diabetic diarrhea. Semin Gastrointest Dis 6:187, 1995

79. Wald A: Incontinence and anorectal dysfunction in patients with diabetes mellitus. Eur J Gastroenterol Hepatol 7:737, 1995

80. Cohen J, West AB, Bini EJ: Infectious diarrhea in human immunodeficiency virus. Gastroenterol Clin North Am 30:637, 2001

81. Mintz E: A riddle wrapped in a mystery inside an enigma: Brainerd diarrhoea turns 20. Lancet 362:2037, 2003

82. Schiller LR: Chronic diarrhea. GI/Liver Secrets, 2nd ed. McNally PR, Ed. Hanley and Belfus, Philadelphia, 2002, p 411

83. Schiller LR: Diarrhea. Med Clin North Am 84:1259, 2000

67 Gastrointestinal Motility and Functional Disorders

Henry P. Parkman, M.D.

Gastrointestinal motility disorders are characterized by acute, recurrent, or chronic symptoms with objective evidence of slow or rapid GI transit or motility in the absence of mucosal disease or obstruction. Some of these disorders include achalasia, diffuse esophageal spasm, gastroesophageal reflux disease (GERD) [*see Chapter 61*], gastroparesis, chronic intestinal pseudo-obstruction (CIP), colonic inertia, and fecal incontinence. Many of these GI motility disorders, especially gastroparesis and fecal incontinence, are being increasingly recognized.

Functional GI disorders are characterized primarily by symptoms suggesting impaired motor or sensory functions in the absence of mucosal or structural abnormality or of known biochemical or metabolic disorders. In the United States, functional GI disorders are estimated to affect 25 million persons. Some of these disorders include functional heartburn, functional dyspepsia, and irritable bowel syndrome (IBS). IBS is the most common of the disorders; it results in abdominal pain and altered bowel movements and is present in 10% to 15% of the population.[1]

Normal Gastrointestinal Motility

GASTRIC MOTILITY

The important motor events related to normal gastric emptying include (1) postprandial receptive relaxation of the gastric fundus, which allows accommodation of food without significantly increasing gastric pressure; (2) rhythmic antral contractions for trituration of large food particles and breakdown into appropriate size; (3) pyloric relaxation, which allows food to enter the duodenum; (4) coordination of antropyloroduodenal motor events; and (5) neural/hormonal inhibitory feedback from nutrients in the small bowel.

Solid and liquid foods empty from the stomach at different rates. Liquids empty from the stomach at an exponential rate; solids are initially retained selectively within the stomach until particles have been triturated to a size smaller than 2 mm, at which point they can be emptied at a linear rate from the stomach.

Normal gastric emptying is regulated by the influences of the central nervous system predominantly through vagal efferent pathways and the enteric nervous system acting on gastric smooth muscle. When a meal is ingested, the proximal portion of the stomach (i.e., the fundus) relaxes to accommodate the food. This response, called gastric accommodation, is mediated by the vagus nerves and involves the activation of intrinsic nitrergic inhibitory nerves in the wall of the stomach. Subsequent fundic and antral smooth muscle contractions result primarily from cholinergically mediated contractions; these contractions result from alterations of the electrical potential of the cell membrane from ions flowing through channels of the cell membrane. The enteric nervous system consists of intrinsic neurons of the GI tract and is organized in ganglionated plexi (primarily the submucosal and myenteric plexi). The enteric nervous system is organized in intricate excitatory and inhibitory circuits. These circuits play essential roles in controlling peristalsis and the migrating motor complex.

Among the enteric plexi are interstitial cells of Cajal, which serve as gastric pacemakers. The afferent enteric nerves are also important in mediating sensation from the stomach.

SMALL INTESTINAL MOTILITY

The small intestine transports solids and liquids at approximately the same rate. Because there is a separation of the two phases in the stomach, liquids may arrive in the colon before the head of the solid phase of the meal. Ileal emptying of chyme is characterized by bolus transfers.

GI motility is characterized by distinct patterns of contractile activity in the fasting and postprandial periods. This is particularly evident in the stomach and small intestine. The fasting period is characterized by a cyclic motor phenomenon called the migrating motor complex. In healthy people, it occurs approximately once every 90 minutes and comprises a period of quiescence (phase I), a period of intermittent pressure activity (phase II), and an activity front, during which the stomach and small intestine contract at their highest frequency (phase III). During phase III of the migrating motor complex, the frequency of contractions reaches three a minute in the stomach and 11 or 12 a minute in the proximal small intestine. The interdigestive activity front migrates a variable distance down the small intestine; there is a gradient in the frequency of contractions during phase III, from 11 or 12 a minute in the duodenum to as low as five a minute in the ileum. The distal small intestine also demonstrates another characteristic motor pattern—a propagated prolonged contraction, or power contraction—that serves to empty residue from the ileum to the colon in bolus transfers.

In the postprandial period, the fasting cyclic activity of the stomach and small intestine is replaced by irregular, fairly frequent contractions in those regions of the stomach and small bowel that come in contact with food. The caloric content of the meal is the major determinant of the duration of this so-called fed pattern. The maximum frequency of contractions is below that noted during phase III of the migrating motor complex.

COLONIC MOTILITY

The colon serves as a reservoir to facilitate the absorption of fluids, electrolytes, and short-chain fatty acids produced by bacterial metabolism of unabsorbed carbohydrates. This reservoir function is centered predominantly in the ascending and transverse colonic regions. The descending colon functions as a conduit for the relatively rapid transit of feces to the sigmoid colon, which acts as a second reservoir. The control and function of contractions in the colon are not fully understood; some irregular contractions serve to mix its contents, whereas high-amplitude propagated contractions (HAPCs), which on average occur four to six times a day, are sometimes associated with mass movement of colonic residue and lead to defecation. After meals of at least 500 kcal, there is a greater propensity for HAPCs to develop and for the tone (i.e., the background state of contractility) of the colon to increase, resulting in bowel movements in the first 2 hours after meals.

Emptying of the sigmoid colon and rectum is largely under volitional control. The defecatory process requires the Valsalva maneuver to raise intra-abdominal pressure, which is transmitted to the rectal contents, and relaxation of the puborectalis (or pelvic floor) and external anal sphincter, which necessitates a coordinated series of functions. This facilitates the opening or straightening of the rectoanal angle and expulsion of stool.

Gastric Motility Disorders

GASTROPARESIS

Gastroparesis is a chronic motility disorder characterized by delayed gastric emptying in the absence of a mechanical cause of obstruction. Most patients with gastroparesis are women.[2]

Gastroparesis is being increasingly recognized, and management of this condition is challenging. Symptoms do not closely correlate with gastric emptying, which is the customary indicator of gastroparesis. Although current management strategies are often suboptimal for improving patients' symptoms, advances are being made in the evaluation and treatment of this disorder.[3,4] New treatments currently under investigation may result in a more favorable outlook for patients with this condition.

Etiologic Variants

Gastroparesis can occur in many clinical settings, with a wide variation in and severity of symptoms [see Table 1]. In one series of 146 patients with gastroparesis, 36% of the cases were idiopathic, 29% were associated with diabetes, and 13% occurred in postsurgical patients; the remaining 22% of cases had miscellaneous causes.[2]

Diabetic gastroparesis Gastroparesis is a well-recognized complication of diabetes mellitus. Classically, gastroparesis occurs in patients with long-standing type 1 diabetes mellitus who have other associated complications of diabetes, such as retinopathy, nephropathy, and peripheral neuropathy.[5] Many affected patients may have other signs of autonomic dysfunction, including postural hypotension. Gastroparesis may also occur in patients with type 2 diabetes.

The prevalence of gastroparesis in patients with either type 1 or type 2 diabetes ranges from 30% to 50%, although the magnitude of gastric delay is modest in many cases.[5] Patients who have had diabetes for a relatively short time may have accelerated emptying. In those with accelerated emptying, impairment of fundic relaxation, which is necessary to accommodate a meal, may be the underlying defect; this may be caused by vagal dysfunction.[6]

Fluctuations in gastric emptying in patients with diabetic gastroparesis appear to influence postprandial blood glucose concentrations.[7] In diabetic patients, delayed gastric emptying contributes to erratic glycemic control because of unpredictable delivery of food into the duodenum.[8] Delayed gastric emptying of nutrients in conjunction with parenteral insulin administration may produce hypoglycemia. Conversely, acceleration of the emptying of nutrients has been reported to cause early postprandial hyperglycemia.[9] Difficulty in the control of blood glucose levels may be an early indication that a diabetic patient is developing gastric motor dysfunction.[2]

Hyperglycemia itself can reversibly interfere with gastric motility in several ways: (1) by decreasing antral contractility; (2) by causing decreases in phase III of the migrating motor complex; (3) by increasing pyloric contractions; (4) by causing disturbances in gastric myoelectric activity; (5) by delaying gastric emptying; and (6) by modulating fundic relaxation.[8] Hyperglycemia also appears to impair vagal efferent function.

Postsurgical gastroparesis Gastroparesis may occur as a complication of a number of abdominal surgical procedures. In the past, most cases resulted from vagotomy performed in combination with gastric drainage to correct medically refractory or complicated peptic ulcer disease. Since the advent of laparoscopic techniques for the treatment of GERD, gastroparesis has become a more common complication of fundoplication (possibly from vagal injury from the surgery). Approximately 5% of patients undergoing vagotomy with antrectomy and gastrojejunostomy (Bilroth I procedure) develop severe postsurgical gastroparesis.[10] In these patients, the antrum is not present to triturate solids, and the proximal stomach is unable to generate sufficient pressure to empty solid food residue.

The combination of vagotomy, distal gastric resection, and Roux-en-Y gastrojejunostomy predisposes to severe gastric stasis resulting from slow emptying from the gastric remnant and delayed small bowel transit in the denervated Roux efferent limb. The Roux-en-Y stasis syndrome—characterized by postprandial abdominal pain, bloating, nausea, and vomiting—is particularly difficult to manage.

Table 1 Causes of Gastroparesis

Diabetes mellitus
Surgical procedures
    Partial gastric resection/vagotomy
    Nissen fundoplication
    Organ transplantation (e.g., lung, heart-lung)
Gastrointestinal disorders associated with delayed gastric emptying
    Diffuse GI motor disorders (e.g., chronic intestinal pseudo-obstruction)
    GERD
    Functional dyspepsia
    Hypertrophic pyloric stenosis
Nongastrointestinal disorders associated with delayed gastric emptying
    Neurologic disorders
        CNS tumors
        Parkinson disease
    Collagen vascular disorders
        Scleroderma
        Systemic lupus erythematosus
    Endocrine and metabolic disorders
        Thyroid dysfunction
        Parathyroid dysfunction
    Eating disorders
        Anorexia nervosa
    Other
        Amyloidosis
        Chronic renal insufficiency
        Gastric infection
        Chronic mesenteric ischemia
        Tumor-associated (paraneoplastic)
        Medication-associated delayed gastric emptying
Idiopathic causes

GERD—gastroesophageal reflux disease

Idiopathic gastroparesis Most patients with idiopathic gastroparesis are women, typically young or middle aged.[11] The anatomic basis of idiopathic gastroparesis is not fully known. In one case of idiopathic gastroparesis, myenteric plexus hypoganglionosis and reductions in the number of interstitial cells of Cajal were observed.[12] A viral etiology has also been postulated for a subset of cases of idiopathic gastroparesis. Some patients with idiopathic gastroparesis report an initial onset of symptoms suggestive of a viral prodrome.[13] In this patient subset, previously healthy patients experience the sudden onset of nausea, vomiting, diarrhea, fever, abdominal cramps, or a combination of these symptoms—suggestive of a GI viral infection; however, the symptoms do not resolve, as would be the case in a viral infection. In these patients, nausea, vomiting, and early satiety become chronic, with resolution of symptoms possibly occurring after several years. The course of idiopathic gastroparesis may fluctuate between acute symptomatic episodes and periods in which symptoms are relatively quiescent. Patients who experience idiopathic gastroparesis without a viruslike onset show less improvement over time. Viruses that have been implicated in idiopathic gastroparesis include cytomegalovirus, Epstein-Barr virus, and varicella-zoster virus.

Diagnosis

The diagnosis of gastroparesis is confirmed by the demonstration of delayed gastric emptying in a symptomatic patient, in the absence of other potential causes.

Clinical manifestations Symptoms of gastroparesis are variable and nonspecific and include early satiety, nausea, vomiting, bloating, and upper abdominal discomfort. In one series of 146 patients with gastroparesis, nausea and vomiting were the most frequently reported symptoms (occurring in 92% and 84% of patients, respectively), followed by abdominal bloating (75%) and early satiety (60%).[2] Patients may also experience distention and anorexia.

Correlation of symptoms with delayed gastric emptying is variable in diabetic gastropathy, idiopathic gastroparesis, and functional dyspepsia. In patients with diabetes, abdominal fullness and bloating were found to be associated with delayed gastric emptying. Symptoms of idiopathic gastroparesis overlap with those of functional dyspepsia; in some patients, it may be difficult to distinguish between the two disorders. In functional dyspepsia, the predominant symptoms typically are abdominal pain and discomfort; in idiopathic gastroparesis, the predominant symptoms are typically nausea, vomiting, early satiety, and bloating. However, early satiety, postprandial fullness, and vomiting have been reported to be associated with delayed emptying in patients with functional dyspepsia.[14]

Medical history Family history and medication history are essential to identify underlying etiologic factors that may result in a motility disorder. In patients with diabetic gastroparesis, diabetes has generally been present for at least 5 years. A careful review of systems will help reveal an underlying collagen vascular disease (e.g., scleroderma) or disturbances of extrinsic neural control that also may be affecting the abdominal viscera. Such symptoms include orthostatic dizziness; difficulties with erection; dryness of mouth, eyes, or vagina; difficulties with visual accommodation in bright lights; and an absence of sweating. Raynaud phenomenon may suggest the presence of scleroderma.

Physical examination On physical examination, the presence of a succussion splash is usually indicative of a region of stasis within the GI tract, typically the stomach. The hands and mouth may show signs of scleroderma. Testing of pupillary responses to light and accommodation, blood pressure in the lying and standing positions, general features of a peripheral neuropathy, and external ocular movements can identify patients with an associated neurologic disturbance, such as those with a long history (usually longer than 10 years) of diabetes mellitus or oculogastrointestinal muscular dystrophy.

Laboratory tests A motility disorder should be suspected whenever undigested solid food or large volumes of liquids are observed during esophagogastroduodenoscopy, which is performed after an overnight fast. Barium studies rarely identify the etiology of the motor disorder except in small bowel systemic sclerosis, which is characterized by megaduodenum and thickened valvulae conniventes in the small intestine. Barium x-ray, however, serves the important function of excluding mechanical obstruction. The diagnosis of a gastric motility disorder, therefore, depends on a careful history and confirmation by transit tests.

If the patient's history includes an obvious etiologic factor, such as long-standing diabetes mellitus, it is usually unnecessary to pursue further investigations.

Routine laboratory testing is not useful for the diagnosis of gastric stasis, although it may help to identify diseases that are associated with delayed gastric emptying or to rule out other disorders [see Table 2]. A complete blood count and metabolic profile (e.g., fasting plasma glucose, potassium, creatinine, serum total protein, albumin, and calcium) are useful to assess the nutritional status of the patient.

Transit tests, which can be performed relatively simply and inexpensively, enable good discrimination between healthy and disease states. The most widely available approach is scintigraphy with scans taken immediately after ingestion of the radiolabeled meal, as well as 1, 2, and 4 hours later.[15,16] Gastric emptying scintigraphy of a solid-phase meal is considered the gold standard for the diagnosis of gastroparesis because this test quantifies the emptying of a physiologic caloric meal.[17] The test meal must have a sufficient caloric content (typically more than 200 kcal) and solid consistency to induce the increased contractions in the stomach and small intestine that occur postprandially. Many centers use a technetium-99m (^{99m}Tc) sulfur colloid–labeled egg sandwich as a test meal.

When the cause of the gastric transit disorder is unclear, referral to a specialized center for upper GI manometry, electrogastrography, and autonomic tests may be needed. Gastroduodenal manometry may identify a myopathic or neuropathic disorder or an unsuspected mechanical obstruction resulting from simultaneous prolonged contractions at several levels of the intestine. Electrogastrography may identify disorders of gastric electrical activity signifying a gastric motility disorder.

Differential Diagnosis

Symptoms of gastroparesis may simulate symptoms of other structural disorders of the stomach and proximal GI tract, such as peptic ulcer disease, partial gastric or small bowel obstruction, gastric cancer, and pancreaticobiliary disorders. There also is an overlap between the symptoms of gastroparesis and those of functional dyspepsia. In fact, idiopathic gastroparesis can be considered one of the causes of functional dyspepsia.

Table 2 Evaluation of Patients Suspected of
Having Gastroparesis[4]

Initial investigation
History, physical examination
Blood tests
Complete blood count
Complete metabolic profile (e.g., glucose, potassium, creatinine, total protein, albumin, calcium)
Amylase, if abdominal pain is a significant symptom
Pregnancy test, if appropriate
Abdominal obstruction series, if vomiting or pain is acute or severe

Evaluate for organic disorders
Upper endoscopy or upper GI barium series to evaluate for mechanical obstruction or mucosal lesions
Biliary ultrasonography if abdominal pain is a significant symptom

Evaluate for delayed gastric emptying
Solid-phase gastric emptying test
Screen for secondary causes of gastroparesis
Thyroid function tests (thyroid-stimulating hormone)
Rheumatologic serologies (e.g., antinuclear antibody, scleroderma antibody)
Glycosylated hemoglobin

Perform treatment trial (i.e., prokinetic agent or antiemetic agent or both)

Consider further investigation (if treatment trial yields no clinical response)
EGG
Antroduodenal manometry
Small bowel evaluation with enteroclysis or small bowel followthrough
Further laboratory tests, if indicated (e.g., ANA, tissue transglutaminase antibody test)

ANA—antinuclear antibody test   EGG—electrogastrogram

Delayed gastric emptying may be caused by conditions other than gastroparesis; the conditions to be differentiated are mechanical obstruction, functional GI disorders such as functional dyspepsia and IBS, and eating disorders such as anorexia nervosa and rumination syndrome. The degree of impairment of gastric emptying in eating disorders is relatively minor compared with diabetic and postvagotomy gastric stasis.

Treatment

The treatment goals for patients with symptomatic gastroparesis are as follows: (1) to control symptoms; (2) to correct fluid, electrolyte, and nutritional deficiencies; and (3) to identify and treat the underlying cause of gastroparesis, if possible. For relatively mild disease, dietary modifications and a low-dose antiemetic or prokinetic agent might provide satisfactory control of symptoms. Patients with severe manifestations of gastroparesis, such as refractory vomiting, pronounced dehydration, or chaotic glucose control, may require hospitalization for intravenous hydration, insulin administration, intravenous administration of antiemetic and prokinetic agents, or a combination of these measures.

Diet modification   In patients with gastroparesis, the liquid nutrient component of the ingested meal should be increased because gastric emptying of liquids often is preserved. The intake of fats and fiber should be minimized because they tend to slow gastric emptying. Indigestible fiber and roughage also may predispose to gastric bezoar formation. Foods that cannot be reliably chewed into small pieces should be avoided. Multiple frequent meals are often recommended to limit the caloric intake with each meal.

Correction of dehydration and electrolyte and nutritional depletion is particularly important during acute exacerbations of gastroparesis. Nutritional support should be tailored to the severity of the deficiencies of trace elements and dietary constituents in each patient. Dietary measures include the use of low-fiber and low-fat caloric supplements that contain iron, folate, calcium, and vitamins D, K, and B_{12}. Patients who have more severe conditions, such as severe diabetic gastroparesis, may need parenteral or enteral nutrition supplementation.

Glycemic control in diabetic patients   To date, no long-term studies have confirmed the beneficial effects of maintenance of near-normal glycemia on gastroparetic symptoms in diabetic patients. Nevertheless, the findings of physiologic studies in healthy volunteers and diabetic patients and other obvious benefits of glycemic control provide a compelling argument for striving to achieve near-normal blood glucose levels in affected diabetic patients.[3]

Antiemetic therapy   Antiemetic agents may be useful in relieving symptoms of gastroparesis. Antiemetic drugs may serve as primary therapy for patients with gastroparesis; they may also be used as adjunctive therapy when combined with medications that promote gastric emptying [*see Table 3*]. Phenothiazines (e.g., prochlorperazine) are commonly prescribed as antiemetic agents; these agents are available in oral, suppository, I.M., and I.V. formulations. For patients with severe symptoms, suppositories or injectable formulations may be more beneficial. Side effects from phenothiazines are common and include sedation and extrapyramidal reactions. Serotonin ($5-HT_3$) receptor antagonists, such as ondansetron, may be helpful in some cases. Ondansetron is available in oral and I.V. formulations.

Prokinetic therapy   Prokinetic medications are often used to enhance gut contractility and promote motility. Some prokinetic agents, notably metoclopramide and domperidone, also exhibit antiemetic properties and may be useful in relieving symptoms of gastroparesis [*see Table 3*]. The response to treatment is usually judged clinically rather than by repeating gastric emptying tests.

Metoclopramide, with its antinausea and indirect cholinomimetic actions, is widely used for the treatment of gastroparesis, though evidence of its efficacy is limited. Controlled trials report that metoclopramide provides symptomatic relief and accelerates gastric emptying of solids and liquids in patients with idiopathic, diabetic, and postvagotomy gastroparesis.[18,19] Metoclopramide is approved for the treatment of diabetic gastroparesis and for the prevention of postoperative and chemotherapy-induced nausea and vomiting. The usual dosage is 10 mg four times a day. Metoclopramide is also available for parenteral use; the usual dose is 10 mg I.M. or I.V. Metoclopramide should be used with caution; it may be useful to administer a test dose (1 to 2 mg) to exclude dystonic reactions resulting from an idiosyncratic reaction. Metoclopramide is effective for the short-term treatment of gastroparesis for up to several weeks; however, symptomatic improvement does not necessarily ac-

Table 3 Therapy for Gastroparesis

Drug	Dose	Comments
Antiemetic agents		
Phenothiazines		
Prochlorperazine	5–10 mg p.o., q. 6–8 hr *or* 5–10 mg I.M. q. 3–4 hr	I.M., I.V., p.o., rectal suppository
Chlorpromazine	10–25 mg p.o., q. 4–6 hr *or* 25–50 mg I.M., I.V. q. 4–6 hr	
Trimethobenzamide	300 mg p.o., q. 6–8 hr *or* 200 mg I.M. q. 6–8 hr	
Butyrophenones		
Droperidol	1.25–5 mg I.M.	
5-HT$_3$ receptor antagonists (e.g., ondansetron)	4–8 mg p.o. or I.V. q. 6–8 hr	Less effective for dysmotility than for chemotherapy-induced emesis
Antihistamines		
Diphenhydramine	25–50 mg p.o., q. 6 hr *or* 10–50 mg I.V. or I.M.	Primarily used for motion sickness
Promethazine	12.5–25 mg p.o. or I.M. q. 4 hr *or* 12.5–25 mg rectally q. 12 hr	
Meclizine	25–50 mg p.o. daily	
Prokinetic agents		
Metoclopramide	10 mg p.o. or I.M. or I.V. q. 6 hr	FDA approved for gastroparesis; prokinetic and antiemetic properties; CNS side effects
Erythromycin	125–250 mg p.o., q. 6–8 hr *or* 100 mg I.M. or I.V. q. 8 hr	GI side effects (i.e., nausea, vomiting, abdominal pain) in many patients; tachyphylaxis with long-term oral administration
Cisapride	10 mg p.o., q. 8 hr	Limited access because of drug interactions and potential for cardiac dysrhythmia
Domperidone	10–30 mg p.o., q. 8 hr	Prokinetic and antiemetic properties; in United States, available through the FDA's IND program but not by prescription
Tegaserod	6 mg p.o., q. 8 hr	Improves gastric emptying; no data on symptoms; FDA approved for constipation in irritable bowel syndrome

IND—Investigational New Drug

company improvement in gastric emptying. The long-term utility of metoclopramide has not been proven. Neuropsychiatric side effects, such as dystonias, are not infrequent, and rare cases of tardive dyskinesia have been reported.

Erythromycin, a macrolide antibiotic that stimulates motilin receptors partly through a cholinergic mechanism, has been shown to stimulate gastric emptying in patients with diabetic gastroparesis, idiopathic gastroparesis, and postvagotomy gastroparesis; however, studies have been small and have not been carefully controlled.[20] In a systematic review of studies on oral erythromycin, improvement in symptoms was noted in 43% of patients.[20] Oral administration of erythromycin should be initiated at low doses (e.g., 125 mg to 250 mg three or four times daily).[3] Intravenous erythromycin (100 mg every 8 hours) is used for hospitalized patients with severe refractory gastroparesis. Side effects of erythromycin at higher doses include nausea, vomiting, and abdominal pain.

Cisapride, a substituted benzamide that acts as a serotonin agonist, has been used to treat altered motility, such as impaired gastric emptying, in patients with both gastroparesis and CIP.[21] The availability of cisapride has been severely restricted in the United States, because it has been associated with important drug interactions (causing cardiac arrhythmias and death).

Domperidone, a peripheral dopaminergic antagonist, has been shown to be efficacious in the treatment of diabetic gastroparesis[22]; symptom improvement was similar to that observed for metoclopramide and cisapride but with fewer CNS side effects. Domperidone is not approved in the United States but may be obtained with the use of a Federal Drug Administration Investigational New Drug Application and Institutional Review Board approval. The usual dosage is 30 to 80 mg/day in three or four divided doses.

Tegaserod is a partial 5-HT$_4$ receptor agonist that has been shown to accelerate gastric and intestinal transit in healthy persons and intestinal transit in patients with constipation-predominant IBS.[23,24] In a preliminary controlled trial, tegaserod was shown to accelerate solid-phase emptying in patients with gastroparesis; gastric emptying normalized in 80% of patients who received 18 mg of tegaserod daily, as compared with 50% of those receiving placebo.[25] Tegaserod is chemically different from the benzamides and does not cause cardiac dysrhythmias.

Pyloric botulinum toxin injection Botulinum toxin is a potent inhibitor of neuromuscular transmission and has been used to treat spastic somatic muscle disorders as well as achalasia. Pilot studies have tested the effects of pyloric injection of botulinum toxin in patients with diabetic and idiopathic gastroparesis. These preliminary studies indicated that treatment with botulinum toxin results in mild improvements in gastric emptying and modest reductions in symptoms for several months.[26,27] Double-blind controlled studies are needed to support the efficacy of this treatment.

Gastric electric stimulation Gastric electric stimulation is an emerging treatment for refractory gastroparesis. It involves an implantable neurostimulator that delivers a high-frequency (i.e., 12 cpm), low-energy signal with short pulses. A randomized, controlled trial indicated that gastric electrical stimulation decreased vomiting frequency and GI symptoms in patients with severe refractory gastroparesis.[28] The gastric electric neurostimulator has been approved by the Food and Drug Administration for the treatment of chronic, refractory nausea and vomiting secondary to diabetic or idiopathic gastroparesis. The response rate to gastric electric stimulation is 50% to 70%. Diabetic patients respond better than patients with idiopathic gastroparesis. In addition, patients with primary symptoms of nausea and vomiting do better than patients with abdominal pain. The main complication of the implantable neurostimulator has been infection, which has necessitated removal of the device in approximately 5% to 10% of cases. Further investigation is needed to confirm the effectiveness of gastric stimulation in the treatment of gastroparesis.

Surgical therapy Surgery is rarely indicated for patients with nonobstructive gastric stasis except for the provision of decompression (e.g., gastrostomy or jejunostomy) or for completion gastrectomy for patients with stasis syndrome after gastric surgery.[29] For patients with gastroparesis who are unable to maintain nutrition with oral intake, surgical or endoscopic placement of a feeding jejunostomy tube may provide adequate nutrition. Switching from oral to small bowel nutrient delivery may decrease symptoms and reduce hospitalizations. Jejunostomy tubes are effective for providing nutrition, fluids, and medications if there is normal small intestinal motor function. Except in cases of profound malnutrition or electrolyte disturbance, enteral feedings are preferable to total parenteral nutrition (TPN) because of the risks of infection, venous thrombosis, and liver disease with TPN. If small bowel dysmotility is suspected, a trial of nasojejunal feedings should precede placement of a permanent jejunostomy tube. Jejunostomy tubes can be placed endoscopically or surgically during laparoscopy or laparotomy. Carefully regulated enteral nutrient infusions may improve glycemic control in diabetic patients with refractory vomiting. Nocturnal feedings may permit daytime employment and functioning.

RAPID GASTRIC EMPTYING (DUMPING SYNDROME)

Rapid gastric emptying (often referred to as dumping) can result from impaired relaxation of the stomach upon ingestion of food. Postprandial intragastric pressure is relatively high and results in active propulsion of liquid foods from the stomach. A high caloric (usually carbohydrate) content of the liquid phase of the meal evokes a rapid insulin response with secondary hypoglycemia. These patients may also have impaired antral contractility and gastric stasis of solids, which may paradoxically result in a clinical picture of both gastroparesis (for solids) and dumping (for liquids).[30]

Symptomatic rapid gastric emptying may also occur as a result of prior gastric surgery, damage to the pylorus, or gastric denervation. Symptoms of the dumping syndrome include sweating, weakness, occasional orthostasis, tachycardia, and diarrhea. The syndrome is often characterized by early dumping or late dumping. Early dumping results from rapid filling of the intestine with hypertonic fluid leading to bloating, crampy abdominal pain, and diarrhea with tachycardia and lightheadedness. Late dumping refers to symptoms primarily of hypoglycemia (i.e., weakness, palpitations, and diaphoresis) occurring 2 to 3 hours after a meal. Although dumping syndromes

can usually be diagnosed clinically, scintigraphic studies using both solid and liquid phase markers can help establish the diagnosis of rapid gastric emptying.[31]

Management of dumping includes patient education (particularly regarding the avoidance of high-nutrient liquid drinks) and, possibly, the addition of guar gum or pectin to retard liquid emptying.[30] If these measures are ineffective, pharmacologic approaches may be effective. For example, the use of subcutaneous octreotide (50 to 100 μg) 15 minutes before meals decreases many of the vasomotor symptoms and also retards gastric emptying and small bowel transit, thereby relieving associated hypoglycemia and diarrhea.[32] Long-term use of octreotide is somewhat limited by side effects, particularly diarrhea and steatorrhea. A long-acting-release octreotide (Sandostatin-LAR) appears to be as effective as octreotide and may be better tolerated.[33]

Disorders of Small Bowel Motility

Motility disorders of the small bowel may be characterized by decreased contractility or by increased or uncoordinated contractility. Symptoms that may arise from the slow propagation of small intestinal contents include postprandial abdominal pain, bloating, nausea, vomiting, and early satiety. These symptoms can also be consistent with mechanical obstruction; the most important question to address initially is whether the symptoms result from obstruction or from a motility disorder. Bacterial overgrowth of the small intestine may occur as a consequence of slow intestinal transit caused by diminished activity during phase III of the migrating motor complex.

Diarrhea is generally the result of rapid intestinal transit; with an accelerated transit time, the amount of time during which the luminal contents are in contact with the mucosa decreases, thereby preventing absorption. Patients may also have maldigestion and malabsorption resulting from poor mixing of the dietary material with the digestive enzymes and bile salts. Accentuated borborygmi may also disturb the patient.

CHRONIC INTESTINAL PSEUDO-OBSTRUCTION

CIP is a syndrome characterized by recurrent clinical symptoms suggestive of intestinal obstruction in the absence of a mechanical blockage of the lumen. The symptoms of pseudo-obstruction are caused by ineffective peristalsis; they are similar to those of gastroparesis and include nausea, vomiting, and abdominal pain with abdominal distension. Radiologic findings consist of air-fluid levels within the small intestinal lumen. CIP is a chronic condition, whereas the syndrome of adynamic ileus is acute and self-limited. The disorder can be caused by several systemic diseases, including scleroderma, amyloidosis, myxedema, and long-standing diabetes. Often, however, there is no known cause; such cases are categorized as chronic idiopathic intestinal pseudo-obstruction (CIIP). The diagnosis of CIIP is often delayed until several years after the onset of symptoms. At one center, a median of 8 years lapsed between onset of symptoms and diagnosis[34]; in these patients, manometry invariably showed abnormal motor patterns. Long-term outcome is generally poor despite surgical and medical therapies.

The two main forms of idiopathic pseudo-obstruction are myopathic (involving the intestinal musculature) and neurogenic (involving the neural apparatus).[35] The bowel wall in patients with the myopathic form (e.g., hollow visceral myopathy) shows thinning and degeneration of the smooth muscle with replacement by fibrous tissue. Patients with the neurogenic form (e.g., visceral neuropathy) have abnormalities in neurons and glial cells within the splanchnic ganglia, the myenteric plexus, or both. In patients with the neurogenic form, the intestinal smooth muscle is normal.

Steps in the evaluation of a patients with suspected CIP include the following: radiographic imaging to eliminate a structural cause of blockage; assessment of the patient's nutritional state; confirmation of dysmotility by means of a transit test; and performance of specialized testing, such as gastroduodenojejunal manometry.[36] In patients with intestinal myopathy, manometry typically reveals low-amplitude contractions that propagate normally. In patients with intestinal neuropathy, individual contractions may be of normal amplitude but are disorganized. Other manifestations include disruption of phase III of the migrating motor complex, bursts of nonpropagating activity during fasting, and failure to convert from the fasting to the fed pattern with a meal.

The natural history of CIP depends on the underlying cause of the syndrome. The management of CIP involves multiple modalities: dietary manipulations, parenteral nutrition, pharmacotherapy, and endoscopic and surgical therapy.[35] Nutritional support by enteral or, if necessary, by parenteral means is an important aspect of management. Pharmacotherapy consists of prokinetic agents and, if indicated, antibiotics for bacterial overgrowth (see below). Venting jejunostomy may be helpful in relieving obstructive symptoms. Small bowel transplantation has been used in some centers.

SMALL INTESTINAL BACTERIAL OVERGROWTH

Normally, gastric acid secretion and intestinal motility play crucial roles in preventing significant numbers of bacteria from accumulating in the upper GI tract. Intestinal dysmotility is an important factor contributing to the development of clinically significant small intestinal bacterial overgrowth. Diarrhea, steatorrhea, and malabsorption are consequences of bacterial overgrowth. Diagnosis can be made with small intestinal aspiration of luminal contents with quantitation of bacteria or by use of the lactulose hydrogen breath test. In the latter test, an early hydrogen peak represents metabolism of the orally administered lactulose by bacteria in the small intestine and indicates bacterial overgrowth. Treatment is with broad-spectrum antibiotics directed against aerobic and anaerobic enteric bacteria.[37] Because of microbial resistance to tetracycline, this agent is no longer effective in many patients. Adequate antimicrobial coverage can be achieved with amoxicillin-clavulanate, metronidazole, rifaximin, and gentamicin.[37]

ILEUS

Ileus is an acute decrease or absence of small bowel motility. Although ileus is most commonly seen in the postoperative setting, it is being increasingly recognized in nonsurgical conditions, usually in the context of severe metabolic or systemic illness. Ileus also occurs in association with peritonitis or following spinal cord injury or pelvic fractures. Postoperative ileus tends to be self-limiting (e.g., lasting up to 3 days after laparotomy). Available evidence suggests that sympathetic inhibitory overactivity from the spinal cord, possibly in conjunction with a decrease in parasympathetic activity, may be important in its development, particularly during the acute postoperative phase.[38] Factors that may prolong postoperative ileus include electrolyte and metabolic abnormalities (especially hypokalemia), medications (such as opiates), and infections (such as peritonitis). Cur-

rently, a multimodal approach (e.g., continuous epidural analgesia with local anesthetics, early feeding, and enforced mobilization) is taken in the prevention and management of postoperative ileus.[39]

RAPID-TRANSIT DYSMOTILITIES OF THE SMALL BOWEL

Rapid transit through the small bowel is a minor component of IBS in some patients. However, it is a major component of other diseases and results in a significant loss of fluid and osmotically active solutes that overwhelm colonic capacitance and reabsorptive capacity and result in severe diarrhea. Examples include postvagotomy diarrhea, short bowel syndrome, diabetic diarrhea, and carcinoid diarrhea.[40] These disturbances of small bowel transit can best be identified by use of scintigraphy or, if scintigraphy is not available, by use of the lactulose-hydrogen breath test.

The objectives of treatment are restoration of hydration and nutrition and retardation of small bowel transit. Dietary interventions include avoidance of hyperosmolar drinks (e.g., virtually all soft drinks), use of iso-osmolar or hypo-osmolar rehydration solutions, and reduction of the fat content in the diet to around 50 g a day to avoid delivery of unabsorbed fat to the colon (where their metabolites are cathartic). Correction of nutritional deficiencies (commonly, calcium, magnesium, potassium, and water- and fat-soluble vitamins) is often required. Pharmacotherapy should be delivered in a stepwise fashion. First, an opioid agent in high dosage (e.g., loperamide, 4 mg) is given one-half hour before each meal and at bedtime to suppress the small bowel transit and colonic response to feeding. Next, verapamil (40 mg b.i.d.) or clonidine (0.1 to 0.2 mg orally or by patch) should be given, and if these are ineffective or produce unacceptable side effects (usually hypotension), subcutaneous octreotide, starting at 50 μg before meals, should be prescribed.[32] A long-acting-release octreotide (Sandostatin-LAR) that is administered intramuscularly is being evaluated as therapy for short bowel syndrome; preliminary evidence suggests that this form of therapy is effective and well tolerated.[41]

Patients with less than 1 m of residual small bowel may be unable to sustain fluid and electrolyte homeostasis without parenteral support. However, it is almost invariably possible to maintain patients with more than 1 m of residual small bowel with oral nutrition, pharmacotherapy, and supplements.

Colorectal Motility Disorders

SLOW-TRANSIT CONSTIPATION

Slow-transit constipation[42] is a motility disorder of the colon that results in prolonged transit. The diagnosis of slow-transit constipation should be made only after exclusion of mucosal diseases, such as tumors and strictures. The diagnosis is most conveniently made by assessing mean colonic transit time through use of abdominal radiography and radiopaque markers. There are two commonly used variations of this method. The first type involves ingestion of 24 radiopaque markers in a soluble medication capsule on 4 successive days; plain abdominal radiography is performed on day 5. The number of markers in the colon approximates the mean colonic transit time in hours (normal: < 72 hours). The second variation requires that the patient ingest 20 markers on day 1; an abdominal x-ray is obtained on day 5. Normally, there should be fewer than five markers remaining in the colon. In all patients with delayed colonic transit, the possibility of outlet obstruction to defecation or a pangastrointestinal motility disorder must be ruled out.

Treatment of slow-transit constipation consists of increasing dietary bulk or fiber and administering osmotic laxatives (e.g., magnesium salts when not contraindicated) and stimulant laxatives or colonic prokinetic agents. A more severe variant of slow-transit constipation is colonic inertia. In this disorder, the colon fails to produce a motor response to physiologic stimuli, such as a meal, or to pharmacologic stimulation, as would occur, for example, after administration of neostigmine, 0.5 mg I.M., or intraluminal bisacodyl, 2 to 4 mg.

MEGACOLON

Megacolon is a cecal dilatation of the colon. Motility disorders arising from dilatation of the colon may be acute (Ogilvie syndrome) or chronic. Chronic megacolon may be congenital (Hirschsprung disease) or may represent the end stage of any form of refractory constipation (e.g., slow-transit constipation or pelvic floor dysfunction).

Acute Megacolon (Ogilvie Syndrome)

In Ogilvie syndrome, colonic dilatation is attributed to a sympathetically mediated reflex response to a number of serious medical or surgical conditions in elderly patients. The initial tasks facing the clinician are to exclude mechanical obstruction (with a hypaque enema), to discontinue enabling medications, and to correct metabolic disturbances.[43] Dilatation of the cecum to a diameter of greater than 12 cm is cause for grave concern. The rectum should be decompressed with an indwelling tube and tap water enemas. Intravenous neostigmine is generally effective and safe for patients with colonic distention that is unresponsive to more conservative therapies. Endoscopic decompression is necessary for patients who do not respond to neostigmine therapy.

Chronic Megacolon

Hirschsprung disease, the congenital form of megacolon, is thought to be caused by the failure of neural crest cells to migrate completely during colonic development. The affected segment of the colon fails to relax, which results in blockage and retention of stool. Hirschsprung disease occurs in one in every 5,000 births. In the majority of patients, the disease is evident in the neonatal period and manifests in symptoms of distal intestinal obstruction such as vomiting, abdominal distension, and failure to pass stool. In patients with less severe disease, the diagnosis may not be made until childhood or adulthood. The clinical presentation usually suggests the diagnosis, which may be supported by findings on abdominal radiography, contrast enema, and anorectal manometry. The gold standard for the diagnosis of Hirschsprung disease is rectal biopsy, which can be performed safely by means of rectal mucosal suction.[44] Surgery is the mainstay of treatment. Various surgical procedures are available; the choice of technique is usually made on the basis of surgeon preference because overall complication rates and long-term results are similar. Enterocolitis is a major complication of surgical repair, affecting as many as 55% of patients.[45] Overall, mortality in patients with Hirschsprung disease is less than 10%.[46]

In chronic idiopathic megacolon, medical measures such as colonic evacuation with enemas, fiber supplementation, and laxatives may suffice. If severe motor dysfunction is confined to the colon, either a subtotal colectomy with an ileorrectal anastomosis or an ileostomy may occasionally be necessary.

FECAL INCONTINENCE

Fecal incontinence is the involuntary passage of fecal material recurring for more than 3 months in a person older than 4 years of age. A review of 16 studies estimated that the prevalence of fecal incontinence ranges from 11% to 15% among community-dwelling adults; however, these values may reflect various biases in the available studies.[47] Fecal incontinence is a common problem in the geriatric population, affecting 12% of community-dwelling adults.[48]

The most common causes of fecal incontinence are the following: (1) weakness of the anal sphincter muscles that restrain passage of a bowel movement; (2) impaired rectal sensation; (3) decreased rectal compliance, which leads to increased frequency and urgency of bowel movements because the ability of the rectum to store fecal matter is reduced; and (4) fecal impaction, which produces constant inhibition of the tone of the internal anal sphincter, permitting leakage of liquid stool around the impaction. The latter is a frequent cause of fecal incontinence in older patients.

Diagnosis

The evaluation of patients with fecal incontinence should begin with the taking of a medical history, followed by a thorough physical examination. Many patients find fecal incontinence a difficult topic to discuss, and specific questioning is often required. True incontinence must be distinguished from a sense of urgency without loss of stool—a symptom that may be associated with such disorders as IBS, pelvic irradiation, and inflammatory disease. The patient should be questioned about the onset, duration, frequency, and severity of symptoms, as well as precipitating events. It is important to determine whether there is a history of prior vaginal delivery, anorectal surgery, pelvic irradiation, diabetes, and neurologic disease, as well as whether symptoms occur in association with diarrhea. The physical examination should include inspection of the perianal area and an internal digital examination with assessment of pelvic floor descent while the patient is bearing down in simulation of a bowel movement.

The history and physical examination may suggest a possible cause of incontinence and thereby direct the choice of diagnostic tests. Sigmoidoscopy and anoscopy may be used to exclude mucosal inflammation, masses, or other pathology as the underlying cause of incontinence. Infrequently, identifying the cause of fecal incontinence requires specialized testing, including anorectal manometry to measure intraluminal pressure, anal endosonography to identify mass lesions, pudendal nerve conduction measurement to diagnose neuropathy, or defecography to define intrinsic lesions.

Treatment

The treatment of fecal incontinence involves three approaches: medical therapy, biofeedback, and surgery. Medical therapy is aimed at reducing stool frequency and improving stool consistency. Limited evidence indicates that antidiarrheal agents (e.g., loperamide and diphenoxylate) and drugs that enhance anal sphincter tone (e.g., valproate sodium) reduce fecal incontinence in patients with watery stool.[49] Stimulant laxatives (e.g., senna and bisacodyl), hyperosmolar laxatives (e.g., sorbitol and lactulose), rectal suppositories (e.g., glycerin and bisacodyl), or enemas (e.g., tap water) are often sufficient to treat constipation. Biofeedback therapy, a noninvasive means of cognitively retraining the pelvic floor and the abdominal wall musculature, is

used to treat fecal incontinence[50]; the American College of Gastroenterology recommends its use in patients with weak sphincter muscles and impaired rectal sensation.[51] Surgery should be considered in patients whose condition does not respond to medical therapy. A number of surgical approaches have been used to treat fecal incontinence, including sphincter repair, implantation of an artificial sphincter, and muscle transfer procedures with or without electrical stimulation. Stoma formation should be reserved for patients who do not respond to any other form of therapy.[52]

Functional Gastrointestinal Disorders

Functional GI disorders share common pathogenetic features, including abnormal motility and heightened visceral sensation. The abnormal motility may be characterized by rapid or slow transit of food or residue through the bowel or abnormal gastric relaxation to accommodate the meal. Abnormal contractile patterns have been described, but more importantly, patients perceive a sensation of excessive gut contractions. In some patients, these syndromes are preceded by an episode of gastroenteritis. In some patients with these conditions, frequently there is evidence of psychological comorbidity, such as anxiety, depression, or both; these symptoms appear to influence the decision of patients to consult their physicians.

FUNCTIONAL DYSPEPSIA

Dyspepsia is characterized by upper abdominal symptoms that occur primarily during the postprandial period; they include nausea, vomiting, pain, bloating, anorexia, and early satiety. Dyspepsia that is not caused by ulcers, obstruction, or cancer is referred to as nonulcer or functional dyspepsia. It affects about 20% of the population of the United States.

An international committee of clinical investigators defined functional dyspepsia (Rome III criteria) as (1) the presence of one or more of four features (i.e., bothersome postprandial fullness, early satiation, epigastric pain, and epigastric burning) for the previous 3 months, with onset of symptoms at least 6 months before diagnosis; and (2) an absence of evidence of structural disease to explain the symptoms.[53]

Pathogenesis

Three main identified factors contribute to the pathophysiologic alterations present in functional dyspepsia: altered gastric emptying, increased gastric sensitivity, and impaired accommodation.[54,55] The pathogenesis in many patients remains unclear. The role that Helicobacter pylori infection plays in dyspepsia is uncertain; current epidemiologic evidence and the results of eradication studies provide insufficient evidence to support a causal relationship.[56,57] A subgroup of patients may suffer nonerosive reflux esophagitis.

Diagnosis

History and physical examination The history usually provides information on the specific symptoms or the spectrum of symptoms experienced by the patient. However, the symptoms appear to have little discriminative value for predicting the physiologic alterations in an individual patient. The symptoms that appear to be most closely related to impaired gastric relaxation or accommodation are early satiety and weight loss.[54] Studies have suggested that the presence of postprandial fullness may be indicative of delayed gastric emptying[54,55]; however, an-

other study found only a weak correlation.[58] Early satiety occurring soon after starting a meal has been associated with reduced gastric accommodation.[54,55] Weight loss of more than 5 kg is more frequent in patients with reduced gastric accommodation than in those with delayed gastric emptying.[54]

The presence of heartburn suggests a component of gastroesophageal reflux.[59] Regurgitation from reflux needs to be differentiated from rumination,[60] which results in the effortless regurgitation of undigested food within 30 minutes after oral ingestion; rumination occurs with virtually every meal and is not associated with nausea.

The physical examination is usually normal. On rare occasions, there may be a succussion splash in the epigastrium from the retention of food in the stomach. An epigastric mass, hepatomegaly, or supraclavicular lymphadenopathy may suggest that the dyspepsia is the result of malignancy. In the presence of alarm features such as dysphagia, bleeding, or weight loss in association with dyspepsia, it is essential to exclude mucosal diseases, such as ulcer or cancer. Cancer may still be present, however, even when these alarm features are absent. Patients are reassured by a negative endoscopic examination.

Laboratory tests In most cases, the underlying cause of dyspepsia will not be obvious from the history and physical examination. For new-onset dyspepsia, endoscopy and testing for H. pylori infection are generally recommended.

Simple, cost-effective tests for mucosal disease, abnormal gastric emptying,[61,62] and impaired gastric accommodation[55,62] provide a rational alternative to the use of sequential empirical trials for identifying the mechanism causing dyspepsia.

There is great interest in identifying ways to demonstrate gastric hypersensitivity before therapy is initiated, because such knowledge would have a bearing on choice of therapy. Tests in which the patient drinks water or a nutrient beverage have been devised to evaluate the maximal tolerated volume and the symptoms of fullness, satiety, bloating, nausea, and pain at a defined period after ingestion (typically 30 minutes).[54,63,64] These tests are noninvasive and inexpensive, and they have been introduced into clinical practice in some centers. However, they do not necessarily differentiate disturbances in the accommodation response from hypersensitivity per se. Until recently, measurement of accommodation required the placement of an intragastric balloon to measure fasting and postprandial volumes[54]; however, gastric accommodation can now be measured noninvasively by means of single-photon emission computed tomography.[55,65]

Treatment

In clinical practice, dyspepsia is often treated with acid-suppressing regimens consisting of proton pump inhibitors or H_2 receptor antagonists; however, the relative efficacy of these drugs remains uncertain.[66] Temporary acid suppression with a proton pump inhibitor or an H_2 receptor agonist may delay diagnosis of cancer.[67]

In cases of dyspepsia associated with H. pylori infection, eradication of the H. pylori infection results in resolution of the syndrome in only a small number of patients (1 in 5 or fewer)[68]; the general consensus is that in the absence of erosions or ulcers, attempted eradication of H. pylori is not indicated for the treatment of dyspepsia, though H. pylori infection is usually attempted anyway because of concern with the development of gastric atrophy or even gastric cancer in the long term.[69]

IRRITABLE BOWEL SYNDROME

IBS is the most commonly diagnosed functional disorder of the GI tract. IBS affects 10% to 15% of the population of the United States, and patients with this disorder account for up to 25% of visits to gastroenterologists.[1,70,71] As generally defined, IBS is characterized by chronic or recurrent abdominal pain associated with altered bowel function (i.e., constipation, diarrhea, or alternating constipation and diarrhea). The diagnosis of IBS is made on the basis of characteristic history, an absence of significant physical findings, an absence of abnormalities on standard laboratory tests, and normal gross and histologic findings on flexible sigmoidoscopy or colonoscopy. The Rome III criteria define IBS as the presence of two or more of the following symptoms occurring for at least 12 weeks in the preceding 12 months: (1) abdominal pain or discomfort that is relieved with defecation; (2) the onset of abdominal pain associated with a change in the frequency of bowel movements; and (3) the onset of pain associated with a change in form (appearance) of stool.[72]

Although classically, motility abnormalities are considered a disorder of the colon, such disorders can also be detected in the small intestine in a majority of patients with IBS. Motor abnormalities in the alimentary tract have been reported in IBS, including altered myoelectric activity and prolonged irregular small bowel and colonic contractions; these abnormalities include duodenal and jejunal clustering, ileal high-pressure waves, and a disturbed postprandial motor response. Abnormal visceral perception, as detected by a lower pain threshold in response to bowel distension, may also represent one of the key physiologic disturbances.

Constipation in patients with IBS may respond to treatment with fiber or simple laxatives, including osmotic agents.[73,74] Serotoninergic agents that activate the 5-HT$_4$ receptor may be approved for the treatment of constipation-predominant IBS. Tegaserod, the first of this class of drugs, appears to be modestly effective in women with constipation-predominant IBS.[75,76] The 5-HT$_3$ antagonist alosetron was found to provide adequate relief of pain, improved stool frequency, decreased urgency, and consistency for many patients whose predominant bowel disturbance was diarrhea.[77] Alosetron was withdrawn from the market because of side effects (e.g., severe constipation and ischemic colitis), but it was reintroduced; the FDA has approved it for the treatment of women with severe diarrhea-predominant IBS whose condition failed to respond to conventional treatment.

IBS patients also tend to use complementary and alternative medicine more frequently than patients with organic bowel diseases.[78] Physicians should be aware of this, both with regard to the potential for adverse interactions and as an indication of emotional unease in these patients.

FUNCTIONAL CONSTIPATION

The Rome criteria III define functional constipation as the presence of two or more of the following symptoms occurring for at least 12 weeks in the preceding 12 months: (1) straining during at least 25% of defecations; (2) lumpy or hard stool in at least 25% of defecations; (3) a sensation of incomplete evacuation in at least 25% of defecations; (4) a sensation of anorectal obstruction or blockage in at least 25% of defecations; (5) manual maneuvers to facilitate defecation used in at least 25% of defecations; and (6) fewer than three bowel movements in a week.[42] The Rome III guidelines also stipulate two additional conditions for the diagnosis of functional constipations, namely: (1) that loose stools are rarely present without the use of laxatives and (2)

that there is insufficient evidence to support a diagnosis of IBS.[42]

Increasing dietary fiber and decreasing dietary fat, as well as the use of biofeedback and medication aimed at symptom relief, may be helpful in the treatment of functional constipation.[42,79] Tegaserod has been approved by the FDA for the treatment of functional constipation; in one randomized trial, 43% of patients taking tegaserod (6 mg twice daily) responded to therapy, compared with 25% of patients taking placebo.[80] Recently, lubiprostone was approved for the treatment of chronic idiopathic constipation. Lubiprostone is a chloride channel opener; its use leads to increased fluid secretion into the small intestine, which in turn leads to an increase in GI transit.

FUNCTIONAL DIARRHEA

The Rome III criteria classify functional diarrhea separately from IBS. The Rome III criteria define functional diarrhea as the presence of loose or watery stool in at least 75% of episodes of stool passage for at least 12 weeks in the preceding 6 months.[42] However, the diagnosis depends upon the evaluation of other potential causes; for this reason, the definition is somewhat limited in guiding clinical evaluation. The appropriate evaluation and treatment of these patients have not been appropriately delineated. Diagnostic measures often include evaluation of the stool for infectious causes and for the presence of fat, which would suggest malabsorption. Blood studies can now screen for celiac sprue and for inflammatory bowel disease. Rectal biopsies are performed during flexible sigmoidoscopy or colonoscopy to evaluate for microscopic colitis.

OUTLET OBSTRUCTION TO DEFECATION

Outlet obstruction to defecation (evacuation disorders) occurs when the patient has difficulty expelling a stool as a result of poorly functioning defecation dynamics.[81]

Diagnosis

The patient may present with constipation or the inability to have spontaneous and complete bowel movements, as well as left-sided abdominal pain. A careful clinical history is useful in identifying failure of evacuation; specifically, patients may experience the need for digital disimpaction of the rectum or digital pressure on the posterior wall of the vagina or the perineum to expel stool. Enemas may not be emptied. The rectal examination identifies an immobile perineum during the process of straining and a tight, unyielding puborectalis sling muscle abutting the rectum posteriorly. This tight pelvic floor persists during attempts to evacuate. In rare instances, the anal sphincter itself is spastic or the entire perineum balloons or herniates down as a result of years of straining or of multiple childbirths, which weaken the ligaments and muscles that normally support the pelvic floor and rectoanal angle.

Treatment

Occasionally, outlet obstruction is caused by an anatomic defect such as a rectocele or rectal internal mucosal prolapse; these are amenable to surgical correction. A spastic pelvic floor or spastic anal sphincter muscles usually respond to biofeedback and muscle relaxation exercises.[82] Some patients with outlet obstruction to defecation have a profound psychological disorder or a history of abuse that requires identification and subsequent therapy.[81]

The author has no commercial relationships with manufacturers of products or providers of services discussed in this chapter.

References

1. Evidence-based position on the management of irritable bowel syndrome in North America. Am J Gastroenterol 97(11 suppl):S1, 2002

2. Soykan I, Sivri B, Sarosiek I, et al: Demography, clinical characteristics, psychological profiles, treatment and long-term follow-up of patients with gastroparesis. Dig Dis Sci 43:2398, 1998

3. Parkman HP, Hasler WL, Fisher RS: American Gastroenterological Association medical position statement: diagnosis and treatment of gastroparesis. Gastroenterology 127:1589, 2004

4. Parkman HP, Hasler WL, Fisher RS: American Gastroenterological Association technical review on the diagnosis and treatment of gastroparesis. Gastroenterology 127:1592, 2004

5. Horowitz M, O'Donovan D, Jones KL, et al: Gastric emptying in diabetes: clinical significance and treatment. Diabet Med 19:177, 2002

6. Frank JW, Saslow SB, Camilleri M, et al: Mechanism of accelerated gastric emptying of liquids and hyperglycemia in patients with type II diabetes mellitus. Gastroenterology 109:755, 1995

7. Gonlachanvit S, Hsu CW, Boden GH, et al: Effect of altering gastric emptying on postprandial plasma glucose concentrations following a physiologic meal in type-2 diabetic patients. Dig Dis Sci 48:488, 2003

8. Rayner CK, Samson M, Jones KL, et al: Relationships of upper gastrointestinal motor and sensory function with glycemic control. Diabetes Care 24:371, 2001

9. Schwartz JG, Green GM, Guan D, et al: Rapid gastric emptying of a solid pancake meal in type 2 diabetic patients. Diabetes Care 19:468, 1996

10. Eagon JC, Miedema BW, Kelly KA: Postgastrectomy syndromes. Surg Clin North Am 72:445, 1992

11. Stanghellini V, Tosetti C, Horowitz M, et al: Predictors of gastroparesis in out-patients with secondary and idiopathic upper gastrointestinal symptoms. Dig Liver Dis 35:389, 2003

12. Zarate N, Mearin F, Wang XY, et al: Severe idiopathic gastroparesis due to neuronal and interstitial cells of Cajal degeneration: pathological findings and management. Dig Dis Sci 52:966, 2003

13. Bityutskiy LP, Soykan I, McCallum RW: Viral gastroparesis: a subgroup of idiopathic gastroparesis: clinical characteristics and long-term outcomes. Am J Gastroenterol 92:1501, 1997

14. Lee KJ, Kindt S, Tack J: Pathophysiology of functional dyspepsia. Best Pract Res Clin Gastroenterol 18:707, 2004

15. Viramontes BE, Kim DY, Camilleri M, et al: Validation of a stable isotope gastric emptying test for normal accelerated or delayed gastric emptying. Neurogastroenterol Motil 12:567, 2001

16. Thomforde GM, Camilleri M, Phillips SF, et al: Evaluation of an inexpensive screening scintigraphic test of gastric emptying. J Nucl Med 36:93, 1995

17. Minocha A, Johnson WD, Abell TL, et al: Prevalence, sociodemography, and quality of life of older versus younger patients with irritable bowel syndrome: a population-based study. Dig Dis Sci 51:446, 2006

18. Perkel MS, Hersh T, Moore C, et al: Metoclopramide therapy in fifty-five patients with delayed gastric emptying. Am J Gastroenterol 74:231, 1980

19. Snape WJ Jr, Battle WM, Schwartz SS, et al: Metoclopramide to treat gastroparesis due to diabetes mellitus: a double-blind, controlled trial. Ann Intern Med 96:444, 1999

20. Magnanti K, Onyemere K, Jones MP: Oral erythromycin and symptomatic relief of gastroparesis: a systematic review. Am J Gastroenterol 98:259, 2003

21. Braden B, Enghofer M, Schaub M, et al: Long-term cisapride treatment improves diabetic gastroparesis but not glycaemic control. Aliment Pharmacol Ther 16:1341, 2002

22. Patterson D, Abell T, Rothstein R, et al: A double-blind multicenter comparison of domperidone and metoclopramide in the treatment of diabetic patients with symptoms of gastroparesis. Am J Gastroenterol 94:1230, 1999

23. Degen L, Petrig C, Studer D, et al: Effect of tegaserod on gut transit in male and female subjects. Neurogastroenterol Motil 17:821, 2005

24. Prather CM, Camilleri M, Zinsmeister AR, et al: Tegaserod accelerates transit in patients with constipation-predominant irritable bowel syndrome. Gastroenterology 118:463, 2000

25. Tougas G, Ghen Y, Luo D, et al: Tegaserod improves gastric emptying in patients with gastroparesis and dyspeptic symptoms (abstr). Gastroenterology 124:A20, 2002

26. Miller LS, Szych GA, Kantor SB, et al: Treatment of idiopathic gastroparesis with injection of botulinum toxin into the pyloric sphincter muscle. Am J Gastroenterol 97:1653, 2002

27. Lacy BE, Zayat EN, Crowell MD, et al: Botulinum toxin for the treatment of gastroparesis: a preliminary report. Am J Gastroenterol 97:1548, 2002

28. Abel T, McCallum R, Hocking M, et al: Gastric electrical stimulation for medically refractory gastroparesis. Gastroenterology 125:421, 2003

29. Jones MP, Maganti K: A systematic review of surgical therapy for gastroparesis. Am J Gastroenterol 98:2122, 2003

30. Hasler WL: Dumping syndrome Curr Treat Options Gastroenterol 5:139, 2002

31. Mariani G, Boni G, Barreca M, et al: Radionuclide gastroesophageal motor studies. J Nucl Med 45:1004, 2004

32. Vecht J, Lamers CB, Masclee AA: Long-term results of octreotide-therapy in severe dumping syndrome. Clin Endocrinal (Oxf) 51:619, 1999

33. Penning C, Vecht J, Masclee AA: Efficacy of depot long-acting release octreotide therapy in severe dumping syndrome. Alimnet Pharmacol Ther 22:963, 2005

34. Stanghellini V, Cogliandro RF, De Giorgio R, et al: Natural history of chronic idiopathic intestinal pseudo-obstruction in adults: a single center study. Clin Gastroenterol Hepatol 3:449, 2005

35. Verne GN, Sninsky CA: Cronic intestinal pseudo-obstruction. Dig Dis 13:163, 1995

36. Stanghellini V, Cogliandro R, Cogliandro L, et al: Clinical use of manometry for the diagnosis of intestinal motor abnormalities. Dig Liver Dis 32:532, 2000

37. Van Citters GW, Lin HC: Management of small intestinal bacterial overgrowth. Curr Gastroenterol Rep 7:317, 2005

38. Bauer AJ, Boeckxstaens GE: Mechanisms of postoperative ileus. Neurogastroenterol Motil 16(suppl 2):54, 2004

39. Holte K, Kehlet H: Prevention of postoperative ileus. Minerva Anestesiol 68:152, 2002

40. von der Ohe MR, Camilleri M, Kvols LK, et al: Motor dysfunction of the small bowel and colon in patients with the carcinoid syndrome and diarrhea. N Engl J Med 329:1073, 1993

41. Nehra V, Camilleri M, Burton D, et al: An open trial of octreotide long-acting release in the management of short bowel syndrome. Am J Gastroenterol 96:1494, 2001

42. Longstreth GF, Thompson WG, Chey WD, et al: Functional bowel disorder. Gastroenterology 130:1480, 2006

43. Fazel A, Verne GN: New solutions to an old problem: acute colonic pseudo-obstruction. J Clin Gastroenterol 39:17, 2005

44. Pini-Prato A, Martucciello G, Jasonni V: Rectal suction biopsy in the diagnosis of intestinal dysganglionoses: 5-year experience with Solo-RBT in 389 patients. J Pediatr Surg 41:1043, 2006

45. Wildhaber BE, Teitelbaum DH, Coran AG: Total colonic Hirschsprung's disease: a 28-year experience. J Pediatr Surg 40:203, 2005

46. Suita S, Taguchi T, Ieriri S, et al: Hirschsprung's disease in Japan: analysis of 3852 patients based on a nationwide survey in 30 years. J Pediatr Surg 40:197, 2005

47. Macmillan AK, Merrie AE, Marshall RJ, et al: The prevalence of fecal incontinence in community-dwelling adults: a systematic review of the literature. Dis Colon Rectum 47:1341, 2004

48. Goode PS, Burgio KL, Halli AD, et al: Prevalence of fecal incontinence in community-dwelling older adults. 53:629, 2005

49. Cheetham M, Brazzelli M, Norton C, et al: Drug treatment for faecal incontinence in adults. Cochrane Database Syst Rev (3):CD002116, 2003

50. Terra MP, Dobben AC, Berghmans B, et al: Electrical stimulation and pelvic floor muscle training with biofeedback in patients with fecal incontinence: a cohort study of 281 patients. Dis Colon Rectum June 15 (Epub ahead of print) 2006

51. Rao SS: Diagnosis and management of fecal incontinence. American College of Gastroenterology Practice Parameters Committee. Am J Gastroenterol 99:1585, 2004 http://www.acg.gi/physicians/guidelines/FecalIncontinence.pdf

52. Maslekar S, Gardiner A, Maklin C, et al: Investigation and treatment of faecal incontinence. Postgrad Med J 82:363, 200653. Tack J, Talley NJ, Camilleri M, et al: Functional gastroduodenal disorders. Gastroenterology 130:1466, 2006

53. Tack J, Talley NJ, Camilleri M, et al: Functional gastroduodenal disorders. Gastroenterology 130:1466, 2006

54. Tack J, Piessevaux H, Coulie B, et al: Role of impaired gastric accommodation to a meal in functional dyspepsia. Gastroenterology 115:1346, 1998

55. Kim DY, Delgado-Aros S, Camilleri M, et al: Noninvasive measurement of gastric accommodation in patients with idiopathic nonulcer dyspepsia. Am J Gastroenterol 96:3099, 2001

56. Danesh J, Lawrence M, Murphy M, et al: Systematic review of the epidemiological evidence on *Helicobacter pylori* infection and nonulcer or uninvestigated dyspepsia. Arch Intern Med 160:1192, 2000

57. Laine L, Schoenfeld P, Fennerty MB: Therapy for *Helicobacter pylori* in patients with nonulcer dyspepsia: a meta-analysis of randomized, controlled trials. Ann Intern Med 134:361, 2001

58. Talley NJ, Locke GR, Lahr B, et al: Functional dyspepsia, delayed gastric emptying and impaired quality of life. Gut 1, 2005 [epub ahead of print]

59. Moayyedi P, Talley NJ, Fennerty MB, et al: Can the clinical history distinguish between organic and functional dyspepsia? JAMA 295:566, 2006

60. Olden KW: Rumination. Curr Treat Options Gastroenterol 4:351, 2001

61. Viramontes BE, Kim DY, Camilleri M, et al: Validation of a stable isotope gastric emptying test for normal, accelerated or delayed gastric emptying. Neurogastroenterol Motil 13:567, 2001

62. Simonian HP, Maurer AH, Knight LC, et al: Simultaneous assessment of gastric accommodation and emptying: studies with liquid and solid meals. J Nucl Med 45:1155, 2004

63. Boeckxstaens GE, Hirsch DP, van den Elzen BD, et al: Impaired drinking capacity in patients with functional dyspepsia: relationship with proximal stomach function. Gastroenterology 121:1054, 2001

64. Chial HJ, Camilleri C, Delgado-Aros S, et al: A nutrient drink test to assess maximum tolerated volume and postprandial symptoms: effects of gender, body mass index and age in health. Neurogastroenterol Motil 14:249, 2002

65. Bredenoord AF, Chial HJ, Camilleri M, et al: Gastric accommodation and emptying in evaluation of patients with upper gastrointestinal symptoms. Clin Gastroenterol Hepatol 1:224, 2003

66. Delaney BC, Ford AC, Forman D, et al: Initial management strategies for dyspepsia. Cochrane Database Syst Rev (4):CD001961, 2005

67. Bramble MG, Suvakovic Z, Hungin AS: Detection of upper gastrointestinal cancer in patients taking antisecretory therapy prior to gastroscopy. Gut 46:464, 2000

68. Moayyedi P, Soo S, Deeks J, et al: Eradication of *Helicobacter pylori* for non-ulcer dyspepsia. Cochrane Database Syst Rev (1):CD002096, 2005

69. Uemura N, Okamoto S, Yamamoto S, et al: *Helicobacter pylori* infection and the de-

velopment of gastric cancer. N Engl J Med 345:784, 2001

70. Saito YA, Locke GR, Talley NJ, et al: A comparison of the Rome and Manning criteria for case identification in epidemiological investigations of irritable bowel syndrome. Am J Gastroenterol 95:2816, 2000

71. Minocha A, Johnson WD, Abell TL, et al: Prevalence, sociodemography, and quality of life of older versus younger patients with irritable bowel syndrome: a population-based study. Dig Dis Sci 51:446, 2006

72. Longstreth GF, Thompson WG, Chey WD, et al: Functional bowel disorders. Gastroenterology 130:1480, 2006

73. Tramonte SM, Brand MB, Mulrow CD, et al: The treatment of chronic constipation in adults: a systematic review. J Gen Intern Med 12:15, 1997

74. Boyce PM, Talley NJ, Balaam B, et al: A randomized controlled trial of cognitive behavior therapy, relaxation training, and routine clinical care for the irritable bowel syndrome. Am J Gastroenterol 98:2209, 2003

75. Müller-Lissner SA, Fumagalli I, Bardhan KD, et al: Tegaserod, a 5-HT4 receptor partial agonist, relieves symptoms in irritable bowel syndrome patients with abdominal pain, bloating and constipation. Aliment Pharmacol Ther 15:1655, 2001

76. Evans BW, Clark WK, Moore DJ, et al: Tegaserod for the treatment of irritable bowel syndrome. Cochrane Database Syst Rev (1):CD003960, 2004

77. Camilleri M, Northcutt AR, Kong S, et al: Efficacy and safety of alosetron in women with irritable bowel syndrome: a randomised, placebo-controlled trial. Lancet 355:1035, 2000

78. Langmead L, Chitnis M, Rampton DS: Use of complementary therapies by patients with IBD may indicate psychological distress. Inflamm Bowel Dis 8:174, 2002

79. Heyman S, Jones KR, Scarlett Y, et al: Biofeedback treatment of constipation: a critical review. Dis Colon Rectum 46:1208, 2003

80. Johanson JF, Wald A, Tougas G, et al: Effect of tegaserod in chronic constipation: a randomized, double-blind, controlled trial. Clin Gastroenterol Hepatol 2:796, 2004

81. Camilleri M, Thompson WG, Fleshman JW, et al: Clinical management of intractable constipation. Ann Intern Med 121:520, 1994

82. Battaglia E, Serra AM, Buonafede G, et al: Long-term study on the effects of visual biofeedback and muscle training as a therapeutic modality in pelvic floor dyssynergia and slow-transit constipation. Dis Colon Rectum 47:90, 2004

Acknowledgment

The author and editors gratefully acknowledge the contributions of the previous author, Michael Camilleri, M.D., to the development and writing of this chapter.

68 Gastrointestinal Bleeding

Elizabeth Rajan, M.D., and David A. Ahlquist, M.D.

Gastrointestinal (GI) bleeding occurs commonly, has many causes, and ranges from trivial to torrential and life-threatening in severity. Practical classification of GI bleeding—based on the presentation, site, and mechanism of the bleed—aids the clinician in selecting an appropriate management algorithm.

GI bleeding is defined as overt when visible red or altered blood is noted in emesis or feces. Overt bleeding is considered major when accompanied by hemodynamic instability and considered minor when not. Occult bleeding is visibly inapparent but is detected directly by stool testing or suggested indirectly by iron deficiency anemia.

GI bleeding occurs when a pathologic process such as ulceration, inflammation, or neoplasia causes erosion of a blood vessel. The size of the eroded artery is an important determinant of the rate of bleeding, the risk of rebleeding, and the clinical outcome. Blood flow and, thus, rate of blood loss vary directly with the diameter of the vessel; small changes in vessel diameter have dramatic effects on bleeding rates. Most GI bleeds result from erosion into small vessels and are trivial and self-limited. Erosion of larger vessels can produce lesions that exceed the capacity of normal hemostasis and result in overt major bleeding. A study of the external diameter of arteries in gastric ulcers that bled recurrently showed a range of 0.1 to 1.8 mm, with a mean of 0.7 mm.[1] Deep, large ulcers are more likely to erode into large blood vessels. Recurrent or persistent bleeding may result from inadequate vasoconstriction because of large vessel size or inflammatory necrosis of the vessel wall, from pseudoaneurysm formation at the bleeding site, or from systemic coagulopathies.

Overt Bleeding

EPIDEMIOLOGY

The reported incidence of GI bleeding varies widely, in part because of varying definitions. Overt minor bleeding, such as from anorectal hemorrhoids, is exceedingly common. Most major bleeding arises from upper GI lesions, and the estimated annual incidence ranges from 40 to 150 episodes per 100,000 population.[2,3] Mortality from upper GI bleeding has remained at 8% to 10% over the past 50 years.[4,5] The fact that, over this period, mortality has failed to decrease substantially despite advances in patient care and technology may reflect the increasing number of elderly patients with complicated comorbidities. Cases in individuals older than 60 years account for 35% to 45% of all cases of acute upper GI bleeding but nearly all of the associated mortality.[6] Lower GI sources account for an estimated 15% to 20% of all major GI bleeds. The incidence of lower GI bleeds increases with age.[7,8]

ETIOLOGY

The causes of GI bleeding are protean [*see Table 1*]. The most common etiologies are briefly elaborated in this subsection.

Upper GI Bleeding

Upper GI bleeding is arbitrarily defined as hemorrhage from a source proximal to the ligament of Treitz (i.e., the esophagus, stomach, or duodenum). Hematemesis essentially always reflects upper GI bleeding, and stools may range from black (melena) to bright red (hematochezia), depending on rates of bleeding and intestinal transit.

Peptic ulcer disease (PUD)   The most common cause of upper GI bleeding is PUD, accounting for 60% of cases found at emergency endoscopy.[9] About 50% of cases have a clean-based ulcer with a low probability of rebleeding, so that only pharmacologic intervention is required.[10] Adherent clots, visible vessels, or active bleeding [*see Figure 1*] portend progressively less favorable outcomes unless endoscopic or surgical treatment is applied. Although nonsteroidal anti-inflammatory drug (NSAID) use and *Helicobacter pylori* infection are the two most important risk factors for bleeding in PUD, heavy alcohol ingestion and smoking are also associated with increased risk.[11-13]

Drugs   Aspirin and other NSAIDs are responsible for most drug-induced GI bleeding. In the United States, more than 30 billion NSAID tablets are consumed annually. Except for sodium salicylate, all NSAIDs can cause bleeding. Acetaminophen is not associated with GI bleeding.

The elderly are especially susceptible to NSAID-induced GI bleeding.[14] NSAIDs may cause bleeding at any level of the GI tract, but they most commonly do so in the stomach or duodenum. Although the bleeding risk increases in proportion to NSAID dose, any amount (including low-dose aspirin taken for

---

Table 1   Major Causes of
Gastrointestinal Bleeding

Inflammatory
  Peptic ulcer disease
  Esophagitis or esophageal ulceration
  Diaphragmatic hernia (Cameron erosions)
  Diverticular disease
  Inflammatory bowel disease
  Meckel diverticulum

Cancers and neoplasms
  Primary lesion at any site
  Metastatic deposits at any site
  Large polyps
  Gastrointestinal stromal tumors

Vascular anomalies
  Gastroesophageal varices
  Angiodysplasia
  Dieulafoy lesion
  Watermelon stomach
  Radiation proctopathy

Drugs
  Aspirin
  Nonsteroidal anti-inflammatory drugs

Miscellaneous
  Postpolypectomy
  Mallory-Weiss tear

cardiovascular prophylaxis) may cause bleeding. Use of selective serotonin reuptake inhibitors (SSRIs) has recently been found to be associated with a higher risk of upper GI bleeding, especially in patients who are also taking NSAIDs or low-dose aspirin.[15] Anticoagulants do not cause GI bleeding per se, but they can unmask or aggravate hemorrhage from preexisting lesions.

Variceal bleeding   Gastroesophageal variceal bleeding accounts for 10% to 30% of all upper GI hemorrhage. Patients present with overt major bleeding that is sudden in onset. Variceal bleeding is distinctive, with large-volume hematemesis of bright-red blood or clots and associated severe hemodynamic instability [*see Figure 2*]. Because of the cathartic nature of blood, patients may also present with hematochezia. A prospective review found that the distribution of bleeding varices was 75% esophageal and 25% gastric.[16] The most common site of bleeding is the distal 5 cm of the esophagus, because of relatively greater variceal distention and thinner supporting tissue surrounding the veins in this region, compared with the upper and the middle esophagus. Varices are present in 40% to 60% of patients with cirrhosis, and hemorrhage occurs in 25% to 35% of them.[17-19] Approximately one third of first variceal bleeds are fatal.[19] Physicians should bear in mind that up to half of patients with portal hypertension bleed from a nonvariceal cause.[16]

Mallory-Weiss tear   Mallory-Weiss tear is a longitudinal mucosal laceration at the gastroesophageal junction or gastric cardia caused by forceful retching or vomiting. Most tears occur within 2 cm of the gastroesophageal junction on the lesser curvature aspect of the cardia. Mallory-Weiss tears account for 5% to 11% of all major upper GI hemorrhages.[20] Most patients present with hematemesis, often associated with alcohol use. Typically, overt bleeding is minor and bleeding ceases spontaneously. Mallory-Weiss tears can also occur with upper GI endoscopy when a patient struggles or retches during the procedure.

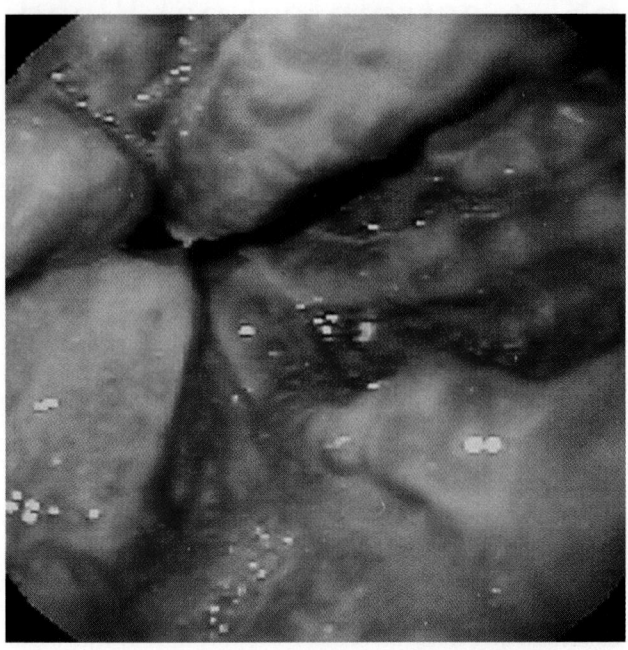

Figure 2   **High-risk esophageal varices with red wale marking.**

Dieulafoy lesions   Dieulafoy lesions account for approximately 5% of cases of major upper GI bleeding.[21] Their characteristic feature is the presence of a large-caliber, tortuous artery in the submucosa close to the mucosal surface, which bleeds upon erosion of the overlying mucosa and artery wall [*see Figure 3*]. They can be extremely difficult to detect endoscopically unless actively bleeding. Dieulafoy lesions are usually single lesions located in the proximal stomach. However, these lesions can occur anywhere throughout the GI tract. A review of 90 Dieulafoy lesions identified 34% of lesions as extragastric.[22]

Lower GI Bleeding

Diverticulosis   Diverticular disease is one of the most common causes of lower GI bleeding, particularly in the elderly. Diverticulosis is uncommon in persons younger than 40 years, but it affects roughly two thirds of persons older than 80 years.[23,24] The mean age period for diverticular hemorrhage is the sixth decade of life. The true incidence of diverticular bleeding is difficult to ascertain, given the different definitions and evaluations used in various studies. Bleeding occurs from an arteriole at either the dome or neck of a diverticulum. Typically, there is no associated diverticulitis. Diverticula are most commonly found in the left colon, but many bleeds arise from diverticula in the right colon. Patients typically present with painless, large-volume hematochezia. Because diverticular bleeding tends to stop spontaneously, the diagnosis is often presumptive and based on exclusion of other sources of bleeding in a patient with diverticulosis.[25]

Angiodysplasia   Angiodysplasia is an acquired vascular ectasia that is considered to be degenerative in origin, given its propensity to occur in the elderly. Typically, patients present between 60 and 80 years of age. The pathogenesis of angiodysplasia remains unclear, but a proposed cause is chronic, intermittent, low-grade obstruction of submucosal veins, leading to dilatation of mucosal capillaries [*see Figure 4*]. The lesions of angiodysplasia are usually small (2 to 5 mm in diameter) and can be single or multiple. These lesions can occur anywhere

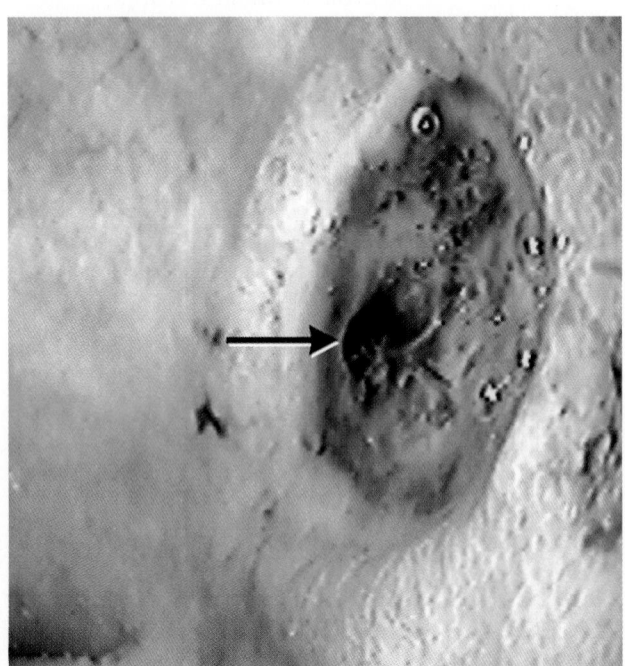

Figure 1   **High-risk posterior duodenal bulb ulcer with nonbleeding visible vessel (arrow).**

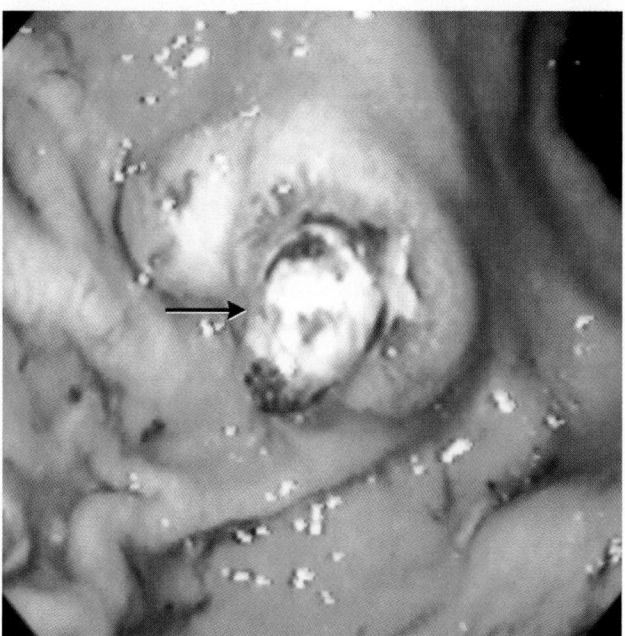

Figure 3 Dieulafoy lesion in gastric fundus (arrow).

along the GI tract but are most commonly found in the proximal colon (approximately 80%), particularly the cecum.[26] Angiodysplasia is an incidental finding at colonoscopy in 2% of nonbleeding patients older than 65 years.[27,28] Fewer than 10% of patients with angiodysplasia will bleed.[27] Bleeding stops spontaneously in the majority of patients, but rebleeding is common.

Polypectomy Colonoscopic polypectomy is generally considered a safe procedure, but hemorrhage is reported to occur in 0.3% to 6.0% of cases.[29] A retrospective study of 83 patients and 274 polypectomy sites found that bleeding occurred at a median

of 5 days (range, 0 to 17 days) after the procedure.[30] Bleeding was associated with advanced age, polyps greater than 1 cm in diameter, sessile polyps, and polyps in the cecum. The prognosis for these patients is favorable. Most cases are managed with observation or endoscopic hemostasis.

Diagnosis

EMERGENT EVALUATION AND MANAGEMENT

Management of GI bleeding is determined by the severity of the bleed; algorithms differ with major bleeding [*see Figure 5*] and minor bleeding [*see Figure 6*]. Patients with overt major bleeding require immediate hospitalization with intensive monitoring. Patients are initially stabilized with fluid and blood component replacement and with correction of any coagulopathy or electrolyte imbalances. Endotracheal intubation may be necessary. Stabilization is followed by immediate endoscopic evaluation and therapy as indicated. If hemorrhage control is ineffective and the patient continues to be hemodynamically unstable, radiologic or surgical interventions are considered.

CLINICAL AND LABORATORY ASSESSMENT

The history and physical examination provide vital information on the location, severity, and duration of bleeding and can help identify patients at increased risk of exsanguination and rebleeding [*see Table 2*]. It is important to remember that patients with overt major bleeding from an upper GI source can present

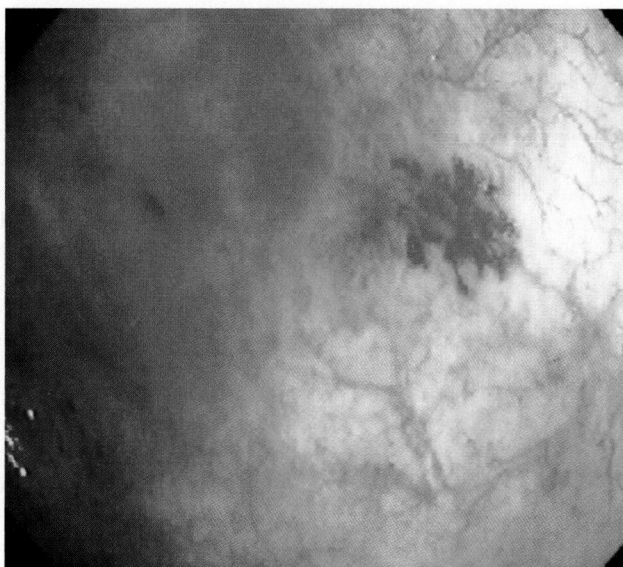

Figure 4 The lesions of angiodysplasia are usually small (2 to 5 mm in diameter) and can be single or multiple. These lesions can occur anywhere along the GI tract but are most commonly found in the proximal colon, particularly the cecum.

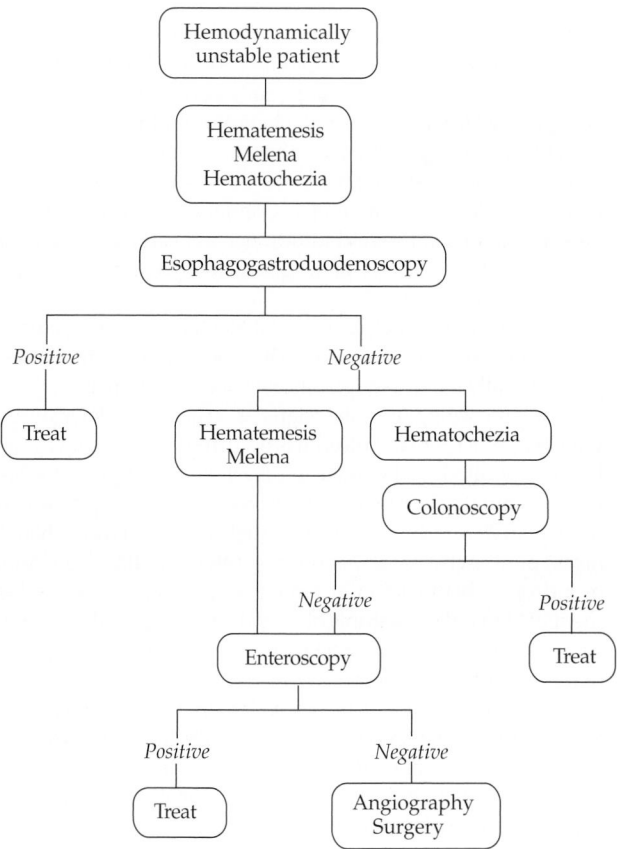

Figure 5 Evaluation and management of overt major gastrointestinal bleeding.

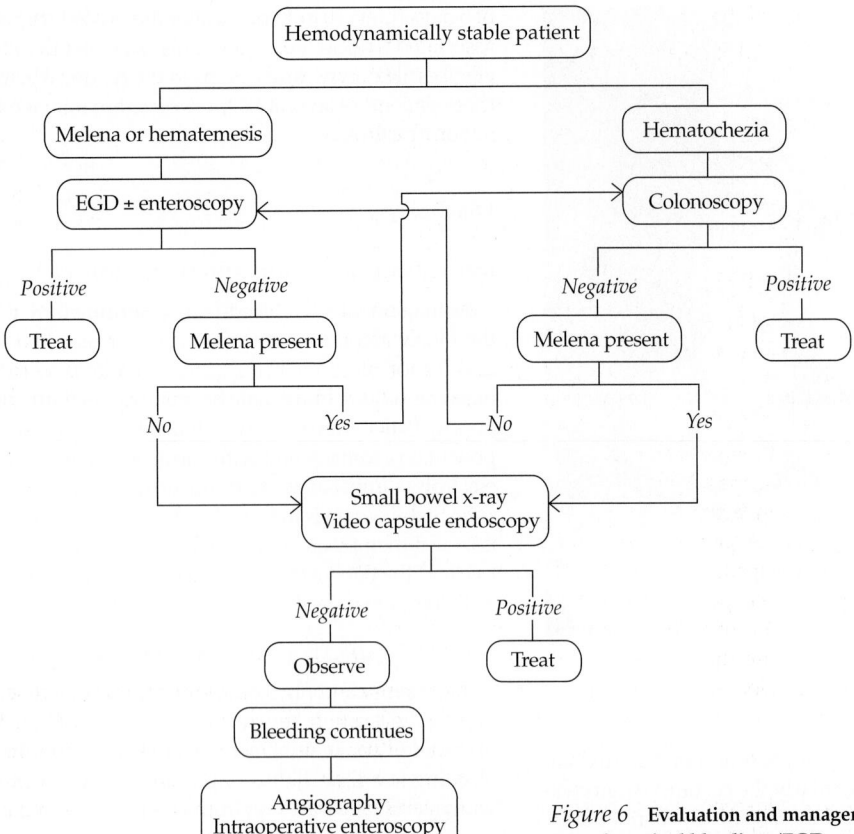

Figure 6 **Evaluation and management of overt minor gastrointestinal bleeding. (EGD—esophagogastroduodenoscopy)**

with hematochezia. These patients can experience visceral discomfort and orthostatic symptoms shortly after the onset of bleeding. Abdominal pain—especially periumbilical cramping and gaseous distention—usually indicates rapid intestinal transit of blood and suggests a major bleed.

The physician should look for evidence of liver disease, PUD, coagulopathy, previous abdominal aortic aneurysm repair, and significant comorbidities such as heart disease and diabetes mellitus. A history of drug or alcohol ingestion may suggest a diagnosis.

After cessation of active upper GI bleeding, patients may experience melena for 2 to 3 days. This does not indicate rebleeding, especially if the hemoglobin level does not decrease.

Serial recording of vital signs is crucial in determining whether an overt major bleed has occurred. Significant volume loss is indicated by hypotension (systolic blood pressure less than 100 mm Hg), orthostasis (a decrease in systolic pressure of more than 20 mm Hg or an increase in heart rate of more than 20 beats/min), tachycardia (heart rate greater than 100 beats/min), or a drop in hemoglobin of more than 2 g/dl. Further assessment of skin pallor, features of liver disease or portal hypertension, and stool color from rectal examination can also help with diagnosis or management.

A nasogastric tube can be placed if there is uncertainty about the location of the bleed in a patient with hematochezia or if bleeding persists in a patient with hematemesis. Aspiration of blood indicates a recent upper GI bleed, but absence of blood in the aspirate does not exclude a recent bleed.

The most important laboratory measurement to assess severity of the initial bleed and to monitor rebleeding is the hemoglobin level. An abrupt drop of more than 2 g/dl indicates a signifi-

cant bleeding episode. An increase in the ratio of blood urea nitrogen to creatinine to more than 25:1 strongly suggests an upper GI source. Measurement of serum electrolyte concentrations, coagulation indices, platelet count, and liver enzyme levels aids in the diagnosis and guides management.

ENDOSCOPY

In most patients, the location of the bleed is identified by upper GI endoscopy or colonoscopy. Endoscopy also provides therapeutic options and essential information on the risk of rebleeding [*see Table 3*]. There are established visual criteria, based on stigmata of recent hemorrhage, that the endoscopist can use to identify patients at high or low risk for rebleeding.

During upper GI endoscopy, if massive active bleeding is encountered, it is prudent to discontinue the procedure and protect the airway by endotracheal intubation before proceeding. If vi-

Table 2 **Clinical High-Risk Criteria for Rebleeding and Mortality**

Advanced age (≥ 70 yr)
Major organ comorbidities
In-hospital bleed
Bright-red hematemesis in patient with liver cirrhosis
Hypotension (systolic blood pressure < 100 mm Hg)
Tachycardia (heart rate >100 bpm)
Orthostasis (BP drop > 20 mm Hg; HR rise > 20 bpm)
Hemoglobin < 10 g/dl or drop of ≥ 2 g/dl
≥ 4 units of blood transfused in 24 hr

Table 3 Endoscopic High-Risk Stigmata for Rebleeding and Indications for Endoscopic Therapy

Nonvariceal bleeding	Arterial spurting Oozing bleed Nonbleeding visible vessel Adherent clot
Variceal bleeding	Large varices (> 5 mm esophageal, > 1 cm gastric) Red wale marks (longitudinal dilated venules resembling whip marks) Cherry-red spots (< 2 mm diameter) Hematocystic spots (> 4 mm diameter)

sualization is impaired, use of large-bore orogastric lavage or a jumbo-channel (6 mm) therapeutic endoscope to evacuate blood and clots may be effective. Erythromycin lactobionate (125 mg intravenously) can also be used to promote quick intestinal transit of blood when active bleeding has stopped.

Before colonoscopy, whenever possible, patients should receive a rapid colonic lavage with 2 to 3 L of a nonabsorbable polyethylene glycol solution administered through a nasogastric tube over 2 hours to cleanse the colon and facilitate adequate visualization.

RADIOLOGY

Selective visceral angiography is considered when endoscopic therapy for an established lesion has failed and surgery is not an option or when the site of an active bleed remains obscure after endoscopy. An optimal examination with a high positive yield is best obtained when there is active bleeding at rates exceeding 0.5 to 1 ml/min. Significant complications—including contrast reaction, acute renal failure, and femoral artery thrombosis—have been reported in approximately 9% of cases.[31,32] The reported sensitivity of angiography varies from 22% to 87%. The specificity approaches 100%.[33]

Radionuclide Technetium Scan

A technetium-99m–labeled red cell scan should be considered when active bleeding is suspected but endoscopy has been negative. Nuclear scans can detect bleeding at rates that exceed 0.1 ml/min. On scans, however, pooled blood may sometimes be mistaken for active bleeding, which contributes to a reported false positive rate of about 22%.[34] Upper GI bleeding may be misdiagnosed as lower because of pooling in the distal ileum or right colon. A positive result is more reliable when the scan is done early rather than delayed (several hours later).

Other Measures

Endoscopic techniques that are currently available for examination of the small bowel include push enteroscopy, wireless capsule endoscopy, and intraoperative enteroscopy. Push enteroscopy typically reaches into the proximal jejunum only, whereas wireless capsule enteroscopy and intraoperative enteroscopy reach the entire small bowel.

Enteroscopy is currently performed using a pediatric colonoscope with or without an overtube. In one study, the diagnostic yield of enteroscopy in overt GI bleeding was 46%; the most common lesions seen were angiodysplasia and ulcers.[35]

Wireless capsule endoscopy represents a new technology involving an easily swallowed 11 × 30 mm capsule. No sedation is required. The capsule contains a color video chip, light source, and transmitter. The patient wears an antenna array on a belt. While transiting through the intestine by peristalsis, the capsule takes color photos and sends them to the antenna array. These images are then downloaded onto a computer after the examination. There is a total of 6 to 8 hours of recording time. This technique may be beneficial in patients with recurrent or occult GI bleeding of obscure origin, but it is not appropriate in unstable patients with major active bleeding.

Intraoperative enteroscopy, performed during exploratory laparotomy, through single or multiple enterotomy sites, is indicated for the occasional patient with active or recurrent major bleeding of obscure origin. Complications include mucosal laceration, intramural hematoma, mesenteric hemorrhage, and intestinal ischemia.[36]

Treatment

NONVARICEAL BLEEDING

Endoscopic Therapy

A variety of endoscopic modalities are currently available for the management of GI bleeding. These can be categorized into thermal, mechanical, and injection devices. Thermal devices are either contact (e.g., heater probe, multipolar electrocautery) or noncontact (e.g., argon plasma coagulator, laser). These devices generate sufficient heat to create a hemostatic bond through tissue desiccation. The heater probe consists of a Teflon-coated hollow aluminum cylinder with a heating coil. Only heat (no electrical current) is delivered to the tissue. Multipolar or bipolar cautery works by completion of an electrical circuit between two electrodes on the probe tip. The argon plasma coagulator utilizes high-frequency monopolar alternating current delivered to target tissue through ionized argon gas. The conduit of argon gas is called the argon plasma. Electrons flow through a channel of electrically activated, ionized argon gas from the probe electrode to the tissue, causing a thermal effect at the interface. In laser photocoagulation, which is less frequently used, the conversion of light to heat results in coagulation or vaporization of tissue. The neodymium:yttrium-aluminum-garnet (Nd:YAG) laser is the one most commonly used. Mechanical devices for hemostasis include metallic clips and rubber-band ligators. An injection solution that is generally used to achieve hemostasis is saline mixed with epinephrine at a 1:10,000 concentration.

These therapeutic modalities are used alone or in combination. A common practice is to start by injecting epinephrine and saline submucosally in the region of active bleeding so as to stop or slow hemorrhaging and therefore allow for adequate inspection. Thermal or mechanical modalities are then used to achieve definitive hemostasis. Prospective, controlled studies have confirmed the benefit of endoscopic intervention in achieving initial hemostasis and in prevention of rebleeding.[37] Combination therapy (i.e., injection plus thermal therapy) has been demonstrated to reduce rebleeding rates more successfully than single therapy.[38,39] Currently, combination therapy using injection followed by either a thermal or a mechanical intervention is the most effective approach. Rebleeding after endoscopic therapy occurs in approximately 20% of cases, typically within 48 to 72 hours after treatment. However, rebleeding can occur as late as 7 days after therapy.

Pharmacotherapy

Initial drug therapy for major nonvariceal upper GI bleeding is directed at gastric acid suppression. In a randomized, double-blind study of high-dose omeprazole versus placebo, rebleeding after endoscopic therapy occurred less frequently in the omeprazole group (7% versus 23%).[40] In general, proton pump inhibitors are administered in doses that reduce gastric acidity. Blood clot stability depends on intragastric pH, with optimum stability at a pH of 6 or higher.[41]

In patients with PUD, long-term acid suppression and eradication of *H. pylori* infection after endoscopic intervention promote ulcer healing, including ulceration at the treatment site, and reduce rebleeding substantially. GI bleeding from NSAIDs is best prevented by avoiding these drugs and by using a high-dose proton pump inhibitor.

Radiologic Intervention

Selective arterial embolization and selective vasoconstriction with intra-arterial infusion of vasopressin are the methods currently available for the control of major nonvariceal GI bleeding. The proponents of embolization favor this form of therapy because it reduces the need for intensive care observation and it eliminates indwelling arterial lines, the risk of catheter dislodgement, and problematic systemic side effects of intravenous vasopressin [see Pharmacotherapy, below]. Advances in catheter design have allowed for superselective embolization of vasa recta; in experienced units, this modality is probably the treatment of choice. A study of superselective embolization in 48 patients with lower GI bleeding showed that embolization was the definitive treatment in 44% of patients, with a 27% technical failure rate.[42] The risks associated with embolization include misplacement of embolic material, inadvertent distal reflux of embolic agent, and excessive devascularization of an organ leading to ischemia and eventual luminal stenosis. Endoscopy can be helpful in determining ischemic injury if suspected. Microcoils (e.g., stainless steel, platinum), gelfoam pledgets, polyvinyl alcohol particles, and collagen suspensions have been used for embolization.

Intra-arterial vasopressin is the drug of choice for selective vasoconstrictive therapy and is generally infused for a minimum of 24 hours. It is associated with a 70% rate of bleeding control and an 18% rate of rebleeding.[43-45] Vasopressin may be ineffective when bleeding arises from large arteries that do not constrict in response to therapy. A study comparing embolization with vasopressin showed similar initial hemostasis rates but a higher rebleeding rate with vasopressin.[2] The use of intra-arterial provocative mesenteric angiography with heparin and tissue plasminogen activator (t-PA) to aid in diagnosis has been described but is still in the experimental stage.

Surgery

Despite the high overall success rate of endoscopic therapy in the treatment of major GI bleeding, surgery is still indicated when (1) initial hemostatic control cannot be achieved, (2) rebleeding occurs despite repeated endoscopic sessions, (3) a large (> 2 cm) penetrating ulcer is present, (4) a vessel larger than 2 mm in diameter is visible within the culprit lesion, (5) the ulcer is located in the posterior duodenal bulb (this location is associated with the large gastroduodenal artery), and (6) the patient requires substantial transfusion (i.e., four or more units of blood over 24 hours). The choice of surgery depends on the location of the bleed and the presence of comorbidities. Localization of the site of bleeding is critical for surgical planning.

Endoscopic Therapy

With variceal bleeding, endoscopic treatment is used primarily for esophageal varices, and the techniques include sclerotherapy and band ligation. Sclerotherapy utilizes a variety of sclerosants to induce variceal thrombosis, with sodium tetradecyl sulfate and ethanolamine oleate used most frequently. Intravariceal injections are more effective than paraesophageal injections in controlling bleeding. Compared with a sham injection, sclerotherapy is significantly more likely to stop bleeding (91% versus 60%), reduce mortality during hospitalization (mortality, 25% versus 49%), reduce rebleeding rates (rebleeding, 20% versus 51%), and reduce transfusion need (four versus eight units).[46] Complications of sclerotherapy include retrosternal chest pain, fever, ulceration (usually deep ulcers that heal within 3 weeks), dysphagia, delayed perforation (1 to 4 weeks later), and stricture formation. Complication rates vary from 19% to 35%.[47-49] The popularity of sclerotherapy has diminished as a result of these complications.

Band ligation is now considered the first-line endoscopic therapy for esophageal varices. The band ligator is readily attached to the distal end of the endoscope, which is advanced to the varix; the endoscopist then suctions the varix into the ligator cap and deploys a rubber band around the varix. This results in the plication of the varices and surrounding submucosal tissue, with fibrosis and eventual obliteration of varices. Comparative studies report a better initial control of bleeding (control rates, 91% versus 77%) and lower rebleeding rates (rebleeding, 24% versus 47%) with band ligation than with sclerotherapy.[47] Complications of banding include retrosternal chest pain, dysphagia from compromise of the esophageal lumen, band ulceration (usually superficial ulcers that heal within 2 weeks), esophageal injury from the overtube, or esophageal perforation. Complication rates vary from 2% to 19%.[50,51]

If bleeding continues despite endoscopic therapy or if endoscopic therapy cannot be initiated, then a modified Sengstaken-Blakemore (Minnesota) tube should be inserted. However, this is only a temporary measure until more definitive treatment—endoscopic, radiologic, or surgical—can be undertaken.

Preventive measures may be indicated in patients with esophageal varices. Preventive measures are generally offered to patients who have a history of a bleed and to those who have large esophageal varices without a prior bleeding event. Currently, the accepted preventive measures for variceal bleeding include endoscopic band ligation, beta-blocker therapy, or a combination of both. Ligation is performed every 14 to 21 days until varices are completely eradicated, which typically requires three or four sessions.

Pharmacotherapy

In acute variceal bleeding, splanchnic blood flow and portal pressure can be reduced by intravenous infusion of vasoconstrictors such as vasopressin, terlipressin, somatostatin, and octreotide. Vasopressin is a potent vasoconstrictor that has a reported overall success rate of 50% but a high rebleeding rate when treatment is discontinued.[52] It has a short half-life and therefore is given as a continuous infusion. Vasopressin-induced hypertension and bradycardia have the potential to confound hemodynamic monitoring and may give false reassurance in the face of active bleeding. Because the systemic vasoconstrictive side effects associated with vasopressin may lead to myocardial

a   *b*

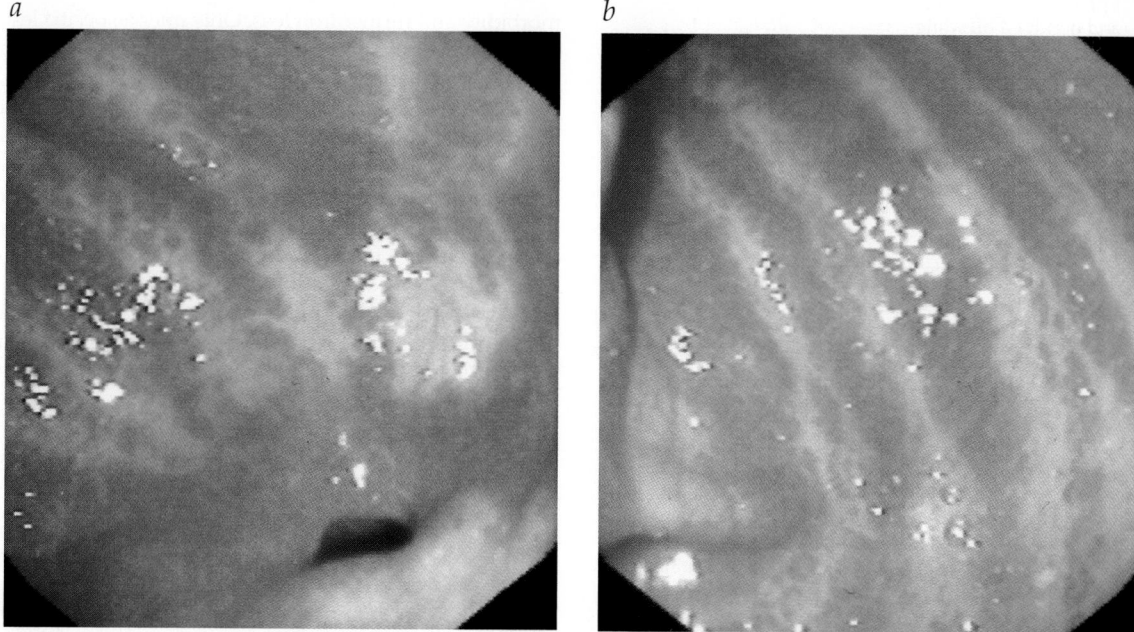

Figure 7   Watermelon stomach (*a*) with typical spokes of vascular ectasia radiating from the pylorus into the antrum and (*b*) close-up view.

or mesenteric ischemia, it is rarely used alone. To minimize these side effects, it is given in conjunction with nitroglycerin. The nitroglycerin can be administered as a continuous infusion, sublingually, or by transdermal patch. Terlipressin is a synthetic analogue of vasopressin that has fewer side effects and a longer half-life and is given in bolus injections; however, terlipressin has not yet been approved for use in the United States.

Somatostatin, a naturally occurring peptide, is reported to stop variceal bleeding in 80% of patients.[17,53] Side effects are few and include hyperglycemia and abdominal pain. Octreotide is a synthetic analogue of somatostatin that is preferred because of its longer half-life. The combination of pharmacologic treatment (e.g., octreotide for 5 days) and endoscopic therapy appear to offer better control of acute bleeding than either alone.

The role of beta blockers is primarily prophylactic. These agents are not used in the acute management of variceal bleeding. The use of isosorbide mononitrate with beta-blocker therapy does not offer a survival advantage and in fact reduces the tolerability of therapy.

Radiologic Intervention

The radiologic intervention available for variceal bleeding is transjugular intrahepatic portosystemic shunt (TIPS). The accepted indications for TIPS are bleeding or rebleeding that cannot be controlled by either pharmacologic or endoscopic therapy. TIPS is contraindicated in patients with severe hepatic failure, chronic heart failure, hepatic encephalopathy, bile duct obstruction, or cholangitis. TIPS is reported to control bleeding in at least 90% of patients, with rebleeding rates of 12% to 26% at 1 year and 16% to 44% at 2 years.[54,55] Patients require close surveillance for shunt dysfunction (evidenced by reduced flow by Doppler ultrasound or reappearance of varices) because primary shunt patency rates are poor (reported cumulative patency rates of 50% at 1 year and 21% at 3 years) but cumulative secondary shunt patency rates can be as satisfactory as 85% and 55% at 1 and 3 years, respectively.[55] TIPS should not be undertaken lightly, because the overall proce-

dure-related mortality can be as high as 1% to 2%,[54] largely from intraperitoneal hemorrhage. Other complications include hepatic encephalopathy, portal vein thrombosis, renal failure, sepsis, and stent migration or stenosis.

Surgical Intervention

Surgical intervention is rarely used for variceal bleeding; it is considered when other measures have proved ineffective. Surgical treatments include portosystemic venous shunt operations and esophageal devascularization. A variety of surgical shunts are available. These are generally classified as total, partial, or selective, depending on the intended impact of portal flow diversion. The end-to-side portacaval shunt is a total shunt that diverts all portal blood flow into the inferior vena cava. The side-to-side portacaval shunt diverts only a part of the portal blood flow. Selective shunts decompress variceal flow while preserving portal blood flow. The distal splenorenal shunt is a selective shunt designed to prevent encephalopathy, which is often seen with total shunts. Surgical shunts are used for both esophageal and gastric varices. Encephalopathy, accelerated progression of liver failure, and perioperative morbidity can occur with surgical intervention. Esophageal devascularization may be an effective means of controlling acute variceal bleeding, but bleeding can recur as additional varices develop.

Occult Bleeding

The critical metabolic sequela of occult GI bleeding is iron deficiency.[56] Occult GI bleeding causes most cases of iron deficiency in adults, especially in men and postmenopausal women.

ETIOLOGY

Most of the many lesions that cause overt bleeding can also produce occult blood loss. However, variceal and diverticular hemorrhage invariably bleed overtly, whereas lesions such as watermelon stomach (gastric antral vascular ectasia) and diaphragmat-

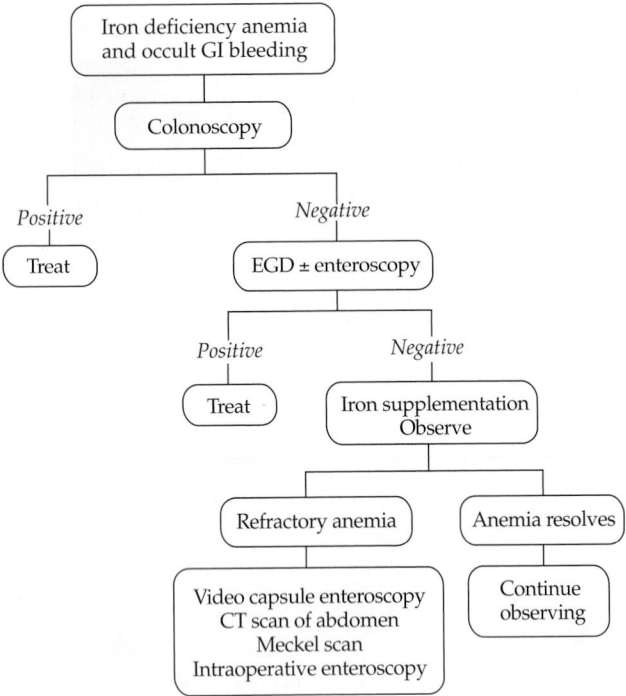

Figure 8 **Evaluation and management of occult gastrointestinal bleeding.**

ic hernia with Cameron erosions tend to bleed occultly. Occult GI bleeding in most patients is suspected only when manifested by fatigue, pallor, or the finding of iron deficiency.

Inflammation

In Western countries, erosive or ulcerative diseases of the esophagus, stomach, and duodenum are the most common GI lesions associated with occult bleeding and iron deficiency anemia. Most peptic disease is caused by either *H. pylori* infection or use of drugs such as aspirin or other NSAIDs. The association between large diaphragmatic hernias and iron deficiency anemia has long been known. A large diaphragmatic hernia is found in about 10% of iron-deficient patients.[57] Blood loss in these patients is generally caused by longitudinal mucosal erosions (Cameron erosions) located proximally in the hernia and believed to be secondary to repeated mechanical trauma from respiration.

Cancers and Neoplasms

In adults from Western countries, GI tumors are second only to PUD as a cause of occult bleeding leading to iron deficiency anemia.[58] Colorectal cancer is currently the most common source of occult bleeding from GI tract malignancies.

Vascular Causes

Vascular malformations are found in approximately 6% of adults with iron deficiency anemia.[59,60] This may be acquired or hereditary (hereditary hemorrhagic telangiectasia). An increasingly recognized and endoscopically treatable vascular lesion is watermelon stomach [*see Figure 7*], which typically presents as iron deficiency anemia in older women.

TREATMENT

When a patient is found to have iron deficiency and occult GI bleeding, it is critical to conduct a thorough GI investigation. Such an evaluation may disclose a health-threatening lesion, in

which case specific therapy can be given to prevent associated morbidity and further iron loss. Only after a specific lesion has been treated or has been ruled out, is it appropriate to place patients on iron therapy and monitor them [*see Figure 8*].

Whatever the culpable lesion, treatment with iron supplementation is important to correct iron deficiency. With conditions such as Cameron erosions, iron supplementation is the mainstay of treatment. Most patients can be managed as outpatients. Oral iron therapy with ferrous sulfate is preferred because it is inexpensive, effective, and, in most cases, well tolerated [*see Chapter 93*]. A maximal adult dose of ferrous sulfate is 325 mg three times a day. Absorption is not appreciably increased with higher doses. Oral iron is as effective as parenteral iron in repleting iron stores, except in patients with a malabsorption syndrome, and is safer.

The authors have no commercial relationships with manufacturers of products or providers of services discussed in this chapter.

References

1. Swain CP, Storey DW, Bown SG, et al: Nature of the bleeding vessel in recurrently bleeding gastric ulcers. Gastroenterology 90:595, 1986

2. Peter DJ, Dougherty JM: Evaluation of the patient with gastrointestinal bleeding: an evidence based approach. Emerg Med Clin North Am 17:239, 1999

3. Vreeburg EM, Snel P, de Bruijne JW, et al: Acute upper gastrointestinal bleeding in the Amsterdam area: incidence, diagnosis, and clinical outcome. Am J Gastroenterol 92:236, 1997

4. Friedman LS, Martin P: The problem of gastrointestinal bleeding. Gastroenterol Clin North Am 22:717, 1993

5. Pianka JD, Affronti J: Management principles of gastrointestinal bleeding. Prim Care 28:557, 2001

6. Farrell JJ, Friedman LS: Gastrointestinal bleeding in the elderly. Gastroenterol Clin North Am 30:377, 2001

7. Gostout CJ, Wang KK, Ahlquist DA, et al: Acute gastrointestinal bleeding: experience of a specialized management team. J Clin Gastroenterol 14:260, 1992

8. Gostout CJ: Acute lower GI bleeding. Current Medicine: Clinical Practice of Gastroenterology. Brandt LJ, Daum F, Eds. Churchill Livingstone, Philadelphia, 1998, p 651

9. Hay JA, Lyubashevsky E, Elashoff J, et al: Upper gastrointestinal hemorrhage—clinical guideline determining the optimal hospital length of stay. Am J Med 100:313, 1996

10. Rockall TA, Logan RF, Devlin HB, et al: Selection of patients for early discharge or outpatient care after acute upper gastrointestinal haemorrhage. National Audit of Acute Upper Gastrointestinal Haemorrhage. Lancet 347:1138, 1996

11. Andersen IB, Jorgensen T, Bonnevie O, et al: Smoking and alcohol intake as risk factors for bleeding and perforated peptic ulcers: a population-based cohort study. Epidemiology 11:434, 2000

12. Bardhan KD, Graham DY, Hunt RH, et al: Effects of smoking on cure of *Helicobacter pylori* infection and duodenal ulcer recurrence in patients treated with clarithromycin and omeprazole. Helicobacter 2:27, 1997

13. Cohen H: Peptic ulcer and *Helicobacter pylori*. Gastroenterol Clin North Am 29:775, 2000

14. Solomon DH, Gurwitz JH: Toxicity of nonsteroidal anti-inflammatory drugs in the elderly: is advanced age a risk factor? Am J Med 102:208, 1997

15. Dalton SO, Johansen C, Mellemkjaer L, et al: Use of selective serotonin reuptake inhibitors and risk of upper gastrointestinal tract bleeding: a population-based cohort study. Arch Intern Med 163:59, 2003

16. Gostout CJ: Patient assessment and resuscitation. Gastrointest Endosc Clin N Am 9:175, 1999

17. Sharara AI, Rockey DC: Gastroesophageal variceal hemorrhage. N Engl J Med 345:669, 2001

18. Cales P, Zabotto B, Meskens C, et al: Gastroesophageal endoscopic features in cirrhosis: observer variability, interassociations, and relationship to hepatic dysfunction. Gastroenterology 98:156, 1990

19. Prediction of the first variceal hemorrhage in patients with cirrhosis of the liver and esophageal varices: a prospective multicenter study. The North Italian Endoscopic Club for the Study and Treatment of Esophageal Varices. N Engl J Med 319:983, 1988

20. Sugawa C, Steffes CP, Nakamura R, et al: Upper GI bleeding in an urban hospital: etiology, recurrence, and prognosis. Ann Surg 212:521, 1990

21. Kasapidis P, Georgopoulos P, Delis V: Endoscopic management and long-term follow-up of Dieulafoy's lesions in the upper GI tract. Gastrointest Endosc 55:527, 2002

22. Norton ID, Petersen BT, Sorbi D: Management and long-term prognosis of Dieulafoy lesion. Gastrointest Endosc 50:762, 1999

23. Buttenschoen K, Buttenschoen DC, Odermath R, et al: Diverticular disease-associated hemorrhage in the elderly. Langenbecks Arch Surg 386:8, 2001

24. Freeman SR, McNally PR: Diverticulitis. Med Clin North Am 77:1149, 1993

25. McGuire HH Jr: Urgent colonoscopy for the diagnosis and treatment of severe diverticular hemorrhage. N Engl J Med 342:1609, 2000

26. Hodgson H: Hormonal therapy for gastrointestinal angiodysplasia. Lancet 359:1630, 2002

27. Imdahl A: Genesis and pathophysiology of lower gastrointestinal bleeding. Langenbecks Arch Surg 386:1, 2001

28. Hochter W, Weingart J, Kuhner W, et al: Angiodysplasia in the colon and rectum: endoscopic morphology, localisation and frequency. Endoscopy 17:182,1985

29. Rosen L, Bub DS, Reed JF 3rd, et al: Hemorrhage following colonoscopic polypectomy. Dis Colon Rectum 36:1126, 1993

30. Sorbi D, Norton I, Conio M, et al: Postpolypectomy lower GI bleeding: descriptive analysis. Gastrointest Endosc 51:690, 2000

31. Lingenfelser T, Ell C: Gastrointestinal bleeding in the elderly. Best Pract Res Clin Gastroenterol 15:963, 2001

32. Egglin TK, O'Moore PV, Feinstein AR, et al: Complications of peripheral arteriography: a new system to identify patients at increased risk. J Vasc Surg 22:787, 1995

33. Koval G, Benner KG, Rosch J, et al: Aggressive angiographic diagnosis in acute lower gastrointestinal hemorrhage. Dig Dis Sci 32:248, 1987

34. Ng DA, Opelka FG, Beck DE, et al: Predictive value of technetium Tc 99m-labeled red blood cell scintigraphy for positive angiogram in massive lower gastrointestinal hemorrhage. Dis Colon Rectum 40:471, 1997

35. Feitoza A, Rajan E, Gostout CJ: Overt gastrointestinal bleeding: diagnostic and therapeutic yield of push-enteroscopy. Am J Gastroenterol 96:S104, 2001

36. Lopez MJ, Cooley JS, Petros JG, et al: Complete intraoperative small-bowel endoscopy in the evaluation of occult gastrointestinal bleeding using the Sonde enteroscope. Arch Surg 131:272, 1996

37. Fullarton GM, Birnie GG, Macdonald A, et al: Controlled trial of heater probe treatment in bleeding peptic ulcers. Br J Surg 76:541, 1989

38. Lin HJ, Tseng GY, Perng CL, et al: Comparison of adrenaline injection and bipolar electrocoagulation for the arrest of peptic ulcer bleeding. Gut 44:715, 1999

39. Bleau BL, Gostout CJ, Sherman KE, et al: Recurrent bleeding from peptic ulcer associated with adherent clot: a randomized study comparing endoscopic treatment with medical therapy. Gastrointest Endosc 56:1, 2002

40. Palmer KR: Intravenous omeprazole after endoscopic treatment of bleeding peptic ulcers. Gut 49:610, 2001

41. Green FW Jr, Kaplan MM, Curtis LE, et al: Effect of acid and pepsin on blood coagulation and platelet aggregation: a possible contributor to prolonged gastroduodenal mucosal hemorrhage. Gastroenterology 74:38, 1978

42. Bandi R, Shetty PC, Sharma RP, et al: Superselective arterial embolization for the treatment of lower gastrointestinal hemorrhage. J Vasc Interv Radiol 12:1399, 2001

43. Rosen RJ, Sanchez G: Angiographic diagnosis and management of gastrointestinal hemorrhage: current concepts. Radiol Clin North Am 32:951, 1994

44. Gostout CJ: The evaluation and management of acute upper gastrointestinal bleeding. Clinical Practice of Gastroenterology. Brandt LJ, Daum F, Eds. Churchill Livingstone, Philadelphia, 1998, p1514

45. Zuccaro G Jr: Management of the adult patient with acute lower gastrointestinal bleeding. American College of Gastroenterology. Practice Parameters Committee. Am J Gastroenterol 93:1202, 1998

46. Sclerotherapy for actively bleeding esophageal varices in male alcoholics with cirrhosis. Veterans Affairs Cooperative Variceal Sclerotherapy Group. Gastrointest Endosc 46:1, 1997

47. Bleau BL: Endoscopic management of the acute variceal bleeding event. Gastrointest Endosc Clin N Am 9:189, 1999

48. Stiegmann GV, Goff JS, Michaletz-Onody PA, et al: Endoscopic sclerotherapy as compared with endoscopic ligation for bleeding esophageal varices. N Engl J Med 326:1527, 1992

49. Lo GH, Lai KH, Cheng JS, et al: Emergency banding ligation versus sclerotherapy for the control of active bleeding from esophageal varices. Hepatology 25:1101, 1997

50. Sarin SK, Govil A, Jain AK, et al: Prospective randomized trial of endoscopic sclerotherapy versus variceal band ligation for esophageal varices: influence on gastropathy, gastric varices and variceal recurrence. J Hepatol 26:826, 1997

51. Laine L, el-Newihi HM, Migikovsky B, et al: Endoscopic ligation compared with sclerotherapy for the treatment of bleeding esophageal varices. Ann Intern Med 119:1, 1993

52. Nader A, Grace ND: Pharmacological intervention during the acute bleeding episode. Gastrointest Endosc Clin N Am 9:301, 1999

53. Double-blind randomized controlled trial comparing terlipressin and somatostatin for acute variceal hemorrhage. Variceal Bleeding Study Group. Gastroenterology 111:1291, 1996

54. McKusick MA: Interventional radiology for the control and prevention of bleeding. Gastrointest Endosc Clin N Am 9:311, 1999

55. Zhuang ZW, Teng GJ, Jeffery RF, et al: Long-term results and quality of life in patients treated with transjugular intrahepatic portosystemic shunts. AJR Am J Roentgenol 179:1597, 2002

56. Ahlquist DA: Approach to the patient with occult gastrointestinal bleeding. Textbook of Gastroenterology, 4th ed. Yamada T, Alpers DH, Kaplowitz N, et al, Eds. Lippincott Williams & Wilkins, Philadelphia, 2003

57. Descamps C, Schmit A, Van Gossum A: "Missed" upper gastrointestinal tract lesions may explain "occult" bleeding. Endoscopy 31:452, 1999

58. Rockey DC, Celo JP: Evaluation of the gastrointestinal tract in patients with iron deficiency anemia. N Engl J Med 329:1691, 1993

59. Kendrick ML, Buttar NS, Anderson MA: Contribution of intraoperative enteroscopy in the management of obscure gastrointestinal bleeding. J Gastrointest Surg 5:162, 2001

60. Gostout CJ, Ahlquist DA, Radford CM, et al: Endoscopic laser therapy for watermelon stomach. Gastroenterology 96:1462, 1989

Acknowledgment

Figures 1 through 4 and 7 © 2003 Mayo Foundation for Medical Education and Research. Used by permission.

69 Acute Viral Hepatitis

Emmet B. Keeffe, M.D., F.A.C.P.

Most cases of acute hepatitis are caused by one of five hepatotrophic viruses: hepatitis A virus (HAV), hepatitis B virus (HBV), hepatitis C virus (HCV), hepatitis D virus (HDV), or hepatitis E virus (HEV).[1,2] In the United States in 1999, 59% of reported cases of acute viral hepatitis were caused by HAV infection and 26.5% by HBV infection; 14.5% were classified as non-A, non-B hepatitis or were unspecified.[3] HDV infection (delta hepatitis) occurs either as a superinfection in chronic HBV carriers or as a coinfection during acute HBV infection. HEV infection occurs predominantly outside the United States, but a few cases have been reported in travelers returning to the United States. All five viruses can cause classic acute viral hepatitis, but only three—HBV, HCV, and HDV—can lead to chronic infection. Finally, drug-induced hepatitis and hepatitis secondary to other viruses that cause systemic illnesses—for example, cytomegalovirus (CMV) and Epstein-Barr virus (EBV)—may mimic typical acute viral hepatitis..

All five types of viral hepatitis are similar and cannot be distinguished reliably by clinical features or routine laboratory tests. Infection either may occur asymptomatically or may be associated with nonspecific flulike symptoms; some patients experience jaundice. The characteristic laboratory abnormality in acute hepatitis is an elevated aminotransferase level, typically greater than 300 IU/L and, occasionally, 1,000 to 3,000 IU/L. The specific etiology of viral hepatitis is determined by serologic testing [*see Table 1*].

Classification and Pathology

HEPATITIS A VIRUS

HAV is a picornavirus similar to poliovirus and rhinovirus.[4] HAV was initially discovered in stool but has also been found in the serum of patients with acute HAV infection and in the cytoplasm of liver cells and bile of animals infected with HAV.[5] It is a nonenveloped, positive-stranded RNA virus that has at least seven genotypes but only one serotype.[4] The antigenic compositions of HAV throughout the world are remarkably similar, which explains the global efficacy of immune globulin and of hepatitis A vaccine. IgM antibody to HAV is detectable at the onset of clinical illness and usually disappears within 60 to 120 days. IgG antibody reaches a high titer during convalescence, persists indefinitely, and confers immunity.

HEPATITIS B VIRUS

HBV, the only member of the family Hepadnaviridae that infects humans, has a diameter of 42 nm and consists of a 28 nm core surrounded by a protein coat; the core contains protein, circular double-stranded DNA, and DNA polymerase [*see Figure 1*].[6] Immunofluorescent antibody studies have detected HBV in the nuclei of infected liver cells. The core moves through the nuclear membrane into the cytoplasm, where it acquires its surface coat. HBV is found in the serum of almost all patients early in the course of acute HBV infection.

Two additional particles appear in the liver cell cytoplasm and serum of patients with HBV: a 22 nm–diameter sphere and a rod-shaped filament of the same diameter. These particles are found at the onset of jaundice in nearly all patients with acute HBV infection. The virion surface coat and the spheres and filaments are composed of pre-S1, pre-S2, and S polypeptides, both glycosylated and unglycosylated. The S polypeptide is the major hepatitis B surface antigen (HBsAg).

Although there is only one major serotype of HBV, HBsAg has five major subtype determinants, termed *a*, *d*, *y*, *w*, and *r*, which are primarily of epidemiologic interest. All HBsAg-positive sera contain determinant *a*; determinants *d* and *y* are mutually exclusive, as are *w* and *r*. Hence, four subtype patterns are possible: *adw*, *ayw*, *adr*, and *ayr*. The first three subtype patterns occur frequently; *ayr* is rare. Many studies have attempted to correlate subtype with clinical course. It appears, however, that subtypes are associated with geographic distributions of HBV rather than with degrees of virulence. Subtype *adw* is most common in the Americas and Europe; *adr* prevails in most of the Far East.

HBV can be classified into eight genotypes (A to H) on the basis of an intergroup divergence of 8% or more in the complete nucleotide sequence.[7,8] Genotypes A (serotype *adw*) and D (*ayw*) are most common in the United States and Europe; genotypes B (*adw*) and C (*adr*) are most frequent in China and Southeast Asia.[9] There are also several variations or mutations in the nucleotide sequence of HBV. Core promoter and precore variants do not produce hepatitis B e antigen (HBeAg); they are most commonly seen with genotypes B, C, and D. Differences in genotypes and variants may account for variations in clinical manifestations of chronic HBV infection throughout the world. For example, genotype C is associated with more severe liver disease and a higher incidence of hepatocellular carcinoma in Asians.

HEPATITIS C VIRUS

HCV is a 9.4 kb, single-stranded, positive-sense RNA virus that accounts for most cases of non-A, non-B hepatitis.[10,11] It is most closely related to the pestiviruses and flaviviruses and is believed to be a distinct genus in the Flaviviridae family. Structural proteins are encoded at the highly conserved 5' end [*see Figure 2*]. Further downstream are the HCV core protein, the envelope proteins, and the four nonstructural proteins at the 3' end. Based on nucleic acid sequence, at least six major genotypes (type 1, 2, 3, etc.) and various subtypes (1a, 1b, 2a, etc.) have been identified

Table 1 Serologic Diagnosis of Acute Viral Hepatitis

Disease	Serology	Comments
Hepatitis A	IgM anti-HAV	Reasonably specific
Hepatitis B	HBsAg IgM anti-HBc	May be negative late Indicates acute hepatitis
Hepatitis C	Anti-HCV HCV RNA	Appears late Appears early
Hepatitis D	HBsAg and anti-HDV + IgM anti-HBc – IgM anti-HBc	Anti-HDV may appear late Coinfection Superinfection
Hepatitis E	Anti-HEV	Not licensed in the United States

HAV—hepatitis A virus HBc—hepatitis B virus core HBsAg—hepatitis B surface antigen HCV—hepatitis C virus HDV—hepatitis D virus HEV—hepatitis E virus

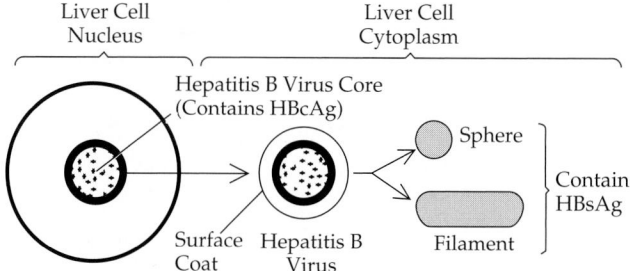

Figure 1 The hepatitis B virus exists in the cytoplasm of parenchymal liver cells of persons with hepatitis B and constitutes the infective virus. The core of this particle is found in the nucleus of parenchymal cells (left), but as it passes through the cytoplasm, it acquires a surface coat (middle). The core contains hepatitis B core antigen (HBcAg). Spheres and filaments, also in the cytoplasm (right), appear to be excess surface coat material. They are the main source of hepatitis B surface antigen (HBsAg) in serum.

worldwide. Specific HCV genotypes exhibit different degrees of responsiveness to interferon therapy. In the United States, genotype 1 is the most common, accounting for 70% to 80% of cases; genotype 2 accounts for about 15% of cases, and genotype 3 accounts for 5%. Other genotypes appear to be uncommon in the United States. Coinfection with more than one genotype may occur, particularly in patients with hemophilia or in others who have been repeatedly exposed to HCV. Quasispecies of HCV also exist. This genetic heterogeneity develops with a longer duration of infection; it may be associated with a poorer response to interferon therapy.

HEPATITIS D VIRUS

HDV, or delta agent, is a single-stranded, circular, negative-polarity, defective RNA virus that requires HBV for its expression.[12] HDV is smaller than any known animal virus and resembles certain plant viruses known as viroids. It circulates in the blood in association with hepatitis D antigen, and the RNA genome has an external coat composed of HBsAg. Although hepatitis D antigen, HDV RNA, and IgM anti–hepatitis D virus (anti-HDV) can be found in the plasma of infected persons, the only commercially available serologic marker for this infection is the total IgG antibody to hepatitis D virus antigen (anti-HDV). When anti-HDV is present in serum, markers of the HBV replication, such as HBeAg and HBV DNA, are usually absent. Although HDV infection is present worldwide, it is most prevalent in Mediterranean countries, the Middle East, and northern Africa. The virus is responsible for epidemics of fulminant hepatitis in South America. HDV infections are uncommon in the United States and northern Europe, ex-

cept in I.V. drug abusers and persons frequently exposed to blood products. HDV is also uncommon in Southeast Asia and China, areas where HBV is common. Successful vaccination against HBV will prevent HDV infection.

HEPATITIS E VIRUS

HEV is a single-stranded, positive-sense RNA virus of approximately 7.5 kb that causes enterically transmitted non-A, non-B hepatitis.[13] The diagnosis of HEV infection can be made by serologic identification of anti-HEV antibodies (not yet commercially available in the United States). HEV has also been identified in the stool of patients with acute HEV infection through use of immune electron microscopy. Strain variation in HEV has been noted in different parts of the world (e.g., the HEV [B or Burma] and HEV [M or Mexico] strains have only 76% sequence similarity), but there is only one serotype. Acute HEV infection is observed in developing countries; sporadic cases in the United States have been diagnosed in travelers returning from endemic areas.

HEPATITIS F AND G VIRUSES

Between 5% and 20% of cases of acute and chronic hepatitis are not caused by the five known hepatitis viruses and have been presumed to be caused by non-A–E agents. A virus identified in stool extracts from French patients with non-A–E hepatitis was tentatively called the hepatitis F virus (HFV),[14] but its existence has never been substantiated. HGV, an RNA virus, was identified as a coinfection in patients with HCV infection and also in persons with non-A–E hepatitis.[15] HGV was found to be similar to a GB virus (GBV).[16] Two viruses, GBV-A and GBV-B, are probably nonhuman virus contaminants of serially passed human serum in tamarins. A third virus, GBV-C, is now identified as HGV. Though closely related to HCV, HGV (GBV-C) does not appear to be pathogenic.[17]

Epidemiology

It is particularly important to consider the epidemiology of types A, B, C, D, and E hepatitis and the special tests that may permit their differentiation, because their prognoses are considerably different [*see Tables 1 and 2*].[1,2]

HEPATITIS A VIRUS

In HAV infection, virus is shed in the stool 14 to 21 days before the onset of jaundice. Although patients may continue shedding virus for the first 1 to 2 weeks of clinical illness, they are usually no longer infectious 21 days after the illness has begun. However, virus may be detected in the stool again if the patient

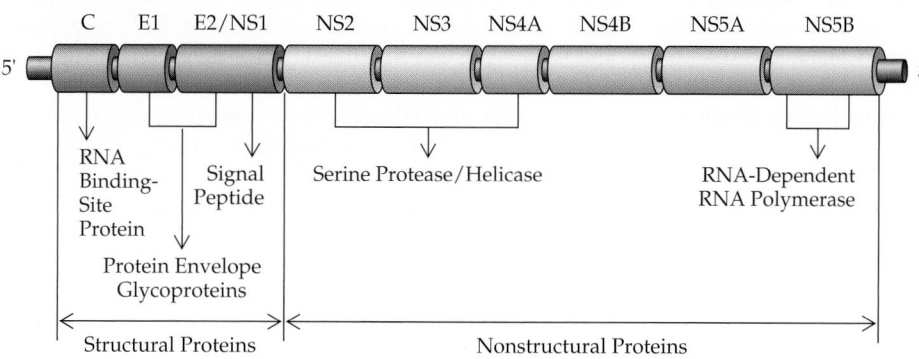

Figure 2 The hepatitis C virus genome consists of a single, long, open reading frame. The three structural proteins (the RNA binding-site protein [C, core protein] and two envelope glycoproteins [E1 and E2]) are encoded on the 5′ end, and the nonstructural proteins (protease, helicase, and RNA-dependent RNA polymerase [NS2, NS3/NS4A, and NS5B]) are encoded on the 3′ end.

Table 2 Features of Type A, Type B, Type C, Type D, and Type E Acute Viral Hepatitis

	Type A	Type B	Type C	Type D	Type E
Mode of transmission	Fecal-oral, sewage-contaminated shellfish	Percutaneous, sexual	Percutaneous and community	Percutaneous	Fecal-oral
Incubation period (days)	20–37 (15–49)*	60–110 (25–160)*	35–70 (21–84)*	Appears to be comparable to type B	10–56
Results of serum antigen and antibody tests	Development of IgM antibody early and IgG antibody in convalescence	Antigen (HBsAg) and antibody (anti-HBc) appear early and persist in carriers	Anti-HCV appears in 6 wk to 9 mo	Anti-HDV appears late and may be short-lived	IgM antibody usually detected within 26 days of jaundice; IgG antibody persists indefinitely
Immunity	45% of the U.S. population has hepatitis A antibodies in serum and is probably immune	5%–15% of the population has anti-HBs	Unknown	Patients immune to hepatitis B are also protected against hepatitis D	Unknown
Prevalence	Seen with increasing frequency in adults	Increasing in the United States	80%–90% of post-transfusion hepatitis; 12%–25% of sporadic acute hepatitis	Unusual in the United States but common in I.V. drug abusers	Rare in the United States
Course	Does not progress to chronic liver disease	Chronic liver disease develops in 1%–5% of adults and 80%–90% of children	Chronic liver disease develops in 85%	> 95% resolution of delta coinfection with acute hepatitis B; chronic infection common if delta superinfection is present in chronic hepatitis B carrier	Does not progress to chronic liver disease
Prevention of the disease after exposure	Pooled γ-globulin (0.02 ml/kg) decreases the occurrence of clinical disease 7- to 8-fold	Hepatitis B immune globulin and hepatitis B vaccine prevent clinical disease in adults and the carrier state in infants	The efficacy of pooled γ-globulin is uncertain	Unknown	Uncertain
Mortality	0%–0.2% with fulminant hepatitis	0.3%–1.5%	Uncertain; may approximate rate for type B	2%–20% for acute icteric hepatitis	1%–2%; may be as high as 10%–15% in pregnant women

*Usual range, with outside limits given in parentheses.

experiences a relapse of the acute illness. HAV is transmitted via food contaminated by feces-soiled hands of infected persons. The disease is quite contagious; transmission in families is common, and several large point-source epidemics have been reported.[18] Outbreaks of HAV infection have been reported in day care centers, with young children being the most commonly infected.[19] Employees of the day care centers and household contacts and close relatives of the infected children contracted the disease with alarming frequency. Ingestion of sewage-contaminated shellfish has resulted in several epidemics of HAV,[20] as has contamination of raw produce.[21] The disease is sexually transmitted in men who have sex with men.[22,23] HAV is also common in I.V. drug abusers, but the method of transmission is uncertain. Viremia is present from 1 to 25 days before the onset of symptoms, but transmission by serum or blood products seldom occurs. Patients with HAV develop immunity to the disease—approximately one third of the population of the United States has serum antibodies to HAV. There is no known human or nonhuman reservoir of HAV.

HEPATITIS B VIRUS

HBV is transmitted primarily through percutaneous inoculation of infected serum or blood products. HBsAg and HBV DNA are found in a wide variety of bodily secretions, but the importance of these factors in the spread of HBV is unknown. The most common mode of transmission in men who have sex with men

may be by oral or genital contact with asymptomatic bleeding lesions in the rectal mucosa. HBV may also be transmitted to the fetus during pregnancy. An appreciable segment of the population has serum antibodies to HBsAg (anti-HBs). Prevalence of anti-HBs varies among subpopulations: middle-class whites have a 5% prevalence; middle-class African Americans, 12%; Chinese Americans, 37%; and white homosexual men, 48%. This antibody confers immunity to HBV.

HEPATITIS C VIRUS

Before the advent of tests that could screen for HCV and thus help eliminate this virus from the blood supply, HCV caused most cases of posttransfusion hepatitis.[24] Since that time, the rate of HCV transmission by transfusion has declined, and the risk of posttransfusion HCV infection is estimated to be between 0.01% and 0.001% per unit transfused.[25] HCV is responsible for more than 80% of non-A, non-B hepatitis.

HCV is transmitted by parenteral means (e.g., transfusions, I.V. drug use, or occupational exposure to blood or blood products).[26] The risk of transmission from a single needle-stick accident averages 1.8% in prospective studies (range, 0% to 7%).[25] It is estimated that the risk of sexual transmission of HCV in monogamous couples is about 5%, well below the risk of sexual transmission of HBV (about 30%) or HIV (about 10% to 15%). However, the rate of HCV infection is higher in persons who have frequent sexual contact with numerous partners, and in this setting, the risk is higher for female partners of men with anti-HCV.[27] Most studies have failed to demonstrate any serologic or virologic evidence of HCV transmission to nonsexual partners within households. Perinatal transmission of HCV infection is unusual, except in babies born to mothers with very high serum HCV RNA, such as mothers with concomitant HIV infection. The risk of perinatal transmission is estimated to be 4% to 7%. There appears to be no increase in HCV infection in breast-fed babies. In summary, barrier precautions are not recommended for monogamous partners, but persons with multiple sexual partners should practice safe sex and use latex condoms. An additional precaution is to avoid shared percutaneous exposures, such as razors and toothbrushes. Finally, there is no reason to advise against pregnancy for a woman with HCV infection, because the rate of perinatal infection is low.

Recipients of organs from donors who have antibodies to HCV have a high probability of becoming infected.[28] Transplantation of an organ from an infected donor is controversial.

HEPATITIS D AND E VIRUSES

HDV occurs only in patients with HBV and is transmitted percutaneously. Simultaneous infection with HBV and HDV may produce a more severe acute hepatitis than that caused by HBV alone.[12]

HEV is a common cause of large epidemics of acute viral hepatitis in developing countries. It characteristically affects adults and may be associated with an unusually high mortality in pregnant women.[13] Epidemics have occurred in rural Mexico, with a high attack rate and with jaundice occurring in more than 5% of the local population. HEV infection has also been found in immigrants to the United States and in travelers to Mexico and the Indian subcontinent.[29]

Diagnosis

CLINICAL MANIFESTATIONS

The onset of viral hepatitis may be gradual or sudden. The symptoms are protean [see Table 3].[1,2] The most common early symptoms are fatigue, lassitude, drowsiness, anorexia, nausea, and dark urine. Dehydration may result from repeated vomiting. Low-grade fever is common; shaking chills are rare. Frank pain

Table 3 Incidence of Symptoms
in Acute Viral Hepatitis

Symptom	Percentage of Patients
Dark urine	94
Fatigue	91
Anorexia	90
Nausea	87
Fever	76
Emesis	71
Headache	70
Abdominal discomfort	65
Light stools	52
Myalgia	52
Drowsiness	49
Irritability	43
Itching	42
Diarrhea	25
Arthralgia	21

may occur in the right upper quadrant, but vague, generalized abdominal discomfort is more common. Itching may occur but is seldom severe. Diarrhea occurs in some cases. About half of patients have myalgias or arthralgias, and some have acute arthritis with local pain, redness, swelling, and effusions. Joint symptoms are usually associated with HBV and HEV infections. Many of these early symptoms abate when jaundice develops or shortly thereafter. In the unusual case of severe hepatitis, confusion, stupor, or even coma may develop; fetor hepaticus and asterixis are usually present.

PHYSICAL EXAMINATION

The sclerae and skin may be icteric. The liver is often enlarged and tender. The spleen is palpable in about 10% of patients. Asterixis, marked peripheral edema, or ascites implies that the disease is unusually severe and suggests a poor prognosis.

LABORATORY TESTS

General Laboratory Findings

Most patients have mild anemia and relative lymphocytosis. The leukocyte count is usually normal but may be greater than 12,000/mm^3. The serum bilirubin level generally does not exceed 15 to 20 mg/dl; levels greater than 30 mg/dl imply severe disease or associated hemolysis. Serum aspartate aminotransferase (AST) and serum alanine aminotransferase (ALT) levels rise 7 to 14 days before the onset of jaundice and begin to fall shortly after jaundice occurs. The degree of aminotransferase elevation does not necessarily parallel severity, but levels less than 500 IU/L usually reflect mild illness.

Serum alkaline phosphatase level is slightly increased but may be markedly elevated in the few patients in whom prominent cholestasis develops later in the course of acute illness. Serum γ-globulin levels are normal or slightly elevated; concentrations greater than 3 g/dl suggest chronic active hepatitis rather than acute viral hepatitis. The serum albumin level and prothrombin time reflect liver cell synthetic capacity and are depressed in patients with severe, acute viral hepatitis.

Serologic and Virologic Assays

Serologic assays are used to identify each type of viral hepatitis [see Table 1].

Hepatitis A virus The IgM antibody to HAV (IgM anti-HAV) appears early and is quite specific for acute HAV infection. It typically persists for an average of 3 months and is then replaced by the IgG anti-HAV, which lasts throughout life and confers immunity to future infection.

Hepatitis B virus A number of serologic tests are useful to physicians who are caring for patients with acute HBV infection [see Table 4]. HBsAg is present on the surface of the hepatitis B virion and in the circulation as spheres and filaments [see Figure 1]. It appears in the serum of infected persons as early as 1 to 2 weeks after parenteral injection of infectious virus and may persist for months. If HBsAg remains in the serum of an infected person for 6 months after an episode of acute HBV infection, it will probably persist indefinitely. The antibody to HBsAg usually appears in the blood 2 to 4 months after an attack of acute HBV infection resolves—in most cases, after HBsAg is no longer detectable. Antibody to the core antigen (anti-HBc) appears promptly in the blood of infected persons and persists indefinitely. High titers of

Table 4   Tests for Hepatitis B Virus Infection

Symbol	Characteristics
HBsAg	Hepatitis B surface antigen; present in surface coat of the hepatitis B virus and in the 22 nm diameter filaments and spheres; purified surface antigen expressed in yeast cells is used in the recombinant hepatitis B vaccines
Anti-HBs	Antibody to HBsAg; present during convalescent phase of acute hepatitis B infection and after successful hepatitis B vaccination; hepatitis B immune globulin derived from serum with high anti-HBs titers is effective in preventing clinical hepatitis B infection
Anti-HBc	Antibody to the hepatitis B virus core; present in all patients with any form of hepatitis B infection; presence of this antibody in the sera is evidence that the patient has been infected in the past or is currently infected with the hepatitis B virus
IgM anti-HBc	Antibody to the hepatitis B core antigen; present in high titers in patients with acute hepatitis B; may be the only marker of acute infection when HBsAg is no longer detectable
Anti-HDV	Antibody to hepatitis D; serologic marker of coinfection or superinfection by hepatitis D of patients with hepatitis B
HBeAg	A soluble protein derived from the hepatitis B virus core; reflects presence in the blood of circulating hepatitis B virus; sera positive for this antigen are highly infectious
Anti-HBe	Anti-HBe appears weeks to months after HBeAg (and the circulating hepatitis B virus) is no longer detectable in the blood; sera positive for this antibody are substantially less infectious

IgM anti-HBc are found in patients with acute disease and may be the only marker of acute HBV infection if HBsAg is no longer detectable. Detection of HBeAg, a soluble protein derived from the core particle, correlates with the presence of HBV DNA and indicates that the HBV is actively replicating. Serum that is positive for HBeAg is highly infectious. A pregnant woman who is positive for HBsAg is much more likely to transmit HBV to her offspring if her blood also contains HBeAg or HBV DNA. The detection of antibody to HBeAg (anti-HBe) in association with the absence of HBV DNA is evidence that viral replication is minimal and the blood is substantially less infectious.

Hepatitis C virus   Detection of antibodies to HCV (anti-HCV) remains the most practical way to diagnose acute and chronic HCV infection.[30,31] Second- and third-generation anti-HCV enzyme-linked immunosorbent assays (ELISA) are now in use. They employ several viral antigens, making them more sensitive and specific than the first-generation test. Recombinant immunoblot assay (RIBA) is the most commonly used supplemental assay for specificity. It incorporates four antigens as separate bands: reaction of two or more of the four bands is considered a positive RIBA test result; reaction of only one band is indeterminate. Third-generation RIBAs appear more specific than earlier generations but are not commonly used because of the widespread availability of HCV RNA assays.

The detection of serum HCV RNA can be used to establish viremia and is widely employed in the management of chronic HCV infection.[30,31] The diagnosis of acute HCV infection can also be established early, before the appearance of anti-HCV, by HCV RNA assays. These assays have become standardized, and serum HCV RNA can be detected both qualitatively and quantitatively. Quantitative HCV RNA assays may help predict the response to interferon: patients with lower levels of viremia respond better than those with higher levels. Finally, in patients with normal serum aminotransferase and RIBA results positive for anti-HCV, serum HCV RNA can distinguish between active infection with viremia and recovery from previous HCV infection.

Hepatitis D and E viruses   HDV infection is diagnosed by the detection of anti-HDV with HBsAg. Patients with acute HDV infection will have HBsAg with IgM anti-HBc along with anti-HDV (i.e., coinfection), whereas patients with chronic HBV infection who are superinfected with HDV will have a negative IgM anti-HBc. HEV is diagnosed by the detection of antibodies to HEV (anti-HEV). Anti-HEV is found in acute and convalescent serum from patients with acute HEV infection. This assay has yet to be licensed in the United States.

Liver Biopsy

Liver biopsy is not usually performed in patients with acute viral hepatitis, because serologic tests are generally diagnostic. Spotty necrosis of liver cells and an inflammatory cell reaction that consists primarily of lymphocytes and histiocytes are the typical histologic findings. Acidophils (dying liver cells) and bile plugs are common. Biopsy performed late in the course of the disease reveals prominent evidence of hepatic cell regeneration (rosette formation and multinucleated cells) and pigment-filled histiocytes. Although usually more marked in the pericentral areas, the inflammatory reaction and cell necrosis appear throughout the parenchyma. In severe hepatitis, necrotic zones link portal areas to one another or to central areas, or they may involve whole lobules (bridging necrosis). The portal tracts contain a mild to moderate mononuclear cell inflammatory reaction, and the limiting plate, which demarcates portal areas from parenchymal cells, may be disrupted.

CLINICAL COURSE

Hepatitis typically produces symptoms for 1 to 2 weeks before the onset of dark urine and jaundice. As icterus deepens, appetite begins to return and malaise lessens. The serum bilirubin level rises for 10 to 14 days and then declines over 2 to 4 weeks. Aminotransferase levels usually begin to decline just before peak jaundice occurs and fall quite rapidly thereafter. The patient often feels much better by the time bilirubin levels have begun to decline. Usually, the clinical course is uneventful and recovery is complete, with liver function returning to normal.

In a small percentage of patients, the clinical course is atypical. Acute viral hepatitis may be protracted in elderly patients or in those infected with either HBV or HCV; the disease may last several months, and full recovery may not occur for a year. Between 6% and 15% of patients with acute viral hepatitis will have recurrent symptoms and worsening of liver function before recovery from the initial attack is complete. This relapse is usually milder than the original attack and is short-lived. In a few patients, the disease has an acute fulminant course leading to hepatic coma and even death. These events appear to be more common in pregnant women infected with HEV. HCV appears to be an unusual cause of fulminant disease.[32] In some countries, a mutant form of HBV that is incapable of encoding for e antigen is associated with fulminant disease.[9] Often, no virus can be identified, leading to speculation that other viruses may be involved—either mutant viruses or as yet unidentified viruses. Some patients do not recover completely from the initial attack, and chronic hepatitis develops. Chronic hepatitis does not occur after HAV or HEV infection. It ensues in 1% to 5% of cases of acute HBV infection and 85% of cases of acute HCV infection.[1,2]

A study in Italy has found that HBsAg carriers who are symptom-free and whose liver function tests are normal have an excellent prognosis. In this study, the risk of hepatocellular carcinoma was low over the mean follow-up period of about 11 years.[33] The natural history of HCV infection is still being studied. Chronic HCV infection appears to progress but does so slowly over many decades.[26,34] In two histologic studies of chronic HCV infection from blood transfusion, the times to the presence of chronic HCV infection averaged 12 years; to the presence of cirrhosis, 21 years; and to the presence of hepatocellular carcinoma, 29 years.[35,36] Both studies reported experiences from tertiary liver centers, however, which may have introduced referral bias. More recent studies suggest that chronic HCV infection is more benign than originally reported and is associated with a low rate of cirrhosis.[37-40] In a large, prospective study of 568 patients with posttransfusion non-A, non-B hepatitis (mostly HCV) who were followed for an average of 18 years, there was no increase in mortality from all causes, but there was a small increase in the number of deaths related to liver disease.[39] Another large, cross-sectional study from Europe of 2,235 patients with chronic HCV infection found the median time from infection to cirrhosis was 30 years,[40] about 10 years longer than the 21-year interval from infection to cirrhosis reported earlier.[35,36] Analysis of liver biopsy specimens showed the rate of fibrosis progression was not normally distributed, with approximately one third of persons progressing to cirrhosis in less than 20 years and another third not appearing to progress to cirrhosis for at least 50 years. Factors associated with an increase in the rate of fibrosis progression were age at which infection occurred (> 40 years), daily alcohol use (> 50 g), and male gender. The role of heavy alcohol abuse in exacerbating the risk of cirrhosis has been confirmed.[41] Once cirrhosis develops in patients with chronic HCV infection, the 10-year rates of decompensation of cirrhosis and development of hepatocellular carcinoma are 29% (3.9% yearly) and 14% (1.4% yearly), respectively.[42] Chronic HBV infection also predisposes the infected person to the development of primary hepatocellular carcinoma, perhaps through the integration of viral DNA into the genome of the host's hepatocytes.[43]

Unusual and sometimes fatal complications of acute viral hepatitis include aplastic anemia, hemolytic anemia, hypoglycemia, and polyarteritis. The risk appears to be higher if infection occurs at a very early age or if chronic liver disease is also present.

Differential Diagnosis

At the time of initial presentation with symptoms and elevated aminotransferase levels, before the results of serologic tests are known, it is worthwhile to consider the differential diagnosis of acute viral hepatitis.

EPSTEIN-BARR VIRUS

EBV, a herpesvirus, usually produces mild hepatitis associated with nausea and vomiting; jaundice occurs in only 10% to 20% of patients.[44] Serum aminotransferase is moderately elevated (300 to 500 IU/L). In most instances, the hepatitis is part of the typical clinical syndrome of infectious mononucleosis. Rarely, hepatic dysfunction is severe and proves to be fatal, particularly in immunodeficient patients.[45] The virus appears to be transmitted during oral-oral contact through infected saliva and may be transmitted parenterally; the incubation period is about 28 days. A rise in titer of specific fluorescent antibodies to EBV or detection and quantitation of viral levels confirm the diagnosis.

CYTOMEGALOVIRUS

CMV, which is also a member of the herpesvirus group, is ubiquitous. About 80% of adults have serum complement-fixation reactivity for CMV. This virus can also produce a disease similar to infectious mononucleosis but without adenopathy or tonsillopharyngeal involvement.[46] Liver involvement may mimic that of the more common forms of viral hepatitis, but it is usually mild and does not progress to chronic liver disease. Diagnosis requires inoculation of an appropriate tissue culture with blood to demonstrate viremia. Polymerase chain reaction to assess quantitative viral loads is the best test and is becoming more widely used.

OTHER VIRUSES

Acute hepatitis caused by herpes simplex virus or varicella-zoster virus, usually accompanied by typical skin lesions, has occurred in immunocompromised patients.

DRUG-INDUCED HEPATITIS

Hundreds of drugs can cause hepatitis that may be indistinguishable from acute viral hepatitis.[47] These idiosyncratic drug reactions are infrequent, unpredictable, and not dose dependent. Clinical onset usually occurs within 2 to 6 weeks after therapy is started but may occur on the first day that the drug is administered or not until 6 months later. The disease may progress despite withdrawal of the drug; failure to withdraw the drug promptly may result in death.

One well-documented drug reaction is the hepatic necrosis that occurs in one in 9,000 to 10,000 patients given halothane. The hepatitis is often fatal and is more common in overweight women or in persons exposed a second time to the anesthetic. Fever, malaise, and elevated aminotransferase levels develop 1 to 12 days after initial exposure to the drug. Onset may be sooner after multiple exposures; the average delay is 3 days. Signs of hepatic necrosis include marked eosinophilia, marked elevation of serum aminotransferase and bilirubin levels, reduced serum albumin levels, and a prolonged prothrombin time. Other common drugs that cause hepatitis are isoniazid, methyldopa, phenytoin, and the sulfonamides. Because most drugs will injure the liver on rare occasions, hepatitis that develops shortly after initiation of a new medication should suggest a drug reaction. The treatment of choice is discontinuance of the medication.

Idiosyncratic drug reactions differ from hepatitis that results from drug overdose. Drug reactions of the latter type are rare because a clear potential for hepatotoxicity usually precludes release of the drug. Acetaminophen, however, is an exception and causes a direct type of liver injury when taken in excessive doses: more than 25 g orally, usually in a suicide attempt, will cause profound hepatocellular necrosis in most persons.[48] Cell injury occurs because the liver produces a toxic metabolite that is usually rendered harmless by conjugation with glutathione. When the drug dose is high, hepatic glutathione stores are depleted and the toxic metabolite accumulates and destroys liver cells.

Oral *N*-acetylcysteine, given in a loading dose of 140 mg/kg followed by 70 mg/kg every 4 hours for a total of 18 doses, reduces hepatotoxicity and mortality in cases of acetaminophen overdose.[49] The drug is most effective when given within 8 hours after the overdose but appears to have some effect as long as 24 hours after the ingestion of acetaminophen. Maximal medical support during the 1- to 2-week illness is mandatory. Acetaminophen can also cause severe hepatotoxicity when taken in high ordinary doses (3 to 4 g daily if hepatic glutathione stores are low as a result of alcoholism with malnutrition (the so-called Tylenol-alcohol syndrome). The beneficial role of *N*-acetylcysteine in this setting is less certain.

Treatment

Many treatments have been recommended for acute viral hepatitis, but it is unlikely that any of them alters the course of the disease. When the patient feels ill, it seems reasonable to reduce physical activity to a tolerable level. For some patients, bed rest may be indicated during the initial phase of illness. Once the patient feels better, there is no reason to restrict activity. Two large, controlled studies of young servicemen with viral hepatitis have shown convincingly that even heavy physical exercise in the recovery period does not result in more frequent relapse or chronic disease.[50,51]

Patients should be encouraged to eat whatever they can; there is no evidence that a low-fat diet is beneficial. At times, nausea and vomiting are so severe that hospitalization and intravenous fluid and electrolyte replacement become necessary. Abstention from alcohol is advised during the acute phase, although alcohol has not been shown to adversely affect the course of viral hepatitis.

Acute HCV infection is usually silent and thus not commonly seen in clinical practice. However, meta-analyses of published studies of interferon-based therapy for acute HCV infection support its efficacy in this setting.[52] In patients who remain viremic at 12 weeks after seroconversion, it is generally recommended that standard doses of peginterferon be administered weekly, with or without ribavirin, for 6 months, which, in comparison with no therapy, increases the likelihood of sustained biochemical (normal ALT levels) and virologic (undetectable HCV RNA) responses.[53]

Many forms of treatment have been recommended for the patient with severe acute viral hepatitis who becomes encephalopathic, but no regimen is clearly effective. In controlled clinical trials, corticosteroids,[54-57] cimetidine,[58] hyperimmune γ-globulin,[59] and exchange transfusions[60] had no effect on the course of acute hepatitis. Although no controlled trials have been completed, liver transplantation improves survival in patients with acute severe viral hepatitis and stage IV hepatic encephalopathy.[61]

Therapy for encephalopathic patients should be supportive, with evaluation for liver transplantation. Bacterial infections should be treated with suitable antibiotics. Bleeding warrants the administration of appropriate clotting factors (fresh frozen plasma, platelets, or both) and transfusions. Clotting abnormalities without bleeding do not justify massive transfusions of fresh frozen plasma, because congestive heart failure can result. Encephalopathy should be treated with oral lactulose (30 ml every 4 hours), although there is little evidence that acute encephalopathy responds to treatment.

Antiviral therapy is available for chronic HBV and chronic HCV infections [*see Chapter 70*].

Screening and Prevention

The U.S. Preventive Services Task Force and the Advisory Committee on Immunization Practices strongly recommend screening for HBsAg in all pregnant women at the first prenatal visit.[62,63] Routine screening of the general population is not recommended. In addition to pregnant women, the American Association for the Study of Liver Diseases recommends screening of high-risk groups: persons born in hyperendemic areas, men who have sex with men, injecting drugs users, patients on dialysis, HIV-infected patients, and family and household contacts of HBV-infected persons.[64]

Prevention of viral hepatitis entails avoidance of exposure to the virus, passive immunization with globulin products, and active immunization with specific vaccines.

PASSIVE IMMUNIZATION

Immune globulin is prepared from human plasma; when given intramuscularly, it decreases the clinical attack rate for HAV by sevenfold to eightfold. The official recommendation of the U.S. Public Health Service is to administer 0.02 ml/kg to contacts as soon as possible after exposure to a confirmed case of HAV infection.[62] Administration more than 2 weeks after exposure is not protective. The usual dose for adults is 2.0 ml; for children weighing up to 25 kg (55 lb), 0.5 ml; and for children between 25 and 50 kg (110 lb), 1.0 ml. Immune globulin should be given to all persons who share a household, hospital room, or dormitory room with an HAV patient. It should also be given to staff and children in day care centers where cases of HAV infection have been identified. When a food handler with acute HAV infection has been identified, immune globulin should be given to coworkers and considered for patrons of the eating establishment if they can be identified and treated within 2 weeks after exposure. Immune globulin need not be given to all contacts at work or school unless there is clear evidence of spread. Classmates and neighborhood children who play together frequently, however, probably should be immunized. Travelers to developing countries are at risk of acquiring HAV, particularly those who plan to visit extensively or to reside in areas with poor sanitation [*see Chapter 8*]. A single dose of 0.02 ml/kg of immune globulin will be protective for as long as 2 months; a dose of 0.06 ml/kg will be protective for 5 months.[65] Individuals who have received one dose of HAV vaccine at 1 month before exposure do not need immune globulin.

Immune globulin contains anti-HBs at low titer (approximately 1:100 by radioimmunoassay), whereas HBV immune globulin has an anti-HBs titer of greater than 1:100,000. When the source is known to be HBsAg positive, persons exposed (by percutaneous or mucous membrane routes) should be given HBV immune globulin (0.06 ml/kg) and HBV vaccine within 24 hours.[63,64] When the HBsAg status of the source is unknown, the first dose of HBV vaccine should be given promptly and the series completed as recommended. If the source is subsequently found to be HBsAg positive, HBV immune globulin (0.06 ml/kg) should be administered, provided that it can be given within 7 days after exposure. Infants who are born to HBsAg-positive mothers should receive 0.5 ml of HBV immune globulin intramuscularly and 0.5 ml of HBV vaccine intramuscularly at another site within 12 hours after birth.

Prophylaxis against HCV infection with γ-globulin is more problematic. Its effect in household or casual contacts and after a needle-stick injury is unknown. The value of immune globulin in the prevention of HEV infection is also uncertain.

Table 5 Administration Schedules and Dosing of Hepatitis B Vaccines[63,64]

Patients	Schedule	Dose Engerix-B	Recombivax
Infants—maternal HBsAg status			
Negative	At birth (before discharge), 1–2, and 6–18 mo	10 µg/0.5 ml	5.0 µg/0.5 ml
Positive or unknown	At birth (≤ 12 hr),* 1–2 mo, and 6 mo	10 µg/0.5 ml	5.0 µg/0.5 ml
Children and adolescents (1–19 yr)	0, 1–2, and 4–6 mo	10 µg/0.5 ml	5.0 µg/0.5 ml
Alternative two-dose regimen for adolescents (11–15 yr)	0 and 4–6 mo	—	10 µg/1.0 ml
Adults (≥ 20 yr)	0, 1–2, and 4–6 mo	20 µg/1.0 ml	10 µg/1.0 ml
Immunocompromised or hemodialysis (< 20 yr)	0, 1, and 6 mo	10 µg/0.5 ml	5.0 µg/0.5 ml
Immunocompromised or hemodialysis (≥ 20 yr)	0, 1, 2, and 6 mo‡ 0, 1, and 6 mos§	40 µg/2.0 ml‡	40 µg/1.0 ml§

*In newborn infants of HBsAg-positive mothers, given with simultaneous administration of hepatitis B immune globulin at a different site.
†Adult formulation.
‡Two 1.0-ml doses administered at one site, on a four-dose schedule at 0, 1, 2, and 6 months.
§Dialysis formulation administered on a three-dose schedule at 0, 1, and 6 months.
HBsAg—hepatitis B surface antigen

ACTIVE IMMUNIZATION

Two HBV vaccines that are produced by recombinant DNA techniques are available (Recombivax HB, Merck & Co., and Engerix-B, SmithKline Beecham Biologicals) [see Table 5].[63,66] Both vaccines are highly effective in inducing antibody to HBV and preventing HBV infection in infants, children, and adults. The recommendations of the Centers for Disease Control and Prevention for the use of HBV vaccine are outlined [see Table 6].

The vaccines are given in three I.M. doses into the deltoid muscle in children and adults, and into the anterolateral thigh muscle in infants and neonates. A suboptimal response has been observed when the vaccine was injected into the buttocks.[67] The second dose is given 1 to 2 months after the first; the third dose is usually given 6 months after the first. For healthy adults, depending on the vaccine preparation, each dose should contain 10 or 20 µg of HBsAg; for patients undergoing hemodialysis and for other immunosuppressed patients, each dose should contain 40 µg; and for infants, children, and adolescents younger than 20 years, each dose should contain 5 to 10 µg. In adolescents aged 11 to 15 years, an alternative two-dose regimen using the adult dose administered at 0 and 4 to 6 months may be considered.

Universal vaccination of all newborns is recommended, regardless of the HBsAg status of the mother. In addition, all children and adolescents younger than 19 years should receive the HBV vaccine series.[63] The vaccine should be given to groups at substantial risk for HBV infection: hospital staff and other health care workers with frequent exposure to blood products, clients and staff of institutions for the mentally retarded, hemodialysis patients, homosexually active males, users of I.V. drugs, recipients of certain blood products, contacts of HBV carriers, special high-risk populations (e.g., emigrants from areas with highly endemic disease), and prisoners. It should be strongly considered for travelers who plan to reside in areas with high levels of endemic HBV infection.

Approximately 3% to 4% of healthy people have little or no antibody response to the vaccine. They appear to lack an immune response gene in the major histocompatibility complex that accounts for the ability to mount a normal antibody response to HBsAg.[68] Repeat vaccination induces a protective level of antibody in less than 50% of such people.[69] Those who do not respond to vaccine and who later become infected with HBV do not have an unusual clinical course.

After successful vaccination, titers of antibody to HBsAg begin to decline, and in 5 years, 20% to 30% of patients lack protective levels.[70] These persons will respond immediately to a booster dose of vaccine, but routine booster vaccination is not recommended.[63] HBV infection may develop in a few persons when the antibody titer falls to low levels, but the infection is invariably asymptomatic and is usually identified only by the development of antibody to the core antigen. However, a booster dose should be given to hemodialysis patients whose anti-HBs level falls below 10 mIU/ml and similarly should be considered in other immunocompromised persons at risk.[63]

Two inactivated HAV vaccines are currently available [see Table 7]. A large, randomized, double-blind efficacy trial demonstrating protection against HAV infection was carried out in Thailand.[71] A total of 40,119 children 1 to 16 years of age received Havrix (Glaxo-

Table 6 Recommendations for Use of Hepatitis B Vaccine[63,66]

Routine immunization
  Universal vaccination of infants beginning at birth
  Vaccination of all previously unvaccinated children and adolescents

Previously unvaccinated adults at increased risk for HBV infection
  Persons with multiple sexual partners
  Sexual partners or household contacts of HBsAg-positive persons
  Men who have sex with men
  Injecting drug users
  Travelers to regions of high HBV endemicity
  Persons with occupational exposure to blood or body fluids
  Clients and staff of institutions for developmentally disabled persons
  Patients with chronic renal failure
  Patients receiving clotting factor concentrates

HBsAg—hepatitis B surface antigen   HBV—hepatitis B virus

Table 7   Administration Schedules and Dosing of Hepatitis A Vaccines

Vaccine	Patients	Dosage	Schedule (months)
Havrix	Children and adolescents (12 mo–18 yr)	720 ELU/0.5 ml	0, 6–12
	Adults (> 18 yr)	1,440 ELU/1.0 ml	0, 6–12
VAQTA	Children and adolescents (12 mo–18 yr)	25 U/0.5 ml	0, 6–18
	Adults (> 18 yr)	50 U/1.0 ml	0, 6–18

ELU—enzyme-linked immunosorbent assay unit

SmithKline) or a control HBV vaccine (Engerix-B) at 0, 1, and 12 months. Patients were crossed over to the alternative vaccine at 18 months. Side effects were minor. The efficacy of Havrix was 94% before the month-12 booster injection and 99% after it. A study of the other inactivated HAV vaccine (VAQTA, Merck & Co.) in 1,037 children in upstate New York found that this vaccine was also safe and 100% effective in preventing HAV infection 50 to 137 days after administration of a single dose.[72] Both Havrix and VAQTA are administered to adults in a 1 ml dose I.M. and to children and adolescents aged 12 months to 18 years in a 0.5 ml dose I.M., followed by a booster in 6 to 12 months (Havrix) or 6 to 18 months (VAQTA).

Compared with the short-term protection afforded by immune globulin, inactivated HAV vaccine will probably induce protection lasting from 5 to 10 years and perhaps much longer.[73] In the United States, the overall incidence of HAV infection has decreased, leading to a higher proportion of adults who are susceptible. Older individuals are known to experience a more severe clinical course, and thus, the costs of HAV infection in the United States remain substantial.[74] These facts underline the importance of ensuring compliance with the current recommendations for HAV vaccination.[65] Routine vaccination of children and adolescents aged 12 months to 18 years is recommended. The vaccine will be particularly useful in preventing HAV infection in persons at high risk for the disease, such as travelers and immigrants to highly endemic regions. The risk of symptomatic HAV infection in travelers staying in Western-style accommodations in high-risk countries is three per 1,000 persons per month.[75] Backpackers or travelers in areas with poor hygienic conditions have a higher risk (20 per 1,000 persons per month). In unprotected travelers from the United States, the incidence of HAV infection is 10 to 100 times that of typhoid fever and 1,000 times that of cholera. Other persons at risk for HAV infection are listed [*see Table 8*].[65] Finally, patients with chronic liver disease may experience a more severe illness with acute HAV infection.[76,77] HAV vaccination has been shown to be safe and effective in patients with chronic viral liver disease.[78]

In addition to single-antigen vaccines for HBV and HAV, three combination vaccines are now available: an HBV–*Haemophilus influenzae* vaccine (Comvax, Merck & Co.), an HBV–diphtheria, tetanus, acellular pertussis–inactivated poliovirus vaccine (Pediarix, Glaxo-SmithKline), and an HAV–HBV vaccine (Twinrix, Glaxo-SmithKline). Comvax and Pediarix are for pediatric use; Twinrix is licensed for persons 18 years of age and older.

The author has no commercial relationships with manufacturers of products or providers of services discussed in this chapter.

References

1. Ryder SD, Beckingham IJ: ABC of diseases of liver, pancreas, and biliary system: acute hepatitis. BMJ 322:151, 2001

2. Younossi ZM: Viral hepatitis guide for practicing physicians. Cleveland Clinic of Medicine. Cleve Clin J Med 67(suppl 1):SI6, 2000

3. Summary of notifiable diseases, United States, 1999. MMWR Morb Mortal Wkly Rep 48:1, 2001

4. Yokosuka O: Molecular biology of hepatitis A virus: significance of various substitutions in the hepatitis A virus genome. J Gastroenterol Hepatol 15(suppl):D91, 2000

5. Feinstone SM, Kapikian AZ, Purcell RH: Hepatitis A: detection by immune electron microscopy of a viruslike antigen associated with acute illness. Science 182:1026, 1973

6. Lee WM: Hepatitis B virus infection. N Engl J Med 337:1733, 1997

7. Norder H, Courouce AM, Magnius LO: Complete genomes, phylogenetic relatedness, and structural proteins of six strains of the hepatitis B virus, four of which represent two new genotypes. Virology 198:489, 1994

8. Stuyver L, De Gendt S, Van Geyt C, et al: A new genotype of hepatitis B virus: complete genome and phylogenetic relatedness. J Gen Virol 81(pt 1):67, 2000

9. Lok AS, Heathcote EJ, Hoofnagle JH: Management of hepatitis B: 2000—summary of a workshop. Gastroenterology 120:1828, 2001

10. Choo QL, Kuo G, Weiner AJ, et al: Isolation of a cDNA clone derived from a blood-borne non-A, non-B viral hepatitis genome. Science 244:359, 1989

11. Bukh J, Miller RH, Purcell RH: Genetic heterogeneity of hepatitis C virus: quasispecies and genotypes. Semin Liver Dis 15:41, 1995

12. Hadziyannis SJ: Review: hepatitis delta. J Gastroenterol Hepatol 12:289, 1997

13. Krawczynski K, Aggarwal R, Kamili S: Hepatitis E. Infect Dis Clin North Am 14:669, 2000

14. Deka N, Sharma MD, Mukerjee R: Isolation of the novel agent from human stool samples that is associated with sporadic non-A, non-B hepatitis. J Virol 68:7810, 1994

15. Linnen J, Wages J Jr, Zhang-Keck ZY, et al: Molecular cloning and disease association of hepatitis G virus: a transfusion-transmissible agent. Science 271:505, 1996

16. Simons JN, Leary TP, Dawson GJ, et al: Isolation of novel virus-like sequences associated with human hepatitis. Nat Med 1:564, 1995

17. Cheung RC, Keeffe EB, Greenberg HB: Hepatitis G virus: is it a hepatitis virus? West J Med 167:23, 1997

18. Hutin YJ, Pool V, Cramer EH, et al: A multistate, foodborne outbreak of hepatitis A. National Hepatitis A Investigation Team. N Engl J Med 340:595, 1999

19. Staes CJ, Schlenker TL, Risk I, et al: Sources of infection among persons with acute hepatitis A and no identified risk factors during a sustained community-wide outbreak. Pediatrics 106:E54, 2000

Table 8   Recommendations for Use of Hepatitis A Vaccine[65]

Routine immunization

All children at age 1 yr (i.e., 12–23 mo). Vaccination should be integrated into the routine childhood vaccination schedule according to the licensed schedules. Children ages 2–18 years who have not been vaccinated by age 2 yr can be vaccinated at subsequent visits.

Persons at increased risk for HAV infection

Persons traveling to or working in countries with high or intermediate HAV endemicity, such as Mexico, the Caribbean, Southeast Asia, South and Central America, and Africa

Men who have sex with men

Users of injection and noninjection illicit drugs

Individuals who work with HAV-infected primates or with HAV in research laboratories

Persons with clotting factor disorders

Outbreaks in communities with high or intermediate rates of HAV infection

Persons at increased risk for more severe disease

Persons with chronic liver disease

HAV—hepatitis A virus

20. Ruddy SJ, Johnson RF, Mosley JW, et al: An epidemic of clam-associated hepatitis. JAMA 208:649, 1969

21. Dentinger CM, Bower WA, Nainan OV, et al: An outbreak of hepatitis A associated with green onions. J Infect Dis 183:1273, 2001

22. Corey L, Holmes KK: Sexual transmission of hepatitis A in homosexual men: incidence and mechanism. N Engl J Med 302:435, 1980

23. Katz MH, Hsu L, Wong E, et al: Seroprevalence of and risk factors for hepatitis A infection among young homosexual and bisexual men. J Infect Dis 175:1225, 1997

24. Kuo G, Choo Q-L, Alter HJ, et al: An assay for circulating antibodies to a major etiologic virus of human non-A, non-B hepatitis. Science 244:362, 1989

25. Alter MJ: Epidemiology of hepatitis C. Hepatology 26(suppl 1):62S, 1997

26. Liang TJ, Rehermann B, Seeff LB, et al: Pathogenesis, natural history, treatment, and prevention of hepatitis C. Ann Intern Med 132:296, 2000

27. Dienstag JL: Sexual and perinatal transmission of hepatitis C. Hepatology 26(suppl 1):66S, 1997

28. Pereira BJ, Wright TL, Schmid CH, et al: A controlled study of hepatitis C transmission by organ transplantation. The New England Organ Bank Hepatitis C Study Group. Lancet 345:484, 1995

29. Hepatitis E among U.S. travelers, 1989–1992. MMWR Morb Mortal Wkly Rep 42:1, 1993

30. Gretch DR: Diagnostic tests for hepatitis C. Hepatology 26(suppl 1):43S, 1997

31. Lok ASF, Gunaratnam NT: Diagnosis of hepatitis C. Hepatology 26(suppl 1):48S, 1997

32. Hoofnagle JH: Hepatitis C: the clinical spectrum of disease. Hepatology 26(suppl 1):15S, 1997

33. de Franchis R, Meucci G, Vecchi M, et al: The natural history of asymptomatic hepatitis B surface antigen carriers. Ann Intern Med 118:191, 1993

34. Seeff LB: Natural history of hepatitis C. Hepatology 26(suppl 1):21S, 1997

35. Kiyosawa K, Sodeyama T, Tanaka E, et al: Interrelationship of blood transfusion, non-A, non-B hepatitis and hepatocellular carcinoma: analysis by detection of antibody to hepatitis C virus. Hepatology 12:671, 1990

36. Tong MJ, el-Farra NS, Reikes AR, et al: Clinical outcomes after transfusion-associated hepatitis C. N Engl J Med 332:1463, 1995

37. Wiese M, Berr F, Lafrenz M, et al: Low frequency of cirrhosis in a hepatitis C (genotype 1b) single-source outbreak in Germany: a 20-year multicenter study. Hepatology 32:91, 2000

38. Rodger AJ, Roberts S, Lanigan A, et al: Assessment of long-term outcomes of community-acquired hepatitis C infection in a cohort with sera stored from 1971 to 1975. Hepatology 32:582, 2000

39. Seeff LB, Buskell-Bales Z, Wright EC, et al: Long-term mortality after transfusion-associated non-A, non-B hepatitis. The National Heart, Lung, and Blood Institute Study Group. N Engl J Med 327:1906, 1992

40. Poynard T, Bedossa P, Opolon P: Natural history of liver fibrosis progression in patients with chronic hepatitis C. The OBSVIRC, METAVIR, CLINIVIR, and DOSVIRC groups. Lancet 349:825, 1997

41. Harris DR, Gonin R, Alter HJ, et al: The relationship of acute transfusion-associated hepatitis to the development of cirrhosis in the presence of alcohol abuse. Ann Intern Med 134:120, 2001

42. Fattovich G, Giustina G, Degos F, et al: Morbidity and mortality in compensated cirrhosis type C: a retrospective follow-up study of 384 patients. Gastroenterology 112:463, 1997

43. Martin P: Hepatocellular carcinoma: risk factors and natural history. Liver Transpl Surg 4(5 suppl 1):S87, 1998

44. Schiff GM: Hepatitis caused by viruses other than hepatitis A, hepatitis B, and non-A, non-B hepatitis viruses. Diseases of the Liver, 7th ed. Schiff L, Schiff ER, eds. JB Lippincott Co, Philadelphia, 1993, p 578

45. Markin RS, Linder J, Zuerlein K, et al: Hepatitis in fatal infectious mononucleosis. Gastroenterology 93:1210, 1987

46. Weller TH: The cytomegaloviruses: ubiquitous agents with protean clinical manifestations. I. N Engl J Med 285:203, 1971

47. Farrell GC: Drug-induced hepatic injury. J Gastroenterol Hepatol 12:S242, 1997

48. Makin AJ, Wendon J, Williams R: A 7-year experience of severe acetaminophen-induced hepatotoxicity (1987–1993). Gastroenterology 109:1907, 1995

49. Smilkstein MJ, Knapp GL, Kulig KW, et al: Efficacy of oral N-acetylcysteine in the treatment of acetaminophen overdose: analysis of the National Multicenter Study (1976 to 1985). N Engl J Med 319:1557, 1988

50. Chalmers TC, Eckhardt RD, Reynolds WE, et al: The treatment of acute infectious hepatitis: controlled studies of the effects of diet, rest, and physical reconditioning on the acute course of the disease and on the incidence of relapses and residual abnormalities. J Clin Invest 34:1163, 1955

51. Repsher LH, Freebern RK: Effects of early and vigorous exercise on recovery from infectious hepatitis. N Engl J Med 281:1393, 1969

52. Quin JW: Interferon therapy for acute hepatitis C viral infection: a review by meta-analysis. Aust N Z J Med 27:611, 1997

53. Heathcote J, Main J: Treatment of hepatitis C. J Viral Hepat 12:223, 2005

54. Gregory PB, Knauer CM, Kempson RL, et al: Steroid therapy in severe viral hepatitis: a double-blind, randomized trial of methyl-prednisolone versus placebo. N Engl J Med 294:681, 1976

55. Redeker AG, Schweitzer IL, Yamahiro HS: Randomization of corticosteroid therapy in fulminant hepatitis (letter). N Engl J Med 294:728, 1976

56. A double-blinded, randomized trial of hydrocortisone in acute hepatic failure (abstr). Acute Hepatic Failure Study Group. Gastroenterology 76:1297, 1979

57. Ware AJ, Cuthbert JA, Shorey J, et al: A prospective trial of steroid therapy in severe viral hepatitis. Gastroenterology 80:219, 1981

58. MacDougall BRD, Bailey RJ, Williams R: H₂-receptor antagonists and antacids in the prevention of acute gastrointestinal hemorrhage in fulminant hepatic failure. Lancet 1:617, 1977

59. Failure of specific immunotherapy in fulminant type B hepatitis. Acute Hepatic Failure Study Group. Ann Intern Med 86:272, 1977

60. Redeker AG, Yamahiro HS: Controlled trial of exchange-transfusion therapy in fulminant hepatitis. Lancet 1:3, 1973

61. Wall W, Adams PC: Liver transplantation for fulminant hepatic failure: North American experience. Liver Transplant Surg 1:178, 1995

62. Screening for hepatitis B virus infection: recommendation statement. U.S. Preventive Services Task Force. AHRQ Pub. No. 05-0550-A:1, 2004
http://www.ahrq.gov/clinic?uspstf/uspshepb.htm

63. A comprehensive strategy to eliminate transmission of hepatitis B virus infection in the United States. MMWR Recomm Rep 54(RR-16):1, 2005

64. Lok AF, McMahon BJ: Chronic hepatitis. Hepatology 39:857, 2004
https://www.aasld.org/eweb/dynamicpage.aspx?site=AASLD3&webcode=ViralHepatitis

65. Prevention of hepatitis A through active or passive immunization: recommendations of the Advisory Committee on Immunization Practices (ACIP). MMWR Recomm Rep 55(RR-07):1, 2006

66. A comprehensive strategy to eliminate transmission of hepatitis B virus infection in the United States. MMWR Morb Mortal Wkly Rep 54(RR-16):1, 2005
Errata: MMWR Morb Mortal Wkly Rep 55:158, 2006

67. Suboptimal response to hepatitis B vaccine given by injection into the buttock. MMWR Morb Mortal Wkly Rep 34:105, 1985

68. Alper CA, Kruskall MS, Marcus-Bagley D, et al: Genetic prediction of nonresponse to hepatitis B vaccine. N Engl J Med 321:708, 1989

69. Weissman JY, Tsuchiyose MM, Tong MJ, et al: Lack of response to recombinant hepatitis B vaccine in nonresponders to the plasma vaccine. JAMA 260:1734, 1988

70. Wainwright RB, McMahon BJ, Bulkow LR, et al: Duration of immunogenicity and efficacy of hepatitis B vaccine in a Yupik Eskimo population. JAMA 261:2362, 1989

71. Innis BL, Snitbhan R, Kunasol P, et al: Protection against hepatitis A by an inactivated vaccine. JAMA 271:1328, 1994

72. Werzberger A, Mensch B, Kuter B, et al: A controlled trial of formalin-inactivated hepatitis A vaccine in healthy children. N Engl J Med 327:453, 1992

73. Lemon SM: Inactivated hepatitis A vaccines (editorial). JAMA 271:1363, 1994

74. Berge JJ, Drennan DP, Jacobs RJ, et al: The cost of hepatitis A infections in American adolescents and adults in 1997. Hepatology 31:469, 2000

75. Steffen R, Kane MA, Shapiro CN, et al: Epidemiology and prevention of hepatitis A in travelers. JAMA 272:885, 1994

76. Keeffe EB: Acute hepatitis A and B in patients with chronic liver disease: prevention with vaccination. Am J Med 118:21S, 2005

77. Vento S, Garofano T, Renzini C, et al: Fulminant hepatitis associated with hepatitis A virus superinfection in patients with chronic hepatitis C. N Engl J Med 338:286, 1998

78. Keeffe EB, Iwarson S, McMahon BJ, et al: Safety and immunogenicity of hepatitis A vaccine in patients with chronic liver disease. Hepatology 27:881, 1998

Acknowledgments

Figure 1   Alan D. Iselin.
Figure 2   Seward Hung.

Peter F. Malet, M.D., F.A.C.P.

Definition

Chronic hepatitis is a term that encompasses an etiologically diverse group of clinical and pathologic diseases. Chronic hepatitis is characterized by the presence of hepatic inflammation on liver biopsy and elevation of serum liver enzymes, especially transaminases.[1] Chronic hepatitis is generally defined as disease that has lasted for 6 months or longer; in many cases, however, the diagnosis can be established earlier.

Etiology

The most important diseases that cause chronic hepatitis are (1) autoimmune hepatitis (AIH) (previously called autoimmune chronic active hepatitis), (2) chronic hepatitis B, which is caused by infection with hepatitis B virus (HBV), and (3) chronic hepatitis C, caused by hepatitis C virus (HCV) [*see Table 1*].

The hepatitis D virus (HDV) may also be present in some patients with HBV infection. Chronic overuse of alcohol may result in chronic hepatic inflammation (alcohol-induced liver disease or alcoholic hepatitis). Nonalcoholic steatohepatitis (NASH) is similar histologically to alcohol-induced liver disease and is discussed more fully elsewhere [*see Chapter 71*]. Less commonly, chronic hepatitis is cryptogenic or caused by drugs. Wilson disease, α_1-antitrypsin deficiency, primary biliary cirrhosis (PBC), and primary sclerosing cholangitis (PSC) are also chronic liver diseases characterized by hepatocellular or bile duct inflammation, but the term chronic hepatitis is not generally used to describe these conditions. Over the past decade, international working groups have substantially modified the terminology of chronic hepatitis to reflect an etiologic basis rather than a pathologic basis.[1] As a result, previously used terms, such as chronic active hepatitis and chronic persistent hepatitis, are no longer used.

Table 1 Major Types of Autoimmune and Chronic Viral Hepatitis

Type/Subtype	Diagnosis
Autoimmune	
Type 1 (classic)	(+) ANA
	(+) ASMA
Type 2	(+) anti-LKM1
Type 3	(+) anti-SLA
	(+) anti-LP
Chronic hepatitis B	(+) HBsAg
	(+) anti-HBc
	(-) anti-HBs
	(+) HBV DNA > 100,000 copies/ml
(+) e antigen	(+) HBeAg
	(-) anti-HBe
(-) e antigen	(-) HBeAg
	(+) anti-HBe
Chronic hepatitis C	(+) anti-HCV
	(+) HCV RNA

ANA—antinuclear antibody ASMA—anti–smooth muscle antibody HBc—hepatitis B c antigen HBeAG—hepatitis B e antigen HBsAG—hepatitis B s antigen HBV—hepatitis B virus HCV—hepatitis C virus LKM—liver/kidney microsome LP—liver/pancreas antigen SLA —soluble liver antigen

Approach to Chronic Hepatitis

DIAGNOSIS

Clinical Manifestations

Clinical manifestations of chronic hepatitis are diverse, ranging from asymptomatic disease characterized by mildly elevated aminotransferase levels to severe, rapidly progressive illness and fulminant hepatic failure. The most common symptoms of chronic hepatitis are fatigue, malaise, and mild abdominal discomfort. Patients with mild chronic hepatitis are usually asymptomatic or have minimal symptoms with no stigma of chronic liver disease on physical examination. In more advanced cases, when hepatic synthetic function begins to diminish (a condition referred to as hepatic decompensation), the symptoms and signs may include anorexia, jaundice, spider angiomas, palmar erythema, ascites, edema, and encephalopathy. Pruritus may occur but is unusual; pruritus is more characteristic of PBC or PSC. A small proportion of patients with AIH have an acute fulminant course and are critically ill at initial presentation. Some extrahepatic manifestations of chronic hepatitis include arthralgias, arthritis, glomerulonephritis, and skin rashes.

Standard Laboratory Tests

The serum alanine aminotransferase (ALT) and aspartate aminotransferase (AST) levels are usually elevated in patients with chronic hepatitis; however, a minority of patients, especially those who have chronic hepatitis B or C, may have either persistently or transiently normal aminotransferase levels. Therefore, even a mild elevation of aminotransferase levels (5 to 10 IU/L higher than the upper limit of normal) should lead physicians to consider the presence of chronic hepatitis. Elevations of more than 400 IU/L are not unusual in cases of AIH and may occasionally be seen with chronic hepatitis B. Aminotransferase levels that are twofold to threefold higher than the upper limit of normal are common with chronic hepatitis C. The serum bilirubin level is usually normal in chronic viral hepatitis, unless hepatic decompensation has occurred. The serum bilirubin level is higher than 3 mg/dl in patients with moderately severe AIH. A characteristic feature of AIH is an increased γ-globulin level (> 1.6 g/dl), which may sometimes be markedly increased (3 to 7 g/dl). In the most severe forms of chronic hepatitis, hepatic synthetic function is impaired; this is manifested by a decreased serum albumin level and a prolonged prothrombin time.

Imaging studies (i.e., ultrasonography and computed tomography) of the abdomen may be normal in early chronic hepatitis or may show variable degrees of hepatomegaly with or without splenomegaly. When more advanced hepatic fibrosis is present, irregularity of liver texture or contour may be seen. Evidence of portal hypertension with portal collateral vessels or ascites may be seen with advanced disease.

Liver Biopsy

The specific etiology of chronic hepatitis can usually be determined by clinical evaluation combined with serologic testing.

Table 2 METAVIR Scoring System for Grading Severity of Chronic Hepatitis

Grade/Stage	Grade of Inflammation	Stage of Fibrosis
1	Minimal	Portal
2	Mild	Periportal, rare bridging
3	Moderate	Bridging
4	Severe	Cirrhosis

Liver biopsy can confirm or exclude certain diagnoses and can establish the grade of inflammatory activity and the stage of fibrosis and cirrhosis.

The grade and stage of chronic hepatitis can be assessed with various semiquantitative scoring systems.[1,2] In the histology activity index (HAI) (also known as the Knodell score), the grades of inflammation range from 0 to 18, and the stages of fibrosis range from 0 to 4. The HAI is sometimes used in clinical research studies but is no longer commonly used in clinical practice.[2] The most popular scoring system for chronic hepatitis is the METAVIR system.[3] This system generates two scores from 0 to 4: one for the degree of inflammation and the other for the degree of fibrosis [*see Table 2*]. Other scoring systems are available but are not commonly used in clinical practice. In addition to the characterization of the degree of inflammation and fibrosis, the evaluation of a liver biopsy specimen from a patient with chronic hepatitis includes a description of all the findings present (e.g., steatosis, bile duct changes, granulomas, type of inflammatory cells, presence of iron, and Mallory hyaline) or a notation of their absence.

DIFFERENTIAL DIAGNOSIS

Primary Biliary Cirrhosis

On liver biopsy, PBC may have features similar to those of AIH but is differentiated by the presence of bile duct inflammation or ductopenia. Marked elevation of serum alkaline phosphatase and high titers of antimitochondrial antibody (AMA) (> 1:160) are useful in making the diagnosis of PBC.

Primary Sclerosing Cholangitis

PSC can sometimes mimic chronic hepatitis. Prominent elevations of the serum alkaline phosphatase level and accompanying inflammatory bowel disease will, in most cases, distinguish this disorder from other types of chronic hepatitis. The definitive diagnosis is made by endoscopic retrograde or magnetic resonance cholangiography.

Alcoholic Liver Disease

Liver enzyme elevations caused by alcohol overuse are very commonly encountered in clinical practice. When the patient admits to the overuse of alcohol, the diagnosis is straightforward; however, careful and repeated questioning of the patient and family members may sometimes be required to obtain an accurate assessment of the patient's alcohol use.

Fatty Liver and Nonalcoholic Steatohepatitis

Fatty liver and nonalcoholic steatohepatitis (NASH) are increasingly common liver diseases that are usually associated with obesity or being overweight. Fatty liver is characterized by macrovesicular and, sometimes, microvesicular steatosis without inflammation; serum transaminase levels may be normal or elevated, sometimes severalfold or more. NASH is characterized by hepatocellular inflammation, steatosis, and, usually, elevated serum transaminase levels. NASH may lead to fibrosis or to cirrhosis. Although radiologic studies are useful in the evaluation of suspected fatty liver and NASH, a definitive diagnosis may only be made with liver biopsy.

Drug-Induced Chronic Hepatitis

Drug-induced chronic hepatitis constitutes a small but important category of chronic hepatitis.[4] α-Methyldopa, nitrofurantoin, and isoniazid are well-recognized causes. In addition, cases have occasionally been reported after therapy with sulfonamides, propylthiouracil, diclofenac, terbinafine, and dantrolene; a number of other drugs have also been implicated. Thus, it is reasonable to discontinue as many medications as possible when chronic hepatitis is first diagnosed. If a patient's hepatitis is drug related, liver function abnormalities and the clinical course of disease frequently improve after the causative agent has been withdrawn, although improvement may take weeks or even months.

Wilson Disease

When neurologic abnormalities are absent, Wilson disease can present as chronic hepatitis. It is critical to establish the diagnosis of Wilson disease, because specific treatment with penicillamine, trientine, or zinc is available. In Wilson disease, the serum ceruloplasmin level is low and the 24-hour urinary copper level is elevated. Slit-lamp examination for Kayser-Fleischer rings should also be performed. Measurement of the hepatic copper content in a needle-biopsy specimen is diagnostic.

α_1-Antitrypsin Deficiency

α_1-Antitrypsin deficiency, which is usually associated with the presence of homozygous ZZ alleles, is associated with progressive liver disease, which evolves into cirrhosis. Liver disease associated with α_1-antitrypsin deficiency can be distinguished from chronic hepatitis by a reduced serum α_1-antitrypsin level and by inclusions in the liver parenchyma that are positive on periodic acid–Schiff (PAS) staining.

Autoimmune Hepatitis

AIH is characterized by portal and periportal inflammation and fibrosis, autoantibodies, and hypergammaglobulinemia.[5] The early recognition of AIH is important because the condition generally responds well to treatment; if left untreated, it can progress to cirrhosis and, occasionally, liver failure and death.

DIAGNOSIS

The diagnosis of AIH rests on the presence of characteristic findings combined with the exclusion of other causes of chronic liver disease. The presentation may be acute or subacute but is more commonly chronic. Other autoimmune diseases may be present concurrently.

Elevated levels of serum transaminase and γ-globulin are typical in AIH. Aminotransferase levels may be slightly elevated or more than 10 times higher than normal. The presence of antinuclear antibody (ANA) or one of the other autoantibodies is common.

A liver biopsy is always useful to establish histologic grading and staging; it is essential in cases in which the diagnosis is not clear on the basis of clinical and laboratory data. Interface hepatitis (formerly called piecemeal necrosis) is the histologic hallmark of AIH; however, this finding is not specific for AIH. The inflammatory component of AIH consists mainly of mononuclear cells; typically, plasma cells are present, but occasionally, they may not be a prominent feature.

In addition to its diagnostic use, liver biopsy is also an important prognostic tool. Patients with portal or mild periportal hepatitis (i.e., hepatitis that extends outside the limiting plate of the portal tract) generally respond well to therapy, whereas those with bridging necrosis (hepatitis that extends or bridges from one portal tract to another), multilobular necrosis, or cirrhosis respond less well to therapy and are at greater risk for progressive liver disease.

The International Autoimmune Hepatitis Group (IAIHG) has published a diagnostic scoring system for atypical AIH for use in adults when the diagnosis is uncertain.[6] The pretreatment score is based on 12 features, and the posttreatment score includes the response to therapy. A pretreatment score of 10 to 15 signifies probable AIH, whereas a score greater than 15 indicates definite AIH. A posttreatment score of 12 to 17 signifies probable AIH, whereas a score greater than 17 indicates definite AIH.

Disease Types

The wide spectrum of clinical and serologic manifestations of AIH has led investigators to propose several types of AIH[5,7] The distinctions in type are based on seropositive findings; however, it should be noted that in some cases of AIH, no serologic markers are present. All the proposed serologic types of AIH respond similarly to immunosuppressive therapy. Type 1, or classic, AIH is the most common form of the disease in the United States. It is characterized by hypergammaglobulinemia and the presence of ANA, anti–smooth muscle antibody (ASMA), or both. Type 2 AIH is characterized by the absence of ANA and ASMA and by the presence of antibody to liver/kidney microsome (anti-LKM1); it is much less common than type 1 and has been observed primarily in Europe. Type 3 is the least well characterized form of AIH, and it is distinguished by the presence of antibody to a soluble liver antigen (anti-SLA), to a recently characterized liver/pancreas antigen (anti-LP), or to both.

Table 3 Typical Regimens for Treatment of Autoimmune Hepatitis

	Schedule	Dose
Monotherapy	Initial dose	Prednisone, 60 mg p.o., q.d.
	Second week	Prednisone, 40 mg p.o., q.d.
	Third and fourth weeks	Prednisone, 30 mg p.o., q.d.
	Thereafter until end point is reached	Prednisone, 20 mg p.o., q.d.
Combination Therapy	Initial dose	Prednisone, 30 mg p.o., q.d. Azathioprine, 50 mg p.o., q.d.
	Second week	Prednisone, 20 mg p.o., q.d. Azathioprine, 50 mg p.o., q.d.
	Third and fourth weeks	Prednisone, 15 mg p.o., q.d. Azathioprine, 50 mg p.o., q.d.
	Thereafter until end point is reached	Prednisone, 10 mg p.o., q.d. Azathioprine, 50–100 mg p.o., q.d.

Overlap Syndromes

Overlap syndromes of AIH and either PBC or PSC have been recognized but are uncommon.[8,9] The term autoimmune cholangitis has been proposed to characterize patients who have biochemical or histologic cholestasis that resembles PBC. These patients test negative for AMA and have a normal IgM level; however, they have high titers of ANA and elevated levels of IgG. Results of cholangiography are normal.

TREATMENT

The standard treatment of AIH is immunosuppressive therapy. Three large randomized, controlled trials evaluated immunosuppressive treatment in patients with severe AIH[10-12]; however, data regarding treatment of patients with mild to moderate AIH are less extensive. The potential benefit of immunosuppressive therapy has to be balanced against the risks, particularly in cases of mild AIH. Most patients who have the clinical, biochemical, and histologic features of AIH should be treated,[5] but treatment may not be appropriate for some patients; for example, patients with advanced cirrhosis and relatively mild abnormalities of serum aminotransferase levels (less than twice the upper limit of normal) are probably not good candidates for such treatment.

The purpose of treatment is to relieve symptoms, decrease hepatic inflammation, and prevent the progression of hepatic fibrosis. The decision whether to initiate treatment can sometimes be problematic, particularly in cases that are atypical (e.g., when test results are negative for all autoantibodies). In such cases, the IAIHG scoring system can be useful in decision making.

Prednisone and Azathioprine Regimens

The usual regimen for most AIH patients consists of a combination of prednisone and azathioprine [see Table 3].[5] The starting doses are usually 30 mg of prednisone daily and 50 mg of azathioprine daily. Maintenance doses (until remission is achieved) are usually 20 mg of prednisone daily and 50 to 150 mg of azathioprine daily. Prednisone alone may be used with equal effectiveness; it is administered at a starting dose of 60 mg daily and is tapered over 4 weeks to a maintenance dose of 20 mg daily. Use of azathioprine may not be appropriate in patients who have severe cytopenia (because of the drug's bone marrow suppressive effect), who are pregnant (because of its potential to cause birth defects), or who have active malignancy (because of its potential to interfere with standard cancer treatment regimens). Azathioprine alone will not induce remission, but long-term azathioprine therapy is effective in maintaining remission.[13]

Response to Therapy

Clinical, biochemical, and histologic remission occurs in 65% of patients within 18 months and in 80% of patients within 3 years after starting treatment. In general, symptoms resolve (i.e., clinical remission) within 3 months, serum transaminase levels improve to normal or less than twice normal (i.e., biochemical remission) within 3 to 6 months, and histologic improvement (i.e., histologic remission) occurs within 18 months to 3 years. The presence of serum autoimmune markers, such as ANA, does not influence the initial response to therapy. Failure to achieve remission may represent either incomplete response to therapy or treatment failure. Patients who have an incomplete response to therapy may experience some improvement in clinical, laboratory, and histologic features when adequate therapy is administered. In cases of treatment failure, patients will experience worsening of disease despite adequate doses and compliance with therapy. Drug toxicities that necessitate the reduction of drug doses may contribute to the failure to achieve remission.

Discontinuance of Therapy

It is not clear-cut when to taper medication doses for the purpose of discontinuance of therapy. One commonly used approach is to begin tapering drugs when clinical and biochemical remissions have been achieved. Some authorities recommend a repeat liver biopsy to determine whether histologic remission has been achieved; however, this approach is not routine practice. When prednisone and azathioprine are used in combination, the dose of prednisone is usually tapered first while that of azathioprine is kept constant at 50 to 150 mg daily. Gradual tapering should occur over several months; however, there is no agreement on the rapidity of the tapering process. Once prednisone is completely discontinued, gradual tapering of azathioprine may begin.

Management of Relapse

Despite every precaution, relapse occurs within 3 to 6 months in approximately 20% to 90% of patients. Relapse is less likely if the histologic findings before tapering show that the hepatic inflammatory activity has completely resolved. If relapse occurs, medication doses should be increased in an attempt to induce remission. Once a patient has a relapse, however, the risk of future relapses is significant.

When a patient has had two or more relapses, a change in treatment approach is warranted[5]; with a change of medications, lower doses can be used to induce remission. After relapse, the aim of therapy is to keep disease activity as quiescent as possible. An acceptable therapeutic end point is a reduction of the serum transaminase level to two times normal or less. Such a serum transaminase level may be achieved with prednisone alone or in combination with azathioprine. Between 80% and 90% of patients can be maintained on a daily dosage of 10 mg of prednisone or less. When both drugs are used, the dose of prednisone can be gradually tapered while that of azathioprine is held constant at approximately 2 mg/kg/day; this combination regimen has a success rate in maintaining disease quiescence that is similar to that of prednisone alone. Limited data are available on the use of drugs such as 6-mercaptopurine and mycophenolate mofetil for the treatment of AIH.

Chronic Hepatitis B

EPIDEMIOLOGY

Chronic hepatitis B is a major global health care problem: 5% of the world's population, or approximately 350 million persons, are chronically infected.[14,15] In the United States, it is estimated that 1.25 million persons are chronically infected.[14] Approximately 0.2% to 0.5% of the United States population is positive for hepatitis B surface antigen (HBsAg); however, chronic HBV infection rates five to 10 times higher have been identified for certain groups, including Asian Americans, immigrants from endemic areas, persons who have received multiple blood transfusions or hemodialysis, intravenous drug users, men who have sex with men, and persons with HIV infection. Age at the time of initial HBV infection is the major determinant of chronicity. As many as 90% of infected neonates develop chronic infection; however, only 3% to 5% of newly infected adults develop

Table 4 Typical Serologic Findings in Hepatitis B Infection

Inactive Carrier State (low viral replication)	Chronic Hepatitis B (high viral replication)
(+) HBsAg	(+) HBsAg
(+) anti-HBc	(+) anti-HBc
(−) anti-HBs	(−) anti-HBs
(−) HBeAg	(+) HBeAg or (−) HBeAg
(+) anti-HBe	(+) HBeAg and (−) anti-HBe
HBV DNA < 100,000 copies/ml	HBV DNA > 100,000 copies/ml, typically in the range of 1 million to 10 million copies/ml
ALT and AST normal	ALT and AST elevated

ALT—alanine aminotransferase   AST—aspartate aminotransferase

chronic infection. Another important risk factor for chronicity is the presence of intrinsic or iatrogenic immunosuppression. Gender is also a well-established but poorly understood determinant of chronicity; women are more likely than men to clear HBsAg. As a result, men predominate in all populations with chronic HBV infection.

Ongoing HBV infection is an important risk factor for the development of hepatocellular carcinoma (HCC). The relative risk of HCC may be 200 times higher in patients with chronic HBV infection than in the general population. Patients with advanced fibrosis and cirrhosis are at highest risk. Evidence suggests that the use of screening tests, including ultrasonography and serum α-fetoprotein, may be useful in the early diagnosis of HCC.[14,16]

DIAGNOSIS

Chronic HBV infection can be readily diagnosed with serologic testing [see Table 4]. The diagnosis of chronic HBV infection is made when HBsAg remains detectable for more than 6 months. In a small percentage of patients with chronic HBV infection, mainly those who are inactive HBsAg carriers (i.e., 1% to 2% of patients a year), HBsAg clears spontaneously.

Categories of Hepatitis Infection

There are two broad categories of chronic HBV infection. The terminology to describe these states varies; the American Association for the Study of Liver Disease (AASLD) practice guidelines refer to these categories as the inactive carrier state and chronic hepatitis B.[14,15] A person who is positive for HBsAg, has normal aminotransferase levels, and has little or no necroinflammatory hepatic activity is an inactive HBsAg carrier. In inactive HBsAg carriers, the serum HBV DNA usually is relatively low ($< 10^5$ copies/ml). However, there are some inactive carriers in whom the serum HBV DNA may be much higher (often in the range of 10^7 to 10^{10} copies/ml), and this has been termed the immune-tolerant state. The immune-tolerant state is most characteristic of patients who were infected perinatally, most commonly in southern Asia.

The other broad disease category defined by AASLD practice guidelines is chronic hepatitis B. A person who is positive for HBsAg, has elevated aminotransferase levels, and has significant necroinflammatory hepatic activity is classified as having chronic hepatitis B. In patients with chronic hepatitis B, the serum HBV DNA usually is relatively high ($> 10^5$ copies/ml). In chronic hepatitis B, the HBeAg is usually positive (and anti-HBe negative); however, there is an increasing prevalence of HBeAg-negative disease. HBeAg is negative in patients with chronic hepatitis B because of a genetic mutation in the HBV DNA genome affecting the production of HBeAg. Chronic hepatitis B is subdivided into HBeAg-positive and HBeAg-negative disease. Typically, HBV DNA levels are somewhat lower in HBeAg-negative disease, and seroconversion from HBeAg to anti-HBe cannot be used as an end point for therapy in these patients.

TREATMENT

The ultimate goal of treatment of chronic hepatitis B is to eradicate HBV infection and prevent the development of cirrhosis or HCC. Interferon, lamivudine, and adefovir dipivoxil [see Table 5] can suppress HBV replication and lead to improvement in the clinical, biochemical, and histologic features of chronic hepatitis B.[14,15] The two oral agents, lamivudine and adefovir, are well tolerated. Interferon has a number of potential side effects, and careful consideration must be given to its use.

All patients with chronic hepatitis B should be considered for treatment.[17] In the majority of patients who are not considered suitable candidates for therapy, the severity of disease will be deemed too mild to warrant treatment. The most severely decompensated cirrhotic patients should be treated with lamivudine because of its extremely good tolerability. For those without severely decompensated cirrhosis, the decision whether to use interferon or oral therapy with lamivudine or adefovir is based on a variety of factors, not the least of which is patient preference. Oral therapy is very well tolerated; however, it typically requires several years of treatment to achieve a seroconversion rate comparable to that which can be achieved by interferon therapy in 6 to 9 months. On the other hand, interferon therapy has many more potential side effects and is considerably more expensive. Generally, interferon treatment is appropriate for those patients able to tolerate its potentially adverse effects.

Terminology Used in Describing Response to Treatment

In HBeAg-positive chronic hepatitis B, the term seroconversion indicates the loss of HBeAg and the appearance of anti-HBe. Seroconversion from HBsAg to anti-HBs can also occur, either spontaneously or after interferon treatment. Response to treatment can be (1) biochemical, as evidenced by the normalization of ALT levels; (2) virologic, as evidenced by a marked decrease in HBV DNA levels ($< 10^5$ copies/ml); or (3) histologic, as evidenced by improvement in or resolution of hepatic necroinflammatory activity. Such responses may be seen either during therapy or after therapy has been stopped. The response to treatment is considered a sustained response if remission is maintained for at least 6 months post treatment.

Interferon Therapy

Therapy with standard interferon has been most extensively studied; however, pegylated interferon (interferon alfa-2a and

alfa-2b) is being used increasingly in clinical practice because of its once-weekly administration and seroconversion rates that are as good as or better than those of standard interferon regimens.

A large number of trials have demonstrated the efficacy of interferon alfa in the treatment of HBeAg-positive chronic hepatitis B.[14] Doses of interferon alfa have been in the range of 5 million units daily to 10 million units three times a week. Treatment for 16 to 24 weeks results in seroconversion from HBeAg to anti-HBe, a low HBV DNA replicative state in about 35% of patients, and loss of HBsAg and the appearance of anti-HBs in approximately 8% of patients.[17] Predictors of a response to interferon therapy include lower pretreatment HBV DNA levels, higher ALT levels (optimally greater than five times the upper limit of normal), and short duration of infection; patients with such characteristics are optimal candidates for treatment with interferon. Relapse and reappearance of HBeAg occur in about 20% of patients. Patients who fail to seroconvert on interferon therapy should be treated with oral agents. It should be noted that interferon therapy is not equally effective in Asian patients, particularly in those whose ALT levels are only minimally elevated.

Patients with mildly decompensated cirrhosis can be treated with low, titrated doses of interferon, although the safety and tolerability of lamivudine or adefovir would make either of these drugs the first choice for treatment. One third of such patients will respond to therapy and have a sustained loss of HBV DNA and HBeAg, which may be associated with resolution of cirrhotic symptoms. These patients must be monitored closely, however, because bacterial infections and exacerbation of hepatitis are potentially serious complications.

Interferon treatment of HBeAg-negative chronic hepatitis B is less well studied. After 12 months of treatment, a sustained response (normalization of ALT levels and low levels of HBV DNA) can be achieved in about 15% to 30% of patients.[17,18]

The use of pegylated interferon has recently been examined in patients with HBeAg-positive and HBeAg-negative chronic hepatitis B.[19,20] In one study, 194 HBeAg-positive patients were randomized to receive 24 weeks of therapy with 90, 180, or 270 µg of pegylated interferon alfa-2a once a week or with standard interferon alfa-2a, 4.5 mIU three times a week.[19] At 24 weeks' follow-up, the HBeAg seroconversion rates were 37%, 35%, and 29%, respectively, for the three pegylated interferon alfa-2a treatment groups and 25% for the standard-interferon group. In another study of HBeAg-negative chronic hepatitis B, 537 patients were randomized to receive 48 weeks of therapy with 180 µg of pegylated interferon alfa-2a; lamivudine, 100 mg daily; or the two regimens combined.[20] At 24 weeks after cessation of therapy, the rates of biochemical and virologic remission were significantly higher in the groups receiving pegylated interferon; the addition of lamivudine did not improve the response rate. The combination of pegylated interferon and lamivudine continues to be studied, but it is too early to draw conclusions about the efficacy of this treatment.[21]

Side effects of interferon therapy Interferon commonly causes side effects, but these are usually manageable. Among these are influenzalike symptoms (i.e., fever, myalgia, arthralgia, and headache), hematologic toxicity (i.e., granulocytopenia, leukopenia, and thrombocytopenia), systemic symptoms (i.e., fatigue and hair thinning), neurologic signs (i.e., decreased concentration, depression, and irritability), and thyroid dysfunction.

Contraindications to interferon therapy Patients with a history of hypersensitivity to interferon, decompensated cirrhosis,

Table 5 Treatment of Chronic Hepatitis B

Drug	Dose
Lamivudine	100 mg p.o., q.d.
Adefovir dipivoxil	10 mg p.o., q.d.
Interferon alfa-2a or alfa-2b	5 million units S.C. daily or 10 million units S.C. three times weekly
Pegylated interferon alfa-2a	180 mg/wk S.C.*
Pegylated interferon alfa-2b	1.5 mg/kg/wk S.C.*

*Optimal dose and duration of treatment are under study.

immunosuppression associated with organ transplantation, active autoimmune disease, or severe psychiatric disease or patients who are elderly or frail are not good candidates for treatment.

Lamivudine Therapy

Lamivudine is a nucleoside analogue that inhibits HBV DNA synthesis. A dose of 100 mg/day achieves maximal suppression of HBV DNA. Lamivudine is cleared mainly in urine, and thus, dose adjustments are required for patients with significant renal failure. It has very few side effects and could be considered for use in virtually any patient with chronic hepatitis B.[14]

Lamivudine and HBeAg-positive chronic hepatitis B In three placebo-controlled studies, improved liver histology occurred in a significantly higher percentage of patients given lamivudine than in patients who received placebo.[22-24] Improvements in liver histology were similar in treatment-naive patients and patients who experienced relapse after interferon therapy or who did not respond to it; the improvements occurred independently of HBeAg seroconversion.[25,26] Serum HBV DNA levels fell rapidly and remained at least 94% below baseline values; serum ALT levels also decreased during therapy, with 50% of patients achieving and maintaining normal ALT levels 2 years post treatment. Patients receiving lamivudine for 1 year experienced a 17% rate of seroconversion from HBeAg to anti-HBe. The seroconversion rate increased progressively with additional years of lamivudine therapy, resulting in 27% seroconversion after 2 years, 33% after 3 years, 47% after 4 years, and 50% after 5 years.[27-30] The cumulative HBeAg seroconversion rate was higher in patients who had elevated baseline ALT levels before treatment. The responses to lamivudine are similar in Asian and non-Asian patients; however, the durability of HBeAg seroconversion appears to be lower in Asian patients (i.e., 60% to 80%). Patients who achieve HBeAg seroconversion can discontinue lamivudine therapy. However, on the basis of limited data, relapse rates may be lower (i.e., seroconversion is more durable) if lamivudine is continued for 3 to 6 months after initial HBeAg seroconversion is documented. The serum levels of ALT and HBV DNA return to pretreatment levels if lamivudine is discontinued before HBeAg seroconversion is achieved. After treatment, some patients may experience serum ALT levels that are transiently higher than pretreatment levels. Generally, no adverse effects have been associated with these elevations, although there are rare reports of severe flares of hepatitis B.

Lamivudine and HBeAg-negative chronic hepatitis B Lamivudine is effective in lowering ALT and HBV DNA levels and improving hepatic histology in patients with HBeAg-negative chronic hepatitis B. Several studies have demonstrated a biochemical and virologic response rate of about 70% at 1 year of therapy[14,17]; however, this response rate decreases to 50% after 2 years and 40% after 3 years. The end point for treatment is unknown, but it is the consensus that treatment beyond 1 year is warranted, provided the patient continues to exhibit a response.[15] The relapse rate after discontinuance of therapy is much higher in these patients than in patients with HBeAg-positive chronic hepatitis B.

Viral resistance to lamivudine therapy Resistant strains of HBV may appear within the first year of lamivudine therapy. The most common mutation imparting resistance occurs near the YMDD (the amino acid sequence tyrosine-methionine-aspartate-aspartate) motif of the HBV DNA polymerase. Resistance to lamivudine therapy occurs in 14% to 32% of patients after 1 year of therapy, 38% after 2 years, 49% after 3 years, 66% after 4 years, and 69% after 5 years.[30] The appearance of lamivudine resistance is manifested by rising HBV DNA and serum transaminase levels. A serologic test detecting HBV mutations imparting lamivudine resistance is available. Generally, patients experiencing lamivudine resistance can be switched to adefovir, which is effective against HBV DNA mutant strains. If patients who develop lamivudine resistance are continued on lamivudine, the initial beneficial effect of treatment on disease activity is usually lost.

Lamivudine and end-stage liver disease Lamivudine plays a role in patients with chronic hepatitis B who have end-stage liver disease. Stabilization and even improvement of biochemical and clinical features of cirrhosis may be seen in a majority of patients. Occasionally, improvement in liver function may result in deferral of liver transplantation.[17,31,32] Lamivudine therapy may serve as a bridge to transplantation for patients with decompensated cirrhosis who are awaiting a donor liver.

Lamivudine and liver transplantation Liver transplantation can be performed for liver failure associated with chronic hepatitis B, but HBV infects the allograft in 80% to 100% of cases if antiviral prophylaxis is not given, and long-term graft survival is only 45% to 50% (compared with 80% to 85% in liver transplant patients with other types of cirrhosis).[32] The HBV reinfection often is accelerated and progresses to cirrhosis. As a result, most transplant centers now implement prophylactic antiviral strategies to reduce reinfection. Before undergoing transplantation, patients should be treated with either lamivudine or adefovir to reduce the HBV viral load. Subsequently, two prophylaxis strategies are (1) the intraoperative, immediately postoperative, and long-term administration of high-dose hepatitis B immune globulin (HBIG) to maintain an anti-HBs level at 100 to 200 mIU/ml or greater, and (2) the administration of HBIG in combination with lamivudine or adefovir.[32] A number of trials suggest that these prophylaxis strategies can reduce the HBV reinfection rate to 10% to 20% and improve 1-year and 3-year graft survival rates.

Adefovir Dipivoxil Therapy

Adefovir dipivoxil is a nucleotide analogue of adenosine monophosphate. Adefovir inhibits HBV DNA polymerase and reverse transcriptase. It is effective against both wild-type and lamivudine-resistant HBV and in both HBeAg-positive and HBeAg-negative chronic hepatitis B.[14,15] Typically, adefovir therapy results in a 3 to 4 $\log_{10}$ drop in serum HBV DNA levels.

In a randomized study involving 515 patients who had HBeAg-positive chronic hepatitis B, treatment with adefovir 10 mg daily for 48 weeks resulted in a 12% HBeAg seroconversion rate.[33] As with lamivudine, the rate of treatment response is higher in patients who have higher pretreatment ALT values. Longer-term studies of adefovir are ongoing, and preliminary results indicate that the HBeAg seroconversion rate increases after 2 years. Adefovir, particularly at higher doses, may result in some renal impairment; therefore, it is prudent to periodically monitor renal function in patients receiving adefovir therapy. Adefovir has not been well studied in patients with chronic hepatitis B and decompensated cirrhosis.

Adefovir therapy in patients with HBeAg-negative chronic hepatitis B results in about a 46% biochemical and virologic response rate after 48 weeks and a 51% response rate after 96 weeks. If therapy is stopped after 48 weeks, relapse occurs in more than 90% of patients.[34,35] Development of drug resistance is much less of a problem with adefovir than with lamivudine. Resistance to adefovir is seen in about 2% of patients after 2 years and 4% of patients after 3 years.

Entecavir Therapy

Entecavir was approved by the Food and Drug Administration in early 2005 for use in the treatment of chronic hepatitis. The efficacy of entecavir is at least comparable to that of lamivudine (at a dose of 0.5 mg orally daily) in previously untreated patients. It is also effective, at a dose of 1 mg orally daily, in patients who develop lamivudine resistance.

Tenofovir Therapy

Tenofovir is related to adefovir. Tenofovir has been approved by the FDA for treatment of HIV infection. Its use in the treatment of chronic hepatitis B is being evaluated, but very limited data have been published.

MANAGEMENT OF HBV REACTIVATION

In some inactive HBsAg carriers, biochemical, clinical, and histologic exacerbations of disease activity have been noted; such exacerbations are characterized by elevated serum transaminase levels, the presence of HBV DNA, and the reversion from anti-HBe to HBeAg. These exacerbations (so-called reactivations) appear spontaneously in about 20% of inactive HBsAg carriers. Repeated reactivations, which are usually asymptomatic, may occur and may lead to progressive fibrosis. Therefore, even inactive HBsAg carriers should be periodically monitored (i.e., every 6 to 12 months) for resurgence of disease activity.

Reactivation may also occur in patients with malignancy during or after cessation of chemotherapy, especially when the chemotherapy regimens include corticosteroids. It is important to be aware of such a possibility because reactivations in these patients, although generally mild, may at times be severe and even fatal. Preemptive therapy with lamivudine in patients with malignancy has been found to decrease the incidence and severity of reactivations.[36,37] Lamivudine therapy should be strongly considered in inactive-HBsAg-carrier patients who are scheduled to have chemotherapy. Patients with chronic hepatitis B who are scheduled to have chemotherapy would presumably already be receiving lamivudine or adefovir; if not, they should be started on lamivudine therapy before initiation of chemotherapy.

Chronic Hepatitis C

EPIDEMIOLOGY

Approximately 30,000 new cases of acute HCV infection are reported annually to the Centers for Disease Control and Prevention. Of these patients, about 80% develop chronic HCV infection.[38] Approximately four million persons in the United States (1.8%) have been infected with HCV, and 74% of these individuals (1.4% of the population) are viremic. The high chronicity rate of HCV infection makes chronic hepatitis C a much more prevalent disease than chronic hepatitis B (0.2% to 0.5% of the general population).

DIAGNOSIS

The diagnosis of chronic hepatitis C is typically made by a positive anti-HCV on enzyme-linked immunosorbent assay and

Table 6 Treatment of Chronic Hepatitis C

HCV Genotypes	Drug Regimen
For HCV genotype 1 (48-wk regimen)	Pegylated interferon alfa-2a, 180 µg/wk S.C., plus ribavirin, 1,000-1,200 mg/day *or* Pegylated interferon alfa-2b, 1.5 µg/kg/wk S.C., plus ribavirin, 800-1,200 mg/day
For HCV genotype 2 or 3 (24-wk regimen)	Pegylated interferon alfa-2a, 180 µg/wk S.C., plus ribavirin, 800 mg/day *or* Pegylated interferon alfa-2b, 1.5 µg/kg/wk S.C., plus ribavirin, 800 mg/day

detectable HCV RNA.[38] Serum transaminase levels are usually elevated; about 20% of patients have persistently normal values. Most infected patients are asymptomatic. Liver biopsy may demonstrate the full spectrum of disease severity, ranging from mild portal tract inflammation and no fibrosis to cirrhosis.

NATURAL HISTORY

After the onset of acute HCV infection, the infection resolves in 15% to 30% of patients and there is a loss of HCV RNA, although anti-HCV remains detectable. The natural history of chronic hepatitis C typically spans several decades. In general, liver disease progresses insidiously, and cirrhosis may not develop for 2 or more decades, if ever. The natural history may be more prolonged when HCV infection occurs earlier in life. In a Japanese study, the mean interval from blood transfusion to development of chronic hepatitis was 10 years; to development of cirrhosis, 21 years; and to development of HCC (a late risk), 29 years.[39] Similar results were found in a population of patients seen in a referral liver center in the United States: the mean interval from transfusion to cirrhosis was 21 years; and for progression to hepatocellular carcinoma, the mean interval was 28 years.[40]

In a European study designed to examine the natural progression of hepatic fibrosis in patients with chronic hepatitis C, the median interval from the presumed time of infection to cirrhosis, identified by liver biopsy, was 30 years.[41] The rate of progression to fibrosis and cirrhosis was not normally distributed; findings suggested at least three populations of patients with chronic hepatitis C: those with rapid progression of fibrosis (median time to cirrhosis < 30 years), those with intermediate progression, and those with no or slow progression of fibrosis. Independent factors associated with an increased rate of progression to cirrhosis are age greater than 40 years at the time of infection, daily alcohol consumption of 50 g or more, and male gender. Fibrosis progression is not related to HCV RNA level or HCV genotype.

TREATMENT

The current standard of care for chronic hepatitis C involves the use of pegylated interferon (interferon alfa-2a or alfa-2b) in combination with ribavirin [*see Table 6*].[38] Polyethylene glycol (PEG) is a water-soluble polymer that is covalently linked to interferon, which markedly increases the half-life, resulting in sustained serum levels and allowing once-weekly administration. Combination therapy with standard (nonpegylated) interferon and ribavirin is still used occasionally. In patients with certain comorbid conditions, monotherapy with interferon (either a pegylated or standard form) is advised because of the risk of severe anemia associated with ribavirin use [see Side Effects of Combination Therapy, below].

Pegylated Interferon and Ribavirin Therapy

The persistence of undetectable HCV RNA for 6 months or more after cessation of therapy is the definition of a sustained virologic response (SVR). The major pretreatment determinant of response is HCV genotype.[38] Patients infected with HCV genotype 1 virus (the most common genotype in the United States) have lower SVR rates (in the range of 42% to 52%) than patients with HCV genotypes 2 and 3 (in the range of 76% to 84%). There are varying responses to treatment of HCV genotypes 4, 5, and 6.

Varying study designs and ribavirin doses have been used to evaluate the efficacy of pegylated interferon (interferon alfa-2a and alfa-2b) and ribavirin combination therapy. Therefore, results of treatment have been reported that often do not reflect comparable treatment regimens, particularly with regard to ribavirin doses. Some studies have used a fixed dose of ribavirin, whereas others have used doses based on weight.[38,42,43] Despite these differences, SVR rates for patients with HCV genotypes 1, 2, and 3 have been similar using either interferon alfa-2a or interferon alfa-2b plus ribavirin at varying doses.

One randomized, double-blind trial clearly addressed the issues of length of therapy and ribavirin doses.[44] In that study, 1,284 patients with HCV genotypes 1, 2, and 3 were randomized to receive pegylated interferon alfa-2a (180 µg/wk) in combination with ribavirin in either a low-dose (800 mg/day) or standard weight-based dose (1,000 or 1,200 mg/day) for 24 or 48 weeks. The SVR for HCV genotype 1 patients was 52% after 48 weeks of treatment using the regimen with 1,000 to 1,200 mg of ribavirin daily versus 41% using the 800 mg ribavirin daily dose; the SVR rates for 24 weeks of treatment were much lower. The SVRs for patients with HCV genotypes 2 and 3 were similar, ranging from 79% to 84%, regardless of which treatment regimen was used. On the basis of the study's findings, 24 weeks of treatment with pegylated interferon and ribavirin at a dosage of 800 mg daily (which resulted in an SVR of 84%) is sufficient to achieve an optimal SVR in patients with HCV genotype 2 or 3. However, patients with HCV genotype 1 must be treated for 48 weeks using pegylated interferon and ribavirin at a dosage of 1,000 to 1,200 mg daily to achieve an optimal SVR. This and other studies have led to the practice of administering treatment for 48 weeks to patients with genotype 1 and for 24 weeks to those with genotype 2 or 3 [see Table 6]. Among factors shown to lessen the likelihood of successful therapy are high viral load ($> 2 \times 10^6$ copies/ml), male gender, African-American ethnicity, long duration of infection, and advanced fibrosis.

Early virologic response Because pegylated interferon and ribavirin combination therapy has many side effects, strategies have been studied to determine whether continuation of treatment after an early virologic response (EVR) will likely result in an SVR.[45,46] Such studies have mostly centered on patients with HCV genotype 1, because the standard treatment length is longer and the SVR rates are lower for genotype 1 than for genotypes 2 and 3. The values of HCV RNA at two time points (12 and 24 weeks) have been closely examined. If a patient with HCV genotype 1 does not have an undetectable level of HCV RNA after 24 weeks of treatment, the chance of achieving an SVR with another 24 weeks of treatment is extremely low (i.e., in the range of 1% or less). It is strongly recommended that treatment be halted in such patients, unless individual circumstances dictate otherwise.

Recent studies have focused on the 12-week HCV RNA value and have examined the negative predictive value for achieving an SVR based on various declines in HCV RNA, as compared with baseline values. For HCV genotype 1 patients, failure to achieve a drop of 2 $\log_{10}$ or greater in HCV RNA values after 12 weeks of treatment has a negative predictive value of approximately 97% to 100% for achieving SVR after a full course of 48 weeks of treatment. Clinical judgment must be used in deciding whether to discontinue therapy after failure to achieve a 12-week SVR. The value of determining a 12-week EVR in patients who have HCV genotype 2 or 3 is unclear because virtually all these patients achieve a response at 12 weeks. The utility of determining a 4-week EVR for HCV genotype 2 or 3 patients is under study.

Side effects of combination therapy Side effects are varied and common with interferon and ribavirin combination therapy[38,47] and may necessitate discontinuance of therapy in 10% to 15% of patients. The major side effect of ribavirin is a dose-dependent hemolytic anemia, which is reversible and usually stabilizes after 6 weeks of treatment. For milder degrees of anemia, the ribavirin dose can be temporarily decreased. If the anemia is not corrected by a reduction in the ribavirin dose, epoetin can be used. If severe anemia develops, ribavirin must be discontinued, either temporarily or permanently.

Patients with preexisting moderate to severe anemia usually cannot tolerate the degree of hemolysis that occurs with ribavirin therapy, which can be dangerous. Moreover, patients with cardiovascular disease are particularly at risk should severe anemia develop during therapy, and very careful consideration would have to be given to the decision to initiate interferon monotherapy because of the drug's side effects. Patients with any degree of symptomatic cardiovascular disease are not candidates for interferon monotherapy. Patients with chronic hepatitis C and comorbid conditions preventing the use of ribavirin can be treated with interferon monotherapy, although this treatment has an SVR rate considerably lower than that of combination therapy. Ribavirin is teratogenic; therefore, patients must be advised against its use during pregnancy. Other side effects attributed to ribavirin are rash and nasal or sinus problems.

Interferon can cause or exacerbate depression and other psychiatric symptoms. Caution is warranted in using interferon therapy for patients with depression; however, these patients can often be managed with antidepressants, with or without reduction in interferon dosage. Interferon has many other potential side effects, including leukopenia and thrombocytopenia, thyroid dysfunction, insomnia, hair thinning, headaches, weight loss, various neurologic dysfunctions, and irritability. Deaths have occurred, usually because of sepsis, suicide, or cardiovascular disease.

Sustained virologic response In 5- to 10-year follow-up studies of patients who had an initial posttreatment 6-month SVR, relapse occurred in 1% to 2 % of patients.[48] Following an SVR, there is usually improvement of liver histology, including significant regression of hepatic fibrosis in about 25% of patients. Interferon therapy may delay or prevent liver decompensation resulting from cirrhosis, as well as the development of HCC, particularly in patients who show a sustained response.[49]

Relapse after Treatment

Relapse after a course of therapy is defined by detectable levels of HCV RNA, which were undetectable during treatment. Relapse usually occurs within the first 6 months after treatment. No effective treatment is available to patients in whom relapse occurs after the standard regimen of pegylated interferon and ribavirin.

Nonresponse to Therapy

Nonresponse to antiviral therapy is defined as detectable serum HCV RNA levels during therapy. A variant of nonresponse called breakthrough is characterized by an initial disappearance of HCV RNA, with subsequent reappearance of HCV RNA while the patient is still being treated. There are no effective treatments available for patients who experience a nonresponse to current therapies.

Liver Transplantation

Cirrhosis caused by chronic hepatitis C is the most common indication for liver transplantation. Although hepatitis C virus reinfects the allograft in nearly all cases, the subsequent illness is usually mild, but a small percentage of cases progress to cirrhosis and liver failure. There is no consensus of opinion regarding guidelines for treatment of chronic hepatitis C after liver transplantation.[38] Usually, posttransplant treatment is more difficult because of more severe cytopenia and complications related to immunosuppression.

The author has received grants for clinical research from Roche Pharmaceuticals and Schering-Plough Corporation.

The drugs pegylated interferon alfa-2a, pegylated interferon alfa-2b, and azathioprine have not been approved by the FDA for uses described in this chapter.

References

1. Desmet VJ, Gerber M, Hoofnagle JH, et al: Classification of chronic hepatitis: diagnosis, grading and staging. Hepatology 19:1513, 1994

2. Brunt EM: Grading and staging the histopathological lesions of chronic hepatitis: the Knodell histology activity index and beyond. Hepatology 31:241, 2000

3. Bedossa P, Poynard T: An algorithm for the grading of activity in chronic hepatitis C. The METAVIR Cooperative Study Group. Hepatology 24:289, 1996

4. Lee WM: Drug-induced hepatotoxicity. N Engl J Med 349:474, 2003

5. Czaja AJ, Freese DK: Diagnosis and treatment of autoimmune hepatitis. AASLD Practice Guidelines. Hepatology 36:479, 2002

6. Alvarez F, Berg PA, Bianchi FB, et al: Review of criteria for diagnosis of autoimmune hepatitis. International Autoimmune Hepatitis Group report. J Hepatol 31:929, 1999

7. Czaja AJ, Manns MP: The validity and importance of subtypes of autoimmune hepatitis: a point of view. Am J Gastroenterol 90:1206, 1995

8. Czaja AJ: Frequency and nature of the variant syndromes of autoimmune liver disease. Hepatology 28:360, 1998

9. Ben-Ari Z, Czaja AJ: Autoimmune hepatitis and its variant syndromes. Gut 49:589, 2001

10. Soloway RD, Summerskill WHJ, Baggenstoss AH, et al: Clinical, biochemical, and histological remission of severe chronic active liver disease: a controlled trial of treatments and early prognosis. Gastroenterology 63:820, 1972

11. Murray-Lyon IM, Stern RB, Williams R: Controlled trial of prednisone and azathioprine in active chronic hepatitis. Lancet 1:735, 1973

12. Cook CG, Mulligan R, Sherlock S: Controlled prospective trial of corticosteroid therapy in active chronic hepatitis. QJ Med 40:159, 1971

13. Johnson PJ, McFarlane IG, Williams R: Azathioprine for long-term maintenance of remission in autoimmune hepatitis. N Engl J Med 333:958, 1995

14. Lok ASF, McMahon BJ: Chronic hepatitis B. AASLD Practice Guidelines. Hepatology 34:1225, 2001

15. Lok ASF, McMahon BJ: Chronic hepatitis B: update of recommendations. AASLD Practice Guidelines. Hepatology 39:1, 2004

16. McMahon BJ, Bulkow L, Harpster A, et al: Screening for hepatocellular carcinoma in Alaska natives infected with chronic hepatitis B: a 16-year population-based study. Hepatology 32:842, 2000

17. Keefe EB, Dietrich DT, Han S-HB, et al: A treatment algorithm for the management of chronic hepatitis B virus infection in the United States. Clin Gastroenterol Hepatol 2:87, 2004

18. Manesis EK, Hadziyannis SJ: Interferon alpha treatment and retreatment of hepatitis B e antigen-negative chronic hepatitis B. Gastroenterology 121:101, 2001

19. Cooksley W, Piratvisuth T, Lee SD, et al: Peginterferon alfa-2a (40 Kda): an advance in the treatment of hepatitis B e antigen-positive chronic hepatitis B. J Viral Hepatitis 10:298, 2003

20. Marcellin P, Lau GK, Bonino F, et al: Peginterferon alfa-2a alone, lamivudine alone, and the two in combination in patients with HBeAg-negative chronic hepatitis B. N Engl J Med 351:1206, 2004

21. Chan HL, Leung NW, Hui AY, et al: A randomized, controlled trial of combination therapy for chronic hepatitis B: comparing pegylated interferon-alpha2b and lamivudine with lamivudine alone. Ann Intern Med 142:240, 2005

22. Dienstag JL, Schiff ER, Wright TL, et al: Lamivudine as initial treatment for chronic hepatitis B in the United States. N Engl J Med 341:1256, 1999

23. Lai CL, Chien RN, Leung NW, et al: A one-year trial of lamivudine for chronic hepatitis B. Asia Hepatitis Lamivudine Study Group. N Engl J Med 339:61, 1998

24. Schalm SW, Heathcote J, Cianciara J, et al: Lamivudine and alpha interferon combination treatment of patients with chronic hepatitis B infection: a randomized trial. Gut 46:562, 2000

25. Honkoop P, de Man RA, Zondervan PE, et al: Histological improvement in patients with chronic hepatitis B virus infection treated with lamivudine. Liver 17:103, 1997

26. Suzuki Y, Kumada H, Ikeda K, et al: Histological changes in liver biopsies after one year of lamivudine treatment in patients with chronic hepatitis B infection. J Hepatol 30:743, 1999

27. Liaw YF, Leung NWY, Chang TT, et al: Effects of extended lamivudine therapy in Asian patients with chronic hepatitis B. Gastroenterology 119:172, 2000

28. Leung NWY, Lai CL, Chang TT, et al: Extended lamivudine treatment in patients with chronic hepatitis B enhances hepatitis B e antigen seroconversion rates: results after 3 years of therapy. Hepatology 33:1527, 2001

29. Chang TT, Lai CL, Liaw YF, et al: Incremental increases in HBeAg seroconversion and continued ALT normalization in Asian chronic HBV (CHB) patients treated with lamivudine for four years. Antiviral Therapy 16(suppl 1):44, 2000

30. Guan R, Lai CL, Liaw YF, et al: Efficacy and safety of 5-years lamivudune treatment of Chinese patients with chronic hepatitis B. J Gastroenterol Hepatol 16(suppl 1):A60, 2001

31. Villeneuve JP, Condreay LD, Willems B, et al: Lamivudine treatment for decompensated cirrhosis resulting from chronic hepatitis B. Hepatology 31:207, 2000

32. Keeffe EB: End-stage liver disease and liver transplantation: role of lamivudine therapy in patients with chronic hepatitis B. J Med Virol 61:403, 2000

33. Marcellin P, Chang TT, Lim SG, et al: Adefovir dipivoxil for the treatment of hepatitis B e antigen-positive chronic hepatitis B. N Engl J Med 348:808, 2003

34. Hadziyannis SJ, Tassopoulos N, Heathcote EJ, et al: Adefovir dipivoxil for the treatment of hepatitis B e antigen-negative chronic hepatitis B. N Engl J Med 348:800, 2003

35. Hadziyannis SJ, Tassopoulos N, Heathcote EJ, et al: Two year results from a double-blind, randomized, placebo-controlled study of adefovir dipivoxil (ADV) for presumed precore mutant chronic hepatitis B. J Hepatol 38(suppl 2):143, 2003

36. Lau GKK, He ML, Fong DYT, et al: Preemptive use of lamivudine reduces hepatitis B exacerbation after allogenic hematopoietic cell transplantation. Hepatology 36:702, 2002

37. Rossi G, Pelizzari A, Motta M, et al: Primary prophylaxis with lamivudine of hepatitis B reactivation in chronic HBsAg carriers with lymphoid malignancies treated with chemotherapy. Br J Haematol 115:58, 2001

38. Strader DB, Wright T, Thomas DL, et al: Diagnosis, management, and treatment of hepatitis C. AASLD Practice Guideline. Hepatology 39:1147, 2004

39. Kiyosawa K, Sodeyama T, Tanaka E, et al: Interrelationship of blood transfusion, non-A, non-B hepatitis and hepatocellular carcinoma: analysis by detection of antibody to hepatitis C virus. Hepatology 12:671, 1990

40. Tong MJ, El-Farra NS, Reikes AR, et al: Clinical outcomes after transfusion-associated hepatitis C. N Engl J Med 332:1463, 1995

41. Poynard T, Bedossa P, Opolon P, et al: Natural history of liver fibrosis progression in patients with chronic hepatitis C. Lancet 349:825, 1997

42. Fried MW, Shiffman ML, Reddy KR, et al: Combination of peginterferon alfa-2a plus ribavirin in patients with chronic hepatitis C virus infection. N Engl J Med 347:975, 2002

43. Manns MP, McHutchison JG, Gordon SC, et al: Peginterferon alfa-2b plus ribavirin compared with interferon alfa-2b plus ribavirin for initial treatment of chronic hepatitis C: a randomized trial. Lancet 358:958, 2001

44. Hadziyannis SJ, Sette H, Morgan TR, et al: Peginterferon-alpha2a and ribavirin combination therapy in chronic hepatitis C: a randomized study of treatment duration and ribavirin dose. Ann Intern Med 140:346, 2004

45. Russo MW, Fried MW: Hepatitis C therapy: guidelines for stopping therapy. Curr Gastroenterol Rep 6:17, 2004

46. Davis GL, Wong JB, McHutchison JG, et al: Early virologic response to treatment with peginterferon alfa-2b plus ribavirin in patients with chronic hepatitis C. Hepatology 38:645, 2003

47. Russo MW, Fried MW: Side effects of therapy for chronic hepatitis C. Gastroenterology 124:1711, 2003

48. Lau DTY, Kleiner DE, Ghany MG, et al: 10-Year follow-up after interferon-alpha therapy for chronic hepatitis C. Hepatology 28:1121, 1998

49. Yoshida H, Shiratori Y, Moriyama M, et al: Interferon therapy reduces the risk for hepatocellular carcinoma: national surveillance program of cirrhotic and noncirrhotic patients with chronic hepatitis C in Japan: IHIT Study Group: inhibition of hepatocarcinogenesis by interferon therapy. Ann Intern Med 131:174, 1999

71 Cirrhosis of the Liver

Ramón Bataller, M.D., and Pere Ginès, M.D.

Cirrhosis is the most advanced stage of most types of chronic liver disease. It is defined as a diffuse disorganization of normal hepatic structure by extensive fibrosis associated with regenerative nodules. Fibrosis is potentially reversible if the causative agent is removed. However, advanced cirrhosis comprises major alterations in the hepatic vascular bed and is usually irreversible.[1] Clinically, cirrhosis is associated with high morbidity and mortality. It leads to a wide spectrum of characteristic clinical manifestations, mainly from hepatic insufficiency and portal hypertension.[2] Major complications include ascites, renal failure, gastrointestinal bleeding, encephalopathy, bacterial infections, and coagulopathy. Cirrhosis is also a risk factor for developing hepatocellular carcinoma (HCC). Decompensated cirrhosis carries a poor prognosis, in both the short and the long term, and orthotopic liver transplantation (OLT) is often indicated.

Epidemiology

Cirrhosis is the ninth leading cause of death in the United States.[3] Chronic liver disease and cirrhosis cause 4% to 5% of deaths in persons 45 to 54 years of age and result in about 30,000 deaths each year. The incidence of newly diagnosed cases of chronic liver disease in the United States is 72.3 per 100,000 population. The prevalence of chronic liver disease and cirrhosis is 5.5 million cases. Over 60% of patients are male. Cirrhosis is more common in Hispanic whites and Native Americans; it is the sixth leading cause of death in those two populations. The economic impact of cirrhosis is considerable, with $1.5 billion in direct costs and $234 million in indirect costs in 2000.[4] In 2002, there were 421,000 hospitalizations for chronic liver disease and cirrhosis.[5]

Etiology and Genetic Factors

In the United States, the main causes of cirrhosis are hepatitis C virus (HCV) infection and alcoholic liver disease, which account for two thirds of all cirrhosis cases. Other major causes are hepatitis B virus (HBV) infection, autoimmune hepatitis, chronic cholestasis (primary biliary cirrhosis [PBC] and primary sclerosing cholangitis [PSC]), and genetic metabolic diseases (hemochromatosis and Wilson disease) [see Table 1]. With the current epidemic of obesity, nonalcoholic steatohepatitis (NASH) is increasingly being recognized as a major cause of cirrhosis. Many patients diagnosed with cryptogenic cirrhosis have a history of metabolic syndrome, suggesting a role for NASH in the pathogenesis of their cirrhosis.

Many genes interact with environmental factors to cause cirrhosis.[6] Nongenetic factors that influence progression to cirrhosis include age, alcohol intake, immunosuppressive therapy, and HIV infection. Genetic factors involved in the pathogenesis of cirrhosis are not well known, but they may explain the broad spectrum of responses to the same etiologic agent found in patients with chronic liver disease. Polymorphisms in genes encoding immunoregulatory proteins, inflammatory cytokines, and fibrogenic mediators influence the occurrence of conditions that may cause chronic liver injury (e.g., alcohol abuse, chronic HCV infection, and autoimmune disorders), as well as modulate the progression of chronic hepatitis to cirrhosis.

Pathogenesis

EARLY PHASE: LIVER FIBROGENESIS

Cirrhosis is the end stage of many forms of chronic liver disease that are characterized by progressive fibrosis. Hepatic fibrosis is the result of the wound-healing response of the liver to repeated injury.[7] It consists of the accumulation of extracellular matrix (ECM) proteins, mainly fibrillar collagen, from both increased ECM synthesis and decreased degradation. Myofibroblasts, mostly derived from hepatic stellate cells, are the main ECM-producing cells in the injured liver. Chronic injury promotes the activation of stellate cells into fibrogenic myofibroblasts [see Figure 1]. Key mediators of this process include inflammatory cytokines, transforming growth factor–1 (TGF-1), and angiotensin II. The pathogenesis of liver fibrosis varies with the underlying cause. In alcohol-induced liver disease, lipopolysaccharide levels are elevated in portal blood; the lipopolysaccharide activates Kupffer cells to release reactive oxygen species and cytokines, activating stellate cells and sensitizing hepatocytes to undergo apoptosis. The pathogenesis of HCV-induced liver fibrosis is poorly understood. HCV infects hepatocytes, causing oxidative stress and inducing the recruitment of inflammatory cells. Both factors lead to stellate cell activation. In chron-

Table 1   Main Causes of Cirrhosis

Viral diseases	Hepatitis B Hepatitis C Hepatitis D
Autoimmune diseases	Autoimmune hepatitis Primary biliary cirrhosis Primary sclerosing cholangitis Graft versus host disease
Hepatotoxic agents	Alcohol abuse Drugs (e.g., methotrexate, α-methyldopa, amiodarone) Vitamin A intoxication
Acquired metabolic diseases	Nonalcoholic steatohepatitis
Vascular diseases	Chronic right-sided heart failure Budd-Chiari syndrome Veno-occlusive disease Inferior vena cava thrombosis
Genetic diseases	Wilson disease Hemochromatosis Type IV glycogen storage disease Tyrosinemia α_1-Antitrypsin deficiency
Miscellaneous	Secondary biliary cirrhosis Cryptogenic

a

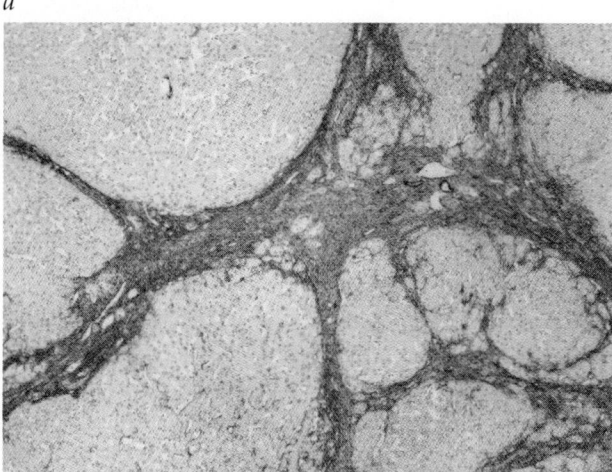

b

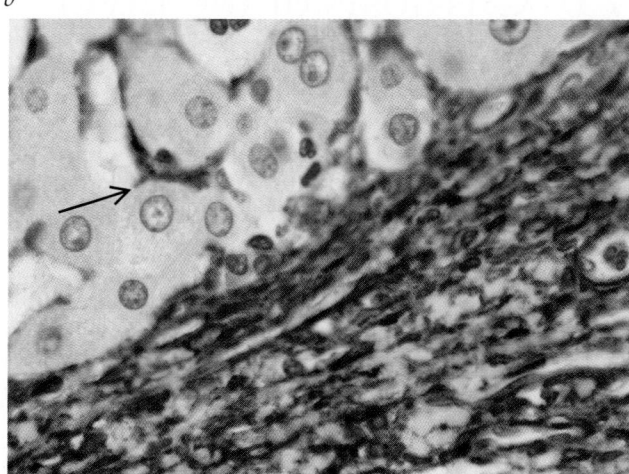

Figure 1 Immunohistochemical analysis of accumulation of fibrogenic myofibroblasts (smooth muscle [α-actin–positive] cells) in a liver biopsy specimen from a 56-year-old man with liver cirrhosis from chronic hepatitis C infection. The patient was admitted for the study of new-onset ascites. Myofibroblasts mainly accumulate in fibrous septa. Some activated hepatic stellate cells can be observed around hepatic sinusoids (arrow). (*a*) Magnification: ×40; (*b*) magnification: ×600.

ic cholestatic disorders, such as PBC, T cells and cytokines mediate persistent bile duct damage. Biliary cells secrete fibrogenic mediators that activate neighboring portal myofibroblasts to secrete ECM. Eventually, perisinusoidal stellate cells become activated and fibrotic bands develop. The pathogenesis of liver fibrosis in NASH is poorly understood, but a so-called two-hit model has been proposed: first, hyperglycemia and insulin resistance lead to elevated serum levels of free fatty acids, resulting in hepatic steatosis; second, oxidative stress and inflammatory cytokines promote hepatocyte apoptosis and the recruitment of inflammatory cells, leading to progressive fibrosis.

CIRRHOSIS

Bridging fibrosis is associated with profound abnormalities in hepatic microcirculation.[8] Capillarization of the hepatic sinusoids occurs, and new vessels form within the fibrous sheath. There is a local predominance of vasoconstrictors over vasodilators, resulting in a tonic contraction of perisinusoidal stellate cells that increases vascular resistance. Moreover, thrombosis in small vessels occurs and intrahepatic arterial shunts develop. Hepatocytes proliferate in ischemic areas in a disorganized manner, forming regenerative nodules. Pressure in the portal venous system progressively increases, leading to the development of portocollateral veins and esophageal varices.[9] The resulting portal hypertension leads to splanchnic vasodilatation, which increases hepatic venous blood flow. Systemic vascular resistance is decreased, and eventually, there is a marked activation of systemic vasoconstrictor systems that worsen portal hypertension and favor ascites formation. Hepatocellular function is progressively impaired, and there is decreased function of the reticuloendothelial system, leading to endotoxemia and the increased risk of bacterial infections. Eventually, hepatocellular function fails, resulting in severe coagulopathy and hepatic encephalopathy. A profound circulatory dysfunction from impaired myocardial function and decreased systemic vascular resistance is frequently seen. In very late stages of cirrhosis, renal vasoconstriction develops, leading to the hepatorenal syndrome (HRS). In this phase of the disease, most patients die unless an OLT is rapidly performed.

Diagnosis

The diagnostic process in a patient with suspected cirrhosis is intended to determine the presence, severity, and cause of the condition. Data obtained from the history, physical examination, laboratory tests, and liver biopsy are used to identify the etiology of cirrhosis [*see Table 2*].

CLINICAL MANIFESTATIONS

Cirrhosis can be clinically silent, and some cases are discovered incidentally at laparotomy or autopsy. In many patients, symptoms are insidious in onset and include generalized weakness, anorexia, malaise, and weight loss. Skeletal muscle mass is frequently reduced. So-called compensated cirrhosis is defined by the absence of symptoms or the presence of only minor symptoms. Eventually, most patients exhibit the clinical manifestations of hepatocellular dysfunction and portal hypertension, including progressive jaundice, bleeding from gastroesophageal varices, ascites, and neuropsychiatric symptoms. The abrupt onset of one of these complications may be the first manifestation of cirrhosis. Coagulopathy and subsequent mucosal bleeding typically occur in patients with advanced cirrhosis. Progressive obstruction to bile flow, which is especially common in patients with PBC and PSC, leads to skin hyperpigmentation, jaundice, pruritus, and xanthelasmas. Patients who have progressed to such conditions often experience malnutrition secondary to anorexia, fat malabsorption, and increased catabolism. Deficiency of fat-soluble vitamins is also frequently found in patients with cirrhosis. In patients with alcohol-induced liver disease, extrahepatic symptoms related to the nervous system, the heart, and the pancreas can also be present.

PHYSICAL EXAMINATION FINDINGS

Physical examination can be normal in patients with early cirrhosis. More commonly, the liver is enlarged initially and is palpable. In advanced cirrhosis, liver size usually decreases. Splenomegaly is a common finding. Ascites, peripheral edema, or both may be present, and collateral venous circulation can be observed in the abdomen. Patients with hepatic encephalopathy have altered mental status, decreased consciousness, and asterixis. Other signs typical of cirrhosis include muscle wasting, palmar erythema, vascular spiders, gynecomastia, axillary hair loss, testicular atrophy, and fetor hepaticus. In alcoholic patients, Dupuytren contractures, parotid gland enlargement, and peripheral neuropathy can be noted. Skin hyperpigmentation is typical of patients with cholestatic disorders (e.g., PBC) or hemochromatosis. Advanced cirrhosis is commonly marked by severe malnourishment, prominent ascites, and neuropsychiatric symptoms [see Figure 2].

LABORATORY STUDIES

Blood Tests

Liver function test results are commonly abnormal in patients with cirrhosis. Serum aspartate aminotransferase (AST) levels are frequently elevated, but levels above 300 U/L are uncommon. Serum levels of alanine aminotransferase (ALT) may be relatively low (AST/ALT ratio greater than 2). Serum prothrombin time is frequently prolonged, reflecting reduced synthesis of clotting proteins, most notably the vitamin K–dependent factors. Serum albumin levels are decreased, mainly because of poor hepatocellular synthesis. Total serum globulin concentration increases in advanced cirrhosis, as a result of poor reticuloendothelial function and increased blood levels of bacterial products. The alkaline phosphatase concentration is usually only moderately increased, except in patients with biliary diseases (i.e., PBC or PSC), who show markedly increased levels of alka-

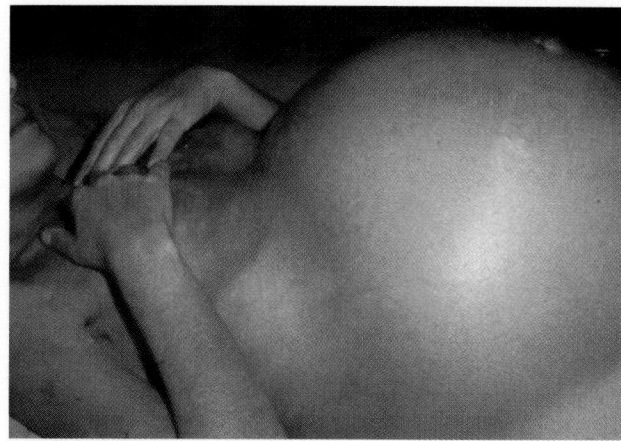

Figure 2 **Photograph of a 45-year-old patient with advanced cirrhosis from alcohol-induced liver disease. The patient was admitted because of tense ascites, and a superimposed acute alcoholic hepatitis was diagnosed. A large-volume paracentesis followed by albumin administration was performed.**

line phosphatase and γ-glutamyl transpeptidase, which in some cases are associated with increased bilirubin levels. Anemia is fairly common; it is usually normocytic, but it may be microcytic, hypochromic from chronic GI bleeding, macrocytic from folate deficiency (in alcoholism), or hemolytic. Hypersplenism can lead to leukopenia and thrombocytopenia. Cholesterol and triglyceride levels may be increased in patients with biliary obstruction, whereas they are low in patients with advanced cirrhosis of nonbiliary origin. Cirrhotic patients may develop glucose intolerance and diabetes mellitus, mainly because of insulin resistance. Central hyperventilation may lead to respiratory alkalosis. Dietary deficiency and increased urinary losses cause hypomagnesemia and hypophosphatemia. Renal failure, as indicated by elevated creatinine and blood urea nitrogen levels, and hyponatremia can be observed in cirrhotic patients with ascites.

Imaging Studies

Real-time ultrasonography, in combination with color flow Doppler, is the most useful tool in the evaluation of patients with cirrhosis.[10] Ultrasonography is useful for demonstrating the morphologic characteristics of cirrhosis, including irregular or nodular liver edges, altered structure, and signs of portal hypertension such as portocollateral veins. It is also useful to detect hepatic steatosis, ascites, splenomegaly, and portal vein thrombosis. In patients with cholestasis, ultrasonography helps rule out extrahepatic causes of jaundice. Doppler ultrasonography provides useful information on portal hemodynamics and can detect reversal of portal blood flow [see Figure 3]. Ultrasound examination is particularly helpful for detecting hepatic tumors such as HCC. Demonstration of tumor vascularization by Doppler ultrasonography, with or without injection of ultrasound contrast, is valuable in the differentiation of regenerating nodules from HCC. Dynamic studies using computed tomography and magnetic resonance imaging are also useful in the assessment of cirrhosis and the diagnosis of hepatic tumors previously detected by ultrasonography. The use of CT or MRI to screen for HCC in patients with cirrhosis is limited by the high cost of these techniques.

Liver Biopsy

Liver biopsy can unequivocally establish the presence of cir-

Table 2 Identification of the Main Causes of Cirrhosis

Cause	Diagnostic Method
Alcohol-related	Medical history (also obtained from relatives), urinary alcohol levels, histologic findings
Hepatitis C virus (HCV)	Anti-HCV antibodies, HCV RNA assay
Hepatitis B virus (HBV)	HBsAg, HBV DNA assay
Hepatitis D virus (HDV)	Anti-delta IgM or IgG
Autoimmune disease	Antitissue antibodies (ANA, LKM, ASMA), hypergammaglobulinemia, histologic findings
Primary biliary cirrhosis	AMA, histologic findings
Primary sclerosing cholangitis	Severe cholestasis; detection of biliary tract abnormalities by magnetic resonance imaging/magnetic resonance cholangiopancreatography (MRI/MRCP) or ERCP; ANCA; presence of inflammatory bowel disease; histologic findings
Wilson disease	Serum ceruloplasmin levels, Kayser-Fleischer rings, copper content in the liver, genetic studies
Hemochromatosis	Serum ferritin levels, total iron binding capacity, iron content in the liver, genetic studies
Nonalcoholic steatohepatitis	Metabolic syndrome, histologic findings (may be absent in cirrhosis), absence of alcohol abuse

AMA—antimitochondrial antibodies ANA—antinuclear antibody ANCA—antineutrophil cytoplasmic autoantibodies ASMA—anti–smooth muscle antibodies ERCP—endoscopic retrograde cholangiopancreatography HBsAg—hepatitis B surface antigen LKM—liver/kidney microsomal antibody

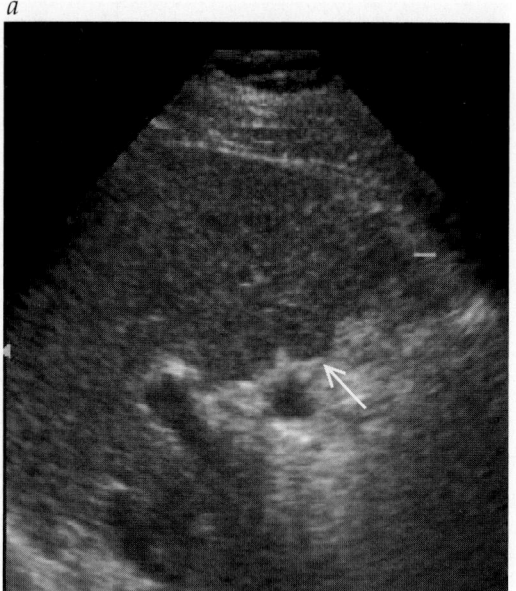 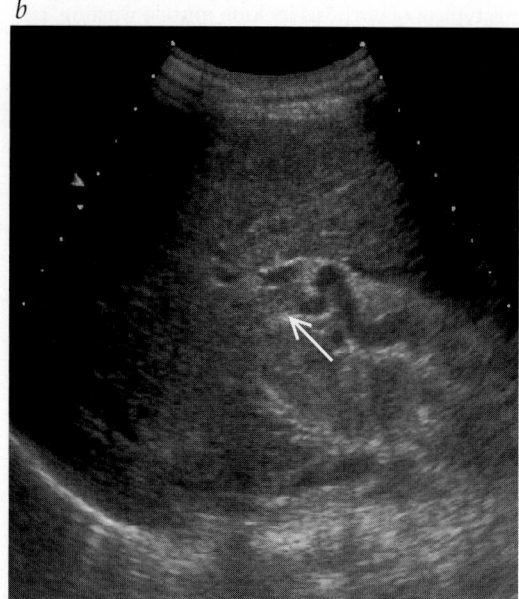

Figure 3   **Real-time ultrasound images of a 56-year-old man with liver cirrhosis from chronic hepatitis C. The patient had a compensated cirrhosis and was undergoing liver ultrasonography plus determination of α-fetoprotein serum levels every 6 months to screen for hepatocellular carcinoma. (*a*) The liver showed irregular edges (arrow) and an altered structure. (*b*) A patent portal vein thrombosis was detected (arrow).**

rhosis.[11] Liver biopsy helps determine the cause of cirrhosis, as well as provides information on the extent of liver damage. The biopsy is usually performed using a percutaneous approach, but percutaneous biopsy should not be used in patients with severe coagulopathy (i.e., those with an international normalized ratio [INR] greater than 1.5 or a platelet count less than 50,000/μl), and it must be used with caution in patients with ascites or severe obesity. Limitations of liver biopsy are that it is an invasive procedure and that sampling error can occur (i.e., false negative results), especially in patients with macronodular cirrhosis.

Transjugular liver biopsy offers an alternative to percutaneous biopsy. Transjugular liver biopsy can be used in patients with ascites; is indicated in patients with severe coagulopathy; and allows the measurement of portal pressure.[12] However, the amount of tissue obtained is limited, and often, the diagnosis of cirrhosis cannot be made. In selected cases, liver biopsy can be performed during laparoscopy. This approach is generally reserved for the staging of cancer or for ascites of unknown origin.

Histologic findings that define cirrhosis include extensive fibrosis and regenerative nodules. The degree of infiltration of inflammatory cells depends on the activity of the underlying disease. Micronodular cirrhosis is characterized by the presence of uniformly small nodules (diameter < 3 mm), whereas in macronodular cirrhosis, nodules vary in size (diameter 3 mm to 5 cm) and contain some normal lobular structure (e.g., portal tracts or terminal hepatic venules).

In some cases, histologic findings help identify the causative agent of cirrhosis, such as periportal lymphocyte infiltration in HCV-induced cirrhosis; Mallory bodies, polymorphonuclear leukocyte (PMN) infiltration, and steatosis in alcohol-induced cirrhosis and NASH; biliary involvement in PBC; and massive iron deposition in hemochromatosis. In advanced cirrhosis, however, different underlying diseases may have similar histologic findings.

Management

GENERAL MEASURES

Cirrhotic patients should undergo regular follow-up. Patients with compensated cirrhosis should be seen two or three times a year. At diagnosis, an extensive medical history should be taken and laboratory tests, including viral serologies, performed to identify the causative agent. Endoscopic examination should be done to assess the presence and size of esophageal varices. Abdominal ultrasonography and α-fetoprotein serum measurements should be performed at diagnosis and every 6 months thereafter to detect early HCC. Criteria for OLT should be reviewed periodically, and major clinical complications (i.e., bacterial infections, renal impairment, and GI bleeding) should be actively prevented.[13] Many patients complain of anorexia, and care should be taken to ensure that patients take in adequate calories and protein. Nutritional supplements are often beneficial. Zinc deficiency is common and should be treated. Zinc sulfate (50 to 200 mg/day) may be effective in the treatment of muscle cramps and is adjunctive therapy for hepatic encephalopathy. Pruritus is a common complaint in cirrhotic patients, especially in those with chronic cholestasis (i.e., PBC and PSC). Drugs that may provide relief for pruritus include cholestyramine, ursodeoxycholic acid, naltrexone, rifampicin, and ondansetron. Some men suffer from hypogonadism; those with severe symptoms can be treated with topical testosterone preparations, although their safety and efficacy are not well studied. Patients with cirrhosis may develop osteoporosis. Supplementation with calcium and vitamin D is important in patients at high risk for osteoporosis, especially patients with chronic cholestasis and those receiving corticosteroids for autoimmune hepatitis. Evidence of decreased bone mineralization from bone densitometry studies also may prompt institution of therapy with a bisphosphonate (e.g., alendronate). Mild exercise, including walking or swimming, should be encouraged in patients with compensated cirrhosis. Debilitated patients frequently benefit from formal exercise programs supervised by a physical therapist. Patients with cirrhosis should be vaccinated against hepatitis A. Other protective measures include vaccination against hepatitis B, pneumococcal infection, and influenza. Potential hepatotoxic medications should be avoided. Patients with ascites should not receive nonsteroidal anti-inflammatory drugs (NSAIDs) or nephrotoxic antibiotics (e.g., aminoglycosides). NSAID use may predispose patients with cirrhosis to development of renal failure or GI bleeding. Surgery and general anesthesia carry increased risks in patients with cirrhosis, particularly those with portal hypertension, and may lead to hepatic decompensation.

COMPENSATED CIRRHOSIS

Specific medical therapies may be applied to different liver diseases to diminish disease progression. However, these therapies may become progressively less effective if chronic liver disease evolves into cirrhosis. In patients with compensated cirrhosis, specific therapies prevent the development of clinical complications and therefore delay the need for liver transplantation. Treatment with pegylated interferon plus ribavirin should be considered in patients with compensated cirrhosis from HCV infection, although the rate of sustained response is lower than in noncirrhotic patients.[14] Moreover, antiviral treatment may worsen existing anemia or thrombocytopenia, and drug discontinuance is frequent. In patients with HBV-related cirrhosis, lamivudine appears to be a safe and effective antiviral agent, which may improve or stabilize liver disease in selected patients with advanced cirrhosis and active HBV replication.[15] However, viral resistance can develop with prolonged treatment. Adefovir and entecavir are newer antiviral agents that have activity against both wild-type and lamivudine-resistant HBV. The most effective measure for patients with alcohol-induced cirrhosis is to stop drinking.[16] Abstinence can stabilize and may dramatically improve liver function. Psychological support is highly recommended to help patients achieve prolonged alcohol abstinence. Nutritional support is advisable in all alcoholic patients. Although small clinical trials have shown improvement in survival and reversal of cirrhosis with colchicine treatment, a randomized, controlled trial found that in patients with advanced alcoholic cirrhosis, there was no reduction in overall or liver-specific mortality with colchicine; although liver histology improved to septal fibrosis in a minority of patients after 24 months of treatment, rates of improvement were similar with placebo and colchicine.[17]

In cases of superimposed alcoholic hepatitis, treatment with glucocorticoids (40 mg/day for 4 weeks followed by tapering of therapy for 1 or 2 weeks) or pentoxifylline (400 mg three times daily) increases short-term survival.[18] In patients with PBC, ursodiol (13 to 15 mg/kg/day) relieves pruritus and improves blood chemistry test results.[19] Although ursodiol may result in a decrease in the need for OLT, its usefulness in cirrhotic patients is limited. Other treatments (e.g., glucocorticoids, colchicine, azathioprine) are not indicated, because they are associated with severe side effects. No specific therapy has been shown to improve the outcome of patients with PSC, but ursodiol does have beneficial effects on biochemical parameters. In patients with cirrhosis resulting from autoimmune hepatitis, immunosuppressant therapy (e.g., glucocorticoids) should be used with caution because it may favor infections, and necroinflammatory injury at this stage of the disease is usually mild. Patients with cirrhosis resulting from hemochromatosis benefit from phlebotomies to reduce iron stores [see

Chapter 91]; those with Wilson disease benefit from treatment with copper chelators (i.e., D-penicillamine or trientine) or zinc [see Chapter 180].

DECOMPENSATED CIRRHOSIS

Ascites

Ascites is the most frequent complication of cirrhosis.[20] It impairs quality of life and increases the risk of bacterial infections. It is caused primarily by splanchnic vasodilatation from increased synthesis of vasodilators (e.g., nitric oxide). Severe splanchnic vasodilatation decreases effective arterial blood volume, which activates systemic vasoconstrictor and sodium-retaining factors. In advanced cirrhosis, solute-free water excretion is also impaired and renal vasoconstriction develops, leading to dilutional hyponatremia and HRS, respectively. Ascites can be graded into three groups: grade 1 ascites is clinically silent and detectable only by ultrasonography; grade 2 ascites is moderate, with patent distention of the abdomen; and grade 3 ascites is tense, with marked abdominal distention.

The first step in the evaluation of patients with new-onset ascites is to rule out extrahepatic causes (e.g., tuberculosis and malignancies). Besides serum tests, ultrasonography is useful to confirm signs of cirrhosis, rule out HCC, and detect portal vein thrombosis. Ascitic fluid should be examined in patients with new-onset ascites, suspected spontaneous bacterial peritonitis (SBP), encephalopathy, or GI bleeding. Measurements should be done of cell counts, albumin and total protein concentrations, and culture in blood culture bottles. Renal function and circulatory status should also be assessed in all patients.

The initial management of ascites includes reduction of sodium intake to 60 to 90 mEq/day. In patients with dilutional hyponatremia (i.e., a serum sodium concentration of 130 mmol/L in the presence of ascites or edema), fluid intake should be restricted to less than 1,000 ml/day, although compliance is problematic. Patients with moderate-volume ascites can achieve a negative sodium balance and loss of ascitic fluid with spironolactone (50 to 200 mg/day) or amiloride (5 to 10 mg/day). Low doses of furosemide (20 to 40 mg/day) may be also added; however, patients should be followed closely to avoid excessive diuresis. The recommended weight loss to prevent renal failure is 300 to 500 g/day in patients without peripheral edema and 800 to 1,000 g/day in those with peripheral edema. Patients with large-volume ascites should be treated initially with large-volume paracentesis. Plasma expanders should be given to prevent paracentesis-induced circulatory dysfunction and renal failure.[21] Albumin is the plasma expander of choice if more than 5 L of ascitic fluid is removed (8 g of I.V. albumin for each 1 L of ascitic fluid removed). Spironolactone (100 to 400 mg/day), with or without furosemide (40 to 160 mg/day), can be given to prevent recurrence of ascites. Doses of diuretics should be adjusted according to diuretic response.

Refractory ascites, which is defined as a lack of response to high doses of diuretics or the occurrence of side effects (e.g., renal failure, encephalopathy, hyponatremia, or hyperkalemia) that preclude the use of diuretics, occurs in 5% to 10% of patients with ascites. Current therapeutic strategies for patients with refractory ascites include repeated large-volume paracentesis with plasma expanders and transjugular intrahepatic portosystemic shunting (TIPS) [see Figure 4]. TIPS is effective in preventing ascites recurrence, but it does not improve survival.[22] The principal drawbacks of TIPS are the high rates of shunt stenosis and hepatic encephalopathy. The use of polytetrafluoroethylene-covered prostheses for TIPS can improve patency rates and decrease clinical relapses and the need for reintervention, without increasing the risk of encephalopathy.[23] TIPS is indicated for patients without severe liver failure or encephalopathy who have loculated fluid that cannot be treated with paracentesis and for those who do not tolerate repeated paracentesis. Patients with ascites should be evaluated for OLT, because their 5-year survival rate is only 30% to 40%. Patients with refractory ascites, SBP, or HRS have a worse prognosis, and prioritization in the waiting list should be considered.

Dilutional hyponatremia is present in 30% to 35% of hospitalized patients with cirrhosis and ascites.[24] It reflects impaired excretion of renal solute free water caused by nonosmotic hypersecretion of antidiuretic hormone. Although dilutional hyponatremia is commonly asymptomatic, it may favor the development of hepatic encephalopathy. Management consists of fluid restriction (1,000 ml/day) and discontinuance of diuretics; however, these measures do not correct hyponatremia in many cases. Vasopressin type 2 receptor antagonists are being evaluated for the management of hyponatremia, but they are not available in the United States.

Hepatorenal Syndrome

HRS is the most severe complication of patients with cirrhosis.[25] It is a functional renal failure resulting from extreme renal vasoconstriction [see Chapter 165]. HRS may occur spontaneously or after precipitating conditions such as SBP, acute alcoholic hepatitis, or large-volume paracentesis without plasma expansion. Diagnostic criteria for HRS have been established [see Table 3].[26]

There are two clinical types of HRS. Type 1 is characterized by progressive oliguria and a rapid rise of the serum creatinine concentration to more than 2.5 mg/dl. Survival of patients with type 1 HRS is extremely poor. Type 2 is defined by a moderate and stable increase in the serum creatinine concentration and is frequently associated with refractory ascites.

In type 1 HRS, the use of vasoconstrictors (e.g., terlipressin, midrodine, and norepinephrine) plus intravenous albumin improves renal function in more than half of patients.[27] TIPS is effective for patients with HRS, but its use is not recommended for patients with severe liver dysfunction. These treatments may serve as a bridge to OLT. Liver transplantation is the treatment of choice, but its applicability is limited by the poor survival of these patients.

Spontaneous Bacterial Peritonitis

SBP is a severe infection found in 15% to 25% of cirrhotic patients hospitalized with ascites.[28] Predisposing factors include severe liver insufficiency and low protein content in ascitic fluid (< 1 g/dl). SBP appears to be related to the translocation of GI tract bacteria from the mesenteric lymph nodes. Clinical manifestations are variable, ranging from no symptoms to a severe picture of peritonitis [see Chapter 128]. SBP should also be suspected in cirrhotic patients with impairment of renal or liver function that has no apparent cause.

The most common causative organisms are Escherichia coli, Streptococcus pneumoniae, Klebsiella species, and other gram-negative enteric organisms. SBP is diagnosed when the ascitic fluid has more than 250 PMNs/μl or is positive for leukocyte esterase (3+ or 4+) on urine dipstick testing. Culture results of ascitic fluid are positive in fewer than 50% of patients.

SBP should be treated empirically. The most commonly used regimen is a 5- to 7-day course of a third-generation cephalosporin (e.g., cefotaxime, 2 g every 8 to 12 hours, or ceftriaxone, 1 g/day).[29] Alternatives include oral ofloxacin and other intravenous antibiotics with activity against gram-negative enteric organisms. Development of renal failure during SBP is common and is the most important predictor of mortality. Administration of albumin at a dose of 1.5 g/kg at diagnosis and 1 g/kg 48 hours later prevents renal failure and reduces mortality from 30% to 10%.[30] Response to therapy is indicated by decreases in the signs of infection and in the PMN count in ascitic fluid. After SBP resolution, patients have a 70% chance of recurrence within 1 year. Prophylactic antibiotic therapy can reduce the recurrence rate of SBP to 20%.[31] Current prophylactic regimens include norfloxacin, 400 mg/day, and trimethoprim-sulfamethoxazole, one double-strength tablet 5 days a week. The 1-year survival probability after an episode of SBP is only 40%. Accordingly, eligible patients should be evaluated for OLT after resolution of SBP.

a

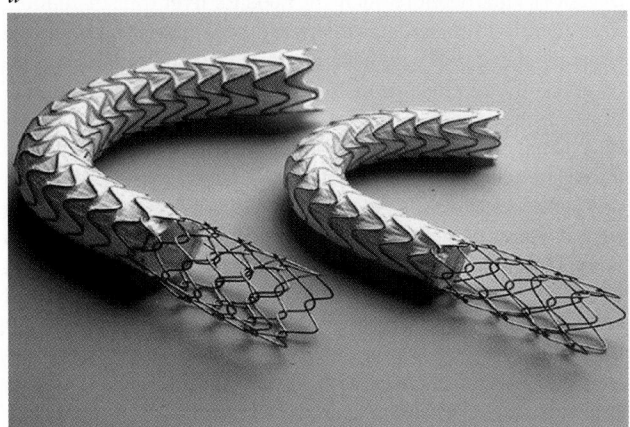

b

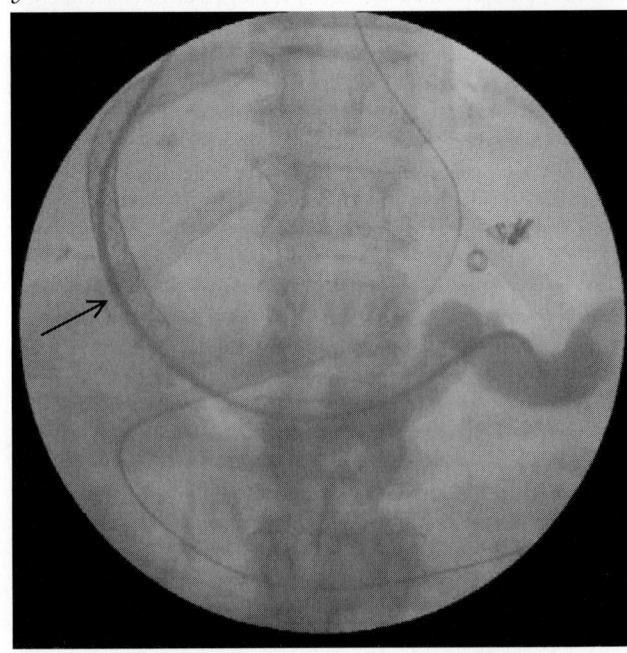

Figure 4 **Transjugular intrahepatic portosystemic shunting is basically indicated for patients with variceal bleeding and refractory ascites. It consists of (*a*) an autoexpandable stent, which is inserted using a transjugular approach. (*b*) The stent (arrow) creates a shunt between a portal vein branch and the inferior vena cava.**

Table 3 Diagnostic Criteria for Hepatorenal Syndrome*

Major Criteria

Low glomerular filtration rate, as indicated by serum creatinine level > 1.5 mg/dl or 24-hr creatinine clearance < 40 ml/min

Absence of shock, ongoing bacterial infection, fluid losses, and current treatment with nephrotoxic drugs

No sustained improvement in renal function (decrease in serum creatinine to ≤ 1.5 mg/dl or increase in creatinine clearance to ≥ 40 ml/min) after diuretic withdrawal and expansion of plasma volume with 1.5 L of a plasma expander

Proteinuria < 500 mg/day and no ultrasound evidence of obstructive uropathy or parenchymal renal disease

Additional Criteria

Urinary volume < 500 ml/day

Urinary sodium level < 10 mEq/L

Urinary osmolality > plasma osmolality

Urinary red blood cells < 50 cells/high-power field

Serum sodium concentration < 130 mEq/L

*According to the International Ascites Club.[26]

Variceal Bleeding

Rupture of gastroesophageal varices because of portal hypertension is a severe and frequent complication of cirrhosis.[32] Portal hypertension is caused by increased intrahepatic vascular resistance, as well as increased portal blood flow secondary to splanchnic vasodilatation. It is recommended that all patients with cirrhosis be screened for gastroesophageal varices and that those with large varices be offered primary prophylaxis. If esophageal varices are very small or absent, it is recommended that an endoscopic examination be performed every 2 years.

Primary prophylaxis of variceal bleeding should be initiated in patients with medium-size to large varices. Nonselective beta blockers (e.g., nadolol or propranolol) are the treatment of choice. They should be given in a stepwise fashion, with the dose being increased until the resting heart rate decreases by 25% of the baseline value. However, there are a number of limitations to the use of beta blockers in such patients (e.g., hypotension).[33] Alternatively, varices can be eradicated by repeated sessions of endoscopic variceal band ligation, although this is more commonly done in Europe than in the United States. Pharmacologic therapy and endoscopic therapy are similarly effective; both reduce the risk of bleeding by 40% to 50%.[34] Endoscopic treatment should be offered to cirrhotic patients in whom the use of beta blockers is contraindicated. The combination of variceal band ligation and beta blockers seems to be more effective than beta blockers alone and is being evaluated in large clinical trials.[35]

Acute variceal bleeding Initial therapy for acute variceal bleeding should be directed at correcting hypovolemia, achieving hemostasis, and preventing severe complications (e.g., renal failure, bacterial infections, and hepatic encephalopathy).[32] Volume replacement, as well as the need for blood transfusion, should be considered. Excessive transfusion should be avoided, because it may increase portal pressure and favor variceal rebleeding. In patients with hepatic encephalopathy and those requiring aggressive sedation for endoscopic examination, endotracheal intubation should be considered. Antibiotics (norfloxacin, 400 mg/day, or cefotaxime, 2 g every 12 hours; both for 7 days) decrease the rate of bacterial infections and improve outcome.[28]

Hemostatic treatments include vasoactive drugs, endoscopic band ligation, and surgical portosystemic shunts or TIPS. Vasoactive drugs that are effective in controlling variceal bleeding include octreotide (100 µg bolus, followed by 50 µg/hr for 5 days); alternatives currently unavailable in the United States are terlipressin (2 mg every 4 hours for the first 48 hours, then 1 mg every 4 hours for up to 5 days) and somatostatin (bolus of 250 µg, followed by an infusion of 250 µg/hr for 5 days).[36]

Pharmacologic therapy controls variceal bleeding in 75% to 80% of cases. Cirrhotic patients with upper gastrointestinal bleeding should be initially treated with a vasoactive drug. If the endoscopic examination confirms that esophageal varices are the source of the hemorrhage, variceal band ligation should be performed and drug therapy maintained for 5 days to prevent early variceal rebleeding. This approach controls bleeding in most patients. In patients with massive bleeding, balloon tamponade may temporarily help in controlling the hemorrhage. A repeat session of therapeutic endoscopy can be performed in patients who rebleed. In patients who are hemodynamically unstable or who experience several rebleeding episodes, TIPS or surgical portosystemic shunts or both should be considered.[37,38] TIPS controls bleeding in more than 90% of cases and is preferred over shunt surgery because it is associated with lower morbidity and mortality. However, TIPS can impair liver function in patients with advanced cirrhosis. Patients with preserved liver function (Child-Pugh class A) may also benefit from shunt surgery (i.e., H-graft portacaval shunt or mesocaval shunt).

Because of the high rate of rebleeding (60%), secondary prophylaxis is recommended. Drug therapy with nonselective beta blockers and repeated sessions of variceal band ligation are similarly effective.[39] The beneficial effect of beta blockers should be confirmed by the hepatic venous pressure portal gradient (HVPG), if this is available. A reduction of HVPG to less than 12 mm Hg or by 20% protects patients from variceal rebleeding.[40] The combination of beta blockers and endoscopic band ligation seems to be more effective than either treatment used alone; this combined approach is being evaluated. TIPS, surgical portosystemic shunting, or both should be considered for patients who rebleed despite drug therapy and endoscopic treatment.

Hepatopulmonary Syndrome

The hepatopulmonary syndrome (HPS), which is characterized by hypoxemia from intrapulmonary shunting, a ventilation-perfusion mismatch, or both, develops in some patients with cirrhosis.[41] Patients with HPS have no apparent parenchymal lung disease but have orthodeoxia, the unusual finding of increased hypoxemia with the change from a supine to a standing position. Other typical manifestations include exertional dyspnea, platypnea, and digital clubbing.[42] The diagnostic workup includes arterial blood gas measurements, contrast-enhanced echocardiography, and scanning with technetium-99m–labeled macroaggregated albumin. Pulmonary angiography may be necessary to detect discrete arteriovenous communications. Pharmacologic agents, such as almitrine bismesylate, prostaglandin $F_{2\alpha}$, indomethacin, somatostatin, and methylene blue, have been used to treat HPS, but results have been disappointing. Although TIPS may improve oxygenation, OLT is the only curative treatment; by 6 months after OLT, about 80% of patients with HPS have improved oxygenation.[43]

Hepatic Encephalopathy

Hepatic encephalopathy is a syndrome observed in patients

with advanced cirrhosis that is marked by personality changes, intellectual impairment, neuromuscular dysfunction, and a depressed level of consciousness.[44] The pathogenesis involves altered brain-energy metabolism and increased permeability of the blood-brain barrier, facilitating the passage of neurotoxins.[45] Putative neurotoxins include short-chain fatty acids, mercaptans, false neurotransmitters (e.g., tyramine, octopamine, and β-phenylethanolamines), ammonia, and γ-aminobutyric acid.[46]

The diagnosis of hepatic encephalopathy is made on the basis of altered mental status and neuromuscular signs in the absence of any specific mental or neurologic disease. Hepatic encephalopathy is classified into five grades, according to clinical severity [see Table 4]. In addition, hepatic encephalopathy can be classified as episodic, persistent, or minimal. Minimal encephalopathy refers to patients with subtle manifestations of hepatic encephalopathy that cannot be detected by standard clinical examination.[47]

Typical findings on physical examination include asterixis and fetor hepaticus. The serum ammonia level (arterial or free venous) is commonly elevated. Electroencephalography usually shows high-amplitude low-frequency waves and triphasic waves. CT scan and MRI studies of the brain may be important in ruling out neurologic diseases.

Common precipitating factors of hepatic encephalopathy include diuretic therapy, renal failure, GI bleeding, bacterial infections, and constipation. Dietary protein overload is an infrequent cause of worsening encephalopathy. Medications—notably opiates, benzodiazepines, antidepressants, and antipsychotic agents—also may worsen encephalopathy symptoms. Surgical portosystemic shunts and TIPS favor the development of encephalopathy. The differential diagnosis for hepatic encephalopathy includes intracranial lesions, central nervous system infections, metabolic encephalopathy, toxic encephalopathy from alcohol or drugs, organic brain syndrome, and postseizure encephalopathy. In the initial management of hepatic encephalopathy, precipitants should be identified and corrected.[48] Lactulose, lactitol (not available in the United States), or both are helpful in patients with the acute onset of severe encephalopathy symptoms and in patients with milder, chronic symptoms.[49] Lactulose stimulates the passage of ammonia from tissues into the gut lumen and inhibits intestinal ammonia production. The initial lactulose dosage is 30 ml orally once or twice a day. The dose is increased until the patient has two to four loose stools a day. The dose should be reduced if the patient complains of diarrhea, abdominal cramping, or bloating. In hospitalized patients with severe encephalopathy, higher doses of lactulose may be administered via either a nasogastric tube or a rectal tube.[50] Neomycin (2 to 6 g/day), metronidazole (250 mg/day), rifaximin (1,200 mg/day), and other antibiotics (e.g., oral vancomycin, paromomycin, and oral quinolones) serve as second-line agents.[51] Antibiotics work by decreasing the colonic concentration of ammoniagenic bacteria. Other chemicals capable of decreasing blood ammonia levels are L-ornithine–L-aspartate (available in Europe) and sodium benzoate. Low-protein diets are not recommended, because they worsen the catabolic status of these patients and may cause malnutrition. In patients with portosystemic shunts, including TIPS, shunt-diameter reduction can be considered when hepatic encephalopathy is severe and does not respond to medical therapy. Because hepatic encephalopathy carries a poor prognosis, patients with episodic or permanent encephalopathy should be evaluated for OLT. The specific prognosis of patients with minimal encephalopathy is still unknown.

Table 4   Grading of Hepatic Encephalopathy

Grade	Clinical Manifestations
0 (subclinical)	Normal mental status, but minimal changes in memory, concentration, intellectual function, and coordination
1	Mild confusion, euphoria or depression, decreased attention, slowing of ability to perform mental tasks, irritability, disorder of sleep pattern (i.e., inverted sleep cycle)
2	Drowsiness, lethargy, gross deficits in ability to perform mental tasks, obvious personality changes, inappropriate behavior, intermittent disorientation (usually for time)
3	Somnolent but arousable, unable to perform mental tasks, disorientation to time and place, marked confusion, amnesia, occasional fits of rage, speech is present but incomprehensible
4	Coma, with or without response to painful stimuli

Hepatocellular Carcinoma

HCC is currently the main cause of mortality in cirrhotic patients.[52] The annual incidence of HCC in cirrhosis from HCV is 3% to 5%. Surveillance to detect early HCC involves the use of ultrasound examination and serum α-fetoprotein measurement every 6 months. In patients with nodules smaller than 1 cm, which are malignant in less than 50% of cases, close follow-up is recommended. HCC diagnosis is based on elevated serum α-fetoprotein levels, ultrasonography, helical CT and MRI findings, and positive cytohistology. The prognosis in patients with early-stage HCC depends on tumor status, liver function, and the treatment applied. Different staging systems (e.g., Barcelona Clinic Liver Cancer [BCLC] or Okuda) use tumor characteristics and liver function to classify patients with HCC.[53] Unfortunately, many HCC patients are diagnosed at advanced stages of disease that preclude the use of curative treatments. The 3-year survival rates of patients at intermediate and advanced stages of HCC are 65% and 16%, respectively. Curative treatments for HCC include surgical resection, OLT, and percutaneous ablation. In well-se-

Table 5   Indications for Liver Transplantation

Disease	Criteria
Hepatocellular liver disease	Serum bilirubin > 3 mg/dl Serum albumin < 2.5 g/dl Prothrombin time > 5 sec above control
Cholestatic liver disease	Serum bilirubin > 5 mg/dl Intractable pruritus Progressive bone disease Recurrent bacterial cholangitis
Both hepatocellular and cholestatic liver disease	Recurrent or severe hepatic encephalopathy Refractory ascites Spontaneous bacterial peritonitis Recurrent portal hypertensive bleeding Progressive malnutrition
Hepatocellular carcinoma	< 3 nodules No nodule > 5 cm No portal invasion

lected patients, resection and OLT achieve the best outcomes, with 5-year survival rates of 60% to 70%, whereas 5-year survival rates with percutaneous treatments are only 40% to 50%. Transplantation is the ideal treatment for patients with one tumor and decompensated cirrhosis or multicentric small tumors.[54] Arterial embolization may improve quality of life and, in some cases, even increase survival. Tamoxifen does not seem to have a significant beneficial effect.

Indications for Liver Transplantation

OLT is a central tool for the management of advanced cirrhosis.[55] In the United States, more than 3,000 liver transplants are performed each year. However, because there are many more candidates for transplantation than there are available donor livers, the selection and timing of patient referral are critical. The general indications for OLT are broadly categorized as clinical and biochemical [see Table 5]. Biochemical indexes vary, depending on whether liver disease is caused by hepatocellular conditions or chronic cholestatic disorders. Patients should be referred for transplant workup if the serum bilirubin level is greater than 3 mg/dl in noncholestatic disease or greater than 5 mg/dl in cholestatic disorders; if the prothrombin time is prolonged by more than 5 seconds; or if the serum albumin level is below 2.5 g/dl. Clinical criteria include HCC, hepatic encephalopathy, refractory ascites, recurrent variceal bleeding, SBP, and intractable pruritus. The clinical complications of cholestatic liver disease, such as intractable pruritus, recurrent bacterial cholangitis, and progressive bone disease, often warrant liver transplantation before hepatic encephalopathy or variceal hemorrhage develops. HCV-infected patients with decompensated cirrhosis awaiting OLT can be treated with pegylated interferon plus ribavirin; in these patients, treatment can be initiated several months before OLT to prevent graft reinfection.[56]

Contraindications for OLT include severe cardiovascular or pulmonary disease, active drug or alcohol abuse, malignancy outside the liver, sepsis, or psychosocial problems that may jeopardize a patient's ability to follow medical regimens after transplantation. The presence of HIV infection was considered a contraindication to transplantation, but successful liver transplantations are now being performed in patients in whom antiretroviral therapy has eliminated any detectable HIV viral load. Additional clinical study is required before OLT can be offered routinely to such patients.

In the United States, the Model for End-Stage Liver Disease (MELD) is the scoring system used by most liver transplant centers for determining priority for OLT.[57] MELD relies primarily on the bilirubin level, INR, and creatinine level to determine a patient's risk of dying within 3 months if OLT is not performed.[58] Patients' scores are calculated continuously while they are on the waiting list for OLT. Scores typically range from 6 (less ill) to 40 (gravely ill). A MELD calculator is available on the Internet (http://www.unos.org/resources/MeldPeldCalculator.asp?index=98).

Advances in surgical technique, organ preservation, and immunosuppression have resulted in dramatic improvements in postoperative survival over the past 2 decades.[59] In the early 1980s, 1-year and 5-year survival after liver transplantation were only 70% and 15%, respectively; the current rates are 85% and more than 70%. In most cases, patients can anticipate a good quality of life after liver transplantation.

Approximately 15% of patients listed as candidates for liver transplantation die before a donor organ becomes available. Strategies to improve the current donor organ shortage include programs to increase public awareness of the importance of organ donation, increased utilization of living-donor liver transplantation for pediatric recipients, and exploration of the efficacy and safety of living-donor liver transplantation in adults.[60]

Prognosis

The prognosis of patients with cirrhosis depends on the underlying disease, the occurrence of major complications (i.e., ascites, GI bleeding, encephalopathy, HRS, or bacterial infections), the degree of liver insufficiency, and the existence of HCC. In patients with compensated cirrhosis, the 10-year probability of major clinical complications is 58% and that of survival is 47%. For patients with decompensated cirrhosis, prognosis can be estimated by the older Child-Pugh classification and by the MELD score.[61] The variables included in the Child-Pugh score reflect the synthetic (albumin and prothrombin time) and elimination (bilirubin) functions of the liver, as well as major complications (ascites and encephalopathy). In contrast, the MELD score includes only numeric variables that reflect liver function (INR and bilirubin level) and renal function (creatinine level). The principal advantages of the MELD score are that it is based on objective variables selected for their influence on prognosis and that continuous recalculation helps in scoring individuals more precisely among large populations.[58] However, the MELD score has not been validated in some clinical situations. For example, in patients with type 1 HRS, the MELD score may underestimate survival.[62]

The authors have no commercial relationships with manufacturers of products or providers of services discussed in this chapter.

References

1. Desmet VJ, Roskams T: Cirrhosis reversal: a duel between dogma and myth. J Hepatol 40:860, 2004

2. Afdhal NH: The natural history of hepatitis C. Semin Liver Dis 24(suppl 2):3, 2004

3. Vong S, Bell BP: Chronic liver disease mortality in the United States, 1990–1998. Hepatology 39:476, 2004.

4. Sandler RS, Everhart JE, Donowitz M, et al: The burden of selected digestive diseases in the United States. Gastroenterology 122:1500, 2002

5. Kozak LJ, Owings MF, Hall MJ: National Hospital Discharge Survey: 2002 annual summary with detailed diagnosis and procedure data. National Center for Health Statistics. Vital Health Stat 13:1, 2005

6. Bataller R, North KE, Brenner DA: Genetic polymorphisms and the progression of liver fibrosis: a critical appraisal. Hepatology 37:493, 2003

7. Bataller R, Brenner DA: Liver fibrosis. J Clin Invest 115:209, 2005

8. Roskams T, Baptista A, Bianchi L, et al: Histopathology of portal hypertension: a practical guideline. Histopathology 42:2, 2003

9. Groszmann RJ, Abraldes JG. Portal hypertension: from bedside to bench. J Clin Gastroenterol 39:S125, 2005

10. Murakami T, Mochizuki K, Nakamura H: Imaging evaluation of the cirrhotic liver. Semin Liver Dis 21:213, 2001

11. Dienstag JL: The role of liver biopsy in chronic hepatitis C. Hepatology 36:S152, 2002

12. McCormack G, Nolan N, McCormick PA: Transjugular liver biopsy: a review. Ir Med J 94:11, 2001

13. Cardenas A, Gines P: Management of complications of cirrhosis in patients awaiting liver transplantation. J Hepatol 42(suppl):S124, 2005

14. Wright TL: Treatment of patients with hepatitis C and cirrhosis. Hepatology 36:S185, 2002

15. Lai CJ, Terrault NA: Antiviral therapy in patients with chronic hepatitis B and cirrhosis. Gastroenterol Clin North Am 33:629, 2004

16. Levitsky J, Mailliard ME: Diagnosis and therapy of alcoholic liver disease. Semin Liver Dis 24:233, 2004

17. Morgan TR, Weiss DG, Nemchausky B, et al: Colchicine treatment of alcoholic cirrhosis: a randomized, placebo-controlled clinical trial of patient survival. Gastroenterology 128:882, 2005

18. O'Shea RS, McCullough AJ: Treatment of alcoholic hepatitis. Clin Liver Dis 9:103, 2005

19. Oo YH, Neuberger J: Options for treatment of primary biliary cirrhosis. Drugs 64:2261, 2004

20. Gines P, Cardenas A, Arroyo V, et al: Management of cirrhosis and ascites. N Engl J Med 350:1646, 2004

21. Gines P, Tito L, Arroyo V, et al: Randomized comparative study of therapeutic paracentesis with and without intravenous albumin in cirrhosis. Gastroenterology 94:1493, 1988

22. Gines P, Uriz J, Calahorra B, et al: Transjugular intrahepatic portosystemic shunting versus paracentesis plus albumin for refractory ascites in cirrhosis. Gastroenterology 123:1839, 2004

23. Bureau C, Garcia-Pagan JC, Otal P, et al: Improved clinical outcome using polytetrafluoroethylene-coated stents for TIPS: results of a randomized study. Gastroenterology 126:469, 2004

24. Cardenas A, Gines P: Pathogenesis and treatment of fluid and electrolyte imbalance in cirrhosis. Semin Nephrol 21:308, 2001

25. Gines P, Guevara M, Arroyo V, et al: Hepatorenal syndrome. Lancet 362:1819, 2003

26. Arroyo V, Gines P, Gerbes AL, et al: Definition and diagnostic criteria of refractory ascites and hepatorenal syndrome in cirrhosis. International Ascites Club. Hepatology 23:164, 1996

27. Ortega R, Gines P, Uriz J, et al: Terlipressin therapy with and without albumin for patients with hepatorenal syndrome: results of a prospective, nonrandomized study. Hepatology 36:941, 2002

28. Garcia-Tsao G: Bacterial infections in cirrhosis. Can J Gastroenterol 18:405, 2004

29. Fernandez J, Bauer TM, Navasa M, et al: Diagnosis, treatment and prevention of spontaneous bacterial peritonitis. Baillieres Best Pract Res Clin Gastroenterol 14:975, 2000

30. Sort P, Navasa M, Arroyo V, et al: Effect of intravenous albumin on renal impairment and mortality in patients with cirrhosis and spontaneous bacterial peritonitis. N Engl J Med 341:403, 1999

31. Gines P, Rimola A, Planas R, et al: Norfloxacin prevents spontaneous bacterial peritonitis recurrence in cirrhosis: results of a double-blind, placebo-controlled trial. Hepatology 12:716, 1990

32. Bosch J, Abraldes JG: Management of gastrointestinal bleeding in patients with cirrhosis of the liver. Semin Hematol 41:8, 2004

33. Bernard B, Lebrec D, Mathurin P, et al: Propranolol and sclerotherapy in the prevention of gastrointestinal rebleeding in patients with cirrhosis: a meta-analysis. J Hepatol 26:312, 1997

34. Jutabha R, Jensen DM, Martin P, et al: Randomized study comparing banding and propranolol to prevent initial variceal hemorrhage in cirrhotics with high-risk esophageal varices. Gastroenterology 128:870, 2005

35. Chalasani N, Boyer TD: Primary prophylaxis against variceal bleeding: beta-blockers, endoscopic ligation, or both? Am J Gastroenterol 100:805, 2005

36. de Franchis R: Somatostatin, somatostatin analogues and other vasoactive drugs in the treatment of bleeding oesophageal varices. Dig Liver Dis 36(suppl 1):S93, 2004

37. Vangeli M, Patch D, Burroughs AK: Salvage tips for uncontrolled variceal bleeding. J Hepatol 37:703, 2002

38. Neuhaus P, Blumhardt G: Surgery for portal hypertension. Hepatogastroenterology 38:355, 1991

39. Patch D, Sabin CA, Goulis J, et al: A randomized, controlled trial of medical therapy versus endoscopic ligation for the prevention of variceal rebleeding in patients with cirrhosis. Gastroenterology 123:1013, 2002

40. Merkel C, Bolognesi M, Sacerdoti D, et al: The hemodynamic response to medical treatment of portal hypertension as a predictor of clinical effectiveness in the primary prophylaxis of variceal bleeding in cirrhosis. Hepatology 32:930, 2000

41. Hoeper MM, Krowka MJ, Strassburg CP: Portopulmonary hypertension and hepatopulmonary syndrome. Lancet 363:1461, 2004

42. Lima BL, Franca AV, Pazin-Filho A, et al: Frequency, clinical characteristics, and respiratory parameters of hepatopulmonary syndrome. Mayo Clin Proc 79:42, 2004

43. Swanson KL, Wiesner RH, Krowka MJ: Natural history of hepatopulmonary syndrome: impact of liver transplantation. Hepatology 41:1122, 2005

44. Ferenci P, Lockwood A, Mullen K, et al: Hepatic encephalopathy—definition, nomenclature, diagnosis, and quantification: final report of the working party at the 11th World Congresses of Gastroenterology, Vienna, 1998. Hepatology 35:716, 2002

45. Butterworth RF: Pathogenesis of hepatic encephalopathy: new insights from neuroimaging and molecular studies. J Hepatol 39:278, 2003

46. Jones EA: Ammonia, the GABA neurotransmitter system, and hepatic encephalopathy. Metab Brain Dis 17:275, 2002

47. Ortiz M, Jacas C, Cordoba J: Minimal hepatic encephalopathy: diagnosis, clinical significance and recommendations. J Hepatol 42(suppl):S45, 2005

48. Blei AT: Treatment of hepatic encephalopathy. Lancet 365:1383, 2005

49. Morgan MY, Hawley KE: Lactitol vs. lactulose in the treatment of acute hepatic encephalopathy in cirrhotic patients: a double-blind, randomized trial. Hepatology 7:1278, 1987

50. Bongaerts G, Severijnen R, Timmerman H: Effect of antibiotics, prebiotics and probiotics in treatment for hepatic encephalopathy. Med Hypotheses 64:64, 2005

51. Mas A, Rodes J, Sunyer L, et al: Comparison of rifaximin and lactitol in the treatment of acute hepatic encephalopathy: results of a randomized, double-blind, double-dummy, controlled clinical trial. J Hepatol 38:51, 2003

52. Llovet JM, Burroughs A, Bruix J: Hepatocellular carcinoma. Lancet 362:1907, 2003

53. Llovet JM, Fuster J, Bruix J: The Barcelona approach: diagnosis, staging, and treatment of hepatocellular carcinoma. Liver Transpl 10:S115, 2004

54. Schwartz M: Liver transplantation for hepatocellular carcinoma. Gastroenterology 127:S268, 2004

55. Brown KA: Liver transplantation. Curr Opin Gastroenterol 21:331, 2005

56. Forns X, Garcia-Retortillo M, Serrano T, et al: Antiviral therapy of patients with decompensated cirrhosis to prevent recurrence of hepatitis C after liver transplantation. J Hepatol 39:389, 2003

57. Freeman RB Jr: MELD and liver allocation: continuous quality improvement. Hepatology 40:787, 2004

58. Kamath PS, Wiesner RH, Malinchoc M, et al: A model to predict survival in patients with end-stage liver disease. Hepatology 33:464, 2001

59. Tra TT, Nissen N, Poordad FF, et al: Advances in liver transplantation: new strategies and current care expand access, enhance survival. Postgrad Med 115:73, 2004

60. White SA, Al-Mukhtar A, Lodge JP, et al: Progress in living donor liver transplantation. Transplant Proc 36:2720, 2004

61. Durand F, Valla D: Assessment of the prognosis of cirrhosis: Child-Pugh versus MELD. J Hepatol 42(suppl):S100, 2005

62. Alessandria C, Ozdogan O, Guevara M, et al: MELD score and clinical type predict prognosis in hepatorenal syndrome: relevance to liver transplantation. Hepatology 41:1282, 2005

72 Gallstones and Biliary Tract Disease

Kimberly M. Persley, M.D., and Rajeev Jain, M.D., F.A.C.P.

Gallstone and biliary tract diseases constitute a common and costly health problem in the United States.[1] The prevalence of gallstones increases with age in all racial groups. Increased body weight, rapid weight loss, pregnancy, alcoholic cirrhosis, and a family history of gallstone disease also appear to be risk factors.[2-4]

Incidence and Prevalence of Gallstones

In one epidemiologic study of persons 30 years of age and older, new gallstones were found to develop in 2.2% of men and 2.9% of women over a 5-year period.[2] In the United States, gallstones occur in approximately 10% of persons older than 40 years, but the prevalence is significantly higher in women, increasing to 20% to 25% in women older than 50 years. Fortunately, only 20% to 30% of gallstones are symptomatic, with biliary colic being the most common symptom. A report from the Third National Health and Nutrition Examination Survey (NHANES III) stated that an estimated 6.3 million men and 14.2 million women 20 to 74 years of age had gallbladder diseases.[5]

Gallstone Formation

Two principal types of stone, the cholesterol stone and the pigment stone, form in the gallbladder and biliary tract. The cholesterol stone is composed mainly of cholesterol (> 50% of stone composition) and comprises multiple layers of cholesterol crystals and mucin glycoproteins. Mixed gallstones contain 20% to 50% cholesterol. The pigment stone contains a wide variety of organic and inorganic components, including calcium bilirubinate (40% to 50% of dry weight). In Europe and the United States, 90% of gallstones are of the cholesterol or mixed type; the remainder are pigment gallstones. Multiple risk factors for cholesterol and pigment gallstone formation have been identified [see Table 1]. In cholesterol gallstone formation, a genetic predisposition has been proposed on the basis of murine models and epidemiologic studies that show ethnic and geographic differences, as well as familial clustering of cholesterol gallstone disease.[6]

PIGMENT GALLSTONE FORMATION

The pathogenesis of pigment gallstones is not completely understood, but bacteria may play a central role.[7] Black pigment stones are most often seen in patients with cirrhosis or hemolytic anemia and are found predominantly in the gallbladder. Brown pigment stones, which are common in Asians, are the most common stone to appear de novo in the bile duct and are associated with biliary tract infection. The prevalence of gallstones and gallbladder disease in Asians ranges from 5% to 20%.[8] Pigment stones, in contrast to cholesterol stones, are often radiopaque and can be seen on plain abdominal x-rays [see Figure 1].

CHOLESTEROL GALLSTONE FORMATION

Cholesterol is a minor but clinically significant component of bile. The other components of bile are bile salts, phospholipids, conjugated bilirubin, fatty acids, water, electrolytes, and other organic and inorganic substances. Cholesterol is a hydrophobic molecule that is relatively insoluble in water and precipitates unless it is maintained in solution by bile salts. Bile salt molecules possess hydrophilic (water-soluble) and hydrophobic (fat-soluble) regions that maintain cholesterol in a soluble state.

When bile salt molecules in water reach concentrations of 2 to 4 mM, they form spherical complexes called micelles; the concentration at which micelles form is known as the critical micellar concentration. In micelles, the negatively charged hydrophilic ends of the molecules face outward, toward the water, and the uncharged hydrophobic regions face the center of the sphere, toward one another. Cholesterol molecules are enclosed in the hydrophobic interiors.

A pure bile salt micelle must comprise at least 50 molecules to enclose a single molecule of cholesterol. The intercalation of phospholipids (principally lecithin) between bile salt molecules of a micelle improve the efficiency with which the micelle solubilizes cholesterol. Such a mixed micelle [see Figure 2], which is the type that exists in bile, needs only seven bile salt molecules to solubilize one cholesterol molecule. Free bile salt molecules exist in equilibrium with mixed micelles in a water solution. The combined molar concentration of bile salt and phospholipid is about 11 times that of cholesterol.

Cholesterol Saturated Bile

Cholesterol gallstone formation is potentiated by hepatic secretion of bile containing excess cholesterol relative to the concentration of bile salt.[3,9] This occurs most often because of an increase in the biliary concentration of cholesterol but may also result from decreased bile acid secretion in certain disease states. Excess cholesterol is solubilized in micelles and in vesicles composed of phospholipid bilayers. Cholesterol crystal formation seems to occur at the surface of these vesicles.

Nucleation of Crystals and Gallbladder Stasis

In addition to supersaturated bile, nucleation of crystals and gallbladder stasis are also important factors in gallstone formation. Microscopic crystals initially precipitate from a supersatu-

Table 1 Risk Factors for Cholesterol and Pigment Gallstone Formation

Cholesterol Gallstones	Pigment Gallstones
Increasing age	Increasing age
Female gender	Chronic hemolysis
Obesity	Alcoholic liver disease
Rapid weight loss	Biliary infection
Native-American heritage	Asian heritage
Hyperalimentation (gallbladder stasis)	Hyperalimentation (gallbladder stasis)
Elevated triglyceride levels	Duodenal diverticulum
Medications (e.g., fibric acid derivatives, estrogens, octreotide)	Truncal vagotomy
Ileal disease, resection, or bypass	Primary biliary cirrhosis

rated bile in a process called nucleation, which is influenced by several pronucleating and antinucleating proteins.[3,9] Protein mucins, which are secreted by the gallbladder, and calcium are crucial promoters of the nucleation process. Prostaglandins stimulate the synthesis and secretion of mucins. Antinucleating factors, such as certain apolipoproteins, have been less well studied. Gallbladder stasis, with concentration and acidification of bile, is also an important factor in gallstone formation, promoting the growth of cholesterol crystals into stones. Cholesterol stones rarely recur in patients after cholecystectomy.

Development of Biliary Sludge

Biliary sludge (or microlithiasis) is a term that is often applied to cholesterol crystals of sufficient number to be visualized on ultrasonography.[10] Biliary sludge, the precursor of most gallstones, is a mix of mucus, cholesterol monohydrate microcrystals, and calcium bilirubinate granules.[4] Gallbladder sludge has been shown to precipitate biliary colic, acute cholecystitis, or pancreatitis and should be regarded as part of the spectrum of gallstone disease.

Gallbladder sludge and gallstones occur in 10% of women during pregnancy and in the early postpartum period, with significant spontaneous regression.[11] Gallbladder sludge is also associated with fasting, rapid weight loss, parenteral nutrition, cirrhosis, and certain medications, such as ceftriaxone, cyclosporine, and octreotide.[10]

Choledocholithiasis

Common bile duct stones may form de novo in bile ducts (so-called primary choledocholithiasis, constituting 5% of bile duct stones) or migrate from the gallbladder to the biliary tract (secondary choledocholithiasis, constituting 95% of bile duct stones). Stones in the biliary tract usually have the same composition as those in the gallbladder, although some are softer and brownish. The brown color is a result of deposition of calcium bilirubinate and other calcium salts as a result of bacterial deconjugation of bilirubin and hydrolysis of phospholipids.

Cholecystitis and Cholelithiasis

Patients who have stones in the gallbladder or the biliary tree display syndromes that range from acute disease to chronic symptomatic or silent disease. Gallstone disease (cholelithiasis) may remain silent throughout a person's lifetime. At any stage of disease, obstruction of the cystic duct or common bile duct by a gallstone that has passed from the gallbladder may cause pain, with or without acute inflammation (cholecystitis).

SYMPTOMATIC CHOLELITHIASIS

With the exception of biliary colic, most symptoms of gallstones are not specific for gallstone disease; a meta-analysis indicated that 80% of patients with gallstones presented with other abdominal symptoms.[12] Biliary colic is a misnomer, because the pain is steady and not colicky. The pain of biliary colic is caused by functional spasm of the cystic duct obstructed by a stone. Biliary colic often develops without any precipitating events. Typically, the pain is localized to the epigastrium, has a sudden onset, and increases rapidly in intensity to a plateau that can last as long as 3 hours before subsiding. Some patients describe the pain as excruciating or lancinating, whereas others describe it as a deep ache or cramp. The pain may radiate to the interscapular region or to the right shoulder, and it may be associated with

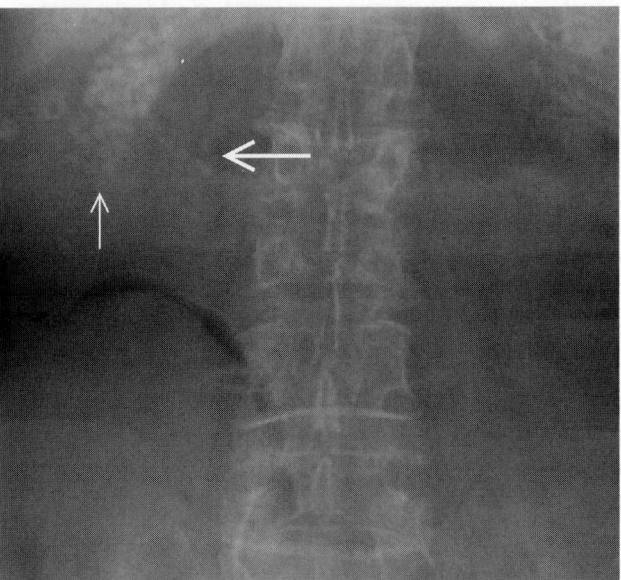

Figure 1 **Radiograph of the right upper abdominal quadrant showing radiopaque stones in the gallbladder (small arrow) and common bile duct (large arrow).**

nausea or vomiting. The pain is less frequently located in the left upper quadrant, precordium, or lower abdomen. Pain lasting longer than 6 hours or pain that is associated with fever suggests acute cholecystitis. Gastrointestinal symptoms, such as dyspepsia, heartburn, bloating, and fatty-food intolerance, are common whether or not gallstones are present. Thus, the diagnosis of biliary colic is based on clinical judgment. Once an episode of biliary colic has occurred, repeated attacks of pain are common.

ACUTE CHOLECYSTITIS

Acute cholecystitis refers to a syndrome of abdominal pain, fever, and leukocytosis associated with gallbladder inflammation, which is usually related to gallstone disease. Cholelithiasis is present in 90% to 95% of patients with acute cholecystitis, and most patients have had previous attacks of biliary colic. Acute cholecystitis may present as an acalculous cholecystitis in 5% to 10% of patients. It is predominantly noted in older men who are critically ill after major surgery, severe trauma, or extensive burn injury.[13] In rare cases, acute cholecystitis can result from a specific infection, such as that caused by *Salmonella* species. *Salmonella* organisms can also colonize the gallbladder epithelium without inflammation (carrier state). Cytomegalovirus and crytosporidia can infect the biliary system, resulting in cholecystitis or cholangitis in immunocompromised patients, such as those with AIDS or those who have undergone bone marrow transplantation.

Diagnosis

Clinical manifestations   An episode of prolonged right upper quadrant pain (> 6 hours), especially if associated with fever, should arouse suspicion of acute cholecystitis, as opposed to simple biliary colic. Clinical features of acute cholecystitis include anorexia, nausea, vomiting, fever, and abdominal pain that initially may localize to the epigastrium before shifting to the right upper quadrant. The severe abdominal pain associated with acute cholecystitis is caused by inflammation of the gallbladder wall.[9] Most patients who present with jaundice have stones in the common bile duct. Patients are ill for several days to a week before the acute attack completely subsides. Acalculous cholecystitis, an acute necroinflammatory disease, is clinically identical to acute cholecystitis but is not associated with gallstones.

Physical examination Physical examination may reveal upper quadrant subcostal tenderness and pain on inspiration, often with inspiratory arrest (the Murphy sign). Of all physical examination findings, the Murphy sign has the highest positive likelihood ratio (LR) for acute cholecystitis (LR, 2.8; 95% confidence interval [CI], 0.8 to 8.6).[14] The gallbladder may be palpable, especially at the time of the first attack, before fibrosis has reduced its distensibility. Tenderness, guarding, and rebound pain in the area of an inflamed gallbladder are important findings. Generalized rebound tenderness in a patient who has been ill for several days may reflect a perforation; however, localized tenderness may indicate secondary pancreatitis or an abscess in the area of the gallbladder.

Laboratory evaluation Laboratory tests frequently reveal leukocytosis and mild hyperbilirubinemia, which may occur in the absence of biliary obstruction secondary to reduced hepatic excretion of bile.[15] In one prospective study, 25% of patients with acute cholecystitis had a serum bilirubin level of 2 to 5 mg/dl and had no common bile duct abnormalities; 4% had an elevated amylase level without pancreatitis.[16] No single laboratory parameter has a sufficient positive or negative LR to establish the diagnosis of acute cholecystitis or rule it out.[14]

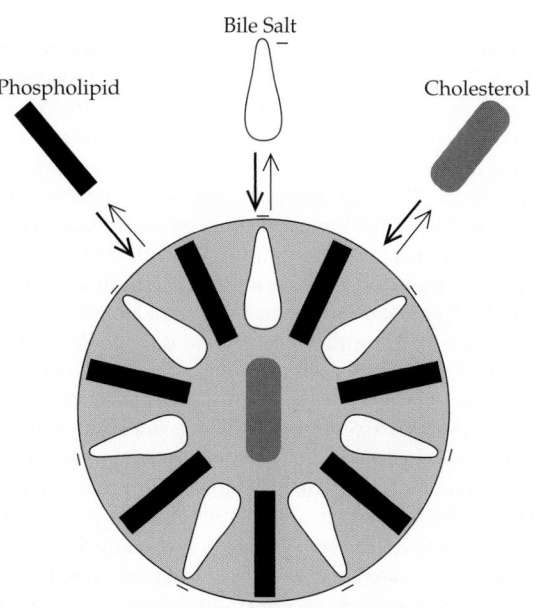

Figure 2 Cholesterol is solubilized in bile by the formation of mixed micelles that consist predominantly of bile salt and phospholipid. Micelles form when the concentration of bile salts in water is between 2 and 4 mM, the so-called critical micellar concentration (CMC). The negatively charged hydrophilic region of the bile salt molecule faces outward into the water phase, whereas the uncharged hydrophobic region is directed inward. These three components—bile salts, phospholipids, and cholesterol—exist in equilibrium between the free state and micelle constituents. At the CMC for bile salts, the equilibrium shifts strongly in the direction of the micelle. If bile salt concentrations are insufficient, the hydrophobic cholesterol molecules will precipitate to form a nidus for a gallstone.

Imaging studies Acute cholecystitis should be suspected when a patient presenting with certain clinical manifestations (see above) is found to have gallstones on an imaging study. However, the mere presence of gallstones is not confirmation of acute cholecystitis, because asymptomatic cholelithiasis [*see* Asymptomatic Cholelithiasis, *below*] is a common condition in the general population. Ultimately, the combination of physical findings and laboratory results suggests the diagnosis of acute cholecystitis, which can then be confirmed by diagnostic imaging.[14]

Transabdominal ultrasonography (TUS) is the diagnostic procedure of choice for a patient with suspected gallstones and acute cholecystitis. Meta-analysis indicates that TUS has a sensitivity of 88% to 90% and a specificity of 97% to 98% for the diagnosis of gallstones larger than 2 mm.[17] Gallbladder ultrasonography should ideally be preceded by an 8-hour fast, because gallstones are best visualized in a distended, bile-filled gallbladder. In addition to detecting gallstones, TUS can be used to identify other causes of right upper quadrant pain, such as hepatic abscess or malignancy, and it may reveal biliary duct obstruction. However, specific evidence of acute cholecystitis (i.e., the presence of pericholecystic fluid, edema of the gallbladder wall, or both) is found infrequently. Occasionally, a sonographic Murphy sign will be elicited when the ultrasound probe is positioned below the right costal margin.

Cholescintigraphy is the best method of confirming the clinical diagnosis of acute cholecystitis.[17] This procedure takes only 60 to 90 minutes and involves the intravenous injection of technetium-99m (^{99m}TC)–labeled hepatoiminodiacetic acid (HIDA, or lidofenin), which is selectively excreted into the biliary tree and enters the gallbladder. In the presence of acute cholecystitis, radiolabeled material enters the common bile duct and duodenum but not the gallbladder. Meta-analysis suggests that radionuclide scanning is the most accurate method of diagnosing acute cholecystitis.[17] Occasionally, the scan gives false positive results in patients who have alcoholic liver disease or who are fasting or receiving total parenteral nutrition; however, false negative results are rare. Radionuclide scanning may not be useful for patients with deep jaundice, because the labeled agent fails to enter the biliary tree.

Direct examination of bile is more sensitive than ultrasonography in the diagnosis of biliary sludge. Ideally, gallbladder bile, rather than hepatic and ductal bile, should be obtained to maximize sensitivity for detecting microlithiasis; gallbladder bile is most reliably obtained by cholecystokinin-induced stimulation of the gallbladder [*see* Chronic Cholecystitis, Bile Collection and Examination, *below*]. Bile collected at endoscopic retrograde cholangiopancreatography (ERCP) after the injection of contrast may lead to false positive findings of crystals.[18] Bile must be centrifuged and examined under polarizing or light microscopy for detection of crystals. Plain abdominal x-rays are much less useful than cholescintigraphy or ultrasonography, because only 15% to 20% of stones are radiopaque; oral cholecystography is also less useful and is now rarely performed because it requires 24 to 48 hours to perform and is less accurate than ultrasonography.

Differential Diagnosis

Because no single clinical or laboratory measurement carries sufficient weight to establish or exclude the diagnosis of acute cholecystitis,[14] the differential diagnosis is broad; it includes diseases that are characterized by severe epigastric symptoms and transient abnormal results on liver function testing.

Severe acute viral hepatitis or alcoholic hepatitis may be associated with moderately severe right upper quadrant pain, fever, and leukocytosis. A history of acute alcoholism, the finding of an enlarged liver, or markedly elevated aminotransferase levels should help distinguish one of these diagnoses from acute cholecystitis.

A patient with a penetrating or perforating ulcer may have severe epigastric pain and usually has a history of ulcer; free air may be evident on a plain abdominal x-ray if the ulcer has perforated. Early in its course, acute appendicitis may produce symptoms similar to those of acute cholecystitis, particularly if the appendix is retrocecal or the cecum is malpositioned in the subhepatic area. Acute pyelonephritis of the right kidney may produce anterior pain similar to the pain that occurs with acute cholecystitis. Pneumonia or infarction of the right lung may also cause abdominal symptoms.

Acute pancreatitis may be nearly impossible to distinguish from acute cholecystitis. Patients with either disorder may exhibit moderate signs on physical examination, with tenderness or localized rebound pain in the epigastrium. Serum amylase and lipase levels can be high in either condition, but the higher these enzyme levels are, the more likely it is that pancreatitis is present. Cholelithiasis occasionally causes pancreatitis, which further complicates the diagnosis. At times, only the clinical course distinguishes pancreatitis from cholecystitis.

Treatment

Medical therapy   Patients with a clinical diagnosis of acute cholecystitis should not be fed and should be given intravenous fluids and electrolytes. It is usually necessary to give a narcotic analgesic such as morphine or meperidine to alleviate severe pain. Febrile patients who have leukocytosis or bandemia (elevated circulating band forms) should be given a broad-spectrum antibiotic, such as a third-generation cephalosporin or, for broader coverage against *Enterococcus*, ampicillin-sulbactam or piperacillin-tazobactam. Nasogastric tube decompression may be required in patients who present with vomiting or with evidence of an ileus. The usual course is one of gradual improvement for several days. Persistence of severe symptoms may indicate pericholecystic abscess or perforation.

Surgery   In acute cholecystitis, laparoscopic cholecystectomy should be performed within 96 hours of onset of symptoms because the increasing inflammatory changes that occur over time have been implicated in bile duct injury; these changes may necessitate converting the procedure to an open cholecystectomy.[19,20] Early laparoscopic cholecystectomy is recommended for acute cholecystitis, because a delay in surgery does not reduce morbidity, mortality, rate of conversion to open surgery, or mean hospital stay.[21,22] In skilled hands, the laparoscopic procedure carries approximately the same risk as that of open cholecystectomy, but it is associated with much less postoperative pain and a shorter convalescence.[19] In patients with cirrhosis, laparoscopic cholecystectomy is performed for more emergent reasons and is associated with higher morbidity; however, the laparoscopic approach offers advantages of less blood loss, shorter operative time, and shorter length of hospitalization in patients with compensated cirrhosis.[23] In addition, laparoscopic cholecystectomy can be safely performed during pregnancy.[24] Laparoscopic cholecystectomy is less expensive than minilaparotomy or open cholecystectomy in high-volume surgery.[25]

In the United States, approximately 75% of all cholecystec-

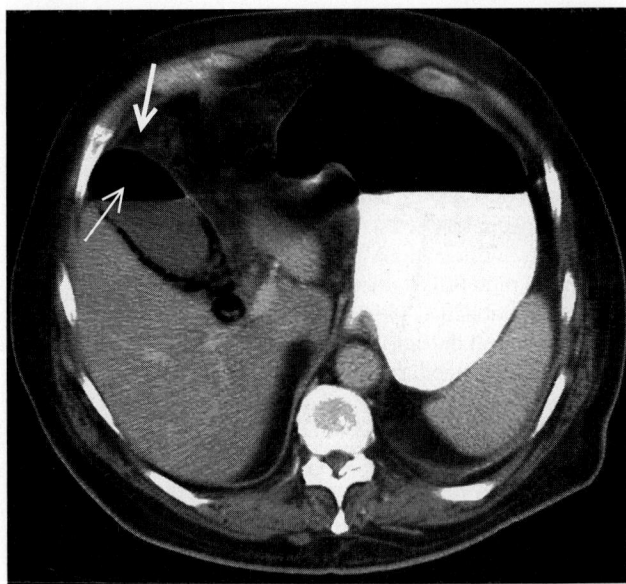

Figure 3   CT scan from an elderly man with nausea and abdominal pain following an acute myocardial infarction, angioplasty, and stent placement. The scan shows air in the wall of the gallbladder and an air-fluid level within the gallbladder, diagnostic of emphysematous cholecystitis. The patient was treated with antibiotics and a percutaneous cholecystostomy tube; laparoscopic cholecystectomy was planned in a few months.

tomies are performed laparoscopically; in 5% to 10% of these patients, the procedure has to be converted to open cholecystectomy.[26] The complication rate of laparoscopic cholecystectomy is less than 5%, which is comparable to the rate reported for conventional cholecystectomy. Complications of laparoscopic cholecystectomy (bleeding and injury to the common bile duct, vasculature, and bowel) are more common when the surgeon is inexperienced.[27] Although mortality appears to be lower for laparoscopic cholecystectomy than for open cholecystectomy, the total number of cholecystectomy-related deaths has not decreased over the years, because more procedures are being performed.[28-30] This suggests that the benefits of laparoscopic cholecystectomy have expanded the indications for cholecystectomy.

Cholangiography can be performed during laparoscopic biliary surgery. However, because 10% to 15% of patients with acute cholecystitis have common duct stones, the physician should consider preoperative ERCP in patients with suspected choledocholithiasis (e.g., patients with jaundice, cholangitis, or a dilated common bile duct, as seen on ultrasonography).[31] Common duct stones can be removed endoscopically. If endoscopic common duct stone removal is not possible, the operative procedure of choice is cholecystectomy, either open or laparoscopic, for common bile duct exploration and stone removal.

Some patients (e.g., patients with septic shock, peritonitis, severe pancreatitis, portal hypertension, or marked clotting disorders) are not candidates for laparoscopic cholecystectomy. These patients should generally undergo either open cholecystectomy, if their condition permits, or simple cholecystostomy. Cholecystostomy, either operative or percutaneous under ultrasound guidance, involves extracting the stones and draining the biliary tree through a catheter left in the gallbladder. Percutaneous cholecystostomy is superior to gallbladder aspiration in severe acute cholecystitis.[32] Cholangiography can be carried out later through this drainage catheter. For patients who respond to cholecystostomy and improve enough to become candidates for elective surgery, interval cholecystectomy is recommended, because the risk of recurrent symptoms is significant.[20]

Surgery is contraindicated for some patients because of the presence of other serious medical problems. In these cases, conservative medical therapy, including the use of antibiotics, may be the only possible approach for the acute attack.

Complications

The major complications of acute cholecystitis are related to severe inflammation and necrosis of gallbladder tissue.[33] Jaundice in the absence of choledocholithiasis can be noted in 15% of patients with acute cholecystitis; the stone impacted in the cystic duct results in edema and swelling, leading to extrinsic compression of the common hepatic duct, the common bile duct, or both [see Mirizzi Syndrome, below].[34]

Localized perforation and abscess Localized perforation and abscess formation are commonly found in patients who have severe symptoms that persist for many days. Such patients usually show localized right upper quadrant tenderness and rebound pain. In patients who have a delayed or subacute presentation, perforation typically occurs in the gallbladder fundus, as a consequence of ischemia that leads to gangrene and necrosis.[35] In patients who present with acute symptoms, the clinical differentiation between uncomplicated cholecystitis and gallbladder perforation is difficult; in this setting, ultrasonography should be the initial diagnostic modality.[36] These patients often have diabetes or other immuncompromising conditions; therefore, acute symptoms in diabetic or immunocompromised patients may heighten the suspicion for perforation. Free perforation extending into the peritoneum occurs in 2% to 10% of patients with acute cholecystitis; it is associated with peritonitis and a mortality of 10% to 30%.[37]

Empyema Empyema of the gallbladder occurs in 2% to 3% of patients with acute cholecystitis.[38] Typically, abdominal pain is severe and lasts for more than 7 days. The physical examination is not distinctive. Mortality approaches 25%; death often occurs as a result of septicemia.

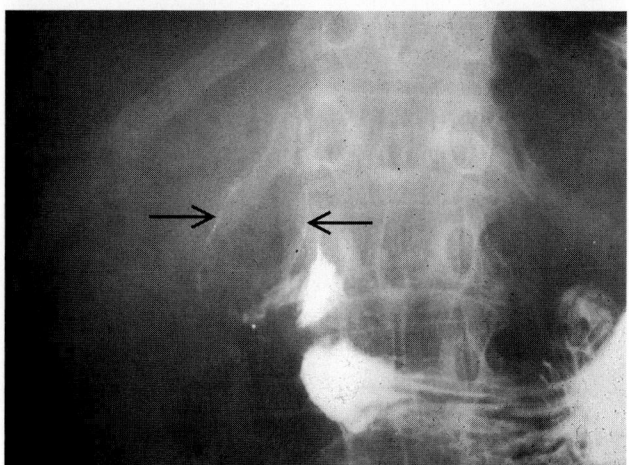

Figure 4 **Radiograph of the right upper abdominal quadrant during upper GI barium study showing a calcified wall of the gallbladder ("porcelain" gallbladder), indicating chronic cholecystitis and a high risk of gallbladder cancer.**

Emphysematous cholecystitis Emphysematous cholecystitis, which has a higher morbidity than uncomplicated acute cholecystitis, is usually caused by gas-forming bacteria, such as *Clostridium perfringens* and other clostridia, *Escherichia coli*, or anaerobic streptococci. Patients who have such infections are often very ill, and up to 50% also have diabetes.[35] Emphysematous cholecystitis occurs three times more often in men than in women.[39] Many cases of this type of cholecystitis are not associated with cholelithiasis. An ultrasound or computed tomography scan frequently reveals gas within the gallbladder; however, one study indicated that a plain abdominal x-ray is not sensitive as a diagnostic study in emphysematous cholecystitis [see Figure 3].[39]

Cholecystenteric fistula Another possible complication of acute cholecystitis is a cholecystenteric fistula, in which the gallbladder is connected either to the duodenum or to the hepatic flexure of the colon. In rare cases, the gallbladder communicates directly with the stomach or jejunum. A large gallstone (> 2.5 cm in diameter) will erode through the gallbladder wall into the duodenum. Subsequently, the stone may become impacted at the terminal ileum, causing small bowel obstruction, or in the duodenal bulb, resulting in gastric outlet obstruction (Bouveret syndrome). A cholecystenteric fistula is suspected when a plain abdominal x-ray shows pneumobilia, an ectopic stone, and mechanical obstruction. A barium upper gastrointestinal series can delineate a fistulous tract between the gallbladder and the intestines. CT scanning can define the site of obstruction and visualize the cholecystenteric fistula in 11% of patients.[40] Treatment of cholecystenteric fistula usually consists of one-stage cholecystectomy, exploration of the common bile duct, closure of the fistula, and extraction of the impacted stone.

Gallstones and malignancy Gallstones are present in 65% to 90% of patients with gallbladder cancer, although it is not clear whether gallstones themselves are the causal factor in oncogenesis.[41] A palpable gallbladder is usually found in malignant obstruction of the common bile duct (Courvoisier's law); however, this sign is uncommon in cases in which obstruction is caused by gallstones.

CHRONIC CHOLECYSTITIS

Chronic cholelithiasis is usually accompanied by evidence of chronic cholecystitis. The wall of the gallbladder is often thickened, fibrotic, and rigid, and the gallbladder is thus prevented from contracting and expanding normally. This condition may arise from a series of attacks of acute cholecystitis, from chronic mechanical irritation by calculi, or from both. The gallbladder wall may calcify and appear as the so-called porcelain gallbladder on plain abdominal x-ray [see Figure 4].

Diagnosis

Clinical manifestations It is difficult to attribute any symptom to chronic cholecystitis per se. Complaints of flatulence, heartburn, and nonspecific postprandial distress are common in patients with chronic cholecystitis, but such symptoms are also common in patients with no evidence of gallbladder disease. It is possible, however, to elicit a history of discrete attacks of abdominal pain resembling those of acute cholecystitis.

Physical examination Findings on physical examination are usually normal unless the patient is experiencing an acute attack of cholecystitis. The gallbladder is rarely palpable because scarring associated with chronic cholecystitis prevents expansion.

Laboratory evaluation   Results of routine laboratory tests are usually normal; occasionally, the serum alkaline phosphatase level is modestly elevated.

Imaging studies   TUS is the procedure of choice for the diagnosis of chronic gallbladder disease. In 90% to 95% of cases of cholelithiasis, ultrasonography demonstrates the echo of the calculus and the acoustic shadow behind the calculus [*see Figure 5*]. When the ultrasound is nondiagnostic, oral cholecystography may still be used to evaluate a patient with suspected gallbladder disease. If a double dose of the oral contrast agent fails to cause gallbladder opacification, cholelithiasis and chronic cholecystitis are almost certainly present. Cholescintigraphy is not helpful in diagnosing chronic cholelithiasis or chronic cholecystitis [*see* Acute Cholecystitis, *above*].

ERCP may reveal gallstones in the gallbladder of patients who have biliary tract pain and whose oral cholecystograms and gallbladder sonograms are normal. In one study, small gallstones were found with ERCP in 29 of 206 such patients (14%); the presence of these stones was confirmed during surgery.[42] CT or magnetic resonance imaging may also detect gallstones, but these techniques are unlikely to demonstrate stones not detected by ultrasonography. Endoscopic ultrasonography (EUS), with or without duodenal bile aspiration, may be a promising diagnostic approach in patients who have typical biliary symptoms but normal findings on transabdominal ultrasound.[43-45]

Bile collection and examination   Gallbladder bile can be obtained by nasogastric tube or by endoscopic aspiration of the duodenum after infusing cholecystokinin intravenously to promote gallbladder emptying. In patients with biliary sludge, examination of bile under light and polarizing microscopy can show cholesterol crystals, which appear as rhomboid plates with a notch in one corner. Bile collected from the common bile duct during ERCP rarely contains precipitate, because hepatic bile transits rapidly through the biliary system,[10] and injection of contrast can lead to false positive results.[18] In one small study, EUS-guided aspiration of gallbladder bile was complicated by bile peritonitis in two of three patients.[46] Although some experts consider bile microscopy to be a gold standard in the diagnosis of biliary sludge, crystal analysis is limited by the need for invasive evaluation, meticulous sample processing, and institutional expertise.

Treatment

Surgery   Elective cholecystectomy is indicated for patients who have symptomatic gallstones and chronic cholecystitis. Recurrent pain is to be expected in these patients if cholecystectomy is not performed. As many as 50% of patients with symptomatic gallstones who do not undergo cholecystectomy experience serious complications within 20 years after initial onset of symptoms.[47]

It is occasionally difficult to determine whether abdominal symptoms are secondary to documented gallbladder disease. A history of typical recurrent pain makes this determination easier. In certain cases, elective cholecystectomy is performed as a last diagnostic procedure when a thorough search for other causes of abdominal symptoms has proved negative. All too often, the symptoms recur postoperatively.

Dissolution therapy   Oral bile acids, such as ursodeoxycholic acid (8 to 12 mg/kg daily) and chenodeoxycholic acid (13 to 15 mg/kg daily), can decrease biliary cholesterol levels; and when administered for months to years, ursodeoxycholic acid and chenodoxycholic acid can result in complete gallstone dissolution in 30% and 14% of patients, respectively.[48] A randomized, controlled trial found that combination therapy using these two agents was not superior to monotherapy with ursodeoxycholic acid.[49] Chenodeoxycholic acid has largely been replaced by the safer ursodeoxycholic acid; however, these drugs are effective only in patients with small cholesterol stones and a functioning gallbladder. A high rate of gallstone recurrence is noted after cessation of therapy. Infusing methyl *tert*-butyl ether through a transhepatic catheter directly into the gallbladder can rapidly dissolve cholesterol stones.[50] The rapid infusion and removal of this ether, which remains liquid at body temperature, results in the dissolution of most cholesterol gallstones within 4 to 31 hours. Dissolution therapy has limited value, except in patients who are poor candidates for surgery.

Extracorporeal biliary lithotripsy   Stones in the gallbladder or common bile duct have been successfully fragmented using extracorporeal shock wave lithotripsy (ESWL), a technique widely employed for the nonsurgical fragmentation of kidney stones. Patients undergoing biliary ESWL are carefully positioned and monitored so that the shock waves are targeted at the gallstones. The highest success rates of biliary ESWL are seen in patients with a radiolucent solitary gallstone less than 2 cm in diameter; 60% to 84% of these patients are free of stones after 6 to 12 months of therapy.[51] ESWL has been associated with low rates of adverse events such as pancreatitis, biliary pain, hepatic hematoma, and hematuria. The administration of oral ursodeoxycholic acid after fragmentation of stones has been associated with an increase in the percentage of patients who are free of gallbladder stones 6 months after ESWL.[52,53] In one study, 21% of patients who received 10 to 12 mg/kg of ursodeoxycholic acid daily for 6 months after ESWL were free of gallbladder stones at the end of the treatment period; in contrast, only 9% of patients who received placebo for 6 months were free of stones.[53] Stone

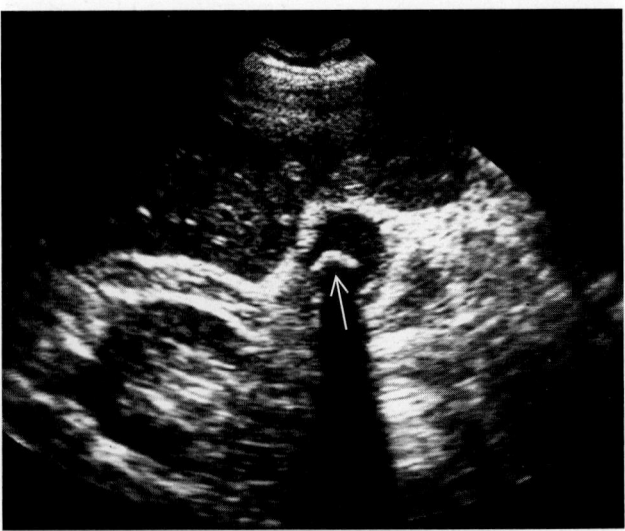

Figure 5   **Ultrasound of the gallbladder showing, in the center of the image, a stone within the gallbladder with a triangular area of acoustic attenuation ("shadowing") behind the gallstone.**

fragments in the common bile duct may pass spontaneously after endoscopic sphincterotomy or can be extracted with a basket. The usefulness of biliary ESWL is limited by its high rate of gallstone recurrence and the widespread availability of laparoscopic cholecystectomy.

ASYMPTOMATIC CHOLELITHIASIS

Most gallstones are asymptomatic (silent gallstones). In one prospective study, gallstones were present or there was evidence of cholecystectomy in 291 of 1,701 persons (17%) at the time of postmortem examination.[54] Of these 291 persons, only 31 had undergone cholecystectomy, presumably because of symptomatic disease. Ten deaths were directly attributable to the gallstones; four of these deaths occurred after cholecystectomy.

Natural History

Silent gallstones seldom lead to problems. In a long-term follow-up study of patients with asymptomatic gallstones, the cumulative risk of the development of symptoms was 10% at 5 years, 15% at 10 years, and 18% at 15 years or later.[55] Nineteen percent of patients who experienced symptoms (2.5% of the patients enrolled in the study) subsequently developed acute cholecystitis or pancreatitis. No patients died of gallbladder disease during a mean follow-up period of more than 10 years.

Diagnosis

Asymptomatic gallstones are usually identified incidentally on transabdominal or pelvic ultrasonography performed for other diagnostic purposes, such as the evaluation of gynecologic symptoms or findings on physical examination.

Treatment

Patients who have asymptomatic gallstones should generally be managed conservatively without surgery. Exceptions may be made for patients at increased risk for gallbladder cancer, such as Pima Indians, patients with calcified gallbladders (porcelain gallbladder), patients with very large gallstones (> 3 cm), and patients with an associated gallbladder polyp greater than 10 mm in diameter.[56]

In the past, prophylactic cholecystectomy was recommended for diabetic patients who had asymptomatic gallstones; anecdotal reports suggested that such patients did poorly when cholecystectomy was performed as an emergency procedure. However, two well-controlled, retrospective studies of patients undergoing surgery for acute cholecystitis and a decision analysis showed that diabetes was not an independent risk factor of operative mortality or serious postoperative complications, and prophylactic cholecystectomy resulted in a shortened life span.[57,58] Thus, prophylactic cholecystectomy cannot be recommended for patients with diabetes.

CHOLEDOCHOLITHIASIS

Choledocholithiasis, a condition in which a stone lodges in the common bile duct after passage from the gallbladder through the cystic duct, develops secondary to chronic cholelithiasis in 15% to 20% of patients.[9,59] Primary common bile duct stones are more commonly seen in Asian populations than in populations of the Western world. This increased incidence of primary common bile duct stones is attributed to the increased prevalence of flukes and parasitic infections (e.g., clonorchiasis, fascioliasis, and ascariasis) in Asia, because of the prevalent use of uncooked seafood in the diet. Other risk factors for choledo-

cholithiasis include the presence of periampullary diverticula and advancing age.[60]

Diagnosis

Clinical manifestations The signs and symptoms associated with choledocholithiasis vary. Some patients have no symptoms, whereas others may present with an acute illness. Pain is a common feature and is often located in the right upper quadrant or midepigastrium, with radiation of the pain to the interscapular region. Pain may be associated with nausea, vomiting, or both; it can be indistinguishable from biliary colic. Cholangitis may present as the Charcot triad (fever, pain, and jaundice) or the Reynold pentad (Charcot triad of symptoms, hypotension, and a change in mental status). Patients may also present with pancreatitis.

Physical examination Vital signs may reveal an elevated temperature. In more acutely ill patients, hypotension and tachycardia may occur. Physical exam may reveal tenderness and guarding in the right upper quadrant and midepigastrium. Hepatomegaly may be found when common bile duct obstruction has been present for some time. Scleral icterus may also be seen.

Laboratory evaluation Both serum bilirubin and alkaline phosphatase levels can be markedly elevated. However, when the stones do not obstruct the duct, the serum bilirubin level may be only slightly elevated or may be normal, and the alkaline phosphatase level may be substantially elevated. Typically, serum aminotransferase levels are only modestly elevated. It would be unusual to see aminotransferase levels higher than 1,000 IU/L. In some instances, aminotransferase levels rise and fall rapidly early in the course of bile duct obstruction.

Imaging studies TUS may detect only 50% of common bile duct stones[61]; however, it can often detect dilatation of common bile duct and intrahepatic ducts. The sensitivity of TUS for detecting common duct stones increases to 76% when ductal dilatation of more than 6 mm is used as the primary end point for choledocholithiasis. CT is no more sensitive or specific than TUS. Cholescintigraphy may show common bile duct obstruction, particularly when symptoms are of recent onset, but not all common bile duct stones will cause complete bile duct obstruction. Magnetic resonance cholangiopancreatography (MRCP) and EUS have similar accuracies in detecting common bile duct stones. MRCP [see Figure 6] is noninvasive and may be preferred in cases where the suspicion of choledocholithiasis is mild to moderate.[62,63]

ERCP allows radiographic visualization of the biliary tree [see Figure 7] and the option of therapeutic intervention.[64,65] EUS has greater sensitivity and specificity than ERCP in the detection of common bile duct stones but lacks the therapeutic option available with ERCP.[66] Therefore, ERCP is the technique of choice if common bile duct stones are highly suspected on the basis of the history, physical examination findings, and laboratory and imaging studies. When ERCP is unavailable or is unsuccessful in detecting bile duct stones, percutaneous transhepatic cholangiography (PTC) allows for direct imaging of bile ducts and offers the potential for therapeutic intervention. PTC involves accessing the bile ducts via a small needle.[67] The success rate of PTC in patients with dilated ducts is close to 100%; nondilated ducts are entered successfully about 70% of the time. Complica-

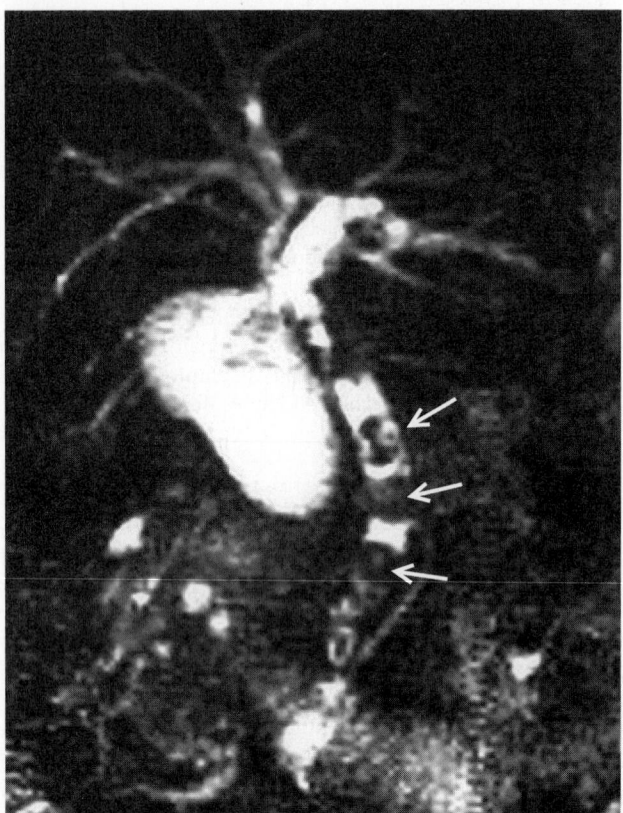

Figure 6 **This magnetic resonance cholangiopancreatogram shows multiple gallstones (arrows) in the common bile duct (choledocholithiasis).**

tion rates for both ERCP and PTC approach 5%. ERCP has replaced PTC as the technique of choice.

Treatment

Endoscopic sphincterotomy is the initial treatment for the patient with choledocholithiasis. In one large study, sphincterotomy was successful in 97.5% of patients with common bile duct stones, although more than one attempt was necessary in some patients. The overall rate of clearance of bile duct stones was 84.5%. The remaining patients required either surgery or permanent placement of a biliary endoprosthesis. The overall complication rate was 6.9%, and the complications included bleeding, cholangitis, pancreatitis, and perforation. The 30-day procedure-related mortality was 0.6%.[68] Follow-up studies have shown a low rate of recurrence of biliary duct problems and a low incidence of papillary stenosis.[69] Operative exploration of the common duct should be reserved for the few patients in whom endoscopic sphincterotomy is unsuccessful. Laparoscopic removal of biliary stones may be an alternative to preoperative ERCP.[70,71]

Endoscopic sphincterotomy is also the treatment of choice for patients with retained bile duct stones after gallbladder or biliary tract surgery. If sphincterotomy fails and if the patient has a T tube in place, instrumental extraction through the mature T-tube tract may be successful. Surgical exploration of the biliary tree is indicated if nonsurgical treatments fail.

MIRIZZI SYNDROME

Mirizzi syndrome refers to an obstruction of the common hepatic duct caused by a stone impacted at the neck of the gall-

bladder or the cystic duct. Mirizzi syndrome is classified into type I and type II.[72] In Mirizzi syndrome type I, there is only an extrinsic compression of the common hepatic duct by the gallstone and accompanying inflammation. In Mirizzi syndrome type II, a cholecystocholedochal fistula is established by the mechanism of pressure-induced necrosis from the gallstone.

Diagnosis

The clinical presentation of individuals with Mirizzi syndrome varies greatly.[73] Obstructive jaundice is commonly seen. However, 20% to 40% of patients may present without jaundice or have normal serum aminotransferase levels.[74] Biliary imaging tests often fail to demonstrate the features of Mirizzi syndrome; therefore, successful management of patients with Mirizzi syndrome is a challenge and relies heavily upon clinical suspicion and early recognition by the treating physician.

Treatment

Nonsurgical treatment of Mirizzi syndrome is limited and suboptimal. Long-term biliary stenting has a relatively high incidence of complications, including cholangitis and secondary biliary cirrhosis.[73] Nonsurgical lithotripsy and stone removal is restricted to patients with Mirizzi syndrome type II.[75] In Mirizzi syndrome type I, the offending stones are not accessible for clearance via bile ducts. Cholecystectomy is the treatment of choice. If the gallbladder is not removed, patients with Mirizzi syndrome are left at significant risk for complications from continued gallstone disease, including acute cholangitis, cholecystitis, suppurative cholangitis, liver abscess, secondary biliary cholangitis, and, perhaps, gallbladder carcinoma.[73,75,76] Nonsurgical treatment of patients with Mirizzi syndrome should be limited to those patients who are unfit for surgery or who have a shortened life expectancy.[34]

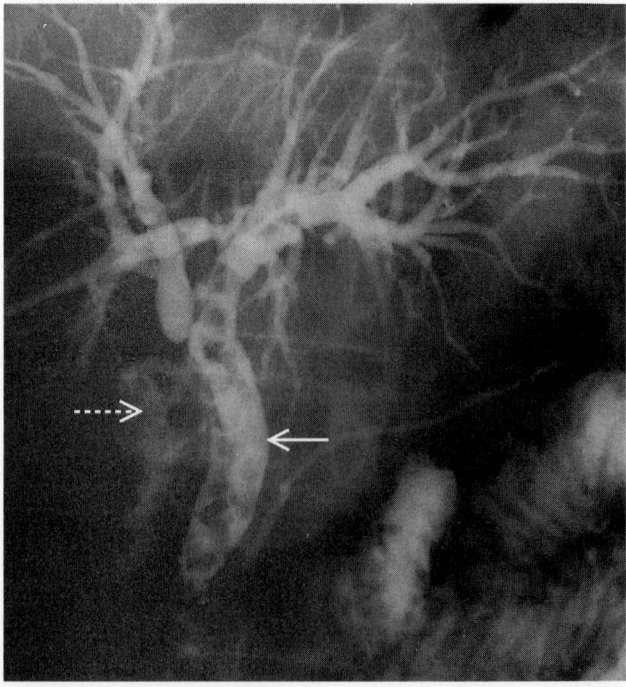

Figure 7 **Endoscopic retrograde cholangiopancreatography reveals abnormalities in a patient with gallstones. Multiple radiolucent areas establish the diagnosis of stones in the gallbladder (broken arrow) and common bile duct (solid arrow).**

Chronic Biliary Tract Disease

Chronic inflammation of biliary ducts is usually caused by partial or complete obstruction of the biliary tree. Some patients with chronic cholelithiasis or other chronic diseases of the biliary ducts will experience associated chronic inflammation or stricturing of the biliary tree.

DIAGNOSTIC OVERVIEW

Clinical Manifestations

Patients with chronic inflammation of the biliary tree may complain of fatigue, intermittent fever and chills, anorexia, pruritus, and weight loss. The physical examination may be fairly unremarkable; jaundice, excoriations of the skin related to marked pruritus, and stigmata of chronic liver disease may raise the level of suspicion.

Laboratory Evaluation

Laboratory tests will often reveal chronically elevated serum alkaline phosphatase levels and increased levels of serum 5´-nucleotidase, leucine aminopeptidase, and γ-glutamyl transpeptidase (GGT). Transient elevations of the total bilirubin level may also been seen.

Imaging Studies

Direct visualization of the biliary tree is important in determining whether the symptoms and signs result from an anatomic defect that can be corrected by endoscopic therapy or surgery. Use of MRCP or ERCP usually leads to identification of the obstructive site.

SPECIFIC PRESENTATIONS

Common Bile Duct Stricture

Benign and malignant strictures are similar in appearance, as imaged by ERCP or MRCP. Epithelial samples of biliary strictures for evaluation can be obtained by brush cytology; fine-needle aspiration; endoscopic pinch biopsy; or a combination of the three. The sensitivity of brush cytology is as high as 70% for the diagnosis of a malignant stricture of the bile duct; specificity is as high as 100%.[77] Simple bile duct aspiration alone is not as reliable. Common bile duct stricture, which may result from biliary tract surgery, can be treated endoscopically with balloon dilatation or with the placement of an endoprosthesis. If these treatments are unsuccessful, surgical intervention may prove beneficial for selected patients.

Primary Sclerosing Cholangitis

Primary sclerosing cholangitis (PSC) is a disease of unknown etiology that is characterized by an irregular inflammatory fibrosis of both the intrahepatic and extrahepatic bile ducts [*see Figure 8*].[78] It usually occurs in men between 20 and 50 years of age.

Patients may present with jaundice, pruritus, nonspecific pain, fever, and weight loss. Approximately 75% of patients will have chronic ulcerative colitis. Liver function tests show cholestatic abnormalities.[78]

Ursodeoxycholic acid therapy will usually result in an improvement in the biochemical markers of cholestasis, but it has not been shown to increase survival.[79] Endoscopic treatment of significant ductal strictures may also improve biochemical markers of cholestasis and reduce the number of episodes of

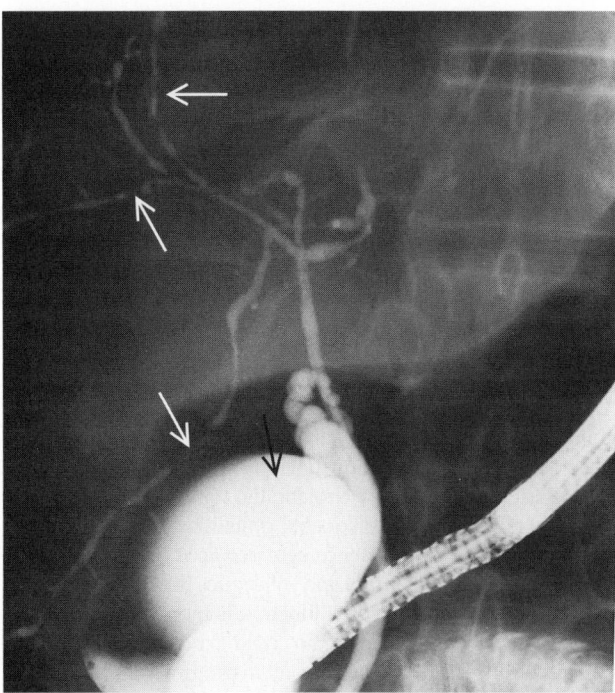

Figure 8 **This cholangiogram, obtained during endoscopic retrograde cholangiopancreatography, shows a normal gallbladder (black arrow) and a narrowed biliary tree with many areas of segmental stenosis (white arrows), diagnostic of primary sclerosing cholangitis.**

cholangitis.[80] A combined approach using therapeutic stricture dilatation and ursodeoxycholic acid therapy may benefit a select group of patients.

Patients with PSC are at increased risk for biliary tract cancer. The incidence of cholangiocarcinoma in patients with PSC is as high as 30%, and there is an increased risk of gallbladder and pancreatic cancer.[81] A substantial number of patients with PSC may have undetected cholangiocarcinoma at the time of liver transplantation.

Recurrent Pyogenic Cholangitis

Recurrent pyogenic cholangitis (RPC), as its name suggests, is a condition characterized by recurrent bouts of inflammation of the bile ducts. It most commonly affects patients of Asian descent. The exact etiology of RPC is unclear. Some experts propose a dietary or infectious cause. The parasites *Opisthorchis sinensis* and *Ascaris lumbricoides* are commonly found in the stools of affected patients.[82]

Patients typically present with repeated attacks of fever, chills, abdominal pain, and jaundice. Laboratory tests usually demonstrate an elevation in serum bilirubin and alkaline phosphatase levels. Elevations in serum aminotransferase levels and the prothrombin time signify hepatocyte injury, although the prothrombin time may also be prolonged because of vitamin K malabsorption.[83]

Imaging studies, such as ultrasonography, may be somewhat confusing in patients with RPC, because there may be areas of intrahepatic biliary dilatation without common bile duct dilatation. Evaluation using CT or MRCP usually defines the areas of intrahepatic and extrahepatic biliary dilatation more clearly than does ultrasonography, and these techniques also provide three-dimensional information.[84] ERCP is often required to confirm areas of stricture and dilatation. ERCP also allows for possible therapeutic intervention. PTC provides access to peripheral ducts that may be inaccessible by ERCP.[85]

Treatment usually consists of antibiotic therapy and endoscopic or surgical stone clearance to improve biliary drainage.

Choledochal Cyst

Biliary cystic disease includes choledochal cyst disease and the less common gallbladder cysts and cystic duct cysts.[86] Choledochal cyst is an ectasia of the common bile duct that may present in late childhood or in adult life as obstructive jaundice. The cause of the disorder is not fully defined, and both congenital and acquired etiologies are postulated.[87]

Diagnosis Clinical manifestations of choledochal cyst in children include abdominal pain, cholangitis, and an abdominal mass. A palpable mass is unusual in adults, because adults tend to present with recurrent cholangitis, pancreatitis, or, rarely, portal hypertension. Choledochal cysts may involve any segment of the bile duct and are categorized according to the classification proposed by Todani and colleagues [see Table 2].[88] An abnormal pancreatobiliary duct junction is more common in patients with choledochal cysts and could expose the bile ducts to pancreatic juices, which could result in progressive injury to the ductal system. Type I cysts are the most common, accounting for 40% to 60% of all cases, followed by type IV. Types II, III, and V are rare.

A combination of imaging studies may establish the diagnosis. Ultrasonography may delineate the cyst and intrahepatic portions of the disease. CT and MRCP may provide useful information in regard to the extent of disease and the potential for malignancy. ERCP, PTC, and intraoperative cholangiography are important for diagnostic evaluation and surgical planning.

Table 2 Modified Classification System for Choledochal Cysts and Surgical Procedure of Choice

Classification	Type	Procedure of Choice
Type IA	Choledochal cyst	Roux-en-Y hepaticojejunostomy
Type IB	Segmented choledochal dilatation	
Type IC	Diffuse or cylindrical duct dilatation	
Type II	Extrahepatic duct diverticulum	Excision of diverticulum
Type III	Choledochocele	Endoscopic sphincterotomy
Type IVA	Multiple intrahepatic and extrahepatic duct cysts	Roux-en-Y hepaticojejunostomy
Type IVB	Multiple extrahepatic duct cysts	
Type V	Intrahepatic duct cysts (Caroli disease and Caroli syndrome)	Hepatic resection, liver transplantation

*All patients with choledochal cysts must undergo cholecystectomy to decrease the risk of malignancy, with the possible exception of patients with type III cysts. For the much rarer gallbladder and cystic duct cysts, treatment is cholecystectomy.

Table 3 Clinical Classification System for Biliary-Specific Abdominal Pain Associated with SOD*

Criteria

A. Typical biliary-type pain
B. Elevated liver enzyme levels (AST, alkaline phosphatase, or both more than two times normal on at least two occasions)
C. Delayed drainage of contrast injection during ERCP (> 45 min)
D. Dilated common bile duct (> 12 mm)

Classification Based on above Criteria

Biliary type I: criteria A through D are present; SOD is present in 80%–90% of patients
Biliary type II : criterion A plus one or two other criteria are present; SOD is present in 50% of patients
Biliary type III: only criterion A is present; SOD is uncommon

---

*A similar classification for SOD and pancreatic-type abdominal pain exists but is not included in this table.
AST — aspartate aminotransferase   ERCP — endoscopic retrograde cholangiopancreatography   SOD — sphincter of Oddi dysfunction

---

Treatment The initial treatment of choledochal cysts depends on the age of the patient, the presentation, and the type of the cyst. In terms of definitive treatment, pharmacologic or endoscopic management offers little benefit in that these forms of therapy do not address the well-described malignant potential of bile duct cysts.[89] Therefore, the primary role of endoscopic procedures is in the initial evaluation and diagnosis of bile duct cysts. However, endoscopic interventions such as lithotripsy, stone extraction, and laser ablation have proved successful in the treatment of intrahepatic and extrahepatic biliary stones in patients with Caroli disease, a congenital disorder associated with renal cystic disease of varying severity.[90] Endoscopic therapy, such as stone extraction, can be a definitive treatment for patients with recurrent pyogenic cholangitis. It would be the chosen therapy in elderly patients or in patients considered to be poor candidates for surgery. The current standard for surgical treatment in the patient who is a reasonable surgical risk is excision of the cyst with free biliary drainage into the gastrointestinal tract. The classical surgical reconstruction is a hepaticojejunostomy with a Roux-en-Y [see Table 2] reconstruction.[91]

Sphincter of Oddi Dysfunction

Sphincter of Oddi dysfunction (SOD) is a benign condition of intermittent or permanent obstruction of biliary drainage, pancreatic drainage, or both that is caused either by a stenosis or by smooth muscle dysfunction of the sphincter muscle.[92] Biliary SOD is classified into three types on the basis of clinical parameters using the modified Milwaukee criteria [see Table 3].

Diagnosis Biliary SOD is usually seen in women in the fourth to sixth decades of life. The symptoms arise typically after cholecystectomy, although SOD may occur in patients with an intact gallbladder.[93,94] The clinical presentation of biliary SOD is episodic abdominal pain in the epigastric region or the right upper quadrant that may radiate to the back or shoulders. It may be associated with nausea or vomiting that worsens with eating. Laboratory tests may reveal elevated liver function. Right upper quadrant ultrasonography and CT may reveal a dilated common bile duct.

ERCP with sphincter of Oddi manometry is the gold standard for diagnosis of SOD. A basal sphincter pressure of more than 40 mm Hg is abnormal and indicative of SOD.[95] Other tests that are noninvaive and less reliable may also indicate the presence of SOD; such tests include a provocation test with morphine (or neostigmine), which produces biliary pain and elevation of the serum aminotransferase level; ultrasound evaluation of dilatation and emptying of the common bile duct after secretin stimulation; or the kinetics of ductal emptying studied by scintigraphy.[96]

Sphincter of Oddi manometry is not required to confirm the diagnosis of type I SOD disease. However, patients classified with type II disease should undergo sphincter of Oddi manometry because only 50% of patients in this group have SOD. In patients classified as having type II disease, only patients whose SOD is confirmed by sphincter of Oddi manometry should undergo endoscopic sphincterotomy. Sphincter of Oddi manometry, endoscopic sphincterotomy, or both have low efficacy in patients with type III disease.

Treatment A low-fat diet may decrease biliary or pancreatic stimulation, although the efficacy of this approach is unknown. Endoscopic sphincterotomy is the primary treatment for patients with SOD type I disease and for patients with types II and III disease in which the presence of SOD has been confirmed by manometry. Over 90% of patients with type I disease will have a favorable response to endoscopic sphincterotomy; therefore, manometry should not be performed in these patients.

Pharmacologic therapies (i.e., calcium channel blockers and nitrates) are primarily used in patients with type III disease, because in these patients, sphincter of Oddi manometry has the greatest risk of complication and the smallest diagnostic yield. Treatment with calcium channel blockers and nitrates decreases pain by relaxing the sphincter smooth muscle.[92]

Other endoscopic therapies such as balloon dilatation, injection of botulinum toxin, temporary stent placement, and surgical sphincteroplasty are not widely used in the treatment of SOD.[97-99]

Kimberly M. Persley, M.D., has no commercial relationships with manufacturers of products or providers of services discussed in this chapter.

Rajeev Jain, M.D., F.A.C.P., is an advisor or consultant for AstraZeneca Pharmaceuticals LP.

References

1. Sandler RS, Everhart JE, Donowitz M, et al: The burden of selected digestive diseases in the United States. Gastroenterology 122:1500, 2002

2. Jensen KH, Jorgensen T: Incidence of gallstones in a Danish population. Gastroenterology 100:790, 1991

3. Donovan JM: Physical and metabolic factors in gallstone pathogenesis. Gastroenterol Clin North Am 28:75, 1999

4. Ko CW, Sekijima JH, Lee SP: Biliary sludge. Ann Intern Med 130(4 pt 1):301, 1999

5. Everhart JE, Khare M, Hill M, et al: Prevalence and ethnic differences in gallbladder disease in the United States. Gastroenterology 117:632, 1999

6. Wang DQ, Afdhal NH: Genetic analysis of cholesterol gallstone formation: searching for Lith (gallstone) genes. Curr Gastroenterol Rep 6:140, 2004

7. Stewart L, Oesterle AL, Erdan I, et al: Pathogenesis of pigment gallstones in Western societies: the central role of bacteria. J Gastrointest Surg 6:891, 2002

8. Shaffer EA: Epidemiology and risk factors for gallstone disease: has the paradigm changed in the 21st century? Curr Gastroenterol Rep 7:132, 2005

9. Johnston DE, Kaplan MM: Pathogenesis and treatment of gallstones. N Engl J Med 328:412, 1993

10. Jain R: Biliary sludge: When should it ot be ignored? Curr Treat Options Gastroenterol 7:105, 2004

11. Ko CW, Beresford SA, Schulte SJ, et al: Incidence, natural history, and risk factors for biliary sludge and stones during pregnancy. Hepatology 41:359, 2005

12. Berger MY, van der Velden JJ, Lijmer JG, et al: Abdominal symptoms: do they predict gallstones? A systematic review. Scand J Gastroenterol 35:70, 2000

13. Owen CC, Jain R: Acute acalculous cholecystitis. Curr Treat Options Gastroenterol 8:99, 2005

14. Trowbridge RL, Rutkowski NK, Shojania KG: Does this patient have acute cholecystitis? JAMA 289:80, 2003

15. Edlund G, Kempi V, van der Linden W: Jaundice in acute cholecystitis without common duct stones. Acta Chir Scand 149:597, 1983

16. Kurzweil SM, Shapiro MJ, Andrus CH, et al: Hyperbilirubinemia without common bile duct abnormalities and hyperamylasemia without pancreatitis in patients with gallbladder disease. Arch Surg 129:829, 1994

17. Shea JA, Berlin JA, Escarce JJ, et al: Revised estimates of diagnostic test sensitivity and specificity in suspected biliary tract disease. Arch Intern Med 154:2573, 1994

18. Parasher VK, Romain K, Sukumar R, et al: Can ERCP contrast agents cause pseudomicrolithiasis? Their effect on the final outcome of bile analysis in patients with suspected microlithiasis. Gastrointest Endosc 51(4 pt 1):401, 2000

19. Zacks SL, Sandler RS, Rutledge R, et al: A population-based cohort study comparing laparoscopic cholecystectomy and open cholecystectomy. Am J Gastroenterol 97:334, 2002

20. Bhattacharya D, Ammori BJ: Contemporary minimally invasive approaches to the management of acute cholecystitis: a review and appraisal. Surg Laparosc Endosc Percutan Tech 15:1, 2005

21. Shikata S, Noguchi Y, Fukui T: Early versus delayed cholecystectomy for acute cholecystitis: a meta-analysis of randomized controlled trials. Surg Today 35:553, 2005

22. Papi C, Catarci M, D'Ambrosio L, et al: Timing of cholecystectomy for acute calculous cholecystitis: a meta-analysis. Am J Gastroenterol 99:147, 2004

23. Puggioni A, Wong LL: A metaanalysis of laparoscopic cholecystectomy in patients with cirrhosis. J Am Coll Surg 197:921, 2003

24. Barone JE, Bears S, Chen S, et al: Outcome study of cholecystectomy during pregnancy. Am J Surg 177:232, 1999

25. Nilsson E, Ros A, Rahmqvist M, et al: Cholecystectomy: costs and health-related quality of life: a comparison of two techniques. Int J Qual Health Care 16:473, 2004

26. Livingston EH, Rege RV: A nationwide study of conversion from laparoscopic to open cholecystectomy. Am J Surg 188:205, 2004

27. See WA, Fisher RJ, Winfield HN, et al: Laparoscopic surgical training: effectiveness and impact on urological surgical practice patterns. J Urol 149:1054, 1993

28. Legorreta AP, Silber JH, Costantino GN, et al: Increased cholecystectomy rate after the introduction of laparoscopic cholecystectomy. JAMA 270:1429, 1993

29. Steiner CA, Bass EB, Talamini MA, et al: Surgical rates and operative mortality for open and laparoscopic cholecystectomy in Maryland. N Engl J Med 330:403, 1994

30. Escarce JJ, Chen W, Schwartz JS: Falling cholecystectomy thresholds since the introduction of laparoscopic cholecystectomy. JAMA 273:1581, 1995

31. Tse F, Barkun JS, Barkun AN: The elective evaluation of patients with suspected choledocholithiasis undergoing laparoscopic cholecystectomy. Gastrointest Endosc 60:437, 2004

32. Ito K, Fujita N, Noda Y, et al: Percutaneous cholecystostomy versus gallbladder aspiration for acute cholecystitis: a prospective randomized controlled trial. AJR Am J Roentgenol 183:193, 2004

33. Abou-Saif A, Al-Kawas FH: Complications of gallstone disease: Mirizzi syndrome, cholecystocholedochal fistula, and gallstone ileus. Am J Gastroenterol 97:249, 2002

34. Gomez G: Mirizzi syndrome. Curr Treat Options Gastroenterol 5:95, 2002

35. Bennett GL, Balthazar EJ: Ultrasound and CT evaluation of emergent gallbladder pathology. Radiol Clin North Am 41:1203, 2003

36. Sood BP, Kalra N, Gupta S, et al: Role of sonography in the diagnosis of gallbladder perforation. J Clin Ultrasound 30:270, 2002

37. Menakuru SR, Kaman L, Behera A, et al: Current management of gall bladder perforations. ANZ J Surg 74:843, 2004

38. Thornton JR, Heaton KW, Espiner HJ, et al: Empyema of the gall bladder: reappraisal of a neglected disease. Gut 24:1183, 1983

39. Gill K, Chapman A, Weston M: The changing face of emphysematous cholecystitis. Br J Radiol 70:986, 1997

40. Lassandro F, Gagliardi N, Scuderi M, et al: Gallstone ileus analysis of radiologic findings in 27 patients. Eur J Radiol 50:23, 2004

41. Misra S, Chaturvedi A, Misra NC, et al: Carcinoma of the gallbladder. Lancet Oncol 4:167, 2003

42. Venu RP, Geenen JE, Toouli J, et al: Endoscopic retrograde cholangiopancreatography. Diagnosis of cholelithiasis in patients with normal gallbladder x-ray and ultrasound studies. JAMA 249:758, 1983

43. Thorboll J, Vilmann P, Jacobsen B, et al: Endoscopic ultrasonography in detection of cholelithiasis in patients with biliary pain and negative transabdominal ultrasonography. Scand J Gastroenterol 39:267, 2004

44. Dill JE, Hill S, Callis J, et al: Combined endoscopic ultrasound and stimulated biliary drainage in cholecystitis and microlithiasis—diagnoses and outcomes. Endoscopy 27:424, 1995

45. Dahan P, Andant C, Levy P, et al: Prospective evaluation of endoscopic ultrasonography and microscopic examination of duodenal bile in the diagnosis of cholecystolithiasis in 45 patients with normal conventional ultrasonography. Gut 38:277, 1996

46. Jacobson BC, Waxman I, Parmar K, et al: Endoscopic ultrasound-guided gallbladder bile aspiration in idiopathic pancreatitis carries a significant risk of bile peritonitis. Pancreatology 2:26, 2002

47. Wenckert A, Robertson B: The natural course of gallstone disease: eleven-year review of 781 nonoperated cases. Gastroenterology 50:376, 1966

48. Broughan TA: Gallstones. Curr Treat Options Gastroenterol 2:154, 1999

49. Petroni ML, Jazrawi RP, Pazzi P, et al: Ursodeoxycholic acid alone or with chenodeoxycholic acid for dissolution of cholesterol gallstones: a randomized multicentre trial. The British-Italian Gallstone Study group. Aliment Pharmacol Ther 15:123, 2001

50. Thistle JL, May GR, Bender CE, et al: Dissolution of cholesterol gallbladder stones by methyl *tert*-butyl ether administered by percutaneous transhepatic catheter. N Engl J Med 320:633, 1989

51. Paumgartner G, Sauter GH: Extracorporeal shock wave lithotripsy of gallstones: 20th anniversary of the first treatment. Eur J Gastroenterol Hepatol 17:525, 2005

52. Tsumita R, Sugiura N, Abe A, et al: Long-term evaluation of extracorporeal shockwave lithotripsy for cholesterol gallstones. J Gastroenterol Hepatol 16:93, 2001

53. Schoenfield LJ, Berci G, Carnovale RL, et al: The effect of ursodiol on the efficacy and safety of extracorporeal shock-wave lithotripsy of gallstones. The Dornier National Biliary Lithotripsy Study. N Engl J Med 323:1239, 1990

54. Godrey PJ, Bates T, Harrison M, et al: Gall stones and mortality: a study of all gall stone related deaths in a single health district. Gut 25:1029, 1984

55. Gracie WA, Ransohoff DF: The natural history of silent gallstones: the innocent gallstone is not a myth. N Engl J Med 307:798, 1982

56. Guidelines for the Treatment of Gallstones. American College of Physicians. Ann Intern Med 119:620, 1993

57. Ransohoff DF, Miller GL, Forsythe SB, et al: Outcome of acute cholecystitis in patients with diabetes mellitus. Ann Intern Med 106:829, 1987

58. Friedman LS, Roberts MS, Brett AS, et al: Management of asymptomatic gallstones in the diabetic patient: a decision analysis. Ann Intern Med 109:913, 1988

59. Ahmed A, Cheung RC, Keeffe EB: Management of gallstones and their complications. Am Fam Physician 61:1673, 2000

60. Houdart R, Perniceni T, Darne B, et al: Predicting common bile duct lithiasis: determination and prospective validation of a model predicting low risk. Am J Surg 170:38, 1995

61. Lichtenbaum RA, McMullen HF, Newman RM: Preoperative abdominal ultrasound may be misleading in risk stratification for presence of common bile duct abnormalities. Surg Endosc 14:254, 2000

62. Kondo S, Isayama H, Akahane M, et al: Detection of common bile duct stones: comparison between endoscopic ultrasonography, magnetic resonance cholangiography, and helical-computed-tomographic cholangiography. Eur J Radiol 54:271, 2005

63. Aube C, Delorme B, Yzet T, et al: MR cholangiopancreatography versus endoscopic sonography in suspected common bile duct lithiasis: a prospective, comparative study. AJR Am J Roentgenol 184:55, 2005

64. Ramesh H: A balanced approach to choledocholithiasis. Surg Endosc 15:1494, 2001

65. NIH state-of-the-science statement on endoscopic retrograde cholangiopancreatography (ERCP) for diagnosis and therapy. NIH Consens State Sci Statements 19:1, 2002

66. Palazzo L, O'Toole D: EUS in common bile duct stones. Gastrointest Endosc 56(4 suppl):S49, 2002

67. Mueller PR, vanSonnenberg E, Simeone JF: Fine-needle transhepatic cholangiography: indications and usefulness. Ann Intern Med 97:567, 1982

68. Vaira D, D'Anna L, Ainley C, et al: Endoscopic sphincterotomy in 1000 consecutive patients. Lancet 2:431, 1989

69. Hawes RH, Cotton PB, Vallon AG: Follow-up 6 to 11 years after duodenoscopic sphincterotomy for stones in patients with prior cholecystectomy. Gastroenterology 98:1008, 1990

70. Hawasli A, Lloyd L, Cacucci B: Management of choledocholithiasis in the era of laparoscopic surgery. Am Surg 66:425, 2000

71. Ponsky JL, Heniford BT, Gersin K: Choledocholithiasis: evolving intraoperative strategies. Am Surg 66:262, 2000

72. Csendes A, Diaz JC, Burdiles P, et al: Mirizzi syndrome and cholecystobiliary fistula: a unifying classification. Br J Surg 76:1139, 1989

73. England RE, Martin DF: Endoscopic management of Mirizzi's syndrome. Gut 40:272, 1997

74. Curet MJ, Rosendale DE, Congilosi S: Mirizzi syndrome in a Native American population. Am J Surg 168:616, 1994

75. Tsuyuguchi T, Saisho H, Ishihara T, et al: Long-term follow-up after treatment of Mirizzi syndrome by peroral cholangioscopy. Gastrointest Endosc 52:639, 2000

76. Redaelli CA, Buchler MW, Schilling MK, et al: High coincidence of Mirizzi syndrome and gallbladder carcinoma. Surgery 121:58, 1997

77. Foutch PG, Kerr D, Harlan JR, et al: Endoscopic retrograde wire-guided brush cytology for diagnosis of patients with malignant obstruction of the bile duct. Am J Gastroenterol 85:791, 1990

78. Angulo P, Lindor KD: Primary sclerosing cholangitis. Hepatology 30:325, 1999

79. Lindor KD: Ursodiol for primary sclerosing cholangitis. Mayo Primary Sclerosing Cholangitis–Ursodeoxycholic Acid Study Group. N Engl J Med 336:691, 1997

80. Johnson GK, Geenen JE, Venu RP, et al: Endoscopic treatment of biliary duct strictures in sclerosing cholangitis: follow-up assessment of a new therapeutic approach. Gastrointest Endosc 33:9, 1987

81. Buckles DC, Lindor KD, Larusso NF, et al: In primary sclerosing cholangitis, gallbladder polyps are frequently malignant. Am J Gastroenterol 97:1138, 2002

82. Fan ST, Choi TK, Wong J: Recurrent pyogenic cholangitis: current management. World J Surg 15:248, 1991

83. Wilson MK, Stephen MS, Mathur M, et al: Recurrent pyogenic cholangitis or "oriental cholangiohepatitis" in occidentals: case reports of four patients. Aust N Z J Surg 66:649, 1996

84. Kim MJ, Cha SW, Mitchell DG, et al: MR imaging findings in recurrent pyogenic cholangitis. AJR Am J Roentgenol 173:1545, 1999

85. Jeyarajah DR: Recurrent pyogenic cholangitis. Curr Treat Options Gastroenterol 7:91, 2004

86. Liu CL, Fan ST, Lo CM, et al: Choledochal cysts in adults. Arch Surg 137:465, 2002

87. Cheney M, Rustad DG, Lilly JR: Choledochal cyst. World J Surg 9:244, 1985

88. Todani T, Watanabe Y, Narusue M, et al: Classification, operative procedures, and review of thirty-seven cases including cancer arising from choledochal cyst. Am J Surg 134:263, 1977

89. Postema RR, Hazebroek FW: Choledochal cysts in children: a review of 28 years of treatment in a Dutch children's hospital. Eur J Surg 165:1159, 1999

90. Shemesh E, Czerniak A, Klein E, et al: The role of endoscopic retrograde cholangiopancreatography in the diagnosis and treatment of adult choledochal cyst. Surg Gynecol Obstet 167:423, 1988

91. Terblanche J, Worthley CS, Spence RA, et al: High or low hepaticojejunostomy for bile duct strictures? Surgery 108:828, 1990

92. Menees S, Elta GH: Sphincter of Oddi dysfunction. Curr Treat Options Gastroenterol 8:109, 2005

93. Black NA, Thompson E, Sanderson CF: Symptoms and health status before and six weeks after open cholecystectomy: a European cohort study. ECHSS Group. European Collaborative Health Services Study Group. Gut 35:1301, 1994

94. Luman W, Adams WH, Nixon SN, et al: Incidence of persistent symptoms after laparoscopic cholecystectomy: a prospective study. Gut 39:863, 1996

95. Toouli J, Roberts-Thomson IC, Dent J, et al: Manometric disorders in patients with suspected sphincter of Oddi dysfunction. Gastroenterology 88(5 pt 1):1243, 1985

96. Pineau BC, Knapple WL, Spicer KM, et al: Cholecystokinin-stimulated mebrofenin (99mTc-Choletec) hepatobiliary scintigraphy in asymptomatic postcholecystectomy individuals: assessment of specificity, interobserver reliability, and reproducibility. Am J Gastroenterol 96:3106, 2001

97. Geenen JE, Hogan WJ, Dodds WJ, et al: The efficacy of endoscopic sphincterotomy after cholecystectomy in patients with sphincter-of-Oddi dysfunction. N Engl J Med 320:82, 1989

98. Wehrmann T, Schmitt TH, Arndt A, et al: Endoscopic injection of botulinum toxin in patients with recurrent acute pancreatitis due to pancreatic sphincter of Oddi dysfunction. Aliment Pharmacol Ther 14:1469, 2000

99. Moody FG, Becker JM, Potts JR: Transduodenal sphincteroplasty and transampullary septectomy for postcholecystectomy pain. Ann Surg 197:627, 1983

Acknowledgments

Figure 1   Courtesy of William E. Stevens, M.D.

Figure 2   Alan Iselin.

Figure 3   Courtesy of Laura Thomas, M.D., and Mark Feldman, M.D.

Figures 4 and 5   Courtesy of Mark Feldman, M.D.

Figure 6   Courtesy of David Riepe, M.D.

Figures 7 and 8   Courtesy of Malcolm F. Anderson, M.D.

73 Diseases of the Pancreas

Peter Draganov, M.D., and Chris E. Forsmark, M.D., F.A.C.P.

Definitions of Disease Presentations

ACUTE AND CHRONIC PANCREATITIS

Acute pancreatitis has traditionally been defined as an acute inflammatory process of the pancreas that (1) is associated with abdominal pain and elevations in serum levels of pancreatic enzymes and (2) disrupts normal pancreatic architecture and function only until the illness resolves. Chronic pancreatitis, on the other hand, is traditionally described as associated with permanent and irreversible damage to the gland. These definitions, which were developed at a series of international meetings, have limited applicability for clinicians. For example, some patients with severe acute pancreatitis develop substantial necrosis of the gland during the acute attack and sustain permanent abnormalities of both pancreatic architecture and pancreatic function. Likewise, many patients with an acute attack of alcoholic pancreatitis have already developed histologic changes of chronic pancreatitis at the onset of symptoms. Both types of patient are at risk for the complications of acute pancreatitis and are best managed as having acute pancreatitis, although they do not fit the traditional classification schemes.

In addressing these problems, the most recent consensus conference, the International Symposium on Acute Pancreatitis,[1] defined acute pancreatitis in a more clinically useful manner—that is, as an acute inflammatory process of the pancreas with variable involvement of regional tissues and remote organ systems. Because it may not be possible at the time of the attack to determine whether permanent architectural or functional changes are present or will develop, the disease may subsequently be reclassified, on the basis of additional clinical information, as chronic pancreatitis or as an acute exacerbation of chronic pancreatitis.

The International Symposium on Acute Pancreatitis also defined severe acute pancreatitis as the presence of organ failure (e.g., shock, pulmonary insufficiency, renal failure, or gastrointestinal bleeding) or pancreatic or peripancreatic complications (e.g., necrosis, abscess, or pseudocyst), or both, along with unfavorable early prognostic signs (e.g., using the Ranson criteria or the APACHE II score) [see Determining Disease Severity, *below*]. Although not perfect, these clinical definitions more closely fit the approach to management.

COMPLICATIONS OF PANCREATITIS

As part of the consensus conference on acute pancreatitis,[1] more precise definitions were developed to describe the local and systemic complications of acute pancreatitis. An acute fluid collection was defined as a collection of fluid occurring in or around the pancreas early in the course of acute pancreatitis. This collection of fluid is composed of both pancreatic juice and inflammatory fluid; it is poorly circumscribed and lacks a visible wall of fibrosis or granulation tissue. On computed tomography, these collections are seen as low-attenuation areas without a visible capsule. They are quite common in acute pancreatitis, occurring in 30% to 50% of cases.[2] Many of these acute fluid collections resolve, but some may persist and develop a visible capsule, at which time they are termed pseudocysts.

Pseudocysts are defined as collections of fluid (pancreatic juice) surrounded by a fibrous capsule. It takes at least 4 to 6 weeks for an acute fluid collection to develop a capsule and become a pseudocyst. Pseudocysts may remain sterile or may become secondarily infected.

Pancreatic necrosis is a pathologic finding but is clinically defined on contrast-enhanced CT (CECT) as areas of pancreatic parenchyma that show no enhancement with the infusion of intravenous contrast. Acute necrotizing pancreatitis (i.e., CECT findings of pancreatic necrosis) may be subclassified as sterile necrosis or infected necrosis on the basis of the presence or absence of bacteria in an aspiration or surgical sample. Acute interstitial pancreatitis is defined by the absence of CECT findings of necrosis. Finally, pancreatic abscess is defined as a circumscribed collection of pus containing little necrotic tissue. What formerly was called infected pseudocyst is now referred to as a pancreatic abscess. The term phlegmon was omitted from the report because there was no consensus on its definition.

Acute Pancreatitis

EPIDEMIOLOGY

Estimates of the incidence of acute pancreatitis range from about 5 to 25 cases per 100,000 population. In the United States, between 166,000 and 224,000 patients are admitted each year with a primary diagnosis of acute pancreatitis.[3] The number of patients discharged from hospitals with a diagnosis of acute pancreatitis has steadily increased over the past 20 years.[4,5] Similar trends have been seen in other developed countries.[6] The reason for the increased incidence of acute pancreatitis in the United States is unclear, but the increase may be related to the increased incidence of gallstones (one of the major causes of acute pancreatitis)[5] in association with the epidemic of obesity.[7] In large series from referral hospitals, the mortality associated with acute pancreatitis has ranged from 5% to 10%; however, this range is probably high because of referral patterns, as recent estimates using more comprehensive hospital databases have documented an overall mortality of about 2%.[8] Mortality varies with etiology, the development of complications or necrosis, and the number and severity of comorbid medical conditions.[9,10] The cost of care is substantial, with estimates of total direct and indirect costs ranging from $3.6 billion to $6 billion annually.[1,5,8]

ETIOLOGY

Many factors have been implicated as causes of acute pancreatitis [see Table 1]. Together, gallstone disease and alcohol abuse account for 70% to 80% of all cases of acute pancreatitis.[1] The prevalence of acute pancreatitis varies from population to population, depending on the relative prevalence of alcohol abuse and gallstone disease.

Gallstone Disease

The exact mechanism by which gallstone disease causes acute pancreatitis is not completely understood. It is clear that the passage of a gallstone through the ampulla of Vater is an important initiating event for gallstone pancreatitis, most likely by the gallstone's causing transient obstruction of the pancreatic duct or by edema resulting after stone passage. The association between obesity and gallstone disease is well established,[4] but abdominal obesity may be a more specific risk factor. A large prospective study indicated that abdominal adiposity in men carries a relative risk of gallstone disease of 2.29.[11]

Alcohol Abuse

The mechanism by which alcohol consumption produces acute (and chronic) pancreatitis remains obscure. In most patients, long-standing abuse of alcohol is required, and in such patients, histologic chronic pancreatitis is usually present at the onset of a clinically apparent acute attack.[12] In a minority of patients, a large alcoholic binge is the initiating event for acute pancreatitis, and no evidence is found of preexisting chronic damage to the gland.

Obstruction of the Pancreatic Duct

A number of disorders appear to cause acute pancreatitis by a process that obstructs the pancreatic duct. The most common of these is the presence of gallstones (see above). The other conditions are relatively uncommon. One such condition is sphincter of Oddi dysfunction, in which elevations of basal pancreatic sphincter pressure (more than 40 mm Hg above duodenal baseline pressures) produce pancreatic duct obstruction and acute pancreatitis. In addition, both benign and malignant strictures of the pancreatic duct can produce acute pancreatitis, as can malignancy of the ampulla of Vater. Given this, a search for underlying pancreatic or ampullary malignancy is warranted in patients at higher risk for malignancy (e.g., those older than 40 to 45 years) with unexplained pancreatitis. Less common causes of pancreatic duct obstruction and acute pancreatitis include choledochal cysts, periampullary duodenal diverticula, and worms migrating through the ampulla (Ascaris lumbricoides, Clonorchis sinensis).

Pancreas divisum, which occurs in 5% to 7% of the population, is a rare cause of acute pancreatitis.[13,14] In this congenital condition, the fetal dorsal and ventral pancreatic buds fail to fuse, and the majority of pancreatic secretions enter the duodenum through the smaller minor papilla. In a small subset of patients with pancreas divisum, the minor papilla may be inadequate to allow free drainage of pancreatic juice, creating a blockage that may lead to acute or chronic pancreatitis.[13-15]

Drugs and Toxins

Drug-induced acute pancreatitis is a relatively rare event and is usually idiosyncratic.[16,17] The antimetabolites 6-mercaptopurine and azathioprine have the highest attack rate, causing acute pancreatitis in up to 4% of patients who take these drugs. Many additional drugs have been reported to cause acute pancreatitis, the most common being pentamidine, didanosine, sulfonamides, valproic acid, furosemide, and aminosalicylates. In addition to ethyl alcohol [see Alcohol Abuse, above], a number of toxins may injure the pancreas and cause acute pancreatitis; these include methyl alcohol, organophosphate insecticides, and the venom from certain Central and South American scorpions. Scorpion venom and insecticides appear to cause acute pancreatitis by hyperstimulating pancreatic secretion via a cholinergic mechanism.

Table 1 Causes of Acute Pancreatitis

Gallstones and microlithiasis
Alcohol abuse
Obstruction of pancreatic duct
　Sphincter of Oddi dysfunction
　Pancreas divisum with stenotic minor papilla
　Ampullary or pancreatic tumors
Trauma
　Post-ERCP trauma
　Blunt or penetrating trauma
Toxins
　Methyl alcohol
　Scorpion venom
　Organophosphate insecticides
Drugs
　Azathioprine
　6-Mercaptopurine (6-MP)
　Pentamidine
　Didanosine
　Sulfonamides
　Valproic acid
　Furosemide
　Aminosalicylates
Infections
　Viral (mumps, rubella, coxsackie B, cytomegalovirus, HIV)
　Bacterial (Klebsiella, Escherichia coli)
　Fungal (Candida)
Hypertriglyceridemia
Genetic mutation
　Hereditary pancreatitis
　Cystic fibrosis
Surgery

ERCP—endoscopic retrograde cholangiopancreatography

Infection

A number of infections have been reported to cause acute pancreatitis; among them are a variety of viral infections such as cytomegalovirus, mumps, rubella, and coxsackie B. Patients with AIDS commonly have increased serum amylase levels in the absence of acute pancreatitis and less commonly develop acute pancreatitis secondary to opportunistic infections (e.g., cytomegalovirus, Cryptosporidium, or Mycobacterium infections) or as a side effect of a medication.[18]

Metabolic Factors

Metabolic causes of acute pancreatitis include hypertriglyceridemia and hypercalcemia. Serum triglycerides generally need to be in excess of 1,000 mg/dl to produce acute pancreatitis.[19] Serum triglyceride levels in excess of 1,000 mg/dl are most commonly seen in type V hyperlipoproteinemia and are usually associated with diabetes mellitus. Acute pancreatitis can itself raise triglyceride levels but not to this degree. The use of estrogens in postmenopausal women with underlying hypertriglyceridemia is associated with increased levels of triglyceride and the induction of pancreatitis, particularly if the fasting triglyceride level before initiating estrogen treatment is more than 750 mg/dl.[20] Hypercalcemia, usually associated with hyperparathyroidism, is a very rare metabolic cause of acute pancreatitis.

Trauma

Trauma to the pancreas or pancreatic duct may cause acute

pancreatitis. Blunt trauma to the abdomen may cause contusion, laceration, or complete transection of the gland. In most cases of major trauma affecting the pancreas, damage occurs at the mid-body of the pancreas, where the pancreas is crushed against the vertebral bodies; acute pancreatitis develops rapidly in most of these patients. Patients with less extensive injuries may experience a delayed onset of symptoms up to several months or even longer after the trauma. Iatrogenic trauma during endoscopic retrograde cholangiopancreatography (ERCP) causes acute pancreatitis in about 3% to 5% of cases, although in certain subgroups (e.g., those suspected of having sphincter of Oddi dysfunction), the risk may be as high as 20% to 25%.[21] ERCP appears to cause pancreatitis as a consequence of obstruction, inflammation, and edema of the pancreatic duct orifice and by barotrauma to the acinar cells. Ischemic injury to the pancreas may occur in the setting of many surgical procedures, because the pancreatic vasculature has very limited ability for vasodilatation. In such cases, postoperative pancreatitis is often quite severe and most commonly occurs after cardiac surgery or cardiopulmonary bypass.

Genetic Factors

A number of mutations have been described in association with acute and chronic pancreatitis. These include mutations in the cationic trypsinogen (PRSS1), cystic fibrosis transmembrane conductance regulator (CFTR), and secretory trypsin inhibitor (or serine protease inhibitor Kazal type 1 [SPINK1]) genes.[22] These conditions are most commonly associated with chronic pancreatitis [see Chronic Pancreatitis, Etiology, below] but in some cases may also produce acute flares. A number of studies have examined polymorphisms in cytokines involved in the inflammatory response to determine whether such polymorphisms might be predictors of the severity of acute pancreatitis. To date, these studies have been unrevealing.

Autoimmune Pancreatitis

Autoimmune pancreatitis is a benign disease characterized by irregular narrowing of the pancreatic duct, swelling of the parenchyma, and lymphoplasmacytic infiltration and fibrosis. Autoimmune pancreatitis can present clinically as an attack of acute pancreatitis. Patients with autoimmune pancreatitis may have high antinuclear antibody and serum IgG4 concentrations, providing a useful means of distinguishing this disorder from other diseases of the pancreas or biliary tract.[23,24] Patients with autoimmune pancreatitis generally have a favorable response to corticosteroid treatment.

Undetermined Causes

After evaluation, about 25% of all patients with acute pancreatitis do not have a specific definable etiology. In fact, after gallstones and alcohol, idiopathic acute pancreatitis is the most common diagnosis. Some of these patients may be surreptitious alcoholics, but many more appear to have a forme fruste of gallstone disease. Two series have documented the presence of microscopic gallstones (so-called microlithiasis) in two thirds to three fourths of patients with apparent idiopathic acute pancreatitis.[25,26] The importance of microlithiasis is underscored by the fact that cholecystectomy, ERCP with sphincterotomy, and agents used to dissolve gallstones (e.g., ursodeoxycholic acid) all reduced the frequency of recurrent attacks of acute pancreatitis in patients participating in these studies. Unfortunately, there is as yet no standardized method to determine the presence of microlithiasis.

The pathophysiology of acute pancreatitis, irrespective of cause, remains poorly understood. All etiologies appear to converge on a final common pathway that allows the premature activation of digestive enzymes within the pancreas.[27,28] The conversion of the inactive proenzyme trypsinogen to its active form trypsin appears to be a critical early step because trypsin can then activate most of the other digestive proenzymes. The release of activated digestive enzymes into the pancreas and surrounding tissues can produce tissue damage and necrosis of the pancreas, its surrounding fat, and adjacent structures. This chemical "burn" of the retroperitoneum leads to substantial fluid loss into this area—so-called third-space fluid losses. Not all patients with acute pancreatitis develop necrosis of the pancreas itself; necrosis is most commonly seen in severe attacks of acute pancreatitis. Substantial pancreatic necrosis (acute necrotizing pancreatitis) is usually distinguished from the milder form in which necrosis is absent (interstitial pancreatitis).

The release of activated digestive enzymes into the systemic circulation can overwhelm normal protective mechanisms (e.g., antiproteases) and cause direct damage to distant organs and other systemic enzyme systems (e.g., complement and kinin systems). Finally, a number of inflammatory mediators and cytokines can be released from inflammatory cells to produce a systemic immune response syndrome (SIRS) or sepsislike syndrome.[29,30] The combination of activated digestive enzymes in the systemic circulation, the activation of other enzyme systems, and the release of inflammatory cytokines can produce the severe systemic complications associated with severe acute pancreatitis [see Table 2]. Recognition of the role of these inflammatory mediators has not only improved our understanding of the pathophysiology of acute pancreatitis but also provided potential new targets for therapy.

DIAGNOSIS

Clinical Findings

The diagnosis of acute pancreatitis is usually suspected on the basis of compatible signs and symptoms and confirmed by laboratory tests and radiographic imaging. Pain is the most common symptom of acute pancreatitis, occurring in up to 95% of patients. The pain of acute pancreatitis is most commonly felt in the epigastrium and radiates to the back in up to two thirds of patients. Pain may be felt more diffusely across the abdomen. The pain is usually quite severe, reaches its maximum intensity within 30 minutes, and lasts hours to days. In some cases, pain may not be the dominant symptom, particularly if it is masked by multiorgan failure, delirium, or coma; in rare cases, pain may be absent altogether. Nausea and vomiting are commonly associated with the pain of pancreatitis. No relief of the abdominal pain is achieved by vomiting.

The physical examination usually reveals epigastric or diffuse tenderness on palpation, with rebound tenderness and guarding present in the most severe cases. The abdomen is often distended and tympanic, and bowel sounds may be decreased or absent. Vital signs may be normal; more commonly, tachycardia, hypotension, tachypnea, and low-grade fever are noted. Orthostatic hypotension, tachycardia, and shock early in the course of acute pancreatitis are markers for substantial third-space fluid losses and indicate both a poor prognosis and probable need for admission to an intensive care unit. Dyspnea or tachypnea may occur because of muscular splinting secondary to abdominal pain, pleural effusions, or a pulmonary capillary leak syndrome (i.e., acute respiratory distress syndrome [ARDS]). Generally, the presence of tachypnea, dyspnea, or oxygen desaturation merits ICU admission. Rare physical findings include ecchymoses of the flank (Grey Turner sign) and umbilicus (Cullen sign) and eruptive xanthomas in patients with hyperlipidemic pancreatitis; signs of alcoholic liver disease may be present in patients with alcoholic pancreatitis. Altered mental status may be present and usually has multiple causes (alcohol withdrawal, hypotension, electrolyte imbalance, and hypoxemia). Jaundice may be present, either from obstruction of the bile duct by a gallstone or from extrinsic compression of the bile duct by a large peripancreatic fluid collection. Purtscher retinopathy presenting as retinal hemorrhage is a very rare complication of acute pancreatitis.

Laboratory Tests

A history and physical examination suggestive of acute pancreatitis may be seen in a wide variety of intra-abdominal diseases. Therefore, the diagnosis is usually confirmed with a combination of laboratory tests and imaging studies.

Serum amylase　The serum amylase level has long been the most widely used confirmatory laboratory measurement for acute pancreatitis. At least 75% of patients with acute pancreatitis will have increased levels of serum amylase at the time of initial evaluation.[31] Levels greater than three times the upper limit of normal are highly suggestive of acute pancreatitis. Amylase is cleared by the kidney; in patients with renal failure, a higher threshold of five times the upper limit of normal should be used. Normal levels of serum amylase, however, do not rule out the presence of pancreatitis. Serum amylase levels may be normal in some patients with acute alcoholic pancreatitis and in patients with hyperlipidemic pancreatitis (marked elevations in triglyceride levels can interfere with the laboratory assay for amylase). More generally, elevated levels of serum amylase may have already returned to normal if testing is delayed until several days after the onset of symptoms. In several large series of fatal pancreatitis, 10% to 30% of patients who died of acute pancreatitis were undiagnosed before autopsy.[32] The diagnosis of acute pancreatitis is generally missed in such patients for one of two reasons: serum amylase levels are normal (or are not measured) or the presenting symptoms are atypical (e.g., coma or multiorgan failure rather than abdominal pain). The true sensitivity of the serum amylase measurement as a diagnostic test for acute pancreatitis is therefore difficult to determine.

Elevations of the serum amylase level are not specific for acute pancreatitis and may be associated with a very wide variety of nonpancreatic conditions [*see Table 3*]. Although many of these other conditions would not be mistaken for acute pancreatitis, a number of intra-abdominal conditions can produce increased serum amylase levels and mimic both the signs and the symptoms of acute pancreatitis. Such disorders include intestinal ischemia and perforation, bowel obstruction, choledocholithiasis, cholelithiasis with cholecystitis, tubo-ovarian disease (ectopic pregnancy, acute salpingitis), and acute appendicitis.

Serum lipase　The serum lipase level is often used as an adjunct to or in place of serum amylase testing as a confirmatory test for acute pancreatitis. Accurate measurement of serum lipase was difficult in the past, but new methods provide high levels of precision. The lipase level is in fact slightly more sensitive and somewhat more specific for acute pancreatitis than the amy-

Table 2　Complications of Acute Pancreatitis

Local complications
　Peripancreatic fluid collection
　Pseudocyst
　Pancreatic necrosis (sterile or infected)
　Abscess
　Duodenal obstruction
　Biliary obstruction
Systemic complications
　Cardiovascular
　　Hypotension and shock
　　Pericardial effusion and tamponade
　　ECG changes
　Pulmonary
　　Hypoxia
　　Atelectasis, pneumonia
　　Pleural effusion
　　Acute respiratory distress syndrome
　Metabolic
　　Hypocalcemia
　　Hypertriglyceridemia
　　Hyperglycemia
　Renal
　　Oliguria and azotemia
　　Acute tubular necrosis
　Hematologic
　　Disseminated intravascular coagulation (DIC)
　　Vascular thrombosis (particularly splenic vein)
　Gastrointestinal bleeding
　Other
　　Encephalopathy
　　Distant fat necrosis
　　Retinopathy

lase level.[31] In addition, serum lipase stays elevated longer and can confirm a diagnosis of acute pancreatitis up to 5 to 10 days after the onset of symptoms, by which time amylase levels have generally returned to normal. Like amylase, lipase may be elevated in other intra-abdominal conditions (with the exception of tubo-ovarian disease) and may be elevated in renal failure. Elevations that are more than three times the upper limit of normal have the greatest diagnostic sensitivity and specificity, but again, this threshold may need to be increased to five times the upper limit of normal in patients with renal failure. Lipase is probably preferable to amylase as a confirmatory test because in addition to its greater specificity, it is no more costly and, in most hospitals, has equally rapid availability.

Other tests　Leukocytosis is frequently present in acute pancreatitis. The hematocrit may be normal, but in patients with severe pancreatitis and substantial third-space fluid loss, hemoconcentration is present. There are a number of methods to gauge the severity of pancreatitis, but the presence of hemoconcentration is a reasonably accurate marker of severe pancreatitis.[33] Hyperglycemia and hypocalcemia may also be present. Tetany is rare because ionized calcium levels are usually normal in pancreatitis despite the presence of hypocalcemia. Liver chemistries may be elevated in persons with gallstone pancreatitis or with intrinsic liver disease (e.g., alcoholic hepatitis). Elevations of alanine aminotransferase levels to three times the normal level strongly suggest gallstone disease as the etiology; however, any significant abnormality of liver chemistries should raise the suspicion of gallstone pancreatitis, particularly if the abnormalities rapidly return to the normal range over the course of a few days.[34] The differentiation of gallstone pancreatitis from other forms of pancreatitis is important because specific therapy may be required [see Removal of Common Bile Duct Stones, below].

Imaging Studies

Imaging studies, particularly ultrasound and CT, can be useful in confirming a diagnosis of acute pancreatitis, determining etiology, and assessing the severity of the attack.

Radiology   Plain abdominal radiographs may help in the evaluation of acute abdominal pain by documenting the presence of conditions (e.g., an ileus or free intraperitoneal air) that cause acute pain, but the findings are never specific enough to confirm a diagnosis of acute pancreatitis. Similarly, barium or water-soluble contrast studies of the upper gastrointestinal tract are not helpful in confirming a diagnosis of acute pancreatitis.

Ultrasonography   Abdominal ultrasonography (US) is a highly useful test in the evaluation of suspected acute pancreatitis. Diagnostic abnormalities of the pancreas, including pancreatic enlargement, changes in echotexture, and peripancreatic fluid collections, can be seen in up to two thirds of patients; in the remaining third, overlying bowel gas limits the ability of sound transmission, thus preventing adequate visualization of the pancreas.

US is the most sensitive test for detecting stones in the gallbladder in patients with gallstone pancreatitis. The presence of gallstones or a dilated bile duct visualized on US is highly predictive of gallstone disease as the etiology of acute pancreatitis. If the gallbladder and biliary tree cannot be imaged on initial ultrasonography, a repeat ultrasound several days later may prove diagnostic of gallstone pancreatitis.

Computed tomography   Computed tomography is much more accurate than US in confirming the presence of acute pancreatitis, although CT is less accurate in evaluating the biliary tree and gallbladder for stones.[35-37] The two tests are therefore often used together in patients with acute pancreatitis. CT results may be normal in a small subset of patients with very mild acute pancreatitis (10% of patients), but the test is reliably diagnostic in moderate or severe disease. CT is also quite useful in assessing conditions that mimic severe acute pancreatitis. In addition, CT plays a very important role in determining severity of the attack [see CT Findings, below].

The use of a rapid bolus of intravenous contrast coupled with rapid scanning of the pancreas by use of CECT can provide a diagnosis of acute pancreatitis and, very importantly, assess the severity of disease and the extent of pancreatic necrosis. As visualized on CECT, viable pancreatic parenchyma is enhanced by uptake of the contrast medium, and necrotic areas of the gland are unenhanced. The extent of necrosis is a very important indicator of prognosis.[35-37]

CT scans are not required in every patient with acute pancreatitis, but they should be performed in patients with a first attack of pancreatitis, with moderate or severe symptoms, with systemic complications, in whom there is a suspicion of a complication (e.g., pancreatic pseudocyst), with smoldering pancreatitis that is slow to improve, or when the diagnosis is unclear.

Magnetic resonance imaging   Gadolinium-enhanced dynamic magnetic resonance imaging can be used to grade the severity of acute pancreatitis if there are contraindications to intravenous contrast–enhanced CT, such as renal failure or iodine sensitivity.[38] Furthermore, magnetic resonance cholangiopancreatography (MRCP) is an accurate way to test for the presence of common bile duct stones.[39] It may be difficult, however, to perform MRI or MRCP in very sick patients.

Endoscopy   ERCP and endoscopic ultrasonography (EUS) are not used as diagnostic tests for acute pancreatitis, although they may be useful in determining etiology. ERCP is accurate in evaluating many of the less common causes of acute pancreatitis, including microlithiasis, sphincter of Oddi dysfunction, pancreas divisum, and pancreatic duct strictures (benign and malignant). As a diagnostic test, ERCP is generally reserved for patients who have experienced a second attack of unexplained pancreatitis, although use of ERCP may be considered as a diagnostic option after a single attack of unexplained pancreatitis in patients at risk for malignant pancreatic duct strictures (e.g., those older than 40 to 45 years). ERCP certainly has value as a therapeutic tool (e.g., for finding and removing common bile duct stones in patients with gallstone pancreatitis).

EUS is also useful in the documentation of gallstones, microlithiasis, pancreatic tumors, and pancreas divisum. Although it is used less frequently than ERCP in patients with acute pancreatitis (primarily because it is not widely available), EUS has a significantly lower risk of complications. EUS is highly accurate in both documenting stones and visualizing tumors (more sensitive than ERCP) and will be used more commonly in the future [see Figure 1].

Table 3   Nonpancreatic Causes of Elevated Amylase and Lipase Levels

Amylase	*Lipase*

Biliary disease
  Common bile duct obstruction
  Acute cholecystitis
	Biliary disease
	  Common bile duct obstruction
	  Acute cholecystitis

Intestinal ischemia, obstruction, or perforation	Intestinal ischemia, obstruction, or perforation
Acute appendicitis	Acute appendicitis

Gynecologic conditions
  Ectopic pregnancy
  Acute salpingitis
  Ovarian cysts and malignancies
	Renal insufficiency

Renal insufficiency	
Macroamylasemia	
Salivary gland disease, including mumps	

Miscellaneous causes
  Anorexia nervosa
  Diabetic ketoacidosis
  Lung cancer
  Head trauma	

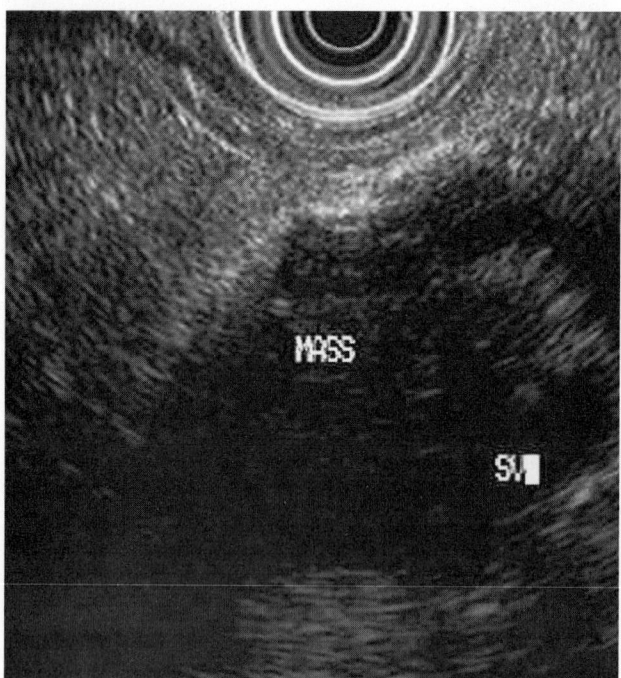

Figure 1   **An endoscopic ultrasound image of a pancreatic mass in a patient with unexplained acute pancreatitis. The mass is labeled and sits on the splenic vein (SV). The mass was not visible on computed tomography.**

Determining Disease Severity

Three quarters of patients with acute pancreatitis have a benign course and recover rapidly. The highest morbidity and mortality are in patients with necrotizing pancreatitis. The mortality associated with acute pancreatitis is 2% to 10%, with the lower estimates of mortality coming from database analyses and the higher estimates coming from more selected or referral populations. Mortality within the first week of the illness is most commonly from ARDS, multiorgan failure, or a sepsislike syndrome. Patients with persisting organ failure are at greatest risk of mortality; transient organ failure is generally not associated with mortality. Mortality after the first or second week is most commonly caused by infection of pancreatic tissue (i.e., pancreatic abscess or infected necrosis).

After making a diagnosis of acute pancreatitis, the clinician's next goal is to estimate prognosis and severity of disease. The accurate assessment of prognosis and severity allows more accurate decision making regarding ICU admission, measurement of central venous pressure or pulmonary capillary wedge pressure, and administration of prophylactic antibiotics. The assessment of severity of acute pancreatitis may be based on clinical features, laboratory tests, or imaging studies or a combination of the three. Frequently, careful evaluation by an experienced clinician is a very helpful method of gauging severity and detecting complications. The presence of delirium or coma, hypoxia, or features suggestive of massive third-space fluid loss (i.e., hypotension, tachycardia, oliguria, azotemia, or hemoconcentration) within the first 24 hours suggests a severe attack and the need for ICU admission.[40] Many patients will not develop such a dramatic illness, and a number of multiple-factor scoring systems are available to assist the clinician in determining severity and estimating prognosis.

Multiple-factor scoring systems   Several multiple-factor scoring systems have been developed that use a combination of clinical and laboratory features to determine disease severity; these include the Ranson criteria [*see Table 4*], modified Glasgow criteria, and APACHE II criteria [*see Table 5*]. The most widely quoted system developed by Ranson utilizes two systems: one for gallstone pancreatitis and one for nongallstone (alcoholic) pancreatitis. In the Ranson system, the presence of one or two criteria is very specific, though not sensitive, for clinically mild pancreatitis.[40,41] The presence of three or four risk factors is associated with a mortality of 15%, although many patients with three or four criteria also recover rapidly without sequelae. The presence of a high number of criteria (e.g., six or seven Ranson criteria) is associated with a high likelihood of substantial morbidity and mortality (> 50% mortality).[40,41] All of the multiple-factor scoring systems suffer from the limitation of a high false positive rate; in other words, the presence of a moderate number of criteria is generally associated with moderate risk of morbidity and mortality, but the scoring systems do not identify whether that individual patient is likely to suffer morbidity or mortality. The APACHE II system has an advantage over the Ranson and Glasgow systems in that it can be applied at any point in the clinical illness; the Ranson and Glasgow scores require up to 48 hours before they can be calculated. Three or more Ranson criteria or eight or more APACHE II points are commonly considered an indication of an unfavorable prognosis.

CT findings   CT is a useful adjunct for estimating disease severity. The initial scoring systems correlated the severity of the pancreatic and peripancreatic inflammatory processes with the prognosis. Subsequently, CT was combined with a rapidly administered bolus of intravenous contrast (CECT) to define the presence and extent of pancreatic necrosis; this technique has become widely used.[36,37,41] The lack of vascular contrast enhancement of the pancreas on CECT corresponds in a general way to the presence of necrosis. Pancreatic necrosis complicates about 25% of all cases of acute pancreatitis and is generally associated with more clinically severe disease; it is particularly associated with the development of the late complications of pancreatic abscess and infected necrosis.[37,41,42]

As with all systems used in assessing severity, CECT produces a significant number of false positive results, in that many patients who have evidence of necrosis on dynamic CT scanning have a mild clinical course.[43] Despite that, the presence of substantial pancreatic necrosis (more than one third of the gland) is a useful marker of severity because nearly all patients with a clinically severe course have necrosis and almost all cases of serious pancreatic infection occurs in this group.[42,43]

At the International Symposium on Acute Pancreatitis, an attempt was made to consolidate the various methods for determining disease severity into a unified approach.[1] The resulting system defines severe pancreatitis by a combination of clinical features (organ failure), multiple-factor scoring systems, and the presence of local pancreatic complications [*see Table 6*]. This system is useful in that it consolidates the various methods, but it does not replace frequent and experienced clinical observation.

MANAGEMENT

The treatment of acute pancreatitis has four goals: (1) provide supportive care; (2) minimize or reduce the local necrosis and the systemic inflammatory process; (3) recognize and treat complications; and (4) prevent subsequent attacks.

Supportive Care

Mild acute pancreatitis The foundations of supportive care include making the patient nil per os (NPO); providing relief from pain and nausea; replacing fluid losses; providing nutrition, if needed; and monitoring for the development of complications. This is relatively straightforward in patients with mild pancreatitis, because fluid losses are modest and complications are rare. Pain and nausea can usually be controlled by the use of moderate dosages of intravenous analgesics and antiemetics. Even in mild pancreatitis, fluid losses may be significant because of third-space fluid losses, vomiting, and insensible losses; appropriate fluid resuscitation is critical in minimizing complications. Patients can generally be fed when bowel sounds have returned and pain has resolved.

Severe acute pancreatitis When pancreatitis is severe or is predicted to be severe (based on CT or CECT findings, multiple-factor scoring systems, early evidence of significant third-space fluid losses, or early respiratory insufficiency), supportive care is more challenging and usually requires the resources of an ICU. Prompt and vigorous fluid replacement is critical in the early phases of severe acute pancreatitis and can minimize or prevent early complications, including renal failure and cardiovascular collapse.[44] The pancreas itself is prone to ischemic injury in the setting of intravascular fluid volume depletion. The pancreatic microcirculation has little capacity to respond to diminished blood supply, and intravascular volume depletion may worsen the degree of pancreatic necrosis. For all these reasons, early and vigorous fluid resuscitation is important in the management of severe pancreatitis.[40,44]

Hemoconcentration is a common and readily available marker of substantial third-space fluid losses. Measurement of central venous pressure or, if required, pulmonary capillary wedge pressure allows accurate assessment of fluid needs. Fluid needs of 5 to 10 L/day are not uncommon. Treatment with crystalloid solutions is usually appropriate, although colloid solutions (albumin or blood) may be appropriate when albumin levels are extremely low (< 2.0 mg/dl) or when the hematocrit is below 25%.

Admission to an ICU, in addition to facilitating the monitoring of fluid resuscitation, allows for intensive monitoring of respiratory and metabolic complications. Pulmonary capillary leak syndrome (i.e., ARDS) is one of the most serious complications of severe pancreatitis. Hypoxia and dyspnea are usually noted, but ARDS must be distinguished from fluid overload or congestive heart failure. This is best done with the use of a Swan-Ganz catheter. A variety of early metabolic complications (e.g., hyperglycemia, hypocalcemia, hypertriglyceridemia, and hypomagnesemia) are also most easily managed in an ICU setting.

Nutritional support is useful for patients with severe pancreatitis and for those with milder pancreatitis who nonetheless are unable to eat for more than 5 to 7 days. The preferred route of providing exogenous nutrients has changed. For years, total parenteral nutrition (TPN) has been the standard practice. Accumulating evidence suggests that enteral feeding is comparable or superior to TPN.[45-47] Prospective, randomized trials have demonstrated that enteral feeding infused distal to the ligament of Treitz is associated with fewer complications (infection and hyperglycemia) and is cheaper than TPN.[45] Although the evidence is not definitive,[47] the accumulating data supporting this method of enteral feeding have led to a shift in the preferred method of providing nutrition to patients with acute pancreatitis. The main practical challenge in using enteral jejunal feeding is placing and maintaining position of the nasojejunal tube.

Treatment of Necrosis and Inflammation

Pancreatic rest No treatment has been proved to interrupt the inflammatory process effectively. Many early studies focused on strategies that were thought to "rest" the pancreas beyond the rest associated with maintaining the patient NPO. These have included nasogastric suction, H_2 receptor antagonists, atropine, somatostatin and its analogue octreotide, glucagon, and even fluorouracil. None of these approaches appear to have any benefit on the outcome of acute pancreatitis, although meta-analyses of somatostatin and octreotide suggest a slight trend toward benefit.[48] That is not to say that nasogastric suction is not useful if the patient has substantial nausea and vomiting or that administration of H_2 receptor antagonists does not prevent stress erosions and ulcers; however, neither of these therapies improves the overall outcome of the acute pancreatitis itself.

Protease removal or inhibition A second strategy to interrupt the inflammatory process is to remove proteases by peritoneal lavage or inhibit circulating proteases by administration of antiproteases (e.g., aprotinin or gabexate). However, neither method of protease control has been shown to be of benefit in acute pancreatitis. One potential reason for lack of efficacy is that these therapies can generally be administered only after the initiation of acute pancreatitis. In animal models, these therapies have been administered before the initiation of pancreatitis and have been shown to be nearly uniformly beneficial.[49] Pancreatitis induced by ERCP offers a unique opportunity to administer therapy in humans before the onset of acute pancreatitis. Although the data are inconclusive, meta-analyses have identified a reduction in post-ERCP pancreatitis in patients receiving the protease inhibitor gabexate or the antisecretory hormone somatostatin (but not, interestingly, its analogue octreotide).[50,51] The effect of these agents is only modest, and they are not available for clinical use in the United States. The effect of other methods, particularly the use of temporary pancreatic duct stents, appears to be far superior.

Anticytokine therapy Some studies have focused on control of the systemic immune response through the modulation of inflammatory cytokines. Because this cytokine cascade is felt to

Table 4 Ranson Prognostic Scoring System for Pancreatitis

Type	On Admission	Within 48 Hours
Nongallstone pancreatitis	Age > 55 yr WBC count > 16,000/mm³ Glucose > 200 mg/dl LDH > 350 IU/L AST > 250 U/L	Decrease in Hct > 10 points Increase in BUN > 5 mg/dl Serum calcium < 8 mg/dl P_aO_2 < 60 mm Hg Base deficit > 4 mmol/L Fluid deficit > 6 L
Gallstone pancreatitis	Age > 70 yr WBC count > 18,000/mm³ Glucose > 220 mg/dl LDH > 400 IU/L AST > 500 U/L	Decrease in Hct > 10 points Increase in BUN > 2 mg/dl Serum calcium < 8 mg/dl Base deficit > 5 mmol/L Fluid deficit > 4 L

AST—aspartate aminotransferase BUN—blood urea nitrogen Hct—hematocrit LDH—lactate dehydrogenase P_aO_2—arterial oxygen tension WBC—white blood cell

Table 5   APACHE II Severity of Disease Classification System*

Physiologic Variable	Physiologic Points								
	Range								
Rectal temperature (°C)	≥ 41°	39.0°–40.9°	—	38.5°–38.9°	36.0°–38.4°	34.0°–35.9°	32.0°–31.9°	30.0°–31.9°	≤ 29.9°
Mean arterial pressure (mm Hg)	≥ 160	130–159	110–129	—	70–109	—	50–69	—	≤ 49
Heart rate (ventricular response)	≥ 180	140–179	110–139	—	70–109	—	55–69	40–54	≥ 39
Respiratory rate (nonventilated or ventilated)	≥ 50	35–49	—	25–34	12–24	10–11	6–9	—	≤ 5
A-aPo$_2$ (mm Hg) F$_I$O$_2$ ≥ 0.5 (record A-aPo$_2$) F$_I$O$_2$ < 0.5 (record only P$_a$o$_2$)	≥ 500 —	350–499 —	200–349 —	— —	< 200 Po$_2$ > 70	— Po$_2$ 61–70	— —	— Po$_2$ 55–60	— Po$_2$ < 55
Arterial pH	≥ 7.7	7.6–7.69	—	7.5–7.59	7.33–7.49	—	7.25–7.32	7.15–7.24	< 7.15
Serum sodium (mmol/L)	≥ 180	160–179	155–159	150–154	130–149	—	120–129	111–119	< 110
Serum potassium (mmol/L)	≥ 7.0	6.0–6.9	—	5.5–5.9	3.5–5.4	3.0–3.4	2.5–2.9	—	< 2.5
Serum creatinine (mg/dl)†	≥ 3.5	2.0–3.4	1.5–1.9	—	0.6–1.4	—	< 0.6	—	—
Hematocrit (%)	≥ 60	—	50.0–59.9	46.0–49.9	30.0–45.9	—	20.0–29.9	—	< 20
White blood cell count 1,000/mm³	≥ 40	—	20.0–39.9	15–19.9	3.0–14.9	—	1.0–2.9	—	< 1
Serum HCO$_3$ (mmol/L)‡	≥ 52	41.0–51.9	—	32.0–40.9	22.0–31.9	—	18.0–21.9	14.0–17.9	< 15
Individual variable points	+4	+3	+2	+1	0	+1	+2	+3	+4

Total acute physiology score = sum of the individual variable points for all 12 variables.
*APACHE II Score = Physiologic points + Glasgow Coma points + Age points + Chronic Health points.

underlie the development of multiorgan failure, cytokines are attractive targets for therapy. Platelet-activating factor (PAF) has been considered to be a major proinflammatory cytokine, and several small randomized trials using an antagonist of PAF have suggested that this agent may reduce the severity of pancreatitis if administered early in the disease course. The results of these small trials, however, have not been confirmed in a large randomized trial.[52] PAF antagonists have also been tested as therapies to prevent post-ERCP pancreatitis but have not shown significant benefit. It is likely that interfering with the cytokine cascade will require multiple agents, and further testing of these and similar therapies will clarify the role they play in the treatment of severe acute pancreatitis.

Removal of common bile duct stones   A therapy that has been tested as a strategy to reduce local or systemic inflammation is the removal of common bile duct stones in patients with gallstone pancreatitis. In the vast majority of patients with gallstone pancreatitis, the offending bile duct stone has already passed into the duodenum at the onset of disease. Evaluation of the common bile duct for stones early in the clinical course of gallstone pancreatitis detects the presence of stones in up to 78% of patients. This level drops to between 3% and 33% if the evaluation is undertaken later in the clinical course.[53] The vast majority of patients thus pass the stone spontaneously; however, in a small subset of patients, a persistent common bile duct stone remains, and anecdotal observations suggest that these patients seem to be at risk for more severe pancreatitis (e.g., more organ failure and a greater degree of necrosis) and concomitant cholangitis. It is well established that cholangitis complicates up to 10% of cases of gallstone pancreatitis. Furthermore, it may be difficult

in some patients to distinguish the presence of concomitant cholangitis from severe pancreatitis, because the two diseases may present similar features (e.g., fever, leukocytosis, abdominal pain, and abnormal liver chemistries). Therefore, the strategy was proposed to remove common bile duct stones in patients with gallstone pancreatitis as a means to reduce severity of disease and to prevent or treat concomitant cholangitis.

Early attempts to remove persistent common bile duct stones by surgery were associated with a mortality higher than that associated with conservative management. Subsequently, endoscopic techniques (e.g., ERCP) were used to remove stones. Three randomized trials assessed the utility of early ERCP and stone removal in patients with suspected gallstone pancreatitis.[54-56]

The initial study reported that the morbidity in patients with gallstone pancreatitis who underwent ERCP and stone removal within 72 hours was lower than the morbidity in a group of patients managed conservatively.[54] This benefit included a reduction in complications (organ failure and others) and a trend (not statistically significant) toward lower mortality. These benefits were restricted to a subgroup of patients who were predicted to have a severe attack. The second randomized trial noted a reduction in biliary sepsis but no reduction in organ failure or other complications associated with severe gallstone pancreatitis.[55] One of the two studies therefore suggested that early ERCP reduced the severity of pancreatitis, whereas the other study found that ERCP had no effect on the severity of pancreatitis but merely prevented or treated concomitant cholangitis caused by common bile duct stones. A third randomized trial attempted to reconcile these results by excluding patients with cholangitis or those at high risk for cholangitis (i.e., patients with jaundice). This study demonstrated no re-

Table 5 (*continued*)

	Glasgow Coma Points	
	Response	*Points*
Eyes open	Spontaneous	+4
	To voice	+3
	To pain	+2
	None	+1
Verbal response	Oriented	+5
	Confused conversation	+4
	Inappropriate words	+3
	Incomprehensible sounds	+2
	None	+1
Best motor response	Obeys commands	+6
	Localizes pain	+5
	Flexion-withdrawal to pain	+4
	Abnormal flexion (decorticate)	+3
	Abnormal extension (decerebrate)	+2
	None/flaccid	+1

Total Glasgow Coma points = 15 – Glasgow Coma score.

Age Points

Age (yr)	Points
< 44	0
45–54	2
55–64	3
65–74	5
≥ 75	6

Chronic Health Points

Hepatic	Biopsy-proven cirrhosis and documented portal hypertension; past episodes of upper GI bleeding attributed to portal hypertension; or prior episodes of hepatic failure, encephalopathy, or coma
Cardiovascular	New York Heart Association class IV status
Respiratory	Chronic restrictive, obstructive, or vascular disease resulting in severe exercise restriction (e.g., unable to climb stairs or perform household duties) or documented chronic hypoxia, hypercapnia, secondary polycythemia, severe pulmonary hypertension (> 40 mm Hg), or respirator dependency
Renal	Recurring long-term dialysis
Immunocompromised	The patient has received therapy that suppresses resistance to infection (e.g., immunosuppression, chemotherapy, radiation, long-term or recent high-dose steroids) or has a disease that is sufficiently advanced to suppress resistance to infection (e.g., leukemia, lymphoma, or AIDS)
	If the patient has a history of severe organ system insufficiency§ or is immunocompromised,§ assign points as follows:
	Nonoperative or emergency postoperative patients, 5 points
	Elective postoperative patients, 2 points

†Double point score for acute renal failure.

‡Venous; not preferred use if there are no arterial blood gases.

§Organ insufficiency or immunocompromised state must have been evident before hospital admission.

A-aPo$_2$—alveolar-arterial oxygen tension difference F$_1$O$_2$—fraction of inspired oxygen P$_a$O$_2$—arterial oxygen tension

duction in morbidity or mortality in patients with gallstone pancreatitis but without jaundice.[56]

Taken together, these three studies suggest that early ERCP is indicated in patients with evidence of biliary sepsis (i.e., fever, jaundice, and right upper quadrant pain) and in those with a high likelihood of developing biliary sepsis. High risk of biliary sepsis might be clinically defined as findings highly suggestive of a persistent obstructing common bile duct stone and could be defined by the presence of a stone in the common bile duct as visualized on radiographic imaging; by persistently abnormal liver chemistries; or by radiographic evidence of a persistently dilated bile duct. Early ERCP may also be considered in patients with early and progressive organ system failure, in whom it may be difficult to determine whether the downhill course is caused by severe pancreatitis or by associated cholangitis. Undertaking ERCP in this situation can be challenging, and sedating these critically ill individuals is not without risk.

Treatment of Complications

Systemic complications Systemic complications of acute pancreatitis can occur in a wide variety of organ systems [*see Table 2*].[44,57] Systemic complications, particularly shock, ARDS, and multiorgan failure, are the most common causes of death from acute pancreatitis within the first week of the illness. In patients with severe pancreatitis, fluid losses into the retroperitoneum can be massive and can produce intravascular volume depletion, hypotension and shock, and renal failure. The development of renal failure, shock, or massive volume depletion is an indication of severe disease and is associated with increased mortality. Most substantial fluid losses occur early in the course of acute pancreatitis; hence, attention must be paid to adequate and aggressive fluid resuscitation early in the disease course.[44]

Hypoxia Hypoxia is not uncommon during the initial stages of acute pancreatitis. A subset of patients will develop more substantial or prolonged hypoxia and go on to develop ARDS. Thus, it is reasonable to monitor patients with acute pancreatitis, especially those with severe acute pancreatitis, by means of pulse oximetry to detect the development of hypox-

Table 6 Atlanta Criteria for Severity

Organ failure
  Shock (supine systolic blood pressure < 90 mm Hg)
  Pulmonary insufficiency (P$_a$O$_2$ < 60 mm Hg)
  Renal failure (serum creatinine > 2 mg/dl)
  Gastrointestinal tract bleeding (> 500 ml in 24 hr)

and/or

Local complications
  Necrosis
  Abscess
  Pseudocysts

and/or

Unfavorable prognostic signs
  Ranson score > 3
  APACHE II score > 8

emia. Because patients who develop hypoxia are also at risk for MOF, persistent hypoxemia merits ICU admission. Fluid management in these patients can be difficult and is best done with monitoring of pulmonary capillary wedge pressure. Mechanical ventilation, usually with positive end-expiratory pressure (PEEP), is often necessary.

Cardiac complications   A variety of cardiac complications may occur in severe acute pancreatitis, including congestive heart failure, myocardial infarction, cardiac arrhythmias, and cardiogenic shock. Hypotension is most commonly caused by third-space fluid losses and intravascular volume depletion. Cardiac dysfunction may, however, occur as part of SIRS seen in severe acute pancreatitis, which is characterized by high cardiac output and low systemic vascular resistance. Hypotension that is not responsive to fluid resuscitation may require the use of pressor agents.

Metabolic complications   A number of metabolic complications may also occur in acute pancreatitis, including hypocalcemia, hyperglycemia, and hyperlipidemia. Hypocalcemia is most commonly the result of hypoalbuminemia and is uncommonly associated with a reduction in ionized calcium or symptoms of hypocalcemia. Calcium replacement is usually not needed in the absence of decreased ionized calcium or signs of neuromuscular instability (e.g., tetany, the Chvostek sign, and the Trousseau sign). Calcium should, nonetheless, be monitored carefully, as it can be a marker of severe pancreatitis.

Hyperglycemia, like hypocalcemia, is one of the Ranson criteria indicating a poor prognosis. Treatment of mild hyperglycemia is not necessary, but significant increases in blood glucose levels (i.e., levels > 200 mg/dl) should be treated with sliding-scale insulin to minimize associated fluid losses caused by glycosuria and to prevent any detrimental effect on white cell function.

Hyperlipidemia is associated with acute pancreatitis, both as an etiologic factor and as a consequence. Many patients with acute pancreatitis may develop a modest elevation in serum triglyceride levels (i.e., levels > 300 to 400 mg/dl) as a consequence of acute pancreatitis. These elevations in triglyceride levels are usually short-lived and do not require therapy. Levels above 1,000 mg/dl indicate hypertriglyceridemia as the cause, rather than a consequence, of acute pancreatitis. These levels will usually drop rapidly while the patient is NPO. Marked elevations in triglyceride levels (> 10,000 mg/dl) or failure of triglyceride levels to drop as expected may occasionally necessitate the use of plasmapheresis to rapidly clear triglycerides from the serum. After recovery from pancreatitis, patients with hyperlipidemic pancreatitis should be started on appropriate medications and dietary therapy to control lipids.

Gastrointestinal bleeding   Gastrointestinal bleeding may complicate acute pancreatitis and is a marker of a severe attack.[57,58] Bleeding may occur from stress erosions, peptic ulceration, pseudoaneurysm, or varices developing as a consequence of splenic vein thrombosis. Splenic vein thrombosis, which may occur as a consequence of inflammatory and neoplastic pancreatic diseases, causes a left-sided portal hypertension characterized by gastric varices out of proportion to esophageal varices. These varices may bleed and, if they do, may be managed by splenectomy, which is curative. Bleeding from a pseudoaneurysm is usually associated with a pseudocyst [see Chronic Pancreatitis, Treatment of Other Complications, below].

Other systemic complications   Rare complications of acute pancreatitis include other vascular thromboses, disseminated intravascular coagulation, distant fat necrosis in the skin (resembling erythema nodosum), encephalopathy, and sudden blindness.

Pancreatic infection and abscess   Infected pancreatic necrosis, the most serious form of pancreatic infection, occurs in about 1% to 4% of patients overall with pancreatic infection and in 15% to 30% of those with pancreatic necrosis.[42,59,60] The mortality of necrotizing pancreatitis is about 10%, but this rate triples when infection supervenes. Most commonly, infection occurs during the second and third weeks of an attack of severe pancreatitis. The patient develops fever (often, temperatures > 102° F [38.9° C]), leukocytosis, and recurrent or worsening abdominal pain. The infecting organisms usually seed the necrotic area from the gut and are most commonly gram-negative rods (e.g., *Klebsiella* or *Escherichia coli*) and *Staphylococcus aureus*. *Candida*, *Enterococcus*, and anaerobic organisms are seen less commonly as causal agents of pancreatic infection. When infection is suspected, a CT scan should be obtained to evaluate the extent of necrosis and identify optimal locations for percutaneous sampling.[40,42,61] The finding of gas within the pancreatic parenchyma is highly specific but quite insensitive for serious pancreatic infection [see Figure 2]. However, a clinical suspicion of infection together with a finding of necrosis is an indication for percutaneous aspiration of suspicious areas, and a Gram stain and a culture of the collected tissue should be done. Experience over the past 15 years has demonstrated that percutaneous aspiration is both highly accurate and safe.[40,42,59,60] If pancreatic infection is demonstrated on percutaneous aspiration, the therapy of choice is prompt surgical debridement. Successful management of necrotic collections by percutaneous or endoscopic catheterization has also been reported,[62] but these techniques require further study because it is difficult to remove the necrotic tissue through catheters and, hence, difficult to cure the infection by this means.

Pancreatic abscess may also complicate severe acute pancreatitis, usually as a consequence of superinfection of a preexisting fluid collection or pseudocyst. Less commonly, an abscess develops secondary to superinfection of necrotic sites in the pancreas. The clinical presentation of pancreatic abscess is indistinguishable from that of infected necrosis, although therapy may differ.

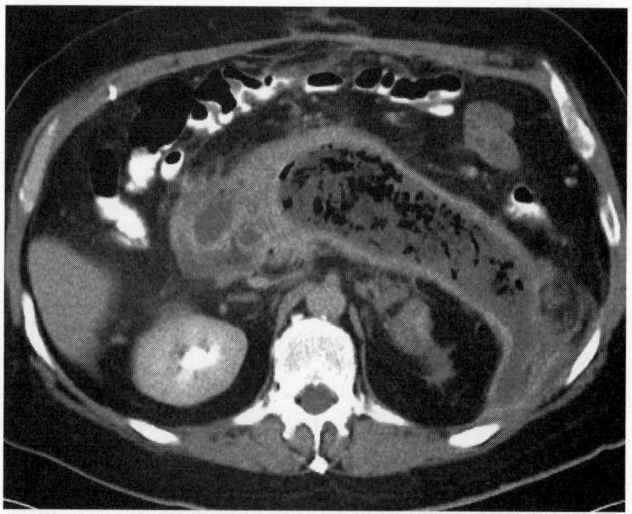

Figure 2   **A CT scan demonstrating a large amount of air within the necrotic pancreas in a patient with infected pancreatic necrosis.**

Therapy for pancreatic abscess usually consists of antibiotics and drainage. Unlike infected necrosis, which is typically treated by surgical debridement, pancreatic abscess may allow treatment by percutaneous or endoscopic tube drainage, because typically there is little solid necrotic tissue in the abscess cavity. The decision whether to treat with tube drainage or surgical exploration depends on whether the collections contain solid necrotic tissue (indicating infected necrosis, which typically necessitates open surgical drainage) or primarily pus (indicating abscess, which may allow drainage by endoscopic or percutaneous tube). However, distinguishing infected necrosis from pus may be difficult, and the most accurate picture of the collection contents is probably provided by MRI and EUS. EUS in particular is valuable because the collection not only can be assessed for the character of its contents but also can be drained safely in the same setting if appropriate. If doubt exists, it is better to err on the side of caution and opt for open surgical drainage.

Because the consequences of abscess and infected pancreatic necrosis are often severe, numerous studies have been directed toward identifying effective measures to prevent these infections. Currently, however, the role of antibiotics in the prevention of pancreatic infection is controversial. Early studies using prophylactic ampicillin demonstrated no reduction in pancreatic infections; it was later demonstrated that ampicillin does not penetrate the necrotic pancreas at adequate concentrations. More recent studies have identified agents that have adequate penetration of the necrotic pancreas; effective therapies include imipenem,[63,64] cefuroxime,[65] ofloxacin and metronidazole,[66] and ciprofloxacin and metronidazole.[67] A Cochrane Database review concluded that intravenous prophylactic antibiotic therapy for 10 to 14 days reduced the risk of superinfection of pancreatic necrosis and mortality.[68] This analysis, however, did not include the only relevant double-blind, randomized trial,[67] which demonstrated that there was no benefit with the use of prophylactic antibiotics for necrotic pancreatitis. These divergent findings have led to a difference of opinion on the overall utility of prophylactic antibiotics.

Generally, antibiotic use should be limited to patients at risk for serious pancreatic infection (i.e., if more than 30% of the gland appears necrotic on CT), and the selected antibiotic should be one that penetrates the necrotic tissue (i.e., imipenem or a fluoroquinolone plus metronidazole). Treatment should be continued for a maximum of 10 to 14 days. Patients receiving these broad-spectrum antibiotics are at risk for infection with resistant bacteria and fungal superinfection. Some researchers have advocated the concomitant use of antifungal agents such as fluconazole to reduce the risk of fungal infection, but the effectiveness of this strategy is unproved.

Fluid collections and pseudocysts Fluid collections in and around the pancreas occur commonly in patients with acute pancreatitis. Peripancreatic fluid collections are generally amorphous and not encapsulated. Most fluid collections resolve spontaneously, but some develop into pseudocysts.[57,69,70] A pseudocyst is a rounded collection of pancreatic fluid enclosed by a wall of fibrous or granulation tissue that can usually be seen on a CT scan. Most collections occur in the lesser sac or pararenal spaces, but they may develop anywhere and may even penetrate adjacent solid organs (e.g., the liver or spleen). Pseudocysts complicate 1% to 8% of all cases of acute pancreatitis.[69,70] Pseudocysts may persist, resolve, be asymptomatic, or be associated with symptoms or complications. The most common symptom associated with a pseudocyst is abdominal pain; however, other symptoms may develop if the pseudocyst obstructs an adjacent hollow viscus. For example, obstruction of the duodenum causes nausea and vomiting, whereas obstruction of the bile duct causes jaundice. Up to two thirds of all pseudocysts ultimately resolve, but spontaneous resolution is unlikely to occur with pseudocysts that are larger than 5 to 6 cm or are present for more than 6 weeks. In addition, pseudocysts larger than 6 cm are somewhat more likely to produce complications, including obstruction of an adjacent hollow viscus (e.g., duodenum or bile duct), infection, bleeding, or rupture. Infection of a pseudocyst (i.e., a pancreatic abscess) is usually relatively easy to manage with antibiotics and endoscopic or percutaneous catheter drainage; however, pseudocysts characterized by bleeding and rupture are associated with much greater morbidity and mortality. Bleeding may occur from a large artery that has formed a pseudoaneurysm from the pressure exerted by a contiguous pseudocyst, and the resulting blood flow can reach the gut through the pancreatic duct or can enter the peritoneum through a rupture of the pseudocyst. An initial bleed may be self-limited, but any unexplained drop in hemoglobin or change in pain pattern in a patient with a pseudocyst is an indication for an emergency CT scan. If any evidence of bleeding is found, emergency angiography with embolization can be lifesaving.[58]

Asymptomatic pseudocysts generally pose little risk of complications, even if they are large.[70] Symptomatic or complicated pseudocysts require therapy, and emergency surgery is required when bleeding or rupture is detected. Otherwise, elective surgical, percutaneous, or endoscopic techniques can be successful, depending on the location of the pseudocyst and the availability of expertise in these modalities. In the past, endoscopic drainage could be applied only to pseudocysts that produced a visible bulging impression in the lumen of the stomach or duodenum. Today, endoscopic pseudocyst drainage can be accomplished by using real-time endoscopic ultrasound guidance without the need of visually observing a bulge.[71] Percutaneous tube drainage can also treat pseudocysts that are farther from the gut lumen; however, tube drainage can produce a chronically draining external pancreatic fistula. Surgical treatment of pseudocysts probably has the best long-term results, but it also carries the most significant morbidity. Endoscopic ultrasound-guided transmural pseudocyst drainage appears to offer the best risk-to-benefit ratio for pseudocysts in anatomically amenable locations, but studies directly comparing surgical, endoscopic, and percutaneous drainage are lacking.

Prevention of Subsequent Attacks

Preventing subsequent attacks of acute pancreatitis requires elimination of the cause of the disease. In patients with acute alcoholic pancreatitis, cessation of alcohol consumption appears to have some benefit in reducing relapse, although unfortunately, the disease may continue to progress to symptomatic chronic pancreatitis despite abstinence. In patients with gallstone pancreatitis, cholecystectomy virtually eliminates recurrence. Similarly, the detection of microlithiasis followed by appropriate therapy (i.e., cholecystectomy, endoscopic biliary sphincterotomy, and possibly the use of ursodeoxycholic acid) can prevent recurrent pancreatitis. Aggressive control of serum lipid levels can prevent recurrent attacks of hyperlipidemic pancreatitis. In patients with a disorder that obstructs the pancreatic duct (e.g., benign or malignant pancreatic duct stricture, pancreas divisum, sphincter of Oddi dysfunction, and ampullary tumor), removal of the obstruction by surgical or endoscopic means is generally effective in preventing relapse.

Chronic Pancreatitis

Chronic pancreatitis is characterized by irreversible damage to the pancreas and the development of histologic evidence of fibrosis and destruction of exocrine (acinar cell) and endocrine (islets of Langerhans) tissue. As with acute pancreatitis, the definition of chronic pancreatitis was developed at international symposia.[72] Several variants of chronic pancreatitis were defined, including chronic calcified pancreatitis (the most common form, which is commonly caused by excessive alcohol intake), chronic obstructive pancreatitis (caused by long-standing pancreatic duct obstruction), and chronic inflammatory pancreatitis (associated with inflammatory and, particularly, autoimmune diseases). Unfortunately, it is often not possible to make the distinction between these variants on the basis of clinical findings or imaging studies, and the distinctions are not very useful to clinicians. Recent classification schemes have focused more on etiology and are somewhat more useful to clinicians.[22]

EPIDEMIOLOGY

The prevalence of chronic pancreatitis varies with the population. Estimates of annual incidence in several studies range from three to nine cases per 100,000 population.[5,73] One study estimated an overall prevalence of 27.4 per 100,00 population. In nonfederal hospitals in the United States, this accounts for 122,000 outpatient visits and more than 20,000 hospitalizations annually.[3,4] The natural history can be quite variable and is clearly affected by the presence of ongoing alcoholism in persons with chronic alcoholic pancreatitis. In one large multicenter study,[74] the standardized mortality ratio was 3.6 (those with a diagnosis of chronic pancreatitis died at 3.6 times the rate of age-matched control subjects). Older persons and those with alcoholic chronic pancreatitis have the lowest survival. Overall, 10-year survival for patients with chronic pancreatitis has been shown to be about 70%, and 20-year survival about 45%.[5,74] Chronic pancreatitis is a strong risk factor for pancreatic adenocarcinoma, which partly explains the increased mortality associated with chronic pancreatitis.

ETIOLOGY

Alcohol Abuse

Alcohol is the cause of chronic pancreatitis in 70% to 90% of all cases. In general, at least 5 years of alcohol intake exceeding 150 g/day is required to develop symptomatic chronic pancreatitis, although some patients develop chronic pancreatitis with less alcohol intake. Only 5% to 15% of heavy drinkers ultimately develop chronic pancreatitis, suggesting that cofactors play an important role in pathogenesis.[12] Predisposing factors may include genetic abnormalities and a diet high in fat and protein. The mechanism by which alcohol causes chronic pancreatitis remains undefined, but it may be related to a change in pancreatic secretion leading to (1) protein plug formation in the pancreatic duct, (2) a direct toxic effect of alcohol or its metabolites, or (3) repeated attacks of acute alcoholic pancreatitis that eventually produce chronic irreversible damage. It has been observed that the vast majority of patients who develop an acute attack of alcoholic pancreatitis already have preexisting chronic damage to the gland.

Tropical Pancreatitis

Tropical pancreatitis is seen in certain areas of Indonesia, India, and Africa. The disease typically presents in childhood, with diabetes, abdominal pain, steatorrhea, malnutrition, and diffuse pancreatic calcifications. Malnutrition appears to be an important cofactor in this disease, as may be the presence of toxic metabolites of the dietary staple cassava. Studies also suggest a strong genetic component, with mutations in the SPINK1 gene occurring in more than one third of patients.[75]

Genetic Factors

Hereditary pancreatitis is an autosomal dominant disease that typically presents in childhood or early adulthood and frequently is accompanied by steatorrhea, diabetes mellitus, and diffuse pancreatic calcifications. Pain and acute episodes of pancreatitis flares may also occur but are somewhat less common in hereditary pancreatitis than in alcoholic chronic pancreatitis. The initially identified genetic abnormality is a defect in the PRSS1 gene on chromosome 7.[22,76] Multiple mutations have been described, but two are more common.[76] The two more common mutations appear to produce a trypsinogen that, once activated, is difficult or impossible to inactivate. The activated enzyme, trypsin, can in turn activate all the other pancreatic enzymes. Chronic pancreatitis appears to be caused in this situation by prolonged low-grade pancreatic injury from the activated proteases. Pancreatic adenocarcinoma frequently complicates the condition; patients with chronic pancreatitis have a 30% risk of developing pancreatic adenocarcinoma by age 70.[77] The risk may be substantially higher in patients with paternal inheritance.

Mutation of the SPINK1 gene increases the propensity to develop chronic pancreatitis,[22,75] although mutation of this gene appears to act as a cofactor. Increased frequency of mutations in SPINK1 is seen in patients with pancreatitis of different etiologies—namely, tropical pancreatitis (> 33% of patients), alcoholic chronic pancreatitis (about 6% of patients), hereditary pancreatitis (in a few kindreds in addition to their PRSS1 mutation), and idiopathic chronic pancreatitis (sometimes in association with additional mutations in the CFTR gene). Mutations in SPINK1 are common in the general population, but in most cases, pancreatic disease does not occur in these individuals; therefore, these mutations provide only a predisposition to chronic pancreatitis and are only some of the many factors contributing to formation of the disease.

CFTR mutations are also associated with chronic pancreatitis. Patients with classic cystic fibrosis commonly develop pancreatic insufficiency that requires supplementation of pancreatic enzyme. Several studies have also suggested that less common cystic fibrosis gene mutations, particularly when they occur as a mixed heterozygote (different mutations on the two alleles), are associated with relapsing pancreatitis and chronic pancreatitis in the absence of obvious sinopulmonary disease.[22,78] Patients with both CFTR and SPINK1 mutations are at exceedingly high risk for chronic pancreatitis.

Undetermined Causes

Some patients may be misdiagnosed as having idiopathic pancreatitis if appropriate genetic studies are not performed or if a careful history of alcohol use is not obtained. Even if genetic studies are done, not all mutations may be identified (e.g., many commercially available screens look for only a few hundred of the more than 1,200 known CFTR mutations), and many identified CFTR and SPINK1 mutations produce only a predisposition to disease (unlike *PRSS1* mutations, which cause disease). Previous studies of patients with so-called idiopathic chronic pancreatitis that did not assess for the presence of genetic mutations appeared to identify two forms: early-onset and late-onset idiopathic chronic pancreatitis. The early-onset form presents just before or during the second decade, and it is typically associated with severe pain in the absence of diabetes, steatorrhea, or pancreatic calcification.[79] The late-onset form presents at a mean age of 56 years and is more commonly associated with exocrine or endocrine insufficiency and less commonly associated with severe pain.[79] The relative role of genetic influences on these two phenotypic variations remains to be determined.

PATHOGENESIS

The pathophysiology of chronic pancreatitis remains poorly understood. The events that occur in hereditary chronic pancreatitis suggest that one common underlying theme may be multiple subclinical episodes of acute injury that ultimately produce chronic pancreatitis.[80] A recent hypothesis (the so-called sentinel acute pancreatitis event [SAPE] hypothesis)[81] suggests that in a patient with an underlying susceptibility (e.g., genetic background), a sentinel event (e.g., alcohol exposure) can trigger the disease process, producing acute inflammation and infiltration of inflammatory cells. The acute pancreatitis may heal or, with repeated episodes, may lead to activation of pancreatic stellate cells and the development of fibrosis (i.e., chronic pancreatitis). This hypothesis, while attractive, is as yet unproved.

DIAGNOSIS

Clinical Findings

The diagnosis of chronic pancreatitis is suspected on the basis of suggestive signs and symptoms and confirmed by further tests of pancreatic structure or function. The disease is usually suspected on the basis of the presence of abdominal pain.

The vast majority of patients with chronic pancreatitis will experience pain at some point during their illness.[73,79] The pain tends to be episodic initially, but it may become more constant or continuous as the disease progresses. During acute attacks, the patient may be thought to have acute pancreatitis until the diagnosis of chronic pancreatitis can ultimately be established. Although there is no pathognomonic character of the pain, it is most commonly felt in the epigastrium, with radiation to the back. In severe episodes, nausea and vomiting are common. The natural history of the pain is quite variable, and it may worsen, stabilize, or even resolve over time. In some patients, the onset is gradual and evolves into constant abdominal pain. However, a minority of patients with chronic pancreatitis have no pain. In these patients, the disease may be suspected on the basis of the development of exocrine insufficiency (steatorrhea, weight loss, and malnutrition) or endocrine insufficiency (diabetes mellitus).

Laboratory Tests

The clinical features suggestive of chronic pancreatitis (e.g., abdominal pain, steatorrhea, weight loss, and malnutrition) are not specific for chronic pancreatitis; the diagnosis requires confirmatory tests. Diagnostic tests are usually separated into tests that detect abnormalities of pancreatic function and tests that detect abnormalities of pancreatic structure [*see Table 7*]. Chronic pancreatitis is a slowly progressive disease, and the abnormalities of pancreatic structure or function may take years to develop or may not develop at all. Hence, all of the diagnostic tests are

Table 7 Diagnostic Tests for Chronic Pancreatitis*

Structural Tests	*Functional Tests*
Endoscopic ultrasonography	Direct hormonal stimulation test (secretin or secretin-CCK test)
Endoscopic retrograde pancreatography	Fecal elastase
Computed tomography	Serum trypsin
Magnetic resonance imaging/magnetic resonance cholangiopancreatography	Fecal fat
Abdominal ultrasound	Serum glucose
Plain abdominal radiograph	—

*Ranked in approximate order of decreasing sensitivity.
CCK—cholecystokinin

most accurate in far-advanced disease, when obvious structural or functional abnormalities have developed.

Structural abnormalities that can be diagnostic of chronic pancreatitis include changes in the main pancreatic duct (dilatation, strictures, irregularity, and pancreatic duct stones), side branches of the pancreatic duct (dilatation and irregularity), or pancreatic parenchyma (diffuse pancreatic calcifications). These findings can be visualized utilizing the diagnostic tests that evaluate pancreatic structure [*see Table 7*].

Functional abnormalities in chronic pancreatitis include a decrease in stimulated secretory capacity, exocrine insufficiency (malabsorption and steatorrhea), and endocrine insufficiency (diabetes mellitus).[82] Patients with alcoholic chronic pancreatitis, hereditary chronic pancreatitis, tropical pancreatitis, and late-onset idiopathic chronic pancreatitis are most likely to develop these abnormalities, although the course of development may take many years. Patients with early-onset idiopathic chronic pancreatitis may not develop these abnormalities at all. This observation has led to a general classification of chronic pancreatitis as either big-duct or small-duct disease [*see Imaging Studies, Disease Classification, below*].

Serum tests Serum amylase or lipase levels may be elevated during acute exacerbations of chronic pancreatitis, but these elevations are usually only modest and are neither routinely present nor diagnostic for chronic pancreatitis. Serum trypsinogen (often called serum trypsin) can also be measured. Low levels of serum trypsinogen (< 20 ng/ml) are highly specific for chronic pancreatitis,[73,83] but such low levels occur only in advanced disease (in the presence of steatorrhea). Very low levels of serum trypsinogen may also be seen occasionally in patients with pancreatic adenocarcinoma. Serum trypsinogen levels are in the normal range in most patients with less advanced chronic pancreatitis.

Stool tests A 72-hour stool collection for fat is the gold standard to detect steatorrhea but is cumbersome and unpleasant to perform. Steatorrhea is seen only in far-advanced chronic pancreatitis. More than 7 g of fat in the stool per 24 hours is considered abnormal. Of note, the patient has to be placed on a diet containing 100 g of fat a day for the results of the stool collection to be valid. At least 90% of the pancreatic enzyme secretory capacity needs to be lost before steatorrhea will develop.[84] Qualitative stool stains for fat (e.g., Sudan III) are far less accurate than a

72-hour collection but are easily performed. They should also be performed only while the patient is on a high-fat diet. Fecal levels of elastase and chymotrypsin may be reduced in patients with chronic pancreatitis, but only in cases of more advanced chronic pancreatitis.[82] Measurement of fecal elastase in a random stool sample is of reasonable accuracy[83,85] in these patients and is now available from reference laboratories in the United States. Values of fecal elastase of less than 200 µg/g of stool are seen in patients with more advanced chronic pancreatitis.

Direct pancreatic function tests   The direct pancreatic function tests involve placing a tube into the duodenum to collect pancreatic juice and are complex and cumbersome. These tests directly measure pancreatic output of enzymes or bicarbonate after stimulation with a secretagogue (e.g., secretin or cholecystokinin or its analogue). Although these tests are able to detect severe decreases in pancreatic secretory output, their strength is in detecting moderate decreases in maximal stimulated secretory capacity. This decrease in maximal stimulated secretory capacity occurs before secretory failure (exocrine insufficiency) in chronic pancreatitis, and the direct function tests are felt to be the most sensitive tests available to detect chronic pancreatitis at an early stage (earlier than any other test).[73,82,86] They are particularly useful in making the diagnosis in patients with small-duct chronic pancreatitis, in whom alternative diagnostic tests (e.g., CT, ERCP) are likely to miss the diagnosis. Unfortunately, direct pancreatic function tests are available only at a few referral centers in the United States. Alternatives to cumbersome traditional pancreatic function testing have been studied. The collection of pure pancreatic juice for 15 minutes at the time of ERCP—the so-called intraductal secretin test—proved to be an inaccurate way to evaluate pancreatic function.[87] Another alternative involves administering a secretagogue (secretin) and collecting pancreatic secretions through an endoscope during upper endoscopy with sedation. Although accurate, the 1-hour collection of pancreatic secretions after secretin stimulation at the time of upper endoscopy appears to be perhaps too impractical for widespread application.[88] It is hoped that refinements will eventually allow these more sensitive tests to be used in a wider population of patients.

Imaging Studies

Radiology   Simple plain abdominal radiographs may detect diffuse pancreatic calcification in very far advanced chronic pancreatitis [*see Figure 3*]. This finding is highly specific but quite insensitive.

Ultrasonography   Abdominal US is most likely to detect advanced abnormalities of pancreatic structure; however, US is diagnostic in only 60% of patients.[73] The pancreas is often not well visualized on transabdominal US. New techniques of contrast-enhanced US and tissue harmonic imaging may provide better diagnostic accuracy.[89]

Computed tomography   CT is much more sensitive than US (CT, 75% to 90%) because of its capacity to detect more focal abnormalities, such as calcification, a dilated pancreatic duct, fluid collections, and focal enlargements. CT may also demonstrate gland atrophy, which is seen in patients of advanced age in the absence of chronic pancreatitis. The use of multislice CT produces images of exceptional quality; this imaging technique should improve diagnostic accuracy, although it has not been

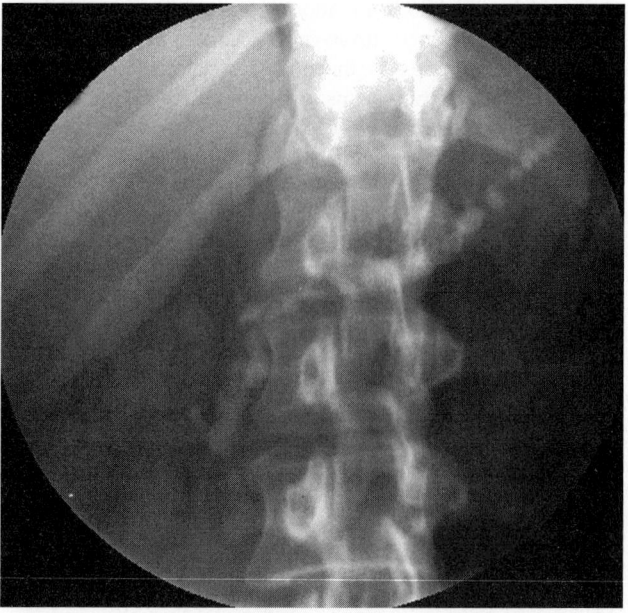

Figure 3   A plain film of the abdomen demonstrating multiple calcified stones in the pancreatic duct in a patient with advanced chronic pancreatitis.

adequately studied.[90] Like US, CT can be falsely negative in early or less advanced chronic pancreatitis.

Magnetic resonance imaging   An improvement in magnetic resonance technology has allowed more accurate imaging of both the pancreatic parenchyma and the pancreatic duct with MRCP. It is not clear whether MRI and MRCP are superior to CT, but they do appear to be at least equivalent to CT in overall accuracy.[90] The use of secretin before MRCP allows improved imaging of the pancreatic duct and, theoretically, calculation of pancreatic secretory volume.[91] Secretin-stimulated MRCP is being used at a number of centers and may improve overall accuracy of MRI for chronic pancreatitis.

Endoscopy   Two endoscopic tests are used to diagnose chronic pancreatitis: ERCP and EUS. ERCP has a reported sensitivity of 75% to 90%.[73,86] With ERCP, radiographic contrast is injected into the pancreatic duct. Changes in the pancreatic duct consistent with chronic pancreatitis include ductal dilatation, strictures, irregularity, and filling defects (stones) in the pancreatic duct [*see Figures 4 and 5*]. The changes associated with chronic pancreatitis that are seen on ERCP are not specific, as they can also be seen in other clinical presentations—namely, (1) in elderly patients with pancreatic duct dilatation caused by aging, (2) in patients with resolving acute pancreatitis, (3) in some patients with pancreatic carcinoma, and (4) in patients who have previously undergone pancreatic duct stenting.[86] In addition to its diagnostic ability, ERCP may have therapeutic application in a subset of patients [*see* Management, Endoscopic and Surgical Therapy, *below*].

EUS, which allows a highly detailed examination of the pancreatic parenchyma and pancreatic duct, routinely detects abnormalities in patients with chronic pancreatitis (high sensitivity). The test is interpreted on the basis of documented changes in both the pancreatic duct and pancreatic parenchyma; a system of grading EUS findings usually assesses nine specific features.[92,93] In addition, a normal EUS examination essentially rules out chronic pancreatitis. The specificity of the test requires some further study in that many patients without clinical chronic pancreatitis may have modest numbers of abnormalities on EUS [*see Figure 6*].[92,93]

Disease classification Depending on the findings on imaging studies, patients may be classified as having so-called big-duct or small-duct chronic pancreatitis. This distinction has both diagnostic and therapeutic implications. Big-duct disease implies substantial abnormalities of the pancreatic duct (gener-

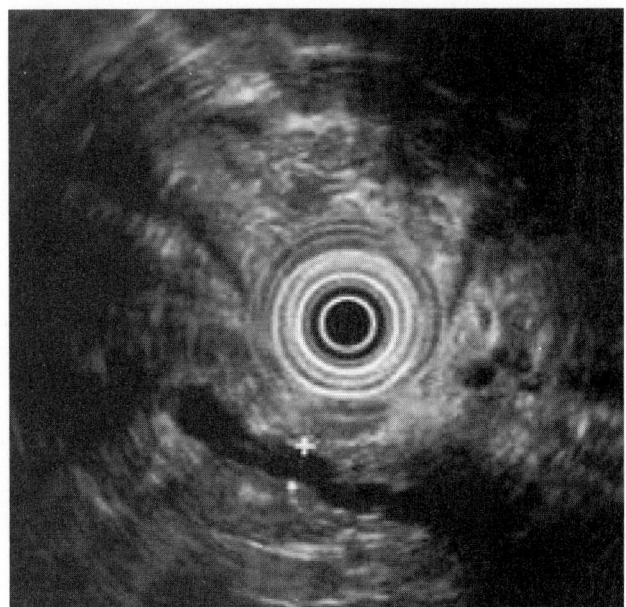

Figure 6 **An endoscopic ultrasound image demonstrating a dilated pancreatic duct (markers) in a patient with advanced chronic pancreatitis.**

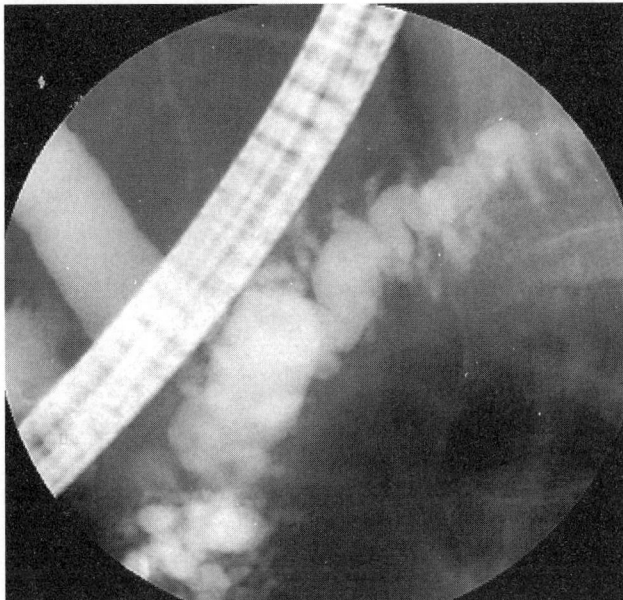

Figure 4 **An endoscopic retrograde cholangiopancreatography image demonstrating massive pancreatic duct dilatation in a patient with big-duct chronic pancreatitis.**

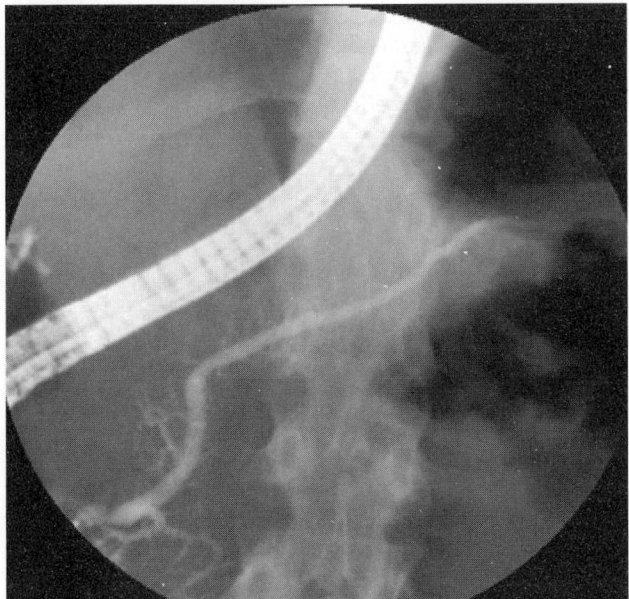

Figure 5 **An endoscopic retrograde cholangiopancreatography image demonstrating minimal pancreatic duct abnormalities in a patient with painful small-duct chronic pancreatitis.**

ally, dilatation visible on US, CT, ERCP, or EUS, often with pancreatic calcifications), and small-duct disease implies the absence of these findings (e.g., a normal or near-normal US, CT, or ERCP) [*see Figures 4 and 5*]. The diagnosis of big-duct disease is much simpler; the disease usually results from alcohol abuse, and the therapeutic options include treatments aimed at decompressing the dilated pancreatic duct. The diagnosis and management of small-duct disease may prove to be more difficult than those of big-duct disease because with small-duct disease, imaging studies may be normal, disease is more commonly idiopathic, and treatment options focus on medical therapy rather than surgical or endoscopic attempts to decompress the pancreatic duct.

Diagnostic Approach

The diagnostic approach to chronic pancreatitis should begin with tests that are safe, inexpensive, and able to detect relatively far advanced disease. Diagnostic tests that fit in this category include serum trypsinogen, fecal elastase, and abdominal US. If these tests do not lead to a diagnosis, riskier or more expensive tests will generally need to be employed (e.g., MRI/MRCP, CT, ERCP, or EUS). Direct pancreatic function testing, if available, logically should be used after the initial tests and before the more expensive or invasive tests, because direct pancreatic function tests are the most sensitive tests available and are lower in cost and less risky than the other options. Because most clinicians do not have access to pancreatic function testing, the riskier, more expensive tests are usually performed, starting with a good-quality CT using pancreatic protocol.

MANAGEMENT

Abdominal Pain

Pain is the most common symptom of chronic pancreatitis requiring medical care. There are a number of potential causes of pain in chronic pancreatitis, including inflammation of pancreatic nerves, pancreatic tissue ischemia, increased pressure in the gland or an associated pseudocyst, obstruction of a surrounding hollow viscus (e.g., duodenum or bile duct), and coexistent pancreatic carcinoma. The initial evaluation should focus on identifying conditions for which specific therapy exists. These conditions include pancreatic pseudocyst, duodenal or bile duct compression, and superimposed pancreatic carcinoma. This evaluation is most commonly done by performing a high-quality CT scan of the abdomen. If such a condition is identified, specific therapy is required [see Treatment of Other Complications, below].

Analgesia and cessation of alcohol use Nonspecific measures to reduce pain in chronic pancreatitis include cessation of alcohol consumption and use of analgesics. Cessation of alcohol consumption can reduce pain in some patients with alcoholic chronic pancreatitis and may prolong life by preventing other alcohol-induced diseases. Unfortunately, abstinence will not halt the progression of chronic pancreatitis, although it may slow it. Analgesics are generally needed, but it is important to start with the least potent agents first (e.g., propoxyphene napsulate or tramadol) because narcotic addiction can occur in up to 30% of patients. Many patients will require more potent narcotics. Adding an antidepressant (a selective serotonin reuptake inhibitor or a tricyclic) may allow potentiation of the narcotic effect. If these simple measures fail, further therapy utilizing medical, endoscopic, or surgical techniques can be considered.

Administration of pancreatic enzymes Several controlled trials have attempted to delineate the effectiveness of orally administered pancreatic enzymes to decrease pain. The concept behind this therapy is that proteases that are present in the duodenum may reduce the stimulus for pancreatic secretion by a negative-feedback mechanism. Only conventional (non–enteric-coated) preparations of pancreatic enzymes can deliver proteases to the duodenum; enteric-coated enzyme preparations deliver proteases too far distally to achieve a negative-feedback effect. Two studies utilizing non–enteric-coated enzymes at high dosages (8 tablets total, in four divided doses with meals and at night, coupled with an agent to suppress gastric acid to prevent premature inactivation of the enzymes) demonstrated a reduction in pain. Four other studies utilizing enteric-coated enzymes showed no effect. A meta-analysis of these studies suggested enzymes are of no benefit in treating pain.[94] In the two studies that demonstrated effectiveness, it appears that persons with less advanced disease (small-duct chronic pancreatitis) respond best, and females with idiopathic chronic pancreatitis seem to have the highest response rate. The role of enzymes in treating pain is controversial, although a consensus review advocated their use.[95] Non–enteric-coated enzyme preparations are of modest effectiveness, but they may be worth a trial in patients with less advanced disease in whom other simple medical measures have failed. A trial of enzymes for pain is generally pointless in patients with advanced or big-duct chronic pancreatitis (mainly alcoholic chronic pancreatitis). These enzyme products are inactivated by gastric acid; thus, concomitant therapy with an agent to reduce gastric acid (H_2 receptor antagonist or proton pump inhibitor) is needed.

Neurolysis Neurolysis via a celiac plexus block or thoracoscopic splanchnicectomy has been evaluated in a number of small studies. The use of percutaneous celiac plexus block has largely been abandoned in patients with chronic pancreatitis be-

cause of its transitory effectiveness. EUS-guided celiac plexus block is simpler and safer than percutaneous techniques and appears to last longer.[96] Thoracoscopic splanchnicectomy involves sectioning the splanchnic nerves at thoracoscopy. The short-term response is good (60% to 80% response), but the long-term response has been disappointing.[97]

Endoscopic and surgical therapy Endoscopic therapy and surgical therapy are most useful in patients with advanced or big-duct chronic pancreatitis. Endoscopic therapy has a general goal of relieving obstruction in the pancreatic duct by dilating or stenting a stricture or by removing an obstructing stone. Only a subset of patients with chronic pancreatitis are candidates for such therapy; generally, endoscopic therapy may be considered an option in patients with a dilated pancreatic duct (big-duct chronic pancreatitis) and an obstructing stricture or stone in the head of the gland. The results of large case series indicate that endoscopic therapy may improve pain in 70% to 80% of carefully selected patients.[73,95,98,99] The only randomized, controlled trial that compared endoscopic therapy with surgery showed that the two therapies provide equivalent short-term pain relief, but surgery provided better long-term pain relief.[100] Even if endoscopic therapy is not possible, however, an ERCP may provide useful information for planning surgical therapy.

Surgical procedures that are commonly used to treat pain include decompression of the main pancreatic duct, with or without resection of a portion of the pancreas. Surgery may also be indicated for treatment of a complication such as a pseudocyst, duodenal or common bile duct obstruction, or pancreatic fistula. For patients with intractable pain and a dilated duct, the most commonly performed procedure is the lateral pancreaticojejunostomy (i.e., modified Puestow procedure), in which the pancreatic duct is widely incised along its length and overlaid with a defunctionalized loop of small intestine for drainage of pancreatic juice directly into the small bowel. In some patients, resection of a portion of the pancreatic head may also be needed to decompress smaller-duct branches in the pancreatic head and uncinate process. Substantial pain relief is obtained in 65% to 85% of patients and appears to be relatively long lasting (in some studies, pain relief was sustained for more than 7 years); over time, the response declines to about 50%.[95,101] Mortality for these procedures is about 3% in experienced hands.

Table 8 Enzyme Supplements for
Chronic Pancreatitis

Preparation	Units of Lipase per Tablet or Capsule
Nonenteric-coated (conventional) preparations	—
Viokase 8, 16	8,000 and 16,000, respectively
Kuzyme-HP	8,000
Generic pancrealipase	8,000
Enteric-coated preparations	—
Creon 10, 20	10,000 and 20,000, respectively
Pancrease MT 4, 10, 16	4,000, 10,000, and 16,000, respectively
Ultrase MT 6, 12, 18, 20	6,000, 12,000, 18,000, and 20,000, respectively

Steatorrhea

The pancreas possesses a 90% functional reserve for the secretion of digestive enzymes.[84] Hence, only 10% of normal maximal output of enzymes is needed to prevent malabsorption of nutrients. Steatorrhea is therefore a late complication of chronic pancreatitis requiring the presence of substantial pancreatic damage. Steatorrhea takes, on average, 13 and 26 years to develop after a diagnosis of alcoholic and idiopathic chronic pancreatitis, respectively.[79] Fat malabsorption tends to occur earlier than protein or carbohydrate malabsorption. Steatorrhea is most precisely established by measuring fecal fat excretion over 72 hours while the patient is on a diet that contains 100 g of fat a day. This test, however, is cumbersome to perform and unpleasant for both patient and staff. In practice, steatorrhea is more commonly diagnosed by identification of clinical features of oily or floating stool, diarrhea, and weight loss and is confirmed by the response to pancreatic enzyme supplementation. Unlike for the treatment of pain, enteric-coated enzyme preparations are commonly selected over non–enteric-coated preparations for the treatment of steatorrhea because of the higher potency and the need for fewer pills with the enteric-coated agents. However, non–enteric-coated enzyme preparations can be used effectively to treat steatorrhea if they are administered in sufficient doses and coadministered with an agent that reduces gastric acid. At least 30,000 units of lipase must be delivered to the small intestine during the prandial and postprandial period to reduce steatorrhea to a manageable level [see Table 8]. The clinical goal of this enzyme replacement therapy is to reduce the diarrhea and the losses in stool of fat, protein, and carbohydrate, thereby allowing maintenance or improvement of weight and nutritional status. In patients who do not achieve these end points, explanations for therapeutic failure need to be considered. Such explanations include patient noncompliance, inadequate dosage of enzyme therapy, destruction of exogenous enzymes by gastric acid (if non–enteric-coated preparations were prescribed), poor diet (particularly in chronic alcoholics), and the presence of a second disease causing malabsorption (e.g., small bowel bacterial overgrowth).[102]

Endocrine Insufficiency

Diabetes mellitus, like steatorrhea, is a late complication of chronic pancreatitis. Progressive destruction of the islets of Langerhans can destroy both insulin- and glucagon-secreting cells. The inadequate glucagon reserves predispose patients with this disorder to treatment-induced hypoglycemia. Complications of diabetes such as neuropathy, retinopathy, and nephropathy occur at the same rate as in other patients with diabetes mellitus.[103] Therapy is usually directed at controlling urinary losses of glucose rather than at maintaining tight control of blood glucose levels. Overvigorous attempts at tight control of blood glucose levels are often associated with disastrous complications of treatment-induced hypoglycemia.[104] However, attempts at tight control of blood glucose levels are indicated in patients with hyperlipidemic pancreatitis because in this group, the diabetes is usually a primary illness and tight control of blood glucose levels makes control of serum lipid levels possible.

Other Complications

Pancreatic pseudocyst In chronic pancreatitis, as in acute pancreatitis [see Acute Pancreatitis, Treatment of Complications, above], asymptomatic pseudocysts less than 6 cm can be safely observed. However, unlike in acute pancreatitis, most pseudocysts that occur in the setting of chronic pancreatitis are generally mature at the time of their diagnosis, and therapy therefore need not be delayed if therapy is indicated. Symptomatic, complicated, or enlarging pseudocysts require therapy by percutaneous, endoscopic, or surgical techniques. Surgical therapy usually involves cyst decompression into a loop of small bowel, and this is often coupled with a pancreatic duct drainage procedure (e.g., modified Puestow procedure). Surgical therapy has a long-term success rate of more than 90%, with an operative mortality of less than 3%.[69,70,73] Percutaneous tube drainage of pseudocysts is also a management option and is immediately successful in 95% of patients. The long-term success rate of percutaneous drainage is still unknown, but it is certainly less than that of surgical techniques. Endoscopic therapy has short-term success rates greater than 90%.[69,70] The limited number of studies that have evaluated the long-term success rate of endoscopic drainage suggest excellent results, with complete resolution of the pseudocyst observed in 90% of patients.[69,70,105]

Complicated pseudocysts may require specific types of therapy. An infected pseudocyst (pancreatic abscess) generally responds to antibiotics and drainage (e.g., endoscopic, percutaneous, or surgical). Bleeding from a pseudocyst may occur in small vessels in its wall or from an associated large arterial pseudoaneurysm. Bleeding from a pseudoaneurysm requires urgent angiography with embolization, sometimes followed by surgical therapy.[58] If no pseudoaneurysm is present on angiography, surgical therapy remains the best choice of therapy for bleeding pseudocysts. Some pseudocysts may rupture and produce a pancreatic fistula that drains into the peritoneal cavity (producing pancreatic ascites) or into the pleural space (producing a pancreatic pleural effusion). In such cases, patients may not complain of symptoms of chronic pancreatitis but may instead note abdominal distention or shortness of breath. The diagnosis can be established by documenting high levels of amylase in the leaked fluid, typically more than 4,000 U/L.[73,106] Treatment may require surgery, and ERCP is used preoperatively to delineate the location of the leak. In many patients, endoscopic therapy and placement of a stent across the fistula site will prove curative.

Other cystic lesions A number of other cystic lesions may occur in the pancreas, including true cysts and cystic neoplasms. Serous cystic neoplasms are benign, but mucin-producing cystic neoplasms may follow a more malignant course. Mucinous cystic neoplasms present as large cystic collections (cystadenomas and cystadenocarcinomas) and may be relatively asymptomatic. Most cystic neoplasms occur in middle-aged patients, particularly in women.[107] They are often mistaken for pseudocysts and inappropriately treated as such. These cystic neoplasms may follow an initially benign course; but when they undergo malignant degeneration, they have poor outcomes equivalent to those of standard adenocarcinoma.

The presence of a pancreatic cystic collection in a middle-aged person (particularly female) without a previous history of pancreatitis should immediately suggest a cystic neoplasm, not a pseudocyst. The diagnosis of a cystic neoplasm requires histologic evidence of epithelial or neoplastic tissue in the cyst wall. Analysis of the cyst fluid obtained by EUS is becoming a highly useful method of differentiating pseudocysts from cystic neoplasms.[108] When these cystic collections are mistaken for pseudocysts, they are treated with drainage, and no tissue is obtained to allow differentiation of a cystic neoplasm from a pseudocyst. Therefore, the therapy of choice for cystic neoplasms is surgical resection, not drainage.

Intraductal papillary mucinous tumors (IPMT, formerly called mucinous ductal ectasia) are characterized by superficially spreading neoplastic tissue along the wall of the pancreatic duct. This neoplastic tissue produces mucin, and patients usually present with a markedly dilated pancreatic duct filled with gelatinous mucin. The appearance is often pathognomonic on ERCP but is occasionally mistaken for chronic pancreatitis. The natural history of the lesions is variable. In general, resection is attempted if the patient is a fit surgical candidate. Depending on the extent of the neoplastic tissue along the pancreatic duct, extensive resection may be needed to eliminate the lesion.[109]

Pancreatic cancer Chronic pancreatitis is a risk factor for pancreatic carcinoma, and the two diseases can be difficult to distinguish in some patients. The risk is about 4% after 20 years of disease.[110] The cancer risk may be as high as 40% in patients with hereditary chronic pancreatitis.[77] There is no effective method of surveillance in these patients and no absolutely reliable method to distinguish cancer from chronic pancreatitis. EUS with directed biopsy, ERCP with cytologic brushings, CT scan, and tumor markers such as CA19-9 are most commonly used.

Common bile duct or duodenal obstruction Fibrosis and inflammation in the head of the pancreas may compress surrounding hollow structures, particularly the common bile duct and duodenum. Compression of the common bile duct produces jaundice, and duodenal compression produces symptoms similar to those of gastric outlet obstruction. Both duodenal compression and gastric outlet obstruction generally require surgical repair with a biliary bypass or gastrojejunostomy, respectively.

Peter Draganov, M.D., has no commercial relationships with manufacturers of products or providers of services discussed in this chapter.

Chris E. Forsmark, M.D., F.A.C.P., has received grants for clinical research from AstraZeneca Pharmaceuticals LP and TAP Pharmaceutical Products, Inc., and has received grants for educational activities from Cook Endoscopy and the Olympus Corporation.

Octreotide acetate and pancreatic enzymes discussed in this chapter have not been approved by the FDA for use in the treatment of chronic pancreatic pain.

References

1. Bradley EL 3rd: A clinically based classification system for acute pancreatitis. Arch Surg 128:586, 1993
2. DiMagno EP, Chari S: Acute pancreatitis. Sleisinger and Fordtran's Gastrointestinal and Liver Disease: Pathophysiology, Diagnosis, Management, 7th ed. Feldman M, Friedman LS, Sleisenger MH, Eds. WB Saunders Co, Philadelphia, 2002, p 913
3. Go VLW, Everhart JE: Pancreatitis. Digestive Diseases in the United States: Epidemiology and Impact. Everhart JE, Ed. (NIH Publication No. 94-1447.) U.S. Dept of Health and Human Services, Public Health Service, National Institutes of Health, Washington, DC, 1994, p 693
4. DeFrances CJ, Hall MJ, Podgornik MN: 2003 National Hospital Discharge Survey. Advance data from vital and health statistics (No. 359). National Center for Health Statistics, Hyattsville, Maryland, 2005 http://www.cdc.gov/nchs/data/ad/ad359.pdf
5. Lowenfels AB, Sullivan T, Fioranti J, et al: The epidemiology and impact of pancreatic diseases in the United States. Curr Gastroenterol Rep 7:90, 2005
6. Lindkvist B, Appelros S, Manjer J, et al: Trends in incidence of acute pancreatitis in a Swedish population: is there really an increase? Clin Gastroenterol Hepatol 2:83, 2004
7. Overweight and Obesity: Obesity Trends: U.S. Obesity Trends 1985–2004 (Online). Centers for Disease Control and Prevention, Atlanta, 2005 http://www.cdc.gov/nccdphp/dnpa/obesity/trend/maps/index.htm
8. Grendell JH: Clinical and economic impact of acute pancreatitis in the United States (abstr). Pancreas 19:422, 1999
9. Mann DV, Hershman MJ, Hittinger R, et al: Multicentre audit of death from acute pancreatitis. Br J Surg 81:890, 1994
10. Talamini G, Bassi C, Falconi M, et al: Risk of death from acute pancreatitis: role of early simple "routine" data. Int J Pancreatol 19:15, 1996
11. Tsai CJ, Leitzmann MF, Willett WC, et al: Prospective study of abdominal adiposity and gallstone disease in U.S. men. Am J Clin Nutr 80:38, 2004
12. Hanck C, Whitcomb DC: Alcoholic pancreatitis. Gastroenterol Clin North Am 33:751, 2004
13. Klein SD, Affronti JP: Pancreas divisum, an evidence-based review: part I, pathophysiology. Gastrointest Endosc 60:419, 2004
14. Klein SD, Affronti JP: Pancreas divisum, an evidence-based review: part II, patient selection and treatment. Gastrointest Endosc 60:585, 2004
15. Lans JI, Geenen JE, Johanson JF, et al: Endoscopic therapy in patients with pancreas divisum and acute pancreatitis: a prospective, randomized, controlled clinical trial. Gastrointest Endosc 38:430, 1992
16. Lankisch PG, Droege M, Gottesleben F: Drug-induced acute pancreatitis: incidence and severity. Gut 37:565, 1995
17. Trivedi CD, Pitchumoni CS: Drug-induced pancreatitis: an update. J Clin Gastroenterol 239:709, 2005
18. Reisler RB, Murphy RL, Redfield RR, et al: Incidence of pancreatitis in HIV-1-infected individuals enrolled in 20 adult AIDS clinical trials group studies: lessons learned. J Acquir Immune Defic Syndr 39:159, 2005
19. Yadav D, Pitchumoni CS: Issues in hyperlipidemic pancreatitis. J Clin Gastroenterol 36:54, 2005
20. Glueck CJ, Lang J, Hamer T, et al: Severe hypertriglyceridemia and pancreatitis when estrogen replacement therapy is given to hypertriglyceridemic women. J Lab Clin Med 123:59, 1994
21. Freeman ML, DiSario JA, Nelson DB, et al: Risk factors for post-ERCP pancreatitis: a prospective, multicenter study. Gastrointest Endosc 54:425, 2001
22. Etemad B, Whitcomb DC: Chronic pancreatitis: diagnosis, classification, and new genetic developments. Gastroenterology 120:682, 2001
23. Hamano H, Kawa S, Horiuchi A, et al: High serum IgG4 concentrations in patients with sclerosing pancreatitis. N Engl J Med 344:732, 2001
24. Lara LP, Chari ST: Autoimmune pancreatitis. Curr Gastroenterol Rep 7:101, 2005
25. Ros E, Navarro S, Bru C, et al: Occult microlithiasis in "idiopathic" acute pancreatitis: prevention of relapses by cholecystectomy or ursodeoxycholic acid therapy. Gastroenterology 101:1701, 1991
26. Lee SP, Nichols JF, Park HZ: Biliary sludge as a cause of acute pancreatitis. N Engl J Med 326:589, 1992
27. Bhatia M, Wong FL, Cao Y, et al: Pathophysiology of acute pancreatitis. Pancreatology 5:132, 2005
28. Halangk W, Lerch MM: Early events in acute pancreatitis. Gastroenterol Clin North Am 33:717, 2004
29. Norman J: The role of cytokines in the pathogenesis of acute pancreatitis. Am J Surg 175:76, 1998
30. Raraty MG, Connor S, Criddle DN, et al: Acute pancreatitis and organ failure: pathophysiology, natural history, and management strategies. Curr Gastroenterol Rep 6:99, 2004
31. Al-Bahrani AZ, Ammori BJ: Clinical laboratory assessment of acute pancreatitis. Clin Chim Acta 362:26, 2005 [Epub July 18, 2005]
32. Lankisch PG, Schirren CA, Kunze E: Undetected fatal pancreatitis. Why is the disease so frequently overlooked? Am J Gastroenterol 86:322, 1991
33. Baillargeon JD, Orav J, Ramagopal V, et al: Hemoconcentration as an early risk factor for necrotizing pancreatitis. Am J Gastroenterol 93:2130, 1998
34. Tenner S, Dubner H, Steinberg W: Predicting gallstone pancreatitis with laboratory parameters: a meta-analysis. Am J Gastroenterol 89:1863, 1994
35. Balthazar EJ, Freeny PC, vanSonnenberg E: Imaging and intervention in acute pancreatitis. Radiology 193:297, 1994
36. Balthazar EJ: Staging of acute pancreatitis. Radiol Clin North Am 40:1129, 2002
37. Balthazar EJ: Complications of acute pancreatitis: clinical and CT evaluation. Radiol Clin North Am 40:1211, 2002
38. Arvanitakis M, Delhaye M, DeMaertelaere V, et al: Computed tomography and magnetic resonance imaging in the assessment of acute pancreatitis. Gastroenterology 126:715, 2004
39. Halla AH, Amortegui JD, Jeroukhimov IM, et al: Magnetic resonance cholangiopancreatography accurately detects common bile duct stones in resolving gallstone pancreatitis. J Am Coll Surg 200:869, 2005
40. Banks PA: Practice guidelines in acute pancreatitis. Am J Gastroenterol 92:377, 1997
41. Papachristou GI, Whitcomb DC: Predictors of severity and necrosis in acute pancreatitis. Gastroenterol Clin North Am 33:871, 2004
42. Baron TH, Morgan DE: Acute necrotizing pancreatitis. N Engl J Med 340:1412, 1999
43. Tenner S, Sica G, Hughes M, et al: Relationship of necrosis to organ failure in severe acute pancreatitis. Gastroenterology 113:899, 1997
44. Tenner S: Initial management of acute pancreatitis: critical issues during the first 72 hours. Am J Gastroenterol 99:2489, 2004
45. McClave SA, Dryden GW: Issues of nutritional support for the patient with acute pancreatitis. Semin Gastrointest Dis 13:154, 2002
46. Kaushik N, O'Keefe SJ: Nutritional support in acute pancreatitis. Curr Gastroenterol Rep 6:320, 2004
47. Al-Omran M, Groof A, Wilke D: Enteral versus parenteral nutrition for acute pancreatitis. Cochrane Database Syst Rev (1):CD002837, 2003
48. Andriulli A, Leandro G, Clemente R, et al: Meta-analysis of somatostatin, octreotide, and gabexate mesilate in the therapy of acute pancreatitis. Aliment Pharmacol Ther 12:237, 1998

49. Steinberg WM, Schlesselman SE: Treatment of acute pancreatitis: comparison of animal and human studies. Gastroenterology 93:1420, 1987

50. Andriulli A, Caruso N, Quitadamo M, et al: Antisecretory vs. antiproteasic drugs in the prevention of post-ERCP pancreatitis: the evidence-based medicine derived from a meta-analysis study. JOP 4:41, 2003

51. Antrulli A, Leandro G, Niro G, et al: Pharmacologic treatment can prevent pancreatic injury after ERCP: a meta-analysis. Gastrointest Endosc 55:100, 2000

52. Johnson CD, Kingsnorth AN, Imrie CE, et al: A double blind, randomized, placebo controlled study of a platelet activating factor antagonist lexipafant in the treatment and prevention of organ failure in predicted severe acute pancreatitis. Gut 48:62, 2001

53. Neoptolemos JP, Ogunbiyi O, Wilson PG, et al: Etiology, pathogenesis, natural history and treatment of biliary acute pancreatitis. The Pancreas. Warshaw AL, Buchler MW, Carr-Locke DL, et al, Eds. Blackwell Science, Malden, Massachusetts, 1998, p 521

54. Neoptolemos JP, London NJ, James D, et al: Controlled trial of urgent endoscopic retrograde cholangiopancreatography and endoscopic sphincterotomy versus conservative management for acute pancreatitis due to gallstones. Lancet 2:979, 1988

55. Fan ST, Lai ECS, Mok FPT, et al: Early treatment of acute biliary pancreatitis by endoscopic papillotomy. N Engl J Med 328:228, 1993

56. Folsch UR, Nitsche R, Ludtke R, et al: Early ERCP and papillotomy compared with conservative management for acute biliary pancreatitis. German Study Group on Acute Biliary Pancreatitis. N Engl J Med 336:237, 1997

57. Forsmark CE, Grendell JH: Complications of pancreatitis. Semin Gastrointest Dis l2:165, 1991

58. Forsmark CE, Wilcox CM, Grendell JH: Endoscopy-negative upper gastrointestinal hemorrhage in a patient with chronic pancreatitis. Gastroenterology 102:320, 1992

59. Gerzof SG, Banks PA, Robbins AH, et al: Early diagnosis of pancreatic infection by computed tomography–guided aspiration. Gastroenterology 93:1315, 1987

60. Beger HG, Bittner R, Block S, et al: Bacterial contamination of pancreatic necrosis: a prospective clinical study. Gastroenterology; 91:433, 1986

61. Kendrick ML, Sarr MG: Pancreatic necrosis and infections in patients with acute pancreatitis. Pancreatitis and Its Complications. Forsmark CE, Ed. Humana Press, Totowa, New Jersey, 2004, p 99

62. Baron TH, Harewood GC, Morgan DG: Outcome differences after endoscopic drainage of pancreatic necrosis, acute pancreatic pseudocysts, and chronic pancreatic pseudocysts. Gastrointest Endosc 56:150, 2002

63. Pederzoli P, Bassi S, Vesenti S, et al: A randomized multicenter clinical trial of antibiotic prophylaxis of septic complications in acute necrotizing pancreatitis with imipenem. Surg Gynecol Obstet 176:480, 1993

64. Nordback I, Sand J, Saaristo R, et al: Early treatment with antibiotics reduces the need for surgery in acute necrotizing pancreatitis—a single-center randomized study. J Gastrointest Surg 5:113, 2001

65. Sainio V, Kemppainen E, Puolakkainen P, et al: Early antibiotic treatment in acute necrotizing pancreatitis. Lancet 346:663, 1995

66. Schwarz M, Isenmann R, Meyer H, et al: Antibiotic use in necrotizing pancreatitis: results of a controlled study. Dtsch Med Wochenschr 122:356, 1997

67. Isenmann R, Runzi M, Kron M, et al: Prophylactic antibiotic treatment in patients with predicted severe acute pancreatitis: a placebo-controlled, double-blind trial. Gastroenterology 126:997, 2004

68. Bassi C, Larvin M, Villatoro E: Antibiotic therapy for prophylaxis against infection of pancreatic necrosis in acute pancreatitis. Cochrane Database Syst Rev (4):CD002941, 2003
http://www.cochrane.org/reviews/en/ab002941.html

69. Baillie J: Pancreatic pseudocysts (part I). Gastrointest Endosc 59:873, 2004

70. Baillie J: Pancreatic pseudocysts (part II). Gastrointest Endosc 60:105, 2004

71. Giovannini M: Endoscopic ultrasound-guided pancreatic pseudocyst drainage. Gastrointest Endosc Clin N Am 15:179, 2005

72. Sarles H, Adler G, Dani R, et al: Classifications of pancreatitis and definition of pancreatic diseases. Digestion 43:234, 1989

73. Forsmark CE: Chronic pancreatitis. Gastrointestinal and Liver Disease. Pathophysiology, Diagnosis, Management, 7th ed. Feldman M, Friedman LS, Sleisenger MH, Eds. WB Saunders Co, Philadelphia, 2002, p 940

74. Lowenfels AB, Maisonneuve P, Cavallini G, et al: Prognosis of chronic pancreatitis: an international multicenter study. Am J Gastroenterol 89:1467, 1994

75. Schneider A: Serine protease inhibitor Kazal type 1 mutations and pancreatitis. Gasteroenterol Clin North Am 33:789, 2004

76. Howes N, Greenhalf W, Stocken DD, et al: Cationic trypsinogen mutations and pancreatitis. Gastroenterol Clin North Am 33:767, 2004

77. Lowenfels AB, Maisonneuve P, Whitcomb DC: Risk factors for cancer in hereditary pancreatitis. International Hereditary Pancreatitis Study Group. Med Clin North Am 84:565, 2000

78. Cohn JA, Mitchell RM, Jowell PS: The role of cystic fibrosis gene mutations in determining susceptibility to chronic pancreatitis. Gastroenterol Clin North Am 33:817, 2004

79. Layer P, Yamamoto H, Kalthoff L, et al: The different courses of early- and late-onset idiopathic and alcoholic chronic pancreatitis. Gastroenterology 107:1481, 1994

80. Stevens T, Conwell DL, Zuccaro G: Pathogenesis of chronic pancreatitis: an evidence-based review of past theories and recent developments. Am J Gastroenterol 99:2256, 2004

81. Whitcomb DC: Genetic predisposition to alcoholic chronic pancreatitis. Pancreas 27:321, 2003

82. Chowdhury RS, Forsmark CE: Pancreatic function testing. Aliment Pharmacol Ther 17:733, 2003

83. Jacobsen DG, Currington C, Connery K, et al: Trypsin-like immunoreactivity as a test for pancreatic insufficiency. N Engl J Med 310:1307, 1984

84. DiMagno EP, Go VLW, Summerskill WHJ: Relations between pancreatic enzyme outputs and malabsorption in severe pancreatic insufficiency. N Engl J Med 288:813, 1973

85. Lankisch PG: Now that fecal elastase is available in the United States, should clinicians start using it? Curr Gastroenterol Rep 6:126, 2004

86. Forsmark CE, Toskes PP: What does an abnormal pancreatogram mean? Gastrointest Endosc Clin N Am 5:105, 1995

87. Draganov P, Patel A, Fazel A, et al: Prospective evaluation of the accuracy of the intraductal secretin test in the diagnosis of chronic pancreatitis. Clin Gastroenterol Hepatol 3:695, 2005

88. Conwell DL, Zuccaro G Jr, Vargo JJ, et al: An endoscopic pancreatic function test with synthetic porcine secretin for the evaluation of chronic abdominal pain and suspected chronic pancreatitis. Gastrointest Endosc 57:37, 2003

89. Kwon RS, Brugge WR: New advances in pancreatic imaging. Curr Opin Gastroenterol 21:561, 2005

90. Del Frate C, Zanardi R, Mortele K, et al: Advances in imaging for pancreatic disease. Curr Gastroenterol Rep 4:140, 2002

91. Ball MA, Sztantics A, Metens T, et al: Quantification of pancreatic exocrine function with secretin-enhanced magnetic resonance cholangiopancreatography: normal values and short-term effects of pancreatic duct drainage procedures in chronic pancreatitis: initial results. Eur Radiol l15:2110, 2005

92. Wallace MB, Hawes RH: Endoscopic ultrasound in the diagnosis and treatment of chronic pancreatitis. Pancreas 23:26, 2001

93. Forsmark CE: The diagnosis of chronic pancreatitis. Gastrointest Endosc 52:293, 2000

94. Brown A, Hughes M, Tenner S, et al: Does pancreatic enzyme supplementation reduce pain in patients with chronic pancreatitis: a meta-analysis. Am J Gastroenterol 92:2032, 1997

95. Warshaw AL, Banks PA, Fernandez-Del Castillo C: AGA technical review: treatment of pain in chronic pancreatitis. Gastroenterology 115:763, 1998

96. Gress F, Schmidt C, Sherman S, et al: A prospective randomized comparison of endoscopic ultrasound– and computed tomography–guided celiac plexus block for managing chronic pancreatitis pain. Am J Gastroenterol 94:900, 1999

97. Bradley EL 3rd, Bem J: Nerve blocks and neuroablative surgery for chronic pancreatitis. World J Surg 27:1241, 2003

98. Delhaye M, Arvanitakis M, Verset G, et al: Long-term clinical outcome after endoscopic pancreatic ductal drainage for patients with painful chronic pancreatitis. Clin Gastroenterol Hepatol 2:1096, 2004

99. Rösch T, Daniel S, Scholz M, et al: Endoscopic treatment of chronic pancreatitis: a multicenter study of 1,000 patients with long-term follow-up. Endoscopy 34:765, 2002

100. Dite P, Ruzicka M, Zboril V, et al: A prospective, randomized trial comparing endoscopic with surgical therapy for chronic pancreatitis. Endoscopy 35:553, 2003

101. Sakorafas GH, Farnell MB, Farley DR, et al: Long-term results after surgery for chronic pancreatitis. Int J Pancreatol 27:131, 2000

102. Pongprasobchai S, DiMango EP: Treatment of exocrine pancreatic insufficiency. Pancreatitis and Its Complications. Forsmark CD, Ed. Humana Press, Totowa, New Jersey, 2004, p 295

103. Levitt NS, Adams G, Salmon J, et al: The prevalence and severity of microvascular complications in pancreatic diabetes and IDDM. Diabetes Care 18:971, 1995

104. Linde J, Nilsson LH, Barany FR: Diabetes and hypoglycemia in chronic pancreatitis. Scand J Gastroenterol 12:369, 1977

105. Giovannini M, Pesenti C, Rolland AL, et al: Endoscopic ultrasound-guided drainage of pancreatic pseudocysts or pancreatic abscesses using a therapeutic echo endoscope. Endoscopy 33:473, 2001

106. Rockey DC, Cello JP: Pancreaticopleural fistula: report of 7 cases and a review of the literature. Medicine (Baltimore) 69:332, 1990

107. Mishra G, Forsmark CE: Cystic neoplasms of the pancreas. Curr Treat Options Gastroenterol 3:355, 2000

108. Levy MJ, Clain JE: Evaluation and management of cystic pancreatic tumors: emphasis on the role of EUS FNA. Clin Gastroenterol Hepatol 2:639, 2004

109. Fernandez-del Castillo C, Warshaw AL: Cystic neoplasms of the pancreas. Pancreatology 1:641, 2001

110. Lowenfels AB, Maisonneuve P, Cavallini G, et al: Pancreatitis and the risk of pancreatic cancer. N Engl J Med 328:1433, 1993

74 Liver and Pancreas Transplantation

Robert L. Carithers, Jr., M.D., F.A.C.P, and James D. Perkins, M.D.

Liver Transplantation

More than 6,000 liver transplantations are performed annually in the United States.[1] Enhancements in patient selection, surgical technique, and the availability of powerful immunosuppressive agents have resulted in steady improvement in patient survival. As a result, liver transplantation has been accepted as the standard of care for patients with severe acute or chronic liver disease in whom conventional modalities of therapy have failed. The major obstacle to the procedure is the critical shortage of donor organs.

CANDIDATES FOR TRANSPLANTATION

Any patient with acute or chronic liver failure is a potential candidate for liver transplantation; there are a number of common indications [see Table 1].[2] The three most important questions addressed during the evaluation of candidates for liver transplantation are the following:

1. Can the patient survive the operation and perioperative hospitalization?
2. Can the patient comply with long-term immunosuppressive therapy?
3. Does the patient have other medical conditions that would severely compromise long-term survival?

The methods of evaluating candidates for transplantation include careful history and physical examination; cardiopulmonary testing, including echocardiography, dobutamine stress testing, pulmonary function testing, and cardiac catheterization; measurement of creatinine clearance; abdominal imaging studies to evaluate portal vein patency and to detect hepatocellular carcinoma; and a thorough evaluation of social factors and support.[2] Echocardiography is useful in assessing left ventricular function and detecting pulmonary hypertension, which is seen in as many as 5% of cirrhotic patients.[3] Color flow Doppler studies of the portal vein are used to gauge the integrity of portal vein flow. If extensive portal vein thrombosis is detected, the transplant surgeon can obtain extra donor vessels to bypass the blockade if necessary. Computed tomographic angiography permits detection of small hepatocellular carcinomas and aberrant arterial blood supply to the liver. Rigorous evaluation of the patient for any addictive behavior and assessment of the patient's social support system allow the transplant team to plan in advance for any needed services, which may include counseling, specialized addiction treatment, housing, transportation, and financial assistance for medications and other expenses.

CONTRAINDICATIONS TO TRANSPLANTATION

Patients with severe neurologic or cardiopulmonary disease cannot withstand the stress of transplantation surgery. Patients with cirrhosis who have severe pulmonary hypertension rarely survive the operation and perioperative period.[4] Other contraindications to transplantation include severe or morbid obesity, extrahepatic malignancies, systemic infection, and cholan-giocarcinoma.[5] The most common surgical contraindication to liver transplantation is thrombosis of the portal vein and other splanchnic veins to such an extent that viable portal blood flow cannot be achieved.[6] Finally, the most frequent contraindications to liver transplantation are ongoing destructive behavior resulting from drug or alcohol addiction and the inability of the patient to comply with the complex medical regimen required after the operation.

TIMING OF TRANSPLANTATION

Determining the optimal time to refer patients for evaluation and to perform the operation can be as important to the outcome as patient selection. A few simple clinical approaches have proved useful in determining the prognosis of patients with liver disease. These include use of the Child-Turcotte-Pugh (CTP) classification [see Table 2]; use of the Model for End-Stage Liver Disease (MELD) for predicting survival in patients with liver disease; determination of the degree of ascites; and identification of other complications of cirrhosis.[7,8]

MELD, which employs a scoring system based on the serum bilirubin level, the serum creatinine level, and the international normalized ratio (INR) for prothrombin time, is now used for the allocation of donor organs in patients on liver transplantation waiting lists in the United States.[9,10] MELD scores range from 6 to 40, with higher scores representing sicker patients, who are granted earlier access to donor organs.[11] The United Network for Organ Sharing provides on their Web site a resource for calculating MELD scores for individual patients.[12] The MELD score can accurately predict 3-month mortality of patients with chronic liver disease who are on the liver waiting list [see Figure 1].[11] The MELD score also is an accurate predictor of survival after liver transplantation.[13] By comparing pretransplantation and posttransplantation outcomes, it has been shown that for patients who undergo liver

---

Table 1 Common Indications for Liver Transplantation

Chronic hepatitis
  Hepatitis C
  Hepatitis B
  Autoimmune hepatitis
Cholestatic liver disease
  Biliary atresia (in children)
  Primary biliary cirrhosis
  Sclerosing cholangitis
Metabolic diseases
  Wilson disease
  α_1-Antitrypsin deficiency
  Hemochromatosis
Malignancy
  Primary hepatocellular carcinoma

Hemangioendothelioma
Alcoholic liver disease
Cryptogenic cirrhosis
Miscellaneous conditions
  Hepatic veno-occlusive disease
  Nonalcoholic steatohepatitis
  Tyrosinemia
  Crigler-Najjar syndrome
Fulminant hepatic failure
  Hepatitis B
  Hepatitis A
  Acetaminophen overdose
  Other drug-induced hepatitis
  Toxin-induced hepatitis
  Other viral hepatitides

Table 2 Child-Turcotte-Pugh (CTP) Classification*

	Score		
	1	2	3
Encephalopathy (grade)	None	1–2	3–4
Ascites	Absent	Slight	Moderate
Bilirubin (mg/dl)	1–2	2–3	> 3
Albumin (g/dl)	> 3.5	2.8–3.5	< 2.8
Prothrombin time (seconds prolonged)	1–4	4–6	> 6

*Minimum CTP score, 5 points; maximum CTP score, 15 points. CTP class A: 5 to 6 points. CTP class B: 7 to 9 points. CTP class C: 10 to 15 points.

transplantation for chronic liver failure, survival is improved only in those with MELD scores greater than 15 at the time of the operation.[14]

The MELD score, CTP classification, and assessment of the complications of cirrhosis are the most useful tools for determining the optimal referral of patients to transplant centers.[8] It is recommended that patients who show evidence of hepatic dysfunction (i.e., a MELD score of 10 or higher and a CTP score of 7 or higher) or who experience their first major complication (e.g., ascites or hepatic encephelopathy) should be referred to centers for potential transplantation.[2] Development of other, more ominous complications of cirrhosis (e.g., hepatocellular carcinoma, spontaneous bacterial peritonitis, and hepatorenal syndrome) indicate the need for immediate referral of patients to a transplant center.

OPERATIVE PROCEDURES

Most liver transplantations are performed using a whole cadaveric liver placed in the orthotopic position. To increase the overall organ supply and especially to aid young children, for whom there is a perennial shortage of donor organs, a cadaveric liver can be divided into parts for more than one recipient [*see Figure 2*]. The same techniques can be used with living donors, with only part of the liver being removed for transplantation. Living related donor transplantation for children is a well-established procedure.[15] Living related donor transplantation for adults is also being performed at many transplantation centers, although donor safety remains a major concern.[16,17]

Liver transplantation is a complex, time-consuming operation that requires vascular reconstruction of the hepatic venous drainage to the inferior vena cava, to the hepatic artery, and to the portal vein. The hepatic vein of the donor organ is anastomosed to the inferior vena cava of the recipient; the donor hepatic artery is anastomosed to the recipient hepatic artery; and the portal vein is reconstructed by a vein graft or patch. Biliary reconstruction is usually accomplished by use of an end-to-end anastomosis of the proximal donor bile duct attached to the distal recipient duct; however, in recipients with diseased ducts, the donor duct is usually anastomosed to the jejunum by way of a Roux-en-Y loop.

A number of complications can be anticipated after liver transplantation, including perioperative and surgical complications, immunologic and infectious disorders, and a variety of medical complications.

COMPLICATIONS OF TRANSPLANTATION

Perioperative and Surgical Complications

The most serious immediate complication seen after liver transplantation is nonfunction of the transplanted liver, which occurs in 5% to 10% of cases. In these cases, patients fail to recover neurologic function; coagulopathy fails to improve spontaneously; and there is progressive jaundice and acidosis. Emergent retransplantation is the only recourse for these patients.

Other important surgical complications encountered after liver transplantation include hepatic artery thrombosis, portal vein thrombosis, and biliary tract complications (e.g., bile leaks and obstruction). Biliary tract complications are the most common; fortunately, most can be managed effectively with endoscopic techniques.[18] Hepatic artery thrombosis is a much more serious complication that can result in the need for retransplantation. A variety of surgical and nonsurgical factors are associated with an increased risk of hepatic artery thrombosis. Included among the nonsurgical factors are immunologic status, hypercoagulable states, tobacco use, and cytomegalovirus infection.[19]

Immunologic Complications (Graft Rejection)

Two types of allograft rejection are seen after liver transplantation: cellular and ductopenic. Cellular rejection, which is usually manifested by elevated aminotransferase levels, is most commonly seen 6 to 10 weeks after transplantation. The diagnosis is confirmed by liver biopsy, which reveals cellular invasion of small bile ducts and vascular endothelium. Most patients respond rapidly to increased immunosuppression. Ductopenic rejection is a more indolent process that usually presents as progressive jaundice months to years after transplantation. Liver biopsies reveal gradual disappearance of intrahepatic bile ducts. Most patients with this condition ultimately require retransplantation.

Infectious Complications

Infections remain among the most serious complications encountered after liver transplantation. Many potential pathogens (e.g., *Pneumocystis jiroveci* and cytomegalovirus) can usually be prevented with aggressive prophylaxis. In the early postoperative period, the most common pathogens are fungal and nosocomial bacterial infections. Candidiasis and aspergillosis, which remain the most serious infections encountered after liver transplantation, often occur in malnourished, critically ill patients.[20] During the first few months after surgery, cytomegalovirus in-

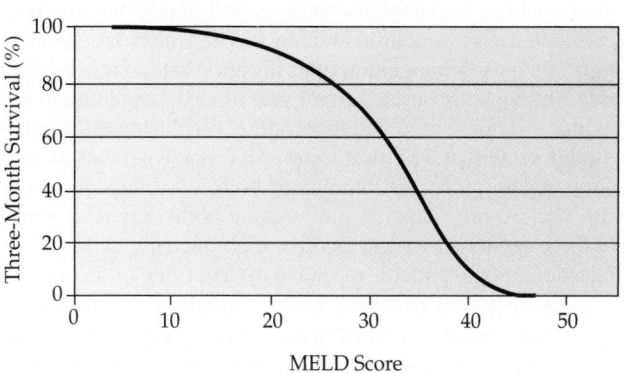

Figure 1 **Estimated 3-month survival as a function of the MELD score.[11]**

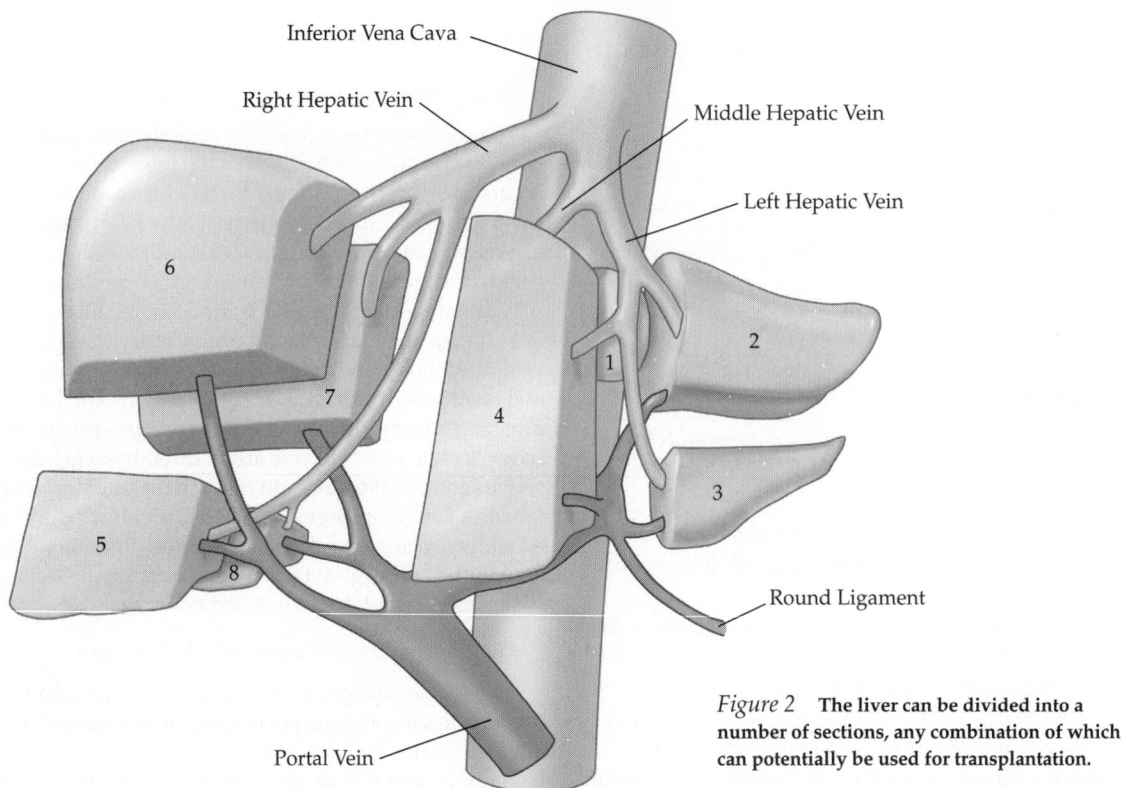

Inferior Vena Cava

Right Hepatic Vein

Middle Hepatic Vein

Left Hepatic Vein

Round Ligament

Portal Vein

Figure 2 **The liver can be divided into a number of sections, any combination of which can potentially be used for transplantation.**

fection and recurrent hepatitis B and C virus infections become much more prominent. Infection with antimicrobial-resistant bacteria, such as methicillin-resistant *Staphylococcus aureus* (MRSA) or vancomycin-resistant *Enterococcus faecium* (VREF), is associated with increased postoperative mortality.[21]

Complications of Immunosuppressive Therapy

A number of immunosuppressive agents are now available for use after solid-organ transplantation. These agents include cyclosporine, tacrolimus, azathioprine, mycophenolate mofetil, sirolimus, and corticosteroids, as well as various polyclonal or monoclonal antilymphocyte preparations.[22] Most liver transplant recipients receive either cyclosporine or tacrolimus in combination with one or more other immunosuppressive agents.

Complications from cyclosporine and tacrolimus Cyclosporine and tacrolimus are both associated with a number of complications, including renal dysfunction, neurologic toxicity, hypertension, pancreatic injury, and a variety of metabolic abnormalities. Renal failure occurs in 10% of patients who take cyclosporine or tacrolimus within 10 years after transplantation.[23] Patients with a glomerular filtration rate of less than 40 ml/min/kg body surface area 1 year after transplantation are at high risk for subsequent renal failure. Replacing calcineurin inhibitors with other immunosuppressive agents, such as mycophenolate mofetil, sirolimus, or both, may improve renal function in some patients, although monotherapy with either of these agents is associated with a slight increase in the risk of rejection.[24] Some patients receiving cyclosporine or tacrolimus experience severe neuropsychiatric complications, including psychosis, seizures, and apraxia.[25] Many patients who take these drugs complain of headaches, tremors, and severe musculoskeletal pains. Hypertension, which is quite common in patients who take either cyclosporine or tacrolimus, is thought

to result from peripheral and renal vasoconstriction.[26] Pancreatic damage with development of type 1 (insulin-dependent) diabetes mellitus is more common after the use of tacrolimus. Patients who take either drug can experience hyperkalemia, hyperuricemia, and elevated cholesterol and triglyceride levels.[27] Switching patients from cyclosporine to tacrolimus appears to reduce the severity of hyerlipidemias in some patients.[28,29] Treatment with low-dose cerivastatin or pravastatin also has been shown to significantly improve lipid profiles without adversely affecting liver function.[30] Cyclosporine, but not tacrolimus, is associated with gingival hyperplasia and excessive hair growth, particularly on the arms and face.

Complications from azathioprine, mycophenolate mofetil, and sirolimus Azathioprine and mycophenolate mofetil can cause bone marrow depression with leukopenia, thrombocytopenia, and anemia. A number of patients who take mycophenolate mofetil also experience gastrointestinal side effects, including nausea, abdominal pain, and diarrhea. Long-term corticosteroid therapy is associated with obesity, hypertension, glucose intolerance, cataracts, osteoporosis, and hypercholesterolemia. Side effects of sirolimus include gastrointestinal symptoms and marked elevations of serum lipids, particularly when sirolimus is used in combination with cyclosporine.[31]

Complications from drug-drug interactions Both cyclosporine and tacrolimus are extensively metabolized in the liver, primarily via the cytochrome P-450 IIIA enzyme. As a result, both drugs are prone to numerous drug-drug interactions.[22] The most dramatic examples include interactions with ketoconazole and phenytoin. Ketoconazole inhibits the P-450 IIIA enzyme and can result in marked increases in circulating levels of cyclosporine and tacrolimus. In contrast, phenytoin induces the enzyme, resulting in enhanced metabolism of cyclosporine and

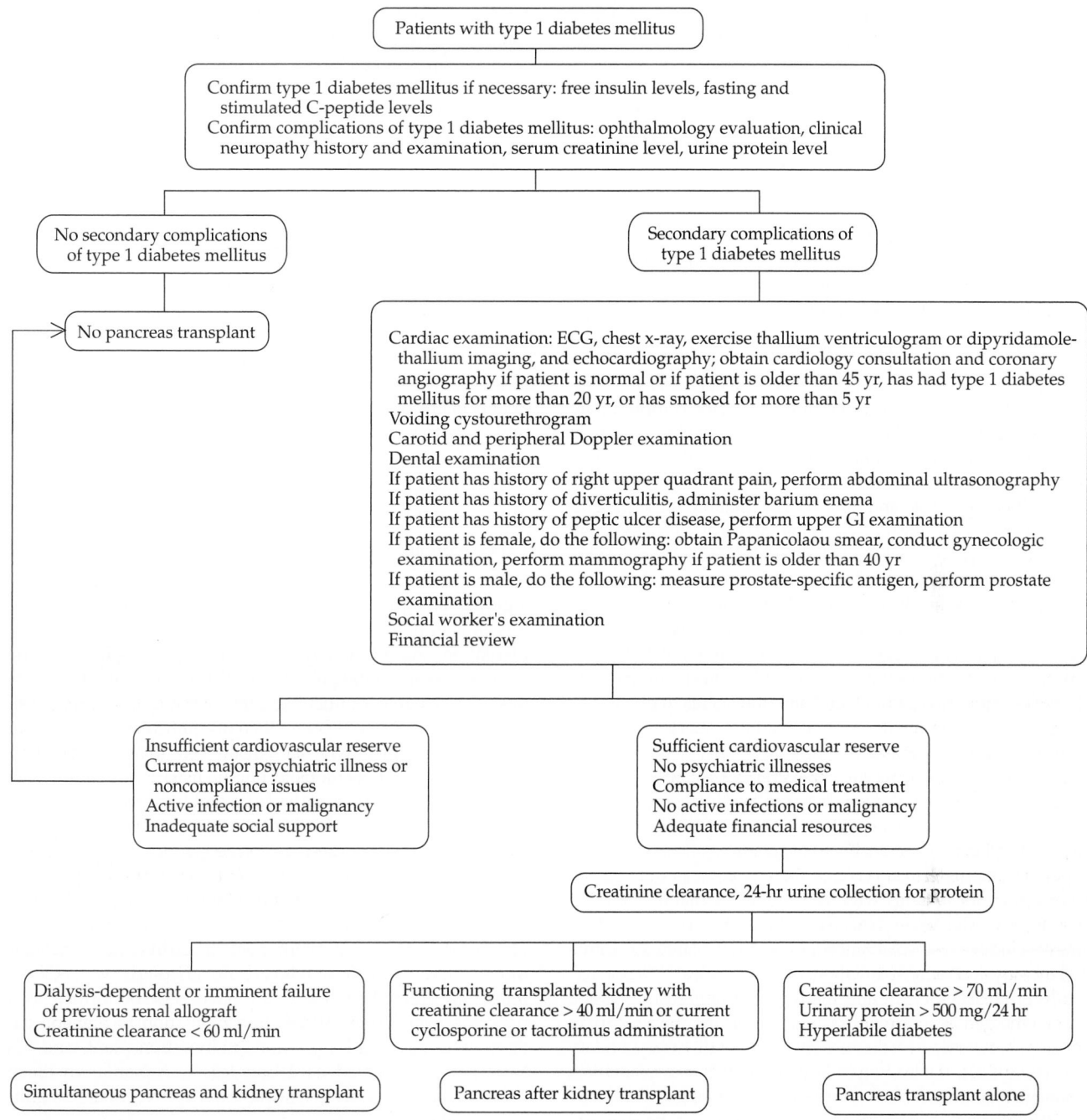

Figure 3 **Algorithm for evaluation of patients with type 1 (insulin-dependent) diabetes mellitus being considered for pancreas transplantation.**

tacrolimus and difficulty maintaining adequate circulating levels of both drugs. A number of other commonly used drugs have lesser but important effects on cyclosporine and tacrolimus metabolism. Awareness of these interactions is important in managing patients after transplantation.

Delayed complications from immunosuppressive drugs
Most of the delayed complications seen after liver transplantation are secondary to the long-term use of immunosuppressive drugs. The most common of these complications include renal dysfunction, hypertension, diabetes, hyperkalemia and hyperuricemia, hyperlipidemia, obesity, and malignancies.[32] Hyper-

tension can usually be effectively managed with a combination of calcium channel blockers and beta blockers.[33] Transient hyperkalemia can be managed effectively with sodium polystyrene sulfonate. If hyperkalemia is sustained, fludrocortisone can be used. Although many patients experience hyperuricemia after liver transplantation, very few experience gout. Treatment of gout is difficult because allopurinol can interfere with azathioprine metabolism, which can result in profound, life-threatening leukopenia, and because nonsteroidal anti-inflammatory drugs often worsen renal dysfunction. The necessity for treatment of hyperlipidemia after liver transplantation remains unclear. Obese patients who have undergone liver transplantation need a regular exercise program, limited caloric intake, and reduction or discontinuance of corticosteroids.[34] After age-related cardiovascular complications, malignancies are the leading cause of late death in liver transplant recipients. The most common tumors seen in these patients are lymphoproliferative disorders associated with chronic viral infections and skin cancers (e.g., squamous cell carcinoma and Kaposi sarcoma).[35] Many more recipients of liver transplantation are now receiving the bulk of their care from general internists, gastroenterologists, and primary care physicians. As a result, recognition of potential long-term complications and the need for appropriate immunizations and regular screening visits have become increasingly important.[36]

Disease-Specific Complications

Certain patients require specific management after liver transplantation because of potential disease-specific complications. For example, progressive liver disease can develop rapidly in patients with hepatitis B and can become fatal within a year after transplantation. However, if they are treated with aggressive antiviral therapy before and after transplantation, these patients have an excellent outcome, with minimal risk of severe recurrent disease.[37] Most potential transplant candidates now receive antiviral therapy with lamivudine, adefovir, or entecavir before the operation to reduce levels of circulating virus. Some patients with decompensated cirrhosis have such a dramatic response that transplantation can be postponed indefinitely.[38] After surgery, most patients now receive continuous treatment with hepatitis B immune globulin and antiviral agents to prevent recurrent disease.[39] There is concern about the emergence of viral mutations after long-term therapy with any of the antiviral agents; however, patients who have strains resistant to one form of therapy have been successfully treated with other agents.[40]

Patients with chronic hepatitis C virus infection who undergo liver transplantation invariably have persistent infection after the operation. Long-term survival of these patients is significantly worse than for patients who receive transplantation for other conditions.[41] The optimal management of these patients, which may include pretransplantation and posttransplantation antiviral therapy and retransplantation, remains unclear.[42] Donor age, early graft dysfunction, and the type of immunosuppression have emerged as important factors influencing the severity of postoperative disease.[43] Because chronic liver disease secondary to hepatitis C is the leading indication for liver transplantation, management of such cases is an issue of increasing importance.

Patients with genetic hemochromatosis also have a significantly worse outcome compared to patients who have undergone liver transplantation for other indications. This is particularly true for patients who are homozygous for the C282Y mutation or heterozygous for the C282Y and H63D mutations. Patients without genetic alterations who have hepatic iron overload at the time of transplantation also have poor outcomes.[44]

Patients with liver disease caused by sclerosing cholangitis often have associated inflammatory bowel disease. Although the transplant effectively addresses their liver disease, these patients remain at high risk for colon cancer. As a result, they require careful monitoring with colonoscopy and biopsies at least annually. If severe dysplasia is detected, these patients can be effectively treated with colectomy.

Liver transplantation has emerged as the optimal treatment for most patients with hepatocellular carcinoma (HCC). Excellent disease-free survival after transplantation is seen in patients who have (1) a single tumor no greater than 5 cm in diameter, or no more than three lesions, none of which are greater than 3 cm in diameter; (2) no radiographic evidence of vascular invasion; and (3) no evidence of metastases on head and chest CT scans and bone scans.[45] The issue of long waiting periods before transplantation has been addressed in the new MELD system for allocation of donor organs, which gives patients with HCC who are optimal candidates for transplantation elevated scores to facilitate early transplantation.[10]

OUTCOMES AFTER TRANSPLANTATION

Survival after liver transplantation has improved steadily over the past 10 years. Most centers now report 1-year survival rates of 85% to 90% and 5-year survival rates of 75% to 80%.[1,2] During the same interval, the costs have progressively decreased as the result of reduced hospitalization for most patients.[46] The quality of life for most patients after successful transplantation is quite good. Most patients have been able to return to work, and physically active recipients have returned to vigorous endeavors, including marathon running and mountain climbing.

Pancreas Transplantation

Pancreas transplantation, which aims at providing physiologic insulin replacement, is a therapy that reliably achieves euglycemia in patients with type 1 diabetes mellitus. Islet transplantation (engrafting only the insulin-producing B cells of the pancreas) is an exciting alternative that is still in its clinical infancy.[47-49] Two major difficulties prevent this technique from becoming widespread: (1) more than one pancreas is required to provide the recipient with enough islet cells to become euglycemic; and (2) the meticulous technique used for obtaining islet cells for transplantation varies from center to center.[50]

Since the first vascularized pancreas transplantation in 1966, more than 23,000 have been performed worldwide.[51,52] Approximately 78% of pancreas transplantations have been performed with simultaneous kidney transplantations from the same donors (i.e., simultaneous pancreas and kidney [SPK] transplantation), with the recipients being those in whom renal failure is imminent or those who are already on dialysis.[52] Of the remaining transplantations, 16% have been performed as a pancreas after kidney (PAK) transplantation in diabetic patients who have had a previous kidney transplant, and 7% have been performed as a pancreas transplantation alone (PTA) in diabetic patients who have not yet experienced significant renal failure.[52]

The goals of pancreas transplantation are to improve the quality of life for patients with type 1 diabetes mellitus, reverse the metabolic abnormalities caused by the disease, and prevent the secondary complications of the disease. Despite these lofty goals, postoperative complications and the need for long-term immunosuppression have rendered pancreas transplantation controversial except in a select subpopulation of patients.

CANDIDATES FOR TRANSPLANTATION

During evaluation, it is essential to confirm the diagnosis of type 1 diabetes mellitus, to confirm that secondary complications of diabetes are present, to determine the candidate's ability to undergo a major operation, and to rule out any contraindications to the operation.[53] The type of procedure to be performed is determined by the renal function status of the potential recipient [see Figure 3].

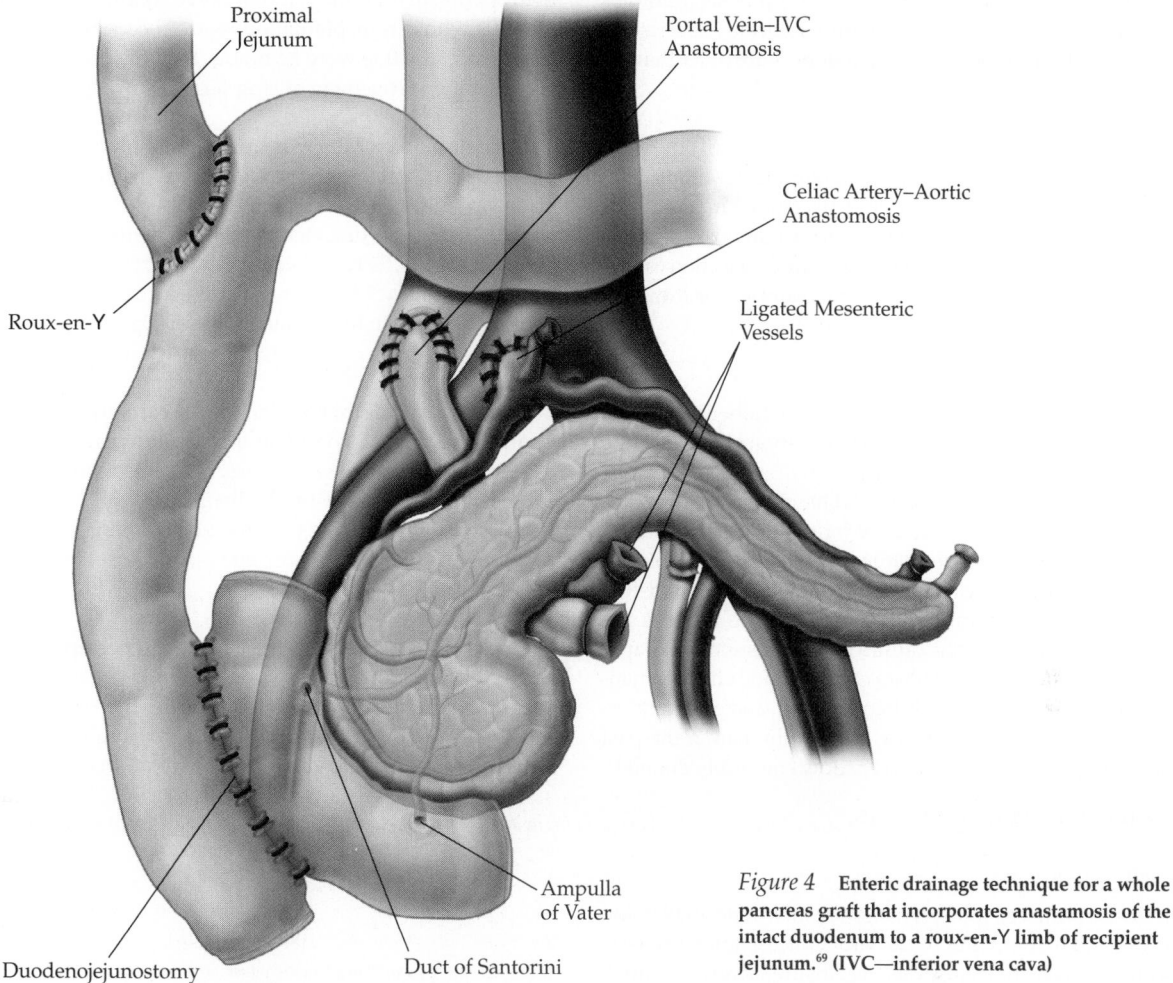

Proximal Jejunum

Portal Vein–IVC Anastomosis

Celiac Artery–Aortic Anastomosis

Roux-en-Y

Ligated Mesenteric Vessels

Duodenojejunostomy

Duct of Santorini

Ampulla of Vater

Figure 4 **Enteric drainage technique for a whole pancreas graft that incorporates anastamosis of the intact duodenum to a roux-en-Y limb of recipient jejunum.[69] (IVC—inferior vena cava)**

CONTRAINDICATIONS TO TRANSPLANTATION

Patients with insufficient cardiovascular reserve (e.g., those who recently had a myocardial infarction), patients with a left ventricular ejection fraction below 50%, or patients with coronary angiographic evidence of significant uncorrectable coronary artery disease should not undergo pancreas transplantation[53] [*see Figure 3*]. Unnecessary loss of pancreas grafts is avoided by excluding patients with current major psychiatric illness or evidence of significant noncompliance. In addition, transplantation should not be considered in patients with an active infection or malignancy.

Other contraindications are controversial and depend on the individual transplantation center. Extremity amputations necessitated by vascular disease usually indicate severe generalized vasculopathy and suggest a condition in which pancreas transplantation would not be beneficial. Patients whose weight is greater than 130% of their ideal body weight often have insulin resistance and, as a result, are not helped by transplantation.[53] Continued cigarette use often indicates poor compliance in patients who have already been strongly encouraged to stop smoking. Severe neurogenic bladder dysfunction usually predicts a complicated postoperative course and is considered a contraindication at some centers.

OPERATIVE PROCEDURES

Pancreas transplantation includes placement of the pancreas graft, usually in the right lower quadrant, with the reconstruct-

ed arteries of the pancreas anastomosed to the common iliac artery [*see Figure 4*].[54] To provide drainage for pancreatic exocrine excretions, the increasingly favored procedure is to anastomose the duodenum of the graft to the recipient's small bowel as opposed to the mobilized urinary bladder.[52,54,55] The venous drainage of the graft is achieved by anastomosing the portal vein either to the mobilized common iliac vein or to the portal vein.[54,55] In SPK transplantation, the kidney is placed in the left lower quadrant.

PERIOPERATIVE CARE

In the immediate postoperative period, specific care should be directed toward monitoring cardiovascular function.[54] Insulin infusions are generally given for a few days to rest the transplanted islets. Because many patients have some form of diabetic gastropathy, a nasogastric tube is required for 4 to 7 days postoperatively. A urinary catheter is required for an extended period to reduce the risk of complications from neurogenic bladder dysfunction.

COMPLICATIONS OF TRANSPLANTATION

Surgical Complications

Surgical complications of pancreas transplantation have recently been analyzed in a large, prospective, multicenter study.[56] Complications can occur within the first 3 postoperative months; such complications include the necessity of reoperation, arterial and venous graft vessel thrombosis, intra-abdominal hemorrhage, and enteric or ureteral leaks. The risk of these complications is increased when donors are older than 45 years of age.[56]

Immunologic Complications (Graft Rejection)

Rejection, which is the leading cause of graft loss after a successful pancreas transplantation, has decreased markedly in the past few years.[52] The gold standard for diagnosis of rejection is histopathologic evaluation of the graft.[57] Rejection can be confirmed histologically, because tissue samples of the graft can be obtained by percutaneous biopsies.[57]

Complications of Medical Therapy

With the increased use of enteric drainage rather than bladder drainage, the complications of dehydration and metabolic acidosis have decreased significantly.[55]

Tacrolimus and mycophenolate acid have become the mainstay of immunosuppressive therapy for pancreas transplantation. In addition, most pancreas transplant centers now use induction immunosuppressive therapy followed by steroid-free maintenance therapy[58]; this preventive measure reduces the risk of medical complications caused by corticosteroid therapy.

Graft pancreatitis, which is also a common side effect, is manifested by hyperamylasemia, abdominal pain, and graft tenderness. This complication occurs less frequently than in the past because most pancreas transplants are now enterically drained.

OUTCOMES AFTER TRANSPLANTATION

Metabolic Outcomes

Successful pancreas transplantation results in normalization of glucose and hemoglobin A_{1c} levels.[53] Glucose tolerance tests are normal or near normal; however, insulin levels are much higher than normal in recipients of pancreas transplantation. The systemic venous drainage of the graft causes elevated plasma levels of insulin, which is known to be a potent regulator of plasma lipoprotein metabolism. As a result, SPK transplantation recipients have a more favorable lipid profile than patients with type 1 diabetes mellitus who have kidney transplants.[59]

Effect on Disorders Associated with Type 1 Diabetes Mellitus

Diabetic nephropathy A transplanted pancreas can prevent or reduce the nephropathy that eventually develops in diabetic patients with a kidney graft. The presence of a transplanted pancreas can also reduce the risk of diabetic nephropathy in the kidneys of SPK transplant recipients.[60] The successful pancreas transplant alone can improve diabetic nephropathy, as evidenced by reduced proteinuria and unchanged creatinine levels and clearance rates at 1 year posttransplantation.[61]

Retinopathy Pancreas transplantation appears to have a stabilizing effect on retinopathy. In a recent study, pancreas transplantation was associated with improvement or stabilization of diabetic retinopathy in more than 90% of patients. Even in patients whose retinopathy was more advanced before they underwent surgery, the majority experienced no further progression after the transplantation.[62]

Neuropathy Reestablishment of the euglycemic state by successful pancreas transplantation halts or reverses diabetic neuropathy. In one study, motor nerve conduction increased in patients whose transplantations were successful.[63] Changes in autonomic function were favorable, but they did not amount to significant improvement at long-term follow-up.[63]

Vasculopathy Pancreas transplantation has at least a partial beneficial effect on the macroangiopathy of the carotid artery in patients with type 1 diabetes mellitus.[64] Also, compared with type 1 diabetes mellitus patients who receive kidney transplants, SPK recipients show improvement of diabetic microangiopathy.[62,65] The progression of coronary atherosclerosis in patients with functioning pancreas grafts is reduced.

Survival Outcomes

Patient survival exceeds 96% at 1 year and 90% at 3 years. Graft survival (i.e., complete insulin independence) exceeds 85% at 1 year and 75% at 3 years.[46] Patients who undergo SPK transplantation have a markedly improved 10-year survival, compared with diabetic patients who undergo kidney transplantation alone.[52,66,67]

Quality of Life

Quality of life in terms of general health perception, physical ability, and sexual activity is higher for SPK transplant recipients than for patients with type 1 diabetes mellitus who receive kidney transplants, and it is far higher for SPK transplant recipients than for patients who remain on hemodialysis.[68]

The authors have no commercial relationships with manufacturers of products or providers of services discussed in this chapter.

References

1. Scientific Registry of Transplant Recipients, accessed August, 2006 www.ustransplant.org

2. Murray KF, Carithers RL Jr: AASLD practice guidelines: evaluation of the patient for liver transplantation. Hepatology 41:1407, 2005

3. Colle IO, Moreau R, Godinho E, et al: Diagnosis of pulmonary hypertension in candidates for liver transplantation: a prospective study. Hepatology 37:401, 2003

4. Krowka MJ, Plevak DJ, Findlay JY, et al: Pulmonary hemodynamics and perioperative cardiopulmonary-related mortality in patients with portopulmonary hypertension undergoing liver transplantation. Liver Transpl 6:443, 2000

5. Nair S, Verma S, Thuluvath PJ: Obesity and its effect on survival in patients undergoing orthotopic liver transplantation in the United States. Hepatology 35:105, 2002

6. Manzanet G, Sanjuan F, Orbis P, et al: Liver transplantation in patients with portal vein thrombosis. Liver Transpl 7:125, 2001

7. Malinchoc M, Kamath PS, Gordon FD, et al: A model to predict poor survival in patients undergoing transjugular intrahepatic portosystemic shunts. Hepatology 31:864, 2000

8. Lucey MR, Brown KA, Everson GT, et al: Minimal criteria for placement of adults on the liver transplant waiting list: a report of a national conference organized by the American Society of Transplant Physicians and the American Association for the Study of Liver Diseases. Liver Transpl Surg 3:628, 1997

9. Kamath PS, Wiesner RH, Malinchoc M, et al: A model to predict survival in patients with end-stage liver disease. Hepatology 33:464, 2001

10. Wiesner RH, McDiarmid SV, Kamath PS, et al: MELD and PELD: application of survival models to liver allocation. Liver Transpl 7:567, 2001

11. Wiesner R, Edwards E, Freeman R, et al: Model for End-Stage Liver Disease (MELD) and allocation of donor livers. Gastroenterology 124:91, 2003

12. Merion RM: When is a patient too well and when is a patient too sick for a liver transplant? Liver Transpl 10(suppl 2):S69, 2004

13. Merion RM, Schaubel DE, Dykstra DM, et al: The survival benefit of liver transplantation. Am J Transplant 5:307, 2005

14. United Network for Organ Sharing (UNOS): Resources: MELD/PELD calculator. http://222.unos.org/resources/MeldPeldCalculator.asp

15. Otte JB, Ville-de-Goyet J, Reding R, et al: Pediatric liver transplantation: from the full-size liver graft to reduced, split, and living related liver transplantation. Pediatr Surg Int 13:308, 1998

16. Trotter JF, Wachs M, Everson GT, et al: Adult-to-adult transplantation of the right hepatic lobe from a living donor. N Engl J Med 346:1074, 2002

17. Surman OS: The ethics of partial-liver donation. N Engl J Med 346:1038, 2002

18. Moser MA, Wall WJ: Management of biliary problems after liver transplantation. Liver Transpl 7(suppl 1):S46, 2001

19. Pastacaldi S, Teixeira R, Montalto P, et al: Hepatic artery thrombosis after orthotopic liver transplantation: a review of nonsurgical causes. Liver Transpl 7:75, 2001

20. Rabkin JM, Oroloff SL, Corless CL, et al: Association of fungal infection and increased mortality in liver transplant recipients. Am J Surg 179:426, 2000

21. Singh N, Gayowski T, Rihs JD, et al: Evolving trends in multiple-antibiotic-resistant bacteria in liver transplant recipients: a longitudinal study of antimicrobial susceptibility patterns. Liver Transpl 7:22, 2001

22. Levy GA: Long-term immunosuppression and drug interactions. Liver Transpl 7(suppl 1):S53, 2001

23. Cohen AJ, Stegall MD, Rosen CB, et al: Chronic renal dysfunction late after liver transplantation. Liver Transpl 8:916, 2002

24. Schlitt HJ, Barkmann A, Boker KH, et al: Replacement of calcineurin inhibitors with mycophenolate mofetil in liver-transplant recipients with renal dysfunction: a randomized controlled study. Lancet 357:587, 2001

25. Beresford TP: Neuropsychiatric complications of liver and other solid organ transplantation. Liver Transpl 7(suppl 1):S36, 2001

26. Textor SC, Taler SJ, Canzanello VJ: Posttransplantation hypertension related to calcineurin inhibitors. Liver Transpl 6:521, 2000

27. Charco R, Cantarell C, Vargas V, et al: Serum cholesterol changes in long-term survivors of liver transplantation: a comparison between cyclosporine and tacrolimus therapy. Liver Transpl Surg 5:204, 1999

28. Manzarbeitia C, Reich DJ, Rothstein KD, et al: Tacrolimus conversion improves hyperlipidemic states in stable liver transplant recipients. Liver Transpl 7:93, 2001

29. Neal DA, Gimson AE, Gibbs P, et al: Beneficial effects of converting liver transplant recipients from cyclosporine to tacrolimus on blood pressure, serum lipids, and weight. Liver Transpl 7:533, 2001

30. Zachoval R, Gerbes AL, Schwandt P, et al: Short-term effects of statin therapy in patients with hyperlipoproteinemia after liver transplantation: results of a randomized cross-over trial. J Hepatol 35:86, 2001

31. Trotter JF, Wachs ME, Trouillot TE, et al: Dyslipidemia during sirolimus therapy in liver transplant recipients occurs with concomitant cyclosporine but not tacrolimus. Liver Transpl 7:401, 2001

32. Sheiner PA, Magliocca JF, Bodian CA, et al: Long-term medical complications in patients surviving > or = 5 years after liver transplant. Transplantation 69:781, 2000

33. Gonwa TA: Hypertension and renal dysfunction in long-term liver transplant recipients. Liver Transpl 7(suppl 1):S26, 2001

34. Reubin A: Long-term management of the liver transplant patient: diabetes, hyperlipidemia, and obesity. Liver Transpl 7(suppl 1):S13, 2001

35. Fung JJ, Jain A, Kwak EJ, et al: De novo malignancies after liver transplantation: a major late cause of late death. Liver Transpl 7(suppl 1):S109, 2001

36. McCashland TM: Posttransplantation care: role of the primary care physician versus transplant center. Liver Transpl 7(suppl 1):S2, 2001

37. Steinmuller T, Seehofer D, Rayes N, et al: Increasing applicability of liver transplantation for patients with hepatitis B-related liver disease. Hepatology 35:1528, 2002

38. Fontana RJ, Hann HW, Perrillo RP, et al: Determinants of early mortality in patients with decompensated chronic hepatitis B treated with antiviral therapy. Gastroenterology 123:719, 2002

39. Multimer D: Review article: hepatitis B and liver transplantation. Aliment Pharmacol Ther 23:1031, 2006

40. Schreibman IR, Schiff ER: Prevention and treatment of recurrent hepatitis B after liver transplantation: the current role of nucleoside and nucleotide analogues. Ann Clin Microbiol Antimicrob 5:8, 2006

41. Forman LM, Lewis JD, Berlin JA, et al: The association between hepatitis C infection and survival after orthotopic liver transplantation. Gastroenterology 122:889, 2002

42. Davis GL: The challenge of progressive hepatitis C following liver transplantation. Liver Transpl 12:19,2006

43. Lake JR, Shorr JS, Steffen BJ, et al: Differential effects of donor age in liver transplant recipients infected with hepatitis B, hepatitis C and without viral hepatitis. Am J Transplant 5:549, 2005

44. Kowley KV, Brandhagen DJ, Gish RG, et al: Survival after liver transplantation in patients with iron overload: the national hemochromatosis transplant registry. Gastroenterology 129:494, 2005

45. Bruix J, Llovet JM: Prognostic prediction and treatment strategy in hepatocellular carcinoma. Hepatology 35:519, 2002

46. Best JH, Veenstra DL, Geppert J: Trends in expenditures for Medicare liver transplant recipients. Liver Transpl 7:858, 2001

47. Worldwide Transplant Center Directory: Islet transplants. Clin Transpl, 2001, p 383

48. Ryan EA, Lakey JR, Paty BW, et al: Successful islet transplantation: continued insulin reserve provides long-term glycemic control. Diabetes 51:2148, 2002

49. Robertson RP: Islet transplantation as a treatment for diabetes: a work in progress. N Engl J Med 350:694, 2004

50. Hakim NS: Recent developments and future prospects in pancreatic transplantation. Exp Clin Transplant 1:26, 2003

51. Kelly WD, Lillehei RC, Merkel FK, et al: Allotransplantation of the pancreas and duodenum along with the kidney in diabetic nephropathy. Surgery 61:827, 1967

52. Gruessner AC, Sutherland DE: Pancreas transplant outcomes for United States (US) and non-US cases as reported to the United Network for Organ Sharing (UNOS) and the International Pancreas Transplant Registry (IPTR) as of June 2004. Clin Transplant 19:433, 2005

53. Robertson RP, Sutherland DE, Lanz KJ: Normoglycemia and preserved insulin secretory reserve in diabetic patients 10–18 years after pancreas transplantation. Diabetes 48:1737, 1999

54. Perkins JD, Fromme GA, Narr BJ, et al: Pancreas transplantation at Mayo: II. Operative and perioperative management. Mayo Clin Proc 65:483, 1990

55. Stratta RJ, Gaber AO, Shokouh-Amiri MH, et al: A prospective comparison of systemic-bladder versus portal-enteric drainage in vascularized pancreas transplantation. Surgery 127:217, 2000

56. Malaise J, Steurer W, Koenigsrainer A, et al: Simultaneous pancreas-kidney transplantation in a large multicenter study: surgical complications. Transplant Proc 37:2859, 2005

57. Laftavi MR, Gruessner AC, Bland BJ, et al: Significance of pancreas graft biopsy in detection of rejection. Transplant Proc 30:642, 1998

58. Kaufman DB, Leventhal JR, Gallon LG: Alemtuzumab induction and prednisone-free maintenance immunotherapy in simultaneous pancreas-kidney transplantation comparison with rabbit antithymocyte globulin induction: long-term results. Am J Transplant 6:331, 2006

59. Foger B, Konigsrainer A, Palos G, et al: Effect of pancreas transplantation on lipoprotein lipase, postprandial lipemia, and HDL cholesterol. Transplantation 58:899, 1994

60. Wilczek HE, Jaremko G, Tyden G, et al: Evolution of diabetic nephropathy in kidney grafts. Transplantation 59:51, 1995

61. Coppelli A, Giannarelli R, Vistoli F, et al: The beneficial effects of pancreas transplant alone on diabetic nephropathy. Diabetes Care 28:1366, 2005

62. Giannarelli R, Coppelli A, Sartini M, et al: Effects of pancreas-kidney transplantation on diabetic retinopathy. Transpl Int 18:619, 2005

63. Navarro X, Sutherland DE, Kennedy WR: Long-term effects of pancreatic transplantation on diabetic neuropathy. Ann Neurol 42:727, 1997

64. Larsen JL, Ratanasuwan T, Burkman T, et al: Carotid intima media thickness decreases after pancreas transplantation. Transplantation 73:936, 2002

65. Jukema JW, Smets YF, van der Pijl JW, et al: Impact of simultaneous pancreas and kidney transplantation on progression of coronary atherosclerosis in patients with end-stage renal failure due to type 1 diabetes. Diabetes Care 25:906, 2002

66. Tyden G, Tollemar J, Bolinder J: Combined pancreas and kidney transplantation improves survival in patients with end-stage diabetic nephropathy. Clin Transplant 14:505, 2000

67. Reddy KS, Stablein D, Taranto S, et al: Long-term survival following simultaneous kidney-pancreas transplantation versus kidney transplantation alone in patients with type 1 diabetes mellitus and renal failure. Am J Kidney Dis 41:464, 2003

68. Gross CR, Limwattananon C, Matthees B, et al: Impact of transplantation on quality of life in patients with diabetes and renal dysfunction. Transplantation 70:1736, 2000

69. Prieto M, Sutherland DE, Goetz FC, et al: Pancreas transplant results according to the technique of duct management: bladder versus enteric drainage. Surgery 102:680,1987

Acknowledgments

Figure 2   Tom Moore.

Figure 4   Alice Y. Chen

75 Enteral and Parenteral Nutrition

Khursheed N. Jeejeebhoy, M.B.B.S., PH.D.

Definitions

Enteral nutrition is the process of nourishing a patient with a liquid diet of defined composition, usually given through a nasogastric, nasointestinal, gastrostomy, or jejunostomy tube. Parenteral nutrition is the administration of nutrients directly into the bloodstream through a central venous catheter or by peripheral infusion. When the only source of nutrient intake is via the parenteral route, it is called total parenteral nutrition (TPN). The term nutritional support refers to the use of enteral or parenteral nutrition rather than to an oral diet, with or without supplements.

Etiology of Malnutrition

In circumstances in which food is available, malnutrition has three main causes: (1) insufficient intake of food, as a result of conditions such as anorexia, coma, dysphagia, gastric lesions, and psychological factors; (2) heightened metabolic requirements, as may occur in burns, trauma, sepsis, and neoplasia; and (3) intestinal failure, which comprises all conditions that prevent the proper intake, digestion, or absorption of a normal oral diet. Malnutrition from reduced food intake or gastrointestinal failure is most amenable to treatment or prevention with nutritional support. Although nutritional support may overcome some of the effects of trauma, burns, sepsis, or cancer, nutritional support alone may be unable to prevent the development of critical malnutrition in such cases.

Effects of Malnutrition

Even in the absence of disease, malnutrition adversely influences function and survival. A study of Irish hunger strikers found a 30% mortality in strikers who lost 35% to 40% of their body weight.[1] Similarly, in patients with cancer, weight loss of about 30% preceded death.[2] In 12 human volunteers, semistarvation (with a 15% to 20% weight loss over 24 weeks) led to a 60% decrease in function on the basis of a fitness score.[1] Even after 20 weeks of refeeding, the fitness score and handgrip strength in these individuals did not return to normal. Other studies have shown that lack of food intake results in substantial loss of muscle function in addition to loss of body mass.[3] Surgical patients who had weight loss greater than 10% and clinical evidence of dysfunction of two or more organ systems (including skeletal and respiratory muscles) preoperatively had significantly more postoperative complications than did normal patients or those with weight loss but no physiologic dysfunction.[4]

The presence of various diseases compounds the effects of malnutrition. In ill patients, malnutrition results in nutritionally associated complications such as poor wound healing, increased infections, delayed rehabilitation, and increased mortality.

Evidence Regarding Nutritional Support

Well-nourished patients are unlikely to benefit from nutritional support. However, in patients with initial malnutrition and poor function who have continued inability to eat or to absorb ingested food, randomized controlled trials have demonstrated that nutritional support favorably influences outcome by reducing nutritionally associated complications.

PARENTERAL NUTRITION

Three large meta-analyses of parenteral nutrition have given inconsistent results. In a comparison of parenteral nutrition with standard care in 26 trials, Heyland and colleagues[5] found that parenteral nutrition did not influence overall mortality but did reduce complications in malnourished patients. Benefit from TPN was observed in studies performed before 1988, in studies deemed to be of less statistical quality, and in patients who did not receive lipid. These researchers found only six trials of parenteral nutrition in critical illness; in these trials, complications and mortality were significantly higher than in trials done in surgical patients. Another meta-analysis showed that in malnourished patients, standard care, compared with parenteral nutrition, was associated with increased mortality and a trend toward increased infectious complications; in well-nourished patients, infections were more frequent with parenteral nutrition than with standard care or enteral nutrition.[6] These authors speculated that the increased infectious complications in patients on parenteral nutrition were attributable to hyperglycemia. Not all the studies included in this meta-analysis mentioned blood glucose, but of the seven that did, six found both hyperglycemia and increased infectious complications.

Koretz and colleagues[7] have done a technical review and made recommendations to the American Gastroenterological Association about parenteral nutrition. They found that overall, mortality with parenteral nutrition was no lower than mortality with standard care. In contrast to the meta-analysis by Heyland and colleagues,[5] this analysis showed that total complications and length of stay were lower only in studies in which lipid was a component of TPN. Infectious complications were increased with TPN, especially in cancer patients. Benefit from parenteral nutrition was seen only in patients with upper GI cancer, who had significantly fewer complications when given perioperative parenteral nutrition.

ENTERAL NUTRITION

Enteral nutrition has not been compared with standard care in the same systematic way as has parenteral nutrition. However, comparisons of enteral nutrition with parenteral nutrition have consistently shown fewer infectious complications with enteral nutrition than with parenteral nutrition.[6] Data from a large controlled trial in intensive care unit patients showed that keeping blood glucose levels below 127 mg/dl (7 mmol/L) significantly reduced mortality from sepsis-related multisystem organ failure.[8] Hyperglycemia probably was more frequent with parenteral nutrition because patients randomized to parenteral nutrition received more calories than those on enteral nutrition,[9] despite the intent to make both groups isocaloric. None of these studies prove that enteral nutrition is better than standard therapy; rather, they show that enteral nutrition is less likely than parenteral nutrition to cause infection. In a 562-patient trial of enteral nutrition versus TPN that mirrored the conventional practice of nutritional support, Woodcock and colleagues[10] concluded that TPN did not increase sepsis, enteral nutrition delivered less than the target nutritional intake, and procedure-related complications were greater with enteral nutrition.

Determining the Need for Nutritional Support

Unfortunately, for many clinical situations there are no data from randomized, controlled trials to help clinicians determine how to identify patients who are likely to progress to critical weight loss and to determine when to start nutritional support in patients who are at risk. In the absence of reliable data, clinicians have to make decisions about nutritional support at the bedside. Obviously, a previously healthy person who does not eat for 1 or 2 days does not need nutritional support. On the other hand, if inadequate nutritional intake persists for weeks, weight loss will continue; the loss will accelerate if there is added trauma or sepsis; and when loss of body weight exceeds 30%, there is an increased likelihood of death.

The risk of malnutrition can be assessed with a clinical tool called the Subjective Global Assessment (SGA).[11] The SGA, which can be used by physicians, dietitians, or nurses after brief training, is based on a focused history and physical examination that includes the degree and progression of any weight loss, dietary intake, ability to take and absorb food (state of the GI tract), the degree of stress from comorbidity, and functional status.[12] This information is used to classify the patient into one of three groups: A (normally nourished and unlikely to

progress to a malnourished state), B (normally nourished but likely to progress to a malnourished state), or C (malnourished and progressing to increasing malnutrition).

The SGA not only provides an assessment of the patient's current nutritional status but also predicts the possible nutritional outcome if nutritional support is not instituted. More important, it allows the clinician to weigh the role of disease severity versus limited nutrient intake as the cause of malnutrition.

Two controlled studies of the SGA have shown that the likelihood of nutritionally associated complications progressively increased from grades A to C. Patients who are classified as SGA C are very likely to develop nutritionally associated complications and therefore should benefit from nutritional support. These studies also found that the SGA grade correlated with other objective measures of nutritional status but was more likely to predict nutritionally associated complications than several of the objective measures taken individually.[13] SGA has been shown to be a valid predictor of nutritionally associated complications in general surgical patients, patients on dialysis, and liver transplant patients. In two large studies, SGA independently identified increased mortality and morbidity from malnutrition, even when the data were adjusted for other factors influencing survival and complications.[14,15]

Nutritional Support in Specific Clinical Conditions

INSUFFICIENT ORAL INTAKE DESPITE A NORMAL GUT

Well-nourished Patients

In general, most patients with serious illness have reduced food intake, partly from the illness itself and partly as a result of iatrogenic factors. Most hospital inpatients eat insufficient food or are prevented from eating. Several studies have indicated that a significant number of hospital patients have signs of malnutrition. Patients likely to have an inadequate intake of food are those with critical illness (e.g., trauma, burns, severe sepsis, respiratory failure); coma and neurologic diseases; or major psychiatric illnesses. Although many hospital patients fit these categories, there are no controlled trials to provide guidelines that can be confidently used to guide nutritional support in such patients and to confirm that nutritional support can reduce the occurrence of nutritionally associated complications. Clinically, it is a common practice to start nutritional support if the period of reduced intake exceeds 7 to 10 days or weight loss exceeds 10%.[16] Unfortunately, this practice has no supporting data except consensus and expert opinion.

Early enteral feeding has been recommended on the basis of a randomized trial in trauma patients who were to undergo a laparotomy and had an abdominal trauma index greater than 15.[17] This subset constituted 20% of all trauma patients admitted during the period of study. These patients, who were well nourished on admission, were randomized to a group who received early (12 to 18 hours after surgery) institution of enteral feeding through a jejunostomy tube inserted at surgery or to a control group in whom TPN was started 5 days after surgery if the patient was not yet on a regular oral diet. There was no difference in overall complications between the groups, but septic complications were significantly lower in the early-fed group (4%, versus 26% in the TPN group). Such data are subject to the criticism that there was no control group receiving standard care. However, there are other reasons to support early feeding. In a randomized trial of postoperative supplemental sip

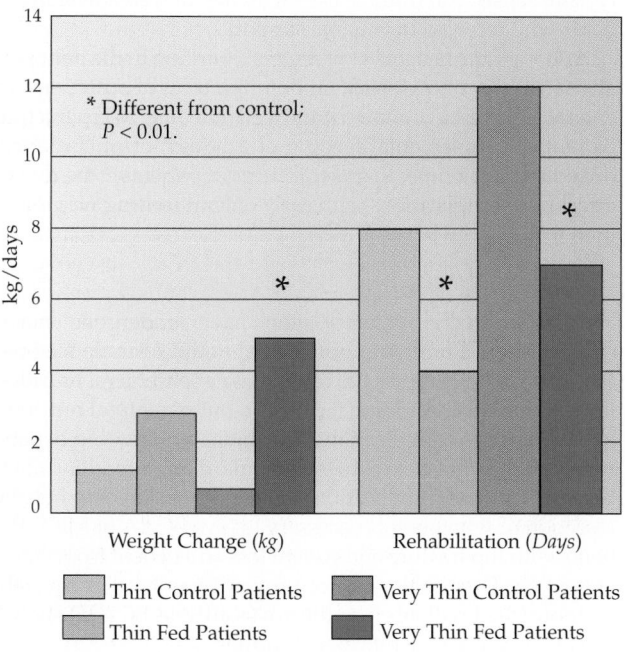

Figure 1 **In elderly women with femoral neck fractures, weight increase was greater and rehabilitation time was shorter in those who received overnight supplementary enteral feeding than in control subjects, who were given a normal hospital diet. The effect was evident in thin patients and was particularly marked in very thin patients.[22]**

feeding of a liquid formulation, grip strength significantly improved and the occurrence of serious infections was reduced.[18] In a trial of 501 hospitalized elderly patients randomized to oral supplements or a ward diet, Larsson and colleagues[19] showed that irrespective of their initial nutritional status, the supplemented patients had lower mortality, better mobility, and a shorter hospital stay. The difference between ward diet and supplementation was even more pronounced in a secondary analysis of patients with weight loss.

Recommendations The available data suggest that well-nourished patients who are admitted with major trauma should receive enteral nutrition. Elderly patients should receive supplemental feeding or enteral nutrition if they are incapable of eating adequately. However, all hospitalized patients should have their SGA assessed so that possible future outcome without nutritional support can be documented and considered. For example, if a previously healthy patient has a severe head injury and is likely to remain comatose (and therefore unable to eat) for an indefinite period, it is easy to predict that malnutrition will occur in the absence of nutritional support. Such a patient should be started on enteral nutrition. Similarly, major burns, the hypermetabolic state, anorexia, and ileus all result in rapid weight loss unless nutritional support is given. Each case needs to be assessed individually, however. Repeated evaluation of the SGA allows the clinician to determine any impediment to the intake of food, the presence of GI dysfunction, and progressive functional loss and weight loss, which signal the need to start nutritional support.

The purely scientific approach would be to avoid nutritional support in all situations for which proof of benefit from randomized, controlled studies is lacking; however, in patients without adequate oral intake, this approach could in some cases result in starvation and death. The pragmatic approach is to evaluate the patient, using the SGA, and start nutritional support if the clinical evidence shows that otherwise the patient is likely to progress to critical malnutrition.[20]

Malnourished Patients

There are no controlled trials to show that nutritional support will reduce complications in all patients classified as SGA C. However, there are several indirect lines of evidence suggesting that nutritional support in such patients will reduce complications and improve outcome.

A multicenter, randomized, controlled trial undertaken by the Veterans Affairs Total Parenteral Nutrition Cooperative Study Group[21] stratified patients into three nutritional groups. In the group of severely malnourished patients, the rate of major noninfectious complications was significantly lower in patients randomized to TPN than in control subjects (5.3% versus 42.9%). Overall rates of complications and infectious complications in TPN-treated patients in this trial were not different from those in control patients, however.

Other studies have shown that nutritional supplementation can significantly reduce rehabilitation time in patients with hip fractures who had severe weight loss [*see Figure 1*][22] and that elderly patients with hip fractures, especially those with weight loss, benefit the most from supplemental feeding.[19]

Recommendations Elderly patients, especially those with weight loss, should receive nutritional supplements in the hospital. Despite the lack of data from well-designed controlled trials, patients who are classified as SGA C should be given nutritional support.

SURGERY

In a meta-analysis of perioperative parenteral nutrition, Detsky and colleagues[23] combined the results of 14 randomized or quasi-randomized trials and showed that absolute morbidity was reduced by 5.2% and the relative risk reduction was 20.7%. These differences were not statistically significant, however ($P = 0.21$). Of the 14 studies, only one showed a significant reduction in complication and fatality rates with TPN. These authors concluded that perioperative TPN did not influence outcome. On the other hand, only three of the 14 trials were limited to malnourished patients (who were the most likely to benefit from TPN), so the negative result may simply reflect the fact that the trials were weighted by patients who were unlikely to benefit from nutritional support. In contrast, Twomey[24] concluded that the pooled estimate in malnourished surgical patients shows a 7.1% reduction in morbidity with TPN. In the VA trial,[21] secondary analysis showed that the severely malnourished patients had a reduction in overall morbidity from 47% to 26% with perioperative TPN.

Fan and colleagues[25] conducted a controlled trial of perioperative nutritional support in 124 patients undergoing major hepatic resection for hepatocellular carcinoma. The patients were randomized to parenteral nutrition plus oral diet or to diet only. Patients in the treatment arm received 1.5 g/kg of amino acids, of which 35% were branched-chain amino acids (BCAA), with 30 kcal/kg of a glucose-lipid mixture for energy. Medium-chain triglycerides (MCT) constituted 50% of the lipid infused. The parenteral formulation was given for 14 days. At least 20% of the patients had a preoperative weight loss of greater than 10% and therefore were likely to be malnourished, but 80% did not have weight loss. Overall morbidity, morbidity from sepsis, and diuretic use for ascites all were lower in patients who received nutritional support.

Although the benefits of parenteral nutrition in the perioperative state are controversial, randomized trials of postoperative enteral feeding have shown improved outcome. In hip fracture patients,[22] supplemental feeding of a liquid formula diet reduced recovery time. In general surgical patients,[26] the rate of infectious complications with early enteral feeding was lower than that with nil per os (NPO).

Recommendations

Postoperatively, patients who have undergone major surgery should receive supplemental liquid formula feeding. The data do not support the routine use of parenteral nutrition for perioperative nutritional support, but parenteral nutrition clearly reduces complications in patients undergoing hepatic resection. It is not clear whether standard parenteral formulations will reduce complications in patients undergoing hepatic resection or whether it is necessary to give BCAA or MCT. Patients with hip fracture and weight loss will benefit from enteral feeding. Despite the lack of proven benefit, other severely malnourished patients (i.e., those classified as SGA C) should receive perioperative nutritional support.

SERIOUS COMPROMISE OF BOWEL FUNCTION

In patients with massive small bowel resection (i.e., less than 60 cm remaining), chronic bowel obstruction, extensive bowel disease, severe radiation enteritis, or end jejunostomy in which oral feeding results in uncontrolled fluid and electrolyte losses, parenteral nutrition is needed because oral feeding is very unlikely to provide sufficient nourishment. An economic analysis of such patients showed that provision of parenteral nutrition at home was associated with improved quality of life and was cost-effective.[27] The outlook was especially good for those with chronic intestinal failure from benign disease.[28]

Recommendations

Initially, all patients with a short bowel (see above) need parenteral nutrition. Later, about 30% (especially those with an intact or partially intact colon) can be treated with oral diet and supplements. Enteral nutrition is not necessary in these patients; controlled studies have shown that enteral nutrition was no better than an oral diet in patients with a short bowel and end jejunostomy.[29] Patients with a massive resection can absorb 50% to 60% of an oral diet.[30] By using oral rehydration solution, supplements, and a high-calorie oral diet, about 30% of such patients can reduce or stop home parenteral nutrition. The remaining patients will require supplemental fluid and electrolytes or parenteral nutrition to maintain a normal weight and electrolyte-fluid status.

BOWEL REST

Parenteral Nutrition

Bowel rest is widely used in pancreatitis, intestinal fistulas, and inflammatory bowel disease. The bowel is rested by keeping the patient NPO. Malnutrition is avoided by instituting parenteral nutrition.

Parenteral nutrition is used in pancreatitis because eating often induces pain in such cases. The only controlled trial of parenteral nutrition versus oral diet in patients with mild pancreatitis showed that TPN did not influence recovery.[31] In two trials comparing parenteral nutrition with enteral nutrition in patients with mild or acute pancreatitis, the trial of patients with mild pancreatitis[32] found no difference in septic complications, whereas the trial of patients with severe pancreatitis[33] found less sepsis with enteral nutrition. However, in the latter trial, twice the number of patients on parenteral nutrition were hyperglycemic, a factor known to increase septic complications.[8] Again, these trials do not prove that enteral nutrition is better than standard care.

Parenteral nutrition is useful in patients with intestinal fistulas, in whom eating increases output and fasting reduces output by 30% to 50%. However, there are no controlled trials comparing the effect of bowel rest plus parenteral nutrition with that of oral intake in the healing of fistulas.

In inflammatory bowel disease, bowel rest reduces abdominal discomfort and diarrhea. Controlled trials have not shown that bowel rest aids recovery in these patients, however.[34]

Recommendations Because pancreatitis, intestinal fistulas, and inflammatory bowel disease may prevent the ingestion or absorption of oral nutrients and result in malnutrition, the use of bowel rest and parenteral nutrition is a reasonable strategy in some of these cases, despite the lack of evidence that bowel rest alters the course of the disease. Specifically, enteral or parenteral nutrition should be given to prevent or treat malnutrition when a patient cannot take in or absorb nutrients for 7 to 10 days, when a patient loses nutrients because of a fistula for 7 to 10 days, or when a patient is clearly malnourished (SGA C).

The route of administration selected should be capable of delivering the ideal nutrient intake successfully. For example, enteral nutrition is unlikely to be successful in a patient with a high jejunal fistula who is putting out large volumes of intestinal contents.

Enteral Nutrition in Crohn Disease

Controlled trials in Crohn disease have shown that enteral nutrition reduces the activity of the disease and, in children, promotes growth.[35] However, a meta-analysis of eight randomized, controlled trials of 413 patients with Crohn disease showed that enteral nutrition was not as effective as corticosteroids in inducing a remission (odds ratio of enteral nutrition/corticosteroids, 0.35; confidence interval, 0.23–0.53). In addition, there was no difference between elemental and polymeric diets in inducing clinical remission.[36] Regrettably, there are no placebo-controlled trials to show whether enteral nutrition is an effective modality for treatment of active Crohn disease.

Recommendations Enteral nutrition is not a replacement for routine drug treatment of active Crohn disease, but under certain circumstances it has definite benefits. Enteral nutrition is especially useful in promoting growth and reducing disease activity in children with growth failure. In such children, enteral nutrition can be given on a long-term basis at home, along with other treatment to promote growth.

In line with other recommendations for nutritional support, patients with active Crohn disease who are SGA C should be treated with enteral nutrition and other modalities as required. However, if they are SGA C and are unable to tolerate enteral nutrition, parenteral nutrition should be used until they can tolerate adequate nutrition by the oral route. Nutritional support is also necessary when serial SGA determinations show evidence of poor intake and the patient has severe GI symptoms and continued functional impairment that could lead to critical malnutrition. The route used depends on the capacity of the GI tract to absorb nutrients.

CANCER MALNUTRITION

Malnutrition in metastatic cancer has been used as an indication for parenteral nutrition. Controlled trials have failed to substantiate that nutritional support is beneficial in patients with metastatic cancer,[37] however, and in fact have suggested that parenteral nutrition may have adverse effects. On the other hand, parenteral nutrition has been shown to favorably influence graft survival in patients receiving a bone marrow transplant.[38]

Recommendations

In cancer patients, nutritional support with enteral or parenteral nutrition is appropriate for preventing or treating malnutrition that is not caused by the tumor per se. For example, patients whose colon cancer has been eradicated but who suffer from short bowel because of extensive radiation enteritis should respond to parenteral nutrition. Criteria for nutritional support in cancer patients are as follows: (1) there is no evidence of tumor or its progression; (2) the patient has a GI complication, such as radiation enteritis or resection; and (3) as a result of this GI complication, critical malnutrition has occurred or will predictably occur (i.e., the patient is SGA C, or serial evaluation of SGA indicates progression toward SGA C).

The most difficult ethical question concerns the use of parenteral nutrition for patients in whom tumor progression causes intestinal obstruction or cachexia. Parenteral nutrition is being increasingly used for this indication [see Home Parenteral Nutrition, below].

RENAL FAILURE

Because patients with renal disease cannot excrete nitrogen normally, parenteral nutrition in which the source of nitrogen is limited to essential amino acids (EAA) has been used to reduce urea production. A meta-analysis has concluded that parenteral nutrition with EAA does not improve survival to discharge; when the trials were adjusted for quality, there was no effect of EAA.[39]

Recommendations

Patients with renal failure who cannot meet their nutritional requirements by the oral route should be given nutritional support and have fluid, electrolytes, and nitrogenous metabolites removed by dialysis or continuous arteriovenous hemofiltration. Fluid intake is minimized by using enteral nutrition with a calorie density of 2 kcal/ml or parenteral nutrition containing 35% dextrose or 20% lipid as the source of energy. Sodium intake should be restricted to 40 to 70 mmol/day, and other electrolytes should be added if their plasma levels fall. Acidosis should be controlled by appropriate dialysis. Trace elements and vitamin supplements need not be curtailed.

HEPATIC FAILURE AND ALCOHOLIC LIVER DISEASE

The discovery that hepatic encephalopathy is associated with reduced BCAAs and increased aromatic amino acids in plasma has led to the use of parenteral nutrition formulas enriched in BCAAs and reduced in aromatic amino acids. Meta-analysis of trials comparing BCAA-enriched mixtures with standard therapy has shown significant improvement in encephalopathy and, possibly, in short-term mortality.[40] On the other hand, there is no evidence that standard amino acid mixtures or enteral nutrition providing 0.8 to 1 g/kg/day of protein or amino acids has precipitated encephalopathy. In fact, 75 g/day of supplementary amino acids with 400 kcal/day of dextrose improved liver function and was tolerated by patients with severe alcoholic hepatitis.[41]

Recommendations

Patients with hepatic failure who are unable to be on a normal diet need enteral or parenteral nutrition. The protein intake should be about 0.8 to 1 g/kg/day of a high-quality protein or balanced amino acids. Carbohydrates and fat should be given in equal proportions because these patients are carbohydrate intolerant but utilize fat well, and fat infusions increase the levels of BCAA in plasma.[42] Because these patients are sodium and water overloaded, they should receive a total of about 1,500 ml of water daily, and their sodium intake should be restricted to 20 mmol/day. Supplemental potassium, vitamins (A, D, and B complex), and zinc should be given.

Practice of Nutritional Support

GENERAL PRINCIPLES OF NUTRITIONAL CARE

At hospital admission, all patients should be interviewed by a dietitian and have their SGA calculated to determine whether they can be maintained on a normal or modified oral diet (with

Table 1 Procedure for Nasogastric or Nasoenteral Tube Placement

1. Explain the procedure to the patient, to obtain cooperation.
2. Seat the patient comfortably at the edge of the bed, sitting upright.
3. Check nostrils for painful lesions and obstruction.
4. Insert stylet into tube and lubricate.
5. Measure approximate length of tube to be passed by the distance between the tip of the nose to the ear and down to the midepigastrium. Add about 25 cm to this distance.
6. Flex neck slightly.
7. Pass tube through an unobstructed nostril. If the patient finds this very uncomfortable, spray nostril with lidocaine 4% topical solution.
8. Ask the patient to swallow water as the tube is passed.
9. If the patient coughs or chokes, withdraw tube into the pharynx and reinsert.
10. Aspirate gastric contents to confirm position of tube.
11. Air may be injected into the tube while auscultating to determine the intragastric location of the tube.
12. For nasogastric feeding, confirm the tube position by x-ray before infusing.
13. For nasoenteral feeding, place the patient in right lateral position and gradually advance tube. Metoclopramide, 10 mg I.V., may be used to propel the tube.
14. If tube has not passed into the bowel by 24 hours, endoscopic or fluoroscopic guidance may be used.

supplements) or whether nutritional support is indicated and, if so, how urgently. In patients requiring nutritional support, the physician and the dietitian should define nutrient intake, route of administration, and goals. The most important objective is maintenance of uninterrupted nutrient intake, to avoid weeks of starvation followed by the urgent institution of parenteral nutrition to an iatrogenically malnourished patient.

Oral Nutrition

In patients who can eat, close attention to maintenance of oral dietary intake—and use of supplements, where required—should be the standard of care. Enteral nutrition should be considered if it becomes clear that this approach does not permit sufficient intake to meet requirements.

Enteral Nutrition

Enteral nutrition is applicable to all patients, but it should be used with caution in patients with (1) clinically significant gastroesophageal reflux; (2) intestinal obstruction; (3) GI fistula or recent surgical anastomosis, unless the tube can be inserted distal to the area in question or threaded at operation past the area; and (4) cardiovascular instability with shock. Gastric retention is a relative contraindication. In patients who accumulate secretions in the stomach and then aspirate, it may be possible to pass a feeding tube into the small intestine and aspirate the stomach with a second tube. However, in such cases the relative discomfort of two tubes versus parenteral nutrition should be considered. A survey of hospitalized patients and outpatients showed that patients preferred parenteral nutrition over enteral nutrition.[43]

Short-term enteral access Nasogastric or nasoenteric placement of a feeding tube provides short-term enteral access. The tube should be small bore (9 to 12 French) and 105 to 110 cm long [see Table 1]. These tubes are usually made of Silastic or polyurethane. The latter become very slippery when wet, thus aiding insertion. I prefer intestinal placement of the tube, because controlled trials have shown better achievement of nutrient intake[44] and, possibly, reduced risk of aspiration when the tube is placed beyond the ligament of Treitz.

Long-term feeding The definition of long-term feeding is arbitrary. Children with Crohn disease have been fed for months by teaching them to pass a nasogastric tube each night, receive a nocturnal feeding, and then remove the tube in the morning before going to school. However, in many instances nasal tubes become uncomfortable, and a gastrostomy tube can be placed endoscopically by a gastroenterologist or an interventional radiologist. This method has been shown to be safer and more cost-effective than a surgically placed gastrostomy. There are two methods of percutaneous endoscopic gastrostomy (PEG): the pull (Ponsky-Gauderer) method and the push (Russell) method.

Feeding into the small bowel can be performed after the insertion of a percutaneous endoscopic jejunostomy (PEJ). After the tract of the PEG tube is established, a PEJ tube with two arms can replace the tube. One arm remains in the stomach and can be used to drain this organ; the other arm is advanced under endoscopic guidance through the pylorus into the small intestine. In this way, the stomach can be decompressed, and simultaneously, the patient can be fed into the small bowel.

To eliminate the inconvenience of the bulky feeding tube, patients with long-term gastrostomies can be fitted with a so-called button device, which lies flush with the abdominal wall. Between feedings, a valve in the device closes off access to the stomach; during feedings, the feeding tube is inserted past the valve, permitting access to the stomach.

Parenteral Nutrition

The intravenous route is used as a supplement to oral or enteral nutrition or is used as the sole source of nutrition (TPN) when it becomes clear that the patient is not receiving sufficient nutrients by the other routes. Regular evaluation of SGA should be performed during TPN to ensure that the patient's nutrient requirements are being met.

Short-term parenteral feeding Short-term infusions are best given through a peripherally inserted central catheter (PICC). These catheters are inserted into an arm or forearm vein and advanced into the superior vena cava. PICCs are comfortable and avoid the risks of subclavian puncture or the difficulties of maintaining sterility of the exit sites of jugular catheters. In addition, full TPN with hypertonic mixtures can be given through these catheters without risk of thrombosis. Despite the designation "short term," these catheters can be used for months.

Long-term parenteral feeding Patients with intestinal failure often require parenteral feeding for years. To permit long-term parenteral feeding, an interventional radiologist advances a specially designed catheter through a subcutaneous tunnel via the jugular vein to the superior vena cava. The tip of this catheter should lie just above the right atrium, to avoid thrombotic complications. Near the exit site, within the subcutaneous tunnel, the catheter is surrounded by a Dacron cuff. Fibroblasts will grow into the cuff, sealing and anchoring the skin exit site.

Protein

Protein requirements are met by giving whole proteins, peptides, or amino acids in enteral nutrition and by infusing an amino acid mixture in parenteral nutrition. The goal is to promote nitrogen retention and protein synthesis. Although limiting glucose and lipid (energy) intake will maximize nitrogen retention, dietary protein has an anabolic effect independent of energy intake, and will reduce nitrogen losses when infused alone.[45] Thus, the amount of amino acids given appears to be a very important determinant of nitrogen balance.

About 1 to 1.5 g/kg of ideal body weight of protein or amino acids will be sufficient for most patients with normal renal function. Additional amounts should be added for losses from prior depletion or current hypercatabolism. In patients with hepatic failure, protein intake should be restricted to 0.8 to 1.0 g/kg a day.

Glutamine

Glutamine is an amino acid released by muscle and used by immune cells and enteral cells for energy. In malnutrition and after trauma, muscle glutamine and muscle protein synthesis are reduced. The infusion of glutamine normalizes muscle glutamine and restores protein synthesis.[46] Clinically, bone marrow transplant patients were noted to have fewer episodes of sepsis and a shorter hospital stay if they received a glutamine-supplemented amino acid solution.[47] Because glutamine does not have a long shelf-life in solution, dipeptides containing glutamine have been used as a substitute. Infusion of solutions containing such dipeptides has been found to increase muscle glutamine and improve protein synthesis.[46]

Immunonutrition

Enteral formulations enriched in arginine, omega-3 fatty acids, and glutamine nucleotides are considered to enhance the immune response; treatment with these formulations is referred to as immunonutrition. These formulations vary in composition, but they are distinguished by high (12 to 15 g/L) or low (4 to 6 g/L) arginine content, presence or absence of glutamine and nucleotides, and different concentrations of omega-3 fatty acids. A summit on immune-enhancing enteral therapy[48] concluded, on the basis of published literature, that imunonutrition should be given to malnourished patients undergoing elective GI surgery and to trauma patients with an injury severity score of 18 or greater or an abdominal trauma index of 20 or greater. Immunonutrition was also recommended, despite lack of evidence, in patients undergoing head and neck surgery or aortic reconstruction, as well as in patients with severe head injury or burns, and in ventilator-dependent nonseptic patients. It was not recommended for patients with splanchnic hypoperfusion or bowel obstruction distal to the access site or after major upper GI hemorrhage.

A systematic review of immunonutrition by Heyland and colleagues[49] showed that it reduced septic complications but did not reduce mortality. Their analysis of 22 randomized, controlled trials covering 2,419 critically ill or surgical patients indicated that only high-arginine formulations reduced infectious complications and length of stay. These authors concluded that in patients undergoing elective surgery, immunonutrition may reduce complications and reduce length of stay. Pending further studies, however, immunonutrition was not recommended in patients with critical illness. Because many trauma and septic patients may be critically ill, these authors' recommendations are at variance with those of the immunonutrition summit (see above). The finding that benefit is seen only with the formulation containing higher amounts of arginine raises the question whether arginine per se or the higher nitrogen intake is responsible for the benefit.

Energy (Glucose and Lipids)

In healthy persons, basal energy expenditure (BEE), or basal metabolic rate (BMR), in kilocalories a day can be predicted with the Harris-Benedict equation:

$$\text{BEE in males} = 66.5 + (13.8 \times \text{weight in kg}) + (5.0 \times \text{height in cm}) - (6.8 \times \text{age in yr})$$

$$\text{BEE in females} = 655.1 + (9.6 \times \text{weight in kg}) + (1.8 \times \text{height in cm}) - (4.7 \times \text{age in yr})$$

A calculator to be used for determining BEE according to the Harris-Benedict equation can be found on the Internet, at www-users.med.cornell.edu/~spon/picu/calc/beecalc.htm.

For patients substantially on bed rest, about 30% should be added to the BEE to meet their metabolic requirements. In practice, this calculates as a daily expenditure of about 31 kcal/kg. An expert group has suggested a daily intake of 25 kcal/kg in ICU patients.[50] Therefore, 25 to 30 kcal/kg/day will meet the needs of most patients, except those with burns. Malnutrition reduces the expected BEE by as much as 35%; injury, sepsis, and, especially, burns increase requirements.[51] Baker and colleagues[52] found that in critically sick patients in respiratory failure, the maximal degree of hypermetabolism was about 30%.

Energy requirements during TPN can be met by infusing glucose or lipid emulsions. These nonprotein energy sources enhance nitrogen retention. The most striking increase in nitrogen balance has been found to occur when energy was increased from 0 kcal/kg to 30 kcal/kg of ideal body weight. Increases above that provided only slight improvement. In obese persons, a high-protein formulation with only about 14 kcal/kg/day meets nitrogen requirements[53] and is associated with satisfactory wound healing.[54]

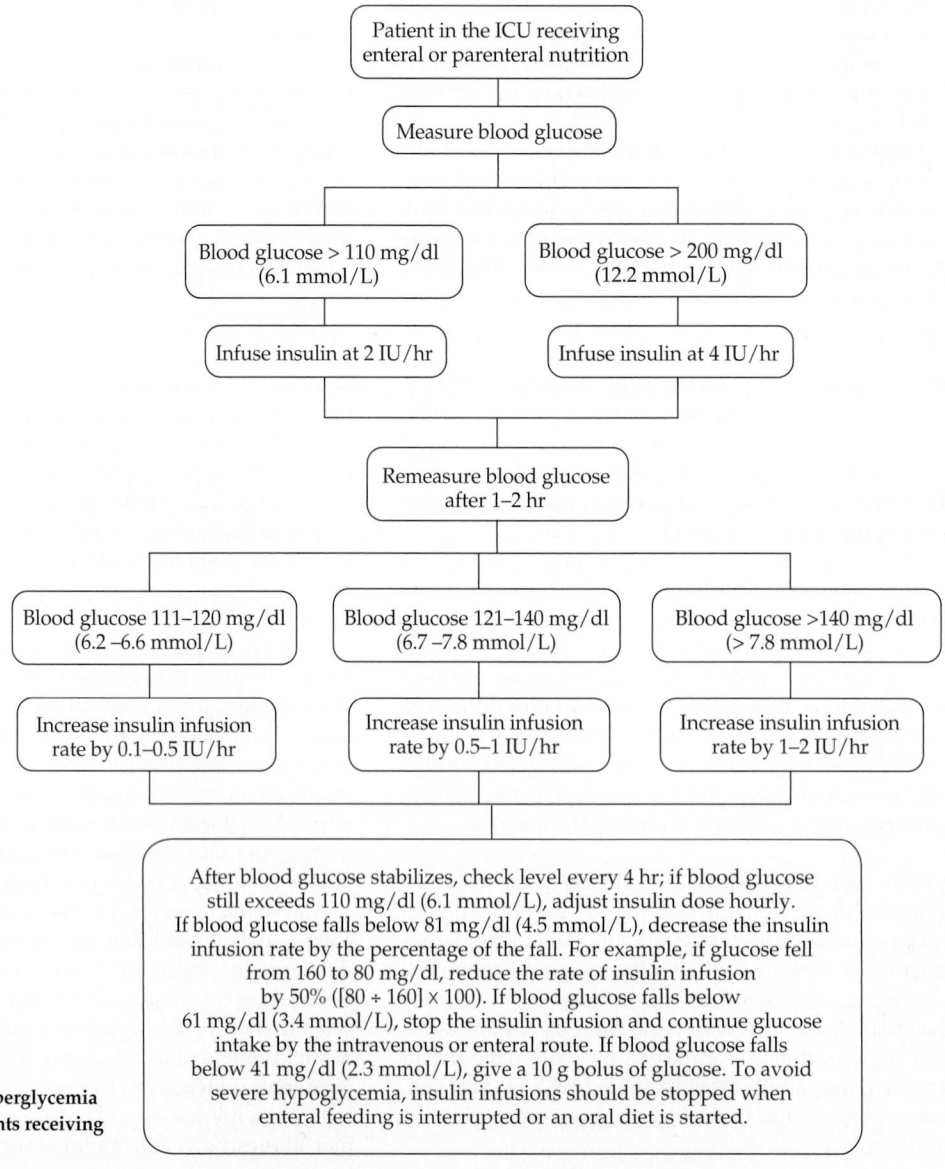

Figure 2 **Controlling hyperglycemia in intensive care unit patients receiving nutritional support.**

Table 2 Daily Electrolyte and Trace Element Requirements for Adults on Total Parenteral Nutrition

Element	Normal	Increased GI Losses	Renal Failure	Comments
Sodium (mmol)	80–120	Meet losses	20–40	Reduce in heart failure
Potassium (mmol)	40–80	80–120	0–20	Correct hypokalemia before starting nutrition
Magnesium (mmol)	5–10	10–20	0–5	Correct hypomagnesemia before starting nutrition
Phosphorus (mmol)	10–15	10–15	0–5	Risk of dangerously low serum levels when feeding patients with severe malnutrition
Zinc (mg)	TPN: 3–4 Enteral: 15–20	TPN: 12–25 Enteral: 50–100	No change	—
Copper (mg)	TPN: 0.25–0.3 Enteral: 2–4	TPN: 0.5–0.7 Enteral: 4–8	No change	Reduce to 0.1 in hepatic failure

Because glucose spares nitrogen in fasting persons, it has been advocated as the main source of energy for parenteral nutrition. However, recent studies have shown that in malnourished patients and septic patients, lipids can promote nitrogen retention and increase total body nitrogen to the same extent as glucose, provided amino acids are given.[55] Fats constitute about 30% of total energy in most enteral formulas. Furthermore, glucose-lipid mixtures facilitate the control of severe hyperglycemia in septic patients with insulin resistance.[50]

Infusion of glucose at rates that exceed energy requirements elevates O_2 consumption, CO_2 production, resting energy expenditure, and urinary norepinephrine excretion. However, the magnitude of increased CO_2 production is small if total calories infused conform to levels recommended for the patient's clinical situation.[51]

The exact amount of lipid to include in the parenteral nutrition regimen is controversial. In a randomized, controlled trial of 512 bone marrow transplant patients receiving TPN, sepsis was no more frequent in patients who received 30% of energy as lipid than in those who received only sufficient lipids to meet essential fatty acid (EFA) needs (6% to 8% of energy intake).[56] In addition, EFA deficiency developed in some of the latter patients, and in some, this small amount of lipid was insufficient to meet energy requirements without induction of hyperglycemia from the glucose component. These authors recommend giving 25% to 30% of energy as long-chain triglycerides (LCTs). In contrast, a study in 57 trauma patients found that TPN with added lipid increased sepsis and hospital stay.[57] It was not clear whether the adverse effect was from the lipid per se or the increased energy intake while on lipid.

Because of their glucose content, both enteral nutrition and TPN enhance the risk of sepsis if the blood glucose level is allowed to rise above 127 mg/dl (7 mmol/L).[8] Therefore, insulin should be infused in patients receiving nutritional support to keep them as close to normoglycemia as possible [see Figure 2].

Whereas the major concern with glucose-based formulations is hyperglycemia, the key concern with lipid emulsions is hypertriglyceridemia, which may induce pancreatitis. Lipid particles also reduce gas diffusion in the lungs and inhibit the reticuloendothelial system. Provided that lipid emulsions are infused continuously at a rate that does not exceed 110 mg/kg/hr, hypertriglyceridemia does not occur. When these principles are followed, 30% to 50% of nonprotein calories can be given as fat, especially in glucose-intolerant patients.

Electrolytes, Trace Elements, and Vitamins

In patients receiving nutritional support, levels of electrolytes and trace elements should be adjusted to fit the clinical circumstances [see Table 2]. Carbohydrate feeding induces sodium retention, resulting in refeeding edema. In malnourished patients, great care should be taken to prevent salt and water overload.

Body potassium is disproportionately reduced relative to nitrogen in malnourished patients. Positive nitrogen balance does not occur unless potassium, phosphorus, and magnesium are given.[58,59] During enteral and parenteral nutrition, serum phosphorus may drop precipitously and cause dangerous neurologic symptoms.[60]

Micronutrients comprise vitamins and trace elements. The former are complex organic compounds; the latter are inorganic elements. Trace elements important to nutritional support include zinc, copper, chromium, and selenium. Diarrhea increases zinc requirements markedly and copper requirements modestly [see Table 2]. Oral chromium requirements have not been precisely determined, but deficiency occurs in patients receiving TPN; in one of my patients, the daily chromium needs were increased to 10 to 20 µg. Patients receiving parenteral nutrition may develop selenium deficiency, with muscle pains and cardiomyopathy. Increased losses of selenium can occur from the GI tract and from wounds. The recommended dose of selenium for stable patients is 40 µg/day. Patients depleted of selenium may require as much a 120 µg/day to regain normal levels.

The current recommendations for vitamins [see Table 3] specify the amounts required to maintain normal plasma or blood levels in patients on long-term home parenteral nutrition. There are no clearly defined recommendations for critically sick or septic patients.

HOME PARENTERAL NUTRITION

Patients with intestinal failure from a short bowel, chronic bowel obstruction, radiation enteritis, or untreatable malabsorption can be nourished by parenteral nutrition given at home. Arteriovenous shunts were initially used for long-term venous access in these patients, but success was limited because of clotting or disruption of the shunt. Long-term success has been achieved with a tunneled silicone rubber catheter or an implanted reservoir. Premixed nutrients are infused overnight. The catheter is then disconnected and a heparin lock applied, leaving the patient free to attend to daily activities. We have used home parenteral nutrition for more than 20 years in

Table 3 Recommendations for Vitamins in Adults
on Total Parenteral Nutrition

Vitamin	Recommended Daily Dose
A	3,300 IU
D_2	200 IU
E	10 IU
K_1	150 mg
Ascorbate	200 mg
Thiamin	6 mg
Riboflavin	3.6 mg
Pyridoxine	6 mg
Niacin	40 mg
Pantothenate	15 mg
Biotin	60 µg
Folate	600 µg
Cobalamin	5 µg

two patients with total jejunoileal resection; one continues to receive it after 30 years. Survival of patients with short bowel from treatment for Crohn disease or pseudo-obstruction is excellent. Home parenteral nutrition increases quality-adjusted years of life in these patients and is cost-effective. On the other hand, mean survival in AIDS patients or those with metastatic cancer who receive home parenteral nutrition is about 3 months. There is no evidence that home parenteral nutrition prolongs their survival or enhances their quality of life. Trials are urgently required to justify the use of home parenteral nutrition in terminal cancer and AIDS.

Complications of Long-term Home Parenteral Nutrition

At the start of nutritional support, patients are vulnerable to complications related to venous and enteral access and to metabolic complications. Careful and frequent monitoring and adjusting of nutrient intake will prevent these complications. Over the longer term, patients receiving TPN are vulnerable to three organ-specific complications: hepatic disease, bone disease, and gallstones.

Hepatic disease   The most serious form of hepatic disease related to TPN is chronic cholestasis with fibrosis. This condition is most common in patients with a very short bowel. The exact cause is unknown, but absorption of endotoxin or alteration in bile salts by bacterial dehydroxylation are possible factors. Successful treatment with metronidazole and with ursodeoxycholic acid has been reported. In some patients, carnitine infusions have corrected cholestasis.

Bone disease   Bone loss during long-term TPN is a complex issue. In a prospective longitudinal study, patients were noted to have a high bone turnover before the institution of home parenteral nutrition, but during TPN this changed to osteomalacia and slow bone turnover. This process has been attributed to aluminum toxicity but occurs in its absence[61] and

seems to respond to withdrawal of vitamin D from the TPN formula. In a prospective 4-year study of patients on home parenteral nutrition, withdrawal of vitamin D increased spinal bone mass.[62] On the other hand, patients on home parenteral nutrition can lose bone mass as a result of factors such as active inflammatory bowel disease, corticosteroid therapy, and inactivity. Some clinicians are treating reduced bone mineral density in these patients with intravenous bisphosphonates such as pamidronate and clodronate (the latter is not available in the United States). Although there are no controlled trials of bisphosphonates in patients receiving home parenteral nutrition, there are anecdotal reports of improvement of bone mass with this therapy.

Gallstones   The short bowel state results in bile salt deficiency and increased biliary cholesterol secretion. In addition, sludge composed of bilirubin and calcium forms in the gallbladder. Consequently, the incidence of gallstones is high in these patients. These stones are mixed cholesterol and pigment.

The author has no commercial relationships with manufacturers of products or providers of services discussed in this chapter.

References

1. Allison SP: The uses and limitations of nutritional support. Clin Nutr 11:319, 1992
2. DeWys WD, Begg D, Lavin PT: Prognostic effect of weight loss prior to chemotherapy in cancer patients. Am J Med 69:491, 1980
3. Jeejeebhoy KN: Rhoads lecture—1988. Bulk or bounce—the object of nutritional support. JPEN J Parenter Enteral Nutr 12:539, 1988
4. Windsor JA, Hill GL: Weight loss with physiologic impairment: a basic indicator of surgical risk. Ann Surg 207:290, 1988
5. Heyland DK, MacDonald S, Keefe L, et al: Total parenteral nutrition in the critically ill patient: a meta-analysis. JAMA 280:2013, 1998
6. Braunschweig CL, Levy P, Sheean PM, et al: Enteral compared with parenteral nutrition: a meta-analysis. Am J Clin Nutr 74:534, 2001
7. Koretz RL, Lipman TO, Klein S: AGA Technical Review on Parenteral Nutrition. American Gastroenterological Association. Gastroenterology 121:970, 2001
8. van den Berghe G, Wouters P, Weekers F, et al: Intensive insulin therapy in the critically ill patient. N Engl J Med 345:1359, 2001
9. Jeejeebhoy KN: TPN: potion or poison. Am J Clin Nutr 74:160, 2001
10. Woodcock NP, Zeigler D, Palmer MD, et al: Enteral versus parenteral nutrition: a pragmatic study. Nutrition 17:1, 2000
11. Baker J, Detsky AS, Wesson DE, et al: Nutritional assessment: a comparison of clinical judgment and objective measurements. N Engl J Med 306: 969, 1982
12. Detsky AS, McLaughlin JR, Baker JP, et al: What is subjective global assessment of nutritional status? JPEN J Parenter Enteral Nutr 11:8, 1987
13. Detsky AS, Baker JP, O'Rourke K, et al: Predicting nutrition-associated complications for patients undergoing gastrointestinal surgery. JPEN J Parenter Enteral Nutr 11:440, 1987
14. Perman M, Crivelli A, Khoury M: Nutritional prognosis in hospitalized patients. Am J Clin Nutr 75:426S, 2002
15. Pirlich M, Schütz T, Gastell S, et al: Malnutrition affects long-term prognosis in hospitalized patients. Gastroenterology 122(suppl):A636, 2002
16. Guidelines for the use of parenteral and enteral nutrition in adult and pediatric patients. JPEN J Parenter Enteral Nutr 26(1 suppl):1SA, 2002
17. Moore EE, Jones TN: Benefits of immediate jejunostomy feeding after major abdominal trauma: a prospective, randomized study. J Trauma 26:874, 1986
18. Rana SK, Bray J, Menzies-Gow N, et al: Short term benefits of post-operative oral dietary supplements in surgical patients. Clin Nutr 11:337, 1992
19. Larsson J, Unosson M, Ek AC, et al: Effect of dietary supplement on nutritional status and clinical outcome in 501 geriatric patients: a randomized study. Clin Nutr 9:179, 1990
20. Detsky AS: Parenteral nutrition: is it helpful? N Engl J Med 325:573, 1991
21. Perioperative total parenteral nutrition in surgical patients. The Veterans Affairs Total Parenteral Nutrition Cooperative Study Group. N Engl J Med 325:525, 1991
22. Bastow MD, Rawlings J, Allison SP: Benefits of supplementary tube feeding after fractured neck of femur: a randomised controlled trial. BMJ 287:1589, 1983
23. Detsky AS, Baker J, O'Rourke K, et al: Perioperative parenteral nutrition: a meta-analysis. Ann Intern Med 107:195, 1987
24. Twomey PL: Cost-effectiveness of total parenteral nutrition. Clinical Nutrition, Parenteral Nutrition. Rombeau JL, Caldwell MD, Eds. WB Saunders Co, Philadelphia, 1993, p 401

25. Fan S-T, Lo C-M, Lai ECS, et al: Perioperative nutritional support in patients undergoing hepatectomy for hepatocellular carcinoma. N Engl J Med 331:1547, 1994

26. Lewis SJ, Egger M, Sylvester PA, et al: Early enteral feeding versus "nil by mouth" after gastrointestinal surgery: systematic review and meta-analysis of controlled trials. BMJ 323:773, 2001

27. Detsky AS, McLaughlin JR, Abrams HB, et al: A cost-utility analysis of the home parenteral nutrition program at Toronto General Hospital: 1970–1982. JPEN J Parenter Enteral Nutr 10:49, 1986

28. Messing B, Lemann M, Landis P, et al: Prognosis of patients with nonmalignant chronic intestinal failure receiving long-term home parenteral nutrition. Gastroenterology 108:1005, 1995

29. McIntyre PB, Fitchew M, Lennard-Jones JE: Patients with a high jejunostomy do not need a special diet. Gastroenterology 91:25, 1986

30. Woolf GM, Miller C, Kurian V, et al: Diet for patients with a short bowel: high fat or high carbohydrate? Gastroenterology 84:823, 1983

31. Sax HC, Warner BW, Talamini MA, et al: Early total parenteral nutrition in acute pancreatitis: lack of beneficial effects. Am J Surg 153:117, 1987

32. McClave SA, Greene LM, Snider HL, et al: Comparison of the safety of early enteral vs parenteral nutrition in mild acute pancreatitis. JPEN J Parenter Enteral Nutr 21:14, 1997

33. Kalfarentzos F, Kehagias J, Mead N, et al: Enteral nutrition is superior to parenteral nutrition in severe acute pancreatitis: results of a randomized trial. Br J Surg 84:1665, 1997

34. Greenberg GR, Fleming CR, Jeejeebhoy KN, et al: Controlled trial of bowel rest and nutritional support in the management of Crohn's disease. Gut 29:1309, 1988

35. Polk DB, Hattner JAT, Kerner JA: Improved growth and disease activity after intermittent administration of a defined formula diet in children with Crohn's disease. JPEN J Parenter Enteral Nutr 16:499, 1992

36. Griffiths AM, Ohlsson A, Sherman PM, et al: Meta-analysis of enteral nutrition as primary treatment of active Crohn's disease. Gastroenterology 108:1056, 1995

37. McGeer AJ, Detsky AS, O'Rourke K: Parenteral nutrition in cancer patients undergoing chemotherapy: a meta-analysis. Nutrition 6:233, 1990

38. Weisdorf SA, Lysne J, Wind D, et al: Positive effect of prophylactic total parenteral nutrition on long-term outcome of bone marrow transplantation. Transplantation 43:833, 1987

39. Naylor CD, Detsky AS, O'Rourke K, et al: Does treatment with essential amino acids and hypertonic glucose improve survival in acute renal failure? A meta-analysis. Ren Fail 10:141, 1987

40. Naylor CD, O'Rourke K, Detsky AS, et al: Parenteral nutrition with branched-chain amino acids in hepatic encephalopathy: a meta-analysis. Gastroenterology 97:1033, 1989

41. Bonkovsky HL, Fiellin DA, Smith GS, et al: A randomized, controlled trial of treatment of alcoholic hepatitis with parenteral nutrition and oxandrolone. I: Short-term effects on liver function. Am J Gastroenterol 86:1200, 1991

42. Glynn MJ, Powell-Tuck J, Reaveley DA: High lipid parenteral nutrition improves portosystemic encephalopathy. JPEN J Parenter Enteral Nutr 12:457, 1988

43. Scolapio JS, Picco MF, Tarrosa VB: Enteral versus parenteral nutrition: the patient's preference. JPEN J Parenter Enteral Nutr 26:248, 2002

44. Montecalvo MA, Steger KA, Farber HW, et al: Nutritional outcome and pneumonia in critical care patients randomized to gastric versus jejunal tube feedings. Crit Care Med 20:1377, 1992

45. Greenberg GR, Marliss EB, Anderson GH, et al: Protein-sparing therapy in postoperative patients: effects of added hypocaloric glucose or lipid. N Engl J Med 294:1411, 1976

46. Hammarqvist F, Wernerman J, von der Decken A, et al: Alanyl-glutamine counteracts the depletion of free glutamine and the postoperative decline in protein synthesis in skeletal muscle. Ann Surg 212:637, 1990

47. Ziegler TR: Glutamine supplementation in bone marrow transplantation. Br J Nutr 87(suppl 1):S9, 2002

48. Proceedings from Summit on Immune-Enhancing Enteral Therapy. May 25-26, 2000, San Diego, California, USA. JPEN J Parenter Enteral Nutr 25(2 suppl):S1, 2001

49. Heyland DK, Novak F, Drover JW, et al: Should immunonutrition become routine in critically ill patients? JAMA 286:944, 2001

50. Applied nutrition in ICU patients. Consensus statement of the American College of Chest Physicians. Chest 111:769, 1997

51. Allard JP, Pichard C, Hoshino E, et al: Validation of a new formula for calculating the energy requirements of burn patients. JPEN J Parenter Enteral Nutr 14:115, 1990

52. Baker JP, Detsky AS, Stewart S, et al: Randomized trial of total parenteral nutrition in critically ill patients: metabolic effects of varying glucose-lipid ratios as the energy source. Gastroenterology 87:53, 1984

53. Choban PS, Burge JC, Scales D, et al: Hypoenergetic nutrition support in hospitalized obese patients: a simplified method for clinical application. Am J Clin Nutr 66:546, 1997

54. Dickerson RN, Rosato EF, Mullen JL: Net protein anabolism with hypocaloric parenteral nutrition in obese stressed patients. Am J Clin Nutr 44:747, 1986

55. MacFie J, Smith RC, Hill GL: Glucose or fat as a non-protein energy source? A controlled clinical trial in gastroenterological patients requiring intravenous nutrition. Gastroenterology 80:103, 1981

56. Lenssen P, Bruemmer BA, Bowden RA, et al: Intravenous lipid dose and incidence of bacteremia and fungemia in patients undergoing marrow transplantation. Am J Clin Nutr 67:927, 1998

57. Battistella FD, Widergren JT, Anderson JT, et al: A prospective, randomized trial of intravenous fat emulsion administration in trauma victims requiring total parenteral nutrition. J Trauma 43:52, 1997

58. Rudman D, Millikan WJ, Richardson TJ, et al: Elemental balances during intravenous hyperalimentation of underweight adult subjects. J Clin Invest 55:94, 1975

59. Freeman JB, Wittime MF, Stegink LD, et al: Effects of magnesium infusions on magnesium and nitrogen balance during parenteral nutrition. Can J Surg 25:570, 1982

60. Silvis SE, DiBartolomeo AG, Aaker HM: Hypophosphatemia and neurological changes secondary to oral caloric intake: a variant of hyperalimentation syndrome. Am J Gastroenterol 73:215, 1980

61. Karton MA, Rettmer R, Lipkin EW, et al: D-Lactate and metabolic bone disease in patients receiving long-term parenteral nutrition. JPEN J Parenter Enteral Nutr 13:132, 1989

62. Verhage AH, Cheong WK, Allard JP, et al: Vars Research Award. Increase in lumbar spine bone mineral content in patients on long-term parenteral nutrition without vitamin D supplementation. JPEN J Parenter Enteral Nutr 19:431, 1995

76 Normal and Abnormal Menstruation

Janet E. Hall, M.D.

Physiology of the Reproductive System in Women

Normal reproductive function requires precise integration of hormonal events involving the hypothalamus, the pituitary, and the ovary, with the uterus, vagina, and breast acting as key end organs for ovarian steroid effects. The number of oogonia peaks at approximately 7 million at approximately 20 weeks' gestation. Thus, at birth, the ovary has its full complement of primary oocytes. Each oocyte is surrounded by a layer of granulosa cells that form a primary preantral follicle. Subsequent to the formation of the primary preantral follicle, an outer layer of theca cells forms a secondary preantral follicle. These preantral follicles remain in a quiescent state until puberty, when complex—and as yet poorly understood—events result in an increase in activation of the hypothalamic component of the reproductive axis, manifested by secretion of gonadotropin-releasing hormone (GnRH), which is also known as luteinizing hormone–releasing hormone (LHRH).

GnRH stimulates pituitary secretion of luteinizing hormone (LH) and follicle-stimulating hormone (FSH). LH and FSH then stimulate the ovary. Although a number of releasing hormones are secreted in pulsatile fashion, GnRH is unique because pulsatile stimulation of the gonadotrope is required for normal synthesis and secretion of LH and FSH. In contrast, continuous infusion of GnRH, or the use of a GnRH agonist that simulates a continuous infusion, results in downregulation of gonadotrope responsiveness to GnRH.

HORMONAL INTEGRATION OF THE NORMAL MENSTRUAL CYCLE

Normal reproductive function in women involves repetitive cycles of follicle development, ovulation, and preparation of the endometrium for implantation should conception occur. The precise signals that govern the transformation of the quiescent hypothalamic-pituitary axis of childhood to the adult reproductive state remain incompletely understood. However, the transformation is known to include a period of nocturnal augmentation of pulsatile LH secretion, which is followed by development of the normal 24-hour pattern of gonadotropin secretion and cyclic ovarian function that is characteristic of adults. This sequence of changes, which is responsible for mature reproductive function, is coordinated through a series of negative and positive feedback loops [see Figure 1] that alter the frequency of the pulsatile secretion of GnRH, the pituitary response to GnRH, and the relative secretion of LH and FSH from the gonadotrope.[1] For most of the cycle, the reproductive system functions in a classic endocrine negative feedback mode, with hypothalamic stimulation of pituitary gonadotropin secretion culminating in ovarian secretion of steroid hormones (i.e., estradiol and progesterone) and peptide hormones (i.e., inhibin B and inhibin A).[2] In turn, ovarian hormones restrain hypothalamic GnRH secretion, pituitary responsiveness, or both. In addition to these negative feedback controls, the menstrual cycle is uniquely dependent on positive feedback to produce an LH surge (the preovulatory or midcycle surge) that is essential for ovulation of a mature follicle.

The menstrual cycle is functionally divided into the follicular and luteal phases [see Figure 2]. In the follicular phase, which begins on the first day of menses, a cohort of ovarian follicles is recruited into active growth under the influence of rising levels of FSH.[3] This cohort of follicles produces estradiol and inhibin B [see Figure 2]; the latter appears to be a marker of functional granulosa cell number. LH is required to stimulate theca cell production of androgen precursors, which then diffuse across the basement membrane into the granulosa cell, where they are aromatized to estradiol under the control of FSH. A dominant follicle emerges, which is distinguished by its size, increasing responsiveness to FSH, and higher concentrations of estradiol and inhibin A; the other follicles in the cohort regress and become atretic. Rising levels of estradiol, and probably inhibin A, restrain FSH secretion from the pituitary during this critical period of development such that only a single follicle matures in the vast majority of cycles. With further growth of the dominant follicle, estradiol and inhibin A secretion increase exponentially and the follicle acquires LH receptors. The growth of the follicle is augmented not only by the increase in cell mass but also by the accumulation of fluid within the antrum of the follicle. Functionally, the antrum serves as a unique environment for the oocyte and its surrounding cells; clinically, the fluid in the antrum is visible on ultrasound and can be used to assess follicle growth. Increasing levels of estradiol secreted by the developing follicle are responsible for proliferative changes in the endometrium. The exponential rise in estradiol also stimulates an LH surge (and a smaller FSH surge), which triggers resumption of meiosis in the oocyte, follicle rupture or ovulation, and luteinization of the granulosa cells. In animal models, positive feedback occurs at the level of both the hypothalamus and pituitary; in women, the role of the hypothalamus in this process has not been established.

The luteal, or postovulatory, phase begins immediately after ovulation, with formation of the corpus luteum from the ruptured follicle. Progesterone and inhibin A are produced from the luteinized granulosa cells that also continue to aromatize theca-derived androgen precursors, producing estradiol. Together, estrogen and progesterone produce the secretory changes of the endometrium that are necessary for implantation. Although the corpus luteum is supported by LH secretion, its sensitivity to LH diminishes over time. With the demise of the corpus luteum, hormonal support of the endometrium declines. Vascular changes in the endometrium occur as a result of either inflammation or local hypoxia and ischemia, leading to the release of cytokines, cell death, and the extravasation of blood into the uterine cavity.

In conjunction with loss of hormonal support of the endometrium, there is also a decline in negative feedback at the pituitary (from estradiol and inhibin A) and the hypothalamus (from estradiol and progesterone), resulting in a selective increase in FSH secretion relative to LH secretion.

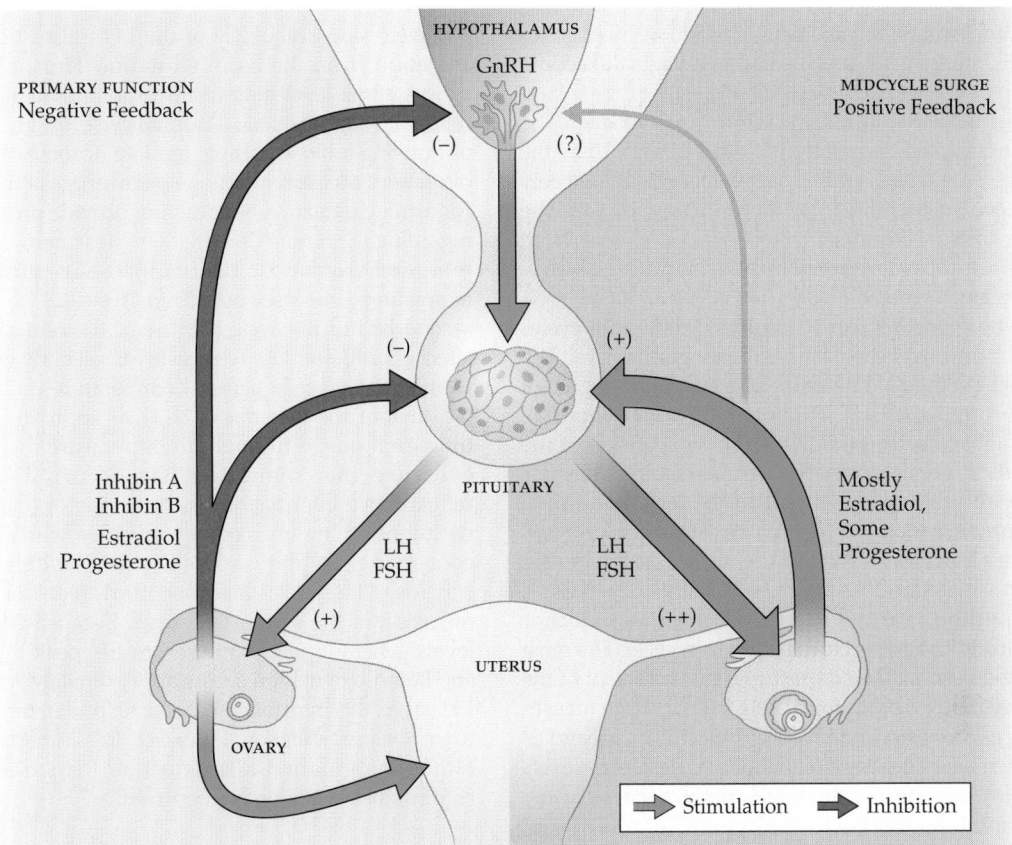

PRIMARY FUNCTION
Negative Feedback

MIDCYCLE SURGE
Positive Feedback

HYPOTHALAMUS
GnRH

(−)   (?)

(−)   (+)

PITUITARY

Inhibin A
Inhibin B
Estradiol
Progesterone

Mostly
Estradiol,
Some
Progesterone

LH
FSH

LH
FSH

(+)   (++)

UTERUS

OVARY

⇒ Stimulation   ⇒ Inhibition

Figure 1   **Normal reproductive function requires the coordinated functioning of the hypothalamus, pituitary, and ovaries. The hypothalamus secretes gonadotropin-releasing hormone (GnRH) in a pulsatile fashion to stimulate the pituitary to secrete luteinizing hormone (LH) and follicle-stimulating hormone (FSH). These gonadotropins stimulate folliculogenesis and secretion of various hormones by the ovaries, including estradiol, progesterone, inhibin A, and inhibin B. In turn, estradiol and progesterone affect the uterus and outflow tract. Rising levels of estradiol and progesterone, along with inhibin A and inhibin B secreted by the ovaries, provide negative feedback that restrains hypothalamic GnRH secretion, pituitary responsiveness to GnRH, or both. This reduces the secretion of FSH and, to a somewhat lesser extent, of LH. Suppression of FSH secretion limits the number of follicles that develop to maturity and the number of eggs that will eventually ovulate.**

At midcycle, a switch from negative to positive feedback occurs. Estradiol levels reach a critical threshold, signaling the pituitary to generate the preovulatory surge of gonadotropins.[1] In animal models, the hypothalamus is also involved in this step, but in women, its role is less clear. The switch from negative to positive feedback is not well understood but relates to the duration and level of exposure to estradiol and, to a lesser extent, progesterone, secreted by a mature ovarian follicle.

FSH secretion begins to rise during the luteal-follicular transition and before the onset of menses, stimulating the development of a new cohort of follicles and the beginning of a new cycle of follicle growth and ovulation.

If conception occurs, the corpus luteum is "rescued" by human chorionic gonadotropin (hCG). hCG, which is produced by the trophoblast, binds to the LH receptors on the corpus luteum, maintaining steroid hormone production and preventing involution of the corpus luteum. The corpus luteum is essential for maintenance of pregnancy for the first 6 to 10 weeks, until the placenta takes over steroid hormone production.

CLINICAL ASSESSMENT OF NORMAL FUNCTION

The first menstrual period, or menarche, occurs relatively late in the series of developmental milestones that characterize normal pubertal development. Menarche is generally preceded by pubic and axillary hair development, which result

from adrenal androgen secretion, and by breast development, which is very sensitive to the low levels of estrogen secreted from the ovary or peripherally converted from adrenal androgens. In the United States, menarche occurs at 12.7 years of age on average; menarche occurs at a younger age in African-American girls.[4]

Anovulatory and irregular cycles are common in the years immediately after menarche, but menstrual bleeding should become regular and predictable within 2 to 4 years. Thereafter, menstrual cycle length is approximately 28 days, with a range of 25 to 35 days considered normal.[5] Although cycle lengths vary considerably between women, cycle-to-cycle variability in an individual woman is much less and is generally thought to be +/− 2 days. Cycle lengths shorten gradually with age, however; by the time a woman has passed the age of 35, her cycles will be noticeably shorter than they were during her younger reproductive years. As women approach menopause, there is an increase in the incidence of anovulatory cycles, and bleeding patterns may become erratic, with an increase or decrease in the interval between episodes of vaginal bleeding or a change in bleeding pattern.

The duration of the luteal phase in normal cycles is relatively constant and ranges from 12 to 14 days. Thus, the variability in cycle length in normal women results largely from variations in the length of the follicular phase. The duration of menstrual bleeding in ovulatory cycles varies from 4 to 6 days in different women, but the duration is fairly consistent in a given woman.

Women who report regular monthly bleeding with cycles that do not vary by more than 4 days generally have ovulatory cycles. Some women experience a minor degree of discomfort around the time of ovulation (mittelschmerz), which is thought to be caused by the rapid expansion of the dominant follicle. Ovulatory cycles are often, but not always, associated with moliminal symptoms; the term molimimal refers to symptoms such as bloating, breast tenderness, and food cravings that may occur in the several days before menses.

Several methods can be used to determine whether ovulation is likely to have occurred in a given cycle. The most reliable method used in clinical practice is measurement of the serum progesterone level approximately 7 days before menses is expected. A progesterone level of 5 ng/ml or greater is generally taken as evidence of ovulation. Progesterone levels exhibit wide swings during the luteal phase, because of the relatively slow frequency of the LH pulses that stimulate its secretion from the corpus luteum. Thus, although a low progesterone level may result from anovulation, it may also reflect a trough value in a normal cycle, or it may be the result of drawing a blood sample too late or too early in relation to ovulation. Measurement of serum progesterone is useful in confirming ovulation but does not provide precise information regarding the timing of ovulation. Measurement of basal body temperature can be useful in this regard. Basal body temperature increases by 0.5° to 1° F (0.28° to 0.55° C) in the second half of the cycle because of the central hypothalamic effect of progesterone. To measure basal body temperature, the woman should take her oral temperature on first awakening (i.e., before she gets out of bed), at approximately the same time each day. Although a temperature increase provides evidence that ovulation has occurred and provides retrospective information on the timing of ovulation, it is not useful for timing intercourse in women who are interested in conceiving. Ovulation kits are now widely used for this purpose. They are designed to detect LH in urine as a reflection of the serum LH surge. Because peak urinary LH levels generally follow the serum LH peak by at least a day and because ovulation occurs approximately 36 hours after the LH surge, this information can be helpful in timing intercourse to just before ovulation. However, it is important to note that although ovulation kits detect an LH surge, they do not confirm that ovulation has occurred.

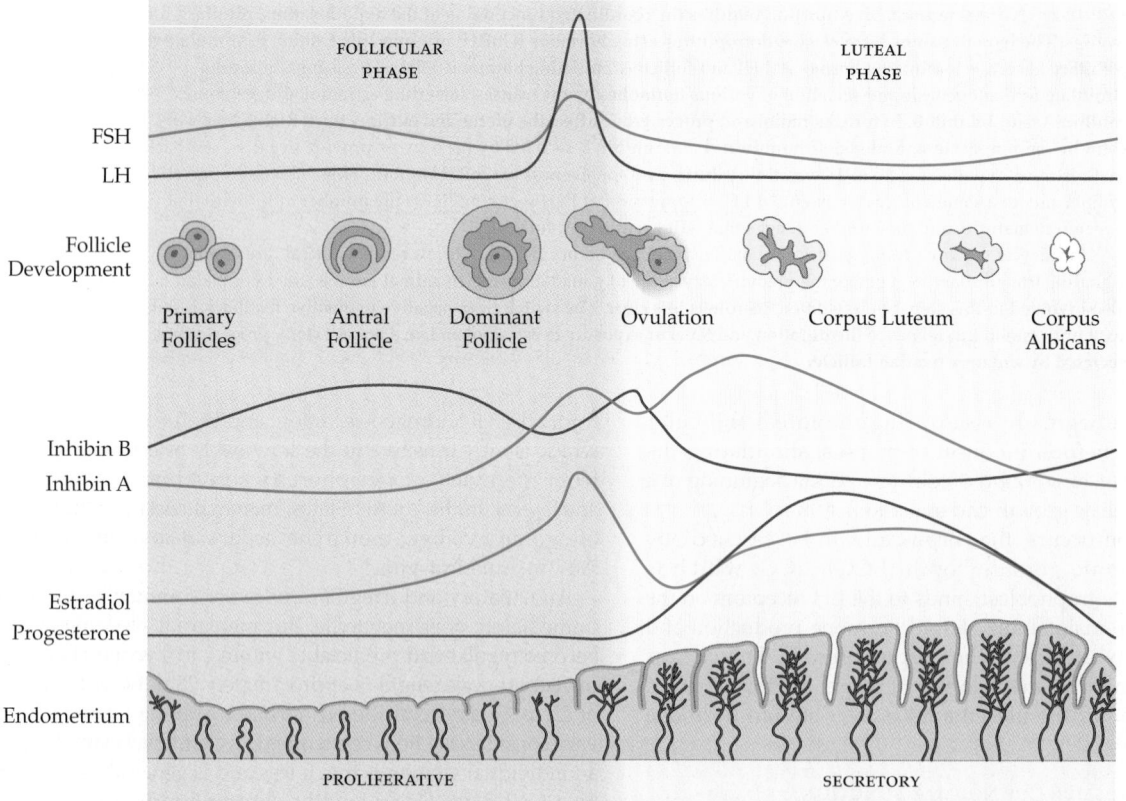

Figure 2 **Normal menstrual cycle function can be divided into the follicular phase and the luteal phase. In the follicular phase, recruitment of a single ovarian follicle and its development into a dominant follicle is associated with endometrial proliferation. In the luteal phase, the secretion of estradiol and progesterone prepares the endometrium for implantation should conception occur.**[1]

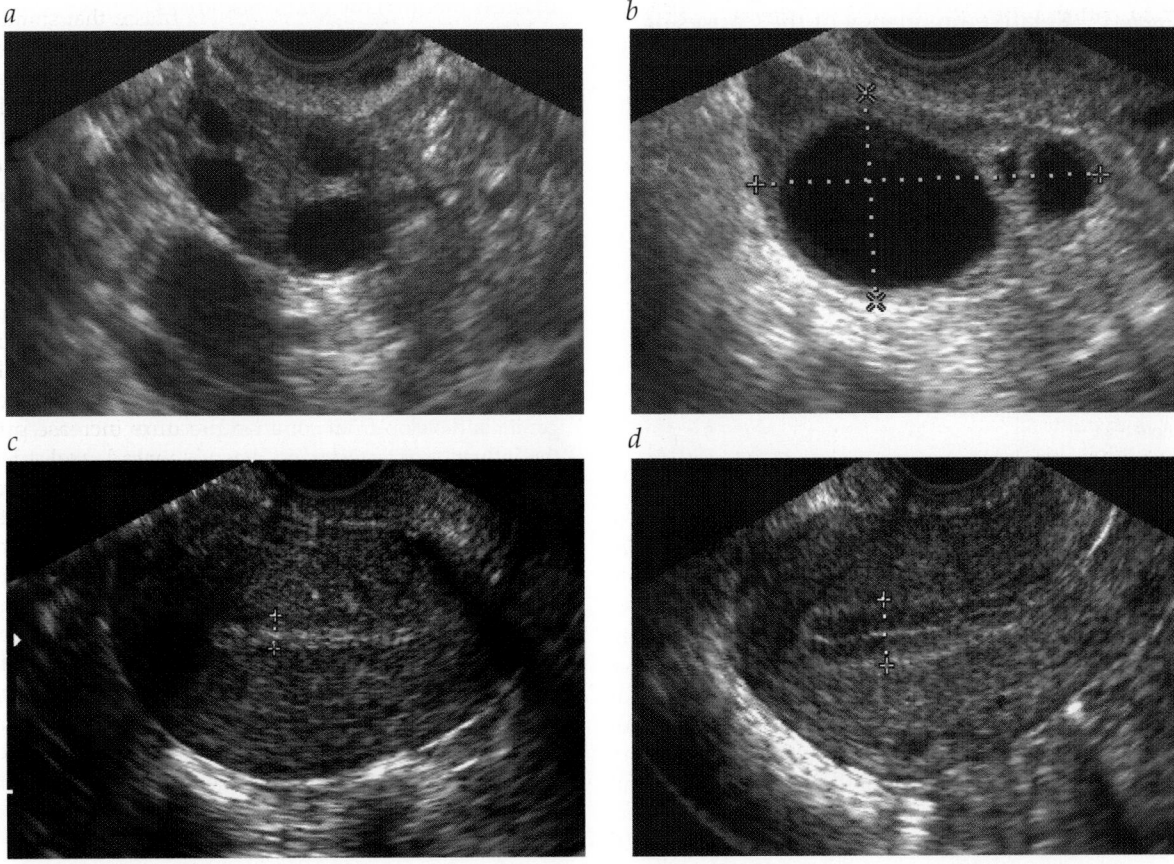

Figure 3   **Pelvic ultrasound can be used to evaluate both follicle growth and the increase in endometrial thickness during spontaneous and induced folliculogenesis. Early stimulation results in recruitment of a cohort of follicles that generally measure less than 1.0 mm in maximum diameter (*a*). In normal cycles, one of these will become dominant and grow to a preovulatory size of between 18 and 24 mm (*b*). The increase in follicle growth and estradiol secretion results in an increase in the thickness of the endometrium from 4 to 5 mm after menstruation (*c*) to 8 to 10 mm before ovulation (*d*).**

Ultrasound Assessment of Reproductive Function

Advances in the use of abdominal and transvaginal ultrasound have aided significantly in the ability to assess the ovary, uterus, and outflow tract in normal women and to use this information for evaluation of patients with menstrual cycle abnormalities. Ultrasound is used to detect the growth of the fluid-filled antrum of the developing follicle [*see Figure 3*]. It can also be used to assess the degree to which the endometrium proliferates in response to increasing estradiol levels during the follicular phase and to determine the presence of the characteristic changes in echogenicity of the secretory endometrium of the luteal phase.

Amenorrhea

DEFINITION

Abnormalities in hypothalamic GnRH secretion, pituitary responsiveness to GnRH stimulation, ovarian function, or endometrial responsiveness can disrupt normal reproductive cycles and lead to absent or irregular menses (i.e., amenorrhea or oligomenorrhea). Amenorrhea can be primary or secondary.

Primary Amenorrhea

Primary amenorrhea is diagnosed by the absence of menses with no evidence of breast development by the age of 14; the absence of menses with breast development by the age of 16; or the absence of menses more than 2 years after the onset of breast development. Girls with primary amenorrhea who are at less than the third percentile for height at age 14 should also be evaluated. Primary amenorrhea is relatively infrequent, occurring in less than 0.1% of girls in the United States.

Secondary Amenorrhea and Oligomenorrhea

Secondary amenorrhea is defined as the cessation of menses once they have begun; oligomenorrhea is defined as the occurrence of fewer than 10 menses a year or a cycle length longer than 35 days. The distinction between oligomenorrhea and amenorrhea is not always clear-cut, but the absence of menses for a period of 3 to 6 months is generally defined as amenorrhea. Approximately 5% of women in the United States experience at least 3 months of secondary amenorrhea in a given year. Both the timing of menarche and the prevalence of secondary amenorrhea are influenced by adequate nutrition and thus vary significantly in different parts of the world.

DIAGNOSIS

Evaluation of primary and secondary amenorrhea depends on an understanding of the factors that can alter function of the four critical components of the reproductive axis. For initial diagnosis, it is convenient to divide menstrual cycle abnormalities into two categories: those stemming from

Table 1 Relative Frequency of the Causes of Amenorrhea

Source of Abnormalities	Percentage of Cases	
	Primary Amenorrhea	Secondary Amenorrhea
Hypothalamus	25	35
Pituitary gland	2	20
Polycystic ovary syndrome	7	30
Ovary	45	10
Outflow tract	21	5

abnormalities of the uterus or outflow tract and those resulting from ovulatory dysfunction. Further diagnosis of ovulatory dysfunction disorders is guided by gonadotropin levels, because of the role of ovarian negative feedback in ovulatory dysfunction [see Figure 1].The relative frequency of presentation of disorders at each level of the reproductive axis is influenced by whether amenorrhea is primary[6] or secondary[7] [see Table 1]. Disorders of the ovary and uterus or of the outflow tract are relatively more common in primary than in secondary amenorrhea. Both oligomenorrhea and frequent bleeding are manifestations of disordered ovulation, and therefore, the pathophysiologic considerations are the same as for secondary amenorrhea. Finally, although a number of the processes that cause primary amenorrhea will not cause secondary amenorrhea, most processes that cause secondary amenorrhea can also produce primary amenorrhea.

A critical point is that pregnancy is the single most common cause of amenorrhea in women of reproductive age. In the early stages of pregnancy, hCG produced by the developing embryo stimulates the secretion of estrogen and progesterone from the corpus luteum. These hormones support the endometrium and provide feedback to the hypothalamus and pituitary so as to inhibit secretion of LH and FSH. Some degree of vaginal bleeding can occur between 10 days and 2 weeks after conception (i.e., around the time of an expected period), although this bleeding is often much lighter or of shorter duration than a normal period. It is therefore essential to rule out pregnancy in all women with reproductive capacity who present with abnormal menses or amenorrhea.

An algorithm for the diagnosis of amenorrhea or oligomenorrhea is presented [see Figure 4].[8] The number of tests required to make an initial diagnosis is relatively small. Although a progestin challenge test was part of many diagnostic algorithms in the past, it is no longer considered diagnostically useful because of its lack of specificity.[9,10] Neuroimaging studies are required only in specific circumstances, such as in patients with hypogonadotropic hypogonadism in the setting of primary amenorrhea or those with elevated prolactin levels or evidence of other abnormalities in hypothalamic or pituitary function. Further workup will be led by findings from the history, physical examination, and initial laboratory tests and may require referral to an endocrinologist or gynecologist.

UTERINE OR OUTFLOW TRACT DISORDERS

Although they comprise a relatively small percentage of all causes of amenorrhea, disorders of the uterus or outflow tract are a critical diagnostic consideration. This is particularly true for primary amenorrhea, but it is also relevant in selected patients with secondary amenorrhea. During embryologic development, the internal genitalia are formed from paired müllerian ducts that fuse in the midline to form the uterus, cervix, and proximal third of the vagina. In the male, secretion of müllerian-inhibiting substance (MIS; also known as antimüllerian hormone) from the developing testes causes regression of the müllerian system, whereas the action of testosterone promotes growth of the wolffian system, from which the male internal genitalia are formed. The external genitalia develop from common precursor structures. Under the influence of testosterone, external male genitalia develop; in the absence of testosterone, the female genital structures are formed, including the distal third of the vagina and the female external genitalia.

Outflow Tract Obstruction

Obstruction of the outflow tract can result from a transverse vaginal septum or an imperforate hymen. In this setting, the obstruction may be readily apparent on bimanual examination, or a tender mass may be palpated because of the accumulation of blood in the uterus or vagina. These patients present with normal pubertal development, normal gonadotropin levels, and possibly cyclic pain. Surgical correction is necessary to relieve the obstruction. There is a significant risk of endometriosis associated with this condition.

Müllerian Agenesis (Mayer-Rokitansky-Kuster-Hauser Syndrome)

Müllerian agenesis is a congenital anomaly characterized by the absence or hypoplasia of the uterus, vagina, or both. The hypothalamic-pituitary-ovarian axis is normal, and hormonal levels are within normal ranges. Mutations in the WNT4 gene have been described in association with this syndrome.[11] The clinical presentation is that of primary amenorrhea but with otherwise normal pubertal development. Patients may experience cyclic pain, depending on whether or not a rudimentary uterus is present, and are likely to need vaginal dilatation or surgical correction of the vagina. A third of patients have urinary tract abnormalities, and over 10% have skeletal abnormalities.[12] Ovarian function is normal; thus, patients are able to have children using in vitro techniques and a surrogate carrier.

Androgen Insensitivity Syndrome

Approximately 10% of all cases of primary amenorrhea result from complete androgen insensitivity syndrome, an X-linked recessive disorder.[13] Such patients have a male karyotype but are phenotypically female. They do not develop wolffian structures or male external genitalia, because of resistance to testosterone.

Diagnosis The presence of gonadally derived MIS causes regression of müllerian ducts. Consequently, affected individuals lack internal female genitalia, including the uterus and cervix, but retain the lower third of the vagina. Patients will therefore have a blind vagina on physical examination. Because of resistance to androgens, axillary and pubic hair are

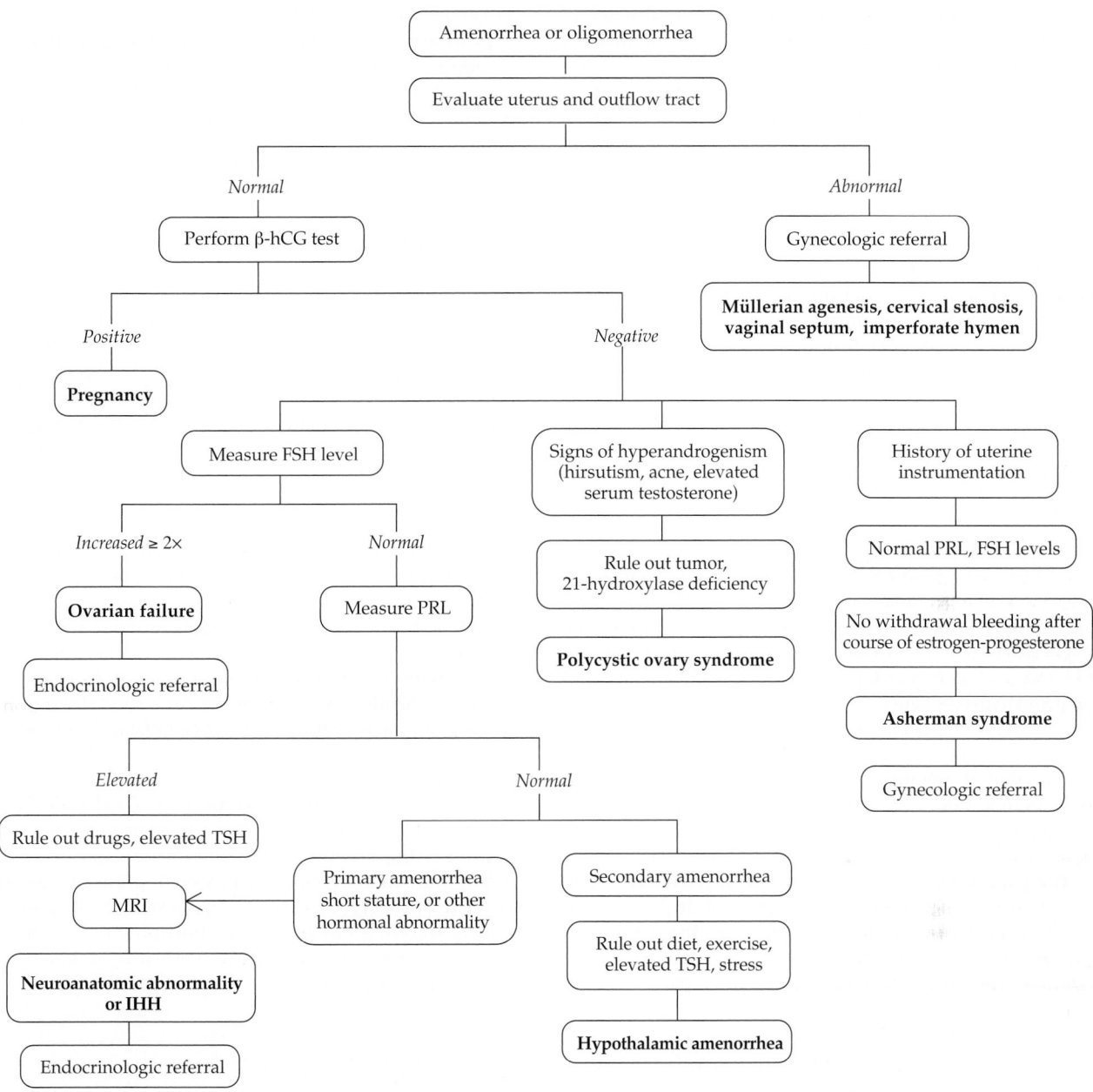

Figure 4 **Evaluation of amenorrhea.**[8] **(FSH—follicle-stimulating hormone; hCG—human chorionic gonadotropin; IHH—idiopathic hypogonadotropic hypogonadism; MRI—magnetic resonance imaging; PRL—prolactin; TSH—thyroid-stimulating hormone)**

absent or scant. Breast development is usually normal, however, because of peripheral conversion of androgens to estrogen and the lack of inhibitory androgen effects on breast tissue. Laboratory investigation reveals the presence of elevated gonadotropin levels, mildly elevated testosterone levels, and high estradiol levels.

Management   Spermatogenesis does not occur in the gonad, but there is a risk of the development of gonadoblastomas. Thus, gonadectomy is required, although whether to perform this procedure early or wait until after puberty remains controversial. After surgery, estrogen replacement is indicated, and patients may require vaginal dilatation for adequate sexual functioning. In addition, bone density should be evaluated and osteoporosis or osteopenia treated as

necessary. The development of a close relationship with the physician or a therapist is important for these patients.

Asherman Syndrome

Asherman syndrome is characterized clinically by secondary amenorrhea or decreased menstrual bleeding; it results from the partial or complete obliteration of the uterine cavity by intrauterine adhesions or synechiae that interfere with normal growth and shedding of the endometrium. The patient's history usually includes infection early in pregnancy or vigorous curettage that has removed the basal epithelial levels. Other infectious causes have also been implicated, including genital tuberculosis, brucellosis, and schistosomiasis.

Diagnosis   The diagnosis of Asherman syndrome is

suspected on the basis of the history and an absence of withdrawal bleeding after treatment with a combination regimen consisting of conjugated estrogens, 2.5 mg daily, for 35 days and medroxyprogesterone acetate, 10 mg daily, for the final 10 days. Hysterosalpingography or hysteroscopy can be used for confirmation of the diagnosis. Hormonal levels remain normal in patients with Asherman syndrome.

Management The preferred treatment of Asherman syndrome is resection of intrauterine adhesions by operative hysteroscopy, followed by estrogen therapy to foster endometrial growth. The outcome is generally excellent, with approximately 75% of patients achieving a successful pregnancy. Repeated treatments may be necessary to restore menses, however. If pregnancy is achieved, abnormalities in placentation are a potential side effect of the disease and its treatment.

DISORDERS OF OVULATION

Hypogonadotropic Hypogonadism

Hypogonadotropic hypogonadism may result from anatomic, congenital (genetic), or functional abnormalities that interfere with the normal pattern of secretion of GnRH or, less commonly, pituitary responsiveness to GnRH. In this setting, hypoestrogenism is associated with normal to low levels of LH and FSH, although the level of FSH is often somewhat higher than that of LH.

Neuroanatomic Causes of Hypogonadotropic Hypogonadism

Differential diagnosis Hypogonadotropic hypogonadism resulting from specific lesions of the hypothalamus and pituitary is much less common than hypogonadotropic hypogonadism resulting from functional causes. However, it is critical that tumors and infiltrative diseases be considered in the differential diagnosis of hypogonadotropic hypogonadism [*see Table 2*]. This is particularly true when the patient has primary amenorrhea and has not experienced puberty or has not progressed through puberty at a normal pace. It is also critical if there are other features suggestive of hypothalamic or pituitary dysfunction, such as short stature, diabetes insipidus, or galactorrhea, or if the patient presents with a history of headache. In these settings, magnetic resonance imaging or enhanced computed tomography scanning will be required.

The most common tumor affecting the hypothalamus is craniopharyngioma. Patients with craniopharyngioma usually present in childhood with short stature (as a result of the tumor's interfering with normal GnRH secretion), diabetes insipidus, or headache. Primary or secondary amenorrhea may be presenting features, however. Other tumors and infiltrative diseases are far less common but must be considered. In addition, the hypothalamus is highly sensitive to external radiation; menstrual dysfunction has been reported in up to 70% of women with such exposure. In contrast, the pituitary is much less radiosensitive. With the exception of highly focused proton-beam radiation therapy, radiation is far likely to interfere with reproductive function through damage to the hypothalamus than through damage to the pituitary.

The most common cause of hypogonadotropic hypogonadism of pituitary origin is hyperprolactinemia. Up to a third of women presenting with secondary amenorrhea can be expected to have a prolactin-secreting microadenoma.[14] Patients with prolactin-secreting microadenomas may also present with less dramatic alterations in menstrual cycle dynamics, including oligoamenorrhea or a short luteal phase. Infertility may also be the presenting complaint. As in patients with tumors that secrete growth hormone or adrenocorticotropic hormone (ACTH), the mechanism of amenorrhea in patients with prolactinomas is not the mass effect but rather the inhibition of hypothalamic GnRH secretion by hormones from the tumor. Importantly, although gonadotropin-secreting tumors were initially reported to secrete primarily inactive gonadotropin subunits,[15] there are now a number of reports of tumors secreting bioactive gonadotropins in patients of reproductive age who presented with elevated estradiol levels and ovarian hyperstimulation or endometrial hyperplasia.[16,17]

Table 2 Neuroanatomic Causes of Hypogonadotropic Hypogonadism

Pathology	Hypothalamus	Pituitary Gland
Tumors	Craniopharyngioma Germinoma Glioma Meningioma Endodermal sinus tumor Metastatic tumors Midline dermoid cyst Teratoma	Prolactinoma Acromegaly Gonadotropin-secreting tumors
Infiltrative diseases	Histiocytosis X Tuberculosis Sarcoidosis Wegener granulomatosis	Lymphocytic hypophysitis Hemochromatosis
Other	Head injury Cranial irradiation Surgery	Infarct (Sheehan syndrome) Empty sella syndrome Pituitary irradiation Surgery

Although hyperprolactinemia is most commonly thought of in association with specific prolactin-secreting tumors of the pituitary (either prolactinomas or growth hormone–secreting tumors), hyperprolactinemia may also be a sign of other neuroanatomic lesions. Both hypothalamic tumors and infiltrative diseases of the hypothalamus can result in destruction of dopamine-producing neurons, with hyperprolactinemia occurring secondary to the loss of this inhibitory regulator of prolactin secretion. Likewise, compression of the pituitary stalk by a space-occupying lesion will cause hyperprolactinemia by interfering with the flow of dopamine from the hypothalamus, which normally mediates control of prolactin secretion. Thus, persistent hyperprolactinemia in the absence of common causes of hyperprolactinemia (e.g., renal or liver disease, medications, and severe hypothyroidism) requires cranial imaging with MRI or enhanced CT.

Breast-feeding may result in amenorrhea. Rarely, postpartum amenorrhea can be caused by Sheehan syndrome, which typically follows severe obstetric hemorrhage and maternal hypotension, or by lymphocytic hypophysitis.[18] Pituitary hypofunction in Sheehan syndrome may be limited to gonadotropin deficiency, but it is generally associated with deficiencies of other pituitary hormones (e.g., prolactin, ACTH, or thyroid-stimulating hormone). In addition to amenorrhea, presenting symptoms may include failure to lactate, fatigue, and hypotension.

Management Patients with hypogonadotropic hypogonadism resulting from neuroanatomic disorders should be managed in collaboration with an endocrinologist and a neurosurgeon; these patients will require evaluation of adrenal and thyroid function, growth hormone secretion, and posterior pituitary function. Long-term replacement of some or all of these hormones will be required. Patients who remain amenorrheic after treatment should receive estrogen and progesterone replacement therapy, unless they have a meningioma, because these tumors may have estrogen and progesterone receptors. If pregnancy is desired, pulsatile GnRH therapy is effective for ovulation induction in the majority of patients.[19] Gonadotropin therapy is also effective and is more commonly available, although care must be taken to avoid multiple gestation. Medications such as clomiphene citrate are unlikely to be effective for ovulation induction in these patients.

The management strategy is somewhat different for patients with hyperprolactinemia.[14] Patients with a macroadenoma should be managed in collaboration with an endocrinologist. For patients with microadenomas who are not interested in pregnancy, oral contraceptives are a safe treatment of amenorrhea and are not associated with significant tumor growth. For patients interested in becoming pregnant, treatment with a dopamine agonist such as pergolide, which is administered daily, or cabergoline, which is administered once or twice a week, is generally effective. Treatment of patients with a microadenoma is usually discontinued once pregnancy is confirmed.

Congenital (Genetic) Causes

Etiology Isolated GnRH deficiency, or idiopathic hypogonadotropic hypogonadism (IHH) causes failure of pubertal development and primary amenorrhea in women. IHH is termed Kallmann syndrome when it is accompanied by anosmia. Although isolated GnRH deficiency is extremely rare in women, significant advances have been made in understanding the specific gene mutations involved, phenotypic variability, and treatment response. Several genes have now been associated with IHH in men and women[20] and can be broadly categorized as influencing migration of GnRH neurons from their site of origin in or near the olfactory bulb (*KAL1* and *FGFR1*), affecting control of GnRH synthesis or secretion (*GPR54, PC1, LEP,* and *LEPR*), or affecting receptivity to GnRH (*GnRHR* and *NROB1* [previously *DAX1*]). Studies of GPR54 are particularly interesting.[21] GPR54 is a G-protein–coupled receptor whose natural ligands include metastin and kisspeptin. Metastin has been shown to profoundly increase LH secretion and is hypothesized to be a mediator of puberty.

Other genetic abnormalities have been shown to cause deficiencies in gonadotropin secretion in addition to abnormalities in other pituitary hormones; these involve the genes *PROP1, HESX1,* and *LHX3.* Thus, researchers are just beginning to define the genes responsible for normal hypothalamic and pituitary function, and it is expected that other genetic causes of hypogonadotropic hypogonadism will be found.

Diagnosis Classically, women with IHH present with primary amenorrhea and an absence of breast development but with some axillary and pubic hair development, because adrenarche is normal in IHH. Patients may demonstrate eunuchoid proportions (i.e., a lower body segment that is longer than the upper and an arm span that is longer than the height) as a result of failure of epiphyseal closure. Anosmia or hyposmia may or may not be present, and there may be evidence of midline facial defects, such as a cleft lip or palate. The levels of LH, FSH, and estradiol are generally very low. The uterus is hypoplastic, as might be expected in the prepubertal state, and may not be clearly identified on ultrasound, but the external genitalia, vagina, and cervix are normal on examination. Patients with genes that influence GnRH receptivity may present with some pubertal development and even with secondary amenorrhea.[22]

Management Induction of secondary sexual characteristics in patients with hypogonadism requires initial exposure to low levels of estrogen before the addition of progesterone or a progestin. Therefore, oral contraceptives cannot be used for initial therapy. Once normal breast development has been achieved, however, these patients should be maintained on oral contraceptives until they are interested in conceiving. Uterine growth will occur with estrogen exposure. For the majority of patients (even some with *GnRHR* mutations), ovulation can be induced by pulsatile GnRH therapy; this form of therapy is the treatment of choice where available.[23,24] Alternatively, exogenous gonadotropin therapy can be used, but it is important to remember that these patients will require LH in addition to FSH for normal steroidogenesis; also, it should be borne in mind that these patients are very responsive to gonadotropin therapy and are at risk for multiple gestation.

Functional Causes

Hypothalamic amenorrhea from functional causes (HA) accounts for a third of the cases of amenorrhea in women of reproductive age. Current theories of its etiology highlight a mismatch between energy expenditure and energy intake.[25]

There is also some indication that the hypothalamic-pituitary-adrenal axis may play a role in some patients,[26] either alone or in combination with issues of energy balance. Some evidence suggests that some patients may have a particular genetic susceptibility to these stressors. Most recent attention has focused on the role of leptin in the GnRH dysfunction of HA. Compared with women with regular menstrual cycles, women with HA have lower leptin levels and the diurnal rhythm of leptin is blunted.[27] The body mass index is similar in both groups. In a study of exogenous leptin treatment, patients who received leptin for up to 3 months demonstrated an increased frequency of pulsatile LH secretion and increased folliculogenesis and ovulation.[28]

Differential diagnosis HA can present as either delayed menarche or secondary amenorrhea. It is commonly associated with exercise, nutritional deprivation, abnormal eating behaviors, and acute weight loss. The prevalence of both anorexia and bulimia in women in the affected age range makes it essential to rule out these eating disorders in the evaluation of HA; this is done by directed history [see Chapter 213]. Acute and chronic illness can lead to menstrual dysfunction; both hypothyroidism and hyperthyroidism have been associated with anovulation and infertility, as has Cushing syndrome.

Gonadotropin levels in patients with HA are generally in the low to low-normal range, and hypoestrogenism is usually present. The FSH level is generally higher than the LH level. However, the pattern of pulsatile LH (and therefore GnRH) secretion is very abnormal, and LH levels are likely to be more variable in patients with HA than in patients with IHH. The diagnosis of hypothalamic amenorrhea from functional causes is made after hypogonadotropic hypogonadism of neuroanatomic cause has been ruled out. Neuroimaging is required in all patients with hypogonadotropic hypogonadism and primary amenorrhea, but it is not required in all patients presenting with low gonadotropin levels and secondary amenorrhea; in particular, neuroimaging is not required in patients with a definite history of an eating disorder, excessive exercise, or chronic illness. Neuroimaging is advised in the absence of such a history, in patients with other forms of endocrine hypofunction, and in patients with headache.

Management Patients with HA require longitudinal follow-up. Normal menstrual function generally resumes when precipitating factors are reversed.[29] However, in a small percentage of women with secondary HA, normal menstrual function does not resume, suggesting that there may be other etiologies underlying their amenorrhea that are as yet poorly understood. Oral contraceptives will provide appropriate estrogen replacement for patients who are not interested in becoming pregnant, but contraceptives may not be sufficient for normalizing bone density in women with inadequate nutritional intake. Periodic assessment of bone density may be required, along with calcium and vitamin D supplementation. For women interested in becoming pregnant, clomiphene citrate is not usually effective, but it can be tried. Pulsatile GnRH therapy is the treatment of choice in these patients, but it is not widely available in the United States. As with treatment of IHH, exogenous gonadotropins are likely to be highly effective, but LH may be required, and risks of multiple gestation must be seriously considered. Patients with eating disorders will need ongoing psychiatric support, because pregnancy and the postpartum period put such patients at increased risk from their eating disorder.

Hypergonadotropic Hypogonadism: The Ovary

Definition and epidemiology Ovarian failure is considered premature when it occurs in women younger than 40 years of age. Premature ovarian failure (POF) occurs in less than 1% of the female population. POF accounts for about 10% of secondary amenorrhea, but it accounts for a considerably higher percentage of primary amenorrhea, because a significant proportion of POF cases are the result of genetic abnormalities.

Differential diagnosis The diagnosis of POF is established by finding gonadotropin levels in the postmenopausal range. FSH is a better marker of ovarian failure than is LH. As with normal menopause, POF may wax and wane, so serial measurements may be required to confirm the diagnosis. Once the diagnosis has been established, a workup to determine the cause is warranted, although a cause can be determined in only a minority of patients.

Turner syndrome accounts for the largest percentage of patients with POF. The streak ovaries and ovarian failure associated with this syndrome result from accelerated atresia. Recognition of Turner syndrome is important, because these patients are at risk for a significant number of other health problems,[30] including gonadal tumors resulting from the presence of Y chromosomal material. POF is also seen in association other chromosomal abnormalities, such as the triple X syndrome, blepharophimosis (resulting from mutations in the transcription factor FOXL2), and dystrophic myotonia. POF is present in premutation carriers of the fragile X syndrome, a severe mental retardation syndrome that results from a mutation in the FMR1 gene.[31] It may be appropriate to offer testing for the fragile X premutation and genetic counseling if the patient is interested in fertility and presents with some evidence of follicle growth or if she has a sister who might be interested in becoming pregnant.[32]

POF can also follow the destruction of oocytes, as occurs in patients with galactosemia; destruction of oocytes also occurs in association with chemotherapy (especially with the use of alkylating agents), radiation therapy, certain viral infections, or autoimmune processes. POF may be seen in polyglandular failure syndromes and is frequently associated with hypothyroidism. From 2% to 10% of women with POF have Addison disease or are at risk for the development of adrenal failure secondary to autoantibodies against adrenal or steroid cells.[33]

Several other disorders that result in varying degrees of hypergonadotropic hypogonadism must be considered in the differential diagnosis of POF. Mutations in the genes for gonadotropin hormones and their receptors are rare, but a number of patients with such mutations have been described.[34,35] Mutations in the FSHβ gene result in primary amenorrhea with LH levels in the menopausal range; FSH levels remain normal. This same pattern of gonadotropin levels has been described in a male patient with an LHβ mutation, but no such mutations have been described in women to date. Both FSH and LH receptor mutations have been associated with primary and secondary amenorrhea; levels of both LH and FSH are increased with FSH receptor mutations, although only LH levels are increased with LH receptor mutations. Aromatase deficiency and 17α hydroxylase deficiency are also associated with hypergonadotropic hypogonadism, in conjunction with hyperandrogenism and hypertension, respectively. Gonadotropin-secreting tumors are often thought of in association with hypergonadotropic hypogonadism; however, case reports have generally described elevated gonadotropin levels in association with high, rather than low, estrogen levels and a clinical presentation of ovarian hyperstimulation or dysfunctional bleeding.[16,17]

Management There are no proven therapies for ovarian failure. Women who are not interested in fertility should be treated with estrogen and progesterone replacement or oral contraceptives to maintain adequate bone density. Patients with Turner syndrome or an autoimmune etiology or patients in whom the initial evaluation does not disclose a cause should be followed longitudinally to monitor for possible development of autoimmune or other disorders. In general, women who are interested in becoming pregnant will be referred for oocyte donation, which has a very high chance of success. However, for patients with recently diagnosed POF, one study has shown that approximately 16% may achieve pregnancy over a 6-month period with monitoring of follicle growth, administration of hCG for ovulation, and intrauterine insemination.[36]

Polycystic Ovary Syndrome

Polycystic ovary syndrome (PCOS) affects approximately 7% of women of reproductive age. The syndrome is characterized by clinical or biochemical evidence of hyperandrogenism and menstrual dysfunction, with symptoms generally beginning shortly after menarche. Abnormalities in gonadotropin secretion and insulin dynamics are often present, and the vast majority of women with this disorder will exhibit the classic polycystic ovarian morphology. An increase in LH levels in the presence of normal FSH levels and low to normal estradiol levels are characteristic in lean patients with PCOS, whereas in obese patients with PCOS, the LH/FSH abnormality is less pronounced and insulin resistance is a more prominent feature. The diagnosis and management of PCOS are discussed in detail elsewhere [see Chapter 79].

Abnormal Vaginal Bleeding

DEFINITION

Women with normal menses bleed for up to 7 days and lose approximately 60 ml of blood during that time. Regular bleeding in excess of this duration or amount is termed menorrhagia, whereas prolonged bleeding at irregular intervals is called menometrorrhagia. A decrease in blood flow, as can be seen in Asherman syndrome, is termed hypomenorrhea.

ETIOLOGY

Abnormal bleeding patterns are often associated with anovulatory cycles, but they may also be caused by disease. The prevalence of abnormal bleeding of different causes varies by age. Bleeding related to pregnancy must be considered in all women from adolescence to menopause.

In adolescents, anovulation is common in the first several years after menarche, but heavy bleeding in this age group is frequently associated with a bleeding diathesis,[37] such as von Willebrand disease, hematologic malignancies, or the use of anticoagulants. Structural lesions or systemic illness (e.g., hypothyroidism) are less common.

The most common cause of menorrhagia in adult women, aside from pregnancy, is structural lesions. These include uterine polyps, fibroids, and adenomyosis. However, it is also critical to consider the possibility of uterine or cervical malignancy. Anovulatory and irregular cycles are associated with an increased risk of endometrial hyperplasia, and the prevalence of uterine cancer is estimated to be from 10 to 40 cases per 100,000 women in the adult age group. A bleeding diathesis and thyroid dysfunction should also be considered. In adult women, intermenstrual bleeding is not uncommon in the first 3 months of oral contraceptive use; intermenstrual bleeding that occurs after the first 3 months of contraceptive use should be evaluated. The most common causes are infections, including endometritis and cervicitis; cervical and endometrial polyps; and cancer, including the rare estrogen-secreting ovarian tumors.

Bleeding in postmenopausal women should almost always be evaluated. The exception is in women on hormone replacement therapy, in whom evaluation is not needed if bleeding begins and resolves within the first 6 to 9 months of treatment. Although the most common cause of bleeding in postmenopausal women is endometrial atrophy,[38] the risk of endometrial cancer increases after age 35. In women on hormone replacement therapy, the risk of endometrial cancer is 0.1% if the endometrial thickness is 5 mm or less on transvaginal ultrasound, but the risk is 1% with an endometrial thickness of greater than 5 mm. In women not on hormone replacement therapy, the estimated risk is 1% with an endometrial thickness of 5 mm or less and 10% with an endometrial thickness of greater than 5 mm.[39]

The specific cause of the bleeding must be recognized so that appropriate treatment can be instituted. Evaluation of all patients presenting with abnormal uterine bleeding will therefore include a careful pelvic examination, assessment of cervical cytology (i.e., a Pap smear), and a pregnancy test. Further evaluation will depend on the age and ovulatory status of the patient but may include a pelvic ultrasound to determine whether fibroids or adenomyosis are present and to assess endometrial thickness; endometrial biopsy should be performed in women older than 35 years and in women 18 to 35 years of age who have particular risk factors. The evaluation will also include a complete blood count, prothrombin time, partial thromboplastin time, and possibly tests for factor VIII and von Willebrand factor antigen. Again, no evaluation is needed for postmenopausal women on hormone replacement therapy if bleeding begins and resolves within the first 6 to 9 months of treatment.

MANAGEMENT

Management will depend on the specific cause identified. Assuming that pregnancy and endometrial cancer and intrauterine pathology have been excluded, medical and hormonal treatments are highly likely to be effective. For severe acute bleeding, high-dose oral estrogen is used, along with a balloon Foley catheter to tamponade bleeding until medical management is effective or surgical therapy is indicated. Minimally invasive procedures such as endometrial ablation may be appropriate in some patients[40]; hysterectomy is indicated only occasionally. Patients with chronic or less severe bleeding may be treated with oral contraceptives, a progesterone-releasing intrauterine device, cyclic progestin therapy, or occasionally GnRH agonists. Nonsteroidal anti-inflammatory drugs (NSAIDs) reduce flow by 20% to 50% and are useful in ovulatory women.[41] Antifibrinolytics (e.g., tranexamic acid) and danazol may also be appropriate, but their use is limited by significant side effects.

Dysmenorrhea

DEFINITION AND EPIDEMIOLOGY

Dysmenorrhea is the term given to painful menstruation. The lower abdominal discomfort is generally described as crampy; it begins with the onset of bleeding and gradually decreases over the next 12 to 72 hours. It may be associated with nausea, diarrhea, fatigue, and headache. The prevalence of dysmenorrhea in adolescents ranges from 60% to 93%, although it is considered severe in only 15%.[42] It generally begins in adolescence, approximately 2 years after menarche, in conjunction with the establishment of ovulatory cycles. Its prevalence diminishes after pregnancy and with the use of oral contraceptives.[43] Dysmenorrhea may be primary or may be secondary to pelvic disorders such as endometriosis, adenomyosis, uterine fibroids, or chronic pelvic inflammatory disease.

ETIOLOGY

Primary Dysmenorrhea

Sequential stimulation of the uterus by estrogen and progesterone results in increased stores of prostaglandin precursors, which are converted to prostaglandins during menstruation. These prostaglandins are responsible for intense uterine contractions that decrease blood flow to the myometrium, resulting in tissue hypoxia, ischemia, and pain. This cascade of events is thought to underlie primary dysmenorrhea.[44]

Secondary Dysmenorrhea

The pain associated with secondary dysmenorrhea is directly related to the specific pathologic process.

Endometriosis In endometriosis, endometrial glands and stroma are present outside of the uterus, causing intra-abdominal hemorrhage, fibrosis, and adhesions in association with hormonal stimulation of the endometriotic tissue and bleeding. Dysmenorrhea generally precedes menstruation by several days and is often also present at the time of ovulation. Painful intercourse, painful bowel movements, nodules in the uterosacral ligament, and lateral displacement of the cervix are common presenting symptoms and signs.[45] Although serum levels of CA125 are increased in endometriosis, the low negative predictive value of this marker limits its utility in evaluating women with dysmenorrhea.

Adenomyosis The presence of ectopic endometrial glands and stroma within the myometrium is termed adenomyosis. The uterus is diffusely enlarged and tender just before menses.

Dysmenorrhea is confined to menses but is often associated with excessive bleeding.

Other causes Other secondary causes of dysmenorrhea include cervical stenosis, which may be a congenital abnormality or may result from trauma, infection, or surgery. Chronic pelvic inflammatory disease causes pain in association with distortion of the pelvic anatomy by adhesions, whereas pelvic congestion originates with engorgement and thrombosis of pelvic veins and causes a burning and throbbing pain that is worse at night and with prolonged standing. Pelvic masses and uterine leiomyomas may result in dysmenorrhea; pelvic ultrasonography is highly sensitive for the detection of these conditions.

MANAGEMENT

Medical management is effective in the majority of women with dysmenorrhea. Local application of heat (i.e., use of a lower abdominal heating pad) and taking supplemental vitamins (B_1, 100 mg a day; B_6, 200 mg a day; and E, 200 to 500 IU a day) may be helpful as first-line treatments. Unless pelvic pathology is suspected, treatment with NSAIDs should be considered; NSAIDs have been associated with a response rate in excess of 80% that is sustained over multiple cycles. One approach is to start with a dose of an NSAID at the upper end of the dose range a day before the expected onset of menses and continue regular administration for 2 to 3 days. Oral contraceptives have also been shown to be effective in the treatment of dysmenorrhea. Combination pills have been most extensively studied. Some patients prefer the long-cycle regimen of 3 months of active pills, then 1 week off; however, breakthrough bleeding is a frequent reason for discontinuing this regimen. Some data indicate beneficial effects from acupuncture, herbs, yoga, and exercise and possibly transcutaneous nerve stimulation.

Patients who do not respond to NSAIDs and oral contraceptives are more likely to have a pelvic disorder, particularly endometriosis. In these patients, diagnostic laparoscopy is warranted to guide further treatment.

The author has been a consultant for Ferring Pharmaceuticals and has received grant or research support from Abbott Laboratories, Berlex, Inc., Ferring Pharmaceuticals, and Serono, Inc.

References

1. Hall JE: Neuroendocrine control of the menstrual cycle. Yen and Jaffe's Reproductive Endocrinology, 5th ed. Strauss JF, Barbieri RL, Eds. Elsevier, Philadelphia, 2004

2. Welt C, Sidis Y, Keutmann H, et al: Activins, inhibins, and follistatins: from endocrinology to signaling: a paradigm for the new millennium. Exp Biol Med (Maywood) 227:724, 2002

3. Strauss JF III, Williams CJ: The ovarian life cycle. Yen and Jaffe's Reproductive Endocrinology, Strauss JF, Barbieri RL, Eds. Elsevier, Philadelphia, 1999

4. Palmert MR, Boepple PA: Variation in the timing of puberty: clinical spectrum and genetic investigation. J Clin Endocrinol Metab 86:2364, 2001

5. Treloar AE, Boynton RE, Behn BG, et al: Variation of the human menstrual cycle through reproductive life. Int J Fertil 12:77, 1967

6. Reindollar RH, Byrd JR, McDonough PG: Delayed sexual development: a study of 252 patients. Am J Obstet Gynecol 140:371, 1981

7. Reindollar RH, Novak M, Tho SP, et al: Adult-onset amenorrhea: a study of 262 patients. Am J Obstet Gynecol 155:531, 1986

8. Seminara S, Hall J: Amenorrhea. Physicians' Information and Educational Resource (PIER). American College of Physicians, Philadelphia, 2006

9. Nakamura S, Douchi T, Oki T, et al: Relationship between sonographic endometrial thickness and progestin-induced withdrawal bleeding. Obstet Gynecol 87:722, 1996

10. Rarick LD, Shangold MM, Ahmed SW: Cervical mucus and serum estradiol as predictors of response to progestin challenge. Fertil Steril 54:353, 1990

11. Biason-Lauber A, Konrad D, Navratil F, et al: A *WNT4* mutation associated with mül-lerian-duct regression and virilization in a 46,XX woman. N Engl J Med 351:792, 2004

12. Pittock ST, Babovic-Vuksanovic D, Lteif A: Mayer-Rokitansky-Kuster-Hauser anomaly and its associated malformations. Am J Med Genet A 135:314, 2005

13. McPhaul MJ: Androgen receptor mutations and androgen insensitivity. Mol Cell Endocrinol 198:61, 2002

14. Molitch ME: Medical management of prolactin-secreting pituitary adenomas. Pituitary 5:55, 2002

15. Daneshdoost L, Gennarelli TA, Bashey HM, et al: Recognition of gonadotroph adenomas in women. N Engl J Med 324:589, 1991

16. Djerassi A, Coutifaris C, West VA, et al: Gonadotroph adenoma in a premenopausal woman secreting follicle-stimulating hormone and causing ovarian hyperstimulation. J Clin Endocrinol Metab 80:591, 1995

17. Maruyama T, Masuda H, Uchida H, et al: Follicle stimulating hormone–secreting pituitary microadenoma with fluctuating levels of ovarian hyperstimulation. Obstet Gynecol 105:1215, 2005

18. Molitch ME: Pituitary diseases in pregnancy. Semin Perinatol 22:457, 1998

19. Hall JE, Martin KA, Whitney HA, et al: Potential for fertility with replacement of hypothalamic gonadotropin-releasing hormone in long term female survivors of cranial tumors. J Clin Endocrinol Metab 79:1166, 1994

20. Seminara SB, Crowley WF Jr: Genetic approaches to unraveling reproductive disorders: examples of bedside to bench research in the genomic era. Endocr Rev 23:382, 2002

21. Seminara SB: Metastin and its G protein-coupled receptor, GPR54: critical pathway modulating GnRH secretion. Front Neuroendocrinol 26:131, 2005

22. Seminara S, Crowley WF Jr: The genetics of IHH: a paradox. Clin Endocrinol (Oxf) 55:159, 2001

23. Seminara SB, Beranova M, Oliveira LM, et al: Successful use of pulsatile gonadotropin-releasing hormone (GnRH) for ovulation induction and pregnancy in a patient with GnRH receptor mutations. J Clin Endocrinol Metab 85:556, 2000

24. Martin K, Santoro N, Hall J, et al: Clinical review 15: management of ovulatory disorders with pulsatile gonadotropin-releasing hormone. J Clin Endocrinol Metab 71:1081A, 1990

25. Warren MP, Fried JL: Hypothalamic amenorrhea: the effects of environmental stresses on the reproductive system: a central effect of the central nervous system. Endocrinol Metab Clin North Am 30:611, 2001

26. Brundu B, Loucks TL, Adler LJ, et al: Increased cortisol in the cerebrospinal fluid of women with functional hypothalamic amenorrhea. J Clin Endocrinol Metab 91:1561, 2006

27. Laughlin GA, Morales AJ, Yen SS: Serum leptin levels in women with polycystic ovary syndrome: the role of insulin resistance/hyperinsulinemia. J Clin Endocrinol Metab 82:1692, 1997

28. Welt CK, Chan JL, Bullen J, et al: Recombinant human leptin in women with hypothalamic amenorrhea. N Engl J Med 351:987, 2004

29. Perkins RB, Hall JE, Martin KA: Aetiology, previous menstrual function and patterns of neuro-endocrine disturbance as prognostic indicators in hypothalamic amenorrhoea. Hum Reprod 16:2198, 2001

30. Sybert VP, McCauley E: Turner's syndrome. N Engl J Med 351:1227, 2004

31. Murray A: Premature ovarian failure and the FMR1 gene. Semin Reprod Med 18:59, 2000

32. Conway GS, Payne NN, Webb J, et al: Fragile X premutation screening in women with premature ovarian failure. Hum Reprod 13:1184, 1998

33. Bakalov VK, Vanderhoof VH, Bondy CA, et al: Adrenal antibodies detect asymptomatic auto-immune adrenal insufficiency in young women with spontaneous premature ovarian failure. Hum Reprod 17:2096, 2002

34. McDonough PG: Molecular abnormalities of FSH and LH action. Ann N Y Acad Sci 997:22, 2003

35. Huhtaniemi IT: LH and FSH receptor mutations and their effects on puberty. Horm Res 57(suppl 2):35, 2002

36. Taylor AE, Adams JM, Mulder JE, et al: A randomized, controlled trial of estradiol replacement therapy in women with hypergonadotropic amenorrhea. J Clin Endocrinol Metab 81:3615, 1996

37. Kadir RA, Economides DL, Sabin CA, et al: Frequency of inherited bleeding disorders in women with menorrhagia. Lancet 351:485, 1998

38. Moodley M, Roberts C: Clinical pathway for the evaluation of postmenopausal bleeding with an emphasis on endometrial cancer detection. J Obstet Gynaecol 24:736, 2004

39. Goldstein SR, Zeltser I, Horan CK, et al: Ultrasonography-based triage for perimenopausal patients with abnormal uterine bleeding. Am J Obstet Gynecol 177:102, 1997

40. DeCherney AH, Diamond MP, Lavy G, et al: Endometrial ablation for intractable uterine bleeding: hysteroscopic resection. Obstet Gynecol 70:668, 1987

41. Lethaby A, Augood C, Duckitt K: Nonsteroidal anti-inflammatory drugs for heavy menstrual bleeding. Cochrane Database Syst Rev CD000400, 2002

42. Andersch B, Milsom I: An epidemiologic study of young women with dysmenorrhea. Am J Obstet Gynecol 144:655, 1982

43. Sundell G, Milsom I, Andersch B: Factors influencing the prevalence and severity of dysmenorrhoea in young women. Br J Obstet Gynaecol 97:588, 1990

44. Proctor M, Farquhar C: Dysmenorrhoea. Clin Evid 2524, 2004

45. Propst AM, Storti K, Barbieri RL: Lateral cervical displacement is associated with endometriosis. Fertil Steril 70:568, 1998

Acknowledgment

Figures 1 and 2   Seward Hung

Figure 3   Images courtesy of J. M. Adams, D.M.U.

77 Premenstrual Syndrome

Sarah L. Berga, M.D.

Premenstrual syndrome (PMS) is a recurrent constellation of affective and physical symptoms that begin during the luteal phase of the menstrual cycle and resolve completely or almost completely during the follicular phase. The number, severity, and duration of symptoms occur along a spectrum. It is estimated that 20% to 40% of women report premenstrual symptoms during the luteal phase, but only 5% to 10% of women report symptoms severe enough to significantly interfere with their lifestyle. The long-term natural history of PMS is unclear.

The fourth edition of the *Diagnostic and Statistical Manual* of the American Psychiatric Association (DSM-IV) defines a related syndrome, premenstrual dysphoric disorder (PMDD), to facilitate an accurate psychiatric diagnosis [*see Table 1*].[1] The criteria for PMDD are also used to define research populations so that therapeutic responses can be quantitated and generalized. PMDD is often considered a variant of depression, an impression buttressed by the treatment efficacy of antidepressants, particularly selective serotonin reuptake inhibitors (SSRIs), in women who meet the criteria for PMDD.[2-4]

Pathogenesis

Most evidence suggests that PMS/PMDD is caused by aberrant responses of target tissues, particularly the brain, to normal fluctuations in serum levels of ovarian gonadal steroids.[5-7] The causes of the untoward central nervous system responses are not firmly established[8] [*see Table 2*], but several pathogenic mechanisms are currently being explored. Altered metabolism of progesterone by the CNS may lead to altered CNS reactivity and neurotransmission. Specifically, one of the principal metabolites of progesterone, allopregnanolone, decreases anxiety. Women with PMS show lower levels of allopregnanolone during their luteal phase[9,10]; they may instead produce a predominance of anxiogenic progesterone metabolites.

PMS/PMDD may involve alterations in CNS neurotransmission that cause heightened reactivity to normal excursions in gonadal steroid levels. This exaggerated reactivity may be inherited or acquired. An acquired cause of altered CNS neurotransmission is chronic stress. Chronobiologic disturbances documented in women with PMDD have been interpreted as evidence of an underlying aberration in CNS function.[11] High levels of estrogen or of estrogen and progesterone may elicit or aggravate this underlying brain dysfunction, which would explain why symptoms are greatest during the luteal phase or at ovulation. In women with PMS/PMDD, but not in women without it, the symptom complex can be replicated by exposure to, followed by withdrawal from, exogenous estrogen and progesterone.[12] There is also an association between PMS and dysmenorrhea, further suggesting that PMS is an exaggerated tissue response to normal hormonal changes.

Diagnosis

To warrant medical attention, evaluation, and intervention, premenstrual symptoms must be recurrent and sufficiently severe to interfere with daily work and social activities. To establish the diagnosis of PMS/PMDD, the clinician must confirm that the patient has the characteristic manifestations of the disorder at the appropriate time in her menstrual cycle.

It is also important to identify any concurrent conditions likely to complicate treatment [*see Table 3*]. Many women with PMS/PMDD have a personal or family history of alcoholism. A history of sexual abuse, particularly in childhood or adolescence, may be common in women with severe PMS/PMDD.[13] This population also has an increased personal and family history of posttraumatic stress disorder, mood disorders, schizophrenia, eating disorders, postpartum depression or psychosis, personality disorders, and anxiety disorders. A positive family history does not necessarily imply an inherited biologic vulnerability, because persistent exposure to dysfunctional family interactions is a chronic stress that can alter underlying CNS function.

Conclusive diagnosis of PMS/PMDD requires the documentation of concordance between symptoms and the luteal or periovulatory phase. The diagnosis of PMS/PMDD cannot be made in an anovulatory patient. Ideally, symptoms and menstrual dates should be followed prospectively to establish synchrony between the luteal phase and increase in symptoms. Two or more cycles and at least five symptoms [*see Table 1*] should be charted before the diagnosis is made. However, with a patient who is suffering severe psychological distress, there may not be time for prospective evaluation. Immediate referral to a psychiatrist may be indicated to prevent suicide or homicide.

If the menstrual cycle is irregular (the menstrual cycle ordinarily lasts from 26 to 30 days) and there is no clear pattern of symptoms, the progesterone level should be measured weekly throughout a cycle to determine whether there is a luteal phase. A progesterone concentration greater than 5 ng/ml, or 15 nmol/L, is generally considered evidence that a woman is in the luteal phase and ovulation is impending. No rise in progesterone indicates anovulation, which may be stress induced. Pa-

---

Table 1   DSM-IV Criteria for Premenstrual Dysphoric Disorder

Symptoms occur in the luteal phase, with prospective confirmation of a 30% increase in symptoms during the luteal phase above the level in the follicular phase

Not an exacerbation of major depression, panic dysthymia, or personality disorder

Marked disturbance in functioning

At least five of the following:

Marked lability	headache, joint or muscle pain, bloating, weight gain)
Marked irritability	
Marked anxiety	
Markedly depressed mood	Avoidance of social activities
Decreased interest	Decreased productivity
Lethargy	Increased sensitivity to rejection
Difficulty concentrating	
Food craving	Feeling overwhelmed
Hypersomnia or insomnia	Feeling out of control
Physical symptoms (breast tenderness or swelling,	Increased interpersonal conflict

---

Table 2 Potential Causes of PMS/PMDD

Aberrant responses of target tissues, especially the brain, to normal gonadal steroid exposures mediated by the following:

    Opioid withdrawal
    Serotonergic imbalance
    Entrainment to endogenous cycles
    Chronobiologic disturbance
    Membrane effects of steroids or steroid metabolites
    Genomic effects of steroids
    Variation in steroid metabolism

---

tients with PMS/PMDD may require further evaluation [*see Chapter 76*]. Symptoms should be charted concurrently with progesterone levels. To meet the diagnostic criteria for PMS/PMDD, the patient's symptoms should become at least 30% more severe during the luteal phase (or when the progesterone concentration is greater than 5 ng/ml) than they were in the follicular phase.

DIFFERENTIAL DIAGNOSIS

If a patient has regular menses and severe dysmenorrhea but no behavioral symptoms, she should be evaluated for possible endometriosis [*see Chapter 79*]. As with all psychiatric diagnoses, it is important to exclude organic causes. In PMS/PMDD, it is especially important to exclude thyroid dysfunction (hyperthyroidism or hypothyroidism) and drug abuse or dependence as contributing factors.

Premenstrual changes in hormone levels can exacerbate underlying medical conditions, including migraine, epilepsy, asthma, irritable bowel syndrome, and diabetes mellitus.[14-16] Such an exacerbation of symptoms is not PMS/PMDD but may resemble it. There is controversy concerning whether depression associated with PMDD represents a premenstrual exacerbation of underlying depression or is a separate clinical entity. However, women with depression often report a premenstrual increase in their dysphoria and depressive symptoms.

If behavioral symptoms are severe and are present throughout the menstrual cycle and if there is no clear pattern of increase in symptom severity during the luteal phase, another psychiatric diagnosis must be considered. The following psychiatric disorders must be excluded: major depression, panic and anxiety disorders, dysthymia, and personality disorder. Such patients should be referred to a psychiatrist for definitive diagnosis and treatment. The most important condition to exclude is depression.

Treatment

Available therapies for PMS/PMDD range from lifestyle modification to surgery. Sustained improvement in a woman with PMS/PMDD generally requires a combination of modalities. The severity of a patient's symptoms and her response to particular modalities should guide the choice of therapies and the pace of their introduction. Mild cases can be treated with lifestyle modification and nonpharmacologic options; severe cases deserve immediate and aggressive intervention.

NONPHARMACOLOGIC THERAPY

Lifestyle interventions for PMS/PMDD include institution of good sleep patterns and regular exercise. The patient should reduce or eliminate the use of tobacco, alcohol, and other drugs.

Dietary treatment helps some patients with PMS/PMDD. Certain vitamin and mineral supplements, including vitamin D, vitamin E, calcium, and magnesium, may be beneficial.[17,18] It has been suggested that diets high in carbohydrates and protein buttress the serotonergic axis.[19] A diet high in tryptophan, a precursor of serotonin, may also be of benefit for patients with mild PMS/PMDD.[20]

Full-spectrum bright-light therapy given in the evening has been shown to markedly reduce symptoms of PMS/PMDD[21,22]; its use can be limited to the luteal phase. Other studies do not support the effectiveness of this form of therapy. A meta-analysis of four small trials found the benefit of bright-light therapy for relief of PMS/PMDD symptoms to be uncertain.[23] Stress management is integral to lifestyle treatment. Biofeedback,[24] massage,[25] and other relaxation methods may be helpful.[26] Education, emotional support, and attention from the physician or therapist are instrumental. However, almost any intervention can be temporarily helpful, as the placebo response is quite high in this disorder.

Some women may wish to treat their PMS/PMDD with herbal remedies, such as oil of primrose, chaste tree berries, or St. John's wort [*see Chapter 9*]. The use of herbal medicine and other complementary and alternative measures for PMS/PMDD has not been strongly validated in randomized, controlled trials.[27] However, a randomized, placebo-controlled trial of 170 women found that fruits of the Vitex agnus castus (i.e., chaste tree) significantly decreased PMS/PMDD irritability, mood variability, anger, headache, and breast fullness, as compared with placebo.[28] More evidence is required to determine the role this agent has in the treatment of PMS/PMDD. Because agnus castus is not controlled by the Food and Drug Administration, it should be used with caution.

Behavioral Therapy

Patients with PMS/PMDD may benefit from cognitive-behavioral therapy or interpersonal therapy.[29] These are formal, structured psychotherapies designed to help patients institute behavioral changes and address cognitive patterns that sustain maladaptive behavior. Response to treatment may take as long as 6 months, but the effects persist indefinitely and the benefits accrue over time. If a patient is having difficulty coping with her symptoms during the early months of psychotherapy, there is no reason not to add pharmacologic treatment. The effects of medication are more rapid in onset than those of psychotherapy, but the effects persist only as long as the patient takes the medication. The model of combined psychotherapy and pharmacotherapy is considered the most effective approach to major depression. In a randomized study comparing psychotherapy, pharmacotherapy (i.e., the use of fluoxetine),

---

Table 3 Pertinent History in PMS/PMDD

Reproductive events	Sleep
Dysmenorrhea	Drug, alcohol, and medication use
Psychosocial adjustments and stressors	
Diet	Endocrine disorders
Exercise	Family and personal history of psychiatric disorders

and psychotherapy combined with pharmacotherapy, significant improvement in PMS/PMDD symptoms was evident in all three treatment groups; no additional benefit was gained by combination therapy.[29]

Disposition

Benefit from nonpharmacologic interventions should be evident within two menstrual cycles. If the patient has shown no improvement at all during that time, the clinician should move on to pharmacotherapy. The frequency and timing of follow-up visits depend on the severity of PMS/PMDD symptoms. Complete resolution of symptoms is rare, regardless of the degree of severity and choice of treatment plan. However, improvement of symptoms can occur with treatment, and the patient should not be robbed of positive expectations.

It is reasonable to wait more than 2 months for a response in a patient who has initiated behavioral therapy in a formal psychiatric setting. On the other hand, with a patient who is in severe psychological distress, 2 months may be too long to wait. The worst-case scenario is that such a patient will interpret a prescription of lifestyle modification and a distant follow-up appointment as a dismissal by her physician and not return for consultation or a change in treatment plan. Clinicians who have limited psychiatric expertise or who practice in a stringent managed-care setting that severely restricts follow-up might consider referring severely distressed patients to a psychiatrist, if one is available and affordable.

Pharmacologic Therapies for Somatic Symptoms

Bromocriptine (2.5 mg/day orally) has been promoted as a treatment for breast tenderness. Spironolactone (25 to 50 mg/day orally) has been given to alleviate bloating. Nonsteroidal anti-inflammatory drugs can be effective treatment for dysmenorrhea.

Progesterone treatment has been shown to be ineffective for PMS/PMDD.[30] Oral contraceptives are likely to aggravate rather than attenuate PMS/PMDD symptoms. Preliminary evidence suggests that a new oral contraceptive pill (Yasmin) containing a combination of low-dose estrogen and the progestin drospirenone can reduce water retention and other symptoms of PMS/PMDD.[31]

Pharmacologic Therapies for Affective Symptoms

Because the pathogenesis of PMS/PMDD probably involves an aberrant CNS response to normal ovarian function, the first-line treatment is to buttress CNS function with antidepressants. The SSRIs fluoxetine (20 mg/day orally), sertraline (50 mg/day), and paroxetine (12.5 mg once daily in the morning; may be increased to 25 mg/day) have been shown to be effective[2-4]; other agents in this class presumably would work but are not as well studied. Although use of SSRIs can be limited to the luteal phase (10 to 14 days), that approach is impractical for many patients, who may have difficulty determining when to start the drug. It is simpler for patients to take the medication every day as long as side effects from the SSRI are not limiting.

Sertraline has a shorter half-life than fluoxetine. The advantage of a shorter half-life is that if the patient experiences unacceptable side effects, the side effects will fade more rapidly once the medication is discontinued. The most prominent side effect of SSRIs in patients with PMS/PMDD—and a common reason for poor compliance with SSRI therapy for the disorder—is sexual dysfunction.[32] Some patients are willing to accept impaired libido as a trade-off for the relief of their symptoms. Buspirone is mildly effective for PMS/PMDD and may be a useful alternative in patients who find the sexual side effects unacceptable.[33] Classified as an atypical antidepressant, buspirone tends to be used for the anxious variety of depression.

Benzodiazepine therapy with alprazolam, taken during the luteal phase, is appropriate for patients whose main symptom is anxiety.[34] However, alprazolam has many more side effects than do SSRIs, even though the dose can be titrated to minimize side effects.

Pharmacologic Interventions that Alter Ovarian Steroid Exposure

Patients with PMS/PMDD who fail to respond adequately to lifestyle modification, oral contraceptive use, and SSRI therapy or who refuse or are unable to follow such measures can be treated with gonadotropin-releasing hormone (GnRH) agonist therapy (e.g., leuprolide, nafarelin, or goserelin).[35-38] GnRH agonists effect a medical oophorectomy. They cannot be continued indefinitely without hormone replacement therapy because of concerns about the long-term deleterious effects of sustained hypoestrogenism, particularly bone loss. Add-back hormone regimens generally involve continuous exposure to small amounts of both estrogen and progestin,[38] thereby obviating the hormonal changes associated with a menstrual cycle.

There is a variety of hormonal preparations available for add-back regimens. It is usually a good idea to administer the estrogen and progestin separately at first, so that the response to each can be monitored. The progestin dose must be large enough to prevent endometrial hyperplasia but below the threshold for triggering PMS/PMDD symptoms. Use of a progestin-containing intrauterine device (IUD) may be considered as an option for minimizing exposure to progestin. Ongoing exposure to even small amounts of progestin (e.g., oral medroxyprogesterone acetate, 2.5 mg daily) may provoke symptoms, however.

The synthetic androgen danazol can be used to temporarily suppress endogenous ovarian function and provide an androgenic environment. However, its side effects may be as problematic as the PMS/PMDD symptoms. The androgenic side effects of danazol include voice changes, hirsutism, and breast regression, all of which may be permanent.

Surgical Therapy

GnRH agonist therapy is expensive; therefore, if a patient is responding well to a GnRH agonist and has completed her childbearing, oophorectomy and hysterectomy may be a reasonable step.[39] Surgery may also be the therapy of choice for patients who have sustained improvement with GnRH-agonist therapy but experience recurrent symptoms with add-back hormone regimens. Postoperatively, these patients are given hormone replacement therapy with continuous estrogen alone. Continuing SSRI therapy may be indicated.

The author has served as a consultant for Berlex, Inc.

References

1. American Psychiatric Association: Diagnostic and Statistical Manual of Psychiatric Disorders, 4th ed. United States Department of Health and Human Services, Washington, DC, 1996, p 714

2. Wyatt KM, Dimmock PW, O'Brien PM: Selective serotonin reuptake inhibitors for premenstrual syndrome. Cochrane Database Syst Rev (4)CD001396, 2002

3. Freeman EW: Luteal phase administration of agents for the treatment of premenstrual dysphoric disorder. CNS Drugs 18:453, 2004

4. Steiner M, Pearlstein T, Cohen LS, et al: Expert guidelines for the treatment of severe PMS, PMDD, and comorbidities: the role of SSRIs. J Womens Health (Larchmt) 15:57, 2006

5. Sundstrom I, Andersson A, Nyberg S, et al: Patients with premenstrual syndrome have a different sensitivity to a neuroactive steroid during the menstrual cycle compared to control subjects. Neuroendocrinology 67:126, 1998

6. Rabin DS, Schmidt PJ, Campbell G, et al: Hypothalamic-pituitary-adrenal function in patients with the premenstrual syndrome. J Clin Endocrinol Metab 71:1158, 1990

7. Epperson CN, Haga K, Mason GF, et al: Cortical gamma-aminobutyric acid levels across the menstrual cycle in healthy women and those with premenstrual dysphoric disorder: a proton magnetic resonance spectroscopy study. Arch Gen Psychiatry 59:851, 2002

8. Berga SL: Understanding premenstrual syndrome. Lancet 351:465, 1998

9. Rapkin AJ, Morgan M, Goldman L, et al: Progesterone metabolite allopregnanolone in women with premenstrual syndrome. Obstet Gynecol 90:709, 1997

10. Lombardi I, Luisi S, Quirici B, et al: Adrenal responses to adrenocorticotropic hormone stimulation in patients with premenstrual syndrome. Gynecol Endocrinol 18:79, 2004

11. Parry BL, Berga SL, Kripke DF, et al: Altered waveform of plasma nocturnal melatonin secretion in premenstrual depression. Arch Gen Psychiatry 47:1139, 1990

12. Schmidt PJ, Nieman LK, Danaceau MA, et al: Differential behavioral effects of gonadal steroids in women with and in those without premenstrual syndrome. N Engl J Med 338:209, 1998

13. Golding JM, Taylor DL, Menard L, et al: Prevalence of sexual abuse history in a sample of women seeking treatment for premenstrual syndrome. J Psychosom Obstet Gynaecol 21:69, 2000

14. Case AM, Reid RL: Menstrual cycle effects on common medical conditions. Compr Ther 27:65, 2001

15. Martin VT, Wernke S, Mandell K, et al: Symptoms of premenstrual syndrome and their association with migraine headache. Headache 46:125, 2006

16. Altman G, Cain KC, Motzer S, et al: Increased symptoms in female IBS patients with dysmenorrhea and PMS. Gastroenterol Nurs 29:4, 2006

17. Bertone-Johnson ER, Hankinson SE, Bendich A, et al: Calcium and vitamin D intake and risk of incident premenstrual syndrome. Arch Intern Med 165:1246, 2005

18. Douglas S: Premenstrual syndrome: evidence-based treatment in family practice. Can Fam Physician 48:1789, 2002

19. Wurtman JJ, Brzezinski A, Wurtman RJ, et al: Effect of nutrient intake on premenstrual depression. Am J Obstet Gynecol 161:1228, 1989

20. Sayegh R, Schiff I, Wurtman J, et al: The effect of a carbohydrate-rich beverage on mood, appetite, and cognitive function in women with premenstrual syndrome. Obstet Gynecol 86:520, 1995

21. Parry BL, Berga SL, Mostofi N, et al: Morning versus evening bright light treatment of late luteal phase dysphoric disorder. Am J Psychiatry 146:1215, 1989

22. Parry BL, Mahan AM, Mostofi N, et al: Light therapy of late luteal phase dysphoric disorder: an extended study. Am J Psychiatry 150:1417, 1993

23. Krasnik C, Montori VM, Guyatt GH, et al: The effect of bright light on depression associated with premenstrual dysphoric disorder. Am J Obstet Gynecol 193:658, 2005

24. Van Zak DB: Biofeedback treatments for premenstrual and premenstrual affective syndromes. Int J Psychosom 41:53, 1994

25. Hernandez-Reif M, Martinez A, Field T, et al: Premenstrual symptoms are relieved by massage therapy. J Psychosom Obstet Gynaecol 21:9, 2000

26. Girman A, Lee R, Kligier B: An integrative medicine approach to premenstrual syndrome. Am J Obstet Gynecol 188:S56, 2003

27. Stevinson C, Ernst E: Complementary/alternative therapies for premenstrual syndrome: a systematic review of randomized controlled trials. Am J Obstet Gynecol 185:227, 2001

28. Schellenberg R: Treatment for the premenstrual syndrome with agnus castus fruit extract: prospective, randomized, placebo-controlled study. BMJ 322:134, 2001

29. Blake F, Salkovskis P, Gath D, et al: Cognitive therapy for premenstrual syndrome: a controlled trial. J Psycosom Res 45:307, 1998

30. Wyatt K, Dimmock P, Jones P, et al: Efficacy of progesterone and progestogens in management of premenstrual syndrome: systematic review. BMJ 323:776, 2001

31. Yonkers KA, Brown C, Pearlstein TB, et al: Efficacy of a new low-dose oral contraceptive with drospirenone in premenstrual dysphoric disorder. Obstet Gynecol 106:492, 2005

32. Sundstrom-Poromaa I, Bixo M, Bjorn I, et al: Compliance to antidepressant drug therapy for treatment of premenstrual syndrome. J Psychosom Obstet Gynaecol 21:205, 2000

33. Landen M, Eriksson O, Sundblad C, et al: Compounds with affinity for serotonergic receptors in the treatment of premenstrual dysphoria: a comparison of buspirone, nefazodone and placebo. Psychopharmacology (Berl) 155:292, 2001

34. Freeman EW, Rickels K, Sondheimer SJ, et al: A double-blind trial of oral progesterone, alprazolam, and placebo in treatment of severe premenstrual syndrome. JAMA 274:51, 1995

35. Freeman EW, Sondheimer SJ, Rickels K: Gonadotropin-releasing hormone agonist in the treatment of premenstrual syndrome with and without ongoing dysphoria: a controlled study. Psychopharmacol Bull 33:303, 1997

36. Brown CS, Ling FW, Andersen RN, et al: Efficacy of depot leuprolide in premenstrual syndrome: effect of symptom severity and type in a controlled trial. Obstet Gynecol 84:779, 1994

37. Mezrow G, Shoupe D, Spicer D, et al: Depot leuprolide acetate with estrogen and progestin add-back for long-term treatment of premenstrual syndrome. Fertil Steril 62:932, 1994

38. Di Carlo C, Palomba S, Tommaselli GA, et al: Use of leuprolide acetate plus tribolone in the treatment of severe premenstrual syndrome. Fertil Steril 75:380, 2001

39. Cronje WH, Vashist A, Studd JW: Hysterectomy and bilateral oophorectomy for severe premenstrual syndrome. Hum Reprod 19:2152, 2004

78 Endometriosis

Robert L. Barbieri, M.D., F.A.C.P.

Definition and Pathophysiology

Endometriosis is a condition in which tissue resembling endometrial glands or stroma occurs outside the uterus. Endometriosis lesions are most often found in the pelvis. Common sites are the peritoneal surfaces posterior to the uterus; the ovary; the peritoneal surfaces anterior to the uterus; the bowel; the bladder; and the appendix. Rarely, endometriosis lesions occur at sites outside the pelvis, such as the respiratory diaphragm.

Endometriosis lesions are heterogeneous, ranging from 1 mm superficial peritoneal lesions to 4 cm deeply invasive lesions in the rectovaginal septum. Ovarian lesions of endometriosis can grow to 4 to 10 cm in size, necessitating surgical resection. Endometriosis lesions undergo cycles of growth and bleeding in tandem with the menstrual cycle. Intraperitoneal bleeding from the lesions elicits an inflammatory response in the pelvis that is associated with pain and infertility.

Epidemiology

Many authorities believe that approximately 5% of women between 15 and 45 years of age have endometriosis.[1] The precise incidence is difficult to determine because there is no inexpensive, highly reliable method for diagnosing endometriosis. The current gold standard for the diagnosis of endometriosis is surgical visualization of endometriosis lesions, usually by laparoscopy, and so (as with any disease that requires expensive and invasive procedures for diagnosis) a significant number of cases may be missed.[2] Collection of definitive data would require selecting a random sample of women and performing laparoscopy on them to determine whether they have endometriosis; understandably, no such study has been done.

Endometriosis is rare before menarche and after menopause, when estrogen production is low. Most cases of endometriosis are diagnosed in women in their 20s who have never had a child. Full-term pregnancy and delivery appear to markedly reduce the risk of developing endometriosis. Multiple full-term pregnancies further reduce the risk. Long periods of amenorrhea (for example, the amenorrhea of athletes) is associated with a reduced risk of endometriosis, as is aerobic exercise for more than 7 hours a week.

Pathogenesis

The pathogenesis of endometriosis lesions involves mechanical, hormonal, immunologic, and genetic factors. The prominence of particular factors may vary from case to case; indeed, it is possible that endometriosis comprises several different diseases with a common clinical outcome.

MECHANICAL FACTORS

In women with a normal uterus, 99.9% of menstrual blood flow occurs in an antegrade direction—that is, from the endometrium through the cervix and into the vagina. Numerous clinical observations as well as experiments in laboratory animals indicate that anatomic changes, such as cervical stenosis, that hinder antegrade flow are associated with an increased risk of endometriosis. In women with cervical stenosis, the relative obstruction at the level of the cervix causes blood to flow from the uterus back through the fallopian tubes and into the peritoneal cavity. This retrograde menstrual flow contains blood, growth factors, and viable bits of endometrial tissue. The greater the amount of retrograde blood flow, the higher the risk of endometriosis. For example, about 80% of women with congenital cervical stenosis and a functioning endometrium will develop endometriosis. Epidemiologic studies suggest that more prolonged menstrual flow (> 8 days) and more frequent menses (cycle length < 27 days) are also associated with an increased risk of endometriosis.[3]

HORMONAL FACTORS

Steroid hormones control the growth and function of endometriosis lesions. Estradiol stimulates growth, and androgens cause atrophy of endometriosis lesions [*see Table 1*]. High doses of progestins induce terminal differentiation in endometriosis lesions, a process called pseudodecidualization. Once endometriosis tissue undergoes pseudodecidualization, it can no longer grow. The reason pregnancy reduces the risk of endometriosis is probably that the extremely high progesterone levels that occur in pregnancy cause pseudodecidualization of endometriosis lesions.

Organochlorine chemicals (e.g., dioxin) can disrupt steroid metabolism; exposure to these pollutants has been proposed as a factor in the development of endometriosis. In animal models, dioxin has been found to increase the incidence and severity of endometriosis,[4] possibly by interfering with the action of progesterone,[5] but the effect in humans has yet to be confirmed.

Table 1 Effects of Different Steroids on Endometrium and Endometriosis Lesions

Steroid	Effect on Endometrium	Effect on Endometriosis Lesions
Estrogen	Growth	Growth
Androgen	Atrophy	Atrophy
Progesterone at physiologic concentrations	Differentiation and secretory changes	No effect on lesions that have no progesterone receptors; differentiation and secretory changes in lesions with progesterone receptors
Progesterone at high concentrations	Decidualization	Pseudodecidualization (a terminal differentiation step)

IMMUNOLOGIC FACTORS

Numerous studies indicate that in women with endometriosis, the pelvic peritoneal environment is immunologically abnormal, with increased concentrations of white blood cells, cytokines, and growth factors. Indeed, elevated levels of cytokines—specifically, tumor necrosis factor–α in peritoneal fluid and interleukin-6 in serum—have been proposed as a potential diagnostic marker for endometriosis.[6] One group of researchers has found an increased incidence of autoimmune disease in women with endometriosis—a finding that supports the concept that immunologic abnormalities play a role in the development of endometriosis.[7]

Some authorities believe that in women with endometriosis, a primary immunologic abnormality prevents the clearance, from the peritoneal environment, of the endometrial tissue fragments deposited by retrograde menstruation.[8] This postulated primary alteration in the immune response allegedly contributes to the development of endometriosis. Other authorities believe that the observed peritoneal immunologic changes are not a cause of endometriosis but a consequence of it: the endometriosis lesions produce a chronic pelvic inflammation, which leads to an increase of immune cells in the peritoneal fluid. Interestingly, factors secreted by these immune cells appear to promote angiogenesis and cause endometriosis lesions to grow. It is likely that there is cross-talk between the immune system and endometriosis lesions: endometriosis lesions cause inflammation, inducing immune cells to enter the peritoneal environment; in turn, immune cells secrete factors that can stimulate the growth of endometriosis lesions.

GENETIC ABNORMALITIES

The risk of endometriosis is approximately doubled in first-degree relatives of women with endometriosis.[9] The heritable aspects of endometriosis may involve alterations in the immune response that predispose women to ectopic transplantation and survival of endometrial tissue.

Ovarian endometriosis cysts (endometriomas) are monoclonal and appear to arise from a somatic mutation in a precursor cell, although those mutations have not been characterized.[10] This finding suggests that a small number of genes play a central role in the pathogenesis of endometriosis.

ENDOMETRIOSIS AND INFERTILITY

An association between endometriosis and infertility in women has long been noted,[11] and many possible mechanisms for the infertility have been identified. Nevertheless, the hypothesis that endometriosis decreases fertility has not been definitively proved by consistent data from rigorous studies.

In advanced endometriosis, infertility can have an anatomic cause: adhesions interfere with the release of the ovum from the ovary and its uptake into the fallopian tube. Although women with early-stage endometriosis often have reduced fertility, a causal link between the endometriosis and the infertility is not clear.

Abnormalities in peritoneal, tubal, and endometrial function caused by endometriosis may inhibit fertility, especially in women with early-stage disease.[11] Numerous investigators have reported peritoneal abnormalities in women with endometriosis, including an increased volume of peritoneal fluid[12] and increased concentrations of activated macrophages,[13] prostaglandin, interleukin-1, tumor necrosis factor, and proteases.[14] Peritoneal fluid from women with advanced endometriosis appears to inhibit sperm function, thereby possibly reducing fertility.[15]

A few investigators have reported that women with endometriosis may have increased levels of antiendometrial antibodies, which may impair endometrial function.[16,17] Some women with early-stage endometriosis have luteal phase dysfunction,[18] abnormal follicle growth,[19] multiple premature luteinizing hormone surges,[20] and luteinized unruptured follicle syndrome.

Intrauterine endometrium may be abnormal in women with endometriosis, which suggests the possibility of a so-called field defect in the müllerian tract. Significant suppression of β_3 integrin has been reported in the endometrium of women with early-stage endometriosis.[21] This decrease in β_3 integrin expression may be associated with an impaired interaction of the embryo with the endometrium. In addition, elevated levels of the müllerian antigen CA-125 have been found on endometrial biopsies taken during the luteal phase of the menstrual cycle from women with advanced endometriosis[22] and in the menstrual discharge of women with endometriosis.[23]

Diagnosis

Although endometriosis is a common disorder, it remains remarkably difficult to diagnose. In one cohort study, women with endometriosis reported that, on average, 4 years elapsed between their first presentation with symptoms caused by endometriosis and their diagnosis.

CLINICAL PRESENTATION

Women with endometriosis typically present because of chronic pelvic pain or infertility. Other possible symptoms include secondary dysmenorrhea, dyspareunia, pain with bowel movements (dyschezia), and pelvic pain not associated with menses. The rare cases of diaphragmatic endometriosis have been associated with chest pain at the onset of menstruation.[24]

PHYSICAL EXAMINATION

In most women with endometriosis, the physical examination is normal. However, certain findings on physical examination suggest the presence of endometriosis. These include tender, thickened, or nodular uterosacral ligaments and fixed adnexal masses. A retroverted, fixed uterus suggests involvement of the cul-de-sac with endometriosis.

The uterosacral ligaments connect the base of the uterus to the sacrum. Nodularity of the ligaments is evident on bimanual pelvic examination as pea-sized nodules palpable at 4 o'clock and 8 o'clock at the base of the cervix. These nodules most often are implants of endometriosis.

Two less common physical findings in endometriosis are cervical stenosis[25] and lateral displacement of the cervix. Lateral displacement of the cervix occurs when one uterosacral ligament becomes severely involved with endometriosis, shortens as a result of scarring, and pulls the cervix to the side.[26]

NONINVASIVE LABORATORY TESTS

A complete blood count, urinalysis, and endocervical cultures for gonococci and *Chlamydia* should be performed to rule out infectious causes of pelvic pain in women. Results of all these tests will be normal in women with endometriosis. In most women with endometriosis, the pelvic sonogram is normal, but other conditions, such as uterine leiomyomas, will be evident on sonography. Although many conditions can cause adnexal masses, including dermoids (mature teratomas), serous and mucinous cysts, and hemorrhagic corpora lutea, endometriomas have classic characteristics on ultrasound, which aids in their diagnosis.

SURGICAL STAGING

The current gold standard for the diagnosis of endometriosis is the surgical visualization of lesions, usually by laparoscopy. The normal peritoneal surface is smooth and glistening, like the inner surface of the oral mucosa. Classic endometriosis lesions are often black, purple, or red and measure 1 to 5 mm in diameter; they stud the surface of the peritoneum. Atypical endometriosis lesions are often translucent or yellow, and they may take the form of either flat plaques or vesicles.

Unfortunately, surgeons vary considerably in their ability to detect endometriosis lesions reliably. One study reported pathologic confirmation rates of visually diagnosed endometriosis at 42%, 65%, and 76% for three different surgeons.[27]

Endometriosis is staged surgically using the American Society of Reproductive Medicine staging system. This system divides the disease into four stages: stage I, minimal; stage II, mild; stage III, moderate; and stage IV, severe. As with detection, however, staging is not always performed consistently. Studies of intersurgeon and intrasurgeon variability in the staging of endometriosis report low reproducibility and a kappa coefficient in the range of 0.28.[28]

HISTOLOGIC DIAGNOSIS

Biopsy and histologic analysis of lesions found on laparoscopy may enable more reliable diagnosis of endometriosis than does visual inspection alone. The criteria for histologic diagnosis of endometriosis include the presence of one of the following components: (1) both endometrial glands and stroma; (2) glandular epithelium with hemosiderin; or (3) endometrial stroma–like tissue with hemosiderin. One weakness of histologic diagnosis for endometriosis is that diagnostic criteria vary among pathologists.[29,30] Furthermore, no study has demonstrated high interobserver reproducibility in the histologic diagnosis of endometriosis.

CLINICAL DIAGNOSIS

An innovative approach to the diagnosis of endometriosis is to use a combination of history, physical examination, and noninvasive laboratory testing.[31] This approach is called clinical diagnosis.

DIFFERENTIAL DIAGNOSIS

Pelvic Pain

Chronic pelvic pain, defined as the presence of pain below the umbilicus for more than 6 months, is a common gynecologic problem. In one study of primary care practices that included 284,162 women 12 to 70 years of age, the reported prevalence of chronic pelvic pain was 3.8%.[32] Along with endometriosis, other common gynecologic causes of chronic pelvic pain include chronic pelvic inflammatory disease, adenomyosis, and uterine leiomyomata. Nongynecologic diseases such as irritable bowel syndrome and fibromyalgia, as well as psychiatric diseases such as somatization, may also contribute to chronic pelvic pain. In populations in which the prevalence of sexually transmitted diseases is low, endometriosis is the most common cause of chronic pelvic pain. In three large studies, 70% to 80% of women with chronic pelvic pain had endometriosis as the cause.[31,33,34]

Infertility

Endometriosis is considered to be responsible for 8% of all cases of infertility. The most common causes of infertility, accounting for about 75% of cases, are ovulatory disorders, tubal disease, and semen abnormalities. Miscellaneous factors, such as cervical or immunologic abnormalities and uterine synechiae, cause 2% of cases; 15% are unexplained.[35-37]

Treatment of Pelvic Pain

Interventions that reduce estradiol production are the most reliable way to cause atrophy of endometriosis lesions and are the most effective in treating pain symptoms. A variety of hormonal and surgical interventions are available for this purpose. Most authorities recommend a stepwise approach to the use of these interventions [see Table 2].

Table 2 Stepwise Treatment of Pelvic Pain

Step	Description	Recommendation
1	Thorough history and physical examination	Detailed history and physical examination forms for evaluating pelvic pain are available on the Internet at www.pelvicpain.org
2	Noninvasive laboratory testing	Pelvic ultrasound, complete blood count, urinalysis, endocervical cultures for gonococci and *Chlamydia*
3	Empirical therapy	Oral contraceptive plus nonsteroidal anti-inflammatory medication
4	Surgical diagnostic procedure	Laparoscopy to determine the cause of pain if empirical therapy does not result in sufficient relief of pain
5	GnRH agonist therapy	For regimens, see Table 3
6	GnRH agonist therapy plus steroid add-back	Consider for reduction of GnRH agonist side effects; for regimens, see Table 4
7	Progestin-only treatment	If GnRH agonists cannot be tolerated because of side effects; for regimens, see Table 5

GnRH—gonadotropin-releasing hormone

HORMONAL TREATMENT FOR RELIEF OF PAIN

Randomized clinical trials have demonstrated that combination estrogen-progestin oral contraceptives, gonadotropin-releasing hormone (GnRH) agonist analogues, danazol, and progestins are all effective in relieving pelvic pain caused by endometriosis. GnRH agonist analogues are the most effective; combination estrogen-progestin oral contraceptives are the least expensive.

Combination Estrogen-Progestin Oral Contraceptives

Oral contraceptives are sometimes effective in the treatment of pelvic pain caused by endometriosis because progestins can block the growth of endometrium and endometriosis lesions. Although estrogen stimulates the growth of endometriosis lesions, modern oral contraceptives are progestin dominant and contain low doses of estrogen.

In the United States, almost all women with chronic pelvic pain are initially treated empirically with a combination of cyclic oral contraceptives and nonsteroidal anti-inflammatory drugs (NSAIDS), such as ibuprofen. In contrast, in some European countries, the standard practice is to perform laparoscopy on women with chronic pelvic pain to determine the cause of the pain before starting hormonal treatment. In one randomized study, women with endometriosis who had not previously undergone hormonal treatment were randomized to receive treatment with either low-dose cyclic oral contraceptives or a GnRH agonist analogue. Both groups experienced significant improvement in pelvic pain and dysmenorrhea. However, the group treated with GnRH agonists had better relief of dyspareunia.[38]

Oral contraceptives can be used in monthly cycles or long-cycle regimens. If a regimen of oral contraceptives taken in monthly cycles does not relieve the pain, many physicians will try a regimen of long-cycle oral contraceptives. In long-cycle regimens, the active pills are taken for 42 to 105 days in a row; no pills are taken for a period of 1 week between cycles.

If oral contraceptives and NSAIDs fail to relieve chronic pelvic pain, most physicians recommend laparoscopy to definitively determine whether endometriosis is present.

GnRH Agonist Analogues

Several GnRH agonists have been approved for use in endometriosis [see Table 3]. These agents are analogues of the native decapeptide GnRH, with substitutions in amino acids 6 and 10. The introduction of D-amino acids at position 6 of native GnRH produces GnRH analogues that are resistant to degradation by endopeptidases and have long half-lives, high affinity for the GnRH receptor, and long receptor occupancy.

Paradoxically, initial treatment with a GnRH agonist analogue stimulates the secretion of luteinizing hormone (LH) and follicle-stimulating hormone (FSH). Prolonged treatment, however, suppresses gonadotropin secretion through the cellular processes of downregulation and desensitization. The suppression of secretion is greater for LH than for FSH. The suppression of pituitary gonadotropin secretion results in suppression of ovarian follicle growth and a 95% decrease in estrogen production. In women treated with many GnRH analogues, the circulating estradiol concentration is suppressed to about 15 pg/ml, which is in the range observed in menopausal women. In essence, this therapy constitutes a reversible medical oophorectomy.

Numerous clinical trials have demonstrated that approximately 85% of women with endometriosis and pelvic pain who are treated with GnRH agonist analogues experience relief of

Table 3 GnRH Agonists Approved for the Treatment of Endometriosis*

GnRH Agonist	Dose
Leuprolide acetate depot	3.75 mg I.M. every 4 wk
Goserelin acetate	3.6 mg subcutaneous implant every 4 wk
Nafarelin acetate	200 μg twice daily as a nasal spray

*Note: In the United States, GnRH agonist therapy is approved for 6 mo as single-agent therapy and for 1 yr when used in combination with a steroid add-back.

their pain. In one placebo-controlled trial, treatment with a GnRH agonist resulted in better relief of pelvic pain than the administration of placebo (85% and 30%, respectively).[39]

GnRH Agonist Analogues plus Steroid Add-Back

GnRH agonist treatment is associated with hypoestrogenic side effects such as vasomotor symptoms (hot flashes), decreased libido, dry vagina, and decreased bone density. Recent trials have demonstrated that use of a steroid (either high-dose progestin or very low dose estrogen) in so-called add-back therapy can minimize these side effects. GnRH agonist treatment combined with low-dose steroid add-back causes atrophy of endometriosis lesions and improves pelvic pain while minimizing hypoestrogenic vasomotor symptoms and bone loss. In one clinical trial, women with endometriosis and chronic pelvic pain were randomized to four different hormone treatment groups: GnRH agonist alone, GnRH agonist plus progestin only (norethindrone, 5 mg daily), GnRH agonist plus low-dose estrogen-progestin (conjugated equine estrogen, 0.625 mg daily, plus norethindrone acetate, 5 mg daily), or GnRH agonist plus high-dose estrogen plus progestin (conjugated equine estrogen, 1.25 mg daily, plus norethindrone acetate, 5 mg daily). All women were treated with the GnRH agonist leuprolide acetate, given in a depot injection of 3.75 mg I.M. every 4 weeks for 1 year. The rate of treatment discontinuance because of continuing pain was significantly higher in the group that received the combination of GnRH agonist and high-dose estrogen than in any of the other treatment groups.[40] The high-dose estrogen probably stimulated continuing function of the endometriosis implants. Consequently, treatment with a combination of GnRH agonist and high-dose estrogen is not recommended for most women with endometriosis and pelvic pain. The women in the three other groups experienced similar decreases in their pelvic pain, suggesting that all three regimens are effective. Bone density de-

Table 4 Steroid Hormone Regimens for Pelvic Pain from Endometriosis

Regimen	Comments
Transdermal estradiol patch, 25 μg daily, plus medroxyprogesterone acetate, 2.5 mg daily[27]	Does not completely prevent bone loss; achieves estradiol concentration in the range of 30 pg/ml
Norethindrone acetate, 5 mg daily[26]	A high dose of progestin; may be associated with symptoms such as bloating and mood changes
Conjugated equine estrogen, 0.625 mg daily, plus norethindrone, 5 mg daily[26]	Preserves bone density and markedly reduces vasomotor symptoms

creased significantly in the women who received the GnRH agonist alone. Bone density was preserved in the groups that were treated with a combination of a GnRH agonist and steroid add-back therapy, and vasomotor symptoms were significantly reduced. This study and others suggest that an optimal treatment of pelvic pain from endometriosis may involve the use of GnRH agonists to suppress ovarian estrogen production, followed by add-back therapy with low doses of estrogen-progestin or progestin alone [see Table 4].

Endometriosis lesions grow when serum estradiol concentration is in the premenopausal range (30 to 300 pg/ml), and they regress when estradiol levels are in the menopausal range (< 20 pg/ml). An important clinical question is, What concentration of estradiol will minimize the growth of endometriosis implants but not cause severe hypoestrogenic side effects? Treatments that achieve estradiol levels in the range of 20 to 30 pg/ml are associated with amenorrhea and regression of endometriosis lesions. In addition, these treatments are associated with fewer side effects than treatments that target estradiol levels to less than 20 pg/ml.[41]

Danazol

The first hormonal treatment of endometriosis was the intramuscular administration of testosterone. High-dose parenteral testosterone therapy was demonstrated to cause regression in endometriosis lesions. Unfortunately, many women became virilized by this treatment. Androgen treatment of endometriosis was resurrected after the development of synthetic oral androgens, such as danazol, which had attenuated androgen properties.[42]

Randomized clinical trials that have directly compared danazol and the GnRH agonists have demonstrated that both treatments improve pelvic pain in approximately 85% of treated women.[43] The side effects of these two treatments are very different. The main side effects of the GnRH agonists are those associated with hypoestrogenism (see above). The main side effects of danazol are weight gain (on average, approximately 4 kg at doses of 800 mg/day), muscle cramps, decrease in breast size, oily skin, and hirsutism.[44] In the United States, these side effects have limited the use of danazol for the treatment of endometriosis.[45] Many of the side effects of danazol are dose dependent. Doses of 50, 100, and 200 mg daily can be effective in relieving pelvic pain caused by endometriosis and are associated with less severe side effects than daily doses of 400 or 800 mg. Doses of danazol of less than 400 mg/day do not reliably suppress ovulation. Danazol crosses the placenta and is a known teratogen, so patients who are taking low doses of danazol must use a reliable method of contraception.

Progestins

High-dose synthetic progestins have been demonstrated to be effective in the treatment of pelvic pain in women with endometriosis [see Table 5]. These agents have multiple mechanisms of action: (1) suppression of LH and FSH secretion, which suppresses estradiol production; (2) direct antiestrogenic effects on endometriosis lesions; and (3) induction of pseudodecidualization. A problem with progestin treatment is that many women gain weight or experience symptoms typical of the premenstrual period, such as mood changes and bloating.

SURGICAL TREATMENT

Surgical treatment of endometriosis is termed either conservative or definitive. In conservative surgery, all the pelvic or-

Table 5 Progestins Effective for Single-Agent Treatment of Endometriosis

Progestin	Dose
Norethindrone acetate	5 mg p.o. daily
Medroxyprogesterone acetate	50 mg p.o. daily; 150 mg I.M. every 90 days
Norgestrel	0.075 mg p.o. daily

gans are preserved; in definitive surgery, both ovaries are removed.

Conservative Surgery

Conservative endometriosis surgery is best accomplished by laparoscopy because postoperative recovery is very rapid, with discharge usually occurring within 1 day. Most surgeons utilize sharp excision to remove endometriosis lesions, electrosurgery to ablate endometriosis lesions, or a combination of the two methods. In one clinical trial, women with pelvic pain caused by endometriosis were randomized to undergo diagnostic laparoscopy and aspiration of peritoneal fluid or to undergo conservative surgery with laparoscopy and resection or ablation of endometriosis lesions. Six months after surgery, 63% of the women treated with surgical resection of endometriosis lesions reported relief of pain, whereas 23% of those treated with diagnostic laparoscopy without surgical resection reported pain relief.[46]

Conservative surgery typically fails to provide permanent relief of endometriosis, however. Within 2 years after surgical treatment, pain recurs in most women with endometriosis.[47] Also, surgical treatment may result in pelvic adhesions, which can become a primary cause of continuing pelvic pain.

Definitive Surgery

Definitive surgery for endometriosis involves removal of both ovaries. Typically, the uterus is removed as well; indeed, in the United States, endometriosis is second only to uterine fibroids as a reason for performing hysterectomy. Many large cohort studies report that about 90% of women with endometriosis and pelvic pain experience long-term relief of their pain through bilateral oophorectomy.[48,49]

After bilateral oophorectomy for endometriosis, patients are typically started on low-dose estrogen replacement. Low-dose estrogen therapy prevents vasomotor symptoms and osteoporosis; pelvic pain usually does not recur.

SURGICAL EXCISION OF OVARIAN MASSES

Endometriomas require surgical excision if they are causing pain or are enlarging. Large ovarian cysts may be the result of ovarian cancer. Surgical removal of the cyst allows a definitive diagnosis of the cause of the cyst to be made. A randomized clinical trial demonstrated that surgical removal of endometriomas resulted in better long-term results than simple aspiration and fenestration of the cyst.[50]

Treatment of Infertility

EARLY-STAGE ENDOMETRIOSIS AND INFERTILITY

Women with minimal or mild (stage I or II) endometriosis and infertility have a baseline fecundity of approximately 0.03

Table 6   Stepwise Treatment of Infertility in Early-Stage Endometriosis

Step	Description	Recommendation
1	Identify and treat all reversible causes of infertility	Proper timing of coitus in relation to ovulation Optimal coital frequency Cessation of cigarette smoking Optimal body mass index Reduce consumption of alcohol and caffeine
2	Laparosocopic surgery to resect endometriosis and remove adhesions	Attempt to restore pelvic anatomy to normal
3	Ovarian stimulation with clomiphene plus intrauterine insemination	Insemination timed to the day before and day of ovulation
4	Ovarian stimulation with gonadotropin injections plus intrauterine insemination	Insemination timed to the day before and day of ovulation; because of increased risk of twin, triplet, and quadruplet pregnancy, some clinicians prefer to skip step 4 and move directly to step 5
5	In vitro fertilization and embryo transfer	—

(3% per cycle, compared with 20% to 36% in normal couples). Numerous randomized studies have demonstrated that a stepwise approach to treatment can increase pregnancy rates in women with early-stage endometriosis [*see Table 6*].

Treatment of Infertility from Other Causes

The first step in the management of early-stage endometriosis and infertility is to identify and treat all reversible causes of infertility in the couple. Many couples have multiple causes of their infertility (e.g., endometriosis in the female partner and a low sperm count in the male partner).

Laparoscopic Surgery

If other causes of infertility have been addressed but the woman is still unable to conceive, the next step is to consider a laparoscopic surgical procedure to ablate or excise endometriosis implants and adhesions and to attempt to restore the pelvis to normal. In one randomized, prospective trial, diagnostic laparoscopy alone was compared with diagnostic laparoscopy combined with surgical resection or ablation of endometriosis in 341 women with early-stage endometriosis. During 36 weeks of post-operative follow-up, fecundity was 0.024 in the diagnosis-only group and 0.047 in the surgically treated group; cumulative pregnancy rates during follow-up were 18% and 31%, respectively.[51]

Intrauterine Insemination

Women who fail to become pregnant after laparoscopic surgery can be treated with intrauterine insemination (IUI) in combination with either clomiphene or gonadotropin injections. Clomiphene is far less expensive than gonadotropins; therefore it is generally used first. These methods are designed to cause multifollicle development and multiple ovulation. In addition, IUI places a large number of motile sperm high in the reproductive tract. Thus, the spermatazoa do not have to travel through the vagina, cervix, and lower portion of the uterus. Both of these methods have been demonstrated to improve pregnancy rates in women with early-stage endometriosis. In one randomized study in 40 women with early-stage endometriosis, fecundity was 0.045 (4.5% per cycle pregnancy rate) in the group that received no treatment and 0.15 in the group treated with three cycles of gonadotropin injections in combination with IUI.[52] Similar findings have been reported by other groups.[53-56]

Table 7   Stepwise Treatment of Infertility in Advanced Endometriosis

Step	Description	Recommendation
1	Identify and treat all reversible causes of infertility	Proper timing of coitus in relation to ovulation Optimal coital frequency Cessation of cigarette smoking Optimal body mass index Reduce consumption of alcohol and caffeine
2	Surgery to resect endometriosis and remove adhesions	Attempt to restore pelvic anatomy to normal
3	Ovarian stimulation with clomiphene plus intrauterine insemination	Insemination timed to the day before and day of ovulation; limited to patients with patent fallopian tubes and no dense ovarian adhesions
4	Ovarian stimulation with gonadotropin injections plus intrauterine insemination	Insemination timed to the day before and day of ovulation; limited to patients with patent fallopian tubes and no dense ovarian adhesions; because of increased risk of twin, triplet, or quadruplet pregnancy, some clinicians prefer to skip step 4 and move directly to step 5
5	In vitro fertilization and embryo transfer	—

Many authorities believe that the per-cycle pregnancy rate drops significantly after three or four cycles of clomiphene or gonadotropin injections in combination with IUI. Consequently, after three cycles of such treatment, the clinician should review with the couple the advantages of proceeding to the next step, which is in vitro fertilization (IVF) with embryo transfer.[57]

In Vitro Fertilization

There are no prospective, large-scale, randomized trials that demonstrate the efficacy of IVF in the treatment of infertility caused by endometriosis. However, the use of IVF in women with endometriosis and infertility routinely results in treatment-cycle pregnancy rates of approximately 0.30, a 10-fold increase over the baseline fecundity seen in such women.[58-60] It should be noted, however, that the outcome of IVF is highly influenced by the woman's age: women younger than 37 years have much better success with IVF than do women older than 37 years.

ADVANCED ENDOMETRIOSIS AND INFERTILITY

In women with moderate or severe endometriosis and infertility, a stepwise approach to treatment is warranted [see Table 7].

Treatment of Infertility from Other Causes

The first step, as in the treatment of early-stage endometriosis, is to identify and correct all other reversible causes of infertility (see above).

Surgical Treatment

The second step is to perform surgical resection for ovarian endometriosis, peritoneal endometriosis, and pelvic adhesions to restore pelvic anatomy and function. There are no randomized, prospective studies that demonstrate the efficacy of surgery in the treatment of advanced endometriosis. However, most authorities believe that surgery improves fertility in these women. One retrospective analysis reviewed the outcome in 130 infertile women with endometriosis who were treated with expectant management, conservative surgery, or expectant management followed by surgery. Although no significant difference was noted between expectant management and surgery in women with mild or moderate endometriosis, women with severe endometriosis appeared to benefit from surgery. Of the 32 women with advanced endometriosis who were observed over 231 months of cumulative follow-up, none became pregnant. Of the 34 women with advanced endometriosis who underwent conservative surgery, 10 became pregnant during 702 cumulative months of follow-up.[61] Similar results have been reported in a meta-analysis of the impact of surgery on fertility in women with endometriosis.[62] These studies suggest that expectant management is not warranted in the treatment of infertility associated with advanced endometriosis and that surgical treatment may improve fecundity.

Pregnancy rates are highest in the 6 to 18 months after the surgical procedure. Additional surgical procedures have not been shown to be effective in increasing fecundity[63]; therefore, if pregnancy does not occur after the first surgery, the clinician should usually move on to intrauterine insemination. Physicians should carefully weigh the limited benefits of second and third operative procedures to enhance fertility against the potential risks of major surgery.

Intrauterine Insemination

Clomiphene or gonadotropin injections in combination with IUI are used empirically in patients with advanced endometriosis and infertility. Most of the clinical trials that have tested these modalities have focused on women with early-stage endometriosis (see above). However, many authorities believe that the benefits of these measures probably extend to women with advanced disease. In patients with severe pelvic adhesions, clinicians may choose to move directly from surgery to in vitro fertilization. Clomiphene or gonadotropins in combination with IUI should not be recommended for women with tubal blockage or dense ovarian adhesions.

In Vitro Fertilization

There are no large, randomized, controlled clinical trials that definitively demonstrate that IVF increases pregnancy rates in women with advanced endometriosis. In one small study involving 21 women with endometriosis and infertility, none of the six women randomized to undergo expectant management became pregnant, whereas five of the 15 women who were treated with IVF became pregnant.[64] Because of the small sample size, however, this study did not have sufficient statistical power to detect true differences between the two groups. One analysis of various infertility treatments demonstrated that for infertile women with advanced endometriosis, rapid progression through the steps to IVF is the most cost-effective treatment approach.[65] In the United States, the median projected cost per IVF cycle in 2001 was $9,226.[66] The cost of having a child with IVF is within the range of the cost of adopting a child. Furthermore, over the past decade, IVF success rates have increased.[67]

IVF is less successful in women with advanced endometriosis who have previously undergone bilateral ovarian surgery; after unilateral oophorectomy and a contralateral ovarian cystectomy, ovarian stimulation is often ineffective, and the pregnancy rate is low. Reduced pregnancy rates for women with advanced endometriosis (compared with women who have early-stage endometriosis or tubal factor infertility) may be the result of a premature depletion of the ovarian follicle pool,[68] abnormal folliculogenesis,[69] or reduced fertilization potential of oocytes.[70]

References

1. Houston DE, Noller KL, Melton LJ, et al: Incidence of pelvic endometriosis in Rochester, Minnesota, 1970–1979. Am J Epidemiol 125:959, 1987

2. Holt VL, Weiss NS: Recommendations for the design of epidemiologic studies of endometriosis. Epidemiology 11:654, 2000

3. Cramer DW, Wilson E, Stillman RJ, et al: The relation of endometriosis to menstrual characteristics, smoking and exercise. JAMA 225:1904, 1986

4. Birnbaum LS, Cummings AM: Dioxins and endometriosis: a plausible hypothesis. Environ Health Perspect 110:15, 2002

5. Bruner-Tran KL, Rier SE, Eisenberg E, et al: The potential role of environmental toxins in the pathophysiology of endometriosis. Gynecol Obstet Invest 48(suppl 1):45, 1999

6. Bedaiwy MA, Falcone T, Sharma RK, et al: Prediction of endometriosis with serum and peritoneal fluid markers: a prospective controlled trial. Hum Reprod 17:426, 2002

7. Sinaii N, Cleary SD, Ballweg ML, et al: Autoimmune and related disease among women with endometriosis: a survey analysis. Fertil Steril 77(suppl 1):S7, 2002

8. Gazvani R, Templeton A: New considerations for the pathogenesis of endometriosis. Int J Gynaecol Obstet 76:117, 2002

9. Simpson JL, Elias S, Malinak LR, et al: Heritable aspects of endometriosis. Am J Obstet Gynecol 137:327, 1980

10. Jimbo J, Hitami Y, Yoshikawa H, et al: Evidence for monoclonal expansion of epithelial cells in ovarian endometrial cysts. Am J Pathol 150:1173, 1997

11. Barbieri RL, Missmer S: Endometriosis and infertility: a cause-effect relationship? Ann N Y Acad Sci 955:23, 2002

12. Haney AF, Muscato JJ, Weinberg JB: Peritoneal fluid cell populations in infertility patients. Fertil Steril 41:122, 1984

13. Halme J, Becker S, Haskill S: Altered maturation and function of peritoneal macrophages: possible role in the pathogenesis of endometriosis. Am J Obstet Gynecol 156:783, 1987

14. Fakih H, Baggett B, Holtz G: Interleukin-1: a possible role in the infertility associated with endometriosis. Fertil Steril 47:213, 1987

15. Oral E, Arici A, Olive DL, et al: Peritoneal fluid from women with moderate or severe endometriosis inhibits sperm motility: the role of seminal fluid components. Fertil Steril 66:787, 1996

16. Badawy SZ, Cuenca V, Stitzel A: Autoimmune phenomena in infertile patients with endometriosis. Obstet Gynecol 63:271, 1984

17. Weed JC, Aquembourg PC: Endometriosis: can it produce an autoimmune response resulting in infertility? Clin Obstet Gynecol 23:885, 1980

18. Cheesman KL, Cheesman SD, Chatterton RT: Alterations in progesterone metabolism and luteal function in infertile women with endometriosis. Fertil Steril 29:270, 1978

19. Wardle PG, McLaughlin EA, McDermott A: Endometriosis and ovulatory disorder: reduced fertilization in vitro compared with tubal and unexplained infertility. Lancet 2:236, 1985

20. Polan ML, Totora M, Caldwell BV, et al: Abnormal ovarian cycles as diagnosed by ultrasound and serum estradiol levels. Fertil Steril 37:342, 1982

21. Lessey BA, Castlebaum AJ, Sawin SW, et al: Aberrant integrin expression in the endometrium of women with endometriosis. J Clin Endocrinol Metab 79:643, 1994

22. McBean JH, Brumsted JR: In vitro CA-125 secretion from women with advanced endometriosis. Fertil Steril 59:89, 1993

23. Takahashi K, Nagata H, Musa AA, et al: Clinical usefulness of CA-125 levels in the menstrual discharge of women with endometriosis. Fertil Steril 54:360, 1990

24. Redwine DB: Diaphragmatic endometriosis: diagnosis, surgical management, and long-term results of treatment. Fertil Steril 77:288, 2002

25. Barbieri RL: Stenosis of the external cervical os: an association with endometriosis in women with chronic pelvic pain. Fertil Steril 70:571, 1998

26. Propst AM, Storti K, Barbieri RL: Lateral cervical displacement: an association with endometriosis. Fertil Steril 70:568, 1998

27. Pardanani S, Barbieri RL: The gold standard for the surgical diagnosis of endometriosis: visual findings or biopsy results. J Gynecol Tech 4:121, 1998

28. Hornstein MD, Friedman AJ, Gleason RE, et al: The reproducibility of the revised American Fertility Society classification of endometriosis. Fertil Steril 59:1015, 1993

29. Jansen RS, Russell P: Non-pigmented endometriosis: clinical, laparoscopic and pathologic definitions. Am J Obstet Gynecol 155:1154, 1986

30. Blaustein A: Pelvic endometriosis. Blaustein's Pathology of the Genital Tract, 2nd ed. Blaustein A, Ed. Springer-Verlag, New York, 1982, p 464

31. Randomized controlled trial of depot leuprolide in patients with chronic pelvic pain and clinically suspected endometriosis. Pelvic Pain Study Group. Obstet Gynecol 93:51, 1999

32. Zondervan KT, Yudkin PL, Vessey MP, et al: Prevalence and incidence of chronic pelvic pain in primary care: evidence from a national general practice database. Br J Obstet Gynaecol 106:1149, 1999

33. Carter JE: Combined hysteroscopy and laparoscopic findings in patients with chronic pelvic pain. J Am Assoc Gynecol Laparoscopy 2:43, 1994

34. Koninckx PR, Lessafre E, Meuleman C, et al: Suggestive evidence that pelvic endometriosis is a progressive disease, whereas deeply infiltrating endometriosis is associated with pelvic pain. Fertil Steril 55:759, 1991

35. Collins JA, Crosignani PG: Unexplained infertility: a review of diagnosis, prognosis, treatment efficacy and management. Int J Gynaecol Obstet 39:267, 1992

36. Templeton AA, Penney GC: The incidence, characteristics, and prognosis of patients whose infertility is unexplained. Fertil Steril 37:175, 1982

37. Guzick DS, Grefenstette I, Baffone K, et al: Infertility evaluation in fertile women: a model for assessing the efficacy of infertility testing. Hum Reprod 9:2306, 1994

38. Vercellini P, Trespidi L, Colombo A, et al: A gonadotropin-releasing hormone agonist versus a low-dose oral contraceptive for pelvic pain associated with endometriosis. Fertil Steril 60:75, 1993

39. Lupron depot (leuprolide acetate for depot suspension) in the treatment of endometriosis: a randomized, placebo-controlled, double-blind study. Lupron Study Group. Fertil Steril 54:419, 1990

40. Leuprolide acetate depot and hormonal add-back in endometriosis: a 12-month study. Lupron Add-Back Study Group. Obstet Gynecol 91:16, 1998

41. Howell R, Edmonds D, Dowsett M, et al: Gonadotropin releasing hormone analogue plus hormone replacement therapy for the treatment of endometriosis: a randomized clinical trial. Fertil Steril 64:474, 1995

42. Barbieri RL, Ryan KJ: Danazol: endocrine pharmacology and therapeutic applica-

tions. Am J Obstet Gynecol 141:453, 1981

43. Henzl MR, Corson SL, Moghissi K, et al: Administration of nasal nafarelin as compared with oral danazol for endometriosis. N Engl J Med 318:485, 1988

44. Barbieri RL, Evans S, Kistner RW: Danazol in the treatment of endometriosis: analysis of 100 cases with a 4-year follow-up. Fertil Steril 37:737, 1982

45. Selak V, Farquhar C, Prentice A, et al: Danazol for pelvic pain associated with endometriosis. Cochrane Database Syst Rev (2):CD000068, 2002

46. Sutton CJ, Ewen SP, Jacobs SA, et al: Laser laparoscopic surgery in the treatment of ovarian endometriosis. J Am Assoc Gynecol Laparoscopy 4:319, 1997

47. Hornstein MD, Hemmings R, Yuzpe AA, et al: Use of nafarelin versus placebo after reductive laparoscopic surgery for endometriosis. Fertil Steril 68:860, 1997

48. Ranney B: Endometriosis. 3. Complete operations. Reasons, sequelae, treatment. Am J Obstet Gynecol 109:1137, 1971

49. Hickman TN, Namnoum AB, Hinton EL, et al: Timing of estrogen replacement following hysterectomy with oophorectomy for endometriosis. Obstet Gynecol 91:673, 1998

50. Beretta P, Franci M, Ghezzi F, et al: Randomized clinical trial of two laparoscopic treatments of endometriomas: cystectomy versus drainage and coagulation. Fertil Steril 70:1176, 1998

51. Laparoscopic surgery in infertile women with minimal or mild endometriosis. The Canadian Collaborative Group on Endometriosis. N Engl J Med 337:217, 1997

52. Fedele L, Bianchi S, Marchini M, et al: Superovulation with human menopausal gonadotropins in the treatment of infertility associated with minimal or mild endometriosis. Fertil Steril 58:28, 1992

53. Tummon IS, Asher LJ, Martin JS, et al: Randomized controlled trial of superovulation and insemination for infertility associated with minimal or mild endometriosis. Fertil Steril 68:8, 1997

54. Nulsen JC, Walsh S, Dumez S, et al: A randomized and longitudinal study of human menopausal gonadotropin with intrauterine insemination in the treatment of infertility. Obstet Gynecol 82:780, 1993

55. Chaffkin LM, Nulsen JC, Luciano AA, et al: A comparative analysis of the cycle fecundity rates associated with combined human menopausal gonadotropin and intrauterine insemination versus either hMG or IUI alone. Fertil Steril 55:252, 1991

56. Guzick DS, Carson SA, Coutifaris C, et al: Efficacy of superovulation and intrauterine insemination in the treatment of infertility. N Engl J Med 340:177, 1999

57. Isaksson R, Tiitinen A: Superovulation with combined insemination or timed intercourse in the treatment of couples with unexplained infertility and minimal endometriosis. Acta Obstet Gynecol Scand 76:550, 1997

58. Olivenenes F, Feldberg D, Liu HC, et al: Endometriosis: a stage by stage analysis: role for in vitro fertilization. Fertil Steril 64:392, 1995

59. Oehninger S, Acosta AA, Kreiner D, et al: In vitro fertilization and embryo transfer: an established and successful therapy for endometriosis. J In Vitro Fertilization and Embryo Transfer 5:249, 1988

60. Chillik CF, Acosta AA, Garcia JE, et al: The role of in vitro fertilization in infertile patients with endometriosis. Fertil Steril 44:56, 1985

61. Olive DL, Lee KL: Analysis of sequential treatment protocols for endometriosis-associated infertility. Am J Obstet Gynecol 154:613, 1986

62. Adamson GD, Pasta DJ: Surgical treatment of endometriosis-associated infertility: meta-analysis compared with survival analysis. Am J Obstet Gynecol 171:1404, 1994

63. Pagidas K, Falcone T, Hemmings R, et al: Comparison of reoperation for moderate and severe endometriosis-related infertility with in vitro fertilization-embryo transfer. Fertil Steril 65:791, 1996

64. Soliman S, Daya S, Collins J: A randomized trial of in vitro fertilization versus conventional treatment for infertility. Fertil Steril 59:1239, 1993

65. Phillips Z, Barraza-Llorens M, Posnett J: Evaluation of the relative cost-effectiveness of treatments for infertility in the UK. Human Reproduction 15:95, 2000

66. Collins J: Cost-effectiveness of in vitro fertilization. Semin Reprod Med 19:279, 2001

67. Cramer DW, Liberman RF, Powers DR, et al: Recent trends in assisted reproductive techniques and associated outcomes. Obstet Gynecol 95:61, 2000

68. Hornstein MD, Barbieri RL, McShane PM: The effects of previous ovarian surgery on the follicular response to ovulation induction in an in vitro fertilization program. J Reprod Med 34:277, 1989

69. Toya M, Saito H, Ohta N, et al: Moderate and severe endometriosis is associated with alterations in the cell cycle of granulose cells in patients undergoing in vitro fertilization and embryo transfer. Fertil Steril 73:344, 2000

70. Pal L, Shifren JL, Isaacson KB, et al: Impact of varying stages of endometriosis on the outcome of in vitro fertilization–embryo transfer. J Assisted Reproduction and Genetics 15:27, 1998

79 Polycystic Ovary Syndrome

Robert L. Barbieri, M.D., F.A.C.P.

The polycystic ovary syndrome (PCOS) is a reproductive and metabolic disorder that is characterized by hyperandrogenism and, in most cases, oligo-ovulation and oligomenorrhea. Many women with PCOS are insulin resistant, obese, and at increased risk for developing type 2 (non–insulin-dependent) diabetes mellitus. The most common presenting problems of women with PCOS are: irregular and infrequent menstrual cycles, hirsutism, anovulatory infertility, obesity, endometrial hyperplasia, and endometrial cancer.

Definition

The definition of PCOS is controversial. The two most widely utilized diagnostic criteria are the NIH criteria and the Rotterdam criteria. The 1990 NIH criteria for PCOS include the presence of both hyperandrogenism (diagnosed by clinical presentation, laboratory testing, or both) and oligo-ovulation (frequently manifesting as oligomenorrhea) in the absence of other causes of hyperandrogenism, such as nonclassic 21-hydroxylase deficiency or an androgen secreting tumor.[1] Oligo-ovulation is defined as a menstrual cycle length greater than 35 days. Most women with PCOS have fewer than nine menses per year. The 2003 Rotterdam criteria for PCOS require the presence of two of the following three conditions: (1) hyperandrogenism, (2) oligo-ovulation, and (3) a multifollicular ovary consistent with PCOS morphology as demonstrated by pelvic ultrasound.[2] The Rotterdam criteria for PCOS morphology are: (1) 12 or more follicles in each ovary measuring 2 to 9 mm in diameter, (2) an increased ovarian volume (> 10 ml) in the absence of a dominant follicle or corpus luteum, or (3) both. Follicle distribution and ovarian stromal echogenicity are not included in the Rotterdam criteria. Both the NIH criteria and the Rotterdam criteria were developed by expert panels; however, neither panel had the benefit of prospective research to determine the clinical and research impacts of the criteria.

The Rotterdam criteria encompass a broader range of clinical presentations than the NIH criteria, yet the Rotterdam criteria have several weaknesses. For example, to fully apply the criteria, all women with either hyperandrogenism alone or oligo-ovulation alone need to receive a transvaginal pelvic ultrasound by a trained expert, which is a potentially expensive use of limited healthcare resources with modest clinical benefit. In addition, as many as 25% of normal ovulatory women without hyperandrogenism or oligo-ovulation have PCOS morphology, indicating that this criterion has a high prevalence in the normal population.[3] Another weakness of the Rotterdam criteria is the inclusion of women who have very mild forms of PCOS—a factor that lessens the usefulness of the criteria in identifying clinically significant PCOS. For example, women with regular ovulatory menses, hyperandrogenism, and PCOS morphology typically have a good clinical prognosis with regards to both their reproductive and metabolic function; many clinicians would diagnose these woman as having so-called idiopathic hirsutism.

The main weakness of the NIH criteria is that a small number of women with PCOS (e.g., women who have hirsutism, multifollicular ovaries, and slightly elevated blood androgen levels) are normo-ovulatory, yet the NIH criteria does not recognize this small group as having PCOS. Most endocrinologists and gynecologists in the United States use the NIH criteria for diagnosing PCOS, and this chapter will do so as well, unless otherwise stated. When the term PCOS is used, it refers to the combination of hyperandrogenism and oligomenorrhea; it does not refer to an ovary with a polycystic appearance on transvaginal ultrasound.

Epidemiology

PCOS is one of the most common endocrine disorders in women. In three population-based studies, the average prevalence of PCOS in women of reproductive age was reported to be about 6%.[4-6] Among anovulatory women, the prevalence of PCOS is approximately 30%.[7] The menstrual irregularity associated with PCOS typically begins before age 18. Signs of clinically significant androgen excess typically follow but may overlap the onset of menstrual irregularity. Adolescents with irregular menses at age 16 are at increased risk for developing PCOS, especially if they are obese or have elevated levels of luteinizing hormone (LH).[8] The peak incidence of PCOS is between 18 and 30 years of age. In the fourth and fifth decades of life, androgen levels in women with PCOS decreased by about 50%, but these levels remain elevated compared with the androgen levels of age-matched normal women.[9]

Ethnic, racial, and other population factors may influence the phenotype and prevalence of PCOS. In a large-cohort study from Kaiser Permanente, the prevalence of PCOS among women 25 to 34 years of age was 2.6%. Women with PCOS were more likely to be obese and have dyslipidemia and diabetes. Among the PCOS cohort, blacks and Hispanics were more likely than whites to be obese, and Asians were less likely to be obese than whites. In this same cohort, blacks were more likely and Hispanics less likely to have hypertension than whites, and Asians and Hispanics were more likely to have diabetes than whites.[10] In another study, Mexican-American women with PCOS were reported to have higher body mass index (BMI) and higher levels of fasting insulin than white women with PCOS.[11]

The risk of PCOS varies among countries. For example, the prevalence of PCOS in Greece (6.8%) and in the Southeast United States (6.6%)[12] appears to be greater than the prevalence in Finland (3.5%).[13] Populations with a low average BMI and a low prevalence of diabetes are probably at reduced risk for developing PCOS.

Family history is a strong risk factor for PCOS. In addition, among women with PCOS, a family history of diabetes is a strong risk factor for the development of impaired glucose tolerance and diabetes. The impact of family history on risk suggests that genetic factors play an important role in the etiology of PCOS.[14]

Etiology and Genetics

The cause of PCOS is not known. PCOS is probably a complex, polygenic disorder whose phenotype is strongly influenced by environmental factors, including obesity. The first-degree relatives of women with PCOS appear to be at increased risk for both hyperandrogenism and menstrual irregularity. In one study, the sisters of 80 women with PCOS were examined for the presence of hyperandrogenism and menstrual irregularity. Of the 115 sisters available for study, 22% fulfilled the NIH criteria for PCOS, and 24% had hyperandrogenemia but regular menstrual cycles.[15] This finding suggests that all first-degree relatives of women diagnosed with PCOS should be screened for the disorder.

There are rare single-gene mutations that are highly associated with hyperandrogenism and menstrual irregularity. For example, women with functional mutations in the alpha or beta subunit of the insulin receptor gene tend to develop severe insulin resistance, acanthosis nigricans, hyperandrogenism, and oligo-ovulation.[16] Several genes have been reported to be associated or linked with the PCOS phenotype, including the insulin gene variable number tandem repeats (VNTR), insulin receptor substrate-1 (IRS-1), insulin receptor substrate-2 (IRS-2), androgen receptor (AR), sex hormone binding globulin (SHBG), cytochrome P450 cyp17, and type 5 17 beta hydroxysteroid dehydrogenase (17 beta-HSD5).[17] In addition, a marker on chromosome 19 near the insulin receptor gene has been strongly associated with PCOS in multiple independent samples.[18]

Preliminary data indicates that the in utero environment of a fetus, especially an environment leading to intrauterine growth restriction or hyperandrogenemia, may increase the likelihood that the newborn will develop hyperandrogenism and insulin resistance as a child or adult.[19-21]

Pathophysiology

Women with PCOS have both reproductive and metabolic abnormalities.

REPRODUCTIVE ABNORMALITIES

The reproductive abnormalities of PCOS include (1) an increase in the hypothalamic pulse frequency of gonadotropin-releasing hormone (GnRH); (2) an increase in pituitary LH secretion (an abnormality present in over 90% of women with PCOS); (3) increased production of ovarian androgens, including testosterone and androstenedione, from the thecal and stromal compartments; (4) dysfunction in ovarian follicle maturation resulting in lack of development of a dominant ovarian follicle, which is a necessary prerequisite to ovulation; and (5) in the absence of ovulation, the accumulation in the ovary of small follicles (2 to 9 mm in diameter). It is the elevated androgen secretion that causes hirsutism in PCOS patients; oligomenorrhea is the consequence of the absence of monthly ovulation.

Women with PCOS show an abnormal increase in both the amplitude and the frequency of LH pulses in the early follicular phase of the menstrual cycle.[22] The elevated LH pulse frequency indicates an underlying increase in the pulse frequency of GnRH secretion by the hypothalamus; this suggests that PCOS may result from a neuroendocrine disorder. The neuroendocrine mechanisms that raise GnRH pulse frequency are poorly characterized but may include alterations in hypothalamic opioid and catecholamine tone.

Ovarian tissue from women with PCOS will continue to over-secrete androgens when cultured in vitro over long periods of time. This suggests that the ovarian tissue has developed a relative independence from stimuli such as LH and insulin.[23]

METABOLIC ABNORMALITIES

The metabolic abnormalities of PCOS include: (1) insulin resistance in both lean and obese women with PCOS, with a higher prevalence in obese women; (2) an increased prevalence of impaired glucose tolerance and impaired fasting glucose; (3) an increased prevalence of diabetes mellitus, especially in obese women with PCOS; and (4) an increased prevalence of the metabolic syndrome as characterized by decreased levels of high-density lipoprotein cholesterol (HDL-C), increased levels of triglycerides, and increased prevalence of hypertension and abdominal obesity.

The pathophysiology of insulin resistance associated with obesity, diabetes, or PCOS is not completely characterized at a molecular level. Disorders of oxidative phosphorylation,[24] insulin receptor defects, and intracellular postreceptor binding defects all appear to contribute to insulin resistance. In women with PCOS, genetic mutations in the insulin receptor and autoantibodies to the insulin receptor are two specific and rare causes of insulin resistance. The most common cause of insulin resistance in PCOS is probably a post-binding defect in insulin signaling that is exacerbated by the development of obesity.[25,26] Another potential mechanism involves a defect in serine phosphorylation of the insulin receptor in women with PCOS; this defect may cause a decrease in receptor function, resulting in insulin resistance.[27] An intriguing hypothesis is that PCOS is a gender-specific form of the metabolic syndrome (i.e., syndrome XX).[28] When pancreatic function is normal, resistance to the action of insulin in the liver, adipose tissue, muscle, and other insulin-sensitive tissues results in a compensatory and chronic hypersecretion of insulin. Laboratory studies suggest that insulin, especially in high concentrations, can stimulate ovarian androgen secretion when combined with LH. Why insulin resistance develops in muscle and fat but not in the ovary remains unclear.[29]

OTHER ABNORMALITIES

In addition to reproductive and metabolic abnormalities, numerous other abnormalities are present in women with PCOS. For example, the levels of SHBG are reduced, as a direct result of the impact of hyperandrogenism and hyperinsulinemia on the liver's production of SHBG. Decreased SHBG and increased androgen secretion result in increased concentrations of bioavailable testosterone. In turn, increased levels of circulating bioavailable testosterone and other androgens stimulate the growth of terminal hairs at androgen-dependent sites. Many women with PCOS have increased adrenal production of androgens such as dehydroepiandrosterone sulfate (DHEAS) and androstenedione. The mechanisms that cause adrenal androgen overproduction in women with PCOS are not fully characterized, but may include mild steroidogenic enzyme defects, such as mildly reduced 21-hydroxylase activity (heterozygotes) or 3-beta hydroxysteroid dehydrogenase activity, increased activity of P450 cyp17, and adrenal overresponsiveness to adrenocorticotropic hormone (ACTH).[30,31]

Diagnosis

The NIH definition of PCOS (see above) requires the presence of both hyperandrogenism and oligo-ovulation and the absence of evidence for another cause of hyperandrogenism, such as nonclassic adrenal hyperplasia resulting from either a 21-hydroxylase deficiency or an androgen-secreting tumor.

The presence of hyperandrogenism is the hallmark of PCOS. Most women with PCOS will show both clinical and biochemi-

Table 1   Characteristics of Common Causes of Androgen Excess

Diagnosis	Cause	Ovulation Status	Testosterone Level	8 A.M. Follicular-Phase 17-Hydroxyprogesterone Level
PCOS	Elevated LH, serum insulin, or both	Anovulation or oligo-ovulation	Elevated (0.75–2 ng/ml) or upper limits of normal	Normal (< 2 ng/ml)
Idiopathic hirsutism	Elevated production of androgen in the pilosebaceous unit, or a mild form of PCOS	Regular ovulation	Normal (< 0.75 ng/ml)	Normal (< 2 ng/ml)
Adrenal hyperplasia	Decrease in 21-hydroxylase activity because of a gene mutation	Anovulation or oligo-ovulation	Elevated (0.75–2 ng/ml)	Elevated (> 2 ng/ml)
Ovarian or adrenal tumor	Disorder of cell growth	Anovulation	Markedly elevated (> 2 ng/ml)	May be elevated

LH—luteinizing hormone   PCOS—polycystic ovary syndrome

cal manifestations. The common clinical signs of hyperandrogenism are hirsutism, acne, and male-pattern baldness. Most women with PCOS do not have signs of virilization, such as clitoromegaly or deepening of the voice. The presence of signs of virilization or the rapid progression of hirsutism should alert the clinician to search for an androgen-secreting tumor or other causes of virilization.

Oligomenorrhea is defined as menstrual cycle lengths greater than 35 days. Most women with PCOS have fewer than nine cycles per year.

HISTORY

The history can provide key information in the differential diagnosis of androgen excess (and heightened androgen sensitivity) in women [*see Table 1*].

Age of Onset

In PCOS, oligomenorrhea, hirsutism, and acne typically begin in the perimenarchal or teenage years. The onset of severe hirsutism in menopause suggests an ovarian neoplasm.

Menstrual History

Patients with PCOS typically experience irregular menstrual cycles starting at menarche. Regular cycles are more consistent with familial or idiopathic hirsutism. A history of initially regular periods followed by onset of oligomenorrhea or amenorrhea and hirsutism with virilization in adult life suggests an androgen-secreting tumor.

Pace of Progression of Hirsutism

In PCOS, hirsutism tends to progress slowly, over many years. Rapid progression to severe hirsutism suggests a virilizing disorder from an androgen-secreting tumor. Patients with androgen-secreting tumors typically report other manifestations of virilization, such as deepening of the voice and secondary amenorrhea. Virilization will be evident on the physical examination (see below).

Family History

Approximately 50% of women with PCOS have a family history of PCOS, type 2 diabetes mellitus, or both.

Medication Use

Some medications appear to cause increased LH secretion and ovarian androgen production; such medication can promote the development of PCOS. In particular, long-term use of the anticonvulsant valproate is strongly associated with the onset of PCOS (see below).[32]

Cigarette Smoking

Women who smoke have higher concentrations of androstenedione and testosterone than do nonsmoking women. Hence, smoking may contribute to hyperandrogenism.[33]

Sleep Apnea

Many women with PCOS are obese and have obstructive sleep apnea (see below). Women with PCOS should be questioned about symptoms of sleep apnea and daytime sleepiness.

PHYSICAL EXAMINATION

Hirsutism

Hirsutism can be assessed objectively with the Ferriman-Gallwey scoring system [*see Figure 1*] [*see Chapter 80*].[34] Along with providing a baseline measurement of hirsutism, this system can also be used to follow the efficacy of treatment. A Ferriman-Gallwey score of 6 or greater and 8 or greater have both been proposed as criteria for defining hirsutism.

Insulin Resistance

Various physical findings point to insulin resistance [*see Table 2*]. Excess weight is a major determinant of insulin resistance and hyperinsulinemia. Relative weight is best assessed by means of the BMI, which is calculated by dividing the patient's weight in kilograms by the square of the patient's height in meters. Women with a BMI of greater than 25 (i.e., those who are overweight) are often insulin resistant and may demonstrate hyperinsulinemia in response to a glucose stimulus. Women with a BMI of greater than 30 (i.e., those who are obese) are almost always insulin resistant. Women with a BMI of less than 22 are unlikely to be insulin resistant unless they have one of a relatively rare group of acquired or inherited lipodystrophic disorders.

Other physical findings that suggest insulin resistance are a waist-to-hip ratio greater than 0.85 and a waist circumference greater than 89 cm (35 in). The presence of acanthosis nigricans or acrochordons (skin tags) suggests the presence of insulin resistance. The syndrome of hyperandrogenism, insulin resistance, and acanthosis nigricans (HAIR-AN syndrome) is the most severe form of the insulin-resistant phenotype of PCOS.

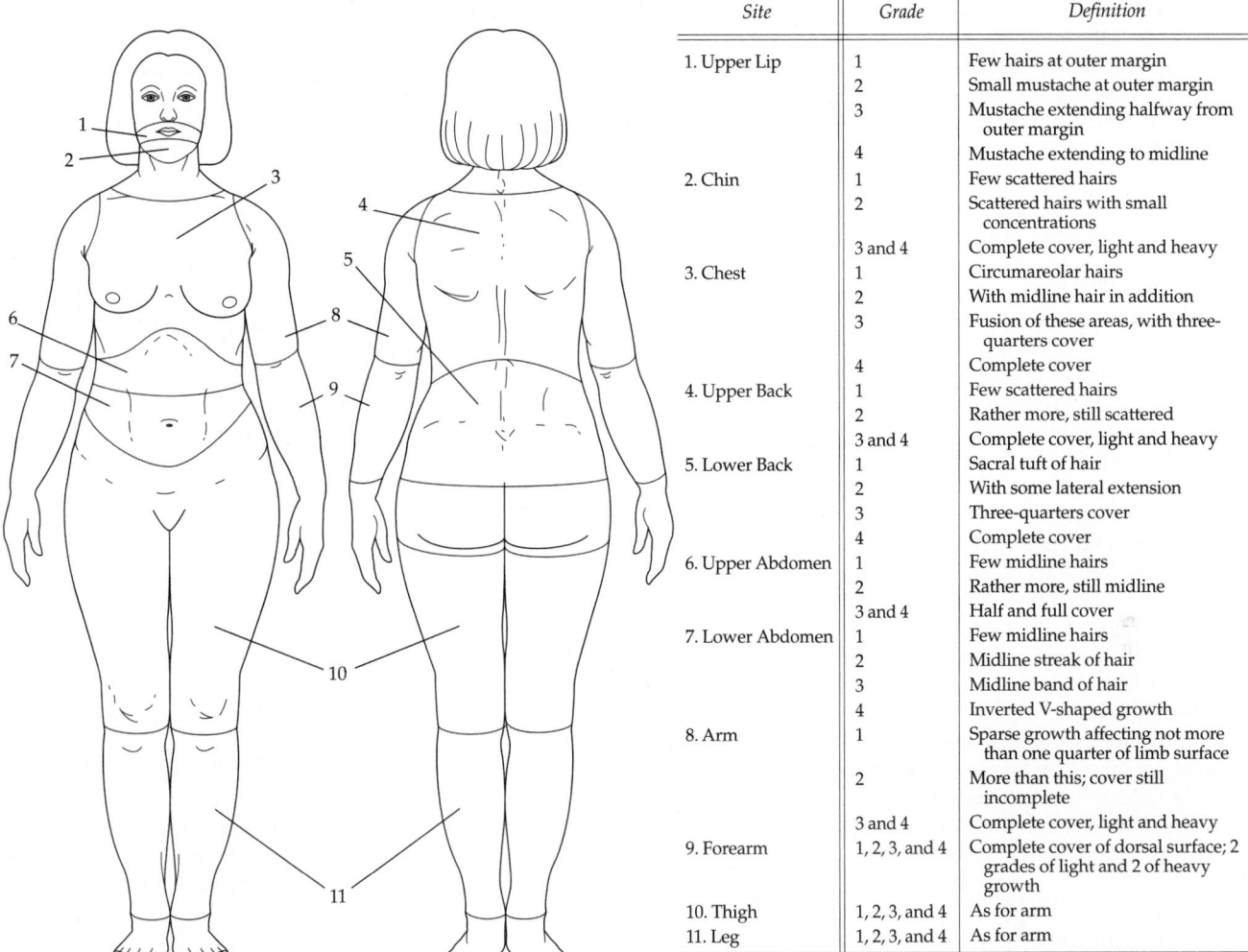

Site	Grade	Definition
1. Upper Lip	1	Few hairs at outer margin
	2	Small mustache at outer margin
	3	Mustache extending halfway from outer margin
	4	Mustache extending to midline
2. Chin	1	Few scattered hairs
	2	Scattered hairs with small concentrations
	3 and 4	Complete cover, light and heavy
3. Chest	1	Circumareolar hairs
	2	With midline hair in addition
	3	Fusion of these areas, with three-quarters cover
	4	Complete cover
4. Upper Back	1	Few scattered hairs
	2	Rather more, still scattered
	3 and 4	Complete cover, light and heavy
5. Lower Back	1	Sacral tuft of hair
	2	With some lateral extension
	3	Three-quarters cover
	4	Complete cover
6. Upper Abdomen	1	Few midline hairs
	2	Rather more, still midline
	3 and 4	Half and full cover
7. Lower Abdomen	1	Few midline hairs
	2	Midline streak of hair
	3	Midline band of hair
	4	Inverted V-shaped growth
8. Arm	1	Sparse growth affecting not more than one quarter of limb surface
	2	More than this; cover still incomplete
	3 and 4	Complete cover, light and heavy
9. Forearm	1, 2, 3, and 4	Complete cover of dorsal surface; 2 grades of light and 2 of heavy growth
10. Thigh	1, 2, 3, and 4	As for arm
11. Leg	1, 2, 3, and 4	As for arm

Figure 1 Ferriman-Gallwey scoring system for quantifying hirsutism. The 11 sites are graded from 0 (no terminal hair) to 4 (severe hirsutism). Women with a total score greater than 8 are considered hirsute.[34]

Unfortunately, the physical findings that are associated with insulin resistance tend to be specific but not sensitive. For example, patients with acanthosis nigricans are almost always insulin resistant, but many women with insulin resistance do not have acanthosis nigricans. Although the identification of severe insulin resistance on the basis of clinical manifestations may be relatively simple, the detection of mild insulin resistance may be difficult.

Metabolic Syndrome

Compared to the general population, women with PCOS are at a twofold greater risk for being diagnosed with the metabolic syndrome.[35] Many authorities recommend that women with PCOS be screened for the presence of the metabolic syndrome. The physical exam findings that are components of the diagnosis of the metabolic syndrome include a waist circumference greater than 35 inches in women and a blood pressure greater than 130/85 mm Hg. The diagnosis of metabolic syndrome requires testing for fasting serum glucose levels, triglyceride levels, and HDL-C levels [see Laboratory Tests, *below*].[36]

Virilization

A key aspect of the physical examination is a search for signs of virilization, such as clitoromegaly, increased upper-body mus-

cle mass, and male pattern baldness. These may indicate the presence of an androgen-secreting tumor.

Women with PCOS have enlarged ovaries, although the ovaries typically are not palpable on pelvic examination, especially in obese women. If pelvic examination discloses a large, complex mass, the patient may have an adrenal or ovarian tumor.

LABORATORY TESTS

The goals of the laboratory evaluation of hyperandrogenism are to rule out an adrenal and ovarian tumor, assess the severity of the androgen excess, determine whether the source of the hy-

Table 2 Physical Findings Associated with Insulin Resistance

Body mass index* > 25	Acanthosis nigricans
Waist-to-hip ratio > 0.85	Numerous acrochordons (skin tags)
Waist > 90 cm	

*Calculated by dividing the patient's weight in kilograms by the square of her height in meters.

perandrogenism is adrenal (nonclassic adrenal hyperplasia resulting from a 21-hydroxylase deficiency) and screen for the presence of the metabolic syndrome.

There are few consensus guidelines on laboratory testing for women with PCOS. In one survey of 176 pediatric endocrinologists, more than 50% of the clinicians recommended testing for the following analytes: testosterone, 17-hydroxyprogesterone, prolactin, DHEAS, LH, follicle-stimulating hormone (FSH), fasting glucose, and fasting insulin.[37] In addition, assessment for the metabolic syndrome is recommended by most authorities.

Testosterone

Serum testosterone concentration provides the best laboratory estimate of the severity of androgen overproduction. Measurement can be taken of total serum testosterone, free serum testosterone, or both. Total serum testosterone measurement is performed by all clinical laboratories; these tests are reasonably well standardized, especially in the range greater than 1.5 ng/ml, and are less expensive than free serum testosterone measurement. Many women with PCOS have a total testosterone concentration in the upper end of the normal range (about 0.60 to 0.80 ng/ml); this range is not well standardized among clinical laboratories. If the total testosterone level is greater than 2 ng/ml (200 ng/dl), the patient probably has ovarian stromal hyperthecosis or an adrenal or ovarian tumor; such a patient needs a detailed evaluation, which should include imaging studies of the ovary and adrenal glands.

Measurement of free serum testosterone concentration is more sensitive than total testosterone measurement in detecting mild androgen overproduction; however, the free serum testosterone assay is not well standardized among laboratories, and is more expensive than a total testosterone assay.

17-Hydroxyprogesterone

Approximately 2% of women who present with hyperandrogenism and oligo-ovulation or anovulation have nonclassic

adrenal hyperplasia resulting from a 21-hydroxylase deficiency. The prevalence of this congenital disorder varies markedly among different ethnic groups, from below 1% in Hispanic populations to as high as 5% to 8% in Ashkenazi Jewish populations. The decision to screen for the disorder depends on the cost-benefit assessment of detection and the baseline prevalence of the disorder in the patient's ethnic group.

If the 17-hydroxyprogesterone level at 8 A.M. (measured in the follicular phase of the menstrual cycle) is greater than 2 ng/ml, the patient probably has nonclassic adrenal hyperplasia resulting from a 21-hydroxylase deficiency. This diagnosis can be confirmed by a 60-minute ACTH stimulation test. The test utilizes a form of synthetic ACTH (cosyntropin) that contains the first 24 of the 39 amino acids of natural ACTH; 0.25 mg ACTH is given intravenously or intramuscularly, and the 17-hydroxyprogesterone level is measured 60 minutes later. An ACTH 17-hydroxyprogesterone level greater than 10 ng/ml after the stimulation test confirms the diagnosis of nonclassic adrenal hyperplasia resulting from a 21-hydroxylase deficiency.

DHEAS

DHEAS, an androgen prohormone that can be converted to testosterone in the periphery, is secreted almost exclusively by the adrenal glands. The normal DHEAS level in premenopausal women is 0.12 to 5.35 µg/dl. A DHEAS level above 10.70 µg/dl—that is, more than twice the upper limit of normal—should raise concern over a possible adrenal tumor.

Serum Prolactin and Thyroid-stimulating Hormone

If the patient has amenorrhea, the laboratory workup should include an assessment of the serum prolactin level to rule out a prolactin-secreting pituitary tumor. Many clinicians also routinely measure serum FSH and serum thyroid-stimulating hormone (TSH) levels in amenorrheic patients.

Serum Luteinizing Hormone and Follicle Stimulating Hormone

The measurement of serum LH presents a special problem in the laboratory evaluation of PCOS. In the research setting—using multiple serum LH measurements (every 10 minutes for at least 8 hours) and a precise and reliable LH assay—elevated LH levels can be documented in more than 90% of women with PCOS. However, because LH secretion is pulsatile and the standard commercial assays are not as precise as research assays, measurement of LH in clinical practice is of only modest utility. An elevated LH level is reasonably specific for PCOS, provided the sample was not taken during a preovulatory LH surge. A normal LH value does not necessarily exclude PCOS, however, because the test sample may have been drawn when the patient was at the nadir of an LH pulse. Another important point is that as BMI increases, the normal range for LH decreases [*see Figure 2*].[38,39] Nomograms that control serum LH for BMI are not widely available. Many women with PCOS have an LH:FSH ratio greater than 2. The ratio of LH:FSH may be a better test for PCOS than a single LH measurement.

Antimullerian Hormone (Mullerian Inhibiting Substance)

Antimullerian hormone (AMH) concentration in the circulation of women with PCOS is elevated to two to three times that of ovulatory women.[40] The number of small antral follicles detected on transvaginal imaging is correlated with serum AMH concentration. Some authorities have recommended replacing

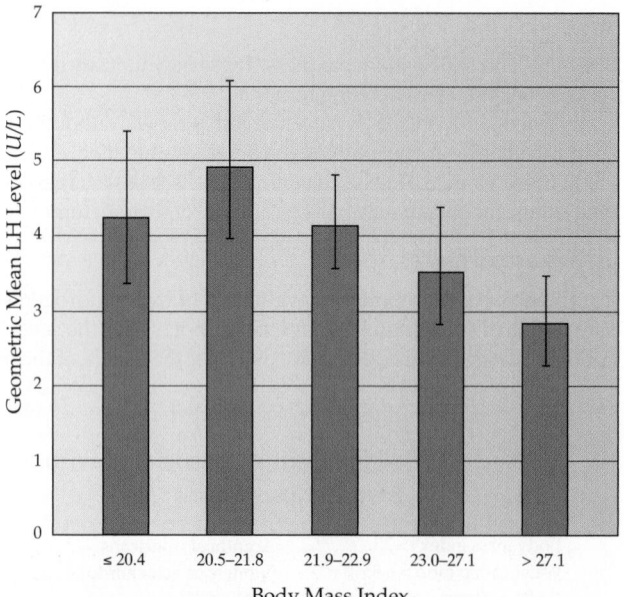

Figure 2 **Relationship between body mass index (BMI) and basal luteinizing hormone (LH) levels in women in the follicular phase of the menstrual cycle.**[38]

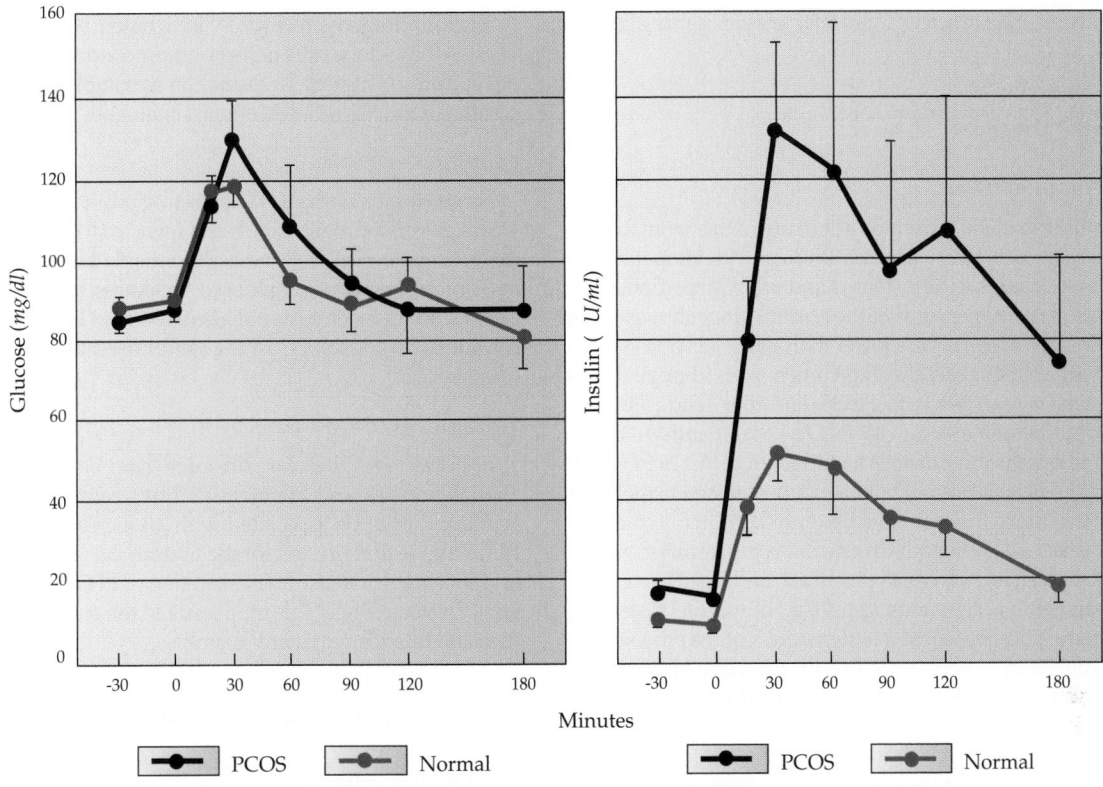

Figure 3 **In response to an oral glucose challenge, nonobese women with PCOS experience an exaggerated increase in circulating insulin compared with weight-matched control subjects; the increase persists for over 3 hours.**[103]

the Rotterdam criteria's method of counting the number of small antral follicles with a serum measurement of AMH.[41]

Pelvic Imaging

Using the NIH criteria, demonstration of polycystic ovaries on pelvic ultrasonography is not essential for the diagnosis of PCOS; however, pelvic imaging is necessary if the Rotterdam criteria are used for the diagnosis of PCOS. Pelvic imaging is clinically indicated if the ovaries are palpable and enlarged on physical examination or the total testosterone concentration is greater than 2.0 ng/ml.

Tests for Detection of the Metabolic Syndrome

The diagnosis of metabolic syndrome requires laboratory testing for HDL-C levels (abnormal, < 50 mg/dl), fasting serum glucose levels (abnormal, > 100 mg/dl), and serum triglyceride levels (abnormal, >150 mg/dl) [*see Chapter 53*].

Screening and Testing for Diabetes Mellitus

The American Diabetes Association recommends screening for type 2 diabetes in women with PCOS.[42] In a population of women with PCOS, approximately 4% have undiagnosed diabetes and 23% have impaired glucose tolerance. There are no clear national guidelines specifying the best method by which to screen and test for diabetes mellitus in women with PCOS. Data suggest that the oral glucose tolerance test may be more sensitive than the fasting serum glucose assay or the hemoglobin A_{1c} assay for the detection of diabetes mellitus in women with PCOS. In one study that compared the oral glucose tolerance test with the fasting serum glucose test, 254 women with PCOS took both tests; 3.2% of women had diabetes on the basis of the fasting

serum glucose test, and 7.5% had diabetes on the basis of the oral glucose tolerance test.[43] Similar findings have been reported in adolescents.[44] The Rotterdam consensus conference recommended screening all obese women with PCOS using an oral glucose tolerance test. Most cases of undiagnosed diabetes occur in obese women with PCOS, not in lean women with PCOS.

Tests for Detection of Insulin Resistance and Hyperinsulinemia

At least 50% of women with PCOS have insulin resistance and hyperinsulinemia. There is no clear consensus on how to detect these two conditions. A major problem is that the least resource-intensive laboratory techniques for diagnosing insulin resistance and hyperinsulinemia are specific but not sensitive. Elevation of the fasting serum insulin level or a fasting serum insulin-to-glucose ratio of less than 4.5 is almost always associated with insulin resistance, but many insulin-resistant women do not have fasting hyperinsulinemia. Laboratory techniques that are both specific and sensitive for detecting insulin resistance, such as euglycemic hyperinsulinemic clamp studies, are too complex and expensive for application in general clinical practice. Until laboratory tests that are both specific and sensitive become widely available for clinical practice, clinicians should determine insulin resistance on the basis of clinical findings and, if necessary, simple laboratory tests—such as assessment of fasting insulin levels or assessment of insulin response to an oral glucose challenge. Even nonobese women with PCOS have marked increases in circulating insulin after a glucose challenge [*see Figure 3*].

The Rotterdam consensus conference concluded that, given limited resources and time, it is preferable to screen for the metabolic syndrome than to screen for insulin resistance using laboratory tests.

Differential Diagnosis

IDIOPATHIC HIRSUTISM

Idiopathic hirsutism is defined as hirsutism in a woman with regular, ovulatory menstrual cycles. Women with idiopathic hirsutism have circulating testosterone and androstenedione concentrations at the upper limit of the normal range; however, in these patients, such levels are lower than the levels observed in women with PCOS [see Table 1]. Women with idiopathic hirsutism often have sisters with PCOS, and they tend to have a lower BMI than their sisters with PCOS.[45] Many authorities believe that idiopathic hirsutism is a mild form of PCOS in which hyperandrogenism is present but has not progressed to the point at which ovulatory menses have become disrupted. Other authorities believe that idiopathic hirsutism is the result of overactive skin conversion of weak precursor androgens (e.g., androstenedione) to potent androgens (e.g., dihydrotestosterone) directly in the pilosebaceous unit. Regardless of the etiology, idiopathic hirsutism is best treated using the same approach as that used for hirsutism in women with PCOS (see below).

VIRILIZATION SYNDROMES

Women with a rapid onset of virilization or a serum testosterone level greater than 2 ng/ml (200 ng/dl) should be evaluated for the presence of an adrenal or ovarian tumor. Magnetic resonance imaging can be used to screen for an adrenal tumor, whereas pelvic sonography may be helpful in detecting an ovarian tumor.

Adrenal carcinoma often presents with rapid-onset virilization; it is often associated with systemic symptoms such as fatigue, weakness, and weight loss. In patients with adrenal carcinoma, the DHEAS concentration is often greater than 8 μg/ml, and 24-hour urinary 17-ketosteroid excretion is markedly increased, to about 30 mg/dl.

OVARIAN HYPERTHECOSIS

Careful histologic examination of ovaries from women with PCOS often reveals islands of luteinized, steroid-secreting stromal cells (stromal hyperthecosis) in the medullary portion of the ovary that are not associated with follicular structures.[46] Severely hyperthecotic ovaries may contain only a small number of follicles, each 4 to 8 mm in diameter. PCOS patients with more severe hyperinsulinemia seem to be at highest risk for hyperthecosis.

Only a small subset of women with hyperandrogenism have stromal hyperthecosis. The diagnosis should be considered in a patient who presents with virilization, a total serum testosterone concentration of greater than 2 ng/ml, a normal LH level, and marked insulin resistance and hyperinsulinemia. Pathologic confirmation of the diagnosis, which requires removal of the ovaries, is not necessary.

Differentiation of ovarian hyperthecosis from PCOS is important because women with ovarian hyperthecosis often do not have significant suppression of circulating testosterone when treated with estrogen-progestin contraceptive alone. Instead, treatment with a GnRH analogue (e.g., leuprolide acetate depot, 3.75 mg intramuscularly every 4 weeks) plus an estrogen-progestin contraceptive, often results in the normalization of circulating androgens.[47] A possible interpretation of this observation is that LH must be profoundly suppressed in order to decrease ovarian androgen production in women with hyperthecotic ovaries. Low-dose estrogen-progestin contraceptives alone do not suppress pituitary LH secretion as completely as they do in combination with a GnRH agonist analogue.

CUSHING SYNDROME

Some women with ACTH-secreting pituitary tumors present with signs of androgen excess and menstrual irregularity. Physical findings such as violaceous abdominal striae larger than 2 cm in diameter and proximal muscle weakness, together with laboratory findings such as hypokalemia, should lead the clinician to consider a diagnosis of Cushing syndrome rather than PCOS [see Chapter 55].

VALPROIC ACID TREATMENT

Epilepsy and bipolar disorder can be associated with oligomenorrhea and hirsutism.[48,49] But treatment with valproic acid appears to be associated with an increased prevalence of PCOS above that present for the underlying condition. Valproic acid increases both pituitary secretion of LH and ovarian secretion of testosterone.[50] This may result in the onset of oligomenorrhea and hirsutism in many women.

Syndromes and Diseases Associated with PCOS

METABOLIC SYNDROME

Many studies report that women with PCOS, especially those who are obese, are at high risk for developing the metabolic syndrome. In the NHANES III cohort, the population-wide risk for metabolic syndrome among women 20 to 29 years of age was 6%; in women with PCOS, it was 45%.[35] In women with PCOS, the most prevalent factors for metabolic syndrome were increased waist circumference (67%) and decreased serum HDL-C (68%). The least prevalent factor was an elevated fasting glucose (4%). Increased levels of triglyceride and low-density lipoprotein cholesterol (LDL-C) and decreased levels of HDL-C are commonly observed in women with PCOS.[51,52]

CARDIOVASCULAR DISEASE

The risk for coronary heart disease among women with PCOS is not precisely characterized. Many surrogate and intermediate markers for coronary heart disease are abnormal in women with PCOS. For example, C-reactive protein[53,54] and endothelin-1[55] are increased in the serum of women with PCOS. In one series, women with PCOS were reported to have more extensive coronary artery disease as demonstrated by cardiac catheterization than ovulatory women.[56] In women older than 45 years of age who have PCOS, the mean thickness of the carotid intima-media was significantly greater than in control subjects, but it was below that observed in women with established carotid artery disease.[57] Women with PCOS appear to have increased coronary artery calcium as shown by computed tomography; however, obesity appears to account for much of the observed association between PCOS and coronary artery calcification.[58] In the Nurses Health Study II cohort, menstrual cycle irregularity was associated with a small and significant increase in the risk for cardiovascular events.[59]

SLEEP APNEA

Obese individuals are at increased risk for sleep apnea. Insulin resistance and the PCOS phenotype appear to increase the

Table 3   Treatment of Hirsutism, Anovulatory Infertility, and Endometrial Hyperplasia in Women with PCOS

Presenting Problem	Standard Treatment	Alternative Treatment
Hirsutism	Oral contraceptive plus spironolactone Weight loss	Oral contraceptive used in a long-cycle regimen, plus spironolactone Oral contraceptive plus GnRH analogue Insulin sensitizer, preferably metformin Finasteride
Acne	Oral contraceptive	Topical agents, oral antibiotics
Infertility	Weight loss Clomiphene Metformin plus clomiphene Clomiphene plus glucocorticoids Low-dose FSH injections Low-dose FSH injections plus metformin	Ovarian surgery IVF-ET
Endometrial hyperplasia	Oral contraceptives High-dose progestins	Weight loss

FSH—follicle-stimulating hormone GnRH—gonadotropin-releasing hormone IVF-ET—in vitro fertilization with embryo transfer

risk for sleep apnea more than obesity alone. Women with PCOS should be screened for the presence of sleep apnea.[60]

NONALCOHOLIC STEATOHEPATITIS

Obese individuals are at increased risk for nonalcoholic steatohepatitis. In one study, 15% of women with PCOS had elevated concentrations of aspartate aminotransferase, elevated alanine aminotransferase, or both. Of the women with elevated liver function tests who underwent liver biopsy, all had nonalcoholic steatohepatitis with fibrosis.[61]

Treatment

Treatment for PCOS can be directed at the chief complaint(s) as well as the other common problems faced by women with the disorder. The most common complaints of women with PCOS are irregular and infrequent menses, hirsutism, and anovulatory infertility [see Table 3]. PCOS should be treated, because it poses long-term risks of endometrial cancer, diabetes mellitus, and possibly cardiovascular disease.

Treatment of PCOS in a woman who smokes cigarettes includes smoking cessation. Discontinuance of smoking may result in a reduction in circulating androgens; also, smoking is a contraindication to the use of oral contraceptives, which are often prescribed for patients with PCOS.

Women with PCOS are frequently overweight or obese. Given the long-term morbidity and mortality associated with excess BMI, weight reduction should be a focus of the treatment plan.[62]

TREATMENT OF IRREGULAR AND INFREQUENT MENSES

The first-line treatment of irregular and infrequent menses, which is the chief complaint of women with PCOS, is a cyclic estrogen-progestin contraceptive. An estrogen-progestin contraceptive can be prescribed as an oral pill, a transvaginal ring, or a transdermal patch. Cyclic estrogen-progestin oral contraceptives produce multiple beneficial effects in patients with PCOS. These effects include the following: (1) decreased LH secretion, which suppresses ovarian androgen production; (2) increased liver pro-

duction of sex hormone–binding globulin, which decreases free testosterone concentration; (3) decreased adrenal androgen production, through an unidentified pathway; (4) prevention of endometrial hyperplasia; and (5) regular uterine withdrawal bleeding. Of course, oral contraceptives also prevent pregnancy. The choice of agent does not seem important; it appears that any oral contraceptive, regardless of the estrogen dose or the progestin employed, can be effective in the treatment of hirsutism. However, most authorities avoid using an androgenic progestin such as norgestrel in treating women with PCOS. Drosperinone, which is a new progestin that has antiandrogenic and antimineralocorticoid properties, may have modest relative benefits in women with PCOS.

The most common regimen of cyclic estrogen-progestin therapy comprises 21 hormone pills and seven placebo pills; however, alternative regimens are available. One such regimen uses 24 hormone pills and three placebo pills. Other regimens use 84 hormone pills and 7 placebo pills; these are referred to as long-cycle regimens. Long-cycle regimens may be associated with better suppression of ovarian testosterone secretion than are standard-cycle regimens, especially in the first few months of treatment.

Many women with PCOS are obese and have multiple risk factors for cardiovascular disease. Some authorities have noted that the risk of cardiovascular complications (e.g., myocardial infarction and stroke) associated with estrogen-progestin contraceptives are approximately twofold greater for women with PCOS than for normo-ovulatory women.[63] However, the attributable risk of the cardiovascular complications is very low (less than one event/10,000 women-years of use) in both groups.

In specific situations where estrogen-progestin therapy is relatively contraindicated, such as in women with PCOS and hypertension, metformin can be used for the induction of regular menses[64]; however, it may take up to 6 months of treatment before metformin induces regular cycles. In one study, after 3 and 6 months of metformin treatment, 55% and 70% of women respectively reported regular menstrual cycles.[65] Metformin induces ovulation, which may increase the risk of pregnancy in women with PCOS using this treatment. Consequently, if the patient is having sexual intercourse and does not desire to become pregnant, a contraceptive is required.

An alternative treatment for irregular menses is to use cyclic progestin, such as medroxyprogesterone acetate (10 mg daily for 14 days each month) to induce a regular cycle. However, this regimen does not provide contraception; in fact, medroxyprogesterone acetate may trigger ovulation by suppressing the elevated GnRH pulse frequency observed in women with PCOS.[66] No high-quality studies directly compare estrogen-progestin versus progestin-only treatment for irregular menses.[67]

TREATMENT OF HIRSUTISM

Recommended treatment of hirsutism combines a hormonal therapy with a nonhormonal therapy [see Chapter 80].

The mainstay of the hormonal treatment of hirsutism resulting from androgen excess is the combination of an estrogen-progestin oral contraceptive (used in regular or long cycles) and an antiandrogen (e.g., spironolactone, 100 mg daily). For patients who prefer monotherapy, estrogen-progestin can be used alone. In a meta-analysis of seven studies, spironolactone, 100 mg daily, was demonstrated to be superior to placebo for subjective improvement of hair overgrowth. In addition, spironolactone, 100 mg daily, was demonstrated to be superior to finasteride, 5 mg daily; finasteride is a blocker of androgen synthesis.[68] Patients should be advised that response to spironolactone tends to be slow; for more immediate results, patients may prefer the use of techniques that directly destroy the hair follicle. The options for nonhormonal therapy of hirsutism include shaving, electrolysis, laser treatment, and the prescription medication eflornithine (Vaniqa),which is an inhibitor of hair growth that is applied topically.[69]

TREATMENT OF ANOVULATORY OR OLIGO-OVULATORY INFERTILITY

Ovulation induction in PCOS follows a stepwise approach, beginning with interventions that require nominal resources (e.g., behavior modification and medical therapy) and escalating to resource-intensive surgical interventions [see Table 4]. If the BMI is greater than 25, weight loss is an important goal. If normalization of the BMI cannot be achieved, clomiphene is often prescribed because it is relatively inexpensive and has an excellent safety profile. Hyperandrogenic, insulin-resistant women are more likely to fail to ovulate and become pregnant with

---

Table 4   A Stepwise Approach to the Induction of Ovulation in Infertile Women with PCOS*

Step 1: if BMI is > 27, weight loss of at least 10%

Step 2: clomiphene

Step 3: if DHEAS > 2 µg/ml (200 µg/dl), clomiphene plus glucocorticoid therapy

Step 4: metformin for 8 to 12 wk

Step 5: metformin plus clomiphene

Step 6: low-dose FSH therapy

Step 7: metformin plus low-dose FSH therapy

Step 8: in vitro fertilization

Step 9: laparoscopic ovarian surgery to reduce ovarian androgen production

*Steps proceed in order of increasing resource intensity.

---

clomiphene than are women who are not insulin resistant. If both weight loss and clomiphene do not induce ovulation and result in pregnancy, the currently available choices for ovulation induction include insulin-sensitizing agents such as metformin, FSH injections, ovarian surgery, and in vitro fertilization with embryo transfer (IVF-ET).

Before initiating ovulation induction for anovulatory infertility, a basic infertility examination should be completed. This should include a semen analysis and possibly a hysterosalpingogram to document tubal patency and a normal uterine contour.

Weight Loss

Many women with PCOS are overweight or obese. In such women, weight loss in the range of 10% of body mass is associated with a decrease in insulin secretion, a decrease in LH secretion, and a decrease in androgen production. The result is often a resumption of regular ovulation and, in some women, pregnancy.[70,71]

Clomiphene

Clomiphene is the most widely used agent for ovulation induction in women with PCOS. Clomiphene is an antiestrogen (or more precisely, a selective estrogen receptor modulator) that blocks estrogen action in the hypothalamus and pituitary, resulting in an increase in pituitary secretion of LH and FSH. In turn, the increased FSH secretion from the pituitary can remove the presence of an intraovarian block prohibiting the development of a dominant follicle, an issue that is often observed in women with PCOS. If clomiphene-induced pituitary secretion of FSH can cause a dominant follicle(s) to grow, that follicle will trigger the pituitary release of LH, and subsequently ovulation will occur.

A meta-analysis of four randomized trials indicates that clomiphene is an effective first-line agent for induction of ovulation in women with PCOS.[72]

The FDA-approved dosage of clomiphene for the induction of ovulation is 50 or 100 mg daily for a maximum of 5 days during each menstrual cycle. After a spontaneous menses or the induction of menses with a progestin withdrawal maneuver (e.g., medroxyprogesterone acetate, 10 mg p.o. daily for 5 days), clomiphene (50 mg daily for 5 days) is started on cycle day 3, 4, or 5. In properly selected women, 50% will ovulate through the use of this clomiphene regimen. Another 25% will ovulate if the dosage of clomiphene is increased to 100 mg daily. During each cycle, determination of ovulation should be attempted by use of basal body temperature charts, ultrasound monitoring of follicle growth and rupture, or luteal-phase progesterone measurements. Some clinicians use endometrial biopsies to document ovulation in cycles where conception is not attempted. In most women, ovulation occurs approximately 5 to 12 days after the last dose of clomiphene. Measurement of the urinary LH surge is recommended to assist the patient in prospectively determining the periovulatory interval.

Although the FDA has approved 100 mg as the maximum daily dosage of clomiphene, many clinicians prescribe clomiphene at doses of 150 mg daily for 5 days, and some give doses of 250 mg daily for 5 days. Women who fail to ovulate after taking clomiphene in doses of 100 mg daily for 5 days may ovulate if they are treated with clomiphene at doses of 150 mg daily for 5 days. Some authorities advocate use of clomiphene at doses up to 250 mg daily for up to 14 days. As many as 70% of the women who fail to ovulate with doses of 100 mg daily will ovulate with higher doses, but fewer than 30% of those become pregnant. In my opinion, there are few data to support the use of clomiphene at doses greater than 150 mg daily. Women who do not become pregnant while taking clomiphene at 150 mg daily should consider other approaches to ovulation induction (see below). Clomiphene treatment can be associated with adverse changes in the reproductive tract, including induction of a luteal-phase defect (delay of endometrial maturation) and the creation of a hostile cervical environment resulting from a low quantity and poor quality of cervical mucus. Some clinicians recommend endometrial biopsy during a test cycle of clomiphene treatment to assess whether clomiphene induces luteal-phase deficiency. Many clinicians recommend that a postcoital test be performed during the first cycle of clomiphene treatment to screen for poor cervical mucus properties.

Multiple pregnancy is a well known outcome of clomiphene use. The absolute risk of high-order multiple gestation with clomiphene treatment was shown to be low in a manufacturer's study of 2,369 clomiphene-induced pregnancies: 7% resulted in twins, 0.5% triplets, 0.3% quadruplets, and 0.13% quintuplets. However, because clomiphene is a heavily prescribed medication, the number of triplets resulting from clomiphene is substantial. The rate of spontaneous abortion after clomiphene-induced ovulation and pregnancy is approximately 15%. The most common side effects of clomiphene include vasomotor symptoms (20%), adnexal tenderness (5%), nausea (3%), headache (1%), and, rarely, blurring of vision or scotomata. Most clinicians permanently discontinue clomiphene in women who experience changes in vision resulting from the drug.

Clomiphene plus Glucocorticoid

Anovulatory women with PCOS who do not ovulate with clomiphene may ovulate if treated with the combination of a short course of dexamethasone followed by clomiphene.[73]

Insulin Sensitizers

A major advance in reproductive endocrinology is the discovery that insulin sensitizers can induce ovulation in infertile women with oligo-ovulation, hyperandrogenism, and insulin resistance. Insulin sensitizers that have been approved for the treatment of diabetes include metformin, rosiglitazone, and pioglitazone. The insulin sensitizer D-chiro-inositol has been demonstrated to induce ovulation in hyperandrogenic insulin-resistant women, but it is currently available for use in research trials only.[74]

Metformin Metformin is an oral biguanide antihyperglycemic agent approved for the treatment of type 2 diabetes mellitus. In women with PCOS, metformin restores regular menstrual cycles, improves hirsutism, increases insulin sensitivity, and improves the lipid profile. In women with PCOS and anovulatory infertility, metformin often restores ovulatory menses, and pregnancy may result.[75,76]

Metformin decreases blood glucose by inhibiting hepatic glucose production and enhancing peripheral glucose uptake. It increases insulin sensitivity at the postreceptor level and stimulates insulin-mediated glucose disposal. Metformin may work through LKB1 (the Peutz-Jegher syndrome tumor suppressor protein) to stimulate adenosine monophosphate-activated protein kinase in the liver.[77] Unlike the sulfonylureas, metformin's mechanism of action does not involve increased insulin secretion.

Metformin is available in immediate-release tablets (500 mg, 850 mg, and 1,000 mg) and extended-release (ER) tablets (500 mg and 750 mg). The typical target dose is approximately 1,500 mg daily; however, doses up to 2,500 mg daily have been utilized. In adolescents, doses as low as 500 mg to 850 mg daily may be effective. The immediate-release formulation is taken in divided doses with breakfast, lunch, and dinner. The ER formulation is taken with dinner (or the largest meal of the day). Many clinicians believe that the ER formulation is associated with fewer gastrointestinal side effects. To minimize gastrointestinal side effects, such as nausea, many clinicians start metformin at 500 mg daily for the first week, then increase the dosage to 500 mg twice daily for the second week, and then increase the dosage again to 500 mg three times daily. Although metformin is not approved by the FDA for the treatment of PCOS, it may be significantly less expensive than FSH injections, ovarian surgery, and IVF-ET; metformin may also have fewer serious side effects than these treatments.

The most common side effects associated with metformin are GI disturbances, including diarrhea, nausea, vomiting, and abdominal bloating. In rare cases, metformin treatment has caused fatal lactic acidosis, but most of these patients had some degree of renal insufficiency or were hypoxic. Before starting treatment with metformin, it is advisable to confirm that the patient's serum creatinine level is less than 1.4 mg/dl.

Metformin increases the number of ovulatory cycles in infertile women with hyperandrogenism and insulin resistance. When used together with clomiphene, metformin significantly increases the rate of ovulation and of pregnancy resulting in live-born singleton births.[78] Metformin has also been shown to enhance the effectiveness of FSH injections to induce ovulation in oligo-ovulatory, hyperandrogenic, and insulin-resistant women.[79]

If a patient has not ovulated after 5 to 10 weeks of metformin treatment, clomiphene can be added (see above). If the patient becomes pregnant, metformin can be discontinued, although it is a category B drug for pregnant women and has been used by some clinicians to treat diabetes in pregnant women.[80]

Metformin versus clomiphene Clomiphene and metformin are both effective first-line agents in the treatment of anovulatory infertility. There is insufficient literature to definitively identify the superior therapy. However, there is concern that clomiphene treatment is associated with a greater risk of spontaneous abortion than metformin.[81] Clomiphene, but not metformin, is approved by the FDA for ovulation induction.

Metformin plus clomiphene In a meta-analysis of 13 clinical trials, the ovulation rates were 46% with metformin alone and 76% with the combination of metformin plus clomiphene.[82] For women who have not ovulated with metformin or clomiphene monotherapy, the combination of the two drugs appears to be effective.

Thiazolidinediones The thiazolidinediones increase cellular sensitivity to the effects of insulin. Agents in this category include pioglitazone, rosiglitazone, and troglitazone. Several studies of troglitazone in women with PCOS reported a decrease in fasting insulin, LH, and testosterone levels, along with an increase in ovulatory cycles.[83,84] Troglitazone was removed from the market because of its association with the risk of death from liver failure. The risk was very small, affecting approximately 1 in 25,000 patients treated with the drug.

Pioglitazone and rosiglitazone, widely used in the treatment of diabetes mellitus, have not been extensively studied for their impact on ovulation. Pilot studies indicate that like troglitazone, both pioglitazone and rosiglitazone are effective for inducing ovulation as monotherapy or in combination with clomiphene.

They are not approved by the FDA for this indication.[85,86] In one study of women with PCOS and anovulatory infertility who had not conceived with clomiphene monotherapy, rosiglitazone plus clomiphene was reported to be associated with a per-cycle pregnancy rate of 21%.[87]

Clomiphene plus Gonadotropin Injection

In women who fail to ovulate after therapy with clomiphene alone, gonadotropin injections can be added to clomiphene treatment to induce ovulation. Typically, the injections are started after clomiphene, 100 to 200 mg daily, has been given for 5 days. The main benefit of this combination is that it tends to reduce the quantity of gonadotropins (an expensive medication) needed to induce ovulation during each cycle, because the rise in endogenous LH and FSH levels induced by clomiphene increases the sensitivity of the follicles to the injected gonadotropins. This regimen has been associated with a 50% decrease in the dosage of gonadotropin required to induce ovulation.[88]

Gonadotropins

The gonadotropins currently available for ovulation induction include (1) FSH produced by recombinant DNA technology and immunopurification and (2) LH plus FSH derived from menopausal urine. The recombinant FSH preparations can be given as subcutaneous injections and are available in ampules of 37.5 or 75 IU. FSH is the primary hormone responsible for follicular recruitment and growth in humans; it can be used as a single agent to induce ovulation in most anovulatory women. Women with PCOS generally do not require exogenous LH to induce follicular development, because their levels of LH secretion are already increased.

In women with PCOS, induction of ovulation with long-term, low-dose FSH treatment appears to result in a high pregnancy rate with a low rate of complications, including high-order multiple gestation and ovarian hyperstimulation.[89] In this approach, 75 units of FSH are given daily for the first 14 days; the dose is then raised by 37.5 units every 7 days until follicular ripening is complete. If FSH treatment fails to result in pregnancy, consideration should be given to the combination of metformin and FSH, ovarian surgery, or IVF-ET.

During gonadotropin induction of ovulation, as many as 20% of patients experience mild to moderate enlargement of the ovaries. Some women treated with gonadotropins develop increased vascular permeability and accumulation of fluid in the peritoneal cavity and pleural space, a condition termed the ovarian hyperstimulation syndrome (OHSS). Clinical manifestations of OHSS include abdominal pain, abdominal distention, nausea, vomiting, diarrhea, and dyspnea. Other physical and laboratory findings of OHSS include weight gain, ovarian enlargement, ascites, pleural effusion, hemoconcentration, electrolyte imbalances, renal dysfunction, and thrombosis.[90] Treatment includes bed rest, maintenance of intravascular volume, prophylaxis against thrombosis, and surgical correction of ovarian torsion.

Before the utilization of repetitive estradiol measurements and sonographic evaluation of follicular development, OHSS occurred in as many as 5% of women receiving gonadotropin treatment. In recent series that employed intense monitoring with these techniques, the rate of OHSS was approximately 0.5%.[91] OHSS may be more severe and have a longer course if a successful pregnancy occurs. Multiple births occur in approximately 15% of pregnancies that take place after ovulation induction with gonadotropins.

Ovarian Surgery

Laparoscopic drilling of the ovary is the most widely studied surgical treatment for ovulation in PCOS[92]; approximately 1,000 cases have been reported. These reports demonstrate that surgery to induce ovulation causes a decrease in circulating LH (50% decline) and testosterone (30% decline) and an increase in FSH (30% increase). The pregnancy rate is in the range of 50% at 12 months and 70% at 24 months. The surgical techniques used for ovarian drilling vary between centers. However, all use a laser or electrosurgery to make multiple millimeter-size punctures in each ovary.

In one randomized, controlled study, 50 women with PCOS and anovulatory infertility were randomized to receive either ovarian surgery for ovulation induction or injections of FSH; at 6 months the cumulative pregnancy rate was 28% in the surgical group and 33% in the FSH injection group (no significant difference).[93] A meta-analysis of six trials concluded that ovarian surgery and FSH injections had similar efficacy for ovulation induction in women with PCOS[94]; however, the long-term effects of ovarian surgery on ovarian function were not well characterized.

In Vitro Fertilization with Embryo Transfer

IVF-ET has been demonstrated to be effective in the treatment of infertile women with PCOS who fail to become pregnant with gonadotropin injections. In preliminary reports, IVF-ET treatment of infertile women with PCOS has been associated with a per-cycle live birth rate of 25% to 35%.[95]

TREATMENT OF OBESITY

Numerous studies have demonstrated the benefits of weight loss in hyperandrogenic, insulin-resistant women.[96] In these studies, mean weight loss ranging from about 10 to 20 kg has been associated with a decrease in insulin levels and testosterone concentration and with ovulation and subsequent pregnancy in many women.[97]

Weight loss is difficult to achieve. A structured program that includes consultation with a nutritionist, encouragement by the physician, a low-calorie diet, and initiation of an exercise program may be the most effective nonsurgical approach in these patients [see Chapter 4]. In select cases, pharmacological adjuvants may be of benefit. Surgical methods of weight reduction can be very effective, especially in women whose BMI is greater than 40 [see Chapter 58].[98]

REDUCTION OF RISK FOR ENDOMETRIAL HYPERPLASIA AND CANCER

Women who are anovulatory, especially those with obesity and insulin resistance, are at increased risk for developing endometrial hyperplasia and cancer. In these women, treatment with cyclic progestin therapy either in the form of an estrogen-progestin contraceptive or as regular cycles of progestin-only therapy can reduce the risk of both endometrial hyperplasia and cancer. For women with PCOS and menorrhagia, an endometrial biopsy is needed to assess the status of the endometrium.[99,100]

TREATMENTS NOT RECOMMENDED

Glucocorticoid Therapy for Hirsutism

Treatment with glucocorticoids may be appropriate in women with ACTH-dependent adrenal androgen overproduction, such as those with nonclassic adrenal hyperplasia resulting from 21-hydroxylase deficiency[101,102]; however, it is not appropriate for the treatment of hirsutism in PCOS. A major problem with glucocorticoid therapy is that the complete suppression of ACTH production often requires giving more glucocorticoid than would normally be produced by the adrenal glands. As a result, patients receiving long-term glucocorticoid treatment are at increased risk for iatrogenic Cushing syndrome, osteoporosis, and diabetes mellitus. In addition, the corticotropin-releasing hormone–ACTH–cortisol axis may become so suppressed that the adrenal response to stress is blunted. For these reasons, it is advisable to avoid using glucocorticoids in the treatment of hirsutism. If the clinician does decide to use glucocorticoid therapy, use of low-dose glucocorticoids (5 or 7.5 mg of prednisone daily) or an alternate-day regimen of glucocorticoids may minimize these risks. Because almost all women treated with glucocorticoids gain weight and many develop osteoporosis, the clinician should carefully monitor weight and bone density in these patients.

Ovarian Surgery for Irregular Menses or Hirsutism

Ovarian surgery can be used to decrease the mass of androgen-secreting thecal and stromal tissue. No randomized, controlled trials have been published concerning the benefits and risks of ovarian surgery for the treatment of irregular menses or hirsutism. In my opinion, the risks of ovarian surgery, such as anesthetic complications, major adhesion formation and ovarian failure are greater than the potential benefits for women with irregular menses or hirsutism. I recommend ovarian surgery only for women with PCOS and anovulatory infertility in whom standard approaches to induction of ovulation such as weight loss, clomiphene, metformin and FSH therapy have failed.

The author has no commercial relationships with manufacturers of products or providers of services discussed in this chapter.

Metformin and rosiglitazone have not been approved by the FDA for uses described in this chapter.

References

1. Zawadski JK, Dunaif A: Diagnostic criteria for polycystic ovary syndrome. Polycystic Ovary Syndrome. Dunaif A, Givens JR, Haseltine FP, et al, Eds. Current Issues in Endocrinology and Metabolism. Blackwell Scientific Publications, Boston, 1992, p 377

2. Revised 2003 consensus on diagnostic criteria and long-term health risks related to polycystic ovary syndrome (PCOS). The Rotterdam ESHRE/ASRM-sponsored PCOS Consensus Workshop Group. Hum Reprod 19:41, 2004

3. Murphy MK, Hall JE, Adams JM, et al: Polycystic ovarian morphology in normal women does not predict the development of PCOS. J Clin Endocrinol Metab Aug 1 (epub ahead of print), 2006

4. Knochenhauer ES, Key TJ, Kahsar-Miller M, et al: Prevalence of PCOS in unselected black and white women of the southeastern United States: a prospective study. J Clin Endocrinol Metab 83:3078, 1998

5. Diamanti-Kandarakis E, Kouli CR, Bergiele AT, et al: A survey of the polycystic ovary syndrome in the Greek island of Lesbos: hormonal and metabolic profile. J Clin Endocrinol Metab 84:4006, 1999

6. Asuncion M, Calvo RM, San Millan JL, et al: A prospective study of the prevalence of the polycystic ovary syndrome in unselected Caucasian women from Spain. J Clin Endocrinol Metab 85:4182, 2000

7. Reindollar RH, Novak M, Tho SP, et al: Adult-onset amenorrhea: a study of 262 patients. Am J Obstet Gynecol 155:531, 1986

8. van Hooff MH, Voorhorst FJ, Kaptein MB, et al: Predictive value of menstrual cycle pattern, body mass index, hormone levels and polycystic ovaries at age 15 years for oligo-amenorrhea at age 18 years. Hum Reprod 19:383, 2004

9. Winters SJ, Talbott E, Guzick DS, et al: Serum testosterone levels decrease in middle age in women with polycystic ovary syndrome. Fertil Steril 73: 724, 2000

10. Lo JC, Feigenbaum SL, Yang J, et al: Epidemiology and adverse cardiovascular risk profile of diagnosed polycystic ovary syndrome. J Clin Endocrinol Metab 91:1357, 2006

11. Kauffman RP, Baker VM, DiMarino P, et al: Polycystic ovarian syndrome and insulin resistance in white and Mexican American women: a comparison of two distinct populations. Am J Obstet Gynecol 187:1362, 2002

12. Azziz R, Woods KS, Reyna R, et al: The prevalence and features of the polycystic ovary syndrome in an unselected population. J Clin Endocrinol Metab 89: 2745, 2004

13. Taponone S, Martikainen H, Jarvelin MR, et al: Hormonal profile of women with self-reported symptoms of oligomenorrhea and/or hirsutism. Northern Finland Birth Cohort 1996 Study. J Clin Endocrinol Metab 88:141, 2003

14. Ehrmann DA, Kasza K, Azziz R, et al: Effects of race and family history of type-2 diabetes on metabolic status of women with polycystic ovary syndrome. J Clin Endocrinol Metab 90:66, 2005

15. Legro RS, Driscoll D, Strauss JF, et al: Evidence for a genetic basis for hyperandrogenemia in polycystic ovary syndrome. PNAS 95:14956, 1998

16. Musso C, Cochran E, Moran SA, et al: Clinical course of genetic diseases of the insulin receptor (type A and Rabson-Mendenhall syndromes): a 30 year perspective. Medicine 83:209, 2004

17. Ehrmann DA: Polycystic ovary syndrome. N Engl J Med 352: 1223, 2005

18. Urbanek M, Woodroffe A, Ewens KG, et al: Candidate gene region for polycystic ovary syndrome on chromosome 19p13.2. J Clin Endocrinol Metab 90:6732, 2005

19. Abbott DH, Dumesic DA, Franks S: Developmental origin of polycystic ovary syndrome—a hypothesis. J Endocrinol 174:1, 2002

20. de Zegher F, Ibanez L: Prenatal growth restraint followed by catch-up of weight: a hyperinsulinemic pathway to polycystic ovary syndrome. Fertil Steril 86:(suppl 1):S4, 2006

21. Ibanez L, Ong K, Dunger DB, et al: Early development of adiposity and insulin resistance after catch-up weight gain in small for gestational age children. J Clin Endocrinol Metab 91:2153, 2006

22. Waldstreicher J, Santoro NF, Hall JE, et al: Hyperfunction of the hypothalamic-pituitary axis in women with polycystic ovary disease: indirect evidence for partial gonadotroph desensitization. J Clin Endocrinol Metab 66:165, 1988

23. Nelson VL, Qin KN, Rosenfield RL, et al: The biochemical basis for increased testosterone production in theca cells propagated from patients with polycystic ovary syndrome. J Clin Endocrinol Metab 86:5925, 2001

24. Peterson KF, Dufour S, Befroy D, et al: GI Impaired mitochondrial activity in the insulin-resistant offspring of patients with type 2 diabetes. N Engl J Med 350:664, 2004

25. Dunaif A, Segal KR, Futterweit W, et al: Profound peripheral insulin resistance, independent of obesity, in polycystic ovary syndrome. Diabetes 38:1165, 1989

26. Venkatesan AM, Dunaif A, Corbould A: Insulin resistance in polycystic ovary syndrome: progress and paradoxes. Recent ProgHorm Res 56:295, 2001

27. Dunaif A, Xia J, Book CB, et al: Excessive insulin receptor serine phosphorylation in cultured fibroblasts in skeletal muscle: a potential mechanism for insulin resistance in the polycystic ovary syndrome. J Clin Invest 96:801, 1995

28. Sam S, Dunaif A: Polycystic ovary syndrome: syndrome XX? Trends Endocrinol Metab 14: 365, 2003

29. Poretsky L: Polycystic ovary syndrome: Increased or preserved ovarian sensitivity to insulin? J Clin Endocrinol Metab 91:2859, 2006

30. Moran C, Reyna R, Boots LS, Azziz R: Adrenocortical hyperresponsiveness to corticotropin in polycystic ovary syndrome patients with adrenal androgen excess. Fertil Steril 81:126, 2004

31. Witchel SF, Kahsar-Miller M, Aston CE, et al: Prevalence of cyp21 mutations and IRS1 variant among women with polycystic ovary syndrome and adrenal androgen excess. Fertil Steril 83:371, 2005

32. Joffe H, Taylor AE, Hall JE: Polycystic ovary syndrome: relationship to epilepsy and antiepileptic drug therapy (editorial). J Clin Endocrinol Metab 86:2946, 2001

33. Sowers MF, Beebe JL, McConnell D, et al: Testosterone concentrations in women aged 25 to 50 years: association with lifestyles, body composition and ovarian status. Am J Epidemiol 153:256, 2001

34. Ferriman D, Gallwey JD: Clinical assessment of body hair growth in women. J Clin Endocrinol Metab 21:1440, 1961

35. Apridonidze T, Essah PA, Iuorno MJ, et al: Prevalence and characteristics of the metabolic syndrome in women with polycystic ovary syndrome. J Clin Endocrinol Metab 90:1929, 2005

36. Grundy SM, Cleeman JI, Daniels SR, et al: Diagnosis and management of the metabolic syndrome: an American Heart Association/National Heart, Lung, and Blood Institute Scientific Statement. Circulation 112:2735, 2005

37. Guttmann-Bauman I: Approach to adolescent polycystic ovary syndrome in the pediatric endocrine community in the United States. J Pediatric Endocrinology 18:499, 2005

38. Bohlke K, Cramer D, Barbieri RL: Relation of luteinizing hormone levels to body mass index in premenopausal women. Fertil Steril 69:500, 1998

39. Pagan YL, Srouji SS, Jimenez Y, et al: Inverse relationship between luteinizing hormone and body mass index in polycystic ovary syndrome: investigation of hypothalamic and pituitary contributions. J Clin Endocrinol Metab 91:1309, 2006

40. Laven JS, Mulders AG, Visser JA, et al: Anti-mullerian hormone serum concentrations in normoovulatory and anovulatory women of reproductive age. J Clin Endocrinol Metab 89:318, 2004

41. Pigny P, Jonard S, Robert Y, Dewailly D: Serum anti-mullerian hormone as a surrogate for antral follicle count for definition of the polycystic ovary syndrome. J Clin Endocrinol Metab 91:941, 2006

42. Screening for type 2 diabetes. American Diabetes Association. Diabetes Care 27(suppl 1):S11, 2004

43. Legro RS, Kunselman AR, Dodson WC, et al: Prevalence and predictors of risk for type 2 diabetes mellitus and impaired glucose tolerance in polycystic ovary syndrome: a prospective controlled study in 254 affected women. J Clin Endocrinol Metab 84:165, 1999

44. Palmert MR, Gordon CM, Kartashov AI, et al: Screening for abnormal glucose tolerance in adolescents with polycystic ovary syndrome. J Clin Endocrinol Metab 87:1017, 2002

45. Escobar-Morreale HF, Serrano-Gotarredona J, Garcia-Robles R, et al: Mild adrenal and ovarian steroidogenic abnormalities in hirsute women without hyperandrogenism: does idiopathic hirsutism exist? Metabolism 46:902, 1997

46. Hughesdon PE: Morphology and morphogenesis of the Stein Leventhal ovary and of so called hyperthecosis. Obstet Gynecol Surv 37:58, 1982

47. Adashi EY: Potential utility of gonadotropin releasing hormone agonists in the management of ovarian hyperandrogenism. Fertil Steril 53:765, 1990

48. Mikkonen K, Vainionpaa LK, Pakarinen AJ, et al: Long-term reproductive endocrine health in young women with epilepsy during puberty. Neurology 62:445, 2004

49. Rasgon NL, Altshuler LL, Fairbanks L, et al: Reproductive function and risk for PCOS in women treated for bipolar disorder. Bipolar Disorders 7:246, 2005

50. Nelson-DeGrave VL, Wickenheisser JK, Cockrell JE, et al: Valproate potentiates androgen biosynthesis in human ovarian theca cells. Endocrinology 145:799, 2004

51. Talbott E, Clerici A, Berga SL, et al: Adverse lipid and coronary heart disease risk profiles in young women with polycystic ovary syndrome. Results of a case control study. J Clin Epidemiol 51:415, 1998

52. Legro RS, Kunselman AR, Dunaif A: Prevalence and predictors of dyslipidemia in women with polycystic ovary syndrome. Am J Med 111:607, 2001

53. Boulman N, Levy Y, Leiba R, et al: Increased C-reactive protein levels in the polycystic ovary syndrome: a marker of cardiovascular disease. J Clin Endocrinol Metab 89:2160, 2004

54. Tarkun I, Arsian BC, Canturk Z, et al: Endothelial dysfunction in young women with polycystic ovary syndrome: relationship with insulin resistance and low-grade chronic inflammation. J Clin Endocrinol Metab 89:5592, 2004

55. Diamanti-Kandarakis E, Spina G, Kouli C, et al: Increased endothelin-1 levels in women with polycystic ovary syndrome and the beneficial effect of metformin therapy. J Clin Endocriniol Metab 86:4666, 2001

56. Birdsall MA, Farquhar CM, White HD: Association between polycystic ovaries and coronary artery disease in women having cardiac catheterization. Ann Intern Med 126:32, 1997

57. Talbott EO, Guzick DS, Sutton-Tyrrell K, et al: Evidence for association between polycystic ovary syndrome and premature carotid atherosclerosis in middle-aged women. Arterioscler Thromb Vasc Biol 20:2414, 2000

58. Christian RC, Dumesic DA, Behrenbeck T, et al: Prevalence and predictors of coronary artery calcification in women with polycystic ovary syndrome. J Clin Endocrinol Metab 88:2562, 2003

59. Solomon CG, Hu FB, Dunaif A, et al: Menstrual cycle irregularity and risk for future cardiovascular disease. J Clin Endocrinol Metab 87:2013, 2002

60. Tasali E, Van Cauter E, Ehrmann DA: Relationships between sleep disordered breathing and glucose metabolism in polycystic ovary syndrome. J Clin Endocrinol Metab 91:36, 2006

61. Setji TL, Holland ND, Sanders LL, et al: Non-alcoholic steatohepatitis and nonalcoholic fatty liver disease in young women with polycystic ovary syndrome. J Clin Endocrinol Metab 91:1741, 2006

62. Adams KF, Schatzkin A, Harris TB, et al: Overweight, obesity and mortality in a large prospective cohort of persons 50 to 71 years old. N Engl J Med 355:763, 2006

63. Baillargeon JP, McCLish DK, Essah PA, et al: Association between the current use of low-dose oral contraceptives and cardiovascular arterial disease: a meta-analysis. J Clin Endocrinol Metab 90:3863, 2005

64. Diamanti-Kandarakis E, Baillargeon JP, Iuorno MJ, et al: A modern medical quandary: polycystic ovary syndrome, insulin resistance and oral contraceptive pills. J Clin Endocrinol Metab 88:1927, 2003

65. Essah PA, Apridonidze T, Iuorno MJ, et al: Effects of short-term and long-term metformin treatment on menstrual cyclicity in women with polycystic ovary syndrome. Fertil Steril 86:230, 2006

66. Chhabra S, McCartney CR, Yoo RY, et al: Progesterone inhibition of the hypothalamic gonadotropin-releasing hormone pulse generator: evidence for varied effects in hyperandrogenemic adolescent girls. J Clin Endocrinol Metab 90:2810, 2005

67. Hickey M, Higham J, Fraser IS: Progestogens versus oestrogens and progestogens for irregual uterine bleeding associated with anovulation. Cochrane Database Syst Rev (2):CD001895, 2000

68. Farquhar C, Lee O, Toomath R, et al: Spironolactone versus placebo in combination with steroids for hirsutism and/or acne. Cochrane Database Syst Rev (4):CD000194, 2003

69. Balfour JA, McClellan K: Topical eflornithine. Am J Clin Dermatol 2:197, 2001

70. Bates GW, Whitworth NS: Effect of body weight reduction on plasma androgens in obese infertile women. Fertil Steril 38:406, 1982

71. Pasquali R, Antenucci D, Casimirri F, et al: Clinical and hormonal characteristics of obese and amenorrheic women before and after weight loss. J Clin Endocrinol Metab 8:173, 1989

72. Hughes E, Collins J, Vandekerckhove P: Clomiphene citrate for ovulation induction in women with oligo-amenorrhea. Cochrane Database Syst Rev (2):CD00056, 2000

73. Elnashar A, Abdelmageed E, Fayed M, et al: Clomiphene citrate and dexamethasone in treatment of clomiphene resistant polycystic ovary syndrome: a prospective placebo-controlled study. Human Reprod 21:1805, 2006

74. Nestler JE, Jakubowicz DJ, Evans WS, et al: Effects of metformin on spontaneous and clomiphene-induced ovulation in the polycystic ovary syndrome. N Engl J Med 338:1876, 1998

75. Vandermolen DT, Ratts VS, Evans WS, et al: Metformin increases the ovulatory rate and pregnancy rate from clomiphene citrate in patients with polycystic ovary syndrome who are resistant to clomiphene citrate alone. Fertil Steril 75:310, 2001

76. Sarlis NJ, Weil SJ, Nelson LM: Administration of metformin to a diabetic woman with extreme hyperandrogenemia of non-tumoral origin: management of infertility and prevention of inadvertent masculinization of a female fetus. J Clin Endocrinol Metab 84:1510, 1999

77. Shaw RJ, Lamia KA, Vasquez D, et al: The kinase LKB1 mediates glucose homeostasis in liver and therapeutic effects of metformin. Science 310:1642, 2005

78. Morin-Papunen LC, Koivunen RM, Ruokonen A, et al: Metformin therapy improves the menstrual pattern with minimal endocrine and metabolic effects in women with polycystic ovary syndrome. Fertil Steril 69:691, 1998

79. DeLeo V, LaMarca A, Ditto A, et al: Effects of metformin on gonadotropin induced ovulation in women with polycystic ovary syndrome. Fertil Steril 72:282, 1999

80. Coetzee EJ, Jackson WU: Metformin in management of pregnant insulin-dependent diabetics. Diabetologia 16:241, 1979

81. Palomba S, Orio F, Falbo A, et al: Prospective parallel randomized, double-blind, double-dummy controlled clinical trial comparing clomiphene citrate and metformin as the first-line treatment for ovulation induction in nonobese anovulatory women with polycystic ovary syndrome. J Clin Endocrinol Metab 90:4068, 2005

82. Lord JM, Flight IHK, Norman RJ: Insulin sensitizing drugs (metformin, troglitazone, rosiglitazone, pioglitazone, D-chiro-inositol) for polycystic ovary syndrome. Cochrane Database Syst Rev (3):CD003053, 2003

83. Dunaif A, Scott D, Finegood D, et al: The insulin-sensitizing agent troglitazone improves metabolic and reproductive abnormalities in the polycystic ovary syndrome. J Clin Endocrinol Metab 81:3299, 1996

84. Ehrmann DA, Schneider DJ, Sobel BE, et al: Troglitazone improves defects in insulin action, insulin secretion, ovarian steroidogenesis and fibrinolysis in women with polycystic ovary syndrome. J Clin Endocrinol Metab 82:2108, 1997

85. Ghazeeri G, Kutteh WH, Bryer-Ash M, et al: Effect of rosiglitazone on spontaneous and clomiphene citrate-induced ovulation induction in women with polycystic ovary syndrome. Fertil Steril 79:562, 2003

86. Romualdi D, Guido M Ciampelli M, et al: Selective effects of pioglitazone on insulin and androgen abnormalities in normo- and hyperinsulinemic obese patients with polycystic ovary syndrome. Hum Reprod 18:1210, 2003

87. Rouzi AA, Ardawi MSM: A randomized controlled trial of the efficacy of rosiglitazone and clomiphene citrate versus metformin and clomiphene citrate in women with clomiphene citrate resistant polycystic ovary syndrome. Fertil Steril 85:428, 2006

88. Jarrell J, McInnes R, Crooke R: Observations on the combination of clomiphene citrate-hMG-hCG in the management of anovulation. Fertil Steril 35:634, 1981

89. Homburg R, Levy R, Ben Rafael Z: A comparative study of conventional regimens with low dose FSH for ovulation in PCOS. Fertil Steril 63:729, 1995

90. Schenker JG, Weinstein D: Ovarian hyperstimulation syndrome: a current survey. Fertil Steril 30:255, 1978

91. Budev MM, Arroliga AC, Falcone T: Ovarian hyperstimulation syndrome. Crit Care Med 3(suppl 10): S301, 2005

92. Donesky BW, Adashi EY: Surgically induced ovulation in the polycystic ovary syndrome: wedge resection revisited in the age of laparoscopy. Fertil Steril 63:439, 1995

93. Farquhar CM, Williamson K, Gudex G, et al. A randomized controlled trial of laparoscopic ovarian diathermy versus gonadotropin therapy for women with clomiphene resistant polycystic ovary syndrome. Fertil Steril 78:404, 2002

94. Farquhar C, Lilford RJ, Marjoribanks J, et al: Laparoscopic drilling by diathermy or laser for ovulation induction in anovulatory polycystic ovary syndrome. Cochrane Database Syst Rev (3):CD001122, 2005

95. Heijnen EM, Eijkemans MJ, Hughes EG, et al: A meta-analysis of outcomes of conventional IVF in women with polycystic ovary syndrome. Hum Reprod Update 12:13, 2006

96. Hoeger KM, Kochman L, Wixom N, et al: A randomized, 48-week, placebo-controlled trial of intensive lifestyle modification and/or metformin therapy in overweight women with polycystic ovary syndrome: a pilot study. Fertil Steril 82:421, 2004

97. Hollman M, Runnebaum B, Gerhard I: Effects of weight loss on the hormonal profile in obese infertile women. Human Reprod 11:1884, 1996

98. Escobar-Morreale HF, Botella-Carretero JI, Alvarez-Blasco F, et al: The polycystic ovary syndrome associated with morbid obesity may resolve after weight loss induced by bariatric surgery. J Clin Endocrinol Metab 90:63643, 2005

99. Pillay OC, Te Fong LF, Crow JC, et al: The association between polycystic ovaries and endometrial cancer. Human Reprod 21:924, 2006

100. Soliman PT, Oh JC, Schmeier KM, Sun CC, et al: Risk factors for young premenopausal women with endometrial cancer. Obstet Gynecol 105: 575, 2005

101. Rittmaster RS, Loriaux DL, Cutler GB: Sensitivity of cortisol and adrenal androgens to dexamethasone suppression in hirsute women. J Clin Endocrinol Metab 81:462, 1985

102. Carmina E, Lobo RA: Ovarian suppression reduces clinical and endocrine expression of late-onset congenital adrenal hyperplasia due to 21-hydroxylase deficiency. Fertil Steril 62:738, 1994

103. Chang JR, Nakamura RM, Judd HL, et al: Insulin resistance in nonobese patients with polycystic ovarian disease. J Clin Endocrinol Metab 57:356, 1983

80 Hirsutism

Robert L. Barbieri, M.D., F.A.C.P.

As an isolated clinical condition, excessive hair growth can significantly detract from a woman's quality of life. Hirsutism that occurs along with certain other clinical findings may also signal significant endocrine disease. For example, hirsutism in the presence of oligomenorrhea is often caused by polycystic ovary syndrome (PCOS) and may be associated with infertility, endometrial hyperplasia, and diabetes mellitus. Hirsutism in the presence of virilization may be caused by androgen secretion from an adrenal or ovarian tumor. Fortunately, almost all cases of hirsutism can be effectively treated with a combination of hormonal and nonhormonal therapies.

Definition

Hirsutism is the presence, in a woman, of coarse, dark terminal hair in a male pattern, often involving the upper lip, chin, sideburns, and chest. Terminal hairs are thick, stiff, and pigmented. In men, they are normally found on the face, chest, abdomen, and back. From a practice perspective, a woman who complains of hirsutism has hirsutism. Clinically, hirsutism is present if the patient's Ferriman-Gallwey score is greater than 8 [see Figure 1].[1,2]

Hirsutism must also be defined in the context of cultural, ethnic, and racial norms. Most Asian and Native American women have less body hair than white women; women from Mediterranean backgrounds have greater numbers of terminal hairs. In some southern European cultures, significant terminal hair on a woman's upper lip is considered normal. In other cultures, a similar amount of terminal hair might be viewed as abnormal.

Hirsutism must be distinguished from hypertrichosis, which is an increase in total body hair, including sites where terminal hair is not usually found, such as the forehead. Most cases of hypertrichosis are associated with the use of drugs such as phenytoin, penicillamine, diazoxide, minoxidil, and cyclosporine. Systemic diseases such as anorexia nervosa, malnutrition, porphyria, and hypothyroidism can also cause hypertrichosis. Treatment of hypertrichosis consists of discontinuance of the inciting drug or treatment of the systemic disease. If these approaches are not successful, treatment with an antiandrogen such as spironolactone (200 mg daily) has been reported to be moderately effective.[3]

Epidemiology

On the basis of a Ferriman-Gallwey score of more than 8, approximately 4% of women have hirsutism; only 1% of women have a Ferriman-Gallwey score above 10.[1,2] Approximately 10% of a population-based cohort of women in Finland self-reported having hirsutism.[4] In this study about 2.5 % of the women reported having both hirsutism and oligomenorrhea, indicating that in the general population, the prevalence of PCOS is lower than the prevalence of hirsutism. However, a greater proportion of women with PCOS seek medical care for their condition than women with hirsutism. Consequently, in a specialty endocrine practice, women with PCOS are overrepresented compared with women with self-reported hirsutism.

Pathogenesis

Hirsutism is caused by an excess of androgen production, androgen action, or both.[5,6] Androgen overproduction can take place in the ovary, the adrenal gland, or the skin itself (specifically, in the hair follicle). In many hirsute women, all three organs overproduce androgens.

There are three types of hair: lanugo, vellus, and terminal. Lanugo is the soft, unmedullated hair seen in the fetus; it is shed in utero in the third trimester or shortly after birth. Vellus hairs are the thin, soft, unpigmented hairs that cover many areas of the body, such as the forehead. Terminal hairs are thick, coarse, and pigmented. Terminal hair is composed of an inner sheath of pigment with an outer sheath of keratin. Androgens stimulate the conversion of vellus hairs to terminal hairs in areas of the body sensitive to androgens, including the face and chest. Paradoxically, androgens cause the loss of terminal hairs in certain areas of the body, such as the frontal and parietal regions of the scalp.

The adrenal gland produces large quantities of the major androgens dehydroepiandrosterone sulfate (DHEAS), dehydroepiandrosterone (DHEA), and androstenedione. The ovary produces androstenedione and testosterone. In end organs, such as the pilosebaceous unit (hair follicle), androstenedione and testosterone can be converted to the potent androgen dihydrotestosterone (DHT) by the enzyme 5-α-reductase type 2. DHT and testosterone are the most potent androgens in humans; both bind with high affinity to the androgen receptor and initiate gene transcription that stimulates the growth of the pilosebaceous units on the face and chest and decreases the growth of pilosebaceous units on the frontal and parietal scalp. DHEA and DHEAS have no inherent androgen activity but can be metabolized to the active androgens testosterone and DHT. In research studies, nearly all hirsute women have been found to have increased production of testosterone, but standard clinical assays may not be sensitive enough to reliably detect the elevations in serum testosterone levels in these patients.[5,7]

Many women with hirsutism have several hormonal defects, including the following: (1) overproduction of adrenal androgens, (2) overproduction of ovarian androgens,[8] (3) increased conversion of androstenedione and testosterone to DHT in the hair follicle, and (4) increased sensitivity of the hair follicle to androgen action. Androgen overproduction in many hirsute women probably arises from multiple pathophysiologic defects, including (1) increased pituitary secretion of luteinizing hormone (LH), which stimulates ovarian production of testosterone and androstenedione; (2) elevated insulin levels, because of insulin resistance, which decrease the production of sex-hormone–binding globulin (SHBG) and thus increase free testosterone levels; (3) mild biochemical defects in the adrenal steroid enzymes that produce cortisol, which increase the ratio of androgen-to-cortisol secretion and result in adrenal androgen overproduction; and (4) increased activity of 5-α-reductase in the hair follicle, which increases the conversion of androgens to DHT in the follicle.

Etiology

The two most common causes of hirsutism are idiopathic hirsutism and PCOS. Idiopathic hirsutism is defined as hirsutism

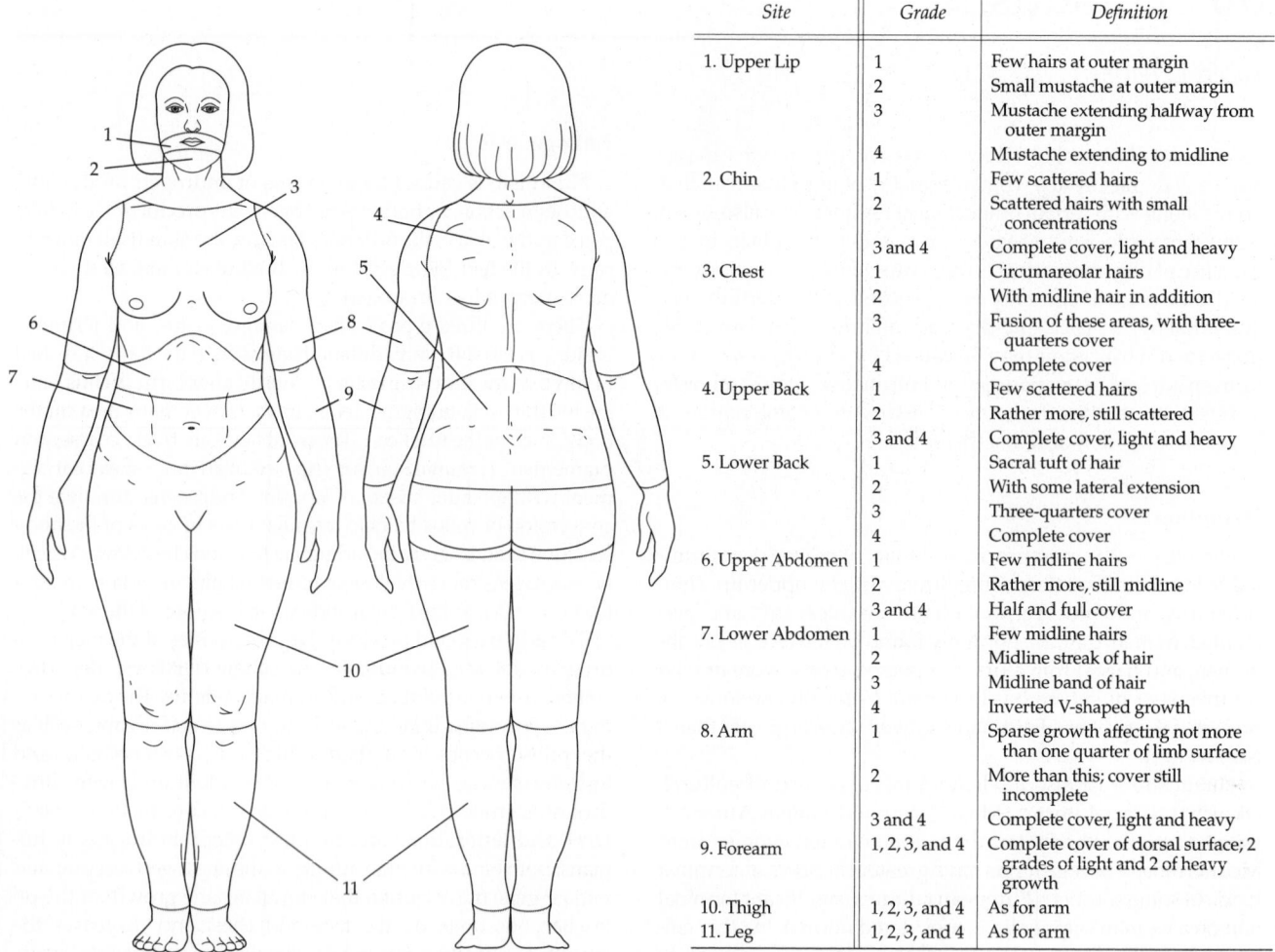

Site	Grade	Definition
1. Upper Lip	1	Few hairs at outer margin
	2	Small mustache at outer margin
	3	Mustache extending halfway from outer margin
	4	Mustache extending to midline
2. Chin	1	Few scattered hairs
	2	Scattered hairs with small concentrations
	3 and 4	Complete cover, light and heavy
3. Chest	1	Circumareolar hairs
	2	With midline hair in addition
	3	Fusion of these areas, with three-quarters cover
	4	Complete cover
4. Upper Back	1	Few scattered hairs
	2	Rather more, still scattered
	3 and 4	Complete cover, light and heavy
5. Lower Back	1	Sacral tuft of hair
	2	With some lateral extension
	3	Three-quarters cover
	4	Complete cover
6. Upper Abdomen	1	Few midline hairs
	2	Rather more, still midline
	3 and 4	Half and full cover
7. Lower Abdomen	1	Few midline hairs
	2	Midline streak of hair
	3	Midline band of hair
	4	Inverted V-shaped growth
8. Arm	1	Sparse growth affecting not more than one quarter of limb surface
	2	More than this; cover still incomplete
	3 and 4	Complete cover, light and heavy
9. Forearm	1, 2, 3, and 4	Complete cover of dorsal surface; 2 grades of light and 2 of heavy growth
10. Thigh	1, 2, 3, and 4	As for arm
11. Leg	1, 2, 3, and 4	As for arm

Figure 1   Ferriman-Gallwey system for clinical scoring of hirsutism.[1,58] **Each of the 11 designated body areas is assigned a score of 0 (absence of coarse dark terminal hairs) to 4 (extensive terminal hair growth). A score higher than 8 indicates hirsutism. Hair scores over the forearms and lower leg do not contribute significantly to the distinction of hirsutism from nonhirsutism.**

(patient self-report or a Ferriman-Gallwey score above 8) in a woman with regular ovulatory menses. PCOS is the combination of oligomenorrhea (oligo-ovulation) and hyperandrogenism, as manifested by hirsutism or elevation in levels of a serum androgen such as androstenedione, testosterone, or DHEA. In many cases, idiopathic hirsutism may be a mild form of PCOS, in which androgen levels are elevated enough to cause hirsutism but not elevated enough to produce oligo-ovulation and oligomenorrhea.[9] In a very small number of women, hirsutism (usually severe hirsutism, the so-called bearded-lady phenomenon) is a manifestation of serious diseases such as adrenal or ovarian tumors. One study of 350 British women who presented with hirsutism or androgenic alopecia found that 68% had idiopathic hirsutism, 30% had PCOS, and 2% had serious underlying disease, including congenital adrenal hyperplasia, ovarian tumors, adrenal tumors, prolactinoma, and acromegaly.[10]

Controversy exists as to a possible relationship between hyperprolactinemia, excess production of adrenal androgens, and hirsutism. Several investigators have reported a relationship between hyperprolactinemia and excess production of DHEAS,[11] but others have not confirmed these observations.[12,13] In one of the most detailed studies, Schiebinger and colleagues[13] found

that in women with hyperprolactinemia, successful treatment decreased the DHEAS production rate from 27 mg to 17 mg a day and increased the metabolic clearance rate from 16 L to 21 L a day. Along with these changes, serum DHEAS decreased from 2.5 μg/ml to 1.8 μg/ml. These results suggest that hyperprolactinemia may play a modest role in stimulating adrenal androgen production and may occasionally contribute to the development of hirsutism.

Diagnosis

The main goal in the evaluation of women with hirsutism is to determine whether idiopathic hirsutism or PCOS is present and to exclude rare, medically serious causes of hyperandrogenism, such as ovarian and adrenal tumors.[14] This can best be done on the basis of the history and physical examination, along with limited laboratory testing [*see Table 1*].

CLINICAL FEATURES

The differentiation between the two most common causes of hirsutism can be made by menstrual history. Women with idiopathic hirsutism have normal menstrual cycles lasting 23 to 35

Table 1   Differential Diagnosis of Hirsutism
in Women of Reproductive Age

Associated Finding	Most Likely Diagnosis
Oligomenorrhea	Polycystic ovary syndrome (PCOS)
Regular ovulatory cycles	Idiopathic hirsutism
Fasting 17-hydroxyprogesterone level > 4 ng/ml	Nonclassic adrenal hyperplasia
Virilization	Ovarian or adrenal androgen-secreting tumor, or ovarian stromal hyperthecosis
Acanthosis nigricans	Severe insulin resistance syndrome, often associated with PCOS or ovarian stromal hyperthecosis
Galactorrhea and elevated serum prolactin level	Hyperprolactinemia

days. Women with PCOS have oligomenorrhea, with some menstrual cycles lasting longer than 35 days. Many women with PCOS have fewer than six spontaneous menstrual cycles a year.

Serious causes of hyperandrogenism (e.g., ovarian or adrenal tumors) typically manifest themselves clinically as virilization, with frontal balding, acne, clitoromegaly, increased upper body muscle mass, and deepening of the voice. Almost all women with signs of virilization are amenorrheic; none have regular ovulatory menstrual cycles. In addition, most women who present with virilization from an ovarian or adrenal tumor report recent onset (within the past year) of their hirsutism and rapid progression of their condition. In contrast, most women with idiopathic hirsutism or PCOS notice the onset of hirsutism many years before presenting for medical care, often during puberty.

When taking the history, the clinician should ask whether the patient has been using androgenic medications such as danazol or testosterone and its derivatives, which is a rare cause of hirsutism. Some female athletes may use anabolic steroids.

LABORATORY TESTING

Serum Androgen Assays

Patients with clinical evidence of hirsutism should undergo measurement of serum testosterone (total or free) and serum 17-hydroxyprogesterone levels. Unfortunately, most of the androgen assays available in clinical practice are designed to differentiate between levels found in normal women and men, and these assays are neither sensitive enough nor specific enough for detecting differences between normal and hirsute women. For example, the mean circulating total testosterone level is approximately 25 ng/dl in normal women, 50 ng/dl in hirsute women, and 600 ng/dl in men. Clinical assays are excellent at differentiating between 25 ng/dl and 600 ng/dl but are poor at differentiating between 25 ng/dl and 50 ng/dl.

Another problem with clinical assays is that testosterone circulates in both free and SHBG-bound forms. Testosterone bound to SHBG is not able to stimulate end organs, such as the pilosebaceous unit. The amount of free testosterone depends on both testosterone production rates and the concentration of SHBG. To complicate the situation, an increase in testosterone production causes a decrease in SHBG production, which re-

sults in a decrease in total testosterone (the form of testosterone that is most often measured in practice) and an increase in free testosterone (a form that is not typically measured in clinical practice).

In most clinical assays, the upper limit of normal for serum testosterone is 80 ng/dl. Almost all women with virilization have serum testosterone levels greater than 150 ng/dl.[15-17] It is probably wise for primary care physicians to seek the help of an endocrinologist if they identify a virilized woman or a woman with a serum testosterone concentration above 150 ng/dl.

Other Tests

In a hirsute woman who has amenorrhea, the serum prolactin level should be measured. Women with PCOS, especially those who are obese, should be screened for diabetes mellitus. This is particularly true of patients in whom physical examination reveals acanthosis nigricans, which suggests significant insulin resistance.

Between 1% and 5% of women who present with hirsutism and oligomenorrhea have nonclassic congenital adrenal hyperplasia (NCAH) from 21-hydroxylase deficiency that was too mild to be detected at birth.[18] All of these women have elevated levels of 17-hydroxyprogesterone (above 4 ng/ml) in the early morning (8 A.M.) during the follicular phase of the menstrual cycle. Consequently, measurement of a follicular-phase 8 A.M. 17-hydroxyprogesterone level can help rule out NCAH. It is not clear whether all women with hirsutism and oligomenorrhea should be screened for NCAH, because the disorder has a low prevalence in many populations. In addition, many women with NCAH respond well to the standard treatments for PCOS. Screening might be warranted in women of ethnic groups that have an increased prevalence of NCAH (e.g., Ashkenazi Jews, Inuits). One middle-of-the-road approach is to screen women for NCAH only if their serum testosterone concentration is above a clearly elevated level, such as 100 ng/dl or 150 ng/dl. This approach will detect the most clinically significant cases of NCAH.

Treatment

The goals of treatment of hirsutism include the following: (1) rule out a serious underlying medical condition such as a virilizing tumor of the adrenal or ovary, (2) slow or stop new hair growth, (3) remove or hide existing hair, (4) evaluate and treat associated hormonal problems such as oligomenorrhea, and (5) anticipate long-term health conditions that can occur in women with hyperandrogenism, such as an increased risk of diabetes.

Hormonal treatment of hirsutism typically does not result in normalization of the Ferriman-Gallwey score (i.e., to below 8). In many studies, patients' Ferriman-Gallwey scores are in the range of 20 to 25 at the initiation of treatment. After 12 months of treatment, the Ferriman-Gallwey scores are in the range of 10 to 15. On the basis of these general observations, clinicians can assure women that treatment is effective but should warn them that treatment is unlikely to reduce facial hair to a level similar to that in nonhirsute women. In addition, clinicians should advise women that it will take at least 6 months for treatment to reach near maximal effects. Finally, most patients report that if they discontinue hormone treatment, the hirsutism recurs over the next 3 to 9 months.

Treatment of hirsutism should be multimodal [*see Table 2*]. It should include hormonal suppression of androgen production or action, along with a nonhormonal method of controlling hair growth. A common strategy is to combine an estrogen-progestin contraceptive formulation with an antiandrogen and to use electrolysis or shaving as a nonhormonal adjuvant. An alternative hormonal approach is treatment with an antiandrogen alone. Alternative nonhormonal treatments include the use of a facial antihair cream or laser destruction of hair follicles [see Nonhormonal Approaches, below].

WEIGHT LOSS

Body mass index (BMI) is a major determinant of insulin resistance and hyperinsulinemia. Women with a BMI greater than 27 kg/m^2 are often insulin resistant.[19] Women with a BMI under 25 kg/m^2 are seldom insulin resistant, unless they have a relatively rare genetic cause of insulin resistance, such as lipodystrophy. Hyperinsulinemia causes hyperandrogenism through several mechanisms. In combination with LH, elevated insulin levels cause the ovarian theca and stroma to produce excess quantities of androstenedione and testosterone.[20] In addition, hyperinsulinemia suppresses hepatic production of SHBG, which causes an increase in free androgens. Excess ovarian production of androgens and decreased SHBG work synergistically to increase the risk of development of hirsutism.

Numerous studies have demonstrated the benefits of weight loss in hyperandrogenic, insulin-resistant women.[21-25] In these studies, mean weight loss ranging from about 10 to 20 kg has been associated with decreases in insulin levels and testosterone concentration and with ovulation and pregnancy in many women.

Weight loss is difficult to achieve. A structured program that includes consultation with a nutritionist, encouragement by the physician, a low-calorie diet, and initiation of an exercise program may be the most effective nonsurgical approach in these patients. Surgical methods of weight reduction can be very effective, especially in women whose BMI is greater than 40 [see Chapter 58].

ESTROGEN-PROGESTIN CONTRACEPTIVES

Combination estrogen-progestin formulations at doses used for contraception (in the form of pills, transdermal patches, or vaginal rings) suppress LH secretion, which in turn suppresses ovarian androgen production.[26,27] In addition, the estrogen in estrogen-progestin combinations increases liver production of SHBG, which binds testosterone and decreases circulating bioavailable testosterone, reducing androgen stimulation of the pilosebaceous units.[28] A further advantage for women with PCOS is that estrogen-progestin combinations, when given cyclically, induce regular withdrawal bleeding.

In a study that examined the effects of 5 years of estrogen-progestin contraceptive treatment for hirsutism, the investigators reported that hirsutism continued to improve through all 5 years of the treatment. Acne improved significantly by 2 years of treatment, but minimal further improvement occurred between 2 and 5 years. Within 6 months of discontinuance of treatment, hirsutism and acne reappeared.[29]

The effectiveness of estrogen-progestin contraceptives may be influenced by body mass. In heavier women, it may be best to select a medication with 35 μg of ethinyl estradiol.

Some estrogen-progestin contraceptive formulations may differ with regard to their effect on hepatic production of SHBG. Norgestrel is an androgenic progestin (derived from 19-nortestosterone) that partially blocks estrogen-induced SHBG

Table 2 Treatment of Hirsutism

Category	Treatment	Potential Toxic Effects
Hormonal	Combination estrogen-progestin contraceptive	Deep vein thrombosis
	Spironolactone, 50–200 mg daily; typical dosage, 100 mg daily	Hyperkalemia in patients with renal disease
	Combination estrogen-progestin contraceptive plus spironolactone, 100 mg daily	—
	Flutamide, 62.5–500 mg daily; typical dosage, 125 mg daily	Liver toxicity
	Finasteride, 2.5–5 mg daily; typical dosage, 5 mg daily	Teratogenicity in male fetuses
	Metformin, 1,500–2,250 mg daily; typical dosage, 2,000 mg daily	Nausea, vomiting; fatal lactic acidosis in patients with renal disease, heart failure, or liver disease
	Gonadotropin-releasing hormone analogue	Hypoestrogenism, including vasomotor symptoms and bone loss, when used as a single agent
Nonhormonal	Shaving; depilatories; bleaching; laser photothermolysis; nonlaser, rapid pulse, intense light therapy; eflornithine cream; electrolysis	—

Note: treatment is best accomplished with the combination of a hormonal treatment and a nonhormonal treatment.

production. Contraceptives that contain androgenic progestins, such as norgestrel, do not result in as great an increase in SHBG production as contraceptives that contain less androgenic progestins, such as drospirenone, desogestrel, ethynodiol diacetate, and norgestimate [see Table 3]. However, for the treatment of hirsutism, any estrogen-progestin contraceptive is superior to no estrogen-progestin contraceptive.

ANTIANDROGENS

Antiandrogens are a cornerstone of therapy for hirsutism. Used alone, antiandrogens appear to be as effective as oral-contraceptive treatment.[30] As with estrogen-progestin treatment, cessation of antiandrogen therapy is followed by recurrence of hirsutism within 1 year in the majority of women.[31]

The antiandrogens with demonstrated efficacy against hirsutism include spironolactone, finasteride, flutamide, and ketoconazole [see Table 2].[32-38] In one high-quality clinical trial, 40 hirsute women were randomized to receive spironolactone (100 mg daily), flutamide (250 mg daily), finasteride (5 mg daily), or placebo. Placebo did not produce a decrease in hirsutism, but all three active treatments were associated with a significant reduction in hirsutism scores. The reductions in the Ferriman-Gallwey score observed after 6 months of treatment were 41% with spironolactone, 39% with flutamide, and 32% with finasteride.[39] Similarly, in a placebo-controlled trial of finasteride (5 mg daily), flutamide (500 mg daily), and estrogen-progestin, the three active treatments resulted in similar decreases in Ferriman-Gallwey scores.[40] A randomized trial that compared flutamide (250 mg daily), finasteride (5 mg daily), ketoconazole (300 mg daily), and estrogen-progestin in 66 hirsute women found that after 1 year of treatment, all three agents significantly decreased the Ferriman-Gallwey score. The magnitude of the reduction in the Ferriman-Gallwey score was 55% with flutamide, 44% with finasteride, 53% with ketoconazole, and 60% with estrogen-progestin; the differences between the agents were not statistically significant.[41]

Individual Antiandrogens

Spironolactone The most widely used antiandrogen for the treatment of hirsutism, spironolactone inhibits the binding of testosterone and DHT to the androgen receptor. Because spironolactone and its active metabolites have very long half-lives, the entire dose can be given once daily. The usual dosage of spironolactone is between 50 and 200 mg daily. Many authorities recommend a dosage of 100 mg daily because it is near the top of the dose-response curve and is associated with fewer side effects than 200 mg daily. Approximately 70% of women treated with spironolactone have reported improvement. In one study of spironolactone (200 mg daily) for the treatment of moderate to severe hirsutism, 19 of 20 women reported improvement, with beneficial effects noticeable within 2 months, peaking at 6 months, and maintained through 12 months of therapy.[42] Because spironolactone may be a teratogen, sexually active patients who are not taking spironolactone along with an estrogen-progestin contraceptive should use barrier contraception.

Finasteride Finasteride inhibits type 1 (skin) and type 2 (prostate) 5-α-reductase, the enzyme that transforms testosterone to the most potent androgen, DHT. The Food and Drug Administration has placed a so-called black-box warning on finasteride, advising that no woman of childbearing age should take the medication or touch a broken pill because of the potential teratogenic effects of an antiandrogen on a male fetus. Consequently, a physician who prescribes finasteride to a hirsute woman may find that the pharmacist refuses to dispense the medication or that the patient's insurance company urges the

patient to stop taking the medicine. These practical considerations argue against prescribing finasteride for the treatment of hirsutism.

Flutamide An androgen receptor antagonist, flutamide is widely used in Europe for the treatment of hirsutism. It is effective at dosages ranging from 67.5 to 500 mg daily. Flutamide is probably a more potent antiandrogen than spironolactone. However, flutamide is much more expensive than spironolactone and can be associated with fatal hepatotoxicity.[43]

Ketoconazole Ketoconazole is an antifungal agent that inhibits cytochrome P-450 enzymes, which are involved in the synthesis of androgens. Treatment with ketoconazole (300 mg daily) inhibits androgen production and is as effective as finasteride, spironolactone, and flutamide in the treatment of hirsutism. However, ketoconazole has more side effects than the other antiandrogens that are commonly used to treat hirsutism.[41] The most commonly reported side effects are nausea, alopecia, headache, and elevated liver enzyme levels. For that reason, I do not recommend the use of ketoconazole to treat hirsutism.

ESTROGEN-PROGESTIN PLUS AN ANTIANDROGEN

The combination of an oral contraceptive and an antiandrogen may be somewhat more effective against hirsutism than either agent used alone. One trial studied the use of an oral contraceptive plus either finasteride (5 mg daily) or placebo for the treatment of hirsutism. After 1 year of treatment, the women who received combination therapy had greater reductions in their Ferriman-Gallwey score than women who received the oral contraceptive alone (48% versus 38%, respectively; $P < 0.05$).[44] On the other hand, a trial comparing an oral contraceptive plus flutamide (250 mg daily) with flutamide alone found the two treatments to be equally effective.[45]

One disadvantage of combined therapy is that it is more expensive than single-agent therapy. Also, the side effects may be additive.

GONADOTROPIN-RELEASING HORMONE ANALOGUES

Long-term administration of a gonadotropin-releasing hormone (GnRH) agonist analogue suppresses pituitary secretion of LH and ovarian secretion of testosterone. Treatment with a GnRH analogue has been demonstrated to reduce Ferriman-Gallwey scores. In head-to-head studies, however, antiandrogens have produced greater reductions in Ferriman-Gallwey scores than GnRH agonist treatment.[46] GnRH agonists are also generally more expensive than antiandrogens, limiting the clinical utility of GnRH agonists as first-line agents in the treatment of hirsutism.

METFORMIN

Many women with hirsutism have insulin resistance, and abnormally elevated concentrations of circulating insulin appear to stimulate ovarian androgen production. Metformin improves insulin dynamics, decreases circulating insulin levels, reduces serum testosterone levels, and reduces the rate of abnormal terminal hair growth. Clinical trials suggest that metformin at a dosage of 1,500 mg daily is effective in the treatment of hirsutism. For example, one randomized study that compared metformin with a cyclic oral contraceptive in 52 women with PCOS and hirsutism found that Ferriman-Gallwey scores after 12 months of treatment were significantly re-

Table 3 Androgenicity of Progestins Used in Oral Contraceptives

Level of Androgenicity	Progestin	Brand Name of Products
High	Norgestrel	LoOvral
	Levonorgestrel	Alesse, Levlite, Nordette, Trilevlen, Tri-Phasil
Moderate	Norethindrone	Genora 1/35, Norinyl 1/35, OrthoNovum 1/35, Ovcon 35
	Norethindrone acetate	Loestrin 1/20 Loestrin 1.5/35
Low	Ethynodiol diacetate	Demulen 1/35
	Norgestimate	Ortho-TriCyclen Ortho-TriCyclen Lo
	Desogestrel	Desogen Ortho-Cept
	Drosperinone	Yasmin

duced in patients taking metformin (25% decrease; $P < 0.01$) but not in those taking oral contraceptives (5% decrease; P = not significant).[47] Mean hair diameter was significantly reduced with both treatments. Similar results have been reported by other investigators.[48]

THIAZOLIDINEDIONES

Like metformin, the thiazolidinediones increase insulin sensitivity. Neither pioglitazone nor rosiglitazone has been extensively studied for its efficacy against hirsutism, however. Before being withdrawn from the market because of hepatic toxicity, troglitazone was demonstrated to be effective in the treatment of hyperandrogenism and hirsutism.[49]

GLUCOCORTICOIDS

Suppression of adrenal gland androgen production with glucocorticoids is effective in the treatment of hirsutism, but long-term glucocorticoid treatment can lead to such serious side effects as weight gain, osteopenia, impaired glucose metabolism, and suppression of adrenal function. Consequently, most endocrinologists do not recommend the long-term use of glucocorticoids for the treatment of hirsutism.

NONHORMONAL APPROACHES

Eflornithine Cream

Topical eflornithine (α-difluoromethylornithine) retards hair growth through mechanisms that are not fully characterized. Eflornithine inhibits ornithine decarboxylase and is active as an anthelmintic agent. Eflornithine is not a depilatory agent; rather, it retards hair growth. The FDA has approved eflornithine for the treatment of hirsutism, and it is available as a 13.9% cream. The standard treatment regimen is application of a thin film to the upper lip and other affected areas of the face twice daily. The applications should be at least 8 hours apart. Patients should not wash the treated areas for 4 hours. To minimize inflammatory side effects, eflornithine should not be applied until at least 5 minutes after plucking, tweezing, cutting, or shaving of hair. In one study, after 24 weeks, approximately 32% of women treated with eflornithine reported marked improvement in facial hirsutism, compared with 8% of women treated with a placebo cream.[50] Improvement is seen within 4 to 8 weeks after starting treatment. Hirsutism may return to pretreatment levels 12 weeks after discontinuing the medication.

The major side effects of eflornithine are stinging and burning at the site of application and inflammation, with reddening of the irritated skin. Less than 1% of the applied dose is absorbed through the skin.

Laser Treatment

Laser therapy can induce selective photothermolysis of the pilosebaceous unit. A brief laser pulse at a wavelength that will be absorbed by the melanin in darkly pigmented hair, but not by lightly pigmented skin, is used to selectively heat the pilosebaceous unit. The use of brief pulses of laser energy minimizes the lateral diffusion of the thermal effect, resulting in maximal delivery of energy to the target and minimal effects in the adjacent skin. Three to six treatments performed every 8 weeks are necessary to control hair growth. Laser hair removal is most successful in patients with lighter skin color and dark hairs. Lasers with ruby and alexandrite generators appear to be most widely utilized.[51] Patients who have undergone laser treatment

of hirsutism report a high degree of satisfaction with the therapy and its results, although many women have recurrence of hirsutism 6 to 12 months after the treatment.[52]

Intense Pulsed Light

An alternative to laser treatment for hirsutism is the use of intense pulsed light that is not coherent (nonlaser). In one form of this treatment, thermal energy is created in hair follicles through the use of broad-spectrum noncoherent radiation with wavelengths from 550 to 1,200 nm administered in macropulses divided into three minipulses. The thermal energy destroys the epithelial cells in the hair follicle and thereby reduces hair growth.[53] In another form of this treatment, nonlaser light with wavelengths of approximately 550 to 585 nm is delivered in energy pulses of 38.7 joules/cm.[54] In small series, many of which had no control group, intense pulsed light has been demonstrated to be effective in reducing facial hirsutism.[55]

Hair Removal and Lightening

Shaving is a safe and useful method for hair removal but may need to be done multiple times each week; depilatory agents and wax can remove hair; and bleaches can lighten hair. These treatments, however, can cause skin irritation and erythema, which is especially troublesome when it occurs on the face. Electrolysis, which destroys the pilosebaceous unit with electrical energy one hair follicle at a time, is effective but labor intensive and expensive. In contrast, laser therapy removes hundreds of hairs simultaneously.

EXPERIMENTAL TREATMENT

Finasteride cream, 0.25%, applied to facial areas has been found superior to placebo in hirsute women. In a small study, administration of finasteride cream for 6 months reduced hair counts by approximately 40%, whereas placebo had no beneficial effects.[56] The FDA has not approved finasteride cream; a compounding pharmacy would need to prepare the medication.

Prognosis

Women with hirsutism should be warned not to expect significant improvement for at least 3 to 6 months after starting hormone therapy. Hair follicles have a life cycle of up to 6 months, and the actively growing hair must reach the end of its life cycle before it will cease to grow. The first response that a patient may observe is that hair is thinner (has a smaller diameter) and lighter in color. This occurs because the pigmented core of the hair shrinks in diameter before the linear growth rate of the hair slows.

Therapy for hirsutism is usually continued indefinitely because increased androgen production or sensitivity may persist for decades. In one study, hormone therapy for 2 years led to a marked decrease in hirsutism, but 80% of patients noted recurrence of hirsutism within 6 months after discontinuing therapy.[57] In most women, excess androgen production begins to decline in the late portion of the fourth decade of life.

The author has no commercial relationships with manufacturers of products or providers of services discussed in this chapter.

None of the oral contraceptives or hormonal agents discussed in this chapter has been approved by the FDA for the specific treatment of hirsutism.

References

1. Ferriman D, Gallwey JD: Clinical assessment of body hair growth in women. J Clin Endocrinol Metab 21:1440, 1961

2. Knochenhauer ES, Key TJ, Kahsar-Miller M, et al: Prevalence of the polycystic ovary syndrome in unselected black and white women of the southeastern United States. J Clin Endocrinol Metab 37:615, 1998

3. Darendeliler F, Bas F, Balaban S, et al: Spironolactone therapy in hypertrichosis. Eur J Endocrinol 135:604, 1996

4. Taponen S, Martikainen H, Jarvelin MR, et al: Hormonal profile of women with self-reported symptoms of oligomenorrhea and/or hirsutism: Northern Finland Birth Cohort 1966 study. J Clin Endocrinol Metab 88:141, 2003

5. Kirschner MA, Samojlik E, Silber D: A comparison of androgen production and clearance in hirsute and obese women. J Steroid Biochem 19:607, 1983

6. Matteri RK, Stanczyk FZ, Gentzschein EE, et al: Androgen sulfate and glucuronide conjugates in nonhirsute and hirsute women with the polycystic ovary syndrome. Am J Obstet Gynecol 167:1807, 1992

7. Samojlik E, Kirschner MA, Silder D, et al: Elevated production and metabolic clearance rates of androgens in morbidly obese women. J Clin Endocrinol Metab 59:949, 1984

8. Escobar-Morreale HF, Serrano-Gotarredona J, Garcia-Robles R, et al: Mild adrenal and ovarian steroidogenic abnormalities in hirsute women without hyperandrogenemia: does idiopathic hirsutism exist? Metabolism 46:902, 1997

9. Carmina E, Lobo RA: Polycystic ovaries in hirsute women with normal menses. Am J Med 111:602, 2001

10. Higuchi K, et al: Prolactin has a direct effect on adrenal androgen secretion. J Clin Endocrinol Metab 59:714, 1984

11. Belisle S, Menard J: Adrenal androgen production in hyperprolactinemic states. Fertil Steril 33:396, 1980

12. Parker LN, Chang S, Odell WD: Adrenal androgens in patients with chronic marked elevation of prolactin. Clin Endocrinol 8:1, 1978

13. Schiebinger RJ, Chrousos GP, Cutler GB Jr, et al: The effect of serum prolactin on plasma adrenal androgens and the production and metabolic clearance rate of dehydroepiandrosterone sulfate in normal and hyperprolactinemic subjects. J Clin Endocrinol Metab 62:202, 1986

14. O'Driscoll JB, Mamtora H, Higginson J, et al: A prospective study of the prevalence of clear cut endocrine disorders and polycystic ovaries in 350 women presenting with hirsutism or androgenic alopecia. Clin Endocrinol 41:231, 1994

15. Friedman CI, Schmidt GE, Kim MH, et al: Serum testosterone concentrations in the evaluation of androgen-producing tumors. Am J Obstet Gynecol 153:44, 1985

16. Meldrum DR, Abraham GE: Peripheral and ovarian venous concentrations of various steroid hormones in virilizing ovarian tumors. Obstet Gynecol 53:36, 1979

17. Derksen J, Nagesser SK, Meidners AE, et al: Identification of virilizing adrenal tumors in hirsute women. N Engl J Med 331:968, 1994

18. Chetkowski RJ, DeFazio J, Shamonki I, et al: The incidence of late-onset congenital adrenal hyperplasia due to 21-hydroxylase deficiency among hirsute women. J Clin Endocrinol Metab 58:595, 1984

19. Weyer C, Bogardus C, Mott DM, et al: The natural history of insulin secretory dysfunction and insulin resistance in the pathogenesis of type 2 diabetes mellitus. J Clin Invest 104:787, 1999

20. Barbieri RL, Smith S, Ryan KJ: The role of hyperinsulinemia in the pathogenesis of ovarian hyperandrogenism. Fertil Steril 50:197, 1988

21. Bates GW, Whitworth NS: Effect of body weight reduction on plasma androgens in obese infertile women. Fertil Steril 38:406, 1982

22. Pasquali R, Antenucci D, Casimirri F, et al: Clinical and hormonal characteristics of obese and amenorrheic women before and after weight loss. J Clin Endocrinol Metab 8:173, 1989

23. Clark AM, Thornley B, Tomlinson L, et al: Weight loss in obese infertile women results in improvements in reproductive outcome for all forms of fertility treatment. Hum Reprod 13:1502, 1998

24. Hollman M, Runnebaum B, Gerhard I: Effects of weight loss on the hormonal profile in obese infertile women. Hum Reprod 11:1884, 1996

25. Clark AM, Ledger W, Galletly C, et al: Weight loss results in significant improvement in pregnancy and ovulation rates in anovulatory obese women. Hum Reprod 10:2705, 1995

26. Givens JR, Andersen RN, Wiser WL: The effectiveness of two oral contraceptives in suppressing plasma androstenedione, testosterone, LH and FSH and in stimulating plasma testosterone binding capacity in hirsute women. Am J Obstet Gynecol 124:333, 1976

27. Givens JR, Andersen RN, Wiser WL, et al: Dynamics of suppression and recovery of plasma FSH, LH, androstenedione and testosterone in polycystic ovary disease using an oral contraceptive. J Clin Endocrinol Metab 38:727, 1974

28. Kullberg G, Hamburger L, Mattson LA, et al: Effects of a low-dose desogestrel-ethinyl estuarial combination on hirsutism, androgens and sex hormone binding globulin in women with polycystic ovary syndrome. Act Obstet Gynecol Scand 64:195, 1985

29. Falsetti L, Gambera A, Tisi G: Efficacy of the combination ethinyl estradiol and cyproterone acetate on endocrine, clinical and ultrasonographic profile in the polycystic ovary syndrome. Hum Reprod 16:36, 2001

30. Spritzer PM, Lisboa KO, Mattiello S, et al: Spironolactone as a single agent for long-term therapy of hirsute patients. Clin Endocrinol 52:587, 2000

31. Yucelten D, Erenus M, Gurbuz O, et al: Recurrence rate of hirsutism after 3 different antiandrogen therapies. J Am Acad Dermatol 41:64, 1999

32. Bayram F, Muderris II, Guven M, et al: Comparison of high-dose flutamide versus low-dose flutamide in the treatment of hirsutism. Eur J Endocrinol 147:467, 2002

33. Falsetti L, Gambera A, Lengrenzi L, et al: Comparison of finasteride versus flutamide in the treatment of hirsutism. Eur J Endocrinol 141:361, 1999

34. Venturoli S, Paradisi R, Banoli A, et al: Low-dose flutamide (125 mg/day) as maintenance therapy in the treatment of hirsutism. Horm Res 56:25, 2001

35. Farquhar C, Lee O, Toomath R, et al: Spironolactone versus placebo or in combination with steroids for hirsutism and/or acne. Cochrane Database Syst Rev (4):CD000194, 2003

36. Muderris II, Bayram F, Guven M: Treatment of hirsutism with lowest dose flutamide (62.5 mg daily). Gynecol Endocrinol 14:38, 2000

37. Petrone A, Civitillo RM, Galante L, et al: Usefulness of a 12-month treatment with finasteride in idiopathic and polycystic ovary syndrome associated hirsutism. Clin Exp Obstet Gynecol 26:213, 1999

38. Barth JH, Cherry CA, Wojnarowska F, et al: Spironolactone is an effective and well-tolerated systematic antiandrogen therapy for hirsute women. J Clin Endocrinol Metab 68:966, 1989

39. Moghetti P, Tosi F, Tosti A, et al: Comparison of spironolactone, flutamide and finasteride efficacy in the treatment of hirsutism: a randomized, double blind, placebo controlled trial. J Clin Endocrinol Metab 85:89, 2000

40. Fruzzetti F, Bersi C, Parrini D, et al: Treatment of hirsutism: comparisons between different antiandrogens with central and peripheral effects. Fertil Steril 71:445, 1999

41. Venturoli S, Marescalchi O, Colombo FM, et al: A prospective randomized trial comparing low dose flutamide, finasteride, ketoconazole and cyproterone acetate-estrogen regimens in the treatment of hirsutism. J Clin Endocrinol Metab 84:1304, 1999

42. Cumming DC, Yang JC, Rebar RW, et al: Treatment of hirsutism with spironolactone. JAMA 247:1295, 1982

43. Wysowski DK, Freiman JP, Touretlot JB, et al: Fatal and nonfatal hepatotoxicity associated with flutamide. Ann Intern Med 119:1150, 1993

44. Sahin Y, Dilber S, Keletimur F: Comparison of Diane 35 and Diane 35 plus finasteride in the treatment of hirsutism. Fertil Steril 75:496, 2001

45. Taner C, Inal M, Basogul O, et al: Comparison of the clinical efficacy and safety of flutamide versus flutamide plus an oral contraceptive in the treatment of hirsutism. Gynecol Obstet Invest 54:105, 2002

46. Pazos F, Escobar-Morreale HF, Balsa J, et al: Prospective randomized study comparing the long-acting gonadotropin-releasing hormone agonist triptorelin, flutamide and cyproterone acetate used in combination with an oral contraceptive in the treatment of hirsutism. Fertil Steril 71:122, 1999

47. Harborne L, Fleming R, Lyall H, et al: Metformin or antiandrogen in the treatment of hirsutism in polycystic ovary syndrome. J Clin Endocrinol Metab 88:4116, 2003

48. Kelly CJ, Gordon D: The effect of metformin on hirsutism in polycystic ovary syndrome. Eur J Endocrinol 147:217, 2002

49. Azziz R, Ehrmann D, Legro RS, et al: Troglitazone improves ovulation and hirsutism in the polycystic ovary syndrome. J Clin Endocrinol Metab 86:1626, 2001

50. Balfour JA, McClellan K: Topical eflornithine. Am J Clin Dermatol 2:197, 2001

51. Sanchez LA, Perez M, Azziz R: Laser hair reduction in the hirsute patient: a critical assessment. Hum Reprod Update 8:169, 2002

52. Loo WJ, Lanigan SW: Laser treatment improves the quality of life of hirsute females. Clin Exp Dermatol 27:439, 2002

53. Sadick NS, Weiss RA, Shea CR, et al: Long-term photoepilation using a broad-spectrum intense pulsed light source. Arch Dermatol 136:1336, 2000

54. Schroeter CA, Raulin C, Thurllimann W, et al: Hair removal in 40 hirsute women with an intense laser-like light source. Eur J Dermatol 9:374, 1999

55. Moreno-Arias GA, Castelo-Branco C, Ferrando J: Side-effects after IPL photodepilation. Dermatol Surg 28:1131, 2002

56. Lucas KJ: Finasteride cream in hirsutism. Endocr Pract 7:5, 2001

57. Kokaly W, McKenna TJ: Relapse of hirsutism following long-term successful treatment with estrogen-progestogen combination. Clin Endocrinol 52:379, 2000

58. Hatch R, Rosenfield RL, Kim MH, et al: Hirsutism: implications, etiology and management. Am J Obstet Gynecol 140:815, 1981

Acknowledgment

Figure 1 Seward Hung.

81 Contraception

Sarah L. Berga, M.D.

Contraception means to prevent conception, but in common medical usage, it also refers to methods that prevent implantation. The goal of contraception is to make every child a wanted child. Some methods of contraception (e.g., barrier methods) also reduce the risk of sexually transmitted infections (STIs), but intrauterine devices (IUDs) may increase the risk of STIs or their consequences.

Contraceptive methods are generally categorized as reversible [see Table 1] or irreversible. Irreversible methods are often referred to as sterilization procedures. Pregnancy termination is not typically regarded as contraception, but the availability of medical methods of abortion has blurred this distinction. Emergency postcoital contraceptive methods are also available.

Most methods of contraception are designed for use by women. Hormonal methods of male contraception are under development, but they are not yet commercially available.[1] Concern remains that side effects will limit acceptance by men.

Historically, methods to prevent or terminate pregnancy have been subject to intense legal regulation. In the United States, legal regulations vary widely from state to state regarding the provision of services to minors, waiting periods for termination and sterilization, husband and parental consent, reporting of complications and deaths, and restrictions on advance directives by pregnant or potentially pregnant women. Some states also have regulations regarding the type of practitioner or the type of facility in which contraceptive and fertility management procedures can be provided, but no state currently bans the use of reversible contraceptives. Some states also permit practitioners to dispense contraceptives to persons under the age of 18 without parental consent. Medical insurance coverage for contraception varies widely.

The percentage of women using a contraceptive method rose from 56% in 1982 to 64% in 1995.[2] A more recent survey indicated that the percentage of women using contraceptive methods in the United States is high, ranging from 75% in Hawaii to 88% in Idaho.[3] The most widely used methods in 2005 were oral contraceptives, vasectomy, tubal ligation, and male condoms.[3] Male condom use is common among unmarried couples; this popularity is due in part to the protection its use affords against certain STIs, particularly HIV infection.

Combined Estrogen-Progestin Contraceptives

Combined estrogen-progestin contraceptives (COCs) are formulated with estrogen (in the form of ethinyl estradiol), in doses ranging from 20 to 35 μg, and a variety of progestins derived from 19-nortestosterone. Individual formulations may have a fixed dose of progestin (monophasic) or may have doses that vary by cycle phase (triphasic). Two preparations contain varying estrogen doses.

EFFICACY AND MECHANISM OF ACTION

COCs are a highly effective method of birth control. Theoretically, efficacy should be about 99.9%, but the typical efficacy is around 97%.[4] The contraceptive effect of COCs derives principally from the suppression of the hypothalamic release of gonadotropin-releasing hormone (GnRH) and the concomitant suppression of the pituitary release of luteinizing hormone (LH) and follicle-stimulating hormone (FSH). The decrease in LH reduces ovarian androgen secretion. The suppression of GnRH is primarily caused by the progestin component. Estrogen also independently suppresses FSH at the pituitary level, thereby retarding folliculogenesis.

COCs are progestin dominant. Progestin exposure causes endometrial decidualization and atrophy, rendering the endometrium unfavorable for implantation and thickening of the cervical mucus, thereby blocking the entry of sperm and bacteria into the upper genital tract. There are three generations of progestins. Third-generation progestins, which are theoretically less androgenic, include desogestrel, gestodene, and norgestimate. The clinical superiority of one progestin over any other has not been demonstrated.

REDUCTION OF ANDROGEN EXPOSURE

All COC preparations reduce androgen exposure by two mechanisms: (1) suppression of ovarian androgen production, as a result of the reduction in LH stimulation of the ovarian theca compartment, and (2) elevation of the level of sex hormone–binding globulin protein, which binds androgens and thereby lowers the unbound fraction of circulating androgens. COCs reduce facial or androgen-dependent hair growth and acne by reducing the circulating concentrations of androgens available to occupy androgen receptors on the pilosebaceous unit. Although women with polycystic ovary syndrome have elevated GnRH and LH levels, COCs containing 30 to 35 μg of estrogen adequately suppress their androgen secretion.[5]

CONTINUOUS VERSUS CYCLIC COC REGIMENS

Traditional COC regimens follow a 28-day cycle, with the woman taking active pills for 21 days and placebos for 7 days. The 7-day placebo window permits significant follicular development, and higher estrogen and progestin doses are then needed to inhibit further folliculogenesis and ovulation. Further, if there is a delay in starting the next pill pack, a so-called escape ovulation may result.

In patients taking COCs to effect ovarian suppression for medical purposes, this 28-day cycle may be less effective. These patients may benefit from a long-cycle regimen—42 to 105 days

---

Table 1 Categories of Commercially Available Reversible Contraceptives

Barrier methods	Progestin preparations
Condoms	Oral
Diaphragms	Injectable
Cervical caps	Implantable
Hormonal	Intrauterine devices
Combined estrogen-	
progestin preparations	
Oral	
Vaginal ring	
Transdermal	
Injectable	

of active pills, and then 1 week off—or a continuous regimen. For long-cycle regimens, patients can use the active pills from several packs or a commercial long-cycle preparation.

In 2003, the Food and Drug Administration (FDA) approved a new contraceptive regimen intended to decrease menstrual bleeding to four times a year. The regimen consists of 84 tablets of ethinyl estradiol and levonorgestrel followed by seven placebo pills. A clinical trial suggested that this formulation provides both high contraceptive efficacy (the failure rate was 0.60 pregnancies per 100 women per year) and endometrial safety.[6]

Available evidence suggests that continuous and interrupted regimens are equivalent in terms of contraceptive efficacy and safety; however, patients on continuous regimens report fewer menstrual symptoms (e.g., headaches, genital irritation, tiredness, bloating, and menstrual pain).[7] It is common to omit the placebo week in women undergoing hormonal treatment for disorders such as polycystic ovary syndrome, endometriosis, or bleeding dyscrasias as well as in those who desire amenorrhea or have headaches or other symptoms provoked by hormonal withdrawal during the placebo week. There are several advantages to a continuous approach, including better suppression of ovarian function. Persistent ovarian cysts may be less likely with a continuous regimen than with a cyclic regimen.

Increased breakthrough bleeding is a potential side effect of a continuous regimen as compared with a cyclic regimen. The increase in breakthrough bleeding is attributable partly to the development of fragile endometrial vessels coursing along the surface of the endometrium and partly to impaired local hemostasis.[8] The only near-continuous COC preparation that may avoid the increase in breakthrough bleeding while increasing follicular suppression is Mircette, whose regimen consists of 2 days of placebo, 5 days of 10 μg of estrogen, and 21 days of a combination of 20 μg of estrogen and 150 μg of desogestrel.[9] One objective of these modifications is to lower overall sex steroid exposure and minimize the unwanted consequences of pill use while minimizing breakthrough bleeding.

NONORAL COMBINED CONTRACEPTIVES

Several combined estrogen-progestin contraceptives that do not use the oral route have been developed. All offer the convenience of less-frequent dosing.

The hormonal vaginal contraceptive ring (NuvaRing) was approved by the FDA in October 2001. This product is a flexible polymer ring, about 2 in. in diameter, which the patient inserts in her vagina. The ring releases a continuous low dose of estrogen and etonogestrel. The ring is left in place for 3 weeks, then removed for the week during which the patient will have her menstrual period. Comparison of the vaginal ring with a COC has shown a lower incidence of irregular bleeding and a higher incidence of a normal intended bleeding pattern with the ring.[10] The continuous use of NuvaRing has not been studied.

The transdermal contraceptive patch (Ortho Evra) was approved by the FDA in November 2001. The patch delivers estrogen and norelgestromin over the course of a week. Patches are applied once a week for 3 consecutive weeks to the skin of the buttocks, the abdomen, the upper torso, or the upper outer arm.[11] In general, the efficacy and cycle control provided by the patch are comparable to those of COCs, but the efficacy of the patch may be lower in women who weigh 198 lb (90 kg) or more.[12] The overall rate of patch detachment is about 4%; about 2% of users experience skin irritation at the site of application. Recently, it was reported that venous thromboembolism rates were higher

Table 2 Potential Side Effects of Oral Contraceptives

Serious side effects	Metabolic changes
	    Decreased insulin action
	    Increase in clotting factors
	    Elevation of triglyceride levels
	    Increase in the metabolic work load
	      of the liver
	    Increase in renin substrate
	Clinical manifestations*
	    Venous thromboembolic events
	    Fatty liver or hepatoma
	    Cholestasis or cholecystitis
	    Diabetes mellitus
	    Hypertension
	    Cardiovascular events
	Exacerbation of depression
	Drug interactions

Nuisance side effects	Mastodynia Reduced libido Reduced vaginal lubrication Increased appetite Weight gain Fatigue Bloating

*These events are rare in healthy women younger than 50 years.

in users of a transdermal patch (i.e., Ortho Evra) as compared with that of COC users. The increase may be caused by variation in the skin's absorption of ethinyl estradiol, a potent procoagulant regardless of route of administration.[13]

An injectable estrogen-progestin contraceptive (Lunelle) is available in the United States. The preparation, which is given intramuscularly once a month, contains medroxyprogesterone acetate and estradiol cypionate in a timed-release form. In clinical trials, efficacy and patient satisfaction have been comparable to that seen with COCs.[14] Other combination injectable contraceptives are available. A meta-analysis reported that norethisterone enanthate formulations generally have lower rates of discontinuance than formulations that contain medroxyprogesterone acetate and estradiol cypionate.[15] However, increased acceptability of injectable contraception most likely depends on methods that allow women to administer their own injections. Injectable contraceptives are also available in progestin-only formulations [see Progestin-Only Contraceptives, below].

SIDE EFFECTS

Myriad serious and nuisance side effects are associated with COCs [see Table 2]. Smoking markedly increases the risk of venous thromboembolism. Smoking is a relative contraindication to COC use, particularly in women older than 35 years.[16] The crucial clinical issue is to convince the woman who smokes to stop smoking rather than deny her access to an acceptable form of contraception. For nonsmokers who take COCs containing 35 μg or less of estrogen, the risk of nonfatal venous thromboembolism is approximately one half that of pregnancy (60 per 100,000 women), but it is greater than that observed in healthy women who do not take oral contraceptives (5 per 100,000 women).[16] The alleged excess mortality from venous thromboembolism attributable to third-generation progestins as compared with other progestins is less than two per million women per year.[17] However, women with familial thrombophilia caused by factor V Leiden or prothrombin mutation 20210A have a greatly increased risk of venous thromboembolism when using any oral contraceptive[18,19] [see Chapter 99]. In white women, the carrier rate of factor V Leiden is approximately 3% and that of prothrombin mutation 20210A is less than 2%, so screening has not been routinely advised.[20] Also, there are other known causes of thrombophilia, but not all thrombophilias can be detected. One study found that the risk of developing deep vein thrombosis was greatest in the first 6 months (threefold higher than the risk associated with prolonged use).[21] Venous thrombosis in the first period of oral contraceptive use may therefore indicate the presence of an inherited clotting defect.

COCs may decrease insulin action, an effect that has been attributed to the progestin component. The use of COCs does not increase the risk of diabetes mellitus in women who do not have other risk factors for the disease. However, in a nonrandomized clinical trial that followed Latin American women with gestational diabetes for 7.5 years post partum, the rate of development of diabetes mellitus was 8.7% for those given nonhormonal contraception, 10.4% for those who used COCs, and 26.5% for those who used progestin-only pills. Life-table analysis showed an increase in diabetes mellitus within 2 years in the progestin-only group.[22] Given these considerations, it is prudent to avoid prescribing any progestin-only form of contraception in women predisposed to diabetes mellitus or in frankly diabetic women. Fortunately, COC use by insulin-dependent diabetic women does not increase the risk of diabetic retinopathy or nephropathy.[23]

COCs have a negligible effect on the overall risk of cancer.[24] Among women who take oral contraceptives for 8 years, the estimated increase in the number of cases of cancer is 125 per 100,000 for cervical cancer and 41 per 100,000 for liver cancer; those increases are offset, however, by decreases in endometrial cancer and ovarian cancer [see Benefits, below].[24] Oral contraceptive use does not appear to increase the risk of breast cancer significantly—regardless of the dose, duration of use, or age at use—even in women with a family history of breast cancer.[25,26] However, COC use may increase breast cancer risk in carriers of BRCA mutations, at least in BRCA1 carriers. In a matched case-control study, BRCA1 carriers who had used oral contraceptives for more than 5 years, before age 30, or before 1975 were at increased risk of breast cancer compared with BRCA1 carriers who had never taken oral contraceptives.[27]

Exposure to high doses of estrogen or progestin may provoke depression and mood disturbances, but this effect is limited to women with an underlying diathesis.[28] It is not known whether oral contraceptive use increases the lifetime risk of depression or hastens its onset in women so predisposed.

Table 3   Contraindications to Oral Contraceptives

Active liver or gallbladder disease
Medically significant hypertriglyceridemia
Active or past venous thromboembolic events
Atherosclerotic heart disease
Undiagnosed vaginal bleeding
Estrogen-dependent neoplasia
   Breast cancer
   Endometrial cancer
Symptomatic mitral valve prolapse
Smoking after 35 years of age

Table 4   Potential Benefits of Oral Contraceptives

Reduced risk of the following disorders:
   Ectopic pregnancy
   Benign breast disease
   Anemia
   Ovarian cysts and cancer
   Endometrial cancer
Lighter and predictable menses
Reduction or elimination of dysmenorrhea
Bone accretion

Progestins have mineralocorticoid activity that results in the retention of up to 2 lb of water in sensitive women. The progestins also increase plasma renin activity; in predisposed women, hypertension may result.

Oral contraceptive use can cause drug interactions by increasing liver production of proteins that bind other drugs, by inhibiting oxidative metabolism in the liver by the P-450 and P-448 cytochrome systems, and by competing for or accelerating conjugation. Conversely, drugs that stimulate the hepatic microsomal system, such as oral antifungal agents or rifampin, may decrease plasma levels of contraceptive steroid and lead to unintended pregnancy. Antibiotics such as ampicillin, tetracyclines, and metronidazole do not interfere with COC efficacy.

CONTRAINDICATIONS

There are specific contraindications to oral contraceptives [see Table 3]. Lactating women should probably not take COCs. Women with hypertension, epilepsy, depression, hepatitis, gallbladder disease, migraine, or premenstrual syndrome (PMS) need to be carefully monitored. Fibroids are not a contraindication to COC use.

BENEFITS

Women use oral contraceptives primarily for birth control. If side effects are tolerable, they are pleased to gain the other benefits [see Table 4]. Women generally appreciate the lighter and predictable menses. Long-cycle regimens and continuous-use regimens offer the option of scheduling or skipping bleeding episodes, which is a major advantage for any busy woman, particularly one who travels or spends time outdoors. Some women use oral contraceptives to treat an underlying disorder, such as polycystic ovary syndrome, dysmenorrhea, endometriosis, or idiopathic hirsutism. In general, the same benefits accrue.

One of the major benefits of COC use is bone accretion. One study showed that as little as 10 µg of estrogen was bone sparing in women older than 40 years, and 5 µg of estrogen plus 1 mg of norethindrone caused bone accretion.[29] Women who are hyperandrogenic but eumenorrheic have greater bone mass than do hyperandrogenic women who are oligomenorrheic. The latter have slightly higher bone mass than eumenorrheic, nonhirsute women. Women with polycystic ovary syndrome or idiopathic hirsutism who take oral contraceptives will have a decrement in endogenous androgen exposure, but COC use in this setting is expected to be bone sparing. Women with hypothalamic hypogonadism, particularly those with an eating disorder, have underlying metabolic disturbances that render their bones less responsive to exogenous steroid exposure. These women may continue to lose or not accrue bone even if they use COCs.[30]

Long-term use of COCs reduces the incidence of endometrial cancer and ovarian cancer. Among women who take oral contraceptives for 8 years, it is estimated that there will be 197 fewer cases of endometrial cancer per 100,000 users and 193 fewer cases of ovarian cancer per 100,000 users.[24] Newer COCs, which contain 20 μg of estrogen, appear to provide identical risk reduction for ovarian cancer as did older formulations, which contained 50 μg or more of estrogen.[31] Studies have shown that oral contraceptives markedly reduce the risk of ovarian cancer in carriers of BRCA1 and BRCA2 mutations (who are at increased risk for ovarian cancer and premenopausal breast cancer); the longer the duration of use, the greater was the protection from ovarian cancer.[32,33] However, another study found that greater parity rather than prolonged use of COCs was the factor responsible for lowering the risk of ovarian cancer in carriers and noncarriers of BRCA1 and BRCA2 mutations.[34] In deciding whether women with germ-line mutations in the BRCA1 gene should use COCs, clinicians should weigh a possible increase in the risk of breast cancer against the convenience of this means of birth control and its potential to reduce the risk of ovarian cancer.

Progestin-Only Contraceptives

EFFICACY AND MECHANISM OF ACTION

Two progestin-only contraceptive methods are commercially available; one involves subdermal implants and the other involves injections. Although several subdermal implant systems have been approved by the FDA, only one (Implanon) is currently available in the United States.

Implanon is a single-rod progestin implant that releases the progestin etonogestrel (40 mg/day); it provides contraception for up to 3 years. A 2-year multicenter study of 330 sexually active women found Implanon to be a safe, highly effective, and rapidly reversible means of contraception.[35]

Norplant, which was the first implant system available in the United States, is composed of six Silastic rods impregnated with the progestin levonorgestrel. The rods are inserted subdermally, generally in the upper arm. Diffusion of levonorgestrel through the wall of each capsule provides a continuous low dose of progestin for at least 5 years. The progestin modestly inhibits the hypothalamic-pituitary-ovarian axis to block ovulation; it also induces endometrial shedding, making implantation unlikely, and thickens cervical mucus, thereby retarding the entry of sperm and bacteria to the upper genital tract. The birth-control efficacy is greater than 99.9%. In 2000, the manufacturer issued an advisory that the contraceptive efficacy of Norplant systems could not be assured; the suspect lots of implants were subsequently found to be effective.[36] Nevertheless, the manufacturer voluntarily withdrew the Norplant system from the market in 2002.

Jadelle, which is a two-rod levonorgestrel implant, was approved by the FDA for 5-year use, although it has not been marketed in the United States. It is as effective as the previous six-rod Norplant system, but it is easier to insert and remove.[37]

Depot medroxyprogesterone acetate (DMPA) is an aqueous suspension of 150 mg designed to be given intramuscularly every 3 months. The birth-control efficacy is greater than 99%. A lower-dose DMPA formulation (DMPA-SC, 104 mg) that is administered subcutaneously every 3 months is also available. Subcutaneous administration is less painful than intramuscular injections and potentially may allow patient self-administration. The risks and benefits of the subcutaneous and intramuscular formulations are similar.[38]

Table 5 Potential Side Effects of Injectable and Implantable Progestin Contraceptives

Breakthrough bleeding	Mastodynia
Headaches	Acne
Mood changes	Bone loss
Weight gain	

SIDE EFFECTS

Subdermal and injectable progestins have side effects [see Table 5]. The principal side effect is breakthrough bleeding caused by the development of fragile endometrial vessels and local derangement of hemostatic mechanisms as a result of excess progestin exposure relative to estrogen exposure.[5] The breakthrough bleeding may respond to the administration of an estrogen such as transdermal estradiol. Progestin implants and injections are relatively contraindicated in women with past or active depression or other psychiatric disorders [see Table 6]. There is some suggestion that progestin-only contraceptives are more mood destabilizing than COCs. The long-term effect on bone accretion depends on the extent of ovarian suppression and its attendant decline in estradiol secretion and on the age of the patient. Younger patients who have not attained peak bone mass may be more adversely affected. Levonorgestrel and etonogestrel implants may be more bone sparing than DMPA. Progestin-only contraceptives have been found to increase the risk of diabetes mellitus in Latin American women who have had gestational diabetes (see above).[22] This may be partly caused by the lack of estrogen, which is an insulin sensitizer.

A recent study indicated that in Latin American women with prior gestational diabetes, use of DMPA conferred a higher risk of diabetes mellitus (19% annual incidence) than that conferred by use of COC (12% annual incidence).[39] The increased risk appeared to be explained by three factors: (1) use in women with increased baseline diabetes risk, (2) weight gain during use, and (3) use with high baseline triglycerides or during breast-feeding, or both. The long-term cardiovascular risks are largely unknown, but in some experimental settings, synthetic progestins provoke vasoconstriction, an effect not seen with progesterone. An epidemiologic analysis from the World Health Organization (WHO) found no excess risk of cardiovascular disease with either combined or progestin-only methods other than an increased risk of stroke in hypertensive women who were given the progestin-only contraceptives.[40]

Another common side effect of progestin-only contraceptives is delay in return of menses. DMPA is given at 90-day intervals, but patients who discontinue this method may not experience immediate return of menses because of variability in the metabolism of the depot form and variable sensitivity of the hypothalamic GnRH pulse generator to low levels of progestin.

Table 6 Contraindications to Injectable and Implantable Progestin Contraceptives

Active liver disease	Active thromboembolic disease
Diabetes mellitus	Active cardiovascular disease
Unexplained vaginal bleeding	Depression
Breast cancer	Other psychiatric disorders

Ovarian cysts or enlarged ovarian follicles during the first year of use of contraceptive implants are common and transient and should not be interpreted as pathologic lesions in the absence of other findings.[41]

Intrauterine Devices

IUDs interfere with sperm migration, fertilization, ovum transport, and implantation, presumably by causing a sterile salpingitis, endometritis, or both. The birth-control efficacy is greater than 97%.

One of the principal benefits of IUDs is that they provide a nonhormonal method of birth control. They are ideal for women who have completed childbearing and who desire a low-maintenance, reversible method of contraception. IUDs are also relatively economical.

Two IUDs are currently available: the Copper T 380A, which lasts 10 years, and the 5-year, levonorgestrel-releasing Mirena. With the copper IUD, both the inert plastic device and the copper contribute to the spermicidal effect and prevention of implantation. With the progestin-containing IUD, part of the efficacy is attributed to the effects of the progestin on the endometrium that retard implantation.[42]

The main side effect associated with IUD use is pelvic inflammatory disease (PID). Most of the increased risk of PID occurs in the first 3 weeks after insertion. Women with more than one sexual partner who are at risk for contracting gonorrhea and chlamydial infection also are at increased risk for PID. Patient selection, rigorous aseptic insertion technique, and screening for STIs may minimize this risk. Routine antibiotic prophylaxis during insertion may not be necessary.[43] Uterine perforation is a rare insertion risk. Dysmenorrhea and menorrhagia have been reported with the copper IUD, whereas decreased menstrual flow, dysmenorrhea, and increased risk of ectopic pregnancy have been reported with the progesterone-releasing IUD.

The primary contraindication to IUD use is a history of PID. Nulligravidity is a relative contraindication. Sexual monogamy should be emphasized as a means of minimizing the risk of STIs and PID.

Barrier Methods

Male and female barrier contraceptives are available. When used correctly, the male condom protects against pregnancy and STIs. The theoretical efficacy of barrier methods for birth control is 98%, but the actual efficacy is about 88%. The efficacy gap results from inconsistent use and condom breakage. The female condom is more difficult to use and has not gained popularity. The diaphragm and cervical cap do not protect against STIs as effectively as condoms. When they are used with spermicides, the birth-control efficacy of diaphragms and cervical caps is theoretically 94%; in practice, however, the efficacy is about 82%. Both cervical caps and diaphragms require fitting and a prescription. They also require user training and diligence. Instructions on their use are provided in the products' package inserts. Spermicides may independently decrease the risk of STIs. When used alone, spermicides have a birth-control efficacy of about 79%.[4] Spermicides that also have antimicrobial activity are in development.

Allergic reactions to latex and hypersensitivity to spermicides occur. Diaphragm use may increase the risk of urinary tract infections because the rim presses against the symphysis pubis and urethra, which may cause incomplete emptying of the bladder and irritation to the urethra during intercourse.

The main contraindication to barrier methods is lack of user motivation and hypersensitivity to spermicides or allergy to latex. The primary benefits of condoms are that they are available without prescription, inexpensive, relatively easy to use, nonhormonal, and protective against STIs. Other barrier methods are only slightly more difficult to use but require fitting and a prescription, so the need for birth control must be anticipated.

Periodic Abstinence

Periodic abstinence, or natural family planning, depends on recognition of the periovulatory window and avoidance of sexual intercourse during that window. As such, it requires that a woman have highly regular menstrual cycles and that both partners be motivated to avoid intercourse when the woman is fertile. There are several methods of detecting the fertile window, including avoiding intercourse on days 9 to 14 of a 28-day cycle, monitoring cervical mucus and body temperature, and monitoring salivary estradiol levels.

Successful use of fertility-awareness methods for birth control requires not only dedication but education. Family health centers, family planning centers, and church-affiliated centers may offer courses on this subject. Information is available on the Internet at sites such as http://my.webmd.com/encyclopedia/article/1819.51010.

Mastering the concepts of menstrual-cycle physiology can be empowering, and couples can use this information to plan a pregnancy, as well as to avoid it. There are no known contraindications. There are no religious prohibitions against periodic abstinence, so it is theoretically available to all women who have predictable cycles.

Periodic abstinence can be frustrating, however, and it is less reliable than other forms of contraception, with an estimated efficacy of 80%. Several factors can interfere with fertility awareness. Even women who usually have very regular cycles may occasionally have a cycle that deviates from what is expected. Vaginitis may obscure the recognition of midcycle mucus. Fever may mimic the progesterone-induced rise in body temperature that normally indicates the onset of the luteal phase, thereby falsely signaling that the fertile period has passed.

Sterilization

Sterilization procedures generally entail occlusion or ligation of the fallopian tubes in women or the vas deferens in men. The birth-control efficacy of sterilization procedures is greater than 99%; they are meant to be permanent. Reversal procedures are available, but the reversibility of tubal ligation or vasectomy is not guaranteed. Sterilization procedures may fail if the fallopian tube is not properly identified or if it recannulates. Vasectomy failures primarily result from not waiting a sufficient length of time after the procedure before having unprotected sexual intercourse. In women, sterilization procedures can be done postpartum, but interval procedures are safer and more effective. Interval procedures employ laparoscopy, with or without general anesthesia. The fallopian tubes are either fulgurated or banded.

Patients may experience feelings of regret after a tubal ligation or vasectomy. Appropriate counseling can minimize this emotional side effect. There is no concrete evidence that vasectomy causes heart disease or prostate cancer. A review of tubal ligation found no evidence of increased rates of premenstrual distress, menorrhagia, dysmenorrhea, or menstrual irregularities in women 30 years of age or older who had undergone interval tubal ligation.[44]

The main contraindication to sterilization is ambivalence. In addition, women who undergo laparoscopic procedures must be suitable surgical candidates. The main benefit of sterilization is its permanence. Because sterilization is a one-time procedure with high efficacy, it is highly cost-effective in appropriately selected candidates. Tubal ligation may decrease the risk of PID and ovarian cancer.

Emergency Contraception

Postcoital contraception aims to desynchronize endometrial development and prevent implantation. Various methods have been proposed.[45] They include high doses of COCs taken within 72 hours after intercourse; levonorgestrel taken within 72 hours after intercourse; high doses of estrogen; danazol; mifepristone, as a single 600 mg dose; and insertion of a copper IUD up to 5 days after ovulation. The contraceptive efficacy of mifepristone or IUDs is at least 99%. A review assessed the efficacy of several methods of emergency contraception (i.e., the Yuzpe regimen, levonorgestrel, mifepristone, danazol, and some combination regimens).[46] The review found that levonorgestrel is more effective than the Yuzpe regimen (200 μg ethinyl estradiol and 2 mg dl-norgestrel, administered in two divided doses) in preventing pregnancy. Levonorgestrel is similar in effectiveness to mid-dose (25 to 50 mg) or low-dose (< 10 mg) mifepristone. The Yuzpe regimen can be used when levonorgestrel and mifepristone are not available.

Scottish and American studies suggested that women given a single emergency contraceptive kit used it correctly without experiencing significant side effects, and they had a lower unintended pregnancy rate.[47,48] In a public health policy initiative, British Columbia allowed pharmacists to distribute emergency contraceptives without a physician's prescription. In all years studied, the frequency of emergency contraceptive use was highest in women aged 20 to 24 years. The analysis of pharmacist treatment consent forms indicated that women tended to obtain emergency contraceptives after a birth control method had failed or when unprotected intercourse occurred at the time of highest risk of safety in their menstrual cycle.[49] Given the safety and efficacy of emergency contraception, many physicians strongly advocate that it be made available over the counter.[50] Patient information on emergency contraception is available on the Internet at http://ec.princeton.edu.

Choosing a Contraceptive Method

There is no perfect contraceptive; all may fail, and all have drawbacks and side effects. Age, motivation, marital status, partner attitude, perceived risk of pregnancy, frequency of intercourse, medical conditions, costs, cultural considerations, and religious beliefs affect the choice of contraceptive methods. The patient's or couple's medical history and preferences must guide the selection of a contraceptive [see Table 7]. Patients should be encouraged to revise their choice on the basis of side effects and changing circumstances.

Patients should be advised to inform the physician of new symptoms before discontinuing a contraceptive method. The physician must remain sensitive to the patient's concerns. Even

Table 7 Contraceptive Characteristics Affecting Choice[44]

Characteristic	Method
High efficacy	Combined oral contraceptives Intrauterine devices Depot medroxyprogesterone acetate Subdermal progestin implants
Limited or no systemic side effects	Barriers Spermicides Periodic abstinence
Minimal effort	Intrauterine devices Subdermal progestin implants Depot medroxyprogesterone acetate
Low cost	Male condom Spermicides Combined oral contraceptives
Nonprescription	Male condom Spermicides Periodic abstinence
No religious prohibitions	Periodic abstinence

Protection against sexually transmitted diseases
  Cervical gonorrhea and chlamydial infection
  Salpingitis
  HIV infection
	
	Barriers
	
	Barriers, hormone contraceptives
	Male and female latex condoms

Other health benefits	Hormone contraceptives
Minimal risk to future fertility	Hormone contraceptives Barriers Periodic abstinence

if a symptom sounds trivial from a medical perspective, it may alarm the patient and cause her to discontinue the method.

The role of condoms and other contraceptives in the reduction of STI transmission must be emphasized so that patients can choose properly from among the available options. Emergency contraception should be discussed and offered to those not seeking long-term contraception.

REVERSIBLE CONTRACEPTIVE METHODS

The first decision point in the choice of a reversible contraceptive method hinges on whether the patient has more than one sexual partner or is in a long-term monogamous relationship. If the patient has more than one sexual partner, condoms with or without hormonal contraception should be recommended. User reluctance and lack of familiarity are the main limitations to condom use. Condoms are ideal for unplanned intercourse.

For healthy women, the ancillary health benefits of combined estrogen-progestin contraceptives should be emphasized. These include a reduced risk of ovarian and endometrial cancer and preservation or accretion of bone mass. The option of using combined hormonal contraceptives to regulate menstrual timing should be discussed as a means of aiding compliance.

COCs, particularly the generic brands, are relatively inexpensive, costing in the range of $10 to $20 a month. COCs work best if taken daily, and some women find it difficult to remember to do so; they may prefer a vaginal ring, transdermal patch, or injectable contraceptive. Women who do not take the pills reliably will have increased rates of pregnancy and side effects, such as breakthrough bleeding. They should be counseled to use a barrier method or spermicide if they miss two consecutive pills or if they start the next package of pills after a hiatus of 8 or more days. In healthy nonsmokers without predisposing medical conditions, the pill is a safe and highly efficacious method of contraception that can be used in women up to 50 years of age. In women who are approaching menopause, COC use not only provides effective contraception but also can regularize menstrual cycles, relieve vasomotor symptoms, and stabilize bone mass.[51] However, the risks of chronic disease associated with long-term use of COCs may outweigh the short-term benefits in this age group.[52]

Women with epilepsy may need to have their antiseizure medications adjusted when they start oral contraceptive therapy, and they may benefit from using a continuous method to avoid fluctuations in antiseizure medication levels. Not all the newer antiseizure drugs interact with oral contraceptives, however,[53] so patients need to be evaluated on a case-by-case basis. Consultation with a pharmacist may be useful.

Follow-up is important in women who choose hormonal contraceptives. Blood pressure should be measured around 3 months after the start of COCs and annually thereafter. If hypertension results, it is prudent to discontinue COCs. Women using hormonal contraception who develop a severe, unremitting headache should be evaluated for possible stroke and cerebral thrombosis.

With prolonged use of COCs—even on a cyclic regimen—some women develop endometrial atrophy and amenorrhea. Once pregnancy has been excluded, it is prudent to recommend a long-cycle or a continuous regimen or one with a shortened placebo window.

Women with active or past PMS and depression, including postpartum depression, should be advised about the potential for negative mood effects associated with COCs. However, a recent formulation (Yasmin), which employs the novel progestin drospirenone, has been shown to reduce PMS symptoms.[54]

Switching to a lower-dosage regimen may reduce nuisance side effects. Physically smaller women or women who metabolize synthetic sex steroids slowly (such as women of Asian descent) should start with a 20 μg pill. Lower-dosage regimens have the benefit of causing fewer estrogen-dependent side effects, such as breast tenderness or nausea. Women with a history of headaches may do better on the lowest dose given in a continuous regimen.

Women who experience exacerbations of migraine headache while taking a COC do not typically have problems on a progestin-only contraceptive; DMPA or subdermal implants may be appropriate for such women.[55] These contraceptive methods may also be appropriate for a patient who has a low risk of depression, PMS, and osteoporosis. The patient must desire extended protection and be willing to undergo the insertion procedure or an injection. Subdermal implants and DMPA are relatively expensive.

Because, unlike an implant, injectable DMPA cannot be removed if a patient experiences adverse effects, many patients fail to continue with this form of contraception. Insertion of subdermal implants requires training and skill. If adverse effects occur with subdermal implants, a surgical procedure is required for their removal. Removal is often more difficult than introduction because of scarring around the capsules. In appropriate patients, however, subdermal implants provide a long-term, low-maintenance birth-control method.

IUDs, barrier methods, or periodic abstinence may be considered if the patient is not a candidate for hormone contraception and is in a long-term monogamous relationship.

Prospective users of IUDs must be made aware of the attendant risks and benefits. To make an informed decision, users need to understand the risks and potential consequences of PID.

Diaphragms and cervical caps are ideal for highly motivated users who desire a nonhormonal method of birth control. Spermicides increase the efficacy of all barrier methods of contraception but also increase cost and bother. Use of barrier methods is increased by public health education and by suggestion that the barrier method be incorporated into foreplay.

Women who report vaginal pruritus, irritation, inflammation, pain, or discharge associated with the use of a barrier method may have a latex allergy or hypersensitivity to spermicide. Latex allergies are particularly common in health care workers, many of whom are women. Formal allergy testing can be done to detect latex allergy, but current tests are not highly reliable. Latex allergy can provoke life-threatening anaphylaxis. Although most spermicides contain nonoxynol-9 as the active contraceptive ingredient, the other constituents may vary. Therefore, it may be possible to minimize irritation by switching to a different preparation. Men may also report allergies to latex or hypersensitivity to spermicides. Latex is preferred for condoms and barrier methods because it is impermeable to HIV.

NONREVERSIBLE CONTRACEPTIVE METHODS

All potential reversible and permanent options must be reviewed before a sterilization procedure is chosen. In general, if a couple seeks sterilization, a vasectomy is recommended because it is safer and less expensive than a laparoscopic tubal ligation. Postpartum tubal ligation is the riskiest, least effective, and most likely to cause regret.

Laparoscopic tubal ligation is expensive and must be performed by a skilled surgeon in an appropriate setting, so availability may be limited by cost or access to an appropriate physician. Many states require mandatory waiting periods. Some require spousal consent. Counseling is the cornerstone of success.

Sarah L. Berga, M.D., has received grants for clinical research and educational activities from Berlex Laboratories, Wyeth-Ayerst Laboratories, Inc., Johnson & Johnson, and Schering-Plough Corporation, Inc.

References

1. Anawalt BD, Amory JK: Male hormonal contraceptives. Expert Opin Pharmacother 2:1389, 2001

2. Piccinino LJ, Mosher WD: Trends in contraceptive use in the United States: 1982–1995. Fam Plann Perspect 30:4, 1998

3. Bensyl DM, Iuliano AD, Carter M, et al: Contraceptive use: United States and territories. Behavioral Risk Factor Surveillance System, 2002. MMWR Surveill Summ 54:1, 2005

4. Trussell J, Hatcher RA, Cates W Jr, et al: A guide to interpreting contraceptive efficacy studies. Obstet Gynecol 76:558, 1990

5. Daniels TL, Berga SL: Resistance of gonadotropin releasing hormone drive to sex steroid–induced suppression in hyperandrogenic anovulation. J Clin Endocrinol Metab 82:4179, 1997

6. Anderson FD, Hait H: A multicenter, randomized study of an extended cycle oral contraceptive. Contraception 68:89, 2003

7. Edelman AB, Gallo MF, Jensen JT, et al: Continuous or extended cycle vs. cyclic use of combined oral contraceptives for contraception. Cochrane Database Syst Rev (3):CD004695, 2005

8. Runic R, Schatz F, Krey L, et al: Alterations in endometrial stromal cell tissue factor protein and messenger ribonucleic acid expression in patients experiencing abnormal uterine bleeding while using Norplant-2 contraception. J Clin Endocrinol Metab 82:1983, 1997

9. Killick SR, Fitzgerald C, Davis A: Ovarian activity in women taking an oral contraceptive containing 20 microgram ethinyl estradiol and 150 microgram desogestrel: effects of low estrogen doses during the hormone-free interval. Am J Obstet Gynecol 179:S18, 1998

10. Oddsson K, Leifels-Fischer B, Wiel-Masson D, et al: Superior cycle control with a contraceptive vaginal ring compared with an oral contraceptive containing 30 μg ethinylestradiol and 150 μg levonorgestrel: a randomized trial. Hum Reprod 20:557, 2005

11. Burkman RT: The transdermal contraceptive patch: a new approach to hormonal contraception. Int J Fertil Womens Med 47:69, 2002

12. Zieman M, Guillebaud J, Weisberg E, et al: Contraceptive efficacy and cycle control with the Ortho Evra/Evra transdermal system: the analysis of pooled data. Fertil Steril 77(suppl 2):S13, 2002

13. Jick SS, Kaye JA, Russmann S, et al: Risk of nonfatal venous thromboembolism in women using contraceptive transdermal patch and oral contraceptives containing norgestimate and 35 µg of ethinyl estradiol. Contraception 73:223, 2006

14. Kaunitz AM: Lunelle monthly injectable contraceptive: an effective, safe, and convenient new birth control option. Arch Gynecol Obstet 265:119, 2001

15. Gallo MF, Grimes DA, Schulz KF, et al: Combination injectable contraceptives for contraception. Cochrane Database Sys Rev (3):CD004568, 2005

16. Farley TM, Collins J, Schlesselman JJ: Hormonal contraception and risk of cardiovascular disease: an international perspective. Contraception 57:211, 1998

17. Drife J: Oral contraception and the risk of thromboembolism: what does it mean to clinicians and their patients? Drug Saf 25:893, 2002

18. Thrombophilic abnormalities, oral contraceptives, and risk of cerebral vein thrombosis: a meta-analysis. Blood 107:2766, 2006

19. Wu O, Robertson L, Langhorne P, et al: Oral contraceptives, hormone replacement therapy, thrombophilias and risk of venous thromboembolism: a systematic review. The Thrombosis: Risk and Economic Assessment of Thrombophilia Screening (TREATS) study. Thromb Haemost 94:17, 2005

20. Bertina RM, Rosendaal FR: Venous thrombosis: the interaction of genes and environment. N Engl J Med 338:1840, 1998

21. Bloemenkamp KW, Rosendaal FR, Helmerhorst FM, et al: Higher risk of venous thrombosis during early use of oral contraceptives in women with inherited clotting defects. Arch Intern Med 160:49, 2000

22. Kjos SL, Peters RK, Xiang A, et al: Contraception and the risk of type 2 diabetes mellitus in Latina women with prior gestational diabetes mellitus. JAMA 280:533, 1998

23. Garg SK, Chase HP, Marshall G, et al: Oral contraceptives and renal and retinal complications in young women with insulin-dependent diabetes mellitus. JAMA 271:1099, 1994

24. Schlesselman JJ: Net effect of oral contraceptive use on the risk of cancer in women in the United States. Obstet Gynecol 85:793, 1995

25. Marchbanks PA, McDonald JA, Wilson HG, et al: Oral contraceptives and the risk of breast cancer. N Engl J Med 346:2025, 2002

26. Silvera SA, Miller AB, Rohan TE: Oral contraceptive use and risk of breast cancer among women with a family history of breast cancer. Cancer Causes Control 16:1059, 2005

27. Narod SA, Dube MP, Klijn J, et al: Oral contraceptives and the risk of breast cancer in BRCA1 and BRCA2 mutation carriers. J Natl Cancer Inst 94:1773, 2002

28. Schmidt PJ, Nieman LK, Danaceau MA, et al: Differential behavioral effects of gonadal steroids in women with and in those without premenstrual syndrome. N Engl J Med 338:209, 1998

29. Speroff L, Rowan J, Symons J, et al: The comparative effect on bone density, endometrium, and lipids of continuous hormones as replacement therapy (CHART study): a randomized controlled trial. JAMA 276:1430, 1996

30. Grinspoon S, Thomas L, Miller K, et al: Effects of recombinant human IGF-I and oral contraceptive administration on bone density in anorexia nervosa. J Clin Endocrinal Metab 87:2883, 2002

31. Risk of ovarian cancer in relation to estrogen and progestin dose and use characteristics of oral contraceptives. SHARE Study Group. Steroid Hormones and Reproductions. Am J Epidemiol 152:233, 2000

32. Narod SA, Risch H, Moslehi R, et al: Oral contraceptives and risk of hereditary ovarian cancer. Hereditary Ovarian Cancer Clinical Study Group. N Engl J Med 339:424, 1998

33. Whittemore AS, Balise RR, Pharoah PD, et al: Oral contraceptive use and ovarian cancer risk among carriers of BRCA1 and BRCA2 mutations. Br J Cancer 91:1911, 2004

34. Modan B, Hartge P, Hirsh-Yechezkel G, et al: Parity, oral contraceptives, and the risk of ovarian cancer among carriers and noncarriers of a BRCA1 or BRCA2 mutation. N Engl J Med 345:235, 2001

35. Funk S, Miller MM, Mishell DR Jr, et al: Safety and efficacy of Implanon, a single-rod implantable contraceptive containing etonogestrel. Contraception 71:319, 2005

36. Important Norplant system (levonorgestrel implants) Update: Back-up contraception no longer required on specified lots. MedWatch, Food and Drug Administration, 2002 http://www.fda.gov/medwatch/SAFETY/2002/norplant.htm

37. Wan LS, Stiber A, Lam LY: The levonorgestrel two-rod implant for long-acting contraception: 10 years of clinical experience. Obstet Gynecol 102:24, 2003

38. Jain J, Dutton C, Nicosia A, et al: Pharmacokinetics ovulation suppression and return to ovulation following a lower dose subcutaneous formulation of Depo-Provera. Contraception 70:11, 2004

39. Xiang AH, Kawakubo M, Kjos SL, et al: Long-acting injectable progestin contraception and risk of type 2 diabetes in Latino women with prior gestational diabetes. Diabetes Care 29:613, 2006

40. Cardiovascular disease and use of oral and injectable progestogen-only contraceptives and combined injectable contraceptives: results of an international, multicenter, case-control study. World Health Organization Collaborative Study of Cardiovascular Disease and Steroid Hormone Contraception. Contraception 57:315, 1998

41. Hidalgo MM, Lisondo C, Juliato CT, et al: Ovarian cysts in users of Implanon and Jadelle subdermal contraceptive implants. Contraception 73:532, 2006

42. Kaunitz AM: Reappearance of the intrauterine device: a "user-friendly" contraceptive. Int J Fertil Womens Med 42:120, 1997

43. Walsh T, Grimes D, Frezieres R, et al: Randomised controlled trial of prophylactic antibiotics before insertion of intrauterine devices. IUD Study Group. Lancet 351:1005, 1998

44. Gentile GP, Kaufinan SC, Helbig DW: Is there any evidence for a post-tubal sterilization syndrome? Fertil Steril 69:179, 1998

45. Glasier A: Emergency postcoital contraception. N Engl J Med 337:1058, 1997

46. Cheng L, Gulmezoglu AM, Oel CJ, et al: Interventions for emergency contraception. Cochrane Database Syst Rev (3):CD001324, 2004

47. Glasier A, Baird D: The effects of self-administering emergency contraception. N Engl J Med 339:1, 1998

48. Raymond EG, Chen PL, Dalebout SM: "Actual use" study of emergency contraceptive pills provided in a simulated over-the-counter manner. Obstet Gynecol 102:17, 2003

49. Soon JA, Levine M, Osmond BL, et al: Effects of making emergency contraception available without a physician's prescription: a population-based study. CMAJ 172:878, 2005

50. Grimes DA, Raymond EG, Jones BS: Emergency contraception over-the-counter: the medical and legal imperatives. Obstet Gynecol 98:151, 2001

51. Kaunitz AM: Oral contraceptive use in perimenopause. Am J Obstet Gynecol 185(2 suppl):S32, 2001

52. Farquhar CM, Marjoribanks J, Lethaby A, et al: Long-term hormone therapy for perimenopausal and postmenopausal women. Cochrane Database Syst Rev (3):CD004143, 2005

53. Hachad H, Ragueneau-Majlessi I, Levy RH: New antiepileptic drugs: review on drug interactions. Ther Drug Monit 24:91, 2002

54. Oelkers W: Drospirenone: a progestogen with antimineralocorticoid properties: a short review. Mol Cell Endocrinol 217:255, 2004

55. Curtis KM, Chrisman CE, Peterson HB, et al: Contraception for women in selected circumstances. WHO Programme for Mapping Best Practices in Reproductive Health. Obstet Gyncecol 99:1100, 2002

82 Infertility

Eric D. Levens, M.D., and Alan H. DeCherney, M.D.

Infertility is defined as the inability to conceive after 1 or more years of regular coitus without contraception. Fecundity is the statistical probability of achieving a pregnancy (resulting in a live birth) within 1 month (one menstrual cycle) of regular unprotected sexual intercourse. Monthly fecundity for a fertile couple ranges from 20% to 35% [*see Table 1*].[1] Within 1 year, more than 85% of all couples trying to conceive will achieve a pregnancy.

The incidence of infertility has been increasing over the past 3 decades. It is estimated that nearly 10% of all couples in the United States have disorders associated with infertility. As a result, about 2.5 million couples seek advice for treatment each year in the United States.[2,3] The common causes of infertility in couples and in women are shown [*see Figures 1 and 2*].

The practitioner needs to approach the infertile couple in a rational and organized manner. After the initial evaluation, all the reproductive factors should be assessed and a treatment plan proposed that addresses the risk,[4] benefit, and cost[5] to the couple [*see Figures 3 and 4*]. Couples who go through this process without success may experience severe emotional and psychological distress. For this reason, patients should be counseled about the probability of their achieving a pregnancy before embarking on this potentially expensive treatment course, and psychological counseling during treatment may be valuable.[6]

Evaluation and Treatment of the Infertile Couple

During the first encounter, both partners should be interviewed. The physician should take note of each partner's age, duration of infertility, past pregnancies, past surgeries, frequency of coital activity, and problems encountered during intercourse (e.g., dyspareunia, impotence, anorgasmia, and lack of libido). All potential problems that are revealed during the initial examination should be addressed and treated accordingly. The initial evaluation should also cover other conditions that can impair fertility in women. Obese and sedentary women are at higher risk for infertility,[7] because obesity promotes anovulation. Cigarette smoking[8] and long-term use of nonsteroidal antiinflammatory drugs (NSAIDs)[9] can contribute to infertility. These effects are most noticeable at the extremes (i.e., marked obesity, heavy smoking, or high NSAID doses).

AGE

Age is an independent risk factor that is instrumental in determining a couple's chance of achieving a successful pregnancy. Nearly 50% of the infertility experienced by couples older than 40 years is caused by problems associated with advancing age.[10] A woman's reproductive capability decreases with advancing age, predominantly because of poor oocyte quality. After women reach 30 years of age, pregnancy rates decrease.[11] By 40 years of age, a woman's monthly fecundity is less than 5%.[12] Male fertility also diminishes with age: sperm quality declines, and the frequency of ejaculation decreases.

The duration of infertility may be just as important a risk factor as the age of the couple. The longer the duration of infertility, the lower is the probability of achieving a successful pregnancy.

MALE INFERTILITY

Infertility in the male partner is the primary cause of infertility in approximately 35% of couples who seek help.[11] Male infertility may be a result of endocrine dysfunction, testicular dysfunction, erectile dysfunction, sperm outlet obstruction, or sperm dysfunction [*see Table 2*]. Although there are numerous causes of male infertility, no identifiable reason for the sperm defect can be found in nearly 50% of men who have abnormal semen analyses.[13] Any previous testicular injury, infection, surgery, radiation, or chemotherapy should be documented during the initial history. The physical examination should focus on penile and testicular anomalies (e.g., hypospadia, cryptorchidism, and varicoceles). If any such anomaly is present, the patient should be referred to a urologist for evaluation and treatment.

After the initial physical examination, a semen analysis should be performed. The specimen is collected after 48 hours of abstinence from ejaculation and evaluated no more than 1 hour after collection.[14] If any parameters are abnormal [*see Table 3*], two additional semen analyses should be performed 2 weeks apart. Persistent abnormalities may warrant urologic evaluation and workup for diabetes mellitus, prolactin elevation, and chromosomal abnormalities.

Numerous tests have been developed to evaluate the functional status of sperm. These tests include cervical mucus testing, which correlates closely with fertilization rates in in vitro fertilization (IVF) but lacks negative predictive value.[15] In addition, the capacity of sperm to bind tightly to the zona pellucida correlates highly with morphology and hyperactivated motility and has excellent positive and negative predictive values.[16] Other tests that can be performed are the sperm penetration assay and the immunobead-binding assay. These tests can detect abnormalities in sperm penetration and motility, respectively, but may not indicate the true nature of the problem. In addition, the development of techniques for microinjection of sperm into egg (i.e., intracytoplasmic sperm injection [ICSI]), which bypasses barriers to fertilization, has limited the utility of the information about sperm binding and fertilization capacity that these tests provide. The future of sperm function testing may lie in postpenetration analysis using molecular techniques such as fluorescence in situ hybridization (FISH).[17]

If the results of semen tests are normal and the female partner's evaluation appears normal, a diagnosis of unexplained infertility is appropriate [*see* Unexplained Infertility, *below*].

Idiopathic oligospermia is the most common cause of infertility in men. Although there is no cure for this problem, treatment may include IVF with ICSI [*see Table 4*]. In severe cases of infertility, this technique can achieve fertilization rates as high as 65%.[18]

Table 1 Fecundity of Normal Couples over Time

Time (Months)	Couples Achieving Pregnancy (%)
1	20–36
3	57
6	72
12	85
24	93

FEMALE INFERTILITY

Tubal and Pelvic Factors

Nearly 35% of the infertility experienced by couples and 40% of the infertility in women is of pelvic origin. Uterine, tubal, and other pelvic abnormalities are responsible for this type of infertility. The clinician should elicit information regarding any history of sexually transmitted diseases, pelvic inflammatory disease, appendicitis with rupture, pelvic tuberculosis, or adnexal surgery. Many patients with tubal or pelvic damage have a history that includes a previous diagnosis of endometriosis, ectopic pregnancy, or submucous myomas. Although uterine myomas seldom cause infertility, they may cause recurrent early pregnancy loss and preterm labor.

Hysterosalpingography (HSG) is one of the initial diagnostic tests used to evaluate uterine, tubal, and pelvic abnormalities. This test is performed during the early proliferative phase, after the cessation of menstrual flow (cycle day 5 to 10). HSG can help identify abnormalities of uterine filling caused by submucous myomas, polyps, uterine synechiae (adhesions), and congenital malformations.

Tubal patency should be evaluated at the time of HSG. A delayed set of radiographs can detect pelvic adhesions and other pelvic abnormalities that prevent the release of contrast material into the pelvis. Once the site of blockage (which may be proximal or distal) has been identified, it can be dealt with accordingly.[19] Patients who are known to be anovulatory may forgo an initial HSG. If ovulation induction is successfully attempted for at least four consecutive cycles and conception does not occur, however, HSG should be performed.

HSG should never be performed on a woman with acute salpingitis, a tender pelvic mass, or allergy to iodine. Women with a known contraindication are better evaluated directly by laparoscopy. Patients who undergo HSG should receive prophylactic treatment for chlamydial infection: oral doxycycline, 100 mg twice daily for 7 days, is effective.

Laparoscopy with chromotubation (intrauterine injection of colored liquid [indigo carmine] to confirm tubal patency) is in-

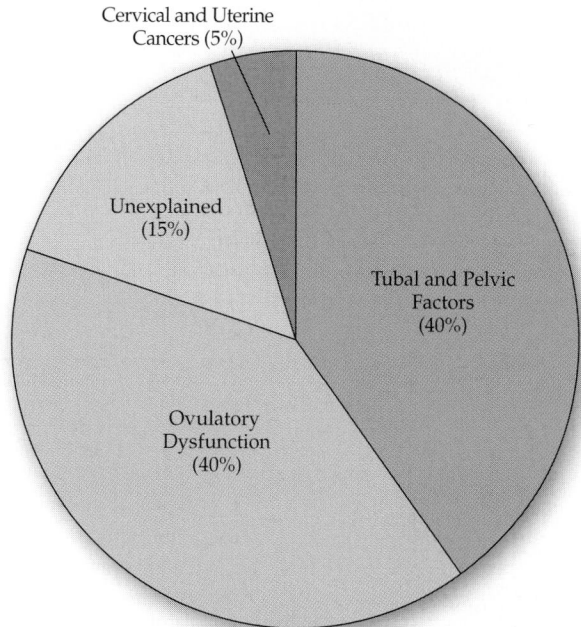

Figure 2 **Causes of infertility in women.**

dicated for patients with abnormal findings on HSG and for patients with unexplained infertility. This procedure may be omitted from the diagnostic workup if IVF is the main focus of treatment. However, surgical resection of the diseased tube should be considered for patients who are diagnosed with a hydrosalpinx on the basis of HSG or laparoscopy. The mere presence of a hydrosalpinx may adversely affect embryo implantation and the success of IVF.[20]

If the laparoscopy and chromotubation reveal tubal occlusion, surgery may be indicated. Isolated proximal or distal tubal occlusions may be treated by various surgical techniques. Combined proximal and distal occlusions are not well corrected with surgery, however, and IVF should be recommended as the treatment of choice to achieve pregnancy in these patients. Age is also important when deciding between tubal surgery and IVF. Older couples should be encouraged to have IVF rather than tubal surgery because the probability of their achieving a pregnancy is higher with IVF.

Cervical Factors

Abnormal cervical mucus is the recognized cause of infertility in 5% to 10% of couples trying to conceive. The postcoital test provides information regarding both the quality of the cervical mucus and its interaction with sperm. This test is performed on cycle day 11 to 13 (24 to 48 hours before ovulation); the male partner must abstain from ejaculation for 48 hours before testing. The cervical mucus is examined 2 to 8 hours after intercourse. The consistency of the cervical mucus is assessed, and the number of motile sperm per high-power field (hpf) is determined. Normal mucus is acellular, clear, thin, and elastic; the mucus should stretch approximately 8 to 10 cm when placed on a glass slide and pulled. This elasticity of the cervical mucus is known as spinnbarkeit. The mucus should also contain at least 5 to 10 progressively motile sperm/hpf.

Cervical mucus that is of poor quality (i.e., thick and nonelastic) will demonstrate a globular rather than a fernlike pattern after drying on a microscope slide. Absent or poor-quality cervical mu-

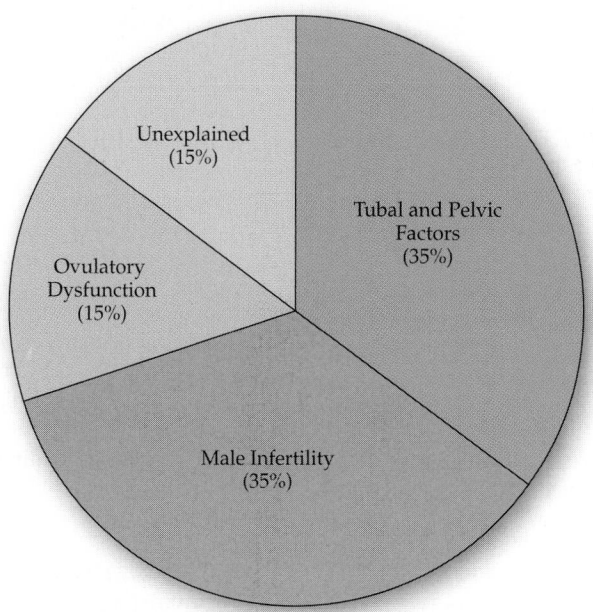

Figure 1 **Causes of infertility in couples.**

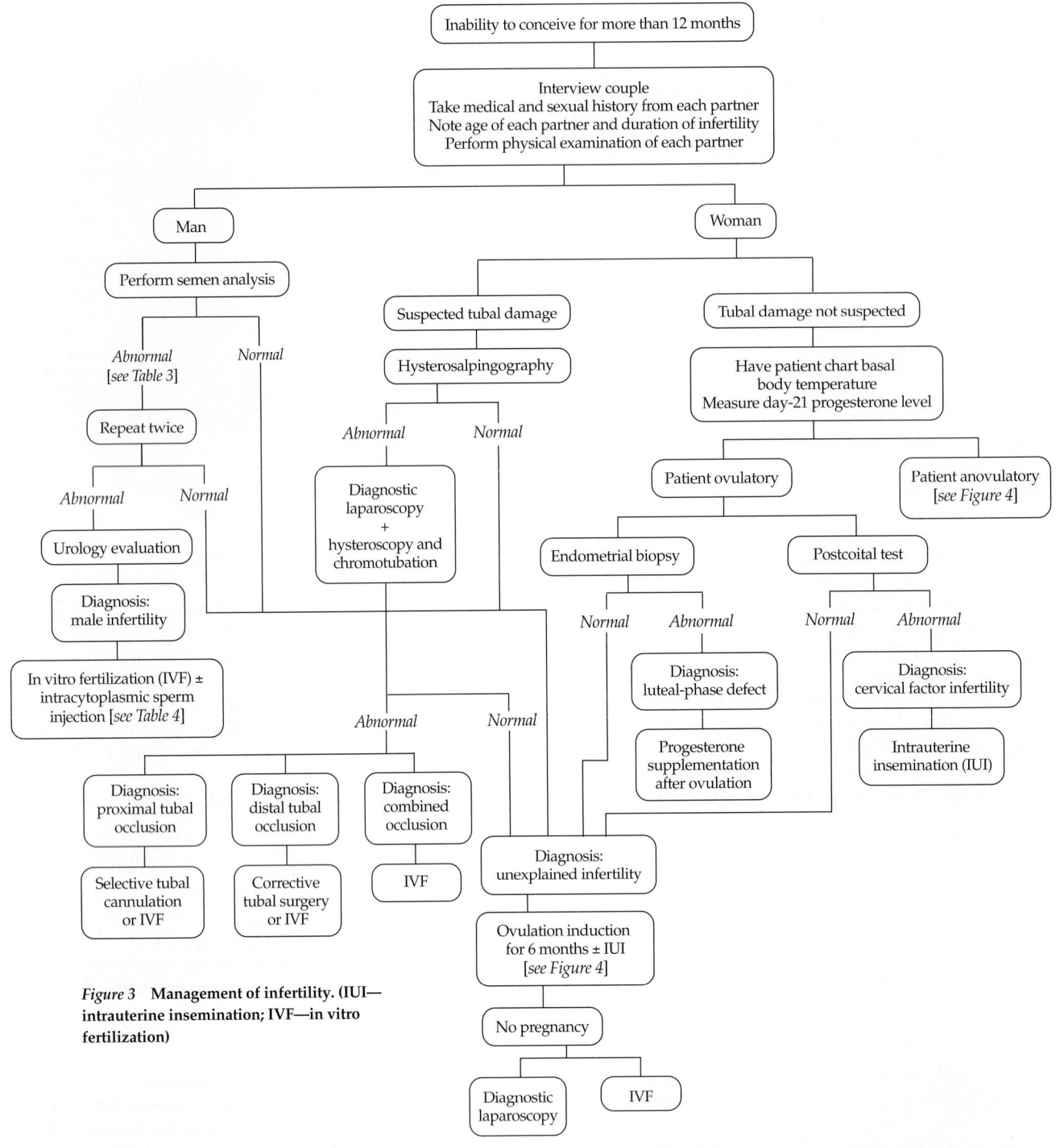

Figure 3 **Management of infertility. (IUI— intrauterine insemination; IVF—in vitro fertilization)**

cus may reflect either inaccurate timing of the test or an abnormality in mucus production. Cervical trauma and infection have been implicated as antecedents to abnormal mucus production.

Both shaky and immotile sperm are found in the cervical mucus of women who produce antisperm antibodies. When all the sperm from a postcoital test are found to be immotile, the patient should be asked whether lubricants or spermicides were used during coitus.

Although the postcoital test has a long history, dating back to 1866, the literature would suggest that its value is limited despite its widespread use. A randomized, controlled clinical trial found that the postcoital test was a poor predictor of fertility.

Moreover, use of the test resulted in an increase in treatments, with additional expense, but had no effect on pregnancy rates.[21] Moreover, postcoital testing has little relevance for patients with probable cervical factor infertility, in whom intrauterine insemination (IUI) is the treatment of choice.[22] IUI bypasses the cervix and allows the physician to place washed sperm directly into the endometrial cavity.[23]

Ovulatory Factors

Ovulatory dysfunction is the cause of 15% of the infertility detected in couples and 40% of the infertility found in women. Anovulation and oligo-ovulation account for most menstrual

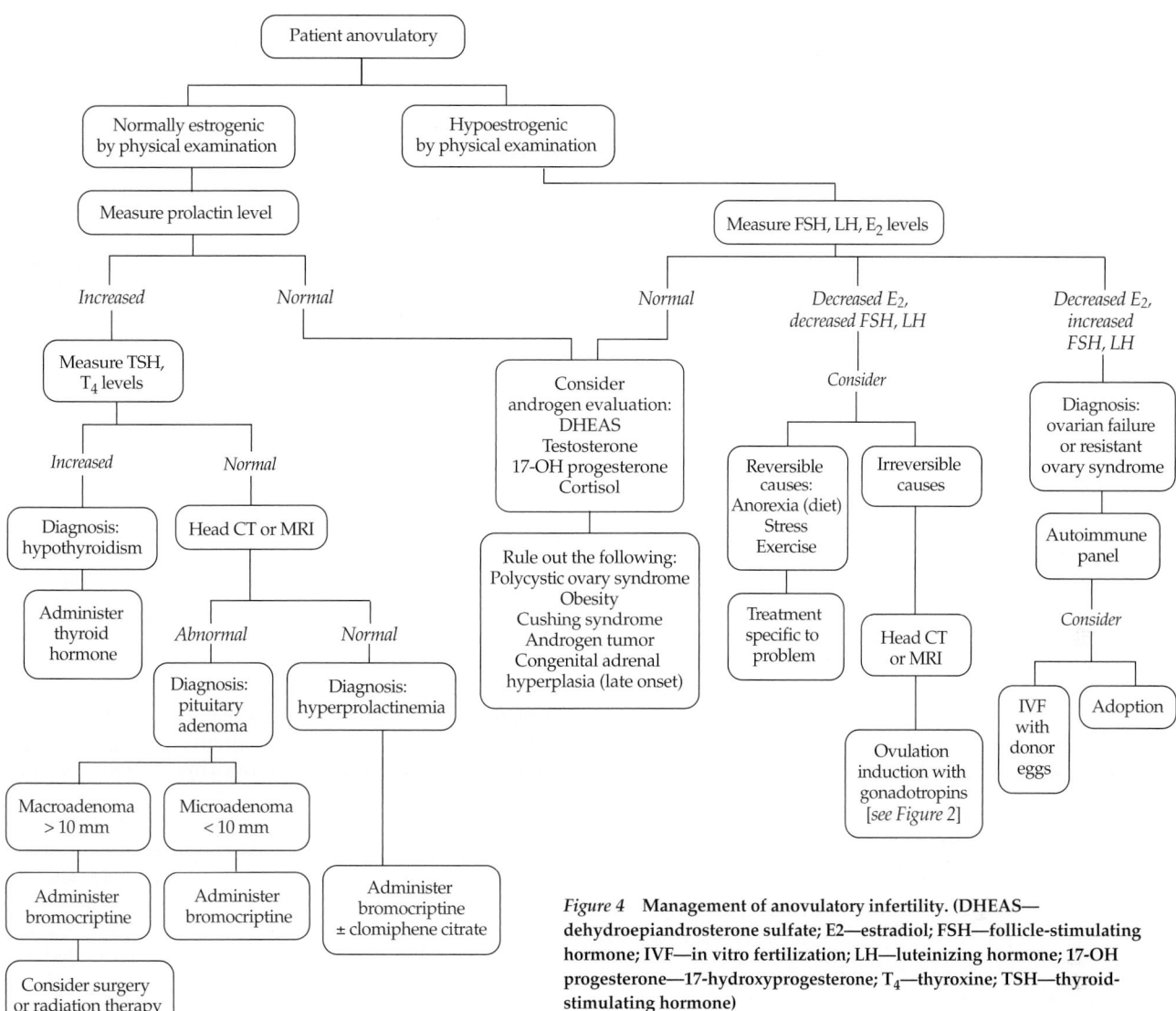

Figure 4 Management of anovulatory infertility. (DHEAS—dehydroepiandrosterone sulfate; E2—estradiol; FSH—follicle-stimulating hormone; IVF—in vitro fertilization; LH—luteinizing hormone; 17-OH progesterone—17-hydroxyprogesterone; T$_4$—thyroxine; TSH—thyroid-stimulating hormone)

abnormalities. Shortened menstrual cycles and luteal phase defects are less common causes of ovulatory dysfunction.

A patient's ovulatory status can be determined by several techniques. The cheapest and least invasive is to have the patient chart her basal body temperature (BBT). To measure BBT, the patient takes her temperature upon awakening each morning, before she gets out of bed. When charting is done correctly, it can aid the clinician by providing indirect evidence of ovulation. A biphasic temperature curve (i.e., an elevated temperature for at least 11 to 16 days) is an indication that ovulation probably occurred. The patient's own assessment of premenstrual molimina further strengthens the indirect evidence of ovulation.

Measurement of the progesterone level on day 21 of the menstrual cycle also provides an indirect assessment of ovulatory status. This method is less time-consuming than BBT charting. Progesterone values of more than 10 ng/ml are consistent with ovulation. A value of less than 3 ng/ml may indicate that ovulation has not occurred. Because progesterone is secreted in a pulsatile manner, only elevated values of progesterone are diagnostically useful. Levels between 3 and 10 ng/ml probably indicate ovulation but give insufficient information regarding the adequacy of the luteal phase.

From 5% to 30% of menstrual cycles in normally menstruating women involve a luteinized unruptured follicle. Although ovulatory symptoms and elevated progesterone levels occur during these cycles, an oocyte is not released and fertilization is impossible. Thus, the predictive value of indirect measures of ovulatory status is limited.

An endometrial biopsy can be performed on cycle days 23 to 26. This test can assess both the ovulatory status of the patient and the adequacy of the luteal phase. A luteal phase defect is defined as a lag in the histologic development of the endometrium by 2 or more days compared with the cycle day of sampling. Luteal phase defects are presumably caused by inadequate progesterone secretion from the corpus luteum.

Treatment has entailed prolonging the luteal phase by administering progesterone, either intramuscularly or intravaginally. The benefit of this approach, however, has not been substantiated.

Anovulation

Measurement of the prolactin level should be done during the initial evaluation of patients who are believed to be anovulatory [see Figure 4].[24] Elevated prolactin levels have a negative feedback effect on the hypothalamus, preventing the pulsatile

Table 2 Causes of Infertility in Men

Endocrine	Hypothalamic-pituitary-gonadal axis dysfunction Pituitary tumors Hypothalamic tumors Gonadotropin deficiencies Exogenous androgens Thyroid dysfunction

Testicular	Primary testicular failure
	 Klinefelter syndrome (47XXY)
	 Y chromosome microdeletions
	Anatomic
	 Varicocele
	 Cryptoorchidism
	 Infections
	  Mumps
	Toxins
	 Drugs
	  Antibiotics (e.g., erythromycins, tetracyclines)
	  Cimetidine
	  Spironolactone
	  Tobacco
	  Marijuana
	  Cocaine
	  Chemotherapeutic drugs (e.g., alkylating
	   agents)
	 Radiation
	 Heat

Erectile dysfunction	Psychosexual Chronic diseases Diabetes Vascular disease Medications Beta blockers
Sperm outlet obstruction	Vasectomy Congenital absence of the vas deferens
Sperm dysfunction	Anti-sperm antibodies Infections (e.g., prostatitis) Sperm binding dysfunction

release of gonadotropin-releasing hormone (GnRH). This, in turn, prevents secretion of follicle-stimulating hormone (FSH) and luteinizing hormone (LH) from the anterior pituitary. Consequently, follicular development and ovulation do not occur.

Hyperprolactinemia is responsible for 15% of all ovulatory disturbances.[25] If the patient has an elevated prolactin level, with or without galactorrhea, the thyroid-stimulating hormone (TSH) level should be measured to rule out primary or secondary hypothyroidism. If the TSH level is normal, a computed tomography scan or magnetic resonance image of the head should be obtained to determine whether the patient has a prolactinoma. Of import is that prolactin levels may also be elevated as a result of the use of certain medications [see Chapter 49]. Pharmacologic agents that deplete dopamine reserves (i.e., antidepressants, antipsychotics, and other psychotropic agents) may also result in hyperprolactinemia and anovulation.

If the CT or MRI findings are abnormal or reveal a pituitary adenoma, the patient should be treated with oral bromocriptine, starting at a dosage of 2.5 to 5 mg daily, or oral cabergoline, 0.25 mg twice weekly. These medications should be titrated until prolactin levels return to normal. When prolactin levels are normalized, restoration of ovulatory function should occur.[26] Pa-

tients with symptomatic macroadenomas may require ablative therapy with either surgery or radiation if medical therapy does not reduce the size of the tumor or if symptoms associated with the tumor persist or worsen.

Patients with hyperprolactinemia and oligomenorrhea (except those with primary and secondary hypothyroidism, who require thyroid hormone replacement) should be treated with bromocriptine only if they are bothered by symptoms (i.e., galactorrhea) or desire fertility. If a patient remains anovulatory despite treatment with bromocriptine, oral clomiphene citrate, starting at a dosage of 50 mg daily for 5 days, can be added as an adjunctive therapy to stimulate ovulation.

If the initial evaluation shows that the patient is hypoestrogenic (i.e., she has an atrophic vagina and perineum and reports hot flashes and lack of lubrication during sexual activity), the physician should obtain serum levels of FSH, LH, and estradiol (E_2). These values will identify patients with hypogonadotropic hypogonadism and those with ovarian failure. Patients with hypogonadotropic hypogonadism should be evaluated with a GnRH stimulation test to determine whether the problem is reversible.

Special attention should be given to anovulatory women who have normal levels of estrogen and prolactin and who have signs of hyperandrogenism and virilization. In these patients, measurements should be made of dehydroepiandrosterone sulfate (DHEAS), total testosterone, 17-hydroxyprogesterone, and 8 A.M. free urine cortisol levels. These tests will help to identify patients with polycystic ovary syndrome (PCOS), ovarian and adrenal neoplasms, congenital adrenal hyperplasia, or Cushing syndrome [see Chapter 79].

Patients with PCOS that is associated with elevated insulin or glucose levels who wish to conceive may benefit from a combined regimen of oral metformin, 850 mg twice daily, and clomiphene citrate. Women treated with this combination have a higher rate of ovulation than those treated with clomiphene citrate alone.[27] Hirsutism and acne should not be treated medically during ovulatory induction cycles.

Elevated levels of both FSH and E_2 on cycle day 3 signify a decrease in ovarian reserve (i.e., a decrease in the total number of follicles present for maturation and ovulation). The diagnosis of premature ovarian failure is reserved for women who are younger than 40 years and have gonadotropin (FSH and LH) levels in the menopausal range.

Depending on the incipient age of ovarian failure, a complete autoimmune profile and possibly a genetic karyotype should be considered to establish a diagnosis.[28] Women with an autoimmune disorder are at increased risk for developing multiple organ failure and should be screened annually. These

Table 3 Semen Analysis Parameters[14]

Parameter	Normal Value
Volume of semen	≥ 2.0 ml
pH	7.2–8.0
Sperm concentration	$\geq 20 \times 10^6$ spermatozoa/ml
Total sperm count	$\geq 40 \times 10^6$ spermatozoa/ejaculate
Motility	$\geq 50\%$ with forward progression
	$\geq 25\%$ with rapid progression
Morphology	$\geq 30\%$ with normal forms
Vitality	$\geq 75\%$ or more living
White blood cell count	$\leq 1 \times 10^6$/ml

Table 4 In Vitro Fertilization

Step 1 Stimulation of ovulation with injectable gonadotropins.
Monitoring of follicular development with vaginal ultrasound.
When mean follicle diameter is ≥ 15 mm, ovulation is triggered with hCG administered intramuscularly.

Step 2 Collection of eggs 34 to 36 hours after hCG injection.

Step 3 Collection of sperm on day of ovum capture or obtain frozen sample.

Step 4 Laboratory (in vitro) incubation of egg(s) with sperm for fertilization and embryo growth.
If sperm are of poor quality, fertilization is facilitated by microinjection (ICSI) of sperm into egg.

Step 5 Transfer of embryo to uterus 3 to 5 days after oocyte aspiration.
Administration of progesterone in oil, 50 to 100 mg/day I.M., or vaginal progesterone suppositories.

Step 6 14-day wait for pregnancy or menstruation.
Measure β-hCG.

hCG—human chorionic gonadotropin   ICSI—intracytoplasmic sperm injection

women should be counseled to consider IVF with donor eggs, or adoption.

UNEXPLAINED INFERTILITY

The incidence of unexplained infertility is estimated to be between 15% and 20%. Couples who do not receive treatment have a monthly fecundity of 3% and a cumulative 3-year pregnancy rate of 60%. However, when a couple has experienced long-standing infertility (> 3 years) and the female partner is older than 35 years, the probability of achieving a pregnancy is markedly reduced.[29]

The treatment for couples with unexplained infertility includes inducement of superovulation with either clomiphene citrate or gonadotropins[30,31] and IUI or one of the assisted reproductive technologies (e.g., IVF, gamete intrafallopian transfer [GIFT], and zygote intrafallopian transfer [ZIFT]).[32] IUI with ovulation induction using gonadotropins produces higher pregnancy rates for couples with male-factor or unexplained infertility than does either procedure performed alone.[22]

Ovulation Induction

To induce ovulation in a woman who has been determined to be anovulatory, clomiphene citrate, 50 mg orally daily, is begun on cycle day 3 to 5 and is continued for a total of 5 days [see Figure 5]. The couple and the physician must decide whether to add IUI to the ovulation induction regimen or have the couple perform timed sexual intercourse.

The couple and physician must also decide whether to monitor follicular development and timing for intercourse or IUI and, if so, whether to use a low-, moderate-, or high-technology method for monitoring. Low-technology monitoring entails charting the BBT. A moderate level of monitoring by the patient can be achieved with an LH kit. The kit enables urinary detection of the LH surge, which usually occurs about 7 days after the last dose of clomiphene citrate. High-technology monitoring entails serial vaginal sonography, with administration of human chorionic gonadotropin (hCG) to trigger ovulation when appropriate; hCG is given in a dose of 10,000 units intramuscularly when the follicle diameter is at least 20 mm.

If the clinician is not monitoring follicular development, the couple is directed to perform timed intercourse every other day, starting on cycle days 12 to 18. Timed intercourse or IUI should begin 24 hours after urinary detection of the LH surge or 36 hours after the administration of hCG. One study has shown that in couples with anovulatory, male, or unexplained infertility, clinical pregnancy rates with IUI and clomiphene citrate did not depend on the method used to establish the timing for IUI.[33] Thus, if cost is a consideration for the couple, urinary LH testing may lower the expense by reducing the number of patient visits and eliminating the midcycle ultrasound study.

If menses does not begin 14 days after timed intercourse or IUI, the hCG level should be checked to determine whether the patient is pregnant. If the patient is not pregnant but did ovulate, as evidenced by an elevation in the progesterone level on day 21 or a biphasic BBT chart, she should undergo another stimulation cycle with the same dosage of clomiphene citrate. This method can be repeated for as long as 6 months. If pregnancy is not achieved by that time, the use of injectable gonadotropins to stimulate ovulation should be considered.

It is important for the clinician to realize that the incidence of multiple gestations (e.g., twins) is nearly 8% in patients taking clomiphene citrate and as high as 35% in patients who use injectable gonadotropins.[22] Therefore, extreme caution and judgment should be exercised with these medications.

For patients who do not ovulate with the initial 50 mg/day dosage of clomiphene citrate (as determined on the basis of a low day-21 progesterone level or a monophasic BBT chart), the dose can be increased to 100 mg or 150 mg daily. If ovulation still does not occur with the higher dosage, ovulation induction with gonadotropins should be employed.[34]

Gonadotropin injections can be given independently of, or in combination with, clomiphene citrate. The addition of gonadotropin injections to clomiphene treatment typically allows the use of lower doses of gonadotropins (an expensive medication) needed to induce ovulation during each cycle.

The gonadotropins currently available for ovulation induction include FSH produced by recombinant DNA technology and immunopurification, and LH in combination with FSH derived from menopausal urine. The recombinant FSH preparations can be given as subcutaneous injections. For combination therapy, FSH injections are generally started after clomiphene citrate has been given for 5 days. Gonadotropins are typically given for 7 to 10 days, with doses adjusted according to follicular growth and E_2 levels.

During gonadotropin induction of ovulation, as many as 20% of patients experience mild to moderate enlargement of the ovaries. A small percentage—perhaps 2%[35]—of women treated with gonadotropins experience increased vascular permeability and the accumulation of fluid in the peritoneal cavity and pleural space, a condition termed ovarian hyperstimulation syndrome (OHSS). Clinical manifestations of OHSS include abdominal pain, abdominal distention, nausea, vomiting, diarrhea, and dyspnea. Other physical and laboratory findings of OHSS include weight gain, ovarian enlargement, ascites, pleural effusion, hemoconcentration, electrolyte imbalances, renal dysfunction, and thrombosis. Treatment includes bed rest, antiemetics, maintenance of intravascular volume, and prophylaxis against thrombosis. Patients with severe OHSS may require hospitalization, paracentesis, and thoracentesis. In rare instances, ovarian torsion may occur and require surgical correction. OHSS may be more severe and have a

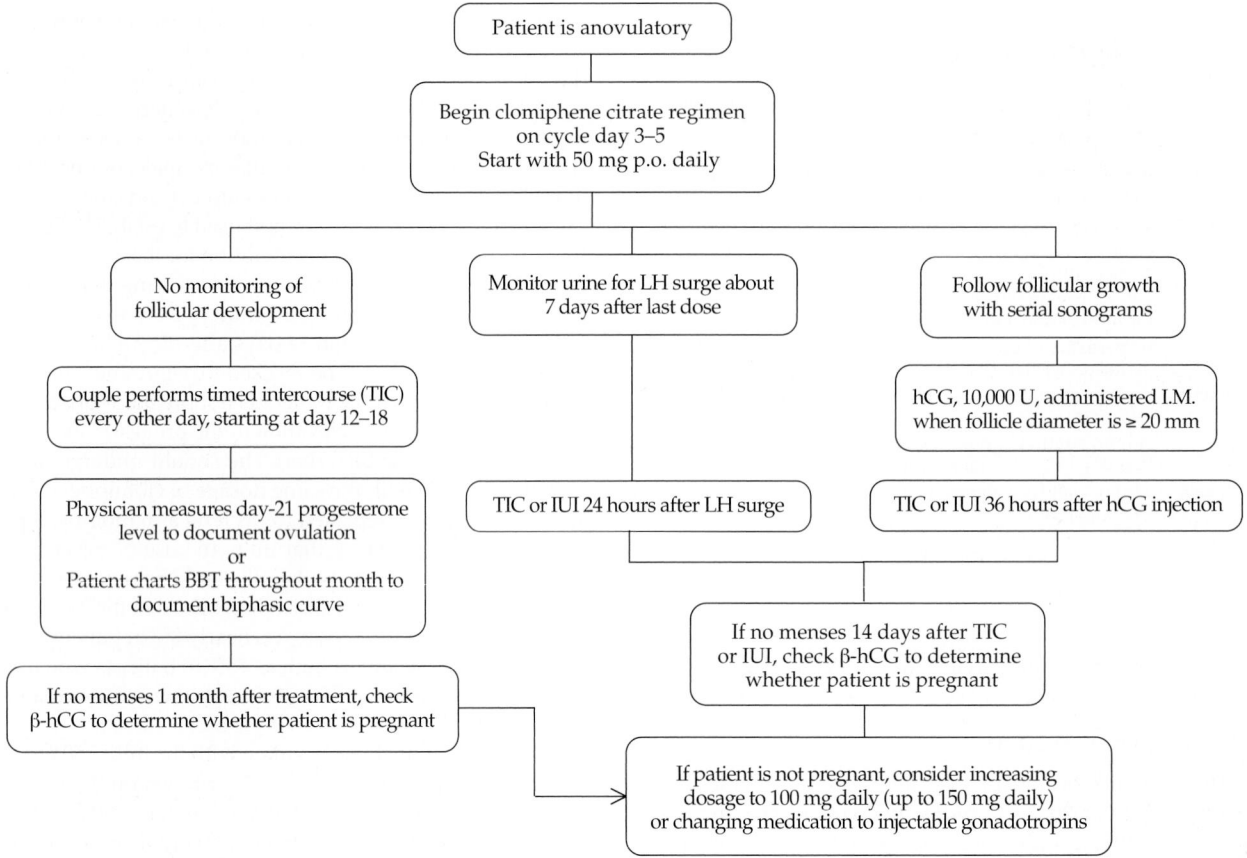

Figure 5 **Ovulation induction with clomiphene citrate. (BBT—basal body temperature; hCG—human chorionic gonadotropin; IUI—intrauterine insemination; TIC—timed intercourse)**

longer course if pregnancy occurs, particularly with multiple gestations.

Advances in Technology

Many advances in infertility therapy have been made in recent years. These include preimplantation genetic diagnosis, in vitro maturation of oocytes, and fertility preservation after treatment for malignancies.

Preimplantation genetic diagnosis (PGD) was developed to test for specific single-gene mutations before implantation of embryos resulting from IVF. This technique is accomplished by removing one to two blastomeres from a 6- to 10-cell embryo and subjecting these cells to either polymerase chain reaction amplification to test for specific mutations or FISH to test for chromosomal abnormalities. Concerns regarding this technology include the possibility of destroying preimplantation embryos or misdiagnosis.[36] In a case-control study, use of PGD was associated with a lower rate of subsequent miscarriage and the possibility of higher pregnancy rates.[37] However, a review has concluded that there are as yet insufficient data to determine whether PGD is an effective intervention in IVF/ICSI for improving live birth rates.[38]

In vitro maturation of oocytes is accomplished by collecting immature oocytes before stimulation and subsequently coculturing them with gonadotropic hormones. These oocytes then develop into mature oocytes. In vitro maturation treatment has been suggested as an alternative to in vivo stimulation of oocytes in infertile women with polycystic ovaries, because it may avoid the risk of OHSS.[39]

With advances in the detection and treatment of cancer, many patients who would once likely have succumbed to their disease are achieving complete remission. Improvements in prognosis place greater importance on the preservation of fertility in patients of reproductive age who are to undergo chemotherapy or radiation. Through sperm cryopreservation, many men who would otherwise be unable to reproduce after therapy are able to do so. Women have had few comparable options; however, studies suggest that the use of GnRH agonists may reduce irreversible ovarian damage from chemotherapy.[40] Other modalities that remain experimental are oocyte cryopreservation and ovarian tissue cryopreservation.

Role of the Generalist

The role of the generalist in the management of the infertile couple cannot be overstated. Although infertility remains a major medical problem, many couples are reluctant to discuss their concerns about infertility. Primary care physicians can open a dialogue on this topic by asking patients about their fertility desires. Such discussion is especially important with patients who have delayed childbearing until later years, particularly those who are older than 35 years. Referral for those patients may be indicated even if conception has been attempted for less than a year. Patients of reproductive age who are diagnosed with malignancies should be queried regarding their desire for future fertility, and appropriate referrals should be made promptly.

When a couple is experiencing difficulty conceiving, the primary care provider should investigate the common causes of infertility and perform a thorough medical and gynecologic history, as well as complete physical examination. A semen analysis is warranted as well. Empirical therapy should not be prolonged if conception is not achieved. Patients in whom abnormalities are found on diagnostic testing and patients older than 35 years who do not conceive promptly should be referred to a fertility specialist.

A primary care provider who gives attention to the reproductive desires of patients, makes a prompt diagnosis of infertility, and engages in open dialogue with the relevant subspecialists can help many patients attain their dreams of a successful live birth.

The authors have no commercial relationships with manufacturers of products or providers of services discussed in this chapter.

References

1. Guttmacher AF: Factors affecting normal expectancy of conception. JAMA 161:855, 1956

2. Chandra A, Mosher WD: The demography of infertility and the use of medical care for infertility. Study Design and Statistics for Infertility Research 64:781, 1994

3. Stephen EH, Chandra A: Use of infertility services in the United States: 1995. Fam Plann Perspect 32:132, 2000

4. Schover LR, Thomas AJ, Falcone T: Attitudes about genetic risk of couples undergoing in-vitro fertilization. Hum Reprod 13:862, 1998

5. Van Voorhis BJ, Stovall DW, Allen BD, et al: Cost-effective treatment of the infertile couple. Fertil Steril 70:995, 1998

6. Kainz K: The role of the psychologist in the evaluation and treatment of infertility. Womens Health Issues 11:481, 2001

7. Rich-Edwards JW, Spiegelman D, Garland M, et al: Physical activity, body mass index, and ovulatory disorder infertility. Epidemiology 13:184, 2002

8. Hull MG, North K, Taylor H, et al: Delayed conception and active and passive smoking. The Avon Longitudinal Study of Pregnancy and Childhood Study Team. Fertil Steril 74:725, 2000

9. Mendonca LL, Khamashta MA, Nelson-Piercy C, et al: Non-steroidal anti-inflammatory drugs as a possible cause for reversible infertility. Rheumatology (Oxford) 39:880, 2000

10. van Kooij RJ, Looman CW, Habbema JD, et al: Age-dependent decrease in embryo implantation rate after in vitro fertilization. Fertil Steril 66:769, 1996

11. Collins JA, Crosignani PG: Unexplained infertility: a review of diagnosis, prognosis, treatment efficacy and management. Int J Gynaecol Obstet 39:267, 1992

12. Menken J, Trussel J, Larsen U: Age and infertility. Science 233:1389, 1986

13. De Kretser DM, Baker HW: Infertility in men: recent advances and continuing controversies. J Clin Endocrinol Metab 84:3443, 1999

14. World Health Organization: WHO Laboratory Manual for the Examination of Human Semen and Semen-Cervical Mucus Interaction, 4th ed. Cambridge University Press, New York, 1999

15. Sharara FI, Illions EH, Coddington CC 3rd, et al: Evaluation of the Tru-Trax cervical mucus penetration test in predicting fertilization and pregnancy rates in in-vitro fertilization. Hum Reprod 10:1481, 1995

16. Oehninger S, Mahony M, Ozgur K, et al: Clinical significance of human sperm–zona pellucida binding. Fertil Steril 67:1121, 1997

17. Carrell DT: Semen analysis at the turn of the century: an evaluation of potential uses of new sperm function assays. Arch Androl 44:65, 2000

18. Hlinka D, Herman M, Vesela J, et al: A modified method of intracytoplasmic sperm injection without the use of polyvinylpyrrolidone. Hum Reprod 13:1922, 1998

19. Penzias AS, Decherney AH: Is there ever a role for tubal surgery? Am J Obstet Gynecol 174:1218, 1996

20. Murray DL, Sagoskin AW, Widra EA, et al: The adverse effect of hydrosalpinges on in vitro fertilization pregnancy rates and the benefit of surgical correction. Fertil Steril 69:41, 1998

21. Oei SG, Helmerhorst FM, Bloemenkamp KW, et al: Effectiveness of the postcoital test: randomised controlled trial. BMJ 317:502, 1998

22. Guzick DS, Carson SA, Coutifaris C, et al: Efficacy of superovulation and intrauterine insemination in the treatment of infertility. National Cooperative Reproductive Medicine Network. N Engl J Med 340:177, 1999

23. Keck C, Gerber-Schafer C, Wilhelm C, et al: Intrauterine insemination for treatment of male infertility. Int J Androl 20(suppl 3):55, 1997

24. Cunnah D, Besser M: Management of prolactinomas. Clin Endocrinol 34:231, 1991

25. Colao A, Annunziato L, Lombardi G: Treatment of prolactinomas. Ann Med 30:452, 1998

26. Shimon I, Melmed S: Management of pituitary tumors. Ann Intern Med 129:472, 1998

27. Nestler JE, Jakubowicz DJ, Evans WS, et al: Effects of metformin on spontaneous and clomiphene-induced ovulation in the polycystic ovary syndrome. N Engl J Med 338:1876, 1998

28. Conway GS, Kaltsas G, Patel A, et al: Characterization of idiopathic premature ovarian failure. Fertil Steril 65:337, 1996

29. Guzick DS, Sullivan MW, Adamson GD, et al: Efficacy of treatment for unexplained infertility. Fertil Steril 70:207, 1998

30. Kousta E, White DM, Franks S: Modern use of clomiphene citrate in induction of ovulation. Hum Reprod Update 3:359, 1997

31. Rust LA, Israel R, Mishell DR Jr: An individualized graduated therapeutic regimen of clomiphene citrate. Am J Obstet Gynecol 120:785, 1974

32. Dodson WC, Haney AF: Controlled ovarian hyperstimulation and intrauterine insemination for treatment of infertility. Fertil Steril 55:457, 1991

33. Deaton JL, Clark RR, Pittaway DE: Clomiphene citrate ovulation induction in combination with a timed intrauterine insemination: the value of urinary luteinizing hormone versus human chorionic gonadotropin timing. Fertil Steril 68:43, 1997

34. ACOG Practice Bulletin: Clinical management guidelines for obstetrician-gynecologists number 34, February 2002. Management of infertility caused by ovulatory dysfunction. American College of Obstetricians and Gynecologists. ACOG Committee on Practice Bulletins–Gynecology. Obstet Gynecol 99:347, 2002

35. Papanikolaou EG, Pozzobon C, Kolibianakis EM, et al: Incidence and prediction of ovarian hyperstimulation syndrome in women undergoing gonadotropin-releasing hormone antagonist in vitro fertilization cycles. Fertil Steril 85:112, 2006

36. Schuppe HC, Schroeder-Printzen I, Lang U, et al: Frontiers in reproductive medicine. Proceedings of the 8th Andrology Symposium/1st Symposium of the Hessian Centre for Reproductive Medicine. Giessen, Germany, November 16, 2002

37. Munne S, Magli C, Cohen J, et al: Positive outcome after preimplantation diagnosis of aneuploidy in human embryos. Hum Reprod 14:2191, 1999

38. Twisk M, Mastenbroek S, van Wely M, et al: Preimplantation genetic screening for abnormal number of chromosomes (aneuploidies) in in vitro fertilisation or intracytoplasmic sperm injection. Cochrane Database Syst Rev 1:CD005291, 2006

39. Chian RC: In-vitro maturation of immature oocytes for infertile women with PCOS. Reprod Biomed Online 8:547, 2004

40. Blumenfeld Z, Dann E, Avivi I, et al: Fertility after treatment for Hodgkin's disease. Ann Oncol 13:138, 2002

83 Ectopic Pregnancy and Spontaneous Abortion

Alan H. DeCherney, M.D.

Ectopic Pregnancy

Ectopic pregnancy is the implantation of an embryo outside the endometrial cavity (i.e., lining of the uterus). The embryo may be implanted in the fallopian tubes, ovaries, abdomen, or cervix. More than 95% of ectopic pregnancies occur in the fallopian tubes, with nearly 80% of ectopic pregnancies occurring in the ampullary portion of the fallopian tube.

Ectopic pregnancies comprise approximately 2% of all reported pregnancies in the United States. If left untreated, ectopic pregnancy can result in rupture of the fallopian tube, which can lead to hemorrhagic shock and death. For that reason, ectopic pregnancy is a major cause of morbidity and mortality in women of reproductive age. It is the third leading cause of maternal mortality and is responsible for nearly 9% of all pregnancy-related deaths.[1] Between 1970 and 1992, the incidence of ectopic pregnancy increased sixfold, which is consistent with the increased prevalence of important risk factors for ectopic pregnancy (see below).[2]

Improvements in diagnostic skills have enabled physicians to treat ectopic pregnancies at an earlier gestational age and by more conservative approaches. Therefore, it is imperative that the primary care physician be able to diagnose and intervene as early as possible to reduce the incidence of irreversible tubal damage and the risk of future infertility [*see Figure 1*].[3]

DIAGNOSIS

Clinical Manifestations

The principal diagnostic task in ectopic pregnancy is distinguishing it from intrauterine pregnancy or threatened abortion. The symptoms of an ectopic pregnancy [*see Table 1*] vary with its location and the rate of its growth. Nearly all women with ectopic pregnancies complain of a colicky abdominal pain that is vague in location. As the pregnancy grows, capillaries are broken and blood spills into the abdominal cavity. The blood that fills the intraperitoneal cavity causes irritation of the left hemidiaphragm, resulting in left shoulder pain; the liver occupies the space directly under the right hemidiaphragm and prevents the blood from reaching the right hemidiaphragm. Almost one quarter of the patients with ruptured ectopic pregnancies have left shoulder pain.

Amenorrhea, the second most common symptom, occurs in more than 75% of patients. The duration of amenorrhea depends on the site of implantation and usually lasts 6 to 8 weeks before the onset of other symptoms.

Vaginal bleeding is also common and may occur a few days to weeks before the patient's initial visit. The pattern of bleeding is most often described as spotting and usually is preceded by the onset and worsening of abdominal pain.

Other symptoms, which occur less frequently, are dizziness, fainting, nausea, vomiting, other signs of pregnancy, the urge to defecate, and passage of tissue through the vagina.

History and Physical Examination

At the initial visit, the patient's medical history should be taken. Patients in whom ectopic pregnancy is suspected often have a history of infertility, pelvic inflammatory disease, endometriosis, or tubal damage [*see Table 2*]. In rare cases, ectopic pregnancy can occur in patients who have undergone tubal sterilization, even many years after the procedure.[4] If the diagnosis of ectopic pregnancy is suspected, a pregnancy test should be performed (e.g., measurement of the human chorionic gonadotropin [hCG] level in urine). The urine hCG test is extremely sensitive; false negative results are very rare.

Patients who have a negative urine hCG test result should be evaluated for other gynecologic problems, including ovarian torsion, a ruptured ovarian cyst, and pelvic inflammatory disease. Gastrointestinal disorders and possible surgical conditions (e.g., appendicitis) should also be investigated.

If the urine hCG test result is positive, a physical examination should be performed and a pelvic sonogram obtained.[5] The physician should assess the degree of abdominal and pelvic pain experienced by the patient and try to elicit signs of peritonitis, which could indicate rupture of an ectopic pregnancy.

Inspection of the patient's cervix with a speculum can help distinguish ectopic pregnancy from spontaneous or threatened abortion. If the cervical os is open, fetal tissue should be observed at the internal cervical os; the diagnosis of an inevitable abortion or incomplete abortion should be made, and a dilatation and curettage (D&C) should be performed. If the cervical os is closed, the examiner should determine both the amount of blood present in the vagina and the amount emanating from the external cervical os. Most women with ectopic pregnancies do not experience heavy vaginal bleeding and have only a light bloody vaginal discharge. In the case of threatened or complete abortion, the patient should be instructed to have pelvic rest and bed rest until the symptoms resolve.

Laboratory Testing

A pelvic sonogram should be obtained to document whether an intrauterine pregnancy (IUP) or extrauterine pregnancy (EUP) exists. The sonographer should focus attention on the uterus, the adnexa, and the cul-de-sac. The endometrium should be inspected, and the presence of a gestational sac and fetal pole should be verified. Attempts should be made to observe the fetal heartbeat to help distinguish normal from abnormal pregnancies. If nothing is present in the uterus, the adnexa should be inspected. If a gestational sac and fetal pole are identified outside the uterus, the diagnosis of an EUP should be made. The ectopic pregnancy can then be treated by medical or surgical means [*see Treatment, below*].

If no IUP or EUP can be documented on sonography, further laboratory evaluation should be pursued. The evaluation should include measurement of the serum β-hCG level, a complete blood count (CBC), and measurement of the prothrombin time (PT) or partial thromboplastin time (PTT). A progesterone assay is optional (see below). A β-hCG value of 1,500 mIU/ml occurs

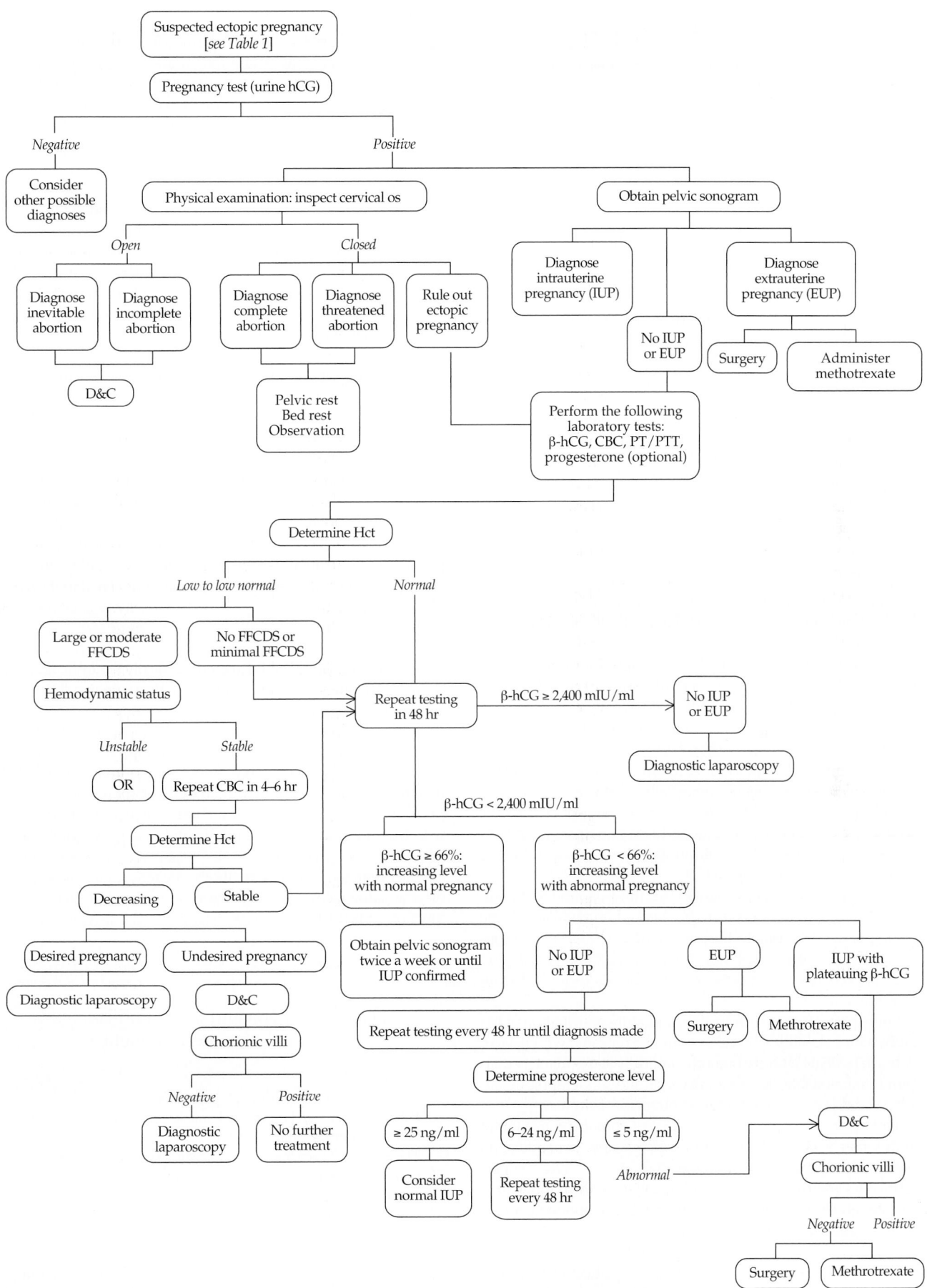

Figure 1 **Management of ectopic pregnancy. (CBC—complete blood count; D&C—dilatation and curettage;**
EUP—extrauterine pregnancy; FFCDS—free fluid in the cul-de-sac; hCG—human chorionic gonadotropin;
Hct—hematocrit; IUP—intrauterine pregnancy; PT—prothrombin time; PTT—partial thromboplastin time)

Table 1   Signs and Symptoms of
Ectopic Pregnancy

Abdominal pain
Amenorrhea
Vaginal bleeding
Dizziness and fainting
Other symptoms of pregnancy

Table 2   Patient History Consistent with
Suspected Ectopic Pregnancy

Prior ectopic pregnancy
History of infertility
Past infection with *Chlamydia* or *Neisseria gonorrhoeae* or history of
  pelvic inflammatory disease
Past or present use of an intrauterine device (IUD)
Current pregnancy conceived with in vitro fertilization (IVF)
History of endometriosis
Current pregnancy conceived while taking oral contraceptives

---

around the time a normal IUP first becomes visible on pelvic sonography. If no IUP is observed and the β-hCG value is 2,400 mIU/ml or higher, an ectopic pregnancy should be suspected.

A baseline hematocrit, along with sonographic evaluation of the patient's cul-de-sac, will provide insight for prognosis and possible treatment options. Free fluid in the cul-de-sac may be blood; this finding increases the likelihood of ectopic pregnancy.[6] Patients with aborting ectopic and early nonruptured ectopic pregnancies may present with blood in the cul-de-sac. If the patient has a normal hematocrit and minimal to no free fluid in the cul-de-sac, repeating pelvic sonography and measurements of the β-hCG level and a CBC in 48 hours is recommended. Patients with low to low-normal hematocrits in conjunction with mild to moderate amounts of free fluid in the cul de sac need further evaluation, including a repeat CBC.

If a moderate to large amount of free fluid is found in the cul-de-sac, blood pressure needs to be checked immediately. If the blood pressure is unstable, the patient should be taken to the operating room for an exploratory laparotomy and transfusion with packed red blood cells and crystalloids to replenish intravascular losses.

Some patients require hospitalization for confirmation of hemodynamic stability. The CBC should be repeated within 4 to 6 hours in patients who are hemodynamically stable. If the hematocrit remains stable, the laboratory tests and sonographic evaluation should be repeated within 48 hours (see below).

Patients with decreasing hematocrits should be evaluated with either a D&C or diagnostic laparoscopy, depending on their desire to maintain the pregnancy. When a D&C is performed for removal of fetal tissue, histology of the removed tissue should show chorionic villi. If no villi are obtained, an ectopic pregnancy should be suspected.

Repeat hCG levels   The doubling time of the β-hCG level in early pregnancies ranges from 48 to 72 hours. A rise in the β-hCG level of at least 66% in 2 days is generally indicative of a

normal IUP. Patients who have normal doubling values of their β-hCG level on repeat evaluation should be followed up in 1 week with a repeat sonogram to confirm a pregnancy in utero.[7]

An abnormally rising β-hCG level (< 66% higher than original values) should be further investigated. Correlation with a repeat sonogram and hematocrit will help guide the clinician to the correct diagnosis and treatment. Although the presence of an ectopic pregnancy should be suspected, an abnormally developing IUP cannot be ruled out. Treatment should be decided not on the basis of only two β-hCG values but, rather, on the entire clinical picture. An abnormally rising β-hCG level that is not substantiated by other laboratory or radiographic evidence should not be treated as an ectopic pregnancy. Surgical or medical treatment of these patients should be considered only when the diagnosis is confirmed and an EUP is documented.

Serum progesterone level   Progesterone values can help the clinician determine the viability of a pregnancy, but only in rare instances can they reveal an ectopic pregnancy.[8] A progesterone level of greater than 25 ng/ml is associated with a normal IUP in nearly 97% of cases. Values of less than 5 ng/ml are associated with abnormal pregnancies, and values between 5 and 25 ng/ml are indeterminate. The usefulness of the progesterone assay is limited because more than 85% of the values obtained are between 5 and 25 ng/ml. Furthermore, most centers are unable to process this test in a timely fashion, with results being unavailable for review and interpretation on the same day that the sample is drawn.

TREATMENT

Ectopic pregnancy can be treated medically or surgically. The choice of treatment should be tailored to the patient's clinical circumstances and preferences.[9,10]

Medical Therapy

Methotrexate should be considered as the primary modality of treatment in all patients who meet the criteria for medical therapy [*see Table 3*].[11,12] Methotrexate is an antimetabolite that interferes with the conversion of dihydrofolic acid to tetrahydrofolic acid, inhibiting DNA synthesis and cell division and thereby terminating the pregnancy. Because methotrexate may, in rare cases, produce hepatotoxicity or bone marrow suppression, baseline liver function tests (LFTs) and a CBC, along with a β-hCG level, must

---

Table 3   Criteria and Contraindications
for Methotrexate Treatment

Criteria
Patient is diagnosed with ectopic pregnancy
Patient is reliable and expected to comply with regimen
Patient is hemodynamically stable
The ectopic pregnancy is no greater than 3.5 to 4 cm in diameter
Contraindications
Absolute
    Hepatic dysfunction
    Moderate to severe anemia
Relative
    Human chorionic gonadotropin concentration ≥ 10,000 mIU/ml
    Fetal cardiac activity detected with sonography

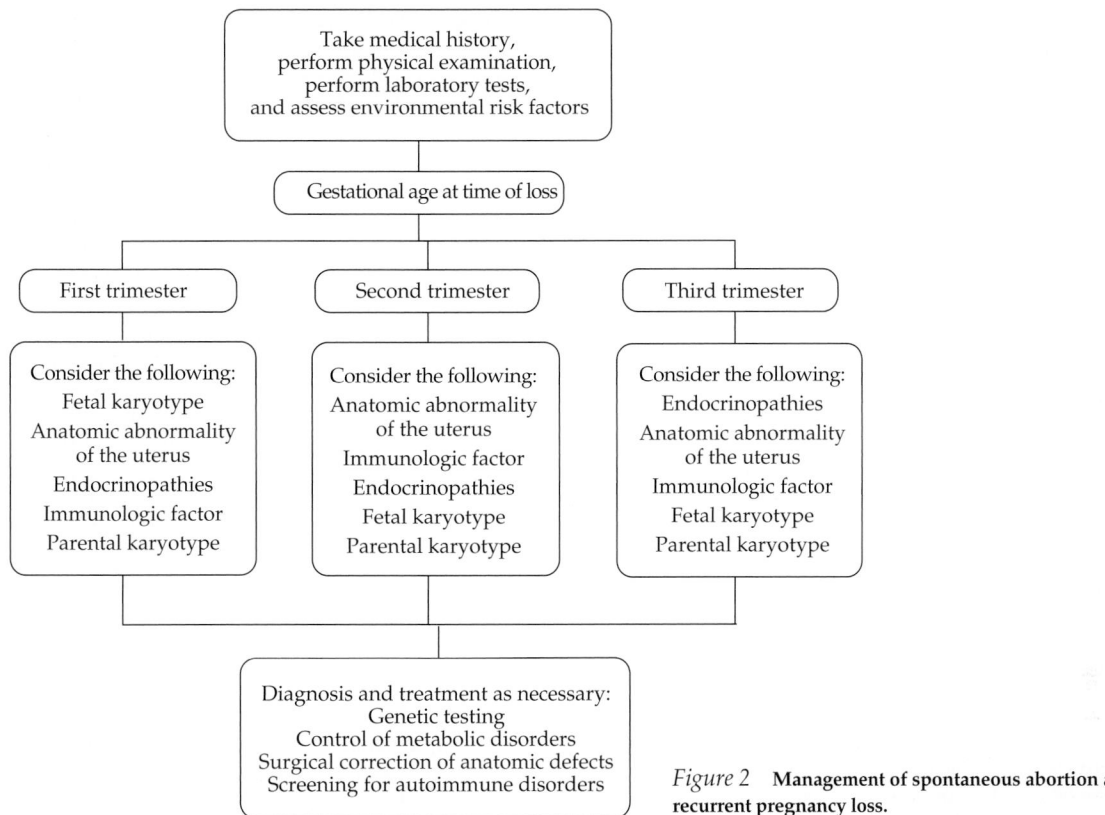

Figure 2   **Management of spontaneous abortion and recurrent pregnancy loss.**

be done in all patients being considered for methotrexate therapy. LFTs and CBCs must be monitored during treatment with repeated doses of methotrexate, and methotrexate should be discontinued if test results become abnormal.

Methotrexate therapy can be given by local injection into the area of the ectopic pregnancy, which requires ultrasound or laparoscopic guidance, or by intramuscular injection as a single-dose or multiple-dose regimen. The multiple-dose regimen is rarely used today, unless the patient fails to respond to the single-dose regimen. The multiple-dose regimen includes citrovorum rescue to protect maternal cells. In the single-dose regimen, 50 mg/m² of methotrexate is given and baseline studies are repeated on day 3 or 4. If the β-hCG level decreases by less than 15%, the treatment can be repeated in 1 week. Of the patients who receive methotrexate, 64% are cured with a single dose.[13] An additional 14% require two or three doses. This gives an overall cure rate of 78%. Patients who are cured with methotrexate have fertility rates equivalent to those of patients who are treated surgically. Unfortunately, 20% of the patients whose ectopic pregnancy is treated pharmacologically will ultimately require surgical intervention.

Surgical Therapy

Surgical modalities for ectopic pregnancy include laparoscopy and laparotomy [see Figure 1]. Laparoscopy with conservative tubal therapy (salpingostomy or salpingotomy) is the preferred surgical method in hemodynamically stable patients, for the following reasons: (1) Less intraoperative blood loss occurs, (2) less postoperative analgesia is required, (3) the hospital stay is shorter, and (4) the cost savings per patient is greater. After laparoscopy, β-hCG levels should be

measured serially until they decrease to nonpregnant levels. If the β-hCG level plateaus, increases, or does not decrease more than 15% in 48 hours, treatment with methotrexate or salpingectomy is required.

In the past, laparotomy and radical tubal surgery (salpingectomy) was recommended for hemodynamically unstable patients. Because of improvements in anesthesia and cardiovascular monitoring, together with advances in laparoscopic surgical skills and experience, operative laparoscopy can now be justified for surgical treatment of ectopic pregnancy even in women with hemodynamic instability.[14] Serial measurement of β-hCG levels is not required after salpingectomy.

Fertility after surgery is not a function of the surgical method employed. Rather, future fertility in these cases depends on three patient factors. The first is a history of infertility; patients with prior infertility have a fourfold lower pregnancy rate than patients without. The second is the status of the contralateral fallopian tube. The third is the extent of adhesions involving the ipsilateral tube.

Spontaneous Abortions

A spontaneous abortion is defined as the spontaneous termination of a pregnancy before 20 weeks' gestation (from the onset of the last menstrual period) or the loss of a pregnancy with a fetal weight of less than 500 g. All pregnancy losses that occur later than 20 weeks' gestational age are termed miscarriages.

Spontaneous abortions occur in about 15% to 20% of all known pregnancies.[15] It has been estimated that more than 50% of all conceptions end in spontaneous abortion. This rate is higher than previous estimates, because spontaneous abortions often

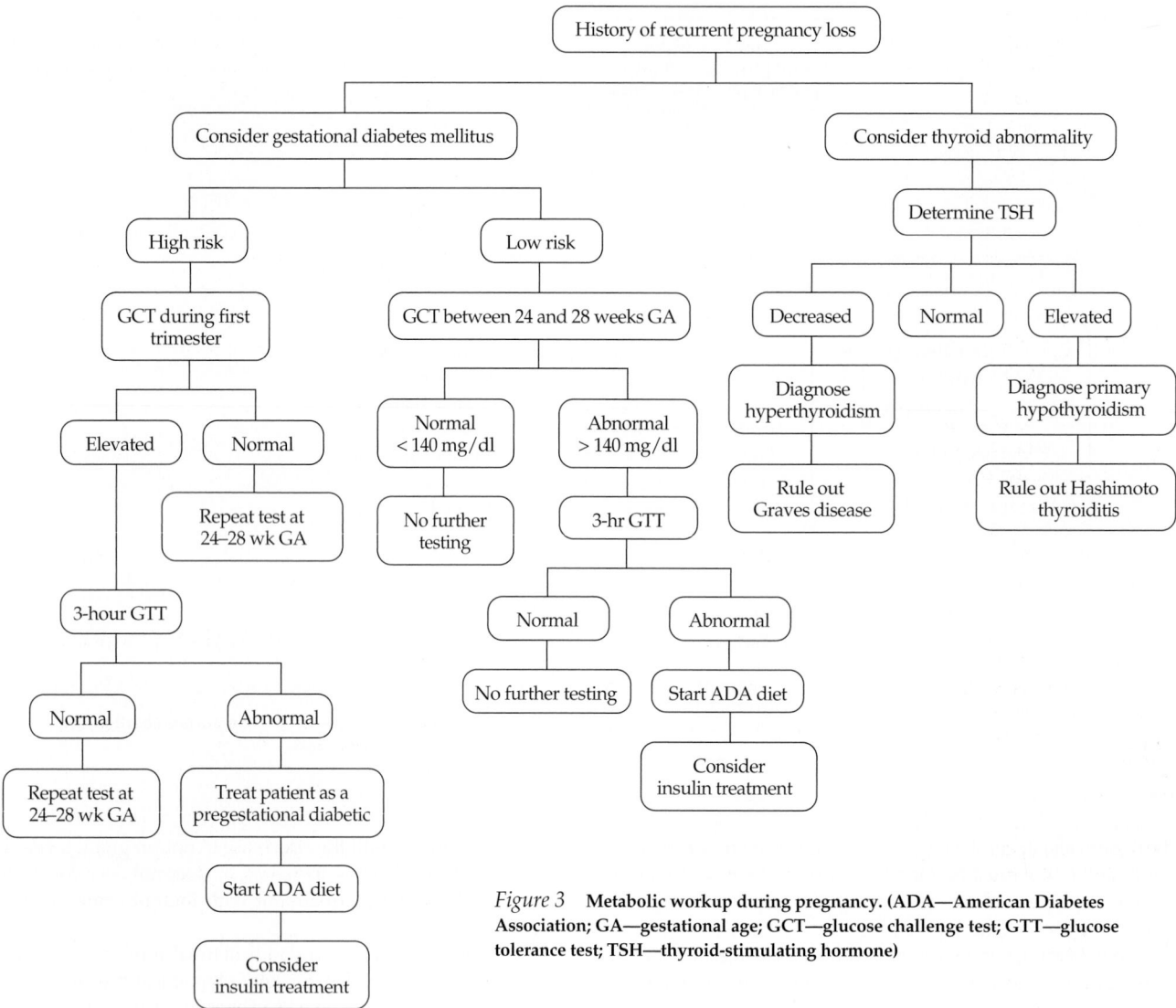

Figure 3 **Metabolic workup during pregnancy. (ADA—American Diabetes Association; GA—gestational age; GCT—glucose challenge test; GTT—glucose tolerance test; TSH—thyroid-stimulating hormone)**

occur around the time of expected menses and are not recognized as abortions.

Traditionally, women who had three or more consecutive pregnancy losses were designated habitual aborters, and it was considered likely that they would continue to have frequent spontaneous abortions. It is now known, however, that in women who have two or more consecutive losses and no history of a live birth, the maximum likelihood that a subsequent pregnancy will result in spontaneous abortion is only about 45%. Women who have at least one live birth before three or more losses have an abortion frequency of less than 30%.[16]

Factors responsible for pregnancy termination vary from one trimester to the next. A strong correlation exists between the gestational age at which the loss occurs and its cause. Therefore, it is important to recognize these potential risks and begin treatment when necessary [*see Figure 2*].

DETERMINING CAUSE OF SPONTANEOUS ABORTION

When a spontaneous abortion has occurred, the physician must investigate the possible causes. A medical history should be taken, possible environmental risk factors should be assessed, and laboratory tests for common infections should be performed.

Depending on whether the abortion occurred during the first, second, or third trimester, the likelihood of genetic, anatomic, or endocrinologic causes varies (see below).

Infections

Organisms that can cause spontaneous abortions include *Ureaplasma, Chlamydia, Listeria,* mycoplasmas, and the TORCH (toxoplasmosis, other [e.g., hepatitis B] rubella, cytomegalovirus, herpes) organisms. Diagnosis is made by cultures of blood or amniotic fluid. Treatments may include antibiotics, γ-globulins, or vaccinations.

Environmental Factors

Cigarette smoking, alcohol consumption, and caffeine consumption can cause spontaneous abortion. The greater the number of cigarettes smoked in a day, the greater the risk of fetal loss. Cleaning solvents and anesthetic gases have been linked to fetal wastage. It is important that pregnant women take precautions and limit their exposure to these agents.

Genetic Factors

Chromosomal abnormalities are responsible for more than 70% of all first-trimester abortions.[17] Aneuploidy problems predominate, with trisomies as a whole constituting the largest group (nearly 50%). Monosomy X (Turner syndrome) is the single most common chromosomal abnormality, accounting for nearly 25% of spontaneous abortions. Maternal nondisjunction during metaphase I is the most common cause of trisomies. It is estimated that only 30% of second-trimester losses and 3% of third-trimester losses are the result of chromosomal defects.

Balanced translocations are the most commonly transmitted parental chromosomal abnormalities responsible for recurrent losses. Thus, genetic testing should be done in couples who have experienced recurrent spontaneous abortion, to determine whether either partner is a carrier. Genetic testing is often done on spontaneously aborted fetuses.

Endocrine Factors

Patients with uncontrolled diabetes mellitus or thyroid disease have an increased risk of fetal demise and spontaneous abortion. Workup for an endocrine disorder should be considered for all patients with recurrent pregnancy losses. Any history or physical examination that is suspect for a metabolic problem should prompt the physician to investigate immediately.

Second- and third-trimester losses are more often the result of a maternal endocrine abnormality. Recognition and control of the metabolic disturbance are the goals of treatment [see Figure 3]. Initial screening begins with a 1-hour glucose challenge test (GCT). This test should be performed in all pregnant women between 24 and 28 weeks' gestational age. A 3-hour glucose tolerance test (GTT) is performed only in women with abnormal GCT values. Evaluation for a thyroid abnormality should be performed at the first prenatal visit. Determining the thyroid-stimulating hormone (TSH) level will distinguish women who have a suspected thyroid dysfunction from those who are euthyroid.[18,19]

Luteal-phase defect is another factor thought to be responsible for early pregnancy loss. Women with this problem characteristically have abnormally shortened secretory phases (< 10 days) or an endometrial lining that is not in phase with the presumed day of the menstrual cycle. An endometrial biopsy that is 2 or more days out of phase with the menstrual cycle is considered diagnostic. Treatment entails the use of progesterone suppositories (25 mg twice daily) to support the luteal phase. However, the benefit of this treatment regimen has not been substantiated.

Anatomic Abnormalities

Uterine cavity malformations are responsible for nearly 15% of recurrent pregnancy losses. Most of these losses occur in the second and third trimesters. Uterine septa are most commonly associated with recurrent abortions. Other causes are submucous myomas, intrauterine adhesions, congenital abnormalities, and cervical incompetence.

A pelvic sonogram and hysterosalpingogram are useful for establishing an initial diagnosis. A magnetic resonance image of the pelvis or a combined laparoscopy and hysteroscopy may be needed for further examination of the uterus. Treatment entails surgical correction of the anatomic defect.

Immunologic Factors

Autoimmune disorders have also been associated with pregnancy losses.[20] These losses commonly occur in the second and third trimesters. Approximately 30% of patients with recurrent pregnancy losses test positive for antinuclear antibodies. Antiphospholipid antibodies, lupus anticoagulants, anticardiolipin antibodies, anti–SS-A (Ro), and anti–SS-B (La) have also been implicated as risk factors. Diagnosis is made by screening the patient for common autoimmune disorders [see Chapter 114].

References

1. Atrash HK, Friede A, Hogue CJ: Ectopic pregnancy mortality in the United States, 1970-1983. Obstet Gynecol 70:817, 1987

2. Ectopic pregnancy—United States, 1990–1992. MMWR Morb Mortal Wkly Rep 44:46, 1995

3. Stovall TG, Ling FW, Carson SA, et al: Nonsurgical diagnosis and treatment of tubal pregnancy. Fertil Steril 54:537, 1990

4. The risk of ectopic pregnancy after tubal sterilization. U.S. Collaborative Review of Sterilization Working Group. N Engl J Med 336:762, 1997

5. Gracia CR, Barnhart KT: Diagnosing ectopic pregnancy: decision analysis comparing six strategies. Obstet Gynecol 97:464, 2001

6. Dart R, McLean R, Dart L: Isolated fluid in the cul-de-sac: how well does it predict ectopic pregnancy? Am J Emerg Med 20:1, 2002

7. Kador N, Romero R: Serial human chorionic gonadotropin measurements in ectopic pregnancy. Am J Obstet Gynecol 158:1239, 1988

8. Stovall TG, Ling FW, Cope BJ, et al: Preventing ruptured ectopic pregnancy with a single serum progesterone. Am J Obstet Gynecol 160:1425, 1989

9. Yao M, Tulandi T: Current status of surgical and nonsurgical management of ectopic pregnancy. Fertil Steril 67:421, 1997

10. Stovall T, Ling FW, Buster JE: Outpatient chemotherapy of unruptured ectopic pregnancy. Fertil Steril 51:435, 1989

11. Stovall TG, Ling FW, Gray LA, et al: Methotrexate treatment of unruptured ectopic pregnancy: a report of 100 cases. Obstet Gynecol 77:749, 1991

12. Carson SA, Buster JE: Ectopic pregnancy. N Engl J Med 329:1174, 1993

13. Stovall TG, Ling FW, Cope BJ, et al: Single-dose methotrexate for treatment of ectopic pregnancy. Obstet Gynecol 77:754, 1991

14. Sagiv R, Debby A, Sadan O, et al: Laparoscopic surgery for extrauterine pregnancy in hemodynamically unstable patients. J Am Assoc Gynecol Laparosc 8:529, 2001

15. Wilcox AJ, Weinberg CR, O'Connor JF, et al: Incidence of early loss of pregnancy. N Engl J Med 319:189, 1988

16. Harger JH, Archer DF, Marchese SG, et al: Etiology of recurrent pregnancy losses and outcome of subsequent pregnancies. Obstet Gynecol 62:574, 1983

17. Byrne J, Warburton D, Kline J, et al: Morphology of early fetal deaths and their chromosomal characteristics. Teratology 32:297, 1985

18. Kjos SL, Buchanan TA: Gestational diabetes mellitus. N Engl J Med 342:896, 2000

19. ACOG Practice Bulletin. Thyroid disease in pregnancy. Obstet Gynecol 98(5 pt 1):879, 2001

20. Coulam CB: Immunologic tests in the evaluation of reproductive disorders: a critical review. Am J Obstet Gynecol 167:1844, 1992

84 Medical Complications in Pregnancy

Ellen W. Seely, M.D., and Jeffrey Ecker, M.D.

Medical complications and intercurrent disease have long presented challenges to obstetricians and other medical providers caring for pregnant women. Contemporary medical practice and treatments have only added to these challenges. Advances in disease management mean that patients with some conditions (e.g., cystic fibrosis) whose life expectancies in the past would have precluded pregnancy are now living to reproductive age. Cures and treatments for other conditions can restore fertility to patients who previously had limited fecundity (e.g., renal transplants in women with renal insufficiency). In vitro fertilization and other assisted reproductive technologies allow the barrier of age, as well as anatomic and genetic barriers, to be surmounted.

All these advances emphasize the need for careful and considered collaboration between clinicians caring for women of reproductive age who are not pregnant and those who care for them during pregnancy. Contraceptive planning and management is vital for patients with significant medical problems, especially those undergoing treatment that is likely to restore fertility (e.g., prescription of metformin for insulin resistance in women with polycystic ovarian syndrome). Primary care clinicians and obstetricians must together evaluate the risk associated with particular diseases in pregnancy and plan for their management, ideally through prepregnancy consultation.

In this chapter, we first review the basic structure and issues for prepregnancy or early pregnancy consultation. We then outline the principles of teratogenesis necessary to evaluate the safety of using medications and other treatments during pregnancy. Next, we discuss the normal physiologic changes of pregnancy. Finally, we discuss specific diseases and conditions that may predate pregnancy or arise as complications of pregnancy and that often require comanagement by obstetricians and medical specialists.

Pregnancy Planning and Counseling

The prognosis for pregnancy complicated by medical conditions is usually improved by pregnancy planning and counseling. In addition, there are a few conditions in which pregnancy may so significantly complicate underlying medical conditions that pregnancy itself is either ill-advised or undertaken only with the greatest of caution. Such conditions include primary pulmonary hypertension and Eisenmenger syndrome (pulmonary hypertension in association with a left-to-right cardiac shunt), each of which carries an approximately 25% to 50% risk of maternal mortality.[1,2] Marfan syndrome with involvement of the aortic root also carries a significant risk of mortality during pregnancy and the puerperium—25% by some estimations.[3] In women with such conditions who have an unplanned pregnancy or who become pregnant in spite of careful contraceptive management, early pregnancy termination should be considered. However, because maternal hormones and physiology change so early in gestation, even early pregnancy interruption does not eliminate all the maternal morbidity and mortality associated with these conditions.

Consultation should also include an evaluation of the risk that a child will inherit the parent's condition. For many disorders, inheritance is defined by mendelian genetics (e.g., autosomal dominant, autosomal recessive, or X-linked disorders). For other conditions that are felt to result from a mix of genetic and environmental exposures (e.g., congenital heart disease), empirical data on inheritance are available. An increasing number of gene defects have been linked to specific disorders, and for many of these, prenatal diagnosis is available. All such diagnoses are facilitated by screening a couple before pregnancy or early in gestation to determine whether genetic testing is informative (i.e., if there is an identifiable mutation or abnormality that can be used in screening DNA from fetal cells). For some couples, family history or ethnic background may indicate the need for screening for specific disorders. The American College of Obstetricians and Gynecologists recommends that white couples with Northern European background be offered screening for cystic fibrosis.[4] Ashkenazi Jews are offered screening for Tay-Sachs disease, Canavan disease, and cystic fibrosis; in addition, Ashkenazi couples may choose screening for an expanded panel of recessive conditions that are more common in this population. Black couples of African background are offered screening to determine whether they are sickle cell carriers. Any fetal testing is facilitated by completing parental screening in advance of pregnancy so that the prospective parents, practitioners, and genetic counselors can anticipate the need for prenatal diagnosis. Such advance planning is essential if couples are considering preimplantation diagnosis, in which embryos created using in vitro fertilization undergo biopsy, their genetic material is studied, and appropriate embryos are transferred for implantation.

Finally, women or couples seeking advice in advance of pregnancy should be counseled about specific dietary or lifestyle changes that may optimize outcome of future pregnancy. Folic acid supplementation of at least 400 µg daily, starting at least 3 months in advance of conception, is recommended to decrease the likelihood of neural tube defects.[5] Planning for a pregnancy may be an impetus to address smoking and the use of alcohol and drugs of abuse. In women with diabetes mellitus (DM), improved glucose control before conception can reduce the risk of birth defects.

Principles of Teratogenesis

Patients and physicians often worry that exposure to medications or environmental agents may increase the risk of birth defects or pregnancy complications. There are, however, few well-designed, prospective studies that address these questions. Such a deficit, while unfortunate, is understandable, because few pregnant women would choose to enroll in prospective, placebo-controlled trials designed simply to examine drug safety. As a result, most of the studies evaluating teratogenesis are retrospective and observational and, therefore, compromised by all the attendant limitations of this approach. In particular, it can be difficult to separate the effect of medications from that of the condition being treated (e.g., determining whether growth restriction in fetuses of women taking beta blockers for hypertension is caused by the hypertension or the beta blocker). Recognizing the inherent difficulty in human studies, some investigators have turned to animal models; with regard to teratogenesis, however, it is clear that mice are not men (or women). Thalidomide, for example, was not recognized as a teratogen in laboratory animals but proved to cause dramatic phocomelia in humans. Conversely, exposure to steroids in early pregnancy has a much stronger association with cleft lips in mice pups than in humans.

There are several other important challenges in determining whether a particular drug or exposure is teratogenic. Potential teratogenic effects may be small (e.g., lithium is associated with Ebstein anomaly in only one in 1,000 exposed pregnancies) or distant from the incident exposure (e.g., clear cell carcinoma in daughters whose mothers used diethylstilbestrol [DES] occurs decades after the mother's use). In addition, many diseases require treatment with multiple medications. As limited as the data are on individual agents, however, information on outcomes associated with combinations of medications and their potential synergistic effects is even more limited.

Given these recognized limitations, several principles can guide counseling regarding medication use or environmental exposure in pregnancy. Because organogenesis begins in early pregnancy, the first trimester is a critical period for teratogenesis. Early exposure is most directly linked with birth defects; however, later exposure may have adverse effects as well. Use of warfarin or ethanol during the second and third trimester, for example, is associated with clear fetal consequences, because brain development continues well into the neonatal period. Good practice, therefore, recommends that throughout pregnancy, physicians should use the fewest number of medications and the lowest doses appropriate to treat the underlying symptoms or conditions.

There are several resources that providers can use to evaluate exposures in anticipation of or during pregnancy. Databases on reproductive risk are available as online references at many hospitals and health care facilities or by subscription (e.g., the Reprorisk system, which is made up of four such databases, is available online [http://www.micromedex.com/products/reprorisk]. The Food and Drug Administration's classification of drugs according to teratogenic potential [see Table 1] and compendia such as the *Physicians' Desk Reference* (PDR) are often used as resources for information on drugs in pregnancy and as guides to patients and providers. Each has important limitations, however. Ratings in the FDA system are often more a reflection of available studies than of evidence of teratogenesis, and the PDR reports all associations between drugs and outcome without rigorously evaluating causality.

The baseline risk of congenital anomalies in the United States is approximately 2% to 3%.[6] To be considered teratogenic, a drug or exposure must be associated with a risk that is higher than threshold, ideally with anomalies clustered in a specific pattern. In fact, only a few drugs are identified teratogens [see Table 2].[7] Family history may also increase the risk that a couple will have a child with birth defects. For example, the risk for congenital heart defects is 0.4% to 0.8% in the general population but rises to 3% to 10% if the mother or father had a heart defect at birth.[8] Other maternal characteristics or behaviors may increase the risk of anomalies; for example, maternal obesity is associated with an increased risk of cardiac and neural tube defects.[9] Finally, environmental exposures, such as exposure to heat or ionizing radiation, especially during the critical first trimester, can increase the risk of miscarriage or birth defects such as spina bifida.[10]

Table 1 The Food and Drug Administration Drug Classification System for Pregnancy

Class A	Controlled studies in women fail to demonstrate a risk to the fetus in the first trimester, and there is no evidence of a risk in later trimesters; the possibility of fetal harm appears remote.
Class B	Either animal-reproduction studies have not demonstrated a fetal risk (and there are no controlled studies in pregnant women) or animal-reproduction studies have shown an adverse effect (other than a decrease in fertility) that was not confirmed in controlled studies in women in the first trimester, and there is no evidence of a risk in later trimesters.
Class C	Either studies in animals have revealed adverse effects on the fetus (teratogenic or embryocidal or other) and there are no controlled studies in women, or studies in women and animals are not available. Drugs should be given only if the potential benefit justifies the potential risk to the fetus.
Class D	There is positive evidence of human fetal risk, but the benefits from use in pregnant women may be acceptable despite the risk (e.g., if the drug is needed in a life-threatening situation or for a serious disease for which safer drugs cannot be used or are ineffective).
Class X	Studies in animals or human beings have demonstrated fetal abnormalities, there is evidence of fetal risk based on human experience, or both, and the risk of the use of the drug in pregnant women clearly outweighs any possible benefit. The drug is contraindicated in women who are or may become pregnant.

Physiologic Changes in Pregnancy

A variety of physiologic adaptations take place over the course of pregnancy. For example, blood volume increases by as much as 50%; red blood cell mass also increases, but to a lesser extent, resulting in a mild dilutional anemia. Cardiac output rises in compensation. The total blood leukocyte count increases to as much as 15,000 cells/ml in the third trimester. The albumin concentration decreases, which tends to increase free levels of protein-bound drugs. The glomerular filtration rate and the renal plasma flow rate increase until midpregnancy, typically by 40%.

Respiratory changes include an increase in tidal volume. The majority of pregnant women experience dyspnea in the first trimester as a paradoxical result of lower carbon dioxide levels.

Placental secretion of hormones, such as placental lactogen, promotes maternal insulin resistance with subsequent postprandial hyperglycemia; glucose is shunted to the fetus, and the mother uses ketones and triglycerides to meet her metabolic needs.

Liver enzyme levels change during pregnancy. Alkaline phosphatase levels double, whereas there is a slight decrease in levels of aspartate aminotransferase, alanine aminotransferase, γ-glutamyl transpeptidase, and bilirubin.

Changes in the coagulation system include marked increases in levels of fibrinogen and factor VIII, with lesser increases in factors VII, IX, X, and XII; protein S levels (both free and bound) decrease. Together with the increase in venous stasis in the lower extremities, these changes can promote thrombosis.

Cardiovascular Disease

HYPERTENSION

Epidemiology

Up to 5% of pregnant women have chronic hypertension.[11] Moreover, the prevalence of chronic hypertension in pregnancy is increasing, for two reasons: (1) women are having children at older ages, when chronic hypertension is more common, and (2) with the increase in obesity in the general population, chronic hypertension is developing at younger ages.

Diagnosis

Chronic hypertension is defined by the Working Group on High Blood Pressure in Pregnancy as a blood pressure greater than 140/90 mm Hg before pregnancy or in the first half of pregnancy.[11]

Management

Blood pressure should be followed closely throughout pregnancy, to guide decision making about initiation or adjustment of medication. In normal pregnancy, blood pressure falls in the late first trimester and returns to prepregnancy ranges near term. Blood pressure in most women with chronic hypertension follows this pattern.

During pregnancy, blood pressure must be kept high enough to maintain placental perfusion. Consequently, blood pressure goals for pregnant women are higher than those for nonpregnant women. The Working Group on High Blood Pressure in Pregnancy recommends antihypertensive treatment for pregnant women with a diastolic blood pressure of 105 mm Hg or higher to decrease risk of maternal stroke and intracerebral hemorrhage.[11] A meta-analysis of existing studies indicates that antihypertensive therapy in women with mild to moderate chronic hypertension does not influence the risk of developing superimposed preeclampsia.[12]

No antihypertensive medications are designated category A in pregnancy, but methyldopa is recommended as first-line therapy, given its long history of use without adverse effects.[11] However, because methyldopa often causes fatigue and has limited potency, labetalol, beta blockers, or calcium channel blockers are often used. Trials of antihypertensive therapies and trials comparing the effectiveness of different agents in pregnancy are very limited; consequently, few data exist to guide choices among these agents.

Angiotensin-converting enzyme (ACE) inhibitors and angiotensin receptor blockers are considered category C in the second and third trimester, because of associated neonatal renal failure.[13,14] Some studies have shown that exposure to ACE inhibitors during the first trimester does not result in ill effects.[13] This finding is important for counseling women who conceive inadvertently while on this class of medication. However, given the number of unplanned pregnancies and the fact that many women do not present for prenatal care in the first trimester, it is prudent that women on these agents be switched to agents of another class when they are planning pregnancy.

Because chronic hypertension in pregnancy is associated with an increased risk of fetal growth restriction and other manifestations of uteroplacental insufficiency, including stillbirth, and because intensive antihypertensive treatment in pregnancy has been associated with intrauterine fetal growth restriction, pregnant women who have chronic hyertension should be carefully monitored. This is usually accomplished by regular evaluation of fetal growth with ultrasonography and, as the pregnancy approaches term, weekly or biweekly evaluation of fetal well-being with nonstress tests (20- to 30-minute evaluations of the pattern of fetal heart rate tracing) or biophysical profiles (ultrasonographic evaluation of fetal movement and amniotic fluid volume). Recognizing the increased risk attendant with these pregnancies, most practitioners plan delivery before the 40th week of gestation even if test results up to that point are reassuring.

Prognosis

Most women with chronic hypertension do well during pregnancy. However, pregnant women with poorly controlled hypertension are at risk for stroke and cerebral hemorrhage, and they are at increased risk for placental abruption.[15] In addition, preeclampsia (exacerbation of hypertension with onset or worsening of proteinuria [see Pregnancy-Specific Conditions, Preeclampsia, below] develops in approximately 25% of women with chronic hypertension, compared with an overall incidence of 5% in the general population.[15] Preeclampsia has the highest risk of maternal and fetal problems associated with essential hypertension. Despite much research, efforts to decrease the incidence of preeclampsia in women at increased risk for it have been unsuccessful. For these reasons, it is important that women with chronic hypertension be followed more closely during pregnancy. Measuring the 24-hour urinary protein level before pregnancy can facilitate the diagnosis of preeclampsia during pregnancy in women with chronic hypertension.

VALVULAR DISEASE

In general, valvular heart diseases such as pulmonic and tricuspid lesions or mitral valve prolapse or regurgitation are well tolerated during pregnancy. Previously undiagnosed and asymptomatic mitral stenosis, however, may become symptomatic during pregnancy as a result of the increased plasma volume. Women with moderate or severe mitral stenosis are at particular risk in the postpartum period, when the fluid previously sequestered in the placenta or lower extremities returns to the systemic circulation, augmenting the existing increased volume. During labor, careful attention to fluid management and judicious diuresis is required for women with mitral stenosis. Epidural anesthesia may help both by providing vascular relaxation,

---

Table 2   Selected Drugs with Suspected or Known Teratogenic Potential[7]

Alcohol	Misoprostol
Androgens	Nonsteroidal anti-inflammatory drugs
Danazol	
Angiotensin-converting enzyme inhibitors	Phenytoin
	Quinolones
Anticholinergic drugs	Retinoids and derivatives
Antithyroid drugs	Acitretin
Methimazole	Etretinate
Propylthiouracil	Isotretinoin
Carbamazepine	Tetracycline
Cyclophosphamide	Thalidomide
Cocaine	Valproic acid
Lithium	Warfarin
Methotrexate	

which slows increases in plasma volume after delivery, and by providing pain relief, which can help slow the patient's heart rate. Lower heart rates in these patients improve the heart's efficiency by promoting adequate atrial filling and the "kick" needed to push blood past the stenotic mitral valve.[16] Symptomatic mitral stenosis has become less common with the fall in the incidence of rheumatic heart disease, but patients who experience critical stenosis can be treated safely during pregnancy with balloon valvuloplasty.[17]

ARRHYTHMIAS

Increased plasma volume may contribute to the onset or worsening of maternal dysrhythmias during pregnancy. Many antiarrhythmic agents are appropriate for use during pregnancy, however, and cardioversion, implantable defibrillators, and pacemakers have all been safely used to control symptomatic dysrhythmias in pregnant women.[18]

PERIPARTUM CARDIOMYOPATHY

Peripartum cardiomyopathy affects one in 1,500 to 15,000 pregnancies and is marked by heart failure in the months before or after delivery. The cause is unknown. Diagnosis is confirmed by echocardiographic demonstration of decreased ejection fraction in the absence of another recognized etiology.[19] Treatment is supportive and focuses on supplemental oxygen, inotropic medication, and diuresis. With such support, 50% of patients improve over a period of weeks. In those who do not improve, cardiac transplantation may be required. In subsequent pregnancies, women who have previously had pregnancies complicated by peripartum cardiomyopathy demonstrate further decline in left ventricular ejection fraction. Death occurs principally in women who enter their next pregnancy with persistent left ventricular dysfunction; mortality in this group can be as high as 20%.[20]

Diabetes Mellitus

EPIDEMIOLOGY

Approximately 1% to 2% of pregnant women have DM that predates their pregnancy (i.e., pregestational DM). In another 2% to 3%, DM develops during the pregnancy (i.e., gestational DM) [see Pregnancy-Specific Conditions, Gestational Diabetes Mellitus, below]. As with chronic hypertension, changes in the demographic profile of women who become pregnant have led to an increase in the frequency of type 2 DM in pregnancy.

MANAGEMENT

Women with pregestational DM should receive preconception care that includes counseling about the importance of preconception glucose control. Preconception care improves glucose control and decreases maternal hospitalizations, the need for neonatal intensive care, birth defects, and fetal and neonatal deaths.[21]

Diet therapy is a mainstay of the management of DM outside of pregnancy and is key in pregnancy. Insulin is the preferred agent for the treatment of DM in pregnancy. Women with type 1 DM will already be on insulin; women with type 2 DM who are on oral agents (e.g., hypoglycemics and insulin sensitizers) should be switched to insulin before conception. Insulin therapy should be intensified before conception to achieve a glycosylated hemoglobin level in the normal range, when possible. Neutral protamine Hagedorn (NPH) and regular insulins have a long track record of use in pregnancy. The short-acting insulins, in particular insulin lispro, have been used increasingly in pregnancy and appear to be safe, but long-term follow-up of infants exposed to these agents in utero is not yet available. The long-acting insulins, such as insulin glargine, have not been extensively tested in pregnancy. Goals for whole-blood glucose levels recommended by the American Diabetes Association (ADA) during pregnancy are fasting levels below 95 mg/dl and 1-hour postprandial levels below 140 mg/dl.

Insulin resistance is a hallmark of normal pregnancy, and it occurs in women with DM as well. As a result, insulin requirements typically increase in pregnancy.

Both type 1 and type 2 DM are associated with an increased risk of fetal growth abnormalities. Women with type 1 DM, particularly those with vascular complications, are at risk for fetal growth restriction. Conversely, women with type 2 DM are at risk for large (macrosomic) newborns. In either case, fetal growth in women with diabetes can be monitored with serial ultrasound scans during pregnancy. DM, particularly when poorly controlled, has also been linked to intrauterine fetal demise; accordingly, for pregnant women with diabetes, most practitioners employ a careful program of fetal surveillance that includes nonstress tests, biophysical profiles, and fetal movement counting. As with pregnancies that are at increased risk from other medical complications, delivery is often planned before the 40th week of gestation.

COMPLICATIONS AND PROGNOSIS

DM is associated with increased risks for both the mother and the fetus. For the mother with DM, there may be acceleration of retinopathy and nephropathy during pregnancy. In addition, women with DM are at increased risk for preeclampsia. For the fetus, poor maternal glycemic control at the time of conception may be associated with a birth defect rate as high as 20%. This rate can be reduced to a rate similar to that of the general population if glycemic control is adequate at conception.

Unless insulin doses are increased to compensate for the insulin resistance of pregnancy, women with type 1 DM may experience diabetic ketoacidosis. In the setting of uncontrolled maternal hyperglycemia, the fetus responds by increasing insulin secretion. Insulin acts as a growth factor for the fetus and can cause macrosomia, which increases the chance of injury during vaginal delivery, as well as the need for cesarean section. This elevation in insulin secretion does not resolve immediately with delivery and can lead to neonatal hypoglycemia. The neonates of women who had DM during pregnancy are also at increased risk for respiratory distress syndrome.

Thyroid Disease

EPIDEMIOLOGY

In general, thyroid disease is more common in women than in men. Both hypothyroidism and hyperthyroidism are common in pregnant women.

HYPERTHYROIDISM

Hyperthyroidism complicates about 0.2% of pregnancies.[22] Graves disease is the most common cause of hyperthyroidism in pregnancy.

Diagnosis

The diagnosis of hyperthyroidism during pregnancy is often complicated by the changes in thyroid function that take place in normal pregnancy. In early pregnancy, the rise in levels of human chorionic gonadotropin, which has thyroid stimulatory activity, results in a compensatory fall in levels of thyroid-stimulating hormone (TSH). Although the fall in TSH concentration is usually within the physiologic range, in some women the TSH falls into the suppressed range. Therefore, the diagnosis of Graves disease should be based not solely on a low TSH level but also on the presence of symptoms of hyperthyroidism and of elevated thyroxine (T_4) levels. Symptoms of hyperthyroidism in pregnancy include weight loss or absence of weight gain, anxiety, and palpitations. Although it is possible that a small degree of thyroid enlargement occurs in normal pregnancy, secondary to increase in plasma volume and thyroid blood flow, a palpable goiter should not be attributed to pregnancy.

Management

Antithyroid medications (thionamides) do cross the placenta, and the fetal thyroid appears to be more sensitive to these agents than the maternal thyroid. Therefore, maternal treatment of euthyroidism is associated with fetal hypothyroidism in about 25% of cases.[23] In addition to fetal and neonatal hypothyroidism, neonatal goiter can be present and can cause respiratory compromise from tracheal compression.

Treatment of maternal hyperthyroidism is recommended only for mothers who are symptomatic. The treatment goal is a T_4 level in the upper range of normal. Hyperthyroidism in pregnancy is one of the few clinical situations in which therapy is guided by the T_4 level rather than the TSH level; normalization of the TSH level is not the goal in these patients.

Propylthiouracil (PTU) and methimazole are the most common drugs used for hyperthyroidism in the United States. There has been some suggestion that PTU crosses the placenta to a lesser degree than methimazole, although the data are limited. Furthermore, methimazole, but not PTU, has been associated with the condition aplasia cutis, a skin defect most commonly involving the scalp. As a result, PTU is the preferred drug for pregnancy. If antithyroid medication does not control the hyperthyroidism and the woman has severe symptoms, thyroidectomy during pregnancy may be required. Radioactive iodine (RAI) ablation is contraindicated during pregnancy, because it can ablate the fetal thyroid and cause congenital hypothyroidism. Concern over uncontrollable hyperthyroidism in pregnancy has led some endocrinologists to recommend RAI thyroid ablation or surgery in women with Graves disease who are planning a pregnancy and in whom control of Graves disease has been difficult, as a result of disease activity or problems with medication. Women with Graves disease who are going to be managed on antithyroid medications should be followed by a clinician with experience in thyroid disease during pregnancy, because the goals of treatment differ from those in nonpregnant patients.

Complications and Prognosis

Severe hyperthyroidism may be associated with stillbirth, preterm delivery, intrauterine growth restriction, preeclampsia, or congestive heart failure.[24] Graves disease usually follows a characteristic course during pregnancy, with exacerbation in the first trimester and improvement or even remission in the third trimester, with exacerbation again about 2 months post partum.

HYPOTHYROIDISM

Maternal hypothyroidism complicates 2% to 5% of pregnancies. For unknown reasons, women with primary hypothyroidism have an increased requirement for thyroid hormone during pregnancy.[25]

Diagnosis

Hypothyroidism is best diagnosed by determination of the TSH level. The upper limit of normal in pregnancy is similar to that outside of pregnancy.

Management

Women with hypothyroidism should have their TSH level measured at the time of a pregnancy test to guide adjustment of their thyroid hormone replacement dose. The TSH level should then be checked at a minimum of each trimester, as well as 4 to 6 weeks after each dose adjustment. Because of the increase in thyroid hormone requirement in pregnancy, some advocate regulating dosing of thyroid hormone before conception to achieve a TSH level of around 1 IU/ml. The increased requirement resolves with delivery, and therefore, the thyroid hormone dose can be reduced to the prepregnancy dose at that time.

Complications and Prognosis

Maternal hypothyroidism has been reported to increase the risk for preeclampsia, placental abruption, and stillbirths. A study of over 400 pregnant women with subclinical hypothyroidism (defined as a TSH level of ≥ 97.5% of the upper range of normal and a T_4 level within normal range) found that rates of hypertension were no different from those in euthyroid pregnant women; however, subclinical hypothyroidism was associated with an increased risk of placental abruption and preterm delivery.[26] The offspring of mothers who were hypothyroid during pregnancy have been reported to have intelligent quotients (IQs) 7 points lower than those of the offspring of euthyroid mothers, although IQs remain in the normal range.[27]

POSTPARTUM THYROIDITIS

The immunologic flare that follows the relative immune suppression of pregnancy may result in thyroiditis. Postpartum thyroiditis is typically transient; it is marked by a period of hyperthyroidism followed by hypothyroidism.

Epidemiology

Postpartum thyroiditis occurs after approximately 8% of pregnancies.[28] Women with type 1 DM are at threefold higher risk; the risk is also higher in women who have had Hashimoto thyroiditis and in those who had postpartum thyroiditis after a previous pregnancy.

Diagnosis

About 2 months after delivery, women with postpartum thyroiditis may experience hyperthyroidism as a result of leakage of thyroid hormone from the inflamed thyroid gland. This phase is often missed because of its short duration (usually 4 weeks or less) and because the patient and her caregivers tend to ascribe its symptoms of anxiety and palpitations to the stress of being a new mother. A TSH level measured at this time will be low. About 6 months after delivery, the hypothyroid phase develops. At this time, patients usually present with fatigue and weight gain or an inability to lose pregnancy-associated weight. Depression can also be a presenting symptom; for that reason, it is important to check the TSH level before making a diagnosis of postpartum depression.

Management

Whether to initiate thyroid hormone therapy in a woman with postpartum thyroiditis depends on the severity of her symptoms. If thyroid hormone replacement therapy is chosen, thyroid hormone can be withdrawn at 1 year post partum to determine whether long-term therapy is indicated. The TSH level should be checked 4 to 6 weeks after stopping therapy, or it should be checked sooner if symptoms of hypothyroidism develop.

Prognosis

In the majority of women with postpartum thyroiditis, thyroid function returns to normal in the ensuing postpartum year. However, some women remain permanently hypothyroid. Overall, approximately 25% of women who have postpartum thyroiditis progress to permanent hypothyroidism in the ensuing 10 years.[28]

Thrombophilia

The risk for thromboembolism during pregnancy is increased, largely as a result of increased venous stasis in the lower extremities and pelvis. In addition, changes in some serum coagulation factors (i.e., elevation of factor VII, factor X, factor VIII, fibrinogen, and von Willebrand factor and decrease of protein S) may contribute to the pregnancy-associated risk for thrombosis. This risk may be particularly prominent in women who have another risk factor for thrombosis, such as inherited or acquired thrombophilia or a history of thrombosis unassociated with trauma—in particular, thrombosis associated with the use of oral contraceptives. Prophylaxis with aspirin or heparin during pregnancy may be indicated for women with any of these risk factors.[29] Although the safety of low-molecular-weight heparin (LMWH) during pregnancy is not definitively established, expert panels have concluded that LMWH may be safely used during pregnancy.[30] Because the timing and course of labor and delivery are not easily predicted and because LMWH has a long duration of action, conversion to unfractionated heparin is generally planned late in the third trimester to minimize bleeding complications from delivery or regional anesthesia. The use of LMWH or unfractionated heparin during pregnancy requires careful monitoring, because changes in plasma volume may affect the usual dosing.[31]

Some studies have suggested that thrombophilias may also be associated with an increased risk of miscarriage and other pregnancy complications, such as stillbirth, growth restriction, and placental abruption.[32] A detailed review of these investigations is beyond the scope of this chapter. Data are, at best, inconclusive, and there is little evidence that intervention (e.g., treatment with heparin, aspirin, or steroids) improves outcome, except possibly in women with antiphospholipid antibody syndrome.[33]

Asthma

As many as 6% of pregnant women have asthma. This disease has a variable course during pregnancy: it is equally likely to worsen, improve, or remain unchanged.[34] In contrast to past reports, current studies indicate that asthma is not associated with an increased risk of preterm delivery and growth restriction.[35] The clinical course in an individual patient may be linked, at least in part, to the patient's and her clinician's willingness to use needed medications during pregnancy. Guidelines from the National Institute of Child Health and Human Development emphasize that continued use of beta agonists and steroids during pregnancy is safe and appropriate.[36] As in nonpregnant women, clinical evaluations such as peak flow measurements can be used to judge disease activity and guide therapy.

Infectious Diseases

Vertical transmission of maternal infection is rare during pregnancy, but some pathogens carry particular pregnancy-associated risks. In addition, infections that are of little or no clinical significance to a woman when she is not pregnant may have serious implications during pregnancy (e.g., parvovirus or cytomegalovirus infection). It is important to note that pregnancy is not a contraindication to most prophylactic measures against infection—including, as appropriate, malaria prophylaxis or vaccination with inactive agents. Seasonal vaccination with influenza is recommended for pregnant women.

HERPES SIMPLEX VIRUS INFECTION

Neonatal infection with herpes simplex virus (HSV) acquired during delivery as a consequence of viral shedding from the cervix and vagina can have devastating consequences for the newborn. Cesarean delivery, especially if performed before active labor when the amniotic membranes are still intact, largely eliminates the possibility of vertical transmission.[37] The risk of delivering an HSV-infected infant is greatest in women with a primary infection with HSV type 1 or 2 at the time of delivery. Although secondary infection carries lower neonatal risk, as a result of the protection afforded by circulating HSV antibodies shared across the placenta with the fetus, cesarean delivery to further limit vertical transmission is still generally recommended when women present in labor with signs or symptoms of secondary infection. To avoid cesarean delivery and reduce neonatal risk, prophylactic treatment with antiviral agents such as acyclovir may be recommended late in the third trimester in an effort to minimize the chances of an outbreak at the time of labor and delivery.[38]

PARVOVIRUS INFECTION

Infection with parvovirus B19, which produces a viral exanthem known as fifth disease, may at times be epidemic in schools or child care settings. Parvovirus infection is usually not of clinical consequence to immunocompetent adults or children. Rarely, fetuses of newly infected pregnant women can develop significant anemia or other complications as a result of transplacental infection. Estimating the precise fetal risk has proved to be challenging, but some series suggest that the risk of the loss of pregnancy when a new maternal infection occurs before the 20th week of gestation may range from 2.5% to 10%.[39] Both early and later infections can result in fetal bone marrow suppression and subsequent anemia; in turn, the anemia leads to pericardial effusion, pleural effusion, and generalized body edema—a condition known as hydrops fetalis. It should be emphasized that such complications are rare, however.[40] Although the anemia is often self-limited, either delivery or in utero fetal red blood cell transfusion may be considered if hydrops fetalis develops.

HIV INFECTION

Although transplacental transmission of HIV infection from mother to fetus has been described, vertical transmission of HIV occurs largely at the time of delivery and is directly linked to maternal viral load. To reduce transmission and optimize maternal health, antiretroviral regimens that were initiated before pregnancy are continued during pregnancy.[41] Because of mitochondrial toxicity, the combination of didanosine and stavudine should be avoided during pregnancy. Additional concern has been raised about teratogenic effects of efavirenz in animals. For women who have not previously been treated with antiviral agents and whose viral loads and CD4+ T cell counts do not themselves dictate treatment, zidovudine is prescribed during the antepartum and intrapartum period, with postpartum treatment for the newborn, because such treatment has been linked to a reduction of vertical transmission.[42] Cesarean delivery has also been shown to protect against vertical transmission in women with HIV infection and high viral loads.[43] Consequently, cesarean delivery should be offered to patients with more than 1,000 copies/ml.[41] Breast-feeding is not recommended for women with HIV infection if appropriate alternatives (e.g., clean water and formula) exist.[44]

HEPATITIS

Women with active hepatitis B or C are at risk for vertical transmission of such infections to their fetus, particularly if either the presence of e-antigen (in the case of hepatitis B) or copy counts indicate high viral loads. Administration of hepatitis B vaccine and immunoglobulin reduces neonatal infection with hepatitis B by 90%. Cesarean delivery is not routinely recommended in the setting of either of these maternal infections. Breast-feeding is not contraindicated in mothers with hepatitis C, nor is it contraindicated in mothers with hepatitis B whose newborns have received appropriate prophylaxis.

GROUP B STREPTOCOCCUS INFECTION

In 20% of women, group B Streptococcus (GBS) can be cultured from the rectovaginal area. Such carriage, of no consequence to adults, can result in early- or late-onset GBS sepsis and mortality in three of 1,000 infants delivered to women who are carriers. Screening for GBS colonization is now recommended during pregnancy; when linked with intrapartum treatment, such screening has reduced neonatal infection to less than one in 1,000 deliveries.[45]

Renal Disease

A 1996 study of the outcomes of 87 pregnancies in 67 women with moderate or severe preexisting renal disease described preterm delivery in 59% and fetal growth restriction in 37%—rates considerably higher than those seen in the general population (11% and 10%, respectively).[46] In addition, pregnancy-related loss of renal function was noted in 43% of these women, although distinguishing natural disease progression from progression caused by the pregnancy is extremely challenging at an individual level and can be difficult even at a population level. Accordingly, careful monitoring of both mother and baby are required during such pregnancies. Some conditions (e.g., autosomal dominant polycystic kidney disease and structural anomalies such as single kidney) increase the risk of fetal renal disease.

Renal transplantation can restore fertility in women with end-stage renal disease. However, it is generally recommended that transplant recipients delay conception until graft function has been stable for 1 to 2 years, blood pressure is well controlled, and the immunosuppressive regimen is optimized. In one review of 2,300 pregnancies in 1,600 women who had had a renal transplant, 13% of patients had a spontaneous abortion

(a rate similar to that in the general population), and 27% elected pregnancy termination; of pregnancies continuing beyond the first trimester, 92% were termed successful, although many of these were complicated by issues of prematurity and growth restriction.[47] Worsening graft function has been noted during posttransplant pregnancies, but whether the deterioration is any worse than that expected outside of pregnancy remains a matter of debate.

Autoimmune Diseases

Whether pregnancy worsens maternal autoimmune disease, such as systemic lupus erythematosus (SLE), remains controversial. Women with such conditions are at risk for preeclampsia and fetal growth restriction. Outcomes for mother and baby are, in general, felt to be best when maternal disease is quiescent.[48] In some cases, continued treatment with steroids may be needed to maintain quiescence and optimize outcomes. Fetuses of women with SLE or other connective tissue diseases and anti-Ro/SS-A or anti-La/SS-B antibodies are at special risk for neonatal lupus, a condition that may be marked by fetal or neonatal heart block, skin disease, and hepatic inflammation.[49] Testing for these serologic markers is important for guiding both fetal and neonatal care. For example, congenital heart block can be detected in utero, and some have suggested that early detection, when linked with steroid treatment of the mother, can improve outcomes.[50]

Recurrent miscarriage, stillbirth, growth restriction, and preeclampsia more frequently complicate pregnancies of women with antiphospholipid antibodies. In small studies, treatment with heparin, aspirin, or both has been shown to improve pregnancy outcome in some women with symptomatic antiphospholipid antibody syndrome.[51] Such data are limited, however, and treatment should carefully be considered on a case-by-case basis.

Cancer

There is no evidence that pregnancy increases the development, hastens the progression, or promotes the recurrence of any cancer. Cancers, particularly those more prevalent in populations of young women (e.g., breast and cervical cancer), will be found during pregnancy, however. Indeed, given that pregnancy may be one of the few times that many young women seek medical care, the examination and screening conducted during pregnancy may improve detection of incidental malignancies. Appropriate diagnostic studies, including mammography, Papanicolaou smear and colposcopy, and endoscopy should not be deferred because of pregnancy.

Management of cancer that is coincident with pregnancy presents many challenges. Because some forms of cancer and its treatment carry risks for both the woman and her fetus, some women may choose pregnancy interruption. In particular, management of invasive cervical cancer requiring surgical excision presents particular challenges. For other cancers in women who choose to continue their pregnancies, surgical and medical management need not be delayed by pregnancy. Several series describe successful chemotherapeutic treatment of malignancies diagnosed early in gestation, in concert with careful fetal monitoring.[52] For malignancies diagnosed later in gestation, early delivery may be considered so as to facilitate treatment.

Neurologic Diseases

EPILEPSY

The management of epilepsy before and during pregnancy demonstrates the careful balance of risks and benefits attendant with treating women of reproductive age, particularly those who require long-term medication. Most antiseizure drugs are associated with an increased risk of congenital anomalies—6% to 9%, compared with the 3% risk for birth defects in the general United States population. These defects cluster in a characteristic pattern that includes facial defects and microcephaly.[53] The risk is further increased by the need for multiple medications or the use of a few particularly teratogenic medications; for example, valproic acid is associated with a 1% to 3% risk of open neural tube defects. Balanced against these risks are the morbidities associated with seizures if medications are discontinued or are inappropriately dosed during pregnancy. Although pregnancy itself does not appear to either lower seizure thresholds or otherwise increase seizure frequency, changes in plasma volume may require increases in dosing to maintain effective drug levels. With careful monitoring, most women with epilepsy can anticipate healthy outcomes for themselves and their babies.[54]

MULTIPLE SCLEROSIS

Multiple sclerosis generally improves during pregnancy—a time of relative immunosuppression. The disease may flare post partum, however.[55] Although steroids might be used during pregnancy if a woman were to have worsening symptoms, many other contemporary treatments are either poorly studied in pregnancy (i.e., glatiramer acetate) or generally discouraged during pregnancy (i.e., interferons).

MYASTHENIA GRAVIS

Infants of women with myasthenia gravis are at risk for a self-limited neonatal myasthenia syndrome that results when antibodies to the acetylcholine receptor cross the placental circulation. Once delivery and cord clamping interrupt the placental circulation, the newborn clears these antibodies and, over a period of weeks, the syndrome improves. In the interval, affected newborns may require ventilatory and nutritional support until muscles involved in breathing and feeding again function normally.

Substance Use

The use of substances, legal and illegal, can have important consequences for pregnancy. Cigarette smoking is associated with an increased risk of intrauterine growth restriction, preterm delivery, and sudden infant death. Although nicotine is labeled class D (i.e., there is positive evidence of its association with human fetal risk) by the FDA, many clinicians use nicotine replacement to help pregnant women quit smoking.[56] In fact, there is reason to believe that nicotine might carry fewer risks when it is absorbed via transdermal patch or chewing gum than when it is delivered together with the carbon monoxide and other toxins contained in inhaled tobacco smoke.

Although the effects of cocaine on the behavior and neural development of newborns have in the past been exaggerated,[57] the use of cocaine during pregnancy may cause placental abruption. Heroin use may cause fetal growth abnormalities, whereas methadone therapy can be initiated and safely maintained during pregnancy.[58] Infants of mothers who use methadone or other prescription and nonprescription narcotics during pregnancy may be born with drug dependence and require careful monitoring after birth to prevent acute withdrawal. In such newborns, tincture of opium is sometimes given and then slowly titrated to minimize the consequences of acute withdrawal.

Fetal alcohol syndrome—marked by abnormal facial features, growth retardation, and central nervous system disturbances—is a consequence of long-term alcohol use. Although higher frequency and volumes of drinking are associated with an increased risk of fetal alcohol syndrome, no safe level of alcohol use during pregnancy can be defined or recommended.[59]

Data examining the effects of caffeine on pregnancy are indeterminate, but some small studies suggest that high exposures (i.e., more than three to five cups of regular coffee a day) may increase the risk of miscarriage. Prudence therefore argues for moderation in women planning to become pregnant.[60]

Both because of the recognized fetal risks and because prenatal care offers a series of regular practitioner contacts, pregnancy may offer an ideal opportunity to address problems of substance use and abuse. Intervention, however, requires a careful balance that encourages treatment without limiting maternal liberties. Mandated screening and reporting may drive women from prenatal care and otherwise limit the therapeutic opportunity that pregnancy presents.

Intrahepatic Cholestasis

Intrahepatic cholestasis appears to result from impaired processing of bile salts and acids in the liver. The etiology remains uncertain, but evidence suggests a genetic predisposition. Intrahepatic cholestasis occurs in 0.1% to 0.01% of pregnant women. The accumulation of these salts in the skin can cause an intense and characteristic pruritus (worse on palms and soles) without associated skin lesions. Jaundice develops in only about 10% of patients.

Liver function tests in women with intrahepatic cholestasis of pregnancy show elevations in levels of γ-glutamyl transpeptidase, alanine aminotransferase, and aspartate aminotransferase. The most specific test is an elevation in the fasting serum total bile acid concentration.

Whether deposition of bile salts in the placenta results in fetal morbidity and mortality is much debated, but some series indicate an increased risk of stillbirth and postpartum hemorrhage in women with cholestasis. Consequently, many practitioners institute a program of fetal monitoring and maternal prothrombin measurement in cholestatic pregnancies and may recommend induced delivery between 36 and 39 weeks of gestation.[61] Ursodeoxycholic acid can relieve pruritus and help normalize liver enzyme levels and may improve fetal outcome.[62]

Pregnancy-Specific Conditions

There are several medical complications of pregnancy that occur only during pregnancy and that resolve once the pregnancy is completed. Three of these pregnancy-specific conditions are hyperemesis gravidarum, preeclampsia, and gestational diabetes.

HYPEREMESIS GRAVIDARUM

Nausea and vomiting complicate as many as 70% of pregnancies. The cause of these symptoms remains obscure but may be related to levels of human chorionic gonadotropin and other hormones that are affected by pregnancy. Older theories suggesting that nausea and vomiting are a psychosomatic reflection of a woman's rejection of her pregnancy have been discredited. Nevertheless, different cultures and individuals may manage symptoms differently, and in any woman, the symptoms may cause stress.

Unless other findings suggest specific causes for nausea and vomiting (e.g., hyperthyroidism, hepatitis or other viral syndromes, or hydatidiform mole), little testing is required; care is supportive. Women may be reassured that the dietary limitations their symptoms require are unlikely to compromise their pregnancy, and in fact, pregnancies accompanied by nausea and vomiting are more likely to be healthful than those without such symptoms.[63] Several randomized, controlled trials have demonstrated that supplementation with vitamin B_6 (10 to 50 mg two or three times a day) may improve symptoms.[64] Some women may require other medications, including antihistamines and dopamine antagonists, to control symptoms.[65]

Fortunately, in most women, nausea and vomiting abate between the 12th and 16th weeks of gestation. Only rarely is hospitalization or enteral nutrition required.

PREECLAMPSIA

Preeclampsia is defined as the onset of hypertension (i.e., blood pressure greater than 140/90 mm Hg) and proteinuria in the second half of pregnancy.[11] Proteinuria in pregnancy is defined as a finding of more than 300 mg of protein on a 24-hour urine collection. Preeclampsia may also be superimposed on chronic hypertension; in these cases, there is an exacerbation of hypertension accompanied by new-onset proteinuria or worsening of preexisting proteinuria. Preeclampsia complicates 3% to 5% of pregnancies. It occurs most commonly in first pregnancies.

Pathogenesis

The cause of preeclampsia is unknown. At the root of the disorder is endothelial dysfunction and placental insufficiency. Several potential factors in preeclampsia include immune dysregulation, genes, insulin resistance, and placental factors such as soluble fms-like tyrosine kinase–1.[66]

Management

Because the cause of preeclampsia is not known, effective interventions have been elusive. The only definitive treatment is delivery of the fetus. Antihypertensive treatment can decrease the maternal risk of stroke but has not been shown to improve pregnancy outcome. Prophylactic treatment with intravenous magnesium sulfate decreases the risk of eclampsia. Preventive efforts to lower the risk for preeclampsia with aspirin or calcium supplementation have been unsuccessful. Close surveillance of both the mother and the fetus is essential and includes more frequent visits or inpatient observation with periodic evaluation of liver and renal function, as well as other blood markers of disease progression (e.g., platelet count), antenatal testing (e.g. nonstress testing, biophysical profile, or evaluation of amniotic fluid alone), and evaluation of fetal growth.

Complications

Complications of preeclampsia affect both the mother and the fetus. Maternal complications include stroke and intracerebral hemorrhage. The HELLP syndrome (hemolysis, elevated liver function, and low platelets) is a life-threatening maternal complication of preeclampsia.

Prognosis

Preeclampsia resolves with delivery or shortly thereafter. Women with a history of preeclampsia are at higher risk for the

disorder in future pregnancies. In addition, these women may be at increased risk for the later development of essential hypertension and other cardiovascular disease.

GESTATIONAL DIABETES MELLITUS

Epidemiology

Gestational diabetes mellitus (GDM) affects about 7% of all pregnancies. The rate of GDM is higher in obese women and in women belonging to certain ethnic groups (e.g., Hispanics).

Pathogenesis

Insulin resistance increases in normal pregnancy. Women who cannot overcome this insulin resistance develop GDM.

Diagnosis

GDM is defined as carbohydrate intolerance diagnosed during pregnancy. However, no universal criteria exist for screening or diagnosis; these criteria differ within and between countries. The ADA recommends screening for GDM in all pregnant women with at least one of the following risk factors: age 25 years or older; ethnicity other than white; family history of DM in a first-degree relative; being overweight before pregnancy or experiencing greater than usual weight gain during pregnancy; or a personal history of either abnormal blood glucose levels or a previous obstetric complication. In the United States, screening is typically performed with a 1-hour glucose tolerance test (GTT) using a 50 g oral glucose load. For women with blood glucose values greater than 140 mg/dl, the next step is a fasting 3-hour 100 g GTT. The diagnosis of GDM is made when patients have two or more GTT values higher than those of either the National Diabetes Data Group or Carpenter-Coustan criteria [see Table 3].[67]

Management

The mainstay of treatment for GDM is diet. The therapeutic goals are fasting whole-blood glucose levels below 95 mg/dl and 1-hour postprandial glucose levels below 140 mg/dl.[67] Women with GDM are taught to perform home glucose monitoring.

If glucose levels remain elevated despite dietary intervention, insulin therapy should be initiated. Although this recommendation has been made routinely for some time, evidence supporting the benefit of treatment for pregnancy outcome was lacking until 2005, when a study demonstrated that perinatal complications were less frequent in newborns of women with GDM who were randomized to management with home glucose monitor-

Table 3 Venous Plasma Glucose Criteria for the Diagnosis of Gestational Diabetes after a 100 g Oral Glucose Tolerance Test*

Time	NDDG Criteria (mg/dl)	Carpenter-Coustan Criteria (mg/dl)
0 (fasting)	105	95
1 hour	190	180
2 hour	165	155
3 hour	145	140

*Gestational diabetes mellitus is diagnosed when two or more results exceed these values.[67]
NDDG—National Diabetes Data Group

ing, dietary therapy, and insulin, compared with the newborns of women who received routine care.[68] A 2004 study suggested that GDM may be effectively managed with oral glyburide rather than insulin,[69] but further studies are needed before this approach is advocated.

Women with GDM who have poor glycemic control or who require insulin or oral agents to regulate blood sugar may benefit from antenatal fetal testing. Clinical or sonographic evaluation for fetal macrosomia may lead physicians to recommend cesarean section rather than vaginal delivery.

Complications

Elevated fasting glucose levels have been associated with fetal demise. Macrosomia risk is also increased. As with preexisting DM, macrosomia increases the chance of shoulder dystocia during vaginal delivery and resultant cesarean section. Like pregestational DM, GDM may result in neonatal hypoglycemia.

Prognosis

GDM is an important risk factor for the future development of type 2 DM. As many as 50% of women who have had GDM will develop type 2 DM over the ensuing 10 years.[70] Obesity further increases this risk. Consequently, questions about GDM should be a standard part of the primary care evaluation in parous women. The ADA recommends yearly screening for DM in women with a history of GDM. Whether screening should entail measurement of a fasting glucose level or a postprandial glucose level has not been established. It seems prudent that women with a history of GDM be advised to reduce weight and to exercise, although studies supporting this recommendation are lacking. Some studies suggest that the use of insulin sensitizers may reduce the rate of conversion of GDM to type 2 DM[71]; these data need to be confirmed in large-scale trials, and cost-effectiveness must be taken into consideration before the use of these agents can be recommended.

The authors have no commercial relationships with manufacturers of products or providers of services discussed in this chapter.

References

1. Gleicher N, Midwall J, Hochberger D, et al: Eisenmenger's syndrome and pregnancy. Obstet Gynecol Surv 34:721, 1979

2. Weiss BM, Hess OM: Pulmonary vascular disease and pregnancy: current controversies, management strategies, and perspectives. Eur Heart J 21:104, 2000

3. Shabetai R: Cardiac Diseases in Maternal Fetal Medicine, 4th ed. Creasy RK, Resnik R, Eds. WB Saunders Co, Philadelphia, 1999, p 793

4. Mennuti MT, Thomson E, Press N: Screening for cystic fibrosis carrier state. Obstet Gynecol 93:456, 1999

5. ACOG practice bulletin. Clinical management guidelines for obstetrician-gynecologists. Number 44, July 2003. Neural tube defects. Obstet Gynecol 102:203, 2003

6. Nelson K, Holmes LB: Malformations due to presumed spontaneous mutations in newborn infants. N Engl J Med 320:19, 1989

7. Koren G, Pastuszak A, Ito S: Drugs in pregnancy. N Engl J Med 338:1128, 1998

8. Whittemore R, Wells JA, Castellsague X: A second-generation study of 427 probands with congenital heart defects and their 837 children. J Am Coll Cardiol 23:1459, 1994

9. Werler MM, Louik C, Shapiro S, et al: Prepregnant weight in relation to risk of neural tube defects. JAMA 275:1089, 1996

10. Milunsky A, Ulcickas M, Rothman KJ, et al: Maternal heat exposure and neural tube defects. JAMA 268:882, 1992

11. Report of the National High Blood Pressure Education Program Working Group on High Blood Pressure in Pregnancy. Am J Obstet Gynecol 183:S1, 2000

12. Abalos E, Duley L, Steyn DW: Antihypertensive drug therapy for mild to moderate hypertension in pregnancy. Cochrane Database Syst Rev (2):CD002252, 2001

13. Hanssens M, Keirse MJ, Vankelecom F, et al: Fetal and neonatal effects of treatment with angiotensin-converting enzyme inhibitors in pregnancy. Obstet Gynecol 78:128, 1991

14. Alwan S, Polifka JE, Friedman JM: Angiotensin II receptor antagonist treatment dur-

ing pregnancy. Birth Defects Res A Clin Mol Teratol 73:123, 2005

15. Sibai BM, Lindheimer M, Hauth J, et al: Risk factors for preeclampsia, abruptio placentae, and adverse neonatal outcomes among women with chronic hypertension. National Institute of Child Health and Human Development Network of Maternal-Fetal Medicine Units. N Engl J Med 339:667, 1998

16. Reimold SC, Rutherford JD: Clinical practice: valvular heart disease in pregnancy. N Engl J Med 349:52, 2003

17. Fawzy ME, Kinsara AJ, Stefadouros M, et al: Long-term outcome of mitral balloon valvotomy in pregnant women. J Heart Valve Dis 10:153, 2001

18. Page RL: Treatment of arrhythmias during pregnancy. Am Heart J 130:871, 1995

19. Pearson GD, Veille JC, Rahimtoola S, et al: Peripartum cardiomyopathy: National Heart, Lung, and Blood Institute and Office of Rare Diseases (National Institutes of Health) workshop recommendations and review. JAMA 283:1183, 2000

20. Elkayam U, Tummala PP, Rao K, et al: Maternal and fetal outcomes of subsequent pregnancies in women with peripartum cardiomyopathy. N Engl J Med 344:1567, 2001

21. Korenbrot CC, Steinberg A, Bender C, et al: Preconception care: a systematic review. Matern Child Health J 6:75, 2002

22. Neale D, Burrow G: Thyroid disease in pregnancy. Obstet Gynecol Clin North Am 31:893, 2004

23. Momotani N, Noh J, Oyanagi H, et al: Antithyroid drug therapy for Graves' disease during pregnancy: optimal regimen for fetal thyroid status. N Engl J Med 315:24, 1986

24. Davis Le, Lucas MJ, Hawkins GD, et al: Thyrotoxicosis complicating pregnancy. Am J Obstet Gynecol 160:63, 1989

25. Mandel SJ, Larsen PR, Seely EW, et al: Increased need for thyroxine during pregnancy in women with primary hypothyroidism. N Engl J Med 323:91, 1990

26. Casey BM, Dashe JS, Wells E, et al: Subclinical hypothyroidism and pregnancy outcomes. Obstet Gynecol 105:239, 2005

27. Haddow JE, Palomaki GE, Allen WC, et al: Maternal thyroid deficiency during pregnancy and subsequent neuropsychological development of the child. N Engl J Med 341:549, 1999

28. Stagnaro-Green A: Postpartum thyroiditis. Best Pract Res Clin Endocrinol Metab 18:303, 2004

29. Bates SM: Treatment and prophylaxis of venous thromboembolism during pregnancy. Thromb Res 108:97, 2003

30. American College of Obstetricians and Gynecologists. ACOG Committee Opinion: safety of Lovenox in pregnancy. Obstet Gynecol 100:845, 2002

31. Sephton V, Farquharson RG, Topping J, et al: A longitudinal study of maternal dose response to low molecular weight heparin in pregnancy. Obstet Gynecol 101:1307, 2003

32. Kupferminc MJ, Eldor A, Steinman N, et al: Increased frequency of genetic thrombophilia in women with complications of pregnancy. N Engl J Med 340:9, 1999

33. Infante-Rivard C, Rivard GE, Yotov WV, et al: Absence of association of thrombophilia polymorphisms with intrauterine growth restriction. N Engl J Med 347:19, 2002

34. Clark SL: Asthma in pregnancy. National Asthma Education Program Working Group on Asthma and Pregnancy. National Institutes of Health, National Heart, Lung and Blood Institute. Obstet Gynecol 82:1036, 1993

35. Dombrowski MP, Schatz M, Wise R, et al: Asthma during pregnancy. Obstet Gynecol 103:5, 2004

36. Managing Asthma During Pregnancy: Recommendations for Pharmacologic Treatment—Update 2004. NIH Publication Number 05-3279. National Institutes of Health, Washington, DC, 2005

37. Brown ZA, Wald A, Morrow RA, et al: Effect of serologic status and cesarean delivery on transmission rates of herpes simplex virus from mother to infant. JAMA 289:203, 2003

38. Corey L, Wald A, Patel R, et al: Once-daily valacyclovir to reduce the risk of transmission of genital herpes. Valacyclovir HSV Transmission Study Group. N Engl J Med 350:11, 2004

39. Young NS, Brown KE: Parvovirus B19. N Engl J Med 350:586, 2004

40. Harger JH, Adler SP, Koch WC, et al: Prospective evaluation of 618 pregnant women exposed to parvovirus B19: risks and symptoms. Obstet Gynecol 91:413, 1998

41. Watts DH: Management of human immunodeficiency virus infection in pregnancy. N Engl J Med 346:1879, 2002

42. Connor EM, Sperling RS, Gelber R, et al: Reduction of maternal-infant transmission of human immunodeficiency virus type 1 with zidovudine treatment. Pediatric AIDS Clinical Trials Group Protocol 076 Study Group. N Engl J Med 331:1173, 1994

43. The mode of delivery and the risk of vertical transmission of human immunodeficiency virus type 1. The International Perinatal HIV Group. N Engl J Med 340:977, 1999

44. Van de Perre P: Postnatal transmission of human immunodeficiency virus type 1: the breast-feeding dilemma. Am J Obstet Gynecol 173:483, 1995

45. American College of Obstetricians and Gynecologists, ACOG Committee Opinion: number 279, December 2002. Prevention of early-onset group B streptococcal disease in newborns. Obstet Gynecol 100:1405, 2002

46. Jones DC, Hayslett JP: Outcome of pregnancy in women with moderate or severe renal insufficiency. N Engl J Med 335:226, 1996

47. Davison JM: Dialysis, transplantation and pregnancy. Am J Kidney Dis 17:127, 1991

48. Cervera R, Font J, Carmona F, et al: Pregnancy outcome in systemic lupus erythematosus: good news for the new millennium. Autoimmun Rev 1:354, 2002

49. Brucato A, Frassi M, Franceschini F, et al: Risk of congenital complete heart block in newborns of mothers with anti-Ro/SSA antibodies detected by counterimmunoelectrophoresis: a prospective study of 100 women. Arthritis Rheum 44:1832, 2001

50. Shinohara K, Miyagawa S, Fujita T, et al: Neonatal lupus erythematosus: results of

maternal corticosteroid therapy. Obstet Gynecol 93:952, 1999

51. Cowchock FS, Reece EA, Balaban D, et al: Repeated fetal losses associated with antiphospholipid antibodies: a collaborative randomized trial comparing prednisone with low-dose heparin treatment. Am J Obstet Gynecol 166:1318, 1992

52. Cardonick E, Iacobucci A: Use of chemotherapy during human pregnancy. Lancet Oncol 5:283, 2004

53. Holmes LB, Harvey EA, Coull BA, et al: The teratogenicity of anticonvulsant drugs. N Engl J Med 344:1132, 2001

54. Richmond JR, Krishnamoorthy P, Andermann E, et al: Epilepsy and pregnancy: an obstetric perspective. Am J Obstet Gynecol 190:371, 2004

55. Confavreux C, Hutchinson M, Hours MM, et al: Rate of pregnancy-related relapse in multiple sclerosis. Pregnancy in Multiple Sclerosis Group. N Engl J Med 339:285, 1998

56. National Institute for Clinical Excellence: Guidance on the use of nicotine replacement therapy (NRT) and bupropion for smoking cessation. Technology Appraisal Guidance No 39. National Institute for Clinical Excellence, London, 2002

57. Singer LT, Arendt R, Minnes S, et al: Cognitive and motor outcomes of cocaine-exposed infants. JAMA 287:1952, 2002

58. Effective medical treatment of opiate addiction. National Consensus Development Panel on Effective Medical Treatment of Opiate Addiction. JAMA 280:1936, 1998

59. Fetal alcohol syndrome and alcohol-related neurodevelopmental disorders. American Academy of Pediatrics, Committee on Substance Abuse and Committee on Children With Disabilities. Pediatrics 106:358, 2000

60. Eskenazi B: Caffeine: filtering the facts. N Engl J Med 341:1688, 1999

61. Mullally BA, Hansen WF: Intrahepatic cholestasis of pregnancy: review of the literature. Obstet Gynecol Surv 57:47, 2002

62. Palma J, Reyes H, Ribalta J, Hernandez I, et al: Ursodeoxycholic acid in the treatment of cholestasis of pregnancy: a randomized, double-blind study controlled with placebo. J Hepatol 27:1022, 1997

63. Weigel RM, Weigel MM: Nausea and vomiting of early pregnancy and pregnancy outcome: a meta-analytical review. Br J Obstet Gynaecol 96:1312, 1989

64. Vutyavanich T, Wongtra-ngan S, Ruangsri R, et al: Pyridoxine for nausea and vomiting of pregnancy: a randomized, double-blind, placebo-controlled trial. Am J Obstet Gynecol 173:881, 1995

65. American College of Obstetricians and Gynecologists: ACOG (American College of Obstetrics and Gynecology) Practice Bulletin: nausea and vomiting of pregnancy. Obstet Gynecol 103:803, 2004

66. Maynard SE, Min Y, Merchan J, et al: Excess placental soluble fms-like tyrosine kinase (sFlt1) may contribute to endothelial dysfunction, hypertension, and proteinuria in preeclampsia. J Clin Invest 111:649, 2003

67. American Diabetes Association Position Statement: Gestational diabetes. Diabetes Care 26:S103, 2003

68. Crowther C, Hiller JE, Moss JR, et al: Effect of treatment of gestational diabetes on pregnancy outcomes. N Engl J Med 352:2477, 2005

69. Langer O, Conway DL, Berkus MD, et al: A comparison of glyburide and insulin in women with gestational diabetes mellitus. N Engl J Med 343:1134, 2004

70. Kim C, Newton KM, Knopp RH: Gestational diabetes and the incidence of type 2 diabetes: a systematic review. Diabetes Care 25:1862, 2002

71. Buchanan TA, Xiang AH, Peters RK, et al: Preservation of pancreatic beta-cell function and prevention of type 2 diabetes by pharmacological treatment of insulin resistance in high-risk Hispanic women. Diabetes 51:2796, 2002

85 Menopause

Susan D. Reed, M.D., M.P.H., *and Eliza L. Sutton,* M.D., F.A.C.P.

Definitions

The female reproductive system matures in a continuous, natural process from menarche to menopause, as the finite numbers of oocytes produced during fetal development are gradually lost to ovulation and senescence. Menopause is defined as the permanent cessation of menses[1]; by convention, the diagnosis of menopause is not made until the individual has had 12 months of amenorrhea. Menopause is thus characterized by the menstrual changes that reflect oocyte depletion and subsequent reduction in ovarian hormone production. However, the manifestations that occur around the time of menopause are caused by the underlying ovarian changes, rather than by the cessation of menstruation itself. Therefore, a woman who has undergone a hysterectomy but who retains her ovaries will experience normal menopausal symptoms as oocyte depletion leads to hypoestrogenism, even though cessation of menstruation occurred with surgery.

Natural menopause occurs at or after 40 years of age and has no underlying pathologic cause [*see* Natural Menopause, *below*]. Induced menopause may occur after chemotherapy, pelvic radiation, or, most commonly, bilateral oophorectomy. Menopause is considered premature when it occurs before 40 years of age but is otherwise natural [*see* Premature Ovarian Failure, *below*].

The climacteric, a term now used infrequently, refers to the time of waning ovarian function associated with menstrual irregularity and vasomotor symptoms. Perimenopause is the time between the onset of the climacteric and the year after the last menses. Menopausal transition is replacing perimenopause and climacteric as the preferred term to describe the time of physiologic change around the cessation of ovarian function [*see Figure 1*].[2] Premenopause is the entire reproductive span before onset of the menopausal transition, and postmenopause is the span of life after menopause.

In the past, natural menopause was considered to be an endocrinopathy, with the ovary depicted as a failing organ and estrogen considered the optimal therapy. Given that menopause is a normal transition in the lives of most women and that significant risks have been associated with postmenopausal hormone "replacement," the viewpoint of menopause as an endocrinopathy is no longer espoused.

Natural Menopause

EPIDEMIOLOGY

The menopausal transition, which precedes menopause, has an average duration of 4 years, with a range of 0 to 10 years.[3-5] The mean age at which menopause occurs in developed countries is 51 years[4,6,7] and may be increasing.[8] The standard deviation around this mean is about 2 years.[4,9] Approximately 95% of women experience menopause by 55 years of age.[4] Several factors appear to influence the age at which women experience menopausal symptoms and the final menstrual period; for example, menopause occurs approximately 1 year earlier in smokers[6,7,10] and nulliparous women.[6,7] Menopause may also occur earlier in women who have had ovarian cystectomies or unilateral oophorectomies.[11]

PHYSIOLOGY AND GENETICS OF REPRODUCTIVE AGING

Ovarian follicular depletion, by means of atresia, is the final common pathway in female reproductive aging. At 5 months of fetal age, the ovaries contain their peak number of primordial follicles, totaling approximately two million. At birth, girls have one million primordial follicles, approximately 25% of which remain at puberty. During the reproductive years, many follicles will begin to develop during each ovulatory cycle; all but one, the dominant follicle, become atretic. An estimated 1,000 follicles remain in the ovaries of a woman 51 years of

Stages of reproductive aging	Reproductive Years			Menopausal Transition		Postmenopause	
	Early	Peak	Late	Early	Late*	Early*	Late
				Perimenopause			
Duration of stage	Variable			Variable		1 yr / 4 yr	Until demise
Menstrual cycles	Variable to regular	Regular		Variable cycle length (> 7 days different from normal)	≥ 2 skipped cycles and an interval of amenorrhea (≥ 60 days)	0 / None	
Endocrine function (FSH levels)	Normal		Elevated or normal	Elevated or normal		↑ / Elevated	

*Stages most likely to be characterized by vasomotor symptoms.

↑ Final Menstrual Period

Figure 1   **The Stages of Reproductive Aging Workshop (STRAW) reproductive staging system showing the relationship of the final menstrual period with menstrual cycle changes and FSH serum concentrations.[2] (FSH—follicle-stimulating hormone, ↑—elevated)**

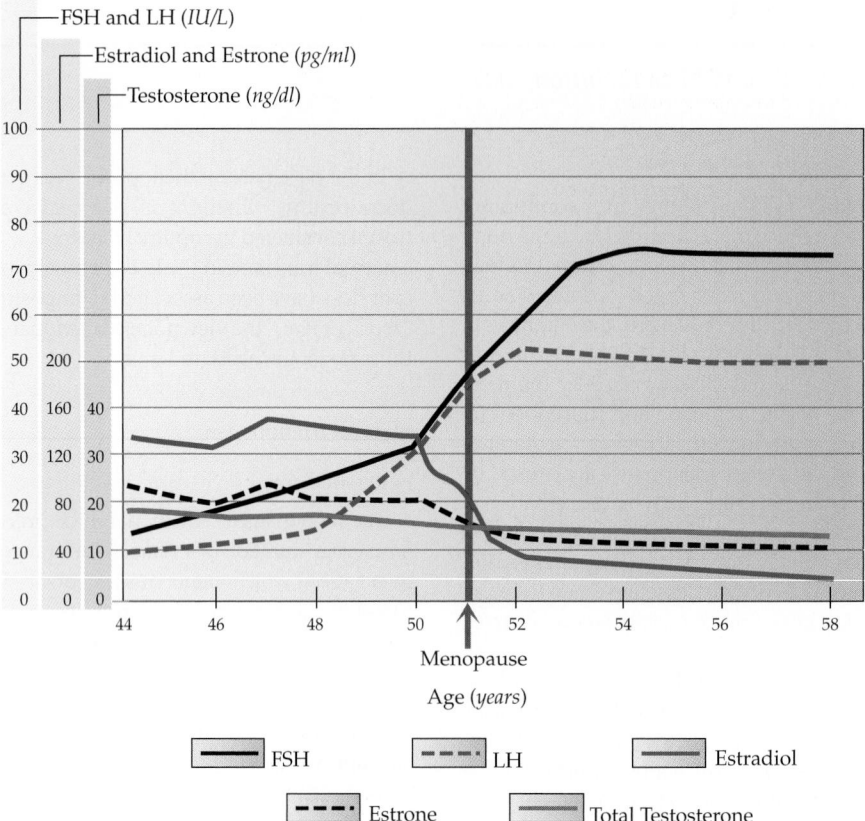

Figure 2 **Approximate average serum concentrations of estradiol, estrone, FSH, LH, and total testosterone during the menopausal transition and postmenopause. A subtle rise in FSH occurs first, followed by a rise in LH and a decline in estradiol and estrone. There are no abrupt changes in testosterone, but a gradual continuous decline occurs that begins before the menopausal transition.[130]**

age.[12] Some poorly responsive follicles persist for a few years after the menopause.[13] This progressive loss of follicles that accompanies aging is characteristic of all mammals studied to date; however, the controlling factors for this process have not been well defined.

Beginning as early as 10 to 15 years before menopause, the length of the menstrual cycle progressively decreases, owing to a shortening of the follicular phase of the cycle. The observed decrease in cycle length continues until the onset of the menopausal transition, when both the average cycle length and the standard deviation of cycle length begin to increase as follicles are depleted and ovulation occurs less frequently.[4,14] Insufficient follicular development results in inadequate estrogen production. With little estrogen available to stimulate the endometrium, amenorrhea results.

There is good evidence that the timing of natural menopause is genetically programmed,[15-17] but the specific genes involved are yet to be well defined. Common allelic variants of the estrogen receptor gene (estrogen receptor–α [ER-α] and ER-β) contribute to the variability in the timing of menopause.[18] In addition, all of the steroid receptors, as well as the proteins and enzymes involved in steroid biosynthesis and metabolism, are known to be coded by polymorphic sites (genetic changes found in at least 1% of the population). This genetic variability adds to the complexity of the actions and interactions of the reproductive steroids and to the timing and extent of menopausal symptoms.

PHYSIOLOGIC CHANGES IN MENOPAUSE

Hormonal Changes

A subtle rise in the concentration of follicle-stimulating hormone (FSH) is the earliest and most consistent clinically measurable hormonal change noted in studies of reproductive aging.[19,20] An FSH level measured during the early follicular stage of the menstrual cycle that is greater than two standard deviations above the mean level in women of reproductive age is a marker of impending menopausal transition.[2] Luteinizing hormone (LH) levels remain normal initially, but they eventually become elevated as ovarian steroid secretion falls and gonadotropin-releasing hormone (GnRH) increases [*see Figures 2 and 3*]. The early selective increase in FSH appears to be caused by decreased secretion of the hormone inhibin B by the ovarian granulosa cells and is a marker of follicular atresia. Inhibin A and B, hormones that are involved in directing follicular development and were first characterized in the 1990s, suppress pituitary FSH production.[21,22] As anovulation predominates, FSH and LH remain chronically elevated (i.e., there is a 10-fold to 20-fold increase in the FSH level and a threefold to fivefold increase in the LH level),[19,21,23] and estradiol levels fall below 50 pg/ml [*see Figure 2*].

The physiologic changes that are associated with menopause are predominantly reflected by changes in circulating levels of estrogens, androgens, and progesterone [*see Figures 2 and 3*]. The hormonal system is made more complex by fluctuations in steroid hormones that alternate between free and bound states. Sex hormone–binding globulin affects serum levels of all steroid hormones, binding preferentially to testosterone, estrogen, and progesterone, in that order.

During the reproductive years, estradiol (E_2) is the principal estrogen, both in quantity and in potency; estrone (E_1) is present in a significant amount but is less potent than estradiol. Estriol (E_3), a weak estrogen, is a metabolite of estrone and estradiol. Despite diminished fertility and ongoing follicular atresia, the ovulatory cycles of women in the menopausal transition have normal to high concentrations of circulating estradiol and estrone. In fact, as women approach the menopausal transition, preovulatory estradiol levels can be higher than those seen in younger women.[24,25]

After menopause, estradiol production drops by 90%,[19,21] owing to follicular atresia [see Figures 2 and 3a]. What little estradiol is produced after menopause comes primarily from peripheral conversion of estrone. Estrone, the dominant estrogen after menopause, is produced through peripheral conversion of adrenal androstenedione by aromatase, primarily in adipose tissues [see Figure 3d]. Fatty breast tissue is a principal site of aromatase activity, but activity is also present in the brain, muscle, liver, and, minimally, the ovary of a postmenopausal woman.

As reproductive aging progresses, serum levels of androgens decrease but not to the extent that estrogen levels diminish. Androstenedione levels drop by approximately 50%,[26-28] ovarian

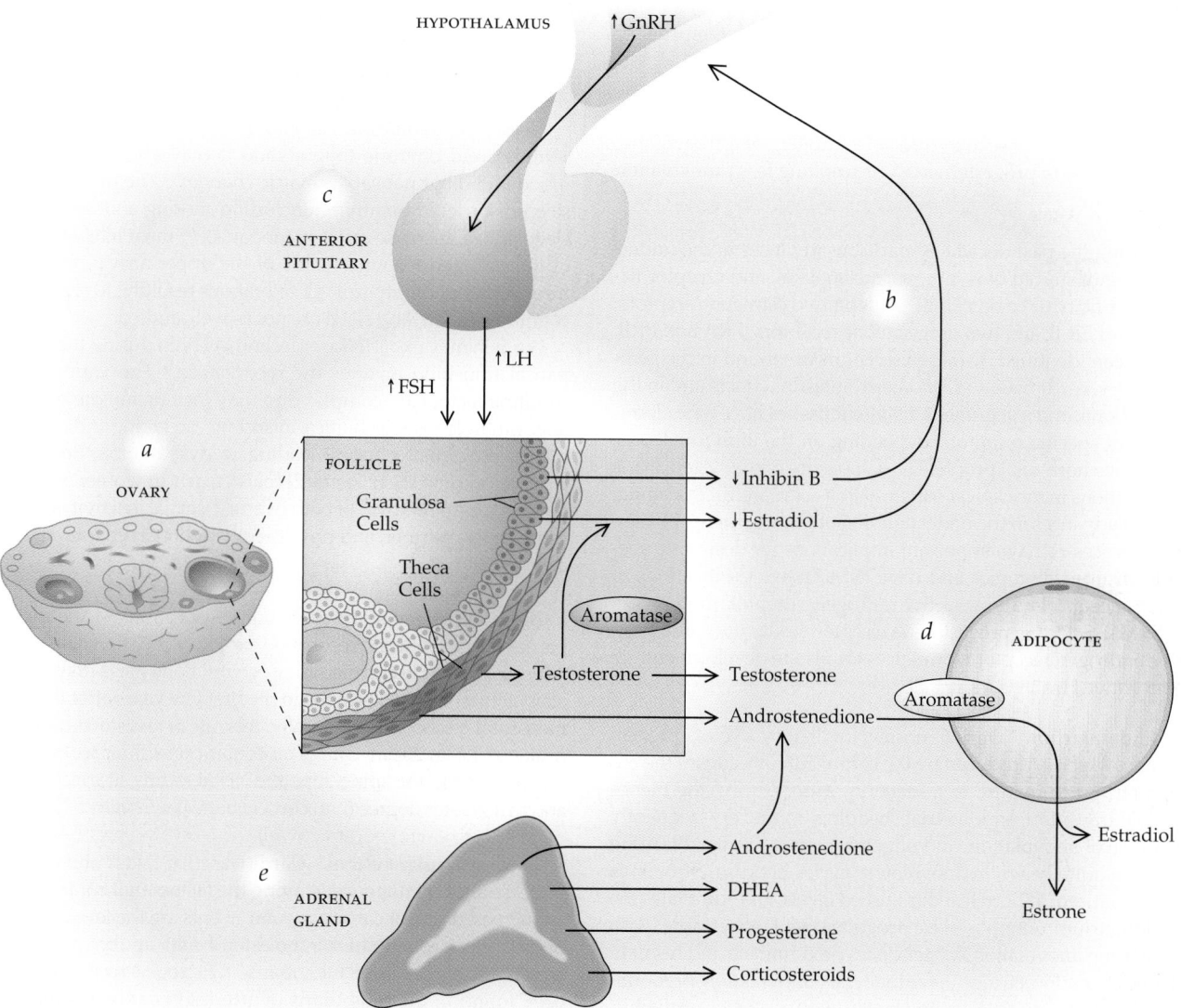

Figure 3   Multiple hormonal changes are associated with reproductive aging. (a) Within the ovary, secretion of inhibin B by granulosa cells decreases when a woman is in her mid-30s, and follicular depletion results in increasing rates of anovulation and diminished ovulatory surges of estradiol and estrone by her early 40s. Ovarian testosterone secretion continues; some ovarian testosterone is converted to estradiol by the enzyme aromatase, and the remainder is secreted as testosterone or the androgen precursor androstenedione. (b) In the menopausal transition, decreased circulating levels of inhibin and, subsequently, decreasing estradiol concentrations result in stimulation of the hypothalamus to increase secretion of GnRH. (c) Elevated circulating GnRH levels stimulate the anterior pituitary to increase secretion of FSH, followed by an increase in LH. Eventually, attempts by the brain to drive the ovary to produce estrogen fail, but production of androstenedione and testosterone by the ovarian theca cells continues in early menopause. (d) With diminished serum estrogen levels, adipocytes are stimulated to convert androstenedione to estrone via the enzyme aromatase. (e) Hormonal synthesis by the adrenal gland remains fairly constant, undergoing changes associated with aging, not menopause per se.

production declines [*see Figure 3a*], and adrenal output remains relatively constant [*see Figure 3e*]. Testosterone decreases by approximately 30% and continues to be secreted by the ovarian stroma, under the influence of LH [*see Figure 3a*].[26-28] Serum concentrations of the adrenal androgen precursor dehydroepiandrosterone (DHEA) decrease with biologic aging, beginning before the final menstrual period [*see Figure 3e*].[26]

During the reproductive years, the principal source of progesterone is the corpus luteum; small concentrations of progesterone continue to be produced by the adrenal gland after the menopause [*see Figure 3e*].

The overall changes in reproductive steroid hormones observed following menopause include the following:

• Negligible estradiol production by the ovary
• A shift from the ovary to the adrenal gland as the primary source of estrogen precursors
• Emergence of estrone as the dominant estrogen
• Continued testosterone production by the ovarian stroma
• An overall increase in the ratio of androgens to estrogens
• A decrease in progesterone levels resulting from anovulation

Target Tissues

During the past decade, remarkable advances in the understanding of steroid biosynthesis, metabolism, and receptor tissue specificity have occurred.[29] At least two estrogen receptors, ER-α and ER-β, and two progesterone receptors, PRA and PRB, have been identified. Estrogen receptors are found in the genitourinary, cardiovascular, and gastrointestinal tracts and in the brain, bone, and integument. Different tissues have a predominance of specific receptors, depending on the individual's endogenous hormonal profile. The complexity of the system leads to variations in the clinical manifestations of reproductive aging. Recent advances in the understanding of these complex physiologic processes have important implications for designing specific targeted therapies and have led to new classifications of pharmaceuticals: the selective estrogen receptor modulators (SERMs). Selective progesterone receptor modulators and selective androgen receptor modulators are also in development [*see Preventive Health Care, below*].

Endometrium During normal ovulatory cycles, progesterone, which is produced by the corpus luteum, causes the endometrium to mature to a secretory state. During the menopausal transition, endometrial shedding occurs less frequently because of anovulation, and oligomenorrhea results.[4] Bleeding may be quite heavy in anovulatory cycles because estrogen is still produced, although at diminished levels, and stimulates the endometrium unopposed by progesterone. Furthermore, with increasing anovulation, longer cycles predominate and result in a thicker endometrium. Eventually, as anovulation predominates and estradiol production by the ovary becomes negligible, amenorrhea results.

Genitourinary epithelium The vagina is a principal target tissue for estrogen. Estrogen matures the vaginal epithelium, making it thicker and rugated. The estrogen-stimulated epithelial cells produce more glycogen, which in turn changes the bacterial flora and increases vaginal acidity.[30] Hypoestrogenism results in thinning of the vaginal and vulvar epithelium. The base of the bladder is also derived from müllerian tissue and likewise is estrogen sensitive. Epithelial changes in the bladder are similar to those occurring in the vagina and vulva and result in thin, pale, friable tissues.

Central and sympathetic nervous systems Fluctuations in estrogen levels are associated with hot flushes.[31] Hot flushes are caused by thermoregulatory dysfunction that is most likely initiated by the hypothalamus in response to estrogen withdrawal. Small elevations in core body temperature are followed by peripheral vasodilation. This results in a sensation of warmth and perspiration, both of which occur at a core body temperature that is lower than normal.[32] To be susceptible to hot flushes, a woman needs to have been exposed to reproductive levels of estrogen and then experience estrogen withdrawal. For example, women with Turner syndrome, who never attain reproductive levels of estrogen, do not experience hot flushes.

Alterations in dopamine, norepinephrine, and serotonin pathways[33-35] associated with systemic estrogen fluctuations may contribute to the vasomotor symptoms experienced during the menopausal transition and postmenopause. In addition to hot flushes and diaphoresis, symptoms may include a sense of prickling of the skin, heart palpitations, and anxiety.

Sleep disruption from vasomotor instability can result in insomnia[36] and daytime fatigue, and it may also contribute to mood and other neuropsychiatric changes.[37] The prevalence of sleep-disordered breathing, including snoring and obstructive sleep apnea, increases after menopause,[38,39] most likely because of the estrogen responsiveness of the upper airway musculature.[40] Other pathophysiologic alterations resulting in changes in cognition, mood, and sleep are not as well studied.

Women may experience a decline in libido during the menopausal transition or after the menopause.[41] The various contributing factors are complex and may include fatigue or stress (e.g., multiple responsibilities, including caretaking and employment), urogenital atrophy leading to dyspareunia, decreased testosterone levels [*see Figure 2*] (particularly in women who undergo surgical removal of both ovaries), sexual inactivity or dysfunction in a partner, and physical or emotional separation from a partner.

Bone Estrogen suppresses bone resorption. At the menopausal transition, bone resorption exceeds formation, and an accelerated loss in bone mass may occur.[42] Bone mass may be lost at an annual rate of 3% to 5% in the first few years after the final menstrual period, but eventually, this rate of loss slows and continues at 1% to 2% a year.[43] Trabecular bone, the predominant type of bone in the spine, hip, and distal radius, is affected first and to a greater degree than cortical bone [*see Chapter 57*].

Cardiovascular system Cardiovascular risks[44] and events[45] increase after menopause. Among the factors that contribute to an increased risk of cardiovascular events are the levels of low-density lipoprotein (LDL) cholesterol and apolipoprotein B, which are higher after menopause.[46] Estrogen receptors have been found in the muscularis of arteries in cardiovascular tissue.[29] Estrogens appear to have a direct vasodilatory effect on the coronary artery, mediated by the formation and release of endothelium-derived relaxing factor, reduction of endothelin levels, and the promotion of prostacyclin production.[47]

Coagulation factors Menopause has been associated with increases in factor VII, factor VIII, plasminogen activator inhibitor–1 (PAI-1), and fibrinogen; all of these changes can lead to hypercoagulable states. Conversely, menopause has been associated with increased levels of antithrombin III and activated protein C, which may be beneficial in that these factors diminish

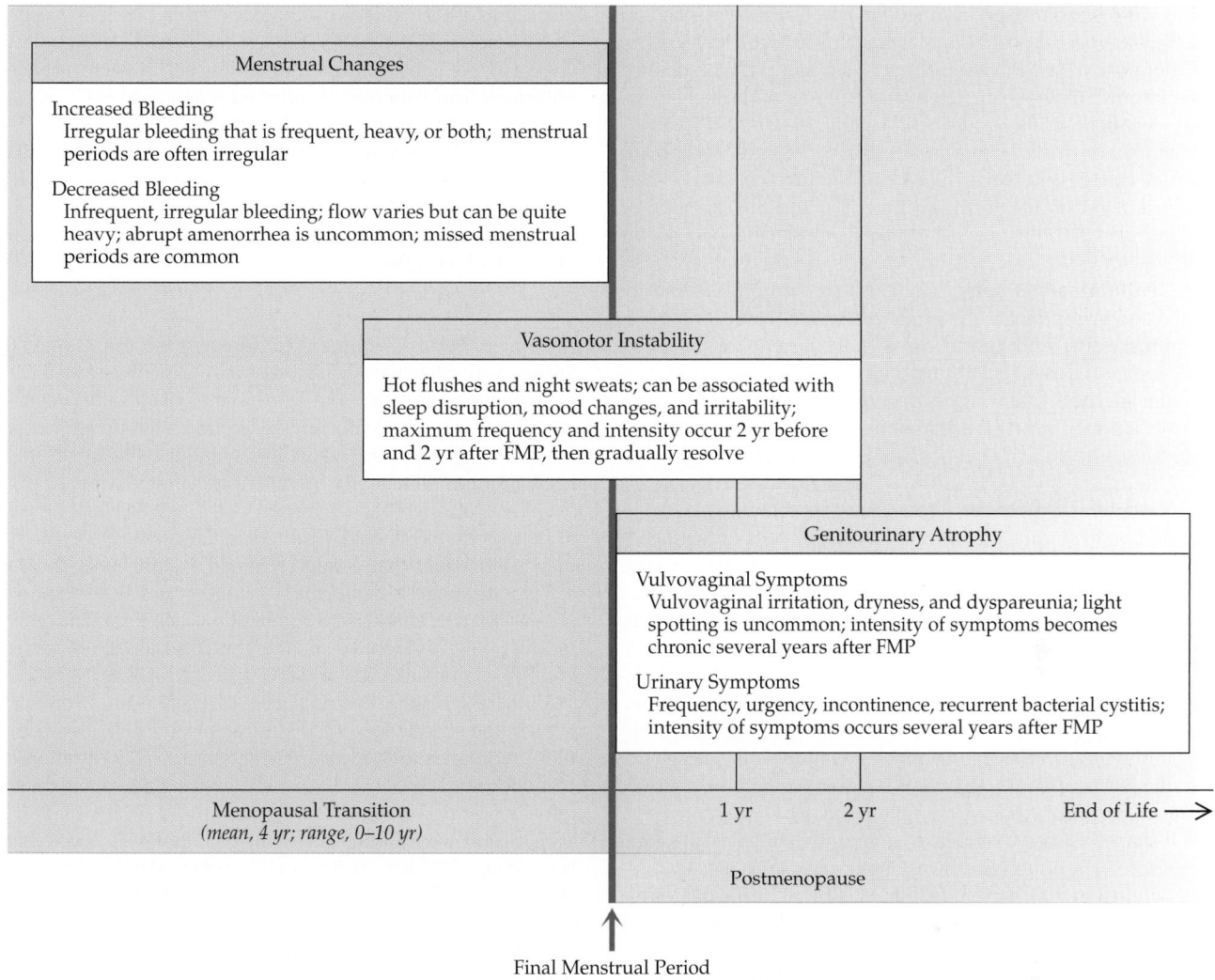

Menstrual Changes
Increased Bleeding Irregular bleeding that is frequent, heavy, or both; menstrual periods are often irregular **Decreased Bleeding** Infrequent, irregular bleeding; flow varies but can be quite heavy; abrupt amenorrhea is uncommon; missed menstrual periods are common

Vasomotor Instability
Hot flushes and night sweats; can be associated with sleep disruption, mood changes, and irritability; maximum frequency and intensity occur 2 yr before and 2 yr after FMP, then gradually resolve

Genitourinary Atrophy
Vulvovaginal Symptoms Vulvovaginal irritation, dryness, and dyspareunia; light spotting is uncommon; intensity of symptoms becomes chronic several years after FMP **Urinary Symptoms** Frequency, urgency, incontinence, recurrent bacterial cystitis; intensity of symptoms occurs several years after FMP

Menopausal Transition
(mean, 4 yr; range, 0–10 yr)

1 yr   2 yr   End of Life ⟶

Postmenopause

Final Menstrual Period

Figure 4   **Characteristic symptoms of the menopausal transition and menopause. Peak vasomotor symptoms occur around the time of the final menstrual period. Menstrual changes are common before the menopause; abrupt amenorrhea preceded by normal cycles is unusual. Genitourinary atrophy is most common in postmenopause.**

coagulation.[48] It is unknown whether these changes are caused by hypoestrogenism alone or by a combination of hormonal changes observed at the time of menopause.

Integument   A decrease in the production of dermal collagen and a subsequent reduction in dermal thickness[49] result in significant changes in women's skin, including wrinkles and dryness. In addition, a reduced rate of cutaneous wound healing has been associated with diminished secretion of transforming growth factor–β1 (TGF-β1) by dermal fibroblasts.[50]

Target-sensitive tissues and neoplastic growth   Changes in the balance of reproductive hormones at the time of menopause have been associated with increased neoplastic growth in specific tissues. Hormonally sensitive neoplasms of the breast, colon, ovary, endometrium, and myometrium (leiomyoma) are widely recognized. Leiomyomas commonly increase in size during the menopausal transition but diminish in the postmenopausal period, presumably as a result of low levels of estradiol and progesterone. Other less common neoplasms occur in the gastrointestinal tract (esophageal and gastric)[51]; blood vessels; adipose and angiolymphatic tissues (angiomyolipoma,[52] lymphangio-

myomatosis)[53]; and the central nervous system (meningioma).[54] All of these neoplastic tissues have been found to have reproductive hormone receptors and appear to be sensitive to steroid hormones. Contrary to previous evidence, recent observations suggest that melanoma is not progesterone sensitive.[55]

DIAGNOSIS

The diagnosis of menopausal transition may be suspected on the basis of symptoms (e.g., menstrual irregularity and vasomotor symptoms) in a woman older than 40 years [*see Figure 4*] well before it can be proven by FSH testing [*see* Laboratory Tests, *below*]. The clinical diagnosis of natural menopause is made if a woman is of an appropriate age and has had 12 months of amenorrhea accompanied by symptoms suggestive of ovarian failure, at which point the FSH serum concentration is so certainly elevated that testing is usually not useful.

Clinical Manifestations

Reproductive system changes   The most common changes in the bleeding pattern in the menopausal transition are shortened cycle length, heavier flow (menorrhagia), and irregular cycle length (metrorrhagia). Intermenstrual bleeding may also occur, but it warrants specific attention because of its association with endometrial neoplasia in women older than 40 years [*see* Laboratory Tests, Biopsy, *below*]. A woman with vasomotor symptoms who has completely missed a menses is likely to experience her final menstrual period within the next 1 to 2 years.[14] Menopause usually occurs several years after the onset of menstrual changes; however, about 10% of women experience abrupt onset of amenorrhea.[3,4] Infertility and the cessation of menses are the only universal manifestations of menopause.

Genitourinary atrophy Genitourinary atrophy is typically mild and asymptomatic during the menopausal transition, but it is progressive and can become quite severe in the postmenopausal years.[3,31] Atrophic vulvovaginitis can present as vaginal dryness, vulvovaginal pruritus, vaginal dyspareunia, or postcoital spotting. Atrophic urethritis and recurrent cystitis can manifest as dysuria, frequency, and incontinence.

Vasomotor symptoms Vasomotor symptoms (i.e., hot flushes and night sweats) are common manifestations of the menopausal transition; for example, 80% of white women experience vasomotor symptoms.[56] Women typically describe hot flushes as a strong sensation of warmth accompanied by flushing, a prickling sensation of the skin, and perspiration that seems to move from the trunk toward the head before it dissipates. These flushes are spontaneous, uncomfortable, and unpredictable, and they can occur any time of the day or night. Each episode is self-limited and typically lasts several minutes. A number of women describe feeling excessively warm in a more continuous pattern. The frequency of vasomotor symptoms may be represented by a bell-shaped curve that peaks around the time of the final menses.[3,37] The occurrence of vasomotor symptoms usually ceases within 4 to 5 years from first onset, although 10% of women may suffer symptoms for much longer (up to 10 years).[14,37]

Changes in libido, sleep, mood, and cognition Changes in mood, libido, and sleep may also occur but are variable in severity[37] and have a wider differential diagnosis. Snoring and daytime sleepiness suggest the possibility of obstructive sleep apnea. Women may complain of mildly diminished cognitive capacity, particularly during the menopausal transition; however, this has not been well studied.

Physical Examination

There are no pathognomonic physical findings in the menopausal transition. However, the physical examination may provide information that suggests the presenting symptoms are the result of an underlying pathologic condition and are not related to normal menopausal transition. Palpation of the thyroid gland and examination for physical signs of hypothyroidism or hyperthyroidism are warranted, particularly if menstrual irregularity, excessive diaphoresis, or neurocognitive changes are present. When intermenstrual bleeding is reported, speculum examination should be performed to rule out cervical or vaginal lesions, such as endocervical polyps. Bimanual pelvic examination is indicated when bleeding is heavy or frequent, to rule out the presence of adnexal masses and evaluate the uterus for fibroids; it is also indicated when pregnancy is possible. When the clinical presentation of oligomenorrhea or amenorrhea is not classic for the menopausal transition, prolactinoma may be suspected, in which case visual-field testing for bitemporal hemianopsia and breast examination for galactorrhea are appropriate. In addition,

inspection of the skin for needle tracks from possible injection use of heroin and evaluation for low body weight or significant weight loss may be useful, because these findings suggest a hypothalamic cause for oligomenorrhea or amenorrhea.

After menopause, vulvovaginal atrophy typically occurs. The vulvovaginal skin may appear pale, thin, and friable and may exhibit a loss of rugae and possible fissuring and erythema. The uterus is smaller, measuring 5 to 6 cm in length, and the ovaries are usually nonpalpable. The cervix may become stenotic and flush with the vagina.

Laboratory Tests

Urine or serum β–human chorionic gonadotropin (β-hCG) testing is crucial in the evaluation of any woman suspected to be in menopausal transition but who has the potential for pregnancy and who presents with a missed period, oligomenorrhea, or irregular vaginal bleeding with or without pain. In addition, testing for high-sensitivity thyroid-stimulating hormone (TSH) should be considered when menorrhagia, excessive diaphoresis, or neurocognitive changes—all potentially associated with the menopausal transition—suggest thyroid dysfunction. If the clinical picture suggests hemorrhagic diathesis, it may be helpful to obtain a platelet count, prothrombin time, and partial thromboplastin time. Additional evaluation for coagulopathies, such as von Willebrand factor, should follow, if appropriate.

With the onset of menstrual irregularity, there are wide variations in the production of FSH, estradiol, and LH.[23] Because of these wide variations, measurement of serum concentrations of these hormones is generally not useful during the menopausal transition and is not indicated unless the clinical situation is atypical and suggests an underlying condition. An elevated follicular-stage FSH level demonstrates that ovarian function is declining, but the FSH level cannot predict when the final menstrual period will occur.[19,21,23] Once a woman has had 12 months without a menses, the FSH is reliably elevated at 25 IU/L, and the estradiol level is less than 50 pg/ml.

Oral contraceptive use during the menopausal transition will treat menopausal symptoms and mask menopause. Oral contraceptives suppress FSH; therefore, the FSH should be drawn on the seventh day of placebo pills or the seventh day of the pill-free week. If menopause has occurred, the serum FSH level will be greater than 25 IU/L when drawn on two separate occasions.

Measurement of FSH serum concentration can assist in the diagnosis of menopause in a woman with vasomotor symptoms who has had a hysterectomy without oophorectomy. FSH testing may also be appropriate in the evaluation of atypical clinical situations; for example, in a case of abrupt-onset amenorrhea in a 40-year-old woman with negative β-hCG testing, measurement of FSH, prolactin, and TSH concentrations should be performed to evaluate for premature ovarian failure, prolactinoma, or thyroid dysfunction [*see* Differential Diagnosis, *below*].

Tests of other body fluids Vaginal fluid pH is elevated after menopause, and vaginal cytology shows a decreased maturation index (increase in parabasal cells).[30] These tests are not typically performed, nor are they necessary, to establish the diagnosis of menopause. In evaluation of vaginal dyspareunia or vulvovaginal pruritus, vaginal fluid pH testing and microscopic examination of vaginal fluid (saline and 10% potassium hydroxide preparations) should be performed to rule out common vaginal infections such as candidiasis, trichomoniasis, or bacterial vaginosis. It should be noted that with genitourinary atrophy, the shift toward a more basic pH can precipitate bacterial overgrowth and concomitant infection.

Imaging Studies

No imaging study is useful in establishing the diagnosis of the menopausal transition or menopause, although pelvic ultrasound may be indicated in the diagnostic evaluation of women with abnormal vaginal bleeding before or after menopause. In women who present with metrorrhagia or menorrhagia during the menopausal transition, pelvic ultrasound can confirm a diagnosis of leiomyomas or endometrial polyps and can suggest a diagnosis of adenomyosis; however, ultrasound cannot rule out endometrial neoplasia in premenopausal women [see Biopsy, below]. In contrast, ultrasound can serve as a screening test for endometrial neoplasia in postmenopausal women who experience bleeding or spotting spontaneously or in conjunction with hormone therapy (HT). In a postmenopausal woman, a homogeneous endometrial thickness of 4 mm or less confers assurance that endometrial hyperplasia or cancer is not present in more than 96% of cases.[57-59]

Biopsy In the menopausal transition, endometrial biopsy should be performed in women who experience intermenstrual bleeding (i.e., bleeding at intervals of fewer than 21 days) or in obese women who present with menometrorrhagia. If the biopsy results are normal or if examination suggests leiomyoma or adenomyosis, ultrasonography should follow. Endometrial biopsy is also indicated in postmenopausal women at heightened risk for endometrial neoplasia (e.g., women with diabetes or obesity) who experience any bleeding after 12 months of amenorrhea or who have an ultrasound result that demonstrates an endometrium at least 4 mm in thickness.

DIFFERENTIAL DIAGNOSIS

Menstrual Changes

For women 45 to 55 years of age who are experiencing progressive oligomennorhea, the most likely diagnosis is the menopausal transition, especially if there are associated vasomotor symptoms. In this setting, a wider differential diagnosis rarely needs to be considered. In younger women who have no vasomotor symptoms or whose menstrual changes are abrupt, a wider differential should be considered [see Premature Ovarian Failure, below]. The differential diagnosis for oligomenorrhea and secondary amenorrhea should always include pregnancy, prolactinoma, thyroid dysfunction, and medication or supplement use.

For women with excessive or intermenstrual bleeding, the differential diagnosis includes hypothyroidism, hyperthyroidism, blood dyscrasias, leiomyoma, adenomyosis, endometrial polyps, endometriosis, endometrial or cervical neoplasia, and hormone-secreting neoplasms such as granulosa cell ovarian cancer. Increased menstrual bleeding induced by medication or supplement use should also be considered.

Genitourinary Atrophy

Multiple conditions can cause genitourinary symptoms similar to those associated with hypoestrogenism occurring in the menopausal transition and menopause. Vulvovaginal symptoms (e.g., vaginal dryness, pruritus, dyspareunia, and postcoital spotting) may be caused by trichomonas vaginitis, yeast vulvovaginitis, bacterial vaginosis, desquamative inflammatory vaginitis, vestibulitis, allergic vulvovaginitis, and vulvar dysplasia or cancer. Urinary symptoms (e.g., dysuria, urinary frequency, and incontinence) may be caused by dietary bladder irritants, detrusor instability, urinary tract infection, and interstitial cystitis. The presence of isolated microscopic hematuria on urinalysis should prompt evaluation for neoplasia of the urinary tract.

Hot Flushes and Night Sweats

Hot flushes and night sweats may be symptoms of a number of disease processes, including hyperthyroidism, pheochromocytoma, carcinoid, and occult infection or neoplasm (e.g., tuberculosis, HIV), and lymphoma with B symptoms. Nonvolitional weight loss or documented fevers suggest a possible underlying disease. On the other hand, weight gain or existing obesity, which provides insulation against loss of body heat, may explain easy perspiration and a sensation of excess warmth in some women.

Changes in Libido, Sleep, Mood, and Cognition

The changes in libido, sleep patterns, mood, and cognition associated with the menopausal transition and menopause may also be induced by mood or anxiety disorders, thyroid dysfunction, and stress. Medications or other substances may cause insomnia, anxiety, mood abnormalities, cognitive changes, and sexual dysfunction. Other symptoms, such as fatigue, may be the result of an unrecognized sleep disorder (e.g., obstructive sleep apnea and restless legs syndrome), an inflammatory or neoplastic process, or multiple sclerosis. New cognitive dysfunction may be the first manifestation of dementia.

MENOPAUSAL TRANSITION AND POSTMENOPAUSAL SYMPTOM MANAGEMENT

Management of women experiencing menopausal symptoms is best approached by (1) defining the reproductive phase[2] of the patient [see Figure 1]; (2) identifying the menopausal symptoms for which treatment is desired [see Figure 4]; and (3) identifying the medical conditions that might influence management options [see Sidebar Internet Resources for Information on Menopause].

The menopausal transition and menopause do not warrant management in and of themselves. However, women who experience bothersome symptoms may want to consider treatment. HT is effective in controlling symptoms of the menopausal transition and menopause, but it carries risks [see Hormone Therapy Risks and Benefits, below].

The Food and Drug Administration has recommended that HT be used only for women with symptoms severe enough to warrant its use and at the lowest dose and for the shortest duration required to ease the menopausal transition. The FDA further recommends that tissue-targeted therapies be used whenever possible.[60]

Because of the potential risks associated with HT, it is recommended that all women taking HT be evaluated on an annual basis. The woman who is taking HT should be instructed to refrain from taking HT 1 week before the annual assessment to allow the physician and patient to evaluate the current severity of symptoms. Women who choose to stop HT may require a slow taper, ranging from 3 to 6 months, for successful cessation. Women on HT are encouraged to attempt cessation after 5 years of use.

Uterine Bleeding

Vaginal bleeding during the menopausal transition is best managed (after appropriate evaluation) with low-dose, combination oral contraceptives (containing 20 μg ethinyl estradiol) or a progestin intrauterine device; both protect against pregnancy and reduce menstrual blood loss. The overall effect of ethinyl estradiol at 20 μg/day is estimated to be three to four times that of 0.625 mg/day of conjugated estrogen; head-to-head trials comparing the clinical effects of the two estrogens do not exist. Although the chance of pregnancy is low (< 1% after age 50),[61] pregnancy may occur during the menopausal transition. Women 40 to 49 years of age have a rate of unintended pregnancy that is now higher than that of any other age group, even teenagers[62]; thus, it is important to address the issue of contraception with every potentially fertile woman until she has experienced 12 months of amenorrhea. Oral contraceptives can be discontinued and symptoms reassessed at approximately age 50 [see Laboratory Testing, above]. Those with persistent and severe vasomotor symptoms and amenorrhea may be transitioned to postmenopausal HT.

Genitourinary Atrophy

Symptoms of genitourinary atrophy may be present during the menopausal transition but typically become more prominent after menopause. Symptoms of genitourinary atrophy usually improve within 2 weeks after initiation of estrogen therapy and should be controlled after 1 to 3 months of use.[63] Estrogen can be administered topically with excellent local effect. Vaginal estrogen creams result in little or no systemic absorption when used at extremely low doses of less than one-eighth applicator (< 0.15 mg conjugated estrogen cream) and one-sixteenth applicator (< 0.025 mg estradiol cream); a full applicator of vaginal estrogen cream can deliver a dose equivalent to that of an oral formulation, although the rate of absorption varies considerably. Initial therapy constitutes nightly application for 2 to 6 weeks; thereafter, maintenance doses can be applied one to three times a week, depending on the severity of symptoms. Use of low-dose vaginal creams does not necessitate the use of a progestin; however, cessation of therapy results in the return of genitourinary atrophy. Low-dose vaginal estrogen rings effectively treat genitourinary atrophy with little or no systemic absorption and no significant endometrial stimulation.

Nonhormonal alternatives include lubricants for use during intercourse and vaginal moisturizers.

Vasomotor Symptoms

Estrogen is highly effective for the treatment of vasomotor symptoms. For women in the menopausal transition who are at risk for pregnancy and who have heavy or frequent menses, treatment with low-dose oral contraceptives provides amelioration of vasomotor symptoms, control of bleeding, and contraception. Cyclical HT is preferable for women in the menopausal transition who are predominantly anovulatory and who do not need contraception, because it provides lower doses of hormones than oral contraceptives. Continuous HT, which is commonly used in women who are approximately 12 months from the final menstrual period, is often associated with bothersome bleeding patterns in women in earlier stages of the menopausal transition.

Low-dose oral contraceptives and HT result in prompt resolution of symptoms within 1 to 2 weeks in 80% of women; they should be titrated to the lowest dose possible to achieve acceptable symptom relief. Systemic administration of estrogen can be achieved orally, transdermally (in the form of a gel or patch), or transmucosally (at a higher dose via the use of a vaginal ring).

Internet Resources for Information on Menopause

General Information about Menopause for Clinicians and Patients

North American Menopause Society
http://www.menopause.org

Women's Health Initiative
http://www.whi.org

Alternative Therapies for Management of Menopausal Symptoms

University of Washington School of Medicine, Department of Family Medicine, on Complementary and Alternative Medicine
http://www.fammed.washington.edu/predoctoral/CAM

ConsumerLab.com
http://www.consumerlab.com

The Longwood Herbal Task Force
http://www.longwoodherbal.org

Natural Medicines Comprehensive Database
http://www.naturaldatabase.com

Some formulations include progestins. Implants and intramuscular injections are less preferable forms of delivery because they release extremely high levels of HT at the time of administration or placement. The lowest doses of estrogens found to be effective for vasomotor symptoms include oral conjugated estrogen 0.03 mg, oral estradiol 0.5 mg, and transdermal estradiol 0.025 mg.

Several nonhormonal alternatives for treatment of vasomotor symptoms may have some efficacy. These include venlafaxine,[64,65] selective serotonin reuptake inhibitors (SSRIs) (e.g., fluoxetine and paroxetine),[66-68] and gabapentin.[69] Less evidence supports the use of clonidine[70,71] and vitamin E[72] as being effective in the control of vasomotor symptoms. Results from controlled clinical trials evaluating the effectiveness of phytoestrogens (including dietary soy) for vasomotor symptoms vary, but most studies indicate that the use of phytoestrogens offers no significant improvement over placebo in reducing the frequency of hot flushes.[73] Black cohosh, a possible phytoestrogen, may be effective, but no large controlled trials have been conducted.[74] Progestin alone is effective[75,76] but is not recommended because of a potential increased risk of breast cancer.[77] Behavioral modification[78,79] and increased exercise[78,80] may diminish the severity of hot flushes. Red clover extract, dong quai, evening primrose oil, and Siberian ginseng have not been found to be effective in small randomized, controlled trials. Other botanicals purported to be effective, including valerian, motherwort, and chasteberry, have not been studied in clinical trials.[81]

Libido, Sleep, Mood, and Cognition

Treatment of sexual dysfunction depends on the underlying etiology. If the cause of decreased libido is not predominantly psychosocial, testosterone therapies have been shown, in some circumstances, to improve sexual function, interest and frequency of desire, and psychological well-being.[82,83] There are no FDA-approved products for diminished libido in women; however, esterified estrogen combined with methyltestosterone is commonly used. Vaginal estrogen therapy, if indicated, can play an important role in the treatment of diminished sexual function resulting from urogenital atrophy.[63]

Vasomotor instability may contribute to disruption of sleep;

thus, estrogen is effective for some women who begin to experience insomnia during the menopausal transition. Alternative therapies include short-term zolpidem and low-dose trazodone.

Estrogen may be beneficial in the treatment of depression in the menopausal transition.[84] Estrogen alone, without an antidepressant, does not appear to be sufficient to treat significant clinical depression in postmenopausal women.[85] However, some investigators support the use of estrogen as an adjunct to other therapies, such as SSRIs, particularly in older women.[86]

MANAGEMENT CONSIDERATIONS

Risks and Benefits of Hormone Therapy

Although the risks and benefits of using HT for the relief or prevention of symptoms in women in the menopausal transition have not been evaluated in clinical trials, information has been established on the risk-to-benefit profile of short-term and long-term use of HT for postmenopausal women 50 to 79 years of age. Historically, it was believed that the estrogen deprivation that accompanies menopause increases the risk of some chronic diseases—specifically, heart disease, osteoporosis, and dementia. On the basis of observational data, long-term postmenopausal HT was recommended during the 1980s and 1990s not only for symptom relief but also to reduce the risk of chronic disease and to prolong life. However, two large randomized, controlled trials (i.e., Heart and Estrogen/Progestin Replacement Study [HERS][87] and the Women's Health Initiative [WHI])[88,89] called this practice into question. HT is no longer recommended for primary or secondary prevention of these conditions in women older than 50 years.

HERS demonstrated no evidence to support the use of HT for the secondary prevention of heart disease[87]; more important, WHI found that HT use conferred an increased risk of cardiovascular disease,[90] stroke,[91] dementia,[92] thromboembolism,[88] and breast cancer[93] in women 50 to 79 years of age. Striking discrepancies in the findings of the randomized trials and the earlier nonrandomized (observational) studies can be explained by selection biases in participants in the observational studies. In the observational studies, women opting for HT therapy tended to be healthier and of higher socioeconomic status than non-HT users. In addition, these women were more likely to be carefully screened for chronic disease before starting HT and, therefore, had a lower risk of developing chronic disease than nonusers of HT.[94] The selection biases inherent in the observational studies were virtually eliminated in the randomized trials.

Counseling about the risks of postmenopausal HT use should now be based on the evidence provided by WHI.[88,89,91-100] The WHI postmenopausal estrogen and progestin therapy (EPT) and estrogen therapy (ET) trials are discussed in greater detail below.

Estrogen and progestin therapy The WHI prematurely halted its clinical trial of EPT in 2002; participants had been followed for an average of 5.2 years. The trial randomized over 16,000 postmenopausal women who were 50 to 79 years of age to take either conjugated equine estrogen (0.625 mg/day) plus medroxyprogesterone acetate (2.5 mg/day) or placebo. The study was halted because the rates of adverse events (i.e., cardiovascular events, stroke, thromboembolism, and breast cancer) were 1% higher in the intervention group and overshadowed the reduced risk of osteoporotic fractures and colon cancer.[88] There was no difference in overall or disease-specific mortality between the HT and placebo groups. The study reported the following risks: (1) thromboembolic events were highest in the first year and remained elevated over 5 years (absolute risk difference, 21/10,000/yr); (2) ischemic cardiac events were highest in the first year and remained elevated and statistically unchanged thereafter (absolute risk difference, 7/10,000/yr); (3) stroke risk was not elevated in the first year, rose slightly in the second year, and remained elevated through year 5 (absolute risk difference, 8/10,000/yr); and (4) breast cancer risk was not appreciably higher in years 1 to 3 but became elevated in year 4 (absolute risk difference, 8/10,000/yr), with the increased breast cancer risk being strongest in the approximately 25% of women who had taken HT before enrolling in the study [*see Table 1*]. The EPT portion of the WHI study showed a

Table 1 WHI Findings: Outcomes Associated with Use of Combined Estrogen and Progestin and Estrogen Alone in Healthy Postmenopausal Women

Outcomes	Combined Estrogen and Progestin*		Estrogen Alone†	
	Relative Risk (95% CI)	Absolute Risk Difference‡	Relative Risk 95% (CI)	Absolute Risk Difference‡
Adverse/neutral				
Deep vein thrombosis[88,89]	2.07 (1.49–2.87)	13	1.47 (1.04–2.08)	6
Pulmonary embolism[88,89]	2.13 (1.39–3.25)	8	1.34 (0.87–2.06)	11
Coronary artery disease[89,90]	1.24 (1.00–1.54)	7	0.91 (0.75–1.12)	5
Ischemic stroke[89,91]	1.44 (1.09–1.90)	8	1.39 (1.10–1.77)	12
Breast cancer[89,93]	1.24 (1.01–1.54)	8	0.77 (0.59–1.01)	7
Probable dementia§[95,98]	2.05 (1.21–3.48)	23	1.49 (0.83–2.66)	12
Beneficial/neutral				
Colorectal cancer[88,89,100]	0.56 (0.38–0.81)	6	1.08 (0.75–1.55)	1
All fractures[88,89,96]	0.76 (0.69–0.85)	44	0.70 (0.63–0.79)	56
Mortality[88,89]	0.98 (0.82–1.18)	1	1.04 (0.88–1.22)	3

*Patients received 0.625 mg/day of conjugated estrogen and 2.5 mg/day of medroxyprogesterone acetate.
†Hysterectomized patients received 0.625 mg/day of conjugated estrogen.
‡Annual per 10,000 women.
§Ages: 65–79 yr.
CI—confidence interval

reduction in the risk of hip fractures (absolute risk difference, 6/10,000/yr)[96] and colorectal cancer (absolute risk difference, 6/10,000/yr).[100]

The Women's Health Initiative Memory Study (WHIMS), a substudy of the WHI continuous combined HT intervention trial, observed the effect of HT on memory and cognition in women 65 to 79 years of age (average age, 73 years).[92,95] A reduction in memory and thinking abilities (as measured by the Modified Mini-Mental State Examination)[95] and an increase in dementia of all types (absolute risk increase, 2/1,000/yr) were observed in women who took HT.[92]

Estrogen therapy The estrogen-only arm of WHI was halted prematurely in early 2004 because of increased risk of stroke; participants had been followed for an average of 6.8 years.[89] Over 10,000 women 50 to 79 years of age were randomized to receive 0.625 mg/day of conjugated equine estrogen or placebo. As in the EPT portion of WHI and HERS, the ET portion of the WHI trial found that estrogen use conveyed an increased risk of deep vein thrombosis (1.47 relative risk; 95% confidence interval [CI], 1.04 to 2.08) and stroke (1.39 relative risk; 95% CI, 1.10 to 1.77) [see Table 1]. Women taking ET had 12 more strokes and six more events of deep vein thrombosis a year than the women taking placebo. The study showed a reduction in the incidence of hip fractures (0.61 relative risk; 95% CI, 0.41 to 0.91) and an unanticipated, though not statistically significant, reduction in breast cancer incidence, a finding that requires further investigation. Observational studies support an increased risk of thromboembolism,[101-103] cholecystitis,[104] and breast cancer[77] in women taking ET.

In contrast to the EPT portion of the WHIMS study, women taking estrogen alone did not have a statistically increased risk of dementia.[98] For women taking ET, as compared with placebo, the risk of having a 10-unit decrease in the Modified Mini-Mental State examination scores (greater than two standard deviations) was 1.47 (95% CI, 1.04 to 2.07). The risk was greater in women with lower cognitive function at initiation of ET.[99]

Type, route of administration, and dose of HT Two observational studies[77,105] and a population-based study from Southern California[106] have increased current understanding of the type, route of administration, and dose of HT with associated breast cancer risk. The findings are as follows: (1) use of estrogen therapy confers greater risk than nonuse[77,107]; (2) use of estrogen plus progestin confers greater risk than use of estrogen alone[77,105,106]; (3) risk increases with duration of estrogen use[77,105,106]; (4) risk with estrogen use is increased in women with low or normal body mass index but not in overweight and obese women[105]; (5) increased risk of breast cancer is associated with any dose and type of commonly used estrogen (i.e., conjugated estrogen and estradiol) and progestin (i.e., medroxyprogesterone acetate, norethisterone, and levonorgestrel/norgestrel); and (6) transdermal formulations of estrogen also confer increased risk.[77] Surprisingly, the use of tibolone, a synthetic steroid with estrogenic, progestogenic, and androgenic properties that is marketed in Europe for its favorable effect on breast symptoms (e.g., tenderness and mastalgia), was also associated with a greater risk of breast cancer than nonuse of steroid hormones.[77] Current evidence indicates that all forms of HT are associated with an increased risk of breast cancer.

Transdermal delivery of estrogen may not be safer if administration is long term; however, transdermal patches and transmucosal delivery systems (including estrogen vaginal rings that provide systemic levels of estrogen for treatment of vasomotor symptoms) avoid the first-pass effect through the liver and may carry a lower risk of thromboembolism,[48,102,108,109] elevation of bile acids,[110] and hypertriglyceridemia[111] than oral estrogen. Studies of moderate- to high-dose regimens suggest that transdermal systems may have a more favorable effect on the coagulation pathway[112] and C-reactive protein[113] than oral products. Transdermal and transmucosal products have been shown to be effective as treatment for vasomotor symptoms[114] and maintenance of bone mineral density.[115]

Given the newly appreciated risks of oral progestins,[77,88] alternative approaches to progestin therapy are gaining popularity. There is a widely held belief that natural progesterone is better than synthetic progestins, but this hypothesis has never been studied. Lower-dose oral micronized progesterone formulations have been widely used in Canada and Europe and were evaluated in the Postmenopausal Estrogen/Progestin Intervention (PEPI) trial.[116] The PEPI study of 596 postmenopausal women found that micronized progesterone combined with estrogen sufficiently diminished the hyperplastic endometrial changes associated with estrogen-only therapy.[116] No other randomized clinical trials exist to better inform us about risks and safety of micronized progesterone, particularly with respect to breast cancer. Likewise, over-the-counter transdermal progesterone creams have not been studied in this regard.

In addition, attention has been directed at nonsystemic therapies. Off-label use of a progestin intrauterine system (IUS) (20 μg/day of levonorgestrel) in postmenopausal women taking estrogen provides low systemic levels of progestin and attenuation of endometrial stimulation by estrogen.[117] Intrauterine levonorgestrel at doses of 10 μg and 14 μg/day have been studied in Europe.[117,118] No increased risk of endometrial hyperplasia or cancer has been observed in women taking estrogen with a progestin IUS in place.[117] Vaginal application of progesterone creams result in local uterine and systemic effects.[119]

Preventive Health Care

The menopausal transition offers women and their health care providers the opportunity to review and focus on preventive health care measures, including basic health habits, such as regular exercise, good nutrition with calcium and vitamin D supplementation, and avoidance of smoking [see Table 2].

WHI demonstrated that HT is effective for the prevention of osteoporotic fractures and colorectal cancer in postmenopausal women, but the risks of HT outweigh the benefits[88] [see Table 1]. The prevalence of certain medical conditions (e.g., dementia, coronary artery disease, breast cancer, colon cancer, and diabetes mellitus) increases with age; it has been demonstrated that prevalence rises more steeply after loss of ovarian function. Recommended management for these conditions is almost always nonhormonal. HT is not indicated for the primary prevention of disease, unless a woman at high risk for osteoporosis chooses HT over other options after consideration of the risks and benefits.[60] Two chronic disease processes associated with hypoestrogenism and aging have a great impact on women's health in the postmenopausal years, namely cardiovascular disease and osteoporosis. Cardiovascular disease is the leading cause of death in women in the United States, and osteoporosis is a major cause of morbidity. The management of these diseases is discussed more fully elsewhere [see Chapter 57].

Table 2 Preventive and Screening Measures for Common Conditions in Postmenopausal Women

Condition	Prevention	Early Detection
Dementia	Participation in cognitive leisure activities Regular exercise Treatment of hypertension Statins and possibly other lipid-lowering agents Long-term NSAID use* Avoidance of HT initiation in postmenopause†	
CAD	Smoking cessation Regular exercise Diet high in nuts, whole-grains, and total fiber (especially water-soluble fiber), folate, and marine n-3 fatty acids Diet low in saturated fat, *trans* fatty acids, and glycemic load Daily, low-dose alcohol Prevention and treatment of hypertension, diabetes mellitus, and hyper-cholesterolemia Consideration of low-dose daily aspirin if risk of CAD events is ≥ 0.7%/yr Avoidance of HT initiation in postmenopause Statins, aspirin, and beta blockers for secondary prevention (underutilized)	
Breast cancer	Minimal exposure to HT (estrogen and/or progestin) Regular exercise Avoidance of increase in weight and waist circumference Weight loss if overweight/obese Reduction of alcohol intake to 0–20 g/day Raloxifene* if at average risk, or tamoxifen if risk ≥ 1.67%/yr	Screening mammography every 1–2 yr, with or without clinical breast exam regardless of age until clinically significant comorbid conditions
Osteoporosis	Adequate calcium and vitamin D intake Weight-bearing exercise Thiazide* diuretics Antiresorptive treatment before first osteoporotic fracture Antiresorptive treatment after osteoporotic fracture HT† if intolerant of or unresponsive to first-line agents	Screening DEXA at age 65 (earlier if risk factors)
Colon cancer	High-fiber diet for primary, but not secondary, prevention of polyps Aspirin* if personal history of adenoma or colon cancer Removal of adenomatous polyps HT* effective but not advised for this indication†	Periodic screening‡ by fecal occult blood testing or sigmoidoscopy
Diabetes mellitus	Regular exercise Weight loss if overweight/obese Metformin, acarbose, and possibly thiazolidinediones for those at high risk HT† effective but not advised for this indication	

*Off-label indication.

†Increased risk of adverse outcomes has been demonstrated for HT initiation in the postmenopausal years. HT is not advised for the primary prevention of disease, because associated risks outweigh benefits for most women; in limited cases, HT may be used for prevention of osteoporosis, after consideration of all other options. HT should be used only for severe and debilitating symptoms, in the lowest dose and most directed therapy possible, and for the shortest time necessary to accomplish symptom control.

‡The United States Preventive Services Task Force (USPSTF) recommends screening for colon cancer starting at age 50 using either annual fecal occult blood testing, sigmoidoscopy (periodicity unspecified), or both.

HT—hormone therapy CAD—coronary artery disease DEXA—dual x-ray absorptiometry NSAID—nonsteroidal anti-inflammatory drug

Premature Ovarian Failure

Premature ovarian failure (POF) is defined as menopause that occurs before 40 years of age that is not iatrogenically induced. The prevalence of POF is approximately 1%.[120] The Study of Women Across the Nation (SWAN) investigated risk factors associated with POF[121] and found that ethnicity influences risk: POF occurs in 1.1% of white women and 1.4% of African-American and Hispanic women, but it occurs in only 0.5% of Chinese-American women and 0.1% of Japanese-American women. Higher body mass index is associated with increased likelihood of POF, especially in African-American

women. Disability and current smoking are associated with greater risk in white women.

ETIOLOGY

There is good evidence to suggest that the timing of the age of menopause is genetically programmed[15,16] and that genes play a significant role in the etiology of premature ovarian failure.[120] Rare genetic and chromosomal causes of premature ovarian failure include familial predisposition, FSH receptor mutations, galactosemia, 17α-hydroxylase deficiency, alterations in gonadotropin structure or function, and structural alterations of the X chromosome (e.g., Turner syndrome mosaicism). A common genetic cause of POF is the fragile X premutation. Up to 3% to 5% of women with POF are carriers of the fragile X premutation, the most common cause of mental retardation in males.[122] Approximately 16% of women who are fragile X premutation heterozygotes have POF.[123]

Premature menopause may be immune-mediated in 30% to 50% of women with POF.[123] Family history is often positive for autoimmune conditions,[124] and other autoimmune diseases may be present in the patient herself,[124] including autoimmune thyroiditis, type 1 diabetes mellitus, autoimmune hemolytic anemia, Addison disease, hypoparathyroidism, idiopathic thrombocytopenic purpura, Crohn disease, myasthenia gravis, rheumatoid arthritis, systemic lupus erythematosus, vitiligo, and polyendocrine failure.

DIAGNOSIS

Clinical Manifestations

The presentation of premature ovarian failure is identical to that observed in natural menopause, with the exception that POF occurs before 40 years of age. It is more common, however, for women with POF to experience waxing and waning of symptoms over longer periods than it is for women who have natural menopause, and some women will ovulate several years after a diagnosis of POF is made.

Physical Examination

A targeted examination for women with oligomenorrhea or secondary amenorrhea is described elsewhere [see Natural Menopause, Physical Examination, above]. Less common etiologies of POF, such as Turner Syndrome (i.e., short stature, webbed neck, shield chest, small fourth metacarpal, and minimal breast development with normal hair distribution), can be detected with a specifically targeted physical examination. Findings of other autoimmune conditions often associated with POF [see Etiology, above] may be present in some women, including signs of thyroid disease (i.e., enlarged, asymmetrical, or nodular thyroid gland; dry skin; lateral eyebrow thinning; delayed relaxation phase on deep tendon reflexes; and myxedema), adrenal dysfunction (i.e., hyperpigmentation and orthostatic hypotension), and systemic lupus erythematosus (i.e., synovitis or malar rash). Galactorrhea suggests an elevated prolactin (PRL) prolactinoma [see Differential Diagnosis, below].

Laboratory Tests

Ovarian failure is most accurately confirmed by measurement of serum FSH. In women with incipient ovarian failure, FSH levels are often between 15 and 25 IU/L and can fluctuate. Complete ovarian failure is associated with repeated serum FSH levels greater than 25 IU/L. Therefore, FSH levels persistently greater than 25 IU/L (drawn on at least two separate occasions) can be useful in making the diagnosis of POF. Testing of urine or serum β-hCG, TSH, and prolactin concentrations should not be deferred if indicated in the evaluation of oligomenorrhea or secondary amenorrhea [see Natural Menopause, Laboratory Tests, above]. If a diagnosis of POF is made, consideration of genetic testing for a premutation allele of fragile X may be advisable, providing that this information would benefit family members and that the patient agrees to testing. If a woman younger than 30 years is diagnosed with POF, a karyotype test should be considered to rule out Turner syndrome mosaicism. When POF

may be caused by autoimmunity, the complete blood count (CBC), erythrocyte sedimentation rate (ESR), rheumatoid factor (RF), antinuclear antibody (ANA), glucose, calcium, and phosphorus levels can point to associated autoimmune conditions that may not otherwise be clinically apparent.

DIFFERENTIAL DIAGNOSIS

Hypergonadotropic amenorrhea can be caused by thyroid dysfunction, hyperprolactinemia, heroin addiction, and the use of some antidepressant and antipsychotic medications.

MANAGEMENT

All women with POF should be treated with exogenous estrogen, either in the form of a low-dose estrogen-progestin combination contraceptive or a postmenopausal HT formulation to manage symptoms and decrease the risk of osteoporosis and osteopenia. Bone mineral density should be obtained at baseline and followed at intervals of 3 to 5 years. It is recommended that women continue estrogen replacement until at least age 50 (approximately the time of natural menopause). Progestin therapy is recommended for women who have a uterus. Women who are at risk for unintended pregnancy should receive exogenous estrogen and progestin in the form of a contraceptive. For those desiring pregnancy, artificial reproductive technology is available. In vitro fertilization utilizing donor eggs and hormonal manipulation to mature the endometrium result in successful pregnancy in women with POF as often as in women with infertility from other causes.[125]

Treatment with oral contraceptives in the general population is associated with an increased risk of thromboembolic disease, cardiovascular disease in smokers, and stroke in women with migraine headaches or hypertension.[126] The risks of using oral contraceptives and postmenopausal HT in women with POF has not been specifically studied.

COMPLICATIONS AND PROGNOSIS

The chance of spontaneous pregnancy in POF is estimated to be less than 10%.[127] Women with POF may be at higher risk for younger onset of cardiovascular disease.[128] It is estimated that women with POF who do not take estrogen have a lower background risk of breast cancer and thromboembolism than the general population.[129] New onset of autoimmune disorders is not uncommon after the diagnosis of POF has been made.

Early-age mortality may occur in women with POF because of autoimmune phenomena, cardiovascular disease, and osteoporosis. A few epidemiologic studies suggest that an earlier age at menopause is associated with substantially increased mortality[128,129]; thus, careful screening for and management of chronic disease processes associated with hypoestrogenism [see Table 2] may be important for sustaining long-term health and quality of life. In addition, careful management of any coexisting autoimmune disorder and reduction, when possible, of potential risks posed by medications used to treat such disorders (e.g., corticosteroids) may be crucial for the long-term health of affected women.

Susan D. Reed, M.D., is a research consultant for Pfizer Inc.

Eliza L. Sutton, M.D., F.A.C.P., has no commercial relationships with manufacturers of products or providers of services discussed in this chapter.

The progestin intrauterine system and esterified estrogen combined with methyltestosterone have not been approved by the FDA for uses described in this chapter.

References

1. Research on the Menopause in the 1990's. Proceedings of a meeting. Geneva, Switzerland, 14–17 June 1994. Maturitas 23:109, 1996

2. Soules MR, Sherman S, Parrott E, et al: Executive summary: Stages of Reproductive Aging Workshop (STRAW). Climacteric 4:267, 2001

3. McKinlay SM, Brambilla DJ, Posner JG: The normal menopause transition. Maturitas 14:103, 1992

4. Treloar AE: Menstrual cyclicity and the pre-menopause. Maturitas 3:249, 1981

5. Kronenberg F: Hot flashes: epidemiology and physiology. Ann N Y Acad Sci 592:52, 1990

6. Kato I, Toniolo P, Akhmedkhanov A, et al: Prospective study of factors influencing the onset of natural menopause. J Clin Epidemiol 51:1271, 1998

7. Gold EB, Bromberger J, Crawford S: Factors associated with age at natural menopause in a multiethnic sample of midlife women. Am J Epidemiol 153:865, 2001

8. Rodstrom K, Bengtsson C, Milsom I, et al: Evidence for a secular trend in menopausal age: a population study of women in Gothenburg. Menopause 10:538, 2003

9. McKinlay SM: The normal menopause transition: an overview. Maturitas 23:137, 1996

10. van Noord PA, Dubas JS, Dorland M, et al: Age at natural menopause in a population-based screening cohort: the role of menarche, fecundity, and lifestyle factors. Fertil Steril 68:95, 1997

11. Cooper GS, Thorp JM Jr: FSH levels in relation to hysterectomy and to unilateral oophorectomy. Obstet Gynecol 94:969, 1999

12. Baker TG: Radiosensitivity of mammalian oocytes with particular reference to the human female. Am J Obstet Gynecol 110:746, 1971

13. Soules MR, Bremmer WJ: The menopause and climacteric: endocrinologic basis and associated symptomatology. J Am Geriatr Soc 30:547, 1982

14. Mitchell ES, Woods NF, Mariella A: Three stages of the menopausal transition from the Seattle Midlife Women's Health Study: toward a more precise definition. Menopause 7:334, 2000

15. Snieder H, MacGregor AJ, Spector TD: Genes control the cessation of a woman's reproductive life: a twin study of hysterectomy and age at menopause. J Clin Endocrinol Metab 83:1875, 1998

16. Treloar SA, Do KA, Martin NG: Genetic influences on the age at menopause. Lancet 352:1084, 1998

17. Torgerson DJ, Thomas RE, Reid DM: Mothers and daughters menopausal ages: is there a link? Eur J Obstet Gynecol Reprod Biol 74:63, 1997

18. Weel AE, Uitterlinden AG, Westendorp IC, et al: Estrogen receptor polymorphism predicts the onset of natural and surgical menopause. J Clin Endocrinol Metab 84:3146, 1999

19. Rannevik G, Jeppsson S, Johnell O, et al: A longitudinal study of the perimenopausal transition: altered profiles of steroid and pituitary hormones, SHBG and bone mineral density. Maturitas 21:103, 1995

20. Cooper GS, Baird DD, Hulka BS, et al: Follicle-stimulating hormone concentrations in relation to active and passive smoking. Obstet Gynecol 85:407, 1995

21. Burger HG, Dudley EC, Hopper JL, et al: Prospectively measured levels of serum follicle-stimulating hormone, estradiol, and the dimeric inhibins during the menopausal transition in a population-based cohort of women. J Clin Endocrinol Metab 84:4025, 1999

22. Klein NA, Battaglia DE, Woodruff TK, et al: Ovarian follicular concentrations of activin, follistatin, inhibin, insulin-like growth factor I (IGF-I), IGF-II, IGF-binding protein-2 (IGFBP-2), IGFBP-3, and vascular endothelial growth factor in spontaneous menstrual cycles of normal women of advanced reproductive age. J Clin Endocrinol Metab 85:4520, 2000

23. Landgren BM, Colllins A, Csemiczky G: Menopause transition: annual changes in serum hormonal patterns over the menstrual cycle in women during a nine-year period prior to menopause. J Clin Endocrinol Metab 89:2763, 2004

24. Dennerstein L, Smith AM, Morse C, et al: Menopausal symptoms in Australian women. Med J Aust 159:232, 1993

25. Santoro N, Brown JR, Adel T, et al: Characterization of reproductive hormonal dynamics in the perimenopause. J Clin Endocrinol Metab 81:1495, 1996

26. Zumoff B, Strain GW, Miller LK, et al: Twenty-four-hour mean plasma testosterone concentration declines with age in normal premenopausal women. J Clin Endocrinol Metab 80:1429, 1995

27. Burger HG, Dudley EC, Cui J, et al: A prospective longitudinal study of serum testosterone, dehydroepiandrosterone sulfate, and sex hormone-binding globulin levels through the menopause transition. J Clin Endocrinol Metab 85:2382, 2000

28. Labrie F, Belanger A, Cusan L, et al: Marked decline in serum concentrations of adrenal C19 sex steroid precursors and conjugated androgen metabolites during aging. J Clin Endocrinol Metab 82:2396, 1997

29. Scobie GA, Macpherson S, Millar MR, et al: Human oestrogen receptors: differential expression of ER alpha and beta and the identification of ER beta variants. Steroids 67:985, 2002

30. Garcia-Closas M, Herrero R, Bratti C, et al: Epidemiologic determinants of vaginal pH. Am J Obstet Gynecol 180:1060, 1999

31. Dennerstein L, Dudley EC, Hopper JL, et al: A prospective population-based study of menopausal symptoms. Obstet Gynecol 96:351, 2000

32. Freedman RR, Krell W: Reduced thermoregulatory null zone in postmenopausal women with hot flashes. Am J Obstet Gynecol 181:66, 1999

33. Berendsen HH: The role of serotonin in hot flushes. Maturitas 36:155, 2000

34. Slopien R, Maczekalski B, Warenik-Szymankiewicz A: Relationship between climacteric symptoms and serum serotonin levels in postmenopausal women. Climacteric 6:53, 2003

35. Warenik-Szymankiewicz A, Meczekalski B: Neuroendocrine aspects of menopause. Ginekol Pol 68:620, 1997

36. Jansson C, Johansson S, Lindh-Astrand L, et al: The prevalence of symptoms possibly related to the climacteric in pre- and postmenopausal women in Linkoping, Sweden. Maturitas 45:129, 2003

37. Moe KE: Reproductive hormones, aging, and sleep. Semin Reprod Endocrinol 17:339, 1999

38. Bixler EO, Vgontzas AN, Lin HM, et al: Prevalence of sleep-disordered breathing in women: effects of gender. Am J Respir Crit Care Med 163:608, 2001

39. Young T, Rabago D, Zgierska A, et al: Objective and subjective sleep quality in premenopausal, perimenopausal, and postmenopausal women in the Wisconsin Sleep Cohort Study. Sleep 26:667, 2003

40. Popovic RM, White DP: Upper airway muscle activity in normal women: influence of hormonal status. J Appl Physiol 84:1055, 1998

41. Dennerstein L, Randolph J, Taffe J, et al: Hormones, mode, sexuality, and the menopausal transition. Fertil Steril 77(suppl 4):S42, 2002

42. Seifert-Klauss V, Mueller JE, Luppa P, et al: Bone metabolism during the perimenopausal transition: a prospective study. Maturitas 41:23, 2002

43. Recker R, Lappe J, Davies K, et al: Characterization of perimenopausal bone loss: a prospective study. J Bone Miner Res 15:1965, 2000

44. Do KA, Green A, Guthrie JR, et al: Longitudinal study of risk factors for coronary heart disease across the menopausal transition. Am J Epidemiol 151:584, 2000

45. Gordon T, Kannel WB, Hjortland MC, et al: Menopause and coronary heart disease. The Framingham Study. Ann Intern Med 89:157, 1978

46. Schaefer EJ, Lamon-Fava S, Cohn SD, et al: Effects of age, gender, and menopause status on plasma low-density lipoprotein cholesterol and apolipoprotein B levels in the Framingham Offspring Study. J Lipid Res 35:779, 1994

47. Wagner JD: Rationale for hormone replacement therapy in atherosclerosis prevention. J Reprod Med 45(3 suppl):245, 2000

48. Peverill RE: Hormone therapy and venous thromboembolism. Best Pract Res Clin Endocrinol Metab 17:149, 2003

49. Bolognia JL: Aging skin. Am J Med 98:99S, 1995

50. Ashcroft GS, Dodsworth J, van Boxtel E, et al: Estrogen accelerates cutaneous wound healing associated with an increase in TGF-beta 1 levels. Nat Med 3:1209, 1997

51. Di Leo A, Messa C, Cavallini A, et al: Estrogens and colorectal cancer. Curr Drug Targets Immune Endocr Metabol Disord 1:1, 2001

52. L'Hostis H, Deminiere C, Ferriere J, et al: Renal angiomyolipoma: a clincopathologic, immunohistochemical, and follow-up study of 46 cases. Am J Surg Pathol 23:1011, 1999

53. Ferrans VJ, Yu ZX, Nelson WK, et al: Lymphangioleiomyomatosis (LAM): a review of clinical and morphological features. J Nippon Med Sch 67:311, 2000

54. Blankenstein MA, Verheijen FM, Jacobs JM, et al: Occurrence, regulation, and significance of progesterone receptors in human meningioma. Steroids 65:795, 2000

55. Pfahlberg A, Hassan K, Wille L, et al: Systematic review of case-control studies: oral contraceptives show no effect on melanoma risk. Public Health Rev 25:309, 1997

56. Keenan NL, Mark S, Fugh-Berman A, et al: Severity of menopausal symptoms and use of both conventional and complementary/alternative therapies. Menopause 10:507, 2003

57. Gull B, Karlsson B, Milsom I, et al: Can ultrasound replace dilation and curettage? A longitudinal evaluation of postmenopausal bleeding and transvaginal sonographic measurement of the endometrium as predictors of endometrial cancer. Am J Obstet Gynecol 188:401, 2003

58. Ferrazzi E, Torri V, Trio D, et al: Sonographic endometrial thickness: a useful test to predict atrophy in patients with postmenopausal bleeding: an Italian multicenter study. Ultrasound Obstet Gynecol 7:315, 1996

59. Tabor A, Watt HC, Wald NJ: Endometrial thickness as a test for endometrial cancer in women with postmenopausal vaginal bleeding. Obstet Gynecol 99:663, 2002

60. Bren L: The estrogen and progestin dilemma: new advice, labeling guidelines. FDA Consum 37:10, 2003

61. Narayan H, Buckett W, McDougall W, et al: Pregnancy after fifty: profile and pregnancy outcome in a series of elderly multigravidae. Eur J Obstet Gynecol Reprod Biol 47:47, 1992

62. Ventura SJ, Abma JC, Mosher WD, et al: Revised pregnancy rates, 1990–97, and new rates for 1998–99: United States. Natl Vital Stat Rep 52:1, 2003

63. Pisani G, Facioni L, Fiorani F, et al: Psychosexual problems in menopause. Minerva Ginecol 50:77, 1998

64. Loprinzi CL, Kugler JW, Sloan JA, et al: Venlafaxine in management of hot flashes in survivors of breast cancer: a randomised controlled trial. Lancet 365:2059, 2000

65. Barton D, La VB, Loprinzi C, et al: Venlafaxine for the control of hot flushes: results of a longitudinal continuation study. Oncol Nurs Forum 29:33, 2002

66. Stearns V, Beebe KL, Iyengar M, et al: Paroxetine controlled release in the treatment of menopausal hot flashes: a randomized controlled trial. JAMA 289:2827, 2003

67. Loprinzi CL, Sloan JA, Perez EA, et al: Phase III evaluation of fluoxetine for treatment of hot flashes. J Clin Oncol 20:1578, 2002

68. Weitzner MA, Moncello J, Jacobsen PB, et al: A pilot trial of paroxetine for the treatment of hot flashes and associated symptoms in women with breast cancer. J Pain Symptom Manage 23:337, 2002

69. Guttuso T Jr, Kurlan R, McDermott MP, et al: Gabapentin's effects on hot flashes in postmenopausal women: a randomized controlled trial. Obstet Gynecol 101:337, 2003

70. Wren BG, Brown LB: A double-blind trial with clonidine and a placebo to treat hot flushes. Med J Aust 144:369, 1986

71. Sonnendecker WY, Polakow ES, Gerdes L: Psycho-endocrine differences and correlations in symptomatic and asymptomatic climacteric women — the possible role of prolactin. S Afr Med J 60:661, 1981

72. Barton DL, Loprinzi CL, Quella SK, et al: Prospective evaluation of vitamin E for hot flashes in breast cancer survivors. J Clin Oncol 16:495, 1998

73. Kronenberg F, Fugh-Berman A: Complementary and alternative medicine for menopausal symptoms: a review of randomized, controlled trials. Ann Intern Med 137:805, 2002

74. Wuttke W, Seidlova-Wuttke D, Gorkow C: The *Cimicifuga* preparation BNO 1055 vs. conjugated estrogens in a double-blind placebo-controlled study: effects on menopause symptoms and bone markers. Maturitas 44:S67, 2003

75. Loprinzi FL, Michalak JC, Quella SK, et al: Megestrol acetate for the prevention of hot flashes. N Engl J Med 331:347, 1994

76. Leonetti HB, Longo S, Anasti JN: Transdermal progesterone cream for vasomotor symptoms and postmenopausal bone loss. Obstet Gynecol 94:225, 1999

77. Beral V, Banks E, Reeves G, et al: Breast cancer and hormone-replacement therapy: the Million Women Study. Lancet 362:1330, 2003

78. Irvin JH, Domar AD, Clark C, et al: The effects of relaxation response training on menopausal symptoms. J Pyschosom Obstet Gynaecol 17:202, 1996

79. Freedman RR, Woodward S: Behavioral treatment of menopausal hot flushes: evaluation by ambulatory monitoring. Am J Obstet Gynecol 167:436, 1992

80. Ivarsson T, Spetz AC, Hammar M: Physical exercise and vasomotor symptoms in postmenopausal women. Maturitas 29:139, 1998

81. Pinn G: Herbs used in obstetrics and gynaecology. Aust Fam Physician 30:351, 2001

82. Shifren J, Braunstein GD, Simon JA, et al: Transdermal testosterone treatment in women with impaired sexual function after oophorectomy. N Engl J Med 343:682, 2000

83. Lobo RA, Rosen RC, Yang HM, et al: Comparative effects of oral esterified estrogens with and without methyltestosterone on endocrine profiles and dimensions of sexual function in postmenopausal women with hypoactive sexual desire. Fertil Steril 79:1341, 2003

84. Schmidt PJ, Nieman LK, Danaceau MA, et al: Estrogen replacement in perimenopause-related depression: a prelimnary report. Am J Obstet Gynecol 183:414, 2000

85. Derman RJ, Dawood MY, Stone S: Quality of life during sequential hormone replacement therapy. Int J Fertil Menopaus Stud 40:73, 1995

86. Schneider LS, Small GW, Clary CM: Estrogen replacement therapy and antidepressant response to sertraline in older depressed women. Am J Geriatr Psychiatry 9:393, 2001

87. Hulley S, Grady D, Bush T, et al: Randomized trial of estrogen plus progestin for secondary prevention of coronary heart disease in postmenopausal women. Heart and Estrogen/progestin Replacement Study (HERS) Research Group. JAMA 280:605, 1998

88. Rossouw JE, Anderson FL, Prentice RL, et al: Risks and benefits of estrogen plus progestin in healthy postmenopausal women: principal results from the Women's Health Initiative randomized controlled trial. JAMA 288:321, 2002

89. Anderson GL, Limacher M, Assaf AR, et al: Effects of conjugated equine estrogen in postmenopausal women with hysterectomy: the Women's Health Initiative randomized controlled trial. JAMA 291:1701, 2004

90. Manson JE, Hsia J, Johnson KC, et al: Estrogen plus progestin and the risk of coronary heart disease. N Engl J Med 349:523, 2003

91. Wassertheil-Smoller S, Hendrix SL, Limacher M, et al: Effect of estrogen plus progestin on stroke in postmenopausal women: the Women's Health Initiative: a randomized trial. JAMA 289:2673, 2003

92. Shumaker SA, Legault C, Rapp SR, et al: Estrogen plus progestin and the incidence of dementia and mild cognitive impairment in postmenopausal women: the Women's Health Initiative Memory Study: a randomized controlled trial. JAMA 289:2651, 2003

93. Chlebowski RT, Hendrix SL, Langer RD, et al: Influence of estrogen plus progestin on breast cancer and mammography in healthy postmenopausal women: the Women's Health Initiative Randomized Trial. JAMA 289:3243, 2003

94. Col NF, Pauker SG: The discrepancy between observational studies and randomized trials of menopausal hormone therapy: did expectations shape experience? Ann Intern Med 139:923, 2003

95. Rapp SR, Espeland MA, Shumaker SA, et al: Effect of estrogen plus progestin on global cognitive function in postmenopausal women: the Women's Health Initiative Memory Study: a randomized controlled trial. JAMA 289:2663, 2003

96. Cauley JA, Robbins J, Chen Z, et al: Effects of estrogen plus progestin on risk of fracture and bone mineral density: the Women's Health Initiative randomized trial. JAMA 290:1729, 2003

97. Anderson GL, Judd HL, Kaunitz AM, et al: Effects of estrogen plus progestin on gynecologic cancers and associated diagnostic procedures: the Women's Health Initiative Investigators. JAMA 290:1739, 2003

98. Shumaker SA, Legault C, Kuller L, et al: Conjugated equine estrogens and incidence of probable dementia and mild cognitive impairment in postmenopausal women. Women's Health Initiative Memory Study. JAMA 291:2941, 2004

99. Espeland MA, Rapp SR, Shumaker SA, et al: Conjugated equine estrogens and global cognitive function in postmenopausal women. Women's Health Initiative Memory Study. JAMA 291:2959, 2004

100. Chlebowski RT, Wactawski-Wende J, Ritenbaush C, et al: Estrogen plus progestin and colorectal cancer in postmenopausal women. N Engl J Med 350:991, 2004

101. Jick H, Derby LE, Myers MW, et al: Risk of hospital admission of idiopathic venous thromboembolism among users of postmenopausal oestrogens. Lancet 348:981, 1996

102. Daly E, Vessey MP, Hawkins MM, et al: Risk of venous thromboembolism in users of hormone replacement therapy. Lancet 348:977, 1996

103. Grodstein F, Stampfer MJ, Goldhaber SZ, et al: Prospective study of exogenous hormones and risk of pulmonary embolism in women. Lancet 348:938, 1996

104. Grady D, Gebretsadik T, Kerlikowske K, et al: Hormone replacement therapy and endometrial cancer risk: a meta-analysis. Obstet Gynecol 85:304, 1995

105. Schairer C, Lubin J, Troisi R, et al: Estrogen-progestin replacement and risk of breast cancer. JAMA 284:691, 2000

106. Ross RK, Paganini-Hill A, Wan PC, et al: Effect of hormone replacement therapy on breast cancer risk: estrogen versus estrogen plus progestin. J Natl Cancer Inst 92:328, 2000

107. Breast cancer and hormone replacement therapy: collaborative reanalysis of data from 51 epidemiological studies of 52,705 women with breast cancer and 108,411 women without breast cancer. Collaborative Group on Hormonal Factors in Breast Cancer. Lancet 350:1047, 1997

108. Scarabin PY, Alhenc-Gelas M, Plu-Bureau G, et al: Effects of oral and transdermal estrogen/progesterone regimens on blood coagulation and fibrinolysis in postmenopausal women: a randomized controlled trial. Arterioscler Thromb Vasc Biol 17:3071, 1997

109. Perez Gutthann S, Garcia Rodriguez LA, Castellsague J, et al: Hormone replacement therapy and risk of venous thromboembolism: population based case-control study. BMJ 314:796, 1997

110. Van Erpecum KJ, Van Berge Henegouwen GP, Verschoor L, et al: Different hepatobiliary effects of oral and transdermal estradiol in postmenopausal women. Gastroenterology 100:482, 1991

111. Sendag F, Karadadas N, Ozsener S, et al: Effects of sequential combined transdermal and oral hormone replacement therapies on serum lipid and lipoproteins in postmenopausal women. Arch Gynecol Obstet 266:38, 2002

112. Chen FP, Lee N, Soong YK, et al: Comparison of transdermal and oral estrogen-progestin replacement therapy: effects on cardiovascular risk factors. Menopause 8:347, 2001

113. Decensi A, Omodei U, Robertson C, et al: Effect of transdermal estradiol and oral conjugated estrogen on C-reactive protein in retinoid-placebo trial in healthy women. Circulation 106:1224, 2002

114. Shulman LP, Yankov V, Uhl K: Safety and efficacy of a continuous once-a-week 17beta-estradiol/levonorgestrel transdermal system and its effects on vasomotor symptoms and endometrial safety in postmenopausal women: the results of two multicenter double-blind, randomized, controlled trials. Menopause 9:195, 2002

115. O'Connell D, Robertson J, Henry D, et al: A systematic review of the skeletal effects of estrogen therapy in postmenopausal women: II. An assessment of treatment effects. Climacteric 1:112, 1998

116. Effects of hormone replacement therapy on endometrial histology in postmenopausal women: the Postmenopausal Estrogen/Progestin Interventions (PEPI) Trial. The Writing Group for the PEPI Trial. JAMA 275:370, 1996

117. Raudaskoski T, Tapanainen J, Tomas E, et al: Intrauterine 10 μg and 20 μg levonorgestrel systems in postmenopausal women receiving oral oestrogen replacement therapy: clinical, endometrial and metabolic response. BJOG 109:136, 2002

118. Wildemeersch D, Schacht E, Wildemeersch P: Performance and acceptability of intrauterine release of levonorgestrel with a miniature delivery system for hormonal substitution therapy, contraception and treatment in peri and postmenopausal women. Maturitas 44:237, 2003

119. Franchin R, De Ziegler D, Bergeron C, et al: Transvaginal administration of progesterone. Obstet Gynecol 90:396, 1997

120. Sherman SL: Premature ovarian failure in the fragile X syndrome. Am J Med Genet 97:189, 2000

121. Luborsky JL, Meyer P, Sowers MF, et al: Premature menopause in a multi-ethnic population study of the menopause transition. Hum Reprod 18:199, 2003

122. Gersak K, Meden-Vrtovec H, Peterlin B: Fragile X permutation in women with sporadic premature ovarian failure in Slovenia. Hum Reprod 18:1637, 2003

123. Hundscheid RD, Sistermans EA, Thomas CM, et al: Imprinting effect in premature ovarian failure confined to paternally inherited fragile X permutations. Am J Hum Genet 66:413, 2000

124. Alper MM, Jolly EE, Garner PR: Pregnancies after premature ovarian failure. Obstet Gynecol 67:59S, 1986

125. Lydic ML, Liu JH, Rebar RW, et al: Success of donor oocyte in vitro fertilization-embryo transfer in recipients with and without premature ovarian failure. Fertil Steril 65:98, 1996

126. Schwingl PJ, Ory HW, Visness CM: Estimates of the risk of cardiovascular death attributable to low-dose oral contraceptives in the United States. Am J Obstet Gynecol 180:241, 1999

127. Rebar RW, Connolly HV: Clinical features of young women with hypergonadotropic amenorrhea. Fertil Steril 53:804, 1990

128. van der Schouw YT, van der Graaf Y, Steyerberg EW, et al: Age at menopause as a risk factor for cardiovascular mortality. Lancet 347:714, 1996

129. Snowdon DA, Kane RL, Beeson WL, et al: Is early natural menopause a biologic marker of health and aging? Am J Public Health 79:709, 1989

130. Rannevik G, Jeppson S, Johnell O, et al: A longitudinal study of the perimenopausal transition: altered profiles of steroid and pituitary hormones, SHBG, and bone mineral density. Maturitas 21:103, 1995

Acknowledgments

Figure 1   Modified from "Executive Summary: Stages of Reproductive Aging Workshop (STRAW)," by M. R. Soules, S. Sherman, E. Parrott, et al., in *Fertility and Sterility* 76:874, 2001.

Figure 3   Seward Hung.

86 Urinary Incontinence and Overactive Bladder Syndrome

Lennox P. Hoyte, M.D., and Robert L. Barbieri, M.D., F.A.C.P.

Definitions

Urinary incontinence falls into two broad categories: stress incontinence, which is leakage related to increases in intra-abdominal pressure, and urge incontinence, which is leakage related to an insuppressible urge to void. Urge incontinence accounts for about half of the incontinence in women.[1]

Overactive bladder syndrome is defined as urinary urgency, with or without urge incontinence and usually with frequency and nocturia.[2] Nocturia, which is often associated with urinary frequency, is defined as a need to urinate that awakens the person during the night.[2]

Epidemiology

The involuntary loss of urine is an extremely common problem in women. Over one third of women in the United States experience urinary incontinence, at an estimated annual cost of $19.5 billion.[3-5] Overactive bladder alone affects approximately 17% of all women and 20% to 30% of women older than 55 years; the prevalence is even higher in residents of nursing homes. Overactive bladder is the third most prevalent chronic condition in the United States, after arthritis and sinusitis.[6,7] The annual cost of overactive bladder is estimated at $12.6 billion.[3,6]

Patients may fail to report these bladder problems, and physicians may fail to address them.[8,9] Many patients do not seek help, because they believe that no effective treatment is available. Two thirds of patients with urinary incontinence report that their bladder symptoms affect daily living, and many patients self-manage their symptoms by voiding frequently, reducing fluid intake, and wearing pads.[2]

Structure and Function of the Lower Urinary Tract

The bladder consists of a smooth muscular reservoir (the detrusor muscle), two inlets (the ureters), and an outlet (the urethra). Urine from the kidneys enters the bladder via the ureters and exits via the urethra, which is itself a muscular tube consisting of smooth and striated muscle. Bladder function has two phases: storage and emptying. During the storage phase, the bladder collects urine; this phase involves relaxation of the detrusor muscle and tightening of the urethral muscle, all of which is under sympathetic and voluntary control. The emptying phase involves relaxation of the urethral muscles and contraction of the detrusor, which is mediated by the parasympathetic system. Under normal circumstances, emptying is voluntarily initiated in the adult.[10]

In women, the bladder and urethra are supported by the anterior vaginal wall, which in turn is suspended by connective tissue attachments from the pelvic floor muscles, specifically the levator ani and the internal obturator muscles.[11,12] Continence is maintained when the urethral closure pressure exceeds the detrusor pressure. Support from the anterior vaginal wall is believed to be required to maintain this relationship during periods of increased intra-abdominal pressure.[11] Consequently, urinary continence depends on the relative relaxation of the detrusor, the contraction of urethral muscles, and the support of the anterior vaginal wall. Incontinence can ensue when these relationships are disrupted.

Mechanisms of Lower Urinary Tract Dysfunction

Stress urinary incontinence is believed to result from a decrease in urethral muscle capability or a loss of vaginal wall support. Urge urinary incontinence usually results when the detrusor contracts at inappropriate times, either overcoming the urethral pressure or triggering a reflex relaxation of the urethral muscles.[13] The overactive bladder syndrome occurs when there are inappropriate detrusor contractions, which may or may not overcome the urethral closure pressure; in the latter instance, the person maintains continence (so-called dry overactive bladder syndrome).[14]

Other, less prevalent structural irregularities can also cause inappropriate urine leakage. These include urinary tract fistulas, urethral obstruction, loss of detrusor contractility, anatomic tract anomalies, and ectopically located ureters. Lower urinary tract infections, medications, pelvic masses, and other conditions can also lead to overactive bladder symptoms or incontinence.

Diagnosis

HISTORY

The clinician should elicit a history of conditions that may cause or contribute to urinary incontinence. These include surgery to the spinal cord, bladder neck, or pelvic floor, which may lead to obstruction; neurologic disease (e.g., multiple sclerosis or a spinal cord lesion); or psychiatric disease (e.g., dementia, which may limit the ability to recognize a need to void). Musculoskeletal function, with emphasis on mobility, should be reviewed. A detailed medication history will identify any medications (e.g., diuretics or alpha blockers) that may affect urine output or bladder function. The patient should be asked about her daily fluid intake (40 to 60 ounces is normal) and number of daily and nightly voids. A range of four to eight voiding episodes a day is considered normal.

Symptoms of dysuria raise the possibility of a bladder infection or painful bladder syndrome. The International Continence Society defines painful bladder syndrome as suprapubic pain related to bladder filling, accompanied by other symptoms, but in the absence of proven urinary infection or other obvious pathology.[2]

Gross hematuria should raise concerns about serious bladder conditions (e.g., neoplasia), which require a specialized workup. The location and quality of the sensation of bladder fullness may be helpful in differentiating overactive

Table 1   Foods and Beverages That May Cause Urinary Frequency and Urgency

Beverages	Alcoholic beverages (all types)
	Carbonated beverages (particularly those with caffeine)
	Milk and milk products
	Coffee (including decaffeinated)
	Tea (excluding herbal teas)
Foods	Citrus fruits
	Tomatoes and tomato-based products
	Highly spiced foods
	Sugar
	Honey
	Chocolate
	Corn syrup
	Artificial sweeteners (e.g., aspartame, saccharine)

bladder from painful bladder syndromes: one study demonstrated that most patients with painful bladder syndrome sense their bladder fullness as urgency and discomfort in the suprapubic and urethral/vulvar regions, as well as occasionally in other body areas, whereas most patients with overactive bladder sense their bladder fullness as urgency in the midline suprapubic area.[15] Associated symptoms (e.g., dyspareunia) may suggest a myofascial etiology. Attention should also be given to the patient's diet, which may contain fluids and foods thought to cause urinary frequency and urgency [*see Table 1*].

Clinical diagnosis of incontinence is facilitated by asking about the dominant feature of the problem [*see Table 2*].[2] The following questions may be helpful:

- Is the leakage preceded by an urge to void? This suggests overactive bladder syndrome. Persistence of leakage during the urge suggests urge incontinence.
- Does the leakage occur only with Valsalva activity (e.g., coughing, laughing, or lifting)? This points to stress incontinence.
- Is there pain associated with bladder fullness or emptying? This suggests painful bladder syndrome.
- Is there bothersome nocturia? If so, possible causes include obstructive sleep apnea and cardiovascular disease (e.g., heart failure).
- Is there continuous urine leakage? This suggests urinary-vaginal fistula.
- Does urine leak from the vagina? This suggests urinary-genital tract fistula

PHYSICAL EXAMINATION

The physical examination should include an evaluation of the patient's mental state, general appearance, and mobility. In the absence of evidence of cystitis, a targeted exam should focus on inspection and palpation of the back, abdomen, urethra, bladder, vagina, uterus, and adnexa. This will permit exclusion of gross abdominal or pelvic masses, pelvic organ prolapse, and urethral diverticula. Inspection of the lower back can reveal anatomic anomalies (e.g., signs of spina bifida) or scars from spinal surgery. A speculum exam may be used to evaluate for atrophic vaginitis, which can be associated with overactive bladder symptoms in postmenopausal women.[16] Prolapse of the vagina or cervix beyond the labia indicates advanced prolapse, which can sometimes be associated with

urinary retention and urinary frequency. Gross fluid collections in the vagina should raise suspicion of a urinary-genital fistula, which requires a specialized workup, especially in the setting of previous pelvic surgery. Transvaginal palpation of the pelvic floor muscles may elicit tenderness of muscle trigger points, which may suggest pelvic myofascial dysfunction or painful bladder syndrome.[16-18]

A neurologic examination focused on the pelvis and lower extremities may be indicated. Such an examination should include perineal sensation, the so-called anal wink reflex (elicited by gently stroking the labia majora posteriorly to anteriorly), patellar reflexes, and extensor and flexor function at the knees and ankles.

The supine cough stress test (CST) may be performed before and after voiding. For the CST, the patient coughs vigorously while in the lithotomy position. Stress urinary incontinence is likely if coughing causes immediate urine leakage from the urethral meatus. On rare occasions, coughing will trigger a detrusor contraction with incontinence (i.e., cough-induced detrusor overactivity incontinence). In these cases, the urine leakage begins seconds after the cough, and the stream continues for some time after coughing stops.

When the type of incontinence is unclear from the history and examination, a bladder diary can sometimes help in clarifying the patient's fluid balance status. The bladder diary can quantify the number and volume of voids, as well as identify cases of excessive fluid intake. Daily fluid intake of 40 to 60 oz is recommended,[19] and urine output should correspond to intake. Two thirds or more of total voided volume should occur during waking hours. Maximum voided volumes greater than 300 ml suggest adequate bladder capacity.[18] Any substantial deviations from these parameters may suggest problems with fluid balance and should prompt further evaluation. For example, the voiding of an abnormally high proportion of urine at night can sometimes indicate postural fluid shifts related to congestive heart failure or indicate transient hypoxia related to obstructive sleep apnea.[20]

LABORATORY TESTING

Patients experiencing incontinence should undergo urinalysis; a negative result is helpful in ruling out cystitis. More detailed office evaluation of the bladder may include measurement of postvoid residual urine, in which the bladder is catheterized within 15 minutes after the patient has spontaneously voided. Postvoid residual amounts of less than 100 ml are considered normal. Postvoid residuals substantially over 100 ml suggest voiding dysfunction and require further workup.

Urodynamic Testing

Advanced bladder testing is usually not obtained if a noninvasive incontinence therapy is planned. When noninvasive therapy fails or when the patient desires invasive therapy, many pelvic floor specialists (i.e., urogynecologists and urologists who specialize in female urinary tract disorders) recommend urodynamic testing in advance of intervention so as to confirm the diagnosis and to rule out associated pathologies. However, some specialists believe that urodynamic testing may be omitted when offering surgical therapy in clear cases of uncomplicated stress incontinence. This approach includes treatment of incontinent patients who

Table 2   Features of Urge Incontinence, Stress Incontinence, and Mixed Incontinence

Feature	Urge Incontinence	Stress Incontinence	Mixed Incontinence
Urgency (sudden strong urge to urinate)	Yes	No	Yes
Frequency with urgency (> seven daytime voids)	Yes	No	Yes
Leakage during physical activities	No	Yes	Yes
Amount of leakage per episode	Large if present	Small	Variable
Ability to reach toilet in time when urge occurs	No	Yes	Variable
Waking up to pass urine at night	Usually	Seldom	Possible

meet the following criteria:

- Symptoms consistent with stress incontinence
- A positive cough stress test
- No evidence of voiding dysfunction
- No prior bladder neck or incontinence surgery
- No advanced pelvic organ prolapse
- No other conditions affecting bladder function (e.g., neurologic disease, diabetes mellitus, or previous pelvic radiation).

Differential Diagnosis

When a patient complains of inappropriate urine leakage, it is important to rule out other readily identifiable causes unrelated to the detrusor or urethral sphincters. For example, cystitis is a common cause of bladder irritation that is often associated with urinary frequency and urgency and sometimes features inappropriate urine leakage.[21] Other, less common causes are medications (e.g., diuretics), diabetes mellitus,[21,22] neoplasia, excessive fluid intake,[23] neurologic disease (e.g., multiple sclerosis[24]), and spinal cord injury.[25] Obstructive sleep apnea and congestive heart failure may cause nocturia.[26,27] Most of these conditions can be eliminated from the differential diagnosis with a history and targeted physical examination.

Management

STRESS INCONTINENCE

Office-Based Treatment

Treatment options available to the primary care provider consist primarily of pelvic floor muscle exercises and incontinence pessaries. These therapies are noninvasive and may be confidently prescribed without the need for advanced bladder testing (i.e., urodynamics).

Pelvic floor muscle therapy   Intensive pelvic floor muscle exercise therapy can yield cure rates of up to 25% at 5 years if the patient practices the exercises diligently.[28] Most patients require supervised training to learn to recognize and contract the appropriate muscles. In this therapy, the patient contracts her pelvic floor muscles for 10 repetitions per cycle, holding each contraction for up to 5 seconds, with a 3-second rest between contractions. Each cycle is repeated up to three times a day. The patient is also encouraged to contract her pelvic floor muscles in advance of coughing, laughing, sneezing, or lifting. Pelvic floor muscle exercise therapy is best applied to the motivated patient who is prepared to keep up the regular schedule of daily exercises.

Incontinence pessaries   Incontinence pessaries are flexible vaginal inserts that compress the bladder neck during Valsalva maneuvers so as to prevent leakage. Most patients are able to insert and remove the pessary, allowing for cleaning and sexual activity. Pessaries are reported to cure stress incontinence in up to 24% of women.[29] About two thirds of patients will try the pessary if it is offered, but up to 45% of those who try a pessary will discontinue its use within 6 months.[30] Pessary treatment is completely reversible and carries only a small risk of urinary retention and vaginal mucosal erosion if left in place for extended periods of time. Most pelvic floor specialists recommend removing the pessary at least every 3 months for cleaning and vaginal inspection to rule out erosion.

The incontinence pessary is most appropriate for patients with mild stress incontinence symptoms who are seeking to avoid or defer surgery for incontinence. Many specialists offer pessaries as a first-line therapy in patients who are unable or unwilling to undergo surgery. Pessaries are reasonably priced, and the cost is covered by many insurance plans.

Pharmacologic therapy   For a time, treatment with norepinephrine-serotonin reuptake inhibitors was considered a promising option for the management of mild stress incontinence. However, after the Food and Drug Administration raised questions about the possible mental health risks, the manufacturer of the leading candidate for such treatment withdrew the agent from FDA consideration for this indication.[31,32] Currently, there is no FDA-approved pharmacologic therapy for stress urinary incontinence.

Surgical Therapy

When conservative therapy for stress urinary incontinence fails, urodynamic testing should be considered to clarify the diagnosis. Therapeutic options for urodynamically confirmed stress incontinence include injected periurethral bulking agents, retropubic urethropexies,[33,34] and suburethral slings.

Bulking agents   Bulking agents can be injected under cystoscopic guidance in the office or the operating room. The procedure requires about 15 to 20 minutes to perform. Bulking agents have success rates (i.e., complete continence) of about 16% to 22% at 3 months and 6% to 18% at 1 year, depending on injection technique.[35] Many patients require repeat injections two or three times annually.

Retropubic urethropexy Retropubic urethropexies (e.g., the Burch procedure) have long-term success rates of approximately 82%.[36] These procedures, however, require general or regional anesthesia and a suprapubic incision and can take 1 to 2 hours to perform.

Suburethral slings Suburethral slings may be constructed from autologous fascial tissues, allografts, or xenografts. Long-term success rates are approximately 85%. Side effects include obstructive urinary retention. The recently introduced synthetic midurethral slings (also called tension-free slings) have demonstrated success rates of about 80% at 2 years, with a 22% complication rate in the hands of experienced operators. Complications of tension-free slings include retropubic hematomas (2%), bladder perforation (9%), postoperative urinary retention (11%), and vaginal wall erosion (2.4%).[36-38] The vast majority of these complications resolve without sequelae.

The most widely used tension-free sling is called the Tension Free Vaginal Tape, or TVT. The TVT is indicated for surgical treatment of stress urinary incontinence. The insertion procedure requires less than 30 minutes of operating time. It may be performed under general or regional anesthesia or under conscious sedation with local anesthesia. Insertion is often performed as an outpatient procedure, and over 95% of patients can be expected to be discharged on the day of surgery, without a urinary catheter. Because of the wide choice of anesthesia options and the short duration of the insertion procedure, the TVT, as well as other minimally invasive midurethral synthetic slings, are considered ideal for older patients, as well as for those with severe comorbidities that might discourage longer, more invasive elective procedures. The tension-free slings also work quite well in healthy younger patients and are favored by patients who need a quick return to work and a short postoperative recovery period.

URINARY FREQUENCY AND URGE INCONTINENCE
(OVERACTIVE BLADDER)

Once the working diagnosis of overactive bladder is made, in a patient who has not had previous bladder neck surgery, therapy can be instituted without urodynamic testing. A variety of noninvasive therapies are available to the primary care physician. Pharmacologic treatment is often a reasonable first choice, provided the patient has no contraindications to it.

Pharmacologic Treatment

Drug therapy is considered a mainstay of therapy for urinary frequency and urgency, with or without incontinence. Muscarinic (M2 and M3) receptors in the bladder wall normally mediate detrusor contractions; antagonism of these receptors reduces bladder irritability.[39] Drugs currently approved by the Food and Drug Administration for the treatment of overactive bladder are anticholinergic compounds with high antimuscarinic activity [see Tables 3 and 4].

Approved antimuscarinic agents appear to be equally effective in reducing the symptoms of overactive bladder, but they have varying degrees of side effects. The side effects are directly related to the anticholinergic activity of these drugs and may involve the central nervous system (somnolence, usually in the elderly), the gastrointestinal tract (constipation), the salivary glands (dry mouth), or the heart (ECG changes). Antimuscarinics are contraindicated in patients with uncontrolled narrow-angle glaucoma. Side effects and medication

Table 3 Currently Available Antimuscarinic Agents[61-64]

Drug (Trade Name)	Dosage
Oxybutynin (Ditropan)	5 mg b.i.d.
Tolterodine (Detrol LA)	2–4 mg q.d.
Trospium (Sanctura)	20 mg b.i.d.
Oxybutynin transdermal (Oxytrol)	One patch twice weekly
Solifenacin (Vesicare)	5–10 mg q.d.
Darifenacin (Enablex)	7.5–15 mg q.d.

cost are probably responsible for the low 18% continuation rate in patients at 6 months.[40]

When cost is a concern, it is reasonable to begin drug therapy with generic oxybutynin, 2.5 mg twice daily. If the bladder symptoms improve satisfactorily within 3 weeks, the patient may continue on this dosage and receive follow-up in about 3 months. If the symptoms do not improve within 3 weeks and the patient is not having bothersome side effects (i.e., dry mouth or constipation), she is instructed to increase the dosage to 5 mg twice daily. If her symptoms do not improve after 3 weeks on this higher dosage, the dosage can be raised further, to 10 mg twice daily. Should this prove unsuccessful, another anticholinergic agent or an alternative therapy should be tried.

Many patients consider twice-daily dosing to be a nuisance. Such patients may prefer a long-acting anticholinergic such as tolterodine, beginning with 2 mg at bedtime. The dosage may be raised to 4 mg after 3 weeks if sufficient symptom improvement is not seen.

Dry mouth from anticholinergic medications can be remedied by having the patient suck on a hard candy (diabetic patients should use sugar-free candies). Constipation can be readily addressed with stool softeners and laxatives. Anticholinergics can sometimes cause mental-state changes in very elderly patients, and the physician must be alert to this possibility.

If anticholinergic agents fail to bring symptom relief or cause intolerable side effects, alternative noninvasive therapies include bladder retraining, pelvic floor physical therapy, and vaginal electrical stimulation. These methods can have good cure rates.

Bladder Retraining

Bladder retraining attempts to recalibrate the central response to bladder filling so as to slowly increase the voiding interval. The clinician first determines the minimum voiding interval (usually from the voiding diary). The patient is then instructed to void on schedule during waking hours, beginning with the minimum voiding interval. The voiding interval is increased by 15 to 30 minutes every 2 weeks, until the patient reaches a voiding interval of 2.5 to 3 hours. It is important that the patient void only at the scheduled times. In clinical trials, timed voiding therapy has produced cure rates of 55% to 60%, as measured by weekly incontinence episodes at 12 weeks[41] and urodynamic testing at 6 months.[42] Despite the proven efficacy of bladder retraining, the demands of the regimen discourage patient adherence, which in one study was only 55%.[43]

Pelvic Floor Muscle Exercises

The micturition cycle is initiated by distention of the bladder wall, which creates a local signal to void; this signal is normally inhibited by the central nervous system until the person chooses to void.[10,13] Pelvic muscle exercise therapy for overactive bladder is based on the theory that tightly held pelvic floor muscles can produce a signal that is received centrally as a sensation of bladder fullness and is interpreted as urgency; according to this theory, releasing the tightness of the pelvic floor muscles may decrease the sensation of bladder fullness. In one study, daily pelvic muscle exercises decreased daily incontinence episodes by up to 82%, with a 67% decrease in nocturia and a 42% decrease in incontinence pad use.[44] Other studies demonstrated less impressive results, with a 40% reduction in weekly leakage episodes and 30% resolution of overactive bladder symptoms.[41] Pelvic floor muscle exercises for overactive bladder are performed in the same way as those for stress incontinence (see above).

Pelvic Floor Physical Therapy

Like pelvic muscle exercises, pelvic muscle physical therapy is intended to decrease urinary urgency by relaxing the pelvic floor musculature. The relationship between urinary urgency and increased muscle tone in the pelvic floor was first noted in patients with interstitial cystitis. Lilihus observed that 81% of interstitial cystitis patients also had levator spasm and tenderness.[45] DeGroat theorized that persistent activation of A-delta and C-fiber nociceptors in the bladder wall exaggerates the so-called guarding reflex, leading to levator ani spasm, pain, and reflex voiding.[13,46] In one study, 8 to 12 weeks of manual physical therapy for the pelvic floor produced moderate to marked improvement or complete resolution in 35 of 42 patients with urinary urgency and frequency; seven of 10 patients with interstitial cystitis also showed improvement.[47] Similar results have been obtained in other studies of pelvic floor physical therapy in women with interstitial cystitis.[17,48,49]

Pelvic floor physical therapy is performed by specially trained physical therapists. The therapy consists of weekly sessions of transvaginal manual myofascial release of tightness and trigger points in the levator ani muscles. Many patients will have substantial improvement of their overactive bladder symptoms after eight weekly therapeutic sessions.

Vaginal Electrical Stimulation

Transvaginal electrical stimulation of the pudendal nerve is believed to lead to inhibition of parasympathetic outflow to the detrusor muscle.[50-52] In well-designed studies, 8 weeks of such therapy cured overactive bladder in 40% to 50% of patients.[53,54] Transvaginal electrical stimulation has Medicare approval for the indication of urinary urgency and frequency, with or without incontinence.

The equipment for vaginal electrical stimulation consists of an external battery-operated pulse generator and a detachable vaginal insert. The therapy is self-administered at home by the patient twice daily for 20 minutes each session.

Advanced Therapy for Overactive Bladder Syndrome

When conservative therapies for overactive bladder syndrome fail, the patient should be referred to a specialist in pelvic floor disorders. Specialists may consider cystoscopic evaluation of the bladder to rule out mucosal anomalies or neoplasia, as well as urodynamic testing to confirm the diagnosis of detrusor overactivity. With the exclusion of intravesical pathology and confirmation of detrusor overactivity, minimally invasive options are available for the management of refractory detrusor overactivity. These options include neuromodulation and intradetrusor injection of botulinum toxin A. More invasive therapies (e.g., urinary diversion and augmentation cystoplasty) are used much less frequently than they once were.

Neuromodulation Neuromodulation is considered in cases of urinary urgency, frequency, and incontinence that is refractory to noninvasive therapies. Neuromodulation is based on the theory that stimulation of sensory afferents can reprogram the central inhibition of the voiding reflex.[50-52] The technique consists of surgically placing an electrical lead into the S3 sacral foramen and stimulating the S3 afferents with a pulsed electrical signal.

Neuromodulation is done as a two-stage procedure. In the first stage, the electrical lead is placed and stimulation is provided via an external pulse generator. Lead placement is performed with the patient under conscious sedation and local anesthesia and requires well under 1 hour. Patients who respond favorably to the test stimulation then undergo permanent subcutaneous implantation of the pulse generator and battery. This second stage requires about 30 minutes. Thereafter, the pulse generator can be programmed using radio-frequency signals via a special programming device. The patient can turn the device on and off and vary the signal intensity with a small portable controller, which is placed on the skin over the implanted battery.

In a prospective, multicenter trial, neuromodulation com-

Table 4 Selectivity, Efficacy, and Side Effects of Antimuscarinic Agents[61-64]

Drug	Selectivity*	↓ Voids (24 hr)	↓ Leaks (24 Hr)	Dry Mouth (%)	Constipation (%)
Oxybutynin	M3 >> M2	2	1.7	30	40
Tolterodine	M3 > M2	2.2	1.7	10	25
Trospium	M3 ? M2	2.3	2.4	22	9
Solifenacin	M3 >> M2	2.6	1.3	21	8
Darifenacin	M3 >> M2	1.7	1.5	31	13

*To muscarinic (M) receptors in the bladder wall.

pletely cured 46% of patients with refractory leakage and eliminated heavy leakage in 65% of patients at 3 years of follow-up; 32% of patients had their number of daily voids reduced to between four and seven, and 56% had their average daily voids reduced by more than half.[55] In a study of 25 community-dwelling residents older than 55 years who had refractory overactive bladder symptoms, however, only 17% achieved total dryness at 1 to 16 months after implantation, although overall, patients had an 80% reduction in heavy leakage, an 80% reduction in pad usage, a 40% reduction in void frequency, and a greater than 50% reduction in number of leakage episodes.[56] The complication rate at test stimulation in 914 procedures was 18% and included lead migration (11.8%), pain (2.1%), and technical problems (2.6%). At 1 year, complications of permanent implants were pain at implantation site (15.3%), new pain (9%), infection (6.1%), transient electrical shock (5.5%), and persistent skin irritation (0.5%).[55]

Botulinum A toxin Botulinum toxin reversibly inhibits neuronal acetylcholine release, leading to decreased neuronal activity at the target organ.[57,58] In bladder applications, this effect is believed to reduce bladder irritability, leading to increased bladder capacities, longer voiding intervals, and a lessening of the urge to void repeatedly. For this procedure, up to 300 units of botulinum A toxin, mixed with 5 ml of normal saline, is injected into multiple sites in the supratrigonal detrusor muscle under cystoscopic guidance. All patients are taught how to self-catheterize, in the unlikely event that urinary retention should occur during the ensuing 1 to 3 weeks.

In a retrospective review of the effects of intradetrusor botulinum A toxin injection, complete continence was achieved in 72% of patients with neurogenic detrusor overactivity from such disorders as multiple sclerosis, spinal cord injury, and meningomyelocele; 27% of patients stopped anticholinergic medication completely, and 72% reduced its use substantially. The effect persisted at 9 months.[59] Similarly, in a multicenter, prospective, randomized, placebo-controlled trial of botulinum A detrusor injection in women with spinal cord injury or multiple sclerosis, urodynamic testing and voiding diaries demonstrated a reduction in leakage of up to 58% at 24 weeks after treatment, with improvement within as little as 2 weeks.[60]

Prognosis

Conservative therapy can provide effective treatment in 50% to 80% of patients with overactive bladder syndrome. When noninvasive therapies fail, specialists can provide minimally invasive therapies. These advanced therapies substantially improve symptoms in a large percentage of refractory cases. Conservative therapies are much less effective in the treatment of stress urinary incontinence, but minimally invasive surgical therapies are quite effective. The short operating times and minimal long-term sequelae associated with these therapies make them well suited to elderly patients and those with comorbidities that would normally preclude elective surgery.

The authors have no commercial relationships with manufacturers of products or providers of services discussed in this chapter.

References

1. Hannestad YS, Rortveit G, Sandvik H, et al: A community-based epidemiological survey of female urinary incontinence: the Norwegian Epincont study. Epidemiology of Incontinence in the County of Nord-Trondelag. J Clin Epidemiol 53:1150, 2000

2. Abrams P, Cardozo L, Fall M, et al: The standardisation of terminology of lower urinary tract function: report from the standardisation sub-committee of the International Continence Society. Neurourol Urodyn 21:167, 2002

3. Hu TW, Wagner TH, Bentkover JD, et al: Costs of urinary incontinence and overactive bladder in the United States: a comparative study. Urology 63:461, 2004

4. The Overactive Bladder: From Basic Science to Clinical Management Consensus Conference. Proceedings. London, England, June 29, 1997. Urology 50(6A suppl):1, 1997

5. Wilson L, Brown JS, Shin GP, et al: Annual direct cost of urinary incontinence. Obstet Gynecol 98:398, 2001

6. Stewart WF, Van Rooyen JB, Cundiff GW, et al: Prevalence and burden of overactive bladder in the United States. World J Urol 20:327, 2003

7. Adams PF, Hendershot GE, Marano MA: Current estimates from the National Health Interview Survey, 1996. Vital Health Stat 10:93, 1999

8. Milsom I, Abrams P, Cardozo L, et al: How widespread are the symptoms of an overactive bladder and how are they managed? A population-based prevalence study. BJU Int 87:760, 2001

9. Stoddart H, Donovan J, Whitley E, et al: Urinary incontinence in older people in the community: a neglected problem? Br J Gen Pract 51:548, 2001

10. De Groat W: Anatomy and physiology of the lower urinary tract. Urol Clin North Am 20:383, 1993

11. Delancey JO: Anatomy and physiology of urinary continence. Clin Obstet Gynecol 33:298, 1990

12. Delancey JO: Structural aspects of the extrinsic continence mechanism. Obstet Gynecol 72:296, 1988

13. De Groat WC: A neurologic basis for the overactive bladder. Urology 50:36, 1997

14. Tubaro A: Defining overactive bladder: epidemiology and burden of disease. Urology 64:2, 2004

15. Fitzgerald MP, Kenton KS, Brubaker L: Localization of the urge to void in patients with painful bladder syndrome. Neurourol Urodyn 24:633, 2005

16. Cardozo LD, Wise BG, Benness CJ: Vaginal oestradiol for the treatment of lower urinary tract symptoms in postmenopausal women—a double-blind placebo-controlled study. J Obstet Gynaecol 21:383, 2001

17. Lukban J, Whitmore K, Kellogg-Spadt S, et al: The effect of manual physical therapy in patients diagnosed with interstitial cystitis, high-tone pelvic floor dysfunction, and sacroiliac dysfunction. Urology 57:121, 2001

18. Fitzgerald MP, Koch D, Senka J: Visceral and cutaneous sensory testing in patients with painful bladder syndrome. Neurourol Urodyn 24:627, 2005

19. Kleiner SM: Water: an essential but overlooked nutrient. J Am Diet Assoc 99:200, 1999

20. Kaynak H, Kaynak D, Oztura I: Does frequency of nocturnal urination reflect the severity of sleep-disordered breathing? J Sleep Res 13:173, 2004

21. McGrother CW, Donaldson MM, Hayward T, et al: Urinary storage symptoms and comorbidities: a prospective population cohort study in middle-aged and older women. Age Ageing 18:18, 2005

22. Lewis CM, Schrader R, Many A, et al: Diabetes and urinary incontinence in 50- to 90-year-old women: a cross-sectional population-based study. Am J Obstet Gynecol 193:2154, 2005

23. Swithinbank L, Hashim H, Abrams P: The effect of fluid intake on urinary symptoms in women. J Urol 174:187, 2005

24. Wollin J, Bennie M, Leech C, et al: Multiple sclerosis and continence issues: an exploratory study. Br J Nurs 14:439, 2005

25. Pesce F, Castellano V, Finazzi AE, et al: Voiding dysfunction in patients with spinal cord lesions at the thoracolumbar vertebral junction. Spinal Cord 35:37, 1997

26. Weiss JP, Blaivas JG: Nocturia. Curr Urol Rep 4:362, 2003

27. Endeshaw YW, Johnson TM, Kutner MH, et al: Sleep-disordered breathing and nocturia in older adults. J Am Geriatr Soc 52:957, 2004

28. Bo K, Kvarstein B, Nygaard I: Lower urinary tract symptoms and pelvic floor muscle exercise adherence after 15 years. Obstet Gynecol 105:999, 2005

29. Robert M, Mainprize TC: Long-term assessment of the incontinence ring pessary for the treatment of stress incontinence. Int Urogynecol J Pelvic Floor Dysfunct 13:326, 2002

30. Donnelly MJ, Powell-Morgan S, Olsen AL, et al: Vaginal pessaries for the management of stress and mixed urinary incontinence. Int Urogynecol J Pelvic Floor Dysfunct 15:302, 2004

31. Fergusson D, Doucette S, Glass KC, et al: Association between suicide attempts and selective serotonin reuptake inhibitors: systematic review of randomised controlled trials. BMJ 330:396, 2005

32. Lenzer J: FDA warns that antidepressants may increase suicidality in adults. BMJ 331:70, 2005

33. Burch JC: Urethrovaginal fixation to Cooper's ligament for correction of stress incontinence, cystocele, and prolapse. Am J Obstet Gynecol 81:281, 1961

34. Burch JC: Cooper's ligament urethrovesical suspension for stress incontinence. Nine years' experience—results, complications, technique. Am J Obstet Gynecol 100:764, 1968

35. Schulz JA, Nager CW, Stanton SL, et al: Bulking agents for stress urinary incontinence: short-term results and complications in a randomized comparison of periurethral and transurethral injections. Int Urogynecol J Pelvic Floor Dysfunct 15:261, 2004

36. Ward KL, Hilton P: A prospective multicentre randomized trial of tension-free vaginal tape and colposuspension for primary urodynamic stress incontinence: two-year follow-up. Am J Obstet Gynecol 190:324, 2004

37. Ward K, Hilton P: Prospective multicentre randomised trial of tension-free vaginal tape and colposuspension as primary treatment for stress incontinence. BMJ 325:67, 2002

38. Wang AC, Lee LY, Lin CT, et al: A histologic and immunohistochemical analysis of defective vaginal healing after continence taping procedures: a prospective case-controlled pilot study. Am J Obstet Gynecol 191:1868, 2004

39. Andersson KE: The overactive bladder: pharmacologic basis of drug treatment. Urology 50(6A suppl):74, 1997

40. Kelleher CJ, Cardozo LD, Khullar V, et al: A medium-term analysis of the subjective efficacy of treatment for women with detrusor instability and low bladder compliance. Br J Obstet Gynaecol 104:988, 1997

41. Wyman JF, Fantl JA, McClish DK, et al: Comparative efficacy of behavioral interventions in the management of female urinary incontinence. Continence Program for Women Research Group. Am J Obstet Gynecol 179:999, 1998

42. McClish DK, Fantl JA, Wyman JF, et al: Bladder training in older women with urinary incontinence: relationship between outcome and changes in urodynamic observations. Obstet Gynecol 77:281, 1991

43. Visco AG, Weidner AC, Cundiff GW, et al: Observed patient compliance with a structured outpatient bladder retraining program. Am J Obstet Gynecol 181:1392, 1999

44. Nygaard IE, Kreder KJ, Lepic MM, et al: Efficacy of pelvic floor muscle exercises in women with stress, urge, and mixed urinary incontinence. Am J Obstet Gynecol 174:120, 1996

45. Lilihus HG, Oravisto KJ, Valtonen EJ: Origin of pain in interstitial cystitis: effect of ultrasound treatment on the concomitant levator ani spasm syndrome. Scand J Urol Nephrol 7:150, 1973

46. Simon LJ, Landis JR, Erickson DR, et al: The Interstitial Cystitis Data Base Study: concepts and preliminary baseline descriptive statistics. Urology 49(5A suppl):64, 1997

47. Weiss JM: Pelvic floor myofascial trigger points: manual therapy for interstitial cystitis and the urgency-frequency syndrome. J Urol 166:2226, 2001

48. Holzberg A, Kellog-Spadts S, Lukban J, et al: Evaluation of transvaginal Theile massage as a therapeutic intervention for women with interstitial cystitis. Urology 57:120, 2001

49. Oyama IA, Rejba A, Lukban JC, et al: Modified Theile massage as therapeutic intervention for female patients with interstitial cystitis and high-tone pelvic floor dysfunction. Urology 64:862, 2004

50. Lindstrom S, Fall M, Carlsson CA, et al: The neurophysiological basis of bladder inhibition in response to intravaginal electrical stimulation. J Urol 129:405, 1983

51. Schmidt RA, Senn E, Tanagho EA: Functional evaluation of sacral nerve root integrity: report of a technique. Urology 35:388, 1990

52. Fall M, Lindstrom S: Electrical stimulation: a physiologic approach to the treatment of urinary incontinence. Urol Clin North Am 18:393, 1991

53. Wang AC, Wang YY, Chen MC: Single-blind, randomized trial of pelvic floor muscle training, biofeedback-assisted pelvic floor muscle training, and electrical stimulation in the management of overactive bladder. Urology 63:61, 2004

54. Brubaker L, Benson JT, Bent A, et al: Transvaginal electrical stimulation for female urinary incontinence. Am J Obstet Gynecol 177:536, 1997

55. Siegel SW, Catanzaro F, Dijkema HE, et al: Long-term results of a multicenter study on sacral nerve stimulation for treatment of urinary urge incontinence, urgency-frequency, and retention. Urology 56:87, 2000

56. Amundsen CL, Webster GD: Sacral neuromodulation in an older, urge-incontinent population. Am J Obstet Gynecol 187:1462, 2002

57. Montecucco C, Schiavo G: Structure and function of tetanus and botulinum neurotoxins. Q Rev Biophys 28:423, 1995

58. Lacy DB, Tepp W, Cohen AC, et al: Crystal structure of botulinum neurotoxin type A and implications for toxicity. Nat Struct Biol 5:898, 1998

59. Reitz A, Stohrer M, Kramer G, et al: European experience of 200 cases treated with botulinum-A toxin injections into the detrusor muscle for urinary incontinence due to neurogenic detrusor overactivity. Eur Urol 45:510, 2004

60. Schurch B, De Seze M, Denys P, et al: Botulinum toxin type A is a safe and effective treatment for neurogenic urinary incontinence: results of a single treatment, randomized, placebo controlled 6-month study. J Urol 174:196, 2005

61. Appell RA: Clinical efficacy and safety of tolterodine in the treatment of overactive bladder: a pooled analysis. Urology 50:90, 1997

62. Zinner N, Gittelman M, Harris R, et al: Trospium chloride improves overactive bladder symptoms: a multicenter phase III trial. J Urol 171:2311, 2004

63. Chapple CR, Rechberger T, Al-Shukri S, et al: Randomized, double-blind placebo- and tolterodine-controlled trial of the once-daily antimuscarinic agent solifenacin in patients with symptomatic overactive bladder. BJU Int 93:303, 2004

64. Haab F, Stewart L, Dwyer P: Darifenacin, an M3 selective receptor antagonist, is an effective and well-tolerated once-daily treatment for overactive bladder. Eur Urol 45:420, 2004

87 Approach to the Patient with a Breast Mass

Valerie L. Staradub, M.D., and Monica Morrow, M.D.

More than half of the patients who present to a breast clinic have the chief complaint of a breast mass.[1] The identification of a breast mass causes a great deal of anxiety in women, although the majority of breast masses are benign. The most important task of the physician who is evaluating a breast mass is to exclude the presence of malignancy. Once malignancy is ruled out, the physician must provide an accurate diagnosis, suitable treatment, and reassurance to the patient.

Assessment of Normal Organ Function

The normal breast is a mixture of epithelial (glandular) elements, stromal tissue, and fat. This heterogeneity is responsible for the lumpiness that is characteristic of normal breasts, particularly in premenopausal women. The upper outer quadrant and the inframammary ridge are usually the most nodular areas of the normal breast. In women older than 40 years, small pealike nodules can often be felt beneath the areola. These nodules represent dilated ducts and are of no clinical concern. Most normal areas of nodularity can be readily identified by their presence in both breasts.

In premenopausal women, the normal hormonal fluctuations of the menstrual cycle often result in changes in breast nodularity that may be mistaken for disease processes. The progesterone surge at ovulation results in mammary duct differentiation and alveolar epithelial cell differentiation into secretory cells. Clinically, this translates to a greater degree of nodularity in the upper outer quadrants of the breasts and may also result in breast tenderness or discomfort. Cyclical nodularity generally decreases after the onset of menses, which is the rationale for the recommendation that a patient perform breast self-examination in the week after her period, when the breasts are the least nodular. These cyclical changes in breast nodularity are often erroneously termed fibrocystic disease, but they are in fact a component of normal physiology.[2] After menopause with its concomitant withdrawal of estradiol and progesterone, the epithelial elements of the breast atrophy, making the breasts softer, less nodular, and easier to examine.

History and Physical Examination of the Patient with a Breast Mass

The key to evaluating the patient who presents with a breast mass is to determine whether a dominant mass is present and to define the level of suspicion for malignancy associated with the mass, should one be detected. These determinations are initially made on the basis of a careful history and physical examination and will direct the approach to diagnosis and management for each patient.

HISTORY

The initial step in obtaining the pertinent history is to characterize the mass by determining the mass's duration, fluctuation with the menstrual cycle, associated tenderness, and whether it has changed in size since the patient first identified it. The pa-

tient should be asked whether she has a history of breast problems, including cyst aspirations and biopsies. A menstrual history is important, including the date of the last period, any recent menstrual irregularities, use of oral contraceptives or hormone replacement therapy, and recent changes in hormone preparation.

An assessment of the patient's level of risk for breast cancer is appropriate [*see Table 1*], although the characteristics of the breast mass rather than the patient's level of risk for cancer should be the primary determinant of the appropriate workup. The characteristics of the breast mass take precedence over the assessment of cancer risk because the majority of women with breast cancer lack identifiable risk factors.[3] When eliciting a family history, it is important to obtain information on both maternal and paternal relatives, because breast cancer on either side of the family is associated with an increased level of risk.

PHYSICAL EXAMINATION

Physical examination is important to confirm the presence of a mass. Often, a mass identified by a patient or a primary care physician is actually an area of normal glandular nodularity or normal breast tissue and underlying structures. In a study of 605 women younger than 40 years, Morrow and colleagues reported that referral by a primary care provider to a surgeon for the evaluation of a breast lump led to confirmation of the presence of a dominant mass in 29% of women, whereas patient-detected masses were confirmed by the surgeon in 36% (a difference that was not statistically significant).[4]

Examination should be carried out with the patient in both an upright sitting position and a supine position. The breasts should be evaluated for symmetry with the arms relaxed and with the arms raised over the head. The presence of skin or nipple retraction, edema, or erythema should be noted. In many women, the breasts are not precisely the same size, and in some women, there may be a significant difference in size. If a size discrepancy is noted, the patient should be questioned regarding its duration. Similarly, many women have bifid or chronically inverted nipples, the latter of which occur particularly after lactation; however, bifid nipples or chronically inverted nipples are of no concern, even if the chronically inverted nipples are present in a patient who has never lactated.

Table 1 Factors Used for Assessment of Breast Cancer Risk

Patient age	Number of relatives with breast and/or ovarian cancer
Patient race	
Age at menarche	
Age at first live birth	Relationship to patient
Age at menopause	Age at diagnosis
History of postmeno-pausal hormone replacement therapy	Number of previous breast biopsies
	Pathologic findings at biopsy

Palpation of both breasts, as well as the axilla, should follow. The axilla should be examined with the patient seated and the ipsilateral arm supported to relax the pectoral muscle. Small palpable nodes are not uncommon in slender women, and any palpable nodes must be assessed for worrisome characteristics such as fixation, large size, or hardness.

Breast palpation should be performed with the patient both in the upright position and in the supine position. In the supine position, the ipsilateral arm should be placed behind the head to spread the breast tissue across the chest wall. The pads, rather than the tips, of the first three fingers should be used for palpation, and pinching of the breast tissue between the fingers should be avoided. The goal of the examination is to determine if a dominant mass is present. Dominant masses are distinguished from nodular breast tissue by having three dimensions and a texture different from the adjacent normal breast. If a mass is identified, it should be measured with a ruler, the consistency should be noted (e.g., soft, rubbery, firm, hard), and the characteristics of its margins described (e.g., well circumscribed, poorly defined) [*see Table 2*]. Fixation of the mass within the breast or to the chest wall should also be noted. If there is uncertainty whether a finding represents a true dominant mass, comparison with the mirror-image location in the opposite breast is often helpful.

Once the examination is complete, regardless of whether a mass is identified, the patient should be asked to indicate the area that concerns her. This ensures that the area of concern to the patient is not overlooked by the physician. At the conclusion of the examination, the patient can be categorized according to four possible assessments: (1) no abnormal finding is appreciated; (2) a prominent nodularity is present, but it does not have the characteristics of a dominant mass; (3) a dominant mass with clinically benign characteristics is present; and (4) a dominant mass suspicious for cancer is present. The appropriate imaging and diagnostic workup is specific to the outcome of the physical examination.

Evaluation of a Breast Mass

NO ABNORMALITY DETECTED BY PHYSICIAN

If no abnormality is detected during a clinical breast examination, even after careful examination of the area of concern, the patient should be reassured of the absence of worrisome findings. Women 40 years of age and older who have not had a mammogram within the past year should receive a mammogram to screen for nonpalpable abnormalities. In younger patients, no imaging should be recommended unless their level of risk for malignancy indicates screening as a prudent measure. To ensure that no worrisome finding was overlooked, a follow-up examination 2 to 3 months after the patient's initial visit is appropriate for physicians who do not have extensive experience in evaluating breast masses. The follow-up visit is also a good time to review the woman's age and cancer risk to determine the appropriate type and frequency of screening tests.

NODULARITY

It can sometimes be difficult to confidently differentiate a nodularity from a dominant mass. In women between 35 and 40 years of age, mammography is usually not helpful in making this determination. Morrow and colleagues reported that in 197 women who were referred for evaluation of a lump but

Table 2 Physical Characteristics of Benign and Malignant Breast Masses

Characteristic	Benign	Malignant
Borders	Well circumscribed	Irregular
Texture	Firm or rubbery	Hard
Mobility	Mobile	Fixed to surrounding tissue
Skin changes	None	Dimpling, retraction
Nipple changes	None	Retraction, bloody discharge, scaling

whose physical examinations were considered by the surgeon to be normal or characterized only by glandular nodularity, only three had a mass identified on mammography that resulted in a breast biopsy, and all three were benign.[4] More commonly, the imaging study led to a recommendation for a 6-month follow-up mammogram to monitor abnormalities that were classified as "probably benign" and were independent of the patient's reason for presentation. None of the abnormalities monitored by follow-up mammograms proved to be carcinoma. Similarly, Harris and Jackson reported that no malignant lesions were identified in their study of 625 women younger than 35 years when mammography was used to examine lumpy breasts and suspected fibrocystic disease.[5]

Directed ultrasound of the area in question is the initial study recommended in young women when there is uncertainty regarding the presence of a dominant mass. If no suspicious findings are revealed on ultrasound, a short-interval follow-up examination in 1 to 2 months is appropriate.

In women older than 40 years, a diagnostic imaging workup should be performed when a dominant mass is identified on physical examination. The mammogram should include placement of a skin marker over the area of interest and extra views of the indicated area, if these are determined to be appropriate by the radiologist. If no abnormality is seen on mammography, a directed ultrasound study should be performed to exclude the presence of mammographically occult carcinoma. If these imaging studies reveal no evidence of a breast mass, then a short-interval follow-up examination constitutes appropriate management.

Attempts at needle aspiration to reassure both the patient and her physician that no worrisome abnormalities are present are not usually helpful in the absence of a dominant mass. Normal breast tissue is significantly less cellular than dominant masses; thus, the rate of nondiagnostic aspirates is significantly higher in cases in which no discrete abnormality is detected than in cases in which a dominant mass is present.[4,6] An aspirate with insufficient material for diagnosis is generally considered an indication for surgical biopsy; therefore, the use of fine-needle aspiration (FNA) for vague areas of nodularity may lead to unnecessary biopsies.

In patients with nodularity on physical examination and a negative imaging workup, a follow-up examination should be performed in 1 to 3 months to ensure the stability and benign nature of the nodularity. If the finding persists, another examination after 6 months is appropriate to ensure that a discrete mass is not evolving [*see Dominant Masses with Clinically Benign Features, below*].

DOMINANT MASSES WITH CLINICALLY BENIGN FEATURES

Imaging Evaluation

In the woman whose physical examination detected a dominant mass with benign clinical features, the initial step in evaluation is to determine whether the mass is cystic or solid. Cysts cannot be reliably diagnosed by physical examination alone, and thus, ultrasound or aspiration of fluid and subsequent resolution of the mass are required for diagnosis [*see Figure 1*].

Ultrasound   In women younger than 35 years, ultrasound is often the only diagnostic study needed for the evaluation of a clinically benign breast mass. Mammography is recommended only if the mass is considered suspicious for malignancy, because cancer is rare in this group and mammograms are usually inconclusive because of breast density. Women older than 35 years who present with a breast mass should be evaluated by mammography and ultrasound.

Ultrasound, unlike mammography, has the capacity to differentiate solid masses from cystic masses. Simple cysts are seen on ultrasound as round or oval with sharply defined margins and posterior acoustic enhancement—that is, the tissue deep to the cyst appears brighter than other breast tissue found at the same level—and without any internal echoes. If a cyst is seen to have a solid component on ultrasound, further workup is warranted.

Aspiration   Complex cysts are defined as those with septations or internal echoes and are traditionally managed by aspiration. However, in a study of 308 complex cysts, the incidence of malignancy was only 0.3%, suggesting that many complex cysts can be managed adequately by short-term follow-up.[7]

Biopsy   Cystic lesions with thick and indistinct walls, thick septations, or any solid component should be biopsied, because some of these masses are malignant. In a study by Berg and colleagues, 18 out of 79 lesions with these characteristics proved to be malignant.[8]

It has been suggested that patients with a palpable breast mass exhibiting normal mammographic and ultrasound findings do not require tissue diagnosis[9]; however, evidence suggests that malignant masses may not be detected by mammography and ultrasonography. Edeiken reported that 22% of 499 women with a palpable breast cancer had a false negative mammogram,[10] and the majority of false negatives were observed in women younger than 50 years (a finding attributed primarily to the prevalence of breast density in young women). Ultrasound is an extremely operator-dependent technique. Although Dennis and colleagues[9] reported that ultrasound has a high sensitivity for the diagnosis of cancer, it is not clear that these results can be generalized to a variety of practice settings.

A patient with a palpable solid mass should be referred to a surgeon for a tissue diagnosis regardless of whether the mass is visualized by imaging studies. Solid masses may be diagnosed with FNA cytology, core-needle biopsy, or excisional biopsy [*see Figure 1*].

Triple Diagnosis Test

The triple diagnosis test uses a combination of physical examination, imaging studies, and FNA cytology as an alternative to surgical excision to establish that a breast mass is benign. The triple test is considered to identify the mass as benign if the physical examination, mammogram, and FNA all indicate a benign process. If the lesion cannot be visualized on mammogram or if the FNA contains insufficient cells for diagnosis, the triple test cannot be confirmatory for a benign lesion. In a study of 191 patients who had confirmatory surgical biopsy, Steinberg and

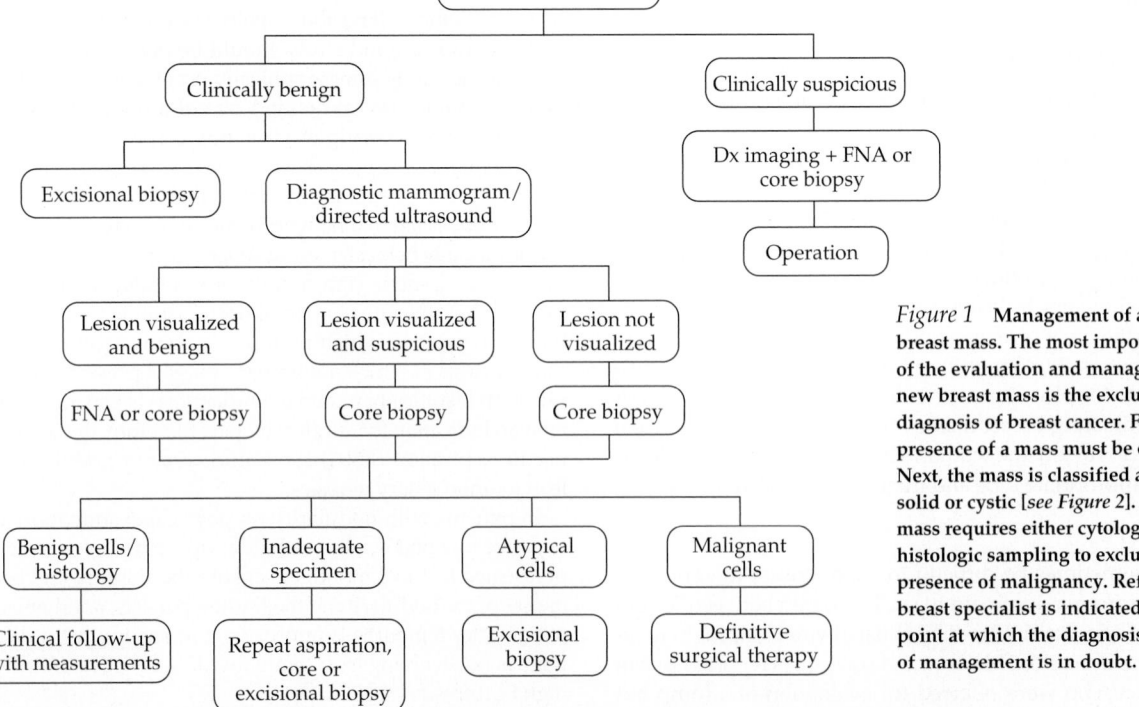

Figure 1   **Management of a solid breast mass. The most important facet of the evaluation and management of a new breast mass is the exclusion of a diagnosis of breast cancer. First, the presence of a mass must be confirmed. Next, the mass is classified as either solid or cystic [*see Figure 2*]. A solid mass requires either cytologic or histologic sampling to exclude the presence of malignancy. Referral to a breast specialist is indicated at any point at which the diagnosis or choice of management is in doubt.**

colleagues reported that the triple test had a sensitivity of 95.5% and a specificity of 100%.[11] Vetto and colleagues reported that the triple diagnosis test is accurate and results in a substantial reduction in the need for surgical excisional biopsies of benign lesions.[12] In their study of 46 breast lesions identified in 43 patients, the triple test produced concordant results in 21 lesions.[12] Twelve triple tests gave concordant benign results, and biopsy was confirmatory in all of these cases (negative predictive value of 100%). In nine cases, there were concordant malignant results, and final pathology on all of these confirmed malignancy (positive predictive value of 100%). There were 25 discordant triple test results (54%): in nine of these cases, the final pathology was benign, and the remaining 16 demonstrated malignancy (positive predictive value of 64%).

No single mode of evaluation used in the triple test is as accurate as the combination of the three.[12] Bicker and colleagues reported that only seven of 2,184 (0.32%) patients assessed as having benign disease by the triple test were subsequently found to have carcinoma, with five of the seven cancers diagnosed within the first year of observation.[13] Overall, FNA has been shown to be quite accurate in the evaluation of benign breast masses [see Table 3].[11,12,14-16] FNA cytology alone has a sensitivity ranging from 65% to 98% and a specificity of 34% to 100%. In a review of 29 studies, the likelihood of identifying malignant cytology in patients with breast cancer ranged from 35% to 92%.[17] Lower sensitivity is associated with smaller tumors and younger patient age; sensitivity is quite high when FNA is performed by trained personnel and interpreted by an experienced cytologist.[18]

Following a benign, concordant triple diagnosis test, an identified mass must be monitored for growth by serial examination and imaging studies, which are generally recommended to be performed every 6 months for 2 years, until stability is documented. Growth of the lesion should prompt surgical excision. Patients opting for observation should be counseled about the small possibility of a delay in the diagnosis of cancer. Particular caution should be used when taking a wait-and-see approach in women 50 years of age or older, because in this group benign breast masses are infrequent and carcinoma is more common.

Core-Needle Biopsy

An alternative approach to the diagnosis of a clinically and radiographically benign lesion is core-needle biopsy. This approach has two advantages: (1) it provides a histologic specimen that can be interpreted by a general pathologist, rather than requiring a specialized cytopathologist, and (2) it provides a specific histologic diagnosis rather than simply classifying the

mass as benign. In one study, 286 breast lesions (232 of which were palpable) were evaluated both by FNA and core-needle biopsy, and the two tests were reported to have equal sensitivity, positive predictive value for malignancy, and equally low rates of samples inadequate for diagnosis.[15] Core biopsy is associated with slightly greater discomfort and higher costs than FNA. Because core biopsies may sample adjacent tissue, rather than the lesion itself, a follow-up evaluation is necessary, even if a benign result is obtained.

Before undertaking an extensive workup to establish with a high degree of certainty that a mass is benign, it is important to ascertain whether the patient will be comfortable with a palpable abnormality left in place in her breast. For the highly anxious patient, the patient in whom follow-up is difficult, or the unreliable patient, excisional biopsy may be the preferred diagnostic strategy, even for lesions felt to be clinically benign.

SUSPICIOUS DOMINANT BREAST MASSES

Imaging Evaluation

If a breast mass has characteristics suggestive of carcinoma, a diagnostic mammogram is the initial step in evaluation. The purpose of the mammogram is to define the absence or presence and extent of nonpalpable disease associated with the mass and to identify additional abnormalities in the ipsilateral or contralateral breast that may influence the choice of local therapy. The purpose of the mammogram is *not* to diagnose the palpable finding. Between 15% and 30% of palpable cancers are not seen on mammography[19]; therefore, a normal mammogram does not ensure the absence of cancer. However, the likelihood of a false negative result can be minimized through the use of a diagnostic mammogram, which may include multiple views in comparison with the two standard views used in screening mammography. In a diagnostic mammogram, a marker is placed on the palpable finding to ensure that the area of the breast containing the mass is included on the films. Failure to visualize lesions in the periphery of the breast is a well-documented cause of false negative mammograms. Extra views are obtained of the tumor site to define the extent of the primary tumor, and these views are critically important to the surgeon when assessing the local therapy options available to the patient. However, regardless of the findings of mammography, women with clinically suspicious breast masses require a histologic diagnosis to exclude the presence of cancer.

Histologic Diagnosis

Needle biopsy, either core biopsy or FNA, is the preferred technique for diagnosing clinically suspicious breast masses.

Table 3 Accuracy of Fine-Needle Aspiration

Study	Number of Patients	Positive Predictive Value (%)	Negative Predictive Value (%)	Sensitivity (%)	Specificity (%)
Morris[14]	261	100	95.5	96	100
Westenend[15]	286	100	—	92	82
Steinberg[11]	191	98	—	49	99.5
Vetto[12]	46	100	95.5	96	100
Patel[16]	731	99.4	85	91	56*

*Included specimens insufficient for diagnosis.

Needle biopsy is more cost-effective than primary surgical excision and does not involve incisions that may interfere with mastectomy incision placement or affect breast skin needed for breast reconstruction, should the patient choose such a treatment option.

False negative rates for core biopsy and FNA, as discussed previously, are similar. A small incidence of false positive findings with FNA has been reported. The likelihood of having a benign final diagnosis after a frankly malignant FNA result is between 0% and 0.2%. However, the likelihood of having a benign final diagnosis after an FNA result reported as suspicious for malignancy is as high as 6.2%; thus, a finding that is suspicious for malignancy on FNA should prompt a surgical excision for definitive diagnosis before proceeding to definitive cancer treatment.[17]

Core biopsy is preferred by many physicians because it provides information about tumor histology and reliably distinguishes invasive from intraductal carcinoma. If needle-biopsy techniques do not provide a definitive diagnosis of malignancy and the mass has suspicious characteristics on physical examination or mammogram, a surgical biopsy should be performed. When surgical excision is undertaken, the procedure should be performed as a lumpectomy that includes excision of some adjacent normal breast tissue and placement of orienting sutures for the pathologist. If the margins are free of cancer, the diagnostic procedure serves as the definitive breast procedure.

Differential Diagnosis and Management of Common Benign Breast Masses

CYSTS

Cysts are most frequent in the perimenopausal years, with 63% of cysts occurring in women between the ages of 40 and 49.[20] Cysts are less common in younger women, accounting for only 10% of breast masses in women younger than 40 years.[4] Cysts are also relatively uncommon in postmenopausal women, except in those receiving hormone replacement therapy. Multiple cysts in the same patient, whether synchronous or metachronous, are not uncommon.[21]

Cysts are usually round or oval and have smooth, well-demarcated borders. They may fluctuate with the menstrual cycle, and they may be tender, especially if they have filled rapidly. Cysts are indistinguishable from solid masses on physical examination and mammography, but they may be suspected because of a history of menstrual-cycle variation and the clinical finding of a well-circumscribed, firm mass. There are two methods to definitively characterize a mass as a cyst: aspiration and ultrasound [see Figure 2]. Aspiration is performed with a 20- to 22-gauge needle and is successful if fluid is obtained and the mass completely resolves. The fluid may be yellow, clear, or a murky greenish-brown. Bloody cyst fluid is an indication for excision, and if blood is identified in the aspirate, the procedure should be promptly halted in an attempt to preserve a part of the mass. Cyst aspiration fluid should not be sent for cytology, because dead epithelial cells are shed into a cyst and atypical findings are likely, despite the low likelihood of malignancy.[20] Additionally, once the cyst has been aspirated, there is no palpable target for the excision mandated by the finding of atypia. In a study of 6,747 cysts with nonbloody aspirates, no cancers were found.[20] If a mass is still pre-

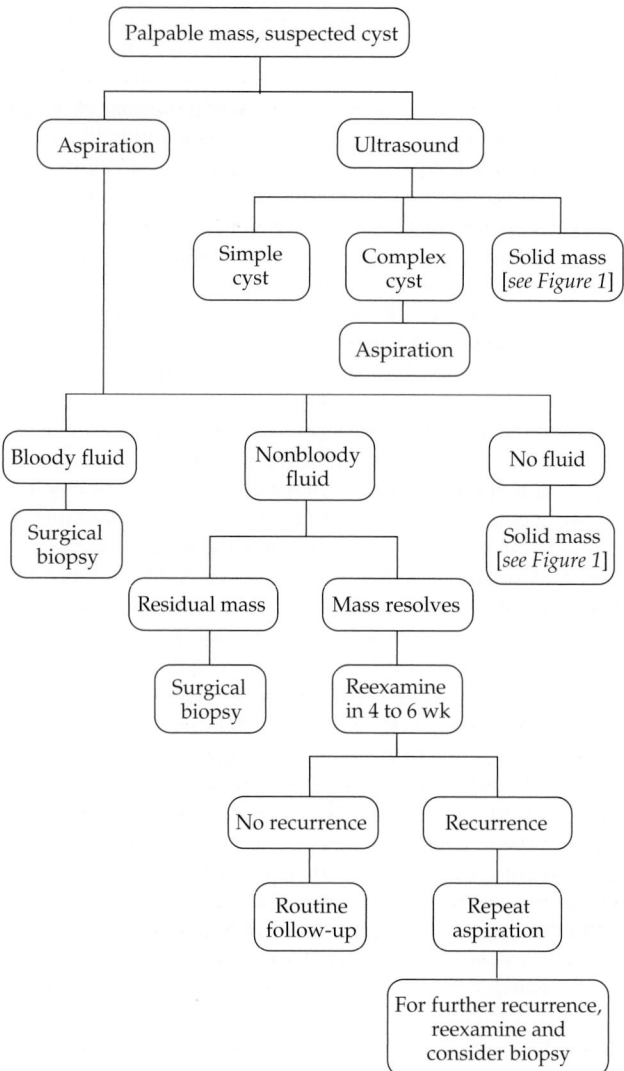

Figure 2 **Management of a breast cyst. Cysts can be identified either by aspiration of fluid or by ultrasound. Prompt diagnosis and management reduce the anxiety level of the patient.**

sent after aspiration, the mass should be evaluated as a dominant solid mass, and a histologic diagnosis should be obtained. If a cyst recurs rapidly (within 1 to 3 weeks) after aspiration, it should be reevaluated. Fewer than 20% of cysts will recur rapidly after aspiration,[22] and rapid refilling of the cyst raises the possibility of a mass resulting in ductal obstruction or a growth within the cyst wall. A second aspiration may be undertaken, but with multiple recurrences, surgical biopsy should be performed to ensure that a cancer with a cystic component is not overlooked.

Patients who do not wish to undergo aspiration of the cyst may opt for targeted ultrasound of the mass. Ultrasound is 98% to 100% accurate in diagnosing simple cysts when careful criteria are used.[23] As previously stated, the criteria for identifying a simple cyst on ultrasound are its round or oval shape, sharply defined margins, posterior acoustic enhancement, and absence of internal echoes. Simple cysts positively identified on ultrasound do not require any treatment, although painful cysts may be aspirated for symptom relief.

SOLID MASSES

Fibroadenomas

Fibroadenomas are a frequent cause of breast mass and occur most commonly in younger women. Fibroadenomas tend to occur at an earlier age in blacks than in whites.[24] A biphasic incidence is reported in white women, with peaks at 25 and 48 years of age[25]; in black women, the peak incidence is between 16 and 25 years of age.[25] Fibroadenoma cannot be definitively diagnosed by clinical examination alone.

Fibroadenomas in young women are usually firm; rubbery; well circumscribed; nontender; and very mobile, because they grow by displacing the surrounding breast tissue. Fibroadenomas can be diagnosed by core biopsy or excisional biopsy, or they may be observed after a benign and concordant triple diagnosis test, whichever is preferable to the patient. Excision is indicated if any aspect of the triple test is discordant or if the lesion enlarges after diagnosis.

Ultrasound is useful to document the stability of a lesion identified as a fibroadenoma that is being managed conservatively. Benign fibroadenomas can change in size. In a study of 1,070 cases diagnosed by FNA and followed for 3 years, a mean change in each of the three dimensions of 20% or less over a 6-month interval was not associated with malignancy.[26] A more significant change in size may be an indication of malignancy or phyllodes tumor.[27,28] Fibroadenomas may increase in size significantly during pregnancy, and younger women considering expectant management of a fibroadenoma should be educated regarding this possibility. Fibroadenomas can also regress entirely or become smaller over time. In a study of 92 fibroadenomas confirmed by FNA and followed for a mean of 47 weeks, 15 (16%) resolved and 30 (33%) enlarged throughout the study.[29] The remaining lesions either remained static or enlarged slightly and then remained unchanged. Tumor resolution is more likely to occur in fibroadenomas in very young women, in new-onset fibroadenomas, in small fibroadenomas, and in fibroadenomas occurring during pregnancy.

Although fibroadenomas themselves are benign, having a fibroadenoma may slightly increase the long-term risk for breast cancer development. For example, a retrospective cohort study showed a 2.17 relative risk for breast cancer in women with fibroadenomas, compared with the study's control subjects.[30] However, in the subset of patients without a family history of breast cancer and with a noncomplex fibroadenoma, no increase in risk was seen, whereas those with complex fibroadenomas had a relative risk between 2 and 4.

Complex fibroadenomas are characterized by epithelial calcification, apocrine metaplasia, and sclerosing adenosis and are larger than 3 mm.[30] Fibroadenomas rarely contain epithelial hyperplasia with atypia, with a frequency of 0.3%.[31] Furthermore, in one study, the presence of such atypia did not correlate with an additional increased risk of future breast carcinoma.[32] Fibroadenomas are regarded by the Cancer Committee of the College of American Pathologists as lesions that do not confer an increased risk for the development of breast cancer.[33]

Phyllodes Tumors

Phyllodes tumors are much less common than fibroadenomas. In one study of 515 benign masses, the ratio of fibroadenomas to phyllodes tumors was 29:1.[34] The majority of phyllodes tumors are benign, but they may grow to a very large size. A rapid change in the size of a mass thought to be a fibroadeno-

---

Table 4 Benign Breast Lesions by Category

Nonproliferative lesions
  Simple cysts
  Mild hyperplasia of the usual type
  Papillary apocrine change
Proliferative lesions without atypia
  Fibroadenomas
  Intraductal papillomas
  Sclerosing adenosis
  Moderate to florid hyperplasia
Proliferative lesions with atypia
  Atypical ductal hyperplasia
  Atypical lobular hyperplasia

---

ma is suggestive of a phyllodes tumor and is an indication for excision. Benign phyllodes tumors have a propensity to recur locally in about 20% of cases unless excised with a 1 to 2 cm margin of normal breast tissue.[35] For very large tumors, adequate resection may necessitate mastectomy.

Other Benign Masses

Hamartomas Hamartomas are uncommon benign breast masses that are usually well circumscribed and contain elements of fat, glandular tissue, and fibrous tissue.[36] Because they contain the same tissues as the normal breast, hamartomas are often difficult to feel and are more typically diagnosed by mammography. Hamartomas do not have specific diagnostic histologic features; thus, tissue diagnosis must be correlated to physical findings and mammographic imaging.[36] The cytologic findings overlap with findings in other benign masses, and they are unlikely to be confused with malignancy.[37] There are extremely rare reports of in situ or invasive carcinoma identified in a breast hamartoma, but for the most part, hamartomas are benign masses.

Fat necrosis Fat necrosis results from trauma to the breast, which can be secondary to operation, accident (e.g., seat-belt injury and falls), or radiation therapy. In up to 50% of cases, the patient cannot recall any antecedent trauma.[38]

Clinically, fat necrosis results in a firm irregular breast mass. Because fat necrosis often occurs superficially in the breast, it may result in skin retraction that mimicks carcinoma. There is a spectrum of imaging findings associated with fat necrosis, including radiolucent oil cysts (which are diagnostic of the condition), dystrophic calcifications, and spiculated masses mimicking carcinoma.[38] It can be difficult to differentiate fat necrosis from malignancy using clinical and radiographic features alone, and biopsy is usually required.

Benign Breast Lesions and Breast Cancer Risk

Much confusion has surrounded the relationship between benign breast disease and breast cancer risk. The seminal work in this area was by Dupont and Page, who reviewed over 10,500 women with benign breast biopsies and reported results based on 3,303 of these women, who were followed for a median of 17 years.[39] Benign disease was categorized into three groups: nonproliferative disease, proliferative disease without atypia, and proliferative disease with atypia [see Table 4].

Women with nonproliferative lesions were not found to be at increased risk for subsequent breast cancer, whereas women with proliferative lesions and no atypia had a relative risk for developing cancer of 1.9. Women with atypical ductal or lobular hyperplasia had a cancer risk 5.3 times that of women with nonproliferative lesions, and women with atypical hyperplasia and a family history of breast cancer had a relative risk for developing cancer of 11. These findings have been validated in a subsequent prospective, case-control study by London and colleagues, who evaluated 121 women with breast cancer who had a prior biopsy for benign breast disease and 448 control subjects (women without cancer matched for year of birth and year of benign biopsy).[40] This study reported a relative risk of 1.6 for patients with proliferative disease and no atypical hyperplasia and a relative risk of 3.7 for patients with proliferative disease and atypical hyperplasia. It is important to recognize that atypical hyperplasia is uncommon in clinically detected lesions, accounting for only 3.6% of patients in the study by Dupont and Page.[39] Although proliferative lesions increase the relative risk of breast cancer development by a factor of 1.5 to 2.0, the absolute risk of breast cancer remains low in the absence of other risk factors. Atypical hyperplasia is a significant risk factor, but the absolute risk of cancer will vary with the individual's age and other risk factors. The modified Gail model is a useful tool for evaluating a woman's overall level of risk after a diagnosis of atypical hyperplasia.[41]

The authors have no commercial relationships with manufacturers of products or providers of services discussed in this chapter.

References

1. Hindle WH: Breast mass evaluation. Clin Obstet Gynecol 45:750, 2002
2. Love SM, Gelman RS, Silen W: Sounding board. Fibrocystic "disease" of the breast—a nondisease? N Engl J Med 307:1010, 1982
3. Madigan MP, Ziegler RG, Benichou J, et al: Proportion of breast cancer cases in the United States explained by well-established risk factors. J Natl Cancer Inst 87:1681, 1995
4. Morrow M, Wong S, Venta L: The evaluation of breast masses in women younger than forty years of age. Surgery 124:634, 1998
5. Harris VJ, Jackson VP: Indications for breast imaging in women under age 35 years. Radiology 172:445, 1989
6. Rimsten A, Stenkvist B, Johanson H, et al: The diagnostic accuracy of palpation and fine-needle biopsy and an evaluation of their combined use in the diagnosis of breast lesions: report on a prospective study in 1244 women with symptoms. Ann Surg 182:1, 1975
7. Venta LA, Kim JP, Pelloski CE, et al: Management of complex breast cysts. AJR Am J Roentgenol 173:1331, 1999
8. Berg WA, Campassi CI, Ioffe OB: Cystic lesions of the breast: sonographic-pathologic correlation. Radiology 227:183, 2003
9. Dennis MA, Parker SH, Klaus AJ, et al: Breast biopsy avoidance: the value of normal mammograms and normal sonograms in the setting of a palpable lump. Radiology 219:186, 2001
10. Edeiken S: Mammography and palpable cancer of the breast. Cancer 61:263, 1988
11. Steinberg JL, Trudeau ME, Ryder DE, et al: Combined fine-needle aspiration, physical examination and mammography in the diagnosis of palpable breast masses: their relation to outcome for women with primary breast cancer. Can J Surg 39:302, 1996
12. Vetto J, Pommier R, Schmidt W, et al: Use of the "triple test" for palpable breast lesions yields high diagnostic accuracy and cost savings. Am J Surg 169:519, 1995
13. Bicker T, Schondorf H, Naujoks H: Long-term follow-up in patients with mammary gland changes found unsuspicious by aspiration cytology. Cancer Detect Prev 11:319, 1988
14. Morris A, Pommier RF, Schmidt WA, et al: Accurate evaluation of palpable breast masses by the triple test score. Arch Surg 133:930, 1998
15. Westenend PJ, Sever AR, Beekman-De Volder HJ, et al: A comparison of aspiration cytology and core needle biopsy in the evaluation of breast lesions. Cancer 93:146, 2001
16. Patel JJ, Gartell PC, Smallwood JA, et al: Fine needle aspiration cytology of breast masses: an evaluation of its accuracy and reasons for diagnostic failure. Ann R Coll Surg Engl 69:156, 1987
17. Giard RW, Hermans J: The value of aspiration cytologic examination of the breast: a statistical review of the medical literature. Cancer 69:2104, 1992
18. Cariaggi MP, Bulgaresi P, Confortini M, et al: Analysis of the causes of false negative cytology reports on breast cancer fine needle aspirates. Cytopathology 6:156, 1995
19. Barton MB, Harris R, Fletcher SW: The rational clinical examination. Does this patient have breast cancer? The screening clinical breast examination: should it be done? How? JAMA 282:1270, 1999
20. Ciatto S, Cariaggi P, Bulgaresi P: The value of routine cytologic examination of breast cyst fluids. Acta Cytol 31:301, 1987
21. Hughes LE, Bundred NJ: Breast macrocysts. World J Surg 13:711, 1989
22. Leis HP Jr: Gross breast cysts: significance and management. Contemp Surg 39:13, 1991
23. Sickles EA, Filly RA, Callen PW: Benign breast lesions: ultrasound detection and diagnosis. Radiology 151:467, 1984
24. Oluwole SF, Freeman HP: Analysis of benign breast lesions in blacks. Am J Surg 137:786, 1979
25. Nigro DM, Organ CH Jr: Fibroadenoma of the female breast: some epidemiologic surprises. Postgrad Med 59:113, 1976
26. Gordon PB, Gagnon FA, Lanzkowsky L: Solid breast masses diagnosed as fibroadenoma at fine-needle aspiration biopsy: acceptable rates of growth at long-term follow-up. Radiology 229:233, 2003
27. Hermann G, Keller RJ, Tartter P, et al: Interval changes in nonpalpable breast lesions as an indication of malignancy. Can Assoc Radiol J 46:105, 1995
28. Sickles EA: Periodic mammographic follow-up of probably benign lesions: results in 3,184 consecutive cases. Radiology 179:463, 1991
29. Wilkinson S, Anderson TJ, Rifkind E, et al: Fibroadenoma of the breast: a follow-up of conservative management. Br J Surg 76:390, 1989
30. Dupont WD, Page DL, Parl FF, et al: Long-term risk of breast cancer in women with fibroadenoma. N Engl J Med 331:10, 1994
31. Kuijper A, Mommers EC, van der Wall E, et al: Histopathology of fibroadenoma of the breast. Am J Clin Pathol 115:736, 2001
32. Carter BA, Page DL, Schuyler P, et al: No elevation in long-term breast carcinoma risk for women with fibroadenomas that contain atypical hyperplasia. Cancer 92:30, 2001
33. Fitzgibbons PL, Henson DE, Hutter RV: Benign breast changes and the risk for subsequent breast cancer: an update of the 1985 consensus statement. Cancer Committee of the College of American Pathologists. Arch Pathol Lab Med 122:1053, 1998
34. Hindle WH, Alonzo LJ: Conservative management of breast fibroadenomas. Am J Obstet Gynecol 164:1647, 1991
35. Mangi AA, Smith BL, Gadd MA, et al: Surgical management of phyllodes tumors. Arch Surg 134:487, 1999
36. Tse GM, Law BK, Ma TK, et al: Hamartoma of the breast: a clinicopathological review. J Clin Pathol 55:951, 2002
37. Herbert M, Schvimer M, Zehavi S, et al: Breast hamartoma: fine-needle aspiration cytologic finding. Cancer 99:255, 2003
38. Bilgen IG, Ustun EE, Memis A: Fat necrosis of the breast: clinical, mammographic and sonographic features. Eur J Radiol 39:92, 2001
39. Dupont WD, Page DL: Risk factors for breast cancer in women with proliferative breast disease. N Engl J Med 312:146, 1985
40. London SJ, Connolly JL, Schnitt SJ, et al: A prospective study of benign breast disease and the risk of breast cancer. JAMA 267:941, 1992
41. Spiegelman D, Colditz GA, Hunter D, et al: Validation of the Gail et al. model for predicting individual breast cancer risk. J Natl Cancer Inst 86:600, 1994

88 Approach to the Patient with a Pelvic Mass

Joseph T. Chambers, M.D., PH.D., and Carolyn D. Runowicz, M.D.

The finding of a pelvic mass may occur in a female patient of any age; fortunately, most masses are associated with a benign neoplasm or process. Nevertheless, each year, between 5% and 10% of women in the United States undergo surgery for a suspected ovarian neoplasm; only 13% to 21% of these women prove to have a malignant ovarian neoplasm.[1]

A pelvic mass may be found on an abdominal or pelvic examination in an asymptomatic patient at a scheduled health maintenance assessment or on examination of a symptomatic patient who presents with a complaint. A mass may also be noted as an incidental finding on imaging studies, usually computed tomographic scans of the abdomen or pelvis or pelvic ultrasonography, obtained either for medical indications unrelated to a suspected pelvic disease or as a screening study for gynecologic malignancies. Increasingly, a pelvic mass is found on imaging studies obtained in the emergency department for the evaluation of vague abdominal pain or trauma.[2]

The differential diagnosis is extensive [see Table 1], because a pelvic mass may be of gynecologic or nongynecologic origin and may be associated with congenital, functional, neoplastic (either benign or malignant), obstructive, or inflammatory processes; a mass may also be associated with pregnancy. When a mass is of gynecologic origin, it may arise from the ovary, fallopian tube, broad ligament, round ligament, uterus, cervix, or uterosacral ligament. Adnexal masses arise from an area comprising the ovary, the fallopian tube, and the ligaments of the uterus. When the mass is of nongynecologic origin, it may arise from the urinary tract system, the gastrointestinal system, or the pelvic vessels or nerves. Rarely, a mass may arise directly from the peritoneum, the retroperitoneum, or the omentum.

The possible etiologies differ markedly, depending on the patient's age and symptoms. Consequently, the complete documentation of symptoms; the past medical, family, and surgical histories; the physical examination; and the initial imaging studies and laboratory tests will narrow the differential diagnosis and direct appropriate evaluation and referral. The overview of the diagnostic evaluation is presented [see Evaluation of the Patient with a Pelvic Mass, *below*], followed by a review of the distinctions in diagnostic workup required for patients of each age group [see Age-Specific Considerations in Patient Evaluation, *below*].

Evaluation of the Patient with a Pelvic Mass

MEDICAL HISTORY

The patient's medical history is essential in the evaluation of a pelvic mass; it includes a complete menstrual history, which establishes menarche and cyclicity of menses. Because ovulation generally occurs midcycle, a new pelvic mass found midcycle could be consistent with a functional cyst, whereas a mass identified later in the cycle would be more consistent with a corpus luteum cyst. A patient with a long history of irregular menses or even secondary amenorrhea with nontender bilateral adnexal masses may have polycystic ovaries. Pelvic inflammatory disease usually presents about a week after menstruation, and

missed menses suggest a pregnancy. Therefore, an accurate menstrual history is useful in directing the patient evaluation.

Menstrual Bleeding

Increased menstrual bleeding often occurs with submucous leiomyomas. Postmenopausal bleeding may be caused by endometrial cancer or, rarely, by hormonally functioning ovarian or fallopian tube neoplasms. Irregular bleeding, pain, and missed menses suggest an ectopic pregnancy.

Although rare, estrogen-producing neoplasms may cause abnormal uterine bleeding, breast tenderness, or hirsutism. In children, precocious puberty may develop.

In women of reproductive age, the medical history must include questions about contraceptive practices, because a patient on oral contraceptive pills is less likely to develop physiologic and functional cysts (e.g., follicular and corpus luteum cysts). In addition, a patient with multiple sexual partners who does not use barrier contraception may develop pelvic inflammatory disease and a chronic tubo-ovarian abscess.

Abdominal Pain

Pain, if present, must be characterized. The onset, pattern of occurrence, and extent or severity of pain may give important indications of the etiology of the suspected pelvic mass. For example, new onset of midcycle pain in premenopausal women suggests the presence of a physiologic cyst. Pain following intercourse may be related to a ruptured cyst, whereas chronic pain during intercourse is suggestive of endometriosis.

Acute pain Acute severe abdominal or pelvic pain accompanies torsion of an adnexal structure or pedunculated leiomyoma (in which case the pain is usually intermittent); hemorrhage or rupture of an ovarian cyst; dilation of the fallopian tube in association with an ectopic pregnancy; or rupture of a pelvic abscess. In addition, a degenerating leiomyoma may also cause acute pain. The rapid stretching of the ovarian capsule by an expanding functional cyst or germ cell neoplasm may produce acute pain. Acute pain associated with nausea, vomiting, and fever suggests an inflammatory process, such as pelvic inflammatory disease, appendicitis, peritonitis from a perforation or infarction of bowel, or diverticulitis.

Chronic, cyclic pain More chronic, cyclic pain, particularly pain associated with dysmenorrhea, dyspareunia, and menorrhagia, suggests endometriosis. In addition, chronic pelvic or abdominal discomfort is often reported with long-standing tubo-ovarian abscesses or chronic hydrosalpinx. Chronic abdominal pain or vague abdominal discomfort accompanied by bloating suggests an ovarian neoplasm.

Changes in Bowel Habits

Changes in bowel habits and constitution, as well as changes in appetite, weight, and energy, may be more consistent with a benign colonic disease or with a cancer arising in any pelvic organ. The medical history of gynecologic cancers or precancerous disease, breast cancer, melanoma, or any cancer may direct the workup. The family history is important, because hereditary cancers, such as those associated with a *BRCA1* or *BRCA2* mutation (e.g., breast, ovary, endometrial cancer), or nonpolyposis colon cancer may present as a pelvic mass.

PHYSICAL EXAMINATION

Before the pelvic examination, the patient should empty her bladder. There must be adequate light for a visual inspection of the external genitalia for signs of androgen excess. The vagina and cervix must be inspected for signs of infection and hormones. A Papanicolaou smear should be obtained if the patient's age and findings on physical examination indicate the need for it. The abdominovaginal examination gives information on the size, shape, consistency, location, mobility, laterality, and tenderness of the mass. This information must be confirmed by the rectovaginal examination, which also evaluates the uterosacral ligaments, the cul-de-sac, and the anorectal area. Physical examination may suggest whether the mass is benign or malignant [*see Table 2*]. When a pelvic mass is identified, a complete physical examination must be performed. Particular attention should be paid to the examination of the breasts, the respiratory system, the nodal areas, and the abdomen.

LABORATORY TESTS

In the evaluation of a pelvic mass, especially in women of reproductive age, a urinary or serum β-human chorionic gonadotropin (β-hCG) test is required. To determine pregnancy, the urinary test is adequate at the time of missed menses. This test, however, is qualitative in nature, and for the management of an ectopic pregnancy or molar pregnancy, a quantitative determination of the β-hCG serum concentration is necessary. In addition to being an indication for pregnancy, elevated levels of β-hCG may be associated with theca-lutein cysts, especially in women with choriocarcinoma, diabetes mellitus, and Rh sensitization; elevated levels of β-hCG are also associated with clomiphene use, human menopausal gonadotropin or human chorionic gonadotropin ovulation induction, and use of gonadotropin-releasing hormone analogues.[3]

A complete blood count will help in assessing anemia; an elevated white cell count suggests an infectious etiology. The erythrocyte sedimentation rate is nonspecific and does not narrow the differential diagnosis.

IMAGING STUDIES

The most important initial diagnostic tool in evaluating a pelvic mass is the pelvic ultrasound, which indicates whether the mass is more likely to be uterine, adnexal, or gastrointestinal in origin. A pelvic ultrasound scan also provides information on the size and consistency of the mass—characteristics that suggest whether the mass is malignant or benign.

Unilocular ovarian cysts are overwhelmingly benign and resolve spontaneously in 3 to 6 months; therefore, observation is the recommended approach to management. If malignancy is suspected on pelvic ultrasound, additional imaging studies such as abdominal pelvic computed tomography or magnetic resonance imaging may assist in confirming the diagnosis. The CT scan may further characterize the malignant potential of the mass and give information regarding evidence of metastatic spread to lymph nodes, the retroperitoneal space, or adjacent structures. If the origin of the pelvic mass is uncertain, an MRI

Table 1 Differential Diagnosis of Pelvic Mass

Ovary	Gastrointestinal tract
Functional cyst	Bowel loops with feces
Endometrioma	Diverticular disease
Benign neoplasm	Inflammatory bowel
Malignant neoplasm	disease
Fallopian tube	Appendicitis
Tubo-ovarian abscess	Benign small bowel
Hydrosalpinx	neoplasm
Paratubal cyst	Colon cancer
Ectopic pregnancy	Urinary tract
Benign neoplasm	Distended bladder
Malignant neoplasm	Pelvic kidney
Uterus	Urachal cyst
Fibroid (pedunculated or	Retroperitoneum
interligamentous)	Abdominal wall
Intrauterine pregnancy	hematoma or abscess
Sarcoma	Sarcoma, lymphoma, or
	teratoma
	Benign neoplasm

may help clarify whether the mass arises from the uterus, adnexa, or another structure (e.g., muscles or nerves).

Ultrasound

Transabdominal and transvaginal ultrasound Two methods of ultrasound provide extensive information about the characteristics of a pelvic mass. Transabdominal ultrasound is better tolerated by patients than is transvaginal ultrasound, and it gives more information about abdominal processes. Transvaginal ultrasound, however, provides better resolution and more precise information of the mass within the pelvic organ. The unique imaging patterns offered by each of these ultrasound modalities frequently help narrow the differential diagnosis.

Physiologic ovarian cysts are usually oval and filled with clear fluid. They may or may not have septations, and they have no echogenic or solid components, with the exception of the corpus luteum. Cystic teratomas are partially cystic and solid with echogenic foci of abnormal tissue from foreign tissues and hemorrhage. Endometriomas are simple cysts with echogenic elements secondary to old and new hemorrhage. Leiomyomas are solid or semisolid, well-circumscribed masses; they are similar in appearance to the myometrium but have no vascular vessels within the mass.

Several morphologic scoring systems have been introduced to predict whether a pelvic mass evaluated by ultrasound is benign or malignant. Most systems agree that the following characteristics are suggestive of malignancy: irregularity in the wall of the mass, the presence of thick septations within the mass, any papillary projection within or emerging from the mass, and a mass containing solid components. Size itself is an important characteristic; a mass larger than 8 cm in diameter raises concern. In general, the more of these characteristics that are present, the greater the chance that the mass is malignant.

Color Doppler ultrasound The use of color flow Doppler imaging may help in determining whether the adnexal mass is malignant or benign, because malignancies have an increased neovascularity and, thus, lower resistance and pulsatile indices. Currently, there is no agreement concerning pulsatile indices that indicate malignancy; nevertheless, specific indices may be less important in suggesting malignancy than overall morphologic pattern, blood flow, and tumor location.

Taking into consideration the findings of regular and color flow ultrasound, the overall sensitivity, using morphologic criteria for malignant disease, ranges from 82% to 100%; specificity ranges from 60% to 95%. It is unclear, however, whether the addition of the color flow Doppler significantly improves these percentages. Two large studies reported that the combined approach (using regular and color flow ultrasound) has a sensitivity of 88% to 97%, a specificity of 97% to 100%, and an accuracy of 83% to 99%.[4]

Computed tomography CT is less frequently used in the initial evaluation of a pelvic mass than other imaging studies. However, the sensitivity, specificity, and accuracy of CT for determining whether the mass is benign or malignant is reported to be comparable to other modalities (i.e., sensitivity, 89%; specificity, 96% to 99%; accuracy, 92% to 94%).[4] CT is better than ultrasound in assessing the retroperitoneal spaces (i.e., nodal systems, pancreas, and spleen) and the omentum. CT is useful in establishing the extent of intra-abdominal and retroperitoneal disease in patients in whom an ovarian malignancy is highly suspected.

Magnetic Resonance Imaging

MRI may be used in the evaluation of a pelvic mass when findings from ultrasound studies are unclear or indeterminate. MRI is particularly useful in clarifying the origin of the mass as either uterine or ovarian. In addition, its accuracy in assessing fatty and hemorrhagic components of a mass can help in the diagnosis of dermoid cysts, hemorrhagic corpus luteum cysts, and endometriosis. This modality may be especially useful in the pregnant patient, if more information is needed than is provided by the pelvic ultrasound.[5]

Positron Emission Tomography

Positron emission tomography (PET) has limited application in the initial evaluation of pelvic masses. It is used primarily to detect recurrent pelvic malignancies.

SERUM TUMOR MARKERS

Serum tumor markers are not used for screening; they are used in the evaluation of patients with suspected malignant pelvic neoplasms. In deciding which serum markers to use, consideration must be given to the patient's age and medical history. For instance, in prepubertal girls and young women, germ cell tumors are the most frequent ovarian malignancy; appropriate serum markers for suspected germ cell tumors include α-fetoprotein (AFP), lactate dehydrogenase (LDH), and β-hCG. In older women with suspected malignancy, it is important to measure epithelial tumor markers, such as CA125. In patients with confirmed malignancy, a significant elevation in the level of a tumor marker may indicate malignant recurrence, whereas decreasing levels reflect response to treatment. Functional genomics and proteomics—the study of human gene sequences and protein sequences, respectively—show promise in identifying novel cellular targets that may be exploited in the future as screening tests for cancer.

Measurement of AFP, LDH, and β-hCG

Dysgerminomas are the most common germ cell tumors and can occur at any age; these malignancies are associated with elevations in AFP, LDH, and β-hCG. Placental alkaline phosphatase and LDH levels are sometimes elevated in patients with dysgerminomas. Endodermal sinus tumors can be monitored by measuring AFP levels, and choriocarcinomas can be monitored by measuring β-hCG levels. Embryonal carcinoma may secrete both AFP and β-hCG. Immature teratomas usually do not secrete any markers. Mixed germ cell tumors may secrete combinations of the above markers. Granulosa cell tumors are associated with elevated levels of inhibin and estradiol in prepubertal and postmenopausal women.

Measurement of CA125

CA125 is a glycoprotein expressed by fetal amniotic and coelomic epithelium and müllerian epithelium. Elevated levels of serum CA125 may suggest an increased risk of malignancy in certain patients; however, elevations of CA125 are also associated with normal and benign conditions. Therefore, CA125 measurement is not useful as a screening test for ovarian cancer. A CA125 serum concentration greater than 35 U/ml is found in 83% of patients with epithelial ovarian cancer, but it is reported to be elevated in only 50% of patients with stage I disease that is limited to the ovary.[6] In addition, CA125 is increased in patients with other malignancies; in those with benign gynecologic conditions; and in patients with diverticulitis and cirrhosis. It is also increased in normal conditions of pregnancy and menstruation [see Table 3].[7] Approximately 1% of healthy women have elevated CA125 serum levels.[8] In women with benign gynecologic conditions, the levels are usually less than 200 U/ml.

In postmenopausal women, CA125 measurement may have some application as a screening test for malignancy but is not a routine screening test. In a prospective Swedish study of 4,290 volunteer women who were at least 50 years of age, the specificity of CA125 measurement for ovarian cancer was reported to be 97% and the positive predictive value was 4.6%, using a CA125 level greater than 30 U/ml.[9] However, an elevated CA125 level in postmenopausal women with a pelvic mass suggests a malignancy. The positive predictive value for elevations of CA125 in this age group has been reported to be 97%.[10] In women of reproductive age, elevations of serum CA125 may raise the suspicion of malignancy when imaging findings (i.e., tumor location, morphologic pattern, and vascularity) are also consistent with malignancy.

Table 2 Physical Findings Associated with Pelvic Mass

Characteristic of Mass	Suggestive of Benign Process	Suggestive of Malignant Process
Unilateral	Yes	Occasionally
Bilateral	Occasionally	Yes
Cystic	Yes	No
Solid	No	Yes
Mobile	Yes	Occasionally
Fixed	Occasionally	Yes
Irregular contour	Occasionally	Yes
Smooth contour	Yes	No
Presence of ascites	No	Yes
Cul-de-sac nodules	Usually no	Yes
Rapid growth rate	No	Yes
Pain	Yes	Usually no
Size	< 5 cm	≥ 10 cm

Table 3 Conditions Associated with an Elevated Serum CA125 Level

Gynecologic malignancies	Epithelial ovarian cancers Germ cell cancers Sex chord stromal tumors Fallopian tube cancers Endometrial cancers Adenocarcinoma of the cervix
Benign gynecologic conditions	Adenomyosis Benign ovarian neoplasms Endometriosis Functional ovarian cysts Leiomyomas Meigs syndrome Menstruation Pregnancy Ovarian hyperstimulation Pelvic inflammation
Nongynecologic conditions	Liver disease and cirrhosis Colitis Congestive heart failure Diabetes Diverticulitis Lupus Mesothelioma Pericarditis Polyarteritis nodosa Surgery Previous irradiation Renal disease Sarcoidosis Tuberculosis
Nongynecologic cancers	Breast Colon Lung Pancreas Lymphoma

Measurement of Other Tumor Markers

CA19-9 and carcinoembryonic antigen (CEA) are commonly used to follow mucinous tumors. However, the sensitivity and specificity of these markers are lower than those found with CA125 measurement.

FINE-NEEDLE ASPIRATION

Fine-needle aspiration (FNA) is not routinely used in the evaluation of pelvic masses. Although it can easily be performed with ultrasound or CT guidance, FNA has limited diagnostic accuracy, especially in the evaluation of cystic structures. In a study of the use of FNA in 235 patients with cystic ovarian masses, 56% of the aspirates were devoid of diagnostic cells. The sensitivity for specific lesions ranged from 35% to 83%, and the specificity approached 100%.[11] Thus, FNA is not accurate, and should rupture of the cyst contents occur, dissemination of malignant cells may result.

BIOPSY

Rarely, a directed biopsy may be indicated in an individual whose imaging studies are consistent with advanced ovarian intra-abdominal disease and in whom surgery is contraindicated because of significant medical problems. A directed biopsy of a peri-toneal tumor implant may be used to identify the histology of the tumor and thus assist in selecting appropriate nonsurgical management (e.g., initial or neoadjuvant chemotherapy) for ovarian cancer. Immunohistochemical staining profiles may provide additional information consistent with ovarian or peritoneal cancer.

Age-Specific Considerations in Patient Evaluation

PELVIC MASS IN PREPUBERTAL GIRLS

Ovarian cysts occur in 2% to 5% of prepubertal girls.[12] During the first months of life, ovarian cysts are generally functional cysts caused by maternal gonadotropin stimulation of the newborn ovary. Persistence of cysts or the finding of a solid or complex component (i.e., a component in which both cystic and solid elements are present) of the adnexal mass suggests other disorders, including Wilms tumors, neuroblastomas, or gastrointestinal tract abnormalities.

The older literature suggests a very high rate of malignancy for ovarian neoplasms in children, with germ cell tumors being the most frequent malignancy and dysgerminomas being the most common germ cell tumor.[13] More recently, it was reported that in girls younger than 10 years who undergo surgery for an adnexal mass, 60% of the masses were not neoplasms, and two thirds of the neoplasms were benign.[14] If there are signs of early sexual development, the child should be evaluated for precocious puberty or a hormonally functioning ovarian neoplasm.

If torsion of the adnexal mass is suspected, pelvic ultrasound may confirm this diagnosis. If a solid component of the adnexal mass is detected, the risk of a germ cell tumor must be considered and serum levels of appropriate tumor markers (i.e., AFP, LDH, and β-hCG) must be obtained.

Because of the rarity of gynecologic diseases in this age group, more common diagnoses, including acute appendicitis, intussusception of the bowel, gastroenteritis, genitourinary disorders, and chronic constipation, must be considered.

PELVIC MASS IN ADOLESCENTS

The differential diagnosis of a pelvic mass in an adolescent girl is broader than that for younger patients because adolescence is accompanied by functioning ovaries and the beginning of sexual activity. A pelvic mass may be caused by a benign neoplasm, a malignant neoplasm, an anatomic abnormality, or an ectopic pregnancy. Sexually transmitted disease (STD) and pelvic inflammatory disease (PID) must be included in the differential diagnosis.

The patient history should include questions about sexual activity, previous history of STD and PID, and use of contraception. Depending on the adolescent's sexual activity, a vaginal examination may also be appropriate. Adolescents deny sexual activity for multiple reasons, but studies show that 50% of adolescent girls have had sexual intercourse by 17 years of age.[15] In adolescents, a pelvic mass that is not associated with pregnancy may require further evaluation by abdominal CT or MRI. When anatomic abnormalities are suspected, the evaluation should include MRI. Genetic studies may also be indicated if a separate adnexal mass is found, because in 25% of the patients with a Y chromosome, dysgenetic gonads are malignant.[16]

Cystic Adnexal Masses

The majority of cystic adnexal masses are related to the normal physiologic ovary; such masses include follicular cysts, corpus luteum cysts, and theca-lutein cysts. Usually unilocular and less than 8 to 10 cm in diameter, cystic adnexal masses commonly resolve within 6 to 8 weeks. Combination monophasic oral contraceptive pills with progestin, as well as estrogen at a dose higher than 50 μg, are reported to reduce the risk of further ovarian cysts. The use of lower-dose oral contraceptives may be less effective.[17,18]

Theca-lutein cysts that occur in pregnancy are usually bilateral, large, and multicystic. They are associated with high β-hCG levels.[3] Spontaneous resolution usually occurs post partum.

Cystic Teratoma

Overall, mature cystic teratomas (dermoid cysts) account for more than half of the ovarian neoplasms in children and adolescents younger than 20 years.[19] These neoplasms usually range from 5 to 10 cm in diameter; 15% are bilateral. Because they arise from pluripotential germ cell lines, they may contain hair, teeth, sebaceous material, neural elements, and other tissues not usually found in the ovary. Some of these elements show unique imaging patterns (e.g., calcified materials on plain radiograph and fat density on pelvic ultrasound).

Malignant Neoplasms

The risk of ovarian malignant neoplasms is lower in adolescents than in younger children.[14] In reports from referral centers, the rate of malignancy in ovarian neoplasms was 35% in prepubertal girls and adolescents; however, in community-hospital centers, the rate of malignancy was 10% in these patients.[20]

Germ cell tumors account for approximately 70% of the malignant ovarian tumors in girls younger than 15 years.[14] Dysgerminomas are the most common such tumors, followed by immature or malignant teratomas, endodermal sinus tumors, embryonal carcinomas, and choriocarcinomas. Stromal tumors and epithelial carcinomas each make up 15% of the ovarian tumors.[14]

Miscellaneous Masses

Pregnancy luteomas, sclerotic ovaries, and endometriotic cysts occur in adolescent girls. These may be incidental findings on physical examination, or they may be associated with symptoms of pain or irregular menses. Torsion, rupture, or leakage of the content of these cysts and subsequent peritoneal irritation may cause the pain. Laparoscopy may be required for full evaluation of the condition that causes the pain.

Anatomic Abnormalities

Around the time of expected menarche, anatomic abnormalities in the development of the müllerian system can cause obstruction of the uterovaginal outflow tract, resulting in a pelvic mass. The anomalies include imperforated hymen, transverse vaginal septa, vaginal agenesis with normal functional endometrium, vaginal duplications with obstructing longitudinal septa, and obstructed uterine horns. If these anomalies cause a blockage of the vagina or the uterus, a mass may develop; such masses may result in cyclic pain, prompting these women to seek treatment.

Ectopic Pregnancy

In women younger than 17 years, approximately 82% of pregnancies are unintended; 75% of pregnancies are unintended in women 18 and 19 years of age.[21] Ectopic pregnancy is associated with pelvic pain, an adnexal mass, and missed or irregular menses. The risk of ectopic pregnancy is increased in women who have a history of STD or PID, as well as in women who fail to use contraception; oral contraceptives lower the risk.

Inflammatory Processes

The differential diagnosis of a pelvic mass in adolescents includes several infectious processes. When a patient presents with fever, an elevated white cell count, and a lower abdominal, pelvic, or adnexal tender mass that is associated with cervical motion tenderness and mucopurulent cervical discharge, a tubo-ovarian abscess or pyosalpinx must be considered. Often, a history of recent unprotected intercourse with a new partner will help establish the diagnosis. Appendicitis must also be considered in this setting. In the less acute setting, a patient with a pelvic mass and a history of STD should be evaluated for PID. Laparoscopy may be useful in confirming the diagnosis of PID; the clinical diagnosis of PID has been reported to be incorrect in up to one third of patients.[22]

PELVIC MASS IN WOMEN OF REPRODUCTIVE AGE

The detection of an asymptomatic pelvic mass is frequent during the reproductive years because women undergo annual examinations for family planning and gynecologic cancer screening. The differential diagnosis includes all the conditions that may cause a pelvic mass in adolescents (i.e., cystic adnexal masses, cystic teratomas, malignant neoplasms, and ectopic pregnancy), as well as leiomyomas, endometriomas, and metastatic neoplasms involving the ovary.

In a series of 100 women undergoing laparotomy for a pelvic mass, the most common diagnoses by age group were cancer, reported in 56% in women 50 years of age or older; endometriosis, reported in 27% of women 31 to 49 years of age; and cystic teratomas, reported in 33% of women younger than 30 years. In women younger than 30 years, only 10% had an ovarian malignancy, and most of these were tumors of low malignant potential. Thus, most pelvic masses that occur during reproductive years will be benign uterine neoplasms or benign ovarian neoplasms.[23]

A pregnancy test is required in all women of reproductive age who present with a suspected pelvic mass. In pregnant women, the use of abdominal and pelvic CT scans must be avoided. If ultrasound studies are inconclusive, an MRI may help identify the source of the mass.[5] If patient age, physical examination, and findings on ultrasound suggest malignancy, it is appropriate to measure epithelial serum tumor markers, such as CA125. However, elevated levels of CA125 may be associated with normal gynecologic conditions, as well as benign uterine and ovarian neoplasms. Risk of malignancy increases with patient age, positive family history, severity of symptoms, and number of imaging findings consistent with malignancy.

Uterine Neoplasms

Epidemiology Leiomyomas (fibroids) are the most common benign uterine neoplasm. They can also rarely arise from the ovary, the cervix, the pelvic ligaments, or other pelvic structures.

Leiomyomas are clinically apparent on examination in approximately 25% of women, but there is a marked difference in racial groups. In the United States, in women 25 to 44 years of age, the incidence rates of leiomyomas that were confirmed by ultrasound or hysterectomy were 8.9 for white women and 30.6 for black women per 1,000 women-years.[24] When uteri are surgically removed for treatment of noncancerous presentations, pathologic examination reveals leiomyomas in 89% of black women and 59% of white women.[25] Similar results are obtained when screening women with ultrasonography: by 50 years of age, more than 80% of black women and 70% of white women will show fibroids.[26]

Leiomyomas are hormonally dependent; thus, these benign neoplasms usually shrink after menopause. They also frequently increase in size during pregnancy, as well as with the use of high-dose exogenous estrogens and, occasionally, with tamoxifen.

Sarcomatous degeneration of leiomyomas is rare. The incidence is reported to range from 0.4% to 1.4%. However, rapid increase in the size of a leiomyoma raises concern, although the definition of rapid growth has not been quantified. In fact, in a retrospective review of 371 patients operated on for rapidly growing leiomyomas, the incidence of leiomyosarcoma was 0.23%. When rapidly growing leiomyoma was defined as an increase of 6 weeks' gestational size over 1 year, none of 198 patients who satisfied this criterion were found to have a sarcoma.[27]

Clinical manifestations Most women with leiomyomas are asymptomatic, but symptoms may occur during the third and fourth decades. Leiomyomas, which are usually nontender, are most frequently found on clinical pelvic examination; but increasingly, they are identified by pelvic ultrasound during evaluation of nonspecific abdominal or pelvic symptoms.

Symptomatic patients may complain of pelvic discomfort, pressure, pain, menorrhagia, and dysmenorrhea. With degeneration or infarction, severe lower abdominal or pelvic pain develops. This may be associated with fever and an elevated white cell count. If the leiomyoma is pedunculated, torsion may cause severe pain, which may be intermittent. The pain may become part of a chronic pelvic pain pattern. Urinary symptoms include urinary frequency from extrinsic pressure on the bladder or, rarely, urinary retention secondary to urethral obstruction from a cervical or lower uterine leiomyoma. Depending on the location and the size of the leiomyoma, rectosigmoid compression and constipation may develop.

Leiomyomas coming through the cervical os can cause severe cramping; if necrotic, a foul vaginal discharge may develop. Abnormal uterine bleeding may be associated with a leiomyoma that disrupts the endometrial lining; the bleeding associated with a leiomyoma is cyclic, occurring in response to ovarian hormones.

Leiomyomas are usually discrete, firm, rounded, rubbery masses; they can vary in size from several millimeters to masses large enough to fill the abdominal pelvic cavity. They can be hard (if calcified) or soft (if cystic). Usually they cause an asymmetrical enlargement of the uterus, but multiple small leiomyomas cause a symmetrically enlarged uterus. Within the uterus, the leiomyoma may be located within the myometrium, beneath the endometrial lining, or on the surface of the uterus. When pedunculated or located posterior in the cul-de-sac, leiomyomas can give the clinical impression of a solid adnexal mass.

Ovarian Neoplasms

About two thirds of all ovarian neoplasms are discovered during the reproductive years; however, in women younger than 45 years, the chance that such neoplasms are malignant is 5% to 18%.[23,28,29] The most common ovarian neoplasms are endometriomas, cystic teratomas, and epithelial ovarian neoplasms. Most ovarian neoplasms produce few specific symptoms, the most common being vague abdominal pelvic pain or discomfort, abdominal distention, pelvic pressure, and urinary or gastrointestinal symptoms. Occasionally, in hormonally active neoplasms, irregular vaginal bleeding may occur.

Endometriomas Endometriomas are benign ovarian masses arising from ectopic endometrial tissue. Their incidence has not been determined. Frequently, endometriomas partially or almost completely replace normal ovarian tissue. Bilateral involvement of the ovaries has been reported in one third to one half of cases.[30] Endometriomas, which are usually less than 15 cm in diameter, may spontaneously rupture or resolve.

Patients who have an endometrioma usually complain of pelvic pain, dysmenorrhea, and dyspareunia; often, patients have an established history of endometriosis and infertility. On imaging evaluation, a mass 6 to 8 cm in diameter may be found. Endometriomas may by characterized by septations, debris, or solid components. These masses may not resolve over time. Endometriomas may be accompanied by an elevation in the CA125 serum level, which may cause concern regarding a malignancy; generally, however, CA125 serum levels associated with endometriomas are less than 200 U/ml.

Cystic teratomas Cystic teratomas, or dermoid cysts, are benign ovarian germ cell tumors. More than 80% of cystic teratomas are diagnosed during the reproductive years.[31] In a 10-year retrospective review, cystic teratomas constituted 62% of all ovarian neoplasms in women younger than 40 years.[29] The malignant transformation of these tumors is less than 2% and mostly occurs in women older than 40 years. There is a 15% risk of torsion and a 10% chance of bilateral presentation.

The risk of epithelial ovarian neoplasms increases with age. Bilateral ovarian neoplasms carry a 2.6-fold increased risk of malignancy, as compared with unilateral neoplasms.[29] Other causes of ovarian enlargement in this age group include metastatic cancer, especially from the breast or the gastrointestinal tract.

PELVIC MASS IN POSTMENOPAUSAL WOMEN

A pelvic mass in postmenopausal women may arise from the gynecologic organs, but increasingly in this age group, a mass may arise from nongynecologic organs. With decreasing ovarian hormone production, leiomyomas should undergo regression, and functional ovarian cysts are less likely. Endometriotic tumors are also not usually found in this age group. Thus, a newly found pelvic mass raises the suspicion of a malignancy.

Epidemiology The incidence of ovarian cancer increases with age, and 30% to 60% of ovarian masses in women older than 50 years are malignant.[23] The average age of a woman when diagnosed with ovarian cancer is 56 to 60 years. The majority of these tumors are epithelial malignancies. Fallopian tube cancer is rare. The differential diagnosis for a pelvic mass in postmenopausal women includes colon cancer, which is the third most common cancer in women.

Ovarian cysts have been reported in 3% to 17% of asymptomatic postmenopausal women undergoing pelvic ultrasound. In a study of 83 patients with thin-walled ovarian cysts less than 5 cm in diameter, 43 underwent surgery; no ovarian cancers were found in this group. In the remaining patients, 32 underwent serial ultrasound studies. In this group, 12 cysts resolved, seven decreased in size, four remained unchanged, and one increased slightly in size. The remaining eight patients underwent cyst aspirations; all the aspirated cysts were benign.[32]

Clinical manifestations   The presentation of ovarian cancer is not specific. Patients may complain of vague gastrointestinal symptoms, including dyspepsia, early satiety, anorexia, bloating, and, occasionally, constipation. In a retrospective survey of 1,725 patients with ovarian cancer, 95% reported symptoms that were categorized as abdominal (77%), gastrointestinal (70%), pain (58%), constitutional (50%), urinary (34%), and pelvic (26%).[33] Fallopian tube cancer may present as uterine bleeding, pelvic pain, and an adnexal mass. Classically, profuse watery vaginal discharge is seen, although this finding is rare.

The findings on examination consistent with advanced disease include abdominal distention with ascites, an abdominal/pelvic mass, and nodularity in the cul-de-sac on rectovaginal examination. An ultrasound of the abdomen and pelvis may show ascites, bilateral complex adnexal masses, and omental implants. In addition, there may be a pleural effusion. Evaluation of these patients should include abdominal and pelvic CT scans and chest x-ray. Again, if imaging studies raise the suspicion of malignancy, it is important to measure serum levels of CA125. An elevated CA125 level in postmenopausal women with a pelvic mass suggests a malignancy, because the positive predictive value for elevated CA125 (i.e., > 65 U/ml) in this age group has been reported to be 97%.[10] Early referral to a gynecologic oncologist is appropriate for patients with a mass that raises suspicion of malignancy.

A pelvic ultrasound may also identify nonmalignant cysts. Studies have suggested that women with simple cysts that are less than 10 cm in diameter and that are without any excrescences, septations, or ascites should undergo serial ultrasound studies.[34,35]

A pelvic mass in a postmenopausal woman with a history of bowel symptoms may suggest colon cancer; the evaluation of the stool may be positive for occult or frank blood. Diverticular disease must also be considered.

Management

The management of a pelvic mass depends on the patient's age, history, tumor characteristics, and likelihood of malignancy. For all age groups, surgery is required for masses that are greater than 10 cm in diameter and for those that are solid, fixed, or bilateral. When these findings are accompanied by significantly elevated levels of tumor markers, the presence of ascites, or a finding on imaging or physical examination that suggests malignancy, the patient should be referred to a gynecologic oncologist.

INFANTS AND PREPUBESCENT GIRLS

Infants and prepubescent girls with suspected physiologic or functional cysts should undergo serial ultrasound studies approximately every 6 weeks. Aspiration of unilocular cysts in prepubescent girls, either with ultrasound guidance or laparoscopy, is associated with a 50% recurrence rate[3] and is usually not recommended. If the mass increases in size, persists after 6 months, or becomes complex, surgery via either laparotomy or laparoscopy is necessary. Conservative management is indicated if the malignancy is confined to one ovary. Consultation with a gynecologic oncologist is necessary.

ADOLESCENT GIRLS

The management of adnexal masses in adolescent girls should have as its aim the preservation of ovarian function. An asymptomatic simple cyst that measures less than 10 cm in diameter may be observed and followed with serial ultrasound studies. To prevent new formation of physiologic cysts, ovarian suppression with oral contraception should begin. If the cyst increases in size, becomes complex, or causes symptoms, then surgery should be performed.

For benign neoplasms, cystectomy is recommended. Because most malignant tumors are unilateral, only the ovary or adnexa need be removed. The contralateral ovary should be inspected. If the ovary appears grossly normal, biopsy need not be performed, nor should the ovary be bivalved (i.e., the surface of the ovary divided and the cortex inspected), because these procedures could lead to peritubal or periovarian adhesions. However, if suspicious areas are identified, biopsies must be performed and a frozen section ordered for histologic analysis during surgery. Histologic analysis will help determine malignancy and indicate the need for consultation with a gynecologic oncologist to establish surgical staging. If the frozen section does not clearly establish malignancy, a second surgery is preferable to performing unnecessary initial surgery. However, the choice of surgery should be undertaken cautiously, because any adnexal surgery may result in tubal adhesions, which could interfere with future fertility.

PID in adolescents should be managed medically. Surgical management of nonmalignant presentations is rarely indicated in adolescents. Surgery, however, may be required to treat a ruptured tubo-ovarian abscess; it may also be required if the disease fails to respond to broad-spectrum antibiotics. Ectopic pregnancy can be managed medically, providing the pregnancy is small and the patient is hemodynamically stable; surgical management is required if these conditions are not met. If surgery is indicated, the procedure should be conservative and aimed at preserving fertility.

WOMEN OF REPRODUCTIVE AGE

The management of a pelvic mass in women of reproductive age will depend on the malignant potential of the mass. Most often, the mass will be a benign uterine leiomyoma. The initial approach will depend on whether the patient is symptomatic and has completed childbearing.

Leiomyomas   Asymptomatic leiomyomas should be followed with periodic pelvic examinations to ensure that there is not a rapid growth in size. The clinical records should document the location; a pelvic ultrasound can more accurately estimate the size. Rapid growth in the postmenopausal years may indicate transformation into a sarcoma. The risk, however, is reported to be less than 2 to 3 per 1,000.

In patients who will soon enter menopause or who are planning to undergo surgery for mildly symptomatic leiomyomas, hormonal therapy using gonadotropin-releasing hormone (GnRH) analogues results in a 40% to 60% decrease in uterine volume. GnRH treatment causes hypoestrogenic states that result in bone loss and hot flashes. Regrowth of the leiomyoma occurs within a few months of treatment cessation in one half of patients. Use of GnRH may be considered (1) as neoadjuvant therapy to shrink the size of the leiomyoma before surgery to permit a vaginal approach, (2) as treatment for anemia secondary to hemorrhage associated with leiomyomas, and (3) as treatment in perimenopausal women in an effort to avoid surgery.

Symptomatic leiomyomas require surgery. The usual indications include abnormal uterine bleeding with anemia that is unresponsive to hormone therapy; chronic pelvic pain with dysmenorrhea and dyspareunia; acute pelvic pain associated with torsion of pedunculated leiomyoma; prolapsing leiomyoma; urinary frequency with hydronephrosis; and symptoms of pelvic or rectal pressure caused by a significantly enlarged leiomyoma. Rarely, infertility caused by a leiomyoma obstructing the fallopian tubes or loss of a pregnancy secondary to a leiomyoma may be an indication for myomectomy. The finding of a mass during pregnancy demands the same management approach as for a nonpregnant patient. If surgery is necessary during pregnancy, the second trimester is the safest period.

Once childbearing is complete, hysterectomy is traditionally the definitive management for symptomatic leiomyomas. However, other treatment options have become available, including laparoscopic myomectomy and hysteroscopic resection of submucosal leiomyoma. In addition, endometrial ablation (e.g., laser, thermal, or chemical ablation, as well as selective arterial embolization) can decrease the bleeding caused by intramural leiomyomas.[36]

Endometriomas Endometriomas that do not spontaneously resolve are managed with surgical excision.

Cystic teratomas In women younger than 45 years, the treatment for a cystic teratoma is ovarian cystectomy, which often can be performed laparoscopically, especially if the mass is less than 10 cm in diameter.

Epithelial ovarian neoplasms Surgical management of epithelial ovarian neoplasms includes removal of the adnexa and surgical staging. Whether the surgery can be conservative (i.e., a unilateral salpingo-oophorectomy) will depend on the extent of the disease and the degree of malignancy (i.e., invasive tumor versus tumor of low malignant potential). These decisions are made in consultation with a gynecologic oncologist.

POSTMENOPAUSAL WOMEN

The risk of a malignancy increases with age, and thus, the threshold for conservative management decreases in postmenopausal women. It has been reported that a suspicious mass seen on ultrasound combined with a CA125 level greater than 65 U/ml has a specificity of 96.1%, a sensitivity of 91.7%, and an accuracy of 94.3% for detecting an ovarian neoplasm in postmenopausal women.[37] On the other hand, a postmenopausal woman with an ovarian simple cyst that is less than 5 cm in diameter and a normal CA125 serum concentration has a 0% risk of malignancy. Thus, the former patient should be referred to a gynecologic oncologist for appropriate management, whereas the latter may be followed with serial ultrasound studies every 4 to 6 months for a year and, provided the tumor remains stable and the patient asymptomatic, annually thereafter.

The authors have no commercial relationships with manufacturers of products or providers of services discussed in this chapter.

References

1. The adnexal mass and early ovarian cancer. Clinical Gynecologic Oncology, 6th ed., DiSaia PJ, Creasman WT, Eds. Mosby, St. Louis, 2001, p 259

2. Slanetz PJ, Hahn PF, Hall DA, et al: The frequency and significance of adnexal lesions incidentally revealed by CT. AJR Am J Roentgenol 168:647, 1997

3. Adams Hillard PJ: Benign diseases of the female reproductive tract: symptoms and signs. Novak's Gynecology, 13th ed. Novak E, Berek JS, Eds. Lippincott Williams & Wilkins, Philadelphia, 2002, p 351

4. Ascher SM, Imaoka I, Hricak H: Diagnostic imaging techniques in gynecologic oncology. Principles and Practice of Gynecologic Oncology, 3rd ed. Hoskins WH, Perez CA, Young RC, et al, Eds. Lippincott Williams & Wilkins, Philadelphia, 2000, p 655

5. Kier R, McCarthy SM, Scoutt LM, et al: Pelvic masses in pregnancy: MR imaging. Radiology 176:709, 1990

6. Jacobs I, Bast RC Jr: The CA 125 tumor-associated antigen: a review of the literature. Hum Reprod 4:1, 1989

7. Rosenthal A, Jacobs I: Ovarian cancer screening. Semin Oncol 25:315, 1998

8. Bast RC Jr, Klug TL, St. John E, et al: A radioimmunoassay using a monoclonal antibody to monitor the course of epithelial ovarian cancer. N Engl J Med 309:883, 1983

9. Einhorn N, Sjovall K, Knapp RC, et al: Prospective evaluation of serum CA 125 levels for early detection of ovarian cancer. Obstet Gynecol 80:14, 1992

10. Brooks SE: Preoperative evaluation of patients with suspected ovarian cancer. Gynecol Oncol 55:S80, 1994

11. Mulvany NJ: Aspiration cytology of ovarian cysts and cystic neoplasms: a study of 235 aspirates. Acta Cytol 40:911, 1996

12. Russell DJ: The female pelvic mass: diagnosis and management. Med Clin North Am 79:1481, 1995

13. Norris HJ, Jensen RD: Relative frequency of ovarian neoplasms in children and adolescents. Cancer 30:713, 1972

14. van Winter JT, Simmons PS, Podratz KC: Surgically treated adnexal masses in infancy, childhood and adolescence. Am J Obstet Gynecol 170:1780, 1994

15. Abma JC, Sonenstein FL: Sexual activity and contraceptive practices among teenagers in the United States, 1988 and 1995. Vital Health Stat 21:1, 2001

16. Schellhas HF: Malignant potential of the dysgenetic gonad. Part 1. Obstet Gynecol 41:74, 1974

17. Holt VL, Daling JR, McKnight B, et al: Functional ovarian cysts in relation to the use of monophasic and triphasic oral contraceptives. Obstet Gynecol 79:529, 1992

18. Lanes SF, Birmann B, Walker AM, et al: Oral contraceptive type and functional ovarian cysts. Am J Obstet Gynecol 166:956, 1992

19. Kozlowski JD: Ovarian masses. Adolesc Med 10:337, 1999

20. Diamond MP, Baxter JW, Peerman GCJ, et al: Occurrence of ovarian masses in childhood and adolescence: a community-wide evaluation. Obstet Gynecol 71:858, 1988

21. Henshaw SK: Unintended pregnancy in the United States. Fam Plann Perspect 30:24, 1998

22. Cibula D, Kuzel D, Fucikova Z, et al: Acute exacerbation of recurrent pelvic inflammatory disease: laparoscopic findings in 141 women with a clinical diagnosis. J Reprod Med 46:49, 2001

23. Hernandez E, Miyazawa K: The pelvic mass: patients' age and pathologic findings. J Reprod Med 33:361, 1988

24. Marshall LM, Spiegelman D, Barbieri RL, et al: Variation in the incidence of uterine leiomyoma among premenopausal women by age and race. Obstet Gynecol 90:967, 1997

25. Kjerulff KH, Langenberg P, Seidman JD, et al: Uterine leiomyomas: racial differences in severity, symptoms and age at diagnosis. J Reprod Med 41:483, 1996

26. Day Baird D, Dunson DB, Hill MC, et al: High cumulative incidence of uterine leiomyoma in black and white women: ultrasound evidence. Am J Obstet Gynecol 188:100, 2003

27. Parker WH, Fu YS, Berek JS: Uterine sarcoma in patients operated on for presumed leiomyoma and rapidly growing leiomyoma. Obstet Gynecol 83:414, 1994

28. Killackey MA, Neuwirth RS: Evaluation and management of the pelvic mass: a review of 540 cases. Obstet Gynecol 71:319, 1988

29. Koonings PP, Campbell K, Mishell DR Jr, et al: Relative frequency of primary ovarian neoplasms: a 10-year review. Obstet Gynecol 74:921, 1989

30. Egger H, Weigmann P: Clinical and surgical aspects of ovarian endometriotic cysts. Arch Gynecol 233:37, 1982

31. Talerman A: Germ cell tumors of the ovary. Blaustein's Pathology of the Female Genital Tract, 5th ed. Blaustein A, Kurman RJ, Eds. Springer Verlag, New York, 2002, p 998

32. Kroon E, Andolf E: Diagnosis and follow-up of simple ovarian cysts detected by ultrasound in postmenopausal women. Obstet Gynecol 85:211, 1995

33. Goff BA, Mandel L, Muntz HG, et al: Ovarian carcinoma diagnosis. Cancer 89:2068, 2000

34. Aubert JM, Rombaut C, Argacha P, et al: Simple adnexal cysts in postmenopausal women: conservative management. Maturitas 30:51, 1998

35. Bailey CL, Ueland FR, Land GL, et al: The malignant potential of small cystic ovarian tumors in women over 50 years of age. Gynecol Oncol 69:3, 1998

36. ACOG committee opinion: uterine artery embolization. Obstet Gynecol 103:403, 2004

37. Maggino T, Gadducci A, D'Addario V, et al: Prospective multicenter study on CA 125 in postmenopausal pelvic masses. Gynecol Oncol 54:117, 1994

89 Approach to the Patient with an Abnormal Pap Smear

Carolyn D. Runowicz, M.D.

Cervical cancer is the third most common gynecologic cancer in the United States. An estimated 10,370 new cases of invasive cervical cancer and 3,710 deaths occur annually, representing 1.4% of cancer deaths in women.[1] In the United States, the incidence of cervical cancer decreased by more than 70% between 1950 and 2000, largely as a result of screening[2]; more than half of the incident cases of invasive cancer are diagnosed in women who have not been adequately screened. Screening cytology methods, such as the Papanicolaou (Pap) smear, are excellent means of identifying preinvasive disease; however, false positive rates are relatively high. Each year, approximately 3.5 million cervical cytologic tests are interpreted as indicating an abnormality requiring additional follow-up or evaluation.[3]

Epidemiology and Risk Factors for Cervical Cancer

The occurrence of invasive cervical cancer is related to age. Premalignant cervical lesions are usually diagnosed in women younger than 40 years, which is 10 to 15 years earlier than in women diagnosed with invasive cervical cancer. This age gap suggests a long latency period for malignant transformation. For example, the diagnosis of cervical intraepithelial neoplasia (CIN) is usually made in women in their twenties, whereas the diagnosis of carcinoma in situ (CIS) is made in women 25 to 35 years of age, and invasive cancer is diagnosed in women older than 40 years.

Infection with high-risk strains of human papillomavirus (HPV) is the most important risk factor for cervical cancer.[4,5] HPV infection is usually transient[6,7]; however, persistent infection by high-risk HPV virus—most commonly, subtypes 16, 18, 31, and 45—is a prerequisite for the development of grade 1 and 2 CIN and invasive cervical cancer.[8]

HPV is usually acquired sexually; high-risk sexual behavior (e.g., having multiple sexual partners and promiscuous sexual partners) increases the risk for exposure to the virus.[9] HPV is a necessary precursor of CIN, but it does not act alone; host factors such as age, immune function,[10] a history of sexually transmitted disease (e.g., *Chlamydia trachomatis*),[11] and smoking[12] are surrogate markers for oncogenesis.

Natural History of Cervical Cancer

Early invasive cervical cancer is frequently asymptomatic, a fact that underscores the importance of routine screening. An abnormal Pap smear is frequently the first indication of a precancerous condition. The abnormalities observed on a cytologic smear or tissue biopsy of the cervix represent alterations in the degree of differentiation of cervical epithelial cells. An understanding of the natural history of low-grade and high-grade CIN lesions is central to the clinical management of patients who have abnormal cervical cytology.

CIN is a preinvasive pathologic intermediate of cervical cancer; it is slow to progress and can be easily detected and treated. The severity of CIN is designated by the extent to which the lesion involves the epithelial thickness. CIN 1 refers to intraepithelial neoplasia in which cellular changes are confined to the basal third of the epithelium; CIN 2 refers to intraepithelial neoplasia in which cellular changes are confined to the basal two thirds of the epithelium; and CIN 3 refers to cellular dysplasia encompassing more than two thirds of the epithelial thickness, including full-thickness lesions. CIS demonstrates full-thickness evidence of neoplasia without invasion of the basement membrane; CIN 3 and CIS may persist unchanged for 10 to 15 years, but eventually the lesion progresses to invasive carcinoma.

Low-grade lesions do not necessarily progress to high-grade lesions. A large cohort study indicated that CIN 1 lesions regressed to normal within 2 years in 44% of patients; they regressed to normal within 5 years in 74% of patients.[13] This series noted that the rates of progression of CIN 1 at 2 and 5 years were 2% and 6%, respectively; rates of progression of CIN 2 were 16% and 25%, respectively.

A primary goal of cervical cytologic screening is to identify women at risk for high-grade lesions; however, cytologic results are often equivocal. To improve the accuracy of cytologic interpretation, a standard system of terminology was adopted to distinguish findings most likely to be precancerous [see Test Interpretation—the Bethesda Reporting System, *below*]. Essentially, this reporting system classified a broad range of atypical findings into two categories: those findings that were more likely to represent high-risk lesions and those whose significance was undetermined.

Screening for Cervical Cancer

WHO SHOULD BE SCREENED?

Abundant evidence indicates that regular gynecologic examinations and cervical cytology decrease cervical cancer incidence and mortality. However, among policy-making organizations, there is some variation in the recommendations concerning the age at which screening should start, the interval of screening, and the age at which routine screening should stop.

Commencement of Screening

The United States Preventive Services Task Force (USPSTF) recommends beginning cytologic screening within 3 years of onset of sexual activity or by age 21, whichever comes first.[14] The recommendations of the American College of Obstetricians and Gynecologists (ACOG)[15] and the American Cancer Society (ACS)[16] are consistent with these guidelines. Other North American organizations, such as the Canadian Task Force on Preventive Health Care (CTFPHC), recommend that screening begin at onset of sexual activity or at 18 years of age.[17]

There is little value in screening women who have never been sexually active; however, many North American organizations recommend routine screening by age 18 or 21 on the basis of the generally high prevalence of sexual activity by that age and concerns that clinicans may not always obtain accurate sexual histories.

Table 1 The 2001 Bethesda System (Abridged)[29]

Table 1 **The 2001 Bethesda System (Abridged)**[29]

Specimen adequacy
> Satisfactory for evaluation *(note presence or absence of endocervical/transformation zone component)*
> Unsatisfactory for evaluation *(specify reason)*
>> Specimen rejected/not processed *(specify reason)*
>> Specimen processed and examined but unsatisfactory for evaluation of epithelial abnormality because of *(specify reason)*

General categorization (optional)
> Negative for intraepithelial lesion or malignancy
> Epithelial cell abnormality
> Other

Interpretation/result
> Negative for intraepithelial lesion or malignancy
>> Organisms
>>> *Trichomonas vaginalis*
>>> Fungal organisms morphologically consistent with *Candida* species
>>> Shift in flora suggestive of bacterial vaginosis
>>> Bacteria morphologically consistent with *Actinomyces* species
>>> Cellular changes consistent with herpes simplex virus
>> Other non-neoplastic findings (optional to report; list not comprehensive)
>>> Reactive cellular changes associated with the following:
>>>> Inflammation (includes typical repair)
>>>> Radiation
>>>> Intrauterine contraceptive device
>>> Glandular cells status post hysterectomy
>>> Atrophy

Epithelial cell abnormalities
> Squamous cell
>> Atypical squamous cells (ASC)
>>> Of undetermined significance (ASC-US)
>>> Cannot exclude HSIL (ASC-H)
>> Low-grade squamous intraepithelial lesion (LSIL) (cellular changes consistent with HPV, mild dysplasia, CIN 1)
>> High-grade squamous intraepithelial lesion (HSIL) (moderate to severe dysplasia, CIN 2, CIN 3, CIS) *(indicate if there are features suspicious of invasion)*
>> Squamous cell carcinoma
> Glandular cell
>> Atypical glandular cells *(specify endocervical, endometrial, or not otherwise specified)*
>> Atypical glandular cells, favor neoplastic *(specify endocervical or not otherwise specified)*
>> Endocervical adenocarcinoma in situ (AIS)
>> Adenocarcinoma
> Other (list not comprehensive)
>> Endometrial cells in a women ≥ 40 years

CIN—cervical intraepithelial neoplasia   CIS—carcinoma in situ

Screening Interval

Because cervical cancer is slow growing, considerable uncertainty surrounds the issue of the screening interval. The USPSTF found no direct evidence that annual screening achieves better outcomes than screening every 3 years. The most direct evidence on which to base a recommendation of a screening interval comes from a prospective cohort analysis of a randomized controlled trial.[18] Among 2,561 women (mean age, 66.7 years) with normal Pap tests at baseline, 110 had an abnormal Pap test within the next 2 years. No woman was found to have CIN 2, CIN 3, or invasive cancer; only one woman had CIN 1 or CIN 2. Thus, the positive predictive value of screening 1 year after a negative Pap test was 0%; after 2 years, the positive predictive value was 0.9%. The authors concluded that Pap tests should not be repeated within 2 years after a negative test. A large study of women younger than 65 years, which included data from the National Breast and Cervical Cancer Early Detection Program and which used a model to estimate the rate at which intraepithelial neoplasia progresses to cancer, found that little further mortality reduction from cervical cancer was achieved by screening every year as compared with every 3 years.[19]

On the basis of the limited evidence, the USPSTF recommends screening at least every 3 years. The ACS guidelines recommend waiting until age 30 before lengthening the screening interval from 1 to 3 years. The ACOG recommends initiating screening with annual smears for 2 or 3 years; if these are negative, intervals of up to 3 years may be appropriate.[20] The ACOG identifies additional risk factors that might justify annual screening, including a history of cervical neoplasia, infection with HPV or other sexually transmitted diseases, or high-risk sexual behavior; however, data by which to determine the benefits of these strategies are limited.[20]

Cessation of Screening

The USPSTF recommendations state that screening can be discontinued in women who have had a total hysterectomy for benign disease (i.e., disease in which there is no evidence of cervical neoplasia or cancer), given the low yield of screening and the potential harms from false positive results in this population.[18] In women with a cervix, the optimal age to discontinue screening is not clear, but the risk of cervical cancer and the yield of screening decline steadily through middle age. However, screening is recommended in older women who have not been previously screened or when information about previous screening is unavailable.[14]

The USPSTF recommends discontinuing routine screening for women older than 65 years who have had adequate recent screening with normal Pap smears and are not otherwise at high risk for cervical cancer.[18] The ACS guidelines recommend that screening can be safely stopped in older women who have had three or more documented, consecutive, technically satisfactory, normal cervical cytologic tests and who have had no abnormal cytologic tests within the past 10 years; routine screening may be discontinued at age 70.[16]

AVAILABLE TESTS

There are several methods for cervical cancer screening: the conventional cytologic Pap smear, the liquid-based Pap smear, and HPV DNA testing in combination with cervical cytology. The purpose of these tests is to screen for cellular abnormalities that are associated with an increased risk of the development of cervical cancer.

Conventional Cytology (Pap Smear)

The Pap smear is the standard screening test for genital tract neoplasia. The reported sensitivity of a single Pap smear varies widely, ranging from 32% to 92%.[21] This low sensitivity prompted the recommendation found in early guidelines that cytologic screening be made annually.[22] False negative rates have been attributed to poor sample preparation, in which precursor cells were obscured by blood, pus, air-drying artifacts, and other cells.[23] A conventional Pap smear costs $25 to $40.

Liquid-Based Cervical Cytology

Liquid-based cytology offers higher sensitivity and comparable specificity to that of the conventional Pap smear.[24] The liquid-based test costs $45 to $60. If used at 3-year intervals, the liquid-based test is cost-effective.[25] Evidence-based reports show that both liquid-based and conventional cytology are acceptable screening tests.[26] One advantage of liquid-based cytology is that HPV testing can be performed on the same preparation (see below).

Cytology and HPV DNA Testing

HPV DNA testing in combination with conventional or liquid-based cytology has been approved by the Food and Drug Administration for primary screening for cervical cancer in women older than 30 years.[27] In this age group, the combination of cytology and HPV DNA testing has been reported to have a sensitivity approximately 10% to 20% greater than that of a single conventional cytologic smear; however, specificity is lower.[28] Because of the high negative predictive value of these combined tests, women who test negative on both the cytologic and HPV DNA testing can increase their screening interval to 3 years.[27]

TEST INTERPRETATION—THE BETHESDA REPORTING SYSTEM

The most common abnormal cervical cytologic result is one of uncertainty. Interpretation of equivocal cytologic findings is complicated by confusion among laboratories and clinicians concerning the use of multiple classification systems and inconsistently defined numerical grading conventions. The Bethesda System, which was introduced in 1988 and is periodically updated (most recently in 2001), was devised as a uniform system of terminology to guide the interpretation of cytologic findings. A significant contribution of the Bethesda System was the standardized laboratory report that includes a description of specimen adequacy (to improve the consistency and quality of reporting) and that uses simplified terminology for the interpretation of equivocal cytologic findings [see Table 1].

Specimen Adequacy

The 2001 update of the Bethesda System qualifies specimens as being either satisfactory or unsatisfactory for evaluation.[29] Minimal squamous cellularity varies with the specimen type: an estimated 8,000 to 12,000 well-visualized squamous cells are acceptable for conventional smears, and 5,000 squamous cells are acceptable for liquid-based preparations. Epithelial cells may be obscured by blood or inflammation and still be considered satisfactory; however, if more than 75% of epithelial cells are obscured, the specimen is unsatisfactory. For specimens containing adequate squamous cellularity, the cytologic report notes the presence or absence of an endocervical/transformation zone component. Adequate endocervical cellularity consists of at least 10 well-preserved endocervical or squamous metaplastic cells.

Interpretaton of Specimen

The Bethesda System stipulates that cervical cytology is primarily a screening test, and the interpretation of morphologic findings described by the cytologic report must be integrated into a clinical context to establish a diagnosis.

Specimens are broadly defined as negative for intraepithelial lesion or malignancy or positive for epithelial cell abnormality.

Epithelial abnormalities include atypical squamous cells, low- and high-grade squamous intraepithelial lesions (LSIL and HSIL), and atypical glandular cells (AGC). A finding of atypical squamous cells that cannot be determined as precancerous is the most common result, and its correct interpretation poses a clinical challenge.

Atypical squamous cells The 2001 Bethesda System qualified a finding of atypical squamous cells (ASC) in two ways: (1) ASC of undetermined significance (ASC-US) and (2) ASC for which HSIL cannot be excluded (ASC-H) [see Table 1]. A finding of undetermined significance emphasizes that some cases of ASC-US are associated with underlying CIN 2,3. ASC-H is used when there are cytologic features suggestive of HSIL but definite evidence is lacking. The ASC-H category constitutes approximately 5% to 10% of all ASC, but it includes women at greatest risk for CIN 2,3.[30,31] HSIL is more often associated with viral persistence and higher risk of progression, whereas LSIL is generally the result of a transient infection of HPV.[32,33]

Squamous epithelial lesions The Bethesda System classifies squamous intraepithelial lesions as low-grade (LSIL) or high-grade (HSIL). Cellular changes consistent with HPV, mild dysplasia, and CIN 1 are combined within the category of LSIL. Moderate to severe dysplasia, CIN 2, CIN 3, and CIS are combined within the category of HSIL. In the Bethesda System, CIN and dysplasia terminology can be used either as substitute terms for squamous intraepithelial lesions or as additional descriptors of intraepithelial lesions.

Atypical glandular cells The Bethesda System classifies glandular cell abnormalities into three types: atypical endocervical cells, endometrial cells, and glandular cells. In the majority of cases, morphologic features permit differentiation between atypical endometrial and endocervical cells. The management of patients with glandular abnormalities may vary significantly, depending on cell type, and distinguishing between these cell types is justified, when possible. The Bethesda System distinguishes AGC (either endocervical, endometrial, or AGC that are not otherwise specified [AGC-NOS]) from AGC (either endocervical or AGC-NOS) that favor neoplasia, because these two categories are associated with different degrees of risk of significant disease. Biopsy-confirmed high-grade lesions, including CIN 2,3, adenocarcinoma in situ, and invasive cancer, have been found in 9% to 41% of women who have AGC-NOS, as compared with 27% to 96% of those who have AGC that favors neoplasia.[34-36]

Management of Cytologic Abnormalities

ATYPICAL SQUAMOUS CELLS

Each year, an estimated two to three million women are diagnosed as having cervical cytology containing ASC.[37,38] The majority of women with ASC do not have a clinically significant lesion. However, 5% to 17% of patients with atypical ASC cytology have CIN 2,3 confirmed by biopsy.[30,39,40] A large, prospective study of routinely screened women reported that 39% of cases of high-grade squamous lesions were detected in women with ASC cytology.[41]

Increased age and a history of treatment of CIN have been reported to increase the risk of CIN in patients with ASC cytology.[42] High viral levels of HPV types known to be associated with cervical cancer have been found to be strongly predictive of high-grade CIN in patients with ASC Pap smears.[43] ASC findings suggestive of neoplastic processes carry a greater risk of high-grade lesions and carcinoma than ASC findings suggestive of reactive processes.

Management Options

The evaluation and management of women with ASC-US cytology is a topic of considerable controversy. The best approach to the management of abnormal cervical cytology is to use the fewest number of tests to resolve the clinical question posed by the presence of ASC. Management options include (1) repeat cytology at a designated interval, (2) high-risk HPV DNA testing, (3) immediate colposcopy, (4) a combination of repeat cervical cytology and HPV DNA testing, (5) direct visual inspection in combination with conventional cytology, (6) referral for colposcopy, and (7) a combination of these strategies.

Repeat cervical cytology A repeat cervical cytology obtained at a later date appeals to many health care providers, because most histologic abnormalities found with ASC-US will be low-grade cervical neoplasia that is likely to regress without definitive therapy. The repeat Pap smear should be obtained 4 to 6 months after the index cytology [see Figure 1]. This is considered the optimal interval; a repeat cytology obtained after less than 4 months is thought to be associated with decreased sensitivity,[40] and after 6 months, 7% of patients with ASC-US smears will have CIN 2,3.[44]

High-risk HPV DNA testing HPV DNA is associated with virtually all cervical cancers and high-grade precursor lesions; the identification of these types of HPV that are associated with a high risk of oncogenesis is useful in identifying patients with ASC-US who are at increased risk for neoplasia.[45]

The probability of HPV expression is influenced by several factors, including age, menstrual cycling, use of exogenous hormones, and immunocompetence.[10,46] The addition of HPV DNA testing to cervical cytologic screening for women with ASC-US may be most effective in women 30 to 35 years of age, who are past the peak of incidence of acute infections [see Table 2].[46] In women whose cytology was classified as ASC-US, those who were 30 years of age or older had a lower prevalence of HPV positivity and a lower referral to colposcopy than younger women (30% versus 65%); this improvement in specificity was not accompanied by a decrement in sensitivity. Establishing age- and population-specific analytic cutoff points for the detection of HPV may further enhance the specificity of HPV DNA testing. Other strategies for improving specificity without compromising sensitivity may include the use of serial HPV DNA testing or lengthening the interval between the index ASC-US cytology and HPV DNA testing.

Of the commercial HPV DNA detection kits, Hybrid Capture 2 (HC2) (Digene Diagnostics, Silver Spring, Maryland) has a higher sensitivity (94.8% versus 84.4% for high-grade precursor lesions) and detects a broader range of high-risk HPV types than other methods.[47] HC2 is a nonradioactive, rapid assay that can detect 18 HPV DNA types,[48] 13 of which convey high risk of oncogenesis. A retrospective study of 398 women showed the HC2 assay to be as sensitive and specific as a single repeat cytologic smear for the detection of CIN.[40] However, it has been argued by some that its use identifies large numbers of low-grade lesions (CIN 1) and transient HPV infections and may lead to

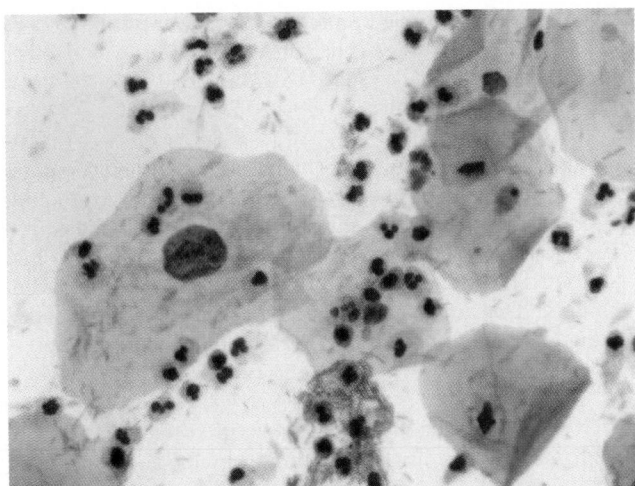

Figure 1 **A Pap smear showing atypical squamous cells of undetermined significance (ASC-US).**

overevaluation and overtreatment because of its low positive predictive value.[47]

Immediate colposcopy Colposcopy would be expected to detect almost all of the cases of high-grade CIN, but it has drawbacks, including expense and the risk of overevaluation and overtreatment in women who do not have CIN. Immediate colposcopy, however, may be indicated for women with a history of CIN, for poorly compliant women, and for women for whom waiting creates undue anxiety.

Studies of the natural history of HPV infection have demonstrated that most HPV infections produce only minor, transient infections.[10,11] A positive HPV DNA test in combination with an ASC-US cervical cytologic finding does not indicate high-grade disease or the presence of cancer, but it does indicate some increased risk of cancer now or in the future. Because of imperfect sensitivity, the initial colposcopy and directed biopsy will not detect about 10% of those women who will have histologically confirmed CIN 2,3 within 2 years of follow-up.[49]

Repeat cytology and direct visualization To compensate for the low sensitivity of a single repeat cervical cytology in women with atypical squamous cells, it has been suggested that repeat cytology be combined with a visual screening method. Direct visual screening methods include cervicoscopy (direct visual inspection of the cervix after an acetic acid wash), speculoscopy (direct visualization of the cervix under low magnification after application of an acetic acid wash), and cervicography (visual inspection of the cervix in which a static photographic image is used to document cervical abnormalities after an acetic acid wash).[50] Several studies that evaluated the combined use of cervicography and repeat cytology reported that this screening approach had a high sensitivity for the detection of CIN 2,3.[51,52] Because the data are limited, more studies are needed before recommending repeat cytology and direct visualization as a screening approach in patients with ASC-US.

Repeat cytology and HPV DNA testing Several studies have reported that the combination of HPV DNA testing and a repeat Pap smear has a sensitivity similar to that of colposcopy for the detection of high-grade CIN.[43,53-55] The negative predictive value of DNA testing for high-risk types of HPV is generally reported to be 98% or greater.[40,56] However, other investigators question the cost-effectiveness of this combined screening strategy in women with ASC-US.[57,58] Use of liquid-based cytology permits the residual transport fluid to be used to test for HPV DNA (a technique referred to as reflex HPV DNA testing).[39] In a large study, Manos and colleagues evaluated HPV DNA testing of residual material from liquid-based cervical cytology using the HC2 assay. An overall sensitivity of 96.9% (95% confidence interval [CI], 88.3% to 99.5%) was achieved when colposcopy of HPV DNA–positive women was performed immediately after the reflex HPV DNA test. The authors concluded that reflex HPV DNA testing of cervical cytology aids in identifying those women at risk for high-grade lesions.[44]

The initial report of the ASC-US/LSIL Triage Study (ALTS) found that reflex HPV DNA testing was more sensitive than a single repeat cytologic smear in detecting CIN 3 in women with ASC-US cytology.[40] The sensitivity of HPV DNA testing for the detection of CIN of grade 3 or higher was 96.3% (95% CI, 91.6% to 98.8%); 56.1% (95% CI, 54.1% to 58.1%) of patients were referred for colposcopy. The sensitivity of a single repeat cytologic specimen for the detection of ASC-US or findings associated with higher risk was 85.3% (95% CI, 78.2% to 90.8%); 58.6% (95% CI, 56.5% to 60.6%) of patients were referred for colposcopy. However, the conventional clinical management strategy for cytologic follow-up is based on a series of repeat cytologic specimens, not on the sensitivity of a single cytologic sampling. A 2-year follow-up of the ALTS showed that a repeat cytologic specimen is as sensitive as HPV DNA testing at an ASC-US referral threshold, but this approach requires two follow-up visits and ultimately more colposcopic examinations than HPV triage (67.1% versus 53.1%).[59]

Reflex HPV DNA testing offers advantages over HPV DNA testing using conventional Pap smears: women do not need an additional clinical examination for specimen collection, and 40% to 60% of women with negative test results are spared a colposcopic examination. However, with this approach, the number of patients needing colposcopies remains high. The combination of HPV DNA testing and cervical cytology increases sensitivity at the expense of specificity, because even potentially oncogenic HPV-type infections are found in women without cervical neoplasia, particularly young, sexually active women. The positive predictive value of HPV DNA testing is similar to that of cytology (18% to 25%), but the negative predictive value is 99.8% to 100%.[60-62]

The drawbacks of reflex HPV DNA testing lie in its tendency to produce false negative and false positive results. A screening

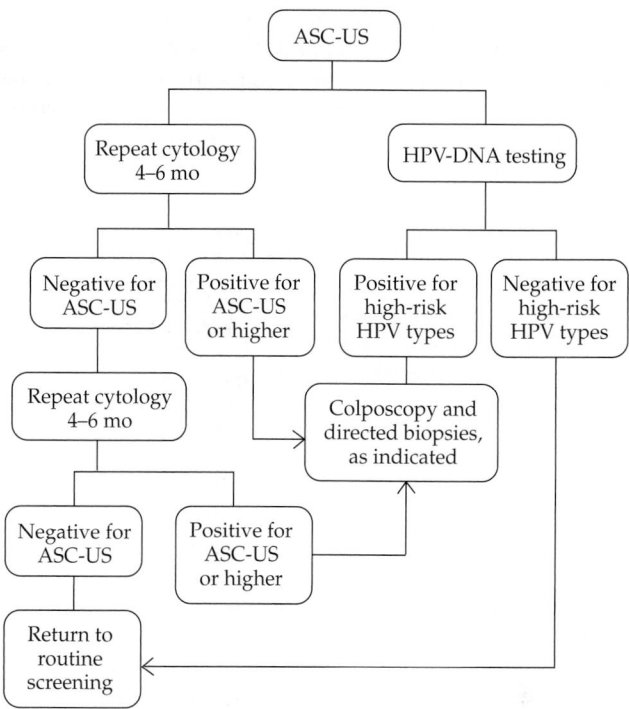

Figure 2 **Management scheme for atypical squamous cells of undetermined significance (ASC-US), based on the consensus guidelines developed by American Society for Colposcopy and Cervical Pathology.[64] (HPV—human papillomavirus)**

study of cervical cytology found a substantial degree of cross-reactivity (6.4%) between the reflex HPV DNA probe and the HPV types not included on the probe; this was detected by retesting all HPV DNA–positive samples with a polymerase chain reaction (PCR) assay. The PCR retest found a significant false positive rate of 3.6% and a false negative rate of 6.1% of all samples defined by the reflex HPV DNA test.[63] Thus, reflex HPV DNA testing has the potential for both overevaluation and underevaluation of high-risk HPV infections. However, the combination of a negative reflex HPV DNA test and a negative cytology indicated the absence of CIN 3 or cancer to a certainty of 100%, with a specificity, positive predictive value, and negative predictive value of 93.8%, 8.6%, and 100%, respectively.[63]

Recommended Management

Different policy-making organizations vary in their recommended approaches to the management of ASC. The American Society for Colposcopy and Cervical Pathology (ASCCP) established consensus guidelines for the management of ASC in 2001. The consensus guidelines classify ASC into two groups: ASC-US and ASC-H (see above).[64] For women with ASC-US cytology, a program of repeat cytologic testing, immediate colposcopy, or DNA testing for high-risk types of HPV are acceptable management options [*see Figure 2*].[64] When liquid-based cytologic is used or when cocollection for HPV DNA testing can be performed, reflex HPV DNA testing is the preferred approach. Women with ASC-US who test negative for high-risk HPV DNA should undergo repeat cytologic testing at 12 months. Women who are managed with immediate colposcopy and who are found not to have CIN should undergo repeat cytologic testing at 12 months.

Table 2 Prevalence of High-Risk HPV Infections Stratified by Age of Women at the First Examination[61]

Age	Women (%)	High-Risk HPV (%)
< 20	418 (5.3)	84 (20.1)
21–30	1,843 (23.2)	435 (23.6)
31–40	2,076 (26.2)	289 (13.9)
41–50	1,925 (24.3)	235 (12.2)
51–60	1,014 (12.8)	110 (10.8)
> 60	656 (8.3)	61 (9.3)
Total	7,932	1,214 (15.3)

HPV—human papillomavirus

When a program of repeat cervical cytologic testing is used, women with ASC-US should undergo repeat cytology (either conventional or liquid-based) at 4- to 6-month intervals until two consecutive results that are negative for intraepithelial lesion or malignancy are obtained. In most instances, women with ASC-H, LSIL, HSIL, and AGC should be referred for immediate colposcopic evaluation [see Squamous Epithelial Lesions, below].[64]

The National Comprehensive Cancer Network guidelines are consistent with the recommendation of the consensus guidelines.[65]

The Society of Obstetricians and Gynecologists of Canada (SOGC) guidelines recommend repeating the cytologic smear every 3 to 6 months until three consecutive negative smears are obtained, after which annual cytologic examinations can be resumed. If cytology continues to demonstrate ASC-US, colposcopy should be performed.[66]

Management of ASC-US in Special Circumstances

Immunosuppressed women with ASC-US are at increased risk for CIN 2,3; high-risk types of HPV are frequently detected in these women. Referral for colposcopy is recommended in all immunosuppressed women who have ASC-US.[64]

In postmenopausal women with ASC-US, the risk of CIN 2,3 is lower than in premenopausal women. Treatment with a course of intravaginal estrogen followed by a repeat cervical cytology 1 week after therapy is an acceptable option.[40] It is also acceptable to manage postmenopausal women who have ASC-US with immediate colposcopy or HPV DNA testing.

ASC-US AND ONCOGENIC HPV DNA

As demonstrated by ALTS and other studies, it is now possible to identify many women with ASC-US who do not need colposcopy. However, women who have oncogenic HPV DNA and ASC-US present a sizable management challenge. It is not known how to manage women with ASC-US who test positive for high-risk HPV DNA but who are not found to have CIN by colposcopy and biopsy. Expert opinion and review of the literature indicate that such women are at low risk for high-grade cervical neoplasia and that repeated colposcopy should not be performed in this setting. Instead, HPV DNA testing along with repeat cytology at 6 and 12 months is recommended.[27] The likelihood that these repeat tests will be negative and that patients will subsequently forgo further surveillance screening is not known.

SQUAMOUS EPITHELIAL LESIONS

For women with LSIL, colposcopy is the recommended management.[64] If the colposcopy results are negative for CIN and cancer, appropriate management entails either repeat cytology at 6 and 12 months or HPV DNA testing at 12 months; subsequent management entails (1) a repeat colposcopy if results are positive for ASC or HPV or (2) a return to routine screening if results are negative. If colposcopy reveals the presence of a lesion, the patient is managed in accordance with the guidelines recommended by the ASCCP.

For women with HSIL, colposcopy with endocervical assessment is the recommended management.[64] If colposcopy reveals no lesion or only biopsy-proven CIN 1, then cytology, colposcopy, and biopsy results should be reviewed; subsequent management depends on the final interpretation of tests. If colposcopy indicates the presence of a lesion, the patient is managed in accordance with the guidelines recommended by the ASCCP.

Management of LSIL and HSIL may vary if the patient is pregnant, postmenopausal, or an adolescent.

ATYPICAL GLANDULAR CELLS

The finding of AGC is significant because AGC is associated with a greater risk of high-grade lesions than the risk associated with ASC. On follow-up evaluation, high-grade lesions (either squamous or glandular) may be seen in 10% to 39% of patients with an AGC cytologic result[35,36]; in comparison, 5% to 17% of patients with atypical ASC cytology have CIN 2,3 confirmed by biopsy.[30,39,40]

Women with atypical endometrial cells should initially be evaluated with endometrial sampling.[64] If no neoplasia is identified, it is recommended that the patient undergo follow-up evaluation using a program of repeat cervical cytologic testing at 4- to 6-month intervals until four consecutive results that are negative for intraepithelial lesion or malignancy are obtained. If a result of ASC or LSIL is obtained on any of the follow-up smears, acceptable options include a repeat colposcopic examination.[64] Continued follow-up evaluation is needed.

The author has no commercial relationships with manufacturers of products or providers of services discussed in this chapter.

References

1. Jemal A, Murray T, Ward E, et al: Cancer statistics, 2005. CA Cancer J Clin 55:10, 2005

2. United States Cancer Statistics: 2000 Incidence. Department of Health and Human Services, Centers for Disease Control and Prevention and National Cancer Institute, Atlanta, 2003

3. Jones BA, Davey DD: Quality management in gynecologic cytology using interlaboratory comparison. Arch Pathol Lab Med 124:672, 2000

4. Schiffman MH, Bauer HM, Hoover RN, et al: Epidemiologic evidence showing that human papillomavirus infection causes most cervical intraepithelial neoplasia. J Natl Cancer Inst 85:958, 1993

5. Human papillomaviruses: Summaries and Evaluations, Vol 64. International Agency for Research on Cancer (IARC), Lyons, 1995
http://www.inchem.org/documents/iarc/vol64/hpv.html

6. Ho GY, Bierman R, Beardsley L, et al: Natural history of cervicovaginal papillomavirus infection in young women. N Engl J Med 338:423, 1998

7. Moscicki AB, Shiboski S, Broering J, et al: The natural history of human papillomavirus infection as measured by repeated DNA testing in adolescent and young women. J Pediatr 132:277, 1998

8. Koutsky LA, Holmes KK, Critchlow CW, et al: A cohort study of the risk of cervical intraepithelial neoplasia grade 2 or 3 in relation to papillomavirus infection. N Engl J Med 327:1272, 1992

9. Shepherd J, Weston R, Peersman G, et al: Interventions for encouraging sexual lifestyles and behaviours intended to prevent cervical cancer. Cochrane Database Syst Rev (2):CD001035, 2000

10. Frisch M, Biggar RJ, Engels EA, et al: Association of cancer with AIDS-related immunosuppression in adults. JAMA 285:3090, 2001

11. Smith JS, Bosetti C, Munoz N, et al: *Chlamydia trachomatis* and invasive cervical cancer: a pooled analysis of the IARC multicentric case-control study. Int J Cancer 111:431, 2004

12. Trimble CL, Genkinger JM, Burke AE, et al: Active and passive cigarette smoking and the risk of cervical neoplasia. Obstet Gynecol 105:174, 2005

13. Holowaty P, Miller AB, Rohan T, et al: Natural history of dysplasia of the cervix. J Natl Cancer Inst 91:252, 1999

14. U.S. Preventive Services Task Force: Screening for Cervical Cancer: Guide to Clinical Preventive Services. AHRQ Publication No. 03-515A, Agency for Healthcare Research and Quality, Rockville, MD, 2003
http://www.ahrq.gov/clinic/uspstf/uspscerv.htm

15. Cervical cancer screening in adolescents: ACOG committee opinion number 300. American College of Obstetricians and Gynecologists Committee on Adolescent Health Care. Obstet Gynecol 104:885, 2004

16. Cervical Cancer: ACS Cancer Detection Guidelines. American Cancer Society, Inc. Atlanta, 2005
http://www.cancer.org

17. Morrison BJ: Screening for cervical cancer. Canadian Task Force on the Periodic Health Examination. Canadian Guide to Clinical Preventive Health Care. Ottawa, 1994, p. 870
http://www.ctfphc.org

18. Sawaya GF, Grady D, Kerlikowske K, et al: The positive predictive value of cervical

smears in previously screened postmenopausal women. The Heart and Estrogen/Progestin Replacement Study (HERS). Ann Intern Med 133:942, 2000

19. Sawaya GF, McConnell KJ, Kulasingam SL, et al: Risk of cervical cancer associated with the interval between cervical-cancer screenings. N Engl J Med 349:1501, 2003

20. Routine cancer screening. ACOG committee opinion number 185. American College of Obstetricians and Gynecologists. Washington DC, 1997

21. Nanda K, McCrory DC, Myers ER, et al: Accuracy of the Papanicolaou test in screening for and follow-up of cervical cytologic abnormalities: a systematic review. Ann Intern Med 132:810, 2000

22. U.S. Preventive Services Task Force: Screening for Cervical Cancer: Guide to Clinical Preventive Services. Agency for Healthcare Research and Quality, Rockville, MD, 1996

23. McGoogan E, Reith A: Would monolayers provide more representative samples and improved preparations for cervical screening? Overview and evaluation of systems available. Acta Cytol 40:107, 1996

24. Abulafia O, Pezzullo JC, Sherer DM: Performance of Thin-Prep liquid-based cervical cytology in comparison with conventionally prepared Papanicolaou smears: a quantitative survey. Gynecol Oncol 90:137, 2003

25. Andy C, Turner LF, Neher JO: Clinical inquiries: is ThinPrep better than conventional Pap smear at detecting cervical cancer? J Fam Pract 53:313, 2004

26. ACOG practice bulletin: clinical management guidelines for obstetrician-gynecologists. Obstet Gynecol 102:417, 2003

27. Wright TC Jr, Schiffman M, Solomon D, et al: Interim guidance for the use of human papillomavirus DNA testing as an adjunct to cervical cytology for screening. Obstet Gynecol 103:304, 2004

28. Ratnam S, Franco EL, Ferenczy A: Human papillomavirus testing for primary screening of cervical cancer precursors. Cancer Epidemiol Biomarkers Prev 9:945, 2000

29. Solomon D, Davey D, Kurman R, et al: The 2001 Bethesda System: terminology for reporting results of cervical cytology. JAMA 287:2114, 2002

30. Malik SN, Wilkerson EJ, Drew PA, et al: Do qualifiers of ASCUS distinguish between low-and high-risk patients? Acta Cytol 43:376, 1999

31. Sherman ME, Tabbara SO, Scott DR, et al: "ASCUS, rule out HSIL": cytologic features, histologic correlates, and human papillomavirus detection. Mod Pathol 12:335, 1999

32. Park TJ, Richart RM, Sun XW, et al: Association between HPV type and clonal status of cervical squamous intraepithelial lesions (SIL). J Natl Cancer Inst 88:355, 1996

33. zur Hausen H: Papillomaviruses causing cancer: evasion from host-cell control in early events in carcinogenesis. J Natl Cancer Inst 92:690, 2000

34. Kennedy AW, Salmieri SS, Wirth SL, et al: Results of the clinical evaluation of atypical glandular cells of undetermined significance (AGCUS) detected on cervical cytology screening. Gynecol Oncol 63:14, 1996

35. Soofer S, Sidawy M: Atypical glandular cells of undetermined significance: clinically significant lesions and means of patient follow-up. Cancer Cytopathol 90:207, 2000

36. Eddy GL, Stumpf KB, Wojtowycz MA, et al: Biopsy findings in five hundred thirty one patients with atypical glandular cells of uncertain significances as defined by the Bethesda System. Am J Obstet Gynecol 177:1188, 1997

37. Kurman RJ, Henson De, Herbst AL, et al: Interim guidelines for management of abnormal cervical cytology. JAMA 271:1866, 1994

38. Davey DD, Woodhouse S, Styer P, et al: Atypical epithelial cells and specimen adequacy: current laboratory practices of participants in the College of American Pathologists Interlaboratory Comparison Program in Cervicovaginal Cytology. Arch Pathol Lab Med 124:203, 2000

39. Wright TC, Lorincz AT, Ferris DG, et al: Reflex human papillomavirus deoxyribonucleic acid testing in women with abnormal Papanicolaou smears. Am J Obstet Gynecol 178:962, 1998

40. Solomon D, Schiffman M, Tarone R: Comparison of three management strategies for patients with atypical squamous cells of undetermined significance: baseline results from a randomized trial. ALTS Study group. J Natl Cancer Inst 93:293, 2001

41. Kinney WK, Manos MM, Hurley LB, et al: Where's the high-grade cervical neoplasia? The importance of the minimally abnormal Papanicolaou diagnoses. Obstet Gynecol 91:973, 1998

42. Wright TC, Sun XW, Koulos J: Comparison of management algorithms for the evaluation of women with low-grade cytologic abnormalities. Obstet Gynecol 85:202, 1995

43. Cox JT, Lorincz AT, Schiffman MH, et al: Human papillomavirus testing by hybrid capture appears to be useful in triaging women with a cytologic diagnosis of atypical squamous cells of undetermined significance. Am J Obstet Gynecol 172:946, 1995

44. Manos MM, Kinney WK, Hurley LB, et al: Identifying women with cervical neopla-

sia using human papillomavirus DNA testing for equivocal Papanicolaou results. JAMA 281:1605, 1999

45. Human papillomaviruses. IARC Monogr Eval Carcinog Risks Hum 64:277, 1995

46. Sherman M, Schiffman M, Cox JT: Effects of age and human papilloma viral load on colposcopy triage: data from the randomized Atypical Squamous Cells of Undetermined Significance/Low-Grade Squamous Intraepithelial Lesion Triage Study (ATLS). J Natl Cancer Inst 94:102, 2002

47. Arbyn M, Buntinx F, Van Ranst M, et al: Virologic versus cytologic triage of women with equivocal Pap smears: a meta-analysis of the accuracy to detect high-grade intraepithelial neoplasia. J Natl Cancer Inst 96:250, 2004

48. Riethmuller D, Gay C, Bertrand X, et al: Genital human papillomavirus infection among women recruited for routine cervical cancer screening or for colposcopy determined by Hybrid Capture II and polymerase chain reaction. Diagn Mol Pathol 8:157, 1999

49. Cox JT, Schiffman M, Solomon D: Prospective follow-up suggests similar risk of subsequent cervical intraepithelial neoplasia grade 2 or 3 among women with cervical intraepithelial neoplasia grade 1 or negative colposcopy and directed biopsy. The ASCUS-LSIL Triage Study (ALTS) Group. Am J Obstet Gynecol 188:1406, 2003

50. Wright TC Jr: Cervical cancer screening using visualization techniques. J Natl Inst Monogr, No 31. National Cancer Institute, Atlanta, 2003, p 66

51. Spitzer M, Krumholz B, Seltzer VL, et al: Comparative utility of repeat Papanicolaou smear, cervicography, and colposcopy in the evaluation of atypical Papanicolaou smears. Obstet Gynecol 69:731, 1987

52. Eskridge C, Begneaud WP, Landweher C: Cervicography combined with repeat Papanicolaou test as triage for low-grade cytologic abnormalities. Obstet Gynecol 92:351, 1998

53. Cox JT, Shiffman MH, Winzelberg AJ, et al: An evaluation of human papillomavirus testing as part of referral to colposcopy clinics. Obstet Gynecol 80:389, 1992

54. Hatch KD, Schneider A, Abdel-Nour MW: An evaluation of human papillomavirus testing for intermediate- and high-risk types as triage before colposcopy. Am J Obstet Gynecol 172:1150, 1995

55. Bergeron C, Jeannel D, Poveda J, et al: Human papillomavirus testing in women with mild cytologic atypia. Obstet Gynecol 95:821, 2000

56. Shlay JC, Dunn T, Byers T, et al: Prediction of cervical intraepithelial neoplasia grade 2–3 using risk assessment and human papillomavirus testing in women with atypia on Papanicolaou smears. Obstet Gynecol 96:410, 2000

57. Kaufman RH, Adam E, Icenogle J, et al: Human papillomavirus testing as triage for atypical squamous cells of undetermined significance and low-grade squamous intraepithelial lesions: sensitivity, specificity, and cost-effectiveness. Am J Obstet Gynecol 177:930, 1997

58. Raab SS, Steiner AL, Hornberger J: The cost-effectiveness of treating women with a cervical vaginal smear diagnosis of atypical squamous cells of undetermined significance. Am J Obstet Gynecol 179:411, 1998

59. Results of a randomized trial on the management of cytology interpretations of atypical squamous cells of undetermined significance. The ASCUS-LSIL Triage Study (ALTS) Group. Am J Obstet Gynecol 188:1383, 2003

60. Cuzick J, Szarewski A, Cubie H, et al: Management of women who test positive for high-risk types of human papillomavirus: the HART study. Lancet 362:1871, 2003

61. Clavel C, Masure M, Bory JP, et al: Human papillomavirus testing in primary screening for the detection of high-grade cervical lesions: a study of 7,932 women. Br J Cancer 84:1616, 2001

62. Sherman ME, Lorincz AT, Scott DR, et al: Baseline cytology, human papillomavirus testing, and risk for cervical neoplasia: a 10-year cohort analysis. J Natl Cancer Inst 95:46, 2003

63. Petry KU, Menton S, Menton M, et al: Inclusion of HPV testing in routine cervical cancer screening for women above 29 years in Germany: results for 8466 patients. Br J Cancer 88:1570, 2003

64. Wright TC, Cox JT, Massad LS, et al: 2001 consensus guidelines for the management of women with cervical cytologic abnormalities. JAMA 287:2120, 2002

65. Cervical Cancer: Clinical Practice Guidelines in Oncology. National Comprehensive Cancer Network, 2004
http://www.nccn.org/professionals/physician_gls/PDF/cervical.pdf

66. Management of the abnormal Papanicolaou smear. SOGC Clinical Practice Guidelines, No. 70, 1998

Acknowledgment

Figure 1   Courtesy of Joan Jones, M.D.

90 Approach to Hematologic Disorders

David C. Dale, M.D., F.A.C.P.

Hematology deals with the normal functions and disorders of the formed elements in the blood (i.e., erythrocytes, leukocytes, and platelets) and the plasma factors governing hemostasis. The blood sustains life by transporting oxygen and essential nutrients, removing waste, and delivering the humoral and cellular factors necessary for host defenses. Platelets and coagulation factors, together with vascular endothelial cells, maintain the integrity of this system. Some hematologic disorders such as anemia, leukocytosis, and bleeding are quite common, occurring secondary to infectious, inflammatory, nutritional, and malignant diseases. Other disorders, including the hematologic malignancies, are far less common. This chapter presents the general principles for understanding the hematopoietic system [*see other chapters under Hematology for a more detailed description of the pathophysiology of specific hematologic diseases and their treatment*].

Hematopoiesis

Hematopoiesis begins in the fetal yolk sac and later occurs predominantly in the liver and the spleen.[1] Recent studies demonstrate that islands of hematopoiesis develop in these tissues from hemangioblasts, which are the common progenitors for both hematopoietic and endothelial cells.[2] These islands then involute as the marrow becomes the primary site for blood cell formation by the seventh month of fetal development. Barring serious damage, such as that which occurs with myelofibrosis or radiation injury, the bone marrow remains the site of blood cell formation throughout the rest of life. In childhood, there is active hematopoiesis in the marrow spaces of the central axial skeleton (i.e., the ribs, vertebrae, and pelvis) and the extremities, extending to the wrists, ankles, and the calvaria. With normal growth and development, hematopoiesis gradually withdraws from the periphery. This change is reversible, however; distal marrow extension can result from intensive stimulation, as occurs with severe hemolytic anemias, long-term administration of hematopoietic growth factors, and hematologic malignancies. The term medullary hematopoiesis refers to the production of blood cells in the bone marrow; the term extramedullary hematopoiesis indicates blood cell production outside the marrow in the spleen, liver, and other locations.

ORGANIZATION OF HEMATOPOIETIC TISSUES

In its normal state, the medullary space in which hematopoietic cells develop contains many adipocytes and has a rich vascular supply [*see Figure 1*].[3] Vascular endothelial cells, marrow fibroblasts, and stromal cells are important sources of the matrix proteins that provide structure to the marrow space; these cells also produce the hematopoietic growth factors and chemokines that regulate blood cell production.[4] The vascular endothelial cells also form an important barrier that keeps immature cells in the marrow and permits mature hematopoietic elements to enter the blood. The abundant adipocytes may influence hematopoiesis by serving as a localized energy source, by synthesizing growth factors, and by affecting the metabolism of androgens and estrogens.[5] Marrow macrophages re-

move effete or apoptotic cells and clear the blood of foreign materials when they enter the marrow. Osteoblasts and osteoclasts maintain and remodel the surrounding cancellous bone and the calcified lattice, which crisscrosses the marrow space.[3]

The thymus, lymph nodes, mucosa-associated lymphatic tissues, and the spleen have multiple hematopoietic functions. Early in development, they are major sites of hematopoiesis. In adulthood, they are principally sites of lymphocyte development, processing of antigens, development of effector T cells, and antibody production [*see other chapters under Immunology, Allergy, and Rheumatology*]. In leukemia and the myeloproliferative disorders, the size and cellular architecture of these tissues are deranged, leading to many of the clinical manifestations of these disorders [*see Chapters 204 and 205*].

Hematopoietic Stem Cells

All cells of the hematopoietic system are derived from common precursor cells, the hematopoietic stem cells. These cells are difficult to identify, in part because they normally represent only about 0.05% of marrow cells. Through self-renewal, this population is maintained at a constant level. Through the use of monoclonal antibodies that recognize specific cell surface molecules expressed selectively on developing hematopoietic cells and other specialized techniques, the stem cells can now be separated from other marrow cells. With these methods, very primitive hematopoietic stem cells have been found to be positive for c-kit and thy-1 but negative for CD34, CD38, CD33, and HLA-DR. For clinical purposes, CD34+ progenitor cell populations, which contain stem cells and some more mature cells, are often used for hematopoietic stem cell transplantation [*see Chapter 101*].

Stem cells give rise to daughter cells, which undergo irreversible differentiation along various hematopoietic cell lineages [*see Figure 2*]. Many aspects of the earliest steps in this differentiation process are not well understood. With lineage commitment, however, differentiation, maturation, and release of cells to the blood come under the control of well-defined hematopoietic growth factors. In the early phases of differentiation, the regulatory roles played by these growth factors overlap. Later in development, some growth factors are lineage specific, meaning that they govern the maturation and deployment of single lineages. Erythropoietin (EPO) (erythrocytes), thrombopoietin (TPO) (platelets), granulocyte colony-stimulating factor (G-CSF) (neutrophils), and macrophage colony-stimulating factor (M-CSF) (monocytes) are the best-characterized lineage-specific factors.

Hematopoietic Growth Factors

The hematopoietic growth factors, also referred to as hematopoietic cytokines, are a family of glycoproteins produced in the bone marrow by endothelial cells, stromal cells, fibroblasts, macrophages, and lymphocytes; they are also produced at distant sites, from which they are transported to the marrow through the blood [*see Table 1*]. The naming of these factors is somewhat confusing. Erythropoietin and thrombopoietin derive part of their names from the Greek word poiesis, meaning "to make." The colony-stimulating factors were first recognized because of their capacity to stimulate early hematopoietic cells to grow into clusters and large colonies in tissue culture systems. The term interleukin denotes factors that are produced by leukocytes and that affect other leukocytes. This is a large family of factors that predominantly govern lymphocytopoiesis, but many members also have broad effects on other lineages. The discovery of new growth factors and of the biologic consequences of deficiencies or excesses of these factors continues to evolve rapidly.

Hematopoietic cells have distinctive patterns of expression of growth factor receptors, and the patterns evolve as the cells differentiate [see Figure 2]. Each growth factor binds only to its specific receptor.[6,7] It is now known that some growth factors share components of the receptor (e.g., interleukin-3 [IL-3], IL-5, and granulocyte-macrophage colony-stimulating factor [GM-CSF] share a common β chain of their receptor); specificity comes from other unique or private components of the receptor. Binding of the ligand to the receptor leads to a conformational change, activation of intracellular kinases, and, ultimately, the triggering of cell proliferation.[8,9] For some growth factors, these pathways are well defined; for others, the pathways are still unclear [see Figure 3].

Hematopoietic growth factors not only stimulate cell proliferation but also prolong cell survival; that is, they have antiapoptotic effects.[10] For some lineages, such as neutrophils and monocytes, growth factor receptors occur on fully mature cells; exposure of these cells to the factors primes the cells for an enhanced responsiveness to bacteria or other stimulators of their metabolic activity. Thus, for cells of the neutrophil lineage, the growth factors G-CSF and GM-CSF can stimulate early hematopoietic cell proliferation, increase the number of cells produced by the marrow, prolong the life span of these cells, and augment cell functions.[11]

Erythropoietin

The peritubular interstitial cells located in the inner cortex and outer medulla of the kidney are the primary site for erythropoietin production.[12] In response to hypoxia, transcription of the erythropoietin gene in these cells increases, resulting in increased secretion of erythropoietin. The protein is then transported through the blood to the marrow to stimulate erythropoiesis. With renal failure, erythropoietin production is severely impaired. In infections and many chronic inflammatory conditions, the erythropoietin response is blunted, and erythropoietin levels are low.[13]

Erythropoietin is a glycosylated protein that modulates erythropoiesis by affecting several steps in red cell development. The most primitive identifiable erythroid cells, the burst-forming unit–erythroid cells (BFU-E), are relatively insensitive to erythropoietin. More mature cells, the colony-forming unit–erythroid cells (CFU-E), are very sensitive. Erythropoietin treatment prolongs survival of erythroid precursors, shortens the time between cell divisions, and increases the number of cells produced from individual precursors.[14]

Erythropoietin can be administered intravenously or subcutaneously for the treatment of anemia caused by inadequate endogenous production of erythropoietin.[15,16] Treatment is maximally effective when the marrow has a generous supply of iron and other nutrients, such as cobalamin and folic acid.[17] For patients with renal failure, who have very low erythropoietin levels, the starting dosage is 50 to 100 units S.C. three times a week. The most easily monitored immediate effect of increased endogenous or exogenous erythropoietin is an increase in the blood reticulocyte count. Normally, as red cell precursors mature, the cells extrude their nucleus at the normal blast stage. The resulting reticulocytes, identified by the supravital stain of their residual ribosomes, persist for about 3 days in the marrow and 1 day in the blood. Erythropoietin shortens the transit time through the marrow, leading to an increase in the number and proportion of blood reticulocytes within a few days.

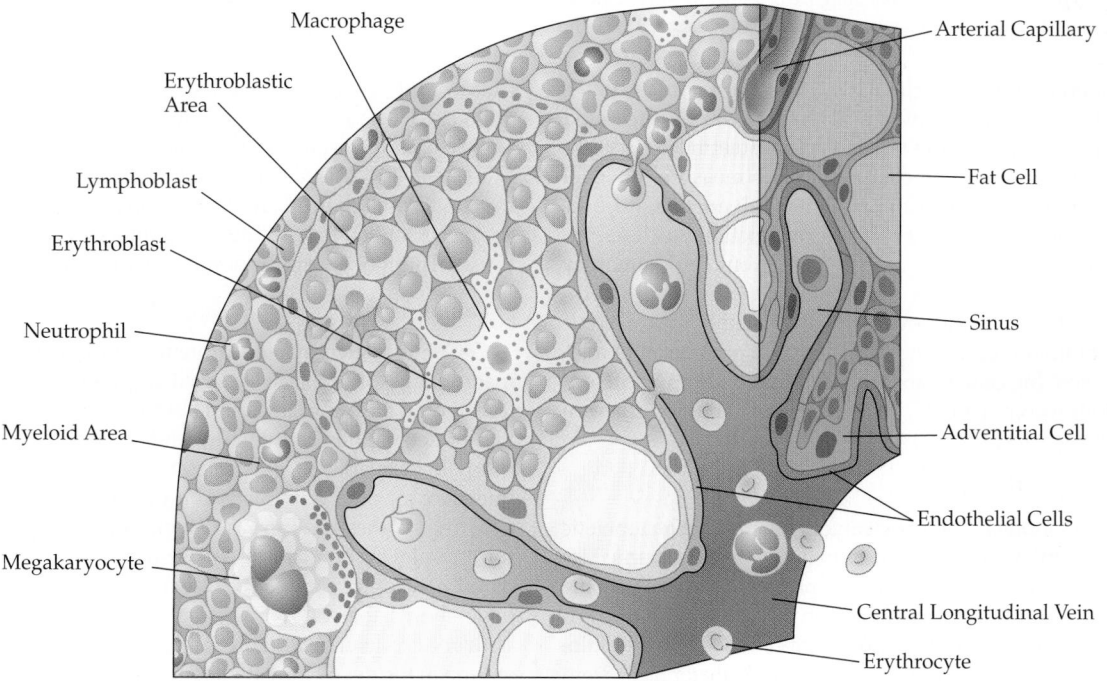

Figure 1   **The architecture of the bone marrow showing the various types of cells.**

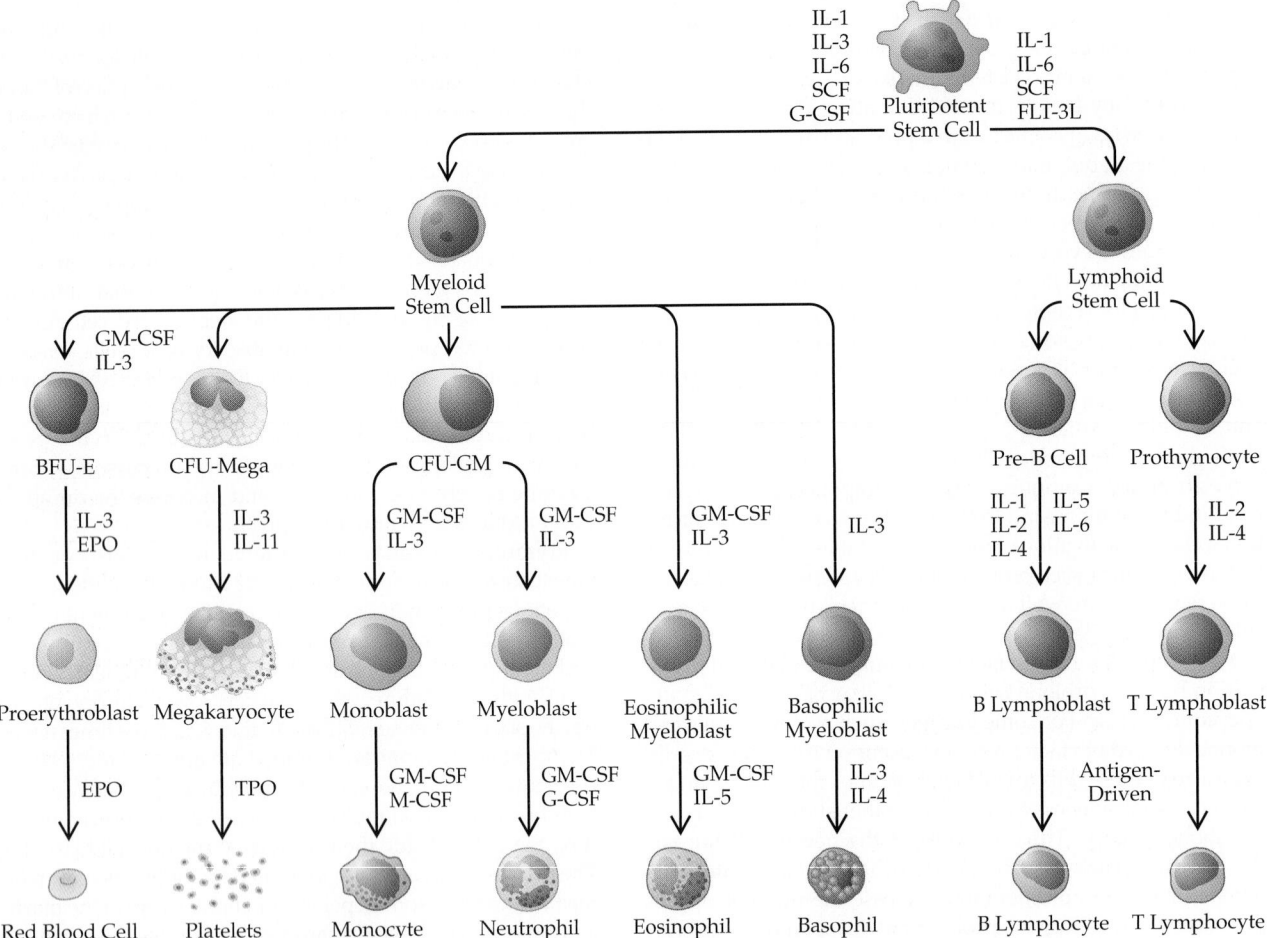

Figure 2   **The pattern for development of various types of blood cells in the bone marrow. (BFU-E—burst-forming unit–erythroid; CFU-GM—colony-forming unit–granulocyte-macrophage; CFU-mega—colony-forming unit–megakaryocyte; EPO—erythropoietin; EPOR—surface component of the erythropoietin receptor; FLT-3L—fms-like tyrosine kinase 3 ligand; G-CSF—granulocyte colony-stimulating factor; GM-CSF—granulocyte-macrophage colony-stimulating factor; IL—interleukin; M-CSF—macrophage colony-stimulating factor; TPO—thrombopoietin; SCF—stem cell factor)**

In some conditions, particularly chronic inflammatory diseases, the effectiveness of erythropoietin can be predicted from measurement of the serum erythropoietin level by immunoassay.[12,13] It may be cost-effective to measure the level before initiating treatment in patients with anemia attributable to suppressed erythropoietin production, such as patients with HIV infection, cancer, and chronic inflammatory diseases. Several studies have shown that erythropoietin treatment decreases the severity of anemia and improves the quality of life for patients with cancer.[18] In patients with anemia caused by cancer and cancer chemotherapy, current guidelines recommend erythropoietin treatment if the hemoglobin level is less than 10 g/dl.[19]

Thrombopoietin

The development of megakaryocytes from hematopoietic stem cells and the level of platelets in the blood are governed by thrombopoietin.[20] Thrombopoietin is produced primarily by the liver and is similar to erythropoietin in structure. However, thrombopoietin has broader biologic effects than erythropoietin, stimulating the proliferation and release of hematopoietic stem cells from the bone marrow and prolonging survival of these cells.[24] Thrombopoietin signals through its specific receptor,

called cMpL, expressed on hematopoietic cells. Plasma thrombopoietin levels are inversely related to the blood platelet count. Deficiencies in thrombopoietin cause thrombocytopenia, and excesses in thrombopoietin cause thrombocytosis. Recombinant human thrombopoietin and related molecules activating cMpL are being studied for treatment of thrombocytopenia of diverse causes. Thrombopoietin is not yet approved for clinical use.

Granulocyte Colony-Stimulating Factor

G-CSF is a glycosylated protein produced by monocytes, macrophages, fibroblasts, stromal cells, and endothelial cells throughout the body.[21] It stimulates the growth and differentiation of neutrophils both in vitro and in vivo. G-CSF levels are normally very low or undetectable but increase with bacterial infections or after administration of bacterial endotoxin.[11] G-CSF (the synthesized form is known as filgrastim or lenograstim) administration causes a dose-dependent increase in the blood neutrophil count in healthy persons. Studies in animals have shown that G-CSF deficiency causes neutropenia.[22] As with erythropoietin, administration of G-CSF leads to an acceleration in the development of neutrophils in the bone marrow, with the neutrophils shifting at an earlier stage than normal from the marrow to the blood.[23]

Table 1   Hematopoietic Growth Factors

Factor	Other Names	Cell Source	Chromosome Location	Function
EPO	Erythropoietin	Juxtaglomerular cells	7q	Stimulates erythrocyte formation and release from marrow
TPO	Thrombopoietin; megakaryocyte growth and development factor (MGDF)	Hepatocytes, renal and endothelial cells, fibroblasts	3q27	Stimulates megakaryocyte proliferation and platelet formation
G-CSF	Granulocyte colony-stimulating factor; filgrastim; lenograstim	Endothelial cells, monocytes, fibroblasts	17q11.2-q21	Stimulates formation and function of neutrophils
GM-CSF	Granulocyte-macrophage colony-stimulating factor	T cells, monocytes, fibroblasts	5q23-q31	Stimulates formation and function of neutrophils, monocytes, and eosinophils
M-CSF	Macrophage colony-stimulating factor; colony stimulating factor–1 (CSF-1)	Endothelial cells, macrophages, fibroblasts	5q33.1	Stimulates monocyte formation and function
IL-1α and IL-1β	Interleukin-1α and -1β, endogenous pyrogen hemopoietin-1	Monocytes, keratinocytes, endothelial cells	2q13	Proliferation of T cells, B cells, and other cells; induces fever and catabolism
IL-2	T cell growth factor	T cells (CD4+, CD8+), large granular lymphocytes (natural killer, or NK, cells)	4q	T cell proliferation, antitumor and antimicrobial effects
IL-3	Multi–colony stimulating factor; mast cell growth factor	Activated T cells; large granular lymphocytes (NK cells)	5q23-q31	Proliferation of early hematopoietic cells
IL-4	B cell growth factor; T cell growth factor II; mast cell growth factor II	T cells	5q23-q31	Proliferation of B cells and T cells; enhances cytotoxic activities
IL-5	Eosinophil differentiation factor; eosinophil colony-stimulating factor	T cells	5q23.3-q32	Stimulates eosinophil formation; stimulates T cell and B cell functions
IL-6	B cell stimulatory factor II; hepatocyte stimulatory factor	Monocytes, tumor cells, B cells and T cells, fibroblasts, endothelial cells	7p	Stimulates and inhibits cell growth; promotes B cell differentiation
IL-7	Lymphopoietin 1; pre–B cell growth factor	Lymphoid tissues and cell lines	8q12-q13	Growth factor for B cells and T cells
IL-11	Plasmacytoma stimulating factor	Fibroblasts, trophoblasts, cancer cell lines	19q13.3-q13.4	Stimulates proliferation of early hematopoietic cells; induces acute-phase protein synthesis
IL-12	Natural killer cell stimulating factor	Macrophages, B cells	5q31-q33; 3p12-q13.2	Stimulates T cell expansion and interferon-gamma; synergistically promotes early hematopoietic cell proliferation
LIF	Leukemia inhibitory factor	Monocytes and lymphocytes; stomal cells	22q	Stimulates hematopoietic cell differentiation
SCF	Stem cell factor; kit ligand; steel factor	Endothelial cells; hepatocytes	4q11-q20	Stimulates proliferation of early hematopoietic cells and mast cells
FLT-3 ligand	fms-like tyrosine kinase 3; STK-1	T cells, stromal cells, and fibroblasts	19q13.3	Stimulates early hematopoietic cell differentiation; increases blood dendritic cells

G-CSF is used primarily to prevent severe neutropenia after cancer chemotherapy, for acceleration of neutrophil recovery after bone marrow transplantation, for mobilization of hematopoietic progenitor cells from the marrow to the blood in hematopoietic transplantation, and for the treatment of severe chronic neutropenia.[24] The usual dosage is 5 μg/kg S.C. daily; higher doses are used to mobilize progenitor cells, and lower doses are used for long-term treatment of neutropenia. A formulation of G-CSF, in which G-CSF is conjugated to polyethylene glycol to reduce renal clearance and prolong the effects of the drug, is also available. Side effects of either form of G-CSF are principally musculoskeletal pain and headaches during the period of rapid marrow expansion soon after therapy is initiated. Other side effects are uncommon. The use of G-CSF to treat chemo-

therapy-induced febrile neutropenia is controversial.[25]

Granulocyte-Macrophage Colony-Stimulating Factor

GM-CSF is a glycosylated protein produced by many types of cells, including T cells. GM-CSF stimulates formation of neutrophils, monocytes, and eosinophils and may also enhance the growth of early cells of other lineages. In contrast to G-CSF, GM-CSF levels generally do not increase with infections or acute inflammatory conditions, and neutropenia does not result from deficiencies of GM-CSF.[26] The marrow effects of G-CSF and GM-CSF are similar, but GM-CSF is less potent in elevating the blood neutrophil count.[27] GM-CSF (the synthesized form is known as sargramostim or molgramostim) is approved in the United States for acceleration of marrow recovery after

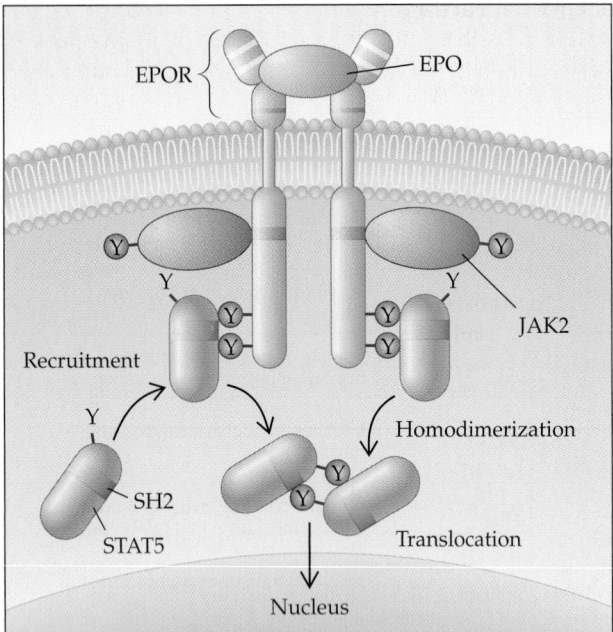

Figure 3   **A model of how hematopoietic growth factors interact with their receptors to initiate cell proliferation. (EPO—erythropoietin; JAK2—Janus kinase 2; SH2—Src homology 2; STAT5—signal transducer and activator of transcription 5)**

bone marrow transplantation or chemotherapy and for mobilization of progenitor cells from the marrow. The usual dosage of GM-CSF is 250 mg/m²/day S.C. The side effects of GM-CSF include bone and musculoskeletal pain, myalgias, and injection-site reactions.

Interleukin-11

IL-11 (oprelvekin) is a pleiotropic cytokine that is expressed by, as well as active in, many tissues. IL-11 acts synergistically with other growth factors, including thrombopoietin, to stimulate megakaryocyte development and platelet formation. The Food and Drug Administration approved it for use in the prevention of severe thrombocytopenia and for patients who need platelet transfusions after chemotherapy. The usual dosage is 50 mg/kg/day S.C. Its side effects include edema, tachycardia, and dyspnea.

Other Growth Factors

Several other hematopoietic growth factors have potential clinical uses. IL-3 acts at an early phase in hematopoiesis to stimulate cell proliferation; however, it has relatively little effect on peripheral counts. Stem cell factor (SCF) and fms-like tyrosine kinase 3 (FLT-3) ligand are other early-acting factors under investigation. M-CSF is a selective factor for monocytes and macrophage formation. IL-5 is a selective factor that is similar to M-CSF but with regard to the generation of eosinophils.

It is presumed that normally, hematopoietic cell formation is governed by combinations of factors, released in a cascade, that closely coordinate the development of these cells. The details of how this process occurs, however, are not yet clear. Numerous laboratory and clinical studies have investigated combinations of factors, but the therapeutic benefit of using multiple growth factors is not yet proved.

DYNAMICS OF HEMATOPOIESIS

In the marrow, blood cells develop in two phases, the proliferative and the maturational phases. During cell proliferation, the precursors of blood cells normally undergo cell division at intervals of about 18 to 24 hours. In the maturational phase, cell division ceases, but final features are added before the cells enter the blood. During this phase, erythrocytes normally lose all their nuclear material, acquire their biconcave shape, and develop their final content of enzymes necessary for maintaining the biconcave shape and resisting destruction by oxidative stress. Normally, it takes 7 to 10 days for erythrocytes to develop from their early precursors, but this process can be accelerated by erythropoietin therapy.

Neutrophils acquire most of their granules (known as the primary, secondary, and tertiary granules), which are necessary for their microbicidal activities, during the proliferative phase. During maturation, their nuclear chromatin condenses, the glycogen content of the cytoplasm increases, and the surface properties governing the circulation, adherence, and migration to tissues are added.[28] Neutrophils reach a fully mature state in the marrow before they are released into the blood. These mature marrow cells are called the marrow neutrophil reserve. Quantitatively, this neutrophil pool is substantially larger—probably

---

Table 2   **Causes of Lymphadenopathy[42]**

Infections

  Bacterial: streptococci,* *Staphylococcus aureus*,* syphilis,*† cat-scratch disease,* *Mycobacterium tuberculosis* and other mycobacteria,† brucellosis,† leptospirosis,† meliodiosis,† chancroid, plague, tularemia, rat-bite fever

  Viral: adenovirus,* HIV,*† infectious mononucleosis,*† herpes simplex,* measles,† rubella,† cytomegalovirus,† hepatitis,† Kawasaki disease

  Mycotic: sporotrichosis, histoplasmosis,† coccidioidomycosis†

  Rickettsial: Rocky Mountain spotted fever,*† scrub typhus†

  Chlamydial: *Chlamydia trachomatis*, lymphogranuloma venereum

  Protozoan: toxoplasmosis,† trypanosomiasis,† kala-azar†

  Helminthic: filariasis,† onchocerciasis

Immunologic Causes

  Stings and bites*

  Drug reactions*†: phenytoin, hydralazine

  Serum sickness*†

  Collagen vascular diseases: rheumatoid arthritis,† dermatomyositis,† angioimmunoblastic lymphadenopathy†

Malignancies

  Hematologic: Hodgkin disease,* acute leukemia,† chronic lymphocytic leukemia,† chronic myelogenous leukemia,† lymphoma,† myelofibrosis†

  Other: metastatic carcinoma, sarcomas

Endocrine Diseases

  Hyperthyroidism†

Histiocytic Disorders

  Lipid storage disease,† malignant histiocytosis,† Langerhans (eosinophilic) histiocytosis

Miscellaneous

  Sarcoidosis, amyloidosis,† chronic granulomatous disease, lymphomatoid granulomatosis, necrotizing lymphadenitis

*Most common causes in general practice in the United States.

†Usually cause generalized lymphadenopathy.

five to 10 times larger—than the total circulating supply of neutrophils. Normally, it takes 10 to 14 days for blood neutrophils to develop from early precursors, but this process is accelerated in the presence of infections and by treatment with G-CSF or GM-CSF [see Chapter 95].

Platelets form from the breaking apart of the cytoplasm of the fully mature megakaryocytes, which are also derived from hematopoietic stem cells.[20] Megakaryocytes undergo reduplication of their nuclear chromatin without cell division, which results in the production of extremely large cells. When marrow damage occurs from chemotherapeutic agents and after hematopoietic transplantation, the megakaryocytes are often the slowest cells to recover, and thrombocytopenia is often the last cytopenia to resolve.

There are important differences in the dynamics or kinetics of erythrocytes, platelets, and leukocytes in the blood. For instance, neutrophils have a blood half-life of only 6 to 8 hours; essentially, a new blood population of neutrophils is formed every 24 hours.[28] Erythrocytes last the longest by far: the normal life span is about 100 days. These differences partially account for why neutrophils and their precursors are the predominant marrow cells, whereas in the blood, erythrocytes far outnumber neutrophils. Similarly, the short half-life and high turnover rate of neutrophils account for why neutropenia is the most frequent hematologic consequence when bone marrow is damaged by drugs or radiation. Finally, transfusion of erythrocytes and platelets is feasible because of their relatively long life span, whereas the short life span of neutrophils has greatly impeded efforts to develop neutrophil transfusion therapy.

Clinical Manifestations of Hematologic Disorders

The following signs and symptoms are frequently observed in patients with hematologic diseases.

WEAKNESS, FATIGUE, AND PALLOR

Weakness and fatigue are common complaints of patients with anemia, especially if it is of recent onset, such as anemia caused by recent blood loss or acute hemolysis.[29] Anemia that develops gradually, particularly in inactive persons, may cause only fatigue. Fatigue is a very common complaint of patients with infections, inflammatory diseases, and malignancies. Other common causes of fatigue include chronic lung diseases, congestive heart failure, endocrine disorders, and depression.

Pallor is recognized by examining the conjunctiva, mucous membranes, nail beds, and palmar creases—tissues lacking melanin pigmentation. The World Health Organization has developed a simple clinical scale to measure pallor for diagnosing anemia when blood counts are not available. The sensitivity and specificity of this scale vary between 70% and 90%, depending on the population and severity of the anemia.[30,31] Other causes of pallor include edema (including myxedema) and vasoconstriction caused by cold temperatures, hemorrhage, hypoglycemia, or shock.

PAIN

Pain, particularly bone pain, is an important marker of hematologic disease. Pain is usually generalized in patients with acute leukemia and multiple myeloma, but most frequently, it is felt in the back or pelvis. With metastatic breast, colon, or lung cancer, the pain is more often localized and asymmetrical. In sickle cell disease, severe bone pain and pain in many other tissues occur with vascular obstruction and infarction caused by obstruction of blood flow by the aggregation of abnormal cells [see Chapter 93]. Bone pain mimicking these disorders occurs with marrow expansion in response to treatment with hematopoietic growth factors.

FATIGUE, PHARYNGITIS, AND FEVER

Fatigue, pharyngitis, and fever are a frequently observed sequence in patients with acutely developing neutropenia, occurring as an idiosyncratic or toxic reaction to many drugs. In cases of severe neutropenia, cough and respiratory symptoms, perianal pain and tenderness, or acute abdominal pain often occurs and necessitates immediate medical assessment [see Chapter 95].

MOUTH ULCERS, GINGIVITIS, AND CERVICAL ADENOPATHY

Mouth ulcers, gingivitis, and cervical adenopathy are common problems of patients with chronic neutropenia [see Chapter 95]. Gingivitis is a serious problem, often leading to periodontal disease and tooth loss.

PERIANAL PAIN, INFLAMMATION, AND BLEEDING

Hemorrhoids are the most common cause of perianal discomfort. Patients with neutropenia readily develop pain and cellulitis in this area. Hemorrhoids, inflammatory bowel disease, and cancer commonly cause rectal bleeding.

LYMPHADENOPATHY AND SPLENOMEGALY

Lymphadenopathy is a common presentation of infectious, inflammatory, and hematologic diseases, particularly the lymphomas and leukemias [see Table 2]. Lymphadenopathy may occur without associated symptoms, but often, fatigue and intermittent fever (e.g., Pel-Ebstein fever) occur. In contrast to acute infectious diseases leading to tender lymphadenopathy, in most hematologic disorders the lymph nodes and spleen are nontender, with a soft to rubbery consistency. Splenomegaly is often more difficult to detect than lymphadenopathy; most of the diseases causing lymphadenopathy can also cause splenic enlargement.

BLEEDING AND BRUISING

Bleeding occurs as a consequence of thrombocytopenia, deficiencies of coagulation factors, or both [see Chapter 97]. Thrombocytopenia usually presents as petechial bleeding that is first observed in the lower extremities. Coagulation factor deficiencies more often cause bleeding into the gastrointestinal tract or joints. Intracranial bleeding, however, can occur with a deficiency of platelets or coagulation factors and can be catastrophic.

THROMBOSIS

Thrombosis can be either venous or arterial [see Chapter 99]. With venous thrombosis, swelling, tenderness, and pain beyond the obstruction usually occur, and embolization to the lungs is a frequent concern. Venous thrombosis usually occurs after inactivity or obstruction of venous flow or with imbalances of coagulation factors. On the other hand, arterial thrombosis usually occurs because of abnormalities of the arterial wall from atherosclerosis or acute vascular injury, as in thrombotic thrombocytopenic purpura, or from thrombocytosis in the myeloproliferative disorders.

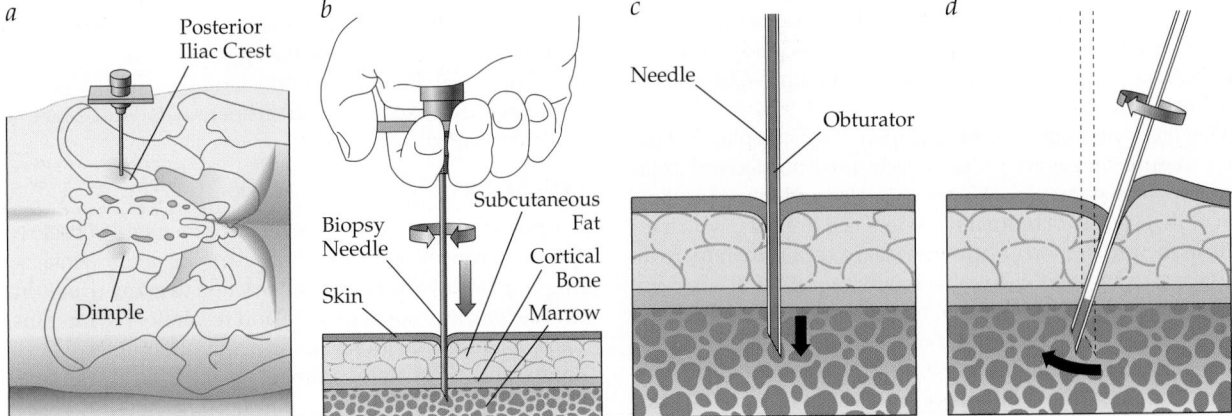

Figure 4   **Bone marrow aspirate and biopsy procedure. (a) The posterior iliac crest is the usual site for sampling; (b) the needle is placed through the skin to the marrow space; (c) the marrow sample is aspirated; and (d) the biopsy sample is carefully removed.**

Laboratory Evaluation

The following basic tests are widely used to diagnose hematologic disorders.

COMPLETE BLOOD CELL COUNTS

CBCs are routinely performed in most laboratories through the use of an electronic particle counter, which determines the total white blood cell and platelet counts and calculates the hematocrit and hemoglobin levels from the erythrocyte count and the dimensions of the red cells. Abnormalities in the CBC are described in other Hematology chapters.

PERIPHERAL BLOOD SMEARS

Peripheral blood smears usually stain with Wright stain. When examined by light microscopy, they reveal the size and shape of blood cells, which allows an estimate to be made of the amount of hemoglobin in erythrocytes. Differential leukocyte counts, enumerating the number of neutrophils, monocytes, lymphocytes, eosinophils, and basophils, are made by manually counting cells on the blood smears or by using an automated cell counter [*see the* Normal Laboratory Values *section*]. The morphology of the leukocytes often provides a clue for the diagnosis of leukemia and for recognizing some disorders of leukocytes that lead to susceptibility to infections [*see Chapter 95*].

RETICULOCYTE COUNTS

Reticulocyte counts are useful for evaluating the marrow response to anemia. Normally, during their first 24 to 36 hours in the circulation, young red cells contain residual ribosomal RNA, which precipitates with certain dyes such as methylene blue. An increase in the proportion or absolute number of reticulocytes occurs a few days after significant blood loss or in response to red blood cell destruction in hemolytic anemias. Low reticulocyte counts in chronic anemia suggest either an endogenous erythropoietin deficiency or a marrow abnormality.

BONE MARROW EXAMINATION

Hematopoietic cells of the bone marrow can be removed by aspiration or by needle biopsy. In adults, the best site is the posterior iliac crest, with the patient in a prone position [*see Figure 4*]. Under special circumstances and in children, other sites can be used, such as the anterior iliac crest, the sternum, or the long bones. With local anesthesia and sterile technique, the patient experiences only transient pain. Bleeding or infection at the injection site is quite uncommon. The aspirate yields cells for morphologic examination, and differential counts reveal the ratio of myeloid cells to erythroid cells (M:E ratio). A biopsy reveals the cellularity of the marrow at the site sampled. Biopsies are particularly useful for examination of the marrow for infiltrative cells (e.g., in lymphomas or carcinomas involving the marrow) and for diagnosing leukemia, characterized by the marrow's being so densely packed with cells that none of the bone marrow can be aspirated. Biopsies take longer for interpretation because they must be decalcified and stained before examination.

Imaging Studies

Radionuclide scanning (e.g., using technetium-99m) reveals the extent of the hematopoietic tissue in the marrow because the phagocytic cells of the marrow take up the radiolabeled particles. Marrow scanning is sometimes used to determine the extensiveness of the hematopoietic tissue; more often, it is useful in determining whether there are localized areas of increased uptake resulting from infection or a malignancy that has metastasized to the marrow. Computed tomography and ultrasonography are useful in determining the size of lymph nodes and the spleen, but they are not particularly useful for marrow examination. The marrow is seen well with magnetic resonance imaging. This technique is principally used to look for infiltrative processes in the marrow space, such as those that occur in malignancies and infections.

The author is a consultant for, receives research support from, and is a member of the speakers' bureau of Amgen, Inc.

References

1. Schatteman GC: Adult bone marrow-derived hemangioblasts, endothelial cell progenitors, and EPCs. Curr Top Dev Biol 64:141, 2004

2. McGrath KE, Palis J: Hematopoiesis in the yolk sac: more than meets the eye. Exp Hematol 33:1021, 2005

3. Verfaillie CM: Anatomy and physiology of hematopoiesis in hematology. Hematology: Basic Principles and Practice, 3rd ed. Hoffman R, Benz EJ, Shattil SJ, et al, Eds. Churchill Livingstone, New York, 2000, p 139

4. Youn BS, Mantel C, Broxmeyer HE: Chemokines, chemokine receptors and hematopoiesis. Immunol Rev 177:150, 2000

5. Dazzi F, Ramasamy R, Glennie S, et al: The role of mesenchymal stem cells in haemopoiesis. Blood Rev Dec 15, 2005 (Epub ahead of print)

6. Thomas D, Vadas M, Lopez A: Regulation of haematopoiesis by growth factors: emerging insights and therapies. Expert Opin Biol Ther 4:869, 2004

7. D'Andrea RJ, Gonda TJ: A model for assembly and activation of the GM-CSF, IL-3 and IL-5 receptors: insights from activated mutants of the common beta subunit. Exp Hematol 28:231, 2000

8. McLemore ML, Grewal S, Liu F, et al: STAT-3 activation is required for normal G-CSF-dependent proliferation and granulocytic differentiation. Immunity 4:193, 2001

9. Haq R, Halupa A, Beattie BK, et al: Regulation of erythropoietin-induced STAT serine phosphorylation by distinct mitogen-activated protein kinases. J Biol Chem 277:17359, 2002

10. Tehranchi R, Fadeel B, Forsblom AM, et al: Granulocyte colony-stimulating factor inhibits spontaneous cytochrome c release and mitochondria-dependent apoptosis of myelodysplastic syndrome hematopoietic progenitors. Blood 101:1080, 2002

11. Hubel K, Dale DC, Liles WC: Therapeutic use of cytokines to modulate phagocyte function for the treatment of infectious diseases: current status of granulocyte colony-stimulating factor, granulocyte-macrophage factor, and interferon-gamma. J Infect Dis 185:1490, 2002

12. Spivak JL: The biology and clinical applications of recombinant erythropoietin. Semin Oncol 25(3 suppl 7):7, 1998

13. Weiss G, Goodnough LT: Anemia of chronic disease. N Engl J Med 10:352:1011, 2005

14. Koury MJ: Erythropoietin: the story of hypoxia and a finely regulated hematopoietic hormone. Exp Hematol 33:1263, 2005

15. Bohlius J, Langensiepen S, Schwarzer G, et al: Erythropoietin for patients with malignant disease. Cochrane Database Syst Rev (3):CD003407, 2004

16. Cody J, Daly C, Campbell M, et al: Recombinant human erythropoietin for chronic renal failure anaemia in pre-dialysis patients. Cochrane Database Syst Rev (3): CD003266, 2005

17. Goodnough LT: The role of iron in erythropoiesis in the absence and presence of erythropoietin therapy. Nephrol Dial Transplant 17(suppl 5):14, 2002

18. Witzig TE, Silberstein PT, Loprinzi CL, et al: Phase III, randomized, double-blind study of epoetin alfa compared with placebo in anemic patients receiving chemotherapy. J Clin Oncol 23:2606, 2005

19. Rizzo JD, Lichtin AE, Woolf SH, et al: Use of epoetin in patients with cancer: evidence-based clinical practice guidelines of the American Society of Clinical Oncology and the American Society of Hematology. Blood 100:2303, 2002

20. Kaushansky K: The molecular mechanisms that control thrombopoiesis. J Clin Invest 115:3339, 2005

21. Roberts AW: G-CSF: a key regulator of neutrophil production, but that's not all! Growth Factors 23:33, 2005

22. Molineux G: Physiologic and pathologic consequences of granulocyte colony-stimulating factor deficiency. Curr Opin Hematol 9:199, 2002

23. Price TH, Chatta GS, Dale DC: Effect of recombinant granulocyte colony-stimulating factor on neutrophil kinetics in normal and elderly humans. Blood 88:335, 1996

24. Lyman GH: Guidelines of the National Comprehensive Cancer Network on the use of myeloid growth factors with cancer chemotherapy: a review of the evidence. J Natl Compr Canc Netw 3:557, 2005

25. Clark OA, Lyman GH, Castro AA, et al: Colony-stimulating factors for chemotherapy-induced febrile neutropenia: a meta-analysis of randomized controlled trials. J Clin Oncol 23:4198, 2005

26. Fleetwood AJ, Cook AD, Hamilton JA: Functions of granulocyte-macrophage colony-stimulating factor. Crit Rev Immunol 25:405, 2005

27. Dale DC, Liles WC, Llewellyn C, et al: Effects of granulocyte-macrophage colony-stimulating factor (GM-CSF) on neutrophil kinetics and function in normal human volunteers. Am J Hematol 57:7, 1998

28. Dale DC, Liles WC: Neutrophils and monocytes: normal physiology and disorders of neutrophil and monocyte production. Blood: Principles and Practice of Hematology. Handin RI, Lux SE, Stossel TP, Eds. Lippincott Williams & Wilkins, Philadelphia, 2003

29. Eichner ER: Fatigue of anemia. Nutr Rev 59:S17, 2001

30. Ingram CF, Lewis SM: Clinical use of WHO haemoglobin colour scale: validation and critique. J Clin Pathol 53:933, 2000

31. Chowdhury ME, Chongsuvivatwong V, Geater AF, et al: Taking a medical history and using a colour scale during clinical examination of pallor improves detection of anaemia. Trop Med Int Health, 7:133, 2002

32. Dale DC: Lymphadenopathy. Outpatient Medicine. Fihn SD, DeWitt DE, Eds. Saunders, Philadelphia, 1998

Acknowledgment

Figures 1 through 4 Seward Hung.

91 Red Blood Cell Function and Disorders of Iron Metabolism

Gary M. Brittenham, M.D.

Red Blood Cell Function

The red blood cell, or erythrocyte, carries oxygen from the lungs to peripheral tissues for utilization and brings carbon dioxide from tissues to the lungs for excretion.[1] The mature erythrocyte dedicates more than 95% of its intracellular protein, as hemoglobin, to these tasks. Hemoglobin, the oxygen transport molecule, binds oxygen molecules at the high oxygen tensions of the pulmonary alveoli and releases oxygen molecules at low oxygen tensions to peripheral tissues.[2,3] Hemoglobin also acts as a carrier of nitric oxide (NO), a third respiratory gas that seems to regulate oxygen delivery.[4] The exact role of NO in the cardiorespiratory cycle is debated,[5] but NO is a potent vasorelaxant that reportedly is released during arteriovenous transit, increasing blood flow and therefore oxygen transport in hypoxic tissue.[4]

The cell membrane of the erythrocyte is a flexible structure composed of a lipid bilayer with integral proteins. These proteins anchor the membrane to an underlying protein skeleton that maintains the biconcave discoid form of the cell.[6] This shape optimizes passage of the cell through the circulatory system and permits apposition of erythrocytes and parenchymal cells across the thin endothelium of capillaries, facilitating exchange of oxygen and carbon dioxide.

In the erythrocyte, a variety of metabolic pathways maintain the iron of hemoglobin in the ferrous state, protect against oxidant damage, generate 2,3-diphosphoglycerate (2,3-DPG) to help regulate oxygen affinity, and maintain osmotic stability through a series of membrane pumps.[7] Without erythrocytes, blood plasma can carry only about 5 ml O_2/L; with erythrocytes containing normal hemoglobin, whole blood can transport about 200 ml O_2/L or more.[1]

STRUCTURE OF HEMOGLOBIN

Hemoglobin is a spherical molecule composed of two pairs of dissimilar globin chains, with a heme group, ferroprotoporphyrin IX, bound covalently at a specific site in each chain.[3] The major adult hemoglobin, hemoglobin A, is formed from a pair of α chains (each containing 141 amino acids) and a pair of β chains (each containing 146 amino acids) and is written as $\alpha_2\beta_2$ [*see Figure 1*].

The configuration of hemoglobin shifts with oxygenation and deoxygenation.[2,8] The deoxy configuration of hemoglobin is stabilized through the binding of protons and 2,3-DPG, a highly charged anion. With oxygenation of one subunit, these bonds are sequentially broken, and the resulting change in tertiary structure increases oxygen affinity of the remaining unliganded subunits.[2] This phenomenon is termed cooperativity or heme-heme interaction. As oxygen is released in the tissues, a reversal of this process decreases oxygen affinity, facilitating the release of oxygen. Conformational changes also contribute to the decrease in oxygen affinity with decreasing pH.[2] This effect, called the Bohr effect, is physiologically beneficial both in the lungs, where elimination of carbon dioxide raises the pH, enhancing

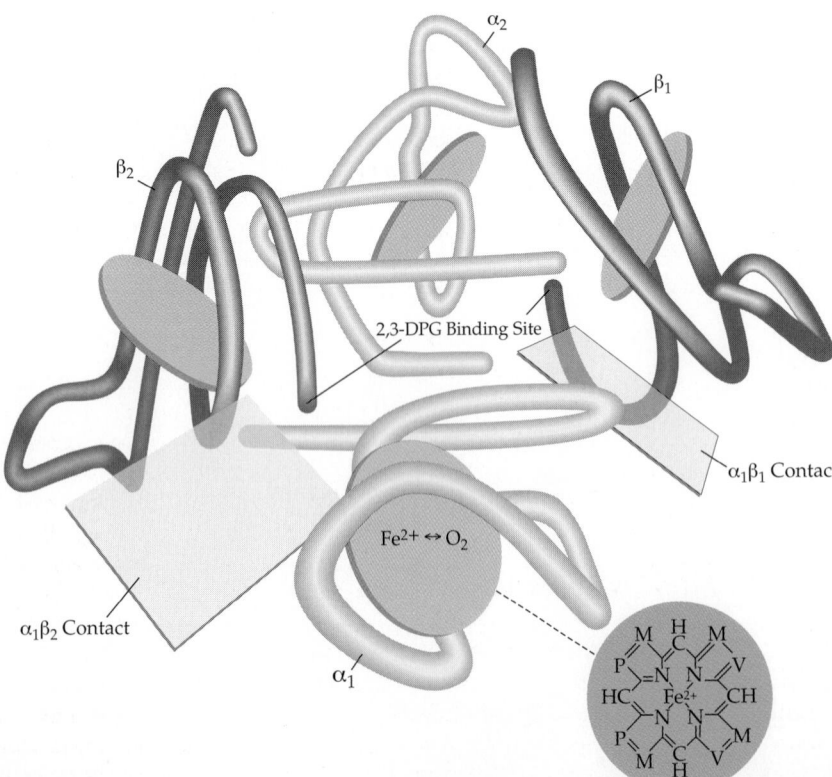

Figure 1 A model of the hemoglobin molecule shows the relative alignment of the α chains (light gray) and β chains (dark gray). 2,3-Diphosphoglycerate (2,3-DPG), a glycolytic intermediate, binds in the central cavity of the hemoglobin and stabilizes the deoxygenated form by cross-linking the β chains, thus reducing the oxygen affinity of hemoglobin. Note that the α and β chains are in contact at two points. On oxygenation, movement of the iron atom into the plane of the heme group (colored disks) apparently triggers other structural changes in the α and β subunits as the molecule assumes the oxygenated conformation. Sliding occurs at the $\alpha_1\beta_2$ interface, and the spacing between the two β chains is reduced in oxyhemoglobin. In the detail showing the structure of heme, M is methyl, V is vinyl, and P is propionic acid.

oxygen affinity and uptake, and in tissues, where carbon dioxide uptake decreases the pH, lowering oxygen affinity and facilitating oxygen release.

FACTORS AFFECTING THE OXYGEN-CARRYING CAPACITY OF HEMOGLOBIN

Oxygen-Hemoglobin Dissociation Curve

The oxygen-hemoglobin dissociation curve [see Figure 2] is a plot of the equilibrium between oxygen and hemoglobin at various oxygen tensions (PO_2).[3] At sea level and at a partial pressure of oxygen of about 90 mm Hg, hemoglobin is 97% saturated in the lungs. After unloading oxygen to tissues, at a PO_2 of about 40 mm Hg in mixed venous blood, the hemoglobin saturation is about 75%. The P_{50} (i.e., the partial pressure of oxygen at which hemoglobin is 50% saturated) is a useful measure of the oxygen affinity of hemoglobin: the higher the affinity, the lower the P_{50}. Under normal physiologic conditions (i.e., a temperature of 37° C [98.6° F]; pH of 7.4; 2,3-DPG level of 5 mmol/L; and carbon dioxide tension [PCO_2] of 40 mm Hg), the P_{50} of normal adult blood is 26 ± 1 mm Hg. The P_{50} is decreased (shifted to the left on the oxygen-hemoglobin dissociation curve) by increasing pH, decreasing 2,3-DPG, or decreasing temperature.

Effects of 2,3-Diphosphoglycerate

The glycolytic intermediate 2,3-DPG, which is present in mature erythrocytes at approximately the same intracellular concentration as hemoglobin, is the most important allosteric regulator of oxygen affinity.[3] With acute hypoxia, 2,3-DPG concentrations increase within hours, which shifts the oxygen-hemoglobin dissociation curve to the right. The increase in the 2,3-DPG concentration promotes delivery of oxygen to tissues but also impedes the acquisition of oxygen in the lungs. Short-term adaptation to hypoxic stress may be helped if the supply of oxygen is plentiful and the cardiopulmonary reserve is robust. At high altitude, with the cardiovascular system unable to effectively meet increased circulatory demands, or in other pathologic circumstances, increased amounts of 2,3-DPG may be counterproductive.[3]

OXYGEN TRANSPORT

Several other physiologic factors function in an integrated manner to provide an adequate supply of oxygen, including blood volume, blood viscosity, pulmonary and cardiac function, and regional blood flow.[9] The concentration of circulating red blood cells depends on the production of erythropoietin by the kidney and the erythropoietic response of the erythroid marrow.[10] Hemoglobin transport of NO, which binds to both heme iron and globin, may help match regional blood flow and oxygen requirements. In peripheral tissues, the erythrocyte may release NO, which would relax the microvasculature, improve blood flow, and enhance oxygen delivery.[4,5] An intriguing development has been the identification of a new class of so-called hexacoordinate hemoglobins (expressed in nerve cells[11] or a wide array of tissues[12]), whose functions are not yet established but which may facilitate oxygen transport, help protect against hypoxia, or scavenge reactive oxygen species.

CARBON DIOXIDE TRANSPORT

After delivering oxygen, hemoglobin binds with carbon dioxide.[13] Deoxyhemoglobin has a higher binding affinity for carbon dioxide than does oxyhemoglobin, facilitating unloading of carbon dioxide from tissues and pulmonary excretion.[13] Most of the

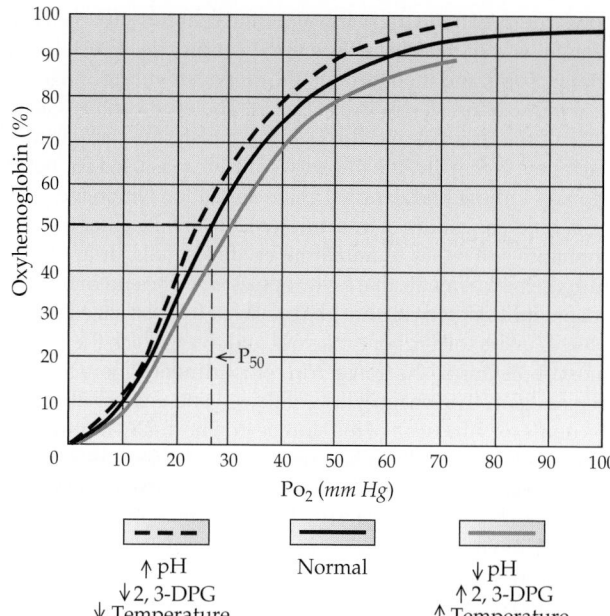

Figure 2 **The normal oxygen-hemoglobin dissociation curve (solid black line) is shifted by changes in temperature, pH, and the intracellular concentration of 2,3-DPG. P_{50} stands for 50% oxygen saturation; PO_2 stands for oxygen tension.**

carbon dioxide from tissue capillaries is transported to the lungs as bicarbonate, with about 10% carried as a carbamino complex reversibly bound to the globin chains.

Iron Metabolism

Remarkable progress continues to be made in understanding disorders of iron metabolism and in improving the diagnosis and management of both iron deficiency and iron overload.[14,15] In the body, iron transports and stores oxygen, carries electrons, catalyzes reactions in oxidative metabolism, and sustains cellular growth and proliferation. With iron deficiency, the body is unable to produce sufficient amounts of heme, other iron-porphyrin complexes, metalloenzymes, and other iron-containing compounds to sustain normal functions. With iron overload, excess iron can catalyze free radical reactions that can damage cellular membranes, proteins, and nucleic acids, resulting in progressive cellular and organ damage and eventual death.

PATTERNS OF IRON BALANCE AND METABOLISM

The concentration of iron in the human body is carefully regulated and is normally maintained at about 40 mg Fe/kg in women and about 50 mg Fe/kg in men. Iron balance is the result of the difference between the amount of iron taken up by the body and the amount lost [see Figure 3]. Because humans are unable to excrete excess iron, iron balance is physiologically regulated by the control of iron absorption. The two major factors that influence iron absorption are the level of body iron stores and the extent of erythropoiesis.[16] If iron stores increase, absorption decreases; if stores decrease, absorption increases. Absorption also increases with increased erythropoietic activity, especially with ineffective erythropoiesis. Most of the iron in the body is located in the erythron, which consists of the totality of circulating erythrocytes and their precursors in the bone marrow. The predominant pathway of internal iron flux is a one-way flow from the plasma iron transport protein, transferrin, to the erythron, and then through the monocyte-macrophage system back to transferrin [see Figure 3]. The erythron uses about 80% of the iron passing through the transferrin compartment each day. Normally, the majority of this iron is used for hemoglobin synthesis and returned to the circulation within red blood cells. Small quantities of iron are stored in ferritin, enter the iron-containing enzymes of immature erythroid cells, or are lost in the products of ineffective erythropoiesis. At the end of their life span, senescent red cells are phagocytized by specialized macrophages in the spleen, bone marrow, and liver, which then return most of the iron to the transferrin compartment, where the cycle begins again. The phagocytosis of flawed and aged erythrocytes accounts for almost all of the storage iron normally found in the macrophages of the liver, bone marrow, and spleen. By contrast, the parenchymal cells of the liver may either take iron from, or give iron to, plasma transferrin. Under normal physiologic conditions, iron recycling is very efficient; less than 0.05% of the total body iron is acquired or lost each day.

MOLECULAR BASIS OF IRON METABOLISM

A number of proteins are now known to be involved in the absorption, transport, utilization, and storage of iron. Some of these proteins have more than one function.

Systemic Iron Transport

Transferrin is the physiologic carrier of iron through the plasma and extracellular fluid.[15] Apotransferrin, transferrin without attached iron, is a single-chain glycoprotein with two structurally similar lobes. Binding of a ferric ion to one of these lobes yields monoferric transferrin; binding of ions to both yields diferric transferrin. The transferrin saturation is the proportion of the available iron-binding sites on transferrin that are occupied by iron atoms, expressed as a percentage. In humans, almost all the circulating plasma apotransferrin is synthesized by the hepatocyte.[17] After delivering iron to cells, apotransferrin is promptly returned to the plasma to again function as an iron transporter, completing 100 to 200 cycles of iron delivery during its lifetime in the circulation.[15]

Cellular Iron Uptake

Specific receptors for transferrin, which are found on the surface membrane of all nucleated cells, provide the route of entry for transferrin-bound iron. The affinity of transferrin receptors is greatest for diferric transferrin, intermediate for monoferric transferrin, and almost negligible for apotransferrin. These differences in affinity contribute to the efficiency of iron delivery. Two forms of the transferrin receptor have now been identified and are designated as transferrin receptor 1 and transferrin receptor 2.[15] Both consist of paired subunits, each of which can

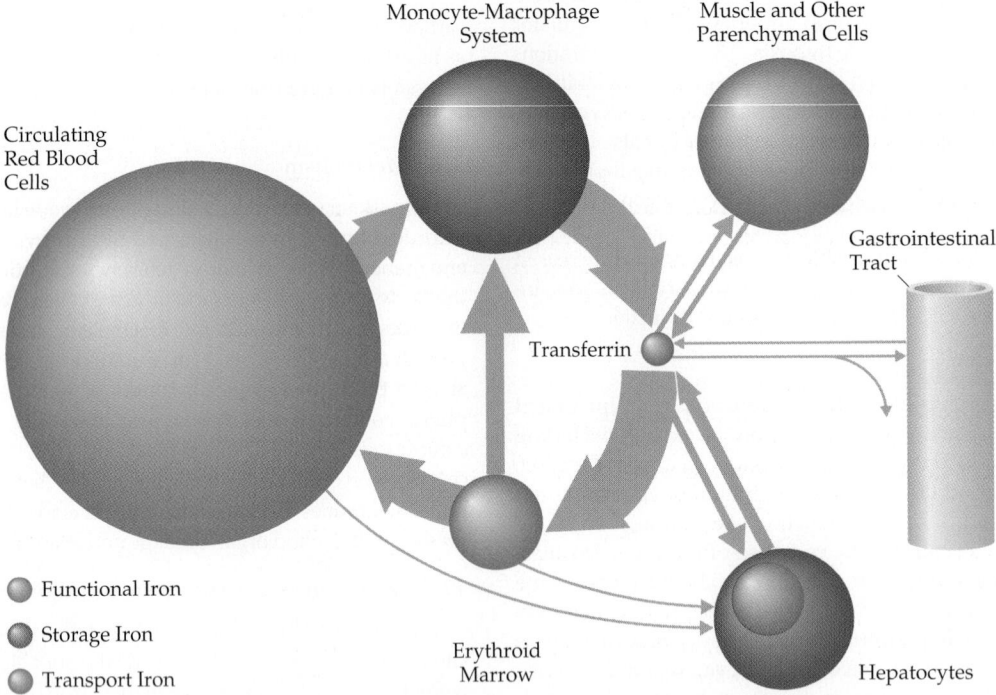

Figure 3 **Body iron supply and storage. The figure shows a schematic representation of the routes of iron movement in the adult.[95] The area of each circle is proportional to the amount of iron contained in the compartment, and the width of each arrow is proportional to the daily flow of iron from one compartment to another. The major portion of iron is found in the erythron as hemoglobin iron (28 mg/kg in women; 32 mg/kg in men) dedicated to oxygen transport and delivery. Small amounts of erythron iron (< 1 mg/kg) are also present in heme and nonheme enzymes in developing red cells. The remainder of functional iron is found as myoglobin iron (4 mg/kg in women; 5 mg/kg in men) in muscle and as iron-containing and iron-dependent enzymes (1 to 2 mg/kg) throughout the cells of the body. Small amounts of iron are deposited within ferritin in erythroid cells, but most storage iron (5 to 6 mg/kg in women; 10 to 12 mg/kg in men) is held in reserve by hepatocytes and macrophages in the liver, bone marrow, spleen, and muscle. The small fraction of transport iron (about 0.2 mg/kg) in the plasma and extracellular fluid is bound to the protein transferrin, which carries iron to meet tissue needs throughout the body.**

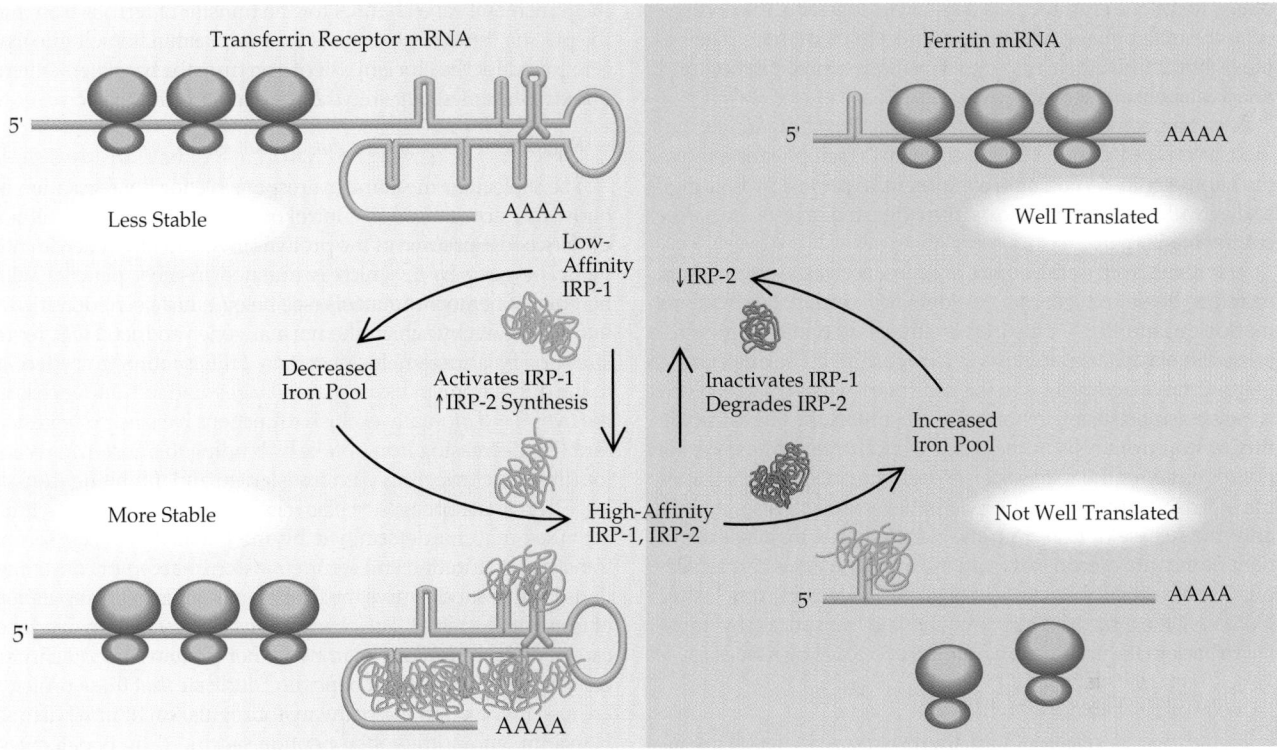

Figure 4 Regulation of transferrin receptor and ferritin expression by the iron regulatory proteins IRP-1 and IRP-2.

bind a molecule of transferrin. Although their extracellular structures are quite similar,[18] the two forms of the receptor have important functional differences. The binding affinity of transferrin receptor 1 for diferric transferrin is about 25-fold to 30-fold greater than that of transferrin receptor 2. Expression of transferrin receptor 1 is regulated by intracellular iron levels (see below), but that of transferrin receptor 2 is not. Transferrin receptor 1 is expressed by all iron-requiring cells, whereas transferrin receptor 2 is most highly expressed on hepatocytes and developing erythroid cells. Transferrin receptor 1 is required for life in mammals[19]; transferrin receptor 2 cannot compensate for the absence of transferrin receptor 1. Transferrin receptor 2 seems to have other functions in maintaining iron homeostasis (see below).

The delivery of transferrin-bound iron begins with the binding of two molecules of monoferric or diferric transferrin to a transferrin receptor on the cell surface.[15] The iron-transferrin–transferrin receptor complex then moves to the interior of the cell within an endosome, where it releases its iron. The dissociated iron is then taken up by the divalent metal transporter–1 (DMT1) and transported across the endosomal membrane for utilization or for storage in the cell.[19] Freed of its iron, the transferrin—now apotransferrin—binds avidly to the transferrin receptor and is carried back to the cell membrane and released into the plasma. [15]

Cellular Iron Storage

Cellular iron storage utilizes ferritin, a protein found in the cytoplasm of virtually all cells. Ferritin is a spherical shell that can store as many as 4,500 atoms of iron in its interior. Ferritin functions both as a safe storage site for iron and as a readily accessible reserve for iron that has been acquired by the cell in excess of its immediate needs.[20] Accordingly, the greatest amounts of ferritin are found in cells dedicated to iron storage (e.g., macrophages and hepatocytes) and in cells with the highest iron requirements

for the synthesis of iron-containing compounds (e.g., developing erythroid cells). Apoferritin, or ferritin without attached iron, is composed of 24 oblong subunits that are designated as H (heavy) and L (light). Ferritin molecules with a greater proportion of H subunits seem to be more active in iron metabolism; ferritin molecules with a greater abundance of L subunits apparently are used for the longer-term storage of iron. A ferritin H–like protein assembled into ferritin shells has been identified within iron-loaded mitochondria of patients with impairment of heme synthesis.[21] In patients with sideroblastic anemia, most of the iron in ringed sideroblasts is sequestered in mitochondrial ferritin.[22]

Regulation of Cellular Iron Uptake and Storage

Cellular iron uptake and storage are regulated through the synthesis of transferrin receptors and ferritin. This synthesis is coordinated by the iron-regulatory proteins IRP-1 and IRP-2 [*see Figure 4*]. When intracellular iron levels are low, IRP-1 and IRP-2 bind to messenger RNA (mRNA) stem-loop elements known as iron-responsive elements (IREs) in transcripts.[23] Transferrin receptor synthesis is regulated by controlling the stability of cytoplasmic transferrin receptor mRNA, whereas ferritin synthesis is regulated by controlling translation of ferritin mRNA without changing the amount of ferritin mRNA in the cytoplasm. As a result, changes in the amounts of the IRPs have opposite effects on the production of transferrin receptor and ferritin, allowing iron to self-regulate its intracellular availability. IRPs also regulate mRNAs for other proteins involved in iron uptake,[24] availability, release,[25] and utilization.[26]

Macrophage Hemoglobin Catabolism and Iron Release

Specialized macrophages in the bone marrow, liver, and spleen selectively recognize and phagocytize erythrocytes that are senescent or damaged.[27] On average, each of these macrophages can phagocytize one erythrocyte a day.[28] After ingesting the erythrocyte, the macrophage lyses the erythrocyte membrane. The hemoglobin within then undergoes oxidative precipitation and rapid catabolism into heme.

Any hemoglobin released into plasma by intravascular hemolysis is rapidly bound by haptoglobin. Macrophages remove the haptoglobin-hemoglobin complex from plasma by binding[29] and endocytosis; the complex is then digested in lysosomes, liberating heme.

The heme from both sources is degraded by the microsomal enzyme heme oxygenase, yielding biliverdin IXa, carbon monoxide, and iron[30,31]; the iron is either stored in ferritin or returned to plasma, apparently via ferroportin.[27,32] The outpouring of iron from macrophages in the bone marrow, liver, and spleen to plasma apotransferrin normally constitutes the largest single flux of iron from cells in the body.[30] Unsaturated transferrin is not required for the release of iron from the macrophages; apotransferrin does not enter the macrophage and accepts iron only after the release of iron from the cell. Rather, a major determinant of the rate of iron exit from the macrophage is ceruloplasmin, which establishes a rate of oxidation of ferrous iron.[33] After oxidation, the ferric iron can be bound and transported by transferrin back to the erythron and other iron-requiring tissues.

Other Pathways of Iron Exchange

Heme that is released into the plasma as a result of intramedullary or intravascular hemolysis is bound by hemopexin. The heme-hemopexin complex is delivered to the hepatocyte via specific receptors and internalized, and the heme is catabolized to liberate the iron.[34] The hepatocyte may either donate iron to plasma transferrin or receive iron from it.[35] At high transferrin saturations, iron moves from the plasma to the liver; at low saturations, iron is mobilized from hepatocyte stores and supplied to plasma transferrin. Normally, the overall magnitude of iron exchange by hepatocytes is only about one fifth that by macrophages. Other pathways of iron movement involve approximately equal exchanges: about 1 mg Fe/day is absorbed and lost, about 3 mg Fe/day is transferred between the plasma and extravascular transferrin compartments, and about 2 mg Fe/day moves between extravascular transferrin and parenchymal tissues.

Intestinal Iron Absorption

The amount of iron in the body is regulated by control of iron absorption in the proximal small intestine. Both heme iron and nonheme iron enter through the brush border of intestinal enterocytes.[36] The exact means by which heme iron is absorbed are still uncertain, but nonheme iron seems to be taken up via the apical iron transporter DMT1 (the same iron transporter that provides an exit for iron from the endosome; see above) and perhaps via other routes.[37] DMT1 is a proton-coupled symporter with a broad substrate range that includes other metallic cations, but its physiologic function appears to be the uptake of Fe^{2+}.[19] DMT1 is a ferrous iron transporter, but most dietary iron is in the ferric form. Duodenal cytochrome b, a heme protein highly expressed in duodenal brush border membrane, reduces luminal iron to the ferrous state for transport into enterocytes via DMT1.[38] Once within the enterocyte, the absorbed iron may be transported across the basolateral membrane into the plasma or stored within ferritin and then lost when the enterocyte is exfoliated. The details of the handling of iron in the enterocyte remain obscure, but as in the macrophage, ferroportin seems to serve as the transmembrane channel for the transfer of ferrous iron into the plasma,[32] and hephaestin is a ceruloplasmin homologue that is required for the efficient exit of iron from the basolateral membrane of the enterocyte into the systemic circulation.[39]

Regulation of Body Iron Absorption and Storage

The molecular mechanisms responsible for the regulation of body iron stores through control of iron absorption are still not understood, but some of the proteins involved have been identified. The gene *HFE*, which is mutated in most patients with hereditary hemochromatosis (see below), has been identified,[40] but the means by which the normal gene product, HFE, regulates iron balance remains uncertain. HFE is found in crypt cells in the duodenum, in tissue macrophages, and in Kupffer cells in the liver. Two mutually exclusive functions have been suggested for HFE: decreasing iron uptake by binding to transferrin receptor (thereby competing with transferrin) and inhibiting iron release from macrophages.[41,42] The relative effects of these offsetting activities may be determined by the balance between serum transferrin saturation and serum transferrin–receptor concentrations.[43] Other models give the liver a central role in the regulation of iron homeostasis.[44] The observations that tissue iron overload can result from mutations in two other proteins, transferrin receptor 2[45] (see above) and hepcidin,[46] indicate that these proteins are also involved in the pathway for regulation of iron balance. Hepcidin, an antimicrobial peptide produced by hepatocytes, seems to act as an iron-regulatory hormone whose expression is inversely related to both iron absorption and macrophage iron release. In HFE-associated hereditary hemochromatosis, expression of hepcidin is not increased despite hepatic iron overload, suggesting that HFE may be involved in the regulation of hepcidin expression in response to changes in body iron stores.[47] Despite these intriguing observations, elucidation of the molecular mechanisms underlying the regulation of body iron absorption and storage will likely await the identification of other key proteins involved.

Iron Deficiency

DEFINITIONS

Iron deficiency designates conditions in which the body's iron requirements exceed iron supply. Iron is needed to restore physiologic loss, which is just under 1 mg/day in men and is about 1.5 mg/day in menstruating women[35]; iron is also needed for growth and pregnancy and to replace pathologic losses. Sequential stages of decreases in body iron can be identified [*see Table 1*]. A decrease in iron stores without a change in the amounts of functional iron compounds is designated as reduced iron stores. When iron stores are exhausted, patients may be described as having iron depletion. Further decrements in the level of body iron result in limited production of hemoglobin and other iron-containing functional compounds; this stage is termed iron-deficient erythropoiesis. Still further decreases in body iron produce iron deficiency anemia.

EPIDEMIOLOGY

Iron deficiency is the most common nutritional deficiency worldwide. Its prevalences are highest in developing countries, where 30% to 70% of the population may be affected[48]; in comparison, the overall prevalence of iron deficiency is less than 20% in the industrialized countries of Europe and North America.[48] In

Table 1   Changes in Iron Stores and Distribution with Increased or Decreased Body Iron Content

Condition	Marrow Iron (0–6+)	Liver Iron (μmol/g, dry weight)	Plasma Ferritin (μg/L)	Plasma Transferrin Receptor (mg/L)	Plasma Iron (μg/dl)	Transferrin Saturation (%)	Protoporphyrin (μg/dl Red Blood Cells)	Red Blood Cells
Iron deficiency anemia	0	< 3.0	< 12	10	< 40	< 10	150	Microcytic, hypochromic
Iron stores depletion	0 to trace amounts	3.0	< 20	5.5	< 115	< 30	30	Normal
Reduced iron stores	1+	< 10.0	< 25	5.5	< 115	30	30	Normal
Normal	2–3+	15.0 ± 5.0	100 ± 60	5.5 ± 1.5	115 ± 50	35 ± 15	30	Normal
Increased iron stores, hereditary hemochromatosis	2–3+	100	1,000	5.5	> 150	> 60	30	Normal
Increased iron stores; transfusional iron overload	4+	200	1,000	5.5	> 150	> 50	30	Normal
Massive iron overload, hereditary hemochromatosis	3–4+	400	4,000	5.5	200	> 60	30	Normal
Massive iron overload; transfusional iron overload	6+	800	4,000	5.5	200	> 90	30	Normal

the United States, the Centers for Disease Control and Prevention estimate that the prevalence of iron deficiency is greatest in toddlers 1 to 2 years of age (7%) and in adolescent girls and adult women 12 to 49 years of age (9% to 16%).[49]

ETIOLOGY

Iron deficiency can result from increased iron requirements, inadequate iron supply, or both [*see Table 2*]. Blood loss is the most common cause of increased iron requirements that lead to iron deficiency. In men and postmenopausal women, iron deficiency is almost always the result of gastrointestinal blood loss.[50] In menstruating women, genitourinary blood loss often accounts for increased iron requirements. Oral contraceptives tend to decrease menstrual blood loss, whereas intrauterine devices tend to increase menstrual bleeding. Other causes of genitourinary bleeding and respiratory tract bleeding can also increase iron requirements [*see Table 2*]. For blood donors, each donation results in the loss of 200 to 250 mg of iron. During periods of growth in infancy, childhood, and adolescence, iron requirements may outstrip the supply of iron available from diet and stores.[51] Iron loss from tissue growth during pregnancy and from bleeding during delivery and post partum averages 740 mg.[35,51] Breast-feeding increases iron requirements by about 0.5 to 1 mg / day.

An insufficient supply of iron may contribute to the development of iron deficiency. In infants and in women with high iron requirements, diets containing inadequate amounts of bioavailable iron increase the risk of iron deficiency.[51] In older children, men, and postmenopausal women, a poor supply of dietary iron is almost never the only factor responsible for iron deficiency; therefore, other etiologic factors must be sought, especially blood loss.[50,52,53] Impaired absorption of iron is an uncommon cause of iron deficiency. In some patients, intestinal malabsorption of iron is only one aspect of more generalized malabsorption[54] [*see Table 2*]. Gastric surgery, especially partial or total gastric resection or gastroenterostomy for bypass of the duodenum, may result in iron deficiency. Although absorption of dietary iron may be poor in such patients, therapeutic iron salts are usually well absorbed, and the iron deficiency can be readily corrected.

The risk of iron deficiency is especially high when iron requirements are increased and the supply of iron is inadequate. For example, infants who are fed cow's milk often become iron deficient because of the combination of increased iron losses from cow's milk–induced gastrointestinal bleeding and the small amounts of bioavailable iron in cow's milk.[51,55] Women with high iron requirements because of menstruation often have diets that contain little bioavailable iron and contain inhibitors of iron absorption, such as calcium. A common mutation of the transferrin gene (designated as G277S) has been associated with a reduction in the circulating transferrin concentration and may predispose menstruating women to iron deficiency.[56] The mechanism underlying this effect is unknown.

DIAGNOSIS

Clinical Manifestations

Patients with iron deficiency may be asymptomatic and their disorder recognized only because of abnormal results of laboratory tests.[51] Other patients may come to medical attention because of the manifestations of the underlying disorder that produced iron deficiency, but they may have no findings resulting from the iron deficiency. Still other patients may present with the signs and symptoms common to all anemias, such as weakness, dizziness, easy fatigability, pallor, irritability, and other indefinite and nonspecific complaints. Iron deficiency may also be associated with signs and symptoms that are unrelated to anemia, such as angular stomatitis, glossitis, postcricoid esophageal stricture or web, and gastric atrophy. In addition, a high prevalence of iron deficiency has been found in patients with the restless legs syndrome, a neurologic disorder characterized by a distressing, irresistible urge to move the legs (akathisia).[57] Finally, some patients present with one or more of the limited number of signs and symptoms thought to be highly specific for iron deficiency, which include blue sclerae[58] and koilonychia. Pagophagia, or pica with ice, is thought to be another highly specific symptom of iron deficiency and disappears shortly after iron therapy is begun.[59] Other types of pica may accompany iron deficiency, but

Table 2 Causes of Iron Deficiency

INCREASED IRON REQUIREMENTS

Blood loss

Gastrointestinal tract

Hemorrhagic lesions (e.g., hiatal hernia, esophageal varices, gastritis, duodenitis, peptic ulcer, cholelithiasis, intrahepatic bleeding, inflammatory bowel disease, diverticulosis, hemorrhoids, or adenomatous polyp)

Occult gastrointestinal malignancy

Chronic ingestion of drugs (e.g., alcohol, salicylates, steroids, and nonsteroidal anti-inflammatory drugs)

Helminthic infections (e.g., hookworm, *Schistosoma mansoni, S. japonicum*, or severe *Trichuris trichiura*)

Other (e.g., vascular purpura with scurvy, aberrant pancreas, Meckel diverticulum, hereditary hemorrhagic telangiectasia, other vascular ectasia of the bowel, or colonic polyposis)

Genitourinary tract

Menstrual blood loss

Other (e.g., uterine malignancies or fibroids, stones, infarction, infection with *S. haematobium*, inflammatory disease, malignancy of the urinary tract, or chronic hemoglobinuria or hemosiderinuria resulting from paroxysmal nocturnal hemoglobinuria or chronic intravascular hemolysis)

Respiratory tract

Chronic recurrent hemoptysis

Idiopathic pulmonary siderosis

Goodpasture syndrome

Blood donation

Growth

Infants, premature infants

Children

Adolescents

Pregnancy and lactation

INADEQUATE IRON SUPPLY

Diets with insufficient amounts of bioavailable iron

Impaired absorption of iron

Intestinal malabsorption (e.g., steatorrhea, sprue, celiac disease, diffuse enteritis, atrophic gastritis with achlorhydria, or pica)

Gastric surgery

---

tration may be increased independently of body iron by infection, inflammation, liver disease, malignancy, and other conditions.[63] Because the serum transferrin receptor concentration seems to be unaffected by these conditions, determination of this value (or the ratio of the serum transferrin receptor concentration to the serum ferritin concentration) provides a means of distinguishing between the anemia of iron deficiency and the anemia associated with chronic inflammatory disorders.[64-66] The concentration ratio of the serum transferrin receptor to serum ferritin can also provide a quantitative estimate of body iron stores that may be useful in monitoring iron status in patients who are highly susceptible to iron deficiency, such as infants, preschool children, and pregnant women.[67] The serum iron level and serum transferrin saturation are decreased in both iron deficiency and infectious or inflammatory states and therefore are of little practical assistance in distinguishing between these conditions. An alternative approach to the detection of an impaired iron supply for erythropoiesis is the use of hematologic indices derived from automated analyzers, such as the proportion of hypochromic cells and reticulocyte cellular indices.[68,69] These measurements of erythrocyte and reticulocyte indices may be particularly useful in the evaluation of iron-restricted erythropoiesis in patients with chronic renal failure or chronic disease who are treated with erythropoietin.[70] An empirical trial of iron therapy may also be an effective means of establishing the diagnosis of iron deficiency.

Although bone marrow examination is now seldom performed solely for the assessment of iron status, the diagnosis of iron deficiency can almost always be verified by direct assessment of marrow iron stores. If no iron stores are present, the diagnosis of iron deficiency is established; if hemosiderin (an intracellular granule that stores iron-containing molecules) is found, iron deficiency is excluded. In addition, with iron deficiency, marrow sideroblasts will be absent or present in low numbers (less than 10% of the number of normoblasts).

TREATMENT

Therapy for iron deficiency anemia should both correct the hemoglobin deficit and replace storage iron [*see Sidebar*, Iron Replacement Therapy]. Oral and parenteral replacement therapies yield similar results,[50,51] but for almost all patients, oral iron is the treatment of choice.[50] Oral iron therapy is effective, safe, and inexpensive.[71] Because of the risk of local and systemic adverse reactions, parenteral iron should be used only in the small number of patients who cannot absorb or tolerate oral iron or whose iron requirements cannot be met by oral therapy because of chronic, uncontrollable bleeding or other blood loss. In severe iron deficiency anemia, red cell transfusions are needed in rare instances to prevent cardiac or cerebral ischemia. Red cell transfusions may also sometimes be necessary for patients whose chronic rate of iron loss exceeds the rate of replacement possible with parenteral therapy. Although the majority of patients take oral iron without difficulty, 10% to 20% experience side effects related to iron—most commonly, gastrointestinal complaints. Despite manufacturers' claims, there are no clinically significant differences between different iron salts.

Iron deficiency can almost always be treated effectively. Alleviation of symptoms often occurs within the first few days of treatment. With uncomplicated iron deficiency, the initial hematologic response—a mild reticulocytosis—usually begins within 3 to 5 days after the start of therapy, reaches a maxi-

none is as specific a symptom as pagophagia. The nonhematologic consequences of iron deficiency are diminished exercise tolerance and work performance and impaired immunity and resistance to infection.[60,61] In children, iron deficiency seems to adversely affect growth, motor development, behavior, and cognitive function[51,62]; these abnormalities may not be reversible with later treatment.

Laboratory Tests

Iron deficiency anemia is the only microcytic hypochromic anemia associated with lack of iron stores. In other microcytic hypochromic disorders, marrow iron stores are normal or increased. Indirect measures of body iron can be used to identify a characteristic sequence of changes that occur as body iron decreases from the iron-replete normal levels to levels found in iron deficiency anemia [*see Table 2*]. Measurement of the serum ferritin concentration is the most useful test for the detection of iron deficiency, because serum ferritin concentrations decrease as body iron stores decline.[50] A serum ferritin concentration below 12 µg/L is virtually diagnostic of absent iron stores. In contrast, a normal serum ferritin concentration does not confirm the presence of storage iron, because serum ferritin concen-

Iron Replacement Therapy

ORAL IRON THERAPY

Indication

Treatment of choice for iron deficiency anemia

Initial therapy to correct iron deficiency anemia

Ferrous iron salt (e.g., ferrous sulfate) given separately from meals in two or three divided doses; for example, ferrous sulfate tablets, 325 mg three times a day, or ferrous gluconate tablets, 300 mg two or three times a day

Continued therapy to replace iron stores

Ferrous iron salt given as a single daily dose of approximately 60 mg of elemental iron until the plasma ferritin concentration is > 50 µg/L (often requires 6 mo or more of treatment)

Management of side effects

Gastrointestinal side effects are the most common (10%–20% of patients) and usually can be managed symptomatically by (1) giving iron with or immediately after meals, (2) reducing the amount of iron in each dose, or (3) reducing the dose frequency to once daily

PARENTERAL IRON THERAPY

Indications

Chronic, uncontrollable blood loss producing iron needs that cannot be met by oral iron therapy

Malabsorption of iron

Intolerance of oral iron despite repeated modifications in dosage regimen

Risks

Immediate, life-threatening anaphylactic reactions

Delayed but severe serum sickness–like reactions with fever, urticaria, adenopathy, myalgias, and arthralgias

Exacerbation of rheumatoid arthritis and related conditions

Local reactions with intramuscular iron (skin staining, muscle necrosis, phlebitis, and persistent pain at injection site)

Precautions

Iron dextran is the only currently available parenteral preparation; a 0.5 ml test dose is to be given at least 1 hr before every intramuscular or intravenous injection of iron dextran, but the value of this precaution is limited because anaphylaxis is not dose dependent and can occur with the test dose

Administration and dosage

Parenteral iron may be administered either intramuscularly (limited to 2 ml or 100 mg of iron per injection) or intravenously (as an undiluted injection, as a total-dose infusion, or as an additive to total parenteral nutrition); because of the risks of therapy, recommendations of the manufacturers and recent-study recommendations for treatment should be reviewed carefully before parenteral iron is given

mum within 8 to 10 days, and declines thereafter. After the first week, the hemoglobin concentration begins to increase and is usually normal within 6 weeks. Microcytosis may not resolve completely for as long as 4 months. If the iron deficiency is treated with oral iron at a dosage of 200 mg/day or less, the serum ferritin concentration remains below 12 µg/L until the anemia is corrected and then gradually rises as storage iron is replenished. If the response to iron therapy is not complete and characteristic, review and reevaluation of the patient is mandatory.[50] One of the most common problems is mistaking the anemia of chronic disease for the anemia of iron deficiency. Recovery may be retarded by coexistent disorders, including other nutritional deficiencies; liver or kidney disease; infectious, inflammatory, or malignant disorders; or continued occult blood loss. In the event of incomplete recovery in a patient who is being treated with oral iron, the form and dosage of iron used should be reviewed, compliance evaluated, and the possibility of malabsorption considered.

Iron Overload

DEFINITIONS

Iron overload arises from a sustained excess of iron supply over iron requirements and causes characteristic patterns of changes in functional, transport, and storage iron. The amount of body iron is normally controlled by regulation of dietary iron absorption. Iron overload develops with conditions that modify or circumvent the regulation of intestinal iron absorption. Because humans have no physiologic means of eliminating excess iron, any persistent increase in intake may eventually result in iron overload. When the extent of iron accumulation exceeds the body's ability to safely sequester the surplus iron, characteristic patterns of tissue damage develop. The precise manifestations of iron overload depend on the underlying abnormality responsible but generally are governed by the magnitude of the body iron burden; the rate at which the increase in body iron has occurred; the distribution of the excess iron between storage sites in macrophages and potentially more harmful deposits in parenchymal cells; and the coexistence of conditions that may ameliorate (e.g., ascorbate deficiency) or worsen (e.g., alcohol use or hepatitis) the outcome. The most common consequences of iron overload are liver disease, pancreatic disease (associated with diabetes mellitus), cardiac dysfunction, endocrine disorders (associated with gonadal insufficiency), arthropathy, and, with some forms of iron overload, specific neurologic abnormalities.

Increased iron absorption may develop because of primary disorders leading to abnormal control of iron absorption, such as hereditary hemochromatosis, or as a secondary consequence of acquired or inherited conditions, such as chronic liver disease or the iron-loading anemias. Iron overload may also result from chronic red blood cell transfusion, which bypasses intestinal control of iron uptake [see Table 3].

PRIMARY IRON OVERLOAD

By far the most common forms of primary iron overload are those related to mutations in the HFE gene. Some of the genes responsible for less common forms of primary iron overload have now been identified, providing valuable insights into the control of iron metabolism. Testing for mutations in the HFE gene has become an essential step in the evaluation of primary iron overload, and continued progress is anticipated in genetic characterization of these disorders.

HFE-Associated Hereditary Hemochromatosis

Epidemiology Hereditary HFE-associated hemochromatosis (hemochromatosis type 1), an autosomal recessive disease, is the most common genetic disorder in persons of northern European descent.[72] Data from the Third National Health and Nutrition Examination Survey (NHANES III) suggest that in the United States, 9.54% of the non-Hispanic white population is heterozygous and 0.30% is homozygous for the most common mutation in HFE, C282Y (see below).[73]

Etiology and genetics The discovery of HFE, the gene on chromosome 6p21.3 that is mutated in most cases of hereditary hemochromatosis,[40] has revolutionized both the understanding and the diagnosis of this disorder. Although the underlying mechanism is still not understood, a defect in the HFE protein results in an inappropriate increase in iron absorption that leads to a progressive buildup of body iron. Initially, the overload has a predominantly parenchymal pattern of deposition, with iron first accumulating in hepatocytes; subsequently, the iron builds up in the pancreas, heart, and other organs.[74,75] Characteristically, macrophage iron levels in the bone marrow may be normal or even decreased despite severe parenchymal iron deposition [see Table 1].

Two missense mutations in the *HFE* gene, usually designated as C282Y and H63D, are responsible for up to 85% of the cases of hereditary hemochromatosis in the United States[73]; in other areas of the world, the percentage ranges from about 60% to almost 100%.[75] In the United States, 15% or more of patients with primary iron overload have neither of these mutations but are clinically indistinguishable from patients who do have one of these mutations.[40] Some of these patients are found to have other mutations in the *HFE* gene. Patients without evidence of mutations on chromosome 6p are classified as having non–HFE-associated hereditary hemochromatosis. The proportion of patients with non–HFE-associated hemochromatosis is higher in populations from southern Europe.[76]

Clinical manifestations   Homozygotes for hereditary hemochromatosis may have no distinctive clinical manifestations, especially at younger ages. In homozygotes who present with hereditary hemochromatosis in middle age or later, the classic tetrad of clinical signs is liver disease, diabetes mellitus, skin pig-

mentation, and gonadal failure.[74,75] Arthropathy may be an early manifestation of the disease and is frequently present in patients with advanced disease. Cardiac failure may develop and may even be the presenting symptom in untreated homozygotes. Body iron stores have usually increased from the normal amount of 1 g or less to 15 to 20 g or more by the time symptoms of parenchymal damage occur, usually in middle or late life. Additional increases in body iron may be fatal, although some patients are able to tolerate a total iron accumulation of as much as 40 to 50 g or more.[77] Men are affected at younger ages than women, presumably because of iron losses during menstruation and childbearing. Environmental factors (e.g., dietary iron content, blood donation or loss, and alcohol use) and coexisting disorders (e.g., viral hepatitis) may greatly influence the rate and severity of organ damage.[74] The penetrance of HFE-associated hereditary hemochromatosis is a subject of controversy. In a study of 41,038 patients attending a health-appraisal clinic in the United States, the results were interpreted as showing that less than 1% of homozygotes develop frank clinical hemochromatosis,[78,79] although this interpretation has been questioned.[80] The Hemochromatosis and Iron Overload Screening (HEIRS) study of more than 100,000 adults should help clarify both the penetrance and the prevalence of HFE-associated hemochromatosis and other forms of iron overload in the United States.[81]

Table 3   Causes of Iron Overload

Primary	Hereditary hemochromatosis
	  HFE associated (type 1)
	  Non–HFE associated
	    Transferrin receptor 2 associated (type 3)
	  Juvenile hemochromatosis (type 2)
	    Chromosome 1q21 associated (type 2A)
	    Hepcidin associated (type 2B)
	  Autosomal dominant hemochromatosis
	    Ferroportin 1 associated (type 4)
	    Ferritin H–subunit mRNA A49U mutation
	      associated
	  Atransferrinemia
	  Aceruloplasminemia

Secondary	Iron-loading anemias (refractory anemias with
	  hypercellular erythroid marrow)
	Chronic liver disease
	Porphyria cutanea tarda
	Insulin resistance–associated hepatic iron overload
	African dietary iron overload*
	Medicinal iron ingestion*
	Parenteral iron overload
	  Transfusional iron overload
	  Inadvertent iron overload from therapeutic
	    injections

Perinatal	Neonatal hemochromatosis Hereditary tyrosinemia (hypermethionemia) Cerebrohepatorenal syndrome GRACILE (Fellman) syndrome

Focal
sequestration
of iron
	Idiopathic pulmonary hemosiderosis
	Renal hemosiderosis
	Associated with neurologic abnormalities
	  Pantothenate kinase–associated neurodegenera-
	    tion (formerly Hallervorden-Spatz syndrome)
	  Neuroferritinopathy
	  Friedreich ataxia

*May have a genetic component.
GRACILE—growth retardation, aminoaciduria, cholestasis, iron overload, lactacidosis, and early death

Screening and diagnostic tests   Screening for hereditary hemochromatosis can use both phenotypic and genotypic methods and is indicated for patients with chronic liver disease or symptoms and signs associated with iron overload.[75,82] Phenotypic screening can provide biochemical evidence of iron overload, but no single test or combination of tests will identify all patients who are genetically susceptible to iron loading.[78] Genotypic screening for the most common *HFE* mutations, C282Y and H63D, in populations of northern European ancestry can identify a majority of those patients at risk for the development of primary iron overload. In pedigree studies, genotyping should replace HLA typing in the assessment of siblings of a C282Y homozygote.[75] In addition, genotyping the spouse of a C282Y homozygote is a cost-efficient strategy that leads to a more selective investigation of children for the hemochromatosis gene. Nonetheless, such limited genetic screening will not detect other mutations associated with iron loading; is less useful in other population groups, such as those originating from southern Europe,[76] Africa,[83] or Asia; and provides no indication of the extent of iron excess. Population screening has been advocated[82,84] but has not been undertaken generally because of uncertainties about disease penetrance[78]; the disease burden and natural history of iron overload; and a variety of ethical, legal, and social concerns.[75,78]

Measurement of the serum transferrin saturation is usually recommended as the initial phenotypic screening determination.[75,82,84,85] Although individual laboratories may have their own reference ranges, a persistent value of 45% or higher is often recommended as a threshold value for further investigation. The serum ferritin concentration is then used as a biochemical indicator of iron overload, and in the absence of complicating factors, increased concentrations suggest increased iron stores.[74] Genetic testing should then be considered in patients with abnormal elevations in transferrin saturation, serum ferritin, or both. The exact role of genetic testing in screening and diagnosis depends in part on the population being examined because of variations in the proportion of patients with hereditary hemochromatosis who have *HFE* mutations.

Once genetic testing has identified a patient as homozygous for the C282Y mutation (i.e., C282Y/C282Y), an elevated transferrin saturation establishes the diagnosis of hereditary hemochromatosis.[85] Liver biopsy, formerly a standard part of the diagnostic process, is no longer needed in most cases. Liver biopsy is indicated to detect cirrhosis if the serum ferritin level is above 1,000 µg/L[86]; biopsy may also be considered in patients with hepatomegaly, patients with abnormal findings on liver function tests, and patients who are older than 40 years.[74,85,87]

Patients who are heterozygous for the C282Y mutation and wild type (i.e., C282Y/wild type) have serum transferrin saturations and serum ferritin concentrations that are similar to those of wild-type homozygotes (i.e., wild type/wild type),[88,89] and these patients do not develop clinically important iron overload.[88] Consequently, finding a persistently elevated level of transferrin saturation, serum ferritin concentration, or both in a C282Y/wild type heterozygote should lead the clinician to search for other causes of iron overload.[85]

In patients who are heterozygous for the C282Y mutation and H63D, the other major *HFE* mutation (i.e., C282Y/H63D), mild to moderate iron overload may develop, but the penetrance of this genotype is even less than that of C282Y/C282Y homozygotes.[74,75,85,87] Heterozygotes for H63D (i.e., H63D/wild type) may have elevated transferrin saturation levels[90] but do not develop iron overload. Homozygotes for H63D (i.e., H63D/H63D) also may have elevated transferrin saturation levels, but the risk of clinically important iron overload is slight.[90] Less common mutations of the *HFE* gene have been identified[91]; S65C heterozygotes with either C282Y (i.e., S65C/C282Y) or H63D (i.e., S65C/H63D) may develop mild iron overload.

Several diagnostic approaches can be pursued in patients with phenotypic evidence of iron overload who are neither homozygous for C282Y (C282Y/C282Y) nor heterozygous for C282Y and H63D (C282Y/H63D). These approaches include further genetic testing for less common *HFE* mutations and for non-*HFE* mutations associated with iron loading; noninvasive assessment of the liver iron concentration[92]; and liver biopsy, which permits a definitive diagnosis of hereditary hemochromatosis regardless of genotype.[74,85,87] Evaluation of the biopsy specimen should include quantitative determination of the non-heme iron concentration, histochemical evaluation of the pattern of iron deposition, and pathologic assessment of tissue injury. Calculation of the hepatic iron index—the hepatic iron concentration (expressed as µmol Fe/g of liver, dry weight) divided by the age of the patient in years—may be helpful in distinguishing homozygotes for hereditary hemochromatosis from heterozygotes or from patients with increased body iron associated with chronic (usually alcoholic) liver disease.[74,87] In the absence of other causes of iron overload, a hepatic iron index greater than 1.9 is evidence for hereditary hemochromatosis. In patients with evidence of increased body iron levels, further evaluation should be directed toward detecting complications of iron overload and may include liver function tests, assessment of glucose tolerance and hormonal function, cardiac examination, joint and bone x-rays, and, especially if cirrhosis is present, screening for hepatocellular carcinoma.[74,85,87]

Treatment The treatment of choice for hereditary hemochromatosis is phlebotomy to reduce the body iron levels to normal or near-normal and maintain them in that range.[74,85,87] In patients with hereditary hemochromatosis who develop cardiac failure, the use of both phlebotomy and chelation therapy has been suggested. Phlebotomy therapy should be started as soon as the diagnosis of the homozygous state for hereditary hemochromatosis has been established; postponement only increases the risk of organ damage from iron overload. The phlebotomy program should remove 500 ml of blood (containing 200 to 250 mg of iron) once weekly or, for heavily loaded patients, twice weekly until the patient is iron deficient.[85] Before each phlebotomy, the hematocrit or hemoglobin concentration should be measured. Initially, the hematocrit and hemoglobin levels will decline by about 10% of their initial values but may then rise as the rate of erythropoiesis increases to match the demands of phlebotomy. Measurements of serum ferritin, iron, and transferrin saturation should be done regularly to follow the progress of iron removal. As iron is removed, the serum ferritin concentration will decrease progressively but the serum transferrin saturation will remain raised until iron stores are almost exhausted. Finally, when all the storage iron has been removed, the ferritin concentration will fall to less than 12 µg/L, the serum iron concentration and transferrin saturation will drop, and the hemoglobin concentration will decrease to less than 10 g/dl for 2 weeks without further phlebotomy. In patients with hereditary hemochromatosis, prolonged treatment is often needed. For example, if the initial body iron burden is 25 g, complete removal of the iron burden with weekly phlebotomy may require 2 years or more. After the iron load has been completely removed, a lifelong program of maintenance phlebotomy is required to prevent reaccumulation of the iron burden.[85] Typically, phlebotomy of 500 ml of blood every 3 to 4 months is needed. The goal of maintenance phlebotomy should be to maintain a serum ferritin concentration of less than about 50 µg/L.

If phlebotomy therapy removes the iron load before diabetes mellitus or cirrhosis develops, the patient's life expectancy is normal.[93] If cirrhosis develops, however, the risk of hepatocellular carcinoma is increased by more than 200-fold.[74] In hereditary hemochromatosis, hepatomas develop almost exclusively in patients with hepatic cirrhosis and are the ultimate cause of death in 20% to 30% of these patients, even after successful removal of the iron burden. Phlebotomy therapy is almost always indicated for patients with hereditary hemochromatosis, even when cirrhosis or organ damage is already present, because further progression of the disease can be stopped and alleviation of some organ dysfunction is possible.

Non–HFE-Associated Hereditary Hemochromatosis

Clinically, non–HFE-associated hereditary hemochromatosis is indistinguishable from hereditary hemochromatosis associated with *HFE* mutations. Genetically, the non-HFE disorder is heterogeneous. One subset of this autosomal recessive disorder, designated as hemochromatosis type 3, is caused by mutations of the gene encoding transferrin receptor 2 on chromosome 7q22.[45]

Juvenile Hemochromatosis

Juvenile hemochromatosis, designated as hemochromatosis type 2, is a rare autosomal recessive disorder in which severe iron overload develops before age 30. The two sexes are affected equally, and patients may present with cardiomyopathy, hypogonadism, impaired glucose tolerance, or some combination of these manifestations.[94] Genetically, two subtypes have so far been distinguished. Type 2A shows linkage to chromosome 1q21, but the responsible gene has not yet been identified.[95] Type 2B is caused by mutations in the gene for hepcidin on chromosome 19q13.[46]

Autosomal Dominant Hemochromatosis

Hemochromatosis with an autosomal dominant pattern of inheritance is also genetically heterogeneous, and at least one variety has been designated as hemochromatosis type 4. Several families have been identified with iron overload associated with mutations in the ferroportin gene (*SLC11A3*) on chromosome 2q32. Characteristically, initial iron accumulation is predominantly reticuloendothelial and the serum ferritin concentration is increased, with relatively low transferrin saturation; mild anemia early in life has been reported in a number of those affected. Some, but not all, of those with ferroportin mutations have also developed parenchymal iron overload.[96] A single Japanese family has been described with autosomal dominant iron overload ascribed to a point mutation (A49U) in the iron-responsive element (IRE) of H-ferritin mRNA.[97] Autosomal dominant hemochromatosis has also been reported in a Melanesian kindred, but the genetic basis has not been determined.[98]

Atransferrinemia and Aceruloplasminemia

Iron overload may also result from two rare autosomal recessive disorders in which the synthesis of plasma proteins vital for iron transport is absent or almost absent. In atransferrinemia, dietary iron is readily absorbed and circulates as nontransferrin plasma iron but cannot be used for erythropoiesis because of the lack of a physiologic means of transport into developing erythroid cells; affected persons die unless they receive transferrin infusion or blood transfusion.[99] In aceruloplasminemia, the deficiency of ceruloplasmin ferroxidase activity results in iron accumulation in the liver, pancreas, and brain, with smaller amounts of excess iron found in the spleen, heart, kidney, thyroid, and retina. Patients present with progressive neurodegeneration of the retina and basal ganglia and with diabetes mellitus in middle age.[100]

SECONDARY IRON OVERLOAD

Secondary iron overload may result from increased gastrointestinal absorption of iron, from transfusion of red blood cells, from inadvertent iatrogenic parenteral administration of iron, or from some combination thereof. Despite the progress made in understanding genetically determined increases in intestinal iron uptake, the pathophysiologic mechanisms responsible for the increased absorption of iron in secondary iron overload are still obscure.

Iron-Loading Anemias

The iron-loading anemias include congenital dyserythropoietic anemia, pyruvate kinase deficiency, thalassemia major (Cooley anemia) and thalassemia intermedia, hemoglobin E–β-thalassemia, a variety of forms of sideroblastic anemia, some myelodysplastic anemias, and other anemic disorders in which the incorporation of iron into hemoglobin is impaired. In patients with iron-loading anemias, severe iron overload may develop as a result of increased gastrointestinal iron absorption. Any red cell transfusions these patients receive will contribute to the iron loading. Because the extent of ineffective erythropoiesis, not the severity of the anemia, seems to determine the rate of iron loading, severe iron overload may develop in patients with only slight or mild anemia.[101] The clinical manifestations and pathology that may develop in patients with iron-loading anemias are similar to those seen in hereditary hemochromatosis, including liver disease, diabetes mellitus, endocrine disorders, and cardiac dysfunction.[102] Suppression of hepcidin synthesis by anemia, hypoxia, or both has been suggested as a potential mechanism for the increased iron absorption,[103] but the distinctive influence of ineffective erythropoiesis remains to be explained.

Other Causes and Forms of Absorption-Related Iron Overload

Chronic liver disease Some patients with chronic liver disease, including those with alcoholic cirrhosis and those with portacaval shunting, may experience minor or modest degrees of iron loading as a result of increased dietary iron absorption.[74] The mechanisms responsible for the increased gastrointestinal iron uptake have not been identified, although ineffective erythropoiesis and hyperferremia associated with alcohol-induced folate and sideroblastic abnormalities have been proposed as etiologic factors.[104] Body iron stores are increased only to a minor degree, typically to 2 to 4 g, but in alcoholic cirrhosis, the higher the liver iron, the shorter the survival.

Porphyria cutanea tarda Symptomatic patients with porphyria cutanea tarda, a hepatic porphyria, usually have a modest increase in body iron levels that almost always is the result of increased gastrointestinal absorption.[102] In patients who are of European ancestry, *HFE* mutations are common and may contribute to the pathogenesis of both the familial and the sporadic forms of the disorder.[105]

Insulin resistance–associated hepatic iron overload An iron-overload syndrome characterized by an increased serum ferritin level with a normal transferrin saturation level in association with glucose or lipid metabolic abnormalities, or both, was first described in 1997[106] and has come to be known as insulin resistance–associated hepatic iron overload.[107] The iron overload is typically mild or moderate, and the histologic appearance is distinct from that of HFE-associated hemochromatosis.

African dietary iron overload In sub-Saharan Africa, iron overload in association with greatly increased dietary iron intake from a fermented maize beverage home-brewed in steel drums has been described. Iron burdens may be as great as those found in hereditary hemochromatosis, and patients may develop liver disease (with cirrhosis and hepatoma), pancreatic disease (with diabetes mellitus), endocrine disorders, and cardiac dysfunction. Although increased dietary iron intake was long considered the sole cause of the increased iron absorption in this disorder, a series of pedigree studies has suggested that a genetic component may be involved and may be common in populations of African ancestry.[83]

Medicinal iron ingestion Ingestion of iron supplements can undoubtedly contribute to the body iron burden of patients with iron-loading disorders, but the extent to which orally administered iron can increase the body iron stores of normal individuals remains uncertain. Although some case reports have described iron accumulation in patients who have taken medicinal iron for long periods, the potential involvement of an unrecognized iron-loading mutation in these individuals cannot be excluded.

Transfusional and Other Parenteral Iron Overload

Etiology and diagnosis An adequate transfusion program can sustain life in patients with severe chronic refractory anemia, but transfusion therapy alone produces a progressive accumulation of the iron contained in transfused red cells.[108] Iron accumulation from transfusion initially occurs predominantly in macrophage sites, followed by redistribution to parenchymal tissues. In patients with severe congenital anemias, such as thalassemia major and the Blackfan-Diamond syndrome, regular transfusions can prevent death from anemia in infancy and permit normal growth and development during childhood. Treatment of acquired transfusion-dependent anemias, such as aplastic anemia, pure red cell aplasia, and hypoplastic or myelodysplastic disorders, among others, may result in the development of marked iron overload. If the transfusion-dependent anemia includes erythroid hyperplasia with ineffective erythropoiesis, increased gastrointestinal iron absorption may add to the iron loading. In such cases, dietary iron uptake may be minimized by suppression of erythropoiesis with an adequate transfusion program. Although sickling disorders (e.g., sickle cell anemia and sickle cell–β-thalassemia) are not transfusion-dependent, these patients may acquire a considerable iron load from repeated transfusions for the prevention of stroke, painful crises, and other recurrent complications.[110] Because humans lack a physiologic means of eliminating excess iron, iron contained in transfused red cells progressively accumulates and eventually damages the liver, heart, pancreas, and other organs; death usually occurs from cardiac failure. In younger patients, the iron burden results in growth failure and, in adolescence, delayed or absent sexual maturation.

Treatment About 200 to 250 mg of iron is added to the body iron load with each unit of transfused red cells. Most transfusion-dependent patients require 200 to 300 ml/kg of blood a year; for example, a 70 kg adult requires about two to three units of blood every 3 to 4 weeks, adding about 6 to 10 g of iron a year. The severity of iron toxicity seems to be related to the magnitude of the body iron burden. Almost all patients who have been treated with transfusion alone and have received 100 or more units of blood (about 20 to 25 g of iron) have developed cardiac iron deposits, often in association with signs of hepatic, pancreatic, and endocrine damage.[108] For patients who are transfusion dependent or severely anemic, the only way to prevent iron overload is treatment with a chelating agent capable of complexing with iron and permitting its excretion. Two chelating agents are available in the United States: deferoxamine, which is administered subcutaneously or intravenously, and deferasirox, which is the first oral agent to receive FDA approval.[109] Clinical trials with deferoxamine have documented the effectiveness of iron chelation as therapy for iron overload, demonstrating that regular iron chelation can decrease the body iron burden, alleviate organ dysfunction, and improve survival.[108] Although toxic side effects can occur, especially with intensive therapy, deferoxamine has been a remarkably safe drug.[108]

Iron chelation therapy should be started early to prevent the accumulation of toxic amounts of iron in vulnerable tissues and to maintain body iron stores at concentrations associated with a low risk of early death and clinical complications. The longer chelation therapy is delayed, the greater the risk of iron toxicity. Because deferoxamine is poorly absorbed after oral administration and rapidly eliminated from the circulation, deferoxamine must be given by slow subcutaneous or intravenous infusion over 9 to 12 hours each day at least 5 days a week to be optimally useful in the treatment of patients with transfusional iron overload.[108] In patients with thalassemia major and other congenital refractory anemias who have been transfusion dependent from early infancy, chelation therapy is best started after about 10 to 20 transfusions, usually when the patient is 3 or 4 years of age.[108] Deferoxamine is administered by slow subcutaneous infusion at a dosage not exceeding 25 mg/kg/day to minimize the risk of growth retardation. In older patients and adults with acquired refractory anemias who require regular transfusion and in patients with sickle cell disease who are chronically transfused for prevention of complications, early therapy also seems prudent, beginning after transfusion of 10 to 20 units of blood. The usual dosage of deferoxamine in these older patients is not more than 50 mg/kg/day, given over 9 to 12 hours by slow subcutaneous infusion at least 5 days a week. Compliance with these near-daily regimens of prolonged parenteral infusions may be difficult, and lack of compliance is the chief obstacle to chelation therapy. Administration of ascorbic acid can enhance deferoxamine-induced iron excretion but carries the risk of an internal redistribution of iron from relatively benign storage sites in macrophages to a potentially toxic pool in parenchymal cells. Although the evidence is anecdotal, large doses of ascorbic acid should be regarded as hazardous in patients with iron overload. Systemic complications of deferoxoxamine use include allergic anaphylactoid reactions, infections, visual abnormalities and auditory dysfunction, and growth retardation.[108] As a result, regular evaluation for drug toxicity should be included in the management of any patient receiving deferoxamine, including annual audiograms, retinal examination, and assessment of growth in children and adolescents. The risk of many of these complications may be minimized by adjusting the deferoxamine dose to the magnitude of the body iron load. In 2005, deferasirox, a once-daily oral iron chelator, received FDA approval for use in the treatment of chronic iron overload resulting from multiple blood transfusions.[109] The utility and safety of deferasirox have been shown in a randomized, multicenter study of patients with β-thalassemia and transfusional iron overload.[111] Although oral chelation therapy would likely improve patient compliance, the cost is high; the estimated annual cost for treatment with this agent in the United States in an adult weighing 60 kg is $39,000 and $58,500 for doses of 20 and 30 mg/kg/day, respectively.[112]

Additional Rare or Uncommon Forms of Iron Overload

Perinatal iron overload occurs in several forms. Neonatal hemochromatosis is a heterogeneous group of disorders associated with severe congenital hepatic disease and deposits of iron in the liver, pancreas, heart, and other extrahepatic sites, with evidence of autosomal recessive inheritance in some cases.[113] Several rare metabolic abnormalities of the neonate may be associated with abnormal iron deposition, including hereditary tyrosinemia (hypermethioninemia); Zellweger cerebrohepatorenal syndrome[114]; the tricho-hepato-enteric syndrome; and the GRACILE (or Fellman) syndrome.[113]

Focal sequestration of iron is found in other rare disorders, including idiopathic pulmonary hemosiderosis and renal hemosiderosis. Such abnormal iron deposition is associated with neurologic abnormalities in Friedreich ataxia, in pantothenate kinase–associated neurodegeneration (formerly Hallervorden-Spatz syndrome), and in neuroferritinopathy.[115] Finally, hyperferritinemia with autosomal dominant congenital cataract[116] is a disorder of iron metabolism in which affected family members present with early-onset, bilateral nuclear cataracts and moderately elevated serum ferritin concentrations.[116] The body iron level is normal in these patients, but overload is often suspected because of the elevated serum ferritin concentrations.

The author has no commercial relationships with manufacturers of products or providers of services discussed in this chapter.

References

1. Klinken S: Red blood cells. Internat J Biochem Cell Biol 34:1513, 2002

2. Yonetani T, Park SI, Tsuneshige A, et al: Global allostery model of hemoglobin: modulation of O(2) affinity, cooperativity, and Bohr effect by heterotropic allosteric effectors. J Biol Chem 277:34508, 2002

3. Hsia CC: Respiratory function of hemoglobin. N Engl J Med 338:239, 1998

4. McMahon TJ, Moon RE, Luschinger BP, et al: Nitric oxide in the human respiratory cycle. Nat Med 8:711, 2002

5. Schechter AN, Gladwin MT: Hemoglobin and the paracrine and endocrine functions of nitric oxide. N Engl J Med 348:1483, 2003

6. Discher DE, Carl P: New insights into red cell network structure, elasticity, and spectrin unfolding—a current review. Cell Mol Biol Lett 6:593, 2001

7. Jacobasch G: Biochemical and genetic basis of red cell enzyme deficiencies. Baillieres Best Pract Res Clin Haematol 13:1, 2000

8. Henry ER, Bettati S, Hofrichter J, et al: A tertiary two-state allosteric model for hemoglobin. Biophys Chem 98:149, 2002

9. Leach RM, Treacher DF: The pulmonary physician in critical care: 2: oxygen delivery and consumption in the critically ill. Thorax 57:170, 2002

10. Fisher JW: Erythropoietin: physiology and pharmacology update. Exp Biol Med (Maywood) 228:1, 2003

11. Trent JT 3rd, Watts RA, Hargrove MS: Human neuroglobin, a hexacoordinate hemoglobin that reversibly binds oxygen. J Biol Chem 276:30106, 2001

12. Burmester T, Ebner B, Weich B, et al: Cytoglobin: a novel globin type ubiquitously expressed in vertebrate tissues. Mol Biol Evol 19:416, 2002

13. Geers C, Gros G: Carbon dioxide transport and carbonic anhydrase in blood and muscle. Physiol Rev 80:681, 2000

14. Andrews NC: Disorders of iron metabolism. N Engl J Med 341:1986, 1999

15. Aisen P, Enns C, Wessling-Resnick M: Chemistry and biology of eukaryotic iron metabolism. Int J Biochem Cell Biol 33:940, 2001

16. Finch C: Regulators of iron balance in humans. Blood 84:1697, 1994

17. Zakin MM, Baron B, Guillou F: Regulation of the tissue-specific expression of transferrin gene. Dev Neurosci 24:222, 2002

18. Trinder D, Baker E: Transferrin receptor 2: a new molecule in iron metabolism. Int J Biochem Cell Biol 35:292, 2003

19. Andrews NC: A genetic view of iron homeostasis. Semin Hematol 39:227, 2002

20. Arosio P, Levi S: Ferritin, iron homeostasis, and oxidative damage. Free Radic Biol Med 33:457, 2002

21. Levi S, Corsi B, Bosisio M, et al: A human mitochondrial ferritin encoded by an intronless gene. J Biol Chem 276:24437, 2001

22. Cazzola M, Invernizzi R, Bergamaschi G, et al: Mitochondrial ferritin expression in erythroid cells from patients with sideroblastic anemia. Blood 101:1996, 2003

23. Rouault TA: Systemic iron metabolism: a review and implications for brain iron metabolism. Pediatr Neurol 25:130, 2001

24. Hubert N, Hentze MW: Previously uncharacterized isoforms of divalent metal transporter (DMT)-1: implications for regulation and cellular function. Proc Natl Acad Sci USA 99:12345, 2002

25. Abboud S, Haile DJ: A novel mammalian iron-regulated protein involved in intracellular iron metabolism. J Biol Chem 275:19906, 2000

26. Cairo G, Recalcati S, Pietrangelo A, et al: The iron regulatory proteins: targets and modulators of free radical reactions and oxidative damage. Free Radic Biol Med 32:1237, 2002

27. Knutson M, Wessling-Resnick M: Iron metabolism in the reticuloendothelial system. Crit Rev Biochem Mol Biol 38:61, 2003

28. Kondo H, Saito K, Grasso JP, et al: Iron metabolism in the erythrophagocytosing Kupffer cell. Hepatology 8:32, 1988

29. Kristiansen M, Graversen JH, Jacobsen C, et al: Identification of the haemoglobin scavenger receptor. Nature 409:198, 2001

30. Wilks A: Heme oxygenase: evolution, structure, and mechanism. Antioxid Redox Signal 4:603, 2002

31. Baranano DE, Wolosker H, Bae BI, et al: A mammalian iron ATPase induced by iron. J Biol Chem 275:15166, 2000

32. Pietrangelo A: Physiology of iron transport and the hemochromatosis gene. Am J Physiol Gastrointest Liver Physiol 282:G403, 2002

33. Hellman NE, Gitlin JD: Ceruloplasmin metabolism and function. Annu Rev Nutr 22:439, 2002

34. Tolosano E, Altruda F: Hemopexin: structure, function, and regulation. DNA Cell Biol 21:297, 2002

35. Bothwell TH, Charlton RW, Cook JD, et al: Iron Metabolism in Man. Blackwell, London, England, 1979

36. Miret S, Simpson RJ, McKie AT: Physiology and molecular biology of dietary iron absorption. Annu Rev Nutr 23:283, 2003

37. Conrad ME, Umbreit JN: Pathways of iron absorption. Blood Cells Mol Dis 29:336, 2002

38. McKie AT, Latunde-Dada GO, Miret S, et al: Molecular evidence for the role of a ferric reductase in iron transport. Biochem Soc Trans 30:722, 2002

39. Anderson GJ, Frazer DM, McKie AT, et al: The expression and regulation of the iron transport molecules hephaestin and IREG1: implications for the control of iron export from the small intestine. Cell Biochem Biophys 36:137, 2002

40. Feder JN, Gnirke A, Thomas W, et al: A novel MHC class I-like gene is mutated in patients with hereditary haemochromatosis. Nat Genet 13:399, 1996

41. Fleming RE, Sly WS: Mechanisms of iron accumulation in hereditary hemochromatosis. Annu Rev Physiol 64:663, 2002

42. Drakesmith H, Sweetland E, Schimanski L, et al: The hemochromatosis protein HFE inhibits iron export from macrophages. Proc Natl Acad Sci USA 99:15602, 2002

43. Townsend A, Drakesmith H: Role of HFE in iron metabolism, hereditary haemochromatosis, anaemia of chronic disease, and secondary iron overload. Lancet 359:786, 2002

44. Frazer DM, Anderson GJ: The orchestration of body iron intake: how and where do enterocytes receive their cues? Blood Cells Mol Dis 30:288, 2003

45. Camaschella C, Roetto A, Cali A, et al: The gene TFR2 is mutated in a new type of haemochromatosis mapping to 7q22. Nat Genet 25:14, 2000

46. Roetto A, Papanikolaou G, Politou M, et al: Mutant antimicrobial peptide hepcidin is associated with severe juvenile hemochromatosis. Nat Genet 33:21, 2003

47. Bridle KR, Frazer DM, Wilkins SJ, et al: Disrupted hepcidin regulation in HFE-associated haemochromatosis and the liver as a regulator of body iron homoeostasis. Lancet 361:669, 2003

48. Ramakrishnan U, Yip R: Experiences and challenges in industrialized countries: control of iron deficiency in industrialized countries. J Nutr 132:820S, 2002

49. Iron Deficiency—United States, 1999–2000. MMWR Morb Mortal Wkly Rep 51:897, 2002

50. Goddard AF, McIntyre AS, Scott BB: Guidelines for the management of iron deficiency anaemia. British Society of Gastroenterology. Gut 46(suppl 3-4):IV1, 2000

51. Recommendations to prevent and control iron deficiency in the United States. MMWR Recomm Rep 47(RR-3):1, 1998

52. Willoughby JM, Laitner SM: Audit of the investigation of iron deficiency anaemia in a district general hospital, with sample guidelines for future practice. Postgrad Med J 76:218, 2000

53. Mukhopadhyay D, Mohanaruban K: Iron deficiency anaemia in older people: investigation, management and treatment. Age Ageing 31:87, 2002

54. Annibale B, Capurso G, Chistolini A, et al: Gastrointestinal causes of refractory iron deficiency anemia in patients without gastrointestinal symptoms. Am J Med 111:439, 2001

55. Sandoval C, Berger E, Ozkaynak MF, et al: Severe iron deficiency anemia in 42 pediatric patients. Pediatr Hematol Oncol 19:157, 2002

56. Lee PL, Halloran C, Trevino R, et al: Human transferrin G277S mutation: a risk factor for iron deficiency anaemia. Br J Haematol 115:329, 2001

57. Earley CJ: Clinical practice. Restless legs syndrome. N Engl J Med 348:2103, 2003

58. Kalra L, Hamlyn AN, Jones BJ: Blue sclerae: a common sign of iron deficiency? Lancet 2:1267, 1986

59. Rector WG Jr: Pica: its frequency and significance in patients with iron-deficiency anemia due to chronic gastrointestinal blood loss. J Gen Intern Med 4:512, 1989

60. Haas JD, Brownlie T 4th: Iron deficiency and reduced work capacity: a critical review of the research to determine a causal relationship. J Nutr 131:676S, 2001

61. Oppenheimer SJ: Iron and its relation to immunity and infectious disease. J Nutr 131:616S, 2001

62. Grantham-McGregor S, Ani C: A review of studies on the effect of iron deficiency on cognitive development in children. J Nutr 131:649S, 2001

63. Cook J: The nutritional assessment of iron status. Arch Latinoam Nutr 49:11S, 1999

64. Cook JD: The measurement of serum transferrin receptor. Am J Med Sci 318:269, 1999

65. Malope BI, MacPhail AP, Alberts M, et al: The ratio of serum transferrin receptor and serum ferritin in the diagnosis of iron status. Br J Haematol 115:84, 2001

66. Beguin Y: Soluble transferrin receptor for the evaluation of erythropoiesis and iron status. Clin Chim Acta 329:9, 2003

67. Cook JD, Flowers CH, Skikne BS: The quantitative assessment of body iron. Blood 101:3359, 2003

68. Brugnara C: Reticulocyte cellular indices: a new approach in the diagnosis of anemias and monitoring of erythropoietic function. Crit Rev Clin Lab Sci 37:93, 2000

69. Thomas C, Thomas L: Biochemical markers and hematologic indices in the diagnosis of functional iron deficiency. Clin Chem 48:1066, 2002

70. Goodnough LT, Skikne B, Brugnara C: Erythropoietin, iron, and erythropoiesis. Blood 96:823, 2000

71. McDiarmid T, Johnson ED: Are any oral iron formulations better tolerated than ferrous sulfate? J Fam Pract 51:576, 2002

72. Milman N, Pedersen P: Evidence that the Cys282Tyr mutation of the HFE gene originated from a population in Southern Scandinavia and spread with the Vikings. Clin Genet 64:36, 2003

73. Steinberg KK, Cogswell ME, Chang JC, et al: Prevalence of C282Y and H63D mutations in the hemochromatosis (HFE) gene in the United States. JAMA 285:2216, 2001

74. Powell LW: Hereditary hemochromatosis and iron overload diseases. J Gastroenterol Hepatol 17(suppl):S191, 2002

75. Bomford A: Genetics of haemochromatosis. Lancet 360:1673, 2002

76. Barosi G, Salvaneschi L, Grasso M, et al: High prevalence of a screening-detected, HFE-unrelated, mild idiopathic iron overload in Northern Italy. Haematologica 87:472, 2002

77. Adams PC, Deugnier Y, Moirand R, et al: The relationship between iron overload, clinical symptoms, and age in 410 patients with genetic hemochromatosis. Hepatology 25:162, 1997

78. Beutler E, Felitti VJ, Koziol JA, et al: Penetrance of 845G→A (C282Y) HFE hereditary haemochromatosis mutation in the USA. Lancet 359:211, 2002

79. Beutler E: The HFE Cys282Tyr mutation as a necessary but not sufficient cause of clinical hereditary hemochromatosis. Blood 101:3347, 2003

80. Ajioka RS, Kushner JP: Clinical consequences of iron overload in hemochromatosis homozygotes. Blood 101:3351, 2003

81. McLaren CE, Barton JC, Adams PC, et al: Hemochromatosis and Iron Overload Screening (HEIRS) study design for an evaluation of 100,000 primary care-based adults. Am J Med Sci 325:53, 2003

82. Niederau C, Strohmeyer G: Strategies for early diagnosis of haemochromatosis. Eur J Gastroenterol Hepatol 14:217, 2002

83. Gordeuk VR: African iron overload. Semin Hematol 39:263, 2002

84. Adams P, Brissot P, Powell LW: EASL International Consensus Conference on Haemochromatosis. J Hepatol 33:485, 2000

85. Brissot P, Guyader D, Loreal O, et al: Clinical aspects of hemochromatosis. Transfus Sci 23:193, 2000

86. Morrison ED, Brandhagen DJ, Phatak PD, et al: Serum ferritin level predicts advanced hepatic fibrosis among U.S. patients with phenotypic hemochromatosis. Ann Intern Med 138:627, 2003

87. Pietrangelo A: Haemochromatosis. Gut 52(suppl 2):ii23, 2003

88. Moirand R, Guyader D, Mendler MH, et al: HFE based re-evaluation of heterozygous hemochromatosis. Am J Med Genet 111:356, 2002

89. Beutler E, Felitti V, Gelbart T, et al: Haematological effects of the C282Y HFE mutation in homozygous and heterozygous states among subjects of northern and southern European ancestry. Br J Haematol 120:887, 2003

90. Gochee PA, Powell LW, Cullen DJ, et al: A population-based study of the biochemical and clinical expression of the H63D hemochromatosis mutation. Gastroenterology 122:646, 2002

91. Pointon JJ, Wallace D, Merryweather-Clarke AT, et al: Uncommon mutations and polymorphisms in the hemochromatosis gene. Genet Test 4:151, 2000

92. Brittenham GM, Badman DG: Noninvasive measurement of iron: report of an NIDDK workshop. Blood 101:15, 2003

93. Niederau C, Fischer R, Purschel A, et al: Long-term survival in patients with hereditary hemochromatosis. Gastroenterology 110:1107, 1996

94. De Gobbi M, Roetto A, Piperno A, et al: Natural history of juvenile haemochromatosis. Br J Haematol 117:973, 2002

95. Roetto A, Totaro A, Cazzola M, et al: Juvenile hemochromatosis locus maps to chromosome 1q. Am J Hum Genet 64:1388, 1999

96. Cazzola M, Cremonesi L, Papaioannou M, et al: Genetic hyperferritinaemia and reticuloendothelial iron overload associated with a three base pair deletion in the coding region of the ferroportin gene (SLC11A3). Br J Haematol 119:539, 2002

97. Kato J, Fujikawa K, Kanda M, et al: A mutation, in the iron-responsive element of H ferritin mRNA, causing autosomal dominant iron overload. Am J Hum Genet 69:191, 2001

98. Eason RJ, Adams PC, Aston CE, et al: Familial iron overload with possible autosomal dominant inheritance. Aust N Z J Med 20:226, 1990

99. Sheth S, Brittenham GM: Genetic disorders affecting proteins of iron metabolism: clinical implications. Annu Rev Med 51:443, 2000

100. Nittis T, Gitlin JD: The copper-iron connection: hereditary aceruloplasminemia. Semin Hematol 39:282, 2002

101. Cazzola M, Beguin Y, Bergamaschi G, et al: Soluble transferrin receptor as a potential determinant of iron loading in congenital anaemias due to ineffective erythropoiesis. Br J Haematol 106:752, 1999

102. Bottomley SS: Secondary iron overload disorders. Semin Hematol 35:77, 1998

103. Nicolas G, Chauvet C, Viatte L, et al: The gene encoding the iron regulatory peptide hepcidin is regulated by anemia, hypoxia, and inflammation. J Clin Invest 110:1037, 2002

104. Conrad ME, Barton JC: Anemia and iron kinetics in alcoholism. Semin Hematol 17:149, 1980

105. Bygum A, Christiansen L, Petersen NE, et al: Familial and sporadic porphyria cutanea tarda: clinical, biochemical and genetic features with emphasis on iron status. Acta Derm Venereol 83:115, 2003

106. Moirand R, Mortaji AM, Loreal O, et al: A new syndrome of liver iron overload with normal transferrin saturation. Lancet 349:95, 1997

107. Chitturi S, George J: Interaction of iron, insulin resistance, and nonalcoholic steatohepatitis. Curr Gastroenterol Rep 5:18, 2003

108. Roberts DJ, Rees D, Howard C, et al: Desferrioxamine mesylate for managing transfusional iron overload in patients with transfusion-dependent thalassaemia. Cochrane Database Syst Rev (4):CD004450, 2005

109. FDA approves first oral drug for chronic iron overload. NDA News. Food and Drug Administration, November 9, 2005 http://www.fda.gov/bbs/topic/NEWS/2005/NEW01258.html

110. Files B, Brambilla D, Kutlar A, et al: Longitudinal changes in ferritin during chronic transfusion: a report from the Stroke Prevention Trial in Sickle Cell Anemia (STOP). J Pediatr Hematol Oncol 24:284, 2002

111. Nisbet-Brown E, Olivieri NF, Giardina PJ, et al: Effectiveness and safety of ICL670 in iron-loaded patients with thalassaemia: a randomised, double-blind, placebo-controlled, dose-escalation trial. Lancet 361:1597, 2003

112. Neufeld EJ: Oral chelators deferasirox and deferiprone for transfusional iron overload in thalassemia major: new data, new questions. Blood 107:3426, 2006

113. Kelly AL, Lunt PW, Rodrigues F, et al: Classification and genetic features of neonatal haemochromatosis: a study of 27 affected pedigrees and molecular analysis of genes implicated in iron metabolism. J Med Genet 38:599, 2001

114. Goldfischer S, Grotsky HW, Chang CH, et al: Idiopathic neonatal iron storage involving the liver, pancreas, heart, and endocrine and exocrine glands. Hepatology 1:58, 1981

115. Ponka P: Rare causes of hereditary iron overload. Semin Hematol 39:249, 2002

116. Cazzola M: Hereditary hyperferritinaemia/cataract syndrome. Best Pract Res Clin Haematol 15:385, 2002

Acknowledgments

Figure 1   Seward Hung.

Figure 2   Marcia Kammerer.

Figure 3   Seward Hung.

Figure 4   Dimitry Schidlovsky.

Stanley L. Schrier, M.D., F.A.C.P.

Classification of Production Defects

Red blood cell production defects cause anemia that is marked by a low absolute reticulocyte count. Examination of the peripheral blood count and the bone marrow aids in classifying these disorders. The marrow characteristically shows one of the following:

1. A normal ratio of myeloid cells to erythroid cells (M:E ratio), normal overall cellularity, and a normal pattern of erythroid maturation.
2. Virtual absence of normal bone marrow elements caused by aplasia (absence of marrow cells) or by replacement of normal marrow elements by fibrosis, solid tumors, granulomas, or leukemia.
3. Erythroid hyperplasia with increased cellularity. Because of defects of erythroid maturation, there is ineffective erythropoiesis or intramedullary hemolysis. Erythroid precursors die in the marrow, and few cells reach the periphery.

Production Defects Associated with Apparently Normal Bone Marrow

ANEMIA OF CHRONIC DISEASE

Definition

The anemia of chronic disease occurs secondary to neoplastic, infectious, and inflammatory diseases and other chronic illnesses, including liver disorders, congestive heart failure, and diabetes mellitus.[1,2] Hematocrit values usually range from 27% to 35%, although 20% of patients have hematocrit values below 25%.[2]

Pathophysiology

The anemia of chronic disease usually results from a combination of slightly shortened red blood cell survival, the sequestration of iron in the reticuloendothelial system, and erythropoietin levels that are less than expected for the degree of anemia.[1,2]

Red blood cells usually have a normal morphologic appearance, although they may occasionally be mildly hypochromic and microcytic. The serum iron and transferrin levels are low, and iron saturation is frequently as low as 15%.[1,2] The serum ferritin level is usually normal or elevated.[2,3] All these changes can be induced by the inflammatory cytokines (e.g., interleukin-1 [IL-1]; tumor necrosis factor–α; interferons alfa, beta, and gamma; and perhaps transforming growth factor–β).[4] Under experimental conditions, these cytokines reduce erythropoietin production, cause hypoferremia, increase serum ferritin levels, impair erythropoiesis, and block release of iron from reticuloendothelial cells.[5] Hepcidin, a newly described mediator of iron metabolism, may be the major mediator of the anemia of chronic disease[6]; hepcidin production is increased up to 100-fold with inflammation. Hepcidin seems to be the long-sought mediator that transmits iron stores to the gut. Hepcidin is secreted when iron stores, primarily in the liver, are increased, and it blocks iron absorption from the gut and causes iron to be trapped in macrophages.[6]

Diagnosis

Mild anemia, with normal or elevated levels of leukocytes and platelets, in a patient with a chronic illness suggests the diagnosis of anemia of chronic disease. This normocytic or hypochromic and microcytic anemia is easily misdiagnosed as iron deficiency anemia, thalassemia trait, or a sideroblastic anemia. If the diagnosis is uncertain after careful examination of the blood smear, the most useful tests for making the diagnosis are measurement of the serum ferritin level and, in rare cases, bone marrow examination that includes an iron stain [see Table 1 and Figure 1]. In some cases, there is more than one cause of the anemia, and thorough examination of the patient may be required to establish the primary cause. For example, a patient who has anemia of chronic disease resulting from carcinoma of the colon may also be iron deficient because of intestinal bleeding. HIV infection produces complex hematologic effects, including Coombs-positive autoimmune hemolytic anemia, but it also

Table 1 Differential Diagnosis of Hypochromic Anemias

	Anemia of Chronic Disorders	*Iron Deficiency Anemia*	*Thalassemia Trait*	*Sideroblastic Anemias*
Smear	Usually normochromic, normocytic but can be mildly hypochromic, microcytic	Varies with the degree of the anemia [see Chapter 91]	Hypochromia, target cells, microcytes, basophilic stippling	May be similar to that of the thalassemia trait
Serum iron level Iron-binding capacity Percent saturation	Low Low 5–16	Low High 0–16	Normal Normal Normal (20–40)	High Normal 60–90
Serum ferritin level	Normal or high	Low	Normal	High
Marrow iron in reticuloendothelial cells	+ + to + + +	0	+ + to + + +	+ + + +
Marrow iron in sideroblasts	0	0	+ + to + + +	+ + + + with ringed sideroblasts
Marrow erythroid precursors	Normal	Generally normal; cytoplasm may be scanty	Usually mild erythroid hyperplasia	Intense erythroid hyperplasia with dyserythropoiesis

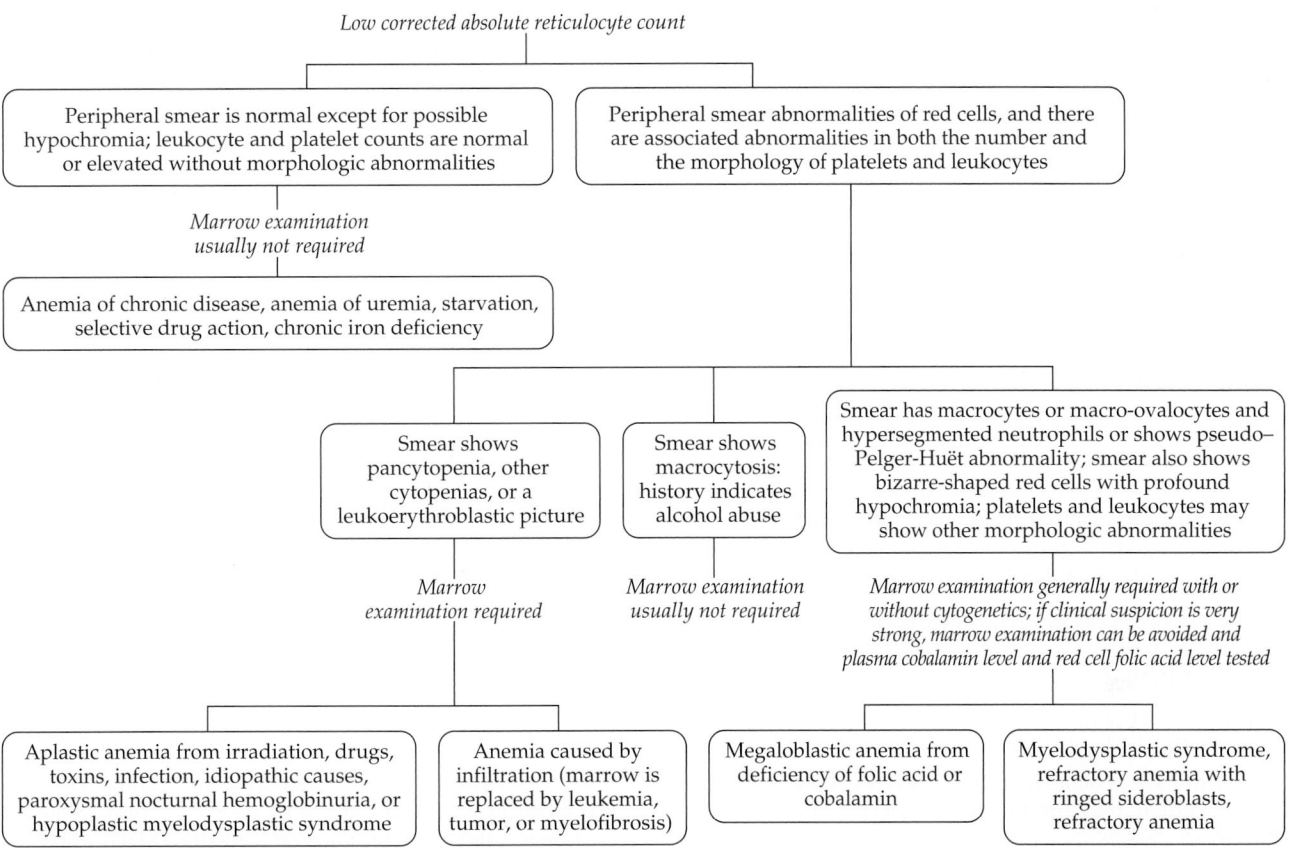

Low corrected absolute reticulocyte count

Peripheral smear is normal except for possible hypochromia; leukocyte and platelet counts are normal or elevated without morphologic abnormalities

Peripheral smear abnormalities of red cells, and there are associated abnormalities in both the number and the morphology of platelets and leukocytes

Marrow examination usually not required

Anemia of chronic disease, anemia of uremia, starvation, selective drug action, chronic iron deficiency

Smear shows pancytopenia, other cytopenias, or a leukoerythroblastic picture

Smear shows macrocytosis: history indicates alcohol abuse

Smear has macrocytes or macro-ovalocytes and hypersegmented neutrophils or shows pseudo–Pelger-Huët abnormality; smear also shows bizarre-shaped red cells with profound hypochromia; platelets and leukocytes may show other morphologic abnormalities

Marrow examination required

Marrow examination usually not required

Marrow examination generally required with or without cytogenetics; if clinical suspicion is very strong, marrow examination can be avoided and plasma cobalamin level and red cell folic acid level tested

Aplastic anemia from irradiation, drugs, toxins, infection, idiopathic causes, paroxysmal nocturnal hemoglobinuria, or hypoplastic myelodysplastic syndrome

Anemia caused by infiltration (marrow is replaced by leukemia, tumor, or myelofibrosis)

Megaloblastic anemia from deficiency of folic acid or cobalamin

Myelodysplastic syndrome, refractory anemia with ringed sideroblasts, refractory anemia

Figure 1   Flowchart shows steps in the diagnosis of anemia caused by production defects. This type of anemia is suggested by a low corrected reticulocyte count or the finding of associated leukocyte or platelet abnormalities on the peripheral blood smear.

causes anemia of chronic disease in the majority of patients with AIDS.[7]

Treatment

Identifying and treating the primary disease is the most important part of managing the anemia of chronic disease. Oral or parenteral iron administration is usually not helpful. Erythropoietin is the standard treatment for patients with anemia of chronic disease. For many patients, administration of pharmacologic doses of erythropoietin corrects the anemia of chronic disease by overriding the defect in erythropoietin production. It is useful to obtain a baseline measurement of the plasma erythropoietin level, because a response to erythropoietin is unlikely in patients whose endogenous levels are above 500 mU/ml. Erythropoietin responses have been reported in patients with rheumatoid arthritis,[8] AIDS,[9] inflammatory bowel disease,[10,11] and cancer.[12] To obtain an optimal response, the patient must have adequate available iron stores (i.e., normal or elevated ferritin level or marrow iron stain) [*see Chapter 90*]. Previously, the recommendation was to start the patient on 100 to 150 U/kg subcutaneously three times weekly; however, most physicians give a single subcutaneous dose of 40,000 units of erythropoietin weekly.[13]

If the hemoglobin level does not rise after 12 weeks, erythropoietin should be discontinued. A longer-acting form of erythropoietin, darbepoietin alfa, can be given subcutaneously at doses of 100 µg weekly or 200 µg every other week.

ANEMIA IN SEVERE RENAL DISEASE

Pathophysiology and Etiology

The predominant cause of anemia in renal disease is a deficiency of erythropoietin production by the diseased kidneys. If underlying inflammatory renal disease is present, there may be a component of anemia of chronic disease.[14] Anorexia and poor iron intake, frequent blood sampling, and loss of erythrocytes during hemodialysis may produce iron deficiency. Folic acid deficiency, hypersplenism, and secondary hyperparathyroidism with marrow fibrosis[4] may also promote anemia.

Anemia in hemodialysis patients can be caused by aluminum toxicity, as well. This anemia was initially identified in patients who had so-called dialysis dementia. Very high plasma aluminum levels probably result from aluminum contamination of the dialysis fluid or gastrointestinal absorption of the aluminum gels taken to bind dietary phosphates. In vitro experiments have shown that aluminum inhibits the growth of the erythroid precursors colony-forming unit–erythroid (CFU-E) and burst-forming unit–erythroid (BFU-E).[15]

Diagnosis

The blood smear should be examined for erythrocyte fragmentation or echinocytosis to exclude other causes of the anemia. The presence of Heinz bodies suggests that oxidative hemolysis has occurred, perhaps caused by oxidants in the hemodialysis fluid.

Treatment

Erythropoietin is the standard treatment for anemic patients with renal disease. Erythropoietin therapy can eliminate the transfusion requirement for patients on hemodialysis and in patients with progressive renal disease who do not yet require hemodialysis. Such treatment significantly improves their quality of life.[16] Side effects, such as hyperkalemia and hypertension, occur infrequently. It is customary to start therapy with 50 U/kg of erythropoietin three times weekly, either intravenously or subcutaneously, and to increase the dosage as necessary to bring the hemoglobin level to the desired value. Parenteral iron supplementation improves the response. ImFed (a form of iron dextran) can be given intramuscularly or intravenously at doses ranging from 100 to 500 mg, with an anticipated frequency of reaction of 4.7%. Ferrlecit (a form of sodium ferric gluconate) can be infused intravenously (125 mg over 1 hour), with the occasional occurrence of hypotension and rash.[12] In a study of patients with anemia caused by aluminum toxicity, treatment with I.V. deferoxamine (30 mg/kg I.V. at the end of each dialysis session) produced substantial improvement.[17]

ANEMIA SECONDARY TO OTHER CONDITIONS

Alcohol Abuse

Excessive alcohol ingestion—either acute or chronic—has profound hematologic effects.[18] Ingestion of about 80 g of alcohol (one bottle of wine, six pints of beer, or one-third bottle of whiskey) daily may produce macrocytosis,[19] stomatocytosis,[20] thrombocytopenia,[21] vacuolization of proerythroblasts, ringed sideroblasts,[20] a sharp drop in serum folic acid levels, and a rise in serum iron levels; it may also impair the reticulocyte response to administered folic acid in a patient known to be folic acid deficient. Acute alcohol ingestion itself does not produce a megaloblastic anemia.[18] It has been postulated that alcohol-induced hematologic toxicity is mediated through acetaldehyde, the major metabolite of ethanol, which is far more toxic and reactive than ethanol. The mechanism for these alcohol-induced abnormalities may be the formation of antibodies against acetaldehyde–hemoglobin adducts.[20] Megaloblasts, macro-ovalocytes, and hypersegmented polymorphonuclear neutrophils (PMNs)

usually appear when concomitant folic acid deficiency is present. Chronic alcohol abuse often results in concomitant folic acid or iron deficiency, severe liver disease, GI bleeding, hypersplenism, and the anemia of chronic disease.

Starvation

Starvation resulting from anorexia nervosa or protein deficiency can cause anemia and even pancytopenia. Hemolysis may also be present [see Figure 2]. The bone marrow biopsy is hypocellular, with a characteristic gelatinous background material consisting of acid mucopolysaccharides. The anemia can occur despite normal folic acid and cobalamin (vitamin B_{12}) levels and can be corrected with proper nutrition.

Hypothyroidism

Hypothyroidism impairs erythrocyte production. The presence of macrocytosis in a hypothyroid patient suggests concomitant dietary folic acid deficiency or pernicious anemia.

Panhypopituitarism

The mild anemia that is associated with severe panhypopituitarism can be corrected by replacement of adrenal, thyroid, and gonadal hormones; the enhancing effect of androgens on the action of erythropoietin is well known.

Aging

The hemoglobin levels, red blood cell indices, and leukocyte and platelet counts of healthy older people are similar to those of younger adults; this finding was confirmed in a study of patients who were 84 years of age or older.[22] Thus, a workup is required when anemia occurs in such older patients. The evaluation and treatment of anemia in the aged has become increasingly important because the presence of anemia (hemoglobin concentration [Hgb] < 12 g/dl in women and < 13 g/dl in men) is an independent risk factor for decline in quality of life.[23]

Production Defects Associated with Marrow Aplasia or Replacement

The combination of anemia and neutropenia or thrombocy-

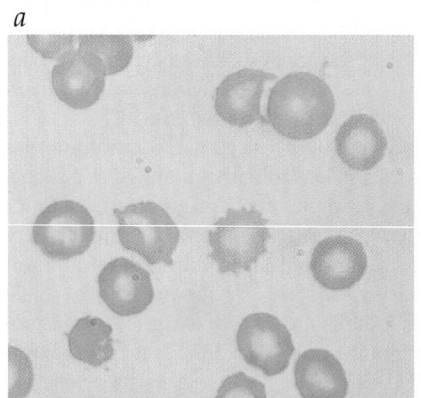
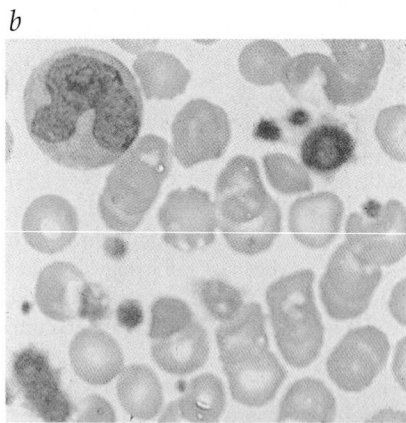
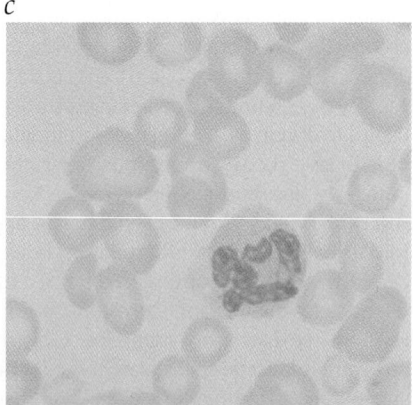

a   *b*   *c*

Figure 2   The peripheral smear changes seen in severe liver disease or starvation (*a*) include distinct variation in size and shape of red blood cells; both sharply spiculed cells (spur cells) and scalloped erythrocytes are prominent. The leukoerythroblastic blood smear (*b*) indicates marrow replacement with extramedullary hematopoiesis. It is characterized by variation in the size and shape of red blood cells, by the presence of nucleated red blood cells in the peripheral blood, by giant platelets, and by immaturity in the myeloid series. In folic acid or cobalamin deficiency (*c*), the smear is characterized by variation in erythrocyte size and by distinct macrocytosis. Occasionally, fish-tailed erythrocytes are present, along with hypersegmented neutrophils.

a *b*

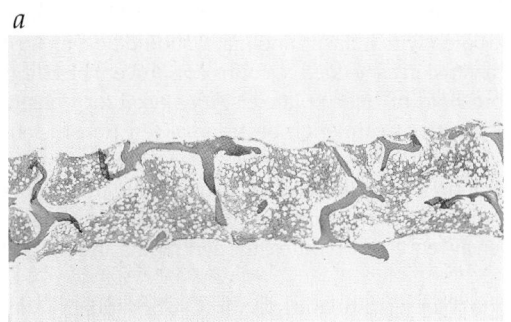 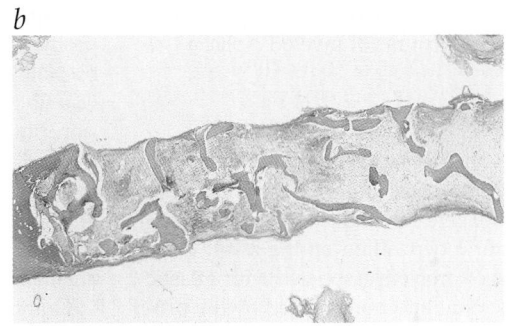

Figure 3 **Shown are (***a***) biopsy of normal bone marrow and (***b***) biopsy of bone marrow from a patient with aplastic anemia showing almost complete aplasia.**

topenia or the combination of all three of these abnormalities (i.e., pancytopenia) usually indicates that the hematopoietic marrow is damaged. If the marrow cavity is infiltrated but pluripotent stem cells are intact, extramedullary hematopoiesis will often develop in the organs of fetal hematopoiesis (i.e., spleen, liver, and distal bones).

Pancytopenia can be congenital or acquired. The finding of combined cytopenias or of immature cells in the blood (myelocytes, metamyelocytes, and erythroblasts)—that is, a leukoerythroblastic blood smear—suggests extramedullary hematopoiesis [*see Figure 2*]. These findings are an indication for bone marrow aspiration and biopsy.

APLASTIC ANEMIA

Definition

Pancytopenia (i.e., anemia, neutropenia, and thrombocytopenia) and aplastic marrow on biopsy examination [*see Figure 3*] establish a working diagnosis of aplastic anemia. The biopsy specimen must not be taken from a marrow site that has been irradiated. It is essential to determine the severity of aplastic anemia. Severe aplastic anemia (SAA) is defined by (1) marrow of less than 25% normal cellularity or marrow of less than 50% normal cellularity in which fewer than 30% of the cells are hematopoietic, and (2) two out of three abnormal peripheral blood values (absolute reticulocyte count < 40,000/μl, absolute neutrophil count [ANC] < 500 μl, or platelet level < 20,000/μl). These criteria have been criticized as being relatively insensitive. Some investigators prefer to identify a cohort of patients with very severe aplastic anemia (VSAA) as those who had an ANC less than 200/μl.[24]

Etiology

Aplastic anemia has a number of causes [*see Table 2*], although in many cases the exact cause cannot be determined.

Ionizing irradiation and chemotherapeutic drugs used in the management of malignant and immunologic disorders have the capacity to destroy hematopoietic stem cells. With careful dosing and scheduling, recovery is expected. Certain drugs, such as chloramphenicol, produce marrow aplasia that is not dose dependent. Gold therapy and the inhalation of organic solvent vapors (e.g., benzene or glue) can also cause fatal marrow failure.

In 2% to 10% of hepatitis patients, severe aplasia occurs 2 to 3 months after a seemingly typical case of acute disease, usually in young men. Often, the hepatitis has no obvious cause, and tests for hepatitis A, B, and C are negative.[25] There is a high incidence of aplastic anemia after liver transplantation in patients with severe non-A, non-B hepatitis.[26]

Several lines of evidence support the possibility that immune disorders can lead to aplasia. Marrow aplasia occurs in graft ver-

sus host disease (GVHD).[27] Immunosuppressive preconditioning improves the chances of successful transplantation of syngeneic marrow into patients with aplastic anemia,[28] and immunosuppressive therapy has been used successfully to treat idiopathic aplastic anemia.[27,28] The blood of some patients with aplastic anemia appears to contain suppressor T cells that suppress the growth of the committed progenitor cells known as colony-forming unit–granulocyte-macrophage (CFU-GM). The suppressor T cells may act by producing interferon gamma.[28] The result of these complex immune mechanisms involving suppressor T cells is a profound decrease in primitive hematopoietic cells as measured by both the long-term culture–initiating cell (LTC-IC) assay and the ability to form secondary colonies from the colonies surviving 5 weeks of marrow culture.[29]

Aplasia can also be part of a prodrome to hairy-cell leukemia [*see Chapter 206*], acute lymphoblastic leukemia [*see*

Table 2 **Causes of Aplastic Anemia**

IRRADIATION

DRUGS

Agents whose use regularly causes myelosuppression

Alkylating agents: melphalan, cyclophosphamide, chlorambucil, busulfan

Antimetabolites: azathioprine, 6-mercaptopurine, hydroxyurea, methotrexate

Other antitumor agents: daunorubicin, doxorubicin, carmustine, lomustine, amsacrine

Agents whose use occasionally causes myelosuppression

Chloramphenicol, gold compounds, arsenic, sulfonamides, mephenytoin, trimethadione, phenylbutazone, quinacrine, indomethacin, diclofenac, felbamate

TOXINS

Benzene, glue vapors

INFECTIONS

Non-A, non-B, non-C hepatitis, infectious mononucleosis, parvovirus infection (attacks erythroid precursors), HIV

MALIGNANT DISEASES

Hairy-cell leukemia, acute lymphocytic leukemia, acute myeloid leukemia (rarely), myelodysplastic syndromes

CLONAL DISORDERS

Paroxysmal nocturnal hemoglobinuria

IMMUNE-MEDIATED APLASIA

Eosinophilic fasciitis

INHERITED DISORDERS

Fanconi anemia

PREGNANCY

Chapter 204], or, in rare cases, acute myeloid leukemia. In addition, aplasia can develop in the course of myelodysplasia [*see Chapter 204*].

Diagnosis

The patient with aplastic anemia may seek medical attention because of fatigue and shortness of breath. Accompanying thrombocytopenia may cause petechiae, oral blood blisters, gingival bleeding, and hematuria depending on the level of the platelet count. By far the major problem associated with aplastic anemia is the recurrent bacterial infections caused by the profound neutropenia. Sepsis, pneumonia, and urinary tract infections are common among patients with aplastic anemia. Invasive fungal infections may cause death, especially in patients with severe neutropenia.

The diagnosis of aplastic anemia requires a marrow aspirate and biopsy [*see Figure 3*], as well as a thorough history of drug exposures, infections, and especially symptoms suggesting viral illnesses and serologic test results for hepatitis, infectious mononucleosis, HIV, and parvovirus [*see Figure 4*]. Measurement of red cell CD59 is helpful in the diagnosis of paroxysmal nocturnal hemoglobinuria.

It is also important to determine the severity of aplastic anemia [*see* Aplastic Anemia, Definition, *above*]. Severe cases are associated with a very low rate of spontaneous remission and a mortality of 70% within 1 year. In contrast, 80% of patients who have milder forms of aplastic anemia survive for 1 year.[24]

Differential Diagnosis

The differential diagnosis of pancytopenia includes chronic lymphocytic leukemia, systemic lupus erythematosus, and congestive splenomegaly. In these diseases, however, the marrow is not aplastic but rather shows hyperplasia of the involved cell lines. Other conditions that cause pancytopenia include hypoplastic myelodysplastic syndrome, acute leukemia, megaloblastosis, and large granular lymphocytic leukemia.[30]

Treatment of Mild Aplastic Anemia

Treatment of milder forms of aplastic anemia involves removing the offending agent and providing supportive therapy, primarily transfusion therapy, anticipating that the remaining pluripotent stem cells will repopulate the marrow.

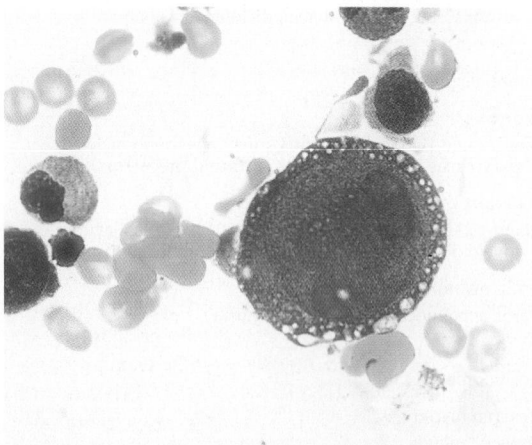

Figure 4   Giant pronormoblast, evident on this marrow smear, strongly suggests a diagnosis of parvovirus infection.

Supportive therapy   Thrombocytopenia is often a major problem associated with aplastic anemia. It should be managed by platelet transfusion as needed to control or prevent bleeding. Usually, a threshold of 10,000 platelets/μl is used for transfusion, but conservative treatment is best, and as few transfusions as possible are given. Extensive platelet replacement may result in allosensitization to platelets and may complicate future allogeneic bone marrow transplantation. Red blood cell transfusions are given as required to control the symptoms and signs of anemia.

Granulocyte colony-stimulating factor (G-CSF) and granulocyte-macrophage colony-stimulating factor (GM-CSF) have been given to patients to raise the absolute neutrophil count and help combat infection. They are usually ineffective when used alone, because of the severe deficiency in precursor cells, which are the target for the actions of G-CSF and GM-CSF.[31] It is generally preferable to proceed to definitive treatment: immuno-suppressive therapy or preferably allogeneic bone marrow transplantation if a matched sibling donor is available [*see Chapter 100*].[32]

Definitive therapy   Transplantation from a matched sibling after a preparative regimen of high-dose cyclophosphamide and antithymocyte globulin, together with the use of methotrexate and cyclosporine for GVHD prophylaxis, is a very effective regimen for patients with aplastic anemia. Current results suggest a cure rate greater than 90%.[33] Results with mismatched or unrelated matched donors are somewhat worse; therefore, patients with aplastic anemia who are without sibling donors are often given a trial of immunosuppressive therapy before transplantation.

Three forms of immunosuppression have been shown to produce partial remission in aplastic anemia.[31,32,34] Antithymocyte globulin (ATG) produced sustained remission in about half of the patients in a randomized trial.[32] High-dose corticosteroids improved blood counts in about 40% of treated patients, and cyclosporine was also shown to be beneficial.[32] (Androgens such as oxymetholone may have a role in the treatment of severe aplastic anemia but are not given alone.[31,34])

Although each of these agents can be used individually or consecutively in the treatment of aplastic anemia, a controlled study suggests that results are better when all three are used simultaneously.[31,32] The combination of ATG, a corticosteroid, and cyclosporine resulted in an actuarial survival of 62% at 36 months. The first signs of response occurred at about 4 weeks; the median time to remission was 60 to 82 days.[32] In this study, patient outcome was related to the quality of hematologic response. An 11-year follow-up report confirmed the effectiveness of the combination of ATG, corticosteroids, and cyclosporine. The relapse rate was 38%, and clonal or malignant diseases developed in 25% of patients.[35]

One recommendation, based on the usual availability of horse ATG in the United States,[31,32] is to administer horse ATG at a dosage of 40 mg/kg/day in 500 ml of saline for 4 days over a period of 4 to 5 hours through an I.V. line equipped with a microaggregate in-line filter. The toxic side effect of ATG is serum sickness, which can usually be controlled with corticosteroids. Prednisone (60 to 100 mg/day) is given orally in divided doses, or methylprednisolone (40 mg) is added to the infusion bottle, and the dose can be increased to 1 mg/kg/day. Corticosteroid therapy is adjusted to control serum sickness, but it can usually be tapered after 2 weeks and stopped after 30 days. Because ATG can lower platelet counts, platelet transfusions are given as needed to maintain the platelet count at more than 20,000 μl.

Cyclosporine (10 to 12 mg/kg/day) is given orally in two divided doses, with the aim of achieving whole blood trough levels of 500 to 800 ng/ml or a serum level of 100 to 200 ng/ml. After 29 days, the cyclosporine dosage can be tapered for a trough whole blood level of 200 to 500 ng/ml.[31,32] The cyclosporine is continued for at least 6 months. Cyclosporine can cause hypertension, renal toxicity, hypomagnesemia, vitiligo, tremors, hypertrichosis, susceptibility to *Pneumocystis carinii* pneumonia (PCP), and gingival hyperplasia.[31,32] In one study, 300 mg of aerosolized pentamidine was given every 4 weeks as PCP prophylaxis.[32]

In another study, G-CSF (5 μg/kg/day) was given subcutaneously for the first 90 days, along with I.V. methylprednisolone (2 mg/kg/day on days 1 through 5, followed by 1 mg/kg/day on days 6 through 10, and tapered off in 30 days), with good results.[36]

In contrast to patients who undergo allogeneic bone marrow transplantation, patients who respond to immunosuppressive therapy are not actually cured. Many of these patients continue to have moderate cytopenia[37]; 20% to 36% experience relapses of aplastic anemia,[31,32,37] and as many as 20% to 36% eventually develop clonal disorders, such as paroxysmal nocturnal hemoglobinuria, myelodysplastic syndrome, and acute leukemia.[31,32] Patients also are at increased risk for the development of solid tumors after treatment of aplastic anemia, but the risk is the same for patients who underwent immunosuppressive therapy as it is for those who underwent allogeneic bone marrow transplantation.[38] More than 50% of patients who have relapses of aplastic anemia after initially responding to immunosuppressive therapy may respond to a second course of therapy.[31,32] For unresponsive patients, a trial of rabbit ATG may work. The rabbit ATG (3.5 mg/kg/day diluted in saline and infused over 6 to 8 hours for 5 consecutive days)[39] is given along with cyclosporine (5 mg/kg/day p.o. on days 1 through 180, then tapered) and G-CSF (5 μg/kg/day on days 1 through 90).

An intriguing report concerns 10 patients with severe aplastic anemia who were treated with high-dose I.V. cyclophosphamide (45 mg/kg/day) for 4 consecutive days.[40] Some patients also received cyclosporine. Only one course of I.V. cyclophosphamide was given. Seven of 10 patients had a complete hematologic response, and six were still alive after a median follow-up of 10.8 years (range, 7.3 to 17.8 years). However, a trial comparing high-dose cyclophosphamide with ATG was ended early because of excessive cyclophosphamide-induced morbidity and mortality.[41] Therefore, the role of high-dose cyclophosphamide in the treatment of aplastic anemia needs extensive clarification.

Treatment of Severe Aplastic Anemia

The choice of appropriate therapy for patients with SAA is influenced by age and disease severity. The European Group for Blood and Marrow Transplantation reported on the results of immunosuppressive therapy in 810 patients subdivided into three age groups: younger than 49, 50 through 59, and older than 60. The 5-year survival rates for those with SAA were 86%, 72%, and 54%, respectively; for those with VSAA, the comparable rates were 49%, 40%, and 21%.[42] Older patients had more bleeding and infections.

Patients younger than 20 years Allogeneic bone marrow transplantation should be performed in patients younger than 20 years if a matched sibling donor is available. Although there

are risks, including chronic GVHD and organ dysfunction caused by the conditioning program,[31] 50% to 80% of patients may be cured; the incidence of later clonal disorders is very low.[34] Allogeneic bone marrow transplantation, along with conditioning programs consisting of cyclophosphamide and ATG, produced an actuarial survival rate of 69% after 15 years.[34] Patients younger than 20 years who do not have a matched sibling donor should consider transplantation from a matched unrelated donor. Allogeneic transplantation from a matched unrelated donor initially produced a 2-year survival rate of only 29% because of severe GVHD.[31] In a study of 15 patients who received unrelated-donor transplantations, all were reported alive at 2 to 86 months (mean follow-up, 51 months); only one patient developed extensive GVHD, and five (33%) developed moderate to acute GVHD. These results suggest that conditioning regimens that contain ATG and cyclophosphamide are improving the treatment outcomes for unrelated donor transplantation in this patient group.[43]

Patients between 20 and 45 years of age Patients between 20 and 45 years of age who are in excellent health and have a fully matched sibling donor may be able to tolerate GVHD and thus benefit from the curative potential of an allogeneic bone marrow transplant. Some experts propose that allogeneic bone marrow transplantation should be considered for patients in this age group,[34] particularly because newer conditioning programs seem to be capable of reducing the severity of GVHD.[31,44] In a study of 154 patients younger than 46 years who received allogeneic transplantation, the median survival was 29 months, and the probability of overall survival at 5 years was 56%.[45]

Patients older than 45 years Previously it was thought that the impact of GVHD was too severe for patients older than 45 years, and it was suggested that these patients receive immunosuppressive therapy.[31,34] However, conditioning programs containing ATG and cyclophosphamide seem to be more tolerable, and even heavily pretreated patients as old as 59 years have done well after allogeneic marrow transplantation.[46]

ACQUIRED PURE RED CELL APLASIA

Definition

In adults, pure red cell aplasia (PRCA) is an acquired disorder. The anemia is severe (hematocrit usually less than 20%), reticulocytopenia is profound (often 0%), the absolute reticulocyte count is usually less than 10,000/μl, and marrow erythroid precursors are virtually absent. Marrow myeloid and megakaryocytic elements are preserved, however, and the peripheral platelet and white blood cell counts are also normal.

Pathophysiology

In PRCA, erythropoiesis is thought to be inhibited primarily by immune mechanisms, including autoantibody-mediated and T cell–mediated suppression of erythroid progenitors, usually at a stage after the CFU-E stage of erythroid differentiation and before formation of proerythroblasts. T cells, particularly of the large granular lymphocyte (T-LGL) class, may be involved in the suppression of erythropoiesis, and in some cases, there is evidence that the suppression is caused by clonal T cells.[47] Autoantibody inhibition of erythropoietin has also been described, but it is quite uncommon.[48] Two other mechanisms probably cause

Table 3 Causes of Acquired Pure Red Cell Aplasia

Primary
Associated with thymoma in 10%–15% of cases[51]
Idiopathic causes

Secondary
Neoplasia: chronic lymphocytic leukemia, chronic myeloid leukemia, Hodgkin and non-Hodgkin lymphomas; large granular lymphocytic proliferative disorders; prodrome to myelodysplastic syndromes[51]
Systemic lupus erythematosus or rheumatoid arthritis
Associated with pregnancy
Associated with autoimmune hemolytic anemia
Drugs: those most commonly associated are phenytoin, chlorpropamide, zidovudine,[57] trimethoprim-sulfamethoxazole, isoniazid[51]
Multiple endocrine gland insufficiency
Primary amyloidosis
Infections: infectious mononucleosis, viral hepatitis, parvovirus infection, HIV[51]
ABO-incompatible bone marrow transplantation

PRCA: (1) a specific attack on erythroid precursors by the parvovirus B19 (one report indicated that 14% of cases were caused by this virus[49]) and (2) an underlying hematopoietic clonal abnormality that may be a prodrome to myelodysplastic syndrome.[48]

Etiology

PRCA may be caused by a variety of processes, including neoplasia, autoimmune disorders, drugs, and infections [see Table 3].

The association of PRCA with LGL proliferation and leukemia is increasingly being recognized.[30] The routine use of T cell receptor gene rearrangement studies in one series showed that nine of 14 patients had a clonal LGL disorder.[50] Presumably, these LGL cells directly mediate inhibition of erythropoiesis.[49,50] In perhaps as many as 20% of cases, PRCA may be a prodrome to the myelodysplastic syndromes or acute myeloid leukemia.[49,51]

Erythroblastopenia also occurs in a small percentage of patients with autoimmune hemolytic anemia [see Chapter 93] and may be caused by autoantibody attack on maturing normoblasts.

The treatment of HIV infection with zidovudine (AZT) produces, in virtually all patients, an anemia that is usually marked by significant macrocytosis.[52] Moderate erythroid hypoplasia is the usual cause of this anemia, which can progress to PRCA.

Parvovirus infection is the cause of the transient aplastic crises that occur in patients who have severe hemolytic disorders. The marrow in patients with such disorders must compensate for the peripheral hemolysis by increasing its production up to sevenfold and thus typically shows an intense erythroid hyperplasia. Although parvovirus can affect all precursor cells, the red cell precursors are the most profoundly affected.[49]

PRCA can complicate ABO-incompatible allogeneic bone marrow transplantation; the recipient's serum continues to express anti-A or anti-B isohemagglutinins against donor A or B antigen expressed on the surface of erythroid progenitors.[51] With PRCA of pregnancy, antibodies against BFU-E usually disappear after delivery, coinciding with clinical remission.[53]

Diagnosis

The patient with PRCA presents with symptoms characteristic of anemia—namely, weakness, fatigue, and shortness of breath. White blood cell and platelet counts are normal morphologically and functionally. A very low reticulocyte count—either a relative reticulocyte value of less than 0.2% or a very low absolute reticulocyte count of less than 10,000 μl—should prompt the physician to order a bone marrow aspirate. In a patient with PRCA, a bone marrow aspirate and biopsy typically show normal myelopoiesis, lymphopoiesis, and megakaryocytopoiesis; erythropoiesis is virtually absent. In the absence of any apparent cause of PRCA, four conditions must be considered: idiopathic PRCA, thymoma, hypoplastic myelodysplastic syndromes (MDS), and LGL leukemia. The workup to diagnose PRCA usually includes computed tomography of the chest to evaluate the possibility of thymoma, immunophenotypic analysis of circulating blood or marrow lymphocytes to identify LGL proliferation, marrow cytogenetics to evaluate the possibility of MDS, and antibody tests for parvovirus.[49] A diagnostic hallmark of parvovirus infection is the appearance of giant pronormoblasts in the marrow [see Figure 4]. The distinction between PRCA associated with the myelodysplastic syndromes and acute myeloid leukemia may be difficult to determine at the time of diagnosis unless a typical myelodysplastic cytogenetic abnormality is detected during a bone marrow examination.

Treatment

Two general principles of management in PRCA are transfusions for symptomatic anemia and cessation of possible offending drugs. No specific therapy is indicated in those forms of PRCA that are self-limited, such as pregnancy, ABO-incompatible bone marrow transplantation, and some cases of parvovirus infection.[51,53] Treatment of PRCA depends on the identified cause. If a thymoma is present, it should be removed surgically[52]; this procedure leads to patient improvement in about one third of such cases.[51] When surgery is impossible, one should consider a course of prednisone combined with octreotide, a somatostatin analogue that binds to thymomas and may inhibit the function of thymic immune cells.[54]

Treatment of other causes of PRCA is based on the supposition that the attack is immune mediated and therefore will respond to immunosuppressive therapy. Treatment can begin with the administration of 60 mg of oral prednisone daily in divided doses; this regimen should be continued for 1 to 3 months.[49] If a patient fails to respond, as indicated by a rise in the reticulocyte count, cyclophosphamide or azathioprine should be added at a dosage of 2 to 3 mg/kg/day orally. Patients with marrow cytogenetic abnormalities suggestive of myelodysplastic syndrome respond poorly.[49,50] Some patients who are refractory to other forms of therapy have responded well to I.V. IgG (0.4 g/kg/day for 5 days).[55]

Patients with LGL proliferation as the underlying cause respond well to cyclophosphamide.[50,56] Usually, low doses of cyclophosphamide (50 to 100 mg/day p.o.) for 3 to 6 months suffice to produce remission, which is sometimes associated with disappearance of LGL proliferation.[50,57] Patients who respond poorly usually respond to oral cyclosporine.[50,57] Cyclosporine (12 mg/kg/day) has been shown to produce responses of approximately 65%, even in patients who did not respond to corticosteroids, plasmapheresis, cyclophosphamide, or azathioprine therapy.[51,58]

For patients in whom parvovirus infection is the cause of PRCA, I.V. IgG works well; the standard dosage is 0.4 g/kg/day for 5 days.[49] For AIDS patients with parvovirus infection and PRCA, I.V. IgG may have to be continued.[57] Recovery from the transient crises of parvovirus infection occurs spontaneously in 1 to 2 weeks after onset of the infection.

ATG therapy for patients with refractory PRCA is similar to that for patients with aplastic anemia (40 mg/kg/day I.V. for 4 days).[51] Other drugs that have been used in refactory cases are azathioprine (2 to 3 mg/kg/day), antilymphocyte globulin, and anti-CD20 monoclonal antibody.[31] In very refractory cases, allogeneic bone marrow transplantation can be effective.[59]

Production Defects with Marrow Erythroid Hyperplasia and Ineffective Erythropoiesis

DEFINITION

Anemia with a low reticulocyte count may occur despite intense marrow erythroid hyperplasia. This paradoxic situation is the hallmark of ineffective erythropoiesis or intramedullary hemolysis. Generalized erythroid impairment may be present, or specific subpopulations of erythroid precursors may be involved. Some of these subpopulations escape death in the marrow, but their progeny are so severely damaged that they are rapidly removed from the circulation; this results in the clinical picture of peripheral hemolysis. Other signs of ineffective erythropoiesis include jaundice, a very high serum lactic dehydrogenase level, and 75% to 90% saturation of serum iron-binding capacity. The classic ferrokinetic picture shows rapid plasma iron clearance, which indicates intense erythroid precursor activity. The delivery of labeled red blood cells to the peripheral circulation, however, is dramatically reduced—a finding that suggests that the precursors are being destroyed by intramedullary hemolysis.

The differential diagnosis includes megaloblastic anemias, sideroblastic anemias, thalassemia [see Chapter 93], myelodysplastic syndromes [see Chapter 204], and agnogenic myeloid metaplasia [see Chapter 205].

MEGALOBLASTIC ANEMIAS

Etiology

Megaloblastic anemias are caused by cobalamin or folic acid deficiency, by drugs that interfere with the synthesis of DNA or with the absorption or metabolism of cobalamin, and by genetic disorders that interfere with DNA metabolism or with the absorption or distribution of cobalamin.

Pathophysiology

Megaloblastic erythropoiesis is characterized by defective DNA synthesis and arrest at the G_2 phase, with impaired maturation and a buildup of cells that do not synthesize DNA and that contain anomalous DNA. This condition leads to asynchronous maturation between the nucleus and cytoplasm.[60] RNA production and protein synthesis continue; thus, larger cells, or megaloblasts, are produced. Ineffective erythropoiesis results, and there is disagreement about the presence of increased apoptosis.[61,62] It is presumed that similar defects in DNA synthesis characterize the mucosal abnormalities of the stomach and tongue. In the granulocytic line, the presence of giant metamyelocytes represents ineffective granulopoiesis.[60]

The role of folic acid and cobalamin The interactions between folic acid and cobalamin are critical in the metabolism of single carbon units, mainly methylene and formyl analogues, which have a key role in the synthesis of DNA and purines [see Figure 5a].[63] There are two major coenzymes of cobalamin, adenosylcobalamin and methylcobalamin. Adenosylcobalamin is the coenzyme for methylmalonyl–coenzyme A mutase, which catalyzes a step in the catabolism of propionic acid [see Figure 5b].[63] Methylcobalamin is the coenzyme for methionine synthase, which functions as a methyltransferase in the reaction that converts 5-methyltetrahydrofolate (CH_3-THF_1) to tetrahydrofolate (THF_1) [see Figure 5a].[63] Cobalamin and folic acid [see Figure 6] combine in the methionine synthase reaction [see Figure 5a], in which the methyl group of CH_3-THF_1 is transferred to cobalamin to form methylcobalamin. Methylcobalamin then transfers its methyl group to homocysteine to form methionine. The monoglutamated THF_1, which is formed by this reaction, is polyglutamated by the enzyme folylpolyglutamate synthase, and a methylene group is added to it by the serine-glycine methyltransferase to form 5,10-methylene THF_n. 5,10-Methylene THF_n provides its methylene to convert deoxyuridylate to thymidylate, a key step in DNA synthesis. 5,10-Methylene THF_n can also be directly converted to CH_3-THF_1 by the enzyme 5,10-methylene tetrahydrofolate reductase, thereby making its methyl group available.

Formyl THF_n (also called leucovorin, folinic acid, or citrovorum factor) has an important role in purine synthesis and DNA metabolism. It can be generated by oxidation of 5,10-methylene THF_n or directly from THF_n by the enzyme formyl THF synthase, with methionine providing the formate group [see Figure 5a].[63] When cobalamin is deficient, CH_3-THF_1 cannot transfer its methyl group to cobalamin; therefore, THF_1 is not free to be polyglutamated by folylpolyglutamate synthase [see Figure 5a]. The polyglutamated form is required for synthesis of either 5,10-methylene THF_n or formyl THF_n; thus, DNA synthesis and purine synthesis are blocked. This hypothesis, the methylfolate trap hypothesis, is supported by the finding of increased levels of CH_3-THF_1 in the plasma of cobalamin-deficient patients. An alternative explanation is the formate starvation hypothesis, wherein cobalamin deficiency impairs methionine generation, which therefore cannot provide the methyl groups needed by the enzyme formyl THF_n synthase to produce formyl THF_n.

Other aspects of folic acid and cobalamin metabolism Neither folic acid nor cobalamin is produced by humans in adequate amounts; both must be absorbed from food. Cobalamin, in particular, is derived from microbial sources and is ingested in the form of meat or eggs.

Most of the dietary folic acid is in the polyglutamate form and is absorbed at the intestinal mucosa. Absorption of radioactively labeled folic acid approaches 80% of a 200 μg dose.[60,63] The serum folic acid level appears to be maintained by folic acid absorbed from food. Enterohepatic circulation of folic acid has been observed in which folic acid passing into the bile and small intestine is quantitatively reabsorbed. In an animal model, ethanol administration blocks the entry of folic acid into the bile. This effect could account, in part, for the sharp fall in the serum folic acid level seen 8 hours after alcohol consumption. A similar fall in serum folic acid level follows phenytoin ingestion. The daily requirement of cobalamin is about 1 μg, and the amount usually provided by the Western diet, which is rich in animal products, is about 5 to 15 μg.[64]

R proteins are a class of cobalamin-binding glycoproteins found in saliva and gastric juice; they are produced by granulocytes and other tissues. Intrinsic factor (IF) is a 45 kd glycopro-

a

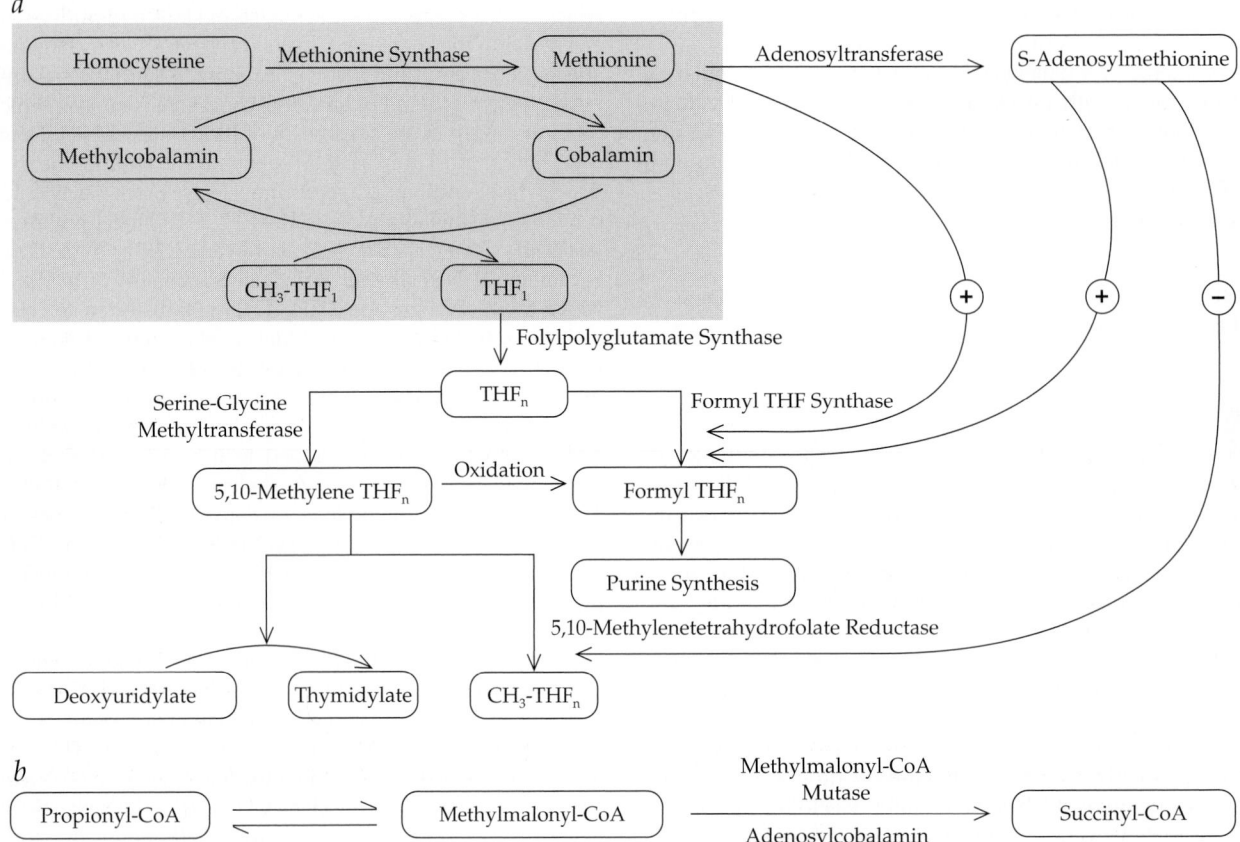

b

Figure 5 (*a*) Intracellular interdependent cofactor activity of cobalamin and folic acid is essential in DNA synthesis and metabolism.[63] (*b*) Adeno-sylcobalamin is a cofactor in the synthesis of succinyl–coenzyme A from methylmalonyl–coenzyme A.[63] (CoA—coenzyme A)

tein, secreted by gastric parietal cells, that is highly specific for unaltered cobalamin. The R protein–cobalamin complex does not bind to ileal receptors and thus is not absorbed. In the stomach, cobalamin binds preferentially to R proteins rather than to IF[60,63,64]; thus, it is the physiologically inactive R protein–cobalamin complex that is discharged into the duodenum. In the duodenum and small intestine, however, the pancreatic proteases along with pepsin degrade the R proteins, freeing cobalamin and allowing it to bind to IF. Thus, gastric atrophy and pancreatic insufficiency contribute to cobalamin malabsorption.[63,64] The IF-cobalamin complex, in the presence of Ca^{2+} and at a pH level greater than 5.4, binds specifically to a limited number of sites on the microvilli of mucosal cells in the terminal portion of the ileum, where absorption takes place [*see Figure 7*].[63,64]

In the plasma, most of the cobalamin is bound to the physiologically unimportant R proteins, transcobalamins I and III (TC-I and TC-III), which are about 70% saturated with cobalamin.[65] The physiologically important transport protein is transcobalamin II (TC-II), which has considerable specificity for cobalamin and is only 5% to 10% saturated with cobalamin. Receptors for the TC-II–cobalamin complex are present on many cell membranes. TC-II binds about 90% of a newly injected dose of cobalamin; and the complex is rapidly cleared, with a half-life of 6 to 9 minutes.[66,67] In persons with congenital TC-II deficiency, which results in severe megaloblastic anemia, both plasma cobalamin transport and cobalamin absorption are impaired. Impaired cobalamin absorption implies that TC-II has a role within the ileal enterocyte, where cobalamin is transferred from IF to TC-II.

The elevation of cobalamin levels seen in patients with chronic granulocytic leukemia or significant granulocytosis is caused by increases in TC-I and, to a lesser extent, TC-III, which are produced in granulocytes.

MEGALOBLASTIC ANEMIA CAUSED BY COBALAMIN DEFICIENCY (PERNICIOUS ANEMIA)

Pathophysiology

Cobalamin deficiency in pernicious anemia is thought to result from an autoimmune gastritis and an autoimmune attack on gastric intrinsic factor. There are two types of anti-IF antibodies: one of these antibodies blocks attachment of cobalamin to IF, and the other blocks attachment of the IF-cobalamin complex to ileal receptors.[66] Clinically, highly specific anti-IF antibodies are found in about 70% of patients with pernicious anemia. A second component of pernicious anemia is chronic atrophic gastritis that leads to a decline in IF production. The chronic atrophic gastritis in pernicious anemia is also associated with an increased risk of intestinal-type gastric cancer and of gastric carcinoid tumors.[67] Pernicious anemia occurs in association with other autoimmune disorders. In one study, autoimmune thyroid disorders were observed in 24% of 162 patients with pernicious anemia.[68]

Diagnosis

Clinical manifestations In addition to macrocytic and megaloblastic anemia, the patient with cobalamin deficiency

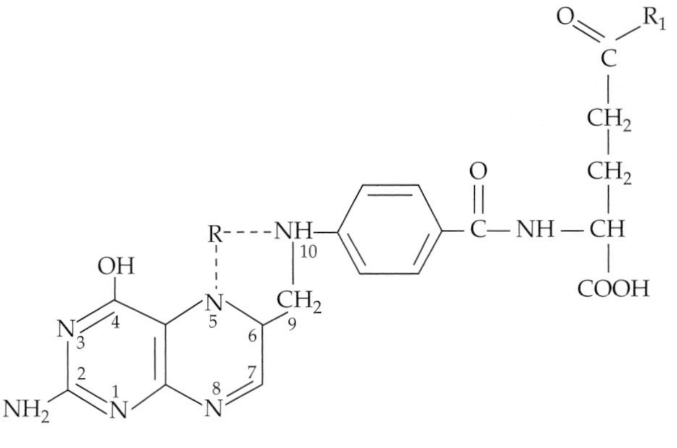

Figure 6 Folic acid functions as a coenzyme in single-carbon transfer reactions. It is not physiologically active until it is reduced at positions 5, 6, 7, and 8 to tetrahydrofolate (THF). Single-carbon groups (R) such as methyl analogues and formate are added at either position 5 or position 10, or they may bridge from 5 to 10, as shown. There may be several glutamates attached in sequence (R$_1$), which convert the monoglutamate to the polyglutamate form. Enzymes of the intestinal mucosa split polyglutamates back to monoglutamate, whereas liver enzymes add glutamate to tetrahydrofolate or to other reduced folic acids.

may present with weakness, lethargy, jaundice, and dementia, as well as atrophy of the lingual papillae and glossitis. Neuropathy is the presenting feature in about 12% of patients with cobalamin (vitamin B$_{12}$) deficiency without concomitant anemia.[69] Patients with severe cobalamin deficiency initially complain of paresthesia. The sense of touch and temperature sensitivity may be minimally impaired. Memory impairment and depression may be prominent.[69] The disease may progress, involving the dorsal columns, causing ataxia and weakness. The physical examination reveals a broad-base gait, Romberg sign, slowed reflexes, and loss of sense of position and feeling of vibration (especially when tested with a 256 Hz tuning fork). If the disorder is not detected and treated, the lateral columns become involved, resulting in weakness, spasticity, inability to walk, sustained clonus, hyperreflexia, and Babinski sign. Because the peripheral nerves, as well as the dorsal and lateral columns, are involved, these neurologic manifestations are sometimes termed subacute combined degeneration or subacute combined system disease.

Cobalamin deficiency appears to be the cause of various neuropsychiatric disorders, with such symptoms as paresthesia, ataxia, limb weakness, gait disturbance, memory defects, hallucinations, and personality and mood changes.[65] These symptoms, however, cannot be easily accounted for by the type of spinal cord lesions that occur in patients with cobalamin deficiency. Investigators have tried to determine whether a defect in methionine synthesis or an abnormality in propionic acid metabolism accounts for the neuropathy associated with cobalamin deficiency [see Figure 5b], but the exact mechanism remains obscure. Accruing evidence supports the impairment of methionine synthase as the cause of the neuropathy.[60,69] A study that measured various metabolites of cobalamin discovered that only high levels of plasma cysteine were predictive of neurologic dysfunction.[70]

Diagnostic workup The evaluation of suspected cobalamin deficiency generally proceeds in two stages: documenting the presence of the vitamin deficiency and determining its cause (e.g., pernicious anemia, malabsorption, dietary lack). The diagnosis can often be established by (1) measurement of the serum cobalamin concentration, (2) evaluation of specific metabolites, and (3) use of the Schilling test to establish malabsorption of cobalamin.

Macrocytosis (mean corpuscular volume [MCV] greater than 100 fl) is a hallmark of cobalamin deficiency, but it may be masked by concurrent disorders, such as iron deficiency. If macrocytocis is not apparent on examination of the peripheral smear, it is easily detected when red blood cell counts are made with an electronic particle counter. The peripheral smear shows macro-ovalocytes, fish-tailed red blood cells, hypersegmented neutrophils, and, occasionally, nucleated red blood cells [see Figure 2]. The finding that a single polymorphonuclear neutrophil has six lobes or that 5% of PMNs have five lobes constitutes strong evidence of megaloblastic anemia. In severe cases, granulocytopenia and thrombocytopenia are present. Examination of the bone marrow is usually not necessary, but if performed, it reveals megaloblastic erythroid hyperplasia and giant metamyelocytes.[60] If severe iron deficiency is concurrent with macrocytosis, the full morphologic expression of megaloblastosis is blocked, although the giant metamyelocytes in the marrow and hypersegmented PMNs in the peripheral blood will still be present.

Plasma cobalamin levels and red blood cell folic acid levels should be measured if the MCV is greater than 100 fl. If performed, a bone marrow aspirate and biopsy typically reveal

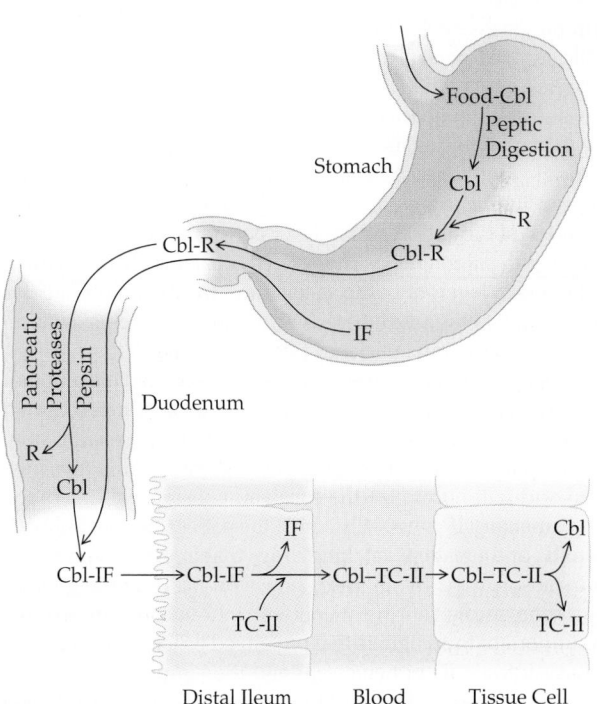

Figure 7 Cobalamin assimilation. Dietary cobalamin (Cbl) enters the stomach and binds to R protein. This physiologically inactive complex enters the duodenum. In the small intestine, pancreatic enzymes and pepsin digest the R protein, and Cbl binds to intrinsic factor (IF). The Cbl-IF complex passes through the intestine until it reaches receptors on the microvilli of mucosal cells in the distal ileum. The Cbl is then transferred to transcobalamin II (TC-II), which circulates in the blood until it binds to receptors on cells in the body and is internalized.

enormous megaloblastic erythroid hyperplasia with giant metamyelocytes.[60] The hypercellularity detected on bone marrow examination can be so dramatic and megaloblasts so immature that clinicians still sometimes make the erroneous diagnosis of leukemia.[60,71]

The standard approach to determining the cause of proven cobalamin deficiency has traditionally relied on the Schilling test, which is becoming difficult to order. The Schilling test measures the absorption of cobalamin labeled with cobalt-57 (^{57}Co). After 1 µg of radioactively labeled cobalamin is given orally, 1,000 µg of unlabeled cobalamin is given parenterally. The parenteral dose saturates transcobalamins I, II, and III, so that a significant portion of the absorbed material is flushed and excreted in the urine. If the amount of ^{57}Co-labeled cobalamin measured in an accurately collected 24-hour urine sample is less than 10% of the dose that was administered orally, cobalamin absorption is poor.

There are increasing numbers of reports of patients with proven pernicious anemia who have low or borderline serum cobalamin levels but normal Schilling test results. As the gastric atrophic lesion of pernicious anemia progresses, the ability to produce acid-pepsin is lost before all IF activity disappears. Thus, the ability to cleave the R protein–cobalamin complex, freeing cobalamin to bind to IF, is impaired. Coexisting infection with *Helicobacter pylori* may further impair production of acid-pepsin.[72] However, there may be sufficient IF to bind the free oral cobalamin administered in the Schilling test and therefore yield a normal value.

Malabsorption of cobalamin can be demonstrated by means of a food Schilling test, which is not available clinically. This test is performed with eggs from chickens that have been injected with radioactive cobalamin[73] and indicates whether there is insufficient acid-pepsin to split the cobalamin-enzyme complex and release free cobalamin to be bound by IF. If pernicious anemia is strongly suspected in a patient whose Schilling test result is apparently normal and whose plasma cobalamin is not diagnostically low, other steps should be taken to confirm the diagnosis, including examination of the blood cell morphology, measurement of the anti-IF antibody, or performance of a therapeutic trial with parenterally administered cobalamin. Measurement of the serum levels of homocysteine and methylmalonic acid is increasingly being used, because both are elevated as a consequence of cobalamin deficiency [*see Figures 5a and b*].[74]

If the initial Schilling test demonstrates reduced excretion of cobalamin, a second phase of the test may be conducted, aimed at correcting cobalamin absorption caused by pernicious anemia. In this phase of the test, supplementary oral IF is administered and will normalize the cobalamin absorption unless the supplementary IF is not fully active, the patient secretes antibodies to IF, or the patient is taking drugs that interfere with cobalamin absorption. In no case, however, will supplementary cobalamin be effective in patients with intestinal malabsorption. It is important to recognize that prolonged cobalamin deficiency impairs intestinal epithelial cells and thus impairs absorption. Therefore, the second stage of the test should only be performed after several weeks of cobalamin replacement therapy. If the result of the second stage of the Schilling test is abnormally low, this suggests the presence of generalized malabsorption, such as may occur in sprue, pancreatic insufficiency, or blind loop syndromes.

Factors affecting test results Concurrent α-thalassemia may minimize the macrocytosis of pernicious anemia.[75] This possibility should be considered particularly in patients of African descent, among whom there is a high incidence of α-thalassemia (about 30%). Anemia of chronic disease or anemia resulting from blood loss and iron deficiency can also reduce the degree of macrocytosis but will not affect the hypersegmentation of neutrophils. In one study, iron deficiency was discovered in 20% of 121 patients with pernicious anemia[76]; in another study, 19% of patients with pernicious anemia were not anemic, and 33% did not have macrocytosis.[77]

Falsely low serum cobalamin levels occur during pregnancy and in folic acid deficiency states.[74] In the past, a decline in the serum cobalamin level was usually not considered important unless the value was very low (i.e., < 150 pg/ml). It has become clear, however, that patients with serum cobalamin levels as high as 250 pg/ml and perhaps higher may have cobalamin deficiency.[73,77,78] Fortunately, the finding of macro-ovalocytes or hypersegmented PMNs on the peripheral smear remains a sensitive indicator for the presence of cobalamin deficiency.

Determining the underlying cause After the presence of macrocytosis and a reduced cobalamin level have been identified, the cause of these conditions must be determined. It is important to remember that macrocytosis can be caused by conditions other than pernicious anemia, including folic acid deficiency, liver disease, alcohol abuse, reticulocytosis, and ingestion of drugs such as antimetabolites, alkylating agents, and zidovudine.[52,75] Cobalamin deficiency can be caused by inadequate absorption resulting from gastric abnormalities (e.g., pernicious anemia, gastritis) and small bowel disease (e.g., tropical sprue, Crohn disease), and pancreatic insufficiency [*see Table 4*].

Gastric surgery in which the IF, pepsin, and acid-secreting components are removed often results in cobalamin deficiency (it occurred in 31% of patients in one study[79]). Patients who have undergone gastric surgery should be regularly screened by measurements of plasma cobalamin or homocysteine levels and supplemented with lifelong cobalamin therapy if the levels are low.[79]

Pancreatic insufficiency can result in malabsorption of cobalamin if the damaged pancreas does not produce enough trypsin and chymotrypsin for digesting the R protein–cobalamin complex and freeing the vitamin to form the complex with IF [*see Figure 7*] [*see Chapter 73*].

There are other causes of cobalamin deficiency. In vegetarians, especially vegans, profound nutritional megaloblastic anemia can develop as a result of very low cobalamin intake. Deficiencies of folic acid and iron have also been observed in vegans.[80] A careful patient history should indicate the possibility of inadequate dietary intake of cobalamin. Infants of vegan mothers can become severely cobalamin deficient, particularly when they are breast-fed.[65] Cobalamin deficiency is surprisingly common in less well developed countries where people are not strict vegans.[65] The incidence is particularly high in pregnant women and in preschool-age children.[65]

Treatment

Specific replacement should be started promptly after the diagnosis has been made and serum samples have been taken to determine cobalamin levels. Patients who have a low serum cobalamin level and macrocytic anemia should undergo a trial of parenteral cobalamin therapy. The diagnosis of cobalamin deficiency is confirmed if cobalamin therapy produces a reticulocytosis in 3 to 4 days that is associated with a rise in the hemoglobin level and a fall in the MCV.

Table 4 Causes of Cobalamin Deficiency

Inadequate Diet
  Strict vegetarianism

Inadequate Absorption
  Gastric abnormalities that produce deficient or defective
    intrinsic factor
    Pernicious anemia
    Total gastrectomy
    Gastritis
  Small bowel disease
    Ileal resection or bypass
    Blind loop syndrome with abnormal gut flora
    Malabsorption
    Tropical sprue
    Crohn disease
  Pancreatic insufficiency

Interference with Cobalamin Absorption
  Drugs
    Neomycin
    Biguanides
    Colchicine
    Ethanol
    Aminosalicylic acid
    Omeprazole
  Fish tapeworm competing for cobalamin

Degradation of Cobalamin Coenzymes
  N_2O anesthesia

Rare Congenital Disorders
  Transcobalamin II deficiency
  Defective intrinsic factor production

If the patient has symptoms of severe anemia, packed red blood cells can be transfused; the transfusion should be administered very slowly to avoid precipitating or aggravating congestive heart failure. This circumstance is one of the few in which a single-unit transfusion may be justified, because it may produce a 25% increase in oxygen-carrying capacity. A large dose of cobalamin should be given because the retention of parenterally administered cobalamin is poor but variable; the vitamin is inexpensive and has no harmful side effects. The reticulocyte response begins in 4 to 6 days, and the granulocyte count, if low, begins to increase at the same time. The hypersegmentation of PMNs disappears after 10 to 14 days, which suggests that in the megaloblastic anemias, granulopoiesis is affected by cobalamin deficiency at two different steps: (1) the lobe number of the PMNs is determined, and (2) granulocytes mature and leave the marrow.[55] Weekly dosages of 1,000 μg of parenteral cobalamin for 6 weeks should be followed by parenteral dosages of 1,000 μg monthly for life. The standard parenteral preparation is cyanocobalamin. For pancreatic insufficiency, cobalamin can be given parenterally or pancreatic enzymes can be administered orally. Specific therapy must be designed for patients with intestinal forms of malabsorption.

Because a small amount of cobalamin is absorbed even in the absence of IF and because only 1 μg/day is required, oral cobalamin has proved adequate for replacement in patients with pernicious anemia, freeing the patient from monthly injections (2,000 μg/day p.o. is recommended).[81]

MEGALOBLASTIC ANEMIA CAUSED BY FOLIC ACID DEFICIENCY

Diagnosis

Clinical manifestations The patient with folic acid deficiency has a clinical presentation that is distinct from that of the patient with cobalamin deficiency.[82] The patient may abuse alcohol or other drugs and have poor dietary intake of folic acid. Patients with folic acid deficiency are more often malnourished than those with cobalamin deficiency. The gastrointestinal symptoms in folic acid deficiency are similar to those in cobalamin deficiency but may be more severe than those in pernicious anemia. Diarrhea is often present. The hematologic manifestations of folic acid deficiency are the same as those of cobalamin deficiency: severe macrocytic anemia, a low absolute reticulocyte count, and a characteristic blood smear showing macro-ovalocytes, occasional megaloblasts, and hypersegmented neutrophils. Patients with megaloblastic anemia who do not have glossitis, a family history of pernicious anemia, or the neurologic features described for cobalamin deficiency may have folic acid deficiency.

Diagnostic workup A meticulous dietary history is important because food faddism, poor dietary intake, and alcoholism are the usual causes of severe folic acid deficiency [see Table 5]. Cobalamin and folic acid deficiencies frequently coexist and are not easily distinguished. In evaluating patients for folic acid deficiency, values for the levels of serum folic acid, serum cobalamin, and red blood cell folic acid must be obtained. The red blood cell folic acid level reflects tissue stores[83] but may be reduced in patients with severe cobalamin deficiency. In isolated cases, the serum folic acid level of cobalamin-deficient patients is usually normal or elevated. Severe, long-standing cobalamin deficiency leads to anorexia and GI disturbances, which may cause dietary folic acid deficiency. As a result, both serum cobalamin and folic acid levels are low, producing a double-deficiency state.

A serum folic acid level less than 2 ng/ml is consistent with folic acid deficiency, as is a red blood cell folic acid level less than 150 ng/ml. If the test results are inconclusive or if it is necessary to distinguish the megaloblastosis of folic acid deficiency from that of cobalamin deficiency, measurements of the serum methylmalonate and homocysteine levels are helpful. If both metabolite tests are normal (i.e., methylmalonate level of 70 to 270 nmol/L and total homocysteine level of 5 to 14 μmol/L), deficiency of both vitamins is ruled out. If the methylmalonate level is normal but the total homocysteine level is increased, folic acid deficiency is likely and investigation into the underlying cause is appropriate.[83]

Determining the underlying cause Folic acid deficiency is most frequently caused by poor dietary intake, but it may also result from inadequate absorption secondary to disease or drug administration [see Table 5]. Ingestion of ethanol by well-nourished individuals does not produce megaloblastosis, but in patients with borderline folic acid stores, ethanol can lower serum folic acid levels and block the reticulocyte response to folic acid administration. Alcohol may block release of folic acid from tissues to the serum.

Megaloblastic anemia occurring as a consequence of drug administration or pregnancy is likely to be caused by folic acid deficiency. Many of the antineoplastic and immunosuppressive agents produce megaloblastosis; these include fluorouracil, hy-

Table 5 Causes of Folic Acid Deficiency

Mechanism	Cause
Absolutely inadequate intake	Alcoholism Nutritional deficiencies
Relatively inadequate intake (resulting from increased folic acid requirements)	Pregnancy Severe hemolysis Chronic hemodialysis or peritoneal dialysis
Inadequate absorption	Tropical sprue Gluten-sensitive enteropathy (nontropical sprue) Crohn disease Lymphoma or amyloidosis of small bowel Diabetic enteropathy Intestinal resections or diversions
Drug-induced interference with folic acid metabolism	Action of dihydrofolate reductase blocked by methotrexate, trimethoprim, pyrimethamine Reduced folate absorption and tissue folate depletion caused by sulfasalazine Interference of unknown mechanism caused by phenytoin, ethanol, antituberculosis drugs, ?oral contraceptives

droxyurea, mercaptopurine, thioguanine, cytarabine, and aza-thioprine. In pregnant women, the presence of megaloblastosis may not be initially apparent. Because the combination of folic acid and iron deficiency is common, full expression of mega-loblastosis is often blocked, and the patient will have a dimor-phic anemia rather than the easily identifiable macro-ovalocyto-sis. Hypersegmentation of PMNs persists.[60,83]

An abnormality in folate metabolism can be caused by a chro-mosomal mutation, and women who are homozygous for this defect are thought to be at higher risk for pregnancies affected by neural tube defects. One of the enzymes that regulates homo-cysteine levels, 5,10-methylenetetrahydrofolate reductase has a genetic variant, C677T. Individuals homozygous for this variant have increased plasma homocysteine levels that are lowered by folate supplementation. About 5% to 10% of the general popula-tion are homozygous for this variant. Both pregnant and non-pregnant women who are homozygous for the C677T mutation have significantly lower red blood cell folic acid levels.[84] These women may be susceptible to cardiovascular disease and stroke and may bear children with neural tube defects.[84,85] It would be advisable to know before pregnancy that a woman is homozy-gous for this variant, and genetic testing would be helpful if a woman has a family history of this defect.

A number of intestinal disorders cause folic acid deficiency. These include severe pancreatic disease and small bowel dis-ease, including malabsorption, ileal disease, Crohn disease, re-section, and bypass [see Table 5]. When there is no apparent cause of cobalamin deficiency, it may be practical to suspect an undiagnosed disease of malabsorption. In one prospective study of patients who had laboratory-defined folate deficiency, 10.9% were positive for celiac disease antibodies and 4.7% had histologically confirmed celiac disease.[86]

Treatment

Standard therapy for folic acid deficiency is 1 mg/day orally. The response, manifested by reticulocytosis in 4 to 6 days, loss of megaloblastosis, and the return of normal blood counts, con-firms the diagnosis of folic acid deficiency. Neutrophil hyper-

segmentation disappears only after 10 to 14 days, however.[60] Pa-tients with megaloblastosis and severe bone marrow depression secondary to administration of drugs that block dihydrofolate reductase, such as pyrimethamine and methotrexate, may be treated with folinic acid. In the case of toxicity after single large doses of methotrexate, a single equivalent dose of I.M. folinic acid (i.e., milligram for milligram) will suffice. For toxicity after chronic pyrimethamine therapy, 1 to 5 mg of folinic acid daily can be given without blocking the antimalarial effects of pyrimethamine. Megaloblastosis caused by anticonvulsant ther-apy can be treated with 1 mg of folic acid daily. Supplementa-tion during pregnancy is advised and may also be useful for pa-tients who have severe chronic hemolysis.

In most patients (i.e., those who do not require a large amount of folic acid because of conditions such as hemolysis or pregnancy), a hematologic response occurs after administration of 200 µg of folic acid daily. The increased demand of folic acid during pregnancy requires administration of about 200 to 300 µg/day.[87] Furthermore, folic acid supplementation seems to pre-vent fetal neural tube defects.[88] Such neural tube defects may oc-cur in the embryo or very early in gestation—even before the pregnancy is confirmed.[89,90] Therefore, it is recommended that women of childbearing age or those who plan to become preg-nant receive about 400 µg of folic acid a day. Women who are homozygous for the C677T mutation should also take folic acid supplements. Staple foods such as flour and cereal grains can be fortified with folic acid. Concern has been expressed, however, that folic acid supplementation may mask the megaloblastosis of pernicious anemia, causing the development of severe neu-ropathy rather than anemia.[89]

SIDEROBLASTIC ANEMIAS

Definition

The sideroblastic anemias are a heterogeneous group of dis-orders characterized by anemia, ringed sideroblasts in the mar-row, and ineffective erythropoiesis.[91] There are hereditary and acquired forms; the latter are subdivided into benign and malig-nant variants. A fairly common form is the myelodysplastic syn-drome called refractory anemia with ringed sideroblasts. Other than alcohol and drugs (e.g., isoniazid), the secondary causes of these diseases remain largely unknown.

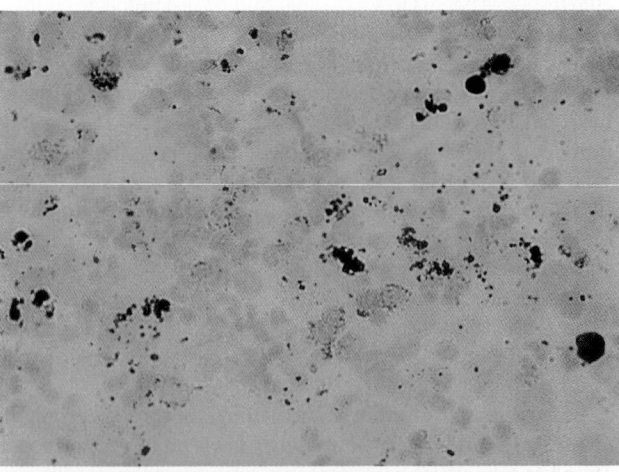

Figure 8 **Prussian blue stain shows ringed sideroblasts in the bone marrow of a patient who has idiopathic sideroblastic anemia.**

Table 6 Sideroblastic Anemias

Type	Disorders
Hereditary variant, probably benign	Sex-linked disorders, autosomal disorders
Acquired variant, probably benign	Mitochondrial DNA deletions (Pearson syndrome)
Probably benign variant	Induced by drugs (e.g., isoniazid or other antituberculosis drugs) or by lead intoxication; alcoholic sideroblastosis; pyridoxine-responsive anemia
Clonal disorder (myelodysplastic syndrome)	Refractory anemia with ringed sideroblasts, acquired idiopathic sideroblastic anemia

Pathophysiology

Abnormalities of heme synthesis are probably the most frequent cause of the hereditary sideroblastic anemias. Molecular defects of the enzyme 5-aminolevulinate synthase have been described as the cause of this abnormality.[90,92] This enzyme initiates the heme synthetic pathway, and its impairment profoundly affects heme synthesis. In other cases, there are major deletions in mitochondrial DNA. Iron enters erythroid precursors, but because heme synthesis is impaired, the iron cannot be incorporated into heme and accumulates on the cristae of mitochondria.[90]

Diagnosis

The principal feature common to all sideroblastic anemias is a refractory or progressive anemia. However, mild, lifelong anemia may go unnoticed. The diagnosis of sideroblastic anemia is established by reticulocytopenia; the red blood cells on smear are frequently profoundly hypochromic and microcytic, and distorted red blood cells and basophilic stippling may be noted.[93,94] Occasionally, Pappenheimer bodies (deposits of iron that stain with the Prussian blue reagent) are present in the red blood cells. There are ringed sideroblasts seen on the marrow aspirate (bone marrow normoblasts with heavy incrustations of nonferritin iron on the mitochondria) [see Figure 8]. Because of ineffective erythropoiesis, there is saturation of serum iron-binding capacity (usually approaching 80%) and elevation of the serum lactate dehydrogenase level. Cytogenetic study of the bone marrow may reveal one of the typical patterns seen in the myelodysplastic syndromes. The sideroblastic anemias can be classified into four groupings: hereditary (probably benign), acquired (probably benign), probably benign, and clonal disorder [see Table 6].

Treatment

For prognostic purposes, it is important to decide whether the patient has a benign or malignant form of sideroblastic anemia. It is also important to recognize reversible forms of sideroblastic anemia (e.g., those caused by alcoholism, folic acid deficiency, and drugs such as isoniazid and chloramphenicol) and to discontinue any potentially offending agents.

Indicators of myelodysplasia include granulocytopenia, thrombocytopenia, dysplastic marrow granulopoiesis, bilobed megakaryocytes, and typical cytogenetic abnormalities. In rare cases, patients have a reticulocyte and hemoglobin response to pyridoxine (200 to 600 mg/day), with or without folic acid.[95]

The author has served as a consultant for Tularik, Inc., and Receptron, Inc.

References

1. Means RT Jr, Krantz SB: Progress in understanding the pathogenesis of the anemia of chronic disease. Blood 80:1639, 1992
2. Cash JM, Sears DA: The anemia of chronic disease: spectrum of associated diseases in a series of unselected hospitalized patients. Am J Med 87:638, 1989
3. Means RT Jr: Pathogenesis of the anemia of chronic disease: a cytokine-mediated anemia. Stem Cells 13:32, 1995
4. Lacombe C: Resistance to erythropoietin. N Engl J Med 334:660, 1996
5. Voulgari PV, Kolios G, Papadopoulos GK, et al: Role of cytokines in the pathogenesis of anemia of chronic disease in rheumatoid arthritis. Clin Immunol 92:153, 1999
6. Ganz T: Hepcidin, a key regulator of iron metabolism and mediator of anemia of inflammation. Blood 102:783, 2003
7. Weiss G: Iron and anemia of chronic disease. Kidney Int 55(suppl 69):12, 1999
8. Pincus T, Olsen NJ, Russell IJ, et al: Multicenter study of recombinant human erythropoietin in correction of anemia in rheumatoid arthritis. Am J Med 89:161, 1990
9. Henry DH, Beall GN, Benson CA, et al: Recombinant human erythropoietin in the treatment of anemia associated with human immunodeficiency virus (HIV) infection and zidovudine therapy. Ann Intern Med 117:739, 1992
10. Dowlati A, R'Zik S, Fillet G, et al: Anaemia of lung cancer is due to impaired erythroid marrow response to erythropoietin stimulation as well as relative inadequacy of erythropoietin production. Br J Haematol 97:297, 1997
11. Schreiber S, Howaldt S, Schnoor M, et al: Recombinant erythropoietin for the treatment of anemia in inflammatory bowel disease. N Engl J Med 334:619, 1996
12. Ludwig H, Fritz E, Leitgeb C, et al: Prediction of response to erythropoietin treatment in chronic anemia of cancer. Blood 84:1056, 1994
13. Goodnough LT, Skikne B, Brugnara C: Erythropoietin, iron, and erythropoiesis. Blood 96:823, 2000
14. Allen DA, Breen C, Yaqoob MM, et al: Inhibition of CFU-E colony formation in uremic patients with inflammatory disease: role of IFN-γ and TNF-α. J Investig Med 47:204, 1999
15. Mladenovic J: Aluminum inhibits erythropoiesis in vitro. J Clin Invest 81:1661, 1988
16. Eschbach JW, Egrie JC, Downing MR, et al: Correction of the anemia of end-stage renal disease with recombinant human erythropoietin: results of a combined phase I and II clinical trial. N Engl J Med 316:73, 1987
17. Altmann P, Plowman D, Marsh F, et al: Aluminum chelation therapy in dialysis patients: evidence for inhibition of haemoglobin synthesis by low levels of aluminum. Lancet 1:1012, 1988
18. Coleman N, Herbert V: Hematologic complications of alcoholism: overview. Semin Hematol 17:164, 1980
19. Lindenbaum J: Folate and vitamin B₁₂ deficiencies in alcoholism. Semin Hematol 17:119, 1980
20. Latvala J, Parkkila S, Melkko J, et al: Acetaldehyde adducts in blood and bone marrow of patients with ethanol-induced erythrocyte abnormalities. Mol Med 7:401, 2001
21. Conrad ME, Barton JC: Anemia and iron kinetics in alcoholism. Semin Hematol 17:149, 1980
22. Baldwin JG Jr: Hematopoietic function in the elderly. Arch Intern Med 148:2544, 1988
23. Penninx BW, Guralnik JM, Onder G, et al: Anemia and decline in physical performance among older persons. Am J Med 115:104, 2003
24. Bacigalupo A, Hows J, Gluckman E, et al: Bone marrow transplantation (BMT) versus immunosuppression for the treatment of severe aplastic anaemia (SAA): a report of the EBMT SAA working party. Br J Haematol 70:177, 1988
25. Brown KE, Tisdale J, Barrett AJ, et al: Hepatitis-associated aplastic anemia. N Engl J Med 336:1059, 1997
26. Tzakis AG, Arditi M, Whitington PF, et al: Aplastic anemia complicating orthotopic liver transplantation for non-A, non-B hepatitis. N Engl J Med 319:393, 1988
27. Young NS: Autoimmunity and its treatment in aplastic anemia. Ann Intern Med 126:166, 1997
28. Young NS, Maciejewski J: The pathophysiology of acquired aplastic anemia. N Engl J Med 336:1365, 1997
29. Maciejewski JP, Selleri C, Sato T, et al: A severe and consistent deficit in marrow and circulating primitive hematopoietic cells (long-term culture-initiating cells) in acquired aplastic anemia. Blood 88:1983, 1996
30. Go RS, Lust JA, Phyliky RL: Aplastic anemia and pure red cell aplasia associated with large granular lymphocyte leukemia. Semin Hematol 40:196, 2003
31. Young NS: Aplastic anemia. Lancet 346:228, 1995
32. Rosenfeld SJ, Kimball J, Vining D, et al: Intensive immunosuppression with antithymocyte globulin and cyclosporine as treatment for severe acquired aplastic anemia. Blood 85:3058, 1995
33. Deeg HJ, Leisenring W, Storb R, et al: Long-term outcome after marrow transplantation for severe aplastic anemia. Blood 91:3637, 1998
34. Doney K, Leisenring W, Storb R, et al: Primary treatment of acquired aplastic anemia: outcomes with bone marrow transplantation and immunosuppressive therapy. Ann Intern Med 126:107, 1997
35. Frickhofen N, Heimpel H, Kaltwasser JP, et al: Antithymocyte globulin with or without cyclosporin A: 11-year follow-up of a randomized trial comparing treatments of aplastic anemia. Blood 101:1236, 2003
36. Bacigalupo A, Bruno B, Saracco P, et al: Antilymphocyte globulin, cyclosporine, prednisolone, and granulocyte colony-stimulating factor for severe aplastic anemia: an update of the GITMO/EBMT study on 100 patients. Blood 95:1931, 2000

37. Frickhoffen N, Kaltwasser JP, Schrezenmeier H, et al: Treatment of aplastic anemia with antilymphocyte globulin and methylprednisolone with or without cyclosporine. N Engl J Med 324:1297, 1991

38. Socié G, Henry-Amar M, Bacigalupo A, et al: Malignant tumors occurring after treatment of aplastic anemia. N Engl J Med 329:1152, 1993

39. Di Bona E, Rodeghiero B, Bruno A, et al: Rabbit antithymocyte globulin (r-ATG) plus cyclosporine and granulocyte colony stimulating factor is an effective treatment for aplastic anaemia patients unresponsive to a first course of intensive immunosuppressive therapy. Br J Haematol 107:330, 1999

40. Brodsky RW, Sensenbrenner LL, Jones RJ: Complete remission in severe aplastic anemia after high-dose cyclophosphamide without bone marrow transplantation. Blood 87: 491, 1996

41. Tisdale JF, Maciejewski JP, Nunez O, et al: Late complications following treatment for severe aplastic anemia (SAA) with high-dose cyclophosphamide (Cy): follow-up of a randomized trial. Blood 100:4668, 2002

42. Tichelli A, Socie G, Henry-Amar M, et al; Effectiveness of immunosuppressive therapy in older patients with aplastic anemia. Ann Intern Med 130:193, 1999

43. Kojima S, Inaba J, Yoshimi A, et al: Unrelated donor marrow transplantation in children with severe aplastic anaemia using cyclophosphamide, antithymocyte globulin and total body irradiation. Br J Haematol 114:706, 2001

44. Paquette RL, Tebyani N, Frane M, et al: Long-term outcome of aplastic anemia in adults treated with antithymocyte globulin: comparison with bone marrow transplantation. Blood 85:283, 1995

45. Kojima S, Matsuyama T, Kato S, et al: Outcome of 154 patients with severe aplastic anemia who received transplants from unrelated donors: the Japan Marrow Donor Program. Blood 100:799, 2002

46. Storb R, Blume KG, O'Donnel MR, et al: Cyclophosphamide and antithymocyte globulin to condition patients with aplastic anemia for allogeneic marrow transplantations: the experience in four centers. Biol Blood Marrow Transplant 7:39, 2001

47. Maung ZT, Norden J, Middleton PG, et al: Pure red cell aplasia: further evidence of T cell clonal disorder. Br J Haematol 87:189, 1994

48. Casadevall N, Dufuy E, Molho-Sabatier P, et al: Brief report: autoantibodies against erythropoietin in a patient with pure red-cell aplasia. N Engl J Med 334:630, 1996

49. Charles RJ, Sabo KM, Kidd PG, et al: The pathophysiology of pure red cell aplasia: implications for therapy. Blood 87:4831, 1996

50. Lacy MQ, Kurtin PJ, Tefferi A: Pure red cell aplasia: association with large granular lymphocyte leukemia and the prognostic value of cytogenetic abnormalities. Blood 87: 3000, 1996

51. Fisch P, Handgretinger R, Schaefer HE: Pure red cell aplasia. Br J Haematol 111:1010, 2000

52. Walker RE, Parker RI, Kovacs JA, et al: Anemia and erythropoiesis in patients with the acquired immunodeficiency syndrome (AIDS) and Kaposi sarcoma treated with zidovudine. Ann Intern Med 108:372, 1988

53. Baker RI, Manoharan A, De Luca E, et al: Pure red cell aplasia of pregnancy: a distinct clinical entity. Br J Haematol 85:619, 1993

54. Palmieri G, Lastoria S, Colao A, et al: Successful treatment of a patient with thymoma and pure red-cell aplasia with octreotide and prednisone. N Engl J Med 336:263, 1997

55. McGuire WA, Yang HH, Bruno E, et al: Treatment of antibody-mediated pure red-cell aplasia with high-dose intravenous gamma globulin. N Engl J Med 317:1004, 1987

56. Yamada O, Mizoguchi H, Oshimi K: Cyclophosphamide therapy for pure red cell aplasia associated with granular lymphocyte-proliferative disorders. Br J Haematol 97:392, 1997

57. Ramratnam B, Gollerkeri A, Schiffman FJ, et al: Management of persistent B19 parvovirus infection in AIDS. Br J Haematol 91:90, 1995

58. Means RT Jr, Dessypris EN, Krantz SB, et al: Treatment of refractory pure red cell aplasia with cyclosporine A: disappearance of IgG inhibitor associated with clinical response. Br J Haematol 78:114, 1991

59. Miller BU, Tichelli A, Passweg JR, et al: Successful treatment of refractory acquired pure red cell aplasia (PRCA) by allogeneic bone marrow transplantation. Bone Marrow Transplant 23:1205, 1999

60. Wickramasinghe S: Morphology biology and biochemistry of cobalamin- and folate-deficient bone marrow cells. Baillieres Clin Haematol 8:441, 1995

61. Koury MJ, Horne DW: Apoptosis mediates and thymidine prevents erythroblast destruction in folate deficiency anemia. Proc Natl Acad Sci USA 91:4067, 1994

62. Igram CF, Davidoff AN, Marais E, et al: Evaluation of DNA analysis for evidence of apoptosis in megaloblastic anaemia. Br J Haematol 96:576, 1997

63. Tefferi A, Pruthi RK: The biochemical basis of cobalamin deficiency. Mayo Clin Proc 69:181, 1994

64. Pruthi RK, Tefferi A: Pernicious anemia revisited. Mayo Clin Proc 69:144, 1994

65. Allen LH: Vitamin B_{12} metabolism and status during pregnancy, lactation and infancy. Adv Exp Med Biol 352:173, 1996

66. Guéant JL, Safi A, Aimone-Gastin I, et al: Autoantibodies in pernicious anemia type I patients recognize sequence 251-256 in human intrinsic factor. Proc Assoc Am Physicians 109:462, 1997

67. Hsing AW, Hansson L-E, McLaughlin JK, et al: Pernicious anemia and subsequent cancer. Cancer 71:745, 1993

68. Carmel R, Spencer CA: Clinical and subclinical thyroid disorders associated with pernicious anemia: observations on abnormal thyroid-stimulating hormone levels and on a possible association of blood group O with hyperthyroidism. Arch Intern Med 142:1465, 1982

69. Weir DG, Scott JM: The biochemical basis of the neuropathy in cobalamin deficiency. Baillieres Clin Haematol 8:479, 1995

70. Carmel R, Melnyk S, James SJ: Cobalamin deficiency with and without neurologic abnormalities: differences in homocysteine and methionine metabolism. Blood 101:3302, 2003

71. Dokal IS, Cox TM, Galton DAG: Vitamin B_{12} and folate deficiency presenting as leukaemia. BMJ 300:1263, 1990

72. Annibale B, Lahner E, Bordi C, et al: Role of *Helicobacter pylori* infection in pernicious anaemia. Dig Liver Dis 32:756, 2000

73. Carmel R, Sinow RM, Siegel ME, et al: Food cobalamin malabsorption occurs frequently in patients with unexplained low serum cobalamin levels. Arch Intern Med 148:1715, 1988

74. Dharmarajan TS, Adiga GU, Norkus EP: Vitamin B_{12} deficiency: recognizing subtle symptoms in older adults. Geriatrics 58:30, 2003

75. Chanarin I, Metz J: Diagnosis of cobalamin deficiency: the old and the new. Br J Haematol 97:695, 1997

76. Carmel R, Weiner JM, Johnson CS: Iron deficiency occurs frequently in patients with pernicious anemia. JAMA 257:1081, 1987

77. Carmel R: Pernicious anemia: the expected findings of very low serum cobalamin levels, anemia, and macrocytosis are often lacking. Arch Intern Med 148:1712, 1988

78. Green R: Screening for vitamin B_{12} deficiency: caveat emptor. Ann Intern Med 124: 509, 1996

79. Sumner AE, Chin MM, Abrahm JL, et al: Elevated methylmalonic acid and total homocysteine levels show high prevalence of vitamin B_{12} deficiency after gastric surgery. Ann Intern Med 124:469, 1996

80. Pippard MJ: Megaloblastic anaemia: geography and diagnosis. Lancet 334:6, 1994

81. Kuzminski AM, Del Giacco EJ, Allen RH, et al: Effective treatment of cobalamin deficiency with oral cobalamin. Blood 92:1191, 1998

82. Carmel R, Green R, Rosenblatt DS: Update on cobalamin, folate, and homocysteine. Hematology (Am Soc Hematol Educ Program) 62:2003

83. Amose RJ, Dawson DW, Fish DI, et al: Guidelines on the investigation and diagnosis of cobalamin and folate deficiencies. Clin Lab Haematol 16:101, 1994

84. Molloy AM, Daly S, Mills JL, et al: Thermolabile variant of 5,10-methylenetetrahydrofolate reductase associated with low red-cell folates: implications for folate intake recommendations. Lancet 349:1591, 1997

85. Wilcken DE: MTHFR 677CT mutation, folate intake, neural-tube defect, and risk of cardiovascular disease. Lancet 350:603, 1997

86. Howard MR, Turnbull AF, Morley P, et al: A prospective study of the prevalence of undiagnosed celiac disease in laboratory defined iron and folate deficiency. J Clin Pathol 55:754, 2002

87. McPartlin J, Halligan A, Scott JM, et al: Accelerated folate breakdown in pregnancy. Lancet 341:148, 1993

88. Wald NJ, Bower C: Folic acid, pernicious anaemia, and prevention of neural tube defects. Lancet 343:307, 1994

89. Carmel R: Subtle cobalamin deficiency. Ann Intern Med 124:338, 1996

90. Cotter PD, May A, Li L, et al: Four new mutations in the erythroid-specific 5-aminolevulinate synthase (ALAS2) gene causing X-linked sideroblastic anemia: increased pyridoxine responsiveness after removal of iron overload by phlebotomy and coinheritance of hereditary hemochromatosis. Blood 93:1757, 1999

91. Alcindor T, Bridges KR: Sideroblastic anaemias. Br J Haematol 116:733, 2002

92. Nakajima O, Takahashi S, Harigae H, et al: Heme deficiency in erythroid lineage causes differentiation arrest and cytoplasmic iron overload. EMBO J 18:6282, 1999

93. Bottomley SS, Healy HM, Brandenburg MA, et al: 5-Aminolevulinate synthase in sideroblastic anemias: mRNA and enzyme activity levels in bone marrow cells. Am J Hematol 41:76, 1992

94. Bottomley SS, May BK, Cox TC, et al: Molecular defects of erythroid 5-aminolevulinate synthase in X-linked sideroblastic anemia. J Bioenerg Biomembr 27:161, 1995

95. Cotter PD, May A, Fitzsimons EJ, et al: Late-onset X-linked sideroblastic anemia: missense mutations in the erythroid-aminolevulinate synthase (ALAS2) gene in two pyridoxine-responsive patients initially diagnosed with acquired refractory anemia and ringed sideroblasts. J Clin Invest 96:2090, 1995

Acknowledgments

Figures 1 and 6 Talar Agasyan.

Figure 5 Alan D. Iselin.

Figure 7 Tom Moore.

93 Hemoglobinopathies and Hemolytic Anemias

Stanley L. Schrier, M.D., F.A.C.P.

Alteration of the erythrocyte membrane usually signals the reticuloendothelial macrophages to remove the damaged red blood cell (RBC) from the circulation. In extraordinary circumstances, however, the damage to the membrane is so great that the erythrocyte undergoes hemolysis, and its intracellular contents, including hemoglobin, are liberated into the plasma. This chapter describes structural and functional features of normal erythrocytes and diseases involving membrane architecture, RBC proteins, and extracorpuscular factors that can lead to shortened RBC survival.

Development, Structure, and Physiology of the Erythrocyte

Erythroid precursor cells undergo four or five cell divisions in the bone marrow and then extrude their nuclei and become reticulocytes. As these enucleate cells mature, hemoglobin synthesis decreases. The cells lose most of their transferrin receptors and enter the peripheral blood; they survive in the circulation for about 4 months.

As they move through the circulation, erythrocytes must withstand severe mechanical and metabolic stresses, deform to traverse capillaries with diameters half their own, resist high shearing forces while moving across the cardiac valves, survive repeated episodes of stasis-induced acidemia and substrate depletion, and avoid removal by the macrophages of the reticuloendothelial system. They must also maintain an internal environment that protects hemoglobin from oxidative attack and sustain the optimum concentration of 2,3-bisphosphoglycerate (2,3-BPG) needed for hemoglobin function.

HEMOGLOBIN

The normal adult RBC contains three forms of hemoglobin (Hb): HbA (96%), HbA_2 (2% to 3%), and HbF (< 2%). Normal HbA ($\alpha_2\beta_2$) is composed of two α chains, coded by four genes on chromosome 16, and two β chains, coded on chromosome 11. HbA_2 is composed of two α chains and two δ chains ($\alpha_2\delta_2$), and fetal hemoglobin (HbF) is composed of two α chains and two γ chains ($\alpha_2\gamma_2$). The genes for the β, δ, and γ chains are closely linked to one another on chromosome 11. The extraordinarily high concentration of hemoglobin in the RBC—33 to 35 g/dl (the mean corpuscular hemoglobin concentration, or MCHC)—produces a viscous solution intracellularly.

NONHEMOGLOBIN CYTOSOL

Erythrocytes principally utilize glucose to maintain the reducing power that protects the cell against oxidative attack, to generate the 2,3-BPG required to modulate the function of hemoglobin, and to control the salt and thus the water content of the RBC by the actions of adenosine triphosphate (ATP) and the transport adenosine triphosphatases (ATPases) [*see Table 1*]. The water and the hemoglobin content of the RBC determine the mean corpuscular volume (MCV) and the MCHC.

PLASMA MEMBRANE

The RBC normally has a discoid shape with a diameter of 7 to 8 μm, an MCV of 85 to 90 femtoliters (fl) (1 fl = 10^{-15} L), and a surface area of 140 μm² [*see Figure 1*]. Its unique shape enables it to squeeze through capillaries as narrow as 3 μm in diameter.

Lipids (phospholipids and cholesterol) account for 50% of the weight of the surface membrane. The phospholipids are distributed asymmetrically in the membrane bilayer, with positively charged ones in the outer half and relatively negatively charged ones predominantly in the inner half. This asymmetry permits the selective intercalation of small charged molecules into either the outer or inner half of the bilayer, producing echinocytes or stomatocytes [*see Figure 1*].

The RBC membrane proteins include integral and peripheral proteins. Integral proteins interact with and span the hydrophobic phospholipid bilayer [*see Figure 2*]. The major integral proteins of the erythrocyte membrane are the glycophorins (which contain most of the membrane sialic acid and carry the MNSs blood group antigens) and band 3, which is the anion and bicarbonate transporter.

Table 1 Erythrocyte Metabolism

Pathway	Product	Functions of Metabolic Products
Glycolysis by Embden-Meyerhof pathway	ATP	Serves as a substrate for all kinase reactions, for the ATPase-linked sodium-potassium pump, for the ATPase-linked calcium efflux pump, and for other ATPases of the RBC membrane, including aminophospholipid translocase Maintains deformable state of RBC membrane
	2,3-DPG	Interacts with deoxyhemoglobin, shifting equilibrium to favor unloading of O_2 from oxyhemoglobin Acts as an intracellular anion that cannot cross the RBC membrane
	NADH	Acts as a substrate for a methemoglobin reductase, enabling it to reduce methemoglobin (Fe^{3+}) to hemoglobin (Fe^{2+})
Pentose phosphate pathway (hexose monophosphate shunt)	NADPH	Serves as a substrate for another methemoglobin reductase in methemoglobin reduction (a fail-safe mechanism) Serves as a coenzyme for glutathione reductase in reduction of oxidized glutathione; reduced glutathione (GSH) protects RBC against oxidative denaturation

ATP—adenosine triphosphate   2,3-DPG—2,3-diphosphoglycerate   NADH—reduced nicotinamide-adenine dinucleotide   NADPH—reduced nicotinamide-adenine dinucleotide phosphate

1107

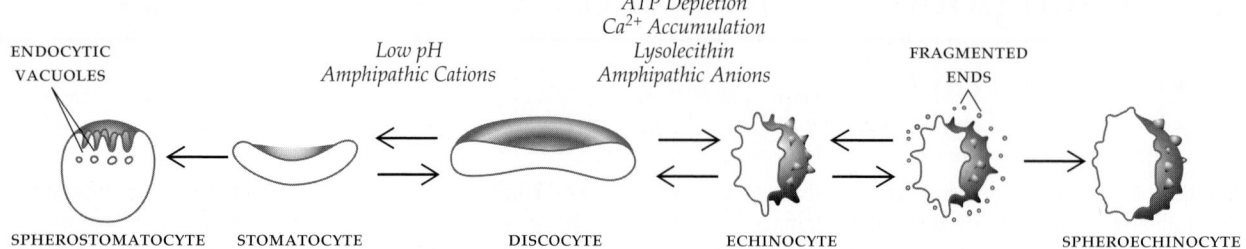

Figure 1   The normal erythrocyte, or discocyte, undergoes shape changes in response to conditions created by treatment with certain agents. Most changes are reversible if inducing agents are removed before the permanent loss of membrane material.

The peripheral proteins are all found at the cytosol face of the membrane. The interaction of these peripheral proteins, which include spectrin and actin, results in the tough but resilient cytoskeleton of the erythrocyte. The peripheral cytoskeleton, in turn, is connected to the integral proteins [*see Figure 2*].[1,2]

The membrane carbohydrates contribute to the external negative charge of the membrane and function partly as blood group antigens. Some of these glycolipids associate with phosphatidylinositol to form a glycolipid anchor, called the glycosylphosphatidylinositol (GPI) anchor. These GPI anchors provide the membrane-anchoring site for several classes of proteins that have important biologic functions at membrane surfaces, including several that serve to control complement action [*see Paroxysmal Nocturnal Hemoglobinuria, below*].[3]

CONTROL OF HYDRATION AND VOLUME

Control of RBC volume has considerable pathophysiologic importance because the water and cation contents of RBCs determine intracellular viscosity and the ratio of surface area to volume. The Na^+ and K^+ content is determined by passive diffusion and by active transport, primarily through Na^+,K^+-ATPase. The major intracellular anion is Cl^-, which enters the RBC with high permeability through band 3. The K^+-Cl^- cotransporter drives the K^+-Cl^- gradient and is activated by RBC swelling and low intracellular pH, causing a net loss of K^+ and Cl^-. The Ca^{2+}-ATPase actively pumps Ca^{2+} out of the RBC, making the free cytosolic Ca^{2+} content less than 0.1 μM—four orders of magnitude lower than the plasma concentration of 1 mM. The Gardos channel, which is a Ca^{2+}-activated K^+ efflux channel, plays an important role in volume regulation. Water enters and exits through a water channel called CHIP 28 (28 kd channel-forming integral membrane protein) or aquaporin. Other important intracellular anions are 2,3-BPG and hemoglobin, neither of which penetrates the cell membrane. When the concentration of free cytosolic Ca^{2+} rises to levels even as low as 0.3 μM, the channel is activated and results in a net loss of K^+. If such a loss is not corrected, the affected RBC becomes dehydrated.[4]

SHAPE CHANGES

ATP depletion, calcium ion accumulation, or treatment with lysolecithin or with anionic amphipathic compounds transforms the normal erythrocyte, or discocyte, into an echinocyte—a crenated spiculated cell sometimes called a burr cell [*see Figure 1*]. Calcium, acting either alone or in concert with the calcium-binding protein calmodulin, can effect the echinocytic shape change. If the echinocytic process persists, fragmentation or budding of the tips of the echinocyte leads to loss of membrane components, particularly of band 3 and phospholipids. This results in loss of surface area, a reduction in the ratio of surface area to volume, and the formation of poorly deformable spheroechinocytes.

PRINCIPLES OF BLOOD FLOW

The major determinants of blood flow are the hematocrit; the plasma concentration of proteins such as fibrinogen and immunoglobulins, which influence the degree of rouleau formation or aggregation; RBC deformability; the caliber of blood vessels; and the shear rate (the ratio of flow rate to tube radius). At the low shear rates that exist in postcapillary venules, the RBCs tend to clump in asymmetrical masses, with a consequent increase in blood viscosity and resistance to flow.

CELL AGING AND DEATH

In the bone marrow, the developing reticulocyte progressively loses its residual RNA over a 4-day period after nuclear extrusion. At the conclusion of this stage, the reticulocyte can no longer engage in protein synthesis. The active K^+-Cl^- cotransporter functions to reduce cell volume. With the membrane protein assembly complete, the resulting mature cell enters the circulation and survives for a period of 100 to 120 days.[5] Erythrocyte death is an age-dependent phenomenon and may be related to mechanical and chemical stresses the cell encounters in the circulation. As the erythrocyte ages, it loses water and its surface area diminishes. The ratio of surface area to volume decreases and the mean corpuscular hemoglobin concentration increases, impairing cell deformability. In addition, decreased enzymatic activity lowers the cell's ability to withstand metabolic stress. Aging may be manifested by changes at the erythrocyte's surface, such as a decrease in the density or type of surface charge or the appearance of a senescence neoantigen, perhaps oxidatively clustered band 3 [*see Figure 2*], that binds specific immunoglobulins and complement components.[6] By such changes, the age-worn erythrocyte signals its incapacity to the reticuloendothelial system, triggering removal by macrophages.

Under physiologic conditions, slightly less than 1% of the RBCs are destroyed each day and are replaced by a virtually identical number of new cells. For a 70 kg (154 lb) man with a blood volume of about 5 L, about 50 ml of whole blood, containing approximately 22 ml of packed erythrocytes, is destroyed and replaced each day. Inasmuch as one third of each erythrocyte is hemoglobin, the replacement of these cells requires the synthesis of about 7 g of hemoglobin each day. Normal adult bone marrow can readily increase its erythroid output fivefold. After extensive and prolonged anemic stress, erythroid production can be raised by as much as seven or eight times. The supply of iron, however, places an important limit on RBC replacement: three fourths of the iron used in the synthesis of cells in a day comes from cells that were destroyed on the previous day.

General Features of Hemolytic Anemias

The severity of anemia is determined both by the rate of RBC destruction and by the marrow's capacity to increase erythroid production. When a person has a healthy marrow, erythrocyte survival time can be reduced from 120 days to 20 days without inducing anemia or jaundice; however, a substantial reticulocytosis will be present in such cases.

Most forms of hemolysis are extravascular; the damaged cell signals its changed status to the reticuloendothelial system via its membrane and is removed. In unusual circumstances in which damage to the erythrocyte is devastating—as in some forms of complement-mediated lysis—or in circumstances in which the reticuloendothelial system cannot cope with the burden of damaged cells, intravascular lysis develops and leads to hemoglobinemia.

Hemoglobin released to the plasma is degraded to αβ dimers, which bind to haptoglobin. The hemoglobin-haptoglobin complexes are removed by the reticuloendothelial system. When the haptoglobin-binding capacity is exceeded, αβ dimers pass into the glomerular filtrate. Some of the αβ dimers are excreted into the urine directly, producing hemoglobinuria, whereas others are taken up by renal tubule cells. Iron-containing renal tubule cells may be excreted for several days after an episode of intravascular hemolysis. Hemosiderinuria can be identified with Prussian blue stain. Free plasma hemoglobin can dissociate into globin and hemin. Hemin may bind to hemopexin and may reach the renal tubule cells in that form, or it may bind to plasma albumin, producing methemalbuminemia.

Intravascular hemolysis may produce severe anemia acutely. In addition, erythrocytic membrane particles released into the plasma may act as potent stimuli for disseminated intravascular coagulation. Acute severe hemolysis is also a cause of acute renal failure [see Chapter 165]. When a patient compensating for a marked increase in hemolysis has an infection that sharply im-pairs marrow erythroid activity,[7] the hemoglobin level may fall dramatically—a condition called aplastic crisis. With chronic hemolysis, pigment stones often develop in the gallbladder.

Causes of hemolysis may be classified as either extracorpuscular or intracorpuscular. The intracorpuscular causes, which are essentially erythrocyte defects, comprise membrane abnormalities, metabolic disturbances, and disorders of hemoglobin structure or biosynthesis. Extracorpuscular causes represent abnormal elements within the vascular bed that attack and destroy normal erythrocytes. Because erythrocytes with intracorpuscular defects that cause hemolysis are intrinsically abnormal, when they are transfused into normal recipients, their survival time is characteristically short. Of the intracorpuscular defects, only one disorder, paroxysmal nocturnal hemoglobinuria, is not hereditary.

Erythrocyte Membrane Defects

DISORDERS OF SALT AND WATER METABOLISM

Hydrocytosis (Hereditary Stomatocytosis)

Hydrocytosis is a hereditary disorder that usually presents early in life as partly compensated hemolytic anemia; occasionally, the spleen is palpable. The MCV is usually elevated. The peripheral smear shows stomatocytes [see Figure 3]. Passive flux of both Na+ and K+ increases greatly. The Na+,K+-ATPase is overwhelmed; the cation concentration and thus the water content of the RBC increase, accounting for the increase in MCV and the decrease in the ratio of surface area to volume. Stomatocytes appear to adhere more avidly than normal RBCs, a finding that may account for the reported increase in thromboembolic events.[8] Perhaps more importantly, the number of RBCs with phosphatidylserine exposed on the outer membrane surface is increased. Phosphatidylserine—a relatively negatively charged

Figure 2 Band 3, the anion transport channel (orange), and the other integral proteins glycophorin A (not shown), glycophorin B (not shown), and glycophorin C (green) span the red cell membrane. Branching external carbohydrate side chains are attached to these proteins. The hydrophilic, polar heads of the phospholipid molecules that make up the bilayer are oriented toward the cell surface, whereas the hydrophobic fatty acid side chains are directed toward the interior of the bilayer. Cholesterol is intercalated between the fatty acid chains. Band 3 binds hemoglobin and glyceraldehyde-3-phosphate dehydrogenase on its cytosol surface. Spectrin (yellow), actin (red), tropomyosin (blue), and band 4.1 (light green) form a latticework on the inner membrane surface. The spectrin heterodimers associate to form heterotetramers. The lower figure depicts the hexagonal cytoskeletal lattice on the inner membrane surface. Band 2.1 (ankyrin) links the integral protein band 3 to the peripheral cytoskeleton through the β chain of spectrin. Additional linkage is provided by glycophorin C and band 4.1.

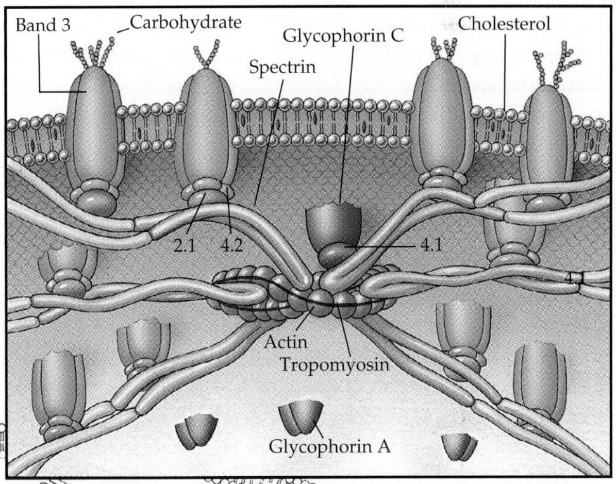

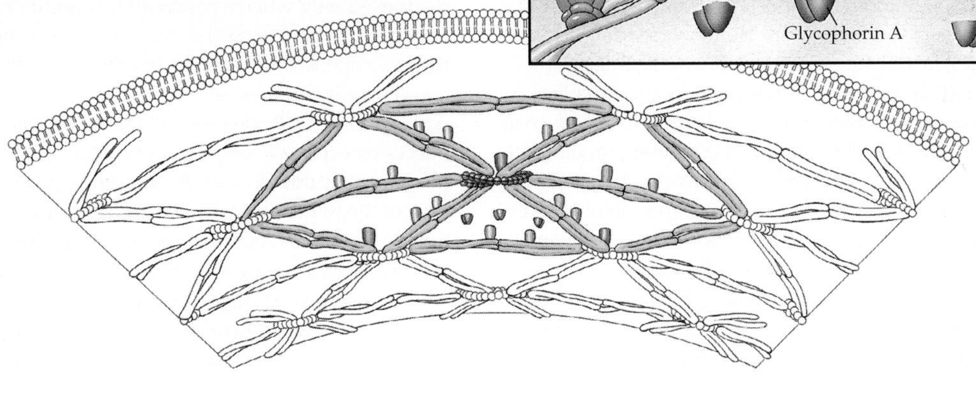

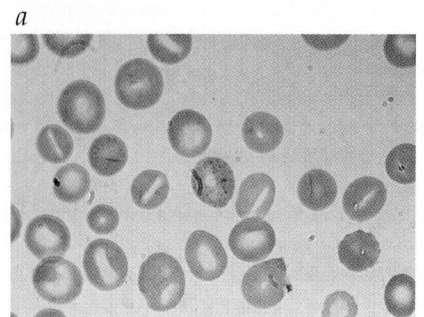 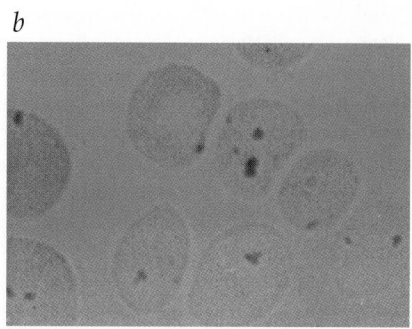 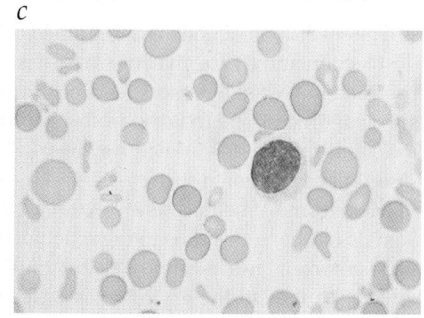

Figure 3 Stomatocytes are identified by slitlike areas of central pallor (*a*); the smear also shows microspherocytes, which are a more advanced stage of stomatocytosis. On scanning electron microscopy or examination of wet preparations, the microspherocytes are shown to be stomatocytes. Microspherocytes are seen in hereditary spherocytosis and in autoimmune hemolytic anemia, as well as in other conditions characterized by relatively selective loss of membrane material or increase in cell volume. Supravital stain of erythrocytes (*b*) shows single and multiple blue-staining Heinz bodies within counterstained erythrocytes. Phase microscopy can also be used to demonstrate Heinz bodies. Elliptocytes are visualized in a smear from a patient with hereditary elliptocytosis (*c*).

phospholipid that is normally found predominantly in the inner membrane layer—provides a nidus for thrombin formation and thus may also contribute to the tendency to thrombosis.[9] Splenectomy may lead to improvement in the anemia. Other therapies may eventually prove useful; vaso-occlusive events were controlled in one patient by long-term RBC transfusion and in another by therapy with pentoxifylline.[8]

Xerocytosis

Xerocytosis, another hereditary hemolytic disorder, is characterized by a membrane defect that leads to loss of cations, particularly K^+. Dehydration of erythrocytes occurs because the K^+ leak exceeds the Na^+ influx, possibly as a result of an overactive K^+-Cl^- cotransporter. Patients present with variably compensated hemolysis. Splenomegaly is not a prominent feature. The peripheral smear is variable, showing target cells, stomatocytes, echinocytes, or so-called hemoglobin puddling (i.e., hemoglobin collected around the circumference of the cell). MCHC is increased. Because these rigid cells are removed in many parts of the reticuloendothelial system, splenectomy is of little benefit.[10] In rare instances, xerocytosis can cause nonimmune hydrops fetalis.[11]

PROTEIN ABNORMALITIES

Hereditary Elliptocytosis

There are perhaps 250 to 500 cases of hereditary elliptocytosis per million population.[10] Three morphologic variants are seen: (1) common hereditary elliptocytosis, (2) spherocytic hereditary elliptocytosis, and (3) stomatocytic hereditary elliptocytosis.[12] Most patients with common hereditary elliptocytosis are heterozygous for this autosomal dominant disorder and have only elliptical RBCs or, at worst, compensated hemolysis. Homozygotes for the disorder may have severe uncompensated hemolytic anemia.

Under applied shear stress, erythrocytes assume an elliptical shape; when the stress is removed, the cell normally recoils to its discoid shape. It has been hypothesized that membrane defects in hereditary elliptocytosis interfere with normal recoil. The membrane defect appears to be a lesion in the membrane cytoskeleton; RBC membranes from patients with hereditary elliptocytosis are almost invariably mechanically fragile.

The diagnosis is made in patients with extravascular intracorpuscular hemolysis who have elliptocytes on the peripheral smear. Elliptocytosis can also be seen in severe iron deficiency,

myeloproliferative and myelodysplastic disorders, and, occasionally, cobalamin and folate deficiencies.[12] Results of the osmotic fragility test are usually normal. Splenectomy has been useful in patients with severe common hereditary elliptocytosis.

Hereditary Propoikilocytosis

The syndrome of hereditary (autosomal recessive) pyropoikilocytosis, a variant of hereditary elliptocytosis, causes severe hemolysis in young children. It is caused by an abnormal α or β spectrin mutation. The blood smear shows extreme microcytosis and extraordinary variation in the size and shape of erythrocytes [*see Figure 3*]. Splenectomy may reduce the rate of hemolysis.

Hereditary Spherocytosis

Hereditary spherocytosis is usually inherited as an autosomal dominant trait and affects about 220 per million people worldwide. A rare autosomal recessive variant of hereditary spherocytosis has been described.

Because of a loss of surface membrane, RBCs assume a microspherocytic shape and thus cannot deform sufficiently to pass through the splenic vasculature; splenic trapping of RBCs, hemolysis, and a compensatory increase in RBC production result. The underlying membrane defects lead to budding of membrane vesicles under conditions of metabolic depletion. These membrane vesicles are enriched in phospholipids from the bilayer, as well as in associated transmembrane proteins [*see Figure 2*]. The underlying molecular lesions appear to consist of deficiencies of spectrin, spectrin-ankyrin, band 3, and band 4.2 (palladin).[12,13]

About 25% of patients with hereditary spherocytosis have completely compensated hemolysis without anemia; their disorder is diagnosed only when a concomitant condition, such as infection or pregnancy, increases the rate of hemolysis or reduces the marrow's compensatory capacity. In other patients, mild anemia, pigmented gallstones, leg ulcers, and splenic rupture may develop. Aplastic crises may be precipitated by ordinary respiratory tract infections, especially by parvovirus infection.[7] It is important to remember that this disease can become apparent during the first year of life, when increased splenic maturation resulting in RBC removal combined with a sluggish erythropoietic response can result in anemia severe enough to require RBC transfusion.[14]

This diagnosis is suggested by a predominance of microspherocytes on the peripheral smear [*see Figure 3b*], an MCHC of 35 g/dl or greater, reticulocytosis, mild jaundice, splenomegaly, and a positive family history, although at least half of newly diagnosed patients have no family history. Confirmation of the diagnosis is made by a 24-hour incubated osmotic fragility test. A negative Coombs test and a family history positive for hereditary spherocytosis rule against a diagnosis of acquired autoimmune hemolytic anemia. Splenectomy eradicates clinical manifestations of the disorder, including aplastic crises.

PAROXYSMAL NOCTURNAL HEMOGLOBINURIA

Paroxysmal nocturnal hemoglobinuria (PNH) is a somatic clonal disorder of hematopoietic stem cells. PNH involves the *PIG-A* gene, which maps to the short arm of the X chromosome.[15] The mutation results in a deficiency of the membrane-anchoring protein phosphatidylinositol glycan class A; the resulting mature hematopoietic cells are usually chimeric. Normal human erythrocytes, and probably platelets and neutrophils, modulate complement attack by at least three GPI membrane-bound proteins: DAF (CD55), C8-binding protein (C8BP), and MIRL (CD59). In the absence of the GPI anchor, all of the proteins that use this membrane anchor will be variably deficient in the blood cells of persons with PNH.[16] Because the defective synthesis of GPI affects all hematopoietic cells, patients with PNH may have variable degrees of anemia, neutropenia, or thrombocytopenia, or they may have complete bone marrow failure.[17]

Diagnosis

Classically, acute episodes of intravascular hemolysis are superimposed on a background of chronic hemolysis. The patient typically notes hemoglobinuria on voiding after sleep.[18,19] Recurrent venous occlusions lead to pulmonary embolism and hepatic and mesenteric vein thrombosis, possibly resulting from release of procoagulant microparticles derived from platelets.[20] A literature review found that thrombotic events accounted for 22% of deaths in patients with PNH.[21] Occasionally, PNH patients with thrombosis are mistakenly thought to have psychosomatic disorders because they complain of recurrent severe pain in the abdomen and back that has no obvious cause. In these cases, the associated anemia and hemolysis may be very mild, and episodes of hemolysis do not necessarily correlate with bouts of pain.

A diagnosis of PNH should be considered in any patient with chronic or episodic hemolysis. The diagnosis should also be considered for patients with recurrent venous thromboembolism, particularly if the thrombus occurs in a site such as the inferior vena cava or the portal mesenteric system or if it produces Budd-Chiari syndrome. Evidence of intravascular hemolysis, such as hemoglobinemia; reduced serum haptoglobin; increased serum methemalbumin; hemoglobinuria; or hemosiderinuria, suggests the diagnosis. The combination of marrow hypoplasia and hemolysis is an important clue. PNH may occur in association with aplastic anemia. Erythrocyte morphology is usually normal. Diagnosis is made by specific tests based on fluorescence-activated cell sorter analysis using antibodies that quantitatively assess DAF (CD55) and particularly MIRL (CD59) on the erythrocyte or on the leukocyte surface.[22]

Treatment

In PNH, the anemia is occasionally so severe (hemoglobin level < 8 g/dl) that the patient needs transfusions regularly[19]; therefore, the choice of transfusion component is critical. It is believed that infusion of blood products containing complement may enhance hemolysis. Infusion of donor white blood cells (WBCs), which are ordinarily present in a unit of packed RBCs, into an HLA-immunized recipient may provide the antigen-antibody reaction that activates complement by the classical pathway. In such a case, the use of special leukocyte-poor units may be helpful [see Chapter 100].

A trial of prednisone (e.g., 60 mg a day with rapid tapering, or 20 to 60 mg every other day) may reduce transfusion requirements and may be helpful in alleviating the anemia. Splenectomy is of very questionable benefit. Surgery is risky in patients with PNH because stasis and trauma accentuate hemolysis and venous occlusion. If surgery is to be performed, prophylactic anticoagulation with warfarin in the perioperative period should be considered.

Patients with PNH are frequently iron deficient. The simple administration of iron to correct this defect, however, often aggravates hemolysis because iron therapy produces a cohort of new cells, many of which are susceptible to complement-mediated lysis. Transfusion before iron therapy may help circumvent this problem because it will decrease the erythropoietic stimulus to the marrow.

Thrombocytopenia resulting from poor platelet production may necessitate platelet transfusions [see Chapter 99].[18] Budd-Chiari syndrome and inferior vena cava thrombosis must be diagnosed and treated quickly with heparin, followed by long-term administration of warfarin. If heparinization is ineffective, thrombolytic therapy (e.g., streptokinase) may be used.[23] Children and adolescents with PNH that is complicated by aplastic anemia should be considered for allogeneic bone marrow transplantation.[19,24] In case reports, the anemia associated with PNH responded to erythropoietin,[25] and four patients with severe neutropenia and thrombocytopenia responded to combinations of granulocyte–colony-stimulating factor (G-CSF) and cyclosporine.[26]

Prognosis

A study of 80 patients with PNH indicated that median survival was 10 years.[18] The causes of PNH-related death were thrombocytopenia, PNH hemolysis, thromboses, or PNH-associated aplastic anemia [see Chapter 92]. Of interest is that 15% of patients experienced spontaneous remission.[18] In rare instances, prolonged and severe iron loss may occur as a result of chronic hemosiderinuria, producing iron deficiency; some patients develop transfusion-associated hemochromatosis.[19]

Acute myeloid leukemia may develop during the course of PNH. In one series, this occurred in three of 80 patients; in another series, of 220 patients, the incidence of myelodysplastic syndromes was 5% and the incidence of acute leukemia was 1%.[19]

Abnormalities of Erythrocyte Metabolism

DEFECTIVE REDUCING POWER

The reducing power of the erythrocyte is provided by reduced glutathione (GSH) and the reduced coenzymes nicotinamide adenine dinucleotide (NADH) and nicotinamide-adenine dinucleotide phosphate (NADPH) [see Table 1]. When erythrocytic stores of these materials are inadequate, hemoglobin and membrane-associated proteins can be oxidized, leading to the production of Heinz bodies, which consist predominantly of oxidative degradation products of hemoglobin [see Figure 3b]. Erythrocytes containing Heinz bodies are rigid and are therefore selectively removed by the reticuloendothelial system.

Defective Glutathione Synthesis

Deficiencies of certain enzymes involved in GSH synthesis lead to oxidative attacks on erythrocytes and to hemolysis. Several reports have described families whose members show almost negligible GSH synthesis and have hemolysis associated with the production of Heinz bodies. Glutathione peroxidase deficiency apparently contributes to hemolysis in newborn infants.

GLUCOSE-6-PHOSPHATE DEHYDROGENASE DEFICIENCY

Glucose-6-phosphate dehydrogenase (G6PD) is the first enzyme in the pentose phosphate pathway, or hexose monophosphate shunt. It catalyzes the conversion of $NADP^+$ to NADPH, a powerful reducing agent. NADPH is a cofactor for glutathione reductase and thus plays a role in protecting the cell against oxidative attack. RBCs deficient in G6PD are therefore susceptible to oxidation and hemolysis.[27,28]

G6PD deficiency is one of the most common disorders in the world; approximately 10% of male blacks in the United States are affected, as are large numbers of black Africans and some inhabitants of the Mediterranean littoral. This disorder confers some selective advantage against endemic malaria. For example, in a study in Ghana on pregnant women (who are highly susceptible to falciparum malaria and its consequences), the prevalence of infection was 66% in normal women, 58% in G6PD heterozygotes, and 50% in homozygotes.[29]

The gene for G6PD is on the X chromosome at band q28; males carry only one gene for this enzyme, so those males that are affected by the disorder are hemizygous. Females are affected much less frequently because they would have to carry two defective G6PD genes to show clinical disease of the same severity as that in males. However, expression of a defective G6PD gene is not completely masked in heterozygous women; in fact, such women exhibit highly variable G6PD enzyme activity. According to the X-inactivation, or Lyon-Beutler, hypothesis,[28] females heterozygous for G6PD have two cell lines: one that contains an active X chromosome with a gene for normal G6PD and another that contains an active X chromosome with a gene for deficient G6PD. Chance partly determines the relative proportions of the two cell lines, which in turn control the clinical severity of the defect.

Classification

There are three clinical classes of G6PD deficiency: class I, which is the uncommon chronic congenital nonspherocytic hemolytic anemia; class II, in which the enzyme deficiency is severe but hemolysis tends to be episodic; and class III, the most common variant, in which the enzyme deficiency is moderate and hemolysis is caused by oxidant attack. The severity of the hemolysis and the anemia is directly related to the magnitude of the enzyme deficiency, which is determined by the half-life of the enzyme. The normal G6PD half-life is 62 days; in class III G6PD deficiency, the enzyme has a half-life of 13 days; and in class II deficiency, G6PD has a half-life of several hours. The cloning and sequencing of the G6PD gene have clarified the classification of G6PD deficiency; before the sequencing of the G6PD gene, more than 300 variants of G6PD deficiency had been described.[28]

Etiology

Hemolysis occurs in persons with class III G6PD deficiency after exposure to a drug or substance that produces an oxidant stress. Ingestion of, or exposure to, fava beans may cause a devastating intravascular hemolysis (known as favism) in G6PD-de-

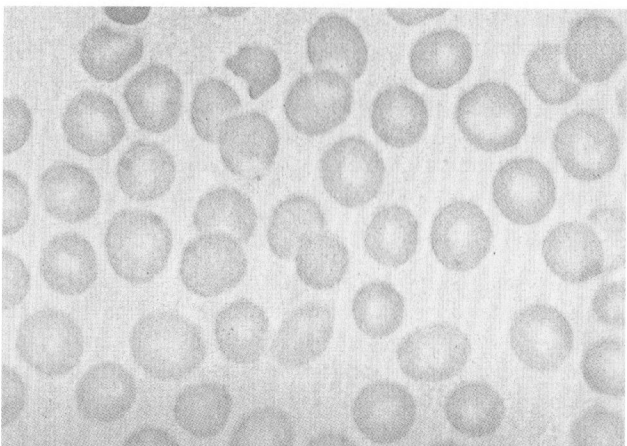

Figure 4 **Bite, hemiblister, or cross-bonded cells are indicative of oxidative attack leading to oxidative hemolysis.**

ficient patients, but it usually occurs only in those with the Mediterranean variant of class II deficiency. Fava beans contain isouramil and divicine, two strong reducing agents whose actions eventuate in the oxidation of membrane proteins. This produces a rigid cell in which hemoglobin is confined to one part of the cytosol; the other part of the cytosol appears as a clear ghost (i.e., the classic bite, hemiblister, or cross-bonded cell) [*see Figure 4*]. These membrane defects cause extravascular and intravascular hemolysis.[27] Severe infections, diabetic ketoacidosis, and renal failure also reportedly trigger hemolysis.

Diagnosis

Hemolytic anemia characterized by the appearance of bite cells and Heinz bodies after administration of certain drugs suggests the possibility of G6PD deficiency [*see Table 2*]. Dapsone, which is capable of inducing oxidant-type hemolysis, has increasingly come into use as prophylaxis for *Pneumocystis carinii* pneumonia in patients infected with HIV [*see Chapter 153*]. Therefore, it is important to screen potential users of dapsone for G6PD deficiency with the standard enzymatic tests. Other agents with oxidative potential, such as amyl nitrite ("poppers"), can cause hemolysis.[30]

Other disorders to be considered in the differential diagnosis of oxidative hemolysis include unstable hemoglobinopathy, he-

Table 2 Drugs That Produce Hemolysis in G6PD-Deficient Patients

Class	Example
Antimalarials	Primaquine Chloroquine
Sulfonamides	Sulfamethoxazole Sulfapyridine
Sulfones	Dapsone
Analgesics	Acetanilid Phenacetin Acetylsalicylic acid (10 g/day)
Nitrofurans	Nitrofurantoin Furazolidone
Water-soluble vitamin K derivatives	Menadiol

moglobin M disease, and deficiencies of other enzymes essential to glutathione metabolism. A G6PD screening test or direct enzyme assay usually resolves the question. Patients with A-type G6PD (class III) deficiency and brisk reticulocytosis, however, may have a near-normal G6PD level because young RBCs have relatively high G6PD levels. In such cases, it is best to repeat the tests when the reticulocyte count returns to normal. Information on genetic testing for G6PD deficiency can be found on the Internet at http://www.geneclinics.org.

Treatment

Avoidance of drugs that may produce hemolysis is critical in management. Acute favism requires circulatory support, maintenance of good renal blood flow, and transfusions with erythrocytes that are not G6PD deficient. The physician must also be alert to the possible onset of disseminated intravascular coagulation.

DEFECTS IN GLYCOLYSIS

The series of reactions constituting the glycolytic pathway generates several products, such as ATP, that have various essential functions in erythrocyte metabolism [*see Table 1*]. Defects involve the major glycolytic pathway (Embden-Meyerhof pathway) and generally interfere with ATP production.

Pyruvate kinase (PK) catalyzes the formation of pyruvate, a reaction associated with ATP synthesis. After G6PD deficiency, PK deficiency (autosomal recessive) is the second most common hereditary enzymopathy. Hemolysis, mild jaundice, and, occasionally, palpable splenomegaly are the presenting problems. The peripheral smear usually reveals normal RBCs, but in a few cases, the RBCs show extreme spiculation. Aplastic crises may occur.[7]

Congenital nonspherocytic hemolysis raises the possibility of PK deficiency. An enzyme assay establishes the diagnosis. Splenectomy should be considered for patients who require transfusions.

Glucose-6-phosphate isomerase deficiency is the third most common enzymopathy that leads to hemolysis. Other enzymopathies are quite rare. Screening tests and specific assays are available for deficiencies of such enzymes as hexokinase, phosphofructokinase, triose phosphate isomerase, phosphoglycerate kinase, and aldolase.

DEFECTS IN NUCLEOTIDE METABOLISM

In hemolytic anemia associated with pyrimidine 5'-nucleotidase deficiency, coarse basophilic stippling persists in mature erythrocytes, presumably because the enzyme deficiency prevents degradation of reticulocyte RNA. This accumulation results in expansion of the total RBC nucleotide pool to a level five times normal. Pyrimidine nucleotides accumulate, and adenine nucleotides are decreased. Glycolysis is impaired by an undetermined mechanism.

Disorders Involving Hemoglobin

CLASSIFICATION OF THE HEMOGLOBINOPATHIES

The clinically important hemoglobinopathies are classified into five categories on the basis of the underlying defect. The defects are as follows:

1. Hemoglobin tends to gel or crystallize (e.g., sickle cell anemia or hemoglobin C disease).
2. Hemoglobin is unstable (e.g., the congenital Heinz body anemias).
3. Hemoglobin has abnormal oxygen-binding properties (e.g., the disorder caused by hemoglobin Chesapeake).
4. Hemoglobin is readily oxidized to methemoglobin (e.g., methemoglobinemia).
5. Hemoglobin chains are synthesized at unequal rates (e.g., the thalassemias).

SICKLE CELL DISEASE

Sickle Cell Anemia

Definition Sickle cell anemia is an autosomal recessive disease caused by the substitution of the amino acid valine for glutamine at the sixth position of the β-hemoglobin chain, which results in the production of HbS.

Epidemiology From 8% to 10% of African Americans and a lesser percentage of persons with eastern Mediterranean, Indian, or Saudi Arabian ancestry have the sickle (HbS) gene. Disease develops in persons who are homozygous for the sickle gene (*HbSS*), in whom 70% to 98% of hemoglobin is of the S type. About 0.2% of African Americans have sickle cell anemia. The fact that the sickle gene occurs in populations living in regions endemic for falciparum malaria suggests that sickle heterozygosity confers a protective advantage against malaria.[31]

Restriction endonuclease analyses indicate that the sickle gene mutation probably arose spontaneously in at least five geographic locations. These variations are called Senegal, Benin, Central African Republic (or Bantu), Saudi-Asian, Cameroon, and Indian (which may be the same as the Saudi-Asian variant). These variants are important clinically because some variants are associated with higher output of γ-globin chains (and thus higher HbF levels); others are associated more often with the gene for α-thalassemia-2 [*see The Thalassemias, below*]. Either of these associations may alleviate some aspects of the sickling process.[31]

Pathophysiology Two major clinical features characterize sickle cell anemia: (1) chronic hemolysis and (2) acute, episodic vaso-occlusive crises that cause organ failure and account for most of the morbidity and mortality associated with the disease.

HbS liganded to oxygen or carbon monoxide shows near-normal solubility. When the molecule gives up its oxygen and changes to the deoxy S form, however, its solubility decreases. In an environment with reduced oxygen, HbS polymerizes into long tubelike fibers that induce erythrocytic sickling.[32]

The deoxyhemoglobin S polymer is in equilibrium with surrounding soluble molecules of deoxyhemoglobin S. An increase in the concentration of HbS, a decrease in pH, or an increase in the concentration of 2,3-BPG tends to stabilize the deoxy S form and enhances gelation.[32] In addition, sickled erythrocytes retain the K^+-Cl^- cotransport function and have sufficient intracellular calcium to activate the Gardos efflux channel[33] [*see Control of Hydration and Volume, above*]. These two mechanisms act together to produce a population of very dense sickled erythrocytes with MCHCs ranging up to 50 g/dl.[33] HbF inhibits polymerization,[33] so patients with high HbF values, such as those with the Saudi-Asian variant of sickle cell anemia, have milder disease.[31] When hypoxemia and the MCHC reach a critical level, polymerization occurs after a variable delay[33]; this delay represents the pe-

a *b* *c*

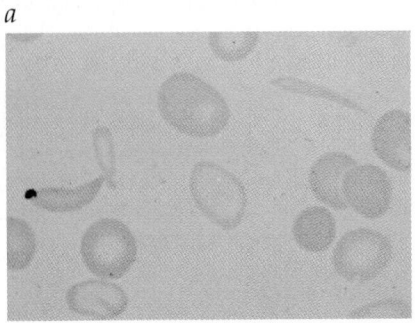 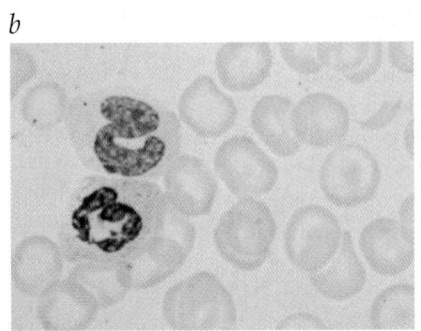 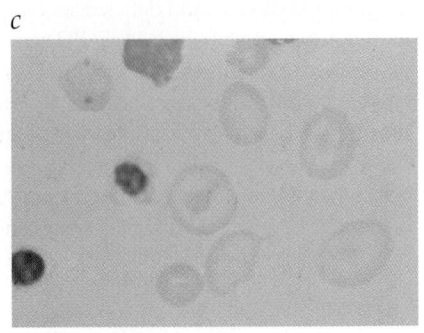

Figure 5 Sickle cell anemia is characterized by markedly distorted sickle cells, including elongated forms (*a*). Target cells (*b*) are seen in a variety of conditions, including hypochromia caused by iron deficiency, hemoglobinopathies such as HbC variants and the thalassemias, and liver disease. Cooley anemia (*c*), or β-thalassemia major, is indicated by profound hypochromia, targeting, variation in size and shape of erythrocytes, and the presence of nucleated red cells.

riod during which the deoxyhemoglobin S tetramers are slowly associating to form a nucleus. When the nucleus reaches a critical size, rapid, almost explosive gelation occurs. Free deoxyhemoglobin S tetramers rapidly attach to the nucleus to produce the long tubelike fibers that align to form parallel tubelike structures that distort the cell and produce the sickle shape [*see Figure 5*].

Most cells in the venous circulation are not sickled. However, sickling will occur if the time to polymerization is shortened to less than 1 second or if RBCs become trapped in the microcirculation. Some RBCs contain polymerized sickle hemoglobin even in the arterial circulation. Another manifestation of membrane damage in sickle cells is the irreversibly sickled cell, which retains its sickle shape even when reoxygenated.[34] Some of these poorly deformable RBCs are directly derived from a subpopulation of reticulocytes that are low in HbF[30] and are removed predominantly in the reticuloendothelial system. The rapid removal of these young cells, as well as older, dense, rigid cells that cannot traverse the monocyte-macrophage system, results in chronic extravascular hemolysis.

Because of the extreme sensitivity of sickling to the local environment, attention has been focused on cellular factors. The extreme hyperosmolality of the renal medulla (1,200 mOsm) dehydrates RBCs and raises the MCHC. Consequently, sickling sufficient to abolish the renal medullary concentrating ability may occur even in patients who have only the sickle trait.

Sickle Crisis and Ischemic Infarction

Sickle crisis is a potentially life-threatening vaso-occlusive complication of sickle disease. The initiating event in the sickle crisis is not known, nor is it clear why some patients have severe crises and others do not.

Clusters of increasingly rigid sickle cells will occlude the microvasculature in the followng circumstances: (1) the pH falls, deoxygenation increases, or the MCHC rises; (2) nitric oxide production decreases or nitric oxide is trapped and removed by free hemoglobin in plasma[35]; (3) microvascular disease is present; or (4) capillary transit time is prolonged. Thrombosis may also play a role in sickle occlusion. There is some disorganization of the membrane phospholipid bilayer, with phosphatidylserine moving to the outer leaflet, possibly enhancing the thromboembolic manifestations of sickle disease.[36] In sickle cell anemia, there also appears to be an increase in circulating endothelial cells, which abnormally express tissue factor and may provide an additional basis for thromboembolism.[37]

Blockage leads to ischemic infarction, the release of inflammatory cytokines, and an amplifying sequence of stasis-induced occlusion, which may progress to sickle crisis. Portal circulations in which oxygen tension is low, such as those in the liver or the kidney, are at particular risk for occlusion.

Risk factors predisposing to painful crises include a hemoglobin level greater than 8.5 g/dl, pregnancy, cold weather, and a high reticulocyte count. Nocturnal hypoxemia is an important risk factor in children.[38] Conversely, the low hematocrit in sickle cell anemia reduces blood viscosity and is protective. Sickle cell patients also characteristically have a high plasma fibrinogen level, which enhances the aggregation of already rigid erythrocytes and increases viscosity, particularly at the low shear rates encountered in the microcirculation.[39] Sickled RBCs also have a greater tendency to adhere to endothelial cells than do normal RBCs.[40] The role of leukocytes in this adhesion process is becoming clearer. Adminstration of G-CSF has led to sickle crises and even death.[41,42] Granulocyte-macrophage CSF (GM-CSF) has caused similar crises. The severity of sickle disease appears to parallel the level of the WBC count, and WBC cell-adhesion molecules seem to be critical to sickle vaso-occlusion.[43,44]

Diagnosis of Sickle Cell Disease

In the past, the diagnosis of sickle cell anemia was usually made on the basis of clinical manifestations occurring in childhood; the affected child was seen to have limitation in exercise tolerance, shortness of breath, tachycardia, frequent severe infections, and episodes of very painful dactylitis. Currently, many cases are identified on screening tests, which may be prompted by the diagnosis in a family member or performed as a routine neonatal procedure; in California and many other states, every fetal cord blood sample is examined by high-performance liquid chromatography (HPLC). Rarely, the disorder is diagnosed in adult life, occasionally during a first pregnancy, when prenatal screening reveals anemia. The general symptoms are limited exercise tolerance, exertional dyspnea, painful crises, bouts of jaundice, and even biliary colic.

The clinical appearance of the patient and a blood smear showing sickled cells, holly leaf cells, and erythrocytes with Howell-Jolly bodies are fairly suggestive of sickle cell anemia. Howell-Jolly bodies represent cytoplasmic remnants of nuclear chromatin that are normally removed by the spleen. Platelet and WBC counts are usually high. Unless an aplastic crisis is in progress, causing a virtual absence of normoblasts, the marrow shows erythroid hyperplasia. Diagnosis is confirmed by performing a sickle preparation: a drop of blood is incubated with fresh 2% sodium metabisulfite, and the proportion of sickle cells is measured immediately and then 1 hour later. Commercial testing sets such as Sickledex rely on the relative insolubility of HbS in 1.0 M phosphate buffers to make the diagnosis. The most definitive tests for sickle cell anemia, however, are hemoglobin electrophoresis or HPLC, which indicate the relative percentages of HbS and HbF. All of these tests are also useful in screening family members for sickle cell trait. Patients who are heterozygous for both the HbS gene and the β-thalassemia gene may appear to be homozygous for HbS. Other varieties of sickling hemoglobin are observed very infrequently. DNA-based methods can also be used to pinpoint the specific genetic abnormality and to identify the subpopulations from which the patient descended[31]; further description and information on diagnostic testing is available online at http://www.geneclinics.org. Persons with sickle cell anemia and α-thalassemia have higher hemoglobin levels, lower reticulocyte counts, a lower MCHC, a lower MCV, and less-dense RBCs than persons who have sickle cell anemia alone. Such patients may have increased life expectancy and perhaps a different pattern of manifestations of veno-occlusive complications.[45] The combination of G6PD deficiency and sickle cell anemia has neither beneficial nor harmful effects.[46,47]

Management of Sickle Cell Disease

Sickle crisis Standard conservative management of sickle crisis centers on rest, hydration, and analgesia. In demonstrably acidotic patients, mild alkalinization should be induced by administration of a bicarbonate solution, which is prepared by addition of an ampule of sodium bicarbonate to 1 L of either 5% dextrose in water or half-normal saline. The bicarbonate solution should be infused at a rate of 5 to 7 ml/kg/hr for the first 4 hours and at 4 ml/kg/hr for the next 20 hours. The role of supplemental oxygen in patients with normal arterial oxygen tension (P_aO_2) and no cardiopulmonary problems is untested.

Pain management Pain [see Chapter 175] is the major concern for 10% to 20% of patients with sickle cell anemia. Avascular necrosis of bone marrow produces excruciating pain that can last as long as 8 to 10 days. The need for pain relief sometimes results in habituation or addiction. Because there are few objective ways to monitor the sickle crisis, the physician may not know whether a demand for narcotics is a manifestation of drug-seeking behavior.

The patient who has sickle cell anemia should be provided with oral analgesics for use at home in an attempt to abort the pain crisis at its onset. Nonsteroidal anti-inflammatory drugs (NSAIDs), such as naproxen (500 mg) and ketorolac (10 mg), can be used initially. If NSAIDs alone are not sufficient, they can be followed by a narcotic-analgesic combination, such as hydrocodone and acetaminophen or oxycodone and aspirin. Adjuvants such as oral diphenhydramine (50 mg) or lorazepam (1 to 2 mg) may calm the patient and perhaps antagonize the actions of released histamine.[48] If these measures, perhaps repeated every 6 hours, do not control the pain, the patient usually requires parenteral treatment. Care from the patient's regular physicians is far preferable to reliance on unfamiliar providers in emergency departments.[48] The patient needs rapid evaluation for possible infection, acute chest syndrome, bone infarction, and other complications, and the pain should be treated either with

10 mg of intravenous morphine along with 50 mg of intramuscular diphenhydramine every 2 hours or with 4 mg of intramuscular hydromorphone along with 50 mg of intramuscular diphenhydramine every 2 hours. If there is no pain relief or inadequate pain relief 30 minutes after the first dose, 50% of the initial dose of opiates can be administered; the respiratory rate should be monitored closely, particularly if it approaches 10 respirations a minute. Some units have used patient-controlled analgesia with good results. It is important to continue to administer parenteral analgesia at regular intervals and to provide increased doses for breakthrough pain. The patient will probably need a laxative and may need an antiemetic, such as prochlorperazine (10 mg p.o. or I.M.). If the patient responds, home therapy with oral controlled-release morphine, such as MS Contin, is usually effective. If pain continues for more than 8 to 12 hours, the patient will probably need to be hospitalized to receive extended therapy with increased doses of analgesia and parenteral fluids, along with observation.[48]

Alteration of sickle cell pathophysiology A clearer understanding of the kinetics of sickling suggests some future prospects for the therapy of sickle cell anemia. Decreasing the MCHC should diminish gelation. An approach that attempts to block the Ca^{2+}-dependent K^+ efflux (Gardos channel) [see Control of Hydration and Volume, above] has been tested in a sickle mouse model and shows promise in preventing RBC dehydration.[49,50]

Therapies to interfere with sickling are being actively pursued. The presence of 20% to 30% HbF in sickle RBCs markedly delays gelation, so a mechanism that would switch on the genes that control fetal hemoglobin synthesis and thus lessen the severity of sickle disease appears feasible.[51,52] Hydroxyurea produces an increase in F reticulocyte and HbF levels. In a phase III trial, patients treated with hydroxyurea (starting dosage, 15 mg/kg/day) had fewer painful crises, admissions for crisis, and episodes of acute chest syndrome, as well as required fewer transfusions, than patients given a placebo.[53] There was no effect on stroke; however, after 8 years of follow-up, mortality was reduced by 40%.[54] The beneficial effect of hydroxyurea accrued after about 8 weeks of therapy and was accompanied by an increase in MCV and an increase in the proportion of F cells; in addition, there was a decrease in neutrophils and a decrease in sickle RBC adhesion to endothelial cells.[55] Trials are also being conducted with butyrate, which can increase γ-chain production, thereby increasing HbF levels and interfering with gelation.[56,57] Demethylating agents such as 5-azacytidine and decitabine can also increase HbF to therapeutically useful levels. Because sickle cells adhere abnormally to the endothelium, attempts have been made to block adhesion; thus far, these efforts have not proved useful.

Inflammatory cytokines appear to play an important role in the sickle crisis, as evidenced by the fact that a predictor of success in hydroxyurea therapy is a decrease in the WBC count.[54,55] Other investigators are studying the possible vasodilatory role of nitric oxide.

Sibling-donor allogeneic bone marrow transplantation can result in cure or can lead to a substitution of sickle trait for sickle cell anemia. Bone marrow transplantation resulted in apparent cure in 15 of 22 carefully selected patients; there were two deaths (9%), and the remaining five patients had complications such as graft failure. Of the 22 patients, 12 had a history of stroke, five had a history of recurrent episodes of acute chest syndrome, and five had recurrent painful crises.[58]

Long-term transfusion therapy   Long-term transfusion therapy has been found to prevent stroke.[59] Some investigators have shown that preventive transfusions reduce or eliminate pain crisis, episodes of acute chest syndrome, bacterial infection, and hospitalization.[60,61] Other authors, however, warn against the dangers of iron overload,[62,63] transfusion hepatitis, problems with venous access, and RBC alloimmunization.[64] Further studies may clarify the role of long-term transfusion therapy.

Complications and Their Management

Skeletal problems   Aseptic necrosis (osteonecrosis) of the femoral head occurs in about 10% of patients, particularly those who also have α-thalassemia. Arthroplasty has been relatively ineffective, partly because of the presence of adjacent hard bone, which interferes with the placement of the prosthesis, and because of the increased risk of infection.[65]

Cardiopulmonary problems   Cardiac complications associated with anemia are the result of a large increase in cardiac output. Such complications include chamber enlargement, cardiomegaly, left ventricular hypertrophy, and flow murmurs.[66] Acute myocardial infarction has occurred in relatively young adults who do not have coronary disease.[67] The incidence of pulmonary hypertension is unknown, but its presence markedly shortens survival.[68]

Acute pulmonary complications are a major cause of morbidity and mortality; such complications include local infection, vascular occlusions in the pulmonary vessels (both in situ thrombosis and embolism), and pulmonary fat embolism from ischemic marrow fat necrosis.[69] A large study of acute chest syndrome found that adult patients were afebrile but had shortness of breath, chills, and pain in the chest and in at least one extremity.[70] Infarctions of the thoracic vertebrae contribute substantially to the pain.[64] Physical examination frequently shows no abnormal chest findings. In one study, the P_aO_2 was found to be low, averaging 71 mm Hg but falling below 60 mm Hg in 25% of patients. In this study, the death rate in adults was 4.3%; death was preceded by a lower hemoglobin value, a higher WBC count, and multilobe involvement. Autopsy of 16 cases showed that nine patients had pulmonary embolism and fat emboli and possibly 20% had bacterial infections. In patients with acute chest syndrome and pulmonary infection, the most common infecting organism was *Chlamydia pneumoniae* (30%), followed by *Mycoplasma pneumoniae* (21%), respiratory syncytial virus (10%), *Staphylococcus aureus* (4%), and *Streptococcus pneumoniae* (3%).[71]

Usually, therapy for acute chest syndrome should include incentive spirometry,[64] antimicrobial therapy for patients with evidence of infection, the cautious use of analgesia, aggressive fluid replacement, and consideration of bronchoalveolar lavage to identify microbial infection or the fat-laden macrophages of fat emboli. Meticulous monitoring is required; repeat measurements of oxygenation should be made, and transfusions should be performed when clinically necessary. One of the most important benefits of hydroxyurea therapy is its ability to reduce the frequency of acute chest syndrome.[53,72] Children may also need supplementary penicillin prophylaxis.[73]

Hepatobiliary disease   Cholelithiasis occurs in 30% to 70% of patients, some of whom exhibit signs and symptoms of cholecystitis.[74] There are conflicting data regarding frequency of cholecystitis or obstruction of the common bile duct.[74,75] If cholecystectomy is to be done, one should wait until the painful crisis is over. Transfusions should be given to raise the hemoglobin to 10 g/dl before surgery, if necessary, and the procedure should be done laparoscopically.[74]

Hepatic complications include congestive hepatopathy secondary to heart failure and viral hepatitis from frequent transfusions. Sickling in the liver can also produce hepatopathy. Often, serum bilirubin levels exceed 30 mg/dl in patients with intrahepatic cholestasis, and coagulation abnormalities may lead to hemorrhagic complications and death.

Renal and urologic complications   Water loss as a result of an inability to concentrate urine may enhance the sickling process. The extremely hypertonic milieu of the renal medulla induces severe sickling and destruction of the vasa recta. Hematuria and papillary necrosis ensue. These complications are also observed in patients with sickle trait and in those who have sickle cell–hemoglobin C disease. The defect in renal concentrating ability appears to depend on the amount of HbS polymer contained in cells and is thus less severe in patients who also have α-thalassemia variants.[76]

Complications include renal tubular acidosis, hyperkalemia, and proteinuria. Treatment with enalapril reduces proteinuria, suggesting the presence of a component of glomerular capillary hypertension.[77] Renal failure, in association with worsening anemia, contributes to the death of about one fifth of patients older than 40 years who have homozygous sickle disease.

Priapism is an extraordinarily painful complication of sickle cell anemia and may result in impotence.[78] A United Kingdom study reported a good response in 13 of 18 patients treated for priapism with the alpha-adrenergic agonist etilefrine; however, this agent is not available in the United States.[79]

Neurologic disorders   Neurologic complications of sickle cell disease include stroke, subarachnoid hemorrhage, and isolated functional losses that suggest a focal occlusion. The pathogenesis of occlusion of the large cerebral arteries is probably different from that of the microvascular occlusive events that occur in hypoxic capillary beds. The most likely underlying causes are damage to the vascular endothelium, followed by extensive intimal proliferation and then thrombosis of the damaged vascular bed.[45] In a multi-institutional study of 4,082 patients, the prevalence of cerebrovascular accidents (CVAs) was 4% to 5%; the incidence was 0.61 per 100 patient-years.[80] Of the CVAs, 54% were infarcts, 34% were hemorrhagic in nature, 11% were transient ischemic attacks (TIAs), and 1% had both infarctive and hemorrhagic features. Of the patients who survived, the recurrence rate of CVA was 14%. Mortality was 11%. Virtually all patients who died had hemorrhagic CVAs.

In a prospective study in which transcranial Doppler ultrasonography was used to pinpoint children at risk for stroke, treatment with standard care or transfusion therapy (to reduce the HbS concentration to < 30%) resulted in only one CVA, compared with 10 CVAs and one intracerebral hematoma in the 65 control subjects (P < 0.002). The trial was terminated early.[59] The success of this trial raises many serious questions about the necessity of ultrasonographic devices for successful management; the optimum duration of transfusion therapy; the inevitable consequences of transfusional hemochromatosis [see β-Thalassemia major (Cooley anemia), *below*] and the necessity for ethnically matched blood to minimize allotransfusion reaction; the willingness of patients and families to accept transfusion therapy; and the role of allogeneic bone marrow transplantation as a potential alternative.[59,81] The risk of recurrent cerebrovascular events is increased in patients receiving long-term transfusion therapy who have multiple cerebral collateral vessels as a result of moyamoya disease (hazard ratio, 2.40).[82]

Ocular complications   The major ocular problems associated with sickle cell anemia are retinopathy, vitreous hemorrhage, and neovascularization. Annual ophthalmologic evaluations are recommended. The efficacy of laser photocoagulation in treating sickle-induced ocular changes is currently being investigated.

Dermatologic complications   Poorly healing leg ulcers can be an important cause of morbidity in patients with sickle cell anemia. The degree of anemia does not seem to correlate with the presence or severity of these ulcers, but incompetence of venous valves and the resulting venous insufficiency have been associated with ulceration.[83] Standard management includes debridement, control of local infection, use of wet-dry dressings, and possibly RBC transfusion. Local treatment with GM-CSF enhances healing, perhaps by stimulating the local growth of macrophages.[84] GM-CSF can be either injected perilesionally or added topically to the wound, but the more successful application method involves the subcutaneous injection of 100 μg of GM-CSF in each of four sites circumferentially around the ulcer at a distance of 5 mm from its edge (resulting in a total dose of 400 μg in the wound). In some circumstances, one treatment sufficed, whereas in others, weekly treatments for 4 to 12 weeks were necessary. This therapy has not been approved by the Food and Drug Administration.

Aplastic crisis   Aplastic crisis rapidly lowers hemoglobin and hematocrit levels and produces reticulocytopenia, as it does in any chronic hemolytic state. Parvovirus infection has been found to cause aplastic crisis,[7] as has bone marrow necrosis.[85]

Susceptibility to infections   Patients with sickle cell anemia are hyposplenic and exhibit complement system abnormalities. Deficient serum opsonizing activity for *Salmonella* organisms may confer an increased susceptibility to those infections, including osteomyelitis.

Anesthesia complications   The hypoxemia and vascular stasis that may occur during general anesthesia enhance sickling and may lead to a sickle crisis in the postoperative period. In an analysis of almost 4,000 patients, 12 deaths were associated with 1,079 procedures, and there were more complications after regional anesthesia than after general anesthesia.[86] A simple transfusion program to raise the hemoglobin level to 10 g/dl was as effective as more aggressive preoperative programs in reducing the rate of complications.[87]

Pregnancy and contraception   The dangers of pregnancy for women with sickle disease include pulmonary problems and an increased incidence of urinary tract infection, hematuria, preeclampsia, and maternal death. Presumably, pelvic hypoxia and the vascular overload associated with pregnancy lead to enhanced sickling, with its attendant complications. Vaso-occlusion in the placenta may account for fetal death and low birth weight.

Experienced clinicians differ in their approach to the pregnant patient with sickle disease. Some advocate only meticulous conservative care, whereas others recommend prophylactic transfu-

sions. A controlled study has indicated that there is no advantage to the use of prophylactic transfusions.[88]

Chorionic villus sampling (which can provide DNA for analysis in the first trimester of pregnancy), DNA amplification techniques, and probes that identify the specific nucleotide change of sickle cell anemia can give a relatively safe and very reliable prenatal diagnosis.[89]

Oral contraceptives may pose a special hazard to women with sickle cell anemia, because they have been associated with a slight increase in the incidence of stroke, venous thromboembolism, and myocardial infarction. However, the emerging evidence that daily use of oral contraceptives containing less than 50 mg of synthetic estrogens is relatively safe suggests that patients with sickle disease can take such medication with reasonable confidence. The use of the Norplant implantable contraceptive device is another alternative for some patients. In any event, pregnancy or abortion in sickle disease carries significant risk.[88]

Genetic Counseling

A key element to be considered in the provision of genetic counseling to patients with sickle trait or sickle disease is the significant morbidity in affected children and adults. Couples with sickle disease or sickle trait may want to have children despite the associated fetal and maternal risks. There are about 4,000 to 5,000 such pregnancies in the United States each year.[89] In one study, 286 of 445 pregnancies (64%) in mothers with sickle cell anemia proceeded to delivery; 21% of the infants were small and thus would be expected to require additional care, which the mother might have difficulty providing. In this study, there was one maternal death caused by sickle cell disease[90] [see Genetic Counseling and Prenatal Diagnosis, *below*].

Prognosis in Sickle Cell Disease

Whereas it was once assumed that most patients with sickle cell anemia would die by 20 years of age, the median age of death is now 42 years for men and 48 years for women.[51] This life expectancy is 25 to 30 years less than that of the general African-American population. Of the identified causes of death, only 18% involved organ failure—predominantly renal disease, heart failure, or the consequences of chronic strokes. Thirty-three percent of patients died during acute pain crises; these crises were frequently associated with the acute chest syndrome and were less often associated with stroke. The presence of α-thalassemia had no measurable effect. Predictors of poor outcome were a white cell count greater than 15,000/μl; a low HbF level; and organ involvement manifested by renal disease, acute chest syndrome, and neurologic events. Taking hydroxyurea had a significant impact on prognosis, with a 40% decrease in mortality and a reduction in painful crises.[91]

SICKLE VARIANTS

Sickle Trait

Heterozygosity for the sickle cell gene results in sickle trait (HbAS). The RBCs of persons with sickle trait have an HbS concentration of less than 50%; frequently, the level is as low as 30%.

Generally, persons with sickle trait lead normal, healthy lives. A few complications occur: hyposthenuria; renal hematuria; and, during pregnancy, bacteriuria and pyelonephritis. Splenic infarction occurs under conditions of hypoxia; it also occurs at high altitudes, predominantly in nonblack persons who have sickle cell anemia.

Sickle trait has been identified as a major risk factor for sudden death during basic training in the military[92]; death has resulted from unexplained cardiac arrest, heatstroke, heat stress, or rhabdomyolysis. Increasing age has been correlated with an increased risk of sudden death. However, these events have occurred under extreme conditions: very strenuous physical activity, usually in untrained persons, occasionally at high altitudes or in extreme heat. Usually, persons with sickle trait who are accustomed to physical activity do not have an increased risk of sudden death. For example, the incidence of sudden death in African-American football players with sickle trait is not higher than in other players.[93]

Therapeutic options for renal hematuria include the administration of diuretics, parenteral bicarbonate, transfusions, or ε-aminocaproic acid.

Sickle Cell–β-Thalassemia

When combined with sickle trait, a defect in the β-thalassemia gene produces a disease very similar to sickle cell anemia. The β-thalassemia gene reduces the rate of synthesis of the β^A chain, resulting in a predominance of β^S in patients with sickle trait. Depending on whether the patient has a β^0 or a β^+ thalassemia, the RBCs contain varying amounts of HbS, HbA, HbA_2, and HbF. Patients with β^0 thalassemia have no HbA, but only HbS, HbF, and HbA_2; thus, disease is severe in these patients. Diagnosis is based on an elevation in the level of HbA_2, HbF, or both on hemoglobin electrophoresis, as well as a positive family history of thalassemia and the sickle gene. In a study of 55 Greek patients, treatment with hydroxyurea resulted in distinct clinical improvement.[94,95] Further description and information on diagnostic testing is available online at http://www.geneclinics.org.

Sickle Cell–Hemoglobin C Disease

In sickle cell–hemoglobin C (HbSC) disease, almost equal amounts of HbS and HbC are formed. Between 1% and 2% of hemoglobin is HbF, and small amounts of HbA_2 are also present; however, HbA is absent. The increased sickling seen in these patients results from the pathologic effect of HbC [see Hemoglobin C Disease, below].[96] As many as 30% to 50% of patients with this disorder are not anemic and have only modest reticulocytosis. Patients may not be identified until the disorder manifests itself in the form of a vaso-occlusive crisis during surgery, pregnancy, or a medical emergency.[97] Splenomegaly, proliferative retinopathy, aseptic necrosis of long bones, and the acute chest syndrome[96] also occur. The peripheral smear [see Figure 5] shows irreversibly sickled cells in addition to target cells, stomatocytes, and erythrocytes with eccentric hemoglobin depositions, probably representing HbC aggregates or crystals. Diagnosis is confirmed by hemoglobin electrophoresis or HPLC.[97] Further information on diagnostic testing is available online at http://www.geneclinics.org.

Management is the same as that for sickle cell anemia. In a study of six patients with HbSC disease, treatment with hydroxyurea at a dosage of 1,000 mg/day resulted in an increase in MCV, a decrease in so-called stress reticulocytes, an increase in hemoglobin, and probably a reduction in cell density. Although not definitive, this small study suggests that hydroxyurea benefits patients with HbSC disease.[98] Life expectancy for patients with HbSC disease is almost 20 years greater than that for patients with HbSS disease.[51]

Hemoglobin C Disease

The HbC molecule is $\alpha_2\beta_2^{6glu\rightarrow lys}$; the gene mutation probably originated at a single site in Burkina Faso, in West Africa.[97] The presence of this hemoglobin produces almost no illness in the heterozygous state but causes mild compensated hemolysis and palpable splenomegaly in the homozygous state.

The relative insolubility of HbC is responsible for the pathologic changes associated with its presence. HbC probably interacts with the K^+-Cl^- cotransporter, which keeps it active, whereas the K^+-Cl^- cotransporter normally shuts off in RBCs after the reticulocyte stage. The result is a loss of K^+, cellular dehydration with elevated MCHC, and then aggregation and crystallization of the poorly soluble HbC.[97] The relative insolubility of HbC causes erythrocytes to become rigid and thereby subject to fragmentation and to loss of membrane material, resulting in the microspherocytes seen on a peripheral blood smear [see Figure 3].

Target cells, an important morphologic finding, constitute about 80% of the erythrocytes. HbC crystals are in the oxyhemoglobin state and dissolve when the RBCs are deoxygenated, probably accounting for the absence of vaso-occlusive episodes.

Diagnosis of hemoglobin C disease is based on blood-smear findings and the absence of evidence of either iron deficiency or thalassemia; the diagnosis is confirmed by hemoglobin electrophoresis. No therapy is required.

Hemoglobin E Disease

In hemoglobin E disease, lysine is substituted for glutamic acid at position 26 of the β-globin chain, resulting in an oxidatively unstable molecule. Hemoglobin E trait is found predominantly in Southeast Asia. It came to clinical attention in the United States as a result of the influx of Southeast Asians, in whom the incidence of this trait is about 10%.

Patients heterozygous for HbE have normal hemoglobin values, microcytosis, and no splenomegaly. Electrophoresis reveals that 70% of the hemoglobin is HbA, 25% is HbE, and the remainder is HbA_2 or HbF. Inexperienced laboratories may mistake HbE for HbA_2; the clue to this error is that HbA_2 never accounts for more than 8% of the total hemoglobin. A laboratory report of an HbA_2 level of 25% should prompt a review of the data.

Patients homozygous for HbE have mild anemia, with a hemoglobin level of about 12 to 13 g/dl, a low mean corpuscular volume, and an elevated RBC count but no reticulocytosis; they exhibit microcytes and target cells. Electrophoresis shows only HbE. Chronic hemolysis does not occur. Oxidant drugs such as dapsone should be avoided in both heterozygotes and homozygotes.

A serious clinical problem occurs when a patient is doubly heterozygous for HbE and β-thalassemia trait. Such patients present with β-thalassemia intermedia, characterized by severe anemia and splenomegaly (see below). These patients occasionally require transfusions of blood and even allogeneic bone marrow transplantation.[99] Further information on diagnostic testing is available online at http://www.geneclinics.org.

Unstable Hemoglobinopathies

Many individual variants make up the unstable hemoglobinopathies. The hemoglobin instabilities stem from amino acid substitutions that deprive the molecule of its heme group, alter the heme pocket, loosen the link between its α and β chains, or weaken the subunit structure [see Chapter 90]. The result of these processes is disruption and precipitation of hemoglobin, particularly when it is subjected to oxidant attack. Precipitated hemoglobin forms Heinz bodies, which are observed even in persons heterozygous for the unstable hemoglobin variant. Because of the deleterious effects of Heinz bodies on the erythrocyte and its membrane, significant hemolysis can occur even in the heterozygous state.

Diagnosis of an unstable hemoglobinopathy is suggested by the presence of a partly compensated chronic nonspherocytic hemolysis. Heinz bodies are observed in the erythrocytes of patients who have undergone splenectomy. Erythrocytes from patients who have not undergone splenectomy demonstrate Heinz bodies on incubation with brilliant cresyl blue dye. The differential diagnosis of a hemoglobinopathy includes G6PD deficiency; this disorder can usually be ruled out by direct assay for the enzyme.

Management includes avoidance of oxidant drugs. Splenectomy may be considered when hemolysis is severe and inadequately compensated.

Hemoglobin with Abnormal Oxygen Affinity

The presence of hemoglobin with increased oxygen affinity should be considered in the differential diagnosis of unexplained erythrocytosis, particularly if there is a familial association [see Chapter 94]. Hemoglobin electrophoresis may reveal the disorder, but in suspected cases, measurement of the oxyhemoglobin dissociation curve [see Chapter 90] is preferable as a basis for diagnosis. Hemoglobin Chesapeake and hemoglobin Rainier are examples of forms with particularly increased oxygen affinity.

The rare instances of hemoglobin with low oxygen affinity, such as hemoglobin Kansas, represent mutations. Patients with low-oxygen-affinity hemoglobinopathy are sometimes cyanotic because of enhanced oxygen unloading.

Methemoglobinemia

Methemoglobin is an oxidation product of hemoglobin in which iron is in the ferric form; thus, the molecule cannot bind oxygen reversibly. Ordinarily, 1% of hemoglobin is in the ferric state. Between 0.5% and 3% of deoxyhemoglobin is normally spontaneously oxidized to methemoglobin every day. The normal reducing power of erythrocytes [see Table 1] maintains the balance between oxidation and reduction. The enzyme system that reduces 95% of methemoglobin to hemoglobin involves two proteins, NADH-cytochrome b_5 reductase and cytochrome b_5, and also requires NADH. As the name suggests, NADH-cytochrome b_5 reductase uses NADH to reduce cytochrome b_5. Reduced cytochrome b_5 then reduces methemoglobin.[100,101] Novel mutations in the affected gene have been described.[102]

Most often, methemoglobinemia is acquired by ingestion of or exposure to oxidants that oxidize Fe^{2+} so fast that the reducing systems are overwhelmed [see Mechanism of Oxidative Attack, below].

There are two congenital forms of methemoglobinemia. In the hereditary enzymopenic form of methemoglobinemia, patients are homozygous or doubly heterozygous for a deficiency of NADH-cytochrome b_5 reductase.[103] These patients appear blue even when only about 10% of their hemoglobin is in the form of methemoglobin, but they are not sick and easily tolerate methemoglobin levels of 25% or more. In contrast, the presence of about 5 g/dl of reduced, deoxygenated hemoglobin produces cyanosis. Patients with this form of methemoglobinemia do not exhibit hemolysis and generally do not require treatment. Assay

of NADH-cytochrome b_5 reductase, done by a special laboratory, can establish the diagnosis. If desired, methylene blue at a dosage of 100 to 300 mg/day orally can be used, but it may produce urinary discomfort.[100] Methylene blue transfers electrons from NADPH to methemoglobin.

The other hereditary form of methemoglobinemia is caused by HbM, of which there are five rare variants. Each of these variants contains an amino acid substitution in the heme pocket, which allows stable bonds to be formed between the heme iron and the amino acid side chains. These bonds keep hemoglobin in the Fe^{3+} form—a form that is unable to bind oxygen and is inaccessible to the reducing enzymes. The disorder is seen only in heterozygotes; about 30% of hemoglobin is abnormal, as detected by electrophoresis. Cyanosis is noted at birth. Hemolysis is minimal, and therapy is not needed.

THE THALASSEMIAS

The thalassemias have a worldwide distribution; in many regions, they are responsible for major medical, social, and economic perturbations. Throughout the world, the regions in which the thalassemias occur are contiguous with regions endemic for malaria, indicating that the heterozygous forms of thalassemia provide protection against malaria.[104] The techniques of molecular biology have helped elucidate the pathophysiology of these syndromes,[104] which in turn has enabled investigators to make unambiguous antenatal diagnoses. Using these data, expectant parents can make thoughtful, informed choices regarding the outcome of pregnancies in which the fetus is severely affected.

Molecular Genetics

Thalassemias have a variety of genetic mechanisms. These include gene deletion, abnormalities in transcription and translation [see Chapter 159], and instability of the mRNA directing globin synthesis or of the globin itself. The genes controlling the synthesis of the α and non-α chains of hemoglobin are located on chromosomes 11 and 16 [see Figure 6].

Pathophysiology

In a healthy person, the synthesis of α and β chains is meticulously coordinated to produce adult HbA ($\alpha_2\beta_2$). In contrast, patients with thalassemia usually demonstrate imbalanced synthesis of normal globin chains. Occasionally, however, thalassemia-like syndromes can result from diminished production of a structurally abnormal chain.[105] Because one of the globin chains is present in reduced amounts, the unpaired chain accumulates in the developing erythroid precursor cell, and toxicity results [see Figure 6]. Consequently, erythroid cells die in the marrow, giving rise to a classic form of ineffective erythropoiesis [see Chapter 92]; affected erythrocytes undergo hemolysis in the peripheral blood.

The β-thalassemias are characterized by diminished production of β-globin chains, causing unmatched α-globin chains to accumulate and aggregate. These aggregates of α chains precipitate, causing decreased ATP synthesis, potassium leak, and reduced amounts of surface sialic acid; the affected erythrocytes are misshapen and relatively rigid. The membrane Ca^{2+} barrier is breached, allowing Ca^{2+} to enter. These α-globin aggregates also appear to keep the K^+-Cl^- cotransporter functioning; as a result, in severe forms of β-thalassemia, dehydration of varying degree is seen.[106] The RBC membranes are unstable and fragment easily; there is evidence of oxidation of RBC membrane proteins 4.1 and

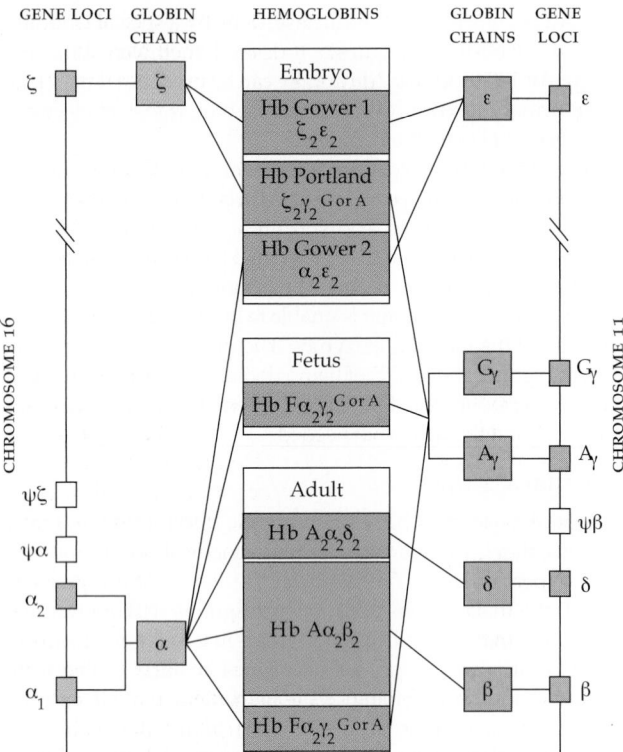

Figure 6   The genes encoding the α and non-α chains that come together to form the hemoglobin tetramer lie on chromosomes 16 and 11, respectively. The α genes are present at duplicated loci. Six distinct species of normal hemoglobin have been described. Three of these hemoglobins are synthesized only during embryonic stages of development (Hb Gower 1, Hb Portland, and Hb Gower 2). HbF predominates during fetal development, and a small amount continues to be synthesized in adult life. HbA and HbA$_2$ constitute the major forms of adult hemoglobin. Different hemoglobin genes are activated at various stages of development. In the embryo, ξ chains combine with ε chains to yield Hb Gower 1 and with γ chains to form Hb Portland; α and ε chains are linked to form Hb Gower 2. There are two varieties of γ chains that are derived from separate loci and that differ in a single amino acid; $^G\gamma$ contains glycine at position 136, whereas $^A\gamma$ contains alanine at this position. The genes coding for the two other non-α chains, β and δ, which are required for the synthesis of adult hemoglobins, are switched on late in fetal development. The factors regulating this precisely coordinated sequence of changes in hemoglobin production are poorly understood; some evidence suggests that DNA segments intervening between the various hemoglobin genes may control the relative rates of synthesis of the adjacent gene products.

spectrin [*see Figure 2*]; and phosphatidylserine migrates to the outer membrane layer, perhaps forming a nidus for thromboembolic events.[107,108] These destructive alterations of the membrane, which can be detected by macrophages, may in part be caused by local oxidation.[109,110] Abnormal accumulations of α chains probably account for the accelerated apoptosis and ineffective erythropoiesis seen in marrow erythroid precursors.[110] The overall decrease in hemoglobin synthesis per cell accounts for the observed hypochromia and target cell formation.

Patients with α-thalassemia demonstrate accumulations of excess β chains that, if present in sufficient amounts, form β_4 tetramers (HbH) [*see Figure 6*]. Such tetramers have high oxygen affinity and are unstable, aggregating in the presence of oxida-

tive stresses such as infection. β-Globin aggregates also become attached to the erythrocyte's membrane skeleton, but they produce lesions different from those produced by α-globin aggregates. In the severe α-thalassemias, ineffective erythropoiesis is less prominent[85]; rather, destruction of peripheral RBCs is the critical characteristic. RBCs in severe α-thalassemia are rigid, but in contrast to those in severe β-thalassemia, the membranes in severe α-thalassemia are more stable than normal.[107,108] Also in contrast to β-thalassemia, the RBCs in severe α-thalassemia are uniformly overhydrated.[106]

Both α-thalassemia and β-thalassemia are characterized by variable degrees of anemia. This variation in the degree of anemia is attributable to varying degrees of ineffective erythropoiesis and hemolysis.[110] When the anemia is severe, the associated hypoxia induces a vigorous compensatory erythropoiesis, leading to expansion of the marrow cavity, osteopenia, and enlargement of reticuloendothelial organs; tumors may arise at sites of extramedullary erythropoietic activity. Destruction of erythroblasts and erythrocytes may predispose to cholelithiasis and obstructive jaundice. Patients with the more severe forms of thalassemia require regular transfusions, which may eventually generate clinically significant iron overload [*see Chapter 91*].

Diagnosis and Treatment of Thalassemia

The HbF and HbA$_2$ measurements that aid in the diagnosis of the β-thalassemias are readily available from clinical laboratories using hemoglobin electrophoresis and, more recently, HPLC. In contrast, the tests required to diagnose the α-thalassemias are quite sophisticated and in the past were performed only in institutions specifically engaged in thalassemia research. Currently, specialized laboratories can detect the number and position of deleted α-globin genes. Further description and information on diagnostic testing is available online at http://www.geneclinics.org.

The clinical diagnostic tools used to assess patients suspected of having α-thalassemia include clinical history, smear evaluation, calculation of indices, brilliant cresyl blue staining, and family studies. In practice, α-thalassemia trait is diagnosed on the basis of a finding of microcytosis in an iron-replete patient who has normal HbA$_2$ and HbF levels.

The diagnosis of either α- or β-thalassemia should be suspected when the MCV is less than 75 fl and the RBC count is greater than 5 million cells/μl. A patient with these two findings has an 85% chance of having a thalassemia syndrome.[111] In one study, diagnosis of thalassemia was not considered in about half of the patients with the disease.

β-Thalassemia

The deficient synthesis of β-globin characteristic of β-thalassemia leads to accumulation of unmatched α chains. A diagnostically significant development in β-thalassemia is the partial compensatory increase of the δ and γ chains that yields elevated levels of HbA$_2$ ($\alpha_2\delta_2$) and HbF ($\alpha_2\gamma_2$), respectively [*see Figure 5*]. The β-thalassemia variants produce three clinical syndromes: β-thalassemia major, β-thalassemia minor, and thalassemia intermedia.

β-Thalassemia major (Cooley anemia) β-Thalassemia major is usually a homozygous or doubly heterozygous condition; both parents of an affected individual carry a β-thalassemia trait. In β^0-thalassemia, the most severe variant, no β chains are synthesized; only HbF and HbA$_2$ are found. β^+-Thalassemia is somewhat less severe. It is characterized by small amounts of β chains and small quantities of HbA in addition to HbF and HbA₂. δβ-Thalassemia is yet milder; it is caused by deletion of the δ-globin and β-globin genes. This mutation prohibits production of HbA₂ and HbA, permitting synthesis of fetal hemoglobin alone.

β-Thalassemia major is characterized by severe anemia that appears in the first year of life. Patients also have jaundice, hepatosplenomegaly, expansion of the erythroid marrow with secondary body changes (including retarded growth), and an increased susceptibility to infection.

Diagnosis is not difficult; no other condition closely resembles Cooley anemia. The peripheral smear shows nucleated RBCs, distorted hypochromic erythrocytes, and basophilic stippling, which represents aggregates of ribosomal RNA [see Figure 5]. Supravital staining reveals accumulations of excess unmatched α chains.

Management consists of aggressive transfusion therapy. The strategy involves transfusing to a hemoglobin level of about 12 g/dl, then allowing the hemoglobin level to fall to about 9 g/dl just before the next transfusion; this prevents such complications as heart failure, fluid overload, and skeletal deformity. Splenectomy is usually necessary to enhance survival of the patient's own RBCs as well as transfused RBCs.[112] Vaccination with pneumococcal vaccine is indicated because of the risk of pneumococcal sepsis after splenectomy.

Long-term transfusions eventually generate iron overload, which if untreated leads to death from cardiac hemochromatosis during adolescence. Iron overload should be managed prophylactically by infusion of subcutaneous deferoxamine, an iron chelator, before iron buildup occurs. Subcutaneous deferoxamine at a dosage of 50 mg/kg/day can effect iron losses of 50 to 200 mg/day but only if infused continuously over 8 to 12 hours for 5 days each week.[113] Such therapy not only prevents left ventricular dysfunction but also reverses already established abnormalities.[114] The beneficial effects of iron chelation have improved the prognosis for persons with Cooley anemia[114]: it is no longer inevitable that patients die in their 20s of arrhythmia and left ventricular failure. With current deferoxamine therapy, 61% of patients born before 1976 have had no cardiovascular disease. Compliant patients whose ferritin levels are mostly below 2,500 ng/ml have a survival rate of 91% after 15 years.[115] However, compliance with deferoxamine is a problem, and the cost of the drug takes it out of reach of most patients in developing countries. In 2005, deferasirox became the first FDA-approved oral iron chelating agent. The utility and safety of deferasirox have been shown in a randomized, multicenter study of patients with β-thalassemia and transfusional iron overload.[117] Although oral chelation therapy promises to improve patient compliance, the annual cost of this therapy is high; ongoing studies continue to examine the efficacy of deferasirox and other oral iron chelators.[118] Bone marrow transplantation has been performed with HLA-matched sibling donors. More than 1,000 patients have now undergone allogeneic bone marrow transplantation from sibling donors who either were normal or had β-thalassemia trait.[119] Some patients with hemoglobin E β-thalassemia have a phenotype fully as severe as β-thalassemia major and require the same therapy, including allogeneic bone marrow transplantation.[99] Experience with cord blood transplantation is more limited.[120] Depending on the condition of the patient at the time of transplantation, the rate of transplantation-related mortality was 5% to 19%; the cure rate was 54% to 90%.[121] Other approaches to the treatment of severe β-thalassemia are still experimental.[56] However, two small clinical trials have shown hydroxyurea to

be of benefit. This treatment probably works by increasing the production of γ chains, which combine with and remove the excess α chains, and by causing an increase in the production of HbF, a useful hemoglobin.[122,123]

β-Thalassemia minor (β-thalassemia trait)   Patients with β-thalassemia minor are usually heterozygous for a β-globin mutation and have either mild or no anemia. The peripheral smear shows distinct hypochromia and microcytosis with basophilic stippling. Splenomegaly is occasionally found.

The HbA₂ level is elevated above 5% in 90% of patients, and the HbF level is raised above 2% in 50% of patients. This increase in fetal hemoglobin occurs in varying proportions per RBC (a phenomenon known as heterocellular distribution), as shown by the Kleihauer-Betke stain. Patients with higher HbF levels have less severe anemia. Heterozygotes for δβ-thalassemia produce increased amounts of HbF but only normal amounts of HbA₂.

Iron deficiency anemia should be excluded from the differential diagnosis of β-thalassemia trait [see Chapter 91]. Generally, it is easy to distinguish the two disorders. Both are associated with hypochromia and microcytosis, but iron deficiency produces hypoproliferation of RBCs, whereas β-thalassemia minor causes only a minimal reduction in their number. At a hemoglobin level of 9 g/dl, an iron-deficient patient has an RBC count of about 3 million cells/μl, whereas a patient with β-thalassemia trait has an RBC count of about 5 million cells/μl. If the diagnosis remains in doubt, measurement of the serum iron and iron-binding capacity or of the serum ferritin level can be used to distinguish these disorders. It is important to remember, however, that a patient with thalassemia trait may also be iron deficient as a consequence of vaginal bleeding, gastrointestinal bleeding, or both.

Thalassemia intermedia   As the term implies, thalassemia intermedia is characterized by clinical manifestations of moderate severity. Patients with this syndrome have distinct anemia, with hemoglobin levels as low as 6 to 7 g/dl; they exhibit variable degrees of hepatosplenomegaly, but they usually do not require regular transfusions. During infections or other erythropoietic insults, however, transfusions may be needed transiently. In two small clinical trials, isobutyramide was found to be of benefit.[124,125]

β-Thalassemia–like variants   The hemoglobinopathy associated with hemoglobin Lepore represents another β-thalassemia variant. Patients who are homozygous for this disorder present with Cooley anemia or thalassemia intermedia, and their RBCs contain only hemoglobin Lepore and HbF.[105]

Hereditary persistence of fetal hemoglobin   The RBCs of patients heterozygous for hereditary persistence of fetal hemoglobin (HPFH) contain about 50% of HbF, whereas homozygotes have 100% of HbF. It was once believed that patients with HPFH were well and had minimal or no anemia, but some clinical variants of HPFH associated with distinct anemia have been described.

α-Thalassemia

The α-globin gene and the β-globin gene differ in two major respects. First, there are no fetal, neonatal, or adult substitutes for the α-globin genes; second, there are only two β-globin genes but four α-globin genes—two α-globin genes on each chromosome 16 [see Figure 6]. The normal α-globin genotype is designated

$\alpha\alpha/\alpha\alpha$. Patients who carry the α-thalassemia–1 variant exhibit a deletion of two α-chain genes from the same chromosome and thus have the --/ or α^0 haplotype; this deletion is common among Asian patients. Patients who have the α-thalassemia–2 variant have lost one α gene on one chromosome and show the -α/ or α^+ haplotype. Although this mutation is particularly frequent among blacks, it is also observed in Asian and Mediterranean populations. Five clinically distinct syndromes have been recognized among patients who carry different genotypes for the α-globin genes: hemoglobin Barts or hydrops fetalis (--/--); hemoglobin H disease (--/-α); heterozygous α-thalassemia–1 (--/$\alpha\alpha$); homozygous α-thalassemia–2 (-α/-α); and the silent carrier syndrome (-α/$\alpha\alpha$).

Hemoglobin Barts (hydrops fetalis)   Children with hemoglobin Barts syndrome are homozygous for α-thalassemia–1 (--/--) and therefore produce no α chains. The unmatched γ chains form γ_4 tetramers (hemoglobin Barts). All infants with this condition are born hydropic, and most die unless rescued by intrauterine stem cell transplantation. The parents are usually heterozygous for α-thalassemia–1 (--/$\alpha\alpha$).

Hemoglobin H disease   The clinical picture of hemoglobin H disease is that of variable hemolytic anemia occurring in patients of Asian, Middle Eastern, or Mediterranean origin. HbH, which precipitates on staining with brilliant cresyl blue, can usually be detected in the patient's freshly drawn RBCs. The molecular mechanisms may involve deletion of three α genes, as would be the case if the patient were doubly heterozygous for α-thalassemia–1 (--/) and α-thalassemia–2 (-α/), yielding a --/-α genotype. Splenomegaly is common. Patients usually do not require regular transfusions, but transient RBC support may be necessary when the patient has infection or experiences other oxidative stresses that lead to the precipitation of the unstable HbH and enhanced hemolysis. During pregnancy, anemia may become clinically severe and require RBC transfusion. Partners of pregnant patients with HbH disease should be screened because if the partner carries an α-thalassemia trait, the fetus may have homozygous α-thalassemia hydrops fetalis. Occasionally there is associated growth retardation and even iron accumulation in the absence of RBC transfusions.[126]

Heterozygous α-thalassemia   Heterozygous α-thalassemia–1 (--/$\alpha\alpha$), a common genotype among Asians, causes mild or no anemia; rather, it engenders distinctly hypochromic, microcytic RBCs. Patients homozygous for α-thalassemia–2 (-α/-α), a common genotype among blacks, lack two α genes; the clinical manifestations of patients with this genotype resemble those of patients heterozygous for α-thalassemia–1. The heterozygous state for α-thalassemia–2 (-α/$\alpha\alpha$) is clinically undetectable and thus represents the silent carrier syndrome.

α-Thalassemia–like syndrome   Hemoglobin constant spring (hemoglobin CS) is a structurally abnormal hemoglobin common in some Asian populations. The α-globin gene contains a mutation in the termination codon, resulting in the synthesis of an α-globin that contains an additional 31 amino acids. Patients heterozygous for this defect have a clinical picture similar to that of a patient homozygous for α-thalassemia–2. Patients homozygous for hemoglobin CS tend to have slightly more severe clinical manifestations than patients heterozygous for α-thalassemia–1. In patients who are doubly heterozygous for α-thalassemia–1 and alpha CS (--/αCS α) and who have HbH/HbCS, disease is slightly more severe than in those with hemoglobin H disease.[110]

Genetic Counseling and Prenatal Diagnosis

Parents who have had a stillborn hydropic infant or a child with Cooley anemia are justifiably reluctant to repeat the experience. Adults from thalassemia families who know themselves to be heterozygous for thalassemia are often eager to receive genetic counseling when starting their own families. Genetic counseling entails screening prospective parents on the basis of routine diagnostic tests and family studies. In addition, advances in molecular genetics can now provide accurate, unambiguous prenatal diagnoses of the thalassemias. In the first trimester, chorionic villus sampling combined with the use of polymorphic DNA markers and synthetic oligonucleotide probes can provide the definitive diagnosis in about 80% of cases of β-thalassemia [*see Chapter 159*].[127,128] Indeed, the incidence of births of infants with thalassemia major has fallen in several parts of the world. Different ethnic groups respond in different ways to genetic counseling.

Extracorpuscular Defects

Erythrocytes can be damaged through trauma or by antibodies, drugs, abnormally functioning organs, and toxins. These causes of an extracorpuscular defect should be considered whenever hemolysis develops in a patient who has no personal or family history of anemia.

MECHANICAL INJURY: MICROANGIOPATHIC HEMOLYSIS

Microangiopathic hemolysis is characterized by the appearance of bizarre, fragmented erythrocytes (e.g., schistocytes, or helmet cells) on a peripheral smear and by signs of intravascular and extravascular hemolysis.

Pathophysiology

The normal erythrocyte can withstand considerable elongation and twisting, but it disintegrates when subjected to strong stretching or shearing forces. Stresses of this magnitude have been observed to occur in jets produced by deformed aortic valves, by arteriovenous shunts, by ventricular septal defects, or by the older valvular prostheses.

Localized intravascular coagulation, in which fibrin strands bridge the arteriolar lumen, is thought to occur in arterioles supplying inflamed or neoplastic tissues. Fibrin strands lop off fragments of RBCs, whose membranes promptly reseal. Some of the erythrocyte contents leak out, however, producing varying degrees of intravascular hemolysis. The distorted RBCs are then removed by the reticuloendothelial system.

Diagnosis

Hemolysis in conjunction with typical blood smear findings is diagnostic of microangiopathic hemolysis [*see Figure 5*]. If the angiopathy is extensive, thrombocytopenia and disseminated intravascular coagulation develop. Causes include hemodynamic jets, vasculitis,[129] giant hemangiomas, thrombotic thrombocytopenic purpura, metastatic cancer,[130] certain infections (especially meningococcemia, rickettsial diseases, and hantavirus infection), hemolytic-uremic syndrome, disseminated intravascular coagulation, drugs (cocaine, cyclosporine, mitomycin, and tacrolimus), and even subclavian catheters.[130,131] Quinine has been identified as a fairly common cause of drug-induced thrombotic thrombocytopenic purpura (TTP) and hemolytic-uremic syndrome.[132] A single case of microangiopathic hemolysis has been described in an infant with cutaneous anthrax.[133]

Treatment

In treating microangiopathic hemolysis, clinicians must focus primary attention on the underlying disease. Patients may become iron deficient and require iron therapy. Supplementation of depleted folate stores may stimulate erythropoiesis. In rare cases, anemia caused by an old prosthetic aortic valve may be severe enough to warrant valve replacement. Plasmapheresis provides effective therapy for TTP [see Chapters 97 and 100].

March hemoglobinuria March hemoglobinuria, a disorder that somewhat resembles microangiopathic hemolysis, usually occurs in young persons after prolonged marching or running or playing on bongo drums. The severe and repetitive trauma to the feet or hands is thought to destroy RBCs circulating in the vessels of the soles and palms. The patient notices red urine that clears in 1 day or less after the activity. Transient hemoglobinemia and hemoglobinuria without anemia, smear abnormalities, or reticulocytosis confirm the diagnosis. The use of padded shoes and the avoidance of paved surfaces may prevent recurrences in persons who continue running.

IMMUNE HEMOLYSIS

General Mechanisms

A classic, well-delineated example of immune (not autoimmune) hemolysis involves fetomaternal incompatibility at Rh locus D, in which the D-negative mother, after contact with D-positive erythrocytes, may produce an IgG anti-D antibody; the antibody crosses the placenta, after which it attacks and destroys fetal erythrocytes. The fetus becomes jaundiced and has spherocytic erythrocytes.

The fetal RBCs, now coated with maternal IgG anti-D antibody, attach to fetal macrophages and monocytes that contain receptors for the Fc portion of these IgG molecules. Macrophagic digestion of portions of the erythrocytic membrane leads to the loss of considerable surface area. The resulting rigid spherocyte returns to the circulation and becomes trapped in the fetal reticuloendothelial system, particularly in the spleen. Hemolysis results. The IgG antibody is maximally active at 37° C; it generally cannot extensively activate the complement pathway, and it cannot agglutinate attacked RBCs suspended in saline.

The direct Coombs antiglobulin test [see Figure 7] is used clinically to detect IgG coating of RBCs. This test is negative in the mother, because her erythrocytes lack D antigen and thus are not coated with anti-D antibody. The indirect Coombs test [see Figure 7], which detects the presence of free serum antibody that reacts with RBCs, is positive for the mother's serum because she has circulating anti-D antibody. In the fetus, in contrast, the direct Coombs test is strongly positive because the fetus's RBCs, which express D antigen, are coated with maternal anti-D antibody. The results of the fetus's indirect Coombs test may be positive or negative, depending on the amount of anti-D antibody that has been transferred by the mother, the avidity of the anti-D antibody for fetal D-positive RBCs, and the availability of D antigen sites on fetal RBCs.

These antibodies are described as warm (maximum activity at 37° C [usually IgG1 or IgG3]) or cold (maximum activity at 5° C [usually IgM]). Antibodies have also been classified as complete (i.e., capable of agglutinating saline-suspended RBCs) and incomplete (i.e., incapable of agglutinating saline-suspended RBCs); their detection requires the use of techniques such as the direct Coombs antiglobulin test [see Figure 7] or enzyme treatment of RBCs.[134] Warm autoantibodies are usually incomplete, whereas cold agglutinins, which are for the most part IgM, are usually complete.[135]

Autoimmune Hemolytic Anemia

Autoimmune hemolytic anemia is generally an acute disorder characterized by extravascular hemolysis. Intravascular hemolysis in this condition is rare and indicates that an extremely rapid rate of erythrocyte destruction is occurring or that the extravascular removal mechanisms have been overwhelmed.

Pathophysiology In autoimmune hemolytic anemia, for reasons that are unclear, autoantibodies form and are directed against central components of the erythrocyte (e.g., Rh antigen, Kell antigen,[134] glycophorin A).[136] Alternatively, the patient's RBCs are sensitized with both an IgG antibody and a complement component, usually C3d. In other circumstances, however, it appears that complement is fixed to the RBC surface by an IgM antibody that is subsequently washed away. Occasionally, the RBCs exhibit only complement components, and no IgG can be detected by the Coombs test. Complement fixation in such cases may be explained by the continued presence of IgG at a level below that detectable in the usual direct antiglobulin test; alternatively, a complement-fixing IgG or IgM antibody had been attached to the cell but was eluted in the testing procedure.[135]

The severity of hemolysis correlates with the number and class of IgG and, in rare cases, IgA molecules attached to the RBC surface. Antibody-coated RBCs attach to the macrophages' receptors (FcRI, FcRII, or FcRIII) by the antibody's Fc portion. The firm binding of RBCs to these macrophage receptors is then followed either by removal of a portion of the RBC membrane, which results in the production of a spherocyte, or by phagocytosis of the entire RBC.[134] Relatively low levels of IgG1 attachment to RBCs produce a positive result on direct Coombs antiglobulin testing without evidence of hemolysis (approximately 1,000 molecules per RBC), whereas much higher levels of IgG1 autoantibody per RBC are associated with frank hemolysis.[134] The combined presence of IgG and complement components may enhance the severity of hemolysis.

Erythrocytes sensitized to IgG alone are usually removed in the spleen, whereas RBCs sensitized to IgG and complement or to complement alone are generally destroyed in the liver, because hepatic Kupffer cells carry receptors specific for complement component C3b.

Differential diagnosis Both an idiopathic variety of autoimmune hemolytic anemia and a variety that occurs secondary to other disorders have been described. Such primary disorders include systemic lupus erythematosus, non-Hodgkin lymphoma (especially chronic lymphocytic leukemia), Hodgkin disease, cancer, myeloma, dermoid cyst, HIV infection, angioimmunoblastic lymphadenopathy with dysproteinemia, hepatitis C,[137] and chronic ulcerative colitis.

Diagnosis Patient presentations vary markedly, from asymptomatic to severe. A person may be found to have a positive Coombs test result when undergoing blood bank or blood

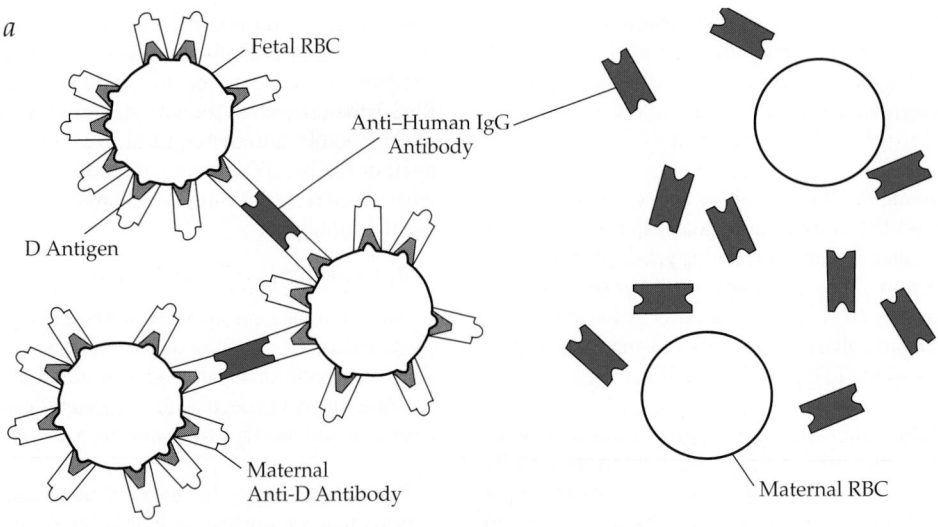

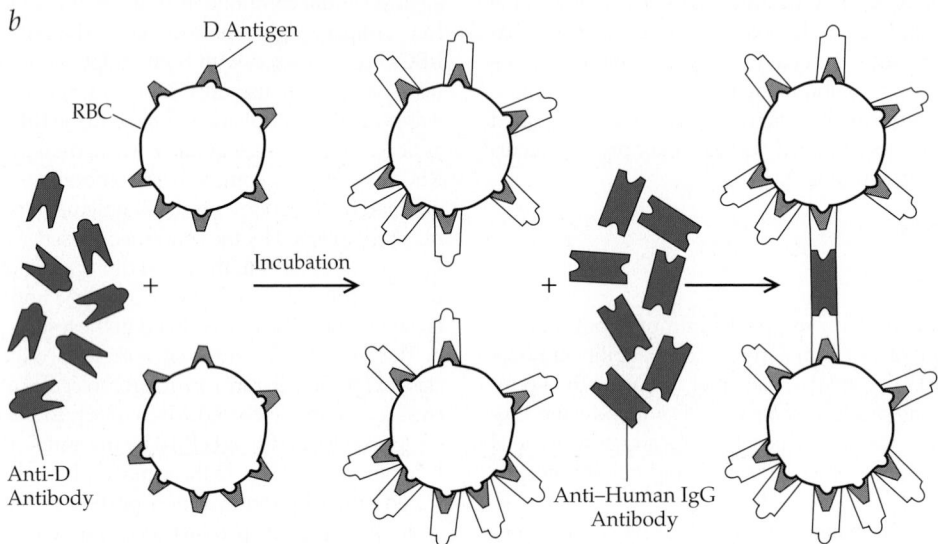

Figure 7 The Coombs test detects the presence of human antibodies or complement components on erythrocytes or the presence of antibodies in serum. The test is useful in diagnosing Rh hemolytic disease of the newborn, autoimmune hemolysis, or potential hemolytic transfusion reactions. The figure illustrates Rh hemolytic disease of the newborn.

In the direct Coombs test (*a*), fetal erythrocytes (RBCs) are shown with D antigen attached to their surfaces. Maternal anti-D antibody binds to the fetal erythrocytes at the D antigen sites in utero. Coombs antiserum, which contains antibody to human IgG, binds to the anti-D antibody on a sample of washed fetal erythrocytes, causing them to clump (a positive reaction). Washed maternal erythrocytes, having no D antigen, will have no attached anti-D antibody and are therefore not clumped by Coombs serum (a negative reaction).

In the indirect Coombs test (*b*), maternal or fetal serum is added to the red cells of another person or to panels of erythrocytes of known antigenic specificity; Coombs antiserum is then added. Clumping in this case occurs only if the test serum, such as the maternal serum, contains anti-D antibody and if the red cells chosen have the D antigen.

The direct Coombs test is used to detect immunoglobulin molecules already attached to erythrocytes, such as those found on the fetal erythrocytes in Rh hemolytic disease of the newborn or in autoimmune hemolytic anemia. Therefore, the test is done on the patient's thoroughly washed erythrocytes. The indirect Coombs test is used for determining whether specific antibodies are present in a serum sample, and it is performed on the patient's serum.

donation screening. Such persons can usually be shown to have complement or the combination of complement and IgG (usually IgG1 or IgG4) on their RBCs, but they are generally not undergoing hemolysis. By contrast, an acute hemolytic episode can lower the hematocrit from 45% to 15% in 2 days. With this extreme presentation, severe fatigue and cardiorespiratory symptoms will develop, together with jaundice, lymphadenopathy, and hepatosplenomegaly.

In severe cases, the blood smear shows macrocytosis, polychromatophilia, variable spherocytosis, and autoagglutination of RBCs. The platelet count is also occasionally depressed (Evans syndrome), and there may be leukopenia. One third of patients may have reticulocytopenia at presentation.[138] The direct Coombs test will be positive. Any or all of these findings may be absent in mild disease.

Whether complement, IgG, or both are present on RBCs should be determined by the use of Coombs reagents that are specifically directed against IgG, IgA, or complement components. Occasionally, an autoimmune hemolytic anemia is suspected, but the direct Coombs test is repeatedly negative; in such cases, the level of autoantibody may be below the level of detectability for very active autoantibodies, such as subclass IgG3 autoantibodies, or the autoantibody may be IgA or IgM.[134]

Patients with evidence of hemolytic anemia should be screened for autoimmune diseases (e.g., systemic lupus erythematosus) and other forms of hemolysis, such as paroxysmal nocturnal hemoglobinuria, cold agglutinin disease, and paroxysmal cold hemoglobinuria.

Treatment Treatment of clinically affected patients is directed at decreasing autoantibody production and reducing the macrophagic attack on the RBCs. Initial therapy usually consists of 60 to 100 mg of prednisone a day, given in divided doses. This therapeutic approach usually produces a slow decrease in antibody coating of RBCs and is thought to interfere with phagocytic attack on coated erythrocytes. A good response to corticosteroid use—indicated by a rise in the reticulocyte count and an improvement in hemoglobin and hematocrit—may be apparent within 1 or 2 days. Supplementation with 1 mg of folic acid a day is recommended.

After the initial response to therapy, which is usually satisfactory, the hemoglobin level and reticulocyte count may return to normal. The Coombs test is then repeated to determine whether the response has become weaker; if so, the prednisone dosage is tapered cautiously. Approximately 20% of patients remain well indefinitely, but the majority suffer from a chronic, treacherous disease that can produce sudden relapses with abrupt anemia. The prednisone should be titrated in accordance with the hemoglobin level, the reticulocyte count (elevation indicates continued hemolysis), and the direct Coombs titer; alternate-day therapy should be considered to minimize steroid side effects. If patients do not respond to standard prednisone therapy, high-dose dexamethasone (e.g., 40 mg/day orally for 4 consecutive days in 28-day cycles[139]) may be effective.

If the corticosteroid dose required for long-term therapy produces significant morbidity, one can proceed empirically either to splenectomy or to the use of immunosuppressive agents. Measurements of splenic sequestration of chromium-51 (^{51}Cr)-labeled erythrocytes do not reliably indicate the benefits of splenectomy. Splenectomy rarely results in extended remission but is valuable as a prednisone-sparing measure. After splenectomy, low-dose prednisone (5 to 10 mg/day) may stabilize the hemoglobin concentration.

The immunosuppressive agent azathioprine or cyclophosphamide can be used as an alternative to splenectomy. There is no reliable evidence to support the use of one of these agents over the other. For patients with very aggressive disease, cyclosporine has been used successfully.[140] Azathioprine should be started at a dosage of 100 to 200 mg a day; the peripheral blood count should be monitored with a view toward preventing reticulocytopenia or neutropenia. Cyclophosphamide is started at a dosage of 100 to 200 mg a day, with monitoring of blood counts and urine; however, because cyclophosphamide can cause ther-

apy-related acute myeloid leukemia or myelodysplastic syndrome, its use should be limited [see Chapter 205].

Azathioprine or cyclophosphamide doses have to be adjusted to reduce the white cell count to about 3,000/mm³. Improvement usually comes in 3 to 4 weeks. When a response occurs, the prednisone dose can be reduced and the hemoglobin level, reticulocyte count, and Coombs titer monitored to determine the minimally required therapy. For patients with very refractory disease, therapy with intravenous cyclophosphamide at doses used for allogeneic bone marrow transplantation has been tried. This approach is clearly myelotoxic, and its usefulness awaits further confirmation. High-dose intravenous IgG has been used to treat autoimmune hemolytic anemia. In one report, only one third of patients had a transient response, and doses larger than those used in idiopathic thrombocytopenic purpura (i.e., 1g/kg/day for 5 days) were required.[141,142]

There are anecdotal reports that rituximab is useful in treating refractory and relapsing cases.[143,144] However, a case of autoimmune hemolytic anemia occurring after rituximab therapy for lymphoproliferative disorder has been reported.[145]

Patients with symptomatic anemia require an RBC transfusion, but often the blood bank reports an incompatibility. Many blood banks regularly perform a direct Coombs antiglobulin test on the recipient's RBCs. A patient who has free antibodies in the serum will exhibit very extensive and broad reactivity against donor panels of RBCs and will usually produce an incompatible major cross-match when tested with the antiglobulin reagent. If transfusions are needed to support cardiorespiratory and central nervous system functions, immediate consultation with the transfusion medicine service is recommended.[135] No patient should be allowed to die because the blood bank does not have a perfectly compatible unit of RBCs. If transfusion is clinically indicated, the physician should administer the best units of blood that are available, because it has been shown that these patients can tolerate even imperfectly matched RBCs.[146]

Drug-Related Immune Hemolysis

Drug-initiated immune hemolysis is often indistinguishable from autoimmune hemolytic anemia. There are two variants: the hapten type and the hemolysis that results from alteration of a membrane antigen.[147]

Hapten type Drugs such as the penicillins and the cephalosporins bind firmly to the erythrocyte membrane. In rare circumstances in which massive dosages of the drug (e.g., more than 10 million units of penicillin a day) are required, the protein-bound drug may act as a hapten and elicit an immune response. An IgG antibody that appears to be directed against the drug–RBC complex is produced[148,149]; this leads to a positive result on direct Coombs testing with the anti-IgG reagent and a negative result with the anti-C3d reagent. When the offending drug is stopped, hemolysis ends in a few days. In contrast, the drug may be bound loosely to produce a neoantigen that generates the immune response.[147] In this circumstance, the result of direct Coombs testing with the anti-C3d reagent is usually positive, and the result of testing with the anti-IgG reagent may be negative.

If the patient's serum is tested against normal cells (i.e., the indirect Coombs test is used), no reaction occurs unless the offending drug and a source of complement are first added to the normal RBCs. Stopping or switching the drug is effective in eliminating the hemolysis because the antibody is usually very specific.

Alteration of a membrane antigen Some drugs may alter a membrane antigen, thereby stimulating the production of IgG antibodies that cross-react with the native antigen. Methyldopa is the classic example of a drug that causes autoimmune hemolytic anemia. Other examples are levodopa, mefenamic acid, and procainamide. Drug administration leads to a positive direct Coombs test with anti-IgG reagents in 15% to 20% of treated patients, but hemolysis occurs in fewer than 1%. The eluted antibody is seen to be a classic IgG autoantibody directed against Rh components. The mechanism of hemolysis is identical to that of autoimmune hemolytic anemia.[150]

The NSAID diclofenac sodium has been reported to cause a devastating acute hemolytic anemia, with evidence of intravascular and extravascular hemolysis accompanied occasionally by shock, organ failure, and even disseminated intravascular coagulation.[151] Patients develop both RBC autoantibodies and drug-dependent antibodies. It is thought that diclofenac sodium binds to the surface of RBCs, forming neoantigens that lead to the generation of true autoantibodies, as well as drug-dependent antibodies. The direct Coombs test is positive with both the IgG and the C3d reagents. Additional antibody reactivity occurs with the addition of diclofenac sodium metabolites obtained from the urine of patients treated with the drug. Therapy consists of recognizing the cause, stopping the diclofenac sodium, and supporting the patient for several days until the process stops.[151]

Delayed Hemolysis of Transfused Erythrocytes

Blood is usually typed only for ABO and Rh-D antigens, but other antigens are also present on RBCs. Thus, a patient who receives extensive transfusions over 1 to 2 weeks may develop an antibody response to one or more of these other antigens. Kell, Duffy, Kidd, and Rh antigens other than D are the usual offenders. When the patient with antibodies receives RBCs expressing these antigens, an acute self-limited hemolysis, usually extravascular, may ensue. Clues are a history of transfusion, spherocytosis on peripheral smear, a positive direct Coombs test, and the recent appearance of an antibody in the patient's serum (positive indirect Coombs test). Usually, no therapy is required, but further transfusions should be cross-matched with the patient's serum [see Chapter 99]. Similar problems arise with transplantation of bone marrow and other tissue.[152]

Cold Agglutinin Disease

Cold agglutinin disease has several variants. One rare variant affects young adults and usually occurs after infection with *Mycoplasma pneumoniae* or infectious mononucleosis, although several cases have also been reported in association with chronic falciparum malaria. A more common variant affects persons about 60 years of age and may present as idiopathic cold agglutinin disease, as a prodrome to a lymphoproliferative or an immunoproliferative disorder, or in association with an already established lymphoproliferative disorder.[153]

Pathophysiology Serologically, cold agglutinin disease is characterized by the presence of high titers of IgM agglutinins (> 1:1,000 and usually > 1:10,000) in serum. These antibodies are maximally active at 4° C, are capable of activating the complement sequence, and are directed against the polysaccharide antigens. Presumably, IgM reacts with erythrocytes circulating in the cooled blood of the nose, ears, and shins, where it fixes complement and then dissociates from the RBCs when they reach warmer areas of the body.

In the postinfectious variety of this disorder, IgM cold agglutinin is oligoclonal and short-lived. Conversely, the IgM is monoclonal in chronic idiopathic cold agglutinin disease or in cases associated with Waldenström macroglobulinemia, chronic lymphocytic leukemia, or other lymphomas. IgM predominantly contains λ light chains in patients with chronic idiopathic cold agglutinin disease or Waldenström macroglobulinemia; in patients with lymphoma, however, the IgM mainly contains κ light chains. Occasionally, the IgM cold agglutinin is detectable as an M protein spike on serum protein electrophoresis [see Chapter 206].

In the post-*Mycoplasma* variant, the mycoplasmas appear to bind to the RBC surface at the Ii antigen site. This receptor-ligand interaction results in the presentation of the I antigen in an immunogenic form.[154] *Listeria monocytogenes* contains the I antigen,[153] further supporting the idea that some infectious agents stimulate the naturally occurring cold agglutinins, as well as cause the postinfectious cold agglutinin disease.

Diagnosis The clinical syndrome of cold agglutinin disease is quite variable. Patients occasionally show only low titers of cold agglutinins and have no other symptoms or have a history of recent pneumonia. In patients with warm-and-cold autoimmune hemolytic anemia, the associated hemolysis tends to be severe and chronic. The RBCs of these patients are coated with IgG and complement components, whereas their serum contains a relatively low titer of cold agglutinin that acts at 30° C and perhaps even at temperatures up to 37° C.

The diagnosis is suggested by hemolytic anemia with acral signs and symptoms. It may be difficult to draw blood, and the RBCs may visibly agglutinate in a cold syringe and on the blood smear. Automated blood cell counters may count the agglutinated RBCs as single cells and thus report absurdly high values for the MCV and MCHC. Usually, the laboratory detects a broadly active cold agglutinin. The direct Coombs test is positive with anticomplement reagents but infrequently positive with anti-IgG.

Findings that support the diagnosis of idiopathic cold agglutinin disease include a high IgM cold agglutinin titer with broad thermal reactivity[134] and I specificity (reacting with erythrocytes from adults but not with cord erythrocytes), pure κ light-chain composition, occasionally an absolute serum IgM elevation, and an M protein pattern on serum protein electrophoresis. Investigation should be directed at discovering a possible lymphoma or other underlying disorder in these patients. Conversely, post-*Mycoplasma* and post–infectious mononucleosis cold agglutinins are polyclonal. The post–infectious mononucleosis antibody is usually directed against i antigens (cord RBCs).

Treatment The post-*Mycoplasma* or the post–infectious mononucleosis variant is usually mild and self-limited and requires no specific treatment. Patients with the idiopathic variety who have acral symptoms must change their way of life, either by moving to a warmer climate or by keeping their ears, nose, hands, and feet covered during cold weather. In severely anemic patients, transfusions with packed RBCs may be required; in such patients, careful cross-matching and warming of the blood is necessary to minimize cold agglutination.

Splenectomy and corticosteroids are generally of no benefit in controlling hemolysis associated with cold agglutinin disease. Presumably, complement-coated cells are removed to a substantial degree by hepatic rather than splenic macrophages, and the cells that produce IgM are relatively insensitive to the effects of corticosteroids. Occasionally, however, high doses of corticosteroids (e.g., 100 mg of prednisone a day) have resulted in a reduction in the hemolytic rate in patients with relatively low titers of cold agglutinins. In the relatively rare variant caused by IgG cold agglutinins, corticosteroids and splenectomy may be of benefit. Use of penicillamine or other reducing agents containing sulfhydryl groups produces no benefit. Good responses are occasionally obtained by the use of chlorambucil at a dosage of 4 to 6 mg/day. Exchange transfusion and plasmapheresis appear to be logical therapies for acute disease, but further clinical studies are needed to evaluate these techniques. Interferon alfa, at a dosage of 3 million U/m² three times weekly, was reported to produce an impressive drop in cold agglutinin titer, with a decrease in serum IgM monoclonal protein and in acral symptoms over a 1-month period.[134] Treatment with rituximab in the doses used to treat non-Hodgkin lymphoma has been beneficial.[155,156]

Paroxysmal Cold Hemoglobinuria

Patients with the rare disorder of paroxysmal cold hemoglobinuria have cold-induced signs and symptoms of intravascular hemolysis. The hemolysis is associated with the presence of an IgG serum antibody that is directed against the RBC's P system. The IgG antibody is best demonstrated by the Donath-Landsteiner test; the serum is mixed either with the patient's own blood cells or with blood cells from a normal person. The mixture is chilled to 4° C. If the IgG antibody associated with this disorder is present, hemolysis occurs after warming to 37° C. In the past, paroxysmal cold hemoglobinuria was usually seen as a complication of syphilis, but it has recently been observed in association with viral infections and non-Hodgkin lymphoma.[157]

HYPERSPLENISM

Hypersplenic disorders constitute a diverse group of clinical conditions sharing the common features of splenomegaly and hemolysis. Splenic enlargement and hemolysis occur in many disorders, including hepatic cirrhosis with congestive splenomegaly, Gaucher disease, lymphoma, connective tissue disorders, Felty syndrome, sarcoidosis, tuberculosis, and other infectious diseases.

Pathophysiology

The spleen's unique structure accounts for several of the pathophysiologic features of hypersplenism. Splenic arterioles have a few direct branches leading to the sinusoids, but most of the terminal arterioles open into the splenic cords. Blood cells pass from the cords to the pulp through slits in the sinus walls; the slits have dimensions of about 1 by 3 μm.[158] Blood cells must squeeze through the longitudinal spaces, which are lined with reticular fibers, and between adventitial cells that are located outside the sinus. Macrophages and endothelial cells line the inside of the sinus. Repeated intimate contact occurs between blood cells and these macrophages.

Blood flow in the spleen is slow. The erythrocyte's pH and oxygen tension level fall, glucose is consumed, and the cell's metabolism is impaired. The hematocrit may increase, further elevating viscosity and resistance to flow. As a consequence, the blood cells are exposed to metabolic and mechanical stresses in the presence of macrophages and other leukocytes that can recognize cell membrane damage. As erythrocytes age, phagocytes remove defective surface areas, transforming the biconcave erythrocytes into rigid spherocytes or RBC fragments; these particles are later trapped and removed by the reticuloendothelial system. A big spleen has a greater than normal blood flow and exposes

an unusually large proportion of blood cells to its culling activities. Thus, the problem in hypersplenism is essentially a quantitative one. A vicious circle may evolve in patients undergoing hemolysis, because hemolysis itself may cause splenomegaly.

Diagnosis

If the spleen is not palpable but the clinical situation is strongly suggestive of splenomegaly, ultrasonography or CT scanning may prove useful. Because blood cells other than erythrocytes are affected by a large spleen, the patient may be pancytopenic. Unless the underlying disease specifically involves the bone marrow, the marrow of patients with hypersplenism is generally hyperplastic because of rapid regeneration of all affected cell lines. The peripheral blood smear is not diagnostic of hypersplenism.

Treatment

If hypersplenism is producing clinically significant complications and if therapy for the patient's primary disease does not shrink the spleen, splenectomy may be necessary. Anemia, however, is not necessarily attributable to hypersplenism, irrespective of the size of the spleen. Hemodilution is another possible mechanism. Patients with massive splenomegaly who have very low hematocrit and hemoglobin values may have a normal RBC mass as assessed with the ⁵¹Cr technique. Massive splenomegaly often is associated with an increase in plasma volume that results in extraordinary hemodilution. Moreover, greatly enlarged spleens may contain a pool of erythrocytes that constitutes as much as 25% of the total RBC mass—in contrast to normal spleens, which have no such RBC pool. In patients with splenomegaly who have a true decrease in RBC mass, the underlying disease may act to reduce RBC production by suppressing erythropoietin production rather than by accelerating destruction. Therefore, it is prudent to determine RBC mass before making the diagnosis of hypersplenism.

DRUGS AND TOXINS AS CAUSES OF HEMOLYSIS

Drugs Causing Oxidative Attack

Pathogenesis Dapsone, sulfasalazine, phenacetin, sodium perchlorate, nitroglycerin, phenazopyridine, primaquine,[100] paraquat, and vitamin K analogues can insert themselves into the oxygen-binding cleft of hemoglobin. By this action, such agents can generate oxidizing free radicals, such as superoxide, hydroxyl free radical, and peroxide. If the erythrocyte's protective reducing mechanisms are overwhelmed [see Table 1], hemoglobin is oxidized to form Heinz bodies and methemoglobin. Sulfhemoglobin is also produced by oxidative attack. The molecule contains a sulfur atom in the porphyrin ring, which gives it a blue-green color. The source of the sulfur atom is not clear, but the presence of sulfur in the heme ring makes it a poor oxygen transporter.[159] The RBC membrane may also suffer from oxidative attack. Damaged cells are removed in the reticuloendothelial system. Hemolysis is usually, but not invariably, extravascular, and Heinz bodies can be seen on a specially stained blood smear. The smear may also show the bite, hemiblister, or cross-bonded cells typical of oxidative attack on erythrocytes [see Figure 4]. Severe oxidative damage apparently causes hemoglobin to puddle at one side of the RBC, leaving a plasma membrane–enclosed hemighost in the remainder. Such hemighosts can be detected in the peripheral blood. Severe oxidative destruction is associated with increased methemoglobin levels and a decrease in RBC levels of GSH. The methemoglobin level is elevated. As little as 1.5 g/dl of methemoglobin or

0.5 g/dl of sulfhemoglobin can produce the physical finding of cyanosis. By contrast, 5 g/dl of reduced deoxyhemoglobin is required to produce comparable cyanosis.[100]

Nitrites can oxidize hemoglobin to methemoglobin. Consequently, the recreational use of butyl and isobutyl nitrites as stimulants, psychedelics, and aphrodisiacs has led to clinical problems. When inhaled in usual amounts, these agents may produce a mild to modest increase in methemoglobin, raising its concentration from the normal level of 1% to 2% to as much as 20%. More extensive inhalation or ingestion of these agents has induced severe methemoglobinemia, characterized by methemoglobin levels approaching 62%. Because methemoglobin does not carry oxygen, these high levels are accompanied by manifestations of tissue hypoxia such as headache, shortness of breath, lethargy, and stupor. Physical examination shows tachycardia, postural hypotension, and cyanosis; the venous blood is purple-brown.[160] If untreated, it is likely to be fatal.

Diagnosis   Diagnosis is based on a history of exposure to an oxidant drug or other toxin, together with characteristic peripheral blood smear findings and elevated methemoglobin measurements.

Treatment   Treatment should restore normal methemoglobin levels. Management starts with the identification and withdrawal of the offending agent. Patients who have severe methemoglobinemia should be treated immediately with 1 to 2 mg/kg of methylene blue; the agent is infused intravenously in a 1 g/dl solution over a 5-minute period. In the presence of the RBC enzyme NADPH-methemoglobin reductase and adequate amounts of the electron donor NADPH [see Table 1], methylene blue is rapidly reduced to leukomethylene blue. This product in turn quickly reduces methemoglobin to hemoglobin. Cyanosis is thereby reversed, and the patient should turn pink immediately after the infusion. Several hours later, however, the patient may again become cyanotic, presumably because nitrates released from tissues reenter the peripheral blood at that time. Readministration of methylene blue at a dosage of 1 mg/kg intravenously over a 5-minute period should restore normal hemoglobin levels.

Successful methylene blue therapy requires adequate supplies of NADPH. Patients who have abnormalities of the pentose phosphate pathway, such as G6PD deficiency, will not respond to this approach and should receive emergency exchange transfusions.[160] Patients with very high levels of methemoglobin (at least 60%) or those whose smears contain many hemighosts should undergo exchange transfusion, perhaps with hemodialysis.[100,160]

Lead-Induced Hemolysis

Lead exposure results in hypertensive encephalopathy, neuropathy, and hemolytic anemia characterized by coarse basophilic stippling in RBCs. The mechanism of lead-induced hemolysis is complex because the metal has several actions: it blocks heme synthesis, thus causing a buildup of RBC protoporphyrin[161]; it produces a deficiency of pyrimidine 5′-nucleotidase[161]; and it attacks erythrocyte membrane phospholipids, producing potassium leak and interfering with Na$^+$,K$^+$-ATPase activity.

Diagnosis   Screening for lead poisoning entails measuring the free erythrocyte protoporphyrin level (sometimes called the zinc protoporphyrin level), which is elevated because lead blocks the last step in heme synthesis. The diagnosis is confirmed by measuring blood and urine lead levels.

Treatment   After the exposure to lead is stopped, use of a chelating agent such as edetate calcium disodium (CaNa$_2$EDTA) may be considered. Treatment is started with 0.5 to 1 g of intravenous CaNa$_2$EDTA, given over a period of 6 to 8 hours; the compound is given daily for 5 days.

After this initial course, 0.5 g of CaNa$_2$EDTA is given as an intravenous bolus or intramuscular injection every 2 days for 2 weeks, during which time the urine lead levels are monitored. Alternatively, the initial 5-day course of CaNa$_2$EDTA can be followed with oral penicillamine: 1 g a day is given for the first 7 days; the drug is withheld for the next 7 days; and during the final 7 days of the regimen, the dosage of 1 g a day is resumed and the urine lead level is measured at the end of the final day. Another study recommends giving 500 mg of penicillamine a day and continuing this dosage for 60 days after the patient has become asymptomatic.[162]

VENOMS AND PHYSICAL AGENTS AS CAUSES OF HEMOLYSIS

Agents Causing Enzymatic Attack

Classic examples of attacking enzymes are the snake-venom or clostridial lecithinases (e.g., phospholipase C). Such enzymes attack the phospholipids of the membrane bilayer and produce RBC fragmentation, spherocytosis, and intravascular and extravascular hemolysis. Disseminated intravascular coagulation and shock may occur. Prompt recognition and management of the primary disorder is critical, as is supportive therapy.

Venom from the brown spider, *Loxosceles intermedia,* releases sphingomyelinases and metalloproteinases that cleave the RBC membrane glycophorins. This in turn facilitates complement activation and lysis of affected RBCs.[163]

Physical Causes of Hemolysis

Freshwater drowning and accidental intravenous administration of sterile water can cause intravascular hemolysis by osmotic lysis. In such cases, RBCs swell and become spheroidal. Saltwater drowning can induce hemolysis by desiccating RBCs. Burns cause temperature-mediated denaturation of erythrocyte membrane polypeptides, resulting in hemolysis.

Infectious Diseases Causing Hemolysis

Malaria is the most important infectious cause of hemolysis. The resulting severe anemia causes the death of large numbers of pregnant women and 2- to 5-year-old children in sub-Saharan Africa. *Plasmodium* species, particularly *P. falciparum*, directly parasitize and destroy RBCs, but the anemia is a complex blend of impaired RBC production, hemolysis of parasitized and non-parasitized[130] RBCs, and ineffective erythropoiesis.[164] The diagnosis is made by pathognomonic findings on the blood smear; treatment is directed against the malarial parasite, with support of the circulation with RBC transfusions if required [see Chapter 157].

Other infectious causes of hemolysis   Infection with *M. pneumoniae* and infectious mononucleosis can cause cold agglutinin hemolysis. Infection with *H. influenzae* type b can cause hemolysis. The major virulence factor of *H. influenzae*, polyribose ribosyl phosphate (PRRP), allows the organism to escape phagocytosis. When PRRP is released into the circulation, it binds to RBCs. The binding of anti-PRRP antibodies then leads to complement-dependent hemolysis.[165] Patients infected with

HIV or cytomegalovirus may have autoimmune hemolytic anemia (see above).[166]

Clostridial sepsis can be devastating; the appearance of free plasma hemoglobin or hemoglobinuria should suggest this often fatal infection. *Clostridium* species are capable of sudden, explosive growth; they can release many enzymes, including phospholipases and proteases, that digest RBCs, producing intravascular hemolysis.

Some infections can cause splenomegaly and hypersplenic hemolysis. Meningococcemia or overwhelming gram-negative septicemia often produces disseminated intravascular coagulation and microangiopathic hemolysis.

Babesiosis is caused by a parasite that invades RBCs and that is transmitted from its rodent reservoir by the same ixodid tick that carries Lyme disease and human granulocytic ehrlichiosis. This disease is being more frequently diagnosed, particularly in New England. Immunocompromised persons, such as those with HIV, are more likely to have chronic and severe infections. The diagnosis has been made on peripheral blood smears, but polymerase chain reaction methods are more sensitive.[167]

HEMOLYSIS ASSOCIATED WITH LIVER DISEASE

Anemia in patients with liver disease is often the result of a production defect rather than hemolysis, but cirrhotic patients may have congestive splenomegaly with hypersplenic hemolysis. Macrocytes (with or without B_{12} or folate deficiency) and target cells (caused by cholesterol elevation) are also common findings in such cases.

Spur cell anemia Severe liver disease, including alcoholic cirrhosis, may result in the formation of irregularly spiculated RBCs known as spur cells (acanthocytes).[168] Spur cells have alterations in their membranes (a decreased ratio of phospholipids to cholesterol[169]) that shorten their survival, resulting in hemolytic anemia.

OTHER CAUSES OF HEMOLYSIS

Copper Accumulation

In rare instances, Wilson disease, a metabolic disorder associated with excessive copper deposition, is first detected during a coincident episode of dramatic, acute hemolysis. The release of free copper into the serum and its subsequent entry into RBCs are thought to be the underlying hemolytic mechanism. In addition to affecting hexokinase levels, the intracellular copper appears to cause formation of oxygen radicals that react with and oxidize membrane components. Although no successful therapeutic intervention has been reported, penicillamine can be given at a dosage of 2 to 4 g once a day orally to reduce the free copper level. The administration of 1,000 to 2,000 IU of vitamin E (α-tocopherol) a day for several days may also be helpful if oxidative attack is an important factor.

Cardiopulmonary Bypass

Free plasma hemoglobin increases after cardiopulmonary bypass. The increase is thought to be caused by activation of the complement pathway. Activation of the complement pathway in turn leads to deposition of the C5b-C9 attack complex on the RBC surface.[170]

The author has served as a consultant for Tularek Corp. and Receptron, Inc., during the past 12 months.

References

1. Liu S-C, Derick LH: Molecular anatomy of the red blood cell membrane skeleton: structure-function relationships. Semin Hematol 29:231, 1992

2. Cohen CM, Gascard P: Regulation and post-translational modification of erythrocyte membrane and membrane-skeletal proteins. Semin Hematol 29:244, 1992

3. Schwartz RS: PIG-A: the target gene in paroxysmal nocturnal hemoglobinuria (editorial). N Engl J Med 330:283, 1994

4. Canessa M: Red cell volume–related ion transport systems in hemoglobinopathies. Hematol Oncol Clin North Am 5:495, 1991

5. Hanspal M, Palek J: Biogenesis of normal and abnormal red blood cell membrane skeleton. Semin Hematol 29:305, 1992

6. Turrini F, Mannu F, Arese P, et al: Characterization of the autologous antibodies that opsonize erythrocytes with clustered integral membrane proteins. Blood 81:3146, 1993

7. Potter CG, Potter AC, Hatton CSR, et al: Variation of erythroid and myeloid precursors in the marrow and peripheral blood of volunteer subjects infected with human parvovirus (B19). J Clin Invest 79:1486, 1987

8. Smith BD, Segel GB: Abnormal erythrocyte endothelial adherence in hereditary stomatocytosis. Blood 89:3451, 1997

9. Gallagher PG, Chang SH, Rettig MP, et al: Altered erythrocyte endothelial adherence and membrane phospholipid asymmetry in hereditary hydrocytosis. Blood 101:4625, 2003

10. Vives Corrons JL, Besson I, Aymerich M, et al: Hereditary xerocytosis: a report of six unrelated Spanish families with leaky red cell syndrome and increased heat stability of the erythrocyte membrane. Br J Haematol 90:817, 1995

11. Ogburn PL Jr, Ramin KD, Danilenko-Dixon D: In utero erythrocyte transfusion for fetal xerocytosis associated with non-immune hydrops fetalis. Am J Obstet Gynecol 185,238, 2001

12. Palek J, Jarolim P: Clinical expression and laboratory detection of red blood cell membrane protein mutations. Semin Hematol 30:249, 1993

13. Dhermy D, Galand C, Bournier O, et al: Heterogenous band 3 deficiency in hereditary spherocytosis related to different band 3 gene defects. Br J Haematol 98:32, 1997

14. Delhommeau F, Cynober T, Schischmanoff, et al: Natural history of hereditary spherocytosis during the first year of life. Blood 95:393, 2000

15. Rosse WF: Hematopoiesis and the defect in paroxysmal hemoglobinuria. J Clin Invest 100:953, 1997

16. Ohashi H, Hotta T, Ichikawa A, et al: Peripheral blood cells are predominantly chimeric of affected and normal cells in patients with paroxysmal nocturnal hemoglobinuria: simultaneous investigation on clonality and expression of glycophosphatidylinositol-anchored proteins. Blood 83:853, 1994

17. Rosti V: The molecular basis of paroxysmal nocturnal hemoglobinuria. Haematologica 85:82, 2000

18. Hillmen P, Lewis SM, Bessler M, et al: Natural history of paroxysmal nocturnal hemoglobinuria. N Engl J Med 333:1253, 1995

19. Socie G, Marie J-Y, de Gramont A, et al: Paroxysmal nocturnal haemoglobinuria: long-term follow-up and prognostic factors. Lancet 348:573, 1996

20. Hugel B, Socié G, Vu T, et al: Elevated levels of circulating procoagulant microparticles in patients with paroxysmal nocturnal hemoglobinuria and aplastic anemia. Blood 93:3451, 1999

21. Ray JG, Burows RF, Ginsberg JS, et al: Paroxysmal nocturnal hemoglobinuria and the risk of venous thrombosis: review and recommendations for management of the pregnant and nonpregnant patient. Haemostasis 30:103, 2000

22. Hall SE, Rosse WF: The use of monoclonal antibodies and flow cytometry in the diagnosis of paroxysmal nocturnal hemoglobinuria. Blood 87:5332, 1996

23. Sholar PW, Bell WR: Thrombolytic therapy for inferior vena cava thrombosis in paroxysmal nocturnal hemoglobinuria. Ann Intern Med 103:539, 1985

24. Saso R, Marsh J, Cevreska L, et al: Bone marrow transplants for paroxysmal nocturnal haemoglobinuria. Br J Haematol 104:392, 1999

25. Balleari E, Gatti AM, Mareni C, et al: Recombinant human erythropoietin for long-term treatment of anemia in paroxysmal nocturnal hemoglobinuria. Haematologica 81:143, 1996

26. Schubert J, Scholz C, Geissler RG: G-CSF and cyclosporine induce an increase of normal cells in hypoplastic paroxysmal nocturnal hemoglobinuria. Ann Hematol 74:225, 1997

27. Arese P, De Flora A: Pathophysiology of hemolysis in glucose-6-phosphate dehydrogenase deficiency. Semin Hematol 27:1, 1990

28. Beutler E: G6PD deficiency. Blood 84:3613, 1994

29. Mockenhaupt FP, Mandelkow J, Till H: Reduced prevalence of *Plasmodium falciparum* infection and of concomitant anaemia in pregnant women with heterozygous G6PD deficiency. Trop Med Int Health 8:118, 2003

30. Neuberger A, Flishman S, Golic A: Hemolytic anemia in G6PD-deficient man after inhalation of amyl nitrite ("poppers"). Isr Med Assoc J 4:1085, 2002

31. Nagel RL, Ranney HM: Genetic epidemiology of structural mutations of the beta-globin gene. Semin Hematol 27:342, 1990

32. Bunn HF: Pathogenesis and treatment of sickle cell disease. N Engl J Med 337:762, 1997

33. Steinberg MH, Rodgers GP: Pathophysiology of sickle cell disease: role of cellular and genetic modifiers. Semin Hematol 38:299, 2001

34. Hebbel RP: Beyond hemoglobin polymerization: the red blood cell membrane and sickle disease pathophysiology. Blood 77:214, 1991

35. Gladwn MT, Lancaster JR Jr, Freeman BA, et al: Nitric oxide's reactions with hemoglobin: a view through the SNO-storm. Nat Med 9:496, 2003

36. Kuypers FA, Lewis RA, Hua M, et al: Detection of altered membrane phospholipid asymmetry in subpopulations of human red blood cells using fluorescently labeled annexin V. Blood 87:1179, 1996

37. Solovey A, Gui L, Key NS, et al: Tissue factor expression by endothelial cells in sickle cell anemia. J Clin Invest 101:1899, 1998

38. Hargrave DR, Wade A, Evans JP, et al: Nocturnal oxygen saturation and painful sickle cell crises in children. Blood 101:846, 2003

39. Singhal A, Doherty JF, Raynes JG: Is there an acute-phase response in steady-state sickle cell disease? Lancet 341:651, 1993

40. Hebbel RP: Adhesive interactions of sickle erythrocytes with endothelium. J Clin Invest 99:2561, 1997

41. Grigg AP: Granulocyte colony-stimulating factor-induced sickle cell crisis and multiorgan dysfunction in a patient with compound heterozygous sickle cell/beta+ thalassemia. Blood 97:3998, 2001

42. Adler BK, Salzman DE, Carabasi MH, et al: Fatal sickle cell crisis after granulocyte colony-stimulating factor administration. Blood 97:3313, 2001

43. Okpala I, Daniel Y, Haynes R, et al: Relationship between the clinical manifestations of sickle cell disease and the expression of adhesion molecules on white blood cells. Eur J Haematol 69:135, 2002

44. Turhan A, Weiss LA, Mohandas N: Primary role for adherent leukocytes in sickle cell vascular occlusion: a new paradigm. Proc Natl Acad Sci USA 99:3047, 2002

45. Francis RB, Johnson CS: Vascular occlusion in sickle cell disease: current concepts and unanswered questions. Blood 77:1405, 1991

46. Steinberg MH, West MS, Gallagher D, et al: Effects of glucose-6-phosphate dehydrogenase deficiency upon sickle cell anemia. Blood 71:748, 1988

47. Nagel RL, Steinberg MH: Role of epistatic (modifier) genes in the modulation of the phenotypic diversity of sickle cell disease. Pediatr Pathol Mol Med 20:123, 2001

48. Ballas SK: Neurobiology and treatment of pain. Sickle Cell Disease: Basic Principles and Clinical Practice. Embury SH, Hebbel RP, Mohandas N, et al, Eds. Raven Press, New York, 1994, p 745

49. Brugnara C, de Franceschi L, Alper SL: Inhibition of Ca^{2+}-dependent K^+ transport and cell dehydration in sickle erythrocytes by clotrimazole and other imidazole derivatives. J Clin Invest 92:520, 1993

50. Bennekou P, de Franceschi L, Pedersen O, et al: Treatment with NS3623, a novel Cl^- conductance blocker, ameliorates erythrocyte dehydration in transgenic SAD mice: a possible new therapeutic approach for sickle cell disease. Blood 97:1451, 2001

51. Platt OS, Brambilla DJ, Rosse WF, et al: Mortality in sickle cell disease: life expectancy and risk factors for early death. N Engl J Med 330:1639, 1994

52. Bunn HF: Induction of fetal hemoglobin in sickle cell disease. Blood 93:1787, 1999

53. Charache S, Terrin ML, Moore RD, et al: Effect of hydroxyurea on the frequency of painful crises in sickle cell anemia. N Engl J Med 332:1317, 1995

54. Steinberg MH, Barton F, Castro O, et al: Hydroxyurea (HU) is associated with reduced mortality in adults with sickle cell anemia (abstr). J Am Soc Hematol 96:485a, 2000

55. Bridges KR, Barabino GD, Brugnara C, et al: A multiparameter analysis of sickle erythrocytes in patients undergoing hydroxyurea therapy. Blood 88:4701, 1996

56. Perrine SP, Ginder GD, Faller DV, et al: A short-term trial of butyrate to stimulate fetal-globin-gene expression in the beta-globin disorders. N Engl J Med 328:81, 1993

57. Atweh GF, Sutton M, Nassif I, et al: Sustained induction of fetal hemoglobin by pulse butyrate therapy in sickle cell disease. Blood 93:1790, 1999

58. Walters MC, Patience M, Leisenring W, et al: Bone marrow transplantation for sickle cell disease. N Engl J Med 335:369, 1996

59. Adams RJ, McKie VC, Hsu L, et al: Prevention of a first stroke by transfusions in children with sickle cell anemia and abnormal results on transcranial Doppler ultrasonography. N Engl J Med 339:5, 1998

60. Vichinsky EP: Understanding the morbidity of sickle cell disease (correspondence). Br J Haematol 99:974, 1997

61. Ohene-Frempong K: Indications for red cell transfusion in sickle cell disease. Semin Hematol 38(1 suppl 1):5, 2001

62. Olivieri NF: Progression of iron overload in sickle cell disease. Semin Hematol 38(1 suppl 1):57, 2001

63. Cohen AR, Martin MB: Iron chelation therapy in sickle cell disease. Semin Hematol 38(1 suppl 1):69, 2001

64. Bellet PS, Kalinyak KA, Shukla R, et al: Incentive spirometry to prevent acute pulmonary complications in sickle cell diseases. N Engl J Med 333:699, 1995

65. Milner PF, Kraus AP, Sebes JI, et al: Sickle cell disease as a cause of osteonecrosis of the femoral head. N Engl J Med 325:1476, 1991

66. Koate P: Cardiovascular pathology in sickle cell anemia. Bull Acad Natl Med 175:1055, 1991

67. Norris S, Johnson CS, Haywood LJ: Sickle cell anemia: does myocardial ischemia occur during crisis? J Natl Med Assoc 83:209, 1991

68. Castro O, Hoque M, Brown BD: Pulmonary hypertension in sickle cell disease: cardiac catheterization results and survival. Blood 101:1257, 2003

69. Vichinsky E, Williams R, Das M, et al: Pulmonary fat embolism: a distinct cause of severe acute chest syndrome in sickle cell anemia. Blood 83:3107, 1994

70. Vichinsky EP, Styles LA, Colangelo LH, et al: Acute chest syndrome in sickle cell disease: clinical presentation and course. Blood 89:1787, 1997

71. Dean D, Neumayr L, Kelly DM, et al: Chlamydia pneumoniae and acute chest syndrome in patients with sickle cell disease. J Pediatr Hematol Oncol 25:46, 2003

72. Styles LA, Schalkwijk CG, Aarsman AJ, et al: Phospholipase A$_2$ levels in acute chest syndrome of sickle cell disease. Blood 87: 2573, 1996

73. Gaston MH, Verter JI, Woods G, et al: Prophylaxis with oral penicillin in children with sickle cell anemia: a randomized trial. N Engl J Med 314:1593, 1986

74. Haberkern CM, Neumayr LD, Orringer EP, et al: Cholecystectomy in sickle cell anemia patients: perioperative outcome of 364 cases from national preoperative transfusion study. Blood 89:1533, 1997

75. Serjeant GR: Sickle-cell disease. Lancet 350:725, 1997

76. Gupta AK, Kirchner KA, Nicholson R, et al: Effects of α-thalassemia and sickle polymerization tendency on the urine-concentrating defect of individuals with sickle cell trait. J Clin Invest 88:1963, 1991

77. Falk RJ, Scheinman J, Phillips G, et al: Prevalence and pathologic features of sickle cell nephropathy and response to inhibition of angiotensin-converting enzyme. N Engl J Med 326:910, 1992

78. Bruno D, Wigfall DR, Zimmerman SA, et al: Genitourinary complications of sickle cell disease. J Urol 166:803, 2001

79. Opkala I, Westerdale N, Jegede T: Etilefrine for the prevention of priapism in adult sickle cell disease. Br J Haematol 118:918, 2002

80. Ohene-Frempong K, Weiner SJ, Sleeper LA, et al: Cerebrovascular accidents in sickle cell disease: rates and risk factors. Blood 91:288, 1998

81. Cohen AR: Sickle cell disease: new treatments, new questions. N Engl J Med 339:42, 1998

82. Dobson SR, Holden KR, Nietert PJ: Moyamoya syndrome in childhood sickle cell disease: a predictive factor for recurrent cerebrovascular events. Blood 99:3144, 2002

83. Mohan JS, Vigilance JE, Marshall JM, et al: Abnormal venous function in patients with homozygous sickle cell (SS) disease and chronic leg ulcers. Clin Sci (Colch) 98:667, 2000

84. Groves RW, Schmidt-Lucke JA: Recombinant human GM-CSF in the treatment of poorly healing wounds. Adv Skin Wound Care 13:107, 2000

85. Serjeant GR, Serjeant BE, Thomas PW, et al: Human parvovirus infection in homozygous sickle cell disease. Lancet 341:1237, 1993

86. Koshy M, Weiner SJ, Miller ST, et al: Surgery and anesthesia in sickle cell disease. Blood 86:3676, 1995

87. Vichinsky EP, Haberkern CM, Neumayr L, et al: A comparison of conservative and aggressive transfusion regimens in the perioperative management of sickle cell disease. N Engl J Med 333:206, 1995

88. Koshy M, Burd L: Management of pregnancy in sickle cell syndromes. Hematol Oncol Clin North Am 5:585, 1991

89. Embury SH: Prenatal diagnosis. Sickle Cell Disease: Basic Principles and Clinical Practice. Embury SH, Hebbel RP, Mohandas N, et al, Eds. Raven Press, New York, 1994, p 485

90. Smith JA, Espeland M, Bellevue R, et al: Pregnancy in sickle cell disease: experience of the Cooperative Study of Sickle Cell Disease. Obstet Gynecol 87:199, 1996

91. Steinberg MH, Barton F, Castro O, et al: Effect of hydroxyurea on mortality and morbidity in adult sickle cell anemia: risks and benefits up to 9 years of treatment. JAMA 289:1645, 2003

92. Kark JA, Posey DM, Schumacher HR, et al: Sickle-cell trait as a risk factor for sudden death in physical training. N Engl J Med 317:781, 1987

93. Sullivan LW: The risks of sickle-cell trait: caution and common sense. N Engl J Med 317:830, 1987

94. Loukopoulos D, Voskaridou E, Kalotychou V, et al: Reduction of the clinical severity of sickle cell/beta-thalassemia with hydroxyurea: the experience of a single center in Greece. Blood Cells Mol Dis 26:453, 2000

95. Rogers ZR: Hydroxyurea therapy for diverse pediatric populations with sickle cell disease. Semin Hematol 34(3 suppl 3):42, 1997

96. Nagel RL, Fabry ME, Steiberg MH: The paradox of hemoglobin SC disease. Blood Rev 17:167, 2003

97. Nagel RL, Lawrence C: The distinct pathobiology of sickle cell–hemoglobin C disease. Hematol Oncol Clin North Am 5:433, 1991

98. Steinberg MH, Nagel RL, Brugnara C: Cellular effects of hydroxyurea in Hb SC disease. Br J Haematol 98:838, 1997

99. Rees DC, Styles L, Vichinsky EP, et al: The hemoglobin E syndromes. Ann NY Acad Sci 850:334, 1998

100. Jaffe ER: Methemoglobinemia in the differential diagnosis of cyanosis. Hosp Pract (Off Ed) 20:92, 1985

101. Charache S: Methemoglobinemia-sleuthing for a new cause (editorial). N Engl J Med 314:776, 1986

102. Manabe J, Arya R, Sumimoto H, et al: Two novel mutations in the reduced nicotinamide adenine dinucleotide (NADH)-cytochrome b5 reductase gene of a patient with generalized type, hereditary methemoglobinemia. Blood 88:3208, 1996

103. Percy MJ, Gillespie MJ, Savage G, et al: Familial idiopathic methemoglobinemia revisited: original cases reveal 2 novel mutations in NADH-cytochrome b5 reductase. Blood 100:3447, 2002

104. Weatherall DJ, Clegg JB: Thalassemia: a global public health problem. Nat Med 2:847, 1996

105. Adams JG III, Coleman MB: Structural hemoglobin variants that produce the phenotype of thalassemia. Semin Hematol 27:229, 1990

106. Schrier SL: Thalassemia: pathophysiology of red cell changes. Annu Rev Med 45:211, 1994

107. Schrier SL: Pathophysiology of thalassemia erythrocytes. Curr Opin Hematol 4:75, 1997

108. Schrier SL: Pathophysiology of thalassemia. Curr Opin Hematol 9:123, 2002

109. Amer J, Goldfarb A, Fibach E: Flow cytometric measurement of reactive oxygen

species production by normal and thalassaemic red blood cells. Eur J Haematol 70:84, 2003

110. Pootrakul P, Sirankapracha P, Hemsorach S, et al: A correlation of erythrokinetics, ineffective erythropoiesis, and erythroid precursor apoptosis in Thai patients with thalassemia. Blood 96:2606, 2000

111. Hansen RM, Hanson G, Anderson T: Failure to suspect and diagnose thalassemic syndromes: interpretation of RBC indices by the nonhematologist. Arch Intern Med 145: 93, 1985

112. Piomelli S: The management of patients with Cooley's anemia: transfusions and splenectomy. Semin Hematol 32:262, 1995

113. Hoffbrand AV: Oral iron chelation. Semin Hematol 33:1, 1996

114. Brittenham GM, Griffith PM, Nienhuis AW, et al: Efficacy of deferoxamine in preventing complications of iron overload in patients with thalassemia major. N Engl J Med 331:567, 1994

115. Olivieri NF, Nathan DG, MacMillan JH, et al: Survival in medically treated patients with homozygous β-thalassemia. N Engl J Med 331:574, 1994

116. Cohen AR, Galanello R, Piga A: Safety and effectiveness of long-term therapy with the oral iron chelator deferiprone. Blood 102:583, 2003

117. Nisbet-Brown E, Olivieri NP, Giardina PJ, et al: Effectiveness and safety of ICL670 in iron-loaded patients with thalassaemia: a randomized, double-blind, placebo-controlled, dose-escalation trial. Lancet 361:1597, 2003

118. Neufeld EJ: Oral chelators deferasirox and deferiprone for transfusional iron overload in thalassemia major: new data, new questions. Blood 107:3426, 2006

119. Winterbourne CC: Oxidative denaturation in congenital hemolytic anemias: the unstable hemoglobins. Semin Haematol 27:41, 1990

120. Issaragrisil S, Visuthisakchai S, Suvatte V, et al: Brief report: transplantation of cord-blood stem cells into a patient with severe thalassemia. N Engl J Med 332:367, 1995

121. Gaziev J, Lucarelli G: Stem cell transplantation for hemoglobinopathies. Curr Opinion Pediatr 15:24, 2003

122. Bradai M, Abad MT, Pissard S, et al: Hydroxyurea can eliminate transfusion requirements in children with severe beta-thalassemia. Blood 102:1529, 2003

123. De Paula EV, Lima CS, Arruda VR, et al: Long-term hydroxyurea therapy in beta-thalassemia patients. Eur J Haematol 70:151, 2003

124. Domenica Cappellini M, Graziadei G, Ciceri L, et al: Oral isobutyramide therapy in patients with thalassemia intermedia: results of a phase II open study. Blood Cells Mol Dis 26:105, 2000

125. Reich S, Buhrer C, Henze G, et al: Oral isobutyramide reduces transfusion requirements in some patients with homozygous beta-thalassemia. Blood 96:3357, 2000

126. Chui DHK, Fucharoen S, Chan V: Hemoglobin H disease: not necessarily a benign disorder. Blood 101:791, 2003

127. Kazazian HH Jr: The thalassemia syndromes: molecular basis and prenatal diagnosis in 1990. Semin Hematol 27:209, 1990

128. Dover GJ, Valle D: Therapy for β-thalassemia: a paradigm for the treatment of genetic disorders. N Engl J Med 331:609, 1994

129. Ross CN, Reuter H, Scott D, et al: Microangiopathic haemolytic anaemia and systemic vasculitis. Br J Rheumatol 35:377, 1996

130. Rytting M, Worth L, Jaffe N: Hemolytic disorders associated with cancer. Hematol Oncol Clin North Am 10:365, 1996

131. Mach-Pascual S, Samii K, Beris P, et al: Microangiopathic hemolytic anemia complicating FK 506 (tacrolimus) therapy. Am J Hematol 52:310, 1996

132. Kojouri K, Vesely SK, George JN: Quinine-associated thrombotic thrombocytopenic purpura–hemolytic uremic syndrome: frequency, clinical features, and long-term outcomes. Ann Intern Med 135:1047, 2001

133. Freedman A, Afonja O, Chang MW, et al: Cutaneous anthrax associated with microangiopathic hemolytic anemia and coagulopathy in a 7-month-old infant. JAMA 287:869, 2002

134. Engelfriet CP, Overbeeke MAM, von dem Borne AEGK: Autoimmune hemolytic anemia. Semin Hematol 29:3, 1992

135. Jefferies LC: Transfusion therapy in autoimmune hemolytic anemia. Hematol Oncol Clin North Am 8:1087, 1994

136. Leddy JP, Falany JL, Kissel GE, et al: Erythrocyte membrane proteins reactive with human (warm-reacting) anti-red cell autoantibodies. J Clin Invest 91:1672, 1993

137. Ramos-Casals M, Garcia-Carrasco M, Lopez-Medrano F, et al: Severe autoimmune cytopenias in treatment-naïve hepatitis C virus infection: clinical description of 35 cases. Medicine 82:87, 2003

138. Liesveld JL, Rowe JM, Lichtman MA: Variability of the erythropoietic response in autoimmune hemolytic anemia: analysis of 109 cases. Blood 69:820, 1987

139. Meyer O, Stahl D, Beckhove P, et al: Pulsed high-dose dexamethasone in chronic autoimmune haemolytic anaemia of warm type. Br J Haematol 98:860, 1997

140. Emilia G, Messora C, Longo G, et al: Long-term salvage treatment by cyclosporin in refractory autoimmune haematological disorders. Br J Haematol 93:341, 1996

141. Collins PW, Newland AC: Treatment modalities of autoimmune blood disorders. Semin Hematol 29:64, 1992

142. Flores G, Cunningham-Rundles C, Newland AC, et al: Efficacy of intravenous immunoglobulin in the treatment of autoimmune hemolytic anemia: results in 73 patients. Am J Hematol 44:237, 1993

143. Gottardo NG, Baker DL, Willis FR: Successful induction and maintenance of long-term remission in a child with chronic relapsing autoimmune hemolytic anemia using rituximab. Pediatr Hematol Oncol 20:557, 2003

144. Trape G, Fianchi L, Lai M, et al: Rituximab chimeric anti-CD20 monoclonal antibody treatment for refractory hemolytic anemia in patients with lymphoproliferative disorders. Haematologica 88:223, 2003

145. Jourdan E, Topart D, Richard B, et al: Severe autoimmune hemolytic anemia following rituximab therapy in a patient with a lymphoproliferative disorder. Leuk Lymphoma 44:889, 2003

146. Salama A, Berghofer H, Mueller-Eckhardt C: Red blood cell transfusion in warm-type autoimmune haemolytic anaemia. Lancet 340:1515, 1992

147. Salama A, Mueller-Eckhardt C: Immune-mediated blood cell dyscrasias related to drugs. Semin Hematol 29:54, 1992

148. Garratty G: Immune cytopenia associated with antibiotics. Transfus Med Rev 7:255, 1993

149. Kopicky JA, Packman CH: The mechanisms of sulfonylurea-induced immune hemolysis: case report and review of the literature. Am J Hematol 23:283, 1986

150. Petz LD: Drug-induced autoimmune hemolytic anemia. Transfus Med Rev 7:242, 1993

151. Salama A, Kroll H, Wittmann G, et al: Diclofenac-induced immune haemolytic anaemia: simultaneous occurrence of red blood cell autoantibodies and drug-dependent antibodies. Br J Haematol 95:640, 1996

152. Ramsey G: Red cell antibodies arising from solid organ transplants. Transfusion 31:76, 1991

153. Silberstein LE: B-cell origin of cold agglutinins. Adv Exp Med Biol 347:193, 1994

154. Loomes LM, Uemura K, Childs RA, et al: Erythrocyte receptors for *Mycoplasma pneumoniae* are sialylated oligosaccharides of Ii antigen type. Nature 307:560, 1984

155. Berentsen S, Tjonnfjord GE, Brudevold R: Favourable response to therapy with the anti-CD20 monoclonal antibody rituximab in primary chronic cold agglutinin disease. Br J Haematol 115:79, 2001

156. Mori A, Tamaru J, Sumi H, et al: Beneficial effects of rituximab on primary cold agglutin disease refractory to conventional therapy. Eur J Haematol 68:243, 2002

157. Sharara AI, Hillsley RE, Wax TD, et al: Paroxysmal cold hemoglobinuria associated with non-Hodgkin's lymphoma. South Med J 87:397, 1994

158. Rosse WF: The spleen as a filter. N Engl J Med 317:704, 1987

159. Lu HC, Shih RD, Marcus S, et al: Pseudomethemoglobinemia: a case and review of sulfhemoglobinemia. Arch Pediatr Adolesc Med 152:803, 1998

160. Coleman MD, Coleman NA: Drug-induced methaemoglobinaemia: treatment issues. Drug Saf 14:394, 1996

161. Valentine WN, Paglia DE, Fink K, et al: Lead poisoning: association with hemolytic anemia, basophilic stippling, erythrocyte pyrimidine 5'-nucleotidase deficiency, and intraerythrocytic accumulation of pyrimidines. J Clin Invest 58:926, 1976

162. Carton JA, Maradona JA, Arribas JM: Acute-subacute lead poisoning: clinical findings and comparative study of diagnostic tests. Arch Intern Med 147:697, 1987

163. Tambourgi DV, De Sousa Da Silva M, Billington SJ, et al: Mechanism of induction of complement susceptibility of erythrocytes by spider and bacterial sphingomyelinases. Immunology 107:93, 2002

164. Nagel RL: Malarial anemia. Hemoglobin 26:329, 2002

165. Shurin SB, Anderson P, Zollinger J, et al: Pathophysiology of hemolysis in infections with *Hemophilus influenzae* type b. J Clin Invest 77:1340, 1986

166. van Spronsen DJ, Breed WPM: Cytomegalovirus-induced thrombocytopenia and haemolysis in an immunocompetent adult. Br J Haematol 92:218, 1996

167. Krause PJ, Spielman A, Telford SR III, et al: Persistent parasitemia after acute babesiosis. N Engl J Med 339:160, 1998

168. Owen JS, Brown DJC, Harry DS, et al: Erythrocyte echinocytosis in liver disease. J Clin Invest 76:2275, 1985

169. Allen DW, Manning N: Cholesterol-loading of membranes of normal erythrocytes inhibits phospholipid repair and arachidonoyl-CoA:1-palmitoyl-sn-glycero-3-phosphocholine acyl transferase: a model of spur cell anemia. Blood 87:3489, 1996

170. Salama A, Hugo F, Heinrich D, et al: Deposition of terminal C5b-complement complexes on erythrocytes and leukocytes during cardiopulmonary bypass. N Engl J Med 318:408, 1988

94 The Polycythemias

Virginia C. Broudy, M.D.

Classification of the Polycythemias

Polycythemia, also called erythrocytosis, is an increase in the number of circulating red blood cells per volume of blood, as reflected by an elevated hematocrit or hemoglobin level. The three major categories of polycythemia are (1) relative polycythemia, (2) secondary polycythemia, and (3) primary polycythemia, or polycythemia vera.

In relative polycythemia, the red blood cell mass is normal but the plasma volume is decreased. Secondary polycythemia is caused by an elevated erythropoietin level. Polycythemia vera is a neoplastic stem cell disorder characterized by an autonomous overproduction of red blood cells and, often, of white blood cells and platelets [*see Chapter 205*].

Initial Evaluation

Patients are often asymptomatic, and the elevated hemoglobin or hematocrit level is usually discovered accidentally. When such an increase in the hemoglobin or hematocrit level is found, it should be promptly evaluated to determine its cause [*see Figure 1*]. Any family history of polycythemia and the results of any previous hematocrit determinations should be obtained. History and physical examination findings suggestive of congenital heart disease, severe chronic obstructive pulmonary disease (COPD), or sleep apnea syndrome should be sought, and the presence or absence of splenomegaly should be determined. The results of the complete blood count, including the platelet count and white blood cell differential, should be critically reviewed for abnormalities. Findings of leukocytosis, thrombocytosis, an occasional circulating immature white blood cell, or increased basophils are suggestive of polycythemia vera and argue against secondary causes of erythrocytosis.

A hematocrit level of 60% or higher in a man or 57% or higher in a woman virtually always indicates a true increase in red blood cell mass (i.e., primary or secondary polycythemia). If the patient's hematocrit is below these values but above normal, a red blood cell mass study is required.[1] To perform this study, a sample of the patient's red blood cells is labeled with radioactive chromium (^{51}Cr) ex vivo and injected back into the patient. A second blood sample is then obtained to quantitate the concentration of ^{51}Cr-labeled red blood cells among the unlabeled red blood cells. In parallel, the patient is given an injection of albumin labeled with radioactive iodine (^{125}I) to measure the plasma volume. If a contraction of plasma volume is noted, the patient has relative polycythemia; if an increase in red blood cell mass is noted, the patient has true (i.e., primary or secondary) polycythemia. Once a relative or an absolute increase in red blood cell mass is documented, an exact diagnosis should be determined [*see Figure 1*].

Relative Polycythemia

Patients with relative polycythemia (Gaisböck syndrome) are often obese, hypertensive men who may also be heavy smokers[2]; such patients often are 45 to 55 years of age—a decade younger than typical for polycythemia vera patients [*see Chapter*

205]. It has been estimated that 0.5% to 0.7% of the healthy male population in the United States have relative polycythemia. Diuretic use for treatment of hypertension may exacerbate the deficit in plasma volume, and smoking-induced high carboxyhemoglobin levels or hypoxemia may also play a role.

Relative polycythemia is usually mild (hematocrit lower than 55%). In patients with a hematocrit lower than 60%, this diagnosis should be considered, and the red blood cell mass and plasma volume should be measured [*see Figure 1*] to avoid an extensive and ultimately frustrating workup for other causes of polycythemia. Patients with relative polycythemia fall into two major groups: (1) those with normal red blood cell mass and clearly decreased plasma volume and (2) those with red blood cell mass and plasma volume at the upper and lower range of normal, respectively. Behavior modification (e.g., an exercise regimen and smoking cessation) is recommended for these patients. Hematocrit returns to normal over time in approximately one third of patients.

Secondary Polycythemia

Secondary polycythemia occurs when erythropoietin production is increased as a result of chronic tissue hypoxia. Causes of tissue hypoxia include life at high altitude, high-affinity hemoglobin, cardiopulmonary disease, obstructive sleep apnea, obesity-hypoventilation syndrome, and high serum levels of carboxyhemoglobin. Polycythemia also occurs in some renal and hepatic disorders, in rare genetic disorders, and from treatment with androgens or erythropoietin.

POLYCYTHEMIA CAUSED BY APPROPRIATE INCREASES IN ERYTHROPOIETIN PRODUCTION

Life at High Altitude

Initial human adaptation to high altitude includes increases in the respiratory rate, cardiac output, and the level of 2,3-bisphosphoglycerate to facilitate oxygen unloading from hemoglobin to the tissues [*see Figure 2*]. Within 6 to 24 hours after a person has ascended to a high altitude, erythropoietin levels increase, resulting in reticulocytosis within 24 to 48 hours. Over several days, serum erythropoietin levels return to normal, but the increase in hematocrit is sustained. In addition to the increase in red blood cell mass, a modest decrease in plasma volume occurs. A patient's travel history should be taken to determine the likelihood of high-altitude effect and thus possibly avoid having to conduct an extensive workup.

Life at high altitude, such as in the Rocky Mountains of North America or the Andes of South America, may result in chronic mountain sickness characterized by headaches, dizziness, mental slowing, dyspnea, and weakness. In such cases, individuals may have a hematocrit as high as 63% and are at risk for the development of pulmonary hypertension, early onset cardiovascular disease, and proteinuria. Treatment with low-dose angiotensin-converting enzyme (ACE) inhibitors (e.g., enalapril, 5 mg orally each day) can improve the hematocrit and renal function over 1 to 2 years.[3]

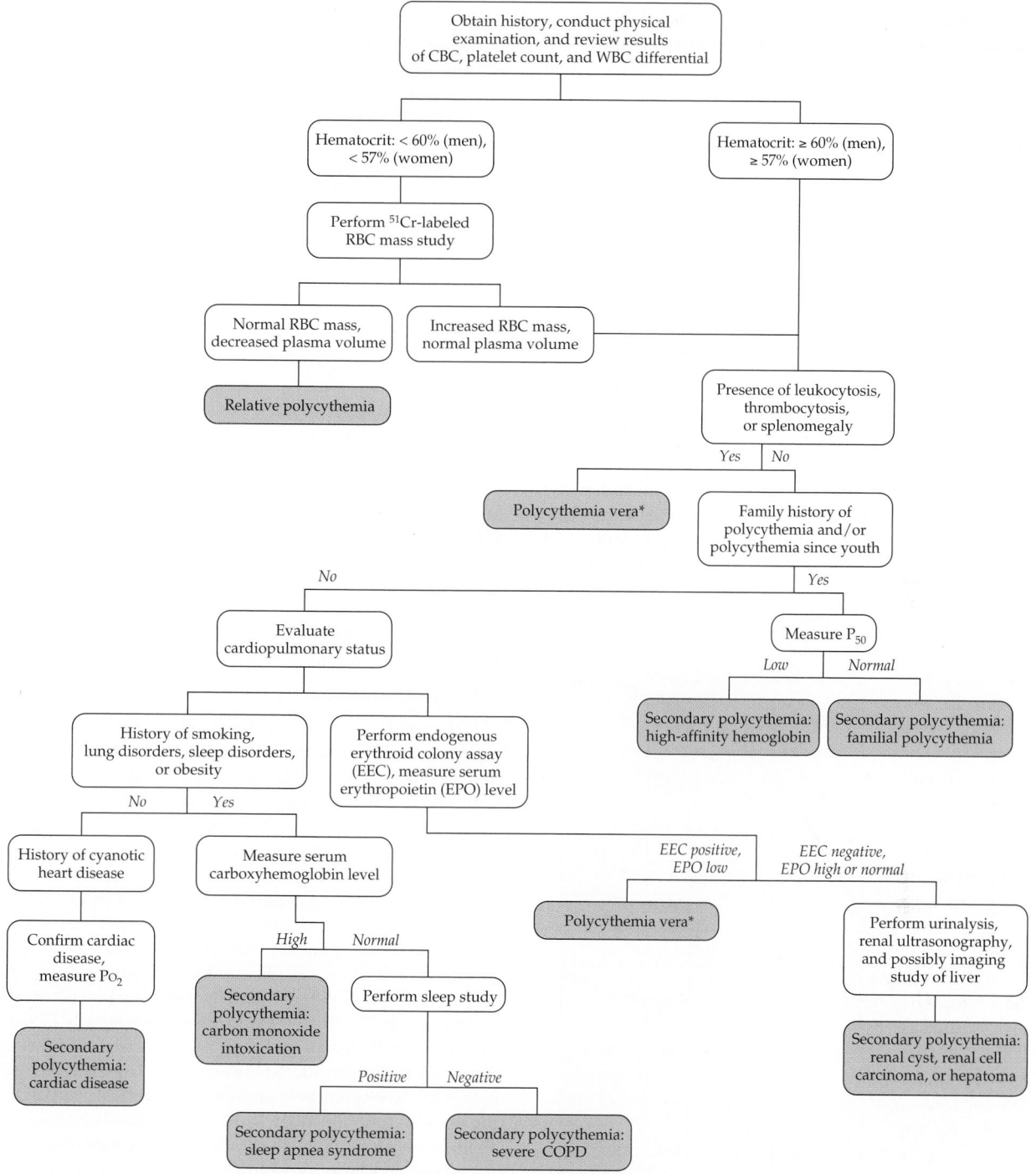

Figure 1 This flowchart depicts an approach to the evaluation of a patient with polycythemia, as evidenced by an elevated hematocrit or hemoglobin level on routine complete blood count. (CBC—complete blood cell count; COPD—chronic obstructive pulmonary disease; EEC—endogenous erythroid colony; EPO—erythropoietin; RBC—red blood cell count; WBC—white blood cell count) *For coverage of polycythemia vera, see Chapter 210.

High-Affinity Hemoglobin

High-affinity hemoglobin is caused by an amino acid substitution in either the α chain or, more commonly, the β chain of globin that impedes the normal conformational change during oxygen loading and unloading. This condition results in an impaired ability to release oxygen in the tissues, causing tissue hypoxia and increased erythropoietin production. More than 100 mutations causing high-affinity hemoglobin have been de-scribed. They are usually familial and are inherited in an autosomal dominant manner but are occasionally the result of spontaneous mutation. A review of the patient's medical history should show evidence of lifelong polycythemia. The hematocrit is usually less than 60%, and the white blood cell and platelet counts are normal. The partial pressure of oxygen at which hemoglobin is 50% saturated (P_{50}) should be measured; it is reduced in patients with high-affinity hemoglobin [see Figure 2].

Hemoglobin electrophoresis is usually not helpful, because many of the mutations that result in high-affinity hemoglobin are electrophoretically silent. However, the mutations can be identified by DNA sequencing. In rare instances, patients have congenital 2,3-bisphosphoglycerate mutase deficiency; the presentations of these patients are similar to those of patients with high-affinity hemoglobin. Patients with high-affinity hemoglobin or congenital 2,3-bisphosphoglycerate mutase deficiency usually have no symptoms of hyperviscosity and require no therapy. Phlebotomy decreases exercise tolerance in these patients and should not be used.

Cardiopulmonary Disease

Polycythemia caused by cardiopulmonary defects (e.g., Eisenmenger complex, univentricular heart, and tetralogy of Fallot) results from a failure to load oxygen onto hemoglobin adequately in the lungs.[4,5] The hematocrit may range from 60% to 75% and cause profound symptoms of hyperviscosity, including headache, dizziness, visual disturbances, fatigue, paresthesias, irritability, and decreased mental acuity. Platelet microparticles are overproduced in cyanotic congenital heart disease, especially when the hematocrit is greater than 60%; overabundance of these microparticles may contribute to the hemostatic abnormalities in these patients.[6] Some adults with cyanotic congenital heart disease have decompensated erythrocytosis, which is characterized by unstable, rising hematocrit and symptomatic hyperviscosity; these patients may benefit from phlebotomy.[5] Other adults with cyanotic congenital heart disease have compensated erythrocytosis, in which a stable (though elevated) hematocrit is maintained without overt symptoms of hyperviscosity; these patients do not require phlebotomy.[5] A practical approach is to cautiously phlebotomize patients whose hematocrits range from 60% to 65% and who have symptoms of hyperviscosity.[5] The extent of phlebotomy should be guided by the patient's symptoms. Acute dehydration, which exacerbates polycythemia, should be excluded from the diagnosis before phlebotomy is performed, and the volume of blood withdrawn should be replaced with isotonic saline. Iron deficiency should be avoided by the use of oral iron therapy if necessary because severe iron deficiency may alter red blood cell rheology and increase the risk of stroke.[7]

Severe COPD can be associated with polycythemia, although the clinical features of COPD usually predominate. In patients who continue to smoke, both hypoxemia and elevated carboxyhemoglobin levels may contribute to the development of polycythemia. Reduction of hematocrit in patients with significant polycythemia caused by COPD results in increased cerebral blood flow, relief from the symptoms of dizziness and headache that are associated with hyperviscosity, and dramatic improvement in mental alertness. In a study of seven patients with severe COPD and pulmonary hypertension, serial phlebotomy reduced pulmonary arterial pressure and improved exercise capacity.[8]

Obstructive Sleep Apnea

Sleep apnea syndrome is estimated to occur in 4% of middle-aged men and 2% of women. The condition is underdiagnosed.[9] Risk factors include obesity, male sex, central body fat distribution, and a family history of obstructive sleep apnea.[10] The prevalence of sleep apnea syndrome increases as the body mass index increases. Recurrent episodes of upper airway collapse during sleep obstruct air movement, resulting in intermittent nocturnal hypoxemia. Patients may have a history of loud snoring, alternating with periods of silence lasting 10 seconds to 1 minute, followed by gasping sounds. Fragmented sleep results in excessive daytime sleepiness and impaired work performance. In addition, the condition may increase the risk of motor vehicle accidents.[11] The hematocrit may be modestly increased in patients with severe obstructive sleep apnea, and this syndrome should be considered in patients with unexplained polycythemia. Nocturnal polysomnography with quantitation of the apnea-hypopnea index can establish the diagnosis. Management of this condition may include weight loss, nasal continuous positive airway pressure, and surgery[12] [see Chapters 189 and 220].

Obesity-Hypoventilation Syndrome

Obesity-hypoventilation syndrome is also known as pickwickian syndrome, in reference to Charles Dickens' astute description of the obese coachboy who had excessive daytime sleepiness. Patients with this syndrome are usually morbidly obese (body mass index of 40 kg/m^2) and have chronic daytime hypoxemia and hypercapnia, in part because of a blunted ventilatory response to these stimuli.[13] Many of these patients also have nocturnal obstructive sleep apnea.[14] Hypoxemia provides the stimulus for increased erythropoietin production and polycythemia. Other clinical features associated with obesity-hypoventilation syndrome are daytime hypersomnolence and cor

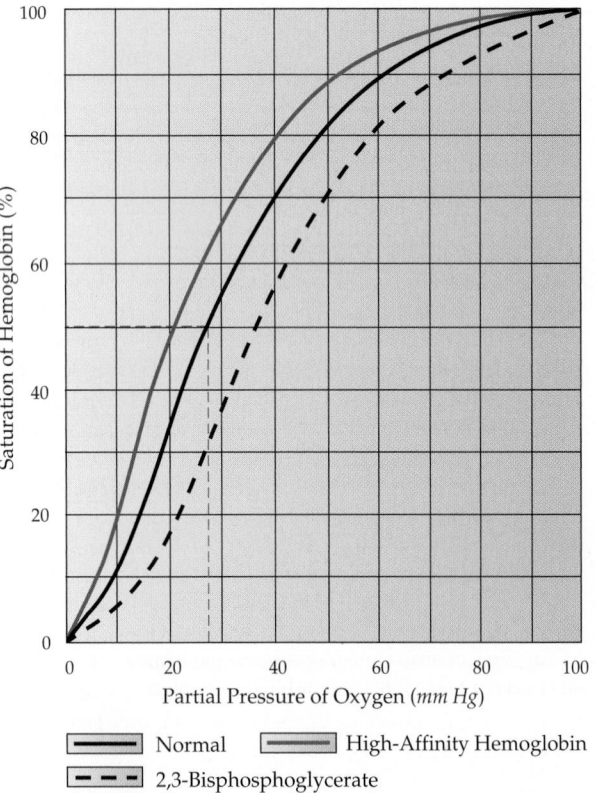

Figure 2 Depicted is the oxygen-hemoglobin dissociation curve (solid black line). The partial pressure of oxygen at which hemoglobin is 50% saturated (P_{50}) is normally 27 mm Hg (broken blue lines). The presence of high-affinity hemoglobin shifts the curve to the left, reflecting impaired oxygen unloading in the tissues (solid blue line). An increase in the level of 2,3-bisphosphoglycerate—a feature of adaptation to high altitude—shifts the curve to the right, reflecting increased oxygen unloading in the tissues (broken black line).

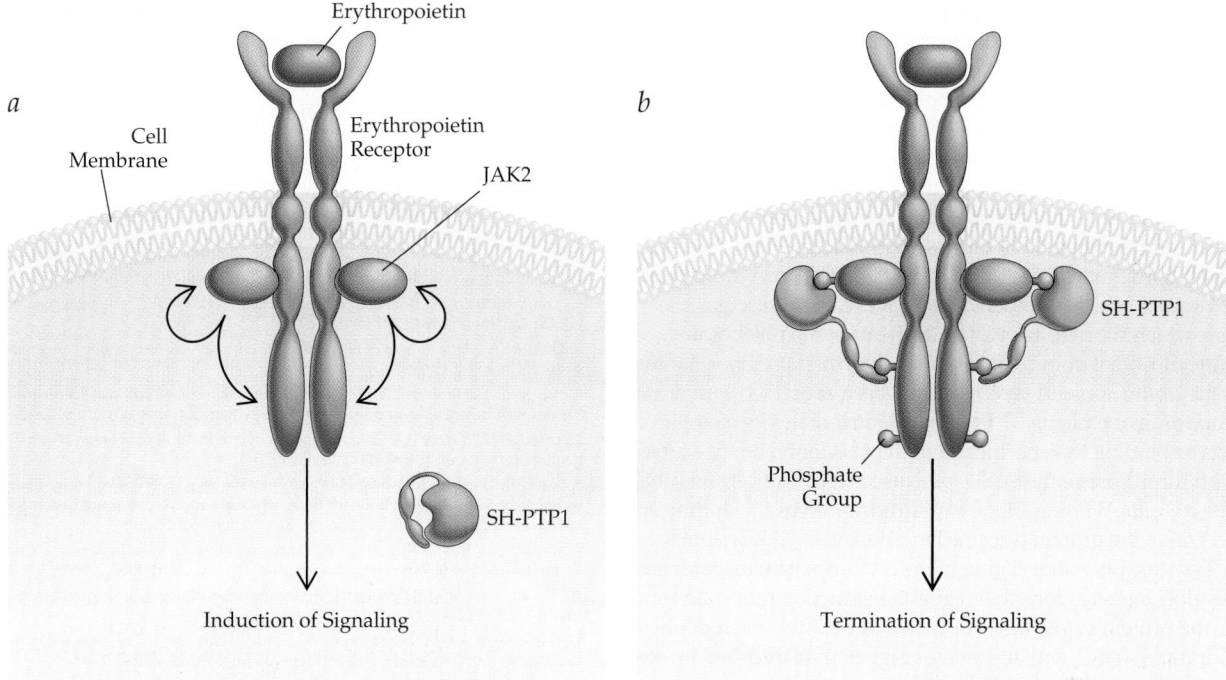

Figure 3 (*a*) Binding of erythropoietin to the erythropoietin receptor on an erythroid progenitor cell triggers association and activation of the protein-tyrosine Janus kinase-2 (JAK2) and the initiation of signal transduction, stimulating growth of the erythroid progenitor cell. (*b*) Binding of the protein-tyrosine phosphatase SH-PTP1 results in dephosphorylation of JAK2 and termination of signal transduction.

pulmonale. Management of this condition includes weight loss and progesterone therapy to stimulate the central respiratory drive [*see Chapter 220*].

High Carboxyhemoglobin Levels

Long-term exposure to carbon monoxide results in chronic high carboxyhemoglobin levels [*see Chapter 15*]. Carbon monoxide binds to hemoglobin with an affinity 210 times greater than that of oxygen, decreasing the quantity of hemoglobin available for oxygen transport. Carbon monoxide binding also increases the affinity of the remaining heme groups for oxygen, shifting the oxygen-hemoglobin dissociation curve to the left [*see Figure 2*] and impairing the unloading of oxygen in the tissues. By these mechanisms, long-term carbon monoxide exposure can cause polycythemia. Cigarette and cigar smokers and persons with long-term occupational exposure to automobile exhaust in poorly ventilated areas (e.g., tollbooth operators, underground-garage attendants, and truck loaders) are at risk. The average carboxyhemoglobin level in the blood of nonsmokers is approximately 1% or less, whereas it is 4% in smokers and as high as 15% in heavy smokers.

Symptoms may include subtle neuropsychiatric abnormalities and exacerbation of angina (likely as a result of impaired myocardial oxygen delivery). The diagnosis can be established by measuring the percentage of carboxyhemoglobin in the blood. Because the half-life of carboxyhemoglobin is approximately 5 hours, the test should be done late in the day, when the patient has smoked the usual number of cigarettes or spent several hours in the work environment. Polycythemic smokers usually have both elevated red blood cell mass and decreased plasma volume. For smokers, the most effective therapy is smoking cessation; abnormal blood and plasma levels revert to normal within 3 months. No therapy is available for persons with occupational polycythemia, with the exception of avoidance of the workplace.

POLYCYTHEMIA CAUSED BY RENAL AND HEPATIC DISORDERS

Polycythemias arise when erythropoietin production is increased because of renal or, less often, hepatic disorders. In adults, approximately 90% of erythropoietin production occurs in the kidney, and 10% occurs in the liver. Because of the intricate regulation of erythropoietin production in the kidney, distortion of renal anatomy can result in polycythemia. Case reports document that renal cysts, hydronephrosis, focal glomerulonephritis, and Bartter syndrome can cause polycythemia. After renal transplantation, approximately 10% to 20% of patients have transient or persistent polycythemia. It is important to identify these patients, because they are at increased risk for arterial or venous thrombotic events and may require phlebotomy or ACE inhibitors.[15] In addition, primary malignancies of the kidney or liver can cause polycythemia. Polycythemia develops in approximately 3% of patients with renal cell carcinoma. Erythropoietin production by primary renal cell carcinoma or hepatoma tissues is the likely cause of polycythemia in these patients. In rare instances, focal nodular hyperplasia of the liver, hepatic or cerebral hemangiomas or hemangioblastomas,[16] uterine fibroids, adrenal adenomas, and pheochromocytomas have been reported to cause polycythemia. Mutations in the von Hippel–Lindau gene have been associated with cerebral hemangioblastomas or renal cell cancer, either as a part of the von Hippel–Lindau syndrome or as an acquired somatic mutation.[17]

FAMILIAL POLYCYTHEMIA

The familial polycythemias are rare diseases resulting from inborn mutations affecting hematopoietic or nonhematopoietic cells. The molecular mechanisms causing familial polycythemia may be different in different families, and mutations may be inherited in an autosomal dominant or recessive fashion.

A high frequency of autosomal recessive familial polycythemia is found in the Chuvash region of Russia.[18] Elegant studies have demonstrated that a point mutation in the von Hippel–Lindau gene results in enhanced stability of hypoxia-inducible factor-1α, which regulates transcription of the erythropoietin gene.[19] Thus, Chuvash polycythemia is a congenital disorder of oxygen homeostasis. Chuvash polycythemia has also been identified in families of European or Asian descent.[20] Patients with Chuvash polycythemia present during the teenage years with headache, dizziness, fatigue, and dyspnea on exertion.[21] Affected members of these families have a high hematocrit (approximately 60%) and elevated levels of erythropoietin, and they have thromboembolism and cerebrovascular disorders, which shorten survival. Treatment is with phlebotomy.

In autosomal dominant familial polycythemia, abnormalities in the erythropoietin receptor have been identified in a small proportion of patients.[22-25] Erythropoietin initiates its biologic effects by binding to a specific receptor that is found on the surface of erythroid progenitor cells, precursor cells, and certain other types of cells. Binding triggers a cascade of events, including activation of the protein tyrosine Janus kinase-2 (JAK2) [see Figure 3]. Tyrosine phosphorylation of the erythropoietin receptor creates docking sites for other signal transduction molecules and for the protein-tyrosine phosphatase SH-PTP1, which dephosphorylates JAK2 and terminates signal transduction. In one large Finnish family with polycythemia, a point mutation in the erythropoietin receptor affecting SH-PTP1 rendered the erythroid progenitor cells hypersensitive to erythropoietin. Interestingly, one member of this family who had a hematocrit of 60% won three gold medals in cross-country skiing at the 1964 Winter Olympics. Another proportion of patients with autosomal dominant familial polycythemia have been found to have mutations in the erythropoietin receptor, resulting in deletion of the carboxyl terminus negative regulatory region of the receptor.[23-25] Individuals with autosomal dominant familial polycythemia have erythrocytosis that remains stable over time; they do not experience leukocytosis or thrombocytosis, and no long-term clinical consequences have been described.

POLYCYTHEMIA CAUSED BY DRUG USE

Androgens (e.g., testosterone) can cause polycythemia by stimulating erythropoietin production.[26] The elevation in hematocrit is usually mild, and hematocrit returns to normal 2 to 3 months after discontinuance of anabolic steroid use. Since recombinant human erythropoietin and darbepoetin have become available, concern has been raised that competitive athletes involved in endurance sports, such as bicycle racing, cross-country skiing, and long-distance running, might surreptitiously self-inject this drug to improve athletic performance.[27-29] Phlebotomy followed by blood doping is known to improve performance in runners and skiers. A similar increase in hematocrit can be achieved with erythropoietin injections, which can increase maximal exercise capacity. The unmonitored increase in red blood cell production may cause significant polycythemia, which, when coupled with exercise-induced dehydration, can have tragic consequences. Erythropoietin abuse has been linked to the deaths of competitive bicyclists.[27] The use of erythropoietin or darbepoetin to improve athletic performance is banned by the International Olympics Committee. Recombinant human erythropoietin can be detected in the urine by isoelectric focusing.[30]

The author has no commercial relationships with manufacturers of products or providers of services discussed in this chapter.

References

1. Pearson TC, Guthrie DL, Simpson J, et al: Interpretation of measured red cell mass and plasma volume in adults: expert panel on radionuclides of the International Council for Standardization in Haematology. Br J Haematol 89:748, 1995

2. Messinezy M, Pearson TC: Apparent polycythaemia: diagnosis, pathogenesis and management. Eur J Haematol 51:125, 1993

3. Plata R, Cornejo A, Arratia C, et al: Angiotensin-converting-enzyme inhibition therapy in altitude polycythaemia: a prospective randomised trial. Lancet 359:663, 2002

4. Vongpatanasin W, Brickner ME, Hillis LD, et al: The Eisenmenger syndrome in adults. Ann Intern Med 128:745, 1998

5. Thorne SA: Management of polycythaemia in adults with cyanotic congenital heart disease. Heart 79:315, 1998

6. Horigome H, Hiramatsu Y, Shigeta O, et al: Overproduction of platelet microparticles in cyanotic congenital heart disease with polycythemia. J Am Coll Cardiol 39:1072, 2002

7. Ammash N, Warnes CA: Cerebrovascular events in adult patients with cyanotic congenital heart disease. J Am Coll Cardiol 28:768, 1996

8. Borst MM, Leschke M, König U, et al: Repetitive hemodilution in chronic obstructive pulmonary disease and pulmonary hypertension: effects on pulmonary hemodynamics, gas exchange, and exercise capacity. Respiration 66:225, 1999

9. Stradling JR, Davies RJO: Sleep 1: Obstructive sleep apnoea/hypopnoea syndrome: definitions, epidemiology, and natural history. Thorax 59:73, 2004

10. Young T, Skatrud J, Peppard P: Risk factors for obstructive sleep apnea in adults. JAMA 291:2013, 2004

11. Teran-Santos J, Jimenez-Gomez A, Cordero-Guevara J: The association between sleep apnea and the risk of traffic accidents. N Engl J Med 340:847, 1999

12. McNicholas WT: Obstructive sleep apnea syndrome: who should be treated? Sleep 23(suppl 4):S187, 2000

13. Martin TJ, Sanders MH: Chronic alveolar hypoventilation: a review for the clinician. Sleep 18:617, 1995

14. Kessler R, Chaouat A, Schinkewitch P, et al: The obesity-hypoventilation syndrome revisited: a prospective study of 34 consecutive cases. Chest 120:369, 2001

15. Vlahakos D, Marathias K, Agroyannis B: Perspectives in renal medicine: posttransplant erythrocytosis. Kidney Int 63:1187, 2003

16. Kuhne M, Sidler D, Hofer S, et al: Diagnosis in oncology: challenging manifestations of malignancies. J Clin Oncol 22:3639, 2004

17. Wiesener MS, Seyfarth M, Warnecke C, et al: Paraneoplastic erythrocytosis associated with an inactivating point mutation of the von Hippel-Lindau gene in a renal cell carcinoma. Blood 99:3562, 2002

18. Sergeyeva A, Gordeuk VR, Tokarev YN, et al: Congenital polycythemia in Chuvashia. Blood 89:2148, 1997

19. Ang SO, Chen H, Hirota K, et al: Disruption of oxygen homeostasis underlies congenital Chuvash polycythemia. Nat Genet 32:614, 2002

20. Percy MJ, McMullin MF, Jowitt SN, et al: Chuvash-type congenital polycythemia in 4 families of Asian and western European ancestry. Blood 102:1097, 2003

21. Gordeuk VR, Sergueeva AI, Miasnikova GY, et al: Congenital disorder of oxygen sensing: association of the homozygous Chuvash polycythemia VHL mutation with thrombosis and vascular abnormalities but not tumors. Blood 103:3924, 2004

22. de la Chapelle A, Traskelin AL, Juvonen E: Truncated erythropoietin receptor causes dominantly inherited benign human erythrocytosis. Proc Natl Acad Sci USA 90:4495, 1993

23. Arcasoy MO, Degar BA, Harris KW, et al: Familial erythrocytosis associated with a short deletion in the erythropoietin receptor. Blood 89:4628, 1997

24. Gregg XT, Prchal JT: Erythropoietin receptor mutations and human disease. Semin Hematol 34:70, 1997

25. Kralovics R, Prchal JT: Genetic heterogeneity of primary familial and congenital polycythemia. Am J Hematol 68:115, 2001

26. Besa EC: Hematologic effects of androgens revisited: an alternative therapy in various hematologic conditions. Semin Hematol 31:134, 1994

27. Tokish JM, Kocher MS, Hawkins RJ: Ergogenic aids: a review of basic science, performance, side effects, and status in sports. Am J Sports Med 32:1543, 2004

28. Vogel G: A race to the starting line. Science 305:632, 2004

29. Noakes TD: Tainted glory: doping and athletic performance. N Engl J Med 351:847, 2004

30. Breidbach A, Catlin DH, Green GA, et al: Detection of recombinant human erythropoietin in urine by isoelectric focusing. Clin Chem 49:901, 2003

Acknowledgments

Figures 1 and 2   Marcia Kammerer.
Figure 3   Jared Schneidman.

95 Nonmalignant Disorders of Leukocytes

David C. Dale, M.D., F.A.C.P.

Leukocytes, or white blood cells, protect the body against infections and participate in many types of immunologic and inflammatory responses. There are two main types of leukocytes: lymphocytes, which are responsible for antibody production and cell-mediated immunity, and phagocytes, which are responsible for the ingestion and killing of microorganisms. Neutrophils, monocytes, macrophages, and eosinophils are all phagocytes [*see Figure 1*]. Leukocytes interact with one another and modulate immune responses through the release of cytokines (interleukins and growth factors), enzymes, and vasoactive substances. This chapter covers the diagnosis of disorders of neutrophils, monocytes, and eosinophils and the treatment of neutropenia; the functions and disorders of lymphocytes are discussed elsewhere [*see Immunology, Allergy, and Rheumatology*].

The White Blood Cell Count

The total white blood cell (WBC) count and differential count are often the first studies performed in evaluating a patient with a suspected infection or with susceptibility to infections. Most laboratories measure the WBC count using automated cell-counting techniques.[1] The normal WBC count ranges from 4,300 to 10,000/mm^3, with a median of 7,000/mm^3 [*see Table 1*]. A differential count gives the percentage for each type of leukocyte. The absolute count is determined by multiplying the total WBC count by this percentage (e.g., WBC × percent neutrophils = absolute neutrophil count). Because the blood level of each type of leukocyte is separately regulated, it is always better to use the absolute count rather than the percentage in assessing abnormalities.

Indications of the Presence of a Phagocytic Cell Disorder

Because the phagocytes, particularly neutrophils, represent the first line of defense against invading microorganisms, disorders in the number or function of these cells often result in an increased susceptibility to infection. A quantitative or qualitative disorder of phagocytic cells should be suspected when a patient has an increased number of bacterial or fungal infections, increasingly severe infections, or infections with unusual organisms.

Neutrophil Physiology

NEUTROPHIL PRODUCTION

Neutrophils are derived from the common stem cell, which also gives rise to erythrocytes, platelets, and other leukocytes. The proliferation and differentiation of the neutrophil precursors are governed by a family of regulatory cytokines. Granulocyte colony-stimulating factor (G-CSF) and granulocyte-macrophage colony-stimulating factor (GM-CSF) are two important cytokines affecting neutrophil production and function. G-CSF selectively stimulates progenitor cells to differentiate into neutrophils and rapidly increases blood neutrophils in hematologically normal individuals [*see Figure 2*].[2,3] GM-CSF stimulates progenitor cells to differentiate into neutrophils, eosinophils, monocytes, macro-

phages, and dendritic cells.[4] The life cycle of the neutrophil consists of bone marrow, blood, and tissue phases. Neutrophil production in the bone marrow takes approximately 10 to 14 days, and the bone marrow produces approximately 1×10^9 neutrophils/kg/day.[5] Most of the body's neutrophils are found in the bone marrow. The mitotic compartment, which contains about 20% of the total neutrophil pool, consists of myeloblasts (the earliest morphologically recognizable precursors), promyelocytes, and myelocytes. The postmitotic pool or maturation compartment—the metamyelocytes, bands, and mature neutrophils—contains about 70% of the body's neutrophils. The marrow neutrophils and bands are sometimes called the storage compartment or marrow reserve. As neutrophils mature, they develop the capacity to enter the blood through increasing deformability and through changes in the adhesion proteins on their surface membranes. Entry into the blood involves interactions of the mature cells and the endothelial cells of the marrow sinusoids that are not yet well understood. Agents that stimulate release of neutrophils from the marrow (e.g., G-CSF, GM-CSF, corticosteroids, or endotoxin administration) can result in a doubling of the blood neutrophil count within 3 to 5 hours. The peripheral blood contains fewer than 10% of the body's neutrophils. In the blood, the neutrophils are divided approximately evenly between the circulating pool and the marginating pool; these pools are in dynamic equilibrium. Cells in the marginating pool can be swept rapidly (within minutes) into the circulation by endogenous or exogenous epinephrine or as a result of exercise or any cause of rapid increase in cardiac output. This response, called demargination, can double the blood neutrophil count very rapidly and is also quickly reversible. The blood half-life of the neutrophils is approximately 6 to 10 hours. Neutrophils leave the blood and enter the tissues by migrating between endothelial cells and penetrating the capillary basement membrane. It is now believed that neutrophils that do not leave the circulatory system die by apoptosis and are removed by mononuclear phagocytes in the spleen, liver, and other tissues.[6]

NEUTROPHIL STRUCTURE

As neutrophil precursors mature, their nuclear chromatin becomes condensed and segmented. Mature cells have no nucleoli, few mitochondria, and very little endoplasmic reticulum. The cytoplasm is filled with granules and glycogen. The primary granules, which appear at the myeloblast and promyelocyte stages, contain myeloperoxidase (MPO), proteases, defensins, and other antibacterial substances.[7,8] Secondary granules, produced primarily during the myelocyte stage, predominate in mature cells. They contain collagenase, lactoferrin, lysozyme, vitamin B$_{12}$–binding protein, and several other proteins. Small tertiary granules are also found in mature neutrophils. Neutrophils also may have cytoplasmic vesicles containing lactases, alkaline phosphatases, and components of nicotinamide-adenine dinucleotide phosphate (NADPH) oxidase.

The surface of the neutrophil is replete with deep folds and ruffles. On the neutrophil surface, there are numerous receptors, including receptors for immunoglobulins (e.g., FcγRII [CD32],

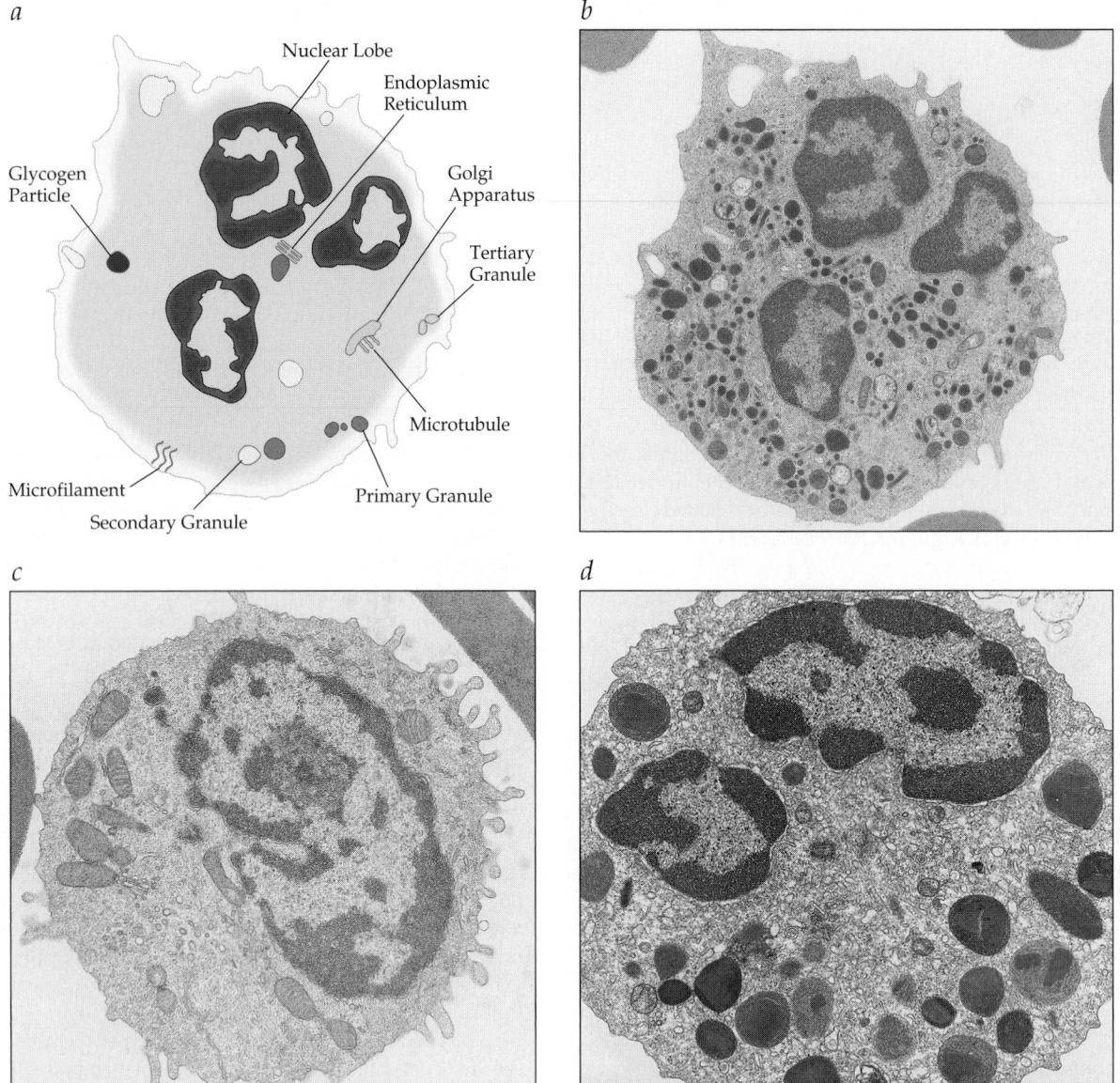

a

Glycogen Particle

Nuclear Lobe

Endoplasmic Reticulum

Golgi Apparatus

Tertiary Granule

Microtubule

Microfilament

Secondary Granule

Primary Granule

b

c

d

Figure 1   Shown are a schematic diagram of a neutrophil (*a*), a corresponding electron micrograph of a neutrophil (*b*), and electron micrographs of a monocyte (*c*) and an eosinophil (*d*).

FcγRIII [CD16]), complement (e.g., CR3 [CD11b18], CR1 [CD35]), chemokines, the colony-stimulating factors G-CSF and GM-CSF, Fas, tumor necrosis factor receptor (TNF-R), and the apoptosis-related receptors.[9]

The cytoskeleton of the neutrophil is composed of microtubules and microfilaments that are critical for phagocytic shape and movement, including migration through the vascular endothelium. The microfilaments, which consist primarily of actin polymers, are dispersed throughout the cytoplasm.[10]

NEUTROPHIL FUNCTION

The major function of neutrophils is to respond rapidly to microbial invasion to kill the invaders. This response has several distinct steps—adherence, migration, recognition, phagocytosis (or ingestion), degranulation, oxidative metabolism, and bacterial killing [*see Figure 3*]. Susceptibility to infection results from abnormalities in any one or a combination of these processes.

Adherence

For neutrophils to move to an inflammatory site, they must first adhere to a capillary wall.[11] Loose adherence is facilitated by L-selectins, such as sialyl-Lewis^x (sLe^x), on the neutrophil and E-selectin and P-selectin on capillary endothelial cells [*see Figure 4*]. Bacterial invasion increases local selectin expression and neutrophil accumulation. Other neutrophil surface proteins, called β_2 integrins, facilitate firmer adhesion to endothelial cells and interact with actin, myosin, and actin-binding proteins to initiate movement of neutrophils to the tissue.[11] The three proteins in this family have a common β subunit (CD18) and a different α subunit (CD11a, CD11b, or CD11c). There is generally increased expression of these proteins (e.g., CD 11b/C18) on neutrophils in response to inflammation. Concomitantly, there is increased expression of the intracellular adherence molecules (ICAMs) on the endothelial cells, with a net result of increased trafficking of neutrophils to the inflammatory focus.

Table 1 Normal Leukocyte Values in Peripheral Blood

Cell Type	Cells/mm³*		Percentage of Total Differential Count
	Median	Range	
All leukocytes (white blood cells)	7,000	4,300–10,000	100
Total neutrophils	4,000	1,800–7,200	55
Band neutrophils	500	100–2,000	10
Segmented neutrophils	3,500	1,000–6,000	45
Lymphocytes	2,500	1,500–4,000	36
Monocytes	450	200–900	6
Eosinophils	150	0–700	2
Basophils	30	0–150	1

*To calculate the number of cells/L, multiply by 10^6.

Chemotaxis

Chemotaxis, the directed movement of cells, occurs when neutrophils detect a chemoattractant at low concentrations and move up the concentration gradient toward its source, which is usually a site in the extravascular spaces.[12] Well-characterized stimulators of neutrophil chemotaxis are the complement proteins C5a, leukotriene B4, interleukin-8 (IL-8), and a family of small peptides, the chemokines. The trafficking of neutrophils from the blood is unidirectional; they do not return from the tissues to the circulation.

Recognition and Phagocytosis

At the site of inflammation, neutrophils utilize their immunoglobulin and complement receptors to recognize bacteria and other particles coated or opsonized by immunoglobulins or complement. Inflammation stimulates neutrophils to express increased numbers of the high-affinity IgG receptor FcγRI (CD64).[13] As the neutrophil internalizes a particle, a phagocytic vesicle, or phagosome, develops around it. This process stimulates degranulation and activates a burst of oxidative metabolism.

Degranulation

When the neutrophil is activated, the granule membranes come in contact with the plasma membranes surrounding the phagosome. The membranes fuse, which leads to the release of granule proteins into the phagosome and to the reorganization of the components of the critical NADPH oxidase system.[14]

Oxidative Metabolism and Bacterial Killing

Resting granulocytes are primarily anaerobic cells that rely on anaerobic glycolysis for adenosine triphosphate (ATP) production. Although chemotaxis, ingestion, and degranulation require

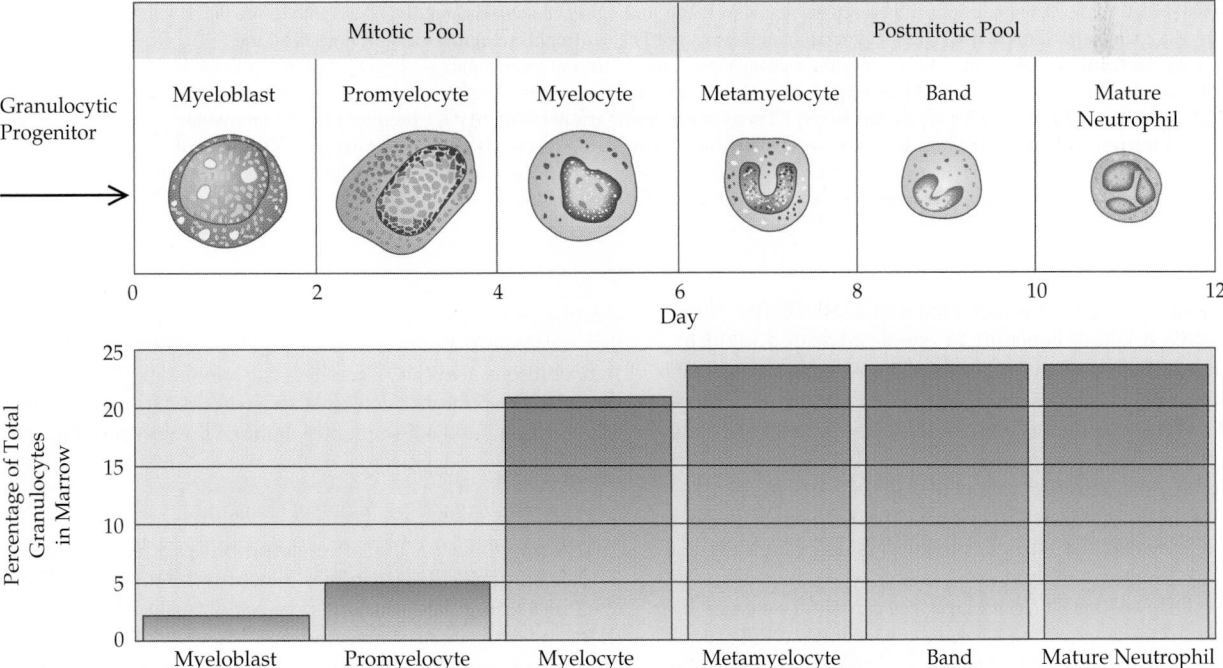

Figure 2 The process of neutrophil maturation begins in the bone marrow (top). After about 12 days, approximately 10% of the mature neutrophils are released into the peripheral blood, where they have a half-life of approximately 6 to 10 hours. Eventually, the neutrophils migrate into the tissues by diapedesis. The percentage of neutrophils at each stage of development (bottom) ranges from about 2% at the myoblast stage to almost 25% at the mature neutrophil stage.

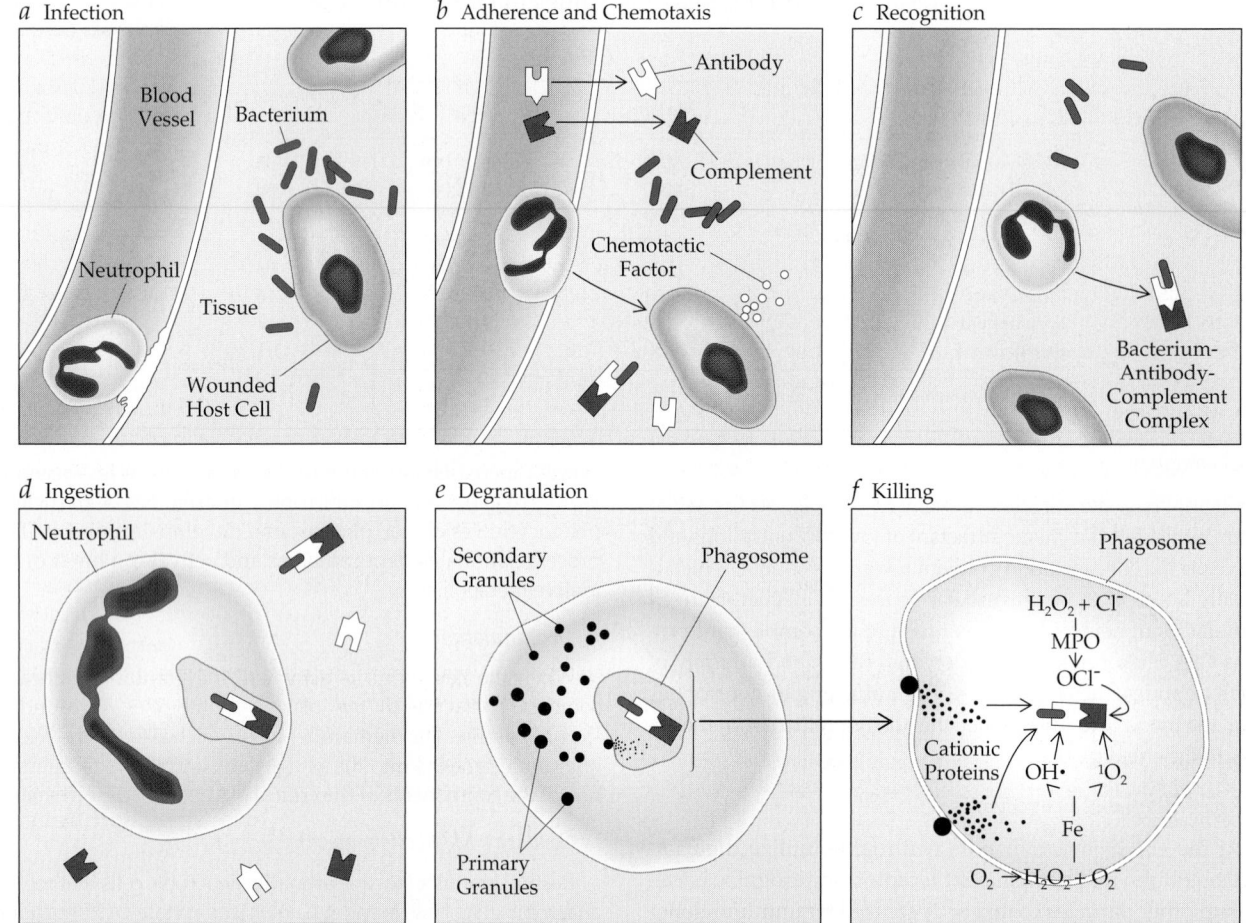

a Infection

b Adherence and Chemotaxis

c Recognition

d Ingestion

e Degranulation

f Killing

Figure 3   The neutrophil response to bacterial invasion involves several stages. A bacterium infects a host cell and injures it (*a*). Bacterial products, antibodies, and complement cause the release of chemotactic factors, which activate a neutrophil in the adjacent blood vessel. The neutrophil adheres to the vessel wall and undergoes chemotaxis and diapedesis into tissue (*b*) to follow the chemoattractants to their sites of generation or expression. The neutrophil recognizes (*c*) and ingests (*d*) the bacterium-antibody-complement complex, forming a phagosome. The neutrophil then undergoes degranulation, a process in which granule membranes fuse with the plasma membrane (*e*). Degranulation releases various enzymes and enhances oxidative metabolism, the products of which are bactericidal (*f*). For example, hydrogen peroxide (H_2O_2), produced from superoxide (O_2^-), can interact with O_2^- in the presence of iron (Fe) to produce hydroxyl radicals (OH•) and singlet oxygen ($^1O_2$), both of which are highly toxic to bacteria. In addition, H_2O_2 and chloride (Cl^-) combine in the presence of the myeloperoxidase (MPO) released in the phagosome to produce hypochlorite (OCl^-), which is also bactericidal.

some energy, they also proceed quite well anaerobically. However, bacterial killing generally is associated with a rapid increase (within seconds) in oxygen use. This respiratory burst occurs as a result of the activation of an NADPH oxidase.[15] Before activation, the components of the oxidase are located separately in the plasma and granule membranes and in the cytosol. The membranes contain two components: gp91[phox] and p22[phox]. The cytosol includes a p47 protein and a p67 protein. When the neutrophil is activated, the cytosolic proteins first associate and then combine with the membrane components to produce the complete NADPH oxidase. NADPH oxidase can reduce oxygen by one electron to superoxide O_2^-; in the process, NADPH is converted to $NADP^+$. The NADPH is then regenerated through the hexose monophosphate shunt. Dismutation of the superoxide in the presence of superoxide dismutase produces hydrogen peroxide (H_2O_2), which can then be converted to hydroxyl radical (OH•). H_2O_2, O_2^-, and OH• are highly toxic. In addition, within

the phagocyte vacuole, hydrogen peroxide and chloride (Cl^-) can combine in the presence of myeloperoxidase to produce hypochlorous acid (HOCl), which is bactericidal.[15] These products of the respiratory burst can also be released from the activated neutrophil and subsequently damage the surrounding cells and tissues.

Responses to and Production of Cytokines

The growth factors that affect neutrophil production, such as G-CSF and GM-CSF, also influence neutrophil function.[16] These cytokines upregulate stimulus-dependent NADPH oxidase activity and can enhance bactericidal and fungicidal activities. Although neutrophils contain very few ribosomes, they can respond to bacterial stimuli by synthesizing and secreting proinflammatory cytokines such as IL-1, IL-6, and tumor necrosis factor–α (TNF-α); monocytes, however, produce much larger quantities of these substances.[17]

Disorders of Neutrophil Number

NEUTROPHILIA

Neutrophilia, or granulocytosis, is usually defined as a neutrophil count greater than 10,000/mm³.

Etiology

Neutrophilia most often occurs secondary to inflammation, stress, or corticosteroid therapy. Cigarette smoking commonly causes neutrophilia as a result of inflammation in the airways and lungs. Malignancies, hemolytic anemia, and lithium therapy are less common causes. Neutrophilia is also associated with splenectomy. Extreme neutrophilia (i.e., neutrophil counts of more than 30,000 to 50,000/mm³), often called a leukemoid reaction, occurs with severe infections, sepsis, hemorrhagic shock, and severe tissue injury of any cause. Neutrophilia is also seen in patients with leukocyte adhesion deficiency (LAD), a rare disease in which neutrophils accumulate in the blood because they lack either the integrin CD11b18 or the selectin sLe˟ (CD15s) required to leave the circulation.[18]

Serious bacterial infections and chronic inflammation are usually associated with changes in both the number of circulating neutrophils and their morphology. Characteristic changes include increased numbers of young cells (bands), of cells with residual endoplasmic reticulum (Döhle bodies), and of cells with more prominent primary granules (toxic granulation). These changes are probably caused by the endogenous production of G-CSF or GM-CSF and are also seen with administration of these growth factors.

Primary neutrophilia (i.e., neutrophilia attributed to defects in proliferation and maturation of neutrophil precursors) occurs in patients with myeloproliferative disorders, such as chronic myeloid leukemia (CML) and polycythemia vera [see Chapter 94]. Hereditary and idiopathic neutrophilias have been described; they are benign and quite rare. One such uncommon idiopathic condition is Sweet syndrome, which is an acute febrile illness with painful cutaneous plaques and associated neutrophilia of any cause.[19] Neutrophilia is also associated with congenital abnormalities. For example, infants with Down syndrome can have transient leukemoid reactions that must be distinguished from congenital leukemia.[20]

Diagnosis

When neutrophilia cannot be readily attributed to an infection or inflammatory condition or to glucocorticosteroid therapy, the possibility of a myeloproliferative disease should be considered. The presence of splenomegaly, metamyelocytes, and myelocytes in the blood, together with increased basophils or eosinophils and a low leukocyte alkaline phosphatase (LAP) score, suggests CML [see Chapter 205]. A high LAP score or the presence of toxic granulations usually suggests an underlying infection. When there is uncertainty, bone marrow aspiration and biopsy, chromosomal analysis, as well as marrow cultures for bacteria (e.g., Salmonella, Brucella, Mycobacterium, and fungi), are warranted. The results of these tests will enable the clinician to make a diagnosis of CML (or another myeloproliferative disorder), a granulomatous infection, inflammatory disease, or metastatic malignancy. If no such cause of neutrophilia can be

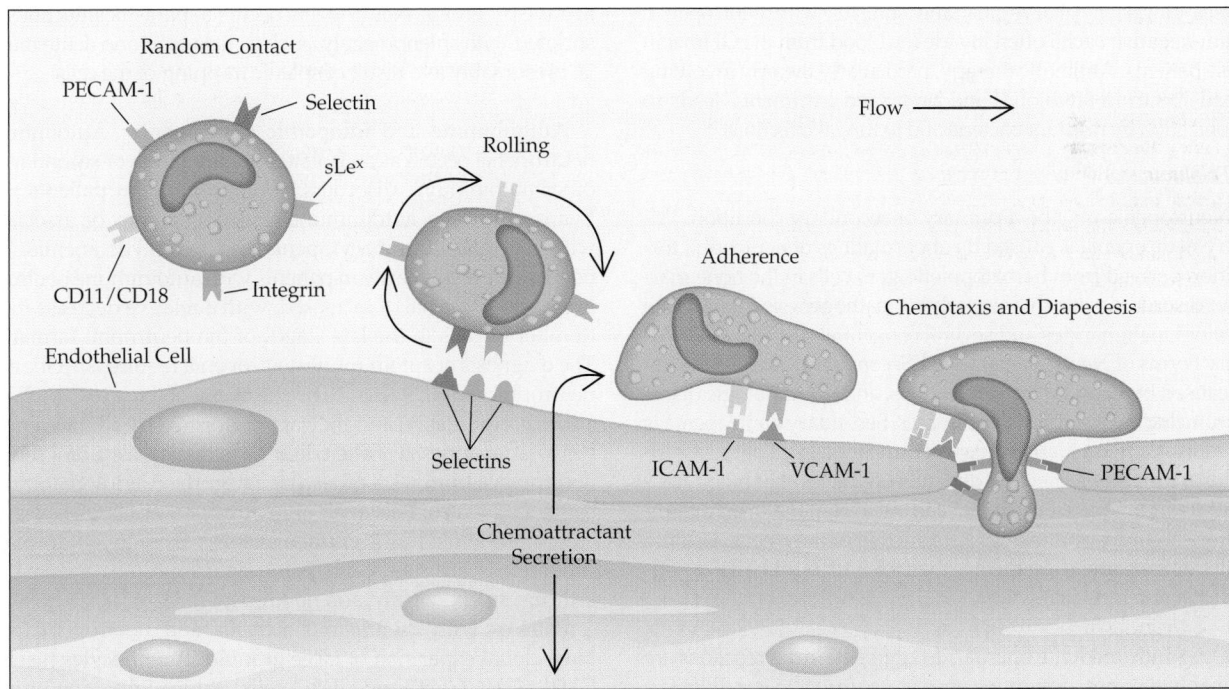

Figure 4 Neutrophils in the peripheral blood exist in either the circulating or the marginating pool. The marginated neutrophils roll along a vessel wall, where their surface carbohydrates interact with selectins on the endothelial cells. After activation by chemotactic agents, the neutrophils change shape and change the affinity of their integrin molecules for endothelial cell intercellular adhesion molecules. The neutrophils then crawl and undergo diapedesis by interacting with platelet–endothelial cell adhesion molecules on the endothelial surface and by liberating hydrolases that permit passage of the neutrophils through the capillary basement membrane. (PECAM-1—platelet–endothelial cell adhesion molecule–1; sLe˟—sialyl-Lewis˟ carbohydrate; ICAM-1—intercellular adhesion molecule–1; VCAM-1—vascular cell adhesion molecule–1)

found in an otherwise healthy-appearing person, a diagnosis of idiopathic or familial neutrophilia may be considered, and repeated neutrophil counts can be performed at monthly intervals until the diagnosis is clarified.

Treatment

Except for the myeloproliferative syndromes, treatment of neutrophilia is not indicated. Neutrophil levels will return to normal when the inflammatory process is resolved.

NEUTROPENIA

Neutropenia is generally defined as a neutrophil count of less than 1,800/mm³, which is two standard deviations below the normal mean. In some populations (e.g., Africans, African Americans, and Yemenite Jews), neutrophil counts as low as 1,000/mm³, or 1.0×10^9/L, are probably normal.[21,22]

In otherwise healthy persons, the risk of bacterial infections is relatively low if the neutrophil count is greater than 500 mm³, or 0.5×10^9/L—the level usually defined as severe neutropenia. When neutropenia develops after myelotoxic chemotherapy, the risk of infection is much greater, particularly in patients whose age and medical history (e.g., diabetes, heart failure, renal failure, previous chemotherapy, and HIV infection) also predispose them to infection.[22,23] Patients with neutropenia are also at greater risk for serious infections if they have disrupted mucosal or cutaneous barriers or are taking corticosteroids. Patients with neutropenia are at risk for infection by those pathogenic organisms that normally colonize body surfaces, particularly the skin, the oropharynx, and the GI tract. Thus, infections from staphylococci occur in neutropenic patients after breaks in the skin. Infection by mixtures of aerobic and anaerobic organisms of the oropharynx frequently causes gingivitis, pharyngitis, and sinusitis with neutropenia. Gram-negative bacilli often invade the blood from the GI tract in these patients. Antibiotic therapy, particularly therapy involving broad-spectrum antibiotics and protracted treatments, leads to colonization by resistant bacteria and to fungal infections.[24]

Etiology

Neutropenia may be a primary or secondary condition. Primary neutropenia is caused by abnormalities of neutrophil formation derived from hematopoietic stem cells in the bone marrow; disorders with this underlying pathogenesis include the myeloid malignancies and several congenital disorders [*see* Primary Forms of Neutropenia, *below*]. Secondary neutropenia may be caused by drug therapy, infections, and immunologic disorders, including autoimmune diseases. Secondary neutropenia is far more common than primary neutropenia. In all of these conditions, the risk of infection depends on the level of blood neutrophils and the capacity of the marrow to respond to an inflammatory stimulus and increase production of these cells. Usually if blood neutrophils are greater than 0.5×10^9/L, the risk of serious infection is relatively low.

Drug-induced neutropenia In aggregate, drug reactions are probably the most common cause of neutropenia in adults [*see* Table 2].[25,26] Many cancer chemotherapy drugs, some of which are also used as cytotoxic immunosuppressive agents (e.g., cyclophosphamide, methotrexate, and azathioprine), predictably cause dose-dependent neutropenia. The use of these agents requires careful attention to medical history, dosages, treatment schedules, and serial neutrophil counts to avoid serious and life-threatening toxicity. Other drugs cause neutropenia idiosyncrat-

ically. Many of these reactions probably occur because drugs can act as immunogens or as haptens, causing immunologic injury to neutrophils and their precursors. Other mechanisms of drug-induced neutropenia may involve direct toxicity of marrow cells in susceptible persons. Most patients recover from drug-induced neutropenia; the time for recovery can vary from 2 days to 2 weeks or more.

Infection-associated neutropenia Viral infections often cause mild neutropenia, especially in children. Such infections include measles and other viral exanthems, infectious mononucleosis, hepatitis, and HIV infection. The mechanisms are diverse. For example, in HIV infection, possible mechanisms include infections of the hematopoietic precursor cells and the marrow stromal cells, which lead to decreased production; induction of autoantibodies, which leads to accelerated turnover of mature neutrophils; and accelerated apoptosis of mature cells.[27] HIV-associated neutropenia generally develops late in AIDS and is often compounded by the use of antiviral agents (e.g., zidovudine, ganciclovir), antibiotics (e.g., sulfonamides), or the presence of hematologic malignancies (e.g., lymphoma, Kaposi sarcoma).[28] With other viral infections, the neutropenia is usually mild and without serious consequences. In rare instances, infectious mononucleosis causes severe hypoplasia, which has more severe consequences.[29] Neutropenia and anemia are common features of human parvovirus B19 infection.[30]

With severe bacterial infections, neutropenia occurs as a consequence of endotoxemia, which results in rapid neutrophil mobilization and turnover, especially in patients with a marrow reserve that is impaired because of previous chemotherapy, other drugs, or alcohol. In this setting, neutropenia generally portends a grave prognosis. Neutropenia occurs in parasitic infections associated with splenomegaly, such as kala-azar and acute malaria, presumably as a result of splenic trapping of the cells.

Autoimmune and idiopathic neutropenia Autoimmune neutropenia occurs as an isolated phenomenon or secondary to other autoimmune disorders.[31] For example, in patients with Evans syndrome, autoimmune neutropenia may be associated with immune thrombocytopenia and hemolytic anemia. The bone marrow cellularity in patients with autoimmune neutropenia is either normal or increased, with a relative decrease in the number of cells in the late stages of the neutrophil formation. The diagnosis of autoimmune neutropenia requires specific antineutrophil antibody tests.[32] The specificity of these tests probably varies considerably, and they are performed by a limited number of laboratories. It is often difficult to distinguish autoimmune neutropenia from cases otherwise categorized as idiopathic neutropenia. Neutropenia with antineutrophil antibodies also occurs in systemic lupus erythematosus,[33] Sjögren syndrome,[34,35] rheumatoid arthritis,[36] and Felty syndrome (i.e., rheumatoid arthritis, splenomegaly, and neutropenia).[37]

Patients with rheumatoid arthritis and neutropenia may have clonal expansion of large granular lymphocytes (usually CD2⁺, CD3⁺, CD8⁺, and CD57⁺ cells), which impair neutrophil production by excessive Fas ligand or interferon-gamma production.[38] Studies indicate that this same mechanism may be involved in cases diagnosed as idiopathic neutropenia.[39] The marrow typically shows increased lymphocytes with reduced neutrophils in the later stages of development. In most patients, the lymphocytosis is clonal and may evolve very gradually into a lymphoid malignancy.[40]

Table 2 Drugs Associated with Neutropenia

ANALGESICS
Aminopyrine
Dipyrone

ANTIBIOTICS
Cephalosporins
Chloramphenicol
Clindamycin
Doxycycline
Flucytosine
Gentamicin
Griseofulvin
Isoniazid
Lincomycin
Metronidazole
Nitrofurantoin
Penicillins
Rifampin
Streptomycin
Sulfonamides
Vancomycin

ANTICONVULSANTS
Carbamazepine
Ethosuximide
Mephenytoin

Phenytoin
Primidone
Trimethadione

ANTIHISTAMINES
Brompheniramine
Cimetidine
Ranitidine
Thenalidine
Tripelennamine

ANTI-INFLAMMATORY AGENTS
Fenoprofen
Gold salts
Ibuprofen
Indomethacin
Phenylbutazone

ANTIMALARIALS
Amodiaquine
Dapsone
Hydroxychloroquine
Pyrimethamine
Quinine

ANTITHYROID DRUGS
Carbimazole

Methimazole
Methylthiouracil
Potassium perchlorate
Propylthiouracil

CARDIOVASCULAR AGENTS
Captopril
Diazoxide
Hydralazine
Methyldopa
Pindolol
Procainamide
Propranolol
Quinidine

DIURETICS
Acetazolamide
Bumetanide
Chlorothiazide
Chlorthalidone
Hydrochlorothiazide
Methazolamide
Spironolactone

HYPOGLYCEMIC AGENTS
Chlorpropamide
Tolbutamide

PHENOTHIAZINES
Chlorpromazine
Methylpromazine
Prochlorperazine
Promazine
Thioridazine
Trifluoperazine
Trimeprazine

SEDATIVES AND
NEUROPHARMACOLOGIC
AGENTS
Chlordiazepoxide
Clozapine
Desipramine
Diazepam
Imipramine
Meprobamate
Metoclopramide

MISCELLANEOUS AGENTS
Allopurinol
Colchicine
Ethanol
Levamisole
Levodopa
Penicillamine

In sarcoidosis, cirrhosis, and congestive splenomegaly of diverse causes, neutropenia and thrombocytopenia often occur concomitantly, presumably because of splenic sequestration. In most instances, the neutropenia is mild and without recognizable consequences.

Other secondary causes of neutropenia Neonates can have severe neutropenia because of transplacental transfer of maternal IgG antibodies to the FcγRIII (CD16) isotype (previously called NA-1 or NA-2) that is inherited from the infant's father.[41] This abnormality is transient, usually lasting less than 3 months. Transient severe neutropenia also can occur in an infant as a result of transplacental transfer of other antibodies (e.g., transfer of IgG) from a mother with autoimmune neutropenia. Pure white cell aplasia is a rare acquired condition characterized by a complete absence of myeloid precursors.[42] Pure white cell aplasia may be associated with a thymoma; if so, the aplasia may respond on removal of the thymoma. The short-term consequences of all these conditions depend primarily upon the level of blood neutrophils and the proliferative response of the marrow when inflammation or infections occur. The causes of other forms of neutropenia in children and adults are often difficult to establish and usually require referral to an expert hematologist.

Primary forms of neutropenia There are a number of congenital and inherited causes of neutropenia [*see Table 3*].

Diagnosis

Neutropenia is easily diagnosed by performing a white blood cell count and differential count. Patients with acute, severe neutropenia are often febrile and are frequently referred to as having acute febrile neutropenia. In this circumstance, attention is immediately focused on determining whether the patient has an infection, as well as focused on instituting empirical antibiotic ther-

apy. Hematologic studies (e.g., bone marrow examination) are generally not necessary, because the cause of neutropenia is recognized from the patient's history, and it will resolve if the inciting cause has been eliminated.

Initial evaluation of patients with chronic neutropenia should include a careful family history and review of the incidence and severity of infections, including oral ulcers, gingivitis, cellulitis, and more serious problems. A complete blood count will reveal whether the neutropenia is isolated or associated with other hematologic abnormalities. Medications should be discontinued if they can be implicated as causes of the neutropenia. A bone marrow biopsy and aspirate are indicated if there is any question of a primary disease affecting the marrow (e.g., metastatic carcinoma, tuberculosis) or if myelodysplasia or a hematologic malignancy is suspected. Serologic testing for infectious mononucleosis, hepatitis, and HIV is often warranted, as is measurement of antinuclear antibodies and rheumatoid factor titers. Broader immunologic assessments (i.e., lymphocyte subtypes and immunoglobulin levels) are warranted if the history suggests a susceptibility to infections by viruses, parasites, or bacteria; and they are also useful to detect clonal proliferation of lymphocytes and to diagnose the large granular lymphocyte syndrome. Neutrophil mobilization with corticosteroids and demargination tests with epinephrine are rarely helpful.

Treatment of Neutropenia

Evidence-based guidelines for management and prevention of acute febrile neutropenia associated with cancer chemotherapy have been developed by the Infectious Diseases Society of America (www.idsociety.org) and the American Society of Clinical Oncology (www.asco.org). Other guidelines are also available (www.guideline.gov) [*see Table 4*]. In general, acute management of severe, idiosyncratic, drug-induced neutropenia should be similarly managed.[43,44]

Table 3 Intrinsic Disorders of Neutrophils That Cause Neutropenia

Disorder	Inheritance	Clinical Features	Diagnosis	Treatment
Congenital neutropenia (also known as infantile genetic agranulocytosis and Kostmann syndrome)	AD, AR, S Locus: 19p13.3	From birth, upper respiratory, lung, liver, and skin infections; mild anemia; thrombocytosis; a normal immune system; possible development of leukemia	Selective, severe neutropenia; marrow promyelocytes but few more mature cells; marrow eosinophils; normal chromosomes; possible G-CSF receptor defect Genetic testing: research only*	G-CSF (effective in most cases); bone marrow transplantation; prophylactic antibiotics
Myelokathexis	AD, S	Recurrent infections; severe leukopenia and neutropenia	Marrow cellularity normal with maturing, often binucleate neutrophils	G-CSF
Cyclic neutropenia (also known as cyclic hematopoiesis)	AD, S Locus: 19p13.3	Regular oscillations of blood cell counts, most prominently of neutrophil and monocyte counts	Serial CBCs show severe neutropenia that recurs regularly, usually every 21 days Genetic testing: research only*	G-CSF
Shwachman-Diamond syndrome	AR Locus: 7q11	Neutropenia with pancreatic insufficiency and sometimes with anemia or thrombocytopenia	Neutropenia with malabsorption caused by pancreatic enzyme deficiency; tests for cystic fibrosis negative Clinical testing available*	G-CSF; pancreatic enzymes
Chédiak-Higashi syndrome	AR, S Locus: 1q42	Recurrent infections; partial albinism; lymphoproliferative syndrome; neutropenia; thrombocytopenia	Giant cytoplasmic granules; defective neutrophil migration and bacterial killing Genetic testing: research only*	Antibiotics; vitamin C; bone marrow transplantation
Reticular dysgenesis and congenital immunodeficiency syndromes with neutropenia	AR, S	From birth, severe infections with severe leukopenia	Neutropenia; hypogammaglobulinemia; T cell and B cell deficiencies	Bone marrow transplantation; immunoglobulin therapy; G-CSF for neutropenia
Dyskeratosis congenita	AR Locus: Xq28; 3q21-q28	Severe infections; skin hyperpigmentation; dystrophic nails; leukoplakia	Skin changes associated with severe neutropenia Clinical testing available*	Prophylactic antibiotics

* See GeneTests (http://www.geneclinics.org) for laboratory directory.

AD—autosomal dominant   AR—autosomal recessive   CBC—complete blood count   G-CSF—granulocyte colony-stimulating factor   S—sporadic cases

Treatments for chronic neutropenia vary with the severity of neutropenia and the pattern of susceptibility to infection. Mild or moderate neutropenia (i.e., counts above 0.5×10^9/L, determined by serial counts over several weeks) rarely requires treatment. The neutropenia in Felty syndrome often responds to splenectomy and weekly doses of methotrexate.[45,46] With few other exceptions, long-term use of corticosteroids, γ-globulin injections, androgens, and splenectomy is not indicated for management of chronic neutropenia. With suspected infections, short-term, broad-spectrum antibiotic therapy is indicated, usually initiated after culture of blood and other body fluids for bacteria. Long-term antibiotic therapy is of unproven benefit in preventing infections, and it carries the risk of colonization by antibiotic-resistant organisms. G-CSF, usually in doses of 1 to 5 mg/kg/day, is of proven benefit for the treatment of congenital, idiopathic, and cyclic neutropenia and hastens the recovery of marrow from neutropenia after cancer chemotherapy.[47] G-CSF and GM-CSF have been widely used to treat other forms of chronic neutropenia, including the neutropenia associated with HIV infection.

Disorders of Neutrophil Function

In patients who have recurrent, severe, or unusual infections but who have a normal number of neutrophils, the presence of a neutrophil function disorder must be considered. Neutrophil function disorders are caused by defects in neutrophil adherence, chemotaxis, degranulation, or oxidative metabolism [see Table 5].

The evaluation of patients with confirmed, recurrent, or un-usual infections is first to review the family history and then to examine the patient [see Figure 5]. A complete blood count and examination of the granulocytes in a blood smear can show neutrophilia or neutropenia, specific granule deficiency, or giant granules such as those that occur in Chédiak-Higashi syndrome. Evaluation of immunoglobulin levels (IgG, IgM, IgA, and IgE) and complement levels (C3 and CH_{50}) are also potentially helpful, especially if there is a pattern of infection by encapsulated bacteria or unusual organisms. After these considerations, neutrophil function should be evaluated with the nitroblue tetrazolium (NBT) test, superoxide production assays, and chemotactic assays. The NBT test and superoxide assays can determine whether a patient has chronic granulomatous disease (CGD), severe glucose-6-phosphate dehydrogenase (G6PD) deficiency, or a glutathione-pathway disorder[14]; chemotactic assays can be used to confirm the diagnosis of Chédiak-Higashi syndrome and acquired chemotactic defects.[12] Leukocyte adhesion deficiency types I and II are diagnosed by flow cytometry.[11] If the results of all of these tests are normal, ingestion assays using the patient's serum and cells and staining for MPO may be helpful. In this manner, all of the known neutrophil function abnormalities can be diagnosed, often with the aid of specialty consultations and a research laboratory.[48]

Monocytes and Macrophage Physiology

Monocytes and macrophages play critical roles in homeostasis and in host defense mechanisms. Monocytes and macro-

Table 4 Guidelines for Management
and Prevention of Febrile Neutropenia[43]

Management

Take careful history and conduct thorough physical examination of the patient

Examine patient carefully for portal for bacterial or fungal infections

Culture blood and other appropriate body fluids

Start antibiotics immediately

Monotherapy (e.g., ceftazidime or imipenem) or duotherapy (e.g., an aminoglycoside, such as gentamicin, with a β-lactam drug that is effective against *Pseudomonas,* such as piperacillin

Add vancomycin if there is a significant risk of gram-positive sepsis

Adjust antibiotic therapy after 3 days, depending on the results of cultures and the patient's clinical status

Switch low-risk patients to oral therapy

Continue broad-spectrum therapy for severely ill patients*

Consider antifungal treatments

Consider colony-stimulating factors as an adjunct to antibiotics for febrile neutropenia in severely ill, high-risk patients†

Prevention

Primary prophylaxis with G-CSF reduces incidence of febrile neutropenia by ~50% when the risk of febrile neutropenia is ~40%‡

Use G-CSF or GM-CSF as a preventive strategy for patients who have had their treatment reduced or experienced a delay in treatment because of an episode of febrile neutropenia or a prolonged period of neutropenia

Consider reducing the intensity of chemotherapy

Note: further information can be found at the following Web sites: www.idsociety.org, www.asco.org, and www.guidelines.gov.
*Resolution of illness generally follows resolution of neutropenia.
†For most patients with febrile neutropenia, CSF therapy has no proven benefit.
‡Administration of G-CSF or GM-CSF is not routinely indicated in previously untreated patients.
G-CSF—granulocyte colony-stimulating factor   GM-CSF—granulocyte-macrophage colony-stimulating factor

phages perform tissue maintenance functions, such as clearance of particles—including bacteria—from the blood and removal of old red blood cells. They process antigens by interacting with T cells and B cells and are essential for containment of mycobacterial, parasitic, fungal, and viral infections.

MONOCYTE-MACROPHAGE DEVELOPMENT

Monocytes develop from hematopoietic progenitor cells in the bone marrow. Once the progenitor cells are committed to a monocyte lineage, they develop morphologically into monoblasts, then promonocytes, and then monocytes. Monocytes are present in the bone marrow and blood. They are the precursors for the tissue mononuclear phagocyte system (including alveolar, peritoneal, and splenic macrophages), Kupffer cells, osteoclasts, dendritic cells, and Langerhans cells. In addition to having phagocytic capabilities, monocytes and macrophages play a central role in the immune response through the generation of numerous cytokines, including growth factors for white blood cells.

With the exception of the alveolar macrophages, which are uniquely dependent on aerobic metabolism for energy production, monocytes and macrophages are facultative anaerobes. Phagocytosis by monocytes and macrophages is associated with an oxidative burst and stimulation of the hexose monophos-

phate shunt. Adhesion, chemotaxis, and activation are similar for monocytes and neutrophils, although macrophages are better than neutrophils at phagocytosis and perform chemotaxis less rapidly and efficiently. Macrophages are also capable of oxygen-independent bactericidal activity that may depend on lytic activity. Stimulated macrophages are capable of producing nitric oxide. Macrophages are capable of secreting many cytokines, growth factors, and acute-phase reactants.

Monocytes and macrophages present antigen to T cells in association with major histocompatibility complex (MHC) class II molecules. This association occurs in the lysosomes of a mononuclear cell before the MHC class II molecules are expressed on the cell surface. Monocytes and macrophages are involved in antibody-dependent and antibody-independent cell-mediated cytotoxicity. The cytotoxicity involves oxidative metabolism, the production of nitric oxide and cytokines, and the secretion of cytotoxic mediators.

Macrophages play a key role in metabolizing high-molecular-weight proteins, glycoproteins, and other material and are intimately involved in the destruction of senescent and killed cells. They also are required for angiogenesis and wound healing and are able to induce neovascularization and endothelial cell proliferation. Given these diverse products and functions, macrophages are involved in many metabolic, infectious, inflammatory, and degenerative diseases.

Increases in blood monocytes (usually less than two times the normal level or less than $1.0 \times 10^9/L$) are a common feature of chronic inflammatory diseases and malignancies. Higher counts of monocytes should raise concern about a hematologic malignancy (e.g., monocytic or myelomonocytic leukemia) [*see Chapter 204*].

Disorders of Monocytes and Macrophages

HISTIOCYTIC SYNDROMES

Histiocytic syndromes are a group of malignant and nonmalignant disorders in which the macrophages and dendritic (Langerhans) cells are the principal cells of abnormality.[49] The malignant disorders include acute monocytic leukemia, monocytic sarcoma, and histiocytic sarcoma. The nonmalignant disorders include the Langerhans cell histiocytosis (LCH) syndromes and the hemophagocytic syndromes, such as sinus histiocytosis with massive lymphadenopathy, hemophagocytic lymphohistiocytosis (HL), and infection-associated hemophagocytic syndrome (IAHS).

Langerhans Cell Histiocytosis Syndromes

The LCH syndromes include solitary eosinophilic granuloma, multifocal eosinophilic granuloma, Hand-Schüller-Christian disease, and Letterer-Siwe disease.[49,50] These disorders predominantly affect children 1 to 15 years of age but also occur in young adults. The LCH syndromes represent a continuum of disease that has been divided on the basis of histologic studies, age at diagnosis, extent of disease, and organ involvement. The signs and symptoms of the LCH syndromes depend on the specific organs involved.[51] The bones, skin, teeth, gingival tissue, ears, endocrine organs, lungs, liver, spleen, lymph nodes, and bone marrow can all be involved and become dysfunctional as a result of cellular infiltration.[52] For example, diabetes insipidus is caused by histocyte infiltration of the pituitary gland,[53] and Erdheim-Chester disease is a multisystem disease characterized by histiocyte infil-

Table 5   Selected Disorders of Neutrophil Function

	Disorder	Inheritance	Clinical Features	Diagnosis	Treatment
Adherence defects	Leukocyte adhesion deficiency I	AR Locus: 21q22.3	Neutrophilia with recurrent severe infections; failure of pus formation; delayed umbilical cord separation	Decreased neutrophil adherence and migration; CD11/CD18 deficiency Clinical testing available*	Bone marrow transplantation; antibiotics
	Leukocyte adhesion deficiency II	S, possibly AR	Neutrophilia with recurrent infections	Neutrophils lack surface sLe^x and have deficient adherence	Bone marrow transplantation; antibiotics
	Actin polymerization defect	AR, S	Recurrent severe infections	Defective neutrophil migration and ingestion of bacteria	Bone marrow transplantation; antibiotics
Granule defects	Chédiak-Higashi syndrome	AR, S Locus: 1q42	Recurrent infections; partial albinism; lymphoproliferative syndrome; neutropenia; thrombocytopenia	Giant cytoplasmic granules; defective neutrophil migration and bacterial killing Genetic testing: research only*	Antibiotics; vitamin C; bone marrow transplantation
	Specific granule deficiency	S, possibly AR	Recurrent infections, especially sinopulmonary and skin infections	Absence of specific (secondary) granules in neutrophils; abnormal neutrophil migration and respiratory burst	Antibiotics
Respiratory burst defects	Chronic granulomatous disease	AR or X-linked CYBA locus: 16q24 CYBB locus: Xp21.1 NCF1 locus: 7q11.23 NCF2 locus: 1q25	Recurrent skin, pulmonary, and liver abscesses	Severely defective respiratory burst; NBT test; abnormality in one of four subunits of NADPH oxidase Clinical testing available*	Interferon gamma; antibiotics
	Glucose-6-phosphate dehydrogenase deficiency	X-linked Locus: Xq28	Recurrent bacterial infections; hemolytic anemia	Reduced levels of glucose-6-phosphate dehydrogenase Clinical testing available*	Antibiotics
	Myeloperoxidase deficiency	AR	Mild, if any, susceptibility to infection	Reduced levels of myeloperoxidase	Generally none indicated

* See GeneTests (http://www.geneclinics.org) for laboratory directory.

AR—autosomal recessive   NADPH—nicotinamide-adenine dinucleotide phosphate   NBT—nitroblue tetrazolium   S—sporadic cases   sLe^x—sialyl-Lewis^x

tration of many tissues.[54] LCH with solitary and multifocal eosinophilic granuloma is found predominantly in older children and young adults; more infiltrative disease is common in younger patients.[55] On presentation, patients with solitary lesions may have an inability to bear weight, or they may have tender swelling caused by tissue infiltrates that overlie a sharply marginated bony lesion. Diagnosis is usually made by demonstration of dendritic cells, eosinophils, and giant cells present in a biopsy specimen; electron microscopy and immunostaining may be helpful for further classification.

Treatment of local LCH is sometimes unnecessary; when it is necessary, surgery or local radiation therapy can be curative.[50-55] LCH syndromes respond to chemotherapeutic agents, including vinblastine, methotrexate, 6-mercaptopurine, etoposide, or 2-chlorodeoxyadenosine (cladribine). There is a long-term risk of secondary or treatment-related malignancies in these patients.

Sinus Histiocytosis with Massive Lymphadenopathy

Sinus histiocytosis with massive lymphadenopathy, or Rosai-Dorfman disease, is characterized by chronic, painless, massive lymphadenopathy that usually involves the cervical nodes and less frequently involves the axillary, hilar, peritracheal, or inguinal nodes.[56] It occurs in both adults and children. Extranodal disease in the respiratory tract, bones, orbits, skin, liver,

and kidneys is present in almost 30% of patients. The disease is usually benign, but significant morbidity and even death may result if massive tissue invasion of the liver, kidneys, lungs, and other critical structures occurs. Patients are usually of African descent, and the incidence of this disease is highest in Africa and the West Indies.

The affected lymph nodes show marked sinusoidal dilatation and follicular hyperplasia with proliferation of foamy histiocytes and multinucleated giant cells in the sinuses. The etiology of this disorder is unknown and may be related to abnormal immune regulation. Attempts at treatment should be reserved for special circumstances that are potentially life threatening. Surgery, irradiation, corticosteroids, vinblastine, and cyclophosphamide have all been administered with varying degrees of success.

Hemophagocytic Lymphohistiocytosis

HL is a rapidly fatal disorder, occurring as a familial or acquired condition; it is characterized by fever, pancytopenia, hepatic dysfunction, and activated macrophages, which overproduce inflammatory cytokines.[57] Family studies suggest that a portion of cases are attributable to mutations in the perforin gene.[58,59] The disease is usually diagnosed in young children; however, secondary forms of HL account for numerous cases in adults and occur in association with bacterial, fungal, and parasitic infections and exposure to various drugs. Treatment is difficult. Chemotherapy may be helpful. If the disease is associated with infection, treatment with appropriate antimicrobials may resolve the disorder.

LYSOSOMAL STORAGE DISEASES

Monocytes and macrophages play a role in tissue remodeling and the removal of senescent cellular debris, and lysosomes are the organelles that perform these functions; therefore, enzymatic abnormalities that involve lysosomal constituents result in disorders of storage that are related to macrophage function. These disorders, usually diagnosed in early childhood, include the mucopolysaccharidoses, the glycoproteinoses, the sphingolipidoses, and the neutral lipid storage diseases [see Table 6]. Enzymatic defects have been described for most of these disorders, and diagnosis depends on demonstrating the enzymatic abnormality in macrophages or histiocytes. Most of these defects result from

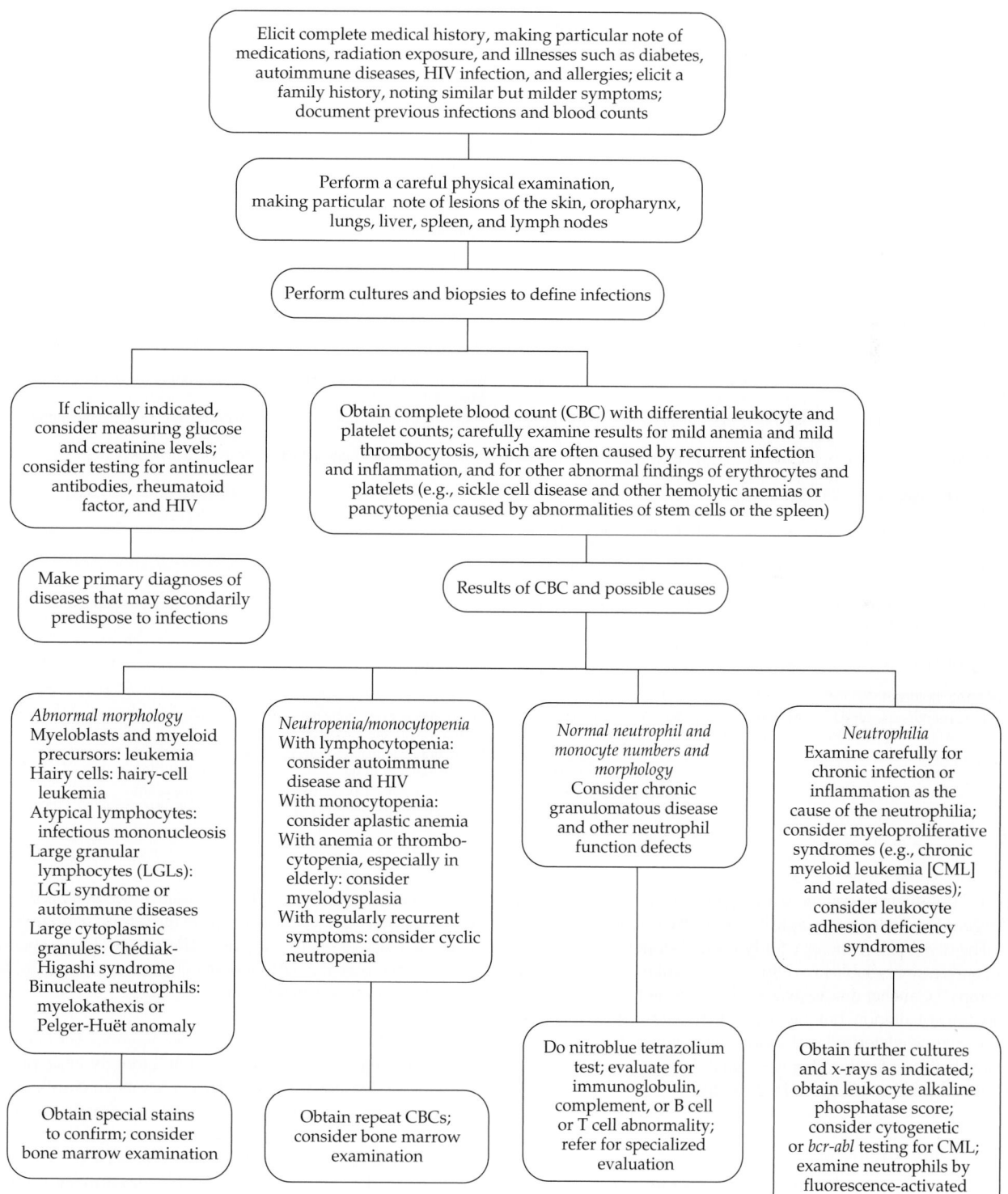

Figure 5   **Steps in the evaluation of a patient with recurrent infections for a phagocytic cell disorder.**

Table 6 Lysosomal Storage Diseases

Disease (Common Name)	Inheritance	Enzymatic Defect	Organs and Tissues Involved	Stored Material
Mucopolysaccharidoses (MPS)				
MPS IH (Hurler syndrome)	AR; locus: 4p16.3	α-L-Iduronidase	Liver, spleen, brain, heart, cornea, bone (mild and severe variants)	Dermatan sulfate, heparan sulfate
MPS II (Hunter syndrome)	Locus: Xq28	Iduronate-2-sulfatase	Liver, spleen, brain, heart, bone	Dermatan sulfate, heparan sulfate
MPS III				
(Sanfilippo A syndrome)	Locus: 17q25.3	Heparan N-sulfatase	Brain, liver, spleen, heart, bone	Heparan sulfate
(Sanfilippo B syndrome)	Locus: 17q21	α-N-Acetylglucosaminidase	Brain, liver, spleen, heart, bone	Heparan sulfate
(Sanfilippo C syndrome)	Chromosome 14	Acetyl-coenzymeA:α-glucosaminide N-Acetyltransferase		
MPS IV				
(Sanfilippo D syndrome)	Locus: 12q14	N-Acetylglucosamine-6-sulfatase		
(Morquio A syndrome)	Locus: 16q24.3	N-Acetylgalactosamine-6-sulfatase	Bone, cornea	Keratan sulfate, chondroitin 6-sulfate
(Morquio B syndrome)	Locus: 3p2	β-Galactosidase	Bone, cornea	Keratan sulfate
MPS VI (Maroteaux-Lamy syndrome)	Locus: 5q11-q13	N-Acetylgalactosamine-4-sulfatase	Bone, cornea, liver, spleen, heart (moderate and severe variants)	Dermatan sulfate
MPS VII (Sly syndrome)	Locus: 7q21	β-Glucuronidase	Brain, liver, spleen, bone, coronary arteries	Dermatan sulfate, heparan sulfate, chondroitin 4-sulfate, chondroitin 6-sulfate
Glycoproteinoses				
Mannosidosis	AR; locus: 19cen-q12	Lysosomal α-mannosidase	Brain, liver, spleen, bone (several variants)	Mannose-rich oligosaccharides
Fucosidosis	Locus: 1p34	Glycoprotein α-fucosidase	Brain, liver, spleen, heart, skin (several variants)	Fucose-containing oligosaccharides
Aspartylglucosaminuria	Locus: 4q32-q33	Aspartylglucosaminidase	Brain, liver, spleen, bone, heart	Aspartylglucosamine-containing peptides
Sialidosis	Locus: 6p21.3	Glycoprotein neuraminidase (sialidase)	Brain, liver, spleen, bone, retina (several variants)	Sialylated glycopeptides
Galactosialidosis	Locus: 20q13	Protector protein deficiency, combined neuraminidase (sialidase) and β-galactosidase deficiency	Brain, liver, spleen, bone (several variants)	GM₁ ganglioside, sialylated glycopeptides
Mucolipidosis II (I-cell disease)	Locus: 4q21-q23	N-Acetylglucosamine-1-phosphotransferase	Brain, bone, connective tissue	Glycoproteins, glycolipids
Mucolipidosis III (Pseudo-Hurler polydystrophy)	?	N-Acetylglucosamine-1-phosphotransferase	Brain, bone, connective tissue	Glycoproteins, glycolipids
Mucolipidosis IV (sialolipidosis)	Locus: 19p13.3-p13.2	Mucolipin 1	?	?
Sphingolipidoses				
(Gaucher disease type I [nonneuronopathic])	AR; locus: 1q21	Acid β-glucosidase, glucocerebrosidase	Liver, spleen, bone, bone marrow (highly variable phenotype)	Glucosylceramide
(Gaucher disease type 2 [acute neuronopathic])		Acid β-glucosidase, glucocerebrosidase	Brain, brain stem, liver, spleen, bone marrow, lungs	Glucosylceramide, glucosylsphingosine
(Gaucher disease type 3 [sub-acute neuronopathic])		Acid β-glucosidase, glucocerebrosidase	Brain, liver, spleen, bone marrow, lungs (variable phenotype)	Glucosylceramide, glucosylsphingosine

(continued)

point mutations or genetic rearrangements at a single locus of the gene that codes for a single lysosomal hydrolase.

The two types of therapy for lysosomal storage diseases that are currently available are cellular transplantation and enzyme therapy.[60] Gaucher disease was formerly treated with bone marrow transplantation, but it is currently treated with alglucerase, an α-mannosyl–terminated glucocerebrosidase. Bone marrow transplantation for the other lysosomal storage diseases is investigational and has yielded mixed results.

Eosinophil Physiology

Eosinophils can enhance or suppress acute inflammatory reactions and mediate responses to helminthic infection, allergy, and certain tumors.[61] Like neutrophils, eosinophils are capable of phagocytosis, but eosinophils are primarily secretory cells. Most of the functions they perform require the release of granule contents or reactive oxygen species. The eosinophils respond to unique chemotactic agents and growth factors that permit their accumulation at sites of inflammation.

EOSINOPHIL STRUCTURE

The granules of eosinophils contain strongly basic proteins and stain intensely with acid dyes. They have a striking and unique appearance on electron microscopy [see Figure 1]. The granules consist of an electron-dense core surrounded by a relatively radiolucent matrix; eosinophil peroxidase is active in the matrix. The dense core has a crystalloid structure and contains eosinophil cationic proteins (ECPs), major basic proteins (MBPs), and eosinophil-derived neurotoxins. MBPs and ECPs are capa-

Table 6   (continued)

Disease (Common Name)	Inheritance	Enzymatic Defect	Organs and Tissues Involved	Stored Material
Metachromatic leuko-dystrophy (MLD)				
Infantile MLD	Locus: 22q13.3-qter	Arylsulfatase A	Brain, peripheral nerves	Sulfatide
Juvenile MLD	Locus: 10q22	Arylsulfatase A	Brain, peripheral nerves	Sulfatide
Adult MLD		Arylsulfatase A, saposin B deficiency	Brain, peripheral nerves	Sulfatide
Pseudodeficiency		Partial arylsulfatase A	Normal	None
Multiple sulfatase deficiency		Unknown primary defect, multiple lysosomal and nonlysosomal sulfatase deficiencies	Brain, liver, spleen, bone	Sulfatide, dermatan sulfate, heparan sulfate
Gangliosidoses				
GM₂ gangliosidoses				
Infantile Tay-Sach disease (TSD)	Locus: 15q23-q24	Hexosaminidase A (α chain)	Brain	GM₂ ganglioside
Juvenile TSD		Hexosaminidase A (α chain)	Brain	GM₂ ganglioside
Adult TSD		Hexosaminidase A (α chain)	Brain	GM₂ ganglioside
Activator deficiency	Locus: 5q31-q33	GM₂ activator	Brain	GM₂ ganglioside
Sandhoff disease		Hexosaminidase B and A (β chain)	Brain, liver, spleen, bone	GM₂ ganglioside, globoside
GM₁ gangliosidoses	Locus: 3p21	β-Galactosidase	Brain, liver, spleen, bone	GM₁ ganglioside, keratan sulfate
Neutral sphingolipidoses				
Fabry disease	Locus: Xq22	α–Galactosidase A	Kidney, vascular endothelial system, heart, central nervous system vessels	Globotriaosylceramide
Schindler disease	Locus: 22q11	α-N-Acetylgalactosaminidase	Brain (probably several variants)	N-Acetylgalactosamine–linked oligosaccharides
Krabbe disease	Locus: 14q31	Galactocerebrosidase	Brain	Galactocerebroside
Niemann-Pick disease				
(Niemann-Pick A disease [infantile])	Locus: 11p15.4-p15.1	Sphingomyelinase	Brain, liver, spleen, lungs	Sphingomyelin
(Niemann-Pick B disease [late-onset])	Locus: 18q11-q12 (C1)	Sphingomyelinase	Liver, spleen, lungs	Sphingomyelin
(Niemann-Pick C disease)	Locus: 18q11-q12 (C2)			
Neutral lipid storage diseases				
Wolman disease	Locus: 10q24-q25	Lysosomal acid lipase	Liver, spleen, adrenal glands, bone marrow	Cholesteryl esters, triglycerides
Cholesterol ester storage disease	Locus: 10q23	Lysosomal acid lipase	Liver, spleen, blood vessels	Cholesteryl esters
Farber disease		Ceramidase	Brain, joints, tendons, skin, liver	Ceramide

ble of inflicting considerable damage to parasites such as schistosomula by binding to and disrupting their cell membranes. In addition, MBPs enhance the adherence of eosinophils and neutrophils to schistosomula.[62]

EOSINOPHIL FUNCTION

Eosinophils respond to a variety of chemotactic factors that enable them to enter tissues and carry out their functions. Some chemokines and chemotactic factors, such as C5a, N-formylmethionyl–containing peptides, and leukotriene B$_4$, stimulate both eosinophils and neutrophils. Several chemotactic stimuli, however, are highly specific for eosinophils. Among these eosinophil-specific stimuli are platelet-activating factor (PAF), eosinophil chemotactic factor of anaphylaxis, and a variety of parasite-derived factors. Responses to PAF, one of the most potent activators of normal eosinophils, include chemotaxis, adherence, enhanced binding of IgE, production of superoxide, release of granule proteins, and synthesis of prostanoids.

Both the production and activation of eosinophils are affected by GM-CSF, IL-5, and IL-3. IL-5 appears to be critical for eosinophil production and deployment.[63] Exposure to low doses of IL-5 also specifically primes eosinophils for later actions by other stimulants. Once activated, the eosinophils have enhanced generation of reactive oxygen species, enhanced glucose utilization and transport, increased oxygen consumption, a reduced cell surface charge, and activation of acid phosphatases in specific granules.

Eosinophils enhance the immune response to helminths. They perform this function by binding to the surface of both larval and adult forms, by damaging target cells through oxygen-dependent mechanisms that are similar to those of neutrophils, and by damaging cell surfaces by releasing granule proteins such as MBP and ECP. Although the release of these proteins similarly damages normal tissues and tumor cells, these interactions between eosinophils and host cells are less well understood. Eosinophils also produce cytokines that enhance the inflammatory response.[64] The presence of eosinophilia in patients with Hodgkin disease appears to be a function of the production of IL-5 by Reed-Sternberg cells. Eosinophils contribute to the fibrosis of the nodular sclerosis type of Hodgkin disease by producing transforming growth factor–β1.

Disorders of Eosinophil Number

EOSINOPHILIA

Evaluation of the patient with eosinophilia (eosinophil count > 700/mm^3) is difficult because the causes of this disorder are multiple and diverse.[65] Common causes of secondary eosinophilia include allergic disorders, infections caused by parasites and other organisms, dermatologic diseases, pulmonary diseases, collagen vascular disease, neoplasms, and immunodeficiency diseases. There are also myriad uncommon causes, such as eosinophilic gastroenteritis, inflammatory bowel disease, chronic active hepatitis, pancreatitis, and hypopituitarism.

HYPEREOSINOPHILIC SYNDROME

The term hypereosinophilic syndrome (HES) is often used for patients with chronic eosinophilia of unknown cause.[66] The criteria used to diagnose HES are an unexplained eosinophil count of greater than 1,500/mm^3 for longer than 6 months and signs or symptoms of infiltration of eosinophils into tissues. Recent evidence points to a mutation in chromosome 4 that results in linkage of the *Rhe* gene and the *PDGFRα* gene.[67]

The clinical features of HES are rash, fever, cough, dyspnea, diarrhea, and peripheral neuropathy. Patients may have chronic congestive heart failure, valvular abnormalities, and distinctive, fibrous, biventricular endocardial thickening with mural thrombi.[66] The blood smear of a patient with HES usually reveals normal mature eosinophils of typical morphology; however, the presence of hypogranulation and cytoplasmic vacuoles has been reported. The total leukocyte count is typically 10,000 to 30,000/mm^3, 30% to 70% of which are eosinophils. The bone marrow is generally hypercellular, with eosinophils constituting 25% to 75% of the marrow elements.

HES can usually be distinguished from malignant disorders associated with eosinophilia, such as acute or chronic eosinophilic leukemias.[68] Allergic reactions must also be excluded; the exclusion of such a reaction is usually based on the history, physical examination, and review of current medications. Because many drugs may generate an allergic reaction accompanied by eosinophilia, all nonessential medication should be discontinued before the patient is evaluated.

Parasitic infections, most commonly with such tissue-invasive helminths as filariae and *Strongyloides, Trichinella, Schistosoma,* and *Toxocara* species, frequently present with eosinophilia. To eliminate parasitosis as the cause of eosinophilia, multiple stool samples and a small bowel aspirate are recommended, particularly in patients who are at particular risk for infection (e.g., those who frequently travel, those who are exposed to animals, and those who have immunodeficiencies). If these test results are negative, serologic assays, radiologic tests, and peripheral blood and bone marrow smears should be performed to exclude the presence of connective tissue diseases, occult lymphoproliferative syndromes and solid tumors, and hematologic malignancies, respectively. In patients with possible cardiac involvement, an echocardiogram should be performed.

Therapy is directed toward lowering the eosinophil count and

Table 7 Causes of Lymphocytosis

Lymphoproliferative disorders (primary lymphocytosis)
  Leukemia
    Acute lymphocytic leukemia
    Chronic lymphocytic leukemia
    Hairy-cell leukemia
    Large granular lymphocyte leukemia
  Lymphoma
  Monoclonal B cell lymphocytosis

Reactive (secondary) lymphocytosis
  Viral infection (most likely with EBV, CMV, HIV, HSV, VZV, rubella, adenovirus, or hepatitis virus)
  Toxoplasmosis
  Pertussis
  Stress
    Acute
      Cardiovascular collapse
      Septic shock
      Sickle cell crisis
      Status epilepticus
      Trauma
      Surgery
      Drugs
      Hypersensitivity
    Chronic
      Autoimmune disorders
      Cancer
      Hyposplenism
      Sarcoidosis
      Cigarette smoking

CMV—cytomegalovirus EBV—Epstein-Barr virus HSV—herpes simplex virus VZV—varicella-zoster virus

correcting specific symptoms. If symptoms involving the lungs or the heart are present, prednisone at a dosage of 1 mg/kg/day should be given for 2 weeks, followed by 1 mg/kg every other day for 3 months or longer. If this treatment fails or if an alternative is necessary to avoid steroid side effects, hydroxyurea at a dosage of 0.5 to 1.5 g/day should be given to lower the WBC count to less than 10,000/mm^3 and the eosinophil count to less than 5,000/mm^3. Study findings suggest that treatment with imatinib mesylate is effective.[69] Alternative agents include interferon alfa, cyclosporine, and etoposide.

Basophil and Mast Cell Physiology

Basophils and mast cells are important in immediate hypersensitivity reactions, asthma, urticaria, allergic rhinitis, and anaphylaxis.[70] They are derived from a common hematopoietic progenitor cell in the bone marrow and are stimulated by soluble mediators, primarily IgE, to release granule contents and arachidonic acid metabolites from their plasma membranes.

The cytoplasmic granules of both basophils and mast cells contain sulfated glycosaminoglycans; in normal basophils, the sulfated glycosaminoglycans are predominantly heparin. The sulfated glycosaminoglycans are the granule contents that are primarily responsible for the intense staining of the basophil. Most, if not all, of the circulating histamine in the body is synthesized by the basophil and stored in its granules. Degranulation causes the release of histamine, which mediates many immediate hypersensitivity effects and which, because it is a potent eosinophil chemoattractant, draws eosinophils to the site of de-granulation. Other substances that are released on basophil de-granulation include additional eosinophil chemotactic factors and a variety of arachidonic acid metabolites, the most impor-tant of which is leukotriene C_4. In addition, the cell membranes of basophils contain high-affinity IgE receptors, the number of which tends to be increased in allergic persons.

Disorders of Basophil Number

BASOPHILIA

Basophilia (basophil count > $150/mm^3$) is seen in myeloprolif-erative disorders, such as CML, polycythemia vera, and myeloid metaplasia; after splenectomy; in some hemolytic anemias; and in Hodgkin disease. The basophil count can also be increased in pa-tients with ulcerative colitis or varicella infection. Although ba-sophils and mast cells are involved in immediate hypersensitivity reactions and basophils are often seen in areas of contact dermati-tis, basophilia is not seen in patients with these disorders.

Lymphocyte Physiology

Lymphocytes (e.g., B cells and T cells) are also derived from hematopoietic stem cells. These cells develop and mature in the bone marrow, thymus, spleen, and lymph nodes and in other spe-cialized lymphoid tissues [see Immunology, Allergy, and Rheumatology].

Disorders of Lymphocytes

LYMPHOCYTOSIS

Lymphocytosis in adults is defined as an absolute lymphocyte count greater than $4,000/mm^3$. In children with the disease, lym-phocyte counts are higher than in adults and may be as high as $20,000/mm^3$ in the first year of life. The blood film of any patient with lymphocytosis should be carefully examined to determine the morphology and diversity of the lymphocytes (e.g., reactive lym-phocytes, large granular lymphocytes, blasts, or smudge cells).

Lymphocytosis can be either primary or secondary. Primary lymphocytosis, often called lymphoproliferative disease, is caused by dysregulation in the production of lymphocytes. The primary lymphocytoses include the leukemias (e.g., chronic lym-phocytic leukemia, acute lymphocytic leukemia, hairy-cell leukemia, or large granular lymphocyte leukemia), the lym-phomas, and monoclonal B cell lymphocytosis [see Table 7].

The reactive, or secondary, lymphocytoses are conditions that involve absolute increases in lymphocytes caused by physiologic or pathophysiologic responses to infection, in-flammation, toxins, cytokines, or unknown agents. The most common causes of reactive lymphocytosis are viral infections: Epstein-Barr virus, cytomegalovirus, herpes simplex virus, varicella-zoster virus, rubella, human T cell lymphotropic virus type I (HTLV-I), HIV, adenovirus, or one of the hepatitis viruses is frequently responsible for the disease. Other pathogens that produce lymphocytosis are Toxoplasma gondii and, in children, Bordetella pertussis (which causes the lympho-cyte count to rise to as high as $70,000/mm^3$). Lymphocytosis is also associated with stress and consequent release of epineph-rine, such as that seen in patients who have had cardiovascu-lar collapse, septic shock, sickle cell crisis, status epilepticus, trauma, major surgery, drug reactions, or hypersensitivity.

Table 8 Causes of Lymphocytopenia

Inherited
  Congenital immunodeficiency diseases
    Severe combined immunodeficiency
      Adenosine deaminase deficiency
      Purine-nucleoside phosphorylase deficiency
      Reticular dysgenesis
    Ataxia-telangiectasia
    Wiskott-Aldrich syndrome
    Cartilage-hair hypoplasia
  Idiopathic CD4$^+$ T lymphocytopenia

Acquired
  Infection
    Viral (e.g., with HIV, a hepatitis virus, influenza virus, or respiratory syncytial virus)
    Bacterial (e.g., typhoid fever, pneumonia, sepsis, or tuberculosis)
  Aplastic anemia
  Autoimmune diseases
  Hodgkin disease
  Sarcoidosis
  Renal failure
  Protein-losing enteropathies
  Chylous ascites
  Zinc deficiency
  Chronic alcohol ingestion
  Immunosuppressive agents (e.g., antithymocyte globulin, corticosteroids, chemotherapeutic agents, and radiation)

Persistent lymphocytosis may be seen in patients with autoim-mune disorders, sarcoidosis, hyposplenism, or cancer and in those who are long-term cigarette smokers.

LYMPHOCYTOPENIA

Lymphocytopenia is defined as a total lymphocyte count less than $1,000/mm^3$. Because in adults 80% of lymphocytes are T cells, most cases of lymphocytopenia are caused by a reduction in the T cell count. The mechanisms of lymphocytopenia are of-ten unknown, and the causes are usually differentiated as inher-ited or acquired.

Inherited lymphocytopenias are usually caused by congenital immunodeficiency diseases. These diseases include severe com-bined immunodeficiency (e.g., adenosine deaminase deficiency, purine-nucleoside phosphorylase deficiency, and reticular dys-genesis), ataxia-telangiectasia, Wiskott-Aldrich syndrome, and cartilage-hair hypoplasia [see Table 8]. In addition, some persons have idiopathic CD4$^+$ T cell lymphocytopenia.

Acquired lymphocytopenia can be seen in patients with viral infections, such as HIV infection, hepatitis, influenza, and respi-ratory syncytial virus infection; in patients with certain bacterial infections, such as typhoid fever, pneumonia, sepsis, and tuber-culosis; and in patients with aplastic anemia, autoimmune dis-eases, Hodgkin disease, sarcoidosis, renal failure, protein-losing enteropathies, and chylous ascites. Zinc deficiency and long-term alcohol ingestion are also associated with lymphocytope-nia. Finally, immunosuppressive agents, such as antithymocyte globulin, corticosteroids, chemotherapeutic agents, and radia-tion, also produce lymphocytopenia.

The author has received grants for clinical research from and served as consul-tant for Amgen, Inc.

References

1. Pierre RV: Peripheral blood film review: The demise of the eyecount leukocyte differential. Clin Lab Med 22:279, 2002

2. Hubel K, Engert A: Clinical applications of granulocyte colony-stimulating factor: an update and summary. Ann Hematol 82:207, 2003

3. Root RK, Dale DC: Granulocyte colony-stimulating factor and granulocyte-macrophage colony-stimulating factor: comparisons and potential for use in the treatment of infections in nonneutropenic patients. J Infect Dis 179:S342, 1999

4. Dranoff G: GM-CSF-based cancer vaccines. Immunol Rev 188:147, 2002

5. Dancey JT, Deubelbeiss KA, Harker LA, et al: Neutrophil kinetics in man. J Clin Invest 58:705, 1976

6. Simon HU: Neutrophil apoptosis pathways and their modifications in inflammation. Immunol Rev 93:101, 2003

7. Gullberg U, Bengtsson N, Bulow E, et al: Processing and targeting of granule proteins in human neutrophils. J Immunol Methods 17:201, 1999

8. Lehrer RI, Ganz T: Cathelicidins: a family of endogenous antimicrobial peptides. Curr Opin Hematol 9:18, 2002

9. Fais S, Malorni W: Leukocyte uropod formation and membrane/cytoskeleton linkage in immune interactions. J Leukoc Biol 73:556, 2003

10. Lindbom L, Werr J: Integrin-dependent neutrophil migration in extravascular tissue. Semin Immunol 14:115, 2002

11. McIntyre TM, Prescott SM, Weyrich AS, et al: Cell-cell interactions: leukocyte-endothelial interactions. Curr Opin Hematol 10:150, 2003

12. Cicchetti G, Allen PG, Glogauer M: Chemotactic signaling pathways in neutrophils: from receptor to actin assembly. Crit Rev Oral Biol Med 13:220, 2002

13. Hogarth PM: Fc receptors are major mediators of antibody-based inflammation in autoimmunity. Curr Opin Immunol 14:798, 2002

14. Babior BM, Lambeth JD, Nauseef W: The neutrophil NADPH oxidase. Arch Biochem Biophys 397:342, 2002

15. Babior BM: Phagocytes and oxidative stress. Am J Med 109:33, 2000

16. Hubel K, Dale DC, Liles WC: Therapeutic use of cytokines to modulate phagocyte function for the treatment of infectious diseases: current status of granulocyte colony-stimulating factor, granulocyte-macrophage colony-stimulating factor, macrophage colony-stimulating factor, and interferon-gamma. J Infect Dis 185:1490, 2002

17. Xing L, Remick DG: Relative cytokine and cytokine inhibitor production by mononuclear cells and neutrophils. Shock 20:10, 2003

18. Bunting M, Harris ES, McIntyre TM, et al: Leukocyte adhesion deficiency syndromes: adhesion and tethering defects involving beta 2 integrins and selectin ligands. Curr Opin Hematol 9:30, 2002

19. Callen JP: Neutrophilic dermatoses. Dermatol Clin 20:409, 2002

20. Creutzig U, Ritter J, Vormoor J: Myelodysplasia and acute myelogenous leukemia in Down's syndrome: a report of 40 children of the AML-BFM Study Group. Leukemia 10:1677, 1996

21. Bain BJ, Phillips D, Thomson K, et al: Investigation of the effect of marathon running on leucocyte counts of subjects of different ethnic origins: relevance to the aetiology of ethnic neutropenia. Br J Haematol 108:483, 2000

22. Scott S: Identification of cancer patients at high risk of febrile neutropenia. Am J Health Syst Pharm 59:S16, 2002

23. Chrischilles E, Delgado DJ, Stolshek BS, et al: Impact of age and colony-stimulating factor use on hospital length of stay for febrile neutropenia in CHOP-treated non-Hodgkin's lymphoma. Cancer Control 9:203, 2002

24. Zinner SH: New pathogens in neutropenic patients with cancer: an update for the new millennium. Int J Antimicrob Agents 16:97, 2000

25. van der Klauw MM, Wilson JH, Stricker BH: Drug-associated agranulocytosis: 20 years of reporting in The Netherlands (1974-1994). Am J Hematol 57:206, 1998

26. van Staa TP, Boulton C, Cooper C, et al: Neutropenia and agranulocytosis in England and Wales: incidence and risk factors. Am J Hematol 72:248, 2003

27. Pitrak DL, Tsai HC, Mullane KM, et al: Accelerated neutrophil apoptosis in the acquired immunodeficiency syndrome. J Clin Invest 15:2714, 1996

28. Kuritzkes DR: Neutropenia, neutrophil dysfunction, and bacterial infection in patients with human immunodeficiency virus disease: the role of granulocyte colony-stimulating factor. Clin Infect Dis 30:256, 2000

29. Sato T, Hirasawa A, Kawabuchi Y, et al: Cellular expressions and serum concentrations of Fas ligand and Fas receptor in patients with infectious mononucleosis. Int J Hematol 72:329, 2000

30. Honda K, Ishiko O, Tsujimura A, et al: Neutropenia accompanying parvovirus B19 infection after gynecologic surgery. Acta Haematol 103:186, 2000

31. Palmblad JE, von dem Borne AE: Idiopathic, immune, infectious, and idiosyncratic neutropenias. Semin Hematol 39:113, 2002

32. Bux J: Molecular nature of antigens implicated in immune neutropenias. Int J Hematol 76:399, 2002

33. Keeling DM, Isenberg DA: Haematological manifestations of systemic lupus erythematosus. Blood Rev 7:199, 1993

34. Ramakrishna R, Chaudhuri K, Sturgess A, et al: Haematological manifestations of primary Sjogren's syndrome: a clinicopathological study. Q J Med 83:547, 1992

35. Starkebaum G: Chronic neutropenia associated with autoimmune disease. Semin Hematol 39:121, 2002

36. Bowman SJ: Hematological manifestations of rheumatoid arthritis. Scand J Rheumatol 31:251, 2002

37. Rosenstein ED, Kramer N: Felty's and pseudo-Felty's syndromes. Semin Arthritis Rheum 21:129, 1991

38. Liu JH, Wei S, Lamy T, et al: Chronic neutropenia mediated by fas ligand. Blood 15:3219, 2000

39. Papadaki HA, Eliopoulos AG, Kosteas T, et al: Impaired granulocytopoiesis in patients with chronic idiopathic neutropenia is associated with increased apoptosis of bone marrow myeloid progenitor cells. Blood 101:2591, 2003

40. Lamy T, Loughran TP Jr: Clinical features of large granular lymphocyte leukemia. Semin Hematol 40:185, 2003

41. Maheshwari A, Christensen RD, Calhoun DA: Immune-mediated neutropenia in the neonate. Acta Paediatr Suppl 91:98, 2002

42. Fumeaux Z, Beris P, Borisch B: Complete remission of pure white cell aplasia associated with thymoma, autoimmune thyroiditis and type 1 diabetes. Eur J Haematol 70:186, 2003

43. Beauchesne MF, Shalansky SJ: Nonchemotherapy drug-induced agranulocytosis: a review of 118 patients treated with colony-stimulating factors. Pharmacotherapy 19:299, 1999

44. Andres E, Kurtz JE, Perrin AE, et al: Haematopoietic growth factor in antithyroid-drug-induced agranulocytosis. QJM 94:423, 2001

45. Rashba EJ, Rowe JM, Packman CH: Treatment of the neutropenia of Felty syndrome. Blood Rev 10:177, 1996

46. Hellmich B, Schnabel A, Gross WL: Treatment of severe neutropenia due to Felty's syndrome or systemic lupus erythematosus with granulocyte colony-stimulating factor. Semin Arthritis Rheum 29:82, 1999

47. Dale DC, Cottle TE, Fier CJ, et al: Severe chronic neutropenia: treatment and follow-up of patients in the Severe Chronic Neutropenia International Registry. Am J Hematol 72:82, 2003

48. Dinauer MC, Lekstrom-Himes JA, Dale DC: Inherited Neutrophil Disorders: Molecular Basis and New Therapies. Hematology (Am Soc Hematol Educ Program) 303: 2000

49. Harris NL, Jaffe ES, Diebold J, et al: The World Health Organization classification of neoplasms of the hematopoietic and lymphoid tissues: report of the Clinical Advisory Committee meeting—Airlie House, Virginia, November, 1997. Hematol J 1:53, 2000

50. Ladisch S: Langerhans cell histiocytosis. Curr Opin Hematol 5:54, 1998

51. Lieberman PH, Jones CR, Steinman RM, et al: Langerhans cell (eosinophilic) granulomatosis: a clinicopathologic study encompassing 50 years. Am J Surg Pathol 20:519, 1996

52. Sundar KM, Gosselin MV, Chung HL, et al: Pulmonary Langerhans cell histiocytosis: emerging concepts in pathobiology, radiology, and clinical evolution of disease. Chest 123:1673, 2003

53. Kaltsas GA, Powles TB, Evanson J: Hypothalamo-pituitary abnormalities in adult patients with Langerhans cell histiocytosis: clinical, endocrinological, and radiological features and response to treatment. J Clin Endocrinol Metab 85:1370, 2000

54. Shamburek RD, Brewer HB Jr, Gochuico BR: Erdheim-Chester disease: a rare multisystem histiocytic disorder associated with interstitial lung disease. Am J Med Sci 321:66, 2001

55. Ghanem L, Tolo VT, D'Ambra P, et al: Langerhans cell histiocytosis of bone in children and adolescents. J Pediatr Orthop 23:124, 2003

56. Pulsoni A, Anghel G, Falcucci P, et al: Treatment of sinus histiocytosis with massive lymphadenopathy (Rosai-Dorfman disease): report of a case and literature review. Am J Hematol 69:67, 2002

57. Ravelli A: Macrophage activation syndrome. Curr Opin Rheumatol 14:548, 2002

58. Goransdotter Ericson K, Fadeel B, Nilsson-Ardnor S, et al: Spectrum of perforin gene mutations in familial hemophagocytic lymphohistiocytosis. Am J Hum Genet 68:590, 2001

59. Feldmann J, Le Deist F, Ouachee-Chardin M, et al: Functional consequences of perforin gene mutations in 22 patients with familial haemophagocytic lymphohistiocytosis. Br J Haematol 117:965, 2002

60. Schiffmann R, Brady RO: New prospects for the treatment of lysosomal storage diseases. Drugs 62:733, 2002

61. Brito-Babapulle F: The eosinophilias, including the idiopathic hypereosinophilic syndrome. Br J Haematol 121:203, 2003

62. Gleich GJ: Mechanisms of eosinophil-associated inflammation. J Allergy Clin Immunol 105:651, 2000

63. Menzies-Gow A, Robinson DS: Eosinophils, eosinophilic cytokines (interleukin-5), and antieosinophilic therapy in asthma. Curr Opin Pulm Med 8:33, 2002

64. Rumbley CA, Sugaya H, Zekavat SA, et al: Activated eosinophils are the major source of Th2-associated cytokines in the schistosome granuloma. J Immunol 162:1003, 1999

65. Rothenberg ME: Eosinophilia. N Engl J Med 338:1592, 1998

66. Roufosse FE, Goldman M, Cogan E: Hypereosinophilic syndrome. N Engl J Med 348:2687, 2003

67. Griffin JH, Leung J, Bruner RJ, et al: Discovery of a fusion kinase in EOL-1 cells and idiopathic hypereosinophilic syndrome. Proc Natl Acad Sci USA 100:7830, 2003

68. Bain BJ: Hypereosinophilia. Curr Opin Hematol 7:21, 2000

69. Cools J, DeAngelo DJ, Gotlib J, et al: A tyrosine kinase created by fusion of the PDGFRA and FIP1L1 genes as a therapeutic target of imatinib in idiopathic hypereosinophilic syndrome. N Engl J Med 348:1201, 2003

70. Prussin C, Metcalfe DD: IgE, mast cells, basophils, and eosinophils. J Allergy Clin Immunol 111:S486, 2003

Acknowledgments

Figure 1 Tom Moore. Electron micrographs courtesy of Dr. E. Chi, University of Washington School of Medicine, Seattle.

Figure 3 Tom Moore.

Lawrence L. K. Leung, M.D.

Hemostasis, the process of blood clot formation, is a coordinated series of responses to vessel injury. It requires complex interactions between platelets, the clotting cascade, blood flow and shear, endothelial cells, and fibrinolysis.

Platelet Plug Formation

Platelets are activated at the site of vascular injury to form a plug to stop bleeding. Physiologic platelet stimuli include adenosine diphosphate (ADP), epinephrine, thrombin, and collagen. ADP and epinephrine are relatively weak platelet stimulators; thrombin and collagen are strong agonists. Thrombin activation is mediated by G protein–coupled protease-activated receptors (PAR),[1] specifically PAR-1 and PAR-4. Thrombin cleaves the external domain of the PAR to initiate transmembrane signaling [*see Figure 1*].[2] Platelet responses to ADP require the coordinated activation of two G–protein–coupled receptors, P2Y1 and P2Y12, which lead to activation of phospholipase C and suppression of cyclic adenosine monophosphate (cAMP) formation, respectively. Antiplatelet drugs such as ticlopidine and clopidogrel block activation of P2Y12.[3] There are also specific receptors for epinephrine, thromboxane A_2, and collagen.

Platelet activation involves four distinct processes: adhesion (deposition of platelets on subendothelial matrix); aggregation (cohesion of platelets); secretion (release of platelet granule proteins); and procoagulant activity (enhancement of thrombin generation) [*see Figure 2*].

ADHESION

Platelet adhesion is primarily mediated by the binding of platelet surface receptor glycoprotein (GP) Ib-IX-V complex to the adhesive protein von Willebrand factor (vWF) in the subendothelial matrix.[4] Deficiency of GPIb-IX-V complex or vWF leads to two congenital bleeding disorders, Bernard-Soulier disease

and von Willebrand disease, respectively [*see Chapter 97*]. Other adhesive interactions (e.g., binding of platelet collagen receptor GPIa-IIa to collagen fibrils in the matrix) also contribute to platelet adhesion.[5]

AGGREGATION

Platelet aggregation involves binding of fibrinogen to the platelet fibrinogen receptor (i.e., the GPIIb-IIIa complex). GPIIb-IIIa (also termed aIIbb3) is a member of a superfamily of adhesive protein receptors, called integrins, which are found in many different cell types. It is the most abundant receptor on the platelet surface. GPIIb-IIIa does not bind fibrinogen on nonstimulated platelets. After platelet stimulation, GPIIb-IIIa undergoes a conformational change and is converted from a low-affinity fibrinogen receptor to a high-affinity receptor in a process termed inside-out signaling. Fibrinogen, a divalent molecule, serves to bridge the activated platelets [*see Figure 3*]. The cytosolic portion of the activated GPIIb-IIIa complex binds to the platelet cytoskeleton and can mediate platelet spreading and clot retraction (in a process termed outside-in signaling).[6] Congenital deficiency of GPIIb-IIIa or fibrinogen leads to Glanzmann thrombasthenia and afibrinogenemia. The GPIIb-IIIa–fibrinogen pathway is the final common course for platelet aggregation. Blockade of this pathway is the basis of an important class of antiplatelet drugs.

PROTEIN SECRETION

After stimulation, platelet granules release ADP and serotonin, which stimulate and recruit additional platelets; adhesive proteins such as fibronectin and thrombospondin, which reinforce and stabilize platelet aggregates; factor V, a component of the clotting cascade; thromboxane, which stimulates vasoconstriction; and growth factors such as platelet-derived growth factor (PDGF), which stimulate proliferation of smooth muscle cells and mediate

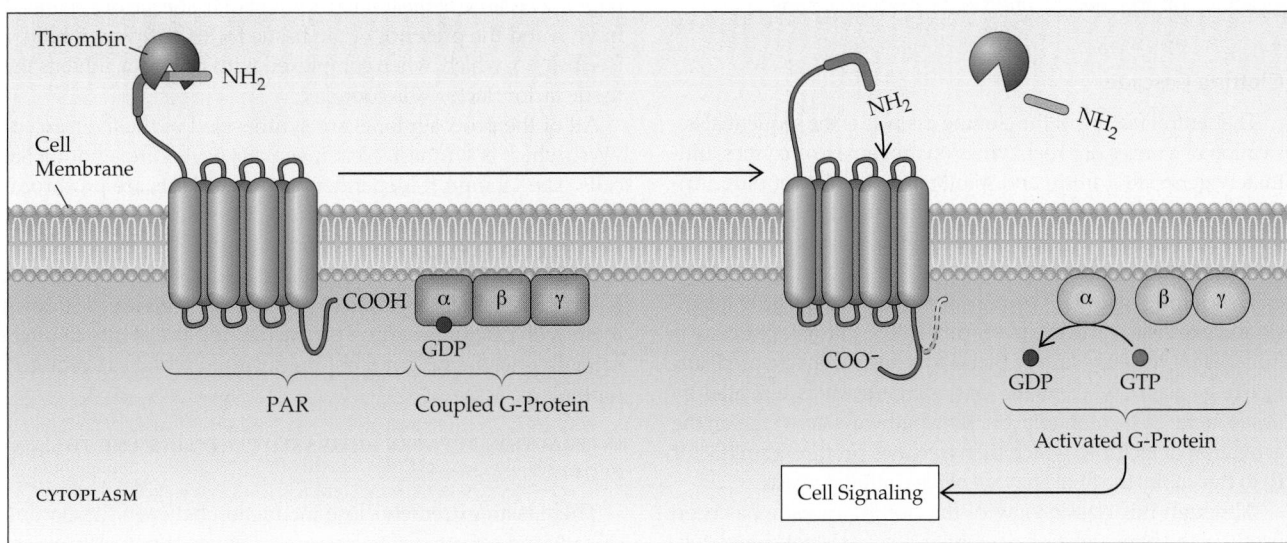

Figure 1 Thrombin activation is mediated by G protein–coupled protease-activated receptor (PAR). Thrombin cleaves the NH_2-terminal exodomain of the PAR, exposing a new NH_2 terminus, which then serves as a tethered ligand to bind intramolecularly to the body of the receptor to initiate transmembrane signaling.

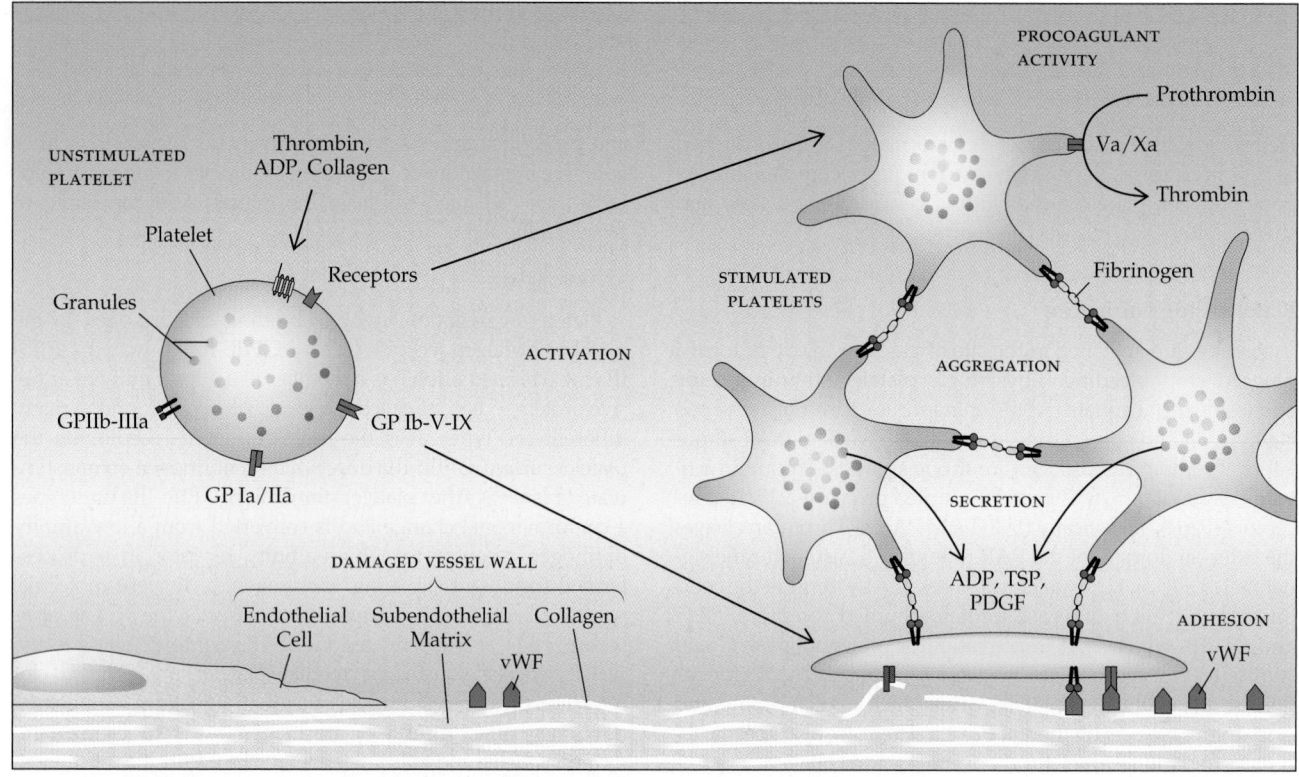

Figure 2 After platelets are activated, they undergo significant morphologic changes, producing elongated pseudopods. They also become extremely adhesive. The functional response of activated platelets involves four distinct processes: adhesion (deposition of platelets on subendothelial matrix); aggregation (cohesion of platelets); secretion (release of platelet granule proteins); and procoagulant activity (enhancement of thrombin generation).

tissue repair. PDGF may also contribute to the development of atherosclerosis and reocclusion after coronary angioplasty.

PROCOAGULATION

Platelet procoagulation involves the assembly of the enzyme complexes of the clotting cascade on the platelet surface. It is an important example of the close interrelationship between platelet activation and the activation of the clotting cascade.

Clotting Cascade

The central feature of the clotting cascade is the sequential activation of a series of proenzymes (zymogens) to enzymes, ultimately generating fibrin and reinforcing the platelet plug. Another key feature, amplification, ensures rapid response for effective hemostasis but demands tight regulation to prevent untoward thrombosis.

The clotting cascade is usually depicted as comprising intrinsic and extrinsic pathways [*see Figure 4*]. The intrinsic pathway is initiated by the exposure of blood to a negatively charged surface (e.g., glass), whereas the extrinsic pathway is activated by tissue factor or thromboplastin. Both pathways converge on the activation of factor X, which then activates prothrombin (factor II) to thrombin, the final enzyme of the clotting cascade.

Although this classic view of the clotting cascade has been useful in the interpretation of clotting times, it is not completely accurate. Patients who are severely deficient in factor XII—as well as many patients deficient in factor XI—do not bleed clinically, which indicates that the initiation part of the intrinsic path-

way (the contact phase) is not important in vivo. It is now established that generation or exposure of tissue factor at the wound site is the primary physiologic event that initiates clotting [*see Figure 4*].[7] Tissue factor functions as a cofactor that is absolutely required by factor VII/factor VIIa to initiate clotting. Factor VIIa activates factor X directly and indirectly via the activation of factor IX. This dual pathway of factor X activation is necessary apparently because of the limited amount of tissue factor generated in vivo and the presence of the tissue factor pathway inhibitor (see below), which, when complexed with factor Xa, inhibits the tissue factor/factor VIIa complex.

All of the procoagulants are synthesized in the liver except vWF, which is synthesized in megakaryocytes and endothelial cells. The vitamin K–dependent procoagulants are prothrombin, factor VII, factor IX, and factor X; the vitamin K–dependent anticoagulants are protein C and protein S. For these factors, the formation of α-carboxyglutamic acid residues by vitamin K–dependent carboxylation of glutamic acid residues endows them with calcium-binding properties and the ability to interact with phospholipid membrane surfaces, which are required for biologic activity.[8]

INTERACTION BETWEEN ACTIVATED PLATELETS AND THE CLOTTING CASCADE

There is an extremely close interaction between the clotting cascade and activated platelet surface in vivo. When platelets are activated, anionic lipids become exposed on the platelet surface, and factor V (stored in platelet granules) is released and bound on the anionic lipids. The factor V on the platelet surface is activated to factor Va and acts as an assembly site for the binding of factor Xa (enzyme) and prothrombin (substrate) known as the prothrombinase complex. At the assembly site, thrombin generation by the prothrombinase complex is approximately 300,000 times more efficient than thrombin generation by fluid-phase factor Xa and prothrombin alone, and the platelet plug keeps the thrombin localized. Factor Xa bound on factor Va is also relatively protected from inhibition by circulating inhibitors such as antithrombin III (AT-III) (see below). Similar enzyme complex assembly applies to the activation of factor X by factor VIIIa (cofactor) and factor IXa (the intrinsic tenase). The result of these processes is efficient amplification and localization of clotting.

Control Mechanisms

Coagulation is modulated by a number of mechanisms: dilution of procoagulants in flowing blood; removal of activated factors through the reticuloendothelial system, especially in the liver; and control by natural antithrombotic pathways. At least seven separate and distinct control systems modulate each phase of hemostasis and protect against thrombosis, vascular inflammation, and tissue damage [see Table 1]. Antithrombin III, protein C, protein S, and tissue factor pathway inhibitor (TFPI) collectively regulate the clotting cascade; prostacyclin and nitric oxide modulate vascular and platelet reactivity; ecto-ADPase inhibits platelet recruitment; and fibrinolysis removes the fibrin clot.

ANTITHROMBIN III–HEPARAN SULFATE SYSTEM

Antithrombin III is a circulating plasma protease inhibitor. It inhibits thrombin and factor Xa, the two key enzymes in the clotting cascade. AT-III also inhibits activated factor XII and factor

XI. In the absence of the glycosaminoglycan heparin, AT-III inhibits thrombin and factor Xa relatively slowly (complete inhibition requires a few minutes). When present, heparin binds to a discrete binding site on AT-III that causes a conformational change in AT-III, which then inhibits thrombin instantaneously and irreversibly. This augmentation of the inhibition of thrombin and factor Xa is the basis for the therapeutic use of heparin as an anticoagulant. Heparan sulfate proteoglycans on the luminal surface of endothelial cells appear to activate AT-III in a manner similar to that of heparin [see Figure 5].[9]

Thus, the endothelial surface is normally coated with a layer of AT-III that is already activated by the endogenous heparan sulfate. Because 1 ml of blood can be exposed to as much as 5,000 cm^2 of endothelial surface, the AT-III–heparan sulfate system is poised to rapidly inactivate any thrombin in the general circulation.

PROTEIN C AND PROTEIN S–THROMBOMODULIN SYSTEM

Thrombomodulin is an integral membrane protein found on the luminal surface of the vascular endothelium in the microcirculation. The binding of thrombin to thrombomodulin results in a remarkable switch in thrombin's substrate specificities: it no longer clots fibrinogen or activates platelets [see Figure 6]. On the other hand, it acquires the ability to activate protein C in plasma.[10] A distinct endothelial receptor for protein C has been found that enhances the activation of protein C by the thrombin-thrombomodulin complex.[11] Activated protein C degrades factor Va and factor VIIIa, the two cofactors responsible for the assembly of the prothrombinase and intrinsic tenase complex in the clotting cascade. Protein S serves as a cofactor for activated protein C. Deficiencies of AT-III, protein C, and protein S are important causes of a hypercoagulable state.

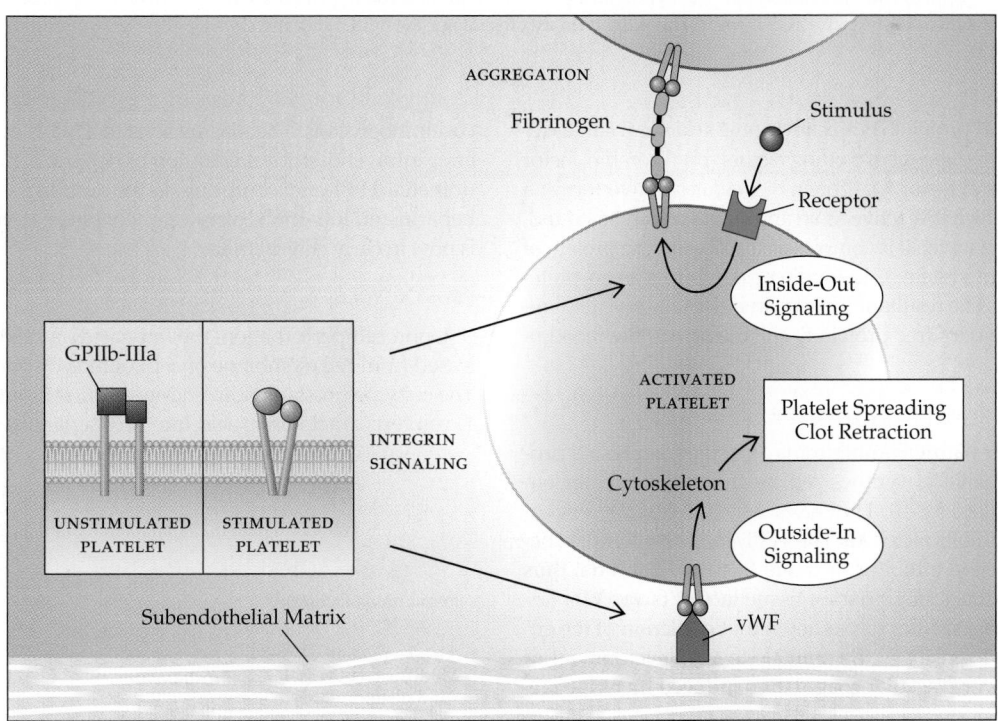

Figure 3 Platelet aggregation involves binding of the divalent molecule fibrinogen to the platelet fibrinogen receptor (the GPIIb-IIIa complex). After platelet stimulation, GPIIb-IIIa is converted from a low-affinity fibrinogen receptor to a high-affinity receptor (inside-out signaling). The cytosolic portion of the activated GPIIb-IIIa complex can mediate platelet spreading and clot retraction (outside-in signaling).

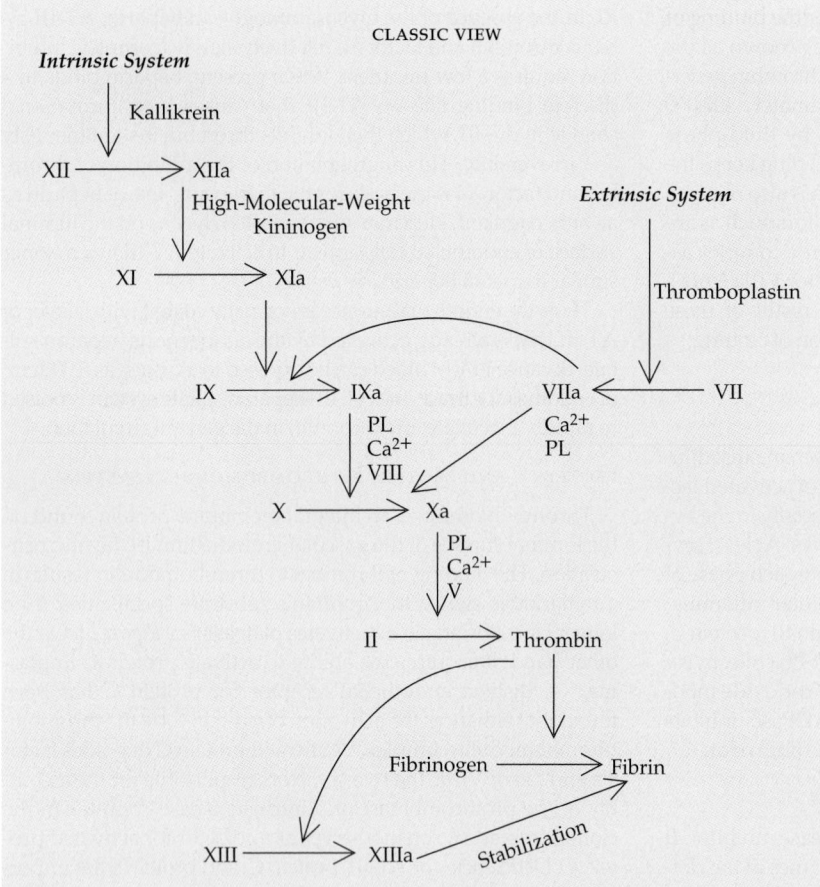
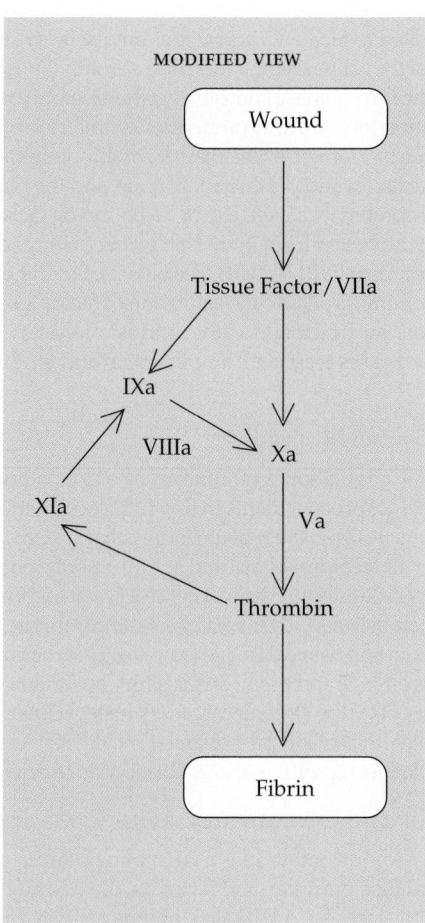

Figure 4 In the classic view of the clotting cascade (*left*), the intrinsic pathway is initiated by the exposure of blood to a negatively charged surface (e.g., glass) and the extrinsic pathway is activated by tissue factor or thromboplastin. In the modified view (*right*), generation or exposure of tissue factor at the wound site is the primary physiologic event that initiates clotting. (PL—phospholipid)

Protein C and protein S both show some structural similarity to the vitamin K–dependent clotting factors (prothrombin, factor VII, factor IX, and factor X). Protein S circulates in two forms: a free form, in which it is active as an anticoagulant, and a bound, inactive form, in which it is complexed to C4b-binding protein of the complement system. C4b-binding protein acts as an acute-phase reactant. The resultant increase in inflammatory states reduces the activity of free protein S, enhancing the likelihood of thrombosis.

TISSUE FACTOR PATHWAY INHIBITOR

Tissue factor pathway inhibitor is a circulating plasma protease inhibitor that is synthesized by the microvascular endothelium. Unlike AT-III, TFPI has a very low plasma concentration. TFPI inhibits factor Xa. The TFPI/factor Xa complex becomes an effective inhibitor of tissue factor/factor VIIa, thus mediating feedback inhibition of tissue factor/factor VIIa [*see Figure 7*]. Animal studies have shown that depletion of the endogenous TFPI sensitizes the animals to the development of disseminated intravascular coagulation induced by tissue factor or endotoxin.[12]

TFPI is primarily synthesized by the microvascular endothelium. Approximately 20% of TFPI circulates in plasma associated with lipoproteins; the majority remains associated with the endothelial surface, apparently bound to the cell-surface gly-

cosaminoglycans. The plasma level of TFPI is greatly increased after intravenous administration of heparin. This release of endothelial TFPI may contribute to the antithrombotic efficacy of heparin and low-molecular-weight heparin. Recombinant TFPI is now in early clinical trials.[13]

PROSTACYCLIN

Upon cell perturbation, the fatty acid arachidonic acid is released from cell membrane phospholipids by phospholipase A_2. The enzyme prostaglandin endoperoxide H synthase-1 (PGHS-1) converts arachidonic acid into prostaglandin endoperoxides

Table 1 Natural Antithrombotic Mechanisms of Endothelial Cells

Regulation of clotting cascade	Tissue factor pathway inhibitor Antithrombin III Protein C/Protein S
Modulation of vessel and platelet reactivity	Prostacyclin Nitric oxide
Inhibition of platelet recruitment	Ecto-ADPase (CD39)
Removal of fibrin clot	Fibrinolysis

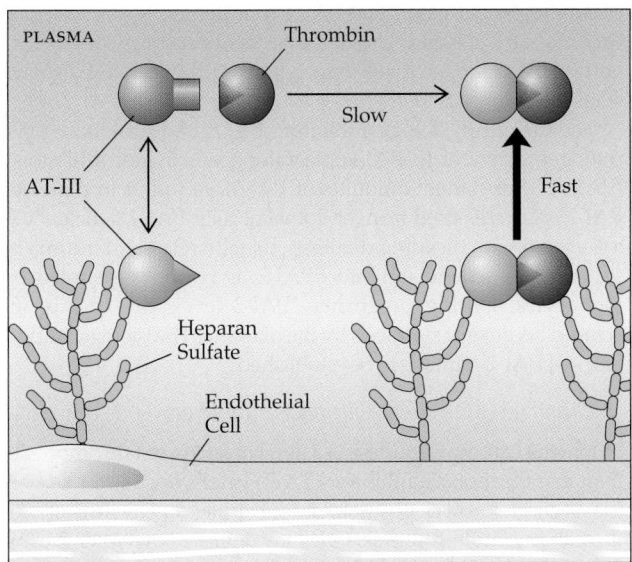

Figure 5 In the absence of heparan sulfate (HS), antithrombin III (AT-III) inhibits thrombin slowly. When HS is present, it binds to a specific site on AT-III that causes a conformational change in AT-III, allowing it to reach the active site of thrombin and inhibit the enzyme instantaneously. HS also binds to a specific site on thrombin, positioning it for optimal inhibition by AT-III.

and finally to thromboxane A_2 (TXA$_2$) in platelets and prostacyclin (PGI$_2$) in endothelial cells. TXA$_2$ and PGI$_2$ have opposite functions. TXA$_2$ is a potent stimulator of platelet aggregation and causes vasoconstriction, whereas PGI$_2$ inhibits platelet aggregation and induces vasodilatation. PGI$_2$ functions by activating adenylate cyclase, which leads to an increase in intracellular cAMP [*see Figure 8*].

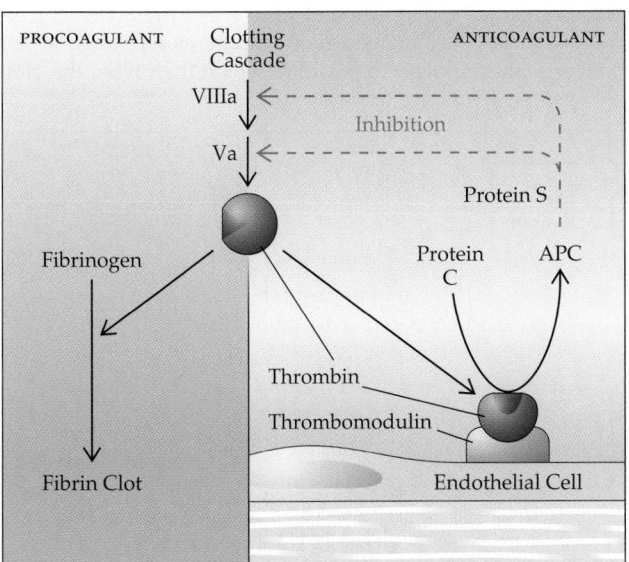

Figure 6 The protein C/protein S pathway is complementary to the AT-III pathway. When thrombin binds to thrombomodulin, thrombin undergoes a conformational change and no longer clots fibrinogen or activates platelets. However, it acquires the ability to activate protein C in plasma. Protein S serves as a cofactor for activated protein C. Activated protein C degrades activated factors V and VIII, the two cofactors in the clotting cascade.

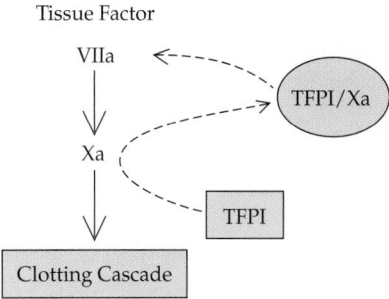

Figure 7 Tissue factor pathway inhibitor (TFPI) binds to and inhibits factor Xa. After binding to factor Xa, TFPI undergoes a conformational change. The TFPI/factor Xa complex then mediates feedback inhibition of tissue factor/factor VIIa.

Cyclooxygenase-1 and Cyclooxygenase-2

Cyclooxygenase-1 (COX-1) is the constitutive isoform of PGHS. Cyclooxygenase-2 (COX-2) is an inducible isoform of PGHS. COX-2 is undetectable in most tissues. However, it can be rapidly induced in response to growth factors, endotoxins, and cytokines in endothelial cells and monocytes (although not in platelets).[14] Evidence indicates that endothelial COX-2 is a major source of PGI$_2$ under physiologic conditions in humans, perhaps because of continual COX-2 induction by hemodynamic shear in the circulation.[15] Aspirin acetylates and irreversibly inhibits both COX-1 and COX-2. Other nonsteroidal anti-inflammatory drugs (NSAIDs) also inhibit COX-1 and COX-2, although not permanently. Selective COX-2 inhibitors are now available as a new generation of NSAIDs.[16]

Because aspirin irreversibly inhibits COX-1 and because platelets cannot make new COX-1, brief exposure to aspirin will permanently inhibit TXA$_2$ production for the life span of affected platelets.

NITRIC OXIDE

Nitric oxide (NO) is formed from L-arginine in endothelial cells. NO stimulates guanylate cyclase, leading to an increase in cyclic guanosine monophosphate (cGMP) in target cells; causes vasodilatation; and inhibits platelet adhesion and aggregation [*see Figure 8*].[17] NO is rapidly destroyed by hemoglobin and thus functions as a local (i.e., paracrine) hormone. Intravenous infusion of an arginine analogue that blocks NO production leads to an immediate and substantial rise in blood pressure. This phenomenon suggests that NO is released continually and basally to regulate vascular tone (in contrast to the production of PGI$_2$, which is more stimulus-responsive). There is significant synergism between NO and PGI$_2$. Formation of NO is catalyzed by NO synthases, which exist in different isoforms in various tissues. In addition to regulating vascular events, NO has a wide range of biologic effects (e.g., neurotransmittal function in the central nervous system).

ECTO-ADPase (CD39)

CD39 is an integral membrane protein found on the endothelial cell surface. It is an active enzyme that rapidly hydrolyzes ADP to AMP, thus functioning as a cell-bound ecto-ADPase. It limits the recruitment of additional platelets into the growing platelet plug by removing ADP released from the dense granules of activated platelets and from damaged erythrocytes and endothelial cells.[18]

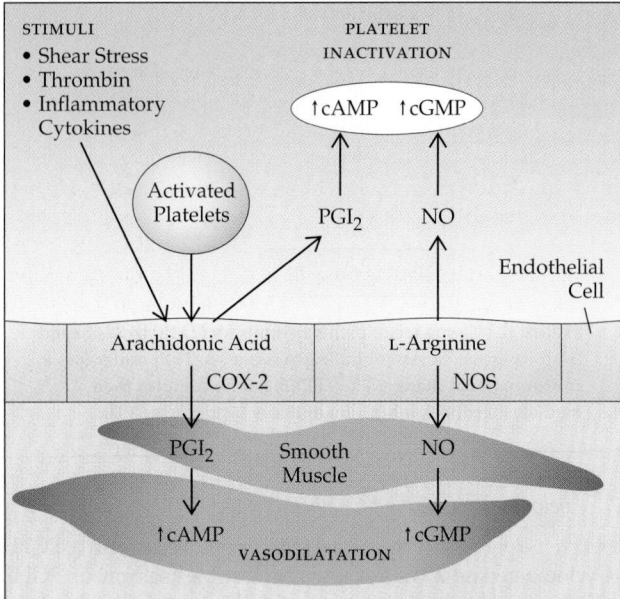

Figure 8   Significant synergism exists between nitric oxide (NO) and prostacyclin (PGI$_2$), leading to platelet inactivation and vasodilatation. The enzyme prostaglandin endoperoxide H synthase–1 (PGHS-1) converts arachidonic acid into PGI$_2$ in endothelial cells. PGI$_2$ activates adenylate cyclase, which leads to an increase in intracellular cyclic adenosine monophosphate (cAMP), inhibiting platelet aggregation and inducing vasodilatation. NO, formed from L-arginine, stimulates production of cyclic guanosine monophosphate (cGMP). Cyclooxygenase-2 (COX-2) is the induced isoform of PGHS; its formation presumably results from hemodynamic shear in the circulation. NO formation is catalyzed by NO synthases (NOS).

FIBRINOLYSIS

Tissue plasminogen activator (t-PA) is released from perturbed endothelial cells near the site of vascular injury. t-PA converts plasminogen to plasmin. Like the AT-III interaction with thrombin, which is accelerated in the presence of endothelial cell surface heparan sulfate, generation of plasmin takes place optimally on a surface (in this case, the fibrin clot). Both t-PA and plasminogen bind to fibrin (via recognition of lysine residues), which facilitates plasmin generation and localized fibrinolysis [*see Figure 9*].

Plasmin cleaves the polymerized fibrin strand at multiple sites, releasing fibrin degradation products. One of the major fibrin degradation products is D-dimer, which consists of two D domains from adjacent fibrin monomers that have been cross-linked by activated factor XIII [*see Figure 10*]. Plasmin has a broad substrate specificity and, in addition to fibrin, cleaves fibrinogen and a variety of plasma proteins and clotting factors. Plasmin bound on the fibrin clot is protected from inactivation, whereas plasmin released into the circulation is rapidly inactivated by plasma α$_2$-antiplasmin. Thus, localized fibrinolysis is achieved, but nonspecific plasmin degradation of plasma proteins is prevented. In rare cases, patients have bleeding problems caused by a congenital deficiency in α$_2$-antiplasmin.

Urokinase is the second physiologic plasminogen activator. It is present in high concentration in the urine. Although t-PA is largely responsible for initiating intravascular fibrinolysis, urokinase is the major activator of fibrinolysis in the extravascular compartment. Urokinase is secreted by many cell types in the form of prourokinase, also termed single-chain urokinase-type

plasminogen activator (scu-PA). Prourokinase is converted to urokinase by plasmin. Urokinase lacks fibrin specificity in converting plasminogen to plasmin, whereas prourokinase displays such specificity.

The major physiologic inhibitor of t-PA and urokinase plasminogen activator (u-PA) is plasminogen activator inhibitor-1 (PAI-1).[19] Substantial amounts of PAI-1 are found in platelets. PAI-1 is also released from endothelial cells. PAI-1 deficiency is associated with bleeding diathesis, usually related to trauma or surgery.[20] A second inhibitor, PAI-2, is normally secreted by monocytes. During pregnancy, PAI-2 levels are greatly increased because of synthesis by the placenta. The biologic importance of PAI-2 remains to be established.

Thrombin-Activatable Fibrinolysis Inhibitor

Plasma carboxypeptidase is a newly recognized thrombin-activatable fibrinolysis inhibitor (TAFI) [*see Figure 11*].[21,22] TAFI is the second known physiologic substrate for the thrombin-thrombomodulin complex. One may envisage that after the initial fibrin clot is formed by thrombin at the site of a vascular wound, thrombin binds to thrombomodulin on the nearby intact endothelial surface. The thrombomodulin-bound thrombin leads to the generation of activated protein C, which dampens the clotting cascade and prevents excessive thrombin generation. At the same time, the thrombomodulin-bound thrombin activates TAFI, thus slowing down the lysis of the existing clot. In hemophilia, the decreased generation of thrombin may lead to suboptimal activation of TAFI and result in premature clot lysis, which contributes to the delayed bleeding observed in these patients.[22] Whether excessive TAFI activity leads to thrombosis is unknown at present.

Overview of Blood Coagulation

The clotting cascade is initiated by the exposure of tissue factor at a vascular wound, which leads to the generation of thrombin and the deposition of a fibrin clot [*see Figure 12*]. Simultaneously, the damaged endothelium releases t-PA, which converts plasminogen to plasmin, which then lyses the clot.

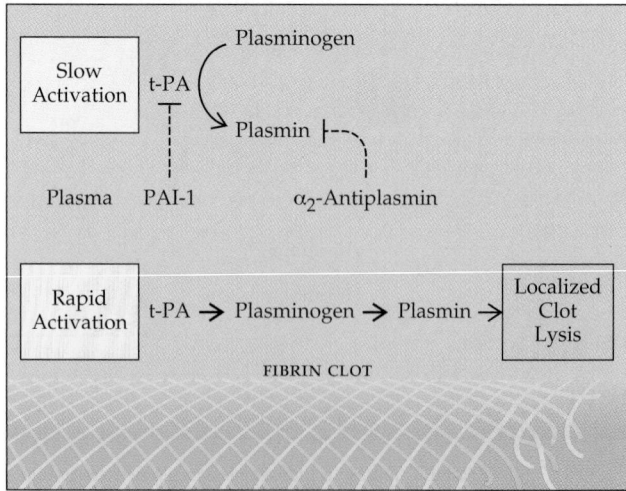

Figure 9   Tissue-type plasminogen activator (t-PA), released from perturbed endothelial cells near an injured blood vessel, converts plasminogen to plasmin. Free plasmin is rapidly inactivated by plasma α$_2$-antiplasmin; plasmin bound to the fibrin clot is protected from inactivation.

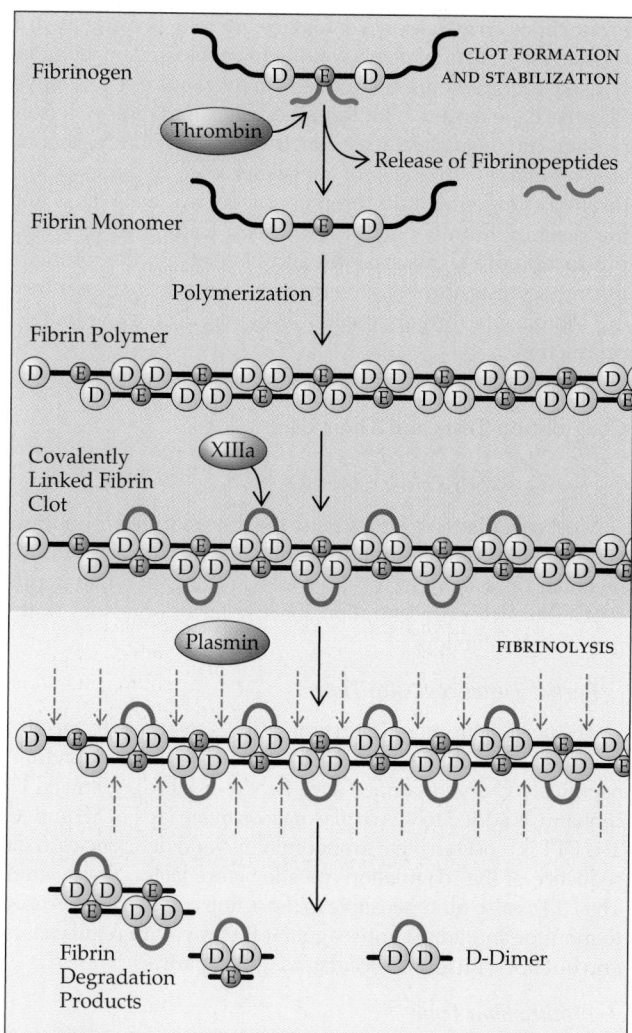

Figure 10 The transformation of fibrinogen to fibrin is initiated by thrombin cleavage of fibrinopeptides A and B from the E domains of fibrinogen to form fibrin monomer. The cleavage apparently changes the overall negative charge of the E domain to a positive charge. This change in charge permits the spontaneous polymerization of fibrin monomers, because the positively charged E domain assembles with the negatively charged D domains of other monomers. The polymer is initially joined by hydrogen bonds. Thrombin activates factor XIII, which catalyzes the formation of covalent bonds between adjacent D domains in the fibrin polymer. Plasmin cleaves the polymerized fibrin strand at multiple sites and releases fibrin degradation products, including D-dimer.

Both pathways are regulated: TF/factor VIIa is regulated by the TFPI/factor Xa complex, and thrombin is regulated by protein C and protein S. Similarly, the activity of t-PA is regulated by PAI-1. Thrombin and plasmin are under the control of their respective inhibitors—AT-III and α_2-antiplasmin, respectively. When these two pathways work in coordinated symmetry, a clot is laid down to stop bleeding, and clot lysis and tissue remodeling then follow. Diminished thrombin generation (as in factor VIII deficiency) or enhanced plasmin production (as in α_2-antiplasmin deficiency) causes hemorrhage [*see Chapter 97*]. Conversely, excessive production of thrombin (as in AT-III or protein C deficiency) leads to thrombosis [*see Chapter 99*].

Heterogeneity of Endothelial Cells and Vascular Bed–Specific Hemostasis

Although the endothelium is generally considered to be a distinct, homogeneous organ system, there are significant differences between arterial, venous, and capillary endothelial cells in terms of morphology and disease susceptibility. Recent studies have shown distinct sets of proteins that mark the arterial and venous endothelial cells from the earliest stages of angiogenesis. Ephrin-B2, an Eph family transmembrane ligand, marks arterial but not venous endothelial cells. Conversely, Eph-B4, a receptor tyrosine kinase for ephrin-B2, marks veins but not arteries.[23]

It is also likely that endothelia from different vascular beds are not identical.[24] For example, the high endothelium in the postcapillary venules of lymph nodes and Peyer patches regulates the circulation of lymphocytes from blood to lymphatics and peripheral tissues. Specific adhesive protein receptors and matrix proteins are highly expressed in these high endothelial venules. The specialized endothelium representing the blood-brain barrier is another example.

These differences between arterial and venous endothelial cells and the vascular bed–specific endothelium may partly account for their different susceptibilities to thrombosis. For example, whereas AT-III and protein C deficiencies are usually associated with deep vein thrombosis of the lower extremities, thrombosis of portal and hepatic veins is frequently associated with myeloproliferative diseases.[25] In both conditions, the underlying defect is a systemic hypercoagulable state, and yet there is a clear predisposition of thrombosis to specific vascular beds. Thus, clinical thrombosis is attributable to an imbalance between systemic prothrombotic stimuli and local antithrombotic mechanisms [*see Chapter 99*].

Platelet Production and Thrombopoietin

Platelets are derived from megakaryocytes, which arise from pluripotent myeloid stem cells. Platelet production is controlled

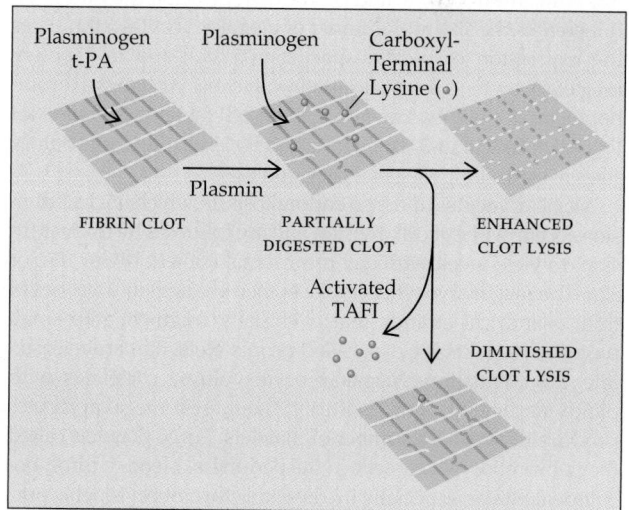

Figure 11 Plasma carboxypeptidase is a thrombin-activatable fibrinolysis inhibitor (TAFI). When fibrin is degraded by plasmin, new carboxyl-terminal lysines are exposed in the partially digested clot. These lysines provide additional sites for plasminogen incorporation and activation in the clot, setting up a positive feedback loop in clot lysis. Thrombin activates carboxypeptidase-B in plasma, which removes the exposed carboxyl-terminal lysines and prevents further plasminogen incorporation into the clot.

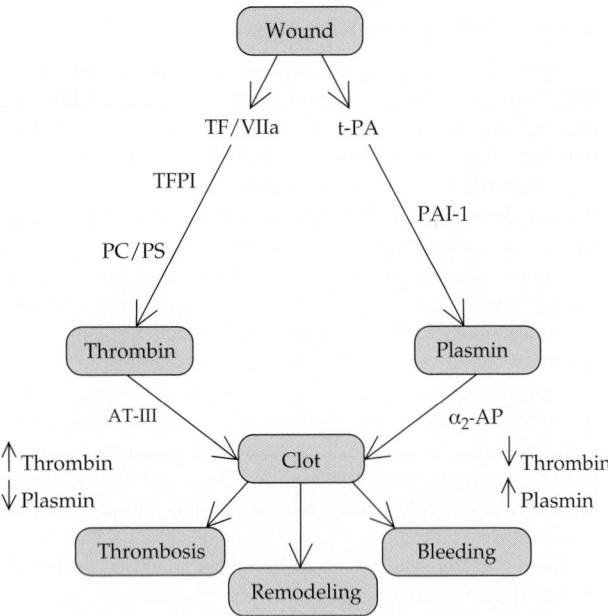

Figure 12 **Exposure of tissue factor at a vascular wound initiates the clotting cascade. Generation of thrombin and deposition of a fibrin clot occur simultaneously with release of t-PA from the damaged epithelium and conversion of plasminogen to plasmin. Plasmin then lyses the clot. When these two pathways work in coordinated symmetry, a clot is laid down to stop bleeding, and clot lysis and remodeling follow. (α_2-AP—α_2-antiplasmin; AT-III—antithrombin III; PAI-1—plasminogen activator inhibitor–1; PC/PS—protein C/protein S; TF—tissue factor; TFPI—tissue factor pathway inhibitor; t-PA—tissue-type plasminogen activator)**

by a thrombopoietin that is involved in the final maturation of the megakaryocyte. Thrombopoietin has multiple actions in megakaryocyte development.[26] It shares some structural homology with erythropoietin and is produced principally by the liver. It increases the size and number of megakaryocytes, stimulates the expression of platelet-specific markers, and is a potent megakaryocyte colony-stimulating factor. Although thrombopoietin is clearly a key factor, stem cell factor (also called kit ligand), interleukin-3 (IL-3), IL-6, and IL-11 all play contributory roles in controlling megakaryocytopoiesis.

Megakaryocytes undergo endomitosis, in which nuclear divisions occur without cell division and are followed by nuclear fusion, to yield a cell with a chromosomal content of 8n, 16n, or 32n. The megakaryocyte cytoplasm then changes into a series of thin, cylindrical strands that eventually fragment into small pieces of megakaryocytes, called proplatelets, that are released into the circulation. Megakaryocyte volume correlates with ploidy and cytoplasmic maturity; the largest megakaryocytes produce the greatest number of platelets. Large platelets called megathrombocytes are seen in the peripheral blood in thrombocytopenic states, especially in idiopathic thrombocytopenic purpura [*see Chapter 97*]. These megathrombocytes probably are young proplatelets and account for the increase in mean platelet volume that occurs during response to or recovery from acute thrombocytopenia.

Platelets entering the circulation survive about 8.5 to 10 days and have a half-life of about 4 days. Approximately 30% to 40% of the platelets are present in a splenic pool that can freely exchange with the circulation. When the need for platelets arises,

production can increase sevenfold to eightfold. Because there is no marrow pool of platelets waiting to be released, meeting increased requirements for platelets may require a few days. Platelets have receptors for thrombopoietin and remove it from plasma, and the platelet mass functions as a major thrombopoietin regulator.[27] In states of megakaryocyte hypoplasia and thrombocytopenia, little thrombopoietin is metabolized and the plasma thrombopoietin level rises, leading to increased production of megakaryocytes and platelets. In the setting of thrombocytosis, thrombopoietin metabolism increases, lowering the plasma thrombopoietin level and decreasing platelet production.

Coagulation Tests and Their Use

TESTS OF COAGULATION CASCADE

Most coagulation tests measure the time required for fibrinogen from plasma to form fibrin strands, which can be detected by either optical or electrical devices. Prolongation may represent a low factor concentration, inactive factor or factors, or the presence of inhibitors.

Partial Thromboplastin Time

The partial thromboplastin time (PTT), sometimes termed the activated PTT (aPTT), tests the intrinsic coagulation system. A negatively charged surface (e.g., kaolin or silica), followed by cephalin, is added to whole plasma to activate factors XII and XI. The PTT is most sensitive to abnormalities and deficiencies in the sequence of the coagulation cascade before factor X activation. The PTT is also quite sensitive to the action of heparin. It is used to monitor and adjust anticoagulant therapy with regular heparin but not with low-molecular-weight heparins.

Prothrombin Time

The prothrombin time (PT) is a test of the extrinsic system. It detects deficiencies in fibrinogen, factor II (prothrombin), factor V, factor VII, and factor X. Tissue factor is added to whole plasma, leading to fibrin formation, normally in 9 to 12 seconds. Results are usually reported using the international normalized ratio (INR). The INR is calculated by using the following equation:

$$INR = (Log\ patient\ PT\ /\ Log\ control\ PT)^C$$

where C represents the international sensitivity index (ISI). In this way, the thromboplastin used in an individual laboratory, with its specific ISI, is calibrated against a standard reference thromboplastin, and the PT is reported as an INR.[28] The presence of a lupus anticoagulant may also interfere with the PT.[29]

Dilute Russell Viper Venom Time

Russell viper venom contains an enzyme that activates factor X; therefore, the dilute Russell viper venom time (DRVVT) measures the common pathway of the clotting cascade. It is sensitive to the presence of a lupuslike anticoagulant that inhibits the phospholipid-dependent prothrombinase complex.

Thrombin Time

The thrombin time (TT) is used to test abnormalities of the conversion of fibrinogen to fibrin. It can be prolonged because of hypofibrinogenemia, abnormal fibrinogen (dysfibrinogen), or the presence of inhibitors (e.g., fibrin degradation products) that interfere with fibrin polymerization. The clinical factors commonly associated with prolonged TT are severe liver disease, disseminated intravascular coagulation, and heparin therapy.

Reptilase Time

Reptilase is a thrombinlike enzyme that converts fibrinogen to fibrin. The reptilase time (RT) is prolonged under conditions similar to those for prolonged TT, with one significant difference: reptilase is not inhibited by the AT-III–heparin complex. Therefore, RT is not prolonged by heparin. A long thrombin time and normal RT suggest a heparin effect.

Fibrinopeptide A

Thrombin activates fibrinogen by splitting off two peptides, fibrinopeptide A (FPA) and FPB, from the Aα and Bβ chain of fibrinogen and converting fibrinogen to fibrin monomer. Measurement of FPA in the blood can be used as an index of thrombin activity in vivo. Because the clotting cascade can be activated during the blood-sample collection, however, precautions are required in the measurement and interpretation of FPA levels.

Fibrinogen

The fibrinogen level in plasma can be measured either antigenically or more commonly by clotting assays. The results are reported in mg/dl.

D-Dimer and Fibrin-Fibrinogen Degradation Products

Fibrinogen degradation products (FDP) and fibrin-fibrinogen split products (FSP) result from plasmin degradation of fibrinogen and fibrin clot [see Figure 9]. D-dimer is released by the plasmin-mediated degradation of fully polymerized fibrin. Plasmin cleavage of fibrinogen or soluble fibrin monomer does not yield the D-dimer. Thus, elevated D-dimer is a specific measure of intravascular fibrin deposition and plasmin degradation characteristic of disseminated intravascular coagulation. The D-dimer test has largely replaced the FSP test.

Factor XIII

Factor XIII is the only clotting factor whose activity is not assessed in PT or PTT because the end point for both tests is the formation of fibrin polymers, irrespective of whether these polymers are cross-linked covalently by activated factor XIII. Factor XIII deficiency may be suspected in an infant who has significant bleeding after circumcision or, more rarely, in an adult patient who has unexplained bleeding.

Plasminogen and α₂-Antiplasmin

The activation of the plasminogen-plasmin system can be inferred from the findings of a long TT, a low plasma fibrinogen level, and an elevated D-dimer level. Another crude test used to measure plasminogen-plasmin activation is the euglobulin lysis time. The sensitivity and specificity of this test is not well defined, however. During extensive thrombosis and fibrinolysis, both plasminogen and α₂-antiplasmin (the physiologic inhibitor of plasmin) are consumed. The direct measurement of plasma levels of plasminogen and α₂-antiplasmin is sometimes useful to assess the extent of fibrinolysis and the requirement for replenishment of these plasma proteins using fresh frozen plasma.

TESTS OF PLATELETS AND OF PLATELET FUNCTION

Peripheral Blood Smear Evaluation

This examination provides quick, definitive information to confirm or question a platelet count. Normally, there are eight to 12 platelets per high-power field (1,000 × magnification), corresponding to a normal platelet count of 150,000 to 300,000/ml. The smear also shows platelet granularity and whether megathrombocytes are present.

Bleeding Time

This test primarily measures platelet function. A spring-loaded device is used to make a standard skin incision on the forearm. A prolonged bleeding time with platelets greater than 100,000/ml suggests impaired function. The bleeding time is difficult to standardize, and a normal bleeding time does not predict the safety of surgical procedures or accurately predict hemorrhage.[30] It should not be used as a general screening test in a preoperative setting. Although once used in the screening of patients for von Willebrand disease or certain platelet function disorders, for these purposes bleeding time has been largely replaced by the platelet function–100 assay (PFA-100).

Platelet Function Assay–100

PFA-100 is a newly developed automated test for platelet function. Citrated whole blood is aspirated through a capillary tube under high shear onto a membrane coated with collagen and epinephrine or collagen and ADP in which a central aperture is made. The time it takes for blood flow through the membrane to stop is denoted as closure time and is a measure of platelet function. The closure time is prolonged in patients with von Willebrand disease or other platelet functional defects.[31] PFA-100 should be considered the first-line test for platelet function disorders.

Platelet Aggregometry

Platelet aggregometers are photometric devices for recording the transmission of light through a suspension of platelets. When platelets aggregate, light passes through the suspension more readily. To test aggregation, dilute concentrations of platelet agonists (e.g., ADP, epinephrine, collagen, and ristocetin) are added to citrated platelet-rich plasma. With the weak agonists, such as ADP and epinephrine, the initial primary wave of aggregation is followed by a secondary wave. The secondary wave reflects the induction of the platelet release reaction, in which platelet granule contents are released to augment further platelet aggregation. A suboptimal secondary wave is seen with platelet storage pool defects in which either platelet granule content is diminished or its release activity is impaired. The latter is commonly associated with aspirin intake or uremia-related thrombocytopathy. Patients with von Willebrand disease will have a suboptimal platelet aggregation response to ristocetin but a normal response to the other agonists. Platelet aggregation testing is labor intensive and expensive and should be performed only in clinical coagulation laboratories that do this test regularly.

TESTS OF INHIBITORS OF HEMOSTASIS

Mixing Studies

A prolonged clotting time (e.g., PTT of 60 seconds [normal, 28 to 30 seconds]) can be caused by either a clotting factor deficiency or an inhibitor. An inhibitor is generally an antibody directed against a specific clotting factor or against a phospholipid-protein complex, the so-called lupus anticoagulant [see Chapter 98]. In a mixing study, one volume of a patient's plasma is mixed with an equal volume of normal plasma. The resulting mixture will provide at least 50% of a deficient factor and correct the abnormality. If the problem is caused by an inhibitor, the resulting plasma mixture still has a prolonged clotting time. A mixing study should always be done when a prolonged clotting time is noted.

Antithrombin III

Bioassays and immunoassays are available for assessing AT-III activity. A functional assay is preferable to an antigenic assay.

Protein C and Protein S

Functional and immunologic methods are available. Because protein C and protein S are vitamin K dependent, their measurement can be problematic in patients taking warfarin. It is best to measure protein C or protein S when the patient has been off warfarin for 3 to 4 weeks.

The author has no commercial relationships with manufacturers of products or providers of services discussed in this chapter.

References

1. Coughlin SR: How thrombin 'talks' to cells: molecular mechanisms and roles in vivo. Arterioscler Thromb Vasc Biol 18:514, 1998

2. Kahn ML, Zheng YW, Huang W, et al: A dual thrombin receptor system for platelet activation. Nature 394:690, 1998

3. Woulfe D, Yang J, Brass L: ADP and platelets: the end of the beginning (commentary). J Clin Invest 107:1503, 2001

4. Clemetson KJ: Platelet GPIb-V-IX complex. Thromb Haemost 78:266, 1997

5. Sixma JJ, Zanten HV, Huizinga EG, et al: Platelet adhesion to collagen: an update. Thromb Haemost 78:434, 1997

6. Shattil SS, Kashiwagi H, Pampori N: Integrin signaling: the platelet paradigm. Blood 91:2645, 1998

7. Rapaport SI, Rao LVM: The tissue factor pathway: how it has become a "prima ballerina". Thromb Haemost 74:7, 1995

8. Furie B, Bouchard BA, Furie BC: Vitamin K-dependent biosynthesis of γ-carboxyglutamic acid. Blood 93:1798, 1999

9. Marcum JA, McKenney JB, Rosenberg RD: Acceleration of thrombin-antithrombin complex formation in rat hindquarters via heparinlike molecules bound to the endothelium. J Clin Invest 74:341, 1986

10. Esmon CT: The roles of protein C and thrombomodulin in the regulation of blood coagulation. J Biol Chem 264:4743, 1989

11. Esmon CT, Ding W, Yasuhiro K, et al: The protein C pathway: new insights. Thromb Haemost 78:70, 1997

12. Morten S, Bendz B: Tissue factor pathway inhibitor: clinical deficiency states. Thromb Haemost 78:467, 1997

13. Bajaj MS, Bajaj SP: Tissue factor pathway inhibitor: potential therapeutic applications. Thromb Haemost 78:471, 1997

14. Smith WL, Garavito RM, DeWitt DL: Prostaglandin endoperoxide H synthases (cyclooxygenases)-1 and -2. J Biol Chem 271:33157, 1996

15. McAdam BF, Mardini IA, Kapoor S, et al: Systemic biosynthesis of prostacyclin by cyclooxygenase (COX)-2: the human pharmacology of a selective inhibitor of COX-2. Proc Natl Acad Sci USA 96:272, 1999

16. Hawkey CJ: COX-2 inhibitors. Lancet 353:307, 1999

17. Moncada S, Higgs A: The L-arginine-nitric oxide pathway. N Engl J Med 329:2002, 1993

18. Marcus AJ, Broekman JM, Drosopoulos J, et al: Thromboregulation by endothelial cells (brief reviews). Arterioscler Thromb Vasc Biol 21:178, 2001

19. Van Meijer M, Pannekoek H: Structure of plasminogen activator inhibitor 1 (PAI-1) and its function in fibrinolysis: an update. Fibrinolysis 9:263, 1995

20. Fay WP, Parker AC, Condrey LR, et al: Human plasminogen activator inhibitor-1 (PAI-1) deficiency: characterization of a large kindred with a null mutation in the PAI-1 gene. Blood 90:204, 1997

21. Bajzar L, Morser J, Nesheim M: TAFI, or plasma procarboxypeptidase B, couples coagulation and fibrinolytic cascades through the thrombin-thrombomodulin complex. J Biol Chem 271:16603, 1996

22. Broze GJ, Higuchi DA: Coagulation-dependent inhibition of fibrinolysis: role of carboxypeptidase-U and the premature lysis of clots from hemophilic plasma. Blood 88:3815, 1996

23. Wang HU, Chen ZF, Anderson DJ: Molecular distinction and angiogenic interaction between embryonic arteries and veins revealed by ephrin-B2 and its receptor Eph-B4. Cell 93:741, 1998

24. Garlanda C, Dejana E: Heterogeneity of endothelial cells: specific markers. Arterioscler Thromb Vasc Biol 17:1193, 1997

25. Dilawari JB, Bambery P, Chawla Y, et al: Hepatic outflow obstruction (Budd-Chiari syndrome): experience with 177 patients and a review of the literature. Medicine (Baltimore) 73:21, 1994

26. Kaushansky K: Thrombopoietin. N Engl J Med 339:746, 1998

27. Kuter DJ, Rosenberg RD: The reciprocal relationship of thrombopoietin (c-Mpl ligand) to changes in the platelet mass during busulfan-induced thrombocytopenia in the rabbit. Blood 85:2720, 1995

28. Hirsh J, Dalen JE, Anderson DR, et al: Oral anticoagulants: mechanism of action, clinical effectiveness, and optimal therapeutic range. Chest 114(suppl):445S, 1998

29. Moll S, Ortel TL: Monitoring warfarin therapy in patients with lupus anticoagulants. Ann Intern Med 127:177, 1997

30. The bleeding time (editorial). Lancet 337:1447, 1991

31. Fressinaud E, Veyradier A, Truchaud F, et al: Screening for von Willebrand disease with a new analyzer using high shear stress: a study of 60 cases. Blood 91:1325, 1998

Acknowledgments

Figures 1, 2, 3, 5, 6, and 8 through 11   Seward Hung.
Figures 4, 7, and 12   Marcia Kammerer.

97 Platelet and Vascular Disorders

Lawrence L. K. Leung, M.D.

Bleeding or bruising that is spontaneous or excessive after tissue injury may be caused by abnormal platelet number or function, abnormal vascular integrity, coagulation defects, fibrinolysis, or a combination of these abnormalities. This chapter addresses hemorrhagic disorders associated with quantitative or qualitative platelet abnormalities and disorders associated with blood vessels. Hemorrhagic disorders associated with abnormalities in coagulation (e.g., von Willebrand disease and hemophilia) are covered elsewhere [*see Chapter 98*].

Approach to the Patient with a Bleeding Disorder

A bleeding disorder may be suspected when a patient complains of excessive bruising or bleeding that often occurs secondary to trauma. The clinical evaluation of a patient with a suspected bleeding disorder begins with a careful history. Assessment of the presenting complaint may suggest where in the hemostatic process a defect is located and whether the defect is inherited or acquired—information that contributes to a rational approach to laboratory evaluation.

PATIENT HISTORY

Bleeding History

Patients suspected of having a bleeding disorder should be questioned about past bleeding problems, bleeding outcomes after surgeries and tooth extractions, character of menses, and dietary habits that might predispose to deficiencies of vitamin K, vitamin B_{12}, and folic acid. The patient should also be questioned about sexual activity, anemia, transfusions, recurrent infections, connective tissue diseases, malignancies, liver and kidney diseases, immunocompromised states, and drug use [*see Medication History, below*].

Many healthy people consider their bleeding and bruising to be excessive, whereas patients with underlying von Willebrand disease, the most common hereditary bleeding disorder, often fail to identify their bleeding symptoms.[1] Given the variability in patients' perceptions of bleeding, as well as the lack of a uniform clinical measure of bleeding severity, a dialogue between the patient and the physician is essential for the evaluation of a bleeding disorder. It is therefore necessary to ask for specific information from patients about bleeding and bruising: (1) If the patient is easily bruised, what size are the bruises? (2) If the patient has had surgery, were blood transfusions needed? (3) If the patient had a wisdom tooth extracted, were return visits required for packing, suturing, or transfusion? The response to trauma is an excellent screening test. A history of surgical procedures, tooth extractions, or significant injury without abnormal bleeding is good evidence against the presence of an inherited hemorrhagic disorder.

The type of bleeding is informative and may suggest the underlying disorder [*see Table 1*]. Active bleeding can be caused by a localized anatomic lesion or an underlying bleeding diathesis. Mucosal bleeding, with recurrent epistaxis, gum bleeding, ecchymoses, and menorrhagia, is suggestive of von Willebrand disease or other platelet disorders. Deep-tissue bleeding (e.g., hemarthrosis and painful muscle hematomas) is more commonly seen in hemophilia and clotting factor deficiencies. Patients with clotting factor deficiencies may have delayed bleeding, presumably because the initial platelet thrombus provides immediate hemostasis but is not properly stabilized by the fibrin clot.

Medication History

A careful history of medication use is a critical aspect of the diagnostic evaluation. The patient should be questioned about use of recreational drugs, prescribed medications, over-the-counter medications, and herbal products. Aspirin use is of particular importance. Aspirin can partially impair platelet function and trigger bleeding symptoms in a patient with mild underlying von Willebrand disease. Because several hundred drug formulations contain aspirin (often with no indication of aspirin content in the product name), identification of aspirin as the cause of a hemorrhagic disorder can be difficult.

LABORATORY EVALUATION

The laboratory evaluation begins with general screening tests, such as platelet count, bleeding time (BT), prothrombin time (PT), activated partial thromboplastin time (aPTT), and thrombin time (TT). These tests are supplemented with specific tests that define platelet or clotting factor abnormalities. Specific tests include examination of the peripheral blood smear; platelet aggregation in response to adenosine diphosphate (ADP), epinephrine, collagen, and ristocetin; platelet release assays; coagulation factor assays; and assessment of factor XIII activity via clot solubility testing [*see Chapter 96*].

In many patients with a bleeding disorder, the likely diagnosis will be suggested from the history and physical examination; the diagnosis can then be confirmed with the appropriate specific tests. When the diagnosis is not immediately apparent, three initial tests should be performed: platelet count, PT, and aPTT. The pattern of results provided by these tests suggests a diagnosis that can then be confirmed with specific testing [*see Table 2*].

Both the PT and aPTT provide a global assessment of the clotting cascade: the PT measures the extrinsic pathway, and the aPTT measures the intrinsic pathway [*see Chapter 96*]. Prolongations of both the PT and the aPTT suggest a clotting defect in the final common portion of the cascade that involves either factor X, factor V, prothrombin, or fibrinogen.

A prolonged PT with a normal aPTT is most commonly seen in a patient taking warfarin; in the absence of warfarin, these test results will indicate either factor VII deficiency or, more rarely, an inhibitor against factor VII.

A prolonged aPTT with a normal PT has a broader differential diagnosis. This combination of test results may denote the presence of an inhibitor against a clotting factor or a deficiency of one of the clotting factors in the intrinsic pathway. It is important to perform a repeat aPTT with equal volumes of the patient's plasma and normal plasma (a mixing study). If the normal plasma does not correct the prolonged aPTT, an inhibitor exists (e.g., a lupuslike anticoagulant or an inhibitor directed against a specific clotting factor). If the normal plasma corrects the prolonged aPTT, the patient has a clotting factor deficiency involving factor XII, factor XI, factor VIII, factor IX, or, more rarely, prekallikrein

Table 1 Clinical Manifestations of Hemorrhagic Disorders

Manifestation	Bleeding Disorder	
	Platelet Defect	Clotting Factor Deficiency
Site of bleeding	Skin, mucous membranes (gingivae, nares, genitourinary tract)	Deep in soft tissues (joints, muscles)
Petechiae	Present	Absent
Ecchymoses	Small, superficial	Large, palpable
Hemarthroses, muscle hematomas	Rare	Common
Bleeding after minor cuts	Common	Rare
Bleeding after surgery	Immediate, mild	Delayed, severe

or high-molecular-weight kininogen. Because the clinical presentations of these clotting factor deficiencies are quite different (e.g., factor VIII and factor IX deficiencies are X linked, frequently with a positive family history), correlation with the clinical setting should be sought and the specific clotting factor levels subsequently determined [*see Chapter 98*]

Thrombocytopenia

Thrombocytopenia, a decreased platelet count, is a common clinical finding that may be caused by decreased platelet production or accelerated platelet removal. Accelerated platelet removal may result from immunologic mechanisms, nonimmunologic mechanisms, or sequestration of platelets in the spleen [*see Table 1*]. Thrombocytopenia can range from a transient, isolated finding to a severe, life-threatening condition.

DIAGNOSTIC EVALUATION

Clinical Manifestations

Patients with thrombocytopenia may be asymptomatic; in these patients, the finding of a low platelet count may be first detected on a routine complete blood count. The most common symptomatic presentation of thrombocytopenia is bleeding—characteristically, mucosal and cutaneous. The hallmark of thrombocytopenia is nonpalpable petechiae, which reflect bleeding probably from capillaries or postcapillary venules [*see Table 1*]. Petechiae usually are only a few millimeters in diameter and occur at sites of increased intravascular pressure, such as over the lower extremities and on the oral mucosa, and at sites constricted by certain types of clothing, such as brassiere straps. Purpura, more extensive subcutaneous bleeding, may occur with a confluence of petechial lesions. Palpable purpura indicates an additional component of vascular inflammation and suggests underlying systemic vasculitis, such as cryoglobulinemia. Thrombocytopenia also leads to mucosal bleeding; deep-tissue bleeding is less common.

Laboratory Tests

Blood count and peripheral smear Laboratory examination should start with the complete blood count and examination of the peripheral smear. The importance of examination of the peripheral smear for estimation of platelet numbers, morphology, and the presence or absence of platelet clumping, as well as evaluation of associated white and red blood cell changes, cannot be overemphasized.

Normally, there are eight to 12 platelets per high-power field (×1,000 magnification), corresponding to a normal platelet count of 15,000 to 30,000/μl. There is no clearly demarcated level of platelets above which patients can be considered safe from bleeding. In general, a platelet count greater than 20,000/μl is considered safe; platelet counts of 10,000/μl or below may be tolerated in nonsurgical patients [*see Chapter 100*]. Patients with idiopathic thrombocytopenic purpura bleed less at a given platelet level than patients with aplastic anemia [*see Idiopathic Thrombocytopenic Purpura, below*]. Presumably, the larger, younger platelets are more effective in hemostasis. The risk of intracranial hemorrhage usually directs therapy.

Elderly patients and patients with coexistent illnesses bleed more than young patients and patients with thrombocytopenia alone. An associated disorder, such as liver dysfunction or connective tissue disease, increases the risk of serious bleeding.

In the initial laboratory evaluation, the complete blood count will establish whether the thrombocytopenia is a single disorder or is associated with anemia or leukopenia, which suggests a production defect as the underlying cause [*see Platelet Production Defects, below*]. If thrombocytopenia is an isolated finding, the physician should confirm the platelet count by repeating the complete blood count. A falsely low platelet count can be the result of in vitro platelet clumping caused by the presence of cold-dependent or ethylenediamenetetraacetic acid–dependent agglutinins. Examination of the blood smear and a repeat platelet count in a citrated or heparin-anticoagulated blood sample will resolve this problem.[2]

The peripheral smear may reveal morphologic abnormalities in platelets and indicate the presence of polychromatophilia, neutropenia, lymphopenia, spherocytosis, blastomycosis, or fragmented microangiopathic erythrocytes. The mean platelet volume, as determined by automated blood cell counters, may provide an additional clue to the cause of the thrombocytopenia. Low platelet volumes (< 6.4 femtoliters) suggest poor production, whereas larger volumes suggest rapid platelet regeneration or dysplastic platelet production.

Bone marrow aspirate and biopsy When accelerated platelet removal appears to be the cause of the patient's thrombocytopenia, a rapid differential diagnosis should be made [*see Table 3*]. A bone marrow aspirate and biopsy will be very helpful in narrowing the diagnosis. Usually, thrombocytopenia with an abundance of normal megakaryocytes in the marrow is the result of accelerated platelet removal.[3] Normally, platelets survive for 10 days and have a half-life of about 4 days; in accelerated-removal states, such as idiopathic thrombocytopenic purpura, the

Table 2 Typical Results of Tests for Hemostatic Function in Bleeding Disorders

Disorder	PC	PT	aPTT
Thrombocytopenia	Low	Normal	Normal
Platelet function abnormalities	Normal	Normal or low	Normal
Vascular purpuras	Normal	Normal	Normal
von Willebrand disease	Normal	Normal	Long
Hemophilia A	Normal	Normal	Long
Disseminated intravascular coagulation	Low	Long	Long

aPTT—activated partial thromboplastin time   PC—platelet count
PT—prothrombin time

platelet half-life may be as short as 30 to 60 minutes. The platelet count will then reflect the balance between accelerated platelet removal and compensatory megakaryopoiesis.

Platelet survival studies are not generally available and are not usually necessary to determine whether accelerated platelet removal is occurring. Infusion of random-donor platelets can be used as a diagnostic and therapeutic procedure. When accelerated platelet removal is responsible for the thrombocytopenia, transfusion with six platelet packs only slightly elevates the platelet count, which then returns to baseline values in less than 24 hours. This therapeutic test becomes unreliable, however, if the patient has been previously alloimmunized by blood or platelet transfusions or by multiple pregnancies.

PLATELET PRODUCTION DEFECTS

Inadequate Platelet Production Due to Stem Cell Destructon

Disorders that injure stem cells or prevent their proliferation frequently cause thrombocytopenia. These disorders affect multi-ple hematopoietic cell lines, and the resulting thrombocytopenia is accompanied by varying degrees of anemia and leukopenia.

Diagnosis   Diagnosis of a platelet production defect is readily established by examination of a bone marrow aspirate and biopsy. The finding of a hypoplastic marrow in which the total cellularity is reduced, along with a decrease in megakaryocytes, implies aplastic or hypoplastic anemia. The first presumption of a cause in these cases is drug toxicity. A marrow that is fibrosed or infiltrated with leukemic or other malignant cells represents the syndrome of pancytopenia from infiltrated marrow.

A marrow aspirate and biopsy sample showing normal cellularity and normal maturation of the erythroid and myeloid precursors, with decreased numbers of apparently normal megakaryocytes, suggest that the patient has ingested a drug, such as ethanol, that specifically affects the megakaryocytic progenitor cells.[4] Ethanol also produces ineffective megakaryopoiesis. In vitamin B_{12} deficiency and folate deficiency, all three marrow cell lines are affected. The marrow smear shows many large hyperlobated megakaryocytes. Some myeloproliferative disorders are characterized by ineffective megakaryopoiesis with bizarre binucleate megakaryocytes.

TREATMENT

If a drug is the suspected cause of the thrombocytopenia, it should be discontinued. Specific replacement is required for deficiencies of vitamin B_{12} and folate. When the thrombocytopenia is causing significant bleeding, platelet transfusion will be required until the situation resolves [*see Chapter 100*].

Interleukin-11 (IL-11), which plays a contributory role in megakaryopoiesis, has been approved for secondary prophylaxis against thrombocytopenia after chemotherapy[5]; however, it has limited efficacy and is associated with moderate toxicity.[6] Two forms of recombinant thrombopoietin—one full length and one with a truncated form—have undergone extensive clinical trials. Both types are potent stimulators of megakaryocyte growth and platelet production and are effective in reducing the thrombocy-

Table 3   Causes of Thrombocytopenia

Type	Disorder	Cause
Platelet production defect	Marrow aplasia or hypoplasia, pancytopenia	Radiation, cytotoxic drugs, idiopathic
	Marrow infiltration, pancytopenia	Cancer (leukemia, lymphoma), fibrosis
	Selective impairment of platelet production	Drugs (ethanol, gold, trimethoprim-sulfamethoxazole, sulfonamides, thiazides, phenylbutazone); infections (childhood rubella, HIV)
	Ineffective megakaryopoiesis	Vitamin B_{12} deficiency, folic acid deficiency, myelodysplastic syndrome, alcohol abuse
Accelerated platelet removal	Immune destruction	Autoantibodies (idiopathic thrombocytopenic purpura, systemic lupus erythematosus, lymphoproliferative disease); proven drug antibodies (quinidine, quinine, heparin, GPIIb-IIIa antagonists); infections (infectious mononucleosis, HIV, gram-negative septicemia, malaria); suspected drug antibodies (thiazide diuretics, acetaminophen, cimetidine, aminosalicylic acid); posttransfusion purpura
	Nonimmunologic removal	Disseminated intravascular coagulation, preeclampsia, vasculitis, thrombotic thrombocytopenic purpura, hemolytic-uremic syndrome, HELLP syndrome, severe bleeding, platelet washout after massive transfusion, giant hemangioma, gram-negative septicemia
	Hypersplenism	Enlarged spleen from various causes

HELLP—hemolysis, elevated liver enzymes, low platelet count

topenia after nonmyeloablative chemotherapy. They have, however, elicited antibody formation; even more worrisome, use of the truncated form has led to the development of functionally neutralizing antibodies that cross-react with the endogenous thrombopoietin.[6] Thrombopoietin mimetics are now in clinical trials.

Inadequate Platelet Production Due to Low Thrombopoietin Level

Moderate thrombocytopenia, generally in the 50,000 to 100,000/µl range, is commonly seen in patients with cirrhosis, which has been conventionally ascribed to platelet sequestration caused by hypersplenism. In addition, there is evidence that low-grade disseminated intravascular coagulation (DIC) occurs in cases of severe liver disease. Impaired clearance of fibrin degradation products may interfere with platelet function and fibrin polymerization. In one study, patients with advanced cirrhosis and thrombocytopenia were found to have low-normal serum levels of thrombopoietin (TPO). Serum TPO levels increased rapidly after orthotopic liver transplantation, and normalization of thrombocytopenia occurred within 14 days after transplantation, irrespective of the change in spleen size.[7] The data indicate that the liver is a major site of TPO production, and decreased hepatic TPO production accounts for a significant part of the thrombocytopenia in liver disease.

ACCELERATED PLATELET REMOVAL DUE TO IMMUNE DESTRUCTION

Idiopathic Thrombocytopenic Purpura

The estimated incidence of idiopathic thrombocytopenic purpura (ITP) is 50 to100 new cases per million persons per year, equally distributed between children and adults.[8,9] ITP typically appears in young women. Predisposing diseases and contributing factors may include infectious mononucleosis and other acute viral illnesses, Graves disease, and Hashimoto thyroiditis,[10] as well as antiphospholipid antibody syndrome.[11] For ITP patients who have antiphospholipid antibody, the outcomes, courses, and response to therapy do not differ from those of other ITP patients.

Pathophysiology ITP is an autoimmune disorder characterized by rapid platelet destruction that is caused by the presence of antibodies against the patient's own platelets. These autoantibodies bind to specific proteins on the platelet surface, and the antibody-coated platelets are removed by the reticuloendothelial system, especially in the spleen. The immunoglobulin on the platelet membrane is usually IgG (most commonly, IgG1). In some patients, only IgG2, IgG3, or IgG4 is present on the platelet surface, suggesting oligoclonality.[12] Immunoglobulin on the platelet membrane is frequently directed against the platelet glycoprotein (GP) IIb-IIIa, the receptor complex that mediates fibrin-ogen binding and platelet aggregation; fortunately, most of these antibodies are not capable of functionally neutralizing the GPIIb-IIIa complex. Less frequently, the immunoglobulin is directed against the GPIb complex.[13] Thrombopoietin levels are normal in ITP, indicating a normal or increased megakaryocyte mass (in contrast to a high thrombopoietin level in aplastic anemia).[14] The marrow may respond to the thrombocytopenia by increasing platelet production. In many cases, however, the marrow response is suboptimal, probably because the antiplatelet antibodies also react with megakaryocyte cell surface antigens. The platelets produced in ITP are usually large and functional, which may account for the clinical observation that most patients with ITP do not have significant clinical bleeding.

Clinical features The onset of ITP is usually insidious. History and physical examination are usually negative except for the presence of petechiae, most commonly in the lower extremities. Clinical bleeding is usually mild, consisting of purpura, epistaxis, gingival bleeding, and menorrhagia. Blood blisters (wet purpura) in the mouth indicate the presence of severe thrombocytopenia. Retinal hemorrhages are uncommon. The spleen is usually not palpable. The presence of a palpable spleen raises the possibility of systemic lupus erythematosus (SLE), lymphoma, infectious mononucleosis, or hypersplenism from underlying chronic liver disease.

Laboratory evaluation The peripheral smear is usually normal; the few platelets that are present are large and well granulated. The presence of hypochromia suggests iron deficiency from chronic blood loss; spherocytes raise the possibility of associated autoimmune hemolysis (Evans syndrome); and red blood cell fragments (schistocytes) suggest DIC, thrombotic thrombocytopenic purpura (TTP), or hemolytic-uremic syndrome (HUS). The marrow shows abundant megakaryocytes; erythroid and myeloid precursors remain normal. Results of tests for SLE are negative. Platelet-associated IgG (PA-IgG) levels are elevated; however, because platelets normally contain IgG in their α-granules, PA-IgG does not distinguish between antiplatelet antibodies, immune complexes deposited on platelet surfaces, and antibodies released from the platelet granules and bound on its surface. Therefore, tests for PA-IgG are not useful in the diagnosis of ITP, unless the tests are performed by special research laboratories that measure platelet antigen-specific antibodies.[15]

Differential diagnosis The differential diagnosis of ITP includes a falsely low platelet count resulting from ethylenediamenetetraacetic acid (EDTA)–dependent or cold-dependent agglutinins that cause in vitro platelet clumping (diagnosed by reexamination of the platelet count in a citrated or heparin-anticoagulated blood sample); the gestational thrombocytopenia of pregnancy (usually a mild problem that is not associated with increased bleeding risk [*see* Idiopathic Thrombocytopenic Purpura in Pregnancy, *below*]); myelodysplastic syndrome (usually associated with anemia and leukopenia); and underlying lymphoproliferative disease.

Course and prognosis ITP is a relatively benign disorder that has a mortality of approximately 1% to 5%; most deaths in adult cases result from intracranial bleeding. Acute ITP is usually confined to children and young adults and is frequently preceded by a viral illness. Permanent spontaneous remission occurs in less than 3 months. Chronic ITP, the usual adult variety, refers to disease that persists for more than 3 months. Although spontaneous remissions and relapses do occur in chronic ITP, long-term spontaneous remissions are uncommon. On the other hand, the long-term prognosis of ITP is benign, even in refractory cases, when these patients are managed properly.[16]

Treatment The treatment of ITP depends on the age of the patient; disease severity; whether petechiae are present alone or with moderate or severe mucosal or central nervous system bleeding; and whether the patient is pregnant.[17]

The American Society of Hematology has released an evidence-based practice guideline for the management of ITP,[15] which can be summarized as follows:

1. Patients with platelet counts above 50,000/μl do not routinely require treatment.
2. Treatment is indicated in patients with platelet counts below 20,000 to 30,000/μl and in patients with platelet counts below 50,000/μl who have significant mucosal bleeding or risk factors for bleeding (e.g., hypertension, peptic ulcer disease, or a vigorous lifestyle).
3. Patients with platelet counts below 20,000/μl need not be hospitalized if they are asymptomatic or if they have only mild purpura.

Patients with asymptomatic mild or moderate thrombocytopenia (i.e., platelet count > 50,000/μl) do not require active therapy. They may be followed and simply alerted to report any mucosal bleeding or crops of new petechiae. Avoidance of aspirin and other nonsteroidal anti-inflammatory drugs (NSAIDs) is strongly advised. The role of Helicobacter pylori eradication in the management of ITP is controversial. It may have a limited value in improving the thrombocytopenia in young patients who have evidence of H. pylori infection and have relatively mild thrombocytopenia (i.e., 30,000 to 70,000/μl) of short duration (< 2 years). H. pylori eradication is not useful in patients with chronic severe ITP.[18]

For patients with moderate mucosal bleeding, therapy is begun with prednisone at a dosage of 60 to 100 mg/day in divided doses. Corticosteroids interfere with the macrophage attack on platelets and eventually reduce the amount of antiplatelet antibody produced by splenic and marrow lymphoid cells. A study showed that a 4-day course of high-dose dexamethasone (40 mg daily) achieved a high remission rate (85%) in newly diagnosed ITP patients; of those patients who responded to therapy, 50% had a sustained response.[19] This remarkably high rate of long-term response after a single course of dexamethasone will require confirmation and longer follow-up.

Unless bleeding is severe, the patient need not be hospitalized. Heavy physical activity, particularly any activity that involves the Valsalva maneuver, should be avoided so as not to increase intracranial pressure. The avoidance of aspirin and other NSAIDs should be emphasized. If required, red blood cell transfusions can be given; however, it is rarely necessary to transfuse platelets in such cases.

The platelet count usually rises several days to 2 to 3 weeks after the start of therapy. When the platelet count reaches normal levels, the prednisone dose can be tapered over a 3- to 4-week period. Although complete long-term remissions with prednisone alone have been reported, sustained complete response after therapy occurs in fewer than 10% of patients.

Splenectomy, usually performed by laparoscopy, is indicated if platelet counts remain below 30,000/μl after 4 to 6 weeks of steroid therapy or when the platelet count begins to fall again after the tapering of steroid. The procedure produces long-standing remission in about 65% of patients with ITP. It is best to administer intravenous immune globulin (IVIg) a few days before splenectomy so that the patient will have a platelet count of at least 30,000 to 50,000/μl at the time of surgery. Generally, a full course of IVIg therapy (1 g/kg/day for 2 days or 0.4 g/kg/day for 5 days) is not required when given as preparation for splenectomy. IVIg will produce a transient increase in the platelet count in the majority of patients, but it is a very expensive thera-

py. The platelet count usually begins to rise on the first postoperative day, often overshooting normal values by the second week. Pneumococcal, Haemophilus influenzae, and meningococcal vaccines should be administered 1 to 2 weeks before surgery.

If the patient is elderly or frail and hence may not survive splenectomy, the disease may be controlled by administration of the minimum amount of corticosteroids required to raise the platelet count to 30,000 to 50,000/μl, a level above which severe bleeding rarely occurs. Because patients with ITP who are classified as therapeutic failures generally do well clinically, the role of such potentially dangerous agents as cyclophosphamide and azathioprine in the management of such cases should be evaluated on a case-by-case basis.

Severe mucosal or CNS bleeding is a true medical emergency requiring hospitalization. Red cells are transfused as required, and prednisone is administered immediately, beginning with a 100 mg dose and then continuing at a level of 25 mg every 6 hours. A full course of IVIg should be administered, and transfusion with 8 to 10 units of random-donor platelets should be carried out when the infusion of the first dose of IVIg, usually given over approximately 60 minutes, is complete. The platelet transfusion after the infusion of IVIg produces a greater and more durable increase in the platelet count. Side effects include generalized aches, headache, flushing, fever, and chills. When severe uterine bleeding occurs, a single 25 mg dose of conjugated estrogen can be administered intravenously to control the hemorrhage. It should be emphasized that the benefit of IVIg is usually transitory and lasts only a few days. Plans for splenectomy should follow this emergency therapy.

The mechanism of action of IVIg is not completely understood. It may produce reticuloendothelial blockade by blocking the IgG-Fc sites on the monocyte-macrophages. Highly specific anti-idiotype antibodies may also block the binding of platelet autoantibodies to the platelet GPIIb-IIIa antigen.[20] Studies indicate that the catabolic rate of IgG is mediated by a new receptor for the Fc component of IgG, termed FcRn (neonatal Fc receptor, so named because it was initially identified in neonatal intestinal epithelium), on the vascular endothelial cells. Normally, IgG, but not IgM, that enters the cell through the process of pinocytosis is protected from catabolic breakdown by binding to the FcRn. After the administration of high-dose IVIg, this receptor is presumably saturated, permitting the degradation of the pathologic antibody to occur in proportion to its concentration in plasma.[21]

Refractory Idiopathic Thrombocytopenic Purpura

About 40% of ITP patients are characterized as refractory; they either remain severely thrombocytopenic after splenectomy and corticosteroid therapy or go into remission but later experience a relapse. Approximately 25% to 40% of patients will have a relapse 5 to 10 years after an initially successful splenectomy.[16] Because serious hemorrhage is uncommon with platelet counts above 30,000/μl, it is often prudent to accept an incomplete response and not proceed to more toxic forms of management. Immunosuppressive agents are generally the mainstay of therapy at this stage. However, it should be emphasized that there are no large randomized studies to address this difficult problem and that generally these patients should be referred to a hematologist.

There are several major treatment alternatives for refractory patients. Rituximab, a chimeric anti-CD20 monoclonal antibody, when administered at 375 mg/m² I.V. once weekly for 4 weeks, produces a lasting and substantial response in approximately one third of patients with chronic refractory ITP; however, long-term follow-up is limited.[22] The majority of the responses occur within 8 weeks after the first infusion. The therapy is generally well tolerated, with most of the side effects (i.e., fever, chills, mild hypotension, and bronchospasm) being infusion related and occurring during or after the first infusion. Rituximab produces a profound and prolonged peripheral B cell depletion in all patients, which can last for more than a year, but serious infection is rare. Azathioprine (100 to 150 mg/day orally) or, alternatively, cyclophosphamide (100 to 150 mg/day orally) plus prednisone (40 to 60 mg/day orally) can be given, but this therapy requires weekly monitoring of complete blood count and platelet count. Prednisone may be tapered and azathioprine or cyclophosphamide adjusted to avoid severe leukopenia. A frequent mistake is to discontinue the therapeutic trial prematurely. Both azathioprine and cyclophosphamide are myelosuppressive and should be given in sufficient dosages to cause a mild leukopenia, with a white blood cell count of approximately 3,000/μl, and both have been associated with development of myelodysplastic syndrome and acute myeloid leukemia. After 1 month, alternate-day prednisone therapy should be considered to avoid steroid side effects. Because of the concern of long-term marrow toxicity associated with azathioprine and cyclophosphamide, rituximab should be considered the first-line therapy in refractory ITP patients, if treatment is indicated.

Another alternative is antibody therapy with intermittent courses of IVIg at the dosage schedules described (see above). The cost of this therapy and the usual short-lived response make it an unattractive choice. Anti-D antibody has been used successfully in Rh⁺(D⁺) patients with ITP; in the presumed mechanism of action, the antibody-coated red blood cells block Fc receptors on macrophages and prevent the accelerated removal of platelets. Other therapeutic options include vincristine, vinblastine,[23] danazol,[24] high-dose dexamethasone, cyclosporine, interferon alfa, and plasmapheresis.

In the refractory splenectomized patient, it is important to check for the continued presence of Howell-Jolly bodies and the possibility of an accessory spleen. The disappearance of Howell-Jolly bodies suggests the presence of a remaining accessory spleen or a regenerated spleen.

Patients with clinically significant thrombocytopenic bleeding can also benefit from fibrinolysis inhibitor ε-aminocaproic acid (EACA). EACA can be given at 2 to 3 g orally four times daily until hemostasis is achieved.

HIV-Related Idiopathic Thrombocytopenic Purpura

HIV-1–related ITP appears to have a pathophysiology that is somewhat different from that of non–HIV-associated ITP, in that the antigenic specificity for the antiplatelet antibody is different. Two major antigenic determinants have been identified—a linear peptide in the platelet membrane GPIIIa and a cleavage product of talin, a platelet cytoskeletal protein, that can be generated by HIV-1 protease.[25,26] In patients with HIV infection, platelets also contain increased amounts of IgG, IgM, complement, and immune complexes. Platelet survival is moderately short, and platelet production is impaired, especially at the later stages of the disease.[27]

The use of immunosuppressive agents in HIV-infected patients is hazardous. If the drop in the platelet count is modest, no therapy is needed. When the thrombocytopenia is severe, a short course of prednisone can be administered, followed by splenectomy.

Acute thrombocytopenic hemorrhage in HIV-associated ITP may be managed with high-dose IVIg, similar to the management of other ITPs. Chronic HIV-associated ITP may respond to oral zidovudine (AZT) or other antiviral therapies [see Chapter 153]. Anti-D antibody, dapsone, and interferon have also been used with some success.[28-30] Patients who refuse splenectomy or who are thought to be poor surgical candidates may respond to low-dose splenic irradiation.[31]

Idiopathic Thrombocytopenic Purpura in Pregnancy

Mild thrombocytopenia, generally in the range of 110,000 to 150,000/μl and seldom below 70,000/μl, occurs in 5% of healthy pregnant women. When thrombocytopenia is observed for the first time during pregnancy, the differential diagnosis must include preeclampsia [see Table 3]. If other diagnoses can be excluded, the diagnosis is gestational thrombocytopenia (incidental thrombocytopenia of pregnancy); it requires no management.[32] If the diagnosis of ITP is made, the the patients is considered to be at high risk for complications. The platelet counts should be monitored regularly and closely, especially in the third trimester, because in many pregnant women with ITP, thrombocytopenia progressively worsens over the course of the pregnancy. The therapeutic choices are limited because splenectomy may cause spontaneous abortion and immunosuppressive agents may damage the developing fetus; therefore, therapy is usually limited to corticosteroids or IVIg. Because corticosteroids increase the risk of preeclampsia and gestational diabetes, IVIg is the drug of choice. Generally, no treatment is required until the platelet count has fallen to 20,000 to 30,000/μl or there is clinical bleeding. Typically, a single dose of IVIg (1 g/kg I.V. over 6 hours) will raise the platelet count to above 50,000/μl in the majority of patients, which will last for 3 to 4 weeks. Repeated doses can be given if necessary. In cases of severe thrombocytopenic hemorrhage, however, all of the available therapies should be used to protect the life and well-being of the mother.

Because the antiplatelet autoantibody in ITP has broad specificity and is almost always an IgG, it can cross the placenta and produce thrombocytopenia in the fetus. During a vaginal delivery, the pressure applied to the head of a thrombocytopenic fetus may induce an intracranial hemorrhage. Concern about this occurrence led many experts in the past to recommend early cesarean sections in women with a history of ITP or active disease. No data exist, however, to support this recommendation, and a much more conservative approach is now generally accepted. Most pregnant women with ITP undergo vaginal deliveries; cesarean sections are performed only for obstetric indications.

There is no correlation between maternal platelet count and the infant's platelet count. A mother with a history of ITP who has a normal platelet count can deliver a thrombocytopenic neonate (~10% incidence). Alternatively, a thrombocytopenic mother can have an infant with a normal platelet count. Measurement of maternal antiplatelet antibody is of no clinical utility. The best predictor of thrombocytopenia in a neonate is the mother's previous experience of giving birth to an infant with neonatal thrombocytopenia.[33] Neonatal severe thrombocytopenia—defined as a platelet count at birth that is less than 20,000/μl—is uncommon (1% to 5% of births), and severe bleeding complications are rare (< 1%).[34,35] The occurrence of neonatal severe thrombocytopenia is also unpredictable. The risk of intracranial hemorrhages in these infants is low (< 1%), and it cannot be reduced by cesarean section.[36] Percutaneous umbilical blood sampling is generally not recommended. Many infants who are born to mothers with ITP will have a decrease in platelet count after delivery, with a nadir on day 2; the infant's platelet count should be monitored daily for several days.[32] Maternal ITP is not a contraindication to breast-feeding.

Thrombocytopenic Purpura with Lymphomas and Systemic Lupus Erythematosus

Patients with SLE, Hodgkin disease, or non-Hodgkin lymphoma can present with a clinical picture identical to that seen in ITP. The diagnostic approach and therapy are the same in these cases as they are in ITP. Splenomegaly with splenic sequestration, marrow infiltration with malignant cells, and recent antineoplastic or immunosuppressive therapy should be excluded. Patients with SLE or lymphoma may have Evans syndrome, in which ITP is associated with autoimmune hemolytic anemia. The management of Evans syndrome is the same as that of ITP and autoimmune hemolytic anemia.

Posttransfusion Purpura

Posttransfusion purpura (PTP) is characterized by acute onset of severe thrombocytopenia, often with a platelet count below 10,000/μl, accompanied by clinical bleeding. It may occur from 2 to 10 days after a transfusion of packed red blood cells or platelet-containing components. Almost all of the affected patients are multiparous women. Such disorders as septic thrombocytopenia, DIC, and heparin-induced thrombocytopenia must be considered in the differential diagnosis. The thrombocytopenia usually lasts for about 4 weeks. Because platelet transfusions are usually futile and sometimes precipitate severe systemic responses, they should be avoided if possible.

The pathophysiology of PTP is not completely understood. In most cases, the patient has been exposed to platelet alloantigens during pregnancy or as a result of a transfusion. Most patients with this disorder have antibodies to the human platelet antigen-1 (HPA-1), a polymorphic epitope present on platelet surface GPIIIa. The HPA-1 has two isoforms, HPA-1a and HPA-1b (previously PLA-1 and PLA-2). In the United States, approximately 98% of the white population, 99% of the African-American population, and 99% of the Asian-American population are homozygous for HPA-1. Patients in whom PTP develops are usually HPA-1a negative and HPA-1b positive. The patient has been sensitized to the HPA-1a antigen, most frequently during pregnancy, and reexposure to HPA-1a platelets during red cell transfusion leads to an anamnestic response and the destruction of the foreign platelets. It is puzzling that alloantibody directed against an antigen present on foreign platelets results in destruction of the patient's autologous platelets, which do not express the HPA-1a antigen. There is evidence suggesting that the HPA-1a antigen becomes soluble and attaches to the HPA-1a–negative platelets. Alternatively, exposure to foreign platelets may induce the formation of a true autoantibody against the endogenous platelets. The HPA-1a/HPA-1b polymorphism accounts for 80% to 90% of PTP. However, the presence of an alloantibody is necessary but insufficient for the development of PTP. Some patients with anti–HPA-1a antibodies become refractory to platelet transfusions but do not have PTP.[37] In addition, the incidence of PTP is far less common than might be predicted by the 1% to 2% of the general population who are homozygous for HPA-1b.

Confirmation of the diagnosis of PTP requires serologic studies demonstrating the presence of anti–HPA-1a antibody and a homozygous HPA-1b genotype. Several rapid platelet genotyping techniques based on the polymerase chain reaction have been developed. Homozygous deficiency of platelet CD36 (glycoprotein IV) occurs in 3% to 5% of Asians and Africans, and alloantibody against CD36 has also been found to be associated with PTP.[38] There are no controlled clinical trials evaluating therapy for PTP because of the limited number of cases. IVIg, used at doses similar to those used in the treatment of ITP, is efficacious in about 80% of cases. Plasmapheresis is also efficacious, but it is more cumbersome than IVIg administration. Use of high doses of corticosteroids is not consistently effective.[39] Transfusion of HPA-1a–negative platelets may provide some transient benefit in life-threatening bleeding situations.[40]

Drug-Induced Immune Platelet Destruction

Drug-induced immune platelet destruction is indistinguishable from ITP. The bone marrow shows abundant megakaryocytes, and special laboratories can detect the presence of antidrug antibodies.

Quinidine and quinine purpura The pathogenic antibodies in cases of quinidine and quinine purpura develop as early as 12 days after exposure to the offending agent. In most cases, drug-dependent antibodies to platelet surface GPIb-IX have been identified in patients' sera.[41] The antibodies are drug dependent because they bind to the platelets only in the presence of quinine or quinidine. Presumably, the binding of the drugs to these platelet surface glycoproteins induces new antigenic sites on the proteins that are recognized by the antibodies.

The agent (quinidine or quinine) should be withdrawn in such cases. Neither corticosteroid therapy nor emergency splenectomy is of documented benefit in purpura induced by these agents. Plasmapheresis to remove the drug and antibodies would appear to be a logical treatment, but there are no systematic studies of its effectiveness. Transfused platelets are removed as rapidly as the recipient's own platelets. Treatment with prednisone and IVIg in a dose similar to that used in ITP is recommended. Platelet transfusion after IVIg infusion may be given to control life-threatening bleeding.

A quinine-induced thrombocytopenia that is closely followed by the development of HUS has been recognized. Quinine-dependent antibodies to platelets, as well as to endothelial cells, have been found in patients' sera.[42] Even the small amount of quinine in tonic water seems to be sufficient to trigger recurrent bouts of the syndrome. Other drugs that may occasionally produce drug-dependent thrombocytopenia include dipyridamole and trimethoprim-sulfamethoxazole.[43]

Heparin-induced thrombocytopenia Heparin-induced thrombocytopenia (HIT) is a frequent cause of drug-induced thrombocytopenia in hospitalized patients. Despite the presence of modest to moderate thrombocytopenia, HIT is rarely associated with bleeding but is associated with significant and sometimes fatal thrombosis [*see Chapter 99*].

Gold-induced thrombocytopenia Gold salt therapy for rheumatoid arthritis produces thrombocytopenia, which is sometimes severe, in 1% to 3% of patients. There are drug-induced autoantibodies that target platelet membrane GPV, but the presence of gold is not required for their reactivity.[44] Most patients respond to therapy with 60 mg of prednisone daily. IVIg is also efficacious.

Cocaine-associated thrombocytopenia An ITP-like syndrome has been reported in intravenous cocaine users. They have been shown to respond to an approach similar to that employed in patients with ITP.[45]

Thrombocytopenia caused by GPIIb-IIIa receptor antagonists Three parenteral GPIIb-IIIa antagonists—abciximab, eptifibatide , and tirofiban—have been approved for use in the treatment of acute coronary artery syndrome and as adjunctive therapy in coronary angioplasty. In contrast to the low platelet counts in other types of drug-induced thrombocytopenia, patients who have low platelet counts resulting from GPIIb-IIIa receptor antagonists can develop acute, often profound thrombocytopenia within a few hours after drug administration. In patients receiving abciximab, thrombocytopenia occurs in about 1% after the first exposure. After a second exposure, the incidence of thrombocytopenia rises to 4%.[46] The incidence of drug-induced thrombocytopenia associated with eptifibatide and tirofiban is probably also about 1% after first exposure.[47]

The abrupt development of severe thrombocytopenia in patients who have never been exposed to these drugs initially suggested that platelets were being destroyed by a nonimmune mechanism. However, accumulating evidence indicates that drug-dependent antibodies, which occur naturally, are the underlying cause. Preexisting anti–GPIIb-IIIa autoantibodies are present in these patients, and after the administration of the anti–GPIIb-IIIa antagonist, the binding of the drug to GPIIb-IIIa induces conformational changes in GPIIb-IIIa such that new epitopes are exposed that are recognized by the autoantibodies. These actions would explain the acute onset of profound thrombocytopenia.[47]

When thrombocytopenia develops (i.e., when platelet counts drop below 100,000/μl), the GPIIb-IIIa antagonist and any other potentially offending medications (e.g., heparin) should be discontinued immediately. Depending on the platelet count, it may not be advisable to discontinue antiplatelet agents such as aspirin or clopidogrel, because in such cases, patients are at high risk for acute coronary artery or stent thrombosis. If the platelet count drops below 10,000/μl, strong consideration should be given to platelet transfusion. In general, only one single-platelet transfusion is sufficient. There are anecdotal reports of acute coronary thrombosis associated with platelet transfusion in this setting when the platelet count climbs over 50,000/μl and the patient is off all antiplatelet agents. Thus, antiplatelet agents may need to be reinstituted. Because eptifibatide and tirofiban have very short half-lives and are cleared from the circulation within hours, the duration of thrombocytopenia is short, once the offending drugs have been discontinued. However, because abciximab has a much longer half-life—with inhibition of platelet function reported up to 1 week after drug discontinuance—thrombocytopenia can persist for 5 to 7 days. Platelet counts should be obtained in all patients before, as well as within 2 to 4 hours after, the initiation of an intravenous GPIIb-IIIa antagonist. It should be noted that a subgroup of patients develop delayed thrombocytopenia 5 to 8 days after abciximab administration. On the basis of limited published experience, it appears to be safe to administer eptifibatide or tirofiban to patients who are sensitive to abciximab, and vice versa.[47]

Thrombocytopenia caused by metabolites of naproxen and acetaminophen Five patients have experienced thrombocytopenia after taking naproxen and acetaminophen. In each case, antibodies that reacted with normal platelets in the presence of a known drug metabolite of naproxen or acetaminophen were

identified.[48] Therefore, the sensitizing agents are drug metabolites that formed in vivo.

ACCELERATED REMOVAL OF PLATELETS BY
NONIMMUNOLOGIC MECHANISMS

There are several nonimmunologic causes for thrombocytopenia. Blood vessel wall injury with increased thrombin generation and increased platelet activation and consumption occurs in several of these conditions.

Thrombotic Thrombocytopenic Purpura and Adult Hemolytic-Uremic Syndrome

TTP and HUS encompass a group of clinical syndromes characterized by widespread platelet-fibrin thrombi deposition in the small arteries and arterioles and capillaries. Thrombotic microangiopathy is a distinct feature of both TTP and HUS; however, the underlying pathogenetic processes in TTP and HUS may differ [see Pathogenesis, below]. Familial TTP/HUS is rare and usually occurs in the immediate postnatal period or infancy, although there are reported cases of delayed onset until the second to third decade of life. More frequently, TTP is either idiopathic or secondary to a variety of conditions [see Etiology, below].

Etiology TTP/HUS occurs spontaneously and is also associated with pregnancy, cancer, bone marrow transplantation, autoimmune diseases, and various drugs. In pregnancy, it resembles severe preeclampsia. In the postpartum period, the CNS manifestations may initially be confused with postpartum depression, with tragic results. Cases have been reported after a normal delivery and with abruptio placentae and preeclampsia.

Several drugs appear to cause TTP/HUS. These include chemotherapeutic drugs (e.g., mitomycin C, bleomycin, and cisplatin), immunosuppressive agents (e.g., cyclosporine and FK506), the antiplatelet agent ticlopidine, oral contraceptives, and quinine. Anecdotal cases of TTP/HUS associated with clopidogrel, which is related to ticlopidine, have also been reported.[49]

Pathogenesis There have been significant advances in the understanding of TTP, showing that the proper processing of von Willebrand factor (vWF) multimers plays a key role in its pathogenesis. vWF is an abundant plasma protein that mediates platelet adhesion to the subendothelium and serves as a carrier molecule for factor VIII [see Chapter 96]. vWF is synthesized by both megakaryocytes and endothelial cells. Monomers of vWF (280,000 daltons) are cross-linked by disulfide bonds to form vWF multimers, which are released into the circulation by endothelial cells and are stored within platelet α-granules and the Weibel-Palade bodies in endothelial cells. The stored vWF multimers can be released upon platelet or endothelial stimulation. These released vWF multimers are larger than plasma vWF multimers and are referred to as ultra-large vWF (ULvWF) multimers, with a molecular size up to 20 million daltons. Functionally, these are the most reactive vWF multimers. In 1982, ULvWF multimers were found in the plasma of patients with chronic relapsing TTP, giving rise to the hypothesis that TTP may result from the deficiency of a vWF-cleaving protease (depolymerase), which causes ULvWF multimers to circulate, contributing to the development of thrombosis.[50] This hypothesis has been proved largely correct with the identification of the vWF-cleaving protease and the demonstration that deficiency of the vWF-cleaving protease activity is associated with TTP.

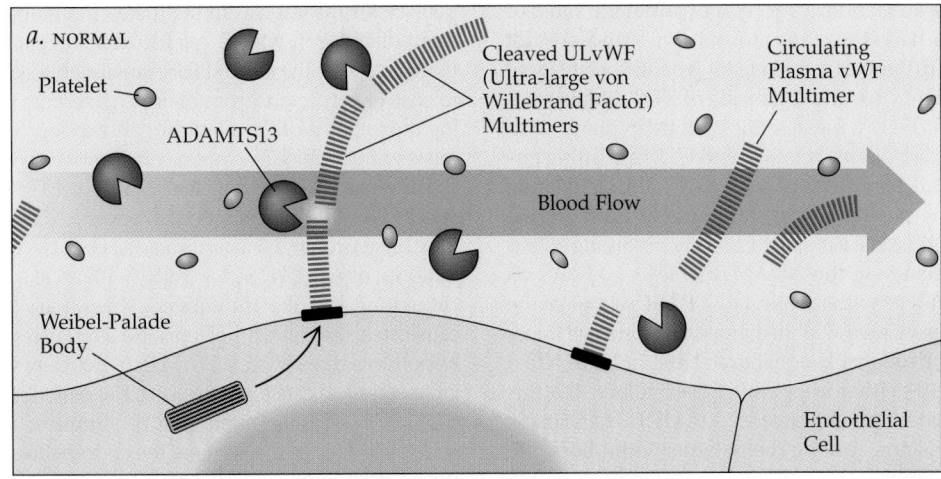

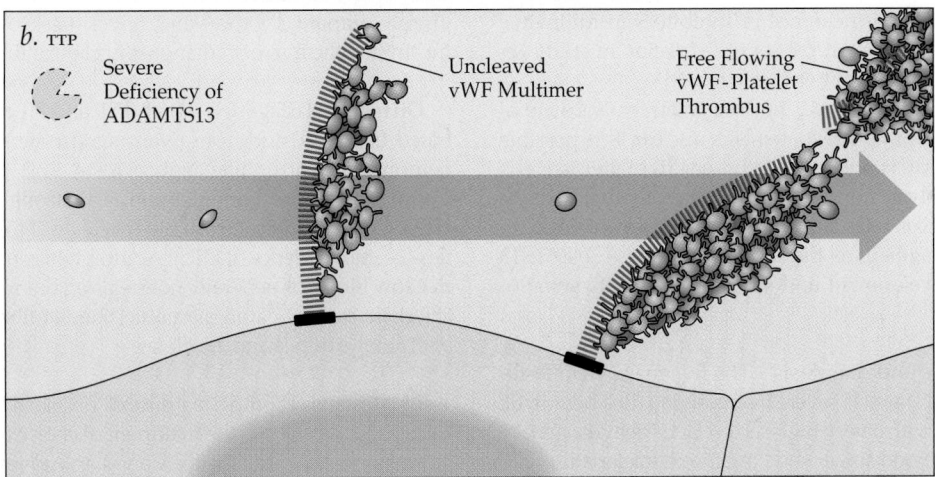

Figure 1 **ADAMTS13 activity in normal and thrombotic thrombocytopenia purpura plasma. (*a*) In normal persons, ADAMTS13 enzyme molecules from the plasma attach to and then cleave the unusually large von Willebrand factor (ULvWF) multimers that are secreted in long strings from stimulated endothelial cells. (*b*) In patients with thrombotic thrombocytopenic purpura (TTP), a deficiency of ADAMTS13 prevents the cleavage of ULvWF multimers secreted by endothelial cells. Platelets carried by flowing blood adhere to the uncleaved ULvWF multimers, resulting in the development of platelet thrombi.**

The vWF-cleaving protease has been identified as ADAMTS13 (a disintegrin-like and metalloprotease with thrombospondin type 1 motif 13).[51] It is a novel metalloprotease that cleaves vWF monomer at a specific site (842Tyr-843Met) in the A2 domain. Current data indicate that ULvWF multimers are secreted from stimulated endothelial cells as a long "string" anchored on the endothelial cell surface. Plasma ADAMTS13 may attach, under flowing conditions within the blood, to the cell surface–bound ULvWF multimers (via the A3 domain in the vWF monomer) and cleave them into the vWF multimers that are normally found in plasma.[52] Partial unfolding of the ULvWF multimers by shear stress forces in the blood presumably enhances the enzymatic cleavage process. Patients with familial TTP have hereditary deficiency of ADAMTS13,[53] whereas patients with acquired idiopathic TTP have antibodies that inhibit the ADAMTS13 activity.[54,55] In either case, the persistence of ULvWF multimers on the stimulated surface of the endothelial cell leads to the adhesion and subsequent aggregation of platelets, which in turn lead to the formation of platelet thrombi [*see Figure 1*]. (Presumably, platelets do not bind to the smaller plasma vWF multimers, be-

cause the platelet binding sites are not exposed in these vWF multimers). In addition to causing ischemic injury at the site of thrombi formation, it is likely that platelet thrombi resulting from aggregation of ULvWF multimers will break up and embolize downstream, resulting in further ischemic tissue damage.

The gene encoding ADAMTS13 is located on chromosome 9q34. More than 50 mutations in this gene have been identified in patients with familial TTP, most of which result in greatly reduced ADAMTS13 secretion in vitro.[51] In many cases of acquired idiopathic TTP, an IgG autoantibody against ADAMTS13 is produced transiently, leading to severe deficiency of ADAMTS13 activity. ULvWF multimers are detectable in the plasma in some patients during the acute episodes but not after recovery.[50]

Although the role of ADAMTS13 in the pathogenesis of TTP has been established, it appears that the majority of patients with HUS do not have severe ADAMTS13 deficiency, strongly suggesting that the pathogenesis of HUS is different.

ADAMTS13 as a screening assay The clinical utility of measuring ADAMTS13 is not established. In part, this is because there is no gold standard for its measurement; most of the current assays have long turnaround times and are not readily available. Furthermore, the sensitivity and specificity of ADAMTS13 deficiency for the diagnosis of TTP remains unclear. Decreased vWF-cleaving activity is found in many clinical conditions that are not associated with TTP, including cirrhosis, chronic renal insufficiency, ITP, DIC, SLE, leukemia, pregnancy, and the postoperative state; it is also associated with advancing age.[56,57] In a prospective study involving 37 patients, severe deficiency in the ADAMTS13 level (< 5%) was found in 80% of patients with idiopathic TTP but in none of the patients with TTP associated with hematopoietic stem cell transplantation, cancer, drugs, or pregnancy.[58] Thus, acquired TTP may be considered as either idiopathic or secondary; the former is generally associated with severe ADAMTS13 deficiency, whereas the latter is not. Among the patients with idiopathic TTP and severe ADAMTS13 deficiency, 44% had inhibitors. Other studies found an incidence of inhibitors in idiopathic TTP of 65% to 95%; however, part of the variation in study results may have to do with patient selection.[59,60]

The reason why an inhibitor is not detectable in a substantial number of the idiopathic TTP patients is unclear. It is possible that the current assay is not sufficiently sensitive; alternatively, the assay may involve a nonneutralizing antibody that binds to ADAMTS13 and accelerates its clearance. New assays using a recombinant vWF fragment as the substrate for the ADAMTS13 protease are in development and should help clarify some of these issues.[61,62]

Clinical features and diagnosis   The five major manifestations (pentad) of TTP are (1) severe microangiopathic hemolytic anemia associated with a very high serum lactic dehydrogenase (LDH) level and a blood smear showing the characteristic schistocytes and helmet cells; (2) moderate to severe thrombocytopenia with increased marrow megakaryocytes, which indicates intravascular platelet activation and consumption; (3) fever, which is occasionally quite high; (4) CNS signs and symptoms that can be quite mild initially with transient agitation, headache, and disorientation but that can sometimes progress explosively to hemiparesis, aphasia, seizures, focal deficits, coma, and death; and (5) renal disease, which is usually mild and produces moderate elevations of serum creatinine and urinary protein levels. It should be emphasized that many patients do not present with all these signs and symptoms. Patients with familial TTP/HUS typically exhibit a chronic relapsing course.

The adult form of HUS has features similar to those of TTP, although the pathophysiology may not be identical [see Pathogenesis, above]. Common features of TTP and HUS include microangiopathic hemolytic anemia, thrombocytopenia, and the presence of platelet fibrin thrombi in the small vessels. Renal involvement is uniformly severe in HUS, whereas CNS disease is less prominent than in TTP. There is a distinct form of HUS that occurs in children after gastrointestinal infection with *Escherichia coli*, usually serotype 0157:H7. These patients present with bloody diarrhea and hemorrhagic colitis. *E. coli* 0157:H7 or other strains elaborate verotoxins (also called Shiga toxins) that bind to specific receptors on the endothelial surface, causing cell damage and even cell death.[63] Verotoxin-1 (VT-1) can induce the upregulation of various prothrombotic and proinflammatory adhesive molecules on endothelial cells.[64] The microvascular endothelial cells are particularly susceptible because they have a high expression of VT-1 receptors, which may explain the propensity for thrombosis in the microcirculation. Antibiotic treatment of children with *E. coli* 0157:H7 infection increases rather than decreases the risk of HUS, presumably because it causes the release of verotoxins from injured bacteria in the intestine, making the toxins more available for absorption. Thus, routine treatment with antibiotics is not recommended.[65]

Whereas a severe deficiency of ADAMTS13 (< 5%) may be specific for TTP,[66] patients with severe ADAMTS13 deficiency may have prolonged asymptomatic periods. It is becoming clear that loss of ADAMTS13 activity, with an associated increase in circulating ULvWF multimers, is necessary but insufficient to cause an acute clinical TTP episode. The current data support the hypothesis that severe ADAMTS13 deficiency, be it from familial or acquired cause, predisposes the patient to thrombosis, and a second vascular inflammatory stimulus, such as infection, surgery, or pregnancy, causes the endothelium to increase its release of the stored UlvWF multimers, which, in the setting of grossly impaired processing, gives rise to ULvWF platelet thrombi in the microcirculation and clinical thrombosis.

Differential diagnosis   Both TTP and HUS must be differentiated from SLE and from Evans syndrome. Microangiopathic hemolysis, neutrophilic leukocytosis, and a negative direct Coombs test (direct antiglobulin test) strongly suggest TTP or HUS. Coagulation tests usually reveal no significant abnormalities (i.e., no evidence of DIC); serum LDH is usually elevated. A marrow biopsy is generally not required but may show the characteristic, but not pathognomonic, platelet-fibrin hyaline thrombi in small arteries and arterioles.

Treatment   Prompt institution of plasma exchange with fresh frozen plasma is the treatment of choice for TTP/HUS. In a large randomized trial by the Canadian Apheresis Group, intensive plasma exchange was more effective than plasma infusion in terms of patient survival (78% versus 63%).[67] In that study, 1.5 times the calculated plasma volume was removed and replaced with fresh frozen plasma during each of the first 3 days of therapy; subsequently, one single-volume exchange a day was performed for a minimum of 7 days. Some investigators obtained good results with a daily single-volume exchange instead of a 1.5-volume exchange.[68] It is reasonable to start with a daily single-volume exchange if the patient is clinically relatively stable, with moderate thrombocytopenia and no significant neurologic impairment. However, if the clinical situation worsens, more intensive double-volume plasma exchange (5,000 to 6,000 ml/day, or approximately 80 ml/kg/day) is indicated. Because vWF multimers are present in cryoprecipitate, cryosupernatant (i.e., fresh frozen plasma from which cryoprecipitate has been removed) can be substituted as replacement fluid when a patient is not responding to routine plasma exchange. One uncontrolled study showed increased benefit from this preparation as compared with fresh frozen plasma.[69] Once therapeutic benefit has been achieved (as measured by restoration of normal CNS function, by rising platelet counts, and by falling LDH levels), the intensity and frequency of plasma exchange can be reduced to single-volume exchanges, first three times weekly and then twice weekly.

Although the importance of prompt plasma exchange has been established, the use of corticosteroids,[70] aspirin, and dipyridamole has not been tested in prospective clinical trials. With the observation of autoantibody against ADAMTS13 as a significant cause of acquired idiopathic TTP, rituximab (375 mg/m²

I.V. once weekly for 4 weeks) has been tried and reported to be effective, although the overall experience is still limited.[71-73] Because pheresis tends to lower the platelet count in a patient who is already thrombocytopenic, the problem of platelet transfusion arises. Some investigators have observed that platelet infusion may lead to exacerbation of TTP,[74] whereas others use platelet transfusions as required.

In the previously described prospective study of patients with severe deficiency in ADAMTS13 activity (see above), plasma exchange proved to be a useful therapy; among the patients with idiopathic TTP and severe ADAMTS13 deficiency without detectable inhibitors, the majority responded to plasma exchange with complete remission and a rise in the ADAMTS13 level.[58] However, in patients with mild ADAMTS13 deficiency and high inhibitor levels, plasma exchange was not effective in reducing the inhibitor titer or in increasing the ADAMTS13 activity. Nevertheless, some of these patients had a favorable clinical response, including resolution of thrombocytopenia and cessation of hemodialysis. Among the patients whose TTP was not idiopathic, response to plasma exchange was variable. Of note, mortality in patients with idiopathic TTP with severe ADAMTS13 deficiency has been shown to be 15% to 20%, whereas mortality in patients with nonidiopathic TTP has been much higher, at 55% to 60%.[58,60] Many of the patients in the latter group have had serious underlying disease and comorbidities, such as hematopoietic stem cell transplantation, which likely has contributed to the high mortality.

Management of acute TTP should therefore depend on the clinical manifestations and course of the disease.[75] In all cases, plasma exchange is first-line therapy. Patients who respond promptly and completely to plasma exchange—which most likely will be those patients with idiopathic TTP and very low or nondetectable levels of inhibitors—may not need any further treatment. For patients who show a suboptimal response—such as an initial rise in platelet counts or a recurrence in thrombocytopenia when the plasma exchange treatments are decreased—glucocorticoid is indicated. For patients who experience a more aggressive course (e.g., those with severe neurologic abnormalities or those who do not respond to the initial plasma exchange with or without steroid therapy), more intensive immunosuppressive therapies, such as rituximab, should be considered.

Microangiopathy may persist for weeks or months after all other evidence of disease has subsided. In a large follow-up study of TTP patients, about one third of patients who entered remission had a relapse over a 10-year period.[76] The risk of recurrence is largely restricted to patients with severe ADAMTS13 deficiency—primarily, patients with idiopathic TTP. Relapse seldom occurs in patients who have TTP in association with hematopoietic stem cell transplantation or drugs. Conflicting data have been reported regarding patients who have had relapses after TTP associated with pregnancy.

Most experts treat adult HUS in a manner similar to that for TTP. However, the response to plasma exchange appears to be less favorable in HUS than in TTP, which may be consistent with the finding that the ADAMTS13 level is generally not diminished in HUS.

Thrombocytopenia Induced by Infection

Severe viral, bacterial, fungal, and parasitic infections can produce DIC and, consequently, thrombocytopenia [see Chapter 99]; however, mechanisms other than DIC may also cause infection-associated thrombocytopenia.

Viral infections Viral infections such as dengue fever and congenital rubella can directly damage the megakaryocytes. Varicella can cause a form of thrombocytopenia that has the characteristics of an immune reaction: increased numbers of megakaryocytes, no evidence of DIC, and the presence of PA-IgG. Usually, no therapy is required. The acute thrombocytopenia in infectious mononucleosis is probably immune mediated, as shown by the increase in marrow megakaryocytes and the favorable response to corticosteroids.

Bacterial septicemia Patients who have severe gram-negative septicemia and platelet counts lower than 50,000/μl usually have evidence of DIC. However, many patients who have both gram-negative and gram-positive septicemia and platelet counts between 50,000 and 150,000/μl have no signs of DIC. The PA-IgG levels are often elevated, which may represent immune complexes deposited on the platelet surface rather than antiplatelet autoantibodies. The key to controlling the thrombocytopenia is establishing appropriate therapy for the infection. If DIC is present, it should be managed with careful control of hypotension and blood volume.

Protozoan infection Thrombocytopenia is common in malaria, although DIC is rare. Platelet survival is short, and elevated PA-IgG has been found to be elevated. The IgG antibody appears to bind to malarial antigens adsorbed to the platelet surface.[77]

Thrombocytopenia during Pregnancy and Peripartum Period

Mild thrombocytopenia, with platelet counts generally in the range of 110,000 to 150,000/μl and seldom below 70,000/μl, occurs in 5% to 8% of pregnant women (gestational thrombocytopenia). It has no clinical significance, but it must be distinguished from ITP, pregnancy-associated TTP, and preeclampsia.

In addition to having hypertension, proteinuria, and evidence of pathologic changes in the kidneys, liver, CNS, and placenta, approximately 15% of patients with preeclampsia have moderate thrombocytopenia. Only a minority of patients with preeclampsia and thrombocytopenia demonstrate laboratory evidence of DIC. The megakaryocyte number is increased, and platelet survival is somewhat shortened. Some patients with preeclampsia and thrombocytopenia also have microangiopathic hemolysis, which suggests that damaged vessels containing fibrin strands are destroying red blood cells and platelets. Intense vasospasm that causes endothelial damage and leads to platelet activation, adherence, and destruction may also play a role. The clinical picture may be indistinguishable from TTP, in which case it should be managed as TTP. Otherwise, management consists of prenatal care for preeclampsia and efforts to detect thrombocytopenia as early as possible.

HELLP syndrome The HELLP syndrome refers to a disorder that occurs during pregnancy and is characterized by hemolysis, elevated levels of liver enzymes, and a low platelet count. It probably represents an extremely severe form of preeclampsia. At some point between the 23rd and 39th week of pregnancy, affected patients present with thrombocytopenia marked by a platelet count of less than 100,000/μl, microangiopathic hemolysis, abnormal liver function test results, and, occasionally, hypertension.[78] The results of the standard coagulation tests for DIC are normal, although there may be some elevation in the level of fibrin degradation products. Patients with the HELLP syndrome are often severely ill, with circulatory, respiratory, and renal failure; postpartum hemorrhage; intrahepatic hemorrhage; and seizures.

The differential diagnosis includes acute fatty liver of pregnancy and TTP/HUS. In acute liver of pregnancy, patients have a prolonged PT and aPTT and low fibrinogen levels; hypertension and proteinuria are usually absent. In TTP/HUS, the liver enzymes are normal or only mildly elevated.

HELLP is treated by terminating the pregnancy, usually by delivery, and by providing meticulous supportive care. In a large series of patients with HELLP, the nadir of thrombocytopenia occurred 1 to 2 days after delivery.[79] It may also develop for the first time within 24 to 48 hours post partum.[80] Treatment of HELLP remains controversial, but corticosteroids appear to be beneficial.[81] Persistent thrombocytopenia with microangiopathy or the presence of organ failure suggests postpartum TTP/HUS; in such patients, plasma exchange therapy should be considered.

Platelet Washout and Vascular Bed Abnormalities

Patients who have brisk bleeding during surgery and who require massive transfusions (e.g., 10 units of packed red cells and multiple units of fresh frozen plasma) frequently develop nonimmune thrombocytopenia. If the platelet level falls below 100,000/μl and the patient is undergoing surgery or another hemostatic challenge, platelets should be administered. Platelets may also be removed by an abnormal vascular bed. In giant hemangiomas, there is sluggish blood flow through improperly endothelialized channels. These surfaces may produce low-grade DIC.

Platelet Sequestration

Another major mechanism of thrombocytopenia is platelet sequestration. Platelet counts of 40,000 to 80,000/μl are common in patients with marked splenomegaly. Clinically significant hemorrhage rarely occurs unless a coexistent hemorrhagic disorder is present. Management is directed toward the primary disease. Splenectomy is rarely necessary.

Platelet Function Disorders

The clue to the existence of a platelet function defect is the finding of clinical hemorrhage in the presence of a prolonged bleeding time and a platelet count higher than 100,000/μl. Petechiae are rare. Platelet morphology and tests of platelet function may be abnormal [see Table 4].

HEREDITARY ABNORMALITIES OF PLATELET FUNCTION

Platelet Membrane Disorders

Bernard-Soulier syndrome is a rare autosomal recessive disease that is characterized by giant platelets, a prolonged bleeding time, moderate thrombocytopenia, and risk of fatal hemorrhage. The defect, which is an absence of the platelet GPIb-IX-V complex (the major vWF binding site of the platelet), causes impaired platelet adhesion to wound surfaces. Ristocetin-induced platelet agglutination is abnormal and is not corrected by the addition of normal plasma containing vWF. Acute hemorrhage is treated by platelet transfusions.

Glanzmann thrombasthenia is a rare autosomal recessive disorder in which platelet morphology and the platelet count are normal but the bleeding time is prolonged. Because the critically

important GPIIb-IIIa complex that forms the platelet binding site for fibrinogen is absent, the platelets do not undergo aggregation after stimulation by ADP, thrombin, or collagen. Ristocetin-induced agglutination, however, is normal. Treatment consists of platelet transfusions when necessary.

Platelet Granule Disorders

Patients with the gray platelet syndrome, a rare disorder, have mucosal bleeding, ecchymoses, and petechiae. Moderate thrombocytopenia is present, and the bleeding time is prolonged. The platelets are larger than normal and appear agranular because of the absence of α-granules. Because the α-granule contents are severely reduced, platelet adhesion and platelet-supported coagulation are deficient. Platelet aggregation with collagen is abnormal. Bleeding episodes should be treated by infusion of normal platelets.

Another rare disorder, the dense granule deficiency syndrome, is characterized by mucosal bleeding associated with a normal platelet count, normal platelet morphology, and variable prolongation of the bleeding time. Platelet aggregation with ADP and collagen are abnormal. The decrease in the dense granular contents of ADP impairs ADP-mediated events. Hemorrhage is treated by platelet transfusion.

1-Desamino-8-D-arginine vasopressin (DDAVP, or desmopressin) is an alternative therapy for patients with primary platelet disorders that require surgery.

ACQUIRED ABNORMALITIES OF PLATELET FUNCTION

Myeloproliferative Diseases and Associated Platelet Abnormalities

Platelet function abnormalities occur in the myeloproliferative diseases: chronic myeloid leukemia, polycythemia vera, essential thrombocythemia, and acute leukemia. The platelet count in chronic myeloproliferative disorders is often very high, but the bleeding time may be prolonged, and clinical bleeding may appear as mucosal hemorrhage and hematomas. The abnormality resembles an acquired storage-pool defect. Megakaryocytes often are abnormal with separated nuclei; the peripheral blood platelets are large and may be degranulated. Management of acute hemorrhage consists of transfusion of normal platelets to bring the level of normal platelets up to 50,000/μl. Aspirin and other NSAIDs should be avoided.

Uremia and Associated Platelet Abnormalities

A prolonged bleeding time associated with clinical bleeding despite a normal platelet count has been well documented in uremia. Uremic platelet dysfunction is presumably caused, in part, by several dialyzable uremic toxins, including phenolic acids and guanidinosuccinic acid.[82] DDAVP (0.3 μg/kg in 50 ml of saline over a 30-minute period) is effective in controlling uremic bleeding for about 4 to 6 hours. DDAVP infusion produces an increase in plasma vWF activity, particularly among the larger multimers of vWF, which may enhance platelet adhesion.

The hematocrit should be maintained above 30% in bleeding uremic patients because the bleeding time is prolonged when the hematocrit falls below 26%.[83] Bleeding may also be controlled by the use of conjugated estrogens. Conjugated estrogen (Premarin) given orally (50 mg/day) or intravenously (0.6 mg/kg/day) for 4 to 5 days shortens the bleeding time by approximately 50% for about 2 weeks.[84] The advantage of conjugated estrogens over DDAVP is the longer duration of their benefi-

Table 4   Classification of Platelet Function Disorders

Type	Characteristic	Cause
Congenital	Membrane abnormalities	Bernard-Soulier disease (GPIb-IX-V defect, impaired adhesion); Glanzmann thrombasthenia (GPIIb-IIIa defect, impaired aggregation)
	Granule abnormalities	Gray platelet syndrome (absent or impaired α-granule release, impaired aggregation); dense granule deficiency (absent or impaired dense granule release, impaired aggregation)
	Deficiency of a plasma factor	von Willebrand disease (deficiency or abnormality of von Willebrand factor, impaired adhesion); afibrinogenemia (deficiency of fibrinogen, impaired aggregation)
Acquired	Production of abnormal platelets	Myeloproliferative disease (essential thrombocytopenia, chronic myelogenous leukemia, polycythemia vera, myelofibrosis, acute myelogenous leukemia); myelodysplasia
	Dysfunction of normal platelets	Systemic disease (uremia, liver disease, paraproteinemias, disseminated intravascular coagulation); drugs (aspirin and other nonsteroidal anti-inflammatory drugs, ticlopidine, clopidogrel, GPIIb-IIIa antagonists, dextran, antibiotics [penicillin, carbenicillin, moxalactam], psychotropic drugs)

cial effect on platelet function, but they have a more delayed onset of action. The two drugs can be used concomitantly.

Patients with end-stage renal disease have complex hemostatic disorders. Despite decreased platelet function (caused by uremic toxins present in the circulating blood), thrombosis of vascular access shunt commonly occurs in patients with end-stage renal failure who are on hemodialysis. Hemostatic parameters suggestive of a hypercoagulable state, such as increased plasma fibrinogen and factor VIII levels, have been described.[82]

Effects of Macroglobulinemia and Other Dysproteinemias on Platelet Function

The presence of high concentrations of viscous proteins produces complicated effects on the entire hemostatic mechanism. The proteins appear to coat platelets and interfere with adhesion and perhaps with aggregation. Management is directed at the primary disease, but if hyperviscosity and bleeding are significant, prompt plasmapheresis may be required to lower the level of abnormal protein and to correct the bleeding disorder.

Drug-Induced Platelet Disorders

Aspirin and other nonsteroidal anti-inflammatory drugs In normal persons, ingestion of 0.6 g of aspirin prolongs the template bleeding time by 2 to 3 minutes. The platelets are irreversibly affected. Thromboxane A_2 (TXA_2) is a potent inducer of platelet release and aggregation [*see Chapter 96*]. Aspirin acetylates and irreversibly inhibits cyclooxygenase-1 (COX-1) and blocks the subsequent generation of thromboxane. Some apparently normal persons display marked sensitivity to the action of aspirin, so that their bleeding times are very much prolonged and they have clinically significant bleeding, particularly during or after surgery or trauma. These patients may have a mild form of von Willebrand disease or storage-pool disease, and their mild bleeding diathesis becomes exacerbated by aspirin's antiplatelet effect.

Uremic patients are especially sensitive to bleeding induced by aspirin. A small dose of aspirin does not prolong the bleeding time of normal persons, but in uremic patients, it produces a significant prolongation, often as much as 15 minutes. The combination of alcohol and aspirin is also dangerous because of aspirin's ability to prolong the bleeding time.

Aspirin-induced bleeding is diagnosed by determining the existence of an acquired platelet function defect (a platelet count above 100,000/μl, abnormal platelet aggregation test results, and no prior bleeding history) and finding evidence of aspirin ingestion. Because approximately 300 compounds on the market contain aspirin, a negative history should be supplemented either by determining a serum salicylate level or by detecting an abnormal collagen aggregation pattern that reverts to normal in 7 days (the typical pattern of aspirin ingestion).

If bleeding is significant, it can be managed by platelet transfusion. Because inhibition of platelet COX-1 by aspirin is irreversible, the hemostatic compromise may last for 4 to 5 days after the aspirin has been discontinued. If the patient needs analgesia, acetaminophen or codeine can be used because neither affects platelet function.

Alcohol In addition to producing thrombocytopenia by suppressing platelet production, alcohol consumption can cause platelet function defects.[85] In vitro studies have shown that alcohol impairs platelet aggregation and TXA_2 release. Platelet function returns to normal after 2 to 3 weeks of abstinence.

Antibiotics Carbenicillin and ticarcillin can inhibit platelet aggregation and contribute to a bleeding disorder, as can massive doses of penicillin. Massive doses of penicillin impair collagen-induced and ristocetin-induced platelet aggregation. Moxalactam, a third-generation cephalosporin, also causes a platelet function disorder. The clinical situation is most important when an acquired platelet function defect develops in a pancytopenic patient being treated for septicemia. Changing the antibiotics usually corrects this problem.

Miscellaneous agents A wide variety of other agents can modify platelet function [*see Table 5*].[86]

Thrombocytosis and Thrombocythemia

DIAGNOSIS

A platelet count higher than 500,000/μl is referred to as reactive thrombocytosis. In reactive thrombocytosis, tests of platelet function (including platelet aggregation studies) are generally normal, and patients do not experience an increased incidence of hemorrhage or thromboembolism even when the platelet count exceeds 1 million/μl.

Elevated platelet counts (often, 1 million to 3 million/μl or more) also occur in chronic myeloid leukemia, agnogenic myeloid metaplasia with myelofibrosis, polycythemia vera, and essential thrombocythemia. In the diagnosis of essential

Table 5   Selected Platelet-Modifying Agents[98]

Anesthetics	Temocillin	Chinese black tree fungus	Tolmetin
General	Ticarcillin	Cloves	Oncologic drugs
Halothane	Antibiotics (other)	Cumin	BCNU
Local	Nitrofurantoin	Ethanol	Daunorubicin
Butacaine	Anticoagulants	Omega-3 fatty acids	Mithramycin
Cocaine	Heparin	Onion extract	Plasma expanders
Cyclaine	Antihistamines	Turmeric	Dextrans
Dibucaine	Chlorpheniramine	Glycoprotein IIb-IIIa	Hydroxyethyl starch
Procaine	Diphenhydramine	antagonists	Psychotropic drugs
Tetracaine	Mepyramine	Abciximab	Phenothiazines
Antibiotics (β-lactam)	Cardiovascular drugs	Eptifibatide	Chlorpromazine
Cephalosporins	Diltiazem	Lamifiban	Promethazine
Cefazolin	Isosorbide dinitrate	Tirofiban	Trifluoperazine
Cefotaxime	Nifedipine	Narcotics	Tricyclic antidepressants
Cefoxitin	Nitroglycerin	Heroin	Amitriptyline
Cephalothin	Nitroprusside	Nonsteroidal anti-inflammatory	Imipramine
Moxalactam	Propranolol	drugs	Nortriptyline
Penicillins	Quinidine	Aspirin*	Miscellaneous agents
Ampicillin	Verapamil	Diflunisal	Clofibrate
Apalcillin	Drugs that increase platelet	Ibuprofen	Clopidogrel
Azlocillin	cAMP concentration	Indomethacin	Ketanserin
Carbenicillin	Dipyridamole*	Meclofenamic acid	Radiographic contrast
Methicillin	Iloprost	Mefenamic acid	agents
Mezlocillin	Prostacyclin	Naproxen	Conray-60
Nafcillin	Fibrinolytic agents	Phenylbutazone	Renografin-76
Penicillin G	Foods and food additives	Piroxicam	Renovist II
Piperacillin	Ajoene	Sulfinpyrazone*	Ticlopidine*
Sulbenicillin		Sulindac	

*Used as a therapeutic antithrombotic agent.
BCNU— bischloronitrosourea (carmustine)   cAMP—cyclic adenosine monophosphate

thrombocythemia, the platelet count is higher than 600,000/μl and other causes of thrombocytosis (e.g., another myeloproliferative disorder or reactive thrombocytosis) have been excluded. A gain-of-function mutation in tyrosine Janus kinase–2 (JAK2) has been found in many patients with myeloproliferative disorders; it is found in about 80% of patients with polycythemia vera and in about 25% to 50% of patients with essential thrombocythemia.[87-89] In myeloproliferative disorders, test results of platelet function are frequently abnormal [see Platelet Function Disorders, above]. Some patients with myeloproliferative disorders seem to show an enhanced propensity for hemorrhage and thromboembolism. Neither platelet number nor measurements of platelet function predict the degree of thrombosis or hemorrhage.

Clinically, the hemorrhagic signs include mucosal, particularly gastrointestinal, bleeding; hematomas; and ecchymoses. There may be splenic vein thrombosis, portal or mesenteric vein thrombosis, and recurrent deep vein thrombosis with or without pulmonary embolism. Arterial thrombosis is less common.

TREATMENT

Patients with essential thrombocythemia and polycythemia vera may have debilitating erythromelalgia (burning and itching of the fingers and toes) that can progress to ischemic acrocyanosis.[90] This symptom complex appears to be caused by occlusion and inflammation of arterioles by platelet aggregates. Aspirin or indomethacin produces relief within hours. Aspirin given at a dosage of 325 mg daily can produce lasting benefit.

Hemorrhage and thrombosis are uncommon events even with platelet counts of 1 million/μl. In a patient with essential thrombocythemia who has clinically significant hemorrhage or thrombosis, good control of the platelet count can be achieved with oral hydroxyurea (15 mg/kg/day), with adjustments in the dosage as needed to lower the platelet count. Hydroxyurea therapy requires careful monitoring of the blood count; thus far, hydroxyurea therapy does not appear to increase the risk of a second malignant disorder. Newer therapies for thrombocythemia include the use of anagrelide, a powerful platelet-lowering agent.[91] A prospective, randomized trial comparing hydroxyurea with anagrelide showed that although the two agents were equally efficacious in long-term control of the platelet count, anagrelide was associated with an increased risk of arterial thrombosis (mostly transient ischemic attacks) and serious hemorrhage.[92] Thus, hydroxyurea (0.5 to 2.0 g daily to maintain the platelet count at less than 400,000/μl) plus low-dose aspirin (81 mg daily) should be the first-line therapy for patients with essential thrombocythemia who are considered at high risk for vascular events.

Vascular Purpuras

Vascular purpuras are a heterogeneous group of disorders [see Table 6] that are characterized by cutaneous hemorrhage and are occasionally associated with mucosal bleeding. The leakage occurs from terminal arterioles, capillaries, and postcapillary venules. The results of tests of platelet number and function and tests of procoagulant function are normal.

HEREDITARY HEMORRHAGIC TELANGIECTASIA

Hereditary hemorrhagic telangiectasia (HHT) is transmitted as an autosomal dominant disease and has an estimated incidence of one in 5,000 to 8,000 persons.[93] Linkage analyses have identified at least three HHT loci, including the genes for endoglin and activinlike receptor kinase. Both proteins are expressed on vascular endothelial cells and may function as receptors for transforming growth factor–β (TGF-β). TGF-β plays a complex role in coordinating responses between endothelial cells and the extracellular matrix. A mutation in the gene for either endoglin or activinlike receptor kinase results in a 50% reduction in the normal quantity of protein on endothelial cells (haploinsufficiency) and leads to the development of abnormal blood vessels and arteriovenous malformations (AVMs).[94]

HHT generally does not present at birth but manifests itself with age. Recurrent epistaxis is typically the earliest sign of disease, commonly occurring in childhood. Pulmonary AVMs, occurring in about 30% of HHT patients, become apparent after puberty and may present as dyspnea, chest pain, and hemoptysis. Physical examination may reveal chest bruits and digital clubbing. Mucocutaneous telangiectasias, which occur in the majority of patients and at characteristic sites (e.g., lips, oral cavity, fingers, and nose), typically become noticeable by the third decade of life and increase in size and number as the patient ages. The diagnosis of HHT should be based on four criteria: (1) spontaneous and recurrent epistaxis, (2) multiple mucocutaneous telangiectasias, (3) evidence of visceral telangiectasias and AVMs (e.g., gastrointestinal tract, pulmonary, hepatic, or cerebral AVMs), and (4) a positive family history of HHT.

Coagulation test results are generally normal. The pulmonary AVMs may be associated with hypoxemia and secondary polycythemia. The diagnosis can be confirmed by pulmonary angiography. If the shunts are large and clinically significant, they can be treated by balloon embolotherapy.[95] Paradoxical embolus with stroke can occur in patients with HHT who have pulmonary arteriovenous shunts and malformations. It has been advocated that asymptomatic HHT patients be screened for AVMs and be treated prophylactically with embolotherapy if AVMs are found.[96] Management of recurrent epistaxis should be conservative and often involves devising methods for obtaining nasal tamponade. Cauterization should be avoided because damage to nasal mucosa may result in vascular regrowth. Gas-

trointestinal bleeding is managed by the use of iron preparations when possible.

ACQUIRED DISORDERS OF BLOOD VESSELS THAT CAUSE BLEEDING

Scurvy

Vitamin C is required for the normal metabolism of collagen, folate, and perhaps iron. The patient with scurvy suffers primarily from impaired collagen synthesis. The lack of proper collagen support for the microvasculature leads to perifollicular hemorrhages, bleeding gums, and even deep tissue hematomas. Presumably, similar collagen defects lead to the so-called corkscrew hair and hyperkeratosis associated with this disorder.[97] The characteristic clinical picture in a malnourished person suggests the diagnosis. Plasma or buffy coat levels of ascorbic acid are low, and other vitamin deficiencies are usually present. Effective therapy consists of 1 g of ascorbic acid daily in divided doses.

Glucocorticoid Excess

Glucocorticoid excess, whether from endogenous or exogenous causes, produces cutaneous hemorrhages, probably because of glucocorticoid-induced catabolism of protein in vascular supportive tissues.

Amyloidosis

Amyloidosis can present as subcutaneous ecchymoses that have a predilection for the neck and upper chest. Biopsy of the site shows the amyloid, which by its infiltration may weaken the vessel walls or interfere with surface activation of platelets, procoagulants, or both. In patients with primary systemic amyloidosis, especially when accompanied by a huge amyloid spleen, the amyloid can in some instances adsorb enough factor X to cause profound factor X deficiency and clinical bleeding. Infusions of fresh frozen plasma are usually ineffective. Recombinant factor VIIa is effective, but it is extremely expensive and provides only temporary benefit. Splenectomy may provide long-term benefit and should be considered in a patient with recurrent serious clinical bleeding.

Immunoglobulin Disorders

The purpuric lesions in patients with immunoglubulin disorders (e.g., cryoglobulinemia, Waldenström macroglobulinemia, Henoch-Schönlein purpura, and multiple myeloma) may be raised (palpable purpura). On biopsy, these lesions may show mast cell degranulation and, when stained appropriately, immune complex deposition. Presumably, the immune complexes provide the chemotactic stimulation that leads to the congregation of neutrophils. Damage to the microvasculature is caused by the complement attack complex and by the release of the contents of the neutrophil granules. This inflammatory component produces the palpable purpura.

Damage to the Microvasculature Due to Emboli

DIC and TTP can cause localized vaso-occlusions leading to microvascular damage and leakage of red blood cells. Similar damage can be caused by emboli that arise from infected heart valves. Fat embolism may complicate fractures of the long bones and pelvis. The syndrome consists of fever; confusion; and petechiae, purpura, or both over the neck, chest, face, and axillae. Cholesterol embolism can also cause petechiae, usually over the lower extremities. It typically occurs in a patient with severe ath-

Table 6 Vascular Purpuras

Congenital disorders	Hereditary hemorrhagic telangiectasia
	Hereditary connective tissue disorders
	  Ehlers-Danlos syndrome
	  Marfan syndrome
	  Pseudoxanthoma elasticum

Acquired disorders	Scurvy
	Amyloidosis
	Glucocorticoid excess
	Immunoglobulin disorders
	Waldenström macroglobulinemia
	  Cryoglobulinemia
	  Hepatitis B
	  Henoch-Schönlein purpura
	Embolism (i.e., microvascular damage from septic and bland emboli from heart valves, fat embolism, and cholesterol embolism)
	Senile purpura

z
z

eroslerosis who has recently undergone an invasive procedure involving the abdominal aorta or renal arteries. Biopsy of the purpura shows cholesterol crystals when an appropriate stain is used.

The author has no commercial relationships with manufacturers of products or providers of services discussed in this chapter.

References

1. Ginsburg D: Molecular genetics of von Willebrand disease. Thromb Haemost 82:585, 1999

2. George JN, el-Harake MA, Raskob GE: Chronic idiopathic thrombocytopenic purpura. N Engl J Med 331:1207, 1994

3. Hirsh J, Dalen JE, Anderson DR, et al: Oral anticoagulants: mechanism of action, clinical effectiveness, and optimal therapeutic range. Chest 114:445S, 1998

4. Gewirtz AM, Hoffman R: Transitory hypomegakaryocytic thrombocytopenia: aetiological association with ethanol abuse and implications regarding regulation of human megakaryocytopoiesis. Br J Haematol 62:333, 1986

5. Tepler I, Elias L, Smith JW II, et al: A randomized placebo-controlled trial of recombinant human interleukin-11 in cancer patients with severe thrombocytopenia due to chemotherapy. Blood 87:3607, 1996

6. Kuter DJ, Begley CG: Recombinant human thrombopoietin: basic biology and evaluation of clinical studies. Blood 100:3457, 2002

7. Peck-Radosavljevic M, Wichlas M, Zacherl J, et al: Thrombopoietin induces rapid resolution of thrombocytopenia after orthotopic liver transplantation through increased platelet production. Blood 95:795, 2000

8. Frederiksen H, Schmidt K: The incidence of idiopathic thrombocytopenic purpura in adults increases with age. Blood 94:909, 1999

9. Cines DB, McMillan R: Management of adult idiopathic thrombocytopenic purpura. Annu Rev Med 56:425, 2005

10. Hofbauer LC, Heufelder AE: Coagulation disorders in thyroid diseases. Eur J Endocrinol 136:1, 1997

11. Stasi R, Stipa E, Masi M, et al: Prevalence and clinical significance of elevated antiphospholipid antibodies in patients with idiopathic thrombocytopenic purpura. Blood 84:4203, 1994

12. Chan H, Moore JC, Finch CN, et al: The IgG subclasses of platelet-associated autoantibodies directed against platelet glycoproteins IIb/IIIa in patients with idiopathic thrombocytopenic purpura. Br J Haematol 122:818, 2003

13. He R, Reid DM, Jones CE, et al: Spectrum of Ig classes, specificities, and titers of serum antiglycoproteins in chronic idiopathic thrombocytopenic purpura. Blood 83:1024, 1994

14. Emmons RV, Reid DM, Cohen RL, et al: Human thrombopoietin levels are high when thrombocytopenia is due to megakaryocyte deficiency and low when due to increased platelet destruction. Blood 87:4068, 1996

15. George JN, Woolf SH, Raskob GE, et al: Idiopathic thrombocytopenic purpura: a practice guideline developed by explicit methods for the American Society of Hematology. Blood 88:3, 1996

16. Stasi R, Stipa E, Masi M, et al: Long term observation of 208 adults with chronic idiopathic thrombocytopenic purpura. Am J Med 98:436, 1995

17. Cortelazzo S, Finazzi G, Buelli M, et al: High risk of severe bleeding in aged patients with chronic idiopathic thrombocytopenic purpura. Blood 77:31, 1991

18. Stasi R, Rossi Z, Stipa E, et al: *Helicobacter pylori* eradication in the management of patients with idiopathic thrombocytopenic purpura. Am J Med 118:414, 2005

19. Cheng Y, Wong RS, Soo YO, et al: Initial management of immune thrombocytopenic purpura with high-dose dexamethasone. N Engl J Med 349:831, 2003

20. Berchtold P, Dale GL, Tani P, et al: Inhibition of autoantibody binding to platelet glycoprotein IIb/IIIa by anti-idiotypic antibodies in intravenous gammaglobulin. Blood 74:2414, 1989

21. Yu Z, Lennon VA: Mechanism of intravenous immune globulin therapy in antibody-mediated autoimmune diseases. N Engl J Med 340:227, 1999

22. Cooper N, Stasi R, Cunningham-Rundles S, et al: The efficacy and safety of B-cell depletion with anti-CD20 monoclonal antibody in adults with chronic immune thrombocytopenic purpura. Br J Haematol 125:232, 2004

23. Facon T, Caulier MT, Wattel E, et al: A randomized trial comparing vinblastine in slow infusion and by bolus I.V. injection in idiopathic thrombocytopenic purpura: a report on 42 patients. Br J Haematol 86:678, 1994

24. Laveder F, Marcolongo R, Zamboni S: Thrombocytopenic purpura following treatment with danazol. Br J Haematol 90:970, 1995

25. Nardi MA, Liu L-X, Karpatkin S: GPIIIa-(49-66) is a major pathophysiologically relevant antigenic determinant for anti-platelet GPIIIa of HIV-1-related immunologic thrombocytopenia. Proc Natl Acad Sci USA 94:7589, 1997

26. Koefoed K, Ditzel HJ: Identification of talin head domain as an immunodominant epitope of the antiplatelet antibody response in patients with HIV-1–associated thrombocytopenia. Blood 104:4054, 2004

27. Najean Y, Rabin JD: The mechanism of thrombocytopenia in patients with HIV infection. J Lab Clin Med 123:415, 1994

28. Scaradavou A, Woo B, Woloski BMR, et al: Intravenous anti-D treatment of immune thrombocytopenic purpura: experience in 272 patients. Blood 89:2689, 1997

29. Durand JM, Lefevre P, Hovette P, et al: Dapsone for thrombocytopenic purpura related to human immunodeficiency virus infection. Am J Med 90:675, 1991

30. Marroni M, Gresele P, Landonio G, et al: Interferon-alpha is effective in the treatment of HIV-1–related, severe, zidovudine-resistant thrombocytopenia. Ann Intern Med 121:423, 1994

31. Needleman SW, Sorace J, Poussin-Rosillo H, et al: Low-dose splenic irradiation in the treatment of autoimmune thrombocytopenia in HIV-infected patients. Ann Intern Med 116:310, 1992

32. Kelton JG: Idiopathic thrombocytopenic purpura complicating pregnancy. Blood Reviews 16:43, 2002

33. Christiaens GC, Nieuwenhuis HK, Bussel JB: Comparison of platelet counts in first and second newborns of mothers with immune thrombocytopenic purpura. Obstet Gynecol 90:546, 1997

34. Burrows RF, Kelton JG: Fetal thrombocytopenia and its relation to maternal thrombocytopenia. N Engl J Med 329:1463, 1993

35. Webert KE, Mittal R, Sigouin C, et al: A retrospective 11-year analysis of obstetric patients with idiopathic thrombocytopenic purpura. Blood 102:4306, 2003

36. Payne SD, Resnik R, Moore TR, et al: Maternal characteristics and risk of severe neonatal thrombocytopenia and intracranial hemorrhage in pregnancies complicated by autoimmune thrombocytopenia. Am J Obstet Gynecol 177:149, 1997

37. Pappalardo PA, Secord AR, Quitevis P, et al: Platelet transfusion refractoriness associated with HPA-1a (Pl (A1)) alloantibody without coexistent HLA antibodies successfully treated with antigen-negative platelet transfusions. Transfusion 41:984, 2001

38. Curtis BR, Ali S, Glazier AM, et al: Isoimmunization against CD36 (glycoprotein IV): description of four cases of neonatal isoimmune thrombocytopenia and brief review of the literature. Transfusion 42:1173, 2002

39. McCrae KR, Herman JH: Posttransfusion purpura: two unusual cases and a literature review. Am J Hematol 52:205, 1996

40. Loren AW, Abrams CS: Efficacy of HPA-1a (PIA1)-negative platelets in a patient with post-transfusion purpura. Am J Hematol 76:258, 2004

41. Burgess JK, Lopez JA, Berndt MC, et al: Quinine-dependent antibodies bind a restricted set of epitopes on the glycoprotein Ib-IX complex: characterization of the epitopes. Blood 92:2366, 1998

42. Glynne P, Salama A, Chaudhry A, et al: Quinine-induced immune thrombocytopenic purpura followed by hemolytic uremic syndrome. Am J Kidney Dis 33:133, 1999

43. Kaufman DW, Kelly JP, Johannes CB, et al: Acute thrombocytopenic purpura in relation to the use of drugs. Blood 82:2714, 1993

44. Garner SF, Campbell K, Metcalfe P, et al: Glycoprotein V: the predominant target antigen in gold-induced autoimmune thrombocytopenia. Blood 100:344, 2002

45. Burday MJ, Martin SE: Cocaine-associated thrombocytopenia. Am J Med 91:656, 1992

46. Tcheng JE, Kereiakes DJ, Lincoff AM, et al: Abciximab readministration: results of the ReoPro Readministration Registry. Circulation 104:870, 2001

47. Aster RH: Immune thrombocytopenia caused by glycoprotein IIb/IIIa inhibitors. Chest 127:53S, 2005

48. Bougie D, Aster R: Immune thrombocytopenia resulting from sensitivity to metabolites of naproxen and acetaminophen. Blood 97:3846, 2001

49. Bennett CL, Connors JM, Carwile JM, et al: Thrombotic thrombocytopenic purpura associated with clopidogrel. N Engl J Med 342:1773, 2000

50. Moake JL: Thrombotic microangiopathies. N Engl J Med 347:589, 2002

51. Levy G, Motto DG, Ginsburg D: ADAMTS13 turns 3. Blood 106:11, 2005

52. Dong JF, Moake JL, Bernardo A, et al: ADAMTS-13 metalloprotease interacts with the endothelial cell-derived ultra-large von Willebrand factor. J Biol Chem 278:29633, 2003

53. Levy GG, Nichols WC, Ian EC, et al: Mutations in a member of the ADAMTS gene family cause thrombotic thrombocytopenic purpura. Nature 413:488, 2001

54. Furlan M, Robles R, Galbusera M, et al: von Willebrand factor–cleaving protease in thrombotic thrombocytopenic purpura and the hemoloytic-uremic syndrome. N Engl J Med 339:1578, 1998

55. Tsai HM, Lian EC: Antibodies to von Willebrand factor–cleaving protease in acute thrombotic thrombocytopenic purpura. N Engl J Med 339:1585, 1998

56. Mannucci PM, Canciani MT, Forza I, et al: Changes in health and disease of the metalloprotease that cleaves von Willebrand factor. Blood 98:2730, 2001

57. Moore JC, Hayward CP, Warkentin TE, et al: Decreased von Willebrand factor protease activity associated with thrombocytopenic disorders. Blood 98:1842, 2001

58. Zheng XL, Kaufman RM, Goodnough LT, et al: Effect of plasma exchange on plasma ADAMTS13 metalloprotease activity, inhibitor level, and clinical outcome in patients with idiopathic and nonidiopathic thrombotic thrombocytopenic purpura. Blood 103:4043, 2004

59. Veyradier A, Obert B, Houllier A, et al: Specific von Willebrand factor–cleaving protease in thrombotic microangiopathies: a study of 111 cases. Blood 98:1765, 2001

60. Vesely SK, George JN, Lammle B, et al: ADAMTS13 activity in thrombotic thrombocytopenic purpura–hemolytic uremic syndrome: relation to presenting features and clinical outcomes in a prospective cohort of 142 patients. Blood 102:60, 2003

61. Kokame K, Matsumoto M, Fujimura Y, et al: VWF73, a region from D1596 to R1668 of von Willebrand factor, provides a minimal substrate for ADAMTS-13. Blood 103:607, 2004

62. Whitelock JL, Nolasco L, Bernardo A, et al: ADAMTS-13 activity in plasma is rapidly measured by a new ELISA method that uses recombinant VWF-A2 domain as substrate. J Thromb Haemost 2:485, 2004

63. Boyce TG, Swerdlow DL, Griffin PM: *Escherichia coli* 0157:H7 and the hemolytic-uremic syndrome. N Engl J Med 333:364, 1995

64. Morigi M, Galbusera M, Binda E, et al: Verotoxin-1–induced up-regulation of adhesive molecules renders microvascular endothelial cells thrombogenic at high shear stress. Blood 98:1828, 2001

65. Wong CS, Jelacic S, Habeeb RL, et al: The risk of the hemolytic-uremic syndrome after antibiotic treatment of *Escherichia coli* O157:H7 infections. N Engl J Med 342:1930, 2000

66. Bianchi V, Robles R, Alberio L, et al: Von Willebrand factor–cleaving protease (ADAMTS13) in thrombocytopenic disorders: a severely deficient activity is specific for thrombotic thrombocytopenic purpura. Blood 100:710, 2002

67. Rock G, Shumak KH, Buskard NA, et al: Comparison of plasma exchange with plasma infusion in the treatment of thrombotic thrombocytopenic purpura. Canadian Apheresis Study Group. N Engl J Med 325:393, 1991

68. George JN, Gilcher RO, Smith JW, et al: Thrombotic thrombocytopenic purpura–hemolytic uremic syndrome: diagnosis and management. J Clin Apheresis 13:120, 1998

69. Rock G, Shumak KH, Sutton DM, et al: Cryosupernatant as replacement fluid for plasma exchange in thrombotic thrombocytopenic purpura. Members of the Canadian Apheresis Group. Br J Haematol 94:383, 1996

70. Bell WR, Braine HG, Ness PM, et al: Improved survival in thrombotic thrombocytopenic purpura–hemolytic uremic syndrome: clinical experience in 108 patients. N Engl J Med 325:398, 1991

71. Zheng X, Pallera AM, Goodnough LT, et al: Remission of chronic thrombotic thrombocytopenic purpura after treatment with cyclophosphamide and rituximab. Ann Intern Med 138:105, 2003

72. Yomtovian R, Niklinski W, Silver B, et al: Rituximab for chronic recurring thrombotic thrombocytopenic purpura: a case report and review of the literature. Br J Haematol 124:787, 2004

73. Fakhouri F, Vernant JP, Veyradier A, et al: Efficiency of curative and prophylactic treatment with rituximab in ADAMTS13 deficient–thrombotic thrombocytopenic purpura: a study of 11 cases. Blood 2005

74. Harkness DR, Byrnes JJ, Lian EC-Y: Hazard of platelet transfusion in thrombotic thrombocytopenic purpura. JAMA 246:1931, 1981

75. Sadler JE, Moake JL, Miyata T, et al: Recent advances in thrombotic thrombocytopenic purpura. Hematology 407, 2004

76. Shumak KH, Rock G, Nair RC, et al: Late relapses in patients successfully treated for thrombotic thrombocytopenic purpura. Ann Intern Med 122:569, 1995

77. Mohanty D, Marwaha N, Ghosh K, et al: Functional and ultrastructural changes of platelets in malarial infection. Trans R Soc Trop Med Hyg 82:369, 1988

78. Van Dam PA, Renier M, Baekelandt M, et al: Disseminated intravascular coagulation and the syndrome of hemolysis, elevated liver enzymes, and low platelets in severe preeclampsia. Obstet Gynecol 73:97, 1989

79. Martin JN Jr, Blake PG, Perry KG Jr, et al: The natural history of HELLP syndrome: patterns of disease progression and regression. Am J Obstet Gynecol 164:1500, 1991

80. Sibai BM, Ramadan MK, Usta I, et al: Maternal morbidity and mortality in 442 pregnancies with hemolysis, elevated liver enzymes, and low platelets (HELLP syndrome). Am J Obstet Gynecol 169:1000, 1993

81. Sibai BM: Diagnosis, controversies, and management of the syndrome of hemolysis, elevated liver enzymes, and low platelet count. Obstet Gynecol 103:981, 2004

82. Boccardo P, Remuzzi G, Galbusera M: Platelet dysfunction in renal failure. Semin Thromb Hemost 30:579, 2004

83. Weigert AL, Schafer AI: Uremic bleeding: pathogenesis and therapy. Am J Med Sci 316:94, 1998

84. Mannucci PM: Hemostatic drugs. N Engl J Med 339:245, 1998

85. Lacoste L, Hung J, Lam JY: Acute and delayed antithrombotic effects of alcohol in humans. Am J Cardiol 87:82, 2001

86. George JN, Shattil SJ: The clinical importance of acquired abnormalities of platelet function. N Engl J Med 324:27, 1991

87. Baxter EJ, Scott LM, Campbell PJ, et al: Acquired mutation of the tyrosine kinase JAK2 in human myeloproliferative disorders. Lancet 365:1954, 2005

88. James C, Ugo V, Le Couedic JP, et al: A unique clonal JAK2 mutation leading to constitutive signalling causes polycythaemia vera. Nature 434:1144, 2005

89. Kralovics R, Passamonti F, Buser AS, et al: A gain-of-function mutation of JAK2 in myeloproliferative disorders. N Engl J Med 352:1779, 2005

90. Layzer RB: Hot feet: erythromelalgia and related disorders. J Child Neurol 16:199, 2001

91. Anagrelide, a therapy for thrombocythemic states: experience in 577 patients. Anagrelide Study Group. Am J Med 92:69, 1992

92. Harrison CN, Campbell PJ, Buck G, et al: Hydroxyurea compared with anagrelide in high-risk essential thrombocytopenia. N Engl J Med 353:33, 2005

93. Begbie ME, Wallace GM, Shovlin CL: Hereditary haemorrhagic telangiectasia (Osler-Weber-Rendu syndrome): a view from the 21st century. Postgrad Med J 79:18, 2003

94. Abdalla SA, Pece-Barbara N, Vera S, et al: Analysis of ALK-1 and endoglin in newborns from families with hereditary telangiectasia type 2. Hum Mol Genet 9:1227, 2000

95. White RI Jr, Lynch-Nyhan A, Terry P, et al: Pulmonary arteriovenous malformation: techniques and long-term outcome of embolotherapy. Radiology 169:663, 1988

96. Shovlin CL: Molecular defects in rare bleeding disorders: hereditary haemorrhagic telangiectasia. Thromb Haemost 78:145, 1997

97. Hirschmann JV, Raugi GJ: Adult scurvy. J Am Acad Dermatol 41:895, 1999

98. George J: Hemostasis and thrombosis. Hematology: Basic Principles and Practice, 3rd ed. Hoffman R, Benz EJ Jr, Shattil SJ, Eds. Churchill Livingstone, Philadelphia, 1999, p 1928

Acknowledgment

Figure 1   Seward Hung.

Lawrence L. K. Leung, M.D.

Bleeding or bruising that is spontaneous or excessive after tissue injury may be caused by coagulation defects, fibrinolysis, abnormal platelet number or function, abnormal vascular integrity, or a combination of these abnormalities. This chapter addresses the various hemorrhagic disorders associated with abnormalities in coagulation. Hemorrhagic disorders associated with quantitative or qualitative platelet abnormalities and disorders associated with blood vessels are discussed elsewhere [*see Chapter 97*].

Disorders of coagulation may be inherited or acquired. Congenital coagulation disorders are rare and are most frequently caused by defects in single coagulation proteins, with the two X-linked disorders—factor VIII and factor IX deficiencies—accounting for the majority of defects. Acquired coagulation disorders are more common than the inherited disorders and are more complex in their pathogenesis. The most common acquired hemorrhagic disorders are vitamin K deficiency, drug-induced hemorrhage, and disseminated intravascular coagulation (DIC).

Hereditary Coagulation Disorders

The coagulation disorders appear clinically as either spontaneous hemorrhage or excessive hemorrhage after trauma or surgery. The patient history usually indicates whether the disorder is congenital or acquired. The hereditary disorders are characterized by their appearance early in life and by the presence of a single abnormality that can account for the entire clinical picture.

VON WILLEBRAND DISEASE

Pathophysiology

von Willebrand disease (vWD), the most common hereditary bleeding disorder, is caused by a deficient or defective plasma von Willebrand factor (vWF). The gene encoding vWF is on chromosome 12. vWF has specific domains for binding clotting factor VIII, heparin, collagen, platelet GPIb, and platelet GPIIb-IIIa. These domains relate directly to the following functions of vWF: (1) its action as a carrier molecule for factor VIII:C, in which it protects the clotting factor from proteolysis and substantially prolongs its plasma half-life; (2) its promotion of primary platelet adhesion at high wall shear rates by linking platelets via their GPIb-IX-V receptor to subendothelial tissues at the wound site; and (3) its support of platelet aggregation by linking platelets via their GPIIb-IIIa receptors.[1] The vWF circulates as multimers that range in size from 0.5 million daltons (the dimer) to 20 million daltons. Even larger noncirculating multimers are present in endothelial cells, where they are stored in the Weibel-Palade bodies. The ultralarge vWF multimers are normally processed by the ADAMTS13 metalloprotease into smaller multimers as they are released from the endothelial cells. The vWF is released either into the circulation or abluminally, where it attaches to subendothelial collagen. Platelet α-granules also contain vWF, which is released when platelets are activated. The vWF multimers that are 12 million daltons or larger are the most effective in supporting platelet adhesion.

Laboratory Evaluation

The many variant forms of vWD differ in their clinical manifestations, laboratory abnormalities, and required therapies. Because vWF is a carrier protein for factor VIII, the activated partial thromboplastin time (aPTT) is prolonged when the vWF level is low. The platelet count is usually, but not invariably, normal. Bleeding time is generally prolonged but not sufficiently reliable to be used for diagnosis. An automated platelet function test utilizing a platelet function analyzer (PFA-100) has been shown to be a better screening test for vWD than the bleeding time.[2,3] In this assay, citrated whole blood is aspirated through a capillary tube under high shear rates onto a membrane coated with collagen in which a central aperture is made. Platelets are activated by either adenosine diphosphate (ADP) or epinephrine. The closure time is a measure of platelet-vWF interaction.

The diagnosis of vWD requires the determination of factor VIII and vWF levels. There are two caveats: (1) laboratory testing is notoriously variable and (2) the patient's blood group affects the vWF level—that is, patients with blood group O have lower vWF levels than those with blood group A, B, or AB, by as much as 30%.[4] The vWF level is measured by either immunologic or functional methods. The former is reported as a percentage of normal vWF antigen. Because vWF circulates in physiologically important multimeric forms, it is sometimes helpful to determine the multimeric composition of the vWF in the patient's plasma. This is especially useful in identifying type 2 vWD (see below). The functional level of vWF is tested by the ristocetin-induced platelet aggregation test. Ristocetin is added to a patient's platelet-rich plasma, where it causes vWF to bind to platelets via the GPIb-IX-V receptor, leading to platelet activation and aggregation. In some laboratories, formalin-fixed platelets are used and, after the addition of ristocetin, agglutination of fixed platelets is measured.

Clinical Variants

The classification scheme for variants of vWD comprises three major groups: type 1 is a partial quantitative deficiency of vWF, type 2 is a qualitative abnormality of vWF, and type 3 is a severe and virtually total quantitative deficiency of vWF [*see Table 1*].[5]

Type 1   Type 1 vWD is the most common form of vWD, accounting for 75% of cases. It is generally an autosomal dominant trait that usually appears in the heterozygous form. In many cases, a mutation in the vWF protein occurs such that the mutant provWF monomers form dimers normally with the wild-type provWF monomers, but the resulting dimers are trapped in the endoplasmic reticulum and cannot be secreted.[6] Patients with classic type 1 vWD have a lifelong history of mild to moderate bleeding, typically from mucosal surfaces. They may be unaware of a bleeding disorder until they undergo surgery or experience trauma, when bleeding may be severe. vWF antigen, factor VIII, and the ristocetin cofactor levels are all decreased.

Type 2   Type 2 vWD is characterized by qualitative abnormalities of vWF and a variable decrease in vWF antigen, factor VIII, and ristocetin cofactor. In type 2A, the largest multimers are absent; in type 2B, multimers bind excessively to platelets be-

Table 1 Classification and Differentiation of von Willebrand Disease

	Type 1	Type 2A	Type 2B	Type 2M	Type 2N	Type 3	Pseudo–von Willebrand Disease
Inheritance	Autosomal dominant	Autosomal dominant	Autosomal dominant	Autosomal dominant	Autosomal dominant	Autosomal recessive	Autosomal dominant
Incidence	~75%	~20%	~5%	Rare	Rare	Uncommon	Uncommon
Cause	Deficiency of normal vWF	Abnormal vWF	Abnormal vWF	Abnormal vWF	Abnormal vWF	Severe deficiency of vWF	Abnormal platelet membrane
Template bleeding time	N or ↑	↑	↑	↑	N or ↑	↑↑	N or ↑
Factor VIII assay	↓	N or ↓	N or ↓	N or ↓	↓↓	↓↓	N or ↓
vWF antigen	↓	Variable	Variable	Variable	N	↓↓	Variable
Ristocetin cofactor (RIPA)	↓	↓	↑	↓	N	↓↓	↑
Plasma vWF multimer analysis	N	Only low-molecular-weight forms present	Only low- and intermediate-molecular-weight forms present	N	N	Variable	Only low- and intermediate-molecular-weight forms present

N—normal   ↓—decreased   ↑—increased   vWF—von Willebrand factor

cause of a gain-of-function mutation; in type 2M, the abnormal vWF does not bind to GPIb-IX-V; and in type 2N, the binding site of vWF for factor VIII is mutated. All type 2 vWD variants, except for the rare type 2M, are characterized by a loss of the high-molecular-weight vWF multimers in the VWF polymer analysis.

Type 3 The rare homozygous or double heterozygous form (type 3 vWD) is characterized by severe hemorrhage, a long aPTT, and factor VIII levels of less than 5%.

Pseudo–von Willebrand disease A platelet form of vWD, which is termed pseudo–von Willebrand disease (pseudo–vWD), has been described in which an abnormal GPIb is present on platelets, causing excessive binding of normal plasma vWF to unstimulated platelets.

The mean level of vWF antigen is 100 IU/dl, but the population distribution of vWF levels is very broad, with the 95% values encompassing 50 IU/dl to 200 IU/dl. The reasons for this broad distribution in vWF levels are not completely understood, but it makes the commonly used threshold (vWF level at 2 SD [standard deviation] below the mean) inadequate for diagnosis of type 1 vWD. This problem with diagnosis is compounded by the fact that mild bleeding symptoms are extremely common in the general population. A recent survey estimates that 25% of men and 46% of women would give a positive history of bleeding symptoms, such as frequent epistaxis, easy bruising, and postpartum bleeding.[7] This suggests that type 1 vWD may be overdiagnosed, and it has been proposed that a more stringent diagnostic criterion be used—namely, limiting the diagnosis of type 1 vWD to patients with a vWF antigen level of less than 20 IU/dl.[6] Patients with modestly reduced vWF antigen levels (i.e., between 30 and 50 IU/dl) usually do not have identifiable vWF gene mutations and rarely cosegregate with a family history of bleeding. Patients with modestly reduced vWF levels (and no history of family bleeding) may have a modestly increased risk of bleeding.

Treatment

Mild or moderate types 1 and 2 1-Desamino-8-D-arginine vasopressin (DDAVP or desmopressin) is effective in the management of traumatic bleeding and before surgery in some patients with mild or moderate type 1 and type 2A vWD. The intravenous administration of DDAVP at a dosage of 0.3 mg/kg over a 15- to 30-minute period causes the release of large amounts of vWF from endothelial cell stores. The peak response usually occurs in 30 to 60 minutes and persists for up to 4 to 6 hours. Repeated DDAVP administrations over a 24-hour period are ineffective; tachyphylaxis follows depletion of the endothelial vWF stores. A DDAVP nasal spray (300 µg) can be used in the ambulatory treatment of patients with vWD, both for the management of bleeding episodes and as preparation for minor surgery.[8] The side effects of intravenous DDAVP are generally mild, including significant water retention and, rarely, thrombosis. Myocardial infarction has been reported. Because of the variability of response to DDAVP, a patient should be given a trial infusion of DDAVP before undergoing a planned procedure to determine whether the patient has an adequate response. Fibrinolysis inhibitor ε-aminocaproic acid (EACA), 3 g four times daily orally for 3 to 7 days, is also useful for dental procedures and minor bleeding events. Aspirin must be avoided.

Moderate and severe types 2 and 3 Patients with severe types 2A and 2B and with type 3 vWD generally require replacement therapy with Humate-P—a pasteurized intermediate-purity factor VIII concentrate that has a substantial amount of large vWF multimers—or with cryoprecipitate infusion containing vWF, factor VIII, and fibrinogen. Cryoprecipitate is generally not recommended. Transfusion of normal platelets can also be attempted on the grounds that platelet vWF can be hemostatically effective.[9]

Treatment during pregnancy Treatment is generally not needed during pregnancy in women with vWD. The plasma vWF level rises during the second and third trimesters but falls rapidly after delivery. Late hemorrhage may occur 2 to 3 weeks post partum.[10] DDAVP is not used before delivery because of the concern that it may initiate contractions. Patients with type 2B vWD may have worsening thrombocytopenia during pregnancy because of the increase of abnormal vWF in plasma.[11]

HEMOPHILIA A

Hemophilia A affects one in 10,000 males and is characterized by a deficient or defective clotting factor VIII. The factor VIII gene, which is located on chromosome X at Xq28, is among the largest known human genes, spanning 186 kb and containing 26 exons. It encodes a protein of about 300,000 daltons, which circulates in plasma at very low concentrations and is normally bound to and protected by vWF. The primary source of factor VIII production is likely the liver, because hemophilia A can be corrected by liver transplantation.

Because the gene for factor VIII coagulant activity is carried on the X chromosome, the disease is manifested in hemizygous males. All of the daughters of a hemophiliac male will be carriers, whereas half of the sons of a mother who carries the hemophilia trait will be hemophiliacs and half of her daughters will be carriers. Families appear to be affected to varying degrees, depending on the specific nature of the genetic defect.

The clinical severity of hemophilia A correlates well with the measured levels of factor VIII coagulant activity. In general, factor VIII levels below 1% are associated with severe hemorrhagic symptoms; levels between 1% and 5%, with moderate hemophilia; and levels between 5% and 25%, with mild hemophilia [see Table 2].

Approximately one third of hemophilia A cases represent new mutations and have a negative family history. More than 300 abnormal factor VIII genes have been found. The abnormalities, which include point mutations, gene insertions, and gene deletions, result in either deficient factor VIII production or the generation of a functionally defective factor VIII. An inversion within intron 22 of the factor VIII gene, which results in a truncated and unstable factor VIII protein, is found in approximately 45% of all severely affected hemophilia A patients (factor VIII levels below 1%).[12]

Diagnosis

Diagnosis is made on the basis of the clinical picture, family history (positive in two thirds of cases), and the factor VIII coagulant activity level. In most cases, the type of bleeding history and a classic family history rule out vWD (which, unlike hemophilia A, is autosomally transmitted). Accurate DNA analysis for the common intron 22 inversion is now available in DNA testing laboratories. This test provides molecular diagnosis in approximately 45% of patients with severe hemophilia. However, it should not be ordered in patients with mild or moderate hemophilia.

Treatment

General principles The psychosocial aspects of hemophilia are complex. A child is often absent from school, is prone to crippling deformities, and runs a risk of drug addiction because of severe pain. Parents are understandably deeply concerned and sometimes troubled by guilt. Treatment should address these issues as well as the specific coagulation problem.

Factor VIII replacement Factor VIII concentrates are effective in controlling spontaneous and traumatic hemorrhage. Currently available factor VIII products derived from plasma have been purified to varying degrees (e.g., Humate-P [intermediate purity], Koate-HP [high purity], and Monoclate [ultrapurity]) and have undergone viral inactivation. There are two forms of full-length recombinant factor VIII (Recombinate and Kogenate), and they are safe and efficacious.[13,14] A second-generation, B-domain–deleted recombinant factor VIII (ReFacto) has also been developed and has been found to be effective and well tolerated.[15] The new recombinant factor VIII has the advantage of considerably higher specific activity, and the final formulation is stable without added human serum albumin, thus further reducing the potential risk of transmission of human infectious agents.

Dental prophylaxis is critically important to reduce the need for dental surgery. Aspirin must be avoided. Revaccination against hepatitis B virus also should be considered.

Genetic counseling should be part of the management program. Because of the difficult life severe hemophiliacs lead, a woman may opt to terminate pregnancy if she is certain of her carrier status or if she knows that her fetus is affected. There are several strategies for detecting carriers. In women who are carriers, factor VIII levels are typically about half of normal, whereas vWF levels are normal. The ratio of factor VIII to vWF for carriers is thus 0.5[16]; however, the error rate for this test is 10% to 17%. A more accurate genetic diagnosis for carriers can be made by a linkage approach. This approach is based on restriction fragment length polymorphisms (RFLPs) within the factor VIII gene. Analysis of the affected male will establish the pattern for the X chromosome carrying the hemophilia allele, without knowledge of the precise mutation. There are a large number of intragenic polymorphisms that allow the two copies of factor VIII genes in a female potential carrier to be distinguished, identifying her carrier state with high accuracy.

These molecular probes for RFLPs are now being used to determine the status of the fetus. Tissue can be obtained by amniocentesis or chorionic villus sampling.

Management of acute hemorrhage Deep tissue bleeding, hemarthrosis, and hematuria are the common forms of clinical bleeding in hemophilia A. Acute threats to life are posed by retroperitoneal hemorrhage; bleeding of the mouth, tongue, or neck that impairs the airway; and intracranial hemorrhage. Both ultrasonography and computed tomography can be used to identify retroperitoneal and intramuscular hematomas.

Table 2 Correlation of Factor VIII Coagulant Activity Level with Bleeding Patterns in Hemophilia

Plasma Factor VIII Level	Bleeding Pattern
< 1%	Severe, presentation in first year of life, bleeding with circumcision, spontaneous hemarthrosis and deep-tissue bleeding
1%–5%	Moderate, presentation in childhood, bleeding after trauma, spontaneous hemarthrosis rare
5%–25%	Mild; may be present in childhood; bleeding after trauma, surgery, or dental extraction
25%–50%	May be undetected, may present in adulthood with bleeding after major trauma or surgery

Principles of replacement therapy   A plasma procoagulant level of 100% means that there is one unit of procoagulant per milliliter of plasma. Most persons have 40 ml of plasma per kilogram of body weight. Thus, from a determination of a patient's plasma volume and procoagulant level, the required amount of factor VIII replacement can be calculated. For example, in the case of a 60 kg boy who has an uncomplicated hemarthrosis of the knee and a baseline factor VIII of less than 1%, raising the factor VIII level to about 25% (0.25 U/ml) for 2 to 3 days should suffice. This patient has a plasma volume of 60 kg × 40 ml/kg, or 2,400 ml; he will need 0.25 U/ml × 2,400 ml, or 600 U of factor VIII, as an initial bolus. Another method of estimation is based on the following effect: the infusion of 1 U of factor VIII per kilogram increases factor VIII levels by 2%. Thus, dividing the desired level of factor VIII increase by 2 will give the number of U/kg required. In the example cited, 25% of factor VIII will require 12.5 U/kg, or 750 U, of factor VIII replacement.

The biologic half-life of factor VIII is approximately 12 hours; the dose can be repeated every 12 to 24 hours as long as needed to control the hemorrhage. In patients with hemarthrosis, the factor VIII level should be maintained for 2 to 3 days.

Elective surgery and dental extraction   Dental work should be performed by a dentist who is experienced in the treatment of hemophiliacs. Before dental extraction, factor VIII is administered to raise the level to approximately 50%. The fibrinolytic inhibitor EACA is started the night before surgery at a loading dose of 3 g orally and continued at 2 to 3 g three or four times daily for 7 to 10 days after the dental work has been completed. Usually, further administration of factor VIII is not required.

Before elective surgery, the factor VIII level should be raised to 50% to 100% (0.5 to 1.0 U/ml) and then maintained above 50% for the next 10 to 14 days. Maintaining a higher concentration of factor VIII does not reduce the frequency of hemorrhage.[17]

DDAVP can be used to treat acute traumatic hemorrhage in patients with mild to moderate hemophilia and even to prepare such patients for minor surgery. DDAVP, which causes the release of vWF from endothelial cell stores, cannot be used repeatedly over many days, because such stores become depleted. DDAVP is infused at a dosage of 0.3 μg/kg in 50 ml of saline over 15 to 30 minutes and produces a prompt increase in factor VIII. The biologic half-life of the released factor VIII is 11 to 12 hours.

Management of an inhibitor   Inhibitors tend to occur in more severely affected patients, who tend to receive the greatest number of factor VIII concentrates. In a recent single-center study of 431 patients over 3 decades, approximately 10% of patients with severe hemophilia A had an inhibitor (about a third were children younger than 10 years).[18] Not all inhibitors produce clinical problems. Assays for factor VIII inhibitors should be performed at regular intervals in all patients who have severe hemophilia.

Hemorrhage in a patient with an inhibitor can be life threatening. In a patient who has an inhibitor titer of less than 5 Bethesda units and who is not a vigorous antibody responder, a large amount of factor VIII concentrate should be administered in an attempt to overwhelm the antibody. Alternative therapies are porcine factor VIII (Hyate:C), prothrombin complex concentrates (e.g., Konyne and Proplex) to circumvent the factor VIII deficiency,[19,20] and activated prothrombin complex concentrates, such as Autoplex-T and FEIBA.

Recombinant activated factor VII (rFVIIa) has been found to be safe and efficacious in 70% to 85% of more than 1,500 bleeding episodes in hemophilia patients with inhibitors.[21,22] Recombinant factor VIIa may compete against the normal plasma unactivated factor VII for tissue factor binding and thus enhance thrombin generation at the bleeding site.[23] In addition, high-dose rFVIIa may bind to activated platelets and activate factors IX and X on the platelet surface in the absence of tissue factor.[24]

High-dose intravenous IgG has been used to treat nonhemophiliacs with acquired factor VIII inhibitors, but it is usually not efficacious in hemophiliacs with inhibitors (alloantibodies).

OTHER HEREDITARY HEMORRHAGIC DISORDERS

Factor IX Deficiency (Hemophilia B)

Factor IX deficiency (hemophilia B, or Christmas disease) is an X-linked hemorrhagic disorder that is clinically indistinguishable from hemophilia A. The factor IX gene is on the X chromosome and produces a clotting factor that, like other vitamin K–dependent factors, has a region rich in γ-carboxylated glutamic acids. Calcium ion bridges link this region to the activated platelet cell surface, where factor IXa interacts with factor VIIIa to form a membrane-associated complex that efficiently converts factor X to factor Xa (intrinsic tenase) [*see Chapter 96*]. A large number of insertions, rearrangements, and deletions have been detected in the factor IX gene, and the hemophilia B syndrome is very heterogeneous.[25]

Diagnosis   Diagnosis of hemophilia B requires a factor IX assay. The management principles are the same as those for hemophilia A. A plasma-derived pasteurized factor IX concentrate preparation (Mononine) displays excellent specific activity and a desirable biologic half-life of 18 to 34 hours. Recombinant factor IX is also commercially available.

Treatment   The level of factor IX that is needed to control hemostasis in patients with hemophilia B is somewhat lower than the level of factor VIII required for the treatment of hemophilia A—about 15% to 20% for the former and 30% to 50% for the latter. Factor IX is a smaller molecule than factor VIII and is distributed in the albumin space. In making replacement calculations, it is assumed that administration of 1 U/kg of factor IX will increase the plasma level by 1%. Factor IX has a biphasic half-life, and plasma levels of this factor can be maintained by infusing the concentrate every 24 hours. Molecular biology techniques can now detect the factor IX deficiency carrier state and permit accurate genetic counseling. Sustained correction of a bleeding disorder in hemophilia B mice has been demonstrated by the gene therapy approach,[26] and clinical trials of factor IX in hemophilia B patients have been initiated.[27]

Factor XI Deficiency

Patients with factor XI deficiency frequently come to medical attention when a prolonged aPTT is detected during preoperative screening. It is most frequently observed in Ashkenazi Jews, although sporadic cases have been described in people of different ethnic origins. Factor XI deficiency is inherited as an autosomal recessive trait, and heterozygous deficiency is not associated with any clinical bleeding. Homozygous or compound heterozygous deficient patients generally have factor XI levels of less than 15%, and most bleeding manifestations in these patients are related to trauma or surgery, especially at sites of high fibrinolytic activity (e.g., the urinary tract, tonsils, and tooth sockets).[28] Factor XI plays a supportive role in the clotting cascade. Factor XI is activated by thrombin and then functions in a positive feedback manner to augment thrombin generation and clot stabilization [see Chapter 96]. Thus, factor XI is primarily required in situations in which there is a significant hemostatic challenge; this explains the mild bleeding diathesis seen in patients with factor XI deficiency.

For patients with severe factor XI deficiency (< 15%) who require surgery, fresh frozen plasma should be used to replenish the plasma level to more than 50%. EACA given orally at a dosage of 3 g three or four times daily is also effective for minor surgical or dental procedures. In a recent retrospective study of 62 women with severe factor XI deficiency, about 70% of the women did not have any postpartum hemorrhage. Of the 30% who did have postpartum hemorrhage, some had a history of recurrent clinical bleeding. Postpartum hemorrhage had no relationship with the particular abnormal factor XI genotype or with the level of factor XI.[29]

Fibrinolytic Abnormalities

Two uncommon congenital hemorrhagic disorders have been ascribed to abnormalities of fibrinolysis. Deficiency of α_2-antiplasmin, the major plasmin inhibitor, has led to uncontrolled plasmin activity with consequent hemorrhage. Enhanced fibrinolytic activity with occasional clinical bleeding has also been linked to deficiency of plasminogen activator inhibitor–1 (PAI-1), the physiologic inhibitor of tissue plasminogen activator (t-PA) and urokinase.[30] Treatment of both types of fibrinolytic abnormalities consists of the antifibrinolytic agents, tranexamic acid, or EACA, all of which block the binding of plasminogen and plasmin to fibrin.

Acquired Hemorrhagic Disorders

In addition to the hereditary coagulation disorders, several acquired disorders have been identified that can lead to generalized hemorrhage.

VITAMIN K DEFICIENCY

A vitamin K–dependent carboxylase in the liver synthesizes γ-carboxyglutamic acid, which is required for the biologic function of prothrombin and factors VII, IX, and X. In the absence of vitamin K, an abnormal prothrombin that lacks γ-carboxyglutamic residues is synthesized. Specific immunoassays performed in patients with vitamin K deficiency reveal a sharp decrease in normal prothrombin levels and a concomitant increased level of the abnormal des-γ-carboxyprothrombin. The same molecular derangement occurs with factors VII, IX, and X.[31]

Clinical Features and Diagnosis

Deficiency of vitamin K, which decreases levels of prothrombin and factors VII, IX, and X, occurs in cases of severe malnutrition, intestinal malabsorption, and obstructive jaundice. In patients with obstructive jaundice, bile salts, which are necessary for the emulsification and absorption of the fat-soluble vitamins (vitamins A, D, E, and K), cannot enter the intestine. Long-term ingestion of oral antibiotics suppresses vitamin K production by intestinal organisms. The effect is especially marked in patients who, because of their illness, are unable to consume a full, nourishing diet. Mucosal bleeding and ecchymoses occur if the procoagulant levels fall below 10% to 15% of normal.

Treatment

Therapy with vitamin K_1 (phytonadione), 10 to 25 mg/day orally for 2 or 3 days—or parenteral vitamin K_1 in cases of obstructive jaundice—usually reverses the abnormality in about 6 to 24 hours. If there is severe bleeding, fresh frozen plasma (approximately 3 units) restores procoagulant levels rapidly [see Principles of Replacement Therapy, above].

DRUG-INDUCED HEMORRHAGE

Warfarin-Induced Hemorrhage

Warfarin overdose or potentiation of its action by other drugs can cause very severe bleeding. The prothrombin time (PT) is prolonged, and mucosal bleeding, gastrointestinal bleeding, or ecchymosis is the usual pattern. If hemorrhage is significant, treatment to restore procoagulant levels to 30% of normal must be started with fresh frozen plasma. If there is no urgency, oral vitamin K_1 may be given. Generally, 1 to 2.5 mg of vitamin K_1 will be sufficient to return anticoagulation (defined as the international normalized ratio [INR]) to therapeutic levels after 16 hours. High doses of vitamin K_1 (10 mg or more) should be avoided because they may cause warfarin resistance for up to a week. Surreptitious warfarin use can be identified by a serum warfarin assay, which is available at special laboratories. Factitious or accidental ingestion of some of the long-acting vitamin K antagonists that are used as rodenticides (superwarfarins) may lead to prolonged bleeding symptoms. The synthesis of vitamin K–dependent clotting factors can be impaired for months after the initial exposure. Repeated administration of fresh frozen plasma, supplemented by massive doses of oral vitamin K_1 (100 to 150 mg/day), may be required to control bleeding symptoms.

Heparin-Induced Hemorrhage

Heparin overdose may not be obvious. It causes subcutaneous hemorrhages and deep tissue hematomas. The aPTT, PT, and thrombin time (TT) are vastly prolonged, but the reptilase time (RT) is normal. Intravenous protamine administration at a dosage of 1 mg/100 U of administered heparin terminates the overdose response. Because the half-life of protamine is shorter than that of heparin, a heparin rebound may occur, necessitating a second administration of protamine. Low-molecular-weight heparin (LMWH) preparations cause as much bleeding as standard unfractionated heparin. The ability of protamine to reverse the actions of LMWH is incomplete. Protamine (1 mg/100 U of anti–factor Xa) can be tried; if protamine treatment is unsuccessful, recombinant factor VIIa should be considered.

Hemorrhage Caused by Thrombolytic Therapy

Thrombolytic therapy is now used for acute myocardial infarction and for some cases of pulmonary embolism. The complications of thrombolytic therapy are essentially all hemorrhagic. In general, bleeding has been confined to relatively trivial oozing at vascular invasion sites, but subdural hematomas, cerebral infarction, and intracranial bleeding have also occurred. The thrombolytic agents, even those designed to be relatively fibrin specific, occasionally cause a significant systemic lytic state, with low levels of fibrinogen, factor V, and factor VIII. Furthermore, the generation of fibrinogen degradation products in turn interferes with the formation of a firm clot and with platelet function.

If thrombolytic therapy is suspected as the cause of bleeding in a particular patient, blood should be drawn quickly for an aPTT, a TT, an RT, and a fibrinogen level. If thrombolytic thera-

Table 3 Causes of Disseminated Intravascular Coagulation (DIC)

Events that initiate DIC
  Septicemia
  Cancer procoagulants (Trousseau syndrome)
  Acute promyelocytic leukemia
  Crush injury, complicated surgery
  Severe intracranial hemorrhage
  Retained conception products, abruptio placentae, amniotic fluid embolism
  Eclampsia, preeclampsia
  Major ABO blood mismatch, hemolytic transfusion reaction
  Burn injuries
  Heatstroke
  Malignant hypertension
  Extensive pump-oxygenation (repair of aortic aneurysm)
  Giant hemangioma (Kasabach-Merritt syndrome)
  Severe vasculitis
Events that complicate and propagate DIC
  Shock
  Complement pathway activation

py is the cause, the aPTT is prolonged, the fibrinogen level is usually below 50 mg/dl, and the TT and RT are both prolonged (as a result of the fibrin degradation products and decreased plasma fibrinogen).

The disorder is treated with cryoprecipitate (to raise the fibrinogen level to approximately 100 mg/dl), fresh frozen plasma, and platelet concentrates. If these measures do not stop the bleeding, the use of a specific antifibrinolytic agent such as EACA should be considered. EACA is given as a 5 g bolus I.V. over 30 to 60 minutes and then in a dosage of 1 g/hr by continuous I.V. infusion.[32]

DYSPROTEINEMIAS

The abnormal proteins associated with myeloma and macroglobulinemia can interfere with platelet function and cause clinical bleeding. These proteins can cause abnormalities in the coagulation tests as well. Both IgG and IgA myeloma proteins can cause prolonged TTs by interfering with the fibrin polymerization process. Less commonly, they may interact with specific clotting factors. Management is directed at the primary disease. Generally, these paraproteins do not cause clinically significant bleeding. If bleeding occurs, plasmapheresis rapidly corrects the defects by abruptly lowering the level of abnormal protein.

DISSEMINATED INTRAVASCULAR COAGULATION

Pathophysiology

Many different circumstances can cause DIC [*see Table 3*]. In each case, massive activation of the clotting cascade overwhelms the natural antithrombotic mechanisms, giving rise to uncontrolled thrombin generation. This condition results in thromboses in the arterial and venous beds, leading to ischemic infarction and necrosis that intensify the damage, release tissue factor, and further activate the clotting cascade. Massive coagulation depletes clotting factors and platelets, giving rise to consumption coagulopathy and bleeding. Tissue damage and the deposition of fibrin result in the release and activation of plasminogen activators and the generation of plasmin in amounts that over-

whelm its inhibitor, α_2-antiplasmin. Plasmin degrades fibrinogen, prothrombin, and factors V and VIII and produces fibrin-fibrinogen degradation products. These substances interfere with normal fibrin polymerization and impair platelet function by binding to the platelet surface GPIIb-IIIa fibrinogen receptor. These fibrin-fibrinogen degradation products thus function as circulating anticoagulant and antiplatelet agents, exacerbating the consumption coagulopathy, and play a significant role in the bleeding diathesis [*see Figure 1*].

Endotoxin released during gram-negative septicemia enhances the expression of tissue factor, thereby accelerating procoagulant activation while suppressing thrombomodulin expression. These actions downregulate the protein C/protein S system, further promoting the tendency to DIC.[33] Experimental-endotoxemia models also showed marked suppression of fibrinolysis activity caused by a sustained increase in plasma PAI-1.[34] In patients with solitary or multiple hemangiomas associated with thrombocytopenia (Kasabach-Merritt syndrome), DIC is presumably initiated by prolonged contact of abnormal endothelial surface with blood in areas of vascular stasis. Platelets and fibrinogen are consumed in these hemangiomas, where fibrinolysis appears to be enhanced,[35] and such consumption can lead to hemorrhage. Certain snakebites can also produce DIC; several mechanisms have been identified. For example, Russell viper venom contains a protease that directly activates factor X and can produce almost instantaneous defibrination.

Clinical Consequences

The clinical consequences of DIC depend on its cause and the rapidity with which the initiating event is propagated. If the activation occurs slowly, an excess of procoagulants is produced, predisposing to thrombosis. At the same time, as long as the liver can compensate for the consumption of clotting factors and

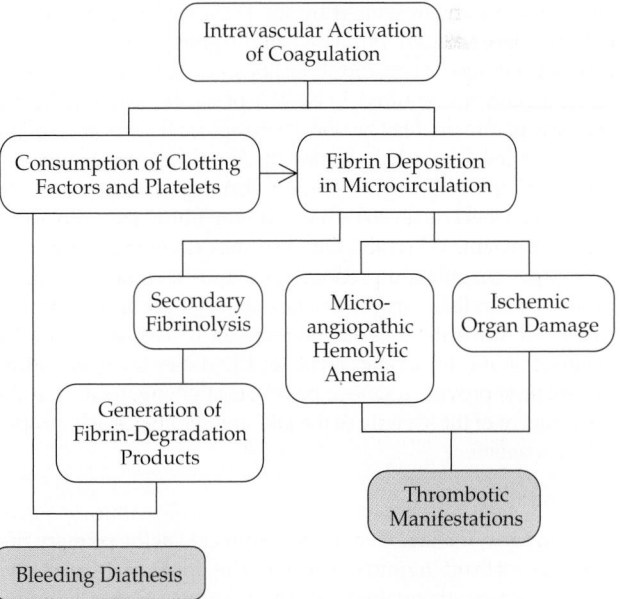

Figure 1 In compensated disseminated intravascular coagulation (DIC), such as that which occurs in Trousseau syndrome, thrombotic manifestations predominate in the clinical presentation. In decompensated DIC, however, fibrin-fibrinogen degradation products exacerbate the consumption coagulopathy and play a significant role in the bleeding diathesis.

the bone marrow maintains an adequate platelet output, the bleeding diathesis will not be clinically apparent. The clinical situation consists of primarily thrombotic manifestations, which can be both venous thrombosis and arterial thrombosis [*see Chapter 99*]. Venous thromboses commonly involve deep vein thrombosis in the extremities or superficial migratory thrombophlebitis. Patients can also experience arterial thrombosis, leading to digital ischemia, renal infarction, or stroke. Arterial ischemia can in part be the result of emboli that originate from fibrin clots in the mitral valve, a condition termed nonbacterial thrombotic endocarditis, or marantic endocarditis. This condition is sometimes known as compensated, or chronic, DIC and accounts for Trousseau syndrome[36] (a chronic DIC caused by an underlying malignancy, most frequently pancreatic or other gastrointestinal cancer). The cancer cells may produce either tissue factor or another procoagulant that activates the clotting system.

If the reaction is brisk and explosive, the clinical picture is dominated by intravascular coagulation; depletion of platelets, fibrinogen, prothrombin, and factors V and VIII; and the production, by plasmin action, of fibrin degradation products, which further interfere with hemostasis. The clinical consequence is a profound systemic bleeding diathesis, with blood oozing from wound sites, intravenous lines, and catheters, as well as bleeding into deep tissues. The intravascular fibrin strands produce microangiopathic hemolytic anemia.

Diagnosis

Microangiopathic red blood cells on smear and a moderate to severe thrombocytopenia suggest the diagnosis. A number of laboratory abnormalities are present in DIC, depending on the stage of the DIC. Because of clotting factor depletion, the aPTT and PT are prolonged and the fibrinogen level is low. Because fibrin degradation products interfere with fibrin polymerization, the TT and RT are also prolonged. The level of fibrin degradation products, as measured by the D-dimer level, is elevated. Plasma plasminogen, protein C, and α_2-antiplasmin levels are also low because of consumption; however, these measurements are generally not required. In the case of compensated DIC, most of these parameters can be normal except for the elevation of the D-dimer level, which indicates the presence of intravascular cross-linked fibrin deposition and fibrinolysis. Sometimes, the fibrinogen level can even be high because fibrinogen is an acute-phase reactant. When the DIC becomes decompensated, consumption coagulation predominates and the other laboratory abnormalities listed are present (see above). Repetition at regular intervals of specific coagulation tests (see above), especially the platelet count, fibrinogen level, and D-dimer level, is critical. These tests provide a kinetic parameter that greatly aids in the assessment of the severity of the DIC and the choice of appropriate management.

Treatment

Currently, management must be directed at the primary disease to switch off the initiating event. This approach may involve chemotherapeutic treatment of an underlying tumor, administration of antibiotics and surgical drainage of an abscess, or emptying the uterus when complications of pregnancy have been the inciting cause. Hemodynamic support is essential. The use of antifibrinolytic agents such as EACA or aprotinin is contraindicated. Despite its bleeding complications, DIC is a severe hypercoagulable state, and these agents block the fibrinolytic system and

may exacerbate its thrombotic complications. The administration of blood products, such as platelets, fresh frozen plasma, or cryoprecipitate, may add fuel to the fire and worsen the consumption coagulopathy. However, if clinical bleeding becomes significant, it is prudent to give vigorous blood product support.

The use of heparin in cases of acute DIC has not been established. Although heparin, by activating antithrombin (AT), is effective in inhibiting thrombin and therefore should be efficacious in the treatment of DIC, its use is generally limited to situations of chronic or compensated DIC. Heparin, given subcutaneously, is effective in the treatment of venous thrombosis in patients with Trousseau syndrome. In the case of decompensated DIC, in which bleeding is the major clinical manifestation, heparin may significantly exacerbate the bleeding and is therefore generally not indicated. The use of high-dose AT infusion has been advocated in this situation, but its efficacy has not been established by randomized studies.[37,38]

Recombinant human activated protein C (APC, or drotrecogin alfa [activated]) has been shown to significantly reduce mortality in patients with severe sepsis (mortality was 24.7% in patients given APC versus 30.8% in patients given placebo).[39] Although it is associated with a slightly increased risk of bleeding, APC appears to be an effective agent in the treatment of severe DIC in patients with sepsis, even for patients with normal protein C levels.[40] In large randomized trials, neither recombinant tissue factor pathway inhibitor (TFPI) nor AT concentrate reduced mortality in septic patients.[41,42] In cases of DIC associated with solitary or multiple hemangiomas, the hemangiomas can be excised when they are localized, and they occasionally show a good response to local irradiation. Attempts to control DIC associated with hemangiomas by the administration of heparin, corticosteroids, aspirin, and estrogens have not been successful. The key to successful management of DIC associated with certain snakebites is identification of the type of snake and prompt administration of appropriate antivenin.

ACQUIRED HEMOPHILIA AND OTHER DISORDERS OF CIRCULATING INHIBITORS

In addition to the hemorrhage caused by the circulating alloantibody inhibitors in severe hemophilias A and B, clinical hemorrhage is occasionally caused by circulating inhibitors directed against specific clotting factors, which seem to appear spontaneously. Because acquired autoantibody to factor VIII, which gives rise to the clinical picture of acquired hemophilia, is the most common of these circulating inhibitors, it will be described here in some detail, but many of the same principles apply to other inhibitors.

Autoantibodies to factor VIII are usually IgGa and, frequently, IgG4 and thus do not fix complement. They are usually directed against the functionally important A2 and C2 domains[43] on factor VIII. About half of the patients with an acquired factor VIII inhibitor have no identifiable associated disorder, but many disease states have been identified in the other patients, including autoimmune disorders such as systemic lupus erythematosus, lymphoproliferative disorders, plasma cell malignancies, drug reactions (e.g., reaction to penicillin), the postpartum state, and skin disorders.[44]

Diagnosis

Patients with an acquired factor VIII inhibitor commonly present with new-onset mucosal hemorrhages, hematomas, and ecchymoses but have a negative bleeding history. Typically, the clinical picture of acquired hemophilia caused by factor VIII inhibitor occurs in an elderly patient or in a young woman during pregnancy or in the postpartum period. The laboratory hallmark of an acquired inhibitor to a clotting factor is a prolonged clotting time that is not corrected by mixing equal parts of the patient's plasma with normal plasma. In the case of factor VIII inhibitor, the PTT is prolonged and the PT and TT are normal. The antibody binds to factor VIII with complex kinetics such that the inhibitory effect becomes apparent only after prolonged incubation. Therefore, if an acquired factor VIII inhibitor is suspected, mixing studies should be performed after 5-minute and 60-minute incubations. The diagnosis can be confirmed by demonstration of a very low factor VIII level when other clotting factor levels are normal. Determination of the titer of the factor VIII inhibitor (expressed in Bethesda units [BU] per milliliter, with 1 BU/ml indicating a sufficient number of inhibitors to cause the complete inhibition of factor VIII in 1 ml of blood) is useful in choosing the appropriate therapy.

Treatment

The hemorrhage caused by circulating inhibitors may be clinically life threatening. Attempts at factor replacement are usually not successful, because the inhibitor inactivates the exogenous factor VIII. Occasionally, if the inhibitor has a low titer (e.g., < 2 to 3 BU/ml), massive factor VIII replacement can overwhelm the inhibitor. However, this treatment may trigger a significant anamnestic response resulting in increased levels of antibody, which complicates further management. Immunosuppressive therapy with a combination of cyclophosphamide (given either as a monthly intravenous pulse therapy or orally on a daily basis) and prednisone has been successful in most cases.[45,46] The inhibitor usually becomes undetectable after three or four monthly cycles of chemotherapy. In the case of severe or life-threatening hemorrhage in which there is insufficient time to reduce the level of inhibitor, porcine factor VIII can be administered, because the antibody usually displays low cross-reactivity.

Another alternative therapy for acute bleeding is the administration of procoagulant complexes, which may bypass the inhibitor block by providing large amounts of factor X and factor VII.[47] Still other therapeutic options include plasmapheresis and high-dose intravenous IgG, although the response rate for intravenous immune globulin (IVIg) appears to be quite low.[48] Recombinant activated factor VII (90 μg/kg given as an I.V. bolus every 2 to 3 hours) has been used successfully in patients with this condition. There is growing evidence that rituximab, given intravenously at 375 mg/m² once weekly for 4 weeks, is effective.[49,50] In patients with a very high titer inhibitor (>100 BU/ml), a combination of rituximab and cyclophosphamide may be required.

ACQUIRED VON WILLEBRAND DISEASE

Diagnosis

Patients with acquired von Willebrand disease, who are generally in their 50s and 60s and do not have a personal or family history of a bleeding disorder, present with mucocutaneous-type bleeding.[51] The workup is the same as that for vWD. The acquired form of the disease frequently occurs in the setting of underlying lymphoproliferative, myeloproliferative, or cardiovascular disease. A study showed that acquired vWD is quite common in patients with severe aortic stenosis. vWF abnormalities are directly related to the severity of aortic stenosis and improve after valve replacement.[52] Acquired vWD is also occasionally associated with angiodysplasia in patients with recurrent gastrointestinal bleeding. Frequently, a small monoclonal gammopathy is found on serum protein electrophoresis. The plasma antibody to vWF is functional in a minority of cases, as demonstrated by inhibition of vWF in a functional assay by mixing studies.[53] However, most cases involve nonneutralizing antibodies to vWF, which can be demonstrated by enzyme-linked immunosorbent assay (ELISA). Presumably, the antibody binds to vWF and causes its rapid clearance, leading to a low plasma vWF level. Nonimmune mechanisms (e.g., adsorption of vWF onto tumor cells) have also been described. Multimeric analysis of plasma vWF typically shows a decrease in the high-molecular-weight multimers, resembling type 2A vWD.

Treatment

DDAVP is useful in correcting the bleeding diathesis in about one third of cases of acquired vWD. High-dose intravenous IgG (1 g/kg I.V. daily for 1 to 2 days) generally garners a good temporary response, with an increase in the vWF level and a shortening of the aPTT, lasting from a few days to 2 weeks. If the patient has a defined lymphoproliferative, myeloproliferative, or autoimmune disease, the underlying disease should be treated. However, the response of acquired vWD to immunosuppressive therapy with cyclophosphamide and prednisone is generally not as favorable as the response in the case of acquired factor VIII inhibitor.

HEMORRHAGE CAUSED BY SEVERE LIVER DISEASE

Patients with severe liver disease may suffer life-threatening hemorrhages. The most frequent types are esophageal and gastrointestinal hemorrhages related to varices, gastritis, or peptic ulcer. There may also be bleeding from biopsy sites and during and after surgery. Mucosal and soft tissue bleeding may occur, but generally, this is not the dominant bleeding problem.

The coagulopathy of severe liver disease is complex and not well delineated. Because the liver is the major site of synthesis for all the clotting factors, decreased levels of multiple clotting factors are observed, including fibrinogen, prothrombin, factor V, and factor VII; factor VIII is excepted, presumably because it is an acute-phase reactant. An increased level of abnormal fibrinogen with reduced clotting capability is also observed in patients with cirrhosis.[54] In addition, there is reduced clearance of activated clotting factors by the liver. DIC appears to occur commonly in patients with cirrhosis[55] (presumably because of triggering of the clotting cascade by hepatic tissue damage), but its precise role in both acute fulminant hepatitis and chronic liver disease has not been firmly established. Moderate thrombocytopenia is common, resulting from a combination of decreased platelet production (from relative deficiency of thrombopoietin [TPO], because the liver is the major site of TPO synthesis) and increased platelet destruction from hypersplenism. Platelet function is generally maintained. There is also evidence of hyperfibrinolysis, but its contribution to the overall hemostatic defect is uncertain. The liver also synthesizes most of the natural anticoagulant proteins. AT, protein C, and protein S levels are decreased. The best screening tests for this disorder include the PT, aPTT, platelet count, fibrinogen level, and D-dimer level. Specific assays that may guide therapy include factor V, factor VII, and AT. Replacement for active bleeding is accomplished by administering fresh frozen plasma, cryoprecipitates, and platelets as required. Prothrombin-complex concentrates are not recommended, because they do not replenish all the deficient clotting factors and may exacerbate the DIC. In general, although the multiple hemostatic defects contribute to the bleeding diathesis in severe liver disease, hemodynamic and anatomic factors are the primary determinants in this situation.

PRIMARY FIBRINOLYSIS

Cases of generalized primary fibrinolysis are rare. Many of the early reports of primary fibrinolysis probably represented secondary fibrinolysis associated with DIC. Postprostatectomy hematuria may constitute a true example of hemorrhage caused by localized fibrinolysis. The high concentration of urokinase in the urine in this condition causes plasminogen to be converted to plasmin with resulting clot lysis. If other causes of persistent postoperative hematuria can be ruled out, the condition can be treated with oral or intravenous EACA. Local instillation of EACA by urethral catheter is also effective.

BLEEDING AFTER CARDIOPULMONARY BYPASS

A mild thrombocytopenia (approximately 100,000/μl) commonly occurs in patients after cardiopulmonary bypass surgery.[56] A significant acquired platelet function disorder develops in some patients, probably caused by contact between the platelets and the oxygenator apparatus, which in turn leads to partial platelet degranulation.[57] In addition to the release of platelet granule contents, activation of fibrinolysis may occur together with modest clotting factor depletion.[58] The hemorrhage in such cases generally responds to platelet transfusions. The use of DDAVP in this setting has been reported to reduce postoperative blood loss; however, a meta-analysis of 17 clinical trials showed only a modest beneficial effect.[59]

The bovine protease inhibitor aprotinin has been shown to reduce bleeding and transfusion requirements in patients undergoing cardiopulmonary bypass.[60] Aprotinin inhibits plasmin and may also attenuate the systemic inflammatory response by inhibition of the proinflammatory mediator kallikrein.[61] It reduces plasmin-mediated proteolysis of platelet membrane proteins and preserves platelet function.[62] Randomized clinical trials showed that the two antifibrinolytic agents EACA and tranexamic acid are equally efficacious as aprotinin in this setting.[63,64] Aprotonin should be reserved for patients who are likely to require blood transfusion, especially those undergoing second operations and those with preexisting hemostatic defects.

Table 4 Differential Diagnosis of Postoperative Hemorrhage

Dilutional thrombocytopenia caused by massive transfusion
Acquired platelet function defect after cardiopulmonary bypass
Inadequate heparin neutralization
Disseminated intravascular coagulation
Coagulopathy caused by shock liver
Acquired antithrombin and anti–factor V inhibitors after exposure to fibrin glue
Heparin-induced thrombocytopenia
Thrombocytopenia caused by GPIIb-IIIa inhibitors (e.g., abciximab)
Hyperfibrinolysis after prostate surgery
Undiagnosed von Willebrand disease or hemophilia
Thrombocytopenia caused by posttransfusion purpura
False abnormalities in coagulation test results

Preoperative testing of hemostasis appears not to be useful.

During bypass surgery, patients are sometimes exposed to topical thrombin (fibrin glue), which is used for local hemostasis control. Generally, bovine thrombin and trace amounts of other clotting factors to which patients may develop antibodies are used in these preparations. The antibodies against bovine thrombin cause a prolongation of the TT but are innocuous in themselves. However, potentially serious complications arise when the antibodies cross-react with human thrombin. Some patients develop antibodies against bovine factor V that cross-react with human factor V and may lead to clinical bleeding.[65,66] A review of reported cases found that bovine thrombin-associated factor V antibodies developed in 40% to 66% of cardiac surgery patients and in 20% of neurosurgery patients, and clinical bleeding complications occurred in about one third of these cases.[67] Mixing studies utilizing the patient's plasma and normal plasma will reveal the presence of the inhibitors, and the measurement of the appropriate factor levels will allow the correct diagnosis to be made. Sometimes, plasmapheresis is required to control the acute bleeding.

EVALUATION OF POSTOPERATIVE BLEEDING

Serious hemorrhage during or after surgery is a complicated clinical problem requiring rapid diagnosis and prompt intervention. The first question is whether the bleeding has a local anatomic cause (e.g., unligated vessel) or is the result of a systemic hemostatic failure. If the patient is bleeding only in the operative area, it would suggest a local anatomic cause, such as an unligated bleeding vessel. The patient's bleeding history, especially with the results of prior surgical procedures, is extremely useful, but the available history may be inadequate or incomplete. A revealing clue to a systemic malfunction is bleeding at multiple sites, particularly areas other than that of the surgical wound. Bleeding around a catheter, from venipuncture sites, and from venous cutdowns is highly indicative of a hemorrhagic disorder.

Rapid assessment of the total clinical setting is imperative. The following questions should be addressed:

• Does the patient have underlying renal, hepatic, or malignant disease?
• Has the surgery required pump bypass techniques or the induction of hypothermia, or has the patient been in shock or been hypothermic?
• How many units of blood and blood products have been given and over what period of time?
• Were baseline screening procoagulant tests obtained before surgery, and is the patient's frozen plasma still available?

The differential diagnosis of postoperative hemorrhage should include a number of bleeding disorders [see Table 4].

Prompt resolution of postoperative bleeding requires a panel of coagulation tests—including aPTT, PT, TT, fibrinogen assay, and D-dimer—a platelet count, and a well-stained blood smear for evaluation of platelet and red cell morphology. This battery of tests should be performed immediately. More specialized studies can be obtained if there is evidence of a specific disorder.

The author has no commercial relationships with manufacturers of products or providers of services discussed in this chapter.

Recombinant factor VIIa has not been approved by the FDA for uses described in this chapter.

References

1. Clemetson KJ: Platelet GPIb-V-IX complex. Thromb Haemost 78:266, 1997

2. Fressinaud E, Veyradier A, Truchaud F, et al: Screening for von Willebrand disease with a new analyzer using high shear stress: a study of 60 cases. Blood 91:1325, 1998

3. Posan E, McBane RD, Grill DE, et al: Comparison of PFA-100 testing and bleeding time for detecting platelet hypofunction and von Willebrand disease in clinical practice. Thromb Haemost 90:482, 2003

4. Triplett DA: Laboratory diagnosis of von Willebrand's disease. Mayo Clin Proc 66:832, 1991

5. Sadler JE, Gralnick HR: A new classification for von Willebrand's disease. Blood 84:676, 1994

6. Sadler JE: New concepts in von Willebrand disease. Annu Rev Med 56:173, 2005

7. Sadler JE: Von Willebrand disease type I: a diagnosis in search of a disease. Blood 101:2089, 2003

8. Rose EH, Aledort LM: Nasal spray desmopressin (DDAVP) for mild hemophilia A and von Willebrand disease. Ann Intern Med 114:563, 1991

9. Castillo R, Monteagudo J, Escolar G, et al: Hemostatic effects of normal platelet transfusion in severe von Willebrand's disease patients. Blood 77:1901, 1991

10. Ito M, Yoshimura K, Toyoda N, et al: Pregnancy and delivery in patients with von Willebrand's disease. J Obstet Gynaecol Res 23:37, 1997

11. Rick ME, Williams SB, Sacher RA, et al: Thrombocytopenia associated with pregnancy in a patient with type IIb von Willebrand's disease. Blood 69:786, 1987

12. Antonarakis SE, Rossiter JP, Young M, et al: Factor VIII inversions in severe hemophilia A: results of an international consortium study. Blood 86:2206, 1995

13. Bray GL, Gomperts ED, Courter S, et al: The Recombinate Study Group: a multicenter study of recombinant factor VIII (Recombinate): safety, efficacy, and inhibitor risk in previously untreated patients with hemophilia A. Blood 83:2428, 1994

14. Seremetis S, Lusher JM, Abildgaard CF, et al: Human recombinant DNA-derived antihemophilic factor (factor VIII) in the treatment of hemophilia A: conclusions of a 5-year study of home therapy. The KOGENATE Study Group. Haemophilia 5:9, 1999

15. Courter SG, Bedrosian CL: Clinical evaluation of B-domain deleted recombinant factor VIII in previously untreated patients. Semin Hematol 38(suppl 4):52, 2001

16. Green PP, Mannucci PM, Briet E, et al: Carrier detection in hemophilia A: a cooperative international study: II. The efficacy of a universal discriminant. Blood 67:1560, 1986

17. Rochat C, McFadyen ML, Schwyzer R, et al: Continuous infusion of intermediate-purity factor VIII in haemophilia A patients undergoing elective surgery. Haemophilia 5:181, 1999

18. Yee TT, Pasi KJ, Lilley PA, et al: Factor VIII inhibitors in haemophiliacs: a single-center experience over 34 years, 1964–97. Br J Haematol 104:909, 1999

19. Hough RE, Hampton KK, Preston FE, et al: Recombinant VIIa concentrate in the management of bleeding following prothrombin complex concentrate-related myocardial infarction in patients with haemophilia and inhibitors. Br J Haematol 111:974, 2000

20. Lusher JM: Controlled clinical trials with prothrombin complex concentrates. Prog Clin Biol Res 150:277, 1984

21. Hedner U, Glazer S, Falch J: Recombinant activated factor VII in the treatment of bleeding episodes in patients with inherited and acquired bleeding disorders. Transfusion Med Rev 7:78, 1993

22. Negrier C, Lienhart A: Overall experience with NovoSeven. Blood Coagul Fibrinolysis 11 (suppl 1):S19, 2000

23. van't Veer C, Golden NJ, Mann KG: Inhibition of thrombin generation by the zymogen factor VII: implications for the treatment of hemophilia A by factor VIIa. Blood 95:1330, 2000

24. Monroe DM, Hoffman M, Allen GA, et al: The factor VII–platelet interplay: effectiveness of recombinant factor VIIa in the treatment of bleeding in severe thrombocytopathia. Semin Thromb Hemost 26:373, 2000

25. Roberts HR, Eberst ME: Current management of hemophilia B. Hematol Oncol Clin North Am 7:1269, 1993

26. Wang L, Takabe K, Bidlingmaier SM, et al: Sustained correction of bleeding disorder in hemophilia B mice by gene therapy. Proc Natl Acad Sci USA 30:3906, 1999

27. White GC II: Gene therapy in hemophilia: clinical trials update. Thromb Haemost 86:172, 2001

28. Salomon O, Seligsohn U: New observation on factor XI deficiency. Haemophilia 10(suppl 4):184, 2004

29. Salomon O, Steinberg DM, Tamarin I, et al: Plasma replacement therapy during labor is not mandatory for women with severe factor XI deficiency. Blood Coagul Fibrinolysis 16:37, 2005

30. Fay WP, Parker AC, Condrey LR, et al: Human plasminogen activator inhibitor-1 (PAI-I) deficiency: characterization of a large kindred with a null mutation in the PAI-1 gene. Blood 90:204, 1997

31. Furie B, Furie BC: Molecular and cellular biology of blood coagulation. N Engl J Med 326:800, 1992

32. Sane DC, Califf RM, Topol EJ, et al: Bleeding during thrombolytic therapy for acute myocardial infarction: mechanisms and management. Ann Intern Med 111:1010, 1989

33. Esmon CT, Fukudome K, Mather T, et al: Inflammation, sepsis, and coagulation. Haematologica 84:254, 1999

34. Levi M: Disseminated intravascular coagulation: what's new? Crit Care Clin 21:449, 2005

35. Hall GW: Kasabach-Merritt syndrome: pathogenesis and management. Br J Haematol 112:851, 2001

36. Rickles FR, Levine MN, Edwards RL: Hemostatic alterations in cancer patients. Cancer Metastasis Rev 11:237, 1992

37. Jochum M: Influence of high-dose antithrombin concentrate therapy on the release of cellular proteases, cytokines, and soluble adhesion molecules in acute inflammation. Semin Hematol 32:14, 1995

38. Fourrier F, Chopin C, Huart JJ, et al: Double-blind, placebo-controlled trial of antithrombin III concentrates in septic shock with disseminated intravascular coagulation. Chest 104:882, 1993

39. Bernard GR, Vincent JL, Laterre PF, et al: Efficacy and safety of recombinant human activated protein C for severe sepsis. N Engl J Med 344:699, 2001

40. Dhainaut JF, Yan SB, Joyce DE, et al: Treatment effects of drotrecogin alfa (activated) in patients with severe sepsis with or without overt disseminated intravasular coagulation. J Thromb Haemost 2:1924, 2004

41. Abraham E, Reinhart K, Opal S, et al: Efficacy and safety of tifacogin (recombinant tissue factor pathway inhibitor) in severe sepsis: a randomized controlled trial. JAMA 290:238, 2003

42. Warren BL, Eid A, Singer P, et al: Caring for the critically ill patient: high-dose antithrombin III in severe sepsis: a randomized controlled trial. JAMA 286:1869, 2001

43. Scandella DH, Nakai H, Felch M, et al: In hemophilia A and autoantibody inhibitor patients: the factor VII A2 domain and light chain are most immunogenic. Thromb Res 101:377, 2001

44. Ludlam CA, Morrison AE, Kessler C: Treatment of acquired hemophilia. Sem Hematol 31:16, 1994

45. Lian C-Y, Larcada AF, Chiu AY-Z: Combination immunosuppressive therapy after factor VIII infusion for acquired factor VIII inhibitor. Ann Intern Med 110:774, 1989

46. Shaffer LG, Phillips MD: Successful treatment of acquired hemophilia with oral immunosuppressive therapy. Ann Intern Med 127:206, 1997

47. Morrison AE, Ludlam CA, Kessler C: Use of porcine factor VIII in the treatment of patients with acquired hemophilia. Blood 81:1513, 1993

48. Crenier L, Ducobu J, des Grottes JM, et al: Low response to high-dose intravenous immunoglobulin in the treatment of acquired factor VIII inhibitor. Br J Haematol 95:750, 1996

49. Wiestner A, Cho HJ, Asch AS, et al: Rituximab in the treatment of acquired factor VIII inhibitors. Blood 100:3426, 2002

50. Stasi R, Brunetti M, Stipa E, et al: Selective B-cell depletion with rituximab for the treatment of patients with acquired hemophilia. Blood 103:4424, 2004

51. Federici AB, Rand JH, Bucciarelli P: Acquired von Willebrand syndrome: data from an international registry. Thromb Haemost 84:345, 2000

52. Vincentelli A, Susen S, Le Tourneau T, et al: Acquired von Willebrand syndrome in aortic stenosis. N Engl J Med 349:343, 2003

53. Mohri H, Motomura S, Kanamori H, et al: Clinical significance of inhibitors in acquired von Willebrand syndrome. Blood 91:3623, 1998

54. Francis JL, Armstrong DJ: Acquired dysfibrinogenemia in liver disease. J Clin Pathol 35:667, 1982

55. Stein SF, Harker LA: Kinetic and functional studies of platelets, fibrinogen, and plasminogen in patients with hepatic cirrhosis. J Lab Clin Med 99:217, 1986

56. Pouplard C, May MA, Regina S, et al: Changes in platelet count after cardiac surgery can effectively predict the development of pathogenic heparin-dependent antibodies. Br J Haematol 128:837, 2005

57. Kestin AS, Valeri CR, Khuri SF, et al: The platelet function defect of cardiopulmonary bypass. Blood 82:107, 1993

58. Bolan CD, Alving BM: Pharmacologic agents in the management of bleeding disorders. Transfusion 30:541, 1990

59. Cattaneo M, Harris AS, Stromberg U, et al: The effect of desmopressin on reducing blood loss in cardiac surgery: a meta-analysis of double-blind, placebo-controlled trials. Thromb Haemost 74:1064, 1995

60. Lemmer JH, Dilling WE, Morton JR, et al: Aprotinin for primary coronary artery bypass grafting: a multicenter trial of three dose regimens. Ann Thorac Surg 62:1659, 1996

61. Khan MM, Gikakis N, Miyamoto S, et al: Aprotinin inhibits thrombin formation and monocyte tissue factor in simulated cardiopulmonary bypass. Ann Thorac Surg 68:473, 1999

62. Day JR, Punjabi PP, Randi AM, et al: Clinical inhibition of the seven-transmembrane thrombin receptor (PAR1) by intravenous aprotinin during cardiothoracic surgery. Circulation 110:2597, 2004

63. Greilich PE, Brouse CF, Whitten CW, et al: Antifibrinolytic therapy during cardiopulmonary bypass reduces proinflammatory cytokine levels: a randomized, double-blind, placebo-controlled study of epsilon-aminocaproic acid and aprotinin. J Thorac Cardiovasc Surg 126:1498, 2003

64. Hekmat K, Zimmermann T, Kampe S, et al: Impact of tranexamic acid vs. aprotinin on blood loss and transfusion requirements after cardiopulmonary bypass: a prospective, randomised, double-blind trial. Curr Med Res Opin 20:121, 2004

65. Zehnder JL, Leung LL: Development of antibodies to thrombin and factor V with recurrent bleeding in a patient exposed to topical bovine thrombin. Blood 76:2011, 1990

66. Berruyer M, Amiral J, French P, et al: Immunization by bovine thrombin used with fibrin glue during cardiovascular operations. J Thorac Cardiovasc Surg 105:892, 1993

67. Streiff MB, Ness PM: Acquired FV inhibitors: a needless iatrogenic complication of bovine thrombin exposure. Transfusion 42:18, 2002

99 Thrombotic Disorders

Lawrence L. K. Leung, M.D.

Thrombosis is more than excessive blood clotting; it also involves vascular inflammation. The classic triad of Virchow identifies three major elements in the pathophysiology of thrombosis: endothelial injury, a decrease in blood flow, and an imbalance between procoagulant and anticoagulant factors.

Endothelial cells can be activated or injured by a variety of stimuli, including mechanical trauma, endotoxins and cytokines, proteases, inflammatory mediators, immune complex deposition, oxygen radicals, and hypoxia. Each of these stimuli affects multiple facets of endothelial cell function, ultimately changing the cell from its natural antithrombotic state to a prothrombotic one.

The vascular endothelium, in its unique location in the vessel wall, is capable of sensing and responding to the different mechanical forces in the blood circulation. The shear stress caused by the friction from blood flow seems to be particularly important in modulating endothelial functions. In areas of linear flow, the blood moves in ordered laminar patterns in a regular pulsatile fashion. Such a steady, laminar blood flow apparently promotes an antithrombotic endothelial phenotype. In areas of disrupted flow, such as at vascular bifurcations or stenoses, the endothelium may be exposed to significant changes in shear gradients, and the cells may become activated and prothrombotic.

Imbalance between procoagulant and anticoagulant factors can be hereditary or acquired [*see Table 1*]. Some clotting factors, such as factor VIII and fibrinogen, are acute-phase reactants: their plasma levels increase significantly with acute inflammation, possibly conferring a transient prothrombotic state. Some hereditary deficiencies of anticoagulant proteins, such as factor V Leiden and antithrombin (AT), are associated with recurrent thrombosis; these are among the best understood clinical hypercoagulable states.

Although the hypercoagulable state is systemic, thrombosis occurs locally (e.g., in the lower extremities). The clinical outcome likely reflects a complex interaction between the systemic prothrombotic predisposition and local hemostatic control mechanisms specific to the vascular bed. Specific and distinctive gene transcript expression patterns in different vascular beds have now been demonstrated.[1]

Assessment of Patients with Thrombotic Disorders

PRIMARY CLINICAL ISSUES IN THROMBOTIC DISORDERS

Important questions in the assessment of thrombosis include the following: (1) How likely is it that the thrombosis is caused by an underlying hypercoagulable state? (2) How extensive a workup is indicated? (3) When should the workup be done? Answers to these questions come from a consideration of the patient's age at the time of the first thrombosis; presence or absence of a provoking factor; family history and past medical history of response to situations associated with high risk of thrombosis; and the site, type, and severity of the thrombosis.

Age of Onset of First Thrombosis

In a retrospective study involving 150 families with an inherited predisposition to recurrent thrombosis (thrombophilia), the mean age at the time of the first thrombosis was 35 to 40 years. However, the first episode of thrombosis can occur as early as the second decade of life if the patient has more than one hereditary risk factor.[2]

Presence or Absence of a Provoking Factor

Common triggers of thrombosis are surgery, trauma, pregnancy, malignancy, prolonged immobilization, and infection. Malignancy or infection can be clinically overt or subclinical. Those circumstances can provoke thrombosis even in persons with a normal coagulation system, and they often uncover a thrombophilia that had been clinically silent.[2] However, sometimes no provoking factors can be identified. Such a spontaneous, idiopathic thrombosis, especially when it occurs in a young person, strongly suggests an underlying hereditary hypercoagulable state.

If thrombosis develops in a patient who has had previous pregnancies or surgeries (especially orthopedic procedures)

Table 1 **Inherited and Acquired Hypercoagulable States**

Inherited
- Resistance to activated protein C/factor V Leiden
- Prothrombin gene mutation 20210A
- Antithrombin III deficiency
- Protein C deficiency
- Protein S deficiency
- Hyperhomocysteinemia

Acquired
- Antiphospholipid antibody syndrome
- Hypercoagulable state associated with physiologic or thrombogenic stimuli:
  - Advancing age
  - Oral contraceptives
  - Pregnancy
  - Surgery
  - Trauma
- Hypercoagulable state associated with other clinical conditions:
  - Malignancy—Trousseau syndrome
  - Heparin-induced thrombocytopenia with thrombosis
  - Nephrotic syndrome
  - Hyperviscosity (polycythemia vera, Waldenström macroglobinemia, multiple myeloma)
  - Myeloproliferative disorders (polycythemia vera, essential thrombocythemia)
  - Paroxysmal nocturnal hemoglobinuria
  - Sickle cell anemia

Rare or not well established
- Dysfibrinogenemia
- Hypoplasminogenemia, dysplasminogenemia
- Abnormal thrombomodulin
- Factor XII deficiency
- Elevated factor VII, factor VIII, fibrinogen, lipoprotein(a), plasminogen activator inhibitor–1

Table 2   Screening Tests for Patients with Suspected Hypercoagulable State

Underlying State	Laboratory Evaluation

Venous thrombosis	Resistance to activated protein C
	  Factor V Leiden (genetic test)
	  Clotting assay (unnecessary if the genetic test for factor V Leiden is positive)
	Prothrombin mutation 20210A (genetic test)
	Antithrombin III (functional assay)
	Protein C (functional assay)
	Protein S
	  Functional assay
	  Antigenic assay for free protein S

Arterial thrombosis	Antibodies associated with heparin-induced thrombocytopenia* Chronic disseminated intravascular coagulation (Trousseau syndrome)* Lipoprotein(a)

Venous thrombosis and/or arterial thrombosis	Plasma homocysteine
	  Fasting level
	  Level after methionine loading (if thrombophilia is strongly suspected)
	Antiphospholipid antibody
	  Clotting assays for lupuslike anticoagulant
	  ELISA for anticardiolipin antibodies IgG and IgM
	Dysfibrinogenemia (if thrombophilia is strongly suspected)
	  Functional assay for fibrinogen level
	  Thrombin time, reptilase time

*In appropriate clinical settings.
ELISA—enzyme-linked immunosorbent assay

without any thrombotic complications, an acquired hypercoagulable state should be considered. Likely conditions in such cases are antiphospholipid antibody syndrome or Trousseau syndrome (see below).

Family History

Objectively documented venous thromboembolism before 50 years of age in a first-degree family member strongly suggests a hereditary thrombotic disorder. However, a negative family history does not exclude a hereditary condition. Clinical thrombosis is frequently the culmination of multiple thrombogenic risk factors, only one of which may be hereditary and irreversible. In patients with symptomatic thrombosis and well-documented hereditary hypercoagulable states, it is not uncommon to find other family members with the same deficiency but no clinical thrombosis.

Recurrent Thrombosis

A patient who experiences recurrent thrombosis likely has a hypercoagulable state (hereditary or acquired). However, if a patient who initially presented with deep vein thrombosis (DVT) in a lower extremity returns with symptoms involving the same leg, the problem may be postphlebitic syndrome rather than recurrent thrombosis. Acute exacerbation of the postphlebitic syndrome, with its increased leg edema and pain, can be difficult to distinguish from recurrent acute DVT. As an anticipatory measure, it is sometimes useful to obtain a repeat compression ultrasound study of the lower extremity after resolution of an acute episode of DVT; the repeat scan can provide a baseline for future comparison.

Site of Thrombosis

Most commonly, thromboses involve the deep veins of the lower extremities. Thrombosis at an atypical site, such as the hepatic, mesenteric, or cerebral veins (or skin necrosis after warfarin administration), increases the likelihood of an underlying hypercoagulable state. Spontaneous axillary vein thrombosis may also indicate the presence of an underlying hypercoagulable state, but this association is controversial.[2-4]

Recurrent thrombosis at arterial sites has a differential diagnosis—and therefore a workup—that is quite different from that for recurrent venous thrombosis [see Table 2]. Most of the common hereditary hypercoagulable states (e.g., AT deficiency or factor V Leiden) are associated with venous thromboses, such as DVT in the lower extremities. They are seldom associated with arterial thromboses, such as transient ischemic attack, stroke, digital ischemia, and myocardial infarction. A few hypercoagulable states, such as the antiphospholipid syndrome and hyperhomocysteinemia, are associated with both types of thrombosis.

The Hypercoagulable Workup

Extent of the workup   On the basis of the above clinical considerations, one may estimate the likelihood of an underlying thrombophilia in a given patient with thrombosis [see Table 3]. Because studies of cost-effectiveness and outcomes are not available, it is difficult to list strict practice guidelines regarding the extent of the hypercoagulable workup. In general, however, if the likelihood of an underlying hypercoagulable state is high, an extensive workup is warranted.

A limited workup is appropriate for mild to moderate DVT of the lower extremities with an obvious provoking factor. For example, in a young woman who experiences DVT in the superficial femoral vein while on an oral contraceptive, evaluation of factor V Leiden, prothrombin mutation 20210A, AT, protein C, protein S, homocysteine, anticardiolipin antibodies, and lupus anticoagulant may be sufficient. On the other hand, an acquired hypercoagulable state should be considered in an elderly patient with a spontaneous DVT and no history of previous thrombosis. Diagnostic possibilities in such cases would include antiphospholipid antibody syndrome, acquired AT deficiency (if the patient has evidence of nephrotic syndrome), or Trousseau syndrome.

When the clinical history strongly suggests thrombophilia—as in a patient with recurrent thrombosis or thrombosis at atypical sites—one may argue that a workup for an underlying hypercoagulable state is unnecessary because the result will not alter the management of the case. However, the identification of any underlying risk factors will improve the understanding of the disease for both the patient and the treating physician; and it will guide the counseling of the patient, especially regarding the need for screening of related family members. In the case of hyperhomocysteinemia and elevated lipoprotein(a) levels, identifi-

---

Table 3   Clinical Features That Suggest Thrombophilia

Age at onset of first thrombosis < 50 yr
No identifiable risk factor
Positive family history
Recurrent thrombosis
Atypical site of thrombosis

cation of risk factors will permit the use of specific therapies (see below).

Timing of the workup The clinician needs to know not only what tests to order but when to order them. In acute thrombosis, many inhibitors of the clotting cascade (e.g., AT and protein C) are consumed. Immediately after the episode, their plasma levels may be decreased, even in patients who do not have a hereditary deficiency. Heparin therapy can reduce antithrombin levels up to 20%, whereas warfarin treatment reduces the levels of protein C and protein S. Usually it is best to postpone measurement of these inhibitors until the acute thrombotic episode is completely resolved, preferably 4 weeks after termination of oral anticoagulation therapy. Tests for specific genotypes (e.g., factor V Leiden) can be performed at any time, however.

Frequency and Relative Risk of Venous Thromboembolism

The frequency of various hypercoagulable states in unselected patients who present with venous thrombosis ranges from 1% to 25% [see Table 4]. It should be recognized that these thrombophilias do not confer equivalent thrombotic risk. Factor V Leiden and prothrombin mutation 20210A, the two most prevalent risk factors, confer only a modest increase in relative risk of thrombosis, approximately threefold to sevenfold above normal. Moderate hyperhomocysteinemia, another common risk factor, also carries a modest increase in risk. Heterozygous deficiencies of AT, protein C, and protein S are generally considered more significant risk factors than factor V Leiden. AT deficiency and the antiphospholipid antibody syndrome are probably the greatest risk factors. The recurrence rate in patients with antiphospholipid antibody syndrome is as high as 50% to 70% in some studies.

Patients with symptomatic thrombosis frequently have more than one risk factor, which may have a synergistic effect in increasing the thrombosis risk. For example, women with factor V Leiden who use oral contraceptives have a risk of venous thromboembolism that is 35-fold higher than that in the general population.

Table 4 Frequency and Relative Risk of Venous Thrombosis in Selected Hypercoagulable States*

Condition	Relative Risk[†]	Frequency[‡]
Antithrombin III deficiency	High	1%–2%
Protein C deficiency	High	3%–4%
Protein S deficiency	High	2%–3%
Factor V Leiden	Modest	20%–25%
Prothrombin mutation 20210A	Modest	10%
Hyperhomocysteinemia	Modest	10%
Oral contraceptive use	Modest	NA

*The incidence of venous thromboembolism in the normal population is estimated to be 0.008% a year (0.03% a year in patients who take oral contraceptives).
[†]Modest risk is defined as an approximate 2.5-fold to fivefold increase in thromboembolism, on the basis of data from the Leiden Thrombophilia Study[146]; high risk is defined as an approximate threefold to fourfold increase over that for factor V Leiden.[2]
[‡]In unselected patients with venous thromboembolism.

Hereditary Hypercoagulable States

ANTITHROMBIN DEFICIENCY

Epidemiology and Etiology

The frequency of symptomatic inherited AT deficiency in the general population has been estimated to be approximately 1 per 2,000 people.[5] The deficiency is transmitted in an autosomal dominant pattern. Homozygous AT deficiency has not been reported, presumably because the condition is incompatible with normal fetal development.

There are two types of inherited AT deficiency. Type I is quantitative, as measured by antigenic and functional assays. A large number of molecular mutations have been characterized in type I AT deficiency, including partial gene deletions and single-nucleotide substitutions that cause nonsense or missense mutations leading to premature stop signals in the protein-translation process.

Type II deficiency is qualitative; plasma levels of AT antigen are normal. The underlying defect is generally a single nucleotide change that causes missense mutations, giving rise to a dysfunctional protein. Many of these proteins have decreased affinity for heparin binding.

In rare cases, AT deficiency is acquired. This condition may occur after administration of intravenous heparin for more than 3 days or after asparaginase therapy. It may also develop in patients with disseminated intravascular coagulation (DIC), severe liver disease, or the nephrotic syndrome.

Pathophysiology

AT inactivates factor Xa and thrombin by forming a stable stoichiometric complex with each of them. AT is present in sufficient amounts in plasma to inactivate all the thrombin formed in a given plasma volume, but it does so slowly unless it is activated by endothelial cell surface heparan sulfate or by administered heparin [see Chapter 97]. Patients with hereditary AT deficiency have evidence of continuous factor X activation and thrombin generation (as supported by elevated plasma levels of prothrombin fragment F1.2) even when they are clinically asymptomatic.

Clinical Presentation

Patients with AT deficiency show an increased incidence of venous thrombosis, usually triggered by a prothrombotic stimulus such as surgery, infection, immobilization, or trauma. This association suggests that the superimposition of a prothrombotic stimulus on an underlying subclinical hypercoagulable state leads to clinical thrombosis.

Typical clinical presentations are DVT of the legs, pulmonary embolism, and occasionally mesenteric vein thrombosis. There is no convincing evidence to suggest that AT deficiency increases the risk of arterial thrombosis.[6]

Affected patients usually have a family history of recurrent thromboses, generally beginning in youth and often associated with surgery or trauma. Pregnancy and the use of oral contraceptives also increase the risk of thromboses in AT-deficient patients. The tendency to thrombosis increases with advancing age: by age 50, only 10% of AT-deficient patients are free of symptoms.

Diagnosis

The AT level should be determined by a functional assay rather than an antigenic assay, so that both type I and type II deficiency can be evaluated. Patients with AT deficiency have a surprisingly modest reduction in the protein: values measured by both bioassay and immunoassay range from 25% to 60% of normal in type I disease.

Treatment

Study of a large AT-deficient kindred indicates that long-term anticoagulant prophylaxis is not warranted in asymptomatic carriers of this deficiency.[7] Asymptomatic carriers should receive prophylactic anticoagulation only in situations known to increase the risk of thrombogenesis, such as abdominal surgery.[7] Once such patients have experienced a thrombotic event, however, they probably require lifelong warfarin therapy. Warfarin is the mainstay of long-term therapy for patients with AT deficiency and recurrent thromboembolism.

Acute episodes of thrombosis must be treated with heparin. Because AT deficiency may render heparin relatively ineffective, the physician should be alert to heparin resistance. In patients receiving unfractionated heparin, resistance is manifested by minimal prolongation of the partial thromboplastin time (PTT) despite the administration of therapeutic doses. If low-molecular-weight heparin (LMWH) is used, as is commonly the case, the level of anti–factor Xa (anti-FXa) should be checked to ensure that a therapeutic anticoagulant effect is achieved [see Chapter 96].

If heparin resistance occurs despite increased doses of heparin, heparin plus purified AT concentrates or fresh frozen plasma should be given. AT has a half-life of about 60 hours. These preparations can be used to carry an AT–deficient patient through surgery or delivery and should bring the AT level up to nearly 100%, depending on the patient's baseline AT level. The AT level should be checked and the infusion repeated at 24-hour intervals to maintain a normal AT level for 5 to 7 days after delivery or surgery.

Pregnancy in an AT–deficient patient is difficult to manage. Because warfarin may cause fetal malformations and neonatal hemorrhage, patients should be treated with full-dose unfractionated heparin or LMWH; those receiving LMWH should be switched to unfractionated heparin 1 to 2 weeks before delivery so that rapid reversal of anticoagulation, if necessary, can be more easily attained. If a therapeutic effect cannot be achieved (as measured by the PTT with unfractionated heparin or the anti-FXa level with LMWH), an AT infusion can be given.[8] Generally, this is not necessary. Anticoagulation should be promptly reinstituted after delivery.

PROTEIN C AND PROTEIN S DEFICIENCY

Pathophysiology and Clinical Presentation

Deficiency or defect in protein C or protein S results in a loss of ability to inactivate excess factor VIIIa and factor Va, the two major cofactors that regulate amplification of the clotting cascade. Protein C levels are low in patients with DIC and liver disease, probably because the activation of hemostasis consumes this factor [see Chapter 97].

Homozygous protein C deficiency causes lethal thrombosis in infants. Heterozygous protein C deficiency probably occurs with a prevalence of 1 per 200 to 300 in the general population. Clinical expression of heterozygous protein C deficiency varies: many persons with heterozygous deficiency, as well as persons with low-normal protein C levels from other causes, do not experience thrombosis,[9] whereas other patients with heterozygous

deficiency exhibit a definite tendency toward venous thrombosis even though their protein C levels are 40% to 50% of normal. This phenotypic variability suggests multiple gene interactions and supports the hypothesis that clinical thrombosis in such patients may result from a combination of protein C deficiency and one or more other prothrombotic mutations.[10] Cerebral venous thrombosis presumably accounts for cases of cerebral hemorrhagic infarction that occur in young adults with protein C deficiency.

Deficiency of protein S also leads to venous thrombosis, including mesenteric vein thrombosis. Pregnancy and the use of oral contraceptives lower the protein S level, which may account for some cases of thromboembolism that occur under such circumstances.[11] Acquired protein S deficiency also occurs in patients with the nephrotic syndrome, who lose protein S in urine.[12] Case reports have associated protein S deficiency with warfarin-induced skin necrosis.[13]

Diagnosis

Functional and antigenic assays for protein C and protein S are now available in most coagulation laboratories. Functional assays are preferable for diagnosis. It is important to measure free protein S because some patients who have low free protein S levels have normal or borderline total protein S levels. Coagulation assays for protein C and protein S can give falsely low values in patients with factor V Leiden.[14]

Treatment

Warfarin is the treatment of choice for preventing thrombosis, even though it lowers protein C levels still further. Because the half-life of protein C is only 6 to 7 hours, much shorter than that of prothrombin and factor X, a period of enhanced hypercoagulability follows initiation of warfarin therapy in patients with protein C deficiency. Heparin should be given along with warfarin during the initiation of anticoagulation; it can be withdrawn afterward. Warfarin-induced skin necrosis is a rare complication of anticoagulation therapy.

FACTOR V LEIDEN

Epidemiology and Etiology

Factor V Leiden is a mutated form of factor V (first identified by researchers in Leiden, The Netherlands) that, once activated, is relatively resistant to the anticoagulant effects of activated protein C (APC). The defect is transmitted as an autosomal dominant trait. Approximately 5% of the general white population is heterozygous for factor V Leiden; the defect is almost absent in other ethnic groups.[15] Factor V Leiden is now considered to be the most common hereditary hypercoagulable state. Its prevalence in patients with thrombophilia is as high as 20% to 50%.[16] In a large cohort study of unselected patients with a first episode of symptomatic DVT, factor V Leiden was found in 16% of patients.[17] In women who have thrombosis while taking oral contraceptives, the frequency of factor V Leiden is about 23%.[18] The relative risk of DVT in a factor V Leiden homozygote (estimated incidence, 0.5% to 1% a year) is approximately 80-fold higher than in a normal person.[19] The risk of thrombosis in persons who are heterozygous for factor V Leiden is estimated to be fourfold to eightfold higher than that in normal persons; the relative risk increases to more than 30-fold when factor V Leiden is combined with oral contraceptive use. The absolute risk of thrombosis, however, is low.[20] Association of factor V Leiden

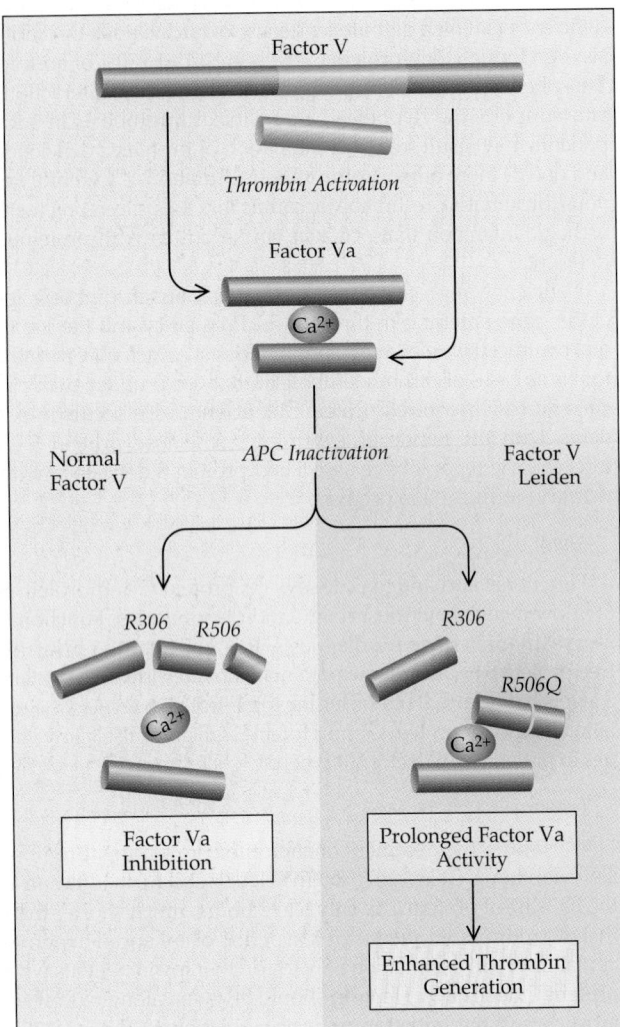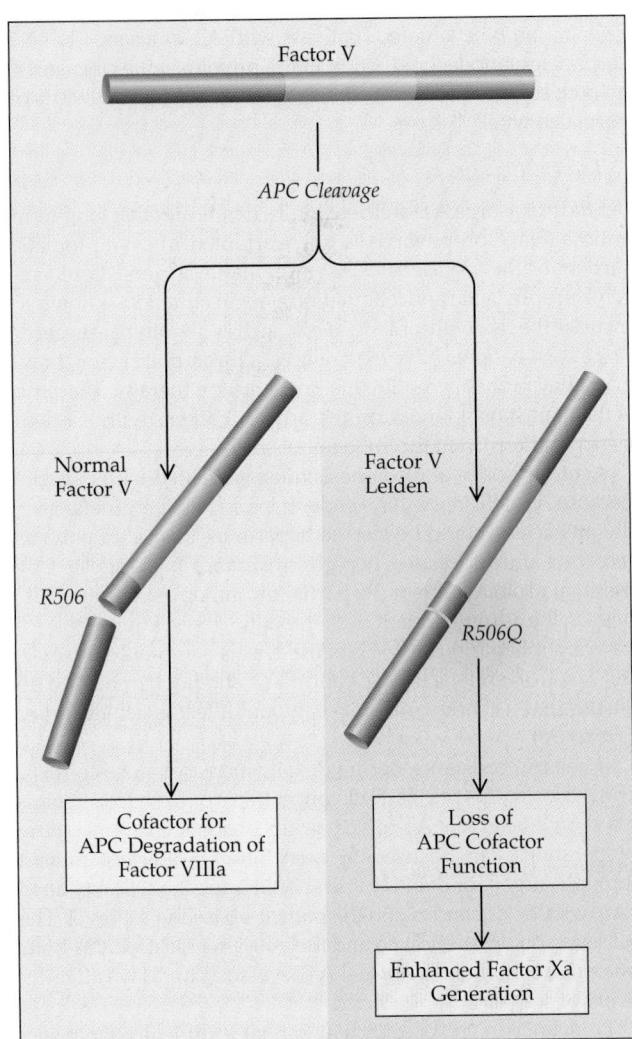

Figure 1   Degradation of thrombin-activated factor V Leiden by activated protein C (APC) is significantly slower than that of normal activated factor V (factor Va), which leads to enhanced thrombin generation (left). Recent evidence suggests that normal factor V, together with protein S, serves as a cofactor of APC in the inhibition of factor VIIIa (right). This APC cofactor function of factor V requires the cleavage of factor V by APC at arginine 506; therefore, factor V Leiden has a poor cofactor function.

with deficiencies of protein C, protein S, or AT has been reported in some families.[21-23] Overall, although factor V Leiden is highly prevalent, it is a relatively weak risk factor for thrombosis.

Approximately 5% of cases associated with inherited resistance to APC are attributable to other mutations and defects.[24-26] Conditions such as factor VIII elevation, pregnancy, oral contraceptive use, and lupus anticoagulant may result in APC resistance.[27] APC resistance that is not caused by factor V Leiden may be a risk factor for stroke[28,29] and venous thrombosis.[30,31] The overall risk of venous thrombosis from APC resistance is similar to or less than that posed by factor V Leiden.[32]

Pathophysiology

Resistance to the anticoagulant effects of APC is caused by a specific mutation in factor V (factor V Leiden or factor V R506Q) that results from a single-nucleotide substitution that leads to the replacement of arginine with glutamine at position 506.[32] Arginine 506 is located at one of the two major APC cleavage sites of activated factor V. Activated factor V Leiden expresses normal procoagulant activity, but its degradation by APC is ap-

proximately 10 times slower than that of normal activated factor V (factor Va). This slowing leads to increased thrombin generation.[33] In addition, evidence suggests that factor V (but not factor Va), together with protein S, serves as a cofactor of APC in the inhibition of the factor VIIIa/factor IXa complex and that factor V Leiden has a poor APC cofactor function [*see Figure 1*].

Clinical Presentation

Clinical manifestations of factor V Leiden are similar to those of deficiencies of AT, protein C, and protein S—mainly, venous thrombosis. However, the first thrombotic manifestation in factor V Leiden often occurs later than in the other hereditary thrombophilic states. Approximately 25% of apparently healthy men older than 60 years who experience a first episode of venous thrombosis have factor V Leiden.[34] There are conflicting data on whether factor V Leiden is associated with an increased risk of recurrent deep vein thrombosis. Several studies reported a slightly enhanced recurrence risk (twofold to fourfold), but more recent studies have shown that the risk of recurrence is similar to that in persons without the mutation.[17,35,36]

Diagnosis

Factor V Leiden can be identified rapidly and precisely with simple DNA-based tests. These tests allow the diagnosis to be made in patients receiving anticoagulation therapy with warfarin and in those who have coexisting antiphospholipid antibodies. Because factor V Leiden is not the sole cause of APC resistance, it may be worthwhile to pursue the diagnosis with an APC-resistance test in selected cases.

Treatment

Management of factor V Leiden is similar to that of AT, protein C, and protein S deficiencies. Patients with a first episode of venous thrombosis should receive anticoagulation therapy for 6 months. Thereafter, they should be given prophylactic anticoagulation therapy in situations known to provoke thrombosis. Long-term anticoagulation should be considered in patients with recurrent thrombosis.[37]

Young women known to be factor V Leiden carriers should avoid the use of oral contraceptives, which increases the relative risk of thrombosis (although the risk remains low in terms of absolute incidence). The optimal treatment of carriers during pregnancy has not been established. The rate of venous thromboembolism is low, about 2% without thrombosis prophylaxis.[20] My practice is not to use thrombosis prophylaxis routinely during pregnancy, but I will consider postpartum prophylaxis for 6 weeks, especially when the family history of thrombosis is strong. Routine screening of family members of patients with factor V Leiden is not cost-effective.[38]

PROTHROMBIN GENE MUTATION 20210A

A G-to-A mutation at nucleotide position 20210 in the 3' untranslated region of the prothrombin gene is associated with an increased incidence of venous thrombosis. The prevalence of the mutation in healthy persons is about 2.3%. Like factor V Leiden, this mutation is very rare in Asians and Africans. Unlike factor V Leiden, it is more common in southern Europeans than in northern Europeans.[39] The relative risk of thrombosis in persons with this mutation is 2.8, which is similar to the relative risk in those with factor V Leiden.[40] The mutation can be found in up to 18% of patients with thrombosis and family histories of thrombosis. The most common presentation is DVT of the lower extremities. Prospective studies have not shown an increased risk of recurrent DVT in patients with this mutation.[41] However, carriers who are heterozygous for both factor V Leiden and the prothrombin mutation have a higher risk of recurrent thrombosis.[35] The combination of oral-contraceptive use and the prothrombin gene mutation is associated with an increased incidence of cerebral vein thrombosis in young women.[42]

HYPERHOMOCYSTEINEMIA

Homocysteine is a highly reactive amino acid that is normally found in blood at levels of 5 to 15 mmol/L. Normally, homocysteine is derived from methionine by a transmethylation process and is remethylated to methionine or converted to cysteine [see Figure 2]. Metabolism of homocysteine requires betaine, cobalamin (vitamin B_{12}), folate, and pyridoxine (vitamin B_6).

Homocysteine can promote oxidation of low-density lipoprotein (LDL) cholesterol and presumably is toxic to vascular endothelium.[43,44] It may also inhibit thrombomodulin expression and protein C activation and suppress endothelial heparan sulfate expression; both of these effects lead to hypercoagulability.[45,46] Homocysteine also enhances the binding of lipoprotein(a) (an atherogenic lipoprotein) to fibrin, which may provide a link between hyperhomocysteinemia, thrombosis, and premature atherosclerosis [see Lipoprotein(a), below].[47] The vascular damage caused by high homocysteine levels leads to arterial and venous thrombosis and, perhaps, accelerated atherosclerosis.

Epidemiology and Etiology

Hyperhomocysteinemia can be divided into three classes: severe (homocysteine plasma concentration > 100 mmol/L), moderate (25 to 100 mmol/L), or mild (16 to 24 mmol/L). Severe hyperhomocysteinemia is usually caused by a homozygous deficiency of the enzyme cystathionine β-synthase. Affected persons have severe mental retardation, ectopic lens, skeletal abnormalities, and severe early-onset arterial and venous thrombotic disease.[48]

Mild or moderate hyperhomocysteinemia results from either hereditary or acquired defects in the homocysteine metabolic pathway. Heterozygous deficiency in cystathionine β-synthase is quite common in the general population, with a frequency of 0.3% to 1.4%.[48] A defect in the remethylation pathway is commonly caused by a thermolabile mutant of the methylenetetrahydrofolate reductase (MTHFR) enzyme whose activity is approximately 50% of normal; the homozygous state has a prevalence of 5% in the general population.[49] However, the homozygous form of the MTHFR thermolabile enzyme isoform is not clinically relevant in patients whose diet includes adequate folate.

Common causes of acquired hyperhomocysteinemia are deficiencies of dietary cobalamin, folate, or pyridoxine. A prospective study found that mild hyperhomocysteinemia is quite common in the elderly, despite normal serum vitamin concentrations.[50] Acquired hyperhomocysteinemia is also common in patients with end-stage renal disease.

Mild to moderate hyperhomocysteinemia is associated with cerebrovascular disease, coronary artery disease, and peripheral vascular disease in persons younger than 55 years and with carotid artery stenosis in the elderly.[51,52] It is found in 10% of patients with a first episode of DVT.[53] In a prospective study, a graded relationship was found between elevated plasma homocysteine levels and mortality in patients with coronary artery disease.[54]

Clinical Presentation

Severe hyperhomocysteinemia should be suspected in patients with the characteristic phenotype (see above). Mild to moderate hyperhomocysteinemia should be suspected in cases of arterial and venous thrombotic disease—including cerebrovascular disease, peripheral arterial disease, and DVT—especially in young persons.

Diagnosis

Plasma homocysteine exists in free and protein-bound forms and is generally measured and reported as total plasma homocysteine (normal range, 5 to 15 mmol/L). Diagnosis of hyperhomocysteinemia is usually made by measuring plasma homocysteine levels after an overnight fast. Because as many as 40% of patients with hyperhomocysteinemia may have a normal fasting level, a methionine-loading test should be considered when indicated.[55] However, methionine is not generally available in most pharmacies. Plasma folate and vitamin B_{12} levels should also be measured to exclude hyperhomocysteinemia caused by folate or B_{12} deficiencies.

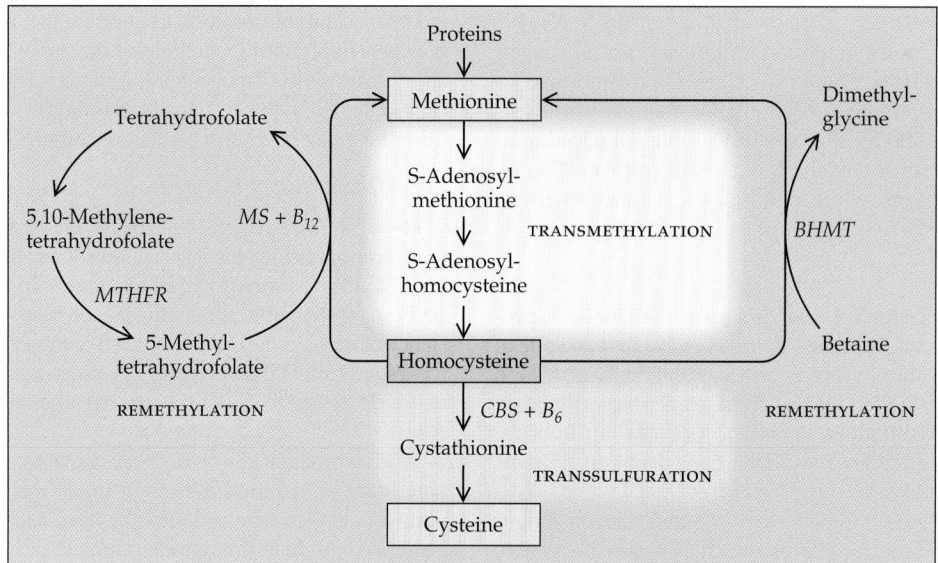

Figure 2   Homocysteine's intracellular metabolism occurs through remethylation to methionine or transsulfuration to cysteine.[142] Elevation in plasma homocysteine levels can result from hereditary deficiency in cystathionine β-synthase (CBS); a thermolabile mutant of methylene-tetrahydrofolate reductase (MTHFR); or low dietary levels of cobalamin (vitamin B_{12}), folate, or pyridoxine (vitamin B_6), which are essential cofactors in the metabolic process. (BHMT—betaine-homocysteine methyltransferase)

Treatment

Daily use of oral pyridoxine (250 mg) and folic acid (5 mg) brings elevated homocysteine levels down to normal in most cases.[56] Patients who have vitamin B_{12} deficiency should be given B_{12} supplements. Repeat measurement of plasma homocysteine levels (generally done 1 month after starting supplementation) may be prudent to ensure that the treatment with pyridoxine and folate is working. Betaine (3 g p.o., b.i.d.) is sometimes effective in patients with hyperhomocysteinemia that is resistant to pyridoxine and folate. It is currently unknown whether correction of hyperhomocysteinemia by these measures leads to clinical benefit.

LIPOPROTEIN(A)

Lipoprotein(a) [Lp(a)] is an independent risk factor for coronary artery thrombosis.[57] A prospective case-control study associated elevated plasma Lp(a) levels with an approximately threefold increase in risk of coronary artery disease in men.[58] The association between high Lp(a) and ischemic stroke in young adults is controversial.[59,60] Distributions of Lp(a) are skewed in the general population—especially among whites, in whom the median is 3.7 mg/dl but the mean is 6.9 mg/dl.[61] The 95th percentile for plasma Lp(a) is estimated to be in the 25 to 30 mg/dl range.

The Lp(a) class of lipoproteins is formed by the assembly of LDL particles and apoprotein(a), a protein that has some structural similarities to plasminogen (specifically, in the kringle domains) and competes with plasminogen for the endothelial cell binding site, thereby displacing plasminogen and downregulating plasmin generation at the endothelial cell surface.[62] High plasma concentrations of Lp(a) may therefore suppress the endothelial fibrinolytic response. Lp(a) is found in the intima of human atherosclerotic vessels, and transgenic mice expressing human Lp(a) develop extensive atherosclerosis.[63] Measurement of Lp(a) levels can be done in commercial laboratories and should be considered in young patients with arterial thrombosis. Elevated LDL cholesterol levels appear to elicit or exacerbate the risk factors associated with high Lp(a), and, therefore, diet,

exercise, and standard pharmacologic approaches should be used in patients with high LDL cholesterol levels.[64] In small studies, niacin at high doses (2 to 4 g p.o. daily) and tamoxifen (20 mg daily) have lowered elevated Lp(a) levels by 30% to 40%.[65,66] High doses of niacin are frequently associated with facial flushing and headaches. These unpleasant side effects can be ameliorated by starting niacin at a low dose (e.g., 300 mg daily) and then increasing the dose incrementally over time or through the use of extended-release niacin. Liver function should be checked periodically.

DYSFIBRINOGENEMIA

Approximately 300 abnormal fibrinogens (dysfibrinogens) have been reported, and about 85 structural defects have been identified in dysfibrinogenemia. These are most commonly characterized by functional defects of fibrinopeptide A release and fibrin polymerization and less commonly by defective plasminogen binding and activation. About half of the fibrinogen mutations are not associated with any clinical symptoms. Mild bleeding or recurrent thrombosis occurs in about equal numbers in the remaining mutations.[67] In rare cases, patients experience both bleeding and thrombosis. Acquired dysfibrinogenemia may complicate hepatocellular carcinoma or chronic liver disease. Evaluation in a general laboratory usually shows a discrepancy between antigenic and functional levels of fibrinogen, because most patients with dysfibrinogens have suboptimal clotting function, with prolonged thrombin time (TT) and reptilase time (RT). The abnormal fibrinogens form fibrin clots that are resistant to clot lysis. Precise identification of the structural defect requires substantial effort in a research laboratory. Management of recurrent thrombosis caused by dysfibrinogenemia is the same as that in other patients with thrombophilia.

DYSPLASMINOGEN AND ABNORMAL FIBRINOLYSIS

In rare cases, abnormal plasminogens (dysplasminogens), which are defective in their activation to plasmin, are associated with thrombosis. Patients with such a disorder have a low plasma plasminogen level on functional assays.[68] Increased levels of plasminogen activator inhibitor–1 (PAI-1) and decreased plasma fibrinolytic activity have been reported in patients with preeclampsia.[69] Acquired impairment of fibrinolytic activity may be associated with postoperative thrombosis.[70] However, more studies are required to establish the role of abnormal fibrinolysis in recurrent clinical thrombosis.[71] Antigenic assays for tissue plasminogen activator (t-PA) and PAI-1 are available in some commercial laboratories, but specific functional assays are available only in research laboratories.

ELEVATED FIBRINOGEN, FACTOR VII, AND FACTOR VIII LEVELS

A high plasma fibrinogen level is an independent risk factor for coronary artery disease.[72] An elevated factor VII level has also been associated with the development of heart disease.[73] A factor VIII level above the 90th percentile of normal is associated with an approximately fivefold increased risk of a first episode of DVT[74,75]; it also increases the risk of recurrence.[76] Additional studies are required to establish the clinical utility of measuring these parameters in patients with thrombosis.

Acquired Hypercoagulable States

ANTIPHOSPHOLIPID ANTIBODY SYNDROME

The antiphospholipid antibody syndrome is caused by autoantibodies to proteins associated with negatively charged phospholipids. The terms antiphospholipid and anticardiolipin are used synonymously. Antiphospholipid antibodies also include lupus anticoagulant, which is an inhibitor that was first identified in patients with systemic lupus erythematosus. Many patients who have this inhibitor do not have lupus, and it is sometimes called lupuslike anticoagulant.

Epidemiology

Antiphospholipid antibody syndrome occurs secondary to systemic lupus erythematosus and, less commonly, to rheumatoid arthritis, temporal arteritis, and other connective tissue disorders. It is also associated with HIV-1 and hepatitis C infections, lymphoproliferative diseases, and certain drugs (e.g., phenothiazine and procainamide). When no risk factor can be identified, the syndrome is regarded as primary. In a large cohort study of 1,000 patients with antiphospholipid antibody syndrome, 53% of patients were classified as having primary antiphospholipid antibody syndrome, and 47% had secondary antiphospholipid antibody syndrome.[77]

Pathophysiology

The two most common protein targets for the antiphospholipid antibodies appear to be β_2-glycoprotein I (β_2-GPI) and prothrombin. β_2-GPI is a plasma protein that binds anionic phospholipids with high affinity. It has weak anticoagulant function in vitro. β_2-GPI can induce cardiolipin from its usual bilaminar form to a hexagonal form that is highly immunogenic.[78] The anticardiolipin antibody enzyme-linked immunosorbent assay (ELISA) usually detects antibodies directed against the cardiolipin/β_2-GPI complex. Lupus anticoagulant antibodies have been purified that specifically react with prothrombin but not thrombin. These purified antibodies can enhance the binding of prothrombin to the cultured endothelial cell surface.[79] Other protein-phospholipid targets may also be involved. Antiphos-

phatidylethanolamine antibodies are found in many patients with antiphospholipid antibody syndrome, and some of these antibodies inhibit activated protein C function.[80] Antibodies to heparin and heparan sulfate, which inhibit the heparin-dependent neutralization of thrombin by AT, have been found.[81] On the basis of this heterogeneity of antiphospholipid antibodies, it seems likely that multiple mechanisms are involved in the pathogenesis of thrombosis in this syndrome.

Clinical Presentation

Thrombotic events occur in approximately 30% of patients with antiphospholipid antibodies (overall incidence, 2.5 events per 100 patient-years).[82] In the cohort study cited above, 37% of patients presented with venous thrombosis, 27% with arterial thrombosis, 15% with both venous and arterial thrombosis, and 12% with fetal loss only[77] [see Chapter 114].

Diagnosis

The diagnosis of antiphospholipid antibody syndrome should be considered in any patient who presents with an idiopathic arterial or venous thrombosis or in a woman with a history of recurrent miscarriages. The diagnosis is confirmed by the presence of anticardiolipin antibodies on ELISA (see above) or lupus anticoagulant on clotting assays.

The general criteria for the diagnosis of lupus anticoagulant are (1) prolongation of at least one phospholipid-dependent clotting assay; (2) proof, by mixing studies, that the prolongation is caused by an inhibitor and not a clotting factor deficiency; and (3) confirmation that the inhibitor is phospholipid dependent [see Table 5]. The clotting tests commonly used are activated PTT (aPTT) and dilute Russell viper venom time (RVVT). The reagents in aPTT are variably sensitive to the lupus anticoagulant and are influenced by concentrations of some plasma clotting factors (e.g., factor VIII). Therefore, an aPTT reagent that is

Table 5 Proposed Clinical and Laboratory Criteria for the Antiphospholipid Antibody Syndrome[93]

Clinical features	Pregnancy morbidity (any of the following): More than one unexplained fetal death at greater than 10 wk Delivery at less than 34 wk, with severe pregnancy-induced hypertension Three or more pregnancy losses at less than 10 wk Thrombosis: Venous (superficial thrombophlebitis; deep vein thrombosis; pulmonary embolism; cerebral and retinal vein thrombosis; renal, splanchnic, and mesenteric vein thrombosis) Arterial (ischemic cerebral infarction, transient cerebral ischemia, amaurosis fugax, migraine, carotid and vertebrobasilar artery thrombosis, aortic arch syndrome, peripheral arterial thrombosis and embolism, renal and mesenteric artery thrombosis, livedo reticularis)
Laboratory features	Lupuslike anticoagulant: Activated partial thromboplastin time, dilute Russell viper venom time, kaolin clotting time, tissue thromboplastin inhibition test Anticardiolipin antibodies (either of the following): IgG anticardiolipin antibodies (> 20 GPL) IgM anticardiolipin antibodies (> 20 MPL) Thrombocytopenia (platelet count < 100,000/µl)

GPL—IgG phospholipid units   MPL—IgM phospholipid units

Table 6   Classification of Antiphospholipid Antibodies[147]

Autoimmune causes

Primary (do not fulfill criteria for systemic lupus erythematosus)

Secondary (fulfill criteria for systemic lupus erythematosus or other connective tissue diseases)

Drug-induced (e.g., phenothiazines, quinidine, quinine, synthetic penicillins, hydralazine)

Alloimmune causes

Infections (viral, bacterial, fungal)

Malignancies (e.g., hairy-cell leukemia, lymphoproliferative disease)

sensitive to the lupus anticoagulant should be used in the screening test. Dilute RVVT is much more sensitive than aPTT but is a manual test and not as well standardized. Other tests, such as kaolin clotting time and the tissue thromboplastin inhibition test, are useful when available. The presence of an inhibitor necessitates a mixing study to demonstrate lack of correction with normal plasma. Correction of the prolongation by addition of phospholipid in the form of platelet lysates or as hexagonal-phase phospholipid will confirm the diagnosis. Clotting factor assays can be carried out in equivocal cases. A lupus anticoagulant will cause functional deficiency of several phospholipid-dependent clotting factors, not just one particular factor.

Anticardiolipin antibodies are reported as IgG (in IgG phospholipid [GPL] units) and IgM (in IgM phospholipid [MPL] units). The prevalence of elevated anticardiolipin IgG and IgM antibodies in normal populations is approximately 5%; with repeated testing, the prevalence is less than 2%.[83] High titers of anticardiolipin IgG antibodies (> 33 GPL) are associated with an approximately fivefold increase in overall thrombotic risk.[82,84] The importance of low titers of IgG antibodies (< 20 GPL), isolated IgM antibodies, and IgA antibodies has not been established.[85,86] Both functional and antigenic assays should be ordered in the evaluation of a patient, because these two assays do not completely overlap. In one study of antiphospholipid antibody syndrome, 88% of patients had anticardiolipin antibodies (IgG, IgM, or both) and 54% of patients had lupus anticoagulant. Lupus anticoagulant was typically found in association with anticardiolipin antibodies, but it occurred in isolation in about 12% of patients.[77] Certain infections and drug exposures may lead to a transient appearance of antiphospholipid antibodies, which disappear after the resolution of infection or discontinuance of the drug [*see Table 6*]. Therefore, laboratory tests should be repeated at least once (6 weeks after the first tests) to confirm the diagnosis. Conversely, approximately 20% of patients with low titers of anticardiolipin IgG antibodies will have higher titers upon repeat testing. Retesting is also warranted in patients with new or recurrent thrombosis.[85]

Treatment

The current therapeutic recommendations for antiphospholipid antibody syndrome are mostly based on observational studies that support an association between antiphospholipid antibodies and thrombosis, particularly recurrent thrombosis.[82-86] In the acute treatment of DVT in patients with antiphospholipid antibody syndrome, monitoring the effect of unfractionated heparin can be problematic because lupus anticoagulant prolongs the aPTT. The use of LMWH circumvents this problem because

LMWH does not require dose titration and monitoring. The patient should be treated with LMWH and warfarin in the usual fashion, with an overlap of at least 5 days before discontinuing LMWH.

Retrospective analysis shows that patients with the antiphospholipid antibody syndrome and a history of thrombosis have a high rate of recurrent thrombosis (in the range of 50% to 70%) if they are not given prolonged warfarin therapy.[87,88] The site of the first thrombotic event (i.e., arterial or venous) tends to predict the site of the recurrent event.[88] High-intensity warfarin therapy, to an international normalized ratio (INR) of 3.0 to 3.5, had been advocated for these patients. This recommendation was based primarily on a retrospective analysis,[87] however, and two prospective clinical trials have now demonstrated that most of these patients can be adequately treated with conventional levels of anticoagulation (i.e., an INR of 2.0 to 3.0).[89] On the other hand, there are clearly some patients with antiphospholipid antibody syndrome who experience recurrent thrombosis with conventional anticoagulation and hence require a higher level of treatment.

The optimal duration of oral anticoagulation therapy for antiphospholipid antibody syndrome has not been fully established. Recurrent venous thrombosis or ischemic stroke usually justifies long-term warfarin. In a patient with a first episode of DVT who is found to have antiphospholipid antibodies, warfarin therapy is indicated for at least 6 months and perhaps for life.[90] The severity of the specific thrombotic episode, the coexistence of any reversible thrombotic risk factors, and the risks of long-term oral anticoagulation therapy should also be considered. It should be noted that the lupus anticoagulant may occasionally increase the prothrombin time (PT) and, in turn, the INR, thus posing a problem for the monitoring of warfarin therapy.[91] When PT and INR increase, use of a lupus anticoagulant–insensitive thromboplastin reagent is helpful.

In asymptomatic patients with anticardiolipin antibodies or lupus anticoagulant but no history of thrombosis, anticoagulation is not required.

Pregnancy Loss in Antiphospholipid Antibody Syndrome

Several prospective studies confirm an association between recurrent miscarriages and antiphospholipid antibodies. The antibodies presumably cause pregnancy loss by promoting placental thrombosis.[92] Antiphospholipid antibodies should be measured in patients with a history of unexplained second- or third-trimester loss, fetal demise, early-onset severe preeclampsia, and intrauterine growth retardation.[93] In contrast, antiphospholipid antibodies are not associated with sporadic early pregnancy loss,[94] which is frequently the result of genetic abnormalities in the fetus. The relationship of antiphospholipid antibodies with infertility is uncertain at present.

The management of pregnant women with antiphospholipid antibody syndrome is difficult because of the syndrome's association with thrombosis and the increased risk of bleeding with antithrombotic therapy. In a prospective, randomized, placebo-controlled trial, a combination of prednisone and aspirin was demonstrated to be ineffective in promoting live birth; in fact, it increased the risk of prematurity.[95] On the other hand, two prospective trials have demonstrated that heparin and low-dose aspirin (81 mg a day) provide a significantly better pregnancy outcome than low-dose aspirin alone, with viable infants being delivered in 70% to 80% of cases.[96,97] Furthermore, low-dose heparin (given initially as 5,000 units subcutaneously twice daily and adjusted to maintain the aPTT within the upper limits of the normal range) seems to be as effective as higher-dose heparin combined with low-dose aspirin.[98] Treatment should begin as soon as pregnancy is confirmed. LMWH is preferable to unfractionated heparin for long-term use because LMWH can be given once or twice daily and may reduce the risk of osteopenia and heparin-induced thrombocytopenia (see below). Enoxaparin (40 mg once daily) and aspirin (100 mg daily) has been given from week 12 of gestation until 6 weeks postpartum with good results.[99]

HEPARIN-INDUCED THROMBOCYTOPENIA AND THROMBOSIS

Epidemiology

Heparin-induced thrombocytopenia (HIT) is a relatively common antibody-mediated drug reaction, occurring in about 1% of patients receiving porcine heparin and 5% of patients receiving bovine heparin.[100] The incidence of HIT is much lower in patients treated with LMWH. In a subset of patients, HIT progresses to a potentially fatal disorder characterized by venous and arterial thrombosis. Interestingly, both the frequency of HIT antibody formation and the clinical manifestations of HIT vary considerably in different patient populations. The incidence of HIT antibody formation is much higher after cardiac surgery than after orthopedic surgery (50% versus 15%); however, the incidence of clinically significant postoperative HIT appears to be lower in cardiac surgical patients than in orthopedic patients, in whom the incidence is 5%.[101,102]

Pathophysiology

The pathogenesis of HIT is attributable to the presence of an IgG antibody that recognizes a complex of heparin and platelet factor 4 (PF4) [see Figure 3].[103] PF4 is a cationic protein found in platelet α-granules; when released from the granules, PF4 binds to the negatively charged heparin molecule with high affinity. The IgG antibody binds to the PF4-heparin complex on platelet membranes, forming a ternary complex that in turn binds to the platelet membrane FcγRII receptor. This binding activates the platelets, leading to further release of PF4 and formation of PF4-heparin complex. The immune complex–coated platelets are cleared rapidly by the reticuloendothelial system, giving rise to thrombocytopenia. The thrombotic complications in HIT are caused by activation of platelets by the immune complex, which leads to the formation of platelet microparticles and enhanced thrombin generation.[104] PF4 also binds to heparinlike sulfated glycosaminoglycans (e.g., heparan sulfate) on the endothelial cell surface. In vitro evidence indicates that the antibody in HIT is able to bind to endothelial cells. The cells may then become activated, giving rise to thrombosis.[105] Given that only a subset of patients who form HIT antibodies experience clinical HIT,[102] the induction of HIT antibodies and the development of thrombocytopenia and subsequent thrombosis should be regarded as a continuum. Concomitant thrombotic risk factors probably play a major role in determining the clinical progression and manifestations of HIT.

Clinical Presentation

HIT typically develops 5 to 10 days after the initiation of heparin therapy. However, in patients who received heparin within the previous 100 days and are being retreated, the onset can be rapid—within hours after starting heparin.[106] Conversely, onset of HIT may not occur until as long as 19 days after heparin therapy is stopped.[107] This delayed-onset HIT appears to be associated with a higher titer of IgG antibodies against the PF4-heparin complex.

HIT is generally defined as a platelet count below $150 \times 10^9/L$ or a drop in the platelet count by more than 50% from the postoperative peak at 5 to 14 days after heparin is started. The mean platelet count in HIT is about $60 \times 10^9/L$. Severe thrombocytopenia, with platelet counts below $20 \times 10^9/L$, occurs in fewer than 10% of patients; in 10% to 15% of patients, despite the 50% drop from peak levels, the platelet count nadir is above $150 \times 10^9/L$.[102]

The risk of HIT-associated thrombosis was once thought to be quite small; however, it is now recognized that thrombosis occurs in about one third to one half of patients with HIT, with venous thrombosis occurring more frequently than arterial thrombosis.[104] Thrombosis can occur at any platelet count, even at a very low one.

DVT, with or without pulmonary embolism, is the most common event leading to the diagnosis of HIT. The disorder may be further complicated by limb gangrene, especially in the setting of warfarin treatment without concomitant alternative anticoagulant coverage (see below). Cerebral vein thrombosis and adrenal hemorrhagic necrosis are uncommon but well-documented complications of HIT, and early diagnosis and urgent therapy can be lifesaving. Arterial thrombosis may present as limb ischemia, stroke, myocardial infarction, or, less commonly, mesenteric thrombosis and renal arterial thrombosis. Some patients have laboratory findings that support a diagnosis of DIC. Heparin-induced skin lesions may occur at heparin injection sites and range from painful erythematous papules to extensive dermal necrosis.[108]

Unlike antibodies induced by quinine, quinidine, or sulfonamides, which can persist for years, heparin-induced antibodies appear to be quite transient. They fall to undetectable levels at a median of 50 to 85 days, depending on the assay performed.[106]

Diagnosis

The diagnosis of HIT is supported by the finding of heparin-induced platelet aggregation in the presence of the patient's serum. However, the sensitivity of this test can be as low as 50%.[109] Sometimes, the patient's serum can cause spontaneous aggregation of donor platelets in the absence of heparin, most likely caused by the presence of immune complexes unrelated to HIT, which makes proper interpretation of the test result impossible. Heparin-induced platelet serotonin release using washed platelets has high sensitivity and specificity for HIT but is available only in a few specialized laboratories. ELISAs to detect antibodies that are reactive to the PF4-heparin complex are commercially available and have become the most commonly used test for HIT. These ELISAs have a higher sensitivity than the platelet aggregation assay and can be more easily performed in a general clinical diagnostic laboratory. However, false positive results (i.e., positive tests in the absence of HIT or thrombocytopenia) occur in 10% to 15% of medical patients and in more than 20% of patients receiving heparin for peripheral vascular surgery. A seroconversion rate as high as 50% has been reported in patients undergoing cardiopulmonary bypass surgery, limiting its usefulness in that situation.[110] Because HIT can be complicated by serious thrombotic problems, however, diagnosis of HIT should be based primarily on appropriate clinical findings, and management should be started while laboratory confirmation is awaited.

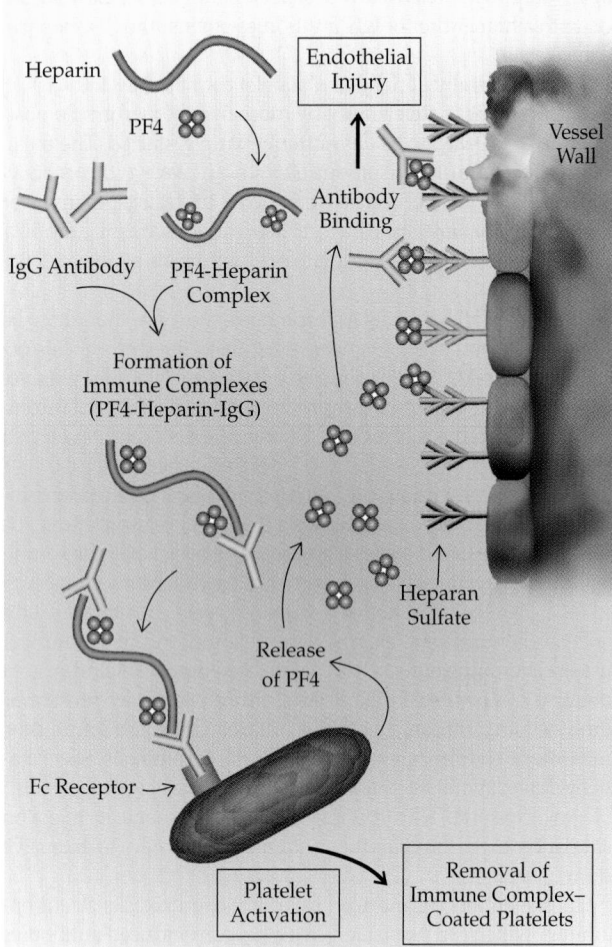

Figure 3 In a proposed explanation for heparin-induced thrombocytopenia, IgG antibodies recognize platelet factor 4 (PF4)–heparin complexes. The resulting PF4-heparin-IgG immune complexes bind to Fc receptors on circulating platelets. Fc-mediated platelet activation releases PF4 from α-granules in platelets, establishing a cycle of platelet activation and formation of prothrombotic platelet microparticles. Removal of immune complex–coated platelets by the reticuloendothelial system results in thrombocytopenia. PF4 also binds to heparan sulfate on the surface of endothelial cells, leading to immune-mediated injury, thrombosis, and disseminated intravascular coagulation.[145]

Treatment

Management of HIT consists of stopping heparin immediately and starting alternative anticoagulation therapy. It is important to discontinue all types of heparin: there are anecdotal reports of HIT caused by trace amounts of heparin used in heparin flushes of intravascular lines. Even if the patient has mild thrombocytopenia alone without any evidence of thrombosis, it is advisable to discontinue heparin and treat the underlying hypercoagulable state with an alternative anticoagulant. This aggressive approach is supported by a retrospective cohort study in which thrombosis developed within 30 days of heparin cessation in approximately half of patients who initially had no clinical symptoms from their HIT.[100]

HIT may develop in patients who were receiving heparin for preexisting thrombosis and are in the process of being switched over to warfarin. If the patient has been on warfarin for 4 or 5 days and the INR has reached an adequate therapeutic range, the clinician may rely on warfarin alone and monitor the patient carefully. However, if the patient has been on warfarin for less than 4 days or has evidence of a thrombotic complication from the HIT, an alternative anticoagulant should be used in addition to warfarin.

Alternative anticoagulant agents include lepirudin, argatroban, and fondaparinux. Although LMWH is much less immunogenic than unfractionated heparin in causing HIT,[104] it cannot be used as a safe substitute when a patient develops HIT caused by unfractionated heparin. LMWH and unfractionated heparin have extensive cross-reactivity (> 90%) in terms of antibody recognition. LMWH is not an appropriate choice in patients with HIT.

Hirudin, a 65-amino-acid protein originally extracted from the salivary gland of the medicinal leech (*Hirudo medicinalis*), is a potent direct thrombin inhibitor. Hirudin binds directly to thrombin's active site, independently of AT. It is not neutralized by PF4. Hirudin's anticoagulant function is monitored by aPTT.

Lepirudin is a recombinant form of hirudin that is approved for treatment of HIT. In two prospective clinical trials, use of lepirudin reduced serious thrombotic complications to about 20% (compared with a rate of about 40% in historical control subjects).[111,112] Lepirudin was given by intravenous bolus (0.4 mg/kg), followed by continuous infusion at 0.15 mg/kg/hr for 2 to 10 days as indicated. The dose was adjusted to maintain a target aPTT of 1.5 to 3 times normal. Patients experienced an increase of minor bleeding (from puncture sites, epistaxis, and hematuria) but no intracranial bleeding. Of note, 40% of patients developed antihirudin antibodies. These are not neutralizing antibodies and may actually enhance the drug's potency, perhaps by delaying its clearance—another reason to monitor aPTT levels. Judging from cardiology intervention trials, bleeding risk would be substantially increased with concomitant use of thrombolytics; therefore, it is not advisable to use the agents in combination. There is no effective antidote for lepirudin. It has a half-life of approximately 1.3 hours and is cleared by the kidneys. Thus, in patients with renal insufficiency, the dose of lepirudin needs to be adjusted carefully on the basis of creatinine clearance values.

Argatroban, a synthetic direct thrombin inhibitor, is approved for prophylaxis or treatment of thrombosis in patients with HIT. It is given by continuous intravenous infusion of 2 mg/kg/min to maintain an aPTT of 1.5 to 3 times baseline (not to exceed 100 seconds or 10 mg/kg/min). In one study, argatroban reduced the serious thrombotic complications of HIT by about 50%, as compared with historical controls, with a major bleeding rate of about 7%.[113] Its half-life is only 40 to 50 minutes. In contrast to lepirudin, argatroban is cleared by the liver and therefore can be used more easily in patients with renal insufficiency. Like lepirudin, argatroban does not have a specific antidote, and bleeding complications need to be watched for carefully.

A third alternative anticoagulant is fondaparinux, a synthetic pentasaccharide that activates AT, leading to thrombin inhibition. Fondaparinux has been approved for prophylaxis against DVT in orthopedic surgery. Because of its small size and reduced negative charge, fondaparinux does not form a complex with PF4 and therefore does not react with the antibody directed against the heparin-PF4 complex in HIT. Case reports describe the successful use of fondaparinux in HIT at a fixed dose of 7.5 mg administered subcutaneously once daily.

Patients who have HIT without associated thrombotic complications should be treated with one of the alternative anticoagulants until the platelet count has returned to normal, which generally takes 5 to 7 days. It is my practice to discontinue the alternative anticoagulant at that time. However, some experienced clinicians choose to continue empirical anticoagulation for up to 1 month, on the rationale that HIT represents an intensive hypercoagulable state. In patients who require prolonged anticoagulation—whether because they have other indications for anticoagulation or because they have had thrombotic complications from HIT—warfarin is used for long-term treatment. Warfarin should be started only after the patient has received adequate anticoagulation therapy with one of the alternative anticoagulants. The two agents should be used concurrently for at least 5 days before the alternative anticoagulant is discontinued. Both lepirudin and argatroban may increase the PT and INR, thus interfering with warfarin dose adjustments. The PT should be rechecked 6 hours after the discontinuance of lepirudin or argatroban to ensure that an INR of 2 to 3 has been achieved. For patients who have had HIT-associated thrombosis, warfarin therapy for 3 months should be adequate.

Some patients with serologically confirmed HIT may, at some point in the future, require surgery that involves cardiopulmonary bypass. The use of recombinant hirudin or argatroban in that situation has been described anecdotally.[112,114,115] Given the transient nature of the heparin-induced antibodies, subsequent reuse of heparin is theoretically reasonable, and indeed, a limited number of patients have been given heparin again after the disappearance of heparin-induced antibodies without any significant clinical sequelae.[106,116] Nevertheless, the use of heparin in this situation should be restricted to patients with a compelling indication for it, such as cardiac or vascular surgery, and only after the absence of detectable heparin-dependent antibodies has been confirmed by a sensitive assay, such as a PF4-heparin ELISA. Also, because reexposure to heparin may elicit a recurrence of heparin-dependent antibodies, heparin should be used only during the procedure itself, and an alternative anticoagulant should be started postoperatively for prophylaxis against recurrence of HIT. The anti–heparin-PF4 antibody should be checked postoperatively.

TROUSSEAU SYNDROME

Epidemiology

Some patients with cancer—especially those with occult solid tumors of the pancreas, ovary, liver, brain, colon, lung, or breast—may experience spontaneous venous thrombosis of the upper and lower extremities, or Trousseau syndrome. These patients also have an increased propensity toward recurrent arterial thrombosis and thromboembolism.[117] In a prospective study of patients who presented with idiopathic symptomatic DVT, cancer was diagnosed in approximately 8% of the patients during a 2-year follow-up (odds ratio, 2.3). In patients with recurrent thrombosis, the incidence of cancer was even higher (17%; odds ratio, 4.3).[118]

Pathophysiology

The underlying cause of Trousseau syndrome is a chronic, compensated form of DIC [see Chapter 97]. The activated procoagulants generated in DIC enhance thrombosis. Immunochemical staining of sections from tumors commonly associated with Trousseau syndrome often reveals tissue factor on the tumor surface.[119,120] A cancer procoagulant has been purified from some

adenocarcinomas and leukemic cells; this procoagulant, identified as a cysteine protease, can activate the clotting cascade by directly activating factor X.[121,122] Interaction of the tumor cells with monocytes, platelets, and endothelial cells may also generate inflammatory cytokines and induce endothelial and monocytic procoagulant activities, further exacerbating the thrombosis. Tumor cells may secrete soluble mucins—complex polysaccharides that can activate leukocytes, leading to platelet-leukocyte microthrombi and thrombin generation.[123] Heparin blocks the tumor mucin activation of leukocytes, which may partially explain heparin's efficacy over warfarin in the treatment of this condition.

Clinical Presentation

Venous thrombosis in Trousseau syndrome usually manifests as migratory superficial thrombophlebitis or DVT of the lower extremities. The recurrent arterial thrombosis in these patients arises from a nonbacterial thrombotic endocarditis in which sterile fibrin is deposited in the mitral valve. The fibrin clot may embolize to cause digital ischemia, transient ischemic attacks, and stroke.

Diagnosis

Coagulation studies in Trousseau syndrome show evidence of chronic, low-grade DIC (i.e., slightly low or even high fibrinogen and platelet levels and high levels of D-dimer). The PT and PTT are generally not prolonged. Overt DIC in such patients is uncommon.

How aggressively should one pursue the diagnosis of an underlying cancer in patients with idiopathic DVT? Research has not yet demonstrated the benefit and cost-effectiveness of an extensive screening approach.[124] In a large cohort study, cancer diagnoses after a primary thrombotic event were highest during the first 6 months of follow-up and declined rapidly to normal levels after the first year. Moreover, 40% of the patients who were diagnosed with cancer in the first year had distant metastases at the time of the diagnosis. It is unclear whether an earlier diagnosis after the thrombotic event would have changed the outcome in these patients. The researchers concluded that an aggressive search for a hidden underlying cancer in such patients is not warranted.[125]

At present, it is prudent to perform a careful history, physical examination, chest x-ray, routine blood counts, and chemistries. Some experts have also recommended multiple tests for fecal occult blood, prostate-specific antigen tests in men, and mammography and pelvic ultrasonography in women.[126,127] Careful follow-up examination and tests should be done as indicated by the initial evaluation.[128]

Treatment

The key to management of Trousseau syndrome is diagnosis and treatment of the underlying tumor. Unfortunately, tumors often present explosively in patients with Trousseau syndrome and may not respond to the usual therapies. In a prospective study, cancer patients had an approximately threefold increase in the rate of recurrent thrombosis and twofold increase in the rate of major bleeding during warfarin treatment of DVT. These complications occurred mostly during the first few months of anticoagulation and did not reflect underanticoagulation or over-anticoagulation but correlated with the extent and severity of the underlying cancer.[129] The likely explanation for the increased thrombosis recurrence in these patients is relative warfarin resistance, whereas the increased bleeding may be related to bleeding at the primary tumor site. A prospective trial found that the risk of recurrent venous thromboembolism was 50% lower in cancer patients who received long-term treatment with the LMWH dalteparin than in those who received oral anticoagulation; there was no significant difference in the risk of major bleeding.[130] If a patient is receiving chemotherapy for the underlying cancer, an exacerbation of the DIC associated with tumor lysis should be anticipated. An increase in the dose of heparin may be required.

THROMBOTIC REACTIONS TO ESTROGENS

Oral contraceptives increase the risk of thromboembolic disease approximately fourfold.[131] Epidemiologic studies indicate that contraceptives containing a third-generation progestin (e.g., desogestrel) carry a twofold greater risk of thrombosis than those with a second-generation drug (levonorgestrel).[132] For that reason, the preferred choice for first-time users of oral contraceptives is a compound containing a second-generation drug (e.g., Alesse, Levlite, Levora, Nordette, Triphasil, Trivora). The risk of venous thromboembolism disappears when the drugs are discontinued.

In postmenopausal women, estrogen replacement increases the risk of venous thromboembolism about threefold. The absolute risk is low, however—it is estimated to be approximately 3.2 per 10,000 patient-years. Therefore, estrogen replacement is not contraindicated in patients who require hormonal treatment to control severe postmenopausal symptoms. However, patients with a previous history of DVT or pulmonary embolism are at increased risk for recurrence and therefore should avoid hormone replacement therapy if possible.[133]

The association between estrogen use and thromboembolic disease remains unexplained.[134] Estrogen treatment is known to produce changes in the plasma levels of many proteins involved in coagulation and fibrinolysis, including decreases in protein S

and AT and increases in plasminogen. The changes are generally quite modest, however, and are not thought to account for the increased risk of thrombosis. On the other hand, in women who are heterozygous for factor V Leiden, oral contraceptive use increases the thrombotic risk synergistically to about 50 times normal.[18] There is also a moderate synergistic increase in thrombotic risk (15-fold) with the combination of factor V Leiden and hormone replacement therapy.[135]

Management of Venous Thromboembolism

The acute management of an initial episode of DVT or pulmonary embolism in patients with proven or presumed underlying risk factors for thrombosis is the same as that in other patients: heparin and then warfarin [*see Chapter 32*].

The optimal intensity and duration of warfarin treatment in DVT have been the subject of many large clinical trials over the past decade. As regards the intensity of oral anticoagulation, an INR of 2 to 3 has proved optimal, with a low rate of thrombosis recurrence and a rate of major bleeding of about 3% a year.[136,137] In comparison, treatment to an INR of 1.5 to 1.9 is less effective in reducing recurrent thrombosis (although it is better than placebo) and provides no significant reduction in bleeding risk.[136,137]

Warfarin therapy usually should be continued for 3 to 6 months. In a prospective study of oral anticoagulation therapy in patients with a first episode of venous thromboembolism, 6 weeks of therapy was adequate for patients with temporary, reversible risk factors for thrombosis (e.g., surgery, trauma, temporary immobilization, or use of oral contraceptives). On the other hand, 6 months of oral anticoagulation therapy was clearly superior for patients with idiopathic venous thromboembolism (who are presumed to have intrinsic risk factors).[138] The recurrence rate was quite high, however—approximately 12% at 2 years. On the basis of this evidence, at least 6 months of oral anticoagulation therapy is indicated in a patient with a first episode of idiopathic DVT or pulmonary embolism.

Further management should depend on results of the hypercoagulable workup (see above). A risk assessment for other predisposing factors will also be relevant.

Unfortunately, even when warfarin treatment is continued for 12 months after a first episode of idiopathic DVT, this does not reduce the risk of recurrent thrombosis once warfarin treatment is discontinued.[139] Generally, there is a rapid rebound phase of recurrent DVT of about 10% during the first 6 to 12 months after warfarin therapy. This suggests that there is a subset of patients (10% to 20%) who have a stronger tendency toward thrombosis and thus experience recurrences fairly soon after discontinuance of oral anticoagulation.

Persistent elevation of D-dimer levels may help identify patients who are more likely to have recurrent thrombosis. In a prospective study, D-dimer levels that remained elevated 1 month after the discontinuance of warfarin were associated with a higher recurrence risk (approximately threefold to eightfold), whereas normal D-dimer levels had a high negative predictive value for recurrence.[140] Thus, patients with elevated D-dimer levels merit more vigilant monitoring and consideration of long-term anticoagulation.

Because the optimal duration of long-term oral anticoagulation therapy for patients with thromboembolism remains undefined, this question is best addressed individually, on the basis of an estimation of the risk of recurrence [*see Table 7*].[141,142] Before undertaking long-term anticoagulation therapy in a high-risk

Table 7 General Guidelines for Management of Patients with Venous Thromboembolism

Recurrence Risk	Management
High Recurrent idiopathic thrombosis One life-threatening thrombosis One spontaneous thrombosis at an unusual site (e.g., mesenteric or cerebral thrombosis) One spontaneous thrombosis associated with antiphospholipid antibody syndrome One thrombosis with two permanent risk factors One thrombosis with Trousseau syndrome	Lifelong oral anticoagulation therapy: INR 2.0 to 3.0
Medium One thrombosis with one permanent risk factor (except Trousseau syndrome) Idiopathic thrombosis with no identifiable risk factor	6 mo of oral anticoagulation therapy after first episode of thrombosis; vigorous prophylaxis in high-risk situations
Low One thrombosis with reversible risk factor	6 wk–3 mo of oral anticoagulation therapy after first episode of thrombosis; vigorous prophylaxis in high-risk situations

INR—international normalized ratio

patient, the clinician must take the patient's risk of bleeding into account.

Of note, none of the published studies shows a significant difference in mortality between patients who receive long-term therapy and those who receive short-term therapy. There is also no evidence to suggest that prophylactic anticoagulation therapy improves overall survival. In historical studies, families with deficiencies of AT and protein C show no higher mortality than the general population displays.[143,144] Current clinical trials are studying the use of full-dose oral anticoagulation therapy for an extended period of time followed by an indefinite period of low-dose anticoagulation therapy. The results of these studies will help define the optimal long-term treatment for patients who are at high risk for recurrence of thromboembolism.

The author has no commercial relationships with manufacturers of products or providers of services discussed in this chapter.

References

1. Chi JT, Chang HY, Haraldsen G, et al: Endothelial cell diversity revealed by global expression profiling. Proc Natl Acad Sci USA 100:10623, 2003

2. Martinelli I, Mannucci PM, De Stefano V, et al: Different risks of thrombosis in four coagulation defects associated with inherited thrombophilia: a study of 150 families. Blood 92:2353, 1998

3. Martinelli I, Cattaneo M, Panzeri D, et al: Risk factors for deep venous thrombosis of the upper extremities. Ann Intern Med 126:707, 1997

4. Prandoni P, Polistena P, Bernardi E, et al: Upper-extremity deep vein thrombosis: risk factors, diagnosis, and complications. Arch Intern Med 157:57, 1997

5. Abilgaard U: Antithrombin and related inhibitors of coagulation. Recent Advances in Blood Coagulation. Poller L, Ed. Churchill Livingstone, Edinburgh, Scotland, 1981, p 151

6. De Stefano V, Leone G, Mastrangelo S, et al: Clinical manifestations and management of inherited thrombophilia: retrospective analysis and follow-up after diagnosis of 238 patients with congenital deficiency of antithrombin III, protein C, protein S. Thromb Haemost 72:352, 1994

7. Demers C, Ginsberg JS, Hirsh J, et al: Thrombosis in antithrombin-deficient persons: report of a large kindred and literature review. Ann Intern Med 116:754, 1992

8. Menache D, O'Malley JP, Schorr JB, et al: Evaluation of the safety, recovery, half-life, and clinical efficacy of antithrombin III (human) in patients with hereditary antithrombin III deficiency. Blood 75:33, 1990

9. Miletich J, Sherman L, Broze G Jr: Absence of thrombosis in subjects with heterozygous protein C deficiency. N Engl J Med 317:991, 1987

10. Miletich JP, Prescott SM, White R, et al: Inherited predisposition to thrombosis. Cell 72:477, 1993

11. Boerger LM, Morris PC, Thurnau GR, et al: Oral contraceptives and gender affect protein S status. Blood 69:692, 1987

12. Vigano-D'Angelo S, D'Angelo A, Kaufman CE Jr, et al: Protein S deficiency occurs in the nephrotic syndrome. Ann Intern Med 107:42, 1987

13. Sallah S, Abdallah JM, Gagnon GA: Recurrent warfarin-induced skin necrosis in kindreds with protein-S deficiency. Haemostasis 28:25, 1998

14. Faioni EM, Franchi F, Asti D, et al: Resistance to activated protein C in nine thrombophilic families: interference in a protein S functional assay. Thromb Haemost 70:1067, 1993

15. Rees DC, Cox M, Clegg JB: World distribution of factor V Leiden. Lancet 346:1133, 1995

16. Svensson PJ, Dahlback B: Resistance to activated protein C as a basis for venous thrombosis. N Engl J Med 330:517, 1994

17. Simioni P, Prandoni P, Lensing AWA, et al: The risk of recurrent venous thromboembolism in patients with an Arg506 Gln mutation in the gene for factor V (factor V Leiden). N Engl J Med 336:399, 1997

18. Vandenbroucke JP, Koster T, Briet E, et al: Increased risk of venous thrombosis in oral-contraceptive users who are carriers of factor V Leiden mutation. Lancet 344:1453, 1994

19. Rosendaal FR, Koster T, Vandenbroucke JP, et al: High-risk of thrombosis in patients homozygous for factor V Leiden (APC-resistance). Blood 85:1504, 1995

20. Middeldorp S, Henkens CMA, Koopman MMW, et al: The incidence of venous thromboembolism in family members of patients with factor V Leiden mutation and venous thrombosis. Ann Intern Med 128:15, 1998

21. Koeleman BPC, Reitsma PH, Allaart RC, et al: Activated protein C resistance as an additional risk factor for thrombosis in protein C–deficient families. Blood 84:1031, 1994

22. Zoller B, Berntsdotter A, Garcia de Frutos P, et al: Resistance to activated protein C as an additional genetic risk factor in hereditary deficiency of protein S. Blood 85:3518, 1995

23. van Boven HH, Reitsma PH, Rosendaal FR, et al: Factor V Leiden (FV R506Q) in

24. Williamson D, Brown K, Luddington R, et al: Factor V Cambridge: a new mutation (Arg306ΔThr) associated with resistance to activated protein C. Blood 91:1140, 1998

25. Chan WP, Lee CK, Kwong YL, et al: A novel mutation of Arg306 of factor V gene in Hong Kong Chinese. Blood 91:1135, 1998

26. Zoller B, Svensson PJ, He X, et al: Identification of the same factor V gene mutation in 47 out of 50 thrombosis-prone families with inherited resistance to activated protein C. J Clin Invest 94:2521, 1994

27. Bertina RM: Laboratory diagnosis of resistance to activated protein C (APC-resistance). Thromb Haemost 78:478, 1997

28. van der Bom JG, Bots ML, Haverkate F, et al: Reduced response to protein C is associated with increased risk for cerebral vascular disease. Ann Intern Med 125:265, 1996

29. Fisher M, Fernandez JA, Ameriso SF, et al: Activated protein C resistance in ischemic stroke not due to factor V arginine506Δglutamine mutation. Stroke 27:1163, 1996

30. Rodeghiero F, Tosetto A: Activated protein C resistance and factor V Leiden mutation are independent risk factors for venous thromboembolism. Ann Intern Med 130:643, 1999

31. de Visser MCH, Rosendaal FR, Bertina RM: A reduced sensitivity to activated protein C in the absence of factor V Leiden increases the risk of venous thrombosis. Blood 93:1271, 1999

32. Bertina RM, Koeleman BPC, Koster T, et al: Mutation in blood coagulation factor V associated with resistance to activated protein C. Nature 369:64, 1994

33. Kalafatis M, Bertina RM, Rand MD, et al: Characterization of the molecular defect in factor V R506Q. J Biol Chem 270:4053, 1995

34. Ridker PM, Hennekens CH, Lindpaintner K, et al: Mutation in the gene coding for coagulation factor V and the risk for myocardial infarction, stroke, and venous thrombosis in apparently healthy men. N Engl J Med 332:912, 1995

35. De Stefano V, Martinelli I, Mannucci PM, et al: The risk of recurrent deep venous thrombosis among heterozygous carriers of both factor V Leiden and the G20210A prothrombin mutation. N Engl J Med 341:801, 1999

36. Eichinger S, Weltermann A, Mannhalter C, et al: The risk of recurrent venous thromboembolism in heterozygous carriers of factor V Leiden and a first spontaneous venous thromboembolism. Arch Intern Med 162:2357, 2002

37. Dahlback B: Resistance to activated protein C caused by the factor V R506Q mutation is a common risk factor for venous thrombosis. Thromb Haemost 78:483, 1997

38. Middeldorp S, Meinardi JR, Koopman MM, et al: A prospective study of asymptomatic carriers of the factor V Leiden mutation to determine the incidence of venous thromboembolism. Ann Intern Med 135:322, 2001

39. Rosendaal FR, Doggen CJ, Zivelin A, et al: Geographic distribution of the 20210 G to A prothrombin variant. Thromb Haemost 79:706, 1998

40. Poort SR, Rosendaal FR, Reitsma PH, et al: A common genetic variation in the 3'-untranslated region of the prothrombin gene is associated with elevated plasma prothrombin levels and an increase in venous thrombosis. Blood 88:3698, 1996

41. The risk of recurrent venous thromboembolism in carriers and non-carriers of the G1691A allele in the coagulation factor V gene and the G20210A allele in the prothrombin gene. DURAC Trial Study Group. Duration of Anticoagulation. Thromb Haemost 81:684, 1999

42. Martinelli I, Sacchi E, Landi G, et al: High risk of cerebral-vein thrombosis in carriers of a prothrombin-gene mutation and in users of oral contraceptives. N Engl J Med 338:1793, 1998

43. Harker LA, Harlan JM, Ross R: Effect of sulfinpyrazone on homocysteine-induced endothelial injury and arteriosclerosis in baboons. Circ Res 53:731, 1983

44. Starkebaum G, Harlan JM: Endothelial cell injury due to copper-catalyzed hydrogen peroxide generation from homocysteine. J Clin Invest 77:1370, 1986

45. Lentz SR, Sadler JE: Inhibition of thrombomodulin surface expression and protein C activation by the thrombogenic agent homocysteine. J Clin Invest 88:1906, 1991

46. Nishinaga M, Ozawa T, Shimada K: Homocysteine, a thrombogenic agent, suppresses anticoagulant heparan sulfate expression in cultured porcine aortic endothelial cells. J Clin Invest 92:1281, 1993

47. Harpel PC, Chang VT, Borth W: Homocysteine and other sulfhydryl compounds enhance the binding of lipoprotein(a) to fibrin: a potential biochemical link between thrombosis, atherogenesis, and sulfhydryl compound metabolism. Proc Natl Acad Sci USA 89:10193, 1992

48. Mudd SH, Levy HL, Skovby F: Disorders of transulfuration. The Metabolic Basis of Inherited Disease. Scriver CR, Beaudet AL, Sly WS, et al, Eds. McGraw-Hill, New York, 1989, p 693

49. Malinow MR: Homocyst(e)ine and arterial occlusive diseases. J Intern Med 236:603, 1994

50. Naurath HJ, Joosten E, Riezier R, et al: Effects of vitamin B12, folate, and vitamin B6 supplements in elderly people with normal serum vitamin concentrations. Lancet 346:85, 1995

51. Clarke R, Daly L, Robinson K, et al: Hyperhomocysteinemia: an independent risk factor for vascular disease. N Engl J Med 324:1149, 1991

52. Selhub J, Jacques PF, Bostom AG, et al: Association between plasma homocysteine concentrations and extracranial carotid-artery stenosis. N Engl J Med 332:286, 1995

53. Den Heijer M, Koster T, Blom HJ, et al: Hyperhomocysteinemia as a risk factor for deep-vein thrombosis. N Engl J Med 334:759, 1996

54. Nygard O, Nordrehaug JE, Refsum H, et al: Plasma homocysteine levels and mortality in patients with coronary artery disease. N Engl J Med 337:230, 1997

55. Bostom AG, Jacques PF, Nadeau MR, et al: Post-methionine load hyperhomocysteinemia in persons with normal fasting total plasma homocysteine: initial results from The NHLBI Family Heart Study. Arteriosclerosis 116:147, 1995

56. Franken DG, Boers GHJ, Blom HJ, et al: Treatment of mild hyperhomocysteinemia in vascular disease patients. Arterioscler Thromb Vasc Biol 14:465, 1994

57. Bostom A, Cupples A, Jenner J, et al: Elevated plasma lipoprotein(a) and coronary heart disease in men aged 55 years and younger. JAMA 276:544, 1996

58. Wild SH, Fortmann SP, Marcovina SM: A prospective case-control study of lipoprotein(a) levels and Apo(a) size and risk of coronary heart disease in Stanford Five-City Project participants. Arterioscler Thromb Vasc Biol 17:239, 1997

59. Nagayama M, Shinohara Y, Nagayama T: Lipoprotein(a) and ischemic cerebrovascular disease in young adults. Stroke 25:74, 1994

60. Ridker PM, Stampfer MJ, Hennekens CH: Plasma concentration of lipoprotein(a) and the risk of future stroke. JAMA 273:1269, 1995

61. Marcovina SM, Albers JJ, Jacobs DR Jr, et al: Lipoprotein(a) concentrations and apolipoprotein(a) phenotypes in Caucasians and African-Americans. The CARDIA study. Arterioscler Thromb 13:1037, 1993

62. Hajjar KA, Gavish D, Breslow JL, et al: Lipoprotein (a) modulation of endothelial cell surface fibrinolysis and its potential role in atherosclerosis. Nature 339:303, 1989

63. Callow MJ, Verstuyft J, Tangirala R, et al: Atherogenesis in transgenic mice with human apolipoprotein B and lipoprotein(a). J Clin Invest 96:1639, 1995

64. Maher VM, Brown BG, Marcovina SM, et al: Effects of lowering elevated LDL cholesterol on the cardiovascular risk of lipoprotein(a). JAMA 274:1771, 1995

65. Gurakar A, Hoeg JM, Kostner G, et al: Levels of lipoprotein(a) decline with neomycin and niacin treatment. Atherosclerosis 57:293, 1985

66. Shewmon DA, Stock JL, Rosen CJ, et al: Tamoxifen and estrogen lower circulating lipoprotein(a) concentrations in healthy postmenopausal women. Arterioscler Thromb 14:1586, 1994

67. Martinez J: Congenital dysfibrinogenemia. Curr Opin Hematol 4:357, 1997

68. Aoki N, Moroi M, Sakata Y, et al: Abnormal plasminogen: a hereditary molecular abnormality found in a patient with recurrent thrombosis. J Clin Invest 61:1186, 1978

69. Estelles A, Gilabert J, Aznar J, et al: Changes in the plasma levels of type 1 and type 2 plasminogen activators in normal pregnancy and in patients with severe preeclampsia. Blood 74:1332, 1989

70. Prins MH, Hirsh J: A critical review of the evidence supporting a relationship between impaired fibrinolytic activity and venous thromboembolism. Arch Intern Med 151:1721, 1991

71. Wiman B: Plasminogen activator inhibitor-1 (PAI-1) in plasma: its role in thrombotic disease. Thromb Haemost 74:71, 1995

72. Meade TW: Fibrinogen in ischemic heart disease. Eur Heart J 16(suppl):31, 1995

73. Meade TW, Mellows S, Brozovic M, et al: Haemostatic function and ischaemic heart disease: principal results of the Northwick Park Heart Study. Lancet 2:533, 1986

74. Koster T, Blann AD, Briet E, et al: Role of clotting factor VIII in effect of von Willebrand factor on occurrence of deep-vein thrombosis. Lancet 345:152, 1995

75. O'Donnell J, Tuddenham EGD, Manning R, et al: High prevalence of elevated factor VIII levels in patients referred for thrombophilia screening: role of increased synthesis and relationship to the acute phase reaction. Thromb Haemost 77:825, 1997

76. Kyrle PA, Minar E, Hirschl M, et al: High plasma levels of factor VIII and the risk of recurrent venous thromboembolism. N Engl J Med 343:457, 2000

77. Antiphospholipid syndrome: clinical and immunologic manifestations and patterns of disease expression in a cohort of 1,000 patients. Euro-Phospholipid Project Group. Arthritis Rheum 46:1019, 2002

78. Rauch J, Janoff AS: Role of antibodies in understanding the interactions between anti-phospholipid antibodies and phospholipids. Phospholipid-Binding Antibodies. N Harris, T Exner, GRV Hughes, et al, Eds. CRC Press, Boca Raton, Florida, 1991, p 108

79. Rao LVM, Hoang AD, Rapaport SI: Mechanisms and effects of the binding of lupus anticoagulant IgG and prothrombin to bound phospholipid. Blood 88:4173, 1996

80. Smirnov MD, Triplett DT, Comp PC, et al: On the role of phosphatidylethanolamine in the inhibition of activated protein C activity by antiphospholipid antibodies. J Clin Invest 95:309, 1995

81. Shibata S, Harpel PC, Gharavi A, et al: Autoantibodies to heparin from patients with antiphospholipid antibody syndrome inhibit formation of antithrombin III–thrombin complexes. Blood 83:2532, 1994

82. Finazzi G, Brancaccio V, Ciavarella N, et al: Natural history and risk factors for thrombosis in 360 patients with antiphospholipid antibodies: a four-year prospective study from the Italian registry. Am J Med 100:530, 1996

83. Vila P, Hernandez MC, Lopez-Fernadez MF, et al: Prevalence, follow-up and clinical significance of the anticardiolipin antibodies in normal subjects. Thromb Haemost 72:209, 1994

84. Ginsburg KS, Liang MH, Newcomer L, et al: Anticardiolipin antibodies and the risk for ischemic stroke and venous thrombosis. Ann Intern Med 117:997, 1992

85. Silver RM, Porter TF, van Leeuwen I, et al: Anticardiolipin antibodies: clinical consequences of "low titers." Obstet Gynecol 87:494, 1996

86. Selva-O'Callaghan A, Ordi-Ros J, Monegal-Ferran F, et al: IgA anticardiolipin antibodies: relation with other antiphospholipid antibodies and clinical significance. Thromb Haemost 79:282, 1998

87. Khamashta MA, Cuardrado MJ, Mujic F, et al: The management of thrombosis in the antiphospholipid-antibody syndrome. N Engl J Med 332:993, 1995

88. Rosove MH, Brewer MC: Antiphospholipid thrombosis: clinical course after the first thrombotic event in 70 patients. Ann Intern Med 117:303, 1992

89. Crowther MA, Ginsberg JS, Julian J, et al: A comparison of two intensities of warfarin for the prevention of recurrent thrombosis in patients with the antiphospholipid antibody syndrome. N Engl J Med 349:1133, 2003

90. Kearon C, Gent M, Hirsh J, et al: A comparison of three months of anticoagulation with extended anticoagulation for a first episode of idiopathic venous thromboembolism. N Engl J Med 340:901, 1999

91. Moll S, Ortel TL: Monitoring warfarin therapy in patients with lupus anticoagulants. Ann Intern Med 127:177, 1997

92. Rand JH, Wu X-X, Andree HAM, et al: Pregnancy loss in the antiphospholipid-antibody syndrome—a possible thrombogenic mechanism. N Engl J Med 337:154, 1997

93. Kutteh WH, Rote NS, Silver R: Antiphospholipid antibodies and reproduction: the antiphospholipid antibody syndrome. Am J Reprod Immunol 41:133, 1999

94. Infante-Rivard C, David M, Gauthier R, et al: Lupus anticoagulants, anticardiolipin antibodies, and fetal loss: a case-controlled study. N Engl J Med 325:1063, 1991

95. Laskin CA, Bombardier C, Hannah ME, et al: Prednisone and aspirin in women with autoantibodies and unexplained recurrent fetal loss. N Engl J Med 337:148, 1997

96. Kutteh WH: Antiphospholipid antibody–associated recurrent pregnancy loss: treatment with heparin and low-dose aspirin is superior to low-dose aspirin alone. Am J Obstet Gynecol 174:1584, 1996

97. Rai R, Cohen H, Dave M, et al: Randomized, controlled trial of aspirin and aspirin plus heparin in pregnant women with recurrent miscarriage asssociated with phospholipid antibodies. BMJ 314:253, 1997

98. Kutteh WH, Ermel LD: A clinical trial for the treatment of antiphospholipid antibody–associated recurrent pregnancy loss with lower dose heparin and aspirin. Am J Reprod Immunol 35:402, 1996

99. Eldor A: Thrombophilia, thrombosis and pregnancy. Thromb Haemost 86:104, 2001

100. Warkentin TE: Heparin-induced thrombocytopenia: a ten-year retrospective. Ann Rev Med 50:129, 1999

101. Bauer TL, Arepally G, Konkle BA, et al: Prevalence of heparin-associated antibodies without thrombosis in patients undergoing cardiopulmonary bypass surgery. Circulation 95:1242, 1997

102. Warkentin TE: Heparin-induced thrombocytopenia: a clinicopathologic syndrome. Thromb Haemost 82:439, 1999

103. Amiral J, Bridey F, Dreyfus M, et al: Platelet factor 4 complexed to heparin is the target for antibodies generated in heparin-induced thrombocytopenia. Thromb Haemost 68:95, 1992

104. Warkentin TE, Levine MN, Hirsh J, et al: Heparin-induced thrombocytopenia in patients treated with low-molecular-weight heparin or unfractionated heparin. N Engl J Med 332:1330, 1995

105. Visentin GP, Ford SE, Scott JP, et al: Antibodies from patients with heparin-induced thrombocytopenia/thrombosis are specific for platelet factor 4 complexed with heparin or bound to endothelial cells. J Clin Invest 93:81, 1994

106. Warkentin TE, Kelton JG: Temporal aspects of heparin-induced thrombocytopenia. N Engl J Med 344:1286, 2001

107. Warkentin TE, Kelton JG: Delayed-onset heparin-induced thrombocytopenia and thrombosis. Ann Intern Med 135:502, 2001

108. Sallah S, Thomas DP, Roberts HR: Warfarin and heparin-induced skin necrosis and the purple toe syndrome: infrequent complications of anticoagulant treatment. Thromb Haemost 78:785, 1997

109. Greinacher A, Amiral J, Dummel V, et al: Laboratory diagnosis of heparin-associated thrombocytopenia and comparison of platelet aggregation test, and platelet factor 4/heparin enzyme linked immunosorbent assay. Transfusion 34:381, 1994

110. Warkentin TE, Greinacher A: Heparin-induced thrombocytopenia and cardiac surgery. Ann Thorac Surg 76:2121, 2003

111. Greinacher A, Volpol H, Potzsch B: Recombinant hirudin in the treatment of patients with heparin-induced thrombocytopenia (HIT). Blood 88(suppl):281a, 1996

112. Schiele F, Vuillemenot A, Kramarz P, et al: Use of recombinant hirudin as antithrombotic treatment in patients with heparin-induced thrombocytopenia. Am J Hematol 50:20, 1995

113. Lewis BE, Wallis DE, Berkowitz SD, et al: Argatroban anticoagulant therapy in patients with heparin-induced thrombocytopenia. Circulation 103:1838, 2001

114. Matsuo T, Yamada T, Yamanashi T, et al: Anticoagulant therapy with MD805 of a hemodialysis patient with heparin-induced thrombocytopenia. Thromb Res 58:663, 1990

115. Gillis S, Merin G, Zahger D, et al: Danaparoid for cardiopulmonary bypass in patients with previous heparin-induced thrombocytopenia. Br J Haematol 98:657, 1997

116. Potzsch B, Klovekorn WP, Madlener K: Use of heparin during cardiopulmonary bypass in patients with a history of heparin-induced thrombocytopenia. N Engl J Med 343:515, 2000

117. Callander N, Rapaport SI: Trousseau's syndrome. West J Med 158:364, 1993

118. Prandoni P, Lensing AWA, Buller HR, et al: Deep-vein thrombosis and the incidence of subsequent symptomatic cancer. N Engl J Med 327:1128, 1992

119. Callander NS, Varki N, Rao LVM: Immunohistochemical identification of tissue factor in solid tumors. Cancer 70:1194, 1992

120. Contrino J, Hair G, Kreutzer DL, et al: In situ detection of tissue factor in vascular endothelial cells: correlation with malignant phenotype of human breast disease. Nat Med 2:209, 1996

121. Falanga A, Gordon SG: Isolation and characterization of cancer procoagulant: a cysteine proteinase from malignant tissue. Biochemistry 24:5558, 1985

122. Falanga A, Consonni R, Marchetti M, et al: Cancer procoagulant and tissue factor are differentially modulated by all-trans-retinoic acid in acute promyelocytic leukemic cells. Blood 92:143, 1998

123. Wahrenbrock M, Borsig L, Le D, et al: Selectin-mucin interactions as a probable molecular explanation for the association of Trousseau syndrome with mucinous adenocarcinomas. J Clin Invest 112:853, 2003

124. Prins MH, Hettiarachchi RJK, Lensing AWA, et al: Newly diagnosed malignancy in patients with venous thromboembolism: search or wait and see? Thromb Haemost 78:121, 1997

125. Sorensen HT, Mellemkjaer L, Steffensen FH, et al: The risk of a diagnosis of cancer after primary deep venous thrombosis or pulmonary embolism. N Engl J Med 338:1169, 1998

126. Silverstein RL, Nachman RL: Cancer and clotting: Trousseau's warning. N Engl J Med 327:1163, 1992

127. Buller H, Ten Cate JW: Primary venous thromboembolism and cancer screening. N Engl J Med 338:1221, 1998

128. Cornuz J, Pearson SD, Creager MA, et al: Importance of findings on the initial evaluation for cancer in patients with symptomatic idiopathic deep venous thrombosis. Ann Intern Med 125:785, 1996

129. Prandoni P, Lensing AW, Picciolo A, et al: Recurrent venous thromboembolism and bleeding complications during anticoagulant treatment in patients with cancer and venous thrombosis. Blood 100:3484, 2002

130. Low-molecular-weight heparin versus a coumarin for the prevention of recurrent venous thromboembolism in patients with cancer. Randomized Comparison of Low-Molecular-Weight Heparin versus Oral Anticoagulant Therapy for the Prevention of Recurrent Venous Thromboembolism in Patients with Cancer (CLOT) Investigators. N Engl J Med 349:146, 2003

131. Vandenbroucke JP, Koster T, Briet E, et al: Increased risk of venous thrombosis in oral-contraceptive users who are carriers of factor V Leiden mutation. Lancet 344:1453, 1994

132. Helmerhorst FM, Bloemenkamp KWM, Rosendaal FR, et al: Oral contraceptives and thrombotic disease: risk of venous thromboembolism. Thromb Haemost 78:327, 1997

133. Hoibraaten E, Qvigstad E, Arnesen H, et al: Increased risk of recurrent venous thromboembolism during hormone replacement therapy—results of the randomized, double-blind, placebo-controlled estrogen in venous thromboembolism trial (EVTET). Thromb Haemost 84:961, 2000

134. Vandenbroucke JP, Rosing J, Bloemenkamp KW, et al: Oral contraceptives and the risk of venous thrombosis. N Engl J Med 344:1527, 2001

135. Rosendaal FR, Vessey M, Rumley A, et al: Hormonal replacement therapy, prothrombotic mutations and the risk of venous thrombosis. Br J Haematol 116:851, 2002

136. Ridker PM, Goldhaber SZ, Danielson E, et al: Long-term, low-intensity warfarin therapy for the prevention of recurrent venous thromboembolism. N Engl J Med 348:1425, 2003

137. Kearon C, Ginsberg JS, Kovacs MJ, et al: Comparison of low-intensity warfarin therapy with conventional-intensity warfarin therapy for long-term prevention of recurrent venous thromboembolism. N Engl J Med 349:631, 2003

138. Schulman S, Rhedin AS, Lindmarker P, et al: A comparison of six weeks with six months of oral anticoagulant therapy after a first episode of venous thromboembolism. N Engl J Med 332:1661, 1995

139. Three months versus one year of oral anticoagulant therapy for idiopathic deep venous thrombosis. Warfarin Optimal Duration Italian Trial Investigators. N Engl J Med 345:165, 2001

140. Palareti G, Legnani C, Cosmi B, et al: Predictive value of D-dimer test for recurrent venous thromboembolism after anticoagulation withdrawal in subjects with a previous idiopathic event and in carriers of congenital thrombophilia. Circulation 108:313, 2003

141. Bauer KA: Management of patients with hereditary defects predisposing to thrombosis including pregnant women. Thromb Haemost 74:94, 1995

142. De Stefano V, Finazzi G, Mannucci PM: Inherited thrombophilia: pathogenesis, clinical syndromes, and management. Blood 87:3531, 1996

143. Rosendaal FR, Heijboer H, Briet E, et al: Mortality in hereditary antithrombin deficiency: 1830 to 1989. Lancet 337:260, 1991

144. Allaart CF, Rosendaal FR, Noteboom WM, et al: Survival in families with hereditary protein C deficiency, 1820 to 1993. BMJ 311:910, 1995

145. Aster RH: Heparin-induced thrombocytopenia and thrombosis. N Engl J Med 332:1374, 1995

146. Koster T, Rosendaal FR, de Ronde H, et al: Venous thrombosis due to poor anticoagulant response to activated protein C: Leiden Thrombophilia Study. Lancet 342:1503, 1993

147. Triplett DA: Protean clinical presentation of antiphospholipid-protein antibodies (APA). Thromb Haemost 74:329, 1995

Acknowledgments

Figures 1 and 2   Seward Hung.

Figure 3   Dr. Rajeev Doshi.

W. Hallowell Churchill, M.D.

Transfusion medicine developed rapidly, owing to several key discoveries and technical advances. These include the discovery of blood group antigens and the understanding of the host immune response to these antigens, the development of methods of anticoagulation and storage of blood, and the creation of plastic bags that allow sterile fractionation of whole blood into components. The potential of blood to act as an agent of disease transmission has heavily shaped both the donation process and transfusion practice.[1] Decisions about whether to transfuse must involve weighing the benefits against the risks. This chapter provides a basis for these decisions, including indications for blood-component use, complications of transfusion therapy, and methods of reducing risks during the collection, processing, and preparation of blood components.

Blood Donation

The donation process for either whole blood or special products, such as single-donor platelets (SDPs) obtained by apheresis, is designed to protect both the donor and the recipient. For example, persons weighing less than 110 lb (49.9 kg) are excluded from donation because they have too small a blood volume to donate blood safely. Donors taking drugs that would impair recovery from a vasovagal donor reaction may also be excluded in some locales. Recipient safety is promoted by excluding donors who are at risk for viral or bacterial infections or are taking medications that could cause reactions or impair the function of donated blood products.

AUTOLOGOUS AND DIRECTED DONATION

Autologous donations and directed donations are two strategies adopted by patients seeking to minimize their real or perceived risk of infection from blood products.

Autologous Donation

In autologous donation, patients deposit their own blood and then receive that blood if they need transfusion therapy. This eliminates the infectious and sensitization risks associated with allogeneic blood. Absolute contraindications to autologous donation are tight aortic stenosis, unstable angina, and active bacterial infection.[2] Low hemoglobin levels and poor venous access frequently limit the number of units that can be collected. With the increasing safety of allogeneic blood, the rationale for autologous donation may ultimately depend on the importance of the possible modulation of recipient immune function associated with allogeneic transfusion rather than the avoidance of blood-borne infections.

Directed Donation

Directed donation is donation for a specific recipient. It usually involves donations made by friends or family members of the intended recipient. It is based on the assumption that transfusions involving donors selected by the recipient carry lower risk of infections than transfusions involving donors from the general population. However, available prevalence data show that the risk of infectious disease from directed donors is no different from that of first-time donors.[3] The current risk of infection via

transfusion is so low [*see Table 1*] that justification for directed donor programs depends primarily on patient preferences or on the need for a selected donor serving as the only source of blood products to reduce the recipient's risk from exposure to multiple donors. The latter form of directed donation is most appropriate for neonatal transfusions, in which one of the biologic parents may provide all the needed blood products.[4]

SCREENING PROCEDURES

The combination of improved donor selection and postdonation testing has greatly decreased the infectious risks of allogeneic blood [*see Table 1*]. Predonation donor screening to identify clinical and lifestyle characteristics associated with higher incidences of infection has produced the biggest decrease in the risk of transfusion-transmitted disease.

POSTDONATION TESTING

Postdonation testing is essential in identifying donors likely to transmit blood-borne infections who are missed in the initial screening process.

Screening for Hepatitis Viruses

Hepatitis C Screening for hepatitis C began in 1990 with the availability of a single antigen-based enzyme-linked immunosorbent assay (ELISA). This assay, together with second- and third-generation assays, their associated confirmatory tests, and nucleic acid testing (NAT) for viral RNA or DNA, has reduced the per-unit risk of hepatitis C virus (HCV) transmission to less than 0.0001% (1 per 1.6 million to 1 per 1.935 million).[5,6] Before these tests were available, the risk per unit was about 4%. Improved hepatitis C testing has eliminated the need for surrogate tests, such as the measurement of alanine aminotransferase (ALT) levels and testing for antibody to hepatitis B virus (HBV) core antigen. However, the test for antibody to HBV core antigen is still used to detect recently infected donors who lack measurable circulating HBV antigen.[7]

The epidemiology of HCV is still poorly understood. Approximately 20% to 25% of persons found to be HCV positive have no known risk factors.[8] Sexual transmission occurs with enough frequency to warrant evaluation of partners and appropriate use

Table 1 Estimated Risk of Infection per Transfused Blood Product[5,6]

Virus	Risk in Year 2000	Risk in Year 2003
Human immunodeficiency virus type 1/type 2 (HIV-1/2)*	1 in 660,000	1 in 2,135,000
Human T cell lymphotropic virus type I/type II (HTLV-I/II)†	1 in 641,000	1 in 2,993,000
Hepatitis B	1 in 63,000	1 in 205,000
Hepatitis C	< 1 in 103,300	1 in 1,935,000

*Risk with p24 antigen testing and HIV antibody testing.
†Approximately 67% of infections resulting from transfused blood products are infections with HTLV-II.

of methods of barrier protection.[9] Heterosexual transmission of HCV may be asymptomatic; a donor who was infected via sexual contact but has not yet developed detectable antibodies is a potential risk to the blood supply. Therefore, persons who are sexual partners of known HCV-infected persons may be excluded from donation. Donors found to be ELISA positive for HCV should have supplemental tests, such as the second-generation and third-generation recombinant immunoblot assays (RIBA-2, RIBA-3). Donors with positive supplemental test results are likely to have a chronic HCV infection and require further clinical evaluation.[10] Donors with negative supplemental test results probably had false positive screening results and may be eligible for reentry into the allogeneic donor pool after 6 months.[11] The infection status of donors with indeterminate supplemental results is best resolved by testing for HCV RNA; those with only a single band on the most sensitive supplemental test (RIBA-3) have a less than 4% chance of having circulating HCV RNA.[12]

Gene amplification methods for detecting HCV RNA are used on all blood products before release for transfusion. These tests directly detect the presence of virus before antibody development and are responsible for the current minuscule risk of HCV transmission.[6] Correlation studies have shown that only 80% of samples with confirmed serologic positive results for HCV are also NAT positive. This is consistent with previous estimates of the prevalence of HCV-positive persons who have cleared the virus.[6]

Hepatitis B Transmission of other forms of hepatitis by blood products is extremely rare. Modern testing methods and eliminating the practice of paying whole blood donors have reduced HBV infections to about one in 205,000 units transfused.

Hepatitis A Because the viremic phase of hepatitis A lasts about 17 days in humans before signs and symptoms develop, hepatitis A transmission from single-donor products is extremely rare. Pooled products, such as factor concentrates, however, carry a substantially higher risk.[13]

Hepatitis D Hepatitis D is a defective virus that requires HBV to produce fulminating hepatitis; it is a concern only for patients already infected with HBV.

Hepatitis G The flavivirus hepatitis G, now shown to include several strains, is present in about 4.5% of normal donors. It is transmitted from mother to infant, sexually, and by blood.[14] Circulating hepatitis G RNA is removed after the recipient develops antibodies, which makes the recipient resistant to further infection.[15] HGV has not been linked to any form of clinical hepatitis in children or adults. It is an example of a blood-borne virus without known pathogenicity; as yet, there is no clear reason to remove it from the blood supply.

Screening for Retroviruses

All blood products are screened for HIV-1, HIV-2, human T cell lymphotropic virus type I (HTLV-I), and HTLV-II. Data obtained nationally from American Red Cross donors indicate that the infection risk has been reduced from two per 100 transfusions to about one per 2 million transfusions because of the exclusion of high-risk donors and the postdonation testing for HIV-1 and HIV-2 antibodies and NAT for viral RNA or DNA.[5]

To have predictive value, the ELISA screening test for HIV must be confirmed by Western blot assay. Studies based on polymerase chain reaction (PCR) data, culture data, and donor review all indicate that donors with negative or indeterminate Western blot results are seldom, if ever, HIV positive.[16] A follow-up study of donors who were ELISA positive and whose Western blot results were indeterminate demonstrated that positive ELISA results persisted in about 45% of cases. Of these, 84% still had indeterminate Western blot results, but none were shown to be HIV positive by PCR.[17,18] There have been occasional false positive results of Western blot assays in low-risk donors.[19] The possibility of a false positive result should be remembered when one is counseling low-risk donors who have had unexplained positive results on Western blot testing; these false positive results must always be confirmed by careful clinical follow-up. Data since the introduction of NAT show that less than 6% of confirmed serologic positive results will be NAT negative. On the other hand, only 1.5% of NAT screen reactives were Western blot indeterminate or negative. Virtually none of these NAT reactives were confirmed by discriminatory NAT testing or PCR.[6]

The prevalence of HTLV-I and HTLV-II in United States donors was about 0.03% in 1995. Data from 2001 suggest that the prevalence has been reduced to about 0.01%; about two thirds of these HTLV-positive patients have HTLV-II.[5] Several longitudinal studies have defined the clinical consequences of HTLV-I/II infection[20-22]; they are useful in advising donors who have had positive or indeterminate test results. In a prospective, longitudinal study comparing seropositive blood donors with seronegative blood donors, both viruses were associated with an increase in the incidence of some infectious diseases. No cases of adult T cell leukemia or lymphoma were identified; myelopathies, though rare, were associated with both HTLV types.[22] The risk of HTLV-I/II transmission by blood products is one per 2,993,000.[5] As with HIV, laboratory studies and epidemiologic investigations of HTLV-I/II indicate that patients with positive screening-test results and negative or indeterminate supplemental-test results are unlikely to have clinical sequelae and that the positive results are most likely false positives.[23]

False Positive Test Results during Donor Screening

The causes of false positive test results for HCV and retroviruses are poorly understood. Flu vaccines administered in 1992 were associated with an increase in false positive results for these viruses.[24] However, the proteins responsible for cross-reactivity have not yet been identified. Tests for low-prevalence infections, even tests with excellent specificity and sensitivity, will always be associated with a substantial proportion of false positive results. Consequently, test characteristics, as well as culture and PCR results, can provide reassurance for donors who are not at risk but who have had positive screening-test results and negative or indeterminate confirmatory-test results. As PCR technology improves, it will probably become the most reliable means of establishing whether a positive result represents infection or is a false positive result.

Emerging Infectious Diseases

Until either screening tests or sterilization procedures become available, epidemiologic considerations are the only possible protective strategy against newly recognized infections.[25] For example, transmission of West Nile virus by blood products has led to new donor questions to eliminate donors at risk for this disease, and a nucleic acid–based test for all donated units was introduced in June 2003.[26] In the case of prion diseases such as variant Creutzfeldt-Jakob disease (vCJD), the restrictions put in place have led to a loss of 4% to 5% of active blood donors and caused transient shortages of certain products such as albumin and immune globulin. In Great Britain, the first case of possible transfusion-transmitted vCJD was reported in December 2003.[27] The report identified 48 recipients of blood from a total of 15 donors who had developed vCJD. In one recipient, symptoms of the disease developed 6.5 years after the possible exposure, a time frame consistent with human-to-human vCJD transmission. The authors estimated the chance of this patient having contracted vCJD independent of the transfusion to be between one in 15,000 and one in 30,000. Estimates of the incidence of new vCJD diagnoses in the United Kingdom suggest that there will be fewer than 200 cases from 2001 to 2005 and fewer than 100 cases from 2006 to 2010.[28] Thus, although the current donor restrictions seem prudent, it is important that donors rejected because of epidemiologic risk for vCJD understand the low probability that they actually have a health problem.

Pretransfusion Testing

ANTIGEN PHENOTYPING

Blood recipients are routinely tested to establish their ABO phenotype and Rh type. Establishing ABO type is essential because isoagglutinins (antibodies) against A or B antigens not present on a person's red cells are acquired during the first 2 years of life. These IgM antibodies will cause an immediate hemolytic reaction if ABO-incompatible red cells are transfused.

The terminal carbohydrate on these antigens determines specificity in the ABO system, with type A being associated with N-acetylgalactosamine and type B being associated with a terminal galactose. Persons with type O lack both of these terminal sugars. These residues are added by a glycosyltransferase, which was thought to be either nonfunctional or absent in type O persons. Yamamoto and colleagues[29] used molecular techniques to prove that glycosyltransferase in type O persons is very similar to the transferase in type A persons. The type O glycosyltransferase is nonfunctional because of a single base deletion that produces a frameshift and a downstream stop codon.

All methods of ABO typing depend on demonstrating that the antigens found on the red cells are consistent with the expected isoagglutinins [see Table 2]. Molecular methods to determine ABO genotype are available.[30] D antigen specificity typing in the Rh system is done because of this antigen's potency as an immunogen. Antibodies to the D antigen are the most important cause of isoimmune hemolytic disease of newborns. Rh antigens are membrane glycolipids or glycoproteins. Antibodies against antigens of this class, which includes the Rh, Duffy, Kell, Kidd, and Lutheran systems, will usually cause shortened red cell survival. In contrast to antigens with carbohydrate-mediated specificity, glycolipid and glycoprotein antigens do not stimulate antibody formation unless the transfusion recipient was previously exposed to allogeneic red cells either from transfusion or from fetal red cells during pregnancy or delivery.

D antigen typing is also done using agglutination techniques. In some cases, less antigenic forms of the D antigen, called weak D, require an antiglobulin reagent to enhance detection. Structural studies of the complementary DNA associated with the major Rh antigens (D, Cc, and Ee) have provided probes for direct genotyping.[31] Molecular methods of prenatal Rh type determination have revealed that most Rh-negative persons lack the D gene.

Some persons with the weak D phenotype have mosaic D genes because of exchange with some of the exons of the CcEe gene.

Because the genotypes of many of the clinically relevant red cell antigens are now known, it should now be possible to predict red cell phenotype by DNA analysis. Reid and colleagues[32] were able to correctly predict the red cell phenotype in 60 multitransfused patients by DNA analysis of each patient's white blood cells. This approach, although not yet generally available, will be useful for recently transfused patients, for whom circulating allogeneic red cells complicate antigen phenotyping.

SCREENING FOR ANTIBODIES

In addition to identifying patient ABO and D red cell phenotypes, blood banks must screen serum for red cell–specific antibodies, which can cause serious reactions with transfused red cells. Screening involves testing serum against indicator type O red cells displaying all the clinically important red cell antigens. Positive reactions are detected by adding an antiglobulin reagent (Coombs reagent) to the incubated mixture of type O red cells after it has been washed free of serum. Any observed agglutination is from the reaction of the antiglobulin reagent with antibody adsorbed on the surface of the indicator red cells [see Chapter 93]. Agglutination of the indicator red cells indicates the presence of other antibodies, which require identification. The absence of agglutination excludes all antibodies except those against antigens so rare that they are not displayed on the indicator red cells.

Use of type-specific blood removes the risk of ABO incompatibility. There is, however, a residual risk of an immunologic reaction from the antibodies to other red cell antigens; such antibodies are present in about 3% to 5% of a random population and in 10% to 15% of persons who were recently transfused or women with a history of pregnancy. Screening for antibodies reduces the frequency of reactions to about 0.06%. Performing a full crossmatch, in which the recipient's serum is tested against the red cells actually being transfused, is of negligible additional benefit, because it excludes only technical errors and the rare antibody that is not detected by the screening. Therefore, a full crossmatch is performed only for persons already known to have made antibodies, because such persons are more likely to form additional antibodies if they are further stimulated by red cell transfusion.

Patients who may receive allogeneic red cells who either have had a transfusion or have become pregnant within the past 3 months must be tested for new antibodies every 3 days. There is no consensus concerning how long the interval should be between patient specimen collection and use of the specimen in pretransfusion testing for patients not recently exposed to red cells. Commonly, specimens are accepted 14 to 28 days before the

Table 2 ABO Typing

Blood Type	Erythrocytes plus Anti-A Serum	Erythrocytes plus Anti-B Serum	Antibodies in Patient's Serum
A	+	0	Anti-B antibodies
B	0	+	Anti-A antibodies
AB	+	+	No antibodies
O	0	0	Anti-A and anti-B antibodies

+—agglutination   0—no agglutination

date for use. However, one study showed that no new antibodies appeared in paired specimens collected up to 1 year apart, suggesting that a longer acceptance interval may be possible.[33]

Blood Components

Most blood donations undergo a fractionation process that allows each component to be used for specific indications. Whole blood can be fractionated into red cells (which contain most of the leukocytes), platelet concentrates (which contain some leukocytes), and plasma [see Table 3]. Plasma can be further subdivided into coagulation components and albumin. Each whole-blood unit can potentially support many recipients and clinical needs, maximizing use of each donation.

After 24 hours' storage, whole blood contains no active platelets, and after 2 days, it is deficient in factors V and VIII. Therefore, except for some autologous blood programs that use whole blood rather than packed red cells, use of whole blood has now been almost completely supplanted by therapy employing specific blood components.

RED BLOOD CELLS

The anticoagulant used determines the shelf life of red cells [see Table 3]. Citrate-phosphate-dextrose (CPD) with the addition of adenine (CPDA-1) increases storage time from 28 days to 35 days. Most red cells are now stored in CPD to which extra nutrients have been added, which increases storage time to 42 days. This additive solution sometimes contains additional saline, which can be removed if units with very high hematocrits (~70%) are needed.

To prevent transfusion reactions or to delay alloimmunization, red cells are further processed by leukocyte reduction (see below) or washing to remove plasma proteins. Current filter technology reduces white cell counts to less than 5×10^6 cells per unit, a concentration that is sufficient to reduce febrile transfusion reactions and delay alloimmunization and platelet refractoriness. Washing red cells removes the plasma, leaving less than 0.5 ml per unit, a degree of plasma depletion usually effective in treating allergic transfusion reactions. Leukocyte filtration and washing red cells usually shorten the product shelf life to 24 hours, because these procedures require breaking the seal on the plastic bag that contains the red cells, thereby increasing the risk of bacterial contamination. Leukocyte reduction can be accomplished during collection, immediately after collection in the blood bank, or at the bedside during product infusion. Prestorage or laboratory filtration is preferred to bedside filtration.[34] Universal leukoreduction has been implemented in Canada and Europe, but it is not yet required in the United States because of concerns regarding cost-effectiveness.

Table 3 Characteristics of Blood Products and Indications for Use

Product	Volume (One Unit)	Hematocrit (Hct) or Platelet Count	White Cell Count	Shelf Life	Donors per Unit	Storage Outside Blood Bank	Indication
Whole blood	450–500 ml (± 10%)	Hct 35–45	$3–5 \times 10^9$	With additive solution, 42 days; with CPDA-1, 35 days; with CPD, 28 days	1	2°–6° C	Massive transfusion if available; exchange transfusions in newborns younger than 3 days
Red cells	With additive solution, 350 ml; with CPD, 250 ml	If additive solution used, Hct 55; if CPD used, Hct 70	$1–2 \times 10^9$	Same as whole blood	1	Same as whole blood	To increase oxygen-carrying capacity; to maintain volume and oxygen-carrying capacity when bleeding
Platelet concentrates	40 ml	$8–9 \times 10^{10}$	$2–6 \times 10^7$	5 days	1/U; given as pool of 5–6 U	Room temperature	For major bleeding or surgical procedures, when platelet count is < 50,000–100,000 μl; for prophylaxis in nonbleeding patients, when platelet count is < 10,000 μl; for bleeding that is refractory to SDPs, when HLA-matched or crossmatched platelets are not available
Single-donor platelets	200–250 ml	$3–5$ ml $\times 10^{11}$	Depends on method of collection	5 days	1	Room temperature	Same as platelet concentrates, but SDPs are preferred because of lower donor exposure
Fresh frozen plasma (FFP)	200–250 ml	—	$< 1 \times 10^5$	1 yr; 24 hr when thawed	1	2°–6° C	Multiple coagulation factor deficiency from bleeding or DIC; reversal of warfarin therapy; factor XI deficiency when factor XI concentrates are unavailable; treatment of TTP
Cryoprecipitate	10–20 ml; pool of 10 U ~ 200 ml	—	$< 1 \times 10^5$	1 yr; 24 hr when thawed	1/U; given as pool of 10 U	2°–6° C wet ice	Replacement of fibrinogen when acutely depleted or when patient cannot tolerate volume load of equivalent amount of FFP (1 pool of cryoprecipitate = 4 FFP); fibrin glue (usually only 1 unit); replacement of von Willebrand factor if concentrate is not available; replacement of factor XIII; replacement for qualitatively abnormal fibrinogen

CPD—citrate-phosphate-dextrose CPDA-1—CPD with adenine DIC—disseminated intravascular coagulation FFP—fresh frozen plasma HLA—human leukocyte antigen SDPs—single-donor platelets TTP—thrombotic thrombocytopenic purpura

Freezing is an alternative method for storing red cells. Red cells can be kept in a cryoprotectant (usually glycerol) for 10 years. Freezing is therefore ideal for storing rare units or autologous units from persons with rare blood types, for whom it is difficult to find compatible allogeneic red cells. When a unit is at the end of its liquid storage shelf life, the cells can be rejuvenated with fresh media and nutrients; they can then be frozen and stored. To be used, frozen red cells must be thawed and the glycerol removed, so preparation time for this product is longer than for products stored in the liquid state. Thawed, deglycerolized red cells generally must be transfused within 24 hours.

PLATELETS

Platelets can be provided either as platelet concentrates from a number of blood donors or from a single donor. SDPs are collected by a continuous apheresis process that removes platelets and returns all other blood components. A single transfusion of platelet concentrates usually consists of platelets derived from four to six units of donated whole blood, which is about the same number of platelets contained in one SDP product. The advantage of SDP therapy is the reduced risk of blood-borne infection and antigen exposure, because the product is from one donor rather than from four to six; disadvantages are a longer collection time, greater cost, and often limited supply. The potential advantages of each of these products have been summarized in a review.[35] ABO Rh–compatible platelets should be used when possible, because studies have shown significantly better therapeutic results from compatible transfusions.[36]

PLASMA

Fresh plasma, frozen within 8 hours of collection (FFP), contains all the procoagulants at normal plasma concentrations. After thawing, it can be kept for 24 hours at 2° to 6° C and will retain 3 to 4 mg/ml of fibrinogen and 1 IU/ml of all the other coagulation components.

Solvent/detergent-treated plasma (S/D plasma) was formerly available as an alternative to FFP with lower infectious risks. However, in 2002 this product was withdrawn from the market by the manufacturer, presumably because of lack of demand for the product and evidence of selective inactivation of certain plasma components. Alternative methods of postcollection sterilization of single units of plasma are becoming available. The main advantage of a postdonation sterilization process is that it protects patients from blood-borne infections, including ones that are not yet recognized. Potential disadvantages are cost and less effectiveness than FFP.

Cryoprecipitate consists of the cryoproteins recovered from FFP when it is rapidly frozen and then allowed to thaw at 2° to 6° C. These cryoproteins include fibrinogen, factor VIII, von Willebrand factor, factor XIII, and fibronectin. About 40% of the components in FFP are recovered. The cryoproteins are suspended in a small amount of plasma that contains ABO isoagglutinin at the concentration found in normal plasma. A pool of 10 units of cryoprecipitate (each derived from one unit of FFP) contains an amount of fibrinogen equivalent to four units of FFP but in one fourth to one fifth the volume. Consequently, a cryoprecipitate pool permits more rapid replacement of fibrinogen than FFP but has the disadvantage of more donor exposures. After the cryoprecipitate is removed from FFP, the residual product is known as cryopoor plasma. Once frozen, cryopoor plasma has the same shelf life as FFP.

Transfusion of Red Cells

INDICATIONS FOR ALLOGENEIC TRANSFUSION

Acute Blood Loss

The decision whether to use red cells depends on the etiology and duration of the anemia, the rate of change of the anemia, and assessment of the patient's ability to compensate for the diminished capacity to carry oxygen that results from the decrease in red cell mass. Management of acute anemia caused by bleeding or operative blood loss will differ from management of chronic anemia to which the patient has adapted. However, the question underlying any red cell transfusion is whether there is sufficient oxygen delivery to tissues for current needs.

Compensatory mechanisms for acute blood loss include adrenergic response, leading to constriction of venous beds, which improves venous return; increased stroke volume, tachycardia, or both; and increased peripheral resistance, which eventually redistributes blood flow to essential organs. Also contributing to the maintenance of intravascular volume is the shifting of fluid to the intravascular space; this shifting occurs relatively rapidly from the extravascular space and more slowly from the intracellular to the extravascular space.[37]

A decrease in blood volume has distinct effects on oxygen delivery, depending on the volume of blood lost and the functioning of the compensatory cardiovascular responses. Restoration of intravascular volume, usually with crystalloid, ensures adequate perfusion of peripheral tissue and is the first treatment goal for a patient with acute blood loss. Whether red cell transfusion is required depends on the extent of blood loss and the presence of comorbid conditions that may limit host response to the blood loss. The American College of Surgeons has correlated blood loss with clinical findings. Loss of up to 15% of total blood volume (class I hemorrhage) usually has little effect; this amount is the maximum permitted in normal blood donation. A class II hemorrhage (15% to 30% loss) results in tachycardia, decreased pulse pressure, and, possibly, restlessness. A class III hemorrhage (30% to 40% loss) leads to obvious signs of hypovolemia; mental status often remains normal. Red cell transfusion is usually indicated when blood loss exceeds 30% in a patient without other significant comorbid conditions. However, the presence of serious cardiac, peripheral vascular, or pulmonary disease can lower this threshold. For example, anemic patients with significant coronary artery disease are more likely to have serious postoperative myocardial complications.

The threshold for red cell transfusion has been evaluated in two randomized, controlled trials. In one study of transfusion after coronary artery bypass, patients who received transfusions for hemoglobin levels below 8 g/dl did no worse than control patients who received transfusions for hemoglobin levels below 9 g/dl.[38] The other trial compared outcomes in critical care patients who received transfusions when their hemoglobin level fell below either 7 g/dl or 10 g/dl.[39] Enrollment in this study was limited to patients who were euvolemic at entry and whose hemoglobin levels were from 7 to 9 g/dl; patients who had undergone routine cardiac procedures or who were actively bleeding upon entry to the intensive care unit were excluded. There was no statistical difference in 30-day mortality for these two groups. However, in the subgroups of patients younger than 55 years and patients whose illness was less severe, as defined by standardized clinical criteria, Kaplan-Meier survival estimates were significantly better in the patients who were not transfused

Table 4 Indications for Platelet Transfusion

Platelet Count (μl)	Indication for Transfusion
< 10,000	All patients, even if asymptomatic
< 20,000	Coagulation disorder or minor bleeding
< 50,000–100,000	Major bleeding or surgical procedure

unless hemoglobin levels dropped below 7 g/dl. These results are provocative, but they must be interpreted cautiously. They do suggest that more restrictive transfusion policies may be safely adopted for selected patients. However, the enrollment criteria may have biased the findings, and this calls into question the applicability of these findings to other settings.

Chronic Anemia

In the chronically anemic patient, an increase in red cell 2,3-diphosphoglycerate leads to a shift in the oxygen dissociation curve and improved delivery of oxygen to tissues. This adaptation augments the mechanisms for improved oxygen delivery described above. Indications for transfusion depend on clinical assessment of the adequacy of oxygen delivery and are also guided by the etiology of the anemia. If the anemia can be reversed with iron, folic acid, or vitamin B$_{12}$, transfusion therapy is indicated only in patients with clinical findings that cannot be tolerated while endogenous red cell mass is being regenerated. Patients with chronic renal disease are typically deficient in erythropoietin. Replacement therapy with exogenous erythropoietin [*see Chapter 92*] often obviates the need for transfusion. Patients with anemia that is a result of chronic disease such as rheumatoid arthritis, malignancy, or AIDS may also respond to erythropoietin.[40,41]

Relatively little is known about transfusion thresholds in specific medical illnesses. An observational trial has addressed the effect of anemia on the 30-day mortality of elderly patients hospitalized with acute myocardial infarction. Mortality was reduced in those patients who were transfused to a hematocrit of 30% to 33%, but transfusion had little or no effect on patients who presented with a hematocrit already in the 30% to 33% range.[42]

INDICATIONS FOR AUTOLOGOUS TRANSFUSION

Whether the criteria for autologous transfusion should be the same as that for allogeneic transfusion remains unresolved. Although the risk associated with autologous blood is less than that associated with allogeneic blood, it is not zero. Errors in labeling, storage, and processing can still occur. For these reasons, many argue that uniform standards based on oxygen delivery should apply, regardless of the blood source. Others, citing the reduced risk, advocate returning most or all of the predeposited units to the patient. There is no clinical evidence that either transfusion policy is associated with better or worse patient outcomes.[43]

Intraoperative and postoperative blood salvage can also help limit allogeneic blood use. Blood salvage is employed in procedures associated with the shedding of large volumes of blood; it involves returning concentrated red cells to the patient after those cells have been washed. Preoperative isovolemic hemodilution (PIH) is a process in which blood collected immediately before surgery is returned as needed postoperatively. This strategy has been shown to be a cost-effective alternative to preoperative autologous donation in patients undergoing radical prosta-tectomy.[44] PIH would be particularly useful if an oxygen-carrying blood substitute were available to replace the autologous blood that is removed. Until it is clear that the cardiovascular risks associated with acute hemodilution do not outweigh the risks associated with allogeneic blood, this approach should be considered with caution.

Transfusion of Platelets

In general, the decision to transfuse platelets rests on the answers to two questions: (1) Is the thrombocytopenia the result of underproduction or increased consumption of platelets? and (2) Do the existing platelets function normally?

INDICATIONS FOR TRANSFUSION

Low Platelet Count

Thrombocytopenia can result from decreased production caused by marrow hypoplasia or from increased consumption caused by conditions such as idiopathic thrombocytopenic purpura (ITP). In a patient with ITP, surviving platelets are larger and younger and function better than would be expected given the platelet count; platelet transfusion is largely avoided or minimized for such a patient. In contrast, with hypoplasia, platelet function is more severely impaired, and the risk of bleeding is relatively higher. Thus, the decision to transfuse patients who have hypoproliferative thrombocytopenia is generally based on their platelet count and is initiated prophylactically when the count drops below a certain threshold. Published consensus guidelines provide an excellent summary of all aspects of platelet therapy.[45]

Studies have shown that the prevalence of bleeding increases significantly below a threshold of about 10,000 platelets/μl in otherwise asymptomatic patients.[46] The desire to avoid allogeneic donor exposure, cost concerns, and increasing platelet demand have encouraged the use of transfusion policies similar to the policy proposed by Wandt and colleagues [*see Table 4*].[45,46]

Nonfunctioning Platelets

Platelet function is the second criterion for the transfusion of platelets. Transfusion is appropriate in a bleeding patient whose platelet count is adequate but whose platelets are nonfunctional as a result of medications such as aspirin or nonsteroidal anti-inflammatory drugs or as a result of bypass surgery. In a bleeding patient, if platelet dysfunction is from inherited or acquired defects, transfusion is indicated to provide a minimum number of normal platelets. Platelet function is abnormal in uremic patients, and definitive treatment requires correction of the uremia. Some studies suggest that interventions that increase von Willebrand factor levels, such as desmopressin (1-desamino-8-D-arginine vasopressin [DDAVP]) conjugated estrogen, or cryoprecipitate, may favorably influence platelet function in uremia.[47] In vitro evidence suggests that DDAVP may improve platelet dysfunction caused by glycoprotein IIb/IIIa (GPIIb/IIIa) inhibitors (e.g., eptifibatide, abciximab, tirofiban) or aspirin.[48]

CONTRAINDICATIONS TO PLATELET TRANSFUSION

Proper investigation of the causes of thrombocytopenia will identify clinical situations in which platelets should be withheld because they contribute to evolution of the illness. These disorders include thrombotic microangiopathies such as TTP, hemolytic-uremic syndrome, and HELLP syndrome (hemolysis, elevated liver enzymes, and a low platelet count). Posttransfusion purpura is usually unresponsive to platelet transfusion but may respond to plasma exchange or intravenous immunoglobulin (IVIg). Platelet transfusions will not help patients with autoimmune thrombocytopenia (e.g., ITP), but they also will not harm them.

RESPONSE TO PLATELET TRANSFUSIONS

Both platelet and host factors influence the response to platelet transfusions. Length of in vitro storage, storage temperature, adequacy of oxygenation, and extent of pretransfusion manipulation all influence in vivo survival. Important host factors that influence survival are temperature, splenomegaly, ABO compatibility, and immune status.

A transfusion of appropriately stored fresh platelets—whether pooled concentrates or SDPs—should contain about $6,000/\mu l$ to $10,000/\mu l$ platelets per unit (5.5×3^{10} platelets). Thus, in an unsensitized 75 kg (165 lb) recipient, each unit should yield an increment of about 60,000 platelets/μl. When needed, a post-transfusion count is usually obtained after 1 hour but can be obtained as early as 10 minutes after transfusion. A patient is considered refractory to platelet transfusions when the 1-hour post-transfusion increment is less than 10,000 platelets/μl after the patient is given 3.3×10^{11} platelets.

PLATELET TRANSFUSIONS IN REFRACTORY CASES

Platelets have platelet-specific antigens, human leukocyte antigens (HLA), and blood group antigens. Immune response to any of these can contribute to platelet unresponsiveness. Platelet surfaces have only class I HLA antigens, of which only HLA-A and HLA-B are clinically important. Polymorphic antigens are found in association with each of the major platelet proteins: HPA1a/2a (formerly called Pl$^{A1/A2}$) and Pen on glycoprotein IIIa, Bak system on glycoprotein IIb, and Br and Ko on glycoproteins Ia and Ib. Each of these antigen groups is associated with isoimmune neonatal thrombocytopenia. The prevalence of antibodies to platelet-specific antigens is increased for patients sensitized to HLA antibodies; therefore, antibodies to both sets of epitopes may contribute to refractoriness in patients who fail to respond to HLA-matched platelets.[49]

Treating a patient refractory to platelet transfusions involves addressing nonimmune causes (e.g., fever, sepsis, bleeding, and disseminated intravascular coagulation [DIC]) and providing recently collected ABO-compatible products. If these strategies fail, minimization of the effects of HLA antibodies or platelet antigens through HLA typing, platelet crossmatching, or both is indicated.[50] Selecting platelets matched at the HLA-A and HLA-B loci may improve responsiveness in about half of patients with positive HLA antibody screens. Unless contraindicated because of transplant considerations, an empirical trial of donations from family members may also be helpful.

In one study undertaken to determine the best method of treating refractory cases, platelet selection by crossmatching was compared with selection by HLA criteria. Selection by crossmatching was equivalent to HLA selection and yielded better results.[51] Another study found that crossmatched platelets provided equivalent platelet increments that were independent of the grade of HLA match.[52] Although these results are promising, the effectiveness of selection either by HLA and crossmatching or by crossmatching alone is often limited by nonimmune host factors. Additionally, these techniques are not yet routinely available.

Modifying the effects of alloimmunization is difficult. IVIg can improve platelet increments but not platelet survival. An analysis of IVIg therapy found that about 50% of alloimmunized patients appeared to benefit from such therapy.[50] Plasma exchange is of limited value because it is difficult to remove IgG antibodies. In some patients, the HLA antibodies responsible for refractoriness may regress over time, so it is important to periodically retest for them. If the HLA antibody screen becomes negative, a trial of non–HLA-matched platelets is warranted.

All in all, the best strategy is prevention, which can be achieved by avoiding unnecessary transfusions and using only leukocyte-depleted products. A randomized, prospective trial of how best to prevent alloimmunization of newly diagnosed patients with acute myeloid leukemia showed equivalent rates of alloimmunization and platelet refractoriness for filtered platelet concentrates, filtered SDPs, and ultraviolet B–irradiated platelets.[53] However, leukocyte reduction did not prevent secondary immune responses in patients already sensitized through either pregnancy or transfusion.[54]

Transfusion of Fresh Frozen Plasma, Plasma Derivatives, and Recombinant Products

FRESH FROZEN PLASMA

Despite a paucity of indications for FFP use, roughly two million units are transfused annually[55] [see Table 3]. FFP is most appropriate for replacing the multiple coagulation deficiencies that result from massive transfusion, liver disease, warfarin toxicity, or acute or chronic DIC. In addition, it can be used to treat thrombotic microangiopathies and specific factor deficiencies when factor concentrates are not available. After one blood volume exchange using only red cells, plasma components are diluted to about 40% of their original concentration; after two blood volume exchanges, plasma components are diluted to 15%. Prothrombin time (PT) and partial thromboplastin time (PTT) become prolonged when coagulation components are lower than 30%, but abnormal bleeding from dilution usually does not occur until these values are less than 17% of normal. Microvascular bleeding associated with a PT and PTT greater than 1.5 times normal is an indication for FFP.[56] Whether FFP replacement is needed when PT and PTT are over 1.5 times normal but not associated with bleeding is less clear-cut; paracentesis and thoracentesis did not cause increased bleeding in patients with PT and PTT that were up to twice normal values.[57]

The FFP dose depends on whether or not a consumptive process is being treated in addition to hemodilution. For hemodilution, 15 ml/kg will usually be sufficient. However, if consumption is occurring, the dose is best guided by the effect of treatment on PT and PTT. If fibrinogen is lower than 80 mg/dl, cryoprecipitate may be required to rapidly increase fibrinogen. However, four units of FFP can be used in most cases to provide the same amount of fibrinogen as one pool of cryoprecipitate. Urgent reversal of the effects of warfarin can usually be accomplished with about 5 to 10 ml/kg of FFP.

Factor XI concentrates, which still have some thrombogenic potential, are available but not yet licensed in the United States.[58] Therefore, FFP is the treatment for factor XI deficiency. FFP is not used to replace antithrombin III, because a purified concentrate is available.[59]

Thrombotic microangiopathies [see Chapter 97] are treated with either FFP transfusions or, more often, plasma exchange with either FFP or cryopoor plasma.[60] Studies suggest that cryopoor plasma may be an alternative to FFP in the treatment of

TTP.[61] The dose of either product is usually equal to a plasma volume exchange of 1.0 to 1.5, which is carried out daily until clinical improvement occurs.

FACTOR VIIA

Recombinant activated factor VII was approved in 1999 for the treatment of bleeding episodes in patients with hemophilia A or B who have antibodies (inhibitors) to factor VIII or IX, respectively. Factor VIIa is also the treatment of choice for the rare patient with factor VII deficiency, whether acquired—as, for example, a consequence of liver disease—or inherited. It is not approved for this purpose, however. In addition, factor VIIa is useful in activation of the coagulation tissue factor pathway. For patients with inhibitors, factor VIIa is given at a dosage of 90 μg/kg as a slow I.V. push over 2 to 5 minutes; the dosage is repeated every 2 hours, as needed. For factor VII deficiency, the dosage is 20 to 30 μg/kg given as a slow I.V. push over 10 minutes; given in this manner, factor VIIa treatment will reduce the PT to normal within 20 minutes after administration. Depending on the clinical setting, the PT will become prolonged again 3 to 4 hours after treatment.

Off-label use of this product to treat uncontrolled hemorrhage in patients who do not have a preexisting bleeding disorder and who are unresponsive to FFP is becoming more common.[62] However, it is important not to use factor VIIa in patients with DIC, because VIIa may exacerbate the DIC. The high cost of this product and its potential for contributing to DIC should limit its use to carefully selected patients for whom other alternatives are not available.

FACTOR VIII CONCENTRATES

The introduction of plasma-derived factor VIII concentrates in the 1960s brought a significant improvement in the treatment of hemophilia A. Unfortunately, these concentrates were derived from large donor pools, and contamination of the factor with HBV, HVC, and, especially, HIV resulted in the widespread transmission of these infections in the hemophilia community. Since 1980, new methods of heat sterilization, solvent/detergent treatment, and immunoaffinity purification have yielded an array of factor concentrates that are highly purified and unable to transmit these infections. The efficacy of these viral-inactivation methods has been validated by using reverse transcription and PCR studies to measure HCV RNA in factor VIII concentrates; HCV RNA was present in 100% of products before treatment but was undetectable after treatment. Besides reducing the risk of infection, use of high-purity factor VIII concentrates may be associated with better preservation of patients' cell-mediated immunity. The 1980s also saw the advent of recombinant factor VIII concentrates.

The factor VIII preparation Humate-P is also rich in von Willebrand factor and is approved for the treatment of von Willebrand disease. This product has the major advantage of being free of the risks of infection associated with cryoprecipitate. If Humate-P is not available, the factor VIII preparations Alphanate or Koate-DVI may be used, but they are not approved for this purpose and their efficacy is uncertain.

The advances in safety and purity of factor VIII concentrates, especially in the case of the recombinant products, have increased the cost per unit fivefold to 10-fold. Recombinant products are used primarily for newly diagnosed patients with hemophilia who have not been exposed to plasma products. Work is just beginning on modifying these recombinant products to make them more effective by reducing immunogenicity and prolonging circulation time.[63]

The possibility that a nonhuman source of factor VIII would be useful in the treatment of patients with acquired factor VIII inhibitors led to the development of a highly purified porcine factor VIII concentrate. This was shown to be effective for patients whose anti–factor VIII antibody does not cross-react with the porcine product.[64] About one third of patients develop antibodies to the porcine product, which limits its usefulness for repeat treatments.

FACTOR IX CONCENTRATES

Factor IX complex concentrates contain about equal amounts of the vitamin K–dependent factors II, VII, IX, and X. These preparations are available in several degrees of purity, but all have the disadvantage of being thrombogenic when used for extended periods or in patients with liver disease. Highly purified factor IX, prepared by immunoaffinity chromatography, is free of this complication and is the product of choice in treating factor IX deficiency.[65] Activated prothrombin complex concentrates (Autoplex-T and FEIBA) have been used to bypass the need for factor VIII in selected patients with hemophilia A and acquired inhibitors. This provides an alternative for patients who do not respond to porcine factor VIII [see Chapter 97].

Transfusion of Granulocytes

Studies have shown granulocyte transfusion to be effective in the treatment of neutropenic patients. Transfusion of granulocytes in doses in the range of 8.3×10^{10} can be obtained by apheresis of donors who have been pretreated with granulocyte colony-stimulating factor (G-CSF) and a single dose of dexamethasone. Granulocyte transfusions at these dose levels have been shown to produce measurable, sustained increments in neutrophils, even into the normal range. The indications and clinical benefits of granulocyte transfusion at these higher doses are still being determined. Randomized trials are required to fully define the clinical efficacy of granulocyte transfusions. After collection, granulocytes must be stored at room temperature and irradiated to prevent transfusion-associated graft versus host disease. Crossmatching should be done to ensure compatibility.[66]

Transfusion of Immune Globulin

Many human immune globulin preparations are available. Immune serum globulin, administered intramuscularly, is used to treat chronic immunodeficiency disease and for prevention or alleviation of measles. Hepatitis A can now be prevented by vaccination [see Chapter 69]. Alternatively, a traveler who will spend less than 3 months in an endemic area can receive 0.02 ml/kg of immune serum globulin. Hepatitis B immune globulin is used for postexposure prophylaxis against HBV infection [see Chapter 5]. It is prepared from plasma with high titers of antibody to hepatitis B surface antigen. $Rh_0(D)$ immune globulin is used to prevent the development of anti-Rh_0 (anti-D) antibodies in Rh-negative women who have just given birth, undergone amniocentesis, or aborted, if the biologic father is thought to be Rh positive.

Intravenous administration of human immune globulin promptly elevates circulating IgG levels; thus, intravenous administration is preferable to intramuscular administration. Several preparations of IVIg are available to treat chronic immunodeficiency disease[67] [see Chapter 102]. The intravenous dosage for such deficiency syndromes is 0.2 g/kg/mo but can be raised to 0.3 g/kg/mo or the agent can be given more often if needed.

The most common side effects of IVIg therapy—headache, nausea, and fever—usually respond to symptomatic treatment and reduction of the infusion rate. Rarer and potentially more severe side effects are anaphylactic reactions, hemolysis from anti-A and anti-B antibodies, and acute renal failure. Renal failure has been attributed to osmotic nephrosis caused by the high sucrose concentration in many IgG preparations.[68,69] In one study, aseptic meningitis was the most common of the serious side effects, with a frequency of 11% (95% confidence interval, 4% to 23%); patients with a history of migraine had a significantly higher incidence of aseptic meningitis.[70]Aseptic meningitis usually occurs within 24 hours after administration and does not respond to a reduction of the infusion rate. Patients may be required to stay in the hospital for symptomatic treatment; if further treatment is needed, changing the lot or preparation of IVIg may alleviate this side effect. Current manufacturing practices eliminate HCV from IVIg preparations.

Transfusion of Stem Cells

Stem cell transplantation was initially pioneered for use in leukemia; currently, it is used to treat a number of life-threatening, malignant, hereditary, and immunologic disorders [see Chapter 206].

Complications of Transfusions

HEMOLYTIC TRANSFUSION REACTIONS

Hemolytic transfusion reactions are classified as immediate or delayed, depending on their pathophysiology. Immediate hemolytic reactions are the result of a preexisting antibody in the recipient that was not detected during pretransfusion testing. Delayed hemolytic reactions are the result of an anamnestic response to an antigen to which the recipient is already sensitized. The renewed antigenic stimulation in a person already primed by previous antigenic exposure results in recrudescence of antibody to levels that can cause hemolysis. This is in contrast to an immune response during primary sensitization, which seldom causes hemolysis, because antibody levels develop at a much slower rate.

Patients with sickle cell disease are more likely than others to become alloimmunized and to have delayed hemolytic transfusion reactions, which often occur in association with recrudescence of an occlusive pain crisis. These reactions are occasionally associated with severe hemolysis involving autologous, as well as allogeneic, red cells. The cause of these episodes is unknown but has been attributed to so-called bystander hemolysis associated with abnormal function of CD59 (MIRL, membrane inhibitor of reactive lysis), transfusion-associated marrow suppression, or both.[71]

Diagnosis of Hemolytic Reactions

The pathophysiologic differences between immediate and delayed hemolytic transfusion reactions account for some of their differences in clinical findings. Fever is a common sign associated with both immediate and delayed hemolytic transfusion reactions.

Clinical evidence of hemolysis is likely to be more severe in immediate hemolytic reactions and may include back pain, pain along the vein into which the blood is being transfused, changes in vital signs, evidence of acute renal failure, and signs of developing DIC. These findings are probably caused by immune complexes activating the complement and kinin systems, by the direct effects of red cell stroma on kidney function, and possibly by the release of inflammatory cytokines such as interleukin-1β (IL-1β), IL-6, and tumor necrosis factor (TNF).[72]

In delayed hemolytic reactions, hemolysis with hemoglobinemia and hematuria (sometimes associated with renal failure) also occurs, but it is less common and generally less severe. In many delayed hemolytic transfusion reactions, the only clinical findings may be a newly positive Coombs test result, the appearance of a new antibody against red cell antigens that are not present on the recipient's red cells, or both. When hemolysis is absent, these reactions are sometimes called delayed serologic transfusion reactions. At the Mayo Clinic, two surveys sought to identify the relative incidence of both kinds of delayed transfusion reactions. The more recent survey, covering the period from 1993 to 1998, revealed a relative increase in delayed serologic transfusion reactions and an associated decrease in delayed hemolytic reactions, with overall increases in the incidence of these reactions. The earlier survey, which covered the period from 1980 to 1992, revealed an association between delayed transfusion reactions and the presence of antibodies to Jk[a] and Fy[a] or antibodies with multiple specificity; this association was not found in the later survey. These changes probably result from improved systems for identifying clinically significant nonhemolytic antibodies.[73]

In some cases, antiglobulin testing may yield positive results after all the transfused cells have been cleared, often with only complement being detected on the red cells. This finding has been attributed to autoimmune hemolysis after the delayed transfusion reaction.

Treatment of Hemolytic Reactions

As soon as a hemolytic transfusion reaction is suspected, the transfusion should be immediately discontinued. The diagnosis can be confirmed or excluded by sending the remaining blood product, together with a freshly drawn posttransfusion specimen, to the blood bank. The blood bank rechecks all records, confirms the patient's type and antibody screen, checks for evidence of hemoglobin in the plasma, and rechecks the crossmatch and antiglobulin test results. These tests will confirm or disprove the diagnosis and identify the antibody causing the immediate hemolytic reaction, when present. Until these studies have been completed, any further blood products can be given only with the approval of the blood bank's medical director.

The side effects of an acute hemolytic transfusion reaction can be managed by supporting renal blood flow with furosemide and supporting tubular urine flow with mannitol; treating shock, if required, with pressors; and giving platelets and FFP as needed to control coagulopathy if DIC develops. Intravenous steroids may be useful. Until the antibody causing the immune hemolysis is identified, only type O red cells and AB plasma should be used.

Managing delayed transfusion reactions is simpler because of the slower tempo at which these reactions develop. The diagnosis requires identifying a new antibody against red cell antigens and searching for clinical evidence of hemolysis. Treatment requires replacement with the appropriate antigen-negative blood products. Acute renal failure and DIC are unlikely but would be managed as described for immediate hemolytic reactions. The severe, atypical delayed transfusion reactions sometimes found in patients with sickle cell disease may require steroids and transfusion support.

Prevention of Hemolytic Reactions

Prevention of immediate and delayed hemolytic transfusion reactions depends on recognizing their respective proximate causes. Immediate hemolytic reactions are usually caused by technical errors made during the procurement or processing of blood specimens, during pretransfusion testing, or during product infusion. In a review of transfusion-related deaths reported to the Food and Drug Administration between 1990 and 1998, approximately 50% were caused by clerical errors that led to transfusion of ABO-incompatible blood, a rate virtually unchanged since reporting began in 1976.[74] Prevention of immediate transfusion reactions is best accomplished by following protocols for obtaining specimens from patients in adequate time before transfusion and checking to see that blood products are appropriate for the intended recipient.

Delayed transfusion reactions are the result of an anamnestic response of antibodies from a previous transfusion (or pregnancy) that are not present in detectable levels at the time the specimen is crossmatched. A careful transfusion history can best prevent delayed hemolytic reactions. Many patients will know whether there were difficulties involving blood obtained for transfusion. If a patient has a history of difficulty with crossmatches, the blood bank can obtain the details from the institution responsible for the previous transfusion. A proper transfusion history can uncover patients likely to have antibodies that the blood bank would not detect. For example, antibodies to Jk^a and Fy^a are characteristically hard to identify because they are quick to rise on stimulation and fall equally rapidly, making later detection difficult.

FEBRILE TRANSFUSION REACTIONS

Nonhemolytic febrile transfusion reactions occur in 1% to 2% of all transfusions and are more likely to occur after platelet transfusions. Until recently, febrile transfusion reactions were attributed to recipient antibody reactions against HLA antigens on donor leukocytes in the transfused product. It is now believed that cytokines produced during storage may also contribute to these reactions.[75] This conclusion is based on observations that platelet products associated with transfusion reactions have higher levels of inflammatory cytokines such as IL-1β, TNF, IL-6, and IL-8 in the supernatant than are found in platelets that do not cause febrile transfusion reactions.[75]

Diagnosis of Febrile Reactions

Febrile reactions are characterized by the development of fever during transfusion or within 5 hours after transfusion. These reactions may be limited to an increase in body temperature of 1° to 2° F but are often associated with chills and rigors.

The differential diagnosis for a patient undergoing a nonhemolytic febrile transfusion reaction should always include unrecognized sepsis. When febrile reaction is suspected, immediate management consists of discontinuing the transfusion, obtaining appropriate cultures, and returning the product to the blood bank. The blood bank obtains cultures from the product and verifies that no errors have occurred in its preparation. The probability that a febrile transfusion reaction has occurred is influenced by the type of product, the number of white cells contained therein, and the transfusion history of the recipient. Febrile reactions to products that have few or no white cells, such as deglycerolized red cells or FFP, are unusual. Unmodified whole blood and red cells contain between 1.3×10^9 and 3×10^9 white cells and are much more likely to cause febrile reactions. In the case of platelets, reactions can be from cytokines made during in vitro storage or from bacterial contamination.

Treatment of Febrile Transfusion Reactions

Febrile transfusion reactions are usually self-limited and respond to symptomatic management with antipyretics. However, symptoms may be of sufficient magnitude to require the use of 50 to 75 mg of meperidine by intravenous bolus. To prevent further occurrences, leukocyte-depleted products are indicated for patients who have had two or more febrile transfusion reactions.

Prevention of Febrile Reactions

Newer designs of filters for leukocyte reduction should decrease the white cell content to below the threshold for febrile transfusion reactions. Because inflammatory cytokines may be involved in febrile transfusion reactions, methods are being implemented to accomplish leukocyte reduction either during or after collection but before storage. In a study comparing products that underwent leukocyte reduction either before storage or at the bedside, significantly fewer febrile reactions occurred in patients receiving prestorage leukocyte-depleted products; there was no difference in the number of allergic reactions.[76]

Prestorage leukocyte reduction is particularly important for platelets because platelets are stored at room temperature and accumulate significantly more cytokines than do red cells, which are refrigerated. Febrile transfusion reactions are also more likely with older products. In one study, platelets that were used after they were in storage for 3 days or less were found to cause significantly fewer febrile transfusion reactions than platelets that were used after longer storage periods.[77] Unfortunately, testing for infectious diseases often takes 2 to 3 days, during which time the product cannot be used. It is therefore impractical to rely on younger products to reduce the risk of febrile transfusion reactions. Other benefits of leukocyte reduction are prevention of HLA alloimmunization; prevention of transmission of leukocyte-bound viruses such as cytomegalovirus (CMV), Epstein-Barr virus, HTLV-I, and HTLV-II; and, possibly, reduction of immune modulation.[78]

Whether these advantages justify leukocyte reduction for all blood products remains an unsettled issue because it is unclear whether the benefits justify the associated increased costs. Managing patients who continue to have febrile reactions after receiving leukocyte-depleted products is a clinical problem for which there are no clear solutions. In addition to premedication with steroids, use of HLA-matched products for patients demonstrated to have HLA antibodies may be helpful. Occasionally, use of washed products is beneficial.

TRANSFUSION-RELATED ACUTE LUNG INJURY

Transfusion-related acute lung injury (TRALI) usually presents as bilateral pulmonary infiltrates within 4 hours after transfusion.[79] The clinical and radiographic picture is that of normal-pressure acute respiratory distress syndrome (ARDS); therefore, the differential diagnosis is sufficiently broad to make the possible causal role of transfusion often go unnoticed. Current evidence suggests that TRALI is associated with the interaction of antibodies (HLA class 1 or class 2 antibodies, antimonocyte antibodies, or antigranulocyte antibodies), with the corresponding antigens on monocytes or granulocytes. A study found such associations in 14 of 16 TRALI patients.[80,81] These interactions cause endothelial injury, alveolar exudation, and the associated clinical findings of ARDS.

A second form of TRALI that involves two clinical events has been proposed.[82-84] In this two-event model, which is based on clinical findings and rat lung studies, the first step is the priming of neutrophils by mediators that arise in certain clinical settings (e.g., recent surgery, massive transfusion, cytokine therapy, or infection).[82] The primed neutrophils adhere to pulmonary endothelium and are activated by a second event, such as exposure to biologically active lipids from blood products.

Diagnosing TRALI depends on excluding cardiac and other causes of ARDS. Demonstration of antileukocyte antibodies helps confirm the diagnosis, but their absence does not exclude TRALI in the appropriate clinical setting. Early diagnosis is important because most patients will improve within 24 hours after conservative treatment is initiated. Unfortunately, a minority of patients develop TRALI associated with severe pulmonary edema and fluid filling the trachea, for which no effective therapy exists.

ALLERGIC TRANSFUSION REACTIONS

Allergic transfusion reactions are more common than febrile nonhemolytic transfusion reactions, occurring in 3% to 4% of transfusions. Allergic transfusion reactions usually present as pruritus and urticaria. A small percentage of patients have anaphylactoid symptoms, including wheezing, bronchospasm, and, occasionally, true anaphylaxis.[85] These reactions had been attributed to an immune response to plasma proteins. However, a 1999 study suggested that they may instead be provoked by increased levels of RANTES (regulated on activation, normal T cell expressed and secreted), an inflammatory chemokine that is stored in platelet alpha granules and accumulates during storage.[86] This is an intriguing hypothesis, because RANTES is known to affect eosinophil and basophil function.

In most cases, symptoms of allergic reactions are local and do not require discontinuance of the transfusion if they are controlled with antihistamines. There is, however, no means as yet to identify the rare patient who will progress to anaphylaxis.[85] It is known that IgA deficiency is associated with an increased likelihood of anaphylaxis, but many patients who are IgA deficient never have any difficulty.

For most patients with urticaria, which seldom progresses to anaphylaxis, management is symptomatic. However, patients known to be IgA deficient should receive cells that have been washed to remove plasma. When plasma products are required, they should be administered in a facility equipped to manage anaphylactic reactions. Using IgA-deficient plasma can minimize the risk, but such plasma is difficult to obtain and may require drawing from a rare donor pool, testing family members, or both.

ATYPICAL TRANSFUSION REACTIONS

Occasionally, patients have reactions that do not fit the categories already defined but clearly seem related to blood transfusion. These reactions have mainly consisted of severe hypotension after platelet infusions. No allergic features are present. The reactions are associated with blood-product infusions through a negatively charged leukocyte reduction filter, and they often occur in patients who are receiving angiotensin-converting enzyme (ACE) inhibitors. A recent study suggests that such reactions may be caused by excessive accumulation of des-Arg9-bradykinin. This metabolite of bradykinin is known to be vasoactive and to be metabolized by ACE.[87] Clinical observations suggest that atypical hypotensive reactions are more likely to occur in patients receiving ACE inhibitors during plasma exchange, hemodialysis, low-density lipoprotein apheresis, IgG-affinity column apheresis, and desensitization immunotherapy. These findings have led to the suggestion that ACE inhibitors should be withheld for 24 hours before any of these procedures are initiated. Such reactions are sufficiently rare that it may be adequate to limit this restriction to patients who have already experienced one of these reactions.[88]

TRANSFUSION-ASSOCIATED GRAFT VERSUS HOST DISEASE

The diagnosis of transfusion-associated graft versus host disease (TA-GVHD) should be considered in any patient who presents after transfusion with fever, skin rash, and diarrhea and has pancytopenia and abnormal results on liver function tests.[89] Signs and symptoms in neonates are similar to those in adults, but fever and rash develop later: in adults, fever occurs after a median of 10 days after transfusion; in neonates, fever occurs after 28 days, with rash appearing 1 to 2 days later.[90] TA-GVHD is a much-feared consequence of transfusion therapy because mortality approaches 100%. It results from transfusing immunocompetent lymphocytes into a recipient who is unable to reject the allogeneic cells. Reaction of the transfused lymphocytes with host antigens leads to the multiple manifestations of TA-GVHD.

TA-GVHD is best prevented by identifying potentially susceptible recipients. Patients who are at significant risk for TA-GVHD include premature infants receiving large doses of allogeneic lymphocytes, patients with congenital defects in cellular immunity or immunity resulting from illness or chemotherapy, and patients who are unable to reject infused cells because of shared antigens with the allogeneic lymphocytes. Patients undergoing autologous or allogeneic bone marrow transplantation are particularly at risk. Many case reports document the association of Hodgkin disease with TA-GVHD, which occurs presumably as a result of acquired defects in T cell immunity. The intensive chemotherapy that is used to treat leukemia, high-grade lymphomas, and solid tumors may also set the stage for TA-GVHD. However, no cases have been identified in AIDS patients. One hypothesis explaining this surprising finding is that the HIV-mediated injury to CD4[+] T cells blocks the development of TA-GVHD.[91]

Patients whose risk for TA-GVHD is a result of receiving transfusions from a homozygous donor of a shared haplotype are the hardest to identify a priori. Donor lymphocytes are not rejected by the recipient but do respond to the nonshared recipient haplotype. This mechanism probably accounts for the majority of cases of TA-GVHD. The chances of receiving haplotype-homozygous blood from an unrelated donor vary with different populations. In Japan, the risk for adults may be as high as 1 in 874; it is estimated to be 1 in 102 in neonates because of the use of fresh whole blood from family members.[92] In France, the risk is estimated to be 1 in 16,835. In the United States, the risk for the white population is thought to be about 1 in 7,147. Risk increases if first-degree relatives are donors.

Once patients at risk are identified [see Table 5], pretreatment of all cellular transfused products with gamma radiation is indicated. On the basis of in vitro studies, the current recommended

Table 5 Patients for Whom Irradiated Blood Products Are Recommended

Fetuses and neonates
Patients with congenital immunodeficiency
Allogeneic and autologous bone marrow transplantation patients
Recipients of some solid-organ transplants*
Patients with hematologic malignancies†
Patients with nonhematologic malignancies, especially if undergoing intensive chemotherapy‡
Recipients who may share haplotypes with donor§

*No consensus, but most agree that heart, liver, and lung recipients should receive irradiated products, whereas recipients of renal allografts do not require irradiated blood.
†Patients with low-grade lymphomas and leukemias in remission may not require irradiated products. Applying restriction to all lymphoma and leukemia patients avoids mistakes.
‡Except for immunosuppression from intensive chemotherapy, there is no consensus.
§Donors in this group include directed donors and first- and second-degree relatives.

dose is 2,500 cGy, which does not affect red cell function or platelet survival if administered immediately before transfusion.[93] However, irradiated red cells stored for 42 days show significant increases in plasma potassium and hemoglobin and a small but significant decrease in cell survival. Consequently, recommended storage after irradiation is only 28 days; most institutions prefer to irradiate immediately before product release when possible. Platelets have normal storage survival 5 days after irradiation and can be irradiated at regional centers before distribution. Leukocyte reduction may provide some protection against TA-GVHD, which is related to the dose of lymphocytes. However, filtration alone is not preventive and must never be used as a substitute for gamma irradiation. Because of the risk associated with a one-way HLA match, blood-bank standards require that family members' blood and blood of directed donors be irradiated.

Treatment of TA-GVHD remains ineffective. Prevention by providing irradiated blood products to all recipients may become the most practical solution to this complication.[94]

BACTERIAL AND PROTOZOAN INFECTIONS

Platelets are associated with the majority of cases of transfusion-related sepsis because the platelets are stored at room temperature.[95] Controlling this problem requires improved disinfection of skin, better detection of subclinical infection, and development of methods for storage at lower temperatures or postcollection sterilization. If sepsis is suspected in patients who have been given red cells, the possibility of *Yersinia enterocolitica* infection should be considered.[96] This organism can grow in the cold, iron-rich environment provided by stored red cells. When such infections occur, the blood is almost always at least 2 weeks old; this period corresponds to the time needed for the usually small initial inoculum to reach clinically significant amounts. Malaria infections have been almost completely eliminated by predonation screening. *Trypanosoma cruzi* can cause a chronic parasitic infection; the incidence of blood-borne transmission has increased to the point that pretransfusion testing for it may soon be needed. Spirochetes cannot be transmitted by products that have been stored longer than 80 hours and are no longer considered a clinically significant source of blood-borne infection.

CYTOMEGALOVIRUS INFECTION

CMV is a common blood-borne infection of no clinical consequence to healthy, immunocompetent recipients, but it can be a severe problem for patients with either acquired or congenital immunodeficiency [see Table 6]. Judged on the basis of screening for antibody to CMV, more than 40% of healthy donors may have the potential to transmit CMV.

There are two approaches to preventing CMV transmission. The first is to use CMV antibody–negative products. The second, more practical approach is to use leukocyte-reduced products, because CMV is transmitted only by leukocytes. On the basis of a prospective, randomized study of more than 500 transplant patients, products that have undergone leukocyte reduction to the current standard of fewer than 0.5×10^6 leukocytes per milliliter are considered to be as effective as seronegative products in preventing CMV infection.[97] It is unclear which product provides the best protection against transfusion-associated CMV infection.[98] Direct comparisons between seroconversion rates after transfusion of prestorage leukocyte-depleted products and seroconversion rates after transfusion of CMV-negative products are required to settle this issue.

IMMUNE MODULATION AS A RESULT OF TRANSFUSION

Evidence that transfusions result in modulation of host immunity has come from studies of transplantation, cancer recurrence, and posttransfusion infection rates. The effect was first observed in cadaver-kidney transplantation; patient survival was shown to increase with increased transfusions. Although this benefit became less important with the introduction of cyclosporine, Opelz and colleagues[99] found increased cadaver-graft survival in transfused recipients whose immunosuppression regimen included cyclosporine.

The hypothesis that immune modulation is related to infused white cells has been supported by studies in animal models and by clinical observations of tumor recurrence and posttransfusion infection rates. Bordin and colleagues[100] have shown in a rabbit model that the number of pulmonary metastases is increased by allogeneic blood transfusions but not by blood from syngeneic littermates. This effect of allogeneic blood is abrogated by prestorage leukocyte reduction but not by poststorage reduction. Randomized clinical studies of posttransfusion infection and cancer recurrence have produced conflicting results.[101] The conflicting data concerning the magnitude and clinical relevance of transfusion-induced immunomodulation need to be resolved. If leukocyte reduction is shown to reduce posttransfusion infections and cancer recurrence, the argument for universal leukocyte reduction of cellular blood products, which is already strong, would become irrefutable. Until this matter is settled, the possible immunomodulatory effect of blood transfusion is another reason to avoid allogeneic blood transfusion whenever possible.

Table 6 Patients for Whom Cytomegalovirus-Negative Blood Products Are Recommended

Neonates, especially if weight is less than 1,200 g
Pregnant women, as a means of preventing primary intrauterine infections
Recipients of solid-organ transplants, especially when the recipient and the organ donor are both CMV negative
Patients with severe combined immunodeficiency

Apheresis

Apheresis therapy is the converse of transfusion therapy; it entails treating disease by removing plasma, specific antibodies, or cells. It has been tried in a broad spectrum of diseases [see Table 7]. Therapeutic apheresis has real risks and may provide little benefit. It is usually an acute intervention that is only transiently effective, unless the underlying problem is being treated effectively. Consequently, it is important to identify criteria for both starting and stopping such treatment. Indications for apheresis that are approved by the American Association of Blood Banks and the American Society for Apheresis have been summarized.[102]

INDICATIONS FOR APHERESIS THERAPY

Neurologic Diseases

Neurologic diseases whose pathogenesis may be antibody mediated are now the most common indications for plasma exchange. Myasthenia gravis occurs when antibodies to acetylcholine receptors cause abnormal neuromuscular transmission. Reductions in these antibody titers from plasma exchange are associated with clinical improvement. A randomized trial compared the use of plasma exchange with the use of IVIg therapy in the treatment of myasthenia gravis; the investigators noted a trend toward better results with plasma exchange, but this trend was not statistically significant.[103] Similar findings were reported from much larger studies of Guillain-Barré syndrome, which is thought to be caused by antibodies to myelin. Two large series comparing plasma exchange with current best therapy showed faster improvement with the addition of plasma exchange. Randomized comparisons of plasma exchange and IVIg in the treatment of Guillain-Barré syndrome have shown these approaches to be equivalent; no additional benefit from using both therapies was shown.[104,105]

Chronic inflammatory demyelinating polyneuropathy (CIDP) is an autoimmune disorder that causes proximal and distal weakness; it has a progressive or relapsing course and is sometimes associated with monoclonal gammopathies. CIDP responds to plasma exchange, except in patients with distal weakness and associated IgM monoclonal gammopathies[106,107]; such patients respond poorly to all modalities of therapy.[108] IVIg therapy and plasma exchange have been shown to be comparably effective in CIDP.[109]

The use of plasma exchange in multiple sclerosis remains controversial. Meta-analysis of six controlled trials of plasma exchange provided some evidence of benefit, but the authors concluded that the subgroups of patients likely to benefit needed further definition.[110] A randomized study of plasma exchange in patients with acute inflammatory demyelinating central nervous system disease showed a significant benefit from the therapy. However, patients continued to have problems with relapse.[111]

Hematologic Diseases

Leukapheresis The hematologic diseases that require apheresis are those associated with obstruction of vascular flow by cells or the blockage of flow by proteins as a result of increased viscosity or cryoprecipitation; antibody-mediated diseases that lead to destruction of the formed elements of the blood; and thrombotic microangiopathies.

Leukostasis is a function of cell number and cell type. Myeloblasts are more likely to cause stasis than are an equivalent number of lymphocytes in a patient with chronic lymphocytic leukemia. Unless pulmonary or cerebral leukostasis is severe enough to cause progression in clinical findings, hydroxyurea is the treatment of choice. It will usually decrease the cell count sufficiently within 24 hours. However, when clinical findings demand improvement within 4 to 8 hours, leukapheresis in addition to hydroxyurea is usually needed.

Red cell exchange Red cell exchange has been used to treat acute chest crises, stroke, and priapism, and it is sometimes used to prepare patients with sickle cell disease for surgery. In these patients, the indications for red cell exchange, versus simple transfusion, are poorly defined. For example, in an analysis of causes and outcomes in acute chest syndrome, simple transfusions were used instead of red cell exchange in about two thirds of patients.[112] Many believe that red cell exchanges should be reserved for patients with progressive pulmonary disease or for those who fail to respond to transfusions. Using Rh and Kell antigen–compatible red cells reduces the incidence of alloimmunization from 7% to 1%[113] and should be standard practice. Red cell exchange leads to less iron accumulation than transfusion therapy, which is an advantage in the treatment of patients with sickle cell disease who require long-term therapy, such as those who have a history of stroke.[114]

Plasma exchange The concentration of paraprotein influences plasma protein viscosity, as does its heavy-chain class. IgM is the largest plasma protein and is nearly 100% intravascular; it is most likely to cause hyperviscosity. IgA and IgG3 are more likely to aggregate and are associated with hyperviscosity more often than other IgG subclasses. As in leukostasis, the choice between plasma exchange and chemotherapy is guided mainly by the clinical symptoms and their rate of progression.

Table 7 Indications for Plasma Exchange

Indications Based on Randomized Trials	Indications Based on Consensus and on Case Reports	Possible Indications
Guillain-Barré syndrome Chronic inflammatory polyneuropathy Peripheral neuropathy associated with MGUS Thrombotic thrombocytopenic purpura	Myasthenia gravis Hyperviscosity Hemolytic-uremic syndrome Persistent HELLP syndrome Posttransfusion purpura Cryoglobulinemia Vasculitis Familial hypercholesterolemia	Pemphigus vulgaris Goodpasture syndrome Autoimmune hemolytic anemia Antibody to coagulation factors Idiopathic thrombocytopenic purpura Cold agglutinin disease

HELLP—hemolysis, elevated liver enzymes, and low platelet count   MGUS—monoclonal gammopathy of unknown significance

Plasma exchange can lower viscosity within hours, whereas most chemotherapy requires days. Acute-onset renal failure caused by myeloma proteins can be improved by lowering the plasma concentration of paraprotein, but more data are needed for this to be considered an established indication.[115]

Despite the role that antibody and immune complexes play in hematologic cytopenia, there are no well-controlled studies supporting the use of plasma exchange. The available case reports usually describe the role of plasma exchange as being that of backup after failure of more established therapies. FFP or cryopoor plasma is used in replacement therapy for thrombotic microangiopathies. Case reports suggest that patients with severe preeclampsia, HELLP syndrome, or both may benefit from plasma exchange with FFP replacement if they fail to improve after delivery.[116]

Antibody-Mediated Renal, Muscular, and Cutaneous Diseases

Despite promising reports from case studies, controlled trials of patients with pemphigus vulgaris,[117] polymyositis, dermatomyositis,[118] and Goodpasture syndrome[119] have raised doubts concerning the value of plasma exchange. However, plasma exchange does appear to be valuable in stopping pulmonary hemorrhage in Goodpasture syndrome.

Immune Complex Diseases

The only indication for plasma exchange in rheumatoid arthritis and systemic lupus erythematosus is severe vasculitis that does not respond to other therapies.

Metabolic Diseases

Plasma exchange and selective removal of low-density lipoproteins (LDLs) have both been used as treatments of familial hypercholesterolemia [see Chapter 59]. Selective removal of LDLs can be accomplished by immunoadsorption, heparin precipitation, or dextran sulfate cellulose absorption, whereas plasma exchange causes significant reduction of both LDLs and HDLs.

COMPLICATIONS OF PLASMA EXCHANGE

The complications associated with plasma exchange are best divided into problems related to apheresis machines and problems related to venous access, type of replacement fluids, and anticoagulant. Apheresis machines accomplish cell and plasma separation by either centrifugation or membrane filtration. All systems monitor air and access pressure, allowing air emboli to be eliminated and access problems to be promptly recognized. Excess transmembrane pressure may cause red cell hemolysis, which leads to increased hemoglobin in the separated plasma. The majority of complications associated with plasma exchange result from the replacement fluid and anticoagulant used. Plasma removed by exchange is commonly replaced with 5% albumin, which carries no risk of infection and does not increase the citrate return but does dilute coagulation factors, causing mild coagulopathy for 24 to 48 hours. On an every-other-day treatment schedule, coagulation abnormalities are usually not clinically significant, but they may become significant if the patient is on a daily treatment schedule. Using FFP prevents dilutional coagulopathy but increases risks of blood-borne infection and allergic reactions. Peripheral venous access is often inadequate to maintain the required flow rates of 45 to 80 ml/min, necessitating central venous access with a large, double-lumen catheter; life-threatening or fatal complications from central catheter placement have been reported.[120] Catheter malfunction should always be considered when a patient shows clinical evidence of hypovolemia, shock, or both while undergoing plasma exchange. The majority of complications, however, are side effects of the citrate anticoagulant. These can include paresthesias, abdominal cramps, and, in rare instances, cardiac arrhythmias or seizures. Citrate toxicity is usually managed easily by slowing the return rate and providing extra calcium, either orally or sometimes intravenously. Patients with renal failure who receive large amounts of citrate may develop a profound metabolic alkalosis.[121]

Future Prospects for Transfusion Therapy

The evolution of transfusion practice has been a steady progression from whole blood to fractionated products designed for specific therapies. The search for a practical replacement for red cells that would allow stable storage, provide adequate oxygen delivery, and be free of significant toxins has been long and filled with substantial obstacles. Hemoglobin-based substitutes are most promising, but they still have problems with purification, adequate oxygen unloading, and potential toxicity. Chemically modified bovine hemoglobin is currently in phase-3 clinical trials and is probably closest to licensure. In the case of coagulation components, recombinant products are beginning to provide highly specific treatment of clinical problems that are poorly managed by current therapy. Bioengineering holds the promise of improving the effectiveness of current recombinant products.[62] Recombinant factor VIIa provides specific therapy for deficiency states and an alternative approach for patients with high-titer factor VIII inhibitors. Recombinant antithrombin III provides specific replacement for patients with congenital deficiency. The off-label use of these products is increasing and brings with it the need for careful studies of cost-effectiveness, which are only beginning to emerge.

A major change in transfusion practice may evolve from the availability of cytokines that can modify endogenous production. Erythropoietin has changed the treatment of anemia associated with chronic renal disease; as a result, many dialysis patients no longer require transfusions. Erythropoietin can also facilitate patients' self-banking their blood for anticipated surgical needs. In some cases, erythropoietin use is accepted by Jehovah's Witness patients, thereby allowing such patients to undergo surgical procedures that would otherwise not be possible. The availability of myeloid growth factors has contributed substantially to the development of methods for collection, and it is possible that mobilizing leukocytes with growth factors can increase the effectiveness of granulocyte transfusions. Thrombopoietin may in time be used to enhance platelet apheresis collections. The immunomodulatory effects of blood transfusion are in the early stages of description. It may be that a better understanding of the mechanisms underlying immunomodulation will permit using these effects to therapeutic advantage, such as to induce tolerance to a transplanted organ or to downregulate antibody production.

Even in an era of accelerating change, certain aspects of transfusion medicine will remain constant. The blood donor remains a kingpin who cannot be replaced by recombinant methodology. Transfusion practice has improved in safety, but there will always be residual risks. Each transfusion will always require careful assessment of whether the risks to the recipient of the transfusion will exceed the risks of going without. Further decrement of these risks will require new systemic approaches for improving the collection of specimens, selecting patients for transfusion of specific products, and continuing education of clinicians who make transfusion decisions.[122]

The author has no commercial relationships with manufacturers of products or providers of services discussed in this chapter.

References

1. Williams AE, Thomson RA, Schreiber GB, et al: Estimates of infectious disease risk factors in US blood donors. JAMA 277:967, 1997

2. Thomas MJG, Gillon J, Desmond MJ: Consensus Conference on Autologous Transfusion: preoperative autologous donation. Transfusion 36:633, 1996

3. Starkey JM, MacPherson JL, Bolgiano DC, et al: Markers for transfusion-transmitted disease in different groups of blood donors. JAMA 262:3452, 1989

4. Strauss RG, Burmeister LF, Johnson K, et al: Randomized trial assessing the feasibility and safety of biologic parents as RBC donors for their preterm infants. Transfusion 40:450, 2000

5. Dodd RY, Notari IV, Stramer SL: Current prevalence and incidence of infectious disease markers and estimated window-period risk in the American Red Cross blood donor population. Transfusion 42:975, 2002

6. Stramer SL: US NAT yield, where are we after 2 years? Transfus Med 12:243, 2002

7. Hening H, Puchta I, Lum J, et al: Frequency and load of hepatitis B virus DNA in first-time blood donors with antibodies to hepatitis B core antigen. Blood 100:2637, 2002

8. Recommendations for prevention and control of hepatitis C virus (HCV) infection and HCV-related chronic disease. MMWR Morb Mortal Wkly Rep 47(RR-19):1, 1998

9. Akahane Y, Kojuma M, Sugai Y, et al: Hepatitis C virus infection in spouses of patients with type C chronic liver disease. Ann Intern Med 120:748, 1994

10. Fried MW: Diagnostic testing for hepatitis C: practical considerations. Am J Med 107:31S, 1999

11. Epstein JS: Clarification of the use of unlicensed anti-HCV supplemental test results in regard to donor notification. FDA memorandum, August 19, 1993. U.S. Food and Drug Administration, Rockville, Maryland http://www.fda.gov/cber/bldmem/081993.pdf

12. Lemaire JM, Courouce AM, Defer C, et al: HCV RNA in blood donors with isolated reactivities by third-generation PCR. Transfusion 40:867, 2000

13. Bower WA, Nainan OV, Han X, et al: Duration of viremia in hepatitis A virus infection. J Infect Dis 182:12, 2000

14. Lefrére JJ, Sender A, Mercier B, et al: High rate of GB virus type C/HGV transmission from mother to infant: possible implications for the prevalence of infection in blood donors. Transfusion 40:602, 2000

15. Sentjens R, Basaras M, Simmonds P, et al: HGV/GB virus C transmission by blood components in patients undergoing open-heart surgery. Transfusion 43:1558, 2003

16. Lackritz EM, Satten GA, Aberle-Grasse J, et al: Estimated risk of transmission of the human immunodeficiency virus by screened blood in the United States. N Engl J Med 333:1712, 1995

17. Jackson JB, Hanson MR, Johnson GM, et al: Long-term follow-up of blood donors with indeterminate human immunodeficiency virus type 1 results on Western blot. Transfusion 35:98, 1995

18. Busch MP, Kleinman SG, Williams AE, et al: Frequency of human immunodeficiency virus (HIV) infection among contemporary anti-HIV-1 and anti-HIV-1/2 supplemental test–indeterminate blood donors. Transfusion 36:37, 1996

19. Sayre KR, Dodd RY, Tegtmeier G, et al: False-positive human immunodeficiency virus type 1 Western blot tests in noninfected blood donors. Transfusion 36:45, 1996

20. Murphy EL, Glynn SA, Fridey J, et al: Increased prevalence of infectious diseases and other adverse outcomes in human T lymphotropic virus types I- and II-infected donors. J Infect Dis 176:1468, 1997

21. Marsh BJ: Infectious complications of human T cell leukemia/lymphoma virus type I infections. Clin Infect Dis 23:138, 1996

22. HTLV-associated myelopathy in a cohort of HTLV-I and HTLV-II infected blood donors. The REDS investigators. Neurology 48:315, 1997

23. Busch MP, Switzer WM, Murphy EL, et al: Absence of evidence of infection with divergent primate T-lymphotropic viruses in United States blood donors who have seroindeterminate HTLV test results. Transfusion 40:443, 2000

24. False-positive serologic tests for human T-cell lymphotropic virus type I among blood donors following influenza vaccination, 1992. MMWR Morb Mortal Wkly Rep 42:173, 1993

25. Dodd RY: Emerging infections, transfusion safety, and epidemiology. N Engl J Med 349:1205, 2003

26. Pealer LN, Marfin AA, Peterson LR, et al: Transmission of West Nile Virus through blood transfusion in the United States in 2002. N Engl J Med 349:1236, 2003

27. Llewelyn CA, Hewitt PE, Knight RS, et al: Possible transmission of variant Creutzfeldt-Jakob disease by blood transfusion. Lancet 363:417, 2004

28. Cooper JD, Bird SM: Predicting the incidence of variant Creutzfeldt-Jakob disease from UK dietary exposure to bovine spongiform encephalopathy for the 1940–1969 and post-1969 birth cohorts. Int J Epidemiol 32:784, 2003

29. Yamamoto FI, Clausen H, White T, et al: Molecular genetic basis of the histo-blood group ABO system. Nature 345:229, 1990

30. Reid ME: Applications of DNA-based assays in blood group antigen and antibody identification. Transfusion 43:1748, 2003

31. Avent ND, Reid ME: The Rh blood group system: a review. Blood 95:375, 2000

32. Reid ME, Rios M, Powell VI, et al: DNA from blood samples can be used to genotype patients who have recently received a transfusion. Transfusion 40:48, 2000

33. Marrosszeky S, McDonald J, Sutherland H, et al: Suitability of preadmission blood samples for pretransfusion testing in elective surgery. Transfusion 37:910, 1997

34. Seftel MD, Growe GH, Petraszko T: Universal prestorage leukoreduction in Canada decreases platelet alloimmunization and refractoriness. Blood 103:333, 2004

35. Chambers LA, Herman JH: Considerations in the selection of a platelet component: apheresis versus whole blood derived. Transfus Med Rev 13:331, 1999

36. Heal JM, Rowe JM, McMican A, et al: The role of ABO matching in platelet transfusion. Eur J Haematol 50:110, 1993

37. Practice guidelines for blood component therapy: a report by the American Society of Anesthesiologists Task Force on Blood Component Therapy. Anesthesiology 84:732, 1996

38. Bracey AW, Radovancevic R, Riggs SA, et al: Lowering the hemoglobin threshold for transfusion in coronary artery bypass procedures: effect on patient outcome. Transfusion 39:1070, 1999

39. A multicenter, randomized, controlled clinical trial of transfusion requirements in critical care. Transfusion Requirements in Critical Care Investigators, Canadian Critical Care Trials Group. N Engl J Med 340:409, 1999

40. Cazzola M, Mercuriali F, Brugnara C: Use of recombinant human erythropoietin outside the setting of uremia. Blood 89:4248, 1997

41. Samol J, Littlewodd TJ: Efficacy of rHuEPO in cancer-related anemia. Br J Haemol 121:3, 2002

42. Wu W, Rathore MPH, Wang Y, et al: Blood transfusion in elderly patients with acute myocardial infarction. N Engl J Med 17:1230, 2001

43. Churchill WH, McGurk S, Chapman RH, et al: The Collaborative Hospital Transfusion Study: variations in the use of autologous blood account for hospital differences in red cell use during primary hip and knee surgery. Transfusion 38:530, 1998

44. Monk TG, Goodnough LT, Birkmeyer JD, et al: Acute normovolemic hemodilution is a cost-effective alternative to preoperative autologous blood donation by patients undergoing radical retropubic prostatectomy. Transfusion 35:559, 1995

45. Guidelines for the use of platelet transfusions. British Committee for Standards in Haematology, Blood Transfusion Task Force. Br J Haematol 122:10, 2003

46. Wandt H, Frank M, Ehniger G, et al: Safety and cost effectiveness of a $10 \times 10^9/L$ trigger for prophylactic platelet transfusions compared with the traditional $20 \times 10^9/L$ trigger: a prospective comparative trial in 105 patients with acute myeloid leukemia. Blood 91:3601, 1998

47. Shemin D, Elnour M, Amarantes B, et al: Oral estrogens decrease bleeding time and improve clinical bleeding in patients with renal failure. Am J Med 89:436, 1990

48. Reiter RA, Mayr F, Blazicek H, et al: Desmopressin antagonizes the in vitro platelet dysfunction induced by GPIIb/IIIa inhibitors and aspirin. Blood 102:4594, 2003

49. Kickler T, Kennedy SD, Braine HG: Alloimmunization to platelet-specific antigens on glycoproteins IIb-IIIa and Ib/IX in multiply transfused thrombocytopenic patients. Transfusion 30:622, 1990

50. Delaflor-Weiss E, Mintz PD: The evaluation and management of platelet refractoriness and alloimmunization. Transf Med Rev 14:180, 2000

51. Moroff G, Garratty G, Heal JM, et al: Selection of platelets for refractory patients by HLA matching and prospective crossmatching. Transfusion 32:633, 1992

52. Friedberg RC, Donnelly SF, Mintz PD: Independent roles for platelet crossmatching and HLA in the selection of platelets for alloimmunized patients. Transfusion 34:215, 1994

53. Leukocyte reduction and ultraviolet irradiation of platelets to prevent alloimmunization and refractoriness to platelet transfusions. The Trial to Reduce Alloimmunization to Platelets Study Group. N Engl J Med 337:1861, 1997

54. Novotny VM, van Doorn R, Witvliet MD, et al: Occurrence of allogeneic HLA and non-HLA antibodies after transfusion of prestorage filtered platelets and red blood cells: a prospective study. Blood 85:1736, 1995

55. Sullivan MT, McCullough J, Schreiber GB, et al: Blood collection and transfusion in the United States in 1997. Transfusion 42:1253, 2002

56. Practice parameters for the use of fresh-frozen plasma, cryoprecipitate, and platelets. Administration Practice Guidelines Development Task Force of the College of American Pathologists. JAMA 271:777, 1994

57. McVay PA, Toy PT: Lack of increased bleeding after paracentesis and thoracentesis in patients with mild coagulation abnormalities. Transfusion 31:164, 1991

58. Mannucci PM, Bauer KA, Santagostino E, et al: Activation of the coagulation cascade after infusion of a factor XI concentrate in congenitally deficient patients. Blood 84:1314, 1994

59. Lechner K, Kyrle PA: Antithrombin III concentrates—are they clinically useful? Thromb Haemost 73:340, 1995

60. George JN: How I treat patients with thrombotic thrombocytopenic purpura–hemolytic uremia syndrome. Blood 96:1223, 2000

61. Rock G, Sutton DM, Nair RC: Cryosupernatant as replacement fluid for plasma exchange in thrombotic thrombocytopenic purpura. Members of the Canadian Apheresis Group. Br J Haematol 94:383, 1996

62. O'Connell NM, Perry DJ, Hodgson AJ, et al: Recombinant FVIIA in the management of uncontrolled hemorrhage. Transfusion 43:1711, 2003

63. Saenko EL, Ananyeva M, Shima M, et al: The future of recombinant coagulation

factors. J Thromb Haemost 1:922, 2002

64. Brettler DB, Forsberg AD, Levine PH, et al: The use of porcine factor VIII concentrate (Hyate:C) in the treatment of patients with inhibitor antibodies to factor VIII: a multicenter US experience. Arch Intern Med 149:1381, 1989

65. Thompson AR: Factor IX concentrates for clinical use. Semin Thromb Hemost 19:25, 1993

66. Price TH: The current prospects for neutrophil transfusions for the treatment of granulocytopenic infected patients. Transfus Med Rev 14:2, 2000

67. Brugnara C, Churchill WH: Plasma component therapy. Thrombosis and Hemorrhage, 2nd ed. Loscalzo J, Schafer AI, Eds. Williams & Wilkins, Baltimore, 1998, p 1135

68. Ahsan N, Weigand LA, Abendroth CS, et al: Acute renal failure following immunoglobulin therapy. Am J Nephrol 16:532, 1996

69. Renal insufficiency and failure associated with immune globulin intravenous therapy —United States, 1985–1998. MMWR Morb Mortal Wkly Rep 48:518, 1999

70. Sekul EA, Cupler EJ, Dalakas MC: Aseptic meningitis associated with high-dose intravenous immunoglobulin therapy: frequency and risk factors. Ann Intern Med 121:259, 1994

71. Garratty G: Severe reactions associated with transfusion of patients with sickle cell disease. Transfusion 37:357, 1997

72. Davenport RD, Kunkel SL: Cytokine roles in hemolytic and nonhemolytic transfusion reactions. Transfus Med Rev 8:157, 1994

73. Pineda AA, Vamvakas EC, Gorden LD, et al: Trends in the incidence of delayed hemolytic and delayed serologic transfusion reactions. Transfusion 39:1097, 1999

74. Lee J-H: Transfusion fatalities reported to the FDA (1990–1998). Bacterial Contamination of Platelets Workshop. Center for Biologics Evaluation and Research, U.S. Food and Drug Administration, Rockville, Maryland, September 24, 1999 http://www.fda.gov/cber/minutes/bact092499.pdf

75. Heddle NM, Klama L, Singer J: The role of plasma from platelet concentrates in transfusion reactions. N Engl J Med 331:625, 1994

76. Federowicz I, Barrett BB, Andersen JW, et al: Characterization of reactions after transfusion of cellular blood components that are white cell reduced before storage. Transfusion 36:21, 1996

77. Kelley DL, Mangini J, Lopez-Plaza I, et al: The utility of ≤3-day-old whole-blood platelets in reducing the incidence of febrile nonhemolytic transfusion reactions. Transfusion 40:439, 2000

78. Dzik S, Aubuchon J, Jeffries L, et al: Leukocyte reduction of blood components: public policy and new technology. Transfus Med Rev 14:34, 2000

79. Popovsky MA, Chaplin HC Jr, Moore SB: Transfusion-related acute lung injury: a neglected, serious complication of hemotherapy. Transfusion 32:589, 1992

80. Kopko PM, Paglieroni TG, Popovsky MA, et al: TRALI: correlation of antigen-antibody and monocyte activation in donor-recipient pairs. Transfusion 43:177, 2003

81. Kao GS, Wood IG, Dorfman DM, et al: Investigations into the role of anti-HLA class II antibodies in TRALI. Transfusion 43:185, 2003

82. Silliman CC, Paterson AJ, Dickey WO, et al: The association of biologically active lipids with the development of transfusion-related acute lung injury: a retrospective study. Transfusion 37:719, 1997

83. Silliman CC, Boshkov LK, Mehdizadehkashi Z, et al: Transfusion-related acute lung injury: epidemiology and a prospective analysis of etiologic factors. Blood 101:454, 2003

84. Silliman CC, Voelkel NF, Allard JD, et al: Plasma and lipids from stored packed red blood cells cause acute lung injury in an animal model. J Clin Invest 101:1458, 1998

85. Sandler SG, Mallory D, Malamut D, et al: Hemagglutination assays for the diagnosis and prevention of IgA anaphylactic transfusion reactions. Transfus Med Rev 9:1, 1995

86. Klüter H, Bubel S, Kirchner H, et al: Febrile and allergic transfusion reactions after the transfusion of white cell–poor platelet preparations. Transfusion 39:1179, 1999

87. Cyr M, Hume HA, Champagne M, et al: Anomaly of the des-Arg9-bradykinin metabolism associated with severe hypotensive reactions during blood transfusions: a preliminary study. Transfusion 39:1084, 1999

88. Owen HG, Brecher ME: Atypical reactions associated with use of angiotensin-converting enzyme inhibitors and apheresis. Transfusion 34:891, 1994

89. Ohto H, Anderson KC: Survey of transfusion-associated graft-versus-host disease in immunocompetent recipients. Transfus Med Rev 10:31, 1996

90. Ohto H, Anderson KC: Posttransfusion graft-versus-host disease in Japanese newborns. Transfusion 36:117, 1996

91. Ammann AJ: Hypothesis: absence of graft-versus-host disease in AIDS is a consequence of HIV-1 infection of CD4+ T cells. J Acquir Immune Defic Syndr 6:1224, 1993

92. Ohto H, Yasuda H, Noguchi M: Risk of transfusion-associated graft-versus-host disease as a result of directed donation from relatives (letter). Transfusion 32:691, 1992

93. Morof FG, Luban NLC: The irradiation of blood and blood components to prevent graft-versus-host disease: technical issues and guidelines. Transfus Med Rev 11:15, 1997

94. Nollet KE, Holland PV: Toward a coalition against transfusion-associated GVHD (editorial). Transfusion 43:1655, 2003

95. McDonald CP, Hartley S, Orchard K, et al: Fatal Clostridium perfringens sepsis from a pooled platelet transfusion. Transfusion 37:259, 1997

96. Red blood cell transfusions contaminated with Yersinia enterocolitica: United States, 1991–1996, and initiation of a national study to detect bacteria-associated transfusion reaction. MMWR Morb Mortal Wkly Rep 46:553, 1997

97. Bowden RA, Slichter SJ, Sayers M, et al: A comparison of filtered leukocyte-reduced and cytomegalovirus (CMV) seronegative blood products for the prevention of transfusion-associated CMV infection after marrow transplant. Blood 86:3598, 1995

98. Nichols WG, Price TH, Gooley T, et al: Transfusion-transmission cytomegalovirus infection after receipt of leukoreduced blood products. Blood 101:4195, 2003

99. Opelz G, Vanrenterghem Y, Kirste G, et al: Prospective evaluation of pretransplant blood transfusions in cadaver kidney recipients. Transplantation 63:964, 1997

100. Bordin JO, Bardossy L, Blajchman MA: Growth enhancement of established tumors by allogeneic blood transfusion in experimental animals and its amelioration by leukodepletion: the importance of the timing of the leukodepletion. Blood 84:344, 1998

101. Vamvakas EC, Blajchman MA: Deleterious clinical effects of transfusion-associated immunomodulation: fact or fiction? Blood 97:1180, 2001

102. Smith JW, Weinstein R, Hillyer C: Therapeutic apheresis: a summary of current indication categories endorsed by the AABB and the American Society for Apheresis. Transfusion 43:820, 2003

103. Gajdos P, Chevret S, Clair B, et al: Clinical trial of plasma exchange and high-dose intravenous immunoglobulin in myasthenia gravis. Myasthenia Gravis Clinical Study Group. Ann Neurol 41:789, 1997

104. Randomised trial of plasma exchange, intravenous immunoglobulin, and combined treatments in Guillain-Barré syndrome. Plasma Exchange/Sandoglobulin Guillain-Barré Syndrome Trial Group. Lancet 349:225, 1997

105. van der Meché FG, Schmitz PI: A randomized trial comparing intravenous immune globulin and plasma exchange in Guillain-Barré syndrome. The Dutch Guillain-Barré Study Group. N Engl J Med 326:1123, 1992

106. Dyck PJ, Low PA, Windebank AJ, et al: Plasma exchange in polyneuropathy associated with monoclonal gammopathy of undetermined significance. N Engl J Med 325:1482, 1991

107. Hahn AF, Bolton CF, Pillay N, et al: Plasma-exchange therapy in chronic inflammatory demyelinating polyneuropathy: a double-blind, sham-controlled, cross-over study. Brain 119:1055, 1996

108. Katz JS, Saperstein DS, Gronseth G, et al: Distal acquired demyelinating symmetric neuropathy. Neurology 54:615, 2000

109. Dyck PJ, Litchy WJ, Kratz KM, et al: A plasma exchange versus immune globulin infusion in chronic inflammatory demyelinating polyradiculoneuropathy. Ann Neurol 36:838, 1994

110. Vamvakas EC, Pineda AA, Weinshenker BG: Meta-analysis of clinical studies of the efficacy of plasma exchange in the treatment of chronic progressive multiple sclerosis. J Clin Apheresis 10:163, 1995

111. Weinshenker BG, O'Brien PC, Petterson TM, et al: A randomized trial of plasma exchange in acute central nervous system inflammatory demyelinating disease. Ann Neurol 46:878, 1999

112. Vichinsky EP, Neumayr LD, Earles AN, et al: Causes and outcomes of the acute chest syndrome in sickle cell disease. N Engl J Med 342:1855, 2000

113. Vichinsky EP, Earles AN, Johnson RA, et al: Alloimmunization in sickle cell anemia and transfusion of racially unmatched blood. N Engl J Med 322:1617, 1990

114. Hilliard LM, Williams BF, Lounsbury AE, et al: Erythrocytapheresis limits iron accumulation in chronically transfused sickle cell patients. Am J Hematol 59:28, 1998

115. Zucchelli P, Pasquali S, Cagnoli L, et al: Controlled plasma exchange trial in acute renal failure due to multiple myeloma. Kidney Int 33:1175, 1988

116. Martin JN, Files FC, Blake PG: Plasma exchange for preeclampsia: I. Postpartum use for persistently severe preeclampsia-eclampsia with HELLP syndrome. Am J Obstet Gynecol 162:126, 1990

117. Guillaume JC, Roujeau JC, Morel P, et al: Controlled study of plasma exchange in pemphigus. Arch Dermatol 124:1659, 1988

118. Miller FW, Leitman SF, Cronin ME, et al: Controlled trial of plasma exchange and leukapheresis in polymyositis and dermatomyositis. N Engl J Med 326:1380, 1992

119. Johnson JP, Moore J Jr, Austin HA III, et al: Therapy of anti-glomerular basement membrane antibody disease: analysis of prognostic significance of clinical, pathologic and treatment factors. Medicine (Baltimore) 64:219, 1985

120. Rizvi MA, Vesely JN, Chandler GL, et al: Complications of plasma exchange in 71 consecutive patients treated for clinically suspected thrombotic thrombocytopenic purpura–hemolytic-uremic syndrome. Transfusion 40:869, 2000

121. Pearl RG, Rosenthal MM: Metabolic alkalosis due to plasmapheresis. Am J Med 79:391, 1985

122. Dzik WH: Emily Cooley Lecture 2002: Transfusion safety in the hospital. Transfusion 43:1190, 2003

Acknowledgment

The author would like to thank Yoriko Saito, M.D., and Siobhan McGurk for their many suggestions and contributions to this chapter.

101 Hematopoietic Cell Transplantation

Frederick R. Appelbaum, M.D.

Hematopoietic cell transplantation can replace abnormal but nonmalignant hematopoietic stem cells with cells from a healthy donor, making transplantation an effective therapy for a variety of nonmalignant diseases of the lymphohematopoietic system. In addition, hematopoietic cell transplantation is used to treat a number of malignancies for two reasons. It allows administration of higher and potentially more effective doses of chemotherapy and radiotherapy that would otherwise cause unacceptable myelosuppression. Further, allogeneic transplantation also confers its own immunologically mediated graft-versus-tumor effect beyond that of chemoradiotherapy. Worldwide, an estimated 45,000 to 50,000 patients underwent hematopoietic cell transplantation in 2005.

Hematopoietic Cell Transplantation for Specific Diseases

TREATMENT OF IMMUNODEFICIENCY STATES

The widest experience in treating immunodeficiency with hematopoietic cell transplantation has been in the treatment of severe combined immunodeficiency disease.[1] When current techniques of supportive care are used, the expected outcome of transplantation from an HLA-identical donor is excellent, with a better than 90% probability of long-term survival.[1] Very good results (approximately 80% survival) can be expected using matched related or unrelated donors. In patients without matched related or unrelated donors, transplantation from a haplotype-mismatched parent results in engraftment and survival longer than 2 years in 50% to 70% of patients. The experience in the treatment of Wiskott-Aldrich syndrome and other immunodeficiency states is limited.[2] Cures have been noted in more than half of patients, with the best results seen in patients who undergo transplantation when they are younger than 5 years.

TREATMENT OF NONMALIGNANT DISEASES OF HEMATOPOIESIS

Aplastic Anemia

Transplantation from matched siblings after a preparative regimen of high-dose cyclophosphamide and antithymocyte globulin, together with the use of methotrexate and cyclosporine for GVHD prophylaxis, is a very effective regimen for patients with aplastic anemia. Current results suggest a cure rate greater than 90%.[3] Results with mismatched or unrelated matched donors are somewhat worse; therefore, patients with aplastic anemia who are without sibling donors are often given a trial of immunosuppressive therapy before transplantation.

Thalassemia

Marrow transplantation from an HLA-identical sibling after a preparative regimen of busulfan and cyclophosphamide can cure from 70% to 90% of patients with thalassemia major.[4] The best results have been obtained in patients who undergo trans-

plantation before they develop hepatomegaly or portal fibrosis and who have been given adequate iron chelation therapy. In one study of 121 such patients, the probabilities of survival and disease-free survival 5 years after transplantation were 95% and 90%, respectively.[4] Prolonged survival can also be achieved with aggressive chelation therapy, but transplantation remains the only curative treatment. Fewer than 30% of patients with thalassemia have an HLA-identical sibling. Outcomes with the use of alternative donors of hematopoietic stem cells (i.e., unrelated persons or HLA-nonidentical family members) have been aided by the establishment of worldwide donor registries, by improvements in the methods of controlling GVHD, and by prevention of fungal and cytomegalovirus infection.

Sickle Cell Anemia

Experience in transplantation for sickle cell disease is small but growing. In a European study of 100 patients with sickle cell disease who received transplants from HLA-matched siblings, the survival rate at 4 years was 88%, and disease-free survival was 80%.[5] In a study of 59 patients in the United States, similar rates were reported—93% and 84%, respectively.[6]

Other Nonmalignant Diseases

Hematopoietic cell transplantation has been used successfully to treat a variety of other nonmalignant but nonetheless fatal diseases. Included in this group are congenital disorders of white cells, including Kostmann syndrome, chronic granulomatous disease, neutrophil actin defects, leukocyte adhesion deficiency, and Chédiak-Higashi syndrome. Congenital anemias, including Fanconi anemia and Blackfan-Diamond anemia, are likewise treatable with hematopoietic cell transplantation.[7]

Osteopetrosis is a rare inherited disorder caused by an inability of the osteoclast to resorb bone. Because the osteoclast is a specialized macrophage derived from the marrow, it follows that osteopetrosis can be treated with marrow transplantation.[8] A final category of treatable nonmalignant diseases are storage diseases caused by enzymatic deficiencies.[8]

TREATMENT OF HEMATOLOGIC MALIGNANCIES

Acute Myeloid Leukemia

Allogeneic marrow transplantation cures 15% to 20% of patients with AML in whom induction therapy fails and, indeed, is the only therapy that can cure such patients.[9] Thus, all patients 60 years of age or younger with newly diagnosed AML should have their HLA type determined, as should their families, soon after diagnosis to enable transplantation for those in whom induction therapy fails. Allogeneic transplantation from matched siblings or matched unrelated donors can cure approximately 30% of patients in second remission and 35% of patients in untreated first relapse—situations that are clear indications for the procedure, because these results are superior to those achieved without transplantation.[10,11]

The role of hematopoietic cell transplantation for patients with AML in first remission remains unsettled. Several large trials have prospectively compared the outcomes of match sibling transplantation, autologous transplantation, and further chemotherapy.[12,13] In general, these trials have suggested a slight advantage in disease-free survival with allogeneic transplantation. For patients categorized according to their cytogenetic risk group, there was no evidence that allogeneic or autologous transplantation offers an advantage for patients categorized as being at good risk. However, allogeneic transplantation was found to provide a sizable benefit for patients categorized as being at poor risk; these patients included those with del(5q)/−5, del(7q)/−7, t(9; 22), inv(3q), or complex karyotypes.[14,15] With continued improvements in chemotherapy and transplantation, as well as the identification of additional risk factors beyond conventional cytogenetics, the comparative roles of chemotherapy and transplantation for AML in first remission will likely continue to be redefined. Nonmyeloablative allogeneic transplantation has recently been reported to result in favorable outcomes in selected older patients with AML in first or second remission.

Acute Lymphocytic Leukemia

As with AML, allogeneic transplantation can cure 15% to 20% of patients with acute lymphocytic leukemia (ALL) in whom induction therapy fails or in whom chemotherapy-resistant disease develops; thus, these patients are candidates for the procedure. The results of transplantation for patients in second remission are better, with cure rates of 30% to 50%. However, further intensive chemotherapy also can cure some patients who suffer an initial relapse, particularly children who experience a relapse more than 18 months after initial induction chemotherapy. In a study comparing allogeneic transplantation in 255 children with chemotherapy in an equal number of children, the rates of disease-free survival at 5 years were found to be 40% in transplant patients and 17% in chemotherapy patients.[16] The relative benefits of transplantation were similar for children with short and long initial remissions. Thus, allogeneic transplantation can be recommended for all patients with ALL in second complete remission who have appropriate donors.

Allogeneic transplantation for ALL in first remission results in long-term disease-free survival in 40% to 70% of adult patients. In a retrospective study comparing these results with those achieved with chemotherapy, no clear advantage could be found for either approach.[17] In the largest prospective, randomized study published to date (involving 572 patients), the 10-year survival rate for patients undergoing allogeneic transplantation was 46%; for those undergoing autologous transplantation, 34%; and for those receiving continued chemotherapy, 31%.[18] In standard-risk patients, there was no difference in outcome between the three approaches (i.e., 10-year survival of 49% with allogeneic transplantation, 49% with autologous transplantation, and 40% with chemotherapy), whereas for high-risk patients, allogeneic transplantation provided the best results (44% versus 10% versus 11%).[18] Because children with ALL, in general, respond well to chemotherapy, there is no role for transplantation at first remission except for those with very high risk disease (e.g., Philadelphia chromosome–positive ALL).[19]

Myelodysplastic Syndromes

The myelodysplastic syndromes are generally considered to be incurable except with marrow transplantation. In some patients, the myelodysplastic syndromes have a relatively indolent course, and transplantation can be safely withheld until the disease progresses. However, once significant granulocytopenia (fewer than 1,000 cells/mm³) or thrombocytopenia (fewer than 40,000 cells/mm³) develops or the proportion of blast cells in the marrow exceeds 5%, transplantation should be seriously considered, because without transplantation, the expected survival time is short. When an HLA-matched sibling is available to serve as a donor, the chance of long-term survival with transplantation is roughly 55%, with better results being obtained in younger patients and in those who receive transplants earlier in the course of their disease.[20] Similar results have been reported with matched unrelated donor transplants.[21] No role has been established for autologous transplantation in the myelodysplastic syndromes.

Myelofibrosis

Allogeneic hematopoietic cell transplantation can cure patients with primary myelofibrosis or myelofibrosis secondary to essential thrombocythemia or polycythemia vera. In one study, 5-year progression-free survival was seen in approximately two-thirds of patients treated with a preparative regimen combining busulfan and cyclophosphamide followed by allogeneic transplantation.[22] Graft failure was rare, despite the presence of splenomegaly and marrow fibrosis.

Chronic Myeloid Leukemia

Allogeneic and syngeneic marrow transplantation are the only forms of therapy known to cure chronic myeloid leukemia (CML). Five-year disease-free survival rates are 15% to 20% for patients who undergo transplantation in blast crisis, 30% to 40% for patients who undergo transplantation during the accelerated phase, and approximately 70% for patients who undergo transplantation during the chronic phase.[23]

Time from diagnosis influences the outcome of transplantation during the chronic phase. The best results are obtained in patients who receive transplants within 1 year of diagnosis; progressively worse results are seen the longer the procedure is delayed.[24] A growing number of patients between 55 and 65 years of age with CML have undergone transplantation, with results not significantly worse than those seen in younger patients.[25] Although the initial experience with the use of unrelated-donor transplantation in CML was substantially worse than the experience with matched-sibling transplantation, subsequent results at some centers have demonstrated a 70% probability of disease-free survival at 3 years.[26]

The overall role of hematopoietic cell transplantation in CML has changed with the introduction of imatinib mesylate, a very effective, relatively nontoxic oral agent used for treatment of CML.[27] Imatinib does not result in complete, molecular-level remissions in most patients, and therefore, some experts would argue that early allogeneic transplantation remains the treatment of choice for younger patients with matched donors. For older patients or those without matched sibling donors, an initial trial of imatinib is generally preferred. Current evidence suggests that exposure to imatinib before transplantation poses no additional risk to the transplant procedure. Strategies of initial therapy with imatinib mesylate combined with careful molecular monitoring and transplantation at the moment of disease progression are being developed.[28]

Chronic Lymphocytic Leukemia

Use of marrow transplantation in chronic lymphocytic leukemia (CLL) has received only limited attention, probably because of the indolent nature of the disease and its propensity to occur in older patients. Of the small number of patients receiving allogeneic transplantation, many have had complete remissions, and approximately half have remained disease free.[29] However, the transplant-related mortality in this group of patients has been substantial. Enduring complete responses with less transplant-related toxicity have been reported with the use of nonmyeloablative allogeneic transplantation.[30] The number of patients treated with autologous transplantation is limited.[31] Complete remissions have been achieved, some of which appear to be sustained.

Non-Hodgkin Lymphoma

Patients with disseminated intermediate or high-grade NHL in whom conventional therapy fails can seldom be cured without transplantation. High-dose therapy followed by autologous or allogeneic marrow transplantation can cure a substantial number of such patients. A number of studies have documented cure rates of 40% to 50% in patients who receive transplants after an initial relapse and whose tumors remain sensitive to chemotherapy.[32] In the initial randomized study testing the role of autologous transplantation in intermediate or high-grade NHL, the 5-year disease-free survival rate for patients who underwent autologous transplantation for chemosensitive disease was 46%, compared with 12% for patients in the chemotherapy group ($P = 0.001$). Cure rates decrease substantially once the disease becomes resistant to conventional-dose chemotherapy.[32] A poor performance status and large tumor bulk are additional adverse risk factors. As in other diseases, patients who receive transplants of allogeneic marrow have a lower relapse rate but a higher risk of nonrelapse mortality than patients who receive autologous transplants.[33] For most categories of intermediate- and high-grade NHL, the outcomes for allogeneic and autologous transplantation appear roughly similar, though an advantage has been suggested for the use of allogeneic transplantation in patients with lymphoblastic lymphoma. The role of transplantation for patients in first remission is unsettled. Of the randomized studies that have thus far been performed, some have found a significant benefit, some have found no benefit, and others have found a benefit only for the subgroup of patients with intermediate- to high-risk disease or high-risk disease.[34]

For patients with recurrent disseminated low-grade NHL, high-dose therapy supported by autologous transplantation results in high response rates and improved progression-free survival compared with standard dose therapy. In a European study, overall survival at 4 years was 46% with chemotherapy compared with 74% with autologous transplantation.[35] The role of autologous transplantation in the initial treatment of patients with indolent lymphomas is under study. Results to date demonstrate higher complete response rates and improved event-free survival, but conclusions about an effect on overall survival remain premature.[36] Myeloablative allogeneic transplantation results in a greater antitumor effect than autologous transplantation, but at the expense of greater toxicity. Nonmyeloablative or reduced-intensity preparative regimens followed by allogeneic transplantation have been reported to result in high response rates with substantially less toxicity than seen with ablative transplants.[37]

Hodgkin Disease

The results of transplantation for Hodgkin disease are similar to those for intermediate and high-grade NHL. For patients with primary progressive Hodgkin disease (defined as progression during induction treatment or within 90 days after completion of therapy), high-dose chemotherapy followed by autologous transplantation resulted in a 5-year disease-free survival rate of 42%—results that appear superior to those achieved with conventional chemotherapy.[38] Prospective randomized trials have similarly shown an advantage for high-dose chemotherapy followed by autologous transplantation, as compared with conventional-dose chemotherapy, for patients with relapsed or refractory Hodgkin disease.[39] There is currently no established role for autologous transplantation as part of the initial treatment strategy for patients with Hodgkin disease, although several trials testing this approach are being performed. As with NHL, patients with Hodgkin disease who are treated with ablative preparative regimens followed by allogeneic transplantation have lower relapse rates but higher nonrelapse mortality.[40] The use of nonmyeloablative or reduced-intensity preparative regimens followed by allogeneic transplantation has been reported to result in complete enduring responses with acceptable levels of toxicity in selected patients who have recurring Hodgkin disease, including some for whom previous autologous transplantation failed.[41]

Multiple Myeloma

High-dose chemotherapy followed by autologous transplantation in patients with recurrent multiple myeloma can result in a substantial reduction in tumor burden and, in many cases, at least temporary complete remissions. Two prospective randomized trials have demonstrated that inclusion of high-dose chemotherapy followed by autologous transplantation in the initial treatment of patients with multiple myeloma results in a significant prolongation in patient survival.[42,43] Prospective randomized trials have suggested that there is a further advantage in treating patients with two cycles of high-dose therapy, each supported by autologous transplantation, compared to a single transplant.[44] Allogeneic hematopoietic cell transplantation following ablative preparative regimens has been used to treat myeloma patients in whom first-line chemotherapy failed; this approach achieved overall survival rates averaging 35% at 5 years.[45] An important finding was that there appeared to be a plateau in the rate of disease-free survival, suggesting that some of these patients were cured. Transplant-associated complications, however, were substantial and occurred more frequently than in most other hematologic malignancies.[46] A decrease in transplant-associated morbidity and mortality without loss of the allogeneic graft-versus-myeloma effect can be achieved with the use of nonmyeloablative or reduced-intensity preparative regimens. A strategy of treating multiple myeloma with a single autologous transplant followed by nonmyeloablative allogeneic transplantation is being tested.[42]

Treatment of Posttransplant Relapse

Patients with malignancies who experience relapse after autologous transplantation occasionally respond to further conventional-dose chemotherapy, particularly when the interval from transplantation to relapse is long. There are more options available to the patient who experiences relapse after allogeneic transplantation. Patients with CML frequently respond to therapy with interferon or imatinib mesylate, and other patients occasionally respond to withdrawal of immunosuppression. Patients who experience relapse after allogeneic transplantation sometimes respond to nonirradiated donor lymphocyte infusions. In a summary of 258 patients reported by a European registry, complete responses were seen in 75% of patients with CML, 38% with myelodysplasia, 24% with AML, and 15% with myeloma.[47] Responses were seldom seen in patients with ALL. The major complications of posttransplant donor lymphocyte infusions have been GVHD and myelosuppression, both of which can be severe or fatal. Starting the transfusion with a low cell dose and then gradually increasing the dose can lessen the risk of severe toxicity. A second hematopoietic cell transplantation can occasionally be effective, particularly in younger patients and in patients who experience a longer interval from first transplant to relapse and who do not have advanced disease.

The author has no commercial relationships with manufacturers of products or providers of services discussed in this chapter.

The FDA has not approved cyclophosphamide, busulfan, antithymocyte globulin, and methotrexate for uses described in this chapter.

References

1. Grunebaum E, Mazzolari E, Porta F, et al: Bone marrow transplantation for severe combined immune deficiency. JAMA 295:508, 2006

2. Ochs HD, Thrasher AJ: The Wiskott-Aldrich syndrome. J Allergy Clin Immunol 117:725, 2006

3. Storb R, Leisenring W, Anasetti C, et al: Long-term follow-up of allogeneic marrow transplants in patients with aplastic anemia conditioned by cyclophosphamide combined with antithymocyte globulin. Blood 89:3890, 1997

4. Lucarelli G, Galimberti M, Giardini C, et al: Bone marrow transplantation in thalassemia: the experience of Pesaro. Ann NY Acad Sci 850:270, 1998

5. Vermylen C, Cornu G, Ferster A, et al: Haematopoietic stem cell transplantation for sickle cell anaemia: the first 50 patients transplanted in Belgium. Bone Marrow Transplant 22:1, 1998

6. Walters MC, Storb R, Patience M, et al: Impact of bone marrow transplantation for symptomatic sickle cell disease: an interim report. Blood 95:1918, 2000

7. Guardiola P, Pasquini R, Dokal I, et al: Outcome of 69 allogeneic stem cell transplantations for Fanconi anemia using HLA-matched unrelated donors: a study on behalf of the European Group for Blood and Marrow Transplantation. Blood 95:422, 2000

8. Nash RA, Bowen JD, McSweeney PA, et al: High-dose immunosuppressive therapy and autologous peripheral blood stem cell transplantation for severe multiple sclerosis. Blood 102:2364, 2003

9. Biggs JC, Horowitz MM, Gale RP, et al: Bone marrow transplants may cure patients with acute leukemia never achieving remission with chemotherapy. Blood 80:1090, 1992

10. Clift RA, Buckner CD, Appelbaum FR, et al: Allogeneic marrow transplantation during untreated first relapse of acute myeloid leukemia. J Clin Oncol 10:1723, 1992

11. Gale RP, Horowitz MM, Rees JK, et al: Chemotherapy versus transplants for acute myelogenous leukemia in second remission. Leukemia 10:13, 1996

12. Cassileth PA, Harrington DP, Appelbaum FR, et al: Chemotherapy compared with autologous or allogeneic bone marrow transplantation in the management of acute myeloid leukemia in first remission. N Engl J Med 339:1649, 1998

13. Harousseau J-L, Cahn J-Y, Pignon B, et al: Comparison of autologous bone marrow transplantation and intensive chemotherapy as postremission therapy in adult acute myeloid leukemia. Blood 90:2978, 1997

14. Slovak ML, Kopecky KJ, Cassileth PA, et al: Karyotypic analysis predicts outcome of preremission and postremission therapy in adult acute myeloid leukemia (AML): a Southwest Oncoloyg Group/Eastern Cooperative Oncology Group study. Blood 96:4075, 2000

15. Suciu S, Mandelli F, deWitt T, et al: Allogeneic compared with autologous stem cell transplantation according to cytogenetic features in AML patients younger than 46 in first complete remission (CR1): an-intention-to-treat EORTIC/GIMEMA AML-10 trial. Blood 102:123, 2003

16. Barrett AJ, Horowitz MM, Pollock BH, et al: Bone marrow transplants from HLA-identical siblings as compared with chemotherapy for children with acute lymphoblastic leukemia in a second remission. N Engl J Med 331:1253, 1994

17. Horowitz MM, Messerer D, Hoelzer D, et al: Chemotherapy compared with bone marrow transplantation for adults with acute lymphoblastic leukemia in first remission. Ann Intern Med 115:13, 1991

18. Thiebaut A, Vernant JP, Degos L, et al: Adult acute lymphocytic leukemia study testing chemotherapy and autologous and allogeneic transplantation: a follow-up report of the French protocol LALA 87. Hematol Oncol Clin North Am 14:1353, 2000

19. Arico M, Valsecchi MG, Camitta B, et al: Outcome of treatment in children with Philadelphia chromosome-positive acute lymphoblastic leukemia. N Engl J Med 342:998, 2000

20. Appelbaum FR, Anderson J: Allogeneic bone marrow transplantation for myelodysplastic syndrome: outcomes analysis according to IPSS score. Leukemia 12 (suppl 1):S25, 1998

21. Deeg HJ, Storer B, Slattery JT, et al: Conditioning with targeted busulfan and cyclophosphamide for hemopoietic stem cell transplantation from related and unrelated donors in patients with myelodysplastic syndrome. Blood 100:1201, 2002

22. Deeg HJ, Gooley TA, Flowers MED, et al: Allogeneic hematopoietic stem cell transplantation for myelofibrosis. Blood 102:3912, 2003

23. Oehler VG, Radich JP, Storer B, et al: Randomized trial of allogeneic related bone marrow transplantation versus peripheral blood stem cell transplantation for chronic myeloid leukemia. Biol Blood Marrow Transplant 11:85, 2005

24. Goldman JM, Szydlo R, Horowitz MM, et al: Choice of pretransplant treatment and timing of transplants for chronic myelogenous leukemia in chronic phase. Blood 82:2235, 1993

25. Clift RA, Appelbaum FR, Thomas ED: Treatment of chronic myeloid leukemia by marrow transplantation. Blood 82:1954, 1993

26. Hansen JA, Gooley TA, Martin PJ, et al: Bone marrow transplants from unrelated donors for patients with chronic myeloid leukemia. N Engl J Med 338:962, 1998

27. O'Brien SG, Guilhot F, Larson RA, et al: Imatinib compared with interferon and low-dose cytarabine for newly diagnosed chronic-phase chronic myeloid leukemia. N Engl J Med 348:994, 2003

28. Baccarani M, Saglio G, Goldman J, et al: Evolving concepts in the management of chronic myeloid leukemia: recommendations from an expert l on behalf of the European Leukemianet. Blood May 18, 2006 [epub ahead of print]

29. Doney KC, Chauncey T, Appelbaum FR: Allogeneic related donor hematopoietic stem cell transplantation for treatment of chronic lymphocytic leukemia. Bone Marrow Transplant 29:817, 2002

30. Sorror ML, Maris MB, Sandmaier BM, et al: Hematopoietic cell transplantation after nonmyeloablative conditioning for advanced chronic lymphocytic leukemia. J Clin Oncol 23:3819, 2005

31. Rabinowe SN, Soiffer RJ, Gribben JG, et al: Autologous and allogeneic bone marrow transplantation for poor prognosis patients with B-cell chronic lymphocytic leukemia. Blood 82:1366, 1993

32. Philip T, Guglielmi C, Hagenbeek A, et al: Autologous bone marrow transplantation as compared with salvage chemotherapy in relapses of chemotherapy-sensitive non-Hodgkin's lymphoma. N Engl J Med 333:1540, 1995

33. Peniket AJ, Ruiz de Elvira MC, Taghipour G, et al: An EBMT registry matched study of allogeneic stem cell transplants for lymphoma: allogeneic transplantation is associated with a lower relapse rate but a higher procedure-related mortality rate than autologous transplantation. Bone Marrow Transplant 31:667, 2003

34. Gianni AM, Bregni M, Siena S, et al: High-dose chemotherapy and autologous bone marrow transplantation compared with MACOP-B in aggressive B-cell lymphoma. N Engl J Med 336:1290, 1997

35. Schouten HC, Qian W, Kvaloy S, et al: High-dose therapy improves progression-free survival and survival in relapsed follicular non-Hodgkin's lymphoma: results from the randomized European CUP trial. J Clin Oncol 21:3918, 2003

36. Lenz G, Dreyling M, Schiegnitz E, et al: Myeloablative radiochemotherapy followed by autologous stem cell transplantation in first remission prolongs progression-free survival in follicular lymphoma: results of a prospective, randomized trial of the German Low-Grade Lymphoma Study Group. Blood 104:2667, 2004

37. Khouri IF, Saliba RM, Giralt SA, et al: Nonablative allogeneic hematopoietic transplantation as adoptive immunotherapy for indolent lymphoma: low incidence of toxicity, acute graft-versus-host disease, and treatment-related mortality. Blood 98:3595, 2001

38. Josting A, Rueffer U, Franklin J, et al: Prognostic factors and treatment outcome in primary progressive Hodgkin lymphoma: a report from the German Hodgkin Lymphoma Study Group. Blood 96:1280, 2000

39. Schmitz N, Pfistner B, Sextro M, et al: Aggressive conventional chemotherapy compared with high-dose chemotherapy with autologous haemopoietic stem-cell transplantation for relapsed chemosensitive Hodgkin's disease: a randomised trial. Lancet 359:2065, 2002

40. Anderson JE, Litzow MR, Appelbaum FR, et al: Allogeneic, syngeneic, and autologous marrow transplantation for Hodgkin's disease: the 21 year Seattle experience. J Clin Oncol 11:2342, 1993

41. Schmitz N, Sureda A, Robinson S: Allogeneic transplantation of hematopoietic stem cells after nonmyeloablative conditioning for Hodgkin's disease: indications and results. Semin Oncol 31:27, 2004

42. Attal M, Harousseau JL, Stoppa AM, et al: A prospective, randomized trial of autologous bone marrow transplantation and chemotherapy in multiple myeloma. N Engl J Med 335:91, 1996

43. Child JA, Morgan GJ, Davies FE, et al: High-dose chemotherapy with hematopoietic stem-cell rescue for multiple myeloma. N Engl J Med 348:1875, 2003

44. Attal M, Harousseau JL, Facon T, et al: Single versus double autologous stem-cell transplantation for multiple myeloma. N Engl J Med 349:2495, 2003

45. Bensinger WI, Buckner CD, Clift RA, et al: Phase 1 study of busulfan and cyclophosphamide in preparation for allogeneic marrow transplant for patients with multiple myeloma. J Clin Oncol 10:1497, 1992

46. Gahrton G, Svensson H, Cavo M, et al: Progress in allogeneic bone marrow and peripheral blood stem cell transplantation for multiple myeloma: a comparison between transplants performed 1983–93 and 1994–98 at European Group for Blood and Marrow Transplantation centres. Br J Haematol 113:209, 2001

47. Kolb HJ, Schattenberg A, Goldman JM, et al: Graft-versus-leukemia effect of donor lymphocyte transfusions in marrow grafted patients. European Group for Blood and Marrow Transplantation Working Party Chronic Leukemia. Blood 86:2041, 1995

Acknowledgment

This work was supported in part by grants CA-18029, CA-47748, and CA-26386 from the National Institutes of Health, U.S. Department of Health and Human Services.

102 Deficiencies in Immunoglobulins and Cell-Mediated Immunity

Fred S. Rosen, M.D.

Immunoglobulin Deficiency Syndromes

Insufficient production of one or more kinds of antibodies characterizes the immunoglobulin deficiency syndromes [*see Table 1*].[1,2] Patients with these deficiencies are subject to recurrent pyogenic infections, such as otitis media, sinusitis, and pneumonia. Repeated episodes of pneumonia can lead to chronic obstructive pulmonary disease. For many of these deficiencies, the genetic basis has now been defined. The primary care physician's role in these disorders is to suspect the diagnosis under the appropriate clinical circumstances—often, unusual susceptibility to certain infections in a patient with a family history of the same—and to order the preliminary laboratory studies. Definitive diagnosis and management is typically the responsibility of the immunologist. Control of the infections to which these patients are susceptible is principally managed by the intravenous administration of large doses of γ-globulin.

X-LINKED AGAMMAGLOBULINEMIA

X-linked agammaglobulinemia, also known as congenital agammaglobulinemia or Bruton disease, was the first immunodeficiency disorder to be described, in 1952.

Genetics and Pathogenesis

The gene responsible for X-linked agammaglobulinemia is located on the long arm of the X chromosome (Xq21.33–q22).[3-5] This gene, termed *btk*, is a member of the *src* family of oncogenes and encodes a unique tyrosine kinase.[4-8] It probably plays a critical role in the maturation of B cells: pre–B cells are present in normal numbers in the bone marrow of males with X-linked agammaglobulinemia, but they do not develop into mature B cells.[2] Because the genes governing the structure of immunoglobulins are on autosomal chromosomes, the mechanism of the disorder must also involve a defect in a regulatory gene.

In patients with X-linked agammaglobulinemia, the lymphoid organs are characterized by a lack of germinal follicles, B cells, and plasma cells. On bone marrow studies, pre–B cells (which contain immunoglobulin μ heavy chains in their cytoplasm and therefore can be identified by immunofluorescence staining with antiserum to the μ chain) are present in normal numbers.

Diagnosis

Clinical manifestations   Because infants are born with IgG from their mother in their blood, boys who have X-linked agammaglobulinemia do not start to show the effects of the disorder

Table 1   Primary Specific Immunodeficiencies Involving Antibodies

Designation	Usual Phenotypic Expression		Presumed Level of Basic Cellular Defect	Known or Presumed Pathogenetic Mechanism	Inheritance
	Antibody Deficiencies	Cellular Abnormalities			
X-linked agamma-globulinemia	All immuno-globulins	↓ B cells	Pre–B cells	Mutations in the gene for Bruton's X-linked tyrosinase (*btk*)	X-linked
Common variable immunodeficiency	All immuno-globulins	Faulty B cell maturation	Immaturity of B cells	↓ Helper T cell function Intrinsic B cell defect Underproduction of B cells Autoantibodies to B cells	Unknown
Selective IgA deficiency	IgA	↓ IgA plasma cells ± ↑ IgA⁺ B cells	Terminal differentiation of IgA⁺ B cells impaired	Unknown	Usually unknown (autosomal recessive more common than autosomal dominant); frequent in families of patients with common variable immunodeficiency
Ig deficiencies, with increased IgM	IgG, IgA, and IgE	↓ IgG and IgA plasma cells ↑ IgM and IgD plasma cells ± ↑ IgM⁺ B cells	Failure of immuno-globulin class switching	X-linked form: mutations in the gene for the CD40 ligand Autosomal recessive form: activation-induced cytidine deaminase	X-linked, autosomal recessive, or unknown
Selective deficiency of IgG subclasses	One or more IgG isotypes	↓ Plasma cells ± ↓ T cells	Unknown	Unknown	Unknown
κ-Chain deficiency	IgG(κ)	↓ κ⁺ B cells	Unknown	Point mutation at 2p11	Autosomal recessive
Transient hypogam-maglobulinemia of infancy	IgG and IgA	↓ Plasma cells B cells normal	Impaired terminal differentiation of B cells	↓ Helper T cells	Frequent in heterozygous individuals in families with various severe combined immunodeficiencies

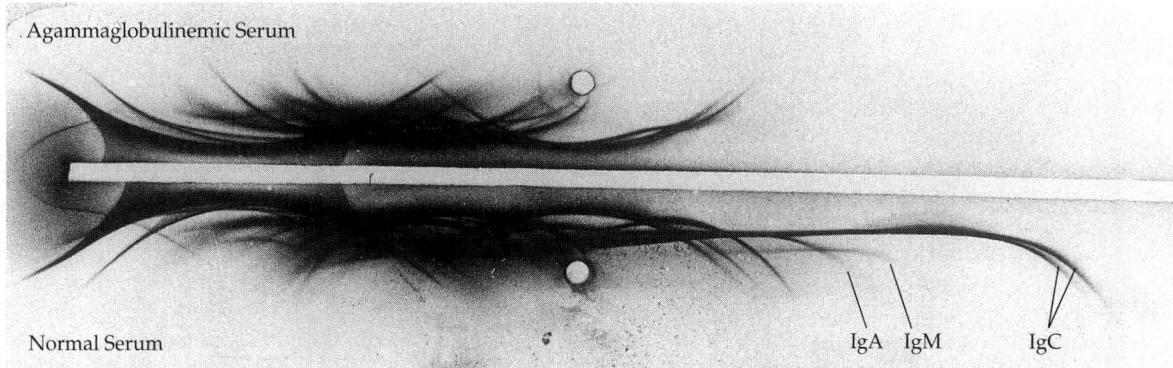

Figure 1   When an immunoelectrophoretic pattern of agammaglobulinemic serum is compared with a normal serum pattern, the absence of IgA, IgM, and IgG—characteristic of the disorder—is clearly demonstrated.

until 6 to 15 months of age. They then demonstrate unusual susceptibility to infections by pyogenic organisms (e.g., otitis media, sinusitis, and pneumonia from *Haemophilus influenzae*, pneumococci, streptococci, staphylococci, and meningococci). Those infections are more frequent and more severe in boys with X-linked agammaglobulinemia than in normal children, and recurrent infection by the same organism is common. Frequently, the infections are slow to respond to antibiotics. Recurrent pulmonary infections often lead to bronchiectasis and pulmonary insufficiency. Affected males have normal resistance to the common viral diseases, fungi, and most gram-negative organisms, but some have developed polio after receiving oral polio vaccine. About one third of patients have symptoms that resemble rheumatoid arthritis, including swollen and painful joints. A severe late complication is a fatal syndrome similar to dermatomyositis but with central neurologic involvement, as well. This syndrome is gradual in onset, usually starting in the second or third decade of life. In several patients with this syndrome, echoviruses have been cultured from the blood, stool, and cerebrospinal fluid.[9]

Laboratory testing   Diagnosis begins with measuring the serum level of each class of immunoglobulin [*see Figure 1*]. Patients with X-linked agammaglobulinemia usually have less than 100 mg/dl of IgG (normal levels are 614 to 1,295 mg/dl), and they have levels of IgA, IgM, IgD, and IgE that are extremely low or undetectable. Such findings should prompt referral of the patient to an immunologist.

In patients with X-linked agammaglobulinemia, analysis of white blood cells by flow cytometry reveals a lack of B cells. These patients are unable to mount an antibody response to antigen challenge, such as routine diphtheria-pertussis-tetanus (DPT) or *H. influenzae* vaccination, and they cannot neutralize the toxin in a Schick test (intradermal injection of diphtheria toxin). In contrast, cell-mediated immune functions, such as delayed hypersensitivity–mediated skin reactions and graft rejection, are essentially normal, and the T cells respond in vitro to phytohemagglutinin and produce lymphokines normally.

Screening   All subsequent male offspring of the mother or maternal aunts of a patient with X-linked agammaglobulinemia should be screened for mutations of the *btk* gene. Because the defect is limited to B cells, female carriers of the gene can be detected by analysis of X-chromosome inactivation in B cells.[10,11] In female carriers, pre–B cells in which the X chromosome bearing the normal gene has been inactivated will not develop into B cells; therefore, all mature B cells will bear an active X chromosome containing only the normal gene.

Treatment

Preparations of 5% or 10% γ-globulin solution are now used as replacement therapy for agammaglobulinemia. Parents can be reassured that these preparations pose no risk of transmitting HIV or other viral infection. Intravenous administration of these preparations is well tolerated; large doses can be given without discomfort or pain. Infants do not require permanent intravenous access.

Dosages of γ-globulin are adjusted according to the patient's health. The minimal effective dosage of intravenous γ-globulin is 300 mg/kg a month; however, higher doses, such as 500 mg/kg a month, are usually optimal.[12] Dividing the monthly dosage of γ-globulin and administering it at 1-week or 2-week intervals is preferable, because it maintains higher immunoglobulin levels. The γ-globulin is infused at a rate of 3 ml/min or slower. Side effects may include headache, shaking chills, flank pain, fever, and hypotension. These can be ameliorated by giving an antihistamine or methylprednisolone before the infusion.

Bacterial infections in patients with X-linked agammaglobulinemia require vigorous antibiotic treatment. Antibiotics should be given in prolonged courses (e.g., 2 weeks) at full doses.

Prognosis   The prognosis is very good for patients whose condition is diagnosed and treated early. A recent study of 31 patients with X-linked agammaglobulinemia found that early and prolonged γ-globulin replacement therapy is effective in preventing bacterial infections and pulmonary insufficiency. Viral infections still developed, however, and one patient died of enteroviral meningoencephalopathy.[13]

COMMON VARIABLE IMMUNODEFICIENCY

Common variable immunodeficiency (CVID) is so called because it accounts for over 50% of cases of immunodeficiency and because patients present with variable clinical manifestations and somewhat inconsistent laboratory findings; disease course varies, as well.

Etiology and Pathogenesis

The cause of CVID is unknown. CVID does not appear to be genetically transmitted—apparently the germ cells are not involved—although some family clusters have been seen. CVID affects males and females equally.

A variety of pathogenetic mechanisms underlie CVID.[2] These include (1) B cells that do not respond to stimulatory signals from T cells, (2) B cells that can synthesize but cannot secrete immunoglobulins, (3) the absence of helper T cells (required for normal B cell function), and (4) the presence of autoantibodies to B cells. In a few cases of CVID, B cells cannot be detected. All patients show markedly low serum levels of all immunoglobulins.

Diagnosis

Clinical manifestations   Onset of CVID can occur at any age, but it usually occurs after puberty. Patients have the same heightened vulnerability to infections as those with X-linked agammaglobulinemia; also, there is chronic involvement of the sinuses and respiratory tract.

CVID is associated with several autoimmune diseases, such as rheumatoid arthritis, idiopathic thrombocytopenia, hemolytic anemia, neutropenia, and, predominantly, pernicious anemia. Infectious diarrhea and malabsorption syndrome are common. CVID is also associated with severe malabsorption syndrome caused by gluten-sensitive enteropathy. It is unclear whether CVID is a cause or an effect of these disorders. Chronic lung disease that produces bronchiectasis is common in CVID; this condition should be differentiated from cystic fibrosis, chronic allergy, and α_1-antitrypsin deficiency. In contrast to X-linked agammaglobulinemia, CVID is often marked by considerable enlargement of regional lymph nodes and splenomegaly.

Laboratory tests   IgG levels in patients with CVID are generally lower than 250 mg/dl, and other immunoglobulins are also markedly decreased. B cells are usually present, but they do not mature normally into plasma cells, which synthesize and secrete immunoglobulins. Tests of cell-mediated immunity also demonstrate defects.

Lymphoid hyperplasia may occur in the gut of patients with CVID. This can be visualized by barium contrast x-ray of the upper GI tract, which is indicated in CVID patients with GI symptoms.

Treatment

Treatment of CVID is essentially the same as that of X-linked agammaglobulinemia: replacement γ-globulin therapy and vigorous use of antibiotics during acute infections. Diarrhea in these patients is frequently caused by *Giardia lamblia* infection, which can be rapidly controlled with quinacrine hydrochloride or metronidazole.[11] Special care must be taken if steroids are used as therapy for the associated autoimmune diseases, because these agents may heighten susceptibility to infection.

Prognosis

Patients with CVID can have a normal life span. Women with the disease can carry a normal pregnancy to term and have normal babies. Although those babies will lack maternal IgG and the passive immunity it confers in the first months of life, they do well without treatment with γ-globulin.

SELECTIVE IMMUNOGLOBULIN DEFICIENCIES

Selective IgA Deficiency

Epidemiology   Selective IgA deficiency is one of the most common immunodeficiencies in whites, occurring in one in 600

to 800 persons in this population. It does not occur in Africans and almost never occurs in Asians.

Genetics and pathogenesis   The genetics of IgA deficiency are unclear. Data on inheritance are conflicting, with some suggesting autosomal dominant inheritance and others suggesting autosomal recessive inheritance.

A few patients lacking serum IgA have secretory IgA, and some patients have monomeric IgM in their secretions. B cells bearing surface IgA are present, indicating that the defect is probably in the terminal differentiation of IgA-secreting cells. In vitro, IgA-bearing cells can be stimulated by mitogens to produce IgA.[14]

Diagnosis   Many patients with IgA deficiency are surprisingly healthy. Nevertheless, IgA deficiency is associated with many clinical syndromes. Patients most often come to medical attention because of recurrent sinus and pulmonary infection by bacteria and viruses. These patients also show a higher incidence of autoimmune, GI, allergic, connective tissue, and malignant diseases. Some patients with IgA deficiency produce antibodies to bovine proteins, suggesting that IgA in the gut normally helps prevent absorption of foreign antigens. IgA deficiency is found in about 70% of patients with ataxia-telangiectasia (see below).

The serum IgA level is less than 5 mg/dl (normal, 60 to 309 mg/dl). Other immunoglobulin levels are normal. Although patients with IgA deficiency usually also have defects in T cell function, most of these patients have normal cell-mediated immunity.

Treatment   There is currently no satisfactory means of supplying adequate levels of IgA. Sinus and pulmonary infections in IgA-deficient patients are treated by standard means.

Complications   In extremely rare instances, patients with IgA deficiency produce IgE antibodies to IgA and will have anaphylactic reactions when given immunoglobulin.[15] Immunoglobulin replacement therapy should be avoided in such patients; blood transfusion can also precipitate an anaphylactic reaction. Patients who require blood should receive red cells from an IgA-deficient donor because anaphylactic reactions may occur even if the red blood cells are washed three times.

Immunoglobulin Deficiency with Elevated IgM

The combination of markedly elevated IgM levels and deficiency of other immunoglobulins is termed the hyper-IgM syndrome. The IgM in these patients is heterogeneous; thus, it is polyclonal and does not emerge from malignant cells.

In 70% of hyper-IgM cases, the syndrome is X-linked; in the remainder, it is autosomal recessive and affects both males and females. The X-linked form of the hyper-IgM syndrome results from a genetic defect in the CD40 ligand, which is found on the surface of activated T cells.[16-18] Normally, this ligand interacts with the CD40 molecule on the B cell surface, inducing isotype switching. The autosomal recessive form of the hyper-IgM syndrome results from a genetic defect in an enzyme called activation-induced cytidine deaminase (AID).[19] This enzyme is involved in RNA editing, but its precise role in immunoglobulin class switching is unknown.

Diagnosis   Patients with hyper-IgM syndrome show increased susceptibility to infection similar to that seen in X-linked agammaglobulinemia (see above). Immunoglobulin assays show an elevated level of IgM (350 to 1,000 mg/dl); the IgD level may also be elevated. IgA is usually undetectable, and the IgG level is normally less than 100 mg/dl. Many plasma cells, as well as lymphocytoid and plasmacytoid cells structurally similar to those of Waldenström macroglobulinemia, are seen in the gut, lymphoid organs, and blood. These plasma cells stain with fluorescein-labeled antibodies to IgM. In the X-linked form of hyper-IgM syndrome, lymph nodes are small and contain no germinal centers. In AID deficiency, lymph nodes are enlarged and contain germinal centers. Lymph node biopsy is not usually obtained for clinical diagnosis, however.

Treatment   Treatment for hyper-IgM syndrome is the same as that for X-linked agammaglobulinemia (see above).

Selective Deficiencies of IgM or the Subclasses of IgG

Selective IgM deficiency is rare. This deficiency may precede the onset of CVID. Patients with selective deficiencies of the IgG subclasses have a decrease in total IgG, the degree of which depends on the subclass involved. The decrease is most profound in the case of IgG1 deficiency because almost three quarters of IgG molecules belong to this subclass. Some patients with IgG deficiency are unable to mount an antibody response to certain antigens. Patients with IgG2 deficiency are especially prone to infection by bacteria with a large amount of surface polysaccharide, such as pneumococci and *H. influenzae*. The diagnosis is confirmed by quantitation of the IgG subclasses and administration of a polysaccharide-antigen vaccine (typically, pneumococcal vaccine); patients with IgG deficiency will fail to produce antibodies in response to vaccination. Patients with selective deficiencies of the IgG subclasses respond to intravenously administered γ-globulin.

Deficiencies of Cell-Mediated Immunity

Extreme susceptibility to opportunistic infection is the most important clinical feature of deficiencies of cell-mediated immunity, or T cell deficiencies. Such deficiencies, which manifest as impairment in delayed hypersensitivity, may be inherited or may be secondary to another disorder [*see Table 2*]. The ac-

---

Table 2   **Conditions Associated with Impaired Delayed Hypersensitivity**

Primary deficiencies of cell-mediated immunity [*see Table 3*]

Chromosomal abnormalities: Bloom syndrome, Down syndrome, Fanconi syndrome

Infections: HIV (AIDS), lepromatous leprosy, Epstein-Barr virus (X-linked lymphoproliferative syndrome), chronic mucocutaneous candidiasis, secondary syphilis, and many other viral and parasitic diseases

Neoplasms: thymoma, Hodgkin disease and other lymphomas, any advanced malignant disease

Connective tissue diseases: systemic lupus erythematosus, advanced rheumatoid arthritis

Physical agents: burns, x-irradiation

Other conditions: sarcoidosis, malnutrition, aging, inflammatory bowel disease, intestinal lymphangiectasia

Iatrogenic causes: chemotherapy, postsurgery, x-irradiation therapy

---

quired immunodeficiency syndrome is discussed elsewhere [*see Chapter 153*].

In general, patients with T cell deficiencies have more frequent and more severe infections than do patients who have pure B cell deficiencies [*see Table 3*].[2] Patients with deficiencies of cell-mediated immunity cannot cope with a number of ordinarily innocuous organisms, such as *Candida albicans* and *Pneumocystis carinii*, and are especially susceptible to enteric bacteria, viruses, and fungi. Live attenuated vaccines are dangerous in these patients: vaccination for smallpox or administration of bacillus Calmette-Guérin (BCG) has led to rapid death.

Determining the defects of cell-mediated immunity requires testing in a specialized immunology laboratory. An extensive array of tests is available at such laboratories [*see Table 4*]. The choice of tests and the order in which they are performed depend on the particular case.

CONGENITAL THYMIC HYPOPLASIA

Pathogenesis

Congenital thymic hypoplasia (DiGeorge syndrome) results from the lack of normal development of the third and fourth brachial, or pharyngeal, pouches, which leads to abnormality in the great vessels and to the absence of the thymus and the parathyroids. Congenital thymic hypoplasia is not inherited; rather, it is thought to result from an intrauterine accident occurring before the eighth week of pregnancy. The absence of the thymus leads to deficiency in cell-mediated immunity.

Diagnosis

Clinical manifestations   Patients with congenital thymic hypoplasia have distinctive facial features, including low-set ears, a shortened philtrum, and ocular hypertelorism. Hypocalcemia from associated parathyroid deficiency is a universal finding and often results in neonatal tetany. There can be a right-sided aortic arch or tetralogy of Fallot or many other cardiac malformations.

Laboratory tests   The T cell defect in children with congenital thymic hypoplasia varies from mild to profound. Severely affected children do not exhibit delayed hypersensitivity reactions; their lymphocytes do not respond to mitogens or antigens in vitro, nor do they produce lymphokines. The lymph nodes lack paracortical lymphocytes. Plasma cells are present, however, and immunoglobulin levels are normal. Although patients with congenital thymic hypoplasia produce specific antibodies when they are immunized with various antigens, the antibody response is not quite normal, because secondary responses are lacking.

As the patient ages, T cell function improves; and usually by the time the child is 5 years of age, skin testing reveals no abnormality in cell-mediated immunity. However, the abnormal T cell phenotype—as indicated by a higher than normal ratio of CD4+ to CD8+ T cells—persists for life. Karyotyping reveals microdeletions at chromosome 22q11 in approximately 90% of patients.

Treatment

Thymus transplantation should be undertaken in those infants with congenital thymic hypoplasia who experience frequent infections. Transplantation of fetal thymus results in rapid acquisition of normal T cell function, which is thought to be secondary to production of a thymic hormone secreted by the thymic epithelium. Rejection appears not to be a problem.

Table 3 Classification of Primary Specific Immunodeficiencies Involving Cell-Mediated Immunity

Designation	Usual Phenotypic Expression		Presumed Level of Basic Cellular Defect	Known or Presumed Pathogenetic Mechanism	Inheritance	Main Associated Features
	Functional Deficiencies	Cellular Abnormalities				
Congenital thymic hypoplasia (DiGeorge syndrome)	CMI, impaired antibody	↓ T cells	Thymocytes	Embryopathy of third and fourth pharyngeal pouch areas	Usually not familial	Hypoparathyroidism Abnormal facies Cardiovascular abnormalities
Severe combined immunodeficiency	CMI, antibody	- T cells, + B cells	LSC	Mutation in γ chain of IL-2R, IL-4R, IL-7R, IL-11R, IL-15R, *JAK3,* or IL-7 receptor α chain	X-linked or autosomal recessive	—
		- T cells, - B cells		Mutation in *RAG1* or *RAG2*	Autosomal recessive	
Adenosine deaminase (ADA) deficiency	CMI, antibody	↓ T cells, ± B cells	LSC or early T cells	Metabolic effects of ADA deficiency	Autosomal recessive	—
Purine nucleoside phosphorylase (PNP) deficiency	CMI ± antibody	↓ T cells	T cells	Metabolic effects of PNP deficiency	Autosomal recessive	Hypoplastic anemia
Reticular dysgenesis	CMI, antibody, phagocytes	↓ T cells, ↓ B cells, ↓ phagocytes	HSC	Unknown	Autosomal recessive	Neutropenia
Wiskott-Aldrich syndrome	Antibody to certain antigens (mainly polysaccharides), CMI (progressive)	↓ T cells, ↑ B cells (progressive)	HSC	Mutations in *WASP* gene	X-linked	Thrombocytopenia Eczema Lymphoreticular cancers
Immunodeficiency with ataxia-telangiectasia	CMI, antibody (partial)	↓ T cells, ↓ plasma cells (mainly those cells producing IgA, IgE, ± IgG)	Defective checkpoints in T and B cell division	Mutations in *ATM* gene	Autosomal recessive	Cerebellar ataxia Telangiectasia Chromosomal abnormalities Raised serum α-fetoprotein levels
MHC class II deficiency	CMI ± antibody	None	T cells, B cells, and antigen-presenting cells	Defects of promoter proteins	Autosomal recessive	Intestinal malabsorption
CD3 deficiency	CMI	None	T cells	Mutations in CD3-ε or CD3-γ	Autosomal recessive	—
CD8 deficiency	CMI	↓ CD8+ T cells, normal number of CD4+ cells	Early T cells	Mutations in *ZAP* genes	Autosomal recessive	—

CMI—cell-mediated immunity   HSC—hematopoietic stem cell   LSC—lymphocytic stem cell

SEVERE COMBINED IMMUNODEFICIENCY

Severe combined immunodeficiency disease (SCID) is characterized by marked depletion of cells that mediate both humoral and cellular immunity—B cells and T cells, respectively. SCID is fatal if left untreated.

Several variants of SCID have been identified. They are designated as T−B− or T−B+, depending on whether B cells are normal or increased (B+) or absent (B−). In addition to the extent of B cell involvement, the variants also differ in the site of the basic cellular defect, the pathogenetic mechanism, and the mode of inheritance [*see Table 3*].

Genetics and Pathogenesis

T−B+ SCID may be transmitted as either an X-linked or an autosomal recessive trait. The specific genetic defect responsible for the X-linked form of T−B+ SCID results from mutations in the γ chain of the interleukin-2 receptor (IL-2R),[20] whose gene is localized to the long arm of the X chromosome at Xq13.[21] This γ chain is also found in the receptors for IL-4, IL-7, IL-11, IL-15, and IL-21.[22] Engagement of the IL-7 receptor by IL-7 is required for T cell maturation, so precursor T cells in these patients do not mature.

When any of those receptors, or IL-2R, are engaged by its ligands, a cytoplasmic tyrosine kinase (Janus-family tyrosine kinase, or JAK3) bound to the γ chain is activated. The gene encoding JAK3 is on an autosome, not the X chromosome. Thus, autosomal recessive T−B+ SCID is caused by mutations in the *JAK3* gene.[23,24]

T−B− SCID is inherited in an autosomal recessive manner. About half of the cases are caused by a deficiency in the enzyme adenosine deaminase (ADA),[25] and another large fraction results from mutations in the recombination-activating genes *RAG-1* and *RAG-2*.[26] These recombinase enzymes are required for the gene rearrangements that occur before T cell receptor or immunoglobulin synthesis. Other patients with autosomal recessive T−B− SCID lack the enzyme purine nucleoside phosphorylase (PNP).[27]

ADA deficiency leads to an accumulation of adenosine, adenosine triphosphate (ATP), and deoxy-ATP (dATP). It has

Table 4 Laboratory Tests Used to Determine Deficiencies of Cell-Mediated Immunity

Skin test: 24- to 48-hr reaction to *Candida*, *Trichophyton*, PPD

Response to nonspecific mitogens: phytohemagglutinin, concanavalin A, pokeweed mitogen

Response to specific mitogens: diphtheria, tetanus, *Candida*

Response to alloantigens: mixed lymphocyte reaction

When responses to alloantigens and nonspecific and specific mitogens are negative: repeat tests while stimulating cells with IL-2

Enumerate T cells with monoclonal antibody to CD3, with or without a cell sorter

Enumerate T cell subsets with monoclonal antibody to CD4 for helper T cells and with monoclonal antibody to CD8

Enumerate T cells positive for Ia (class II) antigens (which measures the number of activated T cells)

Quantitate IL-2 receptors with monoclonal antibody TAC

Quantitate IL-2 and interferon-gamma synthesis

Enumerate NK cells with monoclonal antibodies Leu-7 and Leu-11

Assay NK cell activity using cell line K-562

Assay cytotoxic T cell activity using cell lines of cloned T cells

Enumerate monocytes with monoclonal antibody Mo-1

Assay for IL-1 production by stimulated monocytes

Determine serum level of anti–T cell antibodies

Determine if antibody to HIV is present

HLA typing

Assay erythrocytes for adenosine deaminase and purine nucleoside phosphorylase activity

Detect thymus shadow on x-ray

Note: All patients with defects in cell-mediated immunity should receive all tests listed, except the last three, for optimal examination. The last three tests are for patients suspected of having severe combined immunodeficiency or congenital thymic hypoplasia. HLA typing is needed for prospective recipients of bone marrow transplants.

IL-1—interleukin-1 IL-2—interleukin-2 NK—natural killer
PPD—purified protein derivative of tuberculin

been shown that dATP poisons ribonucleotide reductase, an enzyme required for DNA synthesis. Thus, lymphocytes lacking ADA cannot divide until the dATP overload is decreased or removed. In a similar manner, lymphocytes that lack PNP accumulate guanosine, guanosine triphosphate (GTP), and deoxy-GTP, causing metabolic abnormalities that resemble those seen in ADA deficiency. SCID caused by ADA or PNP deficiency can be diagnosed prenatally by amniocentesis because fibroblasts in the amniotic fluid also show the enzymatic defect.

CD8 deficiency is a rare form of SCID that results from mutations in the *ZAP-70* gene.[28,29] ZAP-70 is a tyrosine kinase that binds to the CD3 ζ chain and is involved in signal transduction from the T cell receptor (the TCR-CD3 complex). CD8+ T cells fail to mature, and mature CD4+ T cells fail to function as a result of the mutations in *ZAP-70*.

Another variant of SCID is reticular dysgenesis, a severe combined immunodeficiency with a generalized granulocyte deficiency. Newborns with this disease lack granulocytes in the blood and bone marrow and die of infection within the first few days of life.

Diagnosis

Clinical manifestations Chronic pulmonary infections, diarrhea, moniliasis, and failure to thrive are the most common manifestations of SCID. The lymph nodes are small to absent despite chronic infections, which usually begin at 3 to 6 months of age.

Laboratory tests Complete blood counts show a low number of lymphocytes. There is absence of a thymic shadow on chest x-ray. (Autopsy in fatal cases has revealed an embryonic thymus that resembles the thymus at 6 weeks of gestation, before invasion with lymphocytes.) Tests for cutaneous delayed hypersensitivity and contact sensitization and in vitro assays of blood lymphocytes are negative, demonstrating the absence of T cells, a phytohemagglutinin response, and lymphokine production. Antibody levels are usually low, although occasionally the IgM level is normal; and sometimes, a myeloma component is seen.

Treatment

Hundreds of cases of SCID have been successfully treated by transplantation of bone marrow cells.[30] By 3 to 8 months after receiving the bone marrow, these patients show normal delayed hypersensitivity and T cell function and are no longer abnormally susceptible to infection.

Immunologic reconstitution with bone marrow cells should be attempted only in specialized centers where comprehensive histocompatibility typing and intensive 24-hour care can be given. If the donor and the recipient are not exceedingly well matched, fatal graft versus host disease (GVHD) will ensue. Even an HLA-mismatched blood transfusion can produce fatal GVHD in such patients: the patient is immunocompromised and thus cannot reject the injected cells, but the histoincompatible cells that have been administered recognize the patient's cells as foreign and react against them.

The manifestations of GVHD include fever, diarrhea, depression of the bone marrow, splenomegaly, and an erythematous rash on the face, trunk, and extremities. The reaction eventually leads to death. GVHD can be avoided by irradiating the blood before transfusion.

It is possible to establish grafts of half-matched (haploidentical) parental marrow in infants with SCID. GVHD can be avoided in those cases if the parental marrow is depleted of T cells before transplantation by passage over lectin columns or by treatment with anti–T cell monoclonal antibody plus complement.

Patients with ADA deficiency have also been treated successfully with infusions of purified adenosine deaminase modified with polyethylene glycol. The ADA gene has been cloned and inserted into a retroviral vector.[31] In a few ADA-deficient children, this vector has been transduced into peripheral blood lymphocytes, which were then reinfused. This gene therapy procedure has corrected the immunodeficiency in these patients, although it must be repeated periodically.[32] Successful gene therapy has also been carried out in X-linked SCID by transducing a Maloney virus vector bearing the gene for the common γ chain into bone marrow cells. Sustained responses have been reported in several of these patients: T cell number and function normalized in these patients, as did B cell function, and infusions of γ globulin were no longer required.[33] Unfortunately, one patient who underwent this treatment subsequently developed a monoclonal lymphocytosis,[34] possibly because the retroviral vector inserted at a site near a gene implicated in T cell leukemias, resulting in increased expression of this gene product.

WISKOTT-ALDRICH SYNDROME

An X-linked recessive disease, Wiskott-Aldrich syndrome (WAS), results from a mutation that has been mapped to the Xp11.3–p11.22 region of the X chromosome. The *WAS* gene has been cloned.[35,36]

The lymphoid system of a patient with WAS appears anatomically intact at birth. Starting in the first months of life, however, there is a decrease in T cells in the paracortical areas of the lymph nodes and a polyclonal expansion of B cells. The T cells in these patients respond poorly to mitogens. The protein encoded by the *WAS* gene appears to be involved in signal transduction that leads to reorganization of the cytoskeleton when lymphocytes are stimulated, which results in defective collaboration between T cells and B cells. Lymphocytes have a markedly abnormal appearance when visualized by scanning electron microscopy. Platelets are abnormally small and few in number.[37] Certain missense mutations in the *WAS* gene lead to a mild disease called X-linked thrombocytopenia.[38]

Diagnosis

Clinical manifestations WAS is characterized by eczema, easy bruising, increased susceptibility to infection (both pyogenic and opportunistic), and bloody diarrhea. These manifestations appear in the first months of life. An increased incidence of hematopoietic malignancies is seen, starting in the second or third decade of life.

Laboratory testing Patients with WAS have normal levels of IgG, high levels of IgE and IgA, and low levels of IgM. Severe thrombocytopenia is universal. Tests of cell-mediated immunity [*see Table 4*] show a variety of abnormalities: WAS patients lack isohemagglutinins and are unable to make antibodies to polysaccharides. They respond to some protein antigens but not to others; in addition, they may exhibit anergy and may not display positive results to skin tests for the usual bacterial or fungal antigens.

Treatment

WAS patients have been treated with marrow transplantation after receiving irradiation or busulfan and antilymphocyte serum to destroy residual lymphocytes; they have then shown normal immune and platelet functions. In WAS patients who do not receive a bone marrow transplant and who experience severe bleeding from thrombocytopenia, splenectomy may be considerably beneficial.[39]

IMMUNOLOGIC DEFICIENCY WITH ATAXIA-TELANGIECTASIA

Ataxia-telangiectasia (A-T) is a disease associated with defects in cell-mediated immunity and with immunoglobulin deficiencies. It is inherited as an autosomal recessive trait. The gene for A-T (*ATM* for A-T mutated) maps to the chromosomal region 11q22.3.[40,41] Normally, the gene appears to function in repair of breaks in double-stranded DNA. Patients with A-T have a disorder of the cell-cycle checkpoint pathway that results in an extreme hypersensitivity to ionizing radiation. Consequently, frequent chromosomal breaks, inversions, and translocations are observed. Postmortem examination may disclose abnormalities in the thymus, which is small and deficient in lymphocytes. There also may be an abnormality in lymph node structure.

Diagnosis

Clinical manifestations A-T presents as a progressive neurologic disease that begins in early childhood. It is characterized by cerebellar ataxia, starting at 18 months of age, followed by increasing tremor and deterioration of mental function. By 5 years of age, progressive telangiectasia is seen in the vessels of the bulbar conjunctiva and is later visible on the skin. The immune deficiencies in these patients leads to recurrent sinus and bronchial infections and subsequent bronchiectasis. An unusually high incidence of lymphoid malignant disorders has been reported in patients with A-T.[42]

Laboratory testing About 70% of patients with A-T have a severe deficiency in IgA. On tests of cell-mediated immunity [*see Table 4*], some A-T patients are anergic and fail to show delayed hypersensitivity responses to common microbial antigens. They may also have abnormal in vitro cell-mediated immune responses and may tolerate allografts.

Treatment and Prognosis

No satisfactory treatment for A-T is currently available. Persons with A-T who survive into their second decade may fail to mature sexually. A-T patients usually die of lymphoid malignancies or other causes by the end of their second decade.

The author has no commercial relationships with manufacturers of products or providers of services discussed in this chapter.

References

1. Rosen FS, Wedgwood RJ, Eibl M, et al: Primary immunodeficiency diseases: report of a WHO Scientific Group. Clin Exp Immunol 109(suppl 1):1, 1997
2. Rosen FS, Cooper MD, Wedgwood RJP: The primary immunodeficiencies. N Engl J Med 333:431, 1995
3. Kwan SP, Terwilliger J, Parmley R, et al: Identification of a closely linked DNA marker, DXS178, to further refine the X-linked agammaglobulinemia locus. Genomics 6:238, 1990
4. Vetrie D, Vorechovsky I, Sideras P, et al: The gene involved in X-linked agammaglobulinaemia is a member of the src family of protein-tyrosine kinases. Nature 361:226, 1993
5. Tsukada S, Saffran DC, Rawlings DJ, et al: Deficient expression of a B cell cytoplasmic tyrosine kinase in human X-linked agammaglobulinemia. Cell 72:279, 1993
6. Hagemann TL, Chen Y, Rosen FS, et al: Genomic organization of the Btk gene and exon scanning for mutations with X-linked agammaglobulinemia. Hum Mol Genet 3:1743, 1994
7. Zhu Q, Zhang M, Winkelstein J, et al: Unique mutations of Bruton's tyrosine kinase in fourteen unrelated X-linked agammaglobulinemia families. Hum Mol Genet 3:1899, 1994
8. Conley ME, Fitch-Hilgenberg ME, Cleveland GL, et al: Screening of genomic DNA to identify mutations in the gene for tyrosine kinase. Hum Mol Genet 3:1751, 1994
9. Misbah SA: Chronic enteroviral meningoencephalitis in agammaglobulinemia: case report and literature review. J Clin Immunol 12:266, 1992
10. Fearon ER, Winkelstein JA, Civin CI, et al: Carrier detection in X-linked agammaglobulinemia by analysis of X-chromosome inactivation. N Engl J Med 316:427, 1987
11. Conley ME, Brown P, Pickard AR, et al: Expression of the gene defect in X-linked agammaglobulinemia. N Engl J Med 315:564, 1986
12. Buckley RH, Schiff RI: The use of intravenous immune globulin in immunodeficiency diseases. N Engl J Med 325:110, 1991
13. Quartier P, Debre M, De Blic J, et al: Early and prolonged intravenous immunoglobulin replacement therapy in childhood agammaglobulinemia: a retrospective survey of 31 patients. J Pediatr 134:589, 1999
14. Conley ME, Cooper MD: Immature IgA B cells in IgA-deficient patients. N Engl J Med 305:495, 1981
15. Burks AW, Sampson HA, Buckley RH: Anaphylactic reactions after gamma globulin administration in patients with hypogammaglobulinemia: detection of IgE antibodies to IgA. N Engl J Med 314:560, 1986
16. Fuleihan R, Ramesh N, Loh R, et al: Defective expression of the CD40 ligand in X chromosome-linked immunoglobulin deficiency with normal or elevated IgM. Proc Natl Acad Sci USA 90:2170, 1993
17. Korthauer U, Graf D, Mages HW, et al: Defective expression of T-cell CD40 ligand causes X-linked immunodeficiency with hyper-IgM. Nature 361:539, 1993
18. Mayer L, Kwan S-P, Thompson C, et al: Evidence for a defect in "switch" T cells in patients with immunodeficiency and hyperimmunoglobulin M. N Engl J Med 314:409, 1986
19. Revy P, Muto T, Levy Y, et al: Activation-induced deaminase (AID) deficiency causes the autosomal recessive form of the hyper-IgM syndrome (HIGM2). Cell 102:565, 2000
20. Noguchi M, Yi H, Rosenblatt HM, et al: Interleukin 2 receptor γ chain mutation results in X-linked severe combined immunodeficiency in humans. Cell 73:147, 1993
21. Puck JM, Conley ME, Bailey LC: Refinements of linkage of human severe combined immunodeficiency (SCDX1) to polymorphic markers in Xq13. Am J Hum Genet 53:176, 1993
22. Puel A, Ziegler SF, Buckley RH, et al: Defective IL7R expression in T(-)B(+)NK(+) severe combined immunodeficiency. Nat Genet 20:394, 1998
23. Macchi P, Villa A, Gillani S, et al: Mutations of Jak 3 gene in patients with autosomal recessive combined immune deficiency (SCID). Nature 377:65, 1995
24. Russell SM, Tayebi N, Nakajima H, et al: Mutation of Jak3 in a patient with SCID: essential role of Jak3 in lymphoid development. Science 270:797, 1995

25. Hirschhorn R: Adenosine deaminase deficiency. Immunodefic Rev 2:175, 1990

26. Schwarz K, Gauss GH, Ludwig L, et al: RAG mutations in human B cell-negative SCID. Science 274:97, 1996

27. Markert ML: Purine nucleoside phosphorylase deficiency. Immunodef Rev 3:45, 1991

28. Arpaia E, Shahar M, Dadi H, et al: Defective T cell receptor signaling and CD8+ thymocyte selection in humans lacking Zap-70 kinase. Cell 76:947, 1994

29. Chan AC, Kadlecek TA, Elder ME, et al: ZAP-70 deficiency in autosomal recessive form of severe combined immunodeficiency. Science 264:1599, 1994

30. Buckley RH, Schiff RI, Schiff SE, et al: Human severe combined immunodeficiency: genetic, phenotypic, and functional diversity in one hundred eight infants. J Pediatrics 130:378, 1997

31. Williams DA, Lemischka IR, Nathan DG, et al: Introduction of new genetic material into pluripotent hematopoietic stem cells of the mouse. Nature 310:476, 1984

32. Blaese RN, Culver KW, Miller AD, et al: T-lymphocyte-directed gene therapy for ADA deficiency SCID: initial trial results after 4 years. Science 270:470, 1995

33. Hacein-Bey-Abina S, Le Deist F, Carlier F, et al: Sustained correction of X-linked severe combined immunodeficiency by ex vivo gene therapy. N Engl J Med 346:1185, 2002

34. Hacein-Bey-Abina S, von Kalle C, Schmidt M, et al: A serious adverse event after successful gene therapy for X-linked severe combined immunodeficiency. N Engl J Med 348:255, 2003

35. Derry JMJ, Ochs HD, Francke U: Isolation of a novel gene mutated in Wiskott-Aldrich syndrome. Cell 78:635, 1994

36. Kwan S-P, Hagemann T, Radke BE, et al: Identification of mutations in the gene responsible for the Wiskott-Aldrich syndrome and characterization of a polymorphic dinucleotide repeat at the DXS 6940 locus adjacent to the disease gene. Proc Natl Acad Sci USA 92:4706, 1995

37. Remold-O'Donnell E, Rosen FS, Kenney DM: Defects in Wiskott-Aldrich syndrome blood cells. Blood 87:2621, 1996

38. Villa A, Notarangelo L, Macchi P, et al: X-linked thrombocytopenia and Wiskott-Aldrich syndrome are allelic diseases with mutations in the WASP gene. Nat Genet 9:414, 1995

39. Mullen CA, Anderson KD, Blaese RM: Splenectomy and/or bone marrow transplantation in the management of Wiskott-Aldrich syndrome: long term follow-up of 62 cases. Blood 82:2961, 1993

40. Gatti RA, Berkel I, Boder E, et al: Localization of an ataxia-telangiectasia gene to chromosome 11q22-23. Nature 336:577, 1988

41. Savitsky K, Barshira A, Gilad S, et al: A single ataxia telangiectasia gene with a product similar to PI-3 kinase. Science 268:1749, 1995

42. Swift M: Genetic aspects of ataxia-telangiectasia. Immunodefic Rev 2:67, 1990

103 Immunologic Tolerance and Autoimmunity

Paul Anderson, M.D., PH.D.

A central concept of immunology is that autoimmune reactions are injurious to the host. Around 1900, Paul Ehrlich postulated that the immune system acquires a state of tolerance to self-antigens; as a corollary to that, he proposed that the breakdown of tolerance would lead to self-destruction, a condition he described as "horror autotoxicus."[1] Subsequent work by mid–20th-century researchers such as Ray Owen,[2] Macfarlane Burnet,[3] and Peter Medawar[4] established the basic mechanism for the development of immunologic tolerance. In recent years, many important advances have been made in our understanding of tolerance at the molecular and cellular levels. These advances are beginning to transform the clinical management of autoimmune diseases and may lead to therapies that prevent rejection of transplanted organs.

Tolerance

Tolerance is defined as a state of immunologic unresponsiveness to antigens, whether self or foreign. Antigens are recognized by specific receptors expressed on the surface of T cells and B cells. Binding of an antigen to the receptor can either activate or inhibit these immune effector cells. The molecular and cellular factors that determine whether receptor ligation induces immunity or tolerance are beginning to be unraveled.

MECHANISMS OF TOLERANCE

Tolerance results from one of three inhibitory influences on T and B cells: (1) clonal deletion, in which antigenic recognition leads to the activation-induced death of specific lymphocytes; (2) clonal anergy, in which lymphocytes are not killed but are rendered unresponsive to the recognized antigen; and (3) T cell–mediated suppression, in which regulatory T cells actively inhibit an immune response to an antigen. Several factors help determine which of those responses will occur.

Immature lymphocytes are more susceptible to induction of tolerance than are mature lymphocytes. Tolerance can be induced in immature lymphocytes either centrally or in the periphery. Central tolerance is acquired when immature lymphocytes encounter antigens in the organs that generate these cells: the thymus (T cells) and the bone marrow (B cells).

T cells recognize antigens that have been processed into peptides and presented in a complex with major histocompatibility complex (MHC) molecules (self-MHC–peptide complexes). Consequently, immature T cells must be screened for their ability to recognize self-MHC. This screening takes place in the thymus gland. T cells bearing receptors that recognize self-MHC are subjected to the processes of positive and negative selection [see Figure 1].[5] Positive selection occurs when T cells bearing receptors with a moderate affinity for self-MHC–peptide complexes receive survival and maturation signals after receptor ligation. Once these cells mature, they are exported to the periphery. Negative selection occurs when T cells bearing receptors with a high affinity for self-MHC–peptide complexes undergo activation-induced death. The thymus gland is capable of presenting many self-antigens that are normally expressed outside of the thymus or during restricted developmental stages.[6,7] This

allows the elimination of most T cells bearing high-affinity receptors for self-MHC–peptide complexes and plays a major role in preventing autoimmunity in peripheral organs. The promiscuous expression of peripheral antigens in thymic epithelial cells is regulated by the autoimmune regulator (AIRE). This transcriptional modulator is mutated in persons with autoimmune polyglandular syndrome type 1 (APS-1), which is characterized by mucocutaneous candidiasis in association with autoimmune tissue damage that variably targets the parathyroid, adrenal glands, ovaries, and other tissues.[6-8] The severity of this syndrome highlights the critical importance of central tolerance to immune homeostasis.

Because positive selection allows the maturation of T cells bearing receptors capable of low-affinity interactions with self-MHC–peptide complexes, potentially self-reactive T cells are normally found in peripheral lymphoid organs. Peripheral tolerance prevents these cells from inducing autoimmune disease.

Peripheral tolerance is achieved in one of three ways.[9] Perhaps the most common mechanism is the failure of T cells bearing low-affinity receptors to recognize self-antigen in the periphery. In this situation, the potentially self-reactive T cell is not activated and remains functionally naive. These cells are functional, however, as is shown by the fact that they can be activated by immunization with self-antigen delivered in the presence of immune adjuvants (e.g., complete Freund adjuvant, which contains microbial products that strongly activate the immune system at many levels). Failure to respond to self-antigen may simply re-

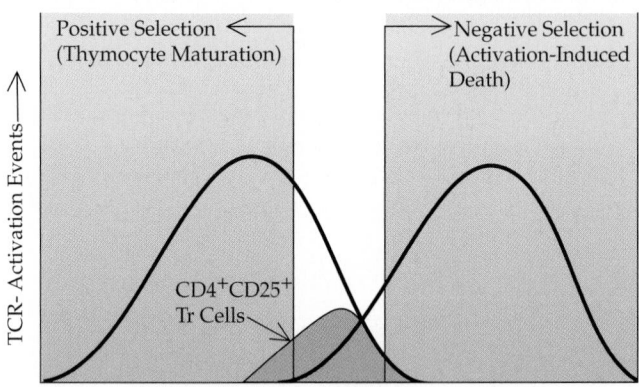

Figure 1 **In the thymus, tolerance is induced through positive and negative selection of immature T cells. The fate of a particular T cell depends on the affinity of its receptor (TCR) for complexes of major histocompatibility complex (MHC) and self-peptides. After ligation, T cells whose receptors have low affinity for self-MCH–peptide complexes receive survival and maturation signals and are exported to the periphery (positive selection); T cells with high affinity undergo activation-induced death (negative selection).**

CD4[+] regulatory T cells (Tr) that express CD25 have intermediate affinity for self-MCH–peptide complexes. This subpopulation of T cells matures in the thymus gland; suppression of their activation takes place in the periphery.

flect a receptor-binding affinity that is below the threshold for T cell activation.

T cells bearing receptors with high affinity for a self-antigen can also remain in an unactivated state if that self-antigen is sequestered from immune effector cells. An example of an antigen that is sequestered from the immune system is myelin basic protein. Because T cells do not normally circulate through the central nervous system, potentially self-reactive cells can persist in an unactivated state in the periphery. Similarly, pancreatic islet cells are normally sequestered from the immune system. In transgenic mice, recombinant proteins expressed on pancreatic islet cells are ignored by high-affinity T cells specific for the recombinant protein. This appears to result from the failure of naive T cells to contact islet cells in the absence of inflammation. In contrast, T cells do become activated in an antigen-specific manner in transgenic mice that express the same recombinant protein in hepatocytes. It therefore appears that circulating lymphocytes contact different tissues in different ways.

A second mechanism of peripheral tolerance involves the elimination of self-reactive T cells by apoptosis. This process is analogous to clonal deletion in the thymus (i.e., negative selection). An example of peripheral deletion is the ability of superantigens (bacterial proteins that bridge selected T cell receptors and selected MHC molecules in an antigen-nonspecific manner) to induce the activation and subsequent death of T cells[10] [see Chapter 124]. Whether peripheral deletion plays an important role in tolerance to self-antigens is not known, however.

A third mechanism of peripheral tolerance involves the acquisition of anergy after ligation of the T cell receptor complex.[11] This antigen-nonresponsive state can be induced in several distinct ways. The most extensively characterized mechanism of anergy induction occurs when the T cell receptor is ligated in the absence of costimulation. In the classic studies of Schwartz and colleagues, T cell clones that were activated by MHC-peptide complexes incorporated into artificial lipid bilayers were rendered nonresponsive to subsequent challenge with peptide-pulsed antigen-presenting cells (APCs).[12] It was subsequently shown that once a T cell has bound with an antigen, the cell requires a so-called second signal delivered by one or more costimulatory molecules to be primed for an immune response. T cells express several surface molecules that can transmit this second signal. These costimulatory receptors are engaged by ligands expressed on the surface of APCs. T cells that are activated in the absence of costimulation acquire defects in the transcriptional control pathways for the production of interleukin-2 (IL-2), an important T cell autocrine growth factor.[13] In vitro anergy can often be overcome by supplying exogenous IL-2 to anergic T cells.

Costimulatory signals can be delivered to T cells by soluble factors or cell surface molecules expressed on APCs. The most potent costimulatory signals are delivered when CD28,[14] CD154,[15] or both are ligated on the surface of T cells [see Figure 2]. Blockade of costimulatory signals by monoclonal antibodies or recombinant receptor antagonists confers potent immunosuppression and allows the acceptance of skin, cardiac, and pancreatic allografts in rodents.[16] Simultaneous blockade of the CD28 and CD154 pathways is significantly more immunosuppressive than blockade of a single costimulatory pathway. The ligand for CD154 is CD40, a protein expressed on the surface of activated B cells, dendritic cells, and macrophages.[15] The ligands for CD28 (B7-1, B7-2, and related proteins[14]) are expressed on the surface of APCs, such as dendritic cells, monocytes, and B cells. Their

expression is induced when APCs are activated in the course of microbial infection. This property heightens the immune response in the setting of perceived danger (i.e., microbial infection). B7-1 and B7-2 have overlapping immunostimulatory roles: mice lacking either protein are only partially deficient in generating an immune response to foreign antigen.[14] Additional costimulatory molecules that are involved in fine tuning the immune response include B7 homologues expressed on APCs (e.g., B7-H1, B7-H2, B7-H3, and B7-DC) that bind to ligands expressed on T cells (ICOS, PD-1, and possibly others).[14]

Ligation of CD28 induces the expression of CTLA-4 (cytotoxic T lymphocyte–associated protein 4), a structurally related protein that turns off activated T cells.[17,18] By this mechanism, the activated T cell initiates a program that will ensure its elimination at the conclusion of the immune response. Compared with CD28, CTLA-4 has a higher affinity for B7-1 and B7-2.[14] The importance of the negative regulatory influence of CTLA-4 is dramatically observed in CTLA-4–null mice. These animals develop a fatal lymphoproliferative syndrome from the uncontrolled activation of self-reactive T cells.[19]

Given the central importance of CD28-B7 interactions in T cell activation and the ability of costimulatory blockade to prevent allograft rejection, it might seem paradoxical that NOD mice (a strain that develops spontaneous diabetes) lacking either CD28 alone or both B7-1 and B7-2 have more severe diabetes.[20] The reason for this appears to be that CD28-B7 interactions are required for the maturation of self-reactive regulatory T cells (Tregs). Tregs, which are generated within the thymus gland, form a distinct class of regulatory T cells that play a major role in ensuring tolerance to self-antigens in the periphery. Just as APS-1 provides a clinical demonstration of the importance of central tolerance to normal immune function, the immune dysregulation, polyendrocrinopathy, enteropathy, and X-linked syndrome (IPEX) dramatically demonstrates the importance of Tregs in the maintenance of self-tolerance.[21] IPEX patients have mutations in the FOXP3 transcription factor that is essential for the maturation and function of Tregs. These patients exhibit hyperactivation of T cells that are reactive with self-antigens, resulting in polyendocrinopathy, inflammatory bowel disease, and allergy.

In rodents, FOXP3-dependent Tregs comprise a subset of peripheral blood CD4+ T cells that express CD25, a subunit of the IL-2 receptor.[22] The selective removal of CD4+ and CD25+ T cells from BALB/c mice results in the development of T cell–mediated autoimmune thyroiditis, gastritis, and diabetes. The CD4+ and CD25+ Treg cells that mature in the thymus gland bear receptors that have an intermediate affinity for self-MHC–peptide complexes [see Figure 1]. In the periphery, antigen exposure confers the ability to suppress the activation of CD4+ and CD25+ T cells in an antigen-independent, cell contact–dependent manner. Although these cells secrete IL-10, a potent anti-inflammatory cytokine, their suppressive activity is cytokine independent. CD4+ and CD25+ T cells can suppress graft versus host disease in allotransplants, and they can prevent autoimmune disease in several different animal models. Consequently, these cells probably play an essential role in maintaining peripheral tolerance to self-antigens.

Although T cells play a dominant role in the maintenance of immune tolerance, non–T cells are also important in this process. Natural killer T (NKT) cells are specialized effectors of innate immunity that are activated by endogenous or microbe-derived lipids bound to CD1.[23] Activated NKT cells express large amounts of interferon gamma and IL-4, allowing them to have profound effects on the immune response. Results of investigations in animal models have implicated NKT cells in the suppression of autoimmune disease.[24] Several autoimmune mouse strains (e.g., NOD, MRL-lpr/lpr, and SJL/J) have reduced the numbers of NKT cells as compared with nonautoimmune strains. In these models, adoptive transfer of NKT cells can ameliorate disease. Moreover, activation of NKT cells by the natural product α-galactosylceramide prevents autoimmune disease in several murine models. Although the role of NKT cells in human autoimmune disease remains to be determined, these results show that components of the innate immune response can have profound effects on discrimination of self from nonself.

Autoimmunity

Despite the multiple and redundant mechanisms that exist to ensure immunologic tolerance to self, autoimmune phenomena are relatively common. In some cases, autoimmune responses accompany a normal immune response to a microbial pathogen. Thus, the appearance of rheumatoid factor (anti-immunoglobulin antibodies) in the serum of patients with bacterial endocarditis is relatively common. In general, these autoantibodies are not pathogenic. The appearance of these antibodies probably results from antigen-nonspecific activation of T cells and B cells bearing low-affinity receptors for self-antigens that are normally held in check by mechanisms of peripheral tolerance. The ability of bacterial products (e.g., lipopolysaccharide) to function as immune adjuvants appears to overcome these repressive influences.

MOLECULAR MIMICRY

Clinical observations have established a link between certain microbial infections and specific autoimmune syndromes. Examples include streptococcal infection and rheumatic fever, *Borrelia burgdorferi* infection and Lyme arthritis, *Trypanosoma cruzi* infection and Chagas disease, and B4 coxsackievirus infection and type 1 diabetes mellitus.[25] These associations suggest that the immune response to a specific microbial peptide may be redirected toward a similar self-peptide, a phenomenon known as molecular mimicry. Although this is an appealing hypothesis, definitive evidence for molecular mimicry has yet to be demonstrated in any of these diseases. The strongest evidence, to date, for molecular mimicry comes from the molecular analysis of the immune response to the tick-borne spirochete *B. burgdorferi*. About 10% of infected patients develop persistent synovitis, despite the eradication of the spirochete by antibiotic therapy.[26] Most patients with treatment-resistant Lyme arthritis have the HLA-DRB1*04041 or HLA-DRB1*0101 major histocompatibility alleles, implicating antigen presentation in disease pathogenesis. These same HLA alleles confer an increased relative risk for rheumatoid arthritis and, perhaps, for synovial disease in general. Treatment-resistant Lyme arthritis is associated with a cellular and humoral immune response to the *B. burgdorferi* outersurface protein OspA, and a computer algorithm predicted that an immunodominant OspA epitope (OspA165-173) should bind to HLA-DRB1*0401. This prediction was confirmed experimentally, and indeed, most patients with treatment-resistant Lyme arthritis have T cells that recognize this immunodominant epitope. The computer algorithm also predicted that a peptide epitope encoded by leukocyte function–associated antigen–1α (LFA-1α) would bind to HLA-DRB1*0401. This binding was

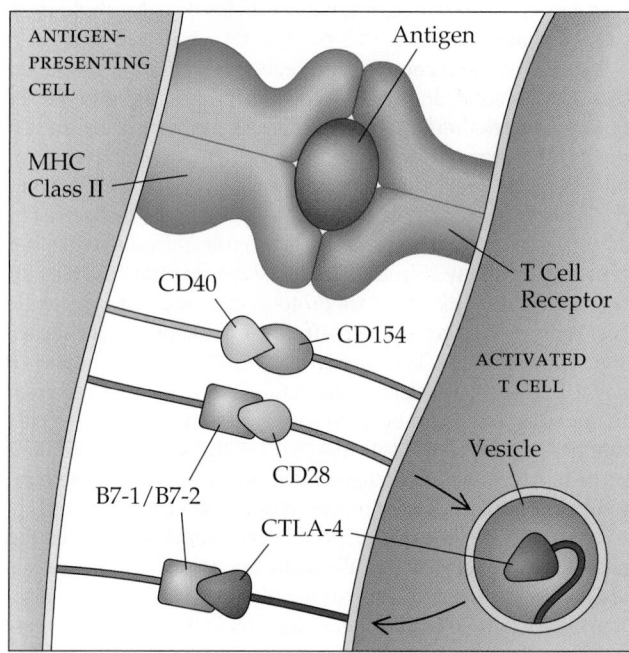

Figure 2   **Activation of T cells begins when the T cell receptor binds with a complex of an MHC molecule and a peptide expressed on the surface of an antigen-presenting cell (APC). Activation is completed by a second signal generated by the ligation of costimulatory molecules expressed on the cell surface of the APC. B7-1/B7-2 interacts with CD28 on the T cell, and CD40 interacts with CD154.**

In unactivated T cells, CTLA-4 (a relative of CD28) is a component of intracellular vesicles. After CD28 ligation, CTLA-4 moves to the cell surface and binds with B7-1/B7-2, generating negative signals that turn off the immune response.

confirmed experimentally, and most patients with treatment-resistant Lyme arthritis have T cells that weakly respond to the LFA-1α peptide epitope. The LFA-1α peptide does not bind to HLA-DRB1*0101, however, indicating that this mechanism cannot explain all cases of treatment-resistant Lyme arthritis. Moreover, it remains to be proved that T cells reactive with LFA-1α are necessary and sufficient for the onset of treatment-resistant Lyme arthritis.[27]

IDENTIFICATION OF AUTOANTIGENS

A common feature of autoimmune diseases is the appearance of autoantibodies in the serum. In some cases, these autoantibodies are directly pathogenic: the clinical syndrome is produced when the antibody binds to its target antigen. The molecular pathogenesis of these autoimmune conditions can be determined with some precision. Unfortunately, the molecular defects that allow the bypass of tolerance to the disease-inducing autoantigen are less well understood.

Pathogenic Autoantibodies

Myasthenia gravis   Nearly all patients with myasthenia gravis have autoantibodies to acetylcholine receptors (ACRs) on skeletal muscle [*see Chapter 182*]. However, the degree of neuromuscular blockade seen in this disease does not always parallel the serum levels of anti-ACR antibodies. The antibodies are polyclonal and bind to several distinct epitopes on the ACR. Although these antibodies can directly inhibit ACR function, they can also promote the endocytosis and accelerated degradation of the ACR or activate complement-mediated destruction of the postsynaptic surface.[28] The supposition that these anti-ACR antibodies have direct pathogenic effects is supported by the fact that injection of ACR antibodies can induce myasthenic weakness in animals and that plasmapheresis is an effective treatment in some patients. Some patients with myasthenia gravis have a coincident thymoma, and thymectomy can be an effective treatment in such patients, suggesting that defects in thymic selection of maturing T cells may play a role in the autoimmune response to the ACR. This could involve impaired negative selection of CD4+ helper T cells reactive with ACR-derived peptides or impaired generation of Tregs specific for ACR-derived peptide epitopes.

Pemphigus Pemphigus vulgaris and bullous pemphigoid are autoimmune skin diseases characterized by the presence of serum autoantibodies that react with adhesion molecules found at the dermoepidermal basement membrane zone [*see Chapter 43*]. In pemphigus vulgaris, a common target antigen is desmoglein 3, a desmosomal adhesion molecule. In bullous pemphigoid, common target antigens are two major hemidesmosomal proteins of 180 kd and 230 kd. Several lines of evidence have implicated autoantibodies targeting these proteins in the pathogenesis of pemphigus. First, autoantibodies are consistently present in patients with pemphigus, levels of those antibodies correlate with disease activity, and the removal of the antibodies by plasmapheresis results in improvement of symptoms. Second, serum from patients with pemphigus vulgaris causes pemphigus-like lesions in mice. Third, newborns of mothers with pemphigus have transient disease resulting from transplacental transmission of maternal antibody.

Autoimmune endocrinopathies Autoantibodies reactive with hormone receptors can contribute to endocrine disorders. High levels of antibody reactive with the peripheral insulin receptor can result in insulin-dependent diabetes mellitus. Paradoxically, low levels of antibody may stimulate the insulin receptor by mimicking insulin, resulting in hypoglycemia.

Autoimmune disease of the thyroid is associated with antibodies directed toward three antigens: microsomal thyroid peroxidase, thyroglobulin, and the thyroid receptor for thyroid-stimulating hormone (TSH). Antibodies to the TSH receptor may mimic the action of TSH, thereby resulting in Graves disease [*see Chapter 50*]. Another apparent autoimmune disease of the thyroid, Hashimoto thyroiditis, is associated with antibodies to the TSH receptor, but the pathogenic role of the antibodies in this disease is unclear. Less commonly, antibodies to the TSH receptor may block the action of TSH and cause hypothyroidism. A pathogenic role for the other two classes of antithyroid autoantibodies has not been established.

Antiphospholipid syndrome The antiphospholipid syndrome (APS) consists of recurrent thrombosis, fetal loss, and thrombocytopenia in association with antibodies to cardiolipin or other negatively charged phospholipids, along with abnormalities of certain clotting tests caused by an inhibitor referred to as the lupus anticoagulant [*see Chapter 99*]. APS can be primary or secondary; secondary APS is usually associated with systemic lupus erythematosus (SLE) or its variants. The antiphospholipid antibodies do not bind to phospholipids alone but to a complex of phospholipids and the plasma proteins β_2-glycoprotein I and prothrombin. These antibodies induce the expression of adhesion molecules on endothelial cells that promote the binding of monocytes and platelets as the first step in a thrombotic cascade.

Nonpathogenic Autoantibodies

Autoantibodies reactive with intracellular targets can serve as markers of specific autoimmune diseases. For example, antibodies reactive with citrullinated peptides are specific markers of rheumatoid arthritis, antibodies reactive with the mitochondrial enzyme 2-oxo acid dehydrogenase are specific markers of primary biliary cirrhosis, and antibodies reactive with the Smith small nuclear ribonucleoprotein (snRNP) complex are specific markers of SLE. Although these autoantibodies are unlikely to be pathogenic, their presence is highly correlated with specific autoimmune diseases. An understanding of the process that promotes the disease-specific bypass of tolerance to a selected antigen is likely to shed light on the pathogenic mechanism underlying individual autoimmune syndromes. An important insight into the mechanism by which tolerance is abrogated in an antigen-specific manner came with the realization that the targets of many autoantibodies found in the serum of patients with autoimmune disease are proteins that are modified in cells undergoing apoptotic cell death.[29] During apoptosis, myriad intracellular proteins, nucleic acids, and lipids are subjected to enzymatic and nonenzymatic modification. These modifications include protease cleavage, phosphorylation, transglutamination, ubiquitination, citrullination, and isoaspartylation.[30] It has been proposed that these modifications create neo-epitopes to which the immune system has not been tolerized.

Although proteins that are modified during apoptosis are preferred targets of the autoantibodies found in the serum of patients with autoimmune disease, it is clear that apoptosis per se is not sufficient to break tolerance to these self proteins. Apoptosis is a ubiquitous process, yet most persons do not develop autoimmune disease. Apparently, the necessary additional element is delay in the execution of the apoptotic program or the clearance of the apoptotic cell. This phenomenon has been demonstrated in mice that lack the first component of complement. C1q functions as an opsonin that binds to apoptotic cells and promotes their clearance by professional phagocytes (neutrophils and macrophages). In the absence of C1q, the clearance of apoptotic corpses is delayed. Delayed clearance of apoptotic cells somehow increases their immunogenicity.[31]

A similar phenomenon occurs when the execution of the apoptotic program is delayed. For example, influenza virus–induced apoptosis in macrophages has been shown to increase the immunogenicity of viral proteins.[32] This phenomenon requires the phagocytosis of infected macrophages by dendritic cells. By a process of cross-priming, the dendritic cell can then present antigens derived from the infected macrophage in a highly efficient manner. Because influenza virus encodes several genes that function to inhibit apoptosis (e.g., *NS1*), virus-induced apoptosis requires many hours to complete. During this delay, the virus replicates within the infected cell, and the virus-infected cell expresses stress-response proteins (heat shock proteins [HSPs]), including HSP70 and HSP90. These HSPs function as natural adjuvants that can deliver peptides to class I MHC molecules expressed by APCs.[33] The generation of modified peptides and the induction of HSPs may account for the increased immunogenicity of apoptotic cells and the generation of autoantibodies reactive with proteins that are modified during apoptotic cell death.

In this model, the autoantibodies that serve as markers of specific autoimmune diseases are generated when the target cell undergoes delayed or aberrant apoptosis. This implies that the primary insult to the target tissue is produced by a stimulus that induces aberrant cell death and modification of the specific autoantigen. Such a process may be initiated by specific environmental factors (e.g., viruses, toxins, or ultraviolet radiation).

The autoantibodies that directly and indirectly contribute to the pathogenesis of autoimmune disease are produced by differentiated B cells. A reduced activation threshold for B cells has been implicated in the pathogenesis of SLE.[34] Moreover, increased activation of B cells may contribute to the predisposition to lymphoma observed in some autoimmune diseases.[34] Finally, preliminary results suggesting therapeutic efficacy of B cell–depleting monoclonal antibodies in patients with rheumatoid arthritis and SLE indicate that B cells play an important role in the pathogenesis of autoimmune disease.[35,36]

GENETICS OF AUTOIMMUNITY

Systemic autoimmunity is a multigenic trait that is significantly influenced by environmental factors. For example, the concordance rate for SLE in monozygotic twins is only 30%, indicating that both genetic and environmental factors contribute to disease onset. The specific genes that promote autoimmunity can be identified in two ways. Most of the genes currently known to promote autoimmunity have been discovered using case-control association methodologies.[37] These studies have linked the expression of specific HLA haplotypes to specific autoimmune diseases. In a similar fashion, case-control studies have linked defects in both classical pathway complement components (C1q, C2, and C4) and Fc receptor alleles to the development of SLE. In families in which two or more members have SLE, genetic linkage analysis has been applied in an attempt to identify disease-susceptibility loci. These studies have identified several chromosomal loci with significant linkage to human SLE.[37] It is likely that future studies will identify a cohort of genes that, alone or in combination, contribute to the autoimmune diathesis.

Studies of transgenic mice that either lack or overexpress specific genes have identified three groups of genes that encode distinct classes of proteins that modify susceptibility to autoimmune disease. Absence of these genes results in autoimmunity. The first group of genes encode proteins involved in the initiation or execution of apoptotic cell death. These proteins include dedicated death receptors and their ligands. Specific members of this family (e.g., Fas and tumor necrosis factor type I [TNF RI]) are required for the clonal elimination of activated T cells after an immune response to microbial infection. Mice lacking either Fas or its ligand develop lymphadenopathy and splenomegaly from the accumulation of previously activated T cells. In some strains of transgenic mice (e.g., MRL), but not in others (e.g., BALB/c), failure to eliminate activated T cells results in an autoimmune disease that resembles SLE. Thus, the absence of Fas or Fas ligand (FasL) promotes the phenotypic expression of an autoimmune diathesis that is intrinsic to the MRL strain (a genetic phenomenon known as epistasis). Although defects in Fas or FasL are not linked to autoimmunity in patients with SLE, mutations in either Fas or FasL produce the autoimmune lymphoproliferative syndrome (ALPS), an autosomal dominant condition characterized by lymphadenopathy, splenomegaly, and autoantibody production.[38] ALPS is also caused by mutations in caspase-10, a component of the effector arm of the apop-

totic death program. Thus, ALPS is an autoimmune disease that results from defective execution of an apoptotic program in activated T cells. The importance of the apoptotic program in determining susceptibility to autoimmune disease is further demonstrated by the autoimmune syndromes observed in mice lacking BIM, a pro-apoptotic protein, or overexpressing BCL-2, an anti-apoptotic protein.

The second group of genes encode proteins involved in the recognition, clearance, or elimination of apoptotic cells. These include proteins that serve as opsonins to promote the phagocytosis of apoptotic cells (e.g., C1q, IgM, SAP/CRP), as well as phagocyte receptors that promote the recognition and ingestion of apoptotic cells (e.g., Mer).

The third group of genes encode proteins that set the threshold for lymphocyte activation. Increased activation of T cells or B cells is likely to disrupt normal mechanisms of tolerance, resulting in autoimmunity. Examples include costimulatory lymphocyte surface molecules (e.g., CD22, PD-1), kinases and phosphatases involved in lymphocyte activation (e.g., Lyn, Cbl-b), and transcription factors (e.g., Foxo3a) that promote lymphocyte activation. These animal studies reveal that genes involved in the regulation of apoptosis or lymphocyte activation are proven modifiers of autoimmune disease in mice and are candidates for the modulation of autoimmunity in humans.

Genome-wide linkage mapping has identified mutations in NOD2 as an etiologic factor in familial Crohn disease, an autoimmune inflammatory process that targets the intestinal mucosa.[39] NOD2 is a cytosolic protein that recognizes muramyl dipeptide (MDP), a metabolite of bacterial peptidoglycan.[40] Recognition of MDP promotes the oligomerization of NOD2, which results in activation of NF-κB and caspase-1—signaling events that lead to the secretion of inflammatory cytokines. Selected patients with Crohn disease possess mutant NOD2 that is unable to promote MDP-mediated activation of NF-κB. The mechanism by which ineffective recognition of bacterial products leads to intestinal inflammation remains to be determined.

ORGAN-SPECIFIC VERSUS SYSTEMIC AUTOIMMUNITY

For many years, organ-specific immunity was thought to result from the activation of lymphocytes bearing receptors specific for a tissue-restricted antigen. In rare cases of molecular mimicry, this may be the case. However, it now appears that the target of an autoimmune attack can shift from one tissue to another in response to defined or undefined genetic modifiers. For example, persons with APS-1 develop various combinations of autoimmune thyroiditis, parathyroid disease, and type 1 diabetes mellitus.[41] Although the factors that determine which tissues become targets of autoimmune attack have not been identified, the fact that different tissues are affected in different persons suggests that unique, tissue-specific autoantigens may not be the primary triggers of disease.

The concept that organ-specific autoimmunity need not be driven by a tissue-specific autoantigen is supported by observations made in two different animal models of autoimmunity. In NOD mice whose MHC locus is replaced with that of another strain, autoimmune thyroiditis develops instead of diabetes.[20] This result suggests that the NOD strain harbors an autoimmune diathesis that can manifest itself as different types of organ-specific autoimmunity. In support of this concept, NOD mice lacking the costimulatory molecule B7-2 develop autoimmune peripheral neuropathy, rather than diabetes.[20] Although the mechanism by which individual tissues are selected for immune attack is not known, these results strongly suggest that factors other than tissue-restricted autoantigens can be the primary determinant of organ-specific autoimmune disease.

Another instructive example of organ-specific autoimmunity that arises in the absence of a defined, tissue-restricted autoantigenic trigger is the inflammatory arthritis that develops in the F1 progeny of K/B×NOD mice.[42] The K/B strain expresses a transgenic T cell receptor that recognizes a self-peptide derived from glucose-6-phosphate isomerase (GPI) presented in the context of Ag7, a class II MHC molecule from the NOD strain. In K/B×NOD mice, T cells bearing the transgene provide help for B cells encoding immunoglobulins that bind to GPI. GPI is an enzyme expressed in all cells, yet anti-GPI antibodies somehow provoke a symmetrical, inflammatory arthritis involving diarthrodial joints in these mice. Although the mechanism by which anti-GPI antibodies provoke arthritis is not fully understood, this model illustrates the potential for an immune response that is directed at a ubiquitous antigen to trigger organ-specific autoimmunity.

One way in which organ-specific autoimmunity can be induced in the absence of a tissue-specific autoantigen is by the pathologic overexpression of inflammatory cytokines. Thus, overexpression of tumor necrosis factor–α (TNF-α) in transgenic mice is sufficient to induce a symmetrical polyarthritis that resembles rheumatoid arthritis.[43] This appears to result from the ability of TNF-α to initiate an inflammatory cytokine cascade within the cells that make up the synovium. The importance of TNF-α in the pathogenesis of rheumatoid arthritis has been dramatically validated by the clinical efficacy of TNF blockers such as infliximab and etanercept[44] [see Chapter 112]. In an analogous fashion, BAFF/Blys, a TNF-α–related protein that promotes the survival and differentiation of B cells, has been proposed to participate in the induction of SLE-like autoimmune syndromes.[45,46] Transgenic mice engineered to overexpress BAFF/Blys develop hypergammaglobulinemia and autoimmune symptoms because of the survival of autoreactive B cells that would normally be deleted from the B cell repertoire. These observations suggest that neutralization of TNF family members may play an important role in the treatment of selected autoimmune diseases.

The author has no commercial relationships with manufacturers of products or providers of services discussed in this chapter.

References

1. Ehrlich P, Morgenroth J: On haemolysis: third communication. Berlin Klin Wochenschr 37:453, 1900
2. Owen R: Immunogenetic consequences of vascular anastomosis between bovine twins. Science 102:400, 1945
3. Burnet F: Clonal selection theory: a modification of Jerne's theory of antibody production using the concept of clonal selection. Aust J Sci 20:67, 1957
4. Billingham R, Brent L, Medawar P: Actively acquired tolerance of foreign cells. Nature 172:603, 1953
5. Nossal GJ: Negative selection of lymphocytes. Cell 76:229, 1994
6. Kyewski B, Derbinski J: Self-representation in the thymus: an extended view. Nat Rev Immunol 4:688, 2004
7. Mathis D, Benoist C: Back to central tolerance. Immunity 20:509, 2004
8. Peterson P, Pitkanen J, Sillanpaa N, et al: Autoimmune polyendocrinopathy candidiasis ectodermal dystrophy (APECED): a model disease to study molecular aspects of endocrine autoimmunity. Clin Exp Immunol 135:348, 2004
9. Fazekas de St. Groth B: DCs and peripheral T cell tolerance. Semin Immunol 13:311, 2001
10. Sundberg E, Li Y, Mariuzza R: So many ways of getting in the way: diversity in the molecular architecture of superantigen-dependent T-cell signaling complexes. Curr Opin Immunol 14:36, 2002
11. Macian F, Im S, Garcia-Cozar F, et al: T-cell anergy. Curr Opin Immunol 16:209, 2004
12. Quill H, Schwartz R: Stimulation of normal inducer T cell clones with antigen presented by purified Ia molecules in planar lipid membranes. J Immunol 138:3704, 1987
13. Nelson BH: IL-2, regulatory T cells, and tolerance. J Immunol 172:3983, 2004
14. Sharpe AH, Freeman GJ: The B7-CD28 superfamily. Nat Rev Immunol 2:116, 2002
15. Quezada SA, Jarvinen LZ, Lind EF, et al: CD40/CD154 interactions at the interface of tolerance and immunity. Annu Rev Immunol 22:307, 2004
16. Sun Y, Subudhi SK, Fu YX: Co-stimulation agonists as a new immunotherapy for autoimmune diseases. Trends Mol Med 9:483, 2003
17. Chikuma S, Bluestone JA: CTLA-4 and tolerance: the biochemical point of view. Immunol Res 28:241, 2003
18. Greenwald RJ, Latchman YE, Sharpe AH: Negative co-receptors on lymphocytes. Curr Opin Immunol 14:391, 2002
19. Tivol E, Borriello F, Schweitzer A, et al: Loss of CTLA-4 leads to massive lymphoproliferation and fatal multiorgan tissue destruction, revealing a critical negative regulatory role of CTLA-4. Immunity 3:541, 1995
20. Lesage S, Goodnow C: Organ-specific autoimmune disease: a deficiency of tolerogenic stimulation. J Exp Med 194:F31, 2001
21. Torgerson T, Ochs H: Immune dysregulation, polyendocrinopathy, enteropathy, X-linked syndrome and immune dysregulation. Curr Opin Immunol 2:481, 2002
22. Sakaguchi S: Naturally arising CD4+ regulatory T cells for immunologic self-tolerance and negative control of immune responses. Annu Rev Immunol 22:531, 2004
23. Brigl M, Brenner MB: CD1: antigen presentation and T cell function. Annu Rev Immunol 22:817, 2004
24. Van Kaer L: α-Galactosylceramide therapy for autoimmune diseases: prospects and obstacles. Nat Rev Immunol 5:31, 2004
25. Rose N, Mackay I: Molecular mimicry: a critical look at exemplary instances in human diseases. Cell Mol Life Sci 57:542, 2000
26. Steere AC, Glickstein L: Elucidation of Lyme arthritis. Nat Rev Immunol 4:143, 2004
27. Benoist C, Mathis D: Autoimmunity provoked by infection: How good is the case for T cell epitope mimicry? Nature Immunol 2:797, 2001
28. Hughes BW, Moro De Casillas ML, Kaminski HJ: Pathophysiology of myasthenia gravis. Semin Neurol 24:21, 2004
29. Hall JC, Casciola-Rosen L, Rosen A: Altered structure of autoantigens during apoptosis. Rheum Dis Clin North Am 30:455, 2004
30. Utz P, Gensler T, Anderson P: Death, autoantigen modifications, and tolerance. Arthritis Res 2:101, 2000
31. Manderson A, Botto M, Walport M: The role of complement in the development of systemic lupus erythematosus. Annu Rev Immunol 22:431, 2004
32. Albert M, Sauter B, Bhardwaj N: Dendritic cells acquire antigen from apoptotic cells and induce class I-restricted CTLs. Nature 392:86, 1998
33. Albert ML: Death-defying immunity: do apoptotic cells influence antigen processing and presentation? Nat Rev Immunol 4:223, 2004
34. Criscione LG, Pisetsky DS: B lymphocytes and systemic lupus erythematosus. Curr Rheumatol Rep 5: 264, 2003
35. Looney RJ, Anolik JH, Campbell D, et al: B cell depletion as a novel treatment for systemic lupus erythematosus: a phase I/II dose-escalation trial of rituzimab. Arthritis Rheum 50:2580, 2004
36. Kotzin BL: The role of B cells in the pathogenesis of rheumatoid arthritis. J Rheumatol Suppl 73:14, 2005
37. Raman K, Mohan C: Genetic underpinnings of autoimmunity—lessons from studies in arthritis, diabetes, lupus and multiple sclerosis. Curr Opin Immunol 15:651, 2003
38. Rieux-Laucat F, Fischer A, Deist FL: Cell-death signaling and human disease. Curr Opin Immunol 15:325, 2003
39. Beutler B: Autoimmunity and apoptosis: the Crohn's connection. Immunity 15:5, 2001
40. Inohara N, Nunez G: NODs: intracellular proteins involved in inflammation and apoptosis. Nat Rev Immunol 3:371, 2003
41. Ruan Q, She J: Autoimmune polyglandular syndrome type 1 and the autoimmune regulator. Clin Lab Med 24:305, 2004
42. Monach PA, Benoist C, Mathis D: The role of antibodies in mouse models of rheumatoid arthritis, and relevance to human disease. Adv Immunol 82:217, 2004
43. Sfikakis P, Kollias G: Tumor necrosis factor biology in experimental and clinical arthritis. Curr Opin Rheumatol 15:380, 2003
44. Vilcek J, Feldmann M: Historical review: cytokines as therapeutics and targets of therapeutics. Trends Pharmacol Sci 25:201, 2004
45. Ramanujam M, Davidson A: The current status of targeting BAFF/BLyS for autoimmune diseases. Arthritis Res Ther 6:197, 2004
46. Cancro M: The BLyS family of ligands and receptors: an archetype for niche-specific regulation. Immunol Rev 202:237, 2004

Acknowledgment

Figure 2 Seward Hung.

104 Allergic Response

Pamela J. Daffern, M.D., and Lawrence B. Schwartz, M.D., PH.D.

Definition of Allergic Response

The word anaphylaxis was coined in 1902 by Charles Richet, in order to contrast the condition with prophylaxis. Richet described anaphylaxis as "the peculiar attribute which certain poisons possess of increasing instead of diminishing the sensitivity of an organism to their action...."[1] One hundred years later, we understand anaphylaxis as the extreme of a spectrum of events mediated by immunoglobulin E (IgE). Persons with IgE-mediated disorders have a genetic propensity to form IgE antibodies against otherwise innocuous environmental antigens (allergens); this propensity is termed atopy (from the Greek *atopos*, meaning "out of place"). In atopic persons, IgE mediates a wide range of reactions, including dermatitis, rhinitis, asthma, urticaria, angioedema, and anaphylaxis.

Confusion arises over the misapplication of the term allergy to describe any untoward reaction to food or medications or to perceived environmental exposures. This confusion is further complicated by the fact that both IgE-mediated and non–IgE-mediated forms of rhinitis, asthma, and atopic dermatitis occur, often in the same person.

In the nonatopic person, exposure to allergen results in immunologic tolerance or neglect, whereas in atopic persons, exposure results in sensitization. On reexposure to the allergen, atopic persons mount an immunologically mediated inflammatory response in the target organ. Other environmental factors—such as tobacco smoke, air pollution, respiratory virus infection, and lack of exposure to certain microbes in childhood—may also promote an allergic inflammatory response.

Epidemiology of Atopic Disorders

Up to 30% of the United States population may be affected by allergic rhinoconjunctivitis, asthma, or atopic dermatitis. This high incidence of atopic disease may reflect societal factors. Fetal development takes place in an intrauterine environment that favors atopic sensitization[2]; the maternal immune system suppresses cell-mediated immune responses in order to prevent rejection of the fetus. Thus, the neonate may enter the world with T cells that are already primed by common environmental and food allergens that have crossed the placenta. It has been proposed that microbial exposure and infections during infancy shift the immune response away from the allergic pattern to a protective immune response.[3] Specifically, after macrophages or dendritic cells ingest microbes, T cells produce cytokines that promote non-IgE responses by B cells. Therefore, the increasing prevalence of atopic disorders in countries that have adopted a Western lifestyle, including overuse of antibiotics, has been attributed to a lack of microbial antigen stimulation.

Humoral and Cellular Mechanisms of Allergic Inflammation Associated with Immediate Hypersensitivity

ANTIGEN-PRESENTING CELLS AND SENSITIZATION

All persons encounter environmental antigens that are capable of inducing an allergic response. Soluble antigens, such as allergens, undergo endocytosis by professional antigen-presenting cells (APCs), which include dendritic cells, such as epidermal Langerhans cells; macrophages; and B cells.[4] However, only dendritic cells and Langerhans cells are able to prime naive T cells and thus are responsible for the sensitization phase.[5,6] Once primary sensitization has been achieved, monocytes and B cells amplify the process. B cells bind allergen through immunoglobulin receptors specific for the allergen, as opposed to nonspecific endocytic pathways used by other APCs. The internalization of antigen results in two processes. The first is general activation of the APC: this includes upregulation of major histocompatibility complex (MHC) and accessory molecules. The second process is fusion of the endocytic vesicle with lysosomes, which results in the formation of specialized antigen-processing vesicles in which antigens are hydrolyzed into protein fragments. The linear peptides that result are incorporated into the antigen-binding groove of a class II human lymphocyte antigen (HLA) molecule during its transport to the cell surface.

In general, APCs will co-express a heterogeneous assortment of allergen-derived peptides and HLA class II molecules on their surface. The efficiency with which processed allergen peptides bind to the HLA class II molecules presumably depends on variations in the HLA loci; these variations are genetically determined. The binding efficiency in turn influences the predisposition of the person to develop allergy to or tolerance of a particular antigen. The APC loaded with processed antigen/HLA class II complexes presents this complex to CD4+,CD8− helper T cells. The genetically determined binding efficiency of an HLA-derived molecule to an antigen also may influence how T cells develop when exposed to that complex.[7] In addition, the quantity of interleukin-12 (IL-12) produced by APCs also influences the type of T cell response.[5]

T CELLS AND MEDIATION OF ALLERGIC INFLAMMATION

The helper T cell response is influenced not only by APCs but also by the age of the person and by the amount, type, duration, and route of allergen exposure.[7,8] Also, the cytokine milieu during lymphocyte differentiation determines the type of effector function of the helper T cell [see Table 1].

For example, bacterial DNA sequences have immunostimulatory regions containing deoxycytidine-phosphate-deoxyguanosine (CpG) repeats. CpG repeats are recognized as foreign by pattern recognition receptors called Toll-like receptor-9 (TLR-9) on APCs.[9,10] These CpG repeats stimulate macrophages and dendritic cells to secrete inflammatory cytokines, including IL-12 and IL-18. These cytokines then induce T cells and natural killer (NK) cells to produce interferon gamma (IFN-γ), a cytokine known to promote nonallergic, protective responses.

Table 1   Cytokines Involved in IgE-Mediated Allergic Inflammation

Cytokine	Source	Function
IL-3	T$_{H2}$ cells,* mast cells, basophils, eosinophils	Promotes granulocyte and macrophage maturation; eosinophil activation and survival
IL-4	T$_{H2}$ cells,* mast cells, basophils	Promotes differentiation of T$_{H0}$ to T$_{H2}$ cells; antagonizes differentiation of T$_{H0}$ to T$_{H1}$ cells; IgE isotype switching
IL-5	T$_{H2}$ cells,* mast cells, eosinophils	Promotes eosinophil development, activation, and survival
IL-13	T$_{H2}$ cells,* mast cells, basophils	IgE isotype switching, eosinophil activation
GM-CSF	T$_{H2}$ cells and activated macrophages,* endothelial and epithelial cells	Promotes granulocyte and macrophage maturation, eosinophil activation, and survival
TNF-α	Monocytes/macrophages,* mast cells	Promotes chemotaxis and activation of leukocytes and vascular endothelium

*Major source.

GM-CSF—granulocyte-macrophage colony-stimulating factor   IL—interleukin   TNF—tumor necrosis factor

This pattern of response by helper T cells is termed a T$_{H1}$ response, because it is associated with differentiation of naive helper T (T$_{H0}$) cells into mature T$_{H1}$ cells. Similarly, the helper T cells of persons without atopy respond to presentation of potentially allergenic peptides by ignoring them or by producing IFN-γ and directing the production of allergen-specific IgG1 and IgG4 antibodies.[11]

In contrast, helper T cells of atopic persons respond to processed aeroallergens by forming IL-4, IL-5, and IL-13 and by directing the production of allergen-specific IgE antibodies. This type of helper T cell response is termed a T$_{H2}$ response. IL-4 and IL-13 share a number of functions, because both cytokines signal through the IL-4Rα/IL-13Rα heterodimer.[12] However, only IL-4 is able to induce the differentiation of T$_{H0}$ cells to T$_{H2}$ cells and to antagonize the differentiation of T$_{H0}$ cells to T$_{H1}$ cells, resulting in IgE-mediated allergic inflammation. In contrast, both IL-12 and IFN-γ induce the differentiation to T$_{H1}$ cells; T$_{H2}$ cell differentiation is inhibited by IFN-γ. Differentiation to T$_{H1}$ cells results in cell-mediated immunity and inflammation.[13] Therefore, the differentiation of T$_{H0}$ cells to either T$_{H1}$ cells or T$_{H2}$ cells appears to be the crucial event that determines which type of immune response will follow.

GENETICS AND THE DEVELOPMENT OF ATOPY

Research has begun to identify specific genetic variants that contribute to the development of the atopic state. For example, a mutation of the IL-12R beta$_2$-chain gene has recently been shown to impair signaling through IL-12. Because IL-12 is a potent inducer of IFN-γ production and because IFN-γ downregulates IgE production (see above), this mutation results in increased IgE production in atopic persons.[14] Polymorphisms in the gene for STAT-6, a transcription factor selectively regulated by IL-4 and IL-13 (cytokines that upregulate IgE production), have also been described.[15] These genetic variations in STAT-6 also appear to be associated with a predisposition to atopy. Finally, an asthma gene (ADAM-33) associated with bronchial hyperresponsiveness but not atopy was recently defined by genetic-linkage analysis of affected sibling pairs. The ADAM-33 gene product, a membrane metalloprotease, may function to modulate the response to cytokines in the lung by solubilizing cytokine membrane receptors, but its precise role still needs to be determined.[16] Like other allergies, however, asthma involves environmental factors. For example, the predisposition to asthma is modified by the presence of allergens and endotoxins.[17]

IgE SYNTHESIS

Once allergen is processed by APCs and presented to T$_{H2}$ cells, a specific sequence of events must follow for IgE production by B cells to occur [*see Figure 1*]. The switch from IgM or IgG production to IgE production by B cells occurs in the genome and requires two signals.[18] The first signal is delivered through the IL-4Rα chain by either IL-4 or IL-13.[12] Signaling through these cytokine receptors initiates transcription from the germline promoter site of the constant portion of the heavy chain of IgE. The IgE heavy-chain gene is located downstream of the IgG and IgM heavy-chain genes and replaces IgG or IgM on the immunoglobulin molecule. The second signal is delivered through activation of the cluster differentiation 40 (CD40) receptor on B cells.[19] Signaling through CD40 activates the recombinases necessary to remove the upstream IgG or IgM heavy-chain constant region and replace it with the corresponding region of IgE. This process switches the type of antibody being produced without altering its antigenic specificity. Stimulation of B cells through CD40 also stimulates growth, differentiation, and survival of these cells.[20]

The ligand for CD40 (CD154, CD40L) is expressed not only on T cells but also on mast cells and basophils. Importantly, all of these cells also secrete IL-4, IL-13, or both, and therefore could potentially play a role in directing B cell production of IgE. However, it seems likely that T cells are responsible for initiating the switch to antigen-specific IgE production. Mast cells and basophils may then amplify deviation of immune responses toward IgE production after the primary IgE sensitization has occurred.[19] It seems likely that binding to CD40 on B cells by mast cells and basophils would enhance polyclonal (i.e., not antigen-dependent or specific) IgE production by B cells, because mast cells and basophils are not dedicated APCs. IgE antibody secreted by B cells circulates briefly, having a serum half-life of 2 to 3 days, before binding to IgE receptors.

IgE RECEPTORS AND REGULATION OF IgE

Receptors for IgE (FcϵR) are expressed on various cells.[21] The high-affinity receptor for IgE, FcϵRI, has two forms that differ by the presence or absence of a beta chain. The beta chain is present in the high-affinity receptor found on mast cells and basophils.[19] The presence of the beta chain amplifies the cellular signaling that occurs when IgE bound to FcϵRI is cross-linked by allergen. Its presence also increases the amount of IgE receptor on the surfaces of mast cells and basophils by up to sixfold.[22]

Levels of FcεRI on the surface of basophils have been shown to correlate with serum IgE levels in various IgE-associated diseases.[23,24] The high-affinity receptor lacking the beta chain is also expressed on monocytes, Langerhans cells, dendritic cells (i.e., APCs other than B cells), activated eosinophils, and epithelial cells.

The low-affinity IgE receptor, FcεRII, bears structural homology to C-type lectins, but not to FcεRI. (Lectin receptors recognize pathogens and also function as adhesion receptors and signaling molecules.) FcεRII, also known as CD23, is expressed on B and T cells, monocytes, eosinophils, and platelets.[25] CD23 expression is increased by IL-4 and IL-13, and increased CD23 expression would presumably facilitate allergen uptake and presentation to T cells by APCs.[26] Furthermore, B cells from allergic asthmatic patients exposed to allergen have increased CD23 expression.[27] Whether allergic inflammation is initiated when IgE is bound to FcεRII is not clear. However, the solubilized form of CD23 may play a regulatory role in IgE synthesis.[26,28]

When a sensitized individual is exposed to allergen, the allergen binds to IgE receptors on mast cells and basophils. If multivalent, the allergen will cross-link a critical number of cell-bound IgE receptors, leading to cellular activation, secretion of media-tors, and production of the symptoms characteristic of early-phase allergic responses.[28]

Clearly, treatment that interferes with IgE activation of mast cells and basophils may be beneficial. Omalizumab, a recombinant, humanized monoclonal antibody directed against the Fcε portion of IgE, has been developed.[29] Important features of this anti-IgE molecule are (1) it does not bind IgE already attached to FcεRI, and therefore does not cause anaphylaxis; (2) it does not activate complement; and (3) it has a much longer half-life than IgE. In phase III trials, omalizumab was administered by subcutaneous injections given every 2 or 4 weeks to patients with allergic rhinitis or with allergic asthma of varying severity.[30,31] All studies showed dramatic reductions in free IgE levels that were dependent on omalizumab dose as well as baseline IgE levels.[32] As levels of serum IgE decreased, so did surface expression of FcεRI on basophils. Moreover, the posttreatment level of free IgE directly correlated with reduced symptom scores, reduced use of rescue medication, and improved quality of life. For asthma, significant reductions in asthma exacerbations, in hospitalizations for asthma, and in the dose of inhaled or oral steroids were also found. A phase II trial of omalizumab in peanut-sensitive children showed a decreased sensitivity to oral peanut challenges.

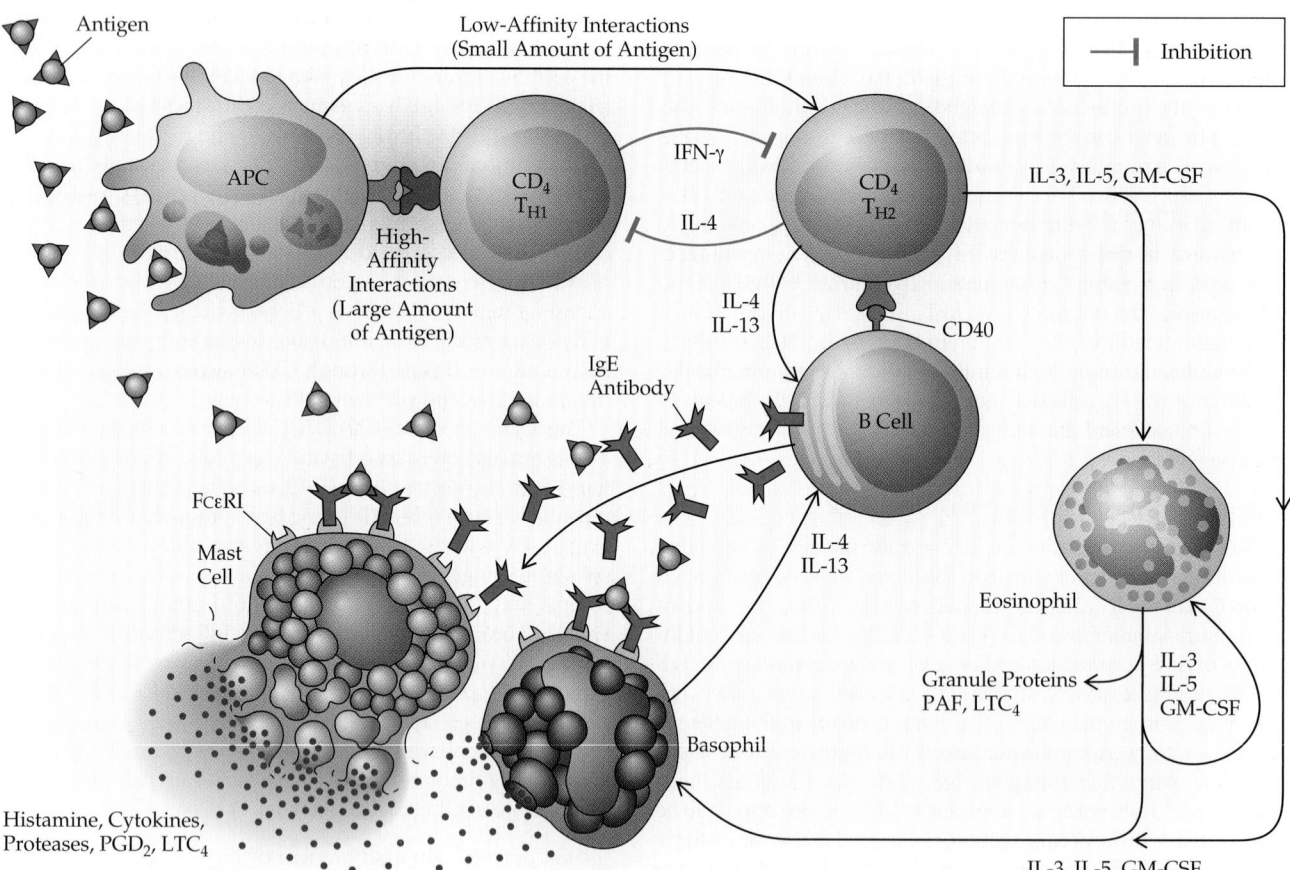

Figure 1 **Inflammatory mechanisms in allergic inflammation. Antigen is taken up by antigen-presenting cells (APCs), processed, and then presented to CD4+ helper T cells (T_H). The strength of interactions between APCs and helper T cells and the quantity of antigen present determine the type of T cell response. Production of interferon gamma (IFN-γ) during T_H1 responses downregulates T_H2 responses, whereas interleukin-4 (IL-4) production by T_H2 inhibits T_H1 responses. IL-4 is also critical for switching B cell antibody production to IgE. Signaling through cluster differentiation 40 (CD40) on the B cell is also required for IgE production. Other T_H2 cytokines, such as IL-3, IL-5, and granulocyte-macrophage colony-stimulating factor (GM-CSF) lead to eosinophil (Eos) and basophil (Baso) production and activation. IgE binds to high-affinity receptors on basophils and mast cells (FcεRI); cross-linking by allergen initiates mediator release. (CpG—deoxycytidine-phosphate-deoxyguanosine; LTC_4—leukotriene C_4; PAF—platelet-activating factor; PGD_2—prostaglandin D_2)**

DEVELOPMENT AND ACTIVATION OF EOSINOPHILS

Eosinophils share a common origin with basophils: a single bone-marrow–derived myeloid progenitor cell has the capacity to give rise to a mixed colony of eosinophils and basophils or to pure colonies of either cell type.[33] A common origin for eosinophils and basophils is further supported by the presence of Charcot-Leyden crystal (CLC) protein and major basic protein (MBP) in both cell types. Eosinophil development is uniquely dependent on the presence of IL-5, a cytokine whose chief source is the T_{H2} helper cell.[34] Along with IL-5, other T cell cytokines—IL-3 and granulocyte-macrophage colony-stimulating factor (GM-CSF)—promote maturation, activation, and prolonged survival of eosinophils.[33] However, only IL-5 potently stimulates the bone marrow to produce eosinophils. In vitro, a low dose of IL-3 favors the development of basophils from progenitors, whereas a high dose of IL-3 favors the development of eosinophils. In contrast, other cytokines may inhibit the growth of eosinophil progenitors. Transforming growth factor–β (TGF-β) contributes to eosinophil apoptosis in vitro and influences progenitor development toward the basophil pathway.[35] IFN-α inhibits progenitor cells in vitro and has been used for treatment of certain patients with eosinophilia refractory to treatment with prednisone.[36]

Eosinophils dwell primarily in tissue. Circulating eosinophils have a short half-life and represent only about 1% of the total number of eosinophils in the body. Epithelial surfaces of mucosal tissues that are exposed to the external environment are heavily inhabited by eosinophils, whereas other tissues are normally devoid of eosinophils.[33] The epithelial tissues of the respiratory tract produce GM-CSF, which is capable of prolonging eosinophil survival in vitro for up to 14 days.

Cell Surface Receptors

Two overlapping populations of circulating eosinophils are thought to represent differing states of eosinophil activation.[37] Nonallergic individuals have greater numbers of eosinophils of normal density and fewer numbers of low-density activated eosinophils. The reverse is true for patients with disorders leading to eosinophilia. This heterogeneity suggests that priming of eosinophils by various cytokines may lead to changes in expression of surface receptors and mediator release [see Table 2]. For example, both high-affinity receptors (FcεRI) and low-affinity receptors (FcεRII) for IgE have been found on peripheral blood eosinophils from patients with hypereosinophilic syndrome. However, eosinophils derived from normal donors or from patients with allergy fail to stain with a panel of monoclonal antibodies directed against IgE receptors.[38] Similar differences have been observed for IgG receptors (FcγR) on eosinophils. Freshly isolated eosinophils express FcγRIIb, a low-affinity IgG receptor that may inhibit mediator release when cross-linked.[34] Both FcγRI and FcγRIII can be induced on eosinophils in vitro when these cells are cultured with IFN-γ, which, in contrast to FcγRIIb, may result in activation. Sera from patients with hay fever contain allergen-specific IgG1 and IgG3, which cause eosinophils to degranulate in vitro in an allergen-dependent manner.[39] Surface receptors for IgA are also present on eosinophils and provide a potent stimulus for release of granule proteins in vitro. The presence of secretory IgA (sIgA) together with eosinophils at mucosal surfaces suggests that IgA-dependent activation also occurs in vivo.[40]

Receptors for complement (C3a and C5a); the lipid mediators platelet-activating factor (PAF), leukotriene C_4 (LTC$_4$), and LTB$_4$; and numerous cytokines and chemokines bind to and activate

Table 2 Receptors on Eosinophils	
IgE receptors	Lipid-mediator receptors
FcεRI (high affinity)	Leukotriene (LT) receptors
FcεRII (low affinity)	LTC$_4$
IgA receptor	LTB$_4$
Complement receptors	Platelet-activating factor (PAF)
C3a	Chemokine receptors
C5a	CCR3
	Others

eosinophils.[33,34] Chemokines of the C-C family play an important chemotactic role for eosinophils. Chemokines of this large family have adjacent cysteine residues (C-C) and have the same receptors. A particular C-C chemokine receptor, CCR3, is found abundantly on eosinophils but not on neutrophils.[41] CCR3 binds at least four chemokines that play crucial roles in the homing of eosinophils to epithelial tissues and that activate eosinophils to release mediators. Another mechanism, which leads to preferential accumulation of eosinophils rather than neutrophils at sites of allergic inflammation, relates to differences in expression of surface adhesion molecules. Eosinophils and neutrophils share several selectins and integrins that initiate the rolling of circulating cells along the endothelium, as well as the subsequent firm adhesion, diapedesis, and transmigration of these cells through the vessel wall. However, eosinophils—but not neutrophils—express an integrin, very late antigen (VLA)-4, whose ligand on endothelial cells (VCAM-1) is upregulated by IL-4 and IL-13, cytokines that are present during T_{H2} responses; consequently, these cytokines promote adherence of eosinophils, but not neutrophils, to endothelium.[42]

Mediators

An array of inflammatory mediators are produced when eosinophils are activated. Preformed mediators are stored in granules and rapidly released once eosinophils are activated. Major basic protein (MBP) is the principal constituent of the granule proteins.[43] Other granule proteins include eosinophil peroxidase (EPO), eosinophil-derived neurotoxin (EDN), and eosinophil cationic protein (ECP). MBP, ECP, and EPO have been shown to damage parasites in vitro; in patients with eosinophil-associated diseases, these proteins are present in high concentrations that can cause toxicity to autologous cells and tissues. Unfortunately, MBP and EPO cause ciliostasis and detachment of respiratory epithelial cells in vitro, and they may contribute to epithelial damage and inflammation in allergic respiratory disorders.[43] However, in one study, treatment of asthmatic patients with anti–IL-5 monoclonal antibody resulted in the selective elimination of eosinophils from the airway, but airway hyperreactivity or the airway response to inhaled allergen were not affected. This leaves open the question of the precise role that eosinophils play in the pathogenesis of atopic asthma.[44] Proteases present in the eosinophils may contribute to airway damage by degrading collagen.[45]

Lipid mediators are rapidly generated by eosinophils after appropriate stimulation. PAF production may lead to activation of platelets, neutrophils, and smooth muscle cells, and thereby induce bronchoconstriction and amplify inflammation. The major eicosanoid product of eosinophils is LTC$_4$, from which LTD$_4$ and LTE$_4$ are derived. These sulfidopeptides are extremely potent at contracting airway smooth muscle, stimulating mucus produc-

a

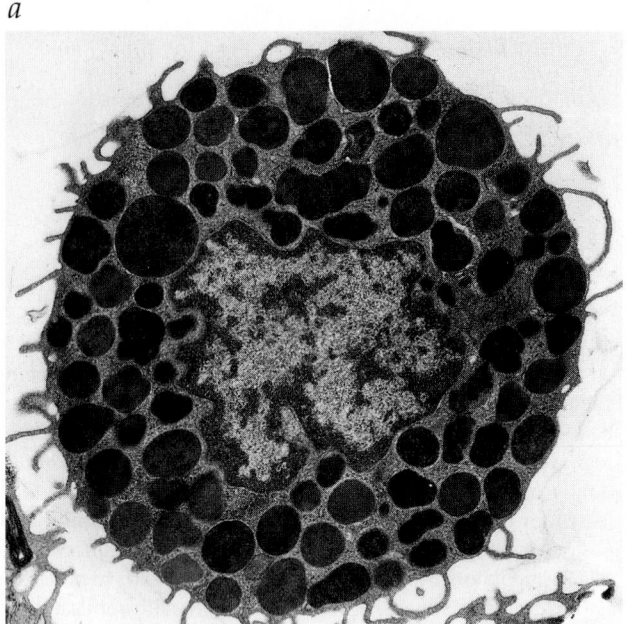

b

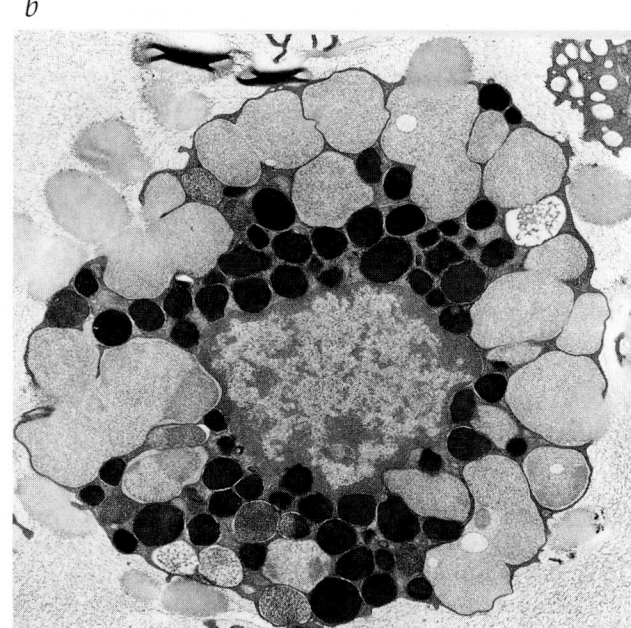

Figure 2 (*a*) Before introduction of antigen, a sensitized mast cell contains many osmotic granules. (*b*) Sixty seconds after treatment with antigen, the peripheral granules have enlarged, neighboring granules have fused, and expulsion of granules from the mast cell has begun.

tion, causing capillary leakage, and promoting chemotaxis of eosinophils.

Numerous cytokines have been identified as potential eosinophil products. Some may function in an autocrine or paracrine manner to activate or prime eosinophils. Others enhance eosinophil development and survival. In addition, eosinophils produce cytokines that regulate immune responses. However, eosinophils elaborate a considerably smaller quantity of cytokines than do lymphocytes. Therefore, the importance of the eosinophil-derived cytokines to allergic inflammation is unclear. Some cytokines that have been demonstrated in vitro have been confirmed in vivo by identifying the protein product in eosinophils infiltrating affected tissues. For example, eosinophils from nasal polyp tissue stain for TGF-β1 and could contribute to the structural pathology.[46] Exposure of allergic patients to allergen revealed eosinophils in nasal mucosal tissues that stain for IL-5 protein; however, much larger contributions of IL-5 are anticipated from T cells in the same tissue.[47]

MAST CELLS AND BASOPHILS AS EFFECTORS OF THE ALLERGIC RESPONSE

Microscopy of mast cells and basophils reveals intensely staining metachromatic granules [*see Figure 2*]. Other common features shared by these cells include the presence of high-affinity receptors for IgE, the release of histamine after cross-linking of the FcεRI by allergen, and common intracellular signaling pathways.[48] There are also numerous differences between the two cell types. Basophils generally complete their maturation in the bone marrow, circulate in the blood, and then are recruited to sites of inflammation.[49] Mast cells that complete their maturation in the bone marrow appear to remain there, whereas those found in peripheral tissues develop from progenitor cells that seed these tissues. Mature mast cells in peripheral tissues may reside there for many months, retaining antigen-specific IgE for periods that exceed the lifespan of IgE in the circulation. Mast cells are strategically distributed in tissues or at mucosal surfaces that interface with the external environment; they are also in proximity to blood vessels and nerves.[50]

All mast cells contain tryptase in their granules; its release is characteristic of mast cell degranulation. However, several additional features further distinguish two types of mast cells [*see Figure 3*].[51] Mast cells of the T type (MC$_T$ cells) are normally the predominant type of mast cell found in the mucosa of the small intestine and in the alveolar wall and epithelium of the respiratory tract. MC$_T$ cells are identified morphologically by a scroll-rich granule structure; they contain tryptase but not chymase, cathepsin G, or mast cell carboxypeptidase. The numbers of MC$_T$ cells in respiratory epithelium are increased in allergic airway inflammation, making them more accessible to inhaled allergens. In a study in asthmatics, increased mast cells predominantly of the MC$_{TC}$ type were localized to the airway smooth muscles but were not present in control subjects or in patients with eosinophilic bronchitis.[52]

In contrast, the MC$_{TC}$ type of mast cell is the dominant type of mast cell in the dermis, conjunctiva, blood vessel walls, and small-intestinal submucosa. Morphologically, MC$_{TC}$ cells display a lattice/grating, scroll-poor granule structure. In addition to tryptase, TC-type mast cells contain chymase, cathepsin G, and mast cell carboxypeptidase. The development of both mast cell types requires stem cell factor (SCF), the ligand for the Kit (tyrosine kinase) receptor. Factors that regulate the recruitment, development, or survival of one mast cell type over the other are not known. Lineage-committing growth factors such as GM-CSF may divert hematopoietic progenitor cells that are capable of forming mast cells when exposed to SCF alone to non–mast cell lineages.[53]

Mediators

Mast cells and basophils form histamine by decarboxylation of histidine. They then store the histamine in their granules. Degranulation releases the histamine, which then interacts with histamine receptors on various tissues. Histamine induces smooth-

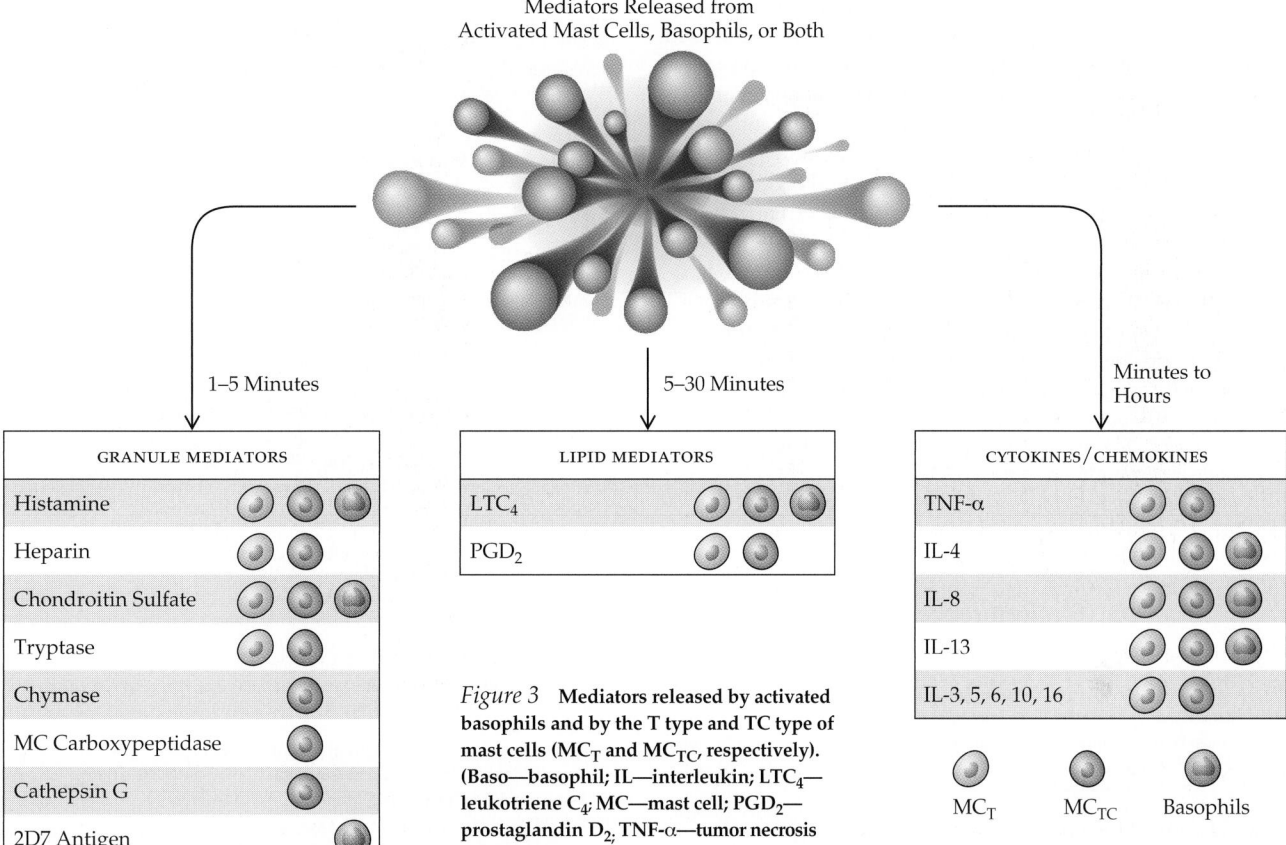

Figure 3 Mediators released by activated basophils and by the T type and TC type of mast cells (MC$_T$ and MC$_{TC}$, respectively). (Baso—basophil; IL—interleukin; LTC$_4$—leukotriene C$_4$; MC—mast cell; PGD$_2$—prostaglandin D$_2$; TNF-α—tumor necrosis factor–α)

muscle contraction, increases mucous secretion in the airway, and stimulates nerve fibers. In addition, it enhances vascular permeability and dilates blood vessels, which results in hypotension if a critical number of cells degranulate. Chondroitin sulfates are proteoglycans that are present in the granules of both basophils and mast cells; heparin proteoglycan is stored exclusively in all mast-cell secretory granules. Both chondroitin sulfate and heparin proteoglycans play a role in packaging of histamine, proteases, and carboxypeptidases in the granules.[54] Heparin is also involved in the processing of chymase and tryptase to catalytically active enzymes. Neutralization of the acidic granule pH during degranulation facilitates the dissociation of histamine from the protease-proteoglycan macromolecular complex.[55] Consequently, histamine appears in the serum within minutes of induction of systemic anaphylaxis by allergen-dependent cross-linking of IgE on mast cells and basophils. Not surprisingly, peak plasma levels of histamine occur 5 minutes after insect-sting–induced anaphylaxis begins and decline to baseline within 20 minutes. Because they are relatively transient, these elevations in histamine levels in plasma are difficult to utilize for the clinical determination of anaphylaxis as a cause of hypotension. However, tryptase diffuses into, and is removed from, the circulation more slowly than histamine. Tryptase levels peak in the circulation 15 minutes to 2 hours after mast-cell degranulation and decline with a half-life of about 2 hours. Peak levels during insect-sting–induced anaphylaxis correlate closely to the drop in mean arterial blood pressure, which is an important measure of clinical severity. For that reason, serum or plasma tryptase levels have been recognized as a clinically useful marker for the diagnosis of systemic anaphylaxis.[55]

Prostaglandin D$_2$ (PGD$_2$) is a newly synthesized cyclooxygenase product of arachidonic acid produced by MC$_T$ and MC$_{TC}$ cells, but not by basophils. PGD$_2$ causes airway smooth muscle to contract, blood vessels to dilate, and platelets to remain unaggregated. In one study of patients with systemic mastocytosis and recurrent episodes of cardiovascular collapse that did not respond to antihistamines, therapeutic success was achieved with cyclooxygenase inhibition that diminished PGD$_2$ production.[56] LTC$_4$ is produced by both mast cells and basophils, as well as by eosinophils, and it is a potent mediator of airway smooth muscle contraction and mucus secretion. Effects of LTC$_4$ are blocked by 5-lipoxygenase inhibition and by leukotriene receptor antagonists.

Mast cells secrete a diverse array of cytokines, including TNF-α, GM-CSF, SCF, and interleukins 3, 4, 5, 6, 10, 13, and 16.[50] TNF-α can reside preformed in mast cell granules and is also synthesized and secreted after mast cell activation. TNF-α causes chemotaxis and activation of many leukocytes, as well as activation of vascular endothelium. IL-4 and IL-13 are central to T$_{H2}$ differentiation, IgE isotype switching, and induction of the adhesion receptors VCAM-1 on endothelium and VLA-4 on eosinophils. Basophils do not synthesize TNF-α and generally produce fewer cytokines than do mast cells. However, activated basophils synthesize more IL-4 and IL-13 on a per-cell basis than any other cell type. In tissues with allergic inflammation that are challenged with allergen, basophils appear to be the predominant source of antigen-specific production of IL-4 and IL-13.[49]

As with eosinophils, a subpopulation of low-density (so-called hypodense) basophils can be detected in peripheral blood samples. This subpopulation is more sensitive to the effects of glucocorticoids than the higher-density basophils. However, functional differences in the hypodense basophils have not been characterized, as they have for eosinophils. Recently, basophil-specific markers have been developed.[57] The monoclonal antibodies named 2D7 and BB1 detect basophil-specific antigens in secretory granules and should prove useful for more precise assessment of basophil involvement in human allergic diseases. For example, substantial numbers of basophils can now be detected in skin and respiratory tissues during the late-phase response to an allergen challenge, and these cells account for a major portion of the IL-4–containing cells in such tissues. Basophils appear to be similar to eosinophils in expression of numerous cytokines and chemokine receptors, including CCR3. Exposure of basophils to most CC chemokines leads to histamine release.

Pamela J. Daffern, M.D., has no commercial relationships with manufacturers of products or providers of services discussed in this chapter.

Lawrence B. Schwartz, M.D., Ph.D., has a licensing agreement with the Pharmacia Corporation for a tryptase assay kit.

References

1. Richet C: Anaphylaxis. The University Press, Liverpool, 1913

2. Prescott SL, Macaubas C, Holt BJ, et al: Transplacental priming of the human immune system to environmental allergens: universal skewing of initial T cell responses toward the Th2 cytokine profile. J Immunol 160:4730, 1998

3. Bjorksten B: The intrauterine and postnatal environments. J Allergy Clin Immunol 104:1119, 1999

4. Klein J, Sato A: The HLA system: first of two parts. N Engl J Med 343:702, 2000

5. Langenkamp A, Messi M, Lanzavecchia A, et al: Kinetics of dendritic cell activation: impact on priming of Th1, Th2 and nonpolarized T cells. Nat Immunol 1:311, 2000

6. Palucka K, Banchereau J: Dendritic cells: a link between innate and adaptive immunity. J Clin Immunol 19:12, 1999

7. Klein J, Sato A: The HLA system: second of two parts. N Engl J Med 343:782, 2000

8. Rogers PR, Croft M: Peptide dose, affinity, and time of differentiation can contribute to the Th1/Th2 cytokine balance. J Immunol 163:1205, 1999

9. Wild JS, Sur S: CpG oligonucleotide modulation of allergic inflammation. Allergy 56:365, 2001

10. Tighe H, Corr M, Roman M, et al: Gene vaccination: plasmid DNA is more than just a blueprint. Immunol Today 19:89, 1998

11. Kay AB: Allergy and allergic diseases: first of two parts. N Engl J Med 344:30, 2001

12. Wills-Karp M, Luyimbazi J, Xu X, et al: Interleukin-13: central mediator of allergic asthma. Science 282:2258, 1998

13. Till S, Durham S, Dickason R, et al: IL-13 production by allergen-stimulated T cells is increased in allergic disease and associated with IL-5 but not IFN-gamma expression. Immunology 91:53, 1997

14. Kondo N, Matsui E, Kaneko H, et al: Reduced interferon-gamma production and mutations of the interleukin-12 receptor beta (2) chain gene in atopic subjects. Int Arch Allergy Immunol 124:117, 2001

15. Tamura K, Arakawa H, Suzuki M, et al: Novel dinucleotide repeat polymorphism in the first exon of the STAT-6 gene is associated with allergic diseases. Clin Exp Allergy 31:1509, 2001

16. Van Eerdewegh P, Little RD, Dupuis J, et al: Association of the ADAM33 gene with asthma and bronchial hyperresponsiveness. Nature 418:426, 2002

17. Gehring U, Bischof W, Fahlbusch B, et al: House dust endotoxin and allergic sensitization in children. Am J Respir Crit Care Med 166:939, 2002

18. Busse WW, Lemanske RF Jr: Asthma. N Engl J Med 344:350, 2001

19. Bacharier LB, Geha RS: Molecular mechanisms of IgE regulation. J Allergy Clin Immunol 105:S547, 2000

20. Doyle IS, Hollmann CA, Crispe IN, et al: Specific blockade by CD54 and MHC II of CD40-mediated signaling for B cell proliferation and survival. Exp Cell Res 265:312, 2001

21. Kinet JP: The high-affinity IgE receptor (Fc epsilon RI): from physiology to pathology. Annu Rev Immunol 17:931, 1999

22. Donnadieu E, Jouvin MH, Kinet JP: A second amplifier function for the allergy-associated Fc(epsilon)RI-beta subunit. Immunity 12:515, 2000

23. Saini SS, MacGlashan DWJ, Sterbinsky SA, et al: Down-regulation of human basophil IgE and Fc epsilon RI alpha surface densities and mediator release by anti-IgE infusions is reversible in vitro and in vivo. J Immunol 162:5624, 1999

24. Saini SS, Richardson JJ, Wofsy C, et al: Expression and modulation of Fc epsilon RI-alpha and Fc epsilon RIbeta in human blood basophils. J Allergy Clin Immunol 107:832, 2001

25. Squire CM, Studer EJ, Lees A, et al: Antigen presentation is enhanced by targeting antigen to the Fc epsilon RII by antigen-anti-Fc epsilon RII conjugates. J Immunol 152:4388, 1994

26. Kisselgof AB, Oettgen HC: The expression of murine B cell CD23, in vivo, is regulated by its ligand, IgE. Int Immunol 10:1377, 1998

27. Bonnefoy JY, Lecoanet-Henchoz S, Aubry JP, et al: CD23 and B-cell activation. Curr Opin Immunol 7:355, 1995

28. Pearlman DS: Pathophysiology of the inflammatory response. J Allergy Clin Immunol 104:S132, 1999

29. Presta LG, Lahr SJ, Shields RL, et al: Humanization of an antibody directed against IgE. J Immunol 151:2623, 1993

30. Milgrom H, Fick RB Jr, Su JQ, et al: Treatment of allergic asthma with monoclonal anti-IgE antibody. rhuMAb-E25 Study Group. N Engl J Med 341:1966, 1999

31. Adelroth E, Rak S, Haahtela T, et al: Recombinant humanized mAB-E25, an anti-IgE mAb, in birch pollen-induced seasonal allergic rhinitis. J Allergy Clin Immunol 106:253, 2000

32. Johansson SG, Haahtela T, O'Byrne PM: Omalizumab and the immune system: an overview of preclinical and clinical data. Ann Allergy Asthma Immunol 89:132, 2002

33. Gleich GJ: Mechanisms of eosinophil-associated inflammation. J Allergy Clin Immunol 105:651, 2000

34. Rothenberg ME: Eosinophilia. N Engl J Med 338:1592, 1998

35. Atsuta J, Fujisawa T, Iguchi K, et al: Inhibitory effect of transforming growth factor beta 1 on cytokine-enhanced eosinophil survival and degranulation. Int Arch Allergy Immunol 108:31, 1995

36. Gratzl S, Palca A, Schmitz M, et al: Treatment with IFN-alpha in corticosteroid-unresponsive asthma. J Allergy Clin Immunol 105:1035, 2000

37. Fukuda T, Dunnette SL, Reed CE, et al: Increased numbers of hypodense eosinophils in the blood of patients with bronchial asthma. Am Rev Respir Dis 132:981, 1985

38. Smith SJ, Ying S, Meng Q, et al: Blood eosinophils from atopic donors express messenger RNA for the alpha, beta, and gamma subunits of the high-affinity IgE receptor (Fc epsilon RI) and intracellular, but not cell surface, alpha subunit protein. J Allergy Clin Immunol 105:309, 2000

39. Kaneko M, Swanson MC, Gleich GJ, et al: Allergen-specific IgG1 and IgG3 through Fc gamma RII induce eosinophil degranulation. J Clin Invest 95:2813, 1995

40. Abu-Ghazaleh RI, Fugisawa T, Mestecky J, et al: IgA-induced eosinophil degranulation. J Immunol 142:2393, 1989

41. Heath H, Qin S, Rao P, et al: Chemokine receptor usage by human eosinophils: the importance of CCR3 demonstrated using an antagonistic monoclonal antibody. J Clin Invest 99:178, 1997

42. Schleimer RP, Sterbinsky SA, Kaiser J, et al: IL-4 induces adherence of human eosinophils and basophils but not neutrophils to endothelium: association with expression of VCAM-1. J Immunol 148:1086, 1992

43. Gleich GJ, Adolphson MS, Leiferman KM: Annual Reviews of Medicine: Selected Topics in Clinical Sciences. Creger WP, Coggins CH, Hancock EW, Eds. Annual Reviews, Inc., Palo Alto, California, 1993, p 85

44. Leckie MJ, ten Brinke A, Khan J, et al: Effects of an interleukin-5 blocking monoclonal antibody on eosinophils, airway hyper-responsiveness, and the late asthmatic response. Lancet 356:2144, 2000

45. Mallya SK, Hall JE, Lee HM, et al: Interaction of matrix metalloproteinases with serine protease inhibitors: new potential roles for matrix metalloproteinase inhibitors. Ann NY Acad Sci 732:303, 1994

46. Bachert C, Gevaert P, Holtappels G, et al: Nasal polyposis: from cytokines to growth. Am J Rhinol 14:279, 2000

47. Lee CH, Lee KS, Rhee CS, et al: Distribution of RANTES and interleukin-5 in allergic nasal mucosa and nasal polyps. Ann Otol Rhinol Laryngol 108:594, 1999

48. Holgate ST: The role of mast cells and basophils in inflammation. Clin Exp Allergy 30:28, 2000

49. Bochner BS: Systemic activation of basophils and eosinophils: markers and consequences. J Allergy Clin Immunol 106:S292, 2000

50. Williams CM, Galli SJ: The diverse potential effector and immunoregulatory roles of mast cells in allergic disease. J Allergy Clin Immunol 105:847, 2000

51. Gurish MF, Austen KF: The diverse roles of mast cells. J Exp Med 194:71, 2001

52. Brightling CE, Bradding P, Symon FA, et al: Mast-cell infiltration of airway smooth muscle in asthma. N Engl J Med 346:1699, 2002

53. Mekori YA, Metcalfe DD: Mast cell–T cell interactions. J Allergy Clin Immunol 104:517, 1999

54. Galli SJ: Mast cells and basophils. Curr Opin Hematol 7:32, 2000

55. Schwartz LB, Irani AM: Serum tryptase and the laboratory diagnosis of systemic mastocytosis. Hematol Oncol Clin North Am 14:641, 2000

56. Roberts LJ 2nd, Sweetman BJ, Lewis RA, et al: Increased production of prostaglandin D2 in patients with systemic mastocytosis. N Engl J Med 303:1400, 1980

57. Kepley CL, Craig SS, Schwartz LB: Identification and partial characterization of a unique marker for human basophils. J Immunol 154:6548, 1995

Acknowledgment

Figures 1 and 3   Seward Hung.

Mitchell H. Grayson, M.D., and Phillip E. Korenblat, M.D., F.A.C.P.

By definition, allergy is an untoward physiologic event mediated by immune mechanisms, usually involving the interaction of an allergen with the allergic antibody, IgE. Common illnesses mediated in this manner include allergic asthma and rhinitis, Hymenoptera hypersensitivity, and certain other causes of anaphylaxis. In addition, a significant proportion of drug, food, and skin reactions are allergic in origin.

Allergic diseases in general, and asthma in particular, have been increasing in prevalence in high-income societies.[1] Although there are undoubtedly many reasons for this increase, one is described in the so-called hygiene hypothesis, which posits that greater exposure to infectious agents (and bacterial endotoxins in particular) early in life reduces the likelihood of subsequent allergy.[2] This hypothesis, which requires further proof of causality, acknowledges an etiologic role for both genetic and environmental factors in allergy: a child with a hereditary predisposition to atopy is more likely to develop clinical allergy if raised in a relatively aseptic environment.

History

In allergic illnesses, the importance of a careful and thorough medical history cannot be overstated. The clinician must dissect the allergic reaction to understand the nature of the event and identify the antigen that was responsible for the reaction. Formal diagnosis of allergy has three elements: characterization of the allergic reaction, correlation with antigen exposure, and demonstration of IgE specific for the suspected allergen. The history is essential for the first two elements, and for practical purposes, the history can sometimes obviate the third element.

The history should begin with a review of the patient's symptoms and their temporal pattern. If the presenting symptoms include wheezing, the clinician should remember the time-honored statement that all that wheezes is not asthma. Furthermore, all that is asthma is not allergy [see Chapter 216].

The presenting symptoms must match the set of features that characterize the suspected allergic illness. For example, patients with perennial allergic rhinitis typically present with sneezing, rhinorrhea, nasal itching, and nasal congestion. Postnasal drainage is not the only symptom of this disease, so postnasal drainage alone—even with evidence of antigen exposure and the presence of specific IgE antibodies—typically would not support the diagnosis of allergic rhinitis.

A central aspect of the history is to establish a link between the time and site of exposure to the presumed allergen and the development of allergic symptoms. Seasonal allergic events are often so characteristic that the diagnosis can be made solely on the basis of the presenting symptoms and their correlation with environmental exposure to the allergen; laboratory evidence may not be needed for the diagnosis. Similarly, symptoms that develop immediately after exposure to animals or their dander often do not need additional supporting evidence for diagnosis.

In the United States, the presence of airborne pollen may vary both temporally and geographically.[3] In general, early spring is characterized by the presence of tree pollen, and late spring is accompanied by grass pollen. Ragweed and other weed pollens are prevalent in the fall, usually until the first hard frost. Mold spores can be found indoors year-round, except possibly in very dry areas. Outdoor mold spores peak during the summer and fall months, and they diminish when snow covers the landscape [see Table 1].

Illnesses such as asthma or rhinitis that occur on a perennial basis, if allergic, should correlate with environmental exposure to a perennial allergen (e.g., dust mites, indoor mold spores, animal dander, or cockroach antigen). Such exposure most often takes place in the household, but the possibility of exposure to allergens in the workplace should not be forgotten. It should be noted that in some warm climates (e.g., that of the southern United States), the pollen season may be nearly year-round and, thus, may be a cause of perennial symptoms.

Allergic reactions to ingested substances typically include skin eruptions, abdominal discomfort, or respiratory symptoms. Severe and life-endangering reactions involving the cardiovascular or respiratory system, or both, may also occur. The list of ingested substances said to cause allergic reactions is seemingly endless. However, foods (particularly peanuts, tree nuts, shellfish, and seeded fruits) and medications are the most common triggers of this type of allergic reaction [see Chapter 109]. Again, the history is essential to establishing a particular substance as the probable cause of an allergic reaction.

The family history is important. Allergic predisposition is genetically mediated, so patients with allergies often report that family members have similar problems. However, in a patient who has both a personal and a family history of angioedema, the disorder may be inherited but not allergic: hereditary angioedema results from the absence of the C1 esterase inhibitor.

Physical Examination

The physical examination of a patient with a suspected allergic illness requires an in-depth focus on the involved organ system or systems. In atopic dermatitis, the skin findings may include patches of lesions that are pruritic, erythematous, papular,

---

Table 1 Inhaled Aeroallergens That Cause Rhinitis, Conjunctivitis, and Asthma

Pollens (tree, grass, and weed pollens)

Dust mites (*Dermatophagoides* species)

Animal proteins (cat, dog, horse, guinea pig, gerbil, mouse, and rat proteins)

Fungal spores (*Alternaria, Aspergillus, Penicillium,* and *Cladosporium* species)

High-molecular-weight proteins (e.g., as derived from insects, insect venoms, and latex)

Low-molecular-weight inorganic and organic chemicals (e.g., toluene diisocyanate and plicatic acid)

scaling, crusting, vesicular, or lichenified—qualities that may occur alone or in combination. Lesions are usually characterized by periodic exacerbations, and it is important to examine these lesions for pyogenic infections.

The distribution of allergic dermatitis lesions varies with the age of the patient. In infants, the dermatitis begins to appear by the sixth to eighth week of life. At this age, the eruptions ordinarily involve the scalp, face (especially the cheeks), ears, and extensor surfaces of the extremities. The trunk, buttocks, and anogenital regions may also be involved. The dermatitis may continue into childhood. Alternatively, allergic dermatitis may first develop at about 2 years of age. Dermatitis in childhood is often found in the antecubital and popliteal fossa, on the neck, and at the flexor and extensor areas of the wrist. In adolescents and adults, the lesions frequently involve the neck and the flexural areas but may occur anywhere on the skin.[4]

Typical urticarial lesions are pruritic, transient (individual lesions resolve within 24 hours), erythematous, and raised; they comprise a wheal with a surrounding erythematous flare. Urticaria can be confused with skin lesions of vasculitis. The presence of hemorrhage or a lesion that lasts longer than 24 hours should raise the specter of urticarial vasculitis. Skin biopsy may be required to differentiate urticarialike lesions.

The hallmarks of allergic rhinoconjunctivitis are bilateral erythema and edema of the conjunctiva, watery ocular discharge, and, often, mild periorbital edema.[5] Allergic shiners (bluish discoloration just below the eye orbits) may be observed. Patients with allergic rhinitis may also have an extra fold in the lower eyelids (Dennie-Morgan lines). On the exterior portion of the nose, a crease may be present as a result of continued upward rubbing of the tip of the nose (the so-called allergic salute). Examination of the nasal cavity often reveals watery secretions and edematous, bluish nasal turbinates that partially occlude the nasal passages [see Chapter 106]. Translucent nasal polyps may be observed, but these are not necessarily a hallmark of allergy; they can be seen in both allergic and nonallergic patients.

The chest examination often may reveal no abnormalities. However, a methodical examination is warranted. The clinician should observe specifically for cyanosis and the use of accessory muscles for respiration. In addition, auscultation is indicated for a prolonged expiratory respiratory phase or for inspiratory and expiratory wheezing. If wheezing is present, it is important to confirm that the sounds emanate from the lungs and not the trachea. All too often, extrathoracic obstruction is missed on the physical examination.

Although cardiovascular findings are not commonly associated with allergic diseases, it is important to remember that hy-

potension, tachyarrhythmia, and—particularly if the patient is using a beta-adrenergic blocking medication—bradycardia may be seen in cases of anaphylaxis.

Assays of IgE

Because allergic diseases result from the interaction of an allergen with specific IgE, analysis for specific IgE in a patient who has clinical allergy is a major diagnostic consideration. Specific IgE can be identified both by in vivo methods (skin testing) and by in vitro methods (e.g., radioallergosorbent testing [RAST]).[6]

SKIN TESTING

Epicutaneous Testing

The most rapid and sensitive test for allergy is skin testing. This in vivo method depends on mast cell–bound or basophil-bound IgE specific for the allergen being tested. Because a positive test requires degranulation of mast cells or basophils and subsequent histamine release, antihistamines will interfere with the outcome. In general, patients should discontinue antihistamines 1 week before skin testing, although certain antihistamines can be discontinued 3 days beforehand [see Table 2]. Corticosteroids do not inhibit this immediate-phase response, and hence, their use is not a contraindication for skin testing.

Skin testing should be performed by a qualified allergist. Initial testing is performed by pricking the epidermis with a small amount of the specific allergen. In patients with IgE specific for the allergen, a wheal-and-flare response will develop at the site within 20 minutes. The areas of edema and erythema are then measured. The results are often reported as wheal size over flare size (both in millimeters) or, alternatively, identified on an arbitrary scale of 1 to 4+, correlating to the size of the wheal, the flare, or both. Histamine is used as a positive control, and because some patients develop hives in response to any strong pressure on the skin (dermatographism), saline is used as a negative control.

Intradermal Testing

If the results of epicutaneous skin testing are negative but the patient's symptoms strongly suggest an allergic etiology, intradermal testing can be performed. This involves injecting 0.02 ml of a dilute allergen solution (usually a 1:100 or 1:1,000 dilution of the concentrated extract) into the dermis. As with epicutaneous testing, the skin is observed for the development of a wheal and flare within 20 minutes. Grading of the results is similar to that for epicutaneous testing.

Intradermal testing has a higher sensitivity but a lower specificity than epicutaneous testing. This means that intradermal testing produces more false positives but fewer false negatives than epicutaneous testing. Although the relevance of isolated positive intradermal tests for aeroallergens is debated, intradermal testing is crucial for the evaluation of drug and insect allergy.

Compared with epicutaneous testing, intradermal testing exposes the body to a significant antigen load and, therefore, poses a higher risk of a systemic reaction. For that reason, intradermal testing is contraindicated in patients who have not had a prior negative result on epicutaneous testing. It is not surprising that five of the six skin-testing fatalities reported from 1945 to 1987 occurred in patients who underwent intradermal testing with-

Table 2 Time before Skin Testing to Stop Antihistamines*

Antihistamine (Trade Name)	Days
Azelastine	7
Cetirizine (Zyrtec)	7
Chlorpheniramine	3
Desloratadine (Clarinex)	7
Diphenhydramine	3
Fexofenadine (Allegra)	7
Loratadine (Claritin)	7

*Note: Other medications (e.g., tricyclic antidepressants) may also have antihistaminic activity.

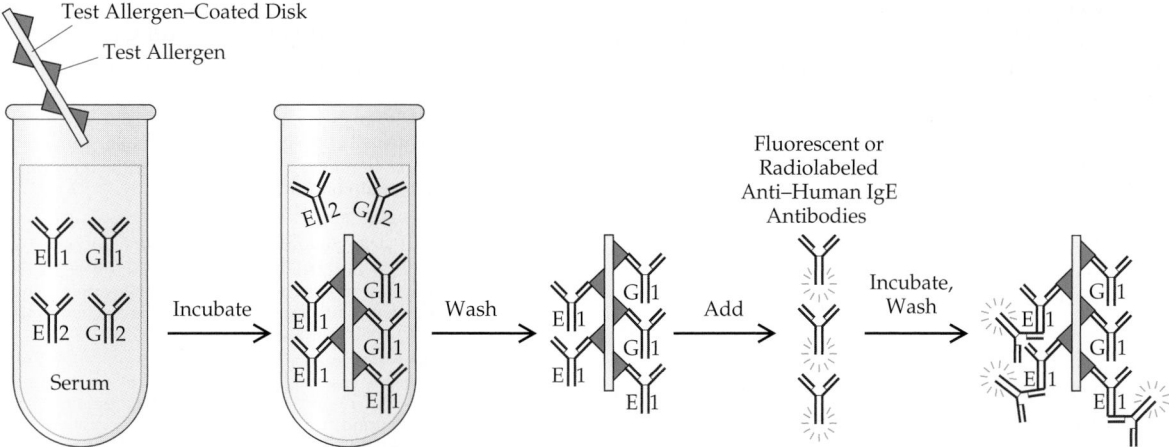

Figure 1　The radioallergosorbent test (RAST). A solid-phase disk coated with the test allergen is incubated with the patient's serum. IgE and IgG antibodies to the test allergen (E1 and G1, respectively) will bind with the allergens on the disk, whereas IgE and IgG antibodies to other allergens (E2 and G2, respectively) will remain free in the serum. After the free antibodies have been washed away, the disk is incubated with antibodies against human IgE that have been labeled with a radioactive or a fluorescent tracer. The tagged anti–human IgE antibodies will then bind IgE attached to the disk; a second washing then removes any unbound tagged antibody. The level of radioactivity or fluorescence is then proportional to the amount of specific IgE against the antigen (E1). IgG against the antigen (G1) does not react with the tagged antibody and therefore is not counted in this test.

out previous epicutaneous testing.[7] Food allergens should never be used for intradermal testing, because they are associated with a high rate of false positive irritant responses. Furthermore, some foods (e.g., peanuts and shellfish) are such potent antigens that they could provoke severe systemic reactions if injected intradermally.

Inaccurate or incorrect skin-testing results can occur for a variety of reasons. For example, the use of low-potency extracts can lead to false negative results, as can certain patient factors, such as (1) age (wheals are small in infants, increase until age 50, and then decline), (2) race (whites produce smaller wheals than African Americans[8]), and (3) antihistamine use (including drugs with antihistaminic properties, such as tricyclic antidepressants). In addition, skin-testing results depend on vascular leak; medications such as adrenergic agents can inhibit this response, leading to false negatives. False positives most often result because of irritant reactions, dermatographism, or a nonspecific reaction from a nearby strong reaction (a so-called bystander reaction).

RADIOALLERGOSORBENT TESTING

RAST and other in vitro tests measure the concentration of nonspecific and allergen-specific IgE in the patient's serum. Because these tests do not depend on IgE-mediated histamine release for their interpretation, they are not adversely affected by the use of antihistamines and other medications (except for anti-IgE, omalizumab [see below]). Although there are circumstances in which high levels of nonspecific IgE can be found, determination of nonspecific IgE is generally of little value, because IgE concentrations vary substantially and there is significant overlap between patients with atopic disease and patients with nonatopic disease. However, the determination of allergen-specific IgE can be useful, especially in patients in whom skin testing cannot be performed (e.g., because of skin disease or inability to stop using antihistamines).

RAST is the most common method of determining allergen-specific IgE in the serum [*see Figure 1*]. This test involves adding the patient's serum to a solid phase (usually a disk) coated with the allergen to be tested. Antibodies in the patient's serum that

are specific for the allergen will bind to the solid phase. After the disk is washed, to remove the unbound antibodies to other allergens, antibodies against human IgE that have been tagged with a radioactive isotope are added. The disk is then washed again, to remove unbound tagged anti-IgE. The level of radiation that is present after washing the disk is directly proportional to the quantity of allergen-specific IgE in the patient's serum. Comparing these values with known standards allows for the determination of allergen-specific IgE. Gaining in popularity is the CAP-RAST system, which is a test for specific IgE that incorporates a solid phase consisting of an encapsulated hydrophilic carrier (in the shape of a cup or "CAP") to which antigen is covalently bonded. This allows for better allergen attachment and much more accurate quantification of specific IgE than can be obtained with traditional RAST testing. Furthermore, CAP-RAST testing is usually performed with fluorescently labeled anti-IgE, as opposed to the radiolabeled anti-IgE in traditional RAST testing. Although the CAP-RAST method is different from traditional RAST testing, some laboratories may refer to both of these modalities as RAST tests.

Although RAST results generally correlate with allergic sensitivity, RAST is more likely than skin testing to produce false positive results. As such, the sensitivity of RAST is lower than that of skin testing. Therefore, skin testing is still the preferred method of identifying the allergens to which a person is sensitive.

INTERPRETATION OF IgE TEST RESULTS

Regardless of the modality used to test for IgE, all results must be correlated with the clinical findings. Only tests whose results fit with the patient's symptoms should be considered relevant for explaining those specific symptoms. In other words, a positive result is useful for therapeutic intervention only if the patient has symptoms when exposed to the allergen, and a negative test is useful only if the patient has no symptoms on exposure to the allergen. An example would be a patient who has a positive skin test to a tree pollen yet has no symptoms in the spring but instead has symptoms in the fall, in a region devoid of tree pollen at that time of the year. Even if tests for weeds and molds were negative, this seasonality of symptoms would still suggest that a fall pollen or untested mold spore is to blame for the symptoms rather than trees, as the testing would suggest. A positive skin test in the absence of exposure or symptoms, however, does not mean that the patient will not develop symptoms to the antigen at some time in the future. In general, the clinician should use the clinical history to guide all testing modalities, rather than using the testing to try to identify unknown triggers.

Treatment

ENVIRONMENTAL CONTROL

The most effective therapeutic intervention for atopic disease is complete removal of the offending allergen or allergens from the patient's environment [*see Table 3*]. For example, environmental control for a patient who is allergic to dust mites would include encasing the pillows and mattress in dust-mite–proof covers, washing all bedding in hot (> 130° F) water weekly, and lowering the ambient humidity in the house to below 45%. Some authorities also recommend the removal of bedroom carpet as an additional control for dust-mite exposure; this recommendation is controversial, however. For pet-allergic patients, the pet should be removed from the household or, at a minimum, should be kept out of the bedroom at all times. Pollen-sensitive individuals will benefit from staying in air-conditioned environments during the time of year when the offending pollen is prevalent.

PHARMACOLOGIC AGENTS

Although environmental control measures constitute the primary treatment for atopic disease, such interventions are sometimes impossible to carry out or do not completely eliminate the allergen and, therefore, do not fully resolve the disease. This is the point at which pharmacotherapy should be added. The medications used in allergic disease are targeted to various components of the allergic cascade [*see Figure 2*]. These medications include antihistamines and decongestants, anti-IgE, long-acting and short-acting bronchodilators, corticosteroids (both topical and systemic), leukotriene receptor antagonists, and theophylline. Although cromolyn and nedocromil sodium have an established tradition of use and favorable safety profiles, their minimal efficacy does not justify their inclusion on this list.

Antihistamines and Decongestants

Antihistamines block the action of histamine at its receptor.[9] Although there are at least four histamine receptors, most allergic symptoms have been attributed to the H_1 receptor. Symptoms mediated by histamine include pruritus, nasal itching, conjunctivitis, and the wheal-and-flare response.

H_1 receptor antagonists can be divided into two broad categories on the basis of their ability to cross the blood-brain barrier and cause sedation. The classic antihistamines, which cause more sedation, include over-the-counter drugs such as diphenhydramine and chlorpheniramine, as well as prescription medications such as cyproheptadine and hydroxyzine. These medications are potent antihistamines, but their usefulness is limited by their central nervous system side effects. Of particular significance is that CNS effects have been shown to last beyond the sedative effects of these medications, leading to decreased reaction time. Therefore, the recommended choice for long-term therapy is a second-generation or third-generation (active me-

---

Table 3 Environmental Control for Allergy Management

General measures

Eliminate irritants, especially cigarette smoke, from home

Keep relative humidity at 45% or less by using air conditioners and dehumidifiers

Specific measures

Pollens: use air conditioner and keep windows of house and car closed; during peak pollen season, avoid outside activities

Molds: outdoor molds can be excluded by keeping windows closed; use exhaust fan in bathroom and kitchen to keep humidity at 50% or less

Dust mites: cover mattresses, box spring, and pillows with impermeable cases; all bedding should be washed in hot water (> 130° F) once a week; if possible, remove carpet; keep the humidity at 45% or less

Feathers: replace feather pillow with Dacron (washable) pillow and wash regularly

Pets: remove the pet from the home; if the patient does not agree to remove the pet, the pet should not be permitted in the bedroom; in addition, to decrease antigen shedding, the pet should be bathed twice weekly

---

tabolite) antihistamine, which will produce minimal sedation. Examples of such agents include over-the-counter loratadine and the prescription drugs cetirizine (Zyrtec), desloratadine (Clarinex), and fexofenadine (Allegra). Also available as a nasal spray is azelastine (Astelin).

Antihistamines do not have a significant effect on nasal congestion. For intermittent congestion, a systemic decongestant may be used. Since phenylpropanolamine (PPA) was taken off the market because of its association with increased frequency of strokes, pseudoephedrine has been the only systemic decongestant available in the United States. Nevertheless, although decongestants provide some relief of the sensation of nasal fullness, they do not alter the underlying etiology.

Anti-IgE Therapy

The allergic response requires the presence of IgE. A newly approved therapeutic modality in the United States is omalizumab, a humanized anti-IgE monoclonal antibody that is administered subcutaneously on a biweekly to monthly schedule and can reduce serum unbound IgE to undetectable levels. This molecule consists of the hypervariable region from a mouse antibody against human IgE that is genetically grafted onto a human IgG molecule—hence the term humanized. Clinically, omalizumab has been shown to significantly reduce symptom scores in patients with allergic rhinitis, as well as to relieve symptoms and modestly improve airway function in patients with moderate to severe asthma.[10-12] This medication has the ability to block the allergic cascade at its initiation and has not been associated with significant side effects.

The appropriate end points for omalizumab therapy remain uncertain. Standard measures of allergic sensitivity are not useful in patients who are taking omalizumab: skin testing will produce negative results, and total IgE will be elevated because IgE is bound to the anti-IgE medication in circulation. Current data support continued administration for a minimum of 12 weeks. Patients with low pulmonary functions, patients who have had emergency department visits within the preceding year, and patients on high-dose inhaled corticosteroids are the most likely to respond to therapy with anti-IgE.[13] The relatively high cost of this medication in the United States may limit its usefulness.

Bronchodilators

Both short-acting and long-acting bronchodilators are available for treatment of asthma. Short-acting bronchodilators relieve bronchoconstriction but have no effect on the underlying inflammatory process, whereas long-acting bronchodilators not only provide symptomatic relief of bronchoconstriction but also may have slight anti-inflammatory properties. Unfortunately, over time there is loss of potency of bronchodilators when they are used alone (subsensitivity). This loss of potency does not occur, however, when bronchodilators are combined with an inhaled corticosteroid. Given the lack of sufficient anti-inflammatory activity and the subsensitivity of bronchodilators, the recommended use of these medications is in combination with an inhaled corticosteroid rather than as monotherapy.[14,15]

Corticosteroids

Corticosteroids inhibit the production of inflammatory cytokines and chemokines, thus reducing the inflammation and cellular recruitment to sites of disease. These medications play a major role in the treatment of allergic disease. They may be given locally (topically) or systemically (orally).

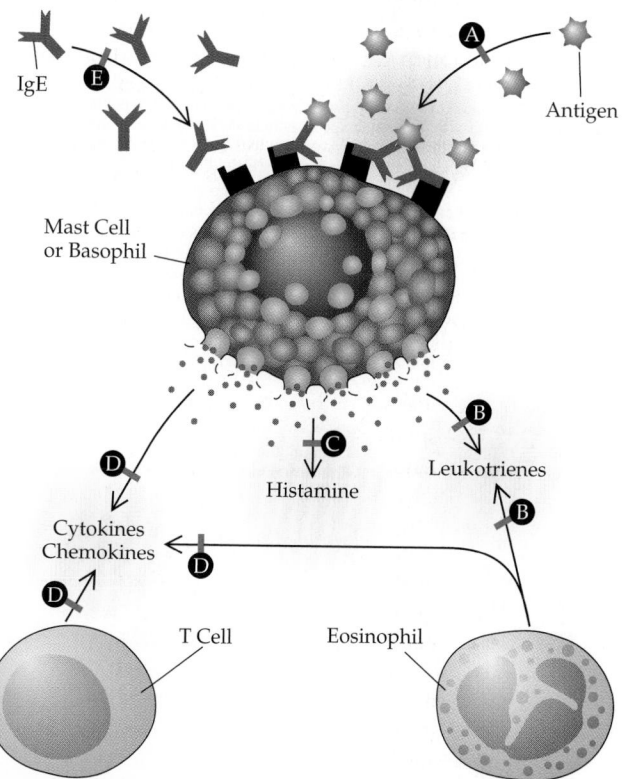

Figure 2 **Mechanisms of action of medications used in allergic diseases. Environmental control (A) minimizes exposure to the antigen to which the patient has specific IgE. If the antigen is present, it binds with specific IgE; cross-linking of the antigen-bound IgE on the surface of a mast cell or basophil starts the allergic cascade, with release of leukotrienes, histamine, cytokines, chemokines, and other mediators such as prostaglandins and proteases (not shown). Leukotriene antagonists (B) block the action of leukotrienes; antihistamines compete with histamine at H$_1$ receptors; corticosteroids (D) inhibit the production of inflammatory cytokines and chemokines. Anti-IgE therapy (e.g., omalizumab) (E) works by directly reducing the amount of IgE in the body. It is unclear at which sites immunotherapy and cromolyn and nedocromil sodium exert their anti-inflammatory action.**

Topical corticosteroids Topical corticosteroids are capable of potent anti-inflammatory effects and are a mainstay of allergic therapy. These medications, which are inhaled for asthma or taken intranasally for rhinitis, have the ability to abrogate the inflammatory response and interfere with multiple aspects of the allergic cascade. However, unlike antihistamines, which provide rapid relief (within 1 to 2 hours), topical corticosteroids may require 3 to 5 days of therapy before full relief is realized. In rhinitis, steroids can relieve the congestion and raise the threshold for the development of symptoms to allergen exposure.[16,17] Significant systemic effects are uncommon with inhaled or intranasal corticosteroids given at the usual recommended doses.

Oral corticosteroids Oral corticosteroids are potent at resolving and preventing most allergic disease. Unfortunately, the usefulness of chronic systemic corticosteroid use is limited by the potentially devastating side effects of these agents, which include weight gain, abnormal fat deposition, adrenal suppression, cataracts, type 2 diabetes mellitus, and osteoporosis.

In general, oral corticosteroids are prescribed only for short bursts and do not require a taper, because therapy for less than 2 weeks is not associated with adrenal suppression. Longer courses are reserved for patients whose condition has been refractory to all other standard therapies.

Leukotriene Antagonists

Leukotriene antagonists (either receptor antagonists or 5-lipoxygenase inhibitors) also have anti-inflammatory properties.[18] Leukotrienes are found at sites of allergic inflammation. Although corticosteroids affect many other inflammatory pathways, they do not seem to have a clinically significant impact on the generation and release of leukotrienes. These molecules are capable of inducing further inflammation by causing the release of additional mediators, as well as the recruitment of inflammatory cells to sites of allergic disease. Consequently, leukotriene antagonists are used in the treatment of both asthma and allergic rhinitis.[19]

Theophylline

Although generally not viewed as a major therapeutic option because of their narrow therapeutic window and significant side effects, methylxanthines still have some usefulness in asthma care. Asthma treatment guidelines suggest theophylline (at a serum concentration of 5 to 15 µg/ml) to be an alternative treatment in mild and moderate persistent asthma.[20] The addition of low-dose theophylline (5 to 10 µg/ml) to inhaled corticosteroids has shown benefit in asthma, with a lower risk of side effects than with higher theophylline doses.[21] As a result, methylxanthines remain worthy of consideration as part of the therapeutic regimen, especially in patients for whom cost is an issue.

IMMUNOTHERAPY

Immunotherapy, or allergy shots, involves injecting increasing doses of the offending antigen or antigens in an attempt to attenuate the specific allergic response. Clinical trials have shown that immunotherapy is successful in treating allergic rhinitis with or without associated asthma.[22,23] An immunotherapy extract is prepared on the basis of skin-testing results. The patient then receives increasing doses subcutaneously on a weekly or twice-weekly schedule for about 5 months. After this so-called build-up phase, the patient is maintained on a stable dose that is administered weekly to monthly for several years. Usually, patients achieve maximal benefit after being on the maintenance dose for 1 year. The duration of treatment is still under investigation; therefore, the discontinuance of immunotherapy must be determined on an individual basis.

Immunotherapy is usually reserved for those patients in whom environmental and pharmacologic interventions have been less than fully successful. The only patients for whom immunotherapy is almost always indicated are those who have systemic symptoms from venom (Hymenoptera) allergy. Immunotherapy is often indicated for allergic rhinitis or asthma that is clearly associated with sensitivity to specific allergens.[24] It is also used in children, because some data suggest that early treatment of allergic rhinitis with immunotherapy may prevent the subsequent development of asthma.[25] Because of the small but real risk of anaphylaxis, immunotherapy should be given only in a medical office or in another carefully screened location, where personnel and supplies are readily available to treat reactions. Similarly, patients with an FEV_1 (forced expiratory volume in 1 second) of less than 70% of predicted or those having an asthma exacerbation should not be given immunotherapy because of the risk of developing even worse bronchospasm. Currently, there is no role for immunotherapy in the treatment of food allergies.

Standard immunotherapy (also known as conventional high-dose immunotherapy) should not be confused with other invalidated and inappropriate methods of immunotherapy. These techniques, which should be avoided, include skin-titration testing and treatment (the Rinkel method), subcutaneous provocation and neutralization, and sublingual provocation.[6]

Mitchell H. Grayson, M.D., is a current recipient of grant/research support and/or member of the speakers' bureaus for Genentech, Merck & Co., Inc., and Novartis.

Phillip E. Korenblat, M.D., F.A.C.P., is a current recipient of grant/research support, a consultant, and/or a member of the speakers' bureaus for the following companies: AstraZeneca, Aventis, Genentech, GlaxoSmithKline, Merck & Co., Inc., Novartis, and Schering.

References

1. Woolcock AJ, Peat JK: Evidence for the increase in asthma worldwide. Ciba Found Symp 206:122,1997
2. Martinez FD: The coming-of-age of the hygiene hypothesis. Respir Res 2:129, 2001
3. Lewis WH, Vinay P, Zenger VE: Airborne and Allergic Pollen of North America. Johns Hopkins University Press, Baltimore, 1983
4. Korenblat PE, Wedner HJ: Allergy, theory and practice, 2nd ed. WB Saunders Co, Philadelphia, 1992, p 210
5. Naclerio R, Solomon W: Rhinitis and inhalant allergens. JAMA 278:1842, 1997
6. Practice parameters for allergy diagnostic testing. Joint Task Force on Practice Parameters for the Diagnosis and Treatment of Asthma. The American Academy of Allergy, Asthma and Immunology and the American College of Allergy, Asthma and Immunology. Ann Allergy Asthma Immunol 75:543, 1995
7. Lockey RF, Benedict LM, Turkeltaub PC, et al: Fatalities from immunotherapy and skin testing. J Allergy Clin Immunol 79:660, 1987
8. Van Niekerk CH, Prinsloo AE: Effect of skin pigmentation on the response to intradermal histamine. Int Arch Allergy Appl Immunol 76:73, 1985
9. Day J: Pros and cons of the use of antihistamines in managing allergic rhinitis. J Allergy Clin Immunol 103:S395, 1999
10. Busse WW: Anti-immunoglobulin E (omalizumab) therapy in allergic asthma. Am J Respir Crit Care Med 164:S12, 2001
11. Casale TB: Anti-immunoglobulin E (omalizumab) therapy in seasonal allergic rhinitis. Am J Respir Crit Care Med 164:S18, 2001
12. Casale TB, Condemi J, LaForce C, et al: Effect of omalizumab on symptoms of seasonal allergic rhinitis: a randomized controlled trial. JAMA 286:2956, 2001
13. Bousquet J, Wenzel S, Holgate S, et al: Predicting response to omalizumab, an anti-IgE antibody, in patients with allergic asthma. Chest 125:1378, 2004
14. Sears MR: Asthma treatment: inhaled beta-agonists. Can Respir J 5(suppl A):54A, 1998
15. Taylor DR, Sears MR, Cockcroft DW: The beta-agonist controversy. Med Clin North Am 80:719, 1996
16. Corren J: Intranasal corticosteroids for allergic rhinitis: how do different agents compare? J Allergy Clin Immunol 104:S144, 1999
17. O'Byrne PM: Inhaled corticosteroids in asthma: importance of early intervention. Inhaled Glucocorticoids in Asthma: Mechanisms and Clinical Actions. Schleimer RP, Busse WW, O'Byrne P, Eds. Marcel Dekker, New York, 1996, p 493
18. O'Byrne PM, Israel E, Drazen JM: Antileukotrienes in the treatment of asthma. Ann Intern Med 127:472, 1997
19. Grayson MH, Bochner BS: New concepts in the pathogenesis and treatment of allergic asthma. Mt Sinai J Med 65:246, 1998
20. National asthma education and prevention program expert panel report 2: guidelines for the diagnosis and management of asthma (NIH Publication No. 97-4051). National Institutes of Health, Bethesda, Maryland, 2002 http://www.nhlbi.nih.gov/guidelines/asthma/asthgdln.htm
21. Evans DJ, Taylor DA, Zetterstrom O, et al: A comparison of low-dose inhaled budesonide plus theophylline and high-dose inhaled budesonide for moderate asthma. N Engl J Med 337:1412, 1997
22. Dykewicz MS, Fineman S, Skoner DP, et al: Diagnosis and management of rhinitis: complete guidelines of the Joint Task Force on Practice Parameters in Allergy, Asthma and Immunology. American Academy of Allergy, Asthma, and Immunology. Ann Allergy Asthma Immunol 81:478, 1998
23. Abramson MJ, Puy RM, Weiner JJ: Is allergen immunotherapy effective in asthma? A meta-analysis of randomized controlled trials. Am J Respir Crit Care Med 151:969, 1995
24. Bousquet J, Lockey R, Malling HJ: Allergen immunotherapy: therapeutic vaccines for allergic diseases. A WHO position paper. J Allergy Clin Immunol 102:558, 1998
25. Jacobsen L: Preventive aspects of immunotherapy: prevention for children at risk of developing asthma. Ann Allergy Asthma Immunol 87(suppl):43, 2001

Acknowledgments

Figure 1   Tom Moore.
Figure 2   Seward Hung.

106 Allergic Rhinitis, Conjunctivitis, and Sinusitis

Raymond G. Slavin, M.D., F.A.C.P.

Allergic rhinitis, conjunctivitis, and sinusitis are closely related disorders. Allergic rhinitis and conjunctivitis share the same causes and pathophysiology; sinusitis typically occurs as a complication of allergic rhinitis.

Allergic Rhinitis

Allergic rhinitis is an allergic inflammatory response in the nose. It can be classified as seasonal or perennial, depending on the allergens triggering the reaction.

EPIDEMIOLOGY

Allergic rhinitis is the most common atopic disorder in the United States. It affects about 24 million Americans—an estimated 8% of the population—with an equal distribution between males and females.[1] The prevalence of allergic rhinitis varies by age: 32% of patients are 17 years of age or younger, 43% are 18 to 44 years of age, 17% are 45 to 64, and only 8% are 65 years of age or older. The costs of treating allergic rhinitis (and indirect costs of the disorder, such as lowered productivity and time lost from work or school) are substantial. The total direct health care cost of treating allergic rhinitis is estimated at $3.4 billion.[1]

ETIOLOGY AND PATHOPHYSIOLOGY

The airborne allergens responsible for allergic rhinitis can be divided into seasonal (trees, grass, weeds, and mold) and nonseasonal or perennial (house dust mites, pets, insects).[2] These aeroallergens land on the nasal mucosa, are processed by antigen-presenting cells, and are then presented to helper T cells. In genetically predisposed persons, this interaction promotes the generation and release of cytokines that induce B cells to produce antigen-specific IgE. The IgE attaches to receptors on mast cells and basophils, and the patient is thereby sensitized. On subsequent exposure, the allergen bridges IgE molecules, resulting in release of mediators, most notably histamine.[3] Histamine causes increased epithelial permeability, vasodilatation, and stimulation of a parasympathetic reflex. As a result, acetylcholine is released, resulting in marked hypersecretion of mucus and increased blood flow. Activation of centers in the central nervous system results in sneezing.

DIAGNOSIS

Clinical Manifestations

Symptoms of allergic rhinitis may include paroxysms of sneezing, nasal congestion, clear rhinorrhea, and itching of the nose and palate. Distinct temporal patterns of symptom production may aid diagnosis. For example, seasonal allergic rhinitis symptoms typically appear during a specific time of the year when aeroallergens are abundant in the outside air. Symptoms of rhinitis that occur whenever the patient is exposed to a pet with fur suggest IgE-mediated sensitivity to that species.[4] Allergic rhinitis may result in fatigue and significant disability.

Physical Examination

The patient with allergic rhinitis may appear uncomfortable, exhibiting mouth breathing. Children in particular may have so-called allergic shiners (dark rings under the eyes). Allergic shiners develop because the edematous nasal tissue compresses the veins that drain the eyes, leading to pooling of blood under the orbits. On the bridge of the nose, a so-called allergic crease may be present—a result of continued upward rubbing of the tip of the nose (the so-called allergic salute). On nasal examination, the mucosa typically appears pale and swollen, with a bluish-gray appearance when the mucosal edema is severe. Many patients have a normal examination, although they often may be sneezing and have rhinorrhea with mucosal edema. The other physical findings tend to be present in the more severely affected patients.

Laboratory Testing

Although a careful history is the most important step toward the diagnosis of allergic disease, skin testing may be useful in pinpointing the offending allergen [*see Chapter 105*]. The simplicity, ease and rapidity of performance, low cost, and high sensitivity of skin testing make such tests preferable to in vitro testing.[5]

DIFFERENTIAL DIAGNOSIS

The two nasal conditions most commonly confused with allergic rhinitis are infectious rhinitis and perennial nonallergic rhinitis (vasomotor rhinitis). Infectious rhinitis is characterized by constitutional symptoms and purulent rhinorrhea. A nasal smear shows a preponderance of neutrophils, whereas in allergic rhinitis, eosinophils predominate. Perennial nonallergic rhinitis is more frequent in women and is precipitated by such nonspecific factors as changes in temperature, humidity, and barometric pressure; strong odors; alcohol; and cigarette smoke. Nasal congestion frequently shifts from side to side and is often alleviated by exercise.[6]

TREATMENT

Therapy for allergic rhinitis comprises three elements: first, minimizing contact with the allergen (environmental control); second, pharmacotherapy; and third, immunotherapy, which is reserved for selected patients. Together, these treatments ensure an excellent prognosis for allergic rhinitis.

Environmental Control

Reducing or completely avoiding the offending allergen is a vital part of allergy management [*see Chapter 105*]. In the case of seasonal allergies, keeping the doors and windows closed and the air conditioning on will reduce the aeroallergen burden manyfold.[7] Measures to avoid house dust mites should focus on the patient's bedroom and include encasing the mattress, box spring, and pillows in occlusive covers; weekly washing of bedding at 130° F or hotter, dehumidification to less than 50%; and removal of reservoirs, such as carpeting. Removal of pets is the optimal approach for pet-sensitive patients. If the patient will not part with the pet, weekly washing of the animal will reduce airborne levels of its allergen.[8] Also, patients with allergic rhinitis appear to be more sensitive to nonspecific irritants, such as cigarette smoke.[9]

Pharmacotherapy

Oral antihistamines are effective in reducing itching, sneezing, and rhinorrhea from allergic rhinitis. A major limitation of the first-generation (classic) antihistamines has been sedation. The second-generation antihistamines—cetirizine (Zyrtec), fexofenadine (Allegra), and loratadine (Claritin) and its metabolite desloratadine (Clarinex)—produce significantly less sedation. In patients with nasal congestion, an antihistamine-decongestant combination can be used.[10] An intranasal antihistamine spray (Astelin) has also proved to be efficacious. In severe cases, a short course of oral corticosteroids may be needed.

The most effective medications for controlling symptoms of allergic rhinitis are nasally inhaled corticosteroids.[11] They include beclomethasone (Beconase), budesonide (Rhinocort), flunisolide (Flonase), mometasone (Nasonex), and triamcinolone (Nasacort). These agents are generally not associated with significant systemic side effects. Local side effects (e.g., nasal irritation and a burning sensation) are minimized if patients are instructed to direct the spray toward the ear and away from the septum.

Leukotriene receptor antagonists have been approved for use in allergic rhinitis and can be considered as a component of combination therapy, particularly if there is associated asthma.

Omalizumab (Xolair) is a recombinant, humanized, monoclonal anti-IgE antibody for treatment of moderate to severe asthma. It has been shown to significantly reduce serum IgE and to have beneficial effects on allergic rhinitis.[12] However, its cost and the present indication by the Food and Drug Administration only for asthma preclude its routine use in allergic rhinitis.

Immunotherapy

Allergen immunotherapy is highly effective in controlling symptoms of allergic rhinitis. It should be considered in patients with severe symptoms that cannot be controlled by other treatment modalities and in those with comorbid conditions such as asthma. Immunotherapy may prevent worsening of asthma or possibly prevent its development.[13] The effectiveness of symptomatic medications, particularly intranasal corticosteroids, has made immunotherapy less necessary.

COMPLICATIONS

There is good evidence that poorly managed allergic rhinitis can result in otitis media[14] and sinusitis.[15] Rhinitis and asthma frequently coexist.[16] More than that, rhinitis appears to be a risk factor for development of asthma,[17,18] and treatment of rhinitis can improve coexisting asthma.[19] Prevention of asthma is an especially important goal in patients with a family history of asthma or atopic disease and early sensitization to aeroallergens.[20]

Allergic Conjunctivitis

Allergic conjunctivitis is the ocular counterpart of allergic rhinitis, and the two often occur together. Approximately 70% of patients with allergic conjunctivitis have an associated atopic disease, such as allergic rhinitis, asthma, or atopic dermatitis.

EPIDEMIOLOGY

Seasonal and perennial allergic conjunctivitis are the most prevalent forms of ocular allergy. Most reports agree that allergic conjunctivitis affects up to 20% of the world's population.[21]

ETIOLOGY AND PATHOGENESIS

Allergic conjunctivitis is triggered by the same aeroallergens and results from the same pathophysiologic processes as allergic rhinitis [see Allergic Rhinitis, Etiology and Pathophysiology, above].

DIAGNOSIS

Clinical Manifestations

Patients with allergic conjunctivitis present with itching of the eyes, accompanied by tearing and a burning sensation. The reaction is usually bilateral, although unilateral conjunctivitis may occur in a patient who has had direct hand-to-eye contact with an allergen such as dog or cat dander.

The periocular tissues are usually swollen and reddened. The conjunctiva is injected, with mild to moderate chemosis, and there is a ropy mucous discharge in the tear film.

Laboratory Tests

Although examination of the ocular discharge in allergic conjunctivitis typically reveals large numbers of eosinophils, this test is almost never done. Instead, allergic conjunctivitis is generally diagnosed clinically. As with allergic rhinitis, skin testing may be performed to identify the offending allergen or allergens [see Allergic Rhinitis, Laboratory Testing, above].

DIFFERENTIAL DIAGNOSIS

The eye condition that is most likely to be confused with allergic conjunctivitis is infectious conjunctivitis (viral or bacterial). Patients with infectious conjunctivitis complain of matting of the eyelids, with a clear to mucopurulent ocular discharge. The conjunctiva is deeply red, and although a burning sensation is common, itching is not as profound as in allergic conjunctivitis. Vernal conjunctivitis, which may also be confused with allergic conjunctivitis, is a severe, bilateral recurrent condition of the eye often occurring in the spring. It is marked by intense pruritus and a typical cobblestone appearance of the upper eyelid.

TREATMENT

Because allergic conjunctivitis results from the same allergens as allergic rhinitis, environmental control measures and immunotherapy are also the same [see Allergic Rhinitis, Treatment, above].

Drug treatment for allergic conjunctivitis typically begins with a topical over-the-counter antihistamine-decongestant combination such as antazoline-naphazoline (Vasocon-A) or pheniramine-naphazoline (Naphcon-A).[21] The next line of therapy would include a selective H_1 receptor antihistamine, a category that includes ketotifen (Zaditor), epinastine (Elestat), levocabastine (Livostin), azelastine (Optivar), and olopatadine (Patanol). Ketotifen, epinastine, and olopatadine also have mast cell-stabilizing properties. A meta-analysis confirms the benefit of topical mast cell stabilizers and antihistamines over placebo for the treatment of allergic conjunctivitis.[22] An additional therapeutic option is a nonsteroidal anti-inflammatory agent such as ketorolac (Acular).[21] For the most severe cases of allergic conjunctivitis, the clinician may consider giving corticosteroid eyedrops—loteprednol etabonate (Lotemax) or rimexolone (Vexol)—for 2 to 3 weeks. Long-term use of these agents has been

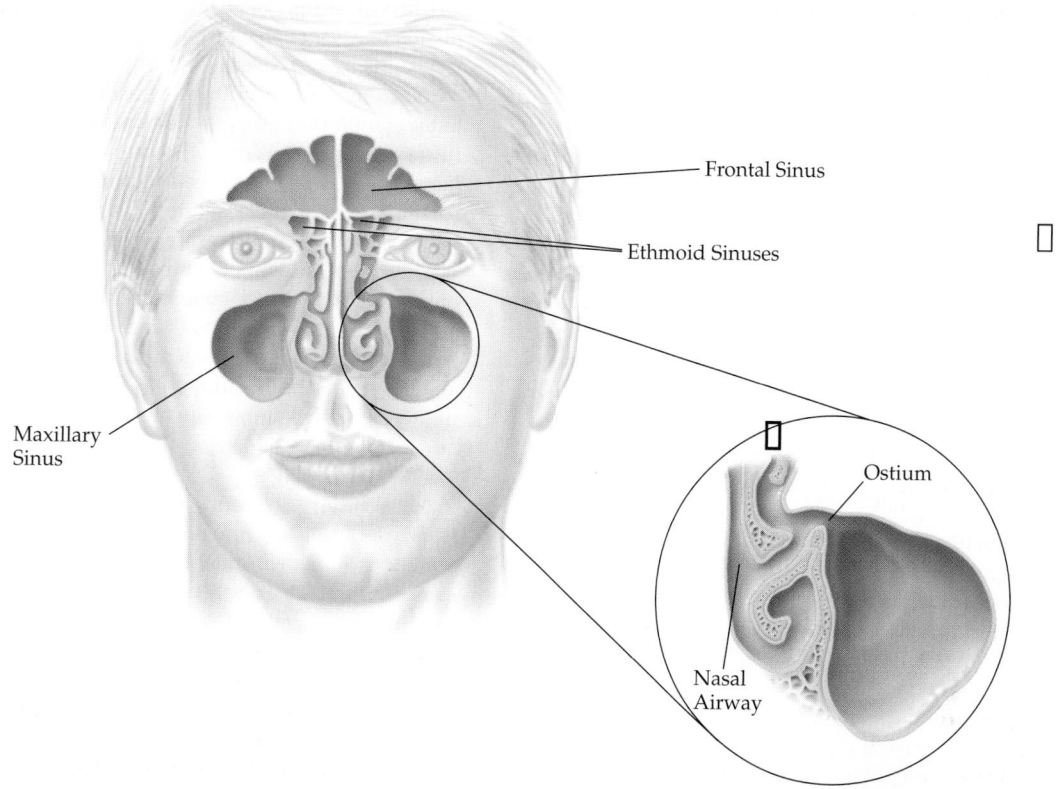

Figure 1   **The paranasal sinuses drain into the nasal passages via narrow ostia. The ostium through which the maxillary sinus drains is on the superior medial wall of the sinus, and hence the maxillary sinuses drain against the force of gravity. Edema of the nasal mucosa from allergic rhinitis can obstruct the ostia, and the resulting accumulation of mucus within the sinuses promotes bacterial infection.**

associated with the development of glaucoma, cataracts, and secondary infection and hence should be managed by an ophthalmologist.

Sinusitis

DEFINITION AND CLASSIFICATION

It has been suggested that the term rhinosinusitis may be more accurate than the term sinusitis, for the following reasons: (1) rhinitis typically precedes sinusitis, (2) sinusitis without rhinitis is rare, (3) the mucosa of the nose and sinuses are contiguous, and (4) symptoms of nasal discharge are prominent in sinusitis.[23]

Rhinosinusitis is classified as acute, recurrent acute, subacute, and chronic. Acute sinusitis is defined as inflammation of the sinuses for less than 4 weeks. Subacute sinusitis, lasting from 4 to 8 weeks, is the development and manifestation of minimal to moderate signs of sinus inflammation without an overt upper respiratory tract infection (URI) or abrupt onset of symptoms. Chronic sinusitis is defined as persistent sinus inflammation for more than 8 weeks. An operational definition of chronic sinusitis is persistent inflammation, documented with imaging techniques, continuing for at least 4 weeks after initiation of appropriate medical therapy in the absence of an intervening acute episode.

EPIDEMIOLOGY

Rhinosinusitis is the most frequently reported chronic disease in the United States, affecting 16% of the adult population.

Chronic rhinosinusitis accounts for 11.6 million physician office visits a year, and the overall direct cost in the United States is estimated to be $4.3 billion annually.[24]

In one study of patients with rhinosinusitis, a 36-item health survey showed significant worsening in several domains, including bodily pain, general health, vitality, and social functioning. Comparison with other chronic diseases (e.g., chronic obstructive pulmonary disease, heart failure, angina, and back pain) revealed significantly worse bodily pain and social functioning in patients with sinusitis.[25]

PATHOGENESIS

The paranasal sinuses are composed of the ethmoid, frontal, maxillary, and sphenoid sinuses [*see Figure 1*]. Microorganisms, pollutants, irritants, and other foreign particles that escape the filtering apparatus of the nose are trapped in the mucus of the sinuses. The steady beating of the cilia that line the sinuses moves mucus out of the sinuses and into the nasal passages via the drainage ostia. This ongoing clearance of the sinuses is important for maintaining health.

The key factors that predispose an individual to rhinosinusitis are local [*see Table 1*]. The most common of these are viral URIs and allergic rhinitis. Edema of the nasal mucosa, which is characteristic of acute infectious or allergic rhinitis, results in obstruction of the ostia, decreased ciliary action in the paranasal sinuses, and increased mucus volume and viscosity. The subsequent accumulation of mucus in the sinus provides an environment for secondary bacterial infection and the conversion of mucus to mucopus.

Cultures from both adults and children with acute sinusitis grow predominantly aerobic organisms, with the heaviest yield being *Streptococcus pneumoniae, Haemophilus influenzae,* and *Moraxella* (formerly *Branhamella*) *catarrhalis.* Although the role of viruses and bacteria in causing acute infectious sinusitis is well established, the role of microbial infection in chronic sinus disease is much less clear. It was once believed that anaerobic organisms were responsible for instances of chronic sinusitis, but aerobes have now been implicated as the major cause. A noninfectious form of chronic rhinosinusitis, sometimes referred to as chronic hyperplastic eosinophilic rhinosinusitis, is marked by a preponderance of eosinophils and mixed mononuclear cells and by a paucity of neutrophils. It is often associated with nasal polyps, asthma, and aspirin sensitivity.[26]

DIAGNOSIS

Clinical Manifestations

Acute sinusitis The most important clinical clue to the diagnosis of acute sinusitis is the failure of symptoms to resolve after a typical cold. The previously clear nasal discharge becomes yellow or green. Fever persists and chills may develop. Pain is often felt in the cheek, or it may be referred to the forehead. The discomfort is often worse on bending over or straining. If the ostium of the maxillary sinus is blocked, pain may be severe and felt in the teeth.

On physical examination, thick, purulent, green or deep-yellow secretions are seen in the nose on the side of the diseased sinus. Because the maxillary sinus is most frequently involved, purulent secretions will be seen most often in the middle meatus, which is the drainage site of the maxillary sinus [*see Chapter 125*]. The middle meatus may be hidden by the middle turbinate; as a result, it may be necessary to shrink the turbinate with a topical decongestant. Once this is accomplished, the nose, particularly the middle meatus, can be examined thoroughly not only for pus but also for underlying problems, such as nasal septal deviation, spurs, and polyps. Frequently, a streak of pus is visible along the lateral wall of the oropharynx. When the diagnosis of sinusitis is in doubt, referring the patient to an otolaryngologist for fiberoptic nasopharyngoscopy can be helpful, because this technique affords a better opportunity for visualization of the drainage ostia of infected sinuses.

Table 1 Factors Predisposing to Sinusitis

Upper respiratory infection	Allergic rhinitis
	Anatomic variants
	Septal deviation
	Haller cells (infraorbital ethmoid cells)
	Hypertrophied adenoids
	Nasal polyps, chronic mucosal thickening
	Nasal or sinus tumors
Foreign bodies	Cigarette smoke
	Swimming and diving; barotraumas
	Rhinitis medicamentosa
	Cocaine abuse
	Nasal intubation
	Periapical abscess in a protruding tooth
	Dental extraction or injections

Chronic sinusitis If mucopus is not evacuated, acute sinusitis may enter a subacute or chronic phase. Chronic maxillary sinusitis may exist alone, but it is usually associated with chronic ethmoid and frontal sinusitis. The lack of pain or systemic symptoms makes chronic sinusitis difficult to diagnose on history alone. A patient may complain of dull pressure in the face or head. Chronic sinusitis generally presents as persistent, sometimes unilateral nasal stuffiness, hyposmia, purulent nasal and postnasal secretions, sore throat, fetid breath, and malaise. The secretions often pool in the hypopharynx at night, and the patient complains of increasing postnasal drainage with resultant cough and, sometimes, wheezing. On physical examination, a patient with chronic sinusitis may display an edematous and hyperemic nasal mucosa bathed in mucopus. Nasal polyps may accompany chronic sinusitis.

Nasal Smear and Sinus Culture

Nasal culture does not give an adequate picture of the organisms responsible for sinusitis. Microscopic examination of nasal secretions, however, may be of great diagnostic value. In instances of sinusitis, one sees sheets of polymorphonucleur neutrophils and bacteria. This is unlike viral URIs, in which polymorphonuclear neutrophils are scanty, or allergic rhinitis, in which a high percentage of eosinophils may be seen. Antral puncture provides a true specimen of the microbiology of the sinus cavity and is generally performed by an otolaryngologist when it is important to determine the pathogen (e.g., if fungal infection is suspected).[27]

Radiology

Two imaging modalities are used for the diagnosis of sinusitis: plain x-rays and computed tomography. In adults, plain films of the sinuses that show mucosal thickening greater than 8 mm, an air-fluid level, or opacification have been shown to correlate with positive bacterial cultures on antral punctures. In children older than 1 year, abnormal findings on maxillary sinus radiographs are generally related to inflammation of the upper airway. Crying has not been shown to be a cause of abnormalities on sinus radiographs in these children.[28]

The diagnostic value of plain films is controversial. Some authorities advise against plain radiographic studies, particularly for diagnosing chronic sinusitis. Conventional radiographs can depict changes of acute sinusitis in maxillary, ethmoid, frontal, and sphenoid sinuses but cannot delineate the status of individual ethmoid air cells or the osteomeatal complex, nor can they accurately show the extent of inflammatory disease in affected patients. For these reasons, CT is the radiographic modality of choice for examining the paranasal sinuses. Coronal CT scans demonstrate the osteomeatal complex and detect subtle disease that is not shown on plain films. The cost of CT scans used to be prohibitive, but through improved technology and the use of limited slices, the price has been reduced to the point where it is quite close to that of plain films in most centers. A limited four-slice coronal CT scan of the sinuses provides much more information than plain films do, and compared with full CT, four-slice coronal CT provides the increased information at a much reduced radiation dose and cost.[29]

Transillumination and ultrasonography are used in the diagnosis of sinusitis. Both are subject to great error, however, and cannot be recommended at the present time.

Ancillary Laboratory Tests

Other laboratory tests may have to be considered in some cases of treatment-resistant sinusitis. Underlying allergy can be determined by appropriate skin testing after a careful history has identified likely allergens. Immunologic testing may be indicated, because patients with refractory sinusitis may have immune dysfunction.[30] Associated immunodeficiency is diagnosed by serum immunoglobulin levels and by antibody responses to specific antigens such as pneumococci, diphtheria, and tetanus. Other considerations in medically resistant sinusitis include cystic fibrosis, fungal infection, and anatomic abnormalities.

DIFFERENTIAL DIAGNOSIS

The condition most often misdiagnosed as rhinosinusitis is a viral URI, which is the most important predisposing cause of acute rhinosinusitis. Rhinosinusitis is probably present if the URI symptoms do not resolve in 3 to 6 days; if the secretions, particularly postnasal secretions, turn yellow or green and persist throughout the day; and if the patient notes fullness of the head and discomfort in the face and teeth.

TREATMENT

Concern has been raised about the overdiagnosis of rhinosinusitis and unnecessary treatment with antibiotics of uncomplicated viral upper respiratory infection. More strict criteria for the use of antibiotics are symptoms for 10 to 14 days or severe symptoms, such as fever with purulent nasal discharge, facial pain or tenderness, and periorbital swelling.[31,32]

The antibiotic of choice for treatment of acute sinusitis is ampicillin or amoxicillin. An appropriate dosage of amoxicillin for acute sinusitis in the adult is 875 mg twice a day for 10 to 14 days. In patients with penicillin sensitivity, trimethoprim-sulfamethoxazole (one double-strength tablet twice a day) is an adequate alternative. More and more cases of β-lactamase–producing organisms are being reported. In penicillin-resistant sinusitis, recommended antibiotics include amoxicillin with clavulanic acid (Augmentin), the quinolones (e.g., levofloxacin [Levaquin]), and telithromycin (Ketek). Antibiotic treatment for chronic sinusitis should be continued for at least 2 weeks. If the patient reports feeling better by the last day of the regimen but still has purulent nasal discharge, the antibiotic can be continued for another 5 to 7 days.

Ancillary treatments for sinusitis, including oral decongestants and mucus thinners, have been advocated, but there are no controlled studies showing their effectiveness. The addition of intranasal corticosteroids may be modestly beneficial in the treatment of patients with recurrent acute or chronic rhinosinusitis.[33]

In some cases of chronic resistant sinusitis, surgical treatment must be considered. A wide array of surgical procedures are available, but functional endoscopic sinus surgery (FESS) has emerged as the technique of choice.[34]

COMPLICATIONS

Complications of sinusitis have decreased in incidence since the introduction of antibiotics. The complications most commonly encountered are cellulitis, abscess, and cavernous sinus thrombosis (all involving the orbit); epidural or subdural abscess; mucocele formation; and osteomyelitis.[35] It is evident in both children[36] and adults[37] not only that there is an association between sinusitis and asthma but also that sinusitis is an important trigger for asthma. In a patient who has both sinusitis and asthma, the asthma will be difficult to manage until the sinusitis is brought under control by either medical or surgical means.

PROGNOSIS

The prognosis for patients with sinusitis should be excellent if the diagnosis is made accurately and promptly and an appropriate antibiotic is administered for a sufficient period of time. Consultation with a specialist should be sought in the following situations:

- If there is a need to clarify the allergic or immunologic basis for sinusitis.
- If sinusitis is refractory to the usual antibiotic treatment.
- If sinusitis is recurrent.
- If sinusitis is associated with unusual opportunistic infections.
- If sinusitis significantly affects performance and quality of life.

Consultation is also appropriate when concomitant conditions are present that complicate assessment or treatment, including chronic otitis media, bronchial asthma, nasal polyps, recurrent pneumonia, immunodeficiencies, aspirin sensitivity, allergic fungal disease, granulomas, and multiple antibiotic sensitivities.

The author has received grants for clinical research from Genentech, Inc., and for educational activities from AstraZeneca Pharmaceuticals LP and has served as a consultant for Dey, Inc., and Aventis.

References

1. Law AW, Reed SD, Sundy JS, et al: Direct costs of allergic rhinitis in the United States: Estimates from the 1996 medical expenditure panel survey. J Allergy Clin Immunol 111:296, 2003

2. Badhwar AK, Druce HM: Allergic rhinitis. Med Clin North Am 76:789, 1992

3. Naclerio RM: Allergic rhinitis. N Engl J Med 325:860, 1991

4. Norman PS: Allergic rhinitis. J Allergy Clin Immunol 75:531, 1985

5. Dykewicz MS, Fineman S: Executive Summary of Joint Task Force Practice Parameters on diagnosis and management of rhinitis. Ann Allergy Asthma Immunol 81:463, 1998

6. Zeiger RS: Allergic and non-allergic rhinitis: classification and pathogenesis (pts 1 and 2). Am J Rhinol 3:21, 113, 1989

7. Nelson HS, Hirsch SR, Ohman JL, et al: Recommendations for the use of residential air-cleaning devices in the treatment of allergic respiratory disease. J Allergy Clin Immunol 82:661, 1988

8. Patel NJ, Bush RK: Role of environmental allergens in rhinitis. Immunol Allergy Clin North Am 20:323, 2000

9. Effect of passive smoking on respiratory symptoms, bronchial responsiveness, lung function, and total serum IgE in the European Community Respiratory Health Survey: a cross-sectional study. European Community Respiratory Health Survey. Lancet 358:2103, 2001

10. Corren J: Allergic rhinitis: treating the adult. J Allergy Clin Immunol 105:S610, 2000

11. Kaszuba SM, Baroody FM, deTineo M, et al: Superiority of an intranasal corticosteroid compared with an oral antihistamine in the as-needed treatment of seasonal allergic rhinitis. Arch Intern Med 161:2581, 2001

12. Casale TB, Condemi J, LaForce C, et al: Effect of omalizumab on symptoms of seasonal allergic rhinitis: a randomized controlled trial. JAMA 286:2956, 2001

13. Durham SR, Walker JM, Varga EM, et al: Long term clinical efficacy of grass pollen immunotherapy. N Engl J Med 341:468, 1999

14. Rachelefsky GS: National guidelines needed to manage rhinitis and prevent complications. Ann Allergy Asthma Immunol 82:296, 1999

15. Skoner DP: Complications of allergic rhinitis. J Allergy Clin Immunol 105:S605, 2000

16. Fox RW, Lockey RF: The impact of rhinosinusitis on asthma. Curr Allergy Asthma Rep 3:513, 2003

17. Greisner WA 3rd, Settipane RJ, Settipane GA: The course of asthma parallels that of allergic rhinitis: a 23-year follow-up study of college students. Allergy Asthma Proc 21:371, 2000

18. Leynaert B, Neukirch C, Kony S, et al: Association between asthma and rhinitis according to atopic sensitization in a population-based study. J Allergy Clin Immunol 113:86, 2004

19. Bousquet J, van Cauwenberge P, Khaltaev N: Allergic rhinitis and its impact on

asthma: area workshop report. J Allergy Clin Immunol 108:147, 2001

20. What are the candidate groups for pharmacotherapeutic intervention to prevent asthma? ETAC Study Group. Pediatr Allergy Immunol 11(suppl 13):41, 2000

21. Bielory L: Allergic and immunologic disorders of the eye. J Allergy Clin Immunol 106:1019, 2000

22. Owen CG, Shah A, Henshaw K, et al: Topical treatments for seasonal allergic conjunctivitis: systematic review and meta-analysis of efficacy and effectiveness. Br J Gen Pract 54:451, 2004

23. Kaliner MA, Osguthorpe JD, Fireman P: Sinusitis: bench to bedside. J Allergy Clin Immunol 99:S829, 1997

24. Anand VK: Epidemiology and economic impact of rhinosinusitis. Ann Otol Rhinol Laryngol Suppl 193:3, 2004

25. Gliklich RE, Metson R: The health impact of chronic sinusitis in patients seeking otolaryngologic care. Otolaryngol Head Neck Surg 113:104, 1995

26. Hamilos D: Chronic sinusitis. J Allergy Clin Immunol 106:213, 2000

27. Orlandi RR: Biopsy and specimen collection in chronic rhinosinusitis. Ann Otol Rhinol Laryngol Suppl 193:24, 2004

28. Kovatch AL, Wald ER, Ledesma-Medina J, et al: Maxillary sinus radiographs in children with nonrespiratory complaints. Pediatrics 73:306, 1984

29. Wippold FJ II, Levitt RG, Evens RG, et al: Limited coronal CT: an alternative screening examination for sinonasal inflammatory disease. Allergy Proc 16:165, 1995

30. Chee L, Graham SM, Carothers DG, et al: Immune dysfunction in refractory sinusitis in a tertiary care setting. Laryngoscope 111:233, 2001

31. Clinical Practice Guidelines: management of sinusitis. American Academy of Pediatrics. Subcommittee on the Management of Sinusitis and Committee on Quality Improvement. Pediatrics 108:798, 2001

32. Snow V, Mottur-Pilson C, Hickner JM, et al: Principles of appropriate antibiotic use for acute rhinosinusitis in adults. Ann Intern Med 134:495, 2001

33. Lund V, Black S, Laszlo ZS, et al: Budesonide aqueous nasal spray is effective as monotherapy in stable patients with chronic rhinosinusitis. J Allergy Clin Immunol 109:290, 2002

34. Kennedy DW: Functional endoscopic sinus surgery technique. Arch Otolaryngol 111:643, 1985

35. Sheffield RW, Cassisi NJ, Karlan MS: Complications of sinusitis: what to watch for. Postgrad Med 63:93, 1978

36. Rachelefsky GS, Katz RM, Siegal SC: Chronic sinus disease with associated reactive airway disease in children. Pediatrics 73:526, 1984

37. Slavin RG: Relationship of nasal disease and sinusitis to bronchial asthma. Ann Allergy 49:76, 1982

Acknowledgment

Figure 1   Alice Y. Chen.

107 Urticaria, Angioedema, and Anaphylaxis

Vincent S. Beltrani, M.D.

Urticaria (hives), angioedema, and anaphylaxis are the prototypical manifestations of mast cell activation. The common denominator in these conditions is the release of potent inflammatory mediators from activated mast cells[1] [*see Chapter 104*]. Urticaria and angioedema are effected primarily by activation of cutaneous mast cells, which are preferentially located around capillaries, lymphatics, appendages, and nerves in the skin. Massive activation of mast cells in the intestinal tract, respiratory tract, and central nervous system produces the multisystemic, potentially catastrophic symptom complex of anaphylaxis.

Although the three conditions have common features and may occur in various combinations, they are more easily understood when discussed individually.

Urticaria

Urticaria is a cutaneous eruption that consists of erythematous, pruritic wheals. Although urticaria is typically transient, it can be persistent, with lesions occurring for weeks to months.

EPIDEMIOLOGY

Urticaria is a common problem, with 15% to 23% of the general population experiencing at least one episode in their lifetime.[2,3] The precise prevalence of urticaria may never be known. Many patients experience transient episodes of hives and do not report them to a health care provider because of their readily identifiable cause, inconsequential nature, and spontaneous resolution. If the papular urticaria that develops after an arthropod bite is included in the spectrum of urticarial lesions, urticaria must be considered a virtually universal human experience.

ETIOLOGY

Injecting histamine into the skin will produce the so-called triple response of Lewis—a prototypical hive. This response comprises the following: (1) erythema, the clinical manifestation of vasodilatation; (2) a wheal, the result of vascular leakage; and (3) pruritus, caused by activation of dendritic itch receptors on nonmyelinated C fibers (neurons) in the epidermis [*see Table 1*]. A fourth feature of intradermally injected histamine is its spontaneous dissipation within 1 hour. Urticaria lasting longer than 1 hour is not caused solely by histamine. Multiple inflammatory mediators have been identified in the effluent of urticarial lesions, and some of these vasoactive mediators (e.g., prostaglandin D_2 and platelet-activating factor) have produced urticaria—with and without pruritus—lasting longer than 1 hour when injected subcutaneously.

PATHOGENESIS

Because histamine plays a leading role in the pathogenesis of urticaria, tracing the source and mechanism of histamine release is the key to understanding urticarial lesions. Most of the body's histamine is stored in tissue mast cells; much smaller amounts are present in basophils and CNS neurons. Mast cells at different anatomic locations, and even at a single site, can vary substantially in mediator content, sensitivity to agents that induce activation, quantity of mediator released, and response to pharmacologic agents.[1] Agents having the ability to initiate the release of mediators from mast cells are called secretagogues. There is debate regarding whether the number of cutaneous mast cells in patients with persistent urticaria increases[4] or remains unchanged.[5] However, it has been generally agreed that these cells have a lower threshold for mediator release. Thus, a more appropriate label for chronic or idiopathic urticaria would be twitchy mast cell syndrome.

A practical categorization of urticaria is a three-part classification based on the etiology and mechanism of mast cell degranulation [*see Table 2*]. The first category comprises cases with an identifiable cause; the second, idiopathic cases; and the third, mastocytosis. Mastocytosis encompasses a wide spectrum of clinical conditions, characterized by a localized or diffuse increase in mast cells in the skin or internal organs. Most cases of mastocytosis are transient, which suggests that this disorder represents a hyperplastic response to abnormal stimuli rather than a true neoplastic process.

DIAGNOSIS

The diagnosis of urticaria is made almost exclusively from an appropriate, complete history. The history should include questions about substances or circumstances that may trigger the urticaria; the clinical features of the urticaria, including its duration, the presence and degree of pruritus, and whether the urticaria is localized or generalized; underlying illnesses; any previous diagnostic procedures or therapy for the condition; and family history of urticaria. A personal or family history of atopy should also be noted. Although the occurrence of urticaria with identifiable triggers is increased in atopic patients, whether the incidence of atopic disease is higher in patients with idiopathic urticaria remains debatable.[6,7]

Many patients presenting with IgE-induced urticaria can identify the cause of their generalized, very pruritic, explosive hives. By merely avoiding that trigger, they remain symptom

Table 1 Pathologic Changes in Urticaria and Their Associated Mediators

Symptom	Pathologic Event	Mediators
Wheal	Vascular permeability	Histamine (H_1) Prostaglandin D_2 Platelet activating factor Bradykinin Leukotrienes C4, D4, E4
Flare	Vasodilatation	Histamine (H_1) Prostaglandin D_2 Platelet activating factor Bradykinin Leukotrienes C4, D4, E4
Pruritus	Sensory nerve stimulation	Histamine (H_1)

Table 2 Classification of Urticarial Lesions

Identifiable cause
  Immunologic
  Nonimmunologic (e.g., cyclooxygenase pathway, opiates)
  Physical urticaria
    Aquagenic urticaria
    Cholinergic urticaria
    Cold urticaria
    Contact urticaria (e.g., jellyfish, nettles)
    Delayed pressure
    Dermatographism
    Solar urticaria
    Vibratory urticaria
Nonidentifiable cause (idiopathic)
  Persistent — occurring almost daily
  Episodic — recurrent, with days of no hives between episodes
  Associated with an underlying disease
    Anaphylaxis (IgE-induced)
    Anaphylactoid (non–IgE-induced)
    Bullous pemphigoid
    Erythema multiforme
    Leukocytoclastic vasculitis
    Serum sickness (via immune complexes)
    Systemic lupus erythematosus
    Viral syndrome (via immune complexes)
Mastocytosis
  Mastocytoma
    Urticaria pigmentosa
    Diffuse cutaneous mastocytosis
    Telangiectasia macularis eruptiva perstans (TMEP)
  Systemic mastocytosis

free. These patients are at greater risk of developing fatal anaphylactic reactions, with or without urticaria.

Common Triggers of Urticaria

Before concluding that urticaria is idiopathic, the clinician must complete a systematic review of possible mast cell secretagogues. These include immunologic and nonimmunologic activators, as well as some whose mechanism is unknown [*see* Table 3].

Drugs Drugs are probably the most easily recognized of the identifiable causes of urticaria because the symptoms usually appear within 36 hours of administration of the drug.[8] The penicillins, aspirin and other nonsteroidal anti-inflammatory drugs (NSAIDs), and sulfa drugs are most commonly involved, but virtually any drug may elicit urticaria. When urticaria develops within 1 to 2 weeks after initiation of therapy with a drug that is known to cause urticaria, that drug must be suspected.

Drugs can cause urticaria via immunologic and nonimmunologic mechanisms. The best understood mechanism involves drug-specific IgE antibodies. These IgE-induced reactions typically arise within 2 weeks after a drug is started, are not dose-related, occur from seconds to minutes after administration of the drug, and may herald an anaphylactic episode [*see* Figure 1].[8] Non-IgE reactions to drugs (e.g., aspirin or other NSAIDs, opioids, and vancomycin) can occur on first exposure or from hours to days after ingestion, are dose related, and may herald an anaphylactoid reaction.[9]

Although urticarial reactions to aspirin and other NSAIDs are rarely induced through IgE, they occur most frequently in atopic persons.[10] Angioedema, with or without urticaria, is the most common symptom of NSAID hypersensitivity. Respiratory symptoms are not more likely to occur in patients who develop an urticarial reaction from an NSAID. Some cyclooxygenase-2 (COX-2) inhibitors, especially rofecoxib, are relatively safe in patients who experience urticaria or angioedema from standard NSAIDs.[11] Patients whose history suggests a non-IgE drug reaction should not undergo routine skin testing and radioallergosorbent testing (RAST) [*see* Chapter 105].

Drug-specific IgE antibodies can be detected by skin testing, but penicillin is the only antibiotic for which reliable skin-test reagents have been developed. Standardized antigens for penicillin include penicilloyl-poly-L-lysine (penicilloyl polylysine), which is considered the major determinant and is commercially available, and several investigational minor determinants. With these reagents, numerous studies have documented the presence of penicillin-specific IgE antibodies in patients who have experienced penicillin-induced urticaria. In contrast, IgE antibodies to other antibiotics have not been demonstrated routinely in patients who have experienced an antibiotic-induced urticaria. Although it is possible that these reactions are not IgE mediated, it is more likely that the IgE antibodies have not been detected because the patients had antibodies directed against a drug metabolite not used in the testing.[12] Consequently, the diagnostic test for confirming drugs (other than the penicillins) as an identifiable cause of an individual's urticaria is to carefully rechallenge the patient, under direct medical su-

Table 3 Mast Cell Secretagogues

Immunologic activators (act on receptors)	IgE antigens (e.g., foods, drugs, latex)
	IgG directed against IgE (autoimmunity)
	  Anti-FcεRI (IgE receptor) antibodies
	Lectins (e.g., strawberries, conconavalin A)
	Neuropeptides (e.g., substance P, somatostatin)
	Complement activators (C3a, C5a)
	Radiocontrast media
	Blood products
	Cytokines
	  IL-1, IL-3, IL-6
	  Granulocyte-macrophage colony-stimulating factor
	  Histamine-releasing factors (HRF)
	  c-*kit* ligand

Nonimmunologic activators	Ionophores (opiates, adrenocorticotropic hormone [ACTH], compound 48/80) Arachidonic acid metabolic pathway inhibition (nonsteroidal anti-inflammatory drugs) Direct effect on cell Opiates (e.g., morphine, codeine) Radiocontrast media Peptides Jellyfish, lobster, eosinophil major basic protein (EMB), polymyxin B, defensins Irradiation Dextran Physical contact (pressure, light, water)
Mechanism unknown	Alcohol, amphetamine, bradykinin, ciprofloxacin, papaverine, rifampin, thiamine, thiopental, tolazoline, vancomycin

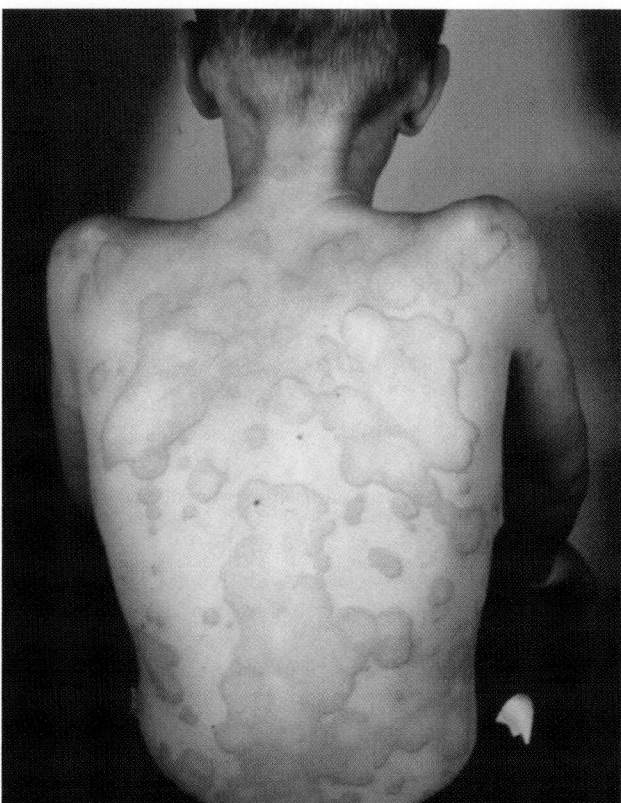

Figure 1 **Generalized, symmetrical, very pruritic urticaria appeared within 10 minutes of an intramuscular injection of penicillin G in this boy. The reaction is polymorphic, with papular urticaria evolving to larger, evanescent urticarial plaques that appear annular because of central clearing. The patient in this photograph subsequently demonstrated a positive prick test to the penicillin allergen penicilloyl polylysine.**

pervision, several weeks after the original episode has resolved. In practice, this is rarely done unless the drug in question is absolutely required to treat a disease.

Foods Foods and additives are the second most easily recognized IgE-induced trigger. Symptoms usually appear within 1 hour after ingestion, and in 80% of these cases, GI symptoms (e.g., cramps, diarrhea, and nausea and vomiting) also occur. Respiratory or, less frequently, cardiovascular symptoms may also accompany or precede cutaneous reactions.[13]

Foods are a common cause of urticaria.[14,15] Although studies of different populations of patients with urticaria provide estimates of the prevalence of food-induced urticaria, prevalence in the general population is unknown. Determining prevalence is complicated by the fact that even in patients with histories of adverse reactions to foods, only about 60% or fewer have reproducible reaction to foods.[16]

Urticarial reactions to foods may result from exposure by ingestion, injection, contact, or inhalation. Eggs, peanuts, milk, nuts, soy, wheat, fish, and shellfish are the foods most often implicated in allergic reactions, but IgE-mediated reactions to numerous other foods and to contaminating substances in foods, such as molds or antibiotics, have been reported.[17] Certain foods, such as egg white, strawberries, and shellfish, have been shown to contain substances that liberate histamine directly through a nonimmunologic mechanism.[18] Urticaria can also result from the ingestion of foods that contain large amounts of histamine, either naturally or as a result of spoilage (e.g., scombroidosis) [*see Chapter 15*].

Some children who experience urticaria after exposure to certain foods such as milk, eggs, soy, or wheat early in life may later tolerate these foods without difficulty. Loss of sensitivity to foods such as peanuts,[19] nuts, or fish may occur less frequently.[20]

The diagnostic tools available to determine whether foods play a role in the production of urticaria in a patient include the history, physical examination, skin testing or RAST, diet and symptom diaries, elimination diets, and food challenges. Although slightly less sensitive than skin-prick test, RASTs for specific IgE antibodies are more widely available; they require only a serum sample and are performed by commercial laboratories, and therefore, they are practical in most primary care practices. As with skin tests, a negative result is very reliable in ruling out an IgE-mediated reaction to a particular food, but a positive result has low specificity.[21] Many patients have positive skin tests and RASTs to several members of a botanical or animal species, indicating immunologic cross-reactivity, but very few patients have symptomatic intrabotanical or intraspecies cross-reactivity. The practice of avoiding all foods within a botanical family when one member is suspected of provoking allergic symptoms generally appears to be unwarranted.[21]

Occupational and hobby exposures Contact urticarial reactions are seen in certain occupational situations, such as health care workers (latex induced) and food handlers (shellfish). Atopic individuals are at a higher risk of developing these immediate-type contact reactions, which may present as pruritus, urticaria, or anaphylaxis.

Latex or natural-rubber latex hypersensitivity is a fairly common identifiable IgE-induced cause of urticaria [*see Chapter 39*]. These patients may experience localized urticaria at the contact area, generalized urticaria with angioedema, or urticaria with systemic involvement (including anaphylaxis). The diagnosis is made from a history of exposure and confirmed by a skin-prick test or RAST.

Systemic illness Urticaria occurs in a variety of autoimmune and infectious diseases. Urticaria is rarely the sole symptom of an underlying disease, however. If the history and physical examination do not suggest an underlying problem, routine laboratory testing is not indicated.

Generalized, urticarial lesions that persist for longer than 24 hours or that burn or sting more than they itch may be a manifestation of rheumatoid arthritis, systemic lupus erythematosus, or other rheumatic disease. Lesions associated with rheumatic illness usually do not blanch on diascopy and may leave ecchymosis and eventually hyperpigmentation. Patients who present in this manner should be assessed for rheumatic disease [*see Chapter 111*].

Approximately 5% to 10% of patients with chronic urticaria have been reported to have antithyroid antibodies but are clinically and biochemically euthyroid.[22,23] For that reason, autoimmune thyroid serologic studies have been recommended for patients with chronic urticaria.[24] There is only anecdotal evidence that treating these patients with exogenous thyroid hormone leads to significant improvement of their urticaria, however.[25,26]

Changes in mast cell reactivity apparently can be part of the immune response to infection. Urticaria reportedly can be a feature of streptococcal pharyngitis, otitis media, infectious mononucleosis, and hepatitis (a slightly higher incidence of hepatitis C antibodies has been reported in patients with urticaria, but whether there is a causal relationship is questionable). Pathogens reportedly associated with urticaria include coxsackievirus, *Mycoplasma*, fungi, and *Candida*. A causative relationship of urticaria with *Helicobacter pylori* has not been confirmed.[27,28] Extensive searches for occult focal infections (e.g., sinusitis) as the cause of urticaria are consistently unsuccessful.[29]

A number of parasitic infestations produce transient urticaria.[30] The urticaria in these patients usually appears from the second to the sixth week of infestation. Random examinations of stool for ova and parasites rarely, if ever, prove positive in patients with urticaria who do not have typical symptoms of parasitic infestation.

Psychological factors Emotional stress can influence mast cell and IgE activity, resulting in the release of vasoactive mediators and exacerbations of chronic urticaria.[31] However, there is no good evidence that psychological factors by themselves can cause urticaria, so urticaria without an identifiable cause should not be dismissed as a psychosomatic illness.

Neoplasms Lymphomas and carcinomas may promote urticaria (paraneoplastic syndrome), but urticaria in patients with neoplasms is usually coincidental. In most cases, the malignancy is known; current evidence does not warrant routinely subjecting patients with unexplained urticaria to an exhaustive evaluation for an occult neoplasm.

Chronic urticaria may occur as part of Schnitzler syndrome, which also includes a monoclonal IgM gammopathy, intermittent fever, joint or bone pain, lymphadenopathy, leukocytosis, and an elevated erythrocyte sedimentation rate (ESR). In 15% of cases, Schnitzler syndrome evolves to lymphoplasmocytic malignancy.[32]

Genetic factors Several of the physical urticarias can be familial. Examples include urticaria induced by cold, heat, light, water, and vibration (see below), as well as urticaria associated with erythropoietic protoporphyria. The Muckle-Wells syndrome is a form of familial urticaria associated with deafness and amyloidosis.[33]

Localized Urticaria

Papular urticaria, some of the physical urticarias, and contact urticaria are the entities to consider when urticaria is restricted to a limited area of the body. Dermatographism, cold urticaria, delayed pressure urticaria, solar urticaria, and aquagenic urticaria are localized wheals produced by specific physical stimuli (i.e., stroking of the skin, cold, sustained pressure, ultraviolet light, and water, respectively).

Papular urticaria Papular urticaria consists of 4 to 8 mm wheals or firm papules, often in grouped clusters and especially on areas of exposed skin. Papular urticaria that is very pruritic, persists longer than typical hives, and is located on exposed parts of the body is often caused by insect bites (fleas, bedbugs, scabies, and other mites). The pattern of the eruption corresponds to the biting habits of the offending insect (e.g., mosquito bites often comprise three quasilinear lesions—referred to as breakfast, lunch, and supper), and the seasonal occurrence corresponds to the peak prevalence of that insect. IgE and IgG antibodies against mosquito antigens have been detected in human sera,[34] but there have been no reported cases of

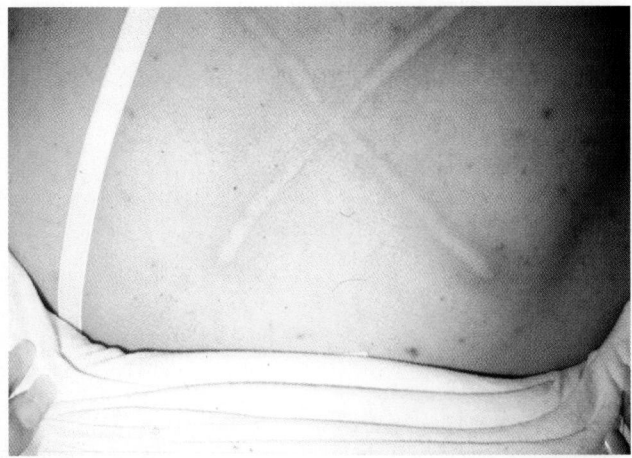

Figure 2 **Dermatographism elicited by gentle stroking of the skin of the back.**

anaphylaxis or death associated with hypersensitivity to mosquitoes. Arthropod bites are the only known cause of bulla on papular urticaria. Papular urticaria persists for 2 to 10 days and may leave postinflammatory hyperpigmentation. Occasionally, healed lesions may recrudesce when fresh crops appear.[35]

Dermatographism Firm stroking of the skin may elicit a wheal and erythema in 5% of a healthy population, but only in a minority of these persons does it also cause any pruritus (socalled symptomatic dermatographism) [*see Figure 2*]. The etiology of dermatographism is uncertain, but passive transfer tests are sometimes positive. Dermatographism (Darier sign) is a common finding in patients with idiopathic urticaria and may be associated with other conditions. For example, dermatographism can be elicited in more than 90% of patients with mastocytosis.[36] Confirmation of mastocytosis always requires biopsy, however. The elicitation of symptomatic dermatographism in patients with urticaria supports the use of both H_1 and H_2 receptor antagonists, which may more effectively reduce wheal size and duration of urticaria.[37]

Delayed pressure urticaria Urticaria that results from localized, continuous (4 to 6 hours) pressure is seen most often in patients with persistent urticaria without an identifiable cause.[38] It may be associated with systemic complaints such as myalgias, arthralgias, and fever. It responds best to aspirin or NSAIDs and poorly to antihistamines.

Cold urticaria The lesions of cold urticaria develop 5 to 30 minutes after exposure to cold and can be caused by wind, bathing, contact, or eating cold foods or drinking cold liquids.[39] Although the urticaria may appear during the period of exposure, more often it develops upon rewarming of the skin. The urticaria usually lasts approximately 30 minutes and resolves spontaneously.

Cold urticaria is often idiopathic and acquired. Patients with these lesions usually have a positive response to an ice-cube–challenge test.[40] Rare forms of acquired cold urticaria include delayed, localized, and reflex cold urticaria. In delayed cold urticaria, lesions develop several hours after exposure; localized cold urticaria lesions occur only at sites of injections or bites; and reflex cold urticaria lesions present as widespread whealing in response to a fall in core body temperature.

Much rarer than acquired forms of cold urticaria is familial cold urticaria. In this autosomal dominant disorder, lesions appear 30 minutes after exposure to generalized cooling, rather than to local application of cold, and may persist for up to 48 hours.

Solar urticaria Solar urticaria is a rare idiopathic disorder in which erythema heralds a pruritic wheal that appears within 5 minutes after exposure to a specific wavelength of light and dissipates within 15 minutes to 3 hours after onset [*see Figure 3*].[41,42] Solar urticaria is usually provoked by light in the visible spectrum, although the specific wavelength that leads to mast cell degranulation may vary from patient to patient. The severity of the reaction depends on the duration of the exposure, the intensity of the irradiation, and the light spectrum.[43] These reactions are believed to result from the development of an antigenic photoproduct, which then triggers an IgE-mediated response. Patients should usually be referred to an allergist or dermatologist for provocative testing.

Aquagenic urticaria Urticaria that appears 2 to 30 minutes after water immersion, regardless of its temperature or source (seawater or tap water) has been reported in a few patients.[44] These pruritic, follicular, cholinergic-like wheals can be reproduced by applying wet compresses to the patient's back for at least 30 minutes. It is believed that aquagenic urticaria occurs when sensitized mast cells are activated by a water-soluble antigen that diffuses through the epidermis, causing the release of acetylcholine and histamine.

Vibratory urticaria Urticaria that follows massage and vigorous toweling has been described in a single family.[45]

Contact urticaria Immediate contact reactions can appear on normal or eczematous skin within minutes to an hour after exposure. The reaction then will disappear within a few hours. Itching, tingling, or burning accompanied by erythema are the mildest form of contact reactions. They are often caused by cosmetics, fruits, and vegetables. Generalized urticaria after a local contact is a rare phenomenon, but it can occur with some allergens.[46]

Contact reactions may have either immunologic or nonimmunologic mechanisms. Immunologic mechanisms require

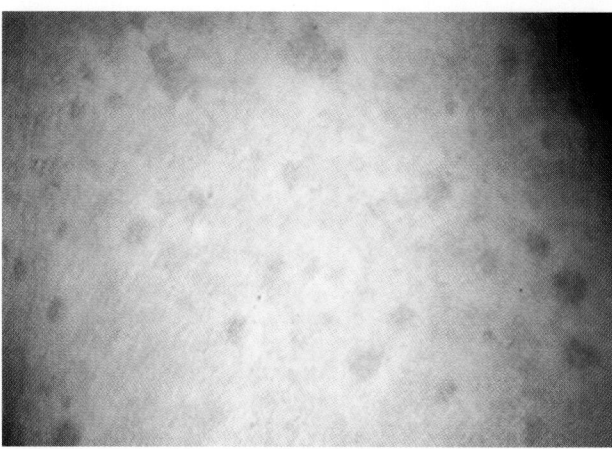

Figure 4 **Lesions of generalized urticaria tend to be symmetrical and sometimes have a halo of pallor surrounding the wheal.**

prior sensitization to the causative agent. The respiratory and gastrointestinal tracts are typically the routes of sensitization, but sensitization to natural latex and some foods may occur through the skin. The substances causing immunologic immediate contact reactions are usually proteins. Foods most commonly involved are fish, shellfish, and wheat flour. Most cases of protein contact dermatitis develop after the person has handled food products for a protracted period. Symptoms usually appear within 30 minutes after direct cutaneous contact with the offending agent.[47] Specific IgE antibodies against the causative allergen can be found by skin testing or RAST.

Most immediate contact reactions are nonimmunologic and occur without previous sensitization. These reactions remain localized. The pathophysiology of nonimmunologic immediate contact reactions has not been established, but it may involve direct influence on dermal vessel walls or a non-IgE release of inflammatory mediators. A list of chemicals that cause occupational allergic contact dermatitis can be found on the Internet at http://www.haz-map.com/allergic.htm.

Generalized Urticaria

The clinical features and natural history of generalized urticaria are as varied and unpredictable as the etiology. Generalized lesions tend to be numerous and symmetrical. Characteristically, they are intensely pruritic, especially at onset. Except for cholinergic papular urticaria, little information about the etiology can be obtained from the morphology. Individual lesions fade completely within 24 hours. Occasionally a halo of pallor surrounds the wheal [*see Figure 4*].

Cholinergic urticaria The lesions of cholinergic urticaria are highly distinctive, consisting of 2 to 3 mm scattered papular wheals surrounded by large, erythematous flares. These lesions are extremely pruritic, and they may affect the entire body but often spare the palms, soles, and axilla.[48] Precipitating stimuli include exercise, warm temperature, ingestion of hot or spicy foods, and possibly emotional stress. The condition often remits within several years but can last for more than 30 years. The diagnosis can be made by provocation with exercise or a hot bath. Cholinergic urticaria can be aborted by the prompt application of cold water or ice to the skin, and a refractory period of up to 24 hours can be induced by a hot bath.

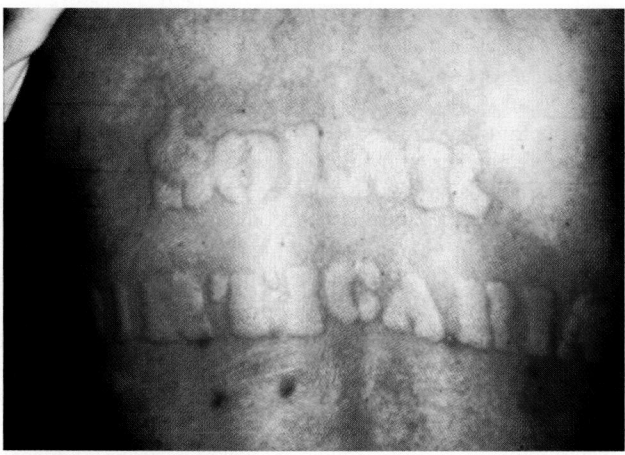

Figure 3 **Solar urticaria.**

Table 4   H$_1$ Antihistamines Available for Treatment of Urticaria

Chemical Group	Agents	Antihistaminic Activity	Sedation	Anticholinergic Activity	Cost
Ethanolamine derivatives	Diphenhydramine	+	++/+++	++	$
	Clemastine	+	++	+	$
Ethylenediamine derivatives	Tripelennamine (PBZ)	++	+	+	$
Piperidine derivatives	Azatadine	+	+	+	$$
	Cyproheptadine	+/++	+/++	+	$
	Fexofenadine (Allegra)*	++/+++	0	0	$$$
	Loratadine (Claritin)*	+/++	0	0	$$$$
Piperazine derivatives	Hydroxyzine	+++	++	+	$
	Cetirizine (Zyrtec)*	+++	+/0	0/+	$$$$
Propylamine derivatives	Acrivastine	++	0/+	0	$$$
	Brompheniramine	+	+	+	$
	Chlorpheniramine	+/++	+	+	$
	Dexchlorpheniramine	+/++	+	+	$$
Phenothiazine derivatives	Promethazine	++/+++	+++	++	$
	Trimeprazine	++	+/++	++	$
Tricyclic antidepressants	Doxepin	+++++	+++	+++	$
	Amitriptyline	+++++	+++/++++	+++	$

*Considered second-generation antihistamines, which are nonsedating (Zyrtec less so) and have other anti-inflammatory properties besides being antihistaminic.

Physical Examination

Recognition of urticaria does not usually present a problem. Unfortunately, except for the contact and physical urticarias, the examination does not facilitate identification of the cause. Episodes of angioedema occur in half the patients presenting with persistent urticaria. The individual swellings of angioedema always last longer than an individual hive and are almost always nonpruritic.

Laboratory Evaluation

The use of laboratory tests in patients with urticaria should be directed toward confirmation of diagnoses suggested by the history and physical examination. Routine laboratory testing should not be performed, because it has consistently proved disappointing for the identification of an etiology. A skin biopsy is indicated if the diagnosis of urticaria is in question. A biopsy should be performed on any urticaria that lasts more than 24 hours, is only mildly pruritic or nonpruritic, is associated with vesicles or bullae, or does not respond to appropriate therapy. The subtleties of the histologic variances demand interpretation by a dermatopathologist.

TREATMENT

Eliminating or avoiding the triggers of mast cell activation is the basis of treatment for urticaria. However, this strategy may be impractical in patients with persistent idiopathic urticaria, which usually has multiple triggers. Any underlying disease should be treated. Idiopathic urticaria is managed symptomatically. Fortunately, the hyperreactive state in patients with idiopathic urticaria eventually resolves spontaneously.

H$_1$ Receptor Antagonists

When used appropriately, antihistamines can offer significant relief to most patients with urticaria. The more the skin lesions resemble the triple response of Lewis, the better they respond to antihistamine treatment. Urticarial vasculitis and delayed pressure urticaria are resistant to antihistamines. Antihistamines compete with histamine for H$_1$ receptor sites on effector cells and thereby prevent, but do not reverse, responses mediated by histamine alone. There are eight recognized chemical groups of H$_1$ receptor antihistamines; all effectively compete for H$_1$ receptor sites [see Table 4]. Among these groups are tricyclic antidepressants, which also have potent antihistaminic activity.

The choice of antihistamine is based on its effectiveness, frequency of administration, and side-effect profile. The dose of the agent selected should be increased to tolerance; if adequate relief is not achieved at the maximal tolerated dose, a drug from another group can be added. Patients do not all respond in the same way to agents from each group. Most of the so-called first-generation (sedative) antihistamines are virtually equivalent in effectiveness, with the major differences being the degree of sedation or anticholinergic effects. Activation of H$_1$ receptors in the brain is responsible for alertness; inhibiting these sites with antihistamines results in sedation. Second-generation (nonsedating) antihistamines tend not to cause drowsiness, because they cross the blood-brain barrier poorly.[49] Many patients find the itching and urticaria to be most troublesome in the evening and at night, so a useful strategy is to combine sedating antihistamines given at bedtime with nonsedating antihistamines during the day. This combination is effective, promotes compliance, and is economical. Tachyphylaxis has not been noted with H$_1$ receptor antagonists.

Because other mediators besides histamine are involved in urticaria, antihistamines are not a panacea. Also, none of the antihistamines have the ability to displace histamine from the H$_1$ receptor site, so the best clinical results are attained when the antihistamines occupy those receptors before the arrival of histamine; hence, round-the-clock dosing is necessary for patients with persistent symptoms.

An effective cocktail for persistent urticaria is fexofenadine (180 mg) or loratidine (10 mg) in the early morning and cetirizine (10 to 20 mg) in the early evening. If this is insufficient, the tricyclic antidepressant doxepin, 10 to 50 mg, can be added at bedtime. (A single dose of doxepin suppresses the histamine-induced wheal and flare for 4 to 6 days.[50]) This cocktail controls symptoms in more than three quarters of patients with persistent urticaria. Prednisone, 0.5 to 1.0 mg/kg/day, should be used only for patients with refractory idiopathic urticaria or with urticarial vasculitis. The goal of treatment should not be to attain a hive-free status but, rather, to minimize compromise of the patient's quality of life from both the disease and its treatment.

In urticaria with an identifiable cause, antihistamines are discontinued once the substance is gone from the body. In persistent urticaria, antihistamines can be sequentially discontinued when patients have been completely free of hives for at least 96 hours. At that point, the morning dose of nonsedating antihistamines can be discontinued. If the patient is still symptom free after another 96 hours, the doxepin dosage can begin to be reduced and, lastly, the cetirizine can be discontinued.

H₂ Receptor Antagonists

Human skin has H_2 receptors as well as H_1 receptors. H_2 receptors are present on the cutaneous arterioles, and their activation can result in vasodilatation (noted as flushing). For that reason, combining H_2 antagonists with H_1 antagonists can be helpful in patients who have prominent flushing, dermatographism, or angioedema.[51] The available evidence does not justify the routine addition of H_2 antagonists to H_1 antagonists in patients with persistent urticaria or urticarial vasculitis.

Beta Agonists

Beta agonists increase intracellular levels of cyclic adenosine monophosphate (cAMP), thereby reducing mediator release by mast cells and promoting vasoconstriction of cutaneous vasculature. Any explosive, generalized urticaria demands the subcutaneous administration of 0.2 ml of aqueous epinephrine 1:1000 (which has combined alpha-agonist and beta-agonist properties), in addition to H_1 antagonists and H_2 antagonists (e.g., doxepin, 10 mg). This is the treatment of choice for anaphylaxis (see below).

Oral beta agonists have been tried for chronic urticaria and angioedema in conjunction with H_1 antagonists and H_2 antagonists. Terbutaline (2.5 to 5.0 mg q.i.d.) deserves a trial in patients not responding to standard treatment. Some studies have demonstrated efficacy, and others have found none.[52,53]

Corticosteroids

Because corticosteroids do not inhibit cutaneous mast cell degranulation, they have no effect on acute urticaria. However, these agents are often used in patients with persistent urticaria whose symptoms are disabling and unresponsive to maximum standard therapy.[54] In these cases, steroids are given in a pulse dose to break the cycle of a resistant episode. The recommended starting dosage of prednisone for persistent urticaria is 0.5 to 1.0 mg/kg/day. This dosage should not be reduced until the patient shows definite clinical improvement.

A protocol for steroid therapy for patients with persistent urticaria has been recommended by the Parameters of Care Committee of the American Academy of Allergy, Asthma and Immunology.[55] Daily steroids are recommended only during the first 1 or 2 weeks for patients with persistent urticaria who have had no relief for a protracted period. The goal is then to utilize an alternate-day regimen with a gradually decreasing dosage over a period of months. Patients should be started on a daily dose of prednisone, 0.5 to 1.0 mg/kg (while continuing the maximum antihistamine regimen). If the symptoms become tolerable, the prednisone dose is decreased by 5 mg every 1 to 3 days until 25 mg a day is reached. The patient's progress is then reassessed every 1 to 2 weeks. Once the patient's condition stabilizes, the dose is decreased by 2.5 to 5 mg every 2 to 3 weeks. When the lowest dose is reached, alternate-day therapy may be tried. Usually, the alternate-day dose is 1.5 times the daily dose. Should some rebound occur on the off day, the alternate-day treatment can be given in divided doses (at 8 A.M. and at 5 P.M.). Once a maintenance dose is reached, the dose of prednisone should be reduced by 1 mg every 1 to 2 weeks.

Other Agents

There are reports of success using the anabolic steroid stanozolol for chronic urticaria,[56] aquagenic urticaria,[57] familial cold urticaria,[58] and cholinergic urticaria. Nifedipine, 20 mg three times daily, has been reported effective for chronic urticaria.[59] This treatment deserves further evaluation. Patients with chronic urticaria are advised to avoid aspirin and all NSAIDs, yet there are anecdotal reports of patients with urticaria who benefit from these drugs. Indomethacin has been used successfully in the management of urticarial vasculitis.[60]

Cyclosporine has proved effective in some cases of chronic idiopathic urticaria refractory to antihistamines, as well as in urticarial vasculitis and solar urticaria.[61] Doses used are 2.5 to 6 mg/kg daily. Higher doses can cause elevation in the blood urea nitrogen (BUN) and serum creatinine levels, but these have returned to normal on discontinuance of the drug.

Leukotriene antagonists have been combined with antihistamines for the management of allergic rhinitis and have been noted to be more effective than the antihistamine alone. Therefore, many allergists have tried this combination for urticaria, with some anecdotal success. There is nothing in the literature to support its use, however, and in my experience, the use of a leukotriene antagonist with an antihistamine offers no advantage for persistent urticaria without angioedema.

PROGNOSIS

Except for IgE-induced urticaria, which may progress to fatal anaphylaxis, the prognosis for the other urticarias is benign, although prolonged episodes of these disorders can be extremely bothersome. To date, there is no evidence that the natural history of any of the urticarial syndromes, whether induced by an identifiable cause or idiopathic, is influenced by treatment. Almost all cases of persistent urticaria eventually resolve, however; even the majority of cases of IgE-induced urticarias (especially those without anaphylaxis) are rarely permanent. Chronic urticaria tends to last longer in elderly persons than in younger ones. Studies of chronic (persistent) idiopathic urticaria have found that with or without treatment, 50% of cases will resolve within 6 to 12 months of onset; 20%, within 12 to 36 months; and another 20%, within 36 to 60 months. Less than 2% of cases persist for 25 years or longer. Over 50% of patients will have at least one recurrence.[62] Interestingly, although anaphylactic or anaphylactoid reactions have been noted in patients with identifiable causes of urticaria, there have been no reports of these reactions ever occurring in patients with persistent urticaria without an identifiable cause. More than 50% of patients with idiopathic urticaria can be made comfortable with appropriate antihistamine therapy. Immunosuppression with corticosteroid dependence occurs in fewer than 5% of patients.

Angioedema

Angioedema is an episodic, asymmetrical, nonpitting swelling of loose tissue (usually skin) [see Figure 5]. It is usually nonerythematous and nonpruritic, and it may be painless. Angioedema rarely lasts less than 2 hours, and it frequently persists for 24 hours or longer. It may occur together with urticaria. Angioedema involving the face can be disfiguring during its course. Laryngeal swelling from angioedema may compromise the airway, leading to stridor and even asphyxiation. Gastrointestinal involvement can cause crampy abdominal pain, followed by watery diarrhea. Most cases of angioedema are a reaction to a food or a drug, but some episodes have no identifiable trigger. There are both hereditary and acquired forms of angioedema.

EPIDEMIOLOGY

It is estimated that approximately 10% of the population will experience at least one episode of angioedema.[63] Angioedema occurs episodically in 50% of patients with urticaria. Of patients who have angioedema as their primary disorder, approximately 20% will also experience episodes of urticaria.[64]

ETIOLOGY

Angioedema can be induced by a variety of mechanisms, including IgE, inhibition of the cyclooxygenase pathway of arachidonic acid metabolism, activation of the kinin-forming system, and activation of complement. In some patients, none of these mechanisms can be identified; these cases are labeled idiopathic.

IgE

IgE-induced angioedema resembles IgE allergy and is typically provoked by foods or drugs. It tends to occur in atopic persons and can be confirmed by prick skin testing or RAST.

Cyclooxygenase Inhibition

There is increasing evidence that the inhibition of the enzyme cyclooxygenase causes the de novo release of leukotrienes, an inflammatory mediator derived from arachidonic acid, in response to injury. Of particular interest in the skin is leukotriene B_4, which can induce neutrophil chemotaxis and increase vascular permeability.[65] Aspirin and other NSAIDs directly inhibit the ability of cyclooxygenase to decrease the formation of prostaglandins and thromboxanes, but not leukotrienes, from arachidonic acid. Angioedema (with or without urticaria) may occur in 100% of patients with hypersensitivity to aspirin or other NSAIDs.[11] Interestingly, not all patients who are hypersensitive to aspirin react to other NSAIDs,[66] and in one study, only 3% of patients sensitive to both aspirin and other NSAIDs reacted to the COX-2 inhibitor rofecoxib.[67]

Activation of the Kinin-Forming System

Bradykinin increases vascular permeability. Angiotensin-converting enzyme (ACE) inhibitors inhibit the kininase enzymes required for degradation of bradykinin, and the resulting elevation in bradykinin levels may lead to angioedema.[68] Angioedema has been reported in approximately 0.1% to

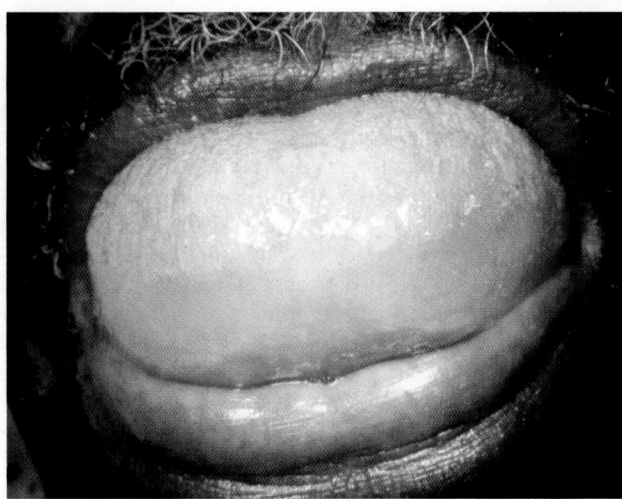

Figure 5 Angioedema of the tongue is evident in this photograph of a 54-year-old man. This episode, the patient's fifth, was unresponsive to epinephrine, antihistamines, and prednisone; his sixth episode required intubation for 92 hours, after which the angioedema resolved spontaneously.

0.5% of patients who take ACE inhibitors.[69] However, because these agents are so widely used, ACE inhibitor–induced angioedema is relatively common.

Angiotensin II receptor blockers (ARBs), such as losartan and valsartan, do not increase bradykinin levels. Nevertheless, rare instances of angioedema have been reported with the use of ARBs.[70]

Complement Activation

Increased susceptibility to angioedema can result from either an inherited defect in C1-esterase inhibitor (C1-INH) activity or an acquired deficiency of C1-INH. The inherited form of the disease, known as hereditary angioedema, is rare. There are two principal types of hereditary angioedema: type 1, which accounts for 80% to 85% of cases and is caused by decreased production of C1-INH, and type 2, in which normal or elevated amounts of functionally deficient C1-INH are produced.[71] A third, very rare form of hereditary angioedema that may be X-linked has recently been described in women.[72]

Acquired angioedema results from increased metabolism or destruction of C1-INH. Two types of acquired angioedema have been described. Type 1, which is caused by excessive activation of complement and subsequent consumption of C1-INH, typically occurs in patients with rheumatologic disorders and B cell lymphoproliferative diseases. Patients with type 2 produce autoantibodies against C1-INH, leading to its inactivation.[73,74]

PATHOGENESIS

Angioedema is consistently described as a variant of urticaria in which the subcutaneous tissues, rather than the dermis, are mainly involved. However, unlike urticaria, which seems to be mediated primarily by histamine, angioedema seems to be mediated primarily by bradykinin and leukotrienes. Anecdotal evidence indicates that although urticaria can be elicited with a histamine prick or intradermal injection, the injection of histamine deeper in the dermis does not produce angioedema. On the other hand, there are patients whose angioedema will dissipate with the administration of antihistamines (especially the combination of H_1 and H_2 receptor antagonists).[75] These observations suggest that several vasoactive mediators are capable of producing angioedema.

Unfortunately, angioedema is almost never biopsied, so there are no documented pathologic descriptions of the disorder. The histopathology is always included with urticaria, and its morphology seems to be assumed. Teleologically, the vasodilatation and vascular leakage occur deeper in the skin, and the specific cellular infiltrate, if any, remains uncertain.

DIAGNOSIS

Diagnosis of angioedema is usually straightforward. Cellulitis, edematous states, trauma (stings), and fasciitis occasionally are considerations in the differential diagnosis. Insights into causes and mechanisms of induction are derived primarily from the history.

The history in a patient with angioedema—especially one who has had repeated episodes—should include the following questions: (1) Is the angioedema always, sometimes, or never associated with urticaria? (2) Is the swelling pruritic? (3) Are there accompanying gastrointestinal symptoms (e.g., pain, nausea and vomiting, or diarrhea)? (4) Is the patient taking any medications? (5) Can the patient identify any apparent triggers for the angioedema?

Patients with IgE-induced angioedema are most likely to present with concomitant urticaria. This form of angioedema may be pruritic and may progress to an anaphylactic reaction. Typically, IgE-induced angioedema occurs within 30 minutes after contact with the IgE antigen. It is most likely to occur in atopic patients. Gastrointestinal symptoms may occur but are uncommon. IgE-induced angioedema often occurs as a drug reaction, with β-lactam antibiotics being the most common trigger.

Cyclooxygenase inhibitors (i.e., aspirin or other NSAIDs) are more apt to cause nonpruritic angioedema. NSAID-induced angioedema is occasionally accompanied by urticaria.

Angioedema induced by ACE inhibitors is nonpruritic and rarely occurs with urticaria. No sex predominance has been noted in patients without gastrointestinal tract involvement, but all patients with GI involvement have been women.[76]

Complement-activated angioedema is never pruritic and is not accompanied by urticaria. In 20% to 25% of patients with hereditary angioedema, there is no family history of the disease (these cases may represent new mutations).[77] Therefore, a positive family history of hereditary angioedema is not a prerequisite for the consideration of this disorder in the differential diagnosis when typical symptoms are present. Symptoms of hereditary angioedema are usually mild or nonexistent during childhood, typically first manifesting during the second decade of life. Acquired angioedema usually develops during or after the fourth decade of life.

Hereditary and acquired angioedema have similar clinical presentations. Episodes can occur without provocation, but some episodes may be associated with trauma, medical procedures, emotional stress, menstruation, oral contraceptive use, infections, or the use of medications such as ACE inhibitors.[71] Manifestations include marked edema of the skin and lining of hollow visceral organs. GI tract involvement results in varying degrees of intestinal obstruction, with severe abdominal pain, nausea, and vomiting. Despite the absence of fever and leukocytosis, these cases are often mistaken for an acute abdomen, which occasionally leads to unnecessary surgical exploration of the abdomen. Typically, the attacks last about 2 to 5 days before resolving spontaneously.

Laboratory Tests

IgE-induced drug reactions are readily identifiable with skin-prick tests or RAST. In complement-activated angioedema, a low level of the complement component C4 is a constant finding and therefore represents a sensitive screening test. A normal level, especially during an attack, rules out both hereditary and acquired angioedema. In patients with suspected complement-activated angioedema, confirmation of the diagnosis can be obtained by measuring antigenic levels of C1-INH, which are low in 85% of patients, or functional levels, which are low in 100% of patients. Hereditary forms of complement-activated angioedema can be distinguished from acquired forms by measurement of C1q complement—levels of which are normal in hereditary forms but decreased in acquired forms.

TREATMENT

Discontinuance of the causative agent is an obvious initial step in angioedema. Emergency measures are necessary to secure the airway if there is airway obstruction by a swollen tongue, uvula, or epiglottis. Monitoring the airway in these patients until the angioedema resolves is imperative. Subcutaneous epinephrine should be given and is helpful in most types of angioedema, except those associated with low levels of C1-INH. Aerosolized epinephrine sprayed on the swollen mucous membrane may at times be helpful.

Antihistamines (both H_1 and H_2 receptor antagonists) are indicated for IgE-induced angioedema (see above). Idiopathic angioedema has been split into those presentations that respond to antihistamine therapy and those that do not.[78] Doxepin (see above) should be given to all patients with idiopathic angioedema, but results are often disappointing if this agent is administered without epinephrine. Leukotriene inhibitors counteract the vasodilation produced by leukotrienes and can reduce the edema.

Intramuscular or intravenous glucocorticoids (prednisone, 0.5 to 1 mg/kg/day, or methylprednisolone, 0.4 to 0.8 mg/kg/day) can be used as adjunctive treatment. However, the anti-inflammatory action of these agents does not affect the underlying cause of the inflammation, and they require hours to take effect. Injectable C1-INH concentrate has been developed and is effective in treating patients with hereditary angioedema,[79] but it is difficult to obtain.

To prevent future episodes of angioedema, patients should avoid identified triggers. ACE inhibitors are contraindicated in patients with idiopathic or C1-INH deficiency, and ARBs should be used only with extreme caution. Patients with idiopathic angioedema should undergo an annual general medical evaluation to identify any underlying occult disease.

Anaphylaxis

Anaphylaxis is an explosive, massive activation of mast cells, with release of their inflammatory mediators in the skin, respiratory tract, and circulatory system resulting in urticaria, wheezing, and hypotension.

The term anaphylaxis has been restricted to IgE-mediated mast cell and basophil activation. Anaphylactoid reactions, although similar in presentation, result from non–IgE-dependent mechanisms and are less likely to have a fatal outcome.[80] For practical purposes, however, it does not matter whether the patient is having true anaphylaxis or an anaphylactoid reaction, because the clinical manifestations and the treatment of these two types of reactions are identical.

EPIDEMIOLOGY

The authors of all epidemiologic reports regarding anaphylaxis believe the incidence to be underestimated because of failure to report or recognize every episode. A Dutch study estimated that only 4% to 8% of anaphylactic reactions were reported.[81] From the combined results of reported series, several significant conclusions can be drawn: First, the occurrence of atopy in anaphylaxis patients can be as high as 53%.[82] Second, the incidence of females predisposed to anaphylactic episodes can be as high as 61%.[83] Third, when the cause of anaphylaxis is found, food and drugs head the list, with peanuts and shellfish being the most common offending foods and NSAIDs and antibiotics being the most common drug offenders.[84] Fourth, cutaneous symptoms are by far the most common manifestation.[85] Fifth, the risk of anaphylaxis in hospitalized patients is reported to be 196 per million population, with the risk being highest in women and in persons younger than 30 years.[86]

ETIOLOGY

A number of substances are known to cause anaphylactic and anaphylactoid reactions [see Table 5]. IgE-mediated anaphylaxis is caused by agents that act as haptens (e.g., β-lactam antibiotics) or by complete antigens (e.g., venoms, foods, allergen extracts). Anaphylatoxins (C3a and C5a) often mediate reactions to human plasma and blood products. The nonimmunologic mast cell activators include radiocontrast media, opiates, and some muscle relaxants. Other anaphylactoid-inducing agents include those agents that modulate arachidonic acid metabolism (i.e., aspirin and other NSAIDs). In a number of cases, the mechanism that leads to anaphylactic or anaphylactoid reactions is unknown (i.e., idiopathic, exercise, and cold urticaria or cholinergic urticaria with anaphylaxis; mastocytosis; and some drug-induced reactions).[87] Patients with idiopathic persistent urticaria or episodic urticaria do not experience anaphylaxis.

PATHOGENESIS

Any of the mast cell secretagogues [see Table 3] have the potential to induce an anaphylactic or anaphylactoid reaction. Activation of the mast cell through the FcεRI receptor by an antigen releases the greatest amount of histamine. The physiologic responses to the release of inflammatory mediators include smooth-muscle spasm in the bronchi and GI tract, vasodilatation, increased vascular permeability, and stimulation of nociceptor nerve endings.

DIAGNOSIS

The classic symptoms of anaphylaxis include flushing, urticaria, angioedema, pruritus, bronchospasm, and abdominal cramping with nausea, vomiting, and diarrhea. Hypotension and shock can result from intravascular volume loss, vasodilatation, and myocardial dysfunction. Symptoms usually begin within 5 to 30 minutes after the causative agent is introduced into the body and within 2 hours after it is ingested. The shorter the latent period, the more ominous the prognosis. In rare cases, symptoms can be delayed in onset for several hours. These are called late reactions. The biphasic reaction, which includes both immediate and late reactions, tends not to be recognized and therefore is more likely to result in a fatal outcome. Least common is the protracted reaction, in which the immediate reaction persists for hours.

Table 5 Estimated Incidence or Prevalence of Acute Anaphylactic Reactions[91]

Cause	Incidence/Prevalence
General cause	1 per 2,700 hospitalized patients
Insect sting	0.4%–0.8% of United States population
Radiocontrast medium	1 per 1,000–14,000 procedures
Penicillin (fatal outcome)	1.0–7.5 per million treatments
General anesthesia	1 per 300 inductions
Hemodialysis	1 per 1,000–5,000 sessions
Immunotherapy (severe reactions)	0.1 per million injections

Table 6 Grading System for Anaphylaxis

Group	Clinical Manifestations
I	Pruritus, flushing, urticaria, or angioedema
II	Pruritus, flushing, urticaria, or angioedema Nausea, dyspnea, tachycardia, or hypotension
III	Pruritus, flushing, urticaria, or angioedema Nausea, dyspnea, tachycardia, or hypotension Bronchospasm and shock
IV	Respiratory arrest Cardiac arrest Other manifestations may be present

Clinical Manifestations

At the onset of anaphylaxis, patients often initially experience a sense of impending doom, accompanied by generalized pruritus and flushing. Almost all patients with anaphylaxis present with cutaneous manifestations that include pruritus, flushing, urticaria, or angioedema.

Anaphylaxis is graded by its clinical presentation [see Table 6]. Cases with signs and symptoms limited to the skin are designated as group I. Group II comprises cutaneous manifestations plus nausea, dyspnea, tachycardia, or hypotension; group III includes all the manifestations of groups I and II plus bronchospasm and true shock. Group IV consists of respiratory arrest, cardiac arrest, or both, with or without other manifestations.

Physical Examination

Cutaneous involvement Flushing, urticaria, and angioedema have been reported in 88% to 100% of patients experiencing anaphylaxis. Pruritus, especially of the scalp, soft palate, palms, soles, and anogenital areas, usually heralds an impending anaphylactic or anaphylactoid reaction or may be the only cutaneous signs of the episode. Conjunctival pruritus, injection, and edema are not unusual.

Respiratory involvement Nasal congestion (occurring in up to 56% of patients), rhinorrhea (16%), laryngeal edema, dyspnea (47%), bronchospasm (24% to 47%), cough, and hoarseness may all be part of the anaphylaxis syndrome.

Cardiovascular involvement Tachycardia and hypotension are common cardiovascular manifestations of anaphylaxis. Uncommon findings include bradycardia (6%), angina (6%), syncope, palpitations, and cardiac arrest (2% to 14%).

Gastrointestinal involvement GI symptoms, including nausea, vomiting, diarrhea, abdominal cramps, and bloating occur in 30% of patients with anaphylaxis.

Neurologic involvement Dizziness or syncope (33%), headache (up to 15%), and seizures (1.5%) may be among the presenting symptoms of anaphylaxis.

Laboratory Evaluation

Anaphylaxis is a clinical diagnosis. Laboratory studies are rarely helpful. Postmortem testing may help clarify the diagnosis in cases of so-called sudden death or in patients who are dead on arrival at the emergency department.

If a patient is seen shortly after an episode, plasma histamine, urinary histamine, or serum tryptase may be helpful in confirming the diagnosis. Plasma histamine levels rise within 10 minutes, but they fall again within 1 hour. Serum β-tryptase levels peak by 1 hour and may remain elevated for as long as 5 hours. However, a negative histamine and tryptase study does not completely rule out the diagnosis of anaphylaxis. Skin testing and RAST for the causative agent (e.g., food, Hymenoptera venom, latex, or drug), if indicated, should be performed 4 to 6 weeks after the episode for greatest sensitivity.

TREATMENT IN THE FIELD

The essential steps in the treatment of anaphylaxis are (1) prevention, (2) recognition, (3) prompt therapy, and (4) early transport to an emergency care facility.

Prevention

Prevention depends on recognition of persons at risk. Use of oral rather than parenteral medications should always be considered in patients at high risk for anaphylaxis. This includes patients with atopy or those with a possible history of allergic reactions to drugs. If drugs are administered parenterally, such patients should remain in a medically supervised area for at least 30 minutes afterward. Patients with known food or drug allergies must read labels to avoid the foods or drugs to which they are allergic. Severely food-allergic patients must be especially careful when dining out and may wish to avoid eating in restaurants altogether. Patients with a history of anaphylactic reaction to Hymenoptera venom should be given information on avoiding future stings and should be referred to an allergist for consideration of venom immunotherapy [see Chapter 110]. Patients with a history of anaphylaxis should always carry an epinephrine autoinjector (Epi-Pen).

Recognition

Immediate diagnosis of a developing reaction is imperative. Because of the risk of respiratory and cardiovascular collapse, the patient's airway, breathing, and circulation (the so-called emergency ABCs) must be rapidly assessed.

Prompt Initiation of Therapy

Anaphylaxis can rarely be overtreated. Treatment must be expeditious and appropriate. A protocol and supplies for prompt treatment should be in place at every medical office or facility. A protocol for diagnosis and management of anaphy-

laxis has been developed by the Joint Task Force on Practice Parameters.[88] The supplies should include oxygen, aqueous epinephrine, injectable antihistamines, intravenous or intramuscular glucocorticoids, oropharyngeal airways, and I.V. fluids. If the clinical assessment even suggests an anaphylactic reaction, it is best to call 911 and initiate therapy.

Whenever possible, decrease the absorption of the antigen. With insect bites and stings on an extremity, for example, apply a tourniquet above the injection site to block venous return and remove the insect stinger. Inject epinephrine (1:1000) locally.

Give supplemental oxygen, 6 to 8 L/min, and administer epinephrine (1:1000) subcutaneously or intramuscularly. The epinephrine dose is 0.2 to 0.5 mg in adults and 0.01 mg/kg in children. If the patient is in cardiopulmonary arrest, epinephrine (1:10,000) should be administered intravenously, in a dose of 0.1 to 1.0 mg for adults and 0.001 to 0.002 mg in children. Patients and their caregivers should recognize that more than one dose of epinephrine may be required.[89]

Intravenous H_1 antihistamines (e.g., diphenhydramine, 50 mg) and H_2 antihistamines (e.g., ranitidine, 50 mg, or cimetidine, 300 mg) should be given. If the patient can swallow, H_2 antihistamines can be given orally. Bronchospasm may be treated with aerosolized beta-adrenergic agonists (albuterol). Severe bronchospasm may require endotracheal intubation or cricothyrotomy. Respiratory failure can occur with or without upper airway compromise. Persistent hypoperfusion and ischemia may lead to myocardial infarction, cerebral ischemia, or renal failure.

Once the acute reaction is under control, systemic corticosteroids (e.g., hydrocortisone sodium phosphate, 100 mg every 2 to 4 hours) may be administered. The patient can be transferred to the emergency department.

PROGNOSIS

Most patients experience only a single episode of anaphylaxis,[82] but some patients have three or more episodes.[90] Death from anaphylaxis is uncommon. Complications are also unusual; most patients recover completely. However, respiratory failure from severe bronchospasm or laryngeal edema can cause hypoxia, which if prolonged could lead to brain injury. Hypotension and hypoxia may lead to cardiac ischemia or arrhythmias.

The author has no commercial relationships with manufacturers of products or providers of services discussed in this chapter.

References

1. Galli SJ: New concepts about the mast cell. N Engl J Med 328:257, 1993

2. Doutre M: Physiopathology of urticaria. Eur J Dermatol 9:601, 1999

3. Longley J, Duffy TP, Kohn S: The mast cell and mast cell disease. J Am Acad Dermatol 32:545, 1995

4. Haas N, Toppe E, Henz BM: Microscopic morphology of different types of urticaria. Arch Dermatol 134:41, 1998

5. Bedard PM, Brunet C, Pelletier G, et al: Increased compound 48/80 induced local histamine release from nonlesional skin of patients with chronic urticaria. J Allergy Clin Immunol 78:1121, 1986

6. Kaplan AP: Urticaria and angioedema. Allergy: Principles & Practice, 5th ed. Middleton E, Reed CE, Ellis EF, et al, Eds. Mosby, St Louis, 1998, p 1104

7. Plumb J, Norlin C, Young PC: Exposures and outcomes of children with urticaria seen in a pediatric practice-based research network: a case-control study. Arch Pediatr Adolesc Med 155:1017, 2000

8. Shipley D, Ormerod AD: Drug-induced urticaria: recognition and treatment. Am J Clin Dermatol 2:151, 2001

9. Bircher AJ: Drug-induced urticaria and angioedema caused by non-IgE mediated pathomechanisms. Eur J Dermatol 9:657, 1999

10. Sanchez-Borges M, Capriles-Hulett A: Atopy is a risk factor for non-steroidal anti-inflammatory drug sensitivity. Ann Allergy Asthma Immunol 84:101, 2000

11. Sanchez Borges M, Capriles-Hulett A, Caballero-Fonseca F, et al: Tolerability to new COX-2 inhibitors in NSAID-sensitive patients with cutaneous reactions. Ann Allergy Asthma Immunol 87:201, 2001

12. Gruchalla RS, Beltrani VS: Drug-induced cutaneous reactions. Allergic Skin Disease. Leung DYM, Greaves MW, Eds. Marcel Dekker, New York, 2000, p 318

13. Sampson HA: Food allergy. Part 2: diagnosis and management. J Allergy Clin Immunol 103:981, 1999

14. Sehgal VN, Rege VL: An interrogative study of 158 urticaria patients. Ann Allergy 31:279, 1973

15. Eggesbo M, Halvorsen R, Tambs K, et al: Prevalence of parentally perceived adverse reaction to food in young children. Pediatr Allergy Immunol 10:122, 1999

16. Bock SA, Sampson HA, Atkins FM, et al: Double-blind, placebo-controlled food challenge as an office procedure: a manual. J Allergy Clin Immunol 82:986, 1988

17. Rockwell WJ: Reactions to molds in foods. Food allergy: a practical approach to diagnosis and management. Chiaramonte LT, Schneider AT, Lifshitz F, Eds. Marcel Dekker, New York, 1988, p 153

18. Anderson JA: Milestones marking the knowledge of adverse reactions to food in the decade of the 1980s. Ann Allergy 72:143, 1994

19. Spergel JM, Beausoleil JL, Pawlowski NA: Resolution of childhood peanut allergy. Ann Allergy Asthma Immunol 85:435, 2000

20. Bock SA: Natural history of severe reactions to foods in young children. J Pediatr 107:676, 1985

21. Sicherer SH, Sampson HA: Food hypersensitivity and atopic dermatitis: pathophysiology, epidemiology, diagnosis, and management. J Allergy Clin Immunol 104:S114, 1999

22. Leznoff A, Sussman GL: Syndrome of idiopathic chronic urticaria and angioedema with thyroid auto-immunity: a study of 90 patients. J Allergy Clin Immunol 84:66, 1989

23. Turktas I, Gokcora N, Demirsoy S, et al: The association of chronic urticaria and angioedema with autoimmune thyroididitis. Int J Dermatol 36:187, 1997

24. Zauli D, Delonardi G, Foderaro S, et al: Thyroid autoimmunity in chronic urticaria. Allergy Asthma Proc 22:93, 2001

25. Rumbyrt JS, Katz JL, Schocket AL: Resolution of chronic urticaria in patients with thyroid autoimmunity. J Allergy Clin Immunol 96:901, 1995

26. Heymann WR: Chronic urticaria and angioedema associated with thyroid autoimmunity: review and therapeutic implications. J Am Acad Dermatol 40:229, 1999

27. Liutu M, Kalimo K, Uksila J, et al: Etiologic aspects of chronic urticaria. Int J Dermatol 37:515, 1998

28. Schnyder B, Helbling A, Pichler WJ: Chronic idiopathic urticaria: natural course and association with Helicobacter pylori infection. Int Arch Allergy Immunol 119:60, 1999

29. Nelson H: Routine sinus roentgenograms and chronic urticaria. JAMA 251:1680, 1984

30. deGentile L, Grandiere-Perez L, Chabasse D: Urticaria and parasites. Allergy Immunol (Paris) 31:288, 1999

31. Picardi A, Abeni D: Stressful life events and skin diseases: disentangling evidence from myth. Psychother Psychosom 70:118, 2001

32. Lipsker D, Veran Y, Grunenberger F, et al: The Schnitzler syndrome: four new cases and review of the literature. Medicine (Baltimore) 80:37, 2001

33. Muckle TJ: The 'Muckle-Wells' syndrome. Br J Dermatol 100:87, 1979

34. Demain JG, Taylor TM: Reactions to stinging and biting arthropods. Cutaneous Allergy. Charlesworth EN, Ed. Blackwell Science Publications, Cambridge, England, 1996, p 299

35. Stibich AS, Schwartz RA: Papular urticaria. Cutis 68:89, 2001

36. Tharp MD, Longley BJ Jr: Mastocytosis. Dermatol Clin 19:679, 2001

37. Kobza-Black A: Management of urticaria. Clin Exp Dermatol 27:328, 2002

38. Sibbald RB: Physical urticaria. Dermatol Clinics North Am 4:57, 1984

39. Wanderer AA: Cold urticaria syndromes: historical background, diagnostic classification, clinical and laboratory characteristics, pathogenesis, and management. J Allergy Clin Immunol 85:965, 1990

40. Neittaanmaki H: Cold urticaria: clinical findings in 220 patients. J Am Acad Dermatol 13:636, 1985

41. Monfrecola G, Masturzo E, Riccardo AM, et al: Solar urticaria: a report of 57 cases. Am J Contact Dermat 11:89, 2000

42. Uetsu N, Miyauchi-Hashimoto H, Okamoto H, et al. The clinical and photobiological characteristics of solar urticaria in 40 patients. Br J Dermatol 142:32, 2000.

43. Ryckaert S, Roelandts R: Solar urticaria. Arch Dermatol 134:71, 1998

44. Luong KV, Nguyen LT: Aquagenic urticaria: report of a case and review of the literature. Ann Allergy Asthma Immunol 80:483, 1998

45. Paterson R, Mellies CJ, Blankenship ML, et al: Vibratory angioedema: a hereditary type of physical hypersensitivity. J Allergy Clin Immunol 50:174, 1972

46. Lahti A: Immediate contact reactions. Curr Probl Dermatol 22:17, 1995

47. Hjorth N, Ree-Peterson J: Occupational protein contact dermatitis in foodhandlers. Contact Derm 2:28, 1976

48. Hirschmann JV, Lawlor F, et al: Cholinergic urticaria. Arch Dermatol 123:462, 1987

49. Lee EE, Maibach HI: Treatment of urticaria: an evidence-based evaluation of antihistamines. Am J Clin Dermatol 2:27, 2001

50. Goldsobel AB, Rohr AS, Siefel SC, et al: Efficacy of doxepin in the treatment of chronic idiopathic urticaria. J Allergy Clin Immunol 78:867, 1986

51. Mansfield LE, Smith JA, Nelson HS: Greater inhibition of dermographia with combination of H1 and H2 antagonists. Ann Allergy 50:264, 1983

52. Kennes B, De Maubeuge J, Delespesse G: Treatment of chronic urticaria with a beta2-adrenergic stimulant. Clin Allergy 7:35, 1977

53. Spangler DL, Vanderpool GE, Carroll MS, et al: Terbutaline in the treatment of chronic urticaria. Ann Allergy 45:246, 1980

54. Kaplan AP: Clinical practice: chronic urticaria and angioedema. N Engl J Med 346:175, 2002

55. The diagnosis and management of urticaria: a practice parameter. Part I: acute urticaria/angioedema; part II: chronic urticaria/angioedema. Joint Task Force on Practice Parameters. Ann Allergy Asthma Immunol 85:521, 2000

56. Parsad D, Pandhi R, Juneja A: Stanozolol in chronic urticaria: a double-blind, placebo controlled trial. J Dermatol 28:299, 2001

57. Fearfield LA, Gazzard B, Bunker CB: Aquagenic urticaria in HIV virus infection treated with stanozolol. Br J Dermatol 137:620, 1997

58. Omerud AD, Smart L, Reid TM, Milford-Ward A: Familial cold urticaria: investigation of a family and response to stanozolol. Arch Dermatol 129:34, 1993

59. Bressler RB, Sowell K, Huston DP: Therapy of chronic idiopathic urticaria with nifedipine: demonstration of beneficial effect in a double blinded, placebo controlled cross-over trial. J Allergy Clin Immunol 83:756, 1989

60. Millins JL, Randle HW, Solley GO, et al: The therapeutic response of urticarial vasculitis to indomethacin. J Am Acad Dermatol 3:349, 1980

61. Grattan CE, O'Donnell BF, Francis DM, et al: Randomized double-blind study of cyclosporin in chronic `idiopathic' urticaria. Br J Dermatol 143:365, 2000

62. Beltrani VS: An overview of chronic urticaria. Clin Rev Allergy Immunol 23:147, 2002

63. Hedner T, Samuelsson O, Lunde H, et al: Angioedema in relation to treatment with angiotensin converting enzyme inhibitors. Br Med J 304:941, 1992

64. Champion RH: Urticaria and angio-edema: a review of 554 patients. Br J Dermatol 81:588, 1969

65. Henig NR, Henderson WR Jr: Anti-leukotriene agents in the treatment of asthma. Current Review of Allergic Diseases. Kaliner MA, Ed. Current Medicine, Philadelphia, 2000, p 71

66. Quiralte J, Bianco C, Castillo R, et al: Intolerance to nonsteroidal anti-inflammatory drugs: results of controlled drug challenges in 98 patients. J Allergy Clin Immunol 98:678, 1996

67. Kelkar PS, Butterfield JH, Teaford HG: Urticaria and angioedema from cyclooxygenase-2 inhibitors. J Rheumatol 28:2553, 2001

68. Agostini A, Cicardi M, Cugno M, et al: Angioedema due to angiotensin-converting enzyme inhibitors. Immunopharmacology 15:21, 1999

69. Hedner T, Samuelsson O, Lunde H, et al: Angioedema in relation to treatment with angiotensin converting enzyme inhibitors. BMJ 304:941, 1992

70. Rodgers JE, Patterson JH: Angiotensin II receptor blockers: clinical relevance and therapeutic role. Am J Health Syst Pharm 58:671, 2001

71. Nzeako UC, Frigas E, Tremaine WJ: Hereditary angioedema: a broad review for clinicians. Arch Intern Med 161:2417, 2001

72. Bork K, Barnstedt SE, Koch P, et al: Hereditary angioedema with normal C1-inhibitor activity in women. Lancet 356:213, 2000

73. Laurent J, Guinnepain MT: Angioedema associated with C1 inhibitor deficiency. Clin Rev Allergy Immunol 17:513, 1999

74. Jackson J, Sims RB, Whelan A, et al: An IgG autoantibody which inactivates C1-inhibitor. Nature 323:722, 1986

75. Black AK, Greaves MW: Antihistamines in urticaria and angioedema. Clin Allergy Immunol 17:249, 2002

76. Chase MP, Fiarman GS, Scholz FJ, et al: Angioedema of the small bowel due to an angiotensin-converting enzyme inhibitor. J Clin Gastroenterol 31:254, 2000

77. Agostini A, Ciccardi M: Hereditary and acquired C-1 inhibitor deficiency: biological and clinical characteristics in 235 patients. Medicine (Baltimore) 71:206, 1992

78. Cicardi M, Bergamaschini L, Zingale LC, et al: Idiopathic nonhistaminergic angioedema. Am J Med 106:650, 1999

79. Bork K, Barnstedt SE: Treatment of 193 episodes of laryngeal edema with C1 inhibitor concentrate in patients with hereditary angioedema. Arch Intern Med 161:714, 2001

80. Luskin AT, Luskin SS: Anaphylaxis and anaphylactoid reactions: diagnosis and management. Am J Ther 3:515, 1996

81. Van der Klauw MM, Stricker BHCH, Herings RMC, et al: A population-based case-cohort study of drug-induced anaphylaxis. Br J Clin Pharmacol 35:400, 1993

82. Yokum MW, Butterfield J, Klein J, et al: Epidemiology of anaphylaxis in Olmsted County, a population-based study. J Allergy Clin Immunol 104:452, 1999

83. Yocum MW, Khan DA: Assessment of patients who have experienced anaphylaxis: a 3-year survey. Mayo Clin Proc 69:16, 1994

84. Kemp SF, Lockey RF, Wolf BL, Lieberman P: Anaphylaxis: a review of 266 cases. Arch Intern Med 155:1749, 1995

85. Perez C, Tejedor MA, Hoz A, et al: Anaphylaxis: a review of 182 patients (abstr). J Allergy Clin Immunol 95:368, 1995

86. Kaufman DW: An epidemiologic study of severe anaphylactic and anaphylactoid reactions among hospital patients: methods and overall risks—abstract from report from the International Collaborative Study of Severe Anaphylaxis. Epidemiology 9:141, 1998

87. Boxer M, Greenberger PA, Patterson R: Clinical summary and course of idiopathic anaphylaxis in 73 patients. Arch Intern Med 147:26, 1987

88. The diagnosis and management of anaphylaxis. Joint Task Force on Practice Parameters, American Academy of Allergy, Asthma and Immunology, American College of Allergy, Asthma and Immunology, and the Joint Council of Allergy, Asthma and Immunology. J Allergy Clin Immunol 101:S465, 1998

89. Korenblat P, Lundie MJ, Dankner RE, et al: A retrospective study of epinephrine administration for anaphylaxis: How many doses are needed? Allergy Asthma Proc 20:383, 1999

90. Weiler JM: Anaphylaxis in the general population: a frequent and occasionally fatal disorder that is under-recognized. J Allergy Clin Immunol 104:271, 1999

91. Sim TC: Anaphylaxis. How to manage and prevent this medical emergency. Postgrad Med 92:277, 1992

Mark S. Dykewicz, M.D., F.A.C.P., and Heather C. Gray, M.D.

Adverse drug reactions are the most common iatrogenic illnesses, occurring in 1% to 15% of drug courses. They are also a frequent presentation in emergency departments. In a large prospective study of 18,820 hospital admissions, 1,225 (6.5%) were related to adverse drug reactions.[1] Most adverse drug reactions result from nonimmunologic or unknown mechanisms (e.g., toxic overdose, toxic side effects, intolerance). Approximately 6% to 10% of drug reactions are caused by proven or suspected immunologic mechanisms mediated by specific antibodies, sensitized T cells, or both.[2] Immunologic reactions develop in patients who have become sensitized by previous exposure or continuous exposure to the same or an antigenically related drug. Although identification of antibodies or sensitized T cells directed against the drug helps confirm the diagnosis of immunologic drug reactions, diagnosis usually is based on clinical presentation.[3] This chapter provides an overview of pathogenesis, discusses recognition of both common and uncommon patterns of allergic drug reactions, and explains the application of diagnostic tests and management techniques.

Pathogenesis

Hypersensitivity drug reactions can be influenced by intrinsic properties of the drug, its administration, and the host. Drug factors that increase risk include a higher molecular weight, the ability of the drug or its reactive metabolites to readily bind to self-proteins to form antigenic hapten-protein conjugates, higher dose, parenteral (as opposed to oral) administration, and repeated exposure to the drug. Host factors that increase risk include adult age, female gender, concurrent infections, and HIV infec-

tion.[4] Phenotypic differences in drug metabolism may also influence risk. For example, rashes from sulfonamides are more likely to occur in patients who are slow acetylator phenotypes, because these patients preferentially metabolize sulfa drugs by alternative oxidative pathways that produce highly reactive metabolites that bind to self-protein carriers.

Although β-lactam antibiotics covalently bind to self-protein carriers to form antigenic conjugates, many non–β-lactam antibiotics require enzyme systems, such as cytochrome P-450, to form reactive products that then bind with self-protein carriers. Consequently, testing with a parent drug may not identify sensitivity to reactive intermediate products.

Classification of Drug Reactions

Classifying drug reactions on the basis of either the temporal relation between drug exposure and adverse manifestations or the presumptive immunologic mechanism may aid in evaluation and management. Temporally, drug reactions are classified as immediate, accelerated, or delayed. Immediate reactions occur within 1 hour of administration and include anaphylaxis. Accelerated reactions, such as urticaria and angioedema, occur within 72 hours of administration. Delayed reactions, which occur 72 hours or more after administration, include urticarial and nonurticarial skin rashes; serum sickness–like reactions; fever; and a variety of cardiopulmonary, hematologic, hepatic, renal, and vasculitic effects.

The Gell and Coombs classification system defines four basic immunologic mechanisms for drug reactions [*see Figure 1*]. However, some clinical presentations may involve several mechanisms, and not all immunologic mechanisms conform to

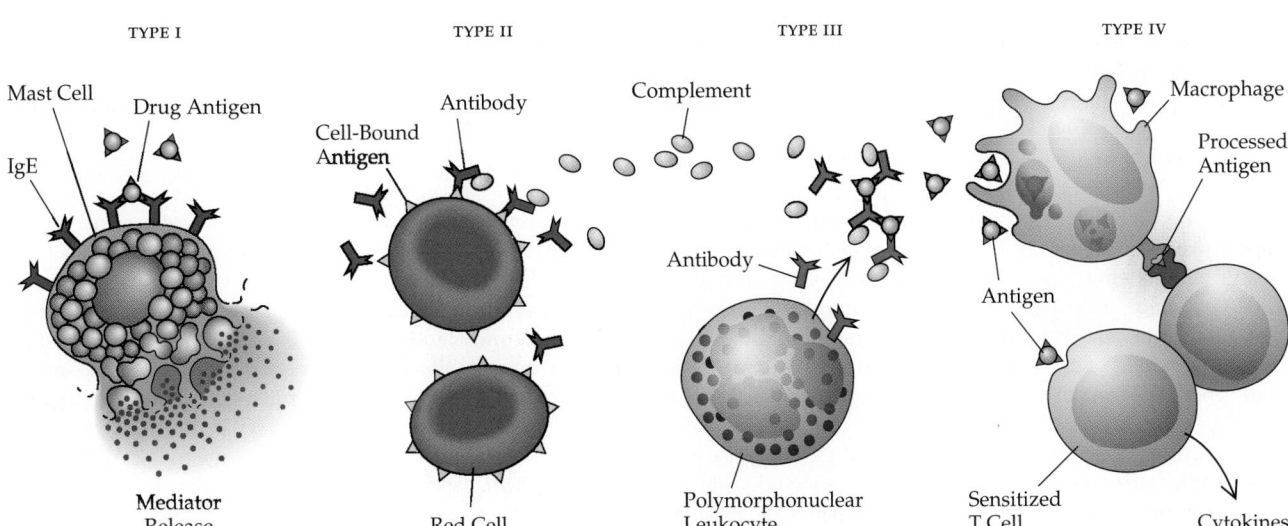

Figure 1   **The Gell and Coombs system defines four basic immunologic mechanisms for drug reactions.[40] Type I reactions (anaphylaxis) result from IgE antibodies binding to drug antigen and cross-linkage of adjacent IgE molecules, leading to mediator release. Type II (cytotoxic) reactions occur when IgG or IgM antibodies recognize drug antigen associated with cell membranes, causing complement activation. Type III (immune complex) reactions involve the formation of antigen-antibody complexes. Type IV (delayed hypersensitivity) reactions are mediated by sensitized lymphocytes.**

Table 1 General Considerations in the Clinical Evaluation of Drug Reactions[9]

Identify drugs that have a history of causing problems in the patient; determine whether there are cross-reacting agents, and avoid them.

If the patient has a late reaction, such as a drug rash, take a careful history of all drugs used in the past month, because it is possible that the causative drug has been discontinued.

Drugs administered with impunity for prolonged periods (e.g., months to years) are rarely responsible for adverse immunologic reactions. Reactions are more likely to result from drugs introduced more recently.

Have a high index of suspicion for drug reactions whenever a patient experiences adverse clinical manifestations. Bear in mind that drug reactions can involve internal organs (e.g., nephritis, hepatitis, isolated lymphadenopathy), often in the absence of eosinophilia.

If an immunologic drug reaction is suspected, stop all nonessential drugs and substitute non–cross-reactive drugs if possible.

the Gell and Coombs classification. Type I (anaphylactic) reactions occur when drug antigen cross-links adjacent IgE antibodies that are bound to the surfaces of mast cells or basophils, with consequent cell activation and release of mediators such as histamine, tryptase, and leukotrienes. Common causes of type I reactions include antibiotics, vaccines, allergen extracts, and proteins (e.g., antisera, insulin). Reactions occur within seconds to minutes of exposure and range from full anaphylaxis to any component thereof, including pruritus, flushing, angioedema, urticaria, bronchospasm, laryngeal edema, rhinoconjunctivitis, hypotension, tachycardia, nausea, vomiting, diarrhea, and abdominal or uterine cramping. In contrast to anaphylaxis, syncope or vasovagal reactions are typically characterized by blanching rather than flushing and by bradycardia rather than tachycardia.

Type II (cytotoxicity) reactions result in cell destruction mediated by an interaction between IgG or IgM antibodies, complement, and a drug antigen associated with cell membranes. Clinical sequelae include immune hemolytic anemia, thrombocytopenia, and granulocytopenia. Heparin-induced thrombocytopenia is mediated by antibodies directed against antigen complexes of heparin and platelet factor 4 on the surface of platelets [*see Chapter 99*].

Type III (immune complex) reactions develop when a drug combines with antibodies to form immune complexes, the deposition of which causes tissue damage. Serum sickness is a type III reaction and may manifest as skin lesions (e.g., urticaria, angioedema, maculopapular or morbilliform rash, palpable purpura), arthralgias and arthritis, lymphadenopathy, fever, nephritis, and hepatitis. Serum sickness usually occurs after 1 to 4 weeks of drug use but may occur sooner in patients with previous exposure. Drug-induced lupus syndromes are also type III reactions. Renal involvement is rare, as is the presence of anti–double-stranded DNA antibodies, but other autoantibodies are common; these autoantibodies include antihistone from procainamide, hydralazine, or phenytoin; perinuclear antineutrophil cytoplasmic antibody (p-ANCA) from minocycline; and SS-A and SS-B from thiazides.[5]

Type IV (delayed hypersensitivity) reactions are mediated by sensitized CD4+ or CD8+ T cells.[6] Allergic contact dermatitis is a classic example and typically develops 24 to 72 hours after topical exposure.

Diagnosis

To identify drug reactions, the physician needs to be familiar with general principles of drug reactions [*see Table 1*] and with the individual drugs the patient has taken.[7] Diagnosis depends largely on the nature of the reaction and its timing in relation to drug use. For example, adverse immunologic reactions to drugs usually occur in the early weeks of drug exposure and become less common with continued drug administration. To confirm the clinical diagnosis, skin testing or drug challenges may be valuable in selected cases [*see Figure 2*].[8]

CLINICAL PRESENTATION

Dermatologic Reactions

Drug reactions involving the skin range from maculopapular and morbilliform rashes to urticaria, angioedema, erythema multiforme, erythema nodosum, bullous eruptions, and exfoliations. Drug eruptions usually occur within days of exposure but may occur after drug cessation. Eruptions are symmetrical and truncal; they are accompanied by pruritus, fever, and, occasionally, eosinophilia. Palm and sole involvement suggests a viral exanthem rather than a drug reaction. Photosensitive drug rashes are of two kinds: phototoxic or photoallergic. Phototoxic reactions are nonimmunologic, generally appear as sunburn 4 to 8 hours after light exposure, and often occur with the first exposure to the drug; tetracycline has been associated with phototoxic reactions. Photoallergic reactions are typically eczematous rashes that occur after days or months of exposure; photoallergic reactions have been associated with some sulfa drugs. Alteration of the drug by ultraviolet light enables conjugation of the drug to self-proteins and T cell–mediated immune responses. Neither type of photosensitive reaction is predictive of other types of adverse reactions to a drug.

Fever

Drug fever may occur by itself or in association with other allergic manifestations, such as a rash. The fever stems from the release of pyrogens by phagocytic cells that have engulfed drug-IgG immune complexes or from cytokine release and other incompletely established processes associated with specific T cell activation. Drug fever usually occurs 7 to 10 days into a treatment course, with prompt defervescence within 48 hours of cessation of the responsible agent.

Systemic Manifestations

Drug reactions can result in systemic involvement, such as interstitial nephritis, nephrotic syndrome, hepatic reactions, myocarditis, and vasculitis. Lung involvement may present as part of a syndrome consisting of malaise, nonproductive cough, chest discomfort, and migratory infiltrates, with or without peripheral eosinophilia (Löffler syndrome). Long-term treatment with penicillin, sulfonamides, or phenytoin can result in generalized lymphadenopathy. Aseptic meningitis has been reported from nonsteroidal anti-inflammatory drugs (NSAIDs), radiocontrast media, and other agents.[4,9,10]

TESTING

Skin Testing

Drug reactions can be identified through immediate-type skin testing only when the process is IgE mediated [*see Figure 2*]. Non–IgE-mediated reactions, such as nonurticarial skin

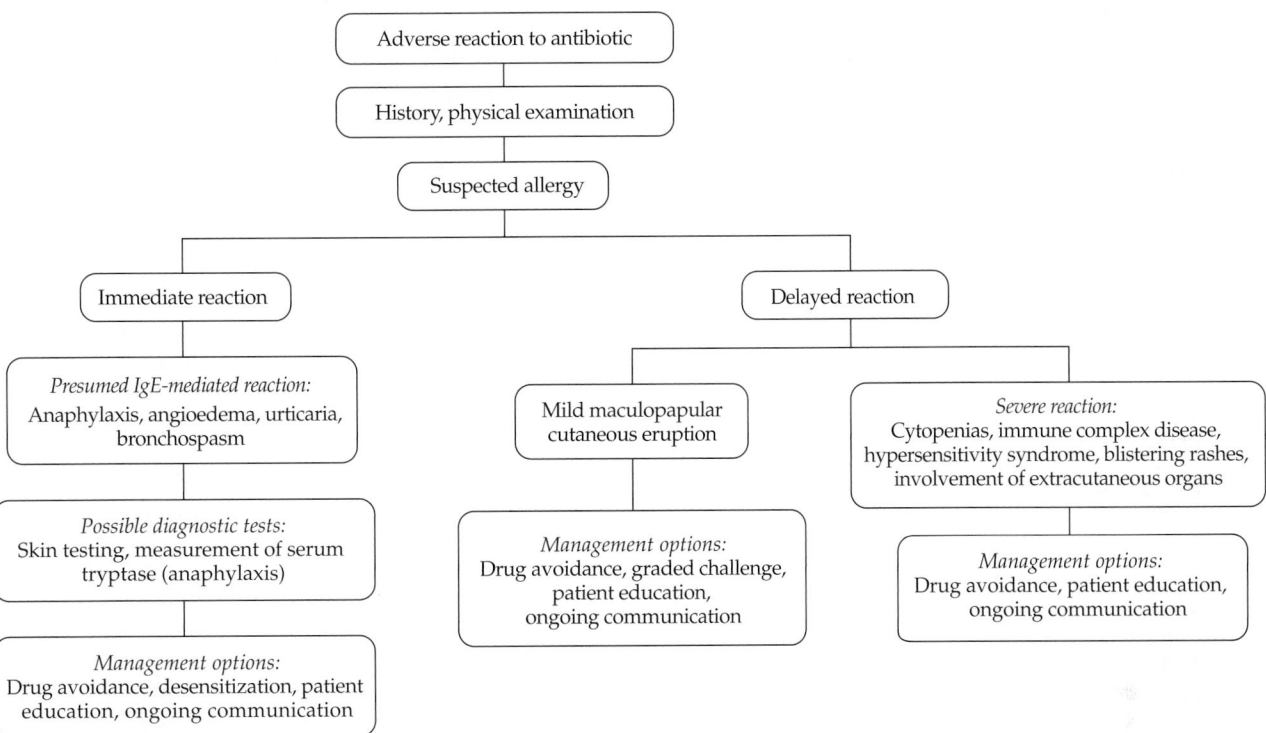

Figure 2 **Management of an immune-mediated antibiotic allergy. The rapidity of a patient's reaction to a drug determines management. An immediate IgE-mediated reaction may require skin testing to identify allergen-specific IgE antibodies; in cases in which the skin test is inconclusive, additional tests may be required. Elevated titers of serum tryptase can confirm the diagnosis in cases of suspected anaphalaxis. Treatment options are determined by the nature and severity of the reaction. In the management of immediate reactions, drug desensitization may be performed if the implicated drug is required for treatment of the patient. For reactions that are not immediate, management depends on the clinical manifestations of the previous reaction. For maculopapular eruptions, readministration of the drug on an incremental-dosing schedule chosen with a specialist (and at dosing intervals ranging from hours to days or even weeks) may allow use of the drug. In all cases, education of the patient and communication with the patient and the referring physician are vital to ensure the success of the management strategy and to prevent a recurrence of antibiotic allergy.[8]**

rashes, cannot be identified in this manner. Skin testing is reliable for protein agents and small-molecular-weight drugs whose allergenic metabolites have been identified and made available for skin testing (e.g., penicillin). Skin testing requires knowledgeable personnel and the use of appropriate concentrations (i.e., concentrations high enough to provoke a reaction but low enough to avoid causing a systemic response).

In Vitro Testing

There are a limited number of radioallergosorbent tests (RASTs) available for detection of IgE antibodies against drugs, including β-lactam antibiotics and anesthetic agents. In vitro tests for drug allergy are generally less sensitive than skin tests but may be useful in certain cases in which skin testing is not possible (e.g., in patients with severe, generalized eczema or in those who must take medications that can suppress skin-test responses).[11]

Drug Challenges

When the probability of a true allergy is remote, a graded challenge can be used to confirm the clinical diagnosis of drug reaction. In graded challenges, the patient is given a test dose at a dose lower than would cause a serious reaction. Subsequent doses are then escalated in large increments, and the patient is observed between doses.[8]

Reactions to Specific Drugs

PENICILLIN

Penicillin, a β-lactam antibiotic, is among the most common causes of immunologic drug reactions. Most deaths from penicillin reactions occur in patients with no history of penicillin allergy. Nonimmunologic rashes are frequently seen with ampicillin or amoxicillin in patients who have concomitant viral infections, chronic lymphocytic leukemia, or hyperuricemia and in patients taking allopurinol. These rashes are typically nonpruritic and are not associated with an increased risk of future intolerance of penicillin antibiotics.

Most immunologic reactions to penicillins are directed against β-lactam core determinants. Less than 5% of penicillin is metabolized to the minor determinants, which include benzyl penicillin G, penicilloates, and benzylpenicilloylamine. IgE antibodies to the minor determinants are usually responsible for severe immediate-type reactions to penicillin. The benzylpenicilloyl moiety, the so-called major determinant, makes up 95% of penicillin metabolites but is less commonly responsible for severe immediate reactions.

Patients who have suffered IgE-mediated penicillin reactions tend to lose their sensitivity over time if penicillin is avoided. By 5 years after an immediate reaction, 50% of such patients have negative results on skin testing. There is contro-

Table 2   Intravenous Desensitization Protocol for
β-Lactam Antibiotics[41]

Dose	β-Lactam Stock Concentration (mg/ml)	Cumulative Dose Given (ml)
1	0.1	0.1
2		0.2
3		0.4
4		0.8
5	1.0	0.15
6		0.3
7		0.6
8		1.00
9	10	0.2
10		0.4
11		0.8
12	100	0.15
13		0.3
14		0.6
15		1.00
16	1,000	0.2
17		0.4

Note: observe patient for approximately 15–40 min after each interval dose and for 30 min after final dose.

versy about whether patients who have lost their sensitivity to penicillin may be more likely than others to be sensitized with subsequent penicillin exposure; accumulating evidence indicates that penicillin resensitization is low.[4,12,13] Skin testing with a major determinant preparation and penicillin G identifies at least 90% to 93% of patients at risk for immediate reaction to penicillin. The negative predictive value of penicillin skin testing is significantly increased by the addition of a minor determinant mixture, but that is not currently commercially available. Penicillin skin testing is usually reliable in identifying patients at risk for immediate reactions to the semisynthetic penicillins,[4,14] but reactions to unique semisynthetic side-chain determinants may occur in special-risk populations, such as cystic fibrosis patients.[15] Skin testing with the side-chain determinants is not commonly done.

Not everyone with a history of a reaction to penicillin should undergo skin testing, but it is important to perform a skin test on patients with a history of anaphylaxis or urticaria associated with penicillin use before they are given penicillin again [*see Figure 2*]. Patients who report a history of maculopapular or morbilliform skin rashes from the use of penicillin are not at higher risk for immediate-type reactions, but skin testing may be considered for these patients because studies have demonstrated that patient histories can be unreliable. A carefully taken patient history can often distinguish patients with credible histories of penicillin allergy (who might benefit from skin testing) from patients whose histories are not credible (who might then be treated with penicillin).[16] However, a large proportion

of patients who report vague histories of penicillin allergy have penicillin-specific IgE antibodies; consequently, patients with vague histories of allergy should undergo penicillin skin testing.[17] Penicillin should not be readministered to patients with a history of penicillin-induced Stevens-Johnson syndrome, toxic epidermal necrolysis (TEN), other exfoliative dermatitis, or bullous skin lesions; therefore, skin testing is not indicated in these cases. Patients with a family history of penicillin allergy but no personal history of penicillin allergy are not at increased risk for allergy to penicillin and, therefore, do not require skin testing. Desensitization is not required in a patient with a history of an immediate reaction and a negative skin test result, but a small test dose may be given as an additional precaution if the previous reaction was life threatening. If there is a compelling indication for a penicillin antibiotic (e.g., neurosyphilis), a rapid desensitization protocol should be used [*see Table 2*].[9,18-20]

Cephalosporins and penicillin have similar bicyclic β-lactam structures and amide side chains [*see Figure 3*]. The degree of immunologic cross-reactivity between these β-lactams is controversial, but patients with penicillin allergy are more likely than the general population to have a reaction to another β-lactam drug. In a large study of patients receiving penicillin followed by a cephalosporin, the unadjusted risk ratio for an allergic-like event for patients who had experienced a prior event, as compared with those who had no such prior event, was 10.1 (confidence interval, 7.4 to 13.8); however, the researchers concluded that cross-reactivity alone is not an adequate explanation for this increased risk.[21] Most experts agree that cephalosporins should be avoided in patients who have a history of an immediate-type reaction to penicillin.[20,22] Immunologic reactions to cephalosporins are more often related to side chains of the cephalosporin antibiotics than to β-lactam core determinants.[23] Cephalosporin skin testing is experimental and has uncertain negative predictive value. There is a lower incidence of immediate-type reactions to third-generation cephalosporins than to the first- and second-generation compounds.[24] Because of its 3-methylthiotetrazole side chain, cefoperazone can cause a nonimmunologic disulfiram-like reaction if taken after ingestion of alcohol. Carbapenems (imipenem) and carbacephems (loracarbef) contain bicyclic β-lactam rings that cause significant cross-reactivity with penicillin.[25] Reactions to monobactams (e.g., aztreonam) are typically directed against side-chain determinants rather than the monocyclic β-lactam nucleus, but cross-reactivity occurs with ceftazidime, which shares an identical side chain with penicillin.[26,27]

SULFA

Drug exanthems from sulfonamide antibiotics are more common than immediate-type reactions, and there is significant cross-reactivity among sulfa compounds. Adverse effects from sulfa antibiotics occur in 2% to 10% of patients who do not have AIDS, whereas 50% of AIDS patients suffer ill effects.[4] The incidence of reactions may be related to the degree of immunodeficiency from HIV infection. The sulfapyridine moiety of sulfasalazine is responsible for most skin rashes from that agent. A 1-month graded challenge protocol is usually successful at inducing tolerance to sulfasalazine in patients who require this agent for treatment of inflammatory bowel disease.[28] Desensitization to sulfonamide antibiotics may be considered to permit the use of these agents for prophylaxis against *Pneumocystis jiroveci* pneumonia in patients with AIDS, toxoplasmosis, and other infections for which there are no good alternatives. A number of protocols have been published. Patients with acute *Pneumocystis* pneumonia may require rapid desensitization protocols that permit therapeutic use of the medication within 6 to 8 hours[29]; those patients receiving a sulfonamide prophylactically can be desensitized with slowly increasing doses. Desensitization protocols should not be attempted in patients with a history of severe drug reactions, such as Stevens-Johnson syndrome or TEN.[20] There is no immunologic cross-reactivity between sulfonamide antibiotics and nonantibiotic agents that have sulfonamide moieties (e.g., thiazides, celecoxib, glyburide, and triptans). However, patients with a history of allergic reactions to sulfonamide or penicillin antibiotics are at increased risk for developing reactions to nonantibiotic sulfonamides.[30] This evidence further demonstrates that patients with a history of drug allergy to some agents are at greater risk than the general population for developing allergic reactions to structurally distinct drugs.

VANCOMYCIN

Vancomycin infusions are commonly associated with the red man syndrome (hypotension, flushing, erythema, pruritus, urticaria, and pain or muscle spasms of the chest and back). The syndrome is caused by non–IgE-mediated histamine release that is more likely with rapid infusion rates (> 10 mg/min). Tolerance of readministration is promoted by reduction of the infusion rate and pretreatment with H_1 (but not H_2) antihistamines. Rarer IgE-mediated reactions to vancomycin can be identified by skin tests.[3,4,9]

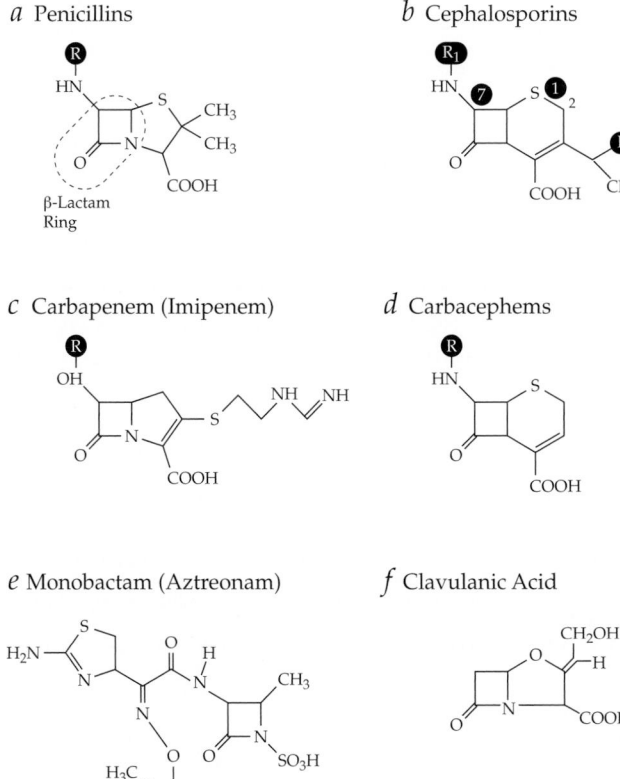

Figure 3 Structure of β-lactam antibiotics. Substitutions at the R position of 6-aminopenicillanic acid create penicillin derivatives. Substitutions at positions 1, R1, R2, and C7 of 7-aminocephalosporanic acid create cephalosporin derivatives.

ACE INHIBITORS

Nonimmunologic adverse effects of angiotensin-converting enzyme (ACE) inhibitors are thought to stem from an accumulation of bradykinin and other vasoactive peptides. The most frequently documented adverse reactions include cough (10% to 25%), rhinitis, and angioedema (0.1% to 0.2%). The onset of cough can occur from 1 day to up to 12 months after starting these drugs and may be associated with increased bronchial reactivity to methacholine. Cough usually resolves within several weeks after drug cessation but may persist for more than a month. In about 60% of cases, angioedema occurs within 2 weeks after patients start the drug, but it can occur months after the initiation of drug therapy. Angioedema usually involves the face and oropharyngeal tissue. It can result in life-threatening upper airway obstruction; for patients with angioedema, particularly of the head and neck, that is unresponsive to usual measures [*see Chapter 107*], fresh frozen plasma administration has been reported to be beneficial.[31] Visceral angioedema can cause abdominal pain. Cough and angioedema do not usually occur in the same patient. Skin testing is of no value. Intolerance to one ACE inhibitor usually predicts intolerance to all drugs of this class. Patients with idiopathic angioedema and urticaria are susceptible to more severe and frequent episodes when given ACE inhibitors. The angiotensin II receptor blockers are generally well tolerated in patients with idiopathic angioedema and urticaria or with ACE inhibitor–related angioedema.[3,9,32]

ASPIRIN AND NSAIDS

Aspirin and other NSAIDs may induce a variety of reactions, ranging from bronchospasm, rhinorrhea, urticaria, and angioedema to anaphylaxis. Aspirin-sensitive respiratory reactions are likely caused by derangement of arachidonic acid metabolism with increased leukotriene production. Mast cell activation may also occur. Patients with respiratory sensitivity to aspirin generally develop dose-dependent reactions to aspirin or structurally distinct NSAIDs that are significant inhibitors of cyclooxygenase-1 (COX-1) but often tolerate agents that have less effect on COX-1 (e.g., salsalate, acetaminophen, sodium or magnesium salicylate). Selective COX-2 inhibitors (e.g., celecoxib, rofecoxib) are well tolerated in these patients.[33] Patients may present with the so-called aspirin triad of concomitant asthma, nasal polyps, and aspirin sensitivity. Between 30% and 40% of patients with polyps and sinusitis and between 8% and 21% of adults with asthma have positive bronchial responses to aspirin.[9,34] Urticarial reactions from aspirin typically occur in a patient subset different from that in which respiratory reactions occur.[35] Some patients with skin reactions to aspirin (often those with a history of idiopathic urticaria and angioedema) have cross-reactivity with NSAIDs, whereas other skin reactors and those who develop anaphylaxis have only specific sensitivity to aspirin or a particular NSAID.[34,36] However, skin testing is not helpful. With appropriate precautions, oral desensitization with aspirin by experienced clinicians can be performed over several days. It is usually effective in patients with respiratory sensitivity but not in those with skin reactions.[37]

ANESTHETIC AGENTS

Adverse reactions to local anesthetic agents are rarely IgE mediated. More commonly, such reactions are toxic responses from inadvertent intravenous administration, overdose, rapid absorption, or anxiety. Symptoms often involve the central nervous system or the cardiovascular system and include hypotension, convulsions, and cardiorespiratory failure. Concurrent administration of epinephrine may be responsible for shakiness and tachycardia. Allergic contact dermatitis and some large local reactions do occur through delayed-type immunologic responses [see Chapter 39]. Local anesthetics are either benzoid acid esters (type I [e.g., procaine, benzocaine]) or nonesters and amides (type II [e.g., lidocaine, bupivacaine, mepivacaine]). There is no cross-reactivity between the two classes, but type I agents cross-react with each other. Management of suspected local anesthetic allergy includes subcutaneous test dosing with the local anesthetic without epinephrine.

Histamine release has been implicated in some reactions from anesthesia-induction agents and muscle relaxants, but the responsible mechanisms for many reactions are not established. During anesthesia, generalized reactions may be caused by muscle relaxants (e.g., succinylcholine, alcuronium, pancuronium), induction agents (e.g., thiopental), opiates, or antibiotics. Narcotics stimulate mast cells directly without an IgE mechanism.

RADIOGRAPHIC CONTRAST MEDIA

Radiographic contrast media cause non–IgE-mediated anaphylactoid reactions that involve direct mast cell and perhaps complement activation; therefore, immediate-type skin testing and test dosing are not helpful. Shellfish allergy results from IgE-mediated reactions to shellfish proteins, and therefore, it is not predictive of risk for contrast reactions. A previous anaphylactoid reaction to contrast at any time in a patient's history is predictive of persistently increased risk of a repeat anaphylactoid reaction, even though the patient may have tolerated contrast without a reaction in the interim. Asthma and allergies are also associated with increased risk.[38]

The use of nonionic contrast media and medication pretreatment can reduce the risk of reaction. One commonly used pretreatment regimen consists of corticosteroids (prednisone, 50 mg, given 13 hours, 7 hours, and 1 hour before contrast administration), H_1 antihistamines (diphenhydramine, 50 mg orally, given 1 hour before administration), and oral adrenergic agents (ephedrine, 25 mg, or albuterol, 4 mg, given orally 1 hour before administration). H_2 receptor blockers are sometimes added. Despite an adequate pretreatment regimen, reactions can still occur. The administration of corticosteroids only 1 to 2 hours before administration of contrast does not reliably prevent reactions in susceptible patients.

Management

MANAGEMENT OF ACUTE REACTIONS

Treatment of acute adverse immunologic drug reactions includes stopping all nonessential suspect drugs and, if necessary, substituting new drugs that should not have cross-reactivity with any of the suspect drugs. Epinephrine, antihistamines, and corticosteroids are the mainstays of treatment of anaphylaxis, and other resuscitative measures may be required [see Chapter 107]. Mild maculopapular rashes may respond to antihistamines alone, but progressing rashes or rashes associated with fever, nausea, or arthralgias should also be treated with systemic corticosteroids. For prolonged, severe reactions, several weeks of prednisone therapy may be required.[3,4,20]

DESENSITIZATION AND OTHER SPECIALIZED APPROACHES

If the probability of a drug allergy is high and drug administration is essential, one may consider desensitization, in which the drug is administered in increasing doses in small increments.[39] Because of the risk of adverse reactions, only experienced physicians should perform desensitization. Once desensitization is achieved, the drug must be continued; otherwise, desensitization will be lost, and the patient will require repeat desensitization before readministration. Pretreatment with antihistamines and corticosteroids is not reliable for preventing IgE-mediated anaphylaxis but can be useful when an anaphylactoid reaction is of concern (as in the use of radiographic contrast media). In extreme circumstances, when continued administration of a drug is essential but the patient is experiencing a reaction such as a late drug rash or interstitial nephritis, continued drug administration may be tolerated if corticosteroids and antihistamines are given to suppress the immunologic reaction. However, in such cases, there is the risk of progression to an exfoliative skin rash, mucocutaneous disorders (e.g., Stevens-Johnson syndrome, TEN), nephritis, hepatitis, or serum sickness.

Mark S. Dykewicz, M.D., F.A.C.P., has received grants for clinical research or educational activities or served as an advisor or consultant to Astra-Zeneca Pharmaceuticals Ltd.; Genentech, Inc.; Novartis AG; GlaxoSmithKline, Inc.; Merck & Co., Inc.; and Schering-Plough Corp.

Heather C. Gray, M.D., has no commercial relationships with manufacturers of products or providers of services discussed in this chapter.

References

1. Pirmohamed M, James S, Meakin S, et al: Adverse drug reactions as cause of admission to hospital: prospective analysis of 18,820 patients. BMJ 329:15, 2004

2. Gruchalla RS: Drug allergy. J Allergy Clin Immunol 111(2 suppl):548, 2003

3. Dykewicz MS: Drug allergy. Comprehensive Therapy 22:353, 1996

4. DeSwarte RD: Drug allergy. Allergic Diseases: Diagnosis and Management, 6th ed. Patterson R, Greenberger PA, Grammer LC, Eds. Lippincott, Philadelphia, 2002, p 295

5. Srivastava M, Rencic A, Diglio G, et al: Drug-induced, Ro/SSA-positive cutaneous lupus erythematosus. Arch Dermatol 139:45, 2003

6. Pichler WJ: Delayed drug hypersensitivity reactions. Ann Intern Med 139:683, 2003

7. Greenberger PA: Drug allergy. J Allergy Clin Immunol 117:S464, 2006

8. Gruchalla RS, Pirmohamed M: Antibiotic allergy. N Engl J Med 354:601, 2006

9. Dykewicz MS: Drug allergy. An Expert Guide to Allergy and Immunology. Slavin RG, Reisman RE, Eds. American College of Physicians, Philadelphia, 1999, p 127

10. DeShazo RD, Kemp SF: Allergic reactions to drugs and biologic agents. JAMA 278:1895, 1997

11. Primeau MN, Adkinson NF Jr: Recent advances in the diagnosis of drug allergy. Curr Opin Allergy Clin Immunol 1:337, 2001

12. Bittner A, Greenberger PA: Incidence of resensitization after tolerating penicillin treatment in penicillin-allergic patients. Allergy Asthma Proc 25:161, 2004

13. Solensky R, Earl HS, Gruchalla RS: Lack of penicillin resensitization in patients with a history of penicillin allergy after receiving repeated penicillin courses. Arch Intern Med 162:822, 2002

14. Sogn DD, Evans R III, Shepherd GM, et al: Results of the National Institute of Allergy and Infectious Diseases collaborative clinical trial to test the predictive value of skin testing with major and minor penicillin determinant derivatives in hospitalized patients. Arch Intern Med 152:1025, 1992

15. Ramesh S: Antibiotic hypersensitivity in patients with CF. Clin Rev Allergy Immunol 23:123, 2002

16. Stember RH: Prevalence of skin test reactivity in patients with convincing, vague, and unacceptable histories of penicillin allergy. Allergy Asthma Proc 26:59, 2005

17. Solensky R, Earl HS, Gruchalla RS: Penicillin allergy: prevalence of vague history in skin test-positive patients. Ann Allergy Asthma Immunol 85:195, 2000

18. Sullivan T, Yecies L, Shatz G, et al: Desensitization of patients allergic to penicillin using orally administered beta-lactam antibiotics. J Allergy Clin Immunol 69:275, 1982

19. Wickern GM, Nish WA, Bitner AS, et al: Allergy to beta-lactams: a survey of current practices. J Allergy Clin Immunol 94:725, 1994

20. Executive summary of disease management of drug hypersensitivity: a practice parameter. Joint Task Force on Practice Parameters, and the Joint Council of Allergy, Asthma and Immunology. Ann Allergy Asthma Immunol 83:665, 1999

21. Apter AJ, Kinman JL, Bilker WB, et al: Is there cross-reactivity between penicillins

and cephalosporins? Am J Med 119:354, 2006

22. Romano A, Gueant-Rogriguez RM, Viola M, et al: Cross-reactivity and tolerability of cephalosporins in patients with immediate hypersensitivity to penicillins. Ann Intern Med 141:16, 2004

23. Kelkar PS, Li JT: Current concepts: cephalosporin allergy. N Engl J Med 345:804, 2001

24. Fonacier L, Hirschberg R, Gerson S: Adverse drug reactions to a cephalosporin in hospitalized patients with a history of penicillin allergy. Allergy Asthma Proc 26:135, 2005

25. Prescott WA Jr, DePestel DD, Ellis JJ, et al: Incidence of carbapenem-associated allergic-type reactions among patients with versus patients without a reported penicillin allergy. Clin Infect Dis 38:1102, 2004

26. Saxon A, Adelman DC, Patel A, et al: Imipenem cross-reactivity with penicillin in humans. J Allergy Clin Immunol 82:213, 1988

27. Adkinson NF Jr: Immunogenicity and cross-allergenicity of aztreonam. Am J Med 88:12S, 1990

28. Purdy BH, Philips DM, Summers RW: Desensitization for sulfasalazine skin rash. Ann Intern Med 100:512, 1984

29. Leoung GS, Stanford JF, Giordano MR, et al: Trimethoprim-sulfamethoxazole (TMP-SMZ) dose escalation versus direct rechallenge for *Pneumocystis carinii* pneumonia prophylaxis in human immunodeficiency virus–infected patients with previous adverse reaction to TMP-SMZ. J Infect Dis 184:992, 2001

30. Strom BL, Schinnar R, Apter AJ: Absence of cross-reactivity between sulfonamide antibiotics and sulfonamide nonantibiotics. N Engl J Med 349:1628, 2003

31. Warrier MR, Copilevitz CA, Dykewicz MS, et al: Fresh frozen plasma (FFP) in the treatment of resistant ACE inhibitor (ACE-I) angioedema. Ann Allergy Asthma Immunol 92:573, 2004

32. Dykewicz MS: Cough and angioedema from ACE inhibitors: new insights into mechanisms and management. Current Opin Allergy Clin Immunol 4:267, 2004

33. Pacor ML, Di Lorenzo G, Biasi D, et al: Safety of rofecoxib in subjects with a history of adverse cutaneous reactions to aspirin and/or non-steroidal anti-inflammatory drugs. Clin Exp Allergy 32:397, 2002

34. Jenkins C, Costello J, Hodge L: Systematic review of prevalence of aspirin induced asthma and its implications for clinical practice. BMJ 328:434, 2004

35. Szczeklik A, Sanak M: The broken balance in aspirin hypersensitivity. Eur J Pharmacol 533:145, 2006

36. Namazy JA, Simon RA: Sensitivity to nonsteroidal anti-inflammatory drugs. Ann Allergy Asthma Immunol 89:542, 2002

37. Berges-Gimeno MP, Simon RA, Stevenson DD: Long-term treatment with aspirin desensitization in asthmatic patients with aspirin-exacerbated respiratory disease. J Allergy Clin Immunol 111:180, 2003

38. Maddox TG: Adverse reactions to contrast material: recognition, prevention, and treatment. Am Fam Physician 66:1229, 2002

39. Solensky R: Drug desensitization. Immunol Allergy Clin North Am 24:425, 2004

40. Grammer LC: Drug allergy. Atlas of Allergies. Slavin RG, Fireman P, Eds. Mosby-Wolfe Publishers, Barcelona, Spain, 1996, p 286

41. Sullivan TJ: Drug allergy. Middleton's Allergy: Principles and Practice, 6th ed. Adkinson NF Jr, Busse WW, Holgate ST, et al, Eds. CV Mosby, Philadelphia, 2003, p 1679

Acknowledgment

Figures 1 and 3   Seward Hung.

109 Food Allergies

A. Wesley Burks, M.D.

Definition

Food hypersensitivity (allergy) and food intolerance constitute the category of adverse reactions to food.[1,2] An adverse food reaction is a clinically abnormal response to an ingested food or food additive. Both food hypersensitivity and food intolerance have often been overdiagnosed, and both terms have been applied incorrectly to all adverse reactions to foods.

FOOD INTOLERANCE

Food intolerance is a general term describing an abnormal physiologic response to an ingested food or food additive. Such reactions are apparently nonimmunologic in nature and have many possible causes, including toxic contaminants (e.g., histamine in scombroid fish poisoning or toxins secreted by *Salmonella, Shigella,* and *Campylobacter*), pharmacologic properties of the food (e.g., caffeine in coffee and tyramine in aged cheeses), characteristics of the host (e.g., metabolic traits such as lactase deficiency), and idiosyncratic responses.

FOOD HYPERSENSITIVITY

Food hypersensitivity is an immunologic reaction resulting from the ingestion of a food or food additive. This reaction can develop after ingestion of a small amount of the substance, and it is unrelated to any physiologic effect of the food or food additive. To most physicians, the term is synonymous with reactions that involve the immunoglobulin E (IgE) mechanism, of which anaphylaxis is the classic example. Although IgE-mediated (type I) hypersensitivity accounts for the majority of well-characterized allergic reactions to food, non–IgE-mediated immune mechanisms are believed to be responsible for a variety of hypersensitivity disorders. This chapter examines adverse food reactions that are IgE mediated, those that are non–IgE mediated, and those that have characteristics of both.

Epidemiology

The true incidence of adverse food reactions is still unknown. Up to 15% of the general population believes that they may be allergic to some food. The best available studies, however, suggest that the actual prevalence of food allergy is 3% to 4% of the adult population.[3] The incidence of adverse food reactions in young children is estimated to be between 6% and 8%. Several well-controlled studies have shown that the vast majority of allergic reactions occur in the first year of life.[3] The foods that commonly cause these reactions in children include eggs, milk, peanuts, and tree nuts. In adults, this list includes fish, shellfish, tree nuts, and peanuts.

Pathophysiology

IGE-MEDIATED REACTIONS

A variety of hypersensitivity responses to an ingested food antigen may result from the lack of development of oral tolerance or a breakdown of oral tolerance in the gastrointestinal tract of a person who is genetically predisposed to such hypersensitivity. Either a failure to develop oral tolerance or a breakdown in oral tolerance results in excessive production of food-specific IgE antibodies. These food-specific antibodies bind high-affinity FcεI receptors on mast cells and basophils and low-affinity FcεII receptors on macrophages, monocytes, lymphocytes, eosinophils, and platelets.[2] After antigen-presenting cells process the food allergen and present the antigen to specific antibodies on mast cells or basophils, the mast cells and basophils release mediators such as histamine, prostaglandins, and leukotrienes [*see Chapter 104*]. These mediators promote vasodilatation, smooth muscle contraction, and mucus secretion, resulting in the symptoms of immediate hypersensitivity. The activated mast cells may also release various cytokines that play a part in the IgE-mediated late-phase response. A rise in plasma histamine levels has been associated with IgE-mediated allergic symptoms after blinded food challenges.

NON–IGE-MEDIATED REACTIONS

Although a variety of non–IgE-mediated immune mechanisms for allergic reactions to food have been proposed, the scientific evidence supporting these mechanisms is limited. Type III (antigen-antibody complex–mediated) hypersensitivity reactions have been examined in several studies. Whereas food antigen–IgE complexes are seen more commonly in patients with food hypersensitivity, there is little evidence supporting disease mediated by other food antigen–immune complexes. Type IV (cell-mediated) hypersensitivity has been suggested as the mechanism for several disorders in which the clinical symptoms do not appear until several hours after the ingestion of the suspected food. This type of immune response may contribute to some adverse food reactions (e.g., enterocolitis), but except in gluten-sensitive enteropathy, significant supporting evidence of a specific cell-mediated hypersensitivity disorder is lacking.

Diagnosis

IGE-MEDIATED HYPERSENSITIVITY

Gastrointestinal Reactions

Food-induced, IgE-mediated GI allergy may manifest itself as a variety of syndromes, including the oral allergy syndrome, immediate GI hypersensitivity, and a small subgroup of cases of allergic eosinophilic gastroenteritis.[4]

Pollen-associated food allergy syndrome The pollen-associated food allergy syndrome is considered a form of contact urticaria that is confined almost exclusively to the oropharynx and rarely involves other target organs [*see Table 1*]. The symptoms include rapid onset of pruritus and angioedema of the lips, tongue, palate, and throat. The symptoms generally resolve quite rapidly. This syndrome is most commonly associated with the ingestion of fresh fruits and vegetables. Interestingly, patients with allergic rhinitis

Table 1   Pollen-Associated Food Allergy Syndrome[27]

Oral manifestations	Burning Swelling Itching Erythema Immediate onset of symptoms
Age at onset	Beyond infancy Typically younger than 5 yr
Proteins implicated	Heat-labile fresh fruit and vegetable allergens Pollen and latex cross-reactivity
Pathology	IgE antibodies
Treatment	Avoidance Cooking
Natural history	Unknown

associated with certain airborne pollens (especially ragweed and birch pollens) are frequently afflicted with this syndrome. Patients with ragweed allergy may experience these symptoms after contact with certain melons (e.g., watermelons, cantaloupe, and honeydew) and bananas. Patients with birch sensitivity often have symptoms after the ingestion of raw potatoes, carrots, celery, apples, and hazelnuts. The diagnosis of this syndrome is based on a suggestive history and positive prick skin tests with the implicated fresh fruits and vegetables, although the sensitivity of these tests may be limited in this disorder [see Prick Skin Tests, below].[5]

Immediate GI hypersensitivity   Immediate GI hypersensitivity may accompany allergic manifestations in other target organs [see Table 2].[6,7] The GI symptoms vary but may include nausea, abdominal pain, abdominal cramping, vomiting, and diarrhea. In children with atopic dermatitis and food allergy, the frequent ingestion of a food allergen appears to induce partial desensitization of GI mast cells, resulting in less pronounced symptoms.

The diagnosis of immediate GI hypersensitivity is based on a suggestive clinical history, positive prick skin tests, resolution of symptoms after complete elimination of the suspected food allergen for up to 2 weeks, and positive results on oral food challenges. After patients have avoided a particular food for 10 to 14 days, it is not unusual for them to experience vomiting during a challenge, even though they were previously able to eat the food without vomiting.

Respiratory and Skin Reactions

Respiratory and ocular symptoms are common manifestations of IgE-mediated reactions to foods.[27] Symptoms may include periocular erythema, periocular pruritus, tearing, nasal congestion, nasal pruritus, sneezing, rhinorrhea, coughing, voice changes, and wheezing. Isolated naso-ocular symptoms are an uncommon manifestation of food hypersensitivity reactions.

The skin is a frequent target organ in IgE-mediated food hypersensitivity reactions. The ingestion of food allergens can either trigger immediate cutaneous symptoms or aggravate chronic cutaneous symptoms. Acute urticaria and angioedema are probably the most common cutaneous manifestations of food hypersensitivity; these hypersensitivity

reactions generally appear within minutes after ingestion of the food allergen. Atopic dermatitis is a chronic skin disorder that generally begins in early infancy and is characterized by typical distribution, extreme pruritus, and a chronically relapsing course; it is associated with asthma and allergic rhinitis [see Chapter 38].[8] Approximately one third of young children with atopic dermatitis have one or more food allergies. The immediate allergic reaction to foods in these patients is IgE mediated. However, their skin disease may be worsened by a mixed IgE-mediated and non–IgE-mediated reaction. Most young children with atopic dermatitis who have food allergy have reactions to milk, eggs, or peanuts.

Systemic Anaphylactic Reactions

Systemic anaphylactic reactions to foods are not uncommon. Systemic symptoms can involve the skin, gastrointestinal tract, and respiratory tract (see above). The foods that most commonly cause anaphylaxis include peanuts, tree nuts, shellfish, and fish, but any food may cause anaphylaxis. Fatal food-induced anaphylaxis occurs most often in adolescents and young adults. Risk factors include asthma and a history of previous severe reactions to food.

MIXED IGE-MEDIATED AND NON–IGE-MEDIATED HYPERSENSITIVITY

Allergic Eosinophilic Gastroenteropathy

Allergic eosinophilic gastroenteropathy is a disorder characterized by infiltration of the gastric or intestinal walls with eosinophils; absence of vasculitis; and, frequently, peripheral blood eosinophilia [see Table 3].[4,9] Patients with this syndrome frequently have postprandial nausea and vomiting, abdominal pain, diarrhea, and, occasionally, steatorrhea; young infants experience failure to thrive, and adults have weight loss. There appears to be a subset of patients with allergic eosinophilic gastroenteritis who have symptoms secondary to food. These patients generally have the mucosal form of this disease, which is characterized by IgE-staining cells in jejunal tissue, elevated IgE levels in duodenal fluids, atopic disease, elevated serum IgE concentrations, positive prick skin tests to a variety of foods and inhalants, peripheral

Table 2   Immediate Gastrointestinal Hypersensitivity[27]

Manifestations	Nausea, abdominal pain, and vomiting within 1–2 hr Diarrhea within 2–6 hr Frequently associated with atopic disease Food-specific IgE antibodies Radiographic: gastric hypotonia and pylorospasm
Age at onset	Infancy, childhood
Proteins implicated	Milk, eggs, peanuts, soy, cereal, fish
Pathology	IgE mediated
Treatment	Protein elimination
Natural history	80% of cases resolve after protein-elimination diet (except in the case of peanut and fish allergy)

blood eosinophilia, iron deficiency anemia, and hypo-albuminemia.

The diagnosis of allergic eosinophilic gastroenteropathy is based on an appropriate history and a GI biopsy demonstrating a characteristic eosinophilic infiltration. Biopsies may need to be performed in multiple sites (up to eight) to effectively exclude eosinophilic gastroenteritis, because the eosinophilic infiltrates may be quite patchy. Patients with the mucosal form of the disease may have atopic symptoms, including food allergy, elevated serum IgE concentrations, and peripheral eosinophilia; they may also have positive skin tests or positive in vitro IgE results. Other laboratory results consistent with this disease include findings of Charcot-Leyden crystals in the stool; anemia; and hypoalbuminemia. Such patients may also have abnormal results on D-xylose testing. An elimination diet for up to 12 weeks may be necessary before complete resolution of symptoms and normalization of intestinal histology.

Some investigators are using the atopy patch test in the diagnosis of allergic eosinophilic gastroenteropathy. Although this practice is interesting from a research standpoint, these studies are not currently proved to be diagnostic.

NON–IGE-MEDIATED HYPERSENSITIVITY

Dietary-Protein Enterocolitis

Enterocolitis from dietary protein (also known as protein intolerance and food protein–induced enterocolitis) occurs most commonly in young infants between 1 week and 3 months of age [see Table 4]. The typical symptoms are isolated to the GI tract and consist of recurrent vomiting, diarrhea, or

Table 3   Allergic Eosinophilic Gastroenterocolitis[27]

Manifestations	Abdominal pain Anorexia Early satiety Failure to thrive Gastric outlet obstruction Gastric or colonic bleeding ±70% of cases atopic Elevated IgE ±Food-specific IgE 50% of cases with peripheral eosinophilia Radiographic Antral obstruction, gastroesophageal reflux, bowel wall edema
Age at onset	Birth to adolescence
Proteins implicated	Cow's milk, eggs, fish, soy, cereals Less than 50% of patients have skin-test specificity
Pathology	Marked eosinophilic infiltration of mucosa and submucosa in gastric antrum, esophagus, duodenum, and colon
Treatment	50% of patients respond to dietary elimination of documented allergen Excellent response to hydrolyzed protein formula in patients younger than 2 yr Excellent response to L-amino acid formula Responsive to steroids
Natural history	Disorder is typically prolonged

Table 4   Dietary-Protein Enterocolitis[27]

Manifestations	Diarrhea with bleeding Anemia Emesis Abdominal distention Failure to thrive Hypotension Fecal leukocytes Normal IgE Food challenge: vomiting in 3–4 hr; diarrhea in 5–8 hr
Age at onset	1 day to 1 yr
Implicated proteins	Cow's milk, soy, rice, poultry, fish
Pathology	Patchy villous injury and colitis
Treatment	80% or more of patients respond to hydrolyzed casein formula; symptoms clear in 3–10 days Up to 20% of patients require L-amino acid formula or temporary intravenous therapy
Natural history	With treatment, 50% of cases resolve by 18 mo and 90% by 36 mo; in soy allergy, illness is often more persistent

both. The symptoms can be severe enough to cause dehydration. Cow's milk and soy protein (particularly in infant formulas) are most often responsible for this syndrome, although egg sensitivity has been reported in older patients. The stools in affected children will often contain occult blood, polymorphonuclear neutrophils (PMNs), and eosinophils and are frequently positive for reducing substances (indicating malabsorbed sugars). Prick skin tests for the putative food protein are characteristically negative. Jejunal biopsies classically reveal flattened villi, edema, and increased numbers of lymphocytes, eosinophils, and mast cells. A food challenge with the responsible protein generally results in vomiting, diarrhea, or both within minutes to several hours; occasionally, patients experience shock.[4,10] It is not uncommon to find children who are sensitive to both cow's milk and soy protein. This sensitivity also tends to be lost by 18 to 24 months of age. Elimination of the offending allergen generally will result in improvement or resolution of the symptoms within 72 hours, although secondary disaccharidase deficiency may persist longer. Oral food challenges, which should be done in a medical setting because they can induce severe vomiting, diarrhea, dehydration, or hypotension, consist of administering 0.3 to 0.6 g/kg body weight of the suspected food allergen.

Dietary-Protein Proctitis

Patients with dietary-protein proctitis generally present in the first few months of life. This disorder is often secondary to cow's milk or soy protein hypersensitivity,[11] but in general, more than 50% of infants with dietary-protein proctitis are exclusively breast-fed at the time that symptoms are observed. Most infants with this disorder do not appear ill and have normally formed stools; they generally come to medical attention because of blood (gross or occult) in their stools. GI lesions are confined to the small bowel. Grossly, the lesions range from patchy mucosal injection to severe friability with small aphthoid ulcerations and bleeding. Microscopically, they are characterized by mucosal edema with eosinophils in the epithelium and lamina propria. If lesions are severe, with crypt destruction, PMNs are also prominent.[12] It is believed that colitis induced by cow's milk or soy protein resolves by 6 months to 2 years after allergen avoidance; however, this belief is not strongly supported by well-controlled studies. Elimination of the offending food allergen leads to resolution of hematochezia within 72 hours, but the mucosal lesions may take up to 1 month to disappear.

Celiac Disease

Celiac disease is an extensive enteropathy leading to malabsorption. Total villous atrophy and an extensive cellular infiltrate are associated with sensitivity to gliadin, the alcohol-soluble portion of gluten found in wheat, oats, rye, and barley. The overall incidence of celiac disease is thought to be one in 4,000 population, but there is wide regional variation; for example, the incidence in Ireland has been reported to be as high as one in 500 population. There is apparently a genetic predisposition to this disease, given that approximately 90% of patients are HLA-B8 positive and nearly 80% have the HLA-DW3 antigen. Patients often present with diarrhea or frank steatorrhea, abdominal distention and flatulence, and weight loss; occasionally, they have nausea and vomiting. Other extraintestinal symptoms and oral ulcers secondary to malabsorption are not common. Laboratory studies for patients with suspected celiac disease include measurement of serum transglutaminase and IgA antiendomysial and antigliadin antibodies.

HISTORY AND PHYSICAL EXAMINATION

As with virtually all medical disorders, the diagnostic approach to a patient with a suspected adverse food reaction begins with the history and physical examination. Depending on the information derived from these initial steps, various laboratory studies may be helpful [*see Table 5*].[13-15]

In cases of suspected adverse food reactions, the value of the history depends largely on the patient's recollection of symptoms and on the examiner's ability to differentiate disorders provoked by food hypersensitivity from disorders with other etiologies. The history may be directly useful in diagnosing food allergy involving acute events (e.g., anaphylaxis after eating fish) but is not always reliable: in many series, less than 50% of reported allergic reactions to food could be substantiated by a double-blind, placebo-controlled food challenge (DBPCFC).[3,7] In chronic disorders such as atopic dermatitis, the history is often an unreliable indicator of the offending allergen.

Several items of information are important in establishing that an allergic reaction to food occurred: (1) the type of food suspected of having provoked the reaction (i.e., typical foods for that age); (2) the quantity of the food ingested; (3) the length of time between ingestion and onset of symptoms; (4) the specific symptoms provoked (e.g., skin, respiratory tract, or gastrointestinal tract); (5) whether similar symptoms developed on other occasions when the same food was eaten; (6) whether other factors (e.g., exercise) were involved in the episode; and (7) the length of time since the last reaction.

Although any food may cause an allergic reaction, only a few foods account for 90% of such reactions. In children, these foods are eggs, milk, peanuts, soy, wheat, and, in Scandinavian countries, fish.

Diet Diary

A diet diary is often a useful adjunct to the medical history. Patients are asked to keep a chronological record of all foods ingested over a specified period of time and to record any symptoms they experience during this period. The diary can be reviewed at a subsequent visit to determine whether there is a relationship between the foods ingested and the symptoms experienced. Uncommonly, this method will reveal an unrecognized association between a food and a patient's symptoms.

Elimination Diet

Elimination diets are often used both in diagnosis and in management of adverse food reactions. If a certain food or foods are suspected of provoking the reaction, they are completely eliminated from the diet. The success of an elimination diet depends on several factors, including the correct identification of the allergen or allergens involved, the ability of the patient to maintain a diet completely free of all forms of the possible offending allergen, and the assumption that other factors will not provoke similar symptoms during the study period. The likelihood of all of these conditions being met is often slim. For example, in a young infant who is reacting to cow's milk formula, resolution of symptoms after substitution of soy formula or casein hydrolysate (e.g., Alimentum, Nutramigen) is highly suggestive of cow's milk allergy but also could reflect lactose intolerance. Avoidance of suspected food allergens before a blinded challenge is recommended so that reactions may be heightened. Elimination diets are rarely diagnostic of food allergy, particularly in chronic disorders such as atopic dermatitis or asthma.

LABORATORY TESTS

Allergy Skin Tests

Prick skin tests Prick skin tests are highly reproducible[16] and are often utilized to screen patients with suspected IgE-mediated food allergies. The glycerinated food extracts (1:10 or 1:20 dilution)[7] and appropriate positive (histamine) and negative (saline) controls are applied by either the prick or puncture technique. A test that elicits a wheal (not including erythema) at least 3 mm greater than the negative control is considered positive; any smaller result is considered negative. Appropriate and good-quality food extracts must be utilized for results to be reliable.

A negative skin test confirms the absence of an IgE-mediated reaction (overall negative predictive accuracy is greater than 95%). However, skin testing with commercial reagents often fails to detect IgE-mediated sensitivity to certain

---

Table 5 **Methods Used in the Evaluation of Allergic Reactions to Food**

Medical history
Diet diary
Elimination diet
Prick skin testing
Radioallergosorbent tests
Open or single-blind challenge
Double-blind, placebo-controlled food challenge (optimal)

Table 6 Diagnostic Levels of Food-Specific IgE in CAP-FEIA Studies

Allergen	Decision Point (kU/L)	PPV (%)
Egg	7 2 (patients < 2 yr)	98 95
Milk	15 5 (patients < 2 yr)	95 95
Peanuts	14	100
Tree nuts	~15	~95

CAP-FEIA—capsulated hydrolic carrier polymer–fluoroenzyme immunoassay
PPV—positive predictive value

fruits and vegetables (e.g., apples, oranges, bananas, pears, melons, potatoes, carrots, and celery), presumably because of the labile nature of the responsible allergens in these foods. In such cases, it may be necessary to use the so-called prick-by-prick method, in which the device used for introducing the allergen into the skin is first pricked into the food. In addition, false negative results are particularly common in very young children, possibly because of lower skin reactivity: children younger than 1 year may have IgE-mediated food allergy without a positive skin test.

A positive skin test to a food is not definitive; it merely indicates the possibility that the patient has symptomatic reactivity to that specific food (overall, the positive predictive accuracy is less than 50%). However, a positive skin test to a food that provokes a severe anaphylactic reaction when eaten by itself may be considered diagnostic. Atopy patch tests for food allergy have been developed, but there is as yet insufficient evidence to support their adoption in clinical practice.

Intradermal skin tests An intradermal skin test is more sensitive than a prick skin test but is much less specific than a DBPCFC.[17] In one study, no patient who had a negative prick skin test but a positive intradermal skin test to a specific food had a positive DBPCFC to that food.[17] In addition, intradermal skin testing is more likely to induce a systemic reaction than is prick skin testing. For those reasons, intradermal skin tests have no role in the diagnosis of food allergy.

In Vitro Assays

Radioallergosorbent tests (RASTs) and similar in vitro assays (including enzyme-linked immunosorbent assays [ELISAs]) are often used to screen for IgE-mediated food allergies. Although RASTs are generally considered slightly less sensitive than skin tests, one study comparing skin tests and Phadebas RAST (a first-generation test for specific IgE) with DBPCFCs found prick skin tests and Phadebas RAST to have similar sensitivity and specificity when a Phadebas score of 3 or greater was considered positive.[18] In this study, lowering the cutoff point for a positive result to a score of 2 brought a slight improvement in sensitivity at the expense of a significant decrease in specificity. In general, in vitro measurements of serum food-specific IgE performed in high-quality laboratories provide information similar to that of prick skin tests. The newest generation of in vitro studies for specific IgE includes the capsulated hydrolic carrier polymer–fluoroenzyme immunoassay (CAP-FEIA). For patients with suspected food allergy, there are now accepted levels of food-specific IgE concentrations on CAP-FEIA testing that can predict a patient's being allergic to that food with greater than 95% certainty.[15] CAP-FEIA is best used for patients with allergic reactions to milk, eggs, peanuts, and, possibly, wheat, soy, and fish [*see Table 6*].

Clinical Cross-reactivity

Certain foods are able to sensitize and elicit reactions after oral exposure and could trigger responses that generalize to related foods (e.g., peanut sensitivity can generalize to legumes). Other foods (e.g., apple) with labile proteins are not strong oral sensitizers. In this latter group of foods, however, sensitization to homologous proteins encountered through respiratory exposure (e.g., birch pollen) may mediate reactions to cross-reacting proteins in the food, with generally mild clinical manifestations. For many of the cross-reactive proteins, lability of proteins in commercial extracts is an issue. Prick skin tests using the prick-prick method with fresh fruits and vegetables may increase sensitivity when evaluating these labile allergens. In general, the cross-reactivity of the major foods is less than 10% for peanuts and other legumes, about 25% for wheat and other grains, about 35% for peanuts and tree nuts, and greater than 50% for tree nuts and other nuts.

Open, Single-Blind and Double-Blind Placebo-Controlled Food Challenges

Open and single-blind food challenges are often the most practical method of diagnosing food allergy. Nevertheless, the DBPCFC has been considered the gold standard for the diagnosis of food allergy.[4] This test has been used successfully by many investigators in both children and adults for the past several years to examine a wide variety of food-related complaints. The selection of foods to be tested in the oral challenge is based on the history or prick skin test (RAST) results.

A DBPCFC is the best means of controlling for the variability of chronic disorders (e.g., chronic urticaria and atopic dermatitis), any potential temporal effects, and acute exacerbations secondary to reducing or discontinuing medications. In particular, psychogenic factors and observer bias are eliminated. Rarely, a false negative DBPCFC occurs when the challenge material a patient receives is not of sufficient quantity to provoke the reaction or when the lyophilization of the food antigen has altered the relevant allergenic epitopes (as may occur with fish antigen). Nevertheless, at present, the DBPCFC has proved to be the most accurate means of diagnosing food allergy.

PRACTICAL APPROACH TO DIAGNOSING FOOD ALLERGY

The diagnosis of food allergy remains a clinical exercise that utilizes a careful history, selective prick skin tests or in vitro IgE results (if an IgE-mediated disorder is suspected), appropriate exclusion diet, and blinded provocation. Other diagnostic tests that do not appear to be of significant value include assessment of food-specific IgG or IgG4 antibody levels, assessment of food antigen–antibody complexes, measures of lymphocyte activation (e.g., ^{3}H uptake, interleukin-2 production, and presence of leukocyte inhibitory factor), and sublingual or intracutaneous provocation. Blinded challenges may not be necessary in suspected GI disorders, which often can be diagnosed on the basis of prechallenge and postchallenge laboratory values and biopsy results.

Table 7 Resources for Patients with Food Allergy

The Food Allergy and Anaphylaxis Network
10400 Easton Place, Suite 107
Fairfax, VA 22030-5647
800-929-4040
http://www.foodallergy.org

National Allergy and Asthma Network/Mothers of Asthmatics
2751 Prosperity Avenue
Suite 150
Fairfax, VA 22031
800-878-4403 / 703-385-4403
http://www.aanma.org

Asthma and Allergy Foundation of America
1125 15th Street, NW, Suite 502
Washington, DC 20005
800-727-8462
http://www.aafa.org

An exclusion diet that eliminates all foods suspected by history or prick skin testing (or, in IgE-mediated disorders, in vitro IgE results) should be conducted for at least 1 to 2 weeks. Some patients with GI disorders may need to have the exclusion diet extended for up to 12 weeks after appropriate biopsies. If no improvement is noted after institution of the diet, food allergy is unlikely. In patients with some chronic diseases, such as atopic dermatitis and chronic asthma, it may be difficult to discriminate the effects of the food allergen from the effects of those diseases (e.g., skin or respiratory tract manifestations).

Open or single-blind challenges in a clinic setting may be helpful to test for allergy to specific foods. Such challenges are less cumbersome and time consuming than DBPCFCs. It is important that the clinician make an unequivocal diagnosis of food allergy; a presumptive diagnosis of food allergy based on a patient's history and prick skin tests or RAST results is no longer acceptable. There are exceptions to this, however, such as the patient who experiences severe anaphylaxis after the isolated ingestion of a specific food. Because of reliance on presumptive diagnoses, over 25% of the United States population have altered their eating habits on the basis of misconceptions about food allergy.

Treatment

The only proven therapy for food allergy is the strict elimination of that food from the patient's diet. In infants, breast-feeding avoids contact with potentially allergenic foods if the mother avoids those foods. In infants with a family history of atopy, moreover, exclusive breast-feeding for at least the first 4 months of life appears to lessen the likelihood of atopic dermatitis.[19] Elimination diets should be supervised because they may lead to malnutrition or eating disorders, especially if they involve the elimination of a large number of foods or are utilized for extended periods of time. Studies have shown that symptomatic food sensitivity generally is lost over time, except for sensitivity to peanuts, tree nuts, and seafood.

Symptomatic food sensitivity is usually very specific; patients rarely react to more than one member of a botanical family or animal species. Consequently, clinicians should confirm that patients are not unnecessarily limiting their diet for fear of allergic reactions. Risk factors for more severe anaphylactic reactions include the following: (1) a history of a previous anaphylactic reaction; (2) a history of asthma, especially if poorly controlled; (3) allergy to peanuts, nuts, fish, or shellfish; (4) current treatment with beta blockers or angiotensin-converting enzyme inhibitors; and, possibly (5) female sex.

It is important to develop a specific, written action plan for patients with food allergy. This plan should include foods to be eliminated; symptoms to watch for; a listing of when and how to use medications, including antihistamines and epinephrine; and when and how to contact emergency medical personnel.

PHARMACOLOGIC THERAPY

Several medications have been used in an attempt to protect patients with food hypersensitivity, including oral cromolyn sodium, H_1 and H_2 antihistamines, ketotifen, corticosteroids, and prostaglandin synthetase inhibitors. Some of these medications may modify food allergy symptoms; overall, however, they have minimal efficacy or are associated with unacceptable side effects.

Epinephrine

The importance of prompt administration of epinephrine when symptoms of systemic reactions to foods develop cannot be overemphasized [see Chapter 107]. Patients with a history of anaphylaxis should always carry an epinephrine autoinjector (Epi-Pen [0.3 mg], Epi-Pen, Jr. [0.15 mg], or Twinject [0.3 mg]). For anaphylaxis, epinephrine is given in a dose of 0.01 mg/kg (generally up to a maximum of 0.3 mg). The route of administration can be intramuscular or subcutaneous, but studies suggest that intramuscular administration is better. If necessary, the dose can be repeated in 15 minutes.

IMMUNOTHERAPY

Blinded, placebo-controlled studies of rush immunotherapy for the treatment of peanut hypersensitivity have demonstrated efficacy in a small number of patients.[20] The adverse-reaction rates have been significant, however, and such reactions preclude general clinical application of rush immunotherapy at this time. Except for patients who are at risk of life-threatening reactions to minuscule amounts of peanut, there is no use for immunotherapy in patients with food allergies. Newer types of immunotherapy for prevention of food-induced anaphylaxis are being developed, such as the following: (1) humanized anti-IgE monoclonal antibody therapy, (2) plasmid-DNA immunotherapy, (3) peptide fragments (so-called overlapping peptides), (4) cytokine-modulated immunotherapy, (5) immunostimulatory sequence-modulated immunotherapy, (6) bacterial-encapsulated allergen immunotherapy, and (7) recombinant protein immunotherapy.[21] A 2003 study of anti-IgE in peanut-allergic patients[22] demonstrated that this medication may eventually be helpful for preventive treatment of food-induced anaphylaxis.

PATIENT EDUCATION

Patient education and support are essential aspects of treatment for patients with food allergy. In particular, adults and older children who are prone to anaphylaxis, as well as parents of pediatric patients, must be informed in a direct but sympathetic way that these reactions are potentially fatal.

When eating away from home, food-sensitive persons should feel comfortable requesting information about the contents of prepared foods. For school-aged children, the American Academy of Pediatrics Committee of School Health has recommended that schools be equipped to treat anaphylaxis in allergic students. Children older than 7 years can usually be taught to inject themselves with epinephrine. The physician must be willing to explain these issues to school personnel and, with the parents, help instruct these personnel in how to deal with them. In the home, the family should eliminate the incriminated allergen or, if this is not practical, place warning stickers on foods with the offending antigens. A variety of groups can help provide patients with support, advocacy, and education about food allergy [see Table 7]. The Food Allergy and Anaphylaxis Network (FAAN) is an excellent resource for patients, families, and other health care professionals.

Prognosis

Children younger than 3 years who are diagnosed with anaphylaxis to foods such as milk, eggs, wheat, or soybeans often outgrow this clinical sensitivity after several years.[9,23,24] Children who develop food sensitivity after 3 years of age are less likely to lose their food reactions over a period of several years. Patients who have very mild reactions (i.e., skin symptoms only) to peanuts during the first 12 to 24 months of life may outgrow their symptoms.[25,26] Allergies to foods such as tree nuts, fish, and seafood are generally not outgrown regardless of the age at which they develop. These persons appear likely to retain their allergic sensitivity for a lifetime. Consequently, new strategies are being evaluated to desensitize patients to these foods.

The author owns stock, stock options, and/or bonds in SEER, Inc.

References

1. Anderson J, Sogn D: Adverse reactions to foods. American Academy of Allergy and Immunology Committee on Adverse Reactions to Foods and the National Institute of Allergy and Infectious Diseases. National Institute of Allergy and Infectious Diseases, Washington, D.C., 1984

2. Sampson HA, Burks AW: Mechanisms of food allergy. Annu Rev Nutr 16:161, 1996

3. Sampson HA: Food allergy. J Allergy Clin Immunol 111(2 suppl):S540, 2003

4. Sampson HA, Anderson JA: Summary and recommendations: classification of gastrointestinal manifestations due to immunologic reactions to foods in infants and young children. J Pediatr Gastroenterol Nutr 30(suppl):S87, 2000

5. Bock SA: Natural history of severe reactions to foods in young children. J Pediatr 107:676, 1985

6. Bock SA, Atkins FM: Patterns of food hypersensitivity during sixteen years of double-blind, placebo-controlled food challenges. J Pediatr 117:561, 1990

7. Sampson HA: Adverse reactions to foods. Allergy: Principles and Practice, 5th ed. Middleton E, Jr, Reed CE, Ellis EF, et al, Eds. Mosby-Year Book, St Louis, 1998, p 1162

8. Eigenmann PA, Sicherer SH, Borkowski TA, et al: Prevalence of IgE-mediated food allergy among children with atopic dermatitis. Pediatrics 101:E8, 1998

9. Bock SA: Prospective appraisal of complaints of adverse reactions to foods in children during the first 3 years of life. Pediatrics 79:683, 1987

10. Goldman AS, Anderson DW, Sellers WA, et al: Milk allergy: I. Oral challenge with milk and isolated milk proteins in allergic children. Pediatrics 32:425, 1963

11. Crowe SE, Perdue MH: Gastrointestinal food hypersensitivity: basic mechanisms of pathophysiology. Gastroenterology 103:1075, 1992

12. Jenkins HR, Pincott JR, Soothill JF, et al: Food allergy: the major cause of infantile colitis. Arch Dis Child 59:326, 1984

13. Burks AW, Sampson HA: Diagnostic approaches to the patient with suspected food allergies. J Pediatr 121:S64, 1992

14. Schwartz HJ: Asthma and food additives. Food Allergy: Adverse Reactions to Foods and Food Additives, 2nd ed. Metcalfe DD, Sampson HA, Simon RA, Eds. Blackwell Science, Oxford, 1997, p 411

15. Sampson HA: Utility of food-specific IgE concentrations in predicting symptomatic food allergy. J Allergy Clin Immunol 107:891, 2001

16. Bock SA, Lee WY, Remigio L, et al: Appraisal of skin tests with food extracts for diagnosis of food hypersensitivity. Clin Allergy 8:559, 1978

17. Bock SA, Buckley J, Holst A, et al: Proper use of skin tests with food extracts in diagnosis of hypersensitivity to food in children. Clin Allergy 7:375, 1977

18. Sampson HA, Albergo R: Comparison of results of skin tests, RAST, and double-blind, placebo-controlled food challenges in children with atopic dermatitis. J Allergy Clin Immunol 74:26, 1984

19. Schoetzau A, Filipiak-Pittroff B, Franke K, et al: Effect of exclusive breast-feeding and early solid food avoidance on the incidence of atopic dermatitis in high-risk infants at 1 year of age. Pediatr Allergy Immunol 13:234, 2002

20. Oppenheimer JJ, Nelson HS, Bock SA, et al: Treatment of peanut allergy with rush immunotherapy. J Allergy Clin Immunol 90:256, 1992

21. Burks AW, Bannon GA, Lehrer SB: Classic specific immunotherapy and new perspectives in specific immunotherapy for food allergy. Allergy 67:121, 2001

22. Leung DY, Sampson HA, Yunginger JW, et al: Effect of anti-IgE therapy in patients with peanut allergy. N Engl J Med 348:986, 2003

23. Bock SA: The natural history of food sensitivity. J Allergy Clin Immunol 69:173, 1982

24. Bock SA, Atkins FM: Patterns of food hypersensitivity during sixteen years of double-blind, placebo-controlled food challenges. J Pediatr 117:561, 1990

25. Skolnick HS, Conover-Walker MK, Koerner CB, et al: The natural history of peanut allergy. J Allergy Clin Immunol 107:367, 2001

26. Hourihane JO, Roberts SA, Warner JO: Resolution of peanut allergy: case-control study. BMJ 316:1271, 1998

27. Zeiger RS: Dietary aspects of food allergy prevention in infants and children. J Pediatr Gastroenterol Nutr 30(suppl):S77, 2000

110 Allergic Reactions to Hymenoptera

David B. K. Golden, M.D., F.A.C.P.

Allergic reactions to insect venom primarily occur as a result of stings by insects of the order Hymenoptera. Allergic swelling can occur at the site of the insect sting, but only rarely does anaphylaxis result. Nonallergic reactions to insect venom have also been reported; these include nephropathy, central and peripheral neurologic syndromes, idiopathic thrombocytopenic purpura, and rhabdomyolysis. These are toxic reactions and are not IgE mediated. Allergic reactions to stings manifest themselves as either late-phase local inflammation (i.e., severe prolonged swelling) or systemic responses (e.g., anaphylaxis).

Epidemiology

Allergic reactions to Hymenoptera stings have been reported in persons of all ages. The reactions may be preceded by a number of uneventful stings. Systemic allergic reactions are reported in up to 1% of children and 3% of adults, although allergic antibodies to Hymenoptera venoms can be detected in 17% to 26% of adults.[1] The frequency of large local allergic reactions is uncertain but is estimated to be about 10% in adults. Fatal allergic reactions to insect stings may occur at any age but are most common in adults older than 45 years.[2] Half of those persons in whom a fatal reaction occurred had no previous history of allergy to insect stings; the other half had previous reactions but failed to take adequate preventive measures. In the United States, at least 40 deaths occur each year as the result of insect stings; other sting fatalities may go unrecognized. In many cases of unexplained sudden death, postmortem blood samples show the presence of both Hymenoptera venom–specific IgE antibodies and elevated serum tryptase levels, indicating the true cause of the fatal reactions.[3]

For 50 years, whole body extracts were used as standard treatment for immunotherapy; such use was based on a lack of knowledge of the natural history of anaphylaxis.[4] We now recognize that the risk of an anaphylactic reaction to a sting varies in accordance with the history of previous stings and is correlated with the results of venom skin testing or radioallergosorbent testing (RAST). The risk declines gradually with time [*see Table 1*]. In high-risk patients, the risk of reaction is 50% to 70%; other persons with a history of insect-sting allergy are at much lower risk. Most affected children have only cutaneous systemic reactions, with no respiratory or vascular symptoms, and have less than a 10% risk of a systemic reaction to a subsequent sting.[5] The risk is also less than 10% in adults or children who have experienced only large local reactions to stings. Furthermore, the allergy is self-limited in many cases. The risk of reaction falls from 50% initially to 33% after 3 to 5 years; the risk is 20% to 25% if more than 10 years have passed since the reaction.[6] However, in some individuals, the risk of anaphylaxis persists for decades, even with no intervening stings.

Etiology

Hymenoptera allergy is directed against the allergenic proteins in the venoms of the stinging insects. Three families of Hymenoptera are important causes of allergy. The bees (i.e., honey-

bees and bumblebees) and vespids (i.e., yellow jackets, hornets, and wasps) are the best known [*see Figures 1 and 2*]. Imported fire ants (*Solenopsis* species) are a rapidly increasing public health hazard in the Southeast and South Central United States, especially on the Gulf Coast [*see Figure 3*].[7] Honeybee stings are more common in agricultural areas. Yellow jackets are the most frequent culprits in the northern areas of North America and Europe, whereas paper wasps (*Polistes* species) are more commonly implicated along the Gulf Coast in the United States and the Mediterranean Coast in Europe.

Knowledge of the behavior of these insects can be helpful in evaluating the history of affected patients. Honeybees are relatively docile and rarely sting or swarm unless provoked. Stings usually occur as a result of garden exposures or from going barefoot outdoors. The barbed stinger of the honeybee remains in the skin, causing the death of the honeybee. Africanized honeybees (killer bees) are more aggressive and are now present in the southern United States.[8] Although an Africanized honeybee is no different from a domestic honeybee with regard to anatomy or venom, Africanized honeybees have a tendency to swarm with little provocation and to sting in large numbers. A large number of stings can cause massive envenomation; the resulting toxic reactions have been fatal to livestock and humans. Bumblebees sting infrequently, but a few cases of systemic reactions have been reported.

Yellow jackets usually nest underground or in the cracks of buildings or wooden ties or logs used in residential landscaping, whereas hornets generally build their nests in shrubs and trees. Paper wasps build an open nest with visible cells; nests are often found on the eaves or windowsills of a home or in the railings of decks or fences. Yellow jackets are scavengers; they are commonly found around food at picnics and in orchards, trash cans, and dumpsters. They are highly aggressive and will sting quite readily. Wasps are less aggressive but will sting readily when disturbed. The vespid stinger usually has finer barbs than the stinger of the bee and does not commonly remain in the skin.

Table 1 Risk of Systemic Reactions and Clinical Recommendations Based on Reaction to Previous Stings and Results of the Venom Skin Test or RAST

Reaction to Previous Sting	Skin Test or RAST	Risk of Systemic Reaction	Clinical Recommendation
None	Positive	10%–20%	Avoidance
Large local	Positive	5%–10%	Avoidance
Cutaneous systemic	Positive, child	1%–10%	Avoidance
	Positive, adult	10%–20%	Venom immunotherapy
Anaphylaxis	Positive	30%–70%	Venom immunotherapy
	Negative	5%–10%	Repeat skin test/RAST

RAST—radioallergosorbent testing

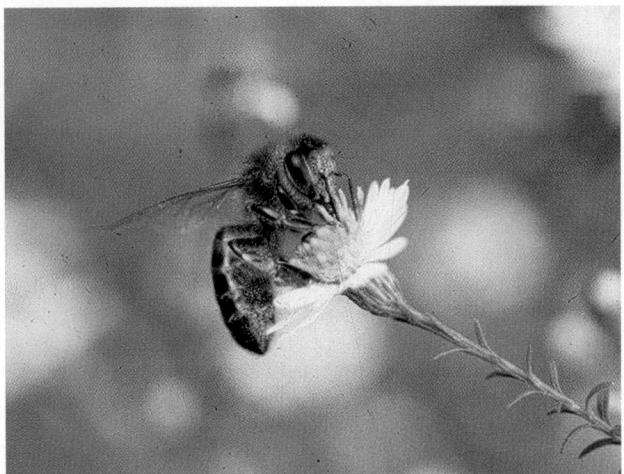

Figure 1   **The honeybee (*Apis mellifera*).**

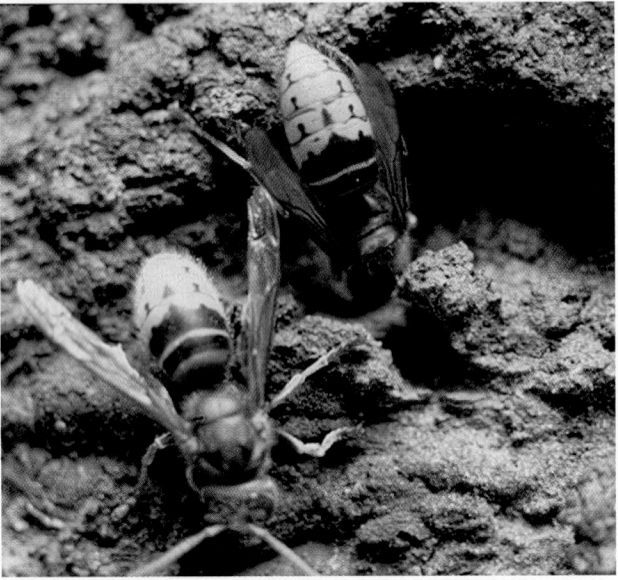

Figure 2   **The European hornet (*Vespa crabro germana*) was introduced into the United States in the mid-19th century. In the United States, its habitat includes most of the eastern United States, Louisiana, and the Dakotas. Although it is a woodland species, its nests can be found in barns, attics, hollow walls, birdhouses, and abandoned beehives.**

Fire ants have stingers, and it is the sting rather than the bite that causes the allergic reaction. Fire ants are widespread in the southeastern United States; in many areas, stings are very frequent, with up to 50% of the population being stung each year. Fire ants build nests in the shape of large mounds; these nests are common in residential and coastal areas. In most cases of fire-ant stings, multiple ants each administer multiple stings, which cause minimal pain. The unique lesions form sterile pustules that can become infected if excoriated [*see Figure 4*].

The allergic sensitivity is directed against proteins in the venoms (but not in the saliva or bodies) of the stinging insects.[9] Honeybee venom contains unique allergens, whereas the vespid venoms cross-react extensively with one another and contain essentially the same allergens. The venom of *Polistes* wasps is less cross-reactive than that of the other vespids. Only 50% of patients who are allergic to yellow-jacket venom experi-ence reactions to wasp venom. The allergenic proteins in fire-ant venom are unique.

Pathogenesis

The pathogenesis of Hymenoptera allergy is the same as that of other forms of anaphylaxis. An initial encounter with a sting in genetically susceptible individuals causes the production of IgE antibodies to the venom allergens. The IgE antibodies become affixed to tissue mast cells and circulating basophils, which thus become armed for response to a later encounter with the same allergen. A subsequent sting can cause cross-linking of these allergic antibodies, leading to the release of mediators (e.g., histamine, leukotrienes, and cytokines) that cause the clinical manifestations of the allergic reaction. There is an association between conditions involving abnormal mast cell number or function and insect-sting anaphylaxis. The allergic reactions to stings are more severe in patients with elevated baseline serum tryptase levels or mastocytosis, and there is a higher incidence of treatment failures and relapse after treatment in these patients.[10-12] Whole body extracts of fire ants are used for diagnostic testing and are effective for immunotherapy, whereas whole body extracts of the other Hymenoptera insects have proved not to contain venom allergens.

Diagnosis

CLINICAL MANIFESTATIONS

Allergic reactions to insect stings may cause local allergic inflammation or the full spectrum of manifestations of anaphylaxis. Large local reactions are late-phase allergic reactions. Progressive swelling begins 6 to 12 hours after the sting, reaching peak size in 24 to 48 hours and resolving in 5 to 10 days. Large local reactions are usually defined as being greater than 6 in. in diameter; they can be massive in size and cause considerable pain. On the extremities, inflammatory lymphangitic streaks occur toward the axillary or inguinal nodes; these streaks are mistaken for signs of infection. Systemic reactions most commonly cause cutaneous signs and symptoms, including generalized flushing, pruritus, urticaria, and angioedema. Other typical manifestations are respiratory (e.g., throat or chest tightness, dyspnea, wheezing) or circulatory (e.g., light-headedness or unconscious-

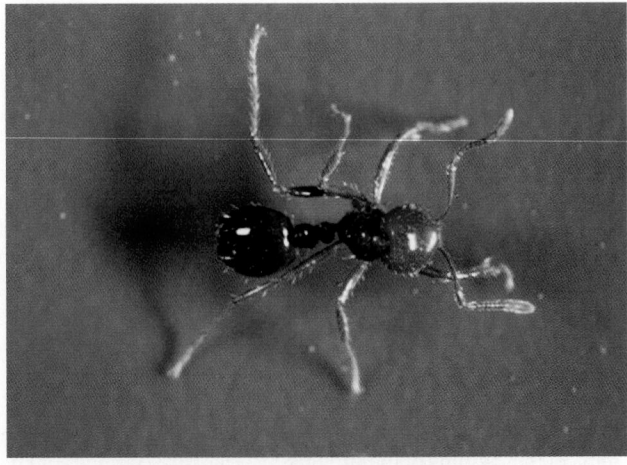

Figure 3   **Red imported fire ant (*Solenopsis invicta*).**

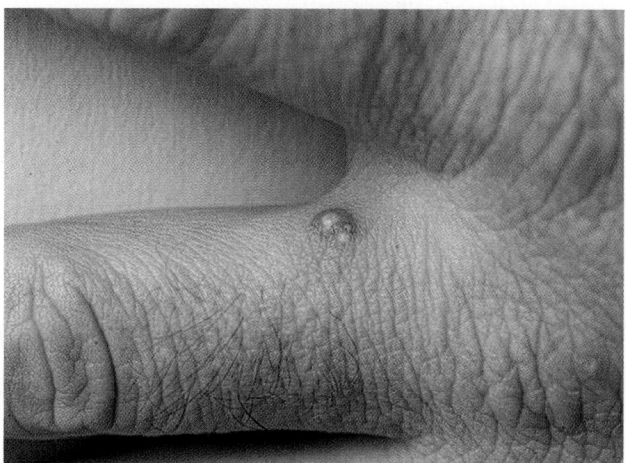

Figure 4   **Appearance of a pustule resulting from the sting of a fire ant. This photograph was taken 24 hours after the patient was stung.**

ness). Less common signs of anaphylaxis include gastrointestinal or uterine cramps, cardiac arrhythmias (e.g., tachycardia or, occasionally, bradycardia), and coronary vasospasm.

In children, systemic reactions to stings usually cause only cutaneous symptoms (e.g., urticaria or angioedema). Respiratory symptoms are less common, and circulatory manifestations are infrequent. Systemic reactions usually follow a predictable and individual pattern in each patient, with worsening of the reaction occurring in less than 10% of cases.[13] Affected individuals commonly do not seek medical attention and usually fail to report having sting reactions unless they are asked.

The diagnosis of insect-sting allergy rests on a history of allergic reactivity, because venom-specific IgE antibodies can be detected in many normal individuals. The positive venom skin test provides confirmation of the allergic nature of the sting reaction and helps define allergenic specificity. The history is most important and should be reviewed in detail with respect to the nature, number, and timing of stings in the past; the time course of the reaction; and all associated symptoms and treatments. The family history, atopic history, and general medical history are also of interest. In addition, it is helpful to know of any medications the patient took before the reaction occurred, as well as any medications the patient is currently using.

PHYSICAL EXAMINATION

It is most important to measure the vital signs, including airflow, when there is dyspnea and to document cutaneous signs. Some patients have symptoms, such as dizziness and dyspnea, that do not correspond to the objective signs (e.g., blood pressure, peak expiratory flow rate) and may be the result of anxiety, panic, and hyperventilation. Any history suggestive of systemic allergic reaction must be taken seriously.

DIAGNOSTIC TESTS

The diagnosis of insect-venom allergy can be confirmed by skin tests or serologic tests using Hymenoptera venoms. Both methods are useful, and they are often complementary in the diagnostic evaluation of affected patients. Both methods require specific experience and training to prevent false interpretations. Diagnostic tests are not usually performed in the absence of a history of a systemic allergic reaction. This is because a positive test occurs in 20% to 30% of adults and is associated with a rela-

tively low 17% chance of a systemic reaction to a future sting.[1]

Intradermal skin tests using serial dilutions of the five Hymenoptera venom protein extracts is the recommended procedure. In the case of fire-ant sensitivity, whole body extracts of imported fire ants give reasonable diagnostic sensitivity and specificity. For Hymenoptera venom testing, intradermal tests are performed with venom concentrations ranging from 0.001 to 1.0 µg/ml to find the minimal concentration that yields a positive result, as compared with a negative diluent control (e.g., human serum albumin saline) and a positive histamine control. Puncture tests with a venom concentration of 0.01 µg/ml may be used initially for patients with a history of very severe reactions.

The diagnosis of insect-sting allergy by detection of allergen-specific IgE antibodies in serum (typically by RAST) is a method of high potential but variable performance.[14] An elevation in the level of venom-specific IgE is certainly diagnostic; but the test is often qualitative and poorly standardized, and it yields negative results in 15% to 20% of patients whose skin-test results are positive.

In the majority of patients who have a definite history of insect-sting reactions, skin-test results are clearly positive; however, in many others, the results are clearly negative. Negative skin-test results in a patient with a history of insect-sting reactions may represent the loss of sensitivity, but it is important to test for venom-specific IgE antibodies in the serum (e.g., by use of RAST).[15] If necessary, the venom skin test may be repeated after several months. A few cases of sting anaphylaxis are non–IgE mediated and may be related to subclinical mastocytosis or simply toxic mast cell hyperreleasability.[12] It is important to note that the degree of sensitivity as detected by skin testing or RAST does not correlate reliably with the degree of sting reaction. The strongest sensitivity to skin tests often occurs in patients who have had only large local reactions, and some patients who have had near-fatal anaphylactic shock show only weak sensitivity on skin testing or RAST. Because of cross-reactivity, skin tests are positive to all three of the common vespid venoms (i.e., yellow jacket, yellow hornet, and white-faced hornet) in 95% of patients allergic to yellow-jacket venom. More than half of patients sensitive to yellow-jacket venom also have positive reactions to testing for sensitivity to *Polistes* wasp venom. It is possible to determine whether the patient has a specific or a cross-reactive sensitivity to wasp venom using a RAST-inhibition test in specialized laboratories.[16]

Differential Diagnosis

Although the diagnosis of insect-sting allergy is relatively straightforward, the history and diagnostic tests can be misleading in some cases. Local swelling may be the result of nonallergic inflammation, but infection is very uncommon and would likely occur many days after the sting. Local cutaneous signs should not be mistaken for systemic eruption. Symptoms of dyspnea, chest discomfort, and dizziness can be the result of hyperventilation associated with anxiety. Patients with asthma who receive a sting may have asthmatic symptoms that are difficult to distinguish from an allergic reaction. Approximately 1% of patients with a history of allergic reactions to insect stings have an underlying abnormality in the release of mediators by mast cells or basophils, as demonstrated by elevated baseline serum tryptase levels. Some of these patients have a form of mastocytosis.[10-12]

Treatment

ACUTE TREATMENT

The treatment of the acute systemic allergic reaction to insect stings is the same as that of other causes of anaphylaxis. The treatment of choice is epinephrine by intramuscular injection.[17,18] The recommended dose is 0.3 to 0.5 mg (0.3 to 0.5 ml of a solution of 1:1,000 weight in volume [w/v]) for adults and 0.01 mg/kg for children. Delay in the use of epinephrine has contributed to fatal reactions. Some persons in anaphylactic shock are resistant to epinephrine. Patients taking beta-blocker medications can also be resistant to the effects of epinephrine. In some cases, anaphylaxis is prolonged or recurrent (biphasic) for 6 to 24 hours and may require intensive medical care.[19] All patients with anaphylaxis should receive full emergency medical attention and remain under observation for 6 hours or longer. Corticosteroids have no role in the treatment of acute anaphylaxis; they are administered to prevent late-phase reactions, but there is no evidence that steroids prevent biphasic anaphylaxis.

Large local reactions may require a burst of corticosteroid, which is most effective if started within 2 hours of the sting. After an initial dose of 40 to 60 mg, the dose is tapered over 3 to 5 days.

PREVENTIVE TREATMENT

General Measures

Patients who are discharged from emergency care after suffering anaphylaxis must receive information on the risk of future reactions. They should also be advised to receive allergy consultation, and they should be given information about prevention. When outdoors, the affected person should avoid bushes and gardens, as well as food and drink that are most likely to attract insects. Drinks, especially in cans, bottles, and straws, can be an unsuspected source of a sting to the tongue or throat. Prescription of an epinephrine autoinjector (e.g., EpiPen and EpiPen Jr., Dey, Napa, California) should be considered in any patient who has experienced a systemic allergic reaction. Some patients may need to use epinephrine immediately after receiving a sting (until they can be immunized); however, most patients can wait for the signs of a developing reaction before using epinephrine. Delay in treatment is reasonable because the majority of persons with a history of mild to moderate systemic reactions do not react to a challenge sting. The age at which a patient should be prescribed an adult-strength autoinjector, rather than a pediatric autoinjector, is uncertain; use of the adult-strength injector may be considered when the child attains a weight of 25 kg.[20] All patients should understand that use of an epinephrine kit is not a substitute for emergency medical attention.

Venom Immunotherapy

Patient selection Current indications for venom immunotherapy are a history of previous systemic allergic reaction to a sting and a positive venom skin test.[21-23] The patients at highest risk are those with a recent history of anaphylaxis and positive skin-test results; in such patients, the risk of a systemic reaction to a subsequent sting is approximately 50%. Children and adults with a history of large local reactions are at low risk for a systemic reaction (i.e., < 10%),[24] as are children whose systemic reactions are limited to cutaneous signs and symptoms.[5] In these low-risk persons, venom immunotherapy is not required, but some patients will still request treatment for reasons related to fear of reaction or frequent exposure. Children with moderate or severe systemic reactions have a relatively high risk of recurrence even 10 to 20 years after allergic reaction to an insect sting.[25] There are some cases of progressively worsening reactions in adults, so all adults with systemic reactions are advised to undergo venom immunotherapy. There is no test that accurately predicts which patients will progress to more severe reactions and which will not.

Initial therapy Initial venom immunotherapy can be completed with a regimen of eight weekly injections or a traditional regimen lasting for 4 to 6 months.[21-23] Rush immunotherapy, typically administered over a period of 2 to 3 days, has been reported to be as safe and effective as the usual regimens.[26,27] The recommended maintenance dose is 100 μg of each of the venoms for which a positive result was seen on skin testing. Standard therapy is 85% to 98% effective in completely preventing systemic allergic reactions, but some patients require higher doses for full protection.[28] The same dose has been recommended for children 3 years of age and older, even though their immune response to venom immunotherapy is twice that of adults.

Adverse reactions Venom immunotherapy causes reactions no more frequently than inhalant allergen immunotherapy.[29] Systemic symptoms occur in 10% to 15% of patients during the initial weeks of treatment, regardless of the regimen used. Most reactions are mild, and fewer than half of the reactions require epinephrine. In unusual cases, there can be repeated problems with systemic reactions to injections. Large local reactions are common but are not predictive of systemic reactions to subsequent injections. All patients must achieve the full 100 μg dose to have optimal clinical protection.

Maintenance and monitoring After reaching the full dose, the same dose is repeated at 4-week intervals for at least 1 year. The dosing interval may then be increased to once every 6 to 8 weeks over several years of treatment. Therapeutic efficacy can be confirmed serologically, but use of only some assays for venom-specific IgG antibodies has correlated strongly with clinical protection.[30] Venom skin testing or RAST is repeated periodically—usually every 2 to 3 years—to determine whether there has been a significant decline in venom-specific IgE.[31] The results of skin testing generally remain unchanged during the first 2 to 3 years but show a significant decline after 4 to 6 years.[6] Fewer than 20% of patients have negative skin-test results after 5 years, but 50% to 60% have negative results after 7 to 10 years.[32]

Duration The package inserts for the commercial venom immunotherapy products available in the United States recommend indefinite immunotherapy. However, the published practice parameters reflect more recent experience and recommendations.[23,31] In most patients, skin-test results and RAST results remain positive after 5 to 10 years of treatment. Studies of several hundred adults and children show that even when skin tests remain positive, venom immunotherapy can usually be stopped after 5 years.[31] Observation of patients for 5 to 10 years after completing a 5- to 8-year course of venom treatment has shown a 5% to 10% risk of systemic symptoms after any sting but only a 2% risk of a reaction requiring epinephrine treatment.[33] Patients who have a higher frequency of relapse include those receiving honeybee-venom therapy, those with a history of very severe pretreatment sting reactions, and those who have had a systemic reaction to a sting or an injection during the period of venom immunotherapy.[22] Several studies have shown that 5 years of therapy is superior to 3 years for suppression of the IgE response and for longer-lasting remission.[34,35] Some patients prefer to continue venom treatment for their continued sense of security. Children who have had a 3- to 5-year course of venom immunotherapy show persistent tolerance even 10 to 20 years after discontinuing treatment.[25]

David B. K. Golden, M.D., F.A.C.P., has no commercial relationships with manufacturers of products or providers of services discussed in this chapter.

References

1. Golden DK, Marsh DG, Kagey-Sobotka A, et al: Epidemiology of insect venom sensitivity. JAMA 262:240, 1989

2. Barnard JH: Studies of 400 Hymenoptera sting deaths in the United States. J Allergy Clin Immunol 52:259, 1973

3. Schwartz HJ, Sutheimer C, Gauerke B, et al: Venom-specific IgE antibodies in postmortem sera from victims of sudden unexpected death. J Allergy Clin Immunol 73:189, 1984

4. Golden DB, Langlois J, Valentine MD, et al: Treatment failures with whole-body extract therapy of insect sting allergy. JAMA 246:2460, 1981

5. Valentine MD, Schuberth KC, Kagey-Sobotka A, et al: The value of immunotherapy with venom in children with allergy to insect stings. N Engl J Med 323:1601, 1990

6. Reisman RE: Natural history of insect sting allergy: relationship of severity of symptoms of initial sting anaphylaxis to re-sting reactions. J Allergy Clin Immunol 90:335, 1992

7. Stafford CT: Hypersensitivity to fire ant venom. Ann Allergy Asthma Immunol 77:87, 1996

8. Schumacher MJ, Egen NB: Significance of Africanized bees for public health: a review. Arch Intern Med 155:2038, 1995

9. King TP, Spangfort MD: Structure and biology of stinging insect venom allergens. Int Arch Allergy Immunol 123:99, 2000

10. Ludolph-Hauser D, Rueff F, Fries C, et al: Constitutively raised serum concentrations of mast-cell tryptase and severe anaphylactic reactions to Hymenoptera stings. Lancet 357:361, 2001

11. Fricker M, Helbling A, Schwartz L, et al: Hymenoptera sting anaphylaxis and urticaria pigmentosa: clinical findings and results of venom immunotherapy in ten patients. J Allergy Clin Immunol 100:11, 1997

12. Oude Elberink J, de Monchy J, Kors JW, et al: Fatal anaphylaxis after a yellow jacket sting, despite venom immunotherapy, in two patients with mastocytosis. J Allergy Clin Immunol 99:153, 1997

13. van der Linden PG, Hack CE, Struyvenberg A, et al: Insect-sting challenge in 324 subjects with a previous anaphylactic reaction: current criteria for insect-venom hypersensitivity do not predict the occurrence and the severity of anaphylaxis. J Allergy Clin Immunol 94:151, 1994

14. Hamilton RG: Responsibility for quality IgE antibody results rests ultimately with the referring physician. Ann Allergy Asthma Immunol 86:353, 2001

15. Golden DB, Kagey-Sobotka A, Norman PS, et al: Insect sting allergy with negative venom skin test responses. J Allergy Clin Immunol 107:897, 2001

16. Hamilton RH, Wisenauer JA, Golden DB, et al: Selection of Hymenoptera venoms for immunotherapy on the basis of patient's IgE antibody cross-reactivity. J Allergy Clin Immunol 92:651, 1993

17. Simons FE, Gu X, Simons KJ: Epinephrine absorption in adults: intramuscular versus subcutaneous injection. J Allergy Clin Immunol 108:871, 2001

18. Nicklas RA, Bernstein IL, Li JT, et al: The diagnosis and management of anaphylaxis. Joint Task Force on Practice Parameters. J Allergy Clin Immunol 101:S465, 1998

19. Lockey RF, Turkeltaub PC, Baird-Warren IA, et al: The Hymenoptera venom study I, 1979–1982: demographic and history-sting data. J Allergy Clin Immunol 82:370, 1988

20. Simons FE, Peterson S, Black CD: Epinephrine dispensing for the out-of-hospital treatment of anaphylaxis in infants and children: a population-based study. Ann Allergy Asthma Immunol 86:622, 2001

21. Golden DB, Schwartz HJ: Guidelines for venom immunotherapy. J Allergy Clin Immunol 77:727, 1986

22. Muller U, Mosbech H: Position paper: immunotherapy with Hymenoptera venoms. Allergy 48:37, 1993

23. Moffitt JE, Golden DB, Reisman RE, et al: Stinging insect hypersensitivity: a practice parameter update. J Allergy Clin Immunol 114:869, 2004

24. Mauriello PM, Barde SH, Georgitis JW, et al: Natural history of large local reactions from stinging insects. J Allergy Clin Immunol 74:494, 1984

25. Golden DBK, Kagey-Sobotka A, Norman PS, et al: Outcomes of allergy to insect stings in children with and without venom immunotherapy. N Engl J Med 351:668, 2004

26. Sturm G, Kranke B, Rudolph C, et al: Rush Hymenoptera venom immunotherapy: a safe and practical protocol for high-risk patients. J Allergy Clin Immunol 110:928, 2002

27. Tankersley MS, Walker RL, Butler WK, et al: Safety and efficacy of an imported fire ant rush immunotherapy protocol with and without prophylactic treatment. J Allergy Clin Immunol 109:556, 2002

28. Rueff F, Wenderoth A, Przybilla B: Patients still reacting to a sting challenge while receiving conventional Hymenoptera venom immunotherapy are protected by increased venom doses. J Allergy Clin Immunol 108:1027, 2001

29. Lockey RF, Turkeltaub PC, Olive ES, et al: The Hymenoptera venom study: III. Safety of venom immunotherapy. J Allergy Clin Immunol 86:775, 1990

30. Golden DB, Lawrence ID, Hamilton RH, et al: Clinical correlation of the venom-specific IgG antibody level during maintenance venom immunotherapy. J Allergy Clin Immunol 90:386, 1992

31. Graft DF, Golden DK, Resiman RE, et al: The discontinuation of Hymenoptera venom immunotherapy. Report from the Committee on Insects. J Allergy Clin Immunol 101:573, 1998

32. Golden DB, Kwiterovich KA, Kagey-Sobotka A, et al: Discontinuing venom immunotherapy: extended observations. J Allergy Clin Immunol 101:298, 1998

33. Golden DB, Kagey-Sobotka A, Lichtenstein LM: Survey of patients after discontinuing venom immunotherapy. J Allergy Clin Immunol 105:385, 2000

34. Keating MU, Kagey-Sobotka A, Hamilton RG, et al: Clinical and immunologic follow-up of patients who stop venom immunotherapy. J Allergy Clin Immunol 88:339, 1991

35. Lerch E, Muller U: Long-term protection after stopping venom immunotherapy: results of re-stings in 200 patients. J Allergy Clin Immunol 101:606, 1998

Acknowledgments

The photographs in Figures 1 and 2 are by Stephen B. Bambara; the photographs in Figures 3 and 4 are by James Baker, Ph.D. All photographs are courtesy of the North Carolina State University Department of Entomology.

Shaun Ruddy, M.D., F.A.C.P.

In 2002, arthritis and chronic joint disease affected one in three adults in the United States, or 70 million persons. Arthritis and musculoskeletal disorders are the leading causes of disability in persons 18 to 65 years of age and are common causes of disability related to employment. Risk factors for these disorders include lower education level, sedentary lifestyle, high body-mass index, and female sex. Age is a major risk factor: the prevalence of these disorders increases with age, with more than 60% of those age 65 and older being affected[1] [*see Figure 1*]. By 2030, when the percentage of the population that is 65 and older will have risen to 20%, the number of people in this age group with arthritis will nearly double, from 21.4 million to 41.1 million.[2]

One in seven patients who visit a physician's office has a complaint regarding the musculoskeletal system.[3] Although many of these patients have benign, self-limited conditions that respond to simple remedies, some patients have serious, complex problems for which timely intervention may be crucial for a successful outcome.

Approach to Diagnosis

Diagnosis of the rheumatic diseases primarily relies on the history and physical examination.[4,5] Expensive laboratory and imaging studies are usually of little use; most have low sensitivity and specificity, and their findings are seldom definitively diagnostic. For example, the serum level of uric acid, a substance intimately involved in the pathogenesis of gout, is of little use in diagnosing gouty arthritis. Uric acid levels are normal in 20% of patients with gout (i.e., false negative results), and most persons with elevated levels will never have gouty arthritis (false positive results) [*see Chapter 118*]. Wide-ranging and expensive investigations often lead to the wrong conclusions. The dearth of useful laboratory aids to diagnose rheumatic disease makes the clinical skills of the physician very important and the diagnosis of such disease an exciting undertaking.

History

A careful and detailed history is the most important part of the evaluation of a patient with arthritis. It focuses the subsequent physical examination and laboratory studies. Relevant factors in the history include the patient's age, sex, and race. In addition, the physician should elicit the location of the pain, which includes both the distribution of affected joints and the point of origin of the pain (i.e., whether it arises from a joint or surrounding structures) [*see Table 1*]. Symmetrical involvement of the small joints of the hands and feet but not the distal interphalangeal joints suggests rheumatoid arthritis. In contrast, distal interphalangeal involvement often occurs in psoriatic arthritis. Bony overgrowth with distal interphalangeal involvement suggests osteoarthritis. Asymmetrical involvement of the large joints accompanied by back pain in a young man is characteristic of spondyloarthropathy. The sudden onset of severe pain in the great toe is a feature of gout (podagra).

Knowing the nature of the pain helps the physician determine whether the disease is inflammatory or noninflammatory [*see Table 1*]. The date of onset and the temporal course of the pain should also be elicited [*see Figure 2*]. The new involvement of joints that had not previously been affected in a patient with joint involvement is common in rheumatoid arthritis and systemic lupus erythematosus (SLE). Migratory polyarthritis, in which one affected joint becomes asymptomatic as another becomes painful, occurs in gonococcal arthritis, Reiter syndrome, and acute rheumatic fever. Intermittent arthritis, in which asymptomatic intervals are punctuated by acute flares, is common in crystal-induced arthritis.

RHEUMATOLOGIC EMERGENCIES

Although rheumatologic emergencies seldom occur, failure to recognize any of a few important symptoms or signs [*see Table 2*] may result in permanent disability or death; thus, the initial contact with the patient requires being alert for these conditions.[5] If a rheumatologic emergency is suspected, prompt initiation of appropriate diagnostic testing and treatment is essential.

After emergencies have been excluded, the approach to diagnosis need not be rushed. Although patients often come to the office with the preconceived notion that they have arthritis and expect quick diagnostic confirmation and treatment, they often must be observed for some time before the diagnosis can be made. Considerable patience and tact may be required in com-

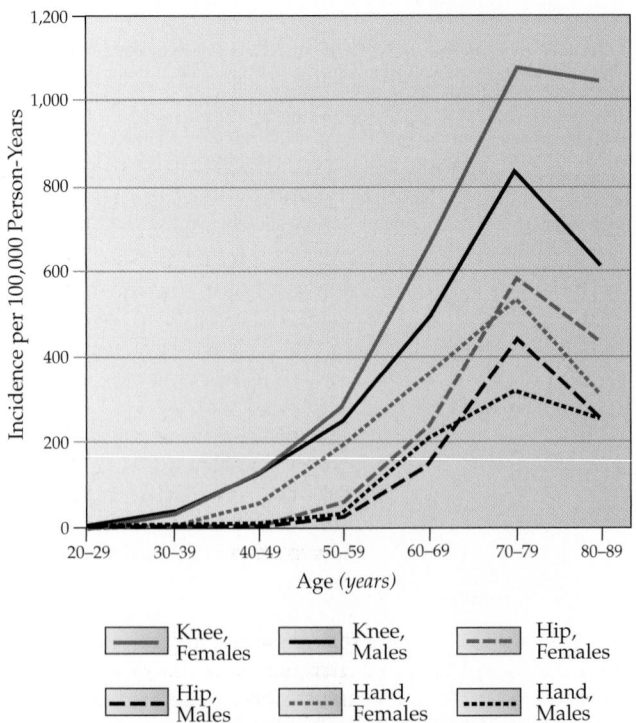

Figure 1 **Incidence of osteoarthritis of the hand, hip, and knee, in members of the Fallon Community Health Plan, 1991–1992, by age and sex.[20]**

Table 1 Common Rheumatic Diseases

	Intra-articular	Extra-articular
Inflammatory	Rheumatoid arthritis Systemic lupus erythematosus Septic arthritis Gout Pseudogout Spondyloarthropathy	Tendinitis Bursitis Polymyositis Vasculitis
Noninflammatory	Osteoarthritis	Fibromyalgia

municating this need to the patient. He or she should be informed that an uncertain diagnosis at presentation is usually a good prognostic sign; the prognosis for patients with clear-cut, easily diagnosed disease is often poor. Temporizing with an indefinite diagnosis—for example, knee pain of uncertain etiology—is better than prematurely classifying a patient's musculoskeletal complaints into a particular diagnostic category. In at least 10% of patients, a diagnosis cannot be made with certainty.

LOCATION OF PAIN

Patients are often not precise in identifying the location of musculoskeletal pain; it helps to ask them to put their hands on the place that hurts. A patient who complains of pain in the hip may point to one of three areas: the inguinal ligament and anterior thigh, suggesting involvement of the true hip joint; the lateral hip girdle, characteristic of trochanteric bursitis; or the buttock, consistent with sacroiliac joint disease or radiation of back pain along the sciatic nerve. During the physical examination, detailed attention to the location of pain helps identify the structures affected. If a specific structure cannot be identified, the pain may be referred from elsewhere. Pain described as diffuse or poorly localized may suggest a serious systemic disease, such

as polymyositis, but more commonly is a manifestation of fibromyalgia or a related pain syndrome.

CHARACTER OF PAIN

Pain that arises from joints and that is dull, alleviated by rest, and worsened by weight bearing or movement of the joint suggests joint damage such as that which occurs in osteoarthritis. Pain that is more intense, accompanied by swelling, and present when the patient is at rest or pain that awakens the patient at night suggests an inflammatory process such as rheumatoid arthritis. Inflammation also causes stiffness after prolonged immobility—the so-called gelling phenomenon, which may last longer than 30 minutes. Patients who have inflammatory joint pain caused by rheumatoid arthritis or SLE typically have significant morning stiffness that lasts as long as several hours and that improves as the day goes on—or at least until they are overwhelmed by the deep fatigue that also accompanies these diseases. The duration of morning stiffness is a rough measure of the activity of the inflammatory disease. Patients who have the noninflammatory joint pain that characterizes osteoarthritis, tendinitis, or bursitis describe focal morning pain that lasts for a few minutes; they are most uncomfortable at the end of the day, after prolonged activity. Shooting, burning, or so-called pins-and-needles discomfort is usually neurogenic.

Symptoms of giving way or locking in a weight-bearing joint generally suggest a mechanical process, such as a cartilage or ligament tear or a loose body within the joint. Locking may also occur when soft tissue inflammation impairs mobility, as when triggering of a finger is caused by a nodule in a flexor tendon as a result of tenosynovitis.

WEAKNESS

A complaint of weakness may reflect one of several disease processes. In patients with focal loss of muscle power in a specific region, indicated by complaints such as, "I can't raise my arm," the obvious possibilities include a neurologic lesion; local

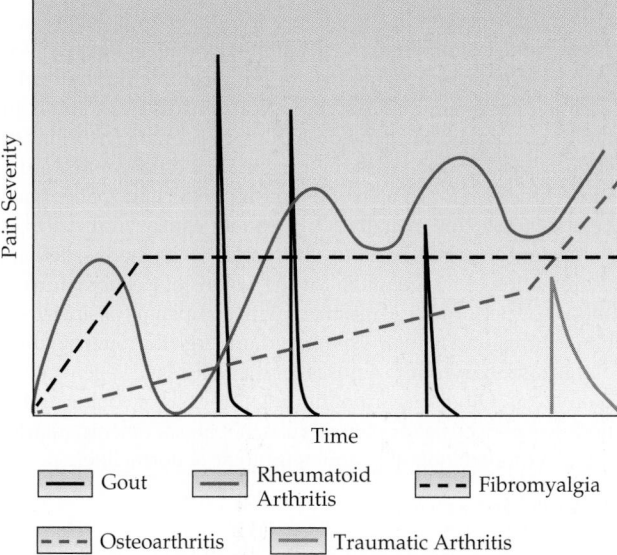

Figure 2 **Variations in the temporal course and severity of pain in the rheumatic diseases. The pain of rheumatoid arthritis may vary in intensity over time. The pain of osteoarthritis tends to be slowly progressive until late in the course of disease, when it may become very severe. The pain of fibromyalgia remains constant. Gout has an intermittent course of high-intensity pain flares. Traumatic arthritis improves more slowly than gout.**[4]

Table 2 Symptoms and Signs of Rheumatologic Emergencies[5]

Symptom or Sign	Condition
History of significant trauma	Fracture, compartmental syndrome, rhabdomyolysis
Systemic symptoms (fever, weight loss)	Infection (septic arthritis, osteomyelitis, endocarditis, necrotizing fasciitis)
Weakness	
Focal	Radiculopathy, entrapment neuropathy, compartmental syndrome, motor neuron disease, mononeuritis multiplex
Global or progressive	Spinal cord compression, myelopathy, transverse myelitis, myositis, response to toxin
Neurogenic pain (burning, numbness, paresthesias)	Radiculopathy, entrapment neuropathy
Point tenderness	Fracture
Red, hot, swollen joint	Septic arthritis, gout, pseudogout
Asymmetrical painful, swollen leg	Deep vein thrombosis
Diffuse shoulder and hip pain, headache in elderly patient	Temporal arteritis
Bowel or bladder dysfunction	Cauda equina syndrome

muscle atrophy; failure of a musculoskeletal unit, such as a ruptured tendon or torn muscle; or weakness secondary to joint pain. A patient who says, "I feel weak all over," should be asked to distinguish true muscle weakness (i.e., loss of power or endurance) from a more generalized sense of asthenia, malaise, or fatigue. The patient with true muscle weakness has difficulty starting or maintaining an activity that requires muscle strength, such as arising from a chair, getting out of bed, or walking up stairs. Physical examination usually confirms the muscular nature of such problems, with the proximal musculature being most affected in myopathies and the distal muscles involved in neuropathies. If the examination shows no objective weakness or other neurologic abnormalities, such as loss of deep tendon reflexes, the patient's report of weakness probably corresponds to asthenia, fatigue, and loss of sense of well-being. If this occurs together with other constitutional symptoms, such as anorexia, weight loss, and low-grade fever, it may indicate an active systemic rheumatic disease such as rheumatoid arthritis or SLE. If the asthenia and fatigue are not accompanied by objective constitutional symptoms, fibromyalgia is more likely.

FUNCTIONAL IMPAIRMENT AND PSYCHOSOCIAL FACTORS

After pain, loss of function is of the greatest concern to patients, making the functional assessment an important part of the history. Exploring this area often affords the physician insights into the way the patient views the disease and what the patient expects. Simple questions asked by the physician may include the following: How has your disease affected you? What can you not

do now that you could do before? What can you not do that you would like to do? Patients with significant functional impairment should be asked more-detailed questions about routine activities of daily living. Explicit questions about sexual function may uncover problems that the patient might otherwise hesitate to describe. The sexual history also identifies risk factors for sexually transmitted joint diseases, such as gonococcal arthritis, Reiter syndrome, and HIV-associated arthropathy. A vocational history may identify specific tasks that exacerbate the disease and that need modification; it may also indicate whether the patient is likely to be exposed to ticks carrying Lyme disease. The history of use of devices such as a cane or crutches and information as to when the patient began using them is helpful in assessing the temporal course of the disease. Claims for workers' compensation or disability or other pending litigation should also be noted.

FAMILY HISTORY

Many rheumatic diseases have strong familial predispositions. Ankylosing spondylitis is the best known, but other autoimmune diseases, such as rheumatoid arthritis and SLE, also have a genetic basis, as do gout and, to a lesser extent, pseudogout.

REVIEW OF SYSTEMS

Once a specific disease is suspected, the patient should be questioned about the presence of other systemic features of the disease. A partial list of clues to systemic disease that can be gleaned from the review of systems is shown [see Table 3].

Physical Examination

GENERAL EXAMINATION

By the time the history is finished, the clinician should have formulated some diagnostic hypotheses that can be used to guide the physical exam. If a patient's complaints are localized and the history elicits no suggestion of a more generalized process, the examination may be limited to the region involved. When systemic symptoms are present, a complete and detailed examination is required. Asymmetrical joint disease and inflammatory back pain raise the possibility of psoriatic arthritis and spondylitis, in which case the physician should very carefully inspect the skin for a patch of psoriasis of which the patient may be unaware. In the sexually active patient with asymmetrical involvement of large joints and a history of conjunctivitis, detailed examination of the genitalia for the lesions of Reiter syndrome should be performed. The patient with complaints of sinus trouble, arthritis, and hemoptysis should undergo thorough scrutiny of the nasopharynx and sinuses for the lesions of Wegener granulomatosis. Other important findings are iritis or conjunctivitis, nodules, pericardial or pleural rubs, hepatic or splenic enlargement, lymphadenopathy, and neurologic abnormalities.

JOINT EXAMINATION

By looking at and palpating the joints, the physician can identify the precise anatomic structures that are the source of the patient's pain and decide whether the pain is caused by inflammation. A goal of the examination is to reproduce the patient's pain, either by motion of the joint or by palpation. Frank redness of the skin overlying a joint is unusual; however, increased temperature, best detected by palpation with the backs of the fingers, is not unusual and, when present, indicates inflammation.

Table 3 Diagnostic Clues from the Review of Systems

Feature	Condition
Facial rash, photosensitivity	Systemic lupus erythematosus
Hair loss	Systemic lupus erythematosus
Uveitis	Spondyloarthropathy, sarcoidosis, Behçet syndrome
Conjunctivitis	Reactive arthritis
Dry eyes and/or mouth	Sjögren syndrome
Oral ulcers	Systemic lupus erythematosus
Nasal discharge, ulcers	Wegener granulomatosis
Diabetes	Diabetic stiff-hand syndrome, Dupuytren contractures, reflex sympathetic dystrophy, carpal tunnel syndrome
Thyroid problems	Osteoporosis, myopathy
Pleurisy	Systemic lupus erythematosus
Hemoptysis	Systemic lupus erythematosus, Wegener granulomatosis
Abdominal pain, bowel dysfunction	Crohn disease, fibromyalgia (with irritable bowel syndrome)
Urethral burning or discharge	Reactive arthritis, septic arthritis
Kidney stones	Gout
Numbness or paresthesias	Carpal tunnel syndrome, vasculitis
Vaginal burning or discharge	Behçet syndrome, septic arthritis

Apparent swelling may be caused by periarticular edema, an effusion in the joint, synovial proliferation, or bony overgrowth; in all cases, it indicates organic disease. Palpation for tenderness may reveal whether the problem lies within the joint or is discretely localized to an overlying bursa or tendon sheath. The finding of fine crepitus with motion of the structure corresponds to the grinding of subchondral bone, denuded of articular cartilage, against opposing bone. Coarser (so-called creaking) crepitus is associated with the fibrinous tendinitis that occurs in scleroderma or traumatic tendinitis. When the examiner is able to move the joint through a passive range of motion that exceeds the active range of motion accomplished voluntarily by the patient, failure of a musculoskeletal unit (e.g., rupture of the rotator cuff in the shoulder) or a neurologic deficit should be suspected. Examination of the spine is the most neglected part of the musculoskeletal examination, probably because it entails moving the patient from the sitting position through the supine and prone positions and then to the standing position. Patients with findings suggestive of a lumbar radiculopathy should have detailed testing of the motor, sensory, and reflex systems in the legs. Reviews of such testing are available on the Internet, at http://www.neuropat.dote.hu/neurology.htm and at http://www.neuroexam.com. An experienced physician can perform a complete musculoskeletal examination in less than 10 minutes.

Laboratory Studies

THE ACUTE-PHASE RESPONSE

The cellular response to inflammation or tissue injury elaborates cytokines such as interleukin-1 (IL-1), IL-6, and tumor necrosis factor (TNF), which have profound effects on the hepatic synthesis of plasma proteins.[6] Concentrations of C-reactive protein (CRP) increase as much as 100-fold within 1 or 2 days after tissue damage; parallel increases in serum amyloid A protein occur. Slower and less marked increases occur in coagulation proteins such as fibrinogen and prothrombin, most of the complement components, normal plasma protease inhibitors, and transport proteins such as ferritin and haptoglobin. Corresponding decreases occur in serum transferrin and albumin, accounting for the low serum iron and albumin levels that accompany inflammatory diseases.

The erythrocyte sedimentation rate (ESR) is the time-honored test used to detect the acute-phase response.[7] The increased rate of fall of the column of erythrocytes is caused by stacking of the cells into rouleaux, induced mainly by increases in the highly asymmetrical fibrinogen molecule; the increased levels of immunoglobulins seen in chronic inflammatory conditions also favor rouleaux formation. The ESR is influenced by many extraneous factors [see Table 4], the most important of which is age. The upper limit of normal for men is obtained by dividing the age in years by 2; for women, it is obtained by adding 10 to the age in years and then dividing that number by 2.

The CRP level is measured by immunoassay and is not influenced by most of the extraneous factors that affect the ESR. It also increases more rapidly than the ESR, which may take several days to increase.

The ESR and CRP tests are nonspecific: ESR and CRP levels may be elevated in a number of inflammatory conditions, such as malignancy, chronic infection, pneumonia, and acute myocardial infarction. Even increases in very low levels of CRP, as detected on a so-called ultrasensitive test, serve as a biomarker

Table 4 Factors That Influence ESR[7]

Factors That Increase ESR	Factors That Decrease ESR
Advancing age	Congestive heart failure
Female sex	Sickle cell disease
Pregnancy	Altered erythrocyte shape
Hypercholesterolemia	(e.g., anisocytosis, spherocytosis, acanthosis, microcytosis)
B cell neoplasm (e.g., myeloma, macroglobulinemia, cryoglobulinemia)	Polycythemia
	Extreme leukocytosis
	Cachexia
Renal failure	Hypofibrinogenemia
	Cryoglobulinemia

ESR—erythrocyte sedimentation rate

for atherosclerosis.[8] These tests are most useful in excluding significant inflammatory disease. For example, in a patient with diffuse pain and tenderness at trigger points, suggesting fibromyalgia, a normal ESR value supports this diagnosis; an ESR of 90 mm/hr dictates close scrutiny for other diseases. If the patient with these symptoms is older than 60 years, polymyalgia rheumatica and temporal arteritis are the primary possibilities. The acute-phase tests are also moderately useful in distinguishing inflammatory from noninflammatory arthritis and in monitoring the course of an inflammatory disease such as rheumatoid arthritis or polymyalgia rheumatica.

IMMUNOLOGIC TESTS

As a class, immunologic tests have low specificity and only moderate sensitivity. They are also more expensive and less reproducible than most other clinical laboratory tests. They should never be used as screening tests; their greatest utility occurs when the pretest probability of disease is high. The misuse of immunologic tests frequently confounds the diagnosis. Two common examples of unnecessary rheumatology referrals are the octogenarian with arthritis of the knees or shoulders who tests positive for rheumatoid factor (unnecessary because positivity in healthy persons increases with age, and osteoarthritis of these joints is common in octogenarians) and the young woman with fatigue; diffuse pains; and a positive, usually low-titer, antinuclear antibody test (unnecessary because low titers of antinuclear antibody are found in as many as 32% of young women[9]; the patient probably has depression or fibromyalgia). The use of so-called arthritis panels, in which many serologic tests are bundled together, increases the likelihood of an abnormal result in a patient without rheumatic disease and should be avoided. Highly specific (and expensive) tests, such as those for antineutrophil cytoplasmic antibody, Lyme disease serology, HLA-B27, antiphospholipid antibody, and antibodies against individual nuclear constituents, should be performed only when the pretest probability of a particular disease is high. In one study of patients with swelling of at least one joint, the rheumatoid factor test had a sensitivity of 65% and a specificity of 87% for the diagnosis of rheumatoid arthritis.[10] At disease onset, a positive test result for rheumatoid factor is predictive of increased severity, as assessed by radiographic evidence of erosions.[11] Antibodies to cyclic citrullinated peptides (anti-CCP) formed by posttranslational modification of arginine residues in proteins such as fillagrin are found in the serum of many patients with rheumatoid arthritis. The 70% sensitivity and 98% specificity of the anti-CCP assays make them very useful in the diagnosis of rheumatoid arthritis, especially during the early

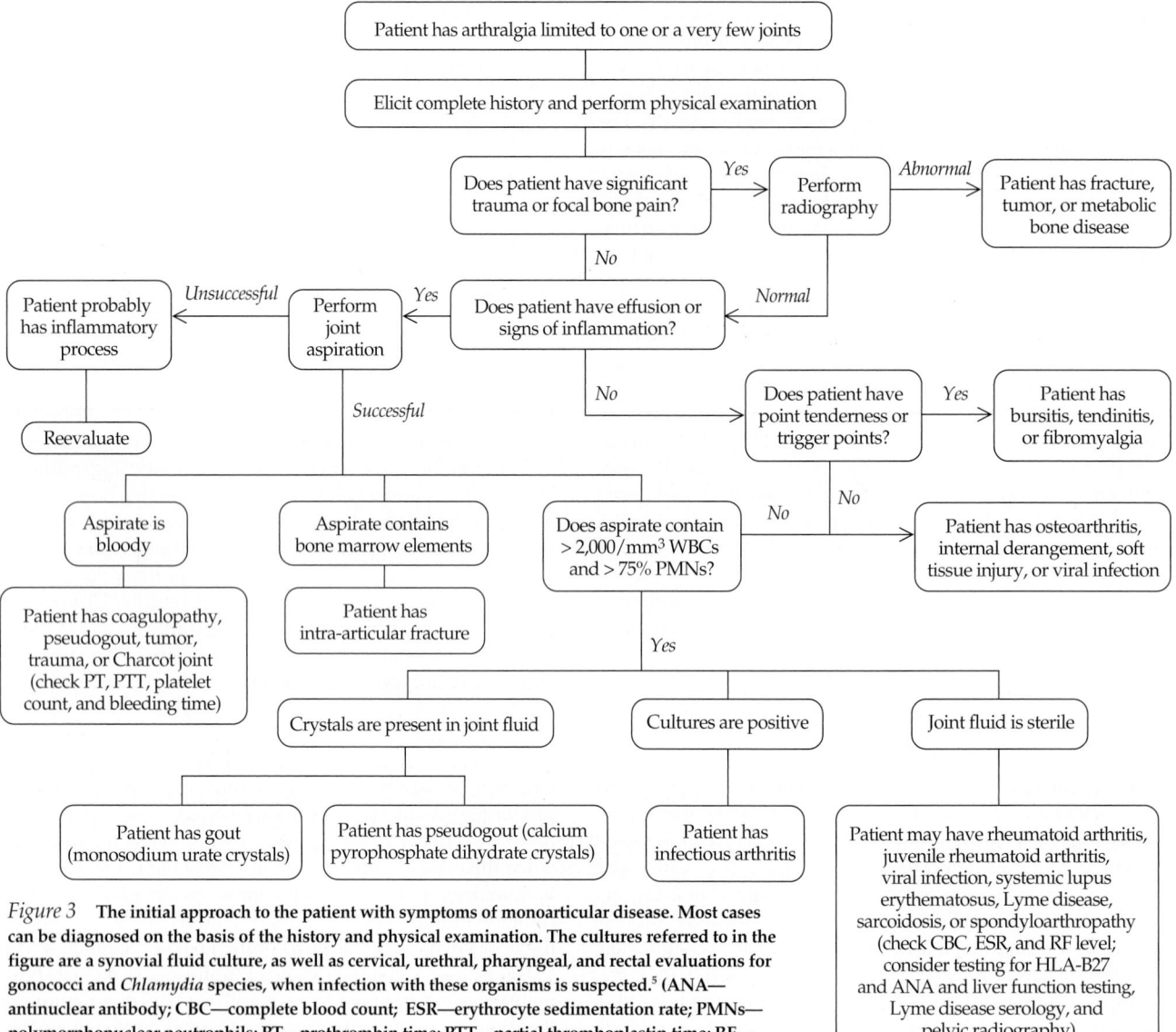

Figure 3 **The initial approach to the patient with symptoms of monoarticular disease. Most cases can be diagnosed on the basis of the history and physical examination. The cultures referred to in the figure are a synovial fluid culture, as well as cervical, urethral, pharyngeal, and rectal evaluations for gonococci and *Chlamydia* species, when infection with these organisms is suspected.[5] (ANA— antinuclear antibody; CBC—complete blood count; ESR—erythrocyte sedimentation rate; PMNs— polymorphonuclear neutrophils; PT—prothrombin time; PTT—partial thromboplastin time; RF— rheumatoid factor; WBCs—white blood cells)**

phases of the disease, when the anti-CCP assay may become positive before the rheumatoid factor test.[12]

SYNOVIAL FLUID ANALYSIS

Examination of synovial fluid is perhaps the most important diagnostic test in rheumatology. It gives the physician one of the few opportunities available for the precise diagnosis of rheumatic disease and permits immediate initiation of specific and effective therapy. In addition, aspiration of synovial fluid is a low-risk procedure: the frequency of iatrogenic infection is less than one in 10,000. Joint aspiration should be performed with aseptic technique as part of the evaluation of every case of acute monoarthritis.

Analysis of the synovial fluid includes a white blood cell count and differential, appropriate cultures and stains for microorganisms, and polarized-light microscopy. The white blood cell count in the synovial fluid is useful in distinguishing inflammatory from noninflammatory arthritis: levels greater than 2,000 cells/mm³ are consistent with inflammation. Patients with crystal-induced arthritis usually have counts in excess of 30,000

cells/mm³. The reliability of the examination of fluid for crystals by polarized-light microscopy depends very much on the laboratory doing the test. The finding of monosodium urate or calcium pyrophosphate dihydrate crystals on polarized-light microscopy is pathognomonic for gout and pseudogout, respectively. The absence of crystals does not exclude these diagnoses, nor does their presence exclude the possibility of coexistent infection. Gram stain and culture may be diagnostic of infection. If patients with established arthritis have fever and an apparent flare, joint infection should be excluded by joint aspiration because septic arthritis occurs more frequently in such patients.

IMAGING

The findings on radiography are unlikely to be abnormal in most patients who have acute arthritis, mechanical back pain, tendinitis, or bursitis; radiography should not be used in these cases. In patients with acute back pain of less than 6 weeks' duration, imaging is not indicated unless there is a high suspicion of systemic disease or progressive neurologic deficit[13] [*see Chapter 120*]. For patients with established arthritis, such as rheuma-

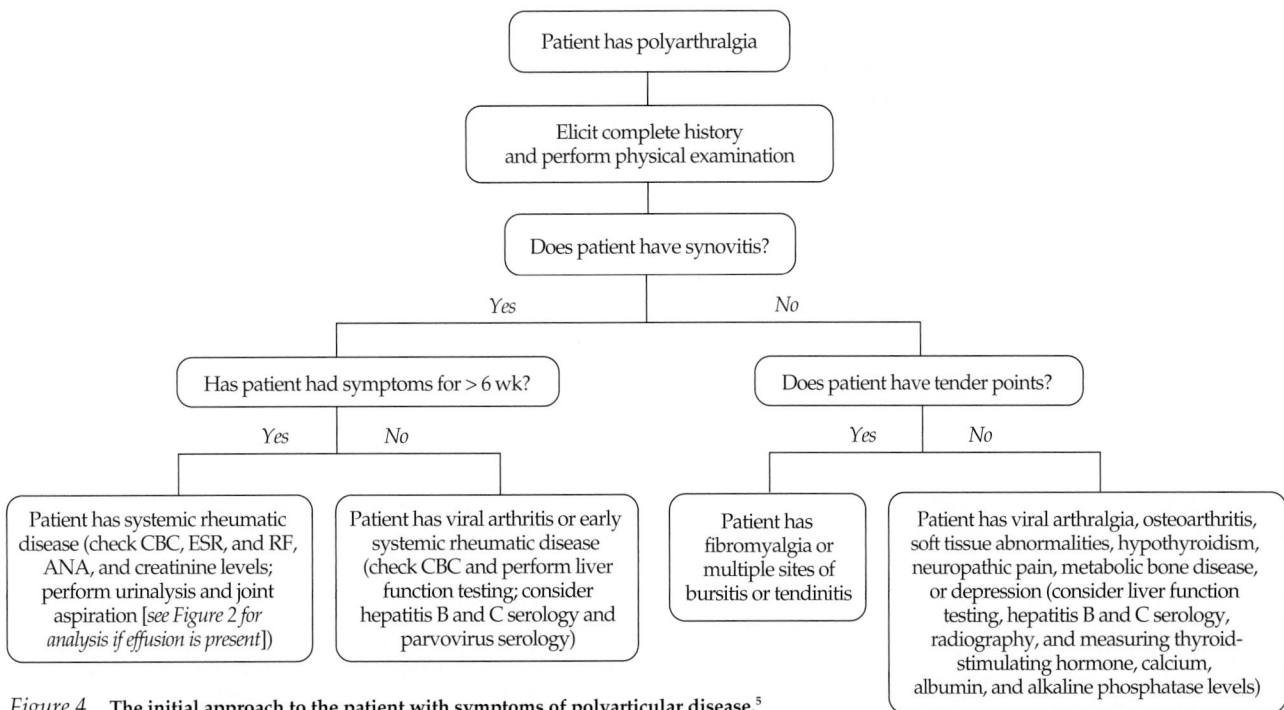

Figure 4   **The initial approach to the patient with symptoms of polyarticular disease.**[5]

toid arthritis, it takes longer than 6 months for radiographic abnormalities such as joint space narrowing and marginal erosions to appear. In patients with osteoarthritis, radiography may be useful in assessing the extent of joint damage, but the correlation between its findings and patients' symptoms is surprisingly poor.

Plain radiography is most useful in patients with significant trauma that suggests the possibility of fracture, in those who experience a sudden loss of function (e.g., an inability to bear weight), in those with symptoms that do not improve despite appropriate treatment, and in those with a suspected infection or neoplastic disease. Computed radiography and digital imaging improve the quality of plain radiographs, make long-distance transmission easy, and eliminate the problem of the lost radiograph. When it is likely that a fracture is present, special views may be required; repeat imaging 7 to 10 days later may detect callus formation at a previously unrecognized fracture site. In patients with chronic disease, repeat radiography is useful in assessing the progress of disease or the necessity of surgical intervention.

Although computed tomography, magnetic resonance imaging, and radionuclide bone scanning are powerful techniques for obtaining information about bones and joints, they should be used only when their results will be used to make important diagnostic or therapeutic decisions. As is true for plain radiography, myelography, and even autopsy, MRI of the spine often reveals abnormalities in people who do not have back pain. In one study, only 36% of patients free of back pain had normal findings on MRI of the lumbar spine.[14] Bone scans are useful in detecting osteomyelitis, stress fractures, and metastases to bone.

Clinical Presentation and Initial Approach

MONOARTICULAR DISEASE

Patients with symptoms that involve one or, at most, a few joints may have posttraumatic syndromes, bursitis, tendinitis, septic arthritis, crystal-induced inflammation (gout or pseudo-

gout), or an atypical presentation of a systemic arthritis such as rheumatoid arthritis [*see Figure 3*]. Arthralgia, in which pain arises from structures surrounding the joint, must be distinguished from arthritis, in which there is evidence of frank involvement of the joint itself. Monoarticular arthritis should be considered to have an infectious etiology until proved otherwise. Prompt aspiration and examination of synovial fluid are usually indicated.

POLYARTICULAR DISEASE

In contrast to monoarticular disease, which often requires an aggressive and invasive diagnostic approach, arthritis involving numerous joints usually requires a more gradual and expectant strategy. The one exception is septic arthritis, which may have a polyarticular onset in up to 20% of patients. In other diseases, there is less urgency in arriving at the diagnosis, and observation for 6 weeks or more may be required. During this period, it is unwise to alarm the patient unnecessarily by musing about the possibility that he or she has a particular systemic rheumatic disease; a wait-and-see attitude is more appropriate. Eventually, most patients with polyarthralgia will prove not to have a systemic rheumatic disease but to have a more benign condition [*see Figure 4*].

DIFFUSE ACHES AND PAINS

Most patients with diffuse aches and pains have a benign, self-limited illness of unknown cause that improves after 1 or 2 weeks of observation. The history often identifies antecedent viral infection or exertional stress as a precipitating factor. Another substantial number of patients prove to have fibromyalgia, which is suggested by an inability to precisely locate the anatomic origins of the pain on physical examination and by the finding of tender trigger points [*see Chapter 121*]. A hemogram and measurements of the ESR or CRP, thyroid-stimulating hormone, creatine kinase (if weakness is an issue), calcium, and phosphate levels are usually sufficient to exclude other diseases [*see Table 5*].

Table 5   Differential Diagnosis
of Diffuse Aches and Pains

Benign postviral syndromes
Postexertional syndromes
Fibromyalgia
Polymyalgia rheumatica
Temporal arteritis
Hypothyroidism
Metabolic bone disease
Hypophosphatemia
Atypical onset of systemic rheumatic disease (e.g., rheumatoid
    arthritis, systemic lupus erythematosus)

Prognosis

Patients who present with complaints of joint pain often express the opinion, "Nothing can be done for my arthritis—I'll just have to learn to live with it." Correcting this misconception is one of the most important things the physician can do during the initial contact. Most kinds of arthritis can be managed quite effectively, and the patient must understand that treatment greatly improves the condition of most patients with arthritis. Even for the most severe diseases, such as rheumatoid arthritis, very effective treatments have been available for 20 years and have brought distinct improvements in long-term outcome.[15,16] New treatments with biologic agents that block the inflammatory cytokines TNF-α and IL-1 are very effective, have a rapid onset of action, and prevent radiographic progression of the disease.[17-19] Educating the patient about the effectiveness of treatment is the first step toward a successful outcome.

The author has no commercial relationships with manufacturers of products or providers of services discussed in this chapter.

References

1. Public health and aging: projected prevalence of self-reported arthritis or chronic joint symptoms among persons aged > 65 years—United States, 2005–2030. MMWR Morb Mortal Wkly Rep 52:489, 2003

2. Prevalence of self-reported arthritis or chronic joint symptoms among adults—United States, 2001. MMWR Morb Mortal Wkly Rep 51:948, 2002

3. Schappert SM: Ambulatory care visits to physician offices, hospital outpatient departments, and emergency departments: United States, 1997. Vital Health Stat 13 143:1, 1999

4. Liang MH, Roberts WN, Robb-Nicholson C, et al: Sorting out musculoskeletal complaints. Rheumatology: Problems in Primary Care. Medical Economics Books, Oradell, New Jersey, 1990

5. Guidelines for the initial evaluation of the adult patient with acute musculoskeletal symptoms. American College of Rheumatology Ad Hoc Committee on Clinical Guidelines. Arthritis Rheum 39:1, 1996

6. Gabay C, Kushner I: Acute-phase proteins and other systemic responses to inflammation. N Engl J Med 340:448, 1999

7. Sox HC, Liang MH: The erythrocyte sedimentation rate: guidelines for rational use. Ann Intern Med 104:515, 1986

8. Labarrere CA, Zaloga GP: C-reactive protein: from innocent bystander to pivotal mediator of atherosclerosis. Am J Med 117:499, 2004

9. Tan EM, Feltkamp TE, Smolen JS, et al: Range of antinuclear antibodies in "healthy" individuals. Arthritis Rheum 40:1601, 1997

10. Saraux A, Berthelot JM, Chales G, et al: Value of laboratory tests in early prediction of rheumatoid arthritis. Arthritis Rheum 47:155, 2002

11. Bukhari M, Lunt M, Harrison BJ, et al: Rheumatoid factor is the major predictor of increasing severity of radiographic erosions in rheumatoid arthritis: results from the Norfolk Arthritis Register Study, a large inception cohort. Arthritis Rheum 46:906, 2002

12. Morrow DA, Ridker PM: C-reactive protein, inflammation, and coronary risk. Med Clin North Am 84:149, 2000

13. Jarvik JG, Deyo RA: Diagnostic evaluation of low back pain with emphasis on imaging. Ann Intern Med 137:586, 2002

14. Jensen MC, Brant-Zawadzki MN, Obuchowski N, et al: Magnetic resonance imaging of the lumbar spine in people without back pain. N Engl J Med 331:69, 1994

15. Fries JF, Williams CA, Morfeld D, et al: Reduction in long-term disability in patients with rheumatoid arthritis by disease-modifying antirheumatic drug-based treatment strategies. Arthritis Rheum 39:616, 1996

16. O'Dell JR, Haire CE, Erikson N, et al: Treatment of rheumatoid arthritis with methotrexate alone, sulfasalazine and hydroxychloroquine, or a combination of all three medications. N Engl J Med 334:1287, 1996

17. Kremer JM: Rational use of new and existing disease-modifying agents in rheumatoid arthritis. Ann Intern Med 134:695, 2001

18. Weinblatt ME, Keystone EC, Furst DE, et al: Adalimumab, a fully human anti-tumor necrosis factor alpha monoclonal antibody, for the treatment of rheumatoid arthritis in patients taking concomitant methotrexate: the ARMADA trial. Arthritis Rheum 48:35, 2003

19. Cohen S, Hurd E, Cush J, et al: Treatment of rheumatoid arthritis with anakinra, a recombinant human interleukin-1 receptor antagonist, in combination with methotrexate: results of a twenty-four-week, multicenter, randomized, double-blind, placebo-controlled trial. Arthritis Rheum 46:614, 2002

20. Oliveria SA, Felson DT, Reed JI, et al: Incidence of symptomatic hand, hip, and knee osteoarthritis among patients in a health maintenance organization. Arthritis Rheum 38:1134, 1995

Acknowledgment

Figures 2 through 4   Marcia Kammerer.

112 Rheumatoid Arthritis

Gary S. Firestein, M.D.

Rheumatoid arthritis (RA) is among the most common forms of chronic inflammatory arthritis. RA affects about 1% of adults, and it is two to three times more prevalent in women than in men. RA may begin as early as infancy, but onset usually occurs in the fifth or sixth decade. There are no specific laboratory tests for RA; diagnosis depends on a constellation of signs and symptoms that can be supported by serology and radiographs. Involvement of the small joints of the hands and feet is often the key to the diagnosis. Specific clinical criteria have evolved [*see Table 1*], but in practice, diagnosis is established by careful observation of the pattern of disease activity over time.

Immunogenetics

Genetic makeup plays a critical role in susceptibility to RA. Identical twins show 12% to 15% concordance for the disease; first-degree relatives of patients with RA have about a twofold to threefold increased incidence. The most prominent genetic linkage in RA involves a unique peptide on the class II major histocompatibility complex (MHC). This susceptibility epitope is associated with the third hypervariable region of DR β chains, which contains a specific sequence of amino acids from 70 through 74 (glutamine-leucine-arginine-alanine-alanine, also known as QKRAA) found in *DRB1*0401*, *DRB1*0404*, and other alleles.[1] This sequence is found in most RA patients; it is associated with increased disease severity, although the disease develops in only a small fraction of patients who have QKRAA. Recent data suggest that the MHC association might not be an independent risk factor for RA; rather, it appears that MHC is associated with the production of anti-citrullinated peptide (CP) antibodies that are, in turn, a true risk factor for disease susceptibility and severity.[2]

Susceptibility to RA is likely polygenic; for instance, certain immunoglobulin genotypes and, perhaps, genetic differences in the galactosylation of immunoglobulin may be predisposing factors. Further studies have identified associations with promoter-region polymorphisms of many cytokines, such as tumor necrosis factor (TNF), interleukin-1 (IL-1), and many others.[3] These

---

Table 1   American Rheumatism Association Criteria
for the Classification of Rheumatoid Arthritis[101]

Criteria

Morning stiffness: morning stiffness in and around the joints lasting at least 1 hr before maximal improvement

Arthritis of three or more joint areas: at least three joint areas have simultaneously had soft tissue swelling or fluid (not bony overgrowth alone) observed by a physician; the 14 possible joint areas (right and left) are proximal interphalangeal (PIP), metacarpophalangeal (MCP), wrist, elbow, knee, ankle, and metatarsophalangeal (MTP) joints

Arthritis of hand joints: at least one joint area swollen as above in wrist, MCP, or PIP joint

Symmetrical arthritis: simultaneous involvement of the same joint areas (as in arthritis of three or more joint areas, above) on both sides of the body (bilateral involvement of PIP, MCP, or MTP joints is acceptable without absolute symmetry)

Rheumatoid nodules: subcutaneous nodules over bony prominences or extensor surfaces or in juxta-articular regions that are observed by a physician

Serum rheumatoid factor: demonstration of abnormal amounts of serum rheumatoid factor by any method that has been positive in fewer than 5% of normal control subjects

Radiographic changes: radiographic changes typical of rheumatoid arthritis on posteroanterior hand and wrist x-rays, which must include erosions or unequivocal bony decalcification localized to or most marked adjacent to the involved joints (osteoarthritis changes alone do not qualify)

Exclusions

The presence of any of the following excludes the diagnosis of rheumatoid arthritis:

Typical rash of systemic lupus erythematosus (SLE)

High concentration of lupus erythematosus cells (four or more in two smears); because of the frequent finding of LE cells in patients with clinically typical rheumatoid arthritis, however, it is suggested that such patients be listed separately

Histologic evidence of polyarteritis nodosa with segmented necrosis of arteries associated with nodular leukocytic infiltration extending perivascularly, including many eosinophils

Persistent muscle swelling of dermatomyositis or weakness of neck, trunk, and pharyngeal muscles

Definite scleroderma (not limited to the fingers)

A clinical picture characteristic of rheumatic fever with migratory joint involvement and evidence of endocarditis, especially if accompanied by subcutaneous nodules, erythema marginatum, or chorea (an elevated antistreptolysin titer will not rule out the diagnosis of rheumatoid arthritis)

A clinical picture characteristic of gouty arthritis with acute attacks of swelling, redness, and pain in one or more joints, especially if responsive to colchicine

Tophi

A clinical picture characteristic of acute infectious arthritis of bacterial or viral origin with an acute focus of infection or a close association with a disease of known infectious origin; chills; fever; acute joint involvement, usually initially migratory (especially if organisms are present in the joint fluid or there is a response to antibiotic therapy)

Tubercle bacilli in joints or histologic evidence of joint tuberculosis

A clinical picture characteristic of reactive arthritis with urethritis and conjunctivitis associated with acute joint involvement, usually initially migratory

A clinical picture characteristic of the shoulder-hand syndrome with unilateral involvement of shoulder and hand and diffuse swelling of the hand, followed by atrophy and contractures

A clinical picture characteristic of hypertrophic osteoarthropathy with clubbing of fingers or hypertrophic periostitis, or both, along the shafts of the long bones, especially if an intrapulmonary lesion is present

A clinical picture characteristic of neuroarthropathy with condensation and destruction of bones of involved joints and associated neurologic findings

Homogentisic acid in the urine grossly detectable by alkalinization

Histologic evidence of sarcoid or a positive Kveim test

Multiple myeloma evidenced by marked increase in plasma cells in the bone marrow or by Bence Jones protein in the urine

Characteristic skin lesions of erythema nodosum

Leukemia or lymphoma with characteristic cells in peripheral blood, bone marrow, or tissues

A clinical picture characteristic of ankylosing spondylitis, psoriasis, ulcerative colitis, or regional enteritis

Note: For classification purposes, a patient is said to have rheumatoid arthritis if he or she has satisfied at least four of the above seven criteria. The first four must be present for at least 6 wk. Patients with two clinical diagnoses are not excluded. Designation as classic, definite, or probable rheumatoid arthritis is *not* to be made.

base substitutions can potentially increase cytokine gene transcription and enhance inflammatory responses. Certain extended haplotypes of peptidylarginine deiminase type 4 (PADI-4), which is one of four *PADI* genes that converts arginine to citrulline, have also been associated with the development of RA in Asian populations[4]; however, this association is not found in Western European populations. A polymorphism in *PTPN22*, a phosphatase gene that regulates T cell function, has also been associated with several autoimmune diseases, including RA.[5] The disease-associated allele (*R620W*) is quite rare in Asia, indicating that different ethnic and racial groups might have distinct genes that predispose them to RA.

Etiology

It is unlikely that a single etiologic factor accounts for all cases of adult RA. A pathogenic organism is often assumed to be responsible, but despite some suggestive data, no conclusive evidence implicates bacteria, including mycoplasmas, or other prokaryotes. Viruslike particles have been isolated from synovial effusions in RA, and some RA patients exhibit evidence of a recent parvovirus B19 infection.[6] Some studies have shown no correlation between RA and serologic evidence of previous infection or the presence of B19 genes in synovial tissue, whereas others have demonstrated presense of parvovirus B19 proteins and infectious virus particles in RA synovium.[7] B19 also can infect cultured synovial fibroblasts and increase invasion into cartilage matrix.[8]

Other viruses that have been isolated from synovial fluid include rubella and Epstein-Barr virus (EBV). Sera from most RA patients contain greater amounts of antibodies to various EBV-derived antigens than normal sera. Suppression of EBV infection by lymphocytes from RA patients is impaired, possibly because T cells mount an insufficient response with low levels of interferon gamma. Although EBV infection is probably not the initial event in RA, it could potentially contribute to persistent immunologic stimulation by acting as a polyclonal activator of B cells, thereby augmenting the production of autoantibodies.

Lymphocytes from some RA patients respond to a region of EBV glycoprotein gp110 that contains the same QKRAA sequence as the susceptibility epitope on DR β chains.[9] Thus, molecular mimicry may lead to autoimmunity in certain EBV-infected individuals. Other xenoproteins, most notably *Escherichia coli* DNA J protein, also contain QKRAA and may contribute to a response against self-MHC.[10]

Retroviruses could serve as infectious causes of RA-like diseases. Synovial human T cell lymphotropic virus type I (HTLV-I) infection is associated with chronic arthritis, and in vitro transduction of synoviocytes with the HTLV-I tax gene leads to increased growth.[11] Retrovirus-like particles have been observed in some synovial samples, and expression of zinc-finger proteins associated with retroviral infections offers some support for this hypothesis.[12]

Many RA patients show evidence of autoimmunity long before the appearance of clinical arthritis. For instance, rheumatoid factors and anti-CP antibodies can be detected in the blood of patients many years before the onset of disease.[13] Both anti-CP antibodies and rheumatoid factors can, in some circumstances, directly contribute to synovial inflammation through complement fixation.[14]

Theories on the initiation of RA remain speculative, but pathogenesis probably involves repeated inflammatory episodes that eventually break tolerance in a person who has the appropriate genetic background.[15] The stimuli that cause inflammation could be related to activation of pattern-recognition receptors known as toll-like receptors (TLRs) located on macrophages, dendritic cells, mast cells, and neutrophils; such activation might then lead to nonspecific articular inflammation.[16] Many products of prokaryotic cells can be detected in the inflamed synovium; these could contribute to the initiation of RA. Endogenous ligands that activate TLRs (e.g., necrotic debris in synovial effusions, heat shock proteins, and fibrinogen) can also contribute to this process. Antigen presenting cells can be "loaded" with articular antigens and migrate to central lymphoid organs where they can activate T cells that, in turn, can stimulate autoreactive B cells. The lymphocytes can then re-enter the circulation, return to the joint, and continue responding to natural and modified articular antigens. In this scenario, no single etiologic agent is required. Instead, nonspecific inflammation in a patient with a particular genetic background can lead to local responses directed at many articular antigens.

Pathogenesis

SYNOVIAL HISTOPATHOLOGY AND INVASION

The synovial tissue in RA becomes markedly hyperplastic, with redundant folds, frondlike villi, and edema. In the earliest stages, blood vessel proliferation and endothelial damage are prominent. Hyperplasia of the synovial intimal lining (the region in direct contact with synovial fluid) can occur, even when sublining inflammatory infiltrate is mild. As the disease progresses, intimal lining hyperplasia becomes more prominent, increasing up to fivefold from the normal thickness of one or two cell layers [*see Figure 1*]. Synovial lining hyperplasia is caused, in part, by local proliferation of the fibroblast-like type B synoviocytes and migration of new macrophage-like type A synoviocytes from bone marrow and blood into the joint. The rate of cell death also determines tissue cellularity. Many cells of the intimal lining contain damaged DNA that normally leads to apoptosis (programmed cell death). Relatively few cells complete this process, possibly as a result of defective apoptosis contributing to hyperplasia.[17]

In chronic RA, inflammatory cells (including T cells, B cells, macrophages, and plasma cells) accumulate in the sublining re-

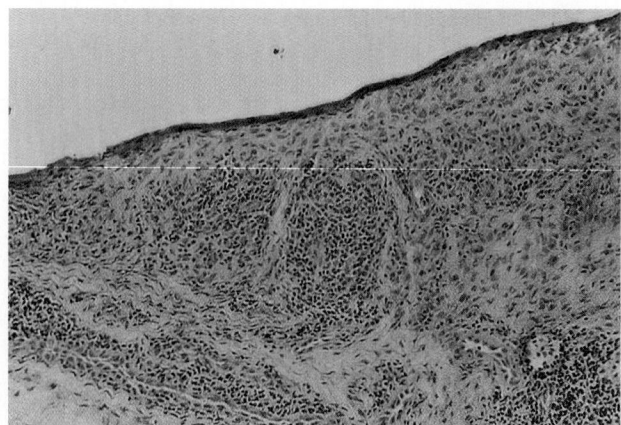

Figure 1 Section of a proliferative synovium from a patient with classic rheumatoid arthritis reveals synovial lining hyperplasia and a sublining lymphocyte infiltration and aggregation.

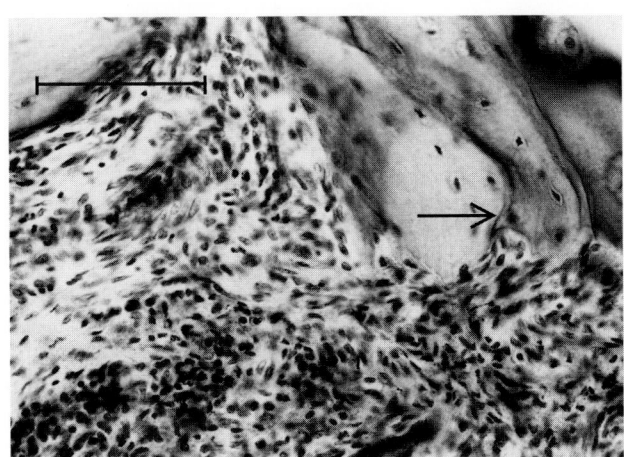

Figure 2 **At the junction between a proliferative inflamed rheumatoid synovium and the bone, scalloped regions of erosion can be seen (arrow). Section is stained with hematoxylin and eosin (bar scale = 100 μm).**

gion. Lymphocytes can organize into discrete aggregates, although diffuse mononuclear cell infiltration or relatively acellular fibrous tissue can also be present. The majority of T cells are CD4+ memory cells with small nuclei and scant cytoplasm. Although the cells are functionally quiescent, many express surface antigens that suggest previous activation. An increase in the number of blood vessels remains a prominent finding in the chronic phase. Capillary morphometry studies suggest that the capillary network is more disorganized than normal, and the tissue bulk outstrips the proliferation of blood vessels.

Rheumatoid synovitis is usually accompanied by increased synovial effusions. The white blood cell (WBC) count in synovial fluid in active RA is about 10,000/mm³ (about 70% neutrophils). In contrast to the synovium, there are more CD8+ T cells than CD4+ T cells in synovial effusions. The polymorphonuclear leukocytes are drawn into the joint fluid along a gradient formed by chemotactic substances that include leukotriene B₄, platelet-activating factor, the C5a fragment of complement, and chemokines such as IL-8. Lymphocytes, macrophages, and shed lining cells are also seen in synovial fluid. Surprisingly, very few neutrophils are present in RA synovium, even though they are abundant in the effusions.

Pannus, which is the invasive region of synovium that erodes into cartilage and bone [*see Figure 2*], contains macrophages and primitive mesenchymal cells but very few lymphocytes. The invasive cells have distinctive characteristics, such as very high expression of vascular cell adhesion molecule–1 and CD55 (decay activating factor).[18] Mesenchymal stem cells have also been described in RA synovial tissue; these cells express distinct surface proteins (e.g., bone morphogenic protein receptors and endoglin) and can migrate into the synovium directly through pores in cortical bone or through the circulating blood.[19]

Damage to bone and cartilage by synovial tissue and pannus is mediated by several families of enzymes, including serine proteases and cathepsins. The most destructive enzymes are the metalloproteinases (e.g., collagenase, stromelysin, and gelatinase) and cathepsins (especially cathepsin K), which can degrade the major structural proteins in the joint. Cytokines such as IL-1 and TNF-α are potent inducers of metalloproteinase gene expression. Although protease inhibitors, like tissue inhibitors of metalloproteinases, are expressed by the rheumatoid synovial

lining, the balance between proteases and inhibitors appears to favor the former in RA.[20] Chondrocytes in the cartilage, synoviocytes in pannus, neutrophils in synovial fluid, and osteoclasts in the bone are the primary sources of proteases. The receptor activator of nuclear factor κB (RANK) and the RANK ligand (RANKL) together play a critical role in local osteoclast activation and bone destruction; contributing roles are also played by TNF-α macrophage colony stimulating factor, IL-6, and other cytokines that support osteoclast maturation. The RANKL/RANK system is counterbalanced by the natural inhibitor osteoprotegerin (OPG); OPG is relatively deficient in RA joints, and this deficiency contributes to bone erosions. In animal models of arthritis, administration of OPG markedly decreases bone destruction, even though inflammation is unaffected.[21]

Destruction of extracellular matrix by rheumatoid synovium mesenchymal cells may occur either as a result of a normal response to the inflammatory cytokine milieu or as a result of abnormal synoviocyte function.[20] RA synoviocytes display an aggressive phenotype characterized by adhesion-independent growth and loss of contact inhibition in vitro. Cultured RA synoviocytes that have been coimplanted with cartilage explants into mice with severe combined immunodeficiency disease invade the cartilage matrix, whereas osteoarthritis synoviocytes and normal dermal fibroblasts do not.[22] Somatic mutations in the genes encoding key regulatory proteins, such as the p53 tumor-suppressor gene, may contribute to the transformed phenotype of synoviocytes.[23] Such abnormalities are likely caused by the high local concentration of oxidants in the rheumatoid joint.

CELLULAR IMMUNITY

Attempts to identify an etiologic agent by determining the proliferative response of synovial T cells to specific antigens have been relatively unrewarding. Articular T cells in RA are often less responsive than peripheral blood cells. For instance, the proliferation of lymphocytes in synovial fluid in response to mitogens or recall antigens (e.g., tetanus toxoid) is significantly lower than the proliferation of blood T cells. Production of cytokines (e.g., interferon gamma and IL-2) by synovial fluid T cells in vitro is also low after stimulation by nonspecific mitogens. The mechanism of defective T cell responses in RA might be related to abnormal intracellular redox balance, which interferes with transduction of the T cell receptor signal.[24]

Mycobacterial antigens and the 60 kd heat shock protein appear to be exceptions to the generally lower T cells responses seen in RA, in that lymphocyte proliferation in response to these antigens is greater in cells from rheumatoid effusions than in peripheral blood T cells. However, the response to these antigens is not specific to RA; in fact, the response is even more prominent in reactive arthritis. Telomere length in rheumatoid T cells is shorter than that in normal T cells, suggesting that the rheumatoid T cells have been cycled through multiple divisions or that they are showing signs of premature "aging." Overactive adaptive immune responses can also be the result of inadequate function of a novel subset of T cells known as regulatory T cells (Tregs) that express CD4 and CD25 on their surface. Some studies suggest that Treg function might be suppressed in RA, partly because of the exposure of Tregs to cytokines such as TNF-α. Treatment with anti-TNF agents appears to correct the defect in some individuals.[25]

Immune dysregulation has been observed in peripheral-blood T cells in patients with RA, especially RA patients with EBV infection. A more specific defect is observed in the autologous mixed lymphocyte reaction, in which RA T cells proliferate and produce cytokines in response to MHC class II antigens expressed on autologous antigen-presenting cells. Autoimmune responses directed toward joint-specific antigens can contribute to synovitis; in some cases, this effect might be enhanced when arginine is converted to citrulline by PADI that is present in the joint. In addition to type II collagen, which is localized to hyaline cartilage, other articular antigens have been implicated. For instance, T cell immunity directed against cartilage protein gp39, cartilage link protein, and proteoglycans have been implicated in RA. Many of these antigens can induce arthritis in mice or rats when the animals are immunized with the antigen in combination with adjuvants. An unusual T cell phenotype (CD4[+], CD28[−]) has been noted in the synovial tissue of patients with RA that might participate in innate and adaptive immunity.[26]

HUMORAL IMMUNITY

Rheumatoid Factors, Anti-Citrullinated Peptide Antibodies, and Other Autoantibodies

Rheumatoid factors are immunoglobulins with antibody specificity for the Fc region of IgG. The standard laboratory tests employed in clinical diagnosis (i.e., latex fixation, sensitized sheep red blood cell agglutination, nephelometry, and enzyme-linked immunosorbent assay) detect only IgM rheumatoid factors. The tests are positive in 70% to 80% of patients with classic RA, depending on the method used. Although patients with classic RA may have negative test results, a high-titer positive result indicates a poorer prognosis—an unremitting course and a greater degree of joint damage.

Rheumatoid factor is not a specific finding for RA. Significant titers are found in patients with related diseases (e.g., systemic lupus erythematosus [SLE], progressive systemic sclerosis, and dermatomyositis) and in patients with nonrheumatic chronic inflammatory disorders and infections. Healthy elderly persons, particularly women, often have positive test results. Rheumatoid factor may be a feature of the early immune response to many proteins, facilitating antigen clearance by macrophages.

IgM rheumatoid factor is most commonly detected; IgG and, less frequently, IgA rheumatoid factors are also sometimes found. The presence of IgG rheumatoid factor is associated with a higher rate of bone erosions and systemic complications (e.g., nodules, necrotizing vasculitis).[27] Clues to the origin of rheumatoid factors in RA are provided by studies evaluating their amino acid and DNA sequences. On the basis of location and types of somatic mutations, as evidenced by polymerase chain reaction, rheumatoid factors in RA appear to result from an antigen-driven immune response.[28] However, it is not certain whether IgG itself serves as the antigen or whether another related epitope is responsible. Rheumatoid factors can be synthesized by B cells and plasma cells that infiltrate the synovium in RA patients, including some seronegative patients.

Antibodies that bind citrullinated peptides are also produced in RA patients and may be more sensitive and specific for RA than rheumatoid factor. Many proteins are citrullinated in synovial tissue, and citrullination also occurs in animal models of arthritis.[29] PADI is the enzyme responsible for posttranslational modification of arginine, and certain isoforms, such as PADI-2 and PADI-4, are overexpressed in inflamed joint tissues; these findings suggest that PADI plays a contributory role in the development of RA. Although CP antigens are com-

monly produced at other sites of inflammation (e.g., the lungs of smokers), antibodies directed against CP are much more specific for RA.[30] B cells that produce these IgG and IgM anti-CP antibodies are present in rheumatoid synovial tissue. High titers of anti-CP antibodies also correlate with more aggressive and destructive disease.

Other autoantibodies might also play a role in RA, including antibodies directed at joint-specific antigens such as gp39, RA33, and p205.[31] Antibodies to glucose-6-phosphate isomerase (GPI), a ubiquitous antigen, can cause arthritis in mice and have also been detected in patients with RA and other inflammatory arthropathies.[32] Anti-GPI antibodies appear to localize in the joints and activate complement, perhaps because GPI can adhere to articular cartilage. The relative contribution of autoantibodies to RA as either a primary or a secondary phenomenon is still uncertain.

The importance of autoantibodies and B cells in RA has recently been supported by studies demonstrating the efficacy of anti-CD20 antibody (rituximab) to deplete B cells.[33] Profound peripheral B cell depletion is accompanied by a modest decrease in rheumatoid factors and anti-CP antibodies. Although there is not a close correlation between autoantibody production and disease activity, recurrence of synovitis after treatment correlates with the return of peripheral B cells and rising titers of potential autoantibodies.

Complement Activation

Complement is activated by the interaction of rheumatoid factors either with normal IgG or with other antibody complexes that form in the joint; activation of complement starts a chain of events that includes production of anaphylatoxins and chemotactic factors. Polymorphonuclear leukocytes then engulf the rheumatoid factor–IgG-complement complexes and release lysosomal enzymes and other products. Complexes of IgG rheumatoid factor that have IgG and complement components are readily detected in the synovium, synovial fluid, and extra-articular lesions. Although the synovium is a rich source of complement production, the levels in rheumatoid synovial fluid are low because of local consumption. Deposits of immunoglobulin and complement have been identified in avascular cartilage and other collagenous tissues of rheumatoid joints and may play a role in the formation of the destructive lesion of RA. These deposits, which are highly specific for RA, may be an attractant for the invasive pannus.

Cytokines

Early studies suggested an unrestricted abundance of cytokines in the rheumatoid joint. However, later experiments demonstrated a relative paucity of many T cell–derived cytokines, including IL-2, IL-4, and TNF-β.[34] One exception is IL-17, which can regulate cartilage metabolism and is produced by CD4[+] T cells in the joint.[35] T cells can also potentially contribute to macrophage and synoviocyte activation by inducing metalloproteinase gene expression via direct cell-cell contact.

T helper cells can be divided into several subsets that mediate distinct functions of the immune system; each subset expresses specific transcription factors. T helper type 1 (Th1) cells produce IL-2, IFN-γ, and IL-6; these cell subsets are characterized by T-bet expression. Th2 cells are characterized by GATA-3 expression; these cells produce the opposite pattern of cytokines (i.e., IL-4, IL-10, IL-13). The Th17 subset produces IL-17 but not IFN-α; this subset can be induced when T cells are exposed to transforming growth factor–β (TGF-β) and either IL-6 or IL-23, each of which is present in the rheumatoid joint.

Th1 and Th17 cell overactivity predominates in most animal models of autoimmunity, whereas Th2 cytokines mediate disease suppression.[36] The relatively small amounts of T cell cytokines that can be detected in RA are biased toward the Th1 and Th17 phenotype; these cytokines include IFN-α and IL-17, for Th1 and Th17, respectively. In contrast, Th2 cytokines (especially IL-4) are virtually absent from the joint. Some IL-10 is present, but it is derived mainly from macrophages, and the amount is not sufficient to suppress Th1 cytokine production. The relative lack of suppressive Th2 cytokines may contribute to the pathogenesis of rheumatoid synovitis. Levels of other suppressive cytokines, such as the natural IL-1 receptor antagonist (IL-1ra), are also low in RA joint tissues.[37]

Macrophage- and fibroblast-derived cytokines (e.g., IL-1, IL-6, IL-12, IL-15, IL-18, IL-32, TNF-α, and granulocyte-macrophage colony-stimulating factor [GM-CSF]) are abundantly expressed in the rheumatoid joint.[38] Many of these cytokines are involved in the pathogenesis of RA; in addition, they regulate the production of proteases—small molecule mediators of inflammation—and recruit additional cells to the joint. TNF-α is especially important because it can induce synoviocyte proliferation, collagenase production, and prostaglandin release. Generalized overexpression of TNF-α can induce arthritis in mice. IL-15 is produced by macrophages but shares many activities with the T cell–derived cytokine IL-2. It increases the ability of T cells to induce TNF-α production by macrophages through an antigen-independent mechanism that involves cell-cell contact.[39] IL-18 is also present in the RA joint and can bias T cell responses toward Th1 or directly activate macrophages to produce proinflammatory mediators.[40] Cytokine networks can potentially establish paracrine or autocrine networks that can perpetuate arthritis long after the etiologic agent has been cleared. Recent studies suggest that anticytokine therapy (including therapy with IL-1, TNF-α, and IL-6) is effective in severe RA and demonstrates the importance of fibroblast and macrophage products in the development of chronic synovitis.

Cytokine-derived macrophages, fibroblasts, and dendritic cells also can help organize the synovial microarchitecture into lymphoid aggregates. For instance, B cell survival and differentiation factors (e.g., BLyS and APRIL) are produced in the rheumatoid synovium.[41] In addition, cytokines (e.g., LIGHT) and chemokines (e.g., CXCL13 and CCL21) orchestrate the recruitment of cells into structures that have germinal centers.[42] Here, antigen presentation can occur and enhance systemic immune response to articular antigens.

Diagnosis

The onset and course of RA can be highly variable, and the lack of a specific biologic marker makes diagnosis difficult. Prolonged observation and the integration of clinical and laboratory data that meet established criteria are often required. Although early diagnosis is important to prevent structural damage and may limit mortality, it is equally important to avoid overdiagnosing RA. Up to 40% of patients with early inflammatory synovitis experience spontaneous remission, and diagnostic criteria generally require at least 6 weeks of continuous signs and symptoms before the diagnosis can be established. Diagnostic criteria have been formulated by the American College of Rheumatology (ACR) [see Table 1].

The onset of RA in adults may be either acute or insidious. In the latter case, systemic manifestations may precede overt symptoms of arthritis by months. In some patients, external events (e.g., major infections, surgical procedures, trauma, or childbirth) precede the clinical onset. How these events relate to pathogenesis is unknown. Small joints of the hands and feet are usually involved at the outset, although large joints (e.g., knees and ankles) are sometimes affected first. In about 10% of cases, monoarthritis of a large joint can presage progression to polyarticular RA.

An insidious onset followed by progression to polyarticular involvement is the most common course. Most patients experience some degree of joint stiffness, especially in the morning after awakening, which may accompany or precede joint swelling or pain. These symptoms are hallmarks of disease activity and help distinguish RA from noninflammatory diseases such as osteoarthritis. However, joint stiffness and swelling are not specific to RA and can occur with other types of inflammatory arthritis. RA patients frequently complain of morning stiffness that lasts more than 30 minutes (often up to several hours).

Examination of the joints reveals varying degrees of swelling, warmth over the involved joint, tenderness to palpation, and limitation of active and passive range of motion. Swelling may be caused by thickening, edema, and increased vascularity of the synovium; by synovial effusions; or by combinations of these factors. In small joints, such as metacarpophalangeal joints, effusions may be difficult to detect: the presence of synovial thickening causes loss of the anatomic landmarks and can obscure the peaks and valleys formed by the joints. In large joints, especially the knees, effusions are usually easy to demonstrate. Unlike acute inflammatory arthritides (e.g., gout or septic arthritis), RA tends not to cause marked erythema, and swelling usually does not extend far beyond the articulation. In elderly patients, the most prominent manifestation may be diffuse swelling of the hands accompanied by aching and marked stiffness in the absence of erythema. This can be difficult to distinguish from polymyalgia rheumatica, especially in patients lacking rheumatoid factor.

Classically, RA is symmetrical. When RA is progressive and unremitting, nearly every peripheral joint may eventually be affected, although the thoracic, lumbar, and sacral spine are usually spared. This clinical presentation is observed in perhaps 10% of patients. In about 75%, the disease waxes and wanes over a period of years. In the remaining patients, complete remissions may be achieved with no evidence of inflammation. Remissions may be only partial, with mild clinical disease persisting despite clear improvement. When the course is progressive, the periods of remission may become shorter, and less impressive decreases in symptoms and findings may occur.

A relatively favorable course with long remissions tends to be associated with age younger than 40 years, acute onset restricted to a few large joints, disease duration less than 1 year, and negative test results for rheumatoid factor and antibodies to citrulline-containing peptides (anti-CP). Conversely, an unfavorable prognosis is often associated with insidious onset, constitutional symptoms (e.g., weight loss, low-grade fever, and profound fatigue), rapid appearance of rheumatoid nodules, and high titers of rheumatoid factor and anti-CP. Homozygosity for the QKRAA sequence in the HLA-DR locus is also associated with more severe disease with extra-articular manifestations. The duration and intensity of inflammation correlates with long-term disability, and there is a significant relationship between persistent elevations in the level of C-reactive protein (CRP) and poor outcome. The appearance of bone erosions early in the course of disease also portends a worse prognosis.

Pregnancy often relieves the symptoms of RA in the second or third trimester through a poorly clarified mechanism. One possible explanation is that the placenta produces large amounts of the α-fetoprotein or suppressive cytokines IL-10 or TGF-β. Recent data suggest a correlation between the presence of fetal DNA in the maternal circulation and subsequent remission during pregnancy.[43] The risk of developing RA appears to be lower in women who have been pregnant. The effect of oral contraceptives on disease susceptibility is controversial; the effect, if any, is probably small. In long-term studies, multiple pregnancies or the use of oral contraceptives did not significantly alter the course of RA.[44]

Mortality is higher in RA patients than in the normal population. For the most part, RA patients die of the same causes as the general public, albeit earlier. In severe RA, mortality can approach that of severe congestive heart failure or Hodgkin disease, thereby justifying aggressive early management. Cardiovascular disease accounts for about 40% to 45% of deaths in RA patients; cancer, about 15%; and infection, about 10%. The inflammatory response, especially when associated with an increase in CRP and the use of proatherogenic treatments such as corticosteroids, correlates with an increased incidence of coronary artery disease.[45] Some data suggest that vigorous treatment of RA might decrease the risk of cardiovascular events.[46] The incidence of lymphoproliferative diseases is increased in patients with RA; non-Hodgkin lymphoma, leukemia, multiple myeloma, and Hodgkin disease account for most excess malignancies.

Specific Joint Disease

Hands and wrists   Involvement of the hands and wrists is the most characteristic finding in RA. Swelling and tenderness are usually noted first at the metacarpophalangeal and proximal interphalangeal joints [*see Figure 3*]. Fusiform swelling at the proximal interphalangeal joints is typical. Distal interphalangeal joints are usually spared. Grip strength is decreased because of pain and mechanical derangement. Flexor tenosynovitis is common; progressive flexion limitation prevents the making of a fist.

Depending on the site and severity of the rheumatoid lesions, varying degrees of ulnar deviation and subluxation at the metacarpophalangeal joints result. These deformities are, in large part, caused by damage and radial deviation at the wrist. As the wrist abnormalities progress, the extensor tendons apply torque across the metacarpophalangeal joints and tend to pull the digits into the classic ulnar deviation position. Other changes in the phalanges include (1) hyperextension at the proximal interphalangeal joint and flexion at the distal interphalangeal joint (so-called swan-neck deformity) and (2) flexion at the proximal interphalangeal joint and extension at the distal interphalangeal joint (boutonnière deformity). Several deformities also affect the thumb and interfere with grasp and pinch. In extreme instances, the fingers are markedly deformed and flail as a result of the destruction of cartilage and bone.

In early RA, relatively painless swelling of the dorsum of the wrist may be noted. Most often, the wrist is painful and is the source of functional limitations (e.g., an inability to remove the lid from a jar). At the volar aspect, median nerve compression caused by synovial expansion can produce carpal tunnel syndrome. On the dorsal surface, synovial proliferation may erode and rupture the extensor tendons of the fingers, rendering the

patient unable to extend the fingers actively at the metacarpophalangeal joints. Decreased dorsiflexion and plantar flexion of the wrist caused by fusion of carpal bones are common in severe disease. Volar subluxation and radial deviation are also common deformities; the ulnar styloid is often one of the first sites of bone erosion.

Elbows and shoulders   Synovitis of the elbow joint and inflammation and nodules in the olecranon bursa are frequent in patients with established RA [*see Figure 4*]. Mild flexion contractures occur early; late in the disease, more severe flexion contractures cause functional disability, especially when associated with decreased shoulder abduction and rotation. Pain with decreased range of motion is commonly caused by synovitis of the glenohumeral joint; occasionally, large anterior effusions are evident. Shoulder pain commonly causes difficulty sleeping at night and functional disability. In chronic RA, the joint space becomes contracted, and rupture of the rotator cuff is very common. True glenohumeral joint arthritis can usually be distinguished from acromioclavicular pain, rotator cuff tendinitis, and subdeltoid bursitis on physical examination.

Hips   The hip is affected later than most other joints. In osteoarthritis, the femoral head tends to migrate superiorly in the acetabulum, but in RA, symmetrical destruction of cartilage leads to axial migration. End-stage rheumatoid disease with typical cartilage loss produces acetabular protrusion of the femoral head [*see Figure 5*].

Knees   Knee arthritis is common and is occasionally a primary manifestation in early RA. Swelling and thickening of the synovium and effusions are usually simple to detect; arthrocentesis readily provides synovial fluid for analysis. Occasionally, large effusions expand into the suprapatellar pouch. Atrophy of muscles around the knee, especially the quadriceps, and resultant weakness can be detected early. Persistent synovitis eventually limits walking because of cartilage destruction, ligament laxity, joint instability, and contractures.

Baker cysts of the popliteal space are lined with synovial membrane and usually communicate with the cavity of the knee joint.

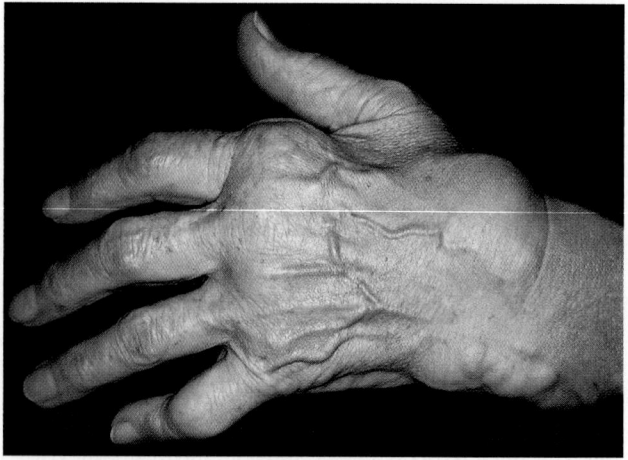

Figure 3   **The hand and wrist are common sites of synovitis in rheumatoid arthritis. Marked swelling in the wrist and metacarpophalangeal joints is caused by synovial proliferation. Modest ulnar deviation of the fingers is also present.**

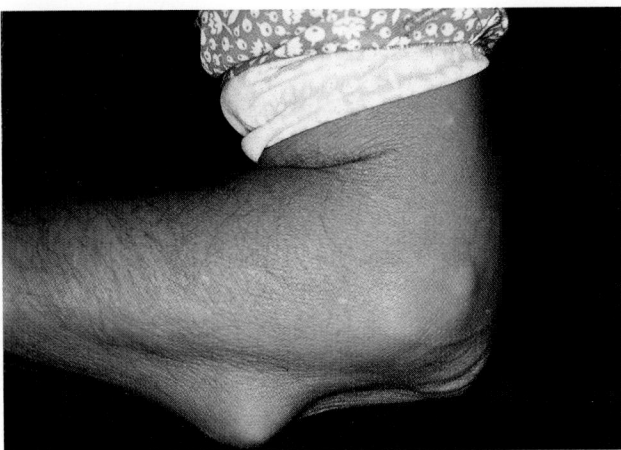

Figure 4 **Rheumatoid nodules commonly form near the extensor surface of the elbow. They can be fixed to the underlying periosteum or can be freely mobile.**

The high pressure generated during knee flexion may be propagated posteriorly and cause rupture or dissection of these cysts. Calf swelling, pain, and erythema result, mimicking thrombophlebitis. Rupture of cysts is not specific to RA, occurring in other forms of inflammatory synovitis as well. Diagnosis of popliteal cysts can be confirmed by ultrasonography or magnetic resonance imaging. Generally, treatment of the cyst is directed to-

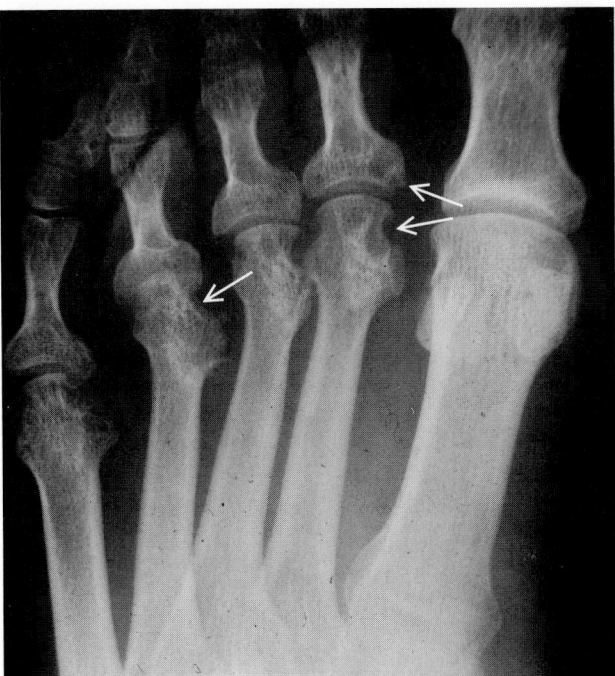

Figure 6 **Erosions (arrows) are visible in the metatarsal heads and in some of the phalanges in this radiograph of the foot of a patient with classic seropositive rheumatoid arthritis.**

ward the underlying knee synovitis. Corticosteroid injections are usually directed into the knee rather than into the cyst.

Ankles and feet   Inflammation of the ankle joints and the small joints of the feet is common. Pain on flexion and extension is a result of tibiotalar arthritis, whereas pain on inversion and eversion is caused by subtalar disease. The metatarsophalangeal joints are sites of early synovitis, which causes pain in the ball of the foot on weight bearing [*see Figure 6*]. Later in the disease, there is subluxation with protrusion of the metatarsal heads, hallux valgus, and collapse of the arch.

Cervical spine   Joints of the thoracic, lumbar, and sacral spine are usually spared in adult RA, but cervical spine disease is frequent and may result in severe pain or neurologic complications.[47] The lesion that has received the most attention is atlantoaxial subluxation and consequent separation at the atlanto-odontoid articulation [*see Figure 7*]. This deformity is best seen on lateral radiographs obtained with the neck flexed, so that the separation of the anterior margin of the odontoid process from the posterior margin of the anterior arch of the atlas can exceed 3 mm. When the separation is severe, the odontoid process may protrude into the foramen magnum and exert pressure on the spinal cord, causing paresthesia or even muscle weakness in the arms and hands. Often, the odontoid process itself is eroded, which minimizes pressure complications but produces instability. Prophylactic surgery to correct subluxation is usually not recommended because of the high morbidity and mortality associated with the procedure. Surgical fixation is indicated in the presence of neurologic signs and symptoms related to spinal cord compression. If the patient requires other surgical procedures, the anesthesiologist should be alerted to the presence of atlantoaxial subluxation to minimize complications of intubation.

a

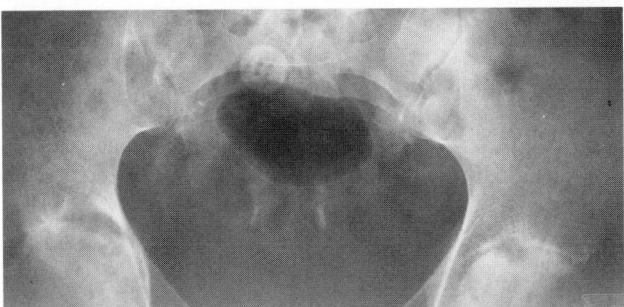

b

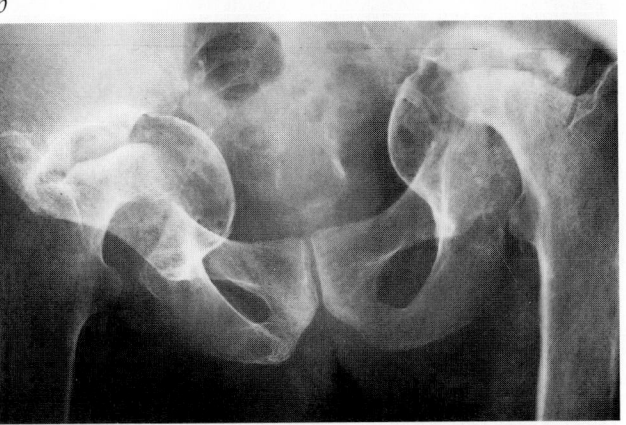

Figure 5 **(*a*) A pelvic radiograph of a patient with classic seropositive rheumatoid arthritis was taken early in the course of the disease. (*b*) Another radiograph taken 4 years later demonstrates marked acetabular protrusion and resorption of the femoral heads, both of which are characteristic of the disease.**

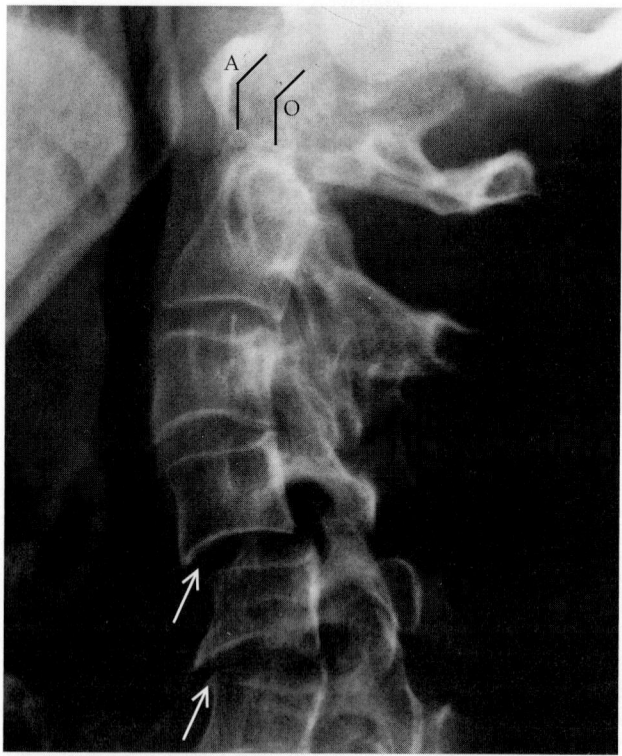

Figure 7 The anterior edge of the odontoid process (O) is abnormally separated from the posterior margin of the arch of the atlas (A) in this lateral radiograph of the cervical spine of a patient with rheumatoid arthritis. Subluxations of the lower cervical vertebral bodies (arrows) are also visible.

Other cervical spine lesions are also seen, including subluxation at multiple levels, erosions at end plates or apophyseal joints, or fusion at these joints. Management of cervical spine pain in the absence of significant subluxation can be frustrating. Traction can be gently applied, but one must always be aware of the instability of these lesions, which necessitates careful monitoring for complications such as cord compression and neurologic dysfunction. Soft collars can provide some temporary relief, but if used excessively, they can exacerbate the problem by weakening the cervical muscles.

Other joints Synovitis of the temporomandibular joints may produce pain on chewing and limit jaw motion. If the joint is sufficiently destroyed, posterior subluxation of the jaw may cause a receding chin. Sternoclavicular arthritis is uncommon but occurs in patients with widespread arthritis. In acute cricoarytenoid arthritis, hoarseness and pain on swallowing may accompany tenderness over the larynx.

Extra-articular Manifestations

RA is a systemic disease, even though it characteristically affects structures in and around the joints. Its systemic manifestations include mild fever, anorexia, weight loss, fatigue, and muscular weakness. Specific organ involvement usually occurs in the context of severe RA, with high titers of rheumatoid factor and nodule formation.

Rheumatoid nodules Rheumatoid nodules are the most common extra-articular manifestation, occurring in about 15% of

patients. Almost all patients in whom nodules develop are seropositive for rheumatoid factor and anti-CP antibodies and have erosive disease [*see Figure 8*]. Nodules are usually subcutaneous and often are found in areas exposed to pressure—for example, over the extensor surfaces of the forearm, the olecranon bursa, the knuckles, the ischial regions, the Achilles tendon, and the bridge of the nose (if glasses are worn). They also occur in viscera. Rheumatoid nodules are firm and are either freely movable or attached to connective tissue (e.g., periosteum or tendons). They range from a few millimeters to more than 2 cm in diameter and often occur in clusters. Nodules typically have a rubbery or gritty feel and can be indistinguishable from gouty tophi on physical examination. The lesion contains a center of fibrinoid necrosis (a mixture of fibrin and other proteins, such as degraded collagen) surrounded by a zone of histiocytes, which tend to be arranged radially. Lymphocytes and plasma cells form an outer layer. The pathogenesis of nodules is likely similar to that of synovitis, with early vascular involvement and local cytokine production.

There is no specific therapy for nodules other than treatment of the underlying arthritis. Surgical removal is often ineffective because nodules can return; it is generally reserved for severe functional impairment or obvious cosmetic problems. The appearance of fresh crops of nodules can indicate active disease. In some cases, exuberant nodule production (rheumatoid nodulosis) is a complication of methotrexate therapy. Rheumatoid nodules are not specific to RA, occurring in other connective tissue diseases (e.g., SLE) or in isolation (e.g., granuloma annulare).

Eyes The sicca syndrome, which is part of Sjögren syndrome, is the most frequent ocular manifestation of RA. Symptoms include sensations of grittiness, accumulation of dried mucoid material (especially in the morning immediately after waking up), and decreased tear production. The relative paucity of tears is demonstrated by decreased wetting of a filter paper strip in a Schirmer test. The dryness is not limited to the eyes and involves other exocrine glands, including those in the nose, the mouth, the rectum, and the vagina. Marked enlargement of lacrimal and salivary glands can occur in severe cases, although this is more common in primary Sjögren syndrome than in RA.

The genetic basis of RA with dry eyes is different from that of primary Sjögren syndrome, which is associated with HLA-DR3

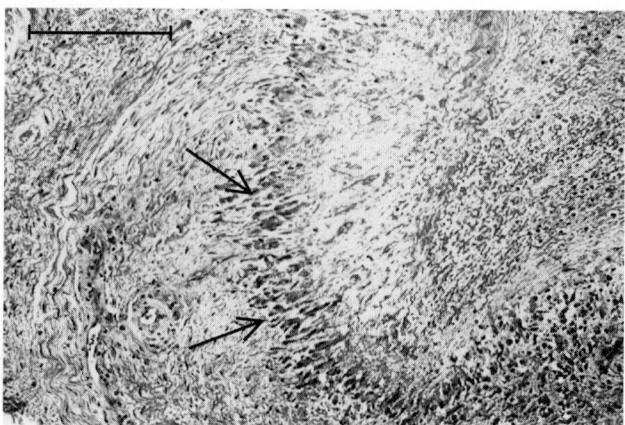

Figure 8 A typical rheumatoid nodule contains an area of fibrinoid necrosis (center) surrounded by palisading histiocytes (arrows). At the periphery are round cells (predominantly lymphocytes). Stain is hematoxylin and eosin (bar scale = 300 μm).

antigen rather than HLA-DR4 antigen.[48] In patients who have the primary syndrome without joint inflammation, there is a greater frequency of recurrent parotitis, Raynaud phenomenon, purpura, lymphadenopathy, myositis, and renal involvement. In all patients with sicca syndrome, lacrimal and salivary glands are characterized histologically by lymphocyte infiltration and distortion of ductal structures. Patients with Sjögren syndrome often have high titers of anti-Ro antibody (also called anti–SS-A). Biopsy of minor salivary glands in the lip can help establish the diagnosis.

Scleritis is painful and may lead to perforation of the sclera and blindness. Episcleritis is common and can often be managed with topical corticosteroids. Matrix loss around the limbus and corneal melting may also lead to perforation. Uveitis and iritis occur no more often in adults with RA than in control populations.

Lungs   The most common form of lung involvement in RA is pleurisy with effusions. Evidence of pleuritis is often found at postmortem examination, but symptomatic pleurisy occurs in fewer than 10% of patients. Clinical features include gradual onset and variable degrees of pain and dyspnea. The effusions generally have protein concentrations greater than 3 to 4 g/dl, as well as glucose concentrations lower than 30 mg/dl; the latter finding has been ascribed to a primary defect in glucose transport. The leukocyte count is rarely higher than 5,000/mm[3] and is dominated by lymphocytes. The lactate dehydrogenase level is often markedly elevated; occasionally, the lipid content is also high. Complement levels are usually low, and rheumatoid factors are present. Pleural biopsy usually reveals nonspecific fibrosis or granulomas. The pleural effusions usually resolve spontaneously within months. Occasionally, repeated aspirations are required to relieve dyspnea; if effusions are troublesome, instillations of glucocorticoids are useful.

Another form of lung involvement is rheumatoid nodules, which occur in the pulmonary parenchyma and on the pleural surface. They range in size from just detectable to several centimeters in diameter. They may be single or multiple, and at times, they cavitate. Such nodules can be difficult to distinguish radiologically from tuberculous or malignant lesions and often require further evaluation, including biopsy.

RA can also be associated with progressive, symptomatic interstitial pulmonary fibrosis; this form of pulmonary fibrosis produces coughing and dyspnea in conjunction with radiographic changes of a diffuse reticular pattern (i.e., honeycomb lung), and it is usually associated with high titers of rheumatoid factor. The lesion is histologically indistinguishable from idiopathic pulmonary fibrosis. Chest radiographs show pleural thickening, nodules, diffuse or patchy infiltrates, and a restrictive ventilatory defect that is characterized by a decreased carbon monoxide diffusion rate. These abnormalities are often associated with cigarette smoking, other extra-articular manifestations, and active disease. Bronchiolitis obliterans, an unusual form of airway obstruction that usually has a viral or toxic etiology, may also develop.

Heart   Cardiac involvement in RA is common but rarely symptomatic. Echocardiographic evidence of pericardial effusion or thickening has been found in about one third of patients studied.[49] Autopsy findings include rheumatoid nodules, healed or active pericarditis, myocarditis, endocarditis, and valvular fibrosis.

Symptomatic pericarditis is most frequent in patients with severe seropositive disease. Overt manifestations include chest pain, friction rub, and associated pleural effusions. The pericardial effusions resemble the pleural effusions in RA. Cardiac tamponade is rare, as is constrictive pericarditis.

Rheumatoid nodules and inflammation in the valves and the conduction system may cause conduction disturbances, including complete heart block. Aortic regurgitation secondary to aortitis and dilation of the aortic root may lead to congestive heart failure.

Blood   Mild anemia of chronic disease is characteristic of active RA, although the hemoglobin level is usually greater than 10 mg/dl. Nonsteroidal anti-inflammatory drugs (NSAIDs) often cause GI blood loss, leading to iron deficiency. Although its levels are not reduced in RA, administration of erythropoietin alleviates anemia.[50]

The constellation of RA with splenomegaly and leukopenia is known as Felty syndrome.[51] The mean serum leukocyte count in such patients is usually 1,500 to 2,000/mm[3], and the mean granulocyte count is 500 to 1,000/mm[3]. Severe thrombocytopenia is uncommon. Infections, particularly of the skin, the perianal region, and the lungs, are frequent and are usually caused by common organisms. Other findings in Felty syndrome include hepatomegaly, lymphadenopathy, and chronic cutaneous ulcerations.

The neutropenia is the result of excessive vascular margination of leukocytes, increased peripheral destruction of leukocytes caused by IgG and IgM antigranulocyte antibodies,[52] and the inhibitory effects of T cells on granulopoiesis. Some cases of Felty syndrome are associated with oligoclonal or monoclonal expansion of large granular lymphocytes in the blood and represent a form of chronic leukemia.[53] Splenectomy usually produces an increase in the leukocyte count, but this increase is sustained in only 30% of patients. Lithium chloride may alleviate the neutropenia, as may treatment of active arthritis with disease-modifying drugs such as methotrexate.[52,54] Treatment with recombinant colony-stimulating factors, such as granulocyte colony-stimulating factor (G-CSF), can increase peripheral granulocyte counts in patients with Felty syndrome.[52] The drug must be given for extended periods because discontinuance leads to relapse.

Neuromuscular involvement   Weakness of muscles adjacent to joints with active synovitis is common. The most common neuropathy is median nerve compression caused by synovitis of the wrist. Entrapment of the ulnar nerve at the elbow or branches of the sural nerve in the tarsal tunnel also occurs.

Mononeuritis multiplex is seen in patients who have severe disease with necrotizing vasculitis and, frequently, deposits of immune complexes in the walls of the blood vessels supplying the involved nerves.[55] In milder cases, only segmental demyelination without vascular abnormalities may be found. Aseptic meningitis resulting from a hypersensitivity reaction to NSAIDs has been documented.[56]

Blood vessels   Vasculitis in small synovial vessels is a hallmark of early RA, but more widespread vascular inflammation of medium-sized muscular arteries also occurs in older men with advanced disease, rheumatoid nodules, and high titers of rheumatoid factor. The involvement of larger vessels is distinct from small vessel disease; such involvement includes leukocytoclastic vasculitis or nail-fold infarcts. The course and prognosis of systemic rheumatoid vasculitis are similar to those of polyarteritis nodosa. Clinically, patients with rheumatoid vasculitis demonstrate polyneuropathy (mononeuritis multiplex), skin ulcerations, purpura, and cutaneous infarctions (sometimes progressing to gangrene). Manifestations of visceral ischemia, including bowel perforations, myocardial infarctions, and cerebral infarctions, are also common. Treatment usually requires cyclophosphamides or high-dose corticosteroids, or both, and still may not be effective. This feared complication has become quite rare, perhaps because of improved therapy for the underlying disease.

Other systems Apart from gastric and duodenal lesions caused by NSAIDs, GI complications are rare in RA. Rheumatoid nodules may involve the pharynx and esophagus. Mild elevations of liver enzymes are common and are usually drug related. Other hepatic abnormalities, particularly elevations in serum alkaline phosphatase and 5'-nucleotidase levels, occur in Sjögren syndrome. These hepatobiliary lesions are ascribed to immune responses to cross-reacting salivary and biliary antigens. Hepatitis C infection is also associated with the development of the sicca syndrome.[57] RA rarely causes specific renal lesions; NSAIDs and amyloid are more often responsible.

IMAGING FEATURES

Because early joint pathology in RA is confined to the synovium, standard radiographs are often not useful. Periarticular osteopenia of the metacarpophalangeal joints and proximal interphalangeal joints in the hand can be evident within months of onset. Joint space narrowing, caused by the loss of articular cartilage, indicates irreversible damage to such cartilage; RA must be active for at least 6 months for such damage to occur. Arthroscopic visualization of articular cartilage (e.g., in the knee) identifies damage to cartilage considerably earlier, but such findings have no value in the management of RA. Subchondral sclerosis is a feature of osteoarthritis but not of RA. Prominent periostitis with new bone formation is much more common in psoriatic arthritis or reactive arthritis syndrome.

Radiographically visualized bone erosions are best seen at the margins of the joint, where the synovium is reflected near the attachment of the capsule. The bone in this region (the so-called "bare area") is not protected by a layer of cartilage and is directly attacked by the invading synovium and osteoclasts. The erosions associated with RA may be difficult to distinguish from those of gout: the latter tend to have sharper borders and overhanging edges of bone, whereas the former are usually small and irregularly shaped. Cystlike radiolucencies may be seen in larger joints. Entire portions of bone adjacent to the joints, such as the metacarpal ends and the ulnar styloid process, may be resorbed. Cartilage destruction caused by RA tends to be evenly distributed within a joint. For instance, both the medial and the lateral compartments of the knee joint are narrowed in RA, whereas the medial compartment is more often affected in osteoarthritis. Progression of erosions takes time in RA; it is rarely necessary to repeat radiographs more often than every 12 months. Damage that is radiographically evident often occurs during the first 2 to 5 years and can progress inexorably in the absence of treatment.

MRI and ultrasound can distinguish synovial pannus from cartilage and synovial fluid and thus can detect pannus as it invades joint structures. The use of intravenous contrast materials, such as gadolinium, permits accurate assessment of synovial invasion and volume. MRI has replaced arthrography for the investigation of large joints, such as the knees.[58] Some studies have shown high-resolution MRI to be effective in evaluat-

ing erosions in small joints[59]; however, the use of MRI and ultrasound to monitor response to therapy is still experimental because of a lack of uniform standards for judging damage. Although most erosions persist or progress, up to one quarter of them heal spontaneously.[60] Because of the lack of standardization, plain radiographs remain the gold standard for following disease progression.

LABORATORY EVALUATION

A mild normochromic, normocytic anemia and an elevated platelet count are usually present in patients with RA. The leukocyte count is generally normal, although neutropenia occurs in association with splenomegaly in Felty syndrome. The erythrocyte sedimentation rate (ESR) and the CRP level are usually elevated in patients with active RA and are useful in monitoring disease activity and response to therapy. Results of serum chemistry studies are normal, although the use of either NSAIDs or methotrexate can lead to elevations in liver enzyme levels. Urinalysis is generally normal.

About 80% to 85% of patients with RA are seropositive for rheumatoid factor. If seropositivity develops, it usually does so before the end of the first year of disease. From 1% to 5% of healthy persons test positive for rheumatoid factor, with the higher percentage noted in the elderly. In the absence of clinical findings of RA, rheumatoid factor does not in itself suggest a diagnosis of RA. Many chronic inflammatory conditions besides RA are associated with positive rheumatoid factor test results, although the titers are usually lower. Compared with rheumatoid factor, testing for antibodies to CP appears to be more specific for RA (85% to 90%) and equally sensitive. Testing for anti-CP could be useful as a diagnostic test, especially in early disease or in patients with hepatitis C in whom rheumatoid factor is usually positive.

Other serologic tests commonly used to diagnose rheumatic diseases are of limited value in RA. Antinuclear antibodies (ANA) are often present in low titer. If anti-DNA antibodies are detected, they are almost always directed against single-stranded DNA rather than native double-stranded DNA. Antibodies to the antigens associated with Sjögren syndrome (SS-A and SS-B) may be positive. Serum complement levels are normal in uncomplicated RA; hypocomplementemia suggests systemic rheumatoid vasculitis. Serologic tests for viruses may help identify patients with postrubella arthritis or parvovirus B19 infection. Hepatitis B and C serologies can also provide useful information, because these infections can cause a self-limited symmetrical polyarthritis that mimics RA.

Analysis of synovial fluid provides supportive data but is rarely diagnostic. Synovial fluid in RA usually appears straw colored and mildly turbid. Bits of fibrin and, occasionally, small fronds of synovium may be aspirated. Leukocyte counts range from 2,000 to 20,000/mm^3. On differential counts, most of the cells (50% to 80%) are neutrophils; the remainder are lymphocytes (mainly T cells) and monocytes. The synovial fluid glucose level is usually normal, which distinguishes RA from acute infection. Synovial fluid complement levels are usually low in inflamed rheumatoid joints despite abundant production of complement proteins by synovium. Tests for rheumatoid factor, antinuclear antibodies, total protein, or lactate dehydrogenase in synovial fluid are not clinically useful. Synovial biopsies, either blind or arthroscopically directed, can be used in clinical trials to assess response to therapy. However, their utility for differential diagnosis or in predicting response to therapy remains limited.

Differential Diagnosis

Patients with other rheumatic diseases often have a symmetrical polyarticular arthritis resembling RA. The presence of high-titer ANA and anti–double-stranded DNA, a low serum complement level, and major organ system involvement (especially nephritis) are clues to the diagnosis of SLE. Careful physical examination often helps the clinician distinguish other rheumatic diseases. Elderly persons with polymyalgia rheumatica can present with peripheral synovitis, although prominent proximal muscle stiffness and a very high ESR (often higher than 80 to 100 mm/hr) are useful differential findings. Viral arthritis mediated by immune complex deposition, as occurs in hepatitis B virus infection or rubella, often has the same distribution as RA but is transient.

Metabolic disorders such as gout and calcium pyrophosphate deposition arthropathies can mimic RA. Radiographs may indicate characteristic gouty erosions or chondrocalcinosis. The finding of crystals in synovial fluid distinguishes these disorders from RA. Septic arthritis is also relatively easy to identify through clinical examination and evaluation of synovial fluid.

Seronegative spondyloarthropathies can present a diagnostic challenge when they exhibit peripheral polyarticular disease. They can generally be distinguished by the lack of symmetry, the distribution of affected joints (usually, lower extremities are affected more than upper, and large joints more than small), the absence of rheumatoid factor, the presence of proliferative bone changes on radiographs, and characteristic skin lesions. However, in some cases, psoriatic arthritis has a clinical picture almost identical to that of RA.

Morning stiffness and involvement of the wrist and metacarpophalangeal joints are uncommon in osteoarthritis, which typically affects the weight-bearing joints and the distal interphalangeal joints. Patients with osteoarthritis usually are seronegative for rheumatoid factor and lack marginal erosions. Synovial effusions are noninflammatory, with a WBC lower than 2,000/mm^3 and a predominance of mononuclear cells.

Rheumatoid joints are more susceptible to bacterial infection than normal joints, and superimposed sepsis may not be readily apparent. The usual signs (e.g., localized erythema, increased pain, and limitation of motion) may be difficult to distinguish from the underlying rheumatoid synovitis or may be suppressed by antirheumatic therapy. Multiple joints may be infected simultaneously; the diagnosis requires arthrocentesis and culture [see Chapter 131].

Management

Optimal management requires an awareness of the variable course of the disorder. Statistical predictions about outcome can be made from clinical features and laboratory abnormalities, but remissions and exacerbations are common, and the risks associated with drugs and surgery must be viewed in the light of this uncertainty. The patient should be aware of the risks both of taking a drug and of not taking it. Active synovitis that persists for a year or more after the onset of RA results in irreversible cartilage damage, joint destruction, and increased mortality. Thus, every effort should be made to suppress the synovitis by pharmacologic methods during the early months.

No specific climate or diet convincingly alters the course of RA. Alternative therapies, including cartilage extracts, do not appear to have more than a placebo effect. However, the power of placebo effects should not be underestimated; most arthritis and pain studies demonstrate a "therapeutic" response in 20% to 30% of patients who receive placebo. Glucosamine and chondroitin sulfate have been studied in osteoarthritis without significant clinical benefit, and few data support their use in RA.

In addition to conveying to the patient an understanding of the disease, management involves efforts to relieve pain and discomfort, preserve strength and joint function, prevent deformities, and attend to systemic complications. Surgical intervention is important not only for replacing destroyed joints but also, at times, for restoring function or preventing further damage.

DRUG THERAPY

Drugs are used to provide pain relief, to control inflammation, and to alter the natural history of disease. Only empirical data support the use of some currently available agents such as sulfasalazine and antimalarial agents; the mechanism of action of these agents is unknown. In formal studies of individual drug therapies, systematic measurements are taken of the number of inflamed joints, the extent of swelling, and the range of joint motion. Laboratory measurements (e.g., ESR, CRP, and hematocrit value) and assessments of subjective features (e.g., pain and morning stiffness) are also made. The information is then assessed globally, although some algorithm-based assessments of laboratory parameters and joint signs are being explored as alternative strategies [see Table 2].

General Recommendations

The appropriate management of RA is rapidly evolving; previous treatment algorithms based on a gradual escalation of treatment (i.e., the traditional pyramid approach) have been replaced by more aggressive treatment approaches.[61] The change has been fomented by a variety of factors, including the following: (1) active RA significantly decreases the life span of affected individuals; (2) active inflammation is associated with increased morbidity and mortality; (3) the development of more effective agents that alter the natural history of RA; (4) the advent of combination therapy; and (5) the recognition that quality of life is a critical determinant of successful management of life of RA patients. No single algorithm thus far has captured the complexity of RA management because of the extensive pharmacopoeia, although broad guidelines can be given [see Figure 9].

Most patients require rapid advancement from NSAIDs to a second-line agent, most often methotrexate. Because symptoms of RA will not be adequately controlled in 70% of patients by methotrexate alone, the clinician is usually faced with the choice of either "add-on" therapy or testing a series of single agents (e.g., sulfasalazine, antimalarials, leflunomide, or a TNF inhibitor). In the United States, most rheumatologists prefer to increase the methotrexate dosage rapidly to 20 to 25 mg/wk and then add another agent within 2 to 3 months if necessary. Morning stiffness lasting longer than 30 minutes, continued pain, or evidence of active synovitis on physical examination is an indication for advancing therapy even if the patient has experienced significant improvement on methotrexate. Typically, one would add either a TNF inhibitor, leflunomide, or sulfasalazine (with or without hydroxychloroquine). Care must be exercised, especially with combinations of methotrexate and leflunomide, because of hepatotoxicity.

Few data demonstrate the superiority of one combination of drugs over another, although there is an increasing bias toward use of TNF inhibitors early in management.[62] In fact, some data suggest that early aggressive management with methotrexate

Table 2 Comparison of Various Antirheumatic Treatments—Small-Molecule and Biologic Drugs

	Drug	Response Rate; Onset of Action	Magnitude of Efficacy (0 to ++++)	Major Toxicities	Dosage
Small Molecule Drugs	Azathioprine	30%–50%; 2–3 mo	++	Hematologic, immunosuppression, cholestasis	100–150 mg/day
	Cyclosporine	30%; 2–3 mo	++	Renal hypertension, hypertrichosis, immunosuppression	2.5–5.0 mg/kg/day
	Hydroxychloroquine	30%–50%; 2–6 mo	++	Retinopathy, myopathy, hyperpigmentation	200 mg b.i.d.
	Leflunomide	50%; 2–3 mo	++	Liver, teratogen, gastrointestinal, skin rash	100 mg/day × 3, then 20 mg/day
	Methotrexate	> 70%; 6–8 wk	+++	Liver, hematologic, oral ulcers	7.5–25 mg/wk
	NSAIDs	> 75%; < 2 wk	+	Gastric and duodenal ulcer, renal	Varied
	Prednisone	> 90%; < 1 wk	+++	Skin atrophy, cataracts, osteoporosis, avascular necrosis	5.0–10 mg/day
	Sulfasalazine	> 30%; 2–3 mo	++	Dyspepsia, hemolysis in glucose-6-phosphate dehydrogenase deficiency, liver	1 g b.i.d. or t.i.d.
Biologic Drugs	Abatacept	50%–70%; 4–12 wk	+++	Injection-site reactions, infections, immune surveillance	500–1,000 mg I.V. q. 4 wk
	Adalumimab	50%–70%; 2–4 wk	+++	Injection-site reactions, infections, immune surveillance	40 mg S.C. every 2 wk
	Anakinra	30%; 1–3 mo	+	Injection-site reactions, infection	100 mg/day S.C.
	Etanercept	50%–70%; 2–4 wk	+++	Injection-site reaction, infection, immune surveillance	25 mg S.C. twice a week
	Infliximab	50%–70%; 2–4 wk	+++	Infusion reaction, infection, immune surveillance	3–10 mg/kg I.V. q. 4–8 wk
	Rituximab	50%–70%; 4–12 wk	+++	Increased infection	500–1,000 mg I.V. q. 2 wk × 2

plus a TNF inhibitor within the first year of disease can lead to long-lasting remission that permits withdrawal of therapy. Prednisone is generally reserved for patients requiring adjunctive "bridge" therapy to improve their ability to perform activities of daily living; the prednisone therapy is maintained until a single-drug or combination therapy permits its use to be tapered or discontinued. The IL-1 inhibitor anakinra is modestly effective; it is usually reserved for patients who do not respond to combinations of methotrexate and TNF inhibitors or other biologics.[63] New agents targeting T cells (abatacept) and B cells (rituximab) are effective and decrease joint destruction.

A variety of treatment strategies are currently under investigation. One strategy involves a step-down protocol of drug therapy; this entails the initial administration of a combination of drugs followed by the scheduled termination, or step down, of individual drugs used in the regimen. Another treatment strategy combines high-dose corticosteroids, which are given in tapered doses over several months, with methotrexate and sulfasalazine, which are given in stable doses; this form of combination therapy has been shown to provide rapid improvement.[64] Some data suggest that early management with triple therapy (e.g., sulfasalazine, hydroxychloroquine, and methotrexate) is very effective.[65]

Although the number of cases of treatment-resistant disease is decreasing, a fraction is recalcitrant to all of the aforementioned drugs. Immunosuppressive agents such as azathioprine or cyclosporine can be used, although the therapeutic ratio is narrow. Experimental approaches can also be considered with appropriate oversight from institutional review boards.

Nonsteroidal Anti-inflammatory Drugs

The use of aspirin for RA has decreased substantially because of the availability of newer NSAIDs. Nonacetylated salicylate compounds, such as choline salicylate and choline magnesium trisalicylate, produce less gastric irritation than aspirin but are more expensive and exert less anti-inflammatory effect.

Other NSAIDs are probably no more effective than aspirin but may have certain advantages (e.g., fewer gastrointestinal effects, better pharmacokinetics, and, usually, fewer pills to be taken daily, which may enhance compliance). The prostaglandin analogue misoprostol, proton pump inhibitors, and, to a lesser extent, H_2 receptor blockers can suppress the GI toxicity of NSAIDs[66] and should be considered for patients who take a nonselective cyclooxygenase inhibitor but have a history of duodenal ulcer or gastritis.[67]

Pharmacokinetics aside, there are a few pharmacologic differences between the various NSAIDs. Sulindac may be associated with less renal toxicity than other NSAIDs, but the clinical relevance is not certain. Most currently available NSAIDs nonselectively block both the constitutively expressed cyclooxygenase-1 (COX-1) and the inducible COX-2, although the relative selectivity for COX-2 can be favorable with some compounds (e.g., meloxicam and diclofenac). The selective COX-2 inhibitor celecoxib is also an effective anti-inflammatory and analgesic agent.[68] It might have fewer GI side effects than nonselective COX inhibitors. In addition, it does not block platelet function and may be used in some situations in which traditional NSAIDs are contraindicated. Both selective and nonselective agents, however, can alter renal blood flow and glomerular filtration rate. Celecoxib is administered in a dosage of 100 to 200 mg orally once or twice daily. The association of cardiovascular events with prolonged use of the COX-2 inhibitor rofecoxib prompted the withdrawal of the drug from the global market in 2004. There is also potential cardiovascular toxicity for nonselective NSAIDs such as naproxen, although this is controversial. However, a recent case-controlled study found that treatment with nonselective NSAIDs was associated with a reduction in the risk of acute myocardial infarction (AMI)[69]; in fact, the reduction in AMI risk was consistent across all disease-modifying antirheumatic drugs, including methotrexate and COX-2 inhibitors, but not in biologic agents. The risk of AMI was increased with the use of glucocorticoids. When prescribing NSAIDs, clinicians should weigh the potential cardiovascular risks against anticipated benefits and consider issues such as dose and comorbid conditions.

Advancement from NSAIDs to second-line agents is recommended if (1) symptoms have not improved sufficiently after a short trial of NSAIDs, (2) the patient has aggressive seropositive disease, or (3) there is radiographic evidence of erosions or joint destruction. The trend today is for more aggressive treatment, and the majority of patients require additional pharmacotherapy.

Methotrexate

Methotrexate is one of the most effective second-line drugs. Methotrexate not only alleviates the signs and symptoms of RA but also decreases the ESR and raises the hematocrit value.[70] It probably also slows the rate of bone erosion in RA, perhaps by decreasing expression of destructive enzymes such as collagenase in synovium.[71]

Methotrexate is usually given in weekly oral doses, usually beginning at 7.5 mg and, if necessary, increasing to 20 to 25 mg over 2 to 3 months. Response to therapy begins in 4 to 6 weeks [*see Figure 9*]. Further increases up to 45 mg/wk administered

parenterally had minimal additional benefit.[72] Over 70% of patients experience some response to methotrexate, and half remain on the drug for at least 5 years. However, two thirds of patients have significant residual synovitis despite maximum methotrexate therapy. Efficacy remains excellent even after years of use.[73] Complete remissions are uncommon, although patients' sense of well-being is often dramatically improved. The benefit requires continuous therapy, and inflammation usually reappears within weeks after stopping therapy. Monitoring of hematologic and liver parameters every 4 to 8 weeks is required. The primary action of methotrexate is anti-inflammatory at the doses used in RA, although immunosuppression resulting in *Pneumocystis* pneumonia has been reported. Improved survival as a result of a reduction in cardiovascular mortality has been reported in patients treated with methotrexate.[74]

Risk factors for toxicity include alcoholism, diabetes, obesity, advanced age, and renal disease. The major concern is hepatic fibrosis, although marrow toxicity and sterility are also important side effects. Methotrexate is a potent teratogen and should not be used in women of childbearing age unless they are using a reliable form of contraception. Idiosyncratic interstitial lung disease can develop even at low doses. Other adverse reactions to methotrexate include nausea, stomatitis, leukopenia, diarrhea, and elevations of serum aminotransferase levels. Some of these toxicities (especially oral ulcers) can be minimized by prophylactic administration of folic acid, 1 mg/day.[75] Hepatotoxicity leading to clinically significant fibrosis or cirrhosis is exceedingly uncommon; accordingly, most centers have abandoned routine monitoring with liver biopsies.[76] A biopsy should be performed if a patient develops persistent abnormalities in blood tests for liver enzymes that do not promptly resolve with discontinuance. Other medications that interfere with folate metabolism (e.g., trimethoprim) should be used with caution in patients taking methotrexate.

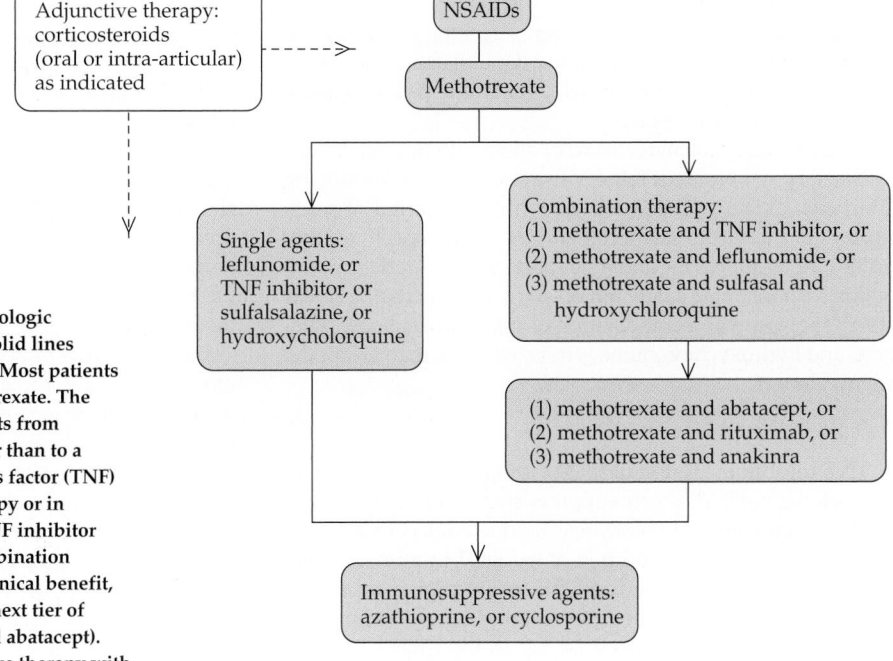

Figure 9 **Proposed algorithm for pharmacologic management of rheumatoid arthritis. The solid lines indicate the standard management options. Most patients require a second-line agent, usually methotrexate. The majority of rheumatologists advance patients from methotrexate to combination therapy, rather than to a series of single agents. If one tumor necrosis factor (TNF) inhibitor is ineffective, either as monotherapy or in combination with methotrexate, another TNF inhibitor may be tried. Similarly, if any first-tier combination therapy option fails to provide sufficient clinical benefit, the patient can be advanced directly to the next tier of combination therapy (e.g., methotrexate and abatacept). In patients with severe symptoms, adjunctive therapy with oral or intra-articular corticosteroids can be added at any stage of management, as indicated by the broken lines.**

Leflunomide

Leflunomide is an effective antirheumatic agent that blocks the pyrimidine synthesis required for stimulated lymphocytes to proliferate. In vitro, it inhibits mitogen-stimulated proliferation of both B cells and T cells. Randomized, controlled trials have demonstrated that leflunomide is approximately as effective as methotrexate in the treatment of active RA.[77] In addition to being clinically effective, leflunomide slows radiographic progression of RA.

The half-life of leflunomide is 2 weeks; for this reason, care must be taken in situations in which toxicity is observed. The usual starting dose is 20 mg/day. Leflunomide can be used in combination with methotrexate, although in this setting the initial dose of leflunomide is usually 10 mg/day; patients must be followed very carefully for hepatotoxicity.[78]

Adverse effects include diarrhea, liver toxicity, rash, oral ulcers, and reversible hair loss. Periodic monitoring of liver enzymes is required. In animal studies, leflunomide has been associated with birth defects; thus, this agent should not be used by pregnant women or women of childbearing age who are not using a reliable form of contraception. Oral cholestyramine can be used to facilitate removal of the drug; cholestyramine accomplishes this by binding the metabolites involved in enterohepatic recirculation.

Antimalarial Drugs and Sulfasalazine as Single and Combination Agents

The antimalarial drug hydroxychloroquine is useful as second-line therapy for RA.[79] Its response rate is lower than that of methotrexate, and less improvement is seen; however, its relative safety makes it an ideal choice for patients with mild early disease or as an additive agent in combination therapy. Adverse reactions to antimalarials occur, particularly retinopathy that may lead to an irreversible decrease in vision; this reaction is rare and can be minimized with regular ophthalmologic examinations.

Sulfasalazine is also useful.[80] It is effective in up to 50% of patients at a dosage of 2 to 3 g/day in divided doses. Only moderate side effects have been reported, especially GI upset. Sulfasalazine is well tolerated; however, screening for glucose-6-phosphate dehydrogenase deficiency (G6PD) deficiency before initiating therapy is recommended. Over 30% of patients continue to take it for at least 5 years.[81]

A significant percentage of RA patients do not experience satisfactory symptomatic relief with a single disease-modifying antirheumatic drug. This lack of response has led clinical investigators to study combination regimens.[82] A prospective study examining azathioprine and methotrexate alone and in combination demonstrated safety but no additive benefits.[83] A 2-year study showed that a combination of methotrexate, sulfasalazine, and hydroxychloroquine is more effective than any of the agents alone.[84]

Biologic Drugs

TNF inhibitors TNF-α blockade using soluble receptors or monoclonal antibodies can suppress signs and symptoms of RA.[85] Recombinant technology was used to engineer the fusion of the receptor to the Fc portion of the IgG1 immunoglobulin molecule to produce etanercept. The fusion protein is entirely human in origin, and antibody formation against it is minimal. Etanercept has been approved for use in the United States in dosages of 25 mg S.C. twice a week or 50 mg S.C. once a week; it has been shown to be beneficial in patients who have only a par-

tial response to methotrexate, used either in combination therapy or as monotherapy.[86]

Two monoclonal antibodies have been approved for use in RA: the human-mouse chimeric monoclonal antibody infliximab and the human monoclonal antibody adalumimab. There are subtle differences in the pharmacology of etanercept and the monoclonal antibodies. Etanercept binds both TNF-α and TNF-β, whereas the monoclonal antibodies have a greater affinity for the TNF-α ligand and bind only to TNF-α. However, the clinical impact of this difference is not clear, and the response rates are similar.

Infliximab is used in combination with methotrexate for treatment of RA; this appears to permit long-term use of infliximab with less formation of neutralizing antibodies.[87] Infliximab is administered by intravenous infusion; the recommended dose is 3 to 10 mg/kg every 8 weeks.

Adalimumab has demonstrated efficacy similar to that of infliximab and etanercept in RA. It is generally administered at a dose of 40 mg S.C. every 2 weeks. In perhaps 10% of patients, the frequency of administration must be increased to once a week. Adalimumab can also used in combination with methotrexate; in a multicenter, randomized, double-blinded study in which patients were given adalimumab and methotrexate combination therapy, 49% of patients with early and aggressive rheumatoid arthritis exhibited disease remission after 2 years.[88]

The clinical response to TNF inhibitors can be dramatic, and an improved sense of well-being can occur within days. Typically, patients who respond to TNF inhibitors will notice decreased pain and stiffness after a few weeks of therapy. About two thirds of patients have at least 20% improvement in the number of swollen and tender joints, and more than half of these patients will have more than 50% improvement. Concomitant with decreased symptoms, serum and synovial cytokine levels decrease, and peripheral blood markers of inflammation (i.e., ESR and the CRP level) decline. Although the clinical effect occurs sooner with the TNF inhibitors than with methotrexate, a significant benefit over methotrexate has not been demonstrated after 3 months of therapy. If a patient fails to respond to one TNF inhibitor or if efficacy declines over time, then it is reasonable to try a second or even a third agent before moving to another class of drugs.

In addition to providing symptomatic improvement, TNF inhibitors prevent or slow bone and cartilage destruction in RA. Perhaps most intriguing is the observation that radiographic progression is prevented even in patients who do not experience clinical improvement. This observation could have important implications for the widespread clinical use of these agents if long-term studies confirm these findings. For now, however, these agents are generally used only after an adequate trial of methotrexate.

Because TNF is important in host defense and possibly in tumor surveillance, impairment of these functions in treated patients could increase the risk of infection and even cancer. The most common adverse reaction to etanercept is local inflammation at the injection site, although serious bacterial and mycobacterial infections have also been observed with TNF inhibitors.[89] When TB occurs, extrapulmonary disease is common and the prognosis is relatively poor. Hence, these agents should be used with caution in patients with active infections. Before therapy with an anti-TNF agent is initiated, a skin test should be performed and a chest x-ray obtained to rule out tuberculosis; prophylactic treatment with isoniazid should be initiated if indicated. This screening process decreases the risk of TB reactivation by up to 90%.[90] More intriguing is the induction of antinuclear and anti-DNA antibodies and, in a few cases, frank SLE in some RA patients treated with anti–TNF-α therapy. Demyelinating syndromes and aplastic anemia have been noted in a small number of patients receiving TNF inhibitors. These agents appear to exacerbate multiple sclerosis; this finding is possibly related to the protective role TNF-α may play in the central nervous system.[91]

Some concerns have been raised regarding an increased risk of lymphoma in patients receiving TNF inhibitors. However, this question is confounded by the fact that the prevalence of lymphoma is higher in patients with RA, compared with that in normal individuals, and it is unclear whether the use of TNF inhibitors further increases the risk of lymphoma. Meta-analysis of anti-TNF antibodies suggests that the risks of solid tumors are increased.[92] However, it is critical to consider whether improved control of disease activity provided by TNF inhibitors diminishes mortality in RA overall, even if their use may be associated with a slight risk of certain malignancies. The data thus far suggest that TNF inhibitors probably will improve survival despite potential toxicity.

T cell targeted therapy: abatacept Activation of naïve T cells requires two signals. First, the T cell receptor engages peptide displayed by class II MHC proteins on antigen presenting cells. Second, a costimulatory signal is provided. There are numerous costimulatory ligand pairs, but perhaps the best characterized is CD80/86 on dendritic cells and CD28 on T cells. Another molecule, cytotoxic T lymphocyte activator–4 (CTLA-4), is also expressed by T cells; because of its high affinity for CD8086, CTLA-4 can compete with CD28 in binding to CD80/86. To take advantage of this characteristic, CTLA-4 was engineered into a fusion protein with the Fc portion of immunoglobulin to create CTLA-4-Ig, or abatacept. This protein interferes with CD80/86-CD28 interactions and blocks T cell activation. Abatacept treatment in combination with methotrexate leads to a 20% improvement in ACR response criteria [see Table 3] in about two thirds of patients, about half of whom have 50% or more improvement.[93] These results are similar to those achieved with TNF inhibitors, although the response tends to be somewhat slower (4 to 12 weeks). Radiographic studies demonstrate that abatacept decreases the rate of bone and cartilage destruction in RA. Because of its distinct mechanism of action, abatacept is nearly as effective in patients who do not respond to TNF inhibitors as in those who do. Combinations of TNF inhibitors and abatacept are contraindicated because this form of combination therapy is associated with markedly increased infections. The major safety issues related to combination therapy using abatacept and methotrexate are an increased risk of infection and, possibly, a failure of immune surveillance, which may carry an increased risk of neoplasia. Abatacept is administered at a dosage 500 to 1,000 mg I.V. every 2 weeks for 1 month and then every 4 weeks thereafter.

B cell targeted therapy: rituximab Mature B cells express the surface molecule CD20 and are depleted when exposed to the anti-CD20 chimeric monoclonal antibody rituximab. This antibody has been widely used for B cell lymphomas and is also effective in RA. The response rates achieved using rituximab in combination with methotrexate are similar to the response rates achieved using abatacept in combination with TNF inhibitors; improvement usually occurs within 2 to 3 months of the first infusion.[33] In addition to improvement in ACR response criteria,

Table 3 American College of Rheumatology (ACR) Definition of Improvement of Rheumatoid Arthritis[102]

20% improvement in tender and swollen joint counts and
20% improvement in three of the five remaining ACR-core set measures:
   Patient global assessments
   Physician global assessments
   Pain
   Disability
   Acute-phase reactant

rituximab also decreases the rate of joint destruction. Like abatacept, rituximab is effective in patients who do not respond to TNF inhibitors. Treatment with rituximab (i.e., two doses of 500 to 1,000 mg/m² I.V. infusion, administered 2 weeks apart) rapidly depletes peripheral blood B cells in RA for up to 1 year. After treatment, levels of rheumatoid factor and anti-CP decline modestly; disease flares are often associated with a temporary increase in titers and the reappearance of B cells in the circulation. Infusion reactions are common and include fever, chills, and hypotension. The possibility of infusion reaction might be decreased by concomitant treatment with corticosteroids (100 mg of methylprednisolone I.V. at the time of infusion). Issues such as the long-term safety of rituximab and the optimal number of treatment cycles are still under investigation. As with other biologics, rituximab use may be associated with an increased risk in patients with bacterial infections.

IL-1 inhibitor: anakinra The natural inhibitor to IL-1, IL-1ra (anakinra), demonstrates modest anti-inflammatory activity in RA.[91] Anakinra also appears to have disease-modifying activity, evidenced by a decrease in radiographic progression. Anakinra is administered subcutaneously at a dose of 100 mg by daily injection, either alone or in combination with methotrexate.[94] The most common side effect is injection-site reaction, although an increased incidence of infections has also been reported. Use of anakinra in combination with TNF inhibitors increases infectious complications; therefore, such combinations should be avoided.

Glucocorticoids

Glucocorticoids are potent anti-inflammatory agents. When used systemically, they decrease joint swelling, pain, and morning stiffness and improve ability to function. Unfortunately, the dosages necessary to maintain such improvement are usually high enough to be associated with long-term side effects (e.g., osteoporosis, osteonecrosis, increased susceptibility to infection, cataracts, myopathy, and poor wound healing). Alternate-day therapy usually cannot be used to reduce these side effects, because RA patients are usually symptomatic on the off days. The conventional wisdom is that glucocorticoids neither alter the course of the disease nor affect the ultimate degree of damage to joints or other structures; however, some evidence indicates that low-dose prednisolone given early in RA can slow the rate of radiographic progression.[95] Although there is considerable difference of opinion regarding the most appropriate use of steroids in RA, they are typically employed as "bridge" therapy for severe disease while awaiting a therapeutic response from other second-line agents. Systemic glucocorticoids, however, even in these low dosages, are associated with accelerated bone loss. Supplemental calcium (1,000 to 1,500 mg daily) and vitamin D (400 to 800 I.U. daily) can be given to postmenopausal women who require daily prednisone therapy, even in low doses. Dual-energy x-ray absorptiometry scans should be used to monitor bone mineral density, and bisphosphonates should be used to treat or prevent osteoporosis in susceptible patients.

Intra-articular glucocorticoids are also useful in limited flares. Administration of such agents requires careful aseptic technique. The procedure involves injection of a local anesthetic agent (e.g., lidocaine) and an insoluble glucocorticoid preparation (e.g., triamcinolone hexacetonide, 20 to 40 mg) into a large joint; smaller amounts (5 to 10 mg) may be injected into small joints, bursae, and tendon sheaths. These local injections usually result in relief of pain and inflammation within days and do not often produce serious side effects. The risk of infection is probably about one in 10,000 procedures. The beneficial effects may last for weeks or months (on average, about 3 to 6 months), but repeated injections may result in increased cartilage destruction, osteonecrosis, and tendon rupture. Thus, intra-articular glucocorticoids are only occasionally useful in relieving inflammation in one or two joints that are particularly symptomatic.

Immunosuppressive Agents

Alkylating agents, particularly cyclophosphamide, and antimetabolites such as azathioprine have been used in patients with severe progressive disease who have not responded to the measures already described. These drugs decrease inflammation and possibly reduce the frequency of new joint erosions. Cyclophosphamide is also effective in controlling rheumatoid vasculitis in some patients. Hematologic toxicity and GI toxicity can be severe; hemorrhagic cystitis is a disturbing complication of oral cyclophosphamide therapy. Azathioprine is safer but has only modest efficacy. The additional potential hazard of inducing neoplasias and chromosomal abnormalities also restricts the usefulness of these agents.

Cyclosporine is a more focused immunosuppressive drug than azathioprine or cyclophosphamide because it targets T cells; it has been used extensively in allograft rejection. Hypertension and decreased creatinine clearance are common side effects, generally related to the cumulative dose. In RA, cyclosporine at a dosage of 2.5 to 5.0 mg/kg/day is an alternative to cyclophosphamide or azathioprine in patients who need immunosuppressive therapy, provided patients are closely monitored for renal toxicity.[96] Despite its potent immunosuppressive effects, a minority of patients have a meaningful clinical response to cyclosporine.

Other Chemotherapeutic Agents

In some studies, minocycline appeared to provide benefit for RA patients.[97] Its mechanism of action is unclear and may be related to the ability of tetracycline analogues to inhibit metalloproteinases. Other novel therapies have had mixed success. Attempts to induce tolerance by oral administration of type II collagen or cartilage protein gp39 have not provided significant benefit, although oral immunization with the susceptibility epitope has demonstrated some evidence of efficacy.[98] A diet supplemented with fish oils, which contain omega-3 fatty acids, reduces synthesis of inflammatory arachidonate metabolites and may be a useful adjuvant therapy for selected patients[99]; a vegetarian diet may augment the effects of fish oil supplement.[100]

PHYSICAL THERAPY

Hospitalization is occasionally helpful in the management of patients with RA, although this approach in an era of managed care and cost constraints is not feasible. Removing the patient from a stressful home environment and instituting a program of rest combined with physical therapy are of great value. Splinting inflamed joints may decrease synovitis.

Physical therapy has a role in the management of RA, although data supporting its ability to change outcome are lacking. Passive range-of-motion exercises help prevent contractures. Isometric exercises build up muscle strength without subjecting inflamed joints to excessive wear, and isotonic exercises further increase muscle strength and help preserve function. Most physical measures, such as whirlpools, heated wax, ultrasonography, and diathermy, make patients feel better during the procedure and perhaps for a short time afterward but offer no significant long-term functional, anti-inflammatory, or disease-modifying benefit; consequently, many patients eventually become disillusioned with them. It is important for patients to maintain an active life, and guidance from physical therapists for range-of-motion exercises and aerobic training is useful. Swimming or other water exercises are especially useful aerobic stresses that minimize the load on the lower extremities.

SURGERY

Indications for surgical intervention include intractable pain and impaired function. Eroded cartilage, ruptured ligaments, and progressive destruction of bone can lead to severe functional derangement that is amenable only to surgical correction. Besides helping restore function to weight-bearing joints, surgery may also restore function in severely deformed hands. In a joint such as the wrist, dorsal synovectomy may prevent extensor tendon ruptures. Although proliferative synovitis often recurs after synovectomy, it may take 1 or 2 years to return and may be less intense than it was initially. Surgery is also useful for removing frayed menisci and other loose bodies that interfere with joint function. In the hands and wrists, operations on periarticular structures (e.g., repair of capsules and replacement of tendons) may restore appearance and function; release of carpal tunnel compression usually relieves pressure on the median nerve. Arthroscopic surgery to remove cartilaginous fragments and to perform a partial synovectomy may be useful when a large, accessible joint (e.g., the knee) is involved with proliferative synovitis.

If gross deformity and joint destruction have occurred, more definitive procedures may be required. In some joints, such as the wrist and ankle, function may be improved by stabilizing the joint through fusion, albeit at the cost of loss of motion. For destroyed joints, total replacement may be necessary. Hip prostheses provide a stable, pain-free joint with a good range of motion in more than 90% of patients. Metal-to-plastic prostheses are also useful in reconstruction of knee, elbow, and shoulder joints. Joint replacement procedures involve a relatively high risk of thromboembolism, but serious infections are rare. Loosening of the components has been observed within several years in as many as 20% of patients.

The author has no commercial relationships with manufacturers of products or providers of services discussed in this chapter.

References

1. Nepom GT, Byers P, Seyfried C, et al: HLA genes associated with rheumatoid arthritis: identification of susceptibility alleles using specific oligonucleotide probes. Arthritis Rheum 32:15, 1989

2. van der Helm-van Mil AH, Verpoort KN, Breedveld FC, et al: The HLA-DRB1 shared epitope alleles are primarily a risk factor for anti-cyclic citrullinated peptide antibodies and are not an independent risk factor for development of rheumatoid arthritis. Arthritis Rheum 54:1117, 2006

3. Cvetkovic JT, Wallberg-Jonsson S, Stegmayr B, et al: Susceptibility for and clinical manifestations of rheumatoid arthritis are associated with polymorphisms of the TNF-alpha, IL-1beta, and IL-1Ra genes. J Rheumatol 29:212, 2002

4. Suzuki A, Yamada R, Chang X, et al: Functional haplotypes of PADI4, encoding citrullinating enzyme peptidylarginine deiminase 4, are associated with rheumatoid arthritis. Nat Genet 34:395, 2003

5. Begovich AB, Carlton VE, Honigberg LA, et al: A missense single-nucleotide polymorphism in a gene encoding a protein tyrosine phosphatase (PTPN22) is associated with rheumatoid arthritis. Am J Hum Genet 75:330, 2004

6. Stahl HD, Pfeiffer R, Von Salis-Soglio G, et al: Parvovirus B19-associated mono- and oligoarticular arthritis may evolve into a chronic inflammatory arthropathy fulfilling criteria for rheumatoid arthritis or spondylarthropathy. Clin Rheumatol 19:510, 2000

7. Takahashi Y, Murai C, Shibata S, et al: Human parvovirus B19 as a causative agent for rheumatoid arthritis. Proc Natl Acad Sci USA 95:8227, 1998

8. Ray NB, Nieva DR, Seftor EA, et al: Induction of an invasive phenotype by human parvovirus B19 in normal human synovial fibroblasts. Arthritis Rheum 44:1582, 2001

9. Albani S, Carson DA: A multistep molecular mimicry hypothesis for the pathogenesis of rheumatoid arthritis. Immunol Today 17:466, 1996

10. Auger I, Roudier J: A function for the QKRAA amino acid motif: mediating binding of DnaJ to DnaK: implications for the association of rheumatoid arthritis with HLA-DR4. J Clin Invest 99:1818, 1997

11. Nakajima T, Aono H, Hasunuma T, et al: Overgrowth of human synovial cells driven by the human T cell leukemia virus type I tax gene. J Clin Invest 92:186, 1993

12. Aicher WK, Heer AH, Trabandt A, et al: Overexpression of zinc-finger transcription factor Z-225/Egr-1 in synoviocytes from rheumatoid arthritis patients. J Immunol 152:5940, 1994

13. Rantapaa-Dahlqvist S, de Jong BA, Berglin E, et al: Antibodies against cyclic citrullinated peptide and IgA rheumatoid factor predict the development of rheumatoid arthritis. Arthritis Rheum 48:2741, 2003

14. Kuhn KA, Kulik L, Tomooka B, et al: Antibodies against citrullinated proteins enhance tissue injury in experimental autoimmune arthritis. J Clin Invest 116:961, 2006

15. Firestein GS, Zvaifler NJ: How important are T cells in chronic rheumatoid synovitis? II. T cell-independent mechanisms from beginning to end. Arthritis Rheum 46:298, 2002

16. Corr M: The tolls of arthritis. Arthritis Rheum 52:223, 2005

17. Firestein GS, Yeo M, Zvaifler NJ: Apoptosis in rheumatoid arthritis synovium. J Clin Invest 96:1631, 1995

18. Zvaifler NJ, Firestein GS: Pannus and pannocytes: alternative models of joint destruction in rheumatoid arthritis. Arthritis Rheum 37:783, 1994

19. Corr M, Zvaifler NJ: Mesenchymal precursor cells. Ann Rheum Dis 61:3, 2002

20. Firestein GS: Invasive fibroblast-like synoviocytes in rheumatoid arthritis: passive responders or transformed aggressors? Arthritis Rheum 39:1781, 1996

21. Gravallese EM, Goldring SR: Cellular mechanisms and the role of cytokines in bone erosions in rheumatoid arthritis. Arthritis Rheum 43:2143, 2000

22. Muller-Ladner U, Kriegsmann J, Franklin BN, et al: Synovial fibroblasts of patients with rheumatoid arthritis attach to and invade normal human cartilage when engrafted into SCID mice. Am J Pathol 149:1607, 1996

23. Tak PP, Zvaifler NJ, Green DR, et al: Rheumatoid arthritis and p53: how oxidative stress might alter the course of inflammatory diseases. Immunol Today 21:78, 2000

24. Gringhuis SI, Leow A, Papendrecht-Van Der Voort EA, et al: Displacement of linker for activation of T cells from the plasma membrane due to redox balance alterations results in hyporesponsiveness of synovial fluid T lymphocytes in rheumatoid arthritis. J Immunol 164:2170, 2000

25. Ehrenstein MR, Evans JG, Singh A, et al: Compromised function of regulatory T cells in rheumatoid arthritis and reversal by anti-TNF-α therapy. J Exp Med 200:277, 2004

26. Warrington KJ, Takemura S, Goronzy JJ, et al: CD4+,CD28- T cells in rheumatoid arthritis patients combine features of the innate and adaptive immune systems. Arthritis Rheum 44:13, 2001

27. Wollheim FA: Predictors of joint damage in rheumatoid arthritis. APMIS 104:81, 1996

28. Ermel RW, Kenny TP, Chen PP, et al: Molecular analysis of rheumatoid factors derived from rheumatoid synovium suggests an antigen-driven response in inflamed joints. Arthritis Rheum 36:380, 1993

29. Vossenaar ER, Nijenhuis S, Helsen MM, et al: Citrullination of synovial proteins in murine models of rheumatoid arthritis. Arthritis Rheum 48:2489, 2003

30. Linn-Rasker SP, van der Helm-van Mil AH, van Gaalen FA, et al: Smoking is a risk factor for anti-CCP antibodies only in rheumatoid arthritis patients who carry HLA-DRB1 shared epitope alleles. Ann Rheum Dis 65:366, 2006

31. Goldbach-Mansky R, Lee J, McCoy A, et al: Rheumatoid arthritis associated autoantibodies in patients with synovitis of recent onset. Arthritis Res 2:236, 2000

32. Benoist C, Mathis D: Autoimmunity provoked by infection: how good is the case for T cell epitope mimicry? Nat Immunol 2:797, 2001

33. Emery P, Fleischmann R, Filipowicz-Sosnowska A, et al: The efficacy and safety of rituximab in patients with active rheumatoid arthritis despite methotrexate treatment: results of a phase IIB randomized, double-blind, placebo-controlled, dose-ranging trial. Arthritis Rheum 54:1390, 2006

34. Firestein GS, Zvaifler NJ: How important are T cells in chronic rheumatoid synovitis? Arthritis Rheum 33:768, 1990

35. Chabaud M, Lubberts E, Joosten L, et al: IL-17 derived from juxta-articular bone and synovium contributes to joint degradation in rheumatoid arthritis. Arthritis Res 3:168, 2001

36. Liblau RS, Singer SM, McDevitt HO: Th1 and Th2 CD4+ T cells in the pathogenesis of organ-specific autoimmune diseases. Immunol Today 16:34, 1995

37. Firestein GS, Boyle D, Yu C, et al: Synovial interleukin-1 receptor antagonist and interleukin-1 balance in rheumatoid arthritis. Arthritis Rheum 37:644, 1994

38. Firestein GS, Alvaro-Gracia JM, Maki R: Quantitative analysis of cytokine gene expression in rheumatoid arthritis. J Immunol 144:3347, 1990

39. McInnes IB, Leung BP, Sturrock RD, et al: Interleukin-15 mediates T cell–dependent regulation of tumor necrosis factor–alpha production in rheumatoid arthritis. Nat Med 3:189, 1997

40. Gracie JA, Forsey RJ, Chan WL, et al: A proinflammatory role for IL-18 in rheumatoid arthritis. J Clin Invest 104:1393, 1999

41. Ohata J, Zvaifler NJ, Nishio M, et al: Fibroblast-like synoviocytes of mesenchymal origin express functional B cell–activating factor of the TNF family in response to proinflammatory cytokines. J Immunol 174:864, 2005

42. Kim WJ, Kang YJ, Koh EM, et al: LIGHT is involved in the pathogenesis of rheumatoid arthritis by inducing the expression of pro-inflammatory cytokines and MMP-9 in macrophages. Immunology 114:272, 2005

43. Yan Z, Lambert NC, Ostensen M, et al: Prospective study of fetal DNA in serum and disease activity during pregnancy in women with inflammatory arthritis. Arthritis Rheum 54:2069, 2006

44. Drossaers-Bakker KW, Zwinderman AH, van Zeben D, et al: Pregnancy and oral contraceptive use do not significantly influence outcome in long term rheumatoid arthritis. Ann Rheum Dis 61:405, 2002

45. Weyand CM, Goronzy JJ, Liuzzo G, et al: T-cell immunity in acute coronary syndromes. Mayo Clin Proc 76:1011, 2001

46. Pham T, Gossec L, Constantin A, et al: Cardiovascular risk and rheumatoid arthritis: clinical practice guidelines based on published evidence and expert opinion. Joint Bone Spine 73:379, 2006

47. Naranjo A, Carmona L, Gavrila D, et al: Prevalence and associated factors of anterior atlantoaxial luxation in a nationwide sample of rheumatoid arthritis. Clin Exp Rheumatol 22:427, 2004

48. Foster H, Stephenson A, Walker D, et al: Linkage studies of HLA and primary Sjögren's syndrome in multicase families. Arthritis Rheum 36:473, 1993

49. MacDonald WJ, Crawford MH, Klippel JH, et al: Echocardiographic assessment of cardiac structure and function in patients with rheumatoid arthritis. Am J Med 63:890, 1977

50. Peeters HR, Jongen-Lavrencic M, Vreugdenhil G, et al: Effect of recombinant human erythropoietin on anaemia and disease activity in patients with rheumatoid arthritis and anaemia of chronic disease: a randomised placebo controlled double blind 52 weeks clinical trial. Ann Rheum Dis 55:739, 1996

51. Balint GP, Balint PV: Felty's syndrome. Best Pract Res Clin Rheumatol 18:631, 2004

52. Hartman KR: Anti-neutrophil antibodies of the immunoglobulin M class in autoimmune neutropenia. Am J Med Sci 308:102, 1994

53. Starkebaum G, Loughran TP Jr, Gaur LK, et al: Immunogenetic similarities between patients with Felty's syndrome and those with clonal expansions of large granular lymphocytes in rheumatoid arthritis. Arthritis Rheum 40:624, 1997

54. Rashba EJ, Rowe JM, Packman CH: Treatment of the neutropenia of Felty syndrome. Blood Rev 10:177, 1996

55. Puechal X, Said G, Hilliquin P, et al: Peripheral neuropathy with necrotizing vasculitis in rheumatoid arthritis: a clinicopathologic and prognostic study of thirty-two patients. Arthritis Rheum 38:1618, 1995

56. Moris G, Garcia-Monco JC: The challenge of drug-induced aseptic meningitis. Arch Intern Med 159:1185, 1999

57. Ramos-Casals M, Loustaud-Ratti V, De Vita S, et al: Sjögren syndrome association with hepatitis C virus: a multicenter analysis of 137 cases. Medicine (Baltimore) 84:81, 2005

58. Poleksic L, Musikic P, Zdravkovic D, et al: MRI evaluation of the knee in rheumatoid arthritis. Br J Rheumatol 35(suppl 3):36, 1996

59. Chen TS, Crues JV 3rd, Ali M, Troum OM: Magnetic resonance imaging is more sensitive than radiographs in detecting change in size of erosions in rheumatoid arthritis. J Rheumatol Aug 1, 2006 [epub ahead of print]

60. McQueen FM, Benton N, Crabbe J, et al: What is the fate of erosions in early rheumatoid arthritis? Tracking individual lesions using x rays and magnetic resonance imaging over the first two years of disease. Ann Rheum Dis 60:859, 2001

61. Guidelines for the management of rheumatoid arthritis: 2002 update. Arthritis Rheum 46:328, 2002

62. Furst DE, Breedveld FC, Burmester GR, et al: Updated consensus statement on tumour necrosis factor blocking agents for the treatment of rheumatoid arthritis (May 2000). Ann Rheum Dis 59(suppl 1):i1, 2000

63. Jiang Y, Genant HK, Watt I, et al: A multicenter, double-blind, dose-ranging, randomized, placebo-controlled study of recombinant human interleukin-1 receptor antagonist in patients with rheumatoid arthritis: radiologic progression and correlation of Genant and Larsen scores. Arthritis Rheum 43:1001, 2000

64. Landewe RB, Boers M, Verhoeven AC, et al: COBRA combination therapy in patients with early rheumatoid arthritis: long-term structural benefits of a brief intervention. Arthritis Rheum 46:347, 2002

65. Neva MH, Kauppi MJ, Kautiainen H, et al: Combination drug therapy retards the development of rheumatoid atlantoaxial subluxations. Arthritis Rheum 43:2397, 2000

66. Raskin JB, White RH, Jackson JE, et al: Misoprostol dosage in the prevention of nonsteroidal anti-inflammatory drug-induced gastric and duodenal ulcers: a comparison of three regimens. Ann Intern Med 123:344, 1995

67. Gabriel SE, Jaakkimainen RL, Bombardier C: The cost-effectiveness of misoprostol for nonsteroidal antiinflammatory drug–associated adverse gastrointestinal events. Arthritis Rheum 36:447, 1993

68. Hinz B, Brune K: Cyclooxygenase-2: 10 years later. J Pharmacol Exp Ther 300:367, 2002

69. Suissa S, Bernatsky S, Hudson M: Antirheumatic drug use and the risk of acute myocardial infarction. Arthritis Rheum 55:531, 2006

70. Alarcon GS: Methotrexate use in rheumatoid arthritis: a clinician's perspective. Immunopharmacology 47:259, 2000

71. Lopez-Mendez A, Daniel WW, Reading JC, et al: Radiographic assessment of disease progression in rheumatoid arthritis patients enrolled in the cooperative systematic studies of the rheumatic diseases program randomized clinical trial of methotrexate, auranofin, or a combination of the two. Arthritis Rheum 36:1364, 1993

72. Lambert CM, Sandhu S, Lochhead A, et al: Dose escalation of parenteral methotrexate in active rheumatoid arthritis that has been unresponsive to conventional doses of methotrexate: a randomized, controlled trial. Arthritis Rheum 50:364, 2004

73. Weinblatt ME, Maier AL, Fraser PA, et al: Longterm prospective study of methotrexate in rheumatoid arthritis: conclusion after 132 months of therapy. J Rheumatol 25:238, 1998

74. Choi HK, Hernan MA, Seeger JD, et al: Methotrexate and mortality in patients with rheumatoid arthritis: a prospective study. Lancet 359:1173, 2002

75. Morgan SL, Baggott JE, Vaughn WH, et al: Supplementation with folic acid during methotrexate therapy for rheumatoid arthritis: a double-blind, placebo-controlled trial. Ann Intern Med 121:833, 1994

76. Erickson AR, Reddy V, Vogelgesang SA, et al: Usefulness of the American College of Rheumatology recommendations for liver biopsy in methotrexate-treated rheumatoid arthritis patients. Arthritis Rheum 38:1115, 1995

77. Cohen S, Cannon GW, Schiff M, et al: Two-year, blinded, randomized controlled trial of treatment of active rheumatoid arthritis with leflunomide compared with methotrexate. Utilization of Leflunomide in the Treatment of Rheumatoid Arthritis Trial Investigator Group. Arthritis Rheum 44:1984, 2001

78. Weinblatt ME, Kremer JM, Coblyn JS, et al: Pharmacokinetics, safety, and efficacy of combination treatment with methotrexate and leflunomide in patients with active rheumatoid arthritis. Arthritis Rheum 42:1322, 1999

79. Conaghan PG, Brooks P: Disease-modifying antirheumatic drugs, including methotrexate, sulfasalazine, gold, antimalarials, and D-penicillamine. Curr Opin Rheumatol 5:276, 1993

80. Plosker GL, Croom KF: Sulfasalazine: a review of its use in the management of rheumatoid arthritis. Drugs 65:1825, 2005

81. McEntegart A, Porter D, Capell HA, et al: Sulfasalazine has a better efficacy/toxicity profile than auranofin-evidence from a 5-year prospective, randomized trial. J Rheumatol 23:1887, 1996

82. Choy EH, Smith C, Dore CJ, et al: A meta-analysis of the efficacy and toxicity of combining disease-modifying anti-rheumatic drugs in rheumatoid arthritis based on patient withdrawal. Rheumatology (Oxford) 44:1414, 2005

83. Willkens RF, Sharp JT, Stablein D, et al: Comparison of azathioprine, methotrexate, and the combination of the two in the treatment of rheumatoid arthritis: a forty-eight-week controlled clinical trial with radiologic outcome assessment. Arthritis Rheum 38:1799, 1995

84. O'Dell JR, Haire CE, Erikson N, et al: Treatment of rheumatoid arthritis with methotrexate alone, sulfasalazine and hydroxychloroquine, or a combination of all three medications. N Engl J Med 334:1287, 1996

85. Moreland LW, Baumgartner SW, Schiff MH: Treatment of rheumatoid arthritis with a recombinant human tumor necrosis factor receptor (p75) fusion protein. N Engl J Med 337:141, 1997

86. Weinblatt ME, Kremer JM, Bankhurst AD, et al: A trial of etanercept, a recombinant tumor necrosis factor receptor:Fc fusion protein, in patients with rheumatoid arthritis receiving methotrexate. N Engl J Med 340:253, 1999

87. Maini R, St Clair EW, Breedveld F, et al: Infliximab (chimeric anti-tumour necrosis factor alpha monoclonal antibody) versus placebo in rheumatoid arthritis patients receiving concomitant methotrexate: a randomised phase III trial. ATTRACT Study Group. Lancet 354:1932, 1999

88. Breedveld FC, Weisman MH, Kavanaugh AF, et al: The PREMIER study: a multicenter, randomized, doubled-blind clinical trial of combination therapy with adalimumab plus methotrexate versus methotrexate alone or adalimumab alone in patients with every, aggressive rheumatoid arthritis who had not had previous methotrexate treatment. Arthritis Rheum 54:26, 2006

89. Keane J, Gershon S, Wise RP, et al: Tuberculosis associated with infliximab, a tumor necrosis factor alpha–neutralizing agent. N Engl J Med 345:1098, 2001

90. Carmona L, Gomez-Reino JJ, Rodriguez-Valverde V, et al: Effectiveness of recommendations to prevent reactivation of latent tuberculosis infection in patients treated with tumor necrosis factor antagonists. Arthritis Rheum 52:1766, 2005

91. Mohan N, Edwards ET, Cupps TR, et al: Demyelination occurring during anti–tumor necrosis factor alpha therapy for inflammatory arthritides. Arthritis Rheum 44:2862, 2001

92. Bongartz T, Sutton AJ, Sweeting MJ, et al: Anti-TNF antibody therapy in rheumatoid arthritis and the risk of serious infections and malignancies: systematic review and meta-analysis of rare harmful effects in randomized controlled trials. JAMA 295:227, 2006

93. Kremer JM, Genant HK, Moreland LW, et al: Effects of abatacept in patients with methotrexate-resistant active rheumatoid arthritis: a randomized trial. Ann Intern Med 144:865, 2006

94. Cohen S, Hurd E, Cush J, et al: Treatment of rheumatoid arthritis with anakinra, a recombinant human interleukin-1 receptor antagonist, in combination with methotrexate: results of a twenty-four-week, multicenter, randomized, double-blind, placebo-controlled trial. Arthritis Rheum 46:614, 2002

95. Wassenberg S, Rau R, Steinfeld P, et al: Very low-dose prednisolone in early rheumatoid arthritis retards radiographic progression over two years: a multicenter, double-blind, placebo-controlled trial. Arthritis Rheum 52:3371, 2005

96. Stein CM, Pincus T, Yocum D, et al: Combination treatment of severe rheumatoid arthritis with cyclosporine and methotrexate for forty-eight weeks: an open-label extension study. The Methotrexate-Cyclosporine Combination Study Group. Arthritis Rheum 40:1843, 1997

97. Stone M, Fortin PR, Pacheco-Tena C, et al: Should tetracycline treatment be used more extensively for rheumatoid arthritis? Metaanalysis demonstrates clinical benefit with reduction in disease activity. J Rheumatol 30:2112, 2003

98. Prakken BJ, Samodal R, Le TD, et al: Epitope-specific immunotherapy induces immune deviation of proinflammatory T cells in rheumatoid arthritis. Proc Natl Acad Sci USA 101:4228, 2004

99. Kremer JM, Lawrence DA, Petrillo GF, et al: Effects of high-dose fish oil on rheumatoid arthritis after stopping nonsteroidal antiinflammatory drugs: clinical and immune correlates. Arthritis Rheum 38:1107, 1995

100. Adam O, Beringer C, Less T, et al: Anti-inflammatory effects of a low arachidonic acid diet and fish oil in patients with rheumatoid arthritis. Rheumatoid Int 23:27, 2003

101. Arnett FC, Edworthy SM, Bloch DA, et al: The American Rheumatism Association 1987 criteria for the classification of rheumatoid arthritis. Arthritis Rheum 31:315, 1988
http://www.rheumatology.org/publications/classification/ra/1987_revised_criteria_classification_ra.asp?aud=mem

102. Felson DT, Anderson JJ, Boers M, et al: ACR preliminary definition of improvement in rheumatoid arthritis. Arthritis Rheum 38:727, 1995
http://www.rheumatology.org/publications/classification/205070.asp

113 Seronegative Spondyloarthritis

Frank C. Arnett, M.D., F.A.C.P.

Definition

The term spondyloarthritis encompasses a family of clinically, epidemiologically, and genetically related inflammatory diseases that primarily affect spinal and peripheral joints. Once considered a variant of rheumatoid arthritis, spondyloarthritis has been shown to differ in such fundamental clinical and pathogenetic ways from rheumatoid disease that the two are now considered distinctly separate entities [see Table 1]. The term seronegative refers to the uniform absence of serum IgM autoantibodies to IgG (rheumatoid factor) in patients with spondyloarthritis. Other distinguishing characteristics are the following:

1. The sacroiliac joints are affected (sacroiliitis); ascending spinal inflammation and bony fusion (spondylitis) often develop after sacroiliitis.
2. Peripheral joints are affected, typically in an oligoarticular and asymmetrical pattern.
3. There is inflammation of sites of ligamentous insertions into bone (entheses), referred to as enthesitis or enthesopathy, as well as inflammation of joint synovium. Inflammation occurs both along the spine and near peripheral joints.
4. There may be inflammation of extra-articular sites, including the eye, the aortic valve, the gastrointestinal tract, the genitourinary system, and the skin.
5. Disease onset typically occurs in young adulthood.
6. There is a strong familial tendency and a striking genetic association with the histocompatibility antigen HLA-B27.
7. Certain bacteria play important pathogenetic roles.

Classification

Spondyloarthritis includes the prototypical spinal arthritis, ankylosing spondylitis; reactive arthritis (formerly known as Reiter syndrome); psoriatic arthritis; enteropathic arthritis (accompanying ulcerative colitis and Crohn disease); juvenile spondyloarthritis (or juvenile ankylosing spondylitis); and such rare disorders as acne-associated arthritis, or SAPHO (synovitis, acne, pustulosis, hyperostosis, osteitis) syndrome, and Whipple disease. The various forms of spondyloarthritis can usually be distinguished from one another by the pattern of joint involvement and associated extra-articular features [see Table 2]. However, some patients have overlapping clinical manifestations that defy categorization; these patients are usually designated as having undifferentiated spondyloarthritis. Because of such patients, the European Spondyloarthropathy Study Group (ESSG) proposed classification criteria for spondyloarthritis that may be useful in clinical diagnosis and epidemiologic studies.[1]

Epidemiology

Estimations of prevalence rates for spondyloarthritis using the ESSG criteria are few.[1-3] Among Germans in Berlin, the prevalence of spondyloarthritis has been reported to be 1.9%; in Inuits in Alaska and Siberia, rates of 2% to 3.4% have been reported. Spondyloarthritis appears to be rare in African and Japanese populations. These differences among ethnic groups are explainable in large part by differences in the frequency of HLA-B27.[1]

Pathogenesis

The various forms of spondyloarthritis appear to be complex disorders resulting from the interplay of several genetic and environmental factors, only a few of which have been identified.

GENETIC FACTORS

Heredity plays a major role in predisposition.[4,5] Family studies have shown that 15% to 20% of patients with ankylosing spondylitis have one or more first-degree relatives with the same disease. In the families of some patients with ankylosing spondylitis, there are relatives with other types of spondyloarthritis or other associated disorders, such as uveitis, psoriasis, and inflammatory bowel disease. Concordance for ankylosing spondylitis in monozygotic twins approaches 63% to 75%, compared with 13% to 23% in dizygotic twins. Genetic modeling in twins and families indicates that ankylosing spondylitis is associated with a multiplicative, polygenic pattern of inheritance, with 97% of the susceptibility to the disease attributed to genetics. These studies suggest that the environmental factors that contribute to development of the disease are probably ubiquitous.

The HLA-B27 allele encoded by the class I HLA-B locus within the major histocompatibility complex (MHC) is the one genetic factor identified thus far that is strongly associated with spondyloarthritis. This allele is present in 90% of patients with ankylosing spondylitis and confers a relative risk for the disease of over 100, but it is found less often in patients with other forms of spondyloarthritis [see Table 2].[5] HLA-B27 shows linkage to ankylosing spondylitis in families and appears to contribute 30% to 50% of the genetic risk; in most cases, it appears essential for disease expression.[4] Other HLA alleles, including HLA-B60, HLA-DR1, and HLA-DR8, also appear to increase the risk of ankylosing spondylitis. In addition, different HLA alleles predispose to psoriasis and psoriatic arthritis, including HLA-B13, HLA-B17, HLA-Cw6, HLA-B38, and HLA-B39.[6] The HLA region shows genetic linkage to inflammatory bowel diseases, but specific HLA alleles show only weak associations.[7] Ongoing human genome searches have revealed additional non-HLA loci linked to ankylosing spondylitis,[4,5] some of which also may be common to Crohn disease[8,9] and psoriasis.[5,10]

Laboratory evidence strongly suggests that the *HLA-B27* gene itself, rather than a linked locus, directly participates in the pathogenesis of ankylosing spondylitis and reactive arthritis. Transgenic rats expressing the human *HLA-B27* and β_2-microglobulin genes spontaneously develop colitis, peripheral and spinal arthritis, enthesitis, skin and nail lesions resembling psoriasis, and genitourinary inflammation.[11] Littermates raised in a germ-free environment do not develop most of these manifestations, however. That finding emphasizes the importance of both the *HLA-B27* gene and gut bacteria, possibly *Bacteroides* species, in pathogenesis and suggests that antibiotics (e.g., sulfasalazine) may be useful in the treatment of reactive arthritis and ankylosing spondylitis in humans. The mechanism by which HLA-B27 promotes disease is unknown, but the following are the prevailing hypotheses[12]: (1) in its function as an MHC class I molecule,

HLA-B27 presents a so-called arthritogenic self-peptide or bacterial peptide to cytotoxic CD8$^+$ T cells, which causes an autoimmune attack on various self-structures; (2) HLA-B27 contains stretches of amino acid sequences that also occur in bacterial proteins, and as a result of this molecular mimicry, a cytotoxic or humoral immune response to these bacterial sequences also involves HLA-B27; (3) HLA-B27, either intracellularly or extracellularly, promotes bacterial persistence or dissemination to joints and other structures; and (4) HLA-B27 is unique among HLA class I molecules in forming so-called homodimers, which may cause misfolding of the protein, resulting in an inflammatory response.[5,13,14]

ENVIRONMENTAL FACTORS

Reactive arthritis provides the strongest evidence of bacterial pathogenesis in spondyloarthritis. Enteric infections by *Shigella flexneri*, *Salmonella* (many species), *Yersinia enterocolitica*, *Y. pseudotuberculosis*, and *Campylobacter jejuni* have all been implicated as triggers of the disease in various epidemics and in sporadic cases, especially in HLA-B27–positive persons.[15,16] Similarly, sexually acquired infections with *Chlamydia trachomatis*[15,16] and perhaps *Ureaplasma urealyticum* may cause reactive arthritis.[17] Pulmonary infection with *Chlamydophila pneumoniae* (formerly known as *Chlamydia pneumoniae*) has also been implicated.[18] Patients with chronic reactive arthritis have been found to have IgA antibodies to the initiating microbe, suggesting a persistent mucosal infection.[19] Moreover, synovial fluid T cells were found to proliferate when challenged with the bacterium that triggered the arthritis.[12] There is no evidence, however, that these microorganisms cause ankylosing spondylitis. Normal gut flora seem more likely to be implicated in ankylosing spondylitis, as suggested by studies of the HLA-B27 transgenic rat[11] and by a high frequency of asymptomatic foci of gut inflammation in patients with ankylosing spondylitis or reactive arthritis.[20]

Pathology

Chronic inflammation with infiltrating mononuclear cells (macrophages, T cells, and B cells) occurs in both peripheral and axial joint structures of patients with spondyloarthritis.[12,21,22] CD4$^+$ helper T cells and CD8$^+$ suppressor-cytotoxic T cells appear to be equally represented. A high concentration of the inflammatory cytokine tumor necrosis factor–α (TNF-α) has been found in the dense cellular infiltrates in synovial portions of sacroiliac joints.[21] When cytokines from the joints and blood of patients with spondyloarthritis were compared with those of patients with rheumatoid arthritis, the cytokines from patients with spondyloarthritis showed a higher ratio of immunosuppressive cytokines, such as interleukin-4 (IL-4) and IL-10, to inflammatory cytokines, such as TNF-α and interferon gamma. This leads to a blunted T helper type 1 (Th1) response in patients with spondyloarthritis.[22] Inherent levels of cytokines, such as TNF-α and IL-10, are determined by genetic polymorphisms in their respective genes.[22] In ankylosing spondylitis, the observed tendency for ligamentous ossification, enthesopathy, and widespread new bone formation is associated with the finding of transforming growth

Table 1   Comparison between Spondyloarthritis and Rheumatoid Arthritis

	Spondyloarthropathies	*Rheumatoid Arthritis*
Distribution	Racial (more prevalent in whites)	Worldwide
Prevalence	0.2%–1.9%	1%–2%
Etiology	Genetic and bacterial	Genetic and unknown
Positive family history	Frequent	Rare
Sex distribution	More frequently diagnosed in males	More common in females
Age at onset	Peak incidence at 20–30 yr	All ages affected; peak incidence 30–50 yr
Joint involvement	Oligoarthritis; asymmetrical; large joints; lower limbs more than upper limbs	Polyarthritis; symmetrical; small and large joints; upper and lower limbs
Sacroiliac involvement	Yes	No
Spinal involvement	Ascending; all segments with fusion	Cervical only; erosions and instability
Subcutaneous nodules	No	Yes
Aortic regurgitation	Yes	No
Ocular involvement	Uveitis, conjunctivitis	Sicca syndrome; scleritis; scleromalacia perforans
Lung involvement	Upper lobe pulmonary fibrosis	Pleural effusions; lower lobe pulmonary fibrosis; nodules; Caplan syndrome
Rheumatoid factor and/or anti-CCP	No	Yes
HLA-B27	Yes	No (normal frequency)
HLA-DR4	25% (normal frequency)	60%–70%
Pathology	Synovitis and enthesopathy	Synovitis
Radiographic findings	Asymmetrical erosive arthritis and periostitis; new bone formation and ankylosis; sacroiliitis, spondylitis	Symmetrical erosive arthritis with bony destruction

anti-CCP—antibodies to cyclic citrullinated peptides

Table 2 Features of Seronegative Spondyloarthritis

	Ankylosing Spondylitis	Reactive Arthritis (Reiter Syndrome)	Psoriatic Arthritis	Enteropathic Arthritis
Sex distribution	Male > female	Male > female	Female > male	Female = male
Age at onset (years)	≥ 20	≥ 20	Any age	Any age
Mode of onset	Gradual	Sudden	Gradual	Peripheral sudden Spinal gradual
Peripheral joints	Often lower limbs Asymmetrical	Usually lower limbs Asymmetrical	Upper > lower limbs Asymmetrical	Lower > upper limbs Symmetrical
Enthesopathy	+	+	+	– Peripheral + Spinal
Heel pain	Occasional	Frequent	Occasional	Infrequent
Spinal involvement	+++ (always)	+ (20%)	+ (20%)	+ (10%)
Symmetry (sacroiliitis and syndesmophytes)	+	+/–	+/–	+
Familial aggregation	++	+	++	++
HLA-B27 positive	90%	63%–75%	20% (50% with sacroiliitis)	10% (50% with sacroiliitis)
Risk for B27-positive person	2% (20% when a relative)	20% (when infected)	?	?
Urethritis	–	+	–	–
Skin involvement	–	+	+++	+
Nail involvement	–	+	+++	–
Mucous membrane involvement	–	++	–	+
Cardiac involvement	+	+	Rare	Rare
Self-limiting	–	+	–	++ Peripheral – Spinal

factor–β (TGF-β) near these sites. TGF-β is a reparative cytokine that stimulates connective tissue matrix formation.

Reactive arthritis was once considered a sterile joint disease triggered in some unknown manner by a distant infection, but more recent studies of synovial fluids and tissues affected by reactive arthritis have consistently revealed the presence of intracellular bacterial antigens from each of the known offending microorganisms.[14,23,24] Moreover, with electron microscopy and polymerase chain reaction, living but dormant *C. trachomatis* has been detected in synovial macrophages and fibroblasts even after many years of disease.[23] It is still unclear whether the enteric pathogens causing reactive arthritis are viable.[14,24] Spinal joint tissue from patients with ankylosing spondylitis is difficult to obtain. Limited studies of sacroiliac joint biopsies have not revealed bacterial antigens.[25]

Ankylosing Spondylitis

EPIDEMIOLOGY

The prevalence of ankylosing spondylitis parallels the frequency of HLA-B27 in different ethnic populations.[1,26] HLA-B27 occurs in 7% to 9% of the white population, and the disease has a prevalence of approximately 0.2% to 0.9%.[2,3,26] One study from Norway, where the frequency of HLA-B27 is twice that seen in the white populations of the United States and the United Kingdom, found that ankylosing spondylitis occurred in 1.9% to 2.2% of men and 0.3% to 0.6% of women.[3] The disease is distinctly rare in African and Japanese populations, in which HLA-B27 is found in low frequency; however, ankylosing spondylitis is common in certain Native-American groups, such as the Haida and Pima, in which the frequency of HLA-B27 is high.[26]

In randomly chosen cohorts of whites possessing HLA-B27, ankylosing spondylitis developed in approximately 2% to 6%.[3] In HLA-B27–positive relatives of patients with ankylosing spondylitis, however, the risk of disease is 20% to 30%. Similar estimates are not available for other ethnic groups, but rates may differ because multiple molecular subtypes of HLA-B27 have been discovered, each with different distributions among various ethnic groups.[5,25-27] HLA-B*2705, followed in frequency by HLA-B*2702, is predominantly found in whites; HLA-B*2704 is found in Chinese; and HLA-B*2703 is found in Africans. Most HLA-B27 subtypes appear to predispose to ankylosing spondylitis, with the possible exceptions of HLA-B*2706, found in Indonesians and Thais, and HLA-B*2709, found in Sardinians.

Ankylosing spondylitis was once considered to be almost exclusively a disease of males, but recent studies suggest a more uniform distribution by sex (the ratio of males to females is 3:1).[1] In females, the disease may be diagnosed less frequently and later in the course of disease because physicians still consider it primarily a disorder of males. Some studies suggest that females have milder disease, with less progressive spinal involvement and more peripheral arthritis. Other studies suggest that the overall pattern of disease is similar in males and females.

Onset typically occurs between 16 and 30 years of age, peaking at around 24 years; ankylosing spondylitis seldom begins in patients older than 40 years. Childhood onset before 16 years

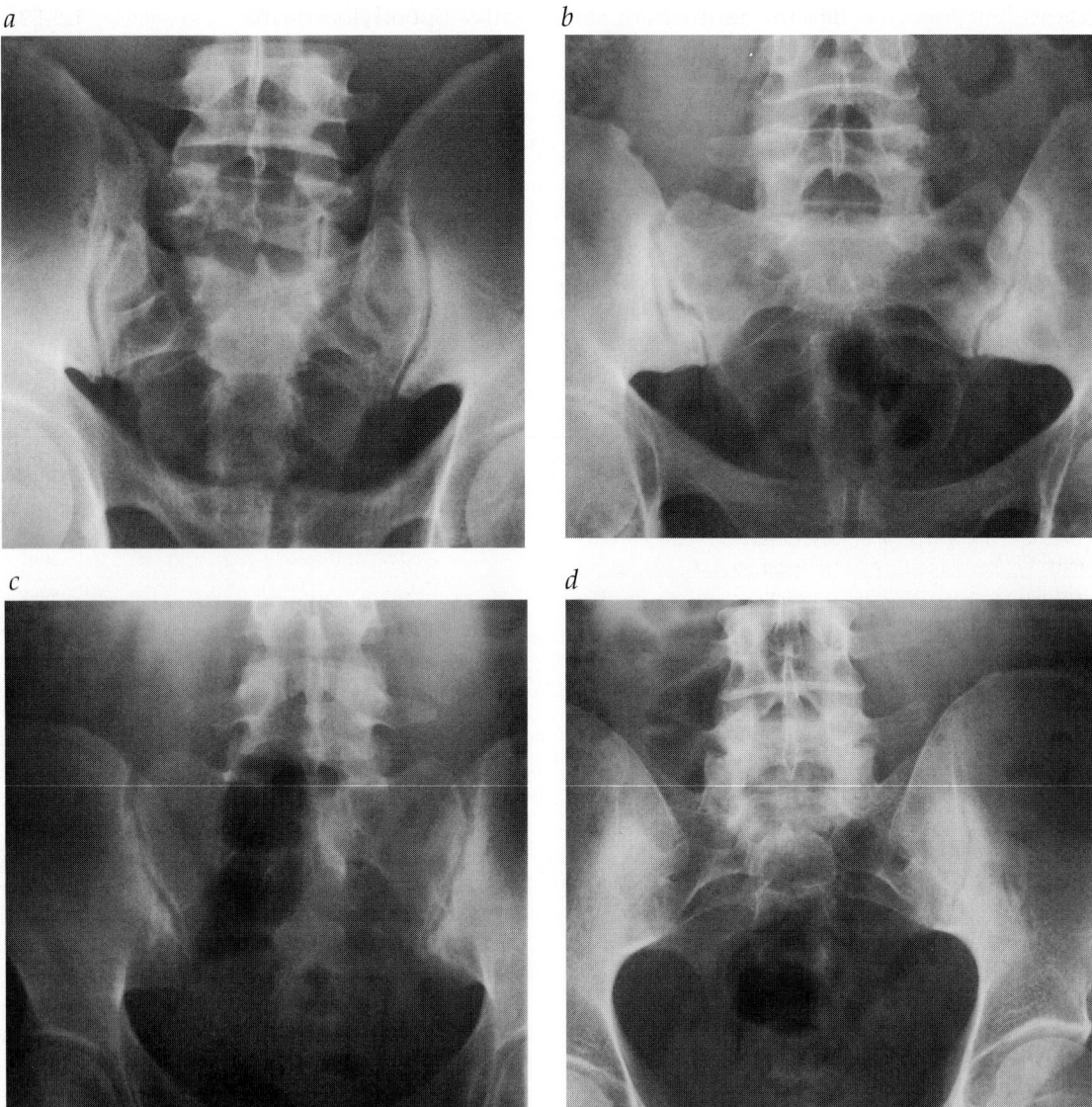

Figure 1 (*a*) **Radiograph of normal sacroiliac joints showing clearly defined joint margins and no sclerosis (grade 0). (*b*) Sclerosis on both margins of each sacroiliac joint but no joint erosions (grade II). (*c*) Sclerosis and erosions of both sacroiliac joints (grade III). (*d*) Complete bony fusion of both sacroiliac joints (grade IV).**

of age occurs in approximately 10% to 20% of cases in the United States and Europe but is more common (54%) in developing countries, suggesting earlier exposure to the environmental triggers.[28]

DIAGNOSIS

The modified New York criteria[1] are currently used to diagnose ankylosing spondylitis. A patient should have one or more of the following clinical criteria:

1. Low back pain of at least 3 months' duration that is alleviated by exercise and is not relieved by rest.
2. Restricted lumbar spinal motion.
3. Decreased chest expansion relative to normal values for age and sex.

In addition, the patient must have definitive radiographic evidence of sacroiliitis (i.e., bilateral sacroiliitis of grade II to IV or unilateral sacroiliitis of grade III or IV) [*see Figure 1*].

A simpler approach in diagnosis is to accept symptomatic sacroiliitis as an adequate definition. Sacroiliitis, as defined radiographically, should be definitive (i.e., grade III or IV changes should be evident) and should be present bilaterally [*see Figure 1*]. In addition, the patient should have no other diseases that could cause sacroiliitis (i.e., reactive arthritis, psoriasis, or inflammatory bowel disease).

Clinical Presentation

Low back pain and stiffness are the usual presenting symptoms of ankylosing spondylitis. Because back pain is such a common complaint in the general population and its causes are myriad, certain characteristics that specifically suggest inflammatory back pain have been formulated:

1. Onset in a person younger than 40 years.
2. Insidious rather than abrupt onset.
3. Persistence of back symptoms for 3 months or longer.
4. Worsening of back pain or stiffness with inactivity.
5. Subsiding of back pain or stiffness with exercise.

Some patients describe buttock pain that often alternates from one side to the other and sometimes radiates down the posterior leg, which is indicative of sacroiliac joint disease. Other patients present with a peripheral arthritis, typically monoarticular or oligoarticular, that affects joints of the lower extremity, often the knee. Careful questioning about subtle musculoskeletal symptoms in such patients is often fruitful. Fatigue can be a major symptom in patients with ankylosing spondylitis and has been found to correlate with level of disease activity, functional ability, global well-being, and mental health status.[29] Elicitation of a history of uveitis or the presence of spondyloarthritic features in family members also strongly suggests the disease. Radiologic evidence of sacroiliitis in any of these clinical presentations, however, is essential in confirming a diagnosis of ankylosing spondylitis [see Radiographic Features, below]. In patients whose sacroiliac radiographs are normal, the presence of HLA-B27 is highly suggestive but not definitive evidence of the disease. Follow-up studies of patients in whom the diagnosis was strongly suspected on the basis of the clinical picture and HLA-B27 positivity showed that sacroiliac joint abnormalities eventually appear on plain x-rays, but the evolution may occur over as many as 10 years. MRI of the sacroiliac joints is a very sensitive method for detecting early sacroiliitis, as well as inflammation elsewhere in the spine.

Patients with juvenile-onset ankylosing spondylitis typically present with peripheral oligoarthritis, often with enthesopathy and infrequently with spinal symptoms.[28] Such patients may be misdiagnosed as having juvenile rheumatoid arthritis [see Juvenile Spondyloarthritis, below]. Spinal involvement usually appears later, in young adulthood.

Physical Examination

Examination of the back may be relatively normal early in the course of the disease. Sacroiliac joints are usually painful when palpated or stressed. When the disease advances into the lumbar spine, the normal lordotic curvature may be lost, and paravertebral muscle spasm is prominent. Forward bending, or flexion, may be restricted, as measured by the Schober test. In this measurement, two points are drawn with the patient standing erect, one at the L5–S1 region and the other 10 cm above this region. With normal flexion, the distance between these two points increases by 4 to 6 cm, but when the lumbar spine becomes fused, there may be little or no increase in distance between the two points. Lateral lumbar bending and extension are also typically restricted.

Thoracic spine involvement causes an exaggerated dorsal kyphosis; in patients with costovertebral joint fusion, chest expansion (as measured circumferentially at the fourth intercostal space from full expiration to inspiration) is reduced to 2.5 cm or less. When the disease ascends into the neck and causes fusion, cervical lordosis is lost and a fixed flexion deformity may occur. Spinal fusion often results in the patient's being severely stooped forward with neck immobile and flexed; the patient has difficulty looking straight ahead.

Peripheral arthritis, especially of the hips, shoulders, and knees, occurs in approximately 30% of patients with ankylosing spondylitis and further increases disability. Peripheral enthesopathic features may include Achilles tendinitis, plantar fasciitis, or costochondritis.[30]

Laboratory Findings

The HLA-B27 histocompatibility antigen is present in more than 90% of ankylosing spondylitis patients. HLA-B27 testing of individual patients, however, is indicated only in atypical cases, when the clinical suspicion is high but the most definitive finding—radiographic evidence of sacroiliitis—is not present. In HLA-B27–positive patients and HLA-B27–negative patients, the patterns and severity of arthritis are similar. HLA-B27–negative patients differ from HLA-B27–positive patients in that in HLA-B27–negative patients, disease onset occurs at an older age, there is no family history of spondylitis, and uveitis or cardiac complications occur infrequently.[1,26] HLA-B27 is found less commonly (50%) in patients with ankylosing spondylitis who are of African ancestry.

Elevation of the erythrocyte sedimentation rate (ESR) occurs in many patients, but it may be normal despite severe disease. C-reactive protein (CRP) levels may be elevated. Serum IgA levels are often elevated.[19] Some patients have a mild normocytic normochromic anemia because of chronic inflammation; in these patients, the platelet count may be high.

Radiographic Features

Bilateral sacroiliitis is the most specific finding that supports a diagnosis of ankylosing spondylitis, and meticulous interpretation of the radiographs is imperative. A grading system that assesses each sacroiliac joint for juxta-articular bony sclerosis, blurring or erosion of joint margins, and bony fusion has been formulated and tested [see Figure 1]. Grade 0 findings are normal. Grade I findings are suspicious but not definitive. Grade II findings show sclerosis on both sides of a joint; such findings are even more suspicious when they occur bilaterally, but they should be interpreted with great caution. Findings of grades III and IV are definitive. Another radiographically defined entity, osteitis condensans ilii, may be misinterpreted as sacroiliitis, and vice versa. Patients with osteitis condensans ilii have sclerosis on the iliac side of both sacroiliac joints; the condition occurs in women who have borne children. Although quantitative radionuclide scans, computed tomography, and MRI have been suggested as superior diagnostic methods, well-performed plain radiographs of the sacroiliac joints (Ferguson view or oblique view) are usually adequate.

An early spinal change seen on radiographs is squaring of the normally concave anterior side of vertebral bodies [see Figure 2]. This phenomenon is caused by inflammation and bony erosion at the site of insertion (enthesitis) of the outer fibers of the annulus fibrosus. Later changes are ossification of ligaments, which are seen on radiographs as syndesmophytes that bridge adjacent vertebral bodies [see Figure 3], producing the classic bamboo-spine appearance [see Figure 4]. Zygapophyseal joints become fused into solid bone. Finally, diffuse osteoporosis may occur, making the spine susceptible to fracture. Bony fusion across joint spaces of affected peripheral joints in ankylosing spondylitis may be the most distinctive change seen on radiographs.

Similar spinal changes are seen in primary ankylosing spondylitis and in the spondylitis associated with inflammatory bowel disease. In spondylitis associated with reactive arthritis and psoriatic arthritis, the sacroiliitis and syndesmophytes tend to be asymmetrical.[31] Another disease that may mimic ankylosing spondylitis is diffuse idiopathic skeletal hyperostosis (DISH).[32] DISH occurs in middle-aged and older persons, especially men; it is characterized by large, flowing syndesmophytes that restrict spinal motion; sacroiliitis is not found, however, and there is no association with HLA-B27.

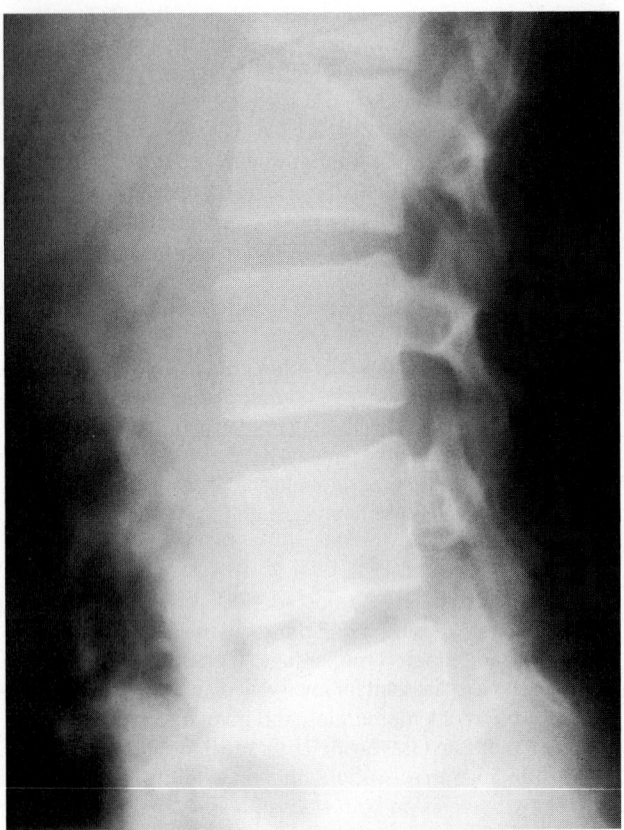

Figure 2 **Loss of the normal anterior concavity of vertebral bodies, resulting in so-called squaring in early ankylosing spondylitis.**

Extra-articular Manifestations

A number of extraskeletal features may complicate the course of ankylosing spondylitis and contribute to morbidity and mortality.

Ocular involvement Acute anterior uveitis, usually occurring episodically and affecting one eye at a time, occurs in 25% of patients. Acute pain, redness, and photophobia are the usual symptoms. Prompt referral to an ophthalmologist for treatment is essential. Uveitis does not correlate with arthritis activity or severity and shows a strong association with HLA-B27, even in patients without spondyloarthritis.[33]

Cardiovascular disease A fibrosing cardiovascular lesion occurs in 2% to 10% of patients with ankylosing spondylitis. The lesion causes the aortic valve and proximal root to thicken, and it often extends into the conducting system, causing aortic regurgitation, atrioventricular block, or both. The lesion probably occurs with a similar frequency in patients with reactive arthritis.[34] In rare instances, mitral regurgitation may also occur. One study emphasized a high prevalence of underlying spondyloarthritis, often undiagnosed, in men requiring cardiac pacemakers for bradyarrhythmias.[34] In addition, this study revealed the strong association of the clinical combination of lone aortic regurgitation and heart block with HLA-B27, with or without apparent arthritis. Fulminant cardiac disease typically appears only after the patient has had spondyloarthritis for many years, but such disease has been described even in very early spondyloarthritis. Echocardiography may detect cardiac abnormalities in some patients without clinical signs.[35] No treatment is known to prevent pro-

gression of spondylitic heart disease; most patients require permanent cardiac pacemakers, aortic valve replacement, or both.

Pulmonary disease Despite restriction of chest wall motion by joint fusion, respiratory function is preserved in most patients with ankylosing spondylitis, owing to good diaphragmatic function. Severe kyphotic deformity, however, may compromise breathing. Approximately 1% of patients with ankylosing spondylitis, usually those with severe disease, also have fibrosis in the upper lung fields that mimics tuberculosis.[36] Cavitation may occur and may be complicated by *Aspergillus* infection. Cough, dyspnea, and even hemoptysis are typical symptoms. Currently available treatment is unsatisfactory.

Renal disease Kidney function is usually normal. The appearance of proteinuria, with or without a nephrotic syndrome, usually indicates complicating amyloidosis or IgA nephropathy. Secondary amyloidosis occurs in approximately 4% of patients and can be diagnosed with abdominal fat-pad or rectal biopsy.[37]

IgA nephropathy is being increasingly recognized. It correlates with high serum IgA levels. Renal function may become impaired, but episodes are usually self-limited.[19]

Neurologic disease Spinal fracture is a major cause of morbidity and mortality in patients with ankylosing spondylitis; cord compression occurs even with seemingly minor trauma.[1] A rigid and osteoporotic cervical spine is most susceptible to fracture, usually at the C6 or C7 level. A high degree of suspicion for fracture is always warranted in patients with localized spinal pain, even when plain x-rays fail to reveal an acute abnormality;

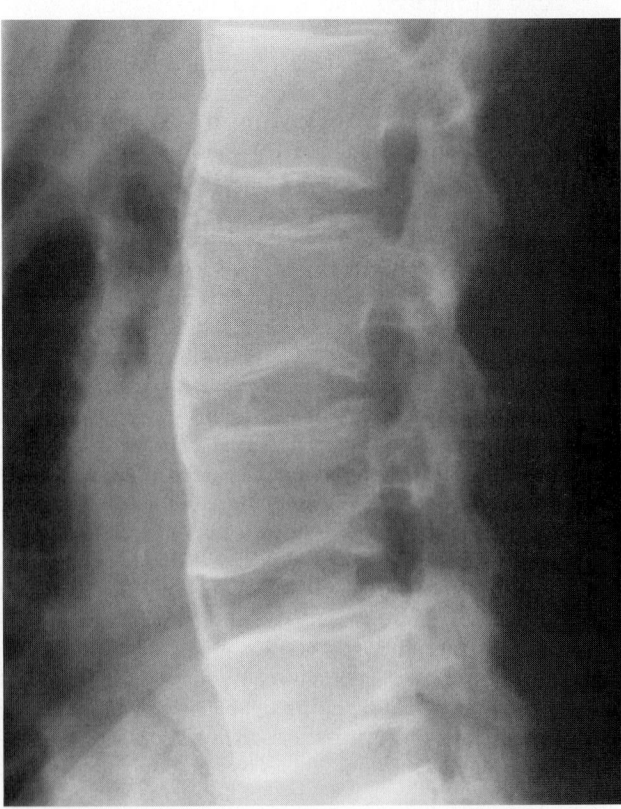

Figure 3 **Progression of ankylosing spondylitis is demonstrated by ossification of the anterior fibers of the annulus fibrosus (syndesmophytes).**

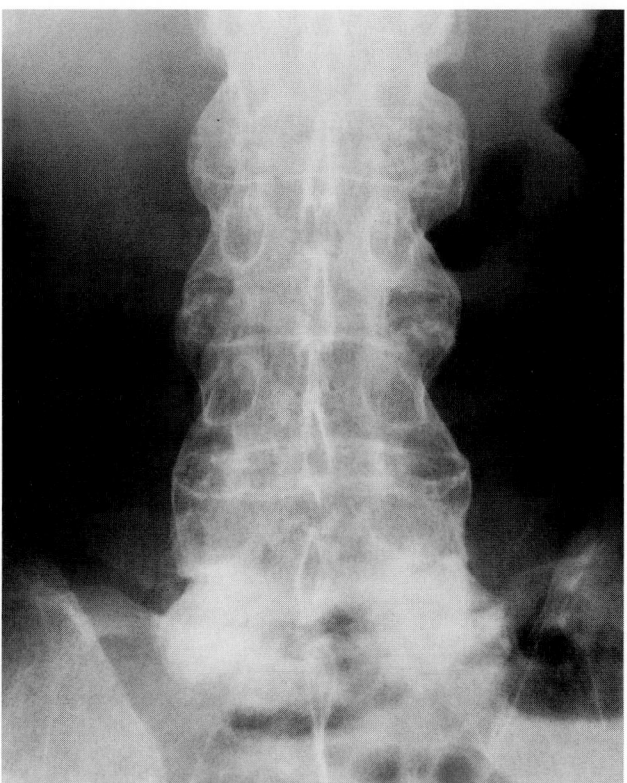

Figure 4   **Patients with severe ankylosing spondylitis may develop the classic bamboo spine, as shown in this radiograph.**

additional imaging with CT is often necessary.

A cauda equina syndrome occurs in rare instances, usually because of arachnoiditis around sacral nerves that leads to progressive leg weakness, paresthesias, and sphincter dysfunction.[38]

Retroperitoneal fibrosis   Fibrosis in the retroperitoneum may be another extra-articular feature of ankylosing spondylitis.[39]

TREATMENT AND PROGNOSIS

Early diagnosis and treatment of ankylosing spondylitis appear to improve functional outcome, but it is not clear whether any drug modifies the disease pathology. Objectives of treatment are pain relief, reduction of inflammation, and maintenance of good posture and spinal function.[40] Patient education is very important. Excellent sources for patient education are available at www.spondylitis.org and www.arthritis.org.

Nonsteroidal anti-inflammatory drugs (NSAIDs) relieve inflammatory symptoms of pain and stiffness and allow patients to engage in an appropriate exercise program. In clinical practice, certain NSAIDs appear to be more often effective than others as treatment for spondyloarthritis [see Table 3]. However, the efficacy of individual agents varies greatly from patient to patient; for that reason, some patients may need to try several NSAIDs before finding one that provides relief. There is no strong evidence that any NSAIDs alter disease progression.

There are now incontrovertible data that selective cyclooxygenase-2 (COX-2) inhibitors, and possibly other NSAIDs, increase a person's risk for cardiovascular disease. Therefore, careful assessment of other risk factors and of the potential benefit compared with risk is essential in all patients. Gastrointestinal intolerance of any of the NSAIDs may present as nausea, gastric discomfort, diarrhea, or, more seriously, gut hemorrhage or perfo-

ration. Concomitant use of a gastroprotective agent, such as misoprostol or a proton pump inhibitor, may significantly reduce GI toxicity in patients treated with NSAIDs. All of these drugs may decrease renal tubular capacity to secrete potassium and can cause an abrupt reduction in renal function when used in patients with renal disease or with renal hypoperfusion resulting from ineffective circulatory volume. Because patients with ankylosing spondylitis will probably take NSAIDs for many years, physicians must diligently monitor for renal and GI tract damage.

In a 6-month randomized, controlled clinical trial, the bisphosphonate pamidronate, given monthly by intravenous infusion, was shown to be effective in improving symptoms and function in patients with ankylosing spondylitis whose disease was refractory to treatment with NSAIDs.[41]

Low-dose corticosteroids (e.g., prednisone, 5 to 10 mg daily) may be necessary to quell inflammation in some patients with highly active disease, but these agents should be used sparingly because they promote osteoporosis and do not improve spinal disease. Injection of repository corticosteroids into affected peripheral joints also may be useful. Injection into the sacroiliac joint, guided by either CT or MRI, may offer relief.

Sulfasalazine, 2 to 3 g daily in two divided doses, has been shown in several placebo-controlled trials to be an effective long-term treatment of ankylosing spondylitis, as well as of other types of spondyloarthritis. Sulfasalazine is very effective for peripheral joint symptoms but not especially effective for axial joint symptoms.[1,40] The drug moiety responsible for the efficacy of sulfasalazine has been proved to be sulfapyridine rather than salicylate; however, it is not clear whether the efficacy results from antimicrobial or other properties of the drug.[42] Because sulfasalazine has been shown to lower acute-phase reactants, such as the ESR and the CRP level, it may modify disease progression; however, this desirable effect has yet to be proved.

Other long-acting agents used to treat rheumatoid arthritis, including gold salts, penicillamine, and hydroxychloroquine, are not effective in ankylosing spondylitis.[40] Methotrexate therapy, which is highly effective for rheumatoid arthritis, is clearly effective in psoriatic arthritis but not in other forms of spondyloarthritis.[6] Administration of radiation therapy to the spine was once used successfully but is no longer recommended because of the risk of subsequent malignancy.

The TNF antagonists etanercept and infliximab have been approved for the treatment of ankylosing spondylitis, as well as psoriatic arthritis. An increasing number of controlled and open-label studies of the use of these agents in each of the forms of spondyloarthritis have shown dramatic and rapid improvement in symptoms; significantly reduced inflammatory changes in the spine and peripheral joints, as evidenced on MRI; and lowered acute-phase reactants such as ESR and CRP. Long-term efficacy and modification of disease progression and outcome have yet to be determined.[5,43-45] Treatment with TNF-α antagonists also has been shown to halt progression of secondary amyloidosis.[46] Because of the high cost of these agents and still-unanswered questions about their long-term safety, guidelines have been developed by international consensus to facilitate the judicious use of TNF antagonists.[5] Many patients with mild disease may never require TNF antagonists.

All patients with ankylosing spondylitis should be informed of potential spinal deformities and how to prevent them. Good posture should be emphasized. A firm mattress and minimal pillow support are recommended. An exercise program of spinal extension and peripheral joint range-of-motion exercises, along

Table 3 Treatment for Spondyloarthritis

Drug	Dose	Efficacy Rating	Comments
Indomethacin*	50 mg t.i.d. or 75 mg SR, q. 12 hr	Effective for symptoms	Side effects: headaches, changes in mentation, peptic ulcers, GI toxicity, intolerance, renal insufficiency
Tolmetin*	600 mg t.i.d.	Effective for symptoms	Side effects: peptic ulcers, GI toxicity, renal insufficiency
Piroxicam*	20 mg q.d.	Effective for symptoms	Side effects: peptic ulcers, GI toxicity, renal insufficiency
Diclofenac*	75 mg b.i.d.	Effective for symptoms	Side effects: peptic ulcers, GI toxicity, renal insufficiency
Sulfasalazine†	1–3 g daily in two divided doses	Long-term efficacy; lowers acute-phase reactants	Side effects: headache, GI intolerance
Methotrexate†	7.5–20 mg weekly	Effective for skin and arthritis in psoriatic arthritis; effectiveness in other diseases unproved	Side effects: GI intolerance, hepatotoxicity, marrow suppression, pulmonary disease
Doxycycline†	100 mg bi.d.	Effective in preventing relapse and in long-term treatment of reactive arthritis only	Side effects: GI intolerance, photosensitivity
Infliximab†	5 mg/kg I.V. every 6–8 wk after loading	Highly effective and immediate response; improved inflammation in joints by MRI; long-term effects unknown	Side effects: allergic reactions; increased susceptibility to infection, especially tuberculosis
Etanercept†	25 mg subcutaneous injections twice a week	Same as infliximab	Injection-site reactions, increased risk of infections

*Concomitant treatment with a proton pump inhibitor or misoprostol recommended for gastric protection.
†Potentially disease-modifying agents.
GI—gastrointestinal   MRI—magnetic resonance imaging   NSAIDs—nonsteroidal anti-inflammatory drugs   SR—slow release

with hydrotherapy, should be prescribed. Swimming is a very effective means of achieving exercise goals.[1,5]

Some patients who experience hip involvement—a major cause of disability—greatly benefit from total hip replacement. Wedge osteotomy for severe spinal kyphosis is available only at a few medical centers. Treatment of spinal fractures is controversial. Pregnancy does not appear to be significantly affected by ankylosing spondylitis.

The prognosis for individual patients is often difficult to ascertain.[47] Worse outcomes have been associated primarily with hip joint involvement and, to a lesser extent, early age at onset. The course of the disease in its first 10 years appears to predict its future course and the functional outcome. Despite long-standing and severe disease, ankylosing spondylitis often does not affect a patient's ability to work. Mortality from the disease is infrequent but may result from cardiac or neurologic complications or amyloidosis.

Reactive Arthritis

Reactive arthritis was originally defined as the triad of nongonococcal urethritis, conjunctivitis, and arthritis. It is now recognized that most patients present with arthritis alone and have no clinical evidence of urethritis or conjunctivitis.[15,16,23,24] The concept of reactive arthritis arose from observations that the disease followed certain enteric infections (such cases are termed epidemic or postenteric) and sexually acquired infections (such cases are termed endemic or postvenereal) [see Pathogenesis, Environmental Factors, above]. Despite this association with previous infection, affected sites were seemingly sterile when cultured for bacteria. It has been found that bacterial antigens, if not viable microorganisms, are present in the joints of affected patients[15,16,26] [see Pathology, above]. Like ankylosing spondylitis, reactive arthritis may be complicated by sacroiliitis, spondylitis, uveitis,

and cardiac lesions. It is also strongly associated with HLA-B27 [see Table 2].

EPIDEMIOLOGY

Reactive arthritis probably has a worldwide distribution, but most epidemiologic and clinical studies have come from Europe and the United States.[15-17] The prevalence of the disease is difficult to ascertain because it changes over time, depending on sexual behavior and the prevalence of enteric pathogens in different populations.[48] It was estimated that from 1950 to 1980 in Rochester, Minnesota, the incidence of reactive arthritis in men younger than 50 years was 0.035%; however, 10- to 20-fold higher rates were reported in homosexual men and in certain Native Americans in whom the frequency of HLA-B27 was high (30% to 40%) and who had endemic exposure to enteric or venereal pathogens.[15]

Reactive arthritis, probably the postvenereal form, is the most common cause of inflammatory arthritis in young men. The disease is recognized in women far less frequently; the reasons for this are unclear, because the ratio of affected men to affected women after epidemics of gastroenteritis is typically 1:1 and, overall, the incidence of reactive arthritis approaches 1% to 2% of persons infected with any of the triggering pathogens.[15,16,26] The incidence appears to have fallen significantly since the HIV epidemic and the adoption of safer sexual practices.[48]

HLA-B27 is found in 63% to 75% of patients with both forms of reactive arthritis and confers a relative risk of approximately 37. Of persons with HLA-B27 who are infected with one of the causative bacteria, reactive arthritis develops in approximately 20%.

DIAGNOSIS

Clinical Presentation

Reactive arthritis typically develops 10 to 30 days after an episode of gastroenteritis or sexual exposure to a venereal pathogen; however, many patients deny any such antecedent events.[15] Episodes of urethritis or conjunctivitis may have been mild and transient or not perceived at all. Thus, recognition of the pattern of musculoskeletal involvement, as well as several other mucocutaneous manifestations, is important in establishing the correct diagnosis.

The arthritis usually is oligoarticular and asymmetrical and predominantly affects lower-extremity joints, most often the knees, ankles, and feet. Diffuse, painful swelling of entire digits (sausaging or dactylitis) occurs frequently. Pain in the heels from Achilles tendinitis or plantar fasciitis, or both, reflects the most common sites of enthesitis; however, enthesopathic pain at other sites is also frequent.[30] Low back pain is a complaint of 60% of patients, and 20% ultimately experience radiographically detectable sacroiliitis. An ascending spondylitis ensues in approximately 10% to 12% of patients.

One or more of the mucocutaneous features can be found on examination in more than 50% of patients, usually early in the disease. Keratoderma blennorrhagica is a papulosquamous skin rash that usually begins on the soles or palms as painless and nonpruritic excrescences resembling mollusk shells [see Figure 5]. With time, these lesions evolve into scaling plaques that may coalesce into a more generalized exfoliative dermatitis. Keratoderma blennorrhagica is clinically and histopathologically the same as the disorder pustular psoriasis [see Chapter 37]. A similar scaling rash on the glans penis in circumcised men is termed circinate balanitis. Moist, shallow ulcers characterize balanitis in uncircumcised men, who may be unaware of the lesions unless the foreskin is retracted [see Figure 6]. Similar painless oral ulcers may be found on the tongue or palate. Nails may become hyperkeratotic, thickened, and deformed, but the characteristic nail

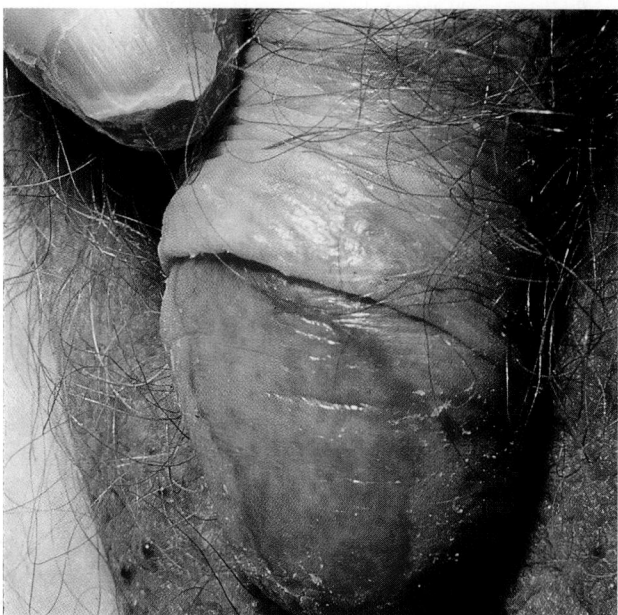

Figure 6 **Superficial penile ulceration of circinate balanitis in an uncircumcised patient with reactive arthritis. Also note dystrophic fingernail.**

pitting of psoriasis is usually absent [see Figure 6]. It is important to search for all of these lesions; they are frequently asymptomatic but are definitive and can establish a diagnosis.

Some patients experience low-grade or high fever at disease onset; malaise—or even prostration—and significant weight loss may ensue. Acute anterior uveitis occurs in approximately 20% of patients with reactive arthritis. Cardiac bradyarrhythmia, aortic regurgitation, or both may also occur during the acute disease phase or may appear later in patients whose illness follows a chronic course.[34] Patients with reactive arthritis who are HLA-B27 positive are more likely to experience sacroiliitis and spondylitis, as well as uveitis, cardiac lesions, or both, and to experience a prolonged disease course.

Reactive arthritis has been frequently described in patients with HIV infection; the joint and skin disease may be more severe than usual in such persons.[15,16,26] This association is now believed to result from sexually acquired enteric and venereal pathogens common to both diseases.

Laboratory Evaluation

Tests of patients with reactive arthritis usually show a modest leukocytosis, thrombocytosis, and anemia, along with elevation of the ESR, reflecting systemic inflammation. Examination of the synovial fluid reveals inflammatory changes of poor mucin clot and leukocytosis; but in contrast to septic arthritis, the glucose level is not low, and bacterial cultures are negative. Polymerase chain reaction (PCR) analysis of synovial fluid or tissue biopsies has been used successfully to detect specific bacterial DNA or RNA in research laboratories; PCR kits should become clinically available soon.[49] Cultures or molecular probes for *C. trachomatis* should be obtained in patients with venereal exposure, genitourinary symptoms, or both.[50] At the same time, tests for concomitant gonorrhea, syphilis, and HIV infection should be performed. In patients with preceding GI symptoms, stool cultures for the triggering organisms are usually negative by the time joint symptoms appear. Serologic tests for *Salmonella* and other enteric pathogens are usually unreliable but may be useful in some cases.[51]

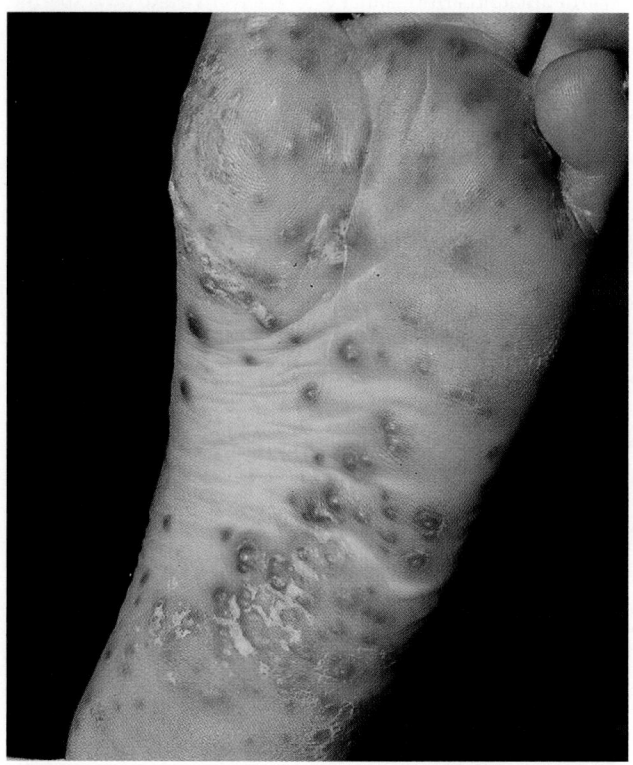

Figure 5 **Typical keratoderma blennorrhagica rash of reactive arthritis on the sole of the foot.**

Radiographic Features

X-rays are of no diagnostic value early in the disease; however, MRI may show inflammatory changes of enthesitis and arthritis. After several months of persistent joint symptoms, enthesopathic symptoms, or both, radiographs may show the distinctive changes of periostitis and bony ankylosis. Patients with chronic heel pain may show a fluffy periosteal reaction or spur formation at the Achilles or plantar tendon insertions.[30] Similar radiographic changes may be seen along metatarsal or phalangeal bones of the feet; bony fusion across joints may be visible. Sacroiliitis, when present, is more often unilateral than bilateral, and large asymmetrical syndesmophytes may be seen in the lumbar spine.[31]

TREATMENT AND PROGNOSIS

Reactive arthritis runs a self-limited course in most patients, lasting 4 to 12 months, although annoying residual musculoskeletal symptoms may persist for years.[51] From 15% to 30% of patients suffer permanent disability.[40] Relapses are not uncommon; it is unclear whether they result from repeat infection or other endogenous mechanisms. The same NSAIDs used to treat ankylosing spondylitis [*see* Ankylosing Spondylitis, Treatment and Prognosis, *above*] [*see* Table 3] are usually effective in quieting inflammatory joint symptoms. Some patients with highly active disease, however, may require short courses of low-dose systemic corticosteroids or repository corticosteroid injections into joints.

Early treatment of genitourinary infections with appropriate antibiotics (e.g., tetracycline or erythromycin) has been shown to reduce the likelihood of subsequent reactive arthritis; however, even early antibiotic use in patients with gastroenteritis does not appear to prevent reactive arthritis.[15,40] A blinded, placebo-controlled trial of the use of tetracycline for the treatment of reactive arthritis demonstrated that the duration of disease was shortened only in patients who had *Chlamydia*-induced disease.[40] Ciprofloxacin has not been shown to shorten the course of chronic reactive arthritis.[40] Controlled studies have shown that sulfasalazine, in dosages similar to those used in the treatment of ankylosing spondylitis, is effective in all forms of spondyloarthritis.[40] Whether any of these antibiotic approaches change the natural history of the disease remains to be proved. Patients with spondyloarthritis that persists despite treatment with NSAIDs and antibiotics may benefit from the use of anti-TNF agents. An increasing number of studies are documenting immediate and dramatic benefit from the use of TNF-α antagonists (e.g., infliximab and etanercept) in such patients.[43] Physical therapy is important in maintaining joint motion and preventing disability.

Psoriatic Arthritis

EPIDEMIOLOGY

The prevalence of cutaneous psoriasis is estimated to be 2% in most white populations; it appears to be lower in populations who are of African or Asian ancestry.[52] An inflammatory arthropathy attributable to psoriasis appears in 5% to 7% of patients with the skin disease, especially in those whose nails are affected.[6] Psoriasis is highly familial, and there is strong evidence that it is a complex genetic disease associated with several HLA alleles and other non–HLA-linked loci[5,53] [*see* Pathogenesis, *above*]. Genomic studies now strongly suggest major but yet unidentified loci for psoriasis susceptibility near HLA-C in the MHC region and on chromosome 17.[5,10] HLA-B27 is only weakly associated with psoriasis and peripheral psoriatic arthritis, but it occurs in 50% of persons who have psoriatic spondylitis. Poten-

tial environmental triggers are streptococcal infection and physical trauma. Psoriatic arthritis is slightly more common in females than in males. Psoriasis frequently first appears in childhood; psoriatic arthritis typically appears in early or middle adulthood, although there are many exceptions. The arthritis may appear before the psoriasis in as many as 40% of children and 15% of adults. Although the incidence of psoriasis and psoriatic arthritis in HIV-positive persons is similar to that in uninfected persons, severe exacerbations of both skin disease and joint disease have been observed in patients with HIV infection, especially as the number of CD4+ T cells declines.

DIAGNOSIS

Clinical Presentation

In general, there is little relation between joint and skin severity. In fact, psoriatic skin lesions may be found only after careful scrutiny of the scalp, the umbilicus, or the gluteal region, and nail pitting or other changes may be the only clues supporting a diagnosis of psoriatic arthritis. Several clinical patterns of joint involvement, often overlapping, have been described:

1. Asymmetrical oligoarthritis of both small and large joints is the most common form of psoriatic arthritis. Involvement of distal interphalangeal joints and sausage-shaped toes or fingers are highly suggestive signs. A disparity is often noted between clinical appearance and subjective symptoms; overtly involved joints may be largely asymptomatic, unlike the concordance usually found in rheumatoid arthritis.
2. Symmetrical polyarthritis may resemble rheumatoid arthritis, although tests for rheumatoid factor and antibodies to cyclic citrullinated peptides (anti-CCP) should be negative. Anti-CCP is a newly discovered autoantibody marker for rheumatoid arthritis that is 65% sensitive and 96% specific. Uncertainty about classification is reasonable because psoriasis and rheumatoid arthritis are both relatively common diseases and are expected to occur together by chance.
3. Arthritis mutilans is the most destructive form of psoriatic arthritis; it occurs in approximately 5% of patients with psoriatic arthritis. Striking bone resorption and telescoping of fingers (opera-glass hand) are characteristic. Affected patients often have concomitant spinal involvement.
4. Psoriatic spondylitis occurs in approximately 20% of patients with psoriatic arthritis, often with unilateral sacroiliitis and large asymmetrical syndesmophytes, similar to the pattern seen in patients with reactive arthritis.
5. Dominant or exclusively distal interphalangeal joint involvement with psoriatic nail changes may occur.

Laboratory Findings

An elevated ESR or CRP level, anemia, and hyperuricemia may be found. Rheumatoid factor, anti-CCP, and antinuclear antibody tests are negative. Synovial fluid shows nonspecific inflammatory changes.

Radiographic Features

A characteristic change is whittling of the distal ends of phalanges, giving the joints a so-called pencil-in-cup appearance, which is radiographically distinctive for psoriatic arthritis. Periostitis—which results in whiskering around joints—bony erosions, and joint fusion in the absence of osteopenia also are common and diagnostically useful findings.

TREATMENT AND PROGNOSIS

NSAIDs similar to those used for ankylosing spondylitis [*see* Ankylosing Spondylitis, Treatment and Prognosis, *above*] [*see Table 3*] are the mainstay of arthritis therapy in most patients but have no effect on the skin disease, which may require separate dermatologic approaches [*see Chapter 37*]. Sulfasalazine, methotrexate, or cyclosporine may be beneficial for both skin and joint disease in NSAID-resistant or severe, progressive disease.[6] Well-controlled studies have demonstrated that TNF-α antagonists (etanercept and infliximab) are highly effective for symptoms and probably modify outcomes for both the arthritis and the skin disease.[43] Gold, penicillamine, and hydroxychloroquine are not useful agents.

Psoriatic arthritis usually runs a more benign course than rheumatoid arthritis does, although clearly there are many patients with severe disease. Many patients with psoriatic arthritis maintain reasonable function, often despite extensive deformities.

Enteropathic Arthritis

Two major clinical patterns of arthritis associated with inflammatory bowel diseases are peripheral arthritis and spondylitis.

PERIPHERAL ARTHRITIS

Approximately 20% of patients with Crohn disease or ulcerative colitis experience an acute peripheral arthritis.[20] Symmetrical swelling of the knees, ankles, or wrists is the most common articular pattern; large effusions may occur. The pathogenesis of the arthritis is unknown, but the disease occurs during periods of active inflammation of the gut and may be the first sign of a bowel flare-up. HLA-B27 is not increased in frequency among inflammatory bowel disease patients with peripheral arthritis, as compared with the normal population. Extraskeletal and extraintestinal manifestations may occur simultaneously and include fever, acute anterior uveitis, painful oral ulcers, erythema nodosum (in Crohn disease), and pyoderma gangrenosum (in ulcerative colitis). Treatment of the arthritis should be aimed at controlling the inflammatory bowel disease. The arthritis seldom results in deformities.

SPONDYLITIS

Sacroiliitis develops in about 10% of patients with inflammatory bowel disease. Clinically, the spondylitis may progress to total spinal ankylosis; radiographically, it is indistinguishable from ankylosing spondylitis.[20,31] There is no correlation of the spondylitis with activity of the bowel disease. HLA-B27 is found in approximately 50% of such patients. Therapy is largely the same as for ankylosing spondylitis [*see* Ankylosing Spondylitis, Treatment and Prognosis, *above*]. Despite the bowel disease, NSAIDs are usually well tolerated.

UNDIFFERENTIATED SPONDYLOARTHRITIS

Inevitably, the presentations of many patients do not conform to the typical presentations described above, and the symptoms and signs defy specific disease classification.[1,54] Examples are a patient with unilateral sacroiliitis, a sausage digit, and uveitis; a patient with typical reactive arthritis who experiences psoriatic arthritis; and a patient with typical ankylosing spondylitis who years later experiences Crohn disease. Such patients are often designated as having undifferentiated spondyloarthritis. The ESSG criteria[1] now make the classification of patients with spondyloarthritis more definitive. There remains, however, a large number of patients with formes frustes that do not fulfill the new crite-

ria but probably fall within the spectrum of spondyloarthritis. Such entities, which are strongly associated with HLA-B27, are chronic inflammatory back and chest pain syndromes (in which radiographs are normal), chronic dactylitis, chronic plantar fasciitis or Achilles tendinitis, pustular psoriasis (keratoderma blennorrhagica), circinate balanitis, acute anterior uveitis, and spondylitic heart disease without evidence of arthritis. In patients suspected of having a limited form of spondyloarthritis, typing for HLA-B27 may prove clinically useful in supporting such a diagnosis.[1,54]

Juvenile Spondyloarthritis

Until recently, the term juvenile rheumatoid arthritis was used, inappropriately, to describe all forms of chronic childhood arthritis. Careful clinical evaluation, autoantibody testing, and HLA typing have revealed a heterogeneous group of diseases in which only a small proportion of affected children truly have rheumatoid arthritis.

Juvenile spondyloarthritis occurs most often in boys; it typically begins in late childhood or adolescence with lower extremity oligoarthropathy and enthesopathy.[28] Spinal symptoms are rare initially but often appear years later. Bony ankylosis of the tarsal bones has been described in some of these patients. Acute anterior uveitis is not uncommon. Such patients are seronegative for rheumatoid factor, anti-CCP, and antinuclear antibodies but are positive for HLA-B27. Less often, a patient may present with chronic polyarthritis with prominent cervical spine fusion rather than lower spine involvement.

Subsets of juvenile arthritis include the following:

1. Oligoarthritis appearing in early childhood, more often in girls; it is associated with antinuclear antibodies, a high risk of chronic iridocyclitis and blindness, and HLA-DR5 (DR11), HLA-DR8, or HLA-DR6, as well as HLA-DP2, but not HLA-B27.
2. Polyarthritis appearing in early childhood, more often in girls who are seronegative for rheumatoid factor and antinuclear antibodies; it is associated with HLA-DR8 and HLA-DP3 but not HLA-B27.
3. Polyarthritis associated with rheumatoid factor, anti-CCP, and HLA-DR4 (but not HLA-B27), which probably represents true juvenile rheumatoid arthritis.
4. Still disease, characterized by high, spiking fever, evanescent rash, hepatosplenomegaly, lymphadenopathy, and polyarthritis in patients who are seronegative and HLA-B27 negative.

Miscellaneous Arthropathies

ACNE-ASSOCIATED ARTHRITIS

A rare inflammatory oligoarthritis may occur in patients with severe forms of acne, including acne conglobata, acne fulminans, hidradenitis suppurativa, and dissecting cellulitis of the scalp.[55] Such patients experience fever and inflamed joints; symptoms resemble those of septic arthritis, but the joints are sterile by culture. Sacroiliitis has been described in some patients.

SAPHO is an acronym for a syndrome that consists of synovitis, severe acne, palmoplantar pustulosis, hyperostosis, and osteitis and that may be a form of spondyloarthritis.[55-57] These arthritides may represent forms of reactive arthritis, but patients are usually HLA-B27 negative. Antibiotic therapy is usually of little or no benefit, but some patients respond to NSAIDs or low-dose corticosteroids. Surgical excision of the affected skin, when possible, has been reported to resolve the arthritis.

WHIPPLE DISEASE

Whipple disease is a rare multisystem disorder that usually affects men (the ratio of affected men to women is 9:1). Patients may present with arthralgias or transient episodes of additive, symmetrical polyarthritis that is nondeforming. Sacroiliitis has been reported in rare instances, and the frequency of HLA-B27 may be increased in patients with Whipple disease. Patients usually have GI symptoms, including diarrhea, steatorrhea, and profound weight loss. Other clues to diagnosis are skin hyperpigmentation, serositis (pleural effusions), lymphadenopathy, uveitis, nervous system disease (ocular palsies or encephalopathy), leukocytosis, and thrombocytosis. The diagnosis traditionally has been based on small-bowel biopsies showing deposits on periodic acid–Schiff staining or electron microscopic demonstration of rodlike bacillary organisms in intestinal macrophages. The causative organism has been identified by RNA sequence analysis and cultured as a gram-positive actinomycete named *Tropheryma whippelii*.[58] Diagnosis can be made on the basis of results from PCR analysis of DNA from affected tissues or blood samples. Long-term treatment with tetracycline usually results in complete remission.

The author has no commercial relationships with manufacturers of products or providers of services discussed in this chapter.

References

1. Khan MA: Update on spondyloarthropathies. Ann Intern Med 136:896, 2002

2. Lawrence RC, Helmick CG, Arnett FC, et al: Estimates of the prevalence of arthritis and selected musculoskeletal disorders in the United States. Arthritis Rheum 41:778, 1998

3. Braun J, Bollow M, Remlinger G, et al: Prevalence of spondyloarthropathies in HLA-B27 positive and negative blood donors. Arthritis Rheum 41:58, 1998

4. Wordsworth P: Genes in the spondyloarthropathies. Rheum Dis Clin North Am 24:845, 1998

5. Reveille JD, Arnett FC: Spondyloarthritis: update on pathogenesis and management. Am J Med 118:592, 2005

6. Gladman DD: Psoriatic arthritis. Rheum Dis Clin North Am 24:829, 1998

7. Hampe J, Shaw SH, Saiz R, et al: Linkage of inflammatory bowel disease to human chromosome 6p. Am J Hum Genet 65:1647, 1999

8. Hugot JP, Chamaillard M, Zouali H, et al: Association of NOD2 leucine-rich repeat variants with susceptibility to Crohn's disease. Nature 411:599, 2001

9. Rioux JD, Daly MJ, Silverberg MS, et al: Genetic variation in the 5q31 cytokine gene cluster confers susceptibility to Crohn's disease. Nat Genet 29:223, 2001

10. Höhler T, Märker-Hermann E: Psoriatic arthritis: clinical aspects, genetics and the role of T cells. Curr Opin Rheumatol 13:273, 2001

11. Taurog JD, Maika SD, Satumtira N, et al: Inflammatory disease in HLA-B27 transgenic rats. Immunol Rev 169:209, 1999

12. Märker-Hermann E, Höhler T: Pathogenesis of human leukocyte antigen B27–positive arthritis: information from clinical materials. Rheum Dis Clin North Am 24:865, 1998

13. Elkman P, Saarinen M, He Q, et al: HLA-B27–transfected (*Salmonella* permissive) and HLA-A2–transfected (*Salmonella* permissive) human monocyte U937 cells differ in their production of cytokines. Infect Immun 70:1609, 2002

14. Lerisalo-Repo M, Hannu T, Mattila L, et al: Microbial factors in spondyloarthropathies: insights from population studies. Curr Opin Rheumatol 15: 408, 2003

15. Amor B: Reiter's syndrome: diagnosis and clinical features. Rheum Dis Clin North Am 24:677, 1998

16. Seiper J: Disease mechanisms in reactive arthritis. Curr Opin Rheumatol 16:110, 2004

17. Vittecoqoq O, Schaeverbeke T, Favre S, et al: Molecular diagnosis of *Ureaplasma urealyticum* in an immunocompetent patient with destructive reactive polyarthritis. Arthritis Rheum 40:2084, 1997

18. Hannu T, Puolakkainen M, Leirisalo-Repo M: *Chlamydia pneumoniae* as a triggering infection in reactive arthritis. Rheumatology 38:411, 1999

19. Montenegro V, Monteiro RC: Elevation of serum IgA in spondyloarthropathies and IgA nephropathy and its pathogenic role. Curr Opin Rheumatol 11:265, 1999

20. De Keyser F, Elewaut D, DeVos M, et al: Bowel inflammation and the spondyloarthropathies. Rheum Dis Clin North Am 24:785, 1998

21. Braun J, Bollow M, Neure L, et al: Use of immunohistologic and in situ hybridization techniques in the examination of sacroiliac joint biopsy specimens from patients with ankylosing spondylitis. Arthritis Rheum 38:499, 1995

22. Rudwaleit M, Höhler T: Cytokine gene polymorphisms relevant for the spondyloarthropathies. Curr Opin Rheumatol 13:250, 2001

23. Gerard HC, Branigan PJ, Schumacher HR, et al: Synovial *Chlamydia trachomatis* in patients with reactive arthritis/Reiter's syndrome are viable but show aberrant gene expression. J Rheumatol 25:734, 1998

24. Nikkari S, Rantakokko K, Ekman P, et al: *Salmonella*-triggered reactive arthritis. Arthritis Rheum 42:84, 1999

25. Braun J, Tuszewski M, Ehlers S, et al: Nested polymerase chain reaction strategy simultaneously targeting DNA sequences of multiple bacterial species in inflammatory joint diseases: examination of sacroiliac and knee joint biopsies of patients with spondyloarthropathies and other arthritides. J Rheumatol 24:1101, 1997

26. Lau CS, Burgos-Vargas R, Louthrenoo W, et al: Features of spondyloarthritis around the world. Rheum Dis Clin North Am 24:753, 1998

27. Blanco-Gelaz MA, Lopez-Vazquez A, Garcia-Fernandez S, et al: Genetic variability, molecular evolution, and geographic diversity of HLA-B27. Hum Immunol 62:1042, 2001

28. Burgos-Vargas R, Pacheco-Tena C, Vazquez-Mellado J: Juvenile-onset spondyloarthropathies. Rheum Dis Clin North Am 23:569, 1997

29. van Tubergen A, Coenen J, Landewe R, et al: Assessment of fatigue in patients with ankylosing spondylitis: a psychometric analysis. Arthritis Rheum 47:8, 2002

30. Francois RJ, Braun J, Khan MA: Entheses and enthesitis: a histopathologic review and relevance to spondyloarthropathies. Curr Opin Rheumatol 13:255, 2001

31. Helliwell PS, Hickling P, Wright V: Do the radiological changes of classic ankylosing spondylitis differ from the changes found in the spondylitis associated with inflammatory bowel disease, psoriasis, and reactive arthritis? Ann Rheum Dis 57:135, 1998

32. Resnick D, Shapiro RF, Wiesner KB, et al: Diffuse idiopathic skeletal hyperostosis (ankylosing hyperostosis of Forestier and Rotes-Querol). Semin Arthritis Rheum 7:153, 1978

33. Banares A, Hernandez-Garcia C, Fernandez-Gutierrez B, et al: Eye involvement in the spondyloarthropathies. Rheum Dis Clin North Am 24:771, 1998

34. Bergfeldt L: HLA-B27–associated cardiac disease. Ann Intern Med 127:621, 1997

35. Roldan CA, Chavez J, Wiest PW, et al: Aortic root disease and valve disease associated with ankylosing spondylitis. J Am Coll Cardiol 32:1397, 1998

36. Casserly IP, Fenlon HM, Breatnach E, et al: Lung findings on high-resolution computed tomography in idiopathic ankylosing spondylitis: correlation with clinical findings, pulmonary function testing and plain radiography. Br J Rheumatol 36:677, 1997

37. Gratacos J, Orellana C, Sanmarti R, et al: Secondary amyloidosis in ankylosing spondylitis: a systematic survey of 137 patients using abdominal fat aspiration. J Rheumatol 24:912, 1997

38. Charlesworth CH, Savy LE, Stevens J, et al: MRI demonstration of arachnoiditis in cauda equina syndrome of ankylosing spondylitis. Neuroradiology 38:462, 1996

39. LeBlanc CM, Inman RD, Dent P, et al: Retroperitoneal fibrosis: an extraarticular manifestation of ankylosing spondylitis. Arthritis Rheum 47:210, 2002

40. Leirisalo-Repo M: Prognosis, course of disease, and treatment of the spondyloarthropathies. Rheum Dis Clin North Am 24:737, 1998

41. Maksymowych WP, Jhangri GS, Fitzgerald AA, et al: A six-month randomized, controlled, double-blind, dose-response comparison of intravenous pamidronate (60 mg versus 10 mg) in the treatment of nonsteroidal antiinflammatory drug–refractory ankylosing spondylitis. Arthritis Rheum 46:766, 2002

42. Taggart A, Gardiner P, McEvoy F, et al: Which is the active moiety of sulfasalazine in ankylosing spondylitis? A randomized, controlled study. Arthritis Rheum 39:1400, 1999

43. Braun J, de Keyser F, Brandt J, et al: New treatment options in spondyloarthropathies: increasing evidence for significant efficacy of anti–tumor necrosis factor therapy. Curr Opin Rheumatol 13:245, 2001

44. Gorman JD, Sack KE, Davis JC Jr: Treatment of ankylosing spondylitis by inhibition of tumor necrosis factor alpha. N Engl J Med 346:1349, 2002

45. Braun J, Brandt J, Listing J, et al: Treatment of active ankylosing spondylitis with infliximab: a randomised controlled multicentre trial. Lancet 359:1187, 2002

46. Fernandez-Nebro A, Tomero E, Ottiz-Santamaria V, et al: Treatment of rheumatic inflammatory disease in 25 patients with secondary amyloidosis using tumor necrosis factor alpha antagonists. Am J Med 118:552, 2005

47. Kerr HE, Sturrock RD: Clinical aspects, outcome assessment, disease course, and extra-articular features of spondyloarthropathies. Curr Opin Rheumatol 11:235, 1999

48. Iliopoulos A, Karras D, Ioakimidis D, et al: Change in the epidemiology of Reiter's syndrome (reactive arthritis) in the post-AIDS era? An analysis of cases appearing in the Greek army. J Rheumatol 22:252, 1995

49. Li F, Schumacher HR, Kieber-Emmons T, et al: Molecular detection of bacterial DNA in venereal-associated arthritis. Arthritis Rheum 39:950, 1996

50. Sieper J, Rudwaleit M, Braun J, et al: Diagnosing reactive arthritis: role of clinical setting in the value of serologic and microbiologic assays. Arthritis Rheum 46:319, 2002

51. Thomson GD, DeRubeis DA, Hodge MA, et al: Post-*Salmonella* reactive arthritis: late clinical sequelae in a point source cohort. Am J Med 98:13, 1995

52. Schon MP, Boehncke WH: Psoriasis. N Engl J Med 352:1899, 2005

53. Gladman DD, Farewell VT: The role of HLA antigens as indicators of disease progression in psoriatic arthritis. Arthritis Rheum 38:845, 1995

54. Olivier I, Salvarani C, Cantini F, et al: Ankylosing spondylitis and undifferentiated spondyloarthropathies: a clinical review and description of a disease subset with older age at onset. Curr Opin Rheumatol 13:280, 2001

55. Olafsson S, Khan MA: Musculoskeletal features of acne, hidradenitis suppurativa, and dissecting cellulitis of the scalp. Rheum Dis Clin North Am 18:215, 1992

56. Winchester R: Psoriatic arthritis and the spectrum of syndromes related to the SAPHO (synovitis, acne, pustulosis, hyperostosis, and osteitis) syndrome. Curr Opin Rheumatol 11:251, 1999

57. Hayem G, Bouchaud-Chabot A, Banali K, et al: SAPHO syndrome: a long-term follow up study of 120 cases. Semin Arthritis Rheum 29:159, 1999

58. Raoult D, Birg ML, La Scola B, et al: Cultivation of the bacillus of Whipple's disease. N Engl J Med 342:620, 2000

114 Systemic Lupus Erythematosus

Michael D. Lockshin, M.D., F.A.C.P.

Disease Definition and Subclassification

Lupus is a chronic autoimmune illness characterized by autoantibodies directed at nuclear antigens and causing a variety of clinical and laboratory abnormalities, including rash, arthritis, leukopenia and thrombocytopenia, alopecia, fever, nephritis, and neurologic disease. Most or all of the symptoms of acute lupus are attributable to immunologic attack on the affected organs. Many complications of long-term disease are attributable both to the disease and to its treatment.[1]

The term lupus applies to several variants of the illness [*see Table 1*], of which systemic lupus erythematosus (SLE) is the most serious and most common. SLE is the prototype of a systemic autoimmune illness, involving multiple organ systems in pathogenically similar ways. Characteristically, patients with SLE progress through periods of active inflammation (flare) and periods of quiescence (remission), both of which may occur spontaneously; periods of flare and quiescence may also be induced. The reasons for the varying course are unknown. Intense sun exposure, drug reactions, and infections are circumstances that are known to induce flare; the aim of treatment is to induce remission.

SLE may occur as an overlap syndrome that shares features with other autoimmune illnesses, such as mixed or undifferentiated connective tissue disease, dermatomyositis, Sjögren syndrome, rheumatoid arthritis, and scleroderma. Organ-specific autoimmune diseases, such as thyroiditis, autoimmune hemolytic anemia, and idiopathic thrombocytopenia, frequently accompany and may be part of SLE.

Lupus may also appear as a skin disease only. Discoid lupus occurs as a destructive, scarring rash, unaccompanied by systemic symptoms or autoantibodies.[2] Subacute cutaneous lupus comprises a characteristic persistent, polycyclic rash; relatively minor visceral symptoms; and strongly positive blood tests.

Drugs such as procainamide and some anticonvulsants induce a lupuslike syndrome, which is called drug-induced lupus.[3] Uncommonly, persons (often relatives of lupus patients) have positive blood tests for lupus but are clinically well. In the absence of symptoms, such persons are not considered to have lupus.

Approximately one third of lupus patients have antiphospholipid antibody, which induces blood clots and fetal death. The presence of this antibody, in the absence of clinical lupus, is referred to as primary antiphospholipid antibody syndrome.[4]

Neonatal lupus is a syndrome consisting of rash, thrombocytopenia, and congenital heart block occurring in infants born of mothers who carry antibody to the SS-A (Ro) and SS-B (La) antigens.[5] It does not evolve into SLE.

Epidemiology and Genetics

SLE is primarily a disease of young women, but the female predominance of SLE has not been explained. Women between 15 and 45 years of age are the most commonly affected; the female-to-male ratio in this age group is between 6:1 and 9:1. African Americans are four times as likely to develop lupus as are whites.[6] The disease incidence in Asians, Hispanics, and Native Americans falls between that of blacks and whites [*see Figure 1*]. No cogent explanation offered to date suggests why African Americans are more frequently affected; racial differences in SLE incidence persist when socioeconomic differences have been controlled. SLE severity in men is similar to that in women. Overall survival is lower in African Americans.[7]

The familial aspects of lupus are striking: approximately 10% of persons with lupus have family members with lupus or other autoimmune disease. Susceptibility to lupus is higher in persons with specific genetic deficiencies [*see Other Genetic Susceptibilities, below*].

Pathophysiology and Pathogenesis

AUTOANTIBODIES

Circulating antibodies to a broad list of autoantigens characterize SLE. Antinuclear antibodies, usually defined by immunofluorescence, are present in almost all lupus patients; tests for antinuclear antibody constitute a screening test (sensitive, but not specific) for the illness. Autoantibodies to nuclear constituents—primarily to double-stranded (native) DNA but also to single-stranded (denatured) DNA, histones, ribonuclear proteins, and other nuclear antigens, such as the Smith (Sm) antigen—confirm the diagnosis and are likely pathogenic. For example, these autoantibodies cause glomerulonephritis by inciting inflammation when deposited as complement-fixing immune complexes on glomerular basement membranes (GBMs) or by binding directly to the GBM.[8] Both animal models and clinical observations suggest that autoantibodies in the presence of complement mediate lupus-associated glomerulonephritis, hemolysis, and thrombocytopenia. Antibodies to phospholipid-binding proteins (beta$_2$-glycoprotein I, prothrombin, and others) mediate thrombosis and fetal loss. Lupus rash and arthritis are less clearly linked to autoantibodies, but immune reactants and inflammation are demonstrable in relevant biopsy specimens, primarily at the GBM.[9] Among lupus manifestations, neurologic lupus is least clearly caused by anti-DNA or other autoantibody; however, anti–ribosomal P antibody may define mood disorders in neurologic lupus.[10] A hypothesis that antibody to a glutamate receptor has diagnostic and pathogenic importance in SLE-associated cognitive dysfunction has proved to be untrue.[11]

ABNORMAL INNATE AND ADAPTIVE IMMUNITY

Genetic defects of immune complex processing are unusually frequent in lupus patients, suggesting that SLE arises because of incomplete or improper disposal of exogenous material.[12] Such defects include abnormalities in complement (deficiencies of C1q, C2, or C4), Fc receptor, apoptotic pathways, and phagocytic cells.[13] Defective clearance of immune complexes may result in their persistence in large quantities,[14] and autoantibodies may be a protective mechanism to neutralize them. Other theories of pathogenesis argue that genetic predispositions that promote T helper type 2 cell (Th2) responses or cytokine dysregulation are the underlying defects leading to the development of SLE.

In animal models, several immune defects that may cause SLE have been identified. These include abnormalities in genes affecting overall immunoreactivity (apoptosis [*Fas, Fas* ligand,

Table 1   Characteristic Features That Distinguish Lupus from Lupuslike Diseases

| Organ System | Lupus | | | | RA | Sjögren Syndrome |
	SLE	Discoid	Drug-Induced	Neonatal		
Skin	Specific rashes, alopecia, mucosal ulcers, periungual telangiectasia	Specific rash, alopecia, mucosal ulcers	Rash	Rash	Subcutaneous nodules	Dry eyes, dry mouth
Joints	Symmetrical nondestructive arthritis	—	Symmetrical nondestructive arthritis	—	Symmetrical destructive arthritis	Symmetrical destructive arthritis
Renal	Glomerulonephritis, renal failure	—	—	—	Amyloidosis (late)	Tubular dysfunction
CNS	Seizures, psychosis, cognitive dysfunction, stroke, myelopathy, neuropathy	—	—	—	Peripheral neuropathy	Peripheral and cranial neuropathy
Cardiac	—	—	—	Heart block	—	—
Blood						
ANA	Strong positive, any pattern	May be positive	Strong positive	Positive	May be positive	Positive
Complement	Low with renal disease or hemolytic anemia	Normal	Normal	Normal or low	Commonly high	Low or high
Diagnostic autoantibodies	Anti-dsDNA, anti-Sm	—	Antihistone	Anti–SS-A, anti–SS-B	Anti-IgG (rheumatoid factor)	Anti–SS-A, anti–SS-B
Other autoantibodies	Anti–SS-A (Ro), anti–SS-B (La), anti-RNP, anti-IgG, anti-ssDNA	Anti-ssDNA	Antihistone	Anti-RNP	—	Anti-IgG
Other abnormalities	Leukopenia, thrombocytopenia, hemolysis	—	Leukopenia	Thrombocytopenia, hemolysis	Leukocytosis, thrombocytosis	Hyperglobulinemia

ANA—antinuclear antibody   CNS—central nervous system   CPK—creatinine phosphokinase   dsDNA—double-stranded DNA   LLD—lupuslike disease   MCTD—mixed connective tissue disorder   PAPS— primary antiphospholipid syndrome   RA—rheumatoid arthritis   RNP—ribonucleoprotein   ssDNA—single-stranded DNA SLE—systemic lupus erythematosus   UCTD—undifferentiated connective tissue disease

(continued)

Bcl-2]), B cell activation (*FcγRIIB, SHP-1, CD22, CD19, PD-1, Lyn, Blys-1*), T cell activation (*TGF-β, TGF- βR, PD-1*), cell proliferation (*p21, Fli-1*), and cytokines (*IFN-γ, IL-4, IL-10, TNF-α*); and genes affecting autoantigen clearance (*C1q, C4, SAP, DNAse-1*).[15,16] Gene array data strongly indicate that interferon genes are markedly upregulated in patients with active SLE. Whether this is causative or a result of disease is not known.[17]

OTHER GENETIC SUSCEPTIBILITIES

Twin and family studies of SLE make it abundantly clear that the illness is highly heritable. HLA types DR3 and DR4 predominate in SLE patients.[18] Specific susceptibility loci on chromosomes 1, 4, and 7, among others, have been identified.[19] Persons with genetic deficiencies of complement appear to be more susceptible to the development of lupus.[20] Specific FcIII gamma receptor alleles increase the severity of lupus nephritis, particularly in whites.[21] The genetics of lupus are extremely complex, however, and no single genetic trait is unequivocally linked to susceptibility to the illness. Several national registries are currently attempting to definitively describe the genetics of lupus.

INFECTIONS

Although an infectious trigger of SLE has long been suspected, no single infection has been found. Universal exposure of children with SLE to Epstein-Barr virus has been noted (at an age when 50% exposure is the norm), suggesting a possible link of this virus to disease.[22] Autoantibodies can be identified in serum specimens up to a decade before the earliest symptoms of SLE. Autoantibodies first appear as one specific antibody, then generalize just before clinical onset. Whether this progression reflects response to infection or autoimmunity is unknown.[23]

ESTROGEN

Some investigators attribute the female predominance of SLE and its occurrence in childbearing years to the upregulating effect of estrogen on the immune system, a phenomenon demonstrable largely in vitro. However, this argument applies to autoimmunity in general, not specifically to lupus, and it fails to explain why other autoimmune diseases have much less striking female-to-male ratios. Furthermore, postmenopausal estrogen replacement and oral contraceptive use do not significantly alter SLE incidence or severity, nor does pregnancy; minor differences in incidence or susceptibility have on occasion been reported.[24-26] Alternative explanations for a high female-to-male ratio include an estrogen-sensitive threshold mechanism[27] or sex differences of exposure to exogenous agents (although none has been convincingly suggested.[28] Reports of patients with Klinefelter syndrome and SLE have prompted investigators to consider the possible involvement of male hypogonadism in the pathogenesis of lupus; patients with Klinefelter syndrome may be unusually susceptible to lupus.

COMPLICATIONS OF CHRONIC ILLNESS

Most current information on SLE pathogenesis focuses on upregulation or downregulation of components of the immune response, genetic controls of immunity, and potential etiologic agents. However, the long-term damage of chronic disease, from tissue injury or treatment, is as important to patients as acute inflammatory disease. Some elements of damage are clearly attributable to therapy: osteoporosis, osteonecrosis, cataracts, and tendon ruptures are all associated with long-term corticosteroid therapy. Other elements of damage result directly from the inflammatory and immunologic aspects of the illness, which lead to tissue necrosis and scarring: progressive renal failure, destruc-

Table 1   (*continued*)

MCTD	UCTD	PAPS	Scleroderma	LLD	Dermatomyositis
Sclerodactyly	—	Livedo reticularis	Scleroderma, periungual telangiectasia	—	Specific rash, periungual telangiectasia
Symmetrical nondestructive arthritis	Symmetrical nondestructive arthritis	—	Transient, symmetrical, early arthritis	Symmetrical nondestructive arthritis	—
—	—	Thrombotic microangiopathy	Angiotensin-driven renal crisis	—	—
—	—	Stroke, myelopathy	Hypertensive crisis	—	Myopathy
—	—	—	—	—	—
Positive, speckled Normal	May be positive Normal	May be positive Normal	Positive, speckled, nucleolar, centromere Normal	May be positive Normal	Positive Normal
Anti-RNP	—	Anticardiolipin, lupus anticoagulant	Anti–Scl-70, anticentromere (topoisomerase I)	—	Anti-Jo-1
—	—	Anti–β_2-glycoprotein I	—	—	—
—	—	Thrombocytopenia	High renin during crisis	—	High CPK and aldolase

tive joint disease, and brain infarcts. Many of these complications are more severe in patients of minority races or lower socioeconomic classes.[29] Still other elements of chronicity bear an uncertain relationship to disease and treatment: accelerated atherosclerosis,[30] valvular heart disease, cognitive dysfunction, and psychosocial dysfunction.

Diagnosis

The American College of Rheumatology (ACR) has defined criteria for the classification of SLE [*see Table 2*].[31] Although the ACR criteria are useful for ensuring uniformity of patients report-

ed in medical journals, the criteria are often mistakenly used as diagnostic criteria. For individual patients, the criteria have high false negative and false positive rates.[32] For instance, a patient with biopsy-proven lupus nephritis, positive antinuclear antibody, and anti-Sm antibody as the only manifestations of disease does not fulfill ACR criteria, whereas a patient with rheumatoid arthritis who has a positive antinuclear antibody, low positive anti-DNA antibody, and leukopenia (e.g., from Felty syndrome) does fulfill ACR criteria. As a rule, characteristic disease of one organ system (kidney, joints, skin) plus a high-titer anti-dsDNA or Sm antibody suffices to make the clinical diagnosis.

In clinical practice, diagnosis of SLE is based on a combination of autoantibody assays, clinical manifestations, and laboratory studies of affected organ systems. The clinical manifestations of lupus are protean. Patients with lupus activity or damage may be asymptomatic or may present with findings that reflect the specific organ systems involved [*see Table 3*].

Symptoms and signs accumulate over time in patients with SLE [*see Table 4*].[33] At any given time, especially at the onset of illness, most often only a few manifestations are present. Arthritis, malaise, cytopenias, and rashes are the most prominent early findings. Nephritis (with renal failure), arthritis, osteoporosis and osteonecrosis (corticosteroid complications), neurologic disease, accelerated atherosclerosis, and cardiac valvular disease dominate the late course. With disease activity and with its treatment, the risk of opportunistic infection is high. For conceptual purposes, it is easiest to consider disease activity and manifestations separately for each affected organ system.

SYSTEMIC SIGNS AND SYMPTOMS

Malaise, arthralgia, myalgias, fever (usually low grade), and weight loss are common manifestations of active SLE. Some patients will have high temperatures (> 40° C [104° F]). Even with very high fever, shaking chills are unusual; when present, they suggest infection. Like the organ-specific manifestations of lupus, the systemic symptoms vary considerably during the day and

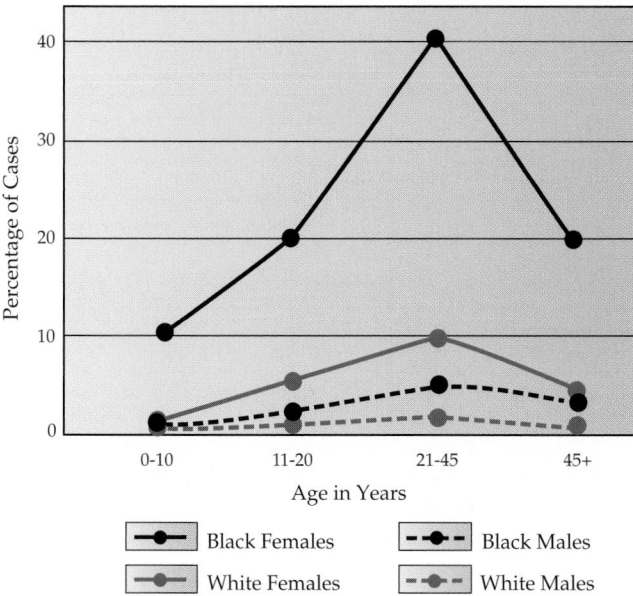

Figure 1   **Age, sex, and race distribution of the incidence of SLE.[6]**

Table 2 American College of Rheumatology Criteria for the Classification of SLE*

Malar rash
Discoid rash
Photosensitivity
Oral ulcers
Arthritis
Serositis (pleuritis or pericarditis)
Renal disorder (proteinuria > 0.5 g/day or cellular casts)
Neurologic disorder (seizures or psychosis)
Hematologic disorder (hemolytic anemia, leukopenia, lymphopenia, or thrombocytopenia)
Immunologic disorder (anti-DNA, anti-Sm, or antiphospholipid antibodies [anticardiolipin, lupus anticoagulant, or biologic false positive test for syphilis])
Antinuclear antibody

Note: these are not diagnostic criteria.
*Four criteria are required to include a patient in an SLE cohort of a research study.

over weeks. In approximately one third of lupus patients, sun exposure, usually intense, will induce systemic flare. Sun exposure that is mild or of short duration does not harm most patients.

SKIN AND MUCOSAL INVOLVEMENT

Up to half of lupus patients manifest some degree of alopecia. Typically, this takes the form of broken frontal hairs and diffuse thinning, which recovers when health is regained. Severe alopecia may occur. Discoid rashes cause focal patches of hair loss.

Most patients develop a rash at some point during their illness. The well-known butterfly rash, on both cheeks and across the bridge of the nose [*see Figure 2*], occurs in only a minority of patients, but most rashes involve the face in some manner. Commonly the tip of the chin, the upper lip, the eyebrows, and the hairline are also involved. The rash may consist of erythema only or may be papular and scaly or deeply pigmented (discoid rash). Discoid rashes, which may scar, are hyperpigmented at the circumference and often depigmented centrally [*see Figure 3*]. Patients with discoid rashes may have either discoid lupus or SLE. Other types of rashes occur only in SLE.

Table 3 Physical Examination Abnormalities in Acute and Chronic SLE *

Organ	Acute Disease		Chronic Disease	
	Common	Uncommon	Common	Uncommon
General	Fever, weight loss	Asthenia	Cachexia	
Skin	Malar rash, rash elsewhere, alopecia	Periungual telangiectasia, vasculitis	Malar rash, rash elsewhere, alopecia, striae, atrophy, pigment change	Periungual telangiectasia, skin ulcers
Nodes	Lymphadenopathy	—	—	—
Breasts	—	—	—	—
Eyes	—	Retinal hemorrhages, exudates	Hypertensive changes	Retinal hemorrhages, exudates
Ears	—	Rash in ear canal, decreased hearing	—	Scarring in ear canal, decreased hearing
Nose	—	Septal ulceration	—	Septal perforation
Throat	—	Mucosal ulcer (hard palate)	—	Mucosal scarring (hard palate)
Chest	—	Rales, pleural rub, effusion	—	Rales, effusion
Heart and vessels	Raynaud phenomenon	Pericardial rub, enlargement	Raynaud phenomenon, valve disease	Enlargement, valve insufficiency, arrhythmia
Abdomen	—	Hepatomegaly, splenomegaly	—	Hepatomegaly, splenomegaly, ascites
Muscles	Weakness, tenderness	—	Weakness, atrophy, tendon rupture	—
Bones	—	—	Fracture (vertebrae, hip), osteonecrosis	—
Joints	Synovitis, restricted motion	—	Synovitis, deformity, restricted motion	Jaccoud deformities
Neuromotor	—	Stroke, mononeuritis multiplex, seizure	—	Stroke, mononeuritis multiplex, seizure
Neurosensory	—	Peripheral neuropathy, mononeuritis multiplex	—	Peripheral neuropathy, mononeuritis multiplex
Cognitive	Depression	Psychosis, dementia	Depression	Psychosis, dementia

*This table is not comprehensive; it does not include rare abnormalities.

Table 4 Frequencies of Various Manifestations of SLE by Disease Stage[33]

Manifestation	Early Disease (%)	Late Disease (%)
Arthritis	46–53	83–95
Rash	9–11	81–88
Fever	3–5	77
Mucosal ulcers	—	7–23
Alopecia	—	37–45
Serositis	5	63
Pulmonary inflammation	—	9
Liver function test abnormalities	1	—
Vasculitis	—	21–27
Myositis	—	5
Osteoporosis	—	High
Osteonecrosis	—	7–24
Leukopenia	41–66	41–66
Thrombocytopenia	2	19–45
Anemia	2	57–73
CNS abnormalities	3	55–59
Nephritis	6	31–53
Renal failure	< 1	20

Diagnostic inflammatory rashes are somewhat raised, scaly, and relatively uniform in appearance across the lesion; they may ulcerate; and they have sharp borders. Less diagnostic rashes occur on the extensor surfaces of the upper arms, the blush area of the neck and shoulders, and the extensor surfaces of the elbows and fingers. These are usually erythematous macular rashes. The erythematous rashes evolve over days to weeks and often leave hyperpigmentation as they recede; they may appear more prominent with fever or pregnancy. Vasculitic rashes (usually small, ulcerating papules) occur on the extensor tips of the elbows; painful, erythematous vascular lesions occur at the distal fingers and palms (lupus pernio). A polycyclic, persistent rash, primarily on the trunk, and specifically associated with anti–SS-A antibody, is known as subacute cutaneous lupus [*see Figure 4*]. A painful subcutaneous lesion that is deeply indurated and tender and may ulcerate is called lupus profundus.

Some patients have only erythema in distributions typical of lupus rashes. Unlike the other rashes, erythematous rashes are not by themselves diagnostic of lupus, but they add to the overall diagnostic information. Lupus rashes are often confused with rosacea (although rosacea is more oily and more papular), polymorphous light eruptions, and allergic reactions.

Chronic nasal ulcers and recurring painless mouth ulcers [*see Figure 5*] (particularly on the hard palate, but also on the gums and buccal mucosa) are characteristic of more severe disease. Mucosal ulcers are irritating rather than severely painful. Periungual telangiectasias and small, ulcerating, vasculitic ulcers on the elbows also occur in more severe disease. A particular type of palmar and digital pulp erythema, known as lupus pernio, is a form of vasculitis. In rare cases, subcutaneous inflammation leads to lupus profundus, consisting of local fat necrosis and painful nodules.

LYMPH NODE INVOLVEMENT

Lymphadenopathy is common in active disease. It is modest in extent and generalized (often noted on computed tomography scans of the abdomen or chest). It resolves rapidly in patients started on corticosteroid therapy for other manifestations of SLE.

CARDIOPULMONARY INVOLVEMENT

SLE is associated with a range of cardiopulmonary disorders [*see Table 5*]. These usually cause symptoms or abnormal physical findings; it is unnecessary to test asymptomatic patients for cardiovascular disease.

Pleuropericarditis is frequently symptomatic but is not usually life-threatening. It causes pain on breathing, as well as elevation of the diaphragm that is evident on physical examination or x-ray. Atelectasis at the bases of the lungs is audible as fine crackling rales or is visible on x-ray as horizontal lines (plate atelectasis). Pulmonary function tests may reflect reduced diffusion capacity, reduced lung volumes, and reduced lung elasticity.

Pleural effusions also occur, but they are not usually large. On thoracentesis, LE cells (polymorphonuclear leukocytes with ingested nuclear debris appearing as a homogeneous round inclusion) may be found on a Wright stain of the fluid buffy coat.

A minority of patients develop respiratory insufficiency from pulmonary fibrosis. A rare manifestation is so-called lupus lung.

a
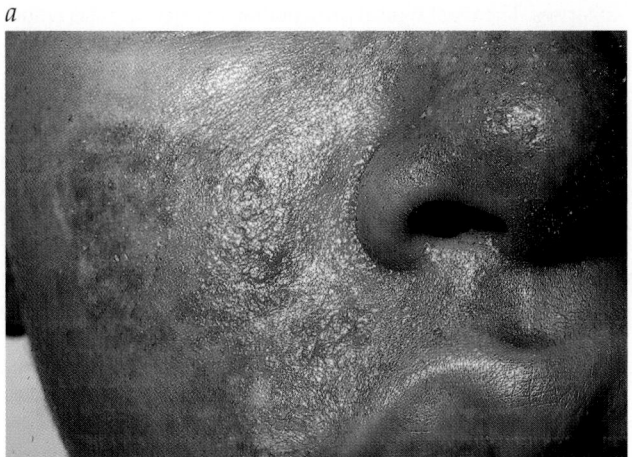

b
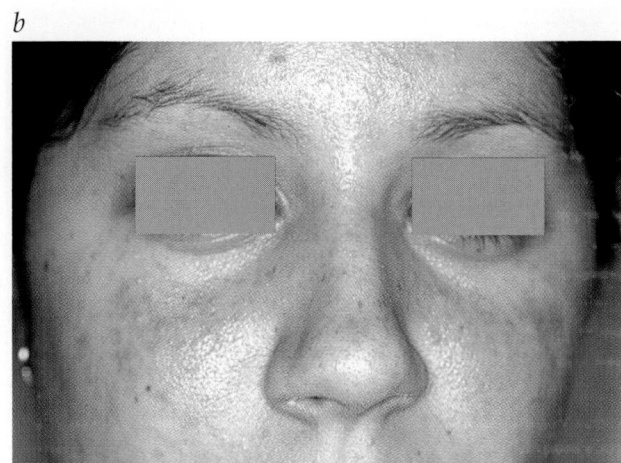

Figure 2 Most lupus rashes involve the face (a). The butterfly rash of lupus, on both cheeks and across the bridge of the nose (b), occurs in only a minority of patients.

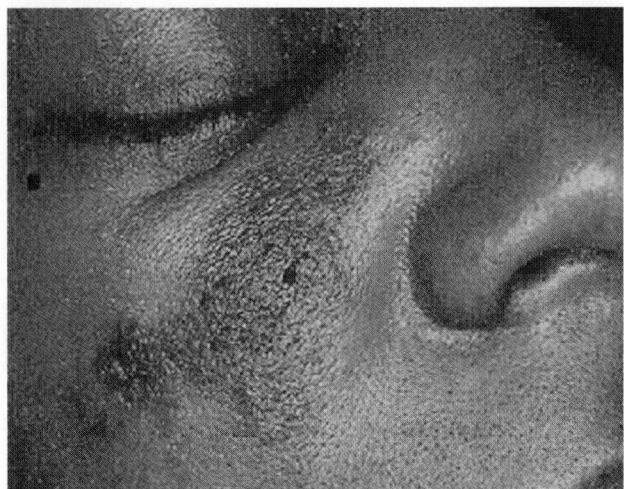

Figure 3   Discoid lupus rashes are hyperpigmented at the circumference and often depigmented centrally.

This consists of inflammatory lung disease or pulmonary hemorrhage, either of which is life threatening.[34] Pulmonary hypertension is uncommon but serious when it occurs, which is most often in patients with intense Raynaud phenomenon, recurrent pulmonary emboli, or pulmonary fibrosis.

Transthoracic echocardiography demonstrates valvular heart disease in up to 30% of patients with long-standing SLE; with transesophageal echocardiography, the frequency is much higher.[35] Libman-Sacks lesions occur primarily on the mitral valve but also occur on the aortic valve and, rarely, on the pulmonic or tricuspid valves. Symptomatic valve disease may be more common in patients with antiphospholipid antibody. Pericardial effusions or thickening occurs during active disease, but otherwise, they are uncommon. Small pericardial effusions, which may be symptomatic or asymptomatic, occur often in patients with active SLE. Life-threatening large effusions are uncommon.

Accelerated atherosclerosis is a risk of long-standing lupus,[36,37] leading to myocardial infarction and other vascular occlusive manifestations before the age of 40. Myocardial infarction may also be caused by coronary vasculitis, but this is less common. It is important to consider atherosclerosis, together with vasculitis

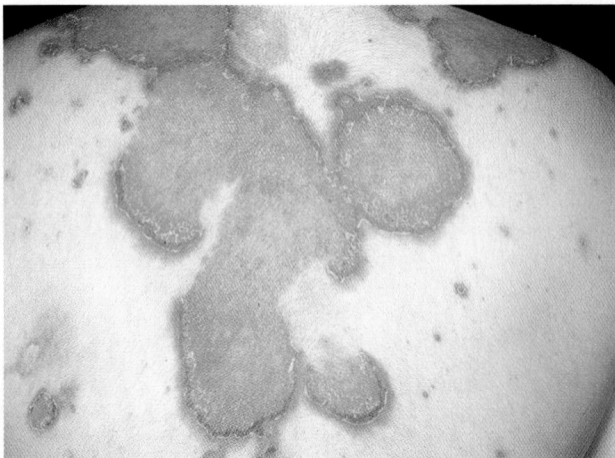

Figure 4   The rash of subacute cutaneous lupus is polycyclic and persistent.

and thrombosis (from antiphospholipid antibody), in patients with long-standing lupus who present with complaints of vascular insufficiency.

Diffuse nonischemic myocarditis may also occur. Newborns suffering the neonatal SLE syndrome may have complete congenital heart block and may die of congestive heart failure.

MUSCULOSKELETAL INVOLVEMENT

The arthritis of SLE is typically painful, transient, and symmetrical, involving the wrists, small joints of the hands, elbows, knees, and ankles. Swelling and redness are modest. Less often, SLE arthritis will present as asymmetrical oligoarthritis or intensely inflamed, sustained polyarthritis resembling that of rheumatoid arthritis. Although deformity may occur as a result of ligamentous laxity (reversible subluxations, Jaccoud arthropathy),[38] rheumatoid-like joint destruction is uncommon.

Inflammatory myositis occurs primarily in patients with overlap features with scleroderma or dermatomyositis. It presents as proximal myopathy; serum levels of muscle enzymes are modestly elevated; and results of electromyography, magnetic resonance imaging, and muscle biopsy, if done, are similar to those seen in dermatomyositis. However, abnormal enzyme levels associated with proximal muscle tenderness or weakness are sufficient for diagnosis in a patient with established SLE.

Lupus does not involve bone directly. However, bone involvement can occur secondary to organ system failure (e.g., renal failure), severe illness (e.g., osteoporosis from inactivity or catabolic state), or treatment (e.g., corticosteroid-induced osteoporosis or avascular necrosis).

Osteoporosis presents as atraumatic fractures of vertebrae or long bones. Its occurrence is a severe threat to SLE patients, even premenopausal women, because of the frequent use of corticosteroids for treatment and because of inactivity attendant upon polyarthritis and systemic illness.

Avascular necrosis (osteonecrosis) most often occurs in patients who have had a severe flare treated with high-intensity corticosteroid therapy, but this complication can develop in patients who have never received corticosteroid treatment. Marked cushingoid features during steroid treatment and Raynaud phenomenon may be predictors of its occurrence.[39] The femoral head is the most commonly involved site, but shoulders, ankles, wrists, metacarpals, and shafts of long bones are also vulnerable.[40] Typically, affected areas become painful at the initial occurrence of infarction and again years later when the necrotic bone collapses. The most typical presentation of osteonecrosis is sudden hip pain 2 or 3 years after a major flare of lupus. Some patients receiving infusions of high-dose intravenous methylprednisolone complain of intense pain at preexisting osteonecrotic sites during and shortly after the infusion. Reducing the corticosteroid dose at the time of occurrence of pain has no effect on the course of the complication.

GASTROINTESTINAL AND HEPATIC INVOLVEMENT

Esophageal dysfunction is rare in SLE; it occurs primarily in patients with severe Raynaud phenomenon or in patients with scleroderma overlap disease. Gastroduodenal ulcer may occur as a result of treatment but is not directly linked to SLE. Ischemia of the small and large intestines may result from systemic vasculitis; it presents as abdominal angina, pneumatosis intestinalis, infarction or perforation, or pseudo-obstruction. Intestinal ischemia is a rare complication, occurring only in the most severely ill patients.[41]

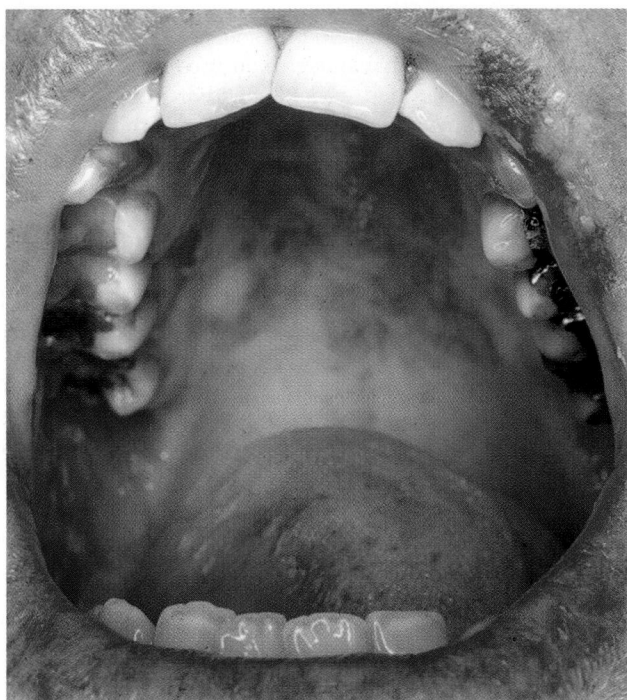

Figure 5 Painless mouth ulcers, most often found on the hard palate but also found on the gums and buccal mucosa, are characteristic of more severe lupus.

Diverticulitis often develops in patients with long-standing SLE, especially after prolonged treatment with corticosteroids. The symptoms of diverticulitis are easily masked by corticosteroid therapy. Consequently, diverticular perforation or abscess is frequently misdiagnosed, especially in young SLE patients.

Chemical hepatitis may follow use of nonsteroidal anti-inflammatory drugs (NSAIDs) (lupus patients appear to be unusually susceptible to this side effect) or other drugs, such as azathioprine.[42] Occasionally, patients suffer concomitant autoimmune hepatitis or primary biliary cirrhosis. In the absence of other causes, abnormalities of liver enzyme levels because of SLE are uncommon.

HEMATOLOGIC INVOLVEMENT

Leukopenia is such a regular feature of SLE that its absence, in untreated disease, should raise suspicion that the diagnosis is incorrect or that infection or tissue necrosis is present. Usually, lymphocyte counts show greater reductions than do granulocyte counts: a leukocyte count of about $3.5/mm^3$, with 10% lymphocytes, is usual. Leukopenia of this degree seldom places patients at serious risk of infection. There is usually no need to administer granulocyte-macrophage colony-stimulating factor (GM-CSF); there are anecdotal reports that administration of this agent may induce lupus flare.

Thrombocytopenia in SLE is usually low grade, with platelet counts greater than $50,000/mm^3$. Severe thrombocytopenia may occur, however; idiopathic thrombocytopenic purpura (ITP) may be an initial presentation of SLE.

SLE may result in anemia of chronic disease and anemia from autoimmune hemolysis. The anemia of chronic disease in SLE patients responds to administration of recombinant erythropoietin.

NEUROLOGIC INVOLVEMENT

Neurologic signs and symptoms represent one of the most serious and least understood aspects of SLE. The primary neurologic manifestations of SLE consist of generalized and focal (usually vascular) brain disease, myelopathy, peripheral neuropathy, mononeuritis multiplex, and cognitive dysfunction. Secondary neurologic events can also occur; these include seizures from hypertension or hemorrhage, delirium from drugs or uremia, brain or spinal cord abscess, and stroke from atheroma or embolus. Attribution of a specific neurologic symptom to active lupus (which is treatable with immunosuppression), as opposed to a complication of lupus or its treatment (which is treatable by ameliorating the offending problem) requires deep investigation and good clinical judgment. Confusion about diagnostic criteria for neurologic lupus led the ACR to publish nomenclature and case-definition criteria for these syndromes.[43]

General Brain Disease

Patients with SLE frequently complain of progressive cognitive dysfunction, such as confusion, forgetfulness, and so-called foggy thinking.[44,45] Retrospective and cross-sectional studies document a high frequency of poor performance on tests of cognitive function, particularly in the executive, short-term memory, and verbal-processing spheres.[46,47] It is not known whether this deficit results from immunologic attack on the brain (by antineuronal or other autoantibodies) or diffuse vascular disease. Cognitive dysfunction may respond to corticosteroid therapy. It seldom progresses to advanced dementia.

Headaches are common in SLE. A special form of migraine called lupus headache has been described, but whether it exists as a definable entity remains a matter of debate.

Focal Brain Disease

Seizures, strokes, cranial neuropathies (including blindness), and cerebellar dysfunction may occur in SLE. These events are assumed to result from vascular occlusion, but they may occur in patients with no known thrombotic diathesis, embolization, atherosclerosis, or vasculitis. Stroke is one of the most common presentations of the antiphospholipid antibody syndrome. Seizures are most common in severely active, febrile, multisystem dis-

---

Table 5 Cardiopulmonary Manifestations of SLE

Pleuropericarditis
Libman-Sacks endocarditis
Valve insufficiency
Valve stenosis
Ischemic cardiomyopathy
    Accelerated atherosclerosis
    Antiphospholipid antibody syndrome
    Hypertensive heart disease
    Vasculitis
Hypertensive heart disease
Pulmonary hypertension
Peripheral arterial insufficiency
    Vasculitis
    Atherosclerosis
    Antiphospholipid antibody syndrome
Peripheral venous thrombosis
Raynaud phenomenon
Complete congenital heart block in newborns with neonatal lupus erythematosus

ease. In this circumstance, they generally do not persist after the disease is brought under control.[48]

Myelopathy

Transverse myelitis occurs in two patterns: (1) abrupt onset, with progression in hours from the first symptom, often heralded by a burning, dysesthetic pain in the legs; and (2) slower progression, in a stuttering fashion, worsening over days. Unless treated immediately and aggressively, both forms may progress to advanced paraparesis or paraplegia. Although few direct data exist to support these hypotheses, it is likely that the first form represents vascular occlusion with spinal cord ischemia and the second form represents inflammatory disease. It is mandatory to exclude a space-occupying mass in all such patients.

A slowly progressive and intermittent myelopathy, very much resembling multiple sclerosis (so-called MS-like or lupoid sclerosis), develops in some lupus patients. There is no definitive way to exclude concomitant MS in these patients except by the association of the myelopathy with SLE and by its failure to progress in the way MS usually does. In this form of lupus myelopathy, cerebrospinal fluid examinations may reveal oligoclonal bands, but MRI studies are atypical for MS.

Peripheral Neuropathy

Stocking-and-glove neuropathy is a slowly progressive lesion that tends to occur in patients with continuing, active disease. Its pathogenesis is unclear; it may result from direct immune attack on peripheral nerves or from vasculitic occlusion of the vasa nervora. Abrupt loss of motor and sensory function, such as sudden occurrence of footdrop or wristdrop, is diagnosed as mononeuritis multiplex. This is a very serious manifestation indicating vasculitis of the vasa nervora; it implies systemic vasculitis, as well.

RENAL INVOLVEMENT

Approximately half of lupus patients develop lupus nephritis, and approximately 10% overall will progress to dialysis or transplantation. Lupus nephritis presents as proteinuria (or an other-wise abnormal urinalysis), hypertension, or a rising serum creatinine level, all of variable degree. In its early stages, lupus nephritis is painless and asymptomatic. In more advanced stages, edema, anemia, symptomatic hypertension, and symptomatic uremia occur. Patients with inflammatory forms of nephritis are usually hypocomplementemic; most have high levels of anti-DNA or anti-Sm antibody. Signs or symptoms of disease active in other organ systems need not accompany lupus nephritis.

The World Health Organization (WHO) pathologic classification of lupus nephritis has been revised. The revised criteria differ from previous classifications by taking into account normal biopsies, scarring, and tubulointerstitial changes; in addition, they incorporate information from immunofluorescence and electron microscopy studies [see Table 6].[49] This classification includes indices of disease activity and chronicity, which delineate acute necrosis, inflammatory infiltrate, crescent formation, scarring, and tubular atrophy to provide further prognostic information.[9] Electron microscopy demonstrates immune complex deposits in subepithelial spaces in membranous lupus nephritis and in subendothelial spaces in proliferative lupus nephritis, as well as in mesangial locations. Characteristic tubuloreticular structures, thought to be RNA degradation products, also appear. Immunofluorescence studies demonstrate IgG, IgM, and C3 deposits in the same distributions. Vascular inflammation or endothelial proliferation is also seen.

Although lupus nephritis may present as anuria, acute hypertension, or fluid retention, most often it is first noted by an abnormal urinalysis. If left untreated, lupus nephritis progresses to renal insufficiency over months to years. Biopsy is necessary primarily when the result will change treatment. Urinalysis and blood chemistry results correlate only roughly with biopsy findings [see Table 7].

SPECIAL PRESENTATIONS

Neonatal Lupus Syndrome

Approximately 25% of infants born to mothers with anti–SS-

Table 6 International Society of Nephrology/Renal Pathology Society (ISN/RPS) 2003 Classification of Lupus Nephritis

Class	Name	Description	Clinical Presentation
I	Minimal mesangial	Normal light microscopy, mesangial immune deposits by immunofluorescence	Normal urinalysis, normal function
II	Mesangial proliferative	Infiltrating cells and proliferation of mesangium	Mild proteinuria, celluria, normal function
III A III A/C III C	Focal active Focal active and chronic Focal chronic	Infiltrating cells and immune complex deposits in portions of the glomerulus and in < 50% of glomeruli (active) or scarring (chronic)	Variable proteinuria, celluria, normal function
IV A IV G IV-S A/C IV-G A/C IV-S C IV-G C	Diffuse and active (A), global (G), segmental (S), chronic (C)	Infiltrating cells and moderate immune complex deposits in entire glomeruli and in ≥ 50% of glomeruli with segmental or global lesions, with or without scarring	Variable proteinuria, celluria; often severe, decreasing function
V	Membranous	Global or segmental subendothelial immune deposits by light, immunofluorescence, or electron microscopy, with or without mesangial lesions	Marked proteinuria, slowly decreasing function
VI	Advanced sclerotic	≥ 90% of glomeruli globally sclerosed without residual activity	Variable proteinuria, decreased function

Table 7   Likely Renal Biopsy Findings According to
Urinalysis and Serum Creatinine Results

Urinalysis		Creatinine Level	Most Likely Pathology
Protein	Cells		
None	None	Normal	Normal or mesangial
Little	WBCs	Normal	Mesangial, focal proliferative
Moderate	WBCs, RBCs	Normal	Mesangial, focal or diffuse proliferative
Moderate	WBCs, RBCs, casts	Normal or elevated	Focal or diffuse proliferative
Severe	WBCs, RBCs, casts	Normal or elevated	Diffuse proliferative, membranoproliferative
Severe	Few	Normal or elevated	Membranous
Moderate	WBCs	Normal or elevated	Interstitial (tubular) disease (in patients with acidosis or electrolyte abnormalities)

A or anti–SS-B antibody will develop a photosensitive rash or thrombocytopenia, both of which are transient. A very small number of these infants will develop complete congenital heart block in utero. Both the cardiac and the skin manifestations constitute the neonatal lupus syndrome. Either can be present independently. The syndrome appears to result from transplacental passage of maternal antibody, and it subsides when the antibody disappears. However, the heart block persists and may be lethal. The antibody likely targets transiently expressed antigens in the fetal conducting system; signals for apoptosis and fibrosis are upregulated.[50]

Antiphospholipid Antibody Syndrome

Between one third and one half of lupus patients have anticardiolipin antibody, lupus anticoagulant, or both. When either of these antibodies is present in high titer, patients are susceptible to recurrent thromboembolic disease, thrombocytopenia, livedo reticularis, and cardiac valvular disease. Women are susceptible to recurrent pregnancy loss. These symptoms, combined with positive blood tests, constitute the antiphospholipid syndrome (APS).[51] In the absence of lupus, the disorder is termed primary APS (PAPS); and when lupus or another rheumatic disease is present, the syndrome is designated secondary APS (SAPS). Current research suggests that the true antigen for the syndrome is the phospholipid binding protein, beta$_2$-glycoprotein I, rather than negatively charged phospholipids themselves. In some patients, antibody to an alternative phospholipid binding protein, such as prothrombin, induces the same syndrome. It is not known what induces clotting events in individual patients, but evidence of endothelial activation or injury, such as circulating endothelial cells, appears to be associated with thromboembolic episodes. The sites of thrombosis are not inflammatory and are best treated by anticoagulation rather than by immunosuppression. However, studies of pregnancy loss in animal models indicate that complement activation is a critical component of fetal injury, suggesting anew the possible involvement of the innate immune system in the development of APS.

LABORATORY TESTS

Tests of a variety of body fluids may be abnormal in patients with SLE [*see Table* 8]. Not all tests are abnormal in all patients. If lupus is suspected, an antinuclear antibody test, a complete blood count, and a urinalysis should be performed; if the results of these tests are all normal, SLE is excluded. However, because lupuslike illnesses are also usually suspected, it is often efficient also to obtain at first visit the following tests: erythrocyte sedimentation rate (ESR) or C-reactive protein level; assays for antibodies against dsDNA, Sm, RNP, SS-A, and SS-B; partial thromboplastin time (or other screening test for lupus anticoagulant) and cardiolipin antibodies; and a chemistry profile that includes liver function tests and serum creatinine level.

The antinuclear antibody (ANA) assay is a screening test for lupus. The ANA assay is almost always positive in high titer (> 1:80) in untreated patients with active disease, but a positive result does not by itself confirm a diagnosis of lupus. Only the anti-dsDNA antibody and anti-Sm antibodies, when present in high titer, are diagnostic of lupus. Anti-dsDNA antibody and complement levels are rough guides to disease activity, but many patients remain well for long periods of time with severely abnormal tests. Hypocomplementemia reflects proliferative lupus nephritis but not other aspects of SLE, including membranous lupus nephritis. The ESR remains elevated in many otherwise well SLE patients, as does the C-reactive protein level.

Brain Imaging Studies

Evaluation of neurologic involvement in SLE is complex. MRI scans, usually with contrast, are indicated for any clinical suspicion of central nervous system disease, such as seizures, cognitive dysfunction, new severe headache, chorea, or stroke symptoms. CT scans are far less definitive, except in stroke. Cerebral angiography or magnetic resonance angiography (MRA) is rarely helpful.

CT and MRI scans of the brain frequently demonstrate atrophy and infarcts (the latter including hyperintense areas in the white matter). These lesions correlate poorly with neurologic disease other than stroke syndromes.[13] Findings on fluorodeoxyglucose positron emission tomography (PET), magnetic resonance spectrography (MRS), and single-photon emission computed tomography (SPECT) are frequently abnormal even in asymptomatic patients and correlate poorly with all but the most severe neuropsychiatric disease.[52] Interpretation of abnormal findings in asymptomatic patients is uncertain.[53,54]

Vascular Evaluation

Vascular evaluation is indicated when there is clinical suspicion of medium-size vascular occlusion. Ultrasound, Doppler studies, angiography, and MRA can demonstrate thromboembolic disease from antiphospholipid antibody or atherosclerosis. The small vessel vasculitis that occurs in SLE is usually beyond the resolution of these technologies.

Table 8 Commonly Abnormal Tests on Body Fluids in SLE

Test	Abnormality	Interpretation
CBC	Normochromic anemia, leukopenia (WBC ~3,000, thrombocytopenia)	Active SLE
ESR and CRP	Elevated	Active SLE
Urinalysis	Proteinuria, hematuria, leukocyturia, cylindruria	Active lupus nephritis
Coombs and reticulocyte count	Positive, high	Hemolytic anemia
APTT, dRVVT	High	If confirmed with mixing test, lupus anticoagulant
Antinuclear antibody	Strongly positive	Positive in almost all patients during active disease; not specific for lupus
Anti-dsDNA antibody	Strongly positive	Positive in two thirds to three quarters of patients during active disease; diagnostic of lupus
Anti-Sm antibody	Positive	Positive in one quarter to one third of patients; diagnostic of lupus
Anti–SS-A, anti–SS-B, and anti-RNP antibodies	Positive	Positive in one third of patients; nonspecific
Anticardiolipin antibody	Positive	Antiphospholipid antibody syndrome
Complement C3, C4, and CH50	Low	Lupus nephritis likely; also hemolytic anemia and cryoglobulinemia
Cryoglobulin	Present	Active SLE
BUN and serum creatinine	Elevated	Severe lupus nephritis, drug toxicity
Liver function tests	Elevated	Drug toxicity (rarely, active SLE)
CSF protein and cells	Elevated	Present in a minority of patients with CNS SLE
Synovial fluid	WBC 5,000–10,000, normal glucose level	Lupus arthritis
Pleural fluid, pericardial fluid	WBC 5,000–10,000, normal glucose level, low complement, LE cells present	Lupus serositis

APTT—activated partial thromboplastin time   BUN—blood urea nitrogen   CBC—complete blood count   CNS—central nervous system   CRP—C-reactive protein   CSF—cerebrospinal fluid   dRVVT—dilute Russell viper venom time   ESR—erythrocyte sedimentation rate   WBC—white blood cells

Renal Evaluation

All lupus patients should have urinalyses performed, preferably at each clinic visit, because renal disease may appear de novo at any time. All patients with any abnormality on urinalysis or with an abnormal blood urea nitrogen (BUN) or serum creatinine level should have monitoring of 24-hour urine protein and creatinine clearance no less often than every 6 months. It is important to consider the results of renal testing in context: a serum creatinine level of 1.2 mg/dl may be within the laboratory range of normal, but in a 110 lb young woman, a level that high is very likely abnormal. Falling creatinine clearance always demands evaluation, even when the patient is clinically well.

Kidney biopsy   The primary indication to perform a kidney biopsy is to help the physician make a treatment decision. Although abnormal biopsy results may be found in asymptomatic patients with normal urinalyses, it is not clear whether treatment of such patients improves outcome. The well patient with normal urinalysis results and normal renal function generally does not need a kidney biopsy, even if the anti-DNA antibody level is high and the complement level is low. The very ill patient with multisystem disease, including abnormal urinalysis results and abnormal renal function, likely will be treated aggressively anyway and does not need a kidney biopsy. The patient with mild systemic disease, mild urinary abnormalities, or both generally should undergo biopsy, because the decision for conservative or aggressive treatment may depend on the result. Occasionally, a biopsy is done to document end-stage, untreatable disease and thereby permit withdrawal of therapy. However, renal ultrasonography can usually provide the same information.

Cardiac Evaluation

Cardiac monitoring with echocardiography or stress tests is unnecessary on a routine basis. Because of the high frequency of accelerated atherosclerosis, however, any occurrence of dyspnea, dyspepsia, or shoulder or arm pain merits consideration of ischemic cardiac disease.

Differential Diagnosis

The differential diagnosis of lupus involves two linked questions: does the patient have a rheumatic disease, and if so, which one?

NONRHEUMATIC ILLNESSES THAT MIMIC SLE

The syndrome of fever, cytopenia, rash, and adenopathy suggests many infections, including HIV, cytomegalovirus, mononucleosis, and bacterial endocarditis. Acute polyarthritis, rash, and cytopenias can result from many viral infections, such as hepatitis, parvovirus, and rubella. These syndromes resolve spontaneously within several weeks. This syndrome also suggests hematologic malignancies, primarily the lymphomas, leukemias, and myelodysplastic syndromes. Although the presence of antinuclear antibody is common in many of these illnesses, the presence of anti-DNA or anti-Sm antibodies is not; also uncommon are the specific rashes of lupus, nephritis, and vascular manifestations such as periungual telangiectasia and vasculitic papules. Photosensitivity and frontal alopecia are also characteristics of lupus that do not occur in these other illnesses.

Non-SLE causes of nephritis include poststreptococcal glomerulonephritis, Goodpasture disease, genetic nephropathies, and toxemia. The rash of rosacea is commonly mistaken for that of lupus. ITP or autoimmune hemolytic anemia may occur as isolated illnesses or as part of the multisystemic involvement of lupus. In these circumstances, full clinical and serologic evaluation for lupus will place the findings in proper context.

RHEUMATIC ILLNESSES THAT RESEMBLE SLE

Lupus may resemble a variety of other rheumatic diseases [see Table 1]. Such diseases include rheumatoid arthritis and Sjögren syndrome [see Chapter 112], as well as scleroderma [see Chapter 115]. The polyarthritic presentation of lupus is very similar to that of rheumatoid arthritis, Lyme disease, and other rheumatic illnesses. In early scleroderma, patients often present with bilateral hand edema that is mistaken for polyarthritis.

Dermatomyositis [see Chapter 116] peaks in three age groups: 5 to 10 years of age, late teens and early 20s, and older than 45 years. The rash of dermatomyositis is similar to that of lupus, but the two rashes tend to involve the eyes differently: in dermatomyositis, telangiectasia causes the so-called heliotrope appearance of the eyelids; lupus rashes involve the eyebrows, but the malar rash stops abruptly at the orbits. Also, the rash in dermatomyositis commonly spares the ear canals, whereas the ear canals are commonly involved in lupus. Periungual telangiectasia is more dramatic in dermatomyositis than in lupus; it also occurs in scleroderma. Rash over the small joints of the hands suggests dermatomyositis; rash between the joints suggests lupus.

Compared with SLE, rheumatoid arthritis occurs in older persons (40 to 60 years of age) and has less of a female predominance (2:1 to 3:1). Although morning stiffness, fatigue, and weight loss are common in patients with rheumatoid arthritis, specific visceral multisystem disease is not. Leukocytosis rather than leukopenia is characteristic of rheumatoid arthritis. Renal disease is very rare, and when it does occur, it is attributable to tubular disease or amyloidosis rather than to glomerulonephritis. High fever does not occur in rheumatoid arthritis. From 10% to 20% of patients with rheumatoid arthritis have antinuclear antibodies; a small percentage have low-titer anti-DNA antibodies, and a minority have anti–SS-A and anti–SS-B antibodies. Complement levels are usually elevated. Rheumatoid factor is present in 80% of patients with rheumatoid arthritis, compared with its presence in 25% of lupus patients.

OVERLAP DISEASE

Some patients have symptoms suggestive of lupus (most commonly, arthritis, pleuritic pain, and cytopenia) but lack the specific diagnostic criteria for lupus (e.g., butterfly rash, glomerulonephritis, and high-titer anti-DNA or anti-Sm antibody). Other patients have lupuslike symptoms together with findings suggestive of rheumatoid arthritis, dermatomyositis, or scleroderma. Patients with no definable serology and a nondescript clinical picture are defined as having undifferentiated connective tissue disease (UCTD). Still other patients have inflammatory myositis, Raynaud phenomenon, and sclerodactyly together with very high titer antibodies to the ribonucleoprotein antigen (U1 RNP) and no anti-DNA or anti-Sm antibody. This set of findings is defined as mixed connective tissue disease (MCTD).

The differentiation of SLE from UCTD, MCTD, and Sjögren syndrome depends on the extent and pattern of different organ involvement (glomerulonephritis is rare in all these disorders except lupus) and on the accompanying serologic abnormalities. High-titer anti-DNA antibody or anti-Sm antibody generally indicates lupus; high-titer anti-RNP antibody with no other positive antibodies indicates MCTD; and anti–SS-A and anti–SS-B antibodies are consistent with Sjögren syndrome but occur in lupus and rheumatoid arthritis, as well. Occasionally, patients have characteristic rheumatoid destructive arthritis, subcutaneous nodules, and high-titer rheumatoid factor and anti-DNA antibody. These patients, as well as those with other overlap features, should be treated as if they have both diseases.

The prognosis in patients with UCTD tends to be more benign than that in patients with SLE. Patients with MCTD do not develop glomerulonephritis, but the long-term prognosis for patients with this disorder is worsened by the eventual development of pulmonary hypertension.

Treatment

ACUTE DISEASE

Management recommendations for the acute symptoms of lupus depend on the severity and organ systems involved. Non–life-threatening manifestations, such as minor arthritis, arthralgia, malaise, myalgias, serositis, and low-grade fever can often be controlled with full doses of NSAIDs. There is no specific preference among the NSAIDs, but lupus patients are unusually susceptible to hepatic and renal toxicities, which must be monitored. Also, in rare cases, lupus patients have developed abrupt high fever and meningitis after taking ibuprofen and similar drugs. Patients who do not respond to NSAIDs usually do respond to low doses (5 to 10 mg/day) of prednisone. As a rule, patients with inflammatory rashes, as well as patients anticipated to be on treatment for months or longer, should receive antimalarial therapy with hydroxychloroquine, 200 mg twice daily. Over a course of 3 months or more, hydroxychloroquine reduces arthralgia, myalgia, rash, fatigue, malaise, and similar symptoms.[55] Patients expected to take corticosteroids for more than a few weeks should strongly consider bone-protective measures [see Osteoporosis, below]. Such patients should also consider the addition of a lipid-lowering agent, such as a statin, to the regimen. Facial rashes, especially erythematous lesions with edema or telangiectasia, may respond to topical therapy with corticosteroid creams.

Alopecia may recover spontaneously, but it is not otherwise easily amenable to therapy. Wigs and falls or hair extenders are useful. Skillful use of makeup can cover most pigment changes caused by discoid lupus.

Low-dose corticosteroid therapy may be appropriate for modest thrombocytopenia or anemia. Leukopenia does not usually require treatment. High-dose corticosteroid therapy (60 mg of prednisone daily) is used for patients with severe systemic symptoms, renal disease, or other visceral disease that is potentially life threatening. Treatment should be initiated in split doses during the day, maintained for 4 to 6 weeks, and then tapered; too early reduction of dose usually results in recurrence of disease activity. If longer-term use of corticosteroids is anticipated, if vasculitis or life-threatening disease is present, or if corticosteroid toxicity is unacceptable, it is generally advisable to add immunosuppressive therapy. Immunosuppressive agents used for lupus include cyclophosphamide administered orally or intravenously, azathioprine, and mycophenolate mofetil. A standard regimen for active lupus nephritis includes a high-dose corticosteroid and intravenous cyclophosphamide. The cyclophosphamide is given at a dosage of 1 g/m^2 monthly for 6 months and then every 3 months for 2 years.

Acute cerebral symptoms (other than stroke) are usually treated with high-dose corticosteroids. Hallucinations and other psychotic symptoms respond to antipsychotic medications such as haloperidol, which is often administered in conjunction with corticosteroids. Because psychosis may also result from the use of a high-dose of a corticosteroid alone, withdrawal of corticosteroids may be necessary in some cases. The distinction between so-called steroid psychosis and lupus psychosis is quite difficult. No single set of criteria distinguishes between the two; evidence of ongoing active lupus in other organ systems is an indication to treat the patient for lupus psychosis. Acute lupus episodes are often treated with bolus doses of a corticosteroid (usually, 1,000 mg of methylprednisolone administered by rapid I.V. infusion [1 hr] once daily for 3 days). Very few formal studies support this practice, but clinical experience suggests its efficacy and relative safety. Bolus corticosteroid treatment may cause abrupt increases in blood pressure, acute vasospasm leading to stroke, cardiac infarct, or intestinal infarct. Transient oliguria and increased serum creatinine levels may also occur. To prevent these complications, bolus therapy should be monitored closely and withheld if hypertension is not controlled. Access to renal replacement therapy must be available in the event that the patient experiences diminished renal function.

Many new therapies are being investigated. These are largely biologic therapies and include the use of drugs directed against receptors of immune-activating cells or recognition cells and the use of modulators of immune response, such as CD154, CTLA-4, and anti-C5b. Removal of antibody by passing patient plasma over an absorptive column is also being studied. Tumor necrosis factor–α (TNF-α) inhibition, which was once thought to be dangerous for SLE patients, is under reconsideration. Attempts at hormone manipulation, as with dehydroepiandrosterone (DHEA), have had only modest success.

No single test informs the physician whether treatment for acute SLE is successful or not. Instead, it is necessary to monitor the entire clinical picture, including symptoms and results of physical examination, routine laboratory tests, and immune function studies.

INDICES OF DISEASE SEVERITY

Flare

Increase of inflammation in any SLE-affected organ system is known as flare. In a subpopulation of SLE patients, flare is a continuous, not a dichotomous, variable. In a given patient, it may occur in different organ systems at different rates and intensities; for instance, rash may become severe while nephritis remains sta-

ble. As a result, several different schemas for measuring flare exist. They differ in giving different weights to individual measures of disease activity (for instance, does new nephritis count more or less than new rash?) and whether serologic measures (antinuclear antibody titer, anti-DNA antibody, complement) do or do not count in the determination. The available indices—SLE Disease Activity Index (SLEDAI), Systemic Lupus Activity Measure (SLAM), and British Isles Lupus Assessment Group (BILAG)[56]—generally agree in identifying flare in populations of patients but often disagree in specifics. There is poor consensus about distinguishing between day-to-day variation of disease activity and a definite flare. Several components of the indices (e.g., quantitation of rash or of arthritis) are sufficiently subjective that investigators in clinical trials must undergo standardization training before they can validate their scores on individual patients.

Flare in pregnancy Proteinuria, thrombocytopenia, and other pregnancy events that occur in the absence of lupus invalidate most scoring systems for pregnant patients. A specific instrument, the SLE Pregnancy Disease Activity Index (SLEPDAI), has been devised for use in pregnant patients.[57]

Damage

Recurring inflammation and vascular occlusion induce irreversible scarring and such permanent deficits as stroke, cataract, skin thinning, osteoporosis, osteonecrosis, and renal failure. It is common practice, therefore, to score SLE patients according to their activity (flare) indices and their damage indices. The most widely used damage index is the Systemic Lupus International Collaborating Clinics (SLICC).[58]

SLE DURING PREGNANCY

Pregnancy in patients with SLE, once thought to be contraindicated, is now a routine event. The complications of pregnancy in these patients are related to three major issues: abnormal renal function, the presence of antiphospholipid antibody, and the presence of anti–SS-A and anti–SS-B antibody. It remains debatable whether lupus is exacerbated by pregnancy, but consensus now exists that pregnant SLE patients do not need prophylactic increases of corticosteroid therapy; rather, they should be treated in the same manner as patients who are not pregnant, except that drugs with fetal toxicity should not be given.

Renal disease, particularly renal insufficiency, strongly predisposes to toxemia of pregnancy. Hypertension, reduced creatinine clearance, and active SLE all threaten the viability of the fetus. Conversely, women who enter pregnancy with no renal disease and no hypertension usually do well. Recurrent pregnancy loss, particularly in the second trimester, is one of the prime clinical manifestations of the antiphospholipid antibody syndrome; for antiphospholipid antibody–positive patients, the peripartum period is one of high risk for thromboembolic disease. Women who have antibody to the SS-A or SS-B antigen are at risk of delivering children with the neonatal lupus syndrome.

CHRONIC DISEASE AND COMPLICATIONS

The major treatment issue for long-term lupus patients is the prevention or management of damage to the arteries, kidneys, bones, and brain rather than the control of immune response and inflammation. The physician must anticipate chronic effects of both the disease and its therapy.

During treatment with high-dose corticosteroids, with or without immunosuppressive agents, avoidance of infections is a primary concern. Herpes zoster, tuberculosis, and a variety of bacterial infections are the primary threats. *Pneumocystis jiroveci* (formerly *Pneumocystis carinii*) infection is seen relatively infrequently; most rheumatologists do not routinely suggest prophylaxis against this organism. Complications of long-term corticosteroid therapy include osteoporosis (see below) and cataracts, cutaneous striae, cutaneous hemorrhage, diabetes, and oral and vaginal candidiasis. In patients with long-standing disease, these complications produce as much morbidity as the disease itself.

Antiphospholipid Antibody Syndrome

Treatment of antiphospholipid antibody syndrome is anticoagulation to an international normalized ratio (INR) of 2.0 to 3.0. Warfarin and low-dose aspirin are used to prevent thrombotic manifestations of the syndrome; heparin or low-molecular-weight heparin is used in pregnant patients.[59] Recent data suggest that the addition of statin drugs, to downregulate endothelial activation, may also be of benefit.[60]

Atherosclerosis

Early-onset, severe atherosclerosis is a common problem in patients with long-standing SLE. Atherosclerosis most commonly presents as coronary and cerebral artery occlusion; peripheral vascular occlusion also occurs. The cause is unknown, but chronic inflammation, corticosteroid therapy, uncontrolled hypertension, diabetes, smoking, and other factors have been implicated. Most specialists in this area recommend early and vigorous treatment of known risk factors in all lupus patients. The atherosclerosis of lupus is managed in the same manner as atherosclerosis in other situations, except that vascular interventions in patients with antiphospholipid antibody syndrome are hazardous.

Osteonecrosis

Although the mechanism of osteonecrosis is not clearly known, many authorities believe that a steroid-induced increase in the volume of lipocytes increases pressure in the bone marrow, cutting off blood flow to the vulnerable areas. Consequently, if osteonecrosis is recognized before the joint has collapsed (usually by bone scan or MRI), trephining the bone to reduce intraosseous pressure (so-called core decompression) has been recommended. However, the validity of this theory and the efficacy of the treatment remain unproved. Usually, joint replacement is eventually required.[61]

Osteoporosis

Osteoporosis follows long-term corticosteroid therapy with sufficient frequency that all patients receiving such therapy should receive prophylaxis for this complication. High-dose oral calcium (i.e., 1,500 mg daily), vitamin D, a bisphosphonate drug, and parathyroid hormone are the primary preventive measures; estrogen replacement may be considered in postmenopausal women who do not have antiphospholipid antibody. Weight-bearing exercise should be encouraged. Other prophylactic measures, including calcitonin and parathyroid hormone, may be appropriate. Because lupus patients are photosensitive, increased sun exposure to prevent osteoporosis is unwise. Bisphosphonates should not be used in women anticipating pregnancy.

Cardiac Disease

Inflammatory cardiomyopathy responds to corticosteroids; ischemic cardiomyopathy does not. Valvular insufficiencies and thromboemboli are late complications of lupus cardiac disease. Bacterial endocarditis rarely complicates this abnormality. Valvulitis generally does not respond to treatment, although it has been reported that acute valvulitis will respond to corticosteroid therapy.[62] Small numbers of patients require valve replacement, usually of the aortic or mitral valve. The mechanism of valvulopathy in SLE is unknown, as are methods of prevention.

PALLIATIVE CARE

A common mistake in the treatment of SLE is to assume that a given complaint reflects ongoing inflammatory disease, rather than irreversible damage, and that it can be controlled with anti-inflammatory and immunosuppressive therapy rather than with palliation. Examples of such symptoms include seizures, dementia, and other neurologic syndromes associated with brain infarcts; cutaneous ulcers caused by long-standing vascular insufficiency; embolic phenomena from atherosclerosis; respiratory insufficiency from pulmonary fibrosis or pulmonary hypertension; arthritis from osteonecrosis, erosive rheumatoid-like arthritis, or tendinosis; and progressive renal insufficiency from arteriolonephrosclerosis, interstitial fibrosis, or glomerulosclerosis.

Dementia

Chronic neurologic disease, often in the form of dementia, is a long-term sequela of SLE. Some causes are stroke (atherosclerotic, hypertensive, or thrombotic associated with antiphospholipid antibody), autoantibody attack on specific brain targets, small vessel occlusive disease, and drugs. Occasionally, patients are severely disabled. No effective prophylaxis is known.

Renal Failure

Patients with renal disease often need angiotensin-converting enzyme inhibitors for proteinuria, antihypertensives for hypertension, erythropoietin for anemia, and diuretics for edema. Renal failure in lupus occurs in three modes. In the first, acute inflammatory nephritis is characterized by distinctly abnormal urinalyses and clinically and serologically evident disease activity. Patients with this type of renal picture have rapidly rising serum creatinine levels and enter renal failure early after diagnosis. If treated aggressively, with high-dose corticosteroids and immunosuppressive drugs, renal failure will be reversible in approximately one third of these patients.[63] In the second mode of renal failure, which occurs only occasionally, patients will have renal failure from drug toxicity—usually NSAIDs—or acute tubular necrosis. Other manifestations of SLE are modified in uremia: rash is less prominent; and fever, cachexia, mucosal ulcers, and cytopenias are more prominent.

In the third mode, which is the most common, lupus patients enter renal failure slowly after many years of disease. Characteristically, at the time renal failure first appears, the patient has little systemic illness and has had months to years of modest renal insufficiency (with creatinine clearance at 10 to 30 ml/min and serum creatinine below 3.5 mg/dl), slowly rising serum creatinine levels, relatively noninflammatory urinary sediments, and progressive anemia. Then, over a few months, the patient develops hypertension and fluid retention with or without cardiac failure. Abdominal pain is frequently present. Ultrasound shows small, fibrotic kidneys or thin, scarred renal cortices. Renal failure is only transiently reversible in such patients. Aggressive immunosuppressive therapy is not helpful at this stage; on the contrary, it may hasten renal deterioration and will complicate initiation of dialysis.

Less commonly, renal failure is caused by antiphospholipid antibody-associated thrombotic microangiopathy. In these cases, the presentation comprises modest proteinuria with bland urine sediment and slowly rising serum creatinine levels, often with moderate hypertension. Lupus vasculitis involving the kidneys tends to be abrupt in onset, with severely abnormal urinalyses, severe hypertension, and rapidly progressive renal failure. This complication is treated with high-dose corticosteroids and immunosuppression. However, full recovery is uncommon.

Lupus patients, particularly those who enter renal failure slowly, tolerate dialysis and renal transplantation well. However, preexisting cardiac, cerebral, and osteoarticular damage may be limiting factors. Patients who enter renal failure acutely often have other active systemic disease, with seizures and cytopenias being the most common. The common belief that lupus becomes inactive in renal failure is likely not true. Rather, in the majority of patients who enter dialysis, the lupus was already inactive systemically and remains so; probably, the renal failure results not from continuing disease but from progressive scarring. In the minority of patients who enter renal failure during an acute systemic flare, usually early in the course of the illness, active systemic disease tends to continue, and it represents a relative contraindication to renal transplantation. Patients on dialysis who have active SLE usually have high anti-DNA antibody levels and low complement levels. They respond to corticosteroid therapy, usually at lower doses than patients who are not on dialysis.

Prognosis

Prognosis in SLE has four elements: immediate prognosis for life, immediate prognosis for individual organ systems, and long-term prognosis for organ systems and for life.

During the early phases of lupus, complete reversal of almost all manifestations (i.e., rash, arthritis, fever, cytopenias, and nephritis) with aggressive therapy is expected. Exceptions include the scarring discoid rash, brain or spinal cord infarcts, and severe nephritis or nephrosis. In rare cases (< 5%), patients have such severe disease that despite treatment, they rapidly progress to death within 2 years. Because most newly diagnosed patients respond to therapy, 5-year survival is 80% to 90%, 10-year survival is 70% to 90%, and 20-year survival is nearly 70%.[6] Determinants of survival are age, renal disease, and race, with African Americans having lower overall survival than whites.[64]

One organ system (e.g., kidneys or platelets) may fail to respond completely to treatment but not directly threaten the patient's life. Such patients may be monitored without intervention. A patient may develop chronic renal insufficiency (e.g., serum creatinine, 3.0 mg/dl) or have persistent thrombocytopenia (platelet count, 30,000/mm³) and be considered to be in remission and in no need of treatment.

Long-term prognosis is a function of organ damage from either SLE or its treatment. Pulmonary fibrosis and pulmonary hypertension respond poorly to therapy, although new protocols, such as bosentan or infusion of prostacyclin, may be useful for pulmonary hypertension. Patients with cardiopulmonary failure who have no other system disease limitations are candidates for heart and lung transplantation. Lupus patients with renal failure are candidates for dialysis and for renal transplantation.

The author has no commercial relationships with manufacturers of products or providers of services discussed in this chapter.

References

1. Zonana-Nacach A, Barr SG, Magder LS, et al: Damage in systemic lupus erythematosus and its association with corticosteroids. Arthritis Rheum 43:1801, 2000

2. Mimouni D, Nousari CH: Systemic lupus erythematosus and the skin. Systemic Lupus Erythematosus, 4th ed. Lahita RG, Ed. Academic Press, San Diego, 2004, p 855

3. Mongey A-B, Hess EV: Drug and environmental lupus: clinical manifestations and differences. Systemic Lupus Erythematosus, 4th ed. Lahita RG, Ed. Academic Press, San Diego, 2004, p 1121

4. Lockshin MD: Antiphospholipid syndrome. Kelley's Textbook of Rheumatology. Ruddy S, Harris ED Jr, Sledge C, Eds.WB Saunders, Philadelphia, 2001, p 1145

5. Buyon JP: Neonatal lupus syndromes. Systemic Lupus Erythematosus, 4th ed. Lahita RG, Ed. Academic Press, San Diego, 2004, p 449

6. Gladman DD: Epidemiology of systemic lupus erythematosus. Systemic Lupus Erythematosus, 4th ed. Lahita RG, Ed. Academic Press, San Diego, 2004, p 697

7. Karlson EW, Daltroy LH, Lew RA, et al: The relationship of socioeconomic status, race, and modifiable risk factors to outcomes in patients with systemic lupus erythematosus. Arthritis Rheum 40:47, 1997

8. Hahn BH: Antibodies to DNA. N Engl J Med 338:1359, 1998

9. Balow JE, Boumpas DT, Austin HA III: Systemic lupus erythematosus and the kidney. Systemic Lupus Erythematosus, 3rd ed. Lahita RG, Ed. Academic Press, San Diego, 1999, p 657

10. Bonfa E, Golombek SJ, Kaufman LD, et al: Association between lupus psychosis and anti–ribosomal P protein antibodies. N Engl J Med 317:265, 1987

11. Harrison MJ, Ravdin LD, Volpe B, et al: Anti-NR2 antibody does not identify cognitive dysfunction in a general SLE population. Arthritis Rheum 50:s596, 2004

12. Walport MJ: Lupus, DNAse, and defective disposal of cellular debris. Nat Genet 25:135, 2000

13. Blanco P, Palucka AK, Gill M, et al: Induction of dendritic cell differentiation by IFN-alpha in systemic lupus erythematosus. Science 294:1540, 2001

14. Davies KA, Robson MG, Peters AM, et al: Defective Fc-dependent processing of immune complexes in patients with systemic lupus erythematosus. Arthritis Rheum 46:1028, 2002

15. Marrack P, Kappler J, Kotzin BL: Autoimmune disease: why and where it occurs. Nat Med 7:899, 2001

16. Davidson A, Diamond B: Autoimmune diseases. N Engl J Med 345:340, 2001

17. Crow MK, Kirou KA: Interferon-alpha in systemic lupus erythematosus. Curr Opin Rheumatol 16:541, 2004

18. Reveille JD: Major histocompatibility complex class II and non–major histocompatibility complex genes in the pathogenesis of systemic erythematosus. Systemic Lupus Erythematosus, 3rd ed. Lahita RG, Ed. Academic Press, San Diego, 1999, p 67

19. Harley JB, Moser KL, Gaffney PM, et al: The genetics of human systemic lupus erythematosus. Curr Opin Immunol 10:690, 1998

20. Abel G, Agnello V: Complement deficiency and systemic lupus erythematosus. Systemic Lupus Erythematosus, 4th ed. Lahita RG, Ed. Academic Press, San Diego, 2004, p 173

21. Zuniga R, Ng J, Peterson MG, et al: Low binding alleles of Fc gamma receptor types IIa and IIIa are inherited independently and are associated with systemic lupus erythematosus in Hispanic patients. Arthritis Rheum 44:361, 2001

22. James JA, Kaufman KM, Farris AD, et al: An increased prevalence of Epstein-Barr virus infection in young patients suggests a possible etiology for systemic lupus erythematosus. J Clin Invest 100:3019, 1997

23. Arbuckle MR, McClain MT, Rubertone MV, et al: Development of autoantibodies before the clinical onset of systemic lupus erythematosus. N Engl J Med 349:1526, 2003

24. Petri M, Robinson C: Review: oral contraceptives and systemic lupus erythematosus. Arthritis Rheum 40:797, 1997

25. Lockshin MD, Sammaritano LR, Schwartzman S: Lupus pregnancy. Systemic Lupus Erythematosus, 4th ed. Lahita RG, Ed. Academic Press, San Diego, 2004, p 449

26. Ruiz-Irastorza G, Lima F, Alves J, et al: Increased rate of lupus flare during pregnancy and the puerperium: a prospective study of 78 pregnancies. Br J Rheumatol 35:133, 1996

27. Bynoe MS, Grimaldi CM, Diamond B: Estrogen up-regulates Bcl-2 and blocks tolerance induction of naive B cells. Proc Natl Acad Sci USA 97:2703, 2000

28. Cooper GS, Dooley MA, Treadwell EL, et al: Hormonal, environmental, and infectious risk factors for developing systemic lupus erythematosus. Arthritis Rheum 41:1714, 1998

29. Alarcon GS, McGwin G Jr, Bartolucci AA, et al: Systemic lupus erythematosus in three ethnic groups: IX. Differences in damage accrual. LUMINA Study Group. Arthritis Rheum 44:2797, 2001

30. Salmon JE, Roman MJ: Accelerated atherosclerosis in systemic lupus erythematosus: implications for patient management. Curr Opin Rheumatol 13:341, 2001

31. Hochberg MC: Updating the American College of Rheumatology revised criteria for the classification of systemic lupus erythematosus (letter). Arthritis Rheum 40:1725, 1997

32. Lockshin MD, Sammaritano LR, Schwartzman S: Brief report: validation of the Sapporo Criteria for antiphospholipid antibody syndrome. Arthritis Rheum 43:440, 2000

33. Lahita RG: The clinical presentation of systemic lupus erythematosus in adults. Systemic Lupus Erythematosus, 4th ed. Lahita RG, Ed. Academic Press, San Diego, 2004, p 435

34. Lawrence EC: Systemic lupus erythematosus and the lung. Systemic Lupus Erythematosus, 4th ed. Lahita RG, Ed. Academic Press, San Diego, 2004, p 961

35. Roldan CA, Shively BK, Crawford MH: Echocardiographic study of valvular heart disease associated with lupus erythematosus. N Engl J Med 335:1424, 1996

36. Lockshin MD, Salmon JE, Roman MJ: Atherosclerosis and lupus: a work in progress (editorial). Arthritis Rheum 44:2215, 2001

37. Roman MJ, Shanker BA, Davis A, et al: Prevalence and correlates of accelerated atherosclerosis in systemic lupus erythematosus. N Engl J Med 349:2399, 2003

38. Bywaters EGL: Jaccoud's syndrome: a sequel to the joint involvement of systemic lupus erythematosus. Clin Rheum Dis 1:125, 1975

39. Mont MA, Glueck CJ, Pacheco IH, et al: Risk factors for osteonecrosis in systemic lupus erythematosus. J Rheumatol 24:645, 1997

40. Nagasawa K, Tsukamoto H, Tada Y, et al: Imaging study on the mode of development and changes in avascular necrosis of the femoral head in systemic lupus erythematosus: long-term observations. Br J Rheumatol 33:343, 1994

41. Dotan I, Mayer L: Nonhepatic gastrointestinal manifestations of systemic lupus erythematosus. Systemic Lupus Erythematosus, 4th ed. Lahita RG, Ed. Academic Press, San Diego, 2004, p 975

42. Mackay IR: Hepatic disease and systemic lupus erythematosus: coincidence or convergence. Systemic Lupus Erythematosus, 4th ed. Lahita RG, Ed. Academic Press, San Diego, 2004, p 993

43. The American College of Rheumatology Nomenclature and Case Definitions for Neuropsychiatric Lupus Syndromes. ACR Ad Hoc Committee on Neuropsychiatric Lupus Nomenclature. Arthritis Rheum 42:599, 1999

44. Hanly JG: Evaluation of patients with CNS involvement in SLE. Baillière's Clin Rheumatol 12:415, 1998

45. Harrison MJ, Gershengorn J: Despite low rate of global impairment in SLE patients, cognitive performance is less than expected (abstr). Arthritis Rheum 44:s197, 2001

46. Kozora E, Thompson LL, West SG, et al: Analysis of cognitive and psychological deficits in systemic lupus erythematosus patients without overt central nervous system disease. Arthritis Rheum 39:2035, 1996

47. Sanna G, Piga M, Terryberry JW, et al: Central nervous system involvement in systemic lupus erythematosus: cerebral imaging and serological profile in patients with and without overt neuropsychiatric manifestations. Lupus 9:573, 2000

48. Gladman DD, Urowitz MB, Slonim D, et al: Evaluation of predictive factors for neurocognitive dysfunction in patients with inactive systemic lupus erythematosus. J Rheumatol 27:2367, 2000

49. Weening JJ, D'Agati VD, Schwartz MM, et al: The classification of glomerulonephritis in systemic lupus erythematosus revisited. Kidney Int 65:521, 2004

50. Clancy RM, Kapur RP, Molad Y, et al: Immunohistologic evidence supports apoptosis, IgG deposition, and novel macrophage/fibroblast crosstalk in the pathologic cascade leading to congenital heart block. Arthritis Rheum 50:173, 2004

51. Wilson WA, Gharavi AE, Koike T, et al: International consensus statement on preliminary classification criteria for definite antiphospholipid syndrome: report of an international workshop. Arthritis Rheum 42:1309, 1999

52. Kozora E, West SG, Kotzin BL, et al: Magnetic resonance imaging abnormalities and cognitive deficits in systemic lupus erythematosus patients without overt central nervous system disease. Arthritis Rheum 41:41, 1998

53. Sibbitt WL Jr, Sibbitt RR, Brooks W: Neuroimaging in neuropsychiatric systemic lupus erythematosus. Arthritis Rheum 42:2026, 1999

54. West SG, Emlen W, Wener MH, et al: Neuropsychiatric lupus erythematosus: a ten-year prospective study on the value of diagnostic tests. Am J Med 99:153, 1995

55. A randomized study of the effect of withdrawing hydroxychloroquine sulfate in systemic lupus erythematosus. Canadian Hydroxychloroquine Study Group. N Engl J Med 324:150, 1991

56. Liang MH, Socher SA, Roberts WN, et al: Measurement of systemic lupus erythematosus activity in clinical research. Arthritis Rheum 31:817, 1988

57. Buyon JP, Kalunian KC, Ramsey-Goldman R, et al: Assessing disease activity in SLE patients during pregnancy. Lupus 8:677, 1999

58. Gladman DD, Goldsmith CH, Urowitz MB, et al: The Systemic Lupus International Collaborating Clinics/American College of Rheumatology (SLICC/ACR) Damage Index for systemic lupus erythematosus international comparison. J Rheumatol 27:373, 2000

59. Khamashta MA, Cuadrado MJ, Mujic F, et al: The management of thrombosis in the antiphospholipid-antibody syndrome. N Engl J Med 332:993, 1995

60. Meroni PL, Raschi E, Testoni C, et al: Statins prevent endothelial activation induced by antiphospholipid (anti-beta$_2$-glycoprotein I) antibodies: effect on the proadhesive and proinflammatory phenotype. Arthritis Rheum 44:2862, 2001

61. Mont MA, Fairbank AC, Petri M, et al: Core decompression for osteonecrosis of the femoral head in systemic lupus erythematosus. Clin Orthop 334:91, 1997

62. Nesher G, Ilany J, Rosenmann D, et al: Valvular dysfunction in antiphospholipid syndrome: prevalence, clinical features and treatment. Semin Arthritis Rheum 27:27, 1997

63. Kimberly RP, Lockshin MD, Sherman RL, et al: Reversible "end-stage" lupus nephritis: analysis of patients able to discontinue dialysis. Am J Med 74:361, 1983

64. Trends in deaths from systemic lupus erythematosus—United States, 1979–1998. MMWR Morb Mortal Wkly Rep 51(17):371, 2002

Acknowledgment

Figure 2b © 2002 Hospital for Special Surgery. http://www.Rheumatology.HSS.edu All rights reserved. Used by permission.

115 Scleroderma and Related Diseases

George Moxley, M.D.

Scleroderma

DEFINITION AND CLASSIFICATION

Scleroderma, or systemic sclerosis, is a rare, slowly progressive rheumatic disease characterized by deposition of fibrous connective tissue in the skin and other tissues. It is accompanied by vascular lesions, especially in the skin, lungs, and kidneys. No cure is known.

Scleroderma may be either systemic or localized, with the systemic illness being either diffuse or limited. The limited form of systemic scleroderma, or CREST syndrome (calcinosis, Raynaud phenomenon, esophageal involvement, sclerodactyly, and telangiectasias), involves internal organs less often than diffuse scleroderma. Except when pulmonary hypertension is present, patients with the limited form have a better prognosis than those with the diffuse form [*see Table 1*]. Systemic scleroderma can be fatal.

Localized scleroderma is confined to the skin, subcutaneous tissue, and muscle and is not accompanied by the Raynaud phenomenon, acrosclerosis, or visceral involvement. There are two forms of localized scleroderma: morphea, which presents as variable-sized plaques of skin induration, and linear, which presents as bands of skin induration on the face or a single extremity. Linear scleroderma may be associated with muscle atrophy and involvement of the underlying bone. It usually afflicts children or young adults and may lead to significant growth impairment of the involved part. In the morphea version, the lesions may persist for months or years, after which improvement may occur [*see Table 1*]. Although there is a possibility of disfigurement, localized scleroderma is not a severe illness, and patients with the disease generally have a normal life span.

EPIDEMIOLOGY

The Raynaud phenomenon is associated with scleroderma [*see* Diagnosis, Clinical Manifestations, *below*]. Primary Raynaud phenomenon (Raynaud phenomenon without underlying illness) is quite common, with up to 30% of young women having episodes. A meta-analysis showed that the transition rate to a defined inflammatory rheumatic disease (e.g., scleroderma or lupus) is 3.2 per 100 patient-years of observation; the eventual development of an inflammatory rheumatic disease occurred in 12.6% of individuals. The best predictor of development of inflammatory disease is an abnormal nailfold capillary pattern, which has a predictive value of 47%; a positive antinuclear antibody test has a predictive value of 30%.[1] Racial, genetic, and environmental factors have been proposed as influences of scleroderma risk and disease pattern.[2]

The overall global incidence of scleroderma is approximately 17 to 19 per one million population per year, with higher rates for women than for men. African Americans experience diffuse scleroderma more often than other ethnic groups; whites are more often diagnosed with the CREST variant.[3] The prevalence in the United States is approximately 24 per 100,000 population[3]—fourfold to ninefold the prevalence in other countries. Mortality factors include diffuse disease, older age at onset, and internal organ involvement, particularly pulmonary and renal involvement. Some investigators have suggested that scleroderma is associated with various environmental expo-

sures.[4] For example, workers exposed to polyvinylchloride may experience the Raynaud phenomenon and scleroderma-like skin thickening.[5] However, no substance has yet been convincingly linked with scleroderma.[5] Silicone breast implants have not been found to be associated with scleroderma.[6]

ETIOLOGY

The etiology of scleroderma is largely unknown. The disease shows familial aggregation consistent with a genetic component, and family history is the strongest risk factor.[3] In the United States, about 1.6% of relatives are affected, an over 60-fold higher prevalence than in the general population (0.026%).[3] One etiologic factor may be a fibrillin defect. Fibrillin is a macromolecule that is a component of elastic fibers, and it is defective in Marfan syndrome. In an animal model (the tight-skin mouse, *tsk1*), a scleroderma-like condition is caused by an insertion into the fibrillin gene that apparently encodes a latent binding region for the transforming growth factor-β (TGF-β) cytokine. One proposed explanation is that the abnormal fibrillin binds an increased number of fibroblast growth factors that influence nearby fibroblasts. The current knowledge extends to Japanese and Oklahoma Choctaw scleroderma patients, who likely have a scleroderma-related genetic defect (e.g., secreted protein acidic and rich in cystein [SPARC]) in the fibrillin chromosomal region either in or near the gene.[7] However, other genes (e.g., *IL-1A, TGF-β,* and *IL-4*) or environmental exposures may also be involved.

PATHOPHYSIOLOGY AND PATHOGENESIS

The common pathologic features of tissues with scleroderma involvement are progressive fibrosis, vascular abnormalities, and inflammation. Fibrosis involves an accumulation of excessive collagen and other extracellular matrix constituents, such as glycosaminoglycans and fibronectin. The vascular abnormalities are intimal hyperplasia with collagen deposition and adventitial fibrosis, capillary dropout, dilatation, tortuosity, and fibrotic atherosclerosis. The inflammatory changes may include cellular infiltration. These pathologic characteristics are believed to be the result of three or more interacting components: autoimmunity, an endothelial abnormality, and a skin fibroblast lesion. An alternative explanation is that these characteristics are the result of a disease process akin to graft versus host disease (GVHD).

Table 1 Classification of Scleroderma

Form	Syndrome
Scleroderma (systemic sclerosis)	Diffuse skin involvement Limited skin involvement (CREST syndrome) Overlapping features of mixed connective tissue disease
Localized scleroderma	Morphea: single or multiple plaques or generalized lesions Linear scleroderma

CREST—calcinosis, Raynaud phenomenon, esophageal involvement, sclerodactyly, and telangiectasias

Immune Cell and Cytokine Abnormalities

Activated thymus-derived lymphocytes predominate among the cells that infiltrate involved tissues; activated inflammatory cells are also present. Such immune and inflammatory cells release a plethora of cytokines and soluble mediators. Of particular note are cytokines influencing fibroblast function: interleukin-1 (IL-1), IL-4, IL-6, IL-8, RANTES (regulated upon activation, normal T cell expressed and secreted), tumor necrosis factor (TNF), and TGF-β. TNF and interferon gamma are antifibrotic,[8] but the action of TGF-β results in a pattern of tissue damage similar to the pattern seen in scleroderma. TGF-β stimulates fibroblasts and vascular smooth muscle cells to make collagen, and it stimulates endothelial cells to make endothelin-1, which, in turn, causes vasoconstriction and collagen production. B cells are also activated in patients with scleroderma, and some autoantibodies are relatively specific for scleroderma. Whether such humoral responses result in scleroderma tissue damage is under investigation.

Fibroblast Abnormalities

As with lymphocytes and macrophages showing activation in scleroderma, fibroblasts are also metabolically activated. Such activated cells overproduce collagen, other extracellular matrix molecules, and cellular adhesion molecules.[9] The reasons why collagen gene expression is increased and sustained have not been fully explained. One possible explanation is that the presence of cytokines such as IL-4 and TGF-β strongly foster collagen production.[8] TGF-β acts in large part through specific receptors that lead to activation of Smads, a family of second messenger/transcription factor proteins.[10] Some genetic studies have supported the proposition that scleroderma is associated with TGF-β markers.[11]

Vascular Abnormalities

Vessels in involved tissues show disrupted pattern and function, characterized by altered endothelial permeability, adhesion of platelets and leukocytes to endothelium, and the presence of inflammatory cells. One current pathogenetic theory is that endothelial homeostasis is disrupted, leading to increased endothelin-1 production, reduced prostacyclin release, and enhanced coagulation.[12] Endothelial cells express increased numbers of adhesion molecules necessary for inflammatory cell adhesion and extravasation. Capillaries become obliterated but are not replaced; involved tissues may become ischemic and then reperfused. The Raynaud phenomenon [see Diagnosis, Clinical Manifestations, below] is a hallmark vascular lesion that likely represents an exaggerated response of a stiff vessel wall to a typical environmental exposure. Microscopic analysis of the nailfolds of patients with scleroderma and Raynaud phenomenon reveals capillary disappearance and dilatation. In scleroderma, small arteries develop concentric intimal fibrosis and thus become narrow; this narrowing in turn greatly increases the vascular reactivity to alpha$_2$-adrenergic agents.

Chimerism and Microchimerism

Chimerism denotes a state in which a person has cells derived from two or more other people. Male DNA consistent with microchimerism has been found more frequently and in higher concentrations in the circulation of women with scleroderma who have had a previous male delivery than in women without scleroderma who have also had a male delivery. In addition, microchimerism has been found in tissues of mothers

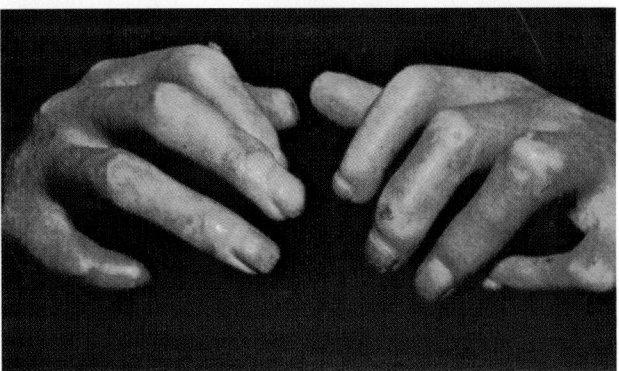

Figure 1   **Severe involvement of the hands in a patient with long-standing scleroderma includes flexion contractures of the fingers related to fibrosis of the skin and of subcutaneous tissues. Increased pigmentation has occurred, and melanin loss (vitiligo) is evident in some areas. The distal aspects of the terminal phalanges in some fingers have undergone resorption or shortening. This process, termed autoamputation, usually occurs without ulceration of the terminal digit; the mechanism is unknown.**

with scleroderma but not in the tissues of healthy mothers.[13] However, cause and effect are not yet established,[14] and parous women are reported to have a reduced scleroderma risk (odds ratio, 0.3).[15]

DIAGNOSIS

Clinical Manifestations

Skin   The first signs of scleroderma in the skin are swelling and thickening of the fingers and hands, with or without involvement of the face; later in the illness, other areas of skin may become thickened. Involvement of the trunk and arms proximal to the elbows is associated with visceral involvement and a poorer prognosis. The skin continues to thicken during the first 2 to 3 years after the onset of disease; the thickening then ceases and may recede, giving the impression that the skin is softening. In subsequent years, skin atrophy occurs, with con-

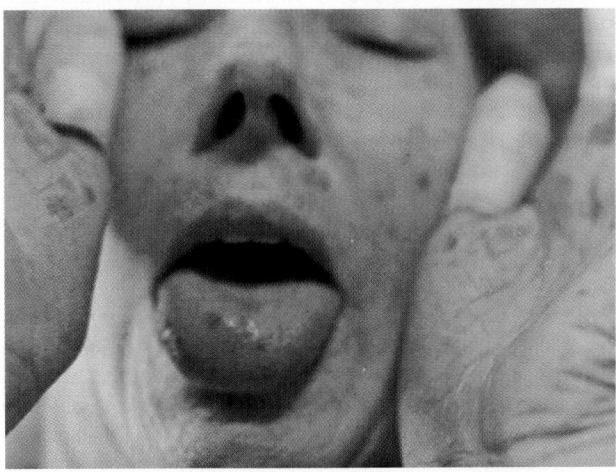

Figure 2   **Telangiectasias appear on the hands, face, and tongue in a patient with the CREST (calcinosis, Raynaud phenomenon, esophageal involvement, sclerodactyly, and telangiectasias) variant of scleroderma. Thumbs are bandaged because of chronic ulcerations associated with the Raynaud phenomenon.**

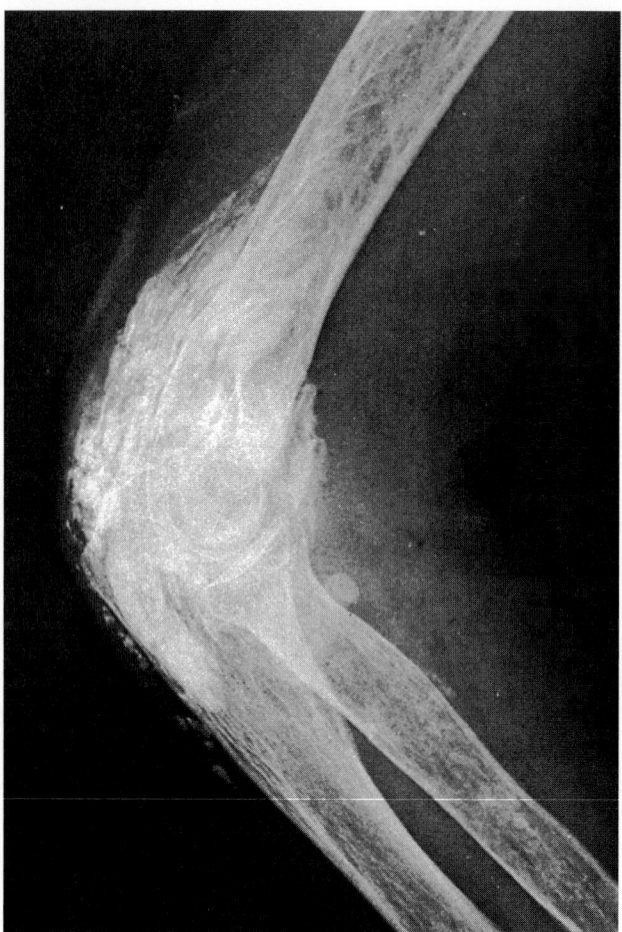

Figure 3 **In scleroderma, extensive calcinosis (hydroxyapatite crystal deposition) may be found in connective tissues and around joints. If extensive, calcinosis is usually associated with at least partial loss of joint motion.**

comitant loss of hair, sebaceous glands, and sweat glands, as well as a loss of pliability. In addition, the skin becomes hide-bound—tightly drawn and bound to underlying structures.

Skin involvement is often most prominent in the hands and fingers (sclerodactyly); frequently, the face is also affected. A tightening of facial skin results in decreased skin lines, a pursed appearance, and a diminution in the oral aperture. The skin tightness may limit mobility, especially in the fingers. Flexion contractures may also develop in the fingers [*see Figure 1*]. Several other skin abnormalities may accompany these changes. Telangiectasias occur frequently and may be numerous [*see Figure 2*]. They are often most prominent on the face, hands, and oral mucosa. Calcinosis—the deposition of hydroxyapatite crystals in subcutaneous areas—may be limited or widespread and is usually located around joint capsules [*see Figure 3*]. Skin ulceration over calcific deposits may lead to drainage of a white material with a consistency resembling toothpaste. A diffuse increase in melanotic pigmentation may extend over the entire skin surface; areas of hypopigmentation are also commonly seen.

The Raynaud phenomenon is an episodic manifestation of numbness or pain accompanied by a two- or three-phase color change in the digits; these changes are triggered by cold temperatures or emotional stress and are relieved by warming the involved part. In severe cases, however, the relation to ambient

temperature is sometimes less obvious. The episode typically begins with pallor, followed by cyanosis and, finally, by redness caused by reactive hyperemia [*see Figure 4*]. Prolonged ischemia may lead to painful digits, ulceration, and even gangrene. Almost all patients (95%) with diffuse or limited scleroderma experience the Raynaud phenomenon. The Raynaud phenomenon is also seen in patients with other disorders, including other autoimmune diseases such as systemic lupus erythematosus (SLE), polymyositis, and several forms of vasculitis; in patients who are receiving certain drugs, such as bleomycin, ergot derivatives, beta blockers, and methysergide; and after occupational exposure to vinyl chloride, cold temperatures, and vibrating tools.

In scleroderma, the Raynaud phenomenon is a manifestation of vasculopathy involving small arteries and capillaries; it occurs not only in the extremities but also in some involved viscera, such as the lungs and kidneys. Patients with scleroderma and the Raynaud phenomenon have characteristic capillary changes on nailfold microscopy. Nailfold microscopy consists of observation of the capillary structure of the periungual tissues with a handheld magnifying lens, such as that used in a standard ophthalmoscope. Patients with underlying scleroderma may exhibit loss of some capillaries and dilatation of capillaries in other nailfold areas. Such changes often occur in asso-

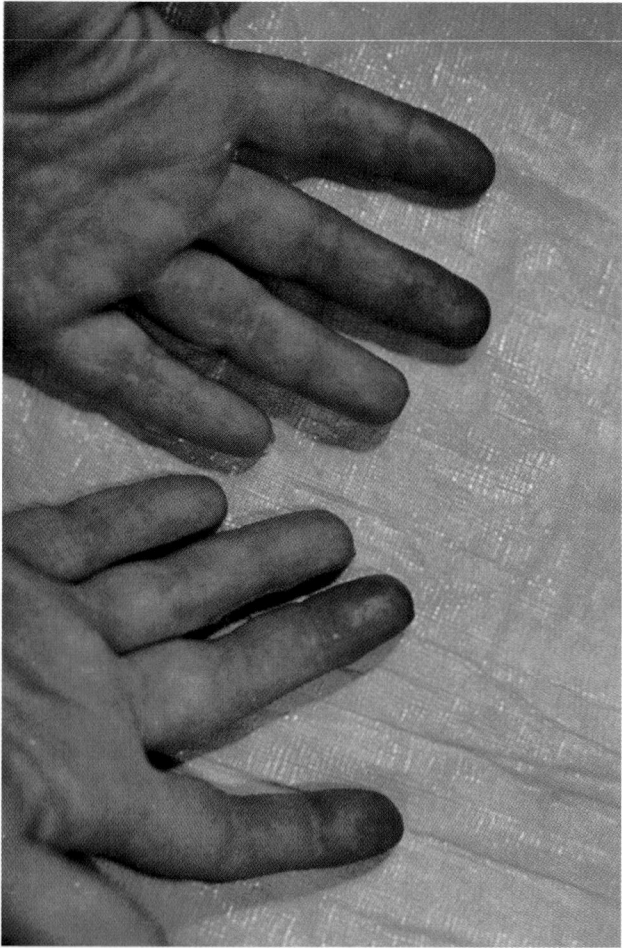

Figure 4 **Vascular pathology usually manifests itself as the Raynaud phenomenon in patients with scleroderma. The cyanotic phase of the Raynaud phenomenon often involves the distal two thirds of the second and third fingers of both hands.**

Table 2   Antinuclear Antibodies in Scleroderma

Immunofluorescent Pattern of Antinuclear Antibody Staining	Antigens	Clinical Pattern	Approximate Frequency (%)	Specificity
Nucleolar	Nuclear ribonucleoproteins (nRNPs)	Diffuse or limited scleroderma	50	Moderate
	RNA polymerases I, II, and III	Diffuse scleroderma	23	High
	Nuclear proteins PM-1 (PM-Scl) and Ku	Scleroderma-polymyositis overlap	< 5	High, for scleroderma and polymyositis
Centromeric (large speckles)*	Centromere proteins (CENP-A, CENP-B, and CENP-C)	Usually in limited scleroderma (CREST syndrome)	50 (of patients with CREST syndrome)	High
Diffuse (fine speckles)	Topoisomerase I (Scl-70)	Diffuse scleroderma	20–33	High
Homogeneous	Histones (mainly H1 and H3)	Localized scleroderma	50	Moderate

*Requires a human epithelial carcinoma cell line (HEp-2).

ciation with internal organ involvement and may be used to predict the development of diffuse scleroderma when visceral involvement is not clinically apparent.

Proposed criteria for early diagnosis of scleroderma include either objective observation or measurement of cold-induced vasospasm, plus either abnormal nailfold microscopy, presence of antibodies directed toward characteristic autoantigens [*see Table 2*],[16] or patient reports of Raynaud phenomenon and the presence of nailfold microscopic changes and autoantibodies.

Musculoskeletal system   A mild, usually symmetrical, inflammatory arthritis can occur in scleroderma. Juxta-articular bone erosions occur frequently, especially in the distal interphalangeal joints, but the degree of destruction is usually less than that seen in rheumatoid arthritis. Flexion contractures of the fingers often develop and are most likely related to fibrosis

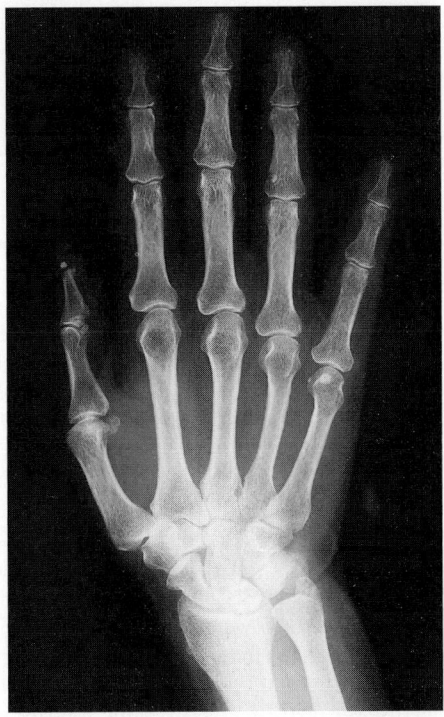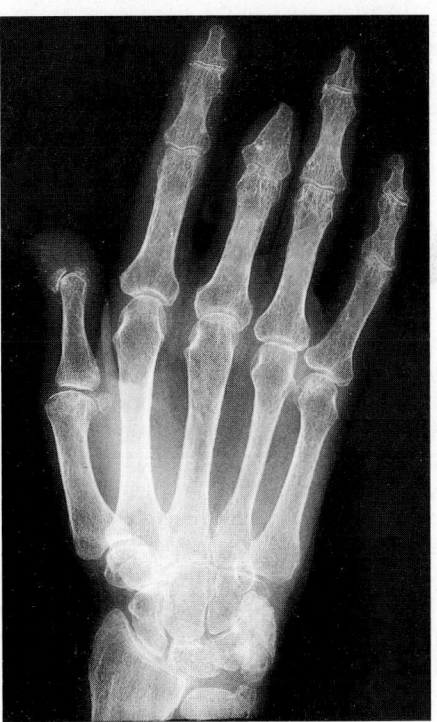

Figure 5   **Over an 8-year period, radiographs taken of the hand of a patient with scleroderma demonstrate a progressive, terminal resorption of the digits. The earlier film (left) shows a loss of the spherical terminal portion of the distal phalanx of the thumb and a small, dense calcific deposit at the terminal aspect of the thumb. After an 8-year period, dramatic changes can be seen (right). An almost complete loss of the terminal phalanx of the thumb and a partial loss of the distal phalanges of the remaining fingers are observed. In addition, the entire distal phalanx of the third finger is lost along with part of the middle phalanx. Loss of the middle phalanx is less common than loss of the distal phalanges. A generalized osteopenia is present in the later stage, which is probably related to osteoporosis of disuse, and a calcific deposit has formed in the ulnar aspect of the wrist. The apparent narrowing of interphalangeal joint spaces may be associated with flexion contractures of the fingers, which are caused by the fibrous thickening of the connective tissues of the hand.**

of the tendons and joint capsules. Crepitus and friction rubs, detected by palpation or auscultation over tendons and bursas, are characteristic findings related to fibrotic changes of underlying tissues. Another skeletal complication is acral osteolysis, which is the resorption of the terminal phalanges and surrounding soft tissue with consequent shortening of the digits [see Figure 5]. It may occur without infection or ulceration. Patients with scleroderma may have one or more of a variety of muscle disorders,[17] such as fatigue without objective evidence of muscle damage, a simple myopathy, or clear-cut inflammatory myositis.

GI tract Almost every part of the GI tract may be involved in scleroderma.[18] Sjögren syndrome, which causes dry eyes and dry mouth, occurs in about one third of patients with scleroderma. Esophageal hypomotility, which is demonstrated by cinefluoroscopic examination and manometric studies, occurs in more than 90% of patients with scleroderma, many of whom are asymptomatic [see Figure 6]. The absence of normal peristaltic waves in the lower two thirds of the esophagus may cause dysphagia; incompetence of the gastroesophageal sphincter leads to reflux esophagitis and sometimes may result in esophageal stricture. Barrett esophagus, esophageal carcinoma, and candidal esophagitis may ensue. Similarly, hypomotility of the stomach, small intestine, colon, and anorectal area may occur, possibly causing gastroparesis, pseudo-obstruction, colonic impaction, or impaired anorectal function. Telangiectasias may be present in the gastric mucosa and the mucosa of the small intestine and colon. Gas may dissect into the intestinal wall (pneumatosis intestinalis) and leak into the peritoneal cavity, simulating a perforated viscus. Characteristic widemouthed diverticula of the colon may develop; these are pathognomonic of scleroderma. The early lesions of the GI tract may be caused by autonomic nerve dysfunction; autonomic nerve dysfunction may in time lead to smooth muscle atrophy and irreversible muscle fibrosis of the gut. Primary biliary cirrhosis and drug-induced hepatitis may also be associated with scleroderma.

Lungs Pulmonary involvement represents an important cause of scleroderma-related morbidity and mortality[19]; lung disease is the most frequent cause of scleroderma-related death. Although scleroderma-related findings may range from associated malignancy and silicosis to calcinosis and hemorrhage, the most common findings are pulmonary vascular disease and interstitial inflammation and fibrosis. Isolated pulmonary hypertension is typically found in the CREST syndrome (prevalence is 50% to 65% in the limited cutaneous subset and up to 35% in the diffuse subset)[20]; interstitial pulmonary fibrosis may be found in both limited and diffuse scleroderma (at postmortem examination, the frequency is about 75%).

Isolated pulmonary hypertension usually results in cough, dyspnea, and syncope; it has a severe prognostic outlook (5-year survival < 10%). Pulmonary hypertension is defined by a resting mean pulmonary arterial pressure greater than 25 mm Hg or an exercise-induced mean pulmonary arterial pressure greater than 30 mm Hg; in addition, pulmonary hypertension is often associated with abnormal diffusing capacity for carbon monoxide. In persons with limited cutaneous involvement, decreasing diffusing capacity of the lung for carbon monoxide ($D_{L_{CO}}$) is an excellent predictor of subsequent pulmonary hypertension; one study of 106 patients reported that at baseline,

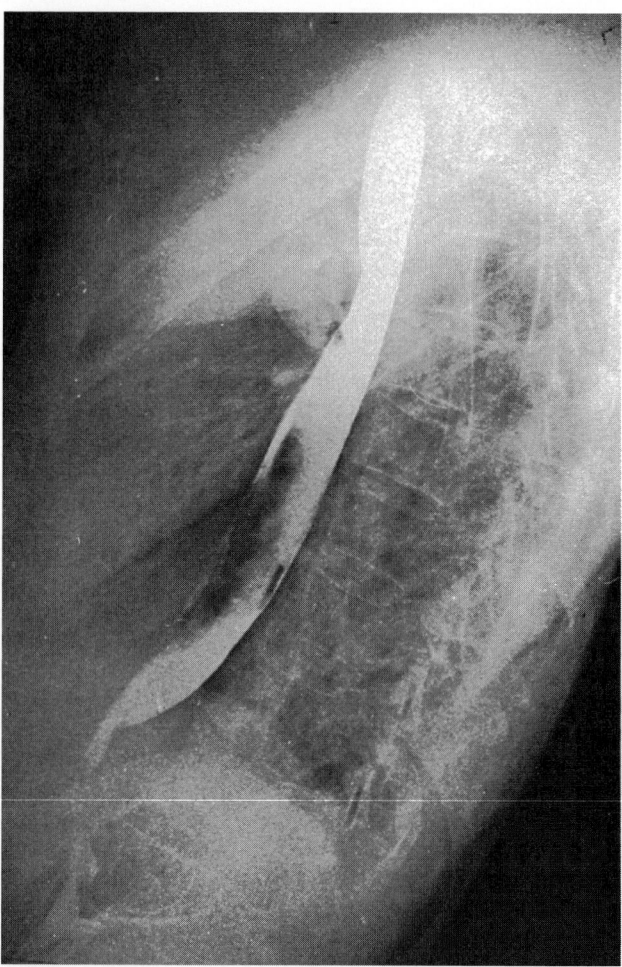

Figure 6 **Hypomotility of the esophagus in scleroderma, which is demonstrated by the lack of peristaltic waves in the barium column, is frequently an asymptomatic finding, but it may be associated with dysphagia and incompetence of the gastric sphincter, which results in reflux esophagitis.**

patients who subsequently developed pulmonary hypertension had a mean pulmonary arterial pressure only slightly higher than patients who did not, but the $D_{L_{CO}}$ in patients with pulmonary hypertension declined from a mean of 80% to a mean of 35%. The early clinical features associated with subsequent pulmonary hypertension included more severe Raynaud phenomenon and digital tip ulcers, as well as positivity for serum autoantibodies directed toward nucleoli.[21]

Interstitial fibrosis is typically accompanied by dyspnea and cough, and the 5-year survival is about 45%. Although chest roentgenograms may show linear and reticular abnormalities, high-resolution CT scanning is favored for the detection of early disease; on CT scans, alveolitis appears as patchy areas with a ground-glass appearance. Interstitial fibrosis appears to result from inflammatory alveolitis: the release of various cytokines and chemokines in the course of the inflammatory process results in fibroblast activation and extracellular matrix remodeling. Association between severe esophageal involvement and interstitial fibrosis suggests that gastroesophageal reflux may contribute to fibrotic changes.[22]

Heart Patients with clinically evident scleroderma-related heart disease have a poor prognosis.[23] The myocardium is involved in approximately 20% to 25% of clinical cases of systemic scleroderma. Scleroderma-associated myocardial disease is typically characterized by patchy areas of myocardial fibrosis replacing normal muscle; this may cause hypertrophy and diminished cardiac output, particularly with exercise. Diastolic dysfunction[24] and atherosclerotic coronary artery disease are common. Myocardial infarctions may develop in patients with scleroderma who have normal findings on coronary artery catheterization. Myocarditis may also occur in patients with scleroderma-associated inflammatory myositis. The patchy myocardial fibrosis and conduction system involvement may result in various arrhythmias and sudden death. Pericardial disease is common at autopsy, but clinically evident pericardial manifestations occur in only 5% to 16% of cases. Such pericardial disease may cause acute pericarditis, arrhythmias, pericardial effusions, or sudden death. In limited cutaneous scleroderma, apart from a similar frequency of cardiac arrhythmias and conduction defects, heart involvement is generally less frequent and less severe than in diffuse scleroderma.

Kidneys Chronic mild proteinuria and mild hypertension are common effects of scleroderma but typically do not result in significant renal dysfunction. The most significant disease process associated with scleroderma is renal crisis,[25] which consists of the rapid development of malignant hypertension, hyperreninemia, microangiopathic hemolytic anemia, and oliguric renal failure. Renal crisis typically occurs in the scleroderma subset characterized by rapidly progressive diffuse skin disease. Renal crisis was formerly the most common cause of death in patients with scleroderma, but aggressive treatment with angiotensin-converting enzyme (ACE) inhibitors early in the course of disease has greatly improved outcome.

Other organ systems Although scleroderma rarely involves the central nervous system, peripheral neuropathy may occur. The most frequent form is unilateral or bilateral trigeminal neuropathy of one or more of the three trigeminal branches; this neuropathy presents as progressive numbness and pain. Widespread autonomic nervous system dysfunction underlies the propensity for the Raynaud phenomenon and intestinal involvement. Hematopoietic consequences of scleroderma are uncommon.

Laboratory Findings

More than 85% of patients with scleroderma have positive test results for antinuclear antibodies[26] [*see Table 2*]. Antibodies to certain nuclear antigens are specific for scleroderma,[27] and each type of antibody is associated with a particular clinical pattern of disease. Antibodies to Scl-70 and to RNA polymerases (usually RNA polymerase III) are seen in patients with systemic scleroderma. In a meta-analysis, anti–Scl-70 antibodies had a positive predictive value of 70% for diffuse cutaneous scleroderma.[28] Anticentromere antibodies are associated with limited scleroderma (the CREST syndrome); the meta-analysis indicated a positive predictive value of 88% for limited cutaneous scleroderma.[28] Antibodies to nuclear ribonucleoprotein (nRNP) are associated with diffuse and limited scleroderma. Antibodies to PM-1 and Ku are infrequent. The presence of these antibodies is usually associated with overlapping clinical features of polymyositis and scleroderma. About 50% of patients with localized scleroderma have antibodies to histones [*see Table 2*].

MANAGEMENT

Management of scleroderma is often a severe challenge,[29] but it includes several potentially lifesaving interventions. Close attention to detecting renal and pulmonary involvement will typically improve eventual outcomes.

Renal Crisis

Renal crisis is a serious scleroderma-related manifestation that is manageable with appropriate therapy. Onset typically is within the first 2 years of the disease course and is more common in diffuse scleroderma than in the limited form of the disease[30]; renal crisis occurs in about 15% of patients with diffuse scleroderma. A clinician should instruct patients with early diffuse scleroderma about daily blood pressure monitoring and initiate antihypertensive therapy if the patient's blood pressure exceeds 130/80 mm Hg. Renal crisis is recognized by diminished renal function with new-onset hypertension (even of modest degree), microscopic hematuria, and proteinuria. Treatment of this medical emergency with ACE inhibitors and other potent antihypertensive drugs appears to arrest the deterioration in renal function. Even in patients who initially require dialysis, ACE inhibitors may restore renal function enough to make dialysis unnecessary.[31] However, this therapy has been shown to be more beneficial when initiated before serum creatinine levels have exceeded 3 mg/dl. In some patients, renal failure progresses despite good control of blood pressure, necessitating dialysis and possibly renal transplantation. Despite reduced frequency with ACE inhibitor therapy and availability of dialysis, renal crisis is associated with poor survival rates.[32]

Pulmonary Involvement

A clinician should be able to detect pulmonary involvement through yearly or twice-yearly pulmonary arterial pressure estimates (from echocardiograms) and measurements of forced vital capacity, carbon monoxide diffusing capacity, and exercise arterial blood gas levels. Patients with pulmonary function abnormalities may then be evaluated with bronchoalveolar lavage, where available, and high-resolution CT to detect the extent of lower respiratory inflammation. Progression is more likely to occur in patients with more extensive lung disease and patients who are positive for anti-Scl-70 antibodies. In diffuse scleroderma, meticulous assessment is warranted, particularly in the first 5 years after onset.[33] In patients with early fibrosing alveolitis, progression of pulmonary fibrosis may be halted by long-term therapy with cyclophosphamide and low-dose prednisone (< 10 mg/day), but this measure is not yet supported by a randomized, controlled trial.[19,33] Cyclophosphamide therapy is a powerful immunosuppressive medication; its use is sometimes associated with adverse events such as bacterial infections, herpes zoster, varicella-zoster virus infection, interstitial cystitis, and malignancies such as bladder transitional cell carcinoma. Often, intravenous cyclophosphamide is effective and somewhat less toxic than oral regimens.[33]

Pulmonary hypertension may be a particularly serious manifestation of scleroderma. In patients with suspected pulmonary arterial hypertension, on the basis of physiologic findings and serial echocardiographic examinations, a right heart catheter measurement of pulmonary arterial pressure should be obtained. Individuals with pulmonary arterial hypertension should receive influenza and pneumococcal immunizations and be counseled regarding cigarette smoking and other important exposures. When hypoxemia is present, supplemental oxygen is appropriate.

If serious pulmonary hypertension occurs, the patient should be referred to a specialist for this condition. Referral is important because current therapy is rapidly evolving, the medications used are not part of the usual formulary, and the specialist's experience will lead to reduced risk of complication and toxicity. Internet resources may prove useful in identifying local specialists and support programs available to scleroderma patients [see Sidebar Internet Resources for Information on Scleroderma].

The therapeutic measures employed for pulmonary arterial hypertension include the use of calcium channel blockers, anticoagulation, prostaglandin medications, phosphodiesterase V inhibitors such as sildenafil, and endothelin receptor antagonists such as bosentan. In a small fraction of patients, high-dose calcium channel blockers will reduce pulmonary arterial pressure and vascular resistance without causing serious adverse effects such as hypotension[34]; in this subset of patients, it is necessary to administer a diuretic to reduce risk of right-sided heart failure. Warfarin therapy (achieving an international normalized ratio of 2.0 to 2.5) increases survival.[34]

Various prostaglandins are helpful for therapy of pulmonary artery hypertension. The currently available prostaglandins include continuous intravenous epoprostanol (2 ng/kg/min) and continuous subcutaneous treprostinil (1.25 ng/kg/min); other oral and inhaled prostaglandins are under study. Epoprostanol has been shown to prolong life and decrease symptoms and improve hemodynamics[35-37]; however, it is exacting in terms of discomfort and disability. Subcutaneous treprostinil therapy is more convenient and improves symptoms and exercise capacity but is sometimes associated with infusion-site pain.[38] Oral sildenafil appears to improve gas exchange[39] and may act synergistically when administered with an inhaled prostaglandin (e.g., iloprost).[40] The most dramatic therapeutic development has been bosentan, an orally administered endothelin-1 antagonist (125 mg twice daily). Bosentan therapy leads to improved exercise capacity, decreased symptoms, and improved hemodynamic effects, but hepatotoxicity is a concern.[41] However, the most beneficial therapies for severe pulmonary arterial hypertension are costly (annual cost of bosentan, $36,000; epoprostanol, $72,000; and treprostinil, $93,000).

Cutaneous Involvement

Most patients with the Raynaud phenomenon may be managed with such measures as avoidance of cold exposure. Instructions to wear warm clothing, gloves, and a hat when exposed to a cold environment may be sufficient. Cigarette smokers have a fourfold risk of digital vascular complications in surgical debridement, amputation, or intravenous vasodilator therapy[42]; smoking cessation is thus a key instruction. In addition, patients should avoid vasoconstrictive agents (e.g., decongestants, caffeine, amphetamines, beta blockers, and ergot alkaloids). For persons with attacks of the Raynaud phenomenon so frequent or so severe as to interfere with daily activities or to put them at risk for skin necrosis, pharmacologic therapy may be employed. Low-dose aspirin (81 mg daily) is recommended.[30] The calcium channel blocking agents promote vasodilatation and generally reduce the frequency and severity of Raynaud phenomenon.[43] Although nifedipine in daily doses of 30 to 60 mg has been effective for most patients, approximately one third do not respond, and some patients experience adverse effects. In double-blind, placebo-controlled trials, other calcium channel blockers have also shown efficacy for the Raynaud phenomenon; these agents include amlodipine, 5 to 10 mg daily, and felodipine, 5 to 10 mg daily. Ischemic digital ulcerations may be difficult to treat and may progress to gangrene of the fingertips. Sympathectomy should be reserved for severe ischemic crises.

GI Tract Involvement

Because gastroesophageal reflux is nearly universal in scleroderma, clinicians typically will instruct scleroderma patients to elevate the head of the bed and will administer proton pump inhibitors. Esophageal motility may be enhanced by use of metoclopramide. Esophageal dilatation may be required if strictures are present. Patients with diminished gastric emptying may be instructed regarding the frequent taking of small meals and may be given prokinetic medications such as metoclopramide. Small bowel motility may present as pain, distention, and vomiting; most episodes can be managed by increasing dietary fiber and avoiding medications that affect motility (e.g., opiates). Octreotide is used for severe small bowel dysmotility. For small bowel bacterial overgrowth with malabsorption, empirical antibiotic therapy with ciprofloxacin, metronidazole, doxycycline, or erythromycin is recommended.

Internet Resources for Information on Scleroderma*

National Institute of Arthritis and Musculoskeletal and Skin Diseases Information Clearinghouse

http://www.niams.nih.gov

This clearinghouse provides information about various forms of arthritis and rheumatic diseases, distributes patient and professional education materials, and refers people to other sources of information.

American College of Rheumatology

http://www.rheumatology.org

This association provides referrals to doctors and health professionals who work on arthritis, rheumatic diseases, and related conditions. The association also provides educational materials and guidelines.

Scleroderma Foundation

http://www.scleroderma.org

The foundation publishes information on scleroderma and offers patient education seminars, support groups, physician referrals, and information hotlines.

Scleroderma Research Foundation

http://www.srfcure.org

The foundation's goal is to find a cure for scleroderma by funding and facilitating the most promising, highest-quality research and by placing the disease and its need for a cure in the public eye. The foundation distributes patient handbooks and a twice-yearly, research-related newsletter.

Arthritis Foundation

http://www.arthritis.org

The foundation is a voluntary organization devoted to supporting research on arthritis and other rheumatic diseases, including scleroderma. It also provides up-to-date information on treatments, nutrition, alternative therapies, and self-management strategies. Chapters nationwide offer exercise programs, classes, support groups, physician referral services, and free literature.

*Descriptions of Web sites are derived from www.niams.nih.gov.

Potential Disease-Modifying Therapies

Potential disease-modifying therapies for scleroderma have also been studied. Penicillamine is no longer recommended because of associated toxicity and minimal efficacy,[44] and methotrexate therapy is of uncertain benefit.[45,46] Stem cell transplants are associated with a higher procedure-related mortality but typically lead to decreased skin manifestations and stabilization of lung function.[47,48] A truly effective disease-modifying therapy is not yet available.

CLINICAL COURSE

In the CREST syndrome, skin involvement is relatively limited, usually affecting only the hands and face; the prognosis for patients with this syndrome is generally favorable unless viscera are involved. However, even the limited CREST variant tends to be unremitting and slowly progressive. Many patients experience an indolent course with little change over several years, although the progression may be more rapid. Diffuse scleroderma is highly variable in its course and manifestations; therefore, its rate of progression is difficult to predict. With the exception of some of the sclerodermatous changes in mixed connective tissue disease, diffuse scleroderma rarely remits completely. Involvement of the viscera, such as the heart, lungs, or, particularly, the kidneys, indicates a poor prognosis. Two other features of scleroderma also indicate a poor outcome: (1) active inflammation, as manifested by an elevated erythrocyte sedimentation rate, and (2) evidence of cardiopulmonary disease, renal disease, or both within 1 year after diagnosis.[49] The life-threatening complications of scleroderma—severe skin involvement, pulmonary fibrosis, and renal crisis—usually occur within the first 2 to 5 years after the onset of disease. After this interval, the disease tends to run an indolent course. The 5-year survival for patients with diffuse scleroderma is approximately 50%, but pediatric patients with the disease have a much better prognosis.[50]

Eosinophilic Fasciitis

Eosinophilic fasciitis can superficially resemble scleroderma. It is characterized by pain, swelling, and tenderness of the extremities, after which induration of the skin and subcutaneous tissues occurs. Joint motion may be limited, but the Raynaud phenomenon, sclerodactyly, and other manifestations of scleroderma are not seen. Laboratory test abnormalities include peripheral blood eosinophilia, which may be marked; elevation of the erythrocyte sedimentation rate; and hyperglobulinemia. Antinuclear antibody and rheumatoid factor test results are negative. Biopsy specimens of involved areas have shown inflammation and thickening of the fascia deep to the subcutaneous tissues. The skin appears normal, but the underlying deep fascia is infiltrated with lymphocytes, plasma cells, histiocytes, and sometimes eosinophils. Eosinophilic fasciitis seems to be either self-limited or responsive to low doses of glucocorticoids. Its etiology remains unknown, but several cases have been reported after strenuous muscle exertion.

Eosinophilia-Myalgia Syndrome

In 1989, a previously unrecognized syndrome associated with ingestion of contaminated L-tryptophan appeared.[51] The eosinophilia-myalgia syndrome is characterized by peripheral eosinophilia, severe and incapacitating myalgias, and fatigue of several weeks' duration. Dyspnea and cough may also be present. Skin involvement consists of variable rashes, edema, and scleroderma-like changes, usually without the visceral manifestations of scleroderma. Interstitial pulmonary infiltrates, hypoxia, pulmonary hypertension, and hypersensitivity pneumonitis may occur. Polyneuropathy has been described in a pattern of mononeuritis multiplex. Neurocognitive disorders, such as memory disturbances and difficulty in concentration, have been reported. Most patients continue to manifest symptoms from 2 to 4 years after onset but have no new signs of inflammation.

The author has no commercial relationships with manufacturers of products or providers of services discussed in this chapter.

References

1. Spencer-Green G: Outcomes in primary Raynaud phenomenon: a meta-analysis of the frequency, rates, and predictors of transition to secondary diseases. Arch Intern Med 158:595, 1998
2. Michet C: Update in the epidemiology of the rheumatic diseases. Curr Opin Rheumatol 10:129, 1998
3. Mayes MD, Lacey JV Jr, Beebe-Dimmer J, et al: Prevalence, incidence, survival, and disease characteristics of systemic sclerosis in a large US population. Arthritis Rheum 48:2246, 2003
4. Nietert PJ, Silver RM: Systemic sclerosis: environmental and occupational risk factors. Curr Opin Rheumatol 12:520, 2000
5. Steen VD: Occupational scleroderma. Curr Opin Rheumatol 11:490, 1999
6. Janowsky EC, Kupper LL, Hulka BS: Meta-analyses of the relation between silicone breast implants and the risk of connective-tissue diseases. N Engl J Med 342:781, 2000
7. Ahmed SS, Tan FK: Identification of novel targets in scleroderma: update on population studies, cDNA arrays, SNP analysis, and mutations. Curr Opin Rheumatol 15:766, 2003
8. Widom RL: Regulation of matrix biosynthesis and degradation in systemic sclerosis. Curr Opin Rheumatol 12:534, 2000
9. Sato S: Abnormalities of adhesion molecules and chemokines in scleroderma. Curr Opin Rheumatol 11:503, 1999
10. Varga J: Scleroderma and Smads: dysfunctional Smad family dynamics culminating in fibrosis. Arthritis Rheum 46:1703, 2002
11. Denton CP, Abraham DJ: Transforming growth factor-beta and connective tissue growth factor: key cytokines in scleroderma pathogenesis. Curr Opin Rheumatol 13:505, 2001
12. Schachna L, Wigley FM: Targeting mediators of vascular injury in scleroderma. Curr Opin Rheumatol 14:686, 2002
13. Johnson KL, Nelson JL, Furst DE, et al: Fetal cell microchimerism in tissue from multiple sites in women with systemic sclerosis. Arthritis Rheum 44:1848, 2001
14. Tan FK, Arnett F: Genetic factors in the etiology of systemic sclerosis and Raynaud phenomenon. Curr Opin Rheumatol 12:511, 2000
15. Pisa FE, Bovenzi M, Romeo L, et al: Reproductive factors and the risk of scleroderma: an Italian case-control study. Arthritis Rheum 46:451, 2002
16. LeRoy EC, Medsger TA Jr: Criteria for the classification of early systemic sclerosis. J Rheumatol 28:1573, 2001
17. Olsen NJ, King LEJ, Park JH: Muscle abnormalities in scleroderma. Rheum Dis Clin North Am 22:783, 1996
18. Sjogren RW: Gastrointestinal features of scleroderma. Curr Opin Rheumatol 8:569, 1996
19. Bolster MB, Silver RM: Assessment and management of scleroderma lung disease. Curr Opin Rheumatol 11:508, 1999
20. Magliano M, Isenberg DA, Hillson J: Pulmonary hypertension in autoimmune rheumatic diseases: where are we now? Arthritis Rheum 46:1997, 2002
21. Steen V, Medsger TA Jr: Predictors of isolated pulmonary hypertension in patients with systemic sclerosis and limited cutaneous involvement. Arthritis Rheum 48:516, 2003
22. Marie I, Dominique S, Levesque H, et al: Esophageal involvement and pulmonary manifestations in systemic sclerosis. Arthritis Rheum 45:346, 2001
23. Deswal A, Follansbee WP: Cardiac involvement in scleroderma. Rheum Dis Clin North Am 22:841, 1996
24. Coghlan JG, Mukerjee D: The heart and pulmonary vasculature in scleroderma: clinical features and pathobiology. Curr Opin Rheumatol 13:495, 2001
25. Steen VD: Scleroderma renal crisis. Rheum Dis Clin North Am 22:861, 1996
26. Okano Y: Antinuclear antibody in systemic sclerosis (scleroderma). Rheum Dis Clin North Am 22:709, 1996
27. Harvey GR, McHugh NJ: Serologic abnormalities in systemic sclerosis. Curr Opin Rheumatol 11:495, 1999
28. Spencer-Green G, Alter D, Welch HG: Test performance in systemic sclerosis: anti-

centromere and anti-Scl-70 antibodies. Am J Med 103:242, 1997

29. Sule SD, Wigley FM: Update on management of scleroderma. Bull Rheum Dis 49:1, 2000

30. Walker JG, Ahern MJ, Smith MD, et al: Scleroderma renal crisis: poor outcome despite aggressive antihypertensive treatment. Intern Med J 33:216, 2003

31. Steen VD, Medsger TA Jr: Long-term outcomes of scleroderma renal crisis. Ann Intern Med 133:600, 2000

32. DeMarco PJ, Weisman MH, Seibold JR, et al: Predictors and outcomes of scleroderma renal crisis: the high-dose versus low-dose D-penicillamine in early diffuse systemic sclerosis trial. Arthritis Rheum 46:2983, 2002

33. Latsi PI, Wells AU: Evaluation and management of alveolitis and interstitial lung disease in scleroderma. Curr Opin Rheumatol 15:748, 2003

34. Rich S, Kaufmann E, Levy PS: The effect of high doses of calcium-channel blockers on survival in primary pulmonary hypertension. N Engl J Med 327:76, 1992

35. Badesch DB, Tapson VF, McGoon MD, et al: Continuous intravenous epoprostenol for pulmonary hypertension due to the scleroderma spectrum of disease: a randomized, controlled trial. Ann Intern Med 132:425, 2000

36. Barst RJ, Rubin LJ, Long WA, et al: A comparison of continuous intravenous epoprostenol (prostacyclin) with conventional therapy for primary pulmonary hypertension. The Primary Pulmonary Hypertension Study Group. N Engl J Med 334:296, 1996

37. Klings ES, Hill NS, Ieong MH, et al: Systemic sclerosis–associated pulmonary hypertension: short- and long-term effects of epoprostenol (prostacyclin). Arthritis Rheum 42:2638, 1999

38. Simonneau G, Barst RJ, Galie N, et al: Continuous subcutaneous infusion of treprostinil, a prostacyclin analogue, in patients with pulmonary arterial hypertension: a double-blind, randomized, placebo-controlled trial. Am J Respir Crit Care Med 165:800, 2002

39. Ghofrani HA, Wiedemann R, Rose F: Sildenafil for treatment of lung fibrosis and pulmonary hypertension: a randomised controlled trial. Lancet 360:895, 2002

40. Ghofrani HA, Wiedemann R, Rose F, et al: Combination therapy with oral sildenafil and inhaled iloprost for severe pulmonary hypertension. Ann Intern Med 136:515, 2002

41. Rubin LJ, Badesch DB, Barst RJ, et al: Bosentan therapy for pulmonary arterial hypertension. N Engl J Med 346:896, 2002

42. Harrison BJ, Silman AJ, Hider SL, et al: Cigarette smoking as a significant risk factor for digital vascular disease in patients with systemic sclerosis. Arthritis Rheum 46:3312, 2002

43. Thompson AE, Shea B, Welch V, et al: Calcium-channel blockers for Raynaud's phenomenon in systemic sclerosis. Arthritis Rheum 44:1841, 2001

44. Clements PJ, Furst DE, Wong WK, et al: High-dose versus low-dose D-penicillamine in early diffuse systemic sclerosis: analysis of a two-year, double-blind, randomized, controlled clinical trial. Arthritis Rheum 42:1194, 1999

45. van den Hoogen FH, Boerbooms AM, Swaak AJ, et al: Comparison of methotrexate with placebo in the treatment of systemic sclerosis: a 24 week randomized double-blind trial, followed by a 24 week observational trial. Br J Rheumatol 35:364, 1996

46. Pope JE, Bellamy N, Seibold JR, et al: A randomized, controlled trial of methotrexate versus placebo in early diffuse scleroderma. Arthritis Rheum 44:1351, 2001

47. Binks M, Passweg JR, Furst D, et al: Phase I/II trial of autologous stem cell transplantation in systemic sclerosis: procedure related mortality and impact on skin disease. Ann Rheum Dis 60:577, 2001

48. Furst DE: Stem cell transplantation for autoimmune disease: progress and problems. Curr Opin Rheumatol 14:220, 2002

49. Bulpitt KJ, Clements PJ, Lachenbruch PA, et al: Early undifferentiated connective tissue disease: III. Outcome and prognostic indicators in early scleroderma (systemic sclerosis). Ann Intern Med 118:602, 1993

50. Foeldvari I: Diffuse and limited cutaneous systemic scleroderma. Curr Opin Rheumatol 12:435, 2000

51. Varga J, Kahari VM: Eosinophilia-myalgia syndrome, eosinophilic fasciitis, and related fibrosing disorders. Curr Opin Rheumatol 9:562, 1997

Nancy J. Olsen, M.D., and Beth L. Brogan, M.D.

Idiopathic inflammatory myopathies, which include polymyositis and dermatomyositis, primarily affect skeletal muscle. The common features of these diseases are weakness of and inflammatory changes in skeletal muscle. In general, the idiopathic inflammatory myopathies are serious disorders that respond variably to therapy. Polymyositis and dermatomyositis may be linked with other rheumatic diseases, notably scleroderma, and with malignancies. Prognosis varies according to the specific syndrome that is expressed.

Classification

Classification of these heterogeneous muscle disorders into subtypes is useful for determining diagnostic and therapeutic approaches.[1,2] Categories are defined on the basis of clinical and histologic features rather than on laboratory or radiologic tests [*see Table 1*].

DERMATOMYOSITIS

Patients with dermatomyositis usually show symmetrical proximal muscle weakness in all extremities, accompanied by a characteristic skin rash. Neck and back muscles may also be weak. Areas of skin most commonly affected by the rash include extensor surfaces of the hands and knees. Subtypes of dermatomyositis include the juvenile form [*see* Juvenile Myositis, *below*]. Another recognized subtype is amyopathic dermatomyositis.[3-5] Patients with this disorder have the characteristic rash but do not have demonstrable muscle abnormalities. One study of such patients has shown that sensitive magnetic resonance imaging techniques can reveal changes after exercise that indicate a metabolic abnormality.[6]

POLYMYOSITIS

Patients with polymyositis have symmetrical proximal muscle weakness similar to that experienced in dermatomyositis, but the rash is absent. Onset of polymyositis may be more difficult to determine, in part because no rash is available as an indicator of possible inflammation. Muscle weakness and atrophy may be more profound than that usually seen in patients with dermatomyositis. However, no formal studies of long-term outcome have been carried out that prove this assertion.

JUVENILE MYOSITIS

Children ranging in age from younger than 5 years through the teen years may be affected by juvenile myositis. Most children have a skin rash, and vasculitis and soft tissue calcifications are much more common in children than in adults.[7] Although residual dermatologic changes, muscle fibrosis, and calcification may occur, the long-term outlook is generally favorable.[8]

MYOSITIS WITH MALIGNANCY

Most, but not all, cases of malignancy-associated myositis are accompanied by the typical rash of dermatomyositis. A recent study showed that patients with dermatomyositis had a relative risk of malignancy of 6.2. For patients with polymyositis or inclusion body myositis, the risk was lower but still significant.[9-11] The incidence of underlying malignancy increases with age[12] and decreases with increasing time from diagnosis.[9] Onset of the myositis may precede or follow discovery of the malignancy. Adults with dermatomyositis should be screened for occult malignancies in the first 2 years after onset of disease.

MYOSITIS WITH OTHER RHEUMATIC DISEASES

Inflammatory myositis may occur with another established rheumatic disease, most commonly scleroderma. Other conditions that can occur with myositis include rheumatoid arthritis, systemic lupus erythematosus (SLE), and Sjögren syndrome. Recent reports have linked scleromyxedema to dermatomyositis[13] and have linked inclusion body myositis to subacute cutaneous lupus.[14,15] Many patients with these overlap conditions have a relatively mild form of muscle inflammation that responds well to treatment. However, a small subset of patients, especially those with coexistent scleroderma, may have a severe and very debilitating muscle weakness that is resistant to therapy.[16]

INCLUSION BODY MYOSITIS

The pattern and severity of muscle weakness in inclusion body myositis (IBM) differs from the pattern of severity seen in the other idiopathic inflammatory myopathies. In addition to the presence of proximal weakness, distal muscles may be involved; and in some cases, muscle abnormalities are asymmetrical. Unlike most of the other muscle disorders discussed in this chapter, IBM afflicts more men than women, with approximately two thirds of affected persons being men. Response to treatment is generally poor.

Epidemiology

PREVALENCE AND INCIDENCE

The estimated prevalence of idiopathic inflammatory myopathies is approximately one case per 100,000 individuals.

Table 1 Classification of Myositis Syndromes

Clinicopathologic Category	Characteristics
Dermatomyositis	Proximal weakness, skin rash; amyopathic variant with rash only
Polymyositis	Proximal weakness without rash
Juvenile myositis	Myositis in childhood, usually with a rash
Myositis with malignancy	Myositis with associated underlying neoplastic disease
Myositis with another connective tissue disease	Coexistent syndrome, usually scleroderma, rheumatoid arthritis, or systemic lupus erythematosus
Inclusion body myositis	Severe weakness with characteristic inclusions on muscle biopsy

This prevalence makes these disorders about 1,000 times less common than rheumatoid arthritis. The rarer syndromes, such as IBM, may constitute 20% or less of all cases. In one study, the annual incidence of idiopathic inflammatory myopathies was 5.5 cases per million population.[17] Incidence rates, however, may be increasing, possibly because of improved methods of detection.

ETHNIC, RACIAL, AND GENDER GROUP DIFFERENCES

No ethnic clustering of the idiopathic inflammatory myopathies has been reported. It has been suggested that incidence rates in North America are increasing faster in African Americans than in whites.[17] In adults, polymyositis is more common than dermatomyositis, whereas in children and young adults, dermatomyositis is the predominant form. It has been suggested that incidence rates are higher in regions that have greater amounts of sun exposure.[18] Polymyositis and dermatomyositis show a female-to-male ratio of approximately 2:1. Risk of underlying malignancy increases significantly after 40 years of age.[12] Malignancies in children are rare but have been reported. The diagnosis of inclusion body myositis is rarely made in persons younger than 50 years.

Etiology and Pathogenesis

The etiology of inflammatory muscle disease remains unknown. The most widely accepted hypotheses suggest multiple factors. One possible scenario is that an initial insult—for example, a virus or another infectious agent or an environmental toxin—leads to muscle damage in a genetically susceptible host. This process in turn triggers an immune response, subsequently causing chronic muscle inflammation.[19]

INFECTIOUS AGENTS

A role for viruses in the etiology of idiopathic inflammatory myopathies has been suggested by seasonal and geographic clustering of new cases. Furthermore, infection with HIV or hepatitis C virus has been associated with the development of myopathy.[20] Most studies looking for evidence of viral genomic material in muscle tissue have failed to find such evidence.[21] Immunoreactivity for hepatitis C in involved muscle tissues has been reported in a single case.[20] Viruses may mediate tissue damage, which may in turn lead to immunologic responses that target or damage muscle tissues.[22] The relative rarity of the myositis syndromes would suggest that if a common infectious agent were involved, coexistent factors would also be required. These factors could include host-specific genetic loci that control the immune response or other noninfectious factors such as drugs or environmental toxins.[18]

NONINFECTIOUS FACTORS

Lipid-lowering agents such as clofibrate and the statin group of drugs have been associated with elevated levels of serum muscle enzymes and with muscle weakness in a small number of patients. However, most patients are asymptomatic. The list of drugs reported to be associated with development of myopathy is very long. For this reason, concomitant medications should be examined closely in any patient with unexplained muscle weakness.[23] Both HIV infection and drugs used in its treatment, such as zidovudine (AZT), have been implicated in the development of myopathy. It is possible that as yet undefined environmental toxins play a role.

GENETIC FACTORS

Familial clustering of inflammatory myositis syndromes occurs, but the great majority of cases are sporadic. Sporadic cases have been linked to HLA-DRB1*0301, whereas familial cases have shown increased prevalence of HLA-DQA1 (DQA1*0501). A form of hereditary IBM has been described in several ethnic groups. Chromosomal links with this disorder have been identified, but candidate genes are as yet undefined.[24] Many of the reported studies of genetic links in inflammatory myopathies have grouped several types of syndromes together. It is probable that future studies that perform separate analyses of the various distinct clinical syndromes will show stronger associations with genetic markers.

AUTOIMMUNE FACTORS

The presence of cellular infiltrates in muscle tissues is a defining feature of inflammatory muscle diseases [see Figure 1]. Light microscopic examination of these infiltrates reveals different patterns of infiltration. In tissues from patients with dermatomyositis, the lymphocytes are generally located around blood vessels and at the periphery of the muscle bundles. Invasion of muscle fibers by mononuclear cells is rarely observed, and there is a relative paucity of necrotic muscle fibers. Complement-mediated capillary damage is also more commonly observed in biopsy samples from dermatomyositis patients, especially those patients with an underlying malignancy. Some studies suggest that dermatomyositis patients with capillary damage who do not have a malignancy have a more acute syndrome that responds better to immunosuppressive treatment. In polymyositis, muscle fibers may be invaded by the mononuclear infiltrates, and focal areas of muscle destruction are seen. Tissues from patients with IBM usually show some degree of inflammation accompanied by intracellular rimmed vacuoles.[25]

Two groups have identified chimeric cells of maternal origin in the peripheral blood and inflammatory lesions of children with myositis. These findings support the hypothesis that

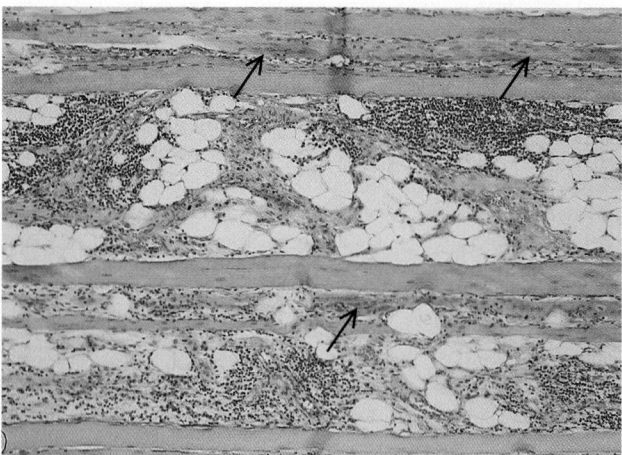

Figure 1 **Extensive pathologic changes can be seen in involved muscle in myositis. These changes include a decrease in the number of striated muscle fibers and a loss of cross-striations in the remaining fibers. Some fibers demonstrate increased numbers of rounded nuclei and basophilic staining (arrows), which suggests attempted regeneration. There is also intense infiltration of the muscle by mononuclear inflammatory cells, predominantly lymphocytes and plasma cells.**

childhood myositis is a manifestation of a graft-versus-host reaction.[26,27]

Differences between polymyositis and dermatomyositis are revealed by immunophenotyping of the cellular infiltrates.[28] Mononuclear cell infiltrates in polymyositis and probably in IBM tissues are predominantly of the CD8+ cytotoxic T cell phenotype. The CD8+ T cells in polymyositis show evidence of clonal expansion, which is most likely driven by muscle-specific antigens.[29] Activated CD8+ T cells probably mediate cytotoxic, immune-mediated, and antigen-specific muscle cell destruction. In dermatomyositis, T cells, predominantly of the CD4+ helper-inducer phenotype, are present along with B cells; restricted clonality is not seen.[29] These differences in histology support the hypothesis that polymyositis and dermatomyositis are distinct disorders with different etiologies.

Diagnosis

Major diagnostic criteria that were proposed by Bohan and Peter in 1975[1,2] remain useful for defining most of the myositis syndromes. However, IBM, which was not recognized at the time these criteria were written, differs somewhat from polymyositis and dermatomyositis. Although sophisticated diagnostic tests, including autoantibody profiles and imaging techniques, are now available, findings obtained through a careful history and physical examination remain indispensable for both making the initial diagnosis and evaluating responses to treatment.

CLINICAL FEATURES

Muscle Weakness

In polymyositis and dermatomyositis, the weakness is predominantly proximal. Distal strength is usually preserved. In IBM, the weakness may be asymmetrical, and diminished distal strength is commonly seen. Muscle strength can be tested in the office or at the bedside and estimated on a semiquantitative scale from 1 to 5. Devices for quantitative assessment of muscle strength, some of which can be used at the bedside, are also available.

Characteristic Skin Rash

The rash of dermatomyositis is a deep-red erythematous eruption, with or without mild scaling and atrophy. It occurs on the face, neck, upper chest, and extensor surfaces of joints such as elbows and those of the hands. Periorbital edema may appear, as may heliotrope erythema, which is characterized by a violet or lilac color, especially of the eyelids. Occasionally, the rash is more widespread or takes different forms [see Figure 2]. Erythema and telangiectasia also occur in periungual areas. In adults, vasculitis is usually confined to the skin and takes the form of urticaria, subcutaneous nodules, periungual infarcts, or digital ulcerations. Cutaneous vasculitis has been associated with underlying malignant disease.

Pulmonary Involvement

Pulmonary involvement occurs in nearly 50% of patients who have myositis, with pneumonia being the most common pulmonary abnormality. Aspiration pneumonia, which is often recurrent, is prevalent in patients who have pharyngeal muscle weakness. Ineffective coughing caused by ventilatory muscle weakness also occurs but is far less common than swallowing

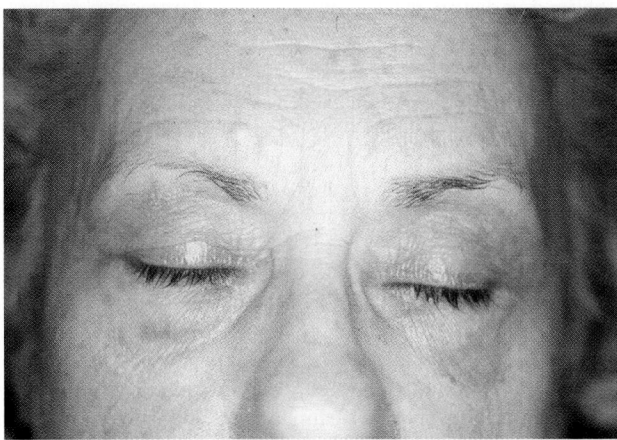

Figure 2 **Skin eruption in a patient with dermatomyositis consists of a deep-red, erythematous, papular rash over the nasal and forehead areas and a lilac-colored, or heliotrope, erythema of the upper eyelid and orbital area.**

problems. In general, the patient with recurrent aspiration pneumonia has a poor prognosis; it indicates marked dysfunction of many muscle groups. Bacterial pneumonia caused by aspiration is a major cause of death in elderly patients.[12] Opportunistic infections may occur in patients undergoing immunosuppressive drug therapy. In addition, some of these drugs, most notably methotrexate, can be associated with the development of pneumonitis, which is usually reversible but is potentially fatal.

Interstitial lung disease (ILD) occurs in up to 30% of myositis patients and in approximately 60% of patients who have antibodies directed against aminoacyl-transfer RNA (tRNA) synthetases. The advent and application of newer, sensitive diagnostic techniques such as high-resolution computed tomography may lead to an increase in the detection of pulmonary abnormalities. The most common presentation is with progressive shortness of breath, which may be accompanied by a nonproductive cough. On physical examination, basilar crepitant rales are usually detected. Progression may be slow, and symptoms may occur in patients with established disease; or onset may be rapid and may occur at the same time as the muscle weakness.[30] Hypoxemia and respiratory alkalosis may be present. In some patients, these abnormalities are detected only after exercise. High-resolution CT scanning is useful for detection of interstitial fibrosis that might not be appreciated on routine chest radiography. Pulmonary function tests may reveal reduced lung volume and diminished diffusion capacity. One of three forms of histology of ILD is usually found: interstitial pneumonia, diffuse alveolar damage, or bronchiolitis obliterans with or without organizing pneumonia. ILD occurs with or without skin involvement. There is no correlation between the development of ILD and the severity of muscle involvement, and ILD may precede or follow the onset of muscle weakness. ILD is associated with a high mortality. Treatment with cyclophosphamide or azathioprine has been reported to be beneficial in some patients.[30] A small number of patients with acute pneumonitis may respond to corticosteroid treatment alone.

Cardiac Abnormalities

Clinically significant involvement of heart muscle is unusual and is probably associated with a poor prognosis. Cardiac abnormalities may take many forms, ranging from rhythm or conduction disturbances to myocardial inflammation or fibrosis. Cardiac muscle abnormalities may be detected by radionuclide scanning studies. However, many histologic and electrical abnormalities are not clinically significant.[31] Therefore, evaluation beyond routine diagnostic studies is rarely indicated.

Calcinosis

Soft tissue calcification is seen most commonly in children. Deposits may be deep along fascial planes or in superficial dermal areas, sometimes with ulceration through the skin. Treatments have been based on largely anecdotal reports; no systematic studies have been carried out.[32] Agents that have been found to be of use in some cases include probenecid, diltiazem, and warfarin. Some patients show spontaneous regression of calcinosis without specific treatment.

Vascular Abnormalities

Raynaud phenomenon is most commonly observed in patients whose myositis is associated with another rheumatic disease (e.g., scleroderma). Clinically significant vasculitis is unusual in adults, although dermatomyositis patients may show vascular changes on histologic examination.

LABORATORY TESTS

Muscle Biopsy

Histologic confirmation of muscle inflammation is required in many, but not all, cases of inflammatory muscle disease. Patients with the characteristic skin rash of dermatomyositis and with elevated serum muscle enzyme levels may be treated without a muscle biopsy, because these two indicators can be used to follow the course of disease. In the absence of a skin rash or elevations in muscle enzyme levels, diagnosis is more difficult; in most patients, a biopsy is needed to confirm the presence of muscle inflammation. Two types of biopsy approaches are used: open surgical and closed needle. The closed-needle approach offers the advantages of decreased morbidity and of lower cost because an operating room is not required. Tissue samples obtained with the closed-needle approach can provide sufficient diagnostic information for interpretation by the muscle pathologist. However, the quality of the specimen obtained is dependent on the skill and experience of the operator. In the absence of such a resource or in special cases in which it is desirable to obtain extra tissue, the open surgical approach is preferable. Imaging studies such as MRI or CT can be used to determine the optimal site for biopsy.

All biopsy specimens require immediate handling by an experienced surgical team working closely with the pathology laboratory to ensure optimal results. Light microscopic analysis is sufficiently informative for most purposes. Because the treatment of polymyositis and that of dermatomyositis are the same, immunophenotyping of cellular infiltrates to distinguish between these two disorders is not indicated for routine diagnostic specimens. Electron microscopy may be required to demonstrate the inclusion bodies that define IBM. Examination of the biopsy specimen by a specialist in neuromuscular pathology may be helpful, because many pathologists do not see these diseases on a regular basis.

Muscle Enzymes

Most patients with inflammatory myopathy have increased muscle enzyme levels at some point during the course of active myositis.[33] The presence of intracellular muscle enzymes in the serum most likely reflects damage to muscle cell membranes. The most commonly used muscle enzyme measurement is the creatine kinase (CK) level. The CK level may rise to many times normal. The MB isozyme of CK may be elevated because of the presence of this isoform in regenerating skeletal muscle. Measurement of CK may be confounded by the presence of naturally occurring inhibitors of this enzyme. Furthermore, racial and gender variations exist for normal levels of CK, with black males generally showing the highest values.[34] Aldolase is another muscle enzyme that may be measured in the serum and may have less variability. However, aldolase is present in tissues other than muscle, and therefore, it is not specific for muscle damage. MRI studies have shown that active muscle inflammation may exist in patients with persistently normal CK serum levels.[35] Reasons for this discordance are not known, but the findings suggest that treatment strategies should be focused on the clinical status of the patient rather than on the muscle enzyme levels.[36]

Autoantibodies

Autoantibodies to nuclear and cytoplasmic antigens are found in as many as 90% of patients with an inflammatory myopathy. These antibodies are often useful in differentiating inflammatory myopathies from diseases that are not autoimmune disorders. Some of these autoantibodies are nonspecific and are seen in several autoimmune disorders. Other autoantibodies are relatively specific for the inflammatory myositis syndromes in general or for specific diagnostic categories. About 25% of patients with inflammatory myositis test positive for antinuclear antibody; in patients with overlapping rheumatic disease syndromes, the percentage is higher. The antinuclear antibody test is generally not helpful in establishing a diagnosis of myositis or one of its subsets. Autoantibodies that are in large part directed against cytoplasmic ribonucleoproteins have been designated as myositis-specific autoantibodies (MSA). Approximately 30% of patients with myositis have one or more of these autoantibodies. They are thus relatively specific but not sensitive to the presence of myositis, and as such, these autoantibodies cannot be used to screen for the presence of disease.

Three groups of patients can be defined by the MSA specificities. These subgroups differ in clinical presentation and prognosis.[37] The first group is defined by the presence of antibodies directed against aminoacyl-tRNA synthetases. The presentation in the first group is generally characterized by an acute onset of muscle disease, with a high incidence of associated interstitial lung disease. Patients in this group may also have arthritis and a hyperkeratotic rash on the hands, known as mechanic's hands. A majority of patients in this group test positive for HLA-DR3. Responses to treatment are variable, and mortality is significant. The second group includes patients with antibodies to the signal recognition particle (SRP). This protein complex facilitates translocation of newly synthesized polypeptides across the endoplasmic reticulum. Patients with anti-SRP have an abrupt onset of muscle weakness and may have associated involvement of cardiac muscle. The majority of patients in this group are African-American women. Responses to treatment are not good, and the prognosis is poor. In one series, the 5-year mortality for anti-SRP patients was 75%. A third group is identified by antibodies to Mi-2, which is a nuclear protein with unknown function. The majority of these patients have the dermatomyositis clinical syndrome with the so-called shawl-sign pattern of rash on the trunk and with cuticular overgrowth. Responses to treatment are generally good, and mortality is lower than that in the other groups. Most of these clinical associations, which were originally described in North American patients, have been confirmed in a large group of European patients.[38] Preliminary reports suggest that antibodies to a novel 155 kd protein may also be useful in identifying patients with amyopathic dermatomyositis.[39]

Electromyography

In most patients, electromyography reveals low-amplitude, polyphasic motor unit potentials, indicating a lack of synchronous contracture in muscle fibers within motor units. This finding correlates with the usually inhomogeneous distribution of muscle degeneration shown by histopathologic examination. Fibrillations and insertional irritability are evidence of membrane abnormalities. These findings are characteristic of, but not specific for, myositis.

IMAGING AND SPECTROSCOPY TECHNIQUES

Conventional radiographs have little value in evaluating skeletal muscle. However, other techniques, including ultrasonography, CT, and MRI, can enhance diagnostic approaches to many myopathies.[40] Of these modalities, MRI has been the most useful in the evaluation and longitudinal management of inflammatory muscle syndromes. However, it may not be the method of choice in all circumstances, and in some of these cases, the alternative modalities of ultrasonography and CT can provide helpful information. Advantages of these three techniques are that they are noninvasive and offer the possibility of examining a volume of muscle larger than that which can be obtained by biopsy. In patients for whom biopsy may be a difficult or traumatic experience, such as young children, imaging may provide sufficient information to proceed with treatment.

Magnetic Resonance Imaging

MRI is a very accurate method for muscle imaging that has been very useful in the diagnosis and management of patients with inflammatory muscle diseases of many kinds. Full assessment requires both T_1- and T_2-weighted images. The T_1 image

is most useful for outlining muscle anatomy because it detects changes in muscle mass caused by atrophy or fat infiltration. Inflammation is readily detected on the T_2-weighted image, where the abnormal areas appear as brightness against the usually dark background of normal muscle [see Figure 3]. Studies using MRI have clearly demonstrated the patchy nature of the muscle inflammation, perhaps explaining why some patients with significant weakness have normal biopsy results. In dermatomyositis, inflammation in the thigh muscles is seen in predominantly anterior muscle compartments, and muscle mass is generally preserved. In patients with polymyositis and inclusion body myositis, extensive fat infiltration and muscle atrophy, which can include all muscle groups, are more likely to be seen. Longitudinal MRI studies can be used to document the effectiveness of immunosuppressive therapy. Patients may be studied in the usual body coil, which allows for visualization of both legs.[41] Other studies have utilized a knee coil positioned over the anterior quadriceps, which provides a greater level of detail.[35] As in all MRI studies, patients must be very carefully questioned for the presence of any indwelling metals before being placed in the magnet.

Ultrasonography

Ultrasonography is a readily available and relatively inexpensive technique that has been used to examine a wide variety of muscle disorders.[42,43] Inflammation within muscle tissues appears on ultrasonography as areas of decreased echogenicity. In addition, blood-flow changes can be measured with related techniques such as color Doppler imaging. Ultrasonography may be useful in guiding the choice of site for needle or open muscle biopsy.

Computed Tomography

CT is not useful for the detection of inflammatory muscle changes. However, areas of atrophy or fat infiltration cause decreased muscle density, which is easily detected by CT. Soft tissue calcifications such as those seen in juvenile dermatomyositis are best visualized with CT. Sometimes, these calcifications are in deep areas that cannot be readily appreciated on physical examination.

a

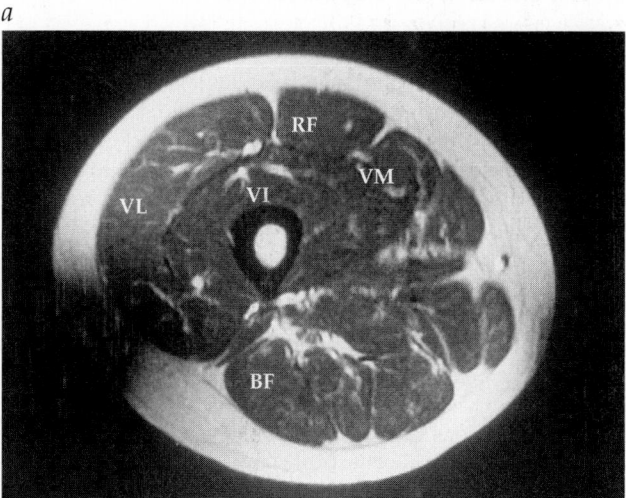

b

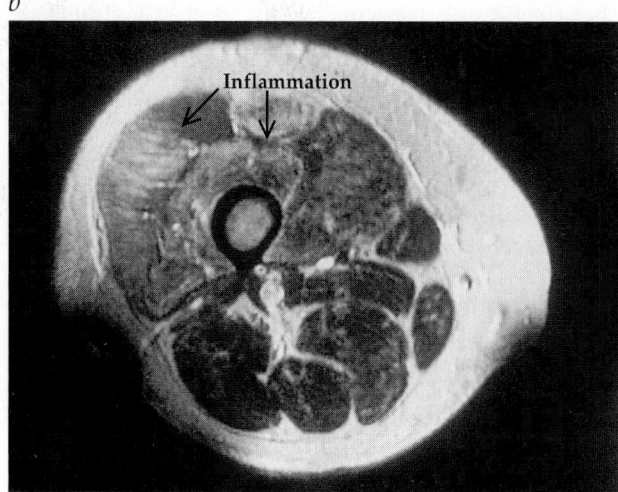

Figure 3 **Magnetic resonance images of thigh muscles in a patient with dermatomyositis. The T_1-weighted image (*a*) shows uniform density in all muscle groups, identified as VL, vastus lateralis; VI, vastus intermedius; VM, vastus medialis; RF, rectus femoris; and BF, biceps femoris. The T_2-weighted image (*b*) illustrates inflammation in muscles of the quadriceps group, shown as areas of brightness or increased signal intensity.[35]**

Magnetic Resonance Spectroscopy

Spectroscopy is primarily a research tool. However, studies have shown the utility of this noninvasive approach for evaluating muscle function, and applications in the clinic may become available in the near future.[35,44] In patients with dermatomyositis, loss of high-energy phosphate compounds needed for efficient muscle contraction has been documented with P-31 magnetic resonance spectroscopy.[44] Longitudinal studies have documented that correction of these metabolic abnormalities may lag behind improvement in muscle inflammation.

EVALUATION FOR UNDERLYING MALIGNANCY

Patients with dermatomyositis and polymyositis are at increased risk for an underlying malignancy. The magnitude of this risk is difficult to determine and varies greatly between reports. One study in a population-based cohort estimated the relative risk of cancer as 1.8 in males and 1.7 in females.[45] A study from Scotland has indicated that the relative risk may be as high as 7.7 in patients with dermatomyositis, with a greater risk in females than in males.[46] In general, the risk is greater in patients with dermatomyositis than in patients with polymyositis and in all patients who are older than 40 years. There is general agreement that routine screening for malignancies should include chest radiography, mammography (in women), examination of stool for occult blood, complete gynecologic examination, and assessment for prostate-specific antigen (in men). Abnormalities seen on these screening tests may suggest the need for additional studies such as endoscopy, colonoscopy, and tissue biopsy. The most difficult malignancies to detect are those arising in the ovary. Uterine transvaginal ultrasonography or CT of the pelvis should be done in women older than 40 years, but some occult ovarian malignancies escape detection even with these tests. Some investigators advocate lower gastrointestinal studies to detect colon cancer in patients older than 65 years.[12] Other, more extensive screening tests for occult malignancies are generally not recommended.

Differential Diagnosis

Diagnosis of dermatomyositis is aided by the presence of the characteristic rash. However, because the rash has features of SLE, this diagnosis may be confused with SLE, especially when the antinuclear antibody test is positive. Patients with polymyositis may be difficult to distinguish from patients with other myopathic disorders [*see Table 2*]. These other disorders include metabolic myopathies, endocrine dysfunction, drug-induced disorders, infections, and miscellaneous syndromes such as sarcoidosis. Some types of dystrophies should also be considered in patients who have muscle weakness and elevated muscle enzyme levels. Myalgia syndromes, such as polymyalgia rheumatica, in which stiffness is a predominant complaint, may confuse the diagnosis in some patients. Fibromyalgia, which is associated with a primary symptom of fatigue rather than muscle weakness, is characterized by the presence of discrete tender points that are not usually present in myositis patients.

Treatment

Guidelines for treatment of the idiopathic inflammatory myopathies are not well established for several reasons. The diseases are uncommon, making it difficult to accumulate suffi-

Table 2 Differential Diagnosis of Inflammatory Myositis

Cause	Effect
Metabolic myopathies	Myophosphorylase deficiency (McArdle disease) Myoadenylate deaminase deficiency Carnitine palmitoyltransferase deficiency Glycogen storage disease Periodic paralysis Hypokalemia, hypomagnesemia
Endocrine disorders	Cushing syndrome Thyroid dysfunction
Drug-induced disorders	Ethanol toxicity Penicillamine toxicity Lipid-lowering drug (statin) toxicity Zidovudine toxicity
Infections	Viral: HIV, coxsackievirus, adenovirus, influenza virus, echovirus
Other rheumatic disorders	Systemic lupus erythematosus (rash) Polymyalgia rheumatica
Miscellaneous disorders	Sarcoidosis, eosinophilia

cient numbers of patients to carry out randomized, controlled trials. In addition, some forms of these diseases have a slow, prolonged course, requiring long periods of observation. Finally, there is as yet no uniformly accepted classification scheme for these disorders; thus, comparisons of therapies administered to different groups of patients at different times and places may not be valid. As examples, in the past, polymyositis and dermatomyositis have been included in the same category, and IBM may not have been recognized. It is now clear that different forms of these diseases vary in prognosis and in response to therapy.

DRUG THERAPY

A table showing drugs for the treatment of inflammatory muscle diseases is provided [*see Table 3*].

Glucocorticoids

Corticosteroids are the mainstay of initial therapy. Most patients with documented muscle inflammation should be started on these drugs at relatively high levels (1 mg/kg/day), given in divided doses. A standard approach has been to maintain this dosage for up to 3 months or until clinical improvement occurs. After this initial period of high-dose therapy, the dose can be consolidated into a single morning dose and then tapered, with the total daily dose being reduced by 20% to 25% each month and a maintenance dose of 5 to 10 mg daily being achieved in about 6 to 8 months. The addition of second-line drugs to the prednisone regimen is now recommended within 3 months after initiation of treatment. Older patients with comorbid conditions such as diabetes and osteoporosis are especially at risk from side effects of steroids. Side effects may include a cushingoid appearance, compression fractures, avascular necrosis, cataracts, and infections. One study has suggested that the side effects of corticosteroid therapy contribute significantly to the morbidity of polymyositis and dermatomyositis.[47] For these reasons, any patient with severe muscle weakness,

Table 3   Drugs for the Treatment of Inflammatory Muscle Diseases

Drug	Dose	Efficacy Rating	Comments
Prednisone	5–60 mg/day	Highly effective for initial treatment	Side effect: cushingoid syndrome Avoid prolonged use at high doses; taper to 10 mg/day or less
Methotrexate	15–25 mg/wk	Effective, steroid-sparing	Side effects: liver abnormalities, pneumonitis Supplement with folate
Azathioprine	100–150 mg/day	Effective, steroid-sparing	Side effect: bone marrow suppression Can be combined with methotrexate
Hydroxychloroquine	200 mg b.i.d.	Effective for skin manifestations	Side effect: retinal toxicity Can be combined with other agents
Cyclophosphamide	100–150 mg daily or as intravenous pulses every 6 wk	Possibly effective for lung involvement	Side effects: bone marrow suppression, hemorrhagic cystitis
Cyclosporine	3 mg/kg/day	Use after other immunosuppressants	Side effects: hypertension, renal dysfunction
Intravenous immunoglobulin	1 g/kg/day, 2 consecutive days monthly	Use in patients in whom other regimens have failed	High cost and limited supply

limited functional status, or underlying conditions that make steroids a high risk (e.g., diabetes mellitus or osteoporosis) should be started on second-line immunosuppressive drugs at the outset.

Methotrexate and Azathioprine

The most commonly used second-line agents for the treatment of inflammatory myopathy are methotrexate and azathioprine. Methotrexate may be given orally or subcutaneously at an initial dosage of 7.5 to 10 mg weekly and then increased gradually to 25 mg weekly. As the dosage of methotrexate is increased, the dosage of prednisone is usually tapered. In general, methotrexate is well tolerated by patients with inflammatory myopathy, but there have been reports of toxicities similar to those seen in patients with rheumatoid arthritis who have taken methotrexate. Regular monitoring of liver function is necessary. Measurement of enzymes other than aminotransferases is required to prevent interference by the ongoing muscle inflammation. γ-Glutamyltranspeptidase is a liver-specific alternative. Methotrexate may be useful in the treatment of interstitial lung disease associated with myositis, but because this drug may in rare cases cause pulmonary toxicity, it is relatively contraindicated in patients with significant lung problems.

Azathioprine has been shown to be effective in patients with myositis in a prospective, controlled, double-blind trial, but treatment for at least 6 months may be required for improvement to occur. Azathioprine therapy should be initiated at a dosage of 50 to 100 mg/day, and the dosage should be increased gradually to a maximum of 150 to 200 mg/day. Side effects include bone marrow suppression and development of infections and, possibly, malignancies. Azathioprine and methotrexate have similar efficacy in these disorders. Patients with myositis in whom therapy with glucocorticoids and either methotrexate or azathioprine has failed may respond to a combination of methotrexate and azathioprine.[48,49]

Other Immunosuppressive Agents

Cyclophosphamide has been given both as intravenous pulse therapy and by daily oral administration. Some data suggest that

it may be useful in adults with the antisynthetase syndrome and in children with vasculitis-related complications of dermatomyositis. Cyclophosphamide may be useful in the treatment of the complication of interstitial lung disease.[30] Other drugs that may be of value in refractory cases include cyclosporine, tacrolimus, anti-TFN agents, anti–B cell agents such as rituximab, and mycophenolate mofetil.[50-52] The adenine analogue fludarabine has also shown some benefit in one study of refractory patients.[53]

Intravenous Immune Globulin

Intravenous immune globulin appears to benefit some patients with either polymyositis or dermatomyositis. A controlled trial of immune globulin in dermatomyositis patients demonstrated efficacy when given at a dosage of 1 g/kg/day for 2 days, repeated monthly for 3 months.[54] The combination of intravenous immune globulin and cyclosporine may be of value.[55] One controlled study suggested that intravenous immune globulin may be of benefit in IBM,[56] but studies by another group failed to show clinical improvements.[57] Treatment with intravenous immune globulin is limited by the restricted supply and very high cost and should be reserved for severe cases not responding to other therapies.

SKIN PROTECTION

The rash of dermatomyositis is usually photosensitive. Therefore, attention to protection from the sun is very important, and patients should be advised to avoid sun exposure as much as possible. Sunscreen preparations, sun-protective clothing, and tinting of windows are often effective. Some dermatologists recommend use of β-carotene, 25 to 30 mg, taken twice daily initially and then increasing to no more than five times a day. Antimalarials may be of benefit, and one report suggests the use of topical tacrolimus.[58]

PHYSICAL THERAPY

Physical therapy plays an important role in the rehabilitation of patients with myositis. During the phase of active inflammatory disease, passive range-of-motion exercises are necessary to prevent contractures. Once the inflammatory component of the disease is controlled, active resistive exercises are useful in regaining muscle strength.

The authors have no commercial relationships with manufacturers of products or providers of services discussed in this chapter.

References

1. Bohan A, Peter JB: Polymyositis and dermatomyositis (pt I). N Engl J Med 292:344, 1975

2. Bohan A, Peter JB: Polymyositis and dermatomyositis (pt II). N Engl J Med 292:403, 1975

3. Euwer RL, Sontheimer RD: Amyopathic dermatomyositis (dermatomyositis sine myositis). J Am Acad Dermatol 24:959, 1991

4. el-Azhara RA, Pakza SY: Amyopathic dermatomyositis: retrospective review of 37 cases. J Am Acad Dermatol 46:560, 2002

5. Caproni M, Cardinali C, Parodi A, et al: Amyopathic dermatomyositis: a review by the Italian Group of Immunodermatology. Arch Dermatol 138:114, 2002

6. Park JH, Olsen NJ, King LE, et al: MRI and P-31 magnetic resonance spectroscopy detect and quantify muscle dysfunction in the amyopathic and myopathic variants of dermatomyositis. Arthritis Rheum 38:68, 1995

7. Pachman LM, Hayford JR, Chung A, et al: Juvenile dermatomyositis at diagnosis: clinical characteristics of 79 children. J Rheumatol 25:1198, 1998

8. Collison CH, Sinal SH, Jorizzo JL, et al: Juvenile dermatomyositis and polymyositis: a follow-up study of long-term sequelae. South Med J 91:17, 1998

9. Buchbinder R, Forbes A, Hall S, et al: Incidence of malignant disease in biopsy-proven inflammatory myopathy: a population-based cohort study. Ann Intern Med 134:1087, 2001

10. Sparsa A, Liozon E, Herrmann F, et al: Routine vs extensive malignancy search for adult dermatomyositis and polymyositis: a study of 40 patients. Arch Dermatol 138:969, 2002

11. Hill CL, Zhang Y, Sigurgeirsson B, et al: Frequency of specific cancer types in dermatomyositis and polymyositis: a population-based study. Lancet 357:96, 2002

12. Marie I, Hatron PY, Levesque H, et al: Influence of age on characteristics of polymyositis and dermatomyositis in adults. Medicine (Baltimore) 78:139, 1999

13. Launay D, Hatron PY, Delaporte E, et al: Scleromyxedema (lichen myxedematosus) associated with dermatomyositis. Br J Dermatol 144:359, 2001

14. Wenzel J, Uerlich M, Gerdsen R, et al: Association of inclusion body myositis with subacute cutaneous lupus erythematosus. Rheumatol Int 21:75, 2001

15. Lindvall B, Bengtsson A, Ernerudh J, et al: Subclinical myositis is common in primary Sjögren's syndrome and is not related to muscle pain. J Rheumatol 29:717, 2002

16. Olsen NJ, King LE Jr, Park JH: Muscle abnormalities in scleroderma. Rheum Dis Clin North Am 22:783, 1996

17. Oddis CV, Conte CG, Steen VD, et al: Incidence of polymyositis-dermatomyositis: a 20-year study of hospital diagnosed cases in Allegheny County, PA 1963-1982. J Rheumatol 17:1329, 1990

18. Reed AM: Myositis in children. Curr Opin Rheumatol 13:428, 2001

19. Englund P, Nennesmo I, Klareskog L, et al: Interleukin-1alpha expression in capillaries and major histocompatibility complex class I expression in type II muscle fibers from polymyositis and dermatomyositis patients: important pathogenic features independent of inflammatory cell clusters in muscle tissue. Arthritis Rheum 46:1044, 2002

20. Kase S, Shiota G, Fujii Y, et al: Inclusion body myositis associated with hepatitis C virus infection. Liver 21:357, 2001

21. Pachman LM, Litt DL, Rowley AH, et al: Lack of detection of enteroviral RNA or bacterial DNA in magnetic resonance imaging–directed muscle biopsies from twenty children with active untreated juvenile dermatomyositis. Arthritis Rheum 38:1513, 1995

22. Ytterberg SR: Infectious agents associated with myopathies. Curr Opin Rheumatol 8:507, 1996

23. Pascuzzi RM: Drugs and toxins associated with myopathies. Curr Opin Rheumatol 10:511, 1998

24. Dalakas MC: Molecular immunology and genetics of inflammatory muscle diseases. Arch Neurol 55:1509, 1998

25. Vogel H: Inclusion body myositis: a review. Adv Anat Pathol 5:164, 1998

26. Reed AM, Picornell YJ, Harwood A, et al: Chimerism in children with juvenile dermatomyositis. 357:887, 2002

27. Artlett CM, Ramos R, Jiminez SA, et al: Chimeric cells of maternal origin in juvenile idiopathic inflammatory myopathies. Childhood Myositis Heterogeneity Collaborative Group. Lancet 356:2155, 2000

28. Engel AG, Arahata K: Mononuclear cells in myopathies: quantitation of functionally distinct subsets, recognition of antigen-specific cell-mediated cytotoxicity in some diseases, and implications for the pathogenesis of the different inflammatory myopathies. Hum Pathol 17:704, 1986

29. Mantegazza R, Andreetta F, Bernasconi P, et al: Analysis of T cell receptor repertoire of muscle-infiltrating T lymphocytes in polymyositis: restricted Vα/β rearrangements may indicate antigen-driven selection. J Clin Invest 91:2880, 1993

30. Schwarz MI: The lung in polymyositis. Clin Chest Med 19:701, 1998

31. Gonzalez-Lopez L, Gamez-Nava JI, Sanchez L, et al: Cardiac manifestations in dermato-polymyositis. Clin Exp Rheumatol 14:373, 1996

32. Spiera R, Kagen L: Extramuscular manifestations in idiopathic inflammatory myopathies. Curr Opin Rheumatol 10:556, 1998

33. Hochberg MC, Feldman D, Stevens MB: Adult onset polymyositis/dermatomyositis: an analysis of clinical and laboratory features and survival in 76 patients with a review of the literature. Semin Arthritis Rheum 15:168, 1986

34. Worrall JG, Phongsathorn V, Hooper RL, et al: Racial variation in serum creatinine kinase unrelated to lean body mass. Br J Rheumatol 29:371, 1990

35. Park JH, Vital T, Ryder N, et al: MR imaging and P-31 MR spectroscopy provide unique quantitative data for longitudinal management of patients with dermatomyositis. Arthritis Rheum 37:736, 1994

36. Dalakas MC: Polymyositis, dermatomyositis, and inclusion-body myositis. N Engl J Med 325:1487, 1991

37. Love LA, Leff RL, Fraser DD, et al: A new approach to the classification of idiopathic inflammatory myopathy: myositis-specific autoantibodies define useful homogeneous patient groups. Medicine (Baltimore) 70:360, 1991

38. Brouwer R, Hengstman GJ, Vree Egberts W, et al: Autoantibody profiles in the sera of European patients with myositis. Ann Rheum Dis 60:116, 2001

39. Sontheimer RD: Would a new name hasten the acceptance of amyopathic dermatomyositis (dermatomyositis sine myositis) as a distinctive subset within the idiopathic inflammatory dermatomyopathies spectrum of clinical illness? J Am Acad Dermatol 46:626, 2002

40. Olsen NJ, Park J: Skeletal muscle imaging for the evaluation of myopathies. Diseases of Skeletal Muscle. Wortmann R, Ed. Lippincott, Williams & Wilkins, New York, 1999, p 293

41. Fraser DD, Frank JA, Dalakas M, et al: Magnetic resonance imaging in the idiopathic inflammatory myopathies. J Rheumatol 18:1693, 1991

42. Reimers CD, Fleckenstein JL, Witt TN, et al: Muscular ultrasound in idiopathic inflammatory myopathies of adults. J Neurol Sci 116:82, 1993

43. Fleckenstein JL, Reimers CD: Inflammatory myopathies: radiologic evaluation. Radiol Clin North Am 34:427, 1996

44. Newman ED, Kurland RJ: P31 magnetic resonance spectroscopy in polymyositis and dermatomyositis: altered energy utilization during exercise. Arthritis Rheum 35:199, 1992

45. Sigurgeirsson B, Lindelof B, Edhag O, et al: Risk of cancer in patients with dermatomyositis or polymyositis. N Engl J Med 326:363, 1992

46. Stockton D, Doherty VR, Brewster DH: Risk of cancer in patients with dermatomyositis or polymyositis, and follow-up implications: a Scottish population-based cohort study. Br J Cancer 85:41, 2001

47. Clarke AE, Bloch DA, Medsger TA, et al: A longitudinal study of functional disability in a national cohort of patients with polymyositis/dermatomyositis. Arthritis Rheum 38:1218, 1995

48. Joffe MM, Love, LA, Leff RL, et al: Drug therapy of the idiopathic inflammatory myopathies: predictors of response to prednisone, azathioprine, and methotrexate and a comparison of their efficacy. Am J Med 94:379, 1993

49. Villalba ML, Hicks JE, Thornton B, et al: A combination of oral methotrexate and azathioprine is more effective than high dose intravenous MTX with leucovorin rescue in treatment-resistant myositis. Arthritis Rheum 38:S307, 1995

50. Vencovsky J, Jarosova K, Machacek S: Cyclosporine A versus methotrexate in the treatment of polymyositis and dermatomyositis. Scand J Rheumatol 29:95, 2000

51. Chaudhry V, Cornblath DR, Griffin JW, et al: Mycophenolate mofetil: a safe and promising immunosuppressant in neuromuscular diseases. Neurology 56:94, 2001

52. Mowzoon N, Sussman A, Bradley WG: Mycophenolate (CellCept) treatment of myasthenia gravis, chronic inflammatory polyneuropathy and inclusion body myositis. J Neurol Sci 185:119, 2001

53. Adams EM, Pucino F, Yarboro C, et al: A pilot study: use of fludarabine for refractory dermatomyositis and polymyositis, and examination of endpoint measures. J Rheumatol 26:352, 1999

54. Dalakas MC, Illa I, Dambrosia JM, et al: A controlled trial of high-dose intravenous immune globulin infusions as treatment for dermatomyositis. N Engl J Med 329:1993, 1993

55. Danieli MG, Malcangi G, Palmieri C, et al: Cyclosporin A and intravenous immunoglobulin treatment in polymyositis/dermatomyositis. Ann Rheum Dis 61:37, 2002

56. Walter MC, Lochmuller H, Toepfer M, et al: High-dose immunoglobulin therapy in sporadic inclusion body myositis: a double-blind, placebo-controlled study. J Neurol 247:22, 2000

57. Dalakas MC, Koffman B, Fujii M, et al: A controlled study of intravenous immunoglobulin combined with prednisone in the treatment of IBM. Neurology 56:323, 2001

58. Jorizzo JL: Dermatomyositis: practical aspects. Arch Dermatol 138:114, 2002

Brian F. Mandell, M.D., PH.D., F.A.C.P.

The diagnosis of a primary vasculitic syndrome is dependent on documentation of vasculitis and the exclusion of diseases that can cause secondary vasculitis. The diagnosis of a specific primary vasculitic disorder depends on the pattern of organ involvement, the histopathology, and the size of affected blood vessels; diagnosis should not be made on the basis of laboratory studies alone (e.g., findings of serum antineutrophil cytoplasmic antibodies [ANCAs] and cryoglobulins).

The major determinants of prognosis and type of therapy include the specific vasculitic disorder, the severity and extent of critical organ involvement, the rate of disease progression, and the etiology, if identifiable. The inflammatory process is often associated with nonspecific symptoms and laboratory abnormalities (e.g., elevated erythrocyte sedimentation rate [ESR], anemia, and fevers) that do not distinguish vasculitic diseases from other inflammatory, infectious, or neoplastic diseases. The toxic nature of the therapies for systemic vasculitis dictates the need for an accurate diagnosis.

Approach to the Patient Suspected of Having Vasculitis

EVALUATION

The physician should not be reluctant to pursue invasive testing in the diagnostic evaluation of patients with a multisystem illness, but biopsy of clinically uninvolved tissue and the use of less specific tests should be eschewed. An approach directed toward "ruling in" a specific form of vasculitis and ruling out reasonable specific alternatives should be pursued.

The first step in the diagnosis of vasculitis is to perform a detailed patient history and physical examination to document specific organ involvement. Special attention should be paid to the skin, eyes, ears, upper airway, joints, urinalysis, lymph nodes, peripheral nerves, and large vessels. A few laboratory tests [see Table 1] should be selectively included in the initial evaluation. Specialized studies, including serologies, are ideally obtained only after a differential diagnosis is formulated. If the urine dipstick test indicates blood, leukocytes, or protein, the physician must promptly examine several fresh urine sediments. Urine that has been sitting for several hours before analysis is not as useful for identification of cellular casts, which rapidly degenerate ex vivo. The presence of red blood cell casts is virtually diagnostic of glomerulonephritis; white cell casts may also be seen. Glomerulonephritis is usually asymptomatic. On the basis of the pattern of organ involvement, a differential diagnosis that includes specific types of systemic vasculitis and other disorders can then be generated, prompting additional, targeted testing.

CLASSIFICATION

Several classification schemes have been proposed for organizing the systemic vasculitic disorders into a consistent paradigm. These classifications are useful in distinguishing the clinical disorders that have distinct differences in prognosis and response to treatment.[1] No scheme is perfect or universally accepted. They all reiterate the characteristics of fulminant or classic disease, placing an emphasis on specificity of diagnosis. If a classification scheme is strictly adhered to, the newly ill patient without fully expressed disease is frequently left without a definitive diagnosis. The physician must recognize that until specific etiologies are defined, these diagnostic entities remain conceptual, and overlap between diseases is not unusual. This must not be a deterrent to instituting therapy in the patient at risk for rapidly progressive organ damage. Nonetheless, classification systems provide useful constructs for communication and the design of research protocols [see Figure 1]. The most widely used classification schemes are based on the caliber of affected blood vessels, the pattern of organ involvement, and the presence or absence of granulomas, significant immune complex deposition, and eosinophilic infiltrates. Some authors have proposed a category of ANCA-associated vasculitis on the basis of the presence or absence of specific serum ANCAs, particularly antibodies to proteinase 3 and myeloperoxidase. At present, the appropriate role of ANCA testing is to support a rationally developed clinical diagnosis. In patients who do not fit perfectly into a well-defined diagnostic category, these serologic tests should not supplant an attempt to obtain a tissue diagnosis. The presence of ANCA is not sufficient to make a diagnosis of a primary vasculitic syndrome; ANCA testing is not a screening test.

When the dominant symptoms and findings (i.e., neuropathy and cutaneous vasculitis) do not suggest a single specific vasculitic disorder, targeted physical examination and serologic testing may be helpful. Most valuable is biopsy confirmation of the specific disorder. The value of indiscriminate testing for antinuclear antibodies, ANCAs, rheumatoid factor, and angiotensin-converting enzyme is arguable. In contrast, infection with hepatitis B or C can be associated with a broad range of vasculitic syndromes; these infections must be routinely excluded in patients with vasculitis involving small or medium-sized vessels when there is no clear-cut evidence of a defined vasculitic disorder, such as Wegener granulomatosis (WG).[2]

OVERVIEW OF TREATMENT

The systemic vasculitides are potentially life threatening and may require potent anti-inflammatory and immunosuppressive therapy. Diagnoses should be made with as much certainty as possible. However, questions regarding alternative diagnoses or coexistent diseases frequently linger. Hence, even after therapy is initiated, physicians should maintain a high degree of vigilance to detect unrelated medical problems, complications of therapy, or both. The signs and symptoms of unrecognized infection may transiently resolve with steroid therapy.[3] With the initiation of potent immunosuppressive therapy, there is a prolonged window of increased susceptibility to opportunistic infection. The greatest risks occur in patients with marked neutropenia or those receiving high doses of corticosteroids. Physicians must be particularly wary about attributing new problems to "flares" in the underlying disease without first excluding a new or recrudescent infection. Patients with varicella-zoster virus may present with fever and pain before the appearance of the vesicles. *Pneumocystis jiroveci*, cytomegalovirus, and systemic fungal infections and reactivation of mycobacterial disease are observed more frequently in patients

Table 1   Selected Laboratory Tests for Patients with Multisystem Disease and Possible Vasculitis

Test	Comments
Platelet count	Thrombocytosis may parallel the acute-phase response Thrombocytopenia is not expected in primary vasculitic syndromes; consider SLE, marrow infiltration, hairy-cell leukemia, TTP, DIC, hypersplenism, APLS, HIV, scleroderma renal crisis, and heparin-induced thrombocytopenia
White blood cell count	Leukopenia is not expected in primary vasculitis; consider SLE, leukemia, hypersplenism, sepsis, myelo-dysplasia, and HIV Eosinophilia is common in Churg-Strauss syndrome; it may occur in WG, rheumatoid arthritis, or normo-tensive scleroderma renal crisis
ESR	Relatively low ESR is seen in DIC, liver failure, and hyperviscosity; ESR is frequently normal in HSP, may be low in Takayasu arteritis, and is normal in ≤ 20% of giant cell arteritis
Transaminases	ALT or AST is elevated in liver disease, myositis, rhabdomyolysis, hemolysis, or myocardial necrosis
Anti–glomerular basement membrane	Useful for evaluation of alveolar hemorrhage, with or without glomerulonephritis; also useful for evaluation of normocomplementemic glomerulonephritis
Antinuclear antibody	Order when there is clinical suspicion of SLE, not as a general screening test for sick patients; negative test makes SLE very unlikely
Antineutrophil cytoplasmic antibody	Order when there is clinical suspicion of WG or MPA; order specific anti-PR3 and antimyeloperoxidase
Drug screen	Order for unexplained CNS symptoms, myocardial ischemia, vascular spasm, panic attacks with systemic features, or tachycardia; urine screen should be done
Blood cultures	Useful for any patient with febrile, multisystem, or wasting illness; pulmonary infiltrates; or focal ischemia/infarction
APLA/PTT/RVVT	Order for unexplained venous or arterial thrombosis or thrombocytopenia
Purified protein derivative (± anergy) skin test	Obtain in any patient who may require steroid therapy or who has unexplained sterile pyuria or hematuria, granulomatous inflammation, chronic meningitis, or possible exposure to tuberculosis
Examination of fresh urinary sediment	Perform in all patients with an unexplained febrile, hypertensive, or multisystem illness
Viral serology tests: hepatitis B, C, and possibly CMV and HIV	Order for abnormal transaminases or elevated hepatic alkaline phosphatase; portal hypertension; PAN or MPA syndrome; or unexplained cryoglobulinemia, polyarthritis, or cutaneous vasculitis
Complement C3, C4	Not a screening test for vasculitis; useful in the differential diagnosis of glomerulonephritis; low in cryo-globulinemia; may be low in endocarditis; usually normal in PAN, MPA, HSP, WG; may be low in viral hepatitis–related glomerulonephritis or vasculitis
Aldolase	Aldolase has no organ specificity; its organ distribution is similar to that of lactic dehydrogenase

ALT—alanine aminotransferase   APLA—antiphospholipid antibody   APLS—antiphospholipid antibody syndrome   AST—aspartate aminotransferase   CMV—cytomegalovirus   DIC—disseminated intravascular coagulation   ESR—erythrocyte sedimentation rate   HSP—Henoch-Schönlein purpura   MPA—microscopic polyangiitis   PAN—polyarteritis nodosa   PR3—proteinase 3   PTT—partial thromboplastin time   RVVT—Russell viper venom test   SLE—systemic lupus erythematosus   TTP—thrombotic thombocytopenic purpura   WG—Wegener granulomatosis

with systemic vasculitides than in the general population. Immunosuppression from steroids and other medications is frequently associated with mucosal candidiasis, less commonly associated with molluscum contagiosum, and rarely associated with Kaposi sarcoma.

Methotrexate, azathioprine, and cyclophosphamide may cause leukopenia and, less often, other cytopenias. In patients with decreased renal function, methotrexate must be used with caution, if at all; the dose of cyclophosphamide should be decreased and carefully monitored because the pro-drug (cyclophosphamide) is renally excreted. Bladder-emptying dysfunction is a relative contraindication to the long-term use of cyclophosphamide, because increased exposure to toxic metabolites of the drug may predispose to bladder cancer or cystitis. The trend in the treatment of patients with certain potentially life-threatening systemic vasculitic syndromes has been to introduce therapy with a short course of high-dose corticosteroids along with a second immunosuppressive agent to induce remission and then, depending on the disease, to taper the corticosteroids and continue immunosuppressive therapy with the safest effective immunosuppressant to maintain re-

mission. The noncorticosteroid agent may initially be cyclophosphamide, which is felt to be the most potent of the noncorticosteroidal immunosuppressants, but cyclophosphamide is then replaced with an agent that has a better safety profile (e.g., methotrexate or azathioprine). Therapy with this agent is then continued for many months. Such an approach has been best evaluated in patients with WG and, in this patient group, has been shown to be effective.

Small Vessel Vasculitis

Vasculitis that affects capillaries and venules is the most common form of vasculitis and almost always involves the skin. It can occur at any age and affects men and women with equal frequency.

ETIOLOGY

Small vessel vasculitis can occur as an idiopathic (primary) disorder or secondary to drug allergy, bacterial endocarditis, viral infections such as those caused by hepatitis B or C, disseminated *Neisseria*, and rickettsiae; it can be part of a defined

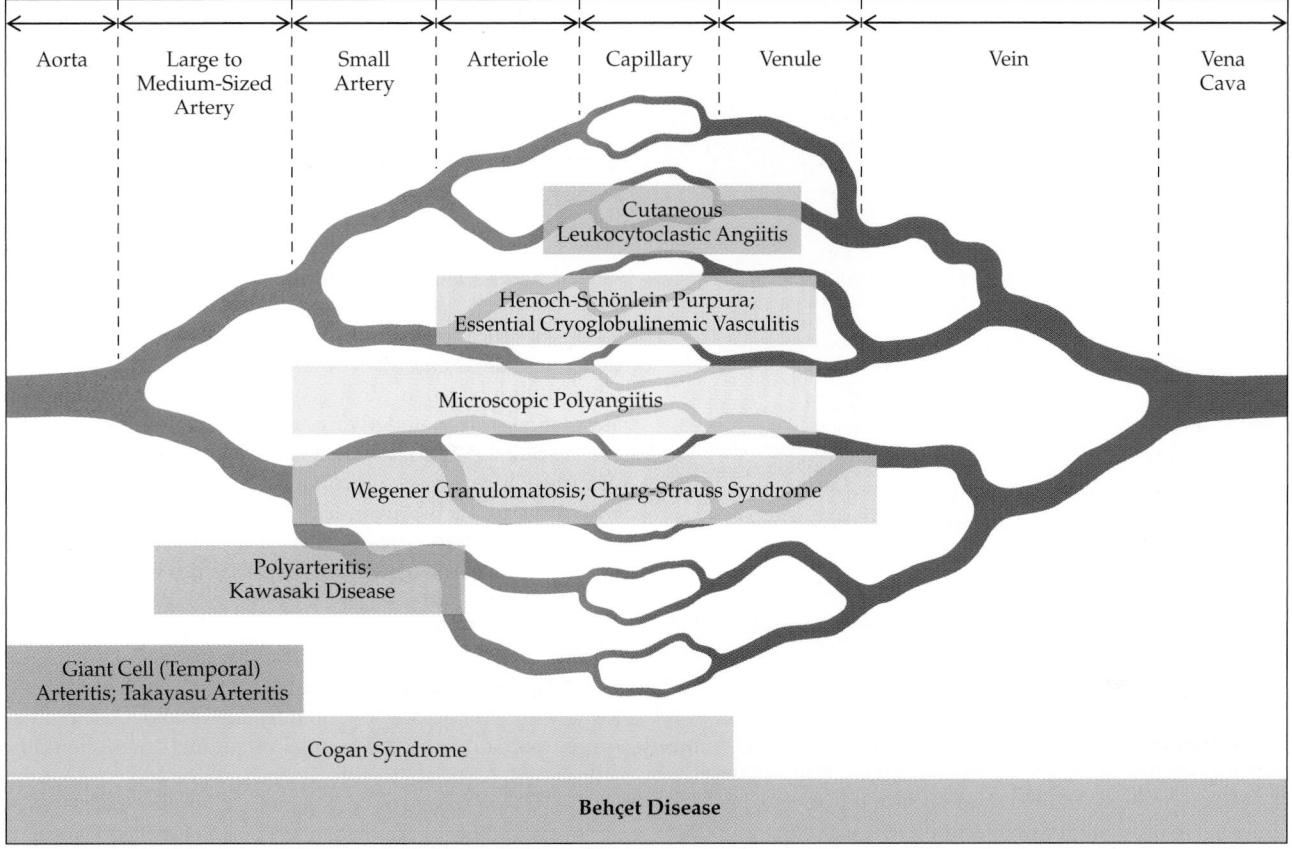

Figure 1 **Classification of the systemic vasculitis syndromes.**[1]

systemic autoimmune disorder such as Sjögren syndrome, systemic lupus erythematosus (SLE), or rheumatoid arthritis; or it can occur in association with hematologic, lymphoid, and solid-organ malignancies [*see Figure 2*]. Small vessel vasculitis can accompany diseases commonly associated with the involvement of larger vessels (e.g., WG).

DIAGNOSIS

Clinical Manifestations

Cutaneous involvement can occur in many of the primary or secondary vasculitic syndromes. Large, medium-sized, or small vessel occlusion can cause livedo, Raynaud phenomenon, or necrosis. Purpuric lesions that partially blanch under pressure are the most common manifestations of small vessel vasculitis. Small vessel vasculitis, particularly when associated with infections, is frequently associated with immune complex deposition. Vasculitis primarily involving the postcapillary venules was termed hypersensitivity vasculitis in older literature.[4] Primary small vessel vasculitis may be limited to the skin or may be associated with visceral involvement, including alveolar hemorrhage, intestinal ischemia or hemorrhage, and glomerulonephritis.

Purpura tends to occur in recurrent crops of lesions of similar age and is more pronounced in gravity-dependent areas [*see Figure 3*]. When purpura is not primarily in gravity-dependent areas, cold agglutinin disease, cryoglobulinemia (which may be associated with an infection such as hepatitis C or with lymphoma), embolism, infiltrative diseases, and self-induced in-

jury should be excluded. Cutaneous vasculitis of any etiology may be associated with striking dependent edema.

In a case series of cutaneous small vessel vasculitis,[4] almost 100% of patients younger than 20 years had disease limited to the skin, whereas approximately 40% of the 172 patients older than 20 years had an associated or underlying systemic disorder. Seventeen adults had a systemic necrotizing vasculitis, four had malignancy, four had a bacterial infection causing the vasculitis, 11 had cryoglobulinemia, and 59 had Henoch-Schönlein purpura. The prevalence of infection with hepatitis C

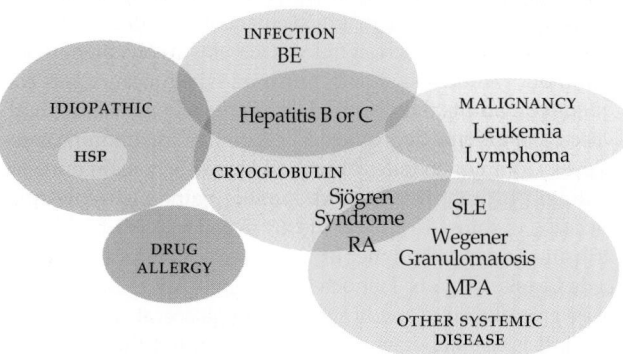

Figure 2 **A Venn diagram illustrates the relations between the causes of small vessel ("hypersensitivity") vasculitis. (BE—bacterial endocarditis; HSP—Henoch-Schönlein purpura; MPA—microscopic polyangiitis; RA—rheumatoid arthritis; SLE—systemic lupus erythematosus)**

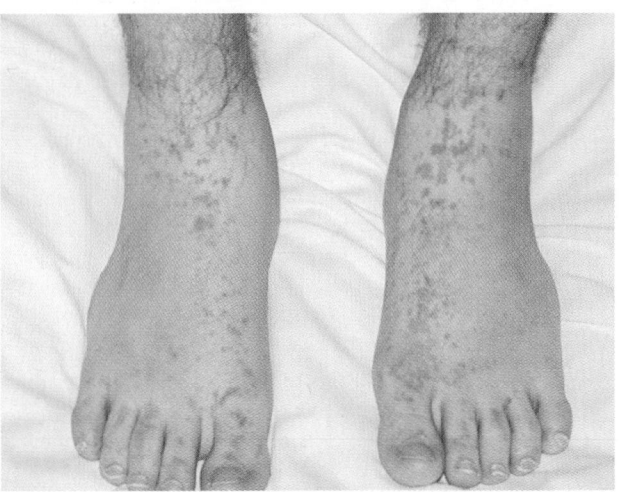

Figure 3 **Palpable purpura of the distal extremities is the most common presentation of small vessel vasculitis.**

virus, likely the most common cause of mixed cryoglobuline-mia,[2] was not reported in this series.

Laboratory Tests

Biopsy is most useful in excluding causes of nonvasculitic purpura such as amyloidosis, leukemia cutis, Kaposi sarcoma, T cell lymphomas, trauma, and cholesterol or myxomatous emboli. Tissue immunofluorescent staining is useful to support the diagnosis of Henoch-Schönlein purpura (specifically, IgA staining), SLE, or infection (the percentage of patients with positive results on immunofluorescent staining is not known). The cells infiltrating and perhaps destroying the vessel wall may be neutrophils or lymphocytes, depending on the etiology. The pathology in most cases of small vessel vasculitis is leukocyto-clastic angiitis (LCA). Hepatitis C infection should be excluded routinely in patients who present with unexplained purpura—an important example of the fact that the presence of LCA does not indicate that a patient's illness is the result of a primary vas-culitic syndrome.

CLINICAL SUBSETS

Henoch-Schönlein Purpura

Henoch-Schönlein purpura is a clinically defined small ves-sel vasculitic syndrome in which cutaneous features are usual-ly striking and in which significant visceral involvement is less common. Henoch-Schönlein purpura, which occurs less fre-quently in adults than in children,[5] is usually associated with vascular and renal deposition of IgA-containing immune com-plexes. Common manifestations of Henoch-Schönlein purpura include purpura; urticaria; abdominal pain; gastrointestinal bleeding or intussusception (mostly in children); arthralgias or arthritis; and glomerulonephritis. Visceral symptoms may pre-cede the skin lesions. Henoch-Schönlein purpura may appear to be precipitated by medications or streptococcal or viral infec-tions. It is usually a self-limited disorder, but the associated glomerulonephritis may, in rare instances (most often in adults), progress to renal failure. In the absence of renal dys-function, Henoch-Schönlein purpura is often a self-limited but frequently recurrent syndrome that may require only symp-tomatic therapy; because some visceral involvement may be

significant, the patient should be periodically monitored until there is a complete resolution of symptoms.

Urticarial Vasculitis

Urticarial vasculitis represents a peculiar subset of small ves-sel vasculitis.[6] The clinical presentation is that of wheals or ser-pentine papules, sometimes with surrounding or geographical-ly separate angioedema. Individual lesions are slow to resolve, often lasting for several days; the disease follows a more pro-longed course than typical urticaria. There is frequently a burn-ing, dysesthetic discomfort from the lesions. Like purpura, the lesions of urticarial vasculitis are frequently located in gravity-dependent areas and often heal with skin hyperpigmentation or an ecchymotic area. Most cases are idiopathic, although an association with an underlying systemic autoimmune disorder such as SLE, IgM paraproteinemia, or a viral infection has been described. In rare cases, urticarial vasculitis has been associated with a syndrome that includes hypocomplementemia and in-terstitial pulmonary disease. This syndrome is distinct from C1 esterase deficiency–associated angioedema, which does not cause urticaria.

TREATMENT

Therapy for cutaneous vasculitis is first directed at eliminat-ing any underlying precipitant. Infectious etiologies should be sought out and treated. Potential offending drugs should be withdrawn. Association with myelodysplasia and myeloprolif-erative disease should be considered, especially if cytopenia or abnormal cell forms are evident on peripheral blood smear. If no precipitants are apparent, low-risk therapy can be attempt-ed with nonsteroidal anti-inflammatory drugs, colchicine, pen-toxifylline, dapsone, or short-term low-dose corticosteroids. These therapies are not uniformly effective at reducing attack frequency or severity. Long-term corticosteroid therapy should be avoided if at all possible. Compressive support stockings or panty hose may be useful in limiting the significant edema that often accompanies cutaneous vasculitis of the legs.

Visceral involvement with organ dysfunction may necessi-tate a more aggressive approach than that used in limited cuta-neous vasculitis. Moderate-dose corticosteroids are generally effective. In the setting of potential complications from chronic corticosteroid use or the setting of severe visceral involvement, methotrexate, azathioprine, cyclophosphamide, or other im-munosuppressive agents may occasionally be required [*see* Table 2]. Apheresis may be effective in the treatment of severe cryoglobulinemic vasculitis. When treating chronic, refractory small vessel disease that is not organ or life threatening, one must pay close attention to the risk-to-benefit ratio of selected therapies.

Wegener Granulomatosis

WG is a relatively uncommon, potentially lethal disease characterized by necrotizing granulomatous inflammation and vasculitis of small and medium-sized vessels.[7,8] Males and fe-males of all ages can be affected.

DIAGNOSIS

Clinical Manifestations

WG is characterized by parenchymal necrosis with a vari-able contributory component of vasculitis. Multiple organs are often involved; there is a predilection for the upper and lower respiratory tracts, eyes, and kidneys.

Upper respiratory tract involvement Upper airway disease may be striking but is often indolent and attributed for months or even years to routine sinus disease until other manifestations of WG are recognized. Even after the diagnosis is made and immunosuppressive treatment is provided, sinus disease may be recalcitrant to therapy. This chronicity may be caused in part by superinfection of damaged tissue by *Staphylococcus aureus*. Anatomic damage can include septal perforations and saddle-nose deformities. Laryngotracheal involvement may result in subglottic stenosis, which is best treated by local corticosteroid injection therapy. Ear involvement is common, particularly otitis media, which may produce conductive hearing loss. Orbital pseudotumors may cause proptosis, ophthalmoplegia, intractable pain, and loss of vision; these inflammatory and fibrous masses may be refractory to anti-inflammatory therapy, immunosuppressive therapy, and even radiation therapy. Conjunctivitis, uveitis, and scleritis alone or in combination commonly occur.

Lower respiratory tract involvement Lung involvement may be absent at the onset of disease, may be asymptomatic, or may present dramatically as diffuse alveolar hemorrhage. One third of pulmonary lesions noted on imaging studies [*see Figure 4*] are asymptomatic (CT scanning is more sensitive than radiography). Nodules may undergo necrosis leading to cavity formation. Bronchospasm is not characteristic of WG. If airway obstruction is suspected, bronchoscopy should be considered to exclude endobronchial or subglottic stenoses. It is frequently necessary to rule out infectious causes of the pulmonary infiltrates, and bronchoscopy with lavage is useful in this regard. However, tissue obtained from transbronchial biopsy is usually of insufficient quantity to confirm the pathologic diagnosis of WG.

Open lung or thoracoscopic biopsy is often the optimal method for demonstrating the typical pathologic findings of WG and for excluding malignancies and atypical infections. Typical open lung biopsy sections[9] may contain areas of necrosis, frequently in a broad pattern; giant cells in the parenchymal tissue; and vasculitis. Not all histopathologic features may be present in the same biopsy section, and vasculitis may not be evident. Because pathology similar to WG may be demonstrated in chronic mycobacterial and fungal infections, special stains and cultures for these agents are essential.

Glomerulonephritis Glomerulonephritis is a common cause of morbidity and mortality in WG. Its presence or absence distinguishes the generalized from the limited forms of the disease. Glomerulonephritis is often aggressive, but it may be relatively indolent. It may be clinically and pathologically indistinguishable from idiopathic, rapidly progressive, crescentic glomerulonephritis, and it is usually clinically silent. The evolution from subclinical to dialysis-dependent renal disease may occur over several weeks. Glomerulonephritis may be present at the outset of the disease, or it may develop only after the patient has been ill with an apparently limited form of the disease. The importance of frequent microscopic urinalyses in the initial and follow-up evaluation of patients with WG cannot be overemphasized. This monitoring can be done by patients at home using routine dipstick analysis to detect occult hematuria. Especially in elderly or debilitated patients, valuable information may be obtained by occasional 24-hour urine

Table 2 Immunosuppressive Therapies for Vasculitis

Drug	Dose	Efficacy Rating	Comments
Prednisone	Often used at 1 mg/kg daily (split doses in severe disease) initially; tapered, with goal of discontinuance by 6 months or sooner if possible; utilize other drugs to enable this if possible	Primary therapy in all forms of life- or organ-threatening forms of vasculitis; probably most rapid-acting therapy	Ideally, check baseline PPD status; consider prophylaxis against *Pneumocystis* (when using high doses) and osteoporosis; monitor for development of glaucoma in elderly patients
Cyclophosphamide	1–3 mg/kg p.o. daily; avoid neutropenia; nadir is usually 9–14 days after initiation of therapy or change in dose; decrease dose in setting of renal insufficiency; monthly "pulse" dosing has been used (0.5–1 g/m²), but there may be greater likelihood of relapse or neutropenia; give pulse dose after dialysis	Most potent nonsteroidal immunosuppressive therapy; unclear onset of action but should be given when severe disease recognized, particularly rapidly progressive glomerulonephritis	Major side effects limit long-term use of this drug: leukopenia, myeloproliferative disease, bladder damage, and malignancy; current trend is to induce remission in WG and other severe forms of vasculitis with prednisone and cyclophosphamide, with tapering of prednisone and change of cyclophosphamide to a less toxic (but likely less effective) medication (e.g., azathioprine or methotrexate)
Azathioprine	2–3 mg/kg daily p.o.	Probably less potent than cyclophosphamide; useful to maintain remission while trying to spare corticosteroid dosing	Not usually given as primary induction therapy; avoid leukopenia; can cause a confusing hypersensitivity reaction that includes high fever, with or without rash and eosinophilia
Methotrexate	Given once weekly (up to approximately 0.3 mg/kg/dose) along with daily folic acid (1 mg)	Less potent than cyclophosphamide; useful to maintain remission while trying to spare corticosteroid dosing; decrease dose for mild renal insufficiency; *avoid in patients with creatinine > 2.5 mg/dl*	Useful in maintaining remission; has been used as primary induction therapy with prednisone in patients with mild WG; significant frequency of relapse in WG patients maintained on this drug alone; monitor WBC, creatinine and transaminase levels (causes hepatitis and can cause cirrhosis; avoid any ethanol ingestion); can be given orally or by weekly injection; folic acid reduces "nuisance" side effects

PPD—purified protein derivative   WBC—white blood cell count   WG—Wegener granulomatosis

a

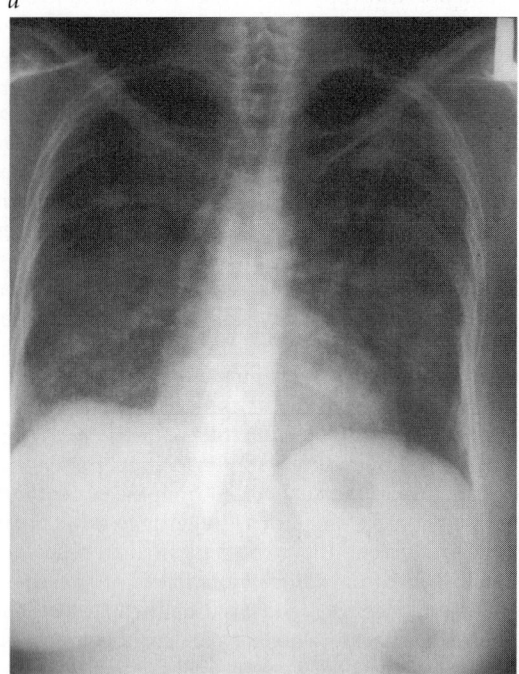

b

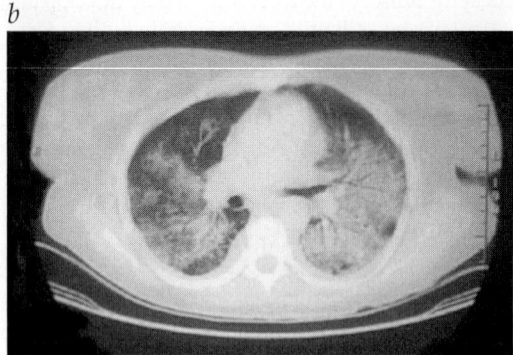

Figure 4   **The nodular infiltrates of the lung in Wegener granulomatosis are shown less extensively in a standard radiograph (*a*) than in a computed tomographic scan (*b*).**

collections, which can establish a more accurate estimate of the glomerular filtration rate (GFR) than that provided by the serum creatinine measurement. Renal biopsy may reveal focal and segmental glomerulonephritis with variable glomerular proliferative changes, crescent formation, and necrosis, in the absence of significant immune complex deposition (so-called pauci-immune glomerulonephritis). Although supportive of the diagnosis of WG, these findings are not diagnostic of the disease, and renal biopsy is not the preferred study to confirm the specific diagnosis of WG [*see Laboratory Tests, below*].

Additional clinical manifestations   Musculoskeletal involvement occurs in over half of patients with WG. Symptoms may include arthralgias or arthritis; these symptoms may be migratory, additive, or of fixed distribution. Rheumatoid factor is frequently present in patients with WG, and it may cause diagnostic confusion with rheumatoid arthritis when joint symptoms are significant. The joint disease of WG only rarely produces bone erosions. Neurologic signs and symptoms occur in

fewer than 50% of patients, peripheral neuropathy in fewer than 20%, and involvement of the central nervous system in fewer than 10%. Oculomotor defects may occur because of impingement by a retro-orbital mass or inflammatory sinus disease. Gastrointestinal ischemia and ulcerations are infrequent but may be confused with inflammatory bowel disease, especially because the latter can be associated with ANCA (usually perinuclear ANCA, or p-ANCA). Up to 50% of WG patients exhibit cutaneous involvement with purpura, panniculitis, or ulcerations. If present, the skin disease generally parallels systemic disease activity. Observations from recent clinical trials suggest that patients with WG are predisposed to develop deep vein thrombosis.[10]

Laboratory Tests

Unexplained chronic inflammation of the respiratory tract or eye or the presence of glomerulonephritis is consistent with the diagnosis of WG. The probability of WG is increased when multiple organ involvement is present, upper airway disease is destructive, and pulmonary nodules (especially with cavities) are demonstrated by radiography. Any combination of organ involvement is possible, but most patients exhibit upper airway involvement at the time of diagnosis.

If the entire clinical picture is compatible with WG and if alternative diagnoses have been appropriately ruled out, the finding of circulating cytoplasmic ANCA (c-ANCA) with anti–proteinase 3 specificity is sufficient to make the provisional diagnosis and initiate therapy without a tissue diagnosis. Approximately 20% of patients with WG may have p-ANCA with antimyeloperoxidase specificity. If there are any atypical features or special concerns regarding the initiation of immunosuppressive therapy or if the patient does not respond appropriately to therapy, histopathologic confirmation of the diagnosis should be aggressively pursued. The presence of ANCA is not equivalent to the presence of vasculitis; ANCA can be found in other diseases.

The ANCA level is not a reliable means to follow disease activity.[11-13] Because WG generally requires therapy with a corticosteroid plus a second agent to induce remission and limit the likelihood of relapse, it should be distinguished from other inflammatory disorders, including other vasculitic syndromes [*see Table 3*], which may be effectively treated with a less toxic regimen.

TREATMENT

Initial treatment of generalized WG warrants dual-drug immunosuppressive therapy. Corticosteroids may produce symptomatic improvement in the upper airway, lungs, skin, and musculoskeletal system, but tapering usually results in a prompt flare in the disease unless a second agent is administered concurrently. Acutely serious disease, particularly renal disease that is progressing, is treated initially with corticosteroids and daily cyclophosphamide with subsequent tapering of the corticosteroids over several months. Many authors now recommend that once remission is achieved, cyclophosphamide therapy should be promptly replaced by methotrexate or azathioprine therapy for at least an additional 12 months of therapy [*see Table 2*]. This approach is now supported by several clinical trials.[14]

There are some strong relative contraindications to the long-term use of cyclophosphamide, including bladder dysfunction (increased risk of drug metabolite–induced cystitis and bladder

Table 3 Clinical Features of Vasculitis

Disorder	Common Target Organs	Special Pathologic Features	Special Laboratory Studies	Comments
Microscopic polyangiitis	Nerve, glomerulus, lung (small vessels), GI tract, skin	No giant cells, vasculitis, proliferative GN (no or rare immune deposits*)	p-ANCA (antimyeloperoxidase)	Rule out hepatitis B and C
Polyarteritis nodosa	Nerve, GI tract	Arteritis of medium muscular arteries, no giant cells, no GN	No ANCA	No small vessel involvement; rule out hepatitis B and C
Wegener granulomatosis	Upper airway, eye, lung (small vessels), glomerulus, nerve, musculoskeletal system	Giant cells, geographic necrosis, mild eosinophilia, vasculitis, proliferative GN (no or rare immune deposits)	c-ANCA (anti-PR3)	Chronic sinus or ear disease
Churg-Strauss syndrome	Nerve, lung infiltrates, heart, skin	Giant cells, eosinophilia, vasculitis, proliferative GN (no or rare immune deposits)	Eosinophilia ± ANCAs	Positive atopic history

*Presence of immune deposits suggests possible hepatitis B or C infection.
ANCA—antineutrophil cytoplasmic antibody c-ANCA—cytoplasmic ANCA GN—glomerulonephritis p-ANCA—perinuclear ANCA PR3—proteinase 3

cancer) and leukopenia; however, even without such contraindications, cyclophosphamide-associated morbidity is significant.[7] In milder or limited WG, weekly doses of methotrexate (0.20 to 0.30 mg/kg, adjusted for renal function) with folic acid or leucovorin may be substituted for cyclophosphamide to induce and maintain remission. Patients undergoing treatment with immunosuppressive agents must be continuously monitored for flares in disease, opportunistic infections, and medication side effects. Flares may be more frequent in patients treated with methotrexate than in those receiving longer courses of cyclophosphamide, and they often occur as the corticosteroids are withdrawn.[13] Side effects of methotrexate include cytopenias and drug-induced pneumonitis. Methotrexate may cause hepatitis, and, on rare occasions, cirrhosis. It should be avoided in the setting of renal insufficiency or alcohol use. Azathioprine can cause a febrile hypersensitivity reaction and leukopenia. Attempts to limit cyclophosphamide side effects by using methotrexate or azathioprine are warranted, but such an approach must be accompanied by careful monitoring for disease flare. Some authors have suggested using trimethoprim-sulfamethoxazole as adjunctive therapy for the treatment of WG because some data suggest that this therapy can decrease the frequency of flares of upper airway disease.[15] However, this approach remains controversial and is not routinely undertaken in conjunction with full-dose methotrexate, because the combination may result in additive antifolate toxicity. Administration of trimethoprim-sulfamethoxazole three times weekly is useful in protecting patients against *P. jiroveci* (formerly *P. carinii*) pneumonia while they are receiving intensive immunosuppressive therapy. Local nasal and sinus toilet and periodic otolaryngoscopic evaluations are a routine part of the care of patients with upper airway disease. Anti–tumor necrosis therapy with etanercept has been shown in a randomized, controlled trial to be ineffective as adjunctive therapy for the treatment of WG.[16]

Prophylactic measures to prevent osteoporosis and regular dual-energy x-ray absorptiometry (DXA) scans to measure bone density should always be considered when corticosteroids are used on a long-term basis.

Churg-Strauss Syndrome

Churg-Strauss syndrome (CSS), or allergic granulomatosis angiitis, is a rare syndrome that affects small to medium-sized arteries and veins in association with bronchial asthma.

DIAGNOSIS

Clinical Manifestations

The inflammatory component of CSS displays clinical similarities to WG in terms of organ involvement and pathology, especially in patients with upper or lower airway disease or glomerulonephritis. CSS differs most strikingly from WG in that the former occurs in patients with a history of atopy, asthma, or allergic rhinitis, which is often ongoing. In the prevasculitic atopy phase, as well as during the systemic phase of the illness, eosinophilia is characteristic and often of striking degree (≥ 1,000 eosinophils/mm³). When eosinophilia is present in WG, it is usually more modest (~ 500 eosinophils/mm³).

Organ-specific features of CSS include some combination of pulmonary infiltrates, cardiomyopathy, coronary arteritis, polyneuropathy (symmetrical or mononeuritis multiplex), ischemic bowel disease, eosinophilic gastroenteritis, ocular inflammation, nasal perforations, glomerulonephritis, cutaneous nodules, and purpura.[17,18]

The patchy pulmonary infiltrates of CSS are often transient and may be associated with alveolar hemorrhage. Pulmonary nodules are uncommon and, unlike WG, rarely cavitate. Pleural effusions often contain abundant eosinophils. Clinical distinction from hypersensitivity pneumonitis, allergic aspergillosis, and pulmonary lymphoma is at times difficult. Several cases of CSS in asthmatic patients have been reported to have occurred after the introduction of inhibitors of 5-lipoxygenase while these patients were being weaned off corticosteroids.

Cardiac disease in CSS can be severe and is a leading cause of mortality. Cardiac infiltration or coronary arteritis can produce heart failure and ischemic syndromes. Valvular heart disease may occur, but it is not as striking or as common in CSS as it is in the idiopathic hypereosinophilic syndrome. Neurologic involvement occurs in more than 60% of patients with CSS. Such involvement may be severe and is generally attributable to arteritis. Cutaneous purpura, urticaria, polymorphous erythematous eruptions, and nodules occur. Gastrointestinal involvement resulting from ischemic vasculitis, eosinophilic gastroenteritis, or both may cause pain, cramping, and diarrhea.

Laboratory Tests

Histopathology typically exhibits extravascular granulomatous inflammation, with a prominent eosinophilic infiltrate, and vasculitis is variably present. Granulomas can be found in tissue at areas separate from the demonstrable vasculitis. Eosinophilic infiltrates in CSS are more striking than those in WG. Abundant eosinophils, granulomas, and giant cells are not found in classic polyarteritis nodosa (PAN) or microscopic polyangiitis (MPA). The pathology of the nodules is not by itself sufficient to make a diagnosis of CSS, because similar pathology can be seen in lymphoma and sarcoidosis. Glomerulonephritis in CSS is frequently not as severe as it is in WG, but when glomerulonephritis is present in CSS, it is usually focal and segmental and indistinguishable from other forms of pauci-immune glomerulonephritis (i.e., glomerulonephritis that is without significant tissue deposition of immune complexes). Circulating ANCAs may be present, and for this reason, CSS is often included as one of the ANCA-associated vasculitides.

TREATMENT

CSS is often responsive to corticosteroid therapy. For most patients, withdrawal of steroids is possible. Bronchial asthma and sinus disease, however, may require ongoing therapy, even if the vasculitic component of the disease has remitted. Patients with severe or refractory visceral organ involvement are empirically treated with additional agents, such as cyclophosphamide, methotrexate, and azathioprine, depending upon the severity of the organ involvement. Corticosteroids are tapered after remission is achieved [see Table 2].

Polyarteritis Nodosa and Microscopic Polyangiitis

CLASSIFICATION

Early reports of PAN and MPA, two forms of necrotizing medium-sized vessel arteritis, did not adequately distinguish the two entities. An international conference proposed that the distinction between these disorders be based on the absence of granulomatous inflammation in both and by involvement of arterioles, capillaries, venules, and glomerular capillaries in MPA but not in PAN.[1] It is now generally accepted that classic PAN is a rare disorder that is linked to arteritis of medium-sized muscular arteries; small vessels are unaffected. Older studies of patients with PAN did not uniformly make this distinction. Even more important, patients with viral hepatitis B or C were not excluded from older studies. The recognition of viral hepatitis is crucially important because chronic hepatitis B or C[2,19] can elicit a secondary vasculitic syndrome indistinguishable from PAN or MPA in presentation but distinct in prognosis and response to therapy.[20]

MPA, unlike PAN, involves smaller vessels ranging in size from capillaries and venules to medium-sized arteries [see Figure 1].[21] Because of the involvement of small vessels, MPA may manifest itself as glomerulonephritis or alveolar hemorrhage, which further distinguishes it from PAN. Clinically, MPA can mimic WG, although some authors have arbitrarily defined MPA as excluding involvement of the upper airway. The recognition that MPA, but not PAN, is an ANCA-associated vasculitis (in which the ANCAs are almost always directed against myeloperoxidase) further clarifies the distinction between these entities.

DIAGNOSIS

Clinical Manifestations

Glomerulonephritis, particularly rapidly progressive glomerulonephritis, and alveolar hemorrhage are common in MPA and absent, by definition, in classic PAN.

PAN affects the medium-sized muscular arteries and, like MPA, is associated with peripheral neuropathy and bowel ischemia.[22-24] Azotemia and hypertension in PAN may occur because of arteritis of the renal arteries and ischemic neuropathy but not because of glomerulonephritis. Microaneurysm formation in medium-sized visceral arteries may be striking in PAN, and the arteries may occasionally rupture.

Constitutional symptoms such as fever, asthenia, and myalgias are common in both PAN and MPA. Elevated acute-phase reactants, thrombocytosis, leukocytosis, and the anemia of inflammatory disease are common, although they are not uniformly present.

When the clinical syndrome of PAN or MPA is suspected, chronic bacterial infection (e.g., endocarditis) and viral infection (e.g., hepatitis B or C) must be excluded. The association with hepatitis B or C infection may not dramatically alter some features of the PAN or MPA syndromes, but membranous glomerulonephritis, cryoglobulinemia, immune complex–associated glomerulonephritis, hepatic failure, and thrombocytopenia are more likely to occur with viral hepatitis–associated vasculitis. Significant immune complex deposition does not occur in PAN or MPA.

Antiphospholipid antibody syndrome (APLS) can mimic PAN by presenting as mesenteric ischemia or renal insufficiency caused by thrombotic occlusion of mesenteric and renal vessels.[25] Features of both APLS and arteritis affecting muscular arteries include livedo reticularis [see Figure 5]. Glomerulonephritis, cryoglobulinemia, immune complex–associated glomerulonephritis, and peripheral neuropathy are not expected to occur in APLS unless the patient also has SLE. Thrombocytopenia can occur with APLS but is usually not present in PAN. Cholesterol embolization should also be considered as a cause of livedo, renal insufficiency, eosinophilia, and constitutional symptoms,[26] particularly if the clinical history includes a recent vascular procedure. Tissue biopsy will often establish the diagnosis

Laboratory Tests

The diagnosis of MPA and PAN should ideally be based on histopathologic demonstration of arteritis and the clinical pattern of disease. A biopsy specimen of clinically involved, nonnecrotic tissue that demonstrates the presence of arteritis of muscular arteries is the ideal supportive finding for the diagnosis of arteritis of a medium-sized vessel, but obtaining such a biopsy sample is not always possible. The presence of serum p-ANCA with antimyeloperoxidase specificity (occurring in approximately 60% of MPA patients) supports the clinical diagnosis of MPA, but p-ANCA is not specific for this disease. ANCAs are not characteristically detected in PAN.

MPA is a form of pauci-immune glomerulonephritis; that is, the renal biopsy tissue in MPA, as in WG and CSS, does not contain extensive immune complexes on immunofluorescent staining or electron microscopy. As opposed to WG, parenchymal inflammation in MPA is not striking (apart from areas of ischemic damage), and giant cells are not found in MPA. Lung biopsy in the setting of pulmonary infiltrates or hemorrhage reveals capillaritis, a histopathologic pattern that can also be seen in WG, SLE, and anti–glomerular basement membrane disease. Lung biopsy in patients with suspected MPA is most useful in ruling out alternative pulmonary diagnoses; open lung and thoracoscopic techniques have a higher yield for vasculitis than transbronchial biopsy does. Classic PAN does not cause glomerulonephritis, lung capillaritis, or pulmonary parenchymal disease.

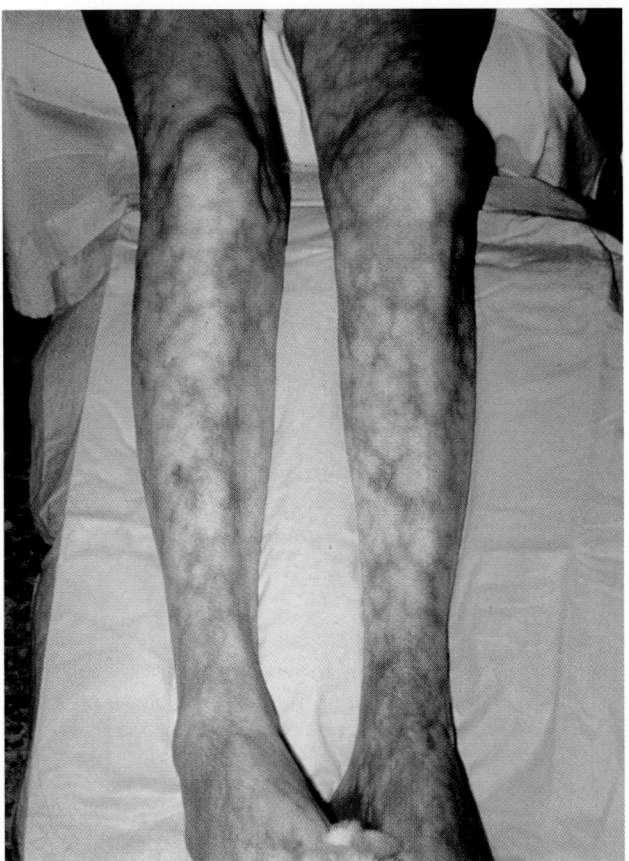

Figure 5   Livedo reticularis is characterized by reddish-blue mottling of the extremities caused by occlusion of the deep dermal arterioles.

The demonstration of arteritis affecting muscular arteries in PAN may be difficult, especially in the patient with dominant constitutional symptoms and the absence of easily accessible, disease-affected tissue. Biopsy efforts should be directed toward tissue that is abnormal as demonstrated by symptoms or objective testing. Sural nerve biopsy has become a popular option when attempting to diagnose an arteritis that is affecting medium-sized muscular vessels. The sural nerve is an accessible pure sensory nerve, and its vasa nervorum contains small as well as medium-sized muscular arteries. Nerve conduction studies can identify a diseased ischemic sural nerve before the appearance of clinical findings.[27] However, multiple reports have emphasized the low diagnostic yield from the biopsy of asymptomatic and electrically normal nerve. Even nerves exhibiting abnormal conduction have reportedly showed no diagnostic pathology 46% of the time.[28] There is notable morbidity associated with sural nerve biopsy; 13 of 60 patients experienced wound infections or delayed healing, and three patients suffered from postprocedure pain in the sural nerve that underwent biopsy.[28] Biopsy of clinically uninvolved tissue (i.e., asymptomatic muscle) has a yield of less than 30% for the diagnosis of PAN.

Abdominal angiography is often performed in the evaluation of patients who may have medium-sized vessel arteritis when biopsy has been unrewarding or is not an option. Arteries affected by polyarteritis nodosa and other disorders of medium-sized muscular arteries may develop microaneurysms or stenoses that can be visualized by angiography. When angiography is used in an effort to diagnose systemic necrotizing vasculitis in the absence of pathologic evidence of the disease, sev-

eral caveats must be noted. Angiography has limited spatial resolution; smaller vessels are not well seen. In patients with primarily smaller vessel disease, the angiogram will not likely be diagnostic. In one study, angiograms were diagnostic in only four of 30 patients with MPA, a disease that affects both small and medium-sized arteries.[21] Different investigators have reported aneurysms in 60% to 90% of patients with PAN. Aneurysms take time to develop and may not be present early in the course of the illness. In addition to being associated with aneurysms, arteritis may be associated with stenoses, which may be longer and smoother than typical atherosclerotic lesions or occlusion. To maximize the yield from the procedure, angiography should include the celiac, renal, and mesenteric vessels. Lack of clinically apparent involvement of an organ (i.e., no intestinal ischemia) does not exclude the possibility of finding abnormal vessels on angiography. It has been suggested that the visualization of aneurysms in PAN denotes more severe disease; it is unclear whether their presence may alternatively relate to the actual duration of the untreated illness. Aneurysms may resolve with successful treatment of primary or viral hepatitis–associated arteritis. The presence of visceral microaneurysms is not diagnostic of PAN. They have also been anecdotally described in patients with WG and MPA, likely representing medium-sized muscular artery involvement in these diseases. Microaneurysms also occur in nonvasculitic disorders. Isolated case reports have described aneurysms in patients with atrial myxoma, bacterial endocarditis, peritoneal carcinomatosis, and severe arterial hypertension, as well as after methamphetamine abuse. Inadequate data are available to assess the sensitivity and specificity or the predictive value of abdominal angiography in the diagnosis of necrotizing arteritis. As is the case when interpreting a biopsy result of suspected vasculitis, imaging studies must be considered in the light of the entire clinical profile. Angiography is generally avoided in the setting of progressive or significant renal insufficiency.

TREATMENT

Treatment of both PAN and MPA is empirical[29] [*see Table 2*]. Corticosteroids in high doses (1 mg/kg/day of prednisone or its equivalent) remain the initial mainstay of therapy for both disorders in the acutely ill patient. Use of corticosteroids alone may be sufficient in patients with PAN who do not have critical organ involvement, defined as renal insufficiency (from renal ischemia, as opposed to glomerular nephritis), gastrointestinal ischemia, cardiomyopathy, or dense peripheral neuropathy. Therapy with corticosteroids alone fails more frequently in MPA than in PAN, given the tendency for frequent relapses in MPA.[21] Patients who require long-term corticosteroid therapy for disease control or patients who have clinical markers of severe disease are usually treated with glucocorticoids and an additional immunosuppressive agent such as cyclophosphamide or methotrexate. The indications for initial combination therapy have not been sufficiently studied.

When active hepatitis B or C infection is present, a relatively short course of steroids should be considered on the basis of extrahepatic disease severity and the organs at acute risk for failure, in conjunction with aggressive antiviral therapy.

Kawasaki Disease

Kawasaki disease (KD) was first described in 1967 as mucocutaneous lymph node syndrome.[30] It typically affects infants and young children, causing dominant cutaneous and oral mucosal manifestations, fever, and coronary arteritis. It can on rare occasions affect adults.

DIAGNOSIS

The presence of characteristic clinical features has permitted the establishment of diagnostic criteria for KD [see Table 4]. Vasculitis may involve vessels ranging in size from venules to the aorta. Prominent inflammation is noted in the larger coronary arteries, which results in aneurysm formation in approximately 25% of untreated patients. The immediate and delayed life-threatening cardiac complications of the disease, coupled with its unique therapy (aspirin and intravenous γ-globulin), mandate prompt clinical diagnosis. Biopsy is generally not necessary, nor is it likely to yield a specific diagnosis.

High spiking fevers may persist for 1 to 2 weeks if left untreated. Rapid defervescence is usually observed with initiation of appropriate therapy. Nonexudative conjunctivitis often appears with the fever. Aseptic (lymphocytic) meningitis is common. Oral involvement includes erythema, dryness and fissuring of the lips, nonexudative pharyngitis, and tongue erythema with very prominent papillae. Mucosal ulcerations are not characteristic of this illness. Distal limb swelling may appear days after the fever, with erythema and tenderness that are not limited to the joints. Desquamation of the hands and feet, often in sheets, may begin days to a few weeks after the onset of fever. When desquamation occurs early in KD, it may appear concurrently with a truncal rash and eye and lip changes; it may mimic a drug reaction or Stevens-Johnson syndrome. The rash is usually diffuse and polymorphous, with urticarial, morbilliform, annular, or plaque components, but it is not vesicular. Adenopathy, which is present in 75% of patients, is most apparent in the cervical region.

The morbidity and mortality (< 3%) of KD is overwhelmingly associated with the development of inflammatory coronary artery aneurysms, most of which are asymptomatic at the time of formation. Aneurysms may be detected by echocardiography. Thrombosis can occur in the aneurysms, resulting in direct or embolic coronary artery occlusion. Coronary events may occur weeks or even many years after the febrile illness. A baseline echocardiogram should be obtained at the time of the acute illness and repeated 2 and 6 weeks later. Early recognition of the disease and treatment with intravenous immunoglobulin and aspirin have significantly decreased the frequency of aneurysm formation and thrombotic coronary events.

TREATMENT

Treatment of KD should be initiated with intravenous immunoglobulin (2 g/kg as a single dose) and aspirin (80 to 100 mg/kg/day every 6 hours) as soon as the disease is seriously suspected.[31] Aspirin is more effective than corticosteroids in preventing aneurysms. Corticosteroid therapy is usually unnecessary, and some authors feel that it is relatively contraindicated. Symptoms tend to respond within several days after the institution of aspirin and intravenous immunoglobulin. In resistant cases, however, corticosteroids are frequently added to the above therapies.

Large Vessel Arteritis

Temporal, or giant cell, arteritis (GCA) of the elderly and Takayasu arteritis (TA) are the most common inflammatory diseases of the aorta and its major branches. Similar vascular

---

Table 4 Diagnostic Criteria for Kawasaki Disease

Persistent fever (> 5 days)

plus

Four of the following five conditions:

Nonpurulent bilateral conjunctivitis

Oral mucosal involvement
  Erythematous pharynx
  Red or fissured lips
  Strawberry tongue

Soft tissue abnormalities of hands and feet
  Edema/erythema
  Desquamation

Polymorphous, nonvesicular rash

Cervical adenopathy

---

targeting may occur in Behçet disease, Cogan syndrome, and sarcoidosis. The last two conditions are distinguished by the pattern of extra-aortic organ involvement. It is uncertain whether TA and GCA are distinct disorders or are the same disorder with modified expression in different age groups.

TEMPORAL OR GIANT CELL ARTERITIS

GCA generally affects persons older than 50 years.[32,33] In many patients, it is associated with the syndrome of polymyalgia rheumatica (PMR). PMR is characterized by proximal muscle pain, with nocturnal and early-morning worsening. There may be a subjective sense of weakness, without true weakness on examination and without elevation of serum muscle enzyme levels. Synovitis may be present, often making it difficult to distinguish between GCA and elderly-onset rheumatoid arthritis.

GCA is variably associated with fever, scalp tenderness, headache, masticatory muscle claudication, peripheral vascular disease, inflammatory aortic aneurysms, and retinal ischemic syndromes. Oligoarticular arthritis, often in the upper extremity, and acute carpal tunnel syndrome can occasionally occur. The ischemic symptoms and signs may be clinically indistinguishable from those occurring in arteriosclerotic obliterative or atheroembolic disease.

Examination for disparate four-extremity pulses, blood pressure readings, abdominal aneurysms, and bruits in the neck, abdomen, and extremities must be part of the routine follow-up visits of patients with GCA or PMR. Pathologic findings of GCA can occur in superficial temporal arteries of patients with PMR, even without any symptoms of GCA. However, routine biopsy of the superficial temporal arteries in patients with PMR, without any other symptoms or findings of GCA, is not warranted, because patients without any physical findings or symptoms to suggest occlusive disease do not generally develop visual loss.

Levels of acute-phase reactants are elevated in more than 80% of patients with GCA but are not completely reliable markers of disease activity during and after therapy. Definitive diagnosis of GCA is generally made by biopsy of the superficial temporal artery. Pathology in GCA usually reveals chronic mononuclear cell infiltrates, destruction of the internal elastic lamina, and giant cells. The presence of giant cells is not requisite to make the diagnosis. The presence of characteristic clinical features such as new headache and jaw claudication, especially with concurrent PMR, may allow for a presumptive diagnosis in the absence of a biopsy or even when the superficial temporal artery biopsy is negative. However, because other conditions can mimic GCA, including atherosclerosis, an attempt to diagnose GCA by biopsy is warranted in most patients.[34] Corticosteroid therapy will not rapidly affect the biopsy results and should not be withheld from a patient who is strongly suspected of having GCA and is awaiting biopsy. Bilateral superficial temporal artery biopsy seems to increase the diagnostic yield.

Differential diagnoses of these inflammatory large vessel occlusive diseases include obliterative atherosclerosis, aortic and branch dissection, antiphospholipid antibody syndrome, fibromuscular dysplasia, sarcoidosis, Buerger disease, and other less common primary vasculitic syndromes (e.g., Behçet disease).

TAKAYASU ARTERITIS

Takayasu arteritis (pulseless disease) is a chronic inflammatory disease affecting the aorta and its major branches.[35] Usually diagnosed in younger, predominantly female patients of reproductive age, TA can also occur in young children and older patients of either sex. TA is more commonly associated with stenoses and aneurysms of the aorta and aortic branch vessels than is GCA.

The presenting clinical syndrome may include a prolonged flulike illness, including a polymyalgia rheumatica pattern of muscle pain. Many patients initially present with symptoms of limb, cerebral, or cardiac ischemia in the absence of any constitutional features. The characteristic features of the disease reflect the ischemia resulting from inflammatory stenoses of the aorta and its major branches. Renal ischemia can elicit high renin hypertension. Predominant sites of stenosis are the aortic arch vessels, particularly the subclavian arteries [see Figure 6]. Arm claudication with supraclavicular or axillary bruits is common. Superficial artery pain and tenderness (e.g., carotidynia) may be found on examination but are not diagnostic of TA. Severe central hypertension caused by renal artery stenosis may be unrecognized because of coexistent arm artery stenosis; thus, four-extremity blood pressure readings must be evaluated initially and

monitored on a frequent basis. Occasionally, stenoses exist in all major vessels of the extremities, and cuff monitoring may be an unreliable measure of central aortic pressures. Stroke is not uncommon and is often related to undetected central hypertension. It is extremely difficult to assess the activity of TA; the presence or absence of constitutional features or elevated acute-phase reactants are poor measures of disease activity. This impression is supported by vessel histopathology obtained during reconstructive surgery. Over 40% of vascular specimens from patients thought to be in remission revealed active inflammation. Thus, regular anatomic monitoring of these vessels by examination and imaging (either on magnetic resonance imaging or angiography) is mandatory.

Diagnosis of TA is usually made by MRI or arteriographic evidence of stenotic lesions; aneurysms are less commonly observed. The entire arch, as well as the abdominal aorta and renal vessels, should be evaluated. It is of paramount importance that central arterial pressure be routinely obtained at the time of angiography and compared with simultaneously obtained arm and leg cuff pressures. The role of sequential vascular MRI and positron emission tomography scanning in the evaluation and follow-up of patients suspected of having TA is currently under investigation; of great interest is whether imaging properties of the vessel wall can contribute to the assessment of disease activity.[36] These imaging techniques may reveal therapy-related changes in vessel wall thickness, inflammation, edema, and changes in lumen size. Pathologic documentation is difficult to obtain in TA, but the histopathology of TA, usually obtained at the time of bypass surgery, is similar to that of GCA. Preoperative discussion with the vascular surgeon is mandatory to ensure that appropriate tissue samples are obtained, if possible.

TREATMENT OF GCA AND TA

Corticosteroids are the initial treatment of both TA and GCA. GCA is generally very responsive to steroid therapy, although the most appropriate initial dose remains controversial. Initial daily doses of between 20 mg and 1 mg/kg have been advocated, with tapering over 8 to 12 months. Most authors are comfortable with a starting dose of 40 mg to 60 mg daily. It is generally recommended (without the support of data from

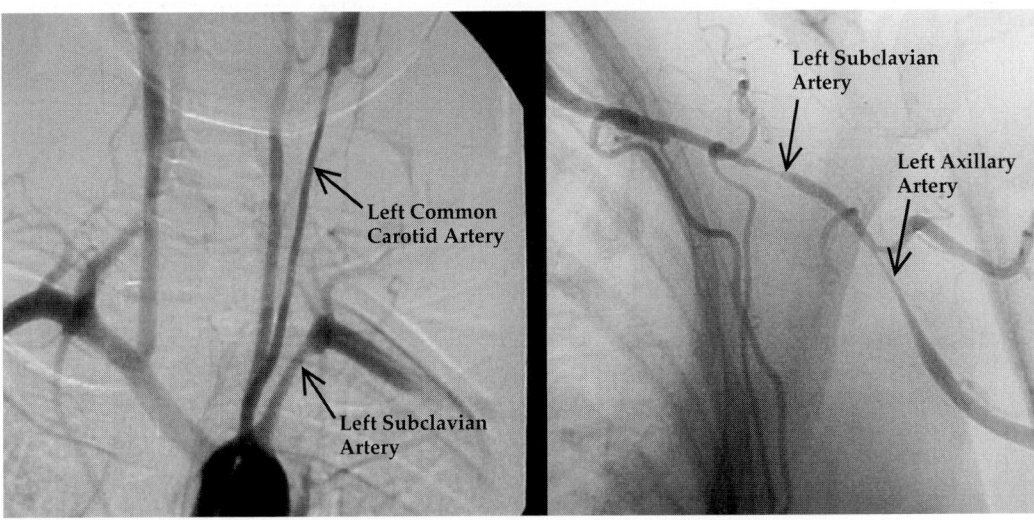

Figure 6 **Angiograms of a patient with Takayasu aortitis demonstrating long, smooth stenotic lesions of the left subclavian artery and involvement of other branches of the aortic arch vessels.**

controlled trials) that patients with any symptoms of ocular ischemia be initially treated with high-dose corticosteroids (at least 1 mg/kg of prednisone or its equivalent, with some authors, predominantly ophthalmologists, suggesting I.V. methylprednisolone in doses of up to 1 g daily for several days). A significant proportion of patients with GCA require several years of therapy.

High-dose corticosteroid therapy, especially in the elderly, is associated with significant morbidity. Measurement of acute-phase reactants provides an imperfect index of disease activity and should not be the sole guide for adjustment of steroid dosing. If significant steroid side effects occur or if patients experience relapses during tapering, a second-line agent such as methotrexate is often given on an empirical basis with the corticosteroid therapy. However, the value of adjunctive steroid-sparing agents in GCA has not yet been proved. A large prospective, randomized trial was unable to demonstrate a positive effect from methotrexate therapy,[37] although a second trial suggested a small benefit.[38] In a recently completed trial, anti–tumor necrosis factor therapy was not shown to provide any additional benefit to corticosteroid therapy.[38] The addition of low-dose aspirin to corticosteroid therapy has been demonstrated to reduce the ischemic complications of temporal arteritis.[39] There have been only anecdotal reports of successful adjunctive use of azathioprine, methotrexate, and mycophenolate in the treatment of resistant TA. Special attention must be paid to the prevention of opportunistic infections, osteoporosis, glaucoma, hyperglycemia, and hyperlipidemia.

Vascular reconstructive surgery, angioplasty, and stent placement are adjunctive therapeutic options for some patients. Very preliminary experience, however, suggests a high degree of stent failure at some centers.[40] The frequent involvement of the subclavian vessels in TA must be taken into consideration when choosing the graft implantation site for coronary or carotid bypass procedures; grafting from these vessels should be avoided.

The author has received educational grants from Abbott Laboratories, Aventis Pharmaceuticals, Inc., and TAP Pharmaceutical Products, Inc., and has received educational grants from and served as advisor or consultant for Sanofi-Aventi and Savient Pharmaceuticals, Inc.

Cytoxan, corticosteroids, methotrexate, azathioprine, pentoxifylline, colchicine, aspirin, and dapsone have not been approved by the FDA for uses described in this chapter.

References

1. Jennette C, Falk RJ, Andrassy K, et al: Nomenclature of systemic vasculitides: proposal of an international consensus conference. Arthritis Rheum 37:187, 1994

2. Vassilopoulos D, Calabrese L: Hepatitis C virus infection and vasculitis. Arth Rheum 46:585, 2002

3. Lawrence EC, Mills J: Bacterial endocarditis mimicking vasculitis with steroid-induced remission. West J Med 124:333, 1976

4. Blanco R, Martinez-Taboada VM, Rodriguez-Valverde V, et al: Cutaneous vasculitis in children and adults: associated disease and etiologic factors in 303 patients. Medicine (Baltimore) 77:403, 1998

5. Gedalia A: Henoch-Schonlein purpura. Curr Rheumatol Rep 6:195, 2004

6. Davis MD, Brewer JD: Urticarial vasculitis and hypocomplementemic urticarial vasculitis syndrome. Immun Allergy Clin North Am 24:183, 2004

7. Hoffman GS, Kerr GS, Leavitt RY, et al: Wegener's granulomatosis: an analysis of 158 patients. Ann Intern Med 116:488, 1992

8. Rheinhold-Keller E, Beuge N, Latza U, et al: An interdisciplinary approach to the care of patients with Wegener's granulomatosis: long term outcome in 155 patients. Arth Rheum 43:1021, 2000

9. Travis WD, Hoffman GS, Leavitt RY, et al: Surgical pathology of the lung in Wegener's granulomatosis. Am J Surg 15:315, 1991

10. Merkel PA, Lo GH, Holbrook JT, et al: Brief communication: high incidence of venous thrombotic events among patients with Wegener's granulomatosis: the Wegener's Clinical Occurrence of Thrombosis Study. Ann Intern Med 142:620, 2005

11. Hoffman GS: Classification of the systemic vasculitides: antineutrophil cytoplasmic antibodies, consensus and controversy. Clin Exp Rheumatol 16:111, 1998

12. Hoffman GS, Specks U: Antineutrophil cytoplasmic antibodies: diagnostic value in systemic vasculitis. Arthritis Rheum 41:1521, 1998

13. Specks U: Methotrexate for Wegener's granulomatosis: what is the evidence? Arthritis Rheum 52:2237, 2005

14. Jayne D, Rasmussen N, Andrassy K, et al: A randomized trial of maintenance therapy for vasculitis associated with antineutrophil cytoplasmic autoantibodies. N Engl J Med 349:36, 2003

15. Stegeman CA, Tervaert JW, de Jong PE, et al: Trimethoprim-sulfamethoxazole (cotrimoxazole) for the prevention of relapses of Wegener's granulomatosis. N Engl J Med 335:16, 1996

16. Seo P, Min YI, Holbrook JT, et al: Damage caused by Wegener's granulomatosis and its treatment: prospective data from the Wegener's Granulomatosis Etanercept Trial (WGET). Arthritis Rheum 52:2168, 2005

17. Guillevin L, Cohen P, Gayraud M, et al: Churg-Strauss syndrome: clinical study and long-term follow up of 96 patients. Medicine (Baltimore) 78:26, 1999

18. Reid AC, Harrison BW, Watts RA, et al: Churg-Strauss syndrome in a district hospital. Q J Med 91:219, 1998

19. Hadziyannis SJ: The spectrum of extrahepatic manifestations in hepatitis C virus infection. J Viral Hepat 4:9, 1997

20. Guillevin L, Lhote F, Cohen P, et al: Polyarteritis nodosa related to hepatitis B virus: a prospective study with long-term observation of 41 patients. Medicine (Baltimore) 74:238, 1995

21. Guillevin L, Durand-Gasselin B, Cevallos R, et al: Microscopic polyangiitis: clinical and laboratory findings in 85 patients. Arthritis Rheum 42:421, 1999

22. Travers RL, Allison DJ, Brettle RP, et al: Polyarteritis nodosa: a clinical and angiographic analysis of 17 cases. Semin Arthritis Rheum 8:184, 1979

23. Guillevin L, Lhote F, Gayraud M, et al: Prognostic factors in polyarteritis nodosa and Churg-Strauss syndrome. Medicine (Baltimore) 75:17, 1996

24. Mandell BF, Hoffman GS: Differentiating the vasculitides. Rheum Dis Clin North Am 20:409, 1994

25. Franchini M, Veneri D: The antiphospholipid syndrome. Hematology 10:265, 2005

26. Om A, Ellahham S, DiScascio G: Cholesterol embolism: an underdiagnosed clinical entity. Am Heart J 124:1321, 1992

27. Wees SJ, Sunwoo IN, Oh SJ: Sural nerve biopsy in systemic necrotizing vasculitis. Am J Med 71:525, 1981

28. Rappaport WD, Valente J, Hunter GC, et al: Clinical utilization and complications of sural nerve biopsy. Am J Surg 166:252, 1993

29. Guillevin L, Lhote F: Treatment of polyarteritis nodosa and microscopic polyangiitis. Arthritis Rheum 41:2100, 1998

30. Yeung RS: Pathogenesis and treatment of Kawasaki's disease. Curr Opin Rheumatol 17:617, 2005

31. Leung DY, Schlievert PM, Meissner HC: The immunopathogenesis and management of Kawasaki syndrome. Arthritis Rheum 41:1538, 1998

32. Weyand CM, Goronzy JJ: Giant-cell arteritis and polymyalgia rheumatica. Ann Intern Med 139:505, 2003

33. Hoffman GS: Treatment of giant cell arteritis: where we have been and why we must move on (review). Cleve Clin J Med 69(suppl II):SII117, 2002

34. Ponge T, Barrier JH, Grolleau JY, et al: The efficacy of selective unilateral temporal artery biopsy versus bilateral biopsies for diagnosis of giant cell arteritis. J Rheumatol 15:997, 1988

35. Kerr GS, Hallahan CW, Giordano J, et al: Takayasu's arteritis. Ann Intern Med 120:919, 1994

36. Tso E, Flamm SD, White RD, et al: Takayasu arteritis: utility and limitations of magnetic resonance imaging in diagnosis and treatment. Arth Rheum 46:1634, 2002

37. Hoffman GS, Cid MC, Hellmann DB, et al: A multicenter, randomized, double-blind, placebo-controlled trial of adjuvant methotrexate treatment for giant cell arteritis. Arthritis Rheum 46:1309, 2002

38. Jover JA, Hernandez-Garcia C, Morado IC, et al: Combined treatment of giant-cell arteritis with methotrexate and prednisone, a randomized, double-blind, placebo-controlled trial. Ann Intern Med 134:106, 2001

39. Nesher G, Berkun Y, Mates M, et al: Risk factors for cranial ischemic complications in giant cell arteritis. Medicine (Baltimore) 83:114, 2004

40. Liang P, Tan-Ong M, Hoffman GS: Takayasu's arteritis: vascular interventions and outcomes. J Rheumatol 31:102, 2004

Acknowledgments

Figures 1 and 2   Seward Hung.

Figure 6   Gary S. Hoffman.

Christopher Wise, M.D., F.A.C.P.

The presence of precipitated crystals in the synovium or synovial fluid can be associated with an inflammatory response that usually manifests itself as an acute arthritis associated with synovial fluid leukocytosis. The identification of monosodium urate (MSU) crystals in the synovial fluid of patients with acute gout in 1961 by McCarty and Hollander represented the initial recognition of arthritis associated with articular crystal deposition.[1] This development was followed in 1962 by the recognition of so-called pseudogout, which is associated with calcium pyrophosphate dihydrate (CPPD) crystals.[2] Since then, a great deal has been learned about these two common types of arthritis. In addition, the role of crystals in the pathogenesis of osteoarthritis and other arthropathies has been further explored. The diagnosis of crystal-induced arthritis requires the identification of crystals in synovial fluid or tissue; in most cases, this acute arthritis is self-limited.

Gout

DEFINITION AND CLASSIFICATION

Gout is defined as an arthritis associated with the presence of MSU crystals in synovial fluid or tissue. Gout is often classified as primary or secondary [*see Table 1*], and both forms are associated with hyperuricemia. Gout associated with an inborn error in metabolism or decreased renal excretion without other renal disease is referred to as primary gout, whereas gout associated with an acquired disease or the use of a drug is called secondary gout. In both primary and secondary gout, chronic hyperuricemia may be the result of overproduction of uric acid caused by increased purine intake, synthesis, or breakdown, or it may be the result of decreased renal excretion of urate.

EPIDEMIOLOGY

Gout is predominantly a disease of middle-aged men, but there is a gradually increasing prevalence in both men and women in older age groups. The annual incidence of gout in men in most studies is in the range of one to three per 1,000, but the incidence is much lower in women. In the Framingham Study, for example, the 2-year incidence of gout was 3.2 per 1,000 men versus 0.5 per 1,000 women.[3] A study of gout in Rochester, Minnesota, over the past 2 decades has suggested that the incidence of gout may be increasing.[4]

The overall prevalence of self-reported gout in the general population is 0.7% to 1.4% in men and 0.5% to 0.6% in women. However, in people older than 65 years, prevalence increases to 4.4% to 5.2% in men and 1.8% to 2.0% in women.[5] In male populations, the prevalence of gout reaches impressive levels by the fifth decade. In a study of male medical students, the prevalence of gout reached 5.8% in whites and 10.9% in African Americans surveyed for a mean of 28 years after graduation.[6] In patients who experience the onset of gout after 60 years of age, the prevalence in men and the prevalence in women are almost equal; in those who experience onset after 80 years of age, the prevalence is greater in women.[7]

The incidence and prevalence of gout are parallel to the incidence and prevalence of hyperuricemia in the general population. Serum urate levels increase by 1 to 2 mg/dl in males at the time of puberty, but females exhibit little change in urate levels until after menopause, when concentrations approach those seen in males.[8] Most patients with elevated serum uric acid levels do not have gout, but hyperuricemia is clearly associated with an increased risk of gout.[9] For example, in persons with serum urate levels greater than 10 mg/dl, the annual incidence of gout is 70 per 1,000 and the 5-year prevalence is 30%, whereas in persons with levels less than 7 mg/dl, the annual incidence is only 0.9 per 1,000 and the 5-year prevalence is 0.6%. Additional factors that correlate strongly with serum urate levels and the prevalence of gout in the general population include serum creatinine levels, body weight, height, blood pressure, and alcohol intake.

PATHOGENESIS AND ETIOLOGY

The development of gout tends to be associated with chronically increased serum levels of uric acid. However, a substantial minority of patients with acute gout have normal uric acid levels, and hyperuricemia does not always lead to the development of gout. Humans are one of the few species with an inactive uricase gene, which results in elevated levels of uric acid. It has been postulated that humans have a propensity to develop hyperuricemia because uric acid confers protection against degenerative diseases by acting as an antioxidant.[10,11] Urate at high levels and under certain conditions will precipitate into MSU crystals, and the deposition of these crystals within the synovium or synovial fluid may lead to the development of gout (see below).

Table 1 Classification of Hyperuricemia and Gout

Primary Hyperuricemia and Gout with No Associated Condition	Secondary Hyperuricemia and Gout with Identifiable Associated Condition
Uric acid undersecretion (80%–90%)	Uric acid undersecretion
Idiopathic	Renal insufficiency (any cause)
Urate overproduction (10%–20%)	Polycystic kidney disease
Idiopathic	Lead nephropathy
HGPRT deficiency	Drugs
PRPP synthetase overactivity	Diuretics
	Salicylates (low dose)
	Pyrazinamide
	Ethambutol
	Niacin
	Cyclosporine
	Didanosine
	Urate overproduction
	Myeloproliferative diseases
	Lymphoproliferative diseases
	Hemolytic anemias
	Polycythemia vera
	Other malignancies
	Psoriasis
	Glycogen storage disease
	Dual mechanism
	Obesity
	Ethanol consumption
	Hypoxemia and tissue hypoperfusion

HGPRT—hypoxanthine-guanine phosphoribosyltransferase
PRPP—phosphoribosylpyrophosphate

Gout has been recognized as a familial disorder since the time of Sir Alfred Garrod. About 40% of patients in most series report a family history of gout, and the hereditary component for serum uric acid levels in the general population has been estimated to be approximately 40%.[8,12] The mechanisms for this association are still not understood, but most available data suggest that serum uric acid levels are controlled by multiple genes involving both production and excretion of uric acid.

Hyperuricemia

The plasma concentration of uric acid is maintained at a relatively constant level in humans because of a balance between production and excretion. Uric acid derives from exogenous and endogenous sources: it is the end product of the metabolism of dietary purines and occurs as a result of the breakdown of purines from nucleic acids during cell turnover. A very small amount of uric acid is passively eliminated through the gastrointestinal tract. Almost all plasma uric acid is filtered at the glomerulus, and 80% is reabsorbed in the proximal tubule. Some of this plasma uric acid is subsequently secreted back into the lumen; a small amount undergoes distal reabsorption.[8,11]

Hyperuricemia can result from decreased renal excretion or increased production of uric acid. In 80% to 90% of patients with primary gout, hyperuricemia is caused by renal underexcretion of uric acid, even though renal function is otherwise normal. The defect in renal excretion of uric acid in patients with primary gout may be attributed to reduced filtration, enhanced reabsorption, or decreased secretion, but it is unclear which of these mechanisms is most important. Even patients with high levels of urate excretion (overproducers) demonstrate a relative decrease in urate clearance compared to patients with normal levels of uric acid production.[13]

Hyperuricemia may develop secondary to numerous conditions (e.g., renal insufficiency, myeloproliferative diseases, obesity, alcohol consumption, and drug intake) [see Table 1]. Patients with secondary gout related to renal disease are hyperuricemic because of a decreased filtered load of uric acid, although decreased tubular secretion may play a role in some patients. Patients with lead nephropathy seem to be particularly prone to the development of gout, and recent studies have suggested that subclinical exposure to environmental lead may contribute to some of the hyperuricemia and gout seen in the general population.[14,15] The hyperuricemia associated with diuretic therapy results from volume depletion, which leads to a decreased filtered load, and from enhanced tubular reabsorption.[16] A renal mechanism is the cause of most other cases of drug-associated hyperuricemia. Low-dose aspirin can cause significant changes in renal handling of urate within a week after therapy is started, particularly in elderly patients.[17] Hyperuricemia and gout may be associated with cyclosporine therapy in renal and cardiac transplantation patients, and it appears to be the result of a combined effect of cyclosporine on renal blood flow and tubular function.[18-20]

Overproduction of uric acid, caused by increased purine synthesis, is seen in about 10% to 20% of patients with primary gout. In addition, four specific heritable defects of purine synthesis have been identified: phosphoribosylpyrophosphate synthetase overactivity, glucose-6-phosphatase deficiency, fructose-1-phosphate aldolase deficiency, and hypoxanthine-guanine phosphoribosyltransferase (HGPRT) deficiency. Of these heritable defects, the best-known is HGPRT deficiency. Complete deficiency of this enzyme is associated with the Lesch-Nyhan syndrome in children, and a partial deficiency has been associated with early-onset gout and nephrolithiasis.

Most diseases that cause secondary hyperuricemia characterized by overproduction of uric acid are associated with increased nucleic acid turnover. These diseases include multiple myeloma, polycythemia, pernicious anemia, hemoglobinopathies, thalassemia, other hemolytic anemias, other myeloproliferative and lymphoproliferative disorders, and other neoplasms. In addition, some critically ill patients may experience hyperuricemia resulting from accelerated breakdown of adenosine triphosphate (ATP).

Uric Acid Precipitation and Crystal-Induced Inflammation

Uric acid dissociates almost completely to the urate anion form at a pH of 7.4. At concentrations greater than 6.5 to 7.0 mg/dl, urate precipitates in the form of MSU crystals. Local conditions in tissues responsible for crystal precipitation and deposition include lower temperature (as is found in peripheral joints), lower pH level in extracellular fluid, and reduced urate binding to plasma proteins. Other local factors that contribute to precipitation and deposition of crystals are trauma and rapid increases in local urate concentration as a result of mobilization of water from peripheral tissues (as occurs when edematous feet are elevated during sleep).

The factors responsible for the inflammatory response to crystals are not completely understood.[8,21] The phlogistic properties of crystals seem to be linked to their ability to bind immunoglobulins and other proteins, particularly complement and lipoproteins. These complexes bind to surface receptors on macrophages and mast cells, leading to activation and release of proinflammatory cytokines, chemotactic factors, and other mediators. An influx of phagocytic cells—particularly neutrophils—follows. Crystals are engulfed, and subsequent disruption of lysosomes releases arachidonate metabolites, collagenases, and oxygen radicals. Several factors have been postulated as contributing to the self-termination of attacks. These factors include digestion of crystals by myeloperoxidase, increased heat and blood flow leading to dissolution and removal of crystals from the joint, alteration of the crystal properties by the inflammatory process itself, and phagocytosis of crystals by more mature macrophages later in the attack.[22,23]

CLINICAL STAGES

Acute Gouty Arthritis

Acute gouty arthritis is usually characterized by a sudden and dramatic onset of pain and swelling, usually in a single joint. This condition occurs most often in lower extremity joints and evolves within hours to marked swelling, warmth, and tenderness. The process often extends beyond the confines of the joint and may mimic cellulitis. The pain of gout is often severe enough to make even the light pressure of bedclothes intolerable, and weight bearing is usually very difficult. Even without treatment, attacks of gout usually subside within a few days, although some attacks may last a few weeks. Early in the course of gout, affected joints usually return to normal after attacks.

The initial attack of gout is monoarticular in 85% to 90% of patients. At least half of initial attacks occur in the first metatarsophalangeal joints (a condition known as podagra), but other joints of the foot may be involved simultaneously or in subsequent attacks. Other lower extremity joints, including the ankles

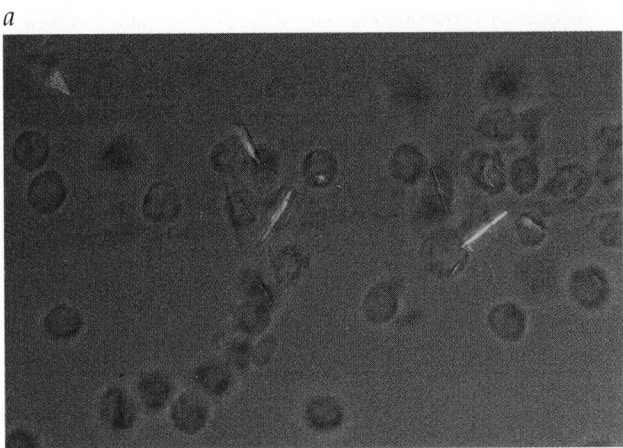 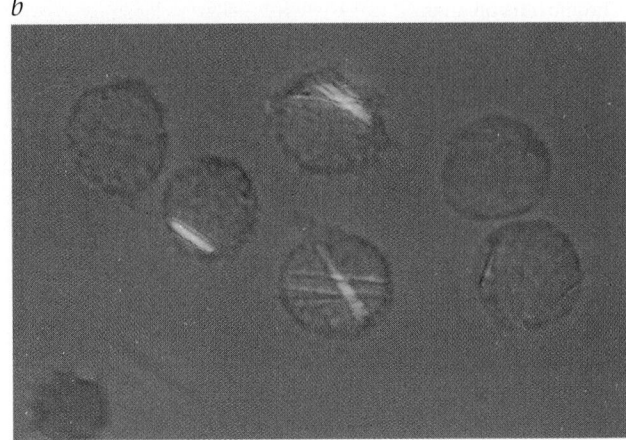

a   *b*

Figure 1   Gout can be diagnosed by demonstration of negatively birefringent monosodium urate crystals in synovial fluid examined by polarized-light microscopy, either free (*a*) or within polymorphonuclear leukocytes (*b*).

and knees, are often affected; in more advanced gout, attacks may occur in upper extremity joints, such as the elbow, wrist, and small joints of the fingers. In older women in particular, involvement of the small joints of the fingers (previously affected by osteoarthritis) is more commonly seen earlier in the course of the disease.[24,25] Acute episodes may also involve the bursae, particularly in the olecranon or prepatellar areas. Polyarticular gout occurs as the initial manifestation in about 10% to 15% of patients and may be associated with fever.[26]

Almost all synovial fluid aspirated early in an acute attack contains typical needlelike crystals, which are negatively birefringent and may be extracellular or may occur within polymorphonuclear leukocytes [*see Figure 1*]. The leukocyte count in most gouty synovial fluid rises to a range of 10,000 to 60,000/mm[3], but it may be much higher in some patients.

Intercritical Gout

After the initial attack of gout subsides, the clinical course of gout may follow one of several patterns. A minority of patients never have another attack of gout, and some may not have an-

other attack for several years. Most patients, however, have recurrent attacks over a period of years. In a study done before the use of hypouricemic agents, 78% of patients had a second attack within 2 years and 93% had a second attack within 10 years.[27] In many patients, symptom-free intervals between attacks become progressively shorter as episodes of acute arthritis increase in frequency. In chronic disease, soft tissue swelling and joint effusions persist for longer periods after each attack. Finally, after 10 to 20 years of recurrent gouty attacks, patients typically develop chronic tophaceous gout.

Chronic Tophaceous Gout

Persistent hyperuricemia with increasingly frequent attacks of gout eventually leads to joint involvement of wider distribution and chronic joint destruction resulting from deposition of massive amounts of urate in and around joints [*see Figure 2a*]. Without therapy to lower serum uric acid levels, the average interval from the first gouty attack to the development of chronic arthritis or tophi is about 12 years.[28] After 20 years, 75% of patients have tophi; patients with the highest urate levels are at highest risk. In

a   *b*

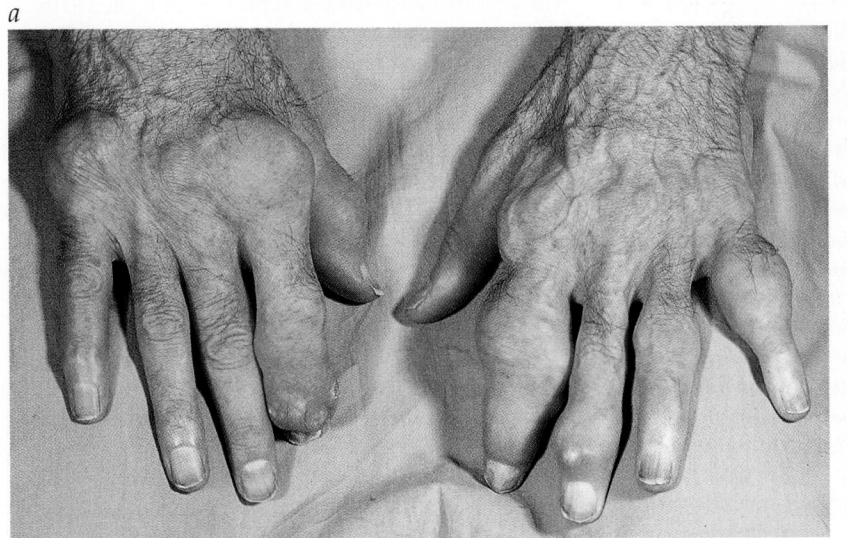 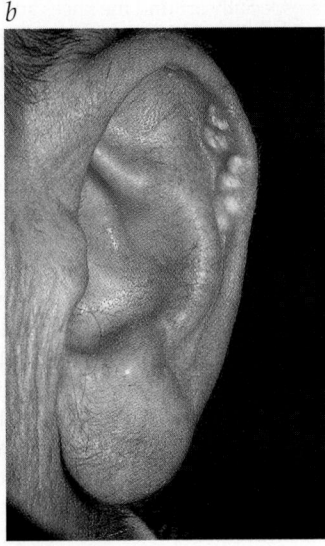

Figure 2   Tophaceous gout, demonstrating chronic swelling in and around the joints of the hand caused by bone destruction and tophaceous deposits in the hands (*a*). Tophi may also be found in extra-articular areas, such as the pinna of the ear (*b*).

Chronic Inflammation in Subchondral Bone   Articular Cartilage   Urate Deposit

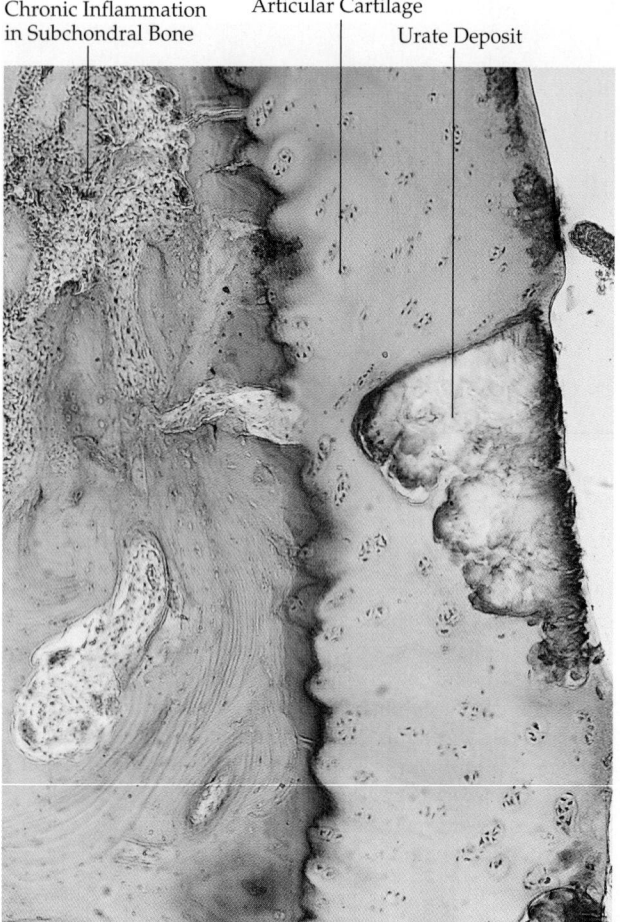

Figure 3 **Microscopic appearance of sodium urate deposits causing a defect in articular cartilage and chronic inflammation in the subchondral bone.**

elderly patients, particularly women, tophi may appear earlier in the course of the disease, sometimes in patients without a history of gouty attacks.[25]

Subcutaneous tophi begin to appear in periarticular and bursal tissues, especially around the knees and elbows, along tendons of the hands and feet, and around the interphalangeal and metacarpophalangeal joints of the hands. Tophaceous deposits are usually firm and movable, and the overlying skin may be normal or thin and reddened. When close to the surface, deposits exhibit a characteristic chalky appearance and may be cream-colored or yellowish. Tophi have also been described in areas not associated with joints, such as the pinna of the ear [*see Figure 2b*], and in unusual visceral locations, such as the myocardium, pericardium, aortic valves, and extradural spinal regions.

Destruction of the articular cartilage and subchondral bone eventually occurs in patients with chronic articular involvement [*see Figure 3*]. Erosive bony lesions may be seen on x-rays as well-defined punched-out lesions in periarticular bone, often associated with overhanging edges of bone.[29] These erosions are usually 5 mm or more in diameter and are larger than those seen in rheumatoid arthritis. Bone mineralization appears to be generally normal in chronic tophaceous gout, and periarticular osteopenia, which is seen in rheumatoid arthritis, is usually not present. The distribution of destructive joint disease in gout is often asymmetrical and patchy.

Associated Conditions

A number of chronic illnesses may be associated with gout and hyperuricemia, either in primary or secondary form. The best-known association is with renal disease, which frequently occurs in patients with gout.[30,31]

Most cases of renal disease in patients with primary forms of gout are believed to be the result of nephrosclerosis related to hypertension. However, experimental evidence suggests that hyperuricemia may play a direct pathogenetic role in the development of renal disease and hypertension.[32] In addition, the presence of intrarenal urate deposits associated with an inflammatory reaction in some patients and the improvement of renal function associated with control of uric acid levels suggest that urate has a causal role in the renal disease seen in patients with chronic tophaceous gout.[33,34]

Renal stones occur in 10% to 25% of patients with gout.[35] Most stones in patients with gout are composed of uric acid. However, some are composed of calcium oxalate and other constituents, and hyperuricemia is believed to contribute to the formation of these stones as well.[36]

An acute urate nephropathy associated with the tumor lysis syndrome has been described in patients with leukemia or lymphoma who are undergoing chemotherapy.[37] This condition is associated with acute oliguria and an elevated urinary urate-to-creatinine ratio (> 1.0) and is usually treated prophylactically with allopurinol and vigorous hydration. An association of gout with renal disease and chronic lead intoxication has been noted in some populations (saturnine gout).[38] In the United States, this association has most often been attributed to the drinking of illicit whiskey produced in lead-lined stills, but it has also been attributed to occupational lead exposure.

Gout has long been associated with obesity, diabetes mellitus, hyperlipidemia, and atherosclerotic cardiovascular disease. The association with diabetes has been variously reported; in lipid disorders, the association is primarily with hypertriglyceridemia, which may in turn be linked to alcohol intake.[39] In addition, a correlation has been found between hyperuricemia and the insulin-resistance syndrome (also referred to as the metabolic syndrome), possibly associated with body-fat distribution and triglyceride levels.[40,41] The association of gout and hyperuricemia with cardiovascular disease appears to be related to the link between these metabolic disorders and hypertension.[42]

Alcohol consumption has long been associated with the precipitation of gouty attacks in susceptible patients. In addition, long-term heavy alcohol consumption promotes hyperuricemia by interfering with renal excretion and increasing production of urate; some alcoholic beverages, particularly beer, serve as a source of dietary purine.[9] Patients with gout have an increased prevalence of hypothyroidism, and urate levels have been shown to decrease with the institution of thyroid replacement therapy, probably through a renal mechanism.[43]

DIAGNOSIS

A diagnosis of gout can be made with certainty only by confirmation of the presence of monosodium urate crystals in synovial fluid or tissue. Elements of the patient's history, physical examination, and laboratory studies can be very helpful in diagnosing gout [*see Table 2*].[44] A typical presentation of podagra in a middle-aged man with known hyperuricemia may be sufficient for an initial tentative diagnosis of gout, particularly if the condition responds well to colchicine. Nodular deposits on the olecra-

Table 2   Diagnosis of Gout

Test	Sensitivity	Specificity	Comments
Microscopic examination of synovial fluid by polarized microscopy	High during acute attacks; some potential between attacks	100% specific	Presence of needle-shaped, negatively birefringent urate crystals is diagnostic
Serum uric acid levels	Unreliable, even during attacks (elevated levels are a risk factor for, but not diagnostic of, gout)	Low in unselected patients (only 30% of people with uric acid > 10 mg/dl will have gout over 5 yr)	Serum levels are lower during attacks in some studies; serial serum levels over months and years may suggest risk of gout and severity
X-rays	Moderate, only in patients with chronic disease; even typical erosions may be difficult to differentiate from other erosions (e.g., as seen in rheumatoid arthritis)	Moderate, depending on nature of changes; otherwise may be difficult to differentiate from other forms	May be useful in patients with chronic disease if interpreted carefully (see text)

non processes, dorsal aspects of the fingers, or finger pads should be sought, particularly in patients with a history of joint problems. Patients with gout may have a normal serum urate level at the time of an attack. With most patients, however, a review of old records reveals a history of chronic hyperuricemia. Radiographs are seldom useful during an acute attack, unless previous attacks have occurred in the area examined and unless, after years of disease, well-defined erosions in or around joints, with characteristic overhanging edges, can be seen.

The detection of needle-shaped, negatively birefringent urate crystals in synovial fluid examined under polarized light microscopy is the definitive diagnostic finding for gout. Although this test is best done on fluid obtained during an acute attack, aspiration of synovial fluid from previously affected joints or aspiration of a subcutaneous nodule suspected of being a tophus may be helpful.[45,46] The synovial fluid should be examined by someone experienced in crystal identification, because an inexperienced person may not recognize the presence of crystals.[47]

Alternative diagnoses should be considered in all patients suspected of having gout. Acute arthritis can be caused by infection, other crystal-induced arthropathies, or other diseases. A Gram stain and culture of the synovial fluid and radiographs may be needed in some patients to rule out these disorders. Gout can be accompanied by fever, particularly during polyarticular attacks, and should be considered in patients suspected of having acute bacterial arthritis whose cultures are negative.[26] In addition, gout and infection can coexist in the same joints, making therapeutic decisions difficult in individual cases. Thus, synovial fluid cultures are essential in any patient who is suspected of having gout and who has fever or purulent-appearing synovial fluid. Pseudogout [see Pseudogout (Calcium Pyrophosphate Dihydrate Deposition Disease), *below*] may cause acute monoarthritis or oligoarthritis that is similar to gout. Radiographs in such patients may show chondrocalcinosis, and CPPD crystals in the synovial fluid are usually easily distinguishable from urate crystals. However, some patients may have both gout and pseudogout in the same joint.

TREATMENT

The goals of therapy for patients with gout include termination of the acute attack, prevention of further attacks during the intercritical period, assessment for associated and contributing factors, and consideration of long-term hypouricemic therapy.[48,49] Each aspect of therapy should be considered separately, and there should be no confusion between efforts to suppress inflammation in acute attacks and efforts to lower serum urate levels, decrease the frequency of attacks, and prevent complications in the future.

Acute Gout

Treatment of acute gout should be initiated as early in the attack as possible. Agents available for terminating the acute attack include colchicine, nonsteroidal anti-inflammatory drugs (NSAIDs), adrenocorticotropic hormone (ACTH), and corticosteroids [see Table 3]. Each agent has a toxicity profile, with advantages and disadvantages applicable to individual circumstances. The patient's overall health and coexistent medical problems, particularly renal disease and gastrointestinal disease, often dictate the choice among these approaches. Corticosteroids and ACTH have been used more often in recent years in patients with multiple comorbid conditions because of the relatively low toxicity profile of these agents.

Colchicine has been used for centuries to treat acute attacks of gout. Given in oral dosages of 0.6 to 1.2 mg initially, followed by 0.6 mg every 2 hours, colchicine begins relieving most attacks of gout within 12 to 24 hours. However, most patients experience nausea, vomiting, abdominal cramps, and diarrhea with these dosages. Colchicine should be given more cautiously in elderly patients and should be avoided in patients with renal or hepatic insufficiency and patients already on long-term colchicine therapy.[50] Intravenous colchicine has been used for acute attacks, but recognition of the potential for bone marrow suppression and other systemic toxicities has resulted in guidelines for restricting dosage and even in a lack of availability in some countries.[51,52]

NSAIDs are useful in most patients with acute gout and remain the agents of choice for young, healthy patients without comorbid diseases. Indomethacin has been the most widely used agent over the years; it usually begins to provide relief within hours after the initial oral dose. Most NSAIDs are comparable in efficacy, although studies comparing NSAIDs in acute gout are few. The use of all NSAIDs is limited by the risks of gastric ulceration and gastritis, acute renal failure, fluid retention, interference with antihypertensive therapy, and, in older patients, problems with mentation. Aspirin is usually avoided because of its dose-related and variable effect on urate excretion. Initial experience with NSAIDs that are selective cyclooxygenase-2 (COX-2) inhibitors suggested that these agents would be useful in treating acute gout, and possibly in long-term prophylaxis, in patients

Table 3   Drug Treatment of Acute Gout

Drug	Dosage	Relative Efficacy	Comments
Colchicine	0.6–1.2 mg p.o. initially, then 0.6 mg p.o., q. 2 hr	Moderate efficacy in high dose, but low threshold for toxicity	Common side effects are nausea, vomiting, cramps, and diarrhea; use with caution in elderly; avoid in patients with renal or hepatic insufficiency and those already on long-term colchicine Reasonably effective in low dose (q.d.–b.i.d.) as prophylaxis for future attacks

NSAIDs
  Indomethacin
  Ibuprofen
  Naproxen
  Diclofenac
  Piroxicam
  Meloxicam
  Nabumetone
COX-2 inhibitor
  Celecoxib
	
	50–75 mg b.i.d., t.i.d.
	600–800 mg t.i.d., q.i.d.
	500 mg b.i.d., t.i.d.
	75 mg b.i.d
	20 mg q.d.
	15 mg q.d.
	1,500 mg q.d.
	
	200 mg q.d., b.i.d.
		Moderately effective; most are comparably effective	NSAIDs carry risk of gastric ulceration, gastritis, acute or chronic renal failure, fluid retention, congestive heart failure interference with antihypertensive therapy; risk of mentation problems in elderly
			COX-2–specific agents reduce risk of GI complications but not other complications; their use increases risk of cardiovascular disease

Corticosteroids
  Triamcinolone acetonide
  (and others)
    Intra-articular
 	
    Intramuscular
    Prednisone (oral)
 	
    ACTH intramuscular
	
	5–10 mg for small joints; 40–60 mg for large joints
	40–60 mg
	40–60 mg p.o. per day to start, taper over 5–14 days
	40–60 mg single dose
		Moderately to extremely effective	Caution in patients with brittle diabetes; some caution in patients with fluid retention or hypertension; overall, safer than NSAIDs or colchicine in these patients

ACTH—adrenocorticotropic hormone   COX-2—cyclooxygenase-2   NSAIDs—nonsteroidal anti-inflammatory drugs

at risk for gastrointestinal toxicity from older nonselective NSAIDs.[53] However, the withdrawal of the COX-2 inhibitors rofecoxib and valdecoxib from the market because of increased risk of myocardial infarction, stroke, and skin reactions with long-term use has clouded the future of these agents.

Corticosteroids have become more widely used in the treatment of acute gout in recent years.[54] Intra-articular steroids after arthrocentesis are extremely useful in providing relief, particularly in large effusions, in which the initial aspiration of fluid results in rapid relief of pain and tightness in the affected joint. The dosage of the steroid triamcinolone depends on the size of the joint, ranging from 5 to 10 mg for small joints of the hands or feet to 40 to 60 mg for larger joints, such as the knee. Systemic corticosteroids may also be useful in patients for whom colchicine or NSAIDs are inadvisable and in patients with polyarticular attacks. Oral prednisone, administered in tapered doses starting at 40 to 60 mg daily, and single intramuscular injections of ACTH (40 units) or triamcinolone (40 to 60 mg) have all been shown to be as effective as NSAIDs in treating acute gout. In most studies of systemic steroids for acute gout, only a small proportion of patients have required repeated therapy for rebound attacks in the first several days after therapy.

Interval Follow-up and Evaluation

Patients remain at increased risk for another attack of gout for several weeks after resolution of the initial attack; prophylaxis with small doses of colchicine or NSAIDs should be used for most patients. Colchicine (0.6 mg one or two times a day) prevents attacks in over 80% of patients. Prophylaxis should be continued for 1 to 2 months after an acute attack and for several months in patients with a history of frequent attacks; it should

also be employed when urate-lowering drugs are initiated.[55] The dose of colchicine should be reduced or the duration of therapy shortened in patients with reduced renal function because bone marrow suppression and myoneuropathy have been reported in patients on long-term low-dose colchicine therapy with a creatinine clearance of less than 50 ml/min.[56]

After an acute attack of gout, a patient can be monitored for recurrent attacks and assessed for potential underlying causes of hyperuricemia. A spot midmorning urine sample to determine the ratio of urinary uric acid per deciliter of glomerular filtrate (urinary urate × plasma creatinine/urinary creatinine) or a 24-hour urine collection helps to classify the patient as an overproducer or underexcretor of urate; this is useful in identifying the optimal drug treatment for lowering serum urate levels, if indicated [see Sidebar Determining Overproducers and Underexcretors of Uric Acid].[1,57] If urinary urate excretion exceeds 0.6 mg/dl of glomerular filtrate or 600 to 700 mg a day, allopurinol is the most appropriate agent for lowering urate levels, by decreasing

---

Determining Overproducers and Underexcretors of Uric Acid

Urinary urate × plasma creatinine/urinary creatinine
   > 0.6 highly suggestive of overproducer
   < 0.6 suggestive of underexcretor
Urate present in 24-hour urine collection
   > 600–700 mg confirms overproducer status
   < 600 mg evidence of underexcretor if serum urate level is elevated

Table 4 Drug Treatment of Chronic Gout (Urate-Lowering Agents)

Drug	Dosage	Relative Efficacy	Comments
Probenecid	1–2 g/day in divided doses	Modest	Limited benefit to patients with decreased renal function; risk of renal stones
Sulfinpyrazone	Up to 400–800 mg/day in divided doses	Modest	Limited benefit to patients with decreased renal function; risk of renal stones
Allopurinol	300–600 mg/day; 200 mg for patients with GFR < 60 ml/min; 100 mg for patients with GFR < 30 ml/min	Extremely effective in lowering serum urate levels	Inhibits metabolism of azathioprine and other drugs; may cause hypersensitivity reaction (discontinue immediately if rash develops)

GFR—glomerular filtration rate

urate production; with lower excretion levels, a uricosuric drug may be useful.

Management after an acute attack should include a review of the patient's overall health, which may reveal important coexistent diseases, medications, and habits that could contribute to hyperuricemia. In particular, alcohol consumption should be discussed as an important factor in hyperuricemia and the precipitation of attacks. A review of the patient's diet may reveal heavy consumption of purine-rich foods, such as organ meats, seafood, or various legumes or other vegetables. In addition, the intercritical period is an excellent time to assess for obesity, hyperlipidemia, and hypertension, which often accompany gout and are correctable risk factors for premature cardiovascular mortality. Although the purine content of the diet usually contributes only about 1.0 mg/dl to the serum urate concentration, a diet that emphasizes calorie reduction, complex carbohydrates, and unsaturated fats will reduce urate levels and improve lipoprotein profiles in patients with gout.[48,58,59] Weight loss and physical activity are important strategies for lowering cardiovascular risk in obese patients; however, evidence suggests that increased physical activity is the perferred treatment[48,58,59]; sedentary, obese patients who have had an acute attack of gout should be strongly encouraged to increase their level of physical activity [*see Chapter 4*].

Chronic Hyperuricemia

In general, patients with asymptomatic hyperuricemia should not be treated with hypouricemic agents. However, patients with persistent marked hyperuricemia (levels > 10 mg/dl) or hyperuricosuria (levels > 1,000 mg/24 hr) should be followed carefully for manifestations of gout or renal stones. Drug therapy to lower urate levels should be considered for patients who have had crystal-proven gout with recurrent attacks and persistent hyperuricemia despite efforts to identify and correct contributing factors [*see Table 4*]. Patients who have had more than two or three attacks, who have tophi or radiographic evidence of joint damage, or who have chronic renal insufficiency and recurrent gout should be treated with hypouricemic therapy if they are willing to comply with a long-term regimen. Reduction of serum urate levels to well into the normal range (i.e., < 6.0 mg/dl) eventually leads to prevention of further attacks and resorption of tophi.[42] Low-dose colchicine or NSAIDs should be used to prevent attacks that can occur for several months after hypouricemic therapy is started.[60]

Agents that increase renal excretion of urate (i.e., uricosuric drugs) can be used in patients with normal renal function who have no history of nephrolithiasis and whose 24-hour excretion of urate is less than 700 mg/day. Probenecid (1 to 2 g/day) is the most commonly used agent in this class, although sulfinpyra-

zone (up to 400 to 800 mg/day) can be used as well. Both agents are of limited use in patients with decreased renal function and carry a risk of precipitating renal stones. High urine volume and alkalinization with bicarbonate intake decrease this risk.

In up to 25% of patients, urate levels are not well controlled with uricosuric drug therapy. Benzbromarone is a uricosuric agent that has been available in Europe for over 20 years but is not available in the United States. Studies have shown that this agent may be useful in lowering uric acid levels in some patients with renal disease.[61]

Allopurinol, the only available inhibitor of xanthine oxidase, reduces serum urate levels in almost all compliant patients and may be used in overproducers or underexcretors. A daily dose of 300 mg is standard in patients with normal renal function, although some patients may require as much as 600 mg to achieve optimal serum urate levels. The dose should be reduced to 200 mg in patients whose glomerular filtration rate (GFR) is less than 60 ml/min and to 100 mg in those whose GFR is less than 30 ml/min. The dose of some other drugs, particularly azathioprine, must be reduced in patients receiving allopurinol, because allopurinol inhibits metabolism. Approximately 2% of patients taking allopurinol develop a hypersensitivity rash that progresses to a severe exfoliative dermatitis.[62] This disorder is more likely to occur in patients taking ampicillin or in those with renal insufficiency. Severe rashes may be accompanied by a syndrome of vasculitis, hepatitis, and interstitial renal disease, with a mortality risk of 20% reported in some series. Because of this risk, allopurinol should be discontinued in any patient who experiences a rash. Allopurinol may be reinstituted in such patients if the rash is mild. Reinitiation of allopurinol therapy should be gradual, starting with oral doses of 50 µg daily and increasing to 100 mg daily over a 4-week period; this strategy effectively desensitizes the majority of patients with prior hypersensitivity reactions to allopurinol therapy.[63]

Pseudogout (Calcium Pyrophosphate Dihydrate Deposition Disease)

DEFINITION AND CLASSIFICATION

CPPD crystals may be found in deposits in and around joints and are characterized by calcification of articular cartilage, menisci, synovium, and other periarticular tissues. McCarty and colleagues first described CPPD crystals in synovial fluids from patients with goutlike attacks in 1962.[2] They used the term pseudogout for this new arthropathy, which is characterized by intra-articular calcifications (chondrocalcinosis), crystals in the synovial fluid, and acute arthropathy. Since then, other clinical presentations and a variety of disease processes have been associated with CPPD crystals. Thus, the term CPPD deposition disease has come to include the various clinical presentations as part of the same general clinical syndrome.

EPIDEMIOLOGY

CPPD deposition disease is generally a disease of the elderly; the average age of patients is approximately 70 years.[64] The prevalence of articular chondrocalcinosis is very low in people younger than 40 years but increases with age and is quite common in older populations. When multiple radiologic studies are obtained, the documented prevalence in the general population is 10% to 15% in those 65 to 75 years of age and over 40% in people older than 80 years.[65,66] CPPD deposition occurs in males and females in differing distribution in different studies, but there does not seem to be a major gender predominance. An increased prevalence of CPPD deposition in certain diseases and familial groups has been reported.

PATHOGENESIS AND ETIOLOGY

The metabolic basis for CPPD formation and deposition is less well understood than that for urate crystals. CPPD crystal formation occurs almost exclusively in the articular and periarticular tissue, most often near the surface of chondrocytes.[64,67] Crystal formation is enhanced by elevated levels of either calcium or inorganic pyrophosphate (PP_i) within local tissues or local factors in the cartilage matrix that promote crystal formation. An abnormal substrate of matrix collagen and proteoglycan, as well as variations in mineral content, may promote crystal deposition. Local elevations of PP_i levels appear to be related to two factors: the overactivity of a cell surface enzyme (ectoenzyme) known as nucleoside triphosphate pyrophosphohydrolase (NTPPH), which catalyzes the extracellular hydrolysis of ATP, and the extracellular transport of PP_i by the transmembrane protein ANK.[68] In addition, some of the excess PP_i production may take place intracellularly through NTPPH or as a by-product of cellular proteoglycan and protein synthesis. Other factors that may contribute to excess PP_i and crystal formation include decreased activity of pyrophosphatase, degenerating cellular debris, abnormal matrix collagen, and even the local influence of growth factors (i.e., transforming growth factor and insulinlike growth factor). The mechanisms by which CPPD crystals induce inflammation are believed to be similar to those observed in gout.

CLINICAL VARIANTS

Most joints with radiographically observed chondrocalcinosis are asymptomatic, although subtle articular symptoms are more common in asymptomatic patients with chondrocalcinosis than in patients without these findings.[69] Clinically symptomatic CPPD deposition disease may take any of several forms that tend to present in acute or chronic fashion, mimicking other arthropathies.

Acute Pseudogout

Acute pseudogout is slightly more common in males than in females. Attacks of this form of CPPD deposition disease are usually acute, increase in intensity over 12 to 36 hours, and last for a few days to a few weeks. Most acute attacks of pseudogout are less intense than attacks of gout. The most commonly involved joint is the knee (seen in over half of patients), followed by the wrist and ankle. In rare cases, attacks in the first metatarsophalangeal joint may be seen.[64] Affected joints previously involved are more likely to be involved in subsequent attacks. At-

tacks may occur in clusters over short periods, and polyarticular attacks occur in a few patients. A moderate synovial fluid leukocytosis is common, and marked elevations in the white blood cell count, mimicking a septic joint, may be seen in some patients. Mild fever and leukocytosis have been described, but not as frequently as in gout.[70] Between attacks, the joint is usually asymptomatic unless there is coexistent osteoarthritis. As in gout, attacks of pseudogout seem to be precipitated in some patients by stressful events, such as surgery, trauma, and acute medical illness. The intra-articular injection of hyaluronate for the symptomatic treatment of osteoarthritis has also been reported to trigger attacks of acute pseudogout.[71]

Chronic Rheumatoid-like Arthritis

About 5% to 10% of patients with CPPD deposition disease experience a polyarticular process resembling rheumatoid arthritis. The disease is indolent, symmetrical in distribution, and characterized by inflammation. Chronic swelling, morning stiffness, and predominant wrist and knee involvement are seen in this group of patients. Because of the relatively high frequency of incidental chondrocalcinosis and positive rheumatoid factors in elderly persons, differentiating CPPD deposition from rheumatoid arthritis can be difficult. A history of acute exacerbations in these patients may help suggest CPPD deposition, whereas the presence of subcutaneous nodules and very high titers of rheumatoid factor favor a diagnosis of rheumatoid arthritis.

Osteoarthritis and CPPD Deposition

About half of patients with CPPD deposition have a chronic degenerative arthritis involving multiple joints, usually in a symmetrical pattern. Women predominate in this group of patients.[64] The knees are most commonly involved, followed by the wrist, metacarpophalangeal joints, hips, spine, and shoulders. CPPD-associated osteoarthritis may be differentiated from typical osteoarthritis by the presence of changes in atypical joints, such as the wrists, elbows, and shoulders. Some patients in this group may not have chondrocalcinosis, but CPPD crystals may be found in the synovial fluid of most of those patients without radiographic findings. In addition, radiographic features of predominantly patellofemoral involvement and femoral cortical erosions in the knee suggest CPPD deposition.[72]

Conditions Associated with CPPD Deposition Disease

Most cases of CPPD deposition disease are sporadic. However, a number of kindreds with familial forms of disease and asso-

Table 5 Conditions Associated with Calcium Pyrophosphate Dihydrate Deposition Disease*

Definite association	Possible or doubtful association
Hemochromatosis	Gout
Hyperparathyroidism	Familial hypocalciuric hypocalcemia
Hypophosphatasia	Acromegaly
Hypomagnesemia	X-linked hypophosphatemic rickets
Probable association	Neuropathic joints
Hypothyroidism	Amyloidosis
	Trauma

See reference 62.
*As pseudogout or radiographic chondrocalcinosis.

118 Crystal-Induced Joint Disease — 1379

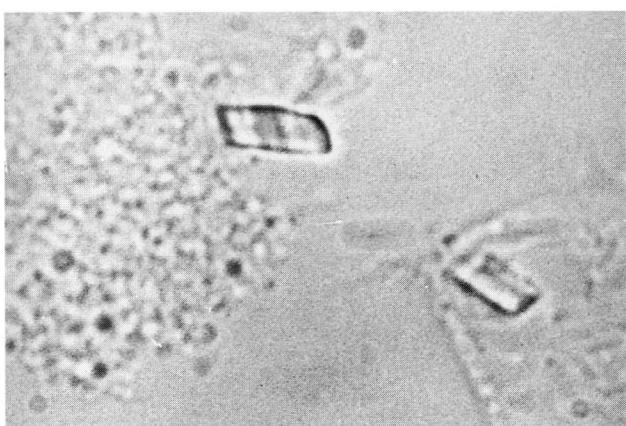

Figure 4   Calcium pyrophosphate dihydrate crystals typical of pseudogout are rhomboid and demonstrate a weakly positive birefringence under polarized light.

ciations with metabolic diseases have been reported. Most of the familial forms have shown an autosomal dominant transmission but have displayed a variety of clinical presentations, and most appear to involve single gene mutations.[73,74] Associations with several endocrine and metabolic conditions have been reported, many of which probably represent no more than a chance occurrence of common age-related conditions [see Table 5].

Definite associations exist between CPPD deposition disease and hemochromatosis, hyperparathyroidism, hypophosphatasia, and hypomagnesemia. A distinct form of arthritis associated with hemochromatosis was first reported in 1964.[75] This arthropathy is similar to osteoarthritis and rheumatoid arthritis and may be the initial presenting feature in some patients. The most frequently involved joints are the metacarpophalangeal joints (primarily the second and third), wrists, and hips; radiologic changes consisting of hooklike osteophytes at the metacarpal heads are a characteristic finding. CPPD deposition has been described in 20% to 30% of patients with primary hyperparathyroidism, more often in older patients.

Attacks of acute pseudogout after parathyroidectomy have been described and are often the first manifestation of CPPD deposition in these patients.[76] Reports have described pseudo-

gout in patients with hypomagnesemia after liver transplantation, possibly related to tacrolimus therapy.[77]

DIAGNOSIS

Synovial fluid aspiration and examination for crystals are essential to the diagnosis. The synovial fluid in pseudogout is usually inflammatory but may be hemorrhagic. A leukocyte count of about 10,000 to 20,000 cells/mm^3 is the rule, but in the small joints, such as the wrist, very high counts may be seen. Synovial fluid should be examined first under regular microscopy, because CPPD crystals are weakly birefringent under polarized microscopy. The crystals are rhomboid or rod-shaped and may be intracellular or extracellular [see Figure 4]. Because of their weak birefringence, CPPD crystals may be missed on initial examination, so it is essential that someone experienced in crystal identification examine the fluid.

Radiographic studies of affected joints often reveal chondrocalcinosis of the articular cartilage. The fibrocartilage of the menisci in the knees [see Figure 5a] or of the triangular ligament at the radioulnar joint at the wrist [see Figure 5b] may have punctate or linear calcifications; similar changes may be seen in the symphysis pubis, shoulder, hip, and intervertebral disks. Linear calcification of the hyaline cartilage in these joints may be seen as well. Other features may include narrowing and sclerosis of the radiocarpal and patellofemoral joints, femoral cortical erosions above the knee, and extra-articular calcifications involving tendons or ligaments.

TREATMENT

Management of the patient with pseudogout is similar to management of the patient with acute gout, with the main goal of therapy being control of the acute inflammatory reaction.[49] Rest of the inflamed joint (or joints) and administration of NSAIDs or intra-articular corticosteroid preparations are the mainstay of therapy. Aspiration of the joint is sufficient to significantly relieve pain and discomfort in some patients. Colchicine is effective in patients with acute pseudogout but should be used cautiously in older patients. At lower doses of 0.6 mg one or two times a day, colchicine can be helpful in preventing further attacks.[78] In some patients, intramuscular or subcutaneous ACTH (40 units) or intramuscular triamcinolone (60 mg) can control the acute inflammatory reaction.[79] For those with chronic pain and inflammation,

a

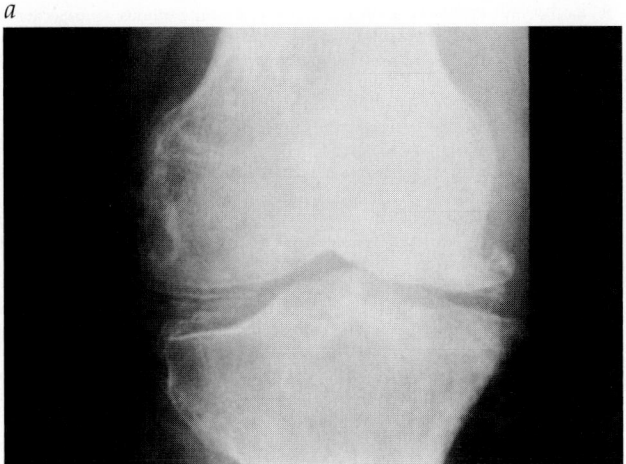

b

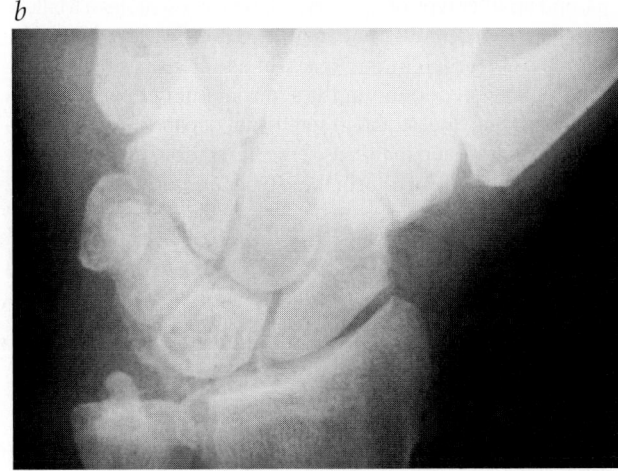

Figure 5   Typical radiographs of chondrocalcinosis seen in CPPD deposition disease, with evidence of intra-articular calcification in the meniscus and hyaline cartilage of the knee (*a*) and the triangular cartilage of the wrist (*b*).

alternatives for management are physiotherapy, analgesics, and NSAIDs. An evaluation of the patient for underlying metabolic abnormalities, particularly hemochromatosis and hyperparathyroidism, should be considered. However, successful treatment of these associated conditions has not been shown to alter the radiographic or clinical course of CPPD deposition disease.

Other Forms of Crystal-Associated Arthritis

BASIC CALCIUM PHOSPHATE DEPOSITION

A group of apatitelike (basic calcium phosphate) crystals has been identified in pathologic synovial fluids and articular and periarticular tissues in a variety of musculoskeletal disorders. These crystals may be found in 30% to 60% of synovial fluids from patients with osteoarthritis and may contribute to the low-grade inflammatory process and cartilage destruction seen in typical osteoarthritis.[80,81] A severe destructive arthropathy of the shoulder and knee, known as the Milwaukee shoulder-knee syndrome, predominantly affects older women.[82] This process is associated with rotator cuff degeneration and rupture, joint instability, and periarticular calcification. The synovial fluid may be serosanguineous and contains few cells; hydroxyapatite crystals may appear as clumps or may look like intracellular shiny coins, but they are not birefringent under polarized-light microscopy. The treatment of this condition is difficult, but joint aspiration and intra-articular corticosteroid injections have been helpful in some patients.

Basic calcium phosphate crystals are also associated with acute calcific periarthritis that may affect the shoulder or other joint areas in periarticular structures. In patients with this condition, periarticular calcific deposits may be found in the shoulder; near the lateral trochanter of the hip; around the wrists, fingers, or knees; or in the ankle and foot. These deposits may be well defined radiographically at the beginning of attacks but often disappear over several weeks. NSAIDs and local corticosteroid injections are usually useful in the treatment of this condition.

OTHER CRYSTALS FOUND IN SYNOVIAL FLUID

A variety of other crystals in synovial fluid have been described. Cholesterol crystals may be seen in some chronic effusions and are most often associated with chronic rheumatoid bursal effusions.[83] Other lipid crystals have been seen after joint trauma, and another type of lipid crystal, which resembles a Maltese cross, has been described and may be responsible for an acute inflammatory reaction in rare cases. In addition, calcium oxalate crystals have been found in the synovial fluid of patients with end-stage renal disease and in soft tissues of patients with primary hyperoxaluria and may cause articular symptoms.[84] The pathogenetic significance of each of these types of crystals is uncertain; they most probably represent incidental secondary phenomena.

The author has received grants for clinical research from Amgen Inc., Abbott Laboratories Inc., Isis Pharmaceuticals, Inc., and Bristol-Myers Squibb Company and has served as a consultant for TAP Pharmaceutical Products Inc.

References

1. McCarty DJ, Hollander JL: Identification of urate crystals in gouty synovial fluids. Ann Intern Med 54:452, 1961

2. McCarty DJ, Kohn NN, Faires JS: The significance of calcium phosphate crystals in the synovial fluid of arthritis patients: the "pseudogout syndrome": I. Clinical aspects. Ann Intern Med 56:711, 1962

3. Abbott RD, Brand FN, Kannel WB, et al: Gout and coronary artery disease: the Framingham Study. J Clin Epidemiol 41:237, 1988

4. Arromdee E, Michet CJ, Crowson CS: Epidemiology of gout: is the incidence rising? J Rheumatol 29:2403, 2002

5. Lawrence RC, Helmick CG, Arnett FC, et al: Estimates of the prevalence of arthritis and selected musculoskeletal diseases in the United States. Arthritis Rheum 41:778, 1998

6. Hochberg MC, Thomas J, Thomas DJ, et al: Racial differences in the incidence of gout. Arthritis Rheum 38:628, 1995

7. Ter Borg EJ, Rasker JJ: Gout in the elderly: a separate entity? Ann Rheum Dis 46:72, 1987

8. Wortmann RL, Kelley WN: Gout and hyperuricemia. Textbook of Rheumatology, 6th ed. Ruddy S, Harris ED, Sledge CB, Eds. WB Saunders Co, Philadelphia, 2001, p 1339

9. Campion EW, Glynn RJ, DeLabry LO: Asymptomatic hyperuricemia: risks and consequences in the Normative Aging Study. Am J Med 82:421, 1987

10. Agudelo CA, Wise CM: Gout: diagnosis, pathogenesis, and clinical manifestations. Curr Opin Rheumatol 13:234, 2001

11. Wortmann RL: Gout and hyperuricemia. Curr Opin Rheumatol 14:281, 2002

12. Wilk JB, Djousse L, Borecki I, et al: Segregation analysis of serum uric acid in the NHLBI Family Heart Study. Hum Genet 106:355, 2000

13. Perez-Ruiz F, Calabozo M, Erauskin GG, et al: Renal underexcretion of uric acid is present in patients with apparent high urinary uric acid output. Arthritis Rheum 47:610, 2002

14. Shadick NA, Kim R, Weiss S, et al: Effect of low level lead exposure on hyperuricemia and gout among middle aged and elderly men: the normative aging study. J Rheumatol 27:1708, 2000

15. Lin JL, Tan DT, Ho HH, et al: Environmental lead exposure and urate excretion in the general population. Am J Med 113:563, 2002

16. Scott JT, Higgens CS: Diuretic induced gout: a multifactorial condition. Ann Rheum Dis 51:259, 1992

17. Caspi D, Lubart E, Graff E, et al: The effect of mini-dose aspirin on renal function and uric acid handling in elderly patients. Arthritis Rheum 43:103, 2000

18. Lin HY, Rocher LL, McQuillan MA, et al: Cyclosporine-induced hyperuricemia and gout. N Engl J Med 321:287, 1989

19. Burack DA, Griffith BP, Thompson ME, et al: Hyperuricemia and gout among heart transplant recipients receiving cyclosporine. Am J Med 92:141, 1992

20. Clive DM: Renal transplant-associated hyperuricemia and gout. J Am Soc Nephrol 11:974, 2000

21. Schiltz C, Liote F, Prudhommeaux F, et al: Monosodium urate monohydrate crystal-induced inflammation in vivo: quantitative histomorphometric analysis of cellular events. Arthritis Rheum 46:1643, 2002

22. Yagnik DR, Hillyer P, Marshall D, et al: Noninflammatory phagocytosis of monosodium urate monohydrate crystals by mouse macrophages: implications for the control of joint inflammation in gout. Arthritis Rheum 43:1779, 2000

23. Landis RC, Yagnik DR, Florey O, et al: Safe disposal of inflammatory monosodium urate monohydrate crystals by differentiated macrophages. Arthritis Rheum 46:3026, 2002

24. Fam AG, Stein J, Rubenstein J: Gouty arthritis in nodal osteoarthritis. J Rheumatol 23:684, 1996

25. Agudelo CA, Wise CM: Crystal-associated arthritis. Clin Geriatr Med 14:495, 1998

26. Hadler NM, Franck WA, Bress NM, et al: Acute polyarticular gout. Am J Med 56:715, 1974

27. Gutman AB: Gout. Textbook of Medicine. Beeson PB, McDermott W, Eds. WB Saunders Co, Philadelphia, 1963, p 1255

28. Gutman AB: The past four decades of progress in the knowledge of gout with an assessment of the present status. Arthritis Rheum 16:431, 1973

29. Barthelemy CR, Nakayama DA, Carrera GF, et al: Gouty arthritis: a prospective radiographic evaluation of sixty patients. Skeletal Radiol 11:1, 1984

30. Yü T-F, Berger L: Renal disease in primary gout: a study of 253 gout patients with proteinuria. Semin Arthritis Rheum 4:293, 1975

31. Yü T-F, Berger L: Impaired renal function in gout: its association with hypertensive vascular disease and intrinsic renal disease. Am J Med 72:95, 1982

32. Johnson RJ, Kang DH, Feig D, et al: Is there a pathogenetic role for uric acid in hypertension and cardiovascular disease and renal disease? Hypertension 41:1183, 2003

33. Tarng D-C, Lin H-Y, Shyong M-L, et al: Renal function in gout patients. Am J Nephrol 15:31, 1995

34. Perez-Ruiz F, Calabozo M, Herrero-Beites AM, et al: Improvement of renal function in patients with chronic gout after proper control of hyperuricemia and gouty bouts. Nephron 86:287, 2000

35. Kramer HM, Curhan G: The association between gout and nephrolithiasis: the National Health and Nutrition Examination Survery III, 1988–1994. Am J Kidney Dis 40:37, 2002

36. Pak CYC, Barilla DE, Holt K, et al: Effect of oral purine load and allopurinol on the crystallization of calcium salts in urine of patients with hyperuricosuric calcium urolithiasis. Am J Med 65:593, 1978

37. Cohen LF, Balow JE, Magrath IT, et al: Acute tumor lysis syndrome: a review of 37 patients with Burkitt's lymphoma. Am J Med 68:486, 1980

38. Reynolds PP, Knapp MJ, Baraf HSB, et al: Moonshine and lead: relationship to the pathogenesis of hyperuricemia in gout. Arthritis Rheum 26:1057, 1983

39. Takahashi S, Yamamoto T, Moriwaki Y, et al: Impaired lipoprotein metabolism in

patients with primary gout: influence of alcohol intake and body weight. Br J Rheumatol 33:731, 1994

40. Bo S, Cavallo-Perin P, Gentile L, et al: Hypouricemia and hyperuricemia in type 2 diabetes: two different phenotypes. Eur J Clin Invest 31:318, 2001

41. Kahn HS, Valdez R: Metabolic risks identified by the combination of enlarged waist and elevated triacylglycerol concentration. Am J Clin Nutr 78:928, 2003

42. Culleton BF, Larson MG, Kannel WB, et al: Serum uric acid and risk for cardiovascular disease and death: the Framingham Heart Study. Ann Intern Med 131:7, 1999

43. Erickson AR, Enzenauer RJ, Nordstrom DM, et al: The prevalence of hypothyroidism in gout. Am J Med 97:231, 1994

44. Wallace SL, Robinson H, Masi AT, et al: Preliminary criteria for the classification of acute arthritis of primary gout. Arthritis Rheum 20:895, 1977

45. Agudelo CA, Weinberger A, Schumacher HR, et al: Definitive diagnosis of gout by identification of urate crystals in asymptomatic metatarsophalangeal joints. Arthritis Rheum 22:559, 1979

46. Pascual E, Batlle E, Martinez A, et al: Synovial fluid analysis for diagnosis of intercritical gout. Ann Intern Med 131:756, 1999

47. Pascual E: Gout update: from lab to the clinic and back. Curr Opin Rheumatol 12:213, 2000

48. Terkeltaub RA: Clinical practice: gout. N Engl J Med 349:1647, 2003

49. Agudelo CA, Wise CM: Crystal deposition diseases. Treatment of the Rheumatic Diseases, 2nd ed. Weisman MH, Weinblatt ME, Louie J, Eds. WB Saunders Co, Philadelphia, 2001, 447

50. Roberts WN, Liang MH, Stern SH: Colchicine in acute gout: reassessment of risks and benefits. JAMA 257:1920, 1987

51. Wallace SL, Singer JZ: Systemic toxicity associated with the intravenous administration of colchicine: guidelines for use (review). J Rheumatol 15:495, 1988

52. Bonnel RA, Villalba ML, Karwoski CB, et al: Deaths associated with inappropriate intravenous colchicine administration. J Emerg Med 22:385, 2002

53. Fam AG: Treating acute gouty arthritis with selective COX 2 inhibitors. BMJ 325:980, 2002

54. Fam AG: Current therapy of acute microcrystalline arthritis and the role of corticosteroids. J Clin Rheumatol 3:35, 1997

55. Yü TF: The efficacy of colchicine prophylaxis in articular gout: a reappraisal after 20 years. Semin Arthritis Rheum 12:256, 1982

56. Wallace SL, Singer JZ, Duncan GJ, et al: Renal function predicts colchicine toxicity: guidelines for the prophylactic use of colchicine in gout. J Rheumatol 18:264, 1991

57. Simkin PA: When, why, and how should we quantify the excretion rate of urinary uric acid? J Rheumatol 28:1207, 2001

58. Dessein PH, Shipton EA, Stanwix AE, et al: Beneficial effects of weight loss associated with moderate calorie/carbohydrate restriction, and increased proportional intake of protein and unsaturated fat on serum urate and lipoprotein levels in gout: a pilot study. Ann Rheum Dis 59:539, 2000

59. Snaith ML: Gout: diet and uric acid revisited. Lancet 358:525, 2001

60. Bull PW, Scott JT: Intermittent control of hyperuricemia in the treatment of gout. J Rheumatol 16:1246, 1989

61. Perez-Ruiz F, Calabozo M, Fernandez-Lopez MJ, et al: Treatment of chronic gout in patients with renal function impairment: an open, randomized, actively controlled study. J Clin Rheumatol 5:49, 1999

62. Rosenthal AK, Ryan LM: Calcium pyrophosphate crystal deposition disease, pseudogout, and articular chondrocalcinosis. Arthritis and Allied Conditions, 14th ed. Koopman WJ, Ed. Williams & Wilkins, Baltimore, 2001, p 2348

63. Fam AG, Dunne SM, Iazzetta J, et al: Efficacy and safety of desensitization to allopurinol following cutaneous reactions. Arthritis Rheum 44:231, 2001

64. Hande KR, Noone RM, Stone WJ: Severe allopurinol toxicity: description and guidelines for prevention in patients with renal insufficiency. Am J Med 76:47, 1984

65. Wilkins E, Dieppe P, Maddison P, et al: Osteoarthritis and articular chondrocalcinosis in the elderly. Ann Rheum Dis 42:280, 1983

66. Doherty M, Dieppe P: Crystal deposition disease in the elderly. Clin Rheum Dis 12:97, 1986

67. Reginato AJ, Reginato AM: Diseases associated with deposition of calcium pyrophosphate or hydroxyapatite. Textbook of Rheumatology, 6th ed. Ruddy S, Harris ED, Sledge CB, Eds. WB Saunders Co, Philadelphia, 2001, p 1377

68. Hirose J, Ryan LM, Masuda I: Up-regulated expression of cartilage intermediate-layer protein and ANK in articular hyaline cartilage from patients with calcium pyrophosphate dihydrate crystal deposition disease. Arthritis Rheum 46:3218, 2002

69. Ellman MH, Levin B: Chondrocalcinosis in elderly persons. Arthritis Rheum 18:43, 1975

70. Bong D, Bennett R: Pseudogout mimicking systemic disease. JAMA 246:1438, 1981

71. Fam AG: What is new about crystals other than monosodium urate? Curr Opin Rheumatol 12:228, 2000

72. Resnick D, Williams G, Weisman MH, et al: Rheumatoid arthritis and pseudorheumatoid arthritis in calcium pyrophosphate dihydrate crystal deposition disease. Radiology 140:615, 1981

73. Jones AC, Chuck AJ, Arie EA, et al: Diseases associated with calcium pyrophosphate deposition disease. Semin Arthritis Rheum 22:188, 1992

74. Timms AE, Zhang Y, Russell RG, et al: Genetic studies of disorders of calcium crystal deposition. Rheumatology (Oxford) 41:725, 2002

75. Schumacher HR Jr: Hemochromatosis and arthritis. Arthritis Rheum 7:41, 1964

76. Rynes RI, Merzig EG: Calcium pyrophosphate crystal deposition disease and hyperparathyroidism: a controlled, prospective study. J Rheumatol 5:460, 1978

77. Perez-Ruiz F, Testillano M, Gastaca MA, et al: "Pseudoseptic" pseudogout associated with hypomagnesemia in liver transplant patients. Transplantation 71:696, 2001

78. Alvarellos A, Spilberg I: Colchicine prophylaxis in pseudogout. J Rheumatol 13:804, 1986

79. Roane DW, Harris MD, Carpenter MT, et al: Prospective use of intramuscular triamcinolone acetonide in pseudogout. J Rheumatol 24:1168, 1997

80. Jaovisidha K, Rosenthal AK: Calcium crystals in osteoarthritis. Curr Opin Rheumatol 14:298, 2002

81. Morgan MP, McCarthy GM: Signaling mechanisms involved in crystal-induced tissue damage. Curr Opin Rheumatol 14:292, 2002

82. Halverson PB, Carrera GF, McCarty DJ: Milwaukee shoulder syndrome: fifteen additional cases and a description of contributing factors. Arch Intern Med 150:677, 1990

83. Wise CM, White RE, Agudelo CA: Synovial fluid lipid abnormalities in various disease states: review and classification. Semin Arthritis Rheum 16:222, 1987

84. Reginato AJ: Calcium oxalate and other crystals of particles associated with arthritis. Arthritis and Allied Conditions. Koopman WJ, Ed. Williams and Wilkins, Baltimore, 2000, p 2393

119 Osteoarthritis

Christopher Wise, M.D., F.A.C.P.

Definition

Osteoarthritis is a common form of arthritis characterized by degeneration of articular cartilage and reactive changes in surrounding bone and periarticular tissue. The disease process results in pain and dysfunction of affected joints and is a major cause of disability in the general population. Osteoarthritis is also frequently referred to as degenerative joint disease; other terms that have been used include osteoarthrosis, hypertrophic arthritis, and atrophic arthritis.

Classification

PRIMARY OSTEOARTHRITIS

Patients without a specific inflammatory or metabolic condition known to be associated with arthritis and without a history of specific injury or trauma are considered to have primary osteoarthritis. However, a number of underlying processes are considered to be important in patients with primary osteoarthritis [*see* Etiologic Factors, Risk Factors, *below*]. In most patients, involvement is limited to one or a small number of joints or joint areas. In some patients, however, multiple joint areas are involved, and these patients are considered to have a separate variant called primary generalized osteoarthritis. Another variant, termed erosive osteoarthritis, is characterized by polyarticular involvement of the small joints of the hand and tends to occur more often in middle-aged and elderly women.

SECONDARY OSTEOARTHRITIS

Secondary osteoarthritis has been associated with several conditions that cause damage to articular cartilage through a variety of mechanisms, including mechanical, inflammatory, and metabolic processes [*see* Table 1]. Acute trauma, particularly intra-articular fractures and meniscal tears, can result in articular instability or incongruity and can lead to osteoarthritis years after an injury.

The role of chronic trauma from certain occupational or avocational activities is not as well established as the role of acute trauma in the development of secondary osteoarthritis. Neurologic disorders that result in the loss of sensory nerve function may be associated with a particularly destructive type of degenerative arthritis (i.e., neuropathic arthritis and Charcot joint) in which cartilage and bone fragmentation are seen with relatively little pain.

Many types of inflammatory arthritis can cause destruction of articular cartilage. The best example of cartilage damage is seen in chronic rheumatoid arthritis, but similar cartilage damage can be seen in postinfectious arthritis, psoriatic arthritis, reactive arthritis, and ankylosing spondylitis.

Congenital and developmental diseases that cause joint incongruity may result in osteoarthritis. This condition is best recognized in epiphyseal dysplasia, Perthes disease, and other processes affecting the femoral head and hip and has also been associated with generalized joint hypermobility, as seen in Ehlers-Danlos syndrome.

Primary bone disorders that affect the mechanics and articular surfaces of nearby joints may also lead to degenerative cartilage changes, particularly around major joints such as the shoulder, hip, and knee. Several metabolic and endocrine disorders have been associated directly or indirectly with the development of osteoarthritis, often with atypical patterns or in unusual locations. In most of these conditions, cartilage damage is associated with the accumulation, in articular cartilage, of a particular substance associated with the metabolic condition (e.g., uric acid or iron). In hemochromatosis, the mechanism of joint damage may also be related to an association with calcium pyrophosphate crystal deposition. In acromegaly, overgrowth of articular cartilage and subsequent mechanical problems appear to be important in the pathogenesis of the disease.

Epidemiology

Osteoarthritis is the most common type of arthritis, and it is one of the most common causes of disability and dependence in the United States.[1,2] Estimating the prevalence of osteoarthritis in the general population is difficult because of the high prevalence of asymptomatic radiographic changes of osteoarthritis and differences in case definition. The prevalence of radiographic changes of osteoarthritis in the population in general, regardless of symptoms, is roughly 30% for the hands, 21% for the feet, and

---

Table 1   Causes of Secondary Osteoarthritis

Trauma
    Acute injury
    Chronic occupational overuse
    Sports overuse
    Neuropathic arthropathy (Charcot joint)

Inflammatory arthritis
    Rheumatoid arthritis
    Infectious arthritis
    Psoriatic arthritis
    Reactive arthritis
    Ankylosing spondylitis

Dysplastic and hereditary conditions
    Congenital hip dysplasia
    Epiphyseal dysplasia
    Chondrodysplasias
    Perthes disease
    Kashin-Bek disease
    Joint hypermobility

Bone disorders
    Osteonecrosis (avascular necrosis)
    Osteochondritis
    Paget disease of bone

Metabolic and endocrine disorders
    Crystal deposition disease (gout, calcium pyrophosphate deposition, basic calcium phosphate)
    Hemochromatosis
    Ochronosis
    Wilson disease
    Bleeding disorders
    Acromegaly

3% for the knees and hips. In persons older than 65 years, changes are seen in the knee in 33% and in the hands in almost 100%. Fortunately, most patients with radiographic changes found in population-based surveys have few symptoms or functional limitations. Men and women 30 to 60 years of age have equal overall prevalence of symptomatic osteoarthritis (approximately 6% have affected knees and 4% have affected hips). For adults older than 60 years, however, the prevalence of symptomatic osteoarthritis (all joints) increases to 17% in men and 30% in women.[1,2]

Men and women tend be affected equally by osteoarthritis in middle age, but after 50 years of age, women are affected more often, particularly in the interphalangeal joints of the fingers.[3] Osteoarthritis is seen in all population groups, although prevalence can vary with certain geographic areas and ethnic groups. For example, osteoarthritis of the hip is least common in Japanese, Saudi Arabian, Chinese, and African populations; and knee involvement is most common in African-American women. Comparisons of osteoarthritis prevalence have shown that hip involvement is less common, but knee involvement is more common, in Chinese men and women than in white men and women in the United States.[4-6]

Etiologic Factors

RISK FACTORS

A number of risk factors are believed to contribute to the development of primary osteoarthritis, including age, obesity, joint malalignment, bone density, hormonal status, nutritional factors, joint dysplasia, trauma, occupational factors, and hereditary factors.[2,7]

Age is the factor most strongly associated with radiographic and clinically significant osteoarthritis, with an exponential increase seen in more severely involved joints. The cellular or biomechanical changes in articular cartilage that occur with aging are not necessarily those seen in osteoarthritis. However, it has been speculated that these changes may facilitate the development of disease.

Obesity is clearly associated with osteoarthritis of the knee. The increased load carried by obese persons and the alterations in gait and posture that redistribute the load contribute to cartilage damage. A study in young men suggested that each increase in weight of 8 kg results in a 70% increase in the risk of symptomatic arthritis of the knee in later years.[8] This association is particularly high in patients with varus malalignment of the knee, and obese patients with malalignment are at risk for more rapid progression of established osteoarthritis in the knee.[9,10] Most of the association of obesity with osteoarthritis of the knee appears to be related to environmental, rather than genetic, factors.[11] The relation of obesity to osteoarthritis in other weight-bearing joints is not as clear-cut and may not be much of a factor at all for hip involvement.

An association between increased bone density and osteoarthritis has been noted in several studies.[12,13] Women with osteoporosis and hip fractures have a decreased risk of osteoarthritis, and those affected by osteoarthritis have significantly increased bone density. This negative association suggests that soft subchondral bone absorbs impact and protects articular cartilage better than dense bone. Paradoxically, however, estrogen deficiency may contribute to the increased prevalence of osteoarthritis in women who have recently entered menopause.[2]

In addition, a study showing that patients with low dietary vitamin D intake have more rapid progression of disease suggests that strong subchondral bone may be particularly important in preventing progression of osteoarthritis once it is established.[14]

Chronic repetitive impact loading is known to cause rapid degenerative changes in articular cartilage in laboratory animals. This mechanism probably accounts for the high frequency of osteoarthritis in certain occupational and athletic settings. In particular, occupational activities that require frequent knee bending increase the risk of knee involvement, and frequent lifting appears to be a risk factor for hip involvement.[15,16] Long-term weight-bearing sports activity is associated with an increased risk of developing radiographic evidence of osteoarthritis. In patients without a history of injury, clinical symptoms do not always correlate well with radiographic changes, and radiographic changes do not often progress significantly, even in older long-distance runners.[17,18] However, a history of specific joint injury, usually related to sports and recreational activities, is an important risk factor for knee and hip disease.[19-21]

Decreased strength and proprioception have been demonstrated in patients with osteoarthritis and likely play a role in pathogenesis of the disease. Patients with radiographic changes of osteoarthritis and no pain have decreased muscle strength in the affected leg, and decreased proprioception has been demonstrated in unaffected knees of patients with unilateral disease.[22,23] In addition, local injection to relieve pain will only partially improve muscle activity and proprioceptive and gait defects.[24] The importance of muscle strength and proprioception to the health of normal cartilage has been further suggested in studies demonstrating cartilage thinning after spinal cord injury.[25,26]

Many patients with osteoarthritis have a family history of the disorder, and multiple genetic factors may be responsible in various forms of osteoarthritis.[27] Osteoarthritis with finger joint involvement in women is probably the best recognized form of arthritis with familial associations,[28] but hereditary factors are also important in osteoarthritis of the hip.[29,30] Metabolic abnormalities related to the hereditary component of osteoarthritis have been found in a number of studies. These abnormalities include associations between variations of collagen genes in familial osteoarthritis and lumbar disk disease; between estrogen and vitamin D receptor genes and osteoarthritis of the knee; and between a gene linked with hemochromatosis in older patients and hand involvement.[31-35] The significance of these findings in relation to osteoarthritis in the general population are uncertain.[36] In addition to the known heritable and acquired joint dysplasias that cause secondary osteoarthritis, subclinical degrees of dysplasia may be a factor in patients with primary osteoarthritis, particularly of the hip.[37] Many different chromosomal markers have been associated with various patterns of osteoarthritis, suggesting that the genetic component in osteoarthritis most likely involves multiple genes.[38-40]

NORMAL ARTICULAR CARTILAGE

Articular cartilage is specialized connective tissue that covers the weight-bearing surfaces of diarthrodial joints. It is composed of sparsely scattered cells (chondrocytes) within an extracellular matrix composed of collagen, proteoglycans, and water, with a very small component of calcium salt.[41]

Most of the collagen in cartilage is type II collagen, which is arranged in thick bundles and is parallel to the surface of the cartilage in outer portions and more perpendicular to the surface in deeper layers. This arrangement of collagen serves as a

a

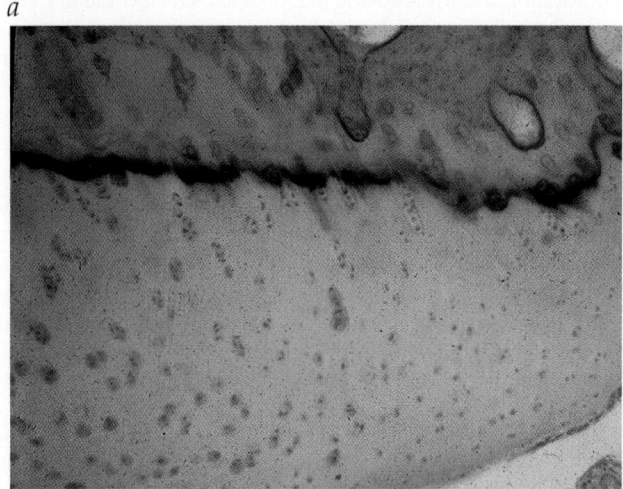

b

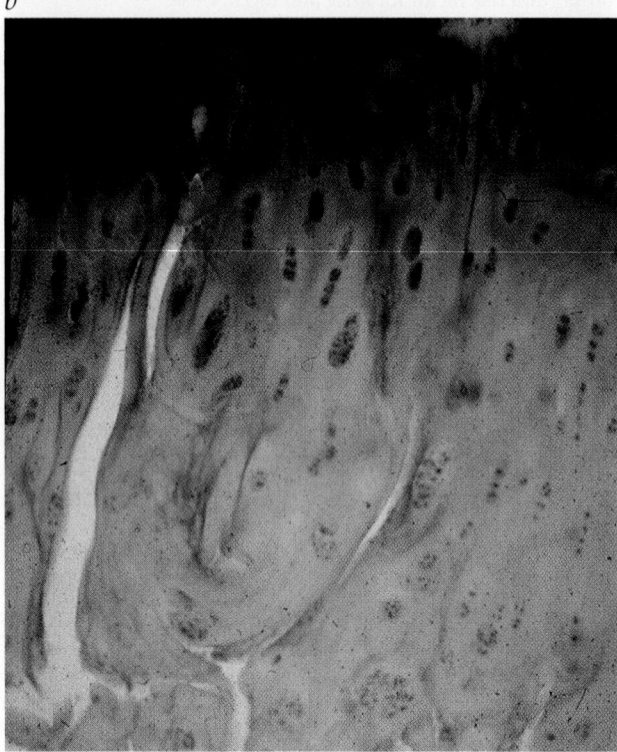

Figure 1 Microscopic appearance of normal articular cartilage (*a*) and osteoarthritic (*b*) articular cartilage. In normal cartilage, the cartilage surface is smooth and chondrocytes are regularly arranged, mostly as single cells; the background proteoglycan staining is homogeneous; and the subchondral bony plate is intact. In osteoarthritis, there is splitting fissuring of the surface, proliferation and clustering of the chondrocytes, and decreased and irregular staining of the background proteoglycan.

limiting membrane, distributes compressive forces, and tethers the uncalcified cartilage to the more basilar calcified cartilage and subchondral bone.

The proteoglycan component of the matrix of articular cartilage is composed predominantly of a large molecule called aggrecan, which consists of a large core protein with covalently attached side chains of glycosaminoglycans, most of which are chondroitin sulfate and keratan sulfate. A link protein connects aggrecan to hyaluronic acid, a long, unbranched polysaccharide molecule that can bind several hundred aggrecan molecules. This aggregate of aggrecan molecules forms a very large molecule with a molecular weight of 100 million daltons or more. The molecule has a high fixed negative charge, which allows the retention of large amounts of water.

The collagen matrix and hydrophilic proteoglycan component form a resilient tissue that holds water under pressure and is capable of dissipating much of the force of weight bearing, protecting soft tissues and subchondral bone.

In normal cartilage, the turnover rate of collagen is relatively slow, whereas proteoglycan turnover is rapid. The normal turnover of these matrix components is mediated by the chondrocytes, which synthesize the components and the proteolytic enzymes responsible for their breakdown. Chondrocytes are, in turn, influenced by a number of factors, including polypeptide growth factors and cytokines, structural and physical stimuli, and even the components of the matrix itself.

CHANGES IN OSTEOARTHRITIC CARTILAGE

Pathologic findings suggest that articular cartilage is the site of the primary abnormality in osteoarthritis. There is a loss of homogeneity, and disruption and fragmentation of the surface occur. Uneven staining for proteoglycans is seen in the matrix, and the deeper layers of cartilage are invaded by capillaries from the calcified cartilage. Chondrocytes, which exist as isolated cells in normal cartilage, begin to proliferate and are found in large clusters and clones, and osteophytes are formed, which are covered by irregular hyaline and fibrocartilage [*see Figure 1*].

In early osteoarthritis, the water content of diseased cartilage increases and the cartilage swells, and the collagen fibers are usually smaller and not as tightly organized. The proteoglycan content of cartilage decreases markedly as disease progresses, with shortening of the glycosaminoglycan chains and impaired molecular aggregation.

Osteoarthritic cartilage is characterized by an increase in anabolic and catabolic activity. In the early stages, the synthesis of collagen, proteoglycans, and hyaluronate is increased and chondrocytes tend to replicate. At the same time, synthesis of degradative enzymes such as collagenase, stromelysin, gelatinase, and hyaluronidase is increased, whereas some of the substances that inhibit cartilage destruction are themselves destroyed or inhibited. In the later stages, the anabolic activities of the chondrocytes become insufficient to keep up with the degradative process. The final result is a matrix that is less structurally sound and less well organized on a macromolecular basis, decreasing its ability to withstand the forces required of articular cartilage.

The biochemical and metabolic changes in cartilage that are considered to be potential etiologic factors in osteoarthritis include abnormalities in collagen structure, crystal deposition, inflammatory mediators, and chondrocyte metabolism. The discovery of a familial form of osteoarthritis associated with a specific genetic defect in collagen has led to speculation that similar abnormalities in collagen or other structural components of cartilage may have etiologic importance. In addition, the association of deposition of hemosiderin, copper, or various crystals with secondary forms of osteoarthritis suggests that substances that alter matrix composition can be responsible for degenerative changes.

The relation of calcium-containing crystals to osteoarthritis is complex.[42] Both calcium pyrophosphate dihydrate and basic calcium phosphate crystals have been associated with osteoarthritic cartilage. In vitro measurement of the by-products of cartilage breakdown suggests that these crystals magnify the degenerative process by stimulation of mitogenesis in fibroblasts and secretion of proteases by cells that ingest the calcium-containing crystals.

The reasons for the increased anabolic and catabolic activities of chondrocytes in osteoarthritis are not well understood.[41] Chondrocytes are influenced by a number of humoral, mechanical, synovial, and cartilage matrix mediators. In particular, prostaglandins, nitric oxide, interleukin-1 (IL-1), transforming growth factor–β, estrogen, and insulinlike growth factor–1 have a variety of stimulatory and inhibitory effects that may be pathogenetically important. In addition, the finding of increased leptin levels in cartilage and synovial fluid of osteoarthritic joints has suggested a role for this substance in the development of osteoarthritis and a role in the relationship between obesity and osteoarthritis.[43,44] Whether the observed abnormalities in these factors are etiologic or merely represent the response of the chondrocyte to other injury is not yet known.[45] The role of inflammation and the potential for damaged cartilage to invoke a more intense inflammatory response than normal cartilage are also areas of ongoing research.[46,47]

The pain of osteoarthritis appears to be derived from inflammation of soft tissue structures surrounding bone, as well as from edema of subchondral bone.[48,49] In addition, edema in subchondral bone is associated with further progression of cartilage damage over time.[50]

Diagnosis

Characteristic radiographic features are usually considered essential for diagnosis but should be corroborated by the presence of compatible symptoms [see Figure 2]. Laboratory studies are useful in the evaluation of patients with osteoarthritis only in that they help to exclude other diagnoses. Thus, the erythrocyte sedimentation rate (ESR), rheumatoid factor, and routine hematologic and biochemical parameters should be normal in patients with osteoarthritis unless the osteoarthritis is attributable to comorbid conditions. Synovial fluid from involved joints is noninflammatory, with leukocyte counts of less than 2,000 cells/mm³ in most patients. The presence of birefringent calcium pyrophosphate dihydrate crystals is diagnostic of a separate process that frequently is concurrent with typical osteoarthritis. Basic calcium phosphate crystals, which are not birefringent, may be seen frequently in typical osteoarthritis if special stains are used.

Even though some patients have multiple joint involvement, specific joints should be considered individually so that no important problem-causing nonarticular or superimposed process is overlooked.

CLINICAL MANIFESTATIONS

General

Typical symptoms of osteoarthritis include pain, stiffness, swelling, deformity, and loss of function. Pain is usually chronic and localized to the involved joint or joints or referred to nearby areas. Pain may be mild or moderate early in the disease but tends to worsen gradually over many years. Most of the pain is made worse with activity and improves with rest. Morning stiffness is not as prolonged as in patients with inflammatory diseases; morning stiffness in patients with osteoarthritis usually

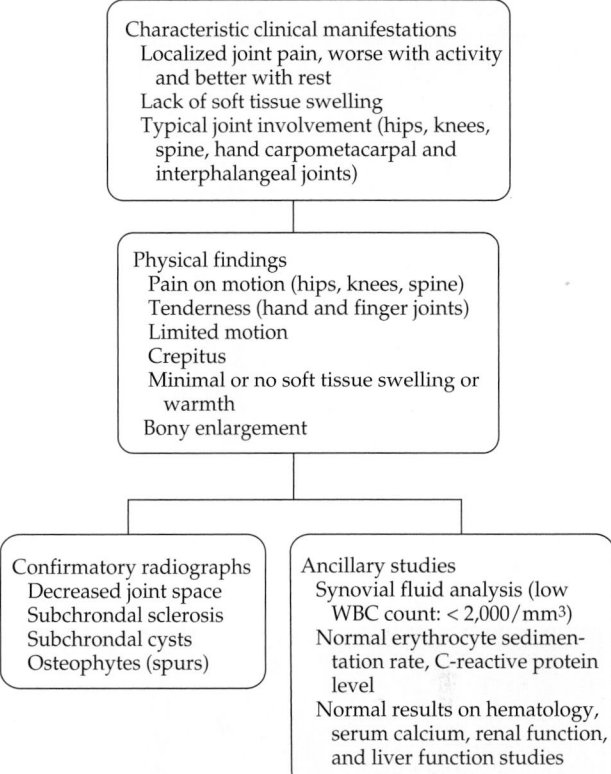

Figure 2 Diagnosis of osteoarthritis.

lasts less than an hour. Many patients complain of stiffening, or so-called gelling, during the day, particularly after sitting for extended periods of time. Swelling tends to be mild or moderate and is often related to bony enlargement rather than soft tissue edema. Deformity and loss of function are later manifestations, occurring after many years of disease.

Physical findings in osteoarthritis include crepitus, pain on motion, bony enlargement, and periarticular tenderness. Synovial effusions may be present, particularly in the knee. Erythema and warmth are unusual and should suggest the presence of coexistent crystal-induced inflammation or other conditions. In more advanced disease, limited range of motion, deformity, and instability may become more prominent findings.

Specific Joint Involvement and Complications

Osteoarthritis has a characteristic pattern of involvement in most patients. Joints frequently involved include the distal and proximal interphalangeal joints, as well as the first carpometacarpal joints in the hands, the cervical and lumbar spines, the hips, the knees, and, less commonly, the small joints of the feet or the acromioclavicular joint. The wrists, metacarpophalangeal joints, elbows, shoulders, and ankles are usually not affected unless there is a history of injury to the specific joint, occupational overuse, or underlying condition that might be a cause of secondary osteoarthritis.

Hands The most commonly affected joints in the hands in patients with osteoarthritis are the distal and proximal interphalangeal joints, in which bony enlargement occurs (i.e., Heberden and Bouchard nodes, respectively) [see Figures 3 and 4]. The progressive enlargement of these joints occurs slowly over many

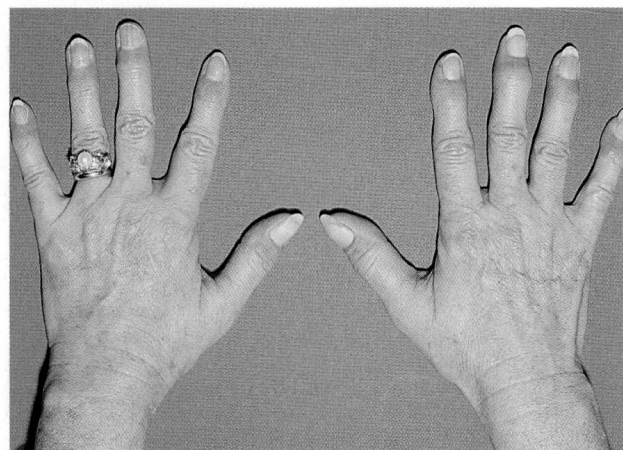

Figure 3   The hands of a patient with typical primary osteoarthritis show bony enlargement of multiple distal interphalangeal joints (Heberden nodes), mostly on the right, and early bony enlargement of the proximal interphalangeal joints (Bouchard nodes) on the left.

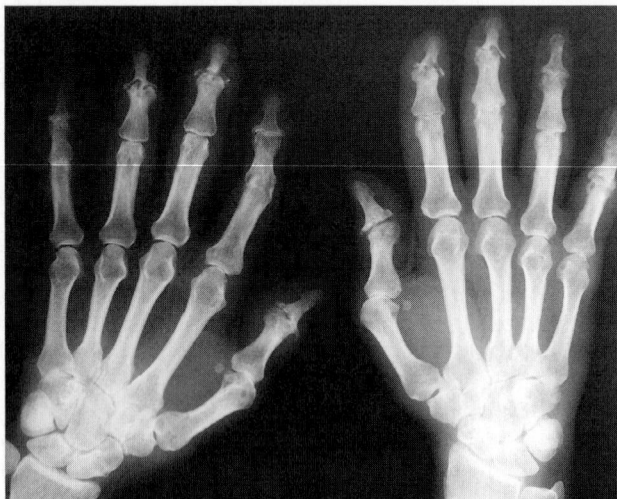

Figure 4   Severe destructive changes involving all of the distal interphalangeal joints and some of the proximal interphalangeal joints are characteristic of erosive osteoarthritis. Osteophytes are present at the margins of involved joints. Sharply demarcated bone erosions are seen in several distal interphalangeal joints, and bony fusion is seen in the proximal interphalangeal joint of the left second digit.

years, is frequently familial, and occurs most often in middle-aged or elderly women. Individual joints may go through inflammatory phases with redness and increased swelling and pain, most of which eventually subsides to a bony enlargement. Small gelatinous cysts may develop over the dorsal aspect of the distal interphalangeal joints and either persist or resolve spontaneously. Many patients with Heberden and Bouchard nodes have very little pain most of the time and therefore may not seek medical attention. The carpometacarpal joint of the thumb is another frequently involved joint, either by itself or along with the more distal joints; in such cases, patients experience pain, bony enlargement, and limited motion of the thumb.

Knees   Osteoarthritis frequently affects the knees and may be a cause of significant disability. Most patients present with pain that is worse with activity and improves with rest; they report

difficulty getting out of chairs or going up steps. Osteoarthritic knees will almost always have crepitus, limited motion, and pain on motion; effusions may or may not be present. In more advanced disease, bony enlargement, instability, and varus angulation may be present. Many patients have involvement of the patellofemoral compartment, but isolated disease in this area should suggest the presence of calcium pyrophosphate deposition disease.

Hips   Osteoarthritis of the hips is another common cause of significant pain and disability [*see Figure 5*]. Most patients experience a progressive disabling pain, usually in the upper thigh or inguinal region, sometimes radiating to the knee. Pain is worse with ambulation and may cause the patient to limp. Patients may also complain of difficulty with activities such as tying shoes, and limited hip motion is found on physical examination.

Spine   Osteoarthritis of the cervical and lumbar spine is referred to as spondylosis. Involvement of the intervertebral disk spaces or the posterior spinal facet joints may cause chronic back or neck pain that worsens with activity and improves with rest. Disk degeneration may be complicated by protrusion of the nucleus pulposus, causing nerve root compression with radicular pain or muscle weakness. In patients with extensive degenerative changes with fibrosis and osteophytes, stenosis of the spinal canal can occur, resulting in chronic cord compression in the cervical spine or compression of the cauda equina in the lumbar region. Lumbar spinal stenosis, causing chronic radicular leg pain that is worse with activity and better with rest (neurogenic claudication), is a common complication in elderly patients. A variant of spinal osteoarthritis occurring in the thoracic spine,

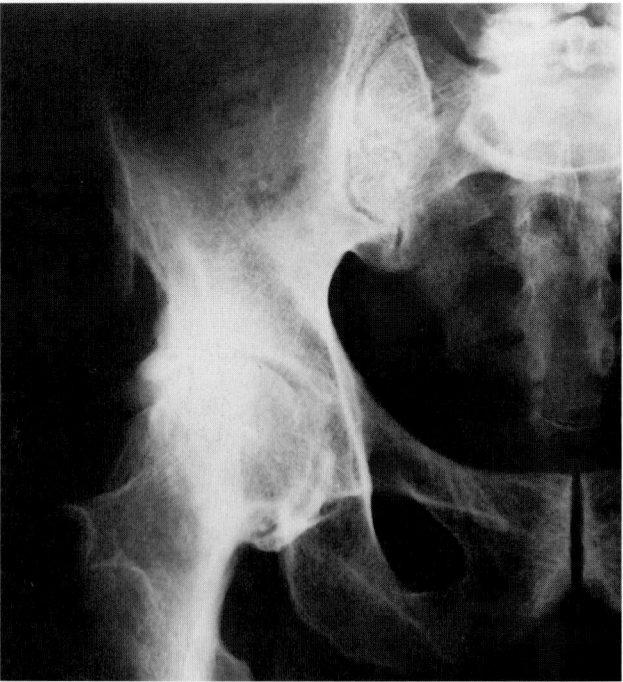

Figure 5   The hip is a common site of involvement in osteoarthritis. Joint space narrowing is most prominent at the superior and lateral aspects of the joint. Increased bony density (sclerosis) is seen in the subchondral bone on both sides of the joint, along with early subchondral cysts and osteophytes (bony spurs) over the superior and inferior aspects of the acetabulum.

known as diffuse idiopathic skeletal hyperostosis (DISH), is characterized by extensive bridging osteophytes and may cause loss of motion but little pain.

Radiologic Features

Typical radiographic findings in osteoarthritis include joint space narrowing, subchondral bone sclerosis, subchondral cysts, and osteophytes (bony spurs) [see Figure 5]. Joint space narrowing, resulting from loss of cartilage, is often asymmetrical and may be the only finding early in the disease process. In weight-bearing joints such as the knees, narrowing may be seen only in a standing view and may be missed in a radiograph obtained with the patient in the recumbent position. In more chronic disease, the hypertrophic features of subchondral sclerosis and osteophyte formation become more prominent, and subluxations or fusion of the joint may become apparent in more severely affected joints. In the small interphalangeal joints of the fingers, central erosions may be seen within the joint space; these erosions should be easily distinguishable from the periarticular erosions of rheumatoid arthritis.

Differential Diagnosis

Because of the high frequency of incidental radiographic changes in the general population, it is important not to attribute all musculoskeletal pain to osteoarthritis, even in patients with radiographic abnormalities. Alternative diagnoses should be made or coexistent conditions suspected in patients who are considered to be at low risk for osteoarthritis (e.g., younger patients) or in those who present with atypical pain patterns or atypical joint involvement. Patients with a relatively sudden onset of pain or with severe pain early in their presentation most often have something other than osteoarthritis. Problems in the wrists, elbows, shoulders, or ankles should raise concerns about other types of arthritis or secondary types of osteoarthritis.

Crystal-induced arthritis should always be considered in patients with acute pain, particularly if swelling and erythema are prominent. Calcium pyrophosphate deposition disease is common in the knees and hips and often coexists with osteoarthritis. Other joints frequently involved are the wrists and shoulders. Detection of chondrocalcinosis on x-ray or of crystals in synovial fluid confirms the diagnosis. Gout usually affects foot and ankle joints in early disease and is not often confused with osteoarthritis, but involvement of the knees is common in later disease. In addition, elderly women with Heberden and Bouchard nodes in the hands may have superimposed attacks in these joints as an initial manifestation of gout. Thus, examination of fluid from these joints for urate crystals may be essential in differentiating gout from an inflammatory flare of erosive osteoarthritis.

Rheumatoid arthritis can usually be distinguished from osteoarthritis on the basis of a different pattern of joint disease, more prominent morning stiffness, and soft tissue swelling and warmth on physical examination. In some patients, the patterns of joint disease may overlap, particularly in the proximal interphalangeal joints, hips, and knees. Thus, in some patients, the presence of an elevated ESR, a high-titer rheumatoid factor, or periarticular erosive changes may be the only way to distinguish these two common conditions.

Polymyalgia rheumatica is a disease of the elderly and is often seen in patients with underlying osteoarthritis. Patients typically have a change in the pattern of pain, more localized to the shoulder and hip girdles, with few peripheral joint symptoms.

Morning stiffness is a prominent feature, and the diagnosis is usually more likely if the ESR is markedly elevated. However, because modest elevations of ESR are seen in many normal elderly individuals, the differentiation of this condition from osteoarthritis is often difficult. In some patients, a rapid response of symptoms to a low dose of corticosteroid is helpful in making a diagnosis.

Ankylosing spondylitis is usually a disease that first manifests in young adulthood and should not be confused with spinal osteoarthritis. However, some patients have only mild levels of pain and may not seek medical attention until later years. In such patients, the radiographic changes in the cervical and lumbar spine in the two conditions should make differentiation between them relatively easy.

Psoriatic arthritis, when present in a classic distribution in the distal interphalangeal joints of the fingers, may mimic Heberden nodes. Psoriatic arthritis usually occurs in younger persons and is more common in males, but differentiation between psoriatic arthritis and Heberden nodes may still be difficult. In young patients with arthritis of the distal interphalangeal joints, a careful search for psoriatic skin lesions and nail changes is essential. On physical examination, the swelling of involved joints is usually greater in the soft tissues, with less bony enlargement. Radiography will usually show more erosive changes and fewer osteophytic changes than in typical osteoarthritis.

Disorders of bone near joints can be confused with osteoarthritis. Osteonecrosis of the hip, knee, or shoulder may cause pain and restricted motion without significant signs of inflammation. Radiographs may be normal initially, and follow-up radiographs or magnetic resonance imaging may be necessary to differentiate this condition from osteoarthritis. Paget disease or osteoporotic fractures may cause pain in the back and hip girdle that is similar to that of osteoarthritis, although the pain is often more severe and acute in patients with fractures.

Nonarticular pain syndromes involving tendons, bursae, peripheral nerves, and internal joint structures may cause pain similar to that of osteoarthritis. Examples include de Quervain tenosynovitis or carpal tunnel syndrome in the hand, trochanteric bursitis or meralgia paresthetica in the hip, anserine bursitis or meniscal tears in the knee, and plantar fasciitis and interdigital neuromas in the feet. Knowledge of nonarticular pain syndromes and the characteristic patterns of symptoms and physical findings in each is essential to diagnosing and differentiating these syndromes from osteoarthritis in the same area.

Management

There is no cure for osteoarthritis and no therapy known to prevent or retard the degenerative biologic process in articular cartilage. Thus, the treatment of osteoarthritis is focused primarily on relieving symptoms and improving function.[51-53] Treatment decisions should be based on the severity and distribution of joint involvement, considered in the light of the patient's other medical problems that might affect the safety and effectiveness of any chosen therapy [see Table 2].

NONPHARMACOLOGIC MEASURES

Nonpharmacologic measures that have the potential to improve outcomes in osteoarthritis include patient education, physical and occupational therapy assessment and interventions, exercise, weight loss, and dietary measures.[7] Exercise, in particular, should be a part of the therapeutic regimen in every

Table 2   Treatment of Osteoarthritis

Treatment Type	Useful for What or Whom?	Measure	Comments
Nonpharmacologic	All patients	Exercise	Range of motion and strengthening of muscles around affected joints
		Weight loss	Particularly valuable in patients with involvement of weight-bearing joints
		Dietary measures	Adequate intake of calcium, vitamin C, and vitamin D
Pharmacologic	Most or all patients	Simple analgesics	Acetaminophen, tramadol, narcotics in selected cases
		NSAIDs	Nonselective NSAIDs for patients at low risk for GI complications; otherwise, consider addition of misoprostol, a proton pump inhibitor, or an H_2 antagonist or use of a cyclooxygenase-2–specific NSAID (coxib)
Ancillary medical and surgical	Selected joints or patients	Splints	Specific for each joint
		Canes or other orthotics	—
		Corticosteroid injections	Knees, fingers; other joints in selected cases
		Hyaluronic acid injections	Knees in some patients
		Arthroscopic surgery	For patients with mechanical symptoms or findings
		Osteotomy	Knees in selected patients
		Total joint replacement	—

NSAIDs—nonsteroidal anti-inflammatory drugs

patient. Quadriceps weakness contributes significantly to disability in patients with osteoarthritis of the knee, and exercises designed to strengthen quadriceps have potential to lessen pain and disability.[54] In addition, aerobic exercise, such as a walking program, can improve function and reduce pain. Most studies of patients with osteoarthritis have found that regular activity is associated with a better outcome.[55-57] However, compliance with exercise programs is often low, and regular supervised follow-up may be helpful.

The role of obesity as an etiologic factor in osteoarthritis of the knee is well established, and some data suggest that weight loss may reduce the risk of development of symptoms in patients predisposed to osteoarthritis. Even though few prospective studies have been done, patients with osteoarthritis of the knees and hips should be encouraged to lose weight if they are above ideal body weight. In addition, epidemiologic studies have suggested a role for adequate dietary vitamin C and D intake in reducing the risk of progression of established osteoarthritis.[14,58] In some patients, measures designed to alter the biomechanical forces on diseased joints should be considered, including patellar taping, wedged insoles, bracing, canes, and crutches.

PHARMACOLOGIC THERAPY

The primary goal of drug therapy in osteoarthritis is to relieve pain. Acetaminophen may be as effective as nonsteroidal anti-inflammatory drugs (NSAIDs),[59] so it should be prescribed initially in most patients. In most cases, up to 3,000 to 4,000 mg of acetaminophen a day can be given. Doses should be limited in patients with exposure to other potentially hepatotoxic substances. In particular, patients who take acetaminophen regularly should be advised to limit alcohol ingestion and be warned about the increased risk of acetaminophen hepatotoxicity in heavy drinkers. Opioids are generally avoided in osteoarthritis but may be useful in selected patients. However, these agents should be used with caution in elderly patients.[60] Tramadol, a

centrally acting analgesic with dual mechanisms, may give relief comparable to that achieved with acetaminophen and codeine. Topical capsaicin may be useful in some patients, especially those with involvement of the knees and hands.

A number of other nutritional supplements and topical therapies have been investigated for the treatment of osteoarthritis.[61,62]

NSAIDs are useful in osteoarthritis mostly for their analgesic effects and, in most patients, are more effective than acetaminophen.[63] Unfortunately, NSAIDs are associated with an increased risk of gastric ulcers and bleeding, particularly in patients with a history of gastrointestinal disease, those on concomitant steroids or anticoagulants, and those older than 65 years. Strategies to reduce this toxicity include the use of lower doses of NSAIDs or concomitant use of misoprostol, histamine$_2$ receptor antagonists, and proton pump inhibitors. The cyclooxygenase-2 (COX-2)–specific NSAIDs (celecoxib and valdecoxib) have been shown to reduce the risk of serious gastrointestinal complications, compared with the nonselective COX inhibitors; however, selective COX-2 inhibitors, with the possible exception of celecoxib, are associated with an increase in the risk of cardiovascular disease. The association of cardiovascular events with the prolonged use of the COX-2 inhibitor rofecoxib (Vioxx) prompted the withdrawal of the drug from the global market in 2004.[66] The Adenomatous Polyp Prevention on Vioxx (APPROVe) study documented that patients taking the drug for 18 months were twice as likely to experience cardiovascular events as patients taking placebo (after 3 years, the rates of cardiovascular events were 1.5% for rofecoxib and 0.7% for placebo).[66] Data from several sources are consistent in finding an increase of hypertension and congestive heart failure in patients taking rofecoxib.[67-69] There is scant evidence to assess the long-term risk of other COX-2 inhibitors. When prescribing COX-2 inhibitors, clinicians should weigh the potential cardiovascular risks against anticipated benefits and consider issues such as dose and comorbid conditions.

Intra-articular corticosteroid injections may be useful in treating selected joints, particularly during exacerbations characterized by increased pain and effusion, and injections in symptomatic knees every 3 months may be a safe and effective means of reducing pain and improving function over longer periods of time.[70] Some animal and in vitro studies have suggested that steroids have a detrimental effect on articular cartilage, but there are few clinical data to support this concern in patients with osteoarthritis. Intra-articular hyaluronic acid derivatives (Hyalgan and Synvisc), given in a series of three to five weekly injections, have been shown to be superior to placebo in most studies and may be useful in relieving pain in selected patients with less advanced disease.[71,72]

SURGERY

In patients with badly damaged knees and hips, total joint replacement is an effective option. Almost all patients experience significant pain relief, and some have improved range of motion. Joint loosening and infection are potential late complications in prosthetic joints but are uncommon. Arthroscopic debridement of affected joints is no better than placebo in unselected patients with osteoarthritis of the knee.[73] Thus, this procedure should be reserved for patients with mechanical symptoms suggesting internal derangement. Realignment of a degenerative knee to allow redistribution of forces is sometimes attempted by a high tibial wedge osteotomy, particularly in younger patients with valgus deformities.

Biologic approaches to the surgical treatment of osteoarthritis have been explored. These include local enhancement of bone marrow progenitor cells and various forms of cartilage transplantation.[51] In addition, stem cell transplantation has been investigated in animal models of osteoarthritis.[74] Most of these approaches are in early stages of development, and none is likely to enter clinical use in the foreseeable future.

PROTECTING CARTILAGE

Therapies with potential to prevent or retard the progression of articular cartilage breakdown have received a great deal of attention in recent years.[75] Agents considered to have so-called chondroprotective potential include tetracyclines, protease inhibitors, glycosaminoglycan compounds, growth factors, and cytokine inhibitors. Oral glucosamine and chondroitin sulfate have been promoted as health food supplements to improve cartilage, but most of the clinical studies with these agents have demonstrated only modest pain relief, compared with placebo, and studies to assess the effect on cartilage are ongoing.[76-79] Inconsistent dosages in studies and lack of standardization of available preparations have complicated assessment of these agents' value.

Tetracyclines have been shown to reduce the severity of osteoarthritis in animals, probably by inhibiting metalloprotease activity, and are being studied in early human trials. Other approaches to disease modification being investigated in animal models include other agents that inhibit metalloproteases or nitric oxide synthase inhibitors.[80]

Biologic therapies designed to augment growth factors or inhibit cytokines have also been investigated in animal models of osteoarthritis. These have included attempts to introduce growth factors or IL-1 receptor antagonist through the use of gene therapy.[81]

Prognosis

Osteoarthritis is a slowly progressive condition with a variable prognosis.[2] Radiographically, most joints will either remain stable or gradually worsen over a 5- to 15-year period. In most patients, symptoms evolve over many years and may spontaneously remit for long periods of time without explanation. Progression of osteoarthritis of the hand is particularly hard to measure because pain levels frequently improve after involved joints become fused. Disease may progress more rapidly in the hips and knees of older women with osteopenic bone. However, in general, predicting the prognosis in patients with osteoarthritis is difficult.

The author has received grants for clinical research from Abbott Laboratories, Amgen, Inc, Bristol-Myers Squibb Co., and Isis Pharmaceuticals, Inc., and has served as advisor or consultant to TAP Pharmaceutical Products, Inc.

References

1. Lawrence RC, Helmick CG, Arnett FC, et al: Estimates of the prevalence of arthritis and selected musculoskeletal disorders in the United States. Arthritis Rheum 41:778, 1998

2. Felson DT, Lawrence RC, Dieppe PA, et al: Osteoarthritis: new insights. I: The disease and its risk factors. Ann Intern Med 133:635, 2000

3. Poole J, Sayer AA, Hardy R, et al: Patterns of interphalangeal hand joint involvement of osteoarthritis among men and women: a British cohort study. Arthritis Rheum 48:3371, 2003

4. Felson DT, Nevitt MC, Zhang Y, et al: High prevalence of lateral knee osteoarthritis in Beijing Chinese compared with Framingham Caucasian subjects. Arthritis Rheum 46:1217, 2002

5. Nevitt MC, Xu L, Zhang Y, et al: Very low prevalence of hip osteoarthritis among Chinese elderly in Beijing, China, compared with whites in the United States: the Beijing osteoarthritis study. Arthritis Rheum 46:1773, 2002

6. Zhang Y, Xu L, Nevitt MC, et al: Comparison of the prevalence of knee osteoarthritis between the elderly Chinese population in Beijing and whites in the United States: the Beijing Osteoarthritis Study. Arthritis Rheum 44:2065, 2001

7. Felson DT, Zhang Y: An update on the epidemiology of knee and hip osteoarthritis with a view to prevention. Arthritis Rheum 41:1343, 1998

8. Gelber AC, Hochberg MC, Mead LA, et al: Body mass index in young men and the risk of subsequent knee and hip osteoarthritis. Am J Med 107:542, 1999

9. Sharma L, Lou C, Cahue S, et al: The mechanism of the effect of obesity in knee osteoarthritis: the mediating role of malalignment. Arthritis Rheum 43:568, 2000

10. Sharma L, Song J, Felson DT, et al: The role of knee alignment in disease progression and functional decline in knee osteoarthritis. JAMA 286:188, 2001

11. Manek NJ, Hart D, Spector TD, et al: The association of body mass index and osteoarthritis of the knee joint: an examination of genetic and environmental influences. Arthritis Rheum 48:1024, 2003

12. Hart DJ, Cronin C, Daniels M, et al: The relationship of bone density and fracture to incident and progressive radiographic osteoarthritis of the knee: the Chingford Study. Arthritis Rheum 46:92, 2002

13. Lane NE, Nevitt MC: Osteoarthritis, bone mass, and fractures: how are they related? Arthritis Rheum 46:1, 2002

14. McAlindon TE, Felson DT, Zhang Y, et al: Relation of dietary intake and serum levels of vitamin D to progression of osteoarthritis of the knee among participants in the Framingham Study. Ann Intern Med 125:353, 1996

15. McAlindon TE, Wilson PFW, Aliabadi P, et al: Level of physical activity and the risk of radiographic and symptomatic knee osteoarthritis in the elderly: the Framingham study. Am J Med 106:151, 1999

16. Coggon D, Croft P, Kellingray S, et al: Occupational physical activities and osteoarthritis of the knee. Arthritis Rheum 43:1443, 2000

17. Spector TD, Harris PA, Hart DJ, et al: Risk of osteoarthritis associated with long-term weight bearing sports: a radiologic survey of the hips and knees in female ex-athletes and population controls. Arthritis Rheum 39:988, 1996

18. Lane NE, Oehlert JW, Bloch DA, et al: The relationship of running to osteoarthritis of the knee and hip and bone mineral density of the lumbar spine: a 9 year longitudinal study. J Rheumatol 25:334, 1998

19. Gelber A, Hochberg M, Mead L, et al: Joint injury in young adults and risk for subsequent knee and hip osteoarthritis. Ann Intern Med 133:321, 2000

20. Biswal S, Hastie T, Andriacchi TP, et al: Risk factors for progressive cartilage loss in the knee. Arthritis Rheum 46:2884, 2002

21. Lievense AM, Bierma-Zeinstra SM, Verhagen AP, et al: Influence of sporting activities on the development of osteoarthritis of the hip: a systematic review. Arthritis Rheum 49:228, 2003

22. Slemenda C, Brandt KD, Heilman DK, et al: Quadriceps weakness and osteoarthritis of the knee. Ann Intern Med 127:97, 1997

23. Sharma L, Pai YC, Holtkamp K, et al: Is knee joint proprioception worse in the arthritic knee versus the unaffected knee in unilateral knee osteoarthritis? Arthritis Rheum 40:1518, 1997

24. Hassan BS, Doherty SA, Mockett S, et al: Effect of pain reduction on postural sway, proprioception, and quadriceps strength in subjects with knee osteoarthritis. Ann Rheum Dis 61:422, 2002

25. Vanwanseele B, Eckstein F, Knecht H, et al: Knee cartilage of spinal cord-injured patients displays progressive thinning in the absence of normal joint loading and movement. Arthritis Rheum 46:2073, 2002

26. Vanwanseele B, Eckstein F, Knecht H, et al: Longitudinal analysis of cartilage atrophy in the knees of patients with spinal cord injury. Arthritis Rheum 48:3377, 2003

27. Holderbaum D, Haqqi TM, Moskowitz RW: Genetics and osteoarthritis: exposing the iceberg. Arthritis Rheum 42:397, 1999

28. Jonsson H, Manolescu I, Stefansson SE, et al: The inheritance of hand osteoarthritis in Iceland. Arthritis Rheum 48:391, 2003

29. Lanyon P, Muir K, Doherty S, et al: Assessment of a genetic contribution to osteoarthritis of the hip: sibling study. BMJ 321:1179, 2000

30. MacGregor AJ, Antoniades L, Matson M, et al: The genetic contribution to radiographic hip osteoarthritis in women: results of a classic twin study. Arthritis Rheum 43:2410, 2000

31. Ross JM, Kowalchuk RM, Shaulinsky J, et al: Association of heterozygous hemochromatosis C282Y gene mutation with hand osteoarthritis. J Rheumatol 30:121, 2003

32. Bergink AP, van Meurs JB, Loughlin J, et al: Estrogen receptor alpha gene haplotype is associated with radiographic osteoarthritis of the knee in elderly men and women. Arthritis Rheum 48:1913, 2003

33. Knowlton RG, Katzenstein PL, Moskowitz RW, et al: Genetic linkage of polymorphism to type II procollagen gene (COL 2A1) to primary osteoarthritis associated with mild chondrodysplasia. N Engl J Med 322:526, 1990

34. Keen RW, Hart DJ, Lanchbury JS, et al: Association of early osteoarthritis of the knee with a Taq I polymorphism of the vitamin D receptor gene. Arthritis Rheum 40:1444, 1997

35. Paassilta P, Lohiniva J, Goring H, et al: Identification of a novel common genetic risk factor for lumbar disc disease. JAMA 285:1843, 2001

36. Baldwin CT, Cupples LA, Joost O, et al: Absence of linkage or association for osteoarthritis with the vitamin D receptor/type II collagen locus: the Framingham Osteoarthritis Study. J Rheumatol 29:161, 2002

37. Lane NE, Lin P, Christiansen L, et al: Association of mild acetabular dysplasia with an increased risk of incident osteoarthritis in elderly white women: the study of osteoporotic fractures. Arthritis Rheum 43:400, 2000

38. Gillaspy E, Spreckley K, Wallis G, et al: Investigation of linkage on chromosome 2q and hand and knee osteoarthritis. Arthritis Rheum 46:3386, 2002

39. Chapman K, Mustafa Z, Dowling B, et al: Finer linkage mapping of primary hip osteoarthritis susceptibility on chromosome 11q in a cohort of affected female sibling pairs. Arthritis Rheum 46:1780, 2002

40. Demissie S, Cupples LA, Myers R, et al: Genome scan for quantity of hand osteoarthritis: the Framingham Study. Arthritis Rheum 46:946, 2002

41. Goldring MB: The role of the chondrocyte in osteoarthritis. Arthritis Rheum 43:1916, 2000

42. Jaovisidha K, Rosenthal AK: Calcium crystals in osteoarthritis. Curr Opin Rheumatol 14:298, 2002

43. Dumond H, Presle N, Terlain B, et al: Evidence for a key role of leptin in osteoarthritis. Arthritis Rheum 48:3118, 2003

44. Loeser RF: Systemic and local regulation of articular cartilage metabolism: where does leptin fit in the puzzle? Arthritis Rheum 48:3009, 2003

45. Clements KM, Price JS, Chambers MG, et al: Gene deletion of either interleukin-1beta, interleukin-1beta-converting enzyme, inducible nitric oxide synthase, or stromelysin 1 accelerates the development of knee osteoarthritis in mice after surgical transection of the medial collateral ligament and partial medial meniscectomy. Arthritis Rheum 48:3452, 2003

46. Pelletier JP, Martel-Pelletier J, Abramson SB: Osteoarthritis, an inflammatory disease: potential implication for the selection of new therapeutic targets. Arthritis Rheum 44:1237, 2001

47. Yuan GH, Masuko-Hongo K, Kato T, et al: Immunologic intervention in the pathogenesis of osteoarthritis. Arthritis Rheum 48:602, 2003

48. Felson DT, Chaisson CE, Hill CL, et al: The association of bone marrow lesions with pain in knee osteoarthritis. Ann Intern Med 134:594, 2001

49. Hill CL, Gale DR, Chaisson CE, et al: Periarticular lesions detected on magnetic resonance imaging: prevalence in knees with and without symptoms. Arthritis Rheum 48:2836, 2003

50. Felson DT, McLaughlin S, Goggins J, et al: Bone marrow edema and its relation to progression of knee osteoarthritis. Ann Intern Med 139:330, 2003

51. Felson DT, Lawrence RC, Hochberg MC, et al: Osteoarthritis: new insights: II. Treatment approaches. Ann Intern Med 133:726, 2000

52. Recommendations for the medical management of osteoarthritis of the hip and knee. American College of Rheumatology Subcommittee on Osteoarthritis Guidelines. Arthritis Rheum 43:1905, 2000

53. Pendleton A, Arden N, Dougados M, et al: EULAR recommendations for the management of knee osteoarthritis: report of a task force of the Standing Committee for the International Clinical Studies Including Therapeutic Trials (ESCIST). Ann Rheum Dis 59:936, 2000

54. Deyle GD, Henderson NE, Matekel RL, et al: Effectiveness of manual physical therapy and exercise in osteoarthritis of the knee: a randomized, controlled study. Ann Intern Med 132:173, 2000

55. Van Baar ME, Assendelft WJJ, Dekker J, et al: Effectiveness of exercise therapy in patients with osteoarthritis of the hip or knee: a systematic review of randomized clinical trials. Arthritis Rheum 42:1361, 1999

56. Penninx BW, Messier SP, Rejeski WJ, et al: Physical exercise and the prevention of disability in activities of daily living in older persons with osteoarthritis. Arch Intern Med 161:2309, 2001

57. Sharma L, Cahue S, Song J, et al: Physical functioning over three years in knee osteoarthritis: role of psychosocial, local mechanical, and neuromuscular factors. Arthritis Rheum 48:3359, 2003

58. McAlindon T, Jacques P, Zhang Y, et al: Do antioxidant micronutrients protect against the development and progression of knee osteoarthritis? Arthritis Rheum 39:648, 1996

59. Bradley JD, Brandt KD, Katz BP, et al: Comparison of an anti-inflammatory dose of ibuprofen, an analgesic dose of ibuprofen, and acetaminophen in the treatment of patients with osteoarthritis of the knee. N Engl J Med 325:87, 1991

60. Peleso PM: Opioid therapy for osteoarthritis of the hip and knee: use it or lose it (editorial)? J Rheumatol 28:6, 2001

61. Hochberg MC: Multidisciplinary integrative approach to treating knee pain in patients with osteoarthritis. Ann Intern Med 139:781, 2003

62. Long L, Soeken K, Ernst E: Herbal medicines for the treatment of osteoarthritis: a systematic review. Rheumatology (Oxford) 40:779, 2001

63. Case JP, Baliunas AJ, Block JA: Lack of efficacy of acetaminophen in treating symptomatic knee osteoarthritis: a randomized, double-blind, placebo-controlled comparison trial with diclofenac sodium. Arch Intern Med 163:169, 2003

64. Schneeweiss S, Solomon DH, Wang PS, et al: Simultaneous assessment of short-term gastrointestinal benefits and cardiovascular risk of selective cyclooxygenase 2 inhibitors and nonselective nonsteroidal anti-inflammatory drugs: an instrumental variable analysis. Arthritis Rheum 54:3390, 2006

65. McGettigan P, Henry D: Cardiovascular risk and inhibition of cyclooxygenase: systematic review of the observational studies of selective and nonselective inhibitors of cyclooxygenase 2. JAMA 296:1633, 2006

66. Singh D: Merck withdraws arthritis drug worldwide. BMJ 329:816, 2004

67. Bombardier C, Laine L, Reicin A, et al: Comparison of upper gastrointestinal toxicity of rofecoxib and naproxen in patients with rheumatoid arthritis. N Engl J Med 343:1520, 2000

68. Solomon DH, Schneeweiss S, Glynn RJ, et al: Relationship between selective cyclooxygenase-2 inhibitors and acute myocardial infarction in older adults. Circulation 209:2068, 2004

69. Solomon DH, Schneeweiss S, Levin R, et al: Relationship between COX-2 specific inhibitors and hypertension. Hypertension 44:140, 2004

70. Raynauld JP, Buckland-Wright C, Ward R, et al: Safety and efficacy of long-term intraarticular steroid injections in osteoarthritis of the knee: a randomized, double-blind, placebo-controlled trial. Arthritis Rheum 48:370, 2003

71. Brandt K, Smith G, Simon L: Intraarticular injection of hyaluronan as treatment for knee osteoarthritis: what is the evidence (review)? Arthritis Rheum 43:1192, 2000

72. Felson DT, Anderson JJ: Hyaluronate sodium injections for osteoarthritis: hope, hype, and hard truths. Arch Intern Med 162:245, 2002

73. Moseley JB, O'Malley K, Petersen NJ, et al: A controlled trial of arthroscopic surgery for osteoarthritis of the knee. N Engl J Med 347:81, 2002

74. Murphy JM, Fink DJ, Hunziker EB, et al: Stem cell therapy in a caprine model of osteoarthritis. Arthritis Rheum 48:3464, 2003

75. Dieppe PA: The management of osteoarthritis in the third millennium. Scand J Rheumatol 29:279, 2000

76. McAlindon TE, LaValley MP, Bulin JP, et al: Glucosamine and chondroitin for treatment of osteoarthritis: a systematic quality assessment and meta-analysis. JAMA 283:1469, 2000

77. Reginster JY, Deroisy R, Rovati CL, et al: Long-term effects of glucosamine sulphate on osteoarthritis progression: a randomised, placebo-controlled clinical trial. Lancet 357:251, 2001

78. Richy F, Bruyere O, Ethgen O, et al: Structural and symptomatic efficacy of glucosamine and chondroitin in knee osteoarthritis: a comprehensive meta-analysis. Arch Intern Med 163:1514, 2003

79. Mengshol JA, Mix KS, Brinckerhoff CE: Matrix metalloproteinases as therapeutic targets in arthritic diseases: bull's-eye or missing the mark? Arthritis Rheum 46:13, 2002

80. Towheed TE: Current status of glucosamine therapy in osteoarthritis. Arthritis Rheum 49:601, 2003

81. Gelse K, Von Der Mark K, Aigner T, et al: Articular cartilage repair by gene therapy using growth factor-producing mesenchymal cells. Arthritis Rheum 48:430, 2003

Acknowledgment

Figure 1   Courtesy of Richard Hard, M.D.

Christopher Wise, M.D., F.A.C.P.

A large proportion of the musculoskeletal problems for which patients seek medical attention are related to periarticular structures and do not represent a true articular process or a more generalized systemic illness.[1] Knowledge of the common nonarticular regional rheumatic disorders is important because of their high prevalence in primary care practice, the dependence on clinical findings for diagnosis, and the high cost that can result from unnecessary laboratory evaluations. The ability to recognize important patterns of pain and associated physical signs is essential to making a correct diagnosis; in most cases, radiographic and laboratory studies are not needed. Diagnostic studies should be utilized judiciously and must be interpreted in the light of existing clinical findings and prestudy suspicion for specific diagnoses.

Most regional rheumatic disorders respond to local measures, such as application of heat or cold, splinting, and injection of glucocorticoids. Nonsteroidal anti-inflammatory drugs (NSAIDs) or mild analgesic medications are often helpful therapeutic adjuncts. Referral for surgical intervention may be indicated for patients with certain conditions. For example, in cases of cervical or lumbar disk disease or spinal stenosis with definite nerve entrapment or spinal cord compression, well-timed decompression may be necessary to restore function or prevent further functional impairment. Arthroscopic intervention is sometimes useful to better define and treat refractory knee and shoulder pain syndromes. Surgical release is indicated for entrapment neuropathies when there is evidence of motor dysfunction. Surgical consultation may be useful for a variety of other syndromes when the response to conservative measures proves to be less than optimal. Physical therapy and occupational therapy are useful for many patients—particularly those patients who have persistent back and shoulder pain—though these therapies may constitute an important part of the treatment of almost any refractory regional pain syndrome.

Definitions

Common regional rheumatic disorders include various types of bursitis, tendinitis, tenosynovitis, myofascial pain, and entrapment neuropathies. Bursitis results from mechanical or inflammatory changes of one of the many bursae in the body. Bursae are synovia-lined sacs around the joints that serve to minimize friction between tendons, ligaments, and bony structures. Tendinitis usually results from trauma or overuse of tissues near sites where tendons attach to bone or at the musculotendinous junction. Myofascial pain originates at sites within muscle groups and surrounding fascial tissues that become tender and painful as a result of localized injury or overuse. Entrapment neuropathies occur at sites where peripheral nerves are compressed as they traverse periarticular areas that allow relatively little room for free movement of the affected nerves.

Neck Pain

Neck pain may result from degenerative changes in the cervical disks and zygapophyseal (facet) joints or from a variety of muscu-

lar, ligamentous, and tendinous conditions.[2] In whiplash injuries occurring after rapid acceleration or deceleration and hyperextension of the head in motor vehicle accidents, a number of structures may be injured.[3] Recovery from whiplash injuries is often incomplete, and a combination of physical and psychosocial factors may contribute to prolongation of pain.[4] Judicious use of analgesics, muscle relaxants, and physiotherapy proves helpful in some patients. The zygapophyseal joints may be the source of pain, and local nerve block with an anesthetic or ablation may be helpful in selected patients.

The term cervical sprain denotes transient neck pain associated with muscle tenderness and spasm. Cervical sprain usually responds to heat, rest, and, occasionally, immobilization and traction. Manual therapy, range-of-motion or strength-training exercises, or acupuncture may provide relief in some patients.[5-7] In cervical disk herniation, nerve root impingement results in pain, paresthesia, and sometimes muscle weakness in the distribution of the affected nerve (usually at the C5 to C7 level). In such patients, radiographic documentation and surgical decompression are sometimes needed if symptoms do not improve with rest or traction or if significant neurologic deficit is present. In some patients with long-standing cervical spondylosis, cervical stenosis may cause chronic compression of the spinal cord (most often at the C3 to C5 level). Surgical decompression is indicated in patients with evolving myelopathy.

Back Pain

Low back pain is the most common musculoskeletal complaint requiring medical attention; it is the fifth most common reason for all physician visits.[8-10] Over half of the general population will seek medical attention for back pain at some point in their lives. An increased risk of back pain is associated with male sex, smoking, frequent lifting of heavy objects, poor general health and conditioning, and certain occupational and sports activities. In addition, preexisting psychological distress, compensation issues, other chronic pain, and job dissatisfaction may play a role in persistent back pain.[11,12] In most patients, the cause of pain cannot be determined with any degree of certainty and is usually attributed to muscular or ligamentous strain, facet joint arthritis, or disk pressure on the annulus fibrosus, vertebral end plate, or nerve roots.[13]

ACUTE BACK PAIN

Diagnosis

For patients with acute back pain, the initial history should be used to identify those who are at increased risk for serious underlying conditions, such as fracture, infection, tumor, or major neurologic deficit[8] [*see Table 1*]. The presence of such factors in patients with acute back pain may indicate the need for radiographic and laboratory studies earlier than in patients without such factors. The initial physical examination should include

Table 1 Indications That Acute Back Pain May Involve Underlying Conditions

Patient demographics	Age > 70 yr History of cancer Glucocorticoid or immunosuppressive drug therapy Alcohol or I.V. drug abuse
Historical features	Weight loss Fever Pain increased by rest
Neurologic symptoms	Bowel or bladder dysfunction Saddle block anesthesia Progressive motor weakness

evaluation for areas of localized bony tenderness and assessment of flexion and straight leg raising. Because acute low back pain will improve within a month in over 90% of patients, further evaluation is usually unnecessary. Plain radiographs should be reserved for patients at high risk for more serious underlying conditions [*see Table 1*], because abnormal findings on plain films are common and do not correlate with back pain. Early use of magnetic resonance imaging or computed tomography has not been shown to change treatment choices or outcomes; consequently, these studies should be reserved for patients with persistent pain and sciatica.[14,15]

Treatment

A number of therapeutic interventions are available for acute back pain, but data supporting efficacy are minimal for most therapies. Strict bed rest should be kept to a minimum (no more than 2 to 4 days), and the continuation of normal activities within the limits permitted by pain should be encouraged. Mild analgesics (including NSAIDs) and muscle relaxants may be useful for early symptom control; opiates should be used sparingly.[16] Spinal manipulation, massage or other physical therapy, graded activity, self-management, or other specific exercise programs may be effective in acute back pain, but most controlled studies suggest little to no advantage of any particular regimen.[17-21] Patient education about the natural history of back pain may result in fewer demands for further diagnostic tests and physician visits and should improve patient satisfaction.

CHRONIC BACK PAIN

Diagnosis

Patients whose pain persists after 4 to 6 weeks of conservative treatment measures should be reassessed. Plain radiography and basic laboratory studies (e.g., complete blood count, erythrocyte sedimentation rate or C-reactive protein level, chemistry profile, and urinalysis) should be considered to screen for systemic illnesses. A herniated lumbar disk should be considered in patients with symptoms of radiculopathy, as suggested by pain radiating down the leg with symptoms reproduced by straight leg raising. MRI may be necessary to confirm a herniated disk, but findings should be interpreted with caution because many asymptomatic persons have disk abnormalities.[22] Electromyography may be useful in differentiating lumbar radiculopathy from other causes of radicular leg pain. Most lumbar disk herniations producing sciatica occur at the L4-L5 and L5-S1 levels.

Surgical intervention is indicated in patients with persistent sciatica and clear-cut evidence of a herniated disk on MRI or myelography–CT scanning.

Treatment

A number of nonpharmacologic approaches to therapy have been studied in patients with chronic low back pain, but no specific regimen appears to be superior to others. Most analyses of prior studies suggest that individualized programs promoting strength and range of motion have modest efficacy.[23-25] Behavioral therapies and using a mattress of medium firmness may provide short-term improvement in some patients, as well.[26,27] Judicious use of analgesics, NSAIDs, and tricyclic antidepressants may help the patient function more fully and may improve outcome.[28] Local therapies in the form of local injections of intradiscal or periarticular steroids, hypertonic irritant solutions (prolotherapy), or acupuncture are no more effective than placebo in most studies.[29-31]

Lumbar Stenosis

Lumbar spinal stenosis, usually a result of extensive degenerative disk disease and osteophytes, should be suspected in elderly patients with chronic back pain associated with sciatica.[32] Patients typically complain of pain, numbness, and weakness in the buttocks that extends to one or both legs. Symptoms are usually brought on by standing or walking and improve when the patient stoops forward, sits, or lies down (i.e., neurogenic claudication or pseudoclaudication). The diagnosis may be confirmed by MRI or myelogram–CT scanning.[33] Conservative measures are helpful in many patients, allowing stable or improved function. Surgical decompression by multilevel laminectomy and fusion should be considered in patients with poor response to conservative measures or progressive functional deterioration.[34-36]

Shoulder Pain

Shoulder pain is one of the most common musculoskeletal problems seen in the outpatient setting.[37] Most shoulder pain results from conditions of the periarticular structures of the joint; true arthritis of the glenohumeral joint is uncommon [*see Figure 1*].

The initial evaluation of shoulder pain should include consideration of pain that may be referred from the neck, thorax, or abdomen. The examination should assess active and passive range of flexion, abduction, and internal and external rotation of the shoulder, along with forward elevation. In addition, areas of localized tenderness may help differentiate the various potential causes of shoulder pain. Plain radiographs are seldom diagnostic but are indicated in patients with a history of trauma or refractory pain or when true glenohumeral joint disease is suspected. For patients who respond poorly to conservative therapy, a variety of specialized tests (e.g., arthrography, arthroscopy, and MRI) are available for further definition of lesions that may require surgery.

ROTATOR CUFF TENDINITIS (IMPINGEMENT SYNDROME)

Rotator cuff tendinitis, or impingement syndrome, is often associated with bursitis of the overlying subacromial bursa and is the cause of most nontraumatic cases of shoulder pain. Rotator cuff tendinitis results from inflammation, degeneration, and attrition of the rotator cuff by mechanical impingement on the acromion, coracoacromial ligament, and sometimes the acromioclavicular joint.

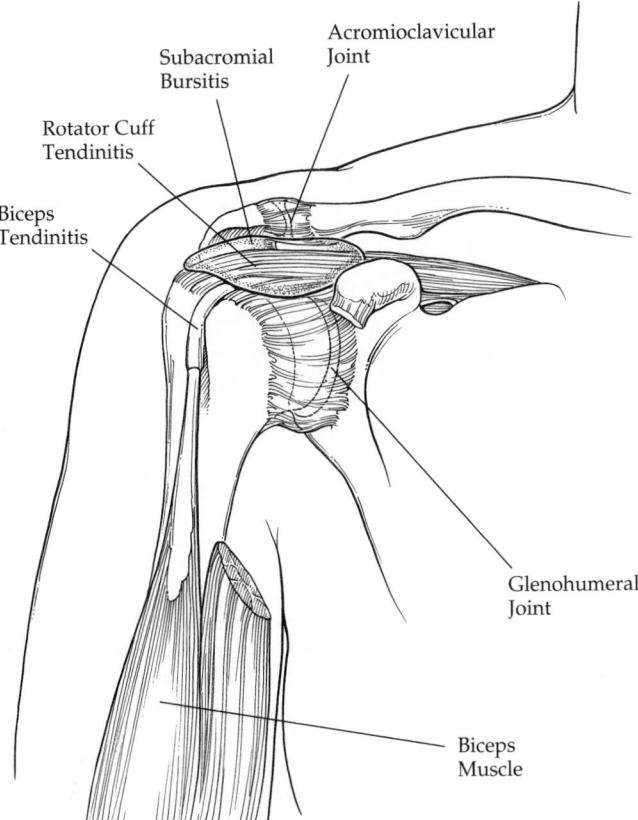

Figure 1 **Tendinitis of the rotator cuff and subacromial bursitis cause pain that is felt over the lateral aspect of the shoulder, whereas bicipital tendinitis, acromioclavicular joint disease, and glenohumeral joint disease cause anterior shoulder pain.**

Rotator cuff tendinitis is seen most commonly in patients 35 to 60 years of age and appears to be partially related to work or activities performed with the arms in highly elevated positions.[38] Younger patients may be affected as a result of athletic activities involving overhand throwing. Patients report an insidious pain that may be diffuse over the lateral deltoid or more localized to the anterior acromial region. Pain worsens with reaching and may be accompanied by a catch as the patient brings the arm into an overhead position. Rotator cuff pain is often particularly bothersome at night and interferes with sleep. On examination, pain may limit movement and may be reproduced by resistance of active movement. The so-called impingement sign is elicited by forced forward elevation of the arm with the scapula stabilized from behind. A coexistent rotator cuff tear may be suspected if the patient cannot hold the arm in a horizontal position against gravity.

The goal of therapy for rotator cuff tendinitis is to relieve pain and maintain or restore range of motion. Treatment should begin with rest and a progressive program of stretching and strengthening exercises, facilitated by an NSAID.[39] Injection of glucocorticoids and local anesthetic into the subacromial space or glenohumeral joint may result in dramatic relief of symptoms and may allow a more rapid, full recovery in some patients.[40,41] Avoidance of repetitive overhead activities of the arms is necessary during recovery, and job modification may be needed to prevent recurrence. In refractory cases, surgical division of the coracoacromial ligament or acromioplasty may be indicated.

CALCIFIC TENDINITIS

Calcific tendinitis is the cause of pain in a subset of patients with apparent rotator cuff disease. In most cases, a more chronic tendinitis is implicated, with associated deposition of calcium in the rotator cuff; calcification in the subacromial space is apparent radiographically. Patients usually have a more acutely painful condition, similar to that seen in crystal-induced arthritis. NSAIDs and local glucocorticoid injections are usually helpful, and surgery is indicated in selected cases. Ultrasound therapy has been shown to provide short-term improvement in symptoms and radiographic signs of calcification, as compared with placebo.[42]

BICIPITAL TENDINITIS

Bicipital tendinitis occurs in the region of the anterior shoulder, where the long head of the biceps tendon passes through the bicipital groove of the humerus and through the joint to insert over the glenoid cavity. Diagnosis is based on the localization of tenderness anteriorly, though this condition may coexist with rotator cuff tendinitis. Rupture of the tendon may occur occasionally, particularly in older patients, and often presents as a bulge in the biceps muscle. Treatment with local measures and range-of-motion exercises is effective, as in rotator cuff disease. Surgical repair of a ruptured tendon is indicated only in younger patients with acute rupture.

FROZEN SHOULDER (ADHESIVE CAPSULITIS)

Frozen shoulder, or adhesive capsulitis, is characterized by progressive pain and global loss of motion in the shoulder. This condition is usually seen in patients with an underlying rotator cuff tendinitis or bicipital tendinitis but has also been associated with stroke, myocardial infarction, cervical radiculopathy, and pulmonary disease. The pathophysiology of frozen shoulder is unclear, and controversy exists as to how significantly capsular inflammation or fibrosis really contributes to the loss of motion that is characteristic of the condition. Treatment is directed toward pain relief and restoration of function, often with a combination of exercises, local heat, ultrasonography, and NSAIDs or mild analgesic medications. Maximal rehabilitation of a frozen shoulder often requires 1 to 2 years. Suprascapular nerve blockade, short courses of systemic steroids, and joint distention with intra-articular steroids have been shown to provide short-term benefit in some studies.[43-45] Manipulative therapy or intra-articular steroid injections combined with physical therapy may provide improvement over longer periods.[46,47] Surgical procedures and capsular distention with saline injection have reportedly proved useful in individual cases.

MYOFASCIAL SHOULDER PAIN SYNDROME

Myofascial shoulder pain syndromes are characterized by pain over the trapezius or medial or lateral scapular borders posteriorly, with the finding of reproducible trigger points. These poorly characterized syndromes usually respond to local injection with glucocorticoids and an anesthetic, though local modalities may be needed in more chronic cases.

Chest Wall Pain

Musculoskeletal chest wall pain syndromes account for about 10% to 15% of cases in which adults are seen for chest pain in the emergency department setting, and they account for about 15% to 20% of patients who have had chest pain but whose coronary angiograms are negative.[48] The diagnosis of musculoskeletal

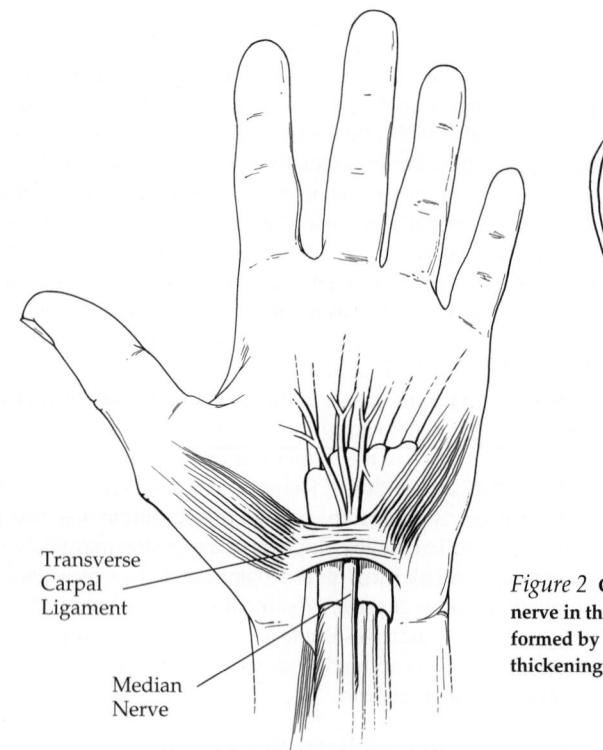

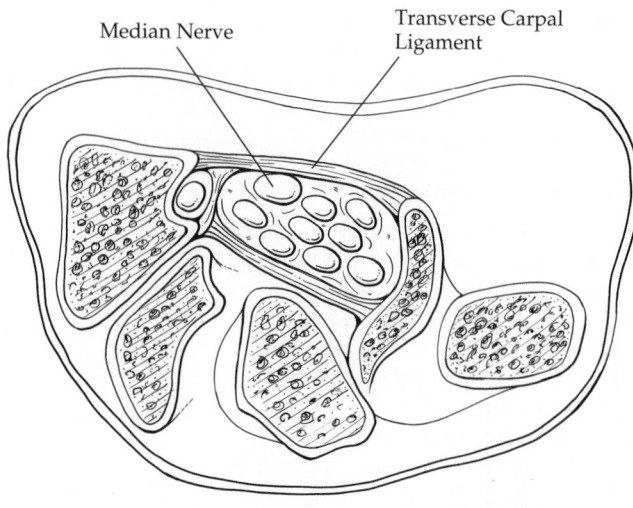

Transverse Carpal Ligament

Median Nerve

Median Nerve

Transverse Carpal Ligament

Figure 2 Carpal tunnel syndrome involves the entrapment of the median nerve in the canal that encloses the nerve and several flexor tendons and that is formed by bones of the wrist and the transverse carpal ligament. Traumatic thickening of the flexor tendon sheaths can compress the median nerve.

chest wall pain requires the finding of consistent areas of tenderness that reproduce the patient's pain. In rare cases, chest pain may result from Tietze syndrome—a benign, painful, nonsuppurative localized swelling of the costosternal, sternoclavicular, or costochondral joints, most often involving the area of the second and third ribs. In most cases, only one area is involved. Young adults are more commonly affected.

More often, patients with musculoskeletal chest wall syndromes have a more diffuse pain syndrome, termed costochondritis or costosternal syndrome, the specific etiology of which is not well understood. Areas of tenderness are not accompanied by warmth, erythema, or swelling; multiple areas of tenderness are found, usually in the upper costochondral or costosternal junctions. A number of less common chest wall syndromes have been described, each defined by the area of tenderness (e.g., xiphoidalgia, sternalis syndrome, and slipping rib syndrome). Musculoskeletal chest wall syndromes are usually self-limited and respond to analgesics, local heat, stretching exercises, and local glucocorticoid injection.

Elbow Pain

The most common nonarticular syndromes of the elbow include epicondylitis, olecranon bursitis, and ulnar nerve entrapment.

EPICONDYLITIS

Epicondylitis is caused by an inflammation at the origin of the tendons and muscles serving the forearm; it is usually caused by overuse or by repetitive activity. Patients typically complain of elbow and forearm pain with activity. When the extensor muscles are involved (i.e., tennis elbow), tenderness is maximal over the lateral epicondyle and aggravated by extension of the wrist against resistance. A similar, less common process may affect the flexor muscles originating at the medial epicondyle (i.e., golfer's elbow).

Epicondylitis usually responds to rest, local heat or ice, NSAIDs, and forearm support to reduce tension at the epicondyle. Local infiltration of glucocorticoids and lidocaine often results in more rapid improvement than other measures in the first month or two but does not appear to affect the outcome over 6 to 12 months.[49,50]

OLECRANON BURSITIS

Olecranon bursitis presents as a discrete swelling with palpable fluid over the tip of the elbow. Traumatic bursitis is characterized by minimal heat or surrounding erythema. The fluid aspirated is noninflammatory and often contains multiple red cells. Infectious bursitis—usually caused by gram-positive skin organisms—is accompanied by heat, erythema, and induration. When infection is suspected, prompt aspiration and culture of the fluid are mandatory. Antibiotics should be started empirically, and the bursa should be reaspirated frequently until the fluid no longer reaccumulates and cultures are negative.[51] Olecranon bursitis may also be part of rheumatoid arthritis or gout, usually in a patient in whom a diagnosis has already been made. On occasion, an initial diagnosis of gout is made by examination of bursal fluid for urate crystals.

ULNAR NERVE ENTRAPMENT

Ulnar nerve entrapment is caused by compression of the ulnar nerve as it passes through the ulnar groove at the elbow[52] [*see Chapter 183*]. Patients with ulnar nerve entrapment typically complain of pain and numbness that radiates from the elbow to the little finger and the medial side of the hand. An increase in paresthesia with elbow flexion is helpful in making the diagnosis, but nerve conduction studies are often needed to confirm the diagnosis. Conservative therapy with a loose cast may help limit elbow flexion and improve symptoms in some patients; surgical decompression is indicated in patients with disabling pain or weakness.

Hand and Wrist Pain

Painful conditions of the tendons and tendon sheaths of the hand and wrist are often related to repetitive or unaccustomed activities. The resultant edema, inflammation, and fibrosis of the structures interfere with the normal function of the tendon as it moves within the sheath.

DE QUERVAIN TENOSYNOVITIS AND FLEXOR TENOSYNOVITIS

De Quervain tenosynovitis affects the abductor pollicis longus and extensor pollicis brevis. Typical symptoms are pain over the radial aspect of the wrist during activities and tenderness that is usually found over the affected tendons proximal to the level of the carpometacarpal joint of the thumb. Pain is reproduced by stretching the tendons with the thumb inside a closed fist (i.e., the Finkelstein maneuver). Flexor tenosynovitis, or trigger finger, is caused by involvement of the flexor tendons of the digits, usually at the level of the metacarpophalangeal joint. Patients complain of locking of the affected digit in a flexed position, often with a sudden painful release on extension. Treatment of de Quervain tenosynovitis and flexor tenosynovitis may require rest, local heat, immobilization with a splint, or local infiltration with glucocorticoids. Surgical release is rarely required.

CARPAL TUNNEL SYNDROME

Carpal tunnel syndrome is caused by compression of the median nerve at the wrist as it courses with the flexor tendons[53] [see Figure 2 and Chapter 183]. Entrapment is usually associated with flexor tenosynovitis related to overuse, vibratory tool use, or trauma.[54] In addition, an association has been observed with cigarette smoking, body weight, and such medical conditions as diabetes mellitus, rheumatoid arthritis, pregnancy, and hypothyroidism, as well as with rare conditions such as amyloidosis, acromegaly, and localized infection.

Carpal tunnel syndrome is relatively common in the general population. A 1999 study found that 14% of the general population has symptoms suggestive of carpal tunnel syndrome; such symptoms were confirmed by clinical examination and electrophysiologic studies in 2% to 3% of the patients studied.[55] In addition, 18% of asymptomatic persons were found to have electrophysiologic evidence of median nerve entrapment. Carpal tunnel syndrome is more common in persons with occupations that require repetitive wrist movements, awkward wrist positions, or the use of vibrating tools or great force. Patients report numbness, tingling, and pain over the palmar radial aspect of the hand; these symptoms are often worse at night or after use. Reproduction of paresthesia with maximal wrist flexion (i.e., the Phalen test) or tapping over the volar aspect of the wrist (i.e., the Tinel sign) are often considered to be helpful clinical findings. However, a review of published studies suggests that the pattern of pain and findings of decreased sensation and weakness of thumb abduction are the most reliable diagnostic findings.[56] Because of the uncertainties in the reliability of diagnostic findings, electrodiagnostic testing is usually necessary to confirm a diagnosis, particularly when surgical intervention is considered.

Conservative treatment measures include use of NSAIDs and placement of a wrist splint in a neutral position. Local injection of glucocorticoids affords short-term relief in most patients, but long-term improvement is less predictable.[57,58] Surgical decompression by sectioning of the volar carpal ligament results in excellent outcome in 67% to 80% of patients; it is indicated in patients whose conditions respond poorly to conservative therapy, patients with chronic or recurrent symptoms, or patients with weakness or atrophy of the thenar muscles.[59] Predictors of less favorable surgical outcome include poor upper extremity function; alcohol use; worse mental health status; and, in workers, involvement of an attorney.[60]

DUPUYTREN CONTRACTURE

Dupuytren contracture is a fibrosing condition of the palmar and digital fascia that results in thickening and puckering of the palmar skin with subcutaneous nodules and often in flexion contracture of the underlying digit. Dupuytren contracture may be associated with other fibrosing syndromes; with an autosomal dominant inheritance pattern; and possibly with liver disease, epilepsy, and alcoholism. Although spontaneous improvement may be seen, surgical intervention to improve function may be useful in individual cases.

STIFF-HAND SYNDROME

The stiff-hand syndrome, resembling scleroderma, is characterized by thickening of the skin and subcutaneous tissues and generalized limitation of hand and wrist motion. This condition is seen almost exclusively in young patients with long-standing type 1 diabetes mellitus.[61]

Hip Girdle Pain

Pain around the hip girdle is a common complaint in clinical practice. Patients with pain resulting from diseases of the hip joint usually describe pain in the anterior thigh or inguinal region that worsens with weight bearing. More commonly, patients with a chief complaint of hip pain have a problem in one of the nonarticular structures of the hip girdle, usually located posteriorly or laterally [see Table 2]. A multitude of bursae have been described in the hip girdle region. Pain in the upper buttock in and around the gluteal muscles is often referred to as myofascial hip pain or gluteal bursitis. Pain in this area is often difficult to differentiate from referred lumbar pain. Local therapy with heat,

Table 2   Differential Diagnosis of Hip Girdle Pain

Clinical Syndrome	Location of Pain	Diagnostic Features and Comments
Acetabular joint pain	Anterior hip (inguinal)	Worse with weight bearing Radiographic confirmation
Ileopectineal bursitis	Anterior hip (inguinal)	Pain with extension Normal radiograph ? Ultrasound or CT scanning
Meralgia paresthetica	Anterior hip (midthigh)	Numbness and tingling Normal hip movement
Trochanteric bursitis	Lateral hip, posterior hip, or both	Normal hip movement Point tenderness Relief with glucocorticoid injection
Myofascial pain	Posterior hip	Localized tenderness Relief with glucocorticoid injection ? Mimics lumbar disease
Gluteal bursitis	Posterior hip	Localized tenderness Relief with glucocorticoid injection ? Mimics lumbar disease
Ischiogluteal bursitis	Posterior hip	Normal hip movement Point tenderness

stretching, or glucocorticoid injection is usually helpful, but many patients require long-term therapy.

TROCHANTERIC BURSITIS (GREATER TROCHANTERIC PAIN SYNDROME)

Trochanteric bursitis is probably the most common cause of hip girdle pain, although a study using MRI suggests that most patients with this pain syndrome may have tendinitis or a partial tear of the gluteus medius tendon.[62] Patients typically complain of pain over the lateral aspect of the hip girdle, sometimes radiating down the thigh, that is worse at night when they lie on the affected side. Pain is sometimes present when the patient arises from a chair, but it tends to improve with ambulation. Point tenderness over the lateral or posterior aspect of the greater trochanter is usually diagnostic, though some patients with referred lumbar facet or disk disease may have a similar presentation. Patients with more severe pain may have a positive Trendelenburg sign on physical examination. Local heat and NSAIDs may be helpful, and a local glucocorticoid injection is curative in most patients. In refractory cases, repeated injections, physical therapy, and, in rare instances, surgical excision of the bursa may be indicated.

ISCHIOGLUTEAL BURSITIS

Ischiogluteal bursitis results from an irritation of the bursa in the area of the attachments of the hamstring and gluteal muscles at the ischial tuberosity. The condition may be brought on by prolonged sitting or by pressure in the area and usually responds to local heat, stretching, or glucocorticoid injection.

ILIOPECTINEAL BURSITIS

Iliopectineal bursitis, which is caused by irritation of the bursa between the iliopsoas muscle and the inguinal ligament, is an uncommon cause of inguinal pain and may mimic true hip joint disease. The diagnosis is suggested by the presence of inguinal pain that is aggravated by extension of the hip (in a patient whose hip x-ray is normal). Confirmation by ultrasonography or CT scanning may be required. Treatment is usually with local measures or, in rare cases, by means of surgical excision.

MERALGIA PARESTHETICA

Meralgia paresthetica is characterized by intermittent paresthesia, hypoesthesia, or hyperesthesia over the upper anterolateral thigh. The syndrome is caused by an entrapment of the lateral femoral cutaneous nerve at the level of the anterosuperior iliac spine where the nerve passes through the lateral end of the inguinal ligament. Causes include local trauma, rapid weight gain, and the wearing of constrictive garments around the hips. Useful therapies include avoidance of pressure in the area, weight loss, and local infiltration of glucocorticoids at the level of the nerve exit.

Knee and Lower Leg Pain

Clinically, the differentiation of articular knee pain from nonarticular pain can be difficult. Most patients with articular knee pain have a relatively diffuse pain that is not well localized to one area of the knee. Physical examination shows loss of motion, crepitus (in osteoarthritis), warmth (in inflammatory arthritis), or the presence of effusion. If knee pain is localized or if the knee has full range of motion without warmth, crepitus, or effusion, one of the following nonarticular syndromes should be considered: infrapatellar tendinitis, Osgood-Schlatter disease, prepatellar bursitis, anserine bursitis, anterior knee pain syndromes, and restless legs syndrome.

INFRAPATELLAR TENDINITIS

Infrapatellar tendinitis, or jumper's knee, causes anterior knee pain below the patella and is often related to athletic activities. Tenderness is localized to the infrapatellar tendon, with no associated swelling, and conservative measures almost always result in resolution of symptoms.

OSGOOD-SCHLATTER DISEASE

Osgood-Schlatter disease is characterized by pain and swelling over the tibial tubercle at the tendon insertion point. This condition is seen predominantly in adolescent males and is thought to represent a traumatic avulsion injury. Symptoms usually resolve with temporary immobilization and slow resumption of activities.

PREPATELLAR BURSITIS

Prepatellar bursitis, or housemaid's knee, causes pain and swelling in the anterior knee superficial to the patella and infrapatellar tendon. An area of localized fluid collection is usually detectable; aspiration is often needed for diagnosis. As in olecranon bursitis of the elbow, prepatellar bursitis may be associated with trauma, localized bacterial infection, and, less commonly, gout, rheumatoid arthritis, and atypical infections. The differentiation between trauma and infection is particularly important for initiation of appropriate therapy.

ANSERINE BURSITIS

Anserine bursitis, which is caused by irritation of the bursa near the attachment of the sartorius and hamstring muscles at the medial tibial condyle, is a common cause of medial knee pain. Patients with this condition complain of pain at night or when climbing stairs, and an area of localized tenderness can be found on examination. Coexistent osteoarthritis of the knee joint is present in many patients, and relief with local heat or injection of glucocorticoids and anesthetic may be helpful both diagnostically and therapeutically.

ANTERIOR KNEE PAIN SYNDROMES

Anterior knee (patellofemoral) pain syndromes usually manifest themselves as pain and crepitus associated with activities that require knee flexion under load conditions (e.g., stair climbing). Physical findings that help with diagnosis include (1) reproduction of pain with pressure over the patella during knee motion and (2) tenderness over the medial surface of the patella. The cause of most anterior knee pain syndromes is uncertain, but the pain may be related to misalignment of the quadriceps with lateral patellar subluxation, patella alta, hypermobility, or findings of chondromalacia of the patella on arthroscopic evaluation. Local measures and an exercise program that emphasizes isometric quadriceps strengthening is helpful in most patients. Some patients require arthroscopic intervention to diagnose and correct articular irregularities or patellar misalignment.

Ankle and Foot Pain

Nonarticular foot and ankle pain is best approached with a consideration of the region affected: the forefoot, midfoot, or hindfoot [see Figure 3].

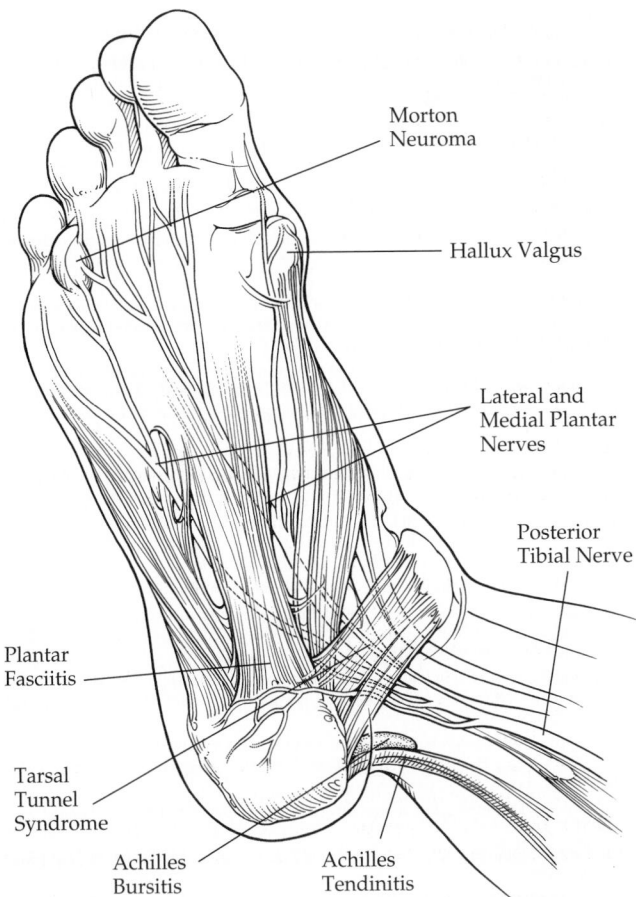

Figure 3 **In the anterior foot, hallux valgus may cause diffuse pain, whereas Morton neuroma is usually localized. Tarsal tunnel syndrome causes paresthesias over the medial and plantar aspects. Plantar fasciitis and Achilles tendinitis are common causes of posterior foot pain.**

FOREFOOT PAIN

Hallux valgus is the leading cause of forefoot pain. It is a common deformity that causes pain because of direct pressure over the first metatarsophalangeal joint resulting from footwear or because of pressure over the lateral toe joints caused by crowding of the toes. In the lateral toes, hammer toe (i.e., plantar flexion of the proximal interphalangeal joint), claw toe (i.e., plantar flexion of the proximal and distal interphalangeal joints), or mallet toe (i.e., isolated flexion contracture of the distal interphalangeal joint) may be associated with a dorsiflexion contracture of the metatarsophalangeal joint. Initial treatment of these problems should begin with adequate footwear that allows ample width for the metatarsal heads, individualized orthoses, and surgical correction (reserved for patients with persistent pain). Morton neuroma is an entrapment neuropathy of the interdigital nerve, with or without an associated plantar neuroma, that is most commonly seen between the third and fourth metatarsal heads. Patients report pain and paresthesia radiating into the affected toes; tenderness between the metatarsal heads that reproduces the described symptoms will also be found. Orthoses to decrease pressure in the area, local glucocorticoid injection, or surgical excision of the neuroma may be needed to relieve symptoms.

MIDFOOT PAIN

Midfoot pain is usually the result of deformities of the arch of the foot or arthritic changes of the midfoot joints. Patients with a cavus foot deformity, peripheral neuropathies, or previous ligamentous injuries from sprains may be predisposed to excessive stresses on the midfoot and early osteoarthritic changes. Tarsal tunnel syndrome is caused by entrapment of the posterior tibial nerve under the flexor retinaculum on the medial side of the ankle. Symptoms of pain and paresthesia over the plantar and distal foot and toes are usually present, and the Tinel sign may be positive. Tarsal tunnel syndrome is much less common and more difficult to diagnose than carpal tunnel syndrome in the wrist. Treatment consists of splinting and NSAIDs. Local glucocorticoid injection and surgical decompression are not as predictably successful as in carpal tunnel syndrome.

HINDFOOT PAIN

Plantar fasciitis is one of the most common causes of hindfoot pain, accounting for up to 15% of all foot symptoms requiring medical attention.[63] The condition is more common in runners and military personnel; other risk factors include obesity, prolonged standing, pes planus, and reduced ankle motion. Patients report pain over the plantar aspect of the heel and midfoot that worsens with walking. Although radiographic spurs in the affected area are common, they may also be seen in asymptomatic persons and are therefore not diagnostic. A majority of patients (approximately 80%) improve regardless of therapy within 12 months of onset. Orthoses, night splints, plantar and heel cord stretching exercises, NSAIDs, and local glucocorticoid injection may be helpful, but few studies have shown conclusive results with any single therapy. Surgical release may be useful for carefully selected patients with poor response to conservative measures. Posterior heel pain is usually caused by Achilles tendinitis or by bursitis of the bursae that lie superficial or deep to the insertion of the Achilles tendon at the calcaneus. Although usually associated with running and other sports activities, Achilles tendinitis may also be part of ankylosing spondylitis and Reiter syndrome and has been reported in association with fluoroquinolone therapy and treatment with systemic or local steroids.[64,65] NSAIDs and orthoses designed to reduce stress on the tendon (e.g., heel lifts) are usually helpful. In most cases, glucocorticoid injections in the Achilles tendon area should be avoided because of the risk of tendon rupture.

The author has no commercial relationships with manufacturers of products or providers of services discussed in this chapter.

References

1. Sheon RP, Moskowitz RW, Goldberg VM: Soft Tissue Rheumatic Pain: Recognition, Management, Prevention, 3rd ed. Lea & Febiger, Philadelphia, 1996

2. Posner J, Glew C: Neck pain. Ann Intern Med 136:758, 2002

3. Eck JC, Hodges SD, Humphreys SC: Whiplash: a review of a commonly misunderstood injury. Am J Med 110:651, 2001

4. Cassidy JD, Carroll LJ, Cote P, et al: Effect of eliminating compensation for pain and suffering on the outcome of insurance claims for whiplash injury. N Engl J Med 342:1179, 2000

5. Hoving JL, Koes BW, de Vet HC, et al: Manual therapy, physical therapy, or continued care by a general practitioner for patients with neck pain: a randomized, controlled trial. Ann Intern Med 136:713, 2002

6. Ylinen J, Takala EP, Nykanene M, et al: Active neck training in the treatment of chronic neck pain in women: a randomized controlled trial. JAMA 289: 2509, 2003

7. White P, Lewith G, Prescott P, et al: Acupuncture versus placebo for the treatment of chronic mechanical neck pain: a randomized, controlled trial. Ann Intern Med 141:911, 2004

8. Deyo RA, Weinstein JN: Low back pain. N Engl J Med 344:363, 2001

9. Carragee EJ: Clinical practice: persistent low back pain. N Engl J Med 352:1891, 2005

10. Manek N: Epidemiology of back disorders: prevalence, risk factors, and prognosis. Curr Opin Rheumatol 17:134, 2005

11. Coste J, Lefrancois G, Guillemin F, et al: Prognosis and quality of life in patients with acute low back pain: insights from a comprehensive inception cohort study. Arthritis Rheum 51:168, 2004

12. Carragee EJ, Alamin TF, Miller JL, et al: Discographic, MRI, and psychosocial determinants of low back pain disability and remission: a prospective study in subjects with benign persistent back pain. Spine J 5:24, 2005

13. Jarvik JG, Deyo RA: Diagnostic evaluation of low back pain with emphasis on imaging. Ann Intern Med 137:586, 2002

14. Jarvik JG, Hollingsworth W, Martin B, et al: Rapid magnetic resonance imaging vs radiographs for patients with low back pain: a randomized controlled trial. JAMA 289:2810, 2003

15. Gilbert FJ, Grant AM, Gillan MG, et al: Low back pain: influence of early MRI imaging or CT on treatment and outcome—a multicenter randomized trial. Radiology 231:343, 2004

16. van Tulder MW, Touray T, Furlan AD, et al: Muscle relaxants for nonspecific low back pain: a systematic review within the framework of the Cochrane collaboration. Spine 28:1978, 2003

17. Assendelft WJ, Morton SC, Yu EI, et al: Spinal manipulative therapy for low back pain: a meta-analysis of effectiveness relative to other therapies. Ann Intern Med 138:871, 2003

18. Cherkin DC, Sherman KJ, Deyo RA, et al: A review of the evidence for the effectiveness, safety, and cost of acupuncture, massage therapy, and spinal manipulation for back pain. Ann Intern Med 138:898, 2003

19. Hayden JA, van Tulder MW, Malmivaara AV, et al: Meta-analysis: exercise therapy for nonspecific low back pain. Ann Intern Med 142:765, 2005

20. Staal JB, Hlobil H, Twisk JW, et al: Graded activity for low back pain in occupational health care: a randomized, controlled trial. Ann Intern Med 140:77, 2004

21. Damush TM, Weinberger M, Perkins SM, et al: The long-term effects of a self-management program for inner-city primary care patients with acute low back pain. Arch Intern Med 163:2632, 2003

22. Kjaer P, Leboeuf-Yde C, Korsholm L, et al: Magnetic resonance imaging and low back pain in adults: a diagnostic imaging study of 40-year-old men and women. Spine 30:1173, 2005

23. Hayden JA, van Tulder MW, Tomlinson G: Systematic review: strategies for using exercise therapy to improve outcomes in low back pain. Ann Intern Med 142:776, 2005

24. Niemisto L, Lahtinen-Suopanki T, Rissanen P, et al: A randomized trial of combined manipulation, stabilizing exercises, and physician consultation compared to physician consultation alone for chronic low back pain. Spine 28:2185, 2003

25. Schonstein E, Kenny DT, Keating J, et al: Work conditioning, work hardening, and functional restoration for workers with back and neck pain. Cochrane Database Syst Rev (1):CD001822, 2003

26. Ostelo R, Tulder M, Vlaeyen J, et al: Behavioural treatment for chronic low back pain. Cochrane Database Syst Rev (1):CD002014, 2005

27. Kovacs FM, Abraira V, Pena A, et al: Effect of firmness of mattress on chronic non-specific low-back pain: randomized, double-blind, controlled, multicentre trial. Lancet 362:1599, 2003

28. Salerno SM, Browning R, Jackson JL: The effect of antidepressant treatment on chronic back pain: a meta-analysis. Arch Intern Med 162:19, 2002

29. Khot A, Bowditch M, Powell J, et al: The use of intradiscal steroid therapy for lumbar spinal discogenic pain: a randomized controlled trial. Spine 29:833, 2004

30. Yelland MJ, Del Mar C, Pirozzo S, et al: Prolotherapy injections for chronic low back pain: a systematic review. Spine 29:2126, 2004

31. Manheimer E, White A, Berman B, et al: Meta-analysis: acupuncture for low back pain. Ann Intern Med 142:651, 2005

32. Arbit E, Pannullo S: Lumbar stenosis: a clinical review. Clin Orthop 384:137, 2001

33. Saint-Louis LA: Lumbar spinal stenosis assessment with computed tomography, magnetic resonance imaging, and myelography. Clin Orthop 384:122, 2001

34. Amundsen T, Weber H, Nordal HJ, et al: Lumbar spinal stenosis: conservative or surgical management? A prospective 10-year study. Spine 25:1424, 2000

35. Atlas SJ, Keller RB, Wu YA, et al: Long-term outcomes of surgical and nonsurgical management of lumbar spinal stenosis: 8 to 10 year results from the Maine lumbar spine study. Spine 30:936, 2005

36. Deyo R, Nachemson A, Mirza SK: Spinal-fusion surgery—the case for restraint. N Engl J Med 350:722, 2004

37. Gomoli AH, Katz JN, Warner JJ, et al: Rotator cuff disorders: recognition and management among patients with shoulder pain. Arthritis Rheum 50:3751, 2004

38. Svendsen SW, Gelineck J, Mathiassen SE, et al: Work above shoulder level and degenerative alterations of the rotator cuff tendons: a magnetic resonance imaging study. Arthritis Rheum 50:3314, 2004

39. Hay EM, Thomas E, Paterson SM, et al: A pragmatic randomized controlled trial of local corticosteroid injection and physiotherapy for the treatment of new episodes of unilateral shoulder pain in primary care. Ann Rheum Dis 62:394, 2003

40. Green S, Buchbinder R, Glazier R, et al: Systematic review of randomised controlled trials of interventions for painful shoulder: selection criteria, outcome assessment, and efficacy. BMJ 316:354, 1998

41. van der Windt DA, Koes BW, Deville W, et al: Effectiveness of corticosteroid injections versus physiotherapy for treatment of painful stiff shoulder in primary care: randomised trial. BMJ 317:1292, 1998

42. Ebenbichler GR, Erdogmus CB, Resch KL, et al: Ultrasound therapy for calcific tendinitis of the shoulder. N Engl J Med 340:1533, 1999

43. Dahan TH, Fortin L, Pelletier M, et al: Double blind randomized clinical trial examining the efficacy of bupivacaine suprascapular nerve blocks in frozen shoulder. J Rheumatol 27:1464, 2000

44. Buchbinder R, Hoving JL, Green S, et al: Short course prednisolone for adhesive capsulitis (frozen shoulder or stiff painful shoulder): a randomized, double blind, placebo controlled trial. Ann Rheum Dis 63:1460, 2004

45. Buchbinder R, Green S, Forbes A, et al: Arthrographic joint distension with saline and steroid improves function and reduces pain in patients with painful stiff shoulder: results of a randomized, double blind, placebo controlled trial. Ann Rheum Dis 63:302, 2004

46. Bergman GJ, Winters JC, Groenier KH, et al: Manipulative therapy in addition to usual medical care for patients with shoulder dysfunction and pain: a randomized, controlled trial. Ann Intern Med 141:432, 2004

47. Carette S, Moffet H, Tardif J, et al: Intraarticular corticosteroids, supervised physiotherapy, or a combination of the two in the treatment of adhesive capsulitis of the shoulder: a placebo-controlled trial. Arthritis Rheum 48:829, 2003

48. Wise CM: Chest wall syndromes. Curr Opin Rheumatol 6:197, 1994

49. Hay EM, Paterson SM, Lewis M, et al: Pragmatic randomised controlled trial of local corticosteroid injection and naproxen for treatment of lateral epicondylitis of elbow in primary care. BMF 319:964, 1999

50. Smidt N, van der Windt DA, Assendelft WJ, et al: Corticosteroid injections, physiotherapy, or a wait-and-see policy for lateral epicondylitis: a randomised controlled trial. Lancet 359:657, 2002

51. Laupland KB, Davies HD: Olecranon septic bursitis managed in an ambulatory setting. The Calgary Home Parenteral Therapy Program Study Group. Clin Invest Med 24:171, 2001

52. Dawson D: Entrapment neuropathies of the upper extremities. N Engl J Med 329:2013, 1993

53. Katz JN, Simmons BP: Clinical practice. Carpal tunnel syndrome. N Engl J Med 346:1807, 2002

54. Nathan PA, Meadows KD, Istvan JA: Predictors of carpal tunnel syndrome: an 11-year study of industrial workers. J Hand Surg (Am) 27:644, 2002

55. Atroshi I, Gummesson C, Johnsson R, et al: Prevalence of carpal tunnel syndrome in a general population. JAMA 282:153, 1999

56. D'Arcy CA, McGee S: The rational clinical examination: does this patient have carpal tunnel syndrome? JAMA 283:3110, 2000

57. O'Gardaigh D, Merry P: Corticosteroid injection for the treatment of carpal tunnel syndrome. Ann Rheum Dis 59:918, 2000

58. Gerritsen AA, de Vet HC, Scholten RJ, et al: Splinting vs surgery in the treatment of carpal tunnel syndrome: a randomized controlled trial. JAMA 288:1245, 2002

59. Ly-Pen D, Andreu JL, deBlas G, et al: Surgical decompression versus local steroid injection in the carpal tunnel syndrome: a one-year, prospective, randomized, open, controlled clinical trial. Arthritis Rheum 52:612, 2005

60. Katz JN, Losina E, Amick BC 3rd, et al: Predictors of outcomes of carpal tunnel release. Arthritis Rheum 44:1184, 2001

61. Jacobs-Kosmin D, DeHoratius RJ: Musculoskeletal manifestations of endocrine disorders. Curr Opin Rheumatol 17:64, 2005

62. Bird PA, Oakley SP, Shnier R, et al: Prospective evaluation of magnetic resonance imaging and physical examination findings in patients with greater trochanteric pain syndrome. Arthritis Rheum 44:2138, 2001

63. Buchbinder R: Clinical practice. Plantar fasciitis. N Engl J Med 350:2159, 2004

64. Paavola M, Kannus P, Jarvinen TA, et al: Achilles tendinopathy. J Bone Joint Surg Am 84:2062, 2002

65. van der Linden PD, Sturkenboom CJM, Herings RMC, et al: Increased risk of Achilles tendon rupture with quinolone antibacterial use, especially in elderly patients taking oral corticosteroids. Arch Intern Med 163:1801, 2003

Acknowledgments

Figures 1 and 3   Susan E. Brust, C.M.I.

Figure 2   Lynn O'Kelley.

121 Fibromyalgia

John Buckner Winfield, M.D.

Definition

Fibromyalgia is a chronic syndrome that occurs predominantly in women and is marked by generalized pain, multiple defined tender points [*see Figure 1*],[1] fatigue, disturbed and nonrestorative sleep, and numerous other somatic complaints. It is not a discrete disease; rather, it lies at the far end of a continuum of psychological distress and chronic pain in the general population. Fibromyalgia largely overlaps with other syndromes, such as chronic fatigue syndrome, irritable bowel syndrome, temporomandibular joint pain, and multiple other regional pain syndromes, all of which feature symptoms that remain unexplained after usual clinical and laboratory assessment and all of which are related to, but not fully dependent on, depression and anxiety.[2] Fibromyalgia frequently coexists with diseases of structurally defined pathology, such as systemic lupus erythematosus (SLE) or rheumatoid arthritis.

Fibromyalgia has been classified as one of a group of disorders that are variously termed symptom-based conditions,[3] functional somatic syndromes,[4] and affective spectrum disorders.[5] Common somatic symptoms in these illnesses are chronic musculoskeletal or abdominal pain, persistent fatigue, disturbed sleep, and cognitive difficulty.[6] Advances in the understanding of the psychophysiologic and neurophysiologic dysregulation in such illnesses is impelling researchers to develop a unifying reclassification of these illnesses as central sensitivity syndromes.[7]

There appear to be discrete subgroups of patients with fibromyalgia vis-à-vis pain sensitivity and psychological factors.[8,9] These subgroups vary in response to therapy and in prognosis.[10]

Epidemiology

Otherwise unexplained widespread pain occurs in about 10% of the general adult population in Western countries, with approximately half of those affected—mostly women—meeting American College of Rheumatology (ACR) classification criteria for fibromyalgia.[11]

Fibromyalgia becomes more common after 60 years of age but occurs not infrequently in children. On a typical day, primary care physicians should expect to interact with several patients with fibromyalgia, many of whom will be seeking care for illness other than fibromyalgia. For example, more than 25% of patients with SLE exhibit painful tender points and other clinical and psychological features of fibromyalgia.

Etiology

The cause of fibromyalgia is unknown. Despite extensive research, no structural pathology has been identified in muscles or other tissues. Although psychological factors associated with chronic distress appear to be important for the development of fibromyalgia in many patients,[12] abundant evidence now indicates that pain in fibromyalgia reflects abnormal pain processing in the central nervous system (i.e., central sensitivity). Clinically, fibromyalgia syndrome is best viewed from a biopsychosocial perspective encompassing multiple variables that contribute to chronic pain and fatigue.

BIOPSYCHOSOCIAL MODEL

At one level, the pain and associated symptoms of fibromyalgia can be viewed according to the Engel biopsychosocial model[13] of chronic illness: health status and outcomes are influenced by the interaction of biologic, psychological, and sociologic variables. Important biologic variables are genetics, gender, sleep, physical condition, stress-related neuroendocrine and autonomic dysregulation, and central sensitization to pain. Psychological (cognitive-behavioral) variables contributing to the chronic pain and fatigue of fibromyalgia include pain beliefs and attributions, mood, depression, anxiety, personality traits and disorders, pain behaviors, hypervigilance, coping strategies, and perceived self-efficacy for pain control. Sociologic (environmental and sociocultural) variables consist of experiences influenced by life and culture that have impact on the course of chronic pain and fatigue, such as psychosocial experiences during childhood, family support, work environment, job satisfaction, and ethnological factors.

Biologic Variables

Genetics Although genetic analyses of community-based populations[14] and twins[15] suggest that somatic symptoms, such as pain and fatigue, are etiologically distinct from symptoms of anxiety and depression, a large family study has established that fibromyalgia and reduced pressure-pain threshold coaggregate with major mood disorder (i.e., major depressive disorder and bipolar disorder).[16] This finding is consistent with the idea that fibromyalgia and major mood disorders share, in part, genetic factors that contribute to the development of these illnesses. One candidate is the short (S) allele of the promoter region of the serotonin transporter gene *5-HTT*, which has been associated with depression and suicidality in response to stressful life events.[17] A higher frequency of the S/S genotype has been reported in patients with fibromyalgia than in healthy control subjects,[18] but an association with *5-HTT* or its alleles is not evident in patients who have fibromyalgia without accompanying depression and psychological distress. Of special interest is the identification of three haplotypes of the gene encoding catechol *O*-methyltransferase—designated low pain sensitivity (LPS), average pain sensitivity (APS), and high pain sensitivity (HPS)—that are strongly associated with variation in the sensitivity to experimental pain and the risk of developing temporomandibular joint disorder, a chronic pain condition closely associated with fibromyalgia.[19] Other susceptibility genes undoubtedly will be discovered in the near future.

Female gender In general, females exhibit higher pain sensitivity than males and are at greater risk for many pain conditions.[20] Central pain-modulatory systems and inflammatory cytokine levels in females are influenced by phasic alterations in reproductive hormone levels; and females and fibromyalgia patients appear to lack certain pain-inhibitory mechanisms that are found in normal males.[21] Stressful or aversive stimuli evoke greater sympathetic nervous system, neuroendocrine, and psychological responses in females than in males. Reporting of unexplained symptoms, independent of psychiatric morbidity, also is more common in females.[22] Certain data suggest that the neural circuits activated by emotional experiences and those involved in encoding of emotional experiences into memory show much more overlap in females than in males.[23] Together with the higher prevalence of abuse in women, these biologic variables may explain, at least in part, the increased susceptibility to fibromyalgia in women.

Sleep disturbance Poor sleep is almost universal in fibromyalgia patients, but fibromyalgia is not primarily a sleep disorder, as had been thought. Pain interferes with sleep, and disturbances in sleep contribute to the experience of pain.[24] In turn, nonrestful sleep and pain underlie the experience of fatigue.

Psychological distress and the stress response system The number of painful tender points in patients with fibromyalgia correlates strongly with patients' levels of psychological distress.[25] Much evidence suggests that there is an association between chronic, unrelieved psychological stress/distress and functional alterations of the stress-response system (the autonomic nervous system and hypothalamic-pituitary-adrenocortical [HPA] axis), which, in turn, contributes to symptoms of anxiety, pain, and fatigue.[26-28] It is unclear, however, whether abnormalities in the stress-response system reflect preexisting vulnerability to fibromyalgia or are a consequence of chronic pain and fatigue.

External triggers Fibromyalgia patients often have fixed beliefs that minor traumatic events, pathogens, chemicals, or other physical agents caused their illness. The available evidence does not support any of those factors as causes, and furthermore, such beliefs can be a barrier to recovery.

Psychological Variables

Cognitive-behavioral variables play a central role in the development and maintenance of persistent pain and functional disability, and psychiatric conditions—especially depression, anxiety, posttraumatic stress disorder (PTSD), and personality disorders—are prevalent in fibromyalgia patients. For example, negative emotions (e.g., depression and anxiety), other negative psychological factors (e.g., loss of control and unpredictability in one's environment), and certain cognitive aspects (e.g., negative beliefs and attributions and catastrophic interpretation of events) can lower pain thresholds and tolerances.[29] Pain behaviors are the actions or expressions by which an individual communicates feelings of pain to the outside world. The response of the outside world (e.g., spouse, physician, or employer) then positively or negatively reinforces the pain experience.

Environmental and Sociocultural Variables

Multiple experiences related to forces in the environment, life, and culture can influence the course of chronic pain and fatigue. These influences can be either positive (e.g., good job satisfaction in a patient with work-related back strain) or negative (e.g., a physician's suggestion that a minor traffic accident may have left the patient with long-term damage). In the United States, negative sociocultural elements include the promotion of fear and suggestibility by the media and by society in general, as well as focus on definable causes by patients, physicians, and attorneys. Adverse experiences during childhood, such as poor family environment or childhood sexual abuse, increase susceptibility to the development of chronic pain in adulthood.[30]

Pathophysiology

There are four principal categories of pain: nociceptive, neuropathic, psychogenic, and chronic pain of complex etiology. Noci-

ceptive pain involves stimulation of peripheral pain receptors during inflammation, injury, or destruction of tissues, and it is characterized by a pain experience that corresponds with the noxious stimulus. Neuropathic pain results from direct injury to nerves, such as the radiculopathic pain of degenerative spondylosis. Psychogenic pain occurs in more strictly psychiatric illness, such as somatization disorder or hysteria. Chronic pain of complex etiology is the type of pain characteristic of fibromyalgia and other central sensitivity syndromes. Shared manifestations are allodynia (pain with stimuli that should not be painful), hyperalgesia, spread of pain, unpleasant sensations after a physical stimulus, and chronicity.

Although chronic pain of complex etiology is as yet incompletely understood, characteristic changes have been observed with functional magnetic resonance imaging of the brain performed during the application of painful pressure in fibromyalgia patients,[31] and many of the biologic elements operant in fibromyalgia and other central sensitivity syndromes have been identified.[32] Such elements include discrete abnormalities in pronociception and antinociception pathways (e.g., increased levels of inflammatory cytokines; decreased availability of serotonin, norepinephrine, and enkephalins; increased levels of substance P in the cerebrospinal fluid; deficiency of biogenic amines that normally regulate the release of substance P; glial activation[33]; and decreased levels of somatomedin C), intrusion of alpha waves into the brain's electrical field during restorative stage 3 and stage 4 non–random eye movement sleep, and dysregulation of the stress response system. Dysregulation of stress response may manifest itself as neurally mediated hypotension, hypofunctional sympathetic reflex response to stressors, or abnormalities of the HPA axis and other neuroendocrine axes, such as growth hormone secretion in response to exercise.

Diagnosis

CLINICAL MANIFESTATIONS

Pain is the hallmark of fibromyalgia. The pain radiates diffusely from the axial skeleton and is localized to muscles and muscle-tendon junctions of the neck, shoulders, hips, and extremities. Fibromyalgia patients describe the pain with such terms as exhausting, miserable, or unbearable. Generalized hyperalgesia is a cardinal feature. Patients frequently complain that even gentle touch is unpleasant, a manifestation of allodynia.

In addition to their persistent widespread pain, fibromyalgia patients experience severe fatigue, insomnia, and low mood or depression [see Table 1]. Fatigue occurring most times of the day on most days, together with subjective weakness and nonrestorative sleep, is almost universal. Cognitive complaints, such as difficulties with concentration and memory, may be prominent. Depression, anxiety disorders, and personality disorders contribute to ongoing psychological distress. Other complaints result from somatization, which can be defined as translating psychological distress into somatic symptoms (which are considered more socially acceptable) and seeking care for those symptoms.

Patients with fibromyalgia have a strong tendency toward external attribution of symptoms, with fixed beliefs that minor trauma, viruses (e.g., Epstein-Barr), *Candida*, mold (e.g., so-called black mold), toxic chemicals, or other physical agents (e.g., silicone breast implants) caused their illness. This can be a barrier to recovery, as can ongoing litigation regarding causation of fibromyalgia, disability-determination proceedings, or workers' compensation claims.

Functional impairment is usually present, at least in patients with fibromyalgia who seek care. Patients report difficulty doing usual activities of daily living and lack of exercise—indeed, they actually fear and avoid exercise.

Regional pain syndromes, such as headache, temporomandibular joint disorder, or irritable bowel syndrome, are often present in fibromyalgia patients. It is essential that the physician not automatically attribute all such symptoms to fibromyalgia, however, because fibromyalgia frequently coexists with other disorders of defined structural pathology, such as SLE and rheumatoid arthritis. Optimum therapy requires recognition of both fibromyalgia and comorbid disease.

In taking the patient history, the physician should inquire about sleep quality, ongoing and past stressors, and feelings of anxiety or depression. Recognition of difficulties in these areas is essential in the overall management of chronic pain and fatigue. Onset of fibromyalgia usually antedates clinical diagnosis by years. Exploration of life events surrounding the onset often reveals major stressors, such as breakup of marriage, loss of job, or bankruptcy. The open-ended question "During your childhood, did you have any bad experiences, such as physical, emotional, or sexual abuse?" not infrequently leads to a catharsis of a significant psychological burden. Current research on the biology of emotion suggests that traumatic experiences during childhood, a period when the brain is still developing, profoundly shape emotions and the subsequent development of functional somatic pain in adulthood. The consequences of abuse are not limited to children; adult domestic violence is an important antecedent of fibromyalgia.[34]

It is valuable to ask whether the patient has previously sought treatment for manifestations of fibromyalgia. Discussion of what treatments have been prescribed and how the patient responded can guide the physician in developing a therapeutic plan. Dependency on opioids and unsuccessful prior referrals to multidisciplinary pain centers suggest a poor prognosis. Fibromyalgia patients are especially likely to use complementary and alternative medicine (CAM), in large part because of disappointing prior encounters with practitioners of traditional medicine. Because some CAM agents are not safe and many have the potential to interact with conventional pharmacologic agents, questions about CAM use are an important part of the history.

PHYSICAL EXAMINATION FINDINGS

A patient with uncomplicated fibromyalgia will have normal results on general physical examination. This reassures both the physician and the patient that a significant alternative cause for the symptoms is unlikely. Evidence of synovitis (i.e., joint effusion, warmth over a joint, and pain on joint motion), objective muscle weakness, or other definite physical or neurologic signs suggests the presence of either comorbid disease or an alternative diagnosis. It is essential to identify concomitant painful diseases such as osteoarthritis of individual joints, degenerative spondylosis, bursitis, or other inflammatory soft tissue conditions, because the nociceptive pain from such common problems is amplified in fibromyalgia. Many patients exhibit signs of regional pain syndromes that are often associated with depression or anxiety, such as tenderness in the jaw area (e.g., temporomandibular joint disorder), subtle lower abdominal tenderness to palpation (e.g., irritable bowel syndrome), psychomotor slowing (e.g., depression), and irritability or hostility (e.g., anxiety, panic disorder, or personality disorder).

Tender Points

Eighteen specific tender points have been identified as a component of the ACR classification criteria for fibromyalgia [see Figure 1].[1] A patient with fibromyalgia will have pain, not just tenderness, on palpation at many of these tender points. Palpation is performed with the thumb, using approximately 4 kg of pressure—about the pressure necessary to blanch the examiner's thumbnail. These tender points represent classification criteria, not diagnostic criteria; attempting to confirm pain at all 18 points is not necessary for diagnosis and may be uncomfortable for patients, who find tender-point palpation quite distressing. An algometer can provide semiquantitative information regarding pressure pain threshold at tender points. Some fibromyalgia patients complain of pain when pressure is applied anywhere on the body, even relatively insensitive areas such as the forehead or thumbnail. Unfortunately, in situations of potential secondary gain (e.g., injury litigation and pending disability determination), the physician must be alert for malingering; some of these patients are well informed regarding the location of tender points. Firm pressure over the trapezii or posterior thorax with a stethoscope, rather than a thumb, can provide insight in such cases.

LABORATORY TESTS

There are no specific laboratory test abnormalities in fibromyalgia. Nevertheless, it is appropriate to conduct limited screening for commonly associated disorders and for other diseases that can cause pain and fatigue.

Blood Tests

Useful tests in fibromyalgia include the following: antinuclear antibody (ANA), complete blood count, erythrocyte sedimentation rate (ESR) or C-reactive protein, thyroid-stimulating hormone (TSH), creatine kinase (CK), aspartate aminotransferase, and alanine aminotransferase. Tests for Lyme disease, Epstein-Barr virus infection, and endocrinologic status (e.g., measure-

Table 1 Symptoms of Fibromyalgia Syndrome[55]

Musculoskeletal	Pain at multiple sites Stiffness "Hurt all over" Swollen feeling in soft tissues
Nonmusculoskeletal	Fatigue (most times of the day) Morning fatigue (symptom of nonrestorative sleep) Poor sleep Paresthesias
Associated symptoms	Self-assessed anxiety Headaches Dysmenorrhea Irritable bowel syndrome Self-assessed depression Restless legs syndrome Sicca symptoms Raynaud phenomenon Female urethral syndrome

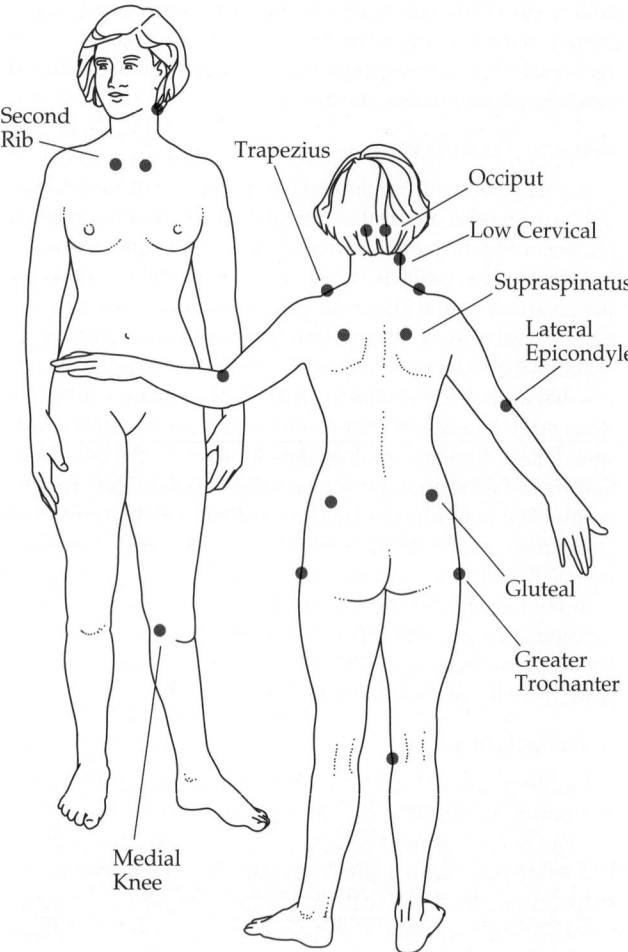

Figure 1   **Tender points in fibromyalgia.**

Labels on figure: Second Rib, Trapezius, Occiput, Low Cervical, Supraspinatus, Lateral Epicondyle, Gluteal, Greater Trochanter, Medial Knee

• Spondyloarthropathy (morning back pain and stiffness, asymmetrical oligoarthritis, sacroiliitis on pelvic x-rays).
• Inflammatory myopathy (muscle tenderness, objective proximal muscle weakness, elevated serum CK).
• Hypothyroidism (myalgias, weight gain, dry skin, fatigue, cold sensitivity, hyporeflexia, elevated TSH level).
• Osteomalacia (diffuse bone pain and tenderness, proximal myopathy with weakness, low serum phosphate and 25-hydroxyvitamin D levels).
• Hemochromatosis (diffuse arthralgias and myalgias are unusual presentations of hemochromatosis, but screening for this disorder with a serum transferrin saturation and a serum ferritin concentration might be considered in patients 40 to 60 years of age, especially if they have small-joint arthropathy in the hands, calcium pyrophosphate dihydrate deposition disease, or both).

It usually is not helpful clinically to distinguish fibromyalgia from chronic fatigue syndrome or the many regional pain syndromes. Giving patients a name for their illness, however, often enables them to concentrate on getting better, rather than continuously searching for a cause and cure.

Treatment

Four principles govern the treatment of fibromyalgia: (1) validation of distress, (2) diagnostic and therapeutic conservatism, (3) an individualized combination of pharmacologic and nonpharmacologic measures, and (4) care rather than cure. Validation of the patient's symptoms and distress begins with the initial history and physical examination, when the physician explores adverse developmental, social, and behavioral variables and past and current stressors. Failure to provide validation, initially or later in the therapeutic relationship, serves only to perpetuate pain and fatigue and may constitute an insurmountable barrier to treatment.

Strong evidence for therapeutic efficacy in fibromyalgia on the basis of randomized, controlled trials has been difficult to obtain. Confounding factors include the incomplete understanding of the syndrome's origin and pathophysiology, the complexity of its symptoms, lack of consensus regarding nosology and clinically meaningful outcome measures, small sample size, short trial duration, and a strong placebo effect because of the close attention patients receive in trials. Much current treatment is empirical and based on proposed, rather than established, models of pathophysiology. Nevertheless, a wealth of published information on treatment of fibromyalgia is now available, including two monographs[35,36] and a series of systematic reviews and meta-analyses of controlled trials.[37-39] Clinical practice guidelines have been developed by the American Pain Society.[40] The available data suggest that the pain, fatigue, nonrestorative sleep, depression, and anxiety respond to a multifaceted therapeutic approach that combines drug therapy with physical, psychological, and behavioral treatments. An overarching goal of therapy is the promotion of self-efficacy—the patient's firmly held belief that he or she can control symptoms of pain and fatigue.

TREATMENT IN GERIATRIC AND PEDIATRIC CASES

Treatment of diffuse pain in older persons[41] and in children[42] requires special approaches. Pain in older persons is often neglected or ignored. Compared with younger persons, older persons exhibit more physical abnormalities, are more sensitive to opioids,

ment of estrogen, testosterone, growth hormone, and dehydroepiandrosterone) are usually unnecessary.

Other Tests

Urinalysis may be useful. Tests for autonomic dysfunction (tilt-table test), studies of nerve conduction velocity and electromyography, and imaging studies should not be done unless there is a specific indication.

Differential Diagnosis

The differential diagnosis of fibromyalgia is very broad [*see Table 2*]. Nevertheless, extensive laboratory testing or imaging studies should not be done unless the patient has objective indications of other disease on physical or neurologic examination. Major causes of diffuse musculoskeletal pain and key clinical and laboratory features are as follows:

• Fibromyalgia (diffuse pain, tenderness, fatigue, stiffness, tender points, normal laboratory findings).
• Rheumatoid arthritis (symmetrical synovitis, presence of rheumatoid factor, elevated ESR and C-reactive protein).
• SLE (constitutional symptoms, rash, arthralgias, presence of ANA and other autoantibodies).
• Polymyalgia rheumatica (age greater than 50 years, shoulder and hip girdle pain, very high ESR).

Table 2 Differential Diagnosis of Fibromyalgia

Major Disorder Group	Selected Specific Disorders
Rheumatologic	Systemic lupus erythematosus* Rheumatoid arthritis, Sjögren syndrome* Polyarticular osteoarthritis, degenerative spondylosis Polymyalgia rheumatica* Polymyositis, statin myopathy Regional pain syndromes* Hypermobility syndromes Spondyloarthropathy
Neurologic	Carpal tunnel syndrome* Cervical radiculopathy* Metabolic myopathies Multiple sclerosis* Cervical cord compression
Chronic infection	Subacute bacterial endocarditis Brucellosis Hepatitis HIV
Endocrine	Hypothyroidism* Diabetes mellitus type 2 Hyperparathyroidism Osteomalacia Hemochromatosis
Neoplastic	Metastatic (e.g., breast, lung, prostate) Myeloma
Psychiatric	Pain disorder associated with psychological factors* (formerly, somatoform pain disorder) Somatization disorder (hysteria, Briquette syndrome)

*Common alternative diagnosis.

have lower self-efficacy, and use fewer cognitive coping methods. There are many barriers to accurate pain assessment in older persons, including fear of diagnostic tests or medications and reluctance to report pain because pain is an expected part of aging.

The general principles of treatment in the elderly are as follows: discuss goals, hopes, and trade-offs openly; start medications at a low dose and raise the dose slowly; pay attention to timing of medications; be aware of economic barriers; include nonpharmacologic treatment as an integral part of management; and educate the patient and caregiver.

In the pediatric population, unexplained diffuse or localized pain is most common in preadolescent to adolescent girls, often in association with incongruent affect, with disproportionate impairment of performance in school, and with psychological distress in the patient, the family, or both. Key aspects of therapy in this population are discontinuance of all medications, psychological evaluation and psychotherapy if necessary, and a program of intense exercise. Prognosis is good for most children with persistent unexplained pain.

PHARMACOLOGIC MANAGEMENT

Diffuse Pain

A well-established conventional approach to initial therapy for fibromyalgia is the use of a tricyclic antidepressant (TCA) at bedtime. Amitriptyline, starting at 10 mg and escalating slowly to 50 mg, is a common choice. In approximately one third of fibromyalgia patients, low doses of amitriptyline produce moderate short-term improvements in pain, disturbed sleep, patient and physician global assessments, physical status, psychological status, and capacity for activities of daily living. Improvements in fatigue, tenderness, and stiffness are more modest. Long-term improvement with TCAs has not been shown to be better than that with placebo, however, and patient acceptance of TCAs is poor because of their anticholinergic and sedative effects and their tendency to cause weight gain. The selective serotonin reuptake inhibitors (SSRIs) fluoxetine[43] and citalopram have proved to be effective in randomized, controlled trials, and the combination of a TCA with an SSRI typically produces greater improvement in pain, sleep, and overall well-being than either drug used alone. Dual-action (i.e., serotonin and noradrenaline) reuptake inhibitors (SNRIs), such as venlafaxine (started at 37.5 mg daily and increased every 4 days to a maximum of 150 to 225 mg daily) and duloxetine (30 to 60 mg daily),[44] have been shown to improve many symptoms in fibromyalgia patients irrespective of comorbid depression. When prescribing antidepressants, the physician should carefully monitor patients for worsening depression and suicidal thoughts. Centrally acting skeletal muscle relaxants (e.g., cyclobenzaprine, baclofen, and tizanidine) generally are not effective as single agents for the diffuse pain of fibromyalgia, although such usage is common practice and is supported by a few clinical trials. Muscle relaxants given at low doses (e.g., cyclobenzaprine, 10 mg at bedtime) in combination with a TCA, SSRI, or SNRI often are beneficial. Topical capsaicin is useful when gently massaged into painful areas twice a day. The patient should be informed that the initial discomfort often encountered with the use of capsaicin will subside with time and that beneficial effects may not be apparent until after 3 to 4 weeks of therapy.

Addition of an antiepileptic drug (AED) frequently is indicated, particularly in patients with severe allodynia and hyperalgesia. AEDs have efficacy for pain sensitivity and as adjunctive medications for disturbed sleep and depression. Many choices are available, including gabapentin, topiramate, tiagabine, and pregabalin[45] [see Table 3]. The dosages of these agents should be escalated slowly over weeks; discontinuance should likewise be done gradually. Adjunctive therapy with anxiolytic drugs that have different durations of action is often beneficial. Combination therapies might include benzodiazepines such as clonazepam (long half-life), lorazepam or temazepam (medium half-life), and alprazolam (short half-life); buspirone; and certain SSRIs [see Chapter 212]. AEDs may have anxiolytic effects, as well.

Table 3 Selected Antiepileptic Drugs for Treatment of Fibromyalgia Pain

Agent (Trade Name)	Dosage
Gabapentin (Neurontin)	300 mg h.s. to 600 mg t.i.d.; escalate over several weeks
Pregabalin (Lyrica)	50 mg t.i.d.; escalate over several weeks to a maximum of 450 mg q.d. in two or three divided doses
Topiramate (Topamax)	25–50 mg h.s. to 200 mg b.i.d.; escalate by 25–50 mg at weekly intervals
Tiagabine (Gabitril)	2–4 mg h.s. to 56 mg q.d. in two to four divided doses; escalate by 4–8 mg at weekly intervals

Several other drugs are useful in special circumstances. Clonidine is of benefit for neuropathic pain and to decrease withdrawal symptoms when tapering opioids. Pramipexole, a D_3 dopamine receptor agonist, has been shown to improve pain scores, reduce fatigue, and increase function in patients requiring opioids for pain control.

Opioids should be avoided if at all possible. Blanket interdiction of all opioid medications in fibromyalgia patients is inappropriate, however, because some patients can achieve a reasonable quality of life and daily functioning in no other way. When opioids prove to be necessary, they must of course be used with extreme caution. Patients must be closely monitored, must agree to seek psychotherapy, and must complete a signed promise to use only one prescribing physician and one dispensing pharmacy. So-called doctor shopping is not uncommon, especially for patients taking fentanyl or oxycodone-containing preparations, which are associated with increased psychological dependency. Tramadol, methadone, and hydrocodone are preferable.

Comorbid Nociceptive or Neuropathic Pain

When patients have discrete sources of pain (so-called peripheral pain generators), such as osteoarthritis, inflammatory arthritis, or degenerative disk disease, treatment should include nonsteroidal anti-inflammatory drugs (NSAIDs), with or without opioid or nonopioid analgesics. Analgesic drugs should be given in a stepwise approach on the basis of pain intensity and response. Clonidine (0.1 mg three times a day) and various AEDs [see Diffuse Pain, above] are helpful in cases of neuropathic pain. Different combinations of corticosteroid injections, activity modification, splints, local heat or cold, and other physical-therapy modalities may be indicated, depending on the specific musculoskeletal disorder.

Fatigue

Fatigue generally improves with effective treatment of pain, depression, and sleep disturbances in combination with a graded aerobic-exercise program. Modafinil may benefit patients in whom overwhelming fatigue is a persistent complaint or may be useful as a bridge therapy during the early phase of an aerobic-exercise program.[46]

Poor Sleep

Sleep disturbances should be managed aggressively, beginning with instruction in the elements of good sleep hygiene, such as avoidance of daytime naps and caffeine. Most patients require medication, such as a single bedtime dose of a TCA. Drugs to be given with or instead of a TCA include al-prazolam, cyclobenzaprine, temazepam, trazodone, and doxipen; these can be given alone or in combination with a non-benzodiazepine hypnotic (e.g., zolpidem, zaleplon, or eszopiclone). Another alternative is the newly released melatonin receptor agonist, ramelteon. Benzodiazepines, such as triazolam, probably are unsuitable for treatment of sleep disturbances in fibromyalgia patients because of associated daytime sedation and cognitive impairment, although they can play a role in treatment of anxiety (see above). Preliminary data suggest that sodium oxybate, a naturally occurring neuromodulator/neurotransmitter, reduces pain and fatigue and improves sleep in patients with disturbed sleep (alpha intrusion and decreased slow-wave sleep).[47] Clonazepam or ropinirole at bedtime is effective for restless legs syndrome, which is very common in patients with fibromyalgia. A formal sleep study to identify sleep apnea and restless legs syndrome is indicated when the above simple measures are ineffective [see Chapter 189].

Depression

Depression requires aggressive pharmacologic treatment. Many well-tolerated drugs are available [see Chapter 208]. Both SNRIs (e.g., venlafaxine and duloxetine) and certain SSRIs (e.g., fluoxetine, citalopram, and fluvoxamine) have been shown to decrease pain and improve overall well-being in fibromyalgia patients independently of the effects of these drugs on depression. Antidepressant drug treatment should be combined with psychotherapeutic management (formal or informal counseling) [see Chapter 208].

NONPHARMACOLOGIC MANAGEMENT

Nonpharmacologic treatments generally have been of greater benefit than pharmacologic treatments in fibromyalgia patients.[38,48] Nondrug treatments may include exercise, meditation, yoga, biofeedback and stress management, counseling, and support groups. Patient education is important [see Sidebar Recommended Internet Sites on Fibromyalgia]. Optimum management of pain and fatigue in many patients is best achieved by interdisciplinary interaction of the primary care physician with allied health professionals and psychologists. Of particular efficacy are such approaches as biofeedback training and water aerobics, which promote active and independent participation by the patient, thereby enhancing self-management and self-efficacy. Conversely, referral of patients to so-called pain clinics that focus on various types of injection therapies and other passive procedures contributes little to the outcome of diffuse pain syndromes.

Biofeedback and Exercise

Significant improvement in physical status and self-reported fibromyalgia symptoms has been achieved by biofeedback training, alone or in combination with relaxation training and aerobic exercise. A systematic review of published trials indicates that supervised aerobic-exercise training has beneficial effects on physical capacity, pain threshold, and global well-being.[49] Unfortunately, prescription of progressive home-based aerobic exercise is of limited efficacy unless the patient is highly motivated and has effective coping skills. Exercise should be of graded intensity; high-intensity fitness programs should be avoided.

Psychological Intervention

Psychotherapeutic counseling is helpful for many patients. Although formal cognitive-behavioral therapy is theoretically attractive, its cost-effectiveness and additional benefit over other interventions have not been established. Other psychological interventions, such as guided imagery, may improve self-reported pain over the short term.

TREATMENTS OF UNCERTAIN BENEFIT

Trigger-point injections, botulinum toxin injections, ultrasound, laser therapy, sphenopalatine blocks, and numerous other interventions have been advocated for fibromyalgia. These modalities either have no place in the treatment of fibromyalgia or are of questionable benefit.

COMPLEMENTARY AND ALTERNATIVE MEDICINE

Complementary and alternative medicine is used almost universally by patients with fibromyalgia, at least in part because of distrust of physicians and frustration with the limited efficacy of much of traditional care. Acupuncture, hypnotherapy, relaxation techniques (e.g., yoga, tai chi, and meditation), certain herbal and nutritional supplements (magnesium, S-adenosylmethionine [SAMe]), and massage may be of benefit [see Chapter 9]. Vegetarian diets, magnet therapies, and chiropractic manipulation are not recommended.[50-52]

WHEN TO REFER

Consultative referral to a rheumatologist familiar with fibromyalgia is indicated when the diagnosis is unclear, when fibromyalgia is complicated by comorbid autoimmune or musculoskeletal disease, and when response to therapy is poor. Psychiatric referral is essential for severe depression with suicidal ideation and for comorbid psychosis.

Complications

Marital and other personal relationships, family health, and capacity to work productively are all threatened by severe fibromyalgia. Addiction to such drugs as opioids, benzodiazepines, and muscle relaxants is a rare but real risk in fibromyalgia patients. Nevertheless, the physician should be cognizant that drug-seeking behavior is often a sign of inadequate symptom control (pseudoaddiction) rather than drug dependency. Abrupt cessation of such medications may be associated with withdrawal symptoms. Exacerbation of symptoms often is iatrogenic—an unsympathetic, uninformed physician who is dismissive of fibromyalgia as a diagnostic entity and who fails to validate suffering can be a major perpetuating factor in this illness.

Prevention

Physicians may unwittingly contribute to the development of chronic pain in patients with acute pain from neck strain—typically incurred in a minor traffic accident—by diagnostic indecision that permits patients to misconstrue the severity of their condition. In these cases, it is important for physicians to avoid such measures as open-ended referral for physical therapy, prolonged release from work, prescription of a neck brace, and failure to reassure the patient that recovery will be rapid and full. The term posttraumatic fibromyalgia should not be used.

Prognosis

Although improved treatment provides optimism for better outcomes in fibromyalgia patients, prospective, long-term, longitudinal studies in academic medical centers have shown little improvement in health status, disease severity, health service utilization, and costs, with approximately 25% of patients with fibromyalgia receiving disability or other compensation payments.[53,54] Persons with fibromyalgia suffer much more than those with other chronic rheumatologic diseases, such as rheumatoid arthritis.

Even though hyperalgesia and allodynia cannot be reversed entirely, most patients can expect substantial improvement in symptoms and in overall quality of life. Resolution of ongoing stress and promotion of the patient's self-efficacy for control of pain are of pivotal importance. Prognoses vary for three fairly distinct subsets of patients: adaptive copers, interpersonally distressed, and dysfunctional.[8,10] Adaptive copers, many of whom do not seek care for fibromyalgia, do well with respect to self-reported pain, disturbed sleep, and fatigue. Interpersonally distressed patients also respond to a comprehensive interdisciplinary therapeutic approach. Dysfunctional patients with high levels of pain, anxiety, and opioid dependence do poorly, as do patients with pending litigation. The treatment goal that responds least to therapy is improvement in daily functioning.

The author has been a member of the speakers' bureau of Wyeth and a member of the advisory committee of Sanofi-Synthelabo, Inc.

References

1. Wolfe F, Smythe HA, Yunus MB, et al: The American College of Rheumatology 1990 Criteria for the Classification of Fibromyalgia: report of the Multicenter Criteria Committee. Arthritis Rheum 33:160, 1990

2. Henningsen P, Zimmermann T, Sattel H: Medically unexplained physical symptoms, anxiety, and depression: a meta-analytic review. Psychosom Med 65:528, 2003

3. Hyams KC: Developing case definitions for symptom-based conditions: the problem of specificity. Epidemiol Rev 20:148, 1998

4. Barsky AJ, Borus JF: Functional somatic syndromes. Ann Intern Med 130:910, 1999

5. Hudson JI, Mangweth B, Pope HG Jr, et al: Family study of affective spectrum disorder. Arch Gen Psychiatry 60:170, 2003

6. Manu P: The Psychopathology of Functional Somatic Syndromes. Haworth Medical Press, Binghamton, New York, 2004

7. Yunus MB: The concept of central sensitivity syndromes. Fibromyalgia and Other Central Pain Syndromes. Wallace DJ, Clauw DJ, Eds. Lippincott Williams & Wilkins, Philadelphia, 2005, p 29

8. Turk DC, Okifuji A, Sinclair JD, et al: Pain, disability, and physical functioning in subgroups of patients with fibromyalgia. J Rheumatol 23:1255, 1996

9. Giesecke T, Williams DA, Harris RE, et al: Subgrouping of fibromyalgia patients on the basis of pressure-pain thresholds and psychological factors. Arthritis Rheum 48:2916, 2003

10. Turk DC, Okifuji A, Sinclair JD, et al: Differential responses by psychosocial subgroups of fibromyalgia syndrome patients to an interdisciplinary treatment. Arthritis Care Res 11:397, 1998

11. Neumann L, Buskila D: Epidemiology of fibromyalgia. Curr Pain Headache Rep 7:362, 2003

12. Winfield JB: Psychological determinants of fibromyalgia and related syndromes. Curr Rev Pain 4:276, 2000

13. The Biopsychosocial Approach: Past, Present, Future. Frankel R, Quill T, McDaniel S, Eds. University of Rochester Press, Rochester, New York, 2003

14. Gillespie NA, Zhu G, Heath AC, et al: The genetic aetiology of somatic distress. Psychol Med 30:1051, 2000

15. Buchwald D, Herrell R, Ashton S, et al: A twin study of chronic fatigue. Psychosom Med 63:936, 2001

16. Arnold LM, Hudson JI, Hess EV, et al: Family study of fibromyalgia. Arthritis Rheum 50:944, 2004

17. Caspi A, Sugden K, Moffitt TE, et al: Influence of life stress on depression: moderation by a polymorphism in the 5-HTT gene. Science 301:386, 2003

18. Offenbaecher M, Bondy B, de Jonge S, et al: Possible association of fibromyalgia with a polymorphism in the serotonin transporter gene regulatory region. Arthritis Rheum 42:2482, 1999

19. Diatchenko L, Slade GD, Nackley AG, et al: Genetic basis for individual variations in pain perception and the development of a chronic pain condition. Hum Mol Genet 14:135, 2005

20. Fillingim RB: Sex-related influences on pain: a review of mechanisms and clinical implications. Rehabil Psychol 48:165, 2003

21. Staud R, Robinson ME, Vierck CJ Jr, et al: Diffuse noxious inhibitory controls (DNIC) at-

tenuate temporal summation of second pain in normal males but not in normal females or fibromyalgia patients. Pain 101:167, 2003

22. Kroenke K, Spitzer RL: Gender differences in the reporting of physical and somatoform symptoms. Psychosom Med 60:150, 1998

23. Canli T, Desmond JE, Zhao Z, et al: Sex differences in the neural basis of emotional memories. Proc Natl Acad Sci USA 99:10789, 2002

24. Moldofsky H: Sleep and pain. Sleep Med Rev 5:385, 2001

25. Wolfe F: The relation between tender points and fibromyalgia symptom variables: evidence that fibromyalgia is not a discrete disorder in the clinic. Ann Rheum Dis 56:268, 1997

26. Okifuji A, Turk DC: Stress and psychophysiological dysregulation in patients with fibromyalgia syndrome. Appl Psychophysiol Biofeedback 27:129, 2002

27. Elenkov IJ, Wilder RL, Chrousos GP, et al: The sympathetic nerve—an integrative interface between two supersystems: the brain and the immune system. Pharmacol Rev 52:595, 2000

28. Crofford LJ: The hypothalamic-pituitary-adrenal axis in the pathogenesis of rheumatic diseases. Endocrinol Metab Clin North Am 31:1, 2002

29. Clauw DJ, Crofford LJ: Chronic widespread pain and fibromyalgia: what we know, and what we need to know. Best Pract Res Clin Rheumatol 17:685, 2003

30. Fillingim RB, Wilkinson CS, Powell T: Self-reported abuse history and pain complaints among healthy young adults. Psychosom Med 61:111, 1999

31. Gracely RH, Petzke F, Wolf JM, et al: Functional magnetic resonance imaging evidence of augmented pain processing in fibromyalgia. Arthritis Rheum 46:1333, 2002

32. Staud R: Fibromyalgia pain: do we know the source? Curr Opin Rheumatol 16:157, 2004

33. Watkins LR, Milligan ED, Maier SF: Glial activation: a driving force for pathological pain. Trends Neurosci 24:450, 2001

34. Walker EA, Keegan D, Gardner G, et al: Psychosocial factors in fibromyalgia compared with rheumatoid arthritis: II. Sexual, physical, and emotional abuse and neglect. Psychosom Med 59:572, 1997

35. Moreland LW, St Clair EW: The use of analgesics in the management of pain in rheumatic diseases. Rheum Dis Clin North Am 25:153, 1999

36. Bennett RM: The rational management of fibromyalgia patients. Rheum Dis Clin North Am 28:181, 2002

37. Arnold LM, Keck PE Jr, Welge JA: Antidepressant treatment of fibromyalgia: a meta-analysis and review. Psychosomatics 41:104, 2000

38. Rossy LA, Buckelew SP, Dorr N, et al: A meta-analysis of fibromyalgia treatment interventions. Ann Behav Med 21:180, 1999

39. Sim J, Adams N: Systematic review of randomized controlled trials of nonpharmacological interventions for fibromyalgia. Clin J Pain 18:324, 2002

40. Burckhardt CS, Goldenberg D, Crofford L, et al: Guideline for the Management of Fibromyalgia Pain in Adults and Children. APS Clinical Practice Guidelines Series, No. 4. American Pain Society, Glenview, Illinois, 2005

41. The management of chronic pain in older persons. American Geriatrics Society Panel on Chronic Pain in Older Persons. J Am Geriatrics Soc 46:635, 1998

42. Schanberg LE: Widespread pain in children: when is it pathologic? Arthritis Rheum 48:2402, 2003

43. Arnold LM, Hess EV, Hudson JI, et al: A randomized, placebo-controlled, double-blind, flexible-dose study of fluoxetine in the treatment of women with fibromyalgia. Am J Med 112:191, 2002

44. Arnold LM, Rosen A, Pritchett YL: A randomized, double-blind, placebo-controlled trial of duloxetine in the treatment of women with fibromyalgia with or without major depressive disorder. Pain 119:5, 2005

45. Crofford LJ, Rowbotham MC, Mease PJ: Pregabalin for the treatment of fibromyalgia syndrome: results of a randomized, double-blind, placebo-controlled trial. Arthritis Rheum 52:1264, 2005

46. Schaller JL, Behar D: Modafinil in fibromyalgia treatment. J Neuropsychiatry Clin Neurosci 13:530, 2001

47. Scharf MB, Baumann M, Berkowitz DV: The effects of sodium oxybate on clinical symptoms and sleep patterns in patients with fibromyalgia. J Rheumatol 30:1070, 2003

48. Williams DA: Psychological and behavioural therapies in fibromyalgia and related syndromes. Best Pract Res Clin Rheumatol 17:649, 2003

49. Busch A, Schachter CL, Peloso PM, et al: Exercise for treating fibromyalgia syndrome. Cochrane Database Syst Rev (3):CD003786, 2002

50. Crofford LJ, Appleton BE: Complementary and alternative therapies for fibromyalgia. Curr Rheumatol Rep 3:147, 2001

51. Ebell MH, Beck E: How effective are complementary/alternative medicine (CAM) therapies for fibromyalgia? J Fam Pract 50:400, 2001

52. Holdcraft LC, Assefi N, Buchwald D: Complementary and alternative medicine in fibromyalgia and related syndromes. Best Pract Res Clin Rheumatol 17:667, 2003

53. Wolfe F, Anderson J, Harkness D, et al: Health status and disease severity in fibromyalgia: results of a six-center longitudinal study. Arthritis Rheum 40:1571, 1997

54. Wolfe F, Anderson J, Harkness D, et al: A prospective, longitudinal, multicenter study of service utilization and costs in fibromyalgia. Arthritis Rheum 40:1560, 1997

55. Yunus MB, Masi AT: Fibromyalgia, restless legs syndrome, periodic limb movement disorder and psychogenic pain. Arthritis and Allied Conditions: A Textbook of Rheumatology. McCarty DJ Jr, Koopman WJ, Eds. Lea & Febiger, Philadelphia, 1993, p 1383

Index

A

Abacavir, for HIV infection, 1831t
  adverse effects of, 1834t
Abatacept, for rheumatoid arthritis, 1308t, 1311
Abciximab, for unstable angina and NSTMI, 309-310, 309t
Abdominal pain, in cancer, 2175
Abdominal surgery, gastroparesis after, 852
Abducens neuropathy, 2294t
Abetalipoproteinemia, 731
  malabsorption in, 832
Abortion
  septic, *C. perfringens* in, 1608
  spontaneous, 1013-1015
    cause of, 1014-1015, 1014f
    management of, 1013f
Abscess. *See also specific anatomic location*
  aortic valve annular, in endocarditis, 1489
  brain. *See* Brain abscess
  cutaneous, 511
  definition of, 429t
  intra-abdominal, 1503-1506
  intraperitoneal, 1504
  liver. *See* Liver abscess
  lung. *See* Lung abscess
  pancreatic, 913, 922-923, 922f, 1505
  perirenal, in urinary tract infection, 1511
  peritonsillar, 1464
  renal, in urinary tract infection, 1511
  retroperitoneal, 1504-1505
  spinal epidural, 1557-1559
    staphylococcal, 1577
  splenic, 1506
  subphrenic, 1504
    fever of undetermined origin in, 1414-1415
Abstinence, as contraceptive, 998
Acanthamoeba infection, 1909, 1910f
Acanthosis nigricans, in diabetes mellitus, 433, 434f
Acarbose, for type 2 diabetes mellitus, 658-659, 658t
Accessory neuropathy, 2294t
Accidents. *See also* Trauma
  alcoholism and, 2627
Acebutolol
  classification of, 267t
  hypersensitivity syndrome reaction due to, 496
  for hypertension, 222t
  toxicity of, 163t
ACE inhibitor(s). *See* Angiotensin-converting enzyme (ACE) inhibitor(s)
Aceruloplasminemia, 1088
Acetaminophen
  hepatotoxicity due to, 878
  metabolites of, thrombocytopenia due to, 1170
  nephropathy due to, 2090
  overdose, 161-162, 162f
    diagnosis of, 161
    treatment of, 161-162, 162f
  for pain, 2183-2184, 2184t
Acetohydroxamic acid, for struvite nephrolithiasis, 2111
Acetylcholine, excessive activity of, 172, 172t
Acetylcysteine, for acetaminophen

overdose, 161-162
Achalasia, 761-763, 761f-762f
  diagnosis of, 762, 762f
  treatment of, 762-763, 761f
Achilles tendinitis, 1397, 1397f
Acid-base disorder(s), 1994-2006
Acid-base physiology
  normal, 1994, 1995f-1997f
  renal acid excretion in, 1994, 1995f-1997f
  renal bicarbonate reabsorption in, 1994, 1995f
Acidemia, hyperkalemia in, 2009
Acid maltase deficiency, 2279, 2279f
Acidosis
  in cardiac arrest, 148t
  hyperchloremic, 1998
  lactic, 1995-1996
    treatment of, 2001
  metabolic. *See* Metabolic acidosis
  respiratory, 2005-2006, 2005t
Acinetobacter species, antimicrobial susceptibilities of, 1421t
Acitretin, for psoriasis, 469
Acne-associated arthritis, 1325-1326
Acne conglobata, 446
Acne cosmetica, 447
Acne excoriee, 447
Acneiform eruptions, as drug reaction, 500
Acne mechanica, 447
Acne vulgaris, 446-451
  chloracne *vs.*, 447
  clinical features of, 446-447, 447f
  clinical variants of, 446-447
  comedonal, 446
    treatment of, 448
  diagnosis of, 446-447
  differential diagnosis of, 447-448
  epidemiology of, 446
  etiology of, 446
  Favre-Racouchot disease *vs.*, 447
  folliculitis *vs.*, 447
  gram-negative folliculitis *vs.*, 447
  hidradenitis suppurativa *vs.*, 447
  inflammatory, 446, 447f
    treatment of, 448-449, 449t
  laboratory tests in, 447, 447t
  milia *vs.*, 447
  in neonates and children, 447
  pathogenesis of, 446
  perioral dermatitis *vs.*, 447
  phototherapy for, 451
  pomade, 447
  rosacea *vs.*, 448, 448f
  treatment of, 448-451, 448t-450t
    antibiotic, 449, 450t
    hormone therapy, 450-451
    isotretinoin in, 449-450, 450t
    systemic, 449-451, 450t
    topical, 448-449, 449t
Acoustic neuroma, in neurofibromatosis, 542
Acquired immunodeficiency syndrome (AIDS), 1819-1846. *See also* Human immunodeficiency virus infection
  acute pancreatitis in, 914
  arthritis in, 1539
  bacillary angiomatosis in, 437-438
  classification of, 1819, 1820t
  condyloma acuminatum in, 437
  cytomegalovirus infection in, 1762
  dementia in. *See* Human immunodeficiency virus infection, dementia

encephalitis in, toxoplasmosis, 1899
  epidemiology of, 1819-1822, 1820f-1821f
    global, 1819-1821
    United States, 1821-1822, 1820f-1821f
  fever of undetermined origin in, 1416
  herpes simplex infection in, 437
  herpes zoster in, 437
  hypogonadism in, 693
  hyponatremia in, 1984
  idiopathic thrombocytopenic purpura in, 1168
  Internet resources for, 1843
  Kaposi sarcoma in, 558-559. *See also* Kaposi sarcoma
  lumbosacral polyradiculopathy in, 2305
  lymphoma in, 2608
  meningitis in, 2352
  molluscum contagiosum in, 437
  neuropathy in, 2304-2305
  neutropenia in, 1142
  opportunistic infections in, cutaneous, 437-438
  oral hairy leukoplakia in, 438
  painful articular syndrome in, 1539
  pain in, 2176
    management of, 2169
  pneumonia in, *Pseudomonas aeruginosa*, 1659
  psoriasis in, 462
  reactive arthritis and, 1323
  scabies in, 438, 516
  seborrheic dermatitis in, 455-456
  sinusitis in, 1457
  skin disorders in, 437-438
  telephone services for, 1843
  therapy for. *See* Human immunodeficiency virus infection, therapy for
  toxoplasmosis in, 1899
Acrocyanosis, 407
Acrodermatitis chronica atrophicans, in Lyme disease, 1713-1714
Acromegaly, 596-597, 596t-597t
  familial, pituitary adenoma in, 591-592
Actinomyces, antimicrobial drugs for, 1427t
Actinomycosis, 1606-1607
  abdominal, 1607
  cervicofacial, 1606-1607
  diagnosis of, 1610
  disseminated, 1607
  epidemiology and etiology of, 1606
  pelvic, 1607
  thoracic, 1607
  treatment of, 1614
Actin polymerization defect, neutrophil function in, 1146t
Acupuncture, 83-84
Acute chest syndrome, in sickle cell anemia, 1116
Acute respiratory distress syndrome (ARDS), 2844-2848
  causes of, 2844, 2845
  definition of, 1443t
  diagnosis of, 2845, 2847
  outcome in, 2847-2848
  pathogenesis of, 2844-2845, 2846f
  respiratory failure in, 2816, 2816f
  in septic shock, 1450, 1452
  treatment of, 2847, 2848t

Acute stress disorder, 2661-2662
Adalumimab
  for psoriasis, 470
  for rheumatoid arthritis, 1308t, 1310
ADAMTS13 screening assay, for thrombotic thrombocytopenic purpura, 1171-1172, 1171f
Adapalene, for acne vulgaris, 449t
Addison disease. *See* Adrenal insufficiency
Adefovir dipivoxil, for chronic hepatitis B, 887-888
Adenocarcinoma, gastrointestinal, in inflammatory bowel disease, 809
Adenoid cystic carcinoma, of lung, 2750
Adenoma sebaceum, in tuberous sclerosis, 440, 441f
Adenomatous polyposis coli (APC). *See also* Familial adenomatous polyposis (FAP)
  genetic testing in, 1958, 1959t, 1961
Adenomyosis, 960
Adenosine, for pharmacologic stress testing, 201t
Adenosine deaminase deficiency, 1230t
Adenovirus, 1781-1782
  encephalitis in, 2352
  enteric, 1800
  laboratory diagnosis of, 1778t
Adhesive capsulitis (frozen shoulder), 1393
Adolescent females, pelvic mass in, 1058-1059, 1061
Adrenal, 679-688
  anatomy of, 679, 679f-680f
  physiology of, 679, 681f
Adrenal cancer, 681-682
Adrenal cortex
  anatomy of, 679, 679f-680f
  hyperfunction of. *See* Cushing disease
Adrenal hyperplasia
  congenital, 685-686, 685f, 687
  idiopathic bilateral, 686
  nonclassic, in polycystic ovary syndrome, 978
Adrenal insufficiency, 682-684, 683t
  diagnosis of, 683, 683t
  hyperkalemia in, 2010
  treatment of, 683-684
Adrenal mass, incidental, 682
Adrenal medulla, anatomy of, 679, 679f-680f
Adrenal tuberculosis, 1683
Adrenocorticotropic hormone (ACTH)
  actions of, 598
  deficiency, 598
  excess. *See* Cushing disease
  synthesis of, 597-598
  synthetic, cortisol levels and, 598
Adrenoleukodystrophy, 2332
Advance directives, 96-97
Advanced-sleep-phase syndrome, 2370
African Americans, renal disease in, 2040
African dietary iron overload, 1088
African tick-bite fever, 1728
Agammaglobulinemia, X-linked, 1226-1227, 1227f, 1226t
Agent Orange, 2378
Aggression, in brain trauma, 2236
Aging. *See* Geriatric patient

exercise and, 35
Agoraphobia, 2658, 2657t
Agranulocytosis, infantile genetic, 1144t
AIDS. See Acquired immunodeficiency syndrome (AIDS)
Aircraft, jet, high altitude and, 80
Airway
advanced, in cardiac resuscitation, 145-146
in cardiac resuscitation, 143
obstruction of
asthma vs., 2705-2706, 2704t
bronchoscopy for, 2693-2695, 2693t, 2695f
pulmonary edema in, 2849
sleep-disordered breathing in, 2797
patency of, 2811-2812, 2812t
in poisoning, 155
Albinism, 584-586
Albuterol, for asthma, 2709, 2711t
Alcohol
isopropyl, poisoning or overdose, 161t, 168t
methyl. See Methanol
Alcohol consumption, 20-21
abusive, 2625
at-risk, 2625
dependence, 2625
diet and, 31
esophageal cancer and, 2490-2491
harmful, 2625
moderate, 2625
oral cancers due to, 2374-2375, 2437
platelet functional effects of, 1175
problem drinking vs. alcohol dependence, 20-21, 20t-21t
as risk factor for stroke, 2211
Alcohol dependence, 20-21, 20t-21t.
See also Alcohol consumption
behavioral-counseling interventions for, 49
Alcoholic cirrhosis. See also Cirrhosis
chronic hepatitis vs., 883
nutritional support in, 944
Alcoholic hepatitis
acute cholecystitis vs., 904
fever of undetermined origin in, 1415
Alcoholic liver disease. See Alcoholic cirrhosis
Alcoholics Anonymous (AA), 2630
Alcoholism, 167-168, 168t, 2625-2634
accidents and injuries in, 2627
alcohol withdrawal syndrome in, 2630-2631
anemia in, 1094
behavior-related problems in, 2627
CAGE questions for, 2627, 2628t
cirrhosis in. See Alcoholic cirrhosis
common problems associated with, 2626-2627
definitions and classification in, 2625-2626
elimination method for, 161t
epidemiology of, 2626
genetics in, 2626
HIV infection in, 2627
management of abuse and dependence in, 2630-2632
medical problems in, 2626
myopathy in, 2284
neuropathy in, 2304
pancreatitis in, 914
chronic, 924
psychiatric problems in, 2626-2627
screening and diagnosis of problems with, 2627-2628, 2628t

self-help groups for, 2630
surgical risk factor management and, 56
tobacco abuse in, 2627
toxic encephalopathy in, 2342
treatment of, 2628-2631, 2629t-2630t
acamprosate, 2632, 2632t
brief intervention therapy as, 2629-2630, 2630t
disulfiram, 2631-2632, 2632t
Internet information for, 2632
naltrexone, 2632, 2632t
pharmacologic treatment for relapse in, 2631-2632
programs for, 2631
psychotherapeutic approaches to, 2631
violence and abuse in, 2627
Alcohol Use Disorder Identification Test (AUDIT), 2628
Alcohol withdrawal states, toxic encephalopathy as, 2342
Alcohol withdrawal syndrome, 2630-2631
Aldosterone
regulation of, 679, 681f
resistance
causes of, 1999t
hyperkalemia in, 2010
Aldosteronism, primary, hypertension in, 217t, 232, 231t
Alefacept, for psoriasis, 471
Alendronate, for osteoporosis, 709
Alfuzosin, for benign prostatic hyperplasia, 2131, 2131t
Alkalosis
contraction, 2003
metabolic. See Metabolic alkalosis
respiratory, 2005-2006, 2005t
Alkylating agent(s), 2413-2414, 2415t-2416t
leukemia due to, 2562
Allergic alveolitis. See also Pneumonitis, hypersensitivity
occupational, 63
Allergic aspergillosis, bronchopulmonary, 2707-2708, 2709f, 2716
segmental pulmonary infiltrates in, 2751, 2750f
Allergic granulomatosis and angiitis (Churg-Strauss syndrome)
cutaneous findings in, 432
multifocal pulmonary infiltrates in, 2749
pulmonary vasculitis in, 2782-2783
Allergic response, 1240-1246
definition of, 1240
immediate hypersensitivity in, 1240-1246. See also Hypersensitivity reaction(s), immediate
Allergic rhinitis. See Rhinitis, allergic
Allergy and atopy. See also specific disorders
allergic contact dermatitis in.
See also Contact dermatitis, allergic
contact dermatitis in, 481-494
diagnostic and therapeutic principles in, 1247-1252
drug, 1271-1277. See also Drug allergy
environmental control for, 1250, 1250t
food, 1278-1284. See also Food allergy
history and physical examination in, 1247-1248, 1247t
IgE assay for, 1248-1250, 1248t, 1249f

immediate hypersensitivity reactions and. See Hypersensitivity reactions, immediate
latex. See Latex allergy
pollen-associated food allergy syndrome, 1278-1279, 1279t
stinging insect. See Stinging insect allergy
treatment in, 1250-1252
anti-IgE therapy, 1250
immunotherapy, 1251-1252
pharmacologic, 1250-1251, 1251f
Allopurinol, for uric acid nephrolithiasis, 2111
Alopecia
androgenic, 563-564, 563f-564f
cicatricial, 568-569, 568t, 568f
diffuse, 564-566, 564t
due to drugs and chemicals, 566, 565t-566t
due to heat, radiation, chemicals, 568
due to pressure and friction, 567
miscellaneous causes of, 569
in syphilis, 569, 569f
traction, 567
traumatic, 567-568
Alopecia areata, 566-568, 567f
nail pathology in, 574, 576f
Alpharetrovirus, 1802t
Altitude, high. See High altitude
Aluminum toxicity, in hemodialysis, dialysis dementia in, 2339
Alveolar cell carcinoma, infiltrates in
chronic diffuse, 2768-2769
focal pulmonary, 2745, 2745f
multifocal pulmonary, 2747, 2746f
Alveolar hemorrhage, diffuse, 2783
in anti-GBM antibody disease, 2783
in idiopathic pulmonary hemosiderosis, 2783
Alveolar hypoventilation
in muscular dystrophy, 2807
primary, 2789
Alveolar overdistention, in mechanical ventilation, 2817-2818, 2817f-2818f
Alveolar proteinosis, 2781-2782, 2782f
Alveolar sarcoidosis, 2771
multifocal pulmonary infiltrates in, 2747, 2746f
Alveolitis
allergic. See also Pneumonitis, hypersensitivity
occupational, 63
fibrosing. See Pulmonary fibrosis, idiopathic
Alzheimer disease, 2217-2223. See also Dementia
anterograde amnesia in, 2217
caregiver support in, 2223
clinical assessment in, 2221
clinical manifestations of, 2220
definitions in, 2217, 2217t
dementia in, 2217
diagnosis of, 2220-2222
epidemiology of, 2217, 2218f
genetic counseling in, 2223
genetics and molecular biology in, 2218-2219, 2219f
laboratory testing and imaging in, 2221-2222, 2221f
pathophysiology of, 2219-2220, 2220f
protective and risk factors in, 2217-2218
treatment of, 2222-2223
Amanita phalloides mushroom poisoning, 175
Amantadine

for influenza, 1786t
for Parkinson disease, 2247
Amebae, free-living, infections due to, 1909, 1910f
Amebiasis, 1903-1906
diagnosis of, 1905, 1903f-1904f
diarrhea due to, 842
differential diagnosis of, 1905-1906
etiology and epidemiology of, 1903-1904
pathogenesis of, 1904-1905, 1904f
treatment of, 1906
Amebic colitis, 1906
Amebic liver abscess, 1904-1905, 1904f
differential diagnosis of, 1906
Amebic lung abscess, 2752
Amenorrhea, 953-959
androgen insensitivity syndrome in, 954-955
Asherman syndrome in, 955-956
breast-feeding and, 957
congenital (genetic) causes of, 957
definition of, 953
diagnosis of, 953-954, 954t, 955f
functional causes of, 957-958
hypergonadotropic hypogonadism in, 958-959
hypogonadotropic hypogonadism in, 956-957, 956t
hypothalamic, 957-958
mullerian agenesis in, 954
outflow tract obstruction in, 954
polycystic ovary syndrome in, 959
primary, 953
secondary, 953
Amikacin, 1432
Amiloride
for hypertension, 221t
for nephrolithiasis, 2109
Amino acid solution(s), for parenteral nutrition, metabolic acidosis due to, 1998
Aminoglutethimide, 2420t
Aminoglycoside(s), 1432-1433. See also individual drugs, e.g., Streptomycin
nephrotoxicity due to, 2032
in pregnancy, 1422t
Amiodarone
for atrial fibrillation, 242t-243t
in cardiac resuscitation, 144t
classification of, 267t
pulmonary disease due to, chronic diffuse infiltrative, 2763-2764
thyrotoxicosis due to, 611
Amlodipine, for hypertension, 221t
Ammonia, renal production of, 1994, 1996f
Amnesia, anterograde, in Alzheimer disease, 2217
Amoxicillin, 1428
exanthematous reaction due to, 495
for Helicobacter infection, 1636t
for Salmonella infection, 1635t
Amoxicillin-clavulanate, 1428
Amphetamine
overdose, 164-165, 164t
seizure due to, 157t
Amphotericin B
as antifungal agent, 1873, 1873t
nephrotoxicity of, 2033
Ampicillin, 1428
exanthematous reaction due to, 495
for Yersinia infection, 1636t
Ampicillin-sulbactam, 1428
Ampulla of Vater, malignancy of, in acute pancreatitis, 914
Amputation, for atherosclerotic peripheral arterial disease, 405

Amylase, serum, in acute pancreatitis, 916, 917t
Amyloidosis, 2593-2594
cardiac, constrictive pericarditis vs., 383t
cutaneous findings in, 436
platelet effects of, 1177
polyneuropathy in, 2302
pulmonary
multiple pulmonary nodules in, 2756-2757
segmental pulmonary infiltrates in, 2751
small intestinal, malabsorption in, 834
tubulointerstitial nephritis in, 2097
Amyloid polyneuropathy(ies), familial, 2302
Amyotrophic lateral sclerosis, 2288-2289
anterior horn cell disease in, 2806
Amyotrophic neuropathy, diabetic, 671
Anaerobic bacteria, 1600
normal flora and, 1600, 1600t-1601t
oxygen tolerance and, 1600
Anaerobic infections, 1600-1616
diagnosis of, 1610-1611
microbiologic, 1610
radiologic and imaging, 1610
management of, 1611-1614
empirical antimicrobial therapy in, 1612-1613, 1613t
hyperbaric oxygen and adjunctive measures in, 1613
predicted antimicrobial susceptibility in, 1611-1612, 1612t
surgical drainage in, 1613
mixed, 1603-1606, 1603t
bacteremia and endocarditis, 1605-1606
clinical presentations in, 1604-1606
female genital tract, 1605
head and neck, 1604
intra-abdominal, 1605
intracranial, 1605
necrotic skin and soft tissue, 1605
pleuropulmonary, 1605
pathogenesis of, 1600-1603
host factors in, 1600
microbial synergy in, 1601
virulence factors in, 1601-1603, 1602t
prevention of, 1615, 1615t
specific infections, 1603-1610, 1603t. See also individual infections
Anagen arrest, 565-566, 565f
Anakinra, for rheumatoid arthritis, 1308t, 1311t
Anal canal, herpes simplex infection of, 1757
Anal cancer, 2506-2507
Analgesic(s). See also Opioid analgesics, Pain
topical, in pain management, 2185
Analgesic nephropathy, 2089-2090, 2089f
Anaphylaxis, 1267-1269
diagnosis of, 1268-1269, 1268t
epidemiology of, 1268
pathogenesis of, 1268, 1268t
treatment and prevention of, 1269
Anaplasma infection
biology and ecology of, 1724-1725
pathophysiology of, 1725
taxonomy of, 1724, 1724f
Anaplasma phagocytophilia infection,

1733
treatment of, 1728t
Anaplasmosis, human granulocytic, 1724, 1733-1734, 1733f
Lyme disease and, 1733
Anastrozole, 2420t
for early (stages I and II) breast cancer, 2465
Andersen syndrome, 2282
Androgen(s)
assay for, in hirsutism, 989
insensitivity to, 694-695
Androgen insensitivity syndrome, 954-955
Anemia, 1092-1106
acute blood loss, red cell transfusion for, 1210-1211
in acute renal failure, 2038
after renal transplantation, 2124
in aging, 1094
in alcohol abuse, 1094
aplastic, 1095-1097. See Aplastic anemia
in cardiac arrest, 148t
chronic, red cell transfusion for, 1211
of chronic disease, 1092-1093
diagnosis of, 1092-1093, 1092t, 1093f
differential diagnosis of, 1092t
pathophysiology of, 1092
treatment of, 1093
in chronic renal failure, 2045, 2045f
hemodialysis and, 2048
due to chloramphenicol, 1095
Fanconi, CNS tumors in, 2310t
hemolytic, 1109-1129. See also Hemolytic anemia
hypochromic, differential diagnosis of, 1092t
iron deficiency, 1082. See also Iron deficiency
epidemiology of, 1082-1083
iron-loading, 1088
megaloblastic, 1099-1104. See also Megaloblastic anemia
in multiple myeloma, 2591
production defects in, 1092-1106
with apparently normal bone marrow, 1092-1094
classification of, 1092
diagnosis of, 1093f
with marrow aplasia or replacement, 1094-1099
with marrow erythroid hyperplasia, 1099-1105
pure red cell aplasia, 1097-1098, 1098t
diagnosis and treatment of, 1098-1099
etiology of, 1098, 1098t
pathophysiology of, 1097-1098
refractory, 2564t
with excess of blasts, 2564t
with ringed sideroblast, 2564t
in rheumatoid arthritis, 1305
in severe renal disease, 1093-1094
sickle cell, 1113-1118. See also Sickle cell anemia
sideroblastic, 1104-1105, 1105t
differential diagnosis of, 1092t
in starvation, 1094, 1094f
Anesthesia, general, in sickle cell anemia, 1117
Anesthetic agents, allergy to, 1275-1276
Aneurysm
aortic. See Aortic aneurysm
cerebral, in endocarditis, 1485-1486
circle of Willis, in polycystic kidney disease, 2098, 2099f

mycotic, in endocarditis, 1485-1486
pulmonary arterial, pulmonary hypertension in, 2862
Angelman syndrome, 1950
Angiitis
allergic. See Churg-Strauss syndrome (allergic granulomatosis and angiitis)
CNS, isolated, encephalopathy in, 2342
Angina, Ludwig, 1465
Angina pectoris, 284-303
causes of, 197
chronic stable, 284
coronary angiography in, 295
diagnosis of, 294
exercise treadmill ECG in, 294
follow-up in, 300-301
follow-up noninvasive testing in, 294-295
left ventricular systolic function testing in, 294
risk stratification in, 294-295
stress testing in, 294-295
therapies for, 300
clinical manifestations of, 285, 285t-286t
coronary atherosclerosis in, 284-285
diagnosis and risk stratification in, 286-295
differential diagnosis of, 285-286, 287t
in differential diagnosis of chest pain, 198t, 197
ECG in, 287-289
exercise, 291-292
epidemiology of, 284
hypertension in, 229
imaging studies in, 289
invasive testing in, 293-294
laboratory tests in, 287-289
noninvasive testing in, 291-293, 291f, 292t
imaging studies under investigation in, 293
patients warranting, 289-290
test selection in, 292-293
pathophysiology and pathogenesis of, 284-285
patient history and risk evaluation in, 286-287, 288f, 289t
physical examination in, 287
preliminary evaluation in, 286-290
stress echocardiography in, 292
stress radionuclide myocardial perfusion imaging in, 292
treatment of, 295-301, 295t
ACE inhibitors for, 298
antihypertensive therapy for, 298
antiplatelet agents in, 296-297
beta blockers for, 299
calcium channel blockers for, 299
in diabetes mellitus, 299-300
dietary modification in, 296
lifestyle modification in, 295-296
lipid-lowering agents for, 297-298
medical therapy in, 296-299
for anginal symptoms, 298-299
for risk reduction, 296-298
nitrates and nitroglycerin for, 299
physical activity in, 296
revascularization in, 300
smoking cessation, 295-296
typical, features of, 289t, 286
unstable, 284, 304-316. See also

Unstable angina and non-ST segment elevation MI
Angiodysplasia, lower GI, 864-865, 865f
Angioedema, 1266-1267, 1266f
diagnosis and treatment of, 1267
epidemiology of, 1266
etiology and pathogenesis of, 1266-1267
urticarial drug reactions and, 497
Angiofibroma, periungual, 576t
Angiography
abdominal, in polyarteritis nodosa, 1367
pulmonary, for pulmonary embolism, 416, 415t
Angiokeratoma, in Fabry disease, 440-441, 442f
Angiolymphoid hyperplasia with eosinophilia, 547
Angioma, spider, 546, 546f
Angiomatosis, bacillary, 1673-1674
in AIDS, 437-438
Angioplasty, coronary. See Coronary angioplasty
Angiosarcoma, 556, 2552-2553
features of, 2550t
treatment of, 2558
Angiostatin, in tumor control, 2394, 2395f
Angiostrongyliasis, 1927-1928
Angiostrongylus cantonensis infection, 1927-1928
Angiotensin-converting enzyme (ACE) inhibitor(s)
allergy to, 1275
for angina pectoris, 298
for heart failure, 342, 343t
for myocardial infarction, acute, 328
nephrotoxicity due to, 2033
for unstable angina and NSTEMI, 314
urticarial drug reactions to, 497
Angiotensin-converting enzyme (ACE) level(s), in sarcoidosis, 2773
Angiotensin receptor blockers, for heart failure, 342, 343t
Animal scabies, 519
Anion gap, 1995. See also Metabolic acidosis
Anisakiasis, 1926
Ankle, rheumatoid arthritis of, 1303
Ankle pain, 1396-1397
Ankylosing spondylitis, 1317-1322
bamboo spine in, 1319, 1321f
cardiovascular disease in, 1320
clinical presentation in, 1318-1319
diagnosis of, 1318-1321, 1318f, 1317t, 1320f-1321f
epidemiology of, 1317-1318
extra-articular findings in, 1320-1321
HLA-B27 in, 1317-1318
in inflammatory bowel disease, 1325
laboratory findings in, 1319
multifocal pulmonary infiltrates in, 2749
neurologic disease in, 1320-1321
ocular findings in, 1320
osteoarthritis vs., 1387
physical examination in, 1319
pulmonary disease in, 1320
radiography in, 1319, 1318f, 1320f-1321f
renal disease in, 1320
respiratory pump dysfunction in, 2802-2803
treatment and prognosis in, 1321-1322
Annelida, 193

Anorectal sexually transmitted disease, in females, 1529-1530
Anorectal tuberculosis, 1682
Anorexia
  in dementia, 103
  palliative treatment of, 102-103
Anorexia nervosa, 2666-2669
  anemia in, 1094
  diagnosis of, 2668
  differential diagnosis of, 2669
  epidemiology of, 2666, 2667
  etiology and genetics in, 2667
  management of, 2668-2669
  medical complications of, 2669
  pathogenesis of, 2667-2668
  prognosis in, 2669
Anorexiant-induced valvular heart disease, 362
Anovulation, in infertility, 1005-1007, 1005f
Anserine bursitis, 1396
Anterior horn cell disease, respiratory dysfunction in, 2806
Anthralin, topical, for psoriasis, 466-467
Anthrax, 127-133, 1593-1596
  classification and epidemiology of, 128
  cutaneous, 131-132, 132f-133f
  diagnosis of, 1594-1595
  etiology and epidemiology of, 1594
  gastrointestinal, 132, 1595
  infection control in, 132-133
  inhalational, 128-131, 129f-131f
    clinical presentation and diagnosis of, 128-129, 129f-131f
    prevention of, 130-131, 132t
    treatment in, 129-130, 131t
    vaccine for, 131
  meningitis in, 1595
  microbiology of, 1594
  oropharyngeal, 132
  pathogenesis of, 1594
  pathophysiology of, 128
  prevention of, 1596
  respiratory, 1595
  skin infection in, 513-514, 513f, 1594-1595, 1594f
  treatment and prognosis in, 1595-1596
Antiandrogen(s), for hirsutism, 990-991, 990t
Antiarrhythmic agent(s), 266-269. See also specific drugs
  for acute myocardial infarction, 329
  classification and mechanism of, 266-268, 267t
  efficacy and outcome of, 268-269
  for prevention of myocardial infarction, 333
  proarrhythmia due to, 268
Antibiotic(s), 1420-1442. See also specific drugs, e.g., Penicillin
  bacterial susceptibility to, 1420, 1421t
  complications of, 1422-1424
    direct toxicity, 1423
      platelets, 1175
    hypersensitivity, 1423
      acute interstitial nephritis, 2087-2088, 2087t
    microbial superinfection as, 1424
  in concurrent illness, 1421
  for COPD, 2730
  dosage and route of administration of, 1420-1421
  in elderly, 1422
  for endocarditis, 1490-1494, 1492t
  identification of infecting organism, 1420, 1421t

for infections in adults, 1425t-1427t
for lung abscess, 1478-1479
for osteomyelitis, 1547-1548, 1547t
overview of, 1420-1424
for pneumonia, 1471-1474, 1472t-1474t
in pregnancy, 1421-1422, 1422t
prophylactic, 1440-1441
  for endocarditis, 1495-1496, 1495t-1497t
  for surgical procedures, 1440-1441
resistance to, public health considerations in, 1424
for septic shock, 1452t, 1452
site of infection and, 1420
topical, 1440
for urinary tract infection, 1512-1516, 1513t
Antibody(ies). See also Immunoglobulin(s)
  monoclonal. See Monoclonal antibody(ies)
Anticancer chemotherapy, 2413-2423, 2415t-2420t. See also individual drugs
  antimicrotubular drugs in, 2421-2422
  for brain tumors, 2313
  combination, 2413
  DNA alkylating and cross-linking agents in, 2413-2414
  DNA topoisomerase inhibitors in, 2414, 2421
  dose-response and schedule in, 2410-2411
  estramustine in, 2422
  gene-based therapies in, 2423
  growth factors, receptors, signal transduction pathways in, 2422-2423
  immunotherapies in, 2423
  metastasis and angiogenesis inhibitors in, 2423
  neurotoxicity due to, 2319-2320, 2319t
  nucleic acid synthesis inhibitors in, 2414
  nucleic acid synthesis or function alteration in, 2413-2414, 2421
  pharmacogenetics of, 2413
  pharmacokinetics of, 2413
  principles of, 2410-2413
  resistance to, 2411-2413, 2412f
    molecular genetics of, 2394-2396, 2395f-2396f
  taxanes in, 2421-2422
  toxicities of, 2413
  vinca alkaloids in, 2421
Anticardiolipin antibody syndrome, 443-444
Anti-CD20 antibody, for non-Hodgkin lymphoma, 2406
Anticholinergic(s)
  for asthma, 2711-2712, 2711t
  overdose, 162
  for Parkinson disease, 2247
Anticholinergic syndrome, in poisoning or drug overdose, 158t
Anticoagulant(s)
  acquired circulating, 1186-1187
  oral, pharmacology of, 417
  overdose, 162-163
  pharmacology of, 416-417
  for prevention of myocardial infarction, 333
  for pulmonary embolism, 420-421
  for unstable angina and NSTMI, 310-312, 311t
  for venous thromboembolism, 420-421
  for venous thrombosis, 420-421

Anticoagulant-induced skin necrosis, 501, 501f, 501t
Anticonvulsant(s)
  for bipolar disorder, 2622, 2621t
  for herpes simplex encephalitis, 2348
  hypersensitivity syndrome reaction due to, 496
Anticytokine therapy, for acute pancreatitis, 919-920
Antidepressant(s). See also specific drugs
  in pain management, 2185
  for panic disorder, 2660
  in terminal illness, 116, 116t
  tricyclic
    for depression, 2617
    overdose, 174, 174t
    seizure due to, 157t
Antiepileptic drugs, in pain management, 2184-2185
Antifungal agent(s), 1870-1873, 1871t-1872t
  amphotericin B as, 1873, 1873t
  azoles as, 1871-1873, 1871t-1872t
    absorption issues of, 1871-1872
    drug-drug interactions of, 1872-1873, 1871t-1872t
    side effects of, 1871
  fluconazole as, 1871-1873, 1871t-1872t
  itraconazole as, 1871-1873, 1871t-1872t
  ketoconazole as, 1871-1873, 1871t-1872t
Anti-GBM antibody disease, 2058-2060, 2058f-2060f
  diffuse alveolar hemorrhage in, 2783
  in nephritic syndrome, 2058-2060, 2058f-2060f
  in renal transplant recipients, 2116
Antigen-presenting cell(s), 1240
Anti-glomerular basement membrane disease, glomerulonephritis in, 2076-2077
Antihistamine(s)
  for allergy, 1250
  overdose, 162
Antihypertensive drug(s)
  for angina pectoris, 298
  drugs that can interfere with, 218t, 218
Anti-IgE therapy, for allergy, 1250
Antimicrobial(s). See Antibiotic(s)
Antimicrotubular agents, 2419t, 2421
Antimullerian hormone, in polycystic ovary syndrome, 978-979
Antineuronal antibody, in paraneoplastic disorders, 2318t, 2318
Antineutrophil cytoplasmic antibody(ies)
  in renal vasculitis, 2075-2076, 2076f
  in Wegener granulomatosis, 2752-2753
Antioncogene(s). See Tumor suppressor gene(s)
Antioxidant(s), colorectal cancer and, 2477
Antiphospholipid antibody syndrome, 1197-1199, 1335, 1329t
  autoimmunity in, 1237
  classification of antibodies in, 1198t, 1198
  clinical presentation in, 1197
  diagnosis of, 1197-1198, 1197t-1198t
  encephalopathy in, 2342-2343
  epidemiology in, 1197
  pathophysiology of, 1197

polyarteritis nodosa vs., 1366, 1367f
pregnancy loss in, 1198-1199
primary, 1335, 1329t
renal involvement in, 2080-2081
treatment in, 1198, 1339
alpha$_2$-Antiplasmin deficiency, 1184
alpha$_2$-Antiplasmin test, 1161
Antiplatelet agent(s)
  for angina pectoris, 296-297
  for stroke, 2206-2208, 2212-2213, 2212t
Antiprotease replacement therapy, for alpha$_1$-antitrypsin deficiency, 2733-2734
Antiprotease therapy, for acute pancreatitis, 919
Antireflux procedures, endoscopic, for gastroesophageal reflux disease, 767-768
Antireflux surgery, for gastroesophageal reflux disease, 767
Antithrombin deficiency, 1192-1193
Antithrombin III assay, 1162
Antithrombin III-heparan sulfate system, in coagulation, 1155, 1157f
Antithrombotic agent(s)
  in atrial fibrillation, 246-248, 246t, 247f
  complications of, 417-418
  for endocarditis, 1495
  pharmacology of, 416-417
  for stroke, 2206-2208, 2212-2213
Antithymocyte globulin, for aplastic anemia, 1096
alpha$_1$-Antitrypsin deficiency, 2732-2734, 2733f
  antiprotease replacement therapy for, 2733-2734
  chest radiography in, 2732, 2732f
  chronic hepatitis in, 883
  diagnosis of, 2733, 2733f
  in emphysema, 2724, 2724f
  genetic variants in, 2732-2733
Antitumor antibody therapy, 2406-2407
Antiviral chemotherapy. See individual drugs
Ants, fire, 191, 1285-1286, 1286f-1287f
Anxiety, in brain trauma, 2235-2236
Anxiety disorder(s), 2657-2665. See also individual disorders
  acute stress disorder, 2661-2662
  conditions confused with, 2659t
  in diagnosis of palpitation, 204t
  FDA-approved drugs for, 2660t
  generalized, 2662
  Internet resources for, 2658
  key symptoms of, 2657t
  management of, 2657
  obsessive-compulsive disorder, 2663-2664
  panic disorder, 2657-2661
  phobia in medical settings, 2664
  posttraumatic stress disorder, 2661-2662
  social, 2662-2663
Aorta
  atheromatous emboli of, 374
  coarctation of, 393-394
    hypertension in, 217t, 234, 231t
  diseases of, 365-376
  normal, 365
  traumatic disease of, 375
Aortic aneurysm, 365-369
  abdominal, 365-368
    clinical presentation in, 365
    diagnostic evaluation in, 365-366
    imaging studies in, 366

physical examination in, 365-366
postoperative risk-factor
    modification in, 368
preoperative evaluation in, 366-
    368, 367f
reducing risk of rupture in, 366
screening for, 365
surgery for, 366-368, 367f
dissecting. *See* Aortic dissection
thoracic, 368-369
    clinical presentation in, 368
    diagnostic evaluation in, 368
    reduction of rupture risk in,
        368-369
    surgical treatment and
        postoperative complications
        of, 369
Aortic dissection, 369-374
    atypical, 373-374
    classification of, 369
    diagnostic evaluation in, 370, 371f-
        373f
    in differential diagnosis of chest
        pain, 198t, 197
    penetrating atherosclerotic ulcer
        in, 373-374
    presentation in, 369-370, 370f
    treatment of, 370-373
        medical, 372-373
        postoperative complications of,
            371-372
        surgical, 371
    without intimal tear, 373
Aortic regurgitation, 357-
    359, 348t, 350t
    clinical manifestations of, 358
    imaging studies of, 358, 358f
    murmur in, 210t
    treatment of, 358-359
Aortic stenosis, 355-357, 348t, 350t
    clinical manifestations of, 355-
        356, 350t
    in differential diagnosis of chest
        pain, 198t, 197
    imaging studies of, 356
    murmur in, 210t
    treatment of, 356-357
Aortic trauma, 385-386, 385f
Aortic valve
    in ankylosing spondylitis, 1320
    annular abscess, in endocarditis,
        1489
    bicuspid, 391-393
APC
    in adenomatous polyposis coli,
        1961
    properties of, 2386t, 2391
Aphasia, progressive, 2222
Apheresis, 1218-1219
    for antibody-mediated renal,
        muscular, and cutaneous
        disease, 1219
    complications of, 1219
    for hematologic disease, 1218-1219
    for immune complex disease, 1219
    indications for, 1218-1219, 1218t
    for metabolic disease, 1219
    for neurologic disease, 1218-1219
Aphthous stomatitis, in inflammatory
    bowel disease, 435, 435f
Aphthous ulcer, in inflammatory
    bowel disease, 435, 435f
Aplastic anemia, 1095-1097
    definition of, 1095, 1095f
    diagnosis of, 1096, 1095f-1096f
    etiology of, 1095, 1095t
    treatment of, 1096-1097
        bone marrow transplantation for,
            1097
        hematopoietic stem cell
            transplantation for, 1222
        immunosuppression for, 1096-1097
        in mild forms, 1096-1097

platelet transfusion for, 1096
    in severe cases, 1097
Apolipoprotein, 729, 730t
Apolipoprotein B-100, familial
    defective, 738-739
Apotransferrin, in iron metabolism,
    1080
Appendectomy, 821
Appendiceal tumor, 819
Appendicitis, 818-821
    acute, acute cholecystitis *vs.*,
        904
    anatomy and pathogenesis of, 818-
        819
    clinical presentation of, 819, 819t
    diagnosis of, 819-820
    diagnostic evaluation in, 819-820
    diagnostic tests in, 820-821
        abdominal CT, 820, 820f
        abdominal ultrasound, 820
        barium enema, 820-821
        treatment of, 821
    epidemiology of, 818
    epiploic, diverticulitis *vs.*, 814-
        815
Appetite control, pro-
    opiomelanocortin peptides and,
    598
Arbovirus infection, encephalitis,
    2352
ARDS. *See* Acute respiratory distress
    syndrome (ARDS)
Arenavirus infections, 1852, 1850t
    meningitis in, 2353
Argatroban, for heparin-induced
    thrombocytopenia, 1200
Aromatase inhibitors, for early
    (stages I and II) breast cancer,
    2465
Aromatherapy, 86t
Arrhythmia. *See also under specific*
    arrhythmia, Tachycardia
    in poisoning, 156, 156t
    in pregnancy, 1019
    ventricular. *See* Ventricular
        arrhythmia(s)
Arsenic, biologic test of exposure
    to, 61t
Arterial occlusive disease. *See*
    Peripheral arterial disease
Arteriosclerosis obliterans. *See*
    Peripheral arterial disease,
    atherosclerotic
Arteriovenous malformation,
    pulmonary, 2756
    pulmonary hypertension in, 2862
Arteritis
    giant cell, 365, 1368-1369
        encephalopathy in, 2342
        fever of undetermined origin in,
            1415
    large vessel, 1368-1370
        Takayasu (pulseless disease), 374-
            375, 1369, 1369f
    temporal, 1368-1369
        fever of undetermined origin in,
            1415
        headache in, 2154t, 2163
Arthralgia, rash, 1857-1858
Arthritis. *See also* Joint infection
    acne-associated, 1325-1326
    enteropathic, 1325
        spondylitis, 1325
    gouty, acute, 1372-1373, 1373f
    in Lyme disease, 1714
    in psoriasis, 464, 1317t, 1324-1325
        osteoarthritis *vs.*, 1387
    reactive, 1317t, 1322-1324
        balanitis in, 1323, 1323f
        diagnosis of, 1322-1324, 1323f
        epidemiology of, 1322
        HIV and, 1323
        HLA-B27 in, 1322

keratoderma blennorrhagicum in,
    1323, 1323f
    treatment and prognosis in, 1325
rheumatoid. *See* Rheumatoid
    arthritis
septic, 1533-1541
    acute, 1536
    anaerobic, 1537
    candidal, 1878t
    clinical subgroups of, 1538-1540
    diagnosis of, 1533-1536
    diagnostic imaging in, 1535-1536
    in elderly patients, 1539
    epidemiology of, 1533
    fungal, 1538
    gram-negative, 1537
    in hemodialysis, 1539
    history in, 1533
    in HIV, 1539
    in intravenous drug abuse, 1539
    in joint prostheses, 1539-1540
    laboratory tests in, 1534-
        1535, 1534f, 1535t
        likely causes of, 1535t
    Mycobacterium marinum, 1538
    Mycobacterium tuberculosis, 1538
    Neisseria gonorrhoeae, 1536-1537
    in organ transplantation, 1539
    Pasteurella multocida, 1538
    pathogenesis of, 1533
    physical examination in, 1533-
        1534
    in rheumatoid arthritis, 1539
    specific infectious agents in,
        1536-1538
    Staphylococcus aureus, 1537
    streptococcal, 1537
    synovial fluid analysis in, 1534-
        1535, 1534f, 1535t
    treatment of, 1540-1541, 1540t
        drainage, 1540
        medical, 1540-1541, 1540t
    Treponema pallidum, 1538
    Ureaplasma urealyticum, 1537-
        1538
    in systemic lupus erythematosus,
        1332
    traumatic, pain in, 1291f
    tuberculous, 1538
Arthritis-dermatitis syndrome,
    gonococcal, 1536, 1622
Arthropathy, enteropathic,
    1317t, 1325
Arthropod-borne encephalitis, 2344t,
    2352
Asbestos
    in lung cancer and mesothelioma,
        2377
    mesothelioma due to, 2554
Asbestosis, chronic diffuse
    pulmonary infiltration in, 2764
Ascites
    in cirrhosis, 895-896. *See also*
        under Cirrhosis
    pleural effusion in, 2828
Asherman syndrome, 955-956
Ash-leaf macule, in tuberous
    sclerosis, 440, 441f
Aspergillosis
    bronchopulmonary, allergic, 1883-
        1884, 1884t-1885t, 2707-
        2708, 2716
        segmental pulmonary infiltrates
            in, 2751, 2750f
    in compromised host, 1882-1887
    invasive, 1885-1887, 1885f, 1885t
        diagnosis of, 1886
        epidemiology and etiology of,
            1885-1886, 1885f
        treatment of, 1886-1887, 1885t
    invasive pulmonary
        large mass in, 2754

multifocal infiltrates in, 2747
Aspiration, of foreign matter,
    segmental pulmonary infiltrates
    in, 2751
Aspiration pneumonia, 1476-1477
Aspirin. *See also* Nonsteroidal anti-
    inflammatory drugs (NSAIDs),
    Salicylate(s)
    allergy to, 1275
    for angina pectoris, 296
    asthma due to, 2706-2707, 2716
    in diabetes mellitus, 674-675
    GI bleeding due to, 863-864
    for myocardial infarction, acute,
        320, 320f
    nephropathy due to, 2090, 2089f
    platelet functional effects of,
        1175
    poisoning or overdose, 172-173
    primary angioplasty and, 326
    for unstable angina and NSTMI,
        309, 309t
Asthma, 2701-2719
    in allergic bronchopulmonary
        aspergillosis, 2707-2708, 2709f
    clinical manifestations of, 2704
    diagnosis of, 2704-2706, 2704t
    differential diagnosis of, 2705-
        2706, 2704t
    due to aspirin or sulfites, 2706-
        2707
    exercise-induced, 2706
    laboratory tests in, 2705
    management of, 2708-2717
        in allergic bronchopulmonary
            aspergillosis, 2716
        in aspirin-induced disease, 2716
        drug therapy in, 2708-2715, 2710t-
            2711t, 2713t
        in exercise-induced disease,
            2716
        in mild intermittent disease,
            2715
        in mild persistent disease, 2715
        in moderate to severe persistent
            disease, 2715-2716
        in occupational disease, 2716
        outpatient care in, 2715-2716
    near-fatal and hyperacute, 2706
    nocturnal, 2706
    occupational, 62-63, 2707, 2708t
    pathogenesis of, 2701-2704
        allergic response in, 2701-
            2702, 2702f
        genetic influence in, 2702-2703
        viral influence in, 2703-
            2704, 2703f
    in pregnancy, 1021, 2707
    respiratory failure in, 2815-2816
    in respiratory viral infection,
        1780
    segmental pulmonary infiltrates
        in, 2751
    sleep-disordered breathing in,
        2797
    specific forms and comorbidities
        of, 2706-2708
    therapy in
        anticholinergic agents in, 2711-
            2712, 2711t
        anti-inflammatory drugs in, 2712-
            2714, 2713t
        beta agonists in, 2709-
            2711, 2711t
        bronchodilators in, 2709-
            2712, 2710t-2711t
        cromolyn and nedocromil in, 2713
        emergency, 2716-2717
        immunotherapy in, 2714-2715
        inhaled glucocorticoids in,
            2712, 2713t
        inpatient, 2717
        leukotriene modifiers in, 2713

omalizumab in, 2714
outpatient, 2715-2716
systemic glucocorticoids in, 2712
theophylline in, 2713-2714
triggers for, 2704
types of reactions in, 2704-2705
Astrocytoma, 2314, 2311t
Astrovirus, enteric, 1800
Asystole
anoxic encephalopathy in, 2336
in cardiac resuscitation, 152, 151f
Ataxia
autosomal recessive
with DNA break repair, 2263t, 2265
with oculomotor apraxia, 2263t, 2265
early-onset, with retained tendon reflexes, 2266
hereditary, 2263-2269
autosomal dominant, 2266-2268, 2264t
diagnosis of, 2267-2268, 2268f, 2268t
genetics and pathogenesis in, 2266-2267, 2264t, 2265f-2267f
autosomal recessive, 2263-2266, 2263t
of Charlevoix-Saguenay, 2265, 2263t
differential diagnosis of, 2268-2269
genotypic classification in, 2263, 2263t-2264t
Internet resources on, 2266
with isolated vitamin E deficiency, 2265, 2263t
management of, 2269
Ataxia-telangiectasia, 2265, 2263t
CNS tumors in, 2310t
immunologic deficiency in, 1232, 1230t
Atazanavir, for HIV infection, adverse effects of, 1834t
Atelectasis
in mechanical ventilation, 2818, 2819f
rounded, 2833
Atenolol
for hypertension, 222t
toxicity of, 163t
Atheroembolism
in peripheral arterial disease, 405-406, 406f
in renal vascular disease, 2083-2084, 2083f
Atheromatous embolus, aortic, 374
Atherosclerosis
coronary, in angina pectoris, 284-285
in dyslipidemia, 732-733
exercise and, 35-36
with normal lipid levels, 736
peripheral arterial. See Peripheral arterial disease, atherosclerotic
in systemic lupus erythematosus, 1332, 1339
Atherosclerotic ulcer, penetrating, 373-374
Athlete. See also Exercise
blood doping (recombinant human erythropoietin abuse) in, 1136
ATM, mechanisms of, 2390-2391
Atopic dermatitis, 474-478
diagnosis of, 475-476, 475t, 476f, 479f
differential diagnosis of, 476, 477t
etiology and pathogenesis of, 474-475

in food allergy, 1279
treatment of, 477-478
Atopic disorders, epidemiology of, 1240
Atopy. See also under Allergy and atopy
definition of, 474, 1240
genetics in, 1241
Atovaquone-proguanil, for malaria chemoprophylaxis, for travelers, 78
Atransferrinemia, 1088
Atrial defibrillator, for atrial fibrillation, 244
Atrial fibrillation, 238-249
in acute myocardial infarction, 248, 330
antithrombotic therapy in, 246-248, 246t, 247f
cardioversion and, 246-247, 247f
in cardiac surgery, 247-248
classification of, 238
diagnosis of, 238-239, 239t
ECG tracing of, 238, 238f
epidemiology of, 238
in hyperthyroidism, 248
in hypertrophic cardiomyopathy, 248
laboratory studies in, 239, 239t
management of, 239-248, 239f-241f
pathophysiology of, 238
in pulmonary disease, 248
sinus rhythm in, 240-244
electrical cardioversion in, 241-243
nonpharmacologic maintenance in, 244
outpatient initiation of antiarrhythmic drugs in, 244
pharmacologic cardioversion in, 240-241, 242t-243t
pharmacologic maintenance in, 243-244, 241f
in thyrotoxicosis, 617
ventricular rate in, 244-245, 245t
Wolff-Parkinson-White syndrome and, 248, 255
Atrial flutter, 256-258, 257f
antithrombotic therapy in, 246
Atrial pacing, for atrial fibrillation, 244
Atrial septal defect, 388-389, 389f
murmur in, 210t
Atrial tachycardia
focal, 256
multifocal, 256
Atrioventricular block
in drug overdose or poisoning, 156t
pacemaker for, 273, 275, 274t
Atrioventricular nodal reentry tachycardia, 251-254, 250f-253f, 254t
classification of, 250-251, 250f-253f
management of, 252-254, 254t
acute therapy, 252-254
catheter ablation, 254
long-term therapy, 254, 254t
pathogenesis and diagnosis of, 251-252, 251f, 253f
Atrioventricular node, 273
Atrioventricular reentry tachycardia, 254-256, 255f. See also Wolff-Parkinson-White syndrome
classification of, 250-251, 250f-253f
Atrioventricular septal defect, 389-390, 390f
Atrophy, definition of, 429t
Atropine, in cardiac resuscitation, 144t

Attention deficit, in brain trauma, 2236
Autoantibody(ies)
in myasthenia gravis, 1236-1237, 2285, 2286f
in myositis, 1354-1355
in systemic lupus erythematosus, 1327
Autoimmune disease, in pregnancy, 1022
Autoimmunity, 1236-1239
autoantigen identification in, 1236-1238
nonpathogenic autoantibodies in, 1237-1238
pathogenic autoantibodies in, 1236-1237
autoantigens from proteins modified during apoptosis in, 1237-1238
genetics of, 1238
molecular mimicry in, 1236
organ-specific, systemic vs., 1238-1239
type 1 diabetes mellitus and, 635
Automatism, in complex partial seizure, 2188
Automobile driving, epilepsy and, 2198
Autonomic neuropathy, diabetic, 671, 2299-2300
Autonomic syndromes, in poisoning or drug overdose, 158t
Avascular necrosis, in HIV infection, 1835
AV block. See Atrioventricular block
Axillary lymph node(s), in breast cancer, 2463
Axillary venous thrombosis, 422
Axonal polyneuropathy, metabolic, 2300
Azathioprine
after liver transplantation, complications of, 934
for autoimmune hemolytic anemia, 1125
for autoimmune hepatitis, 884
for inflammatory bowel disease, 801-802
for myositis, 1357, 1357t
for rheumatoid arthritis, 1308t, 1312
Azelaic acid, for acne vulgaris, 449t
Azithromycin, 1434
for Campylobacter infection, 1635t
in pregnancy, 1422t
for syphilis, 1704, 1704t
Azlocillin, 1428
Azotemia, prerenal, in hospitalized patient, 2027
AZT. See Zidovudine (AZT)
Aztreonam, 1431
in pregnancy, 1422t

B

Babesia microti, 1897
Babesiosis, 1897-1898, 1897f
hemolytic anemia in, 1129
Bacillary angiomatosis, 1673-1674
in AIDS, 437-438
Bacillus(i)
acid-fast, antimicrobial drugs for, 1427t
clinical syndromes caused by, 1596t
gram-negative. See also individual diseases
antimicrobial drugs for, 1425t-1426t
gram-positive, 1584-1599. See also individual diseases, e.g.,

Diphtheria
antimicrobial drugs for, 1425t
Bacillus alvei, 1596t
Bacillus anthracis, 513, 1593-1594
Bacillus Calmette-Guerin (BCG), for tuberculosis chemoprophylaxis, 1694
Bacillus cereus infection, 1596-1597, 1596t
Bacillus sphaericus, 1596t
Bacillus subtilis, 1596t
Bacitracin, 1440
Back pain, 1391-1392
acute, 1391-1392, 1392t
in cancer, 2175
chronic, 1392
Bacteremia
definition of, 1443t
Haemophilus influenzae, 1650
listeriosis, 1591
meningococcal, 1618
Pseudomonas aeruginosa, 1660
staphylococcal, 1577
streptococcal, group A, 1570
Bacterial endotoxin, in sepsis, 1444-1445, 1446f
Bacterial infection. See specific infection
Bacterial overgrowth syndrome, small intestinal, 833-834, 857
Bacterial septicemia, thrombocytopenia due to, 1163
Bacterial superantigens, in sepsis, 1445, 1446f
Bacterial susceptibility, to antimicrobial agents, 1420, 1421t
Bactericidal/permeability-increasing protein, in sepsis, 1445
Bacteroides species, infections, 1603-1606
Balanitis
in arthritis, 1323, 1323f
Candida, 507-508, 1878t
Balanoposthitis, Candida, 1878t
Balantidium coli infection, 1908, 1908t
Balkan nephropathy, 2101
Balloon mitral valvuloplasty, for mitral stenosis, 352-353, 353f
Balo disease, 2328
Balsalazide, for inflammatory bowel disease, 801t
Bamboo spine, in ankylosing spondylitis, 1319, 1321f
Barbiturate(s), overdose, 173
Bariatric (obesity) surgery, 724-725, 725t
Barium enema
in appendicitis, 820-821
in colorectal cancer, 2481
Barium salts, poisoning with, hypokalemia due to, 2007
Barium swallow
in achalasia, 762, 762f
in dysphagia, 759
in esophageal cancer, 772, 772f
in gastroesophageal reflux disease, 765
Barmah Forest virus, 1857
Barotrauma, in mechanical ventilation, 2817-2818, 2818f
Barrett esophagus, 768-769, 768f-769f
diagnosis and surveillance in, 2492t, 2492
esophageal cancer and, 2491
tobacco use and, 2374
Bartonellosis, 1672-1674, 1664t, 1666t
bacteremia and endocarditis in, 1672-1673, 1666t
classic, 1672
Bartter syndrome, 687, 2004
Basal body temperature, in infertility, 1005

Basal cell carcinoma, 549-550, 550f
Basal cell nevus syndrome, 440
Basal energy expenditure (BEE),
   calculation of, 946
Basal ganglia
   cortical degeneration of, 2252
   functional anatomy of, 2239, 2240f
Basal metabolic rate (BMR),
   calculation of, 946
Basophil(s), 1150-1151
   development of, 1072f
   function of, 1150-1151
   in immediate hypersensitivity,
      1244-1246, 1244f-1245f
Basophilia, 1151
Bat bite, 181
B cell(s), development of, 1072f
BCG. See Bacillus Calmette-Guerin
bcl-1, in lymphoma, 2601
bcl-2
   in lymphoma, 2392, 2601, 2602f
   properties of, 2384t
bcr-abl, properties of, 2384, 2384t
bcr-abl-negative chronic myeloid
   leukemia, 2577t
Bcr-Abl tyrosine kinase, new cancer
   therapies and, 2409-2410
Beau line(s), of nails, 573, 573
Becker muscular dystrophy. See
   Muscular dystrophy, Becker
Becker-type myotonia (autosomal
   recessive myotonia congenita),
   2282
Beclomethasone, for asthma,
   2712, 2713t
Bed bugs, 191
Beef tapeworm, 1938, 1939f
Beer potomania, 1983
Bee stings, 1285, 1286f
Behavioral-counseling interventions,
   48-49
Behavior modification, reducing risk
   of injury and disease and, 18
Bell palsy (facial neuropathy), 2293-
   2294, 2294t
Benazepril, for hypertension, 222t
Bence Jones protein, in multiple
   myeloma, 2096-2097, 2097f
Bentiromide test, for malabsorption,
   826, 825t
Benzene, biologic test of exposure
   to, 61t
Benzodiazepine, for premenstrual
   syndrome, 964
Benzodiazepine(s)
   overdose, 173
   overdose of, treatment of, 2642
   for panic disorder, 2660
Benzoyl peroxide, for acne vulgaris,
   449t
Berger disease (IgA nephropathy),
   2056-2057, 2056t, 2057f-2058f
   in ankylosing spondylitis, 1320
Bernard-Soulier syndrome, 1174
Berylliosis, chronic diffuse
   pulmonary infiltration in, 2765
Beryllium disease, chronic (CBD), 63
Beta-adrenergic agonist(s). See also
   specific drugs
   for asthma, 2709-2711, 2711t
   for thyrotoxicosis, 615
   for urticaria, 1265
Beta-adrenergic antagonist(s). See
   also specific drugs, e.g.,
   Propranolol
   for acute myocardial infarction,
      328
   for angina pectoris, 299
   for cardiac arrhythmia, 267t
   for heart failure, 342, 343t
   overdose, 163, 163t
   for unstable angina and NSTMI, 313
Beta blocker(s). See Beta-adrenergic

antagonist(s)
Betaretrovirus, 1802t
Bethlem myopathy, 2276
Bevacizumab, for colorectal cancer,
   2487
Bicalutamide, 2420t
Bicarbonate
   in cardiac resuscitation, 144t
   renal reabsorption of, 1994, 1995f
Bicipital tendinitis, 1393
Bicycle injury, 22
Bifascicular block, pacemaker for,
   274t, 275
Bile acid malabsorption
   diarrhea in, 843
   tests for, 826-827, 827f, 845-846
Bile duct, common
   obstruction of, in chronic
      pancreatitis, 930
   stone in. See Choledocholithiasis
   stricture of, 909
Biliary cirrhosis, primary
   chronic hepatitis vs., 883
   dyslipidemia and, 740-741
Biliary tract cancer, 2505-
   2506, 2506f
Biliary tract disease
   chronic, 908-911
      diagnosis of, 909
   in malabsorption, 824
Biliopancreatic diversion, for
   weight loss, 725t
Billroth I procedure, gastroparesis
   after, 852
Billroth II procedure, steatorrhea
   after, 835
Binge-eating disorder, 2666, 2672-
   2673
   diagnosis of, 2672
   epidemiology of, 2672
   management of, 2672-2673
Biofeedback, 86t
Biologic-based therapies,
   alternative, 85-86, 87t-89t
Biologic response modifier(s). See
   under Interferon, specific types
Biopsy
   bone marrow
      in fever of undetermined origin,
         1417
      in hematologic disease,
         1076, 1076f
      in thrombocytopenia, 1164-
         1165, 1165t
   breast, in mass evaluation, 1050-
      1051, 1050f
   bronchial, bronchoscopy for, 2690
   endometrial, in menopause, 1033
   esophageal, in gastroesophageal
      reflux disease, 765
   in fever of undetermined origin,
      1417
   kidney
      in glomerular disease, 2052-2054
      in lupus nephritis, 1334, 1334t-
         1335t, 1336
   liver
      in cirrhosis, 893-894
      in fever of undetermined origin,
         1417
   lung. See Lung biopsy
   lymph node, in fever of
      undetermined origin, 1417
   muscle, in fever of undetermined
      origin, 1417
   nerve, in peripheral nerve
      disease, 2293
   in pelvic mass, 1058
   pleural, 2698
   skin, in fever of undetermined
      origin, 1417
   small intestine, in gluten-
      sensitive enteropathy,

828, 829f
   temporal artery, in fever of
      undetermined origin, 1417
Bioterrorism, 121-140. See also
   individual diseases
   anthrax, 127-133, 513
   botulism, 134-136
   clinician's role in preparedness,
      121
   communication with authorities
      and, 122
   hemorrhagic fever viruses, 137-138
   Internet resources on, 123
   plague, 133-134
   potential agents for, 121-122, 122t
   smallpox, 122-127
   tularemia, 136-137
Biotin, 29t
Bipolar disorder, 2619-2622
   clinical manifestations of, 2620
   complications of, 2622
   definition of, 2613
   diagnosis of, 2620-2621
   differential diagnosis of, 2621
   epidemiology of, 2619
   etiology and genetics in, 2619
   laboratory tests in, 2621
   management of, 2621-2622, 2621t
      additional therapeutic
         strategies in, 2622
      anticonvulsant medications in,
         2622, 2621t
      atypical antipsychotics in, 2622
      lithium in, 2621-2622, 2621t
      mental-status examination in, 2620-
         2621
   pathogenesis of, 2619-2620
   prognosis in, 2622
Bird fancier's disease, 2765. See
   also Pneumonitis,
   hypersensitivity
Birthmarks, vascular, 544-546
Birt-Hogg-Dube syndrome, 538
Bismuth subsalicylate, for
   Helicobacter infection, 1637t
Bisoprolol, for hypertension, 222t
Bisphosphonate(s), for osteoporosis,
   709
Bite, 180-196
   bat, 181
   cat, 180, 181t-182t
   dog, 180, 181t-182t
   ferret, 180-181
   human, 181, 181t-182t
   insect, 191-192
   mammalian, 180-182, 181t-182t
      domestic, 180-181
      epidemiology of, 180
      nondomestic, 181
      treatment of, 181-182, 181t-183t
   monkey, 181, 182t
   rat, 181, 182t
   snake. See Snakebite
   spider, 187-190
Bitolterol, for asthma, 2709, 2711t
Bivalirudin, for unstable angina and
   NSTMI, 312, 311t
Black patient(s). See African
   Americans
Black widow spider bite, 187-
   188, 188f
Bladder. See Urinary bladder
Blastocystis hominis infection,
   1906, 1907f
Blastomyces dermatitidis, 1865
Blastomycosis, 1865-1866
   clinical presentation in, 1865
   diagnosis of, 1865, 1866f
   differential diagnosis of, 1865-
      1866
   disseminated, 1865
   epidemiology of, 1865
   pathogenesis of, 1865

prognosis in, 1866
   pulmonary, 1865
      large mass in, 2754
   treatment of, 1866
Bleeding disorder. See also
   Platelet(s), Thrombocytopenia
   approach to patient with, 1163-
      1164
Bleeding (hemorrhage). See also
   Thrombocytopenia
   alveolar, diffuse, 2783
   in cardiac arrest, 148t
   diverticular, 817-818
   esophageal. See Esophageal
      varices, bleeding
   gastrointestinal. See
      Gastrointestinal bleeding
   in hematologic disease, 1075
   in hemophilia A. See also
      Hemophilia A
   intracerebral, in stroke,
      2214, 2214t
   menstrual. See Menstrual disorder,
      excessive bleeding
   postoperative, 1188, 1188t
   subarachnoid, in stroke, 2214-2215
   uremic, in chronic renal failure,
      2045
Bleeding time, 1161
Bleomycin, 2419t
   chronic diffuse infiltrative
      pulmonary disease due to, 2762
Blister(s), in vesiculobullous
   disease of skin, 525, 526t-527t
Blister beetles, 191
Blood, fecal occult. See Fecal
   occult blood testing
Blood donation, 1206-1208
   autologous, 1206
   directed, 1206
   postdonation testing for, 1206-
      1208
   emerging infectious diseases
      and, 1207-1208
   false positives in, 1207
   hepatitis and, 1206-1207
   HIV-1 and, 1822-1823
   retroviruses and, 1207
   screening for, 1206, 1206t
Blood doping (recombinant human
   erythropoietin abuse), 1136
Blood flow, principles of, 1108
Blood pH, definition of, 1994, 1994f
Blood pressure
   drugs that can increase, 218t, 218
   high. See Hypertension
   low. See Hypotension
   measurement of, 216t, 216
   monitoring of, ambulatory, 217
   surgical risk factor management
      and, 55
Blood salvage, intraoperative and
   postoperative, 1211
Blood transfusion. See under
   Transfusion
Bloom syndrome, CNS tumors in, 2310t
Blue bloater, 2727, 2725t, 2727f. See
   also Chronic airflow obstruction
   (CAO)
Body-mass index, 714, 714t
Body temperature. See also Fever
   measurement, 1407
   regulation of, 1407
Body water. See Fluid
Bone
   Paget disease of, 711-712
   radionuclide imaging of, in
      osteomyelitis, 1545, 1546t
Bone disease, metabolic, 707-712
Bone infection
   Haemophilus influenzae, 1650
   Pseudomonas aeruginosa, 1661
   staphylococcal, 1576

streptococcal, group A, 1570
Bone loss
  in home parenteral nutrition, 948
  in menopause, 1030
Bone marrow
  biopsy of
    in fever of undetermined origin, 1417
    in hematologic disease, 1076, 1076f
    in thrombocytopenia, 1164-1165, 1165t
    in hematopoiesis, 1070, 1071f
  occupational disease of, 66
Bone marrow transplantation. *See also* Hematopoietic stem cell transplantation
  for aplastic anemia, 1097
  for *beta*-thalassemia, 1121
Bone pain, in cancer, 2175
Bordetella pertussis, 1656, 1656t. *See also* Pertussis
Bornholm disease (epidemic pleurodynia), 2823
Borrelia burgdorferi, 1712
  infection with. *See* Lyme disease
Bortezomib, for multiple myeloma, 2593
Botulinum A toxin, for incontinence, 1046
Botulinum toxin, for achalasia, 763
Botulism, 134-136, 1609-1610
  clinical presentation in, 135
  diagnosis of, 135-136, 1611
  food-borne, 1609
  infant, 1609
  respiratory insufficiency in, 2807
  treatment of, 136, 1614
  wound, 1609
Bouchard nodes, 1385-1386, 1386f
Bovine spongiform encephalopathy (mad cow disease), 2358, 2359
Bowel. *See also* Colon, Small intestine
  irrigation of, for poisoning or drug overdose, 160, 160t
  obstruction of, palliative treatment of, 105
  resection of, chronic diarrhea in, 848
Bowel habits, pelvic mass and, 1055-1056
Bowel rest, nutritional support in, 943
Bowenoid papulosis, 515, 515f
Brachial plexus neuropathy, 2296
Brachytherapy, endobronchial, 2694
Bradyarrhythmia, in acute myocardial infarction, 330
Bradycardia, in drug overdose or poisoning, 156t
Brain
  imaging studies of, in systemic lupus erythematosus, 1335
  radiation injury to, 2320-2321, 2320t
Brain abscess, 1556-1557
  candidal, 1877t
  imaging studies in, 1557, 1558f
  in nocardiosis, 1593
Brain death, definition of, 2337
Brain trauma, 2228-2238. *See also* Coma
  long-term outcome after, 2236
  management of, 2230-2236
    in mild injury, 2230-2232, 2231f, 2230t
    in moderate and severe injury, 2232-2236, 2232f
      agitation in, 2235
      algorithm for, 2232f
      CT in, 2233, 2233f
      initial evaluation and

resuscitation in, 2232-2233, 2232f
      intracranial pressure monitoring in, 2233-2234, 2234t
      MRI in, 2233
    MRI in, 2231, 2231f
    PET in, 2231, 2231f
  neuropsychiatric sequelae of, 2235-2236
    aggression, 2236
    anxiety, 2235-2236
    attention deficit, 2236
    depression, 2235
    irritability, 2236
  pathogenesis of, 2228-2230
    axonal injury in, 2228-2229
    diffuse gray matter dysfunction in, 2230
    focal injury in, 2228
    hypoxia-ischemia in, 2229
    microvascular injury in, 2229
    neuronal vulnerability and excitotoxic injury in, 2229-2230
  posttraumatic epilepsy after, 2236
  rehabilitation for, 2236-2237
  severity of, 2228, 2229t
Brain tumors
  classification of, 2307, 2308t
  diagnosis of, 2311-2312, 2313f
  environmental risk factors for, 2307-2308
  epidemiology of, 2307
  etiology of, 2307-2308, 2309t-2311t
  genetic risk factors for, 2308, 2310t-2311t
  headache in, 2154t, 2166, 2309
  metastatic, 2317, 2431-2432
  MRI in, 2311-2312, 2313f
  pathophysiology of, 2308-2309, 2312f
  prognosis in, 2314
  seizures in, 2310
  specific types of, 2314-2316
  symptoms and signs of, 2309-2311
    false localizing, 2311
    focal, 2310-2311
    generalized, 2309-2310
  treatment of, 2312-2314
    chemotherapy, 2313
    corticosteroid, 2312-2313
    radiation therapy, 2313
    surgery, 2313
BRCA1 gene
  in breast-ovarian cancer syndrome, 2537-2538
  genetic testing for, 1962-1963
  mechanisms of, 2386t, 2391
BRCA2 gene
  in breast-ovarian cancer syndrome, 2537-2538
  genetic testing for, 1962-1963
  mechanisms of, 2386t, 2391
Breast
  cyst of, 1052, 1052f
  normal nodularity in, 1048
  self-examination of, 47, 2460-2461
Breast cancer, 2459-2473
  early (stages I and II), 2461-2468
    diagnosis of, 2461
    follow-up of, 2468, 2469t
    treatment of, 2461-2468
      adjuvant, 2467-2468, 2468t
      aromatase inhibitors, 2465
      axillary dissection, 2463
      breast conservation therapy, 2463
      chemoendocrine therapy, 2467
      chemotherapy, 2465-2467, 2466t
      chemotherapy and ovarian ablation, 2467
      chemotherapy and tamoxifen,

2467
      combination endocrine therapy, 2467
      in ductal carcinoma in situ, 2461, 2463
      in invasive cancer, 2463-2464
      in lobular carcinoma in situ, 2463
      ovarian oblation for, 2464
      radiotherapy for, 2463-2464
      sentinel lymph node mapping as, 2463
      systemic, 2464-2468
      tamoxifen for, 2464-2465
  etiology and epidemiology of, 2459
    environmental factors in, 2377
    genetic risk factors for, 2378-2379
  genetic testing in, 1962-1963
  male, 696
  mammography for, 45-46, 2461
  management of, antitumor antibody therapy for, 2407
  prevention of, 2459-2460, 2460t
    fenretinide for, 2459
    lifestyle modification for, 2459-2460
    prophylactic mastectomy for, 2460
    raloxifene for, 2459
    tamoxifen for, 2459, 2460t
  risk factors for, 1048, 1048t, 2459
  screening for, 44-47, 2460-2461
    breast self-examination, 47
    clinical breast examination, 47
    genetic risk assessment in, 47
    mammography, 45-46
  stage III, 2468
  stage IV or metastatic, 2468-2471
    diagnosis of, 2468
    treatment of, 2468-2471, 2470f-2471f
      biology-based therapy for, 2470
      chemotherapy for, 2469, 2471t
      endocrine therapy for, 2469, 2471f
      supportive care in, 2471
    staging and prognosis in, 2461, 2462t-2463t
Breast cancer syndromes, familial, 2459
Breast-feeding
  amenorrhea and, 957
  HIV transmission and, 1823
Breast mass, 1048-1054
  benign
    breast cancer risk and, 1053-1054, 1053t
    malignant *vs.,* 1049t, 1049
    management of, 1052-1053, 1052f, 1053t
    cystic, 1052, 1052f
    fat necrosis, 1053
    fibroadenoma, 1053
    hamartoma, 1053
    Phyllodes tumor, 1053
    solid mass, 1053
  differential diagnosis of, 1052-1053
  evaluation of, 1049-1052, 1050f, 1051t
    in dominant mass with benign features, 1050-1051, 1050f, 1051t
    no abnormality in, 1049
    nodularity in, 1049
    in suspicious dominant mass, 1051-1052
  history and physical examination in, 1048-1049, 1048t-1049t
  malignant, benign *vs.,* 1049t, 1049
Breast-ovarian cancer syndrome,

2459, 2537-2538
Breathing. *See also* Respiration, Ventilation
  abnormal patterns of, 2789-2792, 2789f-2791f
  apneustic, 2789-2790, 2789f-2790f
  ataxic (Biot), 2789-2790, 2789f-2790f
  in cardiac resuscitation, 143, 146, 146t
  sleep-disordered. *See* Sleep apnea syndrome, Sleep-disordered breathing
Breath test, carbon-13 or -14-labeled urea, for peptic ulcer disease, 782
Brill-Zinsser disease, 1730
Brodie abscess, 1543
Bromocriptine
  for parkinsonism, 2247t
  for premenstrual syndrome, 964
Bronchial brushings, 2690
Bronchial washings, 2689-2690
Bronchiectasis, 1477, 2734-2737
  chest imaging in, 2735, 2736f
  clinical variants of, 2737-2740
  diagnosis of, 2735-2736, 2736f
  etiology and pathogenesis of, 2734-2735
  pulmonary function testing in, 2736
  segmental pulmonary infiltrates in, 2750
  sputum examination in, 2735-2736
  treatment of, 2736-2737
Bronchiolitis, 2740
  viral, 1779-1780
Bronchiolitis interstitial lung disease, respiratory, 2775-2776, 2777f, 2767t-2768t
Bronchiolitis obliterans, 2748
  in hypersensitivity pneumonitis, 2766, 2765f
Bronchiolitis obliterans organizing pneumonia, 2778, 2779f, 2767t-2768t
  multifocal infiltrates in, 2748
Bronchitis
  acute, 1477, 1779
  chronic, 1477. *See also* Chronic obstructive pulmonary disease (COPD)
    chest imaging in, 2728, 2725t
    clinical manifestations of, 2725, 2725t
    definition of, 2720
    epidemiology of, 2720-2721, 2721f
    etiology of, 2721
    natural history of, 2721-2722, 2722f
    pathology in, 2722-2723
      early changes, 2722
      in established disease, 2722
    physical examination, 2725-2726
    treatment of, 2728-2732
Bronchoalveolar lavage, 2690
  in alveolar proteinosis, 2781-2782, 2782f
  in chronic diffuse infiltrative pulmonary disease, 2760-2761
  in *Pneumocystis carinii* pneumonia, 2760
  in sarcoidosis, 2773
Bronchodilator(s)
  for allergy, 1251
  for asthma. *See* Asthma, therapy in
  for COPD, 2728-2730, 2729t
Bronchogenic cyst, single nodule in, 2753, 2754f
Bronchopulmonary sequestration, 2754, 2755f
Bronchoscopy, 2688-2695
  diagnostic, 2688-2692

autofluorescence, 2691-2692
for biopsy, 2690
for bronchial brushings, 2690
for bronchial washings, 2689-2690
for bronchoalveolar lavage, 2690
complications of, 2692
for endobronchial ultrasound, 2691
indications and contraindications for, 2689, 2690t
instrumentation for, 2688-2689, 2689f
navigational, 2692
for transbronchial needle aspiration, 2690-2691, 2691
for visual inspection, 2689
therapeutic, 2692-2695, 2693t, 2695f
for delayed relief of airway obstruction, 2694-2695
for immediate relief of airway obstruction, 2693-2694, 2693t, 2695f
Brown recluse spider bite, 188-190, 189f
Brown-Sequard syndrome, 2321
Brucellosis, 1664-1668
complications and prognosis in, 1667-1668
diagnosis of, 1667, 1664t
epidemiology of, 1664, 1666
etiology of, 1666-1667
pathogenesis of, 1667
treatment of, 1667, 1665t
Brugada syndrome, 265-266
Brugia malayi, 1929t
Brugia timori, 1929t
Budesonide, for asthma, 2712, 2713t
Bulbar muscular atrophy, X-linked, trinucleotide repeat in, 1960t
Bulimia nervosa, 2666, 2669-2672
diabetes mellitus and, 2671
diagnosis of, 2670
differential diagnosis of, 2670
epidemiology of, 2666, 2669
etiology and genetics in, 2669-2670
management of, 2670-2671
pharmacologic therapy in, 2671
psychotherapy in, 2670-2671
medical complications of, 2671
prognosis in, 2672
Bulla, definition of, 426t
Bumblebee stings, 1285
Bumetanide, for hypertension, 221t
Bupropion
for obesity, 724
for smoking cessation, 20
Burkitt lymphoma, 2608
Epstein-Barr virus and, 1763
Burns, hypokalemia in, 2007
Burn wound sepsis, Pseudomonas aeruginosa, 1662
Burrow, definition of, 429t
Bursitis
anserine, 1396
iliopectineal, 1396
ischiogluteal, 1396
olecranon, 1394
prepatellar, 1396
trochanteric, 1396
Buschke-Lowenstein tumor (giant condyloma acuminatum, genital verrucous carcinoma), 515
Buserelin, 2420t
Busulfan, 2415t
for chronic myeloid leukemia, 2578-2579, 2578t
Butterfly rash, in systemic lupus erythematosus, 1330, 1331f

C

c-abl, properties of, 2384
Cachectin. See Tumor necrosis factor alpha
Cadmium
biologic test of exposure to, 61t
tubulointerstitial nephritis due to, 64, 2095
Cafe au lait macules, 539-540
in neurofibromatosis, 440, 441f
Caffeine, in diet, 31
CAGE questionnaire, for alcoholism, 2627, 2628t
Calcific tendinitis, of rotator cuff, 1393
Calcineurin inhibitors
for atopic dermatitis, 477
for prerenal-transplant patient management, 2118
Calcinosis, in scleroderma, 1344, 1343f-1344f
Calciphylaxis, 442, 442f
Calcipotriene, for psoriasis, 465
Calcitonin, for osteoporosis, 710
Calcium. See also Hypercalcemia, Hypocalcemia
dietary, 29, 708, 709t
colorectal cancer and, 2477
measurement of, 699-700
metabolism of, 698-699, 698f
Calcium channel blockers. See also individual drugs, e.g., Verapamil
for acute myocardial infarction, 329
for angina pectoris, 299
overdose, 163-164
for unstable angina and NSTMI, 313
Calcium channel disorders, 2282
Calcium chloride, in cardiac resuscitation, 144t
Calcium-containing stones in nephrolithiasis. See Nephrolithiasis
Calcium monohydrogen phosphate nephrolithiasis. See Nephrolithiasis
Calcium oxalate nephrolithiasis. See Nephrolithiasis
Calcium phosphate deposition, basic, joint disease in, 1380
Calcium pyrophosphate dihydrate deposition disease. See Pseudogout
Calculus(i), renal. See Nephrolithiasis
CA125 levels
in ovarian cancer, 2539
in pelvic mass, 1057, 1058t
Calicivirus infection, in gastroenteritis, 1799-1800
Calories
daily intake of, 25
exercise time and, 36t
restriction of, 720
Cameron ulcer, 778
treatment of, 788
Campylobacter enteritis, 1634, 1637, 1635t
Campylobacter infection, 1634, 1637, 1635t
diarrhea due to, 841
Campylobacter jejuni, 1634
Cancer. See also Carcinogens, Tumor(s), individual anatomic sites
biology of, 2409-2410
cell viability and death in, 2410
invasion and metastases in, 2410
transformation and proliferation in, 2409-2410, 2409f

chemotherapy for. See Anticancer chemotherapy
epidemiology of, 2373-2382. See also Carcinogen(s)
diet in, 2375
environmental carcinogens in, 2373-2378, 2374t
iatrogenic causes in, 2377-2378
infectious agents in, 2376-2377
inherited factors in, 2378-2380, 2379t
high-penetrance, 2378-2379
low-penetrance, 2379-2380
obesity and physical inactivity in, 2375-2376
occupational carcinogens in, 2377
reproductive cancers and, 2377
screening and early detection in, 2380-2381, 2380t
tobacco in, 2374-2375
hypercalcemia in. See Hypercalcemia of malignancy
malnutrition in, nutritional support in, 943-944
molecular genetics of, 1952-1953, 2383-2399
accumulation of genetic lesions, 2391-2392, 2392f-2393f
analysis of
clinical implications of, 2398
expression profile and new therapeutics, 2396-2397, 2397f
cell death and immortality, 2392-2393, 2394f
chemotherapy and drug resistance, 2394-2396, 2395f-2396f
environmental factors and, 2383
metastasis and angiogenesis, 2393-2394, 2395f
microsatellite instability and DNA mismatch repair in, 2391, 2392f
oncogenes in, 2383-2385, 2384t. See also Oncogene(s)
proto-oncogenes in, 2383-2385, 2384t. See also Proto-oncogene(s)
tumor progression, 2391-2396
tumor suppressor genes in, 2386-2391, 2386t. See also Tumor suppressor gene(s)
virus infection and, 2383
in myositis, 1356
occupational, 62, 62t
pain in, 2175
management of, 2179
patient management in, 2408-2409
diagnosis in, 2408
performance status in, 2408, 2408t
staging in, 2408
treatment in, 2408-2409
pharmacology in. See Anticancer chemotherapy
in pregnancy, 1022
preventive health care measures for, 42-47, 47t
in renal transplant recipients, 2115
screening measures for, not recommended, 47-48
treatment principles, 2408-2424
cancer biology, 2409-2410
cancer pharmacology, 2410-2413
scientific basis of, 2409-2413
specific agents in, 2413-2423, 2415t-2420t. See also Anticancer chemotherapy
Trousseau syndrome and, 1201-1202
Cancer pain

abdominal pain in, 2175
back pain in, 2175
bone pain in, 2175
headache, 2175
iatrogenic pain in, 2175
plexopathy in, 2175
Candesartan, for hypertension, 223t
Candida albicans, 1875. See also Candidiasis
Candidiasis
balanitis in, 507-508
in compromised host, 1875-1876, 1880, 1877t-1879t
diagnosis of, 1875-1876
differential diagnosis of, 1876
epidemiology of, 1875
etiology of, 1875
pathogenesis of, 1875
treatment and prognosis in, 1876, 1877t-1879t, 1880
esophageal, 769-770
gastrointestinal, 1875
genital, 1875
hematogenous, 1876
in immunosuppression, chronic mucocutaneous, 1879t
intertrigo, 507, 508f
onychomycosis, 576-577, 575t
oral, 507, 508
oropharyngeal, 1875
paronychia, 508, 508f
vulvovaginitis in, 507-508, 1525, 1524t
Cannabinol(s), abuse of, medication for, 2645
Capecitabine, 2416t
for colorectal cancer, 2487
Capillariasis, 1923
Caplan syndrome, multifocal pulmonary infiltrates in, 2749
Capsaicin, 2186
Captopril, for hypertension, 222t
Carbamate(s), poisoning, 172, 172t
Carbamazepine
in epilepsy, 2193-2194
poisoning or overdose with, elimination method for, 161t
Carbapenem, 1430-1431
Carbenicillin, 1428
Carbidopa-levodopa, for Parkinson disease, 2245, 2244t, 2246t
Carbohydrate malabsorption, tests for, 846
Carbohydrates, dietary, 27, 720-721
Carbon dioxide transport, erythrocyte in, 1079
Carbon monoxide, biologic test of exposure to, 61t
Carbon monoxide poisoning, 164
Carboplatin, 2416t
Carboxyhemoglobin, high levels of, polycythemia due to, 1135, 1134f
Carboxypenicillin, extended-spectrum, 1428
Carbuncle, definition of, 429t
Carcinoembryonic antigen, in colorectal cancer, 2484-2485, 2485t
Carcinogen(s)
environmental, 2373-2378, 2374t
occupational, 62t. See also Occupational disease
Carcinoid syndrome, cutaneous findings in, 435
Carcinoid tumor, pulmonary, segmental infiltrates in, 2750, 2750f
Carcinoma, Merkel cell, 556
Cardiac arrest
comatose survivors of, prognosis in, 2337t, 2336-2337
patient evaluation after, 264-265
treatable conditions in, 148t-149t

Cardiac arrhythmia. *See* Arrhythmia
Cardiac catheterization
  anoxic encephalopathy in, 2337
  pericardial complications of, 381
  in pulmonary hypertension, 2854-
    2855
Cardiac disease. *See* Heart disease
Cardiac dysrhythmia. *See* Arrhythmia
Cardiac electrical system, 273
Cardiac myxoma, 383-384, 383f-384f
  infective endocarditis *vs.*, 1490
Cardiac pacing. *See* Pacemaker
Cardiac resuscitation, 141-154
  chain of survival in, 141-143
    advanced care and, 141-142, 144t
    CPR and, 141, 141t
    defibrillation and, 141, 142t
    emergency medical services and,
      141
    resuscitation outcome and, 142-
      143
  ending, 153
  postresuscitation care, 152-153
  primary survey in, 143-145
    airway in, 143
    breathing in, 143
    CPR in, 143-145
    defibrillation in, 145
  rhythm findings in, 149-152
    asystole, 152, 151f
    pulseless electrical activity,
      152, 151f
    pulseless ventricular
      tachycardia or fibrillation,
      149-152, 150f-151f
  secondary survey in, 145-148
    advanced airway in, 145-146
    breathing and ventilation in,
      146, 146t
    circulation access in, 146
    differential diagnosis and
      definitive care in, 146-
      148, 148t-149t
  technical problems with, 147t
Cardiac tamponade, in cardiac
  arrest, 148t
Cardiac trauma
  blunt, 385-386
  electrical, 386
  penetrating, 386
Cardiac tumor(s), 382-384
  metastatic, 382-383
  primary benign, 383-384, 383f-384f
  primary malignant, 384
Cardiac valvular disease, in
  pregnancy, 1018-1019
Cardioembolism, in stroke, 2203-
  2204, 2205f, 2211-2212
Cardiomyopathy
  dilated
    heart failure in, 338t, 339f
    inherited, in diagnosis of
      palpitation, 204t
    dilated X-linked, in muscular
      dystrophy, 2273
  hypertrophic
    atrial fibrillation in, 248
    in diagnosis of palpitation,
      204t
    in differential diagnosis of
      chest pain, 198t, 197
    heart failure in, 338t, 339f
    murmur in, 210t
  inflammatory, in systemic lupus
    erythematosus, 1339
  peripartum, 1019
  restrictive
    constrictive pericarditis *vs.*,
      383t
    heart failure in, 338t
Cardiopulmonary bypass
  bleeding after, 1188
  hemolytic anemia in, 1129

Cardiopulmonary resuscitation
  ineffective, 147t
  initiation of, 141, 141t, 143-145
Cardiovascular disease. *See also*
  Coronary artery disease, Heart
  disease
  diabetic, 672-675, 669f
  in pregnancy, 1018-1019
  in renal transplant recipients,
    2115
  risk factors for, dietary fatty
    acids and, 26
Cardiovascular patient, 197-213. *See
  also* Heart disease, *specific
  disorders*
  cardiac murmurs in, 208-212, 209t-
    210t, 209f, 211f
    diagnostic evaluation in, 211-
      212, 211f
    history and physical examination
      in, 209-211, 209t-210t
  chest pain in, 197-201, 198t
    diagnostic tests for, 198-
      201, 199t-201t, 199f
    history and physical examination
      in, 197-198, 198t
  dyspnea in, 201-202, 201t, 202f
    diagnostic tests in, 202, 202f
    history and physical examination
      in, 201-202
  Internet information for, 211
  palpitations in, 202-205, 203t-
    204t, 203f
    diagnostic tests in, 204-
      205, 203f, 205t
    history and physical examination
      in, 203-204
  syncope in, 205-208, 205t, 206f
    diagnostic tests in, 206-
      208, 206f
    history and physical examination
      in, 205-206, 204t
Cardiovascular system, exercise and,
  32-33
Cardiovascular trauma, 385-386
Cardioverter-defibrillator,
  implantable
  for acute myocardial infarction,
    333
  for heart failure, 344-345
  for ventricular tachycardia, 269-
    271, 269f, 270t
Carditis, in Lyme disease, 1714
Carmustine, 2415t
  renal complications of, 2091
Carney syndrome, pituitary adenoma
  in, 591
Carnitine deficiency, myopathy in,
  2279-2280
Carnitine palmitoyltransferase
  deficiency, myopathy in, 2280
Carotid artery disease, in stroke,
  2212
Carotid artery dissection, in
  stroke, 2213
Carpal tunnel syndrome, 1395, 1394f,
  2295
Cartilage
  articular, normal, 1383-1384, 1384f
  osteoarthritic, 1384-1385, 1384f.
    See also Osteoarthritis
Carvedilol, for hypertension, 222t
alpha-CAT, properties of, 2386t
beta-CAT, properties of, 2384t
Cat bite, 180, 181t-182t
CATCH 22 syndrome, 395
Catecholamine surge, hypokalemia due
  to, 2006
Caterpillar, puss, 191
Caterpillar stings, 191
Catfish, stings, 194
Cathartics, osmotic, hypernatremia
  and, 1987

Catheter ablation
  of atrial fibrillation, 244
  of ventricular tachycardia, 269
Catheter-related infection
  in neoplasia, 2429
  urinary tract, 1517, 1517t
Caustic alkali, inhalation or
  ingestion of, 165-166, 165t
Cavernous sinus thrombophlebitis,
  1560
  in sinusitis, 1460
Cavitation, pulmonary. *See* Pulmonary
  infiltrate(s), cavitary
CDK4, properties of, 2384t, 2388
Cefaclor, serum sickness-like
  reaction to, 498
Cefotaxime, for septic arthritis,
  1540t
Ceftriaxone
  for meningococcal disease, 1620t
  for *Salmonella* infection, 1635t
  for septic arthritis, 1540t
Celiac disease, 1281
Celiac sprue. *See* Gluten-sensitive
  enteropathy
Cell-cell interactions, antigen
  processing and presentation in.
  See also Antigen(s)
Cell-mediated immunity. *See under*
  Immune mechanisms, *specific
  cells*
Cellulitis
  bacterial, 510-511
  crepitant, 1607
    gas (clostridial myonecrosis)
      vs., 1610
  Haemophilus influenzae, 1650
  orbital, in sinusitis, 1460
  streptococcal, in tinea pedis, 506
Cellulose phosphate, for
  nephrolithiasis, 2110
Centers for Disease Control and
  Prevention (CDC), *Health
  Information for International
  Travel,* 69
Central nervous system
  angiitis of, isolated,
    encephalopathy in, 2342
  bacterial infections of, 1550-
    1562. *See also specific
    infections, e.g.,* Meningitis
  occupational disease of, 64-65
  Pseudomonas aeruginosa infection
    of, 1660-1661
  tuberculosis of, 1682
  tumors of, 2307-2317, 2307t-2308t.
    See also Brain tumors
  viral infections of, 2344-2354.
    *See also specific infections,
    e.g.,* Meningitis
  virus infections of, major, 2344t
Central pontine myelinolysis, 2332
Cephalosporin(s), 1428-1430, 1429t
  first-generation, 1429-1430, 1429t
  in pregnancy, 1422t
  properties of, 1429t
  second-generation, 1430, 1429t
  third- and fourth-generation,
    1430, 1429t
Cerebellar ataxia, vertigo in, 2147-
  2148
Cerebellar degeneration,
  paraneoplastic, 2318
Cerebral aneurysm, mycotic, in
  endocarditis, 1485-1486
Cerebral edema, in herpes simplex
  encephalitis, 2348
Cerebral embolism, in endocarditis,
  1485-1486
Cerebral venous septic
  thrombophlebitis, 1560-1561
Cerebral venous thrombosis, in
  stroke, 2213-2214

Cerebrospinal fluid examination
  low glucose levels in,
    neutrophilia in, 1552t, 1551
  in multiple sclerosis, 2327-2328
Cerebrospinal fluid shunt infection,
  1555-1556
Cerebrovascular disorders, 2201-
  2216. *See also* Stroke
Cerebrovascular syndromes,
  occlusive, 2206t. *See also*
  Stroke
Ceruloplasmin, in iron metabolism,
  1082
Cervical adenopathy, in hematologic
  disease, 1075
Cervical spine, rheumatoid arthritis
  of, 1303-1304, 1304f
Cervix, uterine. *See under* Uterine
Cestode infection, 1936-1941
Cetirizine, in atopic dermatitis,
  478
Cetuximab, for colorectal cancer,
  2487
Chagas disease (American
  trypanosomiasis), 1913-1915. *See
  also* Trypanosomiasis, American
kappa-Chain deficiency, 1226t
Chancre, in syphilis, 1699, 1699f
Chancroid, genital ulcers in, 1528t
Charcoal, activated, for poisoning
  or drug overdose, 160, 160t
Charlevoix-Saguenay, ataxia of,
  2263t, 2265
Chediak-Higashi syndrome
  neutropenia in, 1144t, 1146t
  neutrophil function in, 1146t
Chemotherapy
  anticancer. *See* Anticancer
    chemotherapy
  antimicrobial. *See* Antibiotic(s)
  antiviral. *See individual drugs*
Chest, flail, 2803
Chest pain
  in cardiovascular patient, 197-
    201, 198t
    diagnostic tests for, 198-
      201, 199t-201t, 199f
    history and physical examination
      in, 197-198, 198t
  differential diagnosis of, 285-
    286, 287t
Chest radiography. *See* Radiography,
  chest
Chest wall
  disorders of, 2800-2808. *See also*
    Respiratory pump dysfunction
  pain, 1393-1394
Chicken pox. *See* Varicella
Chikungunya, 1858
Children. *See also* Infant
  acne in, 447
  black widow spider bites in, 188
  death of, 119
  death of parent and, 119
  hematopoiesis in, 1070
  hypercholesterolemia screening
    for, 745-746
  hypertriglyceridemia in, 739
  snakebite in, 187
  syphilis in, 1708
Chinese-herb nephrotoxicity, 2095
Chinese medicine, traditional, 83-84
Chiropractic medicine, 86-87
Chlamydial infection, antimicrobial
  drugs for, 1427t
Chlamydia pneumoniae infection, 1475-
  1476, 1752-1753, 1745t
  pneumonia, 1475-1476
Chlamydia psittaci, 1751-1752, 1745t
Chlamydia species, 1745, 1745t, 1746f
Chlamydia trachomatis, adult
  inclusion conjunctivitis,
  1750, 1748t

Chlamydia trachomatis infection, 1745-1751
  acute urethral syndrome, 1748, 1748t
  epididymitis, 1747, 1748t
  laboratory diagnosis, 1746
  lymphogranuloma venereum, 1749-1750
  mucopurulent cervicitis, 1747-1748, 1748t
  neonatal chlamydial conjunctivitis, 1750
  nongonococcal urethritis, 1747, 1748t
  pelvic inflammatory disease, 1748-1749
  proctitis, 1749, 1748t
  salpingitis, 1748-1749, 1748t
  trachoma, 1750-1751
  urethritis in, male, 1521-1523
Chloracne, 63
  acne vulgaris *vs.,* 447
Chlorambucil, 2415t
  for chronic lymphocytic leukemia, 2587-2588
Chloramphenicol, 1435-1436
  anemia due to, 1095
  in pregnancy, 1422t
Chloride channel disorders, 2282
Chloride depletion, in metabolic alkalosis, 2003, 2003f
Chloridorrhea, congenital, 843
Chloroquine
  for malaria chemoprophylaxis, 77, 77f
  myopathy due to, 2284
  in psoriasis, adverse effects of, 462
Chlorthalidone, for hypertension, 221t
Cholangiography, percutaneous transhepatic, in choledocholithiasis, 907-908
Cholangitis
  autoimmune, autoimmune hepatitis *vs.,* 884
  pyogenic, 909-910
  sclerosing, 909, 909f
    chronic hepatitis *vs.,* 883
    liver transplantation and, 936
Cholecystectomy
  for chronic cholecystitis, 906
  diarrhea after, 849
  laparoscopic, for acute cholecystitis, 904
  open, for acute cholecystitis, 904
  prophylactic, in diabetes mellitus, 907
Cholecystitis, 902-907
  acute, 902-905
    clinical manifestations of, 902-903
    complications of, 905
    differential diagnosis in, 903-904
    imaging studies in, 903
    laboratory evaluation in, 903
    medical therapy in, 904
    physical examination in, 903
    surgery in, 904-905
  chronic, 905-907
    diagnosis of, 905-906, 906f
    imaging studies in, 906, 906f
    treatment of, 906-907
  emphysematous, 905, 904f
Cholecystoenteric fistula, 905
Cholecystostomy, for acute cholecystitis, 904-905
Choledochal cyst, 910, 910t
Choledocholithiasis, 907-908
  clinical manifestations of, 907
  diagnosis of, 907-908, 908f
  treatment of, 908

Cholelithiasis, 902-908. *See also* Gallstone
  asymptomatic, 907
  cholecystitis in, 902-907. *See also* Cholecystitis
  in sickle cell anemia, 1116
Cholera, 1643-1644
  immunization against, 71
  treatment of, 1644, 1636t
Cholescintigraphy, in acute cholecystitis, 903
Cholestasis, intrahepatic, in pregnancy, 1023
Cholesterol. *See also* Lipoprotein
  diet and, 25-26, 25f, 26t
  serum, elevated. *See* Hypercholesterolemia
Cholesterol emboli, tubulointerstitial nephritis in, 2096, 2095f
Cholesterol ester storage disease, 1149t
Cholesterol-lowering-agent myopathy, 2283, 2283t
Cholinergic syndrome, in poisoning or drug overdose, 158t
Chondrosarcoma, 2557-2558
  features of, 2550t
Chordoma, treatment of, 2558
Chorea, 2253, 2254t
Chorionic gonadotropin-mediated hyperthyroidism, 611-612, 612f
Chromium, dietary, 30
Chromosome(s), structure of, 1945-1946, 1948t
Chromotubation, in infertility, 1003
Chronic airflow obstruction (CAO). *See also* Chronic obstructive pulmonary disease (COPD)
  cigarette smoking and, 2720-2721, 2721f
  definition of, 2720
Chronic obstructive pulmonary disease (COPD), 2720-2732. *See also* Chronic airflow obstruction (CAO)
  chest imaging in, 2728, 2725t
  clinical manifestations of, 2725, 2725t
  definition of, 2720
  epidemiology of, 2720-2721
  etiology of, 2721
  gas exchange abnormalities in, 2726-2728, 2727f, 2725t
  natural history of, 2721-2722, 2722f
  oxygen administration for, long-term, 2731-2732
  pathogenesis of, 2724-2725
  pathology in, 2722-2723
    early changes in, 2722
  physical examination in, 2725-2726, 2725t
  pink puffer *vs.* blue bloater in, 2727, 2725t, 2727f
  polycythemia in, 1134
  pulmonary function testing in, 2726, 2726f
  pulmonary rehabilitation in, 2731
  respiratory failure in, 2814-2815
  sleep-disordered breathing in, 2797
  treatment of, 2728-2732
    in acute exacerbation, 2730-2731
    in advanced disease, 2731
    antibiotic, 2730
    bronchodilator, 2728-2730, 2729t
    corticosteroid, 2730, 2730t
    long-term ventilatory support in, 2732
    smoking cessation, 2728
    surgical, 2732
  ventilatory support for, long-

term, 2732
Churg-Strauss syndrome (allergic granulomatosis and angiitis), 1365-1366, 1365t
  cutaneous findings in, 432
  glomerulonephritis in, 2075-2076
  multifocal pulmonary infiltrates in, 2749
  pulmonary vasculitis in, 2782-2783
Chylomicron, 729
Chylomicronemia syndrome, 733
Chylothorax, 2830-2831
Cicatricial alopecia, 568-569, 568t, 568f
Cigarette smoking. *See also* Nicotine, Tobacco
  airflow obstruction due to, chronic, 2720-2721, 2721f. *See also* Chronic airflow obstruction (CAO)
  alcoholism and, 2627
  alcohol use and, in cancer epidemiology, 2374-2375
  bronchitis due to, chronic, 2720
  in cancer epidemiology, 2374-2375
  cessation of, 19-20, 19t, 49
    angina pectoris and, 295-296
    bupropion for, 20
    cancer prevention and, 2375
    for COPD, 2728
    disease risk and, 19, 19t
    lung cancer and, 2443-2444
    nicotine products for, 19
    in chronic renal failure, 2018
  colorectal cancer and, 2479
  in diabetes mellitus, 674
  emphysema due to, 2720-2721, 2722-2723, 2723f. *See also* Emphysema
  in eosinophilic granuloma of lung, 2780
  esophageal cancer and, 2490-2491
  forced expiratory volume in, 2720-2721, 2721f
  high carboxyhemoglobin levels in, polycythemia due to, 1135
  laryngeal cancer due to, 2374, 2437
  lung cancer due to. *See* Lung cancer
  pancreatic cancer and, 2499
  protease-antiprotease imbalance in, 2724, 2724f
  as risk factor for stroke, 2211
  statistics on, 18
Cigar smoking, oral cancers due to, 2374, 2437
Ciguatera poisoning, 175, 175t
Ciliary dyskinesia, primary (Kartagener syndrome), 2739-2740, 2739f
  diagnosis of, 2739
  differential diagnosis of, 2739-2740
Ciprofloxacin, 1438-1439, 1438t
  for *Campylobacter* infection, 1635t
  for *Salmonella* infection, 1635t
  for *Shigella* infection, 1635t
  for *Vibrio* infection, 1636t
  for *Yersinia* infection, 1636t
Ciprofloxin, for meningococcal disease, 1620t
Circadian rhythm, sleep and, 2364, 2370
Circle of Willis, berry aneurysm of, in polycystic kidney disease, 2098, 2099f
Circulatory access, in cardiac resuscitation, 146
Circulatory arrest
  anoxic encephalopathy in, 2336-2337, 2337t
  prognosis in, 2336-2337, 2337t
Cirrhosis, 891-900

  alcoholic. *See* Alcoholic cirrhosis
  biliary. *See* Biliary cirrhosis
  blood tests in, 893
  clinical manifestations of, 892
  diagnosis of, 892-894, 893t, 893f-894f
  edema in, 1989-1990
  epidemiology of, 891
  etiology and genetic factors in, 891, 891t
  fever of unknown origin in, 1415
  hyperkalemia in, 2010
  imaging studies in, 893, 894f
  laboratory studies in, 893-894, 894f
  liver biopsy in, 893-894
  management of, 894-899
    ascites and, 895-896
    in compensated disease, 895
    in decompensated disease, 895-899
    general measures for, 894-895
    hepatic encephalopathy and, 897-898, 898t
    hepatocellular carcinoma and, 898-899
    hepatopulmonary and, 897
    hepatorenal syndrome and, 896, 897t
    liver transplantation and, 899, 898t
    spontaneous bacterial peritonitis and, 896
    variceal bleeding and, 897
  pathogenesis of, 891-892, 892f
    cirrhosis in, 892
    liver fibrogenesis in, 891-892, 892f
  physical findings in, 892-893, 893f
  prognosis in, 899
Cisplatin, 2416t
  nephrotoxicity due to, 2033
  peripheral neuropathy due to, 2319
  renal complications of, 2091
Citrobacter freundii complex, antimicrobial susceptibilities of, 1421t
Cladribine, 2417t
Clarithromycin, 1434
  for *Helicobacter* infection, 1636t
  in pregnancy, 1422t
Claudication
  leg segmental pressure measurements in, 402t
  in peripheral arterial occlusive disease. *See* Peripheral arterial disease
Clavulanate, 1428
Claw toe, 1397
Clay ingestion, hypokalemia and, 2006
Clindamycin, 1435
  for acne vulgaris, 449t
  in pregnancy, 1422t
Clinical decision making, 7-16
  critical evaluation of research reports, 8, 8t
  measures of diagnostic certainty, 8-9
  measures of diagnostic test performance, 9-11, 10t-11t, 11f
  measures of disease frequency, 8, 8t
  measures of treatment effects, 11-12, 12t
  measures of treatment outcome, 12
  medical decision analysis and, 13-15
    cost-effectiveness analysis in, 15
    expected outcome model of, 14-15, 14f
    threshold model of, 13-14, 12f-

13f
Clomiphene, for polycystic ovary syndrome, 982-983
Clomiphene plus glucocorticoid, for polycystic ovary syndrome, 983
Clomiphene plus gonadotropin, for polycystic ovary syndrome, 984
Clonazepam, in epilepsy, 2194
Clonidine, for hypertension, 223t
Clonorchiasis, 1935
Clopidogrel
  for angina pectoris, 296-297
  primary angioplasty and, 326
  for unstable angina and NSTMI, 309-310, 309t
Clostridial infections, 1607-1610
  enterotoxigenic, 1608
  hemolytic anemia in, 1129
  histotoxic, 1607-1608
  neurotoxic, 1608-1610. See also Botulism, Tetanus
Clostridium botulinum. See Botulism
Clostridium difficile, diarrhea due to, 841-842, 1608
  diagnosis of, 1611
  prevention of, 1615
  treatment of, 1614
Clostridium perfringens
  cellulitis, 1607
  food poisoning, 1608
  myonecrosis (gas gangrene), 1607
    treatment of, 1612
    vs. crepitant cellulitis, 1610-1611
  uterine infection, 1608
Clostridium tetani, 1608
Clothing, contact dermatitis due to, 491
Clotting cascade, in coagulation, 1154-1155, 1156f
Cloxacillin, 1424
c-myc, properties of, 2384, 2384t
Coagulation, 1153-1162. See also Hemostasis
  activation of, in sepsis, 1447
  clotting cascade in, 1154-1155, 1156f
    activated platelets and, 1154-1155
    classic vs. modified view of, 1154, 1156f
  control mechanisms of, 1155-1158, 1156t
    antithrombin III-heparan sulfate system as, 1155, 1157f
    cyclooxygenase-1 and cyclooxygenase-2 as, 1157
    ecto-ADPase as, 1157
    fibrinolysis as, 1158, 1158f-1159f
    nitric oxide as, 1157, 1158f
    prostacyclin as, 1156-1157, 1158f
    protein C and protein S-thrombomodulin system as, 1155-1156, 1157f
    thrombin-activatable fibrinolysis inhibitor as, 1158, 1159f
    tissue factor pathway inhibitor as, 1156, 1157f
  disseminated intravascular. See Disseminated intravascular coagulation (DIC)
  overview of, 1158-1159, 1160f
  platelet plug formation in, 1153-1154, 1153f-1155f
    adhesion in, 1153, 1154f
    aggregation in, 1153, 1155f
    procoagulation in, 1154
    protein secretion in, 1153-1154
Coagulation disorder(s), 1180-1189
  acquired, 1184-1188
  drug-induced, 1184-1185

hereditary, 1180-1184. See also Hemophilia; specific disorders, e.g., Hemophilia A
Coagulation factor(s). See under Factor
Coagulation tests, 1160-1162
  antithrombin III assay, 1162
  bleeding time, 1161
  D-dimer and fibrin-fibrinogen degradation products (FDP and FSP), 1161
  dilute Russell viper venom time (DRVVT), 1160
  factor XIII, 1161
  fibrinogen levels, 1161
  fibrinopeptide A (FPA), 1161
  mixing studies, 1161-1162
  partial thromboplastin time (PTT), 1160
  peripheral blood smear evaluation, 1161
  plasminogen and alpha$_2$-antiplasmin, 1161
  platelet aggregometry, 1161
  platelet-function assay-100, 1161
  protein C and protein S test, 1162
  prothrombin time (PT), 1160
  reptilase time (RT), 1161
  thrombin time (TT), 1160-1161
Coal worker's pneumoconiosis, 2765
Cobalamin
  deficiency, in megaloblastic anemia, 1100-1103. See also Megaloblastic anemia
  folate and, in DNA synthesis, 1099-1100, 1100f
Cocaine use
  overdose, 164-165, 164t
  pulmonary edema in, 2850
  seizure due to, 157t
  thrombocytopenia due to, 1169-1170
Cocci
  gram-negative, antimicrobial drugs for, 1425t
  gram-positive, 1563-1583. See also individual organisms, e.g., Pneumococcal infection
    antimicrobial drugs for, 1425t
Coccidioides immitis, 1866-1867
Coccidioidomycosis, 1866-1869
  clinical presentation in, 1867-1868
  diagnosis of, 1868, 1868f
  differential diagnosis of, 1868
  disseminated, 1867-1868
    treatment of, 1869
  epidemiology of, 1866-1867
  pathogenesis of, 1867
  prognosis in, 1869
  pulmonary, 1867
    multiple nodules in, 2755
    treatment of, 1868-1869
  treatment of, 1868-1869
Coccidiosis, 1906-1908
Cockayne-Touraine syndrome, 532
Coelenterates, 192
Cognitive function, in systemic lupus erythematosus, 1333
Colchicine
  for gout, 1375
  myopathy due to, 2284
Cold agglutinin disease, 1126
Colectomy, laparoscopic, for colorectal cancer, 2485-2486
Colistin, 1433
Colitis. See also Enterocolitis
  amebic, 1906
  in Crohn disease, 797
  diverticular, 817
  granulomatous. See Crohn disease
  microscopic colitis syndrome in, 848
  ulcerative. See Ulcerative colitis

Collagenous sprue, 829-830
Collagen vascular disease, chronic diffuse infiltrative pulmonary disease in, 2779-2780, 2767t-2768t
Colon
  cancer of. See Colorectal cancer
  diverticulosis of. See under Diverticulitis, Diverticulosis
  motility in, 851-852
  disorders of, 857-859
Colonoscopy
  for colorectal cancer, 2480-2481
  polypectomy in, bleeding in, 865
  virtual (CT scan), 2481
Colorado tick fever, 1857
Colorectal cancer, 2474-2489
  clinical manifestations of, 2481-2482
  diagnosis of, 2481-2485
  diverticular disease and, 817
  epidemiology of, 2474
    diet and, 2375
  etiology of, 2475-2479
    diet in, 2476-2478, 2477t
    environmental factors in, 2476-2479, 2476t-2477t
    hereditary syndromes and predisposing conditions in, 2475-2476
    lifestyle factors in, 2478-2479
    medications in, 2478, 2478t
  in familial adenomatous polyposis, 2475-2476
  genetic alterations in, 2475
  genetic risk factors for, 2378
  hereditary nonpolyposis, 2476
  inflammatory bowel disease and, 809, 2476
  pathogenesis of, 2474-2475
  polyps in, adenomatous, 2474, 2474f
  risk factors in, 2476t
  screening for, 2479-2481, 2479t-2482t
    barium enema in, 2481
    colonoscopy, 2480-2481
    cost-effectiveness of, 2481
    fecal occult blood testing in, 2479, 2480t
    fiberoptic sigmoidoscopy in, 2480
    implementation of, 2481, 2482t
    molecular detection methods in, 2481
    recommendations, 43-44
    virtual colonoscopy in, 2481
  staging and prognosis in, 2482-2485, 2483f-2484f, 2483t
    carcinoembryonic antigen in, 2484-2485, 2485t
  treatment of, 2485-2487
    in advance disease, 2487
    antitumor antibody therapy for, 2407
    chemotherapy, 2486-2487
    palliative, 2487
    radiation therapy, 2486
    surgical, 2485-2486
Coma. See also Brain trauma
  Glasgow Coma Scale in, 2230, 2230t
  hyperosmolar, hyperglycemic nonketotic, 663
  encephalopathy in, 2340
  in poisoning, 155-156
Comedo, definition of, 426t
Common bile duct. See Bile duct, common
  stone in. See Choledocholithiasis
Common cold, 1778
Common variable immunodeficiency, 1227-1228, 1226t
Complement, activation of, in rheumatoid arthritis, 1300

Complementary and alternative medicine, 82-91
  acupuncture as, 83-84
  biologic-based therapies as, 85, 87t-89t
  definition and classification of, 82, 82t
  energy therapies as, 87-89
  homeopathy as, 84
  information sources for, 90t
  manipulative and body-based therapies as, 86-87
  mind-body interventions as, 84-85, 85f, 86t
  practicing physician and, 89-90
  prevalence and demographics in, 82
  public perception and, 82-83
  research concerns, 83, 84t
  traditional Chinese medicine as, 83-84
  use of, 82-83
Complete blood count (CBC)
  in hematologic disorders, 1076
  in thrombocytopenia, 1164
Compromised host. See Immunocompromised patient
Computed tomography (CT)
  in appendicitis, 820, 820f
  of brain, in systemic lupus erythematosus, 1335
  in brain trauma, 2233, 2233f
  in esophageal cancer, 772
  in herpes simplex encephalitis, 2348
  high-resolution
    in chronic diffuse infiltrative pulmonary disease, 2760, 2760f
    in eosinophilic granuloma of lung, 2760f
    in hilar enlargement, 2837
    in Hodgkin disease, 2598
    in intra-abdominal abscess, 1503
    of lung, in Wegener granulomatosis, 1363, 1364f
    in myositis, 1355
    in osteomyositis, 1546
    in pancreatitis, acute, 917, 918
    in pelvic mass, 1057
    in pleural effusion, 2825
    in pulmonary embolism, 416, 415f
    in pulmonary hypertension, 2854
    in renal disease, 1969t
    in stroke, acute, 2201-2202, 2203f
    in viral encephalitis, 2344, 2345f
Condom
  female, 998
  male, 998
Condyloma acuminatum, 514-515, 514f
  in AIDS, 437
  giant (genital verrucous carcinoma, Buschke-Lowenstein tumor), 515
Condyloma latum, in syphilis, 1700, 1700f
Congenital heart disease. See Heart disease, congenital
Congestive heart failure. See Heart failure, congestive
Conjunctivitis
  adult inclusion, chlamydial, 1750
  allergic, 1254-1255
  gonococcal, 1622, 1624t
  Haemophilus influenzae, 1650
  hemorrhagic, enteroviral, 1797, 1795t
  neonatal chlamydial, 1750
Connective tissue disease
  encephalopathy in, 2342-2343
  mixed, 1337, 1329t
    chronic diffuse infiltrative pulmonary disease in, 2780
  neuropathy in, 2303

pulmonary hypertension in, 2861
undifferentiated, 1337, 1329t
Connective tissue tumor, 543-544
Consciousness, level of, evaluation
of, 2336, 2336t
Constipation
functional, 860
palliative treatment of, 104-
105, 107t-108t
slow-transit, 857-858
Contact dermatitis, 474, 481-494
allergic, 481-486
clinical features of, 483-
484, 484f-485f, 486t
diagnosis of, 483-486
eczematous, 474
environment in, 482, 482t
histopathology of, 484
immunologic status in, 482
misconceptions about, 483t
patch test in, 484-
486, 485f, 486t, 487f, 488t-489t
pathogenesis of, 482-483
predisposing factors, 482, 482t
treatment of, 487-490
systemic, 490
topical, 487
trigger factors in, 487
clothing and textile, 491
etiologic forms of, 490-491
irritant, 474
acute, 481
treatment of, 487-490
systemic, 490
topical, 487
trigger factors in, 487
major types of, 481-490
occupational, 491
photoallergy, 492, 492f
photosensitivity, 491-492, 492t
phototoxicity, 491-492, 492t
systemic, 490
topical medication allergy,
490, 491f
Continuous positive airway pressure
(CPAP), for sleep apnea
syndrome, 2367-2368, 2796
Contraception, 994-1001
abstinence as, 998
barrier, 998
categories of, 994, 994t
choosing, 999-1000, 999t
combined estrogen-progestin, 994-
997
benefits, 996-997, 996t
continuous vs. cyclic, 994-995
contraindications, 996, 996t
efficacy and mechanism of
action, 994
nonoral, 995
reduction of androgen exposure,
994
side effects of, 995-996, 995t
emergency, 999
intrauterine device, 998
nonreversible, 1000
progestin-only, 997-998, 997t
reversible, 999-1000
sterilization as, 998-999
Contraceptive(s)
combined estrogen-progestin, for
endometriosis, 969
estrophasic, for acne vulgaris,
450t
oral
dyslipidemia and, 740
for hirsutism, 990, 991t
plus antiandrogen, for
hirsutism, 991
in sickle cell anemia, 1117
thrombosis and, 1202
in urinary tract infection, 1509
Contraction alkalosis, 2003

Contracture, Dupuytren, 1395
Cooking oils, in diet, 31
Coombs antiglobulin test, for immune
hemolytic anemia, 1123, 1124f
COPD. See Chronic obstructive
pulmonary disease (COPD)
Copper, accumulation of, hemolytic
anemia in, 1129
Copperhead snake, 183, 184f. See also
Snakebite
Coproporphyria, hereditary, 751-
752, 752t, 750f
Coral snakes, 183, 184f. See also
Snakebite
Coronary angiography, in chest pain,
199, 200t, 201
Coronary angioplasty
aspirin therapy and, 326
clopidogrel therapy and, 326
glycoprotein IIb/IIIa inhibitor
therapy and, 326
for myocardial infarction, acute,
325-326, 324f-325f
rescue, 326-327
transfer for, immediate
thrombolytic therapy vs., 321-
322
Coronary artery bypass graft
in angina pectoris, 300
anoxic encephalopathy in, 2337
atrial fibrillation in, 248
diabetes and, 314-315
for myocardial infarction, acute,
326
for unstable angina and NSTEMI,
314-315
Coronary artery disease
angina in. See Angina pectoris
in diabetes mellitus, 675
exercise and, 36
hypertension in, 229
hypothyroidism in, 609
in polycystic ovary syndrome, 980
in preoperative assessment, 51-53
prevention and treatment of, 741-
745
drug therapy in, 744-745, 743t-
744t
primary, 741-742
risk stratification in, 743-744
secondary, 742-743
in renal transplant recipients,
2115
risk of, patient history in, 286-
287, 288f, 289t, 290f
surgical risk factor management
and, 55
valvular heart disease in, 349
Coronary atherosclerosis, in angina
pectoris, 284-285
Coronavirus, 1782
laboratory diagnosis of, 1778t
SARS, 1782-1783
Cor pulmonale, 2855-2857, 2857f
acute, 2855-2856, 2857f
chronic, 2856-2857
Corrosive agent(s), ingestion of,
165-166, 165t
Cortical basal ganglia degeneration,
2252
Corticosteroid(s)
for allergy, 1251
for atopic dermatitis, 477
for autoimmune hemolytic anemia,
1125
for brain tumors, 2312-2313
for COPD, 2730, 2730t
excess, platelet effects of, 1177
for gout, 1376
for hypersensitivity pneumonitis,
2767
for inflammatory bowel disease,
800

inhaled, allergy to, 490
myopathy due to, 2284
for pain, 2184
peptic ulcer disease due to,
NSAIDs with, 778
peripheral neuropathy due to, 2320
for prerenal-transplant patient
management, 2117
for sarcoidosis, 2773
surgical risk factor management
and, 56
topical
allergy to, 490
for atopic dermatitis, 477
for psoriasis, 465, 466t
for urticaria, 1265
Cortisol levels
insulin-induced hypoglycemia and,
598
regulation of, 679, 681f
Corynebacterium diphtheriae, 1584.
See also Diphtheria
Corynebacterium infection,
nondiphtheria, 1587-1589, 1587t
Corynebacterium jeikeium, 1588, 1587t
Corynebacterium ulcerans, 1587t
Corynebacterium urealyticum, 1587-
1588, 1587t
Cost-effectiveness analysis, 15
Cottonmouth snake, 183. See also
Snakebite
Cough
in asthma, 2704
palliative treatment of, 102, 104f
Coumarin, pharmacology of, 417
Cowden disease
breast cancer and, 2459
CNS tumors in, 2310t
cutaneous findings in, 435-
436, 435f
Cowden syndrome, 538
Coxiella burnetii, 1734. See also Q
fever
CPAP. See Continuous positive airway
pressure (CPAP)
Cranial irradiation, pituitary
failure due to, 603
Cranial neuropathy, 2293-2295, 2294t
in diabetes, 671
in diphtheria, 1586
in Lyme disease, 1714
Craniopharyngioma, in
hypogonadotropic hypogonadism,
956
C-reactive protein, in rheumatic
disease, 1293
Creatine kinase, as biochemical
cardiac marker, 305
Creatinine, serum, 1967-1968
in benign prostatic hyperplasia,
2129
Creatinine clearance, 1968
in chronic kidney disease,
2014, 2015t
CREST syndrome, 1342t, 1342,
1347, 1345t, 2780
skin in, 442-443
Creutzfeldt-Jakob disease,
2359, 2359f
genetic, 2359
variant, 2359
blood donation and, 1207-1208
Crimean-Congo hemorrhagic fever,
1850-1851
Critical illness myopathy, 2283
Critical illness polyneuropathy,
2300
Crohn disease, 795-799. See also
Inflammatory bowel disease
clinical manifestations of, 796-
797, 797f, 795t
colitis in, 797
management of, 806-807

complications of, 808-809
adenocarcinoma, 809
extraintestinal, 809
intestinal, 808-809
cutaneous findings in, 435, 435f
differential diagnosis of, 799
of duodenum, 797
treatment of, 806
endoscopy in, 798-799, 798f
enteral nutrition in, 943
of esophagus, 797
histology in, 799, 799f
ileitis in, 797
management of, 806-807
ileocecal, 797
ileocolitis in, 806-807
imaging studies in, 797-799
jejunoileitis in, 797
treatment of, 806
laboratory studies in, 797
maintenance therapy for, 807
malabsorption in, 833
metastatic, cutaneous findings in,
435
perianal, 797, 797f
physical examination in, 797
radiography in, 797-798
of stomach, 797
treatment of, 806
treatment of, 806-808
surgical, 807-808
ulcerative colitis vs., 795t
Cromolyn sodium, for asthma,
2713, 2710t
Croup
acute epiglottitis vs., 1466
viral, 1779
Cruise ships, sanitation issues for,
80
Cryotherapy, endobronchial, 2694-
2695
Cryptococcosis
in compromised host, 1880-
1881, 1880t
in immunosuppression, central
nervous system and, 1880-1881
pulmonary, large mass in, 2754
Cryptococcus neoformans, 1880. See
also Cryptococcosis
Cryptorchidism, 692-693
Cryptosporidiosis, 1907, 1908f
diarrhea due to, 842
Cryptosporidium species, 1907, 1908f
Crystal-induced joint disease, 1371-
1381. See also specific
disorders, e.g., Gout
CT. See Computed tomography
Curling ulcer, 778
Cushing disease. See also Cushing
syndrome
ACTH-secreting adenoma in, 598-
599, 599t
encephalopathy in, 2339-2340
Cushing syndrome, 679-681, 682t. See
also Cushing disease
clinical features of, 599t
diagnosis of, 680, 683f, 682t
hypertension in, 217t, 234, 231t
polycystic ovary syndrome vs., 980
treatment of, 680-681, 683f
Cushing ulcer, 778
Cutaneous disorders. See under Skin,
Skin disorder(s) individual
disorders
drug reactions as. See Drug
allergy, cutaneous
Cyanide poisoning, 166
Cyclin D (CYCD1)
mechanisms of, 2388
properties of, 2384t
Cyclist injury, 22
Cyclooxygenase-1, in coagulation,
1157

Cyclooxygenase-2, in coagulation, 1157
Cyclophosphamide, 2415t
  for autoimmune hemolytic anemia, 1125
  chronic diffuse infiltrative pulmonary disease due to, 2762
  for myositis, 1357, 1357t
  for rheumatoid arthritis, 1312
Cyclophosphamide-doxorubicin-fluorouracil, for breast cancer, 2465, 2466t
Cyclophosphamide infusion, acute hyponatremia due to, 1981t, 1981
Cyclophosphamide-methotrexate-fluorouracil, for breast cancer, 2465, 2466t
Cyclosporiasis, 1907-1908, 1908f
Cyclosporine
  after liver transplantation, complications of, 934
  for aplastic anemia, 1096
  for inflammatory bowel disease, 802
  for prerenal-transplant patient management, 2118-2119
  for psoriasis, 469-470
  renal complications, 2091
  for rheumatoid arthritis, 1312, 1308t
Cyst
  breast, 1052, 1052f
  bronchogenic, 2753, 2754f
  choledochal, 910, 910t
  epidermoid, 537, 537f
  ovarian. See Polycystic ovary syndrome
  pilar, 537
  renal. See also Polycystic kidney disease
    simple, 2097
Cystic adnexal mass, in adolescent female, 1058-1059, 1061
Cysticercosis, 1937-1938, 1937f, 1939f
Cystic fibrosis, 2737-2739
  chronic pancreatitis in, 924
  diagnosis of, 2737-2738
  genetic testing for, 1963
  pathogenesis of, 2736, 2736f
  Pseudomonas aeruginosa infection in, 1659-1660
  treatment of, 2738-2739
Cystic teratoma
  in adolescent female, 1059
  in reproductive age women, 1060, 1062
Cystine nephrolithiasis. See Nephrolithiasis, cystine stones in
Cystinuria, 2111-2112
Cystitis, 1511, 1512t. See also Urinary tract infection
  antimicrobial treatment of, 1513-1514, 1513t, 1514f
  candidal, 1878t
Cystourethrogram, voiding, 1969t
Cytarabine, 2416t
Cytokine(s). See also individual types, e.g., Interleukin
  in IgE-mediated allergic inflammation, 1241t
  in rheumatoid arthritis, 1300-1301
  in sepsis, 1446-1447, 1447t
  T cell subsets and. See also T cell(s)
Cytomegalovirus infection, 1761-1763
  in AIDS, 1762
  clinical syndromes, 1762, 1762f
  diagnosis, prevention, treatment of, 1762-1763, 1763t
  encephalitis in, 1762, 2351
  epidemiology and pathogenesis of, 1761

  esophageal, 770
  fever of undetermined origin in, 1414
  hepatitis in, 877
  in immunocompromised host, 1762
  polyradiculoneuropathy in, 2351-2352
  in renal transplantation, 2121
  retinitis in, 1762, 1762f
    in HIV infection, 1841-1842, 1841t-1842t
  as transfusion reaction, 1217, 1217t
  in transplantation, 1762
Cytopenia, refractory, with multilineage dysplasia, 2564t

D

Dacarbazine, 2416t
Dactinomycin, 2418t
Dairy products, 31
Dalfopristin, 1436-1437
Danazol, for endometriosis, 970
Dapsone, hypersensitivity syndrome reaction due to, 496
Daptomycin, 1437
  in pregnancy, 1422t
Darier disease (keratosis follicularis), 533
Dasatinib, for chronic myelogenous leukemia, 2580
Daunomycin, 2417t
DCC, properties of, 2386t
D-dimer testing, 1161
  for pulmonary embolism, 415, 416f
  for venous thrombosis, 412, 413t
Death
  demographics of, 93
  grief and bereavement in, 117-118
  leading causes of, 92t, 93
Decongestant(s), for allergy, 1250
Deer tick, 1712, 1712f
DEET insect repellent, 75
Defecation, outlet obstruction to, 860
Deferoxamine, for iron poisoning, 169, 1121
Defibrillation
  automatic external, 142t
    in ventricular tachycardia, 271
  emergency, 141, 142t, 145, 149-150, 151f
  manual, 142t
Delavirdine, for HIV infection, 1831t
  adverse effects of, 1834t
Delayed-sleep-phase syndrome, 2370
Delirium
  palliative treatment of, 108-109, 110t
  terminal, 109
Deltaretrovirus, 1802t
Dematiaceous fungal infection, in compromised host, 1890
Dementia
  Alzheimer. See Alzheimer disease
  anorexia in, 103
  dialysis, 2339
  human immunodeficiency virus, 2355-2357. See also Human immunodeficiency virus infection, dementia
  with Lewy bodies, 2224-2225
  non-Alzheimer disease, 2223-2226
  parkinsonism and, 2244, 2252-2253
  semantic, 2222
  in systemic lupus erythematosus, 1339
  vascular, 2223-2224, 2224f
Demyelinating diseases, 2323-2334
  definition of, 2323, 2323f, 2324t
  immune-mediated, 2323. See also

  Multiple sclerosis
    inherited, 2332
    metabolic, 2332-2333
    virus-induced, 2333
Dengue fever, 1847-1848
Dengue hemorrhagic fever, 1849
Dengue virus, 1847
  rash and arthralgia due to, 1858
Dense granule deficiency syndrome, 1174
Dental procedures
  antibiotic prophylaxis for, 351t, 1496, 1495t-1497t
  in hemophilia A, 1183
Dentatorubral-pallidoluysian atrophy, 2264t, 2268t
  trinucleotide repeat in, 1960t
Denture stomatitis, candidal, 1877t
Depressant(s)
  abuse of, 2636
  withdrawal, of, treatment of, 2643
Depression, 2613-2619
  in brain trauma, 2235
  clinical manifestations of, 2615
  definition of, 2613
  diagnosis of, 2615-2616
  differential diagnosis of, 2616
  epidemiology of, 2613
  etiology and genetics of, 2613-2614
  laboratory tests for, 2616
  management of, 2616-2619
    herbal remedies and dietary supplements in, 2618
    inpatient treatment, 2619
    managing therapeutic response in, 2618-2619
    medication selection in, 2618
    monoamine oxidase inhibitors for, 2616-2617
    newer antidepressants for, 2617-2618, 2617t
    nonpharmacologic, 2619
    pharmacologic, 2616-2619
    psychotherapy, 2619
    tricyclic antidepressants for, 2617
  mental-status examination in, 2615-2616
  in Parkinson disease, 2244
  pathogenesis of, 2614
    biogenic amine hypothesis in, 2614
    neuroendocrine and neuropeptide hypothesis in, 2614
    neuroimaging and sleep studies in, 2614
  suicide risk in, 2615-2616
De Quervain tenosynovitis, 1395
De Quervain thyroiditis, 618-619
Dermatitis
  atopic. See Atopic dermatitis
  contact. See Contact dermatitis
  occupational, 63-64
    hardening in, 482
    irritant vs. allergic, 63-64
  perioral, acne vulgaris vs., 447
  pruritic, alopecia areata in, 567
  seborrheic. See Seborrheic dermatitis
  stasis, topical drug allergy in, 490, 491f
Dermatitis herpetiformis, 436, 435f, 530-531, 530f, 526t
  gluten-sensitive enteropathy and, 829
Dermatofibroma, 543, 542f
Dermatofibrosarcoma protuberans, 557
Dermatographism, 1262, 1262f
Dermatomyositis, 442, 442f, 1351. See also Myositis
  systemic lupus erythematosus vs., 1337, 1328t

Dermatophytoses, 504-507. See also entries beginning with Tinea
  annular lesion of, 504, 504f
  anthropophilic, 504
  clinical presentation, 504-506
  diagnosis of, 506
  fungi involved in, 504
  geophilic, 504
  treatment of, 506-507
  zoophilic, 504
Dermatosis, linear IgA, 529, 526t
Dermatosis papulosa nigra, 535, 536f
Dermis, malignant tumors of, 556-559. See also individual types, e.g., Kaposi sarcoma
Dermoid cyst, mediastinal, 2839
Devic disease (neuromyelitis optica), 2328
Dexamethasone, for Salmonella infection, 1635t
Dexfenfluramine, valvular heart disease due to, 362
Dextrose, intravenous, hypokalemia due to, 2006
DHEAS, in polycystic ovary syndrome, 978
Diabetes insipidus, 601-602, 1988-1989
  diagnosis of, 601-602, 1988-1989
  encephalopathy in, 2340
  pathogenesis of, 1988
  treatment of, 602, 1989
Diabetes mellitus
  acanthosis nigricans in, 433, 434f
  after renal transplantation, 2124
  in alcoholic pancreatitis, 929
  angina pectoris in, 299-300
  aspirin in, 674-675
  autoimmunity in, 1237
  bulimia nervosa and, 2671
  cardiovascular complications of, 672-675
  cholecystectomy in, prophylactic, 907
  chronic renal failure in, 2016-2018
  complications of, 666-678. See also individual complications
    intensive in-hospital insulin therapy for, 675-676, 675f
    microvascular, 666-668, 668f
      genetics of, 668
      mechanisms of, 667-668, 668f
      pathogenesis of, 666-668
      screening for, 667t
  coronary artery bypass graft and, 314-315
  coronary artery disease in, 675
  cutaneous findings in, 433-434, 434f
  diarrhea in, 849
  dyslipidemia in, 674
  gastroparesis in, 852
  gestational, 1024-1025, 1024t
  hypertension in, 228-229, 673-674
    in chronic renal disease, 2017-2018
  insulin-dependent (IDDM). See Diabetes mellitus, type 1
  latent autoimmune, 636
  necrobiosis lipoidica in, 433
  neuropathy in. See Polyneuropathy, diabetic
    autonomic, 2299-2300
  non-insulin-dependent (NIDDM). See Diabetes mellitus, type 2
  osteomyelitis in, 1544
  polycystic ovary syndrome and, 979
  polyneuropathy in. See Polyneuropathy, diabetic
  in pregnancy, 1019
  as risk factor for stroke, 2211
  scleredema in, 433-434

smoking in, 674
surgical risk factor management
 and, 55
type 1, 633-650
 chronic renal disease in, 2017
 definition and classification
  of, 633, 633t
 diagnosis of, 639
 emergencies in, 646-648, 646t
  diabetic ketoacidosis, 646-
   647, 646t
  hypoglycemia, 647-648
 epidemiology of, 633
 hormonal regulation of
  metabolism and, 633-634, 634f-
  638f
 malabsorption and, 835
 management of, 639-648
  diabetes control and
   complications trial, 640-
   641
  exercise in, 646
  glycemic control in, 641-644
   glucose meters for, 641-644
   inhaled insulin, 643
   long-acting insulin, 644
  glycemic goals in, 641, 641t
  insulin pumps for, 644-
   645, 643f
  insulin regimens in, 644-
   645, 643f
  nutrition in, 645-646
  pancreas transplantation for,
   645
  pramlintide for, 645
  in pregnancy, 644
 pancreas transplantation and,
  938
 pathogenesis of, 634-638, 638f
  autoimmune factors in, 635
  environmental factors in, 635-
   636
  genetic factors in, 636-638
  insulin deficiency in,
   638, 639f
  temporal sequence of beta cell
   destruction in, 636, 638f
 prevention of, 638-639
type 2, 651-665
 chronic renal disease in, 2017
 definitions, 651, 652t
 diagnosis of, 656
 dyslipidemia in, 737-738
 epidemiology of, 651-652, 652f
 glycemic profiles in, 655, 655f
 hyperosmolar, hyperglycemic
  nonketotic coma in, 663
 encephalopathy in, 2340
 metabolic syndrome, 652-653
 pathogenesis of, 655, 656f
 pathophysiology of, 653-655
  glucose toxicity in, 654-655
  glycemic profiles in, 654-
   655, 655f
  insulin deficiency in,
   653, 653f
  insulin resistance in, 653-
   654, 654f
  metabolic responses to eating
   in, 654, 654f
 prediabetes and, 651, 652t
 prevention of, 655-656
 screening for, 656
 treatment of, 656-663
  during acute illness, 663
  alpha-glucosidase inhibitors
   in, 658-659, 658t
  antihyperglycemic drugs in,
   657-661, 658t-659t
  beta cell stimulants in,
   658, 658t
  gastrointestinal hormone
   agents in, 661, 659t

goals of, 656-657
insulin in, 660-661, 659t
 with oral agents, 662
metformin in, 659, 658t
monitoring glycemic outcomes
 in, 662-663
nutrition and physical
 activity in, 657
oral combination therapy in,
 661-662
oral monotherapy in, 661
principles of pharmacology in,
 661-662
sulfonylureas in, 657-658, 658t
thiazolidinediones in, 659-
 660, 658t
urinary tract infection in, 1508-
 1509
Diabetic ketoacidosis. See
 Ketoacidosis, diabetic
Diabetic truncal neuropathy, 2300
Diagnostic certainty, measures of, 8-
 9
Diagnostic test performance,
 measures of, 9-11, 10t-11t, 11f
Dialysis. See Hemodialysis,
 Peritoneal dialysis
Diaper rash, 1875, 1878t
Diaphragm, contraceptive, 998
 in urinary tract infection, 1509
Diaphragmatic dysfunction,
 postoperative, 2805
Diaphragmatic paralysis, 2804-2805
 bilateral, 2804-2805, 2805f
 unilateral, 2805
Diarrhea, 837-850
 acute, 838-842
  diagnosis of, 838-840
  infectious causes of, 838, 839t
  laboratory testing in, 840, 840f
  normal-anion-gap acidosis in,
   1998
  physical examination in, 839-840
  treatment of, 840-842
   antibiotics as, 841
   diet as, 841
   nonspecific, 840-841, 841t
   in specific infections and
    syndromes, 841-842
  C. difficile, 841-842, 1608
  Campylobacter, 841
 chronic, 842-849, 842t
  in AIDS, 849
  in bowel resection, 848
  classification of, 842, 842t
  diabetic, 849
  diagnosis of, 844-847, 844t, 845f-
   847f
  in dumping syndrome, 848
  fatty, 843-844, 846-847, 847f
  functional, 860
   treatment of, 847-848
  ileostomy, 848-849
  inflammatory, 843, 846, 846f
  in laxative abuse, 848
  in microscopic colitis syndrome,
   848
  of obscure origin, 849
  postcholecystectomy, 849
  postsurgical, 848-849
  in pouchitis, 849
  treatment of, 847-849
   antibiotic, 847
   nonspecific, 847
   in specific diseases and
    syndromes, 847-849
  watery, 843
   in bile acid malabsorption,
    843
   in drug therapy, 843
   idiopathic secretory, 849
   infectious, 843
   in inflammatory bowel disease,

843
  in irritable bowel syndrome,
   843, 847-848
  laboratory tests in, 844
  osmotic, 843, 846, 846f, 847
  other causes of, 843
  physical examination in, 844
  secretory, 843, 845-846, 845f
 classification of, 838
 in congenital chloridorrhea, 843
 definition of, 837
 E. coli
  diffuse-adhering, 1631, 1627t
  enteroaggregative, 1631, 1627t
  enterohemorrhagic, 1627-
   1631, 1627t, 1630f
  enteropathogenic,
   1627, 1627t, 1629f
  enterotoxigenic, 1626-
   1627, 1627t, 1628f
  O157:H7, 841
 Entamoeba histolytica, 842
 epidemiology of, 837
 fecal osmotic gap in, 837-838, 838f
 Giardia lamblia, 842
 nosocomial, 842
 palliative treatment of, 105
 parasitic, 842
 pathophysiology of, 837-838, 838f
 Salmonella, 841
 Shigella, 841
 traveler's, 79-80, 80t
Diazoxide, for hypertensive crisis,
 228t
DIC. See Disseminated intravascular
 coagulation (DIC)
Diclofenac sodium, hemolytic anemia
 due to, autoimmune, 1126
Dicloxacillin, 1424
Didanosine, for HIV infection, 1831t
 adverse effects of, 1834t
Dientamoeba fragilis infection,
 1903, 1903t
Diet, 25-31. See also Obesity
 alcohol in, 31
 angina pectoris and, 296
 caffeine in, 31
 caloric restriction, 720
 in cancer epidemiology, 2375
 carbohydrates in, 27, 720-721
 colorectal cancer and, 2476-
  2478, 2477t
 cooking oils in, 31
 dairy products and eggs in, 31
 elimination, 1281
 energy and, 25
 esophageal cancer and, 2491
 exercise and, 721
 fat and cholesterol in, 25-
  26, 25f, 26t
 fat restriction, 720
 fish in, 31
 flavonoid-rich foods in, 31
 foods in, 30-31
 fruits and vegetables in, 30
 garlic in, 31
 grains in, 31
 health and, 31, 32t
 high-protein, in nephrolithiasis,
  2107-2108
 legumes in, 30-31
 meat and poultry in, 31
 minerals in, 28-30, 30t
 for nephrolithiasis, 2109
 nuts in, 31
 in obesity, 720-721
 protein in, 27-28, 721
 vitamins in, 28, 29t
 water in, 30
Dietary fat, colorectal cancer and,
 2476-2477
Dietary fiber, 27, 27t
 colorectal cancer and, 2477

for weight loss, 721
Dietary supplements
 herbal, 87t-88t
 nonherbal, 89t
 poisoning by, 176
 popular uses for, 89t
Diet diary, 1281
Dieulafoy lesion, 864, 865f
Differentiation antigen(s), 2402
DiGeorge syndrome, 22q11 deletion
 in, 1949
Digitalis, toxicity, 166-167, 167t
Digital rectal exam, for prostate
 cancer, 2529
Digoxin, for heart failure, 342-
 343, 343t
2, 8-Dihydroxyadenine
 nephrolithiasis, 2110
Diltiazem, classification of, 267t
Diltiazem extended release, for
 hypertension, 221t
Dilute Russell viper venom time
 (DRVVT), 1160
Diphenhydramine, seizure due to,
 157t
2, 3-Diphosphoglycerate, in
 erythrocyte function, 1079
Diphtheria, 1584-1587
 clinical manifestations, 1584-1585
 complications of, 1585-1586
  respiratory insufficiency, 2806
 cranial neuropathy in, 1586
 cutaneous, 1585
 diagnosis of, 1584-1586
 etiology and epidemiology of, 1584
 immunization, 1587
  for HIV-infected patients, 1830t
  for travelers, 71
 microbiology of, 1584
 myocarditis in, 1585-1586
 neurologic toxicity in, 1586
 pathogenesis of, 1584, 1585f
 pharyngitis in, 1585, 1586f
 prevention of, 1587
 respiratory tract infection in,
  1585, 1586f
 treatment of, 1586-1587
  antibiotics for, 1586
  carrier state and, 1587
  at various sites, 1585
Dipyridamole, for pharmacologic
 stress testing, 201t
Dirithromycin, 1434
Dirofilaria immitis, 1932
 pulmonary, single nodule in, 2753
Discoid lupus, 1330, 1332f, 1328t
Disease. See also Injury and disease
Disease frequency, measures of, 8, 8t
Disopyramide
 for atrial fibrillation, 242t-243t
 classification of, 267t
Disseminated intravascular
 coagulation (DIC), 1185-
  1186, 1185t, 1185f
 clinical consequences of, 1185-
  1186
 diagnosis of, 1186
 encephalopathy in, 2342
 neoplastic, 2426-2427
 pathophysiology of, 1185, 1185f
 treatment of, 1186
Diuretic(s). See also specific drugs
 chronic hyponatremia due to, 1983
 for edema, 1990-1991, 1991f
 loop
  contraction alkalosis due to,
   2003
  for heart failure, 342, 343t
  hypokalemia due to, 2007
  metabolic alkalosis due to, 2003
  osmotic, hypernatremia and, 1987
 thiazide, metabolic alkalosis due
  to, 2003

Divalent metal transporter-1, in iron metabolism, 1081
Diverticular bleeding, 817-818
Diverticulitis, 813-818
  bleeding in, 817-818
  clinical presentation in, 813-814
  complications of, 816-817
  diagnosis of, 813-814, 814t
  diagnostic tests in, 814
  differential diagnosis of, 814-815
  gynecologic conditions and, 815
  imaging studies in, 814
  in immunocompromised patients, 815
  in systemic lupus erythematosus, 1333
  treatment of, 815-816
    inpatient, 815-816
    outpatient, 815
    preventive, 816
    surgical, 816
Diverticulosis, 813
  bleeding in, 817-818
  diverticular bleeding, 864
  epidemiology of, 813
  pathogenesis of, 813
Dizzy patient, 2135-2149. See also Vertigo, Vestibular
DNA
  replication of, 1944-1945, 1946f-1947f
  structure of, 1944, 1945f
DNA-based testing. See Genetic diagnosis and counseling
DNA topoisomerase inhibitors, 2414, 2417t-2419t, 2421
Dobutamine
  for pharmacologic stress testing, 201t
  for septic shock, 1451
Docetaxel, 2419t
Dofetilide
  for atrial fibrillation, 242t-243t
  classification of, 267t
Dog bite, 180, 181t-182t
Dog tapeworm, 1938-1939
Domestic abuse, alcoholism and, 2627
Domestic violence, 23
Donovanosis, genital ulcers in, 1528t
Dopamine
  for acute renal disease, 2036
  for septic shock, 1451
Dopamine agonist(s), for Parkinson disease, 2244-2245, 2246-2247, 2247t
Dowling-Degos disease, 580-581
Doxazosin
  for benign prostatic hyperplasia, 2131, 2131t
  for hypertension, 223t
Doxorubicin, 2417t
Doxorubicin-cyclophosphamide, for breast cancer, 2465, 2466t
Doxorubicin-cyclophosphamide-paclitaxel, for breast cancer, 2465, 2466t
Doxycycline, 1433
  for acne vulgaris, 450t
  for malaria chemoprophylaxis, for travelers, 78
  for Yersinia infection, 1636t
DPC4, properties of, 2386t
Dracunculiasis, 1929
Dreaming, functions of, 2362
Drinking, problem, 20-21, 20t-21t. See also Alcohol consumption
Drospirenone-ethinyl estradiol, for acne vulgaris, 450t
Drowning
  freshwater, 22
    hemolytic anemia in, 1128
  reducing risk of, 22-23
  saltwater, 22

  hemolytic anemia in, 1128
Drug abuse, 2635-2646. See also Drug dependence
  categories of, 2636-2637, 2636t
  definition of, 2636, 2635t
  diagnosis of, 2640-2641
  epidemiology of, 2637
  etiology of, 2637-2638
  injection, HIV transmission due to, 1822
  intravenous
    endocarditis in, 1486
    osteomyelitis in, 1543
    septic arthritis in, 1539
    septic pulmonary embolism in, 1479-1480
  pathophysiology of, 2638, 2639f, 2640t
  reducing risk of, 21
  rehabilitation in, 2643-2645
    medication for, 2644-2645
  in renal transplant recipients, 2116
  treatment of, 2641-2645
    in acute problems, 2641-2642, 2642t
    guidelines for intervention, 2641
    in intoxication, 2641
    in overdose and toxic reactions, 2641-2642, 2642t
    in substance-abuse depression, anxiety, psychosis, 2642
    in withdrawal states, 2642-2643
    usual clinical course of, 2638-2640, 2640t
Drug addiction. See Drug abuse, Drug dependence
Drug allergy, 1271-1277
  acneiform eruptions, 500
  acute, management of, 1276
  acute generalized exanthematous pustulosis, 500-501, 500f
  acute interstitial nephritis, 2087-2088, 2087t
  adverse, 495
  anticoagulant-induced skin necrosis, 501, 501f, 501t
  blistering, 498-500, 498f-500f
    fixed drug eruptions, 498-499, 498f
  chronic interstitial nephritis, 2089-2091
  classification of, 1271-1272, 1271f
  cutaneous, 495-503, 1272
    diagnosis of, 495
    epidemiology of, 495
    etiology of, 495
  desensitization in, 1276
  diagnosis of, 1272-1273, 1272t
  drug fever, 1272, 1416
  drug-induced linear IgA disease, 499
  erythema multiforme, 500
  exanthematous, 495-497
    complex, 496-497
    simple, 495-496
  hemorrhagic, 1184-1185
  hepatitis as, 877-878
  hyperpigmentation, 579
  hypersensitivity syndrome reaction, 496-497, 496t, 497f
  immune platelet destruction as, 1169-1170
  immunologic mechanisms of, 1271-1272, 1271f
  lichenoid eruptions, 501
  management of, 1276
  nephrotoxic. See Nephrotoxicity
  pathogenesis of, 1271
  pemphigus, 528
  pseudoporphyria, 499
  pustular, 500-501, 500f

  to specific drugs, 1273-1276, 1274t, 1275f
  Stevens-Johnson syndrome, 500
  toxic epidermal necrolysis, 500, 500f
  urticarial, 497-498, 496t, 1260-1261, 1261f
    angioedema and, 497
    serum sickness-like, 498, 496t
    vasculitis, 501-502, 502f
    vertigo as, 2146, 2146t
Drug dependence. See also Drug abuse
  definition of, 2635-2636, 2635t
Drug eruption, fixed, 498-499, 498f
Drug fever, 1272
  as fever of undetermined origin in, 1416
Drug overdose, 155-179. See also individual drugs, Poisoning or drug overdose
Drug reactions. See Drug allergy
Drug therapy
  acute pancreatitis due to, 914
  bereavement and, 119-120
  causing alopecia, 565t
  chronic hepatitis due to, 883
  diarrhea due to, 843
  GI bleeding due to, 863-864
  hypothyroidism due to, 606
  movement disorders due to, 2255t, 2260-2261
  myopathy due to, 2282-2284, 2283t
  parkinsonism due to, 2250, 2242t
  pharmacokinetics in. See Pharmacokinetics
  polyneuropathy due to, 2298, 2299t
  in renal failure. See also Renal disease, drug dosage adjustment in
  teratogenesis and, 1016-1017, 1017t-1018t
  topical, allergic contact dermatitis due to, 490, 491f
  toxic encephalopathy due to, 2341-2342
Duchenne muscular dystrophy. See Muscular dystrophy, Duchenne
Ductus arteriosus, patent, 391
  murmur in, 210t
Duloxetine, 2185
Dumping syndrome, 848, 856
Duodenal ulcer. See Peptic ulcer disease, duodenal
Duodenum
  Crohn disease of, 797
  obstruction of, in chronic pancreatitis, 930
Dupuytren contracture, 1395
Dutasteride, for benign prostatic hyperplasia, 2131-2132
Dysfibrinogenemia, 1196
Dysgerminoma, ovarian, 2541
Dyshidrotic eczema, 474
Dyskeratosis congenita, neutropenia in, 1144t
Dyslipidemia, 729-747
  atherosclerosis in, 732-733
  chylomicronemia syndrome in, 733
  clinical manifestations of, 732-734
  in diabetes mellitus, 674
  endocrine disorders causing, 740
  gastrointestinal disorders causing, 740-741
  hypercholesterolemia screening in children and, 745-746
  nonalcoholic fatty liver disease in, 733-734
  in older patients, 746
  patient approach
    in elevated cholesterol, 734-735
    in elevated triglycerides, 735
  renal disorders causing, 740

  secondary disorders of, 740-741
  secondary to estrogen and progestin therapy, 740
  special issues in, 745-746
  treatment of, 744-745
    with atherosclerosis and normal lipid levels, 736
    drug, 744-745, 744t-745t
    with low HDL, 735-736
    in women, 746
Dysmenorrhea, 960
Dyspepsia
  functional, 859
  peptic ulcer disease vs., 782
Dysphagia, 757-763, 757t, 758f
  in achalasia, 761-763, 761f-762f
  barium swallow in, 759
  in benign esophageal stricture, 759-760, 759f
  clinical evaluation in, 757-758
  diagnostic tests in, 758-759
  in diffuse esophageal spasm, 763
  endoscopy in, 759
  esophageal manometry in, 759
  in esophageal motility abnormalities, 760-763, 761t
  history in, 757-758
  in isolated hypertensive lower esophageal sphincter, 763
  in lower esophageal (Schatzki) ring, 760, 760f
  in nutcracker esophagus, 763
  physical examination in, 758
  in scleroderma, 763
Dysplasminogen, 1196-1197
Dyspnea
  in asthma, 2704
  in cardiovascular patient, 201-202, 201t, 202f
  palliative treatment of, 101-102, 103t
Dysproteinemia
  platelet disorders in, 1185
  tubulointerstitial nephritis in, 2097
Dysrhythmia. See Arrhythmia
Dystonia, 2255-2257
  classification of, 2255-2256
  clinical features of, 2256
  heredodegenerative, 2256
  primary, 2256
  secondary, 2256
  treatment of, 2256-2257
Dystonia-plus syndrome(s), 2256
Dysuria
  acute, in women, 1512t
  in women, 1523

E

EACA, for idiopathic thrombocytopenic purpura, 1168
Ear. See also under Otitis
  swimmer's, Pseudomonas aeruginosa, 1660
Eastern equine encephalitis, 1855
Eating disorder(s), 2666-2673. See also Anorexia nervosa, Bulimia nervosa
  epidemiology of, 2666
  management of, 2666, 2667f
  pregnancy and, 2666
Eaton-Lambert (myasthenic) syndrome, 2287, 2319
  respiratory insufficiency in, 2807
Ebola virus disease, 1853
Ebstein anomaly, of tricuspid valve, 399, 398f
E-CAD, properties of, 2386t
Ecchymosis, definition of, 429t
ECG. See Electrocardiography (ECG)
Echinococcosis, 1940-1941
  cavitary pulmonary infiltrate in,

2752
multiple pulmonary nodules in, 2755-2756
Echinococcus granulosus, 1940
Echinococcus multilocularis, 1940
Echinocyte, 1108, 1108f
Echinodermata, 192-193
Echocardiography
  dobutamine, in chest pain, 200t
  Doppler
    in aortic stenosis, 356
    in mitral stenosis, 351-352, 352f
  exercise, in chest pain, 200t
  in myocardial infarction, acute, 319
  in pulmonary hypertension, 2854, 2856f
  stress, in angina pectoris, 292
Ecstasy (methylenedioxymethamphetamine) (MDMA), 165
  acute hyponatremia due to, 1982
Ecthyma, 510
Ecthyma gangrenosum, *Pseudomonas aeruginosa,* 1661-1662
Ecto-ADPase, in coagulation, 1157
Eczema
  dyshidrotic, 474
  nummular, 474
Eczema herpeticum, 476
Eczematous disorders, 474. *See also* Contact dermatitis, Seborrheic dermatitis
Edema, 1989-1991
  cerebral, in herpes simplex encephalitis, 2348
  chronic hyponatremia in, 1983
  in cirrhosis, 1989-1990
  in congestive heart failure, 1989
  diagnosis of, 1990
  etiology of, 1989-1990
  in extrarenal disease, 1989-1990
  idiopathic, 1990
  in metabolic alkalosis, 2004-2005
  nephritic, 1989
  in nephrotic syndrome, 1989
  pathogenesis of, 1989
  pulmonary. *See* Pulmonary edema
  in renal disease, 1989
  treatment of, 1990-1991
    diuretics for, 1990-1991, 1991f
      clinical use of, 1991
      complications of, 1991
      mechanism of action of, 1990-1991
      resistance to, 1991
Edmonton Symptom Assessment Scale, 100, 101t
Education, food allergy and, 1283-1284, 1283t
Efalizumab, for psoriasis, 471
Efavirenz, for HIV infection, 1831t
  adverse effects of, 1834t
Effusion
  pericardial. *See* Pericardial effusion
  pleural. *See* Pleural effusion
Eflorinithine cream, for hirsutism, 992
EGFR (erb B), properties of, 2384t
Eggs, in diet, 31
Ehrlichia, antimicrobial drugs for, 1427t
Ehrlichia chaffeensis, 1732
Ehrlichia infection
  biology and ecology of, 1724-1725
  pathophysiology of, 1725
Ehrlichial diseases
  diagnosis of, 1727t
  treatment of, 1728t
Ehrlichiosis
  human granulocytic, 1724, 1733-1734, 1733f

Lyme disease and, 1733
  human monocytic, 1732-1733
    diagnosis of, 1732
    epidemiology of, 1732
    treatment of, 1732
Eisenmenger syndrome, 394-395
Elbow(s)
  epicondylitis of, 1394
  golfer's, 1394
  rheumatoid arthritis of, 1302, 1303f
  tennis, 1394
Elbow pain, 1394
Elderly patient. *See* Geriatric patient
Electrical injury, to heart, 386
Electrocardiography (ECG)
  ambulatory, in chest pain, 200t
  in angina pectoris, 287-289
  exercise, in angina pectoris, 291-292
  in hyperkalemia, 2011-2012, 2011f, 2007f
  in hypokalemia, 2008, 2007f
  in myocardial infarction, acute, 318, 318f
  in preoperative assessment, 53
  in pulmonary hypertension, 2854
  in syncope, 206-207
  in unstable angina/NSTEMI, 305
Electroencephalography (EEG)
  in epilepsy, 2191, 2192f
  in herpes simplex encephalitis, 2348
Electrolyte(s). *See also specific substance, e.g.,* Sodium
  in nutritional support, 947, 947t
Electromyography
  in myositis, 1354
  needle, for peripheral nerve disease, 2292
Elliptocytosis, hereditary, 1110
Embolism. *See also* Thromboembolism
  cholesterol, tubulointerstitial nephritis in, 2096, 2095f
  microvasculature damage due to, 1177-1178
  pulmonary. *See* Pulmonary embolism
Embolus, atheromatous, peripheral arterial disease in, 405, 406f
EMLA cream, 2185
Emphysema. *See also* Chronic obstructive pulmonary disease (COPD)
  alpha₁-antitrypsin deficiency in, pathology in, 2724, 2724f
  centriacinar, 2723, 2723f
  chest imaging in, 2728, 2725t
  clinical manifestations of, 2725, 2725t
  definition of, 2720
  epidemiology, 2720-2721, 2721f
  etiology of, 2721
  natural history of, 2721-2722, 2722f
  panacinar, 2723, 2723f
  pathogenesis of, 2724-2725
    alpha₁-antitrypsin deficiency in, 2724, 2724f
    oxidant-antioxidant imbalance in, 2724
  pathology in, 2722-2723
    early changes in, 2722
    in established disease, 2722-2723, 2723f
  physical examination in, 2725-2726
  treatment of, 2728-2732
    lung volume reduction for, 2732
Empty sella syndrome, 603
Empyema
  subdural, 1559-1560
    clinical features in, 1559-1560
    diagnosis in, 1559-1560

etiology in, 1559
    laboratory and imaging findings in, 1560, 1560f
    pathogenesis and pathophysiology in, 1559
    treatment and prognosis in, 1560
  thoracic, 1479, 2831-2832
    classification of, 2831, 2831t
    in hemothorax, 2830
    microorganisms causing, 2831
    treatment of, 2831-2832
    tuberculous, 1680
Emtricitabine, for HIV infection, 1831t
  adverse effects of, 1834t
Enalapril
  for hypertension, 222t
  for hypertensive crisis, 228t
Encephalitis
  adenovirus, 2352
  arboviral, 2352
  arthropod-borne, 2344t, 2352
  aseptic. *See* Encephalitis, viral
  California, 2352
  cytomegalovirus, 1762, 2351
  Eastern equine, 1855, 2352
  enteroviral, 1796, 1794t, 2346
  herpes simplex virus type 1, 2347-2348
    cerebral edema in, 2348
    EEG in, 2348
    imaging studies in, 2348
    treatment of, 2348
  herpes simplex virus type 2, 2347
  herpesvirus type 6, 2352
  HIV, 2352
  influenza, 2347
  Japanese, 1853-1854
    immunization for, 74, 76t
  LaCrosse, 1853
  Murray Valley, 1854
  nonviral causes of, 2346t
  papovavirus BK, 2352
  St. Louis, 1854, 2352
  tick-borne, 1854-1855
    immunization for travelers, 74
  toxoplasmosis, in AIDS, 1899
  Venezuelan equine, 1855-1856
  viral, 1853-1857, 2344-2354
    clinical features of, 2344, 2344t, 2344, 2345f
    diagnosis of, 2344-2345, 2346t
    nonspecific treatment of, 2345-2346
  Western equine, 1856, 2352
Encephalomyelitis
  acute disseminated, 2331-2332
  hepatitis C, 2353
  mumps, 2347
  in poliovirus infection, 2346
Encephalomyelopathy, subacute necrotizing, 2341
Encephalopathy, 2335-2343
  anoxic, 2336-2337
    in cardiac catheterization, 2337
    in cardiac disorders, 2336-2337
    in circulatory arrest, 2336-2337
    in coronary artery bypass surgery, 2337
    in heart transplantation, 2337
  clinical evaluation in, 2335-2336
  in connective tissue diseases, 2342-2343
  in dialysis disequilibrium syndrome, 2339
  in DIC, 2342
  due to anticancer chemotherapy, 2320, 2319t
  due to radiation therapy, 2320, 2319t
  hepatic
    in cirrhosis, 897-898, 898t
    in liver transplantation, 2338

in non-wilsonian hepatocerebral degeneration, 2338
  history in, 2335
  immediate management in, 2335t
  Korsakoff, 2341
  level of consciousness in, 2336, 2336f
  metabolic, 2338-2341
    in central pontine myelinolysis, 2341
    in diabetes mellitus, 2340
    in electrolyte disturbances, 2339
    in gastrointestinal disease, 2338-2339
    in high-altitude sickness, 2338
    in hyperalimentation, 2341
    in hypercalcemia and hypocalcemia, 2339
    in hyperkalemia and hypokalemia, 2339
    in hypocapnia, 2338
    in hypoglycemia, 2340
    in hypomagnesemia and hypermagnesemia, 2339
    in hyponatremia and hypernatremia, 2339
    in hypoxia and hypercapnia, 2338
    in liver disease. *See* Encephalopathy, hepatic
    in nutritional deficiencies, 2340-2341
    in pellagra, 2341
    in pituitary disease, 2339-2340
    in pulmonary insufficiency, 2338
    in renal failure, 2339
    in renal transplantation, 2339
    in thyroid disease, 2340
    in vitamin B$_{12}$ deficiency, 2341
  mitochondrial, 2280-2281
    neurogastrointestinal, 2281
  neurologic examination in, 2335-2336, 2336f
  pancreatic, 2338
  physical examination in, 2335
  portosystemic, 2338
  progressive multifocal, 2333
  pupillary light response in, 2336
  sepsis-related, 2338
  spongiform, 2357-2359
    bovine (mad cow disease), 2358, 2359
    prion hypothesis of, 2358-2359, 2358f-2359f
  toxic, 2341-2342
    iatrogenic, 2341-2342
  uremic, 2339
  in vasculitides, 2342-2343
  Wernicke, 2340-2341
Endobronchial brachytherapy, 2694
Endobronchial cryotherapy, 2694-2695
Endobronchial ultrasound, 2691
Endocarditis
  acute bacterial
    clinical presentation in, 1484, 1484f
    definition of, 1482
    etiology of, 1482
  anaerobic, 1605-1606
  candidal, 1879t
  corynebacterial, antibiotics for, 1493
  enterococcal, antibiotics for, 1491, 1493, 1492t
  in *Erysipelothrix* infection, 1597
  fungal
    antibiotics for, 1494
    etiology of, 1483
  gonococcal, treatment of, 1624t
  gram-negative bacilli, antibiotics for, 1493-1494
  HACEK organisms, antibiotics for, 1493

infective, 1482-1499
  adjunctive laboratory tests in,
    1489
  aortic valve annular abscess in,
    1489
  blood cultures in, 1488-1489
    culture-negative, 1489
    prosthetic valves and, 1489
  cardiac complications of,
    1489, 1489f-1490f
  cardiac conduction abnormalities
    in, 1489, 1490f
  cardiac findings in, 1484
  clinical presentation in, 1483-
    1487
  cutaneous findings in, 439
  cutaneous manifestations of,
    1484, 1484f
  definitions and terminology in,
    1482
  diagnosis of, 1487-1489, 1487t
  differential diagnosis of, 1489-
    1490
  diffuse membranoproliferative
    glomerulonephritis in, 1485
  Duke criteria for, 1487-
    1488, 1487t
  echocardiography for, 1488
  embolic phenomena in, 1485
  epidemiology of, 1482
  etiology of, 1482-1483, 1483t
  fever of undetermined origin in,
    1414
  focal embolic glomerulonephritis
    in, 1485
  multiple pulmonary nodules in,
    2755, 2756f
  musculoskeletal features of,
    1484-1485
  mycotic aneurysms in, 1485
  neurologic manifestations of,
    1485-1486
  ocular findings in, 1485
  in parenteral drug abuse, 1486
  pathogenesis of, 1483
  prognosis in, 1496-1497
  prophylaxis for, 1495-1496, 1495t-
    1497t
    AHA recommendations for, 351t
    esophageal procedures, 351t
    gastrointestinal procedures,
      351t
    genitourinary procedures, 351t
    oral cavity procedures, 351t
    respiratory tract procedures,
      351t
  renal manifestations of, 1485
  splenomegaly in, 1485
  treatment of, 1490-1495
    antimicrobial, 1490-1494, 1492t
    antithrombotic, 1495
    in culture-negative disease,
      1494
    monitoring clinical response
      in, 1494
    surgical, 1494-1495
  Libman-Sacks, valvular heart
    disease in, 349
  marantic, 1482
    infective endocarditis vs., 1490
  nonbacterial thrombotic, 1482
  nosocomial, etiology of, 1483
  prosthetic valve, 1486-1487, 1486t
    bacteremia in, 1489
    Staphylococcus epidermidis, 1581
    surgical intervention for, 1494-
      1495
    Pseudomonas aeruginosa, 1660
  staphylococcal, 1577
    antibiotics for, 1493, 1492t
  Streptococcus, antibiotics for,
    1491, 1492t
  Streptococcus bovis, 1573

subacute bacterial
  clinical presentation in, 1483
  definition of, 1482
  in valvular heart disease, 349
  viridans streptococci, 1573
    antibiotics, 1491, 1492t
Endocervical infection, Neisseria
  gonorrhoeae, 1622, 1624t
Endocrine disease
  autoimmune, 1237
  occupational, 66-67
Endometrial cancer, 2545-2547
  clinical features and evaluation
    in, 2545
  epidemiology of, 2545
  metastatic, 2547
  prognosis and postoperative
    treatment of, 2547, 2546t
  relapsed, 2547
  risk factors in, 2545
  staging and surgical management
    in, 2546-2547, 2546t
  tamoxifen as risk factor in, 2545
Endometrial hyperplasia, in
  polycystic ovary syndrome, 984
Endometrioma, in reproductive age
  women, 1060, 1062
Endometriosis, 960, 966-973
  chronic pelvic pain vs., 968
  definition and pathophysiology of,
    966
  diagnosis of, 967-968
  epidemiology of, 966
  in infertility, 967, 968
    in advanced disease, 972
    treatment of, 970-972, 971t
  pathogenesis of, 966-967, 966t
  pelvic pain in, treatment of, 968-
    970, 968t-970t
    danazol for, 970
    estrogen-progestin oral
      contraceptives for, 969
    GnRH agonist analogues for,
      969, 969t
    GnRH agonist analogues plus
      steroid for, 969-970, 969t
    progestins for, 970, 970t
    surgical, 970
Endometrium, in menopause, 1030, 1033
Endophthalmitis, candidiasis in,
  1879f
Endoscopic retrograde
  cholangiopancreatography (ERCP)
  in acute pancreatitis, 917, 918f
  in choledocholithiasis, 907-
    908, 908f
  in chronic cholecystitis, 906
  in chronic pancreatitis, 926-
    927, 927f
Endoscopic therapy
  for gastroesophageal reflux
    disease, 767-768
  for GI bleeding, 867
  for variceal bleeding, 868. See
    also Esophageal varices
Endoscopy
  in acute pancreatitis, 917, 918f
  in colorectal cancer, 2479-2481
  in Crohn disease, 798-799, 798f
  in dysphagia, 759
  in esophageal cancer, 772, 772f
  in gastroesophageal reflux
    disease, 765
  in GI bleeding, 866-867, 867t
  in peptic ulcer disease, 780, 779f
  in ulcerative colitis, 793-
    794, 793f
Endostatin, in tumor control,
  2394, 2395f
Endothelium-derived relaxing factor.
  See Nitric oxide
Endotoxin, bacterial, in sepsis,
  1444-1445, 1446f

Endotoxin activity assay,
  in sepsis, 1450
Endotoxin tolerance, in sepsis, 1445
Endotracheal intubation
  in cardiac resuscitation, 146t,
    147t
  for upper airway patency,
    2812, 2812t
Enema, barium
  in appendicitis, 820-821
  in colorectal cancer, 2481
Energy therapies, alternative, 87-89
Enoxaparin, for unstable angina and
  NSTMI, 311-312, 311t
Entamoeba histolytica, 1903, 1903f.
  See also Amebiasis
  diarrhea due to, 842
Entecavir, for chronic hepatitis B,
  888
Enteral nutrition. See Nutritional
  support, enteral
Enteric fever. See Salmonella
  infection
Enteric viral infection, 1793-1801
Enteritis. See also under individual
  pathogens
  Campylobacter, 1634, 1637, 1635t
  in males having sex with males,
    1529-1530
  radiation, malabsorption in, 831
  regional. See Crohn disease
Enterobacter cloacae, antimicrobial
  susceptibilities of, 1421t
Enterobacter infections, 1632
Enterococcal infection, 1568t, 1574
Enterococcus faecalis, 1574
Enterococcus faecalis osteomyelitis,
  1548, 1547t
Enterocolitis. See also Colitis
  dietary protein, 1280, 1280t
Enteropathic arthritis, 1317t, 1325
Enteropathy, gluten-sensitive. See
  Gluten-sensitive enteropathy
Enteroscopy
  in GI bleeding, 867
  wireless capsule, 867
Enterovirus infection, 1793-1798
  acute hemorrhagic conjunctivitis,
    1797, 1795t
  of central nervous system, 2344t
  clinical syndromes, 1793-
    1797, 1794t-1795t
  diagnosis and treatment of, 1797
  encephalitis, 1796, 1794t, 2346
  epidemiology of, 1793
  exanthems and enanthems,
    1796, 1794t
  febrile illness, 1794-1795
  immunity to, 1793
  in immunocompromised host,
    1797, 1795t
  meningitis, 2346
    aseptic, 1795-1796, 1794t
  myopericarditis, 1796, 1795t
  neonatal systemic, 1796-1797, 1795t
  other illnesses associated with,
    1797
  pathogenesis of, 1793
  pleurodynia, 1796, 1795t
  poliolike paralytic illness,
    1796, 1794t
  poliomyelitis, 1796, 1794t
  prevention and control of, 1797-
    1798
Environmental carcinogen(s), 2373-
  2378, 2374t
Environmental concerns. See
  Occupational disease
Environmental control, for allergy
  and atopy, 1250, 1250t
Environmental factors
  in allergic contact dermatitis,
    482

in colorectal cancer, 2476-
  2479, 2476t-2477t
Eosinophil(s), 1148-1150
  development of, 1072f
  disorders of, 1150
  function of, 1149-1150
  in immediate hypersensitivity
    reactions, 1243-1244, 1243f
  structure of, 1148-1149, 1138f
Eosinophilia, 1150
  in helminthic infection, 1918
  pulmonary
    with asthma, 2782
    prolonged, without asthma, 2782
    simple (Loffler syndrome), 2782
    tropical, 2782
    multifocal infiltrates in,
      2748
Eosinophilia-myalgia syndrome, 1349
Eosinophilic fasciitis, 443, 1349
Eosinophilic gastroenteritis,
  malabsorption in, 832-833
Eosinophilic gastroenteropathy,
  allergic, 1279-1280, 1280t
Eosinophilic granuloma, of lung,
  2780-2781, 2769t-2770t
  computed tomography in, 2760f
Eosinophilic pneumonia, 2782-2783
  chronic or acute, multifocal
    infiltrates in, 2748
  simple, multifocal infiltrates in,
    2748
Ependymoma, molecular and
  cytogenetic abnormalities in,
  2311t
Epicondylitis, of elbow, 1394
Epidermal appendage, benign tumors
  of, 536-537
Epidermal nevus, 440, 441f, 535-
  536, 536f
Epidermis, malignant tumors of, 549-
  556. See also Skin, Malignant
  tumors of
Epidermoid cyst, 537, 537f
Epidermolysis bullosa, 532-
  533, 533f, 526t
  acquired, 533
  dystrophic, 532-533, 533f
    autosomal recessive, 436
  herpetiformis (Dowling-Meara
    variant), 532
  junctional, 532, 533f
  simplex, 532, 533f
Epididymitis, chlamydial, 1747, 1748t
Epididymo-orchitis, mumps, 1770
Epiglottitis
  acute (supraglottitis), 1465-1466
  Haemophilus influenzae, 1649
Epilepsy, 2187-2200. See also
  Seizure
  benign childhood with
    centrotemporal spikes, 2189
  childhood absence, 2189, 2190f
  classification, 2187-2189, 2187t-
    2188t
  definition, 2187
  diagnosis of, 2190-2191, 2191f-
    2192f
  differential diagnosis, 2191
  EEG in, 2191, 2192f
  generalized seizures in, 2188-
    2189, 2187t-2188t
  juvenile myoclonic, 2189
  management of, 2191-2199
    after first seizure, 2191-2192
    antiepileptic drugs for, 2193-
      2197, 2193t
    drug therapy for, 2192-2197
    surgical, 2197
    vagus nerve stimulation for,
      2197-2198
  nocturnal frontal lobe, 2371
  partial seizures in, 2187-

2188, 2187t
posttraumatic, after brain trauma, 2236
in pregnancy, 1023
pregnancy and, 2198
psychogenic nonepileptic seizure in, 2191
status epilepticus, 2198-2199, 2199f
syndromes, 2189-2190
Epinephrine
for asthma, 2709
in cardiac resuscitation, 144t
in food allergy, 1283
Epiploic appendagitis, diverticulitis vs., 814-815
Epirubicin, 2418t
Epithelium, benign tumors of, 535-536
Eplerenone
for heart failure, 343, 343t
for hypertension, 221t
Eprosartan, for hypertension, 223t
Epsilonretrovirus, 1802t
Epstein-Barr virus infection, 1763-1765
Burkitt lymphoma and, 1763
in cancer epidemiology, 2376
clinical features and complications of, 1763-1764
diagnosis and treatment of, 1764-1765
epidemiology and pathogenesis of, 1763
in hepatitis, 877
Hodgkin disease and, 2596
in immunocompromised host, 1764
in infectious mononucleosis, 1763-1764
in meningoencephalitis, 2351
nasopharyngeal cancer and, 1763, 2437-2438
in renal transplantation, 2122
Eptifibatide, for unstable angina and NSTMI, 309-310, 309t
ERCP. See Endoscopic retrograde cholangiopancreatography (ERCP)
Erectile dysfunction, 696-697
Erosion, definition of, 428t
Ertapenem, 1430
in pregnancy, 1422t
Erysipelas, 510-511, 510f
Erysipeloid, 1597
Erysipelothrix infection, 1597-1598
Erythema, definition of, 429t
Erythema dyschromicum perstans, 579
Erythema marginatum, in rheumatic fever, 433, 434f
Erythema migrans, in Lyme disease, 439, 439f, 1713, 1713f
Erythema multiforme, 531-532, 526t, 531t, 532f
as drug reaction, 500
Erythema nodosum
in inflammatory bowel disease, 435
poststreptococcal, 1572
in sarcoidosis, 2771-2772
Erythrasma, 511-512
Erythrocyte(s)
cell aging and death, 1108, 1109f
control of hydration in, 1108
development, structure, physiology of, 1107-1108
development of, 1072f, 1074
function of, 1078-1079, 1078f-1079f
hemoglobin in, 1107
metabolism of, 1107t, 1107
abnormalities of, 1111-1113
defective reducing power, 1112-1113, 1110f
glucose-6-phosphate dehydrogenase deficiency, 1112-1113

glutathione synthesis, 1112
glycolysis, 1113
nucleotide metabolism, 1113
nonhemoglobin cytosol, 1107, 1107t
plasma membrane, 1107-1108, 1108f-1109f
carbohydrates in, 1108
disorders of, 1109-1111
protein, 1110-1111
salt and water metabolism, 1109-1110
phospholipids and cholesterol in, 1107, 1108f
proteins in, 1107-1108, 1109f
principles of blood flow and, 1108
shape changes in, 1108, 1108f
for transfusion. See Transfusion therapy, red cell
Erythrocyte sedimentation rate, in rheumatic disease, 1293, 1293t
Erythrocytosis. See Polycythemia
Erythroderma, 458-459, 458f
in atopic dermatitis, 475
congenital ichthyosiform, 479, 479f
Erythromycin, 1433-1434
for acne vulgaris, 449t, 450t
for Campylobacter infection, 1635t
in pregnancy, 1422t
Erythromycin-benzoyl peroxide, for acne vulgaris, 449t
Erythromycin estolate, in pregnancy, 1422t
Erythropoietin
in hematopoiesis, 1071-1072, 1073t
recombinant human, abuse of (blood doping), 1136
Escherichia coli
antimicrobial susceptibilities of, 1421t
diffuse-adhering, diarrhea due to, 1631, 1627t
enteroaggregative, diarrhea due to, 1631, 1627t
enterohemorrhagic, diarrhea due to, 1627-1631, 1627t, 1630f
diagnosis of, 1628-1630
epidemiology of, 1627-1628
pathogenesis of, 1628, 1630f
treatment of, 1630-1631
enteropathogenic, diarrhea due to, 1627, 1627t, 1629f
enterotoxigenic, diarrhea due to, 1626-1627, 1627t, 1628f
O157:H7
diarrhea due to, 841
in hemolytic-uremic syndrome, 2079
in urinary tract infection, 1509-1510, 1510f
Escherichia coli infections, 1626-1631, 1627t
extraintestinal, 1631, 1627t
meningitis, 1553t
urinary tract, 1631
Esmolol
classification of, 267t
for hypertensive crisis, 228t
Esophageal cancer, 771-774, 2490-2494
adenocarcinoma
risk factors for, 2491
screening and prevention of, 2491-2492, 2492t
diagnosis of, 771-772, 772f, 2492, 2493f
epidemiology of, 771, 2490
diet and, 2375
tobacco use and, 2374
etiology of, 2490-2491
incidence of, 2490
molecular mutations and pathogenesis of, 2492
risk factors in, 771, 2490-2491

screening and prevention of, 2491-2492
squamous cell
risk factors for, 2491
screening and prevention of, 2491
staging of, 2492-2493, 2493f
treatment of, 772-774, 773f, 2493-2494
in local disease, 2493-2494
in metastatic disease, 2494
Esophageal disorders, 757-775. See also individual disorders, e.g., Dysphagia
Esophageal manometry, for dysphagia, 759
Esophageal motility abnormalities
dysphagia in, 760-763, 761t
in scleroderma, 1346, 1346f
Esophageal ring (Schatzki), in dysphagia, 760, 760f
Esophageal spasm, diffuse, dysphagia in, 763
Esophageal sphincter, lower, isolated hypertensive, 763
Esophageal stricture, in dysphagia, 759-760, 759f
Esophageal varices
bleeding, 864, 864f
endoscopic treatment of, 868
pharmacotherapy for, 868-869
radiologic intervention for, 869
surgical intervention for, 869
in cirrhosis. See under Cirrhosis
Esophagitis
candidal, 769-770, 1877t
cytomegaloviral, 770
herpes simplex, 770
in HIV infection, 770-771
infectious, 769-771
reflux. See Gastroesophageal reflux disease
Esophagus
Barrett, 768-769, 768f-769f
diagnosis and surveillance in, 2492t, 2492
esophageal cancer and, 2491
biopsy of, in gastroesophageal reflux disease, 765
Crohn disease of, 797
nutcracker, 763
pneumatic dilatation of, for achalasia, 762
swallowing disorders of. See Dysphagia
Estramustine, 2422
Estrogen(s)
as cause of gynecomastia, 695
thrombosis and, 1202
Estrogen replacement therapy
cancer epidemiology and, 2377
colorectal cancer and, 2478
dyslipidemia and, 740
for menopause, 1035-1036, 1035t
for postmenopausal osteoporosis, 710
thrombosis and, 1202
Etanercept
for psoriasis, 471
for rheumatoid arthritis, 1308t, 1310
Ethacrynic acid, for hypertension, 221t
Ethambutol, in pregnancy, 1422t
Ethanol abuse. See Alcoholism, Alcohol consumption
Ethical and social issues, 1-6
areas of debate in, 2-3
assessing quality of life, 3
moral limits of medical intervention, 2
when does life begin, 2-3
clinical decision making in,

broader context for, 5
context for decision making in, 2
carrying out decision and, 2
clarifying ethical dilemmas in, 2
information gathering and, 2
on Internet, 4
population-based medicine and rights of individual, 4-5
traditional medical ethics and changing world, 3-5
Ethosuximide, in epilepsy, 2194
Ethylene glycol
nephrotoxicity due to, 2033
poisoning or overdose with, 168, 168t
elimination method for, 161t
metabolic acidosis in, 1996-1997, 2001
Etoposide, 2418t
Euthanasia, 98
Evans syndrome, 1169
Ewing sarcoma, 2558
EWS-FLI1 in, 2385
extraosseous, 2553
features of, 2550t
EWS-FLI1, 2385
Exanthema subitum (roseola infantum), herpesvirus type 6 in, 1765
Exanthematous drug reactions, 495-497
Exanthematous pustulosis, acute generalized, as drug reaction, 500-501, 500f
Exemestane, for early (stages I and II) breast cancer, 2465
Exenatide, for type 2 diabetes mellitus, 661, 659t
Exendin, for type 2 diabetes mellitus, 661, 659t
Exercise, 32-38. See also under Athlete
aging and, 35
angina pectoris and, 296
asthma and, 2706
atherosclerosis prevention and, 35-36
for atherosclerotic peripheral arterial disease, 403
blood lipid effects of, 34
body fluids and, 35
calorie consumption and, 36t
in cancer epidemiology, 2375-2376
cardiovascular response to, 32-33
colorectal cancer and, 2478-2479
complications of, preventing, 38
diabetes
in type 1, 646
in type 2, 657
diet and, 721
hematologic effects of, 34-35
ischemic heart disease and, 36
longevity and, 35-36
medical complications of, 38
hypokalemia, 2007
metabolic effects, 33-34, 34f
musculoskeletal response to, 33
obesity and, 721
physiologic effects of, 32-35
prescribing, 36-38, 37t
psychological effects of, 35
pulmonary response to, 33
in stroke prevention, 2211
Exercise stress testing
in chest pain, 198, 199f, 199t-201t
contraindications to, absolute and relative, 199t
ECG, in chest pain, 200t
noninvasive, 198-199, 199t-201t
pharmacologic, 199, 201t
predischarge, after acute myocardial infarction, 331-

332, 332f
Exfoliation, definition of, 429t
Exostosis, subungual, 576t
Expected-outcome decision analysis, 14-15, 14f
Eyelid disorders. *See entries under* Ocular

F

Fabry disease, 1149t
  cutaneous findings in, 440-441, 442f
Facial neuropathy (Bell palsy), 2293-2294, 2294t
Facies, in Parkinson disease, 2242, 2243f
Factor V Leiden, 1193-1195, 1194f
  genetic testing in, 1960
Factor VII, elevated, 1197
Factor VIIa, for transfusion, 1213
Factor VIII
  activity level of, bleeding patterns in hemophilia and, 1182, 1182t
  deficiency. *See also* Hemophilia A
  elevated, 1197
Factor VIII concentrate, for transfusion, 1213
Factor IX
  deficiency, 1183
  for transfusion, 1213
Factor XI
  deficiency, 1183-1184
  for transfusion, 1212
Factor XIII, tests for, 1161
Falls
  in geriatric patients, 22t, 22
  injury from, 22, 22t
Familial adenomatous polyposis (FAP)
  colorectal cancer in, 2475
  medications and colorectal cancer risk in, 2478
Familial fatal insomnia, 2358, 2359
Familial Mediterranean fever, fever of undetermined origin in, 1416
Familial neoplasms, genetic risk factors for, 2378, 2379t
Fanconi anemia, CNS tumors in, 2310t
Farber disease, 1149t
Farmer's lung, 2758, 2759t, 2765-2766, 2765f. *See also* Pneumonitis, hypersensitivity
Fasciitis
  eosinophilic, 443, 1349
  necrotizing, 512
    cutaneous findings in, 439
    streptococcal group A, 1570
  plantar, of foot, 1397, 1397f
Fascioliasis, 1935-1936
Fasciolopsiasis, 1936
Fat, dietary, colorectal cancer and, 2476-2477
Fat consumption, 25-26, 25f, 26t
  colorectal cancer and, 27
  dietary recommendations for, 26, 26t
  health and, 26
  restriction of, 720
Fat necrosis, of breast, 1053
Fat redistribution syndrome (lipodystrophy syndrome), in HIV infection, 1834-1835
Fatty acids, dietary, cardiovascular risk and, 26
Fatty liver disease, nonalcoholic
  chronic hepatitis *vs.*, 883
  dyslipidemia in, 733-734
Fava bean(s), glucose-6-phosphate dehydrogenase deficiency and, 1112
Favism, 1112
Favre-Racouchot disease, acne

vulgaris *vs.*, 447
Febrile seizures, 1412
Fecal antigen test, in peptic ulcer disease, 782
Fecal fat analysis
  for malabsorption, 825, 825t
  for steatorrhea, 846-847
Fecal impaction, 105
Fecal incontinence, 858-859
Fecal occult blood testing, in colorectal cancer, 2479, 2480t
Fecal testing
  in watery osmotic diarrhea, 845
  in watery secretory diarrhea, 845
Feet. *See* Foot
Felbamate, in epilepsy, 2194
Felodipine, for hypertension, 221t
Felty syndrome, in rheumatoid arthritis, 1305
Female(s)
  acute dysuria in, 1512t
  dyslipidemia management for, 746
  hair loss in, therapy for, 564
  hyperandrogenism in, laboratory evaluation of, 447t
  migraine in, 2159
Fenfluramine, valvular heart disease due to, 362
Fenoldopam, for hypertensive crisis, 228t
Fenretinide, for breast cancer prevention, 2459
Ferret bite, 180-181
Ferritin, in iron metabolism, 1081
Fertilization, in vitro, 1002, 1007t
  for infertility in endometriosis, 972
  for polycystic ovary syndrome, 984
Fetus, hematopoiesis in, 1070
Fever, 1411-1413. *See also specific types, e.g.,* Rheumatic fever
  complications of, 1412
  diagnosis of, 1412
  drug, 1272, 1416
  febrile seizures in, 1412
  hyperthermia *vs.*, 1407-1408, 1407f
  neutropenia and, neoplastic, 2428-2429
  pathophysiology of, 1411-1412
  possible benefits of, 1412
  rat-bite, 181
  in septic shock, 1452
  treatment of, 1412-1413
Fever of undetermined origin, 1413-1418
  in AIDS, 1416
  in alcoholic hepatitis, 1415
  biopsies in, 1417
  causes of, 1413t, 1413
  in cirrhosis, 1415
  in CMV infection, 1414
  in collagen vascular disease, 1415
  diagnosis of, 1416-1417
  in drug fever, 1416
  in elderly patient, 1416
  in endocarditis, 1414
  etiologic classification of, 1413-1416, 1414t
  exploratory laparotomy for, 1417
  factitious, 1416
  in familial Mediterranean fever, 1416
  in giant cell arteritis, 1415
  in granulomatous disease, 1415
  in Hodgkin disease, 1415
  in hypernephroma, 1415
  in infection, 1414-1415, 1414t
    localized, 1414-1415
    systemic, 1414
  in inflammatory bowel disease, 1415
  in inflammatory pseudotumor of intra-abdominal lymph nodes,

1416
    laboratory studies in, 1416-1417
    less common causes of, 1415-1416
    in leukemia, 1415
    in liver abscess, 1414-1415
    in neoplasm, 1415
    in pulmonary emboli, 1415-1416
    radiologic studies in, 1417
    in sarcoidosis, 1415
    in starch peritonitis, 1415
    in Still disease, 1415
    in subphrenic abscess, 1414-1415
    in tuberculosis, 1414
    undiagnosed, 1417-1418
    in Whipple disease, 1416
Fiber, dietary, 27, 27t
  colorectal cancer and, 2477
  for weight loss, 721
Fibrillation
  atrial. *See* Atrial fibrillation
  ventricular. *See* Ventricular fibrillation
Fibrin-fibrinogen degradation products test, 1161
Fibrinogen levels, 1161
  elevated, 1197
Fibrinolysis
  abnormal, 1184, 1196-1197
  in coagulation, 1158, 1158f-1159f
  primary, 1188
Fibrinopeptide A (FPA), 1161
Fibroadenoma, breast, 1053
Fibroelastoma, papillary, cardiac, 384
Fibroleiomyomatous hamartoma, multiple pulmonary, 2756
Fibroma, subungual, in tuberous sclerosis, 440, 441f
Fibromuscular dysplasia
  renal artery stenosis in, 2071-2072
  treatment of, 2073
  in renovascular hypertension, 231
Fibromyalgia, 1399-1406
  clinical manifestations of, 1400-1401
  complications of, 1405
  definition of, 1399
  diagnosis of, 1400-1402, 1401t
  differential diagnosis of, 1402, 1403t
  epidemiology of, 1399
  etiology of, 1399-1400
    biosocial, 1399-1400
    psychological, 1400
  Internet sites on, 1404
  pain in, temporal course of, 1291f
  pathophysiology of, 1400
  physical examination in, 1401, 1402f
  prevention of, 1405
  prognosis in, 1405
  treatment of, 1402-1405
    in geriatric and pediatric cases, 1402-1403
    nonpharmacologic, 1404-1405
    pharmacologic, 1403-1404, 1403t
Fibrosarcoma, 2552
  features of, 2550t
  treatment of, 2558
Fibrosing alveolitis. *See* Pulmonary fibrosis, idiopathic
Fibrosing mediastinitis, 2838-2839
Fibrothorax, in hemothorax, 2830
Filariasis, 1929, 1929-1932
  lymphatic, 1929-1930
  zoonotic, 1932
Filovirus infection, 1852
Finasteride
  for benign hyperplasia of prostate, 2131-2132
  for hirsutism, 991, 992
Fingernail(s). *See* Nail(s)

Fire ants, 191, 1285-1286, 1286f-1287f
Firearms injury, reducing risk of, 23
Fires, prevention of death from, 22
Fish, in diet, 31
Fish poisoning, respiratory insufficiency in, 2806
Fish tapeworm, 1936
Fissure, definition of, 428t
Fistula
  cholecystoenteric, 905
  diverticular, 816
FK506. *See* Tacrolimus
Flail chest, 2803
Flavonoid-rich foods, 31
Flea infestation, 521-522
Flecainide
  for atrial fibrillation, 242t-243t
  classification of, 267t
Flexor tenosynovitis, of hand, 1395
Flinders Island spotted fever, 1728
Flock worker's lung, 63
Flora, normal, anaerobic bacteria in, 1600, 1600t-1601t
Floxuridine, 2416t
FLT-3 ligand, 1073t
Fluconazole
  as antifungal, 1871-1873, 1871t-1872t
  for toenail onychomycosis, 575t
Fludarabine, 2417t
  for chronic lymphocytic leukemia, 2588
Fluid
  compartments of, movement between, 1975-1976
  deficit, disorders of. *See* Hypernatremia
  distribution and composition of, 1975-1976
  excess, disorders of. *See* Hyponatremia
  exercise and, 35
  homeostasis of, 1975-1978
  osmolality of, 1975
  renal processing of, 1976, 1976f, 1978f, 1977t
    glomerular filtration in, 1976
    tubular reabsorption in, 1976, 1976f, 1978f, 1977t
  salt water excess in. *See* Edema
  tonicity of, 1976
  volume
    depletion of. *See* Hypovolemia
    extracellular, 1977, 1979t
    intracellular, 1977, 1979t, 1979f
      in hypotonicity and hypertonicity, 1977-1978
    regulation of, 1976-1977, 1979t, 1979f
Flukes, intestinal, 1936
Flumazenil, for benzodiazepine overdose, 173
Flunisolide, for asthma, 2712, 2713t
Fluoride, biologic test of exposure to, 61t
Fluoroquinolone, 1438-1439, 1438t
  for legionellosis, 1655t
  in pregnancy, 1422t
Fluorouracil, 2416t
  for colorectal cancer, 2486
Fluorouracil-doxorubicin-cyclophosphamide, for breast cancer, 2466t
Fluoxetine, for premenstrual syndrome, 964
Flutamide, 2420t
  for hirsutism, 991
Fluticasone, for asthma, 2712, 2713t
Fogo selvagem, 526t
Folate
  cobalamin and, in DNA synthesis,

1099-1100, 1100f
colorectal cancer and, 2477-2478
Folic acid, 29t
Folic acid deficiency
  causes of, 1103-1104, 1104t
  in megaloblastic anemia, 1103-1104
Folic acid supplement, hypokalemia
  due to, 2006
Folic acid supplementation, neural
  tube defects and, 1016
Follicle stimulating hormone, in
  polycystic ovary syndrome,
  978, 978f
Follicle-stimulating hormone, 599-
  601
Folliculitis
  acne vulgaris vs., 447
  bacterial, 512-513, 513f
  candidal, 1879t
  gram-negative, acne vulgaris vs.,
    447
  Malassezia, 509
  Pseudomonas aeruginosa, 513, 1661
Folliculitis decalvans, 568
Fondaparinux
  for heparin-induced
    thrombocytopenia, 1200
  for venous thromboembolism, 417
Food(s), dietary, 30-31
Food allergy, 1278-1284
  definition of, 1278
  diagnosis of, 1278-1283
  diet diary for, 1281
  elimination diet for, 1281
  epidemiology of, 1278
  history and physical examination
    in, 1281, 1281t
  IgE-mediated, 1278
    gastrointestinal, 1278-
      1279, 1279t
    respiratory and skin, 1279
  laboratory tests for, 1281-1282
    allergy skin tests, 1281-1282
    double-blind placebo-controlled
      food challenge, 1282
    in vitro assays, 1282
  mixed IgE-mediated and non-IgE
    mediated, 1279-1280, 1280t
    allergic eosinophilic
      gastroenteropathy, 1279-
      1280, 1280t
  non-IgE mediated, 1280-1281, 1280t
    celiac disease, 1281
    dietary protein enterocolitis,
      1280, 1280t
    dietary protein proctitis, 1280-
      1281
  non-IgE-mediated, 1278
  pathophysiology of, 1278
  practical approach to diagnosis
    of, 1282-1283
  prognosis in, 1284
  treatment of, 1283-1284
    immunotherapy, 1283
    patient education, 1283-
      1284, 1283t
    pharmacologic, 1283-1284
  urticarial reaction in, 1261
Food challenge, double-blind placebo-
  controlled, 1282
Food hypersensitivity, 1278
Food intolerance, 1278
Food poisoning, 174-176. See also
  specific disorders, e.g.,
  Botulism
  Amanita phalloides mushroom, 175
  Bacillus cereus, 1597
  clostridial, 1608
  dietary supplements, 176
  herbal remedies, 176
  monosodium glutamate, 175-176
  seafood, 175, 175t
  staphylococcal, 1577-1578

Foot
  in diabetes mellitus, 672t, 671, 672
  plantar fasciitis of, 1397, 1397f
  rheumatoid arthritis of,
    1303, 1303f
Foot-and-mouth disease, 1859
Foot pain, 1396-1397, 1397f
Forefoot pain, 1397, 1397f
Foreign matter, aspiration of,
  segmental pulmonary infiltrates
  in, 2751
Formoterol, for asthma, 2709, 2711t
Fosamprenavir, for HIV infection,
  adverse effects of, 1834t
Fosfomycin, 1440
Fosinopril, for hypertension, 222t
Fracture, rib, flail chest in, 2803
Fragile X syndrome, 1950, 1951t,
  1960t
FRAMES counseling, for alcoholism,
  2629, 2630t
Friedreich ataxia, 2263t, 2263-2265
  diagnosis of, 2264
  genetics and pathogenesis in, 2263-
    2264, 2265f
  genetics of, 1950, 1951t
  genetic testing in, 1959, 1960t
  management of, 2264-2265
Frontal bone, osteomyelitis of, in
  sinusitis, 1460
Frontotemporal lobar degeneration,
  2225-2226, 2224f-2225f
Frozen shoulder (adhesive
  capsulitis), 1393
Fruits, dietary, 30
  colorectal cancer and, 2477
Fucosidosis, 1148t
Fukuyama congenital muscular
  dystrophy, 2275
Fundoplication, gastroparesis after,
  852
Fungal infections, in septic
  arthritis, 1538
Fungal organisms, in sepsis, 1445
Fungal pneumonia, multifocal
  infiltrates in, 2747
Furosemide
  for acute renal failure,
    2037, 2037t
  for hypertension, 221t
Furuncle, definition of, 429t
Furunculosis, staphylococcal,
  511, 511f
Fusariosis, in compromised host,
  1888-1890, 1889t
Fusobacterium species, 1604

G

Gabapentin, in epilepsy, 2194
Gaisbock syndrome (relative
  polycythemia), 1132
Gait disturbances, in geriatric
  patients. See also Falls, in
  geriatric patients
Galactosialidosis, 1148t
Gallbladder
  empyema of, in acute
    cholecystitis, 905
  malignancy of, gallstones in, 905
  necrosis of, in acute
    cholecystitis, 905
  porcelain, 905, 905f
Gallium scan, in osteomyelitis, 1545
Gallstone. See also Cholecystitis,
  Choledocholithiasis,
  Cholelithiasis
  cholesterol, 901-902, 901t, 903f
  formation of, 901-902, 901t, 902f-
    903f
  in gallbladder cancer, 905
  in home parenteral nutrition, 948
  incidence and prevalence of, 901

microlithiasis, pancreatitis in,
  915
pancreatitis in. See Pancreatitis,
  gallstone
pigment, 901, 901t, 902f
Gammaretrovirus, 1802t
Gammopathy, monoclonal, of
  undetermined significance
  (MGUS), 2302
Ganglioneuroblastoma, mediastinal,
  2839
Ganglioneuroma, mediastinal, 2839
Gangliosidosis, 1149t
Gangrene
  gas (clostridial myonecrosis),
    1607
    treatment of, 1612
    vs. crepitant cellulitis, 1610-
      1611
  pulmonary, cavitary infiltrates
    in, 2752
Gardner syndrome, 538
Garlic, in diet, 31
Gas gangrene (clostridial
  myonecrosis), 1607
  treatment of, 1612
  vs. crepitant cellulitis, 1610-
    1611
Gastric bypass, for obesity, 724-
  725, 725t
Gastric cancer, 2494-2499
  diagnosis in, 2496-2497, 2497f
  dietary factors in, 2494
  epidemiology of, 2494
    diet and, 2375
  etiology and risk factors in, 2494-
    2496, 2495t, 2495f
  familial, 2495-2496, 2495f
  Helicobacter pylori infection as
    risk factor in, 2376-2377,
    2495
  pathophysiology of, 2496
  screening and prevention of, 2496
  staging and prognosis in,
    2496, 2496t
  treatment in, 2497-2499
    in local disease, 2497-
      2498, 2498f
    in metastatic disease, 2499
Gastric emptying, rapid (dumping
  syndrome), 848, 856
Gastric lavage, for poisoning or
  drug overdose, 159-160, 160t
Gastric lymphoma, 2507-2508
Gastric motility, 851
  disorders of, 852-856
Gastric ulcer. See Peptic ulcer
  disease, gastric
Gastrin, serum, in Zollinger-Ellison
  syndrome, 781
Gastrinoma
  peptic ulcer disease in, 777f, 778
  serum gastrin concentration in,
    781
Gastroenteritis
  eosinophilic, malabsorption in,
    832-833
  Salmonella, 1638-1639
  viral, 1798-1800
Gastroenteropathy, eosinophilic,
  allergic, 1279-1280, 1280t
Gastroesophageal reflux disease
  (GERD), 763-768
  clinical features of, 765
  diagnosis of, 765-766
  in esophageal cancer, 2491
  etiology of, 764-765
    Helicobacter pylori in, 765
    NSAIDs in, 764-765
  pathophysiology of, 764
    antireflux mechanisms and, 764
    esophageal clearance in, 764
    hiatal hernia in, 764

treatment of, 766-768
  antacids and alginic acid, 766
  antireflux surgery, 767
  endoscopic antirefulx
    procedures, 767-768
  H$_2$ receptor blockers, 766
  lifestyle modifications,
    766, 766t
  prokinetic agents, 766
  proton pump inhibitors, 766-767
Gastrointestinal bleeding, 863-871
  in acute pancreatitis, 922
  lower, 864-865, 865f
  in mechanical ventilation, 2819
  occult, 869-870, 869f-870f
  overt, 863-869
    clinical and laboratory
      assessment in, 865-866, 866t
    diagnosis of, 865-867, 865f-866f
    endoscopy in, 866-867, 867t
    epidemiology of, 863
    etiology of, 863-865, 863t, 864f-f
    radiology in, 867
    treatment of, 867-869
      in nonvariceal bleeding, 867-
        868
      in variceal bleeding, 868-869
  upper, 863-864, 864f-865f
Gastrointestinal cancer, 2490-2511.
  See also specific locations,
  e.g., Esophageal cancer
  incidence and mortality of,
    2490, 2490t
Gastrointestinal decontamination,
  after poisoning or drug
  overdose, 159-160, 160t
Gastrointestinal disorders
  encephalopathy in, 2338-2339
  functional, 859-860
Gastrointestinal hypersensitivity,
  immediate, 1279, 1279t
Gastrointestinal motility, 851-862
  disorders of, 852-862
  normal, 851-852
Gastrointestinal stromal tumor,
  2507, 2553-2554
  features of, 2550t
  treatment of, 2556
Gastrointestinal tract procedures,
  antibiotic prophylaxis for, 351t
Gastroparesis, 852-856
  causes of, 852, 852t
  diabetic, 852
  diagnosis of, 853, 854t
  differential diagnosis of, 853-854
  idiopathic, 853
  postsurgical, 852
  treatment of, 854-856, 855t
    antiemetic, 854, 855t
    gastric electrical stimulation,
      855-856
    prokinetic, 854-855, 855t
    pyloric botulinum injection, 855
    surgical, 856
Gastroplasty, vertical banded, 724-
  725, 725t
Gaucher disease, 1148t
Gelling phenomenon, in rheumatic
  disease, 1291
Gemcitabine, 2417t
Gemifloxacin, 1438-1439, 1438t
Generalized anxiety disorder, 2662
Genetic diagnosis and counseling,
  1958-1966
  in breast cancer, 47
  DNA-based testing in, difficulties
    with, 1965
  genetic consultation in, 1964
  genetic-counseling paradigm in,
    1962-1964
    carrier testing and, 1963-
      1964, 1963t
    predictive testing and, 1962-

1963
  prenatal testing and, 1964
  medical testing paradigm for, 1959-
    1962, 1959t
    in asymptomatic at-risk persons,
      1961-1962, 1961t
    in symptomatic persons, 1959-
      1961, 1960t
  molecular testing, 1958, 1958t-
    1959t
    for sequence alteration,
      1958, 1958t
  preimplantation, 1008
Genetic disease, 1946-1951
  abnormal number of chromosomes in,
    1947-1949
  imprinting defects in, 1950
  Internet resources for, 1956
  mitochondrial inheritance in, 1951-
    1952, 1952t
  partial chromosome deletion in,
    1949, 1947f
  privacy issues in, 1956
  single gene mutations in, 1949
  trinucleotide repeat disorders,
    1950-1951, 1951t
Genetics, 1944-1957
  of cancer, 2383-2399
  in hypertension, 215
Genetic testing, preconception, 1016
Genital herpes, 1756-1757, 1756f
Genital infection, meningococcal,
  1619
Genital tuberculosis
  female, 1680
  male, 1680
Genital ulcer disease, 1527-1529,
  1528t
  diagnosis of, 1528-1529, 1528t
  etiology of, 1527-1528
  treatment of, 1529, 1529t
Genital warts, 514-515, 514f
Genitourinary tract
  antibiotic prophylaxis for, 351t
  imaging techniques for, 1968-
    1969, 1969t
  in menopause, 1032, 1033, 1034
Genitourinary tract infection
  chlamydial. See Chlamydia
    trachomatis infection
  gonococcal. See Gonorrhea
  mycoplasmal, 1741-1742
  staphylococcal, 1578
  tuberculous, 1680
Genome
  Human Genome Project, 1953-
    1956, 1954f-1955f
    future applications, 1956
    unresolved questions, 1955-
      1956, 1955f
  structure and function of, 1944-
    1946, 1945f-1947f
Gentamicin, 1432
  for Yersinia infection, 1636t
Geriatric patient
  anemia in, 1094
  antibiotics in, 1422
  common clinical disorders of. See
    also under individual disorder
  dyslipidemia management for, 746
  falls and gait disturbance in,
    22t, 22
  fever of unknown origin in, 1416
  headache in, 2162-2164
  hypertension in, 227-228
  rehabilitation of. See also under
    specific disorder
  septic arthritis in, 1539
  sleep patterns in, 2362
  surgical risk factor management
    and, 56
Germ cell tumor(s)
  in adolescent female, 1059

extragonadal, 2520
  mediastinal, 2839
  ovarian, 2537, 2541
Gerstmann-Straussler syndrome,
  2358, 2359
Gestational diabetes. See Diabetes
  mellitus, gestational
Gestational diabetes mellitus, 1024-
  1025, 1024t
Gestational transient
  thyrotoxicosis, 611-612
GHB (gamma-hydroxybutyric acid),
  poisoning by, 168-169
Ghon lesion, 1678
Giant cell arteritis, 375
  encephalopathy in, 2342
  fever of undetermined origin in,
    1415
  headache in, 2154t, 2163
Giardia lamblia, 1901, 1902f
Giardiasis, 1901-1903
  diagnosis of, 1901-1902, 1902f
  diarrhea in, 842
  differential diagnosis of, 1902
  etiology and epidemiology of,
    1901, 1902f
  pathogenesis of, 1901
  treatment of, 1902-1903
Gingivitis, in hematologic disease,
  1075
Gingivostomatitis, candidal, 1877t
Ginkgo biloba, toxicities of, 176
Gitelman syndrome
  metabolic alkalosis in, 2004
  treatment of, 2005
Glanzmann thrombasthenia, 1174
Glasgow Coma Scale, 2230, 2230t
gli, properties of, 2384t
Glimepiride, for type 2 diabetes
  mellitus, 658, 658t
Glioblastoma, molecular and
  cytogenetic abnormalities in,
  2311t
Glioblastoma multiforme, 2314
Glipizide, for type 2 diabetes
  mellitus, 658, 658t
gamma-Globulin, intravenous,
  hyponatremia in, 1980t
Globus hystericus. See Dysphagia
Glomerular disease, 1970-1972, 1970t,
  2051-2070. See also Nephritic
  syndrome, Nephrotic syndrome
  classification of,
    2051, 2051t, 2053f
  diagnosis of, 2052-2054
  epidemiology of, 2051
  general management of, 2054
  pathogenesis of, 2051-2052, 2053f
  recurrent, in postrenal-
    transplantation, 2120
  renal biopsy in, 2052-2054
  in renal transplant recipients,
    2115-2116
  small vessel, 2075-2082
Glomerular filtration, of body
  fluid, 1976
Glomerular filtration rate (GFR),
  1968
  in chronic renal disease,
    2014, 2014t-2015t, 2042-
    2043, 2042f-2043f
Glomerulonephritis
  acute, 1972, 1970t
  chronic, 1971
  crescentic or rapidly progressive,
    2075-2077, 2075f, 2076t
    ANCA-associated vasculitis in,
      2075-2076, 2076f
    in anti-glomerular basement
      membrane disease, 2076-2077
    in Churg-Strauss syndrome, 2075-
      2076
    immune complex, 2077, 2076t

in Wegener granulomatosis, 1363-
      1364, 2075-2076
  focal embolic, in endocarditis,
    1485
  hepatitis C-associated, 2055
  membranoproliferative, 2067-
    2068, 2067t, 2068f
    in endocarditis, 1485
  postinfectious, 2054-2056
  poststreptococcal, 1572, 2055-
    2056, 2055f-2056f
  rapidly progressive, 1972, 1970t,
    2060, 2061f
Glomerulosclerosis, focal segmental,
  2061-2063, 2062t, 2063f-2064f
Glomus tumor, of nail, 576t
Glossopharyngeal neuralgia, 2294t
Glucagon, in hormonal regulation of
  metabolism, 633-634, 634f-638f
Glucocorticoid(s)
  for asthma, 2712, 2710t, 2713t
  for hirsutism, 992
  for hyperthyroidism, 617
  inhaled, for asthma, 2712, 2713t
  for myositis, 1356-1357, 1357t
  for rheumatoid arthritis, 1311-
    1312
  therapeutic use of, 688
Glucose
  in nutritional support, 946-
    947, 946f
  serum, for hypoglycemia diagnosis,
    627
Glucose meters, 641-644
Glucose-6-phosphate dehydrogenase
  deficiency
  hemolytic anemia in, 1112-1113
    classification of, 1112
    diagnosis and treatment of, 1112-
      1113, 1112t
    drugs producing, 1112t, 1112
    etiology of, 1112, 1112f
    fava beans and, 1112
  neutrophil function in, 1146t
Glucose-6-phosphate isomerase
  deficiency, hemolytic anemia in,
  1113
alpha-Glucosidase inhibitors, for
  type 2 diabetes mellitus, 658-
  659, 658t
Glutamine, for nutritional
  pharmacotherapy, 945
Glutathionine synthesis, defective,
  hemolytic anemia in, 1112
Gluten-sensitive enteropathy, 827-
  829, 828f, 1281
  clinical manifestations of, 827-
    828
  dermatitis herpetiformis and, 829
  diagnosis of, 827-828, 828f
  genetic and etiologic factors in,
    827
  laboratory tests in, 828, 828f
  pathogenesis of, 827
  small intestinal biopsy in,
    828, 829f
  treatment of, 828-829
Glyburide, for type 2 diabetes
  mellitus, 658, 658t
Glyceryl trinitrate, for
  hypertensive crisis, 228t
Glycogenoses, 2278-2279
Glycoprotein IIb-IIIa receptor
  antagonists
  primary angioplasty and, 326
  for unstable angina
    and NSTMI, 310
Glycoproteinoses, 1148t
Glycosuria, hypernatremia and, 1987
Glycylcyclines, 1433
Gnathostomiasis, 1929
Goiter, 619-620. See also entries
  under Thyroid

cervical, 2839
  nodular, colloid, 2839
  toxic. See Graves disease
Gold therapy
  chronic diffuse infiltrative
    pulmonary disease due to, 2764
  thrombocytopenia due to, 1169
Golfer's elbow, 1394
Gonadotropin, for polycystic ovary
  syndrome, 984
Gonadotropin(s)
  deficiency, 600
    in hypogonadism, 692
  testicular synthesis and secretion
    of, 689
Gonadotropin-releasing hormone,
  agonists
  for endometriosis, 969, 969t
  for hirsutism, 991
  plus steroid, for endometriosis,
    969-970, 969t
Gonococcal infection. See also
  Neisseria gonorrhoeae
  disseminated, in septic arthritis,
    1536
Gonorrhea. See also Neisseria
  gonorrhoeae
  clinical features of, in men, 1622
  in males, 1521-1523, 1522f
  treatment of, 1624t
Goodpasture syndrome, 2058
Goserelin, for breast cancer, 2464
Gottron papules, in dermatomyositis,
  442, 442f
Gout, 1371-1377
  chronic tophaceous, 1373-
    1374, 1373f-1374f
  clinical stages of, 1372-1374
  conditions associated with, 1374
  definition and classification of,
    1371, 1371t
  diagnosis of, 1374-1375, 1375t
  epidemiology of, 1371
  intercritical, 1373
  pain in, temporal course of, 1291f
  pathogenesis and etiology of, 1371-
    1372
  renal disease in, 1374
  treatment of, 1375-1377, 1376t-
    1377t
    in acute disease, 1375-1376
      colchicine, 1375
      corticosteroids, 1376
      NSAIDs, 1375-1376
    in chronic disease, 1377
    interval follow-up and
      evaluation in, 1376-1377
Gouty arthritis, acute, 1372-
  1373, 1373f
Graft vs. host disease
  cutaneous findings in, 443, 443f
  as transfusion reaction, 1216-1217
Grains, dietary, 31
Gram-negative bacilli. See also
  individual diseases
  antimicrobials for, 1425t-1426t
  in endocarditis, antibiotics for,
    1493-1494
Gram-negative cocci, antimicrobial
  drugs for, 1425t
Gram-negative organisms
  in sepsis, 1444-1445, 1446f
  in septic arthritis, 1537
Gram-positive bacilli, 1584-1599.
  See also individual diseases,
  e.g., Diphtheria
Gram-positive cocci, 1563-1583. See
  also individual diseases, e.g.,
  Pneumococcal infection
Gram-positive organisms, in sepsis,
  1444-1445, 1446f
Granulocyte(s), for transfusion,
  1213

Granulocyte colony-stimulating factor (G-CSF)
in hematopoiesis, 1072-1073, 1073t
for neoplastic neutropenia, 2429
Granulocyte-macrophage colony-stimulating factor (GM-CSF)
in hematopoiesis, 1073-1074, 1073t
in IgE-mediated allergic inflammation, 1241t
for neoplastic neutropenia, 2429
Granuloma(s)
eosinophilic, of lung, 2760f, 2780-2781, 2769t-2770t
cigarette smoking and, 2780
in hypersensitivity pneumonitis, 2766, 2765f
mediastinal, 2838-2839
pyogenic, 546-547, 546f
in sarcoidosis, 2770, 2771f
Granulomatosis
allergic. See Churg-Strauss syndrome (allergic granulomatosis and angiitis)
lymphomatoid
cutaneous findings in, 432
multiple pulmonary nodules in, 2756
necrotizing sarcoid, 2771
talc-induced, diffuse infiltrative lung disease in, 2764
Wegener. See Wegener granulomatosis
Granulomatous disease
chronic, neutrophil function in, 1146t
fever of undetermined origin in, 1415
Granulomatous mediastinitis, 2838-2839
Granulomatous thyroiditis, 618-619
Granulomatous vasculitis, cutaneous findings in, 432
Granulosa cell tumor, 2541
Graves disease, 610, 611f. See also Thyrotoxicosis
cutaneous findings in, 434
Graves orbitopathy, 617
Gray platelet syndrome, 1174
Great arteries, dextrotransposition of, 396-397
Green-nail syndrome, Pseudomonas aeruginosa, 1661
Grief and bereavement, in terminal illness, 117-118
Griseofulvin, for toenail onychomycosis, 575t
Growth factor(s), in hematopoiesis, 1070-1071, 1073t, 1074f, 1072f
Growth hormone, 594-599
actions of, 594-595
deficiency, adult, 595-596, 596t
insulinlike, 595
synthesis and secretion of, 594
Guanabenz, for hypertension, 223t
Guanfacine, for hypertension, 223t
Guided imagery, 86t
Guillain-Barre syndrome, 2300-2302
apheresis for, 1218
in cytomegaloviral encephalitis, 2351
respiratory insufficiency in, 2806
Guttate hypomelanosis, idiopathic, 586-587
Gynecologic cancer, 2537-2548. See also individual disorders, e.g., Uterine cervical cancer
Gynecomastia, 695-696
Gypsy moths, dermatitis from, 191

H

Haemophilus, non-influenzae species of, 1651

Haemophilus influenzae infection, 1648-1651
antibiotic treatment of, 1651, 1651t
bacteremia, 1650
bone and joint, 1650
cellulitis, 1650
clinical syndromes, 1649-1650
conjunctivitis, 1650
epidemiology of, 1648
epiglottitis, 1649
extrapulmonary, 1650
immunization, 1651
for HIV-infected patient, 1830t
meningitis, 1553t, 1649
microbiologic diagnosis of, 1650
otitis media, 1650
pathogenesis and immunity in, 1648-1649
pneumonia, 1469, 1649-1650
prevention of, 1651
sinusitis, 1650
tracheobronchitis, 1650
Hailey-Hailey disease, 526t, 528
Hair, 563-570
excess. See Hirsutism
growth, physiology and evaluation of, 563
loss. See Alopecia
removal, for hirsutism, 992
Hallucinogenic(s), abuse of, 2637
Hallux valgus, 1397, 1397f
Halothane, hepatic necrosis due to, 877
Hamartoma, pulmonary
multiple fibroleiomyomatous, 2756
single nodule in, 2753
hamartoma, breast, 1053
Hammer toe, 1397
Hand(s)
flexor tenosynovitis, 1395
osteoarthritis, 1385-1386, 1386f
rheumatoid arthritis, 1302, 1302f
Hand pain, 1395
Hantavirus cardiopulmonary syndrome, 1790
Hantavirus disease, 1851, 1849t
Hantavirus pulmonary syndrome, 1851, 1849t
Hard metal disease, 63
Hashimoto thyroiditis. See Thyroiditis, autoimmune (Hashimoto)
HCTZ, for hypertension, 221t
Headache, 2150-2168
in brain tumor, 2154t, 2166, 2309
in cancer, 2175
in cardiac ischemia, 2164
categories of, 2150t, 2150
in cerebrovascular disease, 2162-2163
chronic daily, 2160
clinical classification of, 2151, 2153t-2154t
cluster, 2161-2162
cough, 2164-2165
daily persistent, 2160
diagnostic testing in, 2151-2152, 2155t
drug-induced, 2161
exertional, 2164-2165
first or worst, 2164, 2165t
geriatric, 2162-2164
in head trauma, 2163
history of, 2150, 2151t-2152t
in hypertension, 2166-2167
hypnic, 2164
lupus, 1333
medication-overuse, 2160-2161
migraine, 2152-2159
abdominal, 2156
aura in, 2155
basilar, 2156

clinical features of, 2153-2156
confusional, 2156
epidemiology of, 2152
etiology and pathophysiology of, 2152-2153
familial hemiplegic, 2155
footballers, 2156
intractable, 2157-2158
late-life accompaniments of, 2162
seizure and, 2191
transformed, 2160
treatment of
acute, 2156-2157, 2156t-2157t
preventive, 2158-2159, 2158t
triptans for, 2157, 2157t
triggers of, 2154-2155
variants of, 2155-2156
vestibular, 2146-2147
women and, 2159
in occipital neuralgia, 2167
pain-sensitive structures in, 2150
in paranasal sinusitis, 2166
physical examination in, 2151
in pseudotumor cerebri, 2154t, 2165-2166, 2166t
secondary, 2154t
sexual, 2164-2165
in subarachnoid hemorrhage, 2154t, 2164
tension-type, 2159-2160
thunderclap, 2164
Head and neck, squamous cell carcinoma of, 2437-2441, 2437f
clinical features of, 2438
diagnosis of, 2438-2439
etiology and risk factors in, 2437-2438
examination in, 2438-2439
genetic alterations in, 2438
pathogenesis of, 2438
staging in, 2439
treatment of, 2439-2441
concomitant chemoradiotherapy, 2440
in early disease, 2439
gene therapy, 2440
induction chemotherapy, 2439-2440, 2440f
in locoregionally advanced disease, 2439-2440
in recurrent or metastatic disease, 2440-2441
Head trauma. See also Coma
headache in, 2163
Health care, preventive. See Preventive health care
Health care proxy, 97
Health care workers, HIV-1 transmission to, 1823, 1837
Heart
metastasis to, 382-383
univentricular, 397-399, 397f
Heart block, in acute myocardial infarction, 330
Heart disease. See also Cardiovascular patient, specific disorders
congenital, 388-399. See also specific lesions, e.g., Atrial septal defect
acyanotic, 388-394
shunts, 388-391
valvular, 391-394
cyanotic, 394-399
polycythemia in, 1134
Internet resources for, 388
ischemic. See Coronary artery disease
in rheumatoid arthritis, 1305
valvular, 348-364
anorexiant-induced, 362
aortic. See Aortic

regurgitation, Aortic stenosis
assessment and management of, 349-350, 350t-351t
congenital, 348, 349f
in connective tissue disease, 349
in coronary artery disease, 349
degenerative, 349, 349f
endocarditis in, 349
etiology of, 348-349, 348t, 349f
iatrogenic, 349
in Libman-Sacks endocarditis, 349
mitral. See Mitral prolapse, Mitral regurgitation, Mitral stenosis
myxomatous, 348
prosthetic valves for. See Heart valve replacement
pulmonary, 359
rheumatic, 348-349
in rheumatoid arthritis, 349
secondary, 349
tricuspid, 359
Heart failure, 337-347
classification of, 337, 338t, 339f, 340t, 341f
congestive
edema in, 1989
hyperkalemia in, 2010
pleural effusion in, 2828
definition of, 337
diagnosis of, 340-341
diastolic, 341, 344
epidemiology of, 337-338
etiology of, 338-339, 338t
pathophysiology of, 339-340
in preoperative assessment, 51
prognosis in, 345, 344f
thyrotoxic, 617
treatment of, 341-345, 341t, 343t
biventricular pacing systems, 344
cardioverter-defibrillators, 344-345
medical therapy, 342-344, 343t
revascularization and surgical therapy, 344
Heart rate, modulation of, 273
Heart transplantation, anoxic encephalopathy in, 2337
Heart valve(s), traumatic injury to, 385. See also Heart disease, valvular
Heart valve replacement, prosthetic, 359-362
bioprosthesis, 359-360, 360f
endocarditis in, 1486-1487, 1486t. See also Endocarditis, prosthetic valve
mechanical, 359, 360f
problems and complications of, 360-362
infection, 361
inherent or acquired prosthetic stenosis, 361
in pregnancy, 361-362
thromboembolism, 360
valve failure, 361
valvular thrombosis, 360-361
Staphylococcus epidermidis endocarditis in, 1581
Heatstroke, 1408-1410. See also Hyperthermia
classic, 1408
clinical features of, 1409
diagnosis of, 1409
differential diagnosis of, 1410
exertional, 1408
laboratory findings in, 1409
pathophysiology of, 1409
prevention of, 1409

treatment of, 1410
Heberden nodes, 1385-1386, 1386f
Heerfordt syndrome (uveoparotid
    fever), 2772
Heinz body, in unstable
    hemoglobinopathy, 1119
Helicobacter infection, 1645-
    1647, 1646t, 1636t-1637t
Helicobacter pylori infection, 1645-
    1647, 1646t, 1636t-1637t
  endoscopic biopsy for, 781, 781f
  gastric cancer and, 2376-2377,
    2495
  gastric lymphoma and, 2507-2508
  gastroesophageal reflux disease
    disease and, 765
  laboratory tests for, 1645-
    1646, 1646t
  in peptic ulcer disease, 776, 777f
  serologic tests for, 781-782
Heliotrope erythema, in
    dermatomyositis, 442
HELLP syndrome, 1173-1174
Helminthic infection, 1918-
    1943, 1919f. *See also individual
    disorders, e.g.,* Trichinellosis
Hemangioblastoma, molecular and
    cytogenetic abnormalities in,
    2311t
Hemangioendothelioma, 2552
  features of, 2550t
Hemangioma, 544-545, 544f
  cherry, 546
  strawberry, 545, 544f
Hemangiomatosis, pulmonary
    capillary, pulmonary
    hypertension in, 2863
Hemangiopericytoma, 2553
  features of, 2550t
Hematocrit
  in polycythemia, 1132, 1133f
  surgical risk factor management
    and, 55-56
Hematologic disorder(s), 1070-1077
  bone marrow in, 1076, 1076f
  clinical manifestations, 1075
  complete blood count in, 1076
  imaging studies in, 1076
  laboratory evaluation, 1076, 1076f
  occupational, 66
  peripheral blood smear in, 1076
  reticulocyte count in, 1076
Hematopoiesis, 1070-1075
  bone marrow cells in, 1070, 1071f
  in children, 1070
  dynamics of, 1074-1075
  erythropoietin in, 1071-1072, 1073t
  extramedullary, 1070
  in fetus, 1070
  granulocyte colony-stimulating
    factor in, 1072-1073, 1073t
  granulocyte-macrophage colony-
    stimulating factor in, 1073-
    1074, 1073t
  growth factors in, 1070-
    1071, 1073t, 1074f, 1072f
  medullary, 1070
  stem cells in, 1070, 1072f
  thrombopoietin in, 1072, 1073t
Hematopoietic stem cell
    transplantation, 1214, 1222-
    1225. *See also* Bone marrow
    transplantation
  candidiasis in, 1879t
  for hematologic malignancies, 1222-
    1224
  for immunodeficiency states, 1222
  for leukemia, chronic myeloid,
    2579, 2581f
  for multiple myeloma, 2593
  for nonmalignant diseases of
    hemopoiesis, 1222
  posttransplant relapse and, 1224-

    1225
Hematuria, 1973-1974
  asymptomatic, 1972
  differential diagnosis of, 1974
Heme, synthesis of, 748, 750f
Hemicrania continua, 2160
Hemoccult testing. *See* Fecal occult
    blood testing
Hemochromatosis, 1085-1088
  autosomal dominant, 1088
  clinical findings in, 1086
  epidemiology and etiology of, 1085-
    1086
  juvenile, 1087
  liver transplantation and, 936
  non-HFE-associated, 1087
  screening and diagnostic tests in,
    1086-1087
  treatment of, 1087
Hemodialysis
  in acute renal failure, 2036
  in chronic renal failure, 2046-
    2049
  long-term, 2047-2049, 2047f
    adequacy of, 2047-2048
    anemia and, 2048
    control of concomitant
      conditions in, 2048-2049
    hyperphosphatemia and, 2048
    hypertension and, 2048
    infection and, 2048-2049
    patient management and care
      in, 2047-2049, 2047f
    screening examinations in,
      2049
    secondary hyperparathyroidism
      and, 2048
  planning for, 2046-2047, 2047f
  dialysis dementia in, 2339
  dialysis disequilibrium in, 2339
  pericarditis in, 380
  renal transplantation *vs.*, 2114
  septic arthritis in, 1539
Hemodilution, isovolemic, for blood
    conservation, 1211
Hemoglobin
  with abnormal oxygen affinity,
    1119
  fetal, hereditary persistence of,
    1121
  high-affinity, polycythemia in,
    1133-1134, 1134f
  macrophage catabolism and iron
    release, 1081-1082
  oxygen-carrying capacity of,
    1079, 1079f
  structure of, 1078-1079, 1078f
  synthesis of, 1107
Hemoglobin Barts, 1122
Hemoglobin C disease, 1118
Hemoglobin E disease, 1118
Hemoglobin H disease, 1122
Hemoglobinopathy, 1113-1122. *See
    also specific disorders, e.g.,*
    Sickle cell anemia
  classification of, 1113
  unstable, 1118-1119
Hemoglobinuria
  march, 1123
  paroxysmal cold, 1127
  paroxysmal nocturnal, 1111
Hemolysis, occupational, 66
Hemolytic anemia, 1109-1129. *See
    also specific disorders, e.g.,*
    Sickle cell anemia
  autoimmune, 1123-1125
    diagnosis of, 1123-1125
    pathophysiology of, 1123
    treatment of, 1125
      red cell transfusion, 1125
      splenectomy, 1125
  in babesiosis infection, 1129
  in cardiopulmonary bypass, 1129

  in clostridial sepsis, 1129
  in copper accumulation, 1129
  delayed, in erythrocyte
    transfusion, 1126
  in enzymatic attack on
    erythrocytes, 1128
  in erythrocyte membrane defects,
    1109-1111
  in erythrocyte metabolism
    abnormalities, 1111-1113
  in extracorpuscular defects, 1122-
    1129
  extravascular, 1109
  in freshwater drowning, 1128
  general features of, 1109
  in hemoglobin disorders, 1113-1122
  immune, 1123-1127
    Coombs antiglobulin test for,
      1123, 1124f
    drug-related, 1125-1126
      hapten type, 1125
      membrane antigen alteration
        in, 1126
    pathophysiology of, 1123
  infectious causes of, 1128-1129
  intravascular, 1109
  in lead poisoning, 1128
  in liver disease, 1129
  microangiopathic, 1122-1123
  oxidative attack in, 1127-1128
  physical causes of, 1128-1129
  in *Plasmodium* malaria, 1128
  in saltwater drowning, 1128
  in snake venom poisoning, 1128
Hemolytic-uremic syndrome
  adult, 1170-1173
  E. coli 0157:H7 in, 2079
  neoplastic, 2428
  postpartum, 2035
  in renal transplant recipients,
    2116
Hemophilia A, 1182-1183
  acute hemorrhage in, 1182
  dental surgery and, 1183
  diagnosis of, 1182
  elective surgery and, 1183
  factor VIII replacement in,
    1182, 1182t
  inhibitor management in, 1183
  principles of replacement therapy
    in, 1183
  treatment of, 1182-1183
Hemophilia B, 1183
Hemophilus species. *See under
    Haemophilus*
Hemopneumothorax, 2830
Hemorrhage. *See also* Bleeding
  splinter, 572
Hemorrhagic fever, 1847-1853
  bioterrorism and, 137-138
  clinical presentation in, 137-138
  Crimean-Congo, 1850-1851
  dengue, 1849
  diagnosis and treatment in, 138
  infection control considerations
    in, 138
  Omsk, 1850
  pathophysiology of, 137
  in renal syndrome, 1851
Hemorrhagic telangiectasia,
    hereditary, 1177
Hemosiderosis, pulmonary, alveolar
    hemorrhage in, 2783
Hemostasis, 1153-1162. *See also*
    Coagulation
  vascular-bed specific, endothelial
    heterogeneity and, 1159
Hemothorax, 2830
Henoch-Schonlein purpura, 1362
  IgA nephropathy *vs.*, 2057
  renal involvement in, 2077-2078
Heparin
  intravenous, for acute myocardial

  infarction, 327
  low-molecular-weight
    for acute myocardial infarction,
      327-328
    pharmacology of, 416-417
  overdose, 1184
  pharmacology of, 416-417
  thrombocytopenia due to, 1169,
    1199-1201, 1200f
    clinical presentation in, 1199
    diagnosis of, 1199
    epidemiology of, 1199
    pathophysiology of, 1199, 1200f
    treatment of, 1200-1201
  thrombosis due to, 1199-1201, 1200f
  for unstable angina and NSTMI, 310-
    311, 311t
  for venous thromboembolism, 420
Hepatic cirrhosis. *See* Cirrhosis
Hepatic disease. *See* Liver disease
Hepatic encephalopathy. *See*
    Encephalopathy, hepatic
Hepatitis
  acute, 872-881. *See also under*
    Hepatitis A, Hepatitis B, *etc.*
    active immunization against, 878-
      880, 879t-880t
    acute cholecystitis *vs.*, 904
    classification and pathology of,
      872-873, 873f
    clinical course in, 876-877
    clinical manifestations of,
      875, 875t
    diagnosis of, 875-876
    epidemiology, 873-875, 872t, 874t
    laboratory tests, 875-876, 876t
    liver biopsy in, 876
    passive immunization against,
      878
    prevention of, 878-880
    serologic assays in, 875-
      876, 872t, 876t
    treatment of, 878
  alcoholic
    acute cholecystitis *vs.*, 904
    fever of undetermined origin in,
      1415
  autoimmune, 883-885, 884t
    diagnosis of, 883-884
    major types of, 882t
    overlap syndromes in, 884
    relapse in, 885
    treatment of, 884-885, 884t
    types of, 884
  candidal, 1877t
  chronic, 882-890
    in *alpha*$_1$-antitrypsin
      deficiency, 883
    clinical manifestations of, 882
    definition and etiology of,
      882, 882t
    diagnosis of, 882-883, 883t
    differential diagnosis of, 883
    drug-induced, 883
    laboratory tests for, 882
    liver biopsy in, 882-883, 883t
    major types of, 882t
    METAVIR scoring system for, 883t
    primary biliary cirrhosis *vs.*,
      883
    primary sclerosing cholangitis
      vs., 883
    in Wilson disease, 883
  cytomegaloviral, 877
  drug-induced, 877-878
    in systemic lupus erythematosus,
      1333
  Epstein-Barr, 877
  in pregnancy, 1022
Hepatitis A
  epidemiology of, 874
  features of, 874t
  immunization against

active, 879-880, 880t
  for HIV-infected patients, 1830t
  passive, 878
  preexposure, 880t, 880
  for travelers, 72-73, 73f
  post-blood donation testing for, 1207
  serologic diagnosis of, 872t
  tests for, 875
  viral classification and pathology in, 872
Hepatitis B
  chronic, 885-888
    diagnosis of, 885-886, 885t
    epidemiology of, 885
    hepatocellular carcinoma and, 885, 2376
    reactivation of, 888
    treatment of, 886-888, 886t
      adefovir dipivoxil for, 887-888
      entecavir for, 888
      interferon therapy for, 886-887
      lamivudine for, 887
      tenofovir for, 888
  clinical course in, 876-877
  epidemiology of, 874
  features of, 874t
  immunization against
    active, 878-879, 879t
    for HIV-infected patients, 1830t
    for international travel, 73, 74f
    passive, 878
  liver transplantation and, 936
  post-blood donation testing for, 1207
  in renal transplant recipients, 2115
  serologic diagnosis of, 872t
  tests for, 875-876, 876t
  viral classification and pathology in, 872, 873f
Hepatitis C
  chronic, 888-890
    epidemiology and diagnosis of, 888
    liver transplantation and, 936
    natural history of, 888
    treatment of, 888-890
      interferon and ribavirin combination for, 889, 888t
      liver transplantation for, 890
  clinical course in, 876-877
  encephalomyelitis in, 2353
  epidemiology of, 874-875
  features of, 874t
  glomerulonephritis in, 2055
  immunization against, passive, 878
  post-blood donation testing for, 1206-1207
  in renal transplant recipients, 2115
  serologic diagnosis of, 872t
  tests for, 876
  treatment of, 878
  viral classification and pathology in, 872-873, 873f
Hepatitis D
  epidemiology of, 875
  features of, 874t
  post-blood donation testing for, 1207
  serologic diagnosis of, 872t
  tests for, 876
Hepatitis D virus, classification and pathology of, 873
Hepatitis E
  epidemiology of, 875
  features of, 874t
  serologic diagnosis of, 872t
  tests for, 876
Hepatitis E virus, classification

and pathology of, 873
Hepatitis F virus, classification and pathology of, 873
Hepatitis G, post-blood donation testing for, 1207
Hepatitis G virus, classification and pathology of, 873
Hepatocellular carcinoma, 2503-2505
  in cirrhosis, 898-899
  diagnosis of, 2503
  epidemiology and etiology in, 2503
  hepatitis B in, chronic, 885, 2376
  liver transplantation and, 936
  screening and prevention of, 2503
  staging and prognosis in, 2504, 2504t
  treatment of, 2504-2505
    in advanced, unresectable disease, 2505
    in local, resectable disease, 2504-2505
Hepatocerebral degeneration, chronic non-wilsonian, 2338
Hepatolenticular degeneration. See Wilson disease
Hepatoma. See Hepatocellular carcinoma
Hepatopulmonary syndrome, in cirrhosis, 897
Hepatorenal syndrome
  acute renal failure in, 2034-2035
  in cirrhosis, 896, 897t
Hepatotoxicity
  due to acetaminophen, 878
  due to drug overdose, 877-878
Hephaestin, in iron metabolism, 1082
Herbal dietary supplements, 87t-88t
Herbal remedies
  for atopic dermatitis, 478
  for depression, 2618
  poisoning by, 176
Hernia, hiatal, in gastroesophageal reflux disease, 764
Heroin use, pulmonary edema in, 2849-2850
Herpes gestationis, 530, 526t
Herpes labialis, 1756
Herpes simplex infection, 1755-1758
  in AIDS, 437
  anal, 1757
  central nervous system, 2344t
  diagnosis of, 1758
  encephalitis, 2347-2348
  epidemiology of, 1755-1756
  esophageal, 770
  genital, 1756-1757, 1756f
  genital ulcers in, 1528t, 1529, 1529f
  in immunocompromise, 1757
  meningitis, 2347
  neonatal, 1757-1758
  neurologic complications of, 1757
  neuropathy in, 2348-2349
  ocular, 1756
  oral-labial, 1756
  pathogenesis and clinical features of, 1756-1758, 1756f-1757f
  perianal, 1757, 1757f
  in pregnancy, 1021
  prevention and treatment of, 1758
Herpes simplex virus type 1, 1755-1756
  encephalitis, 2347-2348
Herpes simplex virus type 2, 1755-1756
  encephalitis, 2347
  meningitis, 2347
Herpesvirus(es)
  in human and nonhuman hosts, 2553t
  types of, 1755
Herpesvirus infection, 1755-1767
  Internet information on, 1755
Herpesvirus type 6, 1765

encephalitis in, 2352
Herpesvirus type 7, 1765
Herpesvirus type 8, 1765
  in cancer epidemiology, 2376
Herpes zoster, 1759-1761, 2349-2350
  in AIDS, 437
  clinical features and complications of, 1760, 1760f
  clinical findings in, 2349
  complications of, 2349-2350, 2349f
  diagnosis, prevention, treatment of, 1760-1761
  epidemiology of, 1758-1759
  neuropathy in, 2305
  postherpetic neuralgia in, 1760, 2305-2306, 2349-2350
  treatment of, in acute disease, 2349
  vaccine for, 1760
Herpetic whitlow, 1757, 1757f
Heterophyes heterophyes infection, 1936
Hexamethylmelamine, 2415t
HFE, in iron metabolism, 1082
Hiatal hernia, in gastroesophageal reflux disease, 764
Hidradenitis suppurativa, acne vulgaris vs., 447
High altitude
  jet aircraft and, 80
  metabolic encephalopathy at, 2338
  polycythemia at, 1132, 1134f
  pulmonary edema at, 2849
  pulmonary hypertension at, 2862-2863
High blood pressure. See Hypertension
High-mobility group-1 protein, in sepsis, 1448
Hila, normal anatomy of, 2836
Hilar enlargement, 2836-2837
  in lymphadenopathy, 2836-2837
  in vascular engorgement, 2836-2837
Hindfoot pain, 1397
Hip(s)
  osteoarthritis, 1386
  rheumatoid arthritis, 1302, 1303f
Hip girdle pain, 1395-1396, 1395t
Hip replacement, osteomyelitis after, 1544
Hip surgery, venous thromboembolism in, prophylaxis for, 419
Hirschsprung disease, 858
Hirsutism, 987-993
  clinical features of, 988-989
  definition of, 987, 988f
  diagnosis of, 988-989, 989t
  epidemiology of, 987
  etiology of, 987-988
  idiopathic, polycystic ovary syndrome vs., 980
  laboratory testing in, 989
  pathogenesis of, 987
  in polycystic ovary syndrome, 976-977, 977f
    treatment of, 982
  treatments not recommended, 984-985
  prognosis in, 992
  treatment of, 989-992, 990t-991t
    antiandrogens in, 990-991, 990t
    eflornithine cream in, 992
    estrogen-progestin contraceptives in, 990, 991t
    estrogen-progestin plus antiandrogen in, 991
    experimental, 992
    glucocorticoids in, 992
    gonadotropin-releasing hormone analogues in, 991
    hair removal and lightening in, 992
    intense pulsed light in, 992

laser treatment in, 992
    metformin in, 991-992
    nonhormonal, 992
    thiazolidinediones in, 992
    weight loss in, 990
Hirudin, for heparin-induced thrombocytopenia, 1200
His-Purkinje system, 273
Histamine-receptor antagonist(s)
  H_1, for urticaria, 1264-1265, 1264t
  H_2
    for gastroesophageal reflux disease, 766
    for urticaria, 1265
Histiocytic syndromes, 1145-1147
Histiocytoma, malignant fibrous, 2552
  features of, 2550t
  treatment of, 2558
Histiocytosis X, pulmonary. See Eosinophilic granuloma of lung
Histoplasma capsulatum, 1861
Histoplasmosis, 1861-1864
  clinical presentation in, 1862
  complications of, 1864
  diagnosis of, 1862-1863, 1863f
  differential diagnosis of, 1863
  disseminated, 1862
    treatment of, 1864
  epidemiology of, 1861
  fibrosing mediastinitis in, 1864
  granulomatous mediastinitis, 1864
  pathogenesis of, 1861
  pericarditis in, 1864
  prognosis in, 1864
  pulmonary, 1862
    chronic cavitary, 1862
    multiple nodules in, 2755
    single nodule in, 2753, 2754f
    treatment of, 1864
  treatment of, 1863-1864
HIV infection. See Acquired immunodeficiency syndrome (AIDS), Human immunodeficiency virus infection
HLA antigen(s). See also Major histocompatibility complex (MHC)
HLA-B27
  in ankylosing spondylitis, 1317-1318
  in reactive arthritis, 1322
  in spondyloarthritis, 1315-1316
Hodgkin disease, 2596-2600
  biology of, 2596, 2597f
  clinical features of, 2596-2597
  diagnosis of, 2596-2598
  epidemiology of, 2596
  Epstein-Barr virus and, 2596
  etiology of, 2596
  fever of undetermined origin in, 1415
  histologic classification of, 2596
  history and physical examination in, 2597
  laboratory studies in, 2597-2598
  pulmonary
    focal infiltrates in, 2745
    multifocal infiltrates in, 2747
  Reed-Sternberg cell, 2596, 2597f
  staging and prognosis in, 2598, 2598t-2599t
  treatment of, 2598-2600
    hematopoietic stem cell transplantation for, 1224
    initial
      nodular lymphocyte-predominant disease, 2599
      stage I and II, 2598-2599
      stage III and IV, 2599
    long-term effects of, 2600
    in relapse or refractory disease, 2599-2600

Holter monitoring. *See* Electrocardiography (ECG), ambulatory
Homeopathy, 84
Homicide, psychosocial issues and, 119
Homocysteinemia, as risk factor for stroke, 2211
Honeybee stings, 1285-1286, 1286f
Africanized (killer), 1285
Hookworm infection, 1918-1921, 1920t, 1921f-1922f
canine, 1923-1924
Horn, definition of, 428t
Hornet stings, 1285, 1286f
Hospice, palliative medicine in, 92-93, 94t, 94f
Hospital(s)
antimicrobial resistance in, 1424
palliative medicine in, 92-93
Hospital-acquired infection. *See* Nosocomial infection
Hot flashes, in menopause, 1032, 1033, 1034
Hot-foot syndrome, *Pseudomonas aeruginosa*, 1661
Howell-Jolly bodies, sickle cell anemia, 1114
H-*ras,* properties of, 2384t
HST, properties of, 2384t
hTERT, 2393
HTLV. *See* Human T cell lymphotropic virus
Human bite, 181, 181t-182t
Human Genome Project, 1953-1956, 1954f-1955f
future applications, 1956
unresolved questions, 1955-1956, 1955f
Human immunodeficiency virus
genes and proteins of, 1805t, 1803-1804
structure and life cycle of, 1823-1825, 1824f-1826f
transmission of, 1822-1823
alcoholism and, 2627
injection drug use, 1822
mother-to-child, 1823
occupational, 1823
perinatal, antiretroviral therapy for prevention of, 1838
sexual, 1822
transfusion-related, 1822-1823
type 1 (HIV-1), 1811-1816. *See also* Acquired immunodeficiency syndrome
CD4+ T cells and, 1805-1807, 1806f
genomic diversity of, 1808
laboratory diagnosis of, 1811-1816
antiretroviral genotype and phenotype detection for, 1814-1815
enzyme immunoassays for, 1812
HIV-1 p24 antigen measurement for, 1813
HIV-1 RNA quantitative assays for, 1814
immunoblot for, 1812
rapid serologic testing for, 1812
serologic, 1811-1813
subtype detection in, 1812-1813
viral culture for, 1813
viral nucleic acid detection for, 1813-1814
monitoring of infection in, 1815-1816
discordant viral RNA and CD4+ T cell responses for, 1816

plasma viral RNA for, 1815
viral resistance for, 1815-1816
origin of, 1819
type 2 (HIV-2)
laboratory diagnosis of, 1813
origin of, 1819
Human immunodeficiency virus infection, 1819-1846
acute, 1827-1828
clinical features, 1827
diagnosis of, 1827-1828
laboratory studies in, 1827-1828, 1829t
treatment of, 1828
central nervous system, 2344t
chronic, 1807, 1828-1831
antiretroviral therapy, 1829-1831, 1831f-1832f, 1831t-1832t
initial evaluation in, 1828-1829
overview of management in, 1829-1831
vaccinations in, 1829, 1830t
classification of, 1819, 1820t
cytopathicity in, 1808
dementia, 2355-2357
diagnosis of, 2355-2357, 2357t, 2357f
pathogenesis of, 2355, 2356f
stages of, 2357t
treatment of, 2357
diarrhea in, 849
early events and progression, 1825-1827, 1826f-1827f
epidemiology of, 1819-1822, 1820f-1821f
global, 1819-1821
United States, 1821-1822, 1820f-1821f
esophagitis in, 770-771
hypogonadism in, 693
immune reconstitution syndrome in, 1842
immunization for, 1838-1839
Internet resources for, 1843
latent, 1807
opportunistic infections in, 1839-1843
management of, 1839-1842, 1840t-1841t
prevention of, 1839, 1840t, 1843, 1842t
pain in, management of, 2179-2180
pathogenesis, 1823-1827, 1824f-1827f
peripheral neuropathy in, 2176, 2304-2305
persistent, 1807
pneumococcal infection in, 1565
in pregnancy, 1021-1022
renal transplantation and, 2115
syphilis in, 1708-1709
telephone consultation services for, 1843
therapy for
antiretroviral
adverse reactions to, 1832-1835, 1834t
after sexual activity or needle sharing, 1837
agents, 1830, 1831f, 1831t
bone abnormalities in, 1835
combination therapy for, 1830-1831, 1832f, 1832t
DHHS recommendations for, 1833t
dosing schedules for, 1830
drug selection, 1832-1835
hyperlipidemia in, 1834
hypersensitivity syndrome with, 1833
initiation of therapy, 1831-1832

insulin resistance with, 1833-1834
lactic acidemia with, 1833
lipodystrophy with, 1834-1835
occupational postexposure, 1837
patient adherence in, 1836
to prevent perinatal transmission, 1838
principles of, 1831-1837
regimen selection, 1832, 1833t
resistance and resistance testing in, 1836
RNA levels and CD4+ T cell counts in, 1835-1836
treatment interruptions in, 1836-1837
HIV preventive vaccines for, 1838-1839
prophylactic, 1837-1839
ritonavir boosted protease inhibitor regimens, 1832t
tuberculosis in, 1683-1684
management of, 1839, 1841t
prophylactic measures for prevention of, 1840t
treatment of, 1689-1691, 1689t
Human papilloma virus (HPV)
DNA testing, for cervical cancer, 1065, 1066-1067, 1064t
uterine cervical cancer and, 1063
Human T cell lymphotropic virus(es), 1808-1809
in cancer epidemiology, 2376
classification of subtypes of, 1809
epidemiology of, 1809
laboratory diagnosis of, 1809
latent, 1807
persistent, 1807
Human T cell lymphotropic virus type I (HTLV-I), 1809-1811
ATL and, 1810-1811
acute, 1810
chronic, 1811
lymphomatous, 1810
smoldering, 1811
clinical features and diagnosis of, 1810-1811
epidemiology of, 1809-1810
myelopathy, 1811, 2357
pathogenesis of, 1810
tropical spastic paraparesis, 1811, 2357
Human T cell lymphotropic virus type II (HTLV-II), 1811
Humidifier lung disease, 2765. *See also* Pneumonitis, hypersensitivity
Hunter syndrome, 1148t
Huntington disease, 2253-2254
genetics of, 1950, 1951t
genetic testing in, 1962
trinucleotide repeat in, 1960t
Hurler syndrome, 1148t
Hydatid disease, 1940-1941
Hydralazine
for hypertension, 223t
for hypertensive crisis, 228t
Hydrochlorothiazide, for nephrolithiasis, 2109
Hydrocytosis (hereditary stomatocytosis), 1109-1110, 1110f
Hydrofluoric acid, inhalation or ingestion of, 165t
Hydrogen ion(s)
pH and, 1994, 1994f
renal excretion of, 1994, 1995f-1997f
Hydrothorax. *See* Pleural effusion
gamma-Hydroxybutyric acid (GHB), poisoning by, 168-169
11-Hydroxylase deficiency, 687

17-Hydroxylase deficiency, 687
21-Hydroxylase deficiency, 685-686
17-Hydroxyprogesterone, in polycystic ovary syndrome, 978
Hydroxyurea, 2417t
for chronic myeloid leukemia, 2578-2579, 2578t
for psoriasis, 470
Hymenoptera, allergic reactions to, 1285-1289. *See also* Stinging insect allergy
Hyperadrenocorticism. *See* Cushing disease
Hyperaldosteronism, 686-687, 687f
dexamethasone-suppressible, 686, 687
primary, 686-687, 687f
secondary, 687
Hyperandrogenism, in women, laboratory evaluation of, 447t
Hypercalcemia, 700-705
acute, treatment of, 705, 705t
in acute renal failure, 2038
in calcium nephrolithiasis, 2106-2107
clinical manifestations of, 700
differential diagnosis of, 701, 700t
encephalopathy in, 2339
familial hypocalciuric, 701
history and physical examination in, 700-701, 700t
laboratory studies in, 701
local osteolytic, 704
of malignancy, humoral, 704
metabolic alkalosis in, 2003
in multiple myeloma, 2591
pancreatitis in, 914
parathyroid hormone-independent, 700t, 704-705
diagnosis of, 704
in malignancy, 704
other causes of, 703
treatment of, 705, 705t
parathyroid hormone-mediated, 700t, 701-704
in sarcoidosis, 2772
tubulointerstitial nephritis in, 2094
Hypercalcemia of malignancy, 2429-2431
diagnosis of, 2430
pathophysiology of, 2430
treatment of, 2430-2431
Hypercalciuria
absorptive, 2107
renal, 2106-2107
in sarcoidosis, 2772
tubulointerstitial nephritis in, 2094
Hypercapnia, metabolic encephalopathy in, 2338
Hyperchloremic acidosis, 1998
Hypercholesterolemia
familial, 738
treatment of, 738
polygenic, 739-740
screening, in children, 745-746
Hypercoagulable states. *See also* entries beginning Thrombo-
acquired, 1190, 1190t, 1197-1202
inherited, 1190, 1190t, 1192-1197
patient workup in, 1191-1192, 1191t
venous thrombosis and, 1192t, 1192
Hypercortisolism. *See* Cushing syndrome
Hyperemesis gravidarum, 1023-1024
Hypereosinophilic syndrome, 1150, 2783
Hyperglycemia
in acute pancreatitis, 922
microvascular complications of diabetes and, 666-668, 668f

surgical risk factor management and, 55
untreated, dyslipidemia in, 740
Hyperhomocysteinemia, 1195-1196, 1196f
Hyperinsulinemia, in polycystic ovary syndrome, 979-980, 979f
Hyperkalemia, 2009-2013
  in acute renal disease, 2037
  in acute renal failure, 2036
  in cardiac arrest, 149t
  causes of, 2009-2010, 2009t
  clinical manifestations, 2011
  differential diagnosis, 2012
  ECG manifestations, 2011-2012, 2011f, 2007f
  encephalopathy in, 2339
  in hyperkalemic type I renal tubular acidosis, 2010, 2010t, 1998
  in impaired renal excretion, 2009-2010, 2009t
  in increased cellular release, 2009, 2009t
  in increased potassium intake, 2009, 2009t
  in metabolic acidosis, 1998-1999
  renal defect in, evaluation of, 2010, 2010t
  treatment of, 2012-2013, 2012t
Hyperkalemic periodic paralysis, 2281-2282
Hyperkeratosis, epidermolytic, 479
Hyperlipidemia
  in acute pancreatitis, 922
  after renal transplantation, 2124
  in chronic renal failure, 2019
  definition of, 729
  familial combined, 737
    patient approach in, 737
  in impaired lipoprotein lipase synthesis, 731
  in remnant removal disease, 731
  as risk factor for stroke, 2211
Hyperlipoproteinemia, cutaneous findings in, 433, 433f
Hypermagnesemia, encephalopathy in, 2339
Hypernatremia, 1986-1988
  acute salt poisoning in, 1987
  clinical manifestations, 1987
  diagnosis of, 1987-1988
  encephalopathy in, 2339
  etiology of, 1986-1987
  hypotonic losses in, 1987
    gastric fluid losses in, 1987
    osmotic cathartics in, 1987
    osmotic diuretics and glycosuria in, 1987
    sweat and, 1987
  pathogenesis of, 1986, 1986t
  pure water losses in, 1987
    diabetes insipidus and, 1987
    increased urea excretion, 1987
    insensible, 1987
  recognition of water deficit in, 1987-1988
  treatment of, 1988
    diabetic dehydration and, 1988
    rate of correction in, 1988
Hypernephroma, fever of undetermined origin in, 1415
Hyperoxaluria
  in calcium oxalate nephrolithiasis, 2108
  primary, types I and II, 2108
  treatment of, 2110
  tubulointerstitial nephritis in, 2093-2094
Hyperparathyroidism, 701-704, 703t
  calcium nephrolithiasis in, 2106
  chronic, after renal transplantation, 2124

diagnosis of, 701-702
laboratory tests in, 702
physical examination in, 702
primary, 701
secondary, 701
  in chronic renal failure, hemodialysis and, 2048
tertiary, 701
treatment of, 702-704, 703t
  nonsurgical, 703-704, 703t
  preoperative localization in, 703
  surgical, 703
Hyperphosphatemia
  in acute renal failure, 2038
  in chronic renal failure, 2044
    hemodialysis and, 2048
Hyperpigmentation disorders, 578-581. See also individual types
  confluent and reticulated papillomatosis of Gougerot and Carteaud, 580
  Dowling-Degos disease, 580-581
  drug-induced, 579
  erythema dyschromicum perstans, 579-580
  lentigines, 580
  melasma, 578, 578f
  postinflammatory, 578-579, 579f
Hyperprolactinamia, in hypogonadotropic hypogonadism, 956-957
Hyperprolactinemia, 592-593, 592t
  in infertility, 1006
Hypersensitivity reaction(s)
  to antibiotics, 1423
  to food, 1278. See also Food allergy
  immediate, 1240-1246. See also Allergy and atopy, Atopy
    antigen presenting cells in, 1240
    eosinophils in, 1243-1244, 1243t
    gastrointestinal, 1279, 1279t
    IgE synthesis in, 1241, 1242f
      receptors for and regulation of, 1241-1242
    T cell mediated, 1240-1241, 1241t
    mast cells and basophils in, 1244-1246, 1244f-1245f. See also Basophil(s), Mast cell(s)
  impaired delayed, 1229t, 1229
  to beta-lactam antibiotics, 1431-1432
Hypersensitivity syndrome reaction, drug-related, 496-497, 496t, 497f
Hypersomnia, idiopathic, 2368
Hypersplenism, 1127
Hypertension, 214-237
  after renal transplantation, 2123-2124
  in aldosteronism, 217t, 232, 231t
  ambulatory BP monitoring in, 217
  arterial, in chronic renal failure, 2040-2041
  chronic renal failure in, 2018
    hemodialysis and, 2048
  classification of, 214, 214t
  in coarctation of aorta, 217t, 234, 231t
  complications of, 234-235
  in Cushing syndrome, 217t, 234, 231t
  definition of, 214, 214t
  in diabetes mellitus, 673-674
    in chronic renal disease, 2017-2018
  diagnosis of, 216-219, 216t
  in drug overdose or poisoning, 156-157
  epidemiology of, 214-215

essential, classic features of, 217t, 217
etiology and genetics of, 215
glomerular, in chronic renal failure, 2040-2041
headache in, 2166-2167
history in, 217-218, 218t
initial evaluation in, 217, 217t
laboratory tests in, 218, 219t
malignant, renal involvement in, 2082
nephrosclerosis in, 2095
pathophysiology and pathogenesis of, 215-216
  renal sodium excretion in, 215-216
  sympathetic nervous system activity in, 216
  weight gain and obesity in, 216
in pheochromocytoma, 217t, 232-234, 233t, 231t
physical examination in, 218, 217t
in pregnancy, 1018
prevention of, 219, 220t
prognosis in, 235
pulmonary. See Pulmonary hypertension
renovascular, 231-232
  features of, 217t
  screening options for, 231t, 230
  as risk factor for stroke, 2210-2211
  risk stratification in, 218-219, 219t
secondary, 230-235, 231t
  screening options for, 231t, 230
  specific causes of, 217t, 218
treatment of, 219-230
  in acute stroke, 230
  in chronic kidney disease, 229-230
  combination therapy in, 220, 223
  contraindications to, 225t
  in diabetic patients, 228-229
  drugs for, 221t-223t
  in elderly, 227-228
  in heart disease, 229
  in hypertensive crisis, 226-227, 228t
  improving control rates in, 223-225, 226t
  lifestyle factors in, 220, 220t
  patient condition and, 224t
  pharmacologic, 220-225, 221t-225t, 226f. See also under individual drugs
  in refractory/resistant disease, 225-226
    inappropriate drug regimens and, 225-226
    interfering substances and, 225
    noncompliance and, 225
    office/pseudohypertension, 226
    secondary hypertension and, 226
  white-coat, 226
Hypertensive carotid syndrome, pacemaker for, 274t, 275
Hypertensive crisis, treatment of, 226-227, 228t
Hyperthermia, 1408-1411. See also Heat stroke
  etiology of, 1408, 1408t
  fever vs., 1407-1408, 1407f
  malignant, 158t
    of anesthesia, 1411, 2277-2278
    in poisoning or drug overdose, 157, 158t
Hyperthyroidism. See also Thyrotoxicosis
  atrial fibrillation in, 248
  chorionic gonadotropin-mediated,

611-612, 612f
definitions of, 605
encephalopathy in, 2340
iodine-induced (Jod-Basedow effect), 611
in pregnancy, 1019-1020
surgical risk factor management and, 56
TSH-mediated (central), 612
Hypertonicity, cell volume regulation in, 1977-1978
Hypertriglyceridemia
  in childhood, 739
  drug therapy for lowering, 745
  familial, 738
    patient approach in, 735
  pancreatitis in, 914
Hyperuricemia
  in gout, 1372. See also Gout
  tubulointerstitial nephritis in, 2094
Hyperuricosuria
  in calcium oxalate nephrolithiasis, 2108
  tubulointerstitial nephritis in, 2094
  in uric acid nephrolithiasis, 2108
Hyperventilation, metabolic encephalopathy in, 2338
Hypnotherapy, 86t
Hypoaldosteronism, 687-688
  primary, 687
  secondary, 688
Hypobetalipoproteinemia, 731
Hypocalcemia, 705-706, 706t
  in acute pancreatitis, 922
  in acute renal failure, 2038
  diagnosis of, 706, 706t
  encephalopathy in, 2339
  etiology of, 705-706
  treatment of, 706
Hypocapnia
  metabolic encephalopathy in, 2338
  normal-anion-gap acidosis in, 1998
Hypocitraturia, in calcium oxalate nephrolithiasis, 2108
Hypogammaglobulinemia, of infancy, transient, 1226t
Hypogammaglobulinemic sprue, 830
Hypoglossal neuropathy, 2294t
Hypoglycemia, 626-632, 647-648
  in cardiac arrest, 148t
  classification of, 626, 627t
  clinical manifestations of, 626
  conditions causing, 629-632
  definition of, 626
  diagnosis of, 626-629
  factitious, 630-631
  insulin autoimmune, 631-632
  insulin-induced, cortisol levels and, 598
  in insulinoma, 629-630
  laboratory tests in, 627-629
    beta cell polypeptides and surrogates, 628, 629f
    C-peptide suppression test, 628-629
    glycated hemoglobin, 628
    insulin antibodies, 628
    intravenous tolbutamide test, 629
    mixed-meal test, 628
    oral glucose tolerance test, 628
    prolonged (72-hr) fast, 627-628, 628t
    serum glucose, 627
    sulfonylureas and meglitinides, 628
  metabolic encephalopathy in, 2340
  noninsulinoma pancreatogenous hypoglycemia syndrome, 631
  physical examination in, 626-627
  in poisoning, 155

in type 1 diabetes mellitus
presenting features of, 647
prevention of, 648
severity of episodes, 647-648
treatment of, 648
Hypogonadism
diagnosis of, 600
hypergonadotropic, 958-959
hypogonadotropic, 956-957, 956t
idiopathic, 957
male, 691-694
acquired, 693
congenital, 692-693
diagnosis of, 691-692
diseases causing, 692-693, 689t
etiology of, 691
laboratory findings in, 691-692
primary, 692-693, 689t
secondary, 693-694, 689t
treatment of, 694, 695f
surgically or chemically induced, 693
treatment of, 600
Hypokalemia, 2006-2008
in altered potassium distribution, 2006-2007, 2007t
in cardiac arrest, 149t
causes of, 2006-2007, 2007t
chronic, tubulointerstitial nephritis in, 2094
clinical manifestations of, 2008, 2007f
ECG manifestations, 2008, 2007f
encephalopathy in, 2339
hypomagnesemia and, 2007-2008
in insulin administration, 2006
in low potassium intake, 2006, 2007t
metabolic alkalosis in, 2003-2004, 2003f, 2006
physiologic tests in, 2008
in potassium loss, 2006, 1995f
from bodily sites, 2007-2008
renal, 2007-2008
treatment of, 2008-2009
Hypokalemic periodic paralysis, 2007, 2009, 2282
Hypomagnesemia
in cardiac arrest, 148t
encephalopathy in, 2339
hypokalemia and, 2007-2008
Hypomelanosis of Ito, 440
Hyponatremia, 1978-1986
acute, 1980-1982, 1981t
in cyclophosphamide infusion, 1981t, 1981
diagnosis of, 1982
in ecstasy drug use, 1982
etiology of, 1980-1982
in oxytocin infusion, 1981t, 1981
postoperative, 1981t, 1981
psychotic self-induced, 1981t, 1981-1982
in runners, 1981t, 1982
treatment of, 1982
in acute renal disease, 2037
chronic, 1982-1986
in advanced renal failure, 1982-1983
in AIDS, 1984
in beer potomania, 1983
clinical manifestations of, 1984
diagnosis of, 1984-1985
in diuretic use, 1983
in edema, 1983
etiology of, 1982-1984, 1983t
history and physical examination in, 1984
in hypovolemia, 1983
laboratory tests in, 1984
in SIADH, 1983-1984, 1983t, 1985
therapeutic response in, 1984-1985

treatment of, 1985-1986
complications of, 1986
myelinolysis due to, 1986
osmotic demyelination syndrome due to, 1986
persistent defects in water excretion and, 1985
renal failure and, 1985-1986
reversible defects in water excretion and, 1985
seizures in, 1986
SIADH and, 1985
withdrawal of hyponatremic drugs and, 1984
encephalopathy in, 2339
hyperglycemic, 1980, 1980t
hypotonic, 1978-1980
impaired water excretion in, 1978-1979
nonosmotic release of vasopressin in, 1979
urinary electrolyte losses in, 1979-1980
in intravenous gamma-globulin use, 1980
in intravenous mannitol use, 1980t
in irrigant absorption, 1980, 1980t
nonhypotonic, 1980, 1980t
pseudohyponatremia in, 1980t, 1980
Hypophysitis, lymphocytic, 603
Hypopigmentation disorders, 581-587.
See also individual disorders
albinism, 584-586
idiopathic guttate hypomelanosis, 586-587
piebaldism, 586, 585f
vitiligo, 581-584
Hypopituitarism, encephalopathy in, 2339-2340
Hypotension, in poisoning, 156, 156t
Hypothalamic hormones, 590t
Hypothalamic-pituitary-adrenal axis, 598
Hypothalamus, in thermal control, 1407
Hypothermia
in cardiac arrest, 148t
in poisoning or drug overdose, 157-158
Hypothyroidism, 605-610
acquired, 606
anemia in, 1094
central (secondary), 606
clinical manifestations of, 606-607
complications of, 609
congenital, 605
definitions of, 605
diagnosis of, 606-608
differential diagnosis of, 608
dyslipidemia in, 740
encephalopathy in, 2340
epidemiology of, 605, 606f
etiology and genetics of, 605-606
hair loss due to, 566
laboratory tests in, 607-608, 607t
management of, 608-609
in ischemic heart disease, 609
in mild disease, 609
residual symptoms after therapy in, 609
thyroid hormone therapy in, 608-609
nonthyroid illnesses and drugs in, 608
pathogenesis of, 606
physical examination in, 607
in pregnancy, 1020
prognosis in, 609-610
serum thyroid function tests in, 607, 607t
surgical risk factor management and, 56

Hypotonicity, cell volume regulation in, 1977-1978
Hypoventilation
alveolar
in muscular dystrophy, 2807
primary, 2789
in sleep, 2792
Hypovolemia, 1991-1992
in acute pancreatitis, 921
in cardiac arrest, 148t
chronic hyponatremia in, 1983
diagnosis of, 1992
etiology of, 1992
pathogenesis of, 1991-1992
treatment of, 1992
Hypoxia
in acute pancreatitis, 921-922
in cardiac arrest, 148t
metabolic encephalopathy in, 2338
Hysterosalpingography, in infertility, 1003

I

Ibutilide, for atrial fibrillation, 242t-243t
I cell disease, 1148t
Ichthyosiform erythroderma, congenital, 479, 479f
Ichthyosis, 478-479
acquired, 479, 479f
lamellar, 478
X-linked, 478
Ichthyosis vulgaris, 478
Idarubicin, 2418t
Ifosfamide, 2415t
Ileitis
in Crohn disease, 797
granulomatous. See Crohn disease
Ileocecal tuberculosis, 1682
Ileocolitis, granulomatous. See Crohn disease
Ileostomy diarrhea, 848-849
Ileus, 857
Iliopectineal bursitis, 1396
Imatinib mesylate, for chronic myelogenous leukemia, 2579-2580, 2580t, 2581f
Imipenem, 1430
in pregnancy, 1422t
Imipramine, for panic disorder, 2660
Immotile cilia syndrome (Kartagener syndrome). See Ciliary dyskinesia, primary
Immune complex disease, apheresis for, 1219
Immune globulin
for myositis, 1357, 1357t
for transfusion, 1213-1214
Immune mechanisms
antibody production as. See also Immunoglobulin(s)
antigen processing in. See also Major histocompatibility complex (MHC)
cell-cell interactions in. See also Antigen(s)
cell-mediated. See also specific cells, e.g., T cell(s)
deficiencies in, 1229-1232, 1229t-1231t
in drug allergy, 1271-1272, 1271f
innate, complement in. See also Complement
Immune reconstitution syndrome, in HIV infection, 1842
Immune system, cells of. See individual cell types, e.g., T cell(s)
Immunity, acquired. See also Immune system
Immunization
anthrax, 131

BCG, 1694
diphtheria, 1587
for HIV-infected patients, 1830t
for travelers, 71
Haemophilus influenzae, 1651
for HIV-infected patient, 1830t
hepatitis A
active, 879-880, 880t
for HIV-infected patients, 1830t
passive, 878
hepatitis B
active, 878-879, 879t
for HIV-infected patients, 1830t
for international travel, 73, 74f
passive, 878
hepatitis C, passive, 878
HIV, 1838-1839
for HIV-infected patient, 1829, 1830t
influenza, 1787-1788, 1787t
for HIV-infected patients, 1830t
measles, mumps, rubella, 1771
for HIV-infected patients, 1830t
meningococcal, 1621
pertussis, 1658
pneumococcal, 1567
for HIV-infected patients, 1830t
poliomyelitis
for HIV-infected patients, 1830t
for travelers, 71
as preventive health care measure, 41-42, 46t
smallpox, 125-127, 126f, 1772t
tetanus
for HIV-infected patients, 1830t
for travelers, 71
for travelers, 69-75, 69t
cholera, 71
contraindications, 75
diphtheria, 71
hepatitis A, 72-73, 73f
hepatitis B, 73, 74f
influenza, 71
Japanese encephalitis, 74, 76t
measles, 71
meningococcal, 73-74, 75f
plague, 72
pneumococcal infections, 71
poliomyelitis, 71
rabies, 72
tetanus, 71
tick-borne encephalitis, 74
typhoid, 71-72
yellow fever, 70, 70f
tuberculosis, 1694
uterine cervical cancer, 2542
Immunocompromised patient
aspergillosis in, 1882-1887
candidiasis in, 1875-1876, 1880, 1877t-1879t
cryptococcosis in, 1880-1881, 1880t
cytomegalovirus infection in, 1762
dematiaceous fungal infection in, 1890
diverticulitis in, 815
enterovirus infection in, 1797, 1795t
Epstein-Barr virus infection in, 1764
fusariosis in, 1888-1890, 1889t
herpes simplex infection in, 1757
mycotic infections in, 1875-1891
pneumocystis in, 1881-1882, 1882f, 1883t-1884t
viral pneumonia in, 1780-1781
zygomycosis in, 1887-1888
Immunodeficiency
AIDS. See Acquired immunodeficiency syndrome (AIDS), Human immunodeficiency virus infection
cutaneous findings in, 438
hematopoietic stem cell

transplantation for, 1222
severe combined, 1230-1231, 1230t
hematopoietic stem cell
transplantation for, 1222
Immunoglobulin A (IgA), deficiency,
1226t, 1228
Immunoglobulin A (IgA) nephropathy
(Berger disease), 2056-
2058, 2057f-2058f
in ankylosing spondylitis, 1320
Immunoglobulin deficiency
with elevated IgM, 1226t, 1228-1229
syndromes, 1226-1233, 1226t
Immunoglobulin disorder(s), purpuric
lesions in, 1177
Immunoglobulin E (IgE). See also
under Allergy and atopy
assay for, 1248-1250, 1248t, 1249f
radioallergosorbent, 1249, 1249f
in food allergy, 1278
in immediate hypersensitivity
reactions, 1241, 1242f
skin tests for, 1248-1249, 1248t
Immunoglobulin G (IgG), deficiency,
1229, 1226t
Immunoglobulin M (IgM), deficiency,
1229
Immunologic tolerance, 1234-1236
costimulatory signals in, 1235-
1236, 1236f
mechanisms of, 1234-
1236, 1234f, 1236f
peripheral, 1234-1235
positive vs. negative T cell
selection in, 1234, 1234f
Immunonutrition, 945-946
Immunosuppression. See also
individual types, e.g.,
Neutropenia, individual
infections
herpes simplex infection in, 1757
pneumonia in, 1470, 1780-1781
toxoplasmosis in, 1899
viral-related tubulointerstitial
nephritis in, 2093
Immunosuppressive therapy
cutaneous reactions due to, 438
for rheumatoid arthritis, 1312
Immunotherapy
for allergy, 1251-1252
for asthma, 2714-2715
for food allergy, 1283
tumor. See also under Tumor
venom, 1288-1289
Impetigo, 509, 509f
bullous, 509
Impingement syndrome (rotator cuff
tendinitis), 1392-1393, 1393f
Impotence. See Penile erectile
dysfunction
Incontinence
fecal, 858-859
urinary. See Urinary incontinence
Incontinentia pigmenti, 440
Indapamide, for hypertension, 221t
Indinavir, for HIV infection, 1831t
adverse effects of, 1834t
Indinavir urolithiasis, 2112
Induration, definition of, 429t
Industrial chemicals, polyneuropathy
due to, 2303, 2303t
Infant. See also Children
botulism in, 1609
listeriosis in, 1590
neonatal
acne in, 447
chlamydial conjunctivitis in,
1750
enteroviral infection in, 1796-
1797, 1795t
herpes in, 1757-1758
lupus syndrome in, 444, 1334-
1335, 1328t

sleep patterns in, 2362
streptococcal infection in,
group B, 1573
neutropenia in, 1143
sleep patterns in, 2362
Infarction
myocardial. See Myocardial
infarction
pulmonary, segmental pulmonary
infiltrates in, 2751
Infectious agents, in cancer
epidemiology, 2376-2377
Infectious mononucleosis
CMV, 1762
Epstein-Barr, 1763-1764
Infertility, 1002-1009
age and, 1002
anovulation in, 1005-1007, 1005f
anovulatory or oligo-ovulatory, in
polycystic ovary syndrome,
treatment of, 982-984, 982t
causes of, 1002, 1003f
cervical factors in, 1003-1004
endometriosis in, 967, 968
in advance disease, 972
treatment of, 970-972, 971t
evaluation and treatment in, 1002-
1007
fecundity and, 1002, 1002t
female, 1003-1007
generalist and, 1008-1009
male, 1002, 1006t-1007t
occupational exposures and, 66
management of, 1002, 1004f-1005f
occupational exposures and, 66-67
ovulation induction in, 1007-1008
ovulatory factors in, 1004-1005
technological advances in, 1008
tubal and pelvic factors in, 1003
unexplained, 1007
Inflammatory bowel disease, 790-812.
See also Crohn disease,
Ulcerative colitis
ankylosing spondylitis in, 1325
colorectal cancer and, 2476
complications of, 808-809
adenocarcinoma, 809
intestinal, 808-809
cutaneous findings in, 435, 435f
diarrhea in, 843
differential diagnosis, 799
epidemiology of, 790
etiology of, 790
fever of undetermined origin in,
1415
irritable bowel syndrome in, 803
management of, 799-808
aminosalicylates, 800, 800f, 801t
antibiotics, 802
anti-inflammatory agents, 800-
801, 800f, 801t
azathioprine, 801-802
biologic agents, 802-803
corticosteroids, 800
cyclosporine, 802
immunomodulatory agents, 801-802
6-mercaptopurine, 801-802
mesalamine, 800, 801t
methotrexate, 802
nutritional therapy, 803
omega-3 fatty acids, 803
sulfasalazine, 800, 800f, 801t
supportive, 803-804
tacrolimus, 802
pathogenesis of, 790-791
pregnancy and, 808
prognosis in, 809
Inflammatory myopathy(ies),
idiopathic, 1351-1358. See also
Myositis
Infliximab
for inflammatory bowel disease,
802-803

for psoriasis, 471
for rheumatoid arthritis,
1308t, 1310
Influenza, 1779, 1784-1788, 1786t-
1787t
classification and pathogenesis
of, 1784
complications of, 1785-1786
diagnosis of, 1785
encephalitis in, 2347
epidemiology and transmission of,
1784-1785
immunization for, international
travel and, 71
prevention of, 1787-1788
treatment of, 1786-1787, 1786t
Influenza A, B, laboratory diagnosis
of, 1778t
Influenza immunization, 1787-
1788, 1787t
for HIV-infected patients, 1830t
Infrainguinal bypass, for
atherosclerotic peripheral
arterial disease, 405
Infrapatellar tendinitis, 1396
Inhalant(s), abuse of, 2637
Injury and disease, reducing risk
of, 17-24
accidents and violence and, 21-23
alcohol abuse and, 20-21, 20t-21t
caveats in, 17-18
changing behavior in, 18
domestic violence and, 23
drowning and, 22-23
drug abuse and, 21
falling and, 22, 22t
firearms injury and, 23
fires and, 22
life expectancy and, 18, 18f
motor vehicle injuries and, 21-22
overview of, 17-18
substance abuse and, 18-21
tobacco use and, 18-20, 19t. See
also Cigarette smoking
US Preventive Services Task Force
and, 17t
Insect allergy, stinging. See also
Stinging insect allergy
Hymenoptera, 1285-1289
Insect bites and stings, 191-192
Insect repellents
DEET, 75
mosquito-borne infections and, 75
Insemination, intrauterine, for
infertility in endometriosis,
971-972
Insomnia, 2370-2371, 2365t, 2370t. See
also Sleep disorders
familial fatal, 2358, 2359
Insulin. See also Diabetes mellitus
deficiency
in type 1 diabetes, 638, 639f
hyperkalemia due to, 2009
in type 2 diabetes, 653, 653f
for diabetic ketoacidosis,
hypokalemia due to, 2006
in hormonal regulation of
metabolism, 633-634, 634f-638f
inhaled, 643
intensive in-hospital, 675-
676, 675f
long-acting, 644
regimens for, in type 1 diabetes,
644-645, 643f
resistance
hepatic iron overload in, 1088
in type 2 diabetes, 653-654, 654f
Insulinoma, 629-630
Insulin pump, for type 1 diabetes,
644-645, 643f
Insulin resistance, in polycystic
ovary syndrome, 975, 979-
980, 979f

Insulin sensitizers, for polycystic
ovary syndrome, 983-984
Interferon alfa
for chronic hepatitis B, 886-887
for chronic myeloid leukemia,
2578t, 2580
myopathy due to, 2284
uses of, 2405
Interferon and ribavirin combination
therapy, for chronic hepatitis
C, 889, 888t
Interferon gamma, for atopic
dermatitis, 478
Interleukin-1 (IL-1), in
hematopoiesis, 1073t
Interleukin-2 (IL-2)
in hematopoiesis, 1073t
for metastatic melanoma, 2404-2405
for renal cell carcinoma, 2404-
2405, 2519
Interleukin-3 (IL-3)
in hematopoiesis, 1073t, 1074
in IgE-mediated allergic
inflammation, 1241t
Interleukin-4 (IL-4)
in hematopoiesis, 1073t
in IgE-mediated allergic
inflammation, 1241t
Interleukin-5 (IL-5)
in hematopoiesis, 1073t, 1074
in IgE-mediated allergic
inflammation, 1241t
Interleukin-6 (IL-6), in
hematopoiesis, 1073t
Interleukin-7 (IL-7), in
hematopoiesis, 1073t
Interleukin-11 (IL-11), in
hematopoiesis, 1073t, 1074
Interleukin-12 (IL-12), in
hematopoiesis, 1073t
Interleukin-13 (IL-13), in IgE-
mediated allergic inflammation,
1241t
International travel. See Travel,
international
Internet resources
alcoholism, 2632
anxiety disorders, 2658
biomedical ethics, 4
bioterrorism, 123
cardiovascular disease, 211
CNS neoplasms, 2321
complementary and alternative
medicine, 90t
domestic violence, 23
fibromyalgia, 1404
genetic information, 1956
heart disease, congenital, 388
hereditary ataxia, 2266
herpesvirus, 1755
HIV, 1843
latex allergy, 493
osteoporosis, 711t
palliative medicine, 93
protozoan infections, 1911
respiratory viral infections, 1790
scleroderma, 1348
Intertrigo candidiasis, 507, 508f
Intestinal flukes, 1936
Intestinal lymphangiectasia,
malabsorption in, 832
Intestinal nematode infection, 1918-
1924, 1920t
Intestinal protozoan infections,
1901-1909
Intestinal pseudo-obstruction,
chronic, 856-857
Intra-abdominal abscess, 1503-1506.
See also specific anatomic
location, e.g., Liver abscess
diagnosis of, 1503-1504
prevention of, 1504
treatment of, 1504

Intra-abdominal lymph node(s), inflammatory pseudotumor of, fever of undetermined origin in, 1416

Intracellular fluid, in hypotonicity and hypertonicity, 1977-1978

Intracerebral hemorrhage, in stroke, 2214, 2214t

Intracranial pressure, increased, in brain trauma, 2233-2234, 2234t

Intraperitoneal abscess, 1504

Intrauterine device (IUD), 998

Intravenous drug abuse. See Drug abuse, intravenous

Inulin clearance, 1968

Iodide, for hyperthyroidism, 616-617

Iodine, radioactive, for hyperthyroidism, 616

Iohexol clearance, 1968

Ion channelopathy, 2281-2282

Ipecac, for poisoning or drug overdose, 159, 160t

Ipratropium bromide, for asthma, 2711t, 2811-2812

Irbesartan, for hypertension, 223t

Irinotecan, 2419t
  for colorectal cancer, 2487

Iron
  dietary, 29-30
  storage and supply of
    cellular, 1081, 1081f
    iron regulatory proteins in, 1081, 1081f

Iron absorption
  intestinal, 1082
  regulation of, 1082

Iron deficiency, 1082-1085, 1083t
  clinical manifestations of, 1083-1084
  diagnosis of, 1083-1084
  differential diagnosis of, 1092t
  etiology of, 1083, 1084t
  hair loss due to, 566
  laboratory tests in, 1084
  treatment of, 1084-1085

Iron deficiency anemia, 1082. See also Iron deficiency

Iron exchange, pathways of, 1082

Iron-loading anemia, 1088

Iron metabolism, 1079-1082
  ceruloplasmin in, 1082
  divalent metal transporter-1 in, 1081
  ferritin in, 1081
  hephaestin in, 1082
  HFE in, 1082
  iron regulatory proteins in, 1081, 1081f
  molecular basis of, 1080-1082, 1081f
  patterns of, 1079-1080, 1080f
  transferrin and apotransferrin in, 1080
  transferrin receptor in, 1081, 1081f

Iron overload, 1085-1090
  African dietary, 1088
  causes of, 1086t
  from chronic liver disease, 1088
  definitions of, 1085
  from hemochromatosis, 1085-1088. See also Hemochromatosis
  hepatic, insulin resistance-associated, 1088
  from iron-loading anemias, 1088
  from medicinal iron ingestion, 1088
  perinatal, 1089
  from porphyria cutanea tarda, 1088
  primary, 1085-1087
  secondary, 1088-1090
  transfusional and parenteral, 1088-1089

Iron poisoning, 169, 1121

Iron regulatory protein(s)
  in cellular iron uptake and storage, 1081, 1081f
  in iron metabolism, 1081, 1081f

Iron transport, systemic, 1080

Iron uptake, cellular, 1080-1081
  regulation of, 1081, 1081f

Irritability, in brain trauma, 2236

Irritable bowel syndrome, 860
  diarrhea in, 843, 847-848
  inflammatory bowel disease and, 803

Isaac disease (autoimmune acquired neuromyotonia), 2282

Isaac syndrome (neuromyotonia with K+ channel autoantibodies), 2287-2288

Ischemic heart disease. See Coronary artery disease

Ischiogluteal bursitis, 1396

Isoniazid
  poisoning, 169-170
  in pregnancy, 1422t
  seizure due to, 157t

Isosporiasis, 1906-1907, 1908f

Isotretinoin, for acne vulgaris, 450t, 449-450

Isradipine extended release, for hypertension, 221t

Itraconazole
  as antifungal, 1871-1873, 1871t-1872t
  for toenail onychomycosis, 575t

Ivermectin, for scabies, 518

IVIg, for idiopathic thrombocytopenic purpura, 1167

J

Janeway lesion(s), in endocarditis, 1484, 1484f

Japanese encephalitis, 1853-1854
  immunization for, 74, 76t

Japanese spotted fever, 1728

Jarisch-Herxheimer reaction, 1707

JC virus, in progressive multifocal leukoencephalopathy, 2360

Jejunoileitis, in Crohn disease, 797

Jervell and Lange-Nielsen syndrome, 265

Jet aircraft, high altitude and, 80

Jet lag, 2370

Job, safety and health on. See Occupational disease

Jod-Basedow effect, 611

Joint disease, crystal-induced, 1371-1381. See also specific disorders, e.g., Gout

Joint examination, in rheumatic disease, 1292-1293

Joint infection. See also Arthritis
  Haemophilus influenzae, 1650
  Pseudomonas aeruginosa, 1661
  staphylococcal, 1576
  streptococcal, group A, 1570

Joint prosthesis, septic arthritis in, 1539-1540

Journals, medical. See Medical literature

K

Kallmann syndrome, 957
  hypogonadism in, 693

Kaposi sarcoma, 557-559, 2553, 2553t
  in AIDS, cutaneous findings in, 438, 438f
  classification of, 2553
  complications and prognosis in, 559
  diagnosis of, 558, 558f, 2553, 2553t
  differential diagnosis of, 558
  epidemiology of, 557
  herpesvirus type 8 in, 2376
  etiology of, 557-558
  features of, 2550t
  treatment of, 558-559, 2555-2556

Kartagener syndrome (primary ciliary dyskinesia), 2739-2740, 2739f. See also Ciliary dyskinesia, primary

Kawasaki disease (mucocutaneous lymph node syndrome), 1367-1368, 1368t
  cutaneous findings in, 433
  renal involvement in, 2075

Kayser-Fleischer ring, in Wilson disease, 2258, 2257f

Kearns-Sayre syndrome, 1952, 1952t, 2280-2281

Keloid, 543-544, 543f

Kennedy disease, 694-695

Keratitis
  candidiasis in, 1879t
  Pseudomonas aeruginosa, 1660

Keratoderma blennorrhagicum, in reactive arthritis, 1323, 1323f

Keratolysis, pitted, 512

Keratosis, seborrheic, 535, 535f-536f

Keratosis follicularis (Darier disease), 533

Ketoacidosis, 646-647, 646t, 1996
  diabetic
    encephalopathy in, 2340
    hypokalemia due to insulin in, 2006
    presenting features, 646
    treatment of, 646-647, 646t, 2001
  high-anion-gap metabolic acidosis in, 1996

Ketoconazole
  as antifungal, 1871-1873, 1871t-1872t
  for hirsutism, 991

Ketolides, 1434-1435

Kidney disease. See Renal disease

Kidney stone(s). See Nephrolithiasis

Kidney transplantation. See Renal transplantation

Kimura disease, 547

Kissing bugs, 191

Klebsiella infections, 1632

Klebsiella pneumoniae, antimicrobial susceptibility of, 1421t

Klebsiella pneumoniae meningitis, 1553t

Klinefelter syndrome, 692

Klippel-Trenaunay-Weber syndrome, 545

Knee(s)
  osteoarthritis of, 1386
  rheumatoid arthritis of, 1302-1303

Knee pain, 1396

Knee pain syndrome, anterior, 1396

Knee surgery, venous thromboembolism in, prophylaxis for, 419

Knudson model of tumorigenicity, 2386-2387, 2387f-2388f

Koebner phenomenon, 453, 454f
  in psoriasis, 462

Koilonychia, 573. See also under Nail(s)

Korsakoff encephalopathy, 2341

Kostmann syndrome, neutropenia in, 1144t

Krabbe disease, 1149t

K-ras, properties of, 2384t

Krukenberg tumor, 2539

Kuru, 2358

Kussmaul respiration(s), 1999

Kyphoscoliosis
  measuring scoliotic angle in, 2802, 2802f
  respiratory pump dysfunction in, 2801-2802, 2802f, 2801t

sleep-disordered breathing in, 2798

L

Labetalol
  for hypertension, 222t
  for hypertensive crisis, 228t
  toxicity of, 163t

LaCrosse encephalitis, 1853

beta-Lactam antibiotics, 1431-1432. See also under Penicillin
  acute interstitial nephritis due to, 2087-2088, 2088f
    diagnosis of, 2087-2088, 2088f
    pathogenesis of, 2087
    treatment of, 2087-2088
  allergic reactions to, 1431-1432

Lactic acidosis, 1995-1996
  treatment of, 2001

D-Lactic acidosis, 1996

Lambert-Eaton syndrome. See Eaton-Lambert (myasthenic) syndrome

Lamivudine
  for chronic hepatitis B, 887
  for HIV infection, 1831t
    adverse effects of, 1834t

Lamotrigine
  in epilepsy, 2194-2195
  hypersensitivity syndrome reaction due to, 496

Langerhans cell histiocytosis, 1145-1146

Larva migrans
  cutaneous, 522, 1926, 1927f
  visceral, 1926-1927

Laryngeal cancer
  induction chemotherapy for, 2440f
  tobacco use and, 2374, 2437

Laryngeal sarcoidosis, 2772

Laryngitis, viral, 1778-1779

Laser treatment, for hirsutism, 992

Lassa fever, 1852

Lateral sinus thrombophlebitis, 1560-1561

Latex allergy, 492-493, 497
  at-risk populations and risk factors in, 492-493
  diagnosis and treatment of, 493
  Internet sources for, 493
  urticaria in, 1261

Laxative(s), abuse of, chronic diarrhea in, 848

Lead
  nephropathy due to, 64
  test of exposure to, 61t

Lead poisoning, 170
  hemolytic anemia in, 1128
  tubulointerstitial nephritis in, 2094-2095

Leber hereditary optic neuropathy, 1952, 1952t, 2281

Leflunomide, for rheumatoid arthritis, 1310, 1308t

Leg(s)
  lower, pain in, 1396
  restless legs syndrome, 2368-2369, 2369f

Legionella micdadei infection, 1475

Legionella pneumophila, 1473-1474, 1652-1653. See also Legionnaires disease

Legionella species, 1474-1475
  infections caused by, 1474-1475

Legionellosis, 1652-1656
  clinical syndromes, 1654-1655, 1654t
  epidemiology of, 1652-1653
  microbiologic diagnosis of, 1654-1656, 1655t
  pathogenesis and pathology in, 1653-1654
  treatment and prognosis of,

1656, 1655t
Legionnaires disease, 1474-1475, 1654, 1654t
Legumes, dietary, 30-31
Leigh syndrome, 1952, 1952t
Leiomyoma, 547, 546f
    uterine, 1059-1060, 1061-1062
        benign metastasizing, 2756
Leiomyosarcoma, 2552
    features of, 2550t
Leishmania donovani, 1910
Leishmania mexicana group, 1911, 1912t
Leishmaniasis, 1910-1913
    cutaneous and mucocutaneous, 523, 523f, 1911-1913, 1912t, 1912f-1913f
    diagnosis of, 1911-1912, 1913f
    etiology and epidemiology of, 1911, 1903f
    New World, 1912t, 1911
    pathogenesis of, 1911, 1912f
    treatment of, 1912-1913
    visceral, 1910-1911
Leishmania tropica, 1910
Leishmania viannia group, 1911, 1912t
Lemierre syndrome, 1464-1465
Lennox-Gastaut syndrome, 2190
Lentigines, 580
Lentivirus, 1802t
Lepirudin, for heparin-induced thrombocytopenia, 1200
Leprosy, polyneuropathy in, 2304
Leptomeningeal metastasis, 2317, 2434
Leptospirosis, 1717-1719
    clinical manifestations of, 1718-1719
    diagnosis of, 1718-1719
    epidemiology in, 1717-1718
    laboratory studies in, 1719
    microbiology in, 1717, 1718f
    pathogenesis of, 1718
    treatment and prevention of, 1719
Letrozole, 2420t
    for early (stages I and II) breast cancer, 2465
Leukapheresis, 1218
Leukemia
    acute, 2561-2574
        cytogenetics of, 2565-2566, 2566t
        epidemiology of, 2561
        etiology of, 2561-2562
            chemicals in, 2562
            heredity and genetics in, 2562
            radiation in, 2377-2378, 2561-2562
            viruses in, 2562
        future possibilities, 2573
        hybrid, immunophenotyping in, 2565
        immunophenotyping in, 2565
        morphologic classification of, 2562-2565, 2563t-2564t
        therapy for, general principles of, 2566-2567, 2567t
    acute lymphoblastic, 2571-2573
        Burkitt cell, 2572
        clinical features of, 2571
        cytogenetic abnormalities in, 2571
        diagnosis of, 2571
        immunophenotyping in, 2565
        morphologic classification of, 2564-2565
        Philadelphia chromosome-positive, 2572-2573, 2572t
        treatment of, 2571-2572
            CNS prophylaxis, 2572
            hematopoietic stem cell transplantation for, 1223
            maintenance therapy, 2572
            remission consolidation, 2572

    acute myeloid, 2567-2571
        clinical features of, 2567-2568
        cytogenetic abnormalities in, 2568
        diagnosis of, 2567-2568
        immunophenotyping in, 2565
        morphologic classification of, 2563
        treatment of, 2568-2569
            elderly patients, 2570-2571
            hematopoietic stem cell transplantation for, 1222-1223
            postremission, 2568-2569, 2568t
            in relapsed or refractory disease, 2569
            remission induction, 2568
            WHO classification of, 2562t, 2563
    acute promyelocytic
        PML-RAR-alpha in, 2384t, 2385
        treatment of, 2569
    chronic lymphocytic, 2585-2589
        clinical course and complications in, 2587
        clinical presentation in, 2585
        diagnosis of, 2585-2586
        epidemiology of, 2585
        etiology and pathogenesis of, 2585
        laboratory findings in, 2586, 2586f, 2586t
        staging of, 2586-2587, 2587t
        therapy for, 2587-2588
            biologic, 2588
            combination, 2588
            hematopoietic stem cell transplantation for, 1223-1224
            high-dose therapy with stem-cell support, 2588
            purine analogue, 2588
            in relapsed/refractory disease, 2588-2589
            single agent, 2587-2588
            splenectomy, 2589
            supportive care, 2588-2589
    chronic myelogenous. *See* Leukemia, chronic myeloid
    chronic myeloid, 2575-2580
        bcr-abl-negative, 2577t
        clinical course, 2577-2578, 2576t
        clinical presentation in, 2576
        cytogenetic analysis and molecular assays in, 2577
        cytogenetics of, 2575-2576
        diagnosis of, 2576-2577, 2577t
        differential diagnosis of, 2577, 2577t
        epidemiology of, 2575
        laboratory findings in, 2576-2577
        pathophysiology of, 2575-2576
        peripheral blood and bone marrow assays in, 2576-2577
        Philadelphia chromosome in, 2384
        Philadelphia chromosome negative, 2577t
        prognosis in, 2578
        treatment of, 2578-2580
            conventional agents in, 2578-2579, 2578t
            dasatinib for, 2580
            imatinib mesylate for, 2579-2580, 2580t, 2581f
            interferon alfa for, 2580, 2578t
            novel approaches in, 2580
            stem cell transplantation for, 2579, 2581f, 2579, 2581f
    chronic myelomonocytic, 2564t. *See also* Myelodysplastic syndromes

    fever of undetermined origin in, 1415
    hairy-cell, 2589
    prolymphocytic, 2589
    pulmonary infiltration in, chronic diffuse, 2769
    smoldering myeloid. *See* Myelodysplastic syndromes
    subacute myeloid. *See* Myelodysplastic syndromes
Leukemia inhibitory factor (LIF), 1073t
Leukemia/lymphoma, adult T cell (ATL), HTLV-I and, 1810-1811
    acute, 1810
    chronic, 1811
    lymphomatous, 1810
    smoldering, 1811
Leukocyte. *See also individual cell types, e.g.,* Neutrophil
    nonmalignant disorders, 1137-1152
    types of, 1137, 1138f
Leukocyte adhesion deficiency I, 1146t
Leukocyte adhesion deficiency II, 1146
Leukocyte count, normal, 1137, 1139t
Leukocyte scan, in osteomyelitis, 1545-1546
Leukodystrophy, metachromatic, 2332
Leukoencephalopathy, progressive multifocal, 2359-2360, 2360f
    JC virus in, 2360
Leukonychia, 573-574
Leukopenia
    after renal transplantation, 2124-2125
    in systemic lupus erythematosus, 1333
Leukostasis, apheresis for, 1218
Leukotriene antagonists
    for allergy, 1251
    for asthma, 2713, 2710t
Leuprolide, 2420t
    for breast cancer, 2464
Levalbuterol, for asthma, 2709, 2711t
Levetiracetam, in epilepsy, 2195
Levodopa, for parkinsonism, 2244
Levodopa formulations, for parkinsonism, 2245, 2244t, 2246t
Levofloxacin, 1438-1439, 1438t
    for *Shigella* infection, 1636t
Lewy bodies, in dementia, 2224-2225
Lewy body disease, 2252-2253
Libido, decreased, 697
Libman-Sacks endocarditis, valvular heart disease in, 349
Lice infestation. *See* Pediculosis
Lichenoid eruptions, drug-induced, 501
Lichen planopilaris, 454, 568
Lichen planus, 453-455, 453f
    diagnosis of, 453-454, 454f
    etiology of, 453
    nail pathology in, 576t
    prognosis in, 455
    treatment of, 454-455
        body lesions, 454
        genital and perianal lesions, 454-455
        mouth lesions, 454
Lichenification, 268
Licodaine, transdermal, 2185
Liddle syndrome, hypokalemia in, 2008
Lidocaine
    in cardiac resuscitation, 144t
    classification of, 267t
Lifestyle modification, in hypertension, 220, 220t
Li-Fraumeni syndrome
    breast cancer and, 2459
    CNS tumors in, 2310t
Light, pulsed, intense, for

    hirsutism, 992
Light-chain deposition disease, tubulointerstitial nephritis in, 2097
Limb ischemia, chronic
    clinical categories of, 401t
    Fontaine classification of, 401t
Lindane
    for pediculosis, 520-521
    for scabies, 517-518
Lindsay nails, 573
Linear IgA disease, drug-induced, 499
Linezolid, 1437
Lionfish, 193-194
Lipase
    hepatic, function of, 732, 734f
    serum, in acute pancreatitis, 916, 917t
Lipid(s)
    blood, exercise and, 34
    dietary, cardiovascular risk and, 26
    in nutritional support, 946-947
Lipid-lowering agents
    for angina pectoris, 297-298
    for prevention of myocardial infarction, 332-333
    for unstable angina and NSTMI, 313
Lipid storage disease
    myopathies in, 2279-2280
    neutral, 1149t
Lipodystrophy syndrome (fat redistribution syndrome), in HIV infection, 1834-1835
Lipoid pneumonia, focal infiltrates in, 2746, 2745f
Lipoma, 547
Lipomatosis, mediastinal, 2838
Lipoprotein, 729-732
    assembly and catabolism of, 730
    assembly of, 730-731
    catabolism of, 731-732
    high-density (HDL), 730
        function and regulation of, 732, 733f, 734t
        low levels of, 735-736
    intermediate-density (IDL), 729
    low-density (LDL), 730
        catabolism of, 731-732, 732f
        drug therapy for lowering, 744-745
    metabolism of, 730-732, 731f
        genetic disorders of, 736-740
        secondary disorders of, 740-741
    normal levels of, atherosclerosis in, 736
    structure and classification of, 729-730, 730f
    very low density (VLDL), 729
Lipoprotein(a), 731, 1196
    increased levels of, 739
Liposarcoma, 2551-2552
    features of, 2550t
Lisinopril, for hypertension, 222t
Listeria monocytogenes, 1589, 1590f, 1587t. *See also* Listeriosis
Listeria monocytogenes meningitis, 1590-1591
    antibiotics in, 1553t
Listeria monocytogenes meningoencephalitis, 1590-1591
Listeriosis, 1589-1592
    adult, 1590-1591
    bacteremia in, 1591
    clinical features of, 1590-1591
    etiology and epidemiology of, 1589
    laboratory tests in, 1591
    microbiology of, 1589, 1590f
    miscellaneous infections in, 1591
    neonatal, 1590
    pathogenesis of, 1589-1590

in pregnancy, 1590
prevention of, 1591-1592, 1591t
treatment of, 1591-1592
Literature, medical. *See* Medical
literature
Lithium
for bipolar disorder, 2621-
2622, 2621t
poisoning or overdose, 170-171
elimination method for, 161t
side effects of, renal, 2090
Lithium carbonate, for
hyperthyroidism, 617
Lithotripsy, extracorporeal biliary
for chronic cholecystitis, 906-907
for gallstones, 906-907
Livedo reticularis, in polyarteritis
nodosa, 1366, 1367f
Livedo vasculitis, 444
Liver, cirrhosis of. *See* Cirrhosis
Liver abscess, 1505-1506
amebic, 1904-1905, 1904f
differential diagnosis of, 1906
clinical features of, 1505-1506
diagnosis of, 1506, 1505f
fever of undetermined origin in,
1414-1415
treatment of, 1506
Liver biopsy
in autoimmune hepatitis, 883-884
in cirrhosis, 893-894
in fever of undetermined origin,
1417
Liver cancer. *See also*
Hepatocellular carcinoma
occupational agents causing, 62t
Liver disease
chronic, iron overload in, 1088
coagulopathy in, 1187-1188
encephalopathy in, 2338
hemolytic anemia in, 1129
in home parenteral nutrition, 948
in malabsorption, 824
nutritional support in, 944
occupational, 64
surgical risk factor management
and, 56
Liver necrosis, in halothane
exposure, 877
Liver transplantation, 932-936
candidates for, 932, 932t
for chronic hepatitis C, 890
for cirrhosis, 899, 898t
complications of, 934-936
disease-specific, 936
drug-drug interactions, 934-935
immunologic, 933
immunosuppressive, 934-936
infectious, 933-934
perioperative and surgical, 933
contraindications to, 932
encephalopathy in, 2338
indications for, 932t
operative procedures, 933, 934f
outcomes after, 936
timing of, 932-933, 933f, 933t
Living will, 97
L-*myc*, properties of, 2384t
Loa loa, 1929t
Loffler syndrome (simple pulmonary
eosinophilia), 2782
Löfgren syndrome, 2770
Loiasis, 1932
Lomefloxacin, 1438t
Lomustine, 2415t
Long QT syndrome, congenital, 204t,
265, 2282
Loose anagen syndrome, 567
Lopinavir + ritonavir, for HIV
infection, 1831t
adverse effects of, 1834t
Losartan, for hypertension, 223t
Low blood pressure. *See* Hypotension

LPS signaling, in sepsis, 1444-1445
Ludwig angina, 1465
Lumbar puncture, in headache, 2152
Lumbosacral plexopathy, 2297
Lumbosacral polyradiculopathy, in
AIDS, 2305
Lung
carcinoid tumor of, segmental
infiltrates in, 2750, 2750f
contusion of, focal infiltrates
in, 2746
eosinophilic granuloma of, 2780-
2781, 2769t-2770t
computed tomography in, 2760f
farmer's, 2758, 2759t, 2765-
2766, 2765f. *See also*
Pneumonitis, hypersensitivity
functional assessment of. *See*
Pulmonary function testing
gangrene of, cavitary infiltrates
in, 2752
resection, pulmonary edema in,
2850
rheumatoid nodules in, 1305
torsion of lobe, focal infiltrates
in, 2746
Lung abscess, 1477-1479
amebic, 2752
large mass in, 2754
Lung biopsy
in chronic diffuse infiltrative
pulmonary disease, 2761, 2761t
in hypersensitivity pneumonitis,
2766
open, thoracotomy with, 2696
in pulmonary hypertension, 2855
in sarcoidosis, 2772, 2773f
in Wegener granulomatosis, 1363
Lung cancer, 2443-2456
adenocarcinoma
classification of, 2443t
single nodule in, 2753, 2754f
clinical manifestations and
laboratory studies in, 2445-
2447, 2446t
extrathoracic, 2446-2447, 2446t
intrathoracic, 2445-2446
paraneoplastic syndromes, 2446
pulmonary, 2445
clinical staging in, 2447, 2448f
definition and classification in,
2443, 2443t
diagnosis of, 2445-2448
epidemiology and etiology of, 2443-
2444, 2444t
asbestos in, 2377
tobacco and, 2374-2375
genetic susceptibility and
molecular mechanisms in,
2444, 2444t
large cell
cavitary infiltrates in,
2752, 2752f
classification of, 2443t
large mass in, 2754, 2755f
non-small cell
classification of, 2443t
treatment of, 2448-2454, 2450t
in stage I and II, 2449-2450
in stage III-inoperable, 2451-
2452
in stage III-operable, 2450-
2451
in stage IV disease, 2452-2454
in nonsmokers, 2444
occupational agents causing, 62t
pathophysiology and pathogenesis
of, 2444
prevention of, 2445
prognosis in, 2456
screening in, 48, 2445
small cell
classification of, 2443t

superior vena cava syndrome in,
2425, 2426f-2427f
treatment of, 2454-2456, 2454t
in early-stage disease, 2454
in limited-stage or extensive-
stage disease, 2454-2456
in relapse, 2456
smoking cessation and, 2443-2444
squamous cell, classification of,
2443t
surgical staging in, 2447-
2448, 2448f-2449f
treatment of, 2448-2456
supportive care in, 2456
updates on, 2456
Lung disease. *See* Pulmonary disease
Lung scan, ventilation-perfusion
for pulmonary embolism, 413-
414, 414f
for pulmonary hypertension, 2854,
2857f
Lung transplantation
for chronic bronchitis and
emphysema, 2732
for COPD, 2732
for pulmonary arterial
hypertension, 2859
Lung volume reduction surgery, in
emphysema, 2732
Lupoid sclerosis, 1334
Lupus erythematosus
discoid, 1330, 1332f, 1328t
hair loss in, 568, 568f
drug-induced, 1328t
systemic (SLE), 1327-1341
alveolar hemorrhage in, 2779
brain imaging studies in, 1335
cardiopulmonary involvement in,
1331-1332, 1333f
chronic diffuse infiltrative
pulmonary disease in, 2779
chronic disease and
complications in, 1338-1339
classification of, ACR criteria
for, 1329, 1330t
definition and subclassification
of, 1327, 1328t-1329t
dementia in, 1339
dermatomyositis *vs.*, 1337, 1329t
diagnosis of, 1329-1336, 1330t-
1331t, 1335t-1336t
differential diagnosis in, 1336-
1337, 1328t-1329t
encephalopathy in, 2342
epidemiology and genetics of,
1327, 1329f
flare in, 1338
gastrointestinal involvement in,
1332-1333
hematologic involvement in, 1333
hepatic involvement in, 1332-
1333
laboratory tests in, 1335-
1336, 1336t
lymph node involvement in, 1331
mixed connective tissue disease
vs., 1337, 1329t
musculoskeletal involvement in,
1332
neurologic involvement in, 1333-
1334
nonrheumatic illnesses *vs.*, 1336-
1337
overlap disease *vs.*, 1337
palliative care in, 1339-1340
pathophysiology and pathogenesis
of, 1327-1329
autoantibodies in, 1327
chronic illness in, 1328-1329
estrogen in, 1328
genetic susceptibilities in,
1328
infection in, 1328

innate and adaptive immunity
in, 1327-1328
pneumonitis in, 2779
pregnancy in, 1338
prognosis in, 1340
pulmonary infiltrates in,
multifocal, 2749
renal evaluation in, 1336
renal failure in, 1339-1340
renal involvement in, 1334, 1334t-
1335t
rheumatic illnesses *vs.*,
1337, 1328t-1329t
rheumatoid arthritis *vs.*,
1337, 1328t
Sjogren syndrome *vs.*, 1337, 1328t
skin and mucosal involvement in,
1330-1331, 1331f-1333f
skin lesions in, 443-444, 443f
spontaneous bacterial
peritonitis in, 1500
systemic signs and symptoms of,
1329-1330
thrombocytopenic purpura with,
1169
treatment of, 1337-1340
in acute disease, 1337-1338
indices of disease severity
in, 1338
tubulointerstitial nephritis in,
2100
undifferentiated connective
tissue disease *vs.*,
1337, 1329t
Lupus headache, 1333
Lupus lung, 1331
Lupus nephritis, 1334, 1334t-1335t,
2077
Lupus pernio, in sarcoidosis,
432, 432f, 2771
Lupus syndrome, neonatal, 444, 1334-
1335, 1328t
Luteinizing hormone, 599-601
serum, in polycystic ovary
syndrome, 978, 978f
Lyme disease, 1712-1723
acrodermatitis chronica
atrophicans in, 1713-1714
arthritis in, 1714
carditis in, 1714
clinical manifestations of, 1713-
1714, 1713f
cutaneous findings in, 439-
440, 439f
diagnosis in, 1714-1716
culture in, 1715
microscopy in, 1715
serology in, 1715-1716, 1715f
epidemiology of, 1712-1713, 1712f
erythema migrans in, 439, 439f,
1713, 1713f
history in, 1712
human granulocytic ehrlichiosis
and, 1733
lymphocytoma in, 1713
musculoskeletal features in, 1714
neurologic involvement in, 1714
neuropathy, 2305
prevention of, 1717
treatment of, 1716-1717, 1716t
Lymphadenitis
streptococcal, group A, 1569
tuberculous, 1680
Lymphadenopathy, in Hodgkin disease.
See Hodgkin disease
Lymphangiectasia, intestinal,
malabsorption in, 832
Lymphangioma circumscriptum, 547
Lymphangiomyomatosis, pulmonary
disease in, 2783-2784
Lymphangitic carcinomatosis,
pulmonary, 2768
Lymphatic filariasis, 1929-1930

Lymph node(s), in fever of undetermined origin, 1417
Lymphocyte(s)
  B. *See* B cell(s)
  T. *See* T cell(s)
Lymphocyte infusion, allogeneic, 2405-2406
Lymphocytic hypophysitis, 603
Lymphocytoma, in Lyme disease, 1713
Lymphocytopenia, 1151, 1151t
Lymphocytosis, 1151, 1150t
Lymphogranuloma venereum, 1749-1750
  genital ulcers in, 1528t
Lymphohistiocytosis, hemophagocytic, 1146-1147
Lymphokine-activated killer (LAK) cell(s), 2405
Lymphoma, 2596-2612
  in AIDS, 2608
  anti-CD20 antibody for, 2406
  biology of, 2601-2602, 2602t
  Burkitt, 2608
    Epstein-Barr virus and, 1764
  central nervous system, primary, 2608
  chromosomal translocations in, 2601-2602, 2602t
  CNS, 2316
    incidence of, 2307
  cutaneous, 559-561
    complications of, 561
    diagnosis and differential diagnosis of, 559-560, 560f
    epidemiology and etiology of, 559
    prognosis in, 561
    treatment of, 560-561
  cutaneous T cell, 2609
  diagnosis of, 2603-2605
  diffuse large B cell, 2607-2608
  epidemiology and etiology of, 2600
  epidemiology of, infectious agents in, 2376
  Epstein-Barr virus-associated, 2608
  follicular, 2605-2606
    B cell, *BCL2* in, 2392
  gastric, 2507-2508
  hematopoietic stem cell transplantation for, 1224
  histologic classification of, 2600-2601, 2600t, 2601f-2602f
  Hodgkin. *See* Hodgkin disease
  large cell, anaplastic, 2609
  lymphoblastic, 2608-2609
  mantle cell, 2607
  marginal-zone, 2606-2607
  mucosa-associated lymphoid tissue, 2606-2607
  peripheral T cell, 2609
  pleural effusion in, 2828
  pulmonary
    chronic diffuse infiltration in, 2769
    focal infiltrates in, 2745
  small lymphocytic, 2606
  staging and prognosis in, 2604-2605, 2606f, 2605t
  thrombocytopenic purpura with, 1169
  WHO classification of, 2600-2601, 2600t
Lymphomatoid granulomatosis
  cutaneous findings in, 432
  multiple pulmonary nodules in, 2756
Lymphotoxin. *See* Tumor necrosis factor-*beta* (lymphotoxin)
Lynch syndrome II. *See* Colorectal cancer, hereditary nonpolyposis
Lysosomal storage disease, 1147-1148, 1148t-1149t

M

Machado-Joseph disease (SCA3), 2264t, 2266f, 2268f, 2268t
  genetic testing in, 1959, 1960t
Macleod syndrome, 2740
Macroglobulinemia
  platelet dysfunction in, 1175, 1185
  Waldenstrom, 2593
Macrolide(s), 1433-1434. *See also individual drugs, e.g.,* Erythromycin
  for legionellosis, 1655t
Macrophage(s). *See also* Monocyte-macrophage(s)
Macrophage migration inhibitory factor, in sepsis, 1448
Macule, definition of, 426t
Mad cow disease (bovine spongiform encephalopathy), 2358, 2359
Magnesium
  dietary, 30
  intravenous, for acute myocardial infarction, 329
Magnesium sulfate, in cardiac resuscitation, 144t
Magnetic resonance imaging (MRI)
  in acute pancreatitis, 917
  of brain, in systemic lupus erythematosus, 1335
  in brain trauma, 2231, 2231f, 2233
  in brain tumor, 2311-2312, 2313f
  in epilepsy, 2191, 2191f
  in headache, 2151, 2155t
  in herpes simplex encephalitis, 2348, 2345f
  in multiple sclerosis, 2325-2327, 2326f-2327f
  in myositis, 1355, 1355f
  in osteomyelitis, 1546
  in pelvic mass, 1057
  in pulmonary embolism, 415
  in rheumatoid arthritis, 1306
Magnetic resonance spectroscopy, in myositis, 1356
Major histocompatibility complex (MHC). *See also* HLA antigen(s)
  class II antigens of, deficiency, 1230t
Malabsorption, 824-836
  in abetalipoproteinemia, 832
  bile acid absorption tests for, 826-827, 827f
  clinical manifestations of, 824
  in Crohn disease, 833
  definition of, 824
  in diabetes mellitus, 835
  diseases causing, 827-835
  in eosinophilic gastroenteritis, 832-833
  etiology of, 824, 824t
  fecal fat analysis for, 825, 825t
  in gluten-sensitive enteropathy, 827-829, 828f
  imaging studies for, 825-826, 825t
  in immunoproliferative small intestinal disease, 831-832, 831f
  intestinal lymphangiectasia, 832
  pancreatic exocrine function in, 826, 825t, 824
  in pancreatitis, chronic, 834
  in postgastrectomy steatorrhea, 834-835
  in radiation enteritis, 831
  in short bowel syndrome, 830-831
  in small intestinal amyloidosis, 834
  small intestine biopsy for, 826, 825t
  in stasis (bacterial overgrowth) syndrome, 833-834
  in systemic mastocytosis, 834
  tests for, 825-827, 825t
  in Whipple disease, 831
  xylose absorption test for, 825, 825t
Malaria, 1892-1897
  advice for travelers, 1897
  chemoprophylaxis for, 76-78
    atovaquone-proguanil, 78
    chloroquine, 77, 77f
    doxycycline, 78
    mefloquine, 77-78
    during pregnancy, 78
    primaquine, 78
    proguanil, 78
    sulfadoxine with pyrimethamine, 78
  chloroquine-resistant (CRPF), areas with, 77f, 77
  clinical features of, 1893-1894, 1893t
  diagnosis of, 1893-1895, 1893t, 1895f
  etiology and epidemiology of, 1892
  insect repellents for, 75
  laboratory findings in, 1894-1895, 1895f
  pathogenesis of, 1892-1893, 1894f-1895f
  Plasmodium, hemolytic anemia in, 1129
  resistance, sickle trait erythrocytes and, 1113
  travelers' advisories on, 76-77
  treatment of, 1895-1897, 1896f
Malassezia furfur, 507
Malassezia infections, 509-510
  folliculitis, 509
  tinea versicolor, 508, 509f
Maldigestion. *See* Malabsorption
Male(s)
  having sex with males, sexually transmitted disease in, 1529-1530
  infertility in, 1002, 1006t-1007t
  urethritis in, 1521-1523
Malignancy. *See* Cancer, *specific anatomic sites*
Malignant hyperthermia. *See* Hyperthermia, malignant
Mallet toe, 1397
Mallory-Weiss tear, 864
Malnutrition. *See also* Nutritional support
  effects of, 940
  etiology of, 940
Malta fever, 1664. *See also* Brucellosis
Mammalian bite(s), 180-182, 181t-182t
Mammography, for breast cancer screening, 45-46, 2461
Mammomonogamosis, 1928-1929
Mania. *See* Bipolar disorder
Manipulative therapies, alternative, 86-87
Mannitol, hyponatremia due to, 1980t
Mannometry, esophageal, for dysphagia, 759
Mansonella ozzardi, 1929t
Mansonella perstans, 1929t
Mansonella streptocerca, 1929t
Marburg virus disease, 1853
March hemoglobinuria, 1123
Marie-Unna syndrome, 569
Marine envenomations, 192-194
  annelida, 193
  coelenterates, 192
  echinodermata, 192-193
  porifera, 193
  toxic invertebrates, 192-193
  toxic vertebrates, 193-194
  waterborne infections, 194, 194t

Maroteaux-Lamy syndrome, 1148t
Massage therapy, 87
Mast cell(s), in immediate hypersensitivity, 1244-1246, 1244f-1245f
Mastectomy
  in early invasive breast cancer, with radiotherapy, 2464
  prophylactic, for breast cancer prevention, 2460
Mastocytosis
  cutaneous findings in, 436, 436f
  systemic, malabsorption in, 834
Mastoiditis, candidal, 1877t
Maxacalcitol, for psoriasis, 465-466
Mayaro virus, 1858
Mayer-Rokitansky-Kuster-Hauser syndrome (mullerian agenesis), 954
McArdle disease (muscle phosphorylase deficiency), 2278, 2279f
McCune-Albright syndrome, pituitary adenoma in, 591
MDM-2, properties of, 2384t
Measles, 1768-1769, 1769f
Measles immunization, 1771
  for HIV-infected patients, 1830t
  for travelers, 71
Meat, dietary, 31
  colorectal cancer and, 2477
Mechanical ventilation, 2813-2814, 2813f-2814f
  complications of, 2816-2820
    acute renal failure, 2820
    alveolar overdistention, 2817-2818, 2817f-2818f
    atelectasis, 2818, 2819f
    gastrointestinal bleeding, 2819
    neuromuscular weakness, 2819
    nonpulmonary, 2819-2820
    pneumonia, 1471, 2816-2817
    pressure ulcers, 2819
    pulmonary, 2816-2819
    sinusitis, 2817
    venous thromboembolism, 2819
  pressure-support, 2813, 2813f
  in respiratory failure
    in ARDS, 2816, 2816f
    with asthma, 2815-2816
    with COPD, 2815
  selecting settings for, 2814, 2814f
  terminal wean in, 109-110
  volume-cycled and pressure-cycled, 2813, 2813f
  withdrawal of, 2820-2821, 2820t
Mechlorethamine, 2415t
Median nerve compression, in rheumatoid arthritis, 1305
Mediastinal granuloma, 2838-2839
Mediastinal lipomatosis, 2838-2839
Mediastinal lymph nodes, accessibility of, by diagnostic modes, 2691t
Mediastinal mass, 2838-2839
  anterior, 2839
  middle, 2839
  posterior, 2839
Mediastinitis
  acute, 2837-2838
  fibrosing, 2838-2839
    in histoplasmosis, 1864
  granulomatous, 2838-2839
    in histoplasmosis, 1864
Mediastinoscopy, 2696
Mediastinum
  invasive diagnostic and therapeutic techniques for, 2687-2696, 2687t
  normal anatomy, 2836, 2836f
  widening of, 2838-2839, 2838t
    diffuse, 2838
Medical ethics. *See* Ethical and

social issues
Medical literature, critical appraisal, 8, 8t
Meditation, 86t
Mediterranean fever, 1664. *See also* Brucellosis
  familial, fever of undetermined origin in, 1416
Mediterranean spotted fever, 1728
Medullary sponge kidney, 2100, 2100f
Medulloblastoma, 2316, 2311t
Mee lines, of nails, 573
Mefloquine, for malaria chemoprophylaxis, for travelers, 77-78
Megacolon, 858
  toxic, 792
    treatment of, 805
Megakaryocyte(s), in platelet production, 1159-1160
Megaloblastic anemia, 1099-1104
  cobalamin deficiency, 1100-1103
    causes of, 1102, 1103t
    clinical findings in, 1100-1101
    diagnosis of, 1100-1102
    diagnostic workup in, 1101-1102
    Schilling test for, 1102
    treatment of, 1102-1103
  folic acid deficiency, 1103-1104
    diagnosis of, 1103-1104, 1104t
    treatment of, 1104
Megestrol acetate, 2420t
Melanocytic nevus, 538-539, 539f. *See also under* Nevus
Melanocytic tumor, 538-541
Melanoma, 552-556
  diagnosis of, 553-554, 552f-553f
  differential diagnosis in, 554
  dysplastic nevi, 552-553, 553f, 552t
  epidemiology and etiology of, 552
  familial, CNS tumors in, 2310t
  management of, IL-2 for, 2404-2405
  prognosis in, 555-556, 556t-557t
  risk factors for, 538-539
  staging in, 555, 555t-556t
  treatment of, 554-555
    adjuvant therapy in, 555
    distant metastases, 554-555
    in-transit metastases, 554
    lymph nodes, 554
    primary site, 554
Melanonychia striata, 574-575, 574f
Melanosis, neurocutaneous, 541
Melasma, 578, 578f
MELAS syndrome, 1952, 1952t, 2281
Melioidosis
  multifocal pulmonary infiltrates in, 2747
  multiple pulmonary nodules in, 2755
Melphalan, 2415t
Memorial Symptom Assessment Scale, 100, 102t
MEN1, properties of, 2386t
Menarche, 951
Meniere disease, 2144, 2145f, 2145t
Meningioma, 2315, 2311t
Meningitis
  acute bacterial, 1550-1554
    clinical features of, 1550
    complications and prognosis in, 1554
    epidemiology of, 1550
    etiology of, 1550, 1550t
    laboratory findings in, 1550-1551, 1551f, 1552t
    treatment of, 1551-1554, 1552t-1553t
  after neurosurgery, 1556
  anthrax, 1595
  arenavirus, 2353
  aseptic. *See also* Meningitis, viral

candidal, 1877t
chronic, in sarcoidosis, 2772
cryptococcal, in HIV infection, 1840-1841, 1841t-1842t
enteroviral, 1795-1796, 1794t, 2346
Escherichia coli, 1553t
  gonococcal, treatment of, 1624t
Haemophilus influenzae, 1649
  antibiotics for, 1553t
herpes simplex virus type 2, 2347
HIV, 2352
Klebsiella pneumoniae, 1553t
Listeria monocytogenes, 1590-1591
  antibiotics for, 1553t
in Lyme disease, 1724
meningococcal
  acute, 1618
  antibiotics for, 1553t
Mollaret, 1757
mumps, 2347
nocardial, 1593
nonviral causes of, 2346t
nosocomial, 1556
pneumococcal, 1565
posttraumatic, 1554-1555
Proteus, 1553t
Pseudomonas aeruginosa, 1660-1661
  antibiotics for, 1553t
recurrent nontraumatic, 1555, 1555t
Staphylococcus aureus, 1577
  antibiotics for, 1553t
streptococcal
  group A, antibiotics for, 1553t
  group B, antibiotics for, 1553t
Streptococcus pneumoniae, antibiotics for, 1553t
syphilitic, 1700
tuberculous, 1682
viral, 2344-2354
  clinical manifestations of, 2344, 2344t
  diagnosis of, 2344-2345, 2346t
  nonspecific treatment of, 2345-2346
Meningococcal bacteremia, 1618
Meningococcal infection, immunization for, for travelers, 73-74, 75f
Meningococcal sepsis, 1618
Meningococcemia, 1618, 1619f
  rash in, 439
Meningoencephalitis
  adenovirus, 2352
  arenavirus, 2353
  Epstein-Barr, 2351
  Listeria monocytogenes, 1590-1591
Menopause, 1027-1040
  clinical manifestations of, 1031-1032
  definitions of, 1027, 1027f
  diagnosis of, 1031-1033
  differential diagnosis of, 1033
  epidemiology of, 1027
  hormonal changes in, 1028-1030, 1028f-1029f
  hormone therapy in, 1035-1036, 1035t
  imaging studies in, 1033
  Internet resources for, 1034
  laboratory tests in, 1032-1033
  management considerations in, 1035-1036, 1035t
  natural, 1027-1033
  pelvic mass and, 1060-1061, 1062
  physical examination in, 1032
  physiology and genetics in, 1027-1028
  preventive health care in, 1036, 1035t, 1037t
  symptom management in, 1033-1035
  target tissues in, 1030-1031
    bone, 1030
    cardiovascular system, 1030

central and sympathetic nervous system, 1030
coagulation factors, 1030-1031
endometrium, 1030
genitourinary epithelium, 1030
integument, 1031
neoplastic growth and, 1031
transition to, 1033-1035
urinary tract infection in, 1509
Menstrual cycle, irregular and infrequent, treatment of, 981-982
Menstrual disorder
  excessive bleeding, pelvic mass and, 1055
  in menopause, 1033
Menstruation, 950-961
  clinical assessment of, 951-953, 953f
  hormonal integration of, 950-951, 951f-952f
  physiology of, 950-953
Mental-status examination
  in Alzheimer disease, 2220-2221
  in bipolar disorder, 2620-2621
  in depression, 2615-2616
Meralgia paresthetica, 1396, 2296-2297
Mercaptopurine, 2417t
6-Mercaptopurine, for inflammatory bowel disease, 801-802
Mercury, biologic test of exposure to, 61t
Merkel cell tumors, 556
Meropenem, 1430
  in pregnancy, 1422t
MERRF syndrome, 1952, 1952t, 2281
Mesalamine, for inflammatory bowel disease, 800, 801t
Mesenteric venous thrombosis, 422-423
Mesothelioma, 2554
  asbestos exposure and, 2377, 2554
  features of, 2550t
  treatment of, 2556
MET, properties of, 2384t
Metabolic acidosis, 1994-2002
  in acute renal failure, 2037-2038
  anion gap in, 1994-1999
    high, 1995-1997, 1998t
    normal, 1997-1999, 1998t
  in bicarbonate loss, 1998
  in chronic renal failure, 2044
    treatment of, 2001
  clinical manifestations of, 1999-2000
  diagnosis of, 1999-2000
  due to acid and chloride administration, 1998
  due to ingested agents and toxins, 1996-1997
  in ketoacidosis, 1996. *See* Ketoacidosis
    treatment of, 2001
  laboratory tests in, 2000
  in lactic acidosis, 1995-1996
    treatment of, 2001
  plasma potassium in, 1999
  in reduced renal hydrogen ion excretion, 1999, 1995f
  in renal failure, 1995
  in renal tubular acidosis, type 1, treatment of, 2001-2002
  in rhabdomyolysis, 1996
  treatment of, 2000-2002
Metabolic alkalosis, 2002-2005
  in alkali administration, 2003
  in Bartter syndrome, 2004
  causes of, 2002-2004, 2002t
  chloride depletion in, 2003-2004, 2003f
  clinical manifestations of, 2004
  contraction, 2003

diagnosis of, 2004
effective volume depletion in, 2003, 1995f
in gastrointestinal hydrogen loss, 2002
in Gitelman syndrome, 2004
in hypercalcemia, 2003
in hypokalemia, 2003-2004, 2003f, 2006
in intracellular hydrogen shift, 2003
laboratory tests in, 2004
in renal hydrogen loss, 2002-2003, 2003f, 2002t
treatment of, 2004-2005
Metabolic effects, of exercise, 33-34, 34f
Metabolic syndrome, 652-653, 718, 719t, 736-737, 737t
  diagnosis of, 736-737, 737t
  etiology and risk factors in, 736
  pathophysiology of, 736-737, 734f
  in polycystic ovary syndrome, 977, 980
  tests for, 979
  treatment of, 737
Metabolism, hormonal regulation of, 633-634, 634f-638f
Metachromatic leukodystrophy, 1149t, 2332
Metagonimus yokogawai infection, 1936
Metals, neuropathy due to, 2303-2304
Metapneumonia virus, 1783-1784
Metastasis
  to brain, 2317, 2431-2432
  drugs for inhibition of, 2423
  to heart, 382-383
  to intramedullary spinal cord, 2434
  to leptomeninges, 2317, 2434
  to lung, multiple nodules in, 2756, 2756f
  molecular genetics of, 2393-2394
  to nervous system, 2316-2317
  to pleura, pleural effusion in, 2828
  to spinal cord, 2317
Metformin
  for hirsutism, 991-992
  for polycystic ovary syndrome, 983
  for type 2 diabetes mellitus, 659, 658t
Metformin plus clomiphene, for polycystic ovary syndrome, 983
Methanol, poisoning or overdose with, 168, 168t
  elimination method for, 161t
  metabolic acidosis due to, 1996-1997, 2001
Methemoglobinemia, 171, 1119
  drugs causing, 171
Methionine, colorectal cancer and, 2477-2478
Methotrexate, 2416t
  for asthma, 2710t
  chronic diffuse infiltrative pulmonary disease due to, 2762
  for ectopic pregnancy, 1012-1013, 1012t
  for inflammatory bowel disease, 802
  for myositis, 1357, 1357t
  for psoriasis, 468-469
  for rheumatoid arthritis, 1309, 1308t
Methyldopa
  autoimmune hemolytic anemia due to, 1126
  for hypertension, 223t
Methylenedioxymethamphetamine (MDMA)
  (ecstasy), 165

Methylphenidate (Ritalin) toxicity, 165
Methylprednisolone, for asthma, 2710t
Methyl tert-butyl ether, for gallstones, 906
Metoclopramide, for gastroesophageal reflux disease, 766
Metolazone, for hypertension, 221t
Metoprolol
  toxicity of, 163t
  for unstable angina and NSTMI, 312t
Metoprolol fumarate, for hypertension, 222t
Metoprolol succinate, for hypertension, 222t
Metorchis conjunctus infection, 1936
Metronidazole, 1435
  for Helicobacter infection, 1637t
  for inflammatory bowel disease, 802
  in pregnancy, 1422t
Metyrapone testing, for pituitary function, 598
Mexiletine, classification of, 267t
Mezlocillin, 1428
MHC. See Major histocompatibility complex (MHC)
Mice tapeworm, 1939
Microangiopathy, thrombotic, 2428
Microbial disease, chemotherapy for. See Antibiotic(s)
Microbial flora, of upper respiratory tract, 1456, 1458t
Microbial superinfection, due to antibiotic use, 1424
Microlithiasis, pulmonary, 2784
Microscopic colitis syndrome, 848
Microsporidiosis, 1908-1909, 1909f
Microvolt T wave alternans, in asymptomatic ventricular ectopy, 263
Midfoot pain, 1397
Miglitol, for type 2 diabetes mellitus, 658-659, 658t
Migraine headache. See Headache, migraine
Milia, acne vulgaris vs., 447
Milium, 537, 537f
Milk-alkali syndrome, 2003
Milwaukee shoulder-knee syndrome, 1380
Mind-body interventions, 84-85, 85f, 86t
Mineral(s), dietary, 28-30, 30t
Mineral acids, inhalation or ingestion of, 165t
Mineralocorticoid resistance (pseudohypoaldosteronism), 688
Minimal change disease, 2066-2067, 2066t, 2066f
Minocycline, for acne vulgaris, 450t
Minoxidil, for hypertension, 223t
Mirizzi syndrome, 908
Mitochondrial encephalopathy, 2280-2281
  neurogastrointestinal, 2281
Mitochondrial inheritance, 1951-1952, 1952t
Mitochondrial myopathy, 2280-2281
Mitomycin-C, 2416t
Mitoxantrone, 2418t
Mitral prolapse, 355
  in diagnosis of palpitation, 204t
Mitral regurgitation, 353-355, 348t, 350t
  in acute myocardial infarction, 330-331
  clinical manifestations of, 353, 350t
  imaging studies in, 353
  murmur in, 210t

treatment of, 354-355, 356f
Mitral stenosis, 350-353, 348t, 350t
  balloon mitral valvuloplasty for, 352-353, 353f
  clinical manifestations of, 351, 350t
  imaging studies in, 351-352, 352f
  murmur in, 210t
  surgical commissurotomy for, 353
  treatment of, 352-353, 353f
Mitral valvuloplasty, balloon, for mitral stenosis, 352-353, 353f
MLH1, properties of, 2386t
MMR vaccination, 1771
Moexipril, for hypertension, 222t
Mofetil, after liver transplantation, complications of, 934
Mole, definition of, 535
Mollaret meningitis, 1757
Mollusca, 193
Molluscum contagiosum, 1774, 1773f
  in AIDS, 437
  in atopic dermatitis, 476
Mongolian spot, 540, 540f
Moniliasis. See under Candidiasis
Monkey bite, 181, 182t
Monkey B virus disease, 1858
Monkeypox, 1774
Monoamine oxidase inhibitors (MAOIs), for depression, 2616-2617
Monobactam(s), 1431
Monoclonal antibody(ies), for prerenal-transplant patient management, 2119
Monoclonal gammopathy of undetermined significance, 2590
Monocyte-macrophage(s), 1144-1145
  development of, 1072f, 1145
  functions of, 1145
Monocyte-macrophage colony-stimulating factor, 1073f
Mononeuritis multiplex, in rheumatoid arthritis, 1305
Mononucleosis, infectious
  CMV, 1762
  Epstein-Barr, 1763-1764
Monosodium glutamate (MSG) poisoning, 175-176
Montelukast, for asthma, 2710t, 2713
Moraxella catarrhalis, pneumonia due to, 1469
Moraxella catarrhalis infection, 1651-1652, 1651t
Moricizine, classification of, 267t
Morphea, in scleroderma, 443
Morphine sulfate, for unstable angina and NSTMI, 313, 312t
Morquio syndrome, 1148t
Morton neuroma, 1397, 1397f
Mosquito-borne infections, insect repellents and, 75
Motorcyclist injury, 22
Motor vehicle injury, 21-22
Mouth, dry, palliative treatment of, 106-107, 109t
Movement disorders, 2239-2262. See also individual disorders, e.g., Parkinsonism
  drug-induced and toxin-induced, 2255t, 2260-2261
  hyperkinetic, 2253-2260
  hypokinetic, 2239-2253
  pathophysiology of, 2239, 2240f-2241f
Moxifloxacin, 1438-1439, 1438t
MRI. See Magnetic resonance imaging
MSH2, properties of, 2386t, 2391
mtDNA depletion syndrome, 2281
Mucha-Habermann disease (pityriasis lichenoides), 457-458, 457f
Mucocutaneous lymph node syndrome

(Kawasaki disease), 1367-1368, 1368t
  cutaneous findings in, 433
  renal involvement in, 2075
Mucoepidermoid carcinoma, of lung, 2750
Mucolipidosis, 1148t
Mucopolysaccharidosis, 1148t
Mucormycosis, pulmonary, large mass in, 2754, 2755f
Muehrcke nails, 573
Muir-Torre syndrome, 538
Mullerian agenesis (Mayer-Rokitansky-Kuster-Hauser syndrome), 954
Mullerian inhibiting substance, in polycystic ovary syndrome, 978-979
Multiple chemical sensitivity(ies), 67
Multiple endocrine neoplasia, type I (MEN I)
  CNS tumors in, 2310t
  pituitary adenoma in, 591
Multiple myeloma, 2589-2593
  anemia in, 2591
  Bence Jones protein, 2096-2097, 2097f
  bone disease in, 2590-2591, 2591f
  clinical presentation in, 2590-2591, 2590t, 2591f
  diagnosis of, 2590-2591
  epidemiology of, 2589-2590
  hypercalcemia in, 2591
  hyperviscosity in, 2591
  immunology of, 2590
  infectious disease in, 2591
  monoclonal gammopathy of undetermined significance in, 2590
  neurologic symptoms in, 2591
  osteosclerotic, 2302
  pathogenesis of, 2590
  plasmacytomas in, 2590
  platelet function in, 1185
  renal insufficiency in, 2591
  staging and prognostic factors in, 2591-2592, 2592t
  therapy for, 2592-2593
    indications for, 2592
    in relapsed/refractory disease, 2593
    standard, 2592-2593
    stem cell transplant, 2593, 1224
  tubulointerstitial nephritis in, 2096-2097, 2097f
Multiple organ dysfunction syndrome (MODS)
  definition of, 1443t
  in sepsis, 1448-1449
  in septic shock, 1450, 1450t, 1452
Multiple sclerosis, 2323-2331
  cerebrospinal fluid studies in, 2327-2328
  clinical course of, 2325
  clinical features of, 2324-2325, 2325t
  clinically isolated syndromes in, 2329
  diagnosis of, 2324-2328, 2325t
  differential diagnosis of, 2328
  epidemiology of, 2323
  etiology of, 2323-2324
  evoked response in, 2328
  genetics of, 2324
  laboratory tests for, 2325-2328
  Marburg type, 2328
  MRI for, 2325-2327, 2326f-2327f
  pathology in, 2324
  plasma exchange in, 1218
  in pregnancy, 1023
  prognosis in, 2330-2331
  progressive, 2329-2330
  relapse in, 2328-2329

symptomatic therapy, 2330, 2331t
    ataxia and intention tremor in, 2330
    bladder dysfunction, 2330
    depression and fatigue, 2330
    pain, 2330
    spasticity, 2330
  treatment of, 2328-2331
  variants of, 2328
  vertigo in, 2148
Multiple system atrophy, 2250-2252, 2251f
Mumps, 1769-1770
  encephalomyelitis in, 2347
  immunization against, 1771
    for HIV-infected patients, 1830t
  meningitis in, 2347
  orchitis in, 693
Mupirocin, 1440
  intranasal, for staphylococcal carrier state, 1580
Murmur
  in cardiovascular patient, 208-212, 209t-210t, 209f, 211f
  innocent flow, 210t
Murray Valley encephalitis, 1854
Muscle
  diseases of. See also individual disorders, e.g., Muscular dystrophy
  energy requirements, 2278, 2279f
Muscle biopsy, in fever of undetermined origin, 1417
Muscle-eye-brain disease, 2275-2276
Muscle phosphorylase deficiency (McArdle disease), 2278, 2279f
Muscular dystrophy, 2270-2277
  autosomal dominant, with unique phenotype, 2276-2277
  Becker, 2273, 2271f, 2272t
    genetic testing in, 1960-1961
  classification of, 2270, 2272t
  congenital, 2275-2276
    Fukuyama, 2275
    with joint contractures, 2276
  cytoskeletal protein defects in, 2270, 2271f
  Duchenne, 2270-2273, 2271f, 2272t
    carrier testing in, 1963-1964
    genetic testing in, 1960-1961
    respiratory insufficiency in, 2807
  dystrophinopathy, 2270-2273, 2271f, 2272t
    female carriers and, 2273
    X-linked dilated cardiomyopathy in, 2273
  Emery-Dreifuss, 2273-2274
  facioscapulohumeral, 2277
  intermediate filament protein mutations in, 2276
  limb-girdle, 2274-2276
    autosomal dominant, 2274
    autosomal recessive, 2274-2275
  oculopharyngeal, 1960t, 2277
  rigid spine syndrome, 2276
  X-linked recessive, 2270-2274
Musculoskeletal problem(s), common, 1391-1398. See also individual problems, e.g., Back pain
Musculoskeletal response, to exercise, 33
Musculoskeletal tuberculosis, 1680-1681, 1681f
Mushroom poisoning, 175
Music therapy, 86t
Myasthenia gravis, 2284-2287
  apheresis for, 1218
  autoantibodies in, 1236-1237, 2285, 2286f
  clinical manifestations in, 2286
  diagnosis of, 2286-2287
  epidemiology of, 2285

immunopathogenesis of, 2285-2286, 2286f
immunoregulation in, 2285-2286
in pregnancy, 1023
respiratory insufficiency in, 2806-2807
thymoma in, 2839
treatment of, 2287
Myasthenic syndrome
congenital, 2288
Eaton-Lambert, 2287, 2319
respiratory insufficiency in, 2807
myc, in lymphoma, 2601
Mycobacterial infection. *See also* Tuberculosis
Mycobacterium avium complex infection, in HIV infection
management, 1841t-1842t, 1841
prophylactic measures for prevention of, 1840t
Mycobacterium leprae. See also Leprosy
Mycobacterium marinum, in septic arthritis, 1538
Mycobacterium tuberculosis
prophylactic measures for prevention of, in HIV infection, 1840t
in septic arthritis, 1538
Mycophenolate mofetil
after liver transplantation, complications of, 934
for prerenal-transplant patient management, 2117-2118
for psoriasis, 470
Mycoplasma genitalium, in nongonococcal urethritis, 1741
Mycoplasma hominis
infections caused by, 1742
in nongonococcal urethritis, 1741
in pelvic inflammatory disease, 1742
in postabortion fever, 1742
in postpartum fever, 1742
in pyelonephritis, 1742
Mycoplasmal infection, 1737-1742
antimicrobial drugs for, 1427t
genitourinary, 1741-1742
Mycoplasmal pneumonia, 1737-1741
diagnosis of, 1739-1740, 1740t
epidemiology of, 1737-1738
etiology of, 1737-1738
extrapulmonary manifestations of, 1739-1740
incidence of, 1737
laboratory testing in, 1740, 1740t
pathogenesis, pathology, immunity in, 1738-1739
segmental pulmonary infiltrates in, 2750, 2750f
transmission of, 1737, 1737f
treatment of, 1740-1741, 1741t
Mycoplasma pneumoniae, 1737. *See also* Mycoplasmal pneumonia
Mycoplasma species, 1737
Mycotic infection, 1861-1874. *See also specific infection, e.g.,* Blastomycosis
antifungal therapy for, 1870-1873, 1871t-1872t. *See also Antifungal agent(s)*
in compromised host, 1875-1891
Mydriasis, benign episodic, 2156
Myelinolysis, central pontine, 2332
Myelitis
in Lyme disease, 1714
transverse, 2332
in systemic lupus erythematosus, 1334
Myelodysplastic syndrome, 2563-2564, 2564t
hematopoietic stem cell

transplantation for, 1223
subtypes of, 2564t
treatment of, 2569-2570
Myelofibrosis
hematopoietic stem cell transplantation for, 1223
idiopathic, 2582-2583
Myelokathexis, neutropenia in, 1144t
Myeloma, multiple. *See* Multiple myeloma
Myelopathy
human T cell lymphotropic virus type I (HTLV-I) associated, 1811, 2357
in radiation therapy, 2320
Myeloperoxidase deficiency, neutrophil function in, 1146t
Myeloproliferative disorder(s), 2575-2584. *See also individual disorders, e.g.,* Leukemia
characteristics of, 2575t
platelet dysfunction in, 1174
Myelosis, chronic erythremic. *See* Myelodysplastic syndrome
Myiasis, 522
Myocardial contusion, 385
Myocardial fibrosis, in scleroderma, 1347
Myocardial infarction (MI)
acute, 317-336
ACE inhibitors for, 328
adjunctive medical therapy for, 327-329
antiarrhythmic therapy for, prophylactic, 329
atrial fibrillation in, 248, 330
beta-blocker therapy for, 328
bradyarrhythmia in, 330
calcium channel antagonists for, 329
clinical manifestations of, 317-318
complications of, 329-331
coronary angioplasty for, 325-326, 324f-325f
glycoprotein IIb/IIIa inhibitor and, 326
rescue, 326-327
coronary artery bypass graft for, 326
definitions of, 317, 317t
diagnosis of, 317-319
echocardiography in, 319
electrocardiography in, 318, 318f
emergent therapy in, 319-320
analgesia, 320
aspirin, 320, 320f
oxygen, 320
epidemiology of, 317
heart block in, 330
heparin for
intravenous, 327
low-molecular-weight, 327-328
imaging studies in, 319
laboratory findings, 318-319
magnesium for, 329
mitral regurgitation in, 330-331
myocardial rupture in, 331
nitroglycerin for, intravenous, 329
pacemaker for, 274t, 275
pathogenesis of, 317
physical examination in, 318
predischarge exercise testing after, 331-332, 332f
prognosis in, long-term, 333
radionuclide imaging in, 319
reperfusion therapy for, 320-327
angiography after uncomplicated MI and, 322
strategies and outcomes in, 320-323, 321f, 320t
timing of, 320-321, 321f, 320t

transfer for primary angioplasty *vs.,* 321-322
without ST segment elevation, 322-323, 322t
right ventricular, 331
secondary prevention of, 332-333
antiarrhythmic therapy for, 333
anticoagulant therapy for, 333
implantable cardioverter-defibrillator for, 333
lipid-lowering therapy for, 332-333
risk-factor modulation for, 333
statin therapy for, 329
stroke in, 331
thrombin inhibitors for, direct, 328
thrombolytic therapy for, 323-325, 323f-324f
ventricular arrhythmia in, 329-330
ventricular fibrillation in, 329-330
ventricular septal defects in, 331
ventricular tachycardia in, 330
asymptomatic ventricular ectopy after, 263
in cardiac arrest, 148t
chronic renal failure in, 2016
non-ST segment elevation, 304-316. *See also* Unstable angina and non-ST segment elevation MI
Myocardial ischemia, headache in, 2164
Myocardial perfusion imaging, radionuclide, in angina pectoris, 292
Myocardial rupture, in acute myocardial infarction, 331
Myocarditis, in diphtheria, 1585-1586
Myoclonus, 2259, 2255t
in general medical practice, 2259-2260
Myofascial shoulder pain syndrome, 1393
Myoglobin, as biochemical cardiac marker, 305
Myonecrosis, clostridial (gas gangrene), 1607
treatment of, 1612
vs. crepitant cellulitis, 1610-1611
Myopathy(ies). *See also individual diseases*
in alcoholism, 2284
in carnitine deficiency, 2279-2280
in carnitine palmitoyltransferase deficiency, 2280
cholesterol-lowering agent, 2283, 2283t
critical illness, 2283
drug-induced inflammatory, 2284
due to chloroquine, 2284
due to colchicine, 2284
due to interferon alfa, 2284
due to zidovudine, 2282-2283
inflammatory, idiopathic, 1351-1358
lipid storage, 2279-2280
metabolic, 2278-2280
mitochondrial, 2280-2281
steroid-induced, 2284
toxic, drug-induced, 2282-2284, 2283t
Myopericarditis, enteroviral, 1796, 1795t
Myositis, 1351-1358
autoantibodies in, 1354-1355
autoimmune, 1352-1353, 1352f

chronic diffuse infiltrative pulmonary disease in, 2780
classification of, 1351, 1351t
clinical features of, 1353-1354
calcinosis in, 1354
cardiac abnormalities in, 1353-1354
muscle weakness in, 1353
pulmonary disease in, 1353
skin changes in, 442, 442f
skin rash in, 1353, 1353f
vascular abnormalities in, 1354
computed tomography in, 1355
diagnosis of, 1353-1356
differential diagnosis of, 1356, 1356t
electromyography in, 1355
epidemiology of, 1351-1352
ethnic, racial, gender differences in, 1352
etiology and pathogenesis of, 1352-1353
genetic factors in, 1352
inclusion body, 1351
infectious agents in, 1352
juvenile, 1351
laboratory tests in, 1354-1355
magnetic resonance imaging in, 1355, 1355f
magnetic resonance spectroscopy in, 1356
with malignancy, 1351
muscle biopsy in, 1354
muscle enzymes in, 1354
noninfectious factors in, 1352
with other rheumatic diseases, 1351
prevention and incidence of, 1351-1352
in systemic lupus erythematosus, 1332
treatment of, 1356-1357, 1357t
azathioprine for, 1357, 1357t
cyclophosphamide for, 1357, 1357t
glucocorticoids in, 1356-1357, 1357t
immune globulin for, 1357, 1357t
methotrexate for, 1357, 1357t
skin and physical therapies in, 1357
ultrasonography in, 1355
underlying malignancy in, 1356
Myotonia, paradoxical, 2282
Myotonia congenita
autosomal dominant (Thomsen disease), 2282
autosomal recessive (Becker-type myotonia), 2282
Myotonic dystrophy, 2276-2277
genetics of, 1951
proximal, 2276
respiratory insufficiency in, 2807
trinucleotide repeat in, 1960t
Myxedema, 609. *See also* Hypothyroidism
Myxoid (mucus) cyst, of nail, 576t
Myxoma, cardiac, 383-384, 383f-384f
infective endocarditis *vs.,* 1490

N

Nadolol
for hypertension, 222t
toxicity of, 163t
Naegleria infection, 1909, 1910f
Nafcillin, 1424
Nail(s), 571-577
age-related findings, 572
bacterial and fungal infections of, 575-577, 575t-576t, 574f-575f
bed of, 571-572
brittle, 572

clubbing of, 574
dermatologic disorders affecting, 577, 576t
digital myxoid (mucus) cyst of, 576t
in disease states, 572-575
folds of, 572
glomus tumor of, 576t
half-and-half (Lindsay), 573
longitudinal pigmented bands in (melanonychia striata), 574-575, 574f
matrix of, 571
Mee lines of, 573
Muehrcke, 573
nail-plate pitting (onychia punctata), 574
onychomycosis of, 576-577, 575f
paronychia of
bacterial, 575
Candida, 508, 508f
chronic, 575
periungual angiofibromas of, 576t
plate of, 572
in psoriasis, 464, 464f
splinter hemorrhages of, 572
structure, function, pathophysiology of, 571-572, 571f
subungual exostoses of, 576t
Terry, 573
transverse nail plate depressions (Beau lines), 573, 573
yellow nail syndrome of, 433, 434f, 572
Naloxone, for opioid intoxication, 155-156
Naltrexone, 2644
Naproxen, metabolites of, thrombocytopenia due to, 1170
Narcolepsy, 2368
Nasogastric suction, hypernatremia and, 1987
Nasopharyngeal cancer, 2438
Epstein-Barr virus and, 1764, 2437-2438
Nateglinide, for type 2 diabetes mellitus, 658, 658t
Nausea and vomiting
hypernatremia and, 1987
hypokalemia due to, 2007
palliative treatment of, 103-104, 105t-106t
Neck pain, 1391
Necrobiosis lipoidica, in diabetes mellitus, 433
Necrotizing encephalomyelopathy, subacute, 2341
Necrotizing fasciitis, 512
cutaneous findings in, 439
streptococcal, group A, 1570
Necrotizing sarcoid granulomatosis, 2771
Nedocromil, for asthma, 2713, 2710t
Neisseria
infections due to, 1617-1625, 1617f
other species of, 1624
Neisseria gonorrhoeae. See also Gonococcal infection
chemoprophylaxis for sexual partners, 1624
clinical presentations in, 1622-1623
complications and prognosis in, 1623-1624
diagnosis of, 1522, 1522f, 1623
disseminated, 1622-1623, 1624t
epidemiology of, 1621-1622
infections caused by, 1621-1624
infections due to. See also Gonorrhea
pathogenesis of, 1622
in septic arthritis, 1536

treatment of, 1623, 1624t
Neisseria meningitidis. See also Meningococcal infection, Meningitis
classification of, 1617
clinical presentations in, 1618-1619
complications and prognosis in, 1619
diagnosis of, 1619
differential diagnosis of, 1619-1620
epidemiology and transmission of, 1617
immunization in, 1621
infections caused by, 1617-1621
pathogenesis and immunity in, 1617-1618, 1619f
preventive therapy in, 1620-1621, 1620t
reporting disease, 1621
treatment of, 1620, 1620t
Neisseria meningitidis infection, meningitis, 1553t
Nelfinavir, 1831t
for HIV infection, adverse effects of, 1834t
Nelfinavir urolithiasis, 2112
Nematode infection
intestinal, 1918-1924, 1920t
tissue, 1924-1932
Neonate. See Infant, neonatal
Neoplasia. See Cancer, Tumor(s)
Nephritic syndrome, 2054-2060
anti-glomerular basement membrane disease as, 2058-2060, 2058f-2060f
classification of, 2051, 2051t, 2053f
clinical features of, 2054
edema in, 1989
hepatitis C-associated glomerulonephritis as, 2055
IGA nephropathy, 2056-2057, 2056t, 2057f-2058f
nephrotic syndrome vs., 2051, 2051t, 2053f
postinfectious glomerulonephritis as, 2054-2056
poststreptococcal glomerulonephritis as, 2055-2056, 2055f-2056f
rapidly progressive glomerulonephritis as, 2060, 2061f
Nephritis
acute interstitial
acute renal failure in, 2035
drug-induced, 2086-2089, 2087t
due to antibiotics, 2087-2088, 2088f
due to NSAIDs, 2088
idiopathic, 2100
chronic interstitial
drug-induced, 2089-2091
due to analgesics, 2089-2090, 2089f
due to antineoplastic agents, 2091
due to cyclosporine, 2091
due to lithium, 2090
lupus, 1334, 1334t-1335t, 2077
radiation, 2092
tubulointerstitial. See Tubulointerstitial nephritis
Nephrolithiasis, 2104-2113
active stone passage in, 2104
clinical presentation in, 2104
laboratory studies in, 2104
radiologic studies, 2104, 2105f
treatment in, 2104, 2105f
workup in, 2104
calcium-containing stones in, 2106-

2110
absorptive and renal hypercalciuria, 2107-2108
in distal renal tubular acidosis, 2106
high dietary protein intake and, 2107-2108
hypercalcemia in, 2106-2107
hypercalciuria in, 2106-2107
hyperoxaluria in, 2108
hyperuricosuria in, 2108
hypocitraturia in, 2108
reduced urine volume in, 2108
risk factors for, 2106-2109
stone formation inhibitors in, 2108-2109
treatment of, 2109-2110
amiloride, 2109
cellulose phosphate, 2110
dietary modification, 2109
hydrochlorothiazide, 2109
hyperoxaluria and, 2110
neutral sodium, 2109-2110
potassium citrate, 2110
potassium phosphate, 2109-2110
calcium monohydrogen phosphate stones in, crystallographic analysis of, 2108t
calcium oxalate stones in, crystallographic analysis of, 2108t
chronic and recurrent, 2104-2106
calcium oxalate stones in, 2107f
crystallographic analysis in, 2106, 2108t
cystine stones in, 2107f
diagnosis of, 2105-2106, 2107f, 2108t
laboratory studies, 2105, 2107f
overview of management of, 2106
radiologic studies in, 2105
struvite stones in, 2107f
uric acid stones in, 2107f
cystine stones in, 2111-2112
crystallographic analysis of, 2108t
treatment of, 2111
2, 8-dihydroxyadenine stones in, 2110
drug-induced stones in, 2112
incidence of, 2104
struvite stones in, 2111
crystallographic analysis of, 2108t
treatment of, 2109-2110
uric acid stones in, 2110-2111
crystallographic analysis of, 2108t
in gout, 1374
treatment of, 2110-2111
Nephronophthisis-medullary cystic disease, 2099
Nephropathy
analgesic, 2089-2090, 2089f
Balkan, 2101
diabetic, 670-671, 670f
mechanisms of, 667-668, 668f
pancreas transplantation and, 938
prevention and treatment in, 670-671
screening for, 670
HIV-associated, 2063-2064
IgA (Berger disease), 2056-2057, 2056t, 2057f-2058f
in ankylosing spondylitis, 1320
Henoch-Schonlein purpura vs., 2057
lead, 64
membranous, 2064-2066, 2064t, 2065f-2066f
obstructive, 2091-2092
polyomavirus, 2121-2122

reflux, 2092
uric acid, 1374
Nephrosclerosis, hypertensive, 2095
Nephrotic syndrome, 1971-1972, 1970t, 2060-2067
classification of, 2051, 2051t, 2053f
clinical and laboratory findings in, 2060-2061
complications of, 2061
dyslipidemia and, 740
edema in, 1989
focal segmental glomerulosclerosis as, 2061-2063, 2062t, 2063f-2064f
HIV-associated nephropathy, 2063-2064
membranoproliferative glomerulonephritis as, 2067-2068, 2067t, 2068f
membranous nephropathy as, 2064-2066, 2064t, 2065f-2066f
minimal change disease as, 2066-2067, 2066t, 2066f
nephritic syndrome vs., 2051, 2051t, 2053f
therapeutic principles in, 2061
Nephrotoxicity
of aminoglycosides, 2032
of amphotericin B, 2032-2033
of angiotensin-converting enzyme inhibitors, 2033
cadmium-induced, 2095
Chinese-herb, 2095
of cisplatin, 2033
of ethylene glycol, 2033
lead-induced, 2094-2095
of NSAIDs, 2033
of radiocontrast, 2031-2032
Nerve biopsy, in peripheral nerve disease, 2293
Nerve conduction study(ies), for peripheral nerve disease, 2292
Nervous system
central. See Central nervous system
peripheral. See Peripheral nervous system
Nervous system tumors, 2307-2317, 2307t-2308t. See also Brain tumor
classification of, 2307, 2308t
epidemiology of, 2307
metastatic, 2316-2317
Netilmicin, 1432
NEU (erb B2), properties of, 2384t
Neuralgia
occipital, headache in, 2167
postherpetic, 1760, 2305-2306, 2349-2350
headache in, 2164
trigeminal (tic douloureux), 2294-2295, 2294t
headache in, 2154t, 2163
Neural tube defect, folic acid supplementation and, 1016
Neural tumor, of skin, 541-543
Neuritic plaque, in Alzheimer disease, 2219, 2219f
Neuritis
optic, 2331
vestibular, 2143-2144, 2144t
Neuroblastoma, mediastinal, 2839
Neurocardiogenic syncope, pacemaker for, 274t, 275
Neuroectodermal tumor, peripheral, 2553
features of, 2550t
Neuroepithelial tumor, peripheral, oncogenes in, 2385
Neurofibrillary tangle, in Alzheimer disease, 2219, 2220f
Neurofibroma, mediastinal, 2839

Neurofibromatosis, 542-543
  skin lesions in, 440, 441f
  type 1, 440, 542, 542f
    brain tumors in, 2308, 2310t
  type 2, 440, 542
    brain tumors in, 2308, 2310t
  variants of, 542-543
Neuroleptic malignant syndrome,
    158t, 1410-1411
Neuroma
  acoustic, in neurofibromatosis,
    542
  Morton, 1397, 1397f
Neuromuscular blocking agent(s),
    prolonged muscle paralysis
    after, 2807
Neuromuscular disease, 2270-2290.
    See also individual diseases,
    e.g., Muscular dystrophy
  approach to patient with, 2270
  sleep-disordered breathing in,
    2798
Neuromuscular junction
  diseases of. See also individual
    disorders, e.g., Muscular
    dystrophy
  normal, 2284, 2285f
  transmission at, 2284, 2285f
Neuromuscular transmission,
    disorders of, 2284-2288
Neuromyelitis optica (Devic
    disease), 2328
Neuromyotonia
  autoimmune acquired (Isaac
    disease), 2282
  with K^+ channel autoantibodies
    (Isaac syndrome), 2287-2288
Neuropathy(ies). See also
    Polyneuropathy(ies)
  in AIDS, 2304-2305
  in alcoholism, 2304
  brachial plexus, 2296
  in connective tissue disease, 2303
  cranial, common types of, 2294t
  diabetic. See Polyneuropathy(ies),
    diabetic
  in diphtheria, 1586
  distinctive, 2297t
  drug-induced, 2303, 2299t
  due to radiation injury, 2321
  facial (Bell palsy), 2293-
    2294, 2294t
  herpes simplex virus, 2348-2349
  in Lyme disease, 2305
  metals causing, 2303-2304
  nutritional, 2304
  occupational, 64-65
  oculomotor, 2294t, 2295
  paraneoplastic, 2302
  peripheral. See Peripheral nerve
    disease
  peroneal, 2296
  in rheumatoid arthritis, 1305
  sensory, paraneoplastic, 2318-2319
  stocking-and-glove, in systemic
    lupus erythematosus, 1334
  toxic, 2303-2304, 2303t
  ulnar, 2296
  in uremia, 2300
  in varicella-zoster virus
    infection, 2305-2306
  vasculitic, 2302-2303
Neurosarcoma, 2552
  features of, 2550t
Neurosurgery, meningitis after, 1556
Neurosyphilis, 1700-1701. See also
    Syphilis
  laboratory findings in, 1702
  meningovascular, 1700
  parenchymatous, 1700
  treatment of, 1706, 1705t
Neurotoxicity
  due to anticancer chemotherapy,

2319-2320, 2319t
  due to radiation therapy, 2320-
    2321
Neutropenia, 1141-1144
  autoimmune, 1142-1143
  congenital, 1144t
  cyclic, 1144t
  diagnosis and treatment of, 1143-
    1144
  drug-induced, 1142, 1143t
  fever and, neoplastic, 2428-2429
  idiopathic, 1142-1143
  infection in, 1142
  intrinsic neutrophil disorders in,
    1144t
  neonatal, 1143
Neutrophil(s), 1137-1144
  adherence of, 1138, 1141f
  bacterial killing, 1139-1140, 1140f
  chemotaxis by, 1139, 1140f
  cytokines and, 1140
  cytoskeleton of, 1138
  degranulation in, 1139, 1140f
  development of, 1072f, 1074-1075
  disorders of, 1141-1144. See also
    Neutropenia, Neutrophilia
  functions of, 1138-1140
    disorders of, 1144, 1146t, 1147f
  granules of, 1137
  oxidative metabolism in, 1139-
    1140, 1140f
  production of, 1137, 1139f
  recognition and phagocytosis,
    1139, 1140f
  in sepsis, 1447, 1448f
  structure of, 1137-1138, 1138f
Neutrophil count, absolute, 1137
Neutrophilia, 1141-1142
  in low glucose CSF, 1552t, 1551
  primary, 1141
  secondary, 1141
Nevirapine, for HIV infection, 1831t
  adverse effects of, 1834t
Nevoid basal cell carcinoma
    syndrome, CNS tumors in, 2310t
Nevus
  basal cell, 440
  Becker, 540-541, 541f
  blue, 540, 541f
  congenital giant, pigmented,
    541, 541f
  definition of, 535
  dysplastic, in malignant melanoma,
    552, 552f, 552t
  epidermal, 440, 441f, 535-536, 536f
  halo, 540, 540f
  melanocytic, 538-539, 539f
  spindle cell, 540, 540f
Nevus flammeus (port-wine stain),
    545, 544f
Nevus of Ota, 540
Nevus unius lateris, 535-536, 536f
Newborn. See Infant, neonatal
Newcastle disease virus infection,
    1859
NF-1, properties of, 2386t, 2391
NF-2, properties of, 2386t, 2391
Nicardipine, for hypertensive
    crisis, 228t
Nicardipine extended release, for
    hypertension, 221t
Nicotine, for inflammatory bowel
    disease, 803
Nicotine addiction, 19. See also
    Cigarette smoking, Tobacco
Nicotine gum, 19
Nicotine patch, transdermal, 19
Niemann-Pick disease, 1149t
Nifedipine extended release, for
    hypertension, 221t
Nilutamide, 2420t
Nipah virus, 1857
Nipple, Paget disease of, 556

Nisoldipine, for hypertension, 221t
Nitrate(s)
  for angina pectoris, 299
  for unstable angina and NSTMI, 312-
    313, 312t
Nitric oxide
  in coagulation, 1157, 1158f
  in sepsis, 1447-1448
Nitrofurantoin, 1439-1440
  chronic diffuse infiltrative
    pulmonary disease due to, 2763
  in pregnancy, 1422t
Nitroglycerin
  for angina pectoris, 299
  intravenous, for acute myocardial
    infarction, 329
NMDA receptor channel blockers,
    abuse of, 2637
N-myc, properties of, 2384, 2384t
Nocardia asteroides, 1592, 1592f
Nocardiosis, 1592-1593
  brain abscess in, 1593
  central nervous system, 1593
  cutaneous, 1593
  disseminated, 1593
  meningitis in, 1593
  pulmonary, 1592-1593
    multiple nodules in, 2755
Nocturia, 1041
Nocturnal frontal lobe epilepsy,
    2371
Nocturnal hemoglobinuria,
    paroxysmal. See Hemoglobinuria,
    paroxysmal nocturnal
Nodule, definition of, 426t
Nondysgerminoma, ovarian, 2541
Nonherbal dietary supplements, 89t
Non-Hodgkin lymphoma. See
    Lymphoma
Noninsulinoma pancreatogenous
    hypoglycemia syndrome, 631
Non-rapid eye movement (NREM) sleep,
    2362, 2363f
Nonseminoma, 2519-2520. See also
    Testicular cancer
Nonsteroidal anti-inflammatory drugs
    (NSAIDs). See also Aspirin,
    Salicylate(s)
  acute interstitial nephritis due
    to, 2088
  allergy to, 1275
  asthma due to, 2706-2707
  colorectal cancer and, 2478
  gastroesophageal reflux disease
    disease due to, 764-765
  GI bleeding due to, 863-864
  for gout, 1375-1376
  nephropathy due to, 2090
  nephrotoxicity due to, 2033
  for pain, 2183-2184, 2184t
  peptic ulcer disease due to, 776-
    778, 777f
  platelet functional effects of,
    1175
  for rheumatoid arthritis, 1308-
    1309, 1308t
  urticaria due to, 1260
Norepinephrine, for septic shock,
    1451
Norgestimate-ethinyl estradiol, for
    acne vulgaris, 450t
Norwalk virus infection, 1799-1800
Nosocomial infection
  diarrhea, 842
  Moraxella catarrhalis, 1652
  pneumonia, 1470, 1473-1474
  Pseudomonas aeruginosa, 1659
N-ras, properties of, 2384t
NSAIDs. See Nonsteroidal anti-
    inflammatory drugs (NSAIDs)
Nuclear medicine. See Radionuclide
    imaging
Nucleic acid synthesis inhibitors,

2414, 2416t-2417t
Nucleoside analogue toxicity, 2282-
    2283
Nummular eczema, 474
Nut(s), in diet, 31
Nutcracker esophagus, 763
Nutrient requirements, 945-947
  electrolytes, trace elements,
    vitamins in, 947, 947t-948t
  energy (glucose and lipids) in,
    946-947, 946f
  glutamine in, 945
  immunonutrition in, 945-946
  protein in, 945
Nutrition
  in type 1 diabetes, 645-646
  in type 2 diabetes, 657
Nutritional deficiency(ies)
  metabolic encephalopathy in, 2340-
    2341
  neuropathies in, 2304
Nutritional support. See also
    Malnutrition
  in alcoholic liver disease, 944
  in bowel rest, 943
  in cancer malnutrition, 943-944
  definition of, 940
  determining need for, 941
  enteral, 940-949
    in Crohn disease, 943
    definition of, 940
    evidence regarding, 940-941
    general principles of, 944-945
    long-term, 945
    short-term, 944-945, 944t
  enteral and parenteral, metabolic
    acidosis due to, 1998
  evidence regarding, 940-941
  general principles of, 944-945
  in hepatic failure, 944
  home parenteral, 947-948
  in inflammatory bowel disease, 803
  in insufficient oral intake, 941-
    942
    malnourished patients and,
      942, 941f
    well-nourished patients and, 941-
      942
  metabolic encephalopathy in, 2341
  oral, 944
  parenteral, 940-949
    definition of, 940
    evidence regarding, 940
    general principles of, 945
    long-term, 945
    short-term, 945
  in renal failure, 944
  in septic shock, 1452
  in serious bowel function
    compromise, 942-943
  in specific clinical conditions,
    941-944
  in surgery, 942
  total parenteral, definition of,
    940
Nystagmus, 2140, 2140t

O

Obesity, 714-728. See also Diet
  abdominal, 714
  in cancer epidemiology, 2375-2376
  classification of, 714
    body-mass index in, 714, 714t
    fat distribution in, 714, 714t
  complications of, 725
  definition of, 714
  diagnosis of, 716-718, 718f, 719t
  differential diagnosis of,
    719, 719t
  epidemiology of, 715, 715f-716f
  etiology and genetics of, 715
  history in, 716-718

hypertension and, 216
pathophysiology and pathogenesis of, 716, 717f
physical examination and laboratory tests in, 718, 719t
in polycystic ovary syndrome, 984
prognosis in, 725-726
respiratory pump dysfunction in, 2800-2801, 2801f
treatment of, 720-725
  caloric restriction, 720
  combined diet and exercise, 721-722
  dietary carbohydrate changes, 720-721
  dietary fat restriction, 720
  dietary protein changes, 721
  diet modification, 720-721
  exercise, 721
  nonmedical (lifestyle), 720-722
  pharmacologic, 722-724
    long-term agents, 723-724, 723t
    non-FDA approved, 724
    orlistat, 723-724, 723t
    phentermine, 723, 723t
    short-term agents, 722-723, 723t
    sibutramine, 723, 723t
  surgical, 724-725, 725t
Obesity-hypoventilation syndrome (pickwickian syndrome), polycythemia in, 1134-1135
Obsessive-compulsive disorder, 2663-2664
Obstructive sleep apnea syndrome. See Sleep apnea syndrome
Occipital neuralgia, headache in, 2167
Occupational asthma, 62-63, 2707, 2708t, 2716
Occupational disease
  acute, 60
  basic principles of, 58-61
  cancer as, 62, 62t
  central nervous system, 64-65
  chronic, 60
  clinical evaluation in, 60
  common types, 59t
  dermatologic, 63-64
    contact, 491
    hardening in, 482
  in developed countries, 61-67
  diagnostic decision making in, 61
  dose response in, 58
  endocrine, 66-67
  exposure in, confirming and quantifying, 60-61, 61t
  hematologic, 66
  host factors in, 58-59
  insidious, 60
  liver, 64
  low-level exposures and, 67
  musculoskeletal, 65
  occupational history in, 60
  pathophysiology in, 60
  peripheral nervous system, 64-65
  recurrent, 60
  reproductive, 66-67
  respiratory, 62-63
    acute and recurrent, 62-63
    chronic, 63
  subacute, 60
  temporal relationships in, 58
  urinary tract, 64
Occupational exposure
  in cancer epidemiology, 2377
  chronic diffuse infiltrative pulmonary disease due to, 2758, 2759t
  urticaria in, 1261
Occupational medicine, 58-68
Ocular disorders, in rheumatoid arthritis, 1304-1305

Ocular herpes simplex, 1756
Ocular infection, in *Bacillus cereus* infection, 1597
Ocular toxoplasmosis, 1900
Oculomotor neuropathy, 2295, 2294t
Ofloxacin, 1438-1439, 1438t
Ogilvie syndrome, 858
Oils, cooking, in diet, 31
Olecranon bursitis, 1394
Olfactory neuropathy, 2294t
Oligodendroglioma, 2314-2315, 2311t
Oligomenorrhea, 953
Oligospermia, idiopathic, 1002
Olivopontocerebellar atrophy, infantile-onset, 2265-2266, 2263t
Olmesartan, for hypertension, 223t
Olsalazine, for inflammatory bowel disease, 801t
Omalizumab, for asthma, 2714, 2710t
Omega-3 fatty acids, for inflammatory bowel disease, 803
Omental torsion, diverticulitis *vs.*, 814-815
Omeprazole, for *Helicobacter* infection, 1636t
Omsk hemorrhagic fever, 1850
Onchocerca volvulus, 1929t
Onchocerciasis, 1930-1932, 1931f
Oncogene(s), 2383-2385, 2384t. See also Proto-oncogene(s) and individual genes, i.e., p53
  in vitro and mouse models of, 2385
Oncogene antigen(s), mutated or overexpressed, 2401
Oncologic emergencies, 2425-2435
  bleeding with thrombocytopenia, 2427-2428
  brain metastasis, 2431-2432
  cardiovascular, 2425-2426
  disseminated intravascular coagulation, 2426-2427
  epidural spinal cord compression, 2432-2434, 2433f, 2433t
  fever and neutropenia, 2428
  fever and splenectomy, 2429
  hematologic, 2426-2429
  hemolytic-uremic syndrome, 2428
  hypercalcemia of malignancy, 2429-2431
  intramedullary metastasis, 2434
  leptomeningeal metastasis, 2434
  metabolic, 2429-2431
  neurologic, 2431-2434
  pericardial disease and tamponade, 2425-2426
  superior vena cava syndrome, 2425-2426, 2426f-2427f
  thrombotic microangiopathy, 2428
  tumor lysis syndrome, 2431
Oncoviral protein(s), 2401
Onychia punctata, 574
Onychogryphosis, 572
Onycholysis, 573, 573f
Onychomycosis, 576-577, 574f-575f, 575t. See also under Nail(s)
  candidal, 576-577, 575t, 1879t
  dermatophyte, 576, 574f-575f
Onychoschizia, 572
O'nyong-nyong, 1858
Ophthalmia neonatorum, gonococcal, treatment of, 1624t
Ophthalmoplegia, chronic progressive external, 1952, 1952t
Opioid analgesics, 2180-2183, 2180t
  abuse of, 2636
  administration and formulation of, 2181
  dosing in, 2181-2182
  indications for, 2180, 2180t
  mechanism of, 2180-2181
  opioid conversion and, 2182
  overdose of, treatment of, 2642

  side effects of, 2182-2183
  substitution for, in abuse, 2644
  tolerance and dependency, 2183
  withdrawal of, treatment of, 2643
Opioid intoxication, 171-172
  naloxone for, 155-156
Opisthorchiasis, 1935
Opsoclonus, paraneoplastic, 2318
Optic neuritis, 2331
Optic neuropathy, 2294t
  Leber hereditary, 1952, 1952t, 2281
Oral cancer, epidemiology of, tobacco use and, 2374, 2437
Oral candidiasis, 507, 508
Oral contraception. See Contraceptive(s)
Oral hairy leukoplakia, in AIDS, 438
Oral-labial herpes simplex, 1756
Oral mucosa, lichen planus of, 454
Oral ulcer(s)
  in hematologic disease, 1075
  palliative treatment of, 107
Orbital cellulitis, in sinusitis, 1460
Orbitopathy, Graves, 617
Orchitis, mumps, 693
Orf, 1774, 1773f
Organochlorine(s), biologic test of exposure to, 61
Organophosphate(s)
  biologic test of exposure to, 61t
  poisoning, 172, 172t
Organ transplantation. See Transplantation, individual organs
Orientia tsutsugamushi, 1730-1731
Orlistat, for obesity, 723-724, 723t
Oroya fever, 1672
Orthopnea, in COPD, 2725
Oseltamivir, for influenza, 1786t
Osgood-Schlatter disease, 1396
Osler node(s), in endocarditis, 1484
Osler-Weber-Rendu syndrome. See Telangiectasia, hereditary hemorrhagic
Osmotic cathartics, hypernatremia and, 1987
Osmotic diuretics, hypernatremia and, 1987
Osteoarthritis, 1382-1390
  cartilage in, osteoarthritic, 1384-1385, 1384f
  classification of, 1382
  clinical manifestations, 1385-1387
  definition of, 1382
  diagnosis of, 1385, 1385f
  differential diagnosis, 1387
  epidemiology of, 1382-1383
  etiology of, 1383-1385
  of hands, 1385-1386, 1386f
  of hips, 1386
  of knees, 1386
  management of, 1387-1389, 1388t
    cartilage protection in, 1389
    nonpharmacologic, 1387-1388
    pharmacologic, 1388-1389
    surgery, 1389
  pain in, temporal course of, 1291f
  primary, 1382
  prognosis in, 1389
  pseudogout in, 1378
  radiologic features of, 1387, 1386f
  rheumatoid arthritis *vs.*, 1387
  risk factors in, 1383
  secondary, 1382, 1382t
  of spine, 1386-1387
Osteochondral infection, *Pseudomonas aeruginosa*, 1661
Osteomalacia, 711
Osteomyelitis, 1542-1549
  after hip joint replacement, 1544
  candidal, 1878t
  classification of, 1542

  diagnosis of, 1545-1546, 1546t
  of frontal bone, in sinusitis, 1460
  hematogenous, 1542-1543
    Brodie abscess in, 1543
    clinical features of, 1542-1543
    etiology of, 1542
    in I.V. drug abusers, 1543
    predisposing factors in, 1542
    in sickle cell anemia, 1543
    treatment of, 1548
  pathogenesis, 1544-1545, 1545f
  pneumococcal, 1565
  Pseudomonas aeruginosa, 1661
  secondary to contiguous focus of infection, 1543t, 1543-1544
  treatment of, 1548
  sternal, 1544
  treatment of, 1546-1548, 1547t
    in acute hematogenous disease, 1546-1548
    antibiotic-impregnated acrylic beads for, 1547
    in *Enterococcus faecalis* infections, 1548, 1547t
    in gram-negative infections, 1548
    oral therapy for, 1547
    in *S. aureus* infections, 1547-1548, 1547t
    surgical, 1546-1547
  in vascular insufficiency, 1544
    treatment of, 1548
Osteonecrosis, in systemic lupus erythematosus, 1332, 1339
Osteopenia, in HIV infection, 1835
Osteopetrosis, hematopoietic stem cell transplantation for, 1222
Osteoporosis, 707-711
  after renal transplantation, 2124
  diagnosis of, 707-708
  epidemiology of, 707
  in HIV infection, 1835
  Internet resources for, 711t
  pathogenesis of, 707
  postmenopausal (or postoophorectomy), estrogen replacement therapy for, 710
  risk factors and pathologic causes, 707
  in systemic lupus erythematosus, 1332, 1339
  treatment of, 708-711
    anabolic therapy, 710
    antiresorptive, 709
    bisphosphonates for, 709
    calcitonin for, 710
    combination, 710
    estrogen for, 710
    follow-up, 711
    future, 711
    National Osteoporosis Foundation guidelines for, 710-711
    nutritional, 708-709, 709t
    raloxifene for, 709-710
Osteosarcoma, 2556-2557
  diagnosis of, 2556, 2557f
  features of, 2550t
  staging of, 2556-2557
  treatment of, 2557
Otitis, 1461-1462
Otitis externa, 1462
  malignant, 1462
    Pseudomonas aeruginosa, 1660
Otitis media
  acute, 1461-1462
  chronic, 1462
  Haemophilus influenzae, 1650
  Moraxella catarrhalis, 1652
  pneumococcal, 1565
Ovarian ablation, for breast cancer, 2464
  with chemotherapy, 2467

Ovarian cancer, 2537-2541
in adolescent, 1059
breast-ovarian cancer syndrome
and, 2537-2538
CA125 levels in, 2539
clinical features,
2538, 2538t, 2539f
differential diagnosis, 2538-2539
epidemiology of, 2537-2538
epithelial, 2537, 2537t
clear cell, 2537t
endometrioid, 2537t
mucinous, 2537t
papillary serous
cystadenocarcinoma, 2537t
evaluation of, 2538-2539
familial, 2537-2538
germ cell, 2537, 2541
hereditary nonpolyposis colorectal
cancer (Lynch syndrome II)
and, 2538
Lynch syndrome II and, 2538
in postmenopausal woman, 1060-1061
postoperative treatment of, 2540
relapse in, management of, 2540-
2541, 2541t
risk factors for, 2537-2538
staging and surgical management
of, 2539-2540, 2538t
stromal, 2537, 2541
Ovarian failure, premature, 958-959,
1037-1038
Ovarian hyperthecosis, polycystic
ovary syndrome vs., 980
Ovarian surgery, for polycystic
ovary syndrome, 984
Ovarian tumor(s)
borderline, 2541
dysgerminoma, 2541
immature teratoma, 2541
nondysgerminoma, 2541
in reproductive age women,
1060, 1062
Overactive bladder syndrome, 1041-
1047. See also Urinary
incontinence
Ovulation
determination of, 952
disorders of, 956-959, 956t
induction of, 1007-1008, 1008f
in infertility, 1004-1007
Oxacillin, 1424
Oxaliplatin, 2416t
for colorectal cancer, 2487
Oxazolidinone(s), 1437
Oxcarbazepine, in epilepsy, 2195
Oxygen-hemoglobin dissociation
curve, 1079, 1079f
Oxygen therapy
for acute myocardial infarction,
320
hyperbaric
for anaerobic infections, 1613
for carbon monoxide poisoning,
164
Oxygen transport, erythrocyte in,
1079
Oxytocin infusion, acute
hyponatremia due to, 1981t, 1981

P

p16, properties of, 2386t
p53
in cancer biology, 2410
mechanisms of, 2388-2391, 2390f
Pacemaker, 273-283
for atrioventricular block,
273, 275, 274t
for bifascicular block, 274t, 275
complications of, 279-282, 280t
generator, 280
generator pocket, 279-280

infection, 281-282
lead, 280-281
external interference with,
282, 281t, 282f
future of, 283
for heart failure, 344
for hypertensive carotid syndrome,
274t, 275
implantation, 278-279
indications for, 273-275, 274t
leads, 276, 277f
magnets, 277
for myocardial infarction,
274t, 275
for neurocardiogenic syncope,
274t, 275
programmer, 276-277
programming, 277-278, 277t, 278f
pulse generator, 275-276, 276f
for SA node dysfunction, 274t, 275
systems for, 275-277
for trifascicular block, 274t, 275
Paclitaxel, 2419t
peripheral neuropathy due to, 2319-
2320
Paget disease
of bone, 711-712
extramammary, 556
of nipple, 556
Pain, 2169-2186
ankle, 1396-1397
back, 1391-1392
acute, 1391-1392, 1392t
chronic, 1392
chest, differential diagnosis of,
285-286, 287t
chest wall, 1393-1394
definitions of, 2169
elbow, 1394
epidemiology of, 2169
forefoot, 1397, 1397f
hindfoot, 1397
management of, 2176-2186
antidepressants in, 2185
antiepileptic drugs in, 2184-
2185
assessment in, 2177-2178, 2176t
barriers to effective, 2176-
2177, 2176t
in cancer, 2179
corticosteroids for, 2184
in HIV/AIDS, 2179-2180
new approaches to, 2185-2186
NSAIDs and acetaminophen, 2183-
2184
opioid analgesics, 2180-
2183, 2180t
pharmacologic, 2180-2186
principles of, 2178-2179, 2179f
topical analgesics in, 2185
midfoot, 1397
neck, 1391
neurobiology of, 2169-2175
ascending pathways in, 2173-2174
postsynaptic dorsal column
fibers, 2173
spinocervicothalamic tract,
2173
spinohypothalamic tract, 2173-
2174
spinomesencephalic tract, 2173
spinoreticular tract, 2173
spinothalamic tract, 2173
thalamocortical pathways, 2174
visceral nociceptive tracts,
2173
cancer pain, 2175
central sensitization in, 2172-
2173
descending pathways in, 2174-
2175
dorsal horn in, 2170-2172, 2172f
gate control theory in, 2172

HIV infection and AIDS, 2176
peripheral pain, 2169-2170
nociception, 2169-2170, 2171f
peripheral sensitization, 2170
opioid analgesics for. See Opioid
analgesics
palliative treatment of, 100-101
in rheumatic disease, 1291, 1291f
shoulder, 1392-1393, 1393f
Painful articular syndrome, in AIDS,
1539
Palliative medicine, 92-99
advance directives and, 96-97
anorexia in, 102-103
bowel obstruction in, 105
clinical skills and, 95-96
communication and, 95
constipation in, 104-105, 107t-108t
cough in, 102, 104f
cultural differences and, 96
delirium in, 108-109, 110t
diarrhea in, 105
dyspnea in, 101-102, 103t
ethical issues in, 97-99
assisted suicide or euthanasia,
98-99
futile treatment, 98
legal reprisal, 99
limiting treatment, 97-98
foul-smelling wounds in, 107-108
gastrointestinal symptoms in, 102-
105
history and rationale for, 92
in hospice, 92-93, 94t, 94f
in hospital, 92
mouth symptoms in, 105-107, 109t
nausea and vomiting in, 103-
104, 105t-106t
pain in, 100-101
physical symptoms in, 100-108
pressure ulcers in, 107, 109t
prognosis and, 94-95, 95f
psychiatric symptoms in, 108-
109, 110t
respiratory symptoms in, 101-
102, 104f, 103t
settings for delivery of, 92-93
skin symptoms in, 107-108, 109t
skin ulcers in, malignant, 107
symptom assessment in, 100, 101t-
102t
symptom management and, 95-96
symptom management in, 100-111
symptom management in last hours
of life, 110
terminal wean in, 109-110
Palpitations, in cardiovascular
patient, 202-205, 203t-204t, 203f
Pancolitis, 792
Pancreas, 913-931
abscess of, 913, 922-923, 922f,
1505
necrosis of
definition of, 913
infected, 922-923, 922f
neoplasms of. See also Pancreatic
cancer
cystic, 930
intraductal papillary mucinous,
930
Pancreas divisum, pancreatitis in,
914
Pancreas transplantation, 936-938
candidates for, 936, 935f
complications of, 937-938
immunologic, 938
medical, 938
surgical, 937-938
contraindications to, 937, 935f
diabetic complications and, 938
metabolic outcomes of, 938
operative procedures, 937, 937f
outcomes after, 938

quality of life issues and, 938
for type 1 diabetes, 645
Pancreatic cancer, 2499-2503
in chronic pancreatitis, 930
diagnosis of, 2500-2501, 2501f-
2502f
epidemiology of, 2499
etiology and risk factors in, 2499
familial, 2499, 2499t
molecular mutations and
pathogenesis of,
2500, 2500t, 2501f
screening and prevention of, 2499-
2500
staging of, 2501, 2502t
treatment of, 2501-2503
in local, resectable disease,
2501-2502
in locally advanced,
unresectable disease, 2502-
2503
Pancreatic disease, in
malabsorption, 824
Pancreatic duct, obstruction of,
acute pancreatitis in, 914
Pancreatic function tests, 926
in malabsorption, 826, 825t
Pancreatitis
acute, 913-924
acute cholecystitis vs., 904
APACHE-II classification system
for, 918, 920t-921t
clinical findings in, 915-916
complications in, 921-923
computed tomography in, 917, 918
definition of, 913
diagnosis of, 915-918
disease severity in, 918, 919t-
921t
drug-induced, 914
encephalopathy in, 2338
epidemiology of, 913
etiology of, 913-915, 914t
genetic factors in, 915
idiopathic, 915
imaging studies in, 917, 918f
infection in, 914
interstitial, 913
laboratory tests in, 916-
917, 917t
management of, 918-924
in complications of, 921-923
in necrosis and inflammation,
919-921
in subsequent attacks, 923-924
supportive, 919
microlithiasis in, 915
necrotizing, 913
infected, 922-923
pathogenesis of, 915, 916t
pseudocysts in, 923
Ranson prognostic scoring system
for, 919t, 918
scoring systems for, 918, 919t-
921t
severe, definition of, 913
spontaneous bacterial
peritonitis vs., 1501
alcoholic, 924
diabetes in, 924
pain in, 927-928
steatorrhea in, 929, 928t
autoimmune, 915
chronic, 924-930
big-duct/small-duct, 927, 927f
clinical findings in, 925
common bile duct obstruction in,
930
in cystic fibrosis, 924
cystic lesions in, 929-930
definition of, 913
diabetes in, 929
diagnosis of, 925-927, 925t

duodenal obstruction in, 930
epidemiology of, 924
ERCP in, 926-927, 927f
etiology of, 924-925
idiopathic, 924-925
imaging studies in, 926-927, 926f-927f
laboratory tests in, 925-926
malabsorption in, 834
management of
  analgesia and alcohol cessation, 928
  endoscopic and surgical therapy in, 928
  pancreatic enzymes in, 928
pain in, 927-928
pancreatic cancer in, 930
pancreatic function tests in, 926
pathogenesis of, 925
pseudocysts in, 913, 929
steatorrhea in, 929, 928t
tropical, 924
gallstone, 913-914
  common bile duct stone removal in, 920-921
  microlithiasis in, 915
  Ranson prognostic scoring system for, 917t, 918
hereditary, 924
Panencephalitis, subacute sclerosing, 2333, 2360-2361
Panhypopituitarism, anemia in, 1094
Panic disorder, 2657-2661, 2657t, 2659t
complications of, 2660-2661
diagnosis of, 2659, 2659t
in diagnosis of palpitation, 204t
epidemiology of, 2658
pathophysiology of, 2658-2659
treatment of, 2659-2660, 2660t
Pantothenic acid, 29t
Papanicolaou smear, 2541
Papillomatosis of Gougerot and Carteaud, 580
Papillomavirus infection. See also Warts, Verruca
in head and neck cancer, 2438
in uterine cervical cancer, 2376
Papovavirus BK infection, encephalitis in, 2352
Pap smear, 1063-1069
atypical glandular cells in, 1068
atypical squamous cells in, 1065-1068, 1066f, 1067t
immunosuppressed patient and, 1068
management options in, 1066-1067, 1066f, 1067t
postmenopausal patient and, 1068
recommended management in, 1067-1068, 1067f
Bethesda System for, 1064
conventional, 1064-1065
cytologic abnormalities in, 1065-1068
HPV DNA testing and, 1065
interpretation of, 1065, 1064t
liquid-based, 1065
onogenic HPV DNA in, 1068
squamous epithelial lesions in, 1068
who should be screened, 1063-1064
Papule, definition of, 426t
Papulosis, bowenoid, 515, 515f
Papulosquamous disorder, 452-460
Paragonimiasis, 1934-1935
cavitary pulmonary infiltrate in, 2752
multiple pulmonary nodules in, 2755
Parainfluenza virus, 1778t, 1788
Paralysis, periodic

hyperkalemic, 2281-2282
hypokalemic, 2007, 2009
Paramyotonia congenita, 2281-2282
Paraneoplastic cerebellar degeneration, 2318
Paraneoplastic mixed bullous disease, 526t, 528
Paraneoplastic neuropathy, 2302
Paraneoplastic opsoclonus, 2318
Paraneoplastic sensory neuropathy, 2318-2319
Paraneoplastic syndrome, 2317-2319, 2318t
in lung cancer, 2446
Parapharyngeal infection, 1464-1465
Parapneumonic effusion, 2831-2832, 2831t
tube thoracostomy in, 2699, 2699t
Parapsoriasis, 457-458
large-plaque, 458, 458f
small-plaque, 458, 458f
Paraquat, inhalation or ingestion of, 165t
Parasitic infestation. See also individual disorders
diarrhea in, 842
of skin, 516-524. See also individual disorders, e.g., Scabies
Parasitosis, delusional, 523
Parasomnia, 2366t, 2371
nocturnal frontal lobe epilepsy, 2371
partial arousal disorders, 2371
REM sleep behavior disorder, 2371
Parathyroid hormone
in calcium metabolism, 698-699, 698f
excess. See Hyperparathyroidism
Paravaccinia, 1774
Parenteral nutrition. See Nutritional support, parenteral
Parkinson disease, 2239-2253
advanced
  depression in, 2248
  motor fluctuations and, 2247-2248
  neuroprotective therapy for, 2248-2249, 2249t
  neuropsychiatric symptoms in, 2248
  personality changes and psychosis in, 2248
  surgical treatment of, 2249-2250
treatment of, 2247
bradykinesia in, 2242-2243
clinical features of, 2242-2244
dementia in, 2244
depression in, 2244
differential diagnosis of, 2242t
epidemiology, etiology, genetics in, 2239-2241
facies in, 2242, 2243f
freezing in, 2243-2244
gait in, 2243
muscle rigidity in, 2243
pathogenesis of, 2241-2242, 2243f
sleep disorders in, 2244
treatment of, 2244-2250
  amantadine for, 2247
  anticholinergics for, 2247
  dopamine agonists for, 2244-2245, 2246-2247, 2247t
  initiating, 2245
  levodopa augmentation for, 2246
  levodopa for, 2244
  levodopa formulations for, 2245, 2244t, 2246t
  tremor in, 2242
Parkinsonism
Alzheimer disease vs., 2222
dementia and, 2252-2253
drug-induced, 2250, 2242t

other forms of, 2250-2253
primary tau pathology in, 2252
vascular, 2250
Paronychia, 572. See also Nail(s)
bacterial, 575
candidal, 508, 508f, 1879t
chronic, 575
Paroxysmal nocturnal hemoglobinuria. See Hemoglobinuria, paroxysmal nocturnal
Paroxysmal supraventricular tachycardia. See Supraventricular tachycardia, paroxysmal
Partial thromboplastin time (PTT), 1160
Parvovirus B19, in renal transplantation, 2122
Parvovirus infection, 1771-1772
in pregnancy, 1021
Pasteurella multocida, in septic arthritis, 1538
Patch, definition of, 426t
Patch test, for allergic contact dermatitis, 484-487, 485f, 486t, 487f, 488t-489t
Patent ductus arteriosus, 391
murmur in, 210t
Pearson syndrome, 1952, 1952t
Pectus carinatum, 2803
Pectus excavatum, 2803
Pedestrian injury, 22
Pediculosis, 519-521, 569
diagnosis of, 519-520, 519f-520f
lice species in, 519
treatment of, 520-521, 521t
Pediculosis capitis, 520-521, 521t
Pediculosis corporis, 521, 521t
Pediculosis pubis, 521, 521t
Pel-Ebstein fever, in Hodgkin disease, 2597
Pellagra, metabolic encephalopathy in, 2341
Pelvic floor muscle exercise, for incontinence, 1043, 1045
Pelvic inflammatory disease (PID), 1526-1527, 1527t
chlamydial, 1748-1749
complications of, 1527
microbiology and diagnosis of, 1526
Mycoplasma hominis, 1742
Neisseria gonorrhoeae, 1622
treatment of, 1526-1527, 1527t
Pelvic mass, 1055-1062
in adolescents, 1058-1059, 1061
age-specific considerations in, 1058-1061
biopsy in, 1058
differential diagnosis of, 1055, 1056t
fine-needle aspiration in, 1058
imaging studies in, 1056-1057
in infants, 1061
laboratory tests in, 1056
management of, 1061-1062
medical history in, 1055-1056
patient evaluation in, 1055-1058
physical examination in, 1056, 1057t
in postmenopausal women, 1060-1061, 1062
in prepubertal girls, 1058, 1061
in reproductive-age women, 1059-1060, 1061-1062
serum tumor markers in, 1057-1058, 1058t
Pelvic pain, chronic, endometriosis vs., 968
Pemphigoid
bullous, 529-530, 529f, 526t
cicatricial, 530, 526t
Pemphigus, 525-529

autoimmunity in, 1237
definition and pathogenesis of, 525
drug-related, 499, 499f, 528
endemic, 528
histologic and immunologic findings in, 528
treatment of, 528-529
Pemphigus erythematosus, 526t
Pemphigus foliaceus, 527-528, 526t
Pemphigus vegetans, 526t
Pemphigus vulgaris, 525-527, 527f-528f, 526t
Penicillamine
chronic diffuse infiltrative pulmonary disease due to, 2764
for cystine nephrolithiasis, 2111-2112
Penicillin, 1424, 1428
allergy to, 1273-1274, 1274t, 1275f
in syphilis, 1707
with beta-lactamase inhibitors, 1428
  allergy to, 1431-1432
penicillinase-resistant, 1424
penicillinase-susceptible broad-spectrum, 1428
for pneumococcal infection, 1565-1566, 1566t
in pregnancy, 1422t
for streptococcal infection, 1572-1573
Penicillin G, 1424
Penicillin V, 1424
Penile erectile dysfunction, 696-697
Pentostatin, 2417t
Peptic ulcer disease, 776-789
bleeding, 778-779, 863, 864f
  laboratory studies in, 780
  management of, 786-787, 786f
breath tests for, 782
clinical manifestations of, 778-779
complicated
  laboratory studies in, 780
  physical examination findings in, 779
corticosteroid use in, NSAIDs with, 778
definition of, 776
diagnosis of, 778-781
differential diagnosis, 782, 782t
duodenal
  Helicobacter pylori in. See also Helicobacter pylori infection
    treatment of, 782-784, 783f, 783t
  Helicobacter pylori-negative, treatment of, 784-785, 784t
  intractable, treatment of, 785-786
  uncomplicated, treatment of, 782-785, 783f, 783t
dyspepsia vs., 782
endoscopic tests for, 781, 781f
endoscopy in, 780, 779f
epidemiology of, 776
etiologic tests for, 781-782, 781f
family history in, 779
fecal antigen test in, 782
fistulizing, management of, 788
gastric
  Helicobacter pylori in, treatment of, 785, 783t-785t
  intractable, treatment of, 785-786
  NSAID-related, treatment of, 785, 784t-785t
  uncomplicated, treatment of, 785, 783t, 783t, 784t
in gastrinoma, 777f, 778
Helicobacter pylori in, 776, 777f

treatment of, 782-784, 783f, 783t
idiopathic, 778
imaging studies in, 780-781, 779f-780f
laboratory studies in, 779-780
NSAID use in, 776-778, 777f
treatment of, 785, 784t-785t
obstructing, management of, 787
pathogenesis and etiology of, 776-778, 777f
perforated, management of, 787
physical examination findings in, 779
radiology in, 780-781, 779f-780f
refractory to H₂-receptor blocker, approach to patient with, 779f
serologic tests for, 781-782
stress
acute, 778
management of, 788
surgical diagnosis of, 781
treatment of, 782-788
in bleeding ulcers, 786-787, 786f
in Cameron ulcers, 788
in complicated ulcers, 786-788
in failure to heal, 785-786
in fistulizing ulcers, 788
in frequent recurrence, 786
in intractable disease, 785-786
in obstructing ulcers, 787
in perforated ulcers, 787
in stress ulcers, 788
in uncomplicated disease, 782-785, 783f, 783t
in Zollinger-Ellison syndrome, 778
Peptostreptococcus species, 1604
Pergolide, for parkinsonism, 2247t
Perianal herpes, 1757, 1757f
Periarthritis, calcific, acute, 1380
Pericardial disease, 377-382
neoplastic, 2425-2426
Pericardial effusion, 377-380
after cardiac catheterization, 381
diagnosis of, 378-379, 379f-380f
neoplastic, 380-381
pathophysiology of, 377-378, 379f
radiation-induced, 380
treatment of, 379-380
Pericardial tamponade, neoplastic, 2425-2426
Pericarditis
acute, 377, 378f
after cardiac surgery, 381
candidal, 1879t
constrictive, 381-382
cardiac amyloidosis *vs.*, 383t
diagnosis of, 381-382, 382f, 383t
idiopathic restrictive cardiomyopathy *vs.*, 383t
pathophysiology of, 381, 382f
progression to, 377
treatment of, 382
in differential diagnosis of chest pain, 198t, 197
drug-induced, 381
effusion-constrictive, 2425
in histoplasmosis, 1864
pneumococcal, 1565
purulent, 381
relapsing, 377
in renal dialysis, 380
in renal failure, 380
in rheumatoid arthritis, 1305
tuberculous, 1681-1682
Perilymphatic fistula, 2147
Perindopril, for hypertension, 222t
Perinephric abscess, candidal, 1878t
Periodic limb movements, in sleep, 2369-2370, 2369f
Periodic paralysis
hyperkalemic, 2281-2282
hypokalemic, 2007, 2009, 2282
Perioral dermatitis, acne vulgaris

vs., 447
Peripartum cardiomyopathy, 1019
Peripartum period, thrombocytopenia in, 1173-1174
Peripheral arterial disease, 400-409
acute, 405
in acute arterial thrombosis, 405
atheroembolism in, 405-406
atherosclerotic, 400-405
angiography in, 402, 403f
clinical presentation in, 400-401, 401f, 401t
diagnosis of, 400-402
epidemiology of, 400
noninvasive diagnostic tests in, 401-402, 402f, 402t
risk factors in, 400
treatment of, 402-405
amputation for, 405
antiplatelet therapy in, 402-403
claudication and critical limb ischemia in, 403-404
hygiene in, 403
infrainguinal bypass for, 405
revascularization for, 404-405, 404f
risk-factor modification in, 402-403
popliteal artery entrapment in, 406
Raynaud phenomenon, 406-407, 407t
thromboangiitis obliterans in, 406
Peripheral blood smear
evaluation of, 1161
in thrombocytopenia, 1164
Peripheral blood stem cell transfusion. *See* Hematopoietic stem cell transplantation
Peripheral nerve disease, 2291-2306. *See also* Neuropathy(ies), Polyneuropathy(ies)
clinical manifestations of, 2291-2292
cranial neuropathies in. *See* Cranial neuropathy
diabetic, 671
due to anticancer chemotherapy, 2319-2320
laboratory tests for, 2292-2293
needle electromyography for, 2292
nerve biopsy for, 2293
nerve conduction studies for, 2292
Peripheral nervous system, 2291
anatomy of, 2291, 2292f
occupational disease of, 64-65
regenerative capacities of, 2291
Peripheral neuroepithelial tumor(s), oncogenes in, 2385
Perirenal abscess, in urinary tract infection, 1511
Peritoneal cancer, occupational agents causing, 62t
Peritoneal dialysis
in chronic renal failure, 2046-2049
long-term, 2047-2049
planning for, 2046
peritonitis in, 1502-1503
Peritonitis, 1500-1503
candidal, 1878t
in dialysis patients, 1502-1503
pneumococcal, 1565
secondary, 1501-1502
spontaneous bacterial, 1500-1501
acute pancreatitis *vs.*, 1501
in cirrhosis, 896
in systemic lupus erythematosus, 1500
tuberculous peritonitis *vs.*, 1501
starch, fever of undetermined

origin in, 1415
tuberculous, 1682
spontaneous bacterial peritonitis *vs.*, 1501
Peritonsillar abscess, 1464
Permethrin
for pediculosis, 520
for scabies, 517
Peroneal neuropathy, 2296
Pertussis, 1656-1658
clinical manifestations of, 1657
epidemiology of, 1656
immunization, 1658
microbiologic diagnosis of, 1657
pathogenesis of, 1656-1657, 1656c
treatment and prevention of, 1657-1658
Pesticide, biologic test of exposure to, 61t
PET. *See* Positron emission tomography (PET)
Petechiae
definition of, 429t
in thrombocytopenia, 1164
Peutz-Jeghers syndrome, cutaneous findings in, 436
pH
blood, 1994, 1994f
monitoring, in gastroesophageal reflux disease, 765-766
Phagocytic cell disorder, 1137. *See also under* Neutrophil(s)
Pharmacokinetics, in renal failure. *See also* Renal failure, drug dosage adjustment in
Pharyngitis, 1462-1464
bacterial, 1464
diphtheritic, 1585, 1586f
gonococcal, 1622
streptococcal, 1463-1464
rheumatic fever in, 1571
viral, 1778-1779
Phenacetin, nephropathy due to, 2090
Phenobarbital
in epilepsy, 2195-2196
poisoning or overdose with, elimination method for, 161t
Phenol, inhalation or ingestion of, 165t
Phentermine
for obesity, 722-723, 723t
valvular heart disease due to, 362
Phentolamine, for hypertensive crisis, 228t
Phenytoin, in epilepsy, 2196
Pheochromocytoma, 684-685, 684t
diagnosis of, 684-685, 684t
familial, 233
hypertension in, 217t, 232-234, 233t, 231t
mediastinal, 2839
screening for, 233-234, 233t
treatment of, 685
Philadelphia chromosome, in chronic myeloid leukemia, 2384
Philadelphia chromosome-negative chronic myeloid leukemia, 2577t
Phobias. *See also* Anxiety disorder(s)
in medical settings, 2664
Phosphofructokinase deficiency, 2278-2279
Phosphoglycerate kinase deficiency, 2279, 2279f
Phosphoglycerate mutase deficiency, 2279, 2279f
Photoallergy, 492, 492f
Photodynamic therapy, bronchial, 2695
Photosensitivity, contact dermatitis due to, 491-492, 492t
Phototherapy
for acne vulgaris, 451

for atopic dermatitis, 478
for psoriasis, 467, 468f
Phototoxicity, contact dermatitis due to, 491-492, 492t
Phyllodes tumoe, breast, 1053
Physical activity. *See* Exercise
Physical therapy, for rheumatoid arthritis, 1312
Physician, in terminal illness, 114-115
Pickwickian syndrome (obesity-hypoventilation syndrome), polycythemia in, 1134-1135
Piebaldism, 586, 585f
Pigeon breeder's disease, 2765. *See also* Pneumonitis, hypersensitivity
Pigmentation, disorders of, 578-588. *See also individual disorders*
Pilar cyst, 537
Pimecrolimus, for atopic dermatitis, 477
Pindolol, for hypertension, 222t
Pineal region tumors, 2315-2316
Pink puffer, 2727, 2725t, 2727f. *See also* Chronic airflow obstruction (CAO)
Pinta, 1710, 1705t
Pinworm infection, 1921, 1920t
Piperacillin, 1428
Pittsburgh pneumonia, 1475
Pituitary, 589-604
functional anatomy of, 589-590, 589f, 590t
local mass effect on, 590, 591f
Pituitary adenoma, 590-592, 591t, 2315
ACTH-producing, 598-599, 599t. *See also* Cushing disease
genetic syndromes and, 591-592
in hypogonadotropic hypogonadism, 956-957
in infertility, 1006
nonfunctioning, 600-601
Pituitary apoplexy, 603
Pituitary failure, 602-604, 603t
acquired, 603
developmental, 602-603
diagnosis of, 603-604
treatment of, 604, 604t
Pituitary hormones, 590t. *See also individual hormones*
anterior, disorders of, 592-601
posterior, disorders of, 601-602
Pit vipers, 183, 184f. *See also* Snakebite
Pityriasis lichenoides (Mucha-Habermann disease), 457-458, 457f
Pityriasis rosea, 452-453, 452f
Pityriasis rubra pilaris, 456-457, 456f-457f
Pityrosporum. See Malassezia
Plague, 133-134, 1670-1672
clinical presentation in, 133
communicability and infection control in, 134
complications and prognosis in, 1672
diagnosis of, 133-134, 1671, 1664t
differential diagnosis of, 1671
epidemiology of, 1670, 1670f
etiology of, 1670-1671
immunization, for travelers, 72
pathogenesis of, 1670
pneumonic, postexposure prophylaxis for, 134, 135t
treatment of, 134, 134t, 1671, 1665t
Plantar fasciitis, of foot, 1397, 1397f
Plaque
atherosclerotic. *See* Coronary atherosclerosis
definition of, 426t

Plasma
  fresh frozen, for transfusion,
    1212-1213
  sodium concentration in, 1976
Plasmacytoma, in multiple myeloma,
    2590
Plasma exchange, 1218-1219
Plasminogen activator-1 deficiency,
    1184
Plasminogen test, 1161
Plasmodium falciparum, 1892, 1893t
Plasmodium malariae, 1892, 1893t
Plasmodium ovale, 1892, 1893t
Plasmodium vivax, 1892, 1893t
Platelet(s). *See also*
    Thrombocytopenia
  accelerated removal of
    drug-induced, 1169-1170
    due to immune destruction, 1166-
      1170, 1165t
    due to immune processes. *See
      also* Thrombocytopenic
      purpura
    due to nonimmunologic
      mechanisms, 1170-1174
  in coagulation, 1153-1154, 1153f-
    1155f. *See also* Coagulation
  development of, 1072f, 1075
  drug-induced disorders of, 1175
  functional disorders of, 1174-
    1175, 1175t-1176t
    acquired, 1174-1175, 1176t
    hereditary, 1174
  perioperative washout of, 1174
  production of
    defects in, 1165-1166
    thrombopoietin and, 1159-1160
  sequestration of, thrombocytopenia
    in, 1174
  for transfusion. *See* Transfusion
    therapy, platelet
Platelet aggregometry, 1161
Platelet count, in thrombocytopenia,
    1164
Platelet disorder(s), 1163-1179
  patient approach in, 1163-1164
  thrombocytopenia, 1164-1174. *See
    also* Thrombocytopenia
Platelet-function assay-100, 1161
Platelet glycoprotein IIb-IIIa
    receptor antagonists,
    thrombocytopenia due to, 1170
Platelet granule disorders, 1174
Platelet membrane disorders, 1174
Pleural biopsy, closed, 2698
Pleural calcification, 2833
Pleural cancer, occupational agents
    causing, 62t
Pleural disease, invasive diagnostic
    and therapeutic techniques for,
    2696-2700. *See also individual
    procedures*
  closed pleural biopsy, 2698
  thoracentesis, 2697-2698
  thoracoscopy, 2699-2700
  transthoracic needle aspiration,
    2698
  tube thoracostomy, 2698-2699
Pleural effusion, 2823-2832
  in ascites, 2828
  bloody. *See* Hemothorax
  chest radiography in, 2824-
    2825, 2824f-2826f
  in congestive heart failure, 2828
  CT scan for, 2825
  diagnosis of, 2824-2828
  empyema *vs.,* 1479
  exudative, 2824t, 2826, 2827f
  interlobar, 2825, 2826f
  laboratory studies in, 2825-2828
    amylase level in, 2826
    ANA titer in, 2828
    glucose level in, 2828

pH level in, 2828
  red blood cell count in, 2826-
    2827
  white blood cell count in, 2827
  loculated, 2824, 2825f
  malignant, tube thoracostomy in,
    2699
  in malignant disease, 2828-2829
  massive, 2824, 2825f
  pathophysiology and etiology of,
    2823-2824, 2824t
  in pulmonary embolism, 2829-2830
  in rheumatoid arthritis, 1305
  in sarcoidosis, 2771
  subpulmonary, 2824, 2825f
  in systemic lupus erythematosus,
    1331
  transudative, 2824t, 2826, 2827f
  in tuberculosis, 2829
  ultrasonography for, 2825
Pleural plaque(s), 2832-2833, 2832f
  calcified, 2833, 2832f
Pleural thickening, 2833, 2833f
Pleurisy, 2823
  in rheumatoid arthritis, 1305
Pleuritis
  in rheumatoid arthritis, 1305
  tuberculous, 1678, 1680, 2829
Pleurodesis, chemical, for pleural
    effusion, 2829
Pleurodynia
  enteroviral, 1796, 1795t
  epidemic (Bornholm disease), 2823
Pleuropericarditis, in systemic
    lupus erythematosus, 1331
Plexopathy, in cancer, 2175
PML/RAR-alpha, 2384t, 2385
PMS1, properties of, 2386t
PMS2, properties of, 2386t
Pneumococcal immunization, 1567
  for HIV-infected patients, 1830t
  international travel and, 71
Pneumococcal infection, 1563-1567
  epidemiology of, 1563
  in HIV infection, 1565
  meningitis, 1565
  osteomyelitis, 1565
  otitis media, 1565
  overwhelming postsplenectomy
    infection, 1565
  pathogenesis of, 1563-1564
  pericarditis, 1565
  peritonitis, 1565
  pneumonia, 1564-1565
    epidemiology of, 1469
    focal pulmonary infiltrates in,
      2744, 2745f
    multifocal pulmonary infiltrates
      in, 2746-2747, 2746f
  septic arthritis, 1537
  prevention of, vaccine for, 1567
  septic arthritis, 1565
  treatment of, 1565-1566, 1566t
    penicillin, 1565-1566, 1566t
    in penicillin-resistant *S.
      pneumoniae,* 1565-1566, 1566t
Pneumoconiosis, 63
  chronic diffuse pulmonary
    infiltration in, 2764-2765
  coal worker's, 2765
Pneumocystis carinii pneumonia
  bronchoalveolar lavage in, 2760
  chronic diffuse infiltrative, 2758
Pneumocystis jiroveci
  pneumonia, treatment of,
    1839, 1841t-1842t
  prevention of recurrence of,
    USPHS/IDSA guidelines for,
    1842t
  prophylactic measures for
    prevention of, in HIV
    infection, 1840t
Pneumocystis pneumonia, 1881-

1882, 1882f, 1883t-1884t
  diagnosis of, 1882
  epidemiology of, 1881-1882
  etiology and pathogenesis of, 1882
  treatment of, 1882, 1883t-1884t
Pneumocystosis. *See also
    Pneumocystis carinii* pneumonia
  in compromised host, 1881-
    1882, 1882f, 1883t-1884t
Pneumomediastinum, 2839-2840
  spontaneous, 2840
Pneumonia, 1468-1474
  aspiration, 1476-1477
    antibiotic choices for, 1472-
      1473, 1474t
  bacterial, focal pulmonary
    infiltrates in, 2744, 2745f
  candidal, 1877t
  chlamydial, 1475-1476
  chronic, 1476
  clinical features of, 1470
  community-acquired, 1469-1470
    Pseudomonas aeruginosa, 1659
    treatment of, 1472-1473, 1472t-
      1473t
  diagnosis of, 1470-1471
  differential diagnosis, 1471
  eosinophilic. *See* Eosinophilic
    pneumonia
  epidemiology and etiology of, 1469-
    1470
  fungal, multifocal infiltrates in,
    2747
  gram-negative, epidemiology of,
    1469
  Haemophilus influenzae, 1469, 1649-
    1650
  in HIV disease, *Pseudomonas
    aeruginosa,* 1659
  hospital-acquired, 1470
    treatment of, 1473-1474
  in immunocompromised hosts, 1780-
    1781
  in immunosuppression, 1470
  interstitial
    acute, 2776-2777, 2778f, 2767t-
      2768t
    desquamative, 2775-
      2776, 2777f, 2767t-2768t
    lymphocytic, 2777, 2778f, 2767t-
      2768t
  invasive studies in, 1471
  laboratory studies in, 1470-1471
  lipoid, focal infiltrates in,
    2746, 2745f
  meningococcal, 1618-1619
  Moraxella catarrhalis, 1469, 1652
  mycoplasmal. *See* Mycoplasmal
    pneumonia
  pathophysiology of, 1468-1469
    host defense mechanisms in,
      1468, 1469t
    tissue responses in, 1468-1469
    transmission of organisms to
      lung in, 1468
  Pittsburgh, 1475
  pneumococcal, 1564-1565
    epidemiology of, 1469
    focal pulmonary infiltrates in,
      2744, 2745f
    multifocal pulmonary infiltrates
      in, 2746-2747, 2746f
  *Pneumocystis carinii. See
      Pneumocystis carinii* pneumonia
  recurrent, 1476
  sputum culture in, 1471
  staphylococcal, 1576-1577
    cavitary infiltrates in, 2751
    epidemiology of, 1469
  streptococcal, group A, 1569
  treatment of, 1471-1474
  ventilator-associated, 1471, 2816-
    2817

viral, 1780-1781
Pneumonia/fibrosis, interstitial,
    nonspecific, 2777-
    2778, 2778f, 2767t-2768t
Pneumonitis
  hypersensitivity, 2765f, 2765-2767
    sarcoidosis *vs.,* 2773
  lupus, 2779
  radiation, focal infiltrates in,
    2745-2746
  in rheumatoid arthritis, with
    fibrosis, 2779-2780
Pneumothorax, 2833-2836
  etiology of, 2833-2834
  iatrogenic, 2834
  spontaneous, 2834-2836
    diagnosis of, 2834-2835
    radiography in, 2835, 2835f
    recurrent, 2835-2836
    treatment of, 2835-2836
  tension, 2836
    in cardiac arrest, 149t
  traumatic, 2834
  tube thoracostomy in, 2698-2699
POEMS syndrome, 2302
Poikiloderma, definition of, 429t
Poisoning or drug overdose, 155-179
  activated charcoal, 160, 160t
  acute pancreatitis in, 914
  airway in, 155
  autonomic syndromes in, 158t
  in cardiac arrest, 149t
  cardiac dysrhythmias in, 156, 156t
  ciguatera, 175, 175t
  clinical evaluation in, 158-
    159, 158t-159t
  coma in, 155-156
  complications of, management of,
    155-158
  differential diagnosis in, 159
  enhanced elimination in, 160-
    161, 161t
  fish, respiratory insufficiency
    in, 2806
  food. *See* Food poisoning, *specific
    disorders, e.g.,* Botulism
  gastric lavage for, 159-160, 160t
  gastrointestinal decontamination
    after, 159-160, 160t
  hepatotoxicity due to, 877-878
  hypertension in, 156-157
  hyperthermia in, 157, 158t
  hypotension in, 156, 156t
  hypothermia in, 157-158
  initial stabilization, 155, 155t
  ipecac for, 159, 160t
  laboratory evaluation, 159, 159t
  lead. *See* Lead poisoning
  movement disorders due to, 2255t
  mushroom, 175
  rhabdomyolysis, 158
  salt, hypernatremia and, 1987
  scombroid, 175, 175t
  seafood, 175, 175t
  seizures in, 157, 157t
  shellfish, 175, 175t
  snake venom, hemolytic anemia in,
    1128
  whole bowel irrigation, 160, 160t
Poliolike paralytic illness,
    enteroviral, 1796, 1794t
Poliomyelitis
  anterior horn cell disease in,
    2806
  enteroviral, 1796, 1794t
Poliomyelitis immunization
  for HIV-infected patients, 1830t
  for travelers, 71
Poliovirus infection,
    encephalomyelitis in, 2346
Pollen-associated food allergy
    syndrome, 1278-1279, 1279t
Polyangiitis, microscopic, 1361f,

1365t, 1366-1367
glomerulonephritis in, 2075-2076
Polyarteritis nodosa, 1366-1367
abdominal angiography in, 1367
antiphospholipid antibody syndrome
vs., 1366, 1367f
classification of, 1366, 1361f
clinical manifestations of,
1366, 1367f, 1365t
cutaneous findings in, 441-442
diagnosis of, 1366-1367, 1367f
laboratory tests in, 1366-1367
renal involvement in, 2074-2075
treatment of, 1367
Polychlorinated biphenyl, biologic
test of exposure to, 61t
Polyclonal antibody(ies), for
prerenal-transplant patient
management, 2119
Polycystic kidney disease, 2097-
2099, 2098f-2099f
autosomal dominant, 2097-
2098, 2098f-2099f
berry aneurysm of circle of
Willis in, 2098, 2099f
autosomal recessive, 2099
in renal transplant donor, 2117
secondary hypertension in, 217t
Polycystic ovary syndrome, 959, 974-
986
cardiovascular disease in, 980
definition of, 974
diagnosis of, 975-980, 976t-
977t, 977f-979f
differential diagnosis of, 980
epidemiology of, 974
etiology and genetics of, 974-975
hirsutism in, 976-977, 977f
history in, 976, 976t
in infertility, 1006
laboratory tests in, 977-980, 978f-
979f
antimullerian hormone, 978-979
DHEAS, 978
diabetes mellitus and, 979
17-hydroxyprogesterone, 978
insulin resistance and
hyperinsulinemia and, 979-
980, 979f
metabolic syndrome and, 979
pelvic imaging, 979
serum luteinizing hormone and
follicle stimulating
hormone, 978, 978f
serum prolactin and thyroid-
stimulating hormone, 978
testosterone, 978
metabolic syndrome and, 980
nonalcoholic steatohepatitis in,
981
pathophysiology in, 975
metabolic, 975
reproductive, 975
physical examination in, 976-
977, 977f
sleep apnea in, 980-981
syndromes associated with, 980-981
treatment in, 981-985
for anovulatory or oligo-
ovulatory infertility,
982, 982t
clomiphene, 982-983
clomiphene plus
glucocorticoid, 983
clomiphene plus gonadotropin
injection, 984
gonadotropins, 984
insulin sensitizers, 983-984
metformin, 983
metformin plus clomiphene, 983
metformin vs. clomiphene, 983
ovarian surgery, 984
thiazolidinediones, 983-984

in vitro fertilization, 984
weight loss, 982
for endometrial hyperplasia, 984
for hirsutism, 982
for irregular and infrequent
menses, 981-982
not recommended, 984-985
for obesity, 984
Polycythemia, 1132-1136
appropriate, 1132-1135
in cardiopulmonary disease, 1134
Chuvash, 1135-1136
classification of, 1132
in COPD, 1134
in cyanotic congenital heart
disease, 1134
due to drug use, 1136
due to high carboxyhemoglobin
levels, 1135, 1134f
due to recombinant human
erythropoietin abuse, 1136
evaluation of, flowchart for,
1132, 1133f
familial, 1135-1136, 1135f
with high-affinity hemoglobin,
1133-1134, 1134f
at high altitude, 1132, 1134f
initial evaluation in, 1132, 1133f
in obesity-hypoventilation
syndrome, 1134-1135
in obstructive sleep apnea, 1134
relative (Gaisbock syndrome), 1132
in renal and hepatic disorders,
1135
secondary, 1132-1136
Polycythemia vera, 2580-2582
clinical course, 2581-2582
diagnosis of, 2580, 2581t
differential diagnosis of, 2581
pathophysiology of, 2580
treatment of, 2582
Polymerase chain reaction,
1954, 1954f
Polymyalgia rheumatica, 1387
Polymyositis. See Myositis
Polymyxin B, 1433
Polyneuropathy(ies), 2297-2306. See
also Neuropathy(ies)
in amyloidosis, 2302
axonal, metabolic, 2300
chronic inflammatory
demyelinating, apheresis for,
1218
critical illness, 2300
demyelinating, 2297, 2298t
diabetic, 671-672, 672t, 2298-2299
autonomic, 671, 672, 2299-2300
mechanisms of, 667-668, 668f
pancreas transplantation and,
938
truncal, 2300
differential diagnosis of, 2297-
2298, 2298t
drugs causing, 2298, 2299t
familial amyloid, 2302
immune-inflammatory, 2300-2303
industrial chemicals causing,
2303, 2303t
in infectious disease, 2304-2306
inherited, 2300, 2298t
in leprosy, 2304
monoclonal protein-associated,
2302
Polyomavirus nephropathy, 2121-2122
Polyp(s), adenomatous, in colorectal
cancer, 2474, 2474f
Polypectomy, colonoscopic, bleeding
in, 865
Polyradiculoneuropathy
chronic inflammatory
demyelinating, 2302
cytomegaloviral, 2351-2352
Polysomnographic study

all-night, 2365
in pulmonary hypertension, 2854
Poncet disease (tuberculous
rheumatism), 1678, 1681
Pontiac fever, 1654
Pontine myelinolysis, central,
metabolic encephalopathy in,
2341
Popliteal artery, entrapment of, 406
Porifera, 193
Pork tapeworm, 1937-1938, 1937f, 1939f
Porphyria, 748-756
acute intermittent, 749-
751, 750f, 752t
diagnosis of, 750-751
pathophysiology of, 749-750, 750f
treatment of, 751, 752t
ALAD-deficiency, 752-753, 752t, 750f
classification of, 748, 748f
clinical presentation of, 749-755
with cutaneous photosensitivity,
753-755
erythropoietic, congenital,
437, 437f, 755
hepatoerythropoietic, 754
with neurovisceral attacks, 749-
753, 748f
pathophysiology of, 748-749, 750f
variegate, 751, 752t
Porphyria cutanea tarda, 753-754
cutaneous findings in, 437, 438f
iron overload in, 1088
Portosystemic encephalopathy, 2338
Port-wine stain (nevus flammeus),
545, 544f
Positron emission tomography (PET)
in brain trauma, 2231, 2231f
in osteomyositis, 1546
in pelvic mass, 1057
Postabortion fever, Mycoplasma
hominis and, 1742
Postgastrectomy steatorrhea,
malabsorption in, 834-835
Postherpetic neuralgia, 2349-2350
Postmenopausal disorders. See under
Menopause
Postpartum fever, Mycoplasma hominis
and, 1742
Postpartum hemolytic-uremic
syndrome, 2035
Postpartum infection, streptococcal,
group A, 1570
Postpartum thyroiditis, 1020-1021
Postrenal disease, 1970, 1970t
Postsplenectomy infection,
overwhelming, pneumococcal, 1565
Posttraumatic epilepsy, after brain
trauma, 2236
Posttraumatic stress disorder, 2661-
2662
Potassium
dietary, 30
homeostasis, 2006, 1995f
intake of, low, 2006
plasma, 2006-2013. See also
Hyperkalemia, Hypokalemia
renal regulation of, 2006, 1995f
Potassium channel disorders, 2282
Potassium citrate, for
nephrolithiasis, 2110
Potassium phosphate, for
nephrolithiasis, 2109-2110
Potomania, beer, 1983
Pouchitis, 849
Poultry, dietary, 31
Powassan virus, 1855
Poxvirus infection, 1772-1774
primate, 1859
ruminate, 1859
Prader-Willi syndrome, 1950
Pramipexole, for parkinsonism, 2247t
Pramlintide
for type 1 diabetes, 645

for type 2 diabetes mellitus, 661
Prayer, intercessory, 86t
Prazosin, for hypertension, 223t
Prediabetes and, 651, 652t
Prednisone
for autoimmune hepatitis, 884
for idiopathic thrombocytopenic
purpura, 1167
for rheumatoid arthritis, 1308t
Preeclampsia, 1024
renal involvement in, 2079-2080
Pregabalin, 2186
in epilepsy, 2196
Pregnancy
acute renal failure in, 2035
antibiotics in, 1421-1422, 1422t
in antiphospholipid antibody
syndrome, 1198-1199
arrhythmia in, 1019
asthma in, 1021, 2707, 2716
autoimmune disease in, 1022
black widow spider bites in, 188
cancer in, 1022
cardiac valvular disease in, 1018-
1019
cardiovascular disease in, 1018-
1019
diabetes mellitus in, 1019, 1024-
1025, 1024t
type 1, 644
eating disorders and, 2666
ectopic, 1010-1013, 1011f
in adolescent, 1059
clinical manifestations of,
1010, 1012t
diagnosis of, 1010-1012, 1012t
history and physical examination
of, 1010, 1012t
laboratory testing in, 1010-1012
treatment of, 1012-1013, 1012t,
1011f
epilepsy and, 2198
FDA drug classification system in,
1017t, 1017
gestational diabetes in, 1024-
1025, 1024t. See Diabetes
mellitus, gestational
group B Streptococcus infection
in, 1022
hepatitis in, 1022
herpes simplex infection in, 1021
HIV infection in, 1021-1022
hyperemesis gravidarum in, 1023-
1024
hypertension in, 1018
idiopathic thrombocytopenic
purpura in, 1168-1169
infectious disease in, 1021-1022
inflammatory bowel disease and,
808
intrahepatic cholestasis in, 1023
listeriosis in, 1590
malaria chemoprophylaxis during,
78
medical complications of, 1016-
1026
neurologic disease in, 1023
nicotine medication during, 20
parvovirus infection in, 1021
peripartum cardiomyopathy and,
1019
physiologic changes in, 1017
planning and counseling, 1016
preeclampsia in, 1024
prolactinoma and, 594
prosthetic heart valves and, 361-
362
renal disease in, 1022
in sickle cell anemia, 1117
snakebite in, 186-187
substance abuse in, 1023
syphilis in, 1707-1708
in systemic lupus erythematosus,

1338
teratogenesis and, 1016-1017
thrombocytopenia in, 1173-1174
thrombophilia in, 1021
thyroid disease in, 1019-1021
tuberculosis in, 1691-1692
urinary tract infection in, 1508
treatment of, 1515
venous thromboembolism in, 421-422
venous thrombosis in, 421-422
von Willebrand disease in, 1181-1182
Preleukemia. *See* Myelodysplastic syndrome
Premenstrual syndrome, 962-965, 962t
diagnosis of, 962-963, 962t-963t
differential diagnosis of, 963
pathogenesis of, 962, 963t
treatment of, 963-964
behavioral therapy for, 963-964
nonpharmacologic, 963-964
pharmacologic, 964
surgical, 964
Prenatal testing, DNA-based, 1964
Preoperative assessment, 50-57
approach to consultation in, 50
cardiac risk factor calculation in, 50, 51t-52t
cardiovascular risk in, 51-53
chest x-ray in, 53
clinical evaluation in, 51-54
coronary artery disease in, 51-53
electrocardiography in, 53
endocrine disease in, 54
heart failure in, 51
laboratory testing in, 54-55
liver disease in, 53-54
management of surgical risk factors in, 55-56
advanced age, 56
alcohol abuse, 56
blood pressure, 55
coronary artery disease, 55
corticosteroid therapy, 56
decreased hematocrit, 55-56
diabetes mellitus, 55
hyperglycemia, 55
liver disease, 56
renal insufficiency, 55
thrombosis, 56
thyroid disease, 56
medication review and adjustment in, 54
neurologic disease in, 54
pulmonary function tests in, 53
pulmonary risk in, 53
renal risk in, 53
Prepatellar bursitis, 1396
Prepubertal females, pelvic mass in, 1058, 1061
Prerenal disease, 1969, 1970t
Pressure sore. *See* Pressure ulcer
Pressure ulcer
in mechanical ventilation, 2819
palliative treatment of, 107, 109t
Preventive health care, 41-49
alcohol use, 49
behavioral-counseling interventions, 48-49, 48t
cancer prevention, 42-47, 47t. *See also individual diseases*
breast cancer and, 44-47
cervical cancer and, 42-43
colorectal cancer and, 43-44
cancer screening
lung cancer and, 48
not recommended, 47-48
prostate cancer and, 48
chapters of *ACP Medicine* covering, 41, 42t-43t
immunization, 41-42, 47t. *See also* Immunization
noncancer, 41-42, 46t

noncancer screening, 48, 48t
rationale and evolution of, 41, 44t-45t
reminder systems, 49
smoking cessation, 49
USPSTF evidence ratings in, 41, 46t
Prevotella melaninogenica, 1604
Priapism, in sickle crisis, 1116
Primaquine, for malaria chemoprophylaxis, for travelers, 78
Prion disease
screening for, blood donation and, 1207-1208
in spongiform encephalopathy, 2358-2359, 2358f-2359f
Procainamide
for atrial fibrillation, 242t-243t
classification of, 267t
hypersensitivity syndrome reaction due to, 496
Proctitis
chlamydial, 1749, 1748t
dietary protein, 1280-1281
in males having sex with males, 1529-1530
ulcerative, 791
medical treatment of, 804
Proctocolitis, in males having sex with males, 1529-1530
Proctosigmoiditis, 791-792
Progestins, for endometriosis, 970, 970t
Proguanil, for malaria chemoprophylaxis, for travelers, 78
Prolactin, 592-594
serum, in polycystic ovary syndrome, 978
synthesis, secretion, actions of, 592
Prolactinoma, 593-594, 593t, 595f
pregnancy and, 594
treatment of, 593-594, 593t, 595f
Pro-opiomelanocortin peptides, appetite control and, 598
Propafenone
for atrial fibrillation, 242t-243t
classification of, 267t
Propionibacterium acnes, 1604
Propranolol
classification of, 267t
for hypertension, 222t
toxicity of, 163t
Propranolol extended release, for hypertension, 222t
Prostacyclin, in coagulation, 1156-1157, 1158f
Prostate
benign hyperplasia of, 2126-2134
acute urinary retention in, 2133
clinical features of, 2127
diagnosis of, 2127-2130
epidemiology and risk factors for, 2126, 2126f
history of, 2127-2129, 2128f
International Prostate Symptom Score, 2128, 2128f
laboratory testing in, 2129-2130
management of, 2130-2133, 2130f
medical treatment of, 2130-2132, 2131t
alpha blockers, 2130-2131, 2131t
combination, 2132
finasteride for, 2131-2132
phytotherapy, 2132
pathophysiology of, 2126-2127, 2127f
physical examination in, 2129
surgical treatment of, 2132-2133
transurethral incision of (TUIP), 2132-2133

Prostate cancer, 2528-2536
diagnosis of, 2530
epidemiology of, 2528
environmental factors in, 2377
genetic risk factors for, 2379
natural history of, 2532
pathogenesis of, 2529
prevention of, 2535
risk factors in, 2528-2529
age as, 2528
diet as, 2528
family history as, 2528
hormones and growth factor as, 2528-2529
racial variability as, 2528
screening for, 48, 2529-2530, 2529t-2530t
digital rectal exam, 2529
prostate-specific antigen, 2529-2530, 2529t-2530t
staging in, 2530-2531
clinical, 2530-2531, 2531t
imaging studies in, 2531
multifactorial, 2531, 2532t
treatment of advanced disease, 2533-2535
androgen ablation, 2534
bone pain palliation in, 2535
chemotherapy, 2534-2535
salvage, 2534
treatment of localized disease, 2532-2533, 2532t
adjuvant therapy for, 2533
radiation therapy for, 2533
radical prostatectomy for, 2532
risk of recurrence and, 2533, 2532t
side effects of, 2533
Prostatectomy
open, 2132-2133
transurethral (TURP), 2132-2133
Prostate-specific antigen (PSA), serum
for benign hyperplasia of prostate, 2129
for cancer screening, 2529-2530, 2529t-2530t
Prostatitis, in urinary tract infection, 1511-1512, 1516
Prosthesis
heart valve. *See* Heart valve replacement
joint, septic arthritis in, 1539-1540
Protein(s)
dietary, 27-28
in chronic renal failure, 2044
enterocolitis and, 1280, 1280t
in nephrolithiasis, 2107-2108
obesity and, 721
proctitis and, 1280-1281
as nutrient requirement, 945
Protein C
in coagulation, 1155-1156, 1157f
deficiency, 1193
test for, 1162
Protein intake, in chronic renal failure, 2019, 2019t
Proteinosis, alveolar, 2781-2782, 2782f
Protein S
in coagulation, 1155, 1157f
deficiency, 1193
test for, 1162
Proteinuria, 1972-1973
asymptomatic, 1972
in chronic renal disease, 2014
in chronic renal failure, 2018, 2041
diagnosis of, 1973
glomerular, 1972
orthostatic, 1972
overflow, 1972

persistent, 1972-1973
transient, 1972
tubulointerstitial, 1972-1973
Proteus infections, 1631-1632
Proteus meningitis, 1553t
Proteus mirabilis, 1631-1632
antimicrobial susceptibilities of, 1421t
Prothrombin gene mutation 20210A, 1195
Prothrombin time (PT), 1160
Proton pump inhibitors, for gastroesophageal reflux disease, 766-767
Proto-oncogene(s), 2384-2385, 2384t
activating or gain-of-function mutations, 2383-2385, 2384t, 2385f
chromosomal translocation, 2384-2385
gene amplification, 2384-2385
point mutations, 2383
Protoporphyria, erythropoietic, 754-755
Protozoan infections, 1892-1917. *See also individual disorders, e.g.,* Toxoplasmosis
definitions of, 1892, 1892f
Internet resources for, 1911
intestinal, 1901-1909. *See also individual disorders, e.g.,* Giardiasis
thrombocytopenia due to, 1173
as transfusion reaction, 1217
PSA. *See* Prostate-specific antigen (PSA)
Pseudochylothorax, 2831
Pseudocysts, pancreatic
in acute pancreatitis, 923
in alcoholic pancreatitis, 929
definition of, 913
Pseudogout, 1377-1380
acute, 1378
in chronic rheumatoid-like arthritis, 1378
conditions associated with, 1378-1379, 1378t
diagnosis of, 1379, 1379f
in osteoarthritis, 1378
Pseudo-Hurler polydystrophy, 1148t
Pseudohyperkalemia, 2009t, 2012
Pseudohypertension, 226
Pseudohypoaldosteronism (mineralocorticoid resistance), 688
Pseudohyponatremia, 1980t, 1980
Pseudomonas aeruginosa, antimicrobial susceptibilities of, 1421t
Pseudomonas aeruginosa infection, 1658-1662
antibiotic treatment of, 1662
bacteremia, 1660
central nervous system infections, 1660-1661
clinical syndromes, 1659-1662
cystic fibrosis, 1659-1660
ear infections, 1660
endocarditis, 1660
epidemiology of, 1658
eye infections, 1660
folliculitis, 513
meningitis, 1553t
pathogenesis of, 1658-1659
pneumonia, 1659
community-acquired, 1659
in HIV disease, 1659
nosocomial, 1659
skin infections, 1661-1662
urinary tract infections, 1660
Pseudo-obstruction, intestinal, chronic, 856-857
Pseudopelade, 569

Pseudoporphyria, as drug reaction, 499
Pseudotumor cerebri, headache in, 2154t, 2165-2166, 2166t
Pseudo-von Willebrand disease, 1181
Pseudoxanthoma elasticum, cutaneous findings in, 433, 434f
Psittacosis, 1751-1752
Psoralen and ultraviolet light (PUVA), for psoriasis, 467-468
Psoriasis, 461-473
  arthritis in, 464, 1317t, 1324-1325
    osteoarthritis vs., 1387
  clinical variants in, 462-464, 462f-464f
  diagnosis of, 462-464
  differential diagnosis of, 464-465
  epidemiology of, 461
  erythrodermic, 463, 463f
  etiology of, 461-462
  genetic factors in, 461
  guttate, 462, 463f
  histopathology in, 464
  in HIV infection, 462
  infection and drugs in, 462
  Koebner response in, 462
  nail pathology in, 464, 464f, 574, 576t
  pathogenesis of, 461
  plaque, 462, 462f-463f
  psychological stress and climate in, 461-462
  pustular, 463-464, 464f
  streptococcal infection in, 462
  treatment of, 465-472
    acitretin, 469
    anthralin, topical, 466-467
    biologic therapies for, 470-472
    calcipotriene, topical, 465
    combination therapies in, 470
    corticosteroids, topical, 465, 466t
    cyclosporine, 469-470
    hydroxyurea, 470
    maxacalcitol for, 465-466
    methotrexate, 468-469
    photochemotherapy for, 467-468
    phototherapy, 467, 468f
    prognosis in, 472
    PUVA, 467-468
    systemic therapy, 468-472
    tacalcitol for, 465-466
    tacrolimus (FK506), 470
    tar, topical, 466
    tazarotene, topical, 466
    topical, 465-467, 466t
    vitamin D analogues for, 465-466
Psychiatric disorders
  alcoholism and, 2626-2627
  in dying patients, 108-109, 110t
Psychogenic nonepileptic seizure, 2191
Psychological stress, in psoriasis, 461
Psychosocial issues
  in rheumatic disease, 1292
  in terminal illness, 112-120
    antidepressant medication in, 116, 116t
    breaking bad news and, 112
    communicating with patient and, 113
    family and friends and, 113-114
    grief and bereavement and, 117-118
    helping bereaved in, 118-120
    medications and bereavement, 119-120
    occupation and work and, 114
    patient's response in, 115-117
      anxiety, 115-116
      denial and panic, 115
      depression, 116-117, 116t

despondency, 116
    fear, 115
    personality disorders, 117
    physician's role in, 114-115
      cheerfulness, 114-115
      compassion, 114
      consistency and perseverance, 115
    preliminary considerations in, 112-113
    preparation for end of life, 117
    religion and spirituality and, 114
    specific types of loss, 119
    telling truth and, 112-113
Psychotherapy
  for depression, 2619
  for generalized anxiety disorder, 2662
  for obsessive-compulsive disorder, 2664
  for panic disorder, 2660
  for posttraumatic stress disorder, 2661
  for social anxiety disorder, 2663
Psychotic self-induced hyponatremia, 1981t, 1981-1982
PTCH basal, properties of, 2386t
PTEN, properties of, 2386t, 2391
Puberty, delayed, 694
Public health preparedness, biologic agent categories for, 122t
Pulmonary angiography, in pulmonary embolism, 416, 415t
Pulmonary arterial aneurysm, pulmonary hypertension in, 2862
Pulmonary arterial hypertension, idiopathic, 2857-2859
  diagnosis of, 2858
  epidemiology of, 2857
  etiology and pathogenesis of, 2857-2858
  prognosis in, 2859
  treatment of, 2858-2859
Pulmonary arteriography, in pulmonary hypertension, 2854-2855
  chronic thromboembolic, 2860, 2860f
Pulmonary arteriovenous malformation, 2756
  pulmonary hypertension in, 2862
Pulmonary artery stenosis, pulmonary hypertension in, 2863
Pulmonary blastomycosis, 1865
Pulmonary capillary hemangiomatosis, pulmonary hypertension in, 2863
Pulmonary cavitation. See Pulmonary infiltrate(s), cavitary
Pulmonary coccidioidomycosis, 1867
  treatment of, 1868-1869
Pulmonary disease
  bullous, 2734
  chronic diffuse infiltrative, 2758-2785
    in alveolar hemorrhage, diffuse, 2783
    in alveolar proteinosis, 2781-2782, 2782f, 2769t-2770t
    in anti-GBM antibody disease, 2783, 2769t-2770t
    approach to patient with, 2758-2761, 2759t-2761t, 2760f
    in asbestosis, 2764
    in berylliosis, 2765
    in bronchiolitis obliterans organizing pneumonia, 2778, 2779f, 2767t-2768t
    bronchoalveolar lavage in, 2760-2761
    chest radiography, 2760, 2760t
    in coal worker's pneumoconiosis, 2765

in collagen vascular disease, 2779-2780, 2767t-2768t
    computed tomography in, high-resolution, 2760, 2760f
    in dermatomyositis, 2780
    drug-induced, 2758, 2759t, 2761-2764, 2759t
      amiodarone, 2763-2764
      cytotoxic, 2762-2763
      gold, 2764
      nitrofurantoin, 2763
      noncytotoxic, 2763-2764
      penicillamine, 2764
      talc-induced granulomatosis, 2764
    in eosinophilic granuloma of lung, 2780-2781, 2769t-2770t
    in eosinophilic pneumonia, 2782-2783, 2769t-2770t
    in hypersensitivity pneumonitis, 2765-2767
    infectious, 2758
    laboratory examination in, 2759-2760
    lung biopsy in, 2761, 2761t
    in lymphangiomyomatosis, 2783-2784, 2769t-2770t
    in malignancy, 2767-2769
    in microlithiasis, 2784
    in mixed connective tissue disease, 2780
    occupational, 2758, 2759t
    pathogenesis of, 2758
    physical examination in, 2759
    in pneumoconioses, 2764-2765
    Pneumocystis carinii, 2758. See also Pneumocystis carinii pneumonia
    in polymyositis, 2780
    in progressive systemic sclerosis, 2780
    in pulmonary fibrosis, idiopathic, 2774-2775, 2767t-2768t. See also Pulmonary fibrosis, idiopathic
    pulmonary function testing in, 2760
    in pulmonary hemosiderosis, 2783
    in rheumatoid arthritis, 2779-2780
    in sarcoidosis, 2769-2774. See also Sarcoidosis
    in silicosis, 2764
    in Sjogren syndrome, 2780
    symptoms and history in, 2758-2759
    in systemic lupus erythematosus, 2779
    treatment of, 2761
  chronic obstructive. See Chronic obstructive pulmonary disease (COPD)
  focal and multifocal, 2744-2757. See also Pulmonary infiltrate(s)
  interstitial, sleep-disordered breathing in, 2797
  invasive diagnostic and therapeutic techniques in, 2687-2696, 2687t. See also individual procedures
    diagnostic bronchoscopy, 2688-2692
    mediastinoscopy, 2696
    therapeutic bronchoscopy, 2692-2695
    thoracoscopy, 2696
    thoracotomy with open lung biopsy, 2696
    transesophageal endoscopic ultrasound, 2695-2696
    transthoracic needle aspiration, 2687-2688

Pulmonary edema, 2842-2851
  cardiogenic, 2843, 2844t
    noncardiogenic vs., 2842-2843, 2844t
    treatment of, 2843, 2844t
  in drug administration, 2849-2850, 2850t
  high-altitude, 2849. See also High altitude
  in lung resection, 2850
  in neurologic insults, 2848-2849
  noncardiogenic, 2844-2848. See also Acute respiratory distress syndrome (ARDS)
    cardiogenic vs., 2842-2843, 2844t
  pathogenesis of, 2842
  patient approach, 2842-2843, 2843f, 2842t
  in upper airway obstruction, 2849
Pulmonary embolism, 413-416. See also Thromboembolism, venous, Thrombosis, venous
  anticoagulants for, 420-421
  in cardiac arrest, 149t
  chest radiography for, 413
  clinical features of, 413
  compression ultrasonography for, 415-416
  computed tomography for, 416, 415f
  D-dimer testing for, 415, 416f
  diagnostic approach to, 416f
  diagnostic tests for, 413-416, 414f-415f, 414t-415t
  in endocarditis, 1485
  fever of undetermined origin in, 1415
  magnetic resonance imaging for, 415
  pleural effusion in, 2829-2830
  pulmonary angiography for, 416, 415t
  septic, 1479-1480
  ventilation-perfusion lung scan for, 413-414, 414f
Pulmonary eosinophilia. See Eosinophilia, pulmonary
Pulmonary fibrosis
  idiopathic, 2774-2775, 2767t-2768t
    clinical manifestations of, 2774
    diagnosis of, 2774-2775, 2775f
    lung biopsy in, 2775
    pathogenesis of, 2774, 2776f
    prognosis and treatment of, 2775
  in rheumatoid arthritis, 1305
  in scleroderma, 1346
Pulmonary function, exercise and, 33
Pulmonary function testing, 2674-2686
  airway reactivity, 2683-2684
  in bronchiectasis, 2736
  categories of, 2674-2684
  in chronic diffuse infiltrative pulmonary disease, 2760
  in cigarette smoking, 2720-2721, 2721f-2722f
  in COPD, 2726, 2726f
  diffusing capacity in, 2679-2680, 2680t
  exercise testing, 2682-2683, 2683t
  gas exchange in, 2680-2682, 2682t
    carbon dioxide levels in, 2682
    pulse oximetry in, 2682
  indications for, 2674
  interpretation of, 2684-2686, 2684f
    airway obstruction, 2684-2685, 2685f
    restrictive defects, 2685-2686, 2684f
  in preoperative assessment, 53
  pressure-flow relationships, 2675-2677, 2674f-2677f
    airway resistance in, 2675, 2674f
    spirometry and maximal flow

volume curves in, 2675-2676, 2675f-2677f
pressure-volume relationships, 2677-2678, 2678f-2679f
lung elasticity in, 2678, 2679f
lung volume in, 2677-2678, 2678f
in pulmonary hypertension, 2854
respiratory muscle function in, 2678-2679
Pulmonary hemosiderosis, alveolar hemorrhage in, 2783
Pulmonary histoplasmosis, 1862
treatment of, 1864
multiple nodules in, 2755
single nodule in, 2753, 2754f
Pulmonary hypertension, 2852-2855
chronic thromboembolic, 2859-2861, 2860f
diagnosis of, 2860, 2860f, 2865:XI:2857f
epidemiology of, 2859-2860
pathogenesis of, 2860
prognosis in, 2861
treatment of, 2861
classification of, 2852, 2852t
in connective tissue disease, 2861
diagnosis of, 2853-2855, 2855f-2857f
in hematologic disorders, 2862
imaging and physiologic testing in, 2853-2854, 2856f
pathogenesis of, 2852-2853, 2853t, 2854f
physical examination in, 2853
physiology of, 2852, 2853f
in pulmonary arteriovenous malformation, 2862
in pulmonary veno-occlusive disease, 2861-2862
in scleroderma, 1346
treatment of, 2855
underlying causes of, tests for, 2854-2855, 2857f
venous, pleural effusion in, 2828
Pulmonary infarction, segmental pulmonary infiltrates in, 2751
Pulmonary infection, 1468-1481, 1468t. See also individual disorders, e.g., Pneumonia
major causes of, 1468t
Pulmonary infiltrate(s)
cavitary, 2751-2753, 2751t
in infectious disease, 2751-2752
in lung cancer, 2752, 2752f
in lung gangrene, 2752
in neoplastic disease, 2752, 2752f
in parasitic infection, 2752
in pneumonia, 2751-2752
in suppurative infection, 2752, 2752f
in tuberculosis, 2752, 2752f
in Wegener granulomatosis, 2752-2753, 2752f
focal, 2744-2746, 2744t
in alveolar cell carcinoma, 2745, 2745f
in bacterial pneumonia, 2744, 2745f
chest radiography in, 2744
infectious, 2744, 2745f
in lipoid pneumonia, 2746, 2745f
in lobe torsion, 2746
in lung contusion, 2746
in lymphoma, 2745
neoplastic, 2744-2745, 2744t
noninfectious, neoplastic, 2745-2746, 2744t
in radiation pneumonitis, 2745-2746
multifocal, 2746-2749, 2745t, 2746f
in allergic granulomatosis and angiitis, 2749

in alveolar cell carcinoma, 2746f, 2747
in alveolar sarcoidosis, 2746f, 2747
in ankylosing spondylitis, 2749
in bronchiolitis obliterans organizing pneumonia, 2748
in Caplan syndrome, 2749
chest radiography in, 2744
in chronic or acute eosinophilic pneumonia, 2748
in endemic fungal pneumonia, 2747
in Hodgkin disease, 2747
in infectious disease, 2747
in invasive aspergillosis, 2747
in melioidosis, 2747
in neoplastic disease, 2747, 2746f
in pneumococcal pneumonia, 2746-2747, 2746f
in rheumatoid arthritis, 2749
in silicosis, 2749
in simple eosinophilic pneumonia, 2748
in systemic lupus erythematosus, 2749
in tropical pulmonary eosinophilia, 2748
in tuberculosis, 2747
in Wegener granulomatosis, 2749
segmental, 2749-2751, 2749t
in adenoid cystic carcinoma, 2750
in allergic bronchopulmonary aspergillosis, 2751, 2750f
in amyloidosis, 2751
in asthma, 2751
in bronchiectasis, 2750
in carcinoid lung tumors, 2750, 2750f
in foreign bodies, 2751
in infectious disease, 2750, 2749t, 2750f
in mucoepidermoid carcinoma, 2750
in Mycoplasma pneumonia, 2750, 2750f
in neoplastic disease, 2750-2751, 2749t, 2750f
in pulmonary infarction, 2751
in sarcoidosis, 2751
in tuberculosis, 2750
Pulmonary lymphangitic carcinomatosis, 2768
Pulmonary mass, large, 2754-2755, 2755t
in infectious disease, 2754, 2755f
in neoplastic disease, 2754, 2755f
Pulmonary nodule(s)
multiple, 2755-2757, 2755t
in amyloidosis, 2756-2757
in endocarditis, 2755, 2756f
in endovascular infection, 2755
in infectious disease, 2755-2756
in lymphomatoid granulomatosis, 2756
in neoplastic disease, 2756
in pulmonary arteriovenous malformation, 2756
in sarcoidosis, 2756-2757
in Wegener granulomatosis, 2756, 2756f
single, small, 2753-2754, 2753t
in infectious disease, 2753, 2754f
in neoplastic disease, 2753, 2754f
Pulmonary valve regurgitation, murmur in, 210t
Pulmonary vasculitis, in allergic granulomatosis and angiitis, 2782-2783

Pulmonary veno-occlusive disease, pulmonary hypertension in, 2861-2862
Pulmonic stenosis
congenital, 359, 348t, 350t, 393
murmur in, 210t
Pulsed light, intense, for hirsutism, 992
Pulseless disease (Takayasu arteritis), 374-375
Pulseless electrical activity, in cardiac resuscitation, 152, 151f
Pupillary light response, in encephalopathy, 2336
Pure white cell aplasia, neutropenia with, 1143
Purine nucleoside phosphorylase deficiency, 1230t
Purpura
definition of, 429t
Henoch-Schonlein. See Henoch-Schonlein purpura
thrombocytopenic. See Thrombocytopenic purpura
vascular, 1176-1178, 1177t
in small vessel vasculitis, 1361, 1361f
Puss caterpillar, 191
Pustule, definition of, 426t
Pyelography
intravenous, 1969t
retrograde or antegrade, 1969t
Pyelonephritis
acute
acute cholecystitis vs., 904
Mycoplasma hominis in, 1742
acute bacterial, 2093
acute uncomplicated, management of, 1514-1515, 1515f, 1516t
candidal, 1878t
chronic, 2093
in urinary tract infection, 1511. See also Urinary tract infection
xanthogranulomatous, 2093
Pyoderma gangrenosum, in inflammatory bowel disease, 435, 435f
Pyogenic granuloma, 546-547, 546f
Pyomyositis, tropical, staphylococcal, 1578
Pyrethrin, for pediculosis, 520, 521t
Pyrexia. See Fever, Hyperthermia
Pyropoikilocytosis, hereditary, 1110, 1110f
Pyruvate kinase deficiency, hemolytic anemia in, 1113

Q

22q11 deletion syndrome, 1949
Q fever, 1734-1735
diagnosis of, 1727t, 1734-1735
epidemiology and etiology of, 1734
treatment of, 1728t, 1735
Qigong, 88
QT interval, prolonged, medications causing, 204t
QT syndrome
long, congenital, 204t, 265
short, congenital, 266
Quadriplegia, respiratory dysfunction in, 2806, 2805f
Queensland tick typhus, 1728
Quinapril, for hypertension, 222t
Quinidine
for atrial fibrillation, 242t-243t
classification of, 267t
purpura due to, 1169
Quinine, purpura due to, 1169
Quinupristin, 1436-1437
Quinupristin-dalfopristin, in pregnancy, 1422t

R

Rabies, 1856-1857
Rabies immunization, for travelers, 72
Rabies prophylaxis, postexposure, 182, 183t
Radiation
ionizing
in cancer epidemiology, 2378
leukemia due to, 2377-2378, 2561-2562
ultraviolet (UV), skin cancer and, 549
Radiation enteritis, malabsorption in, 831
Radiation exposure, workplace, leukemia due to, 2561-2562
Radiation nephritis, 2092
Radiation pneumonitis, focal infiltrates in, 2745-2746
Radiation therapy
brain injury due to, late delayed, 2320-2321
for brain tumors, 2313
brain tumors due to, 2321
for breast cancer, 2463-2464
with breast conservation therapy, 2463-2464
with mastectomy, 2464
cranial, pituitary failure due to, 603
encephalopathy due to
acute, 2320
early delayed, 2320
leukemia due to, 2561-2562
for lung cancer. See under Lung cancer
myelopathy or neuropathy due to, late delayed, 2321
neurotoxicity of, 2320-2321
pericardial effusion in, 380
testicular damage in, 693
Radiculitis, in Lyme disease, 1714
Radioallergosorbent (RAST) testing, for IgE, 1249, 1249f
Radiocontrast media
allergy to, 1276
nephrotoxicity of, 2031-2032
Radiography
abdominal
in acute pancreatitis, 917
in renal disease, 1969t
in ankylosing spondylitis, 1319, 1318f, 1320f-1321f
chest
in alpha$_1$-antitrypsin deficiency, 2733, 2733f
in bronchiectasis, 2735, 2736f
in chronic infiltrative pulmonary disease, 2760, 2760t
in focal and multifocal pulmonary infiltrates, 2744
in pleural effusion, 2824-2825, 2824f-2826f
in pneumothorax, 2835, 2835f
in preoperative assessment, 53
in pulmonary embolism, 413
in pulmonary hypertension, 2853-2854
in tuberculosis, 1685
in Wegener granulomatosis, 1363, 1364f
in Crohn disease, 797-798
in fever of undetermined origin, 1417
in osteomyelitis, 1545, 1546t
in rheumatic disease, 1294-1295
in rheumatoid arthritis, 1306
in ulcerative colitis, 794-795, 795f
Radionuclide imaging

in intra-abdominal abscess, 1503-1504
in myocardial infarction, acute, 319
in osteomyelitis, 1545-1546, 1546t
in renal disease, 1969t
in septic arthritis, 1536
technetium-99m perfusion
in chest pain, 200t
in GI bleeding, 867
thallium-201 perfusion, in chest pain, 200t
in ulcerative colitis, 795
Raloxifene, 2419t
for breast cancer prevention, 2459
for osteoporosis, 709-710
Ramipril, for hypertension, 222t
Ramsay Hunt syndrome, 2266
Rapid eye movement (REM) sleep, 2362, 2363f
disorders of, 2371
ras, in cancer biology, 2409, 2409f
Rapid urinary antigen test, for *S. pneumoniae*, 1450
Rash. *See also under* Skin disorder(s)
butterfly, in systemic lupus erythematosus, 1330, 1331f
Rash arthralgia, 1857-1858
Rat bite, 181, 182t
Rat-bite fever, 181, 1721-1722, 1721t
Rat tapeworm, 1939
Rattlesnake, 183, 184f. *See also* Snakebite
Raynaud phenomenon
in peripheral arterial disease, 406-407, 407t
in scleroderma, 1342, 1344-1345, 1344f, 1348
RB1 gene
oncogenic mechanisms of, 2387-2388, 2389f, 2386t
in retinoblastoma, 1961-1962
Rb protein, in cancer biology, 2410
Rectal cancer, chemoradiotherapy for, 2487
Rectal exam, digital, for prostate cancer, 2529
Rectum, *Neisseria gonorrhoeae* infection of, 1622, 1624t
Red cell(s). *See also* Erythrocyte(s)
transfusion. *See* Transfusion therapy, red cell
Red cell exchange, 1218
5alpha-Reductase inhibitors, for benign prostatic hyperplasia, 2131-2132
5alpha-Reductase type 2 deficiency, 695
Reed-Sternberg cell, in Hodgkin disease, 2596, 2597f
Reflux esophagitis. *See* Gastroesophageal reflux disease
Rehabilitation, for brain trauma, 2236-2237
Reiter syndrome, 1317t
Relapsing fever, 1719-1721
clinical manifestations of, 1720
diagnosis and treatment of, 1720-1721, 1720f
epidemiology of, 1720, 1720f
pathogenesis of, 1720
Remnant removal disease, 739
hyperlipidemia in, 731
Renal abscess
candidal, 1878t
macroscopic, in urinary tract infection, 1511
Renal arteriography, 1969t
Renal artery disease, atheromatous, renovascular hypertension in, 232
Renal artery stenosis, 2071-2073

atherosclerotic, 2071
treatment of, 2072-2073
in fibromuscular dysplasia, 2071-2072
treatment of, 2073
pathophysiology and diagnosis in, 2072, 2072f
in postrenal-transplantation, 2120
Renal biopsy
in glomerular disease, 2052-2054
in lupus nephritis, 1334, 1334t-1335t, 1336
Renal calculus(i). *See* Nephrolithiasis
Renal cell carcinoma, 2516-2519
clinical and laboratory findings in, 2516-2517, 2516f
diagnosis of, 2516-2518, 2516f-2517f
epidemiology and etiology of, 2516
imaging studies in, 2517-2518, 2517f
management of, 2518-2519
pathobiology of, 2516
staging in, 2518
treatment of, IL-2 for, 2404-2405
Renal cyst, simple, 2097
Renal cystic disease, acquired, 2099. *See also* Polycystic kidney disease
Renal disease
acute, 2026-2039
acidosis in, 2037-2038
in acute interstitial nephritis, 2035
anemia in, 2038
chronic *vs.*, 2032t
community-acquired, 2031, 2032t
complications of, 2036-2038
cost of care in, 2036
definitions of, 2026, 2026t
dialysis in, 2036
dopamine for, 2036
epidemiology of, 2026
in hospitalized patient, 2026-2031
acute tubular necrosis in, 2027-2028
BUN:creatinine ratio in, 2028
chart review, history, physical examination in, 2028, 2029t, 2030f
diagnosis of, 2028-2031, 2029t, 2030f
etiology of, 2026-2027
imaging studies in, 2030-2031
laboratory tests in, 2028-2030, 2029t
pathophysiology of, 2027-2028
prerenal azotemia in, 2027
renal biopsy in, 2031
urinalysis and urine sediment in, 2029-2030
urinary indices in, 2030, 2031t
urinary volume in, 2028-2029
hyperkalemia in, 2036, 2037
hyperuricemic, 2034
hyponatremia in, 2037
management of, 2035-2038
in mechanical ventilation, 2820
nephrotoxic
aminoglycosides, 2032
amphotericin B, 2032-2033
angiotensin-converting enzyme inhibitors, 2033
cisplatin, 2033
endogenous, 2033-2035
ethylene glycol, 2033
exogenous, 2031-2033
in hepatorenal syndrome, 2034-2035
nonsteroidal anti-inflammatory drugs, 2033

radiocontrast, 2031-2032
in rhabdomyolysis, 2033-2034
in pregnancy, 2035
prevention of, 2026, 2027t, 2036
prognosis in, 2038
in systemic lupus erythematosus, 1339-1340
volume overload in, 2036-2037, 2037t
furosemide for, 2037, 2037t
advanced, chronic hyponatremia in, 1982-1983, 1985-1986
chronic, 2014-2025, 2040-2050
acute *vs.*, 2032t
anemia in, 2023
in arterial hypertension, 2040-2041
calcium and phosphorus imbalance in, 2020-2023, 2022f
in cardiac disease, 2016
comorbidities of, 2015-2016
definition and staging of, 2014, 2014t-2015t
definitions in, 2040
in diabetes mellitus, 2016-2017
diagnosis and clinical course in, 2041-2043, 2041t, 2042f
dialysis in, long-term, 2045-2049. *See also* Hemodialysis, Peritoneal dialysis
differential diagnosis of, 2041, 2041t
dyslipidemia and, 740
epidemiology of, 2040, 2040f
etiology of, 2040, 2041t
evaluation and treatment in, 2015, 2015t-2016t
GFR in, 2042-2043, 2042f-2043f
glomerular filtration rate in, 2014, 2014t-2015t
in glomerular hypertension, 2040-2041
hyperkalemia in, 2160
in hyperlipidemia, 2019
hypertension and, 229-230, 2018
hypertriglyceridemia in, 740
long-term management of, 2044-2045, 2044t
acidosis and, 2044
anemia and, 2045, 2045f
dietary protein and, 2044
hyperphosphatemia and, 2044
uremic bleeding and, 2045
metabolic acidosis in, 1995, 2001, 2020
pathophysiology of, 2040-2041
potassium imbalance in, 2020, 2021f
protein intake and, 2019, 2019t
in proteinuria, 2014, 2018, 2041
referral to nephrologist in, 2024
risk factors for progression of, 2016-2024
in smoking, 2018
sodium and water imbalance in, 2020, 2019t
in stroke, 2015-2016
in systemic lupus erythematosus, 1339-1340
treatment of, 2043-2044
disease duration in, 1967, 1967t
end-stage
cost of, 2049
incidence and prevalence of, 2040, 2040f, 2041t
prognosis in, 2049
in renal transplant recipients, 2115-2116, 2116t
in gout, 1374
imaging techniques in, 1969t, 1968-1969
intrinsic, 1969-1972, 1969f

major syndromes of, 1969-1972, 1970t
nutritional support in, 944
occupational, 64
patient approach in, 1967-1974
pericarditis in, 380
polycystic. *See* Polycystic kidney disease
in pregnancy, 1022
severe, anemia in, 1093-1094
Renal function, assessment of, 1967-1969
Renal insufficiency
in multiple myeloma, 2591
surgical risk factor management and, 55
Renal transplantation, 2114-2125
dialysis *vs.*, 2114
donors for
expanded-criteria, 2114
recipients *vs.*, 2114
encephalopathy in, 2339
living-donor evaluation in, 2116-2117
arterial imaging for, 2117
inherited renal disease and, 2117
laboratory tests for, 2117
medical screening and blood testing for, 2116-2117
psychological assessment for, 2117
long-term management strategies and outcomes in, 2122-2125, 2122f-2123f
coexisting disease, 2123-2124
diabetes mellitus and, 2124
hematologic conditions and, 2124-2125
hyperlipidemia and, 2124
hypertension and, 2123-2124
musculoskeletal conditions and, 2124
prevention of chronic rejection and, 2123, 2123f
posttransplantation complications in, 2120-2122
acute and chronic renal dysfunction, 2120, 2120t
renal parenchymal disorders, 2120
structural disorders, 2120
vascular disorders, 2120
volume depletion, 2120
early diagnosis of, 2120
posttransplantation infections in, 2120-2122, 2121f
cytomegalovirus, 2121
Epstein-Barr, 2122
parvovirus B19, 2122
urinary tract, 2122
pretransplantation patient management in, 2117-2120
antimetabolites for, 2118
calcineurin inhibitors for, 2118-2119
corticosteroids for, 2118
immunosuppression for, 2117-2120, 2118t
strategies for, 2119-2120
polyclonal and monoclonal antibodies for, 2119-2120
TOR inhibitors for, 2119
recipient evaluation in, 2114-2116
cardiovascular disease and, 2115
hepatitis B and, 2115
hepatitis C and, 2115
HIV-positive patients, 2115
infection and, 2115-2116
malignancy and, 2115
medical compliance and substance abuse, 2116
posttransplantation risk factors

in, 2115-2116, 2115t
primary renal disease and, 2115-2116, 2116t
timing of transplantation and, 2116
rejection in
acute, 2101, 2120
chronic, 2120
Renal tubular disorders. *See under* Tubular
Renal tumor(s). *See* Renal cell carcinoma
Renal vascular disease, 1970, 2071-2085, 2071f. *See also individual disease, e.g.,* Renal artery stenosis
atheroembolism and, 2083-2084, 2083f
large vessel, 2071-2074
medium vessel, 2074-2075
sickle cell disease and, 2082-2083
small vessel, 2075-2082
Renal vein thrombosis, 423, 2074
tubulointerstitial nephritis in, 2096
Renovascular hypertension, 231-232
features of, 217t
screening options for, 231t
Repaglinide, for type 2 diabetes mellitus, 658, 658t
Reproduction, female, physiology of, 950-953. *See also* Menstruation
Reproductive disorder(s), occupational, 66-67
Reptilase time (RT), 1161
Respiration. *See also* Breathing, Ventilation
Kussmaul, 1999
Respiratory acidosis, 2005-2006, 2005t
Respiratory alkalosis, 2005-2006, 2005t
in hypokalemia, 2006
Respiratory control system, 2786, 2787f
Respiratory distress syndrome, acute. *See* Acute respiratory distress syndrome (ARDS)
Respiratory failure, 2809-2822
acute, 2809-2814
definition of, 2809, 2810t
diagnosis of, 2811
differential diagnosis of, 2811, 2811t
hypercapnic, 2810, 2810t
diagnosis of, 2811
hypoxemic, 2809-2810, 2810t
diagnosis of, 2811
pathogenesis of, 2809-2810, 2811f
management of, 2811-2814
airway patency in, 2811-2812, 2812t
arterial oxygenation in, 2812-2813
mechanical ventilation in, 2813-2814, 2813f-2814f. *See also* Mechanical ventilation
pathogenesis of, 2809-2810
in acute respiratory distress syndrome, 2816, 2816f
in asthma, 2815-2816
in COPD, 2814-2815
Respiratory infection
in diphtheria, 1585, 1586f
upper, jet travel and, 80
Respiratory pump dysfunction, 2800, 2800t-2801t
in ankylosing spondylitis, 2802-2803
in anterior horn cell disease, 2806

in diaphragmatic paralysis, 2804-2805, 2805f
in flail chest, 2803
in kyphoscoliosis, 2801-2802, 2802f, 2801t
in muscle disorders, 2807
in neuromuscular disorders, 2803-2807, 2800t, 2804t
pathophysiology of, 2803-2804
respiratory compromise in, 2804, 2800t
treatment of, 2804, 2804t
in neuromuscular transmission disorders, 2807
in obesity, 2800-2801, 2801f
in peripheral neuropathy, 2806-2807
in skeletal abnormalities, 2801-2803
in spinal cord syndromes, 2806
in sternal deformities, 2803
Respiratory syncytial virus, 1788-1790
laboratory diagnosis of, 1778t
Respiratory tract
defense mechanisms of, 1468, 1469t
upper
cancer of, occupational agents causing, 62t
microbial flora of, 1456, 1458t
occupational diseases of, 62-63
acute and recurrent, 62-63
chronic, 63
procedures of, antibiotic prophylaxis for, 351t
Respiratory tract cancer. *See* Lung cancer
Respiratory tract infection
lower. *See* Pneumonia
upper, 1456-1467. *See also specific disorders, e.g.,* Sinusitis
complications of, 1456
etiology of, 1456
host defense mechanisms in, 1456
miscellaneous, 1466
pathophysiology, 1456, 1457f, 1458t
streptococcal, group A, 1569
Respiratory viral infection(s), 1776-1792
adenovirus in, 1781-1782
clinical syndromes of, 1778-1781. *See also individual syndromes*
bronchiolitis, 1779-1780
bronchitis, acute, 1779
common cold, 1778
croup, 1779
hantavirus in, 1790
influenza syndrome, 1779
laryngitis, 1778-1779
pharyngitis, 1778-1779
pneumonia, 1780-1781
in immunocompromised hosts, 1780-1781
SARS and, 1780
reactive airway disease exacerbation, 1780
coronavirus in, 1782
diagnosis of, 1778
epidemiology of, 1776, 1776t
human metapneumonia virus in, 1783-1784
infectious agents in, 1776, 1776t
influenza virus in, 1784-1788, 1786t-1787t
Internet resources for, 1790
laboratory tests in, 1777-1778, 1778t
parainfluenza virus in, 1788
pathogenesis of, 1777
pathophysiology of, 1776-1777
respiratory syncytial virus in,

1788-1790
rhinovirus in, 1790
Restless legs syndrome, 2368-2369, 2369f
ret, 2383, 2384t
Reticular dysgenesis
immunodeficiency in, 1230t
neutropenia in, 1144t
Reticulocyte count, in hematologic disorders, 1076
Retinitis, cytomegalovirus
in AIDS, 1762, 1762f
in HIV infection, 1841t-1842t, 1841-1842
Retinoblastoma
CNS tumors in, 2310t
genetic risk factors for, 2378
genetic testing in, 1961-1962
Retinopathy, diabetic, 668-669, 669f, 669t
background, 669, 669t
mechanisms of, 667-668, 668f
pancreas transplantation and, 938
preproliferative, 669, 669t
proliferative, 669, 669t
screening for, 669
treatment of, 669
Retroperitoneal abscess, 1504-1505
Retroperitoneal fibrosis, in ankylosing spondylitis, 1321
Retropharyngeal infection, 1464-1465, 1465f
Retrovirus(es)
biology of, 1802-1805
classification of, 1802, 1802t
definition of, 1802
origins of, 1808
pathogenetic tryptic of, 1804-1805, 1806f
screening for, blood donation and, 1207
structure and replication of, 1802-1804, 1803f-1804f, 1805t
Retrovirus infection, 1802-1818. *See also* Acquired immunodeficiency syndrome (AIDS), Human immunodeficiency virus
cytopathicity in, 1808
genomic diversity in, 1808
latency and persistence in, 1807-1808
pathogenesis of, 1805-1808
viral entry, target-cell tropism, receptor interactions in, 1805-1807
coreceptors in, 1807
receptors in, 1805-1807
Rhabdoid predisposition syndrome, CNS tumors in, 2310t
Rhabdomyolysis
acute renal failure in, 2033-2034
metabolic acidosis in, 1996
in poisoning or drug overdose, 158
Rhabdomyosarcoma, 2552
features of, 2550t
treatment of, 2555
Rheumatic disease
aches and pains in, diffuse, 1295, 1296t
acute-phase response in, 1293, 1293t
common types of, 1291t
C-reactive protein in, 1293
emergency, 1290-1291, 1291t
erythrocyte sedimentation rate in, 1293, 1293t
family history in, 1292
gelling phenomenon in, 1291
history in, 1290-1292
imaging in, 1294-1295
immunologic tests in, 1293-1294
initial approach to, 1295
in monoarticular disease,

1295, 1294f
in polyarticular disease, 1295, 1295f
introduction to, 1290-1296
joint examination in, 1292-1293
laboratory studies in, 1293-1295
pain in
character of, 1291
location of, 1291
temporal course of, 1290, 1291f
physical examination in, 1292-1293
prognosis in, 1295
psychosocial and environmental factors in, 1292
radiography in, 1294-1295
synovial fluid analysis in, 1294
systems review in, 1292, 1292t
weakness in, 1291-1292
Rheumatic fever, 1571, 1571t
cutaneous findings in, 433, 434f
heart disease in, 348-349
infective endocarditis *vs.*, 1490
streptococcal pharyngitis and, 1571
Rheumatic heart disease, 348-349
Rheumatism, tuberculous (Poncet disease), 1678, 1681
Rheumatoid arthritis, 1297-1314
of ankle and foot, 1303, 1303f
ARA classification of, 1297t, 1297
blood in, 1305
blood vessels in, 1305-1306
of cervical spine, 1303-1304, 1304f
clinical features of, 1301-1306
differential diagnosis of, 1307
of elbow and shoulder, 1302, 1303f
encephalopathy in, 2342
etiology of, 1298
extra-articular, 1304-1306
eyes in, 1304-1305
of hand and wrist, 1302, 1302f
heart in, 1305
of hip, 1302, 1303f
immunogenetics in, 1297-1298
of knee, 1302-1303
laboratory evaluation in, 1306
lungs in, 1305
management of, 1307-1312
antimalarial drugs and sulfasalazine for, 1310, 1308t
biologic drugs for, 1310-1311
drug therapy for, 1307-1312, 1308t, 1309f
glucocorticoids for, 1311-1312
immunosuppressive agents for, 1312
leflunomide for, 1310, 1308t
methotrexate for, 1309, 1308t
minocycline for, 1312
NSAIDs for, 1308-1309, 1308t
physical therapy for, 1312
surgery for, 1312
neuromuscular involvement in, 1305
osteoarthritis *vs.*, 1387
other systems in, 1306
pain in, temporal course of, 1291f
pathogenesis of, 1298-1301
cellular immunity in, 1299-1300
complement activation in, 1300
cytokines in, 1300-1301
humoral immunity in, 1300-1301
rheumatoid factors in, 1300
synovial histopathology and invasion, 1298-1299, 1298f-1299f
pneumonitis with fibrosis in, 2779-2780
pulmonary disease in, chronic diffuse infiltrative, 2779-2780
pulmonary infiltrates in, multifocal, 2749

radiography in, 1306
rheumatoid nodules in, 1304, 1304f
septic arthritis in, 1539
systemic lupus erythematosus *vs.*, 1336, 1328t
valvular heart disease in, 349
Rheumatoid factor, 1300, 1306
Rheumatoid nodule(s), 1304, 1304f, 2780
cardiac, 1305
pulmonary, 1305
Rhinitis, allergic, 1253-1254
diagnosis of, 1253
treatment of, 1253-1254
Rhinovirus, 1778t, 1790
Rhodococcus equi, 1588-1589, 1587t
Rib fracture, flail chest in, 2803
Rickettsial infection, 1724-1736, 1724f. *See also specific disorders, e.g.,* Rocky Mountain spotted fever
antimicrobial drugs for, 1427t
biology and ecology of, 1724-1725
pathophysiology of, 1725
taxonomy of, 1724, 1724f
Rickettsialpox, 1727-1728
diagnosis of, 1727t
Rickettsia mongolotimonae, 1729
Rickettsia parkeri infection, 1728-1729
Rickettsia prowazekii, 1729. *See also* Typhus, epidemic (louse-borne)
Rickettsia rickettsii, 1725. *See also* Rocky Mountain spotted fever
Rickettsia typhi, 1729. *See also* Typhus, murine (endemic)
Rifampin, 1440
for meningococcal disease, 1620t
in pregnancy, 1422t
Rifaximin, 1440
Rift Valley fever, 1851-1852
Right ventricular infarction, 331
Rigid spine syndrome muscular dystrophy, 2276
Rimantadine, for influenza, 1786t
Ringworm. *See* Dermatophytoses
Risedronate, for osteoporosis, 709
Ritalin (methylphenidate) toxicity, 165
Ritonavir, for HIV infection, 1831t
adverse effects of, 1834t
Ritonavir boosted protease inhibitor regimens, for HIV infection, 1832t
Rituximab, 2420t
for rheumatoid arthritis, 1308t, 1311
Rocky Mountain spotted fever, 1725-1727, 1727t-1728t
clinical manifestations of, 1725-1726, 1726f
diagnosis of, 1725-1726, 1727t
epidemiology of, 1725
laboratory studies in, 1726
prevention and prognosis in, 1726-1727
rash in, 440, 1725-1726, 1726f
tick vector for, 1725
treatment of, 1726, 1728t
Roentgenography. *See* Radiography
Romano-Ward syndrome, 265
Ropinirole, for parkinsonism, 2247t
Rosacea
acne vulgaris *vs.,* 448, 448f
treatment of, 451
Roseola infantum (exanthema subitum), herpesvirus type 6 in, 1765
Ross River fever, 1858
Rotator cuff tendinitis
calcific, 1393

impingement syndrome, 1392-1393, 1393f
Rotavirus infection, 1798-1799
Roundworm infection, 1918-1921, 1920t, 1922f
Roux-ex-Y stasis syndrome, 852
Rubella, 1770-1771
immunization against, 1771
for HIV-infected patients, 1830t

S

Sacroiliitis, in ankylosing spondylitis, 1318, 1318f. *See also* Ankylosing spondylitis
Sagittal sinus thrombophlebitis, superior, 1561
Salicylate(s). *See also* Aspirin, Nonsteroidal anti-inflammatory drugs (NSAIDs)
poisoning or overdose, 172-173
elimination method for, 161t
metabolic acidosis in, 1996-1997, 2001
Salicylic acid, for acne vulgaris, 449t
Salivary gland tumors, 2441
Salmonella cholerasuis, diarrhea due to, 841
Salmonella enteritidis, diarrhea due to, 841
Salmonella infection, 1638-1641, 1635t, 1636t, 1637t
bacteremia and vascular infection, 1639-1640
carrier state, 1639
enteric fever, 1640-1641, 1639t-1640t, 1642t
epidemiology of, 1638
gastroenteritis, 1638-1639
pathogenesis of, 1638
Salmonella typhi, diarrhea due to, 841
Salmon patch, 545
Salpingitis, acute, chlamydial, 1748-1749, 1748t
Salt poisoning, hypernatremia and, 1987
Salt water
deficiency. *See* Hypovolemia
excess. *See* Edema
Sandhoff disease, 1149t
Sanfilippo syndrome, 1148t
SAPHO, 1325-1326
Saquinavir, for HIV infection, 1831t, 1834t
Sarcoid granulomatosis, necrotizing, 2771
Sarcoidosis, 2769-2774, 2767t-2768t
alveolar, 2771
multifocal pulmonary infiltrates in, 2747, 2746f
angiotensin-converting enzyme levels in, 2773
bone and joint findings in, 2772
calcium nephrolithiasis in, 2107
cardiac findings in, 2772
cutaneous findings in, 432, 432f, 2771-2772
diagnosis of, 2772-2773, 2773f
differential diagnosis of, 2773
endocrine findings in, 2772
epidemiology of, 2769-2770
erythema nodosum in, 2771-2772
extrathoracic, 2771-2772
fever of undetermined origin in, 1415
granuloma formation, 2770, 2771f
hypercalcemia and hypercalciuria in, 2772
hypersensitivity pneumonitis *vs.,* 2773

intrathoracic
clinical findings in, 2770-2771, 2772f
multiple pulmonary nodules in, 2756-2757
segmental infiltrates in, 2751
staging system for, 2770-2771, 2772f
laryngeal, 2772
liver and spleen findings in, 2772
lung biopsy in, 2772, 2773f
lupus pernio in, 432, 432f, 2771
neurologic findings in, 2772
ocular findings in, 2772
pathogenesis of, 2770, 2771f
pleural, 2771
synovial, 2772
treatment of, 2773
tubulointerstitial nephritis in, 2100-2101
upper respiratory findings in, 2772
Sarcoma, 2549-2560
of bone and cartilage, 2556-2558. *See also* Chondrosarcoma, Osteosarcoma
classification of, 2549
epidemiology of, 2549, 2549, 2550t
etiology of, 2549-2550
Ewing, EWS-FLI1 in, 2385
familial, 2549, 2551t
genetic factors in, 2549
Kaposi. *See* Kaposi sarcoma
soft tissue, 2551-2556
diagnosis of, 2551
grading and staging of, 2551, 2551t
histologic variants of, 2551-2554, 2550t
pathophysiology of, 2551
treatment of, 2554-2556
adjuvant chemotherapy for, 2555, 2555t
in advanced disease, 2555
in nonclassic disease, 2555-2556
synovial, 2552
features of, 2550t
translocations diagnostic of, 2549
SARS, pneumonia and, 1780
SARS coronavirus, 1782-1783
Scabies, 516-519
in AIDS, 438, 516
animal, 519
clinical features, 516, 516f-517f
crusted, 516
diagnosis of, 516-517
differential diagnosis of, 517
resistant, 518-519
skin scrapings in, 516-517, 517f
treatment of, 517-519
postscabies itch after, 518
Scalded skin syndrome, staphylococcal
cutaneous findings in, 439
toxic epidermal necrolysis *vs.,* 439
Scar, hypertrophic, 543-544, 543f
Scarlet fever, streptococcal, 1571
cutaneous findings in, 439
Schatzki ring, in dysphagia, 760, 760f
Schilder disease, 2328
Schilling test, for cobalamin deficiency, in megaloblastic anemia, 1102
Schindler disease, 1149t
Schistosoma haematobium, 1932, 1933f-1934f
Schistosoma japonicum, 1932, 1933f-1934f
Schistosoma mansoni, 1932, 1933f-1934f

Schistosoma mekongi, 1932, 1933f-1934f
Schistosomiasis, 1932-1934, 1933f-1934f
Schizophrenia, 2647-2656
clinical course of, 2649
clinical manifestations of, 2649-2650, 2651t
definition of, 2647
diagnosis of, 2649-2651, 2650f, 2651t
differential diagnosis of, 2651-2652, 2652t
epidemiology of, 2647-2648
etiology and genetics of, 2648
laboratory tests in, 2651
management of, 2652-2655
acute treatment, 2653
antipsychotics, 2653-2654, 2653t
electroconvulsive therapy, 2655
future treatment, 2655
maintenance therapy, 2653
pharmacologic, 2653-2655, 2653t
psychosocial, 2655
pathophysiology of, 2648-2649
physical examination in, 2650-2651
subclassification of, 2647
Schwannoma, 2315
malignant, 2552
features of, 2550t
mediastinal, 2839
Scintigraphy. *See* Radionuclide imaging
Scleredema, in diabetes mellitus, 433-434
Scleroderma, 1342-1349
calcinosis in, 1344, 1343f-1344f
chronic diffuse infiltrative pulmonary disease in, 2780
classification of, 1342, 1342t
clinical course in, 1349
clinical features of, 1343-1347
definition of, 1342
diagnosis of, 1343-1347
dysphagia in, 763
epidemiology of, 1342
esophageal hypomotility in, 1346, 1346f
etiology of, 1342
gastrointestinal tract in, 1346, 1346f
heart in, 1346-1347
Internet resources, 1348
laboratory findings in, 1347, 1345t
lungs in, 1346
management of, 1347-1349
in cutaneous involvement, 1348
disease-modifying therapies in, 1349
in GI tract involvement, 1348
in pulmonary involvement, 1347-1348
in renal crisis, 1347
morphea, 443
musculoskeletal system in, 1345-1346, 1345f
pathogenesis of, 1342-1343
chimerism and microchimerism in, 1343
fibroblast abnormalities in, 1343
immune cell and cytokine abnormalities in, 1343
vascular abnormalities in, 1343
pulmonary fibrosis in, 1346
pulmonary hypertension in, 1346
Raynaud phenomenon in, 1342, 1344-1345, 1344f, 1348
renal involvement in, 1347, 2081
skin in, 442-443, 443f, 1343-1345, 1343f-1344f, 1345t
trigeminal neuropathy in, 1347
Sclerosis

amyotrophic lateral, 2288-2289
lupoid, 1334
multiple. *See* Multiple sclerosis
systemic, progressive. *See*
  Scleroderma
tuberous, cutaneous findings in,
  440, 441f
Scombroid poisoning, 175, 175t
Scorpionfish, 193-194
Scorpion stings, 190-191, 190t
Scrapie, 2358, 2358f
Scuba-diving, flying after,
  precautions, 80
Scurvy, 1177
Seabather's eruption, 522, 523f
Seafood poisoning, 175, 175t
Sebaceous hyperplasia, 536, 536f
Seborrheic dermatitis, 455-456, 455f,
  474
  in AIDS, 455-456
Seborrheic keratosis, 535, 535f-536f
Sedative-hypnotic agent(s),
  overdose, 173
Seizure. *See also* Epilepsy
  absence, 2188
  atonic, 2188
  in brain tumor, 2310
  in chronic hyponatremia, 1986
  definition of, 2187
  febrile, 1412
  generalized, 2188-2189, 2187t-2188t
  myoclonic, 2188
  partial, 2187-2188, 2187t-2188t
  in poisoning or drug overdose,
    157, 157t
  tonic-clonic, 2188-2189
  vestibular, 2148
Selenium, dietary, 30
Self-protein(s), abnormal
  posttranslational modification
  of, 2402
Semen analysis, 1002, 1006t
Seminoma, 2519-2520. *See also*
  Testicular cancer
Semustine, 2415t
  renal complications of, 2091
Sensory neuropathy, paraneoplastic,
  2318-2319
Sentinel lymph node mapping, in
  breast cancer, 2463
Sepsis, 1443-1455
  definition of, 1443t, 1443-
    1444, 1443t
  epidemiology of, 1444
  hemodynamic findings in, 1449-
    1450, 1450t
  laboratory values in, 1449-
    1450, 1450t
  meningococcal, 1618
  new therapies for, 1453, 1453t
  pathogenesis of, 1444-1449
    bacterial endotoxin in, 1444-
      1445, 1446f
    bacterial superantigens in,
      1445, 1446f
    bactericidal/permeability-
      increasing protein in, 1445
    coagulation system in, 1447
    cytokine networks, 1446-
      1447, 1447t, 1446f
    endotoxin tolerance and, 1445
    fungal organisms in, 1445
    gram-negative organisms in, 1444-
      1446, 1446f
    gram-positive organisms in, 1444-
      1445, 1446f
    host-derived mediators in, 1446-
      1448
    LPS signaling in, 1444-1445
    microbial factors in, 1444-1446
    multiple organ dysfunction
      syndrome in, 1448-1449
    neutrophil-endothelial cell

interactions in, 1447, 1448f
  nitric oxide in, 1447-1448
  organ dysfunction in, 1448-1449
  Toll-like receptors in, 1444
  severe, 1443t
Sepsis-related encephalopathy, 2338
Septic abortion, *C. perfringens* in,
  1608
Septic arthritis. *See* Arthritis,
  septic
Septic shock. *See also* Sepsis
  acute respiratory distress
    syndrome in, 1450, 1452
  antimicrobial therapy for,
    1452t, 1452-1453
  assessment of tissue perfusion in,
    1452
  blood glucose levels in,
    management of, 1453
  blood transfusion in, 1452
  definition of, 1443t
  diagnostic approach to, 1449-
    1451, 1449t-1450t
  diagnostic techniques in,
    novel, 1450-1451
  fever in, management of, 1452
  fluid resuscitation in, 1451
  general features of, 1449-1450
  management of, 1451-1453, 1452t
  multiple organ dysfunction
    syndrome in, 1450, 1450t, 1452
  nutritional support in, 1452
  vasodilator therapy in, 1451-1452
  vasopressor therapy in, 1451
Serotonin reuptake inhibitors,
  selective, for panic disorder,
  2660
Serotonin syndrome, 158t
Serratia infections, 1632
Serratia marcescens, antimicrobial
  susceptibilities of, 1421t
Sertraline, for premenstrual
  syndrome, 964
Serum sickness-like syndrome, as
  drug reaction, 498, 496t
Sexual activity, HIV transmission
  due to, 1822
Sexually transmitted disease, 1520-
  1532. *See also individual*
  disorders, e.g., Gonorrhea
  anorectal, in females, 1529-1530
  epidemiology and transmission
    dynamics, 1520
  genital ulcer disease, 1527-1529,
    1528t
  lower genital tract infections in
    women, 1523-1526
  in males having sex with males,
    1529-1530
  pelvic inflammatory disease, 1526-
    1527, 1527t
  prevention of, 1521, 1521t
  reporting and sexual partner
    management, 1521, 1521t
  sexual history and counseling in,
    1521
  urethritis
    in females, 1523
    in males, 1521-1523
  vulvovaginitis, 1523-1526, 1524t
Sheehan syndrome, 957
Shellfish poisoning, 175, 175t
  respiratory insufficiency in, 2806
Shift-work sleep disorder, 2370
Shigella infection, 1641-1642, 1635t-
  1636t
  diarrhea due to, 841
Shingles. *See* Herpes zoster
Shock
  drug-induced, 156
  septic, 1443t
Short bowel syndrome, malabsorption
  in, 830-831

Short QT syndrome, congenital, 266
Shoulder
  frozen (adhesive capsulitis), 1393
  rheumatoid arthritis of, 1302
Shoulder pain, 1392-1393, 1393f
Shoulder pain syndrome, myofascial,
  1393
Shwachman-Diamond syndrome,
  neutropenia in, 1144t
Sialolipidosis, 1148t
Siberian tick typhus, 1728
Sibutramine, for obesity, 723, 723t
Sicca syndrome, in rheumatoid
  arthritis, 1304
Sick-building syndrome, 67
Sickle cell anemia, 1113-1118
  complications of, 1116-1117
    aplastic crisis, 1116
    cardiopulmonary, 1116
    dermatologic, 1117
    during general anesthesia, 1117
    hepatobiliary, 1116
    neurologic, 1116-1117
    ocular, 1117
    pregnancy and contraception and,
      1117
    renal and urologic, 1116, 2082-
      2083, 2082f
    skeletal, 1116
    susceptibility to infection,
      1117
  diagnosis of, 1114-1115
  epidemiology of, 1113
  genetic counseling in, 1117
  hemolytic transfusion reaction,
    1214
  Howell-Jolly bodies in, 1114
  malaria resistance and, 1113
  osteomyelitis in, 1543
  pathophysiology of, 1113-
    1114, 1114f
  pregnancy in, 1117
  alpha-thalassemia and, 1115
  therapy for, 1115-1116
    to alter disease
      pathophysiology, 1115
    hematopoietic stem cell
      transplantation for, 1222
    long-term transfusion therapy,
      1116
    for pain management, 1115
    sickle crisis, 1115
  tubulointerstitial nephritis in,
    2095-2096
Sickle cell-hemoglobin C disease,
  1118
Sickle cell *beta*-thalassemia, 1118
Sickle crisis, 1114
  prognosis in, 1117
Sickle trait, 1117-1118
Sigmoidoscopy, in colorectal cancer,
  2480
Signal transduction modulators,
  2419t-2420t, 2422-2423
Silicosis
  chronic diffuse pulmonary
    infiltration in, 2764
  multifocal pulmonary infiltrates
    in, 2749
Simian immunodeficiency virus,
  origin of, 1819
Sinoatrial node, 273
Sinoatrial node dysfunction,
  pacemaker for, 274t, 275
Sinus histiocytosis, with massive
  lymphadenopathy, 1146
Sinusitis, 1255-1257, 1456-
  1461, 1459f
  in AIDS, 1457
  bacteriology of, 1459
  candidal, 1877t
  cavernous sinus thrombophlebitis
    in, 1460

clinical features of, 1457, 1459
clinical variants, 1457, 1459f
complications of, 1257, 1460-1461
diagnosis of, 1256-1257, 1457-1459
differential diagnosis of, 1257,
  1459
etiology of, 1456-1457
Haemophilus influenzae, 1650
intracranial suppuration in, 1460-
  1461
in mechanical ventilation, 2817
Moraxella catarrhalis, 1652
orbital cellulitis in, 1460
osteomyelitis of frontal bone in,
  1460
paranasal, headache in, 2154t,
  2166
pathogenesis of, 1255-
  1256, 1255f, 1256t
treatment of, 1257, 1459-1460
Sinus tachycardia, 258
  in drug overdose or poisoning,
    156t
  inappropriate, 258
Sirolimus
  after liver transplantation,
    complications of, 934
  for prerenal-transplant patient
    management, 2119
Sjogren syndrome
  chronic infiltrative pulmonary
    disease in, 2780
  encephalopathy in, 2342
  systemic lupus erythematosus *vs.,*
    1337, 1328t
  tubulointerstitial nephritis in,
    2101
Skeletal hyperostosis, diffuse
  idiopathic, 1387
Skin
  benign tumors of, 535-548. *See*
    also individual types, e.g.,
    Nevus
    classification of, 535
    connective tissue, 543-544
    epidermal appendage, 536-537
    familial, 537-538
    histologic evaluation of, 535
    melanocytic, 538-541
    neural, 541-543
  biopsy of, in fever of
    undetermined origin, 1417
  in diphtheria, 1585
  malignant tumors of, 549-562. *See*
    also specific histologic
    types, e.g., Melanoma
    epidermal, 549-556
    metastatic, 556
    nonmelanoma, 549-552
    palliative treatment of, 107
    sun exposure and, 549
  palliative care of, 107-108, 109t
  in scleroderma, 1343-1345, 1343f-
    1344f, 1345f
  tags of, 543, 542f
Skin cancer. *See* Skin, malignant
  tumors of, *specific histologic*
  types
Skin disorder(s)
  in AIDS, 437-438
  in cardiopulmonary disease, 432-
    433
  categories of, 429, 430t
  diagnosis of, 425-431
    approach to patient, 425-426
    arriving at, 430-431, 430t
    evaluation in, 425
    scattershot, 426
    "snapshot" approach to, 425-426
    suboptimal methods of, 425-426
    treating symptoms *vs.* disease,
      425
  as drug reactions. *See* Drug

allergy, cutaneous
in endocrinologic disease, 433-434
in food allergy, 1279
in gastrointestinal disease, 434-436
in hematologic disease, 436-437
in immunodeficiency disease, 437-438
in infectious disease, 438-440
lichen planus, 454
maculopapular, in syphilis, 1699-1700, 1700f
morphologic classification of, 426-429
color in, 429
configuration in, 428-429, 430f
distribution in, 428
location in, 428
patterns of presentation, 427-429
primary lesion, 426-427, 426t, 426f-428f
secondary changes in, 427, 428t-429t, 429f
in neurologic disease, 440
in occupational disease, 63-64
in renal disease, 440-442
in rheumatologic disease, 442-444
in systemic disease, 432-445
in systemic lupus erythematosus, 1330-1331, 1331f-1333f
in vascular disease, 432-433
vesiculobullous, 525-534. See also individual disorders, e.g., Pemphigus
blister typology in, 525, 527t
differential diagnosis of, 533-534
differentiating features of, 526t
general clinical assessment of, 525, 526t
Skin infection
abscess in, 511
in anthrax, 513-514, 513f, 1594-1595, 1594f
bacterial, 509-514. See also under Staphylococcal infection, Streptococcal infection
fungal, 504-507. See also Dermatophytoses, Tinea
parasitic, 516-524. See also individual disorders, e.g., Scabies
Pseudomonas aeruginosa, 1661-1662
resident flora in, 511-512
staphylococcal, 1576
streptococcal, group A, 1570
viral, 514-515
yeast, 507-509. See also Candidiasis, Malassezia infections
Skin necrosis, anticoagulant-induced, 501, 501f, 501t
Skin test
for drug allergy, 1272-1273
for fever of undetermined origin, 1417
for food allergy, 1281-1282
for Hymenoptera allergy, 1287
for IgE, 1248-1249, 1248t
SLE. See Lupus erythematosus, systemic (SLE)
Sleep
architecture and stages of, 2362, 2363f
behavioral and physiologic characteristics of, 2364t
circadian rhythms in, 2364
definition of, 2362
functional neuroanatomy in, 2362-2363
hypoventilation in, 2792

in kyphoscoliosis, 2802
non-rapid eye movement (NREM), 2362, 2363f
oxygen saturation in, 2792
patterns, across lifespan, 2362
physiologic changes during, 2363-2364, 2364t
physiology of, 2362-2364
rapid eye movement (REM), 2362, 2363f
respiratory disturbances during, 2791-2792
ventilation in, 2790-2791, 2791f
Sleep apnea, in polycystic ovary syndrome, 976, 980-981
Sleep apnea syndrome, 2366-2368. See also Sleep-disordered breathing
central, 2792-2794
diagnosis of, 2794, 2794f
pathophysiology of, 2792-2793, 2793f
risk factors for, 2793-2794, 2793t
treatment of, 2794
CPAP for, 2367-2368
obstructive, 2794-2797
CPAP for, 2796
diagnosis of, 2795, 2796f
morbidity and mortality in, 2795
oral appliances for, 2796-2797
pathophysiology of, 2794-2795
pharmacologic therapy for, 2797
risk factors in, 2795, 2793t
surgery for, 2797
treatment of, 2795-2797
polycythemia in, 1134
polysomnographic study in, 2367f, 2366
pulmonary hypertension in, 2863
Sleep disorder(s), 2362-2372
all-night polysomnographic study for, 2365
circadian rhythm, 2370
classification of, 2364, 2365t-2366t
diagnosis of, 2364-2365, 2365t-2366t
idiopathic hypersomnia, 2368
insomnia, 2370-2371, 2365t, 2370t
multiple sleep latency test for, 2365
narcolepsy, 2368
nocturnal frontal lobe epilepsy, 2371
parasomnia, 2371, 2366t
in Parkinson disease, 2244
partial arousal, 2371
periodic limb movements in, 2369-2370, 2369f
REM sleep behavior disorder, 2371
restless legs syndrome, 2368-2369, 2369f
shift-work, 2370
sleep apnea syndrome. See Sleep apnea syndrome
Sleep-disordered breathing, 2792. See also Sleep apnea syndrome
in asthma, 2797
in chronic obstructive pulmonary disease, 2797
definition of, 2792
etiology of, 2792
in upper airway disease, 2797
Sleep latency test, multiple, 2365
Sleep study(ies), in depression, 2614
Slow virus infection, 2355-2361
encephalopathies as, spongiform, 2357-2359. See also Encephalopathy, spongiform
HTLV-I myelopathy, 2357
human immunodeficiency virus dementia as, 2355-2357. See

also Human immunodeficiency virus infection, dementia
leukoencephalopathy, progressive multifocal as. See Leukoencephalopathy, progressive multifocal
panencephalitis as, subacute sclerosing, 2360-2361. See also Panencephalitis, subacute sclerosing
Slug, woolly, 191
Sly syndrome, 1148t
SMAD, mechanisms of, 2391
Small cell carcinoma, of lung. See Lung cancer, small cell
Small intestine
adenocarcinoma of, in inflammatory bowel disease, 809
amyloidosis of, malabsorption in, 834
biopsy of
in gluten-sensitive enteropathy, 828, 829f
in malabsorption, 826, 825t
immunoproliferative disease of, malabsorption in, 831-832, 831f
malabsorption in, 824
motility in, 851
disorders of, 856-857
stasis (bacterial overgrowth) syndrome in, malabsorption in, 833-834
Smallpox, 122-127, 1772-1773, 1772t
chickenpox vs., 125t
classification of, 123-124, 123f
diagnosis of, 124-125, 124t-125t
differential diagnosis of, 124-125, 125t
infection control and postexposure isolation in, 125-127
vaccination for, 125-127, 126f, 1772t
SMO, properties of, 2384t
Smoke inhalation, 176
Smoking. See Cigarette smoking, Nicotine, Tobacco
Snakebite, 182-187, 184f
in children, 187
coral, 183, 184f
disposition in, 187
envenomation in, 183-185
pit vipers, 183, 184f
in pregnancy, 186-187
prevention of, 187
treatment in, 185-186
adjunctive therapy in, 186
antivenin therapy in, 185-186
emergency department in, 185
first aid, 185
general management in, 186
venomous, hemolytic anemia in, 1128
Sneddon syndrome, cutaneous findings in, 440
Social anxiety disorder, 2662-2663
Social issues. See Ethical and social issues
Sodium
absorption of, renal, 1976, 1976f, 1978f, 1977t
depletion of. See Hypovolemia
dietary, 28-29
excess. See Edema
excretion of, renal, in hypertension, 215-216
neutral, for nephrolithiasis, 2109-2110
Sodium channel disorders, 2281-2282
Sodium nitroprusside, for hypertensive crisis, 228t
Sodium sulfacetamide-sulfur, for acne vulgaris, 449t
Soft tissue infection

staphylococcal, 1576
streptococcal, group A, 1570
Soft tissue sarcoma, 2551-2556. See also Sarcoma, soft tissue
Somatization disorder, in diagnosis of palpitation, 204t
Sotalol
for atrial fibrillation, 242t-243t
classification of, 267t
Sparganosis, 1940
Specific granule deficiency, 1146t
Spermatogenesis, 690
in hypogonadism, 691-692
stimulation of, in hypogonadism, 694
Spermicide, in urinary tract infection, 1509
Spherocytosis, hereditary, 1110-1111, 1109f-1110f
Sphincter of Oddi dysfunction, 910-911, 910t
in acute pancreatitis, 914
Sphincterotomy, endoscopic, for choledocholithiasis, 908
Sphingolipidosis, 1148t
Spider angioma, 546, 546f
Spider bite, 187-190
black widow, 187-188, 188f
brown recluse, 188-190, 189f
Spinal cord compression, epidural, 2432-2434
diagnosis of, 2432-2433, 2433t
pathophysiology of, 2432, 2433f
treatment of, 2433-2434
Spinal cord syndromes
anterior horn cell disease in, 2806
functional transection in, 2806
respiratory dysfunction in, 2806
Spinal cord tumors, 2316
metastatic, 2317
Spinal epidural abscess, 1557-1559
diagnosis of, 1558-1559
etiology of, 1558
pathogenesis and pathophysiology in, 1557-1558
staphylococcal, 1577
treatment and prognosis in, 1559
Spinal metastasis, intramedullary, 2434
Spinal muscular atrophy
anterior horn cell disease in, 2806
X-linked, trinucleotide repeat in, 1960t
Spine
bamboo, in ankylosing spondylitis, 1319, 1321f
cervical, rheumatoid arthritis of, 1303-1304, 1304f
osteoarthritis of, 1386-1387
Spinocerebellar ataxia, 2264t, 2266-2268, 2268t
trinucleotide repeat in, 1960t
type 3 (Machado-Joseph disease), genetic testing for, 1959, 1960t
Spirillum minus infection, 1721
Spirochetes, antimicrobial drugs for, 1427t
Spironolactone
for heart failure, 343, 343t
for hirsutism, 991
for hypertension, 221t
for premenstrual syndrome, 964
Spleen
anatomy of, 1127
hypersplenism in, 1127
Splenectomy
actual or functional, as oncologic emergency, 2429
for autoimmune hemolytic anemia, 1125

for chronic lymphocytic leukemia, 2589
for idiopathic thrombocytopenic purpura, 1167
Splenic abscess, 1506
Splenic infection, candidal, 1877t
Splenic rupture, in Epstein-Barr virus infection, 1764
Splenic vein thrombosis, in acute pancreatitis, 922
Splenomegaly
in endocarditis, 1485
in hematologic disease, 1075
Spondylitis, ankylosing. *See* Ankylosing spondylitis
Spondyloarthritis
environmental factors in, 1316
juvenile, 1325
pathology in, 1316-1317
seronegative, 1315-1326. *See also individual disorders, e.g., Ankylosing spondylitis*
classification, 1315, 1317t
definition of, 1315, 1316t
epidemiology of, 1315
genetic factors in, 1315-1316, 1317t
pathogenesis of, 1315-1316
undifferentiated, 1325
Sporothrix schenckii, 1869
Sporotrichosis, 1869-1870
lymphocutaneous, 1869, 1870
visceral, 1869-1870
Spouse, death of, 119
Sprue
celiac. *See* Gluten-sensitive enteropathy
collagenous, 829-830
hypogammaglobulinemic, 830
tropical, 829, 829f-830f
Spumavirus, 1802t
Spur cell anemia, in liver disease, 1129
Sputum culture
in bronchiectasis, 2735-2736
in Legionnaires disease, 1475
in lung abscess, 1478
in pneumonia, 1471
Squamous cell carcinoma, 550-552, 551f
of head and neck, 2437-2441, 2437f. *See also under* Head and neck
St. John's wort, 176
St. Louis encephalitis, 1854
Staphylococcal infection, 1574-1581
bacteremic, 1577
bloodstream, 1577
bone and joint, 1576
endocarditis, 1577
antibiotics for, 1493, 1492t
food poisoning, 1577-1578
furunculosis, 511, 511f
genitourinary, 1578
osteomyelitis
antibiotics for, 1547-1548, 1547t
methicillin-resistant, 1547-1548, 1547t
other types of, 1578
pathogenesis of, 1576
pneumonia, 1576-1577
cavitary infiltrates in, 2751
epidemiology of, 1469
respiratory tract, 1576-1577
septic arthritis, 1577
skin and soft tissue, 509-512, 1576
spinal epidural abscess, 1577
treatment of, 1578-1580, 1579t
antibiotic, 1578-1579, 1579t
carrier state and, 1580
tropical pyomyositis, 1578
Staphylococcal scalded skin syndrome
cutaneous findings in, 439

toxic epidermal necrolysis *vs.,* 439, 531, 526t
Staphylococcal toxic-shock syndrome, 1580, 1580t-1581t
cutaneous findings in, 439
Staphylococcus(i), coagulase-negative, antimicrobial susceptibilities of, 1421t
Staphylococcus aureus
antimicrobial susceptibilities of, 1421t
characteristics of, 1575
epidemiology of, 1575-1576
meningitis, antibiotics for, 1553t
methicillin-resistant, 1578-1579
septic arthritis, 1537
vancomycin-resistant, 1579
Staphylococcus epidermidis, 1580-1581
Staphylococcus saprophyticus, 1581
Starch peritonitis, fever of undetermined origin in, 1415
Starling equation, 2842
Starvation, anemia in, 1094, 1094f
Statin therapy, for acute myocardial infarction, 329
Status epilepticus, 2198-2199, 2199f. *See also* Epilepsy
Stavudine, for HIV infection, 1831t
adverse effects of, 1834t
Steatohepatitis, nonalcoholic
chronic hepatitis *vs.,* 883
in polycystic ovary syndrome, 981
Steatorrhea
evaluation of, 846-847, 847f
in pancreatitis, alcoholic, 929, 928t
postgastrectomy, malabsorption in, 834-835
Stem cell(s)
hematopoietic, 1070, 1072f. *See also* Hematopoiesis
for transfusion. *See* Hematopoietic stem cell transplantation
Stem cell factor (SCF), 1073t
Stenotrophomonas maltophilia, antimicrobial susceptibilities of, 1421t
Sterilization, contraceptive, 998-999
Sternal disorders, respiratory pump dysfunction in, 2803
Sternal osteomyelitis, 1544
Steroid(s). *See* Corticosteroid(s), Glucocorticoid(s)
Stevens-Johnson syndrome, 531, 532f
as drug reaction, 500
Stiff-hand syndrome, 1395
Still disease, fever of undetermined origin in, 1415
Stimulant abuse, 2636
treatment of
medication for, 2644
in overdose, 2641-2642, 2642t
in withdrawal, 2643
Stinging insect allergy, Hymenoptera, 1285-1289
diagnosis of, 1286-1287
differential diagnosis of, 1287
epidemiology of, 1285, 1285t
etiology of, 1285-1286, 1286f-1287f
pathogenesis of, 1286
preventive treatment of, 1288-1289
treatment of, 1288-1289
Stingrays, 193
Stings
caterpillar, 191
catfish, 194
insect, 191-192
lionfish, 193-194
mollusca, 193
scorpion, 190-191, 190t
scorpionfish, 193-194

stingray, 193
weeverfish, 194
Stomach
Crohn disease of, 797
watermelon, 869f, 870
Stomach cancer. *See* Gastric cancer
Stomatitis
aphthous, in inflammatory bowel disease, 435, 435f
denture, candidal, 1877t
Stomatocytosis, hereditary (hydrocytosis), 1109-1110, 1110f
Stone(s), kidney. *See* Nephrolithiasis
Stool. *See under* Fecal
Strawberry hemangioma, 545, 544f
Streptobacillus moniliformis infection, 1721
Streptococcal cellulitis, in tinea pedis, 506
Streptococcal infection, 1567-1574, 1568t
anaerobic, 1574, 1568t
endocarditis due to, antibiotics for, 1491, 1492t
group A, 1567-1573, 1568t
bacteremia, 1570
bacteriology in, 1567-1568
bone and joint, 1569
diagnosis and treatment of, 1572-1573
epidemiology of, 1568-1569
erythema nodosum in, 1572
host immune response, 1571
lymphadenitis, 1569
meningitis, 1553t
necrotizing fasciitis, 1570
pathogenesis of, 1569
pharyngitis, 1463-1464
rheumatic fever and, 1571
pneumonia, 1569
postpartum, 1570
poststreptococcal glomerulonephritis in, 1572
rheumatic fever in. *See* Rheumatic fever
scarlet fever in, 439, 1571
skin and soft tissue, 1570
toxic-shock syndrome, 1570
upper respiratory tract, 1569
wound, 1569-1570
group B, 1573, 1568t
meningitis, 1553t
neonatal, 1573
septic arthritis, 1537
group C, 1573, 1568t
group D, 1573, 1568t
group F, 1568t
group G, 1573, 1568t
group H, 1568t
group K, 1568t
non-group A, septic arthritis, 1537
nongroupable, 1573-1574, 1568t
in psoriasis, 462
skin, 509-511
viridans, 1573
endocarditis due to, 1573
antibiotics for, 1491, 1492t
Streptococcus bovis, 1573
Streptococcus infection, group B, in pregnancy, 1022
Streptococcus milleri, 1573
Streptococcus pneumoniae
antimicrobial susceptibilities of, 1421t
characteristics of, 1563, 1567
drug-resistant, 1565-1566, 1566t
meningitis, antibiotics in, 1553t
septic arthritis, 1537
Streptococcus pyogenes. See also Streptococcal infection, group A
characteristics of, 1567

Streptogramin(s), 1436-1437
Streptomycin, 1432
for *Yersinia* infection, 1636t
Streptozotocin, 2415t
Stress disorders
acute, 2661-2662
posttraumatic, 2661-2662
Stress testing. *See* Exercise stress testing
Stress ulcer, acute, 778, 788
Stricture
common bile duct, 909
esophageal, in dysphagia, 759-760, 759f
Stroke, 2201-2216
acute
hypertension in, 230
neuroimaging of, 2201-2202, 2203f-2204f
patient approach, 2201-2202, 2202f
in acute myocardial infarction, 331
chronic renal failure in, 2015-2016
definitions of, 2201
epidemiology of, 2201
headache in, 2162-2163
hemorrhagic, 2201, 2214-2215
intracerebral hemorrhage in, 2214, 2214t
subarachnoid hemorrhage in, 2214-2215
ischemic, 2201, 2202-2214
acute
antiplatelet and antithrombotic treatment for, 2206-2208
diagnosis of, 2204-2206
intra-arterial thrombolysis for, 2208-2209, 2209f
intravenous recombinant tissue plasminogen activator for, 2208, 2208t
neuroprotection for, 2209
prognosis and recovery in, 2210
treatment of, 2206-2210
in arterial dissection, 2213
blood pressure in, 2209
brain and body temperature in, 2209-2210
cardioembolism in, 2203-2204, 2205f
cerebral edema in, 2210
in cerebral venous thrombosis, 2213-2214
deep vein thrombosis in, 2210
diagnostic evaluation of, 2205-2206, 2205f, 2207f
differential diagnosis of, 2204t
etiology of, 2203-2204, 2205f-2206f
hereditary causes, 2213
hyperglycemia in, 2210
idiopathic causes of, 2214
in inflammatory arteriopathy, 2213
large vessel
atherothromboembolism in, 2204, 2206f
lesion localization in, 2204-2205, 2206f, 2206t
medical management of, 2209-2210
prevention of, 2210-2213
antiplatelet and antithrombotic treatment for, 2212-2213, 2213t
cardioembolism risk and, 2211-2212, 2210t
carotid artery disease risk and, 2212
therapy for, 2211-

2213, 2210t, 2213t
respiratory function in, 2209
risk factor reduction for, 2210-2211, 2210t
small vessel occlusive disease in, 2204
uncommon causes of, 2213-2214
volume replacement in, 2209
Strongyloides stercoralis, 1922, 1923f
Strongyloidiasis, 1922-1923, 1923f, 1920t
Struvite nephrolithiasis. *See* Nephrolithiasis, struvite stones in
Sturge-Weber syndrome, port-wine stain in, 545
Subarachnoid hemorrhage
headache in, 2154t, 2164
in stroke, 2214-2215
Subclavian venous thrombosis, 422
Subdural empyema, 1559-1560
Subdural hematoma, headache in, 2154t
Subphrenic abscess, 1504
fever of undetermined origin in, 1414-1415
Substance abuse, in pregnancy, 1023
Substance abuse disorders. *See also under* Drug abuse, Drug dependence
definition of, 2636
depression, anxiety, psychosis in, treatment of, 2642
Subungual fibroma, in tuberous sclerosis, 440, 441f
Suburethral sling, for incontinence, 1044
Suicide
assisted, 98
psychosocial issues and, 119
risk of, in depression, 2615-2616
Sulbactam, 1428
Sulfa allergy, 1274-1275
desensitization in, 1884t
Sulfadoxine with pyrimethamine, for malaria chemoprophylaxis, for travelers, 78
Sulfasalazine
and hydroxychloroquine, for rheumatoid arthritis, 1310, 1308t
for inflammatory bowel disease, 800, 800f, 801t
for psoriasis, 470
Sulfatase deficiency, multiple, 1149t
Sulfite(s), asthma due to, 2706-2707
Sulfonamide(s), 1437
hypersensitivity syndrome reaction due to, 496
in pregnancy, 1422t
Sulfonylureas, for type 2 diabetes mellitus, 657-658, 658t
Sulfur and resorcinol, for acne vulgaris, 449t
Sun exposure
for psoriasis, 467
skin cancer and, 549
Superantigens, bacterial, in sepsis, 1445, 1446f
Superinfection, microbial, due to antibiotic use, 1424
Superior vena cava syndrome, neoplastic, 2425-2426, 2426f-2427f
Supraglottitis (acute epiglottitis), 1465-1466
Supranuclear palsy, progressive, 2252, 2253f
Supraventricular tachycardia, 250-259
paroxysmal, 250

Surgical procedures, prophylaxis for, 1440-1441
Swallowing disorder. *See* Dysphagia
Sweating, hypernatremia and, 1987
Swimmer's ear, *Pseudomonas aeruginosa,* 1660
Swimmer's itch, 522-523
Swyer-James syndrome, 2740
Sympatholytic syndrome, in poisoning or drug overdose, 158t
Sympathomimetic syndrome, in poisoning or drug overdose, 158t
Syncopal spell, 2191
Syncope
in cardiovascular patient, 205-208, 205t, 206f
convulsive, 2191
neurocardiogenic
in anoxic encephalopathy, 2336
pacemaker for, 274t, 275
ventricular arrhythmias and, 264
electrocardiography and, 264
electrophysiologic testing and, 264
history and physical examination in, 264
Syndrome of inappropriate ADH secretion (SIADH)
hyponatremia in, 1983-1984, 1983t
specific cause of, 1985
treatment of, 1985
Syndrome X, 197
Synovial fluid
crystals found in, 1380
in rheumatic disease, 1294
in septic arthritis, 1534-1535, 1534f, 1535t
Synovial sarcoidosis, 2772
Synovial sarcoma, 2550t, 2552
Syphilis, 1697-1711
cardiovascular, 1701
in children, 1708
clinical manifestations of, 1699-1701
complications of, 1707
congenital, 1708
differential diagnosis of, 1702-1703
endemic, 1709-1710, 1705t
epidemiology and etiology of, 1697, 1698f-1699f
genital ulcers in, 1528t
gummatous (benign), 1701, 1701f
in HIV infection, 1708-1709
incidence of, 1697, 1698f
Jarisch-Herxheimer reaction in, 1707
laboratory findings in, 1701-1702
cardiovascular, 1702
in gummatous disease, 1702
in latent disease, 1702
in primary disease, 1701-1702, 1701f
in secondary disease, 1702
latent, 1700
pathogenesis of, 1697-1698, 1699f-1700f, 1699t
penicillin allergy in, 1707
in pregnancy, 1707-1708
primary, 1699
chancre in, 1699, 1699f
secondary, 1699-1700
alopecia in, 569, 569f
condyloma latum in, 1700, 1700f
meningitis in, 1700
skin lesions in, 1699-1700, 1700f
septic arthritis in, 1538
treatment of, 1703-1709, 1704t-1705t
in congenital disease, 1705t
in latent disease, 1705, 1704t
in late symptomatic disease, 1705

in neurosyphilis, 1706, 1705t
in primary and secondary disease, 1703-1704, 1704t
serologic follow-up in, 1706-1707
sexual partners and incubating disease, 1707
Syringoma, 537, 537f
Systemic inflammatory response syndrome (SIRS), definition of, 1443t
Systemic lupus erythematosus. *See* Lupus erythematosus, systemic (SLE)
Systemic sclerosis, progressive. *See* Scleroderma

T

Tacalcitol, for psoriasis, 465-466
Tachycardia
atrial
focal, 256
multifocal, 256
atrioventricular nodal reentrant. *See also* Atrioventricular nodal reentrant tachycardia
atrioventricular nodal reentry, 251-254, 250f-253f, 254t
atrioventricular reentry, 254-256, 255f. *See also* Wolff-Parkinson-White syndrome
sinus, 258
in drug overdose or poisoning, 156t
supraventricular, 250-259
paroxysmal, 250
ventricular. *See* Ventricular tachycardia
Tacrolimus
after liver transplantation, complications of, 934
for atopic dermatitis, 477
for inflammatory bowel disease, 802
for prerenal-transplant patient management, 2118-2119
for psoriasis, 470
Tai Chi, 88
Takayasu arteritis (pulseless disease), 374-375, 1369, 1369f
renal artery in, 2073-2074, 2073t
Talc-induced granulomatosis, diffuse infiltrative lung disease in, 2764
Tamoxifen, 2419t
for breast cancer
with chemotherapy, 2467
in early invasive disease, 2464-2465
preventive, 2459, 2460t
as risk factor in endometrial cancer, 2545
Tamponade
cardiac, in cardiac arrest, 148t
pericardial, neoplastic, 2425
Tamsulosin, for benign prostatic hyperplasia, 2131, 2131t
Tapeworm
beef, 1938, 1939f
dog, 1939-1940
dwarf, 1938-1939
fish, 1936
mice and rat, 1939
other types of, 1939-1940
pork, 1937-1938, 1937f, 1939f
Tar, topical, for psoriasis, 466
Tarantula, 190
Tardive dyskinesia, 2260-2261
Tarsal tunnel syndrome, 1397, 1397f
Taxanes, 2421-2422, 2419t
Tay-Sachs disease, 1149t
Tazarotene

for acne vulgaris, 449t
for psoriasis, 466
Tazobactam, 1428
T cell(s)
CD3, deficiency, 1230t
CD4$^+$
in HIV infection and AIDS, 1805-1807, 1806f
IgE production and, 1240-1241, 1241t
in sepsis, 1446-1447
CD8, deficiency, 1230t
cytotoxic. *See also* T cell(s), CD8
development of, 1072f
helper. *See also* T cell(s), CD4$^+$
TEL-AML1, 2385
Telangiectasia
definition of, 429t
hereditary hemorrhagic, 1177
unilateral, 546
Telithromycin, 1434-1435
Telmisartan, for hypertension, 223t
Telogen effluvium, 564-565, 565t, 565f
Temozolomide, 2416t
Temperature, body. *See also* Fever, Hyperthermia
measurement, 1407
regulation of, 1407
Temporal arteritis, 1368-1369
fever of undetermined origin in, 1415
headache in, 2154t, 2163
Temporal artery biopsy, in fever of undetermined origin, 1417
Tendinitis
Achilles, 1397, 1397f
bicipital, 1393
calcific, of rotator cuff, 1393
infrapatellar, 1396
rotator cuff (impingement syndrome), 1392-1393, 1393f
Teniposide, 2418t
Tennis elbow, 1394
Tenofovir
for chronic hepatitis B, 888
for HIV infection, 1831t
adverse effects of, 1834t
Tenosynovitis
de Quervain, 1395
flexor, of hand, 1395
Tension-type headache, 2159-2160
Teratogenesis, principles of, 1016-1017, 1017t-1018t
Teratoma
cystic
in adolescent female, 1059
in reproductive age women, 1060, 1062
immature, ovarian, 2541
Terazosin
for benign prostatic hyperplasia, 2131, 2131t
for hypertension, 223t
Terbinafine, for toenail onychomycosis, 575t
Terry nails, 573
Testes, 689-697
function throughout life, 690-691, 690f
gonadotropin in, 689
normal function, 689-691
in puberty, 691
in senescence, 691
spermatogenesis in, 690
testosterone in, 689-690
torsion of, 693
undescended, 692-693
in utero, 690
varicocele of, 693
Testicular cancer, 2519-2524
diagnosis of, 2520-2521
epidemiology and etiology of, 2519
management of, 2521-2524, 2522t-

2524t
advanced lymph node involvement and metastases in, 2523, 2523t
in late relapse, 2524
in lymph node metastases of 5 cm or less, 2522-2523
poor-risk and previously treated germ cell tumors in, 2523-2524
in stage I or A disease, 2521-2522
toxicity of chemotherapy in, 2524, 2524t
pathogenesis of, 2519-2520
staging of, 2521, 2521t
tumor markers in, 2521
Testosterone
congenital deficiency of, 693
in hypogonadism, 692
replacement of, in hypogonadism, 694, 695f
serum, in polycystic ovary syndrome, 978
synthesis of, testicular, 689-690
Tetanus, 1608-1609, 1609f
diagnosis of, 1611
prevention of, 1615, 1615t
treatment of, 1614
Tetanus immunization
for HIV-infected patients, 1830t
for travelers, 71
Tetanus prophylaxis, after animal bites, 182t, 182
Tetracycline, 1433
for acne vulgaris, 450t
for *Helicobacter* infection, 1637t
for legionellosis, 1655t
in pregnancy, 1422t
for *Yersinia* infection, 1636t
Tetralogy of Fallot, 395-396, 395f
Textile dye, contact dermatitis due to, 490
TGF-beta II R, properties of, 2386t
Thalassemia, 1119-1112
diagnosis of, 1120
genetic counseling for, 1122
hematopoietic stem cell transplantation for, 1222
molecular genetics, 1120, 1120f
pathophysiology, 1119-1120, 1120f
prenatal diagnosis for, 1122
alpha-Thalassemia, 1121-1122
genetics of, 1949
heterozygous, 1122
molecular genetics, 1121-1122, 1120f, 1949
pathophysiology of, 1120
sickle cell anemia and, 1115
alpha-Thalassemia-like syndrome, 1122
beta-Thalassemia, 1120-1121
bone marrow transplantation for, 1121
intermedia, 1121
major (Cooley anemia), 1120-1121
minor (trait), 1121
sickle trait and, 1117-1118
variants, 1121
Thalassemia trait, 1092t
Theophylline
for asthma, 2713-2714, 2710t
poisoning or overdose, 173-174
elimination method for, 161t
hypokalemia due to, 2007, 2007t
seizure due to, 157t
Therapeutic touch, 89
Thermal control center, hypothalamic, 1407. *See also* Fever, Hyperthermia
Thiazolidinedione, for polycystic ovary syndrome, 983-984
Thiazolidinediones

for hirsutism, 992
for type 2 diabetes mellitus, 659-660, 658t
Thienopyridines, for unstable angina and NSTMI, 309-310
Thioguanine, 2417t
6-Thioguanine, for psoriasis, 470
Thionamide, for thyrotoxicosis, 615-616
Thiotepa, 2415t
Thomsen disease (autosomal dominant myotonia congenita), 2282
Thoracentesis, 2697-2698, 2697t
Thoracic duct, 2830
Thoracoscopy
in lung disease, 2696
in pleural disease, 2699-2700
Thoracostomy, tube, in pleural disease, 2698-2699, 2699t
Thoracotomy, with open lung biopsy, 2696
Thrombin-activatable fibrinolysis inhibitor, in coagulation, 1158, 1159f
Thrombin inhibitors, direct, for acute myocardial infarction, 328
Thrombin time (TT), 1160-1161
Thromboangiitis obliterans (Buerger disease), in peripheral arterial disease, 406
Thrombocythemia, 1175-1176
essential, 2582
Thrombocytopenia, 1163-1174. *See also* Platelet(s)
accelerated platelet removal due to immune processes in, 1166-1170, 1165t. *See also* Thrombocytopenic purpura
blood count and peripheral smear in, 1164
bone marrow aspirate and biopsy in, 1164-1165, 1165t
causes of, 1165t
cocaine-associated, 1169-1170
diagnostic evaluation in, 1164-1165, 1164t-1165t
due to acetaminophen metabolites, 1170
due to naproxen metabolites, 1170
due to platelet glycoprotein IIb-IIIa receptor antagonists, 1170
gold, 1169
heparin-induced, 1169, 1199-1201, 1200f
induced by infection, 1173
bacterial septicemia, 1173
protozoan, 1173
viral, 1173
laboratory tests in, 1164-1165, 1165t
neoplastic, 2427-2428
petechiae in, 1164
platelet production defects in, 1165
in platelet sequestration, 1174
in platelet washout and vascular bed abnormalities, 1174
in pregnancy and peripartum, 1173-1174
in systemic lupus erythematosus, 1333
Thrombocytopenic purpura, 1166-1174
idiopathic, 1166-1169
causes of, 1165t
clinical features of, 1166
course and prognosis in, 1166
differential diagnosis of, 1166
laboratory evaluation in, 1166
pathophysiology of, 1166
treatment of, 1166-1167
antibody therapy with IVIg in, 1167

EACA in, 1168
in HIV patients, 1168
IVIg for, 1167
prednisone for, 1167
in pregnancy, 1168-1169
in refractory disease, 1167-1168
in severe mucosal or CNS bleeding, 1167
splenectomy for, 1167
with lymphoma, 1169
posttransfusion, 1169
with systemic lupus erythematosus, 1169
thrombotic, 1170-1173. *See also* Hemolytic-uremic syndrome
ADAMTS13 screening assay for, 1171-1172, 1171f
clinical features and diagnosis of, 1172
differential diagnosis of, 1172
etiology of, 1170
pathogenesis of, 1170-1171
renal involvement in, 2078-2079, 2078f
treatment of, 1172-1173
Thrombocytosis, 1175-1176
Thromboembolism
in endocarditis, 1485
prosthetic heart valves and, 360
venous, 410-424. *See also* Pulmonary embolism
classification of, 410
diagnosis of, 411-416
frequence and risk of, 1192, 1192t
natural history and prognosis in, 411
pathophysiology of, 410-411
patient management in, 1202-1203, 1202t
in pregnancy, 421-422
prophylaxis for, 418-419, 418t
indications for, 419
risk factors and etiology of, 410
treatment of, 419-421
anticoagulant, 420-421
Thrombolytic agent(s)
complications of, 1184-1185
for myocardial infarction, acute, 323-325, 324f
Thrombophilia, 423
clinical features of, 1191, 1191t
in pregnancy, 1021
Thrombophlebitis
cavernous sinus, 1560
in sinusitis, 1460
lateral sinus, 1560-1561
septic, of cerebral veins, 1560-1561
superior sagittal sinus, 1561
Thrombopoietin
in hematopoiesis, 1072, 1073t
in platelet production, 1159-1160
Thrombosis
arterial
in acute peripheral arterial occlusive disease, 405
screening tests for, 1191t
axillary vein, 422
cerebral venous, in stroke, 2213-2214
due to heparin therapy, 1199-1201, 1200f
in hematologic disease, 1075
mesenteric vein, 422-423
renal vein, 423, 2074
tubulointerstitial nephritis in, 2096
splenic vein, in acute pancreatitis, 922
subclavian vein, 422

venous, 411-412. *See also* Pulmonary embolism
anticoagulants for, 420-421
clinical features, 411, 411t
D-dimer blood testing for, 412, 413t
diagnostic tests in, 411-412, 413t, 412f
in mechanical ventilation, 2819
in pregnancy, 421-422
recurrent, 412-413
screening tests for, 1191t
venography for, 411-412, 412f
venous ultrasonography for, 412, 413t
Thrombotic disorders, 1190-1205
age of onset of, 1190
family history in, 1191
hypercoagulable workup in, 1191-1192, 1191t
patient assessment in, 1190-1192
provoking factors in, 1190-1191
recurrent, 1191
site of, 1191, 1191t
Thrombotic microangiopathy, renal involvement in, 2078, 2078f
Thymic hypoplasia, congenital, 1229, 1230t
Thymoma, 2839
Thyroid, 605-625. *See also* Hyperthyroidism, Hypothyroidism
Thyroid adenoma, toxic, 610-611
Thyroid cancer, 621-623
complications of, 623
diagnosis of, 622
epidemiology of, 605, 621
etiology and pathogenesis of, 621-622
management of, 622-623
prognosis in, 623
Thyroid crisis, 617
Thyroid disease, in pregnancy, 1019-1021
Thyroidectomy, for hyperthyroidism, 616
Thyroid function tests
in hypothyroidism, 607, 607t
in thyrotoxicosis, 613-614, 614t
Thyroid hormone, for hypothyroidism, 608-609
Thyroiditis, 618-619
acute (suppurative), 619
autoimmune (Hashimoto), 606, 618, 1237
encephalopathy in, 2340
de Quervain, 618-619
drug-induced, 619
granulomatous, 618-619
lymphocytic, 618
postpartum, 1020-1021
Reidel, 619
subacute, 618-619
in thyrotoxicosis, 611
Thyroid nodule(s), 620-621
epidemiology of, 605
Thyroid-stimulating hormone, in polycystic ovary syndrome, 978
Thyroid-stimulating hormone (TSH), 601
deficiency, 601
Thyrotoxicosis, 610-618. *See also* Graves disease, Hyperthyroidism
amiodarone-induced, 611
clinical manifestations of, 613
complications of, 617
definitions of, 605
diagnosis of, 613-614, 614t
differential diagnosis of, 614-615
epidemiology of, 605, 606f, 610
etiology, genetics, pathogenesis of, 610-613, 610t, 611f-612f, 612t
exogenous, 612-613

features of, 612t
gestational transient, 611-612
laboratory tests in, 613-614, 614t
management of, 615-617
 antithyroid drugs for, 615-616
 beta-adrenergic blockers in, 615
 other agents for, 616-617
 radioiodine for, 616
 surgery for, 616
physical examination in, 613
prognosis in, 617-618
thyroiditis in, 611
Thyrotropin-secreting adenoma, 601
Thyroxine (T4). See Thyroid function
 tests, Thyroid hormone
TIBOLA (tick-borne lymphadenopathy),
 1727t, 1728-1729
Ticarcillin, 1428
Ticarcillin-clavulanate, 1428
Tic douloureux (trigeminal
 neuralgia), 2294-2295, 2294t
 headache in, 2154t, 2163
Tick(s), 191-192. See also Lyme
 disease
Tick-borne encephalitis
 immunization, for travelers, 74
Tick-borne lymphadenopathy (TIBOLA),
 1727t, 1728-1729
Tick fever, Colorado, 1857
Ticlopidine
 for angina pectoris, 296-297
 for unstable angina and NSTMI, 309-
 310, 309t
Tigecycline, 1433
Timolol, for hypertension, 222t
Tinea barbae, 505-506, 507
Tinea capitis, 504-505, 505f, 507
 endothrix, 569, 569f
Tinea corporis, 505, 504f, 506
Tinea cruris, 506
Tinea faciei, 506
Tinea manuum, 506, 507
Tinea pedis, 506, 505f, 507
 streptococcal cellulitis in, 506
Tinea unguium, 506, 506f, 507, 576
Tinea versicolor, 508, 509f
Tiopronin, for cystine
 nephrolithiasis, 2112
Tipranavir, for HIV infection, 1831t
 adverse effects of, 1834t
Tirofiban, for unstable angina and
 NSTMI, 309-310, 309t
Tissue factor pathway inhibitor, in
 coagulation, 1156, 1157f
Tissue plasminogen activator (t-PA),
 recombinant (rt-PA), for stroke,
 2208, 2208t
Tobacco. See also Cigarette smoking,
 Nicotine
 alcohol use and, in cancer
 epidemiology, 2374-2375
 in cancer epidemiology, 2374-2375
 smokeless
 in cancer epidemiology, 2374
 oral cancer due to, 2374, 2437
Tobramycin, 1432
Toe
 claw, 1397
 hammer, 1397
 mallet, 1397
Toenail(s). See Nail(s)
Toe web syndrome, Pseudomonas
 aeruginosa, 1661
Toll-like receptors, in sepsis, 1444
Toluene, biologic test of exposure
 to, 61t
Topiramate, in epilepsy, 2196
Topotecan, 2419t
Toremifene, 2419t
Torsade de pointes, due to therapy
 for ventricular arrhythmias, 268
Torsemide, for hypertension, 221t
Tourette syndrome, 2258
Toxic encephalopathy, 2341-2342

Toxic epidermal necrolysis, 531, 526t
 as drug reaction, 500, 500f
 staphylococcal scalded skin
 syndrome vs., 439, 531, 526t
Toxic megacolon, 792, 805
Toxic myopathy(ies), drug-induced,
 2282-2284, 2283t
Toxic neuropathy(ies), 2303-
 2304, 2303t
Toxic-shock syndrome
 staphylococcal, 1580, 1580t-1581t
 cutaneous findings in, 439
 streptococcal, 1570
Toxin exposure. See Poisoning or
 drug overdose
Toxoplasma gondii, 1898, 1898f
 in HIV infection
 management of, 1841t, 1839
 prevention of recurrence of,
 1842t
 prophylactic measures for
 prevention of, 1840t
Toxoplasmosis, 1898-1901
 in AIDS, 1899
 clinical syndromes of, 1898-1900
 CNS, in HIV infection, 1840t-
 1842t, 1839
 congenital, 1900
 diagnosis of, 1900
 in immunosuppression, 1899
 ocular, 1900
 primary, 1899
 treatment of, 1900-1901
TP53, properties of, 2386f
Trace element(s), in nutritional
 support, 947, 947t
Tracheobronchitis
 Haemophilus influenzae, 1650
 Moraxella catarrhalis, 1652
Trachoma, 1750-1751
Trandolapril, for hypertension, 222t
Transbronchial needle aspiration,
 2690-2691, 2691t
Transesophageal endoscopic
 ultrasound, 2695-2696
Transferrin, in iron metabolism,
 1080
Transferrin receptor, in iron
 metabolism, 1081, 1081f
Transfusion reaction, 1214-1217
 acute lung injury as, 1215-1216
 allergic, 1216
 atypical, 1216
 bacterial infections as, 1217
 cytomegalovirus infections as,
 1217, 1217t
 febrile, 1215
 graft vs. host disease as, 1216-
 1217
 irradiated blood products for,
 1216-1217, 1217t
 hemolytic, 1214-1215
 diagnosis and treatment of, 1214-
 1215
 immediate vs. delayed, 1214
 prevention of, 1215
 in sickle cell disease, 1214
 immune modulation due to, 1217
 posttransfusion thrombocytopenic
 purpura, 1169
 protozoal infections as, 1217
Transfusion therapy, 1206-1221
 antibody screening for, 1208-1209
 antigen phenotyping, 1208, 1208t
 ABO, 1208, 1208t
 D antigen specificity, 1208
 blood donation for, 1206-1208. See
 also Blood donation
 component, 1209-1214
 characteristics and indications
 for, 1209, 1209t
 cryoprecipitate, 1210, 1209t
 factor VIIa, 1213
 factor VIII, 1213

factor IX, 1213
factor XI, 1212
future prospects of, 1219-1220
granulocyte, 1213
HIV-1 screening in, 1822-1823
HIV-2 screening in, 1822-1823
immune globulin, 1213-1214
infection risks from, 1206t
iron overload in, 1088-1089
irradiated blood products for,
 1216-1217, 1217t
plasma, fresh frozen, 1210, 1209t,
 1212-1213
platelet, 1210, 1209t
 contraindications to, 1211-1212
 indications for, 1211, 1211t
 in low platelet count, 1211
 nonfunctioning platelets and,
 1211
 in refractory patient, 1212
 response to, 1212
pretransfusion testing, 1208-1209
red cell, 1209-1210, 1209t
 for acute blood loss, 1210-1211
 for autoimmune hemolytic anemia,
 1125
 autologous, 1211
 for chronic anemia, 1211
 delayed type hemolysis in, 1126
 frozen, 1210
 indications for, 1210-1211
 intraoperative and postoperative
 blood salvage for, 1211
 isovolemic hemodilution for,
 1211
 leukocyte reduction for, 1209
 washed, 1209
 in septic shock, 1452
 stem cell. See Hematopoietic stem
 cell transplantation
Transient ischemic attack (TIA),
 2201. See also Stroke
Transjugular intrahepatic
 portosystemic shunt (TIPS), for
 variceal bleeding, 869
Transplantation. See also individual
 organs, e.g., Renal
 transplantation
 cytomegalovirus infection in, 1762
 lung. See Lung transplantation
 septic arthritis in, 1539
Transthoracic needle aspiration and
 biopsy
 in lung and mediastinal disease,
 2687-2688, 2688f
 in pleural disease, 2698
Trastuzumab, 2420t, 2464, 2470
Trauma. See also Injury and disease
 aortic, 375, 385-386, 385f
 brain. See Brain trauma
 cardiac, blunt, 385-386
 cardiovascular, 385-386
 head. See also Coma
 headache in, 2163
 pancreatitis in, 914-915
Traumatic arthritis, pain in,
 temporal course of, 1291f
Travel, international
 CDC information for, 69
 health advice for, 69-81
 immunization for, 69-75, 69t
 cholera, 71
 contraindicated, 75
 diphtheria, 71
 hepatitis A, 72-73, 73f
 hepatitis B, 73, 74f
 influenza, 71
 Japanese encephalitis, 74, 76t
 measles, 71
 meningococcal disease, 73-74, 75f
 plague, 72
 pneumococcal infections, 71
 poliomyelitis, 71
 rabies, 72

required, 70, 70f
tetanus, 71
tick-borne encephalitis, 74
typhoid, 71-72
yellow fever, 70, 70f
malaria chemoprophylaxis for, 76-
 78, 1897. See also Malaria
pretravel evaluation for, 69, 69t
Traveler's diarrhea, 79-80, 80t
Travel-related illness, 79-80
Treatment effects, measures of, 11-
 12, 12t
Treatment outcome, measures of, 12
Trematode infection, 1932-1936
Tremor
 essential, 2259
 physiologic, enhanced, 2259
Trench fever, 1672
 urban, 1672-1673
Treponema carateum, 1710
Treponema pallidum, 1697. See also
 Syphilis
 in septic arthritis, 1538
Treponema pallidum pertenue, 1709.
 See also Yaws
Tretinoin, for acne vulgaris, 449t
Triamcinolone, for asthma,
 2712, 2713t
Triamterene, for hypertension, 221t
Trichinella spiralis, 1924
Trichinellosis, 1924-1925
 etiology and epidemiology of, 1924-
 1925
 intestinal phase of, 1925
 laboratory findings and
 differential diagnosis in,
 1925, 1925f
 muscle phase of, 1925
 pathogenesis and clinical features
 of, 1925
 treatment of, 1925
Trichoepithelioma, 537, 537f
Trichomonas vaginalis, in
 vulvovaginitis, 1524-1525, 1524t
Trichomoniasis, 1909-1910
Trichomycosis axillaris, 512
Trichostrongyliasis, 1923
Trichotillomania, 567
Tricuspid regurgitation,
 359, 348t, 350t
 murmur in, 210t
Tricuspid stenosis, 359, 348t
 murmur in, 210t
Tricuspid valve, Ebstein anomaly of,
 399, 398f
Tricyclic antidepressant(s). See
 Antidepressant(s), tricyclic
Trifascicular block, pacemaker for,
 274t, 275
Trigeminal neuralgia (tic
 douloureux), 2294-2295, 2294t
 headache in, 2154t, 2163
Trigeminal neuropathy, in
 scleroderma, 1347
Triglyceride(s)
 drug therapy for lowering, 745
 elevated. See Hypertriglyceridemia
 lipoprotein lipase-mediated
 removal, 731
Triiodothyronine (T3). See Thyroid
 function tests, Thyroid hormone
Trimethaphan, for hypertensive
 crisis, 228t
Trimethoprim, 1437-1438
 in pregnancy, 1422t
Trimethoprim-sulfamethoxazole, 1438
 for acne vulgaris, 450t
 for Salmonella infection, 1635t
 for Shigella infection, 1636t
 for Vibrio infection, 1636t
 for Yersinia infection, 1636t
Trinucleotide repeat diseases,
 genetic testing for, 1959, 1960t
Trochanteric bursitis, 1396

Trochlear neuropathy, 2294t
Trophoblastic tumor, hyperthyroidism in, 611
Tropical pulmonary eosinophilia, 2782
multifocal infiltrates in, 2748
Tropical pyomyositis, staphylococcal, 1578
Tropical spastic paraparesis, HTLV-I and, 1811, 2357
Tropical sprue, 829, 829f-830f
Troponin, as biochemical cardiac marker, 305
Trousseau syndrome, malignancy and, 1201-1202
Truncal neuropathy(ies), diabetic, 2300
Trypanosoma cruzi, 1913
Trypanosomiasis, 1913-1915
African, 1915-1916, 1915f
diagnosis of, 1915-1916
etiology and epidemiology of, 1915, 1915f
treatment of, 1916
American (Chagas disease), 1913-1915
diagnosis of, 1913-1914
etiology and epidemiology of, 1913, 1914f
pathogenesis of, 1913, 1914f
treatment of, 1915
TTG, properties of, 2384t
Tubal factors, in infertility, 1003
Tubal ligation, 998-999
Tuberculin skin testing, 1684, 1685t
Tuberculosis, 1675-1696
abdominal, 1682
acid-fast bacteria smear microscopy for, 1685-1686
adrenal, 1683
arthritis in, 1538
central nervous system, 1682
chest radiography for, 1685
congenital, 1683
contact investigation and reporting in, 1693
diagnosis of, 1685-1687
empyema in, 1680
epidemiology of, 1675-1676, 1676f-1677f
etiology and genetics of, 1676
extrapulmonary, 1679-1683
diagnosis of, 1687
treatment of, 1691, 1691t
genitourinary, 1680
in HIV infection, 1683-1684
management of, 1839, 1841t
prophylactic measures for, 1840t
hospital-based prevention of, 1694
immune response in, 1677-1678, 1677f
incidence of, 1675-1676, 1676f-1677f
latent (LTBI), 1675
new diagnostic tests for, 1684-1685
targeted testing for, 1684-1685, 1685t
treatment of, 1693-1694, 1693t
tuberculin skin testing, 1684, 1685t
lymphadenitis in, 1680
meningitis in, 1682
microbiology studies for, 1685-1687
miliary, 1682-1683
fever of undetermined origin in, 1414
molecular typing for, 1686-1687
musculoskeletal (Pott disease), 1680-1681, 1681f
mycobacterial culture for, 1686
nucleic acid amplification tests

for, 1686
pathogenesis of, 1676-1678, 1677f
pericarditis in, 1681-1682
peritoneal, 1682
pleural, 1680
pleural effusion in, 2829
pleuritis in, 1678, 1680, 2829
pulmonary, 1678-1679
cavitary infiltrates in, 2752, 2752f
imaging studies in, 1679, 1679f
multifocal infiltrates in, 2747
physical findings in, 1679
primary, 1678
reactivation, 1678-1679
secondary, 1678-1679
segmental pulmonary infiltrates in, 2750
sputum induction test for, 1686
susceptibility testing for, 1686
treatment of, 1687-1694
directly observed therapy in, 1687, 1689f
in drug-resistant disease, 1692, 1692t
in drug-susceptible pulmonary disease, 1689, 1689t, 1689f-1690f
in extrapulmonary disease, 1691, 1691t
in HIV-infected patients, 1689-1691, 1689t
initiation of, 1687-1688
for LTBI, 1693-1694, 1693t
monitoring response to, 1692-1693
in pregnancy, 1691-1692
principles of, 1687, 1688t
regimens in, 1688-1692, 1689t, 1691t-1692t, 1689f-1690f
vaccines for, 1694
Tuberculous rheumatism (Poncet disease), 1678, 1681
Tuberous sclerosis
CNS tumors in, 2310t
cutaneous findings in, 440, 441f
Tubular acidosis
incomplete, calcium nephrolithiasis in, 2106
type 1
calcium nephrolithiasis in, 2106
hyperkalemic, 1998, 2010, 2010t
hypokalemic, 1998-1999
normal-anion-gap acidosis in, 1997-1998, 1998t, 1995f
treatment of, 2001-2002
type 2, normal-anion-gap acidosis in, 1998
type 4, 1999, 1995f, 1998t
causes of, 1999t, 2010
hyperkalemia in, 2010
Tubular necrosis, acute, 1970, 1971f, 1970t
in hospitalized patient, 2027-2028
nephrotoxic. *See* Nephrotoxicity
Tubular reabsorption, of body fluid, 1976, 1976f, 1978f, 1977t
Tubulointerstitial nephritis, 2086-2103
in amyloidosis, 2097
in cholesterol emboli, 2096, 2095f
in chronic hypokalemia, 2094
in dysproteinemia, 2097
etiologies of, 2087t
in hypercalcemia and hypercalciuria, 2094
in hyperoxaluria, 2093-2094
in hypertension, 2095
in hyperuricemia and hyperuricosuria, 2094
infectious, 2092-2093
inflammatory, secondary to

systemic infection, 2093
in lead or cadmium exposure, 64, 2094-2095
in light-chain deposition disease, 2097
metabolic and toxic, 2093-2095
in multiple myeloma, 2096-2097, 2097f
in obstructive nephropathy, 2091-2092
from physical factors, 2091-2092
in radiation nephritis, 2092
in reflux nephropathy, 2092
in renal vein thrombosis, 2096
in sarcoidosis, 2100-2101
in sickle cell anemia, 2095-2096
in systemic lupus erythematosus, 2100
in vascular damage, 2095-2096
viral-related, in immunosuppression, 2093
Tubulointerstitial renal disease, 1970, 1971f, 1970t
Tubulointerstitium, normal architecture of, 2086, 2086f
Tularemia, 136-137, 1668-1670
complications and prognosis in, 1670
diagnosis of, 1669, 1664t
differential diagnosis of, 1669
epidemiology of, 1668, 1668f
etiology of, 1668-1669
pathogenesis of, 1669
treatment of, 1670, 1665t
Tumor(s). *See also specific anatomic site*
angiogenesis in
drugs for inhibition of, 2423
molecular genetics of, 2393-2394, 2395f
anticancer chemotherapy for. *See* Anticancer chemotherapy
gene-based therapy for, 2423
immune response to, 2400-2407
cellular, 2402-2403, 2402f
effector mechanisms of, 2402-2403, 2402f
enhancement of, 2403-2407
evading, 2403
host, 2400, 2401f
humoral, 2403
passive, 2405-2407
adoptive cellular immunotherapy for, 2405-2406
antitumor antibody therapy for, 2406-2407
stimulation of, 2403-2405
immunostimulatory cytokines for, 2404-2405
nonspecific, 2403
vaccine therapy, 2404
with dendritic cell vaccines, 2404
with genetically modified tumor cells, 2404
with intact unmodified tumor cells, 2404
with naked DNA vaccines, 2404
with recombinant viral or bacterial vaccines, 2404
with tumor antigens or peptides, 2404
targets for, 2401-2402
abnormal posttranslational modification of self-proteins as, 2402
differentiation antigens as, 2402
mutated or overexpressed oncogene or tumor suppressor gene antigens

as, 2401
oncoviral proteins as, 2401
tumor-associated antigens as, 2401
immunotherapy for, 2423
oncogenes and. *See also* Oncogene(s)
Tumor-associated antigen(s), 2401
Tumor-infiltrating lymphoid (TIL) cell(s), 2405
Tumor lysis syndrome, 2431
Tumor necrosis factor-*alpha* (cachectin), in IgE-mediated allergic inflammation, 1241t
Tumor necrosis factor-*beta* (lymphotoxin), in rheumatoid arthritis, 1310-1311
Tumor suppressor gene(s), 2386-2391, 2386t. *See also individual genes, e.g., p53*
cell cycle progression and *RB1* pathway, 2387-2388, 2389f
genomic stability genes, 2388-2391, 2390f
Knudson model and loss-of-function mutations, 2386-2387, 2387f-2388f
reversion of tumorigenicity and, 2386, 2387f
signaling and differentiation genes, 2391
Tumor suppressor gene antigen(s), mutated or overexpressed, 2401
Tungiasis, 522
Turcot syndrome, CNS tumors in, 2310t
Turner syndrome, 958
Tylenol-alcohol syndrome, 878
Typhoid immunization, for travelers, 71-72
Typhus
epidemic (louse-borne), 1729-1730
diagnosis of, 1727t, 1728
epidemiology and etiology of, 1729
recrudescent, 1730
treatment and prevention of, 1730
treatment of, 1728t
murine (endemic), 1729
diagnosis of, 1727t
scrub, 1730-1732
diagnosis of, 1727t, 1731, 1731f
epidemiology of, 1730-1731
treatment of, 1728t, 1731

U

Ulcer
atherosclerotic, penetrating, 373-374
Cameron, 778
Curling, 778
Cushing, 778
definition of, 428t
duodenal. *See* Peptic ulcer disease, duodenal
foot, in diabetes mellitus, 672
gastric. *See* Peptic ulcer disease, gastric
oral, in hematologic disease, 1075
peptic. *See* Peptic ulcer disease
pressure. *See* Pressure ulcer
stress, acute, 778
Ulcerative colitis, 791-795. *See also* Inflammatory bowel disease
classification of, 791, 792t
clinical manifestations, 791-792
clinical severity of, 792, 792t
complications of, 808-809
adenocarcinoma, 809
extraintestinal, 809
intestinal, 808-809

Crohn disease vs., 795t
diagnosis of, 791-795
differential diagnosis, 799
endoscopy in, 793-794, 793f
extensive, 792
  medical treatment of, 804-805
fulminant, treatment of, 805
histology in, 794, 794f
imaging studies, 794-795, 795f
left-sided, 791-792
  medical treatment of, 804
management of, surgical, 805-806
medical treatment of, 804-805
physical examination in, 792-793
radiography in, 794-795, 795f
scintigraphy in, 795
skin lesions in, 435, 435f
toxic megacolon in, 792, 805
Ulcerative proctitis, 791
Ullrich myopathy, 2276
Ulnar nerve, entrapment of, 1394
Ulnar neuropathy, 2296
Ultrasonography
in acute cholecystitis, 903
in acute pancreatitis, 917
in acute renal failure, 2030-2031
in appendicitis, 820
for breast mass evaluation, 1050
in choledocholithiasis, 907
in chronic cholecystitis, 906, 906f
in cirrhosis, 893, 894f
compression, for pulmonary
  embolism, 415-416
endobronchial, 2691
endoscopic
  in acute pancreatitis, 917, 918f
  transesophageal, 2695-2696
in intra-abdominal abscess, 1503
in myositis, 1355
in pelvic mass, 1056-1057
in pleural effusion, 2825
in renal disease, 1969t
in reproductive function, 953, 953f
venous, in venous thrombosis,
  412, 413t
Ultraviolet (UV) radiation
narrow-band UVB, for psoriasis,
  467
skin cancer and, 549
Undulant fever, 1664. See also
  Brucellosis
Univentricular heart, 397-399, 397f
Unstable angina and non-ST segment
  elevation MI, 304-316
clinical presentation in, 304
definition of, 304
diagnosis of, 304-306
history and physical examination
  in, 304-305, 304t
laboratory tests in, 305
pathophysiology of, 304
risk stratification in, 305-
  306, 305t
treatment in, 306-315
  early invasive vs. early
    conservative, 307-308, 307f-
    308f
  recommendations, 308
  trial results, 308
  initial therapy, 306-307, 306f-
    307f
  mechanical revascularization in,
    314-315
  pharmacologic, 309-314
    angiotensin-converting enzyme
      inhibitors, 314
    anticoagulants for, 310-
      312, 311t
    anti-ischemia, 312-313, 312t
    antiplatelet, 309-310, 309t
    aspirin, 309
    beta blockers, 313
    calcium channel blockers, 313

direct thrombin inhibitors
    for, 312
  fibrinolytic drugs for, 310
  glycoprotein IIb-IIIa receptor
    antagonists, 310
  heparin for, 310-311
  lipid-lowering agents in, 313-
    314
  low-molecular-weight heparin
    for, 311-312
  morphine sulfate, 313, 312t
  nitrates, 312-313, 312t
  thienopyridines, 309-310
  warfarin for, 312
posthospital care in, 315
where to hospitalize, 306
Unverricht-Lundborg disease, 2266
Ureaplasma urealyticum
  infections caused by, 1741
  in nongonococcal urethritis, 1741
  in septic arthritis, 1537-1538
Ureidopenicillins, extended-
  spectrum, 1428
Uremia
  bleeding and platelet function in,
    1174-1175, 2045
  encephalopathy in, 2339
  neuropathy in, 2300
Urethral syndrome, acute,
  chlamydial, 1748, 1748t
Urethritis
  chlamydial, 1747, 1748t
    in males, 1521-1523
    in females, 1523
  gonococcal. See Gonorrhea
  in males, 1521-1523
    diagnosis of, 1522, 1522f
    epidemiology of, 1521
    etiology and microbiology of,
      1521-1522
    recurrent or persistent, 1523
    treatment of, 1522-1523
  Mycoplasma genitalium, 1740
  Mycoplasma hominis, 1740
  nongonococcal, 1741, 1747, 1748t
    in males, 1521-1523
    treatment of, 1741
  Ureaplasma urealyticum, 1740
  in women, 1512t
Uric acid, in gout, 1372. See also
  Gout
Uric acid nephropathy, 1374. See
  also Nephrolithiasis, uric acid
  stones in
Urinalysis
  in acute renal failure, in
    hospitalized patient, 2029-
    2030, 2029t
  in benign hyperplasia of prostate,
    2129
Urinary bladder
  catheter care for, 1517, 1517t
  overactive, 1041-1047. See also
    Urinary incontinence
Urinary bladder cancer, 2512-2516
  clinical and laboratory findings
    in, 2513
  diagnosis of, 2513
  epidemiology and etiology of, 2512
    occupational carcinogens in,
      2377
  management of, 2513-2516, 2514t
    in invasive disease, 2514
    in metastatic disease, 2514-
      2516, 2515f
    in superficial disease, 2513-
      2514
  occupational agents causing, 62t
  pathobiology of, 2512-2513, 2512f
  staging in, 2513, 2512f
Urinary flow rate, for benign
  hyperplasia of prostate, 2129-
  2130

Urinary incontinence, 1041-1047
  definitions in, 1041
  diagnosis of, 1041-1043, 1042t-
    1043t
  differential diagnosis in, 1043
  epidemiology of, 1041
  history in, 1041-1042, 1042t-1043t
  laboratory testing in, 1042-1043
  management in, 1043-1046, 1044t-
    1045t
  mechanisms of, 1041
  physical examination in, 1041
  prognosis in, 1046
  stress, 1041
    management in, 1043-1044
  urge, 1041
    management in, 1044-1046, 1044t-
      1045t
Urinary tract, lower, female, 1041
Urinary tract disorders,
  occupational, 64
Urinary tract infection, 1508-1519
  anatomic abnormalities in, 1510
  bacterial virulence in, 1509-
    1510, 1510f
  catheter-associated, 1517, 1517t
  clinical presentations in, 1511-
    1512
  contraceptive use and, 1509
  cystitis in, 1511, 1512t
  in diabetes mellitus, 1508-1509
  diagnosis of, 1511-1512
  E. coli, 1631
  epidemiology of, 1508-1508, 1508t
  etiology and pathogenesis of, 1509-
    1510, 1510f
  functional abnormalities in, 1510
  genetic factors in, 1509
  incidence of, 1508, 1508t
  kidney infection in. See
    Pyelonephritis
  management of, 1512-1517
    in acute uncomplicated female
      cystitis, 1513-
      1514, 1513t, 1514f
    in acute uncomplicated
      pyelonephritis, 1514-
      1515, 1515f, 1516t
    antimicrobial, 1512-1516
    in complicated infection, 1516
    in males, 1515-1516
    radiologic evaluation in, 1516-
      1517
  in menopause, 1509
  in pregnancy, 1508
    management of, 1515
  prostatitis in, 1511-1512
    management of, 1516
  Pseudomonas aeruginosa, 1660
  pyelonephritis in, 1511
  recurrent
    epidemiology of, 1508
    management of, 1514
    relapsing, management of, 1514
  renal and perirenal abscess in,
    1511
  in renal transplantation, 2122
  Staphylococcus saprophyticus, 1581
  upper. See Pyelonephritis
  vaginal ecology and, 1509
  vesicoureteral reflux in, 1510
Urine
  acute retention of, in benign
    hyperplasia of prostate, 2133
  culture, interpretation of, 1512
  residual, in benign prostatic
    hyperplasia, 2129
  sediment, components of,
    1971, 1971f
Ursodiol, for chronic cholecystitis,
  906
Urticaria, 1259-1266
  aquagenic, 1263

cholinergic, 1263
cold, 1262-1263
common triggers of, 1260-
  1262, 1260t
  drugs as, 1260-1261, 1261f
  foods as, 1261
  genetic factors as, 1262
  neoplasms as, 1262
  occupational and hobby exposures
    as, 1261
  psychological factors as, 1262
  systemic illness as, 1261-1262
contact, 1263
delayed pressure, 1262
diagnosis of, 1259-1264
epidemiology of, 1259
etiology and pathogenesis of,
  1259, 1259t-1260t
generalized, 1263-1264, 1263f
localized, 1262-1263
papular, 1262
physical and laboratory
  examination in, 1264
prognosis in, 1265-1266
solar, 1263
treatment of, 1264-1265, 1264t
vibratory, 1263
Urticarial drug reactions, 497-
  498, 496t
Urticarial vasculitis, 1362
Urticaria pigmentosa, 436, 436f
Uterine bleeding, in menopause, 1033-
  1034
Uterine cancer. See Endometrial
  cancer
Uterine cervical cancer, 2541-2545
  diagnosis and staging of, 2542-
    2543, 2543f
  early detection of preinvasive
    disease in, 2542
  epidemiology and risk factors for,
    1063
  epidemiology and risk factors in,
    2542
  HPV and, 2376
  human papilloma virus and, 1063
  natural history of, 1063
  preventive health care measures
    for, 42-43
  relapse in, management of, 2545
  screening for, 1063-1065
    available tests for, 1064-1065
    test interpretation in,
      1065, 1064t
    who should be screened, 1063-
      1064
  treatment of, 2544-2545, 2543f
    in bulky stage IB disease, 2544-
      2545
    in early stage disease with high-
      risk features, 2544
    in stage IA, 2544
    in stage IB and IIA, 2544, 2543f
    in stage IIB to IVA, 2544
  vaccine for, 2542
Uterine cervical cap, contraceptive,
  998
Uterine cervical mucus, in
  infertility, 1003-1004
Uterine cervicitis, mucopurulent,
  1525-1526
  Neisseria gonorrhoeae, 1622, 1624t
Uterine leiomyoma, 1059-1060, 1061-
  1062
  benign metastasizing, 2756
Uterine outflow obstruction, 954
Uterus, clostridial infection of,
  1608
Uveitis
  in ankylosing spondylitis, 1320
  in sarcoidosis, 2772
Uveoparotid fever (Heerfordt
  syndrome), 2772

V

Vaccination. *See* Immunization
Vaccinia, progressive, 126, 126f
Vaccinia immune globulin, 127
Vaginal bleeding, abnormal, 959-960
Vaginal cervicitis, mucopurulent, chlamydial, 1747-1748, 1748t
Vaginitis, acute dysuria and, 1512t
Vaginosis, bacterial, 1523-1524, 1524t
Vagus nerve stimulation, for epilepsy, 2197-2198
Vagus neuropathy, 2294t
Valley fever, acute. *See* Coccidioidomycosis
Valproate, in epilepsy, 2197
Valproic acid, poisoning or overdose with, elimination method for, 161t
Valproic acid treatment, polycystic ovary syndrome *vs.*, 980
Valsartan, for hypertension, 223t
Valve(s), heart. *See* Heart valve(s), Heart disease, valvular
Valvular heart disease. *See* Heart disease, valvular
Vancomycin, 1436
allergy to, 1275
in pregnancy, 1422t
for septic arthritis, 1540t
Vancomycin-resistant *Staphylococcus aureus*, 1579
Varicella, 1758-1761
clinical syndromes in, 1759
diagnosis, prevention, treatment of, 1760-1761
epidemiology of, 1758
neuropathy in, 2305-2306
rickettsialpox *vs.*, 1728
smallpox *vs.*, 125t
vaccine for, 1760
Varicella-zoster virus, 1758-1761. *See also* Herpes zoster, Varicella
in central nervous system disease, 2344t, 2350-2351
nosocomial transmission of, 1760
prophylactic measures for in HIV infection, 1840t
vaccine for, 1760
in vasculopathy
multifocal, 2350
unifocal, 2350-2351
vasculopathy, 2350-2351
Varicocele, of testes, 693
Varix(ces)
in cirrhosis, 897. *See also under* Cirrhosis
esophageal. *See* Esophageal varices
Vascular birthmarks, 544-546
Vascular purpura, 1176-1178, 1177t
Vascular tumor. *See* Hemangioma
Vasculitis
drug-induced, 501-502, 502f
granulomatous, cutaneous findings in, 432
large vessel, 1368-1370
neuropathy in, 2302-2303
pulmonary, in allergic granulomatosis and angiitis, 2782-2783
renal. *See* Renal vascular disease
in rheumatoid arthritis, 1305-1306
small vessel, 1360-1362
clinical manifestations of, 1361-1362, 1362f
diagnosis of, 1361-1362, 1362f
etiology of, 1360-1361, 1361f
Henoch-Schonlein purpura as, 1362. *See also* Henoch-Schonlein purpura
laboratory tests in, 1362

treatment of, 1362, 1363t
urticarial, 1362
systemic, 1359-1370. *See also specific disorders e.g.,* Polyarteritis nodosa
approach to patient with, 1359-1360
Churg-Strauss syndrome as. *See* Churg-Strauss syndrome
classification in, 1359, 1361f
clinical features of, 1365t
evaluation in, 1359, 1360t
Kawasaki disease as. *See* Kawasaki disease
polyarteritis nodosa as. *See* Polyarteritis nodosa
treatment in, 1359-1360
Wegener granulomatosis as. *See* Wegener granulomatosis
Vasculopathy
acquired, bleeding disorders due to, 1177-1178
in diabetes mellitus, pancreas transplantation and, 938
varicella-zoster virus, 2350
Vasectomy, 998-999
Vasomotor symptoms, in menopause, 1032, 1034, 1033
Vasopressin
in cardiac resuscitation, 144t
deficiency. *See* Diabetes insipidus
for septic shock, 1451
Vegetable(s), dietary, 30
colorectal cancer and, 2477
Velocardiofacial syndrome, 1949
Venezuelan equine encephalitis, 1855-1856
Venography, for venous thrombosis, 411-412, 412f
Venom immunotherapy, 1288-1289
Venous malformation (cavernous hemangioma), 545
Venous thromboembolism. *See* Thromboembolism, venous
Venous thrombosis. *See* Thrombosis, venous
Ventilation. *See also* Breathing, Respiration
in cardiac resuscitation, 146, 146t
mechanical. *See* Mechanical ventilation
physiology of, 2786-2788, 2787f-2788f
brain centers in, 2787, 2788f
chemoreceptors in, 2786
mechanoreceptors in, 2786
in sleep, 2790-2791, 2791f
cardiovascular physiology and, 2791
hypocapnic-apneic threshold and, 2791
load compensation and, 2790-2791, 2791f
upper airway function and, 2790
during wakefulness and sleep, 2786-2799
Ventilatory drive
decreased, 2788-2789
increased, 2788
Ventricular arrhythmia(s), 260-272. *See also* Ventricular tachycardia
in acute myocardial infarction, 329-330
cardiac arrest and, 264-265
heritable, 265-266
nonpharmacologic therapy for, 269-271
pathophysiology of, 260-262
pharmacologic therapy for, 266-269, 267t. *See also individual drugs and* Antiarrhythmic agent(s)
efficacy and outcome, 268-269
extremely wide complex

ventricular rhythm due to, 268
incessant ventricular tachycardia due to, 268
torsade de pointes due to, 268
syncope and, 264
electrocardiography and, 264
electrophysiologic testing and, 264
history and physical examination in, 264
Ventricular ectopy, asymptomatic, 262-264
after myocardial infarction, 263
electrophysiologic studies in, 263-264
microvolt T wave alternans in, 263
prognostic significance of, 262-263
signal-averaged electrocardiography in, 263
Ventricular fibrillation
in acute myocardial infarction, 329-330
anoxic encephalopathy in, 2336
in cardiac resuscitation, 149-152, 150f-151f
antiarrhythmic drugs in, 150-152
defibrillation in, 149-150, 151f
drug therapy in, 150
emergency lab tests in, 150
in drug overdose or poisoning, 156t
Ventricular septal defect, 390-391, 392f
in acute myocardial infarction, 331
murmur in, 210t
Ventricular tachycardia
in abnormal automaticity, 261-262, 261f
in acute myocardial infarction, 330
automated external defibrillators for, 271
in cardiac resuscitation, 149-152, 150f-151f
antiarrhythmic drugs in, 150-152
defibrillation in, 149-150, 151f
drug therapy in, 150
emergency lab tests in, 150
catheter ablation for, 269
in drug overdose or poisoning, 156t
due to triggering, 262
delayed afterdepolarization in, 262
early afterdepolarization in, 262, 262f
implantable cardioverter-defibrillator for, 269-271, 269f, 270t
pathophysiology of, 260-262
reentrant, 260-261, 260f-261f
surgical therapy for, 269
Verapamil, classification of, 267t
Verapamil extended release, for hypertension, 221t
Verruca plana, 514
Verruca plantaris, 514
Verruca vulgaris, 514
Verrucous carcinoma, genital (Buschke-Lowenstein tumor, giant condyloma acuminatum), 515
Vertebral artery dissection, in stroke, 2213
Vertebrobasilar insufficiency, 2145-2146
Vertigo, 2141, 2142t
benign paroxysmal, of childhood, 2156
benign paroxysmal positioning, 2142-2143, 2143f
in cerebellar ataxia, 2147-2148

drug-induced, 2146, 2146t
in multiple sclerosis, 2148
phobic postural, 2144-2145
structural abnormalities in, 2147
Vesicle, definition of, 426t
Vesicoureteral reflux, in urinary tract infection, 1510
Vesicular stomatitis virus infection, 1859
Vesiculobullous disease, of skin, 525-534. *See also individual disorders, e.g.,* Pemphigus
blister typology in, 525, 527t
differential diagnosis of, 533-534
differentiating features of, 526t
general clinical assessment of, 525, 526t
Vestibular disorders, 2142-2148
benign paroxysmal positioning vertigo, 2142-2143, 2143f
drug-induced vertigo, 2146, 2146t
Meniere disease, 2144, 2145f, 2145t
perilymphatic fistula, 2147
phobic postural vertigo, 2144-2145
vertebrobasilar insufficiency, 2145-2146
vestibular migraine, 2146-2147
vestibular neuritis, 2143-2144, 2144t
Vestibular dysfunction, 2136-2142
diagnosis of, 2141-2142, 2141t-2142t
dynamic imbalance, 2138-2139, 2139t
nystagmus, 2140, 2140t-2141t
pursuit eye movements and VOR cancellation, 2139-2140
static imbalance, 2137-2138, 2138f
Vestibular labyrinth, physiology and anatomy of, 2135-2136, 2135f-2138f
Vestibular migraine, 2146-2147
Vestibular neuritis, 2143-2144, 2144t
Vestibular seizure, 2148
Vestibulocochlear neuropathy, 2294t
Vestibulo-ocular reflex, 2135-2136, 2138f
Vestibulospinal reflex, 2135-2136
VHL, properties of, 2386t, 2391
Vibrio cholerae, 1643-1644. *See also* Cholera
non-O1, 1645
Vibrio infection, 1643-1645, 1636t
Vibrio parahaemolyticus infection, 1644
Vibrio vulnificus, cutaneous findings in, 439
Vibrio vulnificus infection, 1645
Vinblastine, 2419t
Vinca alkaloids, 2421, 2419t
Vincristine, 2419t
peripheral neuropathy due to, 2319
Vinorelbine, 2419t
Violence
alcoholism and, 2627
domestic, 23
stress disorders and, 2661
Viral infection. *See also specific infection*
leukemia due to, 2562
thrombocytopenia due to, 1173
Virilization, in polycystic ovary syndrome, 977
Virilization syndrome, polycystic ovary syndrome *vs.*, 980
Visceral larva migrans, 1926-1927
Vitamin(s)
dietary, 28, 29t
in nutritional support, 947, 947t-948t
Vitamin A, 29t
Vitamin B$_1$, 29t
deficiency, neuropathy in, 2304
Vitamin B$_2$, 29t
Vitamin B$_3$, 29t